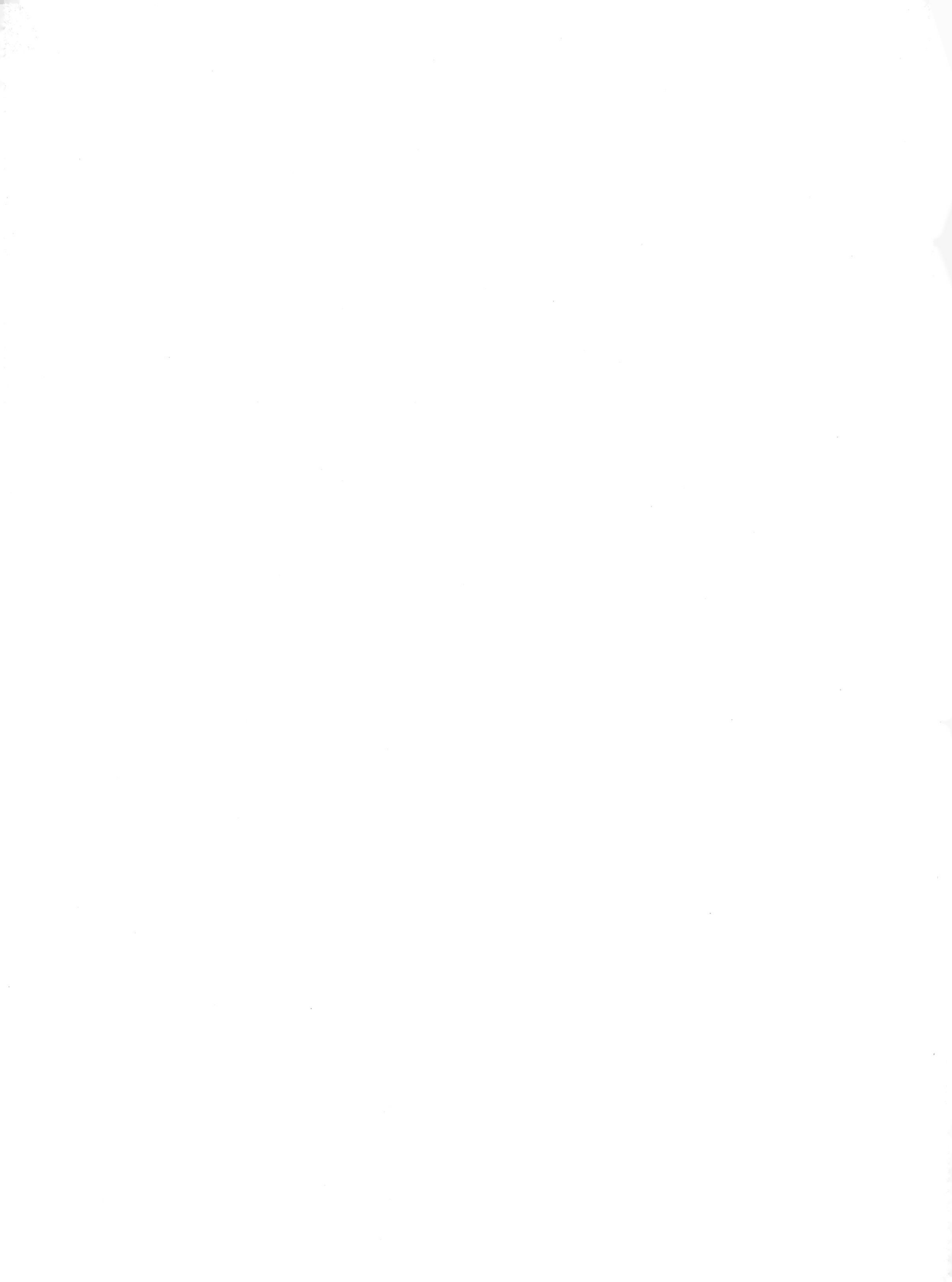

7TH EDITION

Nurse Anesthesia

SASS ELISHA, EdD, CRNA, FAANA, FAAN
Assistant Director, School of Anesthesia
Kaiser Permanente/California State University Fullerton
Southern California Permanente Medical Group
Pasadena, California

JEREMY S. HEINER, EdD, CRNA
Academic and Clinical Educator
Kaiser Permanente/California State University Fullerton
Southern California Permanente Medical Group
Pasadena, California

JOHN J. NAGELHOUT, PhD, CRNA, FAAN
Director Emeritus, School of Anesthesia
Kaiser Permanente/California State University Fullerton
Southern California Permanente Medical Group
Pasadena, California

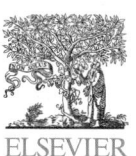

ELSEVIER

Elsevier
3251 Riverport Lane
St. Louis, Missouri 63043

NURSE ANESTHESIA, SEVENTH EDITION

ISBN: 978-0-323-71194-4

Notice

Practitioners and researchers must always rely on their own experience and knowledge in evaluating and using any information, methods, compounds or experiments described herein. Because of rapid advances in the medical sciences, in particular, independent verification of diagnoses and drug dosages should be made. To the fullest extent of the law, no responsibility is assumed by Elsevier, authors, editors or contributors for any injury and/or damage to persons or property as a matter of products liability, negligence or otherwise, or from any use or operation of any methods, products, instructions, or ideas contained in the material herein.

Previous editions copyrighted 2018, 2014, 2010, 2005, 2001, and 1997.

Library of Congress Control Number: 2021939972

Executive Content Strategist: Sonya Seigafuse
Senior Content Development Manager: Lisa Newton
Content Development Specialist: Sara Hardin/Laura Selkirk
Publishing Services Manager: Shereen Jameel
Senior Project Manager: Manikandan Chandrasekaran
Cover Design and Design Direction: Brian Salisbury

Printed in India

Last digit is the print number: 9 8 7 6 5 4 3 2 1

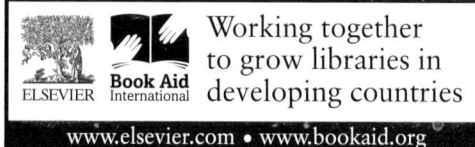

Michael J. Anderson, DNP, ARNP, CRNA
Clinical Associate Professor/Clinical Coordinator
College of Nursing, DNP Anesthesia Nursing Program
University of Iowa
CRNA, Department of Anesthesia
University of Iowa Hospitals and Clinics
Iowa City, Iowa

Jenna Applebee, MSN, CRNA
Certified Registered Nurse Anesthetist
Cardiothoracic and Vascular Anesthesia Institute
Cleveland Clinic
Cleveland, Ohio

Becky J. Ashlock, DNP, CRNA
Certified Registered Nurse Anesthetist
Kaiser Permanente
Panorama City, California

Heather Bair, DNP, CRNA, CHSE
Clinical Assistant Professor/Associate Director
College of Nursing, DNP Anesthesia Nursing Program
University of Iowa
CRNA, Department of Anesthesia
University of Iowa Hospitals and Clinics
Iowa City, Iowa

Kevin Baker, MSNA, CRNA
Cofounder
APEX Anesthesia Review
Maidens, Virginia

Paula J. Belson, PhD, CRNA
CRNA Manager
Children's Hospital Los Angeles
Clinical Instructor of Anesthesia
Keck School of Medicine
Los Angeles, California
Clinical Faculty
California State University, Fullerton
Fullerton, California

Chuck Biddle, PhD, CRNA
Professor Emeritus Nurse Anesthesia
Virginia Commonwealth University
Richmond, Virginia

Laura S. Bonanno, PhD, DNP, CRNA
Nurse Anesthesia Program Director
Professor
Louisiana State University Health Sciences Center
School of Nursing
New Orleans, Louisiana

Sandra K. Bordi, DNP, CRNA
Clinical and Didactic Instructor
School of Anesthesia
Kaiser Permanente
Pasadena, California

Greg Bozimowski, DNP, CRNA
Professor and Chair
Nurse Anesthesia Program
University of Detroit Mercy
Detroit, Michigan

Joni M. Brady, DNP, RN, PMGT-BC, CAPA
Chair, Board of Directors
International Collaboration of PeriAnaesthesia Nurses, Inc.
Alexandria, Virginia

Kurt D. Cao, DNAP, CRNA
Director of CRNA Services
Loma Linda University Health;
Assistant Professor
Nurse Anesthesia Concentration
Loma Linda University School of Nursing
Loma Linda, California

Shawn B. Collins, PhD, DNP, CRNA, FAANA
Professor
Associate Dean, Academic Affairs and Graduate Programs
School of Nursing
Loma Linda University
Loma Linda, California

Richard P. Conley, DNP, CRNA
Assistant Professor and Assistant Director
Nurse Anesthesia Program
University of Maryland
Baltimore, Maryland

Margaret A. Contrera, DNP, CRNA
Assistant CRNA/CAA Director, Cleveland Clinic
Academic and Clinical Faculty, School of Nurse Anesthesia
Cleveland Clinic/Case Western Reserve University
Staff Nurse Anesthetist, Cardiothoracic and Vascular Anesthesia
Cleveland Clinic
Cleveland, Ohio

M. Roseann Diehl, PhD, DNP, CRNA, CHSE-A
Professor Professional Practice
Texas Christian University
Harris College of Nursing and Health Sciences
School of Nurse Anesthesia
Fort Worth, Texas

Michael P. Dosch, PhD, CRNA
Professor
Nurse Anesthesia
University of Detroit Mercy
Detroit, Michigan

Marjorie Everson, PhD, CRNA, FNAP
Faculty Member
Nurse Anesthesia Program
Johns Hopkins University
Baltimore, Maryland
Certified Registered Nurse Anesthetist
Benefis Health System
Great Falls, Montana

Christian R. Falyar, DNAP, CRNA
Professor
Acute Surgical Pain Management Fellowship
Middle Tennessee School of Anesthesia
Nashville, Tennessee

Vincent E. Ford, DNAP, M.Ed., CRNA
Certified Registered Nurse Anesthetist
Duke University Hospital
Durham, North Carolina

Judith A. Franco, EdD, ACNP, CRNA
Assistant Professor of Clinical Anesthesiology
University of Southern California
Los Angeles, California

Daniel Frasca, DNAP, CRNA
Cofounder
APEX Anesthesia Review
Heathsville, Virginia

James S. Furstein, PhD, DNAP, CRNA, CPNP-AC, FAANA
Associate Professor of Clinical Nursing
Assistant Program Director
Nurse Anesthesia Program
University of Cincinnati College of Nursing
Cincinnati, Ohio

Mark H. Gabot, DNP, CRNA
Didactic and Clinical Instructor
School of Anesthesia
Kaiser Permanente
Pasadena, California

Francis Gerbasi, PhD, CRNA
Chief Executive Officer
Council on Accreditation of Nurse Anesthesia
    Educational Programs
Park Ridge, Illinois

Christopher J. Gill, PhD, MBA, CRNA
Assistant Clinical Professor
Nurse Anesthesia
Wayne State University
Detroit, Michigan;
Staff CRNA
Department of Anesthesia
Mount Sinai Hospital
Chicago, Illinois

Sarah E. Giron, PhD, CRNA
Clinical and Didactic Instructor
School of Anesthesia
Kaiser Permanente
Pasadena, California

**Wallena Gould, EdD, CRNA, FAANA,
    FAAN**
Founder and CEO
Diversity in Nurse Anesthesia Mentorship
    Program
Mickleton, New Jersey

Charles Griffis, PhD, CRNA, FAANA
Assistant Clinical Professor
UCLA School of Nursing
Faculty, USC Doctor of Nurse Anesthesia
    Practice Program
Los Angeles, California

Valdor L. Haglund, MS, CRNA
Assistant Professor, Nurse Anesthesia
Wayne State University
Detroit, Michigan

Randolf R. Harvey, BS, CRNA
Chief of Anesthesia
Florida Eye Clinic ASC
Altamonte Springs, Florida

**William O. Howie, BSN, MS, MSNA,
    DNP, CRNA, CCRN**
Staff Nurse Anesthetist
R Adams Cowley Shock Trauma Center
Nurse Anesthesia Adjunct Faculty
University of Maryland Medical Center
Adjunct Associate Professor
Conway School of Nursing
The Catholic University of America
Baltimore, Maryland

Leslie Ann Jeter, DNP, MSNA, CRNA
Senior Clinical Instructor
Nell Hodgson Woodruff School of Nursing
Emory University
Atlanta, Georgia

Vanessa Jones-Oyefeso, PhD, CRNA
Program Director and Assistant Professor
Nurse Anesthesia Concentration
Loma Linda University
Loma Linda, California

Mary C. Karlet, PhD, CRNA
Scottsdale, Arizona

Caroline Killmon, MS, CRNA
Adjunct Faculty
Nurse Anesthesia Program
Wake Forest University School of Medicine
Winston-Salem, North Carolina

Bruce Evan Koch, MSN, CRNA
Partner
Evergreen Anesthesia
Sunnyside, Washington

Mark A. Kossick, DNSc, CRNA, APN
Professor, Director of Graduate Programs
School of Nursing
College of Health and Human Sciences
Western Carolina University
Asheville, North Carolina

**Mary Anne Krogh, PhD, APRN, CRNA,
    FAAN**
Dean, College of Nursing
South Dakota State University
Brookings, South Dakota

Elisabeth Cole McConnell, MSN, CRNA
Staff Certified Registered Nurse Anesthetist
Regional Anesthesia Associates
Bakersfield, California

Andrew Miller, DNP, CRNA
Certified Registered Nurse Anesthetist
Pediatric Anesthesia
University of Iowa Stead Family Children's
    Hospital
Iowa City, Iowa

Nancy A. Moriber, PhD
Assistant Professor, School of Nursing
Fairfield University
Fairfield, Connecticut
Program Director, Nurse Anesthesia
    Program
Fairfield University & Bridgeport Hospital
Bridgeport, Connecticut

**Catherine Y. Morse, EdD, APN-A,
    CRNA, CNE**
Clinical Assistant Professor and Director
Entry to Practice Division: 2+2 Nursing
    Program
School of Nursing, Blackwood Campus
Rutgers, The State University of New Jersey
Newark, New Jersey

**Jan Odom-Forren, PhD, RN, CPAN,
    FASPAN, FAAN**
Associate Professor
College of Nursing
University of Kentucky
Lexington, Kentucky

Cormac O'Sullivan, PhD, MSN, CRNA
Clinical Associate Professor/Director
College of Nursing, DNP Anesthesia
    Nursing Program
University of Iowa
CRNA, Department of Anesthesia
University of Iowa Hospitals and Clinics
Iowa City, Iowa

Nilu G. Patel, DNAP, MSN, CRNA
Faculty, Assistant Clinical Instructor
Anesthesiology
University of Southern California
Senior Nurse Anesthetist
Anesthesiology and Perioperative Care
University of California, Irvine
Orange, California

Joseph E. Pellegrini, PhD, CRNA, FAAN
Adjunct Professor – Nurse Anesthesia
Program
University of Alabama Birmingham
Birmingham, Alabama

Jessica Phillips, MS, CRNA
Assistant Program Director
Assistant Professor–Clinical
Nurse Anesthesia
Wayne State University
Detroit, Michigan

Lee J. Ranalli, DNP, CRNA
Associate Professor
Nurse Anesthesia Program
Midwestern University
Glendale, Arizona

Lynn Reede, DNP, MBA, CRNA, FNAP
Associate Clinical Professor
Bouve College of Health Sciences
School of Nursing, Nurse Anesthesia
    Program
Northeastern University
Boston, Massachusetts

Michael Rieker, DNP, CRNA, FAAN
Professor and Chair of Academic Nursing
Director, Nurse Anesthesia Program
Wake Forest School of Medicine
Winston-Salem, North Carolina

Bernadette T. Higgins Roche, EdD, APN, CRNA, FAANA
Anesthesia Education Consultant
Chicago, Illinois

Bethany K. Seale, MSN, CRNA, APRN
Staff Certified Registered Nurse Anesthetist
Advanced Anesthesia Solutions
North American Partners in Anesthesia
Kingsport, Tennessee

Sarah A. Sheets, MSN, CRNA
Fort Collins, Colorado

Virginia C. Simmons, DNP, CRNA, CHSE-A, FAANA, FAAN
Program Director
Duke University Nurse Anesthesia Program
Duke School of Nursing
Duke University
Durham, North Carolina

Lindsay Shockley, MSN, CRNA
Certified Registered Nurse Anesthetist
Cardiothoracic and Vascular Anesthesia Institute
Cleveland Clinic
Cleveland, Ohio

Renata Sobey, DNP, CRNA
Chief CRNA, Department of Anesthesia
Gottlieb Memorial Hospital
Melrose Park, Illinois
Adjunct Faculty, Department of Nursing
DePaul University
Lincoln Park, Illinois

Greg A. Taylor, MSN, CRNA
Assistant Chief CRNA
The Permanente Medical Group
Roseville/Folsom, California

Andrea J. Teitel, MS, CRNA
Clinical Adjunct Faculty
College of Health Professions, Nurse Anesthesia
University of Detroit Mercy
Detroit, Michigan
Certified Registered Nurse Anesthetist
NorthStar Anesthesia, Huron Valley Sinai Hospital
Commerce Township, Michigan

Darin L. Tharp, MS, CRNA
Certified Registered Nurse Anesthetist
Michigan Medicine
Ann Arbor, Michigan

Jennifer Lynn Thompson, DNP, CRNA
Academic and Clinical Instructor
School of Anesthesia
Kaiser Permanente
Pasadena, California

Andy Tracy, PhD, CRNA
Assistant Director, Nurse Anesthesia
Assistant Professor
The University of Tulsa
Tulsa, Oklahoma

Crystal Trinooson, MS, CRNA
Instructor in Clinical Anesthesiology
Keck Medical Center of USC
Los Angeles, California

Robyn C. Ward, PhD, CRNA
Director, School of Nurse Anesthesia
Associate Professor of Professional Practice
Texas Christian University
Fort Worth, Texas

Richard P. Wilson, MNA, CRNA
Assistant Program Director
Graduate Program in Nurse Anesthesia
University of South Carolina School of Medicine
Columbia, South Carolina

Steven R. Wooden, DNP, NSPM- C, CRNA
President
Wooden Anesthesia PC
Bayou Vista, Texas;
Adjunct Faculty Texas Christian University
Advanced Pain Management Fellowship
Ft. Worth, Texas

We are reprinting the foreword written by John F. Garde from the first edition of *Nurse Anesthesia*, which was published in 1997. John encouraged the publication of the first edition of this text, two decades ago, as an important milestone in the evolution of the specialty of nurse anesthesia. He felt it showcased the breadth and depth of nurse anesthetists' contributions to research and clinical care. John conveyed his enthusiasm for the unique role of nurse anesthetists to everyone he encountered. He believed that anesthesia excellence was manifest when a clinician made a difference in the everyday lives of patients. He was one of the most consequential nurse anesthesia leader of his time. We present the foreword that he wrote for the first edition of this textbook in his honor.

Sass Elisha
Jeremy S. Heiner
John J. Nagelhout

FOREWORD FOR *NURSE ANESTHESIA*, FIRST EDITION

As a new century dawns, nurse anesthetists continue to provide the highest quality anesthesia services to their patients. To put this into perspective, consider that nurse anesthetists safely and compassionately administered anesthesia throughout the entire last century and even prior to that. The writings of Alice Magaw, published between 1899 and 1906, provide a noteworthy benchmark. Magaw detailed the use of chloroform and other anesthesia with the open-drop technique in more than 14,000 surgical cases without a single fatality attributable to anesthesia. She was the first nurse anesthetist to publish articles on the practice of anesthesia and was considered "the mother of anesthesia" during a time when surgeons selected nurses to specialize in anesthesia to provide greater safety for patients requiring anesthesia.

Many pharmacologic and technologic changes in anesthesia have occurred, however, since those noble beginnings. The chapter titles of this textbook serve as an atlas to this expanded knowledge base: "Clinical Monitoring in Anesthesia," "Anesthesia Equipment," "Pharmacokinetics," "Inhalation Anesthetics," "Intravenous Induction Agents," "Local Anesthetics," "Opioid Agonists and Antagonists," and "Neuromuscular Blocking Agents, Reversal Agents, and Their Monitoring," to name a few. Look at the specialty components of anesthesia contained in this book: "Cardiac Anesthesia," "Respiratory Anesthesia," "Thermal Injury and Anesthesia," "Trauma Anesthesia," "Outpatient Anesthesia," "Regional Anesthesia," "Anesthesia for Ophthalmic Procedures,"

"Anesthesia and Orthopedics," "Anesthesia for Ear, Nose, Throat, and Maxillofacial Surgery," "Anesthesia and Laser Surgery," and the list goes on. The continuum for practice in the twenty-first century is that of professionals learning anew how to ensure the best possible care for their patients.

When Agatha Hodgins and other nurse anesthetist pioneers gathered in a classroom in the anesthesia department of the University Hospital of Cleveland on June 17, 1931, they established what was to become the American Association of Nurse Anesthetists (AANA). This group sought to place better-qualified people in the field, to keep those already in nurse anesthesia abreast of modern developments, and to give protection and recognition to this group of professionals.

When the AANA values statement was adopted in 1995, it was not surprising that it reflected this earlier philosophy. The AANA values the following:

- Its members and the advancement of the profession of nurse anesthesia
- Quality service to the public through diverse practice settings based on collaboration and personal choice
- Integrity, accountability, competence, and professional commitment
- Scientific inquiry and contributions to the fields of anesthesiology, nursing, and related disciplines
- Participation in the formation of healthcare policy.

These value statements are supported by knowledgeable practitioners ever in pursuit of their craft.

Nurse Anesthesia is a textbook that builds on a formidable knowledge base and draws on the expertise of CRNAs and other professionals practicing in today's fast-paced, ever-changing environment. I look upon this volume as a means to demonstrate the profession's growth and encourage CRNAs and student nurse anesthetists to read it and reflect upon the dynamic field they have chosen.

I would like to close with one of my favorite quotations from Ralph Waldo Emerson, which I believe reflects all professionals on their prospective journeys:

> *To laugh often and much; to win the respect of intelligent people …;*
> *to earn the appreciation of honest critics …;*
> *to find the best in others …;*
> *to leave the world a bit better. … Bon voyage.*

John F. Garde, MS, CRNA, FAAN

PREFACE

Nurse anesthesia education and clinical practice continue to evolve at a rapid pace. Our professional degree has moved to the doctoral level, and the requisite knowledge needed to provide safe patient care is increasing exponentially. Due to the complexity of modern surgical procedures, ensuring the highest-quality outcomes requires the need for lifelong learning. Anesthesia practice has expanded beyond the traditional surgical settings to include interventional procedures, pain management, and non–operating room anesthetics. The objective of this new edition is to integrate the vast amount of current knowledge to help guide clinical practice.

Technologic innovations that allow this textbook to be used in traditional and various electronic formats are now commonplace. We approach the seventh edition of *Nurse Anesthesia* with a clear intent to bridge these platforms while remaining true to our educational objectives. Since the conception of the first edition of this text more than two decades ago, we continue to be guided by our original vision to fulfill the need for scientifically based, clinically oriented work on which anesthesia practitioners and learners can rely to deliver excellent patient care.

Our intent is to harness the vast knowledge that nurse anesthetists bring to clinical practice and provide a comprehensive, evidence-based resource for continuous learning. We are tremendously gratified that this textbook has become the seminal work for our specialty. *Nurse Anesthesia* is included among the Library of Congress's essential nursing textbooks for medical libraries throughout the United States and in national digital resource databases such as Elsevier's Clinical Key for Nursing. We reach an international audience of nurses and nurse anesthetists and are always pleased when we hear of the positive impact we are having on anesthesia practice worldwide.

We are especially grateful to all of our new and returning authors who bring a wealth of expertise and experience to their respective areas. The majority of clinical anesthesia continues to be provided by nurse anesthetists, and this textbook is a testament to the leadership we bring to academic and clinical nursing. Each chapter has been extensively reviewed and revised to contain the most salient information available. The newest concepts, techniques, and areas of controversy in anesthesia are discussed in detail. Providing effective anesthesia must be viewed as part of a therapeutic continuum of care. For this reason, we have intentionally included the latest medical and surgical information available from the specialties that impact our practice. Integrating new technology and knowledge in the basic sciences into clinical practice has allowed nurse anesthetists to continue to evolve as leaders in providing safe and comprehensive care. We have included new chapters on a wide variety of topics, including patient-centered care, cultural competence and nurse anesthesia practice, infection control and prevention, anesthesia for transplant surgery and organ procurement, chronic pain physiology and management, and crisis resource management and patient safety.

Producing an educational resource of this size and complexity would not be possible without the dedication of our authors and a broad array of experts. We proudly carry over from the previous editions hundreds of anatomic figures that were specially hand-drawn for this text by renowned medical illustrator William E. Loechel. We would like to express our gratitude to the staff at Elsevier who work tirelessly to produce this textbook. This book would not exist without their knowledge, expertise, and enthusiasm. A special thank you to Sonya Seigafuse, Executive Content Strategist; Laura Selkirk, Senior Content Development Specialist; and Manikandan Chandrasekaran, Senior Project Manager.

We would also like to acknowledge the contributions of Karen Plaus, PhD, CRNA, FAANA, FAAN as the coeditor of the first five editions of this text. Dr. Plaus has devoted her career to educating nurse anesthetists and advancing our specialty. Her decades-long achievements on the national and international levels continue to be instrumental in making nurse anesthesia a vital specialty for delivering high-quality health care. Finally, we would like to acknowledge all of the brilliant authors who have contributed to the creation of this book in past editions.

Sass Elisha
Jeremy S. Heiner
John J. Nagelhout

CONTENTS

Nurse Anesthesia: A History of Challenge

Bruce Evan Koch

It is fitting to open a text on nurse anesthesia with a history chapter. Nurses were the first professional group of anesthetists in the United States. Since the discovery of anesthesia in 1846, nurses have provided the majority of anesthetics in this country. Nurses have contributed to incremental progress to improve clinical anesthesia, patient safety, science, education, and public policies supporting anesthesia. Today's American Certified Registered Nurse Anesthetists (CRNAs)* receive state-of-the-art education, are granted a wide scope of practice, and have access to reliable and affordable malpractice insurance. These accomplishments are the result of more than a century of clinical accomplishments and concerted group efforts. By educating others about the history and achievements of CRNAs that created the foundation of our profession, the next generation of nurse anesthetists can learn from the experiences of the past and continue to move our profession toward excellence.

THE DISCOVERY OF MODERN ANESTHESIA

Decades before 1846, people were aware that inhaling nitrous oxide or diethyl ether could produce euphoria. In the late 18th century, the English scientists Joseph Priestley and Humphrey Davy experimented on themselves and even partied with these substances. Davy famously speculated that nitrous oxide "may probably be used with advantage during surgical operations."[1] At the same time, American medical students used ether and nitrous oxide recreationally.

However, almost 40 years would pass before they attempted to use these agents as adjuncts to surgery. A physician from Georgia named Crawford Long used diethyl ether for the removal of a small cyst in 1842, but he did not report his findings. At least two other men, the Massachusetts physician Charles Jackson and the Connecticut dentist Horace Wells, experimented with ether and nitrous oxide. Four years after Long's use of ether, on October 16, 1846, the Boston area dentist William T.G. Morton conclusively demonstrated the use of ether for surgical anesthesia in an operating room (now memorialized as the "Ether Dome") at Massachusetts General Hospital. This event was so important that the surgeon John Collins Warren, who had witnessed many prior failed attempts, reportedly exclaimed, "Gentlemen, *this* is no humbug." Another eminent surgeon who had been in attendance stated, "I have seen something today that will go around the world."[2] From their vantage point, optimism seemed justified; however, another half century would pass before the promise of painless surgery would be substantially fulfilled.

---

*Certified Registered Nurse Anesthetist (CRNA) is the descriptor used throughout this chapter interchangeably with nurse anesthetist and nurse anesthesiologist.

From the outset, Morton's discovery caused problems. People realized its monetary and historic value. Morton attempted to disguise ether so he could profit from it and applied for a patent. Long, Jackson, and Wells all claimed credit for Morton's discovery. The four men battled for years. The physician and writer Oliver Wendell Holmes Sr. (father of the Supreme Court justice) wrote to Morton: "Everybody wants to have a hand in a great discovery… All I want to do is give you a hint or two as to names." Holmes suggested "anesthesia from the Greek for insensible." The term *anesthesia* had been in use before to denote parts of the body benumbed but not paralyzed. Holmes only borrowed the word for the new state of being, though he has received credit for coining it.[3] As the anesthesiologist Robert Dripps noted, "Anesthesia was placed under a cloud."[4]

Nineteenth-century anesthesia was problematic in other, more important ways. Careless anesthetists vexed surgeons and infection-plagued patients and delayed progress in the field of anesthesia for decades. The historian Ira Gunn termed this era "the period of the failed promise."[5]

In the 19th century, physicians wanted to operate but they showed little interest in anesthesia as a medical specialty.[6] James Gather, the pioneer physician anesthetist, gave one explanation for this medical disinterest: "So intense had been the interest in surgery that anesthetics had been used only as a means to an end, and this fully explained the attitude of the profession on this subject in America at the present time." Physicians at the time could not make a living providing anesthesia anywhere outside a major city,[7] and anesthesia was deemed by some as unworthy of a physician's intellect.[8] The historian Marianne Bankert agreed: "Apart from the few physicians who had a genuine intellectual interest in anesthesia, it would also take years for the economics of anesthesia to make it an attractive area for their colleagues—if at first, only as a supplemental source of income."[9]

The work of anesthesia was provided by others: "Students, nurses, newly graduated physicians, specialists in other fields, and even custodians were called upon to be *etherizers*."[10] "Anesthesia could be anybody's business," wrote Virginia S. Thatcher.[11]

Lack of attention led to a degradation of knowledge and technique: The glass inhaler (Fig. 1.1) that Morton commissioned for his 1846 demonstration, and which worked so well, "was abandoned in favor of a small bell-shaped sponge, which was saturated with ether and applied directly over the nose and the mouth of the patient."[11] Not surprisingly, ether pneumonia resulted. Some surgeons turned to chloroform, which had been discovered to have anesthetic properties by James Simpson in England in 1847. "But, very soon, a death occurred from chloroform, then another and another in quick succession. This led to its more careful and restricted use by some surgeons, to its total abandonment by others, but in 1855, the general mass of surgeons and physicians still continued its use…."[12] Thatcher, the first historian of nurses as anesthetists, cited

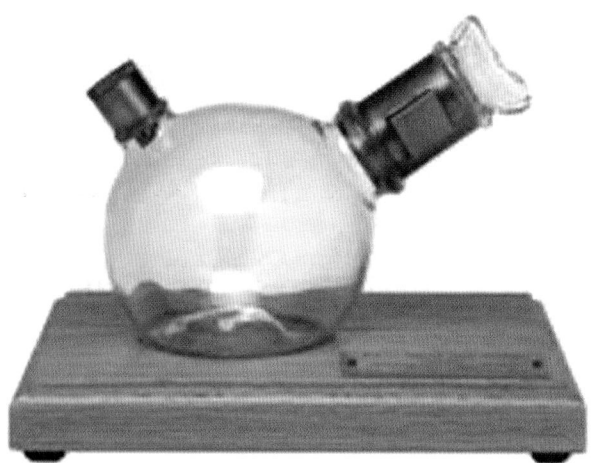

Fig. 1.1 Morton's inhaler, a replica of the inhaler used by William Morton to demonstrate the anesthetizing capacity of ether on October 16, 1846.

one physician who, in 1859, wrote "that most of the fatal cases can be traced to a careless administration of the remedy."[13]

Carelessness in anesthesia persisted for decades. A shocking example was recorded in 1894 by Harvey Cushing, the founder of neurosurgery. Cushing was a student at Harvard Medical School when he wrote:

> My first giving of an anaesthetic was when, a third-year student, I was called down from the seats and sent in a little side room with a patient and an orderly and told to put the patient to sleep. I knew nothing about the patient whatsoever, merely that a nurse came in and gave the patient a hypodermic injection. I proceeded as best I could under the orderly's directions, and in view of the repeated urgent calls for the patient from the amphitheater it seemed to be an interminable time for the old man, who kept gagging, to go to sleep. We finally wheeled him in. I can vividly recall just how he looked and the feel of his bedraggled whiskers. The operation was started and at this juncture there was a sudden great gush of fluid from the patient's mouth, most of which was inhaled, and he died. I stood aside, burning with chagrin and remorse. No one paid the slightest attention to me, although I supposed I had killed the patient. To my perfect amazement, I was told it was nothing at all, that I had nothing to do with the man's death, that he had a strangulated hernia and had been vomiting all night anyway, and that sort of thing happened frequently and I had better forget about and go on with the medical school. I went on with the medical school, but I have never forgotten about it.

Not surprisingly, surgeons began to appreciate the need for professional anesthetists. The need, as Thatcher defined it, was for anesthetists who would "(1) be satisfied with the subordinate role that the work required, (2) make anesthesia their one absorbing interest, (3) not look on the situation of anesthetist as one that put them in a position to watch and learn from the surgeon's technic, (4) accept the comparatively low pay, and (5) have the natural aptitude and intelligence to develop a high level of skill in providing the smooth anesthesia and relaxation that the surgeon demanded."[11] As a result of medical disinterest, poor delivery of anesthesia, and an overwhelming need, nurses were asked to administer anesthesia.

HISTORICAL ANTECEDENTS OF THE NURSE AS AN ANESTHETIST

The Civil War provided the first opportunity for nurses to assume the duties of anesthetist. Evidence is scant but found in three different accounts. Mrs. Harris from Baltimore, Maryland, took chloroform and stimulants to the Battle of Gettysburg. Harris "penetrated as near as possible to the scene of the conflict, ministering as much as in her power to the stream of wounded that filled the cars…."[14] It is not known whether Mrs. Harris was a nurse. A second report connects an unnamed "nurse in attendance" with having administered chloroform to a Union army soldier.[15] The third and most convincing example comes from Catherine S. Lawrence, a native of Skaneateles, New York, who wrote a 175-page autobiography in which she recorded administering anesthesia as a Union army nurse. Lawrence described her duties at a hospital outside Washington, DC, during and after the second battle of Bull Run (1863). She administered medications, resuscitated with restoratives such as ginger, tied sutures around arteries, and administered chloroform. "I rejoice that the time has arrived that our American nurses are being trained for positions so important. A skillful nurse is as important as a skillful physician."[16-18]

The First Civilian Nurses to Practice Anesthesia

Nurses in civilian hospitals began to practice anesthesia during the westward expansion that followed the Civil War. Surgeons taught Catholic hospital Sisters the rudiments of administering ether.[19] Sister Mary Bernard in 1877 entered St. Vincent's Hospital in Erie, Pennsylvania, to train as a nurse and is the earliest known example. Between 1860 and 1900, surgeons throughout the Midwest repeated this practice, training Sisters and secular nurses to administer ether. The Franciscan Sisters, who were active in the building and staffing of St. John's Hospital in Springfield, Illinois, were particularly successful in preparing hospital Sisters to become nurse anesthetists and sending them out to other midwestern hospitals. Having been prepared by another community of the Sisters of St. Francis (Syracuse, New York), Sister Mary Erhard went to Hawaii in 1886, where she administered anesthesia and performed other nursing duties on the island of Maui for approximately 42 years.

The St. Mary's Experience

In the summer of 1883, a very destructive tornado swept through Rochester, Minnesota. In its wake, the tornado "left an idea in the mind of the mother superior of the Sisters of St. Francis." During rescue efforts, she paid a visit to Dr. W.W. Mayo and asked: "Did he not think it would be well to build a hospital in Rochester?" Dr. Mayo thought the town too small to support a hospital, but "Mother Alfred had made up her mind. Quietly, she overruled the Old Doctor's objections and said that if he would promise to take charge of a hospital, the sisters would finance it." St. Mary's Hospital was built and opened, and although hospitals ranked low in the public's mind due to poor anesthesia and deadly infections, by 1904, it had expanded twice to keep up with demand. The hospital has endured until today as the Mayo Clinic. The Mayos (William Sr., William Jr., and Charles) won international acclaim for pioneering surgery.

But how did the Mayos handle the administration of anesthesia? According to Helen Clapsattle, the Mayo family historian, they were aware of its dangers but, unlike their colleagues on the East Coast, they were quick to embrace the open drop method of ether when it was brought to the United States from Germany. They also differed from East Coast physicians in one other respect: "In employing a permanent full-time anesthetist, and that a nurse, the Mayo's were unusual if not unique. In other hospitals anesthetizing was one of the duties of the interns."

Why would they give the job to a nurse? The Mayos had given the job to a nurse "in the first place through necessity; they had no interns. When the interns came, the brothers decided that a nurse was better suited to the task because she was more likely to keep her mind on it, whereas the intern was naturally more interested in what the surgeon was doing."[20]

Nurses won the Mayos' admiration by improving anesthesia care. Alice Magaw could discuss "a hundred and one details as to signs of sufficient anesthesia and ways of recognizing and preventing impending disaster." Magaw, along with her pupil Florence Henderson, refined and advocated the dripping of ether. Ether anesthesia required vigilance and careful attention to detail and to the psychological care of patients to minimize the agitation that often led to disasters like the one previously described by Harvey Cushing.

Henderson described how this was done: "A modified Esmarch inhaler, which is covered with two layers of stockinet, is used…. With the mask held about an inch from the face the ether is dropped upon it, slowly at first, and the patient is asked to breathe naturally through the nose. Then the mask is gradually lowered, and the rapidity of the dropping increased, care being taken not to give the ether fast enough to cause a sensation of smothering or suffocation. As soon as the jaw relaxes the head is turned to one side, because the patient usually breathes more easily with the head in this position." This was quite a contrast to the "crude" methods of most early anesthetizers, and it was successful. Nancy Harris and Joan Hunziker-Dean, who investigated Henderson's life, concluded that "through a delicate balance of interpersonal skills and technical expertise, she was able to essentially eliminate the excitement phase associated with the induction of ether anesthesia and consistently used a fraction of the usual dose. She demonstrated to all who observed that the administration of ether anesthesia could be elevated to an art form."[21]

Magaw and Henderson improved the safety of anesthesia care. Magaw accounted for the delivery of over 14,000 anesthetics "without an accident, the need for artificial respiration or the occurrence of pneumonia or any serious results."[22-26] These were not minor operations. Included were anesthetics for abdominal, intraperitoneal, gynecologic, urologic, orthopedic, ophthalmic, head and neck, and integument operations. Some were even conducted with the patient in the prone position.[23] Magaw and Henderson introduced better teaching methods, too. Early anesthesia education has been described as "on the spot training of any person available."[27] At Mayo, sometimes the "nurses stayed for 2 or 3 months and learned to give ether under supervision."[28] Surgeons who visited from Minneapolis, Baltimore, Chicago, the state of Iowa, and England "sent selected nurses to Rochester to observe Magaw and other nurse anesthetists at St. Mary's Hospital at their work."[11] Charles Mayo was so impressed by Magaw that he named her "The Mother of Anesthesia." To this day, the American Association of Nurse Anesthetists (AANA) confers on an outstanding practitioner an award named for Alice Magaw.

The Great War, a Small Battlefield

Nurse anesthetists played a very large role during World War I. Their involvement began in 1913, just 4 years before the United States became involved militarily, and lasted until the armistice in 1918.

When America entered the war, the Army Nurse Corps numbered 233 regular nurses; it would grow to 3524 nurses by 1918. The number of nurses who actually practiced anesthesia is unknown because at the time nurse anesthetists formed part of the general nursing staff.[28] However, nurse anesthetists were credited with introducing nitrous oxide/oxygen and teaching its administration to the English and the French.[29] As a result of the superior performance of nurse anesthetists, both the army and the navy sent nurses for anesthesia training for the first time.

Several outstanding World War I–era nurse anesthetists have been remembered because they wrote of their work. Nurse anesthetists spent countless hours etherizing wounded soldiers as they arrived in "ceaseless streams for days at a time after battles," wrote Mary J. Roche-Stevenson. "Work at a casualty clearing station came in great waves after major battles, with intervals between of very little to do….

Barrages of gun fire would rock the sector for days, then convoys of wounded would begin to arrive by ambulance. Night and day this ceaseless stream kept coming on…. The seriously wounded, especially the ones in severe shock, were taken to a special ward, given blood transfusions and other treatments in preparation for surgery later. From the receiving tent, the wounded were brought to the surgery, put on the operating tables stretcher and all, given an anesthetic, operated upon, picked up on their stretcher, and loaded on hospital trains for evacuation to base hospitals."[30] Terri Harsch,[28] who described the works of Roche-Stevenson and others such as Sophie Gran Winton, reported that 272 nurses were killed during the war.

In a paper about Miss Nell Bryant from the Mayo Clinic, who was the sole nurse anesthetist stationed at Base Hospital Number 26,[31] we learn that chloroform and ether were in use, the physiology of shock was poorly understood, oxygen and nitrous oxide were given without controlled ventilation, and venipuncture involved a surgical cutdown.

Anne Penland was a nurse anesthetist with the Presbyterian Hospital of New York unit at Base Hospital Number 2. She had the honor of being the first US nurse anesthetist to go officially to the British front, where she so won the confidence of British medical officers that the British decided to train their own nurses in anesthesia, ultimately relieving more than 100 physicians for medical and surgical work. Several hospitals were selected for this training of British nurses, including the American Base Hospital Number 2, with Penland as the instructor.[9]

Commenting in the *Bulletin of the American College of Surgeons*, Frank Bunts wrote: "The (First) World War demonstrated beyond any question the value of the nurse anesthetist."[32] George Crile speculated that "if the Great War had gone on another year, the British army would have adopted the nurse anesthetists right in the middle of the war."[33] Looking back after World War II, Lt. Colonel Katherine Balz, deputy chief of the Army Nurse Corps, credited nurse anesthetists for the fact that 92% of "battle wounded who reached Army hospitals alive were saved."[34]

The Proliferation of Nurse Anesthetists

The first recognition of the value of formalized education also occurred around this time. Isabel Adams Hampton Robb, a leading pioneer in nursing and the first superintendent of the Johns Hopkins School of Nursing, which opened in 1889, had, in 1893, published a nursing textbook titled *Nursing: Its Principles and Practices for Hospital and Private Use*; this textbook included a chapter titled "The Administration of Anaesthetics." By 1917, as a result of the "superior quality of anesthesia performed by nurse anesthetists,"[24] they were given the responsibility for surgical anesthesia at Johns Hopkins Hospital in Baltimore, where a training program was established under the direction of Ms. Olive Berger. Elsewhere, four postgraduate programs were developed: at St. Vincent's Hospital in Portland, Oregon (1909)[25]; at St. John's Hospital in Springfield, Illinois (1912); at New York Postgraduate Hospital in New York City (1912); and at Long Island College Hospital, Brooklyn, New York (1914).[11] Other nurse anesthesia programs were developed as part of the undergraduate nursing curriculum as a specialty option.

The Lakeside Experience

In 1900, Agatha Hodgins (Fig. 1.2), a Canadian nurse, went to Cleveland to work at Lakeside Hospital. Dr. George Crile chose her to become his anesthetist in 1908. Together with Crile, Hodgins pioneered the use of nitrous oxide/oxygen anesthesia, proved its superiority over ether for trauma cases in World War I, and opened and led a prominent school for nurse anesthetists that endured the first major challenge from physician anesthetists. In 1931, Hodgins founded the AANA.

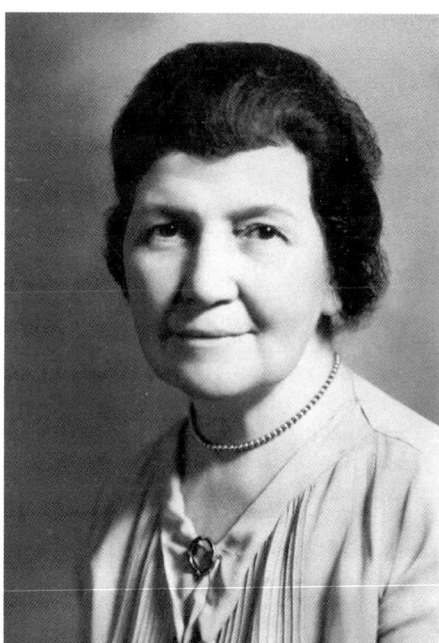

Fig. 1.2 Agatha Hodgins, an educator and founding president of the American Association of Nurse Anesthetists, reintroduced (with other American nurse anesthetists) the use of nitrous oxide for battlefield surgery during World War I in Europe.

Hodgins's primary interest was in education. Like its predecessor, the St. Mary's Hospital in Rochester, Minnesota, the Lakeside Hospital in Cleveland, Ohio, was the recipient of many requests for anesthetist training from both physicians and nurses. According to Thatcher, "Visiting surgeons eager to emulate the Lakeside methods customarily bought a gas machine (the Ohio Monovalve) and then sent a nurse to Cleveland to find out how it worked."[11] Hodgins recalled, "The number of applicants increased so rapidly that we felt some stabilizing of work necessary and the matter of a postgraduate school in anesthesia presented itself." In 1915, Hodgins opened a school at Lakeside Hospital.

The Lakeside School was not the first formal postgraduate anesthesia educational program; that honor belongs to St. Vincent's Hospital in Portland, Oregon. But the Lakeside School is the only program for which original records still exist. There were admission requirements, the course included both clinical and didactic components, tuition was charged, and a diploma was granted. "The department of anesthesia encompassed the school, both being under the charge of Agatha Hodgins as chief anesthetist. She, in turn, worked under the jurisdiction of the superintendent of the hospital and the chief surgeon. For the supervision of the students, she had 1 or 2 assistants until 1922 when the number was increased to 3."[11]

The Lakeside Hospital School prompted the establishment of 54 similar programs at major hospitals across the country.[24] The considerable impact of the Lakeside School on the evolution of nurse anesthesia education into a more formalized, scientifically based discipline can thus be seen.

ANESTHESIA: MEDICINE, NURSING, DENTISTRY, OR WHAT?

Nurse anesthetists appeared to be on the threshold of national acceptance when a New York attorney published a derisive article, titled "The Case Against the Nurse-Anesthetist," in which he introduced the idea that anesthesia was by law exclusively the practice of medicine.

He admonished "self respecting nurses to turn their attention to other matters—perhaps urinalysis."[35] This article, published in 1912, presaged efforts to legislate or litigate nurse anesthetists out of existence. And it set the tone for much of the vitriol directed by physician anesthetists toward CRNAs in the years to come. Although few physicians chose to specialize in anesthesia before World War II, one who did, Francis Hoeffer McMechan—a Cincinnati native—began a crusade around 1911 to claim the field solely for physicians. Through publishing and speaking, McMechan investigated the high-profile Lakeside School and its famous surgeon, George Crile. He alleged that anesthesia was the practice of medicine, and he petitioned the Ohio Medical Board to take action. McMechan considered Ohio a "pivotal state in the national fight for the preservation of the status of the anesthetist as a medical specialist."[36]

In a letter to Crile in 1916, the board claimed that no one other than a registered physician was permitted to administer anesthesia. The board ordered the Lakeside Hospital School of Nursing to cease its anesthesia program or lose its accreditation. Not wanting to be responsible for the loss of the school's accreditation, Crile obeyed the order, pending the outcome of a hearing conducted in 1917. At the hearing, Crile took the position that Lakeside Hospital was only following the lead of many of the major clinics in the country. (Recall Alice Magaw at the Mayo Clinic.) Crile managed to persuade the board of medicine to lift its order, and he was able to reinstitute his nurse anesthesia educational program and his use of nurse anesthetists.

To protect nurse anesthetists, Crile took an additional step. In 1919, together with supporting physicians, he "introduced a bill into the (Ohio) legislature to legalize the administration of anesthetics by nurses."[4,11] An amendment to the legislation stated that nothing in the bill "shall be construed to apply to or prohibit in any way the administration of an anesthetic by a registered nurse *under the direction of and in the immediate presence of* (emphasis added) a licensed physician," provided that such a nurse had taken a prescribed course in anesthesia at a hospital in good standing.[37] Physician supervision of nurse anesthetists, introduced here, would recur many times over.

In 1916, Louisville (Kentucky) Society of Anesthetists passed a resolution proclaiming that only physicians should administer anesthesia. The attorney general concurred, and the Kentucky State Medical Association followed with a resolution stating that it was unethical for a physician to use a nonphysician anesthetist or to use a hospital that permitted nurses to administer anesthesia. These events prompted the surgeon Louis Frank and his nurse anesthetist Margaret Hatfield to ask the state board of health to join them in a lawsuit against the Kentucky State Medical Association. They lost in the lower court, but on appeal they won. In 1917, Judge Hurt of the Kentucky Court of Appeals not only confirmed the right of nurses to administer anesthesia but also enunciated clearly that state licensure was meant to protect consumers, not professionals.

These two cases showed physicians that they could not rely on the courts; however, they were not deterred. Physician anesthetists in California brought suit against Dagmar Nelson, a nurse anesthetist, for practicing medicine without the proper license. The *Chalmers-Francis v. Nelson* case was decided in favor of Nelson at each level of the California civil courts. The California Supreme Court ruled that the functioning of the nurse anesthetist under the supervision of and in the direct presence of the surgeon was the common practice in operating rooms; therefore the nurse anesthetist was not diagnosing and treating within the meaning of the medical practice act.[38,39]

At the time, nurse anesthetists welcomed and embraced the concept of physician supervision because it was couched within statutes that, for the first time, gave them legal status. Gene Blumenreich, who has written extensively on the legal history of anesthesia, noted: "A number of states adopted statutes recognizing the practice of nurse anesthetists. Typically, these statutes followed the formulation in *Frank v. South* and provided that nurse anesthetists were to work under the 'supervision' or 'direction' of a physician." However, the statutes did not define supervision. "It is clear that the legislation was not attempting to create new duties and responsibilities for the supervising physician, but merely to describe what was already occurring practice…to explain why nurse anesthetists were not practicing medicine."[40]

ORGANIZING NATIONALLY: "WE WHO ARE MOST INTERESTED"

In 1926, Agatha Hodgins called together a small group of Lakeside Hospital alumnae to form a national organization. Hodgins had been an educator since World War I, and she sought strength in numbers to address problems related to education. One hundred thirty-three names were submitted, and tentative bylaws were drawn up. According to Ruth Satterfield, who was an eminent CRNA educator and the first nurse appointed as Consultant to the Army Surgeon General, "much of what she (Hodgins) said fell on deaf ears."[41] The association failed to thrive. Five years would pass before several problems would coalesce and force the national organization of nurse anesthetists to come to life.

Physician opposition to nurse anesthetists was one factor in this development. For example, in 1929, the California nurse anesthetists organized after the Board of Medical Examiners alleged that nurse anesthetist Adeline Curtis was practicing medicine illegally. Curtis, a natural public speaker, went on the road with this refrain: "…we can get nowhere without an organization. We're in the minority of course but we must organize."[42] California held its first meeting February 3, 1930.[43] Other states followed suit, and by the end of the 1930s, 23 had established organizations.

Economics brought nurse anesthetists together as well. This era of organization occurred during the Great Depression, and Hodgins noted in 1935 that "the strongest objection of physicians during this period was against those nurse anesthetists who were working on a fee for service basis."[44] Hanchett, who examined the *Chalmers-Francis v. Nelson* case (1933), concluded that the plaintiff California physicians were motivated by economic factors.[45] Thatcher observed that "Miss Hodgins' concept (of an organization) might never have been sparked into action, and organizations of nurse anesthetists might have stayed at the local level if the collapse of the nation's economy had not revived the physician anesthetist's interest in protecting his income by eliminating competition from nurses…."[11]

It was the poor state of anesthesia education that most motivated Hodgins. In 1931, she wrote the following to Curtis, who was embroiled in the California dispute: "My chief interest is in education."[46] So in the face of rising physician opposition, deteriorating economics, and the pressing need to reform education all compounding each other, Hodgins tried again. The National Association of Nurse Anesthetists (NANA) was born on June 17, 1931. Its name would be changed to the American Association of Nurse Anesthetists in 1933. The first meeting was held in a classroom at Lakeside Hospital and was attended by 40 anesthetists from 12 states.[47]

Right away, the new association set its sights on improving the quality of anesthesia by raising educational standards. The new president, in a letter to Marie Louis at the American Nurses Association (ANA), wrote: "It is because of the increasing number of nurses interested in the particular work and growing realization of difficulties existing because of insufficient knowledge of, and proper emphasis on, the importance of education, that we who are most interested are taking the steps to insure our ability to define and help maintain the status of the educated nurse anesthetist."[48] An education committee was formed. Chaired by Helen Lamb, the committee crafted "recommended" curriculum standards for schools and ratcheted them up in 1935 and again in 1936.

The fledgling association was weak with few members and little money. It could not hold its first national meeting for 3 years, much

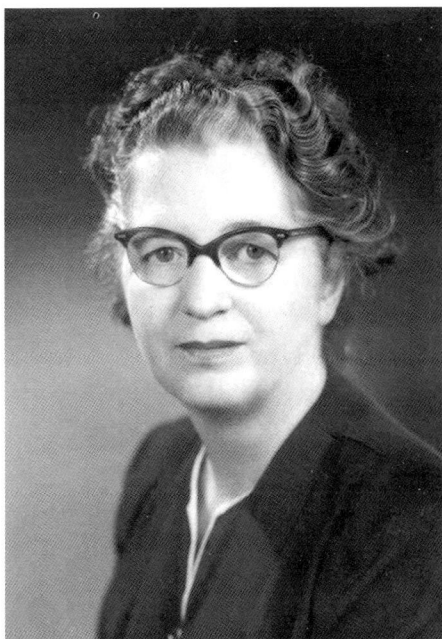

Fig. 1.3 Gertrude Fife and Helen Lamb were among the highly motivated group who built the profession. Fife served as second president (1933–1935) and treasurer (1935–1950) of the National Association of Nurse Anesthetists and edited the *AANA Journal* (1933–1950).

less advance an agenda of education reform. In that period, Hodgins sustained a heart attack and "for all practical purposes bowed out as administrative leader." Gertrude Fife (Fig. 1.3) took over the day-to-day affairs. There grew the realization, attributed by Bankert to Lamb and the education committee, that the problems were of such magnitude that an alliance with a more influential professional association would be required. But which one?

Forming an alliance with a major professional organization would likely prove problematic, as divergent interests could collide and trust would be tested to its limit. The small and newly organized NANA would have to fight to maintain its independence while at the same time obtain much-needed support. According to historian Rosemary Stevens, the AANA "made overtures to the American Board of Anesthesiology (ABA) in 1938 which might have enabled the two movements to combine and the anesthesiologists to take on the responsibility of the nurses' training." But at the time, the ABA was struggling to emerge from under the wing of surgery, and "the nurses were summarily rejected."[49]

So, instead, with the guidance and support of the American Hospital Association, Fife and Lamb planned the first meeting, which was held in Milwaukee in 1933. They also crafted a highly centralized organization to efficiently address the association's concerns. Thatcher listed those concerns: "(1) building up the membership so that there would be a creditable showing at the Milwaukee meeting; (2) arranging a program; (3) getting a constitution and the bylaws revised; and (4) launching the association's educational program."

Membership was to be a privilege, a mark of distinction. The bylaws required that an active member have graduated from an accredited school of nursing, have passed the required state board examination, and maintain an active license. Importantly, an applicant must "have engaged for not less than three years in the practice of the administration of anesthetic drugs prior to 1934 and must be so engaged at the time of making application for membership."[50] As membership surpassed 2500, a survey of schools, using onsite surveyors, evaluated courses being taught. An Anesthesia Records Committee was formed to create a standardized anesthetic record, and the credential "Member

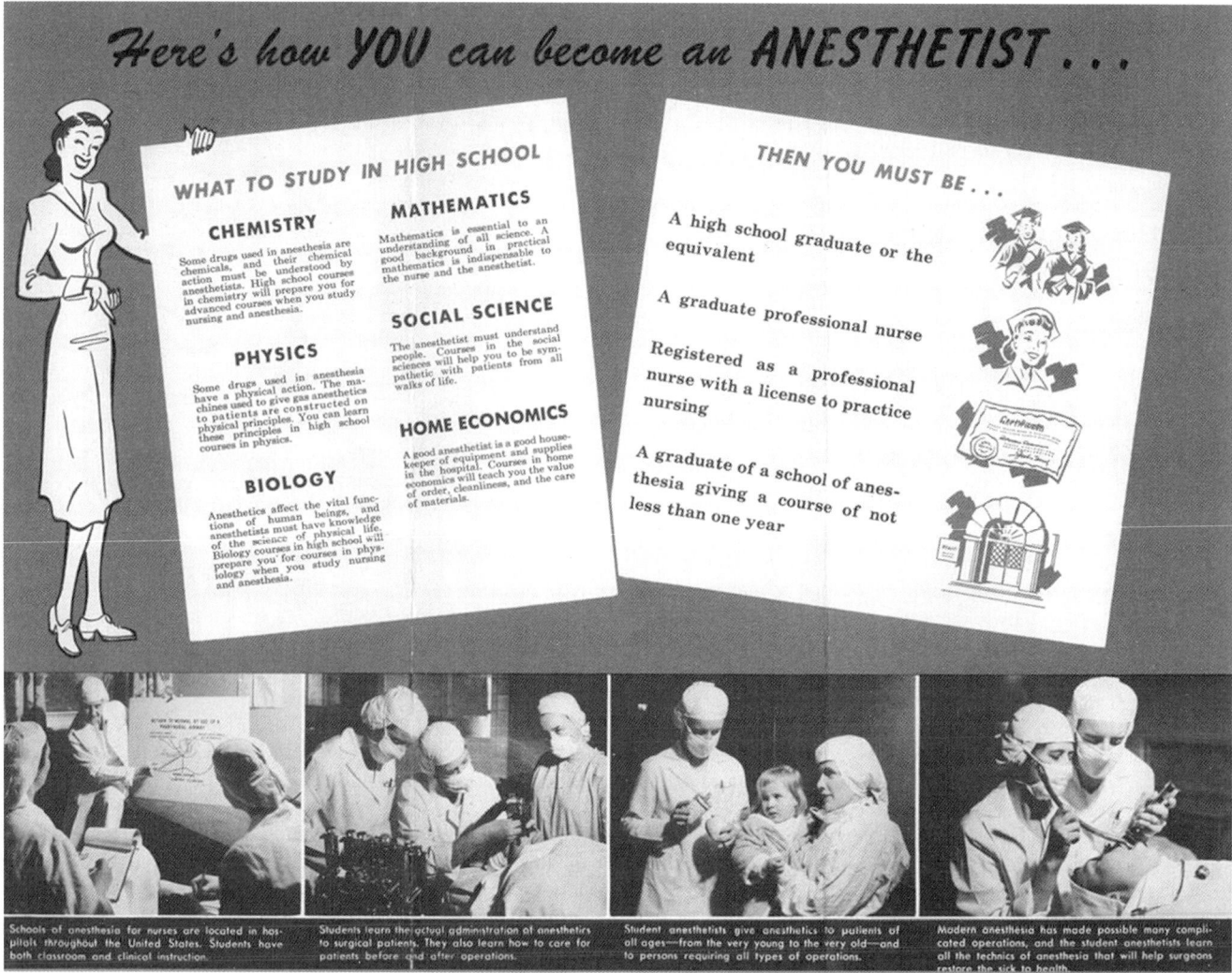

Fig. 1.4 This recruitment brochure was disseminated to schools of nursing to counteract the negative effect of antinurse anesthetist public relations.

of the American Association of Nurse Anesthetists" was implemented. These strides served to show that the profession had left its infancy. Then, World War II erupted and stalled further progress for the nurse anesthesia profession.

WORLD WAR II AND NURSE ANESTHETISTS

When World War II began, nurse anesthetists once again distinguished themselves. They served at home and in all theaters of operations. Mildred Irene Clark, who was originally from North Carolina, joined the army in 1938. Under army auspices, she graduated from Jewish Hospital in Philadelphia, where Hilda Salomon was program director. Clark was on assignment as a nurse anesthetist at the Schofield Barracks Hospital in Hawaii when Pearl Harbor was struck. Clark was among other nurse anesthetists on active duty who set up educational programs for preparing additional nurse anesthetists. Clark completed her career in 1967 as the chief of the Army Nurse Corps, the first nurse anesthetist to hold this position.

Annie Mealer, another notable army nurse anesthetist, was sent from Walter Reed Army Medical Center to the Philippines in 1941. She served as chief nurse and chief nurse anesthetist of the hospital on Corregidor. For 3 years, Mealer was held as a prisoner of war. Among the nurse anesthetists imprisoned with her were Denny Williams, Doris Keho, and Phyllis Arnold Iacobucci. They and 62 other army nurses were imprisoned until February 3, 1945.

Bankert quotes at length a letter Mealer later wrote in which she described her experiences. Mealer recalled housing President Quezon and his family, "giving anesthetics to one casualty after another" who "all needed help that only a nurse could give them." In Japanese custody aboard a troop ship, and sick with dengue fever, Mealer wrote, "I threw my cape down on the deck to lie on it and prayed that the wind would blow the fumes of the stale fish in another direction. I looked around at the nurses in the various uniforms of coveralls and skirts. They had grown slender as reeds but were smiling over some secret rumor about liberation—not realizing they had nearly three more years of hard work and starvation."[9]

The war effort greatly expanded the need for anesthetists in both military and civilian hospitals. Lt. Col. Katherine Balz, education consultant to the army, estimated that "approximately 15,000,000 patients were admitted to Army hospitals during the war, and something had to be done to provide the anesthesia services needed for these patients' care." In 1942, historian Stevens reported that nurse anesthetists outnumbered anesthesiologists by 17 to 1.[51] By the end of World War II, the Army Nurse Corps had educated more than 2000 nurse anesthetists, most (though not all) of whom were given an abbreviated 4- to 6-month curriculum patterned after that required by the AANA (Fig. 1.4).[52] Lt. Col. Balz recalled a situation in which some volunteer nurses were placed into anesthesia service after only 90 days of training! "At the end of that time, these volunteers were thrown into a situation in which 100 operations were being performed every 24 hours...there were not enough hours in the day to care for the patients and at the same time provide for formal instruction. In this hospital, over 5,000 anesthetics were given during a six months' period, and not one death or complication occurred as a result of anesthesia."[53]

The increased needs and the shortened training period posed "extraordinary complications" for the AANA. The questionable quality of newly minted graduates had to somehow be addressed. To maintain standards, the AANA implemented a temporary "program of certification by exam and certification by waiver."[9] Accreditation of programs was postponed entirely.

Despite being ill, Hodgins sent these words of encouragement: "The immense and vital part all branches of medical service will play in this continuing task can—because of its greatness—be now only dimly conceived. They will in very truth be a 'green island' in 'the wide deep sea of misery' now encompassing the earth." These were among her last words. Hodgins passed away in 1945. Her gravesite is located on Martha's Vineyard in Massachusetts.[54]

As World War II drew to a close, the AANA's plans for instituting a certification examination for civilian membership were at last realized. The first examination was given in June 1945. It was completed by "90 women in 39 hospitals in 28 states, plus one in the Territory of Hawaii."[55] It would be hard to conclude that their "high type of service" during the two world wars did not account for this accomplishment. It would also place the AANA firmly in the position of arbiter of quality in nurse anesthesia.

Nationally, World War II was also associated with bringing about certain human rights advances. Jackie Robinson in 1947 played his first game for the Brooklyn Dodgers. President Truman integrated the armed forces in 1948, and the first male nurse was commissioned in 1955, a step attributed to nurse anesthesia. The first two male nurses commissioned in the Army Nurse Corps were nurse anesthetists Edward L.T. Lyon of New York and Frank Maziarski of Washington, and the latter eventually became the 60th president of the AANA.[11,56] The AANA admitted its first black member in 1944 and its first male member in 1947.

A SHORT-LIVED PEACE FOR NURSE ANESTHETISTS AND THE NATION

After the war, the number of physicians in anesthesia greatly increased. In 1940, there were only 285 full-time anesthesiologists, 30.2% of whom were certified; in 1949, there were 1231 anesthesiologists, 38.3% of whom were certified.[57] Gunn attributed the increase to wartime medical experiences "alerting physicians to the potential of anesthesia as a specialty."[58] Bankert listed as causes "the increased complexity of anesthetics, but also...a military structure that encouraged medical specialization and a GI Bill that supported medical residencies."[8] The country produced more physicians, and many were drawn to anesthesiology.

Upon returning from military service, "medical (physician) anesthetists—many of them trained in the Armed Services—(in an effort) to establish themselves in a civilian economy, brought about a resurgence of activity against the nurse anesthetist."[11] One activity was to render "historically invisible" the contributions of nurses. For example, the 1946 centennial celebration of ether at the Massachusetts General Hospital lauded anesthesiologists but made no mention of nurse anesthetists. Thomas Keys published *The History of Surgical Anesthesia,* a widely referenced book that recent analysis has shown was deliberately meant to write nurse anesthesia out of existence.[59] Bankert listed other similar efforts: "a myth is launched of the early superiority of British

anesthetists—a land, so the story goes, which was never so foolish as to allow nurses to administer anesthetics; the national association of physician-anesthetists backdates its founding (from 1936) to 1905; a new word (*anesthesiologist*) is coined in the 1930s to distinguish the work of physician-anesthetists from nurse-anesthetists; 'historical' studies are published with titles such as *The Genesis of Contemporary Anesthesiology,* as though nothing of significance occurred in the field until the 1920s, when physician-anesthesia began to be effectively organized."[8] Anesthesiologists launched a nationwide public relations effort to denigrate nurse anesthetists. In 1947, several "major articles" appeared in *Look Magazine, Hospital Management, Reader's Scope,* and *This Week.* One excerpt railed: "Bad anesthesia causes more operating-room deaths than surgery. Now many hospitals have physician-anesthetists to protect you." Fear was a part of this campaign: "Until the operating rooms of our hospitals are brought into line with the clear requirements of modern anesthesiology, hundreds of Americans will continue to die needlessly on operating tables, sacrificed to ignorance and incompetence."[8] No evidence was offered to support this opinion. The first study of anesthesia-related outcomes would not be conducted until 1954.

These negative public relations efforts did not accomplish their goal. Surgeons, the public, and "often the anesthesiologist himself" were not dissuaded from trusting nurse anesthetists. However, they did "discourage many capable nurses from entering the field," prompting the AANA to promote the profession and recruit nurses who had been frightened away.[11] Anesthesiologists then undertook the first quality of care study in anesthesia. The results, according to Gunn, "shocked and dismayed many anesthesiologists."

The study, which was published in 1954 by Beecher and Todd, was the first prospective analysis of anesthesia outcomes. Ten university hospitals contributed data from approximately 600,000 anesthetics. The death rate for patients treated by nurse anesthetists was half that of anesthesiologists. There was no difference in physical status among the patients treated by the groups of providers. However, that did not stop the authors from surmising (without evidence) that anesthesiologists were anesthetizing more complex surgical cases.[60] Not surprisingly, more quality comparisons would be conducted in the coming decades.

In 1948, for example, Olive Berger at Johns Hopkins reported 480 anesthetics for repair of cyanotic congenital heart disease in infants and children, including tetralogy of Fallot.[61] Betty Lank at Boston Children's Hospital pioneered the use of cyclopropane in pediatric anesthesia.[62] After the United States committed troops to South Korea, the National Women's Press Club named the army nurse as its Woman of the Year (1953). An army nurse anesthetist, Lt. Mildred Rush from Massachusetts, accepted the award on behalf of all army nurses.

It was the Korean War that ultimately led to the accreditation of all nurse anesthesia education programs. During the war itself, the AANA had begun accrediting programs, but it had little authority and no way to reform or close underperforming schools. To enforce proper standards, the AANA successfully appealed to the Department of Health, Education, and Welfare for recognition as the sole accrediting agency.[8] To obtain federal education benefits, returning GIs had to attend an accredited school of anesthesia. Within a few years, civilian schools either brought themselves into compliance with AANA standards or quietly closed. As with certification of graduates, the AANA now found itself as the arbiter of quality in the educating of nurses as anesthetists.

THE NEW AGE AMERICAN HEALTH CARE: THE 1960s

When the 1960s began, the AANA had evolved into a more fully fledged professional organization under the influential leadership of its first full-time executive director, Florence McQuillen, who was hired in 1948. John Lundy, the chairman of anesthesiology at the Mayo Clinic, worked with McQuillen and referred to her as "the best-read person on the literature of anesthesia." McQuillen exerted such a powerful influence at the AANA[8] that in 1965 she was named association executive of the year by the journal *Hospital Management*.

During McQuillen's tenure, membership grew considerably, exceeding 10,000 people. All 50 states had associations affiliated with the AANA. In addition, the members approved the beginnings of a continuing education program in anesthesia.[63]

The decade of the 1960s was a transitional period for everyone in health care. The United States, which had increasingly relied on employer-based health insurance since World War II, extended coverage to elderly and poor people through Medicare and Medicaid in 1965. These programs led to a greater need for health care providers. Educational programs for all health care professionals, including nurse anesthetists, expanded accordingly.

Growth was embraced by anesthesiologists in ways that were not entirely welcomed by CRNAs. Gunn recounted, "Anesthesiologists held meetings to define the future." Some sought an all-physician specialty. Others knew such a goal was unattainable because nurse anesthetists were "providing the majority of anesthesia care in the United States."[64] To resolve the manpower issue, two ideas gained prominence. Some advocated for the support of nurse anesthesia educational programs.[65] Others proposed a second anesthesia practitioner based on a physician assistant model that the anesthesiologists could control.[66,67]

The nationwide expansion of anesthesia prompted communication between anesthesiologists and CRNAs. Since 1947, an American Society of Anesthesiologists (ASA) bylaw precluded anesthesiologists from communicating with the AANA. ASA President Albert Betcher (1963) initiated efforts to establish relations with nurse anesthetists in light of the reality presented by "present and projected personnel needs."[8]

In 1964, the ASA and AANA established a liaison committee that met twice a year. McQuillen wrote that through negotiations, the AANA sought "no interference with the progress of educational programs of the Association, and a curbing of anti-nurse anesthetist activity and publicity."[68] After 3 years of meetings, the *AANA News Bulletin* and the *ASA Newsletter* published a joint statement that read in part: "It is, therefore, highly desirable that continued close liaisons be developed between these organizations for enhancing the quality and quantity of available personnel, for advancing educational opportunities, for determining ethical relationships and for the overall improvement of patient care." C.R. Stephens, a noted anesthesiologist who had worked with nurse anesthetists for many years, wrote in a 1969 report to the ASA: "Progress has not been rapid, but the dialogue has enhanced understanding."[8,69] That progress and understanding would be tested severely during the next decade.

THE 1970s

American involvement in Vietnam (Fig. 1.5) and the era of progressive reforms faded into history during the 1970s. Federal expenditures for health care rose, and in response the government exercised greater scrutiny of health services. In 1974, the US commissioner of education revised the criteria governing nationally recognized accrediting agencies, of which the AANA was one. The new criteria were intended to protect the public's interests by completely separating the professional obligations of a professional association from its proprietary concerns as a trade association.[70] The AANA, which had been widely considered the arbiter of quality in nurse anesthesia, would have to give up its roles in accrediting programs and certifying graduates, roles it had nourished and cherished since 1931. To divest itself of these operations, the AANA undertook a complete reorganization. In 1975, largely through the work of Ira Gunn, Ruth Satterfield, Mary Cavagnaro, and Ed Kaleita, autonomous councils were established and granted accrediting and certifying functions.[55]

This transition provided an opportunity for anesthesiologists to further disrupt CRNA education. Recall that anesthesiologists had turned down a similar opportunity in the 1930s. In the 1970s, the ASA proposed a "Faculty of Nurse Anesthesia Schools" that would replace the AANA as the accrediting agency. However, after strategizing and speaking before the US Office of Education, the Councils on Accreditation and Certification ultimately won the government's approval.

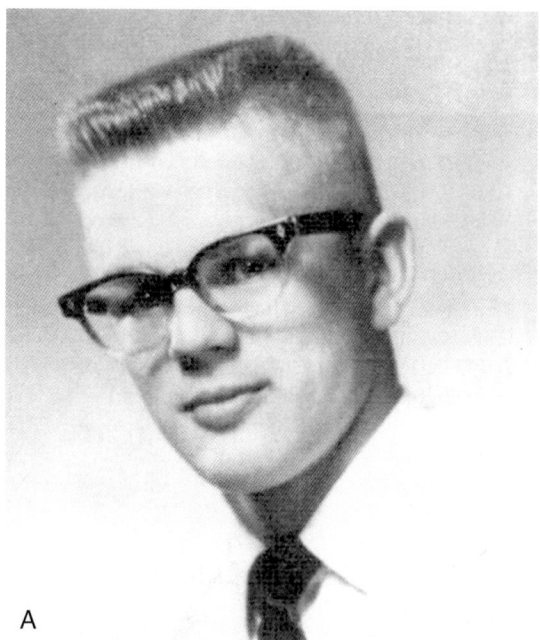
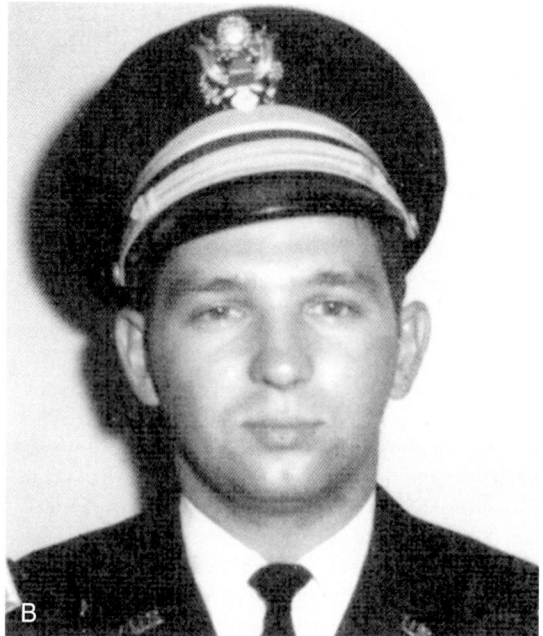

A   B

Fig. 1.5 First Lieutenants Jerome Olmsted (A) and Kenneth Shoemaker (B) were killed in 1967 following the crash of a C47 transport plane carrying wounded soldiers from Pleiku to Qui Nhon, Vietnam.

The struggle over accreditation and certification had several important outcomes. By terminating the AANA's role in accrediting schools and certifying graduates, the AANA became free to pursue laws and policies that would protect CRNAs without fear of creating a conflict between its private interests and its public duties. Second, the struggle between AANA and ASA over accreditation and certification revived the AANA's friendly relationship with the ANA, which had languished since Hodgins had first reached out to the ANA in the 1930s.[8] Third, nurse anesthetist educators saw this episode as an opportunity to upgrade educational programs and move them from hospitals into universities and colleges. John Garde, Ira Gunn, Joyce Kelly, and Sister Mary Arthur Schramm were the CRNAs who pioneered programs in the baccalaureate, and then graduate, frameworks in the early 1970s.[71] In a fourth outgrowth of this era, state nurse anesthetist organizations sought explicit legal recognition, either as a stand-alone law or within the state nurse practice act. This phase of licensure can be traced to a Department of Health, Education, and Welfare committee report from 1971 that "supported an extended scope of function for registered nurses." Higher educational standards, an increased complexity of anesthesia practice, the women's movement, and the increased presence of men in nursing have all been cited as contributing to the greater legal recognition of CRNAs.[72] Nurse anesthetists would soon be listed in the laws or regulations of all 50 states. Legal recognition provided CRNAs greater professional legitimacy. However, Mitch Tobin, the former AANA state legal affairs director, cautioned that from state to state, "the manner, type, and frequency of statutory and regulatory recognition of CRNA practice varies considerably."[73] In the following decade, the AANA would have to issue position statements to clarify and attempt to unify the ways in which CRNAs were treated under different state nurse practice acts and boards of nursing rules.

FEDERAL LEGISLATIVE INITIATIVES IN THE 1980s

By the end of the 1970s, American health care expenditures had grown from $69 billion to $230 billion, and "the reimbursement practices for hospitals and doctors were peculiarly designed to encourage higher costs.[74] Conservatives and some liberals in Congress aimed to cut that back.

Gunn described how cost control played out within anesthesia:

Anesthesiologists billed for services when they were not present in the hospital or even in town. Some chose not to come out at night or on weekends to supervise care provided in emergencies, yet they billed as if they had been present. A number of surgeons, and other providers, complained to both private insurers and Medicare. As a result, some private payers began limiting reimbursement to not more than two concurrent procedures, and Medicare's Inspector General focused on anesthesia reimbursement in the search for potential fraud. Around this time the AANA's Washington counsel, stated that a source in the Inspector General's office of what was then the US Department of Health, Education, and Welfare had told him that approximately 25% of Medicare fraud and abuse investigations were related to anesthesia services.[75]

Two federal efforts to control anesthesia costs and accountability had their genesis in these unjust reimbursement practices.

TEFRA

The first federal effort to control anesthesia costs and accountability was the Tax Equity and Fiscal Responsibility Act (TEFRA), enacted in 1982. TEFRA was designed to control costs and "ensure that an anesthesiologist demonstrated that he or she provided certain services as part of a given anesthetic to qualify for payment."[76] There were seven

services. An anesthesiologist would have to be present for the induction of anesthesia and remain immediately available for consultation. Anesthesiologists could no longer supervise more than four concurrent cases.

TEFRA would have some adverse implications for CRNAs. Its *Guidelines to the Ethical Practice of Anesthesiology* (adopted October 25, 1978; effective February 12, 1979) made this clear.[77] These guidelines separated reimbursement for anesthesiologists based on supervision or medical direction and specified payments on the basis of direction to be limited to not more than two concurrent procedures. Payment took two forms: Where CRNAs were employed by an anesthesiologist, each service was billed as though the anesthesiologist had administered each case. When the CRNAs were hospital employees, the time units for the anesthesiologist were cut in half. When the anesthesiologist's service was supervision and not direction (i.e., supervising three or more CRNAs), the payment was to be made under Part A of Medicare on the basis of a "reasonable charge." The hospital could still bill for the CRNA services of their own employees under Part A if the services were provided within the hospital and under Part B of Medicare if the services were provided in a surgical center.

An Existential Threat Leads to Direct Reimbursement

In early 1983, while the AANA was still dealing with TEFRA, without much fanfare and with less media exposure than usually accompanies such legislation, Congress passed a second cost control bill, the prospective payment system (PPS). The PPS revised the means of calculating Medicare billing from a cost-plus fee-for-service basis to a prospective price based on diagnosis-related groups. This measure posed a much greater threat to CRNAs than did TEFRA.

The PPS legislation was a powerful disincentive to the hiring of nurse anesthetists for the following reasons: (1) It would be impossible for the anesthesia component of payment to cover the full cost of hospital-employed CRNAs; (2) separating CRNA services from the global cost of the surgery (unbundling) was prohibited; and (3) anesthesiologists who had been billing for CRNA services under Medicare Part B could no longer do so. Taken together, these caveats meant "CRNA services were, for all practical purposes, nonreimbursable."[76]

The very real threat posed by PPS mandated action. Either the reimbursement for both anesthesiologists and CRNAs would need to be placed under the same source, Medicare Part A, or AANA would have to seek direct reimbursement rights for CRNAs under Medicare Part B.

In the 1980s, CRNAs were heavily recruited health care professionals. Most CRNAs were employed by hospitals or anesthesiologists, but a growing number of CRNAs practiced privately. Private practice CRNAs were unable to obtain reimbursement directly from Medicare, Medicaid, and many private insurance companies. After a 3-year-long effort that Bankert described as "one of the greatest lobbying achievements not only of the AANA, but of the whole of nursing," President Reagan signed into law the Omnibus Budget Reconciliation Act of 1986.[78]

Since then, Medicare and Medicaid have paid directly for all CRNA services, making nurse anesthetists the first nursing specialty to be so accorded. Of its importance, Dr. Judith Ryan, executive director of the ANA, said, "The American Association of Nurse Anesthetists' achievement to secure direct reimbursement for CRNAs is a singular, notable contribution to identification and payment of the nurse as a provider of care, and nursing services as covered health benefits."[79]

Nonlegislative Legal Problems Arise

In the same decade, events of no less significance took place in civil law pertaining to anesthesia. The courts tested whether a surgeon is liable for the actions of a nurse anesthetist. Traditionally, surgeons have been considered "Captains of the Ship" and were therefore thought to be responsible for everything that occurred inside an operating room. Logically this theory was extended to mean that "nurses (and nurse anesthetists) become the temporary servants or agents of the attending surgeon during the course of an operation, and liability for their negligent acts may thus be imposed upon the surgeon under the doctrine of *respondeat superior*.[8] Blumenreich explained the danger to CRNAs of this theory: "When surgeons work with nurse anesthetists, the surgeons become liable for their mistakes—but when surgeons work with anesthesiologists, the surgeons do not have to worry about what happens at the head of the table." But, in fact, the theory is fallacious. Blumenreich went on to say, "First, surgeons are not always liable for the negligence of nurse anesthetists. Second, surgeons may also be liable for the negligence of anesthesiologists. Third, because a surgeon's liability, whether working with nurse anesthetists or anesthesiologists, depends on the particular facts of the situation, as a practical matter, the surgeon is likely to be included in the suit whether the surgeon is working with a nurse anesthetist or an anesthesiologist." In fact, no surgeon has been held liable in a court of law for the negligence of a nurse anesthetist. Courts have apportioned liability according to the specific facts of a case.[80,81]

A second area of civil law that affected anesthesia in the 1980s was antitrust. Nurse anesthetists, like other professionals, are subject to antitrust laws. However, they can also use those laws when they allege that others have conspired to restrict CRNA practice. Four cases involving CRNAs illustrate this point: *Bhan v. NME Hospitals, Inc.* (1985), *Oltz v. St. Peter's Community Hospital* (1988), *Hyde v. Jefferson Parish Hospital District No. 2* (1983), and *Minnesota Association of Nurse Anesthetists v. Allina Health System Corp.* (2002).

Tafford Oltz's hospital privileges were terminated when the hospital gave an exclusive contract to a group of anesthesiologists. The verdict in Oltz's favor turned on the fact that St. Peter's Community Hospital had significant enough market share within its service area to exert a monopoly, and that by awarding the exclusive contract to the anesthesiologists the hospital damaged competition.[82]

Vinod (Vinnie) Bhan sued his hospital in California after he was terminated and replaced with anesthesiologists. The defendants (both the hospital and the anesthesiologists) asserted that Bhan, as a nurse and nurse anesthetist, did not, in the eyes of the law, compete with physicians because of their different licensure. Bhan lost the case because the hospital that terminated his privileges did not have sufficient market share in the community to restrain competition. However, an appellate court ruling that gave Bhan and CRNAs standing to sue anesthesiologists as competitors set a significant legal precedent for the profession. The Ninth Circuit Court concluded: "No doubt the legal restrictions upon nurse anesthetists create a functional distinction between nurses and MD anesthesiologists. They do not, however, necessarily preclude the existence of a reasonable interchangeability of use or cross-elasticity of demand sufficient to constrain the market power of MD anesthesiologists and thereby to affect competition."[83,84] Blumenreich said, "The Bhan case was important because it gave to some extent the protections of the antitrust laws to nurse anesthetists. Hospitals could not boycott nurse anesthetists." Its results would be more "long-lasting." In a third antitrust case, *Hyde v. Jefferson Parish Hospital* (1983), an anesthesiologist sued the hospital and a group of anesthesiologists that held an exclusive contract with the hospital and worked with hospital-employed CRNAs. Dr. Hyde was denied privileges solely on the basis of the exclusive contract. Hyde claimed that a patient who was admitted for surgery in effect had no choice but to buy anesthesia from the hospital's exclusive group of anesthesiologists. The Jefferson Parish Hospital District won the case at the lower court level, but Hyde appealed all the way to the US Supreme Court.

The ASA filed an *amicus curiae* brief, but in support of Dr. Hyde. The ASA opposed exclusive contracts but attempted to link its opinion to the quality of care, stating that "the elimination of competition through a classic tying arrangement is not simply a matter of dollars and cents. It can adversely affect the quality of medical care. ASA believes that in this setting, it is particularly important that competition be allowed to reward superior performance and innovation, while exposing the indifference to quality that may too often be the hallmark of a monopoly."[85]

The Supreme Court ruled unanimously in favor of the hospital's right to award an exclusive contract for anesthesia services. A footnote in the Court's opinion to the effect that 'there has been no showing that nurse anesthetists provide a lesser quality of care' led Blumenreich to conclude that the AANA accomplished what it set out to do.[86] Gunn wrote that "the Hyde case alerted the AANA to the need to revitalize its public relations program, continue its watch for attempts to discredit CRNAs, and take action either to correct or to prevent further damage."

In a fourth and final antitrust-related case, the Minnesota Association of Nurse Anesthetists (MANA) sued a hospital group and its anesthesiologists alleging restriction of trade and fraudulent billing. Anesthesiologists had forced CRNAs to leave their jobs and return only under restrictive and lesser paying conditions, while at the same time they billed for supervising CRNAs without fulfilling the necessary steps outlined earlier under TEFRA and the PPS conditions for payment. CRNAs across the country donated at least $2.5 million to support the prosecution. The antitrust case was ultimately dismissed, but the fraudulent billing portion resulted in a $10 million out-of-court settlement in favor of MANA. With the settlement money MANA repaid a loan from the AANA and made a significant contribution to the AANA Foundation. Brian Thorson, president of MANA and then-president of AANA during the 10-year-long case, said CRNAs who contemplate using the antitrust laws to right a wrong should think twice:

> Never be afraid to stand up to injustice. With that in mind, the opposition will be extremely well funded, and it is difficult to topple organized medicine.
>
> **Brian Thorson, AANA President**

CRNA ACHIEVEMENTS OF THE 1980s

Although much attention focused on events taking place on the legal front, other important areas of practice were advanced in the 1980s. For example, liability insurance coverage, first offered to CRNAs in 1974 by outside brokerages, was skillfully brought in-house when the AANA bought the Glen Nyhan Agency. Renamed A+, and now called AANA Insurance, the agency has provided a steady stream of insurance to CRNAs since 1988, without which CRNAs would be subject to outside insurance companies, some controlled by physicians.

The AANA Education and Research Foundation was established in 1981; it would be renamed the AANA Foundation in 1995. The foundation has enjoyed enormous support. A current report lists scholarships, grants, poster presentations, fellowships, and health policy research in excess of $4.2 million given to 3800 individuals.[87,88]

The history of nurse anesthesia would be incomplete without remembering CRNA Goldie Brangman (Fig. 1.6). In September 1958 at Harlem Hospital in New York City, Brangman was called to take over at the head of an operating room table by her mentor Helen Mayer, an anesthesiologist. Brangman recalled, "Dr. Mayer stood up, and I sat down." The patient was Dr. Martin Luther King Jr., who had been stabbed while autographing copies of his first book, *March to Freedom*. King would live another 10 years and change history. Brangman, who lived to the age of 102, went on to change anesthesia. She completed 45 years at

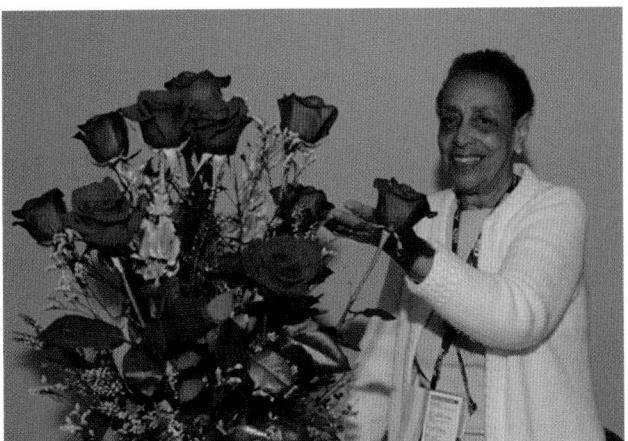

Fig. 1.6 Goldie Brangman.

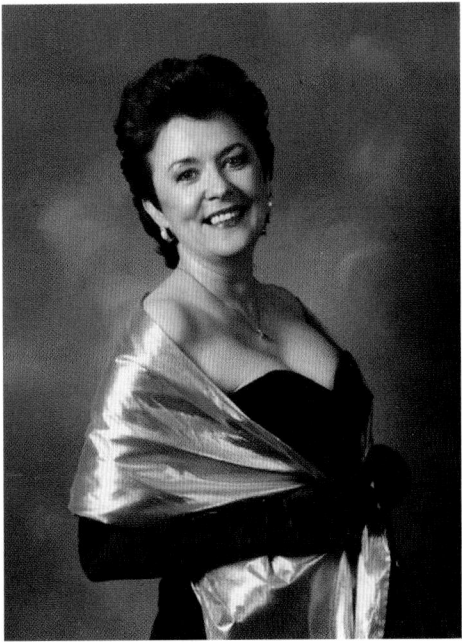

Fig. 1.7 Marianne Downey (nee Bankert).

the Harlem Hospital, 38 of them as director of its school of nurse anesthesia, educating at "least 700 to 750 students. There weren't too many schools at the time that admitted blacks, men, or students from foreign countries. We would hold dinners each weekend and try different foods representing one of our students' diverse ethnic backgrounds."[89]

Between 1967 and 1973, Brangman ascended the AANA hierarchy. As president in 1974, Brangman devoted herself to improving the internal workings of the AANA, which had languished following the 1970 retirement of McQuillen. Her leadership brought on modernized internal and external communications and business methods, and it established an executive committee of the board of trustees. At the same time, the AANA annual meeting was (1) expanded to include concomitant lectures, refresher courses, special activities, and lectures for students and (2) streamlined with written, rather than verbal, committee reports and other important information. Under Brangman's leadership, the members voted to discontinue holding the AANA annual meeting in conjunction with the American Hospital Association. These steps were evidence of dramatic advances in corporate financial and professional maturity.

Brangman was principally an educator who extended the possibility of nurse anesthesia to many who, because of their race, might not otherwise have been admitted to a program. Moreover, she taught regional anesthesia long before it became a standard part of the curriculum and pioneered quality assurance in anesthesia. Brangman was honored with both the Helen Lamb Outstanding Educator Award and Agatha Hodgins Award for Outstanding Accomplishment, the profession's highest attainments. Years later, near the end of her impactful life, Brangman inspired other CRNAs of color to initiate a diversity and inclusion program that would further correct the racial imbalance in nurse anesthesia.[90,91] Marianne Downey (nee Bankert) (Fig 1.7) was an English professor who wrote the vital publication, "Watchful Care: A History of America's Nurse Anesthetists." She had been chair of the English department at the College of Joliet (Illinois) where she took a keen interest in the history of nurses, and nurse anesthetists in particular. Hired by the AANA to follow up the earlier work of Thatcher, Downey showed through astute analysis that early and later CRNAs fought gender-based and economic discrimination to build a nursing specialty that is second to none. "Watchful Care," published in 1989, received very positive reviews from, among other journals, the *American Association for the History of Nursing,*[92] the *Bulletin of the History of Medicine,*[93] and *The Journal of American History.*[94] That Downey conducted her research before the AANA established its own archival program, when 50+ years of books and inactive records were stacked in cardboard boxes in the dusty attic above the association's offices, makes her accomplishment that much more laudable.

In addition, Downey prompted the AANA to preserve its own history by establishing a formal archival program, which lives on today as the John F. Garde Archives.

THE CALL FOR HEALTH CARE REFORM IN THE 1990s

Bill Clinton (whose mother, Virginia Kelly, was a CRNA)[95] was elected president in 1992 with a promise to reform health care. For a variety of reasons, Clinton's health care plan was defeated. In its place, the health insurance industry, in conjunction with the major businesses that provided health insurance to their employees, forced a form of "managed care" on a large portion of the insured population. Managed care, in theory, was intended to (1) move the health care system from a disease treatment to a health maintenance system; (2) do away with incentives found in the fee-for-service system—that is, the more services provided, the more money made—and thereby reduce unnecessary health services[96,97]; (3) promote a cost-effective workforce by emphasizing primary care providers and nonphysician professionals; and (4) promote a shift from independent practice patterns to greater use of salaried personnel. Some anesthesiologist groups found that, under managed care, their workload declined by 40%.[98] Physicians thus scrambled to protect autonomy and income, while patients sought to preserve some choice of provider.

When CRNAs won direct reimbursement rights in 1986, they agreed to accept no more than the amount Medicare assigned for the service as payment in full. In other words, CRNAs would not "balance bill" patients for any portion of their fees. Payment schedules were then devised for anesthesiologists working alone, CRNAs working alone, and anesthesiologists medically directing CRNAs in team practice settings. In the early 1990s, a Government Accounting Office (GAO) study[99] revealed that payments for anesthesia services under the medical direction arrangement were 120% to 140% greater than payments for CRNAs or anesthesiologists working alone. This payment scheme served as a strong incentive for anesthesiologists to employ CRNAs, but it was not budget neutral, which had been the intent of Congress. The GAO recommended payment of only one anesthesia fee, totaling no more than if an anesthesiologist performed the service alone. Furthermore, the study recommended that payment for anesthetic procedures under the medical direction model be split 50% for the

CRNA service and 50% for the anesthesiologist service, a significantly reduced portion for both the anesthesiologists and the CRNAs. The AANA chose to support the single-payment plan. The ASA opposed it. The single-payment reimbursement plan was implemented, and tension between the two groups was exacerbated again.

The reforms of the 1990s, together with the new ability to bill third-party payers for their services, led entrepreneurial CRNAs to venture into the business of anesthesia. At the same time, the Jack Neary Pain Fellowship brought the subspecialty of pain control within the reach of CRNAs. Private CRNA practice had been largely limited to office-based surgery centers and small rural hospitals. Now corporate practices catering to hospitals and larger surgery centers grew, including pain practices. In this scenario, a CRNA businessperson might perform cases but would facilitate and manage a contract for one or more clinical sites.

Attempts to Measure Quality of Care

It was mentioned earlier that during the second half of the 20th century, physicians and then nurses attempted to evaluate the quality of anesthesia care by measuring death rates. In the aforementioned Beecher and Todd study, the anesthesiologist outcomes were inferior to CRNA outcomes.[100] Two decades later, amid complaints about the Veterans Administration (VA) health care system, the US House of Representatives mandated a study by the National Science Foundation regarding the care given to veterans. At the time, CRNAs provided much of the anesthesia administered at VA facilities. The reviewers reported back to Congress in 1977 that there were no significant differences in anesthesia outcomes based on the providers of that care.[101]

In 1980, an anesthesiologist named W. H. Forrest published a portion of an institutional differences study conducted by the Stanford Center for Health Care Research. Forrest divided the institutions between those predominantly served by nurse anesthetists and those predominantly served by anesthesiologists. He concluded—using conservative statistical methods—that there were no significant differences in anesthesia outcomes between the two anesthesia providers.[102]

A North Carolina retrospective study of anesthesia-related mortality from 1969 to 1976, which was performed by a committee from the North Carolina Society of Anesthesiologists, was published in 1981. The findings were similar for all providers (e.g., CRNAs working alone, anesthesiologists working alone, and CRNAs and anesthesiologists working together as a team); however, no test of significance was made in this study.[103]

Between 1992 and 2003, additional studies by Abenstein and Warner, Silber et al., Wiklund and Rosenbaum, and Vila et al. were published and promoted as evidence that "the utilization of anesthesiologists improves anesthesia outcomes." These studies and their rebuttals were summarized in "Quality of Care in Anesthesia," a 2009 publication by AANA.[104] The article by Abenstein and Warner "purported to analyze the quality of care…but failed to mention the key conclusion." For example, the authors claimed that there were "differences in the outcomes of care based on type of provider, *notwithstanding that the actual researchers came to the opposite conclusion*" (emphasis original). The Silbur study "examined the death rate, adverse occurrence rate, and failure rate of 5972 Medicare patients." One analyst concluded that these data were, in fact, not "specific to anesthesia staffing," and "the type of anesthesia provider does not appear to be a significant factor in the occurrence of potentially lethal complications." Two studies attributed to Wiklund and Rosenbaum were also found to be irrelevant. The AANA reviewer pointed out that Wiklund and Rosenbaum, by attributing safer anesthesia to a federal decision to "support training in clinical anesthesiology" had left "the path of unbiased review of the specialty to make unsubstantiated or misleading comments about the unilateral contributions of anesthesiologists to the advancements achieved."

The Silber study stirred up "serious questions of objectivity." "Reportedly, both the *Journal of the American Medical Association* and the *New England Journal of Medicine* declined to publish" it. The timing of its publication led to questions about its motivation. "The abstract was published in the midst of the controversy over the Health Care Financing Administrations (HCFA's) proposal to remove the physician supervision requirement for nurse anesthetists in Medicare cases." The AANA reviewers concluded, "The timing of the publication in the ASA's own journal was politically motivated" to influence the HCFA (now known as the Centers for Medicare and Medicaid Services [CMS]). However, CMS ultimately "dismissed all claims" made by the authors in this study.

The Vila study compared outcomes at ambulatory surgery centers (ASCs) with those in office operating rooms (a practice for many independent CRNAs). It claimed that "the risk of adverse incidents and deaths was approximately 10 times greater in the office setting than in an ASC, and that if all office procedures had been performed in ASCs, approximately 43 injuries and six deaths per year could have been prevented." It concluded with the hopeful remark that "the presence of anesthesiologists in ASCs may be a factor in more favorable outcomes." The AANA analyst pointed out flaws in both the methodology and conclusions of this study. The study "does not specifically mention CRNAs," yet it "makes the unsupportable assertion that office surgery may not be as safe when an anesthesiologist is not present."

Misuse of outcomes research was extensive during this era. Gunn wrote that "in the medical literature in the 1990s, serious questions were raised regarding the quality and relevance of published research, the peer review system, and the selection of articles for publication."[105] A 1993 review concluded that 95% of the medical research being published in journals was either flawed or irrelevant.[106]

The Federal Supervision Regulation

In what past-President Larry Hornsby described as a "message from the grave," Magaw commented that, during the 1890s at the Mayo Clinic, physicians oversaw nurse anesthesia in a "general way." In other words, Magaw and her colleague Henderson were on their own. In the next 20 years, as the acceptance of nurse anesthetists grew, a few physicians sought control over the women who practiced anesthesia. The 1915 challenge to the Lakeside Hospital School made this trend clear. Nurse anesthetists welcomed the legislation sought by Crile and some of his colleagues in Ohio that for the first time codified the practice of nurse anesthesia in law.[11] As noted earlier, the legislation mentioned supervision, but it legitimized their practice.[37,107]

In the 1980s, at the same time TEFRA took effect, the number of anesthesiologists tripled. Increased competition in the anesthesia marketplace prompted Blumenreich to write that supervision became the springboard for yet new attacks. In 1985, H. Ketcham Morrell, president of the ASA, wrote: "…the operating surgeon or obstetrician who purports to provide medical direction of the nurse, in the absence of an anesthesiologist, carries a high risk of exposure, on a variety of legal theories, for the acts of the nurse."[108] An unknown number of surgeons opted for anesthesiologists as a result. Imagined liability among surgeons became such a crisis that Blumenreich wrote: "…no subject has received more of my attention."

For CRNAs, removing supervision from the Medicare Rules was an obvious remedy, because it would impact practice in every state. From 1994 to 2001, HCFA and AANA attempted to do just that. The enormous struggles that ensued were chronicled briefly by Patrick Downey in the *AANA Journal*[109] and in captivating detail by Sandra Larson.[110] Legislation was introduced in both houses of Congress that would remove the supervision requirement and address reimbursement issues. Both the AANA and ASA responded with grassroots public relations campaigns, and the legislation went nowhere. Then, in December 1997, HCFA proposed a major change in its *Hospital Conditions of Participation*, including the elimination of physician supervision of CRNAs. Nursing organizations lined up in support of the change, but medical opposition was fierce. Nullifying legislation was proposed, as were safety studies to delay its consideration. More public relations were deployed, and the controversial claims of the Silbur study (that outcomes are better when CRNAs are supervised by anesthesiologists) were invoked. In March 2000, HCFA ruled that CRNAs could practice without physician supervision, and in its ruling HCFA deemed the Silbur study "irrelevant." But the new rule was not implemented until the final days of the Clinton administration, and the Bush administration, as all new administrations do, placed a moratorium on late-term regulations. In November 2001, the Bush administration, in response to vigorous and costly lobbying by the ASA, "allowed political favoritism" to prevail over rigorous policymaking. The new administration restored the earlier rule containing supervision.

The "final" rule contained an escape clause, a proviso allowing state governors to opt out. Between 20 and 31 states had no laws specifying supervision of CRNAs, which meant governors, if inclined, might provide an opt-out. Before long, some governors did. Iowa was the first, and then a number of rural western states opted out. To date, governors in 19 states have done so. These include Iowa, Nebraska, Idaho, Minnesota, Arizona, New Hampshire, New Mexico, Kansas, North Dakota, Washington, Alaska, Oregon, Montana, South Dakota, Wisconsin, California, Colorado, Kentucky, and Oklahoma. In Michigan, to meet the expanded need for providers during the Covid-19 pandemic, Governor Whitmer suspended the supervision requirement "until the end of the declared emergency." It is unclear what she will do if and when the Covid-19 emergency ends.[111] Depending on one's interpretation of the eligibility rules, this includes between 60% and 90% of eligible states.

Opting out of physician supervision has not altered the safety of anesthesia. Two prominent health economists, Brian Dulisse and Jerry Cromwell, studied Medicare data between 1999 and 2005.[112] They found "no evidence that opting out of the oversight requirement resulted in increased inpatient deaths or complications." This came as no surprise to the AANA and CRNAs. The authors concluded: "We recommend that CMS return to its original intention of allowing nurse anesthetists to work independently of surgeons or anesthesiologist supervision without requiring state governments to formally petition for an exemption."

Other contemporary studies supporting this assertion were collected in the publication *Quality of Care in Anesthesia*.[113] They reported no significant differences between CRNAs and Anesthesiologists with respect to obstetric anesthesia outcomes, similar mortality rates when working individually, and no difference for team versus solo practice. There was also no differences in mortality in hospitals without an Anesthesiologists versus those where they provided or directed anesthesia care. Lastly, the Institute of Medicine—the health arm of the National Academy of Sciences—weighed in with a report, entitled "The Future of Nursing: Focus on Scope of Practice."[114] The report came as a powerful endorsement of nurses as high-quality clinicians. Its conclusion reads, in part:

It is time to eliminate the outdated regulations and organizational and cultural barriers that limit the ability of nurses to practice to the full extent of their education, training, and competence. The U.S. is transforming its health care system to provide quality care leading to improved health outcomes, and nurses can and should play a significant role. The current conflicts between various APRNs scope of practice are based on their education and training. State and federal regulations must be resolved so that they are better able to provide seamless, affordable, and quality care. Scope-of-practice regulations in all states should reflect the full extent not only of nurses but of each profession's education and training. Elimination of barriers for all professions with a focus on collaborative teamwork will maximize and improve care throughout the health care system.

DOCTORAL PREPARATION OF NURSE ANESTHETISTS ACHIEVED

Upgrading Nurse Anesthesia Educational Requirements

Improving academic credentials for CRNA educators and their graduates has always been closely aligned with the goals of the professional association.[115] Nurse anesthesia educators have been responsible for increasing requirements for curricular content, faculty qualifications, and academic credentials for graduates since the early 20th century. Over time, schools of anesthesia have changed from apprenticeships at hospitals into degree-granting institutions fulfilling the vision of early anesthesia leaders for a university education for nurse anesthetists. This movement into academia required identifying the location of schools of anesthesia throughout the nation, determining the essential characteristics of better schools, agreeing on curricular requirements, inspecting schools, and developing a school approval process. Lamb envisioned the bright professional future this upward trend might bring about, writing in 1936 that schools of anesthesia should seek affiliation with universities, and that such affiliation "should eventually result in broadened facilities, both practical and cultural."

Beginning in the mid-1980s, the AANA and the Council on Accreditation (COA) assessed the need for and feasibility of practice-oriented doctoral degrees for nurse anesthetists. In June 2005, the AANA board of directors convened an invitational summit meeting to discuss interests and concerns surrounding doctoral preparation for nurse anesthetists. Following the summit, a Task Force on Doctoral Preparation of Nurse Anesthetists (DTF) was formed and charged with developing options related to doctoral preparation of nurse anesthetists for the AANA board to consider.[116] The DTF's final report and options were presented to the AANA board of directors in April 2007, and in June 2007 the board unanimously adopted the position of supporting doctoral education for entry into nurse anesthesia practice by the year 2025.

Setting a requirement for doctoral education followed in October 2009, when the Council on Accreditation of Nurse Anesthesia Education Programs adopted this position: "The COA will not consider any new master's degree programs for accreditation beyond 2015: and that students accepted into an accredited program on January 1, 2022, and thereafter must graduate with doctoral degrees." The position became part of the Standard on Accreditation of Nurse Anesthesia Educational Programs and the basis for drafting new standards for clinical doctorate programs.[116]

The Changing Face of Nurse Anesthesia

In 2007, President Terry Wicks realized the low visibility of minority CRNAs.[117] AANA had admitted its first black members in 1944, but there had been just one black AANA president, the late Goldie Brangman. Brangman, when she was AANA treasurer, had been excluded from speaking at board meetings; the overall percentage of black CRNAs remained well below 10%, and the number who ascended to state and national positions could be counted on one hand. Wallena Gould and Regina Daniels McKinney developed and implemented a wide-ranging diversity and inclusion effort, including mentorship of candidates and support for students and faculty. Brangman commented that the diversification was a pleasure for her to behold, adding that it builds a better AANA.

MILITARY ANESTHESIA

The US military remains engaged around the world. CRNAs deploy to trouble spots as members of the armed forces. Others work within the Department of Health and Human Services for the US Public Health Service and the VA. CRNAs are versatile, fulfilling more than clinical duties in today's military; they are also leaders and, in some cases, soldiers on the line. CRNAs Maj. Steve McColley and Cpt. Mitchell Bailey earned Bronze Star Medal nominations for acts of courage in Iraq. Maj. Jeffrey Roos, a CRNA stationed at Fort Benning, Georgia, earned a Bronze Star from the army for his lifesaving efforts during Operation Anaconda, the first major US offensive launched in Afghanistan after the September 11, 2001, attacks on the World Trade Center. A CRNA was in the news for extricating Pvt. Jessica Lynch from a hospital in Iraq.

In past wars, CRNA deployments reduced anesthesia staff at stateside hospitals. No data exist to describe the overall impact of the latest escalation on anesthesia services in stateside hospitals. However, the impact of deployments has been mitigated somewhat following a recent policy change in the navy. Navy CRNAs are now considered "licensed independent practitioners" (LIPs), a term coined by The Joint Commission (TJC). According to Cpt. Annette Hasselbeck, NC USN, LIP status has enabled the navy's medical planners to use global sourcing of CRNAs. CRNAs are used interchangeably with anesthesiologists, based on skills, seniority, and availability. This had always been the pattern in practice, but defining CRNAs as LIPs has kept practice in compliance with TJC policy. According to Cpt. Ron Van Nest, NC USN (retired), the policy was changed in 2000 to reflect the fact that CRNAs very often deploy alone and capably make independent clinical decisions that affect anesthetic management. Recognizing CRNAs as LIPs has also kept morale high; all billets are filled, and retention of naval CRNAs is at 100% as of this writing.

INTERNATIONAL FEDERATION OF NURSE ANESTHETISTS

The International Federation of Nurse Anesthetists (IFNA) is a coalition of national associations of nurse anesthetists. It is an affiliate member of the International Council of Nurses and a Nursing Partner of the World Health Organization. The IFNA represents more than 50,000 nurse anesthetists worldwide and is a growing organization with members in both developed and developing countries. The first organizational meeting was held in September 1988, and 11 countries were admitted as charter members in 1989. A World Congress is held every 2 years and is hosted by a member country.

To date, there are 36 member countries. The IFNA has developed international standards for education, standards of practice, standards for patient monitoring, and a code of ethics for nurse anesthetists.[36] An anesthesia approval process for entry-level programs was launched in 2010, offering three levels of awards: registration, recognition, and accreditation. The goal of the Anesthesia Program Approval Process is to encourage programs to comply with the IFNA's *Educational Standards for Preparing Nurse Anesthetists* through an approval process that takes cultural, national, or regional differences into consideration.[118]

PROGRESS IN ANESTHESIA

Since the 1890s, nurse anesthetists facilitated the advancement of modern surgery. Their expertise with ether anesthesia made possible the first successful intracranial, thoracic, adult and pediatric cardiac, and trauma operations.[108] Nurse anesthetists elevated the quality of anesthesia education available to nurses by implementing certification and recently recertification by examination, accreditation of schools, mandatory continuing education, and progressively higher degree standards for entry into practice. Progress in nurse anesthesia attributable to CRNAs has occurred in other areas as well. The AANA Foundation describes hundreds of recent and ongoing CRNA-led research projects.[119] These projects range from basic and applied sciences to clinical anesthesia, education, and economics. Public awareness of CRNAs grew in 2020 as a result of Covid-19. CRNAs are at the forefront of the battle against Covid-19 and frequently appeared in the media during the initial outbreak. This was a marked change from decades in which they were aptly described as "the best kept secret in health care." Notable articles and photographs are listed at "CRNAs in the News."[120]

SUMMARY

Nurses were recruited into the field of anesthesia by surgeons in the latter half of the 19th century because inexpert clinical anesthesia administration by others often resulted in morbidity and mortality. The Civil War was the earliest documented use of nurses as anesthetists, and it became a trend thereafter. By the 1890s, nurse anesthesia, having spread from midwestern Catholic hospitals to cities on both coasts, made anesthesia increasingly safe and thereby facilitated the advancement of surgery. Before the turn of the 20th century, nurse anesthetists provided gratuitous training to others. They opened the first hospital-based anesthesia educational program in 1909. During World War I, nurse anesthetists significantly reduced combat-related surgical morbidity and mortality. By 1920, nurse anesthesia had become well established and well accepted.

Nurse anesthetists formed a national organization in 1931. Dedicating themselves to advancing anesthesia education and patient safety, nurse anesthetists implemented a number of firsts: annual meetings, a monthly bulletin, and a journal. In 1945, the first certification examination for graduates was implemented. As a result of service in the midcentury wars, nurse anesthetists earned officer's status, and men gained the right to join the military's nurse corps. When the military demanded that its nurse anesthetists pass the AANA certification examination, civilian hospitals soon followed suit. By the 1950s, nurse anesthetists worked with surgeons and engineers to pioneer anesthesia machinery, ventilators, and anesthesia for pediatric cardiovascular surgery. During this era, accreditation of anesthesia training programs was achieved.

The second half of the 20th century was marked by a closer involvement between the profession and government. As Medicare paid for a larger proportion of clinical anesthesia services, the government in turn exerted increasing control over how those services were rendered and at what cost to taxpayers. Federal dollars were allocated for nursing education, and the government exerted a measure of control over accreditation. Independent counsels on accreditation, certification, recertification, and public interest evolved.

In the 1960s and 1970s, state governments modernized nurse practice acts to account for new subspecialties in advanced practice nursing. CRNAs had to participate, even though they had long predated other advanced practice nurses. The 1980s and 1990s brought about governmental efforts to "reform" health care by extending services and containing costs. Quality of care entered the debate, and CRNAs ultimately proved what had been shown 50 years earlier: Anesthesia outcomes are no worse and perhaps better when a CRNA administers the anesthetic. For CRNAs, constant vigilance and a presence in federal and state government centers were essential because of each of the aforementioned policy changes.

Progress in nurse anesthesia has occurred over many decades and resulted in an extraordinary record of patient safety. CRNAs have undertaken hundreds of clinical, scientific, and policy research projects to further professional and public understanding of nurse anesthesia.

Patient	Intervention	Comparison	Outcome
61-year-old male, infarction	Streptokinase	Plasminogen activator	Death
31-year-old female, laparoscopy	Ondansetron 4 mg	Droperidol 1.25 mg	Nausea
17-year-old male, arthroscopy	Spinal anesthesia	—	Time in PACU

REFERENCES

For a complete list of references for this chapter, scan this QR code with any smartphone code reader app, or visit the following URL: http://booksite.elsevier.com/9780323711944/.

Nurse Anesthesia Specialty Practice and Education in the United States

Francis Gerbasi, Lynn Reede

NURSE ANESTHESIA EDUCATIONAL REQUIREMENTS

Nurse anesthesia educational requirements form the foundation for the nurse anesthesia profession. The upgrading stringent and robust educational requirements ensure that graduates have the knowledge, skills, and abilities to enter into practice and provide safe anesthesia care. In 1931 the National Association of Nurse Anesthetists (NANA) was established by Agatha Hodgins. A primary goal of NANA was to develop nurse anesthesia educational objectives.[1] In 1939 the NANA changed its name to the American Association of Nurse Anesthesia (AANA). Accreditation standards and processes were established to ensure high-quality nurse anesthesia programs. The accreditation function for nurse anesthesia programs was performed by the AANA until 1975 when the Council on Accreditation of Nurse Anesthesia Educational Programs (COA) was established and assumed responsibility for establishing the standards and accreditation of nurse anesthesia programs. The COA is the only accrediting agency recognized by the US Department of Education (USDE) and the Council for Higher Education Accreditation (CHEA) to accredit nurse anesthesia programs in the United States and Puerto Rico. The scope of the COA's accreditation includes nurse anesthesia programs that award post-master's certificates, master's, or doctoral degrees, including programs offering distance education. The standards (i.e., master's, doctoral, and fellowships) are measures used by the COA to assess the quality of nurse anesthesia education. The COA has been responsible for increasing the requirements for curricular content, faculty qualifications, and academic credentials for graduates. This includes the requirement that all COA-accredited nurse anesthesia programs award a master's degree in 1998 and award doctoral degrees to students entering programs on January 1, 2022, and thereafter.

Nurse Anesthesia Education Today

As of January 1, 2021, there are 124 accredited nurse anesthesia programs and 5 new programs in capability review. There are 103 nurse anesthesia programs approved to offer entry-level doctoral degrees and 25 programs offering post-master's doctoral completion degree programs for Certified Registered Nurse Anesthetists (CRNAs). The remaining 21 programs must be approved by the COA to award doctoral degrees for entry into practice by the deadline of January 1, 2022. The progress made in programs transitioning to award doctoral degrees in the last 10 years is shown in Fig. 2.1.

Nurse anesthesia programs are currently governed by two sets of standards based on the degree the program is awarding. Programs awarding master's degrees are governed by the 2004 *Standards for Accreditation of Nurse Anesthesia Educational Programs.*[2] Programs awarding doctoral degrees are governed by the Standards for Nurse Anesthesia Programs: Practice Doctorate.[3] In 2014 the COA established Standards for Accreditation of Post-Graduate CRNA Fellowships.[4] The processes used to accredit programs and fellowships are focused on ensuring compliance with the *Standards* and the COA *Accreditation Policies and Procedures.*[5]

Accreditation provides a means to assure and improve higher education quality.[6] Revisions to the *Standards* and the accreditation policies occur periodically in order to ensure they continue to reflect the current requirements and prepare graduates for entry into practice, meet USDE and CHEA recognition requirements, and promote improvement in nurse anesthesia education. In 2011, the COA initiated a major revision of its Standards with the purpose of establishing new practice doctorate standards. In 2015 the COA approved the practice doctorate standards.[7] In 2016 the COA established the Programs' Transitions to the Doctoral Level policy.[5] The policy provides the procedural information for programs and reinforces the requirements that all accredited programs must offer a doctoral degree for students entering nurse anesthesia programs by January 1, 2022, and thereafter.

General Educational Requirements for Nurse Anesthesia Programs

Nurse anesthesia programs are required to demonstrate compliance with the *Standards* and the *Accreditation Policies and Procedures* to be accredited by the COA. Programs are required to assess their integrity and educational effectiveness through ongoing evaluation and assessment. Programs must continually monitor and evaluate their didactic and clinical curriculum, including but not limited to curricular content, admissions policies, faculty, and clinical sites used for student educational experiences. In addition to programs' internal assessment processes, programs must submit annual reports to the COA, complete self-studies, and host onsite COA visits.

National Certification Exam Pass Rate

The COA monitors programs' indicators of success and the attainment of their stated outcomes. This includes each program's pass rates on the National Board of Certification and Recertification for Nurse Anesthetists (NBCRNA) National Certification Examination (NCE), students' attrition, and graduates' employment rates.

Programs must demonstrate graduates take the NCE examination and pass it in accordance with the COA's pass-rate requirement. The COA established a certification exam policy for monitoring programs' NCE pass rates in 2003. Major revisions to the policy were made in 2006, 2013, 2016, and 2019. The most recent revised policy establishes three methods that programs can use to meet the mandatory requirement of 80%.[5] Programs must meet or exceed the COA mandatory pass rate using one of the three methods. Programs that fall below the mandatory pass rate will be monitored and must demonstrate improvement. If improvement is not demonstrated within the established

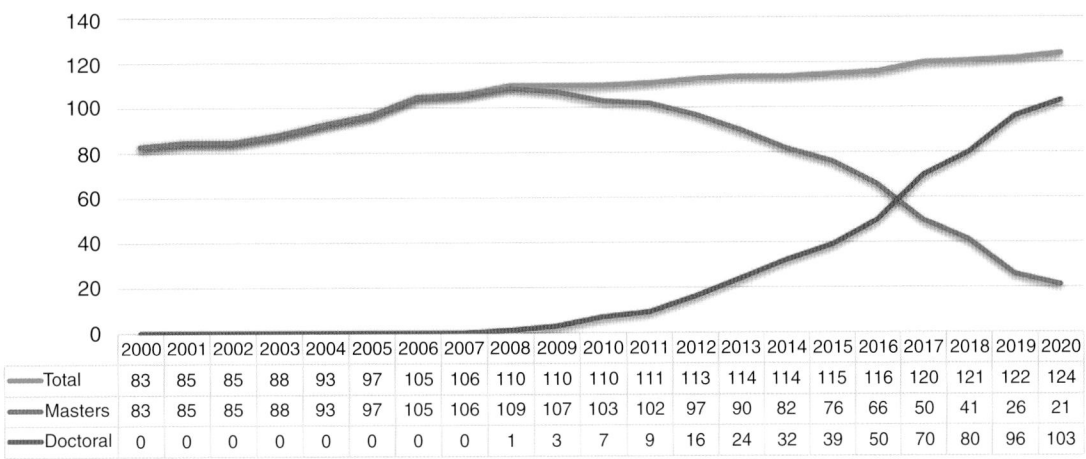

	2000	2001	2002	2003	2004	2005	2006	2007	2008	2009	2010	2011	2012	2013	2014	2015	2016	2017	2018	2019	2020
Total	83	85	85	88	93	97	105	106	110	110	110	111	113	114	114	115	116	120	121	122	124
Masters	83	85	85	88	93	97	105	106	109	107	103	102	97	90	82	76	66	50	41	26	21
Doctoral	0	0	0	0	0	0	0	0	1	3	7	9	16	24	32	39	50	70	80	96	103

Fig. 2.1 Progression of nurse anesthesia programs transitioning to award doctoral degrees.

timeframe, then that specific programs' accreditation is subject to an adverse accreditation action.[8]

In addition, the COA's Public Disclosure of Accreditation Decisions and Performance Data policy requires programs to accurately post their first-time NCE pass rates, attrition rates, and employment rates graduates on their websites, and to link their websites to the COA's list of Accredited Programs.[5,9] These stringent requirements help ensure the effectiveness of nurse anesthesia clinical and didactic education, as well as ensuring that the public is being provided with accurate information related to student achievement.

To assess the overall quality of nurse anesthesia programs, the COA conducts periodic assessment of recent graduates' preparedness for entry into practice. The most recent assessment was conducted in 2015. The results were similar to the previous survey conducted in 2011 that indicated 98% of graduates and 97% of employers identified graduates were prepared for entry into practice. Ninety-six percent of the employers indicated they would hire the same graduates again.[10]

Requirements for an Increase in Class Size

High-quality educational programs must have sufficient resources. In 2013 the COA approved a Program Resources and Student Capacity policy.[5,11] The policy requires programs to submit a request to increase their COA-identified class size verifying there are adequate resources to support the size and scope of the offering to appropriately prepare students for practice and to promote the quality of graduates. Requests to increase class size must be approved prior to the enrollment of additional students.

Nurse Anesthesia Program Administration

The COA has requirements related to the administration of nurse anesthesia programs. The requirements include programs' management of faculty and students, fiscal management, maintenance of COA accreditation and other higher education accreditation requirements of the universities, faculty continuing education, and program evaluations. In 2009 the COA approved a position statement requiring nurse anesthesia programs to employ CRNAs with doctoral degrees in the roles of program administrator and assistant program administrator by January 1, 2018. This was done to support programmatic transition to the doctoral degree for entry in to practice.[12]

Nurse Anesthesia Program Admission Requirements

Programs are required to enroll only students who are of quality appropriate for the profession, and who have the ability to benefit from their education. Minimum admission requirements include graduation from a school of nursing, a baccalaureate or graduate degree in nursing or an appropriate major, current unencumbered license as a registered nurse (RN), and a minimum of 1 year of full-time work experience as a registered nurse in a critical care setting. However, the average critical care experience of RNs entering nurse anesthesia programs is 2.9 years.[13] The critical care experience must have provided the RN with the opportunity to develop as an independent decision maker capable of using and interpreting advanced monitoring techniques based on knowledge of physiologic and pharmacologic principles. Programs determine what types of work experience are acceptable for admission to meet this requirement. Examples of critical care areas include but are not limited to surgical, cardiothoracic, coronary, medical, pediatric, and neonatal intensive care units.

Nurse Anesthesia Education Program Curriculum
Didactic Education

The didactic curricula of nurse anesthesia programs are governed by the master's and doctoral *Standards* and help ensure students are provided with the scientific, clinical, and professional foundations upon which to build sound and safe clinical practice. Programs must demonstrate they provide an extensive educationally sound curriculum combining both academic theory and clinical practice. The curricula must include three separate courses in advanced physiology/pathophysiology, advanced pharmacology, and advanced health assessment. This requirement is consistent with the educational requirements identified in the Advanced Practice Registered Nurse (APRN) Consensus Model.[14] The curricula must also include content areas such as human anatomy, chemistry, biochemistry, physics, genetics, acute and chronic pain management, professional role development, anesthesia equipment, technology, research, clinical correlation conferences, radiology, ultrasound, wellness and substance use disorder, and business of anesthesia/practice management (refer to 2004 Standards, Standard III, Criterion C14 and Practice Doctorate Standards, Curriculum Standards, E.2).[2,3] Courses ensure graduates have the knowledge to provide safe, high-quality anesthesia care. Course content includes the induction, maintenance, and emergence from anesthesia; airway management; anesthesia pharmacology; and anesthesia for special patient populations such as obstetrics, geriatrics, and pediatrics.

Practice Doctorate Scholarly Work

Programs awarding doctoral degrees most commonly award either a Doctor of Nursing Practice (DNP) or Doctor of Nurse Anesthesia

Practice (DNAP). Doctoral programs are required to provide additional content in ethical and multicultural health care, health policy, health care finance, informatics, leadership, and management. Programs also must require students to complete a scholarly work that demonstrates knowledge and scholarship skills within the area of academic focus. In 2020 the COA published a white paper, titled "Scholarly Work for Practice Doctorate Nurse Anesthesia Programs: Current State and Guidance."[15] The purpose of the white paper is to guide programs' development of criteria for scholarly work as defined in the Standards for Accreditation of Nurse Anesthesia Programs: Practice Doctorate.[3]

Student Evaluation

All programs must evaluate students' knowledge and skills to ensure they are meeting the programs' stated objectives as they progress in the program. Evaluations should be anonymous and used to help develop and implement policies and procedures that utilize objective criteria to promote student learning while simultaneously enhancing the programs' quality and integrity.

Educational Methods

The methods used to deliver nurse anesthesia curricula are changing as new technologies are being applied in higher education. Based on COA 2020 Annual Report data and due to Covid-19 restrictions that required programs to discontinue face-to-face classes, 89% of nurse anesthesia programs reported the use of some form of distance education in their provision of didactic instruction.[16] Programs' distance education offerings vary from several core courses to programs in which the majority of the didactic curriculum is provided using distance education. In addition, all of the programs report having access to some form of simulation (e.g., simple models, computer, and full-body patient simulation). Standard E.11 requires programs awarding doctoral degrees to have simulated clinical experiences incorporated in the curriculum.[3] In addition, in 2015 the COA developed a position statement, titled "The Value of Simulation in Nurse Anesthesia Education."[17] The position statement identifies the advantages of simulation and how it relates to actual patient care.

Clinical Education

The clinical curriculum of nurse anesthesia education provides students with an opportunity to apply didactic knowledge in clinical practice. Programs prepare graduates with the knowledge and skills to administer all types of anesthesia, including general, regional, selected local, and moderate sedation to patients of all ages for all types of surgeries. Students use a variety of anesthesia drugs, manage fluid and blood replacement therapy, and interpret data from sophisticated monitoring devices. Additional clinical responsibilities include the insertion of invasive catheters, the recognition and correction of complications that occur during the course of an anesthetic, the provision of airway and ventilatory support during resuscitation, and pain management.

The COA standards require that students engage in a minimum of 2000 clinical hours and a minimum of 650 required cases. The types of cases are listed by age and physical status of the patient, technique, anatomy, and specialty type. These include call experiences and simulation activities. Specific directions are provided regarding how a case may be counted, the difference between administration of a technique and management of a technique, and differentiation between the various types of anesthesia services. Graduates of nurse anesthesia programs have an average of 9369 hours of clinical experience, including 733 hours during their baccalaureate nursing program, 6032 hours as a critical care RN, and 2604 hours (NBCRNA, written communication, May 2017) during their nurse anesthesia program.[18] To provide an authoritative reference for programs in advising students about recording of clinical experiences, in 2015 the COA published *Guidelines for Counting Clinical Experiences*.[19]

The requirements for students who enroll in nurse anesthesia programs on January 1, 2022, and thereafter is to complete a minimum of 650 anesthetics, which must include specialties such as pediatric, obstetric, cardiothoracic, and neurosurgical anesthesia.[2,3] The anesthesia experiences include the care of multiple patient characteristics including healthy patients critically ill patient, and patients of all ages for elective and emergency procedures. In most programs, the minimum number of clinical experiences is surpassed early in their clinical practicum. Based on CY2019 certification transcript data, nurse anesthesia programs provide an average of 851 cases, 1675 hours of anesthesia clinical experience, and 2573 total clinical hours for each student.[12]

Clinical Supervision

In 2019 the COA clarified the requirements for the clinical supervision of students stating CRNAs and/or anesthesiologists are the only individual(s) allowed to supervise nurse anesthesia students. CRNAs and/or anesthesiologists are responsible for the anesthesia care of the patient, and while supervising student, these professionals have the additional responsibilities of providing direct guidance to the student, evaluating the student's performance, and approving a student's plan of care.[20] The clinical faculty evaluates the technical and critical thinking skills of each anesthesia student. The entry into practice competencies for the nurse anesthesia professional are those required at the time of graduation, and focus on providing safe, competent, and ethical anesthesia care to patients for diagnostic, therapeutic, and surgical procedures (refer to 2004 Standards, Standard III, Criterion C21 and Practice Doctorate Standards, Graduate Standards, D1–D51).[2,3] Due to a lack in standardization in clinical assessment, in 2020 the COA developed and completed a Common Clinical Assessment Tool for use on a pilot basis by nurse anesthesia programs.[21]

It is important to note that the entry into practice competencies should be viewed as the structure upon which the nurse anesthetist continues to learn new facts, obtain and refine knowledge, and develop skills along the practice continuum that starts at graduation (proficient) and continues throughout the entire professional career (expert).

Affiliate Organization's Configurations and Relationships

In the 1970s the AANA bylaws were revised to allow for the establishment of four separate autonomous councils under the corporate structure of the AANA: the Council on Accreditation of Nurse Anesthesia Educational Programs (COA), the Council on Certification of Nurse Anesthetists (CCNA), the Council on Recertification of Nurse Anesthetists (COR), and the Council for Public Interest in Anesthesia (CPIA). The councils were established with the intention of informing and assuring the public that accreditation, certification, and recertification activities are within the discipline of nurse anesthesia and are separate from and not unduly influenced by the AANA. In the 2000s there were significant changes in the councils' structure. In 2007 the CCNA and COR separately incorporated to form the NBCRNA. The COA separately incorporated in 2009, and in 2010 the AANA members voted on a AANA bylaws change to not continue to recognize the CPIA. Subsequent to that action the AANA chose to not continue the independent activities of the CPIA and subsequently dissolved the council and subsumed its roles and responsibilities, distributing them across the organization's existing structure. The COA and the NBCRNA are solely responsible for their own internal affairs, including the election of officers, the creation and periodic modification of their bylaws, and the direction of their financial activities. Separate CRNA chief executive officers and boards of directors serve the COA, the NBCRNA, and the AANA. In accordance with their bylaws, membership on the COA and NBCRNA boards include CRNAs, hospital administrators physicians, and members of the public. Membership on the COA also includes university and student representatives, and the NBCRNA has a designated surgeon and anesthesiologist member. To enhance communications, staff and board liaison roles were established in 2013 for the AANA, NBCRNA, and COA. Liaison representatives attend select sessions at the organizations' board meetings. In addition, communication among the AANA, COA, and NBCRNA is facilitated through regularly scheduled leadership meetings that include discussions on issues of mutual concern. More information on the AANA, COA, and NBCRNA can be found at www.aana.com, www.coacrna.org, and www.nbcrna.com, respectively.

Future Trends in Nurse Anesthesia Education

In 2014 a major step forward in specialization occurred when the COA adopted Standards for the Accreditation of Post Graduate CRNA Fellowships and procedures for the accreditation of postgraduate CRNA fellowships.[4] CRNA fellowships contain advanced education and training in a focused area of specialty practice or concentration. As of January 2021, there are five accredited fellowships in pain management and pediatrics.[22] While other specialty groups could eventually avail themselves of this education, the commitment is to focus on the nurse anesthesia community and to expand enrollment to other practice disciplines over time, based on demand and the adequacy of educational resources.

APRN Consensus Model

An important development for the practice of APRNs was the APRN Consensus Model approved in 2008.[14] This is a model for licensure, accreditation, certification, and education. The APRN Consensus Model identifies areas of educational specialization within advanced practice nursing that occur beyond the levels of role and/or practice foci. The APRN Consensus Model is not to be used as a source for regulation of practice, but rather to serve the individual nursing practitioners in their delivery of care and services. The National Council of State Boards of Nursing (NCSBN) has established a campaign for consensus and monitors state progression toward uniformity.[23] The future examination for specialty areas of practice by the CRNA, above the *role of nurse anesthetist* and the population foci of *across the lifespan*, should not be utilized as a gate-keeping mechanism to prevent any CRNA from engaging in any subspecialty practice. As long as CRNAs can demonstrate they have obtained the knowledge, skills, and abilities necessary to engage in a specialized area, individual practitioners should not undergo regulation via additional professional licensure. In 2015 the NBCRNA established a subspecialty credential (NSPM-C) in nonsurgical pain management.[24]

Full Scope of Practice Competency Task Force

In 2018 the AANA and COA supported a Full Scope of Practice Competency Task Force (FSOPCTF). The FSOPCTF's charge was to make evidence-based recommendations intended to continue to prepare nurse anesthetists to meet the needs in all types of practice settings. The task force spent over a year researching, discussing, and formulating its recommendations. It focused on education as the foundation of autonomous and independent CRNA practice. A total of 25 recommendations were made to the AANA, COA, and NBCRNA. To review and evaluate the recommendations, the COA established a Standards Revisions Subcommittee. In 2020 hearings were held and calls of comments distributed on proposed revisions to the Standards reflecting many of the FSOPCTF's recommendations. The COA made revisions to the Standards in 2021.[25]

CERTIFIED REGISTERED NURSE ANESTHETIST PRACTICE

CRNAs are advanced practice registered nurses licensed as independent practitioners who provide holistic, patient-centered comprehensive anesthesia, analgesia, and pain management services for patients across their lifespan, no matter the complexity of their health.[26] As leaders and decision makers, CRNAs work in collaboration with the interprofessional team that includes the patient, other health care professionals, and other qualified practitioners such as physicians (e.g., surgeons, obstetricians, or anesthesiologists), dentists, or podiatrists to provide high-quality anesthesia services.[27-29] Nurse anesthesia practice focuses on each patient's and team member's individual perspective and experience, as well as the importance of diversity, inclusion, and equity. This is described in the AANA's *Diversity, Inclusion and Equity Position Statement* and the *Professional Attributes of the Nurse Anesthetist* core values.[30,31]

Areas of Practice

There are four nurse anesthesia-related practice roles as defined by the NBCRNA. They are clinical practice, administrative, education, and research, or a combination of two or more of the areas of practice.[27,32] In their clinical practice role, nurse anesthetists administer approximately 45 million anesthetics annually for patients in the United States.[32] CRNAs provide comprehensive, patient-specific anesthesia services using anesthesia and analgesia techniques for surgical, obstetric, procedural, diagnostic, and chronic pain management procedures. CRNAs are the direct provider of all elements of anesthesia services in academic and community hospitals, critical access hospitals, ambulatory surgical centers, clinics, and offices, as well as the predominant anesthesia provider in US military, public health services, and Veterans Administration health care facilities. CRNAs are the sole anesthesia providers in nearly 100% of all rural hospitals and their respective communities, providing patients and families access to excellent obstetric, surgical, diagnostic, and trauma stabilization services and care.[32]

CRNAs are an integral part of the health care team, contributing their expertise in perioperative management that may include preanesthesia patient optimization, airway management, critical care, pain management, resuscitation, and other related clinical activities.[26,32] In the face of the opioid crisis, CRNAs have led practice changes to minimize or eliminate single modal opioid analgesia through multimodal pain management during the perioperative period. CRNAs have also integrated ultrasound-guided visualization for regional anesthesia and vascular access along with point-of-care ultrasound (POCUS) to improve the safety of the care they provide and improve patient outcomes. During the Covid-19 pandemic, when elective surgical procedures were canceled, CRNAs were sought and enthusiastically answered the call to lead critical care areas and specialty teams as APRNs. Federal leaders and state governors, in response to the demands of the pandemic, removed scope of practice barriers to allow CRNAs and other APRNs to practice to their full scope of practice and education.

In addition to their clinical practice role, CRNAs are businessowners or administrators, or practice in other leadership positions; participate with the team in quality improvement processes; lead research activities; are educators; collaborate in interdepartmental activities including policy development; and participate on various state and federal governmental agencies.[26,32] CRNAs educate and collaborate with their patients to provide informed, patient-centered health care. Another important role that CRNAs fulfill is that of didactic and clinical educators for nurse anesthesia students, as well as teaching other health care professionals specific skills related to their profession (e.g., flight nurses, medical students, respiratory therapists).

Today, market pressures continue to drive consolidation of health care facilities in local markets and across the country, as well as the growth of health care employment management companies to provide affordable, quality care.[33,34] As health care continues to transition from a reimbursement model based on fee for service to one grounded in value-based care and outcomes, the CRNA offers value and excellence in leadership, holistic patient care, quality, and cost-effective care.[34] To meet the needs of their community, CRNAs may practice in a variety of employment arrangements, such as self-employment, or employment by a health care facility, anesthesia group, health system, practice management company, university, military or clinic, or health care system.[34] In addition, nurse anesthetists practice in various models that include CRNA only, consultative CRNA/anesthesiologist arrangements where each provide anesthesia, or medical direction under an anesthesiologist with the CRNA providing the anesthesia. Each of the models are equally safe and of high quality; however, the CRNA-only and consultative models offer a high degree of cost effectiveness.[34]

CRNA Professional Credential

Professional certification indicates that the individual has met predetermined criteria that measure the knowledge, skills, attitudes, and judgments necessary for entry into the specialty of nurse anesthesia practice. Certification affords the public and employers an awareness of the qualifications and capabilities of health care providers. Consistent with the purpose of professional certification, the CRNA credential indicates that the individual who holds it has evidenced meeting the prescribed criteria necessary to provide the services described within a CRNA's scope of practice.[26,29]

To enter unencumbered practice as a CRNA, an individual must:

1. Comply with all state requirements for current and unrestricted licensure as a registered professional nurse in all states in which he or she currently holds an active license
2. Complete a nurse anesthesia educational program accredited by the COA or its predecessor within the previous 2 calendar years
3. Successfully complete the NCE administered by NBCRNA or its predecessor[29]
4. If applicable, apply for authorization to practice as a CRNA in the state(s)

The NCE eligibility requirements are available in the NBCRNA National Certification (NCE) Handbook, which can be found at www.nbcrna.com/publications/handbooks.

Continued Professional Certification

To maintain the CRNA credential, an individual must meet the requirements set forth by the NBCRNA in the Continued Professional Certification (CPC) Program. The comprehensive and rigorous CPC Program promotes professional development and lifelong learning to address changing accreditation requirements, the evolving health care environment, increasing autonomy of nurse anesthesia practice, and the integration of new technology regardless of practice setting, patients, and conditions. The CPC Program replaced the legacy Recertification Program, beginning in August 2016. The CPC Program is comprised of two 4-year cycles over an 8-year period. During the 8-year period, all elements of the program are repeated every 4 years except for the assessment exam, which is required only once every 8 years. In addition to documentation of practice and licensure, the program components include Class A and Class B credit requirements, completion of the four core modules, and the CPC assessment. In addition to completion of the CPC Program 4-year cycles for maintenance of certification, the CRNA must document his or her anesthesia practice, maintain current state licensure, and certify that he or she has no conditions that could adversely affect the ability to practice anesthesia.[29] Additional information regarding the CPC Program may be found at www.nbcrna.com/continued-certification. It is important to acknowledge that the CPC Program was initially designed to change over time so as to best meet the changing needs of the nurse anesthesia community, the larger health care environment, and the patients who are served by the care and services of the CRNAs in practice.

CRNA Scope of Practice

The AANA *Scope of Nurse Anesthesia Practice* broadly describes the professional roles, functions, and responsibilities as defined by the profession, while the individual CRNA's scope of practice is based on his or her personal education, licensure, experience, and skills.[26,35] The AANA *Nurse Anesthesia Practice Standards, Scope of Nurse Anesthesia Practice* and *Code of Ethics* provide the foundation for nurse anesthesia professional practice.[26,35-37] The *Scope of Practice* and *Nurse Anesthesia Practice Standards* are the foundation for the COA *Standards for Accreditation of Nurse Anesthesia Education Programs* (Table 2.1).[3,26]

The 2019 *Scope of Nurse Anesthesia Practice* addresses the responsibilities associated with clinical anesthesia practice working collaboratively with other health care providers, but is not limited to the services noted in Table 2.2.[26]

The *Scope of Nurse Anesthesia Practice* and the *Standards for Nurse Anesthesia Practice* are the authoritative statements that describe the minimum rules and responsibilities for which the nurse anesthetist is accountable. The standards apply to all anesthetizing locations and are intended to offer guidance for safe and high-quality anesthesia care.[36] Individual state or facility rules and regulations also define CRNA scope of practice. Anesthesia services evolve and change over time as research, evidence, technology, and new medications become available. The CRNA may reference AANA *Considerations for Adding New Activities to Individual CRNA Scope of Practice* to address decision points necessary for addition of new skills to his or her scope of practice.[38] It is also the responsibility of the CRNA to acquire the knowledge, skills, judgment, and experience necessary to safely practice within the scope of practice specific to state and facility policy.[37] More information regarding CRNA practice is available on the AANA website at https://www.aana.com/practice/practice-manual.

AANA ORGANIZATIONAL STRUCTURE AND FUNCTION

The AANA is a professional membership association that represents over 57,000 CRNAs and student registered nurse anesthetists nationwide. According to August 2019 AANA data, nearly 90% of CRNAs in the United States are members of the AANA.[32] The AANA was first incorporated in Ohio on March 12, 1932, as the National Association of Nurse Anesthetists (NANA). It was reincorporated in the state of Illinois on October 17, 1939, and designated as a tax-exempt organization in accordance with subsection 501(c) of the Internal Revenue Code; that same year, the organization's name was changed to the American Association of Nurse Anesthetists.[39] Following an AANA 2020 member resolution, the AANA is in the process of rebranding the association as the American Association of Nurse Anesthesiology.[40]

Information regarding the governance bylaws, policies, and guidelines of the AANA are available at https://www.aana.com/about-us/who-we-are or through the members login page at https://www.aana.com/governance. The bylaws address the classes of membership, decision-making procedures, responsibilities of the AANA's elected

TABLE 2.1   Crosswalk Between AANA Scope of Nurse Anesthesia Practice and COA Standards for Accreditation of Nurse Anesthesia Programs: Practice Doctorate

Element of Scope of Nurse Anesthesia Practice	Standard(s) That Address Element
Provide patient education and counseling	D25, D27, D28, D30, D33, D34, D35
Perform a comprehensive history and physical examination, assessment, and evaluation	D5, D6, D7, D8, D16, D25, D26, D27, D28
Conduct a preanesthesia assessment and evaluation	D5, D6, D7, D15, D16, D25, D26, D28
Develop a comprehensive patient-specific plan for anesthesia, analgesia, multimodal pain management, and recovery	D5, D6, D7, D13, D14, D17, D19, D20, D23, D33, D35, D38
Obtain informed consent for anesthesia and pain management	D5, D6, D7, D25, D28, D32, D35
Select, order, prescribe, and administer preanesthetic medications, including controlled substances	D5, D6, D7, D13, D14, D17, D20, D21, D22, D25, D26, D27, D28, D34
Implement a patient-specific plan of care, which may involve anesthetic techniques such as general, regional, and local anesthesia; sedation; and multimodal pain management	D1, D2, D3, D4, D5, D6, D7, D9, D10, D11, D19, D20, D21, D22, D26, D28, E2.1, E2.2, E2.3, and clinical experience requirements
Select, order, prescribe, and administer anesthetic medications, including controlled substances, adjuvant drugs, accessory drugs, fluids, and blood products	D5, D6, D7, D9, D10, D11, D17, D19, D20, D21, D22, D26, D28, E2.1, E2.2, E2.3, and clinical experience requirements
Select and insert invasive and noninvasive monitoring modalities (e.g., central venous access, arterial lines, cerebral oximetry, bispectral index monitor, transesophageal echocardiogram [TEE])	D5, D6, D7, D8, D13, D14, D17, D19, D21, D22, clinical experience requirements
Select, order, prescribe, and administer postanesthetic medications, including controlled substances	D5, D6, D7, D13, D14, D17, D20, D21, D22, D25, D26, D28, D29, D34
Educate the patient related to recovery, regional analgesia, and continued multimodal pain management	D5, D6, D7, D25, D27, D28, D32, D30, D33, D35
Discharge from the postanesthesia care area or facility	D5, D6, D7, D21, D22, D26, D28, D29
Provide comprehensive patient-centered pain management to optimize recovery	D5, D6, D7, D11, D17, clinical experience requirements, E2.2, E2.3
Provide acute pain services, including multimodal pain management and opioid-sparing techniques	D5, D6, D7, D11, D17, clinical experience requirements, E2.2, E2.3
Provide anesthesia and analgesia using regional techniques for obstetric and other acute pain management	D5, D6, D7, D9, D10, D11, D17, clinical experience requirements, E2.2, E2.3
Provide advanced pain management, including acute, chronic, and interventional pain management	D5, D6, D7, D9, D10, D11, D17, clinical experience requirements, E2.2, E2.3
Perform point-of-care testing	D5, D6, D7, D19
Order, evaluate, and interpret diagnostic laboratory and radiologic studies (e.g., chest x-ray, 12-lead ECG, TEE)	D5, D6, D7, D16, D19, E2.2, E2.3
Use and supervise the use of ultrasound, fluoroscopy, and other technologies for diagnosis and care delivery	D5, D6, D7, D9, D11, E2.2, E2.3, clinical experience requirements
Provide sedation and pain management for palliative care	D1, D2, D3, D4, D5, D6, D7, D9, D10, D11, D19, D20, D21, D22, D26, D28, E2.2, E2.3, clinical experience requirements
Order consults, treatments, or services related to the patient's care (e.g., physical and occupational therapy)	D5, D6, D7, D16, D17, D21, D22, D26, D27, D28, D32
CRNAs provide pivotal health care leadership in roles such as chief executive officer, administrator, manager, anesthesia services director, board member, anesthesia practice owner, national and international researcher, educator, mentor, and advocate	D25, D26, D31, D32, D33, D34, D35, D40
Nurse anesthetists are innovative leaders in the delivery of cost-effective, evidence-based anesthesia and pain management, integrating critical thinking, ethical judgment, quality data, scientific research, and emerging technologies to optimize patient outcomes	D25, D26, D13, D23, D31, D32, D33, D34, D35, D40, D44, D45, D46, D47, D48, D49, D50, D51
CRNAs engage in health care advocacy and policymaking at the institutional, local, state, national, and international levels. They also participate in professional associations focusing on patient access to quality and affordable care.	D25, D26, D13, D14, D33, D34, D35, D36, D38, D40, D41, D42, D43

From American Association of Nurse Anesthetists. Scope of *Nurse Anesthesia Practice*. Park Ridge, IL: AANA; 2020. Retrieved from https://www.aana.com/docs/default-source/practice-aana-com-web-documents-(all)/scope-of-nurse-anesthesia-practice.pdf?sfvrsn=250049b1_6; Council on Accreditation of Nurse Anesthesia Educational Programs. Standards for Accreditation of Nurse Anesthesia Programs: Practice Doctorate, Park Ridge, IL: COA; 2015. Retrieved from https://www.coacrna.org/wp-content/uploads/2020/01/Standards-for-Accreditation-of-Nurse-Anesthesia-Programs-Practice-Doctorate-revised-October-2019.pdf.

TABLE 2.2   Nurse Anesthesia Scope of Practice

Preoperative/ Preprocedure	Intraoperative/ Intraprocedure	Postoperative/ Postprocedure	Pain Management	Other Services
• Provide patient education and counseling • Perform a comprehensive history and physical examination, assessment, and evaluation • Conduct a preanesthesia assessment and evaluation • Develop a comprehensive patient-specific plan for anesthesia, analgesia, multimodal pain management, and recovery • Obtain informed consent for anesthesia and pain management • Select, order, prescribe, and administer preanesthestic medications, including controlled substances	• Implement a patient-specific plan of care, which may involve anesthetic techniques, such as general, regional, and local anesthesia, sedation, and multimodal pain management • Select, order, prescribe, and administer anesthetic medications, including controlled substances, adjuvant drugs, accessory drugs, fluids, and blood products • Select and insert invasive and noninvasive monitoring modalities (e.g., central venous access, arterial lines, cerebral oximetry, bispectral index monitor, TEE	• Facilitate emergence and recovery from anesthesia • Select, order, prescribe, and administer postanesthetic medications, including controlled substances • Conduct postanesthesia evaluation • Educate the patient related to recovery, regional anesthesia, and continued multimodal pain management • Discharge from the postanesthesia care area or facility	• Provide comprehensive patient-centered pain management to optimize recovery • Provide acute pain services, including multimodal pain management and opioid-sparing techniques • Provide anesthesia and analgesia using regional techniques for obstetric and other acute pain management • Provide advanced pain management, including acute, chronic, and interventional pain management	• Prescribe medication, including controlled substances (e.g., pain management, medication-assisted treatment, adjuvants to psychotherapy) • Provide emergency, critical care, and resuscitation services • Perform advanced airway management • Perform point-of-care testing • Order, evaluate, and interpret diagnostic laboratory and radiologic studies (e.g., chest x-ray, 12-lead ECG, TEE) • Use and supervise the use of ultrasound, fluoroscopy, and other technologies for diagnosis and care delivery • Provide sedation and pain management for palliative care • Order consults, treatments, or services related to the patient's care (e.g., physical and occupational therapy)

TEE, Transesophageal echocardiogram; *ECG*, Electrodiogram; *x-ray*, radiograph.
These services are listed in table format for ease of reference. The table is not intended to be all inclusive or limit the services to specified phases of patient care. CRNA scope of practice is dynamic and evolving. CRNA clinical privileges should reflect the full scope of CRNA practice evidenced by individual credentials and performance. TEE - Transesophageal echocardiogram; ECG - Electrodiogram; x-ray - radiograph.
From American Association of Nurse Anesthetists. Scope of Nurse Anesthesia Practice. Park Ridge, IL: AANA; 2020. Retrieved from https://www.aana.com/docs/default-source/practice-aana-com-web-documents-(all)/scope-of-nurse-anesthesia-practice.pdf?sfvrsn=250049b1_6.

officials, the role of the chief executive officer, the configuration of committees, functions of committee members, and the AANA's relationship with state nurse anesthesia associations.[41]

The AANA Board of Directors (BOD) is elected annually by voting-eligible members of the AANA and serves as the governing body for the AANA. The BOD includes the president, president-elect, vice president, treasurer, and seven directors. The BOD is responsible for the leadership and governance of the AANA.[41] The BOD adopts organizational policy and strategic framework, oversees the budget and related financial affairs, adopts clinical standards and guidelines, directs legislative advocacy activities, and serves as a liaison with external governmental and professional organizations. In addition, the BOD collaborates with and considers recommendations for activities that align with the AANA strategic priorities from the AANA staff, the committees of the association, COA, NBCRNA, and AANA Foundation and adopts recommendations as appropriate.

The AANA resides in two offices in Park Ridge, Illinois, and one office in Washington, DC, and employs over 128 staff. The AANA chief executive officer leads and manages the daily activities of the association in collaboration with the executive leadership, senior directors, and staff. Collectively, the AANA staff, committees, and other work groups carry out the strategic priorities as adopted by the elected AANA BOD and consistent with the AANA's mission statement to "advance patient safety, practice excellence, and its members' profession." With this in mind, the

AANA supports advocacy activities at the local, state, and federal levels on behalf of its members and the public in collaboration with the individual state associations of nurse anesthetists. The AANA's organizational structure and resources are available at www.aana.com/about-us.

AANA Foundation

The AANA Foundation serves as the philanthropic arm of the American Association of Nurse Anesthetists. The foundation is a charitable organization devoted to anesthesia research, education, and development. The foundation funds scholarships, doctoral fellowships, postdoctoral fellowships, research grants, general poster sessions, oral "State of the Science" poster sessions and doctoral mentorships. Additional information regarding the AANA Foundation may be found at https://www.aana.com/about-us/aana-foundation.

AANA Association Management Services, Inc.

The AANA owns one subsidiary, the AANA Association Management Services, Inc. (AAMS), which provides non–dues-related sources of revenue and services for the general membership. There are currently two divisions within the AAMS. These divisions provide services related to malpractice insurance and housing (hotel rooms and lodging arrangements in association with meetings and events of the AANA) for both internal and external clients. Additional information is available at www.aana.com/insurance.

SUMMARY

The nurse anesthesia profession along with the American Association of Nurse Anesthetists and affiliate nurse anesthesia organizations (COA and NBCRNA) have grown and evolved for well over a century. As patient and health care delivery systems continue to evolve, CRNAs will continue to be health care leaders well positioned to address the challenges of complex patients and systems of care well into the future. CRNAs in partnership with the AANA have the professional responsibility and opportunity to take an active role to secure their future because a profession and professional organization is only as successful, as its members and their efforts.

REFERENCES

For a complete list of references for this chapter, scan this QR code with any smartphone code reader app, or visit the following URL: http://booksite.elsevier.com/9780323711944/.

Patient-Centered Care, Cultural Competence, and Nurse Anesthesia Practice

Wallena Gould

The nature of health care is transforming, driven in part by landmark recommendations from the National Academy of Medicine (formerly known as the Institute of Medicine [IOM]) for quality and safety in health care systems and health professions.[1] According to the National Academy of Medicine report, health care systems do not consistently provide high-quality care to all Americans, frequently do not translate knowledge into practice, often do not apply new technology safely and appropriately, and do not make the best use of their resources.[1,2] The efforts to become more responsive to improving patient outcomes have resulted in a paradigm shift from the traditional paternalistic provider-centered approach of care delivery to a shared decision-making, patient-centered approach of care delivery. With a patient-centered care perspective, patients are active participants in the decision-making process about their care. Studies have shown that patient-centered care is associated with improvement in care processes, health care utilization, patient satisfaction, self-management, and health outcomes, including decreased mortality.[3-5]

Increasingly, anesthetists are caring for patients who make decisions about health care services based on personal needs and preferences, as well as the advice they receive from physicians, nurses, other care providers, the internet, peer support groups, and a variety of information and communication technologies designed to support care. As anesthetists, it is important that we engage our patients throughout the perioperative period. The provision of quality care is a team activity and, as a member of a team, we must all work well together and efficiently.[6] In this chapter we will (1) discuss health care disparities, (2) review patient-centered care as one of the six domains of health care quality, (3) relate the status of health care quality and health disparities in the United States, and (4) offer considerations for the integration and evaluation of quality patient-centered care into the provision of anesthesia care.

HEALTH CARE DISPARITIES

The changing demographics of the United States in the last 20 years are evident in the racial and ethnic composition in the country's workforce and patient population served. According to the US 2018 census, the population emerges as a more diverse nation. The United States has 328 million people in the country, and the racial and ethnic composition includes White (76%), Hispanic/Latino (18.5%), Black (13.4%), Asian (5.9%), and Pacific Islander (0.2%) American Indian/Alaskan Native (AI/AN; 1.3%).[7] According to the Pew Research Center, there will be a dramatic demographic change in 2050 reports, as Hispanic communities move from a minority to the majority, with 31% of the US population.[8] Studies have revealed that racial and ethnic minorities tend to receive poorer quality of care when compared with non-minorities.[9,10] In light of the current and projected demographics in the population, consideration for applicable measures to reduce race- and ethnic-related disparities in the health care delivery system is warranted.

Nationally, Over 54,000 certified registered nurse anesthetists (CRNAs) administer 49 million anesthetics annually, in various geographic settings, including urban, suburban, rural, military, Veterans Administration (VA), and public health.[11] Using the independent model or team model approach, CRNAs are responsible for the delivery of multispecialty anesthesia care in a variety of practice settings to include hospitals, outpatient surgical clinics, and office-based practices.

According to the American Association of Nurse Anesthetists (AANA) 2018 Race and Ethnicity Profile Survey, for decades the perpetual lack of diversity among anesthesia providers has resulted in an anemic racial and ethnic workforce. Results from the survey revealed the following with regard to the racial and ethnic composition of CRNAs: white (89%), Asian (2.7%), Hispanic/Latino (2.5%), black (1.3%), Asian/Pacific Islander (2.7%), and AI/AN (0.7%).[11,12]

Covid-19

In 2020, both Covid-19 reported cases and death rates were highest among the Hispanic and Black communities. Systemic structural barriers such as high unemployment rates, substandard housing, geographic isolation, lack of access to health care and insurance, and inequities in education contribute to high cases of Covid-19 in communities of color. A comprehensive plan and recommendations for providers for addressing racial and ethnic minorities related to Covid-19 can be found in Box 3.1.

The AI/AN tribal communities as a result of geographic isolation contributed to Covid-19 cases as well as other structural barriers. According to the Centers for Disease Control and Prevention (CDC) website, AI/AN tribal communities that live in multigenerational households may find it difficult to take precautions to protect themselves from Covid-19 or isolate those who are sick, especially if space in the household is limited and many people live in the same household. Public health emergencies can further isolate members of these groups through diminished access to resources needed to prepare or respond to a disease outbreak such as Covid-19.[13]

Prior to Covid-19, black maternal mortality rates were the highest reported national cases. In a 2018 published article, "Reducing Disparities in Severe Maternal Morbidity and Mortality," black women are more likely to die than white women and have higher case-fatality rates from a range of conditions though the leading causes of maternal death for black and white women are similar.[13] According to the CDC, about 700 women die from complications related to pregnancy or childbirth every year, leading all developed nations in terms of maternal mortality. In today's Covid-19 climate, the data suggest an increase in reported black maternal mortality cases during this national crisis.

Like many other health care disciplines, the nurse anesthesia community does not reflect the communities it serves based on the

BOX 3.1 Health Care Provider Recommendations for COVID-19 and At Risk Populations

- Use CDC's standardized protocols and quality improvement guidance in hospitals and medical offices that serve people from racial and ethnic minority groups.
- Provide training to help providers identify their implicit biases, making sure providers understand how these biases can affect the way they communicate with patients and how patients react.
- Train both providers and administrators to understand how biases can affect their decision making, including decisions about resources.
- Provide medical interpreters.
- Work with communities and health care professional organizations to reduce cultural barriers to care.
- Connect patients with community resources that can help older adults and people with underlying medical conditions follow their care plans. For example, help people get extra supplies and medications and remind them to take their medications.
- Learn about social and economic conditions that may put some patients at increased risk for getting sick with Covid-19 (e.g., jobs that require more contact with the public).
- Promote a trusting relationship by encouraging patients to call and ask questions.

CDC, Centers for Disease Control and Prevention.
Adapted from Baptiste DL, Commodore-Mensah Y, Alexander KA, et al. COVID-19: shedding light on racial and health inequities in the USA. *J Clin Nurs.* 2020;29(15-16):2734-2736.

aforementioned 2018 AANA survey and the US population. The nurse anesthesia workforce disparity yields that structural institutional changes within health care systems, nursing and health care professional associations, and colleges and universities in educating and training are needed for a more robust and diverse workforce. Social determinants of health play a significant role in how people access and receive care, and thus require close attention to structural factors that contribute to poor health outcomes among ethnic people.[11] This includes aims to reduce health disparities and inequities as the root causes of persistent poor health outcomes.

PATIENT-CENTERED CARE: WHAT IT IS AND WHY IT IS IMPORTANT

There is a growing demand from patients, policy makers, insurers, regulators, and accreditors to improve health care quality and safety, requiring anesthetists to persistently evaluate the quality of care that they provide.[14] Patient-centered care has been recognized as an effective and efficient health care delivery method that has the potential to improve quality, patient safety, and patient outcomes at both individual and system levels.[15] For this reason, patient-centered care is advocated as a key approach to the design and delivery of services provided by health care professionals (independently or collaboratively) across the health care continuum. Globally, patient-centered care is considered to be the gold standard of health care.[16] Patient-centered care is critical to improving quality, improving safety, and reducing health care cost.[17] However, there is a lack of consensus on what constitutes patient-centered care and how it should be delivered. Although there is disagreement on how patient-centered care is defined, most conceptualizations include the following attributes: (1) education and shared knowledge; (2) involvement of family and friends; (3) collaboration and team management; (4) sensitivity to nonmedical, cultural, and

spiritual dimensions of care; (5) respect for patient needs and preferences; and (6) free flow and accessibility of information.[18] According to the AANA, "patient-centered care is based on the concept of shared decision-making by establishing a patient partnership through sharing information and evidence, acknowledging patient preferences and ideas, identifying choices, and negotiating decisions and agreeing upon an action."[19] Within this context, CRNAs should engage patients in the shared decision-making process, while being respectful of patients' ideas and preferences in the design of a safe, high-quality anesthetic experience. Patients are increasingly demanding a greater input into decision making about their health. Additionally, patients have access to their health information and available options.[20]

Patients report that there is a difference between the care they are seeking and the care that they receive.[21] For example, patients often report significant problems in gaining access to critical information, understanding treatment options, getting explanations regarding medications, and receiving responsive, compassionate service from their providers.[22-25] Outcomes that matter to the patient and that are feasible should guide the delivery of care. In one study, lack of understanding, fear, and anxiety about anesthesia caused one in four patients to postpone surgery, despite anesthesia's long history of quality care and safety.[26] There has been a 97% decrease in anesthesia-related deaths since the 1940s (64/100,000 vs 1/100,000).[27,28]

The Concept of Patient-Centered Care

Most current conceptualizations of patient-centered care are based on research commissioned by the Picker Institute (formerly, Picker Commonwealth Program for Patient-Centered Care).[29] The research identified eight dimensions of patient-centered care:

- Respect for patients' preferences and values
- Emotional support
- Physical comfort
- Information, communication, and education
- Continuity and transition
- Coordination of care
- Involvement of family and friends
- Access to care

This research influenced the landmark National Academy of Medicine report conceptualization and policy initiative.[1] The National Academy of Medicine adopted these categories, but added additional layers of responsibility for health systems, linking quality to patient-centered care.[29] Patient-centered care is one of the six dimensions of high-quality health care identified by the National Academy of Medicine that are essential to the improvement of health care quality. The other dimensions are safety, timeliness, effectiveness, efficiency, and equity (Table 3.1).[1] Patient-centered care is considered the most important dimension because of its close association with safety. The core concepts of patient-centered care are as follows:

- *Dignity and respect.* Anesthetists must listen to and respect the patient's point of view and choices. The anesthesia plan should incorporate the patient and family knowledge, values, beliefs, and cultural background.
- *Information sharing.* Anesthetists should communicate and share complete and unbiased information with patients and families in a useful and affirming way. The information should be timely, complete, and accurate so that shared decision making can occur.
- *Participation.* Patients and families should participate in decision making at the level of their choice.
- *Collaboration.* Patients, families, health care professionals, and health care leaders should collaborate on all aspects of health care (delivery of care, policy and program development, implementation and evaluation, professional education).[30]

TABLE 3.1 Six Dimensions for Improving Health Care Quality as Defined by the National Academy of Medicine

Dimensions	Definitions of Dimensions
Safety	The avoidance, prevention, and amelioration of adverse outcomes or injuries stemming from the processes of health care (errors, deviations, and accidents). Patients should not be harmed by the care that they receive; no harm should come to health care providers. The goal is that *no patient is caused any injury or complication from the effects of the overall anesthesia encounter.*
Timely	There should not be significant delays in treatment or long wait times, especially those that may be harmful.
Effective	Refers to the use of evidence-based care to guide best practices. This includes the underuse of effective care and overuse of ineffective care.
Efficient	The avoidance of waste, including waste of equipment, supplies, ideas, and energy.
Equitable	The provision of care that does not vary in quality based on personal characteristics such as gender, ethnicity, geographic location, or socioeconomic status.
Patient centered	The provision of care that is respectful of and responsive to patient preferences, needs, and values. Making certain that clinical decisions are based on patient values.

Adapted from Longnecker DE, Brown DL, Newman MF, et al. *Anesthesiology.* 3rd ed. New York: McGraw-Hill; 2018; Varughese AM, Hagerman NS, Kurth CD. Quality in pediatric anesthesia. *Pediatr Anesth.* 2010;20(8):684-696.

Berwick et al. further developed these concepts designed to improve health outcomes into the "triple aim."[31] The triple aim includes improving the patient experience (including quality and satisfaction), improving the health of the population, and reducing per capita costs. These aims have been adopted by the Institute for Healthcare Improvement (IHI) and several other organizations. The IHI triple aim concept design includes (1) focus on individuals and families, (2) redesign of primary care services and structures, (3) population health management, (4) cost control platform, and (5) system integration and execution.[32] Other components of patient-centered care that have been identified are coordination and integration of care, holistic care, enhanced provider-patient relationship, health information systems, and sociocultural competence.[33]

The integration of patient-centered care into health care delivery is continuing to evolve, and the methods used to implement patient-centered care into practice vary. The integration of patient-centered care into practice requires a change in organizational culture. At the organizational level, seven key factors contribute to patient-centered care[18]:

- *Leadership.* Chief executive officers (CEOs) and boards of directors must be committed and engaged to sustain patient-centered care.
- *Strategic vision/plan.* This must be clearly communicated to members of the organization. The vision should be consistently communicated. The organization's vision and values should be placed in a high-traffic area to remind health care providers of the patient-centered behaviors expected and to let patients and families know what they can expect.
- *Involvement of patients and families.* This should happen at all levels, from care to key committees of the organization.

- *Supportive work environment for employees.* This includes engagement of employees in all aspects of process design and treating employees with dignity and respect.
- *Systematic measurement and feedback.* Monitoring the impact of changes and interventions.
- *Quality of the built environment.* The provision of a supportive and nurturing physical environment.
- *Supportive technology.* Technology that engages patients and families by facilitating information access and communication.

Policy makers also advocate patient-centered care as a way to improve quality. The three main policy drivers of patient-centered care are:

- Mandatory government requirements for providers to collect and publish patient experience data
- Having information publicly available to enable consumers to choose among service providers
- Incentives for providers who achieve high measures of patient centeredness

The Centers for Medicare and Medicaid Services (CMS) and the Agency for Healthcare Research and Quality (AHRQ) routinely collect data on patient experiences. The Patient Protection and Affordable Care Act of 2010 expanded data collection. The CMS provides financial incentives to health care providers and hospitals that provide information on quality. The Consumer Assessment of Healthcare Providers and Systems (CAHPS) developed standardized surveys to obtain information on patient experiences. Hospitals use CAHPS to assess communication with doctors; communication with nurses; responsiveness of hospital staff; and communication about medicines, pain control, cleanliness and quietness of physical environment, and discharge information.

Patient Engagement

Patient engagement is a strategy used to improve patient-centered care, and it is critical to achieving high-quality care.[34] Patient engagement involves a meaningful participation by patients in different aspects of care (e.g., clinical encounters, guideline development, and research); the health care provider is the expert on medical care, and patients are experts on their own life values and status.[35,36] An important goal of patient engagement is to foster the patient–anesthesia provider relationship through communication, clinical guidance, emotional support, and tailored provision of information. Shared decision making is specifically suited for times when two or more treatment options are available, and both have equally acceptable outcomes.

Patient engagement for anesthetists includes education, risk assessment, intervention, patient questions, and ultimately shared decision making.[37] This type of communication empowers patients to participate in decision making, ask questions, and express feelings and/or concerns. Early patient engagement promotes better outcomes by identifying risks, educating patients, and encouraging shared decision making.

Traditionally, health care information has been exchanged in a face-to-face format. However, health information technology such as eHealth (including web-based interventions, smartphones, and equipment), telephone coaching, and telehealth are dramatically changing how information is exchanged. Clinical decision support is a process designed to provide timely information (usually at the point of care) to assist in clinical decision making for health care providers, staff, patients, or other individuals with knowledge and person-specific information.[38] Greenes defined clinical decision support as "the use of information and communication technologies to bring relevant knowledge to bear on the health care and well-being of a patient."[39]

Tools to assist with decision making include computerized alerts and reminders to providers and patients, clinical guidelines, condition-specific order sets, focused patient data reports and summaries, documentation templates, diagnostic support, and contextually related reference information.[38] Anesthesia clinical decision support tools are characterized as (1) enhancing reimbursement or reducing costs[40,41]; (2) increasing adherence to clinical, compliance, or regulatory protocols[42,43]; (3) improving documentation[44,45]; and (4) monitoring physiologic data in near real time and providing intraoperative recommendations at the point of care.[46-48] Studies show that in anesthesia, clinical decision support tools improve compliance and billing.[49,50]

Cultural Competence and The National Standards for Culturally and Linguistically Appropriate Services in Health and Health Care (The National CLAS Standards)

Patients and health care providers are increasingly diverse and, as a result, more communities are bilingual or speak with limited English proficiency (LEP). CRNAs and nurse anesthesia students are more familiarized with language-specific print, multimedia materials, and signage commonly used by patient populations served. These measures and more were developed from two models by Campinha-Bacote and the US Department of Health and Human Services (HHS) Office of Minority Health. The first model developed was "The Process of Cultural Competence in the Delivery of Health Care Services" with five constructs: cultural awareness, cultural knowledge, cultural skill, cultural encounters, and cultural desire.[51] This model requires health care providers to see themselves as *becoming* culturally competent rather than already being culturally competent. This work led to assumptions regarding cultural competence in the delivery of the health care services model. These assumptions and the model targeted cultural competence that directly impacts delivering optimal health care.

To achieve health equity and reduce health disparities, nurse anesthesia professionals should have the available resources encompassing The National CLAS Standards, the second model designed addressing cultural competence. In 2000, the HHS Office of Minority Health adopted the National CLAS Standards to respond to diverse communities and to respect cultures in the goal to be fully informed in the delivery of health care. By providing a structure to implement culturally and linguistically appropriate services, the National CLAS Standards will improve an organization's ability to address health care disparities. Many racial and ethnic minorities find that language barriers pose a significant problem in their efforts to access health care.[52]

Shared Decision Making

Shared decision making is a strategy to improve patient engagement and is used as a health care quality tool to examine variation in diagnostic procedures. Shared decision making occurs when an anesthesia provider and a patient (and family) work together to make a quality decision about the anesthesia plan that is best. The decision-making process is predicated on evidence-based information about available risk and benefits of each anesthetic option, the anesthetist's experience and knowledge, and patient values and preferences.

Shared decision making has evolved to include interprofessional models of health care delivery.[53] Interprofessional care is defined as "the development of a cohesive practice between professionals from different disciplines to provide an integrated and cohesive answer to the needs of the client and family."[54] The inclusion of an interprofessional model enhances communication among team members, increases patient safety and job satisfaction, and improves patient and process outcomes.[55] Interprofessional collaboration is supported by the AANA.[56]

Barriers to shared decision making include health literacy, lack of familiarity and/or experience with shared decision making, lack of desire to participate in the process, provider lack of knowledge about evidence-based practice, resources, and time.[57,58] Health literacy refers to the skills needed to access, understand, and use information to make an informed decision. Providers will need to consider the patient's ability to understand and apply information.

Health care providers in a fee-for-service environment organization may have a financial disincentive to participate in shared decision making because it may reduce the use of high-cost procedures.[59] Health care providers may also resist the integration of shared decision making into their care because it may interfere with patient workforce.

Benefits of Patient-Centered Care

Patient-centered care has clinical and operational benefits and improves the care experience. When patients and families, providers, and administrators collaborate and partner, patient and provider satisfaction increase, quality and safety of health care increase, and health care costs decrease.[30,60,61] Other benefits associated with patient-centered care include decreased mortality, decreased emergency department visits, fewer medication errors, lower infection rates, higher functional status, improved clinical care, and improved liability claims experience.[62,63] Patient-centered care improves efficiency through a reduction in diagnostic tests, unnecessary referrals, and decreased hospital admission.[64,65] Patient-centered care improves patient satisfaction and trust, which improves provider satisfaction and provider retention rates.[17]

Extensive resources have been allocated to attaining a high-value, high-quality health care system at national, state, and local levels. The HHS is promoting patient-centered care as a way to improve health care quality through the provision of information about local health providers. Others have referred to this high-quality system as value-driven health care.[66] Health care value is defined as the health care outcomes based on the dollars spent.[67] The mantra of value-driven health care is "the right care for every person every time." The focus of value-driven health care is to make care safe, effective, efficient, patient centered, timely, and equitable.

Patient-Centered Care and Cultural Competence

Providing high-quality care to all citizens is the goal of health care reform, but the quality of health care in the United States has drawn concern for many. Although the National Academy of Medicine and the AHRQ have made efforts to reduce health disparities, gaps continue to persist.[68] Some populations experience inequality in health care, decreased patient safety, and poorer health outcomes based on race, ethnicity, socioeconomic status, language, gender, religion, immigrant and refugee status, disability, geography, insurance status, and sexual orientation.[69-72] The National Academy of Medicine (IOM) report, "Unequal Treatment: Confronting Racial and Ethnic Disparities in Healthcare,"[73] found that even with the same socioeconomic status and insurance, and when comorbidities, stage of presentation, and other confounders are controlled for, minorities often receive a lower quality of health care than their white counterparts. The root cause of health disparities is complex and multifactorial and varies across regions and/or populations.

This same report[73] identified several root causes of racial and ethnic disparities that included, among others:
- *Health system factors.* Focuses on issues related to the complexity of the health care system. Minority patients, those with LEP, low health literacy, mistrust, and limited familiarity with the health care system may find it disproportionately difficult to navigate the system.[74] The presence or absence of interpreter services to assist patients with LEP can also cause disparities.

- *Care process variables.* Includes issues related to health care providers' communication, including stereotyping of patients, which may lead to differences in recommendations for treatment and diagnostic procedures, as well as limited skills in communicating with diverse populations, which impacts clinical decision making.
- *Patient-level variables.* Includes difficulty navigating the health care system, such as mistrust of health care provider, refusal of services, poor adherence to treatment, difficulty voicing concerns and asking questions, and delay in seeking care.[74]

Cultural competence of health care providers and the health care systems is a strategy to address disparities and improve outcomes. Culturally competent patient care requires health care providers to be respectful and responsive to the health beliefs, practices, and needs of diverse populations. As health care systems are redesigned to meet the patient-centered care initiative, health care organizations must integrate cultural competence strategies to achieve equity (culture of equity). Cultural competency in health care delivery affects outcomes among diverse populations; therefore it is important that health care professionals understand disparities and take steps to become culturally competent. Increased levels of cultural competency have the potential to improve patient-provider communications, improve the accuracy of diagnoses, prevent patients from exposure to unnecessary risk in diagnostic procedures, enable providers to better obtain true informed consent, and enable patients to participate in shared decision making.[73] Additionally, cultural competency training has also been shown to improve the knowledge and attitudes of health care professionals who care for racial/ethnic and linguistic minority patients.[75]

Patient-centered care and cultural competence have been identified as methods to improve health care quality and reduce disparities.[76] Although these concepts have different foci, they have similarities. The premise is that patient-centered care is culturally competent, and culturally competent care is patient centered. The difference in the two concepts has been defined:

> Both patient-centeredness and cultural competence aim to improve healthcare quality, but each emphasizes different aspects of quality. The primary goal of the patient-centeredness movement has been to provide individualized care and restore an emphasis on personal relationships. It aims to elevate quality for all patients. Alternatively, the primary aim of the cultural competence movement has been to increase health equity and reduce disparities by concentrating on people of color and other disadvantaged populations. Nevertheless, there is significant common ground between the two.[77]

Since publication of the National Academy of Medicine report, several approaches have been used to improve quality, eliminate health care disparities, and improve equity. A Robert Wood Johnson Foundation[78] report outlined six steps involved in the long-term integration and sustainability of efforts to reduce disparities and improve equity:

- *Linking quality and equity.* Focuses on achieving optimal outcomes for all groups of patients, although optimal outcomes of care may differ from person to person and group to group. Linking quality to equity requires implementing a basic quality improvement infrastructure and making equity an integral component of quality improvement. Quality improvement efforts must be tailored to each patient population and target the root causes of inequities and the inclusion of equity into routine quality improvement processes.

A quality improvement infrastructure is essential for the reduction and elimination of disparities. This includes the development of metrics and goals to monitor improvement, shared commitment, and engagement in continuous improvements across all levels of staff, and a process for continuing improvement that supports ongoing adjustment of care. The

collection of health care process and demographic variables (race, ethnicity, and language) is vital to individual quality improvement efforts and efforts to reduce disparities. Equity in the development of quality improvement focuses on improving health outcomes for everyone.

- *Creating a culture of equity.* "A culture of equity means recognizing that disparities may exist in an organization and taking responsibility for reducing them."[69] Cultural competency training improves the patient-provider relationship. The foundation of a culture of equity depends on health care providers and staff recognizing that disparities may exist and taking responsibility for their reduction. Health care organizations must make sure that equity is explicitly reflected in the organizational mission and vision statements. Examples include (1) designating specific leaders who are responsible for disparities reduction; (2) identifying equity champions, individuals who are willing to tackle inequalities in care (passionate and willing to go the extra distance); (3) recruiting and maintaining a diverse workforce that reflects the patient population that is served; (4) creating and maintaining an active patient/community or patient advisory board that is representative of the patient population; and (5) creating and maintaining strong working and consulting relationships with community-based groups and organizations that serve priority populations.
- *Diagnosing the disparity.* The World Health Organization (WHO) defines social determinants of health (SDOH) as "the conditions in which people are born, grow, live, work, and age that impact their health."[79] Nurse anesthetists require a thorough understanding of the SDOH, and health disparity is necessary in the delivery of anesthesia care. Nurses require a comprehensive understanding of social determinants and their associations with health outcomes to provide patient-centered care.[80] A summary of the clinical implications depicting the key health factors of social determinants leading to clinical implications is shown in Box 3.2.

Health inequities among racial minorities are pronounced, persistent, and pervasive.[81] Health disparities are differences in health outcomes that are closely linked with social, economic, and environmental disadvantage—that is, they are often driven by the social conditions in which individuals live, learn, work, and play according to the HHS "Action Plan to Reduce Racial and Ethnic Health Disparities" (HHS Disparities Action Plan). Therefore, affected marginalized groups who have been systematically subjected to policies adversely harming well-being, health care, and workforce are inherently harmed due to racial and ethnic disparities. The

---

BOX 3.2 Clinical Implications of Social Determinants of Health

- Social determinants of health—the conditions in which people are born, grow, play, work, live, and age that affect health and quality of life—are the driving force behind health disparities.
- The chronic stress caused by social determinants such as poverty, racism, inadequate housing, unemployment, and food insecurity damages body systems and is linked to chronic disease and premature aging.
- Implementing social determinants enables nurses to link women to needed resources and assist in program and intervention planning.
- Addressing social determinants requires cross-sector collaboration in which partnerships extend beyond the health care systems.
- Nurses can have the greatest impact on social determinants of health by using their experience and knowledge to advocate for the system-level and policy changes to create health equity.

Adapted from Lanthrop B. Moving toward health equity by addressing social determinants of health. *NWH.* 2020;24(1):36-44.

National Academy of Medicine (IOM) report, "Unequal Treatment: Confronting Racial and Ethnic Disparities in Health Care" identified the lack of insurance as a significant driver of health care disparities.[73] This landmark report identified well over 175 studies documenting racial/ethnic disparities in the diagnosis and treatment of various conditions, even when analyses were controlled for socioeconomic status, insurance status, site of care, stage of disease, comorbidity, and age, among other potential confounders. There is a powerful case to be made for the race-based disparities in health. To reduce health disparities, national intentional strategic plans to increase the diversity of the nation's health care professional workforce, including nurse anesthesia, must be employed. The lack of diversity is a key barrier to ensuring a culturally competent health care system at the provider, organizational, and system levels. Health professional schools are charged with the responsibility of preparing a competent health workforce that can meet the needs of a rapidly changing, racially and ethnically diverse population.[9] The lack of diversity diminishes our nation's capacity to eliminate racial and ethnic health disparities and compromises our national capacity to advance the health sciences.[10] This includes a strategic plan in the recruitment and retention efforts of racial and ethnic nurse anesthesia students, nurse anesthesia faculty, and clinical coordinators at the college and university institutional level. The limited number of minority nurse faculty to serve as role models and mentors creates an additional barrier to the successful recruitment and retention of underrepresented minority groups in nursing. Minority nurses in influential leadership roles are more likely to be better positioned to directly influence resource allocation and the recruitment and retention of a diverse workforce, and shape organizational and national policies aimed at eliminating health disparities.[82] According to the AANA 2018 survey, the racial and ethnic composition data revealed a severely underrepresented workforce of minority nurse anesthetists. To magnify the lack of diversity in the nurse anesthesia profession, only 1.3% account for black CRNAs of the full-time workforce who administer anesthesia to the growing diverse and underserved communities. Fred Reed, DNP, CRNA, has been a leader in nurse anesthesia while working for the Veterans Affairs Administration for decades (Fig. 3.1). A strategic plan to help decrease health disparities should include:

- *Designing the intervention.* Best practices should be used to design the intervention, and the intervention should be based on the findings from the root cause analysis. To be successful, the intervention must be multilevel and target multiple players within the health care system. The Finding Answers Intervention Research (FAIR) database provides a customized list of interventions that address disparities and can be used to facilitate the designing of the intervention. The site has an interactive format, and the interventions are categorized by disease area, racial/ethnic population, organizational setting, and intervention strategy.[83]
- *Securing buy-in.* Buy-in is a critical component for a health disparities intervention to be successful. Buy-in entails a pledge of support/commitment and the provision of resources for interventions and activities from all stakeholders.
- *Implementing change.* If the organizations have analyzed the causes of a targeted disparity (root cause analysis), designed a tailored intervention to address the health disparity identified as most relevant to the patient population, and secured buy-in from all involved stakeholders, then they have laid a strong foundation for success. The implementation process should include regular evaluation of the impact of the intervention. Three types of measures should be used to evaluate the intervention: data evaluation process, outcome, and intervention tracking measures. The long-term goal of an intervention is sustainability.

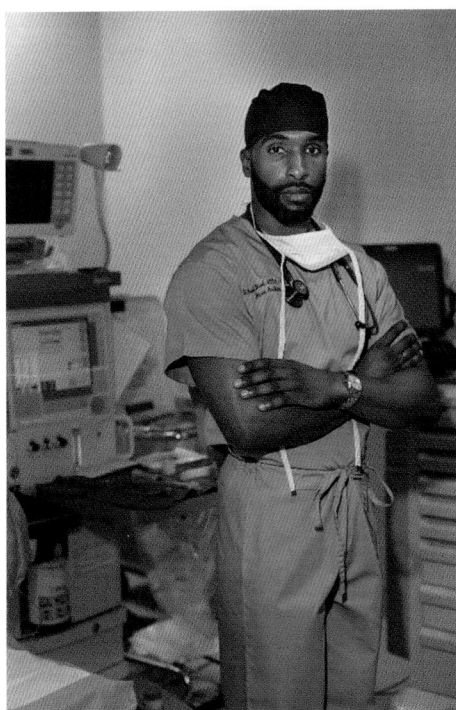

Fig. 3.1 Fred Reed III, DNP, CRNA, nurse anesthesia leader within the Veterans Affairs Administration.

The increased emphasis on cultural competence is driven in part by the increase in minority populations, as well as the passing of the Patient Protection and Affordability Act[84] that increased the number of the newly insured, health care reform, findings indicating that sociocultural differences between patients and providers influence communication and decision making, and the push for value-based health care. These all provide opportunities to reduce disparities and improve equity. The Patient Protection and Affordability Act has components that specifically address disparities; it created accountable care organizations (ACOs), whose aim is to ensure that patients receive the right care at the right time, avoid unnecessary duplication of services, and prevent medical errors. ACOs include groups of doctors, hospitals, and other health care providers that voluntarily come together to provide coordinated, high-quality care. Similarly, the HHS Disparities Action Plan focuses on making "a nation free of disparities in health and health care."[85]

There is overlap between patient-centered care and cultural competence. Patient-centered care and culturally competent care are both needed to improve health outcomes and achieve equity. Every patient and family that has an interaction with health care systems brings with them a subculture that guides their understanding, interpretation, and outcomes of the interaction. Culturally competent care requires that health care systems and health care professionals have the knowledge, attitude, and skills to meet the needs of a diverse population. Table 3.2 provides the key features of a culturally competent health care system and personal interactions. To effectively integrate culturally competent care into a system requires that individuals embrace the differences of populations and consider ways that we are the same, while being respectful of the individual differences. By designing services to a patient's culture and language preference, health professionals can help improve positive health outcomes for diverse populations. As the health care system is redesigned, it is important that health care organizations provide culturally competent care, provide high-quality care to all, eliminate disparities, and assure equity.

TABLE 3.2	Key Features of Cultural Competence of Health Care Systems and Interpersonal Interactions	
Culturally Competent Health Care Systems	**Culturally Competent Health Care Interpersonal Interactions**	
Diverse workforce that reflects the population	Explore and respect patient's values, preferences, and needs	
Having language assistance available	Find common ground	
Ongoing training regarding culturally and linguistically appropriate services	Are aware of biases and assumptions	
	Are aware of health disparities and discrimination	
	Effectively use interpreters as needed	

Patient-Centered Care as a Dimension of Safety and Health Care Quality

Patient safety is the foundation of high-quality health care. There is a growing recognition of the importance of maintaining a culture of safety and quality. The Joint Commission describes a culture of safety as "the summary of knowledge, attitudes, behaviors, and beliefs staff shares about the primary importance of the well-being and care of the patients they serve, supported by systems and structures that reinforce the focus on patient safety." Health care systems that have a culture of safety and provide high-quality care are guided by three principles: trust, reporting, and improvement.

Although the safety of health care has improved, there is still room for improvement. One of the most common types of hospital-acquired infection occurs at the surgical site, accounting for up to 40% of the all hospital-acquired infections.[44,86,87] Surgical site infections increase economic burden (length of stay and hospital cost) and disability-related outcomes. Health care cost doubles for patients with surgical site infection.[88] The Surgical Care Improvement Project, launched by the CMS and the CDC, aimed to reduce perioperative complications (i.e., surgical site infection, perioperative myocardial infarction, postoperative pneumonia, and venous thromboembolism). The initiative mandated that antibiotic prophylaxis be administered with incision, administration of the appropriate antibiotic, and discontinuation of antibiotic within 24 hours. Studies have shown that this initiative has been successful in reducing infection; however, compliance rates range from 60% to 100%.[89-91] Hospitals are given incentives to increase compliance and are required to audit and release Surgical Care Improvement Project data to the CMS and insurance companies.

A culture of safety for nurse anesthesia practice is supported with the document "Patient-Centered Perianesthesia Communication," in which patient-centered care is expressed in more detail. In a literature review aimed to develop a conceptual model of safety culture, Sammer et al.[92] identified seven components that influence a patient safety culture, which includes the following:

- *Leadership.* Leaders seek to align mission and vision, competencies, and resources across all levels of staff.
- *Teamwork.* Collegiality, collaboration, cooperation, and open respectful communication exists among executives and staff.
- *Evidence based.* Patient care processes are standardized and evidence based.
- *Communication.* All staff members, regardless of position, have the right and responsibility to advocate for the patient.
- *Learning.* Learning is valued among staff. The facility strives to learn from mistakes and improve performance.
- *Just.* There is recognition that errors are a system failure, rather than individual failure, while holding individuals accountable for their actions.
- *Patient centered.* Providing care is centered on patients and their family/caregivers. Patients are active participants in their care.

MEASUREMENT OF HEALTH CARE QUALITY IN ANESTHESIA

The main goal of health care quality improvement is to continue what is good about the present health care system while at the same time focusing on the areas that need improvement.[93] The measure of health care quality is not new; however, defining the importance of any given measure is problematic.[94] As established by the Affordable Care Act, the National Quality Strategy (NQS) was created in March 2011 to provide greater clarity on how health care providers and delivery systems could meet the goals of individual experience improvement of care, improved population health, and decreased costs.[31,94] With input from more than 300 stakeholders, the ultimate aim of the NQS is to provide the framework to help focus on the alignment of quality measures and quality improvement activities.[95]

As anesthesia practice enters a new crossroads, patient satisfaction, as a measure of health outcomes and delivery, has emerged as a valuable metric in the evolving system of health care.[96,97] Anesthesia practice has been undergoing change over the last decade; however, in the future, our roles and responsibilities may be called into question and the sustainability of the practice may be in jeopardy if our focus does not continue to evolve. In the era of health reform, it is imperative that nurse anesthesia practice models drive the future of this clinical specialty. Remodeling practice represents a disruptive improvement in which the benefits offered are simpler, less costly, and of equal or higher quality than existing fee-for-service models.[98] As such, clinical practice and patient outcomes will be a more important measure of success as the Affordable Care Act continues to link pay with high-quality care, population health, and reduced expenditures.[98,99]

Further analysis for the benefit of the nurse anesthesia community is sharing multiple supporting resources such as articles, studies, and books on historical need for patient-centered health care, particularly for communities of color. The evidence shows that patient-centered care improves disease outcomes and quality of life, and that it is critical to addressing racial, ethnic, and socioeconomic disparities in health care.[17] Patient-centered health care is a model utilized by health care institutions across the country. The National Academy of Medicine report, "Crossing the Quality Chasm: A New Health System for the 21st Century," defined patient-centered care as care that is "respectful of and responsive to individual patient preferences, needs, and values, and ensuring that patient values guide all clinical decisions."[100]

Decision Making and Patient-Centered Care in Anesthesia

Shared decision making is nothing new in anesthesia practice; it has always been a hallmark of the profession. Anesthesia practice has historically used a form of shared decision making by including physician generalists, physician specialists, nurses, and auxiliary personnel in the course of the perioperative experience. The perioperative experience is successful when is it approached in a way that involves clinicians and patients sharing the best available evidence when making choices that will achieve the most informed decisions regarding the course of the anesthesia experience. The use of interdisciplinary teams is an essential element in the development of quality care measurements. Consensus building between appropriate stakeholders will ensure that risk-benefit trade-offs are thoroughly evaluated.

Health Care Quality and Safety in Anesthesia

Any organization, whether public, private nonprofit, or private for-profit, can develop a measure; however, getting organizational and provider buy-in to adopt a given measure is critical if health plans and payers are to endorse them. Currently, the National Quality Forum (NQF) is the leading organization that reviews and endorses measures. The NQF is a nonprofit, nonpartisan, membership-based organization whose measures and standards serve as a critically important foundation for initiatives to enhance health care value, make patient care safer, and achieve better outcomes.[101] NQF's endorsement process is geared to be a transparent, consensus-based practice that brings together diverse health care stakeholders from the public and private sector to foster quality improvement. At the time of this writing, approximately 300 NQF-endorsed measures are used in more than 20 federal public reporting and pay-for-performance programs, as well as in private sector and state programs.

By setting the example for safe, quality care, the anesthesia professions have been cited as leading the way in patient safety and outcomes. Reductions in anesthesia mortality have been accomplished through using new technologies, standardizing processes, simulation, championing patient safety and quality, and forming the Anesthesia Patient Safety Foundation.[102]

Health care is a shared effort between providers and patients. In 1996, the National Patient Safety Foundation (NPSF) began as an idea at a conference on medical error. The conference was organized by the American Association for the Advancement of Science, the American Medical Association, and the Annenberg Center for Health Sciences at the Eisenhower Medical Center in California. At that meeting, representatives announced plans to form a foundation that would

be "a collaborative initiative involving all members of the health care community aimed at stimulating leadership, fostering awareness, and enhancing patient safety knowledge creation, dissemination, and implementation." NPSF is broader in scope, but similar in concept and mission to its predecessor, the Anesthesia Patient Safety Foundation, which focused on the perioperative arena.

The AANA is continually developing informational sources to aid CRNAs in understanding the complex relationship between quality and value outlined in many of the CMS quality initiatives. These quality initiatives will affect reimbursement. Therefore it is important for CRNAs to build their knowledge base about and become more familiar with these initiatives. The Physician Quality Reporting System (PQRS) program is a CMS quality initiative that affects eligible providers' (EPs') reimbursement rates for covered Physician Fee Schedule (PFS) services furnished to Medicare Part B fee-for-service (FFS) beneficiaries. Although technically a voluntary program, nonparticipation in the PQRS program has financial implications for future Medicare Part B FFS reimbursement. Financial implications exist in the form of payment adjustments based on satisfactory reporting of PQRS measures. Compliance with PQRS reporting requirements also has repercussions beyond the PQRS program; therefore, understanding this program is essential in order to safeguard their Medicare billings.[103]

There are several PQRS reporting mechanisms for single practitioners and group practices. Depending on their specialty, setting, and practice, EPs may choose from the following methods to submit data to CMS: claims based, electronic health record (EHR), Qualified Registry, Qualified Clinical Data Registry (QCDR), or the Group Practice Reporting Option (GPRO).[103] With the passage of the Patient Protection and Affordable Care Act, there is an increased demand for health care providers to accelerate quality improvement and promote transparency through the reporting of clinical quality measures. The CMS, via different quality reporting programs, has been collecting a number of metrics, including performance measures and patient experiences, and is now using them to report on health care provider and group practice performance.[104] A list of QCDRs that support anesthesia measures are available through the AANA.

SUMMARY

Patient-centered care and cultural competence are necessary components when providing high-quality care in nurse anesthesia practice. The importance of viewing the patient as a unique individual with distinct attitudes, values, beliefs, and behaviors exceeds generalizations that can be assumed about various cultural groups. The goal of patient-centered,

culturally competent care is to create an environment free of discrimination, where patients are recognized for their individuality, without regard to race, national origin, color, age, religion, sex (including pregnancy and gender identity), sexual orientation, disability (physical or mental), status as a parent, genetic information, or other factors.

REFERENCES

For a complete list of references for this chapter, scan this QR code with any smartphone code reader app, or visit the following URL: http://booksite.elsevier.com/9780323711944/.

4

Nurse Anesthesia Research: Empowering Decision Making Through Evidence-Based Practice

Elisabeth Cole McConnell, Chuck Biddle

The nurse anesthetist brings a wealth of knowledge and experience to every patient encounter. Evidence-based practice (EBP) guides the safe and effective application of this knowledge in clinical practice by providing the tools necessary to translate high-quality research into successful patient care. EBP provides a systematic and efficient means of assessing the quality of research and applying empirical findings to the clinical setting. Whether selecting an antiemetic, administering an intravenous fluid, deciding on mechanical ventilator settings, or planning postoperative pain control, the nurse anesthetist relies on EBP to guide clinical decision making and improve patient outcomes.

Although there are many approaches to EBP, the essential components common to all include the following:
- Defining the patient's problem
- Proficiently searching the relevant literature
- Critically appraising the discovered literature
- Rationally applying the relevant literature in the context unique to the patient

At the core of EBP is the notion of critical thinking. Critical thinking is applied to the appraisal of the pertinent literature and balanced with clinical experience as the clinician determines whether the evidence is applicable to a particular patient's situation. However, the nurse anesthetist's ability to critically appraise the relevant literature is contingent on the extent of his or her understanding of clinical research. Thus EBP requires the nurse anesthetist to develop a thorough grasp of the process of conducting and evaluating clinical research studies. Such an understanding begins with an exploration of the nature of research and the research process. Mastering these concepts of clinical research is a critical step in practicing successful evidence-based anesthesia.

Research represents a rational approach to making practice choices among initially plausible alternatives and provides a direction and means for validating these choices. The impact of research on the day-to-day activities of the nurse anesthetist has become an especially relevant topic. Before the mid-1970s, the vast majority of nurses functioned without much consideration of research or publication of their ideas. In the late 1970s, nurse anesthesia experienced a period of punctuated evolution. Major driving forces behind this evolution included the movement to a graduate educational framework, a more sophisticated appreciation of the scientific underpinnings of our specialty, national attention to issues of patient outcomes and patient safety, and a growing self-awareness of nurse anesthetists not only as providers of excellent clinical care but also as active participants as scholars in the field. Recognition of the importance of EBP was especially influential in this progression.

Nurse anesthetists primarily function with a practice-oriented perspective, and therefore the recommendations of Brown et al. seem especially relevant.[1] These scholars suggest that four characteristics of research are essential for the development of a scientific knowledge base for a discipline such as nurse anesthesia. First, research should be actively conducted by the members of the discipline. Second, research should be focused on clinical problems encountered by members of the discipline. Third, the approach to these problems must be grounded in a conceptual framework—that is, it must be scientifically based, emphasizing selection, arrangement, and clarification of existing relationships. Finally, the methods used in studying the problems must be fundamentally sound.[1]

METHODS OF KNOWING

The term *research* can be broadly defined as the application of a systematic approach to the study of a problem or question. However, we do not know all the things we claim to know on the basis of systematic inquiry. Other sources of knowledge include authority, personal experience, and logical reasoning.

Perhaps the most advanced way of knowing is reflected in the scientific method. Although it, too, is fallible, the scientific method is more reliable and valid than other methods. It provides for self-evaluation with a system of checks and balances that minimizes bias and faulty reasoning. In essence, it is a systematic approach to solving problems and enhancing our understanding of phenomena. It is, at its foundation, the gathering and interpretation of information without prejudice.

THE NATURE OF RESEARCH

Research is, by definition, a dynamic phenomenon. Whether it is directed purely at the acquisition of knowledge for knowledge's sake (basic research) or at the specific solution of problems (applied research), it is a process that can be conceptualized in terms of at least four characteristics.

First, research can assume many different forms. Second, research must be valid, both internally and externally (Box 4.1). Internal validity is necessary but not sufficient for ensuring external validity. Third, research must be reliable. Reliability refers to the extent to which data collection, analysis, and interpretation are consistent and to which the research can be replicated. Fourth, research must be systematic. The elements of a systematic approach include the identification of the problem(s), the gathering and critical review of relevant information, the collection of data in a highly orchestrated manner, an analysis of the data appropriate to the problem(s) faced, and the development of conclusions within the study's framework.

BOX 4.1 Research Scenario: Internal Versus External Validity

Internal Validity

- The extent to which results can be accurately interpreted and the degree to which the independent variable (that which is manipulated) is responsible for a change in the dependent variable (that which is measured). For example, the patient's blood pressure is measured. A combination of propofol, midazolam, isoflurane, and a new muscle relaxant is used for induction of anesthesia. A postinduction blood pressure is recorded, and the researcher concludes that the new muscle relaxant lowers blood pressure.

Questions

- Has the researcher isolated the effect of the muscle relaxant from those of the other agents?
- Are there plausible or competing alternative explanations?

Analysis

- Internal validity is low because the results cannot be interpreted with any degree of certainty.

External Validity

- The extent to which the results can be generalized; this issue relates to the question, "To whom can the results be applied?" For example, 35 obese men who are nonsurgical volunteers are anesthetized with a standard dose of a new induction drug. The clinical half-life of the drug is determined with plasma drug sampling and brain wave activity monitoring. The researcher concludes that future patients receiving the standard dose of the new drug will experience a clinical half-life of 11 minutes.

Questions

- Is it reasonable to assume that obese patients might respond differently than their nonobese counterparts?
- Might women respond differently than men?
- Could surgical manipulation or other drug therapy have an impact on the pharmacokinetics of the new drug?

Analysis

- External validity is low because the results cannot be generalized to any other individuals except those similar to the subjects in the study.

Scientific knowledge emerges from an enterprise that is intensely human; as a consequence, it is subject to the full spectrum of human strengths and limitations. The scientific discovery and understanding that attend participation in research and its results can be professionally exhilarating and satisfying.

THE EIGHT CRITICAL STAGES IN THE RESEARCH PROCESS

Research accords several personal freedoms to those who engage in it: the freedom to pursue those opportunities in which one is interested, the freedom to exchange ideas with other interested colleagues, and the freedom to be a deconstructionist (i.e., one who challenges existing knowledge). Yet, despite these freedoms, research must be logical, must progress in an orderly manner, and ultimately must be grounded within the framework of the scientific method. If research is a way of searching for truths, uncovering solutions to problems, and generating principles that result in theories, we must come to understand the process of research.

The research process can be described in many different ways. For purposes of simplicity, this process is defined as consisting of eight distinct stages:

1. Identification of the problem
2. Review of the relevant knowledge and literature
3. Formulation of the hypothesis or research question
4. Development of an approach for testing the hypothesis
5. Execution of the research plan
6. Analysis and interpretation of the data
7. Dissemination of the findings to interested colleagues
8. Evaluation of the research report

Stage 1: Identification of the Problem

The selection and formulation of the problem constitute an essential first step in the research process. The researcher decides the general subject of the investigation, guided principally by personal experience and by inductions and deductions based on existing sources of knowledge. The researcher makes the general subject manageable by narrowing the focus of the problem. The following criteria must be met at this phase of the research process:

- The problem area should be of sufficient importance to merit study.
- The problem must be one that is practical to investigate.
- The researcher should be knowledgeable and experienced in the area from which the problem has emerged.
- The researcher should be sincerely motivated and interested in studying the problem.

We constantly encounter problems and situations that can be studied. At clinical anesthesia conferences, one might hear remarks such as the following:

"It seems to me that a small dose of intravenous lidocaine given just before propofol alleviates virtually any pain on injection."

"Do you think there is less nausea and vomiting in outpatients who are deliberately overhydrated?"

"I find that the use of the waveform generated by my pulse oximeter gives me valuable information about depth of anesthesia."

"I believe that the inspiratory pause mechanism on the Ohmeda 7810 ventilator significantly improves arterial oxygen tension in patients with chronic obstructive pulmonary disease."

"I am convinced that sleepiness is a major cause of anesthesia accidents."

A study could emerge from each of these situations, built on ideas, hunches, or curiosity. A problem that lends itself to research often materializes from personal observations and in the sharing of ideas and experiences among those who are familiar with the phenomenon in question.

Once identified, the problem should be stated in terms that clarify the subject and restrict the scope of the study. Defining the terms involved in the problem statement is also critical, as demonstrated in Box 4.2.

The wording of the problem statement sets the stage for the type of study design used. Each step in the research process subsequently influences later steps, and this should be kept in mind at all times. A mistake made early inevitably creates difficulties at some later stage in the process.

Common Mistakes

At this stage of the process, pitfalls can include an overly ready acceptance of the first research idea that comes to mind, as well as a selection of a problem that is too broad or vague to allow effective study.

Stage 2: Review of the Relevant Knowledge and Literature

Once the problem has been identified, information is needed for putting the problem into proper context so that the research can proceed effectively. A well-conducted literature review provides the researcher with the following:

- An understanding of what has already been accomplished in the area of interest

---

BOX 4.2   Research Scenario: Stating the Problem

Poor
- I am unsure of the effectiveness of etomidate in patients.

Better
- I am unsure at what dose etomidate induces unconsciousness in patients undergoing hysterectomy and what impact it has on heart rate, blood pressure, and vascular resistance.

Comments
- The problem should be focused.
- The terms should be clarified.
- The relationships should be understood.
- The problem should not be so narrow as to be trivial.

- A theoretic framework within which the problem can be optimally stated, understood, and studied
- An appreciation for gaps in current understanding of the phenomenon
- Information for avoiding unanticipated difficulties
- Examples of potentially useful or poorly constructed research designs and procedures
- A background for interpreting the results of the proposed investigation
  Effective search strategies are discussed later in the chapter.

Common Mistakes

At this stage in the research process, mistakes include hasty review of the literature, overly heavy reliance on secondary (book) rather than primary (journal) sources, lack of critical examination of the methods by which conclusions were reached, and incorrect copying of references. For example, a mistake in noting the volume number or misspelling an author's name makes it more difficult to locate the source again with ease.

Stage 3: Formulation of the Hypothesis or Research Question

In its most elemental form, a hypothesis is either a proposed solution to a problem or a stated relationship among variables. It establishes and defines the independent variable (the variable that is to be manipulated or is presumed to influence the outcome) and the dependent variable (the outcome that is dependent on the independent variable). The hypothesis is declarative in nature and assumes one of three forms:

1. A *directional hypothesis:* Patients premedicated with midazolam have less anxiety on arrival to the operating room than do those who were not premedicated.
2. A *nondirectional hypothesis:* Patients premedicated with midazolam experience a difference in anxiety on arrival in the operating room when compared with those who were not premedicated.
3. A *null hypothesis:* Patients premedicated with midazolam experience no difference in anxiety on arrival in the operating room compared with those who were not premedicated.

Research questions are generally reserved for investigations that are descriptive or exploratory in nature or for when the relationships among the variables are unclear. A research question might be more appropriate than a hypothesis in a study that proposes to determine the beliefs of anesthesia providers who interact with patients under specific circumstances. For example, consider the following research question: What are the attitudes of nurse anesthetists in the northeastern United States who care for patients with acquired immunodeficiency syndrome (AIDS)?

Common Mistakes

At this point in the process, mistakes include use of a vague or unmanageable hypothesis and development of a research question that cannot be answered reasonably.

Stage 4: Development of an Approach for Testing the Hypothesis

After the research idea has taken shape in the form of a formal hypothesis or research question, a plan of attack is developed. The research proposal represents the stage at which the ideas of the project crystallize into a substantive form. The proposal includes the following:

- A problem statement and clarification of the significance of the proposed study
- The hypothesis or research question
- A sufficient review of the literature for justification of the study
- A description of the research design
- A careful explanation of the sample to be studied
- The type of statistical analysis to be applied

A research proposal is a useful and efficient way for the researcher to determine the completeness of the plan and is usually required if the researcher is to obtain departmental or institutional approval or is applying for financial support.

Research Methods

The research method is the way the truth of a phenomenon is coaxed from the world in which it resides and is freed of the biases of the human condition. A variety of research methods are at our disposal, and researchers are not inflexibly wedded to any particular approach. Researchers do not follow a single scientific method but rather use a body of methods amenable to their fields of study.

Some of the methods available are highly recognizable, permanent components of the researcher's armamentarium, whereas others have evolved not only with respect to time but also in response to the specific needs of a particular problem or discipline. The research method can be influenced by the way a researcher views a problem. For example, a researcher can test a hypothesis, search for a correlation, ask "why" or "how" questions, or probe a phenomenon on the basis of "what would happen if" suppositions. Research methods in the context of EBP will be discussed later in the chapter.

The researcher can view the method on the basis of the fundamental task that it will accomplish. For example, two broad categories into which research efforts can be divided are basic research and applied research. Basic research adds to the existing body of knowledge and may not have immediate, practical use. Applied research is oriented toward solving an immediate, specific, and practical problem.

The research method can be characterized in terms of its temporal relationship to the problem. A retrospective study is the process of surveying the past; the thing in which we are interested has already occurred, and we are simply looking to see what did occur. In contrast, a prospective study looks forward to see what will happen in a given situation; here, the collection of data proceeds forward in time.

It is important to understand several terms fundamental to the research process. As mentioned previously, the dependent variable is the object of the study, or the variable that is being measured. The independent variable is the one that affects the dependent variable and is presumed to cause or influence it. Another way of looking at this relationship is that variables that are a consequence of or are dependent on antecedent variables are considered dependent variables.

Another set of variables consists of control variables, also known as *organismic*, *background*, or *attribute* variables. Control variables are not actively manipulated by the researcher, but because they might influence the relationships under study, they must be controlled, held constant, or randomized so that their effects are neutralized, canceled out, or at least considered by the researcher (Box 4.3).

The term *blinding* or *masking* refers to the process of controlling for obvious and occult bias arising from subjects' or researchers' reactions to what is going on. In a single-blind design, the patients are unaware of which treatment or manipulation is actually being given to them. In the double-blind design, neither the researcher nor the subject is aware of which treatment or manipulation the subject is receiving. Whereas randomization attempts to equalize the groups at the start of the study, blinding equalizes the groups by controlling for psychologic biases that might arise apart from any effect of the treatment. Many factors influence the decision to use a single-blind or a double-blind design. For example, in some situations it may not be feasible to disguise a particular treatment or intervention.

Operationalization is the process of precisely defining a given variable, condition, or process so that it may be replicated in future studies. If researchers do not operationalize the terms, phrases, and manipulations in the study, the net effect could be an ambiguous study. In a study examining the effects of epidural anesthesia in critically ill patients, it would be essential to operationalize the terms *effects* and *critically ill patients*. Without operationalizing these terms, future researchers would not know whether effects referred to patient mortality, paralysis, infection, therapeutic benefit, or some other consequence of epidural anesthesia. Similarly, in a study comparing the quality of inhalation induction with isoflurane and sevoflurane in pediatric patients, it is essential that the researcher operationalize the terms *inhalation induction* and *quality*. Operationalization of terms clearly designates performable and observable acts or procedures in such a way that they can be replicated immutably.

Classifying Research on the Basis of Methodology

The two models or archetypes of research are quantitative and qualitative research. Depending on what is already known about the research question or phenomenon of inquiry, the contextual lens of the researcher, and sometimes the subject being studied itself, research will be conducted using one of these two main models of investigation. There are many classification schemes for research design. Ultimately, the research design is one that is dependent on and inextricably wedded to the study's purpose, scope, and nature of the problem at hand. Study design can be thought of as the architectural plans of the study to answer the research question, whereas the research method is the process and tools necessary to answer the research question. Table 4.1 offers a simplified approach to classifying research methods. Much weight is applied to the type of research method used when assessing its rigor and its relevance to EBP. Fig. 4.1 offers a visual for rank order of evidence from different types of studies and their clinical relevance. Table 4.2 provides a brief synopsis of commonly used study designs.

Quantitative Research designs can be classified into two broad domains: experimental and observational. Observational studies do not involve an investigator-controlled manipulation or intervention, but rather simply track the subjects for a defined period, recording events defined by the researcher's objectives. The independent variable (e.g., a clinical intervention such as a patient who received or did not receive a blood transfusion for aortic valve surgery as part of routine care) is simply a matter of record, and a dependent variable (e.g., an outcome such as the rate of wound infection or fever) is recorded. Such a study can progress forward in time (prospective) or, in the case of a study looking back in time (retrospective), examine an institutional database. Another type of observational study is the cross-sectional study, in which well-defined measures are recorded at predetermined points in time.

BOX 4.3 Research Scenario: Understanding the Types of Variables

Study Group

A new intravenous drug that may be associated with fewer cardiovascular effects than thiopental during induction in pediatric patients is being studied. Fifty children aged 3 to 6 years, undergoing intravenous inductions for hernia repair or eye muscle surgery, are randomized to either the propofol group or the new drug group. Blood pressure, heart rate, and rhythm are measured by a dedicated observer who is unaware of which drug the patients are receiving.

Analysis

The dependent variables are blood pressure, heart rate, and heart rhythm. The independent variable is the drug the child receives, either the propofol or the new drug. A number of control variables are present, including sex, fluid status, time of day, underlying medical history, and concurrent drug therapy. With randomization, such control variables should be equated or neutralized for the two groups, but even randomization is not an absolute guarantee.

TABLE 4.1 Classifying Research by Method

Type	Qualities and Purpose	Example Quantitative
Quantitative		
Experimental	At least one variable manipulated Random assignment to groups Dependent variable is measured Good for determining cause and effect Prospective in nature	Is there more or less pain on injection of one or the other drug? What did the manipulation do?
Ex post facto	Independent variable has already occurred Examines relationships by observing a consequence and looking back for associations Retrospective in nature (Latin for "from a thing done after")	Looking back over 5 years, does a relationship exist between the rate of myocardial infarction and the inhaled anesthetic that was administered?
Descriptive	Describes something as it occurred Incidence, relationships, and distributions are studied Deals more with "what-is?" than "why-is-it-so?" questions	What are the attitudes of nurse anesthetists regarding the care of patients who have AIDS?
Historical	Describes "what was" rather than what effect variables had on others Events are described as accurately as possible through a process of critical inquiry	A test of the hypothesis that Sister M. Bernard was the first nurse anesthetist.
Qualitative Phenomenology Grounded theory Ethnography	Experiences lived by people Perception is viewed as our access to that experience Discovers and conceptualizes the essence of complex processes	What is the nature of the relationship between nurse anesthetists and surgeons in private and in academic settings?

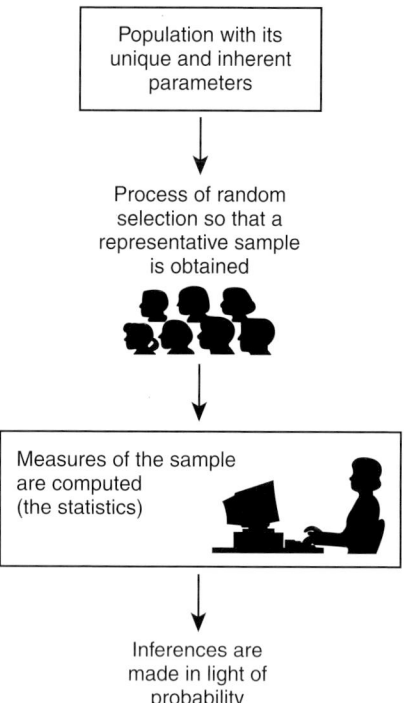

Population with its
unique and inherent
parameters

↓

Process of random
selection so that a
representative sample
is obtained

↓

Measures of the sample
are computed
(the statistics)

↓

Inferences are
made in light of
probability

Fig. 4.1 Conceptual model of inferential statistics.

Case reports are commonly seen in the anesthesia literature and provide an opportunity to vicariously experience the care provided to a patient. These reports describe perioperative events, characteristics of an individual patient (or of a series of similar patients in a case series), and the successes or failures associated with a described management regimen. However, the subjective nature of case reports and studies introduces substantial bias. Due to this bias and because the study design does not allow for the controls necessary for hypothesis testing, this type of design is often used solely to generate a hypothesis.

The case control study is a type of observational study in which a researcher examines a group of patients (the cases) to identify factors that seem to be associated with a past outcome (e.g., blindness following anesthesia). A key component of the design is the identification of a similar group of patients who did not experience the negative outcome (the controls). This component is called matching and is usually conducted with respect to a patient's gender, age, surgical procedure, and other factors. Matching allows the researcher to minimize differences in patient characteristics between the case and control groups that obscure the effect of the variables of interest. For example, in a study of blindness following anesthesia, if the case group contained more patients with type II diabetes mellitus than the control group, a higher incidence of blindness in the case group may be due to complications of diabetes rather than anesthesia. In this example, diabetes would be considered a confounding variable (confounder). Balancing confounding variables between study groups minimizes the risk that extraneous factors are responsible for the association between the variables of interest and the outcome. Traditionally, this type of study is considered sufficiently powered if the ratio of cases to controls is 1:2 or greater (1:3 or 1:4 is optimal). Case control studies are useful for identifying associations between a variable(s) and an outcome but are not powerful enough to allow for cause and effect to be determined.

Observational studies are limited by their inability to control factors that influence the study outcome. In an observational study, the researcher has no control over the treatment assigned to a patient or the numerous variables likely to affect the outcome of interest. As a result, many forms of bias are introduced to the study. At best, the researcher can use observational studies to make associations between described variables. One tool used to improve the validity of conclusions reached by observational studies is the use of propensity score analysis, discussed later in the chapter.

Experimental research designs minimize potential bias by allowing the researcher to control for confounding variables. These studies are prospective and measure the effect of manipulating the independent variable on the dependent variable. Generally, the goal is to describe and assess an intervention for its safety or efficacy or to determine if one approach offers benefits over existing interventions. A cohort study is a prospective study that compares a group of patients either receiving a treatment or having a condition of interest with a control group. Over time, data for the two groups are collected and compared. Cohort studies work well for experiments that might otherwise be unethical or dangerous. For example, such a study might identify two groups of patients scheduled to receive laparoscopic gallbladder surgery: a group of people who are morbidly obese and a comparison group of people who are not. Although researchers cannot randomly assign patients to undergo surgery, cohort studies allow researchers to minimize variability between study groups to compare outcomes of interest. Assessing outcomes such as drug requirements, duration of surgery, positioning-related injury, and ventilator requirements would allow some general conclusions to be reached regarding considerations in caring for patients of different body types undergoing a similar procedure.

The gold standard of clinical experimental research is the randomized controlled trial (RCT). Clinical trials, by definition, involve the use of humans as subjects and require a specific set of criteria (Fig. 4.2). Because powerful controls are established and the influence of bias is reduced, RCTs are better able to reveal the true effect of an intervention on selected measured outcomes. Because of the high quality of the evidence they produce, randomized trials are heavily relied on in EBP. RCTs are discussed in more detail later in the chapter.

Quasi-experimental research differs from experimental research in that it is missing one or more of the key elements required for an experimental design. Either a control group or a randomization procedure may be absent from the design. For example, a practitioner at an institution regularly prescribes ondansetron whereas a fellow practitioner does not. A prospective quasi-experimental trial in which both practitioners use a standard anesthetic technique would allow the two practitioners to use or not use ondansetron as they normally would. The incidence of nausea and vomiting in the first 6 postoperative hours can then be compared between each practitioner's patient groups. Although randomization is not achieved, a study that may not otherwise have been possible because of the inflexibility of the clinicians involved is successfully accomplished. Quasi-experiments, by yielding to one or more of the rigid criteria of the experimental design, offer an attractive alternative in certain circumstances.

Qualitative Research: An Alternative Paradigm

Up to this point, the traditional approach to a problem has been characterized by deductive reasoning, objectivity, manipulation, and control. An alternative approach involves a group of methods characterized by inductive reasoning, subjectivity, exploration, and process orientation. These methods fall under the rubric of qualitative research techniques.

Qualitative techniques include philosophic inquiry, historiography, phenomenology, grounded theory, and ethnography. Qualitative research generally refers to systematic modes of inquiry directed principally at observing, describing, analyzing, interpreting, and understanding the patterns, themes, qualities, and meanings of specific contextual

TABLE 4.2 Synopsis of Major Study Designs		
Study Design	**Advantages**	**Disadvantages**
Survey	• Generally inexpensive and simple • Low risk of ethical problems	• Establishment of association at best; no demonstration of cause and effect • Susceptible to recall bias • Possible unequal distribution of confounders between or among groups • Possible unequal group sizes
Case control study	• Generally quick and inexpensive • Feasible method for studying very rare disorders or disorders with long lag between exposure and outcome • Fewer subjects needed than cross-sectional studies • Ethically safe • Matched subjects	• Reliance on recall or records to determine exposure status • Confounders difficult to identify and control • Possible difficulty in selection of control groups • Large risk of bias: recall, selection
Cohort study	• Can establish timing and directionality of events • Can standardize eligibility criteria and outcome assessments • Administratively easier and less expensive than randomized controlled trials	• Possible difficulty identifying control subjects • Exposure possibly linked to a hidden confounder • Difficulty in blinding • Lack of randomization • For rare disease, large sample or long follow-up necessary
Randomized controlled trial	• Unbiased distribution of confounders • Blinding more likely • Statistical analysis facilitated by randomization	• Costly in terms of time and money • Volunteer bias—not all patients willing to be "randomized"
Observational study	• No random assignment • Generally inexpensive	• Loss of control over the intervention • Loss of control over potential (known and unknown) confounders
Retrospective design	• Cheaper and generally easier to perform than prospective studies • Highly useful for discerning the nature of phenomena, especially in describing associations between or among variables • Improved techniques and statistical methods have made these methods more defensible • Data often housed in existing manual or electronic databases, making access convenient	• Independent variable has already occurred • Loss of control over variables • Cannot ascertain cause-and-effect relationships • Determining which variable is dependent and which variable is independent is not consistently possible when a relationship is revealed
Crossover design	• Smaller sample needed because subjects serve as own controls and error variance is reduced • All subjects receive treatment (at least some of the time) • Statistical tests assuming randomization can be used • Blinding can be maintained • Ethically problematic at times	• All subjects receive placebo or alternative treatment at some point • Lengthy or unknown washout period (recovery from a given intervention) • Not usable for treatments with permanent effects

phenomena. Qualitative research seeks to gain insight by discovering the meanings associated with a given phenomenon and exploring the depth, richness, and complexity inherent in it. The treatise on qualitative approaches by Marshall, Rossman and Blanco is recommended to interested readers.[2]

Sampling

Under most circumstances, studying everyone who might be affected by a particular study is impractical if not impossible. For example, if we want to know how effective intravenous nitroglycerin is in minimizing the rise in blood pressure associated with laryngoscopy in hypertensive patients, we cannot realistically study all hypertensive patients who undergo laryngoscopy. Rather, we would hope to find a smaller group of subjects who are representative of the relevant population at large. By accessing certain information in the sample, we can credibly make inferences or generalizations regarding the population at large.

Similarly, if we want to know how often anesthesia machines in small community hospitals receive preventive maintenance, we cannot visit all the community hospitals in the nation. Instead, we might randomly select a number of hospitals in a number of different states, visit those locations, and inspect the maintenance records. By studying this representative sample, we can make some reasonable and safe generalizations regarding the phenomenon of preventive maintenance at large.

Consider the anecdote about the four blind people who encountered an elephant during one of their daily walks. Each person felt a different part of the elephant. When asked to describe what they had encountered, the first person replied, "a tree trunk" (the elephant's leg). The second reported feeling "a large snake" (the elephant's trunk). The third reported that it was "most definitely a wall" (the elephant's torso). The last person reported that it was "a large, frayed rope" (the elephant's tail). This analogy illustrates that a few discrete sampling points may not be adequate for describing a complex phenomenon. Not only is a random sample best; it should also be large enough and sample a sufficient number of points in the population that a truly representative perspective is gained.

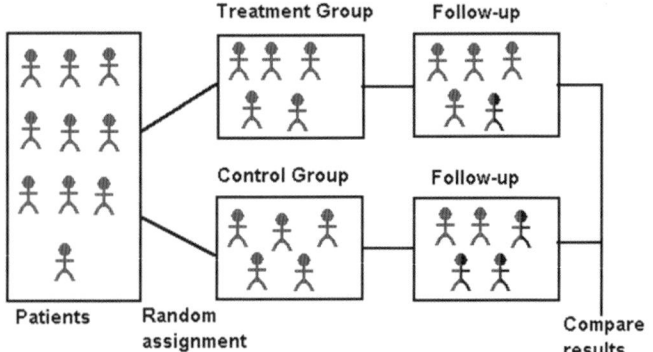

Fig. 4.2 The randomized controlled trial (RCT) is a prospective, longitudinal experimental study in which representative members of the population of interest are randomly assigned to either a treatment group (also called an experimental group) or a control group. Study conditions are carefully controlled so that the only functional difference between the treatment and control groups is the intervention being studied. Ideally, both the subjects and the researchers should be "blinded" to the type of group (treatment or control) to which the subject has been assigned. A sufficiently powered RCT ensures that the study design facilitates the accurate detection of a treatment effect and the size of that effect. Carefully following the study participants and measuring the treatment effect with the appropriate statistical techniques are also essential to a quality RCT. Finally, the RCT should be able to be reproduced by other researchers to confirm the study's findings.

TABLE 4.3	Characteristics of the Four Categories of Measurement	
Category	**Characteristics**	**Examples**
Nominal	Identifies	Male or female
		Diagnosis
Ordinal	Identifies	American Society of Anesthesiologists (ASA) class
	Orders	Order of race finish
Interval	Identifies	Intelligence
	Orders	Calendar years
	Equal intervals	Degrees Fahrenheit or Celsius
Ratio	Identifies	Blood pressure
	Orders	Reaction time
	Equal intervals	Weight
	Has a true zero	Distance
		Degrees Kelvin

Different sampling techniques can be used, depending on the research design. In a true random sample (also known as probability sampling), all members of the population at large have a similar chance of being included in the study. This is rarely the case in clinical research, in which we are confined to dealing with those individuals who present themselves. In this situation, the sample is called a convenience sample. When a convenience sample is used in an experimental study, it is important to ensure that the subjects selected for the study are at least randomized when assigned to treatments or groups. In the ideal situation, the researcher aims for both random selection (from the population at large) and random assignment (to the different groups in the study).

Obtaining a random sample, especially in clinical research, is often a complicated process. Most important is the realization that the concept of randomness is essential to minimizing human biases associated with both selection and assignment. Randomization is discussed in detail later in the chapter.

Instrumentation and Measurement

Two important concepts essential to measurement are validity and reliability. Instrument validity is the degree to which an instrument, such as a blood pressure cuff or a personality inventory, accurately measures what it is intended to measure. Instrument reliability refers to the degree of consistency with which an instrument measures whatever it is measuring, that is, whether the same result is obtained on repeated trials.

Validity and reliability are often easily established for measures of certain physiologic phenomena but may be troublesome in behavioral or psychological evaluations. Imagine trying to determine reliability and validity for a thermometer. Contrast this to trying to establish validity and reliability for a psychological tool that professes to measure a nurse anesthetist's attitude toward euthanasia; obviously, the latter is a much more difficult undertaking. Although a measure must be reliable to be valid, it can be reliable without being valid. For example, a skin temperature probe might reliably (consistently) measure temperature

even in a variety of extreme settings, although it would not be viewed as a valid indicator of core temperature. Both reliability and validity are discussed in degrees rather than in all-or-nothing terms.

Many published instruments have reliability and validity testing reported. When choosing an instrument for a study, it is critical to consider whether the instrument's reliability and validity have been established. For example, if an instrument measures evoked responses in the esophagus as an indicator of depth of anesthesia, it must be determined whether the reliability and validity of the instrument have been established under the conditions of the anesthetic protocol being used in the proposed study. Coefficients of reliability and validity are presented on a scale of 0 to 1, with 1 being perfect.

Occasionally, the researcher may encounter no reasonable measures to use for a study. Instruments for measuring such phenomena as arterial oxygen tension, end-tidal anesthetic concentration, and opioid metabolic by-products are well established. However, a researcher may need to develop a totally new instrument (questionnaire) to determine perceptions regarding the propriety of a given manufacturer's high-pressure promotional campaigns for newly released pharmaceutic products. In developing such a tool, it is helpful to have an expert in the discipline look over the instrument and provide feedback to ensure that the instrument is appropriate.

Researchers have a variety of instruments for measuring phenomena. These include Biospecimen analysis
- Written tests
- Rating scales
- Questionnaires
- Chemical tests
- Physical tests
- Electrical tests
- Visual observation
- Auditory observation
- Psychological inventories

Levels of Measurement. In designing a study, the researcher must decide how to measure a phenomenon such as anxiety level, blood pressure, attitude toward health care, or rate of complications. There are four levels or degrees of measurement: nominal, ordinal, interval, and ratio. The type of data measured determines the kind of statistical analysis that can be done. Table 4.3 characterizes the four levels of measurement.

Nominal-level measurement allows data to be divided into categories, but the only quantifiable measures are the frequencies with which the data fall into each category. For example, in a study assessing the educational level of nurse anesthetists, only the number of nurse anesthetists who fall into each category (certificate, bachelor's degree, master's degree, doctorate) can be reported. No numerical value can be assigned to represent the type of degree received by nurse anesthetists.

Ordinal-level measurement allows for data to be ordered or ranked. For instance, the American Society of Anesthesiologists (ASA) Physical Status system provides for a relative ranking system for patients on the basis of their pathophysiologic status. Although pathophysiologic status cannot be assigned a numerical value, the relative standing of patients can be determined.

Interval-level measurement uses numeric data that are ordered and spaced equally, such as temperature on the Fahrenheit or Centigrade scale, calendar years, or intelligence quotients derived from an intelligence performance test. Here, the distance between adjacent scores is highly meaningful.

Ratio-level measurement uses numeric data that can be ordered and equally spaced. It is based on a scale with an absolute zero point, such as temperature on the Kelvin scale, reaction time, height, and blood pressure. Both interval and ratio level measures can be referred to as *continuous* in nature.

Measurement can also be defined in terms of four broad categories: cognitive, affective, psychomotor, and physiologic. Each can manifest as one of the levels noted earlier. Cognitive measurement addresses the test subjects' knowledge or achievement. For example, what actions should be taken in the face of unexplained bradycardia? Affective measurements determine interests, values, and attitudes, thereby providing behavioral insights. For example, how do nurse anesthetists in different locations feel about anesthetizing patients with AIDS? Psychomotor measurements test the subjects' ability or skill in performing specific tasks, such as evaluating performance with a new laryngoscopic design. Physiologic measurements look at the biologic functioning of the organism, for example, heart rate differences in men and women at basal conditions.

Although researchers sometimes develop unique instruments that must be tested for reliability and validity, many published and acceptable instruments can be located in any number of sources.[3,4]

Measurement of Treatment Effect. Effect size is a measure of the magnitude of the observed relationship between a study treatment and its outcome. Two common measures of effect size are the odds ratio and relative risk. These effect size measures assess the likelihood of an event occurring in two comparison groups. Consider the following fictional data set of all-cause mortality of middle-aged smokers and nonsmokers living in a rural locale. In the modestly sized sample are 462 nonsmokers and 851 smokers. An epidemiologic study tracked these two cohorts for 15 years and reported overall mortality in each group at the end of the study period. The follow-up reveals that 308 nonsmokers were alive and 154 had died. Of the 851 smokers, 142 were alive and 709 had died (Table 4.4).

The data in the table suggest that smokers were more likely to have died during the study period than were nonsmokers. Although it is clear that statistical significance would be demonstrable, the fundamental question is, "How much more likely is a smoker to die than a nonsmoker?" The odds ratio and relative risk can be used to shed light on this question. In a patient population, the odds for a group are calculated by the number of patients who achieve the stated outcome divided by the number of patients who did not. In the current example, the outcome is death. Nonsmokers have 1:2 odds of dying (154/308 = 0.5) during the study. For smokers, the odds of dying are 5:1 (709/142 = 4.993). The odds ratio is the ratio of the odds of the exposure group to the odds of

TABLE 4.4	Outcome for Smokers vs. Nonsmokers in a 15-Year Study		
	Alive	**Dead**	**Total**
Nonsmokers	308	154	462
Smokers	142	709	851
Total	450	863	1313

the nonexposure group. In our example, the "exposure" is smoking. The odds ratio (4.993/0.5 = 9.99) indicates that smokers have almost 10-fold greater odds of dying than nonsmokers in our fictional population.

Relative risk (sometimes called risk ratio) is a measure of probability rather than odds. A group's probability of a stated outcome is measured by the number of patients in the group who achieve the outcome divided by the total number of patients in the group. In our study, nonsmokers have a 33% probability of dying during the study period (154/462 = 0.3333). For smokers, on the other hand, the probability of death is 83% (709/851 = 0.8331). The relative risk (0.8331/0.333 = 2.4995) indicates that the probability of death is 2.5 times greater for smokers than it is for nonsmokers.

The magnitude of these measures is quite different in this example. Although both revealed that smokers were more likely to die during the study period, which of the measures is a more accurate representation of reality? This is not always an easy question to answer, but an important one to consider as one weighs the evidence. In general, relative risk measures events in a way that reflects the directionality of the outcome. For example, if the risk is 1, the exposure is not associated with the outcome—the likelihood of the outcome happening in either the exposure or nonexposure population is equal. With an increased risk, the ratio is greater than 1. The likelihood of the outcome happening in the exposure population is greater than in the nonexposure population. Conversely, if there is a decreased risk, the ratio is less than 1. These two measures are suitable for different purposes and appeal to different people in different ways. The odds ratio is better suited when the outcome of interest is relatively rare, as it tends to overestimate risk in a manner similar to the preceding example.

The Pilot Study

A pilot study is the implementation of a study on a small scale. It includes only a few subjects who will generally not be included in the formal study. Its purpose is to troubleshoot the methodology for any anticipated design problems. The pilot study allows the researcher the opportunity to perform a dry run, ultimately facilitating the progression of the study.

Common Mistakes

At this point in the process, mistakes include failure to adequately operationalize definitions, failure to define the population or sample adequately, unrealistic expectations for subject recruitment and participation, underestimation of the difficulty of design execution, failure to establish instrument reliability and validity, and failure to appreciate the ethical dimensions of the investigation.

Stage 5: Execution of the Research Plan

Up to this point, the research process has involved the acquisition of knowledge regarding the subject, planning the project, and critical thinking about what is to occur. The next stage of the process involves actual data collection and the organization of the data into a format that facilitates data analysis.

Data collection must precisely follow the procedure the researcher previously specified. The real payoff in research comes with the drawing of useful and bona fide conclusions once the data have been collected and precisely analyzed within the framework of the research design. The goal of the previous step—namely, maximization of both internal and external validity—would not be achieved if the researcher were to deviate from the plan.

Maintaining careful records of what was done and what results were recorded is essential. The labeling and sorting of data into the respective categories or chronologies should be extremely precise. No data should be discarded until the researcher knows that they are absolutely unnecessary. Many researchers "stockpile" raw data and their notes because additional uses for the information may not manifest for months or even years after the initial project's completion and publication.

Common Mistakes

The mistakes associated with this stage include drifting from the stated methodology for convenience or administrative purposes, placing excessive demands on subjects, allowing personal bias to creep into the research plan, using observers or research assistants who are improperly trained, failing to obtain a sufficient sample size, and improperly using measurement instruments.

Stage 6: Analysis and Interpretation of the Data

Not only is proper data analysis essential to the design, analysis, and interpretation of the investigation; it is also necessary for understanding and evaluating research studies conducted by other investigators. Analysis has three general phases: the initial mechanical manipulation of the data, the analysis, and the thoughtful formulation of conclusions on the basis of the analysis.

For the purposes of this discussion, the following two questions are posed:
1. What is the rationale for the use of statistical analysis in research?
2. What are the more common statistical procedures used, and under what circumstances are they appropriate?

Descriptive Statistical Techniques

Once the data on the phenomenon under study have been collected, they are often summarized, categorized and described using descriptive statistics. This initial description of the data lays the groundwork for further interpretation of the collected data and inference of the study's external validity (i.e. will this data be appropriately generalizable to the population at large, over time, etc.) This descriptive data is also paramount for appreciating baseline data in studies where an intervention has occurred (i.e. pre- post-test studies or randomized control trials) or the phenomenon is investigated for change over time (i.e. a longitudinal study). For example, if the goal of a study is the determination of the incidence of headache and the change noted in blood pressure in 50 patients undergoing spinal anesthesia, the researcher would describe the number of patients who reported headaches and experienced changes in blood pressure, as well as the pain score and blood pressure values. The study would also report the demographics of the sample of patients in terms of sex, height, weight, or any other relevant variable to summarize the sample characteristics.

The group or set of all the observations of the variable is called a distribution. The distribution yields information about the overall dispersion of the phenomenon within the sample, as well as the exact location of a given measure relative to the group as a whole. In the case of an interval- or ratio-level measurement, such as blood pressure, the distribution of values is probably Gaussian or bell shaped in nature (i.e., some pressures are low, most are intermediate, and some are high). By studying the distribution, the researcher can compare a particular measured value with all the values obtained for the phenomenon.

Alternatively, the researcher might use a technique that clusters data into rational blocks or intervals. For example, in the spinal anesthesia study,

instead of listing all 50 initial blood pressures individually, the researcher could tabulate them according to frequency relative to a given interval. In this case, each measured blood pressure falls within a range, and the frequency of presentation in the sample is tabulated as shown in Table 4.5. Instead of using the tabular form, the researcher could arrange the same data in graphic form, indicating the frequency of the phenomenon on the vertical (y) axis and the blood pressure values on the horizontal (x) axis. In histograms and bar graphs, the width of each bar corresponds to the limits of the interval, and the height of the bar corresponds to the frequency or percent of the cases occurring in a specific interval. A frequency polygram is also a commonly used tool for displaying data. Points are plotted directly over the midpoint of each of the intervals. The data given in Table 4.5 are presented in Fig. 4.3 as a frequency polygram.

Other descriptive statistics include the mean (the arithmetic average of the sample), the median (the point below which one-half of the measurements lie), and the mode (the value occurring most frequently). The range shows the dispersion data from the highest to the lowest value. Variance and standard deviation (SD) must be computed and are based on the concept of deviation (the difference between an observed score and the mean value in the distribution). Variance is the square of the sum of all the deviations divided by the number of scores, and the SD is the positive square root of the variance. Because of variation, investigators describe the data not only in terms of the typical or average value but also the amount of variation that is present. With respect to quantitative data such as blood pressure, number of attempts at intubation, or amount of blood loss, this task is generally a matter of characterizing the distribution of the attribute in terms of its central tendency and dispersion. This is achieved by providing the mean and the SD. In a normal distribution of data, 68% of data will lie within 1 SD from the mean, 95% of data will lie within 2 SDs and 99.7% of data will

TABLE 4.5 Frequency Distribution for Initial Systolic Blood Pressure	
Interval (mm Hg)*	Frequency†
0–60	1
60–90	8
91–120	15
121–150	15
151–180	8
>180	3

*Interval equals the range or band into which a given measure is placed.
†Frequency equals the number of observations falling into that interval.

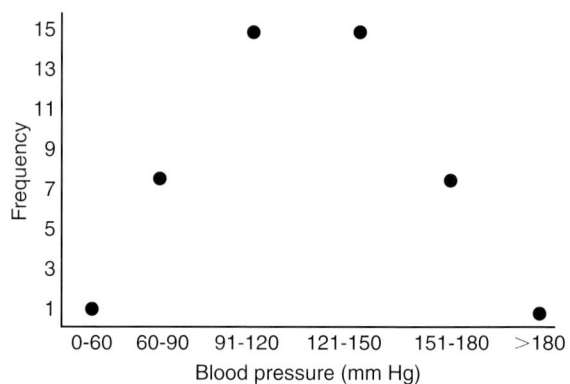

Fig. 4.3 The frequency polygram. Note the bell-shaped configuration the plotted data have assumed; this is typically the "normal" distribution of biologic data (e.g., blood pressure, weight, heart rate, minimum alveolar concentration, intelligence).

lie within 3 SDs. Thus, the normal distribution curve can be thought of as a probability distribution that more data will be closer to to the mean of the data set and less data will lie farther from the mean (Fig. 4.4).

The SD is a tool for describing the variation of individual observations around the mean. Standard error of the mean (SEM) is linked to the SD by the following simple mathematical formula:

$$SEM = SD/\sqrt{n}$$

where $\sqrt{n}$ is the square root of the number of observations in the sample.

The SEM describes the variation of the sample mean (that for the actual data collected) around the true, but unknown, population mean (that for all possible observations). The difficulty with using the SEM is that as the number of subjects or observations increases, the standard error of the mean decreases. In theoretic terms, as n approaches infinity, SEM approaches 0. Researchers are urged to consult with a biostatistician and to develop a rationale before deciding to use the SEM or SD.

In general, the higher the level of measurement used (i.e., ratio > interval > ordinal > nominal), the greater the flexibility in selecting a descriptive statistic. Using the data from the spinal anesthesia study noted earlier, it would be appropriate to compute the SD for initial systolic blood pressure (ratio-level data). However, such a computation would be meaningless for nominal-level information, such as whether subjects are male or female.

Correlational Statistical Techniques

The correlation coefficient is generally used for describing the extent to which two variables are related to each other or for quantifying the degree of that relationship. For example, it would be useful if one were studying the extent to which the level of carbon monoxide in the blood is related to cigarette smoking. Calculated correlations vary from +1.0 (a perfect direct correlation) to −1.0 (a perfect inverse correlation). A correlation of 0 indicates no relationship. Researchers often display the correlations visually in the form of a scattergram, which shows the shape of a relationship between two variables. There are many types of correlational techniques (Table 4.6).

In the hypothetical study of carbon monoxide level and cigarette smoking, a researcher might decide to use the product-moment correlation technique. The numeric value for carbon monoxide in the blood has a true 0 (ratio-level data). A numeric value can also be used to describe daily cigarette smoking (ratio-level data). The correlation between these variables would probably be positive and very high (e.g., 0.8 or even higher), which suggests that heavy use of cigarettes is associated with a high carbon monoxide level in the blood.

Conversely, assume a study examines the relationship between gender (a nominal-level variable) and anesthetic minimum alveolar concentration (a ratio-level variable). In this example, the researcher using the point biserial correlation technique would expect to see near zero correlation because gender has been found to not be associated in any meaningful way with anesthetic requirements.

Inferential Statistical Techniques

Inferential statistical procedures provide a set of techniques that allow the researcher to infer that the events observed in the sample will also occur in the larger unobserved population from which the sample was obtained. There are two basic reasons for using inferential techniques. First, they can assist the researcher who is testing a hypothesis and must decide whether to accept or reject it. For example, a researcher, having a particular value in mind, poses the question, "Is this value reasonable for the population at large in light of the evidence from the sample?" Second, inferential techniques can be used for estimation. For example, a researcher may wants to know what a particular the population value is. Clearly studying an entire population for the certain value would be expensive, time consuming and burdensome for the participants and researcher, so an extrapolation of this information would be more appropriate. The researcher draws a sample, studies it, and makes an inference about the population characteristic (Fig. 4.1). The two classic situations that are addressed by inferential techniques are as follows:

1. *Testing a hypothesis* (Table 4.7): Is there a significant difference in the incidence of nausea between those patients given thiopental and those who receive propofol?
2. *Making an estimation:* What percentage of nurse anesthetists perform a thorough machine check at the start of each day?

Researchers are seemingly preoccupied with the concept of significance. The level of significance (also designated as alpha level or p value) is a criterion used in making decisions regarding a hypothesis. If p is less than 0.05, the probability that the difference observed between the samples was the result of chance alone is less than 5%. Accordingly, the probability that the difference between the samples was real (i.e., it resulted from the treatment) and was not just the result of chance is

TABLE 4.6 **Correlation Techniques Appropriate to Data Type**		
Correlation	**Variable No. 1**	**Variable No. 2**
Product moment	Interval or ratio	Interval or ratio
Spearman rank	Ordinal	Ordinal
Point biserial	Nominal or ordinal	Interval or ratio
Phi	Dichotomy	Dichotomy
Contingency	Nominal	Nominal

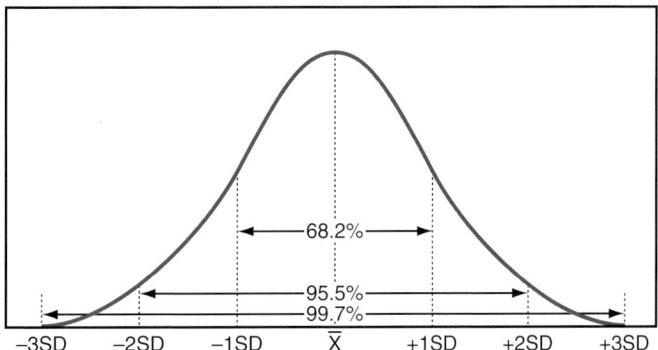

Fig. 4.4 The relationship of standard deviation and mean to a curve of normal distributed data. (From McPherson RA, Pincus MR. Henry's Clinical Diagnosis and Management by Laboratory Methods. 24th ed. St. Louis: Elsevier; 2022.)

TABLE 4.7 Statistical Methods Used for Testing Hypotheses

	TYPE OF EXPERIMENT				
Scale of Measurement	Two Treatment Groups Consisting of Different Individuals	Three or More Treatment Groups Consisting of Different Individuals	Before and After a Single Treatment in the Same Individual	Multiple Treatments in the Same Individual	Association Between Two Variables
Interval (and drawn from normally distributed populations)*	Unpaired t-test	Analysis of variance	Paired t-test	Repeated-measures analysis of variance	Linear regression and Pearson product-moment correlation
Nominal	Chi-squared analysis of contingency table	Chi-squared analysis of contingency table	McNemar test	Cochrane Q	Contingency coefficient
Ordinal	Mann-Whitney rank sum test	Kruskal-Wallis statistic	Wilcoxon signed rank test	Friedman statistic	Spearman rank correlation

*If the assumption of normally distributed populations is not met, the observations should be ranked, and the methods for data measured on the ordinal scale should be used.
Adapted from Glantz SA. *Primer of Biostatistics*. 3rd ed. New York: McGraw-Hill; 1992; Biddle C. *Evidence Trumps Belief: Nurse Anesthetists and Evidence-Based Decision Making in Nurse Anesthesia*. Chicago: AANA Publishing; 2013.

greater than 95%. The type of statistical test used determines the test value that corresponds to a p value of less than 0.05 and indicates a statistically significant result. Statistical tables report these significant test values for each type of statistical test. It is conventional to establish the alpha level before the data analysis is begun; Significance does not prove anything; it does not confer importance or clinical relevance, it simply relays that the results are not likely due to chance at a specified level of probability because it establishes the researchers acceptable risk or probability of committing a type I error (a false positive). Commonly used levels in research are $p < 0.05$ and $p < 0.01$; $p < 0.10$ is sometimes used in preliminary or descriptive studies. More stringent alpha levels ($p < 0.001$) can be used when there is a sufficiently large enough sample to power this analysis or when the results can have serious ramifications (i.e. drug trials), when populations are small, or not much is known about the phenomenon. There is also a trend to simply report the calculated p value and leave the interpretations up to the reader.

In recent years, there has been growing resistance to the exclusive use of the p value in interpreting research findings, despite the still widespread use of the p value in interpreting hypotheses. Fundamentally, the p value was never intended to be a substitute for scientific reasoning. Consumers of the clinical research literature should keep these guidelines in mind:

1. The p value can be distorted by the data's incompatibility with a specific statistic model.
2. The p values do not measure the probability that the studied hypothesis is true or the probability that the data were produced by random chance alone.
3. The p value does not measure the size of an effect or the importance of a result.
4. By itself, the p value does not provide a good measure of evidence regarding a model or hypothesis.

The p value is a dimensionless value that is, at best, only an indicator of the direction of the effect; it in no way speaks to the clinical meaningfulness of the relationship.

Confidence intervals (CIs) provide greater detail about the measured outcome than p values. The purpose of any research study is to provide an estimate of the effect the study treatment would have if it were applied to the entire population of interest—what many call the "true value" of a treatment effect. The confidence interval is the range within which the true value of the treatment effect is expected to fall 95% of the time. In other words, if the study treatment was applied to the entire population of interest, 95 out of 100 times the size of the treatment effect would be within the specified CI range. The 95% CI is most commonly reported, but 90% and 99% CIs are sometimes calculated as well. The CI is very important because it puts an upper and a lower boundary on the likely effect size of any real treatment. In doing so, it also provides an indication of the precision of the treatment effect estimate. A smaller CI indicates greater precision. If a CI is very wide, more data may need to be collected before any definite conclusions can be drawn about the estimate.[5]

Because relative risk and odds ratios are calculated as fractions comparing a treatment group to a nontreatment group, a CI that includes 1 indicates that no statistically significant difference between the groups has been found. Conversely, a CI for relative risk or an odds ratio that does not include 1 is an indication of a statistically significant treatment effect. Research studies often report both p values and CIs, but if only one is reported it should be the CI.[5]

Although explanation and application illustrations are beyond the scope of this chapter, other measures of effect size include, but are not limited to, Pearson's r and Cohen's d. The number needed to treat (NNT) and the number needed to harm are additional examples of metrics that provide clinically applicable "magnitude of effect" information. Some of these metrics are discussed in Table 4.8.

Selecting the Appropriate Statistical Procedure

There are two major categories of inferential procedures: parametric analyses and nonparametric analyses. The major factors that dictate which category should be selected involve the assumptions the investigator makes regarding the data. Parametric procedures are best performed on normally distributed, large interval- or ratio-level data sets in which values are independent and exhibit similar variance. For data that does not fall under these parameters, nonparametric statistical procedures are used. Tables 4.9 and 4.10 provide some guidelines for selecting a statistical procedure.

Power

The sensitivity of the planned experiment and analysis is known as its *power*. The concept of power is important to anyone planning a research project or evaluating a published paper. The estimate of an experiment's ability to accurately test the hypothesis under question

TABLE 4.8 Examples of Effect Size Measures Used in a Meta-analysis

Measure	Attributes
Cohen *d*	Difference between two means divided by the standard deviation (SD) of either group; works when the variances of the two groups are homogeneous. In a meta-analysis, the mean differences are subtracted such that the resultant difference is positive in the direction of improvement. Measurements must be on a continuous scale. Variations exist for data using similar or different measures. Generally, effect size is as follows: $d = 0.2$, small; $d = 0.5$, medium; $d = 0.8$, large.
Correlation measures	Many types, such as phi (Φ), *r*, point biserial, and Kendall tau (τ), depending on the nature of the variables; portray the strength of association between factors under consideration and the outcome.
Number needed to treat (NNT)	Useful measure of an intervention's effectiveness. Describes the active treatment and control/comparison in achieving the desired outcome. NNT = 1 implies a favorable outcome in every patient given the treatment and no patient in the comparison group. NNT = 50 implies that 50 patients must receive the treatment for one of them to experience the desired effect.
Number needed to harm	Similar to NNT; used to examine adverse effects of an intervention.
Odds ratio (OR)	The probability of an event in one group compared with the probability of that event in another. If the OR = 1.0, the likelihood is the same; if the OR > 1.0, the event is more likely in the first group. The calculation puts the odds in the experimental group in the numerator and the odds in the comparison group in the denominator.
Relative risk	The risk of an event happening in a group exposed to a treatment compared with the risk in a nonexposed group. A number >1.0 implies greater risk.
Confidence interval (CI)	Defines a range of values likely to include a measure, generally reported as a 95% CI; implies that 19 times out of 20, the "true" value will be in the specified range of values. Many outcome measures are often reported with their associated 95% CI.

TABLE 4.9 Choice of Statistical Test Based on Assumptions

	Parametric Procedures	Nonparametric Procedures
Nature of the assumptions	Data are interval or ratio level	Data are nominal or ordinal level
	Each value is independent of the other values	Not necessarily distributed "normally" (i.e., data do not "fit" a bell-shaped curve)
	Value is normally distributed	
	Groups have similar variance	
	Usually works best with large population	
Examples of tests	t-test for independent groups*	Chi-squared test
	t-test for dependent samples†	Mann-Whitney test
	Analysis of variance	Kruskal-Wallis test

*For example, two totally unrelated groups are compared.
†For example, a pretest and posttest comparison on one group of people.

TABLE 4.10 Choice of Statistical Test Based on Purpose

Test	Goal
t-test, independent groups	To test the difference between the means of two independent groups
t-test, dependent samples	To test for the difference between dependent, paired samples (e.g., pretreatment and posttreatment outcome)
Analysis of variance	To test the difference among the means of more than two independent groups or more than one independent variable
Chi-squared	To evaluate the difference between observed and expected frequencies
Correlation coefficient	To test whether a relationship exists between two variables (e.g., product moment)
Simple linear regression	Used when one independent variable *(x)* is used to predict a dependent variable *(y)*
Multiple linear regression	To understand the effects of two or more independent variables on a dependent measure
Analysis of covariance	To test for differences between group means after adjustment of the scores on the dependent variable to eliminate the effects of the covariate
Factor analysis	To reduce a large set of variables into a smaller, more manageable set of measures
Canonical correlation	To analyze the relationship between two or more independent variables and two or more dependent variables
Discriminant analysis	To make predictions regarding membership in categories or groups, in contrast to using interval- or ratio-level measures

should be computed before the research is begun. A researcher should ask two critical questions:

1. What is the chance I will incorrectly determine that my treatment had an effect when it really did not (type I error) This is sometimes referred to as a false positive and can be controlled for by the researcher setting the alpha level.
2. What is the chance I will miss an effect that is actually present (type II error) This is sometimes referred to as a false negative and is controlled for by the researcher performing a power analysis to determine the appropriate sample size. Fig. 4.5 depicts the difference between type I and type II errors.

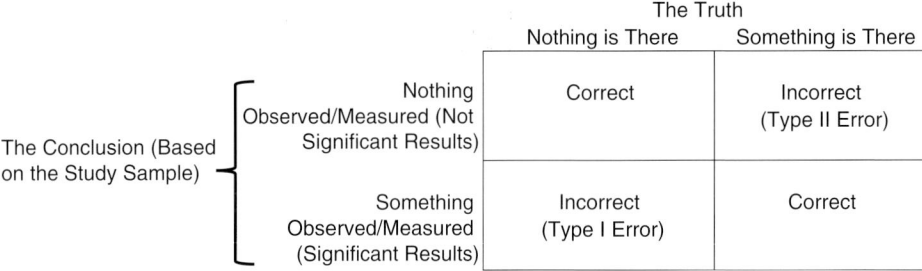

Fig. 4.5 The difference between type I and type II errors.

Power analysis estimates obtained during a study's design stage encourage investigators to thoughtfully enhance the study's sensitivity and strengthens the statistical validity. Making such estimates forces the posing of questions regarding effect size (e.g., how potent is the effect of the independent variable on the dependent variable?) and sample size, both of which are essential in a study. Many adverse outcomes that occur as a result of anesthetic management are rare (e.g., death, postspinal hematoma, blindness, stroke), and studies proposing to measure such outcomes as a function of a particular interventional approach must be "powered" by a large sample size and other methodologic controls.

Common Parametric Tests

Statistical tests are designed to accept or reject the assumed null hypothesis (i.e., there are no differences between groups). Each type of statistical test computes a unique statistical test that reflects the difference between the groups of interest. This test statistic is then reported in terms of significance as a p value, allowing the researcher to conclude whether there is any significant difference between the groups. Any elementary statistics textbook contains tables that list significant values for each type of test statistic.

The t-test is probably the most common parametric test encountered in clinical research studies. Three types of t-tests are used to test the null hypothesis that there is no difference between two group means. A one-sample t-test is used to determine whether the mean of a sample is different from the mean of a known, at-large population. To evaluate whether a study sample in which weight loss interventions were used had a lower body mass index (BMI) than the general population, a one-sample t-test can be conducted to compare the mean BMI of the sample with that of the general population. The resulting test statistic, reported as a p value that falls below 0.05, indicates a 95% probability that the mean sample BMI does not differ from the mean population BMI by chance. That is, the difference between the sample BMI and the population BMI is likely due to the weight loss intervention. An unpaired t-test is used when two independent samples are compared, such as comparing the effect on blood pressure of two different manipulations performed during laryngoscopy. A paired t-test is used on two dependent samples, such as might occur when preintervention and postintervention group scores are compared in the same group of subjects.

The analysis of variance (ANOVA) is another commonly used parametric test that incorporates group means and variances to determine the test statistic. The test statistic is then used to determine whether three or more groups of data vary from one another in a meaningful way. As with other statistical procedures, the ANOVA assumes that the null hypothesis is stated such that all group means are the same. The ANOVA then accepts or rejects the null hypothesis. The test statistic for ANOVA is called the F ratio. As with other statistical tests, statistical tables provide the F ratio values required to achieve statistical significance. The multiple ANOVA (sometimes called *MANOVA*) is used when the effect of multiple grouping factors (e.g., exercise routine, diet, and food journaling) is analyzed. The ANOVA with repeated-measures test is commonly used when all members of a random sample's dependent variable are measured under a number of different conditions or repeatedly measured over time.

Should the ANOVA indicate that a significant difference exists when more than two groups are compared, it cannot localize where the groups differ, only that there is a difference somewhere. In this case, a post hoc test must be used to isolate the between-group or among-group difference. There are many of these tests, and different computer programs and statisticians have their preference; examples include the Fisher, Scheffé, Tukey, Newman-Keuls, and Dunnett tests.

Propensity Score

An increasingly common analysis that is used is called the propensity score (PS). This is particularly important in observational studies where bias may be a powerful confounder. The PS determines the conditional probability, based on a set of baseline metrics such as gender, ASA classification, age, some comorbidity, etc., that a patient would or would not have received a certain intervention. If there is no hidden bias and treatment assignment is thus random, the PS should be indicative. There is considerable movement, using the PS methodology, to elevate the "power" of observational studies to near that of the randomized trial. However, this is a very contentious issue.

Recursive Partitioning

A commonly used tool that has both statistical and methodologic attributes and implications is recursive partitioning. Its roots are in the word *recursive,* meaning to use a rule or procedure that can be applied repeatedly, and *partitioning,* indicating a division into or distribution into portions or shares. This type of approach creates a rule such as "if a patient has finding a, b, or c, then he or she likely has condition x or should be treated with z." Examples of where this kind of rule application has been used include the Goldman Cardiac Risk Stratification, obstructive sleep apnea scales such as STOP-BANG, and the ASA Difficult Airway Algorithm.

Common Mistakes

At this step in the research process, mistakes include selecting an inappropriate statistical procedure, using only one statistical procedure when several should be used, overstating the importance of small differences that are statistically significant but of little clinical importance, interpreting correlational research as evidence of cause-and-effect relationships, and overgeneralizing the findings of the investigation. Some common errors in statistical usage are noted in Box 4.4.

Stage 7: Dissemination of the Findings to Interested Colleagues

The research process is not complete until the results, conclusions, and implications have been adequately communicated to those likely to be interested in the study. Clearly, a study that has been completed

BOX 4.4   Top 10 Common Errors in Statistical Usage

1. No justification for reporting statistical results
   - No control group (when one is possible)
   - Random sampling or random group assignment not performed (or reported)
   - Statistical test not specified
   - Obvious biases or threats to validity
   - No documentation of consent or institutional review board approval
2. Errors in use of the t-test
   - Multiple application without correction
   - Use of independent groups form for paired data and vice versa
   - Use for ordinal data
3. Negative conclusions when statistical test results are not significant
4. Use of a test for independent samples for paired data or repeated measures
5. Inappropriate or no follow-up to analysis of variance
6. Hypotheses generated by the data
7. Use of one-sided tests without justification (or disclosure)
8. Inadequate number for chi-squared analysis
9. Standard error of the mean used for specifying variability
10. Misinterpretation or misrepresentation of p value
    - Small p value called "highly significant"
    - No confidence intervals stated
    - Different interpretation of $p = 0.04$ and $p = 0.06$

but whose results have not been disseminated is of little value. Communication of the research findings can be done through a variety of routes, including publication in journals or newsletters, oral and poster presentations at formal symposia department meetings, or even simply discussion with others interested in the phenomenon.

Researchers fail to publish the results of their work for many reasons. These include such claims as "my findings were not significant," "my results were negative," and "the sample size was small." Negative or insignificant results can be just valuable as positive ones. For example, it has been found that in most circumstances, the by-product of atracurium breakdown, laudanosine, is unlikely to have significant clinical effects.[6] This is an important negative finding that has contributed substantively to clinical understanding.

Similarly, small sample sizes may provide an element of control over variables not present in larger studies or may indicate some preliminary direction as to how to approach a problem. An example is the finding that epidural anesthesia or analgesia in conjunction with light general anesthesia may be preferable to a purely general anesthesia technique and may be associated with lower mortality rates in critically ill patients.[7] Although the sample size in this particular investigation is relatively small, the overall design is acceptable and contributes to our understanding of the issue by stimulating other investigators to pursue answers to the questions raised.

The goal of nurse anesthesia research is the improvement of practice and the dissemination of research findings to clinicians. In a report directed at a highly research-oriented audience, the introduction is usually somewhat detailed, emphasizing the theoretic basis for the research. The introduction is followed by an extensive methodologic section that focuses on establishing the reliability and validity of the instruments used. The findings of the study are presented next, with emphasis on the statistical procedures employed. Finally, the conclusion focuses on the limitations and implications of the study's results.

Writing for a Clinically Oriented Audience

Generally, clinicians find research literature difficult to understand and its clinical application cumbersome. Both authors and journal editors can do much to make research more palatable to the clinical reader, thereby improving the chance that the research findings will be broadly disseminated and integrated into clinical situations. A recipe for successful clinical writing follows.

Clinical readers of research want to extract information applicable to clinical practice as quickly as possible. Therefore the introduction of the research report should be brief, should establish the practical importance of the study, and should present a clear statement of the study's purpose. A deliberate effort should be made to connect the study with the realities of clinical practice.

With respect to the methods section, writing that "a quasi-experimental, Solomon three-group crossover design yielded data that were subjected to canonical and discriminant analysis" does little to satisfy the needs of the average clinical reader. Instead, stating how the subjects were obtained, what manipulations were made, how the measurements were taken, and how the statistical analysis was performed provides the reader with clear straightforward information, allowing him or her to put the study into a clinical context. The methods section should completely describe both the research design and the statistical procedures used, and it should indicate why this approach was selected.

The results of the study should focus on the relevant findings and describe them clearly and fully. Tables or figures, explicitly labeled and simple in design, should be used for representing the findings visually. Admittedly, the more complex the findings, the more difficult it is to avoid a statistical or technical focus.

In the discussion section, the implications of the investigation for theory and future research are somewhat less important to the clinical reader than are the implications for practice. For example, assume that a study demonstrates that the proposed intervention is not ready to be implemented in practice. In this situation, the discussion section should emphasize why this is so and what can be done about it. Encyclopedic comparisons of the results with those of other investigators at this point probably will not contribute materially to the report and may, paradoxically, deter the reader. Alternatively, if a researcher finds that a particular intervention, strategy, or assessment is ready to be introduced into clinical practice, the discussion section should emphasize how and for whom it should be used. It should include considerations such as efficiency and cost, as well as suggestions for clinical implementation.

This recipe for making research reports more palatable to primarily clinically oriented readers is not meant to diminish the importance of highly theoretic research-oriented writing. Many nurse anesthetists continue to generate and publish valuable theoretic manuscripts that contribute to a scientific basis for practice. Researchers and writers must keep the nurse anesthetist audience in mind as they develop and disseminate their findings.

All researchers must understand that the results of their studies, once published, become part of the general knowledge of the scientific community at large. However, the use of this knowledge requires acknowledgment of the original researchers; additionally, published results may be subject to copyright protection laws (i.e., their use may require permission from the publisher). It is not until the information becomes common knowledge that others may use it freely without acknowledgment.

Common Mistakes

At this stage of the research process, common mistakes include not keeping the study focused on the original problem, using an incorrect or improper writing style to address the targeted audience, generalizing the findings too broadly, and failing to address the clinical significance of the study.

Stage 8: Evaluation of the Research Report

Both clinicians (in their reading for application) and researchers (in their writing and analysis) are called on to evaluate research reports despite the fact that many may not have received formal training in reading and interpreting professional literature. Evaluation is the process of appraising the quality of a phenomenon; in this case, it is the findings of research as they bear on the art and science of nurse anesthesia. Outside of the practice settings, humans evaluate hundreds of things every day: Are the apples on the grocery shelves to our liking? Does the description of the program in the television guide entice us to tune in? Is the weather too warm to wear a jacket? Have we cooked the eggs sufficiently? These seem trivial and informal compared with the clinical evaluations the nurse anesthetist must perform daily: Is the patient's anesthesia too deep, too light, or about right? Should I administer more opioid? Is the patient dehydrated, or is the hematocrit level misleading me? Should I perform a rapid-sequence induction? What dose of hypnotic do I use in this 80-year-old patient with a fractured hip? How does the patient's coagulation status affect the choice to place a neuraxial block? Both sets of questions, nonprofessional and professional, are highly evaluative and parallel the evaluative decision making that occurs when anesthesia research literature is read.

Systematic evaluation of the research, which influences the practice of nurse anesthesia, consists of a formal appraisal of the quality and value of the research. This essential step in the research process is multidimensional and can be approached in many ways. The approach outlined in the following subsections involves asking carefully orchestrated, critical questions. The answers to the suggested questions are not necessarily a dichotomous yes or no, but rather are qualitative in nature. An overview of this approach is detailed in Box 4.5.

Evaluating a Study: The Bottom Line

Ultimately, the nurse anesthetist evaluating a study is faced with three questions:

1. Do I disregard the study and its findings entirely, not applying them to either clinical practice or future analysis in any fashion?
2. Do I apply the study only in the sense of expanding my cognitive approach to anesthetic management? (In this scenario, although one may not materially or directly apply the study or its findings to practice, some intellectual growth or understanding is gained from the study, which subsequently is incorporated into one's repertoire.)
3. Do I make a direct application of the study to my practice?

Some questions to ask when one reads a study are listed in Box 4.6.

Common Mistakes

At this stage of the research process, mistakes include failing to adequately evaluate a study's methods and findings, and, in the process, uncritically accepting into practice information that may be misleading or incorrect. Although articles in professional journals should undergo critical review by peers with expertise who can detect mistakes, omissions, and alternative explanations, the ultimate responsibility for evaluating a study and determining the pros and cons of the implementation of its recommendations rests with the clinical reader.

EVIDENCE-BASED PRACTICE: EMPOWERING DECISION MAKING THROUGH RESEARCH

Understanding these concepts of clinical research provides the tools necessary to implement EBP in nurse anesthesia. EBP involves the conscientious and critical use of quality published evidence in making decisions related to the care of a particular patient, considering the caregiver's unique expertise and the setting in which the patient presents. From EBP's very conception, the application of sound empirical evidence to

---

BOX 4.5 Research Scenario: A Guide for Researchers* and Clinicians† in Evaluating Research for Completeness and Clinical Application

Problem
- Is it lucid, researchable, justified, and practical?

Hypothesis
- Is it clear, with the appropriate variables under consideration correctly identified?

Definitions
- Are terms adequately defined and put into context?

Literature
- Is it relevant, current, and organized?

Review
- Is it logical, and does it justify the study?

Methods
- Is the sample representative of the population being considered?
- Is the sample large enough?
- If human subjects were used, was institutional approval granted?
- Is the instrumentation described and valid?
- Is the design compatible with the problem and the hypothesis or research question?
- Is there any evidence of drift from established procedure?
- Are the data-gathering procedures defined?
- Is there enough information for replication of the study, if desired?
- Are the statistical procedures described, and are they appropriate?

Results
- Are results presented clearly, concisely, and without bias?
- Are they organized and displayed logically in tables or figures?
- Are they relevant to the problem or hypothesis?

Discussion
- Is the discussion logically based on the results?
- Is it intimately grounded in the original problem or hypothesis?
- Is there overgeneralization of the findings?
- Is the writing impartial and scientific?
- How can this study be used in the practice setting?
- How similar is the study's environment to the real world?
- What are the risks associated with implementation of the recommendations?

* Researchers should benefit from this by critically asking themselves whether they have included answers to these questions in their report.
† Clinicians should benefit from this by judging the report on the basis of completeness and utility and by finding out whether it contains answers to these questions.

---

clinical practice has had a dramatic impact on patient outcomes. In 1972, Scottish epidemiologist Dr. Archie Cochrane realized that thousands of low-birth-weight premature infants were dying unnecessarily because the results of RCTs documenting the therapeutic effect of corticosteroid therapy in high-risk mothers had not been systematically reviewed and made available to the public. When a rigorous review of existing studies was published, it revealed that corticosteroid therapy reduced the odds of premature infant death from 50% to 30%. Dr. Cochrane's efforts to bring empiric evidence to bear on clinical practice significantly improved premature infant mortality and formed the foundation for modern EBP.

BOX 4.6   Questions to Ask in the Reading of a Study

Object or Hypothesis
- What are the objectives of the study or the questions to be answered?
- What is the population to which the investigators intend to refer their findings?

Design of the Investigation
- Was the study an experiment, planned observations, or an analysis of records?
- How was the sample selected? Do possible sources of selection exist that would make the sample atypical or nonrepresentative? If so, what provision was made for dealing with this bias?
- What is the nature of the control group or standard of comparison?

Observations
- Are there clear definitions of the terms used, including *diagnostic criteria*, *measurements made*, and *criteria of outcome*?
- Was the method of classification or of measurement consistent for all the subjects and relevant to the objectives of the investigation? Do possible biases in measurement exist? If so, what provisions were made to deal with them?
- Are the observations reliable and reproducible?

Presentation of Findings
- Are the findings presented clearly, objectively, and in sufficient detail to enable the reader to judge them for oneself?
- Are the findings internally consistent? That is, do the numbers add up properly, can different tables be reconciled, and so on?

Analysis
- Are the data worthy of statistical analysis? If so, are the methods of statistical analysis appropriate to the source and nature of the data, and is the analysis correctly performed and interpreted?
- Is analysis sufficient for determining whether "significant difference" may be the result of lack of comparability of the group in gender or age distribution, in clinical characteristics, or in other relevant variables?

Conclusions
- Which conclusions are justified by the findings? Which are not?
- Are the conclusions relevant to the questions posed by the investigators?

Constructive Suggestions
- Assume you are planning an investigation to answer the questions put forth in this study. If they have not been clearly asked by the authors, frame them in an appropriate manner. Suggest a practical design, criteria for observations, and type of analysis that would provide reliable and valid information relevant to the questions under study.

Adapted from Colton T. *Statistics in Medicine*. Boston: Little, Brown; 1974.

The Cochrane Center and the Cochrane Collaboration were established shortly thereafter and continue to assist health care providers in bringing EBP to the clinical environment today.[8]

One only needs to examine former "best practices" in the field of anesthesia to understand the importance of informing clinical practice with current, quality research. Many former practices that lacked a foundation in clinical research have since been found to be unsafe or ineffective. Some of these practices include:

- Innovar (a fixed combination of fentanyl and droperidol)
- Chymopapain
- Rapacuronium
- Methoxyflurane (Penthrane)
- Insufflated halothane for tonsillectomy
- "Twilight sleep" for obstetric delivery
- CO_2 gas to increase cerebral blood flow during carotid surgery
- Doxapram (Dopram) to speed anesthetic emergence

The nurse anesthetist can avoid the use of unsafe or ineffective interventions by using EBP. EBP ensures that the safety and efficacy of clinical practices are firmly grounded in systematically reviewed research studies. In the quest to protect patients from harmful or ineffectual practices, EBP is the most powerful weapon in the nurse anesthetist's arsenal.

Clinicians, academics, and the health care environment have much to gain from a structured method to bring scientific advances and the rigor of the clinical research environment to patient care. For the nurse anesthetist, EBP provides a systematic approach to incorporate current research into daily practice. Studies such as those conducted by Shin et al. and Sackett et al. highlight the drastic need to improve the clinical application of recent research findings. These and other studies demonstrate a negative correlation between knowledge of current best practices and length of time in clinical practice.[9-11]

Ely et al.[12] found that clinicians failed to look to current clinical research studies to inform their patient care decisions. The study revealed that clinicians endeavored to seek current best evidence for less than half of the patient management questions they encountered. EBP provides a framework to allow the nurse anesthetist to remain up to date on current best practices throughout a lifetime of clinical practice and to incorporate empirical evidence in everyday patient care decisions.

EBP not only requires knowledge and interventions based on quality research but also facilitates decision making among interventions of apparent equal empiric soundness based on the needs and values of the patient. It is this combination of empiric evidence with patient-centered decision making that renders EBP its greatest value to clinicians and patients alike. With EBP, practitioners are not simply making decisions based on the highest quality evidence; they are making decisions based on the highest quality evidence that is best for the patient. Finally, just as EBP brings the clinician back to the evidence, so too does EBP bring the academic back to clinical practice. Facilitating interaction between the academic and clinical settings provides the optimal environment for accurate and informed patient care.

When solid evidence evolves into sound clinical decision making, patients receive the best possible care; EBP helps the nurse anesthetist choose scientific evidence over confusing (or even unsound) opinion. In addition, EBP complements other foundational approaches to patient care and teaching. Some researchers argue that there is a crucial final step in the EBP model: namely, that clinicians self-evaluate their own EBP. In doing so, clinicians provide an ongoing process of evaluation and sensitivity testing for practice-based decisions.

Clinical research seeks to resolve, refine, and clarify issues involved in the care and management of patients. Each day, the nurse anesthetist is faced with a host of common and uncommon patient scenarios that demand thoughtful, efficient decision making and resultant interventions. How the practitioner comes to decide what course of action to take is in many cases as important as the action itself. Decisions involving the care of patients should be evidence based, a process of considerable complexity involving judging sources of information, evaluating the quality and relevance of information, recognizing the contextual elements that may alter the application of that information in a particular setting, and assessing its impact on the patient.

The Process of Evidence-Based Clinical Practice

What we do in a given circumstance is often more a matter of entrenched belief than a course of action firmly grounded in high-quality research. The published series *Clinical Evidence*, the international source of best available evidence related to common clinical interventions in various disease states, reveals that of 2500 treatments reviewed, 325 (13%) were rated "beneficial," 575 (23%) "likely to be beneficial," 200 (8%) as "a tradeoff between benefit and harm," 150 (6%) "unlikely to be beneficial," 100 (4%) "likely to be ineffective or harmful," and 1150 (46%) as having "unknown effectiveness." One might interpret this in many ways, but it indicates that many treatment decisions are inadequately grounded in firm scientific rationale.[13]

The fundamentals of medicine and nursing have evolved from a time when the teaching and practice of authoritative figures (sages) were simply passed down and uncritically applied to patients. Advances came with clinical evolution, but primarily in the form of case reports, case series, editorials, and other publications that were too often based on preconceived notions and deliberate or unintentional bias. The advent of the RCT some 6 decades ago set the stage for a new era in patient care. Despite advances, practitioners and nurses (in particular) are often resistant in regard to bringing research advances to the bedside. EBP involves a series of consecutive, somewhat overlapping steps that are described in the following sections.

Step 1: Asking a Question That Deserves an Answer

Should we anesthetize and perform elective surgery on a child who presents with an upper respiratory infection on the day of the scheduled procedure? What fluid and glucose management strategy should be used in the diabetic patient recovering from a major peripheral vascular procedure? Is it safe to use ketorolac in the patient just now recovering from a tonsillectomy? What can be done to minimize the risk of ventilator-acquired pneumonia in the postoperative patient receiving mechanical ventilation? Should all patients recovering from general anesthesia receive supplemental oxygen in the postanesthesia care unit? Should obstructive sleep apnea patients recovering from general anesthesia receive continuous positive airway pressure throughout their hospital stay if significant pulmonary hypertension is present? What is the lowest acceptable platelet concentration that permits use of neuraxial anesthesia in the obstetric patient? Such questions are common in practice and merit careful consideration of intervention-related outcomes, but relevant questions can also apply to diagnosis, prognosis, and the potential for harm. It may seem like word play, but the answers to patient care questions are more likely to be important and valid if the questions posed are good. Questions should be focused to the extent that they are both applicable to the patients who are cared for and can be researched.

The "PICO" Approach. A common model used in developing an appropriate clinical question is the PICO approach. PICO is a mnemonic device that describes key components of good question construction, that is, **P**atient, **I**ntervention (or cause), **C**omparison (if appropriate), and **O**utcome. Because clinical circumstances, and their associated questions, vary considerably, not all questions will have a "comparison" group, although many will. Examples of PICO-derived questions follow:

Patient	Intervention	Comparison	Outcome
61-year-old male, infarction	Streptokinase	Plasminogen activator	Death
31-year-old female, laparoscopy	Ondansetron 4 mg	Droperidol 1.25 mg	Nausea
17-year-old male, arthroscopy	Spinal anesthesia	—	Time in PACU

Using the PICO approach, a clinically focused, relevant question emerges from each of the scenarios established above. For example, with respect to the second, a comparison scenario, the following question might emerge:

- In young women undergoing diagnostic laparoscopy for nonspecific pelvic pain and receiving anesthesia with sevoflurane, atracurium, and fentanyl, is there a difference in the rate of postoperative nausea when either ondansetron 4 mg or droperidol 1.25 mg is given 30 minutes prior to emergence?

With respect to the third, noncomparison question, the following question might emerge:

- In adolescents undergoing knee arthroscopy under spinal anesthesia with lidocaine 75 mg and sufentanil 10 mcg, what is the anticipated length of stay in the postanesthesia care unit (PACU) before they are street fit?

Step 2: Searching for Relevant Evidence

Once a question is at hand, the search for information begins; this is a process that can be both time consuming and challenging. Seeking evidence to address the question, "What is the best antiemetic for the postoperative patient?" is much different than asking, "Is isopropyl alcohol inhalation more effective than ondansetron in managing post–general anesthesia nausea in the postpartum tubal ligation patient?" Although providers usually have an opinion about care-related questions, EBP demands that we critically evaluate researchable and meaningful information sources to best address a particular patient's care. Choosing a database is an important first step that can have a significant impact on the studies available to answer patient care questions. *PubMed, Ovid, ScienceDirect, ProQuest, PsycInfo, CINAHL* and *MEDLINE* are familiar, excellent sources[14] but are not applicable in all circumstances, A particularly valuable database specifically related to EBP is the *Cochrane Library*, a collection of well-conducted clinical trials organized into specific topics. Other sources, such as established websites, well-regarded (peer-reviewed, authoritative) textbooks, or even colleagues with a more robust knowledge base may suffice. The crucial aspect of these sources is confidence that the colleague, database, or book chapter is evidence based. The phrase "garbage in, garbage out" has particular application here.

Step 3: What Is It Worth?

EBP is an approach to patient care founded on the belief that clinical decisions must be based on results obtained from rigorously controlled investigations. It is important to recognize that not all evidence that is retrieved or brought to bear on a question has the same value. The pyramid of evidence (Fig. 4.6) demonstrates that the randomized, double-blind, controlled clinical trial has greater worth than the editorial or case report. This hierarchy of value is case and issue sensitive because not all questions have relevant or applicable RCTs. On the other hand, when a number of RCTs are directed toward a similar issue, these can sometimes be combined using rigorous methodology and a common set of statistical procedural processes to produce a meta-analysis (or quantitative systematic review).

The dizzying array of studies in the field of anesthesiology coupled with the complexities and vagaries of this patient population produce an informational tidal wave both frustrating and daunting to clinicians who endeavor to remain on the cutting edge with respect to patient care decisions. EBP cautions against using studies with low external validity (e.g., animal studies) or those based on uncontrolled observations (e.g., case reports, retrospective studies) in rendering decisions that influence or dictate patient care interventions. Here, we will focus on the appraisal of the three study designs that produce the most valuable empiric evidence: the randomized controlled trial, the systematic review, and the meta-analysis.

Randomized Controlled Trials. Among single studies, the RCT is widely considered the gold standard for measuring the effectiveness of clinical interventions. In an RCT, patients are randomly assigned, or "randomized," to one of two or more groups. The aim of randomization is to decrease bias, in part, by equally distributing both known and unknown confounders in the study arms. Any differences in the measured outcomes of each group can thus be attributed to the study's intervention. In an RCT, a control group is used as a baseline for comparison with the intervention groups. The control group may receive a placebo or sham treatment, or it may receive the standard treatment for a particular condition. Among the intervention groups, multiple interventions may be tested, or the same intervention may be tested in different magnitudes. The latter is typical of trials involving drugs, in which different dosages are applied to gauge efficacy, the side effect profile, and safety.

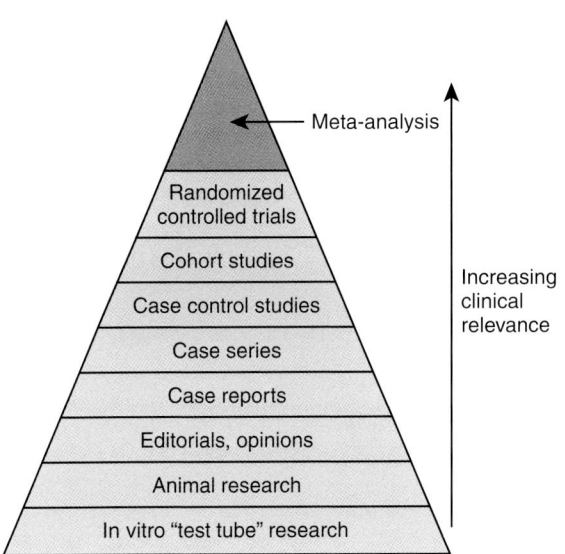

Fig. 4.6 The pyramid of evidence.

Fig. 4.7 illustrates a fictional trial comparing three antifibrinolytic agents used in cardiac surgery to reduce the need for transfusion. Antifibrinolytic B is currently the standard treatment. The starting group of 21 open-heart surgical patients is randomized to receive antifibrinolytic A, B, or C. The patients undergo anesthesia, surgery, and the antifibrinolytic intervention. They are followed for 90 days to assess survival, as well as the number of units of blood transfused postoperatively. Group differences in mortality would be assessed with a nonparametric procedure such as the χ^2 test, and group differences in the amount of blood transfused would be assessed with a parametric tool such as the ANOVA. Using relative risk or odds ratio would allow quantification of the magnitude of the effect of interventions A, B, and C on the outcomes of interest.

The means of randomization is also an important aspect to consider when evaluating an RCT. Alternating assignment or assignment by birth date or hospital admission number are not considered random and are prone to bias. In large clinical trials, simple randomization may be sufficient to eliminate differences in patient characteristics between intervention groups, but other techniques are required for smaller sample sizes. Block randomization and stratification are two strategies used to evenly distribute patient characteristics among small intervention groups. Block randomization groups patients in blocks of two or more. The number of intervention groups determines the number of different patient assignment sequences, which are randomly applied to each block of patients. For example, a study using blocks of three patients with intervention groups A and B would have possible patient assignment sequences of AAA, ABA, AAB, ABB, BBB, BAA, BBA, and BAB. A patient block randomly assigned the ABA sequence would assign the first and third patients to intervention group A and the second patient to intervention group B. Stratification takes the process a step further by first grouping together patients with similar clinical features.[5] Block randomization is then conducted separately on each group to ensure that patients with similar clinical features are randomly distributed into the intervention and control groups.

Additional strategies to reduce bias in the RCT involve the concealment of intervention group assignment and details of the intervention itself. Allocation concealment prevents researchers from consciously

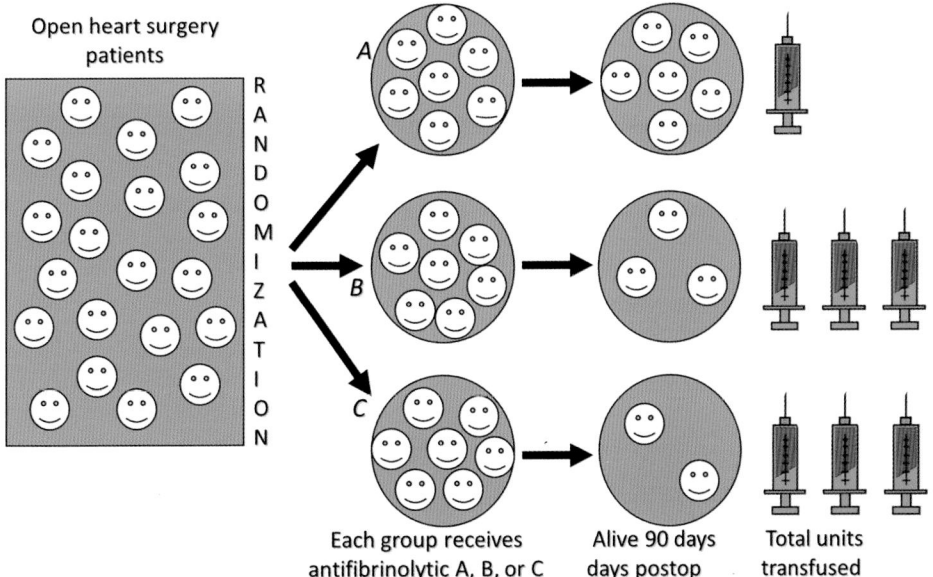

Fig. 4.7 A fictional example of a randomized controlled trial comparing the effects of antifibrinolytics A, B, and C on the need for blood products following cardiac surgery. The total number of units of blood required by the patients in each treatment group who survived 90 days after surgery is then analyzed to determine the treatment effect of the drugs.

or unconsciously assigning a patient to a particular treatment group based on their own personal biases.[5] Blinding (masking) prevents the introduction of bias by participants or investigators who know whether or not they are receiving treatment or are administering the treatment.

Bias may be introduced into the RCT when a study fails to account for patients who do not complete the study. In clinical trials, patients may discontinue treatment for a number of reasons, including unpleasant side effects or burdensome treatment regimens. When these patients are left out of the data analysis process, individual variation is no longer equally distributed between patient groups. Without equivalent treatment and nontreatment groups, the intervention can no longer be said to be the sole determinant of treatment effect. Intention-to-treat analysis incorporates data from all patients regardless of study completion and minimizes bias introduced by patient noncompliance. Published articles should always specify which participants are included in data analysis and use intention-to-treat analysis to evaluate the primary outcome.[5]

It is important to keep in mind that bias inherently exists even in the most rigorously controlled clinical trial, due to the simple fact that no two people (let alone groups of people) are exactly alike. Any small difference between groups has the potential to bias the study results. It is important that the nurse anesthetist critically evaluate the quality of an RCT to determine whether a treatment effect can be reliably determined. A checklist is noted in Box 4.7 to help judge the value of a particular RCT.

Systematic Reviews. We all rely to one extent or another on reviews of primary research to assist us in coming to understand and apply clinical research findings. However, reviews differ substantially in the quality of primary studies included and the methodologic rigor used to assess them. In a traditional narrative review, authors use informal, subjective methods to select and analyze primary studies, often including only those studies that support their hypothesis.[15] By contrast, the authors of a systematic review conduct an exhaustive search of primary studies based on a focused clinical question and use explicit and reproducible methods to select, critically appraise, and synthesize the results of high-quality reports.[15,16] Box 4.8 provides an overview of the methodology of a systematic review.

The title of "systematic review," however, is not in and of itself an indication of quality. It is vital that the nurse anesthetist critically evaluate systematic reviews to determine the validity of the stated results. Box 4.9 provides a list of questions to consider when appraising a systematic review. The validity of the trial methodology, the magnitude and precision of the treatment effect, and the applicability of results to the patient or population of interest should all be considered.[17]

As with any research study, a quality systematic review demands a precisely defined research question. The clinical question should incorporate patients or populations of interest, the intervention, comparisons (if any), and the outcomes of interest. The research question is especially important in a systematic review as it determines the relevance, and therefore inclusion, of associated studies. The search strategy is also critical to the validity of a systematic review. In most cases, searching one database is not sufficient to yield all the important articles on a topic.[18] Moreover, searching only published sources fails to eliminate publication bias, or the underrepresentation of negative results in published reports. A comprehensive search that is not limited to the English language and includes both published and unpublished sources is essential to minimize selection bias. Many authors of systematic reviews also seek out alternative data sources, including "gray literature" (theses, internal reports, pharmaceutic industry files, etc.) and raw unpublished data from primary studies.[16]

A systematic review is only as valid as the poorest quality study it includes. The validity of the incorporated studies is therefore paramount in determining the quality of a systematic review. The authors should specify the quality criteria used to evaluate each study and the quality rating ultimately given to each included study. At least two reviewers should independently assess study quality to reduce the risk of excluding relevant publications and to limit selection bias.[17] The study design should also be appropriate for the clinical question to be answered.

Finally, the results of a systematic review should be an accurate reflection of the aggregated results of each primary publication. Conducting

---

BOX 4.8   The Methodology for a Systematic Review

- State the objectives of the review and define eligibility criteria.
- Search for trials that meet criteria.
- Describe characteristics of each trial; assess methodologic quality.
- Apply eligibility criteria; explain any exclusions.
- Assemble/compile the most comprehensive data set possible.
- Analyze results of eligible RCTs using a common statistical metric.
- Compare alternative analyses if appropriate and possible.
- Prepare a critical summary based on the analysis, stating goals, describing nuances of studies employed, and reporting results.

RTCs, Randomized controlled trials.
The meta-analysis represents a comprehensive, exhaustive survey of high-quality trials on a focused clinical question/objective. There must be clearly articulated and reproducible predetermined criteria for inclusion and a highly critical appraisal of the studies for quality and synthesis.

BOX 4.9   Questions to Ask When Evaluating a Systematic Review

- Did the review address a clearly focused question?
- Was a thorough search done of the appropriate databases?
- Were other potentially important sources explored?
- Did the review include the right type or types of study?
- Did the reviewers try to identify all relevant studies?
- Did the reviewers assess the quality of all the studies included? If so, how?
- If the results of the study have been combined, was it reasonable to do so?
- How are the results presented and what are the main results?
- How precise are the results?
- How sensitive are the results?
- Can the results be applied to your local population?
- Were all important outcomes considered?
- Should practice or policy change as a result of the evidence contained in this review?

Adapted from CASP UK. Critical Appraisal Skills Programme (CASP). *Systematic Review Checklist,* 2020. Accessed at http://media.wix.com/ugd/dded87_a02ff2e3445f4952992d5a96ca562576.pdf.

BOX 4.7   Checklist for Evaluation of the Randomized Controlled Trial

- Is a clear objective for the study stated?
- Is the sample size adequate?
- Is the study population well described?
- Are the interventions clearly described?
- Are randomization and blinding procedures adequate?
- Are valid and reliable outcome measures used?
- Is attrition (dropouts) considered in the analysis?
- Are the statistical methods appropriate?
- Are both clinical and statistical significance reported?
- Are the results generalizable to clinical practice?

a sensitivity analysis is a useful means of assessing the accuracy of the review's results. A sensitivity analysis involves slightly modifying the parameters of the systematic review to account for possible bias. Changing the inclusion criteria, assigning quality ratings differently, incorporating unpublished studies, and including (or excluding) publications of lower quality should not significantly alter the review's overall results. If the key findings disappear when any of these parameters are modified, the review's conclusions should be interpreted with caution.[16]

Whenever possible, the nurse anesthetist should endeavor to use systematic reviews. Systematic reviews are those that incorporate (1) a comprehensive study retrieval process that minimizes publication bias, (2) selection criteria that identify only relevant studies, (3) a critical appraisal of the emergent literature accomplished by knowledgeable and sophisticated clinicians and researchers, and (4) reproducible decisions regarding the relevance and methodologic rigor of the selected primary research. When the results of a systematic review are analyzed quantitatively, it is called a meta-analysis. The meta-analysis is explored next.

Meta-analyses. The meta-analysis has gained an appropriate foothold in the anesthesia literature as the pinnacle of high-quality empiric evidence. A meta-analysis is a systematic review that includes a quantitative statistical analysis of the findings that have emerged from several (or many) discrete studies examining a similar phenomenon. Its purpose is to provide an estimate of the overall benefit or risk of an intervention that has been gleaned from carefully selected RCTs (Fig. 4.8). Rather than simply pooling data from smaller studies, the meta-analysis accounts for differences in sample size, and variability in both study design and determination of the treatment effect.[19] The meta-analysis draws on a heterogeneous group of patients studied in a range of trials and therefore achieves increased power to detect any clinically significant effects. The meta-analysis also provides a precise estimate of the size of any treatment effect that is revealed. A high-quality meta-analysis provides many benefits, including:

- A valid and weighted course of action based on aggregated studies
- Reduced overall risk of bias
- Estimation precision and determination of the effect size of an intervention in a defined patient group
- Transparency in the overall process, improving risk-benefit in a unique patient

Examples of anesthesia-based meta-analyses include those by Tramer, who examined ondansetron as an antiemetic; Ballantyne et al., who studied pulmonary outcomes in patients who had epidural analgesia; Lee et al., who looked at acupuncture and acupressure as alternative approaches in the management of postoperative emetic symptoms; and Biddle, who evaluated the use of nonsteroidal antiinflammatory drugs in the treatment of acute postoperative pain, and later compared the use of ephedrine and phenylephrine on newborn Apgar scores.[20-23]

The steps involved in developing a meta-analysis are described in Box 4.10. The need for rigor in a meta-analysis demands that there be a formal process for conducting it, allowing the researcher to account for the range of relevant findings from high-quality, published research. The primary risk inherent in unsystematic, narrative reviews is that there is a great opportunity for bias in the retrieval, analysis, and critique of selected articles and reports. The meta-analysis overcomes these risks and distinguishes itself from the narrative review through methodologic rigor, producing an unbiased synthesis of the extant literature.

As the distinguishing characteristic of both systematic reviews and meta-analyses is the rigor with which relevant evidence is retrieved, filtered, analyzed, and synthesized, it is especially important that the nurse anesthetist conduct a critical appraisal of these studies before applying the results to clinical practice. Questions that should be asked when evaluating a meta-analysis are similar to those asked in the appraisal of a systematic review:

- Is there a focused, clearly written hypothesis?
- Are there stringent criteria for inclusion of studies in the analysis?
- Are exclusionary criteria justified?
- Are the included studies of high quality?

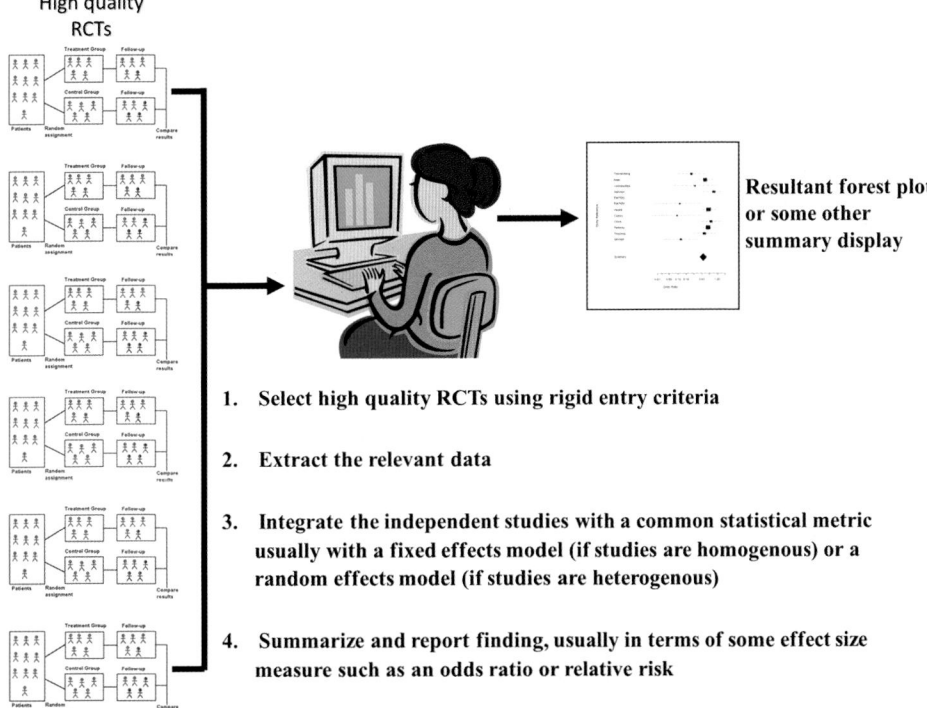

High quality
RCTs

1. **Select high quality RCTs using rigid entry criteria**

2. **Extract the relevant data**

3. **Integrate the independent studies with a common statistical metric usually with a fixed effects model (if studies are homogenous) or a random effects model (if studies are heterogenous)**

4. **Summarize and report finding, usually in terms of some effect size measure such as an odds ratio or relative risk**

Resultant forest plot or some other summary display

Fig. 4.8 A meta-analysis is a systematic review that includes a quantitative statistical analysis of an intervention studied in carefully selected randomized controlled trials (RCTs).

BOX 4.10 Steps Involved in a Meta-analysis

1. List the objectives of the planned review of the randomized control trials.
2. Carefully describe the eligibility criteria for inclusion in the systematic review.
3. Seek research that meets the stated eligibility criteria.
4. Assess each trial or published source individually for its methodologic worth.
5. Assemble the best evidence with oversight (ensuring agreement for inclusion).
6. Analyze the assembled evidence using standard statistical procedures.
7. Compare other analyses, if available.
8. Write up the critical appraisal, carefully describing the previous elements, defining conclusions, and indicating potential applications to the care of patients.

- Is there a systematic approach to evidence retrieval and filtering?
- Are the inclusion criteria strictly adhered to and meticulously described?
- How are the data analyzed and presented?
- Does the effect size measure provide insight into the direction and magnitude of the intervention being studied?
- Are alternative explanations or analyses considered?
- Is bias considered?
- Does the report include a critical examination of the review process?

An important attribute of the meta-analysis is that it is inclusive of all research that meets the established criteria. Unpublished dissertations, theses, and reports may prove to be important sources of information yet can be difficult to track and access. Discussions with acknowledged experts in the domain are often an efficient means by which to access these materials.

A meta-analysis commonly analyzes and reports results using one of several effect size measurements. Table 4.10 (see earlier) presents a list of effect size measures frequently used in a meta-analysis. A common means of displaying data is the use of a pictorial representation, such as a forest plot, and a summary effect size measure such as an odds ratio. The forest plot displays the results of individual studies in comparison with the overall result of the meta-analysis. Squares represent an estimate of the mean result of each study. A horizontal line running through each square indicates the 95% CI boundaries. The overall estimate of the treatment effect revealed by the meta-analysis and its CI are found at the bottom of the plot, usually depicted as a diamond with a horizontal line running through it. In the middle of the plot, a central line represents the threshold of statistical significance. The intervention has achieved a statistically significant treatment effect if the diamond is clear of this line. Generally, at the bottom of the forest plot is a line indicative of the odds ratio that reveals the overall magnitude of the effect (positive or negative), grounding it in clinically practical perspective (Fig. 4.9).

Systematic reviews and meta-analyses are not perfect. Major objections to the meta-analysis and systematic review include the following:
1. The potential to combine studies of great variance in overall quality
2. A possible failure on the researcher's behalf to fully consider variations in subjects, methods, interventions, or outcomes measurement
3. A nonlinear effect of the intervention—a limit (above or below) in which one factor has little or no effect on the other

Careful reading and thoughtful analysis of any published article, whether a case report, a retrospective review, an RCT, or a systematic review, is a responsibility the nurse anesthetist must assume before making direct application of findings to a patient. EBP does not and cannot rely on any one published source. The burden is on the nurse

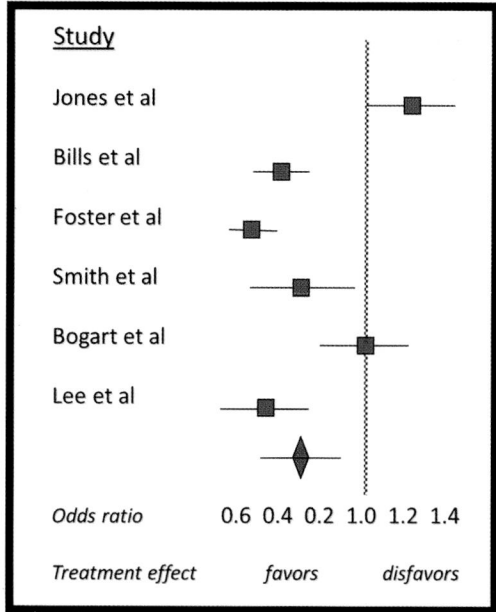

Fig. 4.9 A typical forest plot. A meta-analysis was conducted on the effect of a drug preventing tachycardia. Of the six studies that met the criteria, four found tachycardia less likely to occur in the group receiving the drug compared to the control group. Another way of expressing these results is with an odds ratio, which gives the probability of a given person experiencing an outcome of interest (tachycardia) in a specific circumstance (taking a drug). Because the experimental group (in the numerator) was less likely to experience tachycardia than the control group (in the denominator), the odds ratio is less than 1.0. One of the studies found that people taking the drug were more likely to experience tachycardia, expressed as an odds ratio greater than 1.0. In this example, an odds ratio of less than 1.0 favors a treatment effect of the drug (less tachycardia), whereas an odds ratio of greater than 1.0 disfavors a treatment effect. A square represents the mean effect seen in each study and horizontal lines show the 95% confidence intervals. A diamond indicates the combined odds ratio of all the studies and its confidence interval. A vertical line represents an odds ratio of 1.0, which indicates neither a greater nor lesser likelihood of tachycardia when the drug is taken, and thus neither a favorable nor unfavorable treatment effect.

BOX 4.11 Applying an Intervention to a Patient

- Is the patient well represented by the studies selected?
- Is the planned intervention one with which we are familiar and experienced?
- What are the risks of the intervention: do the benefits outweigh the drawbacks?
- When possible, has the patient been adequately informed and drawn into the decision-making process?

anesthetist to navigate the best possible course of action for the patient's unique circumstance.

Step 4: Applying Evidence to Your Patient

Translating knowledge into practice is the next critical step. If it has been determined that the evidence is valid and important, you must now decide whether you should apply it to the care of your patient. EBP then becomes an ongoing process of inquiry, asking, "Why am I doing it this way?" and "Are there compelling reasons for me to do it differently to achieve a better outcome?" Box 4.11

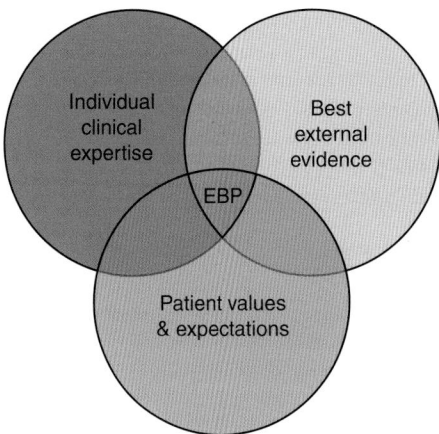

Fig. 4.10 Evidence-based practice (EBP) combines a practitioner's individual experience with the highest quality empiric evidence and the needs of the patient.

provides a list of questions that must be asked when preparing to apply an intervention to a patient. The factors influencing these decisions are complex. Ultimately, the decision to implement an intervention is a blend of experience and science as the value of the evidence is carefully assessed in the context and setting of a particular patient. What is meant by context? Box 4.12 illustrates just a few of the contextual factors that must be considered in the process of EBP.

Often underemphasized in a discussion of EBP is the essential value of clinical experience and clinical judgment, as well as an understanding of individual patients in the context of their personality, culture, and unique experiences. Even with a substantial amount of meaningful evidence to apply, a lack of experience and judgment may result in enormous faltering in its application to individual patients. Experience and judgment are indispensable when considering and ranking interventional options. Certainly, part of the process of EBP is based on consideration of the skill of the clinicians in the studies selected to evaluate and whether all important outcomes have been measured. Similarly, sensitivity to a patient's desires and beliefs is vitally important in taking full advantage of an EBP approach to care.

Most EBP related to anesthesia occurs under circumstances in which the patient's input is likely to be minimal to nonexistent (e.g., choice of neuromuscular blocking drug, intraoperative fluid management, selection of antifibrinolytic, approach to managing body temperature and its measurement, and type and settings of ventilator management). However, many decisions should actively involve patients, especially risk-benefit comparisons (e.g., regional vs. general anesthesia, perioperative blood transfusions, postoperative nausea and pain control, and management of the risks of vision disturbances and peripheral nerve injury).

Although one goal of EBP is to provide the best care possible in the unique contextual situation of a given patient, another is for nurse anesthetists to act as patient advocates. Basing interventions on the triad of the latest research evidence, clinical expertise and experience, and the needs and wishes of the patient (Fig. 4.10) requires nurse anesthetists to act as patient advocates throughout the process. EBP is, by definition, the marriage of excellent clinical science with humanitarianism. Extracting the contextually essential, highest-quality information from the vast, representative research literature and merging it with the art of applying that information to a patient is EBP at its finest. Next, it is time to evaluate the outcome of the intervention.

Step 5: Evaluating the Effect (Outcome) of the Evidence-Based Intervention

A vital component of the process of EBP is evaluation. Here one determines whether the evidence has altered the "usual" practice pattern. If so, has it been associated with improved efficiency and health outcomes, and has it maintained the quality of care? Evaluation allows not only for deciding whether the intervention "works" but also for determining whether variations arise (e.g., dosing, timing, duration, complications, and unexpected occurrences). In doing so, a kind of living, evolving document arises that can be used for purposes of assessing efficacy, quality assurance, and risk.

EVIDENCE-BASED PRACTICE IN NURSE ANESTHESIA

EBP is the hallmark of quality anesthetic care. Whereas nurse anesthetists are increasingly likely to assume the role of primary researcher, all nurse anesthetists regardless of research experience are in a position to read about the latest advances in nurse anesthesia practice and incorporate validated interventions into their clinical practice. Nurse anesthesia research is grounded in solving patient care problems during the preoperative, intraoperative, and postoperative periods. Although much behavioral, educational, and product evaluation–oriented research has been conducted by nurse anesthesia researchers, all nurse anesthesia research is wedded inextricably to patient care. EBP is essential to the professional evolution of nurse anesthesia as nurse anesthetists become increasingly accountable for their own independent basis for practice.

A number of antiscience movements are operative in the world today. At the heart of all these movements is the sophisticated use of the concept of proof by proclamation rather than proof by experimentation. As active consumers and producers of scientific knowledge, nurse anesthetists can do their part by resisting the integration of aberrant and ill-founded thinking into their discipline. This can be achieved if each nurse anesthetist understands the need to maintain a critical dialogue regarding what can be incorporated into nurse anesthesia practice.

All nurse anesthetists are mandated to practice evidence-based care. The American Nurses Association strongly urges even undergraduate nursing students to learn how to read, interpret, and evaluate published research for applicability to nursing practice. Although the evolution of nursing research—and that of nurse anesthesia research in particular—has lagged behind that of many other disciplines, tremendous strides are being made as greater numbers of nurse anesthetists are prepared at both the master's and the doctoral levels. It is essential that nurse anesthetists recognize the need to promote nurse anesthesia as a science-based profession. There is no better way to achieve this end than to continue emphasizing the importance of EBP.[24]

SUMMARY

Basic fluency in research methods is essential to today's anesthesia practice. The ability to evaluate the literature allows the clinician to stay up to date with the rapid advances in medical knowledge. It also gives the anesthetist an avenue to answer questions that arise in daily practice with appropriate evidence to ensure the best patient care and outcomes.

REFERENCES

For a complete list of references for this chapter, scan this QR code with any smartphone code reader app, or visit the following URL: http://booksite.elsevier.com/9780323711944/.

5

General Principles, Pharmacodynamics, and Drug-Receptor Concepts

John J. Nagelhout

The practice of anesthesia requires a full spectrum of drugs from which an anesthetic plan can be implemented to achieve the desired level of surgical anesthesia, analgesia, amnesia, and muscle relaxation. In addition to surgical anesthesia, pain management has evolved as a significant clinical practice component.[1,2] Now that the human genome has been mapped and the field of molecular and cellular proteomics is exploring new concepts, specific receptor-targeted drugs are envisioned, as is a revolution in the way health care is delivered. Likewise, the methods used to provide anesthesia care will undergo a profound change based on this new knowledge. Studies are already challenging long-held concepts of pharmacodynamics and pharmacokinetics that guide the clinical use of anesthetic agents. Target-controlled drug administration that factors in clinical pharmacodynamic and pharmacokinetic information is already being applied.[3,4]

Although the exact mechanism of action of the general anesthetics remains unknown, several targets contribute to the component actions comprising the effects of each anesthetic.[5-7] It remains unclear how the inhalation anesthetic drugs affect the brain to suppress consciousness and movement. The picture that is emerging includes multiple cellular and molecular targets in distinct brain regions that are involved in both the desired and adverse effects of general anesthetics. Consciousness is inhibited in the brain, of course, but movement is likely obtunded at the spinal cord level.[8,9]

Spinal cord receptors are being differentiated from receptors in the brain and targeted with specific drugs. A more in-depth knowledge of the concept of minimum alveolar concentration (MAC), which is used to define inhalation anesthetic dosing, is now coming to light.[10,11] Receptor superfamilies with definable amino acid subunits are the targets of new classes of anesthetic drugs such as α_2-agonists and analgesics.[12] The potentiation of the inhibitory γ-aminobutyric acid (GABA) receptors is considered a primary mechanism of action of inhalation and intravenous anesthetics.[13] The recovery from intravenous anesthesia is described in terms of context-sensitive halftime, which in addition to the usual concept of drug half-life takes into consideration the duration of anesthetic administration rather than just drug redistribution and elimination profiles.[14-16]

The importance of the individual, with a unique genetic profile, is surfacing as a major determinant of anesthesia outcome.[17,18] The number of patients who now make up the portion of the population classified as elderly—those age 60 years and above—is ever increasing. Clinical experience has shown that the response to anesthetic drugs in elderly patients differs from that in younger patients. Age-related changes in drug pharmacokinetics do not totally explain the differences in drug dosing necessary to achieve anesthetic endpoints in elderly patients. Studies to date in elderly patients demonstrate an age-related decline in most receptor populations and an overall decrease in pharmacodynamic responses.[19-22] Preoperative assessment may soon take on an entirely different meaning as patient information becomes more genetically oriented. The choice of anesthetic agents will be based on age-related receptor profiles and the patient's genetic ability to rapidly clear and recover from anesthetic drugs once their administration has been terminated.[23-26] Until that time, anesthetists will continue to administer anesthesia based on age-indexed population drug profiles adjusted for individual pathologies (i.e., general principles of pharmacology).

The current medical economic climate necessitates the optimum selection and use of anesthetic drugs based on their pharmacologic profiles. The term *pharmacology* refers to the study of processes by which a drug produces one or more measured physiologic responses. The concept of a drug-induced tissue response has changed little since Ehrlich first proposed it (circa 1905). What has changed, and continues to change, is our understanding of the processes involved in drug-receptor interactions.[27-29] Attention is now being focused on the biosphere, or the protein receptor site, as not only the locus of drug binding but also a primary regulator of the measured pharmacologic response. Secondary processes, including drug absorption, distribution, biotransformation, and excretion, also influence the pharmacologic response.[30]

RECEPTOR STRUCTURE

A receptor is a protein or other substance that binds to an endogenous chemical or a drug. This coupling causes a chain of events leading to an effect. Receptors have three common properties: sensitivity, selectivity, and specificity. These properties are characterized by the fact that a drug response occurs from a low concentration (sensitivity) produced by structurally similar chemicals (selectivity), and the response from a given set of receptors is always the same because the cells themselves determine the response (specificity). The bonds that form between drugs and receptors typically fall into these categories from weakest to strongest: van der Waals, hydrophobic, hydrogen, ionic, and covalent.

Drug Receptors

The historic concept of a drug-receptor complex (DRC) considers the receptor to be a single protein to which the drug aligned and attached itself. We have now identified multiple mechanisms by which an endogenous substance or drug may complex with a receptor and transmit a signal. There are six classes of drug-receptor proteins based on genetic characterization and similarity of structure and functions.[31] Several examples of different types of receptors are given in Box 5.1.

Drug-receptor proteins may be located within the luminal membrane and at the surface of the ionic channel. They also occupy intracellular sites. The drug lidocaine and other amide and ester local anesthetics, for example, act at intracellular receptor sites near the sodium channel. Studies of acetylcholine and its receptor at the neuromuscular junction indicate that less than 1% of the cell surface binds drug to receptor protein to achieve the tissue response.[32] Complete saturation of available receptors with drug molecules is not necessary for a desired tissue response to be elicited. With recent advances in molecular biology, many receptors have been extensively characterized, with amino acids sequenced and cloned. This is leading to a new and better understanding of receptor pharmacology and new approaches to drug discovery.[33-36]

For intravenously administered drugs, sufficient drug for a maximal tissue response is delivered to the receptor site within the time required for a single complete circulation (~1 minute) provided an adequate drug dose was administered initially. Current understanding of molecular pharmacology suggests that the delay recorded from initial drug administration to the onset of the tissue response reflects the time required for molecular orientation and attachment to the receptor—that is, the time course of the receptor protein conformational change and the tissue response time.[37] As long as both the drug and the receptor are hydrophobic, bonding occurs.[38] Intravenous anesthetics act by binding to membrane receptor channel proteins. The $GABA_A$ (ionotropic receptor family A) inhibitory receptor has been implicated and suggested as a primary site of intravenous anesthetic action, except in the case of ketamine.[39-41] Inhalation anesthetics have long been thought to produce their anesthetic action by dissolving in the lipid bilayer surrounding membrane ion channels and interfering with their ability to open and close. Electrophysiologic evidence gathered since 2011, however, indicates that inhalation anesthetics, like intravenous anesthetics, bind to $GABA_A$ receptor proteins and cause inhibition of signal transduction by increasing the influx of chloride ions through membrane channels.[13,39-41]

Individual agonist drugs have at least three configuration points for attachment to their receptors. With more points of attachment, a more perfect drug-receptor fit occurs. Agonist drugs can induce receptor proteins to alter their topography to achieve a more exacting fit with the drug. The alignment of a drug with its receptor is aided by various bonding forces, of which van der Waals forces and ionic bonding are prominent. Volatile anesthetics (e.g., desflurane, sevoflurane, isoflurane) and nitrous oxide bond to cell receptors by means of a nonspecific hydrophobic bonding mechanism.

Some endogenous proteins provide alternative drug-binding sites. These sites are more correctly termed acceptors; the acceptor reduces the amount of unbound drug available for receptor complexing. Albumin contains numerous acceptor sites and generally binds to acidic drugs. α_1-Acid glycoprotein and β-globulin preferentially bind basic drugs. Drugs bound to these proteins are unavailable to interact with receptors, therefore reducing the available active drug concentration.

Types of Receptors

As previously noted, a variety of receptor types have been isolated and investigated, including GABA, opioid, alpha, beta, acetylcholine, histamine subtypes, and the pain-related capsaicin receptor, in addition to numerous others.[41-45] The nicotinic and muscarinic cholinergic receptors that bind acetylcholine have been studied extensively.[46-48] The acetylcholine receptor protein is a pentamer of five peptide subunits conceptually forming a five-sided ring with the central portion serving as the transduction ion channel. Only two of the five subunits are involved in acetylcholine binding. The remaining three peptide subunits participate in the signal transduction process that involves a protein conformational shift allowing inward movement of sodium ions through the opened ion channel. It is interesting to note that the $GABA_A$ receptor has also been shown to be composed of five peptide subunits arranged to form a pentameric ring.[45,49-51]

Signal Transduction

In biology, signal transduction refers to processes by which a cell converts one kind of signal or stimulus into another. Most often these involve ordered sequences or cascades of biochemical reactions inside the cell. They are commonly referred to as second messenger pathways. An example of a G protein–coupled receptor (GPCR) and its second messenger system is shown in Fig. 5.1.

Many of the actions of the common anesthetic drugs are transduced through cell-surface receptors that are linked to GPCRs. Receptor signaling translates changes to G proteins that are then linked to a second messenger such as cyclic adenosine monophosphate (AMP) or cyclic guanosine monophosphate (GMP). These second messengers regulate enzymes such as protein kinases and phosphatases, which drive their ultimate intracellular actions. Some common second messengers and their physiologic and pharmacology targets are shown in Table 5.1.

Signal transduction for the $GABA_A$ receptor, for example, involves inward chloride ion movement through the opened central channel. The protein compositions of acetylcholine and GABA receptors are remarkably similar, despite their functional differences—specifically, acetylcholine and sodium ions transduce an excitatory signal, and GABA and chloride ions transduce an inhibitory signal.[52,53]

For many drugs, the composition of the receptor protein and the signal transduction process may be identical even though the drug-induced tissue response is not. The primary difference among drug-receptor proteins may be only the selective binding subunits and the ion species moving through the channel.[39,41,43,54,55] The specific peptide subunits are ultimately responsible for the pharmacologic properties of specificity, affinity, and potency.

In addition, specific isomers that have fewer side effects than the racemic mixture have been marketed. Drugs such as dexmedetomidine, ropivacaine, and cisatracurium are selective in their receptor binding and thus achieve a better clinical side-effect profile.[56,57]

DRUG-RESPONSE EQUATION

The drug-response equation is fundamental to pharmacologic principles.[37] It is derived from the law of mass action and is shown in the following equation, where drug (D) combines with receptor (R) to form a DRC that elicits a tissue response (TR).

$$D + R \rightleftharpoons (DRC) \rightleftharpoons TR$$

What remains unique about this equation is that in most cases the DRC represents a highly selective process. Yet the resultant tissue response tends to vary from individual to individual, reflecting each person's unique receptor and genetic profile and physiologic state. The basic drug-response relationship conceptually depends on a common pharmacologic theory of drug action. This is the occupancy theory. Simply stated, the magnitude of a drug's effect is proportional to the number of receptors occupied. Although it is understood that

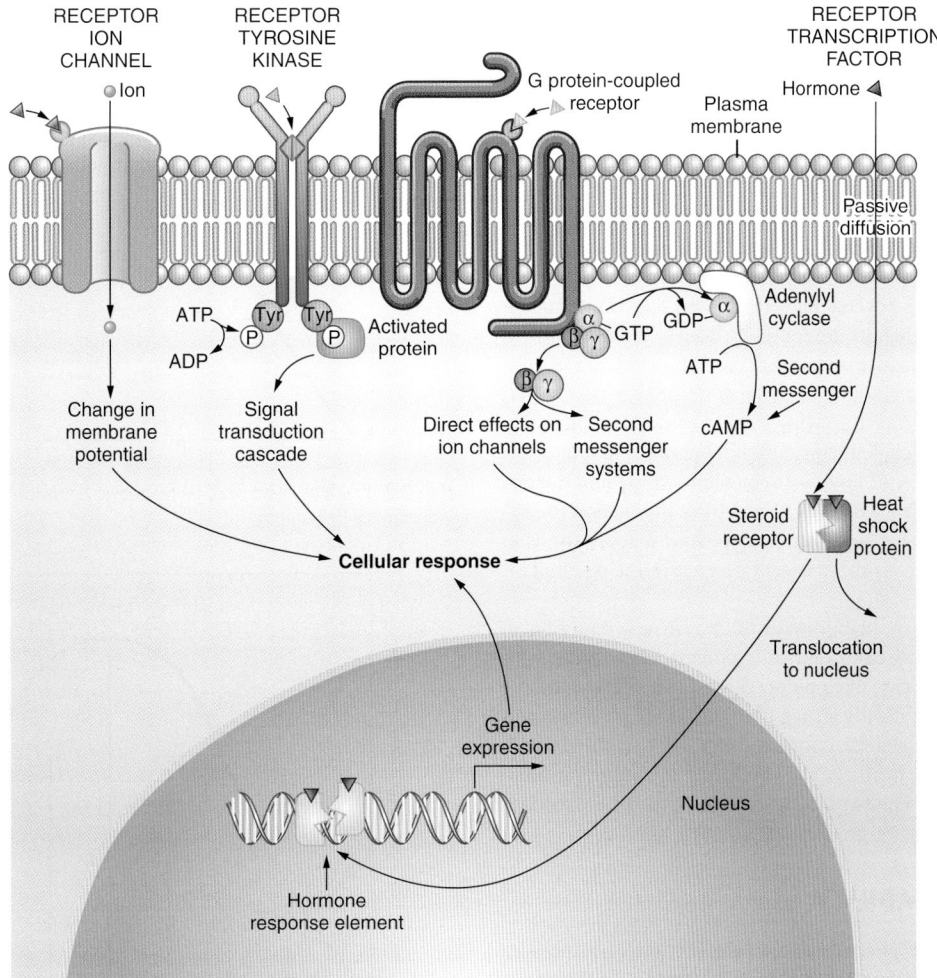

Fig. 5.1 Major modes of signal transduction and intracellular signaling. Binding of an agonist to a receptor ion channel (e.g., GABA$_A$ receptor or nicotinic acetylcholine receptor) leads to opening of a transmembrane pore that permits movement of ions across the plasma membrane. This leads to a change in membrane potential that results in the physiologic response (e.g., change in the firing characteristics of a neuron or muscle contraction). Binding of a ligand to a receptor tyrosine kinase results in receptor dimerization and phosphorylation of the intracellular kinase domain. The activated (phosphorylated) kinase domain is then specifically recognized by proteins such as Src and phospholipase C that in turn activate a network of downstream effectors. These signal transduction pathways ultimately lead to changes in physiologic functioning of the cell such as glucose utilization and cell growth. Binding of a ligand to a seven-transmembrane domain G protein–coupled receptor (GPCR) results in the dissociation of the G protein into the membrane α subunit and the soluble βγ dimer. The α subunit then interacts with downstream effectors such as adenylyl cyclase, which converts ATP into cAMP (a second messenger) that then modifies a number of effector proteins. The βγ dimer can also exert direct cellular effects by modulating activity of a number of ion channels, for example. Effects of steroid hormones are mediated by intracellular receptors, which upon binding their ligand dissociate from a heat shock protein and translocate into the nucleus where they serve to modify gene expression by binding to hormone response elements in the promoter regions. *ADP,* Adenosine diphosphate; *ATP,* adenosine triphosphate; *cAMP,* cyclic adenosine monophosphate; *GDP,* guanosine diphosphate; *GTP,* guanosine triphosphate; *Tyr,* tyrosine. (From Hemmings Jr HC, Egan TD. *Pharmacology and Physiology for Anesthesia.* 2nd ed. Philadelphia: Elsevier; 2019.)

TABLE 5.1 Select Second Messengers

Second Messenger	Target Responses	Common Drug Effectors
Cyclic adenosine monophosphate (cAMP)	Release protein kinases, β-receptor stimulation of energy release, inotropic and chronotropic cardiac effects, production of adrenal and sex steroids, many other endocrine and neural processes	Catecholamines, caffeine, milrinone
Phosphoinositides and calcium	Activate calmodulin	Lithium
Cyclic guanosine monophosphate (cGMP)	Activate protein kinases	Nitroglycerin and sodium nitroprusside

drug-receptor interactions have more complexity than this theory accounts for, it serves as a useful background for many pharmacologic concepts.

PHARMACOGENETICS

Pharmacogenetics is the study of genetically determined variations in response to drugs. This can include variations in how a drug is metabolized and how drugs interact with intended and unintended targets in the body. Pharmacogenetic testing can be useful in ensuring accurate drug dosing, avoiding adverse side effects, and selecting drugs. A variety of pharmacogenetic tests are routinely used to guide treatment of oncology and infectious disease patients based on evidence of clinical benefit. Testing for mutations in patients' tumors is now a part of routine oncologic care for a growing variety of cancers, including breast, colon, lung, stomach, leukemia and lymphoma, and metastatic melanoma. The availability of low-cost sequencing of patient normal and tumor deoxyribonucleic acid (DNA) is driving innovation in cancer care at a very rapid pace, and many more clinical applications of pharmacogenetic testing relevant to cancer care are in the pipeline for clinical release.

Genomic approaches are being used to discover new pathways in common cardiovascular diseases and thus potential new targets for drug development. In the case of clopidogrel, warfarin, and statins, the literature has become sufficiently strong that guidelines are now available describing the use of genetic information to tailor treatment with these therapies, and some health centers are using this information in the care of their patients. Further testing is ongoing to maximize clinical benefit.[58-61]

POPULATION VARIABILITY

Because the objective of pharmacologic intervention is to achieve a desired therapeutic response, anesthetists recognize that a range of responses to a given drug and dosage is possible within a patient population. Therapeutic drug doses reflect average doses of a "normal" population of individuals. Specific therapeutic doses for population subsets (e.g., pediatric, neonatal, geriatric, patients with cardiac or other chronic diseases) are available, thereby narrowing the degree of response variability for a given drug and clinical population. The age, sex, body weight, body surface area, basal metabolic rate, pathologic state, and genetic profile of an individual directly influence the pharmacologic response.

Given the increasing median age of the population in the United States, studies of the influence of age on the responses to anesthetic drugs have increased. Steady-state plasma concentrations of hypnotic drugs such as midazolam and propofol and MAC for inhaled anesthetics (e.g., desflurane, isoflurane, or sevoflurane) required to achieve desired anesthetic endpoints decrease as age increases, independent of any age effect on drug pharmacokinetics.[62-66] Unfortunately, the specifics responsible for the observed age-related decrease in an effective dose of anesthetic drugs are multifaceted. Receptor changes associated with aging and kinetic differences in the elderly are in part responsible for the variation in response. Dose reduction or the use of dosing algorithms for the elderly patient population is indicated.[67]

Mean, Median, and Mode

A graphic description of the dose-response relationship is displayed in Fig. 5.2. The theoretic normal distribution of quantal (desired) responses to increasing drug dose takes the shape of a gaussian curve. Theoretically, the numbers of respondents on both sides of the mean (average dose) are equal, with the greatest percentage of individuals

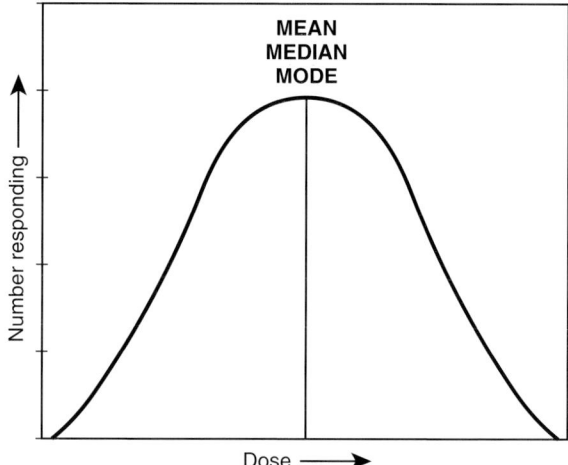

Fig. 5.2 The theoretic normal frequency distribution of a drug response in a normal population.

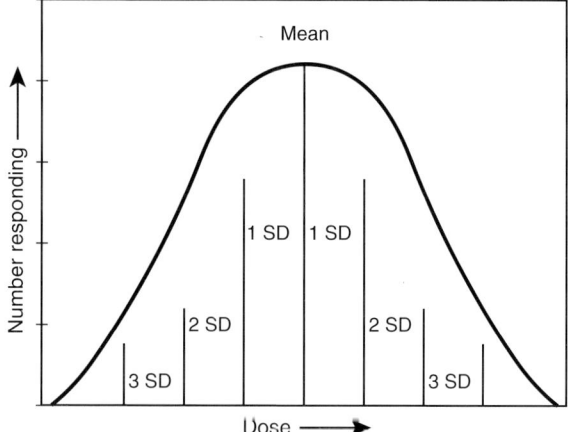

Fig. 5.3 A normal distribution curve showing the standard deviation (SD) in relation to the mean (average) dose value.

responding near the center of the curve. In a gaussian distribution curve, the mean, median, and mode are equidistant from the two extremes.[68] Atypical responders fall at each end of the curve.

On the curve, the mean dose is the arithmetic average of the range of doses that produce a given response. The median dose is that dose on either side of which half of the responses occur. The mode dose is the dose representing the greatest percentage of responses. The mean, median, and mode doses are often close but are rarely the same in actual dose-response curves.

Standard Deviation

The terms *standard deviation* (SD) and *standard error of the mean* (SEM) describe population response variability.[69] The SD provides information regarding the actual responses measured and their difference from the calculated mean. In Fig. 5.3, one SD makes up 68% of the responses (34% to the left and 34% to the right of the mean value); two and three SDs constitute 95% and 99.7% of the responses, respectively. The greater the SD, the less the mean reflects the central tendency of responses.

Standard Error of the Mean

The SEM describes the variance of the mean. It is equivalent to the SD of the mean. By repeating the dose-response measurements on different, normally distributed populations, a slightly different mean dose

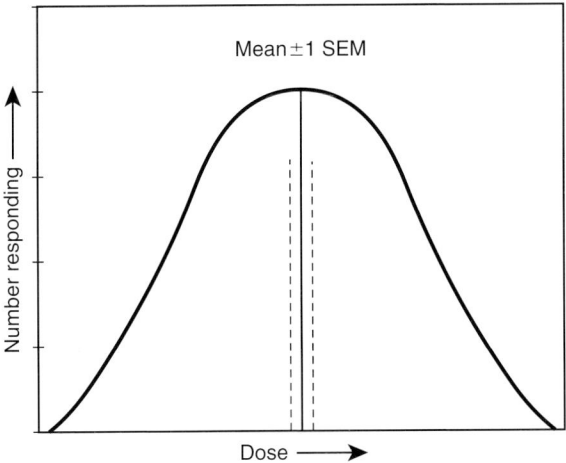

Fig. 5.4 A normal distribution curve showing the relationship of the standard error of the mean *(SEM)* to the mean (average) value.

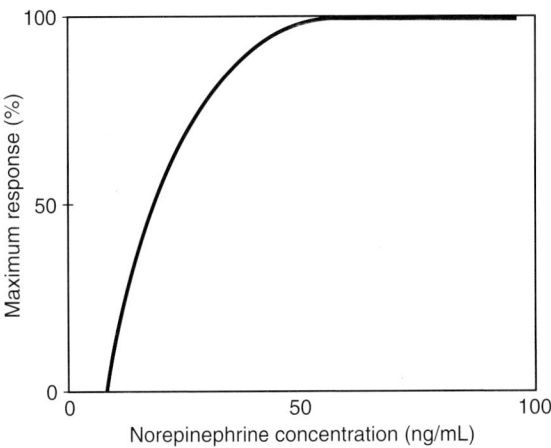

Fig. 5.5 A linear arithmetic graded response curve showing blood vessel constriction to increasing norepinephrine concentrations.

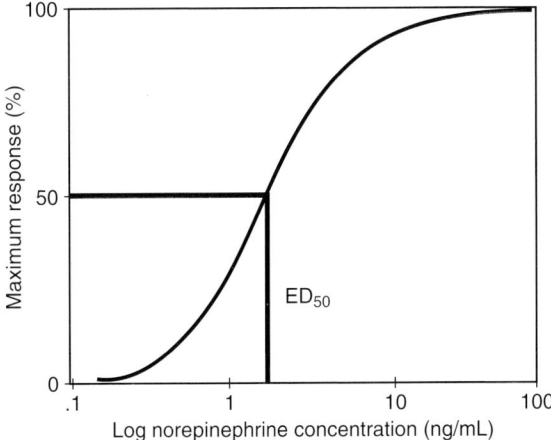

Fig. 5.6 A logarithmic plot of the data from Fig. 5.5 showing blood vessel constriction to increasing concentrations of norepinephrine. The median effective dose *(ED50)* is identified.

value is obtained each time because the mean value is only an arithmetic average of the responses obtained. In Fig. 5.4, one SEM represents the range within which the mean value would occur on repeat testing 68% of the time, and two and three SEMs (not shown) represent the range within which the mean value would occur 95% and 99.7% of the time, respectively. Both the SD and the SEM are important statistical descriptors of observed drug responses in patient care and in research and reflect pharmacologic principles of population variance.[69]

DRUG DOSE RESPONSE

The administration of drugs is largely determined by a mean therapeutic dose per kilogram of body weight or body surface area calculated from a previously determined average dose for the normal population. This approach may be responsible for underdosing and overdosing of patients because population variability is not considered in the calculation. The individual therapeutic response to a fixed mean dose is frequently less than optimal.

Studies that used sensitive quantitative measurement techniques identified a response variability to given drug doses in the normal population that was far greater than previously demonstrated.[27] Clearly, the optimal dosing approach for patients when drugs are administered by the intravenous route is by titration until the desired therapeutic response is attained. This is particularly true in critical care and anesthesia patients in whom drug onset and offset responses are relatively rapid.

Two types of dose-response curves—graded and quantal—describe average drug response and subject variability within a given population.

Graded Dose Response

The graded dose–response curve, which is plotted in linear fashion, characterizes the change in measured response as an administered dose is increased (Fig. 5.5). The response curve has a hyperbolic shape, with the greatest change in response occurring to the left on a small portion of the x-axis. When plotted on a logarithmic scale, the graded dose–response curve takes on an S shape; at the lowest dose, the measured response (e.g., vascular response to norepinephrine) is small or even nonexistent. At the highest doses, the response is maximal and approaches a plateau (Fig. 5.6). Typically, at some point between 20% and 80% of the maximal response, the curve approaches a straight line because changes in dose and response reflect a proportional relationship.

Plotting on a semilogarithmic scale, with the dose in log units, provides a more detailed representation of the entire graded dose–response

curve especially at the two extremes.[27] From a semilogarithmic plot of graded dose responses, the potency of different agonist drugs with similar mechanisms of action (i.e., action through the same receptor) can be compared, or the ability of an antagonist drug to reduce the response to an agonist (e.g., in the alpha receptor blocker, phenoxybenzamine antagonism of norepinephrine-induced vasoconstriction) can be observed. It should be noted that "antagonist" drugs that do not bind to the agonist receptor are not antagonists. For example, neostigmine is not an antagonist of rocuronium because it does not compete with rocuronium for the muscle end-plate receptor site. Neostigmine inhibits acetylcholinesterase, which allows acetylcholine to compete effectively with rocuronium and other nondepolarizing muscle relaxants for the receptor, leading to a recovery of muscle tone. Therefore its effect is at least a partial form of indirect antagonism. Sugammadex is the first and, so far, only drug in a new class of muscle relaxant reversal drugs. Known as a selective relaxant binding agent (SRBA), sugammadex offers a unique mechanism in that it encapsulates the muscle-relaxant molecule, rendering it inactive. The complex formed is eliminated. This is a form of chemical antagonism because no direct receptor action is evident.[70]

Quantal Dose Response

Clinically, a quantal dose–response curve provides information on the frequency with which a given drug dose produces a desired therapeutic

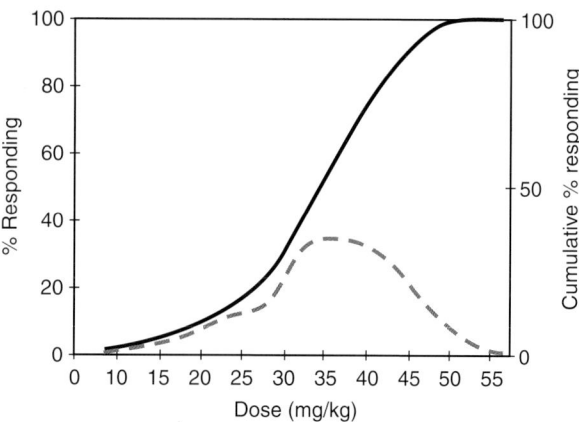

Fig. 5.7 A quantal dose–response curve indicating the frequency of all-or-nothing dose responses. The dashed line represents a histogram of the number of responses measured at each dose. The solid line represents the cumulative response curve of the total number of responses up to and including each dose.

response in a patient population. The response is measured in an all-or-nothing fashion. The quantal response curve describes the variation in response to the threshold dose within a population of seemingly similar individuals (Fig. 5.7). For example, with propofol induction of anesthesia a small number of patients become unconscious after administration of 0.5 mg/kg, more after administration of 1 mg/kg, and virtually all after administration of 2 to 3 mg/kg. Plotting the cumulative number of patients with all-or-nothing responses over a range of doses produces an S-shaped response curve. However, the quantal dose S-shaped curve differs from the graded dose–response S-shaped curve because it reflects population variation for the threshold dose needed to produce a given all-or-nothing desired response.

Descriptive information about population dose-response characteristics can be obtained from quantal dose–response curves.[27] Descriptors such as effective dose, toxic dose, and lethal dose can be identified. The effective dose 99% (ED_{99}) and lethal dose 1% (LD_1) identify the therapeutic safety margin of a drug, as shown in the following equation.

$$\text{Safety margin} = LD_1 - ED_{99}/ED_{99} \times 100$$

When the therapeutic safety margin is great, the risk of drug-induced death is small and the margin of therapeutic safety wide. The opposite is true when the therapeutic safety margin is small.

The term *therapeutic index* (LD_{50}/ED_{50}) describes a drug's median therapeutic safety margin for a particular therapeutic effect.[27] For example, chemotherapeutic drugs have a very narrow margin of safety. Drugs that produce surgical depths of anesthesia, such as sevoflurane and other halogenated anesthetics, also have a relatively narrow margin of safety. Sevoflurane is administered clinically in an amount that is 1.3- to 1.4-fold the MAC, or the dose at which 50% of the patients do not move on surgical stimulation. The MAC can be lethal if the volume percentage delivered is increased to 1.7- to 2.0-fold and maintained for a prolonged period of time.

Another descriptor obtained from the quantal dose–response curve is the median effective dose (ED_{50})—the dose at which 50% of a population responds as desired. The ED_{50} is often used for comparing the potency of drugs within a class. Because the ED_{50} is derived from the linear portion of the quantal dose–response curve (20%–80% of the responders), relatively accurate comparisons of drugs that cause similar responses can be made (see Fig. 5.6). Important in each of these descriptions is the word *median*. Median ED_{50} dose values are derived average response doses from a population of patients.[27] Each individual within the population responds to a median dose based on biologic

variation or, specifically, genetic variations in drug-receptor protein. Confidence limits for a given median dose and its therapeutic response can be calculated. Typically, the proportion of subjects responding to an ED_{50} dose ranges from 45% to 55%. Derived median population dose values provide a point of reference for achieving an individual's optimum therapeutic dose.

For intravenously administered drugs used in anesthesia, the trend is toward drugs that have brief onset-offset times and can be administered by infusion, often with the use of a computer-controlled pump.[71,72] For example, the desired anesthetic response to propofol and remifentanil can be effectively titrated after an initial loading dose.

Future developments related to drugs will include the availability of indwelling drug-analyzing probes similar to the continuous mass spectrometers currently used for analysis of end-tidal anesthetic gas concentrations. Real-time analysis of drug concentration can incorporate feedback control to drug-infusion devices. These target-controlled infusions allow the dose to be set to patient response and automatically maintained with minimal fluctuations in blood and effect site drug concentrations and the tissue response.[73,74] Currently computer-controlled infusion pumps use programs based on pharmacokinetic modeling studies in an attempt to approximate the required effect site drug concentration to achieve and maintain a desired level of anesthesia in patients. The continuing development of ultrafast onset-offset anesthetic drugs such as remifentanil and propofol will simplify titration of the anesthetic endpoint by the anesthetist and minimize undesired effects.

DRUG-RECEPTOR INTERACTIONS

Advances in molecular receptor pharmacology have provided a new understanding of patient drug responses.[28] The drug-receptor interaction describes the formation of a single DRC, which leads to a fractional tissue response (FTR):

$$D + R \underset{k_2}{\overset{k_1}{\rightleftharpoons}} DR \overset{k_3}{\rightarrow} FT$$

The desired tissue response is observed when receptors are sufficiently occupied and activated by free drug. This process obeys the law of mass action: At steady state, equilibrium exists between bound and unbound drug receptors and the concentration of free unbound drug at the site.[75] Specific characteristics of the drug and the receptor determine the association and dissociation of a drug with regard to its receptor and the kinetic, k, rates, which are constants.[37]

Drug Affinity and Efficacy

The terms *affinity* and *efficacy* (intrinsic activity) describe the degree of drug-receptor interaction for a given drug and receptor protein population (e.g., $GABA_A$ and propofol). The observed tissue response reflects the quantity of DRC intact at any given moment. Each drug-receptor interaction elicits a quantum of excitation, and the summation of many individual quanta produces the tissue response.[62] The four concepts derived from a dose-response relationship are potency, efficacy, variability, and slope. Fig. 5.8 shows the overall clinical information derived from determining the dose-response relationships.

The time constant that describes the fractional tissue response after the DRC formation typically has been considered to be near zero or instantaneous. It was believed that the primary time constant thought to influence the onset of tissue response was the duration of the delay in the delivery of drug to the receptor sites. The phrase *pharmacokinetic analysis* of drug absorption and distribution describes onset time and magnitude of drug response. *Drug elimination kinetic analysis* describes the duration of the tissue response.

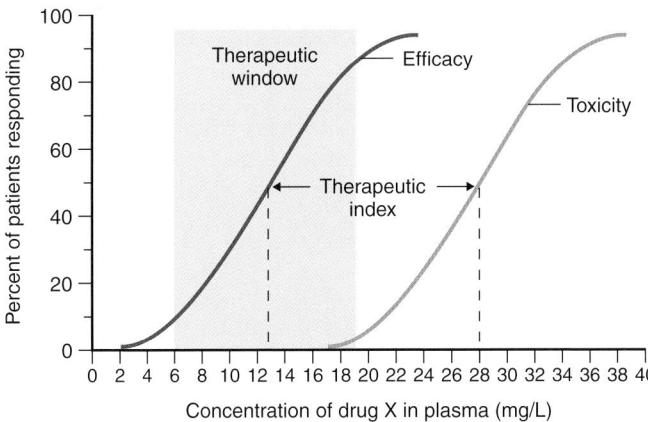

Fig. 5.8 Pattern produced in a dose-response population study in which both effect and toxicity are measured. The therapeutic window is shown as the range of therapeutically effective concentrations, which includes most of the efficacy curve and less than 10% of the toxicity curve. The therapeutic index is calculated by dividing the 50% value on the toxicity curve by the 50% value on the efficacy curve. (From Goldman L, Schafer AI, eds. *Goldman-Cecil Medicine*. 26th ed. Philadelphia: Elsevier; 2020:123.)

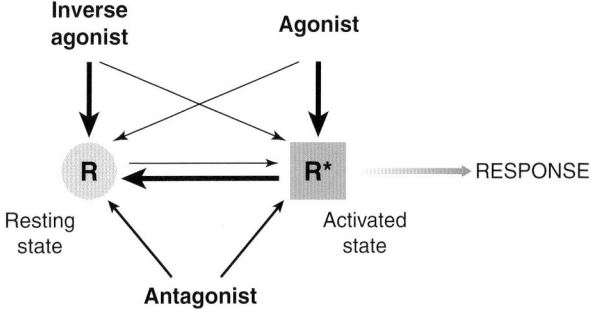

Fig. 5.9 The two-state model. The receptor is shown in two conformational states, "resting" *(R)* and "activated" *(R*)*, which exist in equilibrium. Normally, when no ligand is present, the equilibrium lies far to the left, and few receptors are found in the R* state. For constitutively active receptors, an appreciable proportion of receptors adopt the R* conformation in the absence of any ligand. Agonists have higher affinity for R* than for R, and so shift the equilibrium toward R*. The greater the relative affinity for R* with respect to R, the greater the efficacy of the agonist. An inverse agonist has higher affinity for R than for R*, and so shifts the equilibrium to the left. A "neutral" antagonist has equal affinity for R and R*, and so does not by itself affect the conformational equilibrium but reduces by competition the binding of other ligands. (From Ritter JM, Flower R, Henderson G, et al. *Rang and Dale's Pharmacology*. 9th ed. Edinburgh: Elsevier; 2020:15.)

Drug-Receptor-Response Triad

Current understanding of receptor dynamics has added an additional and possibly the most descriptive component of the drug-receptor-response triad. When a drug combines with its receptor, a conformational change occurs in the receptor protein itself. No tissue response can occur without the structural shift. Evidence does suggest that events within the biosphere after drug association with the receptor are the principal regulatory variables of the response onset-offset time course.[69] An additional theory of drug action is referred to as the two-state model. In this model, the receptor is thought to exist in equilibrium between either an activated or inactivated state. Constitutively active receptors can exist and are shifted toward the activated state even though no agonist or ligand is present. Receptors for benzodiazepines, cannabinoids, and serotonin are examples. Agonists shift the equilibrium toward activation. Antagonists freeze the equilibrium, and inverse agonists shift the equilibrium toward inactivation.[76,77] The two-state model is shown in Fig. 5.9.

Until recently, the terms *drug absorption*, *distribution*, and *elimination* were used solely to describe the tissue-response time course.[78] However, the response may be more complex than was originally thought. It is now known that drug delivery sufficient to occupy 1% of the receptors is in many instances all that is required for a maximum tissue response to occur. Furthermore, the synthesis and destruction of receptor proteins occur at a much more rapid rate than was previously believed—within minutes rather than days. Receptor up-regulation and down-regulation can occur during drug infusion, with new receptor protein being synthesized in response to availability of free unbound drug.[27,28,79,80]

DRUG ANTAGONISM

Pure Antagonists

Pure pharmacologic antagonist drugs are similar in molecular structure to their corresponding agonist drugs. However, owing to the addition or subtraction of one or more chemical moieties, they are unable to initiate the receptor protein conformational shift necessary for eliciting a tissue response. Such antagonist drugs have receptor affinity but lack intrinsic activity or efficacy.

Antagonists that possess the property of weak affinity for the same receptor protein (e.g., atropine, esmolol) are competitive and may be displaced by an agonist. Noncompetitive antagonists, such as

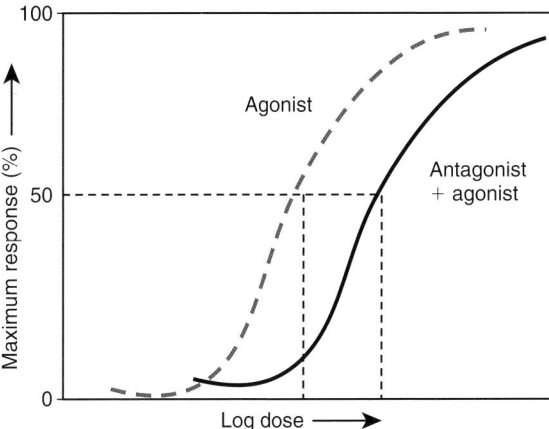

Fig. 5.10 A logarithmic dose-response curve that shows an agonist drug response alone *(dashed line)* and in the presence of an antagonist drug *(solid line)*.

phenoxybenzamine and aspirin, have a strong affinity for the receptor protein, usually via covalent bonds, and cannot be displaced by the agonist.[81] New receptor protein must be synthesized if agonist receptor complexing is to occur.[80,81] As with agonist drugs, not all receptors are bound by antagonists. Antagonists cause a rightward shift in the drug dose response curve. The extent of rightward shift reflects the number of available receptors occupied by the antagonist drug (Fig. 5.10). Comparison of the ED_{50} in Fig. 5.10 shows a reduced affinity of the agonist for its receptor when the antagonist is present.

Agonist-Antagonists

Agonist-antagonists are the second major type of antagonist drugs.[25] As the name implies, agonist-antagonist drugs have receptor protein affinity and intrinsic activity, but often only a fraction of the potency of the pure agonist. Narcotic antagonists are often of the mixed agonist-antagonist type, such as nalbuphine. The mechanism by which agonist-antagonist drugs elicit less of a tissue response is not fully understood. An incomplete receptor protein conformational shift has been suggested.

TABLE 5.2 Drug Interaction Terminology

Drug Interaction	Explanation	Viewed as an Equation
Addition	The combined effect of two drugs acting via the same mechanism is equal to that expected by simple addition of their individual actions. EXAMPLE: midazolam plus diazepam There are infrequent types of interactions such as infraadditive, when the combined effect of both drugs is less than the sum of the effects of either drug alone. Nitrous oxide and sevoflurane have been suggested to be infraadditive.	1 + 1 = 2
Synergism	The combined effect of two drugs is greater than the algebraic sum of their individual effects. EXAMPLE: midazolam plus propofol	1 + 1 = 3
Potentiation	The enhancement of the action of one drug by a second drug that has no detectable action of its own. EXAMPLE: penicillin plus probenecid	1 + 0 = 3
Antagonism	The action of one drug opposes the action of another. EXAMPLE: fentanyl plus naloxone	1 + 1 = 0

Physiologic Antagonism

Physiologic antagonism, another form of antagonism, involves two agonist drugs that bind to different receptors.[27] For competitive antagonism, the agonist and antagonist have affinity for the same receptor protein; in contrast, in physiologic antagonism, both drugs bind to specific unrelated receptor proteins, initiate a protein conformational shift, and elicit individual tissue responses. The responses, however, generate opposing forces such as are observed with isoproterenol-induced vasodilation and norepinephrine-induced vasoconstriction. The net effect on blood pressure is less than it would be if either drug were used by itself. The drug response that predominates depends on the intrinsic activity of each and on the extent of the tissue response that can be elicited.

Chemical Antagonism

Chemical antagonism occurs when a drug's action is blocked, and no receptor activity is involved. For example, protamine is a positively charged protein that forms an ionic bond with heparin, thus rendering it inactive. Sugammadex, mentioned previously, is another example.

Receptor Regulation and Adaptation

Receptors not only initiate regulation of physiologic and biochemical functions but also are themselves subject to many regulatory and homeostatic controls. These controls include regulation of the synthesis and degradation of the receptor by multiple mechanisms, covalent modification, association with other regulatory proteins, and/or relocation within the cell. Modulating inputs may come from other receptors, directly or indirectly, and receptors are almost always subject to feedback regulation by their own signaling outputs.

Continued stimulation of cells with agonists generally results in a state of desensitization, also referred to as refractoriness or down-regulation, such that the effect that follows continued or subsequent exposure to the same concentration of drug is diminished. This phenomenon is very important in therapeutic situations; an example is attenuated response to

BOX 5.2 Anesthetic Drug Combinations

- Inhalation agents when combined are strictly additive, suggesting a common mechanism of action. The exception is nitrous oxide, which has an infraadditive interaction with other inhalation agents.
- Interactions between various intravenous drugs and inhalation agents are synergistic except for nitrous oxide and γ-aminobutyric acid (GABA) sedative hypnotics.
- Interactions between different classes of intravenous drugs such as opioids and sedative hypnotics are also primarily synergistic, except for ketamine and benzodiazepines.

Adapted from Hendrickx JF, Eger II EI, Sonner JM, et al. Is synergy the rule? A review of anesthetic interactions producing hypnosis and immobility. *Anesth Analg.* 2008;107(2):494-506; Lederer S, Dijkstra TMH, Heskes T. Additive dose response models: defining synergy. *Front Pharmacol.* 2019;10:1384; Niu B, Xiao JY, Fang Y, et al. Sevoflurane-induced isoelectric EEG and burst suppression: differential and antagonistic effect of added nitrous oxide. *Anaesthesia.* 2017;72(5):570-579.

the repeated use of β-adrenergic agonists as bronchodilators for the treatment of asthma. Clinically the patient experiences tolerance; increasing doses are required to achieve the same effect.

Chronic administration of an antagonist results in up-regulation as the number and sensitivity of the receptors increase as a response to chronic blockade. Again, the patient develops tolerance, requiring higher doses of the antagonist to counteract the increasing receptor number.

Drug Interaction Terminology

A drug interaction is an alteration in the therapeutic action of a drug by concurrent administration of other drugs or exogenous substances. The common classification is given in Table 5.2.[82] Some drug interactions among the commonly combined anesthetic drugs have been proposed (Box 5.2).

SUMMARY

The pharmacologic principles described in this chapter are essential to understanding drug responses in patients. The drug-receptor subunit site is the primary regulator of onset-offset drug response. More and more evidence suggests that individual genetic variation in receptor proteins accounts for drug-response variation within seemingly normal populations. In clinical anesthesia, the range of patient responses to a given drug dose reflects this variation. The trend toward dosing by titration with rapid onset and offset

anesthetic drugs minimizes the response variability factor by optimizing the use of available receptor proteins.[83] The age-related decline in anesthetic drug dose needed to achieve a desired anesthetic endpoint is related to a change in both pharmacodynamics and pharmacokinetics.

The anesthetist uses pharmacologic intervention to elicit a desired patient response. The site of the intervention is the biosphere, or the protein drug receptor, which is the primary regulator of the therapeutic response.

BOX 5.3   Pharmacodynamic Concepts

- **Agonist:** A substance that binds to a specific receptor and triggers a response in the cell. It mimics the action of an endogenous ligand (such as hormone or neurotransmitter) that binds to the same receptor. In adequate concentrations, it can cause maximal activation of all receptors (a full agonist).
- **Antagonists:** A drug that has affinity for the receptor but no efficacy. It does not activate the receptor to produce a physiologic action. By occupying the receptor, it may block an endogenous chemical response, thereby producing a physiologic consequence. Antagonists commonly have a higher affinity for a given receptor than do agonists. Types of antagonism include pharmacologic, in which competitive is reversible and noncompetitive is irreversible, requiring syntheses of new receptors to reestablish homeostasis. Pharmacokinetic, chemical, and physiologic antagonism may also occur.
- **Affinity or potency:** When considering agonists, the term *potency* is used to differentiate between different agonists that activate the same receptor, and can all produce the same maximal response (efficacy) but at differing concentrations. The most potent drug of a series requires the lowest dose.
- **Efficacy or intrinsic activity:** The efficacy of a drug is its ability to produce the desired response expected by stimulation of a given receptor population. It refers to the maximum possible effect that can be achieved with the drug. The term *intrinsic activity* is often used instead of efficacy, although this more accurately describes the relative maximum effect obtained when comparing compounds in a series.
- **Partial agonist:** Activates a receptor but cannot produce a maximum response. It may also be able to partially block the effects of full agonists. It is postulated that partial agonists possess both agonist and antagonist properties, thus the term *agonist-antagonist* has been used. A partial agonist has a lower efficacy than a full agonist.
- **Inverse agonist:** A drug or endogenous chemical that binds to a receptor, resulting in the opposite action of an agonist. Using the two-state model, they appear to bind preferentially to the inactivated receptor. They may have a theoretic advantage over antagonists in situations in which a disease state is partly due to an up-regulation of receptor activity.
- **Spare receptor concept:** The relationship between the number of receptors stimulated and the response is usually nonlinear. A maximal or almost maximal response can often be produced by activation of only a fraction of the receptors present. A good example can be found in the neuromuscular junction. Occupation of more than 70% of the nicotinic cholinergic muscle receptors by an antagonist is necessary before there is a reduction in response, implying that a maximal response is obtained by activation of only 30% of the total number of receptors.
- **Tolerance:** Individual variation can result in a situation in which an increasing concentration of drug is required to produce a given response. This usually results from its chronic exposure to the agonist. Very rapid development of tolerance, frequently with acute drug administration, is referred to as *tachyphylaxis*. The underlying mechanism may not be clear. Common causes include up- or down-regulation, enzyme induction, depleted neurotransmitter, protein conformational changes, and changes in gene expression.
- **Ligand:** In biochemistry, a ligand is a molecule that binds and forms a complex with a receptor to produce a biologic response. Ligands are endogenous chemicals such as neurotransmitters and hormones that are exogenously administered drugs.
- **Quantal drug response:** Using dose response curves, the actions of a drug can be quantified and expressed as the effective dose ED_{50}, toxic dose TD_{50}, and lethal dose LD_{50}. The therapeutic index is the LD_{50}/ED_{50}.
- **Receptor adaptation or homeostasis:** The number and activity of a receptor population may increase or decrease in response to (usually) chronic drug administration. Up-regulation is the process by which a cell increases the number of receptors to a given drug. Down-regulation is the process by which a cell decreases the number of receptors for a given drug in response to chronic stimulation. β-Adrenergic receptors, for example, up-regulate in the presence of antagonists and down-regulate in the presence of agonists.
- **Tachyphylaxis:** Acute tolerance; the rapid appearance of a progressive decrease in response to a given dose of a drug after continuous or repetitive administration.
- **Efficacy:** The ability of a drug to produce a desired effect or the maximum response. Efficacy is the magnitude of response with respect to the given dose.
- **Ceiling effect:** Refers to the drug dose beyond which there is no increase in effect. Additional dosing often leads to adverse effects.
- **Therapeutic window:** The dosage range of a drug that provides safe, effective therapy with minimal adverse effects.
- **Effect-site concentration:** A mathematically derived virtual location where an anesthetic drug exerts its effect.

Observed variation in patient drug response reflects the functionality of the biosphere and genetics, in addition to physiologic variability.

The mean, median, and mode typically describe the dose-response relationship of a "normally distributed" population. In anesthesia, the patient population is rarely "normal." The drug response of population subsets can be expected to vary around the mean dosage. The trend toward dose titration by infusion allows individualization of the desired drug response, with fewer resultant overresponses and underresponses. The SD, SEM, and median effective dose provide a description of a population's response to a drug. Such descriptors provide only an approximate dosage; the clinician must adjust this dosage for each patient to achieve the desired physiologic response. Viewed at the molecular level, the observed response to a drug represents countless individual drug responses at the biosphere. Each drug-receptor interaction at the protein receptor elicits a fractional tissue response, and the sum of the fractional responses provides the observed response. In accordance with the law of mass action, when free drug binds to a receptor, a conformational shift occurs in the receptor protein. This shift causes a central space or channel to open, allowing specific ions to enter or leave the cell or a G protein to be activated, resulting in a biochemical cascade yielding pharmacologic effects. The resultant tissue response continues until the drug dissociates from the receptor. Antagonist drugs also bind to the receptor but lack the ability to initiate the required protein conformational shift. The sum of fractional tissue responses elicited when an antagonist is present is inadequate for maintaining the desired tissue response. Some common pharmacodynamic concepts are given in Box 5.3.

Molecular pharmacology is identifying site-specific and age-related causes for the observed variation in patient drug response. The fact that we can now sequence and clone many of the receptors and other proteins responsible for a drug's action is rapidly increasing our understanding of pharmacologic events.

REFERENCES

For a complete list of references for this chapter, scan this QR code with any smartphone code reader app, or visit the following URL: http://booksite.elsevier.com/9780323711944/.

6

Pharmacokinetics

John J. Nagelhout

Pharmacokinetics is a term used to describe the study of the changes in the concentration of a drug during the processes of absorption, distribution, metabolism or biotransformation, and elimination from the body. Essentially, it is the study of what the body does to a drug once the medication has been introduced into the system. The knowledge of this discipline is important to understanding the time course and disposition of the anesthetic drugs and the variability of responses from patient to patient. Knowledge of pharmacokinetic concepts is vital for the delivery of serum concentrations that will result in desired effects while minimizing side effects.

Regardless of the route of administration, the vascular system delivers the drug to various tissues. Therefore most kinetic concepts revolve around assessment of blood level over time, even if the correlation with the amount of drug at the effector site is poor. Once in the blood, the drug can either remain within the vascular system and body water, bound to proteins, or cross membranes to enter tissues. The unbound drug enters organs, muscles, fat, and (of greatest importance) the site of activity—the receptors. This transfer of drug to various sites depends on several intrinsic properties of the agent, such as molecular size, degree of ionization, lipid solubility, and protein binding. In addition to these drug properties, uptake also depends on the amount of blood flow to the tissue and the concentration gradient of the drug across membranes.

PROPERTIES THAT INFLUENCE PHARMACOKINETIC ACTIVITY

Molecular Size

The smaller the molecular size of an agent, the better it crosses the lipid barriers and membranes of tissues. When a drug is administered, it must be absorbed across biologic membranes that have very small openings or pores. Generally, molecules with molecular weights greater than 100 to 200 do not cross the cell membranes. Transport across the membranes can occur passively or actively. Passive transport does not require energy and involves transfer of a drug from an area of high concentration to an area of lower concentration. Active transport mechanisms are generally faster and require energy. This transport system uses carriers that form complexes with drug molecules on the membrane surface and can involve movement of the drug molecule against a concentration gradient from an area of low concentration to an area of high concentration.[1] Fig. 6.1 depicts the movement of a drug across cell membranes.

Drug Transporters

Many cell membranes possess specialized transport mechanisms that control entry and exit molecules, such as sugars, amino acids, neurotransmitters, and metal ions. They can be grouped as efflux or uptake transporters depending on the direction in which they flux their drug substrates through membranes. Efflux transporters drive their substrates out of cells, whereas uptake transporters transfer them into cells. Transporters may belong to the ABC (adenosine triphosphate [ATP]–binding cassette), the SLC (solute carrier) transporter, or the OST (organic solute transporter) families.[2,3]

The SLCs control passive movement of solutes down their electrochemical gradient. The ABCs are active pumps requiring energy derived from ATP. Over 300 human genes are believed to code these transporters, most of which act on endogenous substrates; however, some drugs are also transported. Other SLCs are coupled to ATP-dependent ion pumps, and transport can occur against an electrochemical gradient. It may involve exchange of one molecule for another, which is called antiport or transport of two molecules together in the same direction, referred to as symport. The main sites where SLCs, including organic cation transporters (OCTs) and organic anion transporters (OATs), are important are the blood-brain barrier, gastrointestinal (GI) tract, renal tubule, biliary tract, and placenta. Drug transporters are recognized as key players in the pharmacokinetic processes. Transporter proteins have a unique gatekeeper function in controlling drug access to metabolizing enzymes and excretory pathways. This can affect bioavailability, clearance, volume of distribution, and half-life for orally dosed drugs. A classification model referred to as the *Biopharmaceutics Drug Disposition Classification System (BDDCS)* categorizes drug transporter effects.[4,5]

Degree of Ionization and Lipid Solubility

Most drugs are salts of either weak acids or weak bases. When introduced into the body, they behave as a chemical in solution. As acids or bases they exist in solutions in both ionized and nonionized forms. The charged (ionized) form is water soluble, and the uncharged (nonionized) form is lipid soluble. Because the nonionized molecules are lipophilic, they can diffuse across cell membranes such as the blood-brain, gastric, and placental barriers to reach the effect site. On the other hand, the ionized molecules are usually unable to penetrate lipid cell membranes easily because of their low lipid solubility. This results from the electric charges exerted by the ionized drug molecules. These charged drugs are repelled by those sections of the cell membranes with similar charges, preventing their diffusion across the membrane.[1] The higher the degree of ionization, the less access the drug has across tissues such as the GI tract, the blood-brain and placental barriers, liver hepatocytes, and renal reabsorptive membranes. This is important in that ionized drugs are not absorbed well when taken orally and may not be metabolized by the liver to a significant extent. Instead, they are commonly excreted via the renal system.[6]

Whether acidic or basic, the degree of ionization of an agent at a particular site is determined by the dissociation constant (pK_a) of the agent and its pH gradient across the membrane. The pK_a is the negative log of the equilibrium constant for the dissociation of the acid or base.

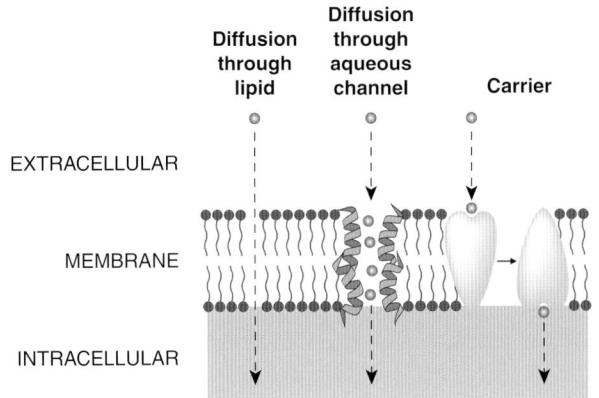

Fig. 6.1 Routes by which solutes can traverse cell membranes. (From Ritter JM, Flower R, Henderson G, et al., eds. *Rang & Dale's Pharmacology*. 9th ed. Edinburgh: Elsevier; 2020:118.)

The relationship between the pK$_a$ of the drug and the pH of the solution may be expressed by two equations. The first equation applies to drugs that are basic in nature:

$$pK_a - pH = \log\frac{(HA^+)}{(A^-)}$$

The second equation applies to acidic drugs:

$$pK_a - pH = \log\frac{(A^-)}{(HA^+)}$$

From these equations, an estimate of the degree of drug absorption can be developed.[6,7] Acids are usually defined as proton donors, whereas bases are made up of molecules that can accept a proton. When the pH is equal to the pK$_a$, the two species exist in equal amounts; for example, because phenobarbital has a pK$_a$ of 7.4 and blood has a pH of 7.4, in the bloodstream the drug is present in equal proportions of charged and uncharged forms.

It is important to note that relatively modest changes in the pH of the environment, when it is close to the pK$_a$, are more significant in changing the ratio of charged to uncharged forms than the same change in pH at some value far removed from the pK$_a$. For example, phenobarbital, with a pK$_a$ of 7.4, is for the most part nondissociated and therefore is nonionized at a pH of 1.4. This results from the fact that the pH is well below the pK$_a$, and when phenobarbital is in a relatively strongly acidic environment with an abundance of protons, it does not give up its protons readily. If a drug is a weak acid and if the pH of the fluid environment is below the pK$_a$, most of the drug's protons are associated with the drug molecule, and the predominant species is uncharged and therefore lipid soluble. Conversely, if the pH is below the pK$_a$ for a drug that is a weak base, an abundance of protons exists, and most of the drug tends to ionize as the proton is donated by the drug molecule, which results in a species that is highly charged and therefore lipid insoluble.[6] The effects of pK$_a$ and pH on ionization are summarized in Box 6.1.[8] The pH ranges in various body compartments are noted in Box 6.2.

Ion Trapping

Ion trapping has several anesthesia-related applications. Influences on oral absorption of drugs, maternal-fetal transfer, and central nervous system toxicity of local anesthetics are commonly cited. The degree of ionization for a specific agent can vary across a membrane that separates fluids with different pH values. For example, morphine sulfate, a base with a pK$_a$ of 7.9 when present in the blood (pH 7.4), exists in appreciable amounts in both ionized and nonionized forms. The uncharged drug fraction moves freely across tissue membranes, and the charged fraction does not. As the drug enters the stomach, a

BOX 6.1 Relationship Among pH, pK$_a$, and Ionization for Weak Acids and Weak Bases*

Weak Acids
- If the pK$_a$ – pH is ≥1 and the pH is lower than the pK$_a$, then the drug is essentially 100% nonionized and in a lipid-soluble form. It will easily cross biologic membranes.
- If the pH – pK$_a$ is ≥1 and the pH is higher than the pK$_a$, then the drug is essentially 100% ionized and in a water-soluble form. It will not cross biologic membranes.

Weak Bases
- If the pK$_a$ – pH is ≥1 and the pH is lower than the pK$_a$, then the drug is essentially 100% ionized and in a water-soluble form. It will not cross biologic membranes.
- If the pH – pK$_a$ is ≥1 and the pH is higher than the pK$_a$, then the drug is essentially 100% nonionized and in a lipid-soluble form. It will easily cross biologic membranes.

For Both Weak Acids and Weak Bases
- If the pK$_a$ – pH is <1, regardless of whether the pH is lower or higher than the pK$_a$, the drug will be partially ionized (water soluble) and partially nonionized (lipid soluble), and if the dose is adequate, the nonionized fraction can cross biologic membranes.

*Rule of thumb for determining ionization: Use absolute values for all calculations.

BOX 6.2 pH of Select Body Fluids

Fluids	pH
Gastric juice	1.0–3.0
Small intestine: duodenum	5.0–6.0
Small intestine: ileum	7–8
Large intestine	7–8
Plasma	7.4
Cerebrospinal fluid	7.3
Urine	4.0–8.0

very acidic environment with a pH of 1.9, morphine accepts protons and becomes ionized, and ion trapping occurs.[6] (Fig. 6.2 illustrates this phenomenon using diazepam as an example.) The drug, however, will be absorbed later, as stomach contents move farther down the GI tract to the more basic and favorable environment of the small intestine.

A similar scenario occurs when agents are transferred between a mother and a fetus, where the placenta is the membrane separating fluids with varying pH values—that of the fetus is more acidic than that of the mother. Again, the lipid-soluble fraction of basic agents such as lidocaine (pK$_a$ 7.9) crosses to the placenta easily. However, once there, because of the lower pH of the fetus, the drug becomes more ionized and cannot easily cross the lipid bilayer of placenta, resulting in accumulation of drug in the fetus. Finally, ion trapping may occur in a local anesthetic overdose situation in which high concentrations of a basic local anesthetic agent have entered the central nervous system and caused toxicity. If the patient experiences respiratory arrest and hypoxia, the resulting acidosis may trap the drug in the brain, resulting in prolonged and possibly more intense toxicity. Ion trapping also plays a role in the use of bicarbonate solutions and carbonated local anesthetics. A discussion of the effects of ion trapping on local anesthetics can be found in Box 10.2.[9,10]

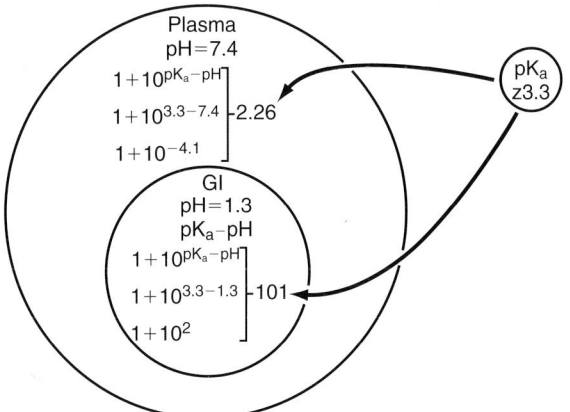

Fig. 6.2 For both weak acids and weak bases, the total concentration of a drug is greater on the side of the membrane where it is more highly ionized. Diazepam, a basic drug with a pK_a of 3.3, is more ionized at gastric pH than it is in plasma. Consequently, it has a greater total concentration in the gastrointestinal (GI) compartment than it does in the plasma.

Protein Binding

Changes in protein binding have long been theorized to influence a drug's clinical effect. Two situations are commonly cited. The first involves a patient with a reduction in proteins, such as that which occurs with severe liver or kidney disease, with protein deficiencies caused by poor nutrition, and during the last trimester of pregnancy, when fluid shifts alter distribution volume. The second situation involves a drug interaction between two or more highly protein-bound drugs.

Potential clinical changes are conceptualized by the following phenomena. Some drugs are bound extensively to proteins in the plasma because of their innate affinity for circulating and tissue proteins. The drug-protein molecule is too large to diffuse through blood vessel membranes and is therefore trapped within the circulatory system. Albumin is quantitatively the most abundant plasma protein, and although it is capable of binding basic, neutral, or acidic drugs, it favors acidic compounds. Two other proteins, α_1-acid glycoprotein (AAG) and β-globulin, favor binding to basic drugs.[11] Lipoproteins bind cyclosporine, and transcortin binds corticosteroids. Protein binding influences how a drug is distributed because a protein-bound drug is not free to act on receptors. High protein binding prevents the drug from leaving the blood to enter tissue, which results in high plasma concentrations. The degree of protein binding for a drug is proportional to its lipid solubility such that the more lipid soluble an agent, the more highly protein bound it tends to be (Box 6.3).[12]

The number of potential binding sites on plasma proteins for drugs is finite; therefore the kinetics for binding behaves like any saturable process in that protein binding can be overcome by adding more agents.[4] The bond between drug and protein is usually weak, and they can dissociate when the plasma concentration of the drug declines or a second drug that binds to the same protein is introduced. For example, when a drug has been in chronic use and is at a steady state, an equilibrium will be reached between free and protein-bound drugs. If a new drug with a high affinity for the same protein sites is introduced, the new drug competes with the chronic drug for binding sites. This leads to displacement of the first drug with an increase in free fraction of that agent. It is important to note that the displaced free drug does become available for biotransformation and elimination, so unless these clearance mechanisms are at capacity, a rise in free fraction will lead to a small change in free plasma concentrations.

Protein binding is expressed in terms of the percentage of total drug bound. Drugs with protein binding greater than 90%, such as warfarin, phenytoin, propranolol, propofol, fentanyl and its analogs, and diazepam, are conceptualized to have an unexpected intensification of their effect if they are displaced from plasma proteins.[13] Drugs that exhibit less than 90% binding have so little change in free active fractions that they are not a concern. The anticoagulant warfarin is commonly used as an example. Because warfarin is approximately 98% bound to plasma proteins, a reduction in bound fraction to 96% causes an increase in the free active fraction of the drug. Furthermore, when hypoalbuminemia exists, decreased albumin levels result in the availability of a greater amount of free drug. These theoretic concerns are rarely clinically relevant, as explained subsequently.

No clinically relevant examples of changes in drug disposition or effects can be clearly ascribed to changes in plasma protein binding. The idea that a drug displaced from plasma proteins increases the unbound drug concentration, increases the drug effect, and perhaps produces toxicity seems a simple and obvious mechanism. Unfortunately, this simple theory, which is appropriate for a test tube, does not work in the body, which is an open system capable of eliminating unbound drugs.[14]

First, a seemingly dramatic change in the unbound fraction from 1% to 10% releases less than 5% of the total amount of drug in the body into the unbound pool because less than one-third of the drug in the body is bound to plasma proteins, even in the most extreme cases (e.g., when warfarin is used). Drug displaced from plasma protein, of course, distributes throughout the volume of distribution, so a 5% increase in the amount of unbound drug in the body produces at most a 5% increase in the pharmacologically active unbound drug at the site of action.

Second, when the amount of unbound drug in plasma increases, the rate of elimination increases (if unbound clearance is unchanged), and, after four half-lives, the unbound concentration returns to its previous steady-state value. When drug interactions associated with protein binding displacement and clinically important effects have been studied, it has been found that the displacing drug is also an inhibitor of clearance, and it is the change in clearance of the unbound drug that is the relevant mechanism explaining the interaction.

The clinical application of plasma protein binding is only to help interpretation of measured drug concentrations. When plasma proteins are lower than normal, total drug concentrations are lowered, but unbound concentrations are not affected.[1]

TABLE 6.1 Routes of Administration

Route	Bioavailability (%)	Comments
Intravenous	100 (by definition)	Most rapid onset; allows for titration of doses; suitable for large volumes
Intramuscular	75 to 100	Moderate volumes feasible; may be painful
Subcutaneous	75 to 100	Smaller volumes than intramuscular; may be painful; suitable for implantation of pellets
Oral	5 to 100	Most convenient and economical; first-pass effect may be significant; requires patient cooperation
Rectal	30 to 100	Less first-pass effect than oral; useful in pediatric patients
Inhalation	5 to 100	Common anesthetic use for inhalation drugs, steroids, bronchodilators, and occasionally resuscitative drugs; very rapid onset (parallels intravenous administration)
Sublingual	60 to 100	Lack of first-pass effect; absorbed directly into systemic circulation
Intrathecal	Low (intentionally)	Specialized application, as with local anesthetics and analgesics, chemotherapy, and antibiotic administration; circumvents blood-brain barrier
Topical	80 to 100	Includes skin, cornea, buccal, vaginal, and nasal mucosa; dermal application results in slow absorption; used for lack of first-pass effect; prolonged duration of action
Intranasal	Up to 95	Rich vascular plexus provides a direct route into the blood; best for lipid soluble agents; mist or atomized formulation is most effective; 0.25–0.3 mL ideal or up to <1 mL of highly concentrated preparation; avoids gastrointestinal destruction and first-pass metabolism; may rapidly achieve therapeutic brain and spinal cord (central nervous system) drug concentrations
Intraosseous	Up to 100 depending on site	Recommended for emergency access when an intravenous line cannot be established such as during resuscitation or in pediatrics

Absorption

Routes of Drug Administration

An important variable in the bioavailability of a drug at its effect site is the route by which the agent is administered. The route of administration determines how much of the drug is delivered to the systemic circulation. When the entire amount of drug given is delivered, the drug is said to have 100% bioavailability. Many routes of drug administration are used; each has advantages and disadvantages (Table 6.1). The routes of drug administration are enteral (involving the GI tract), parenteral (injected subcutaneously, intramuscularly, intravenously, intrathecally, or epidermally), pulmonary, and topical.[15] Absorption mechanisms of relevance to anesthesia are discussed in the following sections.

Enteral Administration. The oral route is the most common and convenient method for administration of drugs. It is relatively inexpensive, does not require a sterile technique, and can be carried out with little skill. However, several disadvantages exist because many conditions, such as emotions, physical activity, and food intake, change the GI environment. Thus orally administered drugs tend to have a lower bioavailability. The stomach has a large surface area, and the length of time a drug remains there is a significant factor in absorption. Because of the low pH in the stomach (1.5–2.5), drugs that are highly acidic, such as barbiturates, tend to remain nonionized and are highly absorbed. Basic drugs that remain intact in the stomach acids can pass through and are more readily absorbed in the intestine. The small intestine is highly vascular and has an alkaline environment (pH 7–8).[15]

The enteral route often results in failure of the drug to be absorbed into the systemic circulation. Alternatively, chemical alteration may occur before entry into the intestines. Presystemic elimination refers to the elimination of drug by the GI system before the drug reaches the systemic circulation. This occurs by means of three mechanisms: the stomach acids hydrolyze the drug (e.g., penicillin), enzymes in the GI wall deactivate the drug, or the liver biotransforms the ingested drug before it reaches the effect site.[6] This liver activity is called first-pass hepatic effect. Drugs absorbed from the GI tract after oral ingestion enter the portal venous blood and pass through the liver first, with subsequent delivery to the tissue receptors. In the liver, they may undergo

BOX 6.4 Drugs That Undergo Substantial First-Pass Elimination

- Aspirin
- Glyceryl trinitrate
- Hydralazine
- Levodopa
- Lidocaine
- Metoprolol
- Morphine
- Cimetidine
- Felodipine
- Verapamil
- Neostigmine
- Midazolam

extensive hepatic extraction and metabolism before they have a chance to enter the systemic circulation (Box 6.4). Agents such as these exhibit large differences between oral and intravenous dosages. To have the desired effect, oral dosages must be exaggerated to compensate for the initial metabolism that occurs before the drug reaches the effect site.

The role transporters play in drug absorption and distribution should be further clarified. The P-glycoprotein transporter is part of a larger family of efflux transporters found in the intestine, liver cells, renal proximal tubular cells, and capillary endothelial cells comprising the blood-brain barrier. Using ATP as an energy source, they transport substances against their concentration gradients. They appear to have developed as a mechanism to protect the body from harmful substances and can influence the ability of a drug to traverse barriers.

The sublingual and buccal routes of administration of drugs bypass the presystemic, portal system first-pass effect and are delivered rapidly to the superior vena cava for transport to the effect site.[1] Nitroglycerin is an example of a sublingual drug that is put under the tongue and absorbed by the rich blood supply there. If ingested, the drug would be hydrolyzed by the stomach; therefore sublingual administration is the

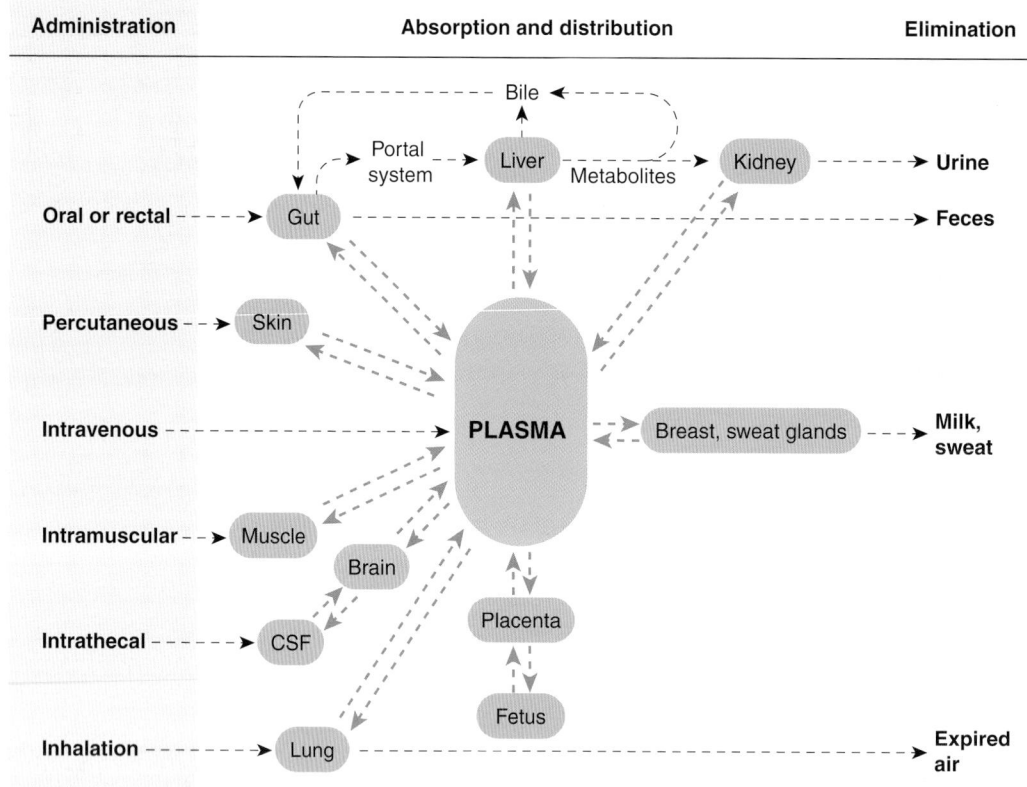

Fig. 6.3 The main routes of drug administration and elimination. *CSF,* Cerebrospinal fluid. (From Ritter JM, Flower R, Henderson G, et al. *Rang and Dale's Pharmacology.* 9th ed. Edinburgh: Elsevier; 2020:125.)

ideal route for this agent. Protein hormones that would also be digested by the stomach are instead placed between the gum and cheek (buccal administration) and enter venous drainage without undergoing hepatic, presystemic elimination.[16,17]

Occasionally, the rectal route of drug administration is the ideal route for prevention of emesis caused by irritation of the GI mucosa by the drug. It is also a preferred method of drug delivery for patients in whom oral ingestion poses difficulty. For example, rectal acetaminophen is administered to infants and young children undergoing general anesthesia for postoperative pain control. Drugs placed in the proximal rectum are absorbed into the portal system via the superior hemorrhoidal vein. They will therefore undergo significant first-pass effect in the liver before entering the systemic circulation, leading to unpredictable responses.[1] Conversely, agents placed in the distal rectum do not undergo presystemic elimination and therefore have more predictable circulatory levels. The disadvantage historically associated with this route was the unpredictability of drug retention and absorption because of rectal contents. However, studies carried out in 2010 have demonstrated that regardless of enema volume, agents are absorbed with consistent plasma concentrations within subjects.[18]

Parenteral Administration. Parenteral administration refers to administration by injection. The most rapid and predictable route to the systemic circulation is the parenteral route. With intramuscular injections, the drug is instilled deep into the muscle among the muscle fascicles.[6] Subcutaneous agents are placed under the skin. With both intramuscular and subcutaneous injections, the systemic absorption of the drug is dependent on the capillary blood flow to the area and the lipid solubility of the agent.[1] Conversely, intravenous injections allow for rapid and accurate delivery of a drug into the systemic circulation. Parenteral administration is the route of choice for anesthetists because it is an exact method of achieving the desired effect from agents delivered.

Pulmonary Administration. The lungs provide a large surface area for drugs administered by inhalation. Bronchodilators and antibiotics are administered via devices such as nebulizers, used to propel aerosols into the alveolar sacs.[18] Anesthetic gases are also effectively administered through the lungs, as described in detail in Chapter 7.

Transdermal (Topical) Administration. The transdermal route is usually chosen for administration of a sustained release agent, providing the patient with a steady therapeutic plasma concentration. Drugs that are administered via this route must possess several characteristics. They usually exist in a combined form; they are both water soluble and lipid soluble. The water solubility is necessary so the drug can penetrate the hair follicles and sweat ducts. Once in the system, the drug must be lipid soluble to traverse the skin and exert effect at the receptors. These agents must have a molecular weight of less than 1000, dose requirements less than 10 mg in a 24-hour period, and a pH of 5 to 9.[1] The area to which the drug is applied must have a relatively thin epidermis with a sufficient blood supply (Fig. 6.3).

Bioavailability

Bioavailability is the extent to which a drug reaches its effect site after its introduction into the body. The rate at which systemic absorption occurs establishes a drug's duration of action and intensity. Many factors play a role in the bioavailability of agents, including lipid solubility, solubility in aqueous and organic solvents, molecular weight, pH, pK_a, and blood flow. For example, drugs given in aqueous solution are more rapidly absorbed than those given in oily solution or solid form because they mix more readily with the aqueous phase at the absorptive site.[19,20]

The environment into which the drug is introduced also has an impact on its bioavailability. The patient's age, sex, pathology, pH, blood flow, and temperature are all factors to consider. For example, pH plays a role when local anesthetic (a weak base) is injected into an infected wound (an acidic environment). In this instance, the local anesthetic is highly ionized (basic agent in acidic environment) and therefore cannot enter the lipid nerve membrane to reach the site of action.

The first-pass effect, which is also referred to as first-pass hepatic metabolism or presystemic metabolism, may occur when a drug is administered orally or, to a lesser extent, rectally. Metabolism occurs in the intestinal wall or the liver prior to the drug entering the systemic circulation. Venous drainage from most portions of the GI tract enters the portal circulation to the liver, which may metabolize a drug, thus reducing the amount available for systemic release.

Therefore the first pass through the liver greatly reduces the bioavailability of the drug. Drugs with a high first-pass effect require a much larger oral dose than sublingual or intravenous doses. Four enzyme systems that are associated with the first-pass effect are located in the GI lumen, gut wall, intestinal bacteria, and liver.[21] Bioavailability ranges with different administration routes are shown in Table 6.1.

Some drugs require metabolism to the active form before a clinical effect is seen. These drugs are administered as prodrugs and are converted from inactive to active form in the liver. This is usually done to improve some selected property of the molecule, such as water solubility or lipid solubility, to improve either absorption or distribution. Common prodrugs include dolasetron, amlodipine, levodopa, and quinapril.[22,23] Some important concepts influencing absorption are listed in Box 6.5.

Distribution

Compartment Models
Compartment models depict the body as composed of distinct sections that represent theoretic spaces with calculated volumes and are used to describe the pharmacokinetics of agents. These models are useful for prediction of serum concentrations and changes in drug concentrations in other tissues. A single-compartment model represents the entire body, through which homogeneous distribution occurs (Fig. 6.4A). Although a one-compartment model is sufficient to describe the

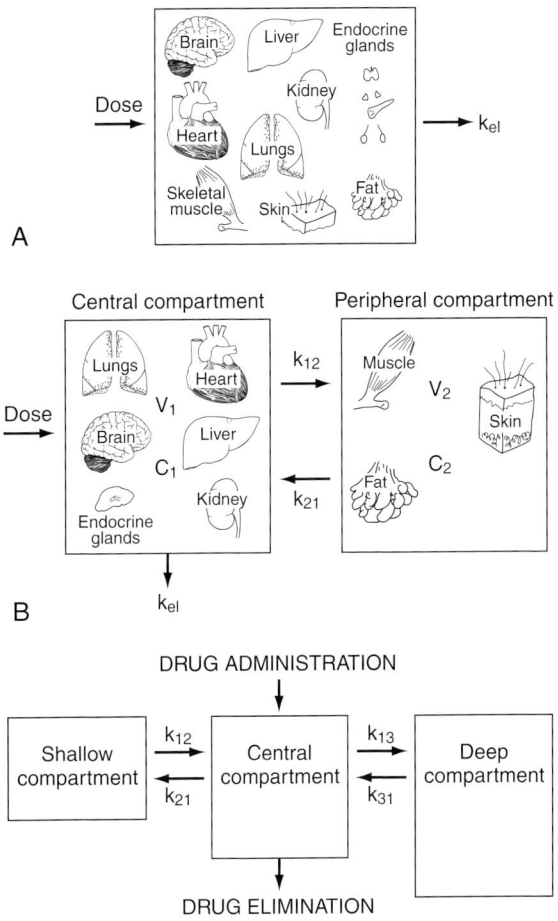

Fig. 6.4 (A) In the one-compartment model, a drug instantaneously and homogeneously is distributed throughout the fluids and tissues that constitute the compartment. When changes in drug concentration occur in any of these tissues, a corresponding quantitative change occurs in drug concentration in all the other tissues. (B) In the two-compartment model, the body is assumed to be made up of two compartments: a central compartment (C_1) made up of a small apparent volume (V_1) and a peripheral compartment (C_2) made up of a larger apparent volume (V_2). (C) The three-compartment model is depicted as having a central compartment into which the drug is administered and two peripheral compartments to which reversible drug distribution occurs. k_{12}, Rate of distribution of drugs to the peripheral compartment; k_{21}, rate of redistribution of drugs back to the central compartment; k_{el}, rate of drug removal or elimination from the body; k_{13}, rate of distribution of drugs from the central compartment to a shallow peripheral compartment; k_{31}, rate of distribution of drugs from the shallow peripheral compartment back to the central compartment (see text for further explanation).

action of many drugs, it is generally insufficient to explain the kinetics of lipid-soluble anesthetic drugs. A two-compartment model is typically used to simplify and explain pharmacokinetic concepts that can be extrapolated to more complex models.[24]

In the two-compartment model, the first compartment is termed the *central compartment* and is composed of intravascular fluid and the highly perfused tissues such as the heart, lungs, brain, liver, and kidneys (see Fig. 6.4B). The central compartment represents only approximately 10% of body mass in an adult; however, it receives approximately 75% of the cardiac output and is also referred to as the vessel-rich group. The peripheral compartment (vessel-poor group) is composed of muscle, fat, and bone and represents 90% of body mass. This second compartment receives approximately 25% of the cardiac

TABLE 6.2	**Tissue Groups Based on Perfusion***			
Characteristic	Vessel Rich	Muscle	Fat	Vessel Poor
Percentage of body weight	10	50	20	20
Percentage of cardiac output	75	19	6	0
Perfusion (mL/min per 100 g)	75	3	3	0

*The vessel-rich group represents the central compartment, and the muscle, fat, and vessel-poor groups are peripheral compartments.

output.[24] The terms *central* and *peripheral compartments* refer to differences in the size of the compartments and the rate at which a drug is distributed to them. The compartments are not true anatomic areas, but instead are conceptual representations of two separate volumes in which a quantitative change in drug concentration occurs.[25]

Drugs leave the central compartment in two phases. Drugs leave by distribution into the tissues or via metabolism and excretion. In the initial phase, after an intravenous bolus dose, those organs with the highest blood flow have the largest amount of drug delivered to them. These highly perfused tissues equilibrate with the initial high serum concentration and attain a high concentration of drug (Table 6.2). As blood flows through the less perfused organs, the drug begins to be deposited in those tissues as well.[19] However, the tissue levels rise more slowly and do not reach as high a concentration as in the vessel-rich group or central compartment, with extraction occurring to a lesser degree. As blood flows through the tissues, serum concentrations drop because of this distribution, and the fall in plasma concentration is described mathematically via the alpha half-life.[26] When the plasma concentration falls below the tissue concentration, the drug reemerges from the highly perfused tissue, enters the plasma serum, and is again redistributed. The drug enters the central compartment for clearance from the body. The degree to which drugs distribute and redistribute from the central compartment to the peripheral compartment, and the resultant concentration of the drug established before elimination occurs, allows for the calculation of the volume of distribution.

Volume of Distribution

The volume of distribution (V_d) is a proportional expression that relates the amount of drug in the body to the serum concentration. It is the apparent volume in which the drug is distributed after it has been introduced into the system.[1] Essentially, it is calculated by dividing the dose of the drug administered intravenously by the plasma concentration before elimination occurs. The V_d is used to calculate the loading dose of a drug that will achieve a steady-state concentration.[24] In practice, a patient's V_d is unknown, and an average V_d is assumed and used to calculate a loading dose that will attain a therapeutic concentration rather than a steady-state concentration.

$$\text{Volume of distribution} = \frac{\text{Dose of drug}}{\text{Plasma concentration of drug}}$$

The theoretical compartments and volumes are envisioned as follows. The plasma compartment contains 4 L. The interstitial fluid (IF) volume contains 10 L. The extracellular fluid (ECF) volume combines the plasma and IF and therefore contains (4 + 10) or 14 L. The intracellular fluid (ICF) volume is 28 L. Total body water is equal to plasma (4 L) + IF (10 L) + ICF (28 L) = 42 L. The typical V_d, normalized for the body weight of a 70-kg adult, would be 42 L/70 kg or 0.6 L/kg. The V_d

gives one the sense of how extensively a drug distributes throughout the body. A drug with a large V_d (>0.6 L/kg) implies that it is widely distributed in the body and likely lipid soluble. A drug with a small V_d (<0.4 L/kg) is largely contained in the plasma and likely water soluble. Other factors such as size, carrier molecules, disease states, and fluid shifts associated with burn injuries or pregnancy may also alter expected distribution volumes.

The V_d of a drug is affected by the physiochemical properties of that drug, such as lipid solubility, plasma protein binding, and molecular size.[6] Drugs that are free, unbound to plasma proteins, and lipid soluble easily cross membranes to tissues and therefore have large calculated volumes of distribution with low plasma concentrations. An example of a drug with a large V_d is propofol.[1] On injection of an induction dose, this highly lipid-soluble drug is distributed quickly to peripheral tissue, thereby ending its action much more rapidly than its elimination half-life would predict. The patient wakes up in just a few minutes because of redistribution from the brain (central compartment) to the peripheral compartment; however, the patient may feel sleepy for hours because of the long elimination half-life of the drug from the whole body (11.6 hours).[6]

The V_d of a drug administered by bolus is also calculated by dividing the total dose administered by the area under the plasma concentration curve. The greater the area under the curve, the longer the drug acts and the drug intensity increases.[6] However, if the drug is infused or given in multiple doses and the amount given equals the amount eliminated, the central and peripheral compartments are in equilibrium. Therefore the V_d at this steady state would differ if the agent were given as a bolus injection.[7]

Structure-Activity Relationship

The affinity of a drug for a specific macromolecular component of the cell and its intrinsic activity are intimately related to its chemical structure.[27] The relationship is frequently quite a rigid one, in that relatively minor modifications in the drug structure may result in major changes in pharmacologic properties. In fact, manipulation of structure-activity relationships often leads to the synthesis of therapeutic agents quite varied in their therapeutic effects, as well as their side effects. Changes in molecular configuration must occur in a manner that leads to alterations of all actions and effects of a drug equally. Therefore it is sometimes possible to develop a congener with a more favorable ratio of therapeutic to toxic effects, enhanced selectivity among different cells or tissues, or more acceptable secondary characteristics than those of the parent drug.[27] Additionally, effective therapeutic agents have been developed by cultivating structurally related competitive antagonists of other drugs or of endogenous substances known to be important in biochemical or physiologic function. Minor modifications of structure can also have profound effects on the pharmacokinetic properties of drugs. The structure of a drug can therefore occasionally supersede all the previously discussed properties, and this structure is of great importance in how a drug behaves in vivo. Important considerations in structure-activity relationships are enantiomerism and isomerism.

Stereochemistry

A carbon-containing compound usually exists as stereoisomers—molecules with the same chemical bonds but different configurations in their fixed spatial arrangements. A specific configuration is achieved either by the presence of double bonds, where there is no freedom of rotation, or by chiral centers, around which varying groups are arranged in a specific sequence.[28] Chiral centers are therefore formed by a carbon atom with four different asymmetric substituents. A molecule with one chiral carbon can have two stereoisomers; however, as the number of carbons in a molecule increases, so does the number of its potential stereoisomers.

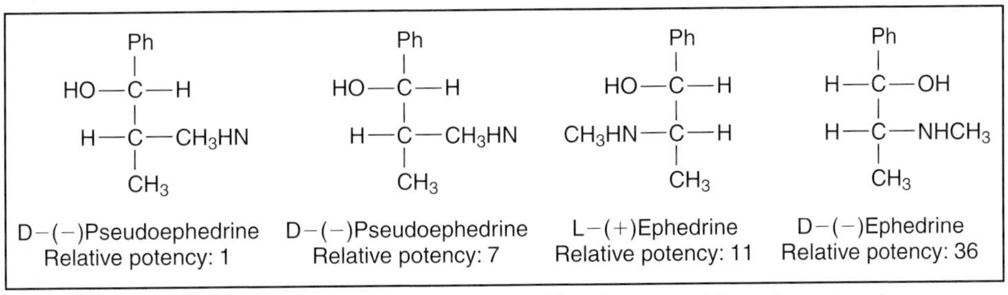

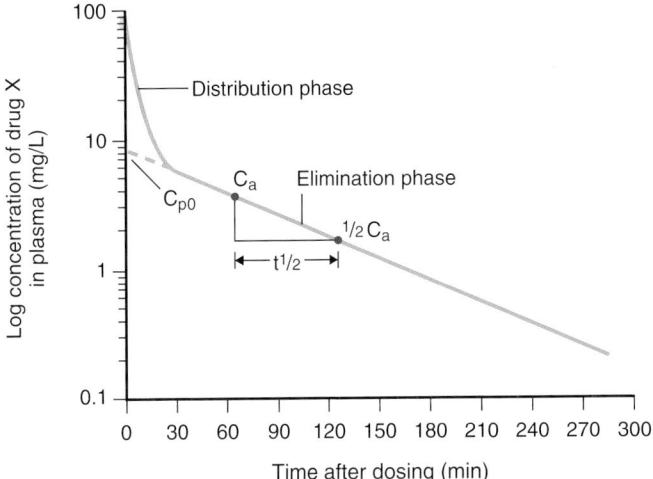

Fig. 6.5 Ephedrine has two chiral centers and four isomers with varying potencies.

Some stereoisomers are nonsuperimposable mirror images of each other called enantiomers. Free rotation about a chiral carbon is not possible, resulting in the existence of two stable forms of the molecule. Two compounds that are enantiomers of each other have the same physical properties, except for the direction in which they rotate polarized light. These concepts become important in that interactions between biomolecules are stereospecific, and interfaces with biologic receptors can differ greatly between two enantiomers, even to the point of no binding. There are numerous examples among drug molecules in which only one isomer exhibits the desired pharmacology. Some isomers may even cause side effects or entirely different effects than their mirror image.[27] For instance, D(−) ephedrine, with a relative potency of 36, is used to a large extent as an antiasthmatic and, by an anesthesia professional, as a pressor amine to restore low blood pressure in the operating arena, whereas L(+) pseudoephedrine, with a relative potency of 7, is used primarily as a nasal decongestant (Fig. 6.5). These drugs therefore have varying activities and potencies, rendering them ideal for varying situations. Cisatracurium, levobupivacaine, ropivacaine, and dexmedetomidine are additional examples of select isomers with improved clinical properties.

Plasma Concentration Curve

A schematic depiction of the decline in plasma concentration of a drug with time after rapid intravenous injection into the central compartment is plotted on a logarithmic graph in Fig. 6.6. The y-axis of the graph represents the plasma concentration, and the x-axis reflects the time after the dose is injected. The first phase of the curve is the α (or distribution) phase, which represents the initial dispersal of drug into the tissue compartments from the central compartment. This slope is usually steep with drugs that are highly lipid soluble, which demonstrates the ability of these agents to cross membrane lipid bilayers and be distributed to the peripheral compartment rapidly, leading to a rapid fall in plasma levels.[1]

The second phase of the curve is a logarithmic plot of the slower elimination, or β phase of the plasma concentration curve. Once equilibrium has been reached, the concentration falls exponentially because of elimination. This portion of the graph is much less steep and has a plateau shape, illustrating the more gradual decline in the drug's plasma concentration. The slope is flatter because it reflects the elimination of the drug from the circulation by the hepatic, renal, and other systems, which is a more gradual process. The plasma concentration curve is an example of a biexponential decay curve because two distinct components of decay exist—a steep slope that describes distribution and a second, less steep slope that depicts the elimination phase.[6]

The elimination phase of the plot is used to determine the elimination half-life of drugs, which becomes important regarding dosing intervals.

Steady State

Theoretically, a steady state occurs when a stable plasma concentration of a drug is achieved. In this instance, all body compartments will have had ample opportunity to equilibrate with the circulating agent, and although tissue concentrations of the drug vary from organ to organ,

Fig. 6.6 Representative drug concentration versus time plot used in pharmacokinetic studies. Concentration of drug is plotted with a logarithmic scale on the ordinate, and time is plotted with a linear scale on the abscissa. The resultant curve has two phases: the distribution phase, which is the initial portion of the plotted line when the concentration of drug decreases rapidly; and the later elimination phase, during which there is an exponential disappearance of drug from the plasma over time. The dotted line extrapolated from the elimination phase back to time zero is used to calculate plasma concentration at a time zero (C_{p0}). During the elimination phase, the half-life (t1/2) can be calculated as the time it takes to decrease the concentration by half (shown here as the time needed to decrease from concentration C_a to ½ C_a). (From Goldman L, Schafer AI. *Goldman-Cecil Medicine.* 26th ed. Philadelphia: Elsevier; 2020:121.)

they are not changing. At this point, drug elimination is equal to the rate at which the drug is made available, so the amount being eliminated in a given time equals the amount being added to the system at the same time.[29] This state is typically reached with chronic administration of a drug or by continuous intravenous administration. Some important distribution concepts are listed in Box 6.6.

Metabolism

Drug metabolism is synonymous with drug biotransformation. Metabolism is an enzyme-catalyzed change in the chemical structure of agents, and it usually involves more than one pathway. The main organ for drug metabolism is the liver, although metabolism can occur in the plasma, lungs, GI tract, kidneys, heart, brain, and skin. The goal of metabolism is to change lipid-soluble agents into more water-soluble forms so the kidneys can then eliminate them from the body. Metabolism usually leads to transformation of active drugs into inactive metabolites; however, numerous consequences can occur. For example, a drug can be metabolized to an active drug with the same or new activity, or an agent can be converted from an inactive prodrug to its active form, as previously noted with dolasetron.[22,23]

BOX 6.6   Drug Distribution

- The major compartments are:
  - Plasma (5% of body weight)
  - Interstitial fluid (16%)
  - Intracellular fluid (35%)
  - Transcellular fluid (2%)
  - Fat (20%)
- Volume of distribution (V_d) is defined as the volume of solvent that would contain the total body content of the drug (Q) at a concentration equal to the measured plasma concentration (C_p): $V_d = Q/C_p$.
- Lipid-insoluble drugs are mainly confined to plasma and interstitial fluids; most do not enter the brain following acute dosing.
- Lipid-soluble drugs reach all compartments and may accumulate in fat.
- For drugs that accumulate outside the plasma compartment (e.g., in fat or by being bound to tissues), V_d may exceed total body volume.

Modified from Ritter JM, Flower R, Henderson G, et al. *Rang and Dale's Pharmacology*. 9th ed. Edinburgh: Elsevier; 2020:130.

BOX 6.7   Common Anesthesia-Related Drugs That Undergo Phase 1 Hydrolysis

Pseudocholinesterase Catalyzed
- Succinylcholine
- Mivacurium
- Cocaine
- Procaine
- Chloroprocaine
- Tetracaine
- Neostigmine (partial pathway)
- Edrophonium (partial pathway)

Nonspecific Esterase Dependent
- Remifentanil
- Atracurium (partial pathway)
- Cisatracurium (partial pathway)
- Esmolol (RBC esterase)
- Aspirin
- Clevidipine

RBC, Red blood cell.

For most drugs administered in therapeutic doses, metabolism occurs as a first-order process, in that the drug is cleared at a rate proportional to the amount of drug present in the plasma. Thus a constant fraction of total drug is metabolized in a set time period. The greatest amount of drug eliminated per unit time occurs when the concentration is highest.[30]

Drugs such as alcohol undergo zero-order kinetics at therapeutic doses. This means that even at therapeutic levels, they exceed the body's ability to excrete or metabolize them. In zero-order kinetics, the available enzyme systems for elimination of drugs are saturated. For these agents, a constant amount of drug is cleared regardless of the plasma concentration, as opposed to a constant percentage as occurs with first-order kinetics. The amount of agent cleared per unit time during zero-order kinetics is the same amount, independent of its plasma concentration.

Drug metabolism occurs in two phases. Phase I reactions are oxidation, reduction, and hydrolysis reactions and generally result in increased polarity of the molecule, transforming a lipid-soluble compound to a water-soluble one. Phase II reactions involve conjugation reactions, in which a drug or metabolite is conjugated with an endogenous substrate such as glucuronic, sulfonic, or acetic acid.[31]

Phase I Reactions

Oxidation reactions generally are reactions in which oxygen is introduced into the molecule, or the oxidative state of a molecule is changed so that its relative oxygen content is increased. The molecule of oxygen is split; one atom oxidizes each molecule of drug, and the other is incorporated into a molecule of water. The loss of electrons results in oxidation. Oxidative metabolism reactions are catalyzed by the enzymes of the cytochrome P-450 system.[31] Reduction pathways of metabolism also use the cytochrome P-450 system. When insufficient amounts of oxygen are present to compete for electrons, these enzymes transfer electrons directly to a substrate rather than to oxygen. Reduction involves the gain of electrons.[32,33]

Hydrolysis is the addition of water to an ester or amide to break the bond and form two smaller molecules. Adding water to these compounds leads to an acid and alcohol, in the case of esters, and to an acid and an amine, in the case of amides. Amide drugs rarely undergo hydrolysis, even though they are formed by removing water. Steric hindrance limits the ability to add water to a drug (hydrolyze it) once the water has been removed. Examples of drugs that are hydrolyzed are listed in Box 6.7.

The result of phase I reactions is typically a more polar compound that is easily excreted by the kidneys. It is also important to note that phase I reactions, by placing hydroxy or carboxy groups on drug molecules, enable phase II reactions to occur.[1]

Phase II Reactions

Phase II reactions are also referred to as synthetic reactions because the body synthesizes a new compound by donating a functional group usually derived from an endogenous acid. The new compound is the conjugate of the drug or the drug product of the phase I reaction with either glucuronic acid, sulfuric acid, glycine, acetic acid, or a methyl group.[29]

The products of phase II reactions almost always have little or no biologic activity. Conjugation always leads to a more polar compound that is more highly ionized at physiologic pH and therefore more easily extractable by the kidney via glomerular filtration. The conjugation proceeds by joining the body's donated group (during phase I reactions) with an OH, COOH, or NH group to form an ester or amide bond. However, many drugs already possess an appropriate functional group for conjugation and therefore do not need to be modified by a prior phase I reaction to be conjugated.

Many intracellular sites exist for drug metabolizing enzymes, such as the endoplasmic reticulum, mitochondria, cytosol, lysosomes, and plasma membrane. Hepatic microsomal enzymes, responsible for biotransformation of numerous agents, reside mainly in the smooth hepatic endoplasmic reticulum. They are termed *microsomal enzymes* because microsomes are fragments of the endoplasmic reticulum that are obtained in vitro by physical disruption of the tissue and differential centrifugation. This microsomal fraction includes proteins called cytochrome (iron-containing hemoprotein) P-450, indicating its peak absorption at 450 nm, when it reacts with carbon monoxide. The cytochrome P-450 is also called the mixed-function oxidase system because it includes both oxidation and reduction steps and has low substrate specificity.[6] Some extrahepatic sites of the P-450 system exist, such as the kidneys, lungs, skin, and intestinal mucosa.

Six well-characterized forms, or isozymes, of the cytochrome P-450 system are involved in drug metabolism in humans: CYP1A2, CYP2D6, CYP2C19, CYP2E1, CYP2C9, and CYP3A.[34] The letters CYP stand for cytochrome P-450; the first number denotes the genetic family, the next letter describes the genetic subfamily, and the second number stands for the specific gene or isozyme.

It is important to note some characteristics of these isozymes. It should be appreciated that small differences in amino acid sequences of the different isozymes lead to differences in drug metabolism and account for genetic variability among individuals' abilities to metabolize agents.[34] Therefore hepatic enzyme activity varies among individuals and is determined genetically. Genetic variability exists in the expression of CYP2C19, CYP2C9, and CYP2D6 and other cytochromes. Genetic variation in the CYP2D6 enzyme, for example, leads to changes in metabolism of β-blockers, which may produce toxicity or their ultrarapid degradation, decreasing efficacy. These polymorphisms in the adrenergic signaling pathway and CYP2D6 gene may influence efficacy, safety, and toxicity of β-blocker therapy in prevention and treatment of perioperative myocardial infarction and the treatment of heart failure and other cardiac diseases.[35-37]

It is possible to increase enzyme activity by stimulating the enzymes over time. This is called enzyme induction and is usually produced by exposure to certain drug or chemical compounds. Alcohol is one such compound; when ingested chronically it induces enzymatic activity. The system can more quickly break down agents that use the same enzymatic system for biotransformation. Other drugs capable of enzyme induction include phenobarbital, phenytoin, rifampin, and carbamazepine. This increased capacity to clear drugs leads to reduction in half-lives of agents and is important regarding dosing intervals.[38,39]

Microsomal enzymes can also be inhibited. This usually occurs through exposure to certain drugs and chemicals, leading to accumulation of the substrate agent, and can cause elevated plasma levels and potentially greater activity and toxicity. For example, erythromycin inhibits the metabolism of theophylline, and cimetidine inhibits the metabolism of many drugs.[34] Box 6.8 contains a summary of important metabolic concepts. A list of cytochrome enzymes, metabolites, inducers, and inhibitors is given in Table 6.3. Some common cytochrome enzyme inducing and inhibiting drugs are listed in Tables 6.4 and 6.5, respectively.

Drug Elimination

Elimination Half-Life

The elimination half-life (t 1/2) is the time necessary for the plasma content of a drug to drop to half of its prevailing concentration after a rapid bolus injection. It takes the same amount of time to reduce a drug's concentration from 100 to 50 mg/L as it does to decrease the concentration from 10 to 5 mg/L. The amount of drug remaining in the body is related to the number of elimination half-lives that have elapsed (Table 6.6). For practical purposes, a drug is regarded as being fully eliminated when approximately 95% has been eliminated from the body. This usually occurs when four or five half-lives have elapsed and is important regarding dosing intervals because drug accumulation occurs if dosing intervals are shorter than this. The body has not been able to rid itself of the initial dose, and subsequent doses will lead to overdose and potential adverse effects. Instances can occur in which, although only 5% of the drug amount remains, it is still somewhat active; however, for most agents, four half-lives is considered sufficient time for the drug's action to be terminated and the agent eliminated from the body. As noted earlier, most drugs leave the body at a constant rate or percentage over time. This is referred to as first-order kinetics

---

BOX 6.8 Drug Metabolism

- Phase I reactions involve oxidation, reduction, and hydrolysis.
  - They usually form more chemically reactive products, which can be pharmacologically active, toxic, or carcinogenic.
  - They often involve a monooxygenase system in which cytochrome P-450 plays a key role.
- Phase II reactions involve conjugation (e.g., glucuronidation) of a reactive group (often inserted during phase I reaction) and usually lead to inactive and polar products that are readily excreted in urine.
- Some conjugated products are excreted via bile, are reactivated in the intestine, and then reabsorbed (enterohepatic circulation).
- Induction of P-450 enzymes can greatly accelerate hepatic drug metabolism. It can increase the toxicity of drugs with toxic metabolites and is an important cause of drug-drug interaction, as is enzyme inhibition.
- Presystemic metabolism in liver or gut wall reduces the bioavailability of several drugs when they are administered by mouth.

Modified from Ritter JM, Flower R, Henderson G, et al. *Rang and Dale's Pharmacology*. 9th ed. Edinburgh: Elsevier; 2020:137.

TABLE 6.3 Common Substrates for Cytochrome Enzymes

1A2	2B6	2C19	2D6	3A4
Amitriptyline	Bupropion	Barbiturates	Codeine	Alprazolam
Nabumetone	Methadone	Topiramate	Tramadol	Midazolam
Desipramine	Ketamine	Diazepam	Meperidine	Cyclosporine
Tizanidine	Testosterone	Amitriptyline	Oxycodone	Sildenafil
Imipramine		Imipramine	Hydrocodone	Indinavir
Acetaminophen	**2C9**	Clomipramine	Dextromethorphan	Verapamil
Cyclobenzaprine	Valproic acid	Sertraline	Amitriptyline	Atorvastatin
Clozapine	Piroxicam	Citalopram	Nortriptyline	Lovastatin
Fluvoxamine	Celecoxib	Phenytoin	Doxepin	Digoxin
Theophylline	Ibuprofen	Carisoprodol	Tamoxifen	Amiodarone
Melatonin	Warfarin	Clopidogrel	Amphetamines	Methadone
Duloxetine			Duloxetine	Erythromycin
Caffeine			Metoclopramide	Trazodone
Lidocaine			Propranolol	Fentanyl
Warfarin			Venlafaxine	Buprenorphine
Methadone				

Metabolism of most currently used drugs occurs by about seven clinically relevant enzymes: *CYP1A2, CYP2C8, CYP2C9, CYP2C19, CYP2D6, CYP2E1*, and *CYP3A4*.
Adapted from Trescot AM. Genetics and implications in perioperative analgesia. *Best Pract Res Clin Anaesthesiol*. 2014;28(2):153-166.

TABLE 6.4   Common Enzyme-Inducing Drugs

1A2	2C9	2C19	2D6	3A4
Carbamazepine	Rifampin	Carbamazepine	Carbamazepine	Carbamazepine
Griseofulvin	Ritonavir	Rifampin	Phenobarbital	Phenytoin
Lansoprazole	Barbiturates	Ginko	Phenytoin	Nevirapine
Omeprazole	St. John wort		Rifampin	Modafinil
Ritonavir			Dexamethasone	Topiramate
Tobacco				Butalbital
St. John wort				St. John wort

Adapted from Trescot AM. Genetics and implications in perioperative analgesia. *Best Pract Res Clin Anaesthesiol.* 2014; 28(2):153-166.

TABLE 6.5   Common Enzyme-Inhibiting Drugs

1A2	2C9	2C19	2D6	3A4
Fluvoxamine	Fluvoxamine	Fluoxetine	Duloxetine	Ketoconazole
Ciprofloxacin	Paroxetine	Fluvoxamine	Cimetidine	Erythromycin
Mexiletine	Amiodarone	Paroxetine	Sertraline	Mifepristone
Verapamil	Modafinil	Topiramate	Fluoxetine	Nefazodone
Caffeine	Tamoxifen	Modafinil	Haloperidol	Grapefruit juice
Grapefruit juice		Birth control pill	Methadone	Indinavir
			Paroxetine	Ritonavir
			Quinidine	Verapamil
			Celecoxib	Diltiazem
			Bupropion	
			Ritonavir	
			Amiodarone	
			Metoclopramide	
			Chlorpromazine	
			Ropivacaine	

Adapted from Trescot AM. Genetics and implications in perioperative analgesia. *Best Pract Res Clin Anaesthesiol.* 2014;28(2):153-166.

TABLE 6.6   Relationship Between Half-Life and Drug Remaining in the Body

Half-Life	Drug Eliminated (%)	Drug Remaining (%)
0	0	100
1	50	50
2	75	25
3	87.5	12.5
4	93.75	6.25
5	96.875	3.125

or dosage independence and is the reason half-life is constant. Other elimination rate kinetic models include zero-order (e.g., alcohol) elimination, in which a constant amount (not a percentage) is eliminated over time, and Michaelis-Menten models (e.g., phenytoin), which are dose dependent and follow zero-order at high doses and first-order elimination once drug levels have fallen.[4]

Context-Sensitive Half-Time

Deficiencies in the use of standard pharmacokinetic parameters such as half-life when describing anesthetic drug administration have led to proposals for the introduction of new models that account for continuous infusion or repeated dosing-induced changes in drug behavior.[40] Context-sensitive half-time was developed through use of computer simulations of typical anesthetic dosing practices to provide a more clinically relevant measure of drug concentrations, taking into consideration the method and duration of administration.[41-43] Advantages and disadvantages of the various elimination models are summarized in Table 6.7.

Other parameters have been introduced, including the relative decrement times. This is the time needed for 80% or 90% decreases in inhalation anesthetic concentration. The major differences in the rates at which desflurane, sevoflurane, and isoflurane are eliminated occur in the final 20% of the elimination process.[44,45]

Newer Kinetic Concepts Related to Anesthesia. The specific practices of drug administration unique to anesthesia have led to the conception of several new pharmacokinetic concepts that are now applied to the understanding of the relationship among drug dose, concentration, and effect (see Table 6.7).

Front-end kinetics refers to the description of intravenous drug behavior immediately following administration. How a drug rapidly moves from the blood into peripheral tissues directly influences the peak plasma drug concentration. Back-end kinetics uses estimates of distribution volume and clearance and is a useful tool to describe the behavior of continuous infusions of intravenous agents. Back-end kinetics provides descriptors of how plasma drug concentrations decrease once a continuous infusion is terminated. An example is

TABLE 6.7 Pharmacokinetic Metrics for Describing Drug Actions

Parameter	Definition	Advantages	Limitations
Terminal half-life	Time taken for drug concentration in the blood to fall by one-half the current value	Easily understood Simple to calculate Useful for describing drug disposition in a one-compartment model	One-compartment models rarely used for describing the kinetics of anesthetic drugs Not "context sensitive" with respect to infusion duration Not informative with respect to actual duration of action
Context-sensitive half-time	A description of the time required for drug concentration to decrease by 50% after termination of drug infusion, based on duration of infusion (context)	Can be calculated for the central (plasma) or a peripheral effect compartment Context sensitivity allows rational drug selection based on anticipated infusion duration	A 50% decrease in central compartment concentration may not be the decrement in drug level required to achieve recovery
Front-end kinetics	A description of intravenous drug behavior immediately following administration	How a drug rapidly moves from the blood into peripheral tissues directly influences the peak plasma drug concentration	Must also consider the drug elimination effects approximately 5 min bolus administration
Back-end kinetics	A description of intravenous drug behavior when administered as continuous infusion, including the time period after termination of infusion	An example is decrement time, which predicts the time required to lower a certain plasma concentration (usually 50%) once an infusion is terminated	Decrement times are dependent on infusion duration

Adapted from Rigby-Jones AE, Sneyd JR. Pharmacokinetics and pharmacodynamics—is there anything new? *Anaesth.* 2012;67(1):5-11; Schnider TW. Pharmacokinetic and pharmacodynamic concepts underpinning total intravenous anesthesia. *J Cardiothorac Vasc Anesth.* 2015;29(1):S7-S10; Bailey JM. Context-sensitive half-times: what are they and how valuable are they in anaesthesiology? *Clin Pharmacokinet.* 2002;41(11):793-799.

decrement time, which predicts the time required to reach a certain plasma concentration (usually 50%) once an infusion is terminated. Decrement times are dependent on infusion duration.[44]

Estimation of Decrement of Drug Effect. Continuous infusions are used to maintain a stable drug concentration and effect without the peaks and troughs associated with bolus dosing. Most of the estimations for duration of effect of anesthetics are based on the value of the terminal half–life of the drug, which is not useful for drugs described by multicompartment models such as most anesthetics. Based initially on pharmacokinetic (PK) models and later on pharmacokinetic/pharmacodynamic (PKPD) models, the concept of context-sensitive decrement time reflects the time required to decrease to a certain plasma concentration once an infusion is terminated. Decrement times are a function of infusion duration. A popular decrement time is 50%, also known as the context-sensitive half-time. The term *context-sensitive* refers to infusion duration and the term *half-time* refers to the 50% decrement time.[44]

Fig. 6.7 shows a graphical description of the time it takes a given drug concentration, in the plasma or effect site, to fall by a given percentage after stopping the infusion. It is not a single number, but a graphical representation and it will always depend on the "context" which is the duration of infusion of drug. The practical application of this concept is that we can estimate the duration of effect as a function of the PKPD of the drug, duration of administration, and intensity of dosing.[41,44]

Clearance

The clearance of a drug is an independent value and is governed by the properties of the drug and the body's capacity to eliminate it. It is defined as the volume of plasma completely cleared of drug by metabolism and excretion per unit of time. Clearance is directly proportional to the dose and inversely related to the agent's half-life, as well as its concentration in the central compartment. Clearance is a very important pharmacokinetic concept because it influences the steady-state concentration for a given drug administered at repeated intervals or by infusion.

The two main organs for clearance are the liver and kidneys. The rate of clearance is determined by the blood flow to these organs, as well as by their ability to extract the drug from the bloodstream.

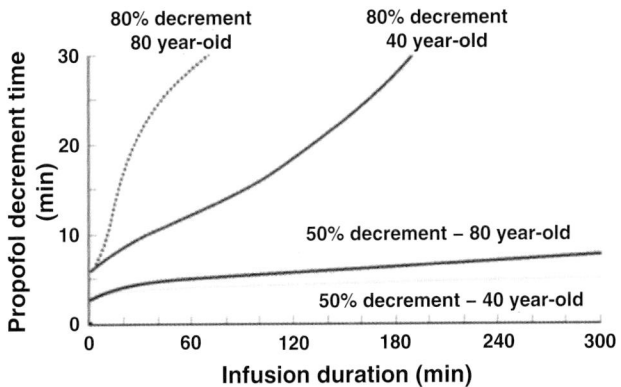

Fig. 6.7 Context-sensitive decrement times for propofol. The graph shows the time it would take for effect site propofol concentration to fall by 80% as a function of infusion duration in an 80–year–old subject as compared with a 40–year–old. Also represented is the time it would take for a decrease of 50% in an 80–year–old vs. a 40–year–old. (From Gambús PL, Trocóniz IF. Pharmacokinetic-pharmacodynamic modelling in anaesthesia. *Br J Clin Pharmacol.* 2015;79[1]:72–84, with permission.)

Mathematically, clearance is equal to the product of the blood flow (Q) and extraction ratio (E):

$$Clearance = Q \times E$$

Total clearance is the sum of all organs' clearance values. The changes in clearance occur when blood flow to the liver or kidney is altered or when their extraction ratios are changed.

Hepatic Clearance. Drugs typically go through perfusion-dependent elimination or capacity-dependent elimination in the liver. Drugs that have a high extraction ratio of 0.7 or greater rely heavily on the perfusion of the liver to be cleared. These drugs are referred to as *high-clearance drugs*. Examples of high-clearance drugs are verapamil, morphine, and lidocaine. Hepatic blood flow for these agents far outweighs enzymatic activity in clearing them from the body, so a decrease in hepatic blood flow decreases the rate of clearance, and a high perfusion state leads to faster clearance. This is termed *perfusion-dependent* elimination.[1]

Capacity-dependent elimination occurs with agents that possess a low extraction ratio of 0.3 or less. When a low extraction rate exists, only a small fraction of the agent is removed per unit of time, and changes in hepatic perfusion do not have significant effect on hepatic clearance. Clearance of these drugs depends on hepatic enzymes and the degree of protein binding. Therefore alterations such as enzyme induction or suppression cause a change in the elimination of these drugs from the body. An increase in enzyme activity causes faster elimination from the body, and enzyme suppression has the opposite outcome. A decrease in protein binding (increase in availability of drug at hepatocytes) also leads to a greater rate of clearance. Examples of drugs with a low hepatic extraction ratio are diazepam and theophylline.[1]

Renal Clearance. The kidneys excrete water-soluble molecules with great ease. The excretion of drugs involves passive glomerular filtration, active tubular secretion, and some reabsorption. Substances that are actively secreted include morphine, meperidine, furosemide, penicillin, and many quaternary ammonium compounds. The amount of drug made available to the renal tubule for elimination depends on the amount of free, unbound drug and the glomerular filtration rate. Water-soluble metabolites are filtered by the glomeruli and eliminated. The kidneys do not excrete lipid-soluble agents as efficiently as water-soluble compounds. For these agents, elimination depends on the liver for metabolism into water-soluble molecules. Indeed, increased water solubility reduces the V_d of agents, leading to their excretion by the kidneys. Conversely, lipid-soluble molecules are reabsorbed from the renal tubules back into the systemic circulation. An example of a lipid-soluble drug that is almost completely reabsorbed (such that little or none of it is excreted unchanged) is propofol.

The pH of the urine can also affect the elimination of drugs. Weak acids are better excreted in alkaline urine; conversely, weak bases are readily excreted in acid urine. The kidneys can use glomerular filtration for elimination of drugs that are highly polar (e.g., aminoglycoside antibiotics). Certain agents (e.g., penicillin) are eliminated via secretion. Some important clearance concepts are noted in Box 6.9.

OTHER FACTORS THAT INFLUENCE PHARMACOKINETICS

Age

Age plays an important role in the manner in which drug disposition occurs. Elderly patients have a decrease in renal function, resulting in impaired excretion of agents that are eliminated in the urine.[8] Creatinine clearance, as an indicator of renal function, parallels the kidneys' ability to excrete drugs and is a useful test in predicting renal pharmacokinetics in the elderly.[6] Liver blood flow decreases with age as well, decreasing the metabolism of agents with moderate to high extraction ratios. The elderly also have an increase in the fat compartment, leading to an increased volume of distribution, which can lead to accumulation of lipid-soluble agents.[17] Liver and renal function are also important in neonates. Elimination of drugs via the kidneys is altered in neonates because of poor renal function in the first year of life. Neonates and premature infants lack the ability to metabolize certain agents because of immature liver enzyme systems.[6] It is therefore important to consider extremes of age when administering any agent that may be highly lipid soluble with a high hepatic extraction ratio or that relies primarily on the kidneys for elimination.

Gender

Gender differences account for some variability in the pharmacokinetics of many agents. In a review of the literature, it was found that female patients had a 20% to 30% greater sensitivity to the muscle relaxant effects

---

BOX 6.9   Elimination of Drugs by the Kidney

- Most drugs, unless highly bound to plasma protein, cross the glomerular filter freely.
- Many drugs, especially weak acids and weak bases, are actively secreted into the renal tubule and rapidly excreted.
- Lipid-soluble drugs are passively reabsorbed along with water by diffusion across the tubular barrier, so are not efficiently excreted in the urine.
- Because of pH partition, weak acids are more rapidly excreted in alkaline urine, and vice versa.
- Several important drugs are removed predominantly by renal excretion and are liable to cause toxicity in elderly persons and patients with renal disease.
- There are instances of clinically important drug-drug interactions due to one drug reducing the renal clearance of another (examples include diuretics/lithium and indomethacin/methotrexate), but these are less common than interactions due to altered drug metabolism.

Modified from Ritter JM, Flower R, Henderson G, et al. *Rang and Dale's Pharmacology.* 9th ed. Edinburgh: Elsevier; 2020:141.

---

of vecuronium, pancuronium, and rocuronium.[46,47] It was also found that male patients were more sensitive to propofol than female patients and that it may be necessary to reduce propofol doses as much as 30% in male patients.[46,48] Gan et al.[49] studied emergence from general anesthesia with propofol, alfentanil, and nitrous oxide. Female patients emerged significantly more quickly than male patients. In fact, female patients were three times more likely than male patients to experience recall under general anesthesia. Females are more sensitive than males to some of the effects of opioid receptor agonists while being more resistant to others.[46-48] Females given opiates may experience respiratory depression and other adverse effects more easily if they are given the same doses as males. These gender differences seem to be more pronounced in premenopausal women, suggesting hormonal mechanisms are a contributing factor.[50,51]

Temperature

Temperature affects tissue metabolism and blood flow, and as such it follows that the pharmacokinetics of agents are also affected by varying temperatures. In general, metabolism and clearance are delayed for almost all drugs during hypothermia and increased with fever.[52]

Knibbe et al.[53] examined the pharmacokinetics of long-term propofol sedation in critically ill patients. Temperature was a significant covariate for clearance of propofol. Warmer temperatures led to faster elimination of propofol, regardless of the concentration of the drug in solution.

Disease States

The incidence of chronic kidney disease (CKD) is growing due to the aging of the population and an increasing incidence of diabetes, hypertension, and obesity, which are leading risk factors of renal failure. CKD is known to impair clearance and elimination of drugs and their metabolites. Uremic toxins, inflammatory cytokines, and parathyroid hormone, which are common in CKD, may be implicated. Altered plasma protein binding of drugs and the activity of several drug-metabolizing enzymes and drug transporters have also been shown to be impaired in chronic renal failure.[54,55]

Hepatic disease may have a large influence on a drug's effect. To predict how hepatic disease will influence drugs in an individual patient may be difficult. Pharmacokinetic alterations vary among acute and chronic hepatic disorders, as well as with the degree to which the liver is impaired. In cirrhosis, all pharmacokinetic phases may be affected, including absorption, distribution, metabolism, and elimination of the drug. Some changes include high portosystemic pressure, which impedes GI absorption. Less first-pass effect in the diseased liver leads to a higher bioavailability of highly extracted drugs administered orally. The V_d for highly protein-bound drugs may be changed secondary to the lowered production of albumin and other plasma proteins. Water-soluble drugs may also exhibit an altered V_d due to volume overload and ascites in patients with cirrhosis. Drug metabolism and elimination are reduced due to impairment of drug-metabolizing enzymes. Phase I mechanisms are affected to a greater extent than phase II processes.[56]

Other disease states can cause variability, as illustrated by a 2003 study that found an increase in the volume distribution of ketamine disproportional to increases in clearance in spinal cord injury inpatients in the intensive care unit, leading to a longer than expected half-life for the drug, again placing the patients at risk for overdose.[57] See Box 6.10 for a summary of some pharmacokinetic principles.

PHARMACOGENETICS AND PHARMACOGENOMICS

Definitions

Pharmacogenetics is the study of variations in human genes that are responsible for different responses to drug therapy. These differences are identified in the pharmacodynamic and pharmacokinetic processes.[58] Pharmacogenomics is an evolution of pharmacogenetics research and involves the identification of drug response markers at the level of disease, drug metabolism, or drug target.[59,60]

Pharmacogenetics and pharmacogenomics take into account the genetic basis for the variability in an individual's drug response. Pharmacogenetics studies variations in genes suspected of affecting drug response, whereas pharmacogenomics encompasses the genome (all genes). The discipline of pharmacogenetics integrates biochemical and pharmacologic concepts and seeks to correlate phenotypic biomarkers with responses. Pharmacogenomics involves DNA sequencing and gene mapping to identify the genetic basis for variations in drug efficacy, metabolism, and transport.[61]

Any clinician can describe the wide variation in patient responses to anesthetic drugs. Much of the variation has been attributed to differences in patient size, age, disease profile, and sex. Advances in pharmacogenetics and pharmacogenomics reveal that genetic differences in drug response also play an important role. We are quickly getting to the point of personalized medicine where genetic testing allows for individualized prevention and therapy. Inherited variations have been identified in approximately 20 genes that affect approximately 80 medications and are clinically actionable. For example, genetic variants now direct the choice of "targeted" anticancer drugs for individual patients. Prevailing efforts are focusing on implementation of an evidenced-based strategy for improving the use of drugs providing a cornerstone for precision medicine.[62,63] Some pharmacogenomic considerations for anesthesia-related drugs are noted in Table 6.8.

History

The history of pharmacogenetics goes back to the days of Pythagoras (510 BC) when he recognized that only some people had fatal responses to ingestion of fava beans, but not all.[64]

Archibald Garrod's 1902 study of alkaptonuria constituted the first genetic link to disease in humans. He later advanced the hypothesis that genetically determined differences in biochemical processes may be the reason for adverse drug reactions.[65]

Familial clustering of toxic drug responses led to suspicion of a biochemical genetic basis for the toxicities.[61] In a seminal article published in 1957, Motulsky[66] outlined many genetic conditions associated with toxic reaction to a specific drug or chemical and proposed that inheritance of certain traits may explain individual variations in drug efficacy and toxic reactions.

Early advances in the field of pharmacogenetics came from research into the biochemical and genetic basis for idiosyncratic drug responses.

BOX 6.10 Summary of Pharmacokinetic Principles

- Clinical pharmacokinetics is the discipline that describes the absorption, distribution, metabolism, and elimination of drugs in patients who require drug therapy.
- Clearance is the most important pharmacokinetic parameter because it determines the steady-state concentration for a given dosage rate. Physiologically, clearance is determined by blood flow to the organ that metabolizes or eliminates the drug and the efficiency of the organ in extracting the drug from the bloodstream.
- The dosage and clearance determine the steady-state concentration.
- The fraction of drug absorbed into the systemic circulation after extravascular administration is defined as its bioavailability.
- Pharmacokinetic models are useful for description of data sets, prediction of serum concentrations after several doses or different routes of administration, and calculation of pharmacokinetic constants such as clearance, volume of distribution, and half-life. The simplest case uses a single compartment to represent the entire body.
- The volume of distribution is a proportionality constant that relates the amount of drug in the body to the serum concentration. The volume of distribution is used to calculate the loading dose of a drug that will immediately achieve a desired steady-state concentration. The value of the volume of distribution is determined by the physiologic volume and how the drug binds in blood and tissues. The volume of distribution determines the loading dose.
- Half-life is the time required for serum concentration to decrease by one-half after absorption and distribution are complete. Half-life is important because it determines the time required to reach steady state and the dosage interval. Half-life is a dependent kinetic variable because its value depends on the values of clearance and volume of distribution.
- The half-life determines the time to reach steady state and the time for "all" of the drug to be eliminated from the body.
- If a drug obeys first-order pharmacokinetics, a simple ratio of dosage to steady-state concentration can be used to estimate a new dosage, if the clearance has not changed.
- Phenytoin is an example of a drug that obeys the Michaelis-Menton model rather than first-order pharmacokinetics. In this case, as plasma concentration increases, the clearance decreases, and the half-life becomes longer.
- *Cytochrome P-450* is a generic term for the group of enzymes responsible for most drug metabolism oxidation reactions. Several P-450 isozymes have been identified, including CYP1A2, CYP2C9, CYP2C19, CYP2D6, CYP2E1, and CYP3A4.
- Factors to be taken into consideration when deciding on the best drug dose for a patient include age, gender, weight, ethnic background, other concurrent disease states, and other drug therapy.
- The importance of transport proteins in drug bioavailability and elimination is now better understood. The principal transport protein involved in the movement of drugs across biologic membranes is P-glycoprotein. P-glycoprotein is present in many organs, including the gastrointestinal tract, liver, and kidney.

Modified from Dipiro JT, Yee G, Posey LM, et al., eds. *Pharmacotherapy: A Pathophysiological Approach.* 11th ed. New York: McGraw-Hill; 2020; Helms RA, Quan DJ, Herfindal ET, et al., eds. *Textbook of Therapeutics: Drug and Disease Management.* 8th ed. Philadelphia: Lippincott Williams & Wilkins; 2006; Schnider TW, Minto CF. Principles of pharmacokinetics. In: Evers AS, ed. *Anesthetic Pharmacology: Basic Principles and Clinical Practice.* 2nd ed. Cambridge, UK: Cambridge University Press; 2011:57–71.

Several independent observations were made. For example, in the 1950s, after reports of prolonged muscle relaxation following administration of succinylcholine during anesthesia, the variation in serum cholinesterase levels was found to be an inherited trait.[67,68] Similarly, hemolytic anemia found in black male soldiers after administration of the antimalarial drug primaquine during World War II led to the discovery of a defect in the gene encoding glucose-6-phosphate dehydrogenase (G6PD).[61]

The term *pharmacogenetics* was coined by Vogel in 1959 and is defined as a "clinically important hereditary variation in response to drugs."[58] In 1962, Kalow wrote a text, *Pharmacogenetics: Heredity and the Response to Drugs.*[69]

In the 1960s, twin studies established the role of genetic factors in individual variations in rates of drug metabolism; however, they did not identify the specific genes involved. Gene identification emerged in the 1980s.[58] Now that the human and many animal genomes have been sequenced, huge strides in genomics and drug therapies are occurring. The development of genomics has led to the hope of individualized drug therapy with increased and targeted efficacy and fewer side effects. The characterization of single nucleotide polymorphisms (SNPs; pronounced "snips") and the effect on drug action has opened new areas of drug research. The emergence of pharmacometabolomics assesses the influence of the metabolic factors and the environment on gene expression. The combination of these disciplines permits factors involving the genetic background of individual and exterior interventions to tailor individual therapies.[70,71]

Polymorphisms

Polymorphic genes relevant to pharmacokinetics (absorption, distribution, metabolism, and excretion) and pharmacodynamics (drug targets: receptors and enzymes) can have a significant impact on pharmacotherapy.[72] Pharmacotherapy may be affected by three types of genetic variation. These include variations in target proteins, enzyme metabolism, or idiosyncratic effects.[73]

Polymorphisms are defined as variations in the DNA sequences that occur in at least 1% of the population.[74-77] There are a number of different types of polymorphisms, but most attention has been focused on SNPs, in which one nucleotide is exchanged for another in a given position.[64] Approximately 10 million SNPs exist, and they can occur anywhere on the genome, but only a fraction are likely to prove relevant to drug response. To matter from a pharmacologic standpoint, the differences generally affect either the function or the amount of target proteins involved in the biochemical pathways of the disease processes the drugs are used to treat.[73]

The genomes of any two individuals are nearly 99.9% identical regardless of race.[73] Most variations in the human genome (polymorphisms) occur in drug-metabolizing enzyme genes. Others occur in the enzyme receptor genes and drug transporter genes.[57] Much of the observed variability in drug response has a basis in pharmacogenetic polymorphisms arising in genetically determined differences in drug absorption, disposition, metabolism, and excretion. The best-characterized pharmacogenetic polymorphisms are those in the cytochrome P-450 family of drug-metabolizing enzymes.[76]

Most drugs are lipophilic and must be metabolized to polar products for excretion. This involves hepatic enzymes and a sequence of steps dependent on the cytochrome P-450 system. Drugs are first metabolized by phase I enzymes (oxidation) and then by phase II enzymes (conjugation that involves sulphation, glucuronidation, or acetylation). Although the effects of polymorphism in phase II enzymes are often less pronounced, the effects of inherited variations in both phase I and II metabolism can be synergistic.

Genetic polymorphisms occur in most, if not all, of the human cytochrome P-450 (CYP) isoenzymes, but functional polymorphisms reside in only four, which account for 40% of all drug metabolism (CYP2A6, CYP2C9, CYP2C19, and CYP2D6). Thus genetically controlled variations are common.[58] As previously noted, cytochrome P-450 (CYP450) is a superfamily of liver enzymes that catalyze phase I drug metabolism. The D6 isozyme of the CYP2 family is particularly affected by genetic variability and currently has 80 identified CYP2D6 alleles, resulting in a

TABLE 6.8 Pharmacogenomic Considerations for Anesthesia-Related Drugs

Drug(s)	Gene	Variant	Clinical Risk
Succinylcholine Succinylcholine Mivacurium	BCHE	Multiple	Prolonged apnea
Desflurane Halothane Isoflurane Sevoflurane	RYR1 CACNA1S	Multiple	Malignant Hyperthermia
Propofol	CYP2B6	rs3745274	Awakening time less
Codeine	CYP2D6	Metabolizer status	↑ Analgesic response ↑ Toxicity in children
Tramadol	CYP2D6	Metabolizer status	↓ Analgesic response ↑ Toxicity in children
Fentanyl	CYP3A4, COMT	Metabolizer status	↓ Drug effect
Lidocaine Prilocaine	G6PD	Deficiency	Methemoglobinemia
Metoprolol	CYP2D6	Metabolizer status	Efficacy, bradycardia
Simvastatin	SLCO1B1	rs4149056	Myopathy
Lansoprazole Omeprazole	CYP2C19	Metabolizer status	Inadequate efficacy

BCHE, butyrylcholinesterase; *COMT,* catechol-O-methyltransferase; *CYP,* cytochrome P; *G6PD,* glucose-6-phosphate dehydrogenase; *SLCO1B1,* solute carrier organic anion transporter family, member 1B1.

variable enzymatic activity ranging from 1% to 200%. Individuals can be classified as having an ultrarapid metabolism, an extensive metabolism, an intermediate metabolism, or a poor metabolism. The distribution of CYP2D6 phenotypes varies according to ethnicity (Table 6.9).

Codeine is a prodrug and requires metabolism by CYP2D6 to be converted into morphine and become analgesic. Morphine is further metabolized into morphine-6-glucuronide and morphine-3-glucuronide; both morphine and morphine-6-glucuronide display opioid activity. Codeine was commonly prescribed because of the belief that, being a weak opioid, it was safe and would not result in adverse outcomes. However, serious morbidity and mortality have occurred in two separate patient populations[63,78] (Fig. 6.8). They include postoperative pediatric tonsillectomy patients and neonates of breast-feeding mothers receiving codeine analgesia. Mothers, neonates, and children who are CYP2D6 ultrarapid or extensive metabolizers may produce toxic levels of active drug from the codeine prodrug. A Food and Drug Administration (FDA) warning and contraindication involving both groups have been added to the package literature. An FDA-approved genetic test (AmpliChip CYP450; Roche Diagnostics, Palo Alto, CA, USA) is commercially available to test genetic variants of CYP2D6.

Individual Drug Response/Genetics

Many variations of pharmacogenetic interest have been elucidated, and with the deciphering of the human genome, many innovative opportunities exist. Genetic variations can modify responses to drugs. Variations in target pathways and metabolic enzymes may render a drug ineffective for some, yet effective for others.[74-77]

Recognition of genetic differences among patients has the potential to allow for individualized drug therapy. Furthermore, with the recognition that certain genetic differences are associated with risk of

TABLE 6.9 Ethnic Distribution of CYP2D6 Activity

Ethnic Group	CYP2D6 PM	CYP2D6 IM	CYP2D6 UM
Caucasian	7–10%		
Asian	1–2%	30%	
African American	2–4%	30%	
Ethiopian			29%
Southern European			10%
Northern European			1–2%

CYP, cytochrome P; *IM*, intermediate metabolizer; *PM*, poor metabolizer; *UM*, ultrarapid metabolizer.
Adapted from Trescot AM. Genetics and implications in perioperative analgesia. *Best Pract Res Clin Anaesthesiol.* 2014;28(2):153-166; Behrooz A. Pharmacogenetics and anaesthetic drugs: implications for perioperative practice. *Ann Med Surg (Lond).* 2015;4(4):470-474.

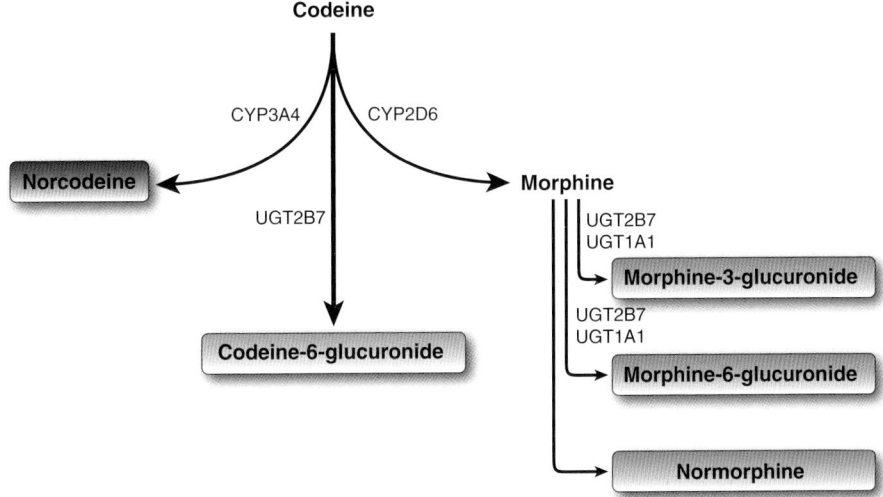

Fig. 6.8 Codeine metabolic pathway.

disease, opportunities to identify these individuals and treat them early may improve efficacy and specificity of their treatment.[58]

Clopidogrel, warfarin, β-blockers, statins, angiotensin-converting enzyme inhibitors, and other cardiovascular medications can now be prescribed by algorithms based on genetic profiles. Rapid advances in characterizing genetic relationships are helping to bring these advances in pharmacokinetics into the clinic.[79] The pharmacogenetic influences on many psychiatric drugs, electroconvulsive therapy, and serotonin syndrome are also being reported.[80-83]

SUMMARY

Pharmacokinetics is an integral part of modern anesthesia clinical practice. Anesthesia providers balance the administration of numerous drugs simultaneously to achieve the necessary drug actions that constitute anesthesia. A thorough understanding of the processes that govern drug kinetics allows for safe and effective practice and facilitates operating room efficiency. This knowledge also allows the clinician to anticipate and avoid potential problems and tailor each anesthetic to specific patient characteristics. Advances in pharmacokinetics and pharmacogenomics will further impact anesthesia care in years to come. Pharmacogenomics has made a significant impact on the direction of drug research and drug therapy. Diseases and drug therapies are complex processes that may challenge the predictive powers of pharmacogenetics. A systems approach may be needed to integrate overall pharmacotherapeutic effects with polymorphisms in multiple genes.[74,75,77]

REFERENCES

For a complete list of references for this chapter, scan this QR code with any smartphone code reader app, or visit the following URL: http://booksite.elsevier.com/9780323711944/.

7

Pharmacokinetics of Inhalation Anesthetics

John J. Nagelhout

The basic action of an anesthetic in the body is largely a function of the drug's chemical structure and the resulting interaction with a cellular receptor complex (Fig. 7.1). A number of heterogeneous compounds exhibit anesthetic properties. The inorganic molecule nitrous oxide and halogenated ethers (e.g., isoflurane, desflurane, and sevoflurane) are all capable of binding to central nervous system and spinal cord neuronal membranes to produce reversible depression. A single specific anesthetic receptor has yet to be found. In fact, multiple sites of action and protein targets probably exist; however, once a critical concentration of drug has entered the brain and spinal cord, loss of consciousness ensues.[1-3]

The administration of inhalation anesthetic gases plays a primary role in modern clinical anesthesia. In anesthesia's early years, administration of a gas such as diethyl ether constituted the entire anesthetic regimen. Now one or two gas anesthetics are combined with a variety of intravenous drugs to produce an anesthetic state. These intravenous drugs include sedative induction agents such as propofol or etomidate, analgesics, neuromuscular blocking drugs, and local anesthetics. This combination allows the use of smaller and more easily manipulated doses of specific receptor agonists and antagonists. Used in the proper combination, the desired amount of anesthesia, analgesia, amnesia, and muscle relaxation can be achieved. Current practice dictates that the anesthetic technique allow for a quick and pleasant induction and recovery with maximum patient safety and efficient caseload management. A sound understanding of inhalation anesthetic pharmacokinetics is essential for safe practice.

PRIMARY FACTORS CONTROLLING UPTAKE, DISTRIBUTION, AND ELIMINATION OF ANESTHETICS

The basic task of anesthetic administration involves taking a drug supplied as a liquid, vaporizing it in an anesthesia machine, and delivering it to the patient's brain and other tissues via the lungs. Therefore the main factors that influence the ability to anesthetize a patient are technical or machine specific, drug related, respiratory, circulatory, and tissue related. The primary factors that influence absorption of the inhalation anesthetics are ventilation, uptake into the blood, cardiac output, the solubility of the anesthetic drug in the blood, and alveolar-to-venous blood partial-pressure difference. Other factors such as the concentration and second gas effects also play a role (Fig. 7.2).[4]

A few assumptions are usually made. The level of anesthesia is related to the alveolar concentrations of anesthetic agents, which can be readily and continuously measured or inferred. The concentration or partial pressure of anesthetic in the lungs is assumed to be the same as in the brain because the drugs are highly lipid soluble and diffusible, and they quickly and easily reach equilibrium among the

highly perfused body compartments. For this reason the dose of an individual drug is expressed in terms of the minimum alveolar concentration (MAC) necessary to produce anesthesia (lack of movement) upon surgical stimulation.[5-8] The definition of MAC is the *minimum alveolar concentration* required to produce anesthesia (lack of movement) in 50% of the population upon surgical stimulation. It is age dependent in that the required dose peaks at approximately 6 months of age and then decreases with increasing age.[9] The faster the alveolar (and therefore brain) concentration rises, the faster anesthesia is achieved. Conversely, the faster the alveolar (brain) concentration falls after discontinuation of the drug, the more quickly the patient emerges.[10] Some factors that can influence MAC are given in Box 7.1.

Machine-Related Factors

Concepts regarding the anesthesia machine and its function are described in detail in Chapter 16. Two factors that may affect uptake early in anesthetic administration are (1) drug solubility in the rubber and plastic machine parts and (2) total machine liter flow of the gases chosen.

The rubber and plastic components of the machine, in addition to the ventilator and absorbent, can retain small quantities of anesthetic gases. Theoretically this could slow administration to the patient at the start of anesthetic delivery. The effect on uptake is minimal in actual clinical practice and essentially ceases after approximately 15 minutes of administration.[11] Nonetheless, sequestration of small amounts of gas in the apparatus has other implications, such as when anesthetizing patients with malignant hyperthermia. All gases except nitrous oxide are potent triggering agents for a hyperthermic episode. To avoid exposure resulting from residual trace amounts of gases, a thorough flush of the anesthesia machine with 100% oxygen at 10 L/min for at least 20 minutes, replacement of breathing circuits and the carbon dioxide canister, and inactivation or removal of vaporizers are advised when

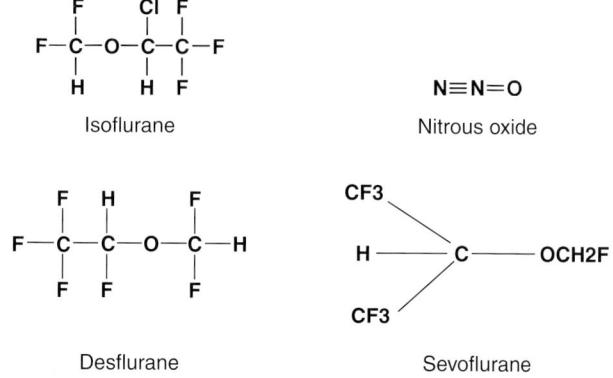

Fig. 7.1 Chemical structure of anesthetic agents. Nitrous oxide is inorganic, and the rest are halogenated ethers.

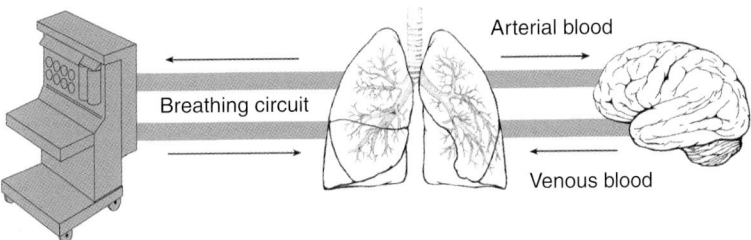

Fig. 7.2 Transfer of an anesthetic gas from the machine through the lungs into the blood and tissues.

BOX 7.1   Factors That Influence MAC

Impact of Physiologic and Pharmacologic Factors on Minimum Alveolar Concentration

Increases in MAC
- Hyperthermia
- Drug-induced increases in central nervous system activity
- Hypernatremia
- Chronic alcohol abuse

Decreases in MAC
- Hypothermia
- Increasing age
- Preoperative sedatives
- Drug-induced decreases in central nervous system activities
- α_2-Agonists
- Acute alcohol ingestion
- Pregnancy
- Postpartum (returns to normal in 24–72 hr)
- Lithium
- Lidocaine
- Hypoxia
- Hypotension
- Cardiopulmonary bypass
- Hyponatremia

MAC, Minimum alveolar concentration.

---

preparing for a patient who is susceptible to malignant hyperthermia. Newer anesthesia workstations may require flowing 10 L/min of fresh gas for up to 104 minutes. For both new and older machines, adding commercially available activated charcoal filters to the circuit will remove anesthetic gases and obviate the need for purging the system as described. However, the anesthesia machine will still need to be flushed with high fresh gas flows (≥10 L/min) for 90 seconds prior to placing the activated charcoal filters on *both* the inspiratory and expiratory ports. These filters are effective in keeping gas concentration below 5 ppm for up to 12 hours with fresh gas flows of at least 3 L/min.[12] Proper preparation may vary with different machines, and consultation with the machine manufacturer is advised.[13,14]

Low liter flows of oxygen and nitrous oxide carrier gas, although economical, deliver the anesthetic more slowly at the start of induction. Increasing liter flows for the first few minutes of the anesthetic minimizes this effect without unduly adding to cost.[15]

Drug-Related Factors

Blood/Gas Solubility

The blood/gas solubility coefficient of an anesthetic is an indicator of the speed of uptake and elimination.[16,17] It reflects the proportion of the anesthetic that will be soluble in the blood, "bind" to blood components, and not readily enter the tissues (blood phase) versus the fraction of the drug that will leave the blood and quickly diffuse into tissues (gas phase). The more soluble the drug (high blood/gas coefficient), the slower the brain and spinal cord uptake and therefore the slower that anesthesia is achieved. Soluble drugs remain in the blood in greater proportion than less soluble agents; therefore less of the drug is released to the tissues during the early, rapid-uptake phase of induction. For example, isoflurane has a blood/gas solubility coefficient of 1.4, or expressed as a ratio, 1.4:1. Therefore 1.4 times as much stays in the blood as a nonreleasable fraction for every 1 molecule that enters the tissues and produces anesthesia. Conversely, agents with low solubility properties (low blood/gas coefficient) leave the blood quickly and enter the tissues, producing a rapid anesthetic state. Desflurane, for example, has a low blood/gas coefficient of 0.42, or expressed as a ratio, 0.42:1. Only 0.42 of a molecule stays in the blood for every 1 molecule (greater than twice as much) that enters the brain. Anesthesia is achieved quickly. Blood/gas solubility coefficients for the inhalation anesthetic agents are listed in Table 7.1.[1,18,19] The rate of rise of an anesthetic in the alveoli relative to the concentration administered is graphically depicted by plotting the fraction in the alveoli over the fraction inspired (Fig. 7.3).

As noted previously, the lower the blood/gas solubility, the faster the rise in lung and brain concentrations. The rate of rise of low-solubility agents such as nitrous oxide and desflurane is greater than moderately soluble drugs such as isoflurane. Note in Fig. 7.3 that nitrous oxide exhibits a slightly faster rate of rise compared with desflurane, despite a higher blood/gas coefficient. This variation in the usual trend is a result of the concentration effect—that is, nitrous oxide is given at much higher concentrations (50%–70%) than desflurane (3%–9%). Fig. 7.4 depicts the effect of anesthetic blood solubility on uptake.

Ventilation Factors

As with all diffusible drugs, anesthetics move down a concentration gradient. Continuous inhalation administration of the agent into the lungs promotes subsequent diffusion into the blood and tissues as the anesthetic progresses. Anesthetic uptake slows throughout the surgical procedure as the tissue compartments become more saturated.[20] The anesthetic is delivered along with the necessary amount of oxygen or an oxygen mix appropriate for the patient's condition. Supplemental nitrous oxide may also be used. Basically, the faster and more deeply a patient breathes or is ventilated, the faster the patient loses consciousness at the start of anesthesia and emerges at the end.[17,21,22] This is often referred to as the ventilation effect.

Ventilation-perfusion deficits or poor lung function hinders inhalation drug administration.[23,24] Rapid-acting (low blood/gas solubility) agents are affected by these deficits to a greater extent than are slower-acting (high blood/gas solubility) drugs.[25] These decreases in speed can be partially compensated for by increasing the concentration of insoluble (fast) agents or increasing ventilation with soluble (slow) drugs.

TABLE 7.1   General Anesthetic Properties of Inhalation Agents

Anesthetic	MAC (%)	Blood/Gas Partition Coefficient (at 37°C)	Oil/Gas Partition Coefficient (at 37°C)
Sevoflurane (Ultane)	2	0.6	50
Isoflurane (Forane)	1.15	1.4	99
Nitrous oxide	105	0.47	1.4
Desflurane (Suprane)	5.8	0.42	18.7

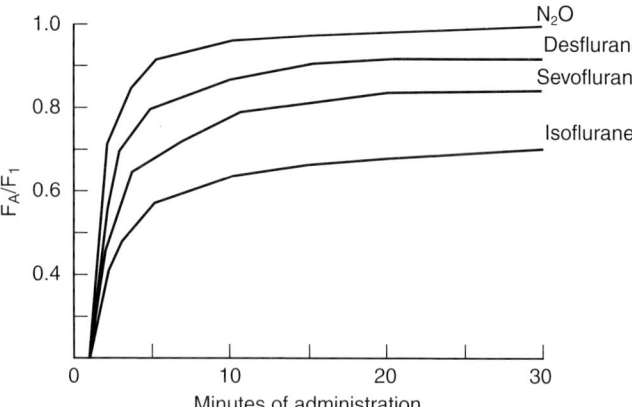

Fig. 7.3 Rate of rise (F_A/F_I) of alveolar concentration of inhalation anesthetics over time. Low blood/gas anesthetics such as nitrous oxide and desflurane achieve a lung concentration much faster than moderate-solubility gases such as isoflurane. Note that nitrous oxide rises in the lungs more quickly than desflurane, in spite of a slightly higher blood/gas solubility. This is the result of the concentration effect.

Concentration or Dose

During the first minutes of gas administration, a higher concentration of the drug than necessary for maintenance, or a loading dose, is delivered to speed initial uptake. This is commonly referred to as overpressuring or the concentration effect.[26] Overpressuring during initial administration is a common clinical practice and is more effective the more soluble the anesthetic. Overpressuring can speed the effect of slower acting agents but has less of an effect on relatively faster acting agents. This practice follows the kinetic standard of using a loading dose to speed onset. After the first few minutes the dose is decreased to normal maintenance levels.[27]

As noted previously, the dose of an anesthetic is expressed in terms of MAC—the relative concentration when the anesthetic is combined with all the other gases in the lungs. Induction and maintenance doses are given as vaporizer settings of partial pressure in Table 7.2.

Second-Gas Effect

Simultaneous administration of a relatively slow agent such as isoflurane and a faster drug such as nitrous oxide (in high concentrations) can speed the onset of the slower agent. This is known as the second-gas effect.[28] The uptake of the slower agent in the alveoli, and to an even greater proportion in the arterial blood, is increased by administering it with a high concentration of the faster acting anesthetic nitrous oxide.[29] For example, sevoflurane, which has low blood solubility (blood/gas solubility coefficient 0.6) is rapidly taken up into tissues. Coadministration of sevoflurane with the slightly faster nitrous oxide produces a small but significant increase in uptake as compared with sevoflurane administration alone.[27,30-32] The mechanism for the second-gas effect is not definitive, but it has traditionally been explained as the large volume uptake of nitrous oxide concentrating the

other alveolar gases. An added effect ventilation/perfusion ratio (V/Q) mismatch and ventilation perfusion scatter on the distribution of blood flow and gas uptake in the lung may play a role.[30] The partial pressure in blood will be 6% greater when nitrous oxide is coadministered, and the effect on blood will not be detected by gas analyzers. Increases in volatile concentrations caused by the second-gas effect persist for the first 15 to 20 minutes of an anesthetic.[30,31]

The second-gas effect also occurs during emergence where the rapid elimination of nitrous oxide produces a clinically significant acceleration in the removal of the accompanying volatile agent.[33]

Tissue-Related Factors

Oil/Gas Solubility

The oil/gas solubility coefficient is an indicator of potency. The higher the solubility, the more potent the drug (see Table 7.1).[34,35] A high solubility coefficient reflects high lipid solubility. Because the anesthetic must traverse the blood-brain barrier and penetrate other lipid membranes to produce its action, highly lipid-soluble drugs tend to be the most potent. Of the current agents, isoflurane (oil/gas partition coefficient 99) is the most potent, and nitrous oxide (oil/gas partition coefficient 1.4) is the least potent. Remember that two factors are at play: how fast the drug is delivered to the tissues (blood/gas solubility) and how efficiently it can access and affect the sites of action (oil/gas solubility). Investigations suggest that polarity along with lipophilicity play important yet not fully understood roles in the mechanism of inhalation anesthetics.[36-38]

Circulatory Factors

The cardiovascular system exerts two major influences on anesthetic uptake and distribution.[39] First, the majority of the blood leaving the lungs with anesthetic is normally distributed to the vital organs or high–blood-flow areas, commonly referred to as the vessel-rich group or central compartment. Organs such as the heart, liver, kidneys, and brain receive proportionately more anesthetic sooner than the muscle and fat areas (Table 7.3). The longer the anesthetic is given, the greater the saturation of all body compartments.

Second, during induction, increases in cardiac output slow onset. All anesthetics are affected; however, the more soluble the agent (higher blood/gas coefficient, and therefore slower), the greater the effect. An increased cardiac output removes more anesthetic from the lungs, which slows the rise in lung and brain concentration.[40-42] This effect dissipates as the anesthetic proceeds.

Metabolism

The modern anesthetics are minimally metabolized (Table 7.4).[43] Possible toxic metabolite formation is not currently a clinical issue.[44] Drug metabolism has historically been associated with various anesthetic-related toxicities. These include hepatotoxicity from halothane[45] and other agents, and nephrotoxicity from methoxyflurane. Nitrous oxide, desflurane, and isoflurane are the least metabolized and do not result in metabolism-related toxicity. Although sevoflurane is

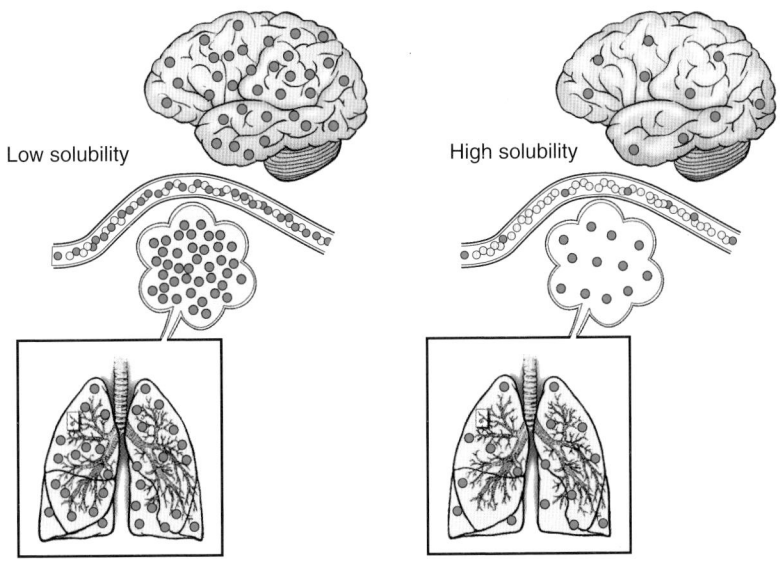

Fig. 7.4 Effect of anesthetic blood/gas solubility on uptake. *(Left)* An anesthetic gas with a low blood/gas solubility is not taken into the blood *(lightly shaded circles)*; therefore the alveolar (thus brain) concentration rises rapidly *(darkly shaded circles)*, and the patient achieves anesthesia quickly. *(Right)* An anesthetic gas with a high blood/gas solubility is taken up and held in the blood *(lightly shaded circles)*, resulting in a slower rise in alveolar (thus brain) concentration *(darkly shaded circles)* and a slower onset of anesthesia.

TABLE 7.2	Inhalation Anesthetic Doses*	
Anesthetic	**Induction (%)**	**Maintenance (%)**
Nitrous oxide	50–70	Same
Isoflurane (Forane)	1–4	0.5–2
Desflurane (Suprane)	3–9	2–6
Sevoflurane (Ultane)	4–8	1–4

*Doses vary according to patient status, procedure, and types of medications coadministered. Doses are given as vaporizer setting or partial pressures.

TABLE 7.3	Tissue Compartments and Perfusion Comparisons			
Characteristic	**Vessel Rich**	**Muscle**	**Fat**	**Vessel Poor**
Body weight	10%	50%	20%	20%
Cardiac output	75%	19%	6%	0%
Perfusion	75 mL/min/ 100 g	3 mL/min/ 100 g	3 mL/min/ 100 g	0 mL/min/ 100 g

TABLE 7.4	Anesthetic Metabolism	
Agent	**Average Metabolism (%)**
Sevoflurane	5–8
Nitrous oxide	<1
Isoflurane	<1
Desflurane	<0.1

tissue/blood partition coefficients are maintained relatively constant; however, there is an enlargement of tissue anesthetic capacity. The decrease in the perfusion of tissues tends to slow drug delivery to the brain and retard induction. However, these effects are balanced by a decrease in anesthetic requirement and an increase in potency of the anesthetics during hypothermia. Overall induction tends to be slower during hypothermia. This can be somewhat overcome by increasing concentrations. During recovery from anesthesia the increased tissue capacity of anesthetics and slower perfusion during hypothermia appear to slow recovery. Hyperthermia increases anesthetic requirement and cardiac output, which also leads to a slower induction.[50-53] Some factors that can affect induction rate are noted in Box 7.2.

Emergence

When the anesthetic is discontinued, the same principles that influence onset apply. The anesthetic leaves the tissues via the blood and exits the lungs with ventilation. Routine practice is to administer 100% oxygen to assist recovery. If nitrous oxide was given, 100% oxygen prevents diffusion hypoxia. Anesthetics redistribute out of the tissues in a more uniform manner compared with the way they distribute during onset. An equilibrium is approached among tissues during the anesthetic period, so recovery tends to be smoother than induction with respect to the excitatory stage responses. In general, the longer an anesthetic is administered, the slower the patient emerges. This effect is greatest with the most soluble isoflurane and less with sevoflurane and desflurane, respectively. Differences among anesthetics are small but significant and are seen primarily during the final 10% of the elimination

metabolized approximately 5% to 8% releasing free fluoride ions, no related clinically significant toxicity has been noted.[46-49]

Temperature

Inhaled anesthetics are often administered to patients during hyperthermic or hypothermic conditions. The rate of induction of anesthesia depends on a balance among alveolar ventilation, cardiac output, tissue perfusion, anesthetic solubility in blood and tissues, anesthetic requirement, and potency. As temperature falls both solubility and potency increase, thereby tending to cancel each other as factors affecting the rate of induction. Decreases in alveolar ventilation and perfusion of brain and other tissues tend to slow induction. Under hypothermia

BOX 7.2 Factors That Can Affect Induction Rate

Faster Induction
Low blood gas solubility
Low cardiac output
High minute ventilation
High fresh gas flows
High concentration (overpressuring)
Second-gas effect

Slower Induction
High blood gas solubility
High cardiac output
Low minute ventilation
Low fresh gas flow rates
Low concentrations
Ventilation perfusion deficits
Hypothermia

BOX 7.3 Emergence From General Anesthesia

General Anesthesia
- Stable administration of anesthetic drugs
- Arousal not possible, unresponsive; eyes closed, with reactive pupils
- Analgesia, akinesia
- Drug-controlled blood pressure and heart rate
- Mechanically controlled ventilation
- Electroencephalogram (EEG) patterns ranging from δ and α activity to burst suppression

Emergence, Phase 1
- Cessation of anesthetic drugs
- Reversal of peripheral-muscle relaxation (akinesis)
- Transition from apnea to irregular breathing to regular breathing
- Increased α and β activity on EEG

Emergence, Phase 2
- Increased heart rate and blood pressure
- Return of autonomic responsiveness
- Responsiveness to painful stimulation
- Salivation (7th and 9th cranial nerve nuclei)
- Tearing (7th cranial nerve nuclei)
- Grimacing (5th and 7th cranial nerve nuclei)
- Swallowing, gagging, coughing (9th and 10th cranial nerve nuclei)
- Return of muscle tone (spinal cord, reticulospinal tract, basal ganglia, and primary motor tracts)
- Defensive posturing
- Further increase in α and β activity on EEG
- Extubation possible

Emergence, Phase 3
- Eye opening
- Responses to some oral commands
- Awake patterns on EEG
- Extubation possible

Adapted from Brown EN, Lydic R, Schiff ND. General anesthesia, sleep, and coma. *N Engl J Med.* 2010;363(27):2638-2650.

process.[54] As expected, the least soluble desflurane exhibits the fastest clinical recovery, with sevoflurane and isoflurane following in that order. Residual anesthetic has been shown to remain in the body for several days following a routine anesthetic.[55] Research from 2015 indicates that emergence may also be influenced by the release of neuropeptides such as orexins A and B, which are important factors regulating sleep-wake cycles and a current target for pharmacologic manipulation.[56,57] Box 7.3 shows several signs and phases of emergence.

Diffusion Hypoxia

During emergence, when high concentrations of a rapid (insoluble) anesthetic such as nitrous oxide have been given, the drug exits the body quickly through the lungs and is replaced by less soluble nitrogen in air. This may result in a transient dilution of normal respiratory gases such as oxygen and carbon dioxide. This phenomenon is referred to as diffusion hypoxia. Administration of 100% oxygen for several minutes when anesthesia is terminated entirely avoids this potential problem.

Diffusion of Nitrous Oxide Into Closed Spaces

Nitrous oxide diffuses into air-containing cavities in the body during an anesthetic procedure. These air-containing spaces are normally rich in nitrogen, which is 34 times less soluble than nitrous oxide. If the space is expandable, it increases in volume. Examples of expandable air cavities include air embolism, pneumothorax, acute intestinal obstruction, intraocular air bubbles produced by sulfur hexafluoride gas injection, and pneumoperitoneum. Rigid air-containing spaces will undergo an increase in pressure. This includes tympanic membrane grafting after tympanomastoid procedures and intracranial air during diagnostic or surgical intracranial procedures. Nitrous oxide should be avoided in these situations. The endotracheal tube cuff, laryngeal mask airway, and balloon-tipped pulmonary artery catheters may expand during nitrous oxide anesthesia, and appropriate precautions and adjustments should be considered.[58-60]

Some characteristics and time courses for air expansion are noted in Table 7.5.[61]

PEDIATRICS

The uptake of inhalation anesthetic drugs is faster in children than in adults, leading to a more rapid induction.[62,63] The child's higher alveolar ventilation specifically related to their increased respiratory rate accounts for this effect.

Infants and children have a higher cardiac output per weight than adults. As noted previously, the higher the cardiac output, the slower the onset. This effect is minimized, however, by the increased cardiac output distributed to the vessel-rich group in children. The infant's lower muscle mass allows more of the agent to concentrate in the vital organs. This overall effect is to promote uptake to the brain.

Finally, anesthetics appear to be less blood soluble (i.e., they work faster) in children than in adults. This effect varies with age and the agent.[64-66] The MAC or required dose of anesthetics is higher in infants and children and decreases with increasing age. Infants aged 6 months have a MAC 1.5 to 1.8 times higher than a 40-year-old adult.[67]

Occasionally, during recovery from anesthesia with inhalation agents, especially sevoflurane and to a lesser extent desflurane, emergence reactions and agitation may occur in infants, children, and young adults.[68-70] It usually occurs within the first 10 minutes of recovery. Emergence agitation typically resolves quickly and is followed by uneventful recovery. Evidence suggests that this phenomenon is not pharmacokinetic or related to rapidity of emergence.[71] Major risk factors include preschool age 2 to 5 years, difficult parental separation behavior, anxiety, and postoperative pain. Minor risk factors include male gender and type of procedure, including tonsillectomy, strabismus surgery, and neurosurgery.[70-72] Administration of propofol, fentanyl, midazolam, dexmedetomidine, or ketamine reduce the incidence of emergence agitation.[72-74] A glossary of pharmacokinetic concepts is given in Table 7.6.

TABLE 7.5 Nitrous Oxide–Induced Space or Compartment Change*

Air Space	Nitrous Oxide–Induced Change
Pneumoencephalogram	CSF pressure increases to three times baseline in 5 min
Intraocular hexafluoride gas	2–18 mm Hg increase in pressure in 20 min
Middle ear pressure	Increased 1–7 mm Hg in 1 hr
Pneumothorax	2–3 times the volume in 5–20 min
Intestinal gas	Double in 150 min
Air bubble	Immediate increases in size occur

*The rate at which the pressure changes depends on the perfusion of surrounding tissue, compliance of the space, and the concentration of nitrous oxide.
CSF, Cerebrospinal fluid.
Data adapted from Evers AS, Maze M, Kharasch ED, et al., eds. *Anesthetic Pharmacology.* 2nd ed. Cambridge: Cambridge University Press; 2011:393.

OTHER FACTORS

Obesity

Obesity has a minimal clinically significant effect on the uptake of the inhalation anesthetics. Some clinicians prefer desflurane because of its low solubility and lipophilicity, which appear to promote a slightly faster recovery. Long procedures and morbid obesity allow for an increase in deposition of anesthetics into fat and may prolong recovery.[75-77]

Pregnancy

Pregnant women have a higher minute ventilation than nonpregnant women, which would predict a faster uptake. Conversely, they also have a higher cardiac output, which tends to slow uptake. Overall, these actions oppose each other so that the uptake of anesthetics in pregnant women will be similar to that in nonpregnant women.[78] Maternal-to-fetal transfer of the nitrous oxide has been studied, and data suggest that placental transfer during cesarean section is slower than maternal uptake and time dependent.[79]

Shunts

Right-to-Left Shunt

A right-to-left shunt may be pathophysiologic or produced as part of the anesthetic technique such as one lung ventilation. With a

TABLE 7.6 Inhalational Anesthetic Pharmacokinetic Concepts

Concept	Comments
Minimum alveolar concentration (MAC)	The MAC required to achieve surgical anesthesia (immobility) in 50% of patients exposed to a noxious stimulus.
MAC awake	The MAC suppressing appropriate response to commands in 50% of patients; memory is usually lost at MAC awake; approximately 0.3–0.5 MAC.
MAC—block adrenergic responses (MAC-BAR)	The alveolar concentration of anesthetic that blunts the autonomic response to noxious stimuli; approximately 1.6–2.0 MAC.
Ventilation effect	The greater the alveolar ventilation, the faster the patient achieves anesthesia.
Concentration effect	The higher the concentration of anesthetic delivered, the faster anesthesia is achieved; this is also referred to as overpressuring; as with any drug, the larger the initial dose administered, the faster the onset of action.
Blood/gas solubility coefficient	The blood/gas solubility coefficient is the indicator of an anesthetic's speed of onset and emergence: the higher the coefficient, the slower the anesthetic; conversely, the lower the coefficient, the faster the anesthetic.
Oil/gas solubility coefficient	The oil/gas solubility coefficient is the indicator of an anesthetic's potency: the higher the coefficient, the more potent the agent.
Second-gas effect	The second-gas effect is a phenomenon in which two anesthetics of varying onset speeds are administered together: a high concentration of a fast anesthetic such as nitrous oxide is administered with a slower second anesthetic gas; the slower gas achieves anesthetic levels more quickly than if it had been given alone.
Diffusion hypoxia	Diffusion hypoxia occurs when high concentrations of nitrous oxide are administered; at the end of the procedure, when nitrous oxide is discontinued, it leaves the body very rapidly, causing a transient dilution of the oxygen and carbon dioxide in the lungs; hypocarbia and hypoxia may occur; administration of 100% oxygen for approximately 3–5 min when nitrous oxide is discontinued alleviates this problem.
Cardiac output effect	Increases in cardiac output decrease the speed of onset of all anesthetics; the more soluble anesthetics are affected to a much greater extent than the insoluble anesthetics.
Ventilation-perfusion abnormalities	Ventilation-perfusion abnormalities reduce the speed of onset of all anesthetics and affect the insoluble agents to a much greater degree than the soluble agents.
Pediatrics	Children achieve anesthesia more rapidly than adults because of a higher ventilatory rate and vessel-rich group blood flow; this occurs despite the fact that the required dose and cardiac output are higher in children.
Obesity	Obesity has minimal clinical effects on anesthetic induction; however, emergence may be slower because of deposition of anesthetics in fat.
Pregnancy	The kinetics of the inhalation anesthetics are similar in pregnant women and nonpregnant women; placental transfer is time dependent as expected.

right-to-left shunt, the shunted blood mixes with and dilutes the blood coming from the ventilated alveoli, resulting in a reduction of alveolar partial pressure of the anesthetic. The decrease in the rise in alveolar concentration slows induction of anesthesia. The extent of slowing in the rise of the alveolar concentration produced by a right to left shunt varies according to the solubility of the anesthetic. The rate of rise of the alveolar concentration of an insoluble agent (low blood/gas coefficient) will be affected more than that of a soluble anesthetic (high blood/gas coefficient). This occurs because uptake of a soluble anesthetic offsets dilutional effects of shunted blood on the alveolar concentration. Uptake of an insoluble drug is minimal, so dilutional effects on the alveolar concentration are unopposed. The impact of a right-to-left shunt is opposite to that observed with changes in cardiac output and alveolar ventilation. When considering these opposing forces, there is no clinically significant effect on the speed of induction.[80,81]

Left-to-Right Shunts

Left-to-right tissue shunts result in the blood delivered to the lungs containing a higher partial pressure of anesthetic than that present in blood that has passed through tissues. Systemic left-to-right shunting causes the anesthetic partial pressure in mixed venous blood to increase more rapidly than it would in the absence of such shunts. When blood flow to other tissues remains normal and the left-to-right shunt simply represents excess cardiac output, the resulting increase in anesthetic uptake is offset by the increase in anesthetic partial pressure in mixed venous blood. The result is a slight increase in the rate of anesthetic delivery or uptake into the brain, muscle, and other tissues. In cases

where large left-to-right shunts result in reduced blood flow to other tissues, anesthetic equilibration in those tissues will be relatively slow.

Left-to-right shunts offset the dilutional effects of a right-to-left shunt on the alveolar concentration. The effect of a left-to-right shunt on the rate of increase in the alveolar anesthetic concentration is detectable only if there is a concomitant right-to-left shunt. Likewise, the effect of a right-to-left shunt on the rate of increase in the arterial anesthetic concentration is maximal in the absence of a left-to-right shunt.[80,81]

Cardiopulmonary Bypass

The transfer characteristics of modern membrane oxygenators are more limited than the lungs. During bypass it is necessary to administer a relative higher concentration of the volatile agent compared to that which is required when administered by normal lung inhalation. This will ensure the adequate transfer across the membrane of the oxygenator and an adequate depth of anesthesia. The uptake of volatile agents administered by the oxygenator is dependent on three factors: blood/gas solubility, which increases as temperature falls; tissue/gas solubility, which increases as temperature falls; and oxygenator uptake.

Like the intact circulation, the uptake and elimination of volatile anesthetic agents during cardiopulmonary bypass (CPB) is inversely proportional to blood/gas solubility. Whereas increasing gas flow to the oxygenator increases uptake of inhalation agents, changes in pump flow rate have no impact. This is likely because of a relatively small blood volume and large pump flow at the oxygenator. This is quite different from the intact circulation where cardiac output has a major impact on the pulmonary uptake of inhalation anesthetic agents.[82,83]

SUMMARY

A thorough understanding of the basic pharmacokinetic principles involved in administering anesthetic gases and the development of clinical skills in their use are the cornerstones of modern anesthesia practice. Adults are generally induced with one of the several available intravenous agents and maintained with a combination of inhalation and intravenous drugs. Better anesthesia machines and more sophisticated monitoring have greatly facilitated the quantification of clinical anesthetic levels and depth, contributing to the remarkable safety of modern anesthesia practice.

REFERENCES

 For a complete list of references for this chapter, scan this QR code with any smartphone code reader app, or visit the following URL: http://booksite.elsevier.com/9780323711944/.

8

Inhalation Anesthetics

John J. Nagelhout

In the span of almost two centuries, major advances have been made in the development and clinical use of inhalation anesthetics (Table 8.1); this continuum includes the investigation of nitrous oxide (N_2O) in 1800 by Humphry Davy[1] following its preliminary discovery by Dr. Priestly in 1786[2] with what was termed *dephlogisticated air*. Then, 195 years later, in 1995, the most current inhaled anesthetic (sevoflurane) was approved by the US Food and Drug Administration (FDA).

The present-day use of N_2O can be credited to Edmund Andrews, a professor of surgery in Chicago. In 1868 he declared that a safer anesthetic could result from combining oxygen (O_2) with N_2O.[3] Before that time, N_2O was administered through a mouthpiece with a nose clamp to prevent the rebreathing of air.

One of the earliest "complete" anesthetic agents used was diethyl ether ($C_2H_5-O-C_2H_5$). The first ether anesthetic was administered in Georgia on March 30, 1842, when Crawford Long anesthetized a patient for a minor operation (excising a tumor).[4] However, the recognition of numerous unfavorable characteristics (excessive secretions with inhalation induction, laryngospasm, excessive depths of anesthesia) prompted its disappearance from clinical practice as newer agents were subsequently developed.

In the 1930s research into potential anesthetic agents was based on the principle of a structure-activity relationship.[5] One of the earliest inhalation anesthetics developed in this manner was divinyl ether. Halothane was introduced into clinical practice in 1956 by Bryce-Smith and O'Brien in Oxford[6] and Johnstone in Manchester,[7] and represented a significant advancement in inhalation anesthesia. Its sweet odor, nonflammability, and high potency offered clinical characteristics that were absent from the previously available inhaled anesthetics. The search for newer and improved inhalation anesthetics persisted, as concerns with the hepatotoxicity and arrhythmogenicity of this alkane derivative began to be documented.

The two most recently released inhalation agents, sevoflurane (synthesized by Regan in the late 1960s) and desflurane (the 653rd compound of more than 700 synthesized by Terrell and colleagues between 1959 and 1966), are commonly used today for a diverse surgical population, based on their pharmacokinetic and pharmacodynamic profiles. Although desflurane and sevoflurane do not possess all of the properties of an ideal inhalation agent, anesthesia providers routinely select one or the other for most surgical procedures due to the sufficient number of clinical benefits attributed to these agents.

Only four new anesthetics have been approved by the FDA over the past 30 years (1985–2014), compared to ten during the preceding 30 years (1955–1984). Investigational anesthetics are almost exclusively intravenous anesthetics, and only one has been approved. None demonstrate a truly novel mechanism of action. The lack of new anesthetics may be due to multiple reasons, including the dramatic improvement in anesthesia safety (which decreases the pressure to develop new drugs with better safety margins), lack of pharmaceutic industry profit, lack of academic interest, and the fact that the mechanism of action of general anesthetics is poorly understood.[8]

RELATIONSHIP BETWEEN CHEMICAL STRUCTURE AND AGENT CHARACTERISTICS

An understanding of the chemical structure of inhalation agents provides insight into their physical properties (e.g., flammability). However, the relationship between the pharmacologic characteristics (e.g., arrhythmogenic properties) and chemical structure of agents is not as predictable. This section reviews the structure-activity relationship of inhalation anesthetics and their clinical relevance. Some selected physical and chemical properties of the anesthetics are listed in Table 8.2.

All commonly used inhalation agents are ethers (R–O–R) or aliphatic hydrocarbons (straight-chain or branched nonaromatic hydrocarbons) with no more than four carbon atoms (Fig. 8.1). The length of the anesthetic molecule is significant in that immobility (anesthetic effect) is attenuated or lost if the chain length exceeds four or five carbon atoms (5 angstroms [Å]).[9] The molecular shape of the agents is spherical or cylindrical with a length less than 1.5 times the diameter.[10]

Of primary importance to the development of inhalation agents was the discovery of the impact of halogenation of organic compounds. Halogenation of hydrocarbons and ethers (the addition of fluorine [F], chlorine [Cl], bromine [Br], or iodine [I]) influences

TABLE 8.1 History of the Introduction of Inhalation Anesthetics	
Anesthetic	**Year Anesthetic Properties Demonstrated/Introduced**
Ether (Crawford Long)	1842
N_2O (Horace Wells)	1845
Chloroform (James Simpson)	1847
Cyclopropane (George Lucas, Velyien Henderson)	1934
Fluroxene	1951
Halothane	1956
Methoxyflurane	1960
Enflurane	1973
Isoflurane	1981
Desflurane	1993
Sevoflurane	1995

TABLE 8.2 Select Characteristics of Inhalation Anesthetics

Characteristics	Nitrous Oxide	Isoflurane	Desflurane	Sevoflurane
Molecular formula	N_2O	$C_3H_2ClF_5O$	$C_3H_2F_6O$	$C_4H_3F_7O$
Ostwald blood/gas partition coefficient (37°C)	0.47	1.43	0.42	0.68
Oil/gas partition coefficient	1.4	99	18.7	50
Saturated vapor pressure (mm Hg, at 20°C)	Gas	238	669	157
Molecular weight (g/mol)	44.01	184.49	168.04	200.05
Preservative	None	None	None	None

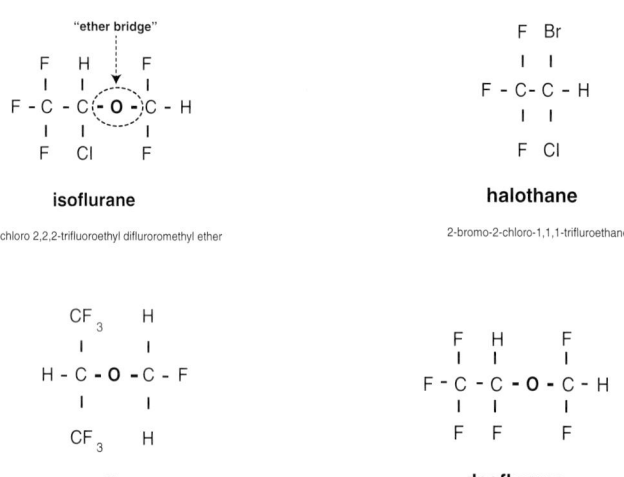

isoflurane

1-chloro 2,2,2-trifluoroethyl difluoromethyl ether

halothane

2-bromo-2-chloro-1,1,1-trifluroethane

sevoflurane

fluoromethyl 2,2,2,-trifuoro-1-(trifluoromethyl) ethyl ether

desflurane

difluoromethyl, 1,2,2,2-tetrafluoroethyl ether

Fig. 8.1 Chemical structure of inhalation agents. The "ether bridges" (R–O–R) are seen with sevoflurane, desflurane, and isoflurane. *R* refers to an alkyl group. Halothane (no longer used) is an example of a halogenated hydrocarbon.

anesthetic potency, arrhythmogenic properties, flammability, and chemical stability (e.g., oxidation during storage and reactions with bases).

Anesthetic potency has been shown to increase when a halogen with a lower atomic mass unit (amu) is replaced by a heavier halogen (e.g., bromine at 80 amu substituted for fluorine at 19 amu).[11–13] Nonetheless, a ceiling effect exists with halogenation of anesthetic compounds. For example, adding F atoms to ether results in a continuum in which the ether becomes more potent, then acts as a strong convulsant, and finally changes to an inert compound with full fluorination.[14]

In general, the potency of inhalation agents has also been found to correlate with the physical property of lipid solubility. A decline in potency (meaning an increase in the minimum alveolar concentration [MAC] of inhalation agents) is associated with a proportional decrease in oil/gas partition coefficient values. Exceptions to this principle exist and demonstrate that the correlation between potency and lipid solubility is not perfect.

With regard to arrhythmogenic properties, increasing the number of halogen atoms within an inhalation agent favors the genesis of cardiac dysrhythmias.[14] Nevertheless, alkanes that contain five halogens (e.g., halothane) are more prone to induce arrhythmias than ethers with six halogen atoms (e.g., isoflurane). This may be due to the lack of an oxygen molecule in halothane as compared to the ethers.[15]

Inhalation anesthetics interact with the main repolarizing cardiac potassium channels (hERG) and IKs channels, as well as with calcium and sodium channels at slightly higher concentrations. Inhibition of these ion channels alters both action potential shape (triangulation) and electrical impulse conduction, which may facilitate arrhythmogenesis by inhalation anesthetics per se and is potentiated by catecholamines. Action potential triangulation by regionally heterogeneous inhibition of calcium (Ca^{2+}) and potassium (K^+) channels will facilitate catecholamine-induced afterdepolarizations, triggered activity, and enhanced automaticity. Inhibition of cardiac sodium channels will reduce conduction velocity and alter the refractory period; this is potentiated by catecholamines and promotes reentry arrhythmias.[16]

Flammability is reduced and chemical stability enhanced by substituting hydrogen atoms with halogens. The epitome of this relationship is demonstrated with desflurane, a compound that contains fluorine as its only halogen and thus strongly resists biodegradation; desflurane is metabolized one tenth as much as isoflurane.[17,18]

PHARMACODYNAMICS

Mechanisms of Action

The exact mechanism of action of inhalation anesthetics remains elusive. A favored hypothesis proposes that general anesthesia results from direct multisite interactions with multiple and diverse ion channels in the brain. Neurotransmitter-gated ion channels and two-pore K^+ channels are key players in the mechanism of anesthesia; however, new information has also implicated voltage-gated ion channels. A variety of ligand-gated ion channels, receptors, and signal transduction proteins are modulated by anesthetics at myriad levels of the central nervous system (CNS). Recent biophysical and structural studies of Na+ and K^+ channels strongly suggest that halogenated inhalational general anesthetics interact with the gates and pore regions of these ion channels to modulate function. A combination of many different mechanisms could be responsible for general anesthetic action. Evidence indicates that no single universal receptor explains the actions of general anesthetics. The multiple components of the anesthetic state, amnesia, sedation/unconsciousness, analgesia, and immobility are mediated by separate effects on different receptors and neuronal pathways.[19–22]

The following properties of anesthetics must be taken into account when developing a theory that attempts to explain their mechanism of action[23]:

- Lipid solubility is directly proportional to potency (Meyer-Overton rule).
- Reversal of anesthetic effect can be achieved with the application of pressure, with some exceptions (animal species variation).

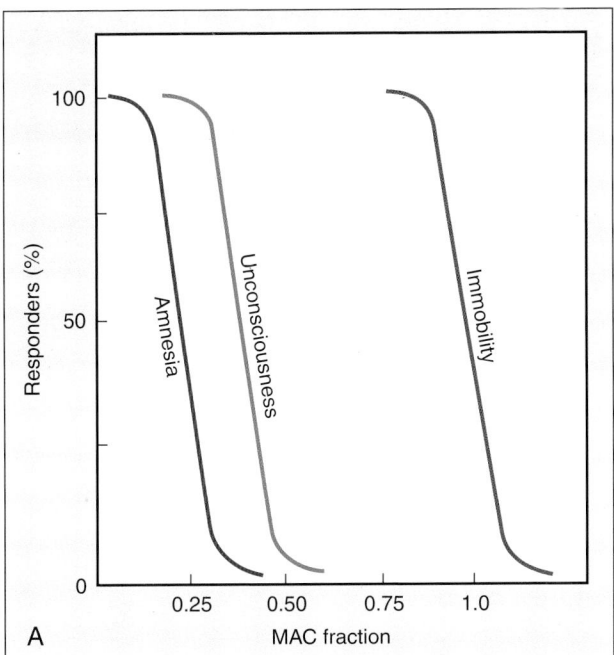
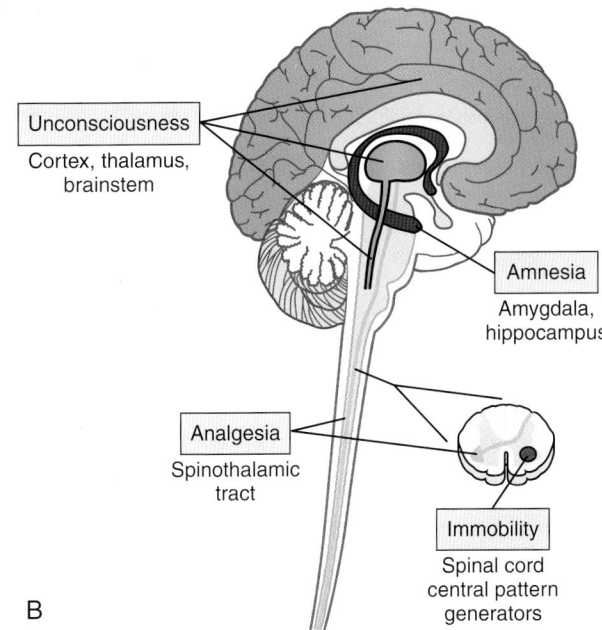

Fig. 8.2 Multiple sites of inhalation anesthetic action. A, Inhalation anesthetics lead to multiple dose-dependent behavioral end points. Cardiovascular responses occur at even greater doses (not shown). B, Amnesia, the most sensitive anesthetic end point, probably involves the hippocampus, amygdala, medio-temporal lobe, and possibly other cortical structures involved in learning and memory. Unconsciousness likely involves the cerebral cortex, thalamus, and brain stem reticular formation essential to consciousness and arousal. Immobility occurs by anesthetic action on the spinal cord central pattern generators. Anesthetic effects on the spinal cord blunt ascending impulses arising from noxious stimulation, leading to analgesia, and might indirectly contribute to anesthetic-induced unconsciousness. (From Hemmings Jr. HC, Egan TD. *Pharmacology and Physiology for Anesthesia.* Philadelphia: Elsevier; 2019:220.)

- No common chemical structure for the variety of compounds is capable of producing anesthesia.
- The molecular and structural changes responsible for producing anesthesia must occur within seconds and be reversible.
- A reduction in body temperature lowers anesthetic requirements.

The unitary hypothesis was previously offered as an attempt to meet these prerequisites. This theory proposed that all inhalation anesthetics work via a similar (undefined) mechanism of action, but not necessarily at the same site of action. One factor that supported this hypothesis was the Meyer-Overton correlation, which recognized that the more lipid soluble the agent, the greater its potency (the lower its MAC value). The Meyer-Overton theory postulated that even though the anesthetic agents have a wide variety of structures, they share the ability to alter the lipid environment of proteins, thus changing their function. Though elegant, this theory has not been supported by research, which instead points to anesthetics binding to specific pockets in proteins and altering their function.[24,25]

In vitro, in vivo, animal, and human subject research has permitted the description of the mechanism of action of inhaled anesthetics relative to distinct anatomic regions of the body (including the cellular level) and molecular changes. The spinal cord is known to mediate immobility to a painful stimulus via several mechanisms, including (1) enhancing background K^+ currents in tandem-pore-domain, weak inward-rectifying K^+ channels (TWIK, TASK [TWIK-related acid-sensitive K^+ channel])[26-28] and (2) reducing spontaneous action potential firing of spinal neurons via glycine receptors and γ-aminobutyric acid type A ($GABA_A$) receptors.[29] Investigators have also demonstrated that nonimmobilizers with lipophilic characteristics (e.g., perfluoropentane) are able to produce amnesia but not immobility to noxious stimuli, which suggests two separate sites and

mechanisms of anesthetic action for some drugs.[30] In contrast with other research, spinal and cerebral $GABA_A$ receptors (which have the same receptor-clinical effect) were shown to contribute to the ability of inhalation anesthetics to produce immobility; therefore, the anesthetic effect of immobility is modulated at the spinal cord and supraspinal level.[31,32]

The CNS effects of amnesia and loss of consciousness are likely produced separately from immobility, as conceptualized in the theory of MAC. The concept of MAC refers to the concentration required to prevent movement in response to a surgical situation. This is probably the result of an effect at the spinal cord level via glycine, sodium, and N-methyl-D-aspartate (NMDA) receptor action. K^+, $GABA_A$, opioid, $α_2$, $5HT_3$, and acetylcholine receptors are likely not involved in producing immobility.[33] They may be involved in varying degrees in the amnestic and anesthetic effects in the CNS.[34,35] The CNS effects are dose related, with amnesia requiring the lowest dose, followed by sedation, unconsciousness, and immobility. These effects are produced at varying anatomic sites (Fig. 8.2). A summary of the mechanisms of action of inhalation anesthetics reviewed in this chapter is provided in Box 8.1.

MINIMUM ALVEOLAR CONCENTRATION

A useful means of comparing the potencies of inhalation agents is to use the concept of MAC, defined as the MAC at equilibrium (expressed as a percentage of 1 atmosphere), where 50% of subjects will not respond to a painful stimulus (i.e., initial surgical skin incision).[36] A response is defined as gross, purposeful movement of the head or extremities. The MAC represents the required dose of the anesthetic. The MAC values for the modern inhalation agents are listed in Table 8.3.[37-40]

BOX 8.1 Mechanisms of Action of Inhalation Anesthetics

- Anesthesia consists of separable and independent components, each of which involves distinct, but possibly overlapping, mechanisms at different sites in the central nervous system.
- The potencies of general anesthetics correlate with their solubility in oil.
- Mutations made to render putative protein targets insensitive to inhaled anesthetics have been expressed in mice but have not generated breakthroughs analogous to the success of this strategy with intravenous anesthetics.
- The effects of inhaled anesthetics cannot be explained by a single molecular mechanism.
- The immobilizing effect of inhaled anesthetics involves actions in the spinal cord, whereas sedation/hypnosis and amnesia involve supraspinal mechanisms that interact with endogenous memory, sleep, and consciousness pathways and networks.
- Inhaled anesthetics suppress excitatory synaptic transmission presynaptically by reducing glutamate release (inhalation anesthetics) and postsynaptically by inhibiting excitatory ionotropic receptors activated by glutamate (gaseous and to some extent inhalation anesthetics).
- There is as yet no comprehensive theory of anesthesia that describes the sequence of events leading from the interaction between an anesthetic molecule and its targets to the behavioral effects.
- Previously, gene deletion studies demonstrated important roles for both ligand- and voltage-gated ion channels in producing anesthetic-induced loss of consciousness. In silico modeling now provides evidence for simultaneous anesthetic modulation of both channel families in thalamocortical neurons as being necessary and sufficient to produce the electroencephalogram signature associated with such unconsciousness.
- Distinct circuits and networks in the brain contribute to anesthetic-induced loss of consciousness while others govern emergence.
- Anesthetic effects can persist beyond the immediate perioperative period with adverse impact on memory, learning, and possibly cognitive function.

Adapted from Perouansky M, Pearce RC, Hemmings HC. Inhalation anesthetics: mechanisms of action. In: Gropper MA, et al., eds. *Miller's Anesthesia*. 9th ed. Philadelphia: Elsevier; 2020:487–508; Hemmings Jr HC, Riegelhaupt PM, Kelz MB, et al. Towards a comprehensive understanding of anesthetic mechanisms of action: a decade of discovery. *Trends Pharmacol Sci*. 2019;40(7):464–481.

The MAC of inhalation agents can be affected by numerous factors, even hair color.[41] With increasing age, the MAC of all inhaled anesthetics is reduced; in humans with a mean age of 18 to 30 years, the MAC of desflurane is 7.25%, in contrast to 6% in humans 30 to 55 years of age.[39,40] Infants represent an exception to the MAC age concept, in that their anesthetic requirements exceed those of neonates. In general, the duration of anesthesia is believed not to affect MAC; however, one group of investigators found that the MAC of isoflurane was reduced over time during surgery.[42] Box 8.2 lists variables shown to reduce and increase MAC.

Two other areas related to MAC are MAC-awake and MAC-BAR (block adrenergic response). MAC-awake is defined as the MAC at which 50% of subjects will respond to the command "open your eyes." It has also been described as the anesthetic concentration that falls between the end-tidal values that allow and prevent response to a command.[43] This end-tidal concentration is usually associated with a loss of recall and encompasses approximately one-third of MAC values. MAC-awake can also be used in combination with MAC values to evaluate the potency of each agent with regard to amnestic properties. This is done by dividing MAC-awake by MAC (to calculate the MAC-awake/MAC ratio). Agents with MAC-awake/MAC ratios between 0.3

TABLE 8.3 Minimum Alveolar Concentrations of Inhalation Anesthetics in Humans With and Without N_2O, Expressed as MAC Values

Anesthetic	MAC* (Expressed as a % of 1 Atmosphere)	MAC in 60–70% N_2O
Nitrous oxide	104	—
Isoflurane	1.17	0.56
Desflurane	6	2.38
Sevoflurane	2	0.66

*For patients aged 30 to 60 years.
MAC, Minimum alveolar concentration; N_2O, nitrous oxide. **MAC-awake** is the minimum alveolar concentration of anesthetic that inhibits responses to command in half of patients. It is approximately one-third of MAC. **MAC-BAR** is the minimum alveolar concentration of anesthetic that blunts the autonomic response to noxious stimuli. It is approximately 1.6 times higher than MAC.

BOX 8.2 Relationship of Physiologic and Pharmacologic Factors to the MAC of Inhaled Anesthetics

Factors That Reduce MAC
- Increased age
- Hypothermia
- Administration of sedative hypnotics
- Coadministration of other anesthetic agents
- α_2 agonists
- Opioids
- Acute ethanol consumption
- Hypoxemia
- Hyponatremia
- Hypermagnesemia
- Anemia (<4.3 mL O_2/dL blood)
- Hypotension (MAP <50 mm Hg)
- Pregnancy
- Lithium

Factors That Increase MAC
- Young age
- Hyperthermia
- Hyperthyroidism
- Hypernatremia
- Acute administration of CNS stimulant drugs
- Red hair in females
- Chronic alcohol abuse

Factors With No Effect on MAC
- Duration of anesthesia
- Gender
- Hypocapnia and hypercapnia
- Metabolic alkalosis
- Hypertension
- Hyperkalemia or hypokalemia

CNS, Central nervous system; *MAC*, minimum alveolar concentration; *MAP*, mean arterial pressure; O_2, oxygen.

and 0.4 (e.g., desflurane, sevoflurane, and isoflurane) are considered potent anesthetics. In contrast, N_2O, which has a ratio of 0.64, is considered a weak amnestic agent.

The MAC-BAR parameter represents the MAC necessary to block the adrenergic response (e.g., changes in plasma norepinephrine concentration, heart rate [HR], rate-pressure product, and mean arterial pressure [MAP]) to skin incision. It can be expressed as a MAC-BAR$_{50}$ or MAC-BAR$_{95}$. The former value is similar to AD$_{95}$ values, which represent the anesthetic dose that inhibits somatic evidence of light anesthesia in 95% of subjects in response to skin incision. Established MAC-BAR$_{50}$ values for inhalation agents (in 60% N_2O) include 1.85 MAC for both isoflurane and desflurane. The MAC-BAR$_{50}$ value of desflurane can be reduced by 85% by administering 1.5 mcg/kg of fentanyl intravenously (IV) 5 minutes before skin incision.[44] When investigating desflurane in 60% N_2O combined with remifentanil at a target plasma concentration of 1 ng/mL (via a computer-driven infusion device), the MAC-BAR$_{50}$ is reduced by 60%, and with a target concentration of 3 ng/mL can be reduced by a further 30%.[45]

The MAC-BAR$_{50}$ for sevoflurane in 66% N_2O is 2.2.[46] It should be emphasized that MAC-BAR values exceed the requirements for ablation of skeletal muscle movement with surgical stimulation; therefore blocking an adrenergic response requires a greater depth of anesthesia than preventing skeletal muscle movement. Clinically, patients usually require anesthetic concentrations that exceed the MAC by 20% to 30% (1.2–1.3 times MAC). At this alveolar concentration, somatic evidence of light anesthesia will typically be abated, and fewer patients will have an adrenergic response to the stresses of surgery.[47]

The concept of MAC has limitations when applied clinically to determine adequacy of anesthesia.[48] It should be viewed as a general guide to the overall depth of anesthesia. Anesthetic requirements vary throughout surgery and from patient to patient and should be titrated to the desired physiologic response. Efforts have attempted to correlate MAC with the bispectral index monitor (BIS) to aid in anesthesia administration. The data show that equipotent doses of the inhalation anesthetics yield different BIS values, and the clinical correlation is directly related to a specific value. The MAC and BIS values are likely measuring different activities.[49] A 2012 outcome study noted that a triple low state, defined as an intraoperative MAP of 75 mm Hg, MAC less than 0.8, and a BIS value less than 45, was associated with an increased length of stay and increased 30-day mortality.[50] Subsequent studies have not replicated these findings.[51,52]

INFLUENCE OF INHALATION AGENTS ON ORGANS AND SYSTEMS

Central Nervous System

The CNS is the primary site of action of the inhalation agents, which exhibit important dose-dependent effects with significant clinical considerations. Such effects include intracranial compliance, autoregulation of cerebral blood flow (CBF; e.g., cerebrovascular reactivity to carbon dioxide [CO_2]), cerebral metabolic rate, cerebrospinal fluid pressure (CSFP), and neurologic assessment. Their typical actions, as well as their effects in patients with CNS pathology, are considered in the following sections.

Cerebral Metabolic Rate and Cerebral Blood Flow

In general, inhalation agents, including isoflurane, sevoflurane, and desflurane, decrease cerebral metabolic rate of O_2 consumption ($CMRO_2$) in a dose-dependent manner, whereas their effect on CBF varies with dose.[53-55] Inhalation anesthetics also produce a dose-dependent increase in CBF. This effect depends on the balance between vasoconstrictive properties, due to flow-metabolism coupling, and the direct cerebral vasodilatory action of the anesthetics. When vascular resistance is decreased, CBF, cerebral blood volume, and CSFP increase. The order of potency for increasing CBF varies; it is affected by the dose of inhalation anesthetic, the administration of other drugs (e.g., propofol, N_2O), and the rate of change in end-tidal concentration of agent.[56-58]

Uncoupling of Cerebral Blood Flow and Metabolism

When decreases in $CMRO_2$ are accompanied by increases in CBF, uncoupling is said to occur. As noted earlier, inhalation anesthetics are capable of producing this effect. This paradoxic response (decreased $CMRO_2$ occurring in conjunction with increased CBF) seems not to occur with 1.0 MAC or less of desflurane or isoflurane.[59] The magnitude of change is variable and dose dependent, meaning some flow-metabolism coupling mechanism is preserved.[60]

Nitrous oxide reduces cerebrovascular tone significantly. This effect is unmasked and enhanced when N_2O is combined with an inhalation anesthetic (decreased autoregulation).[61] The mechanism for increased CBF may be related to a sympathoadrenal-stimulating effect of N_2O. The changes produced by N_2O in the $CMRO_2$ are the reverse of what takes place with inhalation agents (i.e., increased $CMRO_2$). Thus N_2O increases $CMRO_2$ and CBF. Nevertheless, the combination of elevated CBF and $CMRO_2$ still results in an uncoupling between flow and metabolism because the increase in $CMRO_2$ exceeds, albeit slightly, the elevation in CBF. In summary, N_2O use in neurosurgical procedures is acceptable as long as the anesthesia provider recognizes that its vasodilatory effects might adversely affect surgical outcome in patients with reduced intracranial compliance. Mild hyperventilation to low normal ranges of CO_2 helps attenuate the increase in CBF that accompanies the use of N_2O.[62]

Cerebral Vasculature Responsiveness to CO_2

The normal physiologic response of the cerebral vasculature to CO_2 is to vasoconstrict in the presence of hypocapnia and vasodilate with hypercarbia. This reflex is effective in the acute setting when used during neurosurgical procedures to counteract drug-induced vasodilation and to reduce brain bulk within a closed compartment (cranial vault). The usual goal for patients in whom a reduction in intracranial volume is desired is a partial pressure of arterial carbon dioxide ($PaCO_2$) of approximately 30 to 35 mm Hg, with a duration of effectiveness being perhaps no more than 4 to 6 hours.[63]

Differences exist among the inhalation agents in their ability to interfere with the cerebral vasculature's responsiveness to CO_2. Variables that affect the reported differences include the type of surgical procedure the patient is undergoing, associated pathophysiology, and the presence of any coexisting disease(s). In general, however, the concentrations of isoflurane, sevoflurane, and desflurane that are used clinically preserve the reactivity to changes in carbon dioxide and flow-metabolism coupling.[64,65] One study showed that neither isoflurane nor desflurane increases intracranial pressure in normocapnic patients undergoing removal of supratentorial brain tumors. The cerebral perfusion pressure declined in parallel with MAP, as did the cerebral arteriovenous oxygen content difference. The investigators concluded that flow-metabolism coupling may be preserved during anesthesia with isoflurane and desflurane.[66] These findings suggest that the increase in CBF produced by isoflurane, desflurane, and sevoflurane can be effectively prevented by very mild hyperventilation and using concentrations less than 1.5 MAC.

Electroencephalogram and Evoked Potentials

The inhalation agents produce a dose-related suppression of electroencephalography (EEG) activity (an initial increase [and a later decline] in amplitude and decreased frequency), and at high concentrations produce electrical quiescence. At deeper levels of anesthesia, the EEG may temporarily stop recording; at such time, burst suppression is said to have occurred. This is usually achieved at 1.5 to 2 MAC desflurane, and 2 MAC isoflurane or sevoflurane.[58,67]

For those procedures requiring monitoring of the integrity of the spinal cord or mapping of cortical regions of the brain, the anesthetist should be aware that inhalation agents have an inhibitory effect on cortical somatosensory-, motor-, brainstem-, auditory-, and visual-evoked potentials. Isoflurane, desflurane, sevoflurane, and N_2O produce a dose-dependent reduction in these evoked potentials, with visual-evoked potentials being most sensitive and brainstem-evoked potentials most resistant. Two evoked-potential variables commonly assessed are latency and amplitude. An increase in latency or decrease in amplitude of evoked potentials can reflect ischemia or may be secondary to the inhalation agent. Latency is the time between the initiation of a peripheral stimulus (e.g., electrical stimulation of the median nerve at the wrist) and onset of the evoked potential (e.g., cortical) recorded by scalp electrodes.[58,67–70] Sevoflurane can augment epileptic activity. Sevoflurane is the preferred anesthetic for pediatric anesthesia; however, precautions may be advisable in children with a history of epileptic activity.[71,72] The effects of the commonly used anesthetic drugs on sensory- and motor-evoked potentials and some advantages and disadvantages for their use are listed in Table 8.4. The effects of the inhalation anesthetics on EEG are listed in Chapter 19 and Table 19.3.

Emergence and Neurologic Assessment in Adults

Although a smooth and rapid emergence from a general anesthetic is desirable for all surgical patients, it is especially important for neurosurgical patients. Delayed emergence in this specialty of anesthesia can have devastating consequences. A slow return of consciousness makes it difficult to perform the initial postoperative neurologic examination. It can also lead to unnecessary therapeutic or diagnostic intervention and predispose the patient to respiratory complications.[73]

Research has focused on recovery profiles following anesthesia techniques with or without an inhalation agent. Some investigators report a more rapid awakening (after approximately 2 hours of anesthesia) from total intravenous anesthesia (TIVA) in nonneurosurgical patients compared with patients who have received sevoflurane and desflurane combined with N_2O.[74] In side-by-side comparisons of desflurane and sevoflurane, desflurane allows for a more rapid awakening than sevoflurane in volunteers after 8 hours of exposure.[75] One study also found no difference in early postoperative recovery and cognitive function between a balanced sevoflurane-fentanyl technique versus propofol-remifentanil (TIVA) management in patients undergoing supratentorial intracranial surgery.[76] Similarly, a multicenter randomized controlled trial of patients scheduled for elective supratentorial craniotomy surgery found no significant difference between sevoflurane-remifentanil and propofol-remifentanil techniques.[77] The inhalation agents continue to be widely used in most neurosurgical procedures.

Cerebral Neuroprotection

An area of ongoing research has been the application of inhalation anesthetics via preconditioning and postconditioning techniques for neuroprotection following global and/or focal ischemia/hypoxia. Although a growing body of preclinical data suggests that anesthetic agents such as inhalation anesthetics and propofol might have neuroprotective properties, clinical evidence is lacking. There are differences in baseline conditions, comorbidities, the severity of ischemia, and affected brain regions among patients, which may interfere with evaluating the neuroprotective effect of inhalation anesthetics. The goal of neuroprotective treatments is to reduce the clinical effects of cerebral damage through two major mechanisms: increased tolerance of neurologic tissue to ischemia and changes in intracellular responses to energy supply deprivation. Of the various preconditioning strategies, remote ischemic preconditioning (RIPC) and pharmacologic preconditioning appear to be the most clinically promising. Anesthetic preconditioning is a phenomenon of transient organ exposure to anesthetics, within clinical concentrations, that triggers endogenous cellular protection. Anesthetic postconditioning is a concept based on modulation of reperfusion after ischemia that includes the introduction of anesthetics immediately at the onset of reperfusion. RIPC shows potential and is noninvasive, inexpensive, and reasonably well tolerated. Brief episodes of ischemia are induced in an arm or leg by inflation of a blood pressure or tourniquet cuff to more than 20 or 30 mm Hg above systolic blood pressure for 5 to 10 minutes in two to five cycles prior to the potentially injurious cerebral insult.

Magnesium also shows promise, although timing and dosing require clarification. Given the complex pathophysiology of cerebral ischemia and hypoxia, a multimodal approach to neuroprotective strategies may prove the best approach.[78–80] Proposed mechanisms for the neuroprotective effects of the anesthetics are shown in Box 8.3.

Developmental Neurotoxicity

A great deal of concern has arisen regarding the safety of anesthesia in infants and children. There is a growing body of evidence in rodents and nonhuman primates that anesthetics in common clinical use are toxic to the developing brain. Proposed mechanisms of anesthetic-induced neurodegeneration in the newborn involve activation of the intrinsic and extrinsic apoptotic cell death pathways. In the United States alone, more than 1 million children 4 years of age or younger undergo surgical procedures requiring anesthesia each year. The most common procedures required for young children include insertion of pressure equalizing (PE) tubes for chronic ear infection, tonsillectomy, hernia repair, and circumcision, all procedures that typically last less than 60 minutes.[81–84]

Three large-scale clinical studies further address this issue. The Pediatric Anesthesia and NeuroDevelopment Assessment (PANDA) study is a multisite, ambidirectional sibling-matched cohort study conducted at four sites in the United States. Researchers enrolled a total of 105 sibling pairs. Anesthesia consisted of a single exposure to general anesthesia during inguinal hernia surgery in the exposed sibling and no anesthesia exposure in the unexposed sibling, before age 36 months. Among healthy children with a single anesthesia exposure before age 36 months, compared with healthy siblings with no anesthesia exposure, there were no statistically significant differences in IQ scores in later childhood.[84]

Another large-scale study is the General Anaesthesia Compared to Spinal Anesthesia (GAS) Trial, which compares the neurodevelopmental outcome between two anesthetic techniques. It is an international randomized trial comparing general sevoflurane anesthesia with regional anesthesia. A total of 363 infants were randomly assigned to receive awake-regional anesthesia and 359 to receive sevoflurane-based general anesthesia. Outcome data were available for 238 children in the awake-regional group and 294 in the general anesthesia group. Researchers found no evidence that less than 1 hour of sevoflurane anesthesia in infancy increases the risk of adverse neurodevelopmental outcome at 2 years of age compared with awake-regional anesthesia.[85]

TABLE 8.4   The Effect of Various Anesthetic Agents on Neurophysiologic Monitoring of Evoked Potentials

Drug Name	Drug Class	Effect on SSEPs	Effect on MEPs	Length of Emergence	Approximate CST1/2 (min) at 2/4/6 hr and B:GC for Inhalation Agents	Clinical Advantages Relating to Intraoperative Neurophysiologic Monitoring	Disadvantages
Propofol	GABA agonist	↓	↓	+++	15/20/30	Titratable, smooth emergence	Accumulation, slow wakeup
Etomidate	GABA agonist	↑↑	–	++	5/10/20	Titratable, hemodynamically stable	Adrenal suppression, PONV, myoclonus seizures
Midazolam	Benzodiazepine	↓	–	+++	40/60/65	Amnestic	Prolonged emergence
Ketamine	NMDA antagonist	↑	–/↓	+++	15/30/40	Analgesic, amnestic, sympathomimetic, hemodynamically stable	Hallucinations
Fentanyl	Opioid synthetic	–/↓	↓	+++	40/160/240	Analgesic	Accumulation, respiratory depression
Remifentanil	Opioid synthetic	–/↓	–/↓	+	7/7/7	Potent analgesic	Hyperalgesic effect after discontinuation
Sufentanil	Opioid synthetic	–/↓	↓	++	15/20/30	Potent analgesic	Respiratory depression
Dexmedetomidine	α₂ agonist	–/↓	–/↓	+++		Sedative-hypnotic with preserved respiratory drive, awake intubation	Bradycardia and heart block
Isoflurane	Inhalational	↓↓	↓↓↓	+++	1.4	Low cost	Reduced $CMRO_2$ of CNS
Sevoflurane	Inhalational	↓↓	↓↓	++	0.65	Mask induction	Emergence delirium
N₂O	Inhalational	↓↓	↓↓	+	0.47	Rapid elimination, analgesic effect	Synergistic effect on signal depression, PONV
Desflurane	Inhalational	↓↓	↓↓	+	0.42	Rapidly titratable, fast elimination	Emergence delirium, bronchospasm
Rocuronium	NDMR	–	↓↓↓	N/A	N/A	Relatively short half-life and quick elimination after IOA with low doses	Interindividual variability of elimination, risk of residual NMB
Succinylcholine	Depolarizing muscle relaxant	–	↓↓↓	N/A	N/A	Rapid elimination after IOA	Contraindicated in MH and muscular dystrophies, pseudo-cholinesterase deficiency leads to long half-life

Arrows indicate an increase or decrease in the parameter. + MILD, ++ MODERATE, +++ MARKED EFFECT; *B:GC*, Blood:gas partition coefficient (the higher the value, the more agent is dissolved in blood and the longer it takes for the inhalation anesthetic to be eliminated); *CNS*, central nervous system; $CMRO_2$, cerebral metabolic rate for oxygen; *CST1/2*, context-sensitive half-time (elimination half-life as a function of duration of infusion); *GABA*, γ-aminobutyric acid; *IOA*, induction of anesthesia; *MH*, malignant hyperthermia; *MEPs*, motor evoked potentials; *NDMR*, nondepolarizing muscle relaxant; *NMB*, neuromuscular blockade; *NMDA*, N-methyl-D-aspartate; *PONV*, postoperative nausea and vomiting; *SSEPs*, somatosensory evoked potentials.
From Rabai F, Sessions R, Seubert CN. Neurophysiological monitoring and spinal cord integrity. *Best Pract Res Clin Anaesthesiol.* 2016;30(1):53–68.

Finally, a population-based cohort study assessing developmental outcomes at primary school entry (ages 5–6) in more than 28,000 children exposed to general anesthesia was reported. The anesthesia group was compared with more than 55,000 matched controls. They found no evidence of adverse developmental outcomes in children exposed to anesthesia before age 2 or in those with multiple exposures to anesthesia. While there was a very small risk of adverse developmental outcomes in children exposed after age 2, the significance and cause of this finding was unclear. The authors noted that it was reassuring that no adverse effects were seen in such a large group of children exposed to anesthesia under age 2, which is a vulnerable period of human neurodevelopment.[81]

BOX 8.3 Mechanisms Underlying the Neuroprotective Effects of IV and Inhalation Anesthetics

- Inhibition of glutamate release and postsynaptic glutamate receptor-mediated responses
- Stimulation of $GABA_A$ receptors
- Inhibition of the peripheral sympathetic response to ischemia
- Prevention of apoptosis
- Antioxidative effect
- Direct scavenging of free radicals and decrease in lipid peroxidation
- Preconditioning (activation of sarcolemmal and mitochondrial K_{ATP} channels, activation of adenosine receptors, and activation of signaling cascades such as Akt and PKC signaling pathways)
- Antiinflammatory activity

From Jovic M, Unic-Stojanovic D, Isenovic E, et al. Anesthetics and cerebral protection in patients undergoing carotid endarterectomy. *J Cardiothorac Vasc Anesth.* 2015;29(1):178–184.
Akt, Serine/threonine kinase; *GABA_A,* γ-aminobutyric acid A; *IV,* intravenous; *PKC,* protein kinase C.

BOX 8.4 Possible Etiologic Factors of Pediatric Emergence Agitation/Delirium

- Intrinsic characteristics of the anesthetics desflurane and sevoflurane
- Postoperative pain
- Surgery type (ear, nose, and throat surgery)
- Age (preschool-age children)
- Preoperative anxiety
- Previous hospital experience
- Child temperament and personality
- Adjunct medication
- Behaviors (including nonpurposefulness; eyes averted, staring, or closed; and unresponsiveness during early emergence)

The FDA is warning that repeated or lengthy use of general anesthetic and sedation drugs during surgeries or procedures in children younger than 3 years or in pregnant women during their third trimester may affect the development of a child's brain.[82] This is based on animal studies. The FDA notes that recent human studies suggest that a single, relatively short exposure to general anesthetic and sedation drugs in infants or toddlers is unlikely to have negative effects on behavior or learning.[82] In the Unites States clinicians can recommend that parents visit the website for SmartTots (www.smarttots.org), which is a collaboration between the International Anesthesia Research Society and the FDA to coordinate and fund research on the topic of anesthesia and neurodevelopment. This website contains useful resources and a consensus statement created by experts in the field on this topic for both parents and professionals.

The FDA has approved previously announced label changes regarding the use of general anesthetic and sedation medicines in children younger than 3 years. These changes include:

- A new warning stating that exposure to these medicines for lengthy periods of time or over multiple surgeries or procedures may negatively affect brain development in children younger than 3 years.
- Addition of information to the sections of the labels about pregnancy and pediatric use to describe studies in young animals and pregnant animals that showed exposure to general anesthetic and sedation drugs for more than 3 hours can cause widespread loss of nerve cells in the developing brain; studies in young animals suggested these changes resulted in long-term negative effects on the animals' behavior or learning.

General anesthetic and sedation drugs are necessary for patients, including young children and pregnant women, who require surgery or other painful and stressful procedures. In the United States, surgeries during the third trimester of pregnancy requiring general anesthesia are performed only when medically necessary and rarely last longer than 3 hours. Pregnant women should not delay or avoid surgeries or procedures during pregnancy, as doing so can negatively affect themselves and their infants. Similarly, surgeries or procedures in children younger than 3 years should not be delayed or avoided when medically necessary. Consideration should be given to delaying potentially elective surgery in young children where medically appropriate.[82]

Postoperative Cognitive Dysfunction

Postoperative cognitive dysfunction (POCD) as a result of surgery and anesthesia is a concern, especially in the elderly. In a recent study of 8503 twins, a negligible but statistically significant decrease in a sensitive composite cognitive score was present in twins where only one of the twins underwent at least one major surgery, but there was no difference by intrapair analysis. There was no clinically significant association of major surgery and anesthesia with long-term cognitive dysfunction, suggesting that factors other than surgery and anesthesia are more important. A discussion of POCD can be found in Chapter 54.[86]

Emergence Delirium in Children

Emergence delirium (ED) occurs after the use of sevoflurane and desflurane in preschool-aged children in the postanesthesia care unit. Symptoms usually last approximately 10 to 15 minutes and resolve spontaneously once the child eliminates more of the anesthetic. A variety of factors have been suggested to play a potential role in ED. Restless behavior upon emergence causes discomfort to the child, postanesthesia recovery nurses, and parents. Some suggested factors related to transient emergence delirium are noted in Box 8.4. A dose-dependent effect of sevoflurane, which increases seizurelike EEG activity, has also been proposed.[87,88] These children may require analgesics or sedatives, which can delay discharge. It also places patients at increased risk of falls, disruption of surgical repairs, and removal of lines and tubes. ED is self-limiting and devoid of apparent sequelae as long as the child is protected from self-injury. Preventive measures include reducing preoperative anxiety and postoperative pain and providing a quiet, stress-free environment for postanesthesia recovery. Treatment may include small doses of midazolam, ketamine, fentanyl, propofol, or dexmedetomidine. Reuniting the child with the parents is also helpful.[89–91] ED is discussed further in Chapter 55.

Cardiovascular System

All inhalation agents are capable of altering hemodynamics, and the extent is related to various preoperative and intraoperative factors (e.g., ASA physical status classification; coadministration of vasoactive drugs, opioids, benzodiazepines, and propofol). This section reviews the influence of inhalation agents on the cardiovascular system.

Systemic Hemodynamics

Isoflurane, desflurane, and sevoflurane reduce MAP (Fig. 8.3), cardiac output (CO), and cardiac index (CI) in a dose-dependent fashion.[92,93] For example, desflurane, sevoflurane, and isoflurane predominantly reduce MAP via a reduction in systemic vascular resistance (SVR); sevoflurane has the lowest dose-response relationship (Fig. 8.4).[94] N_2O activates the sympathetic nervous system and increases SVR,[95] which

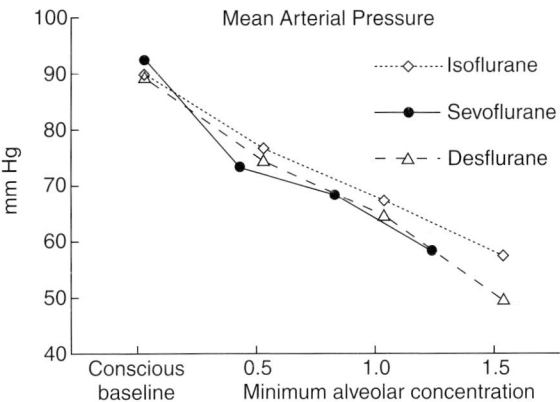

Fig. 8.3 Mean arterial pressure response to the administration of isoflurane, sevoflurane, and desflurane in healthy volunteers. With increasing minimum alveolar anesthetic concentration, progressive decreases
in blood pressure occurred with each of the inhalation anesthetics.
(Adapted from Ebert TJ, Muzi M. Sympathetic hyperactivity during desflurane anesthesia in healthy volunteers: a comparison with isoflurane.
Anesthesiology. 1993;79[3]:444–453; Ebert TJ, Muzi M, Lopatka CW.
Neurocirculatory responses to sevoflurane anesthesia in humans: a
comparison to desflurane. *Anesthesiology.* 1995;83[1]:88–95.)

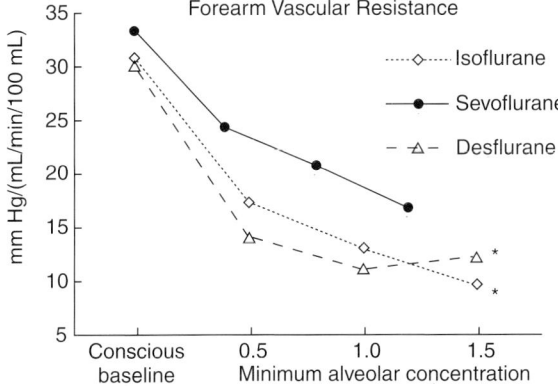

Fig. 8.4 Forearm vascular resistance response to the administration of
isoflurane, sevoflurane, and desflurane in healthy volunteers. In general,
forearm vascular resistance was progressively decreased with increasing minimum alveolar anesthetic concentrations of each of the inhalation anesthetics; however, this decline was less in the group receiving
sevoflurane. (Adapted from Ebert TJ, Muzi M, Lopatka CW. Sympathetic
hyperactivity during desflurane anesthesia in healthy volunteers: a comparison with isoflurane. *Anesthesiology.* 1993;79[3]:444–453; Ebert TJ,
Lopatka CW. Neurocirculatory responses to sevoflurane anesthesia in
humans: a comparison to desflurane. *Anesthesiology.* 1995;83[1]:88–95.)

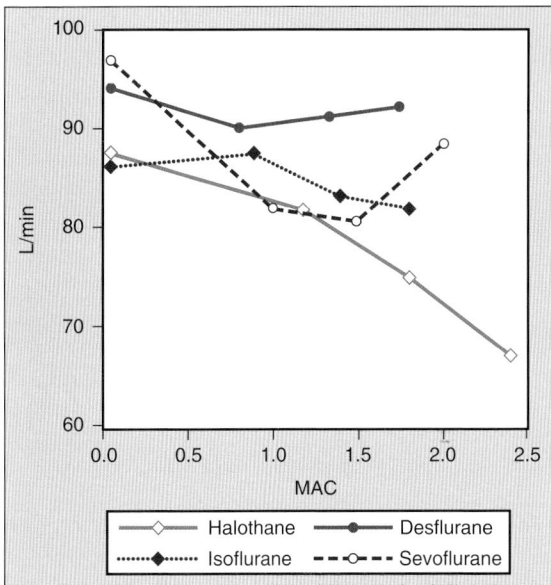

Fig. 8.5 The effects of increasing concentrations (MAC) of halothane,
isoflurane, desflurane, and sevoflurane on cardiac index (L/min) when
administered to healthy volunteers. MAC, Minimum alveolar concentration. (From Cahalan MK. *Hemodynamic Effects of Inhaled Anesthetics.
Review Courses.* Cleveland: International Anesthesia Research Society;
1996:14–18.)

can also lead to an increase in central venous pressure and arterial pressure. This sympathetic nervous system response appears to be intact
during coadministration of inhalation agents.[96]

In general, N_2O used in combination with inhalation agents
increases SVR and helps support arterial blood pressure. Desflurane
supports CI better than sevoflurane and isoflurane at both low and high
MAC levels (i.e., 0.5–1.66 MAC) (Fig. 8.5).[97] With light levels of anesthesia, desflurane maintains CI without an accompanying elevation in
HR. For deeper levels of anesthesia, the CI is probably supported by the
associated rise in HR. Some investigators believe the favorable circulatory profile of desflurane, isoflurane, and sevoflurane results from their
ability to attenuate the body's circulatory compensatory mechanisms
in a dose-related manner.[98,99] In summary, there is no appreciable

difference in the ether anesthetics' ability to produce dose-dependent
depression in arterial pressure and CO.[92,93]

Regarding the impact of the duration of anesthesia on hemodynamics, isoflurane, sevoflurane, and desflurane produce a similar response;
specifically, as MAC-hours of anesthesia increase, CI and HR increase
slightly.[97] The CI effect may be secondary to a continued reduction in
SVR and increase in HR following prolonged exposure to each of the
agents. Protracted anesthesia (8 hours) in healthy volunteers anesthetized with desflurane and sevoflurane led to an increase in pupil size
and HR independent of surgery.[100] These changes are not associated
with increases in plasma catecholamines, blood pressure, or CO_2 production; therefore mydriasis and tachycardia as signs of anesthetic
depth could be misleading at times.

Although anesthetic changes produced at the cellular level have
already been discussed, it is sensible to review the cellular effects of
inhaled anesthetics on the aforementioned areas of the cardiovascular system. In vitro and in vivo studies have revealed that isoflurane,
sevoflurane, and desflurane reduce intracellular free Ca^{2+} concentrations in cardiac and vascular smooth muscle. The mechanism for this
is believed to be a reduction in Ca^{2+} influx through the sarcolemma
and a depression of depolarization-activated Ca^{2+} release from the sarcoplasmic reticulum.[92,93,101] The end result is a depression in the contractile state of the myocardium, along with dilation of the peripheral
vasculature. Other reported cellular effects of inhalation agents include
augmentation and attenuation of endothelium-derived relaxation
factor, inhibition of acetylcholine-induced vascular relaxation,[102] and
attenuation of sodium (Na^+)/Ca^{2+} exchange that leads to a reduction in
the quantity of intracellular Ca^{2+}.[103]

Heart Rate

Inhalation agents and N_2O induce changes in HR relative to the concentration of the anesthetic being used. Alterations in HR are a result of
several variables: antagonism of sinoatrial (SA) node automaticity,[104]
modulation of baroreceptor reflex activity,[105] and sympathetic nervous

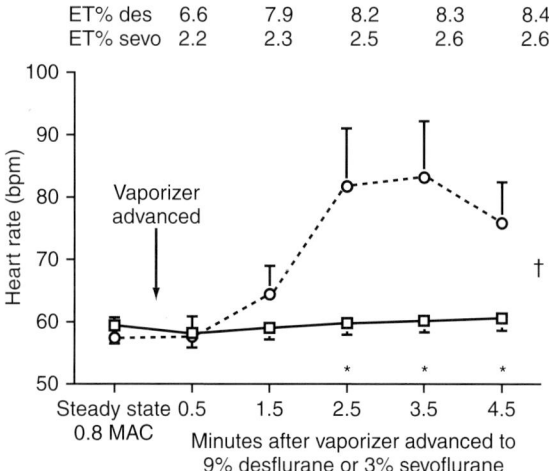

| ET% des | 6.6 | 7.9 | 8.2 | 8.3 | 8.4 |
| ET% sevo | 2.2 | 2.3 | 2.5 | 2.6 | 2.6 |

Fig. 8.6 The effects of sevoflurane *(solid line with squares)* and desflurane *(dashed line with circles)* on heart rate in healthy young volunteers when the inspiratory concentration is rapidly increased from a steady-state value of 0.83 MAC to 1.25 MAC. *Bpm,* Beats per minute; *ET,* end-tidal; *MAC,* minimum alveolar concentration. (Reprinted with permission from Ebert TJ, Muzi M, Lopatka CW. Neurocirculatory responses to sevoflurane in humans: a comparison to desflurane. *Anesthesiology* 1995; 83[1]:88–95.)

system activation via activation of tracheopulmonary and systemic receptors.[106]

Rapid increases in inhaled concentrations of isoflurane, and especially desflurane, can lead to increases in HR and blood pressure secondary to sympathetic activation, due to an irritant effect (Fig. 8.6). Sevoflurane has minimal HR effects. HR increases are accelerated when the concentration is increased rapidly.

Coronary Blood Flow

The term *coronary steal* is defined as a reduction in the perfusion of ischemic myocardium with simultaneous improvement of blood flow to nonischemic tissue. Simply stated, blood has been taken from the "poor" and given to the "rich" (a "reverse–Robin Hood" syndrome). In addition, this phenomenon has been demonstrated to occur more easily with "coronary steal–prone anatomy" (i.e., in multivessel disease models).[107] Reduced SVR is most prominent with isoflurane, leading to suggestions that it could promote a steal phenomenon in patients with coronary artery disease and should be avoided. However, there is no convincing clinical evidence that isoflurane produces a greater risk than other inhaled anesthetics in patients with coronary artery disease as long as perfusion pressure is maintained.[108]

An important qualifier to isoflurane's ability to maldistribute coronary blood flow is the presence of hypotension; when normotension is maintained, a steal phenomenon is abated.[109]

To summarize the effects of isoflurane, desflurane, and sevoflurane on the coronary circulation, each produces vasodilation, with sevoflurane doing so the least. In the presence of hypotension, a steal phenomenon can occur, as it can with inappropriate use of many coronary dilators, and this effect is reversible if normotension is reestablished. Any of these three inhalation anesthetics can be used in patients with a history of ischemic heart disease.

As mentioned previously, inhalation agents may produce a neuroprotective effect; similarly, the heart appears to benefit from the isoflurane, sevoflurane, and desflurane inhaled anesthetics via the initiation of the phenomenon of preconditioning.[110] Anesthetic preconditioning (APC) results in a cascade of intracellular events that help protect the myocardium from ischemic and reperfusion insult, potentially limiting infarct size. The mechanism for this effect is multifactorial and includes such elements as improving contractile function, which prevents the down-regulation of major sarcoplasmic reticulum Ca^{2+} cycling proteins, thereby reducing Ca^{2+} overload in the myocardial cells. The latter effect has been shown to be independent of K^+-sensitive adenosine triphosphate (K_{ATP}) channels, and confers 30% to 40% of the cardioprotective effect produced by inhalational anesthetics.[111,112] On the molecular level, sevoflurane has been found to produce late preconditioning in healthy male volunteers (24–48 hours after sevoflurane administration), as evidenced by altered gene expression in white blood cells (e.g., reduced proinflammatory L-selectin [CD62L] expression on granulocytes).[113] A theoretic application of APC along with other cardioprotective substances such as insulin and adenosine would include administering preconditioning drugs during early coronary artery reperfusion, as is currently done with antiplatelet and antithrombotic therapies. Research has shown that the administration of inhalation agents during myocardial reperfusion activates a group of prosurvival kinases called the Reperfusion Injury Salvage Kinase (RISK) pathway. These prosurvival kinases produce potent cardioprotective effects. The RISK pathway has also been found to be activated during ischemic preconditioning (a brief stimulus of myocardial ischemia/occlusion leading to cardioprotection).[114]

Other factors that have been identified with preconditioning include protein kinase C activation of K_{ATP} channel opening, adenosine receptors (α_1 and α_2 subtypes), and inhibitory G proteins.[115–117] The American College of Cardiology/American Heart Association Guidelines on Perioperative Cardiac Evaluation and Care note that it can be beneficial to use inhalation anesthetic agents during noncardiac surgery for the maintenance of general anesthesia in hemodynamically stable patients at risk for myocardial ischemia.[118] This is due to a protective effect on the myocardium associated with preconditioning.

It has been advocated that sulfonylurea oral hyperglycemic drugs be discontinued 24 to 48 hours prior to elective surgery, due to their ability to close K_{ATP} channels. The glitazones and the nonsteroidal antiinflammatory drugs (NSAIDs) also exhibit an anticonditioning effect. Insulin is recommended as replacement therapy during this time period to abate the negative impact of hyperglycemia on preconditioning.[119,120] A recent multicenter trial of upper limb RIPC performed while patients were under propofol-induced anesthesia did not show a relevant benefit among patients undergoing elective cardiac surgery.[121]

Arrhythmias

The inhalation anesthetics have complex effects on cardiac conduction, including both proarrhythmic and antiarrhythmic actions. Isoflurane, desflurane, and sevoflurane all prolong the electrocardiographic QT interval, potentially increasing the risk of torsades de pointes. Prolongation of the QT interval is likely due to inhibition of the delayed rectifier K^+ current through hERG channels that normally contribute to cardiomyocyte repolarization.[122,123] The arrhythmogenic potential of inhalation agents has long been recognized. All of the agents, with the exception of isoflurane and probably desflurane, are conducive to the development of bradycardia and disturbances in atrioventricular (AV) nodal conduction (excluding second- or third-degree AV block). The mechanism for this is their ability to depress slow-response (SA and AV nodal tissue) and fast-response (atrial or ventricular musculature, Purkinje fibers) action potentials. When fibers become ischemic or injured, the inhalation agents are prone to producing reentrant excitation.[124] In addition, desflurane and sevoflurane[94] have been shown to prolong action potential duration. This effect is consistent with the clinical finding of a prolonged QTc interval in healthy adults and in children receiving desflurane.[125,126]

TABLE 8.5 Cardiovascular Effects of Inhalation Anesthetics

	Cardiac Output	System Vascular Resistance	Mean Arterial Pressure	Heart Rate
Isoflurane	↓ slight	↓	↓	↑
Desflurane	↔	↓	↓	↑
Sevoflurane	↔	↓	↓	↔
Nitrous Oxide	↓	↑	↔	↑

Arrows indicate an increase, decrease, or no change in the parameter. All effects are dose dependent.

The ability of the inhalation agents to reduce the quantity of catecholamines necessary to evoke arrhythmias is commonly, but inaccurately, called sensitization. It is more accurate to describe this phenomenon as an adverse drug interaction. Researchers have determined the nasal and oral submucosal ED_{50} dosage (median effective dose) of epinephrine for inhalation agents to be 2.11 ± 0.15 mcg/kg for halothane and 6.72 ± 0.66 mcg/kg for isoflurane.[127] With these dosages, 50% of subjects experienced three or more premature ventricular contractions or developed ventricular tachycardia during or immediately after a single injection of epinephrine (which required 3.5–11 minutes to complete). Variables that may influence epinephrine ED_{50} values are differences in systemic absorption, route of administration, genetic polymorphisms and mutations, and preexisting atrial or ventricular arrhythmias.[128] When these variables are taken into consideration, it is not surprising that data regarding inhalation agent sensitization are conflicting. Desflurane and sevoflurane both appear to be similar to isoflurane in their epinephrine-arrhythmogenic potential, meaning they also do not promote epinephrine-induced arrhythmias.[129,130]

In general, it is reasonable to anticipate the fewest difficulties with arrhythmias in ASA physical status I and II patients if the subcutaneous epinephrine dose remains 10.0 mcg/kg or less with desflurane, sevoflurane, or isoflurane.[129,130] Additional protection may be achieved by combining a local anesthetic with epinephrine, the net effect being an increase in the minimum threshold dose of epinephrine.[127] Another commonly used method for calculating the "safe" concentration of epinephrine to inject during general anesthesia with a inhalation anesthetic is as follows:
Maximum 10 mL of 1:100,000 epinephrine in a 10-minute period; or a Maximum of 30 mL per hour

Isoflurane and sevoflurane have been shown to be associated with an attenuation of arrhythmias associated with digitalis toxicity occlusion/reperfusion ischemia and a decreased risk of postmyocardial infarction. Isoflurane has also been demonstrated to increase the effective refractory period of the accessory pathway with preexcitement syndrome. These inhaled anesthetics may be preferred agents if a significant concern exists for the appearance of intraoperative arrhythmias related to these pathologic states.[131-133] A summary of the cardiovascular effects of the anesthetics is shown in Table 8.5.

Pulmonary Circulation

Pulmonary vascular resistance (PVR) is also affected by the inhalation agents and N_2O. The effects of N_2O on PVR vary with age and preexisting levels of PVR. In adults with normal PVR, the addition of N_2O results in a small increase in PVR, presumably due to an increase in sympathetic nervous system tone. If a subject has preexisting pulmonary hypertension, the addition of N_2O results in larger increases in

PVR, which may become clinically significant.[134] Inhalation agents decrease pulmonary artery pressure.[96,97]

The pulmonary vasculature also minimizes changes in alveolar-arterial oxygen tension gradient via hypoxic pulmonary vasoconstriction (HPV). HPV helps to match regional ventilation and perfusion, although it has little effect in normal lungs. In patients with lung pathology and any patient having one-lung ventilation, HPV contributes to maintaining oxygenation. It is mildly depressed by inhaled anesthetics, with isoflurane showing the greatest effect.[135] Consistent with this finding, one group of researchers noted only minimal impairment in oxygenation (an approximately 20% reduction in HPV at 1 MAC) in patients having one-lung ventilation performed during thoracotomy procedures. Desflurane and sevoflurane delivered at 1 MAC without N_2O have also been shown to only slightly affect arterial oxygenation in patients placed in a lateral position while undergoing esophagogastrectomy.[136,137]

Respiratory System

As seen with other systems of the body, the inhalation agents exert a dose-response effect on the respiratory system, primarily tidal volume (TV), followed by the depression of respiratory rate (RR). Responsiveness to CO_2 is depressed, and the TV reduces as concentrations of the agents are increased. The compensatory mechanism for the diminished TV with isoflurane, sevoflurane, desflurane, and N_2O is an increase in RR.[138-140] However, the increase in RR is not sufficient to prevent elevations in arterial CO_2 tension. Nevertheless, surgical stimulation is a variable that helps to overcome the respiratory-depressant effects of inhalation agents.[141]

Emergence from an anesthetic can be associated with hypercarbia if the minute volume (MV) is not adequately supported, owing to an inhalation agent's capacity to depress the ventilatory response to $PaCO_2$ and partial pressure arterial oxygen (PaO_2).[140,142,143] Hypercarbia also represents an increase in the apneic threshold (higher $PaCO_2$ values are required for spontaneous ventilation to occur). Patients should be closely monitored during emergence from an anesthetic and following adequate reversal of muscle relaxants to avoid acidosis or hypercarbia. During this phase of the anesthetic, significant end-tidal values of residual inhalation anesthetic may persist, particularly if there was recent administration of an opioid (synergistic effect). It is important to recognize that impairment of the hypoxic ventilatory response by inhalation agents is not abated with CNS arousal or acute pain[144]; even as little as 0.1 MAC of an inhalation agent (excluding desflurane) can suppress ventilatory drive to hypoxia.[145] These findings have implications for patients whose MVs are maintained via a hypoxic drive (e.g., emphysematous patients with depressed central chemoreceptors).

The effectiveness of an inhalation induction is directly related to the ability of an inhalation agent to avoid provoking an irritant response. N_2O and sevoflurane are considered the standards by which other agents are measured because of the low incidence of breath withholding, coughing, secretions, and laryngospasm encountered during inhalational induction.[146] In contrast, desflurane is considered a respiratory irritant when used for mask induction in concentrations greater than 6%[146,147]; therefore it is generally not used to induce anesthesia in pediatric[148] and adult patients. Lastly, the inhalation agents have been shown to relax airway smooth muscle and produce bronchodilation. They have also been used in the treatment of refractory status asthmaticus.[149]

Kidneys

In general, autoregulation of renal circulation remains intact during the administration of inhalation agents. Reductions in systolic blood pressure are accompanied by decreases in renal vascular resistance.[150]

Nevertheless, compensatory reductions in renal vascular resistance can still lead to a decline in the glomerular filtration rate. This may contribute to the commonly observed intraoperative reduction in urinary output.

The potential for an inhalation agent to produce renal damage is commonly assessed by the extent to which it elevates creatinine, blood urea nitrogen, and serum inorganic fluoride concentrations.[151] With the older inhalation agent methoxyflurane, a "toxic threshold" for peak serum concentration was established (50 μmol/L)[152]; at this value, vasopressin-resistant polyuric renal insufficiency occurs.[153]

Of the inhalation agents currently in use, desflurane has been shown in both healthy and chronic renal disease patients[154] to alter indices of renal integrity the least, including no change in the renal function tests of urinary retinol-binding protein and *N*-acetyl-β-glucosaminidase (NAG).[155] In contrast to studies involving desflurane[156] and isoflurane,[157] early research with sevoflurane generated concerns about compromised renal function. Most researchers now accept that levels associated with sevoflurane administration do not represent a significant risk to patients, including those with compromised renal function.[158–160] Millions of sevoflurane anesthetics worldwide have failed to demonstrate any significant untoward renal outcomes in the general surgical population, including patients having coronary artery surgery.[161] Nevertheless, FDA guidelines recommend that sevoflurane be used with caution in patients with renal insufficiency (creatinine >1.5 mg/dL). Researchers have found no appreciable difference in sevoflurane's biotransformation and subsequent fluoride levels in morbidly obese patients compared to nonobese patients.[162]

There was a past concern regarding sevoflurane's degradation within anesthesia circuits by older CO_2 absorbents, producing potential toxins referred to as compound A and others. The development of newer formulations of CO_2 absorbents that do not contain strong bases (NaOH or KOH), which are substituted instead with Ca^{2+} or lithium hydroxide, has removed that concern. In the absence of the newer CO_2 granules, current FDA dosing guidelines recommend that sevoflurane exposure not exceed 2 MAC-hours at flow rates of 1 to less than 2 L/min.[163] Fresh gas flow rates less than 1 L/min are not recommended.

Liver

It has long been known that inhalation anesthetics have the potential to impair liver function. Halothane in particular is associated with significant risk of postoperative liver failure, termed *halothane hepatitis*. Due to the fatal outcome, liver toxicity of inhalation anesthetics has been a longstanding issue over the years. For halothane, immunologic mechanisms and metabolism via reductive pathways may be involved in the underlying pathology; halothane hepatitis occurs several hours or days after anesthesia. Fever, jaundice, and elevation of transaminases (alanine transaminase [ALT], aspartate transaminase [AST]) in the postoperative setting should bring anesthetic-associated hepatitis into discussion.[159] A better understanding of the pathophysiology of this phenomenon has improved diagnostic capabilities for inhalation-agent–induced liver damage.[164,165] It is extremely rare for isoflurane, sevoflurane, and desflurane to produce clinically significant liver damage.[161] Their molecular structure (increased fluorination) resists hepatic degradation, and their pharmacodynamic profile is associated with no changes or slight reductions in hepatic blood flow.[166–169] In summary, the current inhalation agents have an extremely low risk for evoking hepatic injury.

As stated previously, the chemical structure of each inhalation agent determines the extent to which it is metabolized. The agents currently in use undergo metabolism at the following rates: sevoflurane at 5% to 8%, and isoflurane, desflurane, and N_2O in trace amounts.

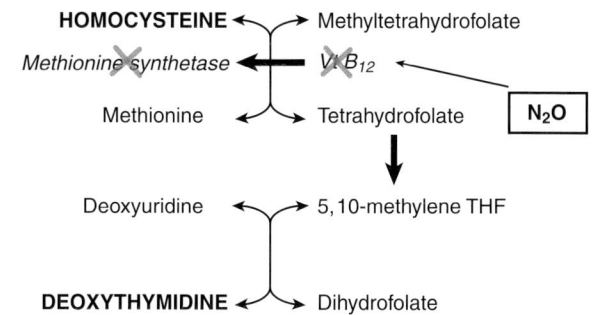

Fig. 8.7 Nitrous oxide (N_2O) oxidizes the cobalt atom on vitamin B_{12}, inhibiting methionine synthetase and causing accumulation of homocysteine and disruption of deoxythymidine synthesis. *THF,* Tetrahydrofolate. (From Fleisher LA. *Evidence-Based Practice of Anesthesiology.* 3rd ed. Philadelphia: Elsevier; 2013:250.)

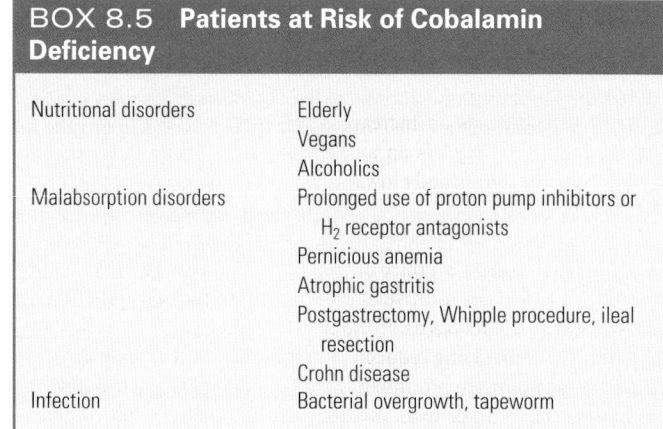

BOX 8.5 **Patients at Risk of Cobalamin Deficiency**

Nutritional disorders	Elderly
	Vegans
	Alcoholics
Malabsorption disorders	Prolonged use of proton pump inhibitors or H$_2$ receptor antagonists
	Pernicious anemia
	Atrophic gastritis
	Postgastrectomy, Whipple procedure, ileal resection
	Crohn disease
Infection	Bacterial overgrowth, tapeworm

From Sanders RD, Weimann J, Maze M. Biologic effects of nitrous oxide: a mechanistic and toxicologic review. *Anesthesiology.* 2008;109(4):707–722.

All currently used inhalation anesthetics are predominantly biodegraded by hepatic metabolism through cytochrome P-450 oxidation (phase I).

Nitrous Oxide

N_2O currently has a niche role as a supplement to the more potent anesthetics and as a component of many IV anesthesia techniques. Its use has declined in recent years in the United States. It was used in 33% of all general anesthetics given in 2009, but only 21% of those given in 2011, as safety questions have arisen.[170,171] In vitro research suggests that N_2O is metabolized minimally (0.004%) by intestinal microflora, yielding molecular nitrogen (N_2).[172] The limited metabolism does not necessarily mean that N_2O is an inert substance within the body. On the contrary, studies have demonstrated that chronic exposure to N_2O can lead to inactivation of the vitamin B_{12} cofactor for the enzyme methionine synthetase.[173] This may disrupt deoxyribonucleic acid (DNA) synthesis and is thought to be related to the teratogenic and immune suppression effects (Fig. 8.7).[174,175] For routine surgical cases, this is generally not an issue, but caution should be exercised with patients who are at risk for cobalamin deficiency (Box 8.5).[176] The contraindications to the use of N_2O are listed in Box 8.6. The safety of N_2O was assessed in several large-scale studies, including the Nitrous oxide anaesthesia and cardiac morbidity after major surgery (ENIGMA-II) and Perioperative Ischemic Evaluation (POISE) trials. These studies noted that N_2O in major noncardiac surgery did not increase mortality, cardiovascular complications, surgical site infections, or adverse

BOX 8.6 Contraindications to the Use of Nitrous Oxide

Indications	Inhalational Analgesia/Sedation
Absolute contraindications	Known deficiency of enzyme or substrate in methionine synthase pathway
	Potential toxicity from expansion of gas-filled space (e.g., emphysema, pneumothorax, middle ear surgery, pneumocephalus, air embolus, bowel obstruction) (see Chapter 7)
	Increased intracranial pressure
Relative contraindications	Pulmonary hypertension
	Prolonged anesthesia (>6 hr)
	First trimester of pregnancy*
	High risk of postoperative nausea and vomiting

*Based on the theoretical (but unproven) detrimental effects.
From Sanders RD, Weimann J, Maze M. Biologic effects of nitrous oxide: a mechanistic and toxicologic review. *Anesthesiology.* 2008;109(4):707–722.

outcomes. There was an increased risk of postoperative nausea and vomiting.[171,177,178] N_2O is an antagonist of the NMDA receptor and may produce a significantly lower risk of chronic pain after surgery.[179]

Neuromuscular System

All inhalation agents produce a dose-dependent relaxation of skeletal muscle, as well as an additive effect with the depolarizing and nondepolarizing muscle relaxants.[180] The mechanism by which this occurs is multifactorial, involving reduced neural activity within the CNS and a presynaptic and more prominent postsynaptic effect at the neuromuscular junction.[181] In general, nondepolarizing muscle relaxant dosages are decreased by approximately 25% to 50% of that required with TIVA when they are used in combination with an inhalation agent.[182]

The inhalation agents have also been shown to delay recovery from the nondepolarizing muscle relaxants. For example, after 30 minutes of exposure to sevoflurane, recovery from vecuronium to 25% of baseline neuromuscular function is prolonged by 89%, and after 60 minutes, prolongation exceeds 100%.[183] The inhalation agents have also been implicated in impairing reversal of nondepolarizing neuromuscular block.[184,185]

Malignant Hyperthermia

All of the potent inhalation agents are capable of triggering malignant hyperthermia. These agents should not be used in malignant hyperthermia–susceptible patients. N_2O may be used in malignant hyperthermia–susceptible patients. Overall, the clinical use of N_2O, in combination with many other agents (e.g., propofol, ketamine, etomidate, opiates, and local anesthetics), is considered acceptable in patients susceptible to malignant hyperthermia.[186,187]

Modern anesthetic techniques have resulted in a change in the clinical presentation of malignant hyperthermia: In some cases, it may present as less fulminant and develop more slowly. The shift in typical clinical presentation is possibly due to the lower triggering potency of modern inhalation anesthetics, the mitigating effects of several IV drugs (neuromuscular blocking agents, α_2-adrenergic receptor agonists, β-adrenergic blockade) or techniques (neuraxial anesthesia), and the routine use of end-tidal CO_2 monitoring, leading to the early withdrawal of triggering drugs.[188]

The FDA has approved a new IV formulation of dantrolene (Ryanodex) for prevention and treatment of malignant hyperthermia in adults and children. The new formulation requires fewer vials, less fluid volume, and less time for preparation and administration than the older IV dantrolene products. Ryanodex is easier and faster to reconstitute and requires less fluid volume for administration, but it is more expensive, has a shorter shelf-life, and requires supplementary doses of mannitol.[189] A complete discussion of malignant hyperthermia can be found in Chapter 36.

INHALATION ANESTHETICS AND PREGNANCY

The incidence of nonobstetric surgery performed during pregnancy ranges from 0.3% to 2.2%, accounting for approximately 100,000 cases per year in both the United States and countries of the European Union. Surgery may be necessary during any stage of pregnancy. Indications for non–pregnancy-related surgery include the presence of acute abdominal disease, most commonly, appendicitis and cholecystitis, ovarian procedures, malignancies, and trauma. In a Swedish Registry of 5405 women who had undergone operations during pregnancy, 42% occurred during the first trimester, 35% during the second trimester, and 23% during the third trimester.[190] In general, no anesthetic agents or drugs commonly used in anesthesia are listed as human teratogens. Non–drug-related maternal conditions, such as severe hypoglycemia, prolonged hypoxia and hypercarbia, and hyperthermia, may be teratogenic in humans.[191] N_2O inhibits methionine synthetase, an enzyme necessary for DNA synthesis, and teratogenic effects have been shown in animals after administering high concentrations for prolonged periods. The conditions required for N_2O teratogenicity are not encountered in clinical practice; however, some clinicians still avoid N_2O in pregnant women. In current practice, it is never necessary to use N_2O in a pregnant patient, as there are many alternatives.[176] Exposure to N_2O has been of greatest concern in dental workers, due to the lack of effective scavenging. Most of the epidemiologic evidence points to a significant relationship between exposure to N_2O and both spontaneous abortion and reduced fertility in these workers.[192] As discussed previously, there is also emerging evidence that inhaled anesthetics may have neurodevelopmental effects in animals, but the effect on a developing human fetus is not clear. The American Congress of Obstetricians and Gynecologists (ACOG) has issued a Committee Opinion on Nonobstetric Surgery during Pregnancy. They note that a pregnant woman should not be denied indicated surgery, but elective surgery should be delayed until after delivery, and nonurgent surgery should be performed in the second trimester.[193,194] This topic is further discussed in Chapter 51.

SUMMARY

Inhalation agents remain the most common class of drugs used to maintain a general anesthetic. The pharmacokinetic and pharmacodynamic profiles of desflurane and sevoflurane facilitate meeting the anesthetic goals of an ever-increasing same-day surgery population. The ease of administration of all ether-based inhalation anesthetics, with or without N_2O, lends itself to common use among a diverse surgical population. Continued research will help guide anesthetists in the selection and application of a variety of inhalation anesthetic techniques. A summary of the systemic effects of the major inhalation anesthetics is given in Table 8.6. Some advantages and disadvantages of selected inhalation anesthetics are given in Table 8.7.

TABLE 8.6 Select Effects of the Inhalation Anesthetics

Variable	Isoflurane	Desflurane	Sevoflurane
Kinetics			
Alveolar equilibration	Moderate	Fast	Fast
Recovery	Moderate	Very fast	Fast
Liver			
Hepatotoxicity	No	No	No
Metabolism (%)	0.2	0.02	5–8
Musculoskeletal relaxation	Moderate	Moderate	Moderate
Respiratory System			
Respiratory irritation	Significant	Significant	No
Central Nervous System			
Seizure activity on EEG	No	No	Yes
Renal System			
Renal toxic metabolites	No	No	No

EEG, Electroencephalogram.
Modified from Thompson J, Moppett I, Wiles M, eds. In: *Smith and Aitkenhead's Textbook of Anaesthesia.* 7th ed. Edinburgh: Elsevier; 2019:49–69.

TABLE 8.7 Clinical Advantages and Disadvantages of Selected Inhalation Anesthetics

Anesthetic	Advantages	Disadvantages
Nitrous oxide	Analgesia Rapid uptake and elimination Little cardiac or respiratory depression Nonpungent Reduces MAC of the more potent agents Minimal biotransformation	Expansion of closed air spaces Requires high concentrations Amount of oxygen delivered is reduced Diffusion hypoxia, increase in teratogenicity, PONV Supports combustion Immune suppression Especially negative climate impact as a greenhouse gas
Isoflurane	Moderate muscle relaxation Decreases cerebral metabolic rate Minimal biotransformation No significant systemic toxicity Inexpensive Possible neurologic and cardiac protection	Pungent odor Airway irritant Trigger for malignant hyperthermia Slower induction and emergence
Desflurane	Rapid uptake and elimination Stable molecular structure, minimal biotransformation No significant systemic toxicity Possible neurologic and cardiac protection	Airway irritant Expensive compared to the other agents Needs special electrically heated vaporizer Rapid increases in inspired concentration can lead to reflex tachycardia and hypertension Trigger for malignant hyperthermia Especially negative climate impact as a greenhouse gas
Sevoflurane	Rapid uptake and elimination Nonpungent Excellent for inhalation induction Cardiovascular effects broadly comparable to those of isoflurane Possible neurologic and cardiac protection	Reacts with soda lime Trigger for malignant hyperthermia Some biotransformation

MAC, Minimum alveolar concentration; *PONV,* postoperative nausea and vomiting.

REFERENCES

For a complete list of references for this chapter, scan this QR code with any smartphone code reader app, or visit the following URL: http://booksite.elsevier.com/9780323711944/.

9

Intravenous Induction Agents

John J. Nagelhout

A historic milestone in anesthesia was reached in 2011 with the decision to cease marketing sodium pentothal, a thiobarbiturate, in the United States and many other countries. Thiobarbiturates, when they were introduced in the 1930s, changed the way anesthesia was delivered. Although their use has declined dramatically in recent decades with the introduction of propofol, the practice of using intravenous push boluses of sedatives to initiate anesthesia remains the standard. Induction refers to the start of anesthesia when the patient is rendered unconscious. The intravenous induction agents allow the patient to experience a pleasant loss of consciousness while also rapidly achieving surgical levels of anesthesia.

Desirable properties for an induction agent include rapid and smooth onset and recovery, analgesia, minimal cardiac and respiratory depression, antiemetic actions, bronchodilation, lack of toxicity or histamine release, and advantageous pharmacokinetics and pharmaceutics. A single ideal intravenous anesthesia induction drug has yet to be developed; however, the agents currently available can be exploited to select an appropriate drug for all surgical and anesthetic requirements. Propofol is the current standard agent and is widely used for induction of general anesthesia and intravenous sedation. Etomidate and ketamine are valuable agents for select anesthetics when propofol use is undesirable. Dexmedetomidine is gaining popularity for niche uses as well. This chapter discusses the advantages and limitations of the currently used intravenous anesthesia induction agents.

NONBARBITURATE INTRAVENOUS ANESTHETICS

Propofol

Chemical Structure and Pharmaceutics

Propofol is a 2,6-diisopropylphenol (Fig. 9.1). It is prepared as a 1% solution in a lipid emulsion of 10% soybean oil, 2.25% glycerol, and 1.2% purified egg lecithin. The pH of propofol (Diprivan) is 7 to 8.5, and the pK_a (negative logarithm of the acid ionization constant) is 11. The pH of the generic form of propofol is 4.5 to 6.4, and the pK_a is 11.[1] This unique vehicle is especially favorable to bacterial contamination. The original trade product, Diprivan, contains 0.005% disodium edetate (EDTA [ethylenediaminetetraacetic acid]) as a preservative to inhibit bacterial and fungal growth. Generic forms of propofol contain 0.025% sodium metabisulfite or benzyl alcohol depending on the manufacturer.[2] Clusters of infections reported after mishandling of earlier preservative-free preparations prompted the addition of these preservatives.[3-5] Careful handling is still important. It is recommended that aseptic conditions be maintained and the drug be used immediately upon withdrawal from a vial for a single patient. Any remaining drug should be discarded. Syringes or vials should never be used for more than one patient. Opened vials or syringes should be discarded within 6 hours if propofol was transferred from the original container.

The pharmaceutic preparations are shown in Table 9.1.

Reformulations of Propofol

Newer formulations of propofol are being investigated that have a more favorable vehicle than the lipid emulsion. These include other soybean and albumin emulsions, micelles, and nanoemulsion cyclodextrins, among others.[1,2,6]

Although propofol has many advantages, such as rapid onset and offset when given for minor procedures such as colonoscopy or bronchoscopy, it can also present some challenges. It has a narrow therapeutic index, and hemodynamic and respiratory depression are troublesome in compromised patients. General anesthesia can easily result from minor dose adjustments. There are propofol supply shortages partly related to difficulties with manufacture of the lipid emulsion formulation. Propofol causes pain on injection, and its use for long-term sedation in the intensive care unit is compromised by propofol infusion syndrome, which may be lethal. It accumulates with longer infusions.[7] Unlike narcotics and benzodiazepines, there is no pharmacologic antagonist.

Pharmacokinetics

Propofol exhibits a generally favorable kinetic profile, which is one of its main clinical benefits in comparison with other induction drugs (Table 9.2).[8-10] Rapid distribution following an intravenous bolus dose into the brain and other highly perfused areas results in a fast onset of generally one circulation time. Rapid redistribution from the central to the peripheral compartments as the drug more evenly distributes to the entire body produces a quick initial decline in blood levels. As distribution continues, the drug is circulated to less well perfused tissues such as muscle, and the brain concentration falls. This effect leads to a rapid reawakening after sedative and anesthetic doses. The time to awakening is dose and patient dependent but is usually in the range of 5 to 15 minutes. The movement of propofol through various body compartments over time is depicted in Fig. 9.2. A visual conceptualization of the redistribution of drugs given by rapid push bolus is shown in Fig. 9.3.

Metabolism plays little role in the initial awakening of the patient but is important in the eventual clearance of the drug. Propofol is metabolized in the liver by CYP2B6, UGTHP4, and CYP2C6.[11] An interesting characteristic of propofol is its rapid metabolic clearance, which exceeds hepatic blood flow.[12] These extrahepatic sites of metabolism probably account for the lack of changes in elimination seen in patients with severe cirrhosis.[13] Less than 1% of propofol is excreted unchanged. The drug's kinetics are also influenced by age, with the elderly requiring lower doses.[14] Children require a higher dose based on body weight because they have an increased volume of distribution compared to adults. Their rate of clearance is also higher.[15] Some accumulation can occur with prolonged infusion secondary to tissue saturation as propofol is extremely lipid soluble.[16] The elimination half-life is 1 to 2 hours.

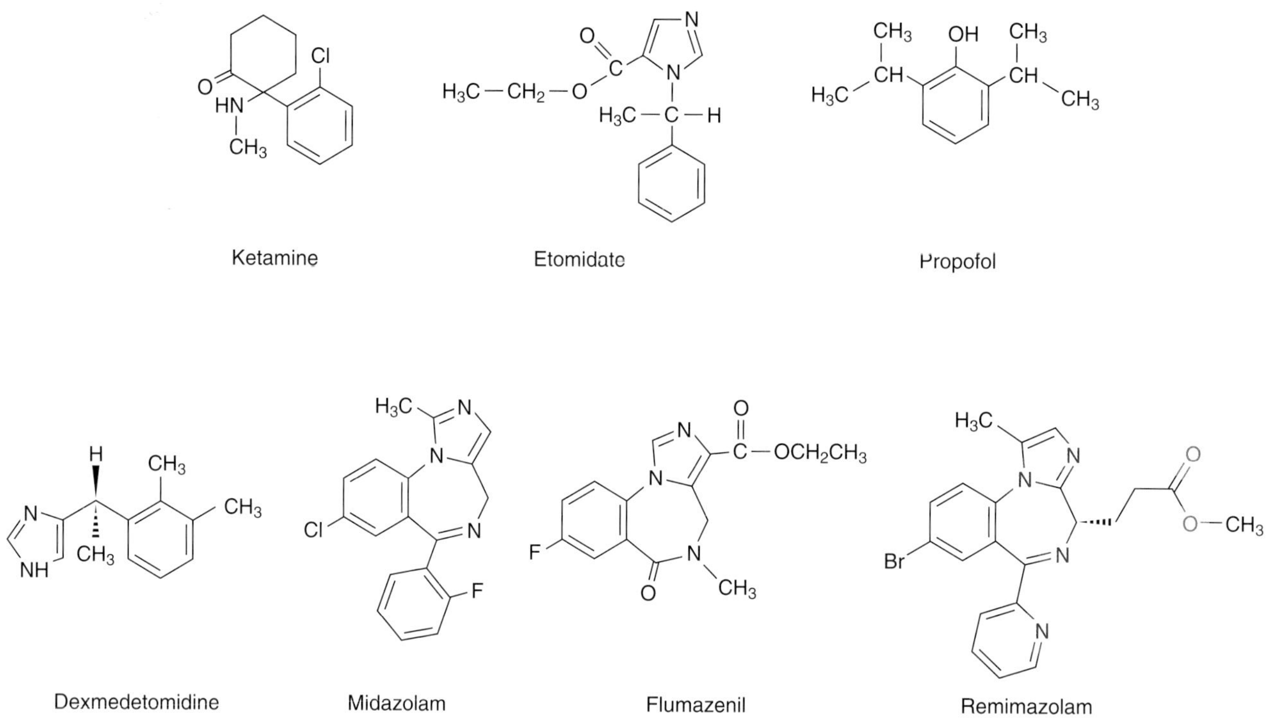

Ketamine   Etomidate   Propofol

Dexmedetomidine   Midazolam   Flumazenil   Remimazolam

Fig. 9.1 Agents used for the induction of general anesthesia, sedation, and benzodiazepine reversal.

TABLE 9.1 Pharmaceutic Preparation of Intravenous Anesthetic Agents

Class	Drug Name	Available Solution	Pain on Injection*
Benzodiazepines	Diazepam (Valium)	0.5% in 40% propylene glycol and 10% alcohol	+++
	Lorazepam (Ativan)	0.4% in propylene glycol	+
	Midazolam (Versed)	0.5% buffered aqueous solution (pH 3.5)	0
Imidazoles	Etomidate (Amidate)	Water soluble at acidic pH, lipophilic at physiologic pH (pK$_a$ 4.24); 0.2% solution in 30% propylene glycol (pH 5)	+++
	Dexmedetomidine (Precedex)	Dexmedetomidine HCl is freely soluble in water and has a pK$_a$ of 7.1 with a pH of 4.5–7.0. The solution is preservative free. Prepare by adding 2 mL of dexmedetomidine (100 mcg/mL) to 48 mL of 0.9% sodium chloride injection for a total of 50 mL. The final concentration is 4 mcg/mL.	0
Alkylphenol	Propofol (Diprivan)	1% solution in an aqueous emulsion containing 10% soybean oil, 2.25% glycerol, and 1.2% egg phosphatide, EDTA (pK$_a$ 11)	++
	Generic propofol	Generic formulations vary; may contain metabisulfite (use with caution in patients with allergies and asthma); formulations that contain benzyl alcohol pH 7–8.5 should be avoided in infants	++
Arylcyclohexylamines	Ketamine (Ketalar)	White crystalline salt 1% or 10% aqueous solution (pH 3.3–5.5; pK$_a$ 7.5)	0

EDTA, Disodium ethylenediamine tetraacetic acid.
*0, None; +, mild; ++, moderate; +++, marked.

TABLE 9.2 Select Pharmacokinetic Values for Intravenous Anesthetic Agents

Drug Name	Distribution Half-Life (min)	Elimination Half-Life (hr)	Clearance (mL/kg/min)	Volume of Distribution (L/kg)	Protein Binding (%)
Diazepam	10–15	20–50	0.3	0.8–1.3	98
Lorazepam	4–5	10–16	0.8–1.8	0.8–1.3	90
Midazolam	7–15	2–4	7–11	1–1.7	94
Etomidate	2–4	2–5	22.5	2.5–4.5	75
Propofol	2–4	1–5	25	2–8	98
Ketamine	11–17	2–3	14.5	2.5–3.5	12
Dexmedetomidine	6–8	2–2.6	8.9	1.54	94

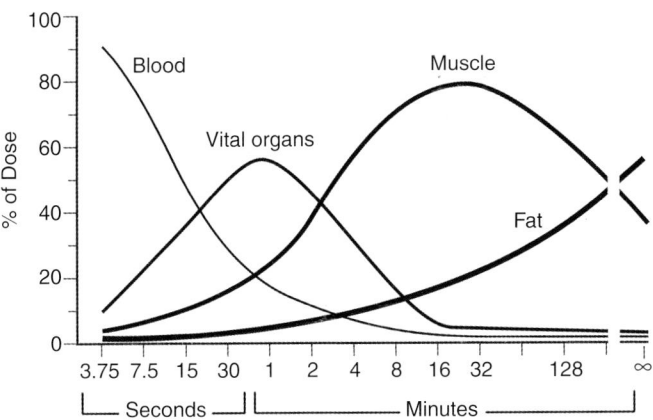

Fig. 9.2 Propofol kinetics. Note that propofol rapidly enters the brain and other vital organs, with peak effects at 1 minute after bolus injection. The brain concentration then falls rapidly over the next 10 to 15 minutes as the drug redistributes more evenly throughout the body to muscle and fat.

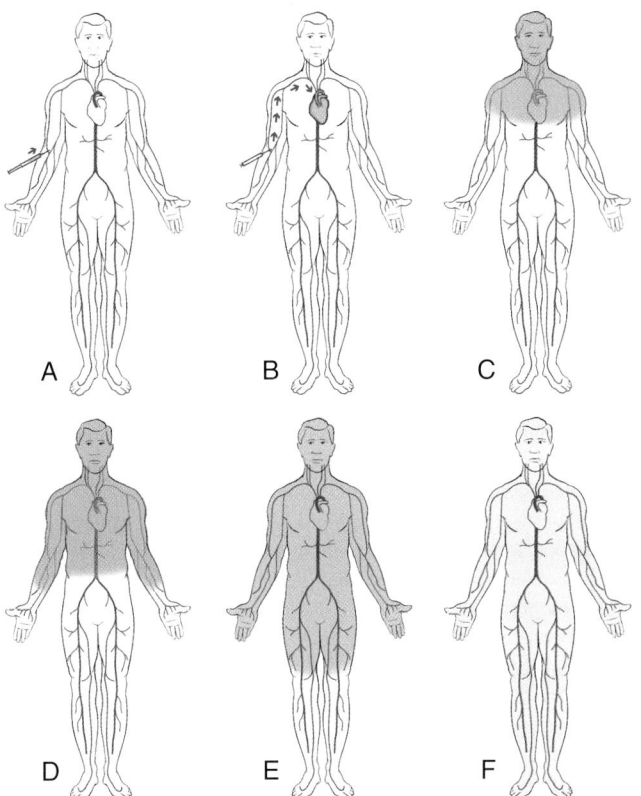

Fig. 9.3 Redistribution of intravenous drugs is shown. (A and B) A drug is administered in the arm and follows the venous circulation to the heart. (C) The high cardiac output and circulatory flow initially distribute the drug to the brain and upper body, and rapid central nervous system effects begin. (D–F) As time passes, usually minutes, the drug more evenly distributes throughout the body, lowering the initial high brain concentration, and the patient awakens.

Concerns that the traditional concept of half-life is misleading when drugs are given for prolonged periods by infusion led to the introduction of context-sensitive half time. The context is the duration of the infusion.[17] It is the time required for a 50% decrease in plasma concentration after an infusion. Further refinements have described decrement times that include the 20% and 80% declines.[18] The decrement time is from the end of the infusion to 50% recovery and

TABLE 9.3 **Factors That Alter Protein Binding**	
Factors	**Percent Bound**
Decreased lipid solubility	Decreases binding
Increased pH (≤8.0)	Increases binding
Increased drug concentration	Decreases binding
Increased protein concentration	Increases binding
Increased competition for binding sites with other drugs	Decreases binding

includes pharmacokinetic data related to concentration decrease and pharmacodynamic data correlating with recovery. These concepts are discussed in Chapter 6.

Propofol reversibly binds to erythrocytes (50%) and plasma proteins; it binds most commonly to plasma albumin (48%). The free concentration is less than 2%.[19] Decreased plasma protein levels resulting from severe renal or hepatic disease and in those patients in the third trimester of pregnancy may lower drug binding and increase the free active fraction. This may increase the effects of propofol. Clinically, this may be a factor when prolonged infusions are used.[20] Factors that can alter protein binding are noted in Table 9.3. Drugs that are highly lipid soluble cross cell membranes rapidly, including the blood-brain and placental barriers. Propofol, being highly soluble, easily enters all body compartments.[21]

Mechanism of Action

Like many other sedatives and anesthetics, propofol appears to exert its effect via an interaction with the inhibitory neurotransmitter γ-aminobutyric acid (GABA) and the $GABA_A$ glycoprotein receptor complex.[22] GABA is a major inhibitory transmitter in the central nervous system (CNS). The $GABA_A$ receptor, which is a ligand-gated ion channel receptor, is activated by the binding of the neurotransmitter GABA. This binding of GABA to the $GABA_A$ receptor initiates the movement of chloride (Cl−) through ion channels into the cell. This results in hyperpolarization of the postsynaptic cell membrane and the inhibition of neuronal cell excitation. A model has been developed that includes sites of action for GABA on the postsynaptic membrane, as well as sites for numerous other drugs. Propofol directly stimulates $GABA_A$ receptors and potentiates the actions of endogenous GABA.[23,24] The GABA receptor and its functions are depicted in Fig. 9.4.

Pharmacodynamics

Central nervous system effects. Propofol produces a rapid and pleasant loss of consciousness and emergence from anesthesia. Low-dose infusions for conscious sedation result in dose-dependent anxiolysis, sedation, and amnesia.[25] There are dose-dependent reductions in cerebral blood flow (CBF), cerebral metabolic rate of oxygen consumption ($CMRO_2$), intracranial pressure (ICP), and cerebral perfusion pressure (CPP).[26] These effects result in part from the decreased mean arterial pressure, depressed metabolic rate, and cerebral vasoconstriction produced by standard doses in a manner comparable to the effects of barbiturates and etomidate.[27,28] Cerebral autoregulation and reactivity to changes in carbon dioxide (CO_2) are preserved with propofol.[29,30]

Electroencephalogram (EEG) data produced a delta rhythm without evidence of epileptiform activity and burst suppression with higher doses.[31] Propofol has been used successfully to manage status epilepticus.[32] Even with these findings, controversy exists over the use of propofol in the patient with epilepsy.[33] Studies in patients with epilepsy showed no epileptogenic activity in any of the sites monitored.

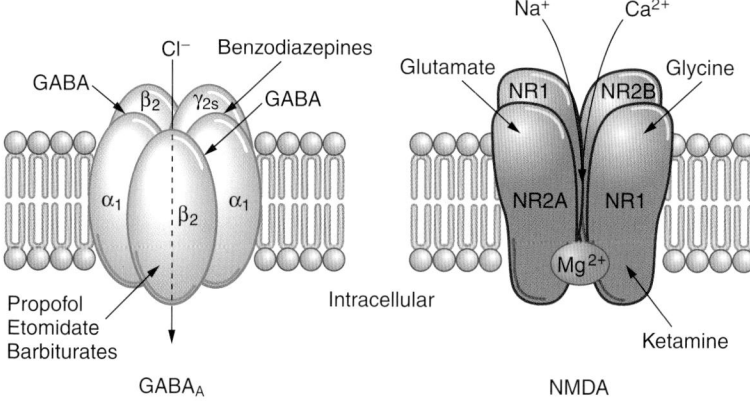

Fig. 9.4 Key targets of intravenous anesthetics. (From Hemmings HC, Egan TD. *Pharmacology and Physiology for Anesthesia: Foundations and Clinical Application.* 2nd ed. Philadelphia: Elsevier; 2019.)

However, in another study, three epileptic patients were reported to experience increased epileptiform activity on EEG after the administration of propofol 2 mg/kg.[34] Studies in patients with epilepsy demonstrated a different response in that the EEG showed no increase in epileptogenic activity at any of the sites monitored.[35] It was also found that activation or extension of EEG activity was greater with thiopental than with propofol (although not statistically significant).[36] Myoclonia induced by propofol results in spontaneous excitatory movements secondary to selective disinhibition of subcortical centers. Adequate dosage may prevent the occurrence of these movements. Myoclonia may occur on induction, but the incidence appears to be lower than that with etomidate. Intraocular pressure is decreased by propofol.[37,38] Evidence for a neuroprotective effect is controversial because studies in both animals and humans have not been consistent. Propofol cannot be indicated as a clinical neuroprotectant alone, but it might play an important role in multimodal neuroprotection. Beneficial effects include preservation of cerebral perfusion, temperature control, prevention of infections, and tight glycemic control.[39,40]

The use of propofol for electroconvulsive therapy (ECT) has been somewhat controversial as a result of the drug's effects on seizure duration. Several studies have shown that propofol reduces the duration of the ECT-induced seizure when compared with barbitures. Evaluating the efficacy of ECT as an antidepressant was typically based on the duration of the seizure: A shortened seizure implied a less effective therapy; however, researchers have found that a reduction in seizure duration does not decrease the efficacy of the ECT. Propofol is associated with shorter seizures than other anesthetics, but that antidepressant efficacy does not seem to be compromised. It is commonly used due to the rapid recovery profile.[41-43]

CNS effects of the intravenous induction drugs are shown in Table 9.4.

Cardiovascular effects. Propofol usually results in a mild to moderate transient decrease in blood pressure in healthy adults and children during anesthesia induction. The decrease in blood pressure is not usually clinically significant. The effects are more pronounced than those seen with equivalent doses of etomidate or midazolam. It can, however, result in significant hypotension in usual induction doses in select patients. Predictors of hypotension during induction are age greater than 50 years, American Society of Anesthesiologists (ASA) class III to IV, baseline mean arterial pressure less than 70 mm Hg, and coadministration of high doses of fentanyl. Hypotension usually occurs within 10 minutes after induction and is more prevalent in the second half of the 0- to 10-minute interval.[44] As with most cardiovascular-depressing sedatives, these effects result from varying degrees of a combination of CNS, cardiac and baroreceptor

TABLE 9.4 Central Nervous System Effects of Intravenous Anesthetics

Agent	CBF	CPP	CMRO$_2$	ICP	IOP
Etomidate	↓↓	↓↓	↓↓	↓↓	↓
Propofol	↓↓	↓↓	↓↓	↓↓	↓↓
Ketamine	↑↑	↑	↑	↑	↑
Midazolam	↑↓	↓	↓	↓	↓
Dexmedetomidine	↓	↑↓	0	↓	↓

CBF, Cerebral blood flow; *CPP*, cerebral perfusion pressure; *CMRO$_2$*, cerebral metabolic rate of oxygen consumption; *ICP*, intracranial pressure; *IOP*, intraocular pressure.
↓, Decreases; ↑, increases; 0, no effect.

depression, and decreases in sympathetic tone and systemic vasodilation. The primary reasons for propofol-induced hypotension are decreased sympathetic tone and vasodilation.[45] Central nervous system and direct cardiac depression play less of a role. A decrease in dose or alternative agents should be considered in the elderly or cardiac-compromised patients. Propofol has been used successfully for cardiac anesthesia when combined with fentanyl in low-dose or infusion regimens (Table 9.5).[46]

Respiratory effects. Transient respiratory depression, more prominent than that seen with etomidate, is common with induction doses of propofol. Decreases in tidal volume are greater than decreases in respiratory rate, although apnea is common on initial administration of induction doses.[47] The frequency and duration of apnea are dependent on the dose, speed of injection, patient characteristics, and the presence of other respiratory depressant medications.[48] Dose-dependent respiratory depression is also common with maintenance infusions. This appears to result from a decreased sensitivity of the respiratory center to carbon dioxide.[49]

Propofol has a minimal bronchodilating effect in patients with or without asthma and in patients who smoke. It does not cause histamine release and has been used successfully for anesthesia induction in asthmatic patients. After tracheal intubation, respiratory resistance is lower, and the incidence of wheezing is decreased, compared with the effects of etomidate.[50,51] Propofol or ketamine are the preferred induction agents in patients with asthma.[52-54]

Other pharmacologic actions. Propofol possesses mild antiemetic effects that are most prominent when given by continuous infusion.[55,56] The mechanism for the antiemetic effects is unclear. It also exhibits antipruritic effects against opioid-induced pruritus.[57,58]

TABLE 9.5	**Cardiac and Respiratory Effects of Intravenous Anesthetic Agents**						
Drug Name	Mean Arterial Pressure	Heart Rate	Cardiac Output	Venous Dilation	Systemic Vascular Resistance	Respiratory Depression	Bronchodilation
Etomidate	0	0	0	0	0	0/–	0
Propofol	– –	–	–	++	– –	– –	0/+
Ketamine	++	++	+	0	+/–	0	+
Diazepam	0/–	–/+	0		–/0	0	0
Midazolam	0/–	–/+	0	+	–/0	0	0
Dexmedetomidine	–	– –	0/–	0	0	0	0

–, Mild decrease; – –, moderate decrease; +, mild increase; ++, moderate increase; 0, no effect.

Patients experience mild to moderate pain on injection with propofol. The incidence is approximately 60% and is most frequently related to the use of smaller veins for injection. The two most effective interventions to reduce pain on injection are the use of the antecubital vein or pretreatment with lidocaine 20 to 40 mg in conjunction with venous occlusion when the hand vein was chosen. Other effective pretreatments are using a lidocaine-propofol admixture, opioids, ketamine, and nonsteroidal antiinflammatory drugs.[59] Intraarterial injection of propofol does not cause vascular injury.

Obstetric use. Propofol easily passes the placental barrier when administered to a pregnant woman due to its high lipid solubility. Sedative effects occur in the neonate when propofol is used for cesarean delivery. Lower 1- and 5-minute Apgar scores have been noted.[60]

The antiemetic effects of propofol may be an advantage in these patients. It is also used for sedation and hypnosis in postpartum tubal ligations and assistive reproductive techniques.

Contraindications and Precautions

Few absolute contraindications exist for propofol other than cases in which a known hypersensitivity exists to propofol or its components or the patient has a disorder of lipid metabolism.[61,62] New generic formulations of propofol, which contain sodium metabisulfite, should not be used in sulfite-sensitive patients. The sulfite may cause allergic-type reactions such as anaphylactic symptoms and life-threatening or less severe asthmatic episodes in certain susceptible people. Sulfite sensitivity is more common in patients with asthma than in patients without asthma.[63] As noted, caution is advised in elderly, debilitated, and cardiac-compromised patients.

Pediatric patients with cardiac mitochondrial disease may receive small bolus doses of propofol, but large bolus doses or continuous infusions are contraindicated due to propofol's effect of inhibiting adenosine triphosphate (ATP) synthesis. Specifically, propofol inhibits mitochondrial acylcarnitine transferase and thus oxidative phosphorylation, which is believed to be responsible for these negative effects.

Allergy

Propofol lipid emulsion formulations have been scrutinized because of their lecithin content. Lecithin (from the Greek *lekithos*, meaning "egg yolk") is a phospholipid compound composed of a range of phosphatidyl esters such as phosphatidylcholine, phosphatidylethanolamine, and phosphatidylserine. These are combined with varying amounts of triglycerides and fatty acids. Lecithin was originally obtained from eggs, although soybeans and other vegetables with high lecithin content have also become useful sources. Apart from its use as an antioxidant synergist, lecithin has important surfactant properties and is used as an emulsifying agent.[64]

Controversy exists regarding whether propofol should be avoided in patients who are allergic to eggs, soy, or peanuts. Egg allergy is most common in children and is usually outgrown by adulthood.[65,66] Experts claim that there is little evidence that propofol should be avoided in egg- or soy-allergic patients.[67-69] The warning labels differ among countries for the same formulation of propofol supplied by the same company. The product information for Diprivan 1% warns of its use in egg- or soy-allergic individuals in Australia, soy/peanut (but not egg) in the United Kingdom, and lists no food allergy warnings in the United States. This is despite all three formulations being supplied by the same company.[67]

A retrospective case review of 28 egg-allergic patients was reported in 2011. Two of the 28 patients had documented egg anaphylaxis. All but the two children with a history of egg anaphylaxis safely received propofol.[68] Data on the two children with documented egg anaphylaxis were not conclusive. The authors suggest propofol is likely to be safe in most egg-allergic children; however, propofol should not be administered to any child with a history of egg anaphylaxis until further evidence is available. Other authors note that there are no confirmed reports of propofol-induced anaphylaxis in egg-allergic patients. They generally demonstrate immediate hypersensitivity to proteins from egg whites. Lecithin is from egg yolks, so there is no reason to contraindicate propofol in egg-allergic patients.[70-72]

Soy allergy is a common early-onset food allergy in children. Many children outgrow the allergy by age 7.[73,74] Refined soy oil of the types used in propofol has the allergenic proteins removed during refining and is therefore safe in patients with soy allergy. The suggestion that peanut-allergic patients may exhibit propofol allergy is due to cross reactivity between these leguminous plants; therefore, just as with soy allergy, there are no data to support the avoidance of propofol in patients with peanut allergy.[70]

Propofol Infusion Syndrome

Propofol is frequently used in adult critical care units for prolonged sedation. Numerous case reports describe findings of various metabolic derangements and organ system failures known collectively as propofol infusion syndrome (PRIS) with long-term high-dose infusions of propofol.[75] This seems to require long-duration infusions of high doses, as encountered in critical care units.[76] This syndrome is associated with significant morbidity and mortality. A precise mechanism of action of PRIS has yet to be demonstrated.[77] Risk factors include doses greater than 5 mg/kg/hour, duration greater than 48 hours, critical illness, high-fat low-carbohydrate intake, inborn errors of mitochondrial fatty acid oxidation, concomitant catecholamine infusion, and steroid administration. Many of the patients who developed this syndrome have been children, but cases in adults

TABLE 9.6 Clinical Features of Adult and Pediatric Patients With Propofol Infusion Syndrome

	Children (*n*=44)	Adults (*n*=124)
Males/females	18/16 (missing in 10 cases)	62/41 (missing in 21 cases)
Age (yr), median (range)	3.92 (0.08–15) (missing in 2 cases)	33 (16–73) (missing in 23 cases)
Body weight (kg), median (range)	15 (1.38–44) (missing in 15 cases)	70 (33–192) (missing in 105 cases)
Duration of propofol infusion (hr), median (range)	66 (0.67–144) (missing in 1 case)	72 (2–229) (missing in 4 cases)
Mean infusion rate (mg kg^{-1} hr^{-1}), median (range)	7.8 (3–70) (missing in 6 cases)	5.1 (1.5–13.68) (missing in 29 cases)
Cumulative propofol dose (mg kg^{-1}), median (range)	493.8 (4.09–1697) (missing in 6 cases)	380.4 (12–1368) (missing in 30 cases)
Number of deaths	23 (52%)	59 (48%)

From Hopkins PM. Propofol infusion syndrome: a structured literature review and analysis of published case reports. *Br J Anaesth.* 2019;122(4):448-459.

are more common. Long-term propofol infusions are no longer used in children because of this risk. It is recommended to always limit the infusion rate to the lowest possible by the use of multimodal sedation.

The syndrome has occurred in patients with acute inflammatory disease with infection or sepsis or acute neurologic disease. One common denominator was the presence of impaired systemic microcirculation with tissue hypoperfusion and hypoxia. Propofol seemed to be a triggering agent when catecholamines and corticosteroids were also administered. Fatty acid metabolism and mitochondrial activity are impaired, creating an oxygen supply-and-demand mismatch that results in cardiac and peripheral muscle necrosis. The current theories propose that propofol inhibits oxidative phosphorylation by (1) inhibition of the transportation of long-chain fatty acids into the cell, as well as (2) inhibitory effects on the mitochondrial respiratory chain and (3) blockage of β adrenoreceptors and cardiac calcium channels. When considering all of these possible mechanisms, the evidence points to a defect in the production of ATP as the probable causative mechanism of this syndrome. While the exact pathophysiology is unclear, it is the mitochondria and, more specifically, the respiratory chain that currently represent the most interesting pathway.[77] Symptoms include severe high anionic gap metabolic acidosis, refractory cardiac failure, persistent bradycardia refractory to treatment, fever, and severe hepatic and renal disturbances.[78] The clinical features are noted in Table 9.6. In a 2015 analysis of 153 available case reports, several factors were evident.[79,80] The typical patient who died with PRIS in the early 1990s was a child with respiratory infection who developed PRIS after having received a high dose of propofol. Nowadays, PRIS is more likely to be seen in an adult or elderly patient sedated with propofol in a critical care unit in whom mild unexplained acidosis and elevation of creatine kinase is noted, sometimes with worsening of acute kidney injury and arrhythmia, but other features of PRIS are often missing. Patients with a creatine kinase measurement of greater than 5000 U/L represent a high-risk population for the development of PRIS. Independent predictors of death are the cumulative dose of propofol, being represented by both mean infusion rate and the duration of infusion, the presence of traumatic brain injury, and fever. Symptoms of propofol infusion syndrome are noted in Table 9.7.

Treatment is supportive and includes discontinuing the propofol, improving gas exchange, cardiac pacing for bradycardia, phosphodiesterase inhibitors, glucagon, extracorporeal membrane oxygenation, and renal replacement therapy.[77] Recommended limits of propofol include administration for no more than 48 hours and no more than 4 mg/kg/hour or 67 mcg/kg/minute.[79,80]

Key points regarding propofol are listed in Box 9.1. Induction doses of the intravenous anesthetics are shown in Table 9.8.

TABLE 9.7 Symptoms of Propofol Infusion Syndrome

Organ System	Adverse Effect
Cardiac disorders	Cardiac failure including pulmonary edema; widening of the QRS complex; bradycardia; ventricular tachycardia or fibrillation; asystole
Vascular disorders	Hypotension
Renal and urinary disorders	Acute kidney injury; change in urine color
Musculoskeletal and connective tissue disorders	Rhabdomyolysis
Metabolism and nutrition disorders	Metabolic acidosis; hyperkalemia; lipidemia
Hepatobilliary disorders	Hepatomegaly; elevated liver transaminases

Adapted from Hopkins PM. Propofol infusion syndrome: a structured literature review and analysis of published case reports. *Br J Anaesth.* 2019;122(4):448-459.

BOX 9.1 Key Points for Propofol Anesthesia

- Propofol is the most commonly used intravenous anesthetic as an induction drug and for sedation.
- Respiratory effects include transient respiratory depression or apnea, depending on dose. Although not a bronchodilator, safe use in asthmatics has been well established.
- Propofol is unique among induction agents in that it exhibits mild antiemetic properties.
- Propofol has a rapid onset and emergence after bolus or continuous infusions of the drug.
- Patients emerge with a mild euphoria followed by rapid dissipation of the sedative effects.
- Propofol reduces cerebral blood flow, $CMRO_2$, and ICP.
- Propofol decreases blood pressure, cardiac output, and systemic vascular resistance to a greater extent than etomidate at equipotent doses.
- The induction dose is 1–2 mg/kg followed by a maintenance infusion of 100–200 mcg/kg/min. Conscious sedation doses are 25–75 mcg/kg/min.

CMRO₂, Cerebral metabolic rate of oxygen consumption; *ICP*, intracranial pressure.

Etomidate

Etomidate (1-[1-phenylethyl]-1*H*-imidazole-5-carboxylic acid ethyl ester) is an intravenous induction agent whose current clinical niche is as an alternative to propofol with little if any cardiorespiratory effects. No intrinsic analgesic properties are associated with the use of

TABLE 9.8 Induction Doses of the Intravenous Anesthetics

Agent	Dose (mg/kg)
Etomidate	0.2–0.3
Propofol	1–2
Ketamine	(see Box 9.4)
Dexmedetomidine	1 mcg/kg infused over 10 min followed by 0.2–0.7 mcg/kg/hr
Midazolam	0.1–0.2

this drug.[81] Side effects such as pain on injection, myoclonia, nausea, vomiting, and adrenocortical suppression, however, have limited wider acceptance of the drug. Etomidate is a carboxylated imidazole derivative that was synthesized in 1965 and introduced to European anesthesia practice in 1972.[82] Etomidate has two isomers, but the (+) isomer is the only one with hypnotic properties (see Fig. 9.1 for the chemical structure of etomidate).[83]

Etomidate is currently supplied as a 2-mg/mL preparation; each milliliter contains 35% propylene glycol as a solvent and has a pH of 8.1 and a pK$_a$ of 4.2. This formulation has been changed over the years to decrease the incidence of pain on injection and spontaneous muscle movements or myoclonia. New formulations are being tested that are designed to maintain the favorable clinical features of etomidate while reducing the primary undesirable effect of prolonged inhibition of adrenal steroidogenesis.[84,85]

Pharmacokinetics

Etomidate is rapidly metabolized in the liver by hepatic microsomal enzymes and plasma esterases. Ester hydrolysis is the primary mode of metabolism in the liver and plasma. Etomidate is hydrolyzed to form inactive carboxylic acid metabolites. Approximately 10% of the administered dose can be recovered in bile, 13% can be recovered in feces, and the remainder of the metabolites are eliminated by the kidney.[86]

The rapid redistribution of etomidate accounts for its extremely short duration of action (see Table 9.2). The drug is lipid soluble and has a volume of distribution that is several times greater than its body weight. Shortly after intravenous injection (within 1 minute), the brain concentration rises rapidly because of the drug's lipid solubility, and over the next several minutes extensive redistribution to other organs and tissues occurs, and the patient regains consciousness.

The total body clearance of etomidate is rapid. The hepatic extraction ratio is 67%. Studies examining dose-response relationships have found a lack of accumulation with this compound.[81] The terminal half-life is 2 to 5 hours.[84]

Awakening occurs 5 to 15 minutes after bolus administration. Like other intravenous induction drugs, this occurs secondary to rapid redistribution to nonnervous sites. Etomidate is 76% protein bound, mostly to albumin. Variations in the amount of available plasma protein alter the amount of free drug available to exert pharmacologic actions. Disease states that produce alterations in plasma protein content could theoretically affect the action, although this rarely happens clinically. Compensatory increases in metabolism and elimination can readily compensate for changes in protein binding.

The mechanism of action of etomidate, like many other CNS depressants, involves GABA modulation (see Fig. 9.4).[87,88] In a clinical investigation of 2500 cases, Doenicke et al.[89] confirmed that no histamine is released by etomidate.

Pharmacodynamics

CNS effects. Etomidate produces a dose-dependent CNS depression within one arm-brain circulation. Its duration of action is also dose dependent,[81] with awakening occurring 5 to 15 minutes after a dose of 0.2 to 0.4 mg/kg. The drug is devoid of analgesic properties.

Cerebral blood flow and cerebral metabolic rate of oxygen consumption are both decreased by etomidate.[90,91] In a study of fully alert patients without neurologic deficit or impaired consciousness, an etomidate induction was followed by an infusion of 2 to 3 mg/minute. Cerebral blood flow decreased 34%, and cerebral metabolism was also reduced (mean decrease of 45%). Decreased oxygen consumption and the associated decrease in carbon dioxide production can cause cerebrovascular vasoconstriction, decreased cerebral blood flow, and decreased intracranial pressure. Also noted during this trial was the maintenance of cerebral blood vessel responsiveness to changes in carbon dioxide levels.[90]

In a study of patients with intracranial pathology, etomidate (0.2 mg/kg given intravenously) was shown to decrease intracranial pressure while maintaining cerebral perfusion pressure. Because of the cardiovascular stability of this drug, mean arterial pressure did not decrease below cerebral autoregulation values at which cerebral blood flow would become pressure dependent. Cerebral perfusion pressure was maintained adequately in all study subjects.[91]

The EEG changes that follow administration of etomidate are similar to those that follow administration of other intravenous induction anesthetics. When compared with thiopental, a lack of beta-wave activity was present during induction, along with a longer duration of stages III and IV.[92]

One negative characteristic of etomidate is its excitatory phenomenon of muscle movements and tremors.[92,93] Referred to as myoclonia, this phenomenon is defined as sudden, generalized, asynchronous muscle contractions.[94] Myoclonia can affect many muscle groups or a single muscle. The movements can be so severe that they resemble, and are often mistaken for, seizures. In EEG patterns monitored during etomidate anesthesia, no specific EEG disturbances occurred during or after myoclonic episodes.[92] The origin of these muscle movements is thought to be related to uneven drug distribution into the brainstem or deep cerebral structures and not to CNS stimulation.[92,95] The incidence of myoclonia ranges between 10% and 60% and varies with the type and the amount of premedication given. Pretreatment with small doses of dexmedetomidine, midazolam, rocuronium, and lidocaine are all effective in reducing myoclonia.[92,96–100] Etomidate is shown to decrease intraocular pressure.

EEG changes with etomidate are similar to those of other intravenous induction drugs. Bispectral index (BIS) monitor values decrease after a bolus of etomidate and correlate well with sedation scores. Etomidate decreases the amplitude and increases latency of auditory evoked potentials (AEPs). The duration of epileptiform activity after ECT is longer after induction with etomidate versus propofol. Somatosensory-evoked potential amplitudes are enhanced by etomidate, and motor-evoked potential amplitudes are suppressed less by etomidate than propofol.[101–103]

Cardiovascular effects. The primary clinical advantage of etomidate over propofol is the hemodynamic stability upon induction in healthy or modestly debilitated patients. In patients with compensated heart disease, changes in heart rate, pulmonary artery pressure, cardiac index, systemic vascular resistance, and systemic blood pressure were not significant.[104] In one study of high-risk patients with significant cardiac disease, hemodynamic stability was maintained with induction doses of 0.3 mg/kg. Also, minimal changes in heart rate, blood pressure, central venous pressure, and intrapulmonary shunting have been demonstrated after etomidate administration.[105] Patients with aortic and mitral valve disease, however, are noted to have significant decreases in systemic blood pressure (17%–19%), pulmonary artery pressure (11%), and pulmonary capillary wedge pressure (17%).[106] Slight decreases in blood pressure are thought to be caused by decreases in systemic vascular resistance. The hemodynamic stability seen with etomidate has been attributed to a unique lack of depression of sympathetic nervous system and baroreceptor function.[107] Etomidate acts as an agonist at α_{2B}-adrenoceptors, which mediates an increase in blood pressure. This effect contributes to the cardiovascular stability of patients with etomidate.[104]

Myocardial oxygen supply and demand are kept constant by a balance of decreased myocardial blood flow and decreased oxygen consumption.[108] No significant cardiac dysrhythmias are associated with etomidate administration. Both renal and hepatic blood flows are maintained by the stability of cardiac output (see Table 9.5). In summary, at equivalent anesthetic doses, propofol depresses cardiorespiratory function to the greatest degree and etomidate depresses it the least.

Respiratory effects. Etomidate affects the respiratory system in a dose-dependent manner. Minute volume decreases, but respiratory rate increases. The respiratory depression seen with propofol use is significantly greater than that seen with etomidate.[108] The ventilatory response to CO_2 is decreased, and etomidate administration may cause brief periods of apnea following induction. Etomidate has little effect on bronchial tone and does not cause histamine release (see Table 9.5).[109,110]

Adrenocortical effects. Adrenal cortical suppression by etomidate has been widely studied, and this effect significantly limits it clinical use. It is useful as a single-dose anesthesia induction agent, but infusions are no longer used. The issue elicited widespread concern after 10 years of use in Europe. Researchers found an increased mortality rate in critically ill patients who received etomidate infusions. This phenomenon was attributed to adrenocortical hypofunction, demonstrated by decreased levels of plasma cortisol.[111] Multiple studies have shown adrenal hormone levels to be decreased for up to 8 to 24 hours after a single induction dose or more than 24 hours with infusion.[112–118] These effects are caused by a reversible dose-dependent inhibition of adrenal steroidogenesis. The enzymes inhibited are the cytochrome P-450–dependent mitochondrial enzymes and 11β-hydroxylase. To a lesser degree, 17α- and 18-hydroxylases are also affected. This results in an increase in cortisol precursors but a decrease in cortisol, aldosterone, and corticosterone levels. This enzyme inhibition results in decreased ascorbic acid synthesis, which is necessary for steroid production.[119] In summary, these effects are primarily caused by a reversible dose-dependent inhibition of the adrenocortical enzyme 11β-hydroxylase. The mechanism for the adrenocortical hypofunction following administration of etomidate is shown in Fig. 9.5.

There have been several reports of single doses of etomidate resulting in patient morbidity caused by adrenocortical suppression. Steroid administration after induction of anesthesia with etomidate did not reduce mortality or cardiovascular morbidity.[120] A widespread controversy exists involving the likelihood of increases in morbidity and mortality from adrenal suppression when etomidate is used for intubation in septic patients.[121,122] The mortality benefit of corticosteroids appears to be greatest in septic shock patients with high vasopressor requirements, evidence of multiorgan failure, and primary lung infections. Corticosteroids consistently lead to a faster reversal of shock and may shorten the duration of mechanical ventilation. Corticosteroids do not seem to increase the risk of superinfection at low doses but frequently lead to a higher frequency of hyperglycemia. They should be used judiciously in other settings as it comes without a demonstrated benefit in mortality and increased potential for adverse effects. There remains a need for improved therapy for patients in septic shock. Corticosteroids

have shown some potential in improving mortality rates and clinical markers.[123,124] The duration of adrenal insufficiency after single-dose etomidate and its effect on outcomes in this population is longer than 24 hours and may last up to 72 hours.[125] The administration of supplemental steroids to counter this effect is controversial. It did not appear effective in septic patients[124]; however, others suggest that the empiric use of steroid supplementation for 48 hours after a single dose of etomidate in critical patients without septic shock should be considered.[125] Further research is needed to define the safe use of single boluses of etomidate in critical patients. It has been suggested that an alternative sedative induction agent should be considered for use in rapid sequence intubation in septic patients on multiple vasopressors or with abdominal source of infection.[112]

Adverse Effects

Other than the adrenal suppression and myoclonia that were discussed previously, the primary adverse effects of etomidate are pain on injection, thrombophlebitis, nausea, and vomiting. Etomidate has been formulated in various solvents in an effort to decrease pain on injection and also thrombophlebitis. The current formulation containing propylene glycol results in burning and pain on injection in up to 90% of patients.[127–129] The incidence of subsequent venous sequelae up to 7 days postoperatively is 50%.[126] Some of the variables identified as contributing to pain on injection include site and speed of injection, size of vessel used, and type of premedication. As with other venous irritating drugs, injection pain can be decreased with lidocaine 20 to 40 mg pretreatment and use of larger veins. No vascular injury occurs after intraarterial injection of etomidate.

Nausea and vomiting are common with etomidate (30%–40%).[82] Opioids also increase the susceptibility to nausea and vomiting.

Contraindications

Etomidate is contraindicated in patients with a known sensitivity, adrenal suppression, and acute porphyrias.

The porphyrias are a group of rare metabolic conditions caused by deficiencies in the enzymes involved in the biosynthetic pathway of heme, a building block of hemoglobin. They can be inherited or acquired. The hereditary porphyrias comprise a group of eight metabolic disorders of the heme biosynthesis pathway. Each porphyria is caused by abnormal function at a separate enzymatic step resulting in a specific accumulation of heme precursors. Porphyrias are classified as hepatic or erythropoietic, based on the organ system in which heme precursors (δ-aminolevulinic acid [ALA], porphobilinogen, and porphyrins) are overproduced.[130–132]

Depending on deficient enzymatic steps, various porphyrins and their precursors accumulate in tissues and may lead to toxicity. They are considered either acute or nonacute and according to the specific biosynthetic step deficiency. The acute types of porphyria are inducible by various enzyme-inducing drugs that may precipitate an attack. The acute forms are acute intermittent porphyria; variegate porphyria; hereditary coproporphyria, and plumboporphyria. The nonacute forms are porphyria cutanea tarda; erythropoietic porphyria; congenital erythropoietic porphyria, and erythropoietic protoporphyria.

The rate-limiting enzyme in the biosynthetic pathway of porphyrins is ALA-synthetase. Drugs that induce this enzyme must be avoided. Symptoms of an attack may include skin lesions and neurovisceral symptoms such as abdominal and nonabdominal pain, vomiting, psychological symptoms, convulsions, muscle weakness, sensory loss, hypertension, tachycardia, and hyponatremia.

Etomidate and barbiturates are contraindicated. General anesthesia can be readily accomplished, however, with the current agents.

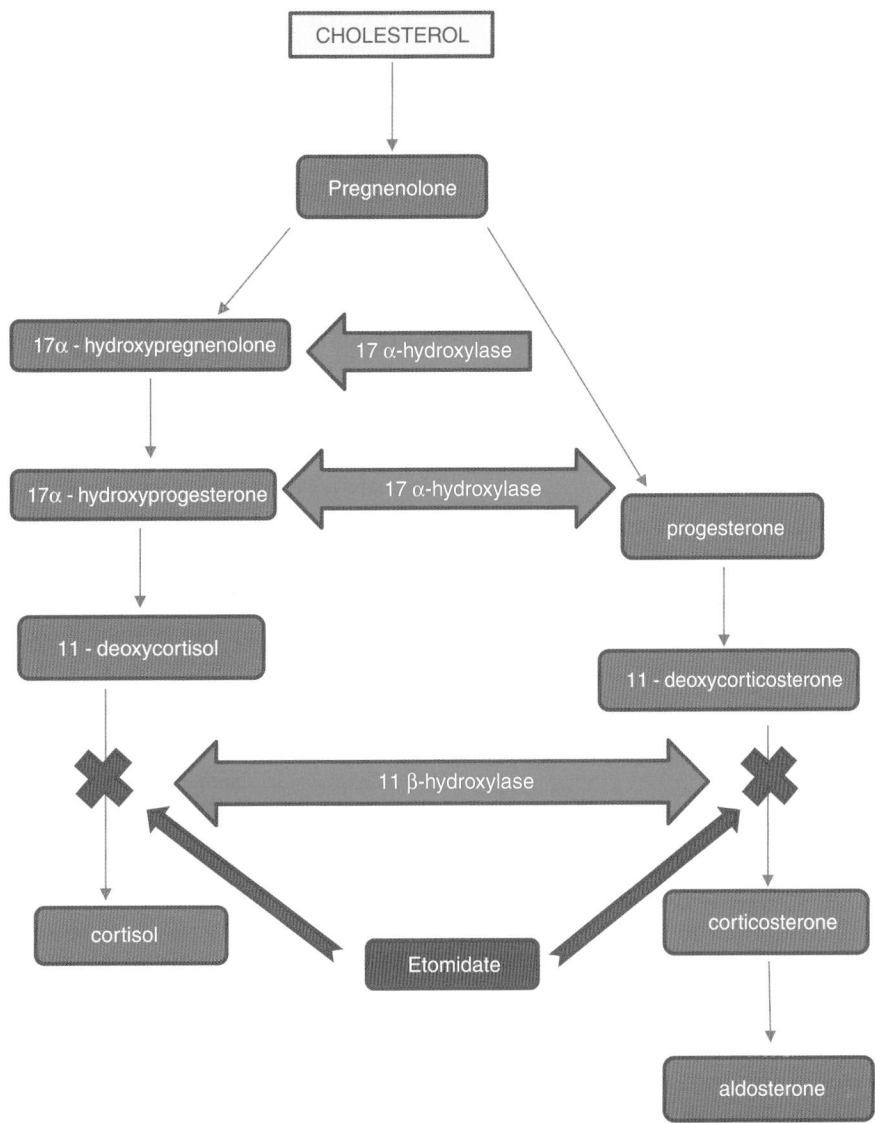

Fig. 9.5 Cortisol production decreases when 11β-hydroxylase is inhibited by etomidate. (From Devlin RJ, Kalil D. Etomidate as an induction agent in sepsis. *Crit Care Nurs Clin North Am.* 2018;30[3]:e1-e9.)

Propofol is the induction agent of choice. Ketamine can also be administered safely. Most muscle relaxants appear to be reasonably safe, and all of the current inhalational agents may be used. Analgesia can be provided with any of the currently used opiates. Local anesthetics may also be safely used.[130-132]

Key points of etomidate pharmacology are shown in Box 9.2.

Ketamine

Ketamine has a long history of anesthetic use, although its popularity has varied over the years. In modern practice, several specific situations exist in which it has unique advantages as an alternative to the more commonly used drugs. Research has led to new uses, as well as a renewed interest in possible untoward effects. It can be very useful for anesthesia and sedation in high-risk, pediatric, and asthmatic patients. Ketamine also has excellent analgesic properties that can be exploited for treatment of perioperative pain.

Ketamine was introduced into clinical practice in 1970 and has a mechanism of action and pharmacologic effects that differ greatly from the classic anesthetic drugs. The anesthetic state is unique because it does not encompass the usual signs and stages of anesthesia with a typical CNS depressant. It produces a catatonic state in which the

---

BOX 9.2 Key Points for Etomidate

- Etomidate is used in compromised patients when the use of the other intravenous anesthetics may be problematic.
- The major advantage of etomidate is minimal cardiorespiratory depression.
- Etomidate reduces intracranial pressure, cerebral blood flow, and $CMRO_2$.
- The mechanism of action of etomidate appears to be GABA-mimetic.
- Involuntary movements or myoclonia during onset is common.
- Etomidate frequently causes burning on injection.
- Etomidate inhibits the enzyme 11β-hydroxylase, which is essential in the production of both corticosteroids and mineralocorticoids. Clinically significant reductions in steroid production may occur with a single dose.
- Etomidate increases postoperative nausea and vomiting.
- The induction dose is 0.2–0.3 mg/kg.

$CMRO_2$, Cerebral metabolic rate of oxygen consumption; *GABA*, γ-aminobutyric acid.

---

patient feels separated from the environment and has profound analgesia and amnesia yet retains most protective reflexes. This ketamine-induced anesthetic state was coined "dissociative anesthesia," a concept described by Corssen and Domino.[132]

Chemical Structure

The structural formula for ketamine is shown in Fig. 9.1. The chemical structure of ketamine is 2-(O-chlorophenyl)-2-(methylamino)cyclo-hexanone. It has a pK$_a$ of 7.5, is partially water soluble, and is slightly acidic (pH 3.5–5.5). Ketamine is an optically active drug with a chiral center that exists as two optical isomers.[133] A racemic mixture is available in the United States and the S(+) isomer is available elsewhere. The S(+) isomer was believed to have a better safety profile, but the advantages of this pure enantiomer are minor.[134]

Mechanisms of Action

Ketamine causes antagonism at N-methyl-D-aspartate amino acid (NMDA) receptors in the brain, resulting in a selective depressant effect on the medial thalamic nuclei that is responsible for blocking afferent signals of pain perception to the thalamus and cortex. The primary site of the analgesic action of ketamine is the thalamoneocortical system. Ketamine has been shown to enhance opioid-induced analgesia and prevent hyperalgesia.[135] The NMDA receptor is a ligand-gated ion channel where anions Ca^{2+} and Na$^+$ are voltage dependent. L-glutamate, an amino acid, is probably the most important excitatory neurotransmitter in the CNS. At the NMDA receptor, it causes the opening of the ion channel. A rapid influx of Na$^+$, Ca^{2+}, and K$^+$ results in the depolarization of the normally negative postsynaptic membrane that initiates the action potential. Ketamine is a noncompetitive antagonist at this receptor.[136,137] Afferent impulses are transmitted to cortical regions of the brain but are not interpreted, so responses to visual, auditory, and pain stimuli are inappropriate.[138] Although cortical association areas are depressed, the limbic system, which is thought to cause excitatory behavior, is simultaneously activated. Ketamine also has effects on opiate, monoamine, cholinergic, purinergic, and adenosine receptors.[139,140] It inhibits tumor necrosis factor-α (TNF-α) and interleukin-6 (IL-6) gene expression, which may account for the antiinflammatory and antihyperanalgesic effects.[141] The NMDA receptor is shown and described in Fig. 9.4.

The analgesia produced by ketamine has a spinal cord component. By injecting bradykinin intraarterially as a noxious stimulus, Nagasaka et al.[142] were able to demonstrate that ketamine blocked the stimulated excitatory activity of wide-dynamic-range neurons in the dorsal horn, thereby preventing transmission of noxious stimuli to the brain.

Metabolism

Hepatic microsomal enzyme systems are responsible for the biotransformation of ketamine. The primary pathway for ketamine metabolism by the cytochrome P-450 system is demethylation to form the metabolite I, norketamine. Hydroxylation of norketamine occurs at one of two positions in the cyclohexone ring to form hydronorketamine metabolites I, II, and III. These metabolites form a glucuronide derivation via conjugation to produce a more water-soluble compound that is eliminated primarily via renal excretion. Thermal dehydration forms dehydroxynorketamine, a cyclohexene derivative (metabolite II).[68,143]

The pharmacologic activity of the metabolite norketamine is approximately 20% to 30% of the activity of ketamine. The activity of the other metabolites is unknown.[144]

Pharmacokinetics

The distribution kinetics of ketamine follow a two-compartment model. Ketamine is able to cross the blood-brain barrier quickly to achieve rapid pharmacologic effect.[145] The onset of a standard 2- to 2.5-mg/kg dose is slower than propofol or etomidate, and it can take 3 to 5 minutes to achieve clinical anesthesia. Reawakening usually occurs within 15 to 30 minutes; however, there is wide patient variability. A much longer duration can be seen with high or repeat doses. Ketamine

is approximately 12% protein bound. Like other induction drugs, brain concentrations decrease rapidly as ketamine is redistributed from the central compartment to peripheral tissue compartments. Redistribution to low-blood-flow tissue compartments accounts for the termination of drug effect and return to consciousness. The slow elimination half-life of the drug is the result of hepatic metabolism and excretion. A large amount of ketamine remains in peripheral tissues as an active drug and may be responsible for prolonged or cumulative effects.[81] The elimination half-life is 2 to 3 hours. Hepatic extraction of ketamine is high because the mean total body clearance is approximately the same as the hepatic blood flow.[146] Ketamine elimination is therefore dependent on hepatic blood flow. Pharmacokinetic values remain consistent with analgesic and anesthetic doses of ketamine, which implies that distribution of ketamine is not dose dependent. Anesthetic levels are present with plasma levels of 640 to 1000 mcg/mL, and analgesic levels are present with plasma ketamine concentrations of 100 to 150 mcg/mL (see Table 9.2).[143]

Intramuscular and oral route. Given intramuscularly, ketamine reaches peak plasma concentrations within 22 minutes.[147] Dosages range from 4 to 6 mg/kg.[136] The onset of anesthetic effects is seen within 5 to 15 minutes depending on dose. Analgesic doses of ketamine (0.44 mg/kg) can be used for painful procedures without causing loss of consciousness and psychic disturbances.[68] After intramuscular administration, approximately 93% of the drug is bioavailable.[81] A consideration with the intramuscular route is the delayed onset of anesthesia. Ketamine can also be used orally in doses of 10 mg/kg. It is usually mixed in cherry syrup or soda to facilitate ingestion. Onset is 10 to 20 minutes. Box 9.3 gives complete dosing information.

Pharmacodynamics

CNS effects. Ketamine produces a dissociative state of anesthesia, so called because the patient appears to be dissociated from the environment. The onset of anesthesia is slower than with propofol or etomidate and may make judgments regarding the onset of sleep and analgesia difficult. In the dissociative state, as originally described by Corssen and Domino,[132] the patient is cataleptic (i.e., the eyes remain open, the pupils are reactive to light, the corneal reflexes are intact, and horizontal nystagmus is present). Lacrimation and eye blinking continue, and salivary gland secretions are increased. Airway reflexes also remain intact (e.g., laryngeal reflex, pharyngeal reflex, coughing, sneezing, and swallowing). Skeletal muscle tone is increased, and occasional purposeless movements occur that are unrelated to painful stimuli.

BOX 9.3   Recommended Doses of Ketamine

Premedication
- A benzodiazepine such as midazolam is administered if patient status allows. An antisialagogue may also be given to decrease secretions.

Induction of Anesthesia
- Ketamine 2–4 mg/kg IV, or 4–6 mg/kg IM (oral dose is 10 mg/kg).

Maintenance of Anesthesia
- Ketamine 15–45 mcg/kg/min (1–3 mg/min) by continuous IV infusion or 0.5–1.0 mg/kg supplemental IV doses as needed.

Sedation and Analgesia
- Ketamine 0.2–0.8 mg/kg IV (over 2–3 min) followed by a continuous ketamine infusion (5–20 mcg/kg/min) 10–20 mg may produce preemptive analgesia.

IM, Intramuscular; *IV*, intravenous.

Because the usual signs of anesthesia are not evident with ketamine, movement in response to painful stimuli is often required for judgments of adequate anesthesia. After administration of a single dose, full reorientation to person, place, and time takes place in 15 to 30 minutes, though, as previously noted, wide variability in durations has been noted.[148] Ketamine is a moderate analgesic that has a preference for skin, bone, and joint pain. Analgesia occurs with subanesthetic doses, and it is widely used for sedation in combination with low doses of benzodiazepines, propofol, and other analgesics.[149]

CBF and regional and possibly global $CMRO_2$ and ICP are increased by ketamine. The effect on glucose utilization varies by brain region.[151-153] The response of cerebral vessels to CO_2 is left intact. For these reasons ketamine has traditionally been thought to be contraindicated in patients with a head injury or an increased ICP. However, it has been noted that ketamine can be used safely in neurologically impaired patients under conditions of controlled ventilation, coadministration of a GABA receptor agonist such as midazolam or propofol, and avoidance of nitrous oxide.[151] Trauma patients with multiple injuries may still benefit from the favorable cardiovascular effects while avoiding untoward neurologic adverse actions.[153] Ketamine produces atypical anesthesia; thus EEG patterns also differ from standard anesthetics. On loss of consciousness and onset of analgesia, ketamine induces a transition from alpha to theta waves (slow waves with moderate to high amplitude) on the EEG. Alpha waves do not reappear until after consciousness returns and analgesia is lost.[154] Ketamine alone does not decrease the BIS even when patients are unconscious. Several researchers have in fact noted an increase in BIS levels when ketamine is added to propofol, fentanyl, or sevoflurane anesthetic. Ketamine does not alter AEPs, midlatency AEP (MLAEP), or A-line autoregressive index monitors based on MLAEPs.[155,156] Ketamine appears advantageous for use in ECT.[157]

Ketamine anesthesia emergence is associated with psychic disturbances immediately on return of consciousness.[158] These emergence reactions are the result of visual, auditory, proprioceptive, and confusional illusions. Descriptions of this phenomenon include vivid illusions, sensations of drunkenness, delirium, restlessness, altered states of consciousness, extracorporeal sensations, and combativeness.[159] The onset occurs with the first verbal contact and usually resolves in a few hours with full return of orientation to person, place, and time. The incidence of emergence reactions is approximately 12%.[160] The incidence appears to be influenced by age, dose, gender, and psychological predisposition and concurrent medications. Recurrent dreams have been reported to occur weeks after a ketamine anesthetic. The benzodiazepines diazepam, lorazepam, and midazolam were found to significantly decrease the incidence of these reactions. Subanesthetic doses of ketamine are being used for short-term treatment of acute and chronic pain. Low doses of ketamine are being used for sedation, postoperative pain relief, analgesia during regional or local anesthesia, and opioid-sparing effect.[161] Emergence reactions with low-dose ketamine are less frequent, but vivid dreaming may still occur. The use of positive mood elevating suggestion helps reduce the recall of unpleasant dreaming.[162] Ketamine has little effect on postoperative nausea and vomiting (PONV). Subanesthetic doses used for analgesia may reduce opioid requirements.[163]

Cardiovascular effects. Ketamine, unlike other intravenous anesthetics, acts as a circulatory stimulant, producing increases in systemic blood pressure, heart rate, cardiac contractility and output, and central venous pressure.[164] Systemic vascular resistance responded differently among patients undergoing cardiac catheterization and angiography (±25%), possibly because of patient variability in autonomic tone and disease states. Other studies have failed to show significant effects in systemic vascular resistance but have found evidence of an increase in pulmonary vascular resistance (42%), pulmonary artery pressure (47%), and right ventricular stroke work. These values persisted throughout the 12-minute measurement period, although they were somewhat decreased (pulmonary vascular resistance 42% at 3–5 minutes and 25% at 12 minutes; mean pulmonary arterial pressure 47% at 3–5 minutes and 23% at 12 minutes). In patients with congenital heart disease and increased pulmonary pressure and resistance, ketamine administration did not adversely affect myocardial function (ejection fractions remained constant).[165]

Ketamine administration causes an increase in myocardial contractility, thereby affecting the myocardial oxygen balance. This increase in myocardial oxygen consumption has not been shown to cause inadequate myocardial perfusion because a concomitant rise in coronary artery perfusion occurs.[166]

Ketamine-induced activation of the sympathetic nervous system that results in endogenous catecholamine release is believed to be one of the mechanisms for the cardiostimulatory properties experienced after administration of the drug. The positive inotropic effect of ketamine also results from an inhibition of neuronal and extraneuronal uptake of norepinephrine.[166] The in vitro negative inotropic effects of ketamine are the result of a decrease in the available calcium ions (Ca^{2+}) intracellularly, caused by an interference with Ca^{2+} delivery mechanisms (net transsarcolemmal Ca^{2+} influx).[167] When the positive inotropic effects of ketamine are blocked, the negative inotropic effects predominate and may result in decreased blood pressure and cardiac output. This phenomenon may be seen clinically in the critically ill patient who, as a result of protracted illness, has decreased catecholamine stores and limited ability to compensate. With an intact sympathetic nervous system, the positive inotropic effects dominate and counteract the negative inotropic effects. By decreasing sympathetic responses, some inhalation anesthetics are able to block the cardiovascular effects of ketamine to produce a decrease in systemic blood pressure and cardiac output.[168] The cardiovascular stimulation produced by ketamine may be deliberately decreased by the prior administration of benzodiazepines in patients in whom that response should be avoided.[169]

Ketamine has been used successfully in patients who are hemodynamically compromised because of shock, trauma, debilitation, or hypovolemia.

Changes in systemic blood pressure are dose related; systolic and diastolic blood pressures increase when larger doses of ketamine are administered (0.5–2.0 mg/kg). However, the heart rate response to different dosages reaches a plateau, with no significant change in rate occurring between doses of 0.5 and 2 mg/kg.

Ketamine has been used successfully for both pediatric and adult cardiac surgery patients with congenital and acquired disease processes.[164] The cardiac and respiratory actions of ketamine are summarized in Table 9.5.

Respiratory effects. The effects of ketamine on the respiratory system are minor and of short duration. Ventilation is generally preserved, as are normal respirations. Transient apnea upon initial administration may occur with rapid administration of larger doses, although it is rare. Arterial blood gases remain within normal limits, and the central response to CO_2 is maintained.[164]

Ketamine increases pulmonary compliance and decreases pulmonary resistance in patients with bronchospastic disease. It is the only active bronchodilating induction agent and the agent of choice in any patient with active asthma who requires surgery. Increased catecholamine levels stimulated by ketamine, along with bronchial smooth muscle relaxation and vagolytic actions, are thought to be the reason for the bronchodilating effects of the drug. Tracheal, bronchial, and salivary muscle gland secretions are increased with ketamine, which may require the use of an antisialagogue. Atropine is superior to glycopyrrolate for this application.[170] The muscle tone of the tongue and jaw is retained, and protective pharyngeal and laryngeal reflexes are left intact. Coughing, gagging, swallowing, and vomiting reflexes remain intact in response to airway stimulation, although some diminution may be present, and silent pulmonary aspiration has occurred in some patients (see Table 9.5).

Intraocular effects. Research into the effects of ketamine administration on intraocular pressure (IOP) has yielded varied results.[172-175] Measurement techniques and adjunctive anesthetics may play a role in the conflicting reports. Ketamine usually increases IOP, but the effect appears dose dependent.[175] A 6-mg/kg dose raises IOP, but a 3-mg/kg dose does not. Ketamine causes nystagmus, increased muscle tone, and muscle spasms, which may not be appropriate for some ophthalmic procedures.[176] When used for procedural sedation in the emergency department at doses of 4 mg/kg or less, there are no clinically meaningful increases in IOP.[177] It blocks oculocardiac reflex–induced arrhythmias better than propofol during sevoflurane anesthesia for strabismus surgery.[178] The common clinical effects of ketamine are shown in Box 9.4.

Obstetric and pediatric use. Ketamine can be used in obstetrics for analgesia or anesthesia. It is highly lipid soluble and readily crosses the placenta into fetal tissue. As an induction agent, ketamine in doses of 0.5 to 1 mg/kg produces rapid anesthesia without compromising uterine tone, uterine blood flow, or neonatal status at delivery. For analgesia, 0.25 mg/kg of ketamine provides pain-related relief, airway stability, and a sustained maternal blood pressure and uninhibited uterine contractions. Use of doses reserved for surgical procedures (2–2.5 mg/kg) results, however, in a depressed neonate on delivery.[179,180] Decreasing this dose to 0.2 to 1 mg/kg spares the newborn this CNS depression because of the rapid redistribution of the drug in the mother and less fetal transfer.

Ketamine can be administered to neonates and children. Sedation, analgesia, amnesia, cardiac and respiratory stability, and a short duration offer advantages in many procedures in these patients.[181] Clinicians have noted it may be the agent of choice for children with a difficult airway or reactive airway diseases such as asthma. It can be used intramuscularly or orally for an uncooperative child requiring intravenous access.[182]

A controversy exists with regard to anesthetic neurotoxicity caused by ketamine. Neuroapoptosis has been noted in several animal models when ketamine is used in the developing brain.[183] How this relates to the use of ketamine and other anesthetics in newborns and children is unclear. This is an area of intense research interest.[186-188]

Clinical uses of ketamine are given in Box 9.5. Recommendations for using ketamine as a sedative, analgesic, or anesthetic during the postoperative period are listed in Box 9.3. Key points of ketamine pharmacology are given in Box 9.6.

BOX 9.5 Clinical Uses of Ketamine

Induction of Anesthesia in High-Risk Patients
- Shock or cardiovascular instability
- Hypovolemia
- Cardiomyopathy
- Trauma
- Bronchospasm

Obstetric Patients
Induction of General Anesthesia
- Severe hypovolemia/trauma
- Acute hemorrhage
- Acute bronchospasm

Low Dose for Analgesia
- To supplement regional anesthetic techniques
- As an additive to opioids in patient-controlled analgesia
- For use in therapy for chronic pain and depression

Adjunct to Local and Regional Anesthetic Techniques
- For sedation and analgesia during intravenous sedation or when a regional block is used
- To supplement an inadequate block

Outpatient Surgery
- For brief diagnostic and therapeutic procedures
- To supplement local and regional block techniques

Use Outside the Operating Room
- In burn units (e.g., debridement, dressing changes)
- In emergency rooms for minor procedures
- In intensive care units (e.g., sedation, painful procedures)
- During radiology procedures

BOX 9.4 Primary Clinical Characteristics and Effects of Ketamine

- Phencyclidine derivative
- Causes unconsciousness; amnesia referred to as dissociative anesthesia
- Increases cerebral metabolic rate, cerebral blood flow, and intracranial pressure
- Causes nystagmus; increased intraocular pressure
- Moderate analgesic
- Increases blood pressure and pulse
- Potent bronchodilator
- Maintains respirations and airway reflexes (NOTE: A period of initial apnea may occur, especially with high doses and rapid administration.)
- Increases salivation and respiratory secretions
- Increases muscle tone
- Associated with emergence delirium, nightmares, and hallucinations
- Requires caution in patients with hypertension, angina, congestive heart failure, increased intracranial pressure, increased intraocular pressure, psychiatric disease, and airway problems

---

BOX 9.6 Key Points for Ketamine Anesthesia

- Site of action of ketamine appears to be the NMDA receptor, where it inhibits glutamate as a noncompetitive antagonist. Other actions are likely.
- Ketamine produces an anesthetic state referred to as dissociative anesthesia.
- Onset of effect is relatively slow compared to other induction drugs (2–5 min).
- Ketamine produces a rise in cerebral perfusion pressure.
- Ketamine is a bronchodilator, preserves airway reflexes, and increases secretions.
- Emergence phenomena—including vivid dreams, floating sensations, and delirium—can occur after ketamine administration. They are more common in adults than children and are reduced by benzodiazepine or other sedative administration.
- Ketamine is an indirect sympathomimetic, releasing catecholamines. This action accounts for the cardiac stimulation and bronchodilation.
- Ketamine is a moderate analgesic and is used preoperatively as an analgesic.

NMDA, N-methyl-D-aspartate.

BENZODIAZEPINES

Benzodiazepines are used in many clinical situations due to their desirable pharmacologic properties, including sedation, hypnosis, muscle relaxation, anxiolysis, anticonvulsant effects, and amnesia. They also have a low incidence of side effects. Benzodiazepines used clinically in the United States are listed in Table 9.9.

Although similar compounds were first synthesized in 1933, the first benzodiazepine synthesized was chlordiazepoxide (Librium) in 1955. It was not introduced into clinical practice until 1960, when it was found to have antianxiety and hypnotic effects. Diazepam was synthesized in 1959, and its metabolite, oxazepam (Serax), was synthesized in 1961. Lorazepam (Ativan) was derived from oxazepam in 1971.[188] The last benzodiazepine to be developed was midazolam (in 1976, by Fryer and Walser), which was the first of the benzodiazepine group to be formulated with anesthesia as its target clinical use. The benzodiazepines available for clinical use have many similarities, but there are differences in potencies, pharmacokinetics, and intensities of clinical properties. Midazolam is widely used in anesthesia and other areas as an anxiolytic, sedative, hypnotic, and amnestic drug. It is rarely used to induce anesthesia due to a prolonged effect at the high doses required. Diazepam and lorazepam, which are also available as intravenous preparations, are occasionally used as well. They are usually reserved for inpatients requiring prolonged sedation. Remimazolam is an ultrashort-acting benzodiazepine currently being developed for procedural sedation and induction, and maintenance of anesthesia. It combines the properties of two unique drugs already established in anesthesia. It is a benzodiazepine like midazolam and has organ-independent metabolism like remifentanil. The incorporation of a carboxylic ester moiety into the benzodiazepine core of remimazolam renders it susceptible to nonspecific tissue esterases, and it is rapidly metabolized into its pharmacologically inactive metabolite.[189,190]

Chemical Structure and Pharmaceutics

The chemical structures of the benzodiazepines share some common features: (1) the benzodiazepine ring system, (2) the presence at positions 1 and 4 of two nitrogen atoms, (3) a phenyl group at position 5, and (4) an electronegative group at position 7 (see Fig. 9.1).[191]

Midazolam has a unique chemical structure in comparison with the other benzodiazepines. The imidazole ring is responsible for its basic formulation, which permits the preparation of salts that are water soluble at a pH of 4.0. In a chemical reaction that depends on the environmental pH, the diazepine ring opens reversibly between positions 4 and 5. Midazolam is water soluble and does not require a lipoidal vehicle (such as propylene glycol) for parenteral use. It is minimal if any side effects of venous irritation or phlebitis occur. Once in physiologic solution with a pH greater than 4.0, the diazepine ring closes, and midazolam becomes lipophilic, an effect that accounts for its rapid onset of action.[190-192]

Injectable midazolam is compounded with 0.8% sodium chloride and 0.01% disodium edetate and 1% benzyl alcohol as a preservative. A pH of 3 is adjusted with hydrochloric acid and, if necessary, sodium hydroxide. Each milliliter of preparation contains 1 mg or 5 mg of midazolam. An oral solution is also available for pediatric sedation.

In each milliliter of solution of diazepam, 0.4 mL of propylene glycol and 0.1 mL of ethyl alcohol are present as solvents, 0.015 mL of benzyl alcohol is present as a preservative, and sodium benzoate or benzoic acid in water is present as a buffer. Each milliliter contains 5 mg of diazepam, and the pH is 6.2 to 6.9.[191]

Each milliliter of lorazepam solution contains 0.18 mL of polyethylene glycol and 2% benzyl alcohol, a preservative. Lorazepam is available in solutions of 2 mg/mL or 4 mg/mL (see Table 9.1 for the preparations of the benzodiazepines).[191]

Mechanisms of Action

The clinical effects of benzodiazepines are a result of an agonist action at what are termed benzodiazepine receptor binding sites on the $GABA_A$ receptor throughout the CNS. GABA is the major inhibitory neurotransmitter in the CNS. The receptor complex is composed of a pentameric array of protein subunits that contain binding sites for GABA itself, benzodiazepines, barbiturates, ethanol, propofol, and many other sedatives. The $GABA_A$ receptor exerts its actions by modulating chloride channels. Many different families of the $GABA_A$ receptors exist, and these subtypes vary in location, function, and pharmacologic effects. When these binding sites are occupied by an agonist, GABA receptor modulation increases the frequency of chloride channel opening, which results in postsynaptic membrane hyperpolarization, and neuronal transmission is inhibited.[193-195]

Three classes of ligands that bind to the benzodiazepine receptors have been identified: agonists, antagonists, and inverse agonists. Midazolam, diazepam, and lorazepam are receptor agonists that allosterically increase binding affinity for GABA, resulting in the opening of the

TABLE 9.9 Benzodiazepines Used Clinically in the United States

Generic Name	Trade Name	Half-Life (hr)	Clinical Application
Alprazolam	Xanax	12–15	Anxiolysis
Chlordiazepoxide	Librium	8–18	Treatment of alcohol withdrawal, etc.
Clonazepam	Klonopin	18.7–39	Treatment of epilepsy
Clorazepate	Tranxene	2.4	Treatment of epilepsy and alcohol withdrawal
Diazepam	Valium	36–50	Sedation; induction and maintenance of anesthesia
Estazolam	ProSom	14	Treatment of insomnia
Flurazepam	Dalmane	2–3	Treatment of insomnia
Lorazepam	Ativan	10–22	Anxiolysis and sedation
Midazolam	Versed	1.7–2.6	Sedation; induction and maintenance of anesthesia
Oxazepam	Serax	3–21	Anxiolysis
Quazepam	Doral	25–41	Treatment of insomnia
Temazepam	Restoril	10–21	Treatment of insomnia
Triazolam	Halcion	2–3	Treatment of insomnia
Flumazenil	Romazicon	0.7–1.3	Reversal of benzodiazepine agonists

chloride channels. Antagonists (e.g., flumazenil) form reversible bonds with the agonist receptor but produce no agonist activity. Inverse agonists cause CNS stimulation by interfering with GABA transmission, which is inhibitory.[195,196] Because the benzodiazepines work allosterically to enhance endogenous GABA binding and not directly, there is a physiologic ceiling to their effect. Their safety and low toxicity are attributed to this built-in limit on their effect.[191] Peripheral benzodiazepine binding sites, not associated with the $GABA_A$ receptor, exist in the mitochondrial membranes of many cells and may modulate cardiovascular and immune function.[197]

Pharmacokinetics

The introduction of new generations of benzodiazepines since their initial release in the 1960s has largely focused on chemical alterations that improve the clinical pharmacokinetics. These changes have resulted in simplified metabolism with fewer active metabolites and thus more predictable time courses. The elimination pharmacokinetics of benzodiazepines can be examined in both two- and three-compartment models. Benzodiazepines have been classified according to their elimination half-lives. These classifications take into account the elimination half-lives of both the parent drug and the active metabolites. Diazepam is long acting ($T_{1/2}$ >24 hours), lorazepam is intermediate ($T_{1/2}$ 6–24 hours), and midazolam is short acting ($T_{1/2}$ <6 hours).[81] The pharmacologic effects of the benzodiazepines, as with the other anesthesia induction drugs, are terminated primarily by redistribution of the drug out of the CNS.

Their pharmacokinetics are influenced by age, gender, obesity, race, and hepatic and renal status to varying degrees. The pharmacokinetics of the three intravenous benzodiazepines are similar with a few important differences. Midazolam exhibits a higher clearance rate and therefore is shorter acting. Lorazepam is less dependent on hepatic cytochrome enzymes for metabolism because it undergoes phase 2 conjugation to a significant extent. Liver disease, as well as hepatic enzyme induction or inhibition, therefore does not influence lorazepam as much as other drugs. Diazepam has a very slow distribution half-life, which limits its usefulness as an acceptable induction agent. Diazepam is extremely lipid soluble, a characteristic that promotes extensive distribution to the tissues. The volume of distribution is large, a characteristic of all benzodiazepines. Also characteristic is extensive protein binding, which theoretically may be affected by disease states that decrease plasma protein levels. All three drugs are primarily bound to albumin. Diazepam is 99% protein bound, lorazepam 85% to 90%, and midazolam 95%. The total body clearance of diazepam is 0.24 to 0.53 mL/min/kg and is totally dependent on hepatic metabolism.

Diazepam exhibits a near-linear relationship between elimination half-life and patient age. Pharmacokinetics in the elderly are altered as a result of slowed drug absorption; increased percentage of adipose tissue in body mass; decreased plasma proteins, hepatic blood flow, and metabolism; and decreased cardiac output and circulation time. A prolonged circulation time allows for a slower onset and a higher plasma drug level that remains in the CNS longer before it redistributes; this phenomenon exaggerates the effects of the drug.[81]

Hepatic microsomal enzymes are responsible for the metabolism of diazepam. Diazepam is demethylated to dimethyl diazepam (nordiazepam), which is an active metabolite that, although less potent, is responsible for prolonged drug effect as a result of its slower metabolism. Diazepam can also be hydroxylated to 3-hydroxydiazepam, which is then demethylated to oxazepam, which is also pharmacologically active and commercially marketed. The termination of action of diazepam is caused by redistribution and eventual metabolism. The terminal half-life is 20 to 50 hours, much longer than that of other benzodiazepines and induction agents.

Pharmacodynamics

CNS effects. All three intravenous drugs produce the characteristic dose-dependent CNS depressant effects of the benzodiazepines, from anxiolysis to sedation, sleep, and with high enough doses of anesthesia. They all produce anticonvulsant effects, amnesia, and muscle-relaxing properties and are useful for inhibiting alcohol withdrawal symptoms. They are not antiemetic; however, lorazepam is used for its sedative, amnestic, and anxiolytic effects in reducing anticipatory chemotherapy-induced nausea and vomiting.

At higher doses they reduce $CMRO_2$ and CBF. They increase the threshold to local anesthetic-induced seizure activity, and midazolam is frequently used as a premedicant in patients having regional anesthesia requiring large volumes of local anesthetics.

All benzodiazepines produce dose-related anterograde amnesia. They generally do not produce reliable retrograde amnesia. Intravenous administration of midazolam produces anterograde amnesia in low doses. Amnesia occurs within 2 to 5 minutes of administration and remains for 20 to 30 minutes.[199-202] Deficits are seen in both short- and long-term memory. These include interfering with episodic, semantic, and iconic memory function.

Benzodiazepines also possess anticonvulsant activity and are effective in the treatment of status epilepticus and sedative-hypnotic withdrawal syndromes. EEG changes include disappearance of the alpha rhythm and the onset of higher frequency beta-rhythm activity.[202] Tolerance, dependence, and withdrawal symptoms occur and vary among the benzodiazepines. Midazolam produces synergistic CNS, cardiovascular, and respiratory effects with fentanyl (see Table 9.4).

Cardiovascular effects. In commonly used clinical doses, the benzodiazepines have minimal cardiovascular effects. A decrease in blood pressure is occasionally seen when midazolam is given with opioids in patients with heart disease or the elderly.

Respiratory effects. Benzodiazepines produce dose-dependent respiratory depression. Midazolam is the most respiratory depressing. Some respiratory depression occurs with diazepam, as evidenced by a decrease in minute ventilation and slope of the CO_2 response curve.[203] Increased respiratory depression and apnea are possible when benzodiazepines are combined with other CNS depressants such as opioids.

Contraindications and Precautions

The most common adverse effects of the benzodiazepines are unexpected respiratory depression and oversedation, and they have been implicated for contributing to postoperative cognitive dysfunction (especially in elderly patients). In the doses used currently, other adverse actions are rare. They should be avoided in patients with acute porphyrias.

Uses

Midazolam is the standard drug given for preoperative medication. Its rapid onset, short duration and half-life, and lack of adverse effects make it ideal for use as a preoperative anxiolytic, sedative, and amnestic.[204] Key points for the use of benzodiazepines are shown in Box 9.7.

Flumazenil

Flumazenil is the sole benzodiazepine antagonist available in the United States (see Fig. 9.1). It is a competitive antagonist with a high affinity for the receptor site. It produces prompt and effective specific reversal of benzodiazepine agonist effects after anesthesia and overdose.[205,206] As with any drug antagonist, its antidotal efficacy depends on the amount of free benzodiazepine at the receptor sites. Its relatively short duration and half-life make the possibility of resedation clinically relevant, especially in overdose situations. A slow titration of 0.2-mg

BOX 9.7 Key Points for Benzodiazepines

- Benzodiazepines act by an agonist effect on the $GABA_A$ receptor, which enhances the inhibitory effect of GABA. Flumazenil is an antagonist at these receptors and reverses the clinical effect of the agonists. Inverse agonists (not used clinically) are anxiogenic.
- Benzodiazepines cause:
  Reduction of anxiety and aggression
  Sedation, leading to improvement of insomnia
  Muscle relaxation and loss of motor coordination
  Suppression of convulsions (antiepileptic effect)
  Anterograde amnesia
- Differences in the pharmacologic profile of different benzodiazepines are minor; clonazepam appears to have more anticonvulsant action in relation to its other effects.
- Benzodiazepines are active orally and differ mainly in respect to their duration of action and half-lives. Some long-acting agents (e.g., diazepam and chlordiazepoxide) are converted to a long-lasting active metabolite nordazepam.
- Midazolam, diazepam, and lorazepam are available intravenously.
- Zolpidem (Ambien) is a short-acting drug that is not a benzodiazepine but acts similarly and is used as a hypnotic.
- Remimazolam is an experimental benzodiazepine with an ester linkage that allows for rapid metabolism to inactive metabolites. It is administered by continuous infusion and may prove useful as a fast-onset, short-duration induction drug.

GABA, γ-aminobutyric acid.

BOX 9.8 α_2-Receptor Subtypes and Functions

α_{2A}-Receptors	α_{2B}-Receptors	α_{2C}-Receptors
• Presynaptic feedback	• Presynaptic feedback	• Presynaptic feedback
• Inhibition of norepinephrine release	• Inhibition of norepinephrine release	• Inhibition of norepinephrine release
• Sedation	• Vasoconstriction, antishivering	• Learning and stress responses
• Hypnosis	• Analgesia	• Feedback inhibition of adrenal epinephrine release
• Analgesia	• Analgesic effect of nitrous oxide	• Modulation of insulin secretion
• Neuroprotection	• Hypertension	
• Hyperglycemia	• Placenta angiogenesis	
• Diuresis		
• Sympatholysis		
• Hypotension		
• Anticonvulsant		
• Hypothermia		
• Modulation of insulin secretion		

doses (2 mL) is given intravenously (up to 1 mg) until the desired level of consciousness is achieved. Doses rarely exceed 1 mg for the reversal of midazolam-induced sedation and 3 mg for suspected benzodiazepine overdose. Onset is 1 to 2 minutes, and duration of action is 45 to 90 minutes depending on total flumazenil dose and the amount of agonist requiring reversal. Withdrawal reactions are possible in patients who are benzodiazepine dependent, and its use in these patients is contraindicated. Flumazenil does not reverse the actions of ethanol or barbiturates.[207] Side effects are rare, although mild anxiogenic effects have been reported.[208] Seizures have been reported in patients with suspected tricyclic and antidepressant overdose, and the use of flumazenil in these situations and in patients with a known history of seizures should be avoided.[209,210]

Dexmedetomidine

The sedative and analgesic effects of α_2-receptor agonists were long recognized from the use of clonidine and the veterinary anesthetic xylazine. Dexmedetomidine was developed as a more selective α_2-agonist, which allows for greater sedation. There are three main chemical classes of α_2-receptor agonists: the phenylethylates such as methyldopa and guanabenz; the imidazolines such as clonidine, dexmedetomidine, mivazerol, and azepexole; and the oxaloazepines. The imidazolines are used in anesthesia. Stimulation of imidazoline receptors account for the hypotensive side effects. The primary effects of dexmedetomidine are sedation, analgesia, anxiolysis, reduced postoperative shivering and agitation, and cardiovascular sympatholytic actions.[212]

Mechanism of Action

α_2-adrenoreceptors are involved in various physiologic functions, particularly in the cardiovascular and central nervous systems. There are three subtypes of α_2-receptors. The subtypes and their putative functions are noted in Box 9.8.[213,214] Dexmedetomidine is highly specific for α_2- versus α_1-receptors at a ratio of 1600:1. α_2-presynaptic receptors function as autoreceptors in the negative feedback loop controlling

neurotransmitter release. When α_2-receptors are stimulated by an agonist such as dexmedetomidine, it results in a decreased catecholamine release. The main site of action for the sedative actions of dexmedetomidine is the pontine noradrenergic nucleus, the locus coeruleus. The α_2-receptors are G protein–coupled receptors, which when activated result in the inhibition of calcium channels, the activation of potassium channels, and the direct modulation of the exocytic release of proteins. This produces hyperpolarization of the cells and thus inhibition.[215,216]

Chemistry and Pharmaceutics

Precedex (dexmedetomidine hydrochloride injection) is a sterile, nonpyrogenic solution for intravenous infusion following dilution. Dexmedetomidine hydrochloride is the S-enantiomer of medetomidine and is chemically described as (+)-4-(S)-[1-(2,3-dimethylphenyl)ethyl]-1H-imidazole monohydrochloride. Dexmedetomidine HCl is freely soluble in water and has a pK_a of 7.1. Its partition coefficient (n-octanol/water) at pH 7.4 is 2.89. Precedex is supplied as a clear, colorless, isotonic solution with a pH of 4.5 to 7.0. Each milliliter of Precedex contains 118 mcg of dexmedetomidine HCl (equivalent to 100 mcg dexmedetomidine base) and 9 mg of sodium chloride in water. The solution is preservative free and contains no additives or chemical stabilizers. Prepare by adding 2 mL of dexmedetomidine (100 mcg/mL) to 48 mL of 0.9% sodium chloride injection for a total of 50 mL. The final concentration is 4 mcg/mL. The loading dose is 1 mcg/kg infused over 10 minutes followed by maintenance infusions of 0.2 to 0.7 mcg/kg/hour. It is approved for up to 24 hours of use for sedation in critical care and for nonintubated patients requiring sedation for short-term surgical procedures. It is used for numerous off-label applications.[211]

Pharmacokinetics

Dexmedetomidine exhibits a rapid distribution phase with a distribution half-life ($T_{1/2}$) of approximately 6 minutes, a terminal elimination half-life ($T_{1/2}$) of approximately 2 hours, and steady-state volume of distribution (Vss) of approximately 118 L. Clearance is estimated to be approximately 39 L/hour. The mean body weight associated with this clearance estimate was 72 kg. Dexmedetomidine exhibits linear kinetics in the dosage range of 0.2 to 0.7 mcg/kg/hour when administered by intravenous infusion for up to 24 hours. Target concentrations are usually in the range of 0.3 to 0.6 mg/mL. Protein binding to both albumin and α_1-acid glycoprotein is 94%.[215] Dexmedetomidine undergoes almost complete biotransformation with very little unchanged in urine and feces. Biotransformation involves both direct glucuronidation as well as cytochrome P-450–mediated metabolism. There are no active metabolites. Similar kinetic data were noted in pediatric patients.[217,218] Onset of action with loading infusion is 10 to 20 minutes, and the duration of action after the infusion is stopped is 10 to 30 minutes.

CNS effects. Dexmedetomidine produces a dose-dependent sedation that resembles natural sleep, unlike the classic GABA receptor agonists. Patients do not experience respiratory depression and are readily arousable.[219] An advantage of this type of sedation is that procedures requiring "wake-up" tests can be more readily accomplished compared to usual anesthetic regimens.[221-223] Dexmedetomidine does not interfere with electrophysiologic monitoring, allowing brain mapping during awake craniotomy and microelectrode recording during implantation of deep-brain stimulators.[223] Motor and somatosensory evoked potentials are maintained when added to a desflurane and remifentanil technique.[224] Decreases in the amplitude of motor evoked potentials may occur at high doses.[225] BIS values are decreased in a dose-dependent manner to a greater extent than with propofol.[226]

Dexmedetomidine does not change cerebral metabolism (CMRO$_2$). CBF is decreased due to cerebral vasoconstriction. This suggests uncoupling between cerebral metabolism and flow due to decreases in central catecholamine turnover. Effects on intracranial pressure are not clinically significant.[227]

The central sympatholytic effects also result in an antishivering action, hypothermia, and a reduction in the neuroendocrine stress response to surgery.[228] A reduction in postoperative agitation and emergence delirium in children and adults is an increasingly used clinical action.[229] A neuroprotective effect has been proposed, but benefits in patients with head injuries remain to be clarified. Reductions in the withdrawal symptoms from sedatives, opioids, and alcohol have been noted. Analgesic- and anesthetic-sparing effects are well documented and are produced at both the brain and spinal cord level. Dexmedetomidine enhances the analgesic effects of nitrous oxide.[230]

Cardiovascular effects. The main cardiovascular effects of dexmedetomidine are hypotension and bradycardia. These result from CNS α-receptor stimulation and systemic vasodilation. Occasionally transient hypertension is seen with rapid initial loading doses or administration of high maintenance doses due to peripheral vasoconstriction; however, dose-dependent hypotension most commonly occurs during general anesthesia. There is no direct effect on myocardial contractility. There is a reduction in myocardial oxygen demand, an antianginal effect. Transient profound hypertension was noted when using glycopyrrolate to treat dexmedetomidine-induced bradycardia in children, and caution is advised when coadministering these drugs.[215]

Respiratory effects. A unique advantage of dexmedetomidine sedation is that respirations are maintained. Brain respiratory responsiveness to CO$_2$ is normal. Airway patency and reflexes are present or only slightly diminished. These properties allow for convenient use in out-of-operating room procedures and difficult airway situations. Dexmedetomidine completely blocked histamine-induced bronchoconstriction in dogs. It appears beneficial to decrease airway reactivity in patients with chronic obstructive pulmonary disease or asthma.[231]

The Sedation Practice in Intensive Care Evaluation (SPICE III) trial is the largest study ever to examine dexmedetomidine sedation in the critically ill. The primary finding is that early sedation with dexmedetomidine is not associated with a reduction in mortality. However, SPICE III does confirm some previously identified characteristics regarding dexmedetomidine use as a sedative agent in patients receiving

mechanical ventilation. First, dexmedetomidine as a sole agent does not reliably provide adequate sedation in all patients and may be insufficient as a sole agent when light sedation is targeted. Second, there are a greater number of adverse events associated with the use of dexmedetomidine when compared with alternative sedatives. In other instances, the findings from SPICE III contradicted the results of prior studies. The presumed benefit of a decrease in the incidence of delirium with dexmedetomidine use was also not seen in SPICE III. Additionally, SPICE III did not find a difference in duration of ICU length of stay. The accumulated efficacy and safety data suggest that current guidelines will need to be updated to address the limitations of dexmedetomidine, and its place as an option of first choice in the management of sedation in all patients receiving mechanical ventilation needs to be reconsidered.[233-235]

Other effects. Dexmedetomidine has a mild diuretic effect mediated via α$_2$-receptor stimulation. Additional beneficial actions include renal, gastroprotective, and antiinflammatory effects. Dexmedetomidine is being widely used for many surgical and diagnostic procedures in both adults and children. It is thought to decrease the incidence of emergence delirium after general anesthesia in pediatric patients. Which clinical situations become established as the best places to use this unique drug is still evolving. Some key points for the clinical use of dexmedetomidine are noted in Box 9.9.

ANESTHETIC NEUROTOXICITY

General anesthetic and sedative drugs are administered to millions of infants and children each year. Data from animal and observational human studies have raised concerns that general anesthetics may cause neurotoxic changes in the developing brain that lead to adverse neurodevelopmental outcomes later in life. To address this concern, in 2009 the Food and Drug Administration (FDA) established a public-private partnership with the International Anesthesia Research Society (IARS) called Strategies for Mitigating Anesthesia Related Neurotoxicity in Tots, or Smart Tots.[235]

Studies have confirmed that commonly used anesthetics and sedatives that either increase inhibitory GABA receptor activity (e.g., propofol, etomidate, sevoflurane, desflurane, and isoflurane) or block excitatory glutamate receptors (e.g., ketamine) produce profound neurotoxic effects in laboratory animals. Factors that influence the extent of injury include age at the time of drug exposure and cumulative anesthetic dose. Histologic changes include widespread apoptosis and cell death, a reduction in the number of synapses, changes in neuronal morphology, and impaired neurogenesis in the hippocampus.[236]

In June 2014, Smart Tots convened a meeting to review the accumulated data. The participants concluded that the current data from animal studies are now sufficiently convincing that large-scale clinical studies are warranted. The group produced a new statement recommending

---

BOX 9.9 Key Points for Clinical Use of Dexmedetomidine

- Dexmedetomidine is an α$_2$-receptor agonist that results in central sympatholysis.
- Dexmedetomidine sedation allows for an arousable patient to ascertain neurologic status.
- Dexmedetomidine does not interfere with neurologic monitoring.
- Hypotension and bradycardia are the most frequent cardiovascular adverse effects.
- Respirations are maintained.
- It may reduce postoperative agitation and emergence reactions.

that surgical procedures performed under anesthesia be avoided in children under 3 years of age unless the situation is urgent. The statement also emphasizes the need to determine whether anesthetic and sedative drugs cause brain damage in infants, toddlers, and children. In particular, randomized clinical trials are needed to determine whether general anesthetics impair neurocognitive development. In December 2015, Smart Tots released a supplemental consensus statement on a recent general anesthesia study (GAS). The GAS study is the first prospective clinical trial to explore the effects of anesthetics on the developing brain in humans. The secondary outcome data, based on 532 subjects, indicated that children who had undergone either general anesthesia or regional anesthesia in a surgical procedure lasting less than 1 hour showed no difference in cognitive development at the 2-year time point.[237]

Smart Tots has taken a first step by establishing an international working group of experts who will generate data on animal models that can inform the design and execution of appropriate clinical trials. In the meantime, parents and care providers should be made aware of the potential risks that anesthetics pose to the developing brain. Further clinical studies may clarify whether anesthetics cause injury in humans. Surgeons, anesthesiologists, and parents should consider carefully how urgently surgery is needed, particularly in children under 3 years of age.[238,239] Anesthetic neurotoxicity is discussed further in Chapter 8.

SUMMARY

The availability of a variety of unique intravenous drugs that contain the necessary properties for use in induction has allowed the clinician to tailor the induction to fit the needs of the patient and surgeon. This characteristic has made it much easier to care for an increasingly diverse and complex patient population. Intravenous anesthetics can be chosen with consideration for the health status of the patient, the type of procedure to be performed, and the patient's susceptibility to possible adverse effects to produce the remarkably safe techniques and excellent outcomes achieved today.

REFERENCES

For a complete list of references for this chapter, scan this QR code with any smartphone code reader app, or visit the following URL: http://booksite.elsevier.com/9780323711944/.

10

Local Anesthetics

John J. Nagelhout

Local anesthetics are drugs that reversibly block the conduction of electrical impulses along nerve fibers. Their ability to perform this function depends on various factors, including the anatomy and physiologic state of the nerve(s) being anesthetized and physicochemical properties of the local anesthetic. These drugs have always been used as a major component of clinical anesthesia and they are increasingly being used to treat acute and chronic pain in new and innovative ways.

ANATOMY OF THE PERIPHERAL NERVE

To fully address the action of local anesthetics, a brief review of the anatomy and physiology of nerve fibers is warranted. The axon, an extension of a centrally located neuron, is the functional unit of peripheral nerves. A cell membrane, or axolemma, and intracellular contents, or axoplasm, are the major components of the axon. Schwann cells, whose functions are support and insulation, surround each axon. In unmyelinated nerves, single Schwann cells cover several axons. Conversely, in larger nerves the Schwann cell sheath covers only one axon and has several concentric layers of myelin.

Between Schwann cells are periodic segments of nerve that do not contain myelin. These areas, known as nodes of Ranvier, are where conduction is propagated. Voltage-gated sodium channels (Na_v) are located in these nonmyelinated segments, the primary site at which local anesthetics exert their inhibitory action. Action potentials jump from node to node, a phenomenon known as saltatory conduction, which significantly facilitates the speed of conduction along the axon.[1,2] Myelinated nerves are larger, conduct impulses faster, and are more difficult to anesthetize with local anesthetics than are unmyelinated nerves[3,4] (Fig. 10.1).

Peripheral nerves have structures containing bundles of axons called fasciculi. Three layers of connective tissue—the endoneurium, perineurium, and epineurium—also are components of a peripheral nerve.[4,5] The endoneurium, which is a delicate connective tissue composed of longitudinally arranged collagen, surrounds and embeds the axons in the fasciculi. The perineurium, which consists of layers of flattened, overlapping cells, binds a group of fascicles together. The epineurium, which surrounds the perineurium, is composed of areolar connective tissue that functionally holds the fascicles together to form a peripheral nerve.[5] These layers of connective tissue are important because they serve as barriers through which local anesthetics must diffuse if they are to exert their pharmacologic action (Fig. 10.2).

NEURON ELECTROPHYSIOLOGY AND THE ACTION MECHANISM OF LOCAL ANESTHETICS

Electrophysiology

Measurement with an electrode placed in the axoplasm of a resting peripheral nerve demonstrates a negative membrane potential of −70 mV to −90 mV.[3,5] This voltage difference across the neuronal membrane at steady state is called the resting membrane potential (Fig. 10.3). An ionic imbalance between the axoplasm and the extracellular fluid causes the electrical potential. Several physiologic mechanisms create the ionic gradient; the primary one is an active, energy-dependent process executed by a sodium-potassium pump (Na^+-K^+/ATPase) located in the axolemma.[6,7]

Although the membrane is relatively permeable to the outward diffusion of K^+, an intracellular-to-extracellular K^+ ratio of 150:5 mmol, or 30:1, exists. An important contributor to this concentration difference is the impermeability of the membrane to other cotransported ions such as Na^+.[7] In addition, the movement of K^+ out of the neuron leaves an excess of intracellular negatively charged organic ions. The negative charge results in an electrostatic counterforce that limits K^+ movement out of the neuron.

Two opposing forces influence K^+ movement into and out of the neuron. First, a concentration gradient pushes K^+ outward. Second, an electrostatic gradient, created by the impermeability of the membrane to cations, tends to keep the K^+ in the cell. The net effect of these counterforces is modest movement of K^+ out of the cell, and this movement creates an intracellular negative charge. The Nernst equation expresses the charge created by the K^+ concentration gradient[3]:

$$\text{Membrane potential} = -58 \log \frac{(K^+ \, 30 \, \text{inside})}{(K^+ \, \text{outside})}$$

Determination of the resting membrane potential is not as simple as the Nernst equation for K^+ indicates, because Na^+ and chloride ($Cl-$) ions also have a minor role in establishing the intracellular resting potential.[3]

When an electrical impulse is applied to a resting nerve, the membrane potential is reversed because of the intracellular movement of Na^+. This occurs because of the higher concentration of Na^+ outside the cell and the stimulation-induced increase in membrane permeability to this ion. The sudden influx of Na^+ that occurs in response to stimulation overrides the efflux of K^+ directed at maintaining the resting membrane potential. Once the process has reversed the membrane potential to 20 mV, an outward electrochemical gradient develops; this gradient resists the concentration-dependent, inward diffusion of Na^+.[5] This state of equilibrium causes the Na^+ channels to close. Shortly after Na^+ enters the cell, K^+ channels begin to open, and the ion rapidly diffuses out of the neuron according to its concentration gradient. The active removal of intracellular Na^+ by the Na^+-K^+ pump and the passive diffusion of K^+ back into the cell restore the resting membrane potential. During repolarization, three Na^+ ions leave the cell for each two K^+ ions that enter[8] (Fig. 10.4).

The sequence of events that causes an action potential results from the passage of ions through pores or channels located in the axolemma. These channels, which are composed of globular proteins, have

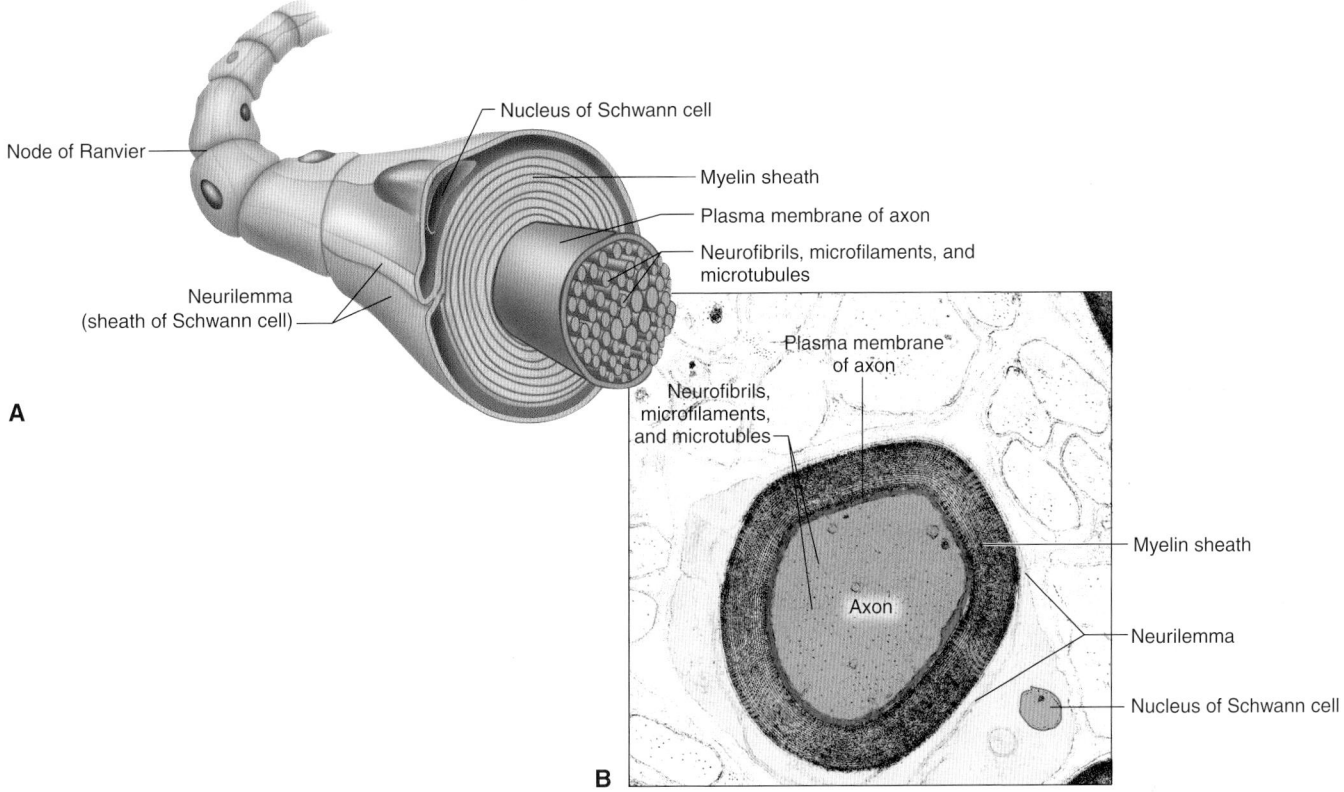

Fig. 10.1 Myelinated axon. (A) The diagram shows a cross section of an axon and its coverings formed by a Schwann cell: the myelin sheath and neurilemma. (B) Transmission electron micrograph showing how the densely wrapped layers of the Schwann cell's plasma membrane form the fatty myelin sheath. (From Patton KT, Thibodeau GA. *Anatomy & Physiology*. 10th ed. St. Louis: Elsevier; 2019:397.)

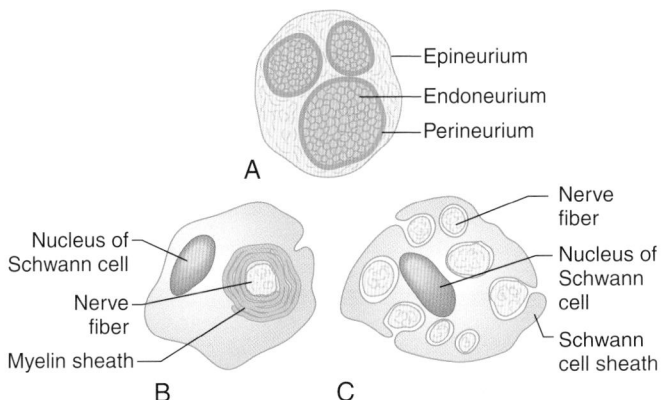

Fig. 10.2 Transverse sections of a peripheral nerve (A) showing the outermost epineurium; the inner perineurium, which collects nerve axons in fascicles; and the endoneurium, which surrounds each myelinated fiber (B), and is encased in the multiple membranous wrappings of myelin formed by one Schwann cell, each of which stretches longitudinally over approximately 100 times the diameter of the axon. The narrow span of axon between these myelinated segments, the node of Ranvier, contains the ion channels that support action potentials. Nonmyelinated fibers (C) are enclosed in bundles of 5 to 10 axons by a chain of Schwann cells that tightly embrace each axon with but one layer of membrane. (From Gropper MA. *Miller's Anesthesia*. 9th ed. Philadelphia: Elsevier; 2020:869.)

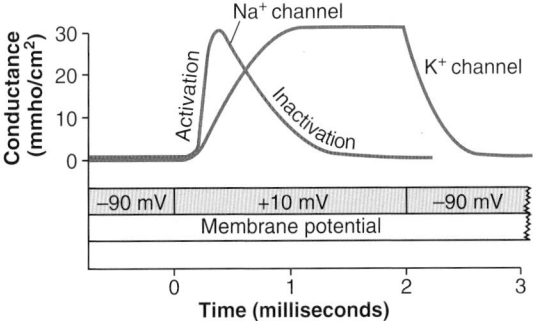

Fig. 10.3 Typical changes in conductance of sodium and potassium ion channels when the membrane potential is suddenly increased from the normal resting value of −90 mV to a positive value of +10 mV for 2 milliseconds. This figure shows that the sodium channels open (activate) and then close (inactivate) before the end of the 2 milliseconds, whereas the potassium channels only open (activate), and the rate of opening is much slower than that of the sodium channels. (From Hall JE. *Guyton and Hall Textbook of Medical Physiology*. 14th ed. Philadelphia: Elsevier; 2021:66.)

Mechanism of Action

As noted earlier, local anesthetics work by reversibly binding to the Na_v. Sodium channels have three functional states: resting (closed), open, and inactive. The resting state exists when the membrane is at its resting membrane potential. When a nerve is stimulated, reversal of the membrane potential occurs until the threshold potential is reached. When this happens a conformational change in the proteins that compose the channel occurs resulting in the open state. An inactive state,

transmural orientation to the phospholipid molecules that constitute the axolemma.[9] Although K^+ and calcium (Ca^{2+}) channels are important, the Na^+ channels are the most significant and best understood with respect to the initiation and propagation of the action potential.[3,10–14]

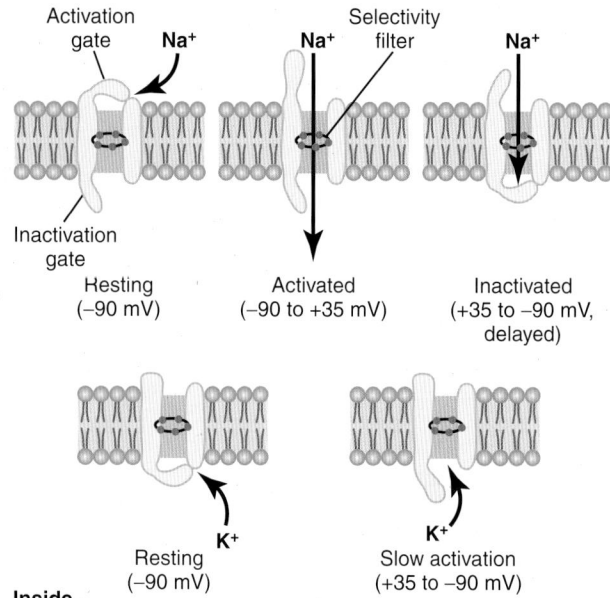

Fig. 10.4 Characteristics of the voltage-gated sodium *(top)* and potassium *(bottom)* channels, showing successive activation and inactivation of the sodium channels and delayed activation of the potassium channels when the membrane potential is changed from the normal resting negative value to a positive value. (From Hall JE. *Guyton and Hall Textbook of Medical Physiology.* 14th ed. Philadelphia: Elsevier; 2021:72.)

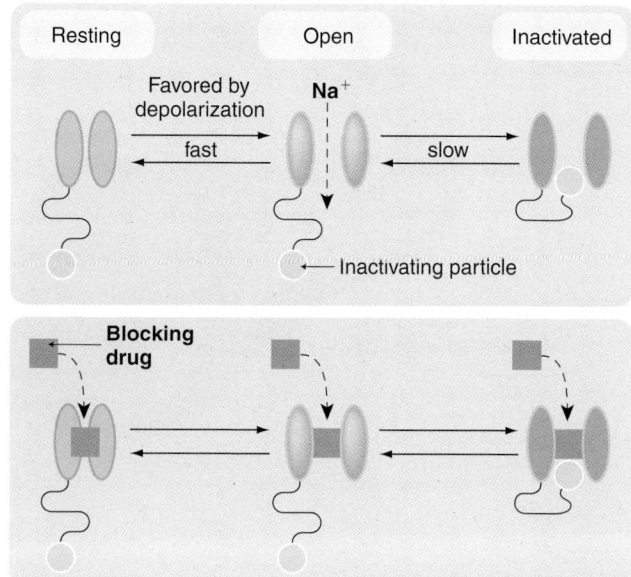

Fig. 10.5 Resting, activated, and inactivated states of voltage-gated channels, exemplified by the sodium channel. Membrane depolarization causes a rapid transition from the resting (closed) state to the open state. The inactivating particle (part of the intracellular domain of the channel protein) is then able to block the channel. Blocking drugs (e.g., local anesthetics and antiepileptic drugs) often show preference for one of the three channel states and thus affect the kinetic behavior of the channels with implications for their clinical application.

characterized by the return of the Na^+ channel to an impermeable state, follows the open state. This state, which prevents initiation of an action potential, lasts until the restoration of the resting membrane potential.[10] This three-state concept describes the changes in the Na_v that occur during depolarization and repolarization. Local anesthetics preferentially bind to receptors both in the open or inactivated states and not to the closed state. This is referred to as the guarded receptor or modulated receptor hypothesis of local anesthetic action. The open or inactive state may increase the affinity for binding the physical access of the drug to the receptor, or both.[11,15] In addition, it should be noted that local anesthetics work faster as the Na_v is repetitively depolarized, which is called use-dependent or phasic block. The more frequently the channel is depolarized, the more time it is available in the open and inactive states and thus available to local anesthetic blockade[16] (Fig. 10.5).

Local anesthetics inhibit the propagation of the action potential by binding reversibly to specific receptors within or adjacent to the internal opening of the Na_v channel.[17] Studies have indicated that these receptors, located on the intracellular side of the cell membrane, have a greater affinity for the charged or ionized form of the local anesthetics.[8,10,18] The uncharged or nonionized portion of the local anesthetic must first penetrate the cell membrane entering the axoplasm before it produces its effects. Fig. 10.6 shows the penetration of local anesthetic into a nerve and subsequent access to the receptor. The sequence is as follows:

1. Almost all clinically useful local anesthetics (except benzocaine) are tertiary amines and when injected will exist in both nonionized (lipid soluble) and ionized (water soluble) forms according to their pK_a (negative logarithm of the acid ionization constant), and the pH of the tissue or compartment.
2. Local anesthetics must gain access to the interior of the neuron to reach their receptor. This occurs by the diffusion of the lipid soluble nonionized fraction across the cell membrane.
3. Once inside the neuron, a new equilibrium forms between ionized and nonionized fractions. The ionized fraction binds to the receptor on the inside of the Na_v.

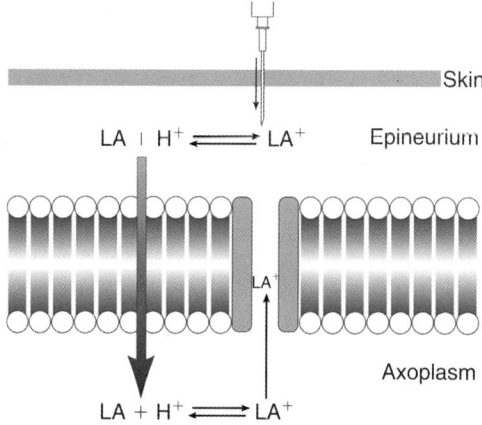

Fig. 10.6 Schematic conceptualization of local anesthetic action. Equilibrium forms outside the nerve between the ionized and nonionized portions. The nonionized portion *(LA)*, which is lipid soluble, enters the nerve. Once inside the axoplasm, the drug equilibrates, and the ionized fraction *(LA+)* attaches to the local anesthetic receptor on the inside of the sodium channel.

Benzocaine is a secondary amine and thus is permanently nonionized or neutral. It penetrates the lipid bilayer and can directly inhibit the Na_v without entering the axoplasm first.[12]

Local anesthetics have additional effects on G protein–coupled receptors affecting intracellular calcium signaling pathways. The inflammatory modulating action of local anesthetics may result from interruptions in these pathways. The antiinflammatory response to local anesthetics also occurs resulting from suppression of polymorphonuclear leukocyte priming, which prevents overactive inflammatory responses without impairing host defenses or suppressing normal inflammation.[16,19]

It must be noted that many questions remain as to the mechanism of the clinical effects of local anesthetics in different types of nerve

TABLE 10.1 Nerve Fiber Characteristics and Sensitivity to Local Anesthetics

Fiber Type	Function	Diameter (µm)	Myelination	Anesthetic Block Onset
Type A				
Alpha (Aα)	Proprioception, motor	6–22	Heavy	Last
Beta (Aβ)	Touch, pressure	6–22	Heavy	Intermediate
Gamma (Aγ)	Muscle tone	3–6	Heavy	Intermediate
Delta (Aδ)	Pain, cold temperature, touch	1–5	Heavy	Intermediate
Type B	Preganglionic autonomic vasomotor	<3	Light	Early
Type C				
Sympathetic	Postganglionic vasomotor	0.3–1.3	None	Early
Dorsal root	Pain, warm and cold temperature, touch	0.4–1.2	None	Early

blocks. Different receptors may be involved in their action in peripheral nerves as opposed to spinal or epidural effects.[20]

Nerve Fiber Sensitivity and Differential Block

It has been observed that nerve functionally has different sensitivity or rates of effect when exposed to local anesthetics. For example, in most major nerve blocks loss of autonomic function occurs first, followed in sequence by perception of superficial pain, touch, and temperature, motor function, and proprioception.[21] This phenomenon is called differential blockade. A clinical example of differential blockade occurs with the use of bupivacaine. When administered by epidural for labor pain, this local anesthetic spares motor function while providing analgesia.[22,23]

Essential to the understanding of differential block is the concept that the diameter and myelination of nerve fibers influence the sensitivity to local anesthetics. For simplicity, nerve fibers are separated into three groups—A, B, and C—on the basis of diameter.[24,25]

The A fibers are further divided into four subgroups known as alpha, beta, gamma, and delta fibers. The alpha fibers are the largest in diameter (12–20 µm) and the most heavily myelinated; they have the fastest conduction velocity of all the fibers, including B and C fibers. Alpha fibers are responsible for motor functions and proprioception. The A beta (5–12 µm) and A gamma fibers (3–6 µm) have conduction velocities second only to A alpha fibers. The A beta fibers provide motor function, touch, and pressure sensation; the A gamma fibers innervate muscle spindles and are responsible for reflexes. The A delta fibers provide pain and temperature sensation. These fibers have a smaller diameter (1–5 µm) and slower conduction velocity than other A fibers. The beta, gamma, and delta fibers are all myelinated to a similar extent.[26]

B fibers have a similar diameter (<3 µm) to A delta fibers; however, they exhibit slower conduction velocity and less myelination than the A fibers. These fibers constitute the preganglionic autonomic nerves. The C fibers, which conduct pain and temperature impulses, are the smallest of all fibers (0.3–1.3 µm) and have the slowest speed of conduction. These are the only fibers that are unmyelinated.[8] Nerve fiber characteristics and local anesthetic sensitivity are summarized in Table 10.1.

It was first believed that nerve fiber diameter was the sole determinant of differential blockade.[27] This assumption came from the results of isolated in vitro studies performed only on myelinated nerves. Subsequent isolated studies on the small, unmyelinated C fibers revealed that they were more resistant to blockade than the larger A delta or B fibers.[8]

This apparent inconsistency can possibly be explained by the concept of conduction safety. This concept refers to the voltage change needed for the propagation of the action potential along the nerve.

This voltage change is significantly greater than the action potential threshold and provides a safety factor for impulse conduction. Gissen et al.[28] defined this safety factor as the "ratio between the magnitude of the action potential and the magnitude of the critical membrane potential." Research has indicated that the margin of safety for transmission is greater in small, slow fibers than in large, fast fibers.

Lastly, differential block may be influenced by the rate of diffusion of local anesthetic molecules across multilayered lipoprotein membranes of the myelin sheath. For example, clinically the resistance to blockade observed in A fibers may be the result of a slower onset resulting from a greater diffusion barrier. As discussed in more detail later, diffusion can be influenced by such factors as the pK_a and the concentration of the local anesthetic, in addition to the pH of the surrounding tissue and nerve fiber.[28]

As the preceding discussion indicates, the concept of differential block is more complex than originally proposed. Recent theories for differential blockade include length of the nerve fiber (in epidural space), frequency of firing (motor fibers fire slower, they need higher concentration of drug), and use of dependent blockade. Currently, a combination of factors is deemed responsible for the differential blockade, including voltage-dependent sodium channel isoforms, use of dependent blockade, and the particular local anesthetic used.[27]

CHEMICAL STRUCTURE OF LOCAL ANESTHETICS

The local anesthetics used clinically for neural blockade are aminoesters or aminoamides and are similar in chemical structure. In general, these drugs have three characteristic segments: (1) an intermediate ester or amide carbon group separates (2) an unsaturated (aromatic) ring system from (3) an amine end (Fig. 10.7). The aromatic ring provides lipophilic characteristics, whereas the tertiary/quaternary amine gives hydrophilicity to the molecule. The amine portion is able to become ionized in physiologic pH and thus is hydrophilic.

Chemically, the major difference among local anesthetics is in their ester or an amide linkage that binds the aromatic ring to the amine group. This linkage is responsible for the classification of these drugs as either esters or amides. The type of linkage is important clinically because it has implications for metabolism, duration, and allergic potential (Fig. 10.8). Box 10.1 lists the local anesthetics according to chemical class. A method for remembering to which chemical class a local anesthetic drug is assigned is esters have one letter *i* in their generic name and the amides have two. The chemical structures are important in determining the pharmacologic effects of these drugs. Minor chemical alterations to drugs within these two bond-related groups can result in

significant changes in drug potency, speed of onset, duration of action, and potential for producing differential block (Fig. 10.9).[5,16,29] These changes are discussed in detail as the specific pharmacologic factors associated with local anesthetics are noted. Table 10.2 summarizes the clinical differences between the ester and amide local anesthetics.

PHARMACODYNAMICS AND PHARMACOKINETIC CONCEPTS

An important difference to note when describing the pharmacokinetics of local anesthetics is intuitive yet bears discussion. Unlike most medications, these agents are intended to remain localized in the area of injection or application. The higher the concentration (number of molecules) of drug injected that remains in the area of the nerve(s) to

be blocked, the faster the onset of action. If multiple nerves are being blocked, a greater intensity may also be evident. Therefore systemic absorption away from the deposition site results in the offset and termination of drug effect rather than the onset as with most other drugs. Factors that affect absorption, such as the vascularity and blood flow of the injection area, lipid and protein binding, and addition of

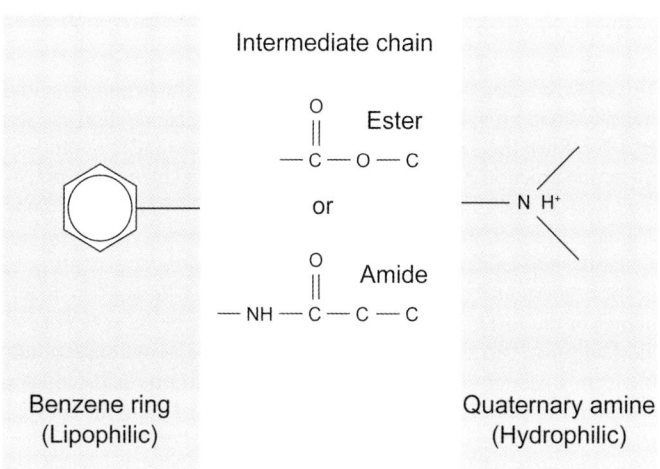

Fig. 10.7 Core structure for local anesthetics, which includes a benzene ring and a quaternary amine separated by an intermediate carbon group. The bond between the benzene ring and the carbon group determines whether the drug is an amide or an ester.

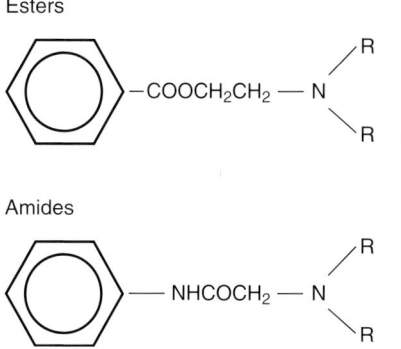

Fig. 10.8 Representative chemical formula for ester and amide local anesthetic drugs.

BOX 10.1	**Ester and Amide Local Anesthetics**
Esters	**Amides**
Procaine	Lidocaine
Chloroprocaine	Mepivacaine
Tetracaine	Prilocaine
Cocaine	Bupivacaine
Benzocaine	Ropivacaine
	Articaine

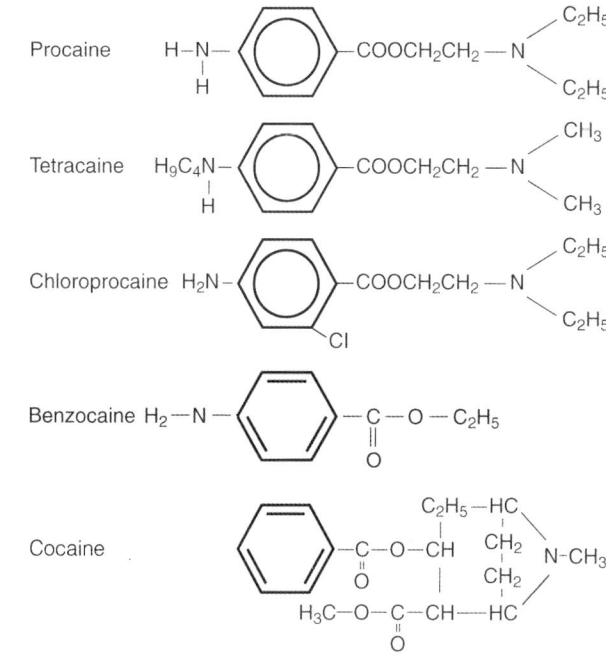

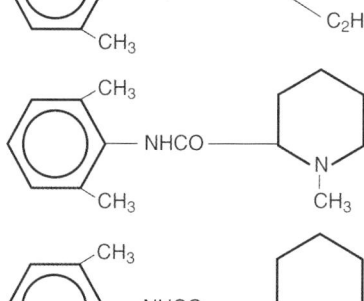

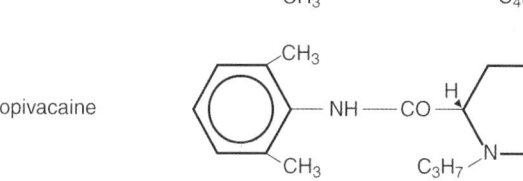

Fig. 10.9 Chemical structure of the most commonly used local anesthetics. Note the chemical substitutions on the benzene ring and the amine end of the molecules.

vasoconstrictors, greatly influence duration of action. The same local anesthetic dose and concentration injected in different areas of the body, with or without added epinephrine, can result in a vastly different duration of action. Absorption also influences toxicity. The slower a local anesthetic is systemically absorbed, the less likely that high blood levels and therefore central nervous system (CNS) or cardiac toxicity will result. Drug metabolism and elimination more readily keep up with absorption, ensuring that toxic blood levels are avoided. A conceptual kinetic depiction of the fate of an injected local anesthetic is shown in Fig. 10.10.

Potency

There is a strong relationship between the lipid solubility of local anesthetics and their potency.[28,29] This finding is understandable considering that the axolemma and myelin sheath are composed primarily of lipids[29,30]; therefore lipid-soluble drugs pass more readily through the nerve membrane. More potent, more lipid-soluble local anesthetics are relatively water insoluble, highly protein bound, and less readily washed out from nerves and surrounding tissues. They bind to Na_v channels with a higher affinity than agents with lower lipid solubility. Increased lipid solubility correlates with increased protein binding, increased potency, longer duration of action, and a higher tendency for severe cardiac toxicity.[12,29] It follows that fewer molecules or lower concentrations of these drugs are required for the production of blockade than if nonlipid-soluble anesthetics are used.[31] Changes in either the aromatic or amine moieties of the local anesthetic molecule can affect the lipid-water partition coefficient. In the amide series, for example, the addition of a butyl group to the amine end of mepivacaine leads to the formation of bupivacaine. Bupivacaine is 26-fold as lipid soluble and 4-fold as potent as mepivacaine. In the case of the esters, the addition of a butyl group to the aromatic end of procaine produces tetracaine, which is considerably more lipid soluble and potent than procaine.[16]

Factors other than lipid solubility can affect potency. For example, the potency of local anesthetics as demonstrated in isolated in vitro studies is not always the same as that observed in vivo. The discrepancy between in vitro and in vivo findings may be the result of many factors, including the vascular and tissue distribution properties of the drug.[32–35]

Duration of Action

The duration of action of local anesthetics demonstrates a relationship to protein binding and lipid solubility.[29,36] In theory, drugs that have a high affinity for protein and lipids attach more firmly to these

substances in the vicinity of the Na_v channel receptor. This means that the drug remains in the channel and surrounding areas for a longer time producing prolonged conduction blockade.[29]

It appears that there is a correlation between the degree of protein binding and duration of the local anesthetic. The addition of larger chemical radicals to the amide or aromatic end of the drugs results in greater protein binding. The duration is directly proportional to plasma protein binding, presumably because the local anesthetic receptor on the neural membrane is also composed of protein.[35,37] It has been theorized that local anesthetics that have increased protein-binding properties (e.g., ropivacaine 94%, bupivacaine 97%) produce a longer duration of anesthesia as a consequence of more efficient binding of the anesthetic to the Na_v channel.[38] For example, bupivacaine is more than 90% bound to plasma protein; however, its homologue, mepivacaine, is only 65% bound.[36] The duration of action of bupivacaine is significantly longer than for mepivacaine. Local anesthetics are weak bases and bind mainly to α_1-acid glycoprotein (AAG). Secondary binding to albumin also occurs.

As in the case of potency, the effect local anesthetics have on the vasculature at the injection site influences the duration of action. This is discussed in detail in the section on vasomotor action and absorption.

Onset of Action

As noted previously, local anesthetics must diffuse through the axolemma before they can interact with receptors. How readily they diffuse through the nerve membrane depends on their chemical structure, lipid solubility, and state of ionization. Of these, ionization is the

TABLE 10.2 **Clinical Differences Between the Ester and Amide Type Local Anesthetics**	
Esters	**Amides**
Ester metabolism is catalyzed by plasma and tissue cholinesterase via hydrolysis; occurs throughout the body and is rapid.	Amides are metabolized in the liver by CYP1A2 and CYP3A4 and thus a significant blood level may develop with rapid absorption.
Although local anesthetic allergy is uncommon, esters have a higher allergy potential, and if patients exhibit an allergy to any ester drug, all other esters should be avoided.	Allergy to amides or between the ester and amide agents is extremely rare.
Ester drugs tend to be shorter acting due to ready metabolism; tetracaine is the longest-acting ester.	Amides are longer acting because they are more lipophilic and protein bound and require transport to the liver for metabolism.

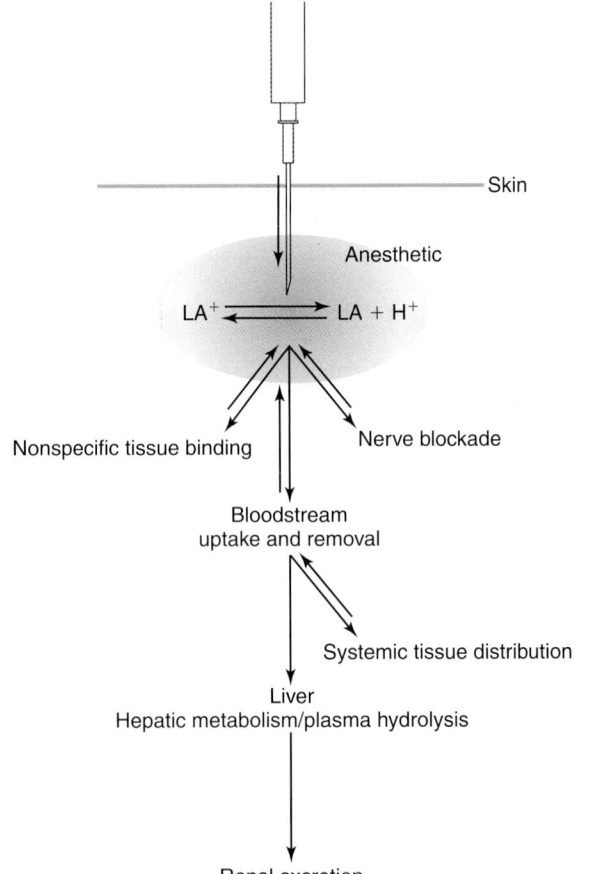

Fig. 10.10 Representation of the fate of a local anesthetic injected into tissue.

most important because the charged or ionized form of a drug does not penetrate membranes effectively.[30,32,37] Thus the more ionized a local anesthetic, the slower it will penetrate a nerve.

Local anesthetics are weak bases. The pK_a of a drug is the pH at which 50% of the drug is in the charged (or ionized) and water-soluble form, whereas the remaining half is uncharged (or nonionized) and lipid soluble. A basic drug becomes predominantly ionized if it is placed in an environment with a pH that is significantly less than its pK_a. Therefore drugs that have a higher pK_a (relative to pH 7.4) are ionized to a greater extent at body pH than those with a lower pK_a. For example, if lidocaine (pK_a 7.74) is placed in plasma (pH 7.4), 65% of the drug is ionized, and 35% remains nonionized. Similarly, if tetracaine (pK_a 8.6) is placed in plasma, 95% of the drug becomes ionized, and 5% remains nonionized.[29]

Because their ionization is less, local anesthetics with lower pK_a (7.6–7.8), such as lidocaine, mepivacaine, and prilocaine, tend to have a more rapid onset of action than drugs with a greater pK_a (8.1–8.6), such as bupivacaine, tetracaine, and procaine. Chloroprocaine is one exception; it has a high pK_a but retains a rapid onset, probably because of the clinical use of high concentrations of the drug, which attenuates the ionization effect. In general, the closer the pK_a is to pH 7.4, the more rapid the onset. Some researchers downplay the role of pK_a on onset. They note that onset is slower the more lipid soluble the drug.[30]

The classification presented in Table 10.3 assists in the selection of an appropriate drug with respect to pharmacokinetic properties.[39]

Vasomotor Action and Absorption

All local anesthetics except cocaine and in some doses and sites of administration ropivacaine and lidocaine produce relaxation of vascular smooth muscle.[33,40] The resultant vasodilation increases blood flow to the tissue in which the drug is deposited. This results in an increase in the drug's absorption, which limits its duration of action and increases the probability of toxic effects. It is interesting to note that ropivacaine and lidocaine are the only parenterally administered local anesthetics with mild vasoconstrictive properties.[40] Cocaine also has vasoconstrictive properties because of its ability to block reuptake of norepinephrine. It is only administered topically.

All local anesthetics are not affected equally when epinephrine is added to the solution. There is a definite benefit in extending the duration of analgesic effects with both short- and intermediate-acting agents. The prolongation of the duration with long-acting drugs is less well defined.[40]

The speed of absorption and entry of the local anesthetic into the systemic circulation obviously has significant implications for toxicity. Absorption of drugs generally occurs in the following order of rapidity: interpleural blocks greater than intercostal greater than caudal greater than epidural greater than brachial plexus greater than sciatic-femoral

and subcutaneous blocks.[16] In general, the more vascular the injected site, the more drug will be absorbed, the higher the blood level that will result, and the greater the possibility for systemic toxicity.

The total dose of local anesthetic, rather than the volume or concentration, linearly determines the peak plasma concentration.[41] For example, 400 mg of lidocaine yields the same peak plasma concentration regardless of whether 40 mL of a 1% or 80 mL of a 0.5% is injected.

Local anesthetic additives include many adjuvants, including the α_2-adrenergic agonists clonidine and dexmedetomidine, opioids, sodium bicarbonate, ketorolac, dexamethasone, and hyaluronidase. These are variously added to increase the safety, quality, intensity, duration, and rate of onset of anesthesia. α_2-adrenergic agonists such as clonidine and dexmedetomidine have local anesthetic properties and can alter the nerve block characteristics.[41–43] The addition of 100 μg of clonidine to a local anesthetic solution prolongs the duration of the long-acting agents approximately 100 additional minutes with minimal side effects. The effect is produced by inhibition of the hyperpolarization-activated cation current (I_h current). This current normally restores nerves from the hyperpolarized state to resting potential. The effect is more pronounced in C fibers (sensory) than A delta (motor). That makes the effects mostly sensory specific. Cost has limited the routine use of clonidine. The use of dexmedetomidine for peripheral nerve blockade is currently being investigated and is not approved for use in the United States.[40]

The addition of a vasoconstrictor (e.g., epinephrine) to local anesthetics can reduce the rate of vascular absorption allowing more of the drug to stay in the local area where it was injected. The availability of the drug for neuronal uptake is increased resulting in a longer and more profound block. Of importance, the slower rate of absorption also attenuates the peak plasma concentration of the drug, thereby reducing systemic toxicity. The magnitude of this effect depends on the drug, dose, and concentration of both the local anesthetic and the vasoconstrictor, in addition to the site of injection.[7] For example, addition of epinephrine to mepivacaine prolongs the time to maximum arterial plasma drug concentration in all situations; however, adding epinephrine to a 2% solution used for an intercostal block has the greatest effect.[44]

Epinephrine does not prolong the duration of blockade to the same extent with all local anesthetics. For example, it prolongs the duration for local infiltration, peripheral nerve block (PNB), and epidural anesthesia with procaine, mepivacaine, and lidocaine.[30,45–48] Research indicates that adding epinephrine to lidocaine solutions increases the intensity and duration of block.[48] The early increase in intensity is not matched with an increase in intraneural lidocaine content at these early times, although the prolonged duration of block by epinephrine appears to correspond to an enlarged lidocaine content in a nerve at later times, as if a very slowly emptying "effector compartment"

TABLE 10.3 Classification of Local Anesthetics Based on Onset, Duration of Action, and Potency

Characteristics	Drug (Generic Name)	Common Brand Name	Onset	Duration of Action (min)
Low potency, short duration of action	procaine	Novocainc	Slow	60–90
	chloroprocaine	Nesacaine	Fast	30–60
Intermediate potency, duration	mepivacaine	Carbocaine	Fast	120–240
	lidocaine	Xylocaine	Fast	90–120
High potency, long duration	tetracaine	Pontocaine	Slow	180–600
	bupivacaine	Marcaine, Sensorcaine	Slow	180–600
	ropivacaine	Naropin	Slow	180–600

received a larger share of the dose. The increase in early analgesia without increased lidocaine content may be explained by a pharmacodynamic action of epinephrine that transiently enhances potency of lidocaine, but also by a pharmacokinetic effect that alters the distribution of the same net content of lidocaine within the nerve. In the case of prilocaine and bupivacaine, infiltration and PNBs are prolonged with epinephrine, whereas no significant effect occurs with epidural anesthesia.[49] The rationale for this discrepancy might be that epidural fat significantly absorbs ropivacaine and bupivacaine because of their high lipid solubility. These drugs are released slowly from the fat deposit, which could prolong the block.[47,49-51] This process overrides the effects of epinephrine on duration of action. In addition, the drug concentration can contribute to the differential effect seen with epinephrine. For example, epinephrine can prolong epidural blocks with 0.125% or 0.25% bupivacaine when used in patients in labor.[50,51] Conversely, epinephrine has less effect with the epidural administration of 0.5% or 0.75% bupivacaine.[52,53]

The addition of epinephrine does not attenuate the peak plasma level of all local anesthetics; for example, epinephrine significantly reduces the peak plasma concentration of lidocaine and mepivacaine regardless of the site of administration. On the other hand, epinephrine does not significantly affect the peak plasma level of prilocaine or bupivacaine after epidural anesthesia. The lack of effect seen with prilocaine may be explained by its slower absorption and rapid tissue redistribution. In the case of bupivacaine, it may be explained by the significant lipid solubility and uptake in the epidural adipose tissue.[28] There is some controversy as to whether epinephrine may produce neurotoxicity when added to local anesthetics. Some clinicians recommend its use only for nerve blocks done without ultrasound guidance or where the needle tip and local anesthetic spread are not adequately visualized as a safety measure to detect intravascular injection.[40,41]

Studies that have compared vasoconstrictors conclude that epinephrine is superior to drugs such as phenylephrine and norepinephrine in producing vasoconstriction with local anesthetics.[54,55] The usual concentration of epinephrine used for this purpose is 1:200,000 or 5 µg/mL.

Miscellaneous Factors That Influence Onset and Duration

Local anesthetics are basic drugs. As discussed previously, they have both water- and lipid-soluble properties. Factors that raise the pH of their environment increase their lipid solubility, and, conversely, lower pH environments result in increased water solubility. These changes to pH result in altered proportions of lipid- and water-soluble fractions of the drugs, which may have clinical consequences. At times the term used for this phenomenon is *ion trapping*. Ion trapping results from changes in pH in relationship to the pK$_a$ of the agent. Instances in which ion trapping may have clinical consequences are noted in Box 10.2.

Local anesthetics have been carbonated to speed onset. In isolated nerve preparations, carbonation gives a more rapid onset and greater intensity of block.[56] Diffusion of carbon dioxide through the nerve membrane can lower the intracellular pH. When local anesthetics accompany this process, they become more ionized within the neuron; this results in an increase in the concentration of the drug in the ionized form at the intracellular binding site.

Controversy exists concerning whether carbonation improves onset time in the in vivo situation.[57] Separate double-blind studies of lidocaine and bupivacaine have failed to yield positive results.[58] This inconsistency may exist because the injected carbon dioxide is rapidly buffered in vivo, so intracellular pH is not greatly affected.[57,58] This practice has been largely abandoned in modern clinical practice.

The addition of sodium bicarbonate to local anesthetics is widely used in epidural anesthesia to speed onset of sensory and motor block.[59-61] The effects of the addition of sodium bicarbonate to peripheral blocks is unclear.[40] In theory the mechanism is that addition of bicarbonate increases the pH of the local anesthetic solution resulting in the presence of more drug in the nonionized state. As stated previously this form of the drug readily diffuses across the cell membranes and would therefore speed onset. Studies done with bupivacaine and lidocaine have indicated that this alteration does facilitate the onset and prolong duration of action.[59,60] Other researchers, however, have noted variable effects on onset and duration depending on whether epinephrine was contained in the solution.[61]

The major limitation to the addition of bicarbonate is the precipitation that can occur in the local anesthetic solution. It also should be noted that the amount of bicarbonate that can be added without precipitation depends on whether the epinephrine is commercially or "freshly" mixed.[59] Manufacturers acidify local anesthetic solutions to increase solubility and stability (the free base is more susceptible to photodegradation and aldehyde formation), which results in a longer shelf life. For example, the pH range of plain lidocaine is 6.5 to 6.8, compared with 3.5 to 4.5 for preparations that contain epinephrine. The lower pH is used with epinephrine because of the instability of this compound in alkaline solutions.

BOX 10.2 Ion Trapping: Clinical Situations in Which Differences Between pK$_a$ and pH May Affect Patient Response

- In the event of local anesthetic overdose, associated respiratory depression may occur resulting in hypoxia and acidosis. The acidosis resulting from hypoxia may increase the ionized fraction of local anesthetic within the cerebral circulation, thereby decreasing the ability of the anesthetic to cross the blood-brain barrier, leave the brain, and reenter the systemic circulation. This phenomenon may prolong and enhance the central nervous system toxicity of local anesthetics.
- Local anesthetic accumulation in the fetal circulation is enhanced by the fact that fetal pH is lower than maternal pH, which may result in high fetal levels of local anesthetics.
- Local anesthetics injected into acidotic, infected tissues are rendered ineffective because of the loss of lipid solubility. The lipid solubility of local anesthetics is diminished in an acidotic environment because of an increased concentration of the ionized, water-soluble form of the drug. The loss of lipid solubility prevents absorption into the nerve, thereby preventing access to the site of action.
- Carbonation of local anesthetics speeds the onset and intensity of action of neural blockade. Carbon dioxide readily diffuses into the nerve, lowering the pH within the nerve. The lipid-soluble form of local anesthetic, after passing through the neuronal membrane, receives protons from the intraneuronal environment and ionizes. An increase in the ionized fraction within the neuron produces a higher concentration of the active form of the anesthetic available at the sodium channel, the site of action. This practice has been largely abandoned in modern clinical practice.
- Commercially available local anesthetics are prepared in a slightly acidic formulation that improves the stability of the drug by increasing the concentration of the ionized, water-soluble form of the drug. Addition of sodium bicarbonate to the local anesthetic mixture increases the pH of the solution, thereby increasing the concentration of the nonionized, lipid-soluble form of the drug. Improving the lipid solubility of the local anesthetic improves diffusion of the local anesthetic through the neuronal membrane, leading to a more rapid onset of action. This seems to be most effective in epidural blocks and least effective in peripheral blocks.

Another benefit of alkalization is that it may result in less pain or stinging on injection. The mechanism of action for this effect could be more complex than just an increase in pH. It may be that the nociceptive nerve fibers may not be as sensitive to the nonionized form of the drug. It also is possible that the nonionized drug diffuses so rapidly through the tissue and axolemma that a sensory block occurs almost instantaneously.[62,63]

The addition of hyaluronidase to local anesthetics as a spreading factor facilitates the diffusion of the drugs in tissues. This additive accomplishes this effect via the hydrolysis of hyaluronic acid, which is a glycosaminoglycan found extensively in the interstitial matrix and basement membranes of tissue. Hyaluronic acid is the main component of interstitial gel, which inhibits the spread of substances through tissue.[64] It is has long been used in ophthalmic blocks to improve quality, speed onset, limit the acute increase in intraocular pressure with periocular injections, and reduce the incidence of postoperative strabismus.[65] It has also been suggested that hyaluronidase reduces hematoma size if a needle that is used with the regional technique punctures a major blood vessel. Other common uses are to facilitate the spread of fluids during hypodermoclysis and radiopaque agents in subcutaneous urography.[64] The addition of hyaluronidase can result in undesirable effects, such as the initiation of allergic reactions, a shortening of the duration of anesthetic action, and an increase in drug toxicity.[66-68] A new human recombinant product, Hylenex, is now available that may improve the safety profile.[69] Currently available hyaluronidase products are listed in Table 10.4. Off-label use for cosmetic applications to reduce edema, epidural adhesions, and chronic lower back pain have led to an increased interest in this agent.[64]

Most current local anesthetics possess either a fast onset but intermediate duration or a slow onset and long duration. Clinicians frequently mix local anesthetics to obtain a more rapid onset and a long duration of action. The use of intermediate-acting mepivacaine combined with long-acting bupivacaine for an ultrasound-guided interscalene block has been reported.[70] Onset was not improved compared to bupivacaine alone, but duration was longer than mepivacaine alone. The duration was shorter than bupivacaine alone. In general, studies indicate a faster onset can be achieved but duration of the block may be decreased.[71,72] Some clinicians have suggested that the use of combinations reduces the risk of toxicity; however, drug errors may increase when using more complex dosing schemes. In addition, the toxicity of local anesthetic combinations appears to be additive.[73-75] The authors suggest that the increased use of ultrasound-guided techniques allows for the use of lower doses and more precise deposition of drug, which may diminish the use of combined local anesthetics.[70]

Distribution

The absorption or injection of local anesthetics into the systemic circulation results in rapid distribution throughout the body. Distribution results in a rapid decrease in the plasma concentration as the drug moves into highly perfused tissue. Rapid distribution into the brain and heart can be a concern because this can lead to systemic toxicity. A secondary, slower disappearance follows, which reflects a combination of distribution into tissues with a more limited blood supply, drug metabolism, and excretion.

Although local anesthetics are distributed throughout the body, their concentration varies in different tissues. Immediately after vascular uptake, more greatly perfused tissues, such as the brain, heart, and lungs, receive more of these drugs than do less perfused tissues. Once equilibration occurs, the local anesthetic leaves the highly perfused tissue and is deposited in tissue with less perfusion. As with many drugs, as they redistribute in the body over time, muscle tissue receives the greatest amount of local anesthetic from redistribution.[64]

The distribution process varies significantly with different local anesthetics. For example, the disappearance rate of prilocaine is more rapid than that of mepivacaine or lidocaine. Ropivacaine also has a shorter half-life than bupivacaine. Distribution of the ester local anesthetics is similar to the amides; however, their rate of metabolism in plasma is very rapid, resulting in much lower and shorter duration systemic plasma concentrations.[16]

Metabolism

The metabolism of local anesthetics differs according to their chemical structure as either amides or esters. Plasma cholinesterase catalyzes the hydrolysis of ester local anesthetics. The hydrolysis occurs through the action of cholinesterase in plasma, red blood cells (RBCs), and the liver.[76-78] The plasma half-lives of procaine and chloroprocaine are shorter than 1 minute. The rapid rate of clearance of these drugs significantly reduces the potential of toxicity. Conversely, hydrolysis of tetracaine is slower and it has limited clinical use (Table 10.5). Saturated, inhibited, or genetically atypical plasma cholinesterase can significantly prolong the plasma half-life of ester local anesthetics.[76,79] This would have little effect on duration of the ester agent because absorption away from the site of injection would occur as usual; however, this effect could theoretically increase the potential for systemic toxicity. For example, atypical plasma cholinesterase has been shown to significantly reduce the rate of procaine metabolism.[80]

Metabolism of the amide local anesthetics occurs primarily in the liver predominantly by microsomal cytochrome P-450 enzymes CYP1A2 and CYP3A4.[81] Table 10.6 presents pharmacokinetic data for the amide local anesthetics.[16]

TABLE 10.4 Available Formulations of Hyaluronidase

Drug	Source	Dosing
Vitrase	Lyophilized, Bovine	A wide range of doses are used depending on the type of regional block and the goals; the dose can vary from 0.75–300 units/mL.
Amphadase	Bovine	
Hydase	Bovine	
Hylenex	Human (recombinant)	

Data from Dunn AL, et al. Hyaluronidase: a review of approved formulations, indications, and off-label use in chronic pain management. *Expert Opin Biol Ther.* 2010;10:127–131; Adams L. Adjuvants to local anaesthesia in ophthalmic surgery. *Br J Ophthalmol.* 2011;95:1345–1349.

TABLE 10.5 Clearance Half-Life of Local Anesthetics

Drug	Clearance (L/min)	Half-Life (min)
Chloroprocaine	N/A	6
Procaine	N/A	6
Tetracaine	N/A	20
Cocaine	N/A	42
Prilocaine	2.84	90
Lidocaine	0.95	90
Mepivacaine	0.78	114
Bupivacaine	0.47	210
Ropivacaine	7.2	114

N/A, Not applicable. The ester compounds are rapidly broken down in the plasma and tissue, so clearance is not a factor.
Adapted from Malamed SF, ed. *Handbook of Local Anesthesia.* 7th ed. St. Louis: Elsevier; 2020:29.

Hepatic clearance is a function of the hepatic extraction ratio and hepatic blood flow and is the primary factor that determines the rate of elimination of amide local anesthetics. The hepatic extraction ratio is dependent on the ratio of free to protein-bound drug and represents the activity level specific to the liver for removing a drug from plasma. This ratio indicates the percentage of drug removed with each pass through the liver. The clearance of drugs that have higher hepatic extraction ratios depends on adequate hepatic blood flow. Hepatic enzyme activity is important when drugs with lower ratios such as bupivacaine are used.[82] Pathologic conditions that influence hepatic function may prolong the elimination half-life of these drugs by a reduction in hepatic blood flow, enzyme activity, or both. For example, lidocaine has a plasma half-life of 1.6 hours; however, in severe hepatic disease, its half-life is 4.9 hours. This probably results from both an enzymatic and a perfusion effect. Flow-limited clearance is affected by upper abdominal and laparoscopic surgery, inhalation anesthetics, hypovolemia, and congestive heart failure. Heart failure significantly reduces the rate of elimination of lidocaine because of a concomitant reduction in hepatic blood flow.[83] Clinically, hepatic dysfunction does not necessitate a reduction of dose for a single injection nerve block. Doses of amides used in continuous infusions or repeat blocks should be reduced 10% to 50%.[84]

Only 1% to 5% of the injected dose of local anesthetic is accounted for by unchanged renal and hepatic excretion. However, the inactive, more water-soluble metabolites of local anesthetics appear in the urine. Although renal dysfunction affects the clearance far less than hepatic failure, it can result in the accumulation of potentially toxic metabolites.[85] It may also affect protein binding to both AAG and albumin. Some authors have suggested a 10% to 20% reduction in patients with severe renal disease.[86]

Pregnancy

The use of local anesthetics in pregnancy deserves some special pharmacokinetic and pharmacodynamic consideration. Both clinical observations and studies indicate that the spread and depth of spinal and epidural anesthesia are increased in pregnant women. Spread of neuraxial anesthesia increases during pregnancy as a result of decreases in thoracolumbar cerebral spinal fluid (CSF) volume and increased neural susceptibility to local anesthetic. At first this was thought to be the result of only mechanical factors produced by a gravid uterus. For example, mechanical factors result in dilation of epidural veins, which leads to narrowing of the epidural and subarachnoid space, thereby reducing the dose requirement.[87] However, hormonal changes appear to also play a role because there is a greater segmental spread of local anesthetics administered in the epidural space during the first trimester of pregnancy when little compression is evident.[88] A relationship appears to exist between the progesterone level in CSF and an increased segmental spread and sensitivity of nerves to these drugs. Studies performed on isolated nerves taken from pregnant animals demonstrate more sensitivity to local anesthetic block than in nonpregnant animals.[89,90]

Local Anesthetics and Tumor Recurrence

It has been suggested, after several retrospective and prospective studies, that regional or local anesthesia may improve patient survival and the disease-free interval after cancer surgery. The potential mechanisms of the antimetastatic effects include both direct and indirect effects of local anesthetics. Direct effects include interference with tumor-promoting pathways and direct toxic effects on tumors when used for local infiltration. Indirect effects result from a reduction of the perioperative stress response and the preservation of the immune response. Surgical resection of primary tumors remains a cornerstone of cancer treatment; however, the surgical process can trigger an immune-suppressing sympathetic response, which promotes tumor growth of any residual cancerous cells postsurgery. It is believed that by blocking afferent pain signals, the body does not mount as large of a sympathetic response that contributes to the perpetuation of disease after surgical treatment.[91–93]

LOCAL ANESTHETIC SYSTEMIC TOXICITY

Local anesthetic systemic toxicity (LAST) is a serious but rare consequence of regional anesthesia. It most commonly results from an inadvertent vascular injection or absorption of large amounts of drug from certain nerve blocks requiring large-volume injections. It can also result from continuous infusion and accumulation of drug and metabolites over many days. Lastly, inadvertent injection into the venous system causes local anesthetic plasma concentrations to peak rapidly. The subsequent high systemic blood levels lead to LAST.

When inadvertent systemic delivery or rapid absorption of large quantities of local anesthetic occurs, the voltage-gated sodium, potassium, and calcium channels in excitable tissues of the central nervous and cardiac systems are depressed. Normal functioning of the CNS involves both excitatory and inhibitory neurons. As LAST progresses, the inhibitory neurons are blocked first. This lack of inhibition on the excitatory neuron is thought to be the mechanism of the observed seizure. The functioning of the heart depends on mechanisms similar to a neuron. Blockade of the cardiac ion channels will affect initiation and propagation of the contraction, and repolarization. A toxic level of local anesthetic results in decreased contractility and several arrhythmias, most commonly bradycardia. The toxicity may manifest initially as hypertension and tachydysrhythmias that progress to depressed cardiac conduction and performance, reduced cardiac output, bradycardia, and hypotension.

With respect to the extent of compromise, the type of local anesthetic plays a role. Shorter-acting lidocaine is less cardiotoxic than the longer-acting and more potent bupivacaine. The greatest number of reported deaths related to LAST involve bupivacaine. The difference between short-acting and longer-acting agents may be related to their physical properties. The more potent agents are more lipid soluble and protein bound. As such, the duration of blockade of any voltage-gated

TABLE 10.6 Pharmacokinetics of Amide Local Anesthetics

Drug	Half-Life Alpha (min)	Half-Life Beta (min)	V_{dss} (L)	Clearance (L)
Prilocaine	0.5	90	261	2.84
Lidocaine	1	90	91	0.95
Mepivacaine	0.7	114	84	0.75
Bupivacaine	2.7	210	72	0.47
Ropivacaine	2.7	114	66.9	0.73

V_{dss}, Volume of distribution at steady state.

channel is probably longer and thus the recovery is delayed. The newer agents ropivacaine and levobupivacaine were developed to address this issue of cardiotoxicity. These agents are accepted as safer; however, care should be taken when using large doses of any local anesthetic.[94]

Widespread attention to this adverse effect is attributed to Albright, who wrote an editorial in 1979 outlining the risks of bupivacaine use in intravenous regional blocks.[95] Subsequently, cases of cardiac toxicity from local anesthetics were reported to the Food and Drug Administration (FDA).[96] Worldwide concern followed with a renewed research and clinical interest and safety recommendations.[84] The American Society of Regional Anesthesia and Pain Medicine (ASRA) Panel on Local Anesthetic Systemic Toxicity has reevaluated the available research and clinical data from 1979 to 2009 and issued recommendations regarding prevention, diagnosis, and treatment of this complication. A review of local anesthetic systemic toxicity cases since publication of the ASRA recommendations was reported in 2015.[97] Many traditional concepts were reevaluated in light of new data, and practice advisories were formulated.

The Third ASRA Practice Advisory on Local Anesthetic Systemic Toxicity published in 2018 noted several new findings.[98] There is an enhanced understanding of the mechanisms that lead to lipid emulsion reversal of LAST, including rapid partitioning, direct inotropy, and postconditioning. Data have emerged that suggest a lower frequency of LAST as reported by single institutions and some registries; nevertheless, a considerable number of events still occur within the general community. Contemporary case reports suggest a trend toward delayed presentation, which may be caused by the increased use of ultrasound guidance (fewer intravascular injections), local infiltration techniques (slower systemic uptake), and continuous local anesthetic infusions. Small patient size and sarcopenia are additional factors that increase potential risk for LAST. An increasing number of reported events occur outside of the traditional hospital setting and involve nonanesthesia providers such as in circumcision procedures.[98]

Incidence and Clinical Presentation

Standard randomized controlled trials of LAST are obviously not ethical, therefore our knowledge is primarily derived from epidemiologic studies, case reports, and animal research. Data from animal and laboratory studies can vary widely depending on the model used, so comparisons and extrapolation to clinical situations can be difficult.

There has been a significant reduction in the incidence of LAST since the 1980s.[99] The estimate of clinically important LAST is approximately 0.03% or 0.27 occurrences per 1000 PNBs and approximately 4 per 10,000 epidurals.[84] This is a dramatic drop, for example, from the previously reported toxicity of 100 per 10,000 epidurals.[100] PNBs traditionally have a higher incidence of LAST because of the large volumes of local anesthetic drugs administered compared to epidurals. A 2016 evaluation of 80,661 PNBs was reported.[101,102] This represents the largest cohort of these regional blocks ever analyzed. There were no cases of cardiac arrest and three cases of seizures caused by LAST. The incident rate of 0.4 per 10,000 demonstrated a pattern of continually improving patient safety for regional anesthesia. This safety improvement is attributed to the widespread adoption of enhanced safety measures, namely ultrasound-guided regional anesthesia, aspirating before injection, incremental injection, use of vascular markers, lower local anesthetic doses, and use of a test dose. Added safety measures included performing the blocks with the patients either awake or sedated with meaningful contact maintained to allow early identification of LAST and the use of midazolam, which may have increased the potential seizure threshold.[101–103]

As mentioned earlier, ASRA has evaluated data from 1979 to 2009 and identified 93 separate LAST events. The classic typical clinical presentation of LAST is a progression of subjective symptoms of CNS excitation such as agitation, tinnitus, circumoral numbness, blurred vision, and a metallic taste followed by muscle twitching, unconsciousness, and seizures; with very high drug levels, cardiac and respiratory arrest occur as well (Fig. 10.11). The sequence occurs because the inhibitory pathways in the brain are affected first, leaving unopposed excitation. This is sometimes referred to as disinhibition. As the blood (therefore brain) levels increase, the more resistant excitatory pathways are inhibited, leading to unconsciousness and coma.[84] A 2018 update notes that this was the presentation in approximately 43% of cases, although the types of CNS symptoms varied. An atypical presentation was evident in approximately 24% of the patients. This was defined as LAST with isolated cardiovascular (CV) symptoms alone. Most of the atypical presentations were for delayed symptoms.[84,98,99,104] Combined CNS and CV system occurred in 33% of cases.[84]

The most common regional block techniques associated with LAST occurred during circumcision procedures performed by nonanesthesia providers. Additional types and frequencies of blocks leading to LAST are noted in Table 10.7. Of 58 cases, 53 followed a single injection and 3 occurred with continuous infusion. Two cases involved both continuous infusions with a supplementary single injection. Bupivacaine was implicated most often with 17 events (36%) followed by lidocaine

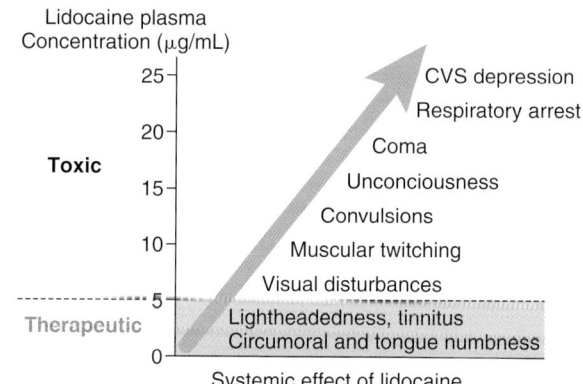

Fig. 10.11 Classically reported sequence of clinical signs after increased central nervous system concentration of lidocaine. *CVS*, Cardiovascular system.

TABLE 10.7 Type and Frequency of Block Resulting in LAST

Block Type	Frequency %
Penile (circumcision)	23
Local infiltration analgesia	17
Neuraxial	13
Upper extremity (including brachial plexus)	8.5
Paravertebral	8.5
Lower extremity (including sciatic femoral)	8.5
Head and neck	8.5
Topical	6
Transabdomims plane	4
Intravenous	2

Total cases 58, 2 reported deaths.
Total <100% due to missing data.
Adapted from Gitman M, Barrington MJ. Local anesthetic systemic toxicity: a review of recent case reports and registries. *Reg Anesth Pain Med.* 2018;43(2):124–130.

(26%), ropivacaine (21%), and others (17%). The patient ages spanned from 4 months to 88 years and American Society of Anesthesiologists (ASA) class from 1 to 4.[84] The timing of the onset of symptoms after a single injection varied from 30 seconds to 60 minutes (Fig. 10.12). It is usually very rapid. In 40% of cases the onset occurred in less than 50 seconds, and in 75% of cases it occurred within 10 minutes of injection. The onset of symptoms following continuous infusion occurred hours or days after starting the drug.[84]

As noted, the most common signs and symptoms of LAST involved the CNS and the CV system. Seizures and loss of consciousness were the most frequent CNS manifestations, and these findings are consistent with the data from the past 3 decades. When CNS and CV symptoms were combined, they most commonly progressed from CNS to CV abnormalities, but this was not the rule, confirming that toxicity may take different forms.[98]

Central Nervous System and Cardiovascular Signs of Toxicity

There are varied presentations of toxicities. Symptoms of CNS toxicity occurred in 83% of cases either alone (43%) or together with significant CV symptoms (33%) (Fig. 10.13). The spectrum of CNS signs of toxicity is given in Fig. 10.14. It is interesting to note that the most frequent symptom was seizures (68%), whereas only 11% exhibited the typical prodromal symptoms. The spectrum of CV signs of toxicity are given in Fig. 10.15. The most common involved various arrhythmias.[84,104]

Prevention of Local Anesthetic Systemic Toxicity

Adaption of suggested safety steps such as the use of test doses, incremental injection with frequent aspiration, and the use of pharmacologic markers such as epinephrine or fentanyl has lowered the incidence of LAST in recent years. Additional practices that have been suggested to improve safety include limiting the total dose of local anesthetic. The clinical principle in any regional technique is to use the lowest dose possible (the product of the concentration and volume) to produce a satisfactory block.[105] The use of generalized maximum recommended doses has been questioned.[86] Systemic blood levels of the same dose of

anesthetic vary greatly depending on the area of blockade, technique, and specific drug. Blood levels are difficult to predict when dosing on a milligram per kilogram basis. Body weight as a guide should be used only in pediatric patients (Table 10.8). The use of ultrasound-guided techniques has been evaluated with regard to improved patient safety. Evidence supports the concept that ultrasound guidance is effective in reducing the incidence of local anesthetic systemic toxicity. There is

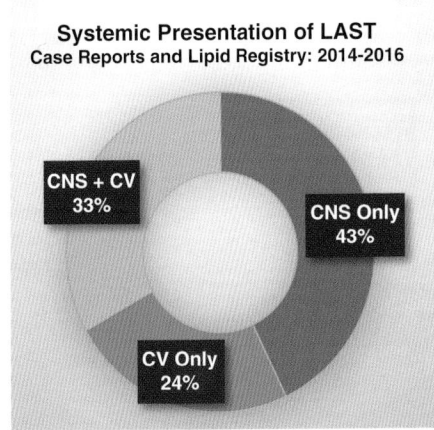

Fig. 10.13 The frequency of local anesthetic systemic toxicity *(LAST)* symptoms and signs referable to cardiovascular *(CV)*, central nervous system *(CNS)*, or both. (Data from Gitman M, Barrington MJ. Local anesthetic systemic toxicity: a review of recent case reports and registries. *Reg Anesth Pain Med.* 2018;43[2]:124–130; Neal JM, Barrington MJ, Fettiplace MR, et al. The third American Society of Regional Anesthesia and Pain Medicine practice advisory on local anesthetic systemic toxicity: executive summary 2017. *Reg Anesth Pain Med.* 2018;43[2]:113–123; Gitman M, Fettiplace MR, Weinberg GL, et al. Local anesthetic systemic toxicity: a narrative literature review and clinical update on prevention, diagnosis, and management. *Plast Reconstr Surg.* 2019;144[3]:783–795.)

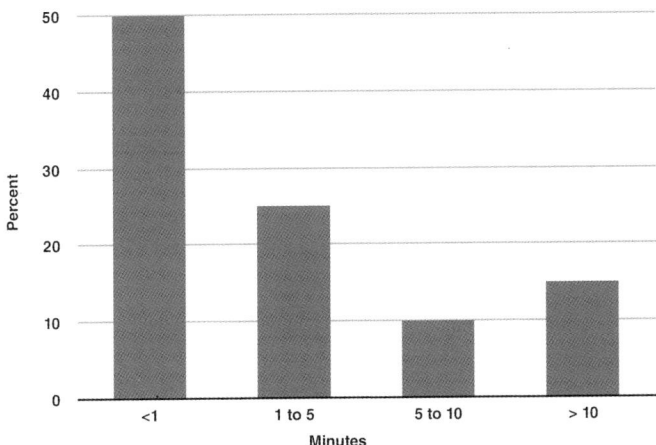

Fig. 10.12 The timing for onset of signs of local anesthetic systemic toxicity after a single injection of local anesthetic (from a total of 77 incidents). (Data from Gitman M, Barrington MJ. Local anesthetic systemic toxicity: a review of recent case reports and registries. *Reg Anesth Pain Med.* 2018;43[2]:124–130; Neal JM, Barrington MJ, Fettiplace MR, et al. The third American Society of Regional Anesthesia and Pain Medicine practice advisory on local anesthetic systemic toxicity: executive summary 2017. *Reg Anesth Pain Med.* 2018;43[2]:113–123; Mercado P, Weinberg GL. Local anesthetic systemic toxicity: prevention and treatment. *Anesthesiol Clin.* 2011;29:233–242.)

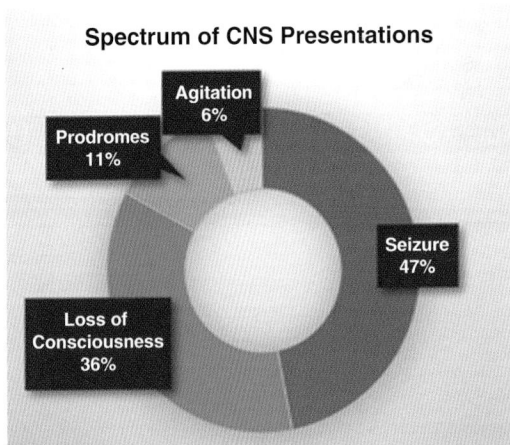

Fig. 10.14 The spectrum of reported signs of central nervous system *(CNS)* toxicity among published cases of local anesthetic systemic toxicity. (Data from Gitman M, Barrington MJ. Local anesthetic systemic toxicity: a review of recent case reports and registries. *Reg Anesth Pain Med.* 2018;43[2]:124–130; Neal JM, Barrington MJ, Fettiplace MR, et al. The third American Society of Regional Anesthesia and Pain Medicine practice advisory on local anesthetic systemic toxicity: executive summary 2017. *Reg Anesth Pain Med.* 2018;43[2]:113–123; Gitman M, Fettiplace MR, Weinberg GL, et al. Local anesthetic systemic toxicity: a narrative literature review and clinical update on prevention, diagnosis, and management. *Plast Reconstr Surg.* 2019;144[3]:783–795.)

also a lower predicted frequency of pneumothorax. Ultrasound guidance does not affect the incidence of peripheral nerve injury associated with regional anesthesia. There is a reduced incidence and intensity of hemidiaphragmatic paresis with ultrasound-guided supraclavicular blocks.[106,107] The current ASRA recommendations for recognizing, preventing, and treating LAST are given in Box 10.3.[105] Risk factors for LAST are listed in Box 10.4. Further recommendations for preventing LAST are noted in Box 10.5.

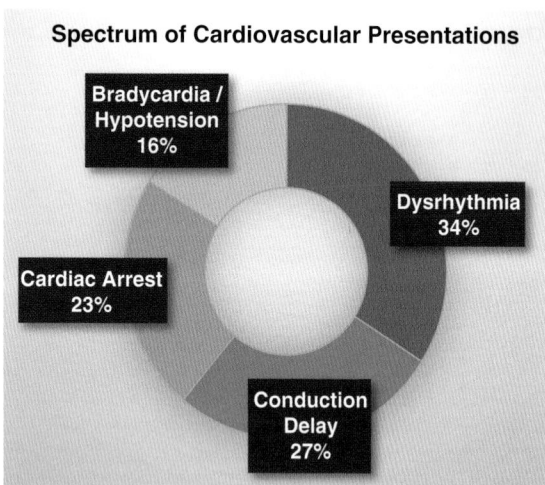

Fig. 10.15 The spectrum of reported signs of cardiovascular toxicity during local anesthetic systemic toxicity. *VF,* Ventricular fibrillation; *VT,* ventricular tachycardia. (Data from Gitman M, Barrington MJ. Local anesthetic systemic toxicity: a review of recent case reports and registries. *Reg Anesth Pain Med.* 2018;43[2]:124–130; Neal JM, Barrington MJ, Fettiplace MR, et al. The third American Society of Regional Anesthesia and Pain Medicine practice advisory on local anesthetic systemic toxicity: executive summary 2017. *Reg Anesth Pain Med.* 2018;43[2]:113–123, Gitman M, Fettiplace MR, Weinberg GL, et al. Local anesthetic systemic toxicity: a narrative literature review and clinical update on prevention, diagnosis, and management. *Plast Reconstr Surg.* 2019;144[3]:783–795.)

Diagnosis and Treatment of Local Anesthetic Systemic Toxicity

Prompt recognition and treatment are essential to minimizing adverse outcomes of LAST. Airway management remains the primary intervention because preventing hypoxia and acidosis are essential first steps. As noted in Box 10.2, acidosis may enhance toxicity by ion trapping local anesthetic in the brain. Seizure suppression is essential to facilitate immediate airway control and prevent or reduce metabolic acidosis. Benzodiazepines are considered the drugs of choice because they are anticonvulsants without causing significant cardiac depression. When benzodiazepines are not available, small doses of propofol are appropriate. Succinylcholine may be useful to suppress intractable seizure-induced tonic-clonic muscle activity despite the lack of CNS effects. Cardiovascular support is essential to maintaining adequate coronary perfusion. The local anesthetics do not irreversibly damage the cardiac cells. Avoiding tissue hypoxia is essential in reversing the progression of toxic cardiac events.[108] Local anesthetic cardiotoxicity, especially with bupivacaine, involves both electrophysiologic disturbances and depression of contractility. The electrical disturbances appear to occur at lower doses and are more contributory to poor outcomes than contractile depression, but differences among specific local anesthetics exist.[109] Lipid emulsion therapy is recommended as a standard part of LAST resuscitation. There is some evidence that it is able to restore spontaneous circulation without the use of vasopressors. In fact, large doses of vasopressors may decrease the effectiveness of lipid emulsions.[110] Vasopressors may be required to maintain adequate blood pressure, but they can worsen local anesthetic-induced arrhythmias. Small doses of epinephrine (<1 μg/kg) are recommended. Vasopressin should be avoided even though it can be used as part of the Advanced Cardiac Life Support guidelines.[108]

As noted previously, lipid emulsion therapy for LAST is the most promising therapy that has emerged. Both laboratory and clinical use have shown it to be instrumental in facilitating successful recovery. The exact mechanisms for the beneficial effects are not clear; however, new theories have been proposed.[111,112] Lipid emulsion reversal of LAST is ultimately linked to cellular mechanisms that are affected by local anesthetics. Under normal circumstances, local anesthetics block nerve conduction by inhibiting transduction of sodium, calcium, and potassium

TABLE 10.8	Local Anesthetic Agents Used Commonly for Infiltrative Injection	
Agent	**Duration of Action**	**Maximum Dosage Guidelines (Total Cumulative Infiltrative Injection Dose Per Procedure*)**
Esters		
Procaine (Novocain)	Short (15–60 min)	7 mg/kg; not to exceed 350–600 mg
Chloroprocaine (Nesacaine)	Short (15–30 min)	Without epinephrine: 11 mg/kg; not to exceed 800 mg total dose
		With epinephrine: 14 mg/kg; not to exceed 1000 mg
Amides		
Lidocaine (Xylocaine)	Medium (30–60 min)	Without epinephrine: 4.5 mg/kg; not to exceed 300 mg
Lidocaine with epinephrine	Long (120–360 min)	With epinephrine: 7 mg/kg
Mepivacaine (Polocaine, Carbocaine)	Medium (45–90 min) Long (120–360 min with epinephrine)	7 mg/kg; not to exceed 400 mg
Bupivacaine (Marcaine)	Long (120–240 min)	Without epinephrine: 2.0 mg/kg; not to exceed 175 mg total dose
Bupivacaine with epinephrine	Long (180–420 min)	With epinephrine: 3 mg/kg; not to exceed 225 mg total dose
Prilocaine (Citanest)	Medium (30–90 min)	Body weight <70 kg: 6 mg/kg; not to exceed 500 mg
Ropivacaine (Naropin)	Long (120–360 min)	3 mg; not to exceed 200 mg for minor nerve block with or without epinephrine

*Nondental use; administer by small incremental doses; administer the smallest dose and concentration required to achieve desired effect; avoid rapid injection.

through voltage-gated ionotropic channels located in the cell membrane. Acute local anesthetic cardiotoxicity negatively impacts myocardial contractility, cardiac conduction, and systemic vascular resistance through a complex and widespread set of events that involve channel blockade, metabolic signaling, and intracellular energy production resulting in inhibition of oxidative phosphorylation. The clinical effects of these cellular events manifest initially as hypertension and tachydysrhythmias that progress to depressed cardiac conduction and performance (reduced cardiac output), bradycardia, and hypotension. Similarly, local anesthetic toxicity on CNS ionic channels manifests initially as altered mental status

BOX 10.3 American Society of Regional Anesthesia and Pain Medicine Checklist for Managing Local Anesthetic Systemic Toxicity

For patients experiencing signs or symptoms of local anesthetic systemic toxicity (LAST), the pharmacologic treatment of LAST is different from other cardiac arrest scenarios.
- Get help.
- Initial focus:
  - *Airway management:* ventilate with 100% oxygen.
  - *Seizure suppression:* benzodiazepines are preferred.
  - *Basic and Advanced Cardiac Life Support (BLS/ACLS) will require adjustments of medications and perhaps prolonged effort.*
- Infuse 20% lipid emulsion.
- Patient <70 kg:
  - IV bolus 1.5 mL/kg over 2–3 min (ideal body weight).
  - Continuous IV infusion at 0.25–0.5 mL/kg/min (ideal body weight).
  - Repeat bolus up to three times for persistent cardiovascular collapse.
  - Continue infusion for at least 10 min after attaining circulatory stability.
  - Recommended upper limit: approximately 12 mL/kg lipid emulsion over the first 30 min.
- Patient >70 kg:
  - IV bolus 100 mL over 2–3 min.
  - Continuous IV infusion 200–250 mL over 10–20 min.
  - Avoid vasopressin, calcium channel blockers, β-blockers, or local anesthetic.
  - Reduce epinephrine doses to <1 mcg/kg.
  - Alert the nearest facility having cardiopulmonary bypass capability.
  - Avoid propofol in patients having signs of cardiovascular instability.
  - Post LAST events and report use of lipid at www.lipidrescue.org.

Be Prepared
- We strongly advise that those using local anesthetics (LAs) establish a plan for managing LAST. Making a LA toxicity kit and posting instructions for its use are encouraged.

Risk Reduction (Be Sensible)
- Use the lowest dose of LA necessary to achieve the desired extent and duration of block.
- Local anesthetic blood levels are influenced by site of injection and dose. Factors that can increase the likelihood of LAST include advanced age, heart failure, ischemic heart disease, conduction abnormalities, metabolic (e.g., mitochondrial) disease, liver disease, low plasma protein concentration, metabolic or respiratory acidosis, and medications that inhibit sodium channels. Patients with severe cardiac dysfunction, particularly very low ejection fraction, are more sensitive to LAST and are more prone to receive "stacked" injections (with resulting elevated LA tissue concentrations) because of slowed circulation time.
- Consider using a pharmacologic marker and/or test dose (e.g., epinephrine 5 µg/mL of LA). Know the expected response, onset, duration, and limitations of a "test dose" in identifying intravascular injection.
- Aspirate the syringe prior to each injection while observing for blood.

- Inject incrementally, observing for signs and querying frequently for symptoms of toxicity between each injection.
- Use ultrasound guidance for the local anesthetic injection.

Detection (Be Vigilant)
- Use standard American Society of Anesthesiologists (ASA) monitors.
- Monitor the patient during and after completing the injection, as clinical toxicity can be delayed up to 30 min or longer after tumescent procedures.
- Consider LAST in any patient with altered mental status, neurologic symptoms, or cardiovascular instability following a regional anesthetic.
- Central nervous system signs (may be subtle or absent):
  - Excitation (agitation, confusion, muscle twitching, seizure)
  - Depression (drowsiness, obtundation, coma, apnea)
  - Nonspecific (metallic taste, circumoral numbness, diplopia, tinnitus, dizziness)
- Cardiovascular signs (often the only manifestation of severe LAST):
  - Initially may be hyperdynamic (hypertension, tachycardia, ventricular arrhythmias), then:
  - Progressive hypotension
  - Conduction block, bradycardia, or asystole
  - Ventricular arrhythmia (ventricular tachycardia, torsades de pointes, ventricular fibrillation)
- Sedative hypnotic drugs reduce seizure risk, but even light sedation may abolish the patient's ability to recognize or report symptoms of rising LA concentrations.

Treatment
- Maintain and secure the airway; 100% oxygen.
- Timing of lipid infusion in LAST is controversial. The most conservative approach, waiting until after ACLS has proven unsuccessful, is unreasonable because early treatment can prevent cardiovascular collapse. Infusing lipid at the earliest sign of LAST can result in unnecessary treatment because only a fraction of patients will progress to severe toxicity. The most reasonable approach to implement lipid therapy is dependent on the clinical severity and rate of progression of LAST.
- There is laboratory evidence that epinephrine can impair resuscitation from LAST and reduce the efficacy of lipid rescue. Therefore it is recommended that one avoid high doses of epinephrine and use smaller doses (e.g., <1 µg/kg) for treating hypotension.
- Propofol should not be used when there are signs of cardiovascular instability. Propofol is a cardiovascular depressant with lipid content too low to provide benefit. Its use is discouraged when there is a risk of progression to cardiovascular collapse.
- Consider drawing blood to measure LA plasma concentration if there is no delay to definitive treatment.
- Transfer to a clinical area with appropriate monitoring, equipment, and staff for >12-hr monitoring.
- Regular clinical review to exclude pancreatitis, including serial amylase or lipase for 2 days.
- Report cases and use of IV lipid emulsion to www.lipidrescue.org.

Data from Neal JM, Barrington MJ, Fettiplace MR, et al. The Third American Society of Regional Anesthesia and Pain Medicine Practice Advisory on local anesthetic systemic toxicity: executive summary 2017. *Reg Anesth Pain Med.* 2018;43(2):113–123; Fettiplace MR, Weinberg G. The mechanisms underlying lipid resuscitation therapy. *Reg Anesth Pain Med.* 2018;43(2):138–149; El-Boghdadly K, Chin KJ. Local anesthetic systemic toxicity: continuing professional development. *Can J Anaesth.* 2016;63:330–349.

BOX 10.4 Risk Factors for Local Anesthetic Systemic Toxicity (LAST)

- Patient characteristics
  - Extremes of age—<16 or >60 yr
  - Low muscle mass—particularly with neonates, infants, and the debilitated elderly
  - Female > male
  - Comorbidities
- Cardiac disease, especially arrhythmias, conduction abnormalities, ischemia, and congestive heart failure
- Liver disease
- Metabolic disease, especially diabetes mellitus, isovaleric acidemia, mitochondrial disease, and carnitine deficiency
- Central nervous system diseases
- Low plasma protein binding—liver disease, malnourishment, infants, pregnancy
- Local anesthetic characteristics
  - Bupivacaine has a lower safety margin and resuscitation is more difficult in the event of LAST, but local anesthetics such as ropivacaine and lidocaine still account for a significant proportion of LAST events.
  - Block site, total local anesthetic dose, test dosing, and patient comorbidities are more predictive of high plasma levels of local anesthetic, body weight, or body mass index.
  - Local anesthetic infusions are particularly problematic after 1–4 days and in patients of small body mass.
  - Seizures are up to five times more likely after peripheral nerve block than epidural block.
- Practice setting
  - Up to 20% of LAST cases occur outside of the hospital setting.
  - Nonanesthesiologists are involved in up to 50% of LAST cases.

Adapted from Neal JM, Barrington MJ, Fettiplace MR, et al. The Third American Society of Regional Anesthesia and Pain Medicine Practice Advisory on local anesthetic systemic toxicity: executive summary 2017. *Reg Anesth Pain Med.* 2018;43(2):113–123.

BOX 10.5 Recommendations for Preventing Local Anesthetic Systemic Toxicity (LAST)

- There is no single measure that can prevent LAST in clinical practice.
- Use the lowest effective dose of local anesthetic (dose = product of volume × concentration).
- Use incremental injection of local anesthetics—administer 3–5 mL aliquots, pausing 15–30 sec between each injection.
  - When using a fixed needle approach (e.g., landmark paresthesia seeking or electrical stimulation), time between injections should encompass one circulation time (approximately 30–45 sec); however, this ideal may be balanced against the risk of needle movement between injections. Circulation time may be increased with lower extremity blocks. Use of larger dosing increments would dictate the need for longer intervals to reduce the cumulative dose from stacked injections before an event of LAST. Incremental injection may be less important with ultrasound guidance given that frequent needle movement is often used with the technique.
- Aspirate the needle or catheter before each injection, recognizing that there is approximately a 2% false-negative rate for this diagnostic intervention.
- When injecting potentially toxic doses of local anesthetic, use of an intravascular marker is recommended. Although epinephrine is an imperfect marker and its use is open to physician judgment, its benefits likely outweigh its risks in most patients:
  - Intravascular injection of epinephrine 10–15 µg/mL in adults produces a ≥10-beat heart rate increase or a ≥15 mm Hg systolic blood pressure (SBP) increase in the absence of β-blockade, active labor, advanced age, or general/neuraxial anesthesia.
  - Intravascular injection of epinephrine 0.5 µg/kg in children produces a ≥15 mm Hg increase in SBP.
  - Appropriate subtoxic doses of local anesthetic can produce subjective symptoms of mild systemic toxicity (e.g., auditory changes, excitation, metallic taste) in unpremedicated patients.
  - Fentanyl 100 µg produces sedation if injected intravascularly in laboring patients.
- Ultrasound guidance may reduce the frequency of intravascular injection, but actual reduction of LAST remains unproven in humans. Individual reports describe LAST despite the use of ultrasound-guided regional anesthesia. The overall effectiveness of ultrasound guidance in reducing the frequency of LAST remains to be determined.
- Caregivers should be aware of the additive nature of local anesthetic toxicity and adjust accordingly local anesthetic redosing and/or administration by different perioperative providers.
- The risk of LAST associated with truncal blocks may be reduced by using lower concentrations of local anesthetics, dosing on lean body weight, adjunctive epinephrine, and observation for at least 30–45 min after the block.
- Patients receiving liposomal bupivacaine (LB) should receive the same level of vigilance afforded to any patient receiving a local anesthetic.
- Include local anesthetic dosing parameters and at-risk patient concerns as part of the preincision surgical pause.

Data from Mulroy MF, Hejtmanek MR. Prevention of local anesthetic systemic toxicity. *Reg Anesth Pain Med.* 2010;35:177–180; Neal JM, Barrington MJ, Fettiplace MR, et al. The Third American Society of Regional Anesthesia and Pain Medicine Practice Advisory on local anesthetic systemic toxicity: executive summary 2017. *Reg Anesth Pain Med.* 2018;43(2):113–123; El-Boghdadly K, Chin KJ. Local anesthetic systemic toxicity: continuing professional development. *Can J Anaesth.* 2016;63:330–349.

and/or mild prodromal symptoms such as paresthesias, tinnitus, and agitation and progress to seizure and possible coma. A number of potential mechanisms of action have been offered, the most prominent of which involved the hypothesis that lipid emulsion infusion effectively created an intravascular lipophilic "sink" into which lipid soluble local anesthetics such as bupivacaine partitioned and were ultimately removed from the body.[98] Twenty years later, the lipid sink theory is no longer believed to be relevant. Lipid emulsion therapy is believed to involve multiple mechanisms that involve active shuttling of local anesthetic away from the heart and brain, cardiotonic effects that involve the heart and/or vasculature, and postconditioning cardioprotective effects.[84,111,112]

Shuttling Effects

Rather than acting as a static lipid sink, current research supports the concept that lipid emulsion works as a dynamic carrier to scavenge local anesthetic away from high blood flow organs that are most sensitive to LAST, such as the heart and brain, and redistribute it to organs that store and detoxify the drug, such as muscle and liver, respectively. The precise mechanisms of local anesthetic binding to lipid droplets are not understood fully but are believed to combine thermodynamic effects (e.g., electrostatic attraction) and physicochemical characteristics (e.g., lipophilicity, acid-base ionization) as positively charged, fat-soluble local anesthetic molecules bind to negatively charged lipid particles. These observations appear to support lipid emulsion having greater efficacy in shuttling the more lipophilic local anesthetics such

BOX 10.6 Recommendations for Diagnosing Local Anesthetic Systemic Toxicity (LAST)

- Classic descriptions of LAST depict a progression of subjective symptoms of central nervous system (CNS) excitement (e.g., agitation, auditory changes, metallic taste, or abrupt onset of psychiatric symptoms) followed by seizures or CNS depression (e.g., drowsiness, coma, or respiratory arrest). Near the end of this continuum, initial signs of cardiac toxicity (e.g., hypertension, tachycardia, or ventricular arrhythmias) are supplanted by cardiac depression (e.g., bradycardia, conduction block, asystole, decreased contractility). However, there is substantial variation in this classic description, including the following:
  - Simultaneous presentation of CNS and cardiac toxicity
  - Cardiac toxicity without prodromal signs and symptoms of CNS toxicity
- The practitioner must be vigilant for atypical or unexpected presentation of LAST.
- The timing of LAST presentation is variable. Immediate (<60 sec) presentation suggests intravascular injection of local anesthetic (LA) with direct access to the brain, whereas presentation that is delayed 1–5 min suggests intermittent or partial intravascular injection, delayed circulation time, or delayed tissue absorption. Because LAST can present >15 min after injection, patients who receive potentially toxic doses of LA should be closely monitored for at least 30 min after injection.
- Case reports associate LAST with underlying cardiac, neurologic, pulmonary, renal, hepatic, or metabolic disease. Heightened vigilance is warranted in these patients, particularly if they are at the extremes of age.
- The overall variability of LAST signs and symptoms, timing of onset, and association with various disease states suggests that practitioners should maintain a low threshold for considering the diagnosis of LAST in patients with atypical or unexpected presentation of CNS or cardiac signs and symptoms after receiving more than a minimal dose of LA.

Data from Neal JM, Barrington MJ, Fettiplace MR, et al. The Third American Society of Regional Anesthesia and Pain Medicine Practice Advisory on local anesthetic systemic toxicity: executive summary 2017. *Reg Anesth Pain Med.* 2018;43(2):113–123; Mercado P, Weinberg GL. Local anesthetic systemic toxicity: prevention and treatment. *Anesthesiol Clin.* 2011;29:233–242; El-Boghdadly K, Chin KJ. Local anesthetic systemic toxicity: continuing professional development. *Can J Anaesth.* 2016;63:330–349.

BOX 10.7 Recommendations for Treating Local Anesthetic Systemic Toxicity (LAST)

- If signs and symptoms of LAST occur, prompt and effective airway management is crucial to preventing hypoxia and acidosis, which are known to potentiate LAST.
- If seizures occur, they should be rapidly halted with benzodiazepines. If benzodiazepines are not readily available, lipid emulsion and small doses of propofol are acceptable.
- Although propofol can stop seizures, large doses further depress cardiac function; propofol should be avoided when there are signs of cardiovascular compromise.
- If seizures persist despite benzodiazepines, small doses of succinylcholine or similar neuromuscular blocker should be considered to minimize acidosis and hypoxemia.
- If cardiac arrest occurs, we recommend standard advance cardiac life support with the following modifications:
  - If epinephrine is used, small initial doses (10–100 µg boluses in adults) are preferred (<1 µg/kg).
  - Vasopressin is not recommended.
  - Avoid calcium channel blockers, β-adrenergic receptor blockers, and sodium channel blockers.
  - If ventricular arrhythmias develop, amiodarone is preferred; treatment with local anesthetics (lidocaine or procainamide) is not recommended.
- Lipid emulsion therapy:
  - Consider administering at the first signs of LAST, after airway management.
  - Timeliness of lipid emulsion is more important than the order of administration modality (bolus vs. injection)
  - 20% lipid emulsion BOLUS
  Patient <70 kg:
  - IV bolus 1.5 mL/kg over 2–3 min (ideal body weight).
  - Continuous IV infusion at 0.25–0.5 mL/kg/min (ideal body weight).
  - Repeat bolus up to three times for persistent cardiovascular collapse.
  - Continue infusion for at least 10 min after attaining circulatory stability.
  - Recommended upper limit: approximately 12 mL/kg lipid emulsion over the first 30 min.
  Patient >70 kg:
  - IV bolus 100 mL over 2–3 min.
  - Continuous IV infusion 200–250 mL over 10–20 min.
- Propofol is not a substitute for lipid emulsion.
- Failure to respond to lipid emulsion and vasopressor therapy should prompt institution of cardiopulmonary bypass. Because there can be considerable lag in beginning cardiopulmonary bypass, it is reasonable to notify the closest facility capable of providing it when cardiovascular compromise is first identified during an episode of LAST.
- Patients with a significant cardiovascular event should be monitored for at least 4–6 hr. If the event is limited to CNS symptoms that resolve quickly, they should be monitored for at least 2 hr.
- Use written or electronic checklists as cognitive aids during the management of LAST. A dedicated reader improves adherence to the checklist.

Data from Neal JM, Barrington MJ, Fettiplace MR, et al. The Third American Society of Regional Anesthesia and Pain Medicine Practice Advisory on local anesthetic systemic toxicity: executive summary 2017. *Reg Anesth Pain Med.* 2018;43(2):113–123; Mercado P, Weinberg GL. Local anesthetic systemic toxicity: prevention and treatment. *Anesthesiol Clin.* 2011;29:233–242; El-Boghdadly K, Chin KJ. Local anesthetic systemic toxicity: continuing professional development. *Can J Anaesth.* 2016;63:330–349.

as bupivacaine. Nevertheless, even the less lipophilic local anesthetics such as lidocaine or mepivacaine are highly lipid soluble and carry a positive charge at physiologic pH. Therefore lipid emulsion should be effective at reversing toxicity after overdose with most local anesthetics. Lipid emulsion also has nonscavenging effects that manifest as cardiotonic and postconditioning effects. Several lines of evidence support the concept that lipid increases cardiac performance, which enhances the shuttling effect. The direct cardiotonic effects of lipid emulsion increase cardiac contractility, which increases cardiac output and blood flow through affected organs. Together, these mechanisms serve to improve both cardiac output and blood pressure. Recent laboratory experiments support the concept that adverse cellular effects of LAST overlap with mechanisms of cardiac ischemia-reperfusion injury. Coupled with the observation that infused lipid emulsion activates cardioprotective pathways, this provides an additional mechanism of postconditioning benefit to the local anesthetic-toxic heart.[111-114]

Lipid emulsion is also recommended if pregnant patients develop LAST.[115] It is also being used for a variety of drug overdoses in emergency situations.[116] The recommendations for diagnosing LAST are given in Box 10.6.[98] Treatment recommendations are given in Box 10.7.[106]

Other Adverse Effects

Allergic Reactions

True allergic reactions to local anesthetics are rare, making up no more than 1% of reactions.[117] The frequency is decreasing with the lower use of the ester-type local anesthetics. Adverse reactions are most commonly a result of anxiety, panic attacks, intravascular injection, vasovagal responses, or epinephrine. A 2012 literature review of local anesthetic reactions identified 23 case series involving 2978 patients, and 29 of these patients had true immunoglobulin E (IgE)–mediated reactions to local anesthetics resulting in a prevalence of 0.97%.[118] Local anesthetics can, however, produce allergic, hypersensitivity, and anaphylactic reactions. The use of ester local anesthetics is associated with a greater incidence of allergic reactions than the use of amides. This is likely because esters are derivatives of and metabolized to para-aminobenzoic acid (PABA), which is an allergenic compound.[119] Allergy to local anesthetics may be caused by methylparaben, paraben, or metabisulfite used as preservatives. In 1984 the FDA mandated removal of methylparaben from single-dose local anesthetic cartridges commonly used in dentistry, which greatly reduced allergic reactions. Sulfites are antioxidants used to stabilize epinephrine in local anesthetic solutions. They are not typically used when the local anesthetic does not contain epinephrine. Sulfites have been involved in non-IgE-mediated hypersensitivity reactions, particularly in patients with asthma. Because testing is very inconsistent, it is difficult to know the role sulfites may play in reactions attributed to a local anesthetic preparation.[120,121] Preservative-free solutions are available. Cross-reactivity among the ester-type local anesthetics is high. Allergy to the amides remains extremely rare. Cross-reactivity within the amides as a class is extremely rare and between esters and amides is absent.[122] A thorough history of allergy may be difficult because patients call many local anesthetic drugs Novocaine. They may not be aware of the specific agent administered. Clinicians use amides when possible because the incidence of allergy is extremely low, and they are not cross-reactive with other amides or esters. If a true allergy is suspected, referral to an allergist for skin testing and incremental dose challenges is prudent. Diphenhydramine (1%) with 1:100,000 epinephrine may be an alternative to local anesthetics.[117,123,124]

Methemoglobinemia

Methemoglobinemia is a disorder characterized by high concentrations of methemoglobin (MetHb) in the blood, which can lead to tissue hypoxia. The ferrous form of hemoglobin (Fe^{2+}) is oxidized to the ferric form (Fe^{3+}). Methemoglobin is an oxidized form of hemoglobin with reduced capacity to carry oxygen, which causes a shift to the left of the oxygen-hemoglobin dissociation curve (Fig. 10.16). Normal methemoglobin levels are less than 1%. Signs and symptoms of developing methemoglobinemia are shown in Table 10.9. Decreasing oxygen saturation via pulse oximetry, which is unresponsive to oxygen supplementation, may occur. Clinical clues to the diagnosis of methemoglobinemia in the anesthetized patient are noted in Box 10.8. It can be diagnosed by CO-oximetry, laboratory testing, or implied by symptoms.[125–127] Clinically, methemoglobinemia can be diagnosed by a discrepancy between the SpO_2 and SaO_2 that is refractory to oxygen therapy, signs of cyanosis, decreased SpO_2 hovering at 85%, chocolate-colored blood, acidosis and tachycardia, and most effectively with use of CO-oximetry. Medications are the most common cause of MetHb in clinical practice, and of these local anesthetics (benzocaine and prilocaine), antibiotics (dapsone), and nitrites (nitroglycerin/nitric oxide) are the most common.[128]

Benzocaine and benzocaine-containing mixtures are widely used for topical anesthesia. The FDA has issued multiple safety bulletins warning of benzocaine-induced methemoglobinemia.[129] In a 2006 communication, the FDA reported 247 cases of methemoglobinemia from benzocaine sprays, including three deaths. Since then the number of cases has continued to rise. The development of methemoglobinemia does not seem to be dose related. Symptoms appear within minutes up to 2 hours after benzocaine use. Benzocaine sprays are marketed as different brand names such as Cetacaine, Hurricaine, Exactacain,

Normal Oxyhemoglobin Equilibrium

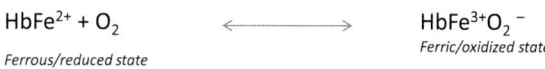

$HbFe^{2+} + O_2$ ⟷ $HbFe^{3+}O_2^-$

Ferrous/reduced state   *Ferric/oxidized state*

Formation of Methemoglobin

$HbFe^{2+}$ + oxidizing substance ⟶ $HbFe^{3+}OH$
methemoglobin

Fig. 10.16 Normal oxyhemoglobin equilibrium and methemoglobin formation. (From Cortazzo JA1, Lichtman AD. Methemoglobinemia: a review and recommendations for management. *J Cardiothorac Vasc Anesth.* 2014; 28:1043–1047.)

TABLE 10.9 Signs and Symptoms Associated With Methemoglobinemia

Methemoglobin Concentration	% Total Hemoglobin	Symptoms
<1.5 g/dL	<10	None
1.5–3.0 g/dL	10–20	Cyanotic skin discoloration
3.0–4.5 g/dl	20–30	Anxiety, lightheadedness, headache, tachycardia
4.5–7.5 g/dL	30–50	Fatigue, confusion, dizziness, tachypnea, increased tachycardia
7.5–10.5 g/dL	50–70	Coma, seizures, arrhythmias, acidosis
>10.5 g/dL	>70	Death

From Cortazzo JA, Lichtman AD. Methemoglobinemia: a review and recommendations for management. *J Cardiothorac Vasc Anesth.* 2014; 28:1043–1047.

BOX 10.8 Clinical Clues to the Diagnosis of Methemoglobinemia in the Anesthetized Patient

1. Hypoxia that does not improve with increased fraction of inspired oxygen (FiO_2)
2. Abnormal coloration of blood
3. Physiologically appropriate partial pressure of arterial oxygen (PaO_2) on blood gas sample with low pulse oximeter saturation—"saturation gap"
4. New-onset cyanosis and/or hypoxia after ingestion of an agent with oxidative properties

From Cortazzo JA, Lichtman AD. Methemoglobinemia: a review and recommendations for management. *J Cardiothorac Vasc Anesth.* 2014;28:1043–1047.

and Topex. A 2011 safety bulletin warned of serious adverse events associated with over-the-counter benzocaine gels, sprays, and liquids. They are applied to the throat and gums for pain relief. The cases were primarily in teething children less than 2 years old. Benzocaine gels and liquids are marketed under the names Anbesol, Hurricaine, Orajel, Baby Orajel, Orabase, and some store brands. Benzocaine should not be used in children under 2 years old.[129]

Prilocaine can produce methemoglobinemia because of one of its metabolites o-toluidine, which oxidizes hemoglobin to methemoglobin. The tendency of prilocaine to produce methemoglobin is dose related. Current recommendations are that prilocaine should not be used in children younger than 6 months old, in pregnant women, or in patients taking other oxidizing drugs. The dose should be limited to 2.5 mg/kg.[130,131]

The treatment for elevated methemoglobin is methylene blue, which is initiated at a rate of 1 to 2 mg/kg intravenously over 3 to 10 minutes. If the methemoglobin level is greater than 50% or the clinical condition worsens, then the higher dose of methylene blue 2 mg/kg can be given initially. In severe cases (i.e., a level of methemoglobin >70%) treatments may include ascorbic acid, riboflavin, hyperbaric oxygen therapy, and even RBC transfusion for refractory cases. Methylene blue is used for cases primarily caused secondary to drug exposure. Recognition is critical because a delay in treatment can lead to cardiopulmonary compromise, neurologic sequelae, and even death.[128,132]

Local Tissue Toxicity

Cauda equina syndrome (CES) manifests as bowel and bladder dysfunction with various degrees of bilateral lower extremity weakness and sensory impairment. There are multiple causes for CES, ranging from neural element compression from hematoma, abscess, or herniated intervertebral discs to poorly understood presentations associated with normal clinical settings. Known risk factors for anesthetic-related CES are supernormal doses of intrathecal local anesthetic and/or the maldistribution of local anesthetic spread within the intrathecal space. Cases of CES have been associated with previously undiagnosed spinal stenosis. In theory, a narrow spinal canal may lead to pressure-induced spinal cord ischemia or limit normal local anesthetic distribution within the intrathecal sac thereby exposing the cauda equina to high drug concentrations. Either of these conditions could promote local anesthetic neurotoxicity and could be exacerbated by additional compromise of the spinal canal, as may occur with nonneutral surgical positioning. Box 10.9 shows the ASRA recommendations regarding CES.[133] Past formulations of chloroprocaine were reported to produce prolonged CES when large doses were given by inadvertent intrathecal injection.[16,134-136] The neurotoxicity was thought to be caused by a combination of large intrathecal doses, low pH, and the preservative sodium metabisulfite. Controversy remains as to whether transient neurologic symptoms (TNS) after spinal anesthesia are a form of local anesthetic neurotoxicity with the use of preservative-free intrathecal 2-chloroprocaine. Spinal 2-chloroprocaine remains off-label in the United States.[137-139]

Lidocaine has been associated with CES when used for continuous spinal anesthesia, and it is no longer used in this anesthetic technique in the United States.[140,141] Single-dose spinal administration of lidocaine has also been implicated in TNS, which results in back and lower extremity pain for up to 5 days postoperatively. No permanent problems occur. Symptoms include a burning, aching, cramplike, and radiating pain in the anterior and posterior aspect of the thighs. Pain radiates to the lower extremities, and lower back pain is common. Other anesthetics have been implicated, but it is much more prevalent following spinal lidocaine.[142] Surgical positioning may be a factor as

well.[143] The exact mechanism is unclear. Newer techniques and agents other than lidocaine are being used now, which has diminished this problem as a clinical issue.[144] Treatment is supportive and should include nonsteroidal antiinflammatory agents when possible.

CLINICAL USE OF LOCAL ANESTHETICS

Topical Anesthesia

Anesthesia with several diverse topical formulations is used for a variety of clinical applications. These include decreasing the pain of venipuncture, circumcision, dressing changes, dentistry, minor surgical procedures, laser procedures, and multiple-injection regional blocks. Some available products are listed in Table 10.10 and described hereafter.[145,146]

Cocaine

Cocaine is derived from the coca plant and is the only naturally occurring local anesthetic. Other unique properties include the ability to block the monoamine transporter in adrenergic neurons. The neuronal transporter is responsible for the termination of the action of catecholamines. This catecholamine reuptake blockade results in significant vasoconstriction. This action in the CNS also accounts for cocaine's analeptic actions. It is used primarily for topical anesthesia of the nose and throat. The clinical use is declining. A maximum of 5 mL of 4% solution or 200 mg should be used. It is frequently administered with other epinephrine-containing preparations so arrhythmias, hypertension, and tachycardia may occur. Caution is advised for possible drug interactions in patients taking other catecholamine-enhancing drugs such as tricyclic antidepressants or monoamine oxidase inhibitors.[147,148]

> ### BOX 10.9 American Society of Regional Anesthesia Recommendations for Minimizing Cauda Equina Syndrome (CES)
>
> These recommendations are intended to encourage optimal patient care but cannot ensure the avoidance of adverse outcomes. As with any practice advisory recommendation, these are subject to revision as knowledge advances regarding specific complications.
> - Initial dosing or redosing of subarachnoid local anesthetic in addition, maldistribution (usually sacral) of local anesthetic spread should be ruled out before redosing single-injection or continuous subarachnoid blocks (Class I).
> - The risks and benefits of neuraxial techniques should be considered in patients known to have moderate-to-severe spinal stenosis, especially if within the vertebral territory of the intended injection (Class II).
> - The incidence of TNS after 40–50 mg intrathecal 2-chloroprocaine seems to be remarkably low. The number of 2-chloropocaine spinal anesthetics reported in the literature is insufficient to determine the risk for CES or other manifestations of neurotoxicity (Class III).
> - Physically and temporally separate disinfectant use from block trays and instruments during neuraxial procedures. Allow the solution to completely dry on skin before needle placement (2–3 min). Care should be taken to avoid needle or catheter contamination from chlorhexidine spraying or dripping, or from applicator device disposal, onto aseptic work surfaces (Class II).

From Neal JM, et al. The second ASRA practice advisory on neurologic complications associated with regional anesthesia and pain medicine: executive summary 2015. *Reg Anesth Pain Med*. 2015;40:401–430. *TNS*, Transient neurologic symptoms.

TABLE 10.10   Topical Anesthesia Products

Product	Composition	Time to Efficacy	Occlusion	Potential
TAC	0.5% tetracaine, 1:2000 epinephrine, and 11.8% cocaine	30 min	No	Hypertension, tachycardia, seizures; cardiac arrest
LET	0.5% tetracaine, 1:2000 epinephrine, and 4% lidocaine	15–30 min	No	None
Topicaine	4% lidocaine	30 min	No	Contact dermatitis
EMLA	2.5% lidocaine and 2.5% prilocaine	30 min–2 hr	Yes	Contact dermatitis; methemoglobinemia
LMX 4/5	4% or 5% liposomal lidocaine	15–40 min	No	None
BLT	20% benzocaine, 6% lidocaine, and 4% tetracaine	15–30 min	No	None

BLT, Benzocaine, lidocaine, tetracaine; *EMLA,* eutectic mixture of local anesthetics; *LET,* lidocaine, epinephrine, and tetracaine; *LMX,* lidocaine mixture; *TAC,* tetracaine, epinephrine, and cocaine.

Data from Kaweski S. Plastic Surgery Educational Foundation Technology Assessment Committee: topical anesthetic creams. *Plast Reconstr Surg.* 2008;121:2161–2165; Lee HS. Recent advances in topical anesthesia. *J Dent Anesth Pain Med.* 2016;16(4):237–244.

Eutectic Mixture of Local Anesthetics

Eutectic mixture of local anesthetics (EMLA) is a mixture of lidocaine and prilocaine that is applied to the skin as either a cream or patch. A eutectic mixture of chemicals has a lower melting point and solidifies at a lower temperature when combined. Pharmacokinetic studies indicate that satisfactory dermal analgesia is achieved 1 hour after application with an occlusive dressing; maximal analgesia occurs 2 to 3 hours after application.[145] When EMLA is applied to areas of abnormal skin (e.g., where psoriasis or eczema is present), absorption is faster, plasma levels are higher, and the duration of anesthesia is shorter. Systemic absorption of lidocaine and prilocaine is dependent on the duration and surface area of application. Toxicity is more likely to occur in infants and small children than in adults. Guidelines for the use of EMLA are given in Table 10.11.

Tetracaine, Epinephrine, and Cocaine

Three available agents—tetracaine, epinephrine, and cocaine (TAC)—have been combined for use on traumatic lacerations. The relative concentration of each component is as follows: tetracaine 0.5%, epinephrine 1:2000, and cocaine 11.8%. This combination has been as effective as infiltration of local anesthetics for the closure of certain types of laceration. Tetracaine and cocaine can produce excellent topical anesthesia, and cocaine and epinephrine result in vasoconstriction at the site of application. TAC is much more expensive to administer than lidocaine. The drug combination in TAC can produce significant toxicity.[145]

Local Wound Infiltration

Pain can be effectively alleviated with local anesthetics; however, their clinical usefulness is limited by their relatively short duration of action. Even long-acting local anesthetics such as bupivacaine and ropivacaine have durations less than 8 to 16 hours. Wound infiltration prior to closing is a common practice for immediate short-term postoperative pain relief. Direct application of local anesthetic and opiate drugs via continuous infusion indwelling catheters provides long-term analgesia. Wound catheters are commonly placed in the subcutaneous, fascial, intraarticular, pleural, and periosteal areas. Local anesthetic systemic toxicity has not been reported.[149–151] Problems associated with the use of indwelling catheters are blockage or breakage, migration away from the intended area, and infection. When intraarticular bupivacaine is used in high concentrations for long periods, chondrotoxicity has been reported.[152]

Sustained Release of Local Anesthetics

Liposomal Bupivacaine (Exparel)

A sustained-release formulation of the local anesthetic bupivacaine that does not require an indwelling catheter to achieve a long duration of action is available. Bupivacaine extended-release liposome injection (Exparel) consists of bupivacaine encapsulated in DepoFoam. It provides continuous and extended postsurgical analgesia for up to 96 hours and is indicated for administration into the operative site to produce postsurgical analgesia.[153]

Liposomal bupivacaine in its current formulation is available in vials of 10 and 20 mL with a 13.3-mg/mL formulation for a total of 133 mg and 266 mg per vial, respectively. Currently the maximum dose per the manufacturer is 266 mg or 20 mL. However, the total dose depends, too, on other factors such as patient comorbidities, size of the surgical site, and volume needed to cover the affected area. Importantly, if used at a peripheral nerve site, the total dose is halved to 133 mg to avoid local anesthetic toxicity. Different formulations of bupivacaine are not bioequivalent even if the milligram dosage is the same. Therefore it is not possible to convert dosing from any other formulations of bupivacaine to Exparel, and vice versa. Doses are additive, therefore caution must be exercised to avoid LAST.[154]

It is recommended that liposomal bupivacaine be used for only FDA-approved indications until future studies are completed that validate broader indications. Table 10.12 lists the FDA-approved blocks for liposomal bupivacaine use. Despite a favorable analgesic profile, liposomal bupivacaine is currently not indicated for use in the obstetric population. Until more evidence supports its use in patients less than 18 years of age, it should be avoided.[154]

Liposomal bupivacaine, when used in total knee arthroplasty, was not associated with a clinically relevant improvement in inpatient opioid prescription, resource utilization, or opioid-related complications in patients who received modern pain management, including a PNB.[155]

Tumescent Anesthesia

Tumescent local anesthesia (TLA) involves the use of lidocaine, sodium bicarbonate, and epinephrine diluted in normal saline to provide anesthesia for liposuction and other procedures. Tumescent lidocaine anesthesia consists of subcutaneous injection of relatively large volumes (up to 4 L or more) of dilute lidocaine (≤1 g/L) and epinephrine (≤1 mg/L). The term *tumescent* refers to the physical appearance of tissues after the instillation of large volumes. Very low concentrations (0.05–0.1%) of lidocaine mixed with epinephrine are used. Common preparations involve the dilution of 500 to 1000 mg to 1000 mL of normal saline. The volume of tumescent anesthesia solution used is determined by the achievement of palpable tumescence (uniform swelling) of the surgical field. Preliminary estimates for

TABLE 10.11 Guidelines for Application of EMLA

Age and Body Weight Requirement	Maximum Total Dose of EMLA	Maximum Application Area
0–3 mo or <5 kg	1 g	10 cm²
3–12 mo and >5 kg	2 g	20 cm²
1–6 yr and <10 kg	10 g	100 cm²
7–12 yr and >20 kg	20 g	200 cm²

EMLA, Eutectic mixture of local anesthetics.
Data from Kaweski S. Plastic Surgery Educational Foundation Technology Assessment Committee: topical anesthetic creams. *Plast Reconstr Surg.* 2008;121:2161–2165; AstraZenaca. EMLA® product monograph; 2017.

TABLE 10.12 Food and Drug Administration (FDA)–Approved Indications for Liposomal Bupivacaine

FDA-Approved Uses	Non-FDA-Approved Uses
Hemorrhoidectomy	Peripheral nerve blocks
Bunionectomy	Intercostal nerve blocks
Transversus abdominis plane block	Epidural injection
Mammoplasty: local infiltration	Total knee arthroplasty: intraarticular
Total knee arthroplasty: local infiltration	
Inguinal hernia repair: local infiltration	

Adapted from Prabhakar A, Ward CT, Watson M, et al. Liposomal bupivacaine and novel local anesthetic formulations. *Best Pract Res Clin Anaesthesiol.* 2019;33(4):425–432.

maximum safe dosages of tumescent lidocaine are 28 mg/kg without liposuction and 45 mg/kg with liposuction. As a result of delayed systemic absorption, these dosages yield serum lidocaine concentrations below levels associated with mild toxicity and are a nonsignificant risk of harm to patients.[156,157]

The maximum dose of lidocaine in TLA can approach 35 to 55 mg/kg. After tumescent infiltration for liposuction, serum lidocaine concentrations peak between 12 and 16 hours after injection. When tumescent lidocaine without epinephrine is used for endovenous laser therapy, peak serum lidocaine concentrations are observed much earlier, between 1 and 2 hours after injection. Slow administration of more dilute concentrations of local anesthetic decreases the risk of local anesthetic systemic toxicity.[156] Strict adherence to liposuction guidelines has minimized adverse reactions from this technique.[94,158] Specific regional anesthetic techniques and blocks are discussed in detail in Chapters 49 and 50.

SUMMARY

Local anesthetic techniques are becoming more commonplace in outpatient procedures, obstetrics, and pain services. A thorough understanding of the pharmacologic properties of local anesthetics is essential to administer and manage local, topical, and regional anesthesia appropriately. The selection of a drug with an appropriate dose, concentration, time to onset, and duration of action for a selected regional technique is critical for a clinically successful block. A thorough evaluation of the data on local anesthetic systemic toxicity has led to new insights into the clinical presentation, prevention, and treatment of this adverse event. Lipid resuscitation offers a new and efficacious approach to clinical management of this problem. Continued efforts to develop new drugs and formulations of existing agents will broaden our ability to address pain management needs.

REFERENCES

For a complete list of references for this chapter, scan this QR code with any smartphone code reader app, or visit the following URL: http://booksite.elsevier.com/9780323711944/.

11

Opioid and Nonopioid Analgesics

John J. Nagelhout

In the past, opium was used as a topical, intravenous, and inhaled analgesic. One of the earliest uses of opium is found in Greek literature dating from 300 BC. Opium sponges, referred to as soporific sponges, were used for the control of pain as early as the 14th century. An attempt to administer opioids by the intravenous route was attributed to Elsholtz in 1665, approximately 200 years before the invention of the syringe and needle. The first attempt to administer an opium vapor by inhalation was documented in 1778. It was not until 1853, when the syringe and needle were introduced into clinical practice by Wood, that an accurate dose of opioid could be administered intravenously.[1,2]

In 1803, Sertürner reported the isolation of a pure substance from opium that he named morphine, after Morpheus, the Greek god of dreams. Other opium alkaloids were soon discovered: codeine by Robiquet in 1832 and papaverine by Merck in 1848. Abuse of opium and isolated alkaloids led to the synthetic production of potent analgesics. The goal of synthetic manufacture of analgesics was the creation of potent analgesics that would have high specificity for receptors, were not addictive, and were free of side effects. Synthetic production led to the development of opioid agonists, partial agonists, agonists-antagonists, and antagonists.[1,2]

OPIOIDS

Opioid is a term used to refer to a group of drugs, both naturally occurring and synthetically produced, that possess opium- or morphine-like properties. Opioids exert their effects by mimicking naturally occurring endogenous opioid peptides or endorphins. The term *narcotic* is derived from the Greek word *narkõtïkos*, meaning "benumbing," and refers to potent morphine-like analgesics with the potential to produce stupor, insensibility, and dependence. Narcotic is not a useful term in a pharmacologic or clinical discussion because of its legal connotations.

Several systems of classification are used to describe opioids. One common method divides the opioids into four categories: agonists, partial agonists, agonists-antagonists, and antagonists. Another system of categorization is based on the chemical derivation of the opioids and divides them into naturally occurring, semisynthetic, and synthetic compounds, with each group having subgroups (Box 11.1).[3] Other classification systems describe the drugs as either weak or strong or hydrophilic and lipophilic.

The term *opioid* is derived from the word *opium* (from *opos*, Greek for "sap"), an extract from the poppy plant *Papaver somniferum*. The properties of opium are attributable to the 20 different isolated alkaloids, and the alkaloids are divided chemically into two types: phenanthrene (from which morphine and codeine are derived) and benzylisoquinoline (from which papaverine, a nonanalgesic drug, is derived). Modification of the morphine molecule with retention of the five-ring structure results in the semisynthetic drugs heroin and hydromorphone. When the furan ring is removed from morphine, the resulting four-ring synthetic opioid levorphanol is formed. The

phenylpiperidines (e.g., fentanyl) and the diphenylheptane derivatives (e.g., methadone) all have only two of the original five rings of the basic morphine molecular structure. A close relationship exists between the stereochemical structure and potency of opioids, with the levo-isomers being the most potent. All opioids, despite the diverse molecular structures, share an *N*-methylpiperidine moiety, which seems to confer analgesic activity.[1] Fig. 11.1 illustrates the structures of the commonly used opioids.

Opioid drugs produce pharmacologic activity by binding to opiate receptors primarily located in the central nervous system (CNS), supraspinal and spinal, and in several peripheral sites. These include the gastrointestinal (GI) system, vasculature, lung, heart, and immune systems. Supraspinal analgesia occurs through activation of opioid receptors in the medulla, midbrain, and other areas, which causes inhibition of neurons involved in pain pathways. Spinal analgesia occurs by activation of presynaptic opioid receptors, which leads to decreased calcium influx and decreased release of neurotransmitters involved in nociception. Clinically, supraspinal and spinal opioid analgesic mechanisms are synergistic.[3] This explains why opioids such as fentanyl and sufentanil produce more profound analgesia when delivered epidurally than when delivered systemically, despite the similar blood concentrations measured with both routes of administration.[1,4]

Opiate Receptors

Opiate receptors have been deoxyribonucleic acid (DNA) and amino acid sequenced and cloned. The discovery of opioid receptors can be traced back to the 1950s, when pharmaceutic companies were involved in research in anticipation of the development of an effective nonaddictive analgesic. In 1973, the examination of vertebrate species led to the discovery of three opiate receptor classes that mediate analgesia.[5] Questions emerged as to why the receptors existed, and further research led to the hypothesis that the receptors possess endogenous functions.

After the discovery of opiate receptors in the early 1970s, the search began for endogenous substances that were their agonists. In 1975, three such agonists were identified: enkephalins, endorphins, and dynorphins.[5] Each group is derived from a distinct precursor polypeptide and has a characteristic anatomic distribution. By the early 1980s, three precursor molecules to these agonists were identified: proenkephalin, pro-opiomelanocortin, and prodynorphin.[1,5] Opioid peptides share the common amino-terminal sequence of Try-Gly-Gly-Phe-(Met or Leu), which has been labeled the opioid motif or message and is necessary for interaction at the receptor site. The peptide selectivity resides in the carboxy-terminal extension, providing the address.[1] Since then, an additional precursor, pronociceptin, that results in nociception, has been identified. Endomorphins 1 and 2, which are agonists at mu (μ) receptors, have been identified, but the precursor's molecule has not yet been defined.[3] In 1975 Hughes and Kosterlitz[6] identified the first endogenous substance with opioid activity.

BOX 11.1   Classification of Opioids Based on Chemical Class

Naturally Occurring Opium Alkaloids
Phenanthrene Derivatives
Morphine
Codeine
Thebaine

Semisynthetic Phenanthrenes
Oxymorphone (Opana)
Hydromorphone (Dilaudid)
Diacetylmorphine (Heroin)
Hydrocodone (Vicodin)
Oxycodone (Oxycontin)

Antagonist Phenanthrenes
Naloxone
Naltrexone
Methylnaltrexone

Benzylisoquinoline Derivatives
Papaverine

Thebaine Derivatives
Buprenorphine
Oxycodone

Synthetic Opioids
Morphinans
Levorphanol
Nalbuphine (Nubain)
Butorphanol (Buprenex)
Dextromethorphan

Diphenylheptanes (Methadones)
Methadone

Benzomorphans
Pentazocine (Talwin)
Phenazocine

Piperidines
Anilinopiperidine
Loperamide

Phenylpiperidines
Meperidine (Demerol)
Alfentanil
Fentanyl
Sufentanil
Remifentanil

Martin et al.[7] were the first to provide evidence for opiate receptor subtypes (Table 11.1). Their findings provided evidence for the existence of three opiate receptors: mu, kappa (κ), and sigma (σ), named after their respective agonists—morphine, ketocyclazocine, and SK&F 10047. The sigma receptor was later determined not to be an opiate receptor. A delta (δ) receptor was subsequently identified. Each major opioid receptor has a unique anatomic distribution in the brain, spinal cord, and periphery.[8] Their diversity is greatest in their extracellular loops.[1] A fourth receptor has been cloned and named opiate receptor-like (ORL1) or the nociceptin orphanin FQ peptide receptor (NOP). Because this receptor family awaits further clarification as to its role in pain signaling and does not display opioid pharmacology, discussion of this category is not included here.

Opioid receptors are expressed by central and peripheral neurons and by pituitary, adrenal, immune, and ectodermal cells.[9] As noted previously, there are three main types of opioid receptors in the CNS: the mu, delta, and kappa receptors; the endogenous ligands for each receptor are noted in Table 11.2.[10] They are not generally selective to one receptor subtype.[11] Additional receptor types were proposed (sigma, epsilon, orphanin) but are no longer considered opioid receptors. They have several cellular mechanisms. There are seven transmembrane G protein–coupled receptors (GPCR) that show 50% to 70% homology between their genes.[12] They either act to inhibit adenylyl cyclases and cyclic adenosine monophosphate (cAMP) production or they directly interact with different ion channels in the membrane. Opioid receptors can modulate pre- and postsynaptic calcium channels, suppressing calcium influx. This causes attenuation of the excitability of neurons and/or reduces the release of pronociceptive neuropeptides. In addition, opioid receptor activation leads to opening of G protein–coupled inwardly rectifying K+ (GIRK) channels, thereby preventing neuronal excitation and/or propagation of action potentials.[13]

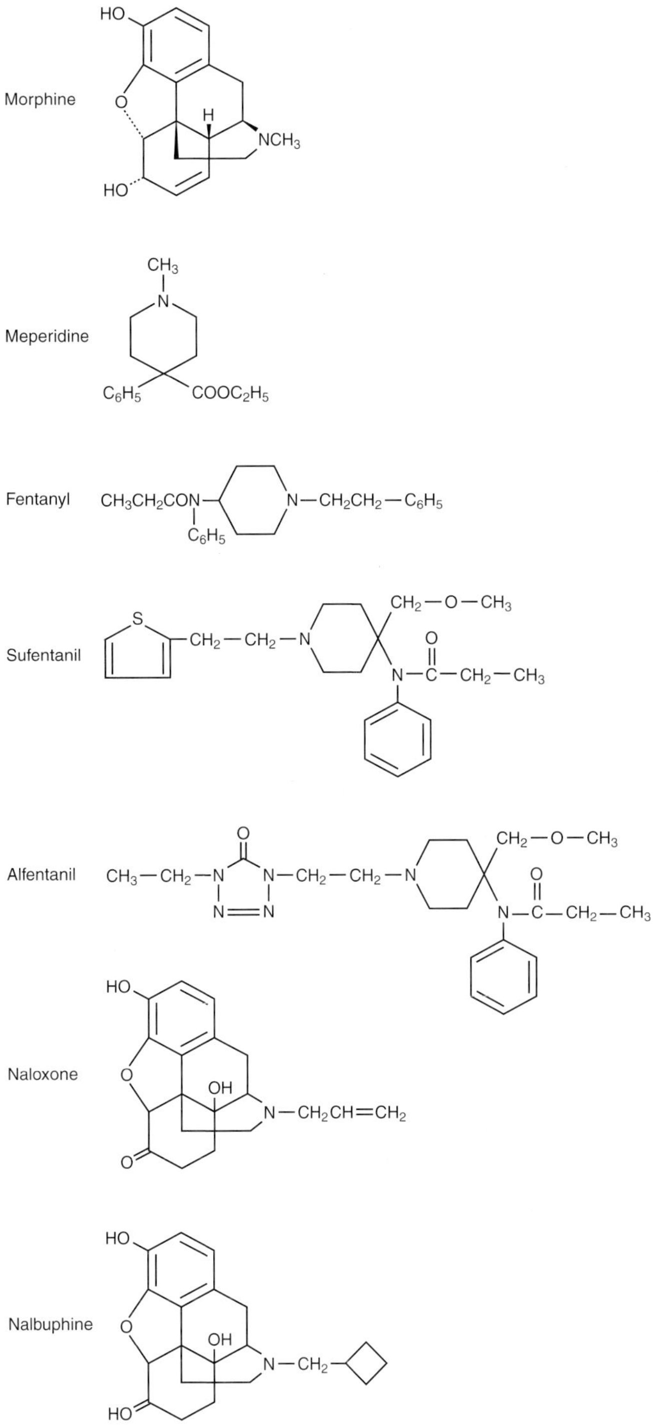

Fig. 11.1 Selected opioid agonists and antagonists used as anesthesia adjunct drugs.

Stimulation of the mu receptor produces supraspinal analgesia, euphoria, a decrease in ventilation, and most of the classic clinical actions of the opioid agonists. Kappa receptor stimulation produces spinal analgesia, sedation, and miosis. Currently, κ-opioid drugs are being investigated for antiinflammatory actions that reduce disease severity of arthritis and other inflammatory diseases.[14–18] The delta receptor is responsible for spinal analgesia, responds to enkephalins, and serves to modulate activity of the mu receptors.[3] Various subtypes of each of the three opiate receptors have been proposed but have not been well defined.[8]

TABLE 11.1   Actions Produced at Each Opioid Receptor Subtype

Effects	Mu (μ) Receptor	Kappa (κ) Receptor	Delta (δ) Receptor
IUPHAR name	MOP	KOP	DOP
Analgesia	Supraspinal, spinal	Supraspinal, spinal	Supraspinal, spinal; modulates mu receptor activity
Cardiovascular	Bradycardia		
Respiratory	Depression	Possible depression	Depression
Central nervous system	Euphoria, sedation, prolactin release, mild hypothermia, catalepsy, indifference to environmental stimulus	Sedation, dysphoria, psychomimetic reactions (hallucinations, delirium)	
Pupil	Miosis	Miosis	
Gastrointestinal	Inhibition of peristalsis, nausea, vomiting		
Genitourinary	Urinary retention	Diuresis (inhibition of vasopressin release)	Urinary retention
Pruritus	Yes		Yes
Physical dependence	Yes	Low abuse potential	Yes
Antishivering		Yes	

DOP, Delta opiate peptide; IUPHAR, International Union of Basic and Clinical Pharmacology; KOP, kappa opiate peptide; MOP, mu opiate peptide.

TABLE 11.2   NC-IUPHAR-Approved Nomenclature for Opioid Peptide Receptors

Current NC-IUPHAR-Approved Nomenclature	Presumed Endogenous Ligand(s)
μ, mu or MOP	β-endorphin enkephalins
	Endomorphin-1 Endomorphin-2
δ, delta or DOP	Enkephalins β-endorphin
κ, kappa or KOP	Dynorphin A Dynorphin B
	α-neoendorphin
NOP	Nociceptin/orphanin FQ
	(N/OFQ)

Receptors activated by opiate drugs respond physiologically to endogenous opioid peptides; they are therefore opioid peptide receptors, the receptor family being designated by the two-letter abbreviation OP. The well-established Greek terminology for opioid receptor types using the descriptors μ, δ, and κ is recommended, but where Greek symbols are not permitted or impractical, the use of mu, delta, or kappa, or MOP, DOP, or KOP is permissible.

No mechanism for the endogenous synthesis of endormorphins has been identified; their status as endogenous ligands for the mu receptor is tentative.

NC-IUPHAR, International Union of Basic and Clinical Pharmacology Committee on Receptor Nomenclature and Drug Classification.
Adapted from Alexander SPH, Christopoulos A, Davenport AP, et al. The concise guide to pharmacology 2019/20: G protein-coupled receptors. Br J Pharmacol. 2019;176(1):S21–S141.

The mechanism of action of opioid drugs is shown in Fig. 11.2. The endogenous ligands for opioid receptors are noted in Table 11.2.

Pharmacokinetics

Pharmacodynamic and pharmacokinetic considerations must be combined to reach an ideal analgesic clinical state. Surgical requirements for analgesic drugs are very different from nonoperative uses. These differences include a much higher analgesic requirement, the coadministration of potent anesthetic and sedative drugs, and the ability to support respiratory effort so that respiratory depression is not an issue until the patient emerges from anesthesia.

In anesthesia, opioids are most commonly administered by the parenteral, intrathecal, and epidural routes. They may also be given by oral, nasal, intramuscular, and transdermal administration. Physiochemical properties of opioids influence their pharmacokinetics. To reach effector sites in the CNS, opioids must cross biologic membranes from the blood to receptors on neural cell membranes. The ability of opioids to cross the blood-brain and placental barriers depends on molecular size, ionization, lipid solubility, and protein binding.[19] The physicochemical characteristics, pharmacokinetic variables, and partition coefficients (octanol and water as a measure of lipid solubility) for several of the commonly used opioid analgesics are summarized in Table 11.3.

The wide variation in dosing of the opioids in anesthesia, depending on the patient and surgical situation, leads to vastly different durations even with the same drug. Fentanyl, for example, can last from 30 minutes to 18 to 24 hours, depending on how it is administered and how much is given. The pharmacokinetic parameters are important, but the context of how they are used in clinical practice is a major factor in the ultimate patient response.

Opioids are modestly absorbed orally. Some opioids undergo extensive first-pass metabolism in the liver, greatly reducing their bioavailability and therapeutic efficacy after oral dosing. Orally administered morphine has limited absorption from the GI tract. Drugs with greater lipophilicity are better absorbed through nasal and buccal mucosa and the skin.

When small doses of the opioids are used, the effects are usually terminated by redistribution rather than metabolism. Larger or multiple doses or continuous infusions are much more dependent on metabolism for offset.[19] Like most drugs, opioids are usually metabolized in the liver to more polar and less active or inactive compounds by both phase 1 and phase 2 processes. Some opioids such as morphine have active metabolites such as morphine-6-glucuronide that can prolong the therapeutic effects of the parent compound. The meperidine metabolite, normeperidine, is neurotoxic and may accumulate in the elderly or in patients with decreased renal or hepatic function. This has led to a decline in its use. It is avoided in the elderly or patients with renal or hepatic dysfunction and where chronic use may be needed.[1]

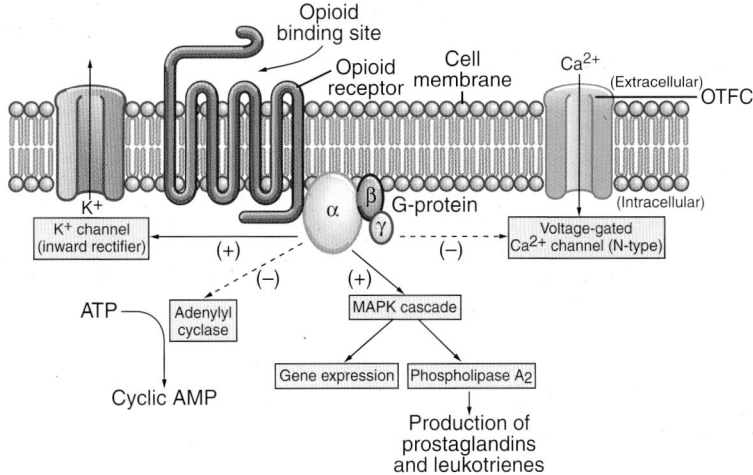

Fig. 11.2 Opioid mechanisms of action. The endogenous ligand or drug binds to the opioid receptor and activates the G protein (three distinct protein subunits), resulting in multiple effects that are primarily inhibitory. The activities of adenylate cyclase and the voltage-dependent Ca^{2+} channels are depressed. The inwardly rectifying K^+ channels and mitogen-activated protein kinase (MAPK) cascade are activated. *AMP*, Adenosine monophosphate; *ATP*, adenosine triphosphate; *OTFC*, oral transmucosal fentanyl citrate. (From Hemmings Jr. HC, Egan TD. *Pharmacology and Physiology for Anesthesia.* 2nd ed. Philadelphia: Elsevier, 2019:334.)

TABLE 11.3 Physicochemical Characteristics and Pharmacokinetics

Opioids	pK_a	Percent Nonionized	Protein Binding (%)	V_c (L/kg)	V_d (L/kg)	Clearance (mL/min/kg)	Elimination Half-Life (hr)	Partition Coefficient (Octanol/Water)
Morphine	7.9	23	35	0.23	2.8	15.5	1.7–3.3	1
Meperidine	8.5	7	70	0.6	2.6	22.7	3–5	21
Methadone	9.3	N/A	85	0.15	3.4	1.6	23	115
Fentanyl	8.4	8.5	84	0.85	4	13	2–4	820
Sufentanil	8	20	93	0.1	2	12	2–3	1750
Alfentanil	6.5	89	92	0.12	0.6	5	1–2	130
Remifentanil	7.26	58	93	0.1–0.2	0.39	41	0.1–0.3	N/A
Butorphanol	8.6	17	80	0.1	5	38.6	2.65	140
Nalbuphine	8.71	N/A	N/A	0.45	4.8	23.1	3.7	N/A

N/A, Not applicable; V_c, volume of distribution central compartment; V_d, volume of distribution.

The opioid drugs are metabolized by the usual cytochrome enzymes, including CYP3A4, CYP2D6, and CYP2B6.[20–22] Remifentanil was designed with an ester group in its structure and is metabolized by hydrolysis in the plasma and tissues by nonspecific esterases. Remifentanil has a low volume of distribution and a large clearance, which results in a short half-life of approximately 10 minutes. Opioids and their metabolites are excreted primarily by the kidneys and secondarily by the biliary system and GI tract.[23] Clinicians become very adept in the art of administering opioids by bolus, incremental injection, or infusion to maximize analgesia during surgery as needed, yet allowing for safe and rapid recovery and residual postoperative analgesia.

Pharmacogenetics

The wide variations in dosing and patient responses have both pharmacodynamic and pharmacokinetic causes. Pharmacogenetics appears to be an important factor as well. Opioids have a narrow therapeutic index, calling for a fine balance between optimizing pain control and sedative effects (without causing respiratory depression), while at the same time recognizing great variability from patient to patient in response and dose requirements. Genetic factors regulating their pharmacokinetics (metabolizing enzymes, transporters) and pharmacodynamics

(receptors and signal transduction) contribute to this variability and to the possibility of adverse drug effects, toxicity, or therapeutic failure of pharmacotherapy. Significant variation in conversion of the prodrug codeine into the active metabolite morphine has been noted.[24] Polymorphisms in CYP2D6 are responsible for the wide variations among different populations.[25]

The clinical use of opioids involves knowledge regarding patient characteristics, their perception, severity, and likely duration of pain, lifestyle variables such as smoking habits and alcohol intake, and opioid drug and dosing regimen selection.[25] Other factors affecting pharmacokinetics and pharmacodynamics of opioids include age, body weight, renal failure, hepatic failure, cardiopulmonary bypass, acid-base changes, and hemorrhagic shock.

In adults, advancing age requires lower opioid doses for the treatment of postsurgical pain. Pediatric doses can vary widely as well. In addition, in relatively similar patient groups, dosage requirements vary. Aubrun et al.[26] reported that in more than 3000 patients morphine dosage requirements for postoperative hip replacement therapy varied almost 40-fold. Large variabilities have been reported in cancer patients receiving morphine via various routes.[25] Variability is contributed to by inherent pain sensitivity, tolerance, and other factors,

BOX 11.2 Pharmacogenetics and Opiates

Cytochrome Enzyme Subtype	Clinical Outcome
CYP2D6	Codeine is a prodrug that is metabolized to its active form, morphine. Extensive metabolizers may produce dangerously high levels of morphine. See Chapter 6. Tramadol is metabolized to its M1 metabolite, which is six times more potent than the parent compound. Hydrocodone effectiveness can vary widely depending on the genetic status of the patient, which influences mu receptor binding. Oxycodone has significant variation and effectiveness depending on the metabolic genotype.
CYP3A4	Fentanyl, buprenorphine, and methadone metabolism vary according to the activity of this enzyme group.
CYP3B6	Women generally have a higher activity of these enzymes, which may alter the metabolism of methadone and propofol.
Mu and kappa receptor variants	Influence the dosing and efficacy of several clinical opioids.

Adapted from Trescot AM. Genetics and implications in perioperative analgesia. *Best Pract Res Clin Anaesthesiol.* 2014;28(2):153–166; Gray K, Adhikary SD, Janicki P. Pharmacogenomics of analgesics in anesthesia practice: a current update of literature. *J Anaesthesiol Clin Pharmacol.* 2018;34(2):155–160.

BOX 11.3 Common Clinical Effects of Opioid Agonists

Acute	Chronic
Analgesia	Tolerance
Respiratory depression	Physical dependence
Sedation	Constipation
Euphoria	
Dysphoria	
Vasodilation	
Bradycardia	
Cough suppression	
Miosis	
Nausea and vomiting	
Skeletal muscle rigidity	
Smooth muscle spasm	
Constipation	
Urinary retention	
Biliary spasm	
Pruritus, rash	
Antishivering (meperidine only)	
Histamine release	
Hormonal effects	

including pharmacogenetics influencing the clinical pharmacology of opioids.[27,28] Some pharmacogenetic influences on the clinical performance of opioids are noted in Box 11.2.

Clinical Effects of Opioids

The common clinical effects of opioid agonists are listed in Box 11.3.

Central Nervous System Effects: Analgesia, Sedation, and Euphoria

Opiate analgesia results from actions in the CNS, spinal cord, and peripheral sites. They are most effective for visceral continuous dull pain; however, at high doses they will relieve any pain. They are less effective against neuropathic pain that requires chronic multimodal therapy.[29–31] The sedative and euphoric actions contribute to the feeling of well-being in awake patients. The analgesic effects of opioids come from their ability to (1) directly inhibit the ascending transmission of nociception information from the spinal cord dorsal horn and (2) activate pain control pathways that descend from the midbrain, via the rostral ventromedial medulla to the spinal cord dorsal horn.[1] The effect of opioids on electroencephalographic and evoked-potential activity is minimal, therefore neurophysiologic monitoring can be conducted during opioid anesthetic techniques. Opiate administration can indirectly cause an increase in intracranial pressure if respiratory depression-induced hypercarbia occurs. They have variable effects on cerebral vascular tone depending on the background anesthetic present. Possible untoward CNS effects when the opioids are used in neurosurgery are easily managed by controlling ventilation and maintaining adequate blood pressures.[32] The comparative potency of the opioid agonists that are used in anesthesia is as follows: sufentanil > fentanyl = remifentanil > alfentanil.

The sedative and euphoric effects of the opiates vary depending on the agent. Patients will exhibit sedation and euphoria that are different with μ- versus κ-agonists. Dysphoria can occur and appears more prominent with drugs that have strong kappa receptor effects or when opioids are taken in the absence of pain. Physical and psychological dependence occur with repeat administration as evidenced by physical withdrawal with abstinence and drug-seeking behaviors.[1,33] The opiates are not anesthetics, so awareness under anesthesia is a concern when even high doses of opiates are used.[34,35] Both acute and chronic tolerance occur with the opiates. Cross-tolerance among μ-agonists will occur. Usually a decrease in duration is noted first, followed eventually by a decrease in effect. The mechanism of tolerance is complex and does not appear to be due to a change in receptor number. Receptor internalization, activation of N-methyl-D-aspartate (NMDA) receptors, second messenger changes, and G protein uncoupling may all play a role. Hyperalgesia, which may result from chronic administration, may be related to these same mechanisms.[1,33]

Respiratory Depression

All opiate agonists produce a dose-dependent depression of respirations via effects on mu and delta receptors in the respiratory centers in the brainstem. They reduce the responsiveness within the respiratory centers to increasing carbon dioxide and decreasing oxygen levels. Thus higher partial pressure of carbon dioxide (PCO_2) levels are required to maintain adequate respiration. Stated in pharmacologic terms, they produce a shift to the right in the CO_2 response curve for respiration. Respiratory rate is affected first, and a classic "narcotized" patient will take slow deep breaths. As doses increase, apnea is produced. Because both analgesia and respiratory depression are mediated via the same receptors, reversal of respiratory depression with antagonists such as naloxone also reverses analgesia. The goal of most clinical anesthetics is to leave some residual analgesia without respiratory depression upon emergence to address postoperative pain.[1]

Miosis

Miosis, or pinpoint pupils, is a prominent action of opioids and is usually present under general anesthesia as a result of the high doses of high-potency opiates used. Minimal tolerance develops to this effect. It is produced by effects in the pupillary reflex arc. Opiate depression of inhibitory γ-aminobutyric acid (GABA) interneurons leads to stimulation of the Edinger-Westphal nucleus, which sends a parasympathetic signal via the ciliary ganglion to the oculomotor nerve to constrict the pupil.[1] Clinicians note the degree of miosis as somewhat indicative of the presence of opiates.

Antitussive Effects

The opiates produce cough suppression via a depressant effect on the cough center in the medulla. Protective glottal reflexes are not affected. Although they all produce this effect, codeine and heroin are especially good suppressants. D-isomers such as dextromethorphan are also effective. The clinical use of opiates can help patients better tolerate airway devices and ventilators.[36]

Nausea and Vomiting

The emetic effect of the opioids is complex. They elicit nausea and vomiting by stimulating the chemoreceptor trigger zone in the area postrema of the medulla. The dominant receptors in this area are serotonin type 3 (5-HT3) and dopamine type 2 (D2). A vestibular component is also probable because the incidence is much higher in ambulatory patients. Nausea and vomiting are rare in the preoperative area and operating room where patients are recumbent. A separate action with higher repeat doses can have an antiemetic effect by depressing the vomiting center. Clinically, when opiates are used as part of the anesthetic plan, there is an increased incidence of postoperative nausea and vomiting.[37] The effect is less frequent with repeat doses although individual patient response is highly variable. Fig. 11.3 depicts the centers in the brain involved with nausea and vomiting and the types of receptors involved.

Cardiac Effects

The usual result of anesthetic use of opioids in healthy patients is bradycardia with little effect on blood pressure. Bradycardia results from medullary vagal stimulation.[1] All opioids induce some degree of dose-dependent peripheral vasodilation. Myocardial contractility, baroreceptor function, and autonomic responsiveness are not affected. Opiate anesthesia is often used in patients with cardiovascular compromise because of this minimal depression. Much of the hypotension produced by morphine, codeine, and meperidine is attributed to histamine release, which is absent with fentanyl, sufentanil, alfentanil, and remifentanil. Histamine$_1$ (H$_1$) and H$_2$ antagonists, when combined, block the cardiovascular effects of vasodilation, tachycardia, and hypotension that result.[19]

Opioids usually produce an antidiuretic effect. Opioids that are agonists at kappa receptors can cause diuresis. They decrease tone at the bladder detrusor muscle and constrict the urinary sphincter. This results in urinary retention. Urinary retention is a common side effect with intrathecal and epidural opioid administration.

Muscle Rigidity

Opioids have no major effects on nerve conduction at the neuromuscular junction or at the skeletal muscle membrane. A generalized hypertonus of skeletal muscle can be produced by large intravenous doses of most opioid agonists. Although morphine can produce rigidity, the problem is most often associated with fentanyl, alfentanil, sufentanil, and remifentanil. The difficulty is caused in part by loss of chest-wall compliance and by constriction of pharyngeal and laryngeal muscles. It becomes very difficult to ventilate the patient unless the rigidity is reversed. It is commonly referred to as tight chest or truncal rigidity. This effect most often occurs during anesthesia induction when high doses of potent opiates are administered rapidly. Remifentanil, which is administered by infusion, may be especially prone to producing this effect. Administration of nitrous oxide may increase the frequency.[38] Opioid-induced muscle rigidity is thought to be mediated by central mu receptors interacting with dopamine and GABA pathways. This

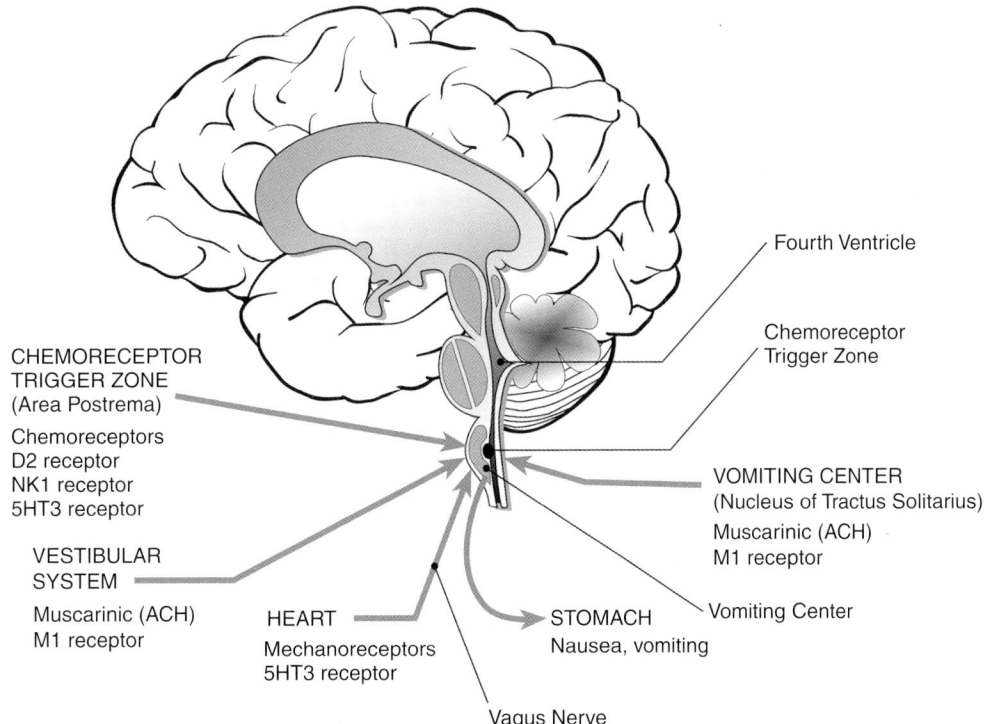

Fig. 11.3 The vomiting center and chemoreceptor trigger zone are shown. Inputs from sites outside the central nervous system are noted. Type and location of various receptors involved in nausea and vomiting are given. Antiemetic drugs act on these receptor targets. *5HT3*, Serotonin; *ACH*, acetylcholine; *D2*, dopamine receptors; *M1*, muscarinic; *NK1*, neurokinin.

rigidity is easily reduced or eliminated by the administration of neuro-muscular blocking agents or naloxone.[39]

Pruritus

Opiates frequently produce a rash, itching, and a feeling of warmth in the "blush" area of the face, upper chest, and arms. This occurs with both histamine and nonhistamine-releasing drugs and is especially prominent with neuraxial administration. The mechanism appears to be through central mu receptors and not local histamine release.[40] Pruritus can be treated with antagonists such as naloxone or naltrexone; however, they also reverse analgesia. Nalbuphine, droperidol, antihistamines, and ondansetron may also be effective. Many clinical pain services have established protocols to treat this problem.[41,42] The mixed μ/κ-opioid partial agonists seem to be the most effective medications that relieve neuraxial opioid-induced itch while preserving analgesia.[43] In a 2016 review it was noted that nalbuphine is superior to placebo, diphenhydramine, naloxone, or propofol in treating opioid-induced pruritus and should be used as a first-line treatment.[44]

Gastrointestinal Effects

Opioids have multiple effects on GI function. They decrease gastric motility and intestinal propulsive activity, prolong gastric emptying time, and reduce secretory activity throughout the GI system. This leads to the common problems of opiate-induced constipation and postoperative ileus. The pharmacologic treatment approach to this problem led to the development of peripherally acting μ-opioid receptor antagonists (PAMORAs). Naldemedine (Symproic), alvimopan (Entereg), methylnaltrexone (Relistor), and naloxegol (Movantik) are locally acting opiate receptor antagonists approved for use in treating these GI side effects. They do not cross biologic compartments due to solubility barriers and therefore work locally in the GI system but do not affect centrally produced analgesia.[45,46] Lubiprostone (Amitiza), a bicyclic fatty acid that activates intestinal chloride channel-2 (ClC-2) in the small intestine, helps to increase fluid secretion and gut motility.[47–49]

Opioids produce a dose-dependent increase in biliary duct pressure and sphincter of Oddi tone via opioid receptor–mediated mechanisms. They also increase urinary sphincter tone. This has led to a few clinical concerns. The use of opiates for the treatment of biliary or renal colic may be compromised by this action. Meperidine, which produces this effect the least among opiate agonists or nonsteroidal antiinflammatory drugs (NSAIDs), is considered the agent of choice for this situation.[50] In anesthesia, the use of opiates during surgery may produce false-positive cholangiograms. The clinical relevance of this effect is questionable since opiates are used routinely without problems.

Endocrine Effects

Opiates reduce the stress response to surgery and have an immunosuppressant effect.[3] Endocrinologic effects of opioids include the release of vasopressin and inhibition of the stress-induced release of corticotropin and gonadotropins from the pituitary. Release of thyrotropin (i.e., thyroid stimulating hormone) from the adenohypophysis is also inhibited. Basal metabolic rate and temperature may also be decreased in patients receiving chronic opioids, although animal data indicate that acute administration can either systemically or intrathecally increase temperature. Opioids slightly decrease body temperature by resetting the equilibrium point of temperature regulation in the hypothalamus.[1]

Opioids and Cancer

Although controversial, mounting data have implicated inhalational anesthesia and opioid analgesia as independent risk factors for cancer recurrence. Conversely, local-regional anesthesia and propofol-based total intravenous anesthesia have been promoted as having potential "chemopreventative" effects. The immune system plays an important role in controlling cancer. Factors that influence protective antitumor immunity have a significant impact on the course of malignant disease. Opioids are essential for the management of cancer pain, and preclinical studies indicate that opioids have the potential to influence tumor immune surveillance mechanisms. It has been suggested that opioids have a protumor action and may have negative effects on cancer survival. This is due to actions that may promote cancer cell proliferation and migration, immunosuppression, inflammation, and angiogenesis or neovascularization. Opioids also inhibit the function of natural killer cells. A definitive conclusion has not been reached. Opioid type and dose, the underlying disease pathology, and organs involved are important factors.[51–53] See Chapter 46 for a further discussion of anesthesia and cancer recurrence.

Neuraxial Effects

The epidural and intrathecal routes have become common for the administration of pain medication. Opioids delivered by epidural or subarachnoid routes behave differently in onset, duration, and side effects than the same drugs given systemically. Pain that is unresponsive to systemic opioids may respond to the same drugs given centrally, reducing some side effects while increasing the incidence of others. Systemic opioids suppress nociception in lamina II and V cells of the dorsal horn of the spinal cord, leaving lamina IV and VI cells (which mediate nonnociceptive information) relatively unaffected.[54]

Spinal administration of opioids is a selective and potent means of producing analgesia. Intrathecal administration allows injection of the opioids directly into the cerebrospinal fluid (CSF), a more efficient method of delivering the drug to the spinal cord opiate receptors. The analgesic response is the result of activity at spinal opiate receptors, especially kappa receptors in the substantia gelatinosa, lamina II of the dorsal horn.[54] Opioids can be given with local anesthetics or other adjuncts intraoperatively at the initiation of spinal anesthesia or postoperatively for pain control.[55] Side effects with spinal administration are similar to those described previously with systemic administration, except that pruritus and urinary retention occur with much greater frequency. Less lipid-soluble agents such as morphine and hydromorphone produce a delayed ventilatory depression, the result of migration of opioid via the CSF to the midbrain vestibular centers.

Respiratory depression is the most common serious complication associated with intrathecally and epidurally administered opioids. Two different levels of respiratory depression can occur after neuraxial morphine administration. An early phase observed soon after administration reflects rapid systemic absorption and is similar to parenteral dosing. A later, more insidious depression that occurs over a period of 8 to 12 hours has been related to rostral flow of CSF and delivery of morphine to the brainstem respiratory center.[56] Awareness of delayed respiratory depression has resulted in increased monitoring of patients and dose reductions, thereby greatly reducing the incidence of serious respiratory depression to that seen with patient-controlled analgesia (PCA) opioids.

Generalized pruritus has been observed with neuraxial morphine and to a lesser extent with other opioids. Mild itching, usually involving the face or chest, is common; however, the intensity of itching can become so annoying that it interferes with sleep. Pruritus is commonly seen with opioids that do not release histamine, such as fentanyl and sufentanil. Pruritus can be treated with antihistamines or with opiate receptor partial agonists or antagonists. The incidence of postoperative nausea and vomiting increases for patients treated with neuraxial opioids. Nausea may result either from the rostral spread of the drug in the spinal fluid to the brainstem or vascular uptake and delivery to the chemoreceptor trigger zone in the area postrema of the medulla.

Urinary retention after spinal opioid analgesia has been related to inhibition of sacral parasympathetic outflow, which results in relaxation of the bladder detrusor muscle and an inability to relax the sphincter.[54]

Opioids with a higher lipid solubility (see Table 11.3) tend to be rapidly absorbed into the spinal tissues after central administration, resulting in a faster onset of action. However, higher lipid solubility is associated with a small area of distribution of the drug along the length of the spinal cord and therefore a more limited area of analgesia.[4] Higher lipid solubility is also associated with faster clearance of the drug out of the epidural and intrathecal space, resulting in a shorter duration of action and higher blood concentrations of the opioid.[54,56] Spinal opioids are advantageous in selective analgesia, which occurs in the absence of motor and sympathetic blockade.

Epidural anesthesia and analgesia have been successfully used in obstetric patients and surgical patients. Epidural doses of opioids, however, are much higher than doses of opioids for intrathecal use. Small portions of epidural opioids cross the dura, enter the CSF, and penetrate spinal tissue in amounts proportional to their lipid solubility. The remaining drug is absorbed by the vasculature, producing plasma levels comparable to those after intramuscular injections and providing supraspinal analgesia.[56] Neuraxial administration of opioids is a selective and potent means of producing analgesia in many surgical and obstetric procedures.[57] Table 11.4 gives neuraxial opioid dosages.[54,56]

Opioid Techniques and Delivery

In clinical practice, opioids are used to relieve pain during monitored anesthesia care, as regional anesthesia, and as a component of balanced anesthesia, as well as a primary component of general anesthesia. The inclusion of opioids reduces pain and anxiety, decreases somatic and autonomic responses to airway manipulation, improves hemodynamic stability, lowers requirements for inhaled anesthetic agents, and provides postoperative analgesia.[58]

The most common method of administering opioids in the practice of anesthesia is intermittent bolus injection, which, although effective for many procedures, produces wide swings in drug plasma concentration. Intermittent periods of deep and light anesthesia are produced. Continuous opioid infusion results in plasma concentration that can be maintained more accurately and consistently. Continuous infusion of opioids is associated with hemodynamic stability, reduces the total necessary dose of opioids, and decreases the need for opioid reversal agents.

Continuous intravenous administration involves the infusion of a loading dose that fills the volume of distribution, followed by continuous drug replacement that keeps the volume of distribution filled as the drug is eliminated.[59]

$$\text{Loading dose (mcg/kg)} = V_d \text{ (mL/kg)} \times C_p \text{ (mcg/mL)}$$

$$\text{Loading dose (mcg/kg)} = V_d \text{ (mL/kg)} \times C_p \text{ (mcg/mL)}$$

where V_d is volume of distribution, C_p is plasma concentration, and Cl is drug clearance. See Table 11.3 for the V_d and Cl of various opioids.

The rate of continuous infusion does not remain constant, but rather is adjusted to meet the patient's needs and to control varying surgical stimuli. The volume of distribution is decreased for patients with hypovolemia and trauma, and for geriatric patients. Factors such as enzyme induction, hepatic failure, and adjunctive drug use are also considered. Table 11.5 provides dose ranges for continuous infusions.

Continuous intravenous infusion can be administered by gravity flow with a manual control device (e.g., Buretrol), an infusion pump, or a syringe pump. Syringe pumps are advantageous because they are programmed to administer drug in units of micrograms per kilogram per minute. Some advantages of continuous infusion techniques are listed in Box 11.4.

Nonparenteral routes of opioid delivery are also used. Fentanyl is the prototypic opioid for transdermal application. Transdermal administration of fentanyl does not require cooperation from the patient; in addition, first-phase hepatic metabolism is not a factor, and the route does not produce discomfort. Currently available formulations permit delivery of 25 to 100 mcg/hour for 24 to 72 hours. The transdermal fentanyl patch provides a relatively constant plasma concentration for 72 hours. It is not currently recommended for use in managing postoperative pain.

Rapid-onset opioids provide new options for effective management of pain. There are various formulations of transmucosal immediate-release fentanyl and, although they were originally developed and approved for use in children before painful procedures, are now used in opioid-tolerant adult patients with breakthrough cancer pain. The formulation options include oral lozenge, buccal tablet, buccal film, sublingual tablet, nasal spray, and a sublingual spray; each has practical considerations that

TABLE 11.4 Doses of Neuraxial Opioids*

Opioid	Single Dose	Infusion Rate
Epidural		
Morphine	2–5 mg	0.1–1 mg/h
Meperidine	25–50 mg	5–20 mg/h
Methadone	5 mg	0.3–0.5 mg/h
Fentanyl	50–100 mcg	25–100 mcg/h
Sufentanil	25–50 mcg	10–50 mcg/h
Butorphanol	2–4 mg	0.2–0.4 mg/h
Subarachnoid		
Morphine	0.25–0.3 mg	
Meperidine	10 mg	
Fentanyl	10–20 mcg	
Sufentanil	5–10 mcg	

*Doses adjusted for age and level of regional injection.

TABLE 11.5 Infusion Rates*

Opioid	Induction (mcg/kg)	Maintenance (mcg/kg/min)
Fentanyl	5–10	0.01–0.05
Sufentanil	1–30	0.005–0.015
Alfentanil	8–100	0.5–3
Remifentanil	0.5–1	0.05–2

*Doses will vary depending on coadministered drugs, patient characteristics, and surgical procedure.

BOX 11.4 Advantages of Continuous Opioid Infusion

- Hemodynamic stability
- Decreased side effects
- Reduced need for opioid-reversal agents
- Reduced use of vasopressor drugs
- Suppression of cortisol and vasopressin response to cardiopulmonary bypass: stress-free anesthesia
- Reduced total dosage of opioids
- Decreased recovery time

vary with the product and route of administration.[60,61] All have the common advantage of rapid entry into the systemic circulation via transmucosal absorption, avoiding hepatic and intestinal first-pass metabolism, which allows for a rapid onset of action that rivals intravenous injections. A high incidence of pruritus is a problematic side effect with transmucosal administration. Fentanyl buccal tablet (Fentora) is indicated for the management of breakthrough pain in cancer patients who are tolerant to 60 mg or greater of oral morphine equivalents.[62]

The Food and Drug Administration (FDA) has approved a nasal spray formulation of fentanyl (Lazanda) for management of breakthrough pain in adult cancer patients who are already receiving and are tolerant to opioid therapy. Nasal administration of sufentanil preoperatively in the pediatric patient has also been studied. After administration, the children remained calm, and some experienced somewhat decreased ventilatory compliance. Recovery room time was not increased, and the highest incidence of nausea and vomiting occurred in the group that received the highest dose of sufentanil. Nasal butorphanol is currently available and is widely used in the management of migraine headaches. Table 11.6 compares dosages for various routes of opioid administration.[63]

INDIVIDUAL OPIOIDS

Agonists
Naturally Occurring Opioids

Morphine. Morphine, the prototype for opioid agonists, is the most abundant alkaloid in raw opium. The primary therapeutic use

TABLE 11.6   Opioid Dose Comparisons

Opioid	Route	Onset	Peak	Duration of Action	Half-Life
Morphine`	PO	60 min	30–60 min	4–5 hr	Neonates 4.5–13 hr
	IM	30–60 min	30–60 min	4–5 hr	Adults 3–5 hr
	IV	20 min	30–60 min	4–5 hr	
	Epidural	60–90 min	30–60 min	8–24 hr	
Codeine	PO	30–60 min	60–90 min	4–6 hr	2.5–3.5 hr
	IM	10–30 min	30–60 min	4–6 hr	2.5–3.5 hr
Hydromorphone	IV	15–30 min	30–90 min	4–5 hr	1–3 hr
Oxycodone	PO	10–15 min	30–60 min	4–5 hr	3.2–4.5 hr
Methadone	PO	30–60 min	30–60 min	6–8 hr	15–30 hr
	IV	5–10 min	15–20 min	4–6 hr	15–30 hr
Meperidine	PO	10–15 min	30–60 min	2–4 hr	2.5–4 hr
	IM	10–15 min	30–60 min	2–4 hr	2.5–4 hr
	IV	5 min	30–60 min	2–4 hr	2.5–4 hr
Alfentanil	IV	Immediate	Immediate		1.5 hr
Fentanyl	Transmucosal	5–15 min	20–30 min	Related to blood levels	6.6 hr
	IM	7–15 min	20–30 min	1–2 hr	2–4 hr
	IV	2–5 min	20–30 min	0.5–1 hr	2–4 hr
	Epidural	20–30 min		2–3 hr	2–4 hr
Remifentanil	IV	1 min	1 min	5–10 min	9 min
Sufentanil	IV	1–3 min		Dose dependent	6 hr
Tramadol	PO	60 min	120 min	9 hr	2–3 hr
Buprenorphine	IM	10–30 min	60 min	6 hr	2–3 hr
	IV	10–30 min	60 min	6 hr	2.5–4 hr
Butorphanol	IM	10–15 min	30–60 min	3–4 hr	2.5–4 hr
	IV	Immediate	30–60 min	3–4 hr	2.6–2.8 hr
Dezocine	IM	15–30 min	60 min	4–6 hr	2.6–2.8 hr
	IV	15–30 min	60 min	4–6 hr	3.5–5 hr
Nalbuphine	IM		30 min		3.5–5 hr
	IV		1–3 min		2–3 hr
Pentazocine	PO	15–30 min		4–5 hr	2–3 hr
	IM	15–30 min		2–3 hr	2–3 hr
	IV	2–3 min		2–3 hr	Neonates 1.2–3 hr
Naloxone	IM	5 min	5–15 min	20–60 min	Adults 1–1.5 hr
	IV	2 min	5–15 min	20–60 min	10.8 hr
Nalmefene	IM	5–15 min	120 min	8 hr	10.8 hr
	IV	2 min	2–3 min	8 hr	6–10 hr
Naltrexone	PO	45–60 min	60 min	24–72 hr	

IM, Intramuscularly; *IV,* intravenously; *PO,* by mouth.

of morphine is the abatement of moderate to severe pain. It is more effective in relieving continuous dull pain than sharp intermittent pain. Morphine can be administered via the intramuscular, intravenous, subcutaneous, oral, intrathecal, and epidural routes. Effects of intravenous morphine on the time course of sedation and analgesia occur with sedation first, followed by analgesia.[64] Morphine-induced sedation therefore should not be considered as an indicator of appropriate analgesia. When given intrathecally, morphine has the longest duration of action of the specific opioids. Morphine is among the least lipophilic of the opioids, resulting in slow penetration of biologic membranes, less accumulation in lipid membranes or fatty tissues, and slower onset.

Morphine undergoes phase 2 glucuronide conjugation in the liver at both the 3 position (which produces morphine-3-glucuronide [M3G]) and the 6 position (which produces morphine-6-glucuronide [M6G]).[65] As a result of the active metabolite, M6G, morphine appears to produce a more prolonged effect, often excessive sedation, in the patient with renal failure. Within the CNS, M6G metabolite is more potent than the parent drug, whereas M3G metabolite is inactive.[65,66] The greater hydrophilicity of M6G than the parent drug normally impedes its passage into the CNS. However, after chronic administration or in patients with renal failure, M6G (at a high blood level) can enter the CNS.

Morphine produces a nonimmunologic release of histamine from tissue mast cells, resulting in local itching, redness, or hives near the site of intravenous injection or generalized flushing. When sufficient histamine is released, the patient may exhibit signs of decreased systemic vascular resistance, hypotension, and tachycardia. Localized histamine release after a morphine injection is not uncommon. Morphine is primarily used for preoperative or postoperative pain relief. The delayed onset and peak effects and large patient variability make it less useful for intraoperative use than fentanyl and its analogs.

Codeine. Considered a weak opioid, codeine is generally not used for treatment of severe pain. Approximately 10% of the administered dose of codeine is O-demethylated to morphine, which accounts for most of its analgesic activity.[57] It has good antitussive activity, but on a weight basis, codeine is a less potent antitussive than morphine. Combinations of codeine with acetaminophen remain very popular as prescribed analgesics. Codeine is contraindicated in children due to the possibility of excessive respiratory depression. Codeine toxicity due to extensive conversion of the prodrug into morphine is discussed in the pharmacogenetics section and in Chapter 6.

Semisynthetic Opioids

Hydromorphone. Derived from morphine in the 1920s, hydromorphone has a pharmacokinetic profile similar to that of morphine, but it is more potent. Hydromorphone is absorbed from the oral, rectal, and parenteral sites. Because of its lipid solubility, it is sometimes used instead of morphine for epidural or spinal administration when a wide area of analgesia is needed.[67] Studies performed on parenteral hydromorphone relative to morphine tend to demonstrate similar analgesia and side effect profiles. Because of the lack of any known active metabolites, it is often recommended for patients with renal failure.[1] It is available in high potency and sustained release preparations.

Synthetic Opioids

Methadone. Introduced in the 1940s, methadone is used primarily for relief of chronic pain, treatment of opioid abstinence syndromes, and treatment of opioid use disorders. Compared to other common opioids, it is well absorbed orally and produces less euphoria. Supplied as a racemic mixture of two optical isomers, most of methadone's

activity comes from the l-isomer. Unlike most opioids, it has a long half-life, allowing for less frequent dosing. It has a prolonged effect in part due to extensive protein binding (90%) with slow release and a lower intrinsic ability of the liver to metabolize it. It also has the advantage of a high bioavailability and no active metabolites. Disadvantages include accumulation and a longer time to reach steady state than other opioids.[68]

Meperidine. Meperidine is a synthetic mu receptor agonist. It is structurally similar to atropine and has an atropine-like antispasmodic effect. After demethylation in the liver, meperidine is partially metabolized to normeperidine, which is half as analgesic as meperidine but lowers the seizure threshold and induces CNS excitability. Normeperidine's elimination half-life is significantly longer than that of meperidine. With accumulation of normeperidine, subjects may experience a CNS excitation characterized by tremors, muscle twitches, and seizures. Due to accumulation of normeperidine, limitations on its use should be considered in patients with renal failure, the elderly, and for chronic use in cancer patients who may require high doses. There is a significant drug interaction that can occur between meperidine and the first-generation monoamine oxidase (MAO)–inhibiting drugs isocarboxazid (Marplan, others), phenelzine (Nardil, others), and tranylcypromine (Parnate, others). Hyperthermia, seizures, and death have been reported.[60–71] See Chapter 14 for further discussion of meperidine drug interactions.

Meperidine is effective in reducing shivering from diverse causes, including general and epidural anesthesia.[72] This appears to result from kappa receptor stimulation. It reduces or eliminates visible shivering and the accompanying increase in oxygen consumption.[33] Anesthetic uses of meperidine have declined in recent years due to the availability of safer, more convenient techniques.

Alfentanil. After bolus injection, alfentanil has a more rapid onset of action and shorter duration than fentanyl, even though it is less lipid soluble. The high nonionized fraction (90%) of alfentanil at physiologic pH and its small volume of distribution increase the amount of drug available for binding in the brain. Although alfentanil is effective epidurally, the duration of analgesia is short, and for this reason it has never achieved popularity. Alfentanil is metabolized in the liver by oxidative N-dealkylation and O-demethylation in the cytochrome P-450 system, and the inactive metabolites are excreted in the urine. Alfentanil has great patient-to-patient variability as seen in the original studies, in which a high coefficient of variation was reported. Erythromycin has been shown to prolong the metabolism of alfentanil and interact with alfentanil to produce clinical symptoms of prolonged respiratory depression and sedation. Its popularity in current practice is limited.[33]

Fentanyl. Fentanyl is the most widely used opioid analgesic in anesthesia. A single administered dose of fentanyl has a short duration of action (approximately 20–40 minutes). It produces a profound dose-dependent analgesia, ventilatory depression, and sedation. The action of a single dose of fentanyl is terminated by redistribution. The high lipid solubility of fentanyl allows for rapid tissue uptake.[19] Fentanyl and its derivatives all undergo significant first-pass uptake in the lungs with temporary accumulation before release. When fentanyl is given in multiple doses or as a continuous infusion, the termination of action reflects elimination but not redistribution. Clearance of fentanyl is dependent on hepatic blood flow. Fentanyl is metabolized by N-dealkylation and hydroxylation to inactive metabolites that are eliminated in urine and bile. Fentanyl elimination is prolonged in the elderly and the neonate.

Initially used intravenously during surgery, fentanyl has many other uses. It is administered for intrathecal, epidural, and postoperative PCA intravenous use. Fentanyl transdermal patches deliver 75 to

100 mcg/hour, resulting in peak plasma concentrations in approximately 18 hours because a subcutaneous depot of drug must be saturated before the drug is consistently absorbed into the bloodstream.[19] The dose remains stable during the presence of the patch. After removal, the decline in blood concentration follows an apparent 17-hour half-life; the true elimination half-life of fentanyl remains at approximately 3 hours, but continued absorption from the subcutaneous depot during elimination makes it appear longer.

Remifentanil. Remifentanil use in anesthesia has increased as new applications are being discovered for its unique profile.[73,74] Its rapid onset and ultrashort duration, titratability, and simple metabolism make it very convenient for many modern clinical perioperative situations. Remifentanil is a moderately lipophilic, piperidine-derived opioid with an ester link. The addition of the ester group allows the drug to be easily and rapidly metabolized by blood and tissue esterases. Kinetic studies indicate that the drug has a small volume of distribution (V_d 0.39 ± 0.25) and an elimination half-life of 8 to 20 minutes. It is metabolized by hydrolysis catalyzed by general esterase enzymes to a less active compound. It is not dependent on cholinesterase enzyme for metabolism, and therefore it is not influenced by quantitative or qualitative changes in cholinesterase. Succinylcholine metabolism does not influence remifentanil breakdown.

Due to the potential for respiratory depression and muscle rigidity, bolus dosing in the preoperative or postoperative care unit is not recommended. Due to its unique metabolic pathway, remifentanil has a short duration of action, a precise and rapid titratable effect because of rapid onset, and noncumulative effects and results in rapid recovery after discontinuation of its administration by infusion. However, because remifentanil has such a prompt offset, it is important to begin alternative analgesic therapy in the postoperative period.[75]

The commercial preparation of remifentanil is a water-soluble, lyophilized powder that contains a free base and glycine as a vehicle to buffer the solution. Because of potential glycine neurotoxicity, remifentanil should not be administered epidurally or intrathecally.[1]

Sufentanil. Sufentanil is the most potent of the phenylpiperidines and is used for situations in which profound analgesia is required, such as in cardiac or other major surgical procedures. The patients are usually in-hospital patients requiring significant analgesia and postoperative care. Sufentanil is a μ-agonist that produces effective analgesia via both the intravenous and intrathecal routes. It is highly lipophilic and potent, with a shorter elimination half-life than fentanyl. Hepatic clearance of sufentanil approaches liver blood flow. Sufentanil metabolism involves O-demethylation and N-dealkylation, with minimal amounts being excreted unchanged in the urine.

The effects of age on the distribution and elimination of sufentanil are reflected in a decrease in the initial volume of distribution for the elderly. The reduced volume of distribution of sufentanil in elderly patients is associated with increased respiratory depression.[33]

Tramadol. Tramadol is a synthetic codeine analog that is a weak μ-opioid receptor agonist, with analgesic effects produced by inhibition of norepinephrine and serotonin neuronal reuptake, as well as presynaptic stimulation of 5-hydroxytryptamine release. Tramadol is a racemic mixture; the (+) enantiomer binds to the mu receptor and inhibits serotonin uptake, whereas the (−) enantiomer inhibits norepinephrine uptake and stimulates $α_2$-adrenergic receptors. It has an elimination half-life of 5 to 6 hours and is an effective analgesic for the treatment of mild to moderate pain. Tramadol can not only cause seizures, but also potentially exacerbate them in patients with predisposing factors. Tramadol-induced analgesia is not entirely reversed by naloxone; however, the respiratory depression caused by tramadol can be reversed. In overdose situations, most of the toxicity is related to the amine uptake inhibition rather than to opioid effects.[1]

Partial Agonists and Agonists-Antagonists

Buprenorphine. Buprenorphine, a synthetic derivative, is a potent partial agonist opioid that binds mainly to the mu receptors.[76] Its slow dissociation from the receptor is a result of its long duration of action (approximately 8 hours). Its high affinity for the mu receptor accounts for the reduced ability of naloxone to reverse the effects of buprenorphine. Clinically significant respiratory depression can occur with therapeutic doses. Buprenorphine exhibits a ceiling effect in which an increase in the dose does not increase respiratory depression; this is believed to result from the fact that the drug's antagonistic effects become more apparent at higher doses. It also has minimal effect on GI motility and smooth muscle sphincter tone. A transdermal system of buprenorphine was developed for treatment of moderate to severe cancer pain.[77] Administered transdermally, it provides analgesia with a low incidence of adverse events. One common application is in opioid use disorder treatment plans.[78]

Butorphanol. Butorphanol, a highly lipophilic opioid, acts as an agonist at the kappa receptors and a weak antagonist at mu receptors. It has the ability to produce substantially more analgesia than morphine. It does produce respiratory depression, but its ceiling effect is below that of μ-agonists. Intranasal butorphanol is used for the treatment of migraine headaches and postoperative pain. Butorphanol has also been studied for epidural use, although it tends to produce significant sedation. It has been shown to be effective in the treatment of postoperative shivering, but the mechanism of this effect is unknown.[78]

Nalbuphine. Nalbuphine has the ability to reverse respiratory depression that results from opioid use while retaining analgesic properties. Nalbuphine acts as both an agonist and an antagonist at the opioid receptors. Nalbuphine's analgesic response is equal to that of morphine. Nalbuphine provides an agonist effect at the kappa receptors and an antagonist effect at the mu receptors. A ceiling effect for respiratory depression and difficulty with reversal with naloxone has been demonstrated with both nalbuphine and butorphanol. Nalbuphine has been used to antagonize pruritus induced by epidural and intrathecal morphine. Nalbuphine effectively antagonizes fentanyl-induced respiratory depression, maintains analgesia, and does not produce adverse circulatory changes.[78]

Antagonists

Naloxone. Naloxone, an oxymorphone derivative, is a pure opioid antagonist. Naloxone blocks the opioid receptor sites and reverses respiratory depression and opioid analgesia. The reversal of respiratory depression and analgesia occurs as a result of competitive antagonism at the mu, kappa, and delta receptors. The duration of action of naloxone is less than that of most opioid agonists, allowing the return of respiratory depression in some patients treated with naloxone.

Naloxone may antagonize intrinsic analgesic systems, as evidenced by its ability to blunt the placebo effect and inhibit the analgesia of electroacupuncture. Studies have demonstrated that naloxone's effect on reversing the effects of morphine is, in fact, titratable. Administration of low doses of naloxone can reverse the side effects of epidural opioids while preserving some of the analgesic effects.

The effects of naloxone use range from discomfort to pulmonary edema to sudden death. Pulmonary edema after naloxone administration has been observed in patients with a documented history of cardiovascular disease. Some cases of acute onset of pulmonary edema have been reported in young male patients who received either 100 or 200 mcg of naloxone.[79] It is believed that the ability of naloxone to inhibit endogenous pain suppression pathways, while allowing unopposed noradrenergic transmission from medullary centers, produces the neurogenic pulmonary edema. Neurogenic pulmonary edema results from an increase in catecholamine levels in healthy patients, as well as in patients with a history of cardiovascular disease. Cautious titration of naloxone is of paramount importance. There are also cases of sudden death reported after naloxone administration.[80] These reports suggest that naloxone produces an increase in blood catecholamine levels that predispose patients to ventricular fibrillation and subsequent cardiac arrest.

Naloxone is undergoing renewed interest as a rescue drug for opioid overdose. The recent increase in deaths from opioid overdose has led to new formulations and delivery vehicles, which can be used by first responders and friends and relatives of intravenous drug abusers. The FDA has approved an intranasal formulation of naloxone (Adapt) for emergency treatment of opioid overdose. It is also available as an autoinjector formulation (Evzio) for intramuscular or subcutaneous administration.[81]

Nalmefene. Structurally similar to naloxone, nalmefene (Revex) is a long-acting parenteral opioid antagonist primarily used in alcohol use disorder programs. It has an elimination half-life of approximately 10 hours (compared with naloxone's half-life of 1 hour) and a duration of action of 8 hours when it is given in the usual doses.[82] The clinical effects of nalmefene are similar to those of naloxone.

In acute opioid overdose, it is recommended that 0.5 to 1.6 mcg be given intravenously. Administration of doses higher than 1.6 mcg does not elicit additional effects and is not recommended. As with all antagonists, slow titration of small doses may minimize side effects. As with naloxone, nalmefene should not be administered to opioid-dependent patients.[83]

Naltrexone. As a synthetic congener of oxymorphone, naltrexone has antagonist and receptor-binding properties similar to those of naloxone but higher oral efficacy and longer duration of action. Its activity is the result of both the parent drug and its 6-beta metabolite. The parent and metabolite have half-lives of 6 and 13 hours, respectively. Naltrexone has a duration of action of approximately 24 hours. An extended release formulation is routinely used in alcohol use disorder programs.[84]

Naltrexone is administered to patients addicted to opioids so that the euphoric effects of opioids can be prevented. When doses greater than 100 mg are administered to the opioid-addicted patient, plasma concentrations are reached within 2 hours, and the agent's half-life is approximately 10 hours. Naltrexone produces an active metabolite with a half-life even longer than that of naltrexone.[1]

Nonnarcotic Analgesics

The NSAIDs and acetaminophen (paracetamol outside the United States) are primarily used in anesthesia as postoperative pain medications. Aspirin is used as an antiplatelet drug for cardiac patients and is rarely given as an analgesic. They are effective for mild to moderate pain. Acetaminophen, ibuprofen, and ketorolac are available as intravenous preparations and are used for select intraoperative and postoperative applications. The mechanism of both the NSAIDs and acetaminophen is inhibition of the cyclooxygenase enzymes, which prevents the production of prostaglandins and thromboxanes. Some important differences exist. The NSAIDs have analgesic, antipyretic, and antiinflammatory properties; acetaminophen, however, provides both analgesic and antipyretic mechanisms but only minimal antiinflammatory actions. It is rare that more than one or two doses are given during anesthesia, so many of the adverse effects of chronic administration are not a concern.[85,86] Table 11.7 lists the doses of the commonly used oral NSAIDs.

Ketorolac. Ketorolac (Toradol) is an intravenous NSAID that has been used for many years in anesthesia. It is very effective for mild to moderate pain. It can be administered via both intramuscular and intravenous routes. The primary advantages over the opioids are the

TABLE 11.7   Commonly Used Oral Nonsteroidal Antiinflammatory Drugs

Generic Name	Trade Name	Adult Dosage
Acetaminophen	Tylenol	500–1000 mg q4h
Acetylsalicylic acid	Aspirin	325–650 mg q4h
Celecoxib	Celebrex	200 mg q12h
Choline magnesium trisalicylate	Trilisate	500–750 mg q8-12h
Diclofenac sodium	Voltaren	25–75 mg q8-12h
Diflunisal	Dolobid	250–500 mg q8-12h
Etodolic acid	Lodine	200–400 mg q6h
Fenoprofen calcium	Nalfon	200 mg q4-6h
Flurbiprofen	Ansaid	100 mg q8-12h
Ibuprofen	Motrin	400–800 mg q6-8h
Indomethacin	Indocin	25–50 mg q8-12h
Ketoprofen	Orudis	25–75 mg q6-8h
Ketorolac	Toradol	10 mg q6-8h
Meclofenamate sodium	Meclomen	50 mg q4-6h
Meloxicam	Mobic	7.5–15 mg QD prn
Naproxen	Naprosyn	275–500 mg q8-12h
Phenylbutazone	Butazolidin	100 mg q6-8h
Piroxicam	Feldene	10–20 mg once daily
Salsalate	Disalcid	500 mg q4h
Sulindac	Clinoril	150–200 mg q12h
Tolmetin	Tolectin	200–600 mg q8h

From Daroff RB, Jankovic J, Mazziotta JC, et al. *Bradley's Neurology in Clinical Practice.* 7th ed. London: Elsevier; 2016.

very low incidence of nausea and vomiting and lack of respiratory depression. It is frequently given near the end of surgical procedures such as laparoscopy to provide postoperative analgesia. It is also used for minor procedures where avoiding opioids is desirable. The usual dose is 30 to 60 mg either intramuscularly or intravenously. The onset is 30 minutes, and the duration of action is 4 to 6 hours.[87] It should not be used in atopic or asthmatic patients, in the elderly, or in patients with renal or GI dysfunction or bleeding disorders.

Bone healing is delayed by the NSAIDs, and many clinicians do not use them as analgesics in orthopedic procedures. Prolonged administration of NSAIDs has been shown to interfere with a successful bone healing response, but prevailing evidence supports the view that NSAID administration is safe in the setting of anticipated primary bone healing (absolute stability) and during the first week of healing via callous formation (secondary bone healing). NSAIDs inhibit bone formation via blockage of mesenchymal stem cell chondrogenic differentiation, which is an important intermediate phase in normal endochondral bone formation.[64] Bleeding may also be a problem in intracranial surgery.[88,89]

Ibuprofen. An intravenous formulation of ibuprofen (Caldolor) is available as an analgesic and antipyretic. Its clinical effects are similar to ketorolac. The usual dose is 400 to 800 mg intravenously over 30 minutes. Onset is 30 minutes, and duration is 4 to 6 hours.[90,91] Contraindications and precautions are similar to ketorolac.

Acetaminophen. Acetaminophen (Ofirmev) is available as an intravenous analgesic and antipyretic drug for use in both adults and children over 2 years old. It also has a significant opiate-sparing effect.

Acetaminophen does not exhibit the significant GI and cardiovascular side effects associated with NSAIDs. The dose in patients over 13 years old is 1000 mg infused over 15 minutes. The dose in children is 15 mg/kg. Onset is approximately 10 minutes with a peak effect in 1 hour. The duration of action is 4 to 6 hours.[92,93] Side effects are rare. Hepatotoxicity is a concern with acetaminophen but not expected with doses less than 4000 mg/day.

OPIOID-SPARING ANESTHESIA

Prompted by the societal opioid epidemic, clinicians are exploring the practicality of providing opioid-sparing or opioid-free anesthesia. These approaches attempt to minimize or eliminate the short- and long-term adverse effects of opioids used perioperatively. The suggestion is that the potential benefits of opioid-free anesthesia may include shorter discharge times, fewer unplanned hospital admissions, and a significant decrease in opioid use in the postanesthesia care unit. Strategies include the use of nonopioid adjuncts in multimodal analgesia techniques with combinations of agents with varying modes of action. Regional techniques and neuraxial anesthesia are commonly included.

Some of the challenges of opioid-sparing techniques include the potential for adverse drug effects and drug interactions with nonopioid medications, as well as inadequate pain control. Neuraxial and peripheral nerve blocks require the skills, equipment, and personnel to administer and monitor the patients closely postoperatively. A collaboration among surgeons, anesthesia providers, patients, and their caregivers is necessary to effectively personalize plans of postoperative care. Research indicates that patients continue to receive opioids after discharge from postanesthesia care. However, the initial opioid effects may be enhanced. There is some evidence that longer-term opioid consumption (>6 hours after surgery) may not be decreased. Future work is needed to determine the impact of transient postoperative opioid reductions resulting from opioid-sparing anesthesia protocols. Whether opioid-sparing anesthesia is beneficial and whether these techniques can improve short- and long-term patient outcomes remain unknown.[94-97] Some drugs and techniques used in opioid-sparing protocols are described in Table 11.8.

TABLE 11.8 Drugs and Techniques Used in Opioid-Sparing Anesthesia

Agent/Technique	Advantages	Disadvantages
Local anesthetic wound infiltration	Easy to perform with minimal risk	Limited duration
Regional blocks	Analgesia, opioid sparing	Invasive procedure, motor block, unwanted side effects
NSAIDs	Analgesia, opioid sparing	Platelet dysfunction, GI irritation, renal dysfunction
Acetaminophen	Analgesia, opioid sparing	Hepatic toxicity
Dexmedetomidine, clonidine	Analgesia, opioid sparing, avoids respiratory depression	Sedation, hypotension, hypertension, bradycardia, postoperative sedation
Gabapentinoids (gabapentin, pregabalin)	Analgesia, opioid sparing	Sedation, dizziness, peripheral edema, blurred vision
Intravenous lidocaine	Analgesia, opioid sparing	Systemic toxicity, dosing uncertain, postoperative sedation
Magnesium	Opioid sparing, some analgesia	Sedation, systemic toxicity, potentiation of neuromuscular blockers, postoperative sedation
Ketamine	Analgesia, opioid sparing, avoids respiratory depression	Hypertension, psychic disturbances, tachycardia, salivation, dosing uncertain, postoperative sedation
Dexamethasone, methylprednisolone	Analgesia, ↓ length of stay in postanesthesia care unit	Hyperglycemia, anxiety

GI, Gastrointestinal; *NSAIDs*, nonsteroidal antiinflammatory drugs.

SUMMARY

Opioids are a group of drugs that bind to receptor sites in the CNS, supraspinal and spinal, and at peripheral sites, producing morphine-like effects. Opioid analgesia results from the inhibition of nociceptive reflexes and the release of neurotransmitters. Because of their multiplicity of sites and mechanisms of action, opioids are a uniquely valued means for analgesia and anesthesia. Opioids are used for preoperative medication, as induction agents, as maintenance anesthetics, and for treatment of postoperative pain. The newer methods of opioid delivery have been growing in popularity. Opioids provide the anesthesia practitioner with a multitude of delivery modalities.

REFERENCES

For a complete list of references for this chapter, scan this QR code with any smartphone code reader app, or visit the following URL: http://booksite.elsevier.com/9780323711944/.

Neuromuscular Blocking Agents, Reversal Agents, and Their Monitoring

John J. Nagelhout

The neuromuscular blocking drugs (NMBDs) are an integral part of anesthesia practice. They allow for easy airway and operative field manipulation, which is essential in today's sophisticated and complex surgical environment. As with many other types of anesthetic drug components, no single agent or agents are ideal in all situations. For example, the development of a rapid onset, ultrashort-acting, nondepolarizing replacement for succinylcholine has eluded researchers for decades. In addition, reversal of the NMBDs is complex, and residual paralysis in the postanesthesia care unit (PACU) remains a problem. Despite these challenges, our knowledge regarding the safe use of these drugs in anesthesia continually evolves. This chapter updates the clinician with the latest information and concepts on the use of these drugs in modern clinical practice.

HISTORY

In the 19th century, Claude Bernard, a famous French physiologist and philosopher, carried out experiments with curare. At this time it was being used by the Amazonian Indians of South America.[1] He noted that animals the Indians hunted for food were paralyzed by arrows poisoned with curare and subsequently died of asphyxiation.[2] Bernard's experiments with the poison the Indians tipped their arrows with formed the basis for our ideas of the neuromuscular junction, neuromuscular transmission, and neuromuscular pharmacology.[3] Indeed, curare had been used since 1857 as an anticonvulsant treatment in tetany and other types of spastic disorders.[4]

Laewen also described the use of curare in anesthetized humans in a German report in 1912.[3] For readers who are interested in historical aspects of this topic, a fascinating and more complete report of the earliest work of these and other researchers, beginning as early as the year 1548, is available in an outstanding review article by Bisset.[5]

In 1936, Dale et al. found that acetylcholine (ACh) was the chemical neurotransmitter that activated the postjunctional muscle membrane receptors after excitation of the nerve terminal.[5] This finding contradicted the once widely held theory that direct electrical transmission from the nerve to the muscle occurs.[6] This discovery provided the impetus for further research concerning pharmacologic agents that could either enhance the action of ACh or prevent it, thereby causing a temporary and reversible state of therapeutic paralysis.

Griffith and Johnson[7] of Montreal, Canada, are universally acknowledged as the persons responsible for the introduction of neuromuscular blockers into anesthetic practice. Their groundbreaking report laid the foundations for other studies that followed. Within a year of their study, Cullen reported on the use of curare in 131 general anesthetic procedures. His only report of an adverse reaction dealt with a 44-year-old woman who experienced "complete paralysis and severe salivation," accompanied by muscular twitching.[4]

Despite initial successes with the neuromuscular blockers, an early study nearly doomed their use before they became widely accepted. Henry Beecher and Donald Todd, two physicians in the anesthesia department of Harvard Medical School, reviewed 599,548 anesthetic procedures administered at 10 institutions between 1948 and 1952. As part of this review, they examined the death rate in patients receiving *curares* (the term by which they described any neuromuscular blocking agent, including tubocurarine chloride, decamethonium bromide, succinylcholine chloride, gallamine triethiodide, and dimethyltubocurarine [*d*-tubocurarine] iodide). Beecher and Todd[8] found that the overall death rate for persons treated with neuromuscular blockers was 1:370, compared with a death rate of 1:2100 in patients who did not receive these agents.

After reviewing the conditions of the patients; the educational background and training of the practitioners who administered the anesthetic (e.g., physician, nurse anesthetist, or physician-in-training); the size of the institution; the sexes, races, and ages of the patients; and numerous other combinations of these factors, the investigators reached the following conclusions:

> [I]n our judgment the situation is one where neither experience of individual nor experience of institution appears to protect. This adds up to evidence that neither mistakes nor preventable error of any kind are involved in the main, but rather the inherent toxicity of the "curares" themselves.[8]

In the litigious environment of modern anesthetic practice, such a statement may have ended the administration of these agents. It would certainly have slowed their development. The positive attributes of the agents, however, were discussed later in the same paper, as Beecher and Todd added this caveat:

> Having presented the foregoing evidence and comment, one can ask what, then, is to be done about these agents? Are they to be banned as a practical solution of the problem? We believe not. These data strongly suggest that great caution in the use of muscle relaxants should be exercised, that the agents available at present be considered as on trial, and that they be employed only when there are clear advantages to be gained by their use, that they not be employed for trivial purposes or as a corrective for generally inadequate anesthesia.[8]

Beecher and Todd's admonition still echoes through the halls of anesthetic practice today. Although the safety and efficacy of neuromuscular blocking agents have markedly increased, the sage advice is still germane for the practitioner: Neuromuscular blocking agents, like all anesthetic agents, are best used where and when they are indicated. Nevertheless, as one leg of the anesthetic objectives that includes anesthesia, analgesia, amnesia, and muscle relaxation, neuromuscular

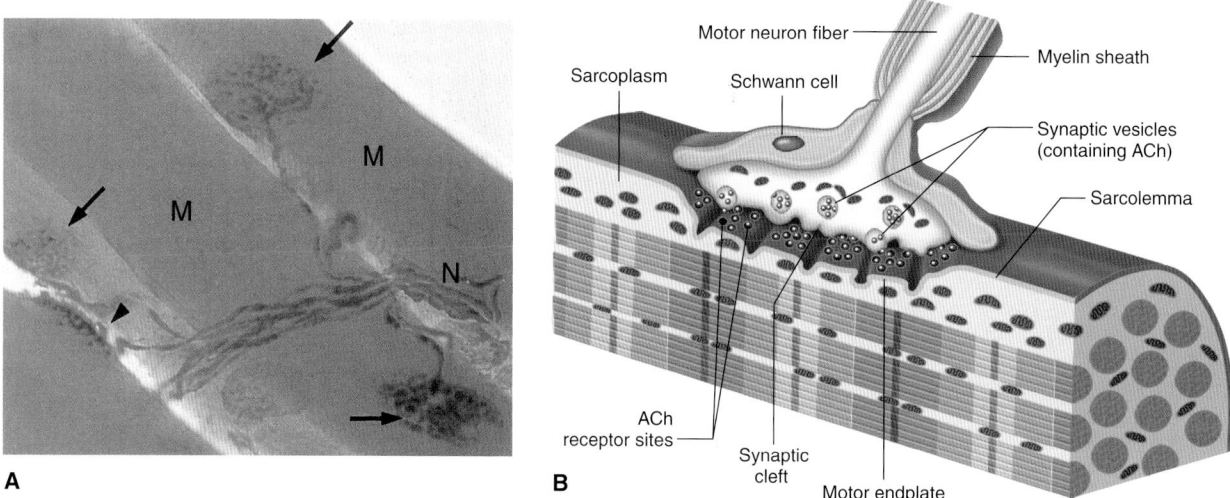

Fig. 12.1 Neuromuscular junction (NMJ). (A) Micrograph showing four NMJs. Three are surface views *(arrows)* and one is a side view *(arrowhead)*. (B) This sketch shows a side view of the NMJ. Note how the distal end of a motor neuron fiber forms a synapse, or "chemical junction," with an adjacent muscle fiber. Neurotransmitter molecules (specifically, acetylcholine [ACh]) are released from the neuron's synaptic vesicles and diffuse across the synaptic cleft. There they stimulate receptors in the motor endplate region of the sarcolemma. *N,* Nerve fibers; *M,* muscle fibers. (From Patton KT. *Anatomy & Physiology.* 10th ed. St. Louis: Elsevier; 2019:362.)

blockade (NMB) has become an integral part of most modern anesthetic techniques. A broad spectrum of these agents now exists, although no single agent has all of what would be the ideal properties. Their individual pharmacokinetic and pharmacodynamic attributes enable the anesthetist to tailor the use of the agent to the physiologic needs of the patient and the requirements of the surgeon.

MONITORING OF NEUROMUSCULAR BLOCKADE

Monitoring of NMB should be the standard of practice during anesthesia when paralysis is administered. Combining objective data from nerve monitoring with clinical signs of paralysis offers obvious advantages when dosing relaxants intraoperatively and assessing postoperative recovery. An important anesthetic discussion has been taking place on the gap between the scientific knowledge of effective monitoring and use of muscle relaxants in anesthesia and actual current clinical practice.[9–12] Expert consensus strongly recommends the routine monitoring of neuromuscular block in the perioperative period as a safety issue. They feel this guides intraoperative relaxant dosing by avoiding overparalysis and helps reduce the incidence of residual weakness in the PACU. An extensive survey of clinicians in the United States[13] and Europe indicate that many practitioners are not using these monitors in everyday practice.[14–16] Several explanations are given: The current quantitative monitors are cumbersome and difficult to use, qualitative monitoring is unreliable, residual paralysis is not a problem in their practice, and clinical signs can be used to assess paralysis in most patients, among others. Survey respondents felt that the incidence of residual paralysis in their practice was usually less than 1%. Objective studies estimate that patients recover safely in spite of residual paralysis and that this problem frequently goes unnoticed. Many patients may have had some difficulty or discomfort but manage to compensate until full recovery occurred and did not need specific interventions. There is no question however, that residual paralysis in the PACU represents a significant potential hazard for airway complications and aspiration. A complete discussion of NMB reversal occurs later in this chapter.

The response to a peripheral nerve monitor indirectly infers the relaxation of musculature. The neuromuscular monitor is an electrical device that delivers a series of electric shocks or impulses to the patient through electrodes applied to the skin near a nerve. There are several methods for monitoring NMB intensity, including acceleromyography (AMG), electromyography (EMG), phonomyography (PMG), mechanomyography (MMG), and kinemyography (KMG). Visual and tactile response to evoked electrical stimulus as assessed by the clinician, or by qualitative monitoring, is the most common method. On activation of the stimulator, various predictable muscle contraction patterns are visible in the presence and absence of neuromuscular blockers. Quantitative monitoring, in which the stimulator is coupled with a displacement transducer as a movement measuring device and a number value is displayed, is preferred but less common. Quantitative monitoring can be accomplished with MMG, AMG, KMG, or EMG.[9]

Depolarization and contraction of a muscle are caused by an action potential traveling along the course of a nerve. As the impulse reaches the motor endplate, ACh is released across the synaptic cleft. It subsequently travels toward the receptor sites on the muscle membrane, resulting in depolarization and subsequent contraction of the muscle.[2] The stimulator elicits the same activity, which makes it useful for the monitoring of NMB (Fig. 12.1).

The proper administration of neuromuscular blocking agents (NMBAs) is essential for patient safety and efficient perioperative workflow. Inadequate doses of NMBAs may result in complications during surgical procedures because of unexpected patient movement and a less than ideal operative field. In contrast, overdosage may result in residual paralysis in the postoperative period, increasing morbidity and the need for labor-intensive interventions (e.g., mechanical ventilation).

Contraction of the adductor muscle of the thumb via stimulation of the ulnar nerve is the preferred site for determining the level of NMB. It is usually accessible and convenient. Disposable electrodes are applied over the ulnar nerve. The distal electrode is placed over the proximal flexor crease of the wrist, and the other electrode is placed over and parallel to the carpi ulnaris tendon. On stimulation of these

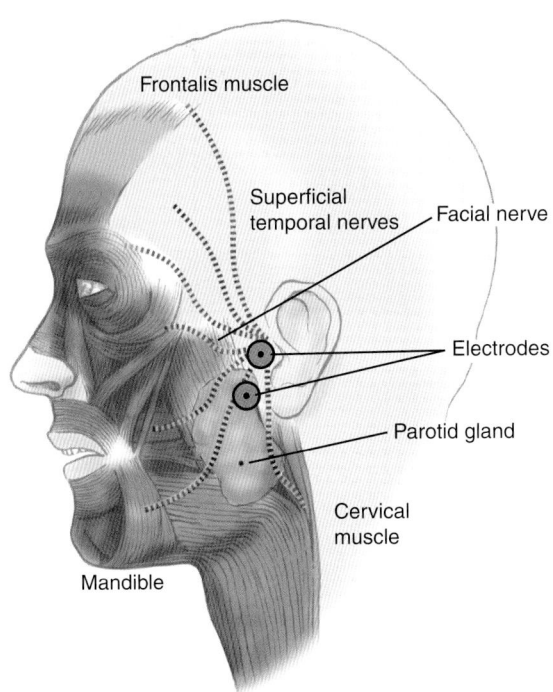

Fig. 12.2 Facial neuromuscular blockade testing.

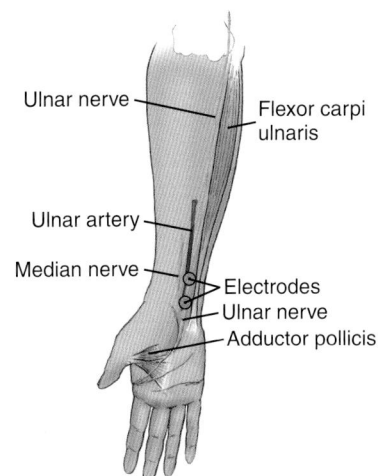

Fig. 12.3 Ulnar neuromuscular blockade testing.

electrodes with the monitoring device, adduction of the thumb is visible. When access to the arm and hand is not practical, other monitoring sites include the nerves of the foot and the facial nerve. Facial nerve monitoring generally involves stimulation of the temporal branch of the facial nerve that supplies the orbicularis oculi muscle around the eye or the corrugator supercilii that moves the eyebrow when frowning.[17,18] The facial and ulnar nerves sites are shown in Figs. 12.2 and 12.3, respectively. Table 12.1 gives a comparison of the ulnar and facial nerve monitoring sites.

A few contrasting factors involving blood flow versus muscle sensitivity must be considered when assessing paralysis and interpreting responses from the ulnar nerve or face. During onset of a relaxant, the muscle group sensitivity exhibits the following pattern: The eye muscles are the most sensitive and are the first group to be affected, followed by the extremities, the trunk of the body (with the neck and chest first), then abdominal muscles, and, lastly, the diaphragm. During recovery, muscle function returns in the opposite pattern with the diaphragm first and the eye muscles last. Blood flow, however, is greater to the head, neck, and diaphragm, so more of the drug is distributed to these areas upon initial distribution and onset. Additionally, there is a difference in sensitivity to relaxants between various muscles surrounding the eye. The corrugator supercilii is more resistant than the orbicularis oculi to NMBAs. Distinguishing between the effects of drugs on these two muscles is very difficult clinically. When monitoring in the face, with its many small nerves and muscles, it is difficult to ensure that only a single nerve is being stimulated and, accordingly, that only one muscle is contracting. This may lead to twitches of the relatively resistant corrugator supercilii muscle to be counted, even in the absence of a twitch by the orbicularis oculi muscle.[17]

Due to these conflicting influences, the facial nerves should be used when assessing relaxant onset. Blood, thus drug, distribution to the facial muscles mirrors distribution in the larynx and diaphragm where relaxation is required for intubation and airway manipulation. Recovery is best measured in the hand. The hand muscles are more sensitive to relaxant than the diaphragm, so if recovery is evident in the

hand, the larynx, and the diaphragm, the upper airway muscles will be recovered as well.[17–19]

Tests of Neuromuscular Function

There are five clinical tests of neuromuscular function: single twitch, train-of-four (TOF), double-burst stimulation (DBS), tetanus, and posttetanic count (PTC). The TOF, DBS, and tetanic stimulation are the most commonly used.[20] The ability to evaluate muscle function with each mode of stimulation varies (Table 12.2).

A brief explanation of the concept called fade is required to understand the responses to nerve monitoring. Fade is the inability to sustain a response to repetitive nerve stimulation and is seen in several of the clinically used monitoring tests. This is a sign of drug-induced muscle paralysis. Fade occurs because the nondepolarizing drugs block presynaptic ACh receptors (AChRs) in addition to their classic antagonist effect at postsynaptic ACh neuromuscular junction sites. The function of presynaptic AChRs is to facilitate the release of ACh from the nerve terminal via a positive feedback mechanism. During high impulse rates of nerve stimulation, this positive feedback mechanism prevents the decrease (fade) of transmitter release. The facilitated ACh release associated with this positive feedback mechanism is blocked by the relaxants.[21] This inhibition is detected as fade during the use of the monitoring tests as described hereafter.

Single Twitch

The first (and simplest) type of stimulation is a single twitch at 0.1 to 1 hertz (Hz) for 0.1 to 0.2 milliseconds (ms). These impulses can be delivered automatically every second, every 10 seconds, or manually, depending on the sophistication of the neurostimulating apparatus.

Unless you have a comparison twitch response before any relaxant is given, this test simply indicates whether 100% paralysis is present. If the patient's muscle moves when stimulated, less than 100% muscle paralysis exists. If no movement is detected, 100% paralysis is present.

Train-of-Four

The second and most widely used means of stimulation is the TOF, which delivers four separate stimuli every 0.5 seconds at a frequency of 2 Hz for 2 seconds. A comparison is made of the four stimulated responses. Each of the four twitch responses are referred to as T_1 through T_4, respectively. Upon the onset of paralysis with a nondepolarizing relaxant, there is a progressive diminution of the twitch responses with visible fade. Fade refers to the fact that each of the successive twitch responses from T_1 through T_4 is smaller. When partial

TABLE 12.1   A Comparison of Neuromuscular Monitoring Sites

Monitoring Site	Response	Comments
Ulnar nerve innervation of the adductor pollicis	Thumb adduction	Usually have easy access Best site to measure recovery
Facial nerves	Eyelid and eyebrow movement	Easily accessed when arm is not available Best site to measure onset Corrugator supercilii (eyebrow) is more resistant to relaxants than the orbicularis oculi (eyelid)

TABLE 12.2   Common Neuromuscular Monitoring Tests

Monitoring Test	Definition	Comments	Stimulation Characteristics
Single twitch	A single supramaximal electrical stimulus ranging from 0.1–1.0 Hz	Requires baseline before drug administration; generally used as a qualitative rather than quantitative assessment	
Train-of-four	A series of four twitches at 2 Hz every 0.5 sec for 2 sec	Reflects blockade from 70–100%; useful during onset, maintenance, and emergence Train-of-four ratio is determined by comparing T_1–T_4	$T_1\ T_2\ T_3\ T_4$
Double-burst simulation	Two short bursts of 50-Hz tetanus separated by 0.75 sec	Similar to train-of-four; useful during onset, maintenance, and emergence; may be easier to detect fade than with train-of-four; tactile evaluation	
Tetanus	Generally consists of rapid delivery of a 30-, 50-, or 100-Hz stimulus for 5 sec	Should be used sparingly for deep block assessment; painful	
Posttetanic count	50-Hz tetanus for 5 sec, a 3-sec pause, then single twitches of 1 Hz	Used only when train-of-four and double-burst stimulation are absent; count of less than eight indicates deep block, and prolonged recovery is likely	

paralysis is present, yet all four twitch responses can be elicited with fade from T_1 through T_4, an assessment can be made regarding the size of T_4 compared to T_1. This T_4:T_1 ratio is referred to as the train-of-four ratio (TOFR). TOF testing can aid in approximating the degree or percent of paralysis present. It is most sensitive between 70% and 100% paralysis. The fourth twitch (T_4) disappears first, which represents a block of 75% to 80%. Progressive disappearance of the third twitch (T_4 and T_3 absent) indicates 80% to 85% block. When three twitches are abolished (T_4, T_3, and T_2 are absent), 90% to 95% NMB is present. When 100% paralysis is achieved, no responses can be elicited. Fig. 12.4 correlates the responses to TOF stimulation with the approximate degree of paralysis present. Intraoperatively, the ideal degree of paralysis necessary for any procedure with sufficient anesthetic depth is 85% to 95%. That correlates with one to two twitch responses present upon TOF stimulation. Avoiding total 100% paralysis intraoperatively ensures a successful operative procedure while avoiding overdosing of the relaxant. Less total relaxant administered lessens the chances of residual paralysis upon reversal.[22]

A representative assessment of the TOF test during onset and recovery of a nondepolarizing relaxant is shown in Figs. 12.5 and 12.6, respectively.

Double-Burst Stimulation

Double-burst stimulation was conceptualized as an analog to TOF with some improvements. It consists of two short bursts of a 50-Hz tetanus separated by 0.75 second. The use of DBS seems to improve the ability to detect residual paralysis during recovery. The suggestion is that DBS relies on the direct comparison of the muscle contraction in response to two rapidly sequential minitetanic bursts, rather than the indirect comparison of the fourth twitch with the first twitch as in the TOFR. It is thought that the comparison of the fourth to the first twitches when assessing the TOFR is hindered by the second and third twitches, which provide no useful information. Evaluating two rather than four twitch responses facilitates detection of fade. Tactile evaluation is suggested to improve the ability to detect fade. Responses are similar to the TOF. Fade of the second impulse is comparable to a TOFR of less than 0.6 and indicates significant paralysis.[19] A comparison is shown in Fig. 12.7.[20,23,24]

Tetanus

Tetanus consists of continuous electrical stimulation for 5 seconds at 50 or 100 Hz. The 100-Hz current is more reliable for detecting fade but is not always specific.[19,25] If the muscle contraction produced is sustained for the entire 5 seconds of stimulation without fade, significant paralysis is unlikely. If fade is present, clinically significant block remains.[20,26] The higher intensity of stimulation produced by tetanic frequencies as compared to TOF, DBS, or a single twitch makes it useful when other tests such as TOF or DBS are equivocal. The test is painful and should not be repeated too often, to avoid muscle fatigue.

Train-of-four suppression | | **Percent neuromuscular block**

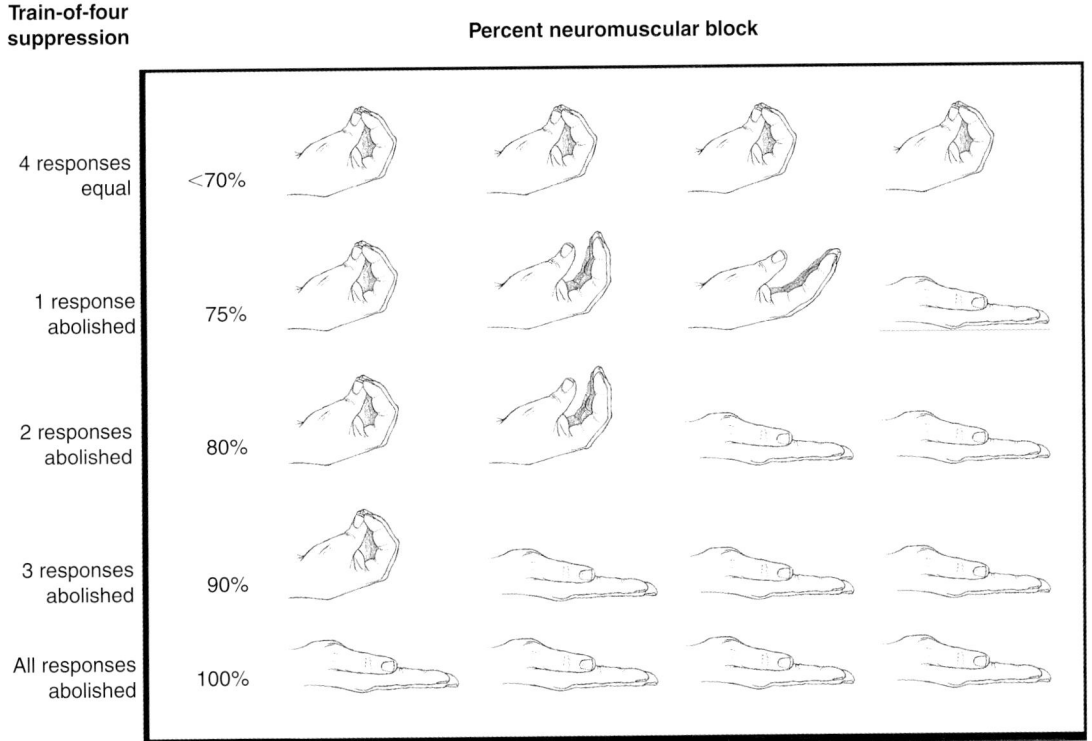

Fig. 12.4 Train-of-four test.

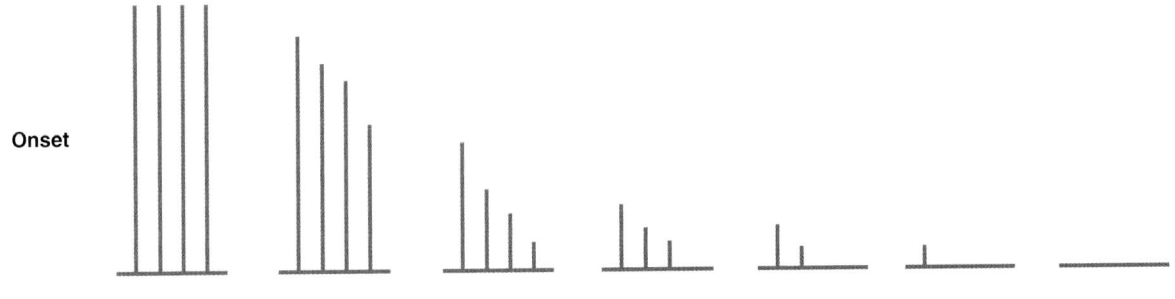

Nondepolarizing Drug

Fig. 12.5 Characteristic train-of-four response during onset of a nondepolarizing muscle relaxant.

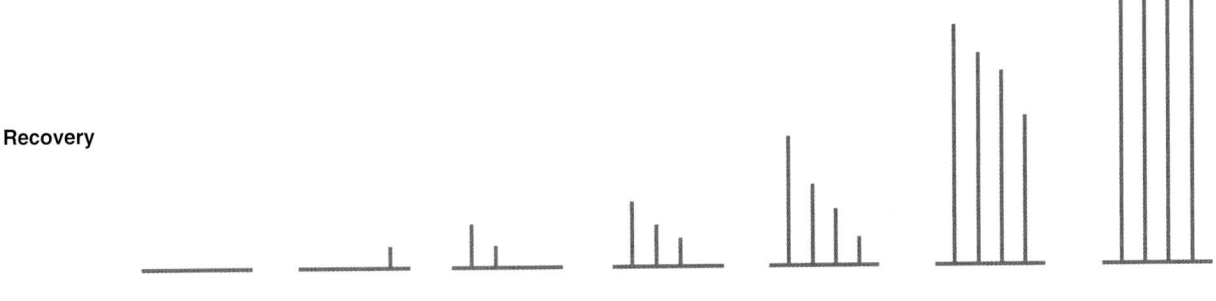

Nondepolarizing Drug

Fig. 12.6 Characteristic train-of-four response during recovery from a nondepolarizing muscle relaxant.

Posttetanic Count

The PTC was rarely used clinically but is undergoing a newfound interest since the introduction of sugammadex. Several sugammadex dosing regimens are based on the PTC and will be discussed under reversal drugs. It is performed only when there is no response to any of the commonly used tests due to the presence of 100% paralysis.

Because you are already aware that the patient is completely paralyzed, the value of the PTC is to attempt to give a rough time estimate as to when recovery may occur. The PTC mode involves the use of a 50-Hz tetanic stimulation for 5 seconds, followed in 3 seconds by a series of single 1-Hz twitch stimulations.[24] An understanding of the phenomenon of posttetanic potentiation (also referred to as posttetanic

TOF   DBS$_{3,3}$

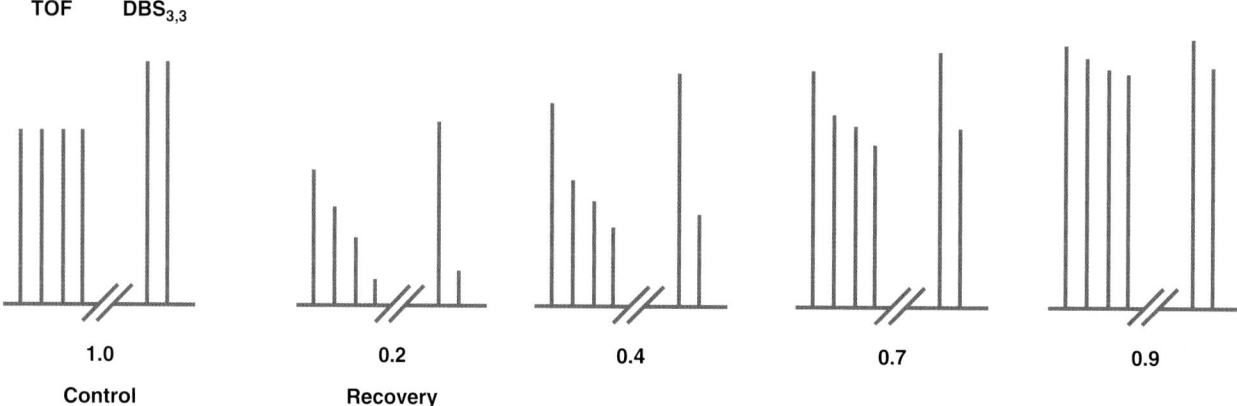

| 1.0 | 0.2 | 0.4 | 0.7 | 0.9 |

Control   Recovery

Fig. 12.7 A comparison of responses to double-burst *(DBS)* and train-of-four *(TOF)* stimulation during recovery from a nondepolarizing muscle relaxant.

stimulation or facilitation) is necessary to comprehend the PTC test. When the 50-Hz tetanus is applied, there is no response because the patient is completely blocked. Application of the 50-Hz tetanus, however, transiently mobilizes excesses of ACh so that after a 3-second pause you are able to produce a short series of single-twitch responses in the hand. Because they occur only after a tetanic stimulation and not before, this single-twitch response is called posttetanic potentiation. This extra ACh will, in effect, "transiently reverse" the relaxant by competing for the receptor at the local monitoring site. This augmented response will only last several seconds until the excess ACh dissipates. The number of twitches elicited is counted. The higher the count, the less intense the block. The usual count is between 0 (deep block) and 8 (less intense block where TOF response should return). With rocuronium, for example, neostigmine reversal of an intense block where the PTC was 1 to 2 takes more than 50 minutes.[27,28] At a PTC of 6 to 8, reversal should occur in less than 10 minutes.

Neuromuscular monitoring terminology and tests are summarized in Box 12.1, Fig. 12.2 (earlier), and Table 12.3. Some key points related to successful use of tests of neuromuscular transmission are given in Box 12.2.[29]

DEPOLARIZING AGENTS

Succinylcholine Chloride

Succinylcholine chloride (Anectine, Quelicin, and others) is very familiar to every clinician, having been a standard for several decades of practice. Although its widespread use in clinical anesthesia represents the standard of care for a variety of situations, opinions regarding its use remain divided because of some of its untoward effects.

Stephen Thesleff at the Karolinska Institute in Stockholm was one of the pioneers who introduced the drug into clinical practice. Initial description of the neuromuscular blocking properties of succinylcholine is credited to Daniel Bovet. (Bovet was awarded the Nobel Prize for Physiology and Medicine in 1957 for his discovery of synthetic compounds that act on the vascular system and skeletal muscle.[30]) The first use of succinylcholine in the United States occurred in 1952. Foldes et al.[31] described this agent in the following manner:

> Compared to other muscle relaxants used in anesthesiology, succinylcholine possesses several advantages, the outstanding one, in our experience, being its easy controllability, which permitted almost instantaneous changes in degree of muscular relaxation. With succinylcholine, both increasing and decreasing muscular relaxation took less than a minute.[31]

The disadvantages of succinylcholine have been well recorded through years of clinical experience. It has no action in the ganglionic nicotinic receptors but may cause bradycardia by an action on cardiac cholinergic muscarinic receptors.[32,33] Prolonged NMB can result from excessive doses of succinylcholine in patients with atypical, inhibited, or deficient levels of plasma cholinesterases.[3,32]

Succinylcholine is the only remaining depolarizing muscle relaxant licensed for use in the United States. Remembering the composition of the drug is helpful in better understanding its effects and side effects. Succinylcholine results from the joining of two ACh molecules and is represented by the chemical formula $C_{14}H_{30}N_2O_4$. Although succinylcholine mimics the action of ACh by depolarizing the motor endplate, its degradation is distinct. In contrast with the degradation of ACh by acetylcholinesterase (AChE), succinylcholine is hydrolyzed by plasma cholinesterase (pseudocholinesterase). The popularity of this muscle relaxant is rooted in its unique ability to provide a quick onset and short duration of effect. A bolus of 0.5 to 1.5 mg/kg is the recommended dose for adequate adult paralysis and relaxation for intubation.[34] The dose of succinylcholine that provides the desired paralytic effect in 95% of the population (i.e., effective dose, 95% response [ED$_{95}$]) is approximately 0.30 mg/kg.[35]

Pharmacokinetics

Onset. Succinylcholine has an extremely rapid onset and remains the gold standard against which other agents are compared. In general, muscle relaxants exhibit an inverse relationship between potency and onset speed. The lower the potency, the faster the speed. A lower potency drug requires larger doses so a muscle gradient will be achieved more quickly.[36] A typical intubating dose of 1 to 1.5 mg/kg results in a maximum suppression of muscle twitch and good to excellent

TABLE 12.3   Key Points Related to Tests of Neuromuscular Transmission and Reversal

Test	Acceptable Clinical Result to Suggest Normal Function	Approximate Percent of Receptors Occupied When Response Returns to Normal Value	Comments, Advantages, and Disadvantages
Tidal volume	At least 5 mL/kg	80	Necessary, but insensitive as an indicator of neuromuscular function
Single-twitch strength	Qualitatively as strong as baseline	75–80	Uncomfortable; need to know twitch strength before relaxant administration; insensitive as an indicator of recovery, but useful as a gauge of deep neuromuscular blockade
Train-of-four (TOF)	No palpable fade	70–75	Uncomfortable, but more sensitive as indicator of recovery than single twitch; used as a gauge of depth of block by counting the number of responses perceptible
Sustained tetanus at 50 Hz for 5 sec	At least 20 mL/kg	70	Very uncomfortable, but a reliable indicator of adequate recovery
Vital capacity	At least 20 mL/kg	70	Requires patient cooperation, but is the goal for achievement of full clinical recovery
Double-burst stimulation	No palpable fade	60–70	Uncomfortable, but more sensitive than TOF as an indicator of peripheral function; no perceptible fade indicates TOF of at least recovery of 60%
Inspiratory force	At least –40 cm H_2O	50	Difficult to perform with endotracheal intubation, but a reliable gauge of normal diaphragmatic function
Head lift	Must be performed unaided with patient supine and sustained for 5 sec	50	Requires patient cooperation, but remains the standard test of normal clinical function
Hand grip	Sustained at a level qualitatively similar to preinduction	50	Sustained strong grip, though also requires patient cooperation; is another good gauge of normal function
Sustained bite	Sustained jaw clench on tongue blade	50	Very reliable with patient cooperation; corresponds with TOF of 85%

Modified from Miller RD. Neuromuscular blocking drugs. In Miller RD, Pardo M, eds. *Basics of Anesthesia*. 7th ed. Philadelphia: Elsevier; 2018:156.

intubating conditions within 1 to 1.5 minutes of administration.[34,37,38] Onset of action of succinylcholine at the larynx with administration of 1 mg/kg is 34 seconds.[39,40] The onset as measured at peripheral sites such as the adductor pollicis is slightly longer at 1 minute.[41] The rapid onset of succinylcholine is based on its action as an initial agonist at the nicotinic receptor, rather than as a competitive antagonist. Succinylcholine works by activating the muscle-type nicotinic cholinergic receptors, followed by desensitization.[33] This action results in the need for significantly less drug at the receptor site to produce neuromuscular block. In contrast, most NMBAs require 75% or more receptor occupancy for clinically useful paralysis to result. Variable onset must be considered in patients with altered physiology. Patients with atypical plasma cholinesterase may exhibit prolonged onset after succinylcholine administration.[42] A summary of the doses, onsets, and durations of the neuromuscular blocking drugs is given in Table 12.4.

Duration. The plasma half-life of succinylcholine is 2 to 4 minutes.[43] The clinical duration of succinylcholine (i.e., the length of time during which its clinical effects can be recognized) is generally 5 to 10 minutes, with full recovery evident at 12 to 15 minutes. Twitch recovery of 25%, as measured by the laryngeal adductor pollicis responses, is 4.3 minutes, whereas 90% to 95% twitch recovery has been reported to occur in 8 minutes.[39] In a 2015 study of 1630 patients given a 1-mg/kg dose, average duration was 7.3 minutes. A duration greater than 10 minutes was noted in 16% of patients. Independent risk factors

associated with prolonged duration included physical status, sex, age, hepatic disease, pregnancy, history of cancer, and use of etomidate or metoclopramide.[44]

Elimination. Succinylcholine is degraded via hydrolysis by plasma cholinesterases. These enzymes, although found in the plasma, are produced by the liver. Initially, hydrolysis results in the transformation of succinylcholine into succinylmonocholine and choline (Fig. 12.8). Succinylmonocholine is further degraded by plasma cholinesterase into succinic acid and choline. Succinylcholine metabolism is so rapid that only 10% of the injected dose ever reaches the neuromuscular junction.[30] A summary of the elimination routes for the neuromuscular blocking drugs is given in Table 12.5.

Central Nervous System

Like all muscle relaxants, succinylcholine contains a quaternary ammonium in its structure, rendering it water soluble in the body. It does not therefore pass the blood-brain barrier and has no direct central nervous system (CNS) effects. Succinylcholine indirectly increases intracranial pressure (ICP), and therefore concern has always existed as to the appropriateness of its use in certain neurosurgical procedures and in patients with brain pathology and increased ICP.[39] Research conducted in animals shows a small and transient rise of 10 to 15 mm Hg for 5 to 8 minutes after administration.[43] The rise is associated with an increased cerebral blood flow, muscle spindle afferent activity, and electroencephalogram arousal. Fasciculation of the neck muscles causing jugular vein stasis appears to be a factor.[45] The ICP effects are blocked by pretreatment with a small dose of nondepolarizing relaxant.[46] In clinical practice, the administration of succinylcholine is preceded by an anesthetic induction agent that lowers ICP, so that may help counteract this effect as well. Nevertheless, the routine use of succinylcholine in neurosurgery has declined.[47] It remains widely used, with nondepolarizing relaxant and lidocaine pretreatment, for emergency procedures requiring rapid airway control via rapid sequence induction (RSI).[32]

BOX 12.2 General Guidelines for Successful Neuromuscular Monitoring

- Objective (quantitative) monitoring of neuromuscular function should be used when possible.
- Peripheral nerve stimulator units should display the delivered current output, which should be at least 30 mA.
- During onset, paralysis begins with the eye muscles, followed by the extremities, trunk (from the neck muscles downward through the intercostals), abdominal muscles, and finally the diaphragm. Recovery returns in the opposite manner. Protective reflex muscles of the pharynx and upper esophagus recover later than the diaphragm, larynx, hands, or face.
- Monitoring of the facial nerve for determination of onset and readiness for intubation may be preferable to monitoring of the ulnar nerve.
- Monitoring of the offset and recovery from neuromuscular blockade is probably better at the ulnar nerve.
- Tactile evaluation of train-of-four (TOF) and double-burst stimulation (DBS) fade reduces but does not eliminate the incidence of postoperative residual paralysis compared with the use of clinical criteria to assess readiness for tracheal extubation.
- Adequate spontaneous recovery should be established before pharmacologic antagonism of neuromuscular blocking drug (NMDD) block with anticholinesterases. This requirement does not apply to reversal with sugammadex.
- When there is only one response to TOF stimulation, successful reversal may take as long as 30 min.
- At a TOF count of two or three responses, recovery usually takes 4 to 15 min after intermediate-acting drugs.
- When the fourth response to TOF stimulation appears, adequate recovery can be achieved within 5 min of reversal with neostigmine or 2 to 3 min after use of edrophonium.
- When the fourth twitch of the TOF returns, the TOF ratio may be determined. Compare the size of the fourth twitch (T_4) with the size of the first twitch (T_1), using T_4:T_1 as a ratio. The timing of tracheal extubation should be guided by quantitative monitoring tests such as TOF >0.9 or DBS_3 >0.9.

Cardiovascular System

Succinylcholine usually results in slight tachycardia; however, sudden abrupt bradycardia may result from repeat dosing in adults and any dose in children. Many types of arrhythmias have been reported. The bradycardia results from autonomic ganglia and parasympathetic muscarinic receptor stimulation. Another possible mechanism for the bradycardia associated with succinylcholine administration is thought to be related to its metabolite, succinylmonocholine, which causes stimulation of cholinergic receptors in the sinoatrial node.[48]

An intubating dose of succinylcholine increases serum potassium levels by 0.5 to 1 mEq/L.[43] Although this may not be significant in the normokalemic patient, it may be life threatening in patients with preexisting hyperkalemia.[49] Gronert[50] presents a case that involved an 11-year-old girl who experienced cardiac arrest after receiving succinylcholine. Her cardiac arrest and eventual death were directly attributed to a high potassium release after the succinylcholine administration (10.2 mEq/L). The exaggerated potassium release after the succinylcholine administration in this case was determined to be related to a familial myopathy evidenced by extremely high patient levels of creatine kinase. Succinylcholine administration, hyperkalemia, and myopathy are discussed later. Some clinicians believe that a second dose of succinylcholine indicated by any event should be preceded by intravenous atropine or glycopyrrolate for its anticholinergic effects; however, others do not.[49]

Hepatic System

Cholinesterase enzyme subtypes are produced in the liver. Pseudocholinesterase (PChE) degrades succinylcholine, therefore certain types of liver damage may prolong the effects of the drug.[48] Ester compounds such as succinylcholine are metabolized by adding water in a process referred to as hydrolysis. The basic reaction is ESTER + H_2O ↔ ACID + ALCOHOL. Three esterase enzymes that can act as catalysts for these hydrolysis reactions exist in the plasma: cholinesterase, paraoxonase, and albumin esterase. Paraoxonase and albumin esterase are frequently referred to as nonspecific esterases. Additionally, red blood cells (RBCs) contain two esterase enzymes in their cytosol: One is referred to as RBC esterase, esterase D, or S-formylglutathione; the other is AChE in small amounts.[51]

Cholinesterase is a generic term used for a family of related enzymes that hydrolyze choline esters at a faster rate than other esters under optimal conditions. The major function of cholinesterase is to terminate the action of ACh at cholinergic nerve endings in synapses or in effector organs.[52] Two subtypes of cholinesterase exist in the human body, with several variations and a confusing set of names. One type of cholinesterase is AChE, also known as true, specific, genuine, and type I cholinesterase. This enzyme is found in erythrocytes, nerve endings, the lungs, the spleen, and gray matter of the brain. It is a

---

TABLE 12.4 Neuromuscular Blocking Agents: Dose, Onset, and Duration*

Agent	ED_{95} (mg/kg)	Intubating Dose (mg/kg)	Time to Onset	Duration of Action (min)
Succinylcholine (Anectine)	0.3	1–1.5	30–60 sec	Ultrashort, 5–15
Mivacurium (Mivacron)	0.08	0.25	2–3 min	Short, 15–20
Atracurium (Tracrium)	0.15	0.5	2–4 min	Intermediate, 30–60
Cisatracurium (Nimbex)	0.05	0.1	2–4 min	Intermediate, 30–60
Rocuronium (Zemuron)	0.3	0.6–1	1–1.5 min	Intermediate, 30–60
Vecuronium (Norcuron)	0.05	0.1	2–4 min	Intermediate, 30–60

*All data for adult patients without significant disease.
ED_{95}, Effective dose for 95% paralysis.

membrane-bound glycoprotein and exists in several molecular forms. The other subgroup is PChE, also known as plasma, serum, benzoyl, false, butyryl, nonspecific, and type II cholinesterase. It exists in plasma and has more than 11 isoenzyme variants. PChE is also present in the liver, smooth muscle, intestines, pancreas, heart, and white matter of the brain.

Measurements of PChE activity can serve as a sensitive measure of the synthetic capacity of the liver. In the absence of known inhibitors, any decrease in activity reflects impaired synthesis of the enzyme. A moderate decrease (30%–50%) is seen in acute hepatitis and

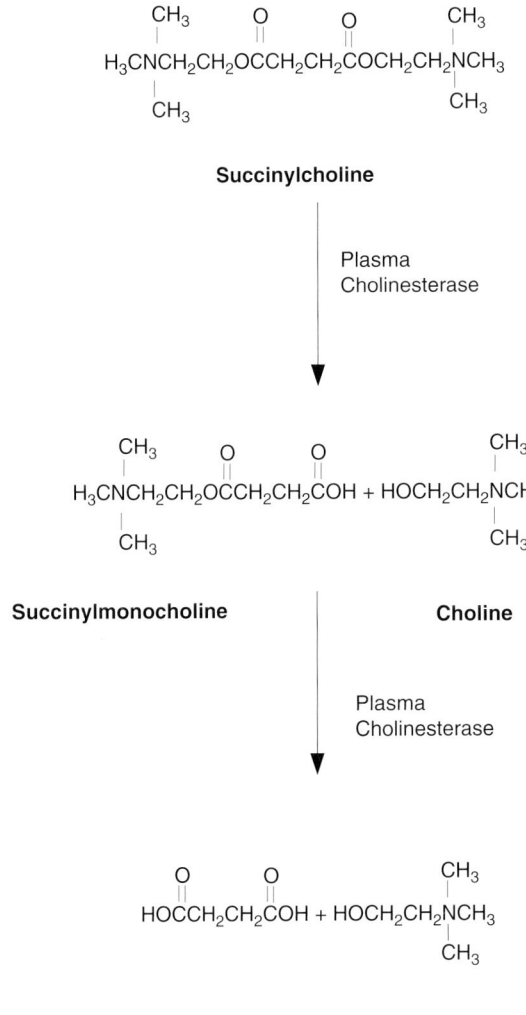

Succinylcholine

Plasma Cholinesterase

Succinylmonocholine   **Choline**

Plasma Cholinesterase

Succinic Acid   **Choline**

Fig. 12.8 Metabolism of succinylcholine.

long-standing chronic hepatitis, whereas a severe decrease (50%–70%) is seen in advanced cirrhosis and in some carcinomas with metastases to the liver. Decreased levels of PChE are also found in pregnant women and newborns and in patients with acute infections, pulmonary embolism, muscular dystrophy, myocardial infarction, and after certain surgical procedures.[48] Essentially normal levels are noted in patients with mild cirrhosis or obstructive jaundice. Increased levels have been observed in cases of nephrotic syndrome, thyrotoxicosis, and hemochromatosis, in obese patients with diabetes, and in patients with anxiety and other psychiatric states. Patients generally develop neuromuscular symptoms at approximately 60% of normal activity, and serious neuromuscular effects are seen at approximately 20% of normal activity.[53]

Table 12.6 lists some common anesthesia-related drugs that undergo hydrolysis, along with the enzyme catalyst involved.

Genetic Variants of Pseudocholinesterase and the Dibucaine Inhibition Test

Some patients exhibit genetic variations in PChE that result in a prolonged response and apnea when the patient is exposed to succinylcholine. Although such individuals may lead a normal life in every other respect, their atypical variants of cholinesterase are unable to hydrolyze certain ester-containing drugs in the usual fashion. The most frequent variations in the PChE gene are the atypical (A) and Kalow (K) variants. The K variant is the most common mutation and is present in 25% of whites.[54] Over 75 mutations in the coding sequence have been reported; however, most are extremely rare.[53,55,56] The fluoride resistant (F), silent (S), and K variants are not tested for clinically because of assay difficulty and lack of clinical relevance. Phenotype-genotype concordance studies have been reported that allow detailed genetic mapping and clinical data to be evaluated.[53]

In the usual clinical scenario, a patient completes surgery and is unable to breathe. Muscle relaxation cannot be successfully reversed. If succinylcholine was used to facilitate intubation, differential diagnosis leads the anesthesia provider to conclude that a potential atypical pseudocholinesterase may be present.[57-59] The patient is taken to the PACU, placed on a ventilator, sedated, and monitored until the succinylcholine wears off. Sedation is important because these patients have a high risk of being awake and paralyzed.[60] The patient recovers and is subsequently discharged, but prior to discharge a blood sample is taken to perform a dibucaine inhibition test to help determine (1) whether an atypical enzyme was present and (2) the cause of the prolonged apnea. The dibucaine number and enzyme activity are both determined. By treating the patient's serum with dibucaine and measuring the residual PChE activity compared with the PChE of an untreated sample, the metabolic sensitivity to succinylcholine can be measured. The patient is contacted postdischarge and counseled as appropriate, according to the findings. The administration of whole blood, fresh frozen plasma,

TABLE 12.5	Neuromuscular Blockers: Elimination Mechanism	
Agent	**Elimination Mechanism**	**Comments**
Atracurium	Hofmann elimination; nonspecific esterases	Nonorgan-dependent elimination produces consistent duration in patients with significant hepatic and renal disease, as well as the elderly
Cisatracurium	Hofmann elimination; nonspecific esterases	Similar to atracurium but without the histamine release
Rocuronium	Hepatic; renal	May be prolonged with hepatic and renal disease
Vecuronium	Renal (20–30%); hepatic (40–80%)	May be prolonged with hepatic disease
Succinylcholine	Plasma cholinesterase	Prolonged in patients with cholinesterase deficiency
Mivacurium	Plasma cholinesterase	Prolonged in patients with cholinesterase deficiency

TABLE 12.6 Common Esterase-Dependent, Anesthesia-Related Drugs

Drug	Enzyme
Succinylcholine	Pseudocholinesterase
Mivacurium	Pseudocholinesterase
Ester local anesthetics:	Pseudocholinesterase
Cocaine	
Procaine	
Chloroprocaine	
Tetracaine	
Neostigmine	Pseudocholinesterase
Edrophonium	Pseudocholinesterase
Atracurium	Nonspecific esterases (plasma)
Cisatracurium	Nonspecific esterases (plasma)
Remifentanil	Nonspecific esterases (plasma)
Esmolol	Nonspecific (RBC esterases) plasma
Clevidipine	Nonspecific esterases (plasma)

MOC, Methoxycarbonyl; *RBC,* red blood cell.

BOX 12.3 Dibucaine Inhibition Test Outcomes

1. Low dibucaine number + slightly lower activity = atypical enzyme and prolonged apnea
2. Normal dibucaine number + low activity = normal enzyme with low levels present and prolonged apnea
3. Low dibucaine number + very low activity = possible rare variant-type enzyme with very low levels present and prolonged apnea
4. Normal dibucaine number + normal activity = normal enzyme and amount. (Another reason for the prolonged apnea to be investigated.)

or purified human cholinesterase has been suggested as a treatment for the prolonged apnea. Although they may be successful, there are additional transfusion risks and cost issues.[48] It is safer to let the effects of succinylcholine dissipate on their own with sedation and ventilation as noted earlier.

Dibucaine is an amide local anesthetic that inhibits typical or usual PChE but not atypical PChE. For example, the normal dibucaine number of 80 means that 80% of the PChE activity was inhibited by dibucaine. If a dibucaine number of 20 is obtained, the patient has atypical enzyme because dibucaine did not inhibit the patient's enzyme activity. If a patient experiences prolonged apnea after succinylcholine administration, it is imperative to differentiate between an atypical genetic variant of PChE or simply low levels of normal PChE enzyme. Possible interpretations of a dibucaine test are given in Box 12.3.

Patients with acute or chronic liver disease, organophosphate poisoning, or chronic renal disease; patients in the late stages of pregnancy; and those undergoing estrogen therapy may have markedly decreased PChE activities but normal enzyme. PChE phenotype interpretation is based on the total PChE activity and the percent of inhibition caused by dibucaine (Table 12.7).

Gene sequencing combined with biochemical testing can provide patients and their families with a comprehensive assessment of the likelihood of this type of event.[53,54,56]

Renal System

Succinylcholine may be used in surgical patients with renal disease when preoperative potassium levels are normal. The use of succinylcholine in patients with elevated preoperative potassium levels is contraindicated.[61] Patients with renal failure and end-stage renal disease are frequently dialyzed prior to surgery; so as long as the serum potassium is within normal limits, succinylcholine may be used safely.[62] Patients with renal disease may have lower cholinesterase levels.[63]

Effects in Special Populations

Elderly patients. The onset of succinylcholine may be slightly prolonged in the elderly due to a slower circulation time, but the clinical relevance is minimal.[64] Reduced plasma cholinesterase levels in elderly men may allow for a reduced dose of succinylcholine. A unique possible

drug interaction has been noted in elderly patients taking donepezil (Aricept), rivastigmine (Exelon), or galantamine (Razadyne). These are anticholinesterase drugs used to treat Alzheimer disease and select forms of dementia. They increase ACh levels in the CNS and are referred to as cognitive enhancers. Theoretically the inhibition of cholinesterase produced by these agents may prolong the action of succinylcholine. The amount of systemic cholinesterase inhibition, however, does not produce clinically significant prolongation of succinylcholine[65] (Box 12.4).

Obese patients. No contraindication to the use of succinylcholine exists in obese patients. The utility of RSI in anesthetic management of the obese patient makes its use common.[66] The recommended dose of succinylcholine is 1.0 mg/kg, based on total body weight, to produce excellent intubating conditions.[67] In a 2003 study by Brodsky and Foster,[68] succinylcholine was given to 14 morbidly obese patients (body mass indices 35.8–58) who underwent laparoscopic gastric bypass surgery. The authors administered doses ranging from 120 to 140 mg and successfully intubated all of the patients. Only 2 of the 14 patients complained of postoperative myalgia. Dosing should be based on total body weight. Because succinylcholine is water soluble, it would seem that doses based on lean body weight would suffice. However, morbidly obese patients have increased fluid compartments and pseudocholinesterase levels and require higher doses to ensure adequate paralysis.[69,70]

Pediatrics. In children, succinylcholine is used only in emergency situations to secure an airway. Routine use in elective procedures was abandoned in the early 1990s, owing to several widely reported cases of severe hyperkalemia and rhabdomyolysis in what appeared to be healthy children. The cases involved routine procedures in children with undiagnosed Duchenne muscular dystrophy (DMD).[71–75] This is an X chromosome–linked disorder with onset of symptoms usually around 5 years of age. Patients exhibit a typical progression of weakness and atrophy that starts in the legs and pelvis, spreads to the shoulders and neck, and finally involves the upper extremities and respiratory muscles. Life expectancy is rarely more than 30 years; death is often a consequence of cardiac and respiratory diseases. Children with DMD frequently require orthopedic surgery for repair of scoliosis or contractures.[76,77]

The Food and Drug Administration (FDA), in conjunction with the anesthesia community, placed the following warning on the use of succinylcholine:

RISK OF CARDIAC ARREST FROM HYPERKALEMIC RHABDOMYOLYSIS.

There have been rare reports of acute rhabdomyolysis with hyperkalemia followed by ventricular dysrhythmias, cardiac arrest, and death after the administration of succinylcholine to apparently healthy children who were subsequently found to have undiagnosed skeletal muscle myopathy, most frequently Duchenne muscular dystrophy.

TABLE 12.7 Select Inherited Variants of Cholinesterase

PChE Variant	Genetic Label	Frequency (%)	Population Incidence	Enzyme Activity	Duration of Succinylcholine
Usual	Homozygote U	96	Normal	Normal	Normal; dibucaine number 70–80
—	Heterozygote U/A	3	1 in 480	Decreased	Slightly prolonged; dibucaine number 50–69
Atypical	Homozygote A	0.3	1 in 3200	Decreased by 70% or more	Significantly prolonged; dibucaine number 16–30
Fluoride	Homozygote F	0.03	Extremely rare	Decreased by 60%	Moderately prolonged
Silent	Homozygote S	0.04	Extremely rare	No activity	Significantly prolonged

PChE, Plasma cholinesterase.

BOX 12.4 Drugs That May Inhibit Cholinesterase

Agents Used to Treat Alzheimer Disease
- Donepezil (Aricept)
- Rivastigmine (Exelon)
- Galantamine (Razadyne)—herbal medicine also available over the counter

This syndrome often presents as peaked T-waves and sudden cardiac arrest within minutes after the administration of the drug in healthy appearing children (usually, but not exclusively, males, and most frequently 8 years of age or younger). There have also been reports in adolescents.

Therefore, when a healthy appearing infant or child develops cardiac arrest soon after administration of succinylcholine not felt to be due to inadequate ventilation, oxygenation, or anesthetic overdose, immediate treatment for hyperkalemia should be instituted. This should include administration of intravenous (IV) calcium, bicarbonate, and glucose with insulin, with hyperventilation. Due to the abrupt onset of this syndrome, routine resuscitative measures are likely to be unsuccessful. However, extraordinary and prolonged resuscitative efforts have resulted in successful resuscitation in some reported cases. In addition, in presence of signs of malignant hyperthermia, appropriate treatment should be instituted concurrently.

Since there may be no signs or symptoms to alert the practitioner to which patients are at risk, it is recommended that the use of succinylcholine in children should be reserved for emergency intubation or instances where immediate securing of the airway is necessary (e.g., laryngospasm, difficult airway, full stomach) or for intramuscular use when a suitable vein is inaccessible.[78]

Because neither succinylcholine nor halothane is routinely used in children, the incidence of masseter spasm and malignant hyperthermia has decreased. Older studies have been reported in which jaw-opening ability and the presence or absence of masseter spasm, often considered a precursor of malignant hyperpyrexia, were studied. Research was conducted on 63 children anesthetized with halothane, then relaxed with succinylcholine, pancuronium, or vecuronium. Although vecuronium and pancuronium did not cause problems with jaw opening, succinylcholine was associated with this problem, and some of the

succinylcholine patients were difficult to intubate.[78] Masseter spasm was noted to be more frequent in children administered succinylcholine concomitantly with halothane, compared with children who received succinylcholine and thiopental.[36,79]

A random sample of 6500 anesthetic records (53% of 12,169 anesthetic procedures performed) was reviewed. Fifteen cases of masseter spasm were identified. In each case, the patient underwent halothane induction and was then given succinylcholine intravenously. Seven of the 15 cases of masseter spasm developed in children between ages 8 and 10 years.[80] Researchers noted an increased incidence of masseter spasm in children with strabismus who were anesthetized with halothane and received intravenous succinylcholine. Of 1468 halothane anesthetic procedures, 15 cases of masseter spasm were discovered, and of these 15 cases 6 occurred in the 211 patients with strabismus.[81]

In current practice, masseter spasm, although rare, is seen in adults during anesthesia induction and often in emergency rooms or critical care units during emergency airway management.[82,83] Common side effects of succinylcholine and contraindications for its use are noted in Table 12.8 and Box 12.5, respectively.

Other Factors

Intraocular pressure. Intraocular pressure (IOP) is known to increase by 5 to 15 mm Hg for as much as 10 minutes after succinylcholine administration.[43,84] The average is approximately 10 mm Hg for approximately 6 minutes. The exact mechanism of this increase is unknown. Some feel that tonic contractions of the extraocular muscles via fasciculation may explain this IOP increase. It is now thought, however, that succinylcholine-induced IOP increase is a vascular event, with choroidal vascular dilation or a decrease in drainage secondary to elevated central venous pressure temporarily inhibiting the flow of aqueous humor through the canal of Schlemm.[84]

This rise in IOP with succinylcholine administration is significantly less than the IOP increase associated with coughing or bucking. Patients who receive succinylcholine and are intubated 1 minute after its administration had IOPs that were not significantly higher than baseline. There are no documented reports of the extrusion of globe contents following the use of succinylcholine in open-eye emergency procedures. A 2006 review has essentially refuted the issue of eye damage after succinylcholine administration in open-globe injuries. It appears to be a theoretical concern only. Securing the airway remains the primary issue.[36,43,84] A thorough discussion of the use of succinylcholine and eye injuries is found in Chapter 44.

Hyperkalemia. Succinylcholine administration results in a transient hyperkalemia. A 0.5- to 1-mEq/L increase in serum potassium levels

TABLE 12.8   Side Effects of Succinylcholine

Side Effect	Probable Cause
Hyperkalemia	Normally, serum K^+ is increased by up to 0.5 mEq/L secondary to potassium leaking from the depolarized muscle; in up-regulated patients, levels may rise much higher
Dysrhythmias	Tachycardia (usually mild) is the most common effect; bradycardia secondary to hyperkalemia, especially with repeat doses, can occur (wide electrocardiographic complexes leading to cardiac arrest have been seen in children with Duchenne muscular dystrophy and other muscle disorders)
Myalgia	Secondary to fasciculation, even though some patients complain of muscle pain without having shown visible evidence of fasciculation
Myoglobinemia	Rare complication after extensive fasciculation or in malignant hyperthermia
Elevated intragastric pressure	Secondary to transient contraction of abdominal muscles during fasciculation; however, elevations of intragastric pressure seen after succinylcholine are not clinically relevant; less significant than occur with CO_2 insufflation during laparoscopic procedures
Elevated intracranial pressure (ICP)	Postulated to be secondary to fasciculation, increased central venous pressure; associated with increased cerebral blood flow secondary to muscle-spindle afferent activity and actions on peripheral neuromuscular junctions (ICP effects can be blocked by pretreatment with a small dose of nondepolarizing relaxant and the usual initial administration of an induction agent; may safely be used in neurosurgical procedures)
Elevated intraocular pressure (IOP)	Increases within 1 min and peaks at an increase of 9 mm Hg within 6 min after administration; increase is a vascular event, with choroidal vascular dilation or a decrease in drainage secondary to elevated central venous pressure, temporarily inhibiting the flow of aqueous humor through the canal of Schlemm; generally considered safe in ocular emergencies
Malignant hyperthermia	Associated with a genetic predisposition; mechanism by which succinylcholine triggers the syndrome is not understood
Masseter spasm	Seen in anesthetic and emergency use; sometimes followed by malignant hyperthermia

CO_2, Carbon dioxide; K^+, potassium.
Modified from Freid EB. Succinylcholine. In: Fleisher L, Rosenbaum SH. *Complications in Anesthesia*. 3rd ed. Philadelphia: Elsevier; 2018:391–394; Atlee JL. *Complications in Anesthesia*. 2nd ed. Philadelphia: Elsevier; 2007.

BOX 12.5   Contraindications to the Use of Succinylcholine

- Hyperkalemia
- Burn patients with injuries of over 35% total body surface area (TBSA), third-degree burn
- Severe muscle trauma
- Neurologic injury (e.g., paraplegia, quadriplegia)
- Hyperkalemia resulting from renal failure
- Severe sepsis (e.g., abdominal)
- Muscle wasting, prolonged immobilization, extensive muscle denervation
- Malignant hyperthermia
- Duchenne muscular dystrophy
- Selected muscle disorders (see Table 12.9)
- Should be used in children under 8 years old only in emergency situations; not for routine intubation
- Genetic variants of pseudocholinesterase
- Allergy

within 3 minutes after administration is usual. The effects were reported as lasting fewer than 10 to 15 minutes.[61]

A muscle receives signals to perform various functions from action potentials. As the action potential traverses the neuron, an influx of sodium and release of potassium occur. This mechanism of potassium release during normal muscle signaling is the same mechanism by which serum potassium increases because of the depolarization associated with receiving succinylcholine.[61]

Hyperkalemia may be profound in certain patients. In a review, Martyn and Richtsfeld[85] noted that lethal hyperkalemic responses to succinylcholine continue to be reported, although the mechanisms have not been completely elucidated. In the normally innervated mature muscle, AChRs are located only in the junctional area. But in certain pathologic states—including upper or lower motor denervation, infection, direct muscle trauma, muscle tumor, muscle inflammation, burn injury, immobilization, and prolonged chemical denervation by muscle relaxants, drugs, or toxins—there is an up-regulation (increase) of AChRs spreading throughout the muscle membrane. There is also an additional expression of two new isoforms of AChRs. The depolarization of these AChRs by succinylcholine and its metabolites leads to potassium efflux from the muscle and severe hyperkalemia. The nicotinic (neuronal) α7 AChRs, which are also in muscle, are depolarized not only by Ach and succinylcholine but by choline. Persistent choline stimulation may play a critical role in the hyperkalemic response to succinylcholine in patients with up-regulated AChRs.[85] Pathologic conditions with the potential for producing hyperkalemia associated with succinylcholine use are listed in Box 12.6.

Succinylcholine has been implicated in hyperkalemia after its administration to burn patients; therefore it is contraindicated in these patients.[86] Receptor up-regulation resulting from thermal trauma has been associated with several documented cases of cardiac arrest involving succinylcholine administration.[50] Indeed, plasma potassium levels as high as 15 mEq/L have been reported after the administration of succinylcholine, with this effect occurring 4 to 10 days after the burn and lasting for years.[87] The burn injury–related increase of AChRs is probably related to inflammation and local denervation of muscle.

- Upper or lower motor neuron defect
- Spinal cord trauma
- Prolonged chemical denervation (e.g., muscle relaxants, magnesium, clostridial toxins)
- Direct muscle trauma, tumor, or inflammation
- Select muscular dystrophies and myopathies
- Thermal trauma
- Disuse atrophy
- Stroke
- Tetanus
- Severe infection

Major third-degree burns involving extensive body surface area may up-regulate AChRs throughout the body because of the extent and direct inflammation and injury to muscle. Hyperkalemia after burn injury to a single limb (8% body surface area) has been observed, indicating that burn size alone is not the only contributing factor. It is generally reported that the administration of succinylcholine to a burn patient more than 24 hours after the burn is unsafe; however, others note that succinylcholine can be safely used with burn patients for several days after the burn, because receptor up-regulation does not begin until 24 to 48 hours after the burn.[88,89] Some researchers recommend avoidance of succinylcholine, starting 48 hours after injury.[89] Changes in responses to both succinylcholine and the nondepolarizing agents have been noted for years after a major burn injury. Immobilization due to contractures may play a role. Succinylcholine should never be used in these patients, regardless of the time postburn.[84,90]

Treatment of succinylcholine-induced hyperkalemia involves the emergency administration of drugs that promote the cellular uptake of potassium; these include insulin with glucose, catecholamines, and sodium bicarbonate.

The use of various muscle relaxants in patients with muscle disorders is reviewed in Table 12.9.

Malignant hyperthermia. Malignant hyperthermia (MH) is a pharmacogenetic skeletal muscle disorder triggered by volatile anesthetics, succinylcholine, and stress. Succinylcholine is absolutely contraindicated in patients with known or suspected MH or who have MH in their families.[91] The exact mechanism for the possible triggering action remains unclear.[92] Mutations in the skeletal muscle ryanodine receptor gene may result in altered calcium release from sarcoplasmic reticulum stores, giving rise to MH. Patients who develop MH show signs such as muscle rigidity, rhabdomyolysis, increased carbon dioxide production, convulsions, metabolic acidosis, tachycardia, and a rapid increase in temperature.[93–95] A complete discussion of the physiologic and treatment aspects of MH can be found in Chapter 36.

Myalgias and fasciculations. Postoperative muscle pain, particularly in the face, subcostal region, trunk, neck, upper abdominal muscles, and shoulders, is a common occurrence after succinylcholine administration.[96] A meta-analysis that included 52 randomized clinical trials found several interesting results.[97] The incidence of succinylcholine-induced myalgia is high, and symptoms sometimes last for several days. Small doses of nondepolarizing muscle relaxants, approximately 10% to 30% of the ED_{95}, reduce the incidence of fasciculations and myalgia, although pretreatment side effects occur. Higher doses of succinylcholine decrease the risk of myalgia compared with lower doses, and opioids do not have any impact. Pretreatment with sodium channel blockers (i.e., lidocaine) or nonsteroidal antiinflammatory drugs (diclofenac and aspirin) may prevent myalgia.

Myalgias are generally attributed to the occurrence of fasciculations resulting from the shearing forces and repetitive firing of the motor nerve terminals, which causes uncoordinated muscle contractions. Patients who experience muscle pain most often are women and those persons who rarely participate in muscular activity. Conversely, patients at extremes of age, as well as pregnant patients, are least affected. Postoperative myalgias associated with succinylcholine increase in severity with early ambulation, which may consequently delay postoperative healing.[96]

Prevention is the key to avoiding postoperative muscle pain. Although not always effective, the incidence of myalgia is greatly reduced with nondepolarizer pretreatment. Use of no more than 10% of the ED_{95} is safe and effective and will avoid most of the difficulties of the patient experiencing weakness prior to loss of consciousness. Effective and equivalent doses have been reported as 0.04 mg/kg rocuronium, 1.5 mg atracurium, and 0.3 mg vecuronium.[98,99]

Phase II block. Administration of large doses of succinylcholine results in an alteration in the characteristics of the block.[49] Succinylcholine produces specific unique responses to nerve stimulation when compared with the nondepolarizing agents. These include a sustained response to tetanic stimulation, no fade with TOF or DBS, and no posttetanic potentiation. Figs. 12.9 and 12.10 show the characteristic TOF responses during onset and recovery from succinylcholine-induced block, respectively. Box 12.7 compares the characteristics of depolarizing and nondepolarizing NMB. Large doses of succinylcholine cause changes that resemble more of a nondepolarizing block, as evidenced by fade in response to tetanic stimuli, TOF, and DBS, the appearance of posttetanic potentiation, and, theoretically, antagonism with drugs such as neostigmine. This is commonly referred to as a desensitization, dual, or phase II block. Some experts do not use these terms interchangeably.[48]

As explained earlier, tetanic fade is caused by an interaction with cholinergic presynaptic receptors mediating positive feedback–induced ACh release from the motor nerve end.[33,85] The finding that high doses of succinylcholine inhibited presynaptic $\alpha_3\beta_2$ AChRs (i.e., the compound behaved like a nondepolarizing relaxant) may help explain how high or repeated doses of succinylcholine result in a nondepolarizing type of block (phase II block) characterized by fade and posttetanic potentiation.[100] The exact mechanism is unclear; however, an electrical imbalance caused by repeated opening of junctional channels has been proposed.[48] Development of a desensitization block is a historic discussion because doses exceeding 6 to 8 mg/kg are required, and high doses, as seen with succinylcholine infusions, are no longer used in current practice.

NONDEPOLARIZING AGENTS

The efficacy of the nondepolarizing relaxants is similar, so the choice of one drug over another is largely made on other factors. Specific patient characteristics, type of surgical procedure, pharmacokinetics, and side effect profile guide the selection of an individual relaxant for a given situation. The intermediate duration nondepolarizing relaxants are almost exclusively used in current clinical practice.

Rocuronium Bromide

Rocuronium is the most widely used nondepolarizing relaxant in the United States.[13] The introduction of vecuronium and atracurium, both of which were marketed as intermediate-acting NMBAs, improved the flexibility of the clinician in matching the agent to the expected duration of surgery.[101] Slow onset, solution stability, and histamine release remained problems to be overcome.[102] Rocuronium (Zemuron) has been developed to partially fill this void. It combines a duration and

TABLE 12.9 Anesthetic Considerations in Patients With Muscle Disorders

Muscle Disorder	Succinylcholine	Nondepolarizing Muscle Relaxant	Regional Anesthesia	Volatile Anesthetic	Malignant Hyperthermia (MH) Risk	Comments
Dystrophinopathies (Duchenne and Becker muscular dystrophy)	Contraindicated	Increased sensitivity	Yes	No: may produce significant rhabdomyolysis	Weak evidence of susceptibility	Consider sugammadex for reversal; intravenous (IV) drugs if general anesthetic required
Myasthenia gravis	Prolonged duration if anticholinesterase (AChE) continued; sensitive if AChE discontinued	Increased sensitivity	Yes	Yes	Not susceptible	Thymoma may cause airway difficulties; cardiac dysfunction, conduction disorders and myocarditis; potential for cholinergic crisis; administer neostigmine cautiously
Amyotrophic lateral sclerosis (ALS); Lou Gehrig disease	Contraindicated	Increased sensitivity	Yes	Yes	Not susceptible	Bulbar dysfunction; assess for respiratory reserve, avoid drugs that prolong QT interval
Lambert-Eaton syndrome	Contraindicated	Increased sensitivity	Yes	Yes	Not susceptible	Autonomic dysfunction common
Guillain-Barré syndrome	Contraindicated	Increased sensitivity	Yes	Yes	Not susceptible	Severe autonomic dysfunction common
Charcot-Marie-Tooth disease	Contraindicated	Increased sensitivity	Controversial	Yes	Not susceptible	May have increased sensitivity to IV sedatives; response to atracurium and mivacurium normal
Mitochondrial myopathy	Contraindicated	Variable sensitivity	Yes	Yes	Not susceptible	Avoid propofol infusion; avoid opiate induced respiratory depression; prone to hypoglycemia and lactic acidosis; prepare pacemaker
Myotonic dystrophy	Contraindicated	Increased sensitivity	Yes	Controversial	Not susceptible	Very sensitive to anesthetics; significant cardiac disease common; avoid anticholinesterases and hypothermia
Multiple sclerosis	Contraindicated	Increased sensitivity	Epidural safe; spinal controversial	Yes	Not susceptible	Avoid emotional stress; minimize changes in fluid or hemodynamic dynamics; thromboprophylaxis may be needed
Critical illness polyneuropathy and critical illness myopathy	Contraindicated	Variable resistance	Avoided unless major risk for gen. anesthesia	Yes	Not susceptible	Avoid aminoglycosides, hyperglycemia; treat sepsis aggressively; prone to liver and kidney failure
Central core disease	Contraindicated	Increased sensitivity	Yes	Avoid	Susceptible	Scoliosis and cardiomyopathies common
Hyperkalemic periodic paralysis	Contraindicated	Increased sensitivity	Yes	Avoid	Not susceptible	Neostigmine and succinylcholine contraindicated; monitor potassium
McArdle disease	Contraindicated	Variable sensitivity	Yes	Avoid	Weak evidence of susceptibility	Avoid drugs that cause sympathetic stimulation; infuse glucose solutions
Friedreich ataxia	Contraindicated	Variable sensitivity	Yes, but may be difficult due to severe scoliosis	Yes	Not susceptible	High incidence of heart failure, cardiac assessment mandatory
Chronic inflammatory demyelinating polyneuropathy	Contraindicated	Increased sensitivity	Avoid	Yes	Not susceptible	Assess respiratory reserve
Huntington disease	Yes, but may have low levels or fluoride-resistant genotype pseudocholinesterase	Normal response	Yes	Yes	Not susceptible	Bulbar muscle dysfunction increases aspiration risk; avoid metoclopramide; may be taking multiple psychotropic medications so be aware of potential drug interactions

Adapted from Romero A, Joshi GP. Neuromuscular disease and anesthesia. *Muscle Nerve.* 2013;48(3):451–460; Schieren M, et al. Anaesthetic management of patients with myopathies. *Eur J Anaesthesiol.* 2017;34(10):641–649; Gurnaney H, et al. Malignant hyperthermia and muscular dystrophies. *Anesth Analg.* 2009;109(4):1043–1048.

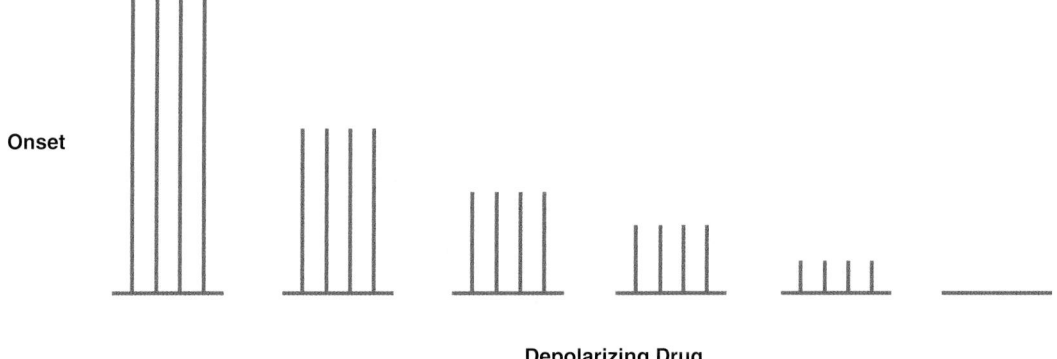

Fig. 12.9 Characteristic train-of-four response during the onset of succinylcholine.

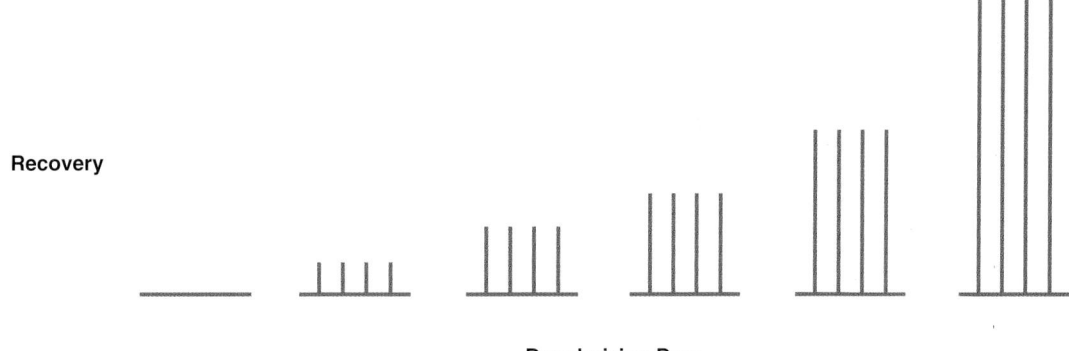

Fig. 12.10 Characteristic train-of-four response during recovery from succinylcholine.

BOX 12.7   Characteristics of Neuromuscular Blockade

Depolarizing (Phase I) Block
- Muscle fasciculation precedes onset of neuromuscular blockade
- Sustained response to tetanic stimulation
- Absence of posttetanic potentiation, stimulation, or facilitation
- Lack of fade to tetanus, train-of-four, or double-burst stimulation
- Block antagonized by prior administration of nondepolarizer as pretreatment (approximately 20% more succinylcholine required)
- Block potentiated by anticholinesterase drugs

Nondepolarizing (Phase II) Block
- Absence of muscle fasciculation
- Appearance of tetanic fade and posttetanic potentiation, stimulation, or facilitation
- Train-of-four and double-burst fade
- Reversal with anticholinesterase drugs
- In rare cases may be produced by an overdose and desensitization with succinylcholine at doses >6 mg/kg

---

cardiovascular profile comparable to those of vecuronium, with an onset that is only slightly longer than that of succinylcholine.[101–103]

A derivative of vecuronium, rocuronium bromide is chemically designated as 1-[17β-(acetyloxy)-3α-hydroxy-2β-(4-morpholinyl)-5α-androstan-16β-yl]-1-(2-propenyl) pyrrolidinium bromide, and it has one-seventh to one-eighth the potency of its derivative.[38,49,103] It is a monoquaternary structure that also shares its aminosteroid structure with pancuronium[104] (Fig. 12.11). The pH of rocuronium is adjusted to

4.0, and the agent contains no preservative. It exists in a solution that is stable at room temperature for up to 30 days.[105]

Results of clinical studies of both healthy children and healthy adults suggest an ED_{95} of approximately 0.3 mg/kg.[37] Its steady-state volume of distribution in healthy adults is 207 (14) mL/kg and is slightly smaller for children ages 4 to 8 years. Rocuronium is approximately 46% bound to human plasma proteins, somewhat less than other neuromuscular blockers. This decreased plasma protein binding may lead to a slightly more rapid onset because more unbound drug is readily available at the neuronal binding sites.[106]

Pharmacokinetics

Onset. Rocuronium is the NMBA of choice for RSI when succinylcholine is either contraindicated or otherwise not used. A disadvantage of using rocuronium during RSI is its long duration of action.[107,108]

Administration of rocuronium with doses ranging from 0.6 to 1.2 mg/kg provides good to excellent intubating conditions within 45 to 90 seconds.[39,109,110] A meta-analysis noted that although rocuronium 1.2 mg/kg produces excellent intubating conditions, succinylcholine is superior in achieving excellent and clinically acceptable intubating conditions. It also has a shorter duration of action, which is clinically advantageous.[111,112] The onset of muscle relaxants is related to potency: The less potent an agent, the faster the onset. Rocuronium has an onset of action that is inversely proportional to its potency,[103] and it is less potent than other steroidal-based neuromuscular blockers.[113,114] This decreased potency allows a larger mass of drug at the prejunctional and postjunctional cholinoreceptors.[39,113] This large drug mass at the receptor site yields a faster onset.[115,116]

One method used clinically to accelerate the onset of rocuronium when administering it to intubate during RSI is referred to as priming.

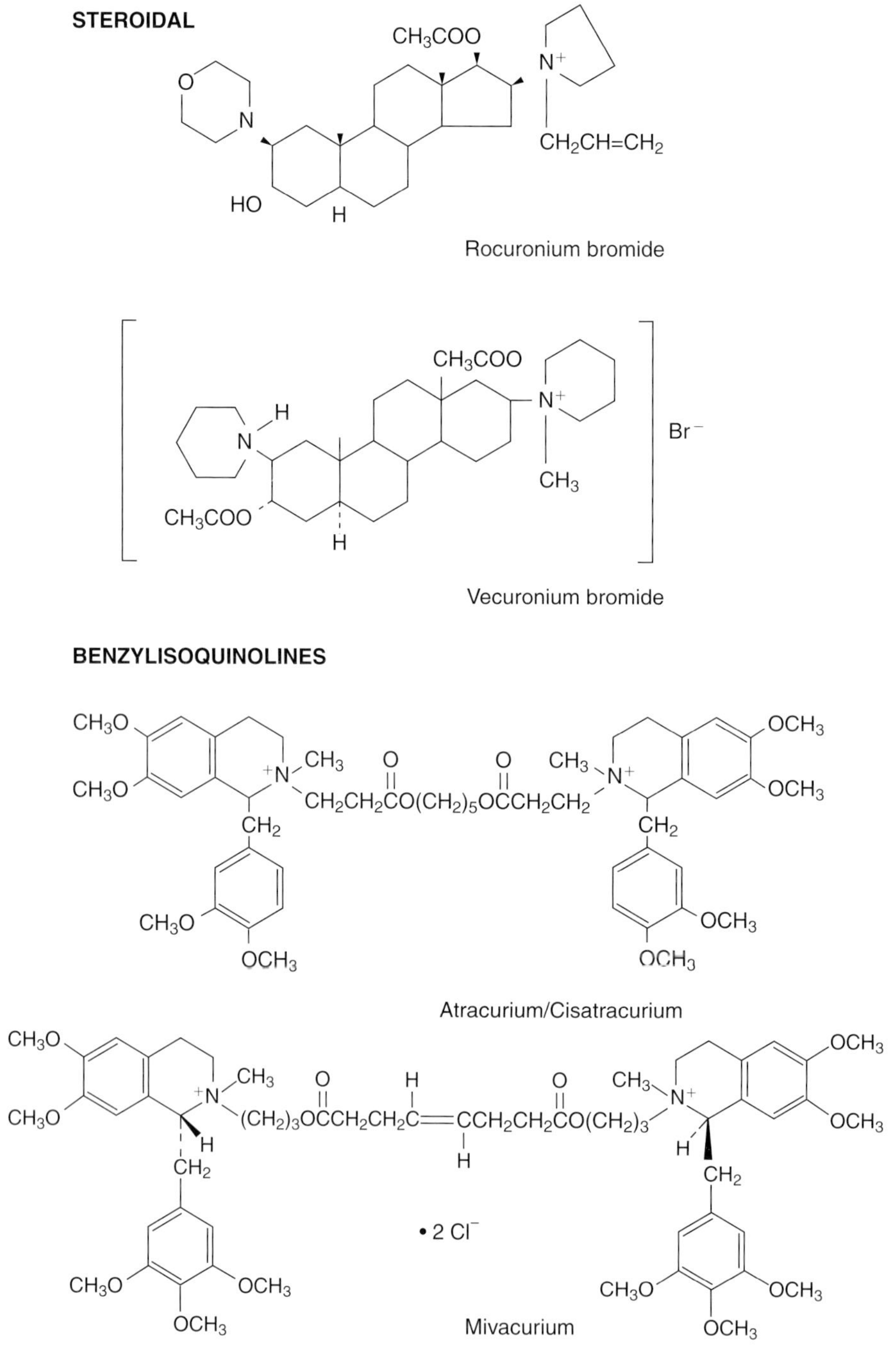

STEROIDAL

Rocuronium bromide

Vecuronium bromide

BENZYLISOQUINOLINES

Atracurium/Cisatracurium

Mivacurium

Fig. 12.11 Chemical structures of nondepolarizing muscle relaxants.

Priming involves giving 10% of the calculated intubating dose prior to inducing anesthesia. After a period of 1 to 3 minutes, the patient is anesthetized, and the remaining rocuronium is given. Giving a small portion of the relaxant dose in this manner speeds the onset by valuable seconds.[117–119] Priming, however, produces respiratory distress in 10% of the patients in which it is used.[120]

Duration. Rocuronium is classified as an intermediate duration relaxant.[41] In usual ED_{95} doses, it lasts 30 to 60 minutes. The duration of action is similar to that of vecuronium, and its duration depends, like that of any other agent, on the dose administered.[38] An intubating dose of 0.6 to 1 mg/kg provides a clinical duration of 30 to 90 minutes.[38,39] The administration of 0.6 mg/kg resulted in 10% recovery of T_1 within

27.2 (5.5) minutes, whereas 25%, 75%, and 90% recovery of T_1 occurred in 31.1 (5.6) minutes, 39.3 (6.2) minutes, and 41.2 (6.1) minutes, respectively.[121] Recovery of the TOFR to 0.8 when rocuronium was administered with sevoflurane, isoflurane, and propofol occurred in 103 (30.7), 69 (20.4), and 62 (21.1) minutes, respectively.[122]

Elimination. Rocuronium undergoes both hepatic and renal elimination. Biliary elimination of unchanged drug is the primary method of rocuronium elimination. It also undergoes deacetylation via the liver.[121–123] Renal excretion accounts for 33% of elimination.[49] Plasma levels of rocuronium follow a three-compartment open model. This results in extensive redistribution after intravenous injection. Therefore, before elimination occurs, serum levels of the drug are low enough to result in substantial recovery.[37] The elimination half-life of rocuronium is 60 to 120 minutes. The elimination half-lives of the agent in children, normal adults, and elderly persons are 38.3 minutes, 56 minutes, and 137 minutes, respectively.[113,124] Patients with significant liver or kidney disease will have a prolonged effect.[52,63]

Vecuronium Bromide

Vecuronium bromide (Norcuron) is a potent nondepolarizing neuromuscular blocker. Studies comparing vecuronium with pancuronium, its predecessor, found vecuronium to be 1.5 times more potent than its parent compound.[125] Both agents were developed by manipulation of the steroid nucleus. The molecule was successfully altered from bisquaternary pancuronium to a monoquaternary compound, creating an agent with a more rapid onset and a shorter duration. Vecuronium is more lipophilic than pancuronium, although it is still predominantly a hydrophilic compound. This change in its solubility is thought to be the cause of its differing pharmacokinetic profile.[126–128]

It is chemically designated as piperidinium 1-[(2β, 3α, 5α, 16β, 17β)-3, 17-bis(acetyloxy)-2-(1-piperidinyl) androstan-16-yl]-1-methyl bromide[127](see Fig. 12.11).

Vecuronium is available as a 10- or 20-mg, sterile, nonpyrogenic powder for intravenous use only. Once reconstituted, the solution has a pH of 4.0 and is stable for 24 hours at 25°C.[127] The dose-response curve to derive the ED_{95} was found to be 0.03 mg/kg.[126] The agent has a steady-state volume of distribution of 0.21 to 0.27 L/kg.[128]

Pharmacokinetics

Onset. Vecuronium has an onset of action that is 1.5 times that of pancuronium, a proportion similar to that of its potency.[129,130] The induction dose of vecuronium is 0.1 mg/kg (more than two times the ED_{95}), which produces a maximum suppression of muscle twitch within 3 minutes of administration. The onset varies with the concurrent anesthetic administered and is inversely proportional to the dose.[131] With balanced anesthesia, a 0.1-mg/kg dose of vecuronium resulted in an onset of 3.1 minutes, whereas in patients receiving isoflurane, nitrous oxide–oxygen (N_2O-O_2) anesthesia, the onset time decreased to 1.8 minutes.[128,132–134]

Duration. Duration of action varies with the type of anesthetic being administered and the dose of the agent. This phenomenon has been noted with other nondepolarizing agents, as well as with vecuronium.[134] The duration is 36.2 ± 6.4 minutes after a dose of 0.1 mg/kg in patients undergoing intravenous anesthesia.[132] The time from 25% twitch recovery to 75% twitch recovery at a dose of 0.1 mg/kg was 11 to 12 minutes and the duration 30 to 45 minutes.

Elimination. Vecuronium is eliminated via hepatic and renal mechanisms. Vecuronium undergoes elimination via an orthodox three-compartment model. Because it is more lipophilic than other agents in its class, vecuronium does not depend solely on the kidneys for elimination. Only 20% to 30% of the administered dose is recovered unchanged in the urine within 24 hours.[126] A major portion of the dose (40%–80%) is taken up by the liver and excreted in bile.[130] Small amounts of its metabolites (3-hydroxy, 17-hydroxy, and 3,17-hydroxy) can be detected by thin-layer chromatography. The 3-desacetyl metabolite is thought to have approximately 50% the potency of vecuronium.[9] It is avoided in critical care units for long-term administration because of accumulation. Reported elimination half-lives range from 51 to 90 minutes in healthy adults. Total clearances have been reported from 3 to 5.6 mL/kg/min.[125,135,136]

Pancuronium Bromide

Pancuronium has little use in anesthesia practice today because of its long duration of action. The chemical designation of pancuronium bromide is 2β, 16β-dipiperidine-5α-androstane-3α, 17-β-diol diacetate dimethobromide (see Fig. 12.11). It has a volume of distribution of 0.18 to 0.26 L/kg; is an odorless, white, crystalline powder; and has a melting point of 215°C. Extensive testing revealed an effective dose of 0.02 to 0.05 mg/kg in mice, rats, rabbits, cats, and dogs.[6] Further research determined the ED_{95} of pancuronium to be 0.075 mg/kg in humans with an induction dose of roughly twice that value (0.1–0.15 mg/kg).[135,136]

Pharmacodynamic Summary

The mean onset time is 2 to 2.5 minutes. The average duration of action is 60 to 90 minutes. Pancuronium is primarily excreted via the kidney. Therefore pancuronium will have a prolonged duration of action in patients with renal failure. Thirty-five percent of the drug is also released in the bile.[93]

Atracurium Besylate

Atracurium (Tracrium) was developed as a result of a joint venture between the Department of Pharmaceutical Chemistry at the University of Strathclyde and Wellcome Research Laboratories. The objective of the investigators was to develop an agent with the following characteristics:

- Competitive bisquaternary neuromuscular blocker
- Highly selective in action
- Degradable without renal or hepatic intervention[137,138]

The resulting agent was a bisquaternary competitive neuromuscular blocker in the form of a besylate salt.[126,137] Atracurium is classified as a benzylisoquinoline and is designated as 2,2′-[1,5-pentanediylbis[oxy(3-oxo-3,1-propanediyl)] bis[1-[(3,4-dimethoxyphenyl) methyl]-1,2,3,4-tetrahydro-6,7-dimethoxy-2-methyl-isoquinolinium] dibenzenesulfonate. The pH of atracurium is adjusted to 3.25 to 3.65, and the agent contains the preservative benzyl alcohol. Atracurium loses potency at the rate of 6% per year when it is refrigerated at 5°C. At room temperature, the agent degrades approximately 5% per month, and its recommended unrefrigerated shelf life is 14 days. It was developed with an intermediate duration in mind, and it spontaneously degrades to inactive products. It is well absorbed intravenously, with an ED_{95} of 0.10 to 0.25 mg/kg.[126,139]

Atracurium is rapidly distributed throughout the extracellular space after intravenous injection and has a volume of distribution of 153 (13) mL/kg. It is approximately 82% protein bound and does not distribute into the fat because it is ionized.[140] Obese patients who received atracurium according to ideal body weight demonstrated no difference in recovery indices or recovery times when compared with control patients of normal weight because of the agent's lack of organ dependency for elimination.[141–143] The chemical structure of atracurium besylate is shown in Fig. 12.11.

Pharmacokinetics

Onset. As expected, atracurium has an onset time that is inversely proportional to dosage, in the range of 1.2 to 2.8 minutes. When various doses of atracurium were given to 70 patients anesthetized with fentanyl, thiopental, and N_2O-O_2 anesthesia, clinical effects were seen at doses of 0.3 to 0.6 mg/kg. Other investigators, however, have found the onset to be longer, in the range of 2.31 to 3.55 minutes.[131,132,144]

Duration. The duration of atracurium increases as its dose increases. Duration of maximum effect and duration to 95% recovery of peak contraction are reported in the range of 5.6 to 69.5 minutes.[132,145,146] On average, as an intermediate relaxant, the duration of action is 30 to 60 minutes.

Elimination. The development of atracurium arose from the discovery of the plant *Leontice leontopetalum* and one of its components, designated petaline. This component was similar to tubocurarine and was observed to undergo an unexpectedly facile degradation in mild alkali by the well-known Hofmann elimination pathway, with loss of water and formation of a tertiary base.[139] Stenlake's pursuit of this research led to the development of atracurium, which does not rely on any organ system for its breakdown and elimination. Study of the clinical pharmacology of atracurium reveals that its molecules decompose by Hofmann elimination, as well as by nonspecific ester hydrolysis.[137,139,141,147]

Hofmann elimination is a temperature- and pH-dependent breakdown of the drug molecule. In the vial, atracurium is at room temperature in an acidic medium. When injected, the pH rises to blood pH of 7.4, and the temperature increases to body temperature. These increases in pH and temperature allow the Hofmann elimination to ensue. Atracurium degrades via Hofmann elimination (10%–40%). In mild alkaline states, fission occurs at the quaternary nitrogen position, and laudanosine is subsequently released.[147,148] The agent then degrades further. Ester hydrolysis also occurs, and it is catalyzed by nonspecific esterases into a quaternary alcohol and a quaternary acid.[137,147] These metabolites are excreted primarily in bile and urine. A summary of some select properties of neuromuscular blockers is given in Table 12.10.

Cisatracurium Besylate

The most notable of the 10 stereoisomers of atracurium, cisatracurium besylate (Nimbex) has gained popularity in the clinical arena since the mid-1990s. It is a nondepolarizing muscle relaxant, three times more potent than atracurium with a slower onset of action. The agent is available as a sterile, nonpyrogenic aqueous solution in 5-, 10-, and 20-mL vials. The pH is 3.25 to 3.65, and the concentration is 2 mg/mL (except in the 20-mL vial, in which the concentration is 10 mg/mL for convenience in the intensive care unit setting).[149] Advantages of cisatracurium include maintenance of cardiovascular stability, nonorgan-dependent elimination, and a lack of histamine release after injection.[150,151]

Pharmacokinetics

Onset. Cisatracurium is regarded as intermediate in its onset and duration of action. In adults the ED_{95} is 0.05 mg/kg during N_2O-O_2 opioid anesthesia.[152] It has been noted to be five times more potent than rocuronium, with a slower onset of action, longer duration, and slower spontaneous recovery.[153,154] An intravenous bolus of 0.1 mg/kg (twice the ED_{95}) produces desired levels of relaxation within 3.1 minutes.[155] Doses of three to four times the ED_{95} (0.15–0.2 mg/kg) decrease the mean time of onset to 3.4 and 2.8 minutes, respectively.[156]

Duration. After doses of three to four times the ED_{95}, the average time for the first twitch in a TOF to recover to 25% of control is 65 minutes.[157] Further studies report that the duration of cisatracurium with an intubating dose of 0.25 mg/kg is 55 to 75 minutes. Full recovery at the aforementioned dose occurs in 75 to 100 minutes. Additional sources report the duration as 55 to 61 minutes.[158]

Elimination. Cisatracurium, like atracurium, undergoes Hofmann elimination (which is pH and temperature dependent) in the plasma and tissues. Hofmann elimination accounts for 77% of total body clearance, and nonspecific esterases are responsible for 23% of total body clearance. Of the organ-dependent clearance, 16% occurs through renal pathways.[159] Studies have demonstrated a half-life of approximately 26 to 36 minutes, with an increase in the rate of degradation as pH increases.[160] As with atracurium, one of the metabolites of cisatracurium is laudanosine along with acrylates. However, cisatracurium liberates one-fifth as much laudanosine as atracurium.[161] A summary of some select properties of neuromuscular blockers is given in Table 12.10.

Mivacurium Chloride

Mivacurium (Mivacron) was marketed as the first "short-acting" NMBA. The drug company that marketed it in the United States stopped in 2006 due to manufacturing issues. It was reintroduced in 2016. Its chemical formula is [R-(R*, R*-[E])]-2,2′-[(1,8-dioxo-4-octene-1,8-diyl) bis(oxy-3,1-propenediyl) bis(1,2,3,4-tetrahydro-6,7-dimethoxy-2-methyl-1-(3,4,5-trimethoxyphenyl) methyl) isoquinolinium] chloride. Mivacurium is classified as a benzylisoquinolinium and consists of a mixture of three different isomers. Perioperative relaxation is achieved with a dose of 0.05 mg/kg. The ED_{95} of mivacurium is 0.08 mg/kg. Its degradation by plasma cholinesterase provides it with a short duration[48,162] (see Fig. 12.11).

Pharmacodynamic Summary

The onset time of mivacurium is dose dependent and ranges from 1.5 minutes with 0.25 mg/kg up to 4 minutes with 0.15 mg/kg.[163,164] Mivacurium chloride was developed specifically to fill the niche between the ultrashort-acting succinylcholine and intermediate-acting agents. The duration of mivacurium is 15 to 20 minutes. Like that of succinylcholine, mivacurium's degradation by plasma cholinesterase results in its short action. The metabolites of mivacurium are excreted in the bile and urine, after the agent itself has been broken down by plasma cholinesterases.[165] Any disease process that interferes with the production of this enzyme results in the prolongation of action of this agent.[166,167] Thus mivacurium should not be administered to patients with atypical plasma cholinesterase. Prolonged paralysis after a test dose of 30 mcg/kg in a patient with a previously known plasma cholinesterase deficit has been reported.[60]

Nondepolarizing Agents' Effect on Various Organ Systems

Central Nervous System

All muscle relaxants are quaternary ammonium compounds and therefore water soluble at physiologic pH. As such, they are unable to cross physiologic barriers such as the blood-brain, placental, and gastric, and therefore have no CNS effects.

Cardiovascular System

The NMBAs have no direct effect on cardiac muscle. Any cardiovascular changes that occur with the administration of a muscle relaxant are caused by indirect actions such as histamine release or effects on the autonomic nervous system. Of the current nondepolarizing relaxants, only atracurium and mivacurium exhibit any cardiac effects. Atracurium and mivacurium are associated with increases in heart rate and decreases in blood pressure at usual clinical doses due to histamine release.[168,169] Systolic and diastolic pressures significantly decrease, and cardiac output was significantly increased at 2, 5, and 10 minutes after a bolus dose. The increase in cardiac output is the result of a markedly decreased systemic vascular resistance. Nearly all of the hemodynamic changes associated with the administration of atracurium and mivacurium have been linked to the release of histamine.[48] Administration of cisatracurium does not result in histamine release. The effects of stimulation of histamine receptors and the resulting effects are listed in Box 12.8.

The steroidal relaxants, vecuronium and rocuronium, have no significant cardiac effects at clinical doses.[48] The cardiovascular effects of the neuromuscular blocking agents are summarized in Box 12.9.

Hepatic System

The steroidal relaxants rocuronium and vecuronium are affected by changes in hepatic status. They are primarily eliminated by a combination of liver metabolism and biliary and renal excretion, and therefore

TABLE 12.10 Summary of Select Properties of Neuromuscular Blocking Agents

Classification	ED$_{95}$ (mg/kg)	Intubating Dose Usually 2–3 × ED$_{95}$ (mg/kg)	Onset	Duration	Metabolism	Elimination Kidney (%)	Liver (%)	Automatic Ganglia Effect (SNS and PNS)	Cardiac Muscarinic Effect (Vagal Block)	Histamine Release	Resulting Cardiac Action
Ultrashort											
Succinylcholine (Anectine, Quelicin)	0.3	1–1.5	30–60 sec	5–10 min	Plasma cholinesterase	<2	0	Stimulates	Stimulates and/or blocks	0?	Usually tachycardia, bradycardia with repeat doses
Intermediate											
Atracurium (Tracrium)	0.15	0.5	2–4 min	30–60 min	Hofmann elimination, nonspecific esterase hydrolysis	10–40 metabolites	0	0	0	Yes	Hypotension, tachycardia, flushing
Cisatracurium (Nimbex)	0.05	0.1	2–4 min	30–60 min	Hofmann elimination, nonspecific esterase hydrolysis	Up to 77 metabolites	0	0	0	0	0
Rocuronium (Zemuron)	0.3	1	1–3 min	30–60 min	Hepatic and renal	10–30	70–90	0	0	0	0
Vecuronium (Norcuron)	0.05	0.1	2–4 min	30–60 min	Hepatic and renal	40–50	50–60	0	0	0	0

BOX 12.8 Effects of Stimulation of Histamine Receptors by Neuromuscular Blockers

H_1 Receptors	H_2 Receptors
Increased capillary permeability	Increased gastric acid production
Bronchoconstriction	Systemic and cerebral vasodilation
Intestinal contraction	Positive inotropic effects
Negative dromotropic effects	Positive chronotropic effects

Atracurium and mivacurium release modest amounts of histamine. Slight histamine release may occur with succinylcholine. The amount of histamine release is dependent on dose and speed of injection.

With endogenous histamine release, all receptor responses are elicited.

Prophylaxis against histamine release requires administration of both H_1- and H_2-receptor blockers.

H, Histamine.

BOX 12.9 Cardiac Effects of Neuromuscular Blocking Drugs

- Atracurium and mivacurium cause histamine release and may produce hypotension and tachycardia.
- Succinylcholine usually results in slight tachycardia. Repeat dosing in adults and any dose in children may produce sudden, abrupt bradycardia. Many types of arrhythmias have been reported.

their duration of action is prolonged in patients with hepatic disease. Vecuronium, which is metabolized in the liver, has been administered to patients with hepatic disease.[170-174] Lebrault et al.,[170] for example, compared patients with cirrhosis who received 0.2 mg of vecuronium per kilogram with healthy control patients and found that elimination half-life was prolonged approximately 60%. This effect resulted in a time to return of 50% twitch height of 130 minutes in the cirrhotic group, compared with 62 minutes in healthy patients. Differences in clearance among alcoholic patients with liver disease are dose dependent and usually not significant.[174] Rocuronium has an increased volume of distribution and elimination times, resulting in significantly longer durations.[170-173] The duration of action of rocuronium, as well as the onset, is typically prolonged in patients with hepatic disease such as cirrhosis. Patients with hepatic dysfunction demonstrate an elimination half-life that is increased to 173 minutes, compared with the normal 60 to 120 minutes. This supports the finding that the route of plasma clearance of rocuronium is predominantly hepatic with much of the drug excreted being unchanged in bile.[175] Cautious dosing is warranted, along with vigilant monitoring of neuromuscular function in these patients.

An active desacetyl metabolite results from the breakdown of each of the steroidal relaxants. These metabolites exhibit relaxant activity and accumulate with prolonged use. Although this does not pose a problem perioperatively, prolonged paralysis and myopathies in patients with multiorgan failure in critical care units has been a problem with multiday use. Practice guidelines for sustained NMB in critically ill adults and children have been published.[176-178] Nondepolarizing relaxants are used in intensive care to immobilize patients for procedural interventions, decrease oxygen consumption, facilitate mechanical ventilation, reduce intracranial pressure, prevent shivering, and manage tetanus and acute respiratory distress syndrome (ARDS). Emerging data may support the use of cisatracurium in select patients with ARDS.[179,180] Cisatracurium may be kinetically preferred

for patients with organ dysfunction. Close monitoring with peripheral nerve stimulation is recommended, with sustained use of nondepolarizing relaxants to avoid drug accumulation and minimize the risk for adverse drug events. Reversal of paralysis is best achieved by discontinuing therapy.[170]

Atracurium and cisatracurium are not affected by changes in liver function and are the agents of choice for use in patients with liver disease because of their unique method of metabolism, specifically their breakdown pathway via Hofmann elimination and nonesterase-dependent hydrolysis.[126] Cisatracurium is preferred for its lack of histamine release. The pharmacokinetics of atracurium in patients with hepatic and renal disease were compared with those in nonimpaired control subjects. No differences in plasma elimination half-lives were noted.[181] The effect of atracurium infusions in patients with fulminant hepatic failure who were awaiting liver transplantation, as well as during liver transplantation, has been studied. Plasma clearances and half-lives were similar to those reported in healthy individuals, and no cumulative effects were noted.[173,174]

Renal System

The steroidal relaxants rocuronium and vecuronium are affected by changes in renal status. Because both drugs depend to varying degrees on renal and hepatic elimination, their duration of action is prolonged in patients with decreases in renal function. A small portion of rocuronium is excreted unchanged in the urine, resulting in a prolonged elimination half-life in patients with renal disease.[175] The onset time of rocuronium is not affected by renal failure.[182]

Atracurium and cisatracurium are considered the agents of choice in patients with renal disease. Onset and duration are not affected by changes in renal function. Doses of three times the ED_{95} (0.15 mg/kg) of cisatracurium were given to 39 patients with decreased renal function, all of whom were induced with fentanyl and thiopental. Onset time, mean arterial blood pressure, heart rate, and time to recovery of 25% T_1 were assessed, and there was no significant variation in the drug effects compared with patients with normal renal function.[183]

Effects in Special Populations

Elderly patients. The onset times of the NMBAs are generally delayed in the elderly due to slower circulation times and other kinetic changes associated with aging.[184] This is true for all relaxants. The dosing interval and duration of action of the steroidal relaxants rocuronium and vecuronium are prolonged in the elderly due to decreased hepatic and renal clearance and an increased volume of distribution.[184-187] The duration of atracurium and cisatracurium is not affected by aging, making these the most predictable NMBAs in the elderly.

Obese patients. The use of the NMBAs in obese patients raises some special clinical considerations. Obese patients require a rapid-sequence induction more frequently than nonobese patients, owing to their higher risk for gastroesophageal reflux disease and pulmonary aspiration. A difficult airway is more often encountered. It is especially important to ensure full reversal of the relaxant actions in this patient group because of the higher occurrence of breathing abnormalities and lung compromise. Sleep apnea syndrome and the associated anesthetic management must be considered.[188-191] The duration of action of the steroidal relaxants rocuronium and vecuronium is prolonged likely due to a decrease in elimination.

The kinetics of atracurium and cisatracurium are not significantly changed in obese patients, making these the most reliable agents. Cisatracurium is preferred for its lack of histamine release. Several authors recommend that to avoid overdosing, NMBAs should be dosed at ideal body weight, except for succinylcholine, which is given according to total body weight.[69,70,190,192-195]

Pediatrics. When compared with adults, several differences exist among neonates, infants, and children in relation to their response to NMBAs. A more complete discussion of neonatal and pediatric pharmacology is given in Chapters 52 and 53. A few general observations can be made here. The neuromuscular junction is incomplete at delivery and continues to mature throughout infancy.[196] The sensitivity to any relaxant may change from birth through childhood. Neonates and infants have a higher volume of distribution and differences in redistribution, elimination, and metabolic rates, which vary with age. Young children appear to be more sensitive to nondepolarizing drugs than adults. There is age-related variability in the required dose of an NMBA. The ED_{95} is the lowest in neonates due to the immaturity of the neuromuscular junction. It is higher in children 3 to 10 years old and increases further toward adult doses in children 13 years and older. The increased volume of distribution from an expanded extracellular fluid volume in neonates means a similar initial dose (per kilogram) is given to neonates and teenagers. Children tend to require larger doses than adults. The reason for the larger dose requirement in children is unclear but may be the result of increased muscle bulk.[197,198]

The onset of action for NMBAs is faster in neonates than it is in older children and adults due to a greater cardiac output per kilogram. The duration of action of the intermediate NMBAs is longer in infants younger than 10 months of age than in children 1 to 5 years of age. Recovery is faster in children than adults.[197,198]

Other Factors

Hypothermia. The importance of keeping the patient's core body temperature normothermic cannot be overstated. Hypothermic patients exhibit a prolonged duration of action to all muscle relaxants due to decreased metabolism and delayed hepatic and renal clearance.[48] Severe (but not mild) hypothermia makes it more difficult to antagonize a neuromuscular block.[199–201]

Allergy. The role of muscle relaxants in perioperative anaphylaxis is well established. It primarily follows anesthetic induction but may occur during emergence with sugammadex. It is an immunoglobulin E (IgE)–mediated pathologic mechanism. Neuromuscular blocking agents and antibiotics are the most common drugs involved. Latex allergy now occurs infrequently. The initial diagnosis is presumptive, whereas the etiologic assessment is linked to the clinical presentation, tryptase levels, and skin test results. Because anaphylaxis presents with significant hypovolemia and vasoplegia, aggressive fluid therapy and epinephrine are the cornerstones of management.[202–205]

Succinylcholine and rocuronium are the NMBAs that are most frequently involved, and cisatracurium is the least. Cross-sensitization among the different agents is common and is more frequent with aminosteroid than with the benzylisoquinoline drugs. Estimates of the incidence of perioperative anaphylaxis vary between 1:6000 and 1:20,000 anaesthetics.[206,207] Quaternary and tertiary ammonium ions in the relaxant molecules are the main component of the allergenic sites on the reactive drugs. The flexibility of the chain between the ammonium ions, as well as the distance between the substituted ammonium ions, might be of importance during the elicitation phase of IgE-mediated reactions. Flexible molecules, such as succinylcholine, are considered more potent in stimulating sensitized cells than rigid molecules, such as the older relaxant pancuronium.[208] The rate of NMBA anaphylaxis shows marked geographic variation, suggesting that there may be external or environmental factors involved. Ammonium ions are found in a wide variety of chemical structures, including prescription and over-the-counter medications and common household chemicals. Epidemiologic studies have shown a possible link to the consumption of pholcodine, a nonprescription antitussive drug used outside of the United States, which contains a tertiary ammonium ion, and an increased incidence of NMBA anaphylaxis. This link has prompted the withdrawal of pholcodine in some countries.[209,210] Skin testing and follow-up guidelines have been published.[211–213] A complete discussion of anaphylaxis management and anesthesia is given in Chapter 46.

REVERSAL OF NEUROMUSCULAR BLOCKADE

Complete and effective reversal of the action of the muscle relaxants is one of the most important aspects of clinical practice. Incomplete relaxant reversal and the resulting difficulties continue to be a challenge. The use of nerve stimulators and our knowledge of relaxant pharmacology continue to evolve; however, a significant incidence of postoperative residual paralysis stubbornly remains. Three anticholinesterase agents for reversal of the relaxants are available, although neostigmine is used overwhelmingly. Edrophonium may be used when a faster onset is desired, or if there are shortages of neostigmine, but its efficacy is less than that of neostigmine. The reduced effectiveness limits its use to situations where significant recovery has already occurred. Because of this lower potency, the degree of spontaneous recovery from neuromuscular block at the time of edrophonium administration should be at least a TOF count of 4. Pyridostigmine is largely historical and rarely used. It is available for treatment of myasthenia gravis. Fortunately a new paradigm is unfolding with the introduction of the selective relaxant binding agent (SRBA) sugammadex.[214]

A thorough evaluation of the current data on the clinical use of relaxants and their reversal has been reported and discussed in several publications.[214–217] The criteria for determination that successful recovery has taken place have been clarified, and factors that can affect recovery have been noted. The decision faced by the clinician at the end of a procedure involves determining when the relaxant effects have dissipated and the patient can safely control his or her own airway. A number of factors combining objective monitoring with clinical signs must be obtained to assure safe recovery. Several studies have indicated that the incidence of residual paralysis may be as high as 63.5%. The RECITE (Residual Curarization and its Incidence at Tracheal Extubation) study was a prospective observational study completed in 2015 at eight hospitals in Canada investigating the incidence and severity of residual NMB. They found that the incidence of residual NMB, defined as a TOFR less than 0.9, was 63.5% at tracheal extubation and 56.5% at arrival at the PACU.[215] Other studies have noted similar results.[216] Residual paralysis may be evident even up to 4 hours after use of an intermediate relaxant.[217,218] This phenomenon is frequently referred to as recurarization, implying that adequate reversal was obtained but the drug effect was reestablished. This term is a misnomer because the noted effect is most likely unrecognized residual paralysis. Reversal should not be attempted unless spontaneous recovery of one to two twitches of the TOF has occurred because the block may be too deep to obtain adequate reversal.[9–12] Many clinicians recommend that four twitches or the TOF be evident prior to reversal.[218] A TOFR of 0.9 should be the standard attained because even small degrees of residual block increase the incidence of adverse respiratory events and may increase longer-term morbidity as well.[219,220] This is due to previously unrecognized decreases in airway patency and swallowing unless a TOFR of 0.9 is present. An increased incidence of adverse effects such as hypoxia, hypercarbia, atelectasis, and airway obstruction may occur in the PACU.[202,221,222] This is especially true in higher risk or elderly patients. A study by Murphy et al.[223] suggests the incidence of significant respiratory adverse events in the PACU is 0.8%. Quantitative monitoring should be the gold standard because qualitative assessments of the signs of recovery are frequently misinterpreted by even the most experienced clinicians. It can be difficult to detect subtle differences in fade of TOF and tetanus with subjective qualitative

BOX 12.10 Adverse Effects of Residual Neuromuscular Block

Volunteer Studies

- Impairment of pharyngeal coordination and force of contraction
- Swallowing dysfunction/delayed initiation of the swallowing reflex
- Reductions in upper esophageal sphincter tone
- Increased risk of aspiration
- Reductions in upper airway volumes
- Impairment of upper airway dilator muscle function
- Decreased inspiratory airflow
- Upper airway obstruction
- Impaired hypoxic ventilatory drive
- Symptoms of muscle weakness (visual disturbances, severe facial weakness, difficulty speaking and drinking), generalized weakness

Clinical Studies in Surgical Patients

- Increased risk of postoperative hypoxemia
- Increased incidence of upper airway obstruction during transport to the postanesthesia care unit (PACU)
- Higher risk of critical respiratory events in the PACU
- Symptoms and signs of profound muscle weakness
- Delays in meeting PACU discharge criteria and achieving actual discharge
- Prolonged postoperative ventilatory weaning and increased intubation times (cardiac surgical patients)
- Increased risk of postoperative pulmonary complications (atelectasis or pneumonia)
- Intraoperative awareness

From Murphy GS, Brull SJ. Residual neuromuscular block: lessons unlearned. Part I: definitions, incidence, and adverse physiologic effects of residual neuromuscular block. *Anesth Analg.* 2010;111(1):120–128; Brull SJ, Kopman AF. Current status of neuromuscular reversal and monitoring: challenges and opportunities. *Anesthesiology.* 2017;126(1):173–190.

BOX 12.11 Reversal Considerations in Clinical Practice

Considerations When Return of Muscle Function Is Incomplete

- As with any reversal agent, the ability to counteract a nondepolarizing blocking agent depends on the amount of spontaneous recovery before the administration of a reversal drug.
- Has enough time been allowed for the anticholinesterase to antagonize the block (at least 15–30 min)?
- Is the neuromuscular blockade too intense to be antagonized?
- Even if recovery appears clinically adequate, a small dose of neostigmine may be prudent if the time since relaxant administration is <4 hr.
- Has an adequate dose of antagonist been given?
- Are the other anesthetics and adjunctive agents contributing to patient weakness?
- Has metabolism or excretion of the relaxant been reduced by a possibly unrecognized process?
- Have acid-base and electrolyte status, temperature, age, drug interactions, and other factors that may prolong relaxant action been contemplated?
- The safest approach when any question as to successful reversal remains is to provide proper sedation and controlled ventilation until adequate recovery is ensured.

tests.[224] Interestingly, many clinicians speculated that the introduction of sugammadex with its high efficacy may reduce the need for neuromuscular monitoring. The opposite has happened. Quantitative monitoring for degree of residual blockade at the end of a procedure is essential for proper administration of sugammadex reversal. Assessment of TOF, and, if no response, the PTC, guide dose selection.

Some adverse effects of residual neuromuscular block are noted in Box 12.10.

General principles for avoiding residual paralysis are given in Box 12.11. Factors influencing the incidence of postoperative residual NMB are shown in Box 12.12.

CHOLINESTERASE INHIBITORS

The mechanism of action of the cholinesterase inhibitors is primarily the result of its structural relationship and interaction with AChE, a protein with a molecular weight of approximately 320,000 and the capacity to hydrolyze an estimated 300,000 molecules of ACh per minute.[225]

Edrophonium and neostigmine contain an ionized center that actively combines either at the active center or at the site specifically removed from the active center of AChE. Edrophonium is a simple alcohol that contains a quaternary ammonium group.[225] It is considered a reversible inhibitor of cholinesterase because it electrostatically attaches to the anionic site of AChE and is stabilized by hydrogen binding at the esteratic site of the enzyme. Because a true chemical bond is

not formed, ACh competes with edrophonium for the binding site of AChE, and therefore it has a shorter duration of action than those of compounds that form a bond.[226]

Neostigmine is a carbamic acid ester of alcohol and contains a quaternary or tertiary ammonium group.[225] It forms a carbamyl-ester complex at the esteratic site of cholinesterase. This drug-enzyme complex then degrades in the same manner as the ACh-cholinesterase complex. The carbamate group is transferred to AChE, leaving it unable to hydrolyze ACh.[49]

The indirect-acting cholinesterase inhibitors exert their effect by inhibiting AChE, thereby increasing the concentration of endogenous ACh around the cholinoreceptors.[225] They act as alternative substrates for the enzyme. This provides a twofold mechanism in the reversal of NMB. First, increasing the concentration of ACh in the junctional cleft changes the agonist-antagonist ratio, thereby increasing the likelihood that the ACh will reoccupy the receptor site once occupied by the neuromuscular blocker, as well as occupying sites not previously engaged. Second, the life of the ACh within the cleft is increased. The increased concentration of ACh prolongs the time it remains in the cleft, allowing time for the antagonist dissociation and the reactivation of the receptor site. Evidence also suggests that these agents have direct influences on neuromuscular transmission independent of enzyme inhibition. These include at least three distinct although possibly interacting mechanisms, including a weak agonist action, the formation of desensitized receptor complex intermediates, and the alteration of the conductance properties of active channels.[227]

Although the result of inhibition of AChE is the same when edrophonium or neostigmine is administered, the means by which these agents accomplish the task varies. Edrophonium binds reversibly with the negatively charged enzyme site by electrostatic attraction of its positively charged nitrogen. This effect prevents catalytic binding with ACh for the short time that edrophonium occupies the binding site. Although the duration of receptor site occupation is short for edrophonium, the duration of its effects is prolonged by the fact that once it leaves the receptor site, it finds another to occupy and continues with this process until eliminated.[228]

BOX 12.12   Factors Influencing the Incidence of Postoperative Residual Neuromuscular Blockade

Definition of Residual Neuromuscular Blockade
- Objective train-of-four (TOF) measurements (TOF ratio <0.9)
- Clinical signs or symptoms of muscle weakness

Type and Dose of Neuromuscular Blocking Drug (NMBD) Administered Intraoperatively
- Intermediate-acting NMBD
- Long-acting NMBD
- Bolus vs infusion

Use of Neuromuscular Monitoring Intraoperatively
- Qualitative monitoring (TOF and double-burst stimulation studied)
- Quantitative monitoring (acceleromyography studied)
- No neuromuscular monitoring (clinical signs)

Degree of Neuromuscular Blockade Maintained Intraoperatively
- TOF count of 1–2
- TOF count of 2–3

Amount of Spontaneous Recovery at Time of Reversal
- The greater the extent of spontaneous recovery present, the more effective the reversal

Type of Anesthesia Used Intraoperatively
- Inhalation drugs
- Intravenous anesthesia (total intravenous anesthesia [TIVA])

Type and Dose of Anticholinesterase Reversal Drug
- Neostigmine
- Edrophonium
- Sugammadex

Duration of Anesthesia
Time Interval Between Anticholinesterase Administration and Objective Monitoring
- TOF measurements

Patient Factors
- Metabolic derangements in the postanesthesia care unit (PACU) (acidosis, hypercarbia, hypoxia, electrolyte imbalance or hypothermia)
- Organ dysfunction such as renal hepatic cardiac or neuromuscular disease

Drug Therapy in PACU
- Opioids
- Antibiotics
- Lithium
- Magnesium
- Local anesthetics

From Murphy GS, Brull SJ. Residual neuromuscular block: lessons unlearned. Part I: definitions, incidence, and adverse physiologic effects of residual neuromuscular block. *Anesth Analg.* 2010;111(1):120–128; Brull SJ, Kopman AF. Current status of neuromuscular reversal and monitoring: challenges and opportunities. *Anesthesiology.* 2017;126(1):173–190.

Enzymatic inactivation is accomplished by neostigmine. Electrostatic interaction between the ionized centers of drug and enzyme takes place initially as with edrophonium. This phenomenon then leads to a hydrolytic chemical reaction in which a shift in covalent bonds occurs, resulting in the formation of a carbamylated enzyme. This methyl-carbamyl AChE is much more stable and resistant to hydrolysis than the acetyl enzyme, resulting in an enzyme that is incapable of inactivating ACh.

These differences in chemical deactivation of AChE result in differing pharmacokinetic profiles. Edrophonium and neostigmine are quaternary ammonium compounds that are poorly lipid soluble. At moderate doses, penetration through lipid barriers (e.g., gastrointestinal tract, placenta, and blood-brain barrier) is minimal if present at all.

Edrophonium is the most rapid acting of these agents, with an onset time of 30 to 60 seconds after intravenous administration and a duration of 5 to 10 minutes. Intramuscular administration results in an onset of 2 to 10 minutes.[229] Renal excretion accounts for approximately 75% of the edrophonium eliminated, although in the absence of renal function, hepatic metabolism accounts for the inactivation of 30% of the injected dose; this amount undergoes conjugation to inactive edrophonium glucuronide. The elimination half-life of edrophonium is 110 minutes in the healthy patient and 304 minutes in the anephric patient. The volume of distribution is 1.1 and 0.7 L/kg in normal and anephric patients, respectively.

After intravenous administration of neostigmine, onset occurs within 4 to 8 minutes. Duration of action is 0.5 to 2 hours, although other sources suggest durations from 60 minutes to 4 hours. Renal excretion accounts for roughly 50% of the neostigmine eliminated, primarily by glomerular filtration. The remaining 50% of the neostigmine dose is hydrolyzed by plasma esterases and hepatic metabolism to 3-hydroxyphenyltrimethyl ammonium (3-OH PPM) and conjugated

3-OH PPM. These metabolites have approximately one-tenth the activity of the parent compounds and are renally eliminated. The elimination half-life of neostigmine is 70 to 80 minutes, increasing to 181 to 183 minutes in anephric patients. The volume of distribution of 0.7 L/kg in healthy patients increases to 0.8 L/kg in those with renal failure.[225,228] Successful reversal is usually attained in 10 to 30 minutes. In a much discussed report published in 2015, it was noted that there is a dose-dependent increase in postoperative respiratory complications when doses of neostigmine exceed 60 mcg/kg. These doses are in the upper range of recommended neostigmine dosing. Neostigmine-induced partial neuromuscular transmission block may explain adverse respiratory outcomes in patients who received high-dose neostigmine after recovery of neuromuscular transmission. They caution that neostigmine does not reverse deep NMB. Administration to patients who present with deep NMB can result in incomplete reversal. Furthermore, it may lead to anesthesia providers falsely believing their patients to have safe return of muscular function.[220,231]

The pharmacology of the reversal agents is summarized in Table 12.11. The common clinical signs of muscle recovery after administration of a muscle relaxant are listed in Box 12.13. Some considerations that apply when reversal is incomplete are noted in Box 12.10. Factors that may prolong paralysis are listed in Box 12.14.

ANTICHOLINERGICS

Atropine or glycopyrrolate are used in combination with neostigmine or edrophonium to prevent the parasympathomimetic side effects of the anticholinesterase drugs. If given alone, neostigmine and the other anticholinesterase drugs would cause severe vagal effects due to the systemic buildup of acetylcholine. These would include bradycardia and arrhythmias, hypotension, bronchoconstriction, hypersalivation,

TABLE 12.11   Commonly Used Anticholinesterase, Anticholinergic, and Select Relaxant Binding Agents

Agent	Dose Range	Onset (min)	Duration	Comments
Neostigmine	25–75 mcg/kg	5–15	45–90 min	Most commonly used reversal agent; may increase incidence of postoperative nausea and vomiting
Edrophonium	500–1000 mcg/kg	5–10	30–60 min	Not recommended for deep block; rapid onset, short duration, incremental injection advised
Atropine	15 mcg/kg	1–2	1–2 hr	Should be combined with edrophonium because of more rapid onset
Glycopyrrolate	10–20 mcg/kg	2	2–4 hr	Less initial tachycardia than atropine; no central nervous system effects; most frequently used
Sugammadex	2–16 mg/kg	1–2	2–16 hr	Selective relaxant binding agent; up to 16 mg/kg has been safely used

BOX 12.13   Common Clinical Signs of Recovery From Neuromuscular Blockers

- Adequate tidal volume and rate
- Respirations smooth and unlabored
- Opens eyes widely on command; no diplopia
- Sustained protrusion and purposeful movement of tongue
- Effective swallowing and sustained bite
- Able to sustain head or leg lift for at least 5 sec (in small children, a strong knee-to-chest movement is equivalent.)
- Arm lift and touch the opposite shoulder
- Strong, constant hand grip
- Effective cough
- Adequate vital capacity of at least 15 mL/kg
- Adequate inspiratory force of at least 25–30 cm H_2O negative pressure
- Sustained tetanic response to 50 Hz for 5 sec
- Train-of-four ratio >0.9 with no fade
- No fade to double-burst stimulation

diarrhea, and an increase in postoperative nausea and vomiting. Glycopyrrolate is used more often because it produces less initial tachycardia and has no CNS effects. The antimuscarinic can be given first, or the glycopyrrolate and neostigmine may be mixed in the same syringe.

Anticholinergic, *antimuscarinic*, and *parasympatholytic* are three common terms used to describe compounds that originate from alkaloids of the belladonna plant. Each group name divides these compounds into subgroups that have a more similar mechanism of action. For the purposes of this section, all of the compounds are referred to as antimuscarinics. Atropine (*dl*-hyoscyamine) is the prototype of this group, and many of the currently available products are structural derivatives obtained both naturally and synthetically.[232] Atropine is found in the plant *Atropa belladonna*, or deadly nightshade, and in *Datura stramonium*, also known as jimsonweed.[140] Preparations of these plants have been used by clinicians for centuries; belladonna was used as a poison during the time of the Roman Empire and in the Middle Ages. In 1867 Bezold and Bloebaun began to study the cardiac effects of belladonna's vagal inhibition, and in 1931 Mein isolated atropine in the pure form.[24]

Atropine and scopolamine are naturally occurring tertiary amines. Semisynthetic congeners of the belladonna alkaloids represented by glycopyrrolate are usually quaternary ammonium derivatives. These quaternary ammonium derivatives often have potent peripheral effects without CNS activity.

All the antimuscarinics are absorbed orally to some extent, although this route is often unpredictable. Intramuscular or intravenous administration is usually the route used. Scopolamine has the additional advantage of transdermal absorption. Atropine is well absorbed from the gastrointestinal tract, by inhalation via endotracheal administration, and by intravenous and intramuscular routes. Given orally, 90% of the dose is absorbed and reaches peak plasma levels within 1 hour. Intramuscular and intravenous administration results in peak plasma levels within 30 minutes and 2 to 4 minutes, respectively. Atropine is well distributed throughout the body. It crosses both the blood-brain barrier and the placental barrier. Both the kidneys and liver aid in the elimination of atropine. Although elimination is biphasic, the terminal half-life is 2 to 3 hours. Metabolism by the liver results in several metabolites: tropic acid, tropine, and glucuronide conjugates. Approximately 30% to 50% of a dose is excreted unchanged in the urine. Small amounts of atropine may also be eliminated in expired air as carbon dioxide and in feces.[232]

Glycopyrrolate is a quaternary ammonium compound whose ionization limits gastrointestinal absorption, blood-brain barrier, and placental penetration. After intravenous administration, glycopyrrolate has an onset of 1 minute. Intramuscular and subcutaneous administration results in an onset of 15 to 30 minutes. Vagal blockade can persist for 2 to 3 hours. Serum levels of glycopyrrolate decline quickly, and less than 10% of the drug remains in the serum after 5 minutes. Glycopyrrolate is excreted in feces and urine, primarily as an unchanged drug. Small amounts are metabolized to inactive metabolites. Eighty-five percent of an intravenous dose is excreted in the urine within 48 hours.[140]

Atropine and glycopyrrolate are commonly administered to prevent the muscarinic effects of anticholinesterase inhibitors. Atropine induces its vagolytic effect more rapidly than glycopyrrolate. Atropine appears to be somewhat better suited for use with edrophonium, whereas the onset times of glycopyrrolate and neostigmine are more closely matched. When administered with edrophonium, the usual recommended dose of atropine is 7 mcg/kg.[140] With 0.5 to 2.5 mg of neostigmine, the recommended dose of atropine is 0.6 to 1.2 mg, and that of glycopyrrolate is 0.2 to 0.6 mg.[232] (See Chapter 13, Table 13.6 for a comparison of the anticholinergics.)

Selective Relaxant Binding Agents—Sugammadex

Sugammadex (Bridion) is the first SRBA to be introduced as a reversal for clinical NMB. The name *sugammadex* is a contraction of sugar and γ-cyclodextrin. It is a modified γ-cyclodextrin that works by encapsulating

BOX 12.14 Factors That May Prolong Paralysis

Pathophysiologic Causes
Acid maltase deficiency
Adrenocortical dysfunction
Acute intermittent porphyria
Amyotrophic lateral sclerosis
Anoxia and ischemia
Carcinomatous polyneuropathy
Cholinesterase deficiency or genetic variance
Compressive neuropathy
Critical illness polyneuropathy
Diphtheria
Eaton-Lambert syndrome
Guillain-Barré syndrome
Hypokalemia and hypocalcemia
Hypomagnesemia
Hypophosphatemia
Hypothermia
Motor neuron disease
Multiple sclerosis
Muscular dystrophy
Myasthenia gravis
Myotonic syndromes
Neurofibromatosis
Nonspecific nutritional deficiency
Poliomyelitis
Pyridoxine abuse
Polymyositis
Renal failure (variable prolongation)
Respiratory acidosis
Sepsis
Thiamine deficiency
Tick bite paralysis
Trauma

Vitamin E deficiency
Wound botulism

Pharmacologic Causes
Aminoglycoside toxicity
Penicillin toxicity
Steroid myopathy

Antihypertensives
Calcium channel blockers
β-blockers
Furosemide

Antidysrhythmics
Quinidine
Procainamide
Local anesthetics in large doses

Antibiotics
Aminoglycoside antibiotics
Polymyxin B
Clindamycin
Tetracycline

Miscellaneous Drugs
Cyclosporine
Steroids
Volatile anesthetics
Dantrolene
Magnesium
Lithium
Azathioprine
Organophosphate (poisoning)

Modified from Kirby RR et al., eds. *Clinical Anesthesia Practice.* 2nd ed. Philadelphia: Elsevier; 2002.

and forming very tight water-soluble complexes at a 1:1 ratio with steroidal neuromuscular blocking drugs. Once encapsulation occurs, it does not dissociate, and the sugammadex-relaxant complex is excreted in the urine. Reversal occurs independent of the depth of block, therefore even deep blockade can be reversed with the appropriate dose. The concentration of free muscle relaxant falls rapidly, and muscle strength is reestablished. It is most effective reversing rocuronium and vecuronium, in that order. It does not affect the benzylisoquinolines atracurium and cisatracurium.[233,234] Used in appropriate doses, sugammadex can reverse any depth of rocuronium or vecuronium block within 3 minutes.

Pharmacokinetics

Sugammadex is biologically inactive. The pharmacokinetics of sugammadex show a linear dose relationship in doses up to 8.0 mg/kg. Clearance is approximately 120 L/min and the volume of distribution is 18 L. The elimination half-life is 2.3 hours. Up to 80% of an administered dose of sugammadex is eliminated in the urine within 24 hours. Sugammadex does not bind to plasma proteins or erythrocytes. Due to the dependence on renal elimination, the drug should be avoided in patients with significant renal disease.[228,234]

Clinical Use

The dosage range of sugammadex varies from 2 to 16 mg/kg according to the depth of blockade at the time of reversal. Sugammadex comes

in 2- or 5-mL vials as 100 mg/mL. Monitoring for twitch responses to determine the timing and dose for sugammadex administration is essential. The drug is administered as a single bolus injection. A dose of 2 mg/kg is recommended if spontaneous recovery has reached the reappearance of the second twitch or more in response to TOF stimulation. A dose of 4 mg/kg is recommended if spontaneous recovery of the twitch response has reached 1 to 2 PTC and there are no twitch responses to TOF stimulation. A dose of 16 mg/kg is recommended if there is a clinical need to reverse NMB soon (approximately 3 minutes) after administration of a single dose of 1.2 mg/kg of rocuronium.[235-237] A suggested dosing strategy for reversal is given in Table 12.12.

Sugammadex appears to be safe and well tolerated. The most commonly reported adverse drug reactions include nausea, vomiting, allergy, hypertension, and headache.[235] Anaphylaxis has been reported and is the reason approval was initially delayed by the FDA.

Hypersensitivity reactions to all anesthetics during the perioperative period have an incidence between 1:3500 and 1:20,000 exposures, and the associated mortality approaches 9%. Hypersensitivity to sugammadex appears to be relatively low, with only 15 cases being reported in a recent review. In the majority of the reported cases, the anaphylactic reactions were evident within the first 4 minutes after administration of sugammadex. Cardiovascular collapse was treated successfully with fluid resuscitation and epinephrine therapy.[214,238]

Nerve Stimulator Test	Response and Depth of Block	Reversal Sugammadex (mg/kg)	Reversal Neostigmine (mcg/kg)
Posttetanic count	Profound (count <3)	4–16 mg/kg	Delay reversal
	Deep (count >0)	4–16 mg/kg	Delay reversal
TOF count	Intermediate (TOF count 1–4)	2–4 mg/kg	70 mcg/kg
	Recovery (TOF count 4)		
	With fade	2 mg/kg	35 mcg/kg
	No fade	1 mg/kg	35 mcg/kg
TOF ratio	Recovery (TOF count 4)		
	TOF ratio 0–0.8	2 mg/kg	30–60 mcg/kg
	TOF ratio >0.9	No reversal	No reversal

TABLE 12.12   **Reversal Dosing Strategy**

TOF, Train-of-four.

Sugammadex binds oral contraceptives, and women of childbearing age should be counseled about using alternative contraceptive methods for 1 week after exposure to sugammadex. In many institutions, this potential side effect is disclosed as part of the preoperative anesthesia consent.[216]

The other major factor that delayed the approval by the FDA has been the potential effect of sugammadex on coagulation. In patients receiving sugammadex, the activated partial thromboplastin time and the prothrombin time were increased by 5.5% and 3.0% after a 4-mg/kg dose or higher, respectively; however, these increases returned to normal values within 60 minutes. Likely as a consequence of these being relatively minor and short-lived effects on coagulation parameters, the incidence of bleeding events in patients receiving sugammadex (2.9%) and those not exposed to sugammadex (4.1%) was comparable. Additionally, effects on the various coagulation assays are likely an in vitro artifact.[214,238–240] Sugammadex is not recommended for use in patients with severe renal impairment, including those requiring dialysis.[241]

In the rare event that neuromuscular block needs to be reestablished, a benzylisoquinoline such as atracurium, mivacurium, or cisatracurium should be given. Succinylcholine is not affected.[237] Recurrence of paralysis is rare but has been reported and is usually related to an inadequate sugammadex dose.[241]

SUMMARY

Like every other agent used in the practice of anesthesia, neuromuscular blocking agents are useful tools in the hands of skilled clinicians. It should go without saying that these agents should never be administered without first appropriately sedating the patient. The exception is if the patient's condition is so marginal that even the most careful use of sedation could increase the chance for morbidity or death. The decision to use neuromuscular blockers in the absence of sedation should be made only after the most careful and thorough consideration. Prevention of movement should provide the surgeon with the optimum field on which lifesaving skills can be practiced.

REFERENCES

For a complete list of references for this chapter, scan this QR code with any smartphone code reader app, or visit the following URL: http://booksite.elsevier.com/9780323711944/.

13

Autonomic and Cardiac Pharmacology

John J. Nagelhout

Cardiovascular medicine continues to be one of the most rapidly changing specialties in modern clinical practice. Management guidelines are continuously being refined as data from large-scale clinical trials are reported. The number of patients requiring noncardiac surgery who have had coronary interventions is increasing. Many patients have complex management plans that require consultation with their cardiologists. Providing high-quality anesthetic care involves continuous monitoring of all the body's systems, with a special emphasis on the cardiovascular status of the patient. Complex anesthetic plans and invasive surgical intervention can produce profound stress on patients' cardiovascular balance and require careful manipulation of vital signs. The array of diagnostic tests, monitors, and drugs available makes a thorough understanding of autonomic and cardiac pharmacology essential. A well-devised treatment plan will make the anesthetic course flow smoothly. Intraoperative planning for the immediate and late postoperative periods is critical to avoiding untoward outcomes. The number and variety of medications in a patient's profile require a delicate balance between the anesthetic requirements and maintaining a successful continuum of therapy for the long-term needs of the patient. This chapter presents a broad overview of the many autonomic and cardiovascular medicines that may be encountered during the perioperative period and their important anesthetic considerations.

AUTONOMIC DRUGS—SYMPATHOMIMETIC AMINES

The sympathomimetic amines include the three naturally occurring catecholamines epinephrine, norepinephrine, and dopamine and a number of synthetic agents such as ephedrine, phenylephrine, and dobutamine. These drugs are used in a variety of situations, including the treatment of anesthesia-induced hypotension, bradycardia, anaphylaxis, shock, heart failure, and cardiac resuscitation.

The basic structure of the sympathomimetic amines is β-(3,4-dihydroxyphenyl)-ethylamine. This structure consists of a substituted benzene ring and an ethylamine side chain.[1] The effects elicited by this pharmacologic class are the result of the stimulation of β-adrenergic, α-adrenergic, and dopamine-adrenergic receptors. The innervation of the effector organs by the autonomic system is outlined in Table 13.1.

The efficacy of a particular sympathomimetic amine depends on its concentration at the receptor site, its affinity for specific receptors, and the population of receptors available for binding. The physiologic effects vary dramatically as to the amount of natural catecholamine release or dose of drug administered. Medications that affect the autonomic nervous system are summarized in Table 13.2.

Epinephrine

Epinephrine, one of the naturally occurring catecholamines, is the final product in the chain of catecholamine synthesis. (See Chapter 37 for a complete description of catecholamine synthesis.) Although both epinephrine and norepinephrine are agonists at both alpha and beta receptors, norepinephrine has minimal beta$_1$ activity in low doses, whereas epinephrine strongly stimulates both beta$_1$ and beta$_2$ receptors.

Epinephrine is useful not only in the treatment of anaphylaxis and cardiopulmonary resuscitation, but also its combination of alpha and beta effects makes it an appropriate choice for the treatment of some shock states that involve both poor tissue oxygen delivery and hypotension. In small doses, epinephrine may well be useful as a sympathomimetic agent in patients unresponsive to indirect-acting agents and in those in whom simultaneous beta$_1$ (cardiac stimulation) and beta$_2$ receptor stimulation (vasodilation) may be helpful. With epinephrine, the dominance of alpha or beta effects is dose related.

Epinephrine's beta$_1$ effect produces marked positive inotropic (force of contraction), chronotropic (heart rate), and dromotropic (conduction velocity) actions. It should be noted that as heart rate, left ventricular stroke work, stroke volume, and cardiac output increase, so does myocardial oxygen consumption. In addition, the corresponding increased automaticity of all foci, including ectopic foci, may lead to arrhythmia. Marked vigilance must be maintained in an effort to ensure that myocardial oxygen demand does not exceed supply. It should be recalled that epinephrine administration can both increase myocardial demand and decrease myocardial supply. However, in low doses used to treat hypotension, epinephrine can improve coronary artery perfusion by increased mean arterial pressure (MAP).

Beneficial effects of beta$_2$ stimulation include bronchodilation, vasodilation, and stabilization of mast cells, with a resultant decrease in histamine release. Concurrently, alpha stimulation promotes a decrease in bronchial secretion. The net effect is a decrease in airway resistance with an improvement in oxygenation.

With low doses of epinephrine (10 mcg/min), the peripheral vasculature promotes the redistribution of blood flow to skeletal muscle, thereby producing a decrease in systemic vascular resistance. As the dose of epinephrine is increased, the alpha effect predominates, with resultant vasoconstriction and an increase in systemic pressures. The systolic pressure is increased, whereas the diastolic pressure remains relatively unchanged, with a resultant increase in pulse pressure. It should be noted that, if the coronary arteries are not obstructed, autoregulation increases oxygen delivery to meet the increased demand.[2] However, in the presence of a coronary artery lesion, oxygen delivery may be insufficient to meet demand, and myocardial ischemia results.[3]

The increased alpha effect that occurs with greater doses of epinephrine also results in renal and splanchnic vasoconstriction. Renal vascular resistance and, ultimately, renal blood flow are decreased. Beta stimulation leads to activation of the renin-angiotensin system (RAS) and to an increase in lipolysis, glycogenolysis, gluconeogenesis, ketone production, and lactate release by skeletal muscle. Insulin secretion is inhibited by an overriding beta$_2$ stimulation. Epinephrine-induced

TABLE 13.1   Typical Autonomic Influences on Peripheral Effector Organs

Organ System	Sympathetic Effect	Adrenergic Receptor Type	Parasympathetic Effect	Cholinergic Receptor Type
Eye				
Radial muscle, iris	Contraction (mydriasis)	α_1		
Sphincter muscle, iris			Contraction (miosis)	M_3, M_2
Ciliary muscle	Relaxation for far vision	β_2	Contraction for near vision (accommodation)	M_3, M_2
Heart				
Sinoatrial node	Increase in heart rate	β_1	Decrease in heart rate	M_2
Atria	Increase in contractility and conduction velocity	β_1	Decrease in contractility	M_2
Atrioventricular node	Increase in automaticity and conduction velocity	β_1	Decrease in conduction velocity; atrioventricular block	M_2
His-Purkinje system	Increase in automaticity and conduction velocity	β_1	Little effect	M_2
Ventricle	Increase in contractility, conduction velocity, automaticity	β_1	Slight decrease in contractility	M_2
Blood Vessels				
Arteries				
Coronary	Constriction; dilation	α; β_2	None	—
Skin and mucosa	Constriction	α_1; β_2	None	—
Skeletal muscle	Constriction; dilation	α_1; β_2	None	—
Cerebral	Constriction (slight)	α_1	None	—
Pulmonary	Constriction; dilation	α_1; β_2	None	—
Abdominal viscera	Constriction; dilation	α_1; β_2	None	—
Salivary glands	Constriction and reduced secretions	α_1; α_2	Dilation and increased secretions	M_3
Renal	Constriction; dilation	α_1, α_2; β_1, β_2	None	—
Veins	Constriction; dilation	α_1, α_2; β_2	None	—
Lung				
Tracheal and bronchial smooth muscle	Relaxation	β_2	Contraction	M_2, M_3
GI Tract				
Motility and tone	Decrease	α_1, α_2; β_1, β_2	Increase	M_2, M_3
Sphincters	Contraction	α_1	Relaxation	M_3, M_2
Secretion	Inhibition	α_2	Stimulation	M_3, M_2
Gallbladder and ducts	Relaxation	β_2	Contraction	M
Kidney				
Renin secretion	Increase	β_1	None	—
Urinary Bladder				
Detrusor	Relaxation	β_2, β_3	Contraction	M_3, M_2
Trigone and sphincter	Contraction	α_1	Relaxation	M_3, M_2
Uterus	Contraction (pregnant)	α_1	None	—
	Relaxation (pregnant and nonpregnant)	β_2		
Liver	Glycogenolysis and gluconeogenesis; increased blood sugar	α_1; β_2		
Pancreas				
Islets (β cells)	Decreased insulin secretion	α_2	None	—
	Increased insulin secretion	β_2	None	—
Adipocytes	Lipolysis	α_1; β_1, β_2, β_3	None	—

α, Alpha receptor; β, beta receptor; *GI*, gastrointestinal; *M*, muscarinic receptor.

TABLE 13.2 Effects of Autonomic Drugs

Organ Systems	α-Agonists	α-Blocker	β-Agonists	β-Blocker	Cholinergic Agonists	Anticholinergic
Eye	Mydriasis	Miosis (slight)	NCRE	↓ Intraocular pressure	Miosis, ↓ intraocular pressure	Mydriasis, cycloplegia, ↑ intraocular pressure
Heart						
Rate	Bradycardia (reflex)	Tachycardia (reflex)	Tachycardia	Bradycardia	Bradycardia	Tachycardia
Contractility	NCRE	Slight increase (reflex)	↑	↓	↓ (slight)	↑ (slight)
Conduction velocity	NCRE	NCRE	↑	↓	↓	↑
Blood (vessels)	Vasoconstriction	Vasodilation	Vasodilation	Vasoconstriction	NCRE	NCRE
Lungs	NCRE	NCRE	Bronchodilation	Bronchoconstriction	Bronchoconstriction	Bronchodilation (slight)
GI Tract	↓ Motility and secretion	NCRE	↓ Motility and secretion	NCRE	↑ Motility and secretion	↓ Motility and secretion
Uterus	Contraction	NCRE	Relaxation	NCRE	NCRE	NCRE
Liver	↑ Blood sugar	NCRE	↑ Blood sugar	Hypoglycemia	NCRE	NCRE

↑, Increase; ↓, decrease; *GI*, gastrointestinal; *NCRE*, no clinically relevant effect.

beta$_2$ stimulation also can cause transient hyperkalemia as potassium follows glucose out of hepatic cells. This is followed by a longer hypokalemia as beta$_2$ stimulation then forces this extracellular potassium into red blood cells.[4]

Norepinephrine

Norepinephrine is a potent vasopressor. Although it is not as potent as epinephrine in stimulating alpha receptors in equal doses, it has little beta$_2$ activity at low doses, and the end result is, for the most part, unopposed alpha stimulation. The chronotropic effect seen with beta$_1$ stimulation is generally absent with norepinephrine in low doses because of the increase in systemic vascular resistance, which induces reflex vagal activity.

The aforementioned combination of adrenergic stimulation results in a decrease in vital organ flow; however, coronary artery perfusion may be increased because of the increase in diastolic pressure. Renal vascular resistance is increased, and urine output may fall. An increase in preload may be seen because norepinephrine is a venoconstrictor.[5,6]

Both norepinephrine and dopamine are used as first-line therapy for shock. There is an ongoing debate as to whether either one is superior. A 2016 meta-analysis suggests that they are equally effective, although dopamine produces more adverse events such as arrhythmias and possibly increased mortality.[7] Norepinephrine is generally used in patients with adequate cardiac output but low systemic vascular resistance. In this group of patients, however, the underlying problem of peripheral tissue perfusion-oxygenation may be exacerbated by the intense norepinephrine-induced peripheral vasoconstriction, even if adequate blood pressure has been achieved.

Norepinephrine does have some generalized metabolic effects, such as a decrease in insulin production, but these metabolic effects are present to a lesser degree than those seen with epinephrine. Adverse effects are usually a result of the intense vasoconstriction.

Dopamine

Dopamine is an endogenous central and peripheral neurotransmitter that is derived from dopa in the chain of catecholamine synthesis. Pharmacologically, dopamine stimulates dopamine receptors, beta receptors, and alpha receptors in a dose-dependent manner because of differing receptor affinities. Dopaminergic receptors are stimulated with low doses of less than 1 to 4 mcg/kg/min. At moderate doses of 5 to 10 mcg/kg/min, beta effects are elicited. Lastly, at infusion rates of 11 to 20 mcg/kg/min, alpha stimulation is predominant. Dopamine also has an indirect sympathomimetic effect, eliciting the release of norepinephrine via beta$_1$ stimulation.[8]

Norepinephrine is now considered first-line therapy for a patient in septic or vasodilatory shock. Some clinicians have found dopamine to have a poor response in cases of gram-negative sepsis because the sensitivity of beta receptors is diminished due to a down-regulation.[9,10]

During surgery and anesthesia, dopamine is administered for its dopaminergic effect. The stimulation of dopamine receptors in the renal artery promotes an increase in renal blood flow and a resultant increase in glomerular filtration rate and urine output. However, the benefits of so-called renal dopamine are in doubt, and many clinicians have abandoned the practice.[11–13] The urine output increases, but long-term morbidity and mortality do not improve. Dopamine also inhibits aldosterone resulting in an increase in sodium excretion and urine output.

Dopamine has been implicated in several cases of severe limb ischemia. If dopamine is administered through a peripheral line, increased vigilance in pediatric patients and in patients with any type of vascular disease such as diabetes, atherosclerosis, or Raynaud phenomenon is advised. The presence of an arterial line in the affected limb also increases the incidence of limb ischemia with concurrent dopamine infusion. Other metabolic and central nervous system (CNS) effects, similar to those seen with epinephrine but less extensive, have been attributed to dopamine administration.[4]

The monoamine oxidase enzymes metabolize dopamine, therefore the effects of dopamine can be prolonged in patients receiving a monoamine oxidase inhibitor. Tricyclic antidepressants may also augment the activity of sympathomimetic drugs.

Isoproterenol

Isoproterenol is a synthetic catecholamine with the same underlying chemical structure as the endogenous catecholamines. It is a potent nonselective agonist of beta$_1$ and beta$_2$ receptors but has no agonistic activity at alpha receptors or dopamine receptors. The use of isoproterenol has been limited since the emergence of dobutamine and milrinone. In current practice it is occasionally used in the treatment of bradycardia with heart block and torsades de pointes ventricular tachycardia.[14] Isoproterenol is also used after heart transplant for chronotropic support.[15]

The profound beta$_1$ stimulation induced by isoproterenol results in positive inotropic and chronotropic effects. In combination with the peripheral beta$_2$-induced vasodilation and resultant drop in systemic vascular resistance, an increase in cardiac output is seen. However, the positive inotropic and chronotropic effects dramatically increase myocardial oxygen consumption, which may already be compromised by the beta$_2$-induced peripheral vasodilation, causing a decrease in diastolic blood pressure and ultimately a decrease in coronary artery perfusion. These effects are especially detrimental in patients with coronary artery disease. Isoproterenol is also a potent bronchodilator and pulmonary vasodilator.

The detrimental effects of isoproterenol on the heart, such as excessive tachycardia, induction of myocardial ischemia, and arrhythmia production, are the major factors limiting its use for the treatment of significant heart block unresponsive to atropine. Other side effects are similar to those seen with epinephrine but occur to a lesser extent.

Dobutamine

Dobutamine is a synthetic sympathomimetic amine. It is a modification of isoproterenol, but its use is much more widespread. Dobutamine is used primarily as a β$_1$-agonist, and has mild beta$_2$ effects.[16,17] Dobutamine induces a strong inotropic response with minimal chronotropy. The beta$_2$ receptors located on the vasculature produce a vasodilatory effect and result in a decrease in systemic vascular resistance (SVR) and blood pressure. The resultant increase in cardiac output compensates for the decrease in SVR, and the blood pressure increases or, at low doses, remains relatively unchanged. Pulmonary artery pressure decreases, and an increase in left ventricular stroke work index is observed.[18]

The positive inotropic effects, coupled with the lack of chronotropy and maintenance of normal blood pressure, have made this agent an option in cardiogenic and septic shock and in select patients with mild heart failure.[19] It is also frequently used for heart stimulation for cardiac stress testing.[14] Evidence indicates significant adverse effects when dobutamine is used in cardiac surgery, and clinicians have stopped using it for inotropic support in this situation.[20]

DIRECT-ACTING α-AGONISTS

α$_1$-agonists

Phenylephrine

Phenylephrine (Neo-Synephrine) is the most commonly used pure α-agonist. Phenylephrine has strong alpha-stimulating effects, with virtually no beta receptor stimulation. A sharp rise in blood pressure is produced as a result of a significant increase in peripheral resistance secondary to the alpha$_1$ stimulation. A reflex bradycardia is commonly elicited secondary to baroreceptor stimulation. Careful titration of intravenous (IV) phenylephrine boluses is necessary to avoid large changes in blood pressure and decreases in heart rate. The onset of action of IV phenylephrine is immediate, with the duration of action ranging from 5 to 20 minutes. Due to the potent vasoconstricting effects, phenylephrine is used topically to prevent nosebleeds during nasal intubation or to reduce bleeding during ear, nose, and throat surgery. It is also used as a mydriatic in ophthalmology. Severe hypertension may occur, however, and careful dose titration should be observed. Judicious use of other agents such as oxymetazoline or epinephrine is an alternative.[21–23]

Other Inotropes

Vasopressin

Arginine vasopressin is an endogenous hormone that is produced in the hypothalamus, stored in the posterior pituitary, and released from the magnocellular neurons of the hypothalamus. It functions to control osmoregulation, and its release is stimulated by increased osmolality and hypovolemia. Arginine vasopressin is also referred to as antidiuretic hormone. Vasopressin deficiency and down-regulation of vasopressin receptors are common in septic shock.[24] Vasopressin is a potent vasoconstrictor; however, it selectively dilates renal afferent, pulmonary, and cerebral arterioles. Low-dose vasopressin infusion (0.03–0.04 units/min) increases blood pressure, urine output, and creatinine clearance and decreases the dosage of norepinephrine required to maintain blood pressure in patients with septic shock. It is mostly used as an add-on therapy with catecholamine vasopressors. Increases in blood pressure occur in the first hour of administration, and the catecholamine vasopressor can then be titrated down. In a randomized trial, low-dose vasopressin added to norepinephrine was not significantly better than as-needed norepinephrine alone, although added vasopressin may be useful in patients with less severe shock. Complications of vasopressin include gastrointestinal ischemia, decreased cardiac output, skin or digital necrosis, and cardiac arrest (especially at doses >0.04 units/min).[25–27] Vasopressin agonists such as terlipressin and desmopressin have a variety of uses, including bleeding reduction, antidiuresis in diabetes insipidus, and treatment of enuresis.[28]

Phosphodiesterase Inhibitors

Milrinone. The phosphodiesterase 3 (PDE-3) inhibitors, also known as nonglycoside noncatecholamines, include milrinone (Primacor). They differ structurally and functionally from catecholamines and are generally used as alternatives or adjuncts to the standard inotropes in cardiac surgery and heart failure.[29–32]

Phosphodiesterases are a group of enzymes that play a role in a variety of physiologic actions. Eleven subfamilies have been identified.[33] They break down the second messenger cyclic adenosine monophosphate (cAMP) or cyclic guanosine monophosphate (cGMP) in various cells. PDE-3 inhibitors such as milrinone prevent the breakdown of cAMP and thus enhance its action. Milrinone induces positive inotropic action and vasodilation without producing tachycardia. It is occasionally referred to as an inodilator.[34] Milrinone substantially improves left ventricular function in association with an acceleration of calcium uptake by the sarcoplasmic reticulum. This acceleration appears to result from an inhibition of membrane-bound PDE-3 in the sarcoplasm, which induces a local elevation of cAMP. This allows for the buildup of cAMP and a subsequent increase in the uptake of intracellular calcium. Adrenergic receptors are not used to achieve the inotropic effect. It follows that these drugs retain their inotropic effect even in the presence of β-blocking agents or during beta receptor down-regulation, situations that are frequently encountered in patients with heart failure. Therefore, by virtue of their alternative pathway, PDE-3 inhibitors may be used to augment the effect of direct-acting β-agonists such as dobutamine or dopamine. Milrinone improves weaning of high-risk patients from cardiopulmonary bypass.[31,32]

These agents act as vasodilators because of the differential mechanism of cAMP action in the smooth muscle versus the myocardium. In the smooth muscle, cAMP causes an efflux of calcium, with a resultant relaxation of the muscle and vasodilation. The clinical result is a decrease in both preload and afterload. This effect, along with the absence of an associated increase in heart rate, probably contributes to the absence of an increase in myocardial oxygen consumption. Sildenafil (Viagra, Revatio) is a PDE-5 inhibitor that produces vasodilation and is used to treat pulmonary arterial hypertension. Pulmonary vasodilation reduces the workload of the right ventricle and improves symptoms of right-sided heart failure.

Milrinone enhances diastolic function, increases cardiac output, and decreases pulmonary capillary wedge pressure. Side effects can include arrhythmias. Elimination is via the kidney, therefore milrinone should be used with caution in patients with renal failure because of the potential for life-threatening arrhythmias. The current manufacturer's recommendation for the administration of milrinone is an IV loading dose of 50 mcg/kg, administered slowly over 10 minutes to avoid hypotension, followed by an infusion of 0.5 mcg/kg as needed. Table 13.3 outlines the current vasopressors and some of their uses.

MIXED FUNCTION AGONISTS

Ephedrine

Ephedrine is a synthetic noncatecholamine sympathomimetic commonly used in anesthesia practice. It stimulates both alpha and beta receptors directly, and it indirectly causes release of endogenous catecholamines. It has both central and peripheral actions. Ephedrine's effects are similar to those seen with epinephrine; however, they are more moderate and are not accompanied by a dramatic increase in serum glucose concentrations. The duration of action of ephedrine is also longer than that of epinephrine, owing to its lack of a basic catechol structure; this characteristic makes it resistant to metabolism by monoamine oxidase.[14]

Ephedrine produces dose-related increases in blood pressure, cardiac output, heart rate, and systemic vascular resistance. Ephedrine

is often the first sympathomimetic chosen to alleviate hypotension because of the cardiac-depressant effects of anesthetic agents and the vasodilation resulting from spinal anesthesia. Ephedrine, when administered intravenously in doses ranging from 5 to 25 mg, has an immediate onset and a duration of action of 15 minutes to 1.5 hours, depending on dose. This drug should be used cautiously in patients with questionable coronary perfusion because myocardial oxygen consumption may increase more dramatically than anticipated as a result of ephedrine's positive inotropic effect. Ephedrine also causes bronchodilation due to beta$_2$ receptor agonism in the lungs. In obstetrics, ephedrine had long been considered the drug of choice to address maternal hypotension after regional anesthesia because it was felt to maintain uterine blood flow better than phenylephrine. Newer data are questioning this long-standing practice, and phenylephrine is now recommended over ephedrine.[35–37] Ephedrine produces increases in fetal metabolic rate, leading to fetal acidosis due to beta stimulation, and phenylephrine does not.[38] As with any indirect-acting agent, tachyphylaxis may develop with subsequent dosing, because catecholamine stores become depleted.[39] Ephedrine also may be administered by oral, intramuscular, or subcutaneous routes.

SELECTIVE β$_2$-AGONISTS

The β$_2$-agonists include albuterol (Proventil, Ventolin, others), levalbuterol (Xopenex), pirbuterol (Maxair), and salmeterol (Serevent). These selective β$_2$-agonists are effective in treating obstructive airway diseases such as asthma, chronic obstructive pulmonary disease, and acute bronchospasm. Long-acting β-agonists (LABA) formulations include

TABLE 13.3 Vasopressor Agents

| Agent | Dose Range | PERIPHERAL VASCULATURE | | CARDIAC EFFECTS | | | Typical Use |
		Vasoconstriction	Vasodilation	Heart Rate	Contractility	Dysrhythmias	
Dopamine	1–4 mcg/kg/min	0	1+	1+	1+	1+	"Renal dose" does not improve renal function; may be used with bradycardia and hypotension
	5–10 mcg/kg/min	1–2+	1+	2+	2+	2+	
	11–20 mcg/kg/min	2–3+	1+	2+	2+	3+	Vasopressor range
Vasopressin	0.04–0.1 units/min	3–4+	0	0	0	1+	Septic shock, post–cardiopulmonary bypass shock state, no outcome benefit in sepsis
Phenylephrine	20–200 mcg/min	4+	0	0	0	1+	Vasodilatory shock, best for supraventricular tachycardia
Norepinephrine	1–20 mcg/min	4+	0	2+	2+	2+	First-line vasopressor for septic shock, vasodilatory shock
Epinephrine	1–20 mcg/min	4+	0	4+	4+	4+	Refractory shock, shock with bradycardia, anaphylactic shock
Dobutamine	1–20 mcg/kg/min	1+	2+	1–2+	3+	3+	Cardiogenic shock, septic shock
Milrinone	37.5–75 mcg/kg bolus followed by 0.375–0.75 mcg/min	0	2+	1+	3+	2+	Cardiogenic shock, right heart failure, dilates pulmonary artery; caution in renal failure

From Angus DC. Approach to patient with shock. In Goldman L, Schafer AI, eds. *Goldman's Cecil Medicine*. 26th ed. Philadelphia: Elsevier; 2020:646.

formoterol (Foradil), arformoterol (Brovana), indacaterol (Arcapta), olodaterol (Striverdi Respimat), and salmeterol (Serevent).[40,41]

The selectivity of these agents for beta$_2$ receptors results in the desired response of bronchodilation and a lower incidence of the undesired beta$_1$ responses of tachycardia and arrhythmia. None of these agents, however, are completely selective. These agents are available in aerosol form, and it is widely accepted that aerosol delivery is as effective as subcutaneous or other means of administration. Drugs of this class also have an increased duration of action because of their noncatecholamine structure; this renders them resistant to methylation by catechol-O-methyltransferase (COMT). Two puffs of nebulized or metered-dose inhaler–administered albuterol or salmeterol 10 to 15 minutes before exercise have been shown to have similar efficacy in preventing exercise-induced asthma.[42]

Chronic use of these agents can result in tachyphylaxis secondary to down-regulation (i.e., diminished quantity) of beta receptors. Increased hyperresponsiveness of the airway also has been suspected with chronic use of these agents. A black box warning about a higher risk of asthma-related death was added to the package inserts of all preparations containing a long-acting β$_2$-agonist. If the addition of formoterol or salmeterol to an inhaled corticosteroid is found to improve symptomatic control, it is safer to give formoterol or salmeterol in the form of a combination inhaler.[43,44]

The β$_2$-agonists have been administered to delay premature labor, although their use has declined dramatically because of a high frequency of adverse events and a lack of efficacy. This is referred to as a tocolytic effect. Uterine relaxation is achieved through an increase in cAMP levels; this decreases intracellular calcium levels and ultimately diminishes the level of actin-myosin coupling.[45–47] Doses of selected vasoactive drugs are listed in Table 13.4. For a complete discussion of tocolysis, see Chapter 51. Mirabegron (Myrbetriq) is a β$_3$-agonist that inhibits the detrusor muscle and is used for overactive bladder.

α$_2$-agonists
Clonidine
Clonidine (Catapres) is a presynaptic α$_2$-agonist. Clonidine decreases blood pressure by acting as an agonist at peripheral presynaptic alpha$_2$ receptors and central alpha$_2$ receptors. Stimulation of the peripheral presynaptic alpha$_2$ receptors causes inhibition of catecholamine release, with subsequent vasodilation. Stimulation of the central alpha$_2$ receptors, which is considered the main antihypertensive mechanism of action, results in diminished sympathetic outflow and a resultant decrease in circulating catecholamines and renin activity. It is usually

TABLE 13.4   Doses of Select Vasoactive Drugs

Drug	Bolus Dose	Infusion Dose Rate	Comments
Calcium chloride (CaCl$_2$) or gluconate	500–1000 mg (chloride)		Onset: <1 min Peak effect: <1 min Duration: 10–20 min
Dobutamine (Dobutrex)	500–2000 mg (gluconate)	2–20 mcg/kg/min	Onset: 1–2 min Peak effect: 1–10 min Duration: 10 min
Dopamine		1–2 mcg/kg/min (renal doses) 2–10 mcg/kg/min (cardiac doses) 10–20 mcg/kg/min (vasopressor doses)	Onset: 2–4 min Peak effect: 2–10 min Duration: <10 min
Ephedrine	5- to 10-mg incremental doses		Dilute to 5 or 10 mg/mL Onset: <1 min Peak effect: 2–5 min Duration: 10–60 min
Epinephrine	10–100 mcg	0.01–0.03 mcg/kg/min (β doses) 0.03–0.15 mcg/kg/min (α and β doses) 0.15–0.3 mcg/kg/min (α doses)	Onset: <1 min Peak effect: 1–2 min Duration: 5–10 min
Glucagon	1–5 mg over 2–5 min		
Milrinone (Primacor)	50 mcg/kg	0.375–0.75 mcg/kg/min	
Norepinephrine (Levophed)		0.01–0.2 mcg/kg/min	Onset: <1 min Peak effect: 1–2 min Duration: 2–10 min
Phentolamine	5 mg (50–100 mcg/kg); repeat as required	1–10 mcg/kg/min	Onset: 1–2 min Peak effect: 2 min Duration: 10–15 min
Phenylephrine (Neo-Synephrine)	40–100 mcg	0.15–0.75 mcg/kg/min	Onset: <1 min Peak effect: 1 min Duration: 15–20 min
Sodium nitroprusside (Nitropres)		0.1–10 mcg/kg/min	Onset: <1 min Peak effect: 1–2 min Duration: 1–10 min
Vasopressin (Pitressin)	10–20 units	0.1–1.0 units/min	Onset: 1–5 min Peak effect: 5 min Duration: 10–30 min

reserved for short-term oral treatment of severe hypertension as an add-on drug.[48] Rebound hypertension, seen after abrupt discontinuation of clonidine use, is a major concern. The resultant increase in catecholamine levels manifests as tachycardia and hypertension. Continuing the medication throughout the perioperative period is essential. Tapering the dose and discontinuation may occasionally be indicated. Patches may also be used during surgery to prevent withdrawal.

Clonidine is available in oral, transdermal, and epidural forms. The transdermal form is frequently encountered and is administered at a fixed rate for a period of 1 week. Additional uses of clonidine include use as a premedicant sedative, as an analgesic in combination with opiates for epidural treatment of severe pain (Duraclon), and for suppression of alcohol withdrawal symptoms.[49] Clonidine is used as part of a catecholamine suppression test in the diagnosis of pheochromocytoma.

Dexmedetomidine

Dexmedetomidine is an α_2-agonist that is marketed for short-term sedation in critical care. It is used as an adjunct to anesthesia in a variety of situations.[50] Dexmedetomidine provides dose-dependent sedation, analgesia, sympatholysis, and anxiolysis without significant respiratory depression. The side effects are predictable from the pharmacologic profile of α_2-adrenoceptor agonists and include hypotension, bradycardia, oversedation, and delayed recovery. Dexmedetomidine is discussed in detail in Chapter 9. The mechanism of presynaptic α_2-agonism is shown in Fig. 13.1.

α-RECEPTOR ANTAGONISTS

The α-receptor antagonists are used for treatment of hypertension, benign prostatic hyperplasia (BPH), pheochromocytoma, Raynaud phenomenon, and ergot alkaloid toxicity.[39] Common side effects include orthostatic hypotension and baroreceptor-mediated reflex tachycardia, which may make them somewhat difficult to use in the treatment of hypertension in the ambulatory patient. In addition, because of the significantly longer duration of action of the alpha-receptor antagonists,

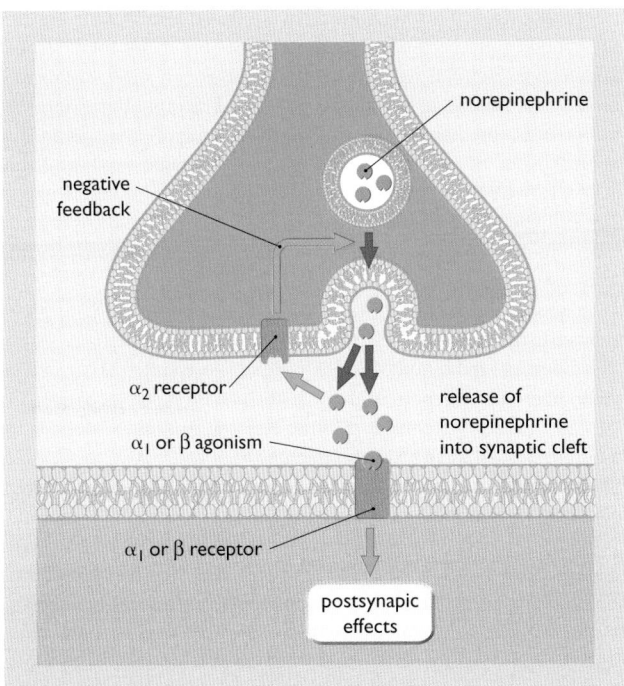

Fig. 13.1 Presynaptic α_2-agonism. (From Page C, et al. *Integrated Pharmacology.* 3rd ed. Edinburgh: Mosby; 2006:420.)

other agents are considered more predictable for treating emergent episodes of hypertension.

Phenoxybenzamine

Phenoxybenzamine (Dibenzyline) is a halo alkylamine with both α_1- and α_2-blocking activity. Phenoxybenzamine binds to alpha receptors noncompetitively and irreversibly, and its action is terminated only by metabolism of the drug and generation of new alpha receptors. Clinically this drug is used preoperatively in patients with pheochromocytoma to decrease the response to endogenous catecholamines. The preoperative course is started 1 to 3 weeks before surgery, with the oral dosage titrated up to 40 to 120 mg in two or three divided daily doses. It may be combined with the tyrosine hydroxylase inhibitor metyrosine (Demser). Phenoxybenzamine also prevents the sympathomimetic response expected from phenylephrine. The response to norepinephrine is limited to its β_1-agonist activity, and treatment with epinephrine may show "epi-reversal," which is an enhanced beta$_2$ response with a worsening of hypotension and tachycardia. The primary side effect is orthostatic hypertension. Nasal stuffiness has been frequently associated with phenoxybenzamine use.[14,51]

Phentolamine

Phentolamine, an imidazole, is a competitive antagonist of alpha$_1$ and alpha$_2$ receptors. It has a rapid onset after IV administration and a much shorter duration of action when compared with phenoxybenzamine. It can be used for the short-term control of hypertension in patients with pheochromocytoma. The recommended dose is 1 to 5 mg by slow IV push. Phentolamine has also been used to treat local infiltrations of vasoconstricting agents. Phentolamine (5–10 mg) can be mixed with 10 mL of normal saline and injected directly into the site of the infiltration.[51]

Prazosin and Other Alpha-Receptor Antagonists

Prazosin (Minipress), doxazosin (Cardura), and terazosin (Hytrin) are selective α_1-antagonists used in the treatment of chronic hypertension and BPH. Their lack of α_2-blocking activity indicates that they have no effect on norepinephrine levels. Therefore selectivity for alpha$_1$ receptors leaves the inhibitory action of alpha$_2$ receptors on norepinephrine release intact, and less norepinephrine-induced tachycardia results than when a nonselective α-antagonist is used. Prazosin induces vasodilation in both arterioles and veins. Peripheral vascular resistance and cardiac preload and afterload are diminished. The drugs are administered orally, and orthostatic hypotension can be a major side effect.

Tamsulosin (Flomax), alfuzosin (Uroxatral), and silodosin (Rapaflo) are alpha$_1$-selective antagonists that produce relaxation of the bladder neck and prostate, helping relax smooth muscle tone and relieve obstructive urinary symptoms. They are commonly used with 5α-reductase inhibitors such as finasteride (Proscar) and dutasteride (Avodart) for the treatment of BPH. Because they do not antagonize beta receptors there is a decreased risk of hypotension.[52] Tamsulosin, and other α-antagonists, have been noted to produce floppy iris syndrome, which may complicate cataract surgery. Discontinuing them prior to surgery is not required as long as the ophthalmologist is aware of their administration.[53,54]

Droperidol

Droperidol (Inapsine), a butyrophenone, is used as an antiemetic in anesthesia practice. It produces both dopamine and α-adrenergic blockade, and thus small reductions in blood pressure may occur especially in volume-depleted patients. The use of droperidol has decreased markedly as a result of the black box warning required by the US Food and Drug Administration (FDA) as part of the package insert for this drug. Use of droperidol has been associated with prolongation of the corrected QT interval in certain patients, increasing the probability of the development of torsades de pointes, which has led to serious morbidity and death. There has been considerable debate regarding the relationship between the anesthetic administration of droperidol in very low doses as an antiemetic and the complications described.[55] Little doubt remains, however, that the potential for administrative and legal difficulties, added to issues of patient safety, have led to significant changes in the pattern of use of this drug.[56,57] A 12-lead electrocardiogram is required by the FDA prior to the use of droperidol. Off-label use of very low doses as an antiemetic may still be useful. Evidence suggests that the serotonin type 3 receptor antagonists have a similar frequency of QT interval prolongation.[55,58]

β-ADRENERGIC BLOCKING AGENTS

The β-blockers are one of the most widely prescribed classes of drugs. Common applications for these agents include the treatment of angina pectoris, hypertension, postmyocardial infarctions (post-MIs), supraventricular tachycardias (including Wolff-Parkinson-White syndrome), and atrial fibrillation (AF); the suppression of increased sympathetic activity (e.g., as occurs with intubation); the management of hypertrophic obstructive cardiomyopathies and congestive heart failure (CHF); the treatment of migraine headaches; and the preoperative preparation of hyperthyroid patients. They are also effective in the treatment of digitalis-induced arrhythmias and in the management of select atrial and ventricular arrhythmias.[59] β-blockers also prevent the detrimental effects associated with cardiac remodeling, which occurs in many cardiac diseases.[60]

The use of perioperative β-blockade in high-risk patients is discussed as follows and in Chapter 28.

The β-blockers are structurally related to isoproterenol. They bind beta receptors in a competitive manner and prevent the actions of catecholamines and other β-agonists. Because these agents are competitive antagonists, if an agonist is present in sufficient concentration at the receptor, the blocking actions of the β-antagonists can be overcome.

The β-blockers are subdivided on the basis of their selectivity for cardiac beta$_1$ receptors and other notable clinical differences, such as their ability to induce vasodilation by additional mechanisms or whether they have partial agonist activity. Table 13.5 lists the β-blockers according to classification subtype.[61]

The degree of receptor selectivity is important because antagonism of beta$_1$ receptors results in lowered heart rate, decreased myocardial contractility, and diminished atrioventricular (AV) conduction velocity; it also has beneficial effects with regard to decreasing myocardial oxygen consumption and the treatment of arrhythmias. However, antagonism of beta$_2$ receptors can result in adverse effects such as bronchoconstriction, hypoglycemia, and peripheral vasoconstriction. It is important to note that, as the dose of the selective β-blockers is increased, the degree of selectivity is diminished.

Some of the β-blockers act as partial agonists, and as such possess intrinsic sympathomimetic activity (ISA). A partial agonist does not stimulate beta receptors to the extent that a full agonist does, and in the presence of a full agonist the partial agonist acts as a competitive antagonist. It follows that β-blockers with ISA competitively antagonize the effects of a full agonist (e.g., endogenous catecholamines released during times of maximal sympathetic tone) down to the activity level of its partial agonist component. ISA minimizes the risk of bronchoconstriction in patients with reactive airway disease who require β-blockade. Pindolol, acebutolol, penbutolol, and carteolol are β-adrenergic blocking agents that possess ISA.

Membrane-stabilizing activity is another property of some β-blockers. These agents diminish arrhythmogenicity by exerting a quinidine-like effect in the heart. However, membrane-stabilizing activity is seen only with high drug concentrations.[62] Propranolol and pindolol are two β-blockers with membrane-stabilizing activity. Labetalol and carvedilol are mixed beta- and alpha-receptor antagonists; the added alpha-receptor blockade makes them vasodilators. Nebivolol (Bystolic) is a new cardioselective β-blocker approved for the treatment of hypertension. It is unique in that it has nitric oxide (NO)–mediated vasodilating properties.[63]

Some potential problems with β-adrenergic blocking agents have already been mentioned. β-blockade can result in both bronchospasm and the development of overt cardiac failure in some high-risk patients receiving high doses or IV administration. Other potential problems arise with beta$_2$-receptor blockade in patients with peripheral vascular disease and Raynaud phenomenon because of the possible potentiation of peripheral vasoconstriction. In diabetic patients, signs of hypoglycemia may be masked, and the patient's ability to increase serum glucose levels may be impaired. Serum potassium levels may also become elevated with β$_2$-blockade because uptake into skeletal muscle is inhibited. In patients whose heart rate is controlled to maintain cardiac output, β-blockade may have a significant impact on blood pressure.

The beta receptors are considered labile receptors—that is, they are subject to significant up- and down-regulation. Long-term therapy with β-blockers leads to up-regulation of beta receptors or an increase in the absolute number and activity of receptors. This phenomenon is suspected to be the underlying cause of the withdrawal syndrome seen with abrupt discontinuation of β-adrenergic antagonist use. Raynaud phenomenon is characterized by increased sympathetic activity for up to 2 days. Obviously this means the patient receiving β-blockers should continue to receive them without interruption throughout the perioperative period. The effects of the β-blocking agents on the ischemic heart are summarized in Fig. 13.2.

Anesthetic Uses

Metoprolol, Esmolol, and Labetalol

Three β-adrenergic blocking agents that are available in IV form are especially useful in the perioperative period. They are metoprolol, esmolol, and labetalol. Esmolol has replaced propranolol in most instances of β-blocker application in anesthesia because of its rapid onset and short duration of action. Esmolol has an onset time of 2 minutes and an elimination half-life of approximately 9 minutes. Its rapid onset and short half-life, as well as its duration of action of 10 to 15 minutes, make it easily and reliably titratable in acute care situations. The recommended IV loading dose of esmolol is 500 mcg/kg; this is followed by an infusion of 100 to 300 mcg/kg/min as needed. Small boluses of 10 to 20 mg may be given, and administration can be repeated according to patient response. Esmolol is metabolized by nonspecific plasma esterases found in the cytosol of red blood cells. Metoprolol is used after MI or in some types of angina and hypertension once the patient is stable to normalize vital signs. IV administration of 5-mg doses at 5-minute intervals to a maximum dose of 15 mg is recommended.[23,61]

Labetalol (Normodyne, Trandate) is classified as a nonselective β-blocker but is unique in that it also possesses an α-blocking component. It provides β-blockade along with α-blockade in a ratio of 7:1. Unlike the standard β-blocker, labetalol produces vasodilation secondary to its α-blocking properties. This action can be extremely beneficial in situations in which an acute rise in blood pressure could be devastating to the clinical outcome. The usual IV dose of labetalol is 0.25 mg/kg; this dose can be repeated every few minutes as indicated and followed by an infusion, if indicated, at a rate of 2 mg/min. In clinical practice a

TABLE 13.5 Antihypertensive Drugs

Drug	Daily Adult Maintenance Dosage	Frequent or Severe Adverse Effects
Angiotensin-Converting Enzyme (ACE) Inhibitors		
Benazepril (Lotensin)	10–80 mg in one or two doses	Cough; hypotension, particularly with a diuretic or volume depletion; rash; acute renal failure with bilateral renal artery stenosis or stenosis of the artery to a solitary kidney; angioedema; hyperkalemia if also taking potassium supplements or potassium-sparing diuretics; loss of taste, usually not severe; blood dyscrasias and renal damage rare, except in patients with renal dysfunction; increased fetal mortality with second- and third-trimester exposure; may decrease excretion of lithium
Captopril (Capoten)	12.5–150 mg in two or three doses	
Enalapril (Vasotec)	2.5–40 mg in one or two doses	
Fosinopril (Monopril)	10–80 mg in one or two doses	
Lisinopril (Prinivil or Zestril)	5–40 mg in one dose	
Moexipril (Univasc)	7.5–30 mg in one or two doses	
Perindopril (Aceon)	4–8 mg in one or two doses	
Quinapril (Accupril)	5–80 mg in one or two doses	
Ramipril (Altace)	1.25–20 mg in one or two doses	
Trandolapril (Mavik)	1–8 mg in one or two doses	
Angiotensin-Receptor Antagonists		
Azilsartan (Edarbi)	80 mg once a day	Similar to ACE inhibitors, but do not cause cough
Candesartan (Atacand)	8–32 mg in one dose	
Eprosartan (Teveten)	400–800 mg in one or two doses	
Irbesartan (Avapro)	150–300 mg in one dose	
Losartan (Cozaar)	25–100 mg in one or two doses	
Olmesartan (Benicar)	20–40 mg in one dose	
Telmisartan (Micardis)	40–80 mg in one dose	
Valsartan (Diovan)	80–320 mg in one dose	
β-Adrenergic Blocking Drugs		
Atenolol (Tenormin)	25–100 mg in one or two doses	Fatigue; depression; bradycardia; decreased exercise tolerance; congestive heart failure; aggravated peripheral arterial insufficiency; aggravated allergic reactions; bronchospasm; mask symptoms of and delay in recovery from hypoglycemia; Raynaud phenomenon; insomnia; vivid dreams or hallucinations; acute mental disorder; impotence; increased serum triglycerides
Betaxolol generic	5–40 mg in one dose	
Bisoprolol (Zebeta)	5–20 mg in one dose	
Metoprolol (Lopressor, Toprol-XL)	50–200 mg in one or two doses Extended release 25–400 mg once	
Nadolol (Corgard)	20–320 mg in one dose	
Propranolol (Inderal)	40–240 mg in two doses	
Timolol generic	10–60 mg in two doses	
β-Adrenergic Blocking Drugs With Intrinsic Sympathomimetic Activity		
Acebutolol (Sectral)	200–1200 mg in one or two doses	Similar to other β-adrenergic blocking drugs but with less resting bradycardia and fewer lipid changes; acebutolol has been associated with positive antinuclear antibody test and occasional drug-induced lupus
Penbutolol (Levatol)	10–80 mg in one dose	
Pindolol generic	10–60 mg in two doses	
α- and β-Blockers		
Carvedilol (Coreg)	12.5–50 mg in two doses	Similar to other β-adrenergic blocking drugs, but more orthostatic hypotension; no effect on serum lipids
Labetalol generic	200–1200 mg in two doses	

Continued

TABLE 13.5   Antihypertensive Drugs—cont'd

Drug	Daily Adult Maintenance Dosage	Frequent or Severe Adverse Effects
β-Blocker With Vasodilating Nitric Oxide Mediated Activity		
Nebivolol (Bystolic)	5–40 mg once	Vasodilator due to nitric oxide–mediated action
Thiazide-Type Diuretics (Usually Once Daily)		
Chlorothiazide (Diuril)	125–500 mg once	Hyperuricemia; hypokalemia; hypomagnesemia; hyperglycemia; hyponatremia; hypercholesterolemia; hypertriglyceridemia; pancreatitis; rashes and other allergic reactions; sexual dysfunction; photosensitivity reactions; may decrease excretion of lithium
Hydrochlorothiazide (Microzide)	12.5–50 mg once	
Chlorthalidone (Thalitone)	12.5–50 mg once	
Indapamide, generic	1.25–5 mg once	
Metolazone (Zaroxolyn)	1.25–5 mg once	
Loop Diuretics		
Bumetanide generic	0.5–2 mg in two doses	Dehydration; circulatory collapse; hypokalemia; hyponatremia; hypomagnesemia; hyperglycemia; metabolic alkalosis; hyperuricemia; blood dyscrasias; rashes; lipid changes as with thiazide-type diuretics
Ethacrynic acid (Edecrin)	25–100 mg in two or three doses	
Furosemide (Lasix)	20–320 mg in two doses	
Torsemide (Demadex)	5–20 mg in one or two doses	
Potassium-Sparing Diuretics		
Amiloride (Midamor)	5–10 mg in one or two doses	Hyperkalemia; GI disturbances; rash; headache
Triamterene (Dyrenium)	50–150 mg in one or two doses	Hyperkalemia; GI disturbances; nephrolithiasis
Aldosterone Antagonists		
Spironolactone (Aldactone)	12.5–100 mg in one or two doses	Hyperkalemia; hyponatremia; mastodynia; gynecomastia; menstrual abnormalities; GI disturbances; rash
Eplerenone (Inspra)	25–100 mg in one or two doses	Hyperkalemia; hypernatremia
Calcium Channel Blockers		
Diltiazem (Cardizem CD)	120–360 mg in one dose	Dizziness; headache; edema; constipation (especially verapamil); AV block; bradycardia; heart failure; lupus-like rash
(Tiazac)	120–540 mg in one dose	
Verapamil (Calan)	120–480 mg in one or two doses	
(Calan SR)	120–480 mg in one or two doses	
(Isoptin SR)	120–480 mg in one or two doses	
(Verelan)	120–480 mg in one dose	
(Covera HS)	180–540 mg in one dose	
Dihydropyridines		
Amlodipine (Norvasc)	2.5–10 mg in one dose	Dizziness; headache; peripheral edema (more than with verapamil and diltiazem; more common in women); flushing; tachycardia; rash; gingival hyperplasia
Felodipine (Plendil)	2.5–10 mg in one dose	
Isradipine (DynaCirc, DynaCirc CR)	5–10 mg in two doses	
Nicardipine, generic Nicardipine, extended release (Cardene SR)	60–120 mg in two or three doses	
Nifedipine (Adalat CC, Procardia XL)	30–90 mg once	
Nisoldipine (Sular)	17–34 mg once	
α-Adrenergic Blockers		
Prazosin (Minipress)	1–20 mg in two or three doses First dose is 1 mg at bedtime	Syncope with first dose; dizziness and vertigo; headache; palpitations; fluid retention; drowsiness; weakness; anticholinergic effects; priapism
Terazosin (Hytrin)	Maintenance: 1–20 mg once First dose is 1 mg at bedtime	Both similar to prazosin, but with less hypotension after first dose

TABLE 13.5   Antihypertensive Drugs—cont'd

Drug	Daily Adult Maintenance Dosage	Frequent or Severe Adverse Effects
Doxazosin (Cardura)	1–2 mg in one dose First day: 1 mg at bedtime	
Central α-Adrenergic Agonists		
Clonidine (Catapres)	0.1–0.6 mg in two or three doses	CNS reactions similar to methyldopa, but more sedation and dry mouth; bradycardia; heart block; rebound hypertension (less likely with patches); contact dermatitis from patches
(Catapres TTS)	One patch weekly (0.1–0.3 mg/day)	Similar to clonidine
Guanfacine generic	1–3 mg in one dose	Drowsiness; sedation, fatigue; depression; dry mouth; heart block; autoimmune disorders, including colitis, hepatitis, hepatic necrosis; Coombs-positive hemolytic anemia; lupuslike syndrome; thrombocytopenia; red cell aplasia; impotence
Methyldopa generic	250 mg to 2 g in two doses	
Direct Vasodilators		
Hydralazine generic	40–200 mg in two to four doses	Tachycardia; aggravation of angina; headache; dizziness; fluid retention; nasal congestion; lupuslike syndrome; hepatitis
Minoxidil generic	2.5–40 mg in one or two doses	Tachycardia; aggravation of angina; marked fluid retention; pericardial effusion; hair growth on face and body
Renin Inhibitor		
Aliskiren (Tekturna)	150–300 mg once daily	First direct renin inhibitor for treatment of hypertension; avid binding of renin and long half-life could lead to hypotension unresponsive to discontinuing drug

AV, Atrioventricular; *CNS*, central nervous system; *GI*, gastrointestinal.
From Drugs for hypertension. *Med Lett Drugs Ther.* 2020;62(1598):73–80.

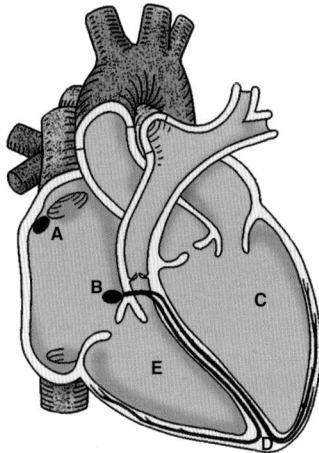

Fig. 13.2 Cardiac effects of β-adrenergic blocking drugs. (A) Negative chronotropic. (B) Negative dromotropic. (C) Negative inotropic. (D) Antiarrhythmic. (E) Antiischemic.

bolus dose of labetalol (5–10 mg) is titrated and repeated on the basis of patient response. Labetalol can have a duration of action ranging from 2 to 6 hours depending on dose. Because labetalol provides beta-receptor antagonism, preexisting bradycardia is a contraindication for the use in acute management of hypertension. It is recommended for hypertensive episodes in obstetric patients. Uterine blood flow is not affected in obstetric patients even in the event of a dramatic decrease in systemic blood pressure. Labetalol undergoes hepatic metabolism and renal elimination.[61,63,64]

There is a major controversy as to the use of prophylactic use of perioperative β-blockers. Studies are conflicting, and several major studies have been retracted. In 2008 the largest randomized controlled

trial of perioperative β-blocker use, PeriOperative ISchemic Evaluation (POISE), indicated that β-blockade offered cardiac protection in coronary heart disease. However, there was a significant increase in all-cause mortality, particularly in patients who became septic or hypotensive. There was also a significant increase in strokes, contributed to by hypotension. Hypotension and bradycardia were much more frequent in the β-blocked patients. A meta-analysis of randomized controlled trials (including POISE) showed that some subgroups of patients could benefit from perioperative β-blockade, including those at high risk and those in whom β-blockade was strictly titrated.[65] The increased mortality risk associated with perioperative β-blockade resulted in a reappraisal of their perioperative use. β-blocker initiation decreased sharply in the second half of 2008 and continued to decrease afterwards. A number of clinicians feel that until we have new clinical trials showing definitive benefit, their use should be minimal.[66–68] In 2014 new guidelines were introduced by the American College of Cardiology/American Heart Association (ACC/AHA) Task Force.[69,70] The European Society of Cardiology/European Society of Anaesthesiology (ESC/ESA) offered similar guidelines.[71] Both sets of guidelines strongly recommend continuing treatment in patients currently taking β-blockers. The new guidelines recommend considering starting β-blockers in patients with known ischemic heart disease or myocardial ischemia and in patients with multiple cardiac risk factors (two [according to the ESC/ESA guidelines] and three [according to the ACC/AHA guidelines]). The ACC/AHA guidelines suggest that initiating β-blockers in patients with a compelling indication for β-blockers but with no other cardiac risk factor is of uncertain benefit. Both sets of guidelines recommend starting β-blocker therapy well in advance of surgery, between 2 and 30 days prior (ESC/ESA). The possibility of harm is emphasized. The ACC/AHA guidelines consider starting β-blockers the day of surgery as potentially harmful, a view endorsed by the ESC/ESA guidelines, with another caveat against initiation of β-blockers in patients undergoing low-risk surgery. The ESC/ESA guidelines recommend using atenolol or bisoprolol as a first choice.[72]

β-blockers may reduce the risk for perioperative MI but with the side effect of increasing stroke risk and with no evidence for a reduction in overall mortality. In patients who do not have a very high risk for perioperative MI, β-blockers probably increase risk. Whether it is helpful to start β-blockers before surgery in patients with intermediate- to high-risk ischemia on stress testing or with three or more Revised Cardiac Risk Index (RCRI) risk factors is unknown, and data to support this option are insufficient. Furthermore, any benefits are more likely to be seen when β-blockers are started at least 1 week before surgery at a low dose and titrated to a heart rate of 55 to 70 beats per minute. Until more evidence is available, it seems prudent to avoid starting β-blockers immediately before surgery and to avoid them in the settings of emergency surgery, prior cerebrovascular disease, or sepsis, but to continue β-blockers in patients who are already taking them.[70–74]

Perioperative application of β-blockers still plays a pivotal role in cardiac surgery. They can substantially reduce the high burden of postoperative supraventricular and ventricular arrhythmias. Their influence on mortality, acute MI (AMI), stroke, congestive heart failure, hypotension, and bradycardia in this setting remains unclear. In noncardiac surgery, evidence shows an association of β-blockers with increased all-cause mortality. Data from low risk of bias trials further suggest an increase in stroke rate with the use of β-blockers. The substantial reduction in supraventricular arrhythmias and AMI in this setting seems to be offset by the potential increase in mortality and stroke.[73,74] A recommendation for the management of perioperative β-blockade is shown in Box 13.1. β-blockers are contraindicated in patients with asthma, bradyarrhythmias, acute heart failure, or advanced heart block. Researchers investigated whether an α_2-adrenergic agonist such as clonidine or dexmedetomidine may have some benefit in reducing activation of the sympathetic nervous system during and after noncardiac surgery. They found that administration of low-dose clonidine in patients undergoing noncardiac surgery did not reduce the rate of the

---

> ### BOX 13.1   Suggestions for Managing Perioperative β-Blockers
>
> β-blockers should be continued in patients undergoing surgery who have been on β-blockers chronically.
>
> It is reasonable for the management of β-blockers after surgery to be guided by clinical circumstances, independent of when the agent was started.
>
> In patients with intermediate- or high-risk myocardial ischemia noted in preoperative risk stratification tests, it may be reasonable to begin perioperative β-blockers.
>
> In patients with three or more Revised Cardiac Risk Index (RCRI) risk factors (e.g., diabetes mellitus, heart failure, coronary artery disease, renal insufficiency, or cerebrovascular accident), it may be reasonable to begin β-blockers before surgery.
>
> In patients with a compelling long-term indication for β-blocker therapy but no other RCRI risk factors, initiating β-blockers in the perioperative setting as an approach to reduce perioperative risk is of uncertain benefit.
>
> In patients in whom β-blocker therapy is initiated, it may be reasonable to begin perioperative β-blockers far enough in advance to assess safety and tolerability, preferably more than 1 day before surgery.
>
> β-blocker therapy should not be started on the day of surgery.

Adapted from Fleisher LA. 2014 ACC/AHA guideline on perioperative cardiovascular evaluation and management of patients undergoing noncardiac surgery: a report of the American College of Cardiology/ American Heart Association task force on practice guidelines. *J Am Coll Cardiol.* 2014;64(22):e77–e137.

composite outcome of death or nonfatal MI. There was, however, an increased risk of clinically important hypotension and nonfatal cardiac arrest.[75] The 2014 ACC/AHA guidelines are quite clear that alpha$_2$-receptor agonists are not recommended for the prevention of cardiac events. The ESC/ESA guidelines make no specific recommendation, but state that alpha$_2$-receptor agonists should not be administered to patients undergoing noncardiac surgery.[70,71]

STATINS

Statins have documented benefits for primary and secondary prevention of cardiovascular disease and are thought to improve perioperative outcomes in patients undergoing surgery. Statins reduce endovascular inflammation and stabilize endothelial plaque. Compliance with both antiplatelet and statin therapy in vascular surgical patients is associated with significantly improved long-term survival. There are insufficient data to support a recommendation on perioperative statin therapy for patients undergoing noncardiac surgery.[76–78] The ACC/AHA guidelines recommend continuing statins perioperatively for patients who are currently taking them. The ESA/ESC guidelines agree and add that continuation of statins should favor drugs with a long half-life or extended release to maintain some of statins' effects until oral administration can resume postoperatively.[70,71]

ANTIPLATELET DRUGS

Many patients with cardiovascular disease or significant risk factors are taking lifelong aspirin. Whether aspirin should be continued or withheld in patients undergoing noncardiac surgery is a common clinical question. Clinicians must balance discontinuing the beneficial antithrombotic effect of aspirin against the possibility of increasing perioperative bleeding. Results from the POISE-2 trial of over 10,000 patients suggest that aspirin administration during the perioperative period does not change the risk of a cardiovascular event and may result in increased bleeding.[79] A focused review published in 2015 of the available data suggests that aspirin should not be administered to patients undergoing surgery unless there is a definitive guideline-based primary or secondary prevention indication. Aside from closed-space procedures such as intracranial, middle ear, or posterior eye surgery, intramedullary spine surgery, or possibly prostate surgery, continuation of aspirin administration throughout the perioperative period may be warranted for moderate-risk patients taking lifelong aspirin for a guideline-based secondary but not primary prevention.[80] An evidence-based update was recently published on perioperative aspirin management for elective surgery.[81] They noted the following three recommendations:

1. For the majority of patients using aspirin for primary cardiovascular disease prevention, preoperative aspirin cessation is safe. Importantly, many patients start aspirin without seeking a physician's opinion, hence careful attention to identifying self-prescribing of aspirin should be part of routine perioperative assessment. In these patients, the drug may be safely discontinued 7 days preoperatively if it is being used for primary prevention, and there should be full return of platelet function in this time frame.

2. For patients prescribed aspirin for secondary prevention but without a coronary stent, it is not fully clarified as to the safety of preoperative aspirin cessation. The limited data that do exist suggest that continuing aspirin might be prudent. Noncoronary stented patients with high cardiovascular disease risk should likely have aspirin continued throughout the perioperative period unless undergoing closed-spaced procedure or procedure with high bleeding. In the context of recent acute coronary syndrome (ACS), patients should

ideally be on dual antiplatelet therapy (DAPT) for 1 year, but if surgery is urgent (i.e., cancer operation) it should proceed while continuing aspirin monotherapy at a minimum. Recent data suggest that, in the absence of noncardiac surgery, a shortened duration of DAPT appears safe with the continuation of monotherapy.

3. For patients with cerebrovascular disease and/or peripheral arterial disease there are also minimal prospective data, but the totality of observational data and guideline recommendations suggests stopping preoperative aspirin is associated with significant risk.[81]

CHOLINERGICS

Cholinergic agents mimic the actions of the neurotransmitter acetylcholine but have been developed to differ in terms of comparative nicotinic and muscarinic activity and duration of action. Acetylcholine (Miochol) has no clinical application, owing to its generalized enhancement of cholinergic effects throughout the body and its extremely short duration of action (approximately 1 msec), which is a result of its rapid metabolism by acetylcholinesterase.

Methacholine (Provocholine), carbachol (or carbamylcholine chloride), and bethanechol (or carbamylmethylcholine) are choline esters that have limited clinical application. Methacholine can be used as an aerosol in the diagnosis of reactive airway disease, whereas carbachol, because of its significant muscarinic and nicotinic activity, is used only as a topical ophthalmic solution in the treatment of narrow-angle glaucoma and for inducing miosis during diagnostic testing and surgery. Bethanechol is theoretically useful in instances of ileus and urinary retention, such as in postvagotomy and postpartum patients, respectively. Bethanechol's relative lack of nicotinic activity makes it the most attractive of these three agents, and it is the agent most frequently encountered in clinical practice. Potential side effects of these agents include any cholinergic-induced response such as bradycardia, varying degrees of heart block, hypotension, bronchoconstriction, and an increase in gastric secretions.[82]

ANTICHOLINERGICS

The anticholinergics are familiar agents in anesthesia practice. Atropine, scopolamine, and glycopyrrolate are the three anticholinergics used in anesthesia practice. These agents are competitive antagonists of acetylcholine at muscarinic receptors. A comparison of the basic properties of the anticholinergic agents is provided in Table 13.6. Subtypes of muscarinic and nicotinic receptors are summarized in Tables 13.7 and 13.8.

Atropine

Atropine, a belladonna alkaloid, is the prototype anticholinergic. The anesthetist can use atropine for its antisialagogue effects, for the prevention or treatment of bradycardia, and concurrently with anticholinesterase agents in the reversal of muscle relaxants for preventing the resultant bradycardia from anticholinesterase-induced acetylcholine buildup. The usual adult IV dose for increasing heart rate during anesthesia is 0.4 to 0.6 mg, with the time to onset being 1 to 2 minutes. Atropine is a tertiary amine; this allows it to cross the blood-brain barrier freely and may result in transient bradycardia during onset when low doses are given. However, significant CNS effects are rarely evident at usual clinical doses. Hepatic metabolism accounts for approximately half of a dose of atropine, with the remainder being eliminated unchanged in the urine. The elimination half-life of atropine is

TABLE 13.6 Comparative Effects of Anticholinergic Drugs

Effect	Atropine	Scopolamine	Glycopyrrolate
Sedate	+	+++	0
Antisialagogue	+	+++	++
Increase heart rate	+++	+	++
Relax smooth muscle	++	+	++
Mydriasis, cycloplegia	+	+++	0
Prevent motion-induced nausea	+	+++	0
Decrease gastric hydrogen ion secretion	+	+	+

TABLE 13.7 Properties of Muscarinic (M₁-M₅) Receptors

	M₁	M₂	M₃	M₄	M₅
Location	CNS Stomach	Heart CNS	Glands GI, CNS	CNS Heart	CNS
Important clinical effects	Increased cognition and memory; gastric acid production	Bradycardia, smooth muscle contraction	Salivary secretions, bladder contraction	Promotes dopamine release	Promotes dopamine release, dilation of cerebral arteries

CNS, Central nervous system; GI, gastrointestinal.

TABLE 13.8 Characteristics of Subtypes of Nicotinic Acetylcholine Receptors (nAChRs)

Receptor Subtype	Main Synaptic Location	Membrane Response
Skeletal muscle (N_M)	Skeletal neuromuscular junction (postjunctional)	Excitatory; endplate depolarization; skeletal muscle contraction
Peripheral neuronal (N_N)	Autonomic ganglia; adrenal medulla	Excitatory; depolarization; firing of postganglion neuron and secretion of catecholamines
Central nervous system (CNS)	CNS; pre- and postjunctional	Pre- and postsynaptic excitation
		Prejunctional control of transmitter release

approximately 4 hours. Atropine should be avoided in patients with narrow-angle glaucoma because it increases intraocular pressure. *Central anticholinergic syndrome, atropine poisoning,* and *belladonna alkaloid toxicity* are various terms to describe extreme antimuscarinic effects associated with atropine and scopolamine overdose. This event can progress to CNS depression and coma. The decades-old mnemonic "red as a beet, blind as a bat, dry as a bone, mad as a hatter, and hot as a hare" was devised to be an easy way to remember the signs and symptoms of belladonna overdose. These include flushing ("red as a beet"), extreme mydriasis ("blind as a bat"), lack of secretions and dry mouth ("dry as a bone"), confusion ("mad as a hatter"), and hyperthermia ("hot as a hare").[82]

Scopolamine

Scopolamine (Isopto Hyoscine) is another belladonna alkaloid with anticholinergic effects. Scopolamine is a tertiary amine. Compared with atropine, the CNS effects of scopolamine are much more pronounced at lower doses, and it does not substantially increase heart rate. It can be used as a preoperative medication, with sedation and amnesia being a desirable effect. Scopolamine is also used to diminish the incidence of postoperative nausea and vomiting. A scopolamine patch (Transderm-Scop) containing a total dose of 1.5 mg is ideally applied behind the ear 4 hours prior to anesthesia. The clinical duration of action is 3 days.[82]

Tiotropium

Tiotropium (Spiriva) is a long-acting inhaled muscarinic antagonist that is used as a bronchodilator for patients with chronic obstructive pulmonary disease (COPD) and asthma. Tiotropium improves lung function and quality of life and decreases COPD exacerbations but does not significantly reduce the rate of decline in the forced expiratory volume.[83]

Glycopyrrolate

Glycopyrrolate (Robinul), a synthetic quaternary ammonium compound, has become the most frequently used anticholinergic in anesthesia practice. It has excellent antisialagogue activity[82] and a longer duration of action than belladonna alkaloids. It prevents bradycardia without inducing significant levels of tachycardia. The quaternary ammonium structure of glycopyrrolate prevents it from crossing the blood-brain barrier to any significant degree, therefore CNS effects are not seen. This is an important advantage of glycopyrrolate because atropine and scopolamine cross the blood-brain barrier and have CNS effects that can contribute to postoperative delirium.[84] This property also makes it the agent of choice in obstetrics because it does not pass the placental barrier. Adult IV doses are generally 0.1 to 0.2 mg for antisialagogue activity and for the treatment of bradycardia. Onset of action is rapid, and the duration of action is up to 4 hours. It is used in combination with neostigmine for the reversal of nondepolarizing neuromuscular blockers. Glycopyrrolate produces less tachycardia than atropine in the period leading up to the onset of neostigmine administration for reversal of neuromuscular blockade.[82]

DIRECT VASODILATORS

Within the category of direct vasodilators, sodium nitroprusside, nitroglycerin, and hydralazine are the three drugs most commonly used (Table 13.9). All three produce direct vasodilation: Sodium nitroprusside produces arterial and venous relaxation, nitroglycerin has a greater effect on venous relaxation than on arterial relaxation, and hydralazine produces primarily arterial relaxation. The mechanism of action of all three agents is believed to be primarily an induced increase in the concentration of vascular NO, although that mechanism has not been confirmed with hydralazine.[85] The mechanism of action is depicted in Fig. 13.3. The vasodilators nitroprusside and nitroglycerin

TABLE 13.9	**Parenteral Drugs for Treatment of Severe Hypertension**					
Drug	**Class**	**Route and Dose**	**Onset**	**Duration**	**Comments**
Labetalol (Trandate, Normodyne)	α- and β-adrenergic blocker	Generally used in 5- to 10-mg incremental doses titrated to effect in the perioperative period	≤5 min	3–6 hr	Not for patients with bronchospasm, congestive heart failure, first-degree heart block, cardiogenic shock, or severe bradycardia
Nicardipine (Cardene IV)	Calcium channel blocker	IV: 5 mg/hr, increased by 2.5 mg/hr every 15 min up to 15 mg/hr	1–5 min	3–6 hr	May cause reflex tachycardia
Clevidipine (Cleviprex)	Calcium channel blocker	IV infusion: 1–2 mg/hr initially; double the dose at 90-s intervals until desired results are achieved (16 mg/hr max)	2–4 min	5–15 min	Rapidly degraded by tissue and blood esterases; contraindicated with allergy to soy or eggs; may cause reflex tachycardia
Nitroglycerin	Venous arteriolar vasodilator	IV infusion pump: 5–100 mcg/min	2–5 min	5–10 min	Headache, tachycardia can occur; tolerance may develop with prolonged use
Sodium nitroprusside	Arteriolar and venous vasodilator	IV infusion pump: 0.3–10 mcg/kg/min	Seconds	3–5 min	Thiocyanate or cyanide toxicity with prolonged or too rapid infusion
Esmolol	β-blocker	IV: 500 mcg/kg/min for 1 min titrated to effect, usually 50 mcg/kg/min	1–2 min	5–10 min	Cardioselective; however, use with caution in patients with asthma

IV, Intravenous.

Adapted from Victor RG. Arterial hypertension. In: Goldman L, Schafer AI, eds. *Goldman's Cecil Medicine.* 26th ed. Philadelphia: Elsevier; 2020:443–456; Victor RG, Libby P. Systemic hypertension: management. In: Zipes DP, et al., eds. *Braunwald's Heart Disease.* 11th ed. Philadelphia: Elsevier; 2019:928–955; Lewek J, et al. Pharmacological management of malignant hypertension. *Expert Opin Pharmacother.* 2020;21(10):1189–1192.

are frequently used for controlled hypotension under anesthesia. Combined with the inhalation and IV anesthetics, they facilitate a reduction in blood loss and the need for transfusions during a variety of surgical procedures.[86] Hydralazine is used in combination with isosorbide dinitrate for the treatment of systolic heart failure in blacks. It may also serve as an alternative for patients with an intolerance to angiotensin antagonists.[87]

Nitrovasodilators

Sodium Nitroprusside

Sodium nitroprusside is frequently used for the emergent control of hypertension, for inducing hypotension to decrease blood loss during surgical procedures, and for the treatment of acute cardiac disorders. Its rapid onset (within seconds) and its short duration of action (1–3 min) make it unique among agents for the rapid control of blood pressure. Sodium nitroprusside reduces both afterload and preload, which results in a decrease in cardiac filling pressures and an increase in stroke volume and cardiac output. Left ventricular volumes are decreased, and diminished myocardial wall tension should contribute to a decrease in myocardial oxygen consumption.

Usually sodium nitroprusside is started as an infusion at 0.3 mcg/kg/min and is titrated until a response occurs. An infusion rate of 3 mcg/kg/min is rarely exceeded, but young, normotensive patients may require up to 5 mcg/kg/min to achieve the desired response.[88,89] The maximum recommended infusion rate is 10 mcg/kg/min. Sodium nitroprusside is mixed with 5% dextrose in water, and the bottle and tubing are covered in a protective wrap as light causes the sodium nitroprusside to decompose. An infusion pump should always be used with sodium nitroprusside because of its potency and the associated risk of cyanide toxicity.

Cyanide toxicity. The chemical structure of sodium nitroprusside contains five cyanide ions, which are released upon metabolism by plasma hemoglobin. One cyanide ion binds methemoglobin to form cyanmethemoglobin, whereas the other four cyanide ions undergo rhodanese-catalyzed conversion to thiocyanate in the liver, with the thiocyanate undergoing renal elimination. This conversion to thiocyanate requires the cofactor thiosulfate B_{12}. Cyanide toxicity results when this metabolic pathway is quantitatively overwhelmed. Preventing cyanide toxicity from sodium nitroprusside begins with awareness of maximum doses and lengths of administration. In general, when more than 500 mcg/kg of sodium nitroprusside is administered faster than 2 mcg/kg/min, cyanide is generated faster than the patient can eliminate it. Chronic administration should not exceed 0.5 mcg/kg/min. Clinically the development of metabolic acidosis, increased mixed venous oxygen content, tachycardia, and tachyphylaxis during sodium nitroprusside use are signs of cyanide toxicity.

Treatment of cyanide toxicity consists of discontinuing the sodium nitroprusside infusion, administering oxygen, and treating metabolic acidosis. Sodium nitrite 3% at 4 to 6 mg/kg can be administered over 3 to 5 minutes to promote the production of methemoglobin so that excess cyanide ions can be bound. Sodium thiosulfate at 150 to 200 mg/kg over 15 minutes can be administered every 2 hours as needed; vitamin B_{12} also can be administered. Hydroxycobalamin can be very effective. Methylene blue at 1 to 2 mg/kg may also be useful. A new prodrug, sulfanegen sodium, is also being tested.[90,91]

Nitroglycerin

Nitroglycerin is used in the treatment of angina pectoris and ischemia under anesthesia and can be used for lowering blood pressure. It has a rapid onset and short duration, so it is easily titratable. Nitroglycerin causes venodilation, with an increase in venous capacitance and a resultant decrease in preload. This results in a lowering of cardiac filling pressures, a lessening of myocardial wall tension, and ultimately a decrease in myocardial oxygen requirements. Nitroglycerin's primary mechanism of action in the relief of angina is a decrease in preload and cardiac work. Some of the larger coronary vessels may become dilated, with a resultant redirection and increase in blood flow to ischemic myocardium. It also relieves coronary spasm. At higher concentrations of nitroglycerin, arterial vasodilation also can occur.[92]

Use of sublingual nitroglycerin (0.3-mg tablets) up to a total of three tablets is the most efficient treatment for acute angina. Relief is generally achieved in 1 to 2 minutes and lasts up to 30 minutes. IV nitroglycerin also has an onset time of 1 to 2 minutes and duration of action of up to 10 minutes. Nitroglycerin is extensively metabolized in the liver and has a half-life of only 3 minutes.[87] IV nitroglycerin is used for "unloading" of the heart in CHF and MI.[93] Guidelines suggest that IV infusions should be instituted following three sublingual doses of 0.4 mg every 5 minutes in patients having an ST-segment elevation MI (STEMI). Nitroglycerin infusions are usually started at 10 to 20 mcg/min and are titrated up until effective. IV nitroglycerin can also be used for controlled hypotension but is not as effective as an infusion of sodium nitroprusside. Because nitroglycerin exerts its main effect on venous capacitance, any decrease in blood pressure is more volume dependent when compared with sodium nitroprusside–induced hypotension. Nitrates should be avoided in patients with a blood pressure less than 90 mm Hg and a heart rate less than 50 bpm or above 100 bpm, and in patients with right ventricular infarction. Of note to the anesthesia provider is the ability of nitroglycerin to relax the smooth muscle of the biliary tract and provide relief from narcotic-induced biliary spasm. Generally, 50 mg of nitroglycerin is mixed with 250 mL of dextrose 5% in water.[94] For extended coverage, nitroglycerin patches and ointments are also available. A summary of antihypertensive agents dosing information is found in Table 13.5.

Hydralazine

Hydralazine causes direct relaxation of arterial smooth muscle. It can be administered intravenously for the control of hypertension in

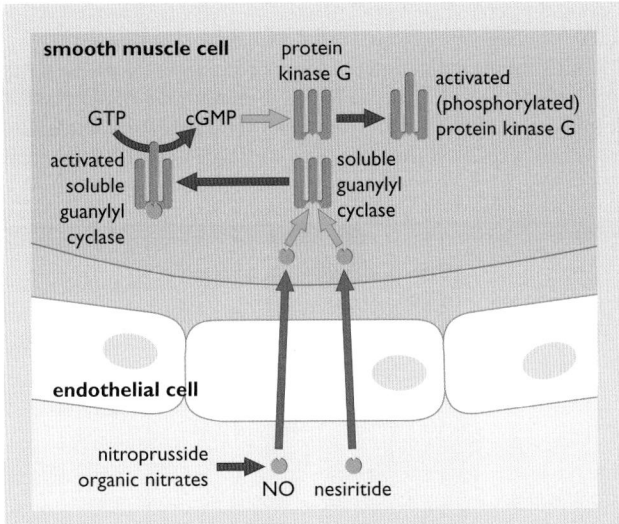

Fig. 13.3 Molecular and cellular mechanisms of action of nitrate and nitrite vasodilators, nitric oxide (NO), and nesiritide. The primary molecular target, soluble guanylyl cyclase, is accessed by drug or NO diffusion between cells. The product, phosphorylated protein kinase, causes vascular smooth muscle relaxation by phosphorylating (and inactivating) myosin light chain kinase. *cGMP*, Cyclic guanosine monophosphate; *GTP*, guanosine-5′-triphosphate. (From Page C, et al. *Integrated Pharmacology.* 3rd ed. Elsevier: Edinburgh; 2006:391.)

doses ranging from 2.5 to 20 mg. Tachycardia frequently accompanies the decrease in blood pressure, secondary to the preferential reduction in afterload. It is important to remember that the onset of action can occur from 2 to 20 minutes after administration depending on the depth of anesthesia, therefore adequate time should be allowed before the initiation of repeat dosing so that profound decreases in blood pressure can be prevented. The elimination half-life in plasma is approximately 1 hour, but the duration of vasodilating action can be as long as 12 hours.[95–97] Hydralazine undergoes hepatic metabolism with renal excretion. Acetylation is partly responsible for the metabolism of hydralazine. Slow acetylators may be more prone to a drug-induced lupus syndrome that can result from high serum concentrations of hydralazine during chronic treatment. Hydralazine is used for hypertensive episodes during pregnancy.[98]

CALCIUM CHANNEL BLOCKERS

The calcium channel blockers (CCBs) are useful pharmacologic agents for the treatment of angina, hypertension, arrhythmias, peripheral vascular disease, esophageal spasm, cerebral vasospasm, and controlled hypotension.[99] There are three chemical classes of CCBs: 1,4-dihydropyridine derivatives such as nifedipine (Adalat, Procardia); diltiazem (Cardizem), which is a benzothiazepine derivative; and verapamil (Calan, Isoptin), which is a phenylalkylamine derivative.

All CCBs have negative inotropic and chronotropic actions. They are class 4 antiarrhythmics that block calcium channels, therefore they depress electrical impulses in the sinoatrial (SA) and AV nodes. They produce coronary and systemic vasodilation. Different drugs in the three classes vary as to their individual ability to produce each of these effects.[62]

A discussion of the generalized mechanism of action of the calcium antagonists is necessary for a better understanding of their role. Depolarization of the SA and AV nodes is dependent on the inward flux of calcium during the depolarization phases of the cardiac action potential. Calcium channel antagonists "block" these channels, diminishing the inward flux of calcium and prolonging phase 2, and in this way exert a negative chronotropic effect on the heart. Ventricular pacemaker foci are dependent on the inward flux of sodium, which is minimally (if at all) affected by the calcium antagonists. It then follows that the calcium antagonists are effective in patients with atrial tachyarrhythmias. Verapamil and diltiazem are the most commonly used CCBs as antiarrhythmics. They are effective in treating atrial tachyarrhythmias (including Wolff-Parkinson-White syndrome) and in controlling the ventricular response to AF and flutter. Verapamil is not indicated for the treatment of AF associated with Wolff-Parkinson-White syndrome, nor is it indicated for the treatment of "simple" atrial tachycardia, for which β-blockers may be a better choice.

CCBs also exert a negative inotropic effect on the heart, which can be beneficial in patients with angina. Cardiac contractility is dependent on the influx of calcium into cardiac cells, and this is slowed by the CCBs. This negative inotropic effect then leads to a decrease in myocardial oxygen consumption. Calcium channel antagonists produce relaxation of vascular smooth muscle, resulting in vasodilation. Systemic vasodilation of both arteries and veins results in a decreased preload and afterload, which contributes to an increase in cardiac output and a decrease in myocardial work and oxygen consumption. The negative inotropic action and vasodilation account for the antihypertensive effect.[100] Coronary arteries also are affected, with an increase in coronary blood flow. The CCBs are especially beneficial in the prevention of angina resulting from spasm of the coronary arteries, such as Prinzmetal angina.

Nimodipine has been a long-standing treatment of cerebral vasospasm associated with neurologic emergencies such as ruptured

aneurisms and neurosurgery.[1] Nimodipine is a dihydropyridine agent thought to inhibit voltage-gated calcium channels in the arterial wall smooth muscle cells, which results in vasodilatation, It is the only FDA-approved oral agent for vasospasm. Milrinone, nicardipine, verapamil, dantrolene, and fasudil are other agents used for chemical angioplasty.[101–103]

Verapamil at 2.5 to 10 mg IV (dose can be repeated every 30 min) can be given for the treatment of atrial tachyarrhythmias. The onset time is up to 10 minutes, and the duration of action ranges from 2 to 4 hours. Verapamil is metabolized hepatically, has an elimination half-life of 4 to 7 hours, and is renally eliminated. Verapamil has been largely replaced by adenosine as the first-line drug of choice in the treatment of supraventricular tachycardias. Nicardipine is also useful as an IV preparation for the treatment of perioperative hypertension.[104,105] The effects of CCBs on the ischemic heart are summarized in Fig. 13.4.

Varying degrees of AV block, myocardial depression, and hypotension are associated with the use of the calcium antagonists. An additive effect should be anticipated if the calcium channel antagonists are used with other cardiodepressant agents such as anesthetics.[106]

Clevidipine (Cleviprex) is a dihydropyridine L-type CCB indicated as an IV antihypertensive. It is highly selective for vascular muscle and does not affect myocardial contractility or conduction. Its antihypertensive effect is largely due to arterial vasodilation. Clevidipine is rapidly metabolized by nonspecific esterases in the blood. The terminal half-life is approximately 15 minutes. It is formulated as a lipid emulsion, so careful handling is essential. The starting dose is 1 to 2 mg/h, titrated up to 16 mg/h or less, according to patient response. Onset is 2 to 4 minutes, and duration is 5 to 15 minutes (see Table 13.9).[107,108]

ANGIOTENSIN-CONVERTING ENZYME INHIBITORS

Angiotensin-converting enzyme (ACE) inhibitors are widely prescribed for the treatment of hypertension, angina, diabetic neuropathy, and CHF, and in the management of the post-MI patient.[109,110] These drugs exert their action by inhibiting ACE. Along with the angiotensin receptor blockers (ARBs), they are often described as angiotensin axis–blocking drugs (AABs). A brief description of the RAS is necessary for a full understanding of the actions of ACE inhibitors (Fig. 13.5).

Renin, a proteolytic protein, is released from the juxtaglomerular apparatus in the kidney in response to diminished blood pressure. Renin is responsible for the conversion of precursor angiotensinogen, which is released from the liver, to the decapeptide angiotensin

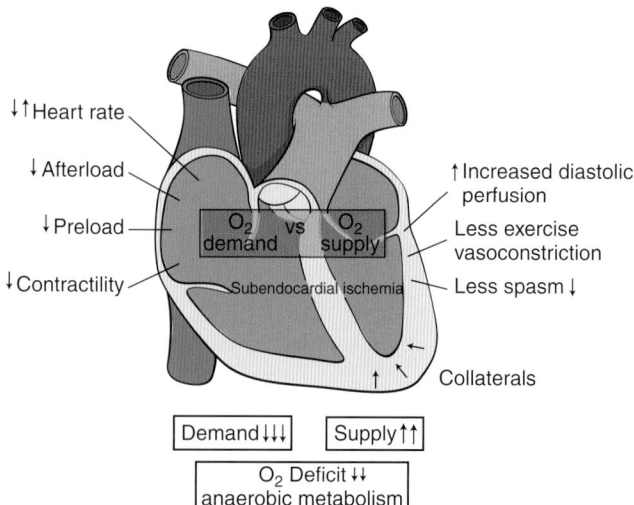

Fig. 13.4 Effects of calcium channel blockers on the ischemic heart.

I. Angiotensin I is then converted to the octapeptide angiotensin II by the ACE. ACE is primarily located in the endothelial tissue of the lung. Angiotensin II is a potent vasopressor that also stimulates the release of endogenous norepinephrine and aldosterone. The end result is an increase in peripheral vasoconstriction, with an increase in blood pressure and a resultant decrease in cardiac output. The higher aldosterone level results in increased sodium and water reabsorption, with concomitant secretion of potassium.[109] The ACE inhibitors block this action and produce vasodilation. Common ACE inhibitors are listed in Table 13.5. Enalapril is a prodrug, and it undergoes hepatic metabolism to its active form of enalaprilat. Enalaprilat is available for IV administration for use in perioperative hypertension, but it is rarely used. All of these agents are renally eliminated, and their elimination half-lives can be expected to be prolonged in renally compromised patients.

Adverse effects associated with the ACE inhibitors include cough, angioedema, renal failure, hyperkalemia, neutropenia, and proteinuria. The dry cough resulting from the ACE inhibitors occurs in up to 25% of patients and is the most common reason for discontinuation of the drug. If an ACE inhibitor cannot be tolerated, an ARB is substituted. The reason for the cough has been determined, as ACE is also responsible for the metabolism of bradykinin, which is blocked by these drugs. The resulting buildup of bradykinin contributes to the cough.[111,112]

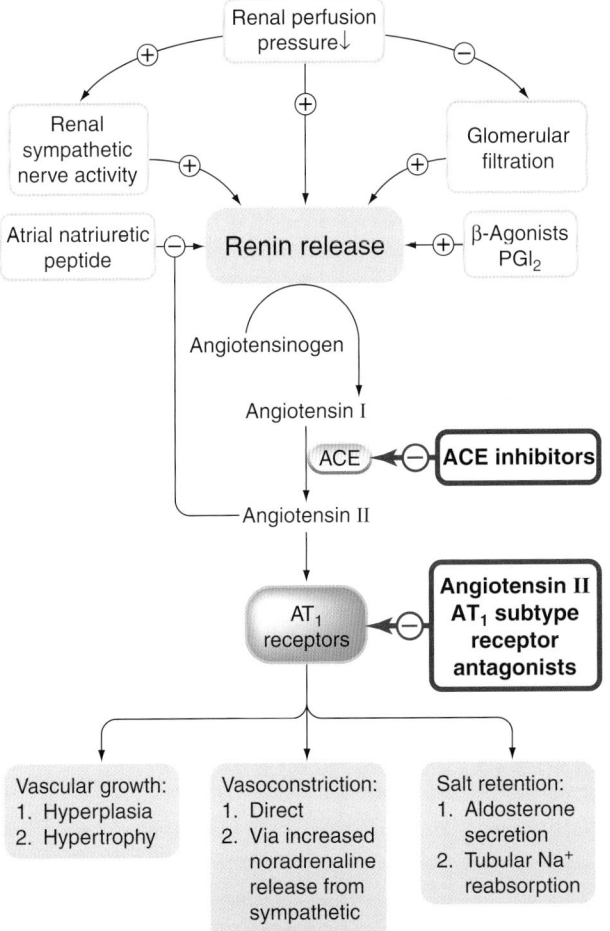

Fig. 13.5 Control of renin release and formation, and action of angiotensin II. Sites of action of drugs that inhibit the cascade are shown. *ACE*, Angiotensin-converting enzyme; *AT₁*, angiotensin II receptor subtype 1. (From Rang HP, et al. *Rang and Dale's Pharmacology.* 9th ed. Edinburgh: Elsevier; 2020:295.)

ANGIOTENSIN II RECEPTOR BLOCKERS

ARBs are a class of drugs that are useful for the treatment of hypertension and CHF. Their pharmacologic actions are similar to the ACE inhibitors, but their mechanism of action is competitive blockade of type 1 angiotensin II (AT_1) receptors (see Table 13.5 and Fig. 13.5).[113] They are effective for lowering blood pressure without the cough and angioedema associated with ACE inhibitors. Unlike the ACE inhibitors, they do not prevent the breakdown of bradykinin and therefore do not produce cough. There are no IV preparations currently marketed. The ARBs are often reserved for patients who cannot tolerate an ACE inhibitor.[63]

ANESTHESIA MANAGEMENT OF PATIENTS TAKING ANGIOTENSIN AXIS BLOCKERS

There has been a controversy for many years about whether ACE inhibitors or ARBs should be withheld the morning of surgery. The long-term clinical consequences of continuing versus withholding preoperative ACE inhibitors/ARBs are controversial. Most, if not all, cardiac medications are continued preoperatively up to and including the day of surgery.[114] The ACE inhibitors may result in an increase in refractory hypotension during induction and maintenance of anesthesia if not discontinued prior to surgery. Hypotension usually occurs within 30 minutes of induction of anesthesia. Concurrent diuretic therapy increases hypotensive frequency.[115] Even though withholding these medications may decrease hypotensive episodes intraoperatively, some argue that it could lead to a loss of their established long-term benefits and increase the risk for precipitating a withdrawal hypertensive crisis on the day of surgery.[116] There are conflicting data regarding the association between perioperative angiotensin blockers and the development of end-organ damage. There is an increased incidence of acute kidney injury (AKI) in patients on perioperative ACEs or ARBs undergoing vascular surgery, thoracic surgery, and orthopedic surgery. However, the incidence of AKI in patients on perioperative ARBs following cardiac surgery has been shown in certain studies to be increased, unchanged, and even decreased.[117] Additionally, in a 2015 large retrospective Veterans Hospital study, researchers reported that in patients who had their ACE withheld prior to surgery, a postoperative delay in resuming the ACE or ARBs past 2 days postoperatively is strongly associated with an increased 30-day mortality rate, especially in younger patients.[118]

This phenomenon is sometimes referred to as vasoplegic syndrome (VS). VS is defined as unexpected refractory hypotension under general anesthesia with a MAP less than 50 mm Hg, a cardiac index greater than 2.5 L/min/m², and a low systemic vascular resistance, despite adrenergic vasopressor administration. It is most commonly seen with cardiac surgery but can occur during any anesthetic. The incidence of VS in cardiac surgical patients is 8% to 10% but may increase to upwards of 50% in patients taking AABs. In cardiac surgical patients with persistent hypotension into the postoperative period, the associated mortality approaches 25%. The proposed mechanism involves selective depression of the three blood pressure support systems: the sympathetic nervous system, renin angiotensin, and vasopressin systems. Sympathetic nervous system depression under anesthesia leaves maintenance of blood pressure dependent on the renin-angiotensin and the vasopressinergic systems. ACE inhibitors and Angiotensin Receptor Antagonists (ARA) inhibit the RAS, leaving only vasopressin to maintain blood pressure. Other proposed mechanisms for developing refractory hypotension include cytokine and NO-mediated smooth muscle relaxation, catecholamine receptor down-regulation, cell hyperpolarization, and endothelial injury.[119]

Conventional therapies include decreasing the anesthetic agent, inducing volume expansion, and administering phenylephrine, ephedrine, or glycopyrrolate, as indicated. High doses may be required. If further therapy is needed, then norepinephrine, epinephrine, and dopamine may be used. If they are not effective, the administration of vasopressin may increase blood pressure. A 0.5- to 1.0-unit bolus of vasopressin may be given, followed by an infusion dose of 0.03 units/min of vasopressin or 1 to 2 mcg/kg/hour of terlipressin, as needed. Methylene blue is suggested as a last resort when other interventions fail. A bolus dose of 1 to 2 mg/kg over 10 to 20 minutes followed by an infusion of 0.25 mg/kg/hour for 48 to 72 hours is recommended, with a maximum dose of 7 mg/kg. Methylene blue is believed to interfere with the NO-cGMP pathway, inhibiting the vasodilating effect on smooth muscle. It is prudent to withhold the ACE or ARB the morning of surgery and reinstitute it immediately postoperatively to minimize this effect.[120]

CATECHOLAMINE-DEPLETING AGENTS

Catecholamine-depleting agents are rarely encountered in modern anesthesia practice, but the anesthetist should be familiar with their mechanism of action. The classic member of this group is reserpine. Reserpine blocks the uptake of catecholamines into storage vesicles within the presynaptic adrenergic neuron by inhibiting the vesicular monoamine transporter. This exposes the catecholamines to metabolism by monoamine oxidase in the axoplasm. This "catecholamine depletion" is responsible for the antihypertensive action of reserpine.[121]

TYROSINE HYDROXYLASE INHIBITORS

Metyrosine (Demser) is a tyrosine hydroxylase inhibitor. Tyrosine hydroxylase is responsible for catalyzing the conversion of tyrosine to dopa and is considered the rate-limiting step in catecholamine synthesis. Inhibition of tyrosine hydroxylase results in a decrease in circulating catecholamine levels. It is used as an add-on drug to the α- and β-blockers for the control of the blood pressure in patients with pheochromocytoma.[122]

CATECHOL-*O*-METHYLTRANSFERASE INHIBITORS

Tolcapone (Tasmar), Opicapone (Ongentys), and entacapone (Comtan) are used for the treatment of Parkinson disease as an adjunct to levodopa or carbidopa therapy. A third drug, nebicapone, is in clinical trials. These drugs are selective and reversible inhibitors of COMT. They enhance the action of levodopa and produce less fluctuation in drug response. There are concerns that COMT inhibitors may interact with various cardiac drugs by reducing their metabolism. Tolcapone administration is associated with fatal cases of drug-induced liver damage. Caution should be taken when administering drugs such as isoproterenol, dobutamine, dopamine, norepinephrine, and epinephrine. Reduced doses should be started initially until the response can be assessed.[123,124]

CARDIAC GLYCOSIDES

Characterized by the digitalis preparations, the cardiac glycosides have been used to treat CHF for 2 centuries. The most common preparation used is digoxin. The primary inotropic effect of digitalis is achieved by binding to the alpha subunit of the sodium-potassium adenosine triphosphatase (Na/K ATPase) in cardiac cells (the Na/K ATPase is somewhat erroneously referred to as the sodium-potassium pump).[34] This results in an increase in the concentration of intracellular calcium during systole, which augments myocardial contractility. Normally, the Na/K ATPase exchanges intracellular sodium for extracellular potassium against their concentration gradients. Inhibition of this exchange results in an increase in intracellular sodium, which results in decreased calcium exchange and a higher level of intracellular calcium. The mechanism of action of digitalis is shown in Fig. 13.6. The additional calcium enhances contraction. Digitalis produces an increase in both the diastolic filling and ejection fractions.

Electrophysiologically, enhancement of vagal tone, another prominent effect of digitalis, results in slowing of the heart rate and prolongation of AV conduction. Because of its vagal effects, digitalis is also used to control the ventricular response to AF and other atrial tachyarrhythmias. The digitalis-induced enhancement of vagal tone leads to slowing of impulse conduction through the AV node and prolongation of the effective refractory period of the AV node. Its use as both an

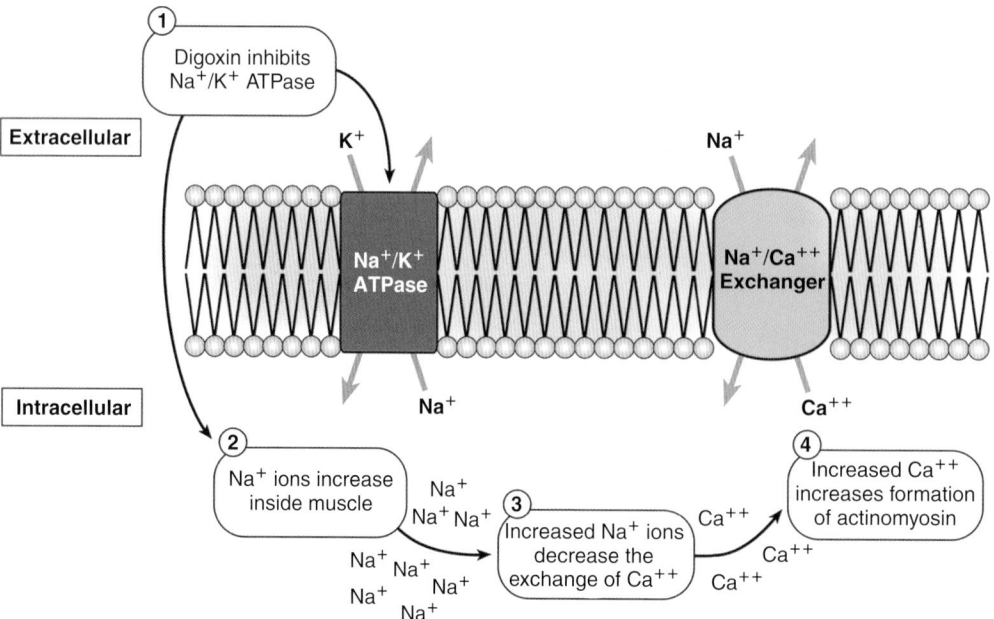

Fig. 13.6 The mechanism of action of digitalis. *(1)* The sodium-potassium ATPase is inhibited, resulting in increased intracellular sodium; *(2)* increased intracellular sodium produces a decrease in the exchange of sodium and calcium; *(3)* intracellular calcium increases; and *(4)* muscle contraction is enhanced.

antiarrhythmic and an inotrope has decreased significantly with the introduction of more efficacious and safer drugs.

Digitalis preparations have a narrow therapeutic index, significant variability in action among patients, and several serious side effects. Hypokalemia greatly enhances the effects of digoxin, whereas hyperkalemia has the opposite effect.[125] A patient with hypokalemia receiving digitalis level within a therapeutic range may show toxic effects. Digoxin serum levels are also mediated by the P-glycoprotein transporter. All known arrhythmias have been attributed to digitalis toxicity. Other signs and symptoms of digitalis toxicity include nausea, vomiting, diarrhea, headache, fatigue, and colored vision. Under anesthesia, the first sign is usually an arrhythmia, frequently premature ventricular contractions. Close monitoring of electrolytes should be performed in digoxin-treated patients receiving preoperative bowel preparation. Calcium administration is contraindicated in digoxin-treated patients because it may lead to cardiac arrest. The serum levels of potassium and digitalis can be monitored preoperatively in select patients.[126]

Some common mechanisms for drugs affecting the sympathetic nervous system are shown in Fig. 13.7.

MANAGEMENT OF SPECIFIC DISEASES

In past decades, treatment of cardiovascular diseases under anesthesia was difficult, and options were limited. The lack of specific cardiac drugs and the limited selection of anesthetic agents warranted symptomatic therapy designed to facilitate surgery until the patient was in the postanesthesia care unit. Currently, with the vast array of cardiac drugs, the improved sophistication of anesthetic management, and monitoring that provides extensive hemodynamic information, the anesthesia

provider is able to treat patients in a manner that is appropriate for management of their diseases. Therapies can be chosen that fit into a patient's plan of care. The anesthetic process can safely and effectively continue the care management of the individual patient. To assist in predicting possible poor outcomes, ACC/AHA and the ESC have classified the cardiovascular and surgical risks (Boxes 13.2 and 13.3).[127,128]

The drugs listed for therapy of the cardiovascular disorders that follow are presented not so much for their specific intraoperative use but as a means of continuing the patient's current drug profile. Patient treatment mirrors general nonoperative indications and considerations. Anesthetic techniques take into account the combined effects of cardiac drugs and anesthetic agents when administered together.

Congestive Heart Failure

More than 40% of people older than age 85 years have heart failure, and more than 8 million people in the United States will have heart failure by 2030. In the United States, heart failure is the leading cause of hospitalization in patients older than age 65 years, and once a patient is hospitalized for heart failure, the 30-day risk of rehospitalization is 25%, with a 10% risk of 30-day postdischarge mortality. Although survival has improved, the absolute mortality rates for heart failure remain approximately 50% within 5 years of diagnosis.[129] CHF is the only major cardiovascular disorder that is increasing in prevalence, with an estimated annual cost of $40 billion. Fortunately, data suggest that hospitalization and mortality rates are declining, which may indicate that aggressive intervention and management are yielding positive results.[130] The classification of heart failure is given in Box 13.4.

Heart failure is a major independent predictor of adverse perioperative outcomes in noncardiac surgery.[131] Mortality estimates range

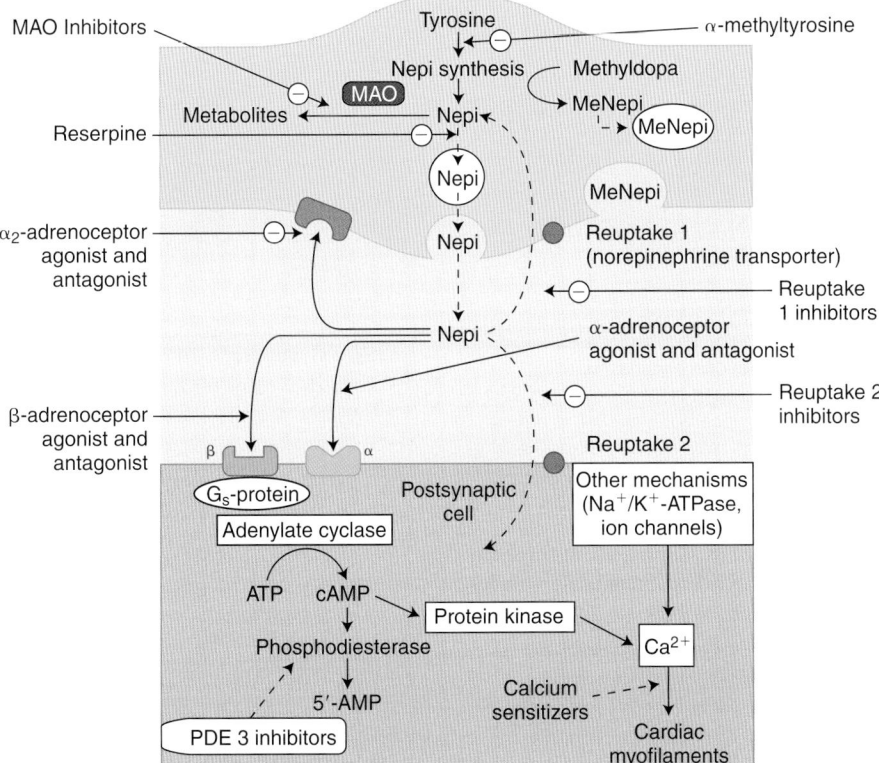

Fig. 13.7 Common mechanisms for drugs affecting the sympathetic nervous system. *ATP*, Adenosine triphosphate; *5'-AMP*, 5' adenosine monophosphate; *cAMP*, cyclic guanosine monophosphate; *MAO*, monoamine oxidase; *MeNepi*, methylnorepinephrine; *Nepi*, norepinephrine; *PDE-3*, phosphodiesterase 3.

BOX 13.2 Clinical Predictors of Increased Perioperative Cardiovascular Risk

Major Risk Factors

Unstable Coronary Syndromes
- Acute or recent myocardial infarction with evidence of important ischemic risk by clinical symptoms or noninvasive study*
- Unstable or severe angina (Canadian class III or IV)

Decompensated Heart Failure
- New York Heart Association functional class IV; worsening or new-onset heart failure

Significant Arrhythmias
- High-grade atrioventricular block
- Mobitz II atrioventricular block
- Third-degree atrioventricular block
- Symptomatic ventricular arrhythmias
- Supraventricular arrhythmias, including atrial fibrillation with an uncontrolled ventricular rate >100 at rest
- Symptomatic bradycardia
- Newly recognized ventricular tachycardia

Severe Valvular Disease
- Severe aortic stenosis with mean pressure gradient >40 mm Hg; aortic valve area <1 cm²; or exhibiting symptoms
- Symptomatic mitral stenosis; progressive dyspnea on exertion; exertional presyncope; or heart failure

Intermediate Risk Factors
- Mild angina pectoris (Canadian class I or II)
- Previous myocardial infarction identified by history or pathologic Q waves
- Compensated or previous heart failure
- Diabetes mellitus (particularly insulin dependent)
- Renal insufficiency

Minor Risk Factors
- Advanced age
- Abnormal ECG (left ventricular hypertrophy, left bundle-branch block, ST-T abnormalities)
- Rhythm other than sinus (e.g., atrial fibrillation)
- Low functional capacity (e.g., inability to climb one flight of stairs with a bag of groceries)
- History of stroke
- Uncontrolled systemic hypertension

*The American College of Cardiology National Database Library defines recent myocardial infarction as having occurred >7 days, but ≤1 month (30 days), previously; acute myocardial infarction is defined as having occurred within the last 7 days; may include "stable" angina in patients who are unusually sedentary.
ECG, Electrocardiogram.

BOX 13.3 Cardiac Risk Stratification for Noncardiac Surgical Procedures

High (Very Elevated) Risk (Cardiac Risk >5%)
- Major vascular surgery
- Emergent major operations
- Prolonged procedures with large fluid shifts or significant blood loss

Intermediate (but Elevated) Risk (Cardiac Risk Generally 1%–5%)
- Carotid endarterectomy
- Endovascular aortic aneurysm repair
- Head and neck surgery
- Intraperitoneal and intrathoracic surgery
- Orthopedic surgery
- Prostate surgery

Low Risk (Cardiac Risk <1%)
- Superficial procedures
- Cataract surgery
- Breast surgery
- Ambulatory surgery

From Cohn SL. Preoperative evaluation. In: Goldman L, Schafer AI, eds. *Goldman's Cecil Medicine.* 26th ed. Philadelphia: Elsevier; 2020:2578–2583.

BOX 13.4 New York Heart Association Functional Classification for Heart Failure

Class I (Mild)
- No limitation of physical activity
- Ordinary physical activity does not cause undue fatigue, palpitation, or dyspnea.

Class II (Mild)
- Slight limitation of physical activity
- Comfortable at rest, but ordinary physical activity results in fatigue, palpitation, or dyspnea.

Class III (Moderate)
- Marked limitation of physical activity
- Comfortable at rest, but less than ordinary activity causes fatigue, palpitation, or dyspnea.

Class IV (Severe)
- Unable to carry out any physical activity without discomfort
- Symptoms of cardiac insufficiency at rest
- If any physical activity is undertaken, discomfort is increased.

Adapted from Januzzi JL, Mann DL. Approach to the patient with heart failure. In: Zipes DP, et al., eds. *Braunwald's Heart Disease.* 11th ed. Philadelphia: Elsevier; 2019:403.

from 10% for elective surgery to as high as 30% in patients undergoing abdominal surgery. In patients with CHF and renal failure undergoing emergency surgery, mortality rates as high as 76% have been reported.[132–134] In a multicenter cohort study of patients undergoing noncardiac surgery from 2005 to 2010, conducted as part of the American College of Surgeons National Surgical Quality Improvement Program, worsening preoperative heart failure was associated with a significant increase in postoperative morbidity and mortality when controlling for other comorbidities. Although these likely have a multifactorial etiology, patients are much more likely to suffer from respiratory, renal, and infectious complications than from cardiac complications.[135]

CHF is a syndrome resulting from a cardiac malfunction that impairs the ability of the heart to eject blood and meet the circulatory demands of the body. It is defined as a complex clinical syndrome that can result from any structural or functional cardiac disorder that interferes with the ability of the ventricle to fill with or eject blood. Alterations associated with CHF include impairment-induced complex changes in the structure of the ventricle, called ventricular remodeling, along with hormonal and physiologic alterations.[136] The chamber dilates, hypertrophies, and becomes more spherical. Substantial evidence suggests that activation of the body's endogenous neurohormonal systems, such as the RAS, plays an important role in cardiac remodeling and the progression of heart failure. Treatment is complex and tailored to the patient's age, current disease state, and associated concurrent disorders. It involves a polypharmaceutic approach that is referred to as triple therapy. This includes ACE inhibitors, β-blockers, and diuretics. Statins are usually added as well. Other agents useful in select patients may include digoxin, ARBs, nitrates, aldosterone, and hydralazine. Mechanical support devices may be added as well.[129]

In the perioperative period, anesthesia providers are faced with managing therapy for all degrees of CHF severity. The goal can range from prevention of symptom progression to surviving an emergency procedure in life-threatening cases. When appropriate, regional nerve block techniques should be considered, but patients may have difficulty lying flat during surgery. No single general anesthetic technique has proven superior. Invasive arterial blood pressure monitoring and transesophageal echocardiography (TEE) are useful for guiding intraoperative decision making and fluid management. TEE is especially useful in diagnosing whether hypotensive episodes are the result of inadequate circulating blood volume, worsening ventricular function, or arterial vasoconstriction.

Drugs such as the inotropes, phosphodiesterase inhibitors, diuretics, and vasodilators are commonly used intraoperatively in acute episodes (see Tables 13.3 and 13.9).[126,132,137]

Arrhythmias

The incidence of serious arrhythmias requiring intervention during general anesthesia is relatively low. A large multicenter study found that, not counting simple tachycardia, bradycardia, or clinically minor rhythm disturbances, the frequency of serious arrhythmias was 1.6% in a series of more than 17,000 patients who underwent general anesthesia.[138] It is surprising that the incidence is not higher because several contradictory factors are involved. Most drugs given during anesthesia are cardiac depressants, therefore they tend to be antiarrhythmic. However, patients with multiple drug profiles in combination with the anesthetics may experience drug interactions that lead to rhythm disturbances. Add to these pharmacologic factors the stresses of surgery and anesthesia, and a multitude of effects on cardiac rhythms may be expected.

A report on perioperative arrhythmias noted that the incidence of postoperative arrhythmia after cardiothoracic surgery is approximately 30% to 40%, with postoperative AF being most common.[139] In noncardiothoracic procedures, the incidence ranges from 4% to 20% depending on the type of surgery performed. Bradyarrhythmias are common after cardiac surgery and occur most frequently in the early postoperative period. These arrhythmias, in part, are related to the fluctuation in vagal tone caused by direct surgical injury and local edema. The initial management of patients with perioperative atrial arrhythmia depends on the hemodynamic effect of the arrhythmia on the patient's clinical status. The first step in managing these patients is to eliminate any potential precipitating factors. Multiple studies have demonstrated that β-blockers reduce the risk of AF by up to 61% compared with placebo. Therefore routine administration of β-blockers after cardiac surgery should be the standard of care to prevent AF. Sustained monomorphic or polymorphic ventricular arrhythmias are uncommon and occur in approximately 1% to 3% of patients usually within the first week after surgery.[139]

In recent years new pharmacologic and nonpharmacologic management approaches for cardiac arrhythmias have emerged. New drugs, implantable cardiac devices (ICDs), and ablation therapy are available for managing these disorders. The use of antiarrhythmic drugs in the United States is declining because of the increasing use of ablation therapy and ICDs.[62] Some causes of intraoperative rhythm disturbances are listed in Box 13.5.

BOX 13.5 Causes of Intraoperative Rhythm Disturbances

General Factors
- Advanced age
- Left atrial enlargement
- Heightened adrenergic state
- Drug toxicity (proarrhythmic)
- Hypoxia
- Hypovolemia
- Hemodynamic instability
- Reperfusion after cessation of bypass
- Hypertension
- Hypoglycemia or hyperglycemia
- Pulmonary disease
- β-blocker withdrawal

Structural Heart Disease
- Coronary artery disease
- Myocardial infarction
- Valvular and congenital heart disease
- Cardiomyopathy
- Sick sinus or long QT interval syndrome
- Wolff-Parkinson-White syndrome
- Heart disease secondary to systemic disease (e.g., uremia, diabetes)
- Sinus bradycardia
- Atrioventricular node heart block

Transient Imbalance
- Stress: electrolyte or metabolic imbalance
- Laryngoscopy, hypoxia, hypercarbia
- Device malfunction, microshock
- Diagnostic or therapeutic intervention (pacemakers, cardioverter-defibrillators)
- Surgical stimulation
- Central vascular catheters

Adapted from Fleischer LA, Rosenbaum SH. *Complications in Anesthesia.* 3rd ed. Philadelphia: Elsevier; 2018:625–630; Melduni RM, et al. Management of arrhythmias in the perioperative setting. *Clin Geriatr Med.* 2012;28(4):729–743.

The goal of drug therapy for arrhythmias during anesthesia should be to treat immediate hemodynamic problems and prevent progression of serious arrhythmias. Treatment is similar to that in the nonoperative setting, with the caveat that most therapies should be carefully titrated to avoid unexpected proarrhythmic or excessive hypotensive outcomes. Some cautionary statements should precede any discussion on the use of antiarrhythmic agents during anesthesia:

- The cause of the arrhythmia should be explored before any treatment is instituted. A cardiology consult should be obtained when possible.
- Adequacy of ventilation, depth of anesthesia, acid-base balance, and fluid and electrolyte balance must be verified before appropriate therapy can be formulated.
- Multiple-drug administration, which constitutes modern anesthesia practice, may result in unexpected drug interactions. Analysis of complex arrhythmias with the commonly used three- or five-lead electrocardiograph system during a surgical procedure is less than ideal for proper diagnosis and treatment. Nonetheless, rhythm disturbances that compromise hemodynamic stability or may progress to more severe dysfunction must be addressed.

Classification of antiarrhythmic drugs is given in Table 13.10. Characteristics and treatment for the common arrhythmias are given in Table 13.11.

Hypertension

Hypertension is a major health problem in the United States; an estimated 78 million Americans have hypertension or should be monitored for elevated blood pressure.[48] Hypertension is the most common condition seen in primary care and leads to MI, stroke, renal failure, and death if not detected early and treated appropriately. The classification of hypertension is given in Table 13.12. Age as a factor in defining hypertension was the major change in recent guidelines. The optimal blood pressure is believed to be less than 120 systolic and less than 80 diastolic, although many clinicians consider less than 130 systolic to be adequate. Patients are categorized as having elevated blood pressure at levels of 120-129 systolic and below 80 diastolic. Stage 1 or 2 hypertension has been redefined as well.[140]

A large number of drugs are available for the treatment of high blood pressure. The main classes of drugs used to treat hypertension include diuretics, CCBs, ACE inhibitors, and ARBs.[141,142] β-blockers are frequently included as initial therapy but may not be preferred in some hypertensive patients.[143,144]

JNC 8 notes that there is moderate evidence to support initiating drug treatment with an ACE inhibitor, ARA, CCB, or thiazide-type diuretic in the nonblack hypertensive population, including those with diabetes. In the black hypertensive population, including those with diabetes, a CCB or thiazide-type diuretic is recommended as initial therapy. There is moderate evidence to support initial or add-on antihypertensive therapy with an ACE inhibitor or ARA in persons with chronic kidney disease to improve kidney outcomes.[140]

Many patients with hypertension are taking two or more drugs to control their blood pressure. The most important aspect of treatment is to reduce blood pressure to goal levels, and the specific drug combination appears to be less important. Unfortunately, despite the remarkable progress in therapy, blood pressure remains inadequately controlled in more than half of patients with hypertension in the United States.[145,146]

Drugs available for the treatment of hypertension are listed in Table 13.5. Antihypertensive drugs that are safe for use during pregnancy are listed in Table 13.13.

Manipulation of the patient's blood pressure is an ongoing task during anesthesia, and many drugs are available to increase and decrease blood pressure when indicated. Improved monitoring and more sophisticated anesthetic techniques have made control of blood pressure almost routine.

The problem of hypertension has varying significance in preoperative, intraoperative, and postoperative situations. Mild to moderate hypertension probably represents only a minor risk for anesthesia and surgery.[147] Patients with more severe hypertensive episodes are at greater risk and will benefit from acute therapy combined with postoperative long-term follow-up.[148] Hypertensive episodes during the perioperative period occur most often during emergence from anesthesia and may be associated with pain, airway stimulation, hypoxia-hypercarbia, hypothermia and shivering, bladder distention, withdrawal from preoperative medications, and intraoperative use of vasopressors. Drugs useful for the treatment of perioperative hypertension are listed in Table 13.9.

Coronary Heart Disease

An estimated 15 million Americans currently have coronary heart disease. Among individuals aged 45 and older, the incidence of stable angina pectoris is approximately 500,000 per year; approximately 65% of these patients are men. Nearly 8 million Americans have prevalent angina pectoris. Although deaths attributable to coronary disease have declined in the United States during the past several decades, ischemic heart disease is now the leading cause of death worldwide, and it is expected that this rate of rise will continue to accelerate as a consequence of the epidemic rise in obesity, type 2 diabetes, and metabolic syndrome. An estimated 7 million patients went to emergency departments in 2010 for chest pain, and approximately 1.5 million of them were hospitalized with ACS.[149,150]

The goal of any anesthetic in a cardiac-compromised patient is hemodynamic optimization, tailored to each patient's unique disease and surgical profile. No single anesthetic technique or agent has been shown to be superior.[151] Finding a balance that avoids increases in myocardial work while maintaining proper perfusion is essential.[152,153]

The causes of coronary artery disease and management of patients with the disorder are discussed in detail in Chapters 25 and 26. The classification of angina pectoris is given in Table 13.14.

Usual pharmacotherapy includes nitrates, β-blockers, CCBs, aspirin, and lipid-lowering or statin drugs (Table 13.15). Nitrates are given for symptomatic relief of acute anginal episodes. Positive benefits have been noted for perioperative statin use.[154] Preoperative statin use is associated with reduced cardiac mortality after primary elective coronary artery bypass grafting. Postoperative statin discontinuation is associated with increased in-hospital mortality.[155] The β-blockers, ACE inhibitors, and CCBs are listed in Table 13.5. The HMG-CoA (3-hydroxy-3-methylglutaryl–coenzyme A) reductase inhibitors (statins) are listed in Table 13.16.

PREOPERATIVE ADMINISTRATION OF CARDIAC DRUGS

Continuation of the patient's cardiac medications throughout the perioperative period is now considered routine practice. This also includes aspirin, which adds little bleeding risk to surgical procedures.

TABLE 13.10   Classification of Antiarrhythmic Drugs

Class	Electrophysiologic Effect	Drug
I	Depression of phase 0 depolarization (block sodium channels)	
IA	Moderate depression and prolonged repolarization	Quinidine, procainamide, disopyramide
IB	Weak depression and shortened repolarization	Lidocaine, mexiletine, phenytoin, tocainide
IC	Strong depression with little effect on repolarization	Flecainide, propafenone, moricizine
II	β-adrenergic blocking effects	Esmolol, propranolol, metoprolol, timolol, pindolol, atenolol, acebutolol, nadolol, carvedilol
III	Prolongs repolarization (blocks potassium channels)	Amiodarone, bretylium, sotalol, ibutilide, dofetilide
IV	Calcium channel–blocking effects	Verapamil, diltiazem
Other		Adenosine, adenosine triphosphate, digoxin, atropine

TABLE 13.11 Characteristics of Arrhythmias*

Type of Arrhythmia	P WAVES Rate (beats/min)	Rhythm	Contour	QRS COMPLEXES Rate (beats/min)	Rhythm	Contour	Ventricular Response to Carotid Sinus Massage	PHYSICAL EXAMINATION Intensity of S$_1$	Splitting of S$_2$	A Waves	Treatment
Sinus rhythm	60–100	Regular†	Normal	60–100	Regular	Normal	Gradual slowing and return to former rate	Constant	Normal	Normal	None
Sinus bradycardia	<60	Regular	Normal	<60	Regular	Normal	Gradual slowing and return to former rate	Constant	Normal	Normal	None, unless symptomatic; atropine
Sinus tachycardia	100–180	Regular	May be peaked	100–180	Regular	Normal	Gradual slowing‡ and return to former rate	Constant	Normal	Normal	None, unless symptomatic; treat underlying disease
AV nodal reentry	150–250	Very regular except at onset and termination	Retrograde; difficult to see; lost in QRS complex	150–250	Very regular except at onset and termination	Normal	Abrupt slowing caused by termination of tachycardia or no effect	Constant	Normal	Constant cannon A waves	Vagal stimulation, adenosine, verapamil, digitalis, propranolol, DC shock, pacing
Atrial flutter	250–350	Regular	Sawtooth	75–175	Generally regular in absence of drugs or disease	Normal	Abrupt slowing and return to former rate; flutter remains	Constant; variable if AV block changing	Normal	Flutter waves	DC shock, digitalis, quinidine, propranolol, verapamil, adenosine
Atrial fibrillation	400–600	Grossly irregular	Baseline undulation, no P waves	100–160	Grossly irregular	Normal	Slowing; gross irregularity remains	Variable	Normal	No A waves	Digitalis, quinidine, DC shock, verapamil, adenosine
Atrial tachycardia with block	150–250	Regular; may be irregular	Abnormal	75–200	Generally regular in absence of drugs or disease	Normal	Abrupt slowing and return to normal rate; tachycardia remains	Constant; variable if AV block changing	Normal	More A waves than C-V waves	Stop digitalis if toxic; digitalis if not toxic; possibly verapamil
AV junctional rhythm	40–100§	Regular	Normal	40–60	Fairly regular	Normal	None; may be slight slowing	Variable‖	Normal	Intermittent cannon waves	None, unless symptomatic; atropine
Reciprocating tachycardias using an accessory (WPW) pathway	150–250	Very regular except at onset and termination	Retrograde; difficult to see; monitor the QRS complex	150–250	Very regular except at onset and termination	Normal	Abrupt slowing caused by termination of tachycardia or no effect	Constant but decreased	Normal	Constant cannon waves	See AV nodal reentry earlier
Nonparoxysmal AV junctional tachycardia	60–100‖	Regular	Normal	70–130	Fairly regular	Normal	None; may be slight slowing	Variable‖	Normal	Intermittent cannon waves‖	None, unless symptomatic; stop digitalis if toxic
Ventricular tachycardia	60–100‖	Regular	Normal	110–250	Fairly regular, may be irregular	Abnormal, >0.12 sec	None	Variable‖	Abnormal	Intermittent cannon waves‖	Lidocaine, procainamide, DC shock, quinidine, amiodarone

Continued

TABLE 13.11   Characteristics of Arrhythmias*—cont'd

Type of Arrhythmia	P WAVES			QRS COMPLEXES			Ventricular Response to Carotid Sinus Massage	PHYSICAL EXAMINATION			
	Rate (beats/min)	Rhythm	Contour	Rate (beats/min)	Rhythm	Contour		Intensity of S_1	Splitting of S_2	A Waves	Treatment
Accelerated idioventricular rhythm	60–100||	Regular	Normal	50–110	Fairly regular; may be irregular	Abnormal, >0.12 sec	None	Variable||	Abnormal	Intermittent cannon waves||	None, unless symptomatic; lidocaine, atropine
Ventricular flutter	60–100||	Regular	Normal; difficult to see	150–300	Regular	Sine wave	None	Soft or absent	Soft or absent	Cannon waves	DC shock
Ventricular fibrillation	60–100||	Regular	Normal; difficult to see	400–600	Grossly irregular	Baseline undulations; no QRS	None	None	None	Cannon waves	DC shock
First-degree AV block	60–100¶	Regular	Normal	60–100	Regular	Normal	Gradual slowing caused by sinus	Constant, diminished	Normal	Normal	None
Type 1 second-degree AV block	60–100¶	Regular	Normal	30–100	Irregular**	Normal	Slowing caused by sinus slowing and an increase in AV block	Cyclical decrease, then increase after pause	Normal	Normal; increasing A-C interval; A waves without C waves	None, unless symptomatic; atropine
Type II second-degree AV block	60–100¶	Regular	Normal	30–100	Irregular¶	Abnormal, >0.12 sec	Gradual slowing caused by sinus slowing	Constant	Abnormal	Normal; constant A-C interval; A waves	Pacemaker
Complete AV block	60–100||	Regular	Normal	<40	Fairly regular	Abnormal, 0.12 sec	None	Variable¶	Abnormal	Intermittent cannon waves¶	Pacemaker
Right bundle branch block	60–100	Regular	Normal	60–100	Regular	Abnormal, 0.12 sec	Gradual slowing and return to former rate	Constant	Wide	Normal	None
Left bundle branch block	60–100	Regular	Normal	60–100	Regular	Abnormal, >0.12 sec	Gradual slowing and return to former rate	Constant	Paradoxical	Normal	None

*In an effort to summarize these arrhythmias in tabular form, generalizations have to be made. For example, the response to carotid sinus massage may be slightly different from what is listed. Acute therapy to terminate a tachycardia may be different from chronic therapy to prevent recurrence. Some of the exceptions are indicated in the footnotes; the reader is referred to text for a complete discussion.

†P waves initiated by sinus node discharge may not be precisely regular because of sinus arrhythmia.

‡Frequently, carotid sinus massage fails to slow a sinus tachycardia.

§Any independent atrial arrhythmia may exit or the atria may be captured retrogradely.

\|\|Constant if the atria are captured retrogradely.

¶Atrial rhythm and rate may vary, depending on whether sinus bradycardia, sinus tachycardia, or another abnormality is the atrial mechanism.

**Regular or constant if block is unchanging.

From Miller JM, et al. Therapy for cardiac arrhythmias. In: Zipes DP, et al., eds. *Braunwald's Heart Disease.* 11 ed. Philadelphia: Elsevier; 2019:670–705.

TABLE 13.12 Classification and Management of Blood Pressure for Adults

Blood Pressure Classification	Systolic Blood Pressure (mm Hg)	Diastolic Blood Pressure (mm Hg)
Normal	<120	and <80
Elevated	120–129	or <80
Stage 1 hypertension	130–139	or 80–89
Stage 2 hypertension	≥140	or ≥90

From Whelton PK, Carey RM, Aronow WS, et al. 2017 ACC/AHA/AAPA/ABC/ACPM/AGS/APhA/ASH/ASPC/NMA/PCNA guideline for the prevention, detection, evaluation, and management of high blood pressure in adults: executive summary: a report of the American College of Cardiology/American Heart Association task force on clinical practice guidelines. *Circulation*. 2018;138(17):e426–e483.

TABLE 13.13 Antihypertensive Drugs Used in Pregnancy*

Suggested Drug	Comments
Central α-agonists	Methyldopa is the drug of choice
β-blockers	Metoprolol (Atenolol and labetalol have been associated with an increased incidence of low and very-low birthweight infants)
Diuretics	Diuretics recommended for chronic hypertension if prescribed before gestation or if patients appear to be salt sensitive; diuretics not recommended in patients with preeclampsia
Direct vasodilators	Hydralazine is the parenteral drug of choice, based on its long history of safety and efficacy

*Angiotensin-converting enzyme (ACE) inhibitors and angiotensin II receptor blockers should not be used. Fetal abnormalities and death have been reported.
From Bellos I, et al. Comparative efficacy and safety of oral antihypertensive agents in pregnant women with chronic hypertension: a network metaanalysis. *Am J Obstet Gynecol*. 2020;S0002-9378(20)30338-0.

TABLE 13.14 Classification of Angina Pectoris

Class	New York Heart Association Functional Classification	Canadian Cardiovascular Society Functional Classification	Specific Activity Scale
I	Patients with cardiac disease but without resulting limitations of physical activity. Ordinary physical activity does not cause undue fatigue, palpitation, dyspnea, or anginal pain.	Ordinary physical activity, such as walking and climbing stairs, does not cause angina. Angina with strenuous or rapid or prolonged exertion at work or recreation.	Patients can perform to completion any activity requiring ≥7 metabolic equivalents (e.g., can carry 24 lb up eight steps; carry objects that weigh 80 lb; do outdoor work [shovel snow, spade soil]; do recreational activities [skiing, basketball, squash, handball, jog or walk 5 mph]).
II	Patients with cardiac disease resulting in slight limitation of physical activity. They are comfortable at rest. Ordinary physical activity results in fatigue, palpitations, dyspnea, or anginal pain.	Slight limitation of ordinary activity. Walking or climbing stairs rapidly, walking uphill, walking or stair climbing after meals, in cold, in wind, or when under emotional stress, or only during the few hours after awakening. Walking more than two blocks on the level and climbing more than one flight of ordinary stairs at a normal pace and in normal conditions.	Patient can perform to completion any activity requiring ≥5 metabolic equivalents but cannot and does not perform to completion activities requiring ≥7 metabolic equivalents (e.g., have sexual intercourse without stopping, garden, rake, weed, roller skate, dance foxtrot, walk at 4 mph on level ground).
III	Patients with cardiac disease resulting in marked limitation of physical activity. They are comfortable at rest less than ordinary physical activity causes fatigue, palpitations, dyspnea, or anginal pain.	Marked limitation of ordinary physical activity. Walking one or two blocks on the level and climbing more than one flight in normal conditions.	Patient can perform to completion any activity requiring ≥2 metabolic equivalents but cannot and does not perform to completion any activities requiring ≥5 metabolic equivalents (e.g., shower without stopping, strip and make bed, clean windows, walk 2.5 mph, bowl, play golf, dress without stopping).
IV	Patients with cardiac disease resulting in inability to carry on any physical activity without discomfort. Symptoms of cardiac insufficiency or of the anginal syndrome may be present even at rest. If any physical activity is undertaken, discomfort is increased.	Inability to carry on any physical activity without discomfort—anginal syndrome may be present at rest.	Patient cannot or does not perform to completion activities requiring ≥2 metabolic equivalents; cannot carry out activities listed previously (Specific Activity Scale, class III).

From Goldman L, et al. Comparative reproducibility and validity of systems for assessing cardiovascular functional class: advantages of a new specific activity scale. *Circulation*. 1981;64:1227–1234.

It is better to have the patient's disease state under proper control than to discontinue any medications before surgery and risk having the patient in an unstable condition. Withdrawal after abrupt discontinuation of β-blockers and clonidine is especially severe.

Aspirin is recommended as a lifelong therapy that in general should not be interrupted for patients with cardiovascular disease. The abrupt withdrawal of aspirin can cause a platelet rebound phenomenon and prothrombotic state, leading to a major adverse cardiovascular event.

TABLE 13.15 Drug Therapy for Angina

Drug	Comments
Nitrates	First-line therapy for acute attacks; mechanism is a decrease in oxygen demand via a reduction in preload and some beneficial redistribution in blood flow
β-blockers	Cornerstone therapy for chronic prophylaxis; decrease cardiac demand via lower heart rate, blood pressure, and contractility
Calcium channel blockers	Especially effective in variant angina and in patients intolerant to β-blockers; reduce preload and afterload, and increase coronary flow
Antiplatelet drugs	Aspirin inhibits platelet and endothelial cyclooxygenase; reduces coronary thrombosis; clopidogrel (Plavix) may be substituted in patients with contraindications to aspirin
Statins	HMG-CoA reductase inhibitors, commonly referred to as statins; reduce C-reactive protein, thrombogenicity, and adverse cardiac events
Angiotensin-converting enzyme inhibitors	May be useful in patients with coronary artery disease and diabetes or other vascular diseases
Ranolazine	Ranolazine (Ranexa) is usually given in conjunction with the standard antianginal agents; blocks the late inward sodium current reducing intracellular calcium overload

HMG-CoA, 3-hydroxy-3-methylglutaryl-coenzyme A.

A complete discussion of this phenomenon can be found in the earlier section on anesthetic uses of β-blockers.[79,80]

An estimated 600,000 coronary artery stents are placed annually in the United States for the management of acute and chronic coronary artery disease, and the use of stents continues to grow. The frequency of noncardiac surgery after coronary stenting is estimated to be more than 10% at 1 year and 20% at 2 years.[156] Dual antiplatelet therapy (DAPT) with aspirin and a $P2Y_{12}$ inhibitor such as clopidogrel (Plavix), prasugrel (Effient), ticagrelor (Brilinta), or cangrelor (Kengreal) is standard at least 6 weeks after placement of bare-metal stents (BMS), 3 to 6 months after MI, and at least 12 months after placement of drug-eluting stents (DES). Some patients remain on dual antiplatelet therapy for longer periods. The 2016 update by the ACC/AHA recommends the following: (A) Elective noncardiac surgery should be delayed 30 days after BMS implantation and optimally 6 months after DES implantation because of the risk of in-stent thrombosis and/or bleeding from DAPT during surgery. (B) In patients treated with DAPT after coronary stent implantation who must undergo surgical procedures that mandate the discontinuation of $P2Y_{12}$ inhibitor therapy, it is recommended that aspirin be continued if possible and the $P2Y_{12}$ platelet receptor inhibitor be restarted as soon as possible after surgery. (C) When noncardiac surgery is required in patients currently taking a $P2Y_{12}$ inhibitor, a consensus decision among treating clinicians as to the relative risks of surgery and discontinuation or continuation of antiplatelet therapy can be useful. (D) Elective noncardiac surgery after DES implantation in patients for whom $P2Y_{12}$ inhibitor therapy will need to be discontinued may be considered after 3 months if the risk of further delay of surgery is greater than the expected risks of stent thrombosis. (E) Elective noncardiac surgery should not be performed within 30 days after BMS implantation or within 3 months after DES implantation in patients in whom DAPT will need to be discontinued perioperatively.[157]

In surgical patients, antiplatelet therapy should be maintained in all situations in which the risk of surgical bleeding is low, which is usually the case in an ambulatory setting. If this is not possible, aspirin should be continued in the perioperative period, although the management of $P2Y_{12}$ inhibitors should be individualized according to the individual patient and type of surgery. The exception is surgery in a closed space, such as intracranial procedures; procedures in the posterior eye chamber, middle ear, or intramedullary spine; and possibly transurethral prostatectomy or surgeries associated with massive bleeding and difficult hemostasis.[158-160] A complete discussion of the anesthesia management of patients on antiplatelet drugs can be found in Chapter 38.

TABLE 13.16 HMG-CoA Reductase Inhibitors (Statins)

Drug	Initial Dosage	Maximum Dosage	Comments
Atorvastatin (Lipitor)	10 mg once	80 mg once	Statins are generally tolerated better than other lipid-lowering drugs. Mild transient gastrointestinal disturbances, muscle pain, rash, and headache have occurred. Some patients have reported sleep disturbances. An increase in liver enzymes and creatine phosphokinase may occur with significant myalgia and muscle weakness.
Fluvastatin (Lescol)	20 mg once	40 mg bid	
Lovastatin (Mevacor)	20 mg once	80 mg once	
Pitavastatin (Livalo)	2 mg once	4 mg once	
Pravastatin (Pravachol)	40 mg once	80 mg once	
Rosuvastatin (Crestor)	10 mg once	40 mg once	
Simvastatin (Zocor)	20 mg once	80 mg once	

HMG-CoA, 3-hydroxy-3-methylglutaryl-coenzyme A.
Adapted from Lipid lowering drugs. *Med Lett Drugs Ther.* 2019;61(1565):17–24.

SUMMARY

Both advances in diagnostic and screening tests for heart disease and improvements in cardiac disease management continue to make impressive strides. Angioplasty is more effective and widely available, and electrophysiologic treatment of rhythm disorders is now considered routine. The number and diversity of cardiac medications we encounter in the perioperative period continues to grow. These advances require that anesthesia clinicians stay abreast of ever more complex clinical techniques but at the same time improve anesthesia quality and safety for patients.

REFERENCES

For a complete list of references for this chapter, scan this QR code with any smartphone code reader app, or visit the following URL: http://booksite.elsevier.com/9780323711944/.

14

Additional Drugs of Interest

John J. Nagelhout

PERIOPERATIVE ANTIBIOTICS

Surgical site infections (SSIs) are a significant burden to the patient and the health care system. They are the most common perioperative infection and the most frequent cause of hospital readmission after surgery, accounting for nearly 20% of unplanned readmissions.[1] There are an estimated 157,000 SSIs annually in the United States. They prolong hospitalization an average of 7 to 10 days and have an estimated annual incremental cost of $3.3 billion. The mortality rate associated with SSI is 3%, with approximately three-quarters of deaths being directly attributed to the infection.[2] Estimates from 2013 indicate that the average added cost of an SSI is approximately $21,000.[3] Costs can exceed $41,000 for more complicated deep infections.[4] An SSI is an infection that occurs somewhere in the operative field following surgery. The Centers for Disease Control and Prevention (CDC) define SSIs to include both incisional SSI and organ space SSI. Incisional SSI is subdivided into superficial and deep SSI, depending on whether the infection is limited to the skin and subcutaneous tissue only (superficial SSI) or extends into the deeper tissues, such as the fascial and muscular layers of the body wall (deep SSI). Organ/space SSI is an infection that occurs anywhere within the operative field other than where the body wall tissues were incised. Examples include intraabdominal abscess developing after an abdominal operation, empyema developing after a thoracic operation, and osteomyelitis or joint infection developing after an orthopedic procedure.[5,6] The CDC National Healthcare Safety Network is the nation's most widely used healthcare-associated infection tracking system. Risk factors for developing an SSI are listed in Box 14.1. The 10 most common isolates in surgical site and nosocomial infections are listed in Table 14.1. Surgical wound classification is noted in Table 14.2. For a complete discussion of infection control procedures see the information presented in Chapter 61.

Choosing the proper antimicrobial agent is essential. Prophylaxis should be directed against the most likely organism without covering all possible pathogens to decrease drug resistance. A drug for surgical prophylaxis should (1) prevent SSI, (2) prevent SSI-related morbidity and mortality, (3) reduce the duration and cost of health care, (4) produce no adverse effects, and (5) have no adverse consequences for the microbial flora of the patient or the hospital. To achieve these goals, an antimicrobial agent should be (1) active against the pathogens most likely to contaminate the surgical site, (2) given in an appropriate dosage and at a time that ensures adequate serum and tissue concentrations during the period of potential contamination, (3) safe, and (4) administered for the shortest effective period to minimize adverse effects, the development of resistance, and costs.[7] Some common antimicrobials and their mechanism of action are listed in Table 14.3. Antibiotics may be classified as β-lactams or non–β-lactams. The β-lactam drugs include penicillins, cephalosporins, and carbapenems. β-lactam antibiotics contain a four-membered β-lactam ring and consist of several classes: the penicillins (penams), cephalosporins (cephems), and the carbapenems, monobactams, oxacephems, and clavams. Non–β-lactam antibiotics, such as macrolides, sulfonamides, quinolines, and aminoglycosides, are different chemically.

The Surgical Care Improvement Project (SCIP) is a national quality partnership of organizations interested in improving surgical care by significantly reducing surgical complications.[8] Since 2006 they have been setting core measures designed to reduce SSIs. The SCIP National Quality Core Measures are evidence-based clinical care guidelines that are audited and reported to a national database and have been used as a quality measure to compare hospitals. Even though they have increased the focus on SSI, there has not been a measurable improvement in infection rates to date.[9] The SCIP core performance measures are listed in Table 14.4.

Bundled interventions are an approach that attempts to group the best evidence-based measures into routine care for all patients. It involves preoperative screening, decolonization, and targeted prophylaxis. It includes methods for preoperative removal of hair (where appropriate), rational antibiotic prophylaxis, avoidance of perioperative hypothermia, management of perioperative blood glucose, and effective preoperative bathing and skin preparation.[10,11] A recent report (2015) from a tertiary medical center on a bundled program in eight intensive care units noted impressive reductions in catheter-based infections. They implemented a catheter bundle that included hand hygiene, provider education, chlorhexidine skin preparation, use of maximum barrier precautions, a dedicated line cart, checklist, avoidance of the femoral vein for catheter insertion, chlorhexidine-impregnated dressings, use of antiinfective catheters, and daily consideration of the need for the catheter.[12] The development of 30-day postoperative infections has been directly linked to bacterial transmission events originating from anesthesia workstation reservoirs. Anesthesia providers should consider implementation of measures designed to target attenuation of bacterial transmission occurring during the routine administration of all anesthetics. Evidence suggests that a multimodal approach, including double gloving during airway instrumentation, intraoperative hand hygiene, patient screening and decolonization, and environmental equipment decontamination, may reduce the risk of postoperative infections.[13]

Drug Administration

β-lactams work primarily via time-dependent killing, which means the time that the drug concentration exceeds the minimum inhibitory concentration (MIC) of the target organism is the primary determinant of its efficacy. In contrast, fluoroquinolones exhibit concentration-dependent killing. Vancomycin exhibits both types of effects.[14] It is recommended that administration of the first dose of the prophylactic antibiotic should be 60 minutes before the initial surgical incision to ensure adequate serum and tissue levels. If vancomycin or a fluoroquinolone is used, the infusion should begin

BOX 14.1 Risk Factors for Surgical Site Infections

Patient Related
- Age
- Nutritional status
- Diabetes
- Smoking
- Obesity
- Coexistent infections at a remote body site
- Colonization with microorganisms
- Altered immune response
- Length of preoperative stay
- Hypothermia

Operation
- Duration of surgical scrub
- Skin antisepsis
- Preoperative shaving
- Duration of operation
- Antimicrobial prophylaxis
- Operating room ventilation
- Inadequate sterilization of instruments
- Foreign material in the surgical site
- Surgical drains
- Surgical technique
- Poor hemostasis
- Failure to obliterate dead space
- Tissue trauma

Adapted from Young PY, et al. Surgical site infections. *Surg Clin North Am.* 2014;94(6):1245–1264.

TABLE 14.2 Surgical Wound Classification

Class	Type	Description
I	Clean	An uninfected operative wound in which no inflammation is encountered and the respiratory, alimentary, genital, or uninfected urinary tract is not entered. In addition, clean wounds are primarily closed and, if necessary, drained with closed drainage. Operative incisional wounds that follow nonpenetrating (blunt) trauma should be included in this category if they meet the criteria.
II	Clean—contaminated	An operative wound in which the respiratory, alimentary, genital, or urinary tracts are entered under controlled conditions and without unusual contamination. Specifically, operations involving the biliary tract, appendix, vagina, and oropharynx are included in this category, provided no evidence of infection or major break in technique is encountered.
III	Contaminated	Open, fresh, accidental wounds. In addition, operations with major breaks in sterile technique (e.g., open cardiac massage) or gross spillage from the gastrointestinal tract, and incisions in which acute, nonpurulent inflammation is encountered are included in this category.
IV	Dirty—infected	Old traumatic wounds with retained devitalized tissue and those that involve existing clinical infection or perforated viscera. This definition suggests that the organisms causing postoperative infection were present in the operative field before the operation.

From Young PY, et al. Surgical site infections. *Surg Clin North Am.* 2014;94(6):1245–1264.

TABLE 14.1 National Nosocomial Infections Surveillance Top 10 Most Common Isolates (Percentage Distribution) in Surgical Site Infections and Nosocomial Infections

Pathogen	Surgical Site Infections (n = 17,671) %
Staphylococcus aureus	30
Escherichia coli	9
Coagulase-negative *Staphylococci*	11
Enterococcus sp	11
Pseudomonas aeruginosa	8
Enterobacter sp	4
Candida albicans	3
Klebsiella pneumoniae	4
Gram-positive anaerobes	1
Proteus mirabilis	3

Data from National Nosocomial Infections Surveillance (NNIS) System Report, data summary from January 1992 through June 2004, issued October 2004. *Am J Infect Control.* 2004;32(8):470–485; Sievert DM, et al. Antimicrobial-resistant pathogens associated with healthcare-associated infections: summary of data reported to the National Healthcare Safety Network at the Centers for Disease Control and Prevention, 2009-2010. *Infect Control Hosp Epidemiol.* 2013;34(1):1–14.

within 60 to 120 minutes before the incision because of the prolonged infusion times required for these drugs.[7] Redosing of antibiotics is recommended at approximately two half-lives of the drug. For cefazolin (Ancef), for example, with an elimination half-life of 1.4 to 2 hours, that would be approximately 4 hours. Because β-lactam antibiotics work on time-dependent killing, some clinicians have suggested continuous intravenous (IV) infusion after an initial loading dose as the suggested method of administering antibiotic prophylaxis.[15] Procedures associated with significant blood loss and replacement may require more frequent redosing. Suggested redosing may occur after every 1500 mL of blood loss, or possibly after exchange of every 30% loss of blood volume.[15,16] The duration of antimicrobial prophylaxis should be less than 24 hours for most procedures. Table 14.5 lists the common antimicrobial prophylaxis for various surgical procedures.[17]

Antibiotic Allergy

Antibiotics account for approximately 15% of anesthesia-related anaphylactic reactions, with penicillins and cephalosporins being responsible for 70% of these. Penicillin allergy is the most commonly reported drug allergy in the United States. The prevalence of reported penicillin allergy is 10% in the general population. However, more than 90% of these patients are found not to be allergic to penicillin after skin testing. In patients found to have a penicillin allergy, the

TABLE 14.3 Select Antibiotic Classes and General Mechanisms

Target and Group	Drugs	Mechanisms
Cell Wall		
ß-lactams	Penicillins, cephalosporins, carbapenems, monobactams	Inhibition of transpeptidases responsible for peptidoglycan cross-linking -' loss structural integrity
Glycopeptides	Vancomycin	Inhibition of peptidoglycan cross-linking by steric inhibition -' loss of structural integrity
Cell Membrane		
Polymyxins	Colistin, polymyxin B	Disruption of outer cell membrane of gram-negative bacteria -' altered cell membrane permeability
Ribosome		
Aminoglycosides	Gentamicin, tobramycin, amikacin, streptomycin	Binding to 30S ribosomal subunit -' inhibition of protein synthesis production of mistranslated proteins
Macrolides	Azithromycin, clarithromycin, erythromycin	Binding to 50S ribosomal submit -' inhibition of protein synthesis
Tetracyclines and glycylcyclines	Doxycycline, tigecycline	Binding to 30S ribosomal submit -' inhibition of protein synthesis
Lincosamides	Clindamycin	Binding to 50S ribosomal submit -' inhibition of protein synthesis
DNA Synthesis and Structure		
Fluoroquinolones	Ciprofloxacin, levofloxacin, moxifloxacin	Inhibition of bacterial topoisomerases, preventing DNA uncoiling -' DNA strand breakage
Antifolates	Trimethoprim/ sulfamethoxazole	Sequential inhibition of nucleotide precursors -' interruption of DNA synthesis
Nitroimidazoles	Metronidazole	Generation of free radicals -' DNA destabilization and strand breakage

Adapted from MacDougall et al. Antimicrobial therapy. In Evers AS, et al. *Anesthetic Pharmacology Basic Principles and Clinical Practice*. Cambridge: Cambridge University Press; 2011:964; Bryan CS. Infectious diseases. In Rakel RE, Rakel DP. *Textbook of Family Medicine*. Philadelphia: Elsevier; 2016;183–235; Bratzler DW, et al. Clinical practice guidelines for antimicrobial prophylaxis in surgery. *Am J Health Syst Pharm*. 2013;70(3):195–283.

TABLE 14.4 Surgical Care Improvement Project Performance Measures

SCIP INF-1	Prophylactic antibiotic received within 1 hr before surgical incision
SCIP INF-2	Proper prophylactic antibiotic selected
SCIP INF-3	Prophylactic antibiotics discontinued within 24 hr after surgery end time
SCIP INF-4	Cardiac surgery patients with controlled postoperative blood glucose
SCIP INF-6	Surgery patients with appropriate hair removal
SCIP INF-7	Colorectal surgery with immediate postoperative normothermia measures
SCIP INF-9	Urinary catheter removed on postoperative day 2
SCIP INF-10	Appropriate perioperative temperature management
SCIP VTE-1	Patients with recommended venous thromboembolism prophylaxis ordered
SCIP VTE-2	Patients who received appropriate venous thromboembolism prophylaxis within 24 hr prior to surgery to 24 hr after surgery

INF, Infection measure; *SCIP*, Surgical Care Improvement Project; *VTE*, Venous thromboembolism.
From Surgical Care Improvement Project. https://manual.jointcommission.org/releases/archive/TJC2010B/SurgicalCareImprovementProject.html.2020.

frequency of positive results on skin testing decreases by 10% per year of avoidance. Therefore 80% to 100% of patients may test negative for penicillin allergy by 10 years after their reaction. Skin testing for penicillin allergy is safe and reliable for type 1 immunoglobulin E (IgE)–mediated reactions. The rate of cephalosporin allergy is approximately 1%. The rate of cross-reactivity between penicillin and cephalosporins has been reported to be 3%. Cephalosporins and other nonpenicillin β-lactams are widely, safely, and appropriately used in individuals, even in those with a confirmed penicillin allergy. There is little, if any, clinically significant immunologic cross-reactivity between penicillins and other β-lactams.[18–20] Cross-sensitivity occurs when the R1 side chains of the penicillins and cephalosporins are similar. That is not the case with cefazolin, which is why many clinicians consider it safe in patients with a penicillin allergy. Cephalosporins with R1 side chains similar to penicillins include cephalexin, cefaclor, and cefadroxil.[14] Reactions to antibiotics can be classified according to the interval between the last administration of the drug and the onset of symptoms. Immediate reactions occurring within an hour of exposure are almost always either IgE mediated or due to direct stimulation of mast cells. Reactions occurring later than 1 hour probably have multiple mechanisms, including being IgE mediated or involving cell-mediated reactions. The latter are likely caused by drug-specific T lymphocytes.[21,22]

Antibiotic-Anesthetic Drug Interactions

Most antibiotics can cause neuromuscular blockade in the absence of neuromuscular blocking agents (NMBAs). The aminoglycosides, polymyxins (lincomycin and clindamycin), and tetracycline antibiotics can potentiate neuromuscular blockade. An interaction between the cephalosporins and penicillins and NMBAs has not been reported. If prolonged skeletal muscle weakness occurs, ventilation should be controlled until strength spontaneously returns. Calcium should not be given in an attempt to reverse the interaction because the antagonism it produces is not sustained, and it may diminish the antibacterial effect of the antibiotics.[23]

TABLE 14.5 Antimicrobial Prophylaxis for Surgery

Type of Surgical Procedure	Common Pathogens	Recommended Antibiotics	Usual Adult Dosage[1]
Cardiac			
Coronary artery bypass grafting, valve repairs, device implantation	Staphylococcus aureus, Staphylococcus epidermidis	Cefazolin	2 g IV[4,5]
		or cefuroxime	1.5 g IV[5]
Gastrointestinal			
Esophageal, gastroduodenal; entry into the GI lumen or patients at high risk for infection[6]	Enteric gram-negative bacilli, gram-positive cocci	Cefazolin[3,7]	2 g IV[4]
Biliary tract; open or high-risk laparoscopic[8]	Enteric gram-negative bacilli, enterococci, clostridia	Cefazolin[3,7,9]	2 g IV[4]
Colorectal[10]	Enteric gram-negative bacilli, anaerobes, enterococci	Cefazolin	2 g IV[4]
		+ metronidazole[3,7]	0.5 g IV
		or cefoxitin or cefotetan[3,7]	2 g IV
		or ampicillin/sulbactam[3,7,11]	3 g IV
		or ceftriaxone	2 g IV
		+ metronidazole[3,7,12]	0.5 g IV
		or ertapenem[3,7,13]	1 g IV
Appendectomy, nonperforated	Enteric gram-negative bacilli, anaerobes, enterococci	Cefoxitin or cefotetan[3,7]	2 g IV
		or cefazolin	2 g IV[4]
		+ metronidazole[3,7]	0.5 g IV
Hernia	Gram-positive cocci	Cefazolin[2,3]	2 g IV[4]
Genitourinary			
Cystoscopy alone	Enteric gram-negative bacilli, enterococci	High-risk[14] only: ciprofloxacin[11]	500 mg PO or 400 mg IV
		or trimethoprim/sulfamethoxazole[11]	160/800 mg (1 DS tab) PO
Cystoscopy with manipulation or upper tract instrumentation[15]	Enteric gram-negative bacilli, enterococci	Ciprofloxacin[11]	500 mg PO or 400 mg IV
		or trimethoprim/sulfamethoxazole[11]	160/800 mg (1 DS tab) PO
Open or laparoscopic surgery[16]	Enteric gram-negative bacilli, enterococci	Cefazolin[3,7]	2 g IV[4]
Gynecologic and Obstetric			
Vaginal, abdominal, or laparoscopic hysterectomy	Enteric gram-negative bacilli, anaerobes, group B strep, enterococci	Cefazolin[3,7]	2 g IV[4]
		or cefoxitin or cefotetan[3,7]	2 g IV
		or ampicillin/sulbactam[3,7,11]	3 g IV
Cesarean section	Same as for hysterectomy	Cefazolin[3,7]	2 g IV[4]
Abortion, surgical	Same as for hysterectomy	Doxycycline 300 mg	PO[17]
Head and Neck Surgery			
Incisions through oral or pharyngeal mucosa	Anaerobes, enteric gram-negative bacilli, S. aureus	Cefazolin	2 g IV[4]
		+ metronidazole[3,18]	0.5 g IV[4]
		or ampicillin/sulbactam[3,11,18]	3 g IV
Neurosurgery			
Craniotomy, spinal and CSF-shunting procedures, intrathecal pump placement	S. aureus, S. epidermidis, Propionibacterium acnes	Cefazolin[2,3]	2 g IV[4]
Ophthalmic[19]	S. epidermidis, S. aureus, streptococci, enterococci, P. acnes, Corynebacterium spp., enteric gram-negative bacilli, Pseudomonas spp.	Neomycin-gramicidin-polymyxin B, gatifloxacin, or moxifloxacin	1 drop q5-15 min × 5 doses
		± cefazolin	100 mg subconjunctivally at the end of the procedure
Orthopedic			
Spinal, hip fracture, internal fixation, total joint replacement	S. aureus, S. epidermidis, P. acnes (shoulder)	Cefazolin[2,3,20]	2 g IV[4]
Thoracic (Noncardiac)			
Lobectomy, pneumonectomy, lung resection, thoracotomy	S. aureus, S. epidermidis, streptococci, enteric gram-negative bacilli	Cefazolin[2,3]	2 g IV[4]
		or ampicillin/sulbactam[2,3,11]	3 g IV

Continued

TABLE 14.5   Antimicrobial Prophylaxis for Surgery—cont'd

Type of Surgical Procedure	Common Pathogens	Recommended Antibiotics	Usual Adult Dosage[1]
Vascular			
Arterial involving a prosthesis, the abdominal aorta, or a groin incision	S. aureus, S. epidermidis, enteric gram-negative bacilli	Cefazolin[2,3]	2 g IV[4]
Lower extremity amputation for ischemia	S. aureus, S. epidermidis, enteric gram-negative bacilli, clostridia	Cefazolin[2,3]	2 g IV[4]

[1]Parenteral prophylactic antimicrobials can be given as a single IV dose begun within 60 min before the initial incision. For procedures that exceed 2 half-lives of the drug or those with major blood loss, or in patients with extensive burns, additional intraoperative doses should be given at intervals of about two times the half-life of the drug (ampicillin/sulbactam every 2 hr, cefazolin every 4 hr, cefuroxime every 4 hr, cefoxitin every 2 hr, clindamycin every 6 hr, vancomycin every 12 hr) for the duration of the procedure in patients with normal renal function. If vancomycin or fluoroquinolone is used, the infusion should be started within 60–120 min before the initial incision to have adequate tissue levels at the time of incision and to minimize the possibility of an infusion reaction close to the time of induction of anesthesia.

[2]Vancomycin (15 mg/kg IV) or clindamycin (900 mg IV) is a reasonable alternative for patients who are allergic to β-lactams. They only provide coverage against gram-positive organisms; for procedures in which enteric gram-negative bacilli are common pathogens, many experts would add an aminoglycoside (gentamicin, tobramycin, or amikacin), aztreonam, or a fluoroquinolone.

[3]A dose of vancomycin (15 mg/kg) can be given in addition to the recommended antimicrobial(s) in patients colonized with MRSA or in hospitals in which methicillin-resistant S. aureus and S. epidermidis are a frequent cause of postoperative wound infection. Vancomycin is less effective than cefazolin in preventing surgical site infections due to methicillin-susceptible Staphylococcus aureus (MSSA). Vancomycin has activity only against gram-positive bacteria; for procedures in which enteric gram-negative bacilli are common pathogens, many experts would add another drug such as an aminoglycoside (gentamicin, tobramycin, or amikacin), aztreonam, or a fluoroquinolone. Rapid IV administration of vancomycin may cause hypotension, which could be especially dangerous during induction of anesthesia. Even when the drug is given over 60 min, hypotension may occur; treatment with diphenhydramine (Benadryl, others) and further slowing of the infusion rate may be helpful. An infusion rate of 10–15 mg/min (≥1 hr/1000 mg) has been recommended (Crawford T, et al. Clin Infect Dis 2012;54:1474).

[4]Dose for patients who weigh <120 kg; the recommended dose is 3 g for those weighing ≥120 kg. Morbidly obese patients may need higher doses.

[5]Some experts recommend an additional dose when patients are removed from bypass during open-heart surgery.

[6]Morbid obesity, GI obstruction, decreased gastric acidity or GI motility, gastric bleeding, malignancy or perforation, or immunosuppression.

[7]For patients who are allergic to β-lactams, clindamycin (900 mg IV) or vancomycin (15 mg/kg IV) with either gentamicin, aztreonam, or a fluoroquinolone is a reasonable alternative. Fluoroquinolones should not be used for prophylaxis in cesarean section.

[8]Age >70 years, acute cholecystitis, nonfunctioning gallbladder, obstructive jaundice, common bile duct stones, duration >120 min, diabetes, pregnancy, or immunosuppression.

[9]Cefotetan, cefoxitin, and ampicillin/sulbactam are reasonable alternatives.

[10]In addition to mechanical bowel preparation, 1 g of neomycin plus 1 g of erythromycin at 1 PM, 2 PM, and 11 PM or 2 g of neomycin plus 2 g of metronidazole at 7 PM and 11 PM the day before an 8 AM operation.

[11]Due to increasing resistance of Escherichia coli, local sensitivity profiles should be reviewed before use.

[12]Where there is increasing resistance of gram-negative isolates to first- and second-generation cephalosporins, a single dose of ceftriaxone plus metronidazole may be preferred over routine use of carbapenems.

[13]Ertapenem is FDA approved for prophylaxis in colorectal surgery. It was more effective than cefotetan in one study, but it was associated with an increased risk of Clostridium difficile infection and other adverse effects (Itani KM, et al. N Engl J Med 2006;355:2640). Routine use could promote carbapenem resistance.

[14]Urine culture positive or unavailable, preoperative catheter, transrectal prostatic biopsy, or placement of prosthetic material.

[15]Shock wave lithotripsy, ureteroscopy.

[16]Including percutaneous renal surgery, procedures with entry into the urinary tract, and those involving implantation of a prosthesis. If manipulation of bowel is involved, prophylaxis is given according to colorectal guidelines.

[17]Divided into 100 mg before the procedure and 200 mg after.

[18]For patients who are allergic to β-lactams, clindamycin (900 mg IV) is a reasonable alternative.

[19]Preoperative application of povidone-iodine to the skin and conjunctiva is recommended.

[20]If a tourniquet is to be used during the procedure, the entire dose of antibiotic must be infused before its inflation.

DS, Double strength; GI, gastrointestinal; OR, operating room; PO, per os.

Reprinted with permission from Treatment Guidelines from The Medical Letter, 2016;58(1495):65–66.

Antibiotic Prophylaxis for Surgical and Dental Procedures

The routine use of antibiotic prophylaxis (AP) to prevent endocarditis in patients undergoing surgical or dental procedures is an area of long-standing controversy. Significant differences in recommendations from experts in the United States, United Kingdom, and other countries exist. The National Institute for Health and Care Excellence (NICE) in the United Kingdom issued recommendations, which eliminated AP altogether. The American Heart Association (AHA) significantly narrowed the indications to high-risk groups only.[24–28] Patients at increased risk of developing infective endocarditis are listed in Box 14.2. Consensus recommendations differ as to the type of procedure, such as gastrointestinal (GI) or dental. Box 14.3 notes the type of procedures in which AP may be appropriate. Table 14.6 lists common antibiotic recommendations for dental AP.[29,30]

ANTIEMETICS AND PERIOPERATIVE NAUSEA AND VOMITING

The anesthesia community has put tremendous effort into addressing the issue of postoperative nausea and vomiting (PONV) and

BOX 14.2   Patients at Increased Risk of Developing Infective Endocarditis

High Risk

- Patients with a previous history of infective endocarditis
- Patients with any form of prosthetic heart valve (including a transcatheter valve)
- Those in whom prosthetic material was used for cardiac valve repair
- Patients with any type of cyanotic congenital heart disease
- Patients with any type of congenital heart disease repaired with prosthetic material, whether placed surgically or by percutaneous techniques, for the first 6 mo after the procedure or lifelong if a residual shunt or valvular regurgitation remains
- Cardiac transplantation recipients who develop cardiac valvulopathy

Moderate Risk

- Patients with a previous history of rheumatic fever
- Patients with any other form of native valve disease (including the most commonly identified conditions: bicuspid aortic valve, mitral valve prolapse, and calcific aortic stenosis)
- Patients with unrepaired congenital anomalies of the heart valves

Adapted from Thornhill MH, et al. Guidelines on prophylaxis to prevent infective endocarditis. *Br Dent J.* 2016;220(2):51–56; Habib G, et al. 2015 ESC guidelines for the management of infective endocarditis: the Task Force for the Management of Infective Endocarditis of the European Society of Cardiologist (ESC). Endorsed by: European Association for Cardio-Thoracic Surgery (EACTS), the European Association of Nuclear Medicine (EANM). *Eur Heart J.* 2015;36(44):3075–3128.

BOX 14.3   Recommendations for Prophylaxis of Infective Endocarditis in the Highest-Risk Patients According to the Type of At-Risk Procedure

Recommendations

Dental Procedures

Antibiotic prophylaxis should considered only be for dental procedures regarding manipulation of the gingival or periapical region of the teeth or perforation of the oral mucosa.

Antibiotic prophylaxis is not recommended for local anesthetic injections in noninfected tissues, treatment of superficial caries, removal of sutures, dental x-rays, placement or adjustment of removable prosthodontic or orthodontic appliances or braces, or following the shedding of deciduous teeth or trauma to the lips and oral mucosa.

Respiratory Tract Procedures

Antibiotic prophylaxis is not recommended for respiratory tract procedures, including bronchoscopy or laryngoscopy or transnasal or endotracheal intubation.

Gastrointestinal or Urogenital Procedures or TOE

Antibiotic prophylaxis is not recommended for gastroscopy, colonoscopy, cystoscopy, vaginal or cesarean delivery, or TOE.

Skin and Soft Tissue Procedure

Antibiotic prophylaxis is not recommended for any procedure.

TOE, Transesophageal echocardiography.
From Habib G, et al. 2015 ESC guidelines for the management of infective endocarditis: the Task Force for the Management of Infective Endocarditis of the European Society of Cardiologist (ESC). Endorsed by: European Association for Cardio-Thoracic Surgery (EACTS), the European Association of Nuclear Medicine (EANM). *Eur Heart* J. 2015,36(44):3075–3128.

postdischarge nausea and vomiting (PDNV). These undesirable responses to anesthesia unfortunately persist as a clinical problem and make the anesthetic experience unpleasant for the patient and provider, and greatly reduce patient satisfaction. This complication may result in incisional stress and significant postoperative problems, especially after certain procedures such as oral/facial surgery, neurosurgical procedures, and upper GI surgery. Bleeding, fluid and electrolyte disturbances, cardiovascular stress, and aspiration may occur. In addition, postanesthesia care unit (PACU) discharge may be delayed with PONV, or hospital readmission may be necessary from PDNV. This increases use of resources and personnel with the resulting increases in cost.[31–33] In a widely reported study on the risk for PDNV, it was noted that the incidence of nausea and vomiting was higher after discharge than in the PACU. Apfel et al. conducted a prospective multicenter study of 2170 adults undergoing general anesthesia. In the PACU, 19.9% of patients had nausea and 3.9% had vomiting. The incidence of severe nausea was 3.6% and severe vomiting 0.2%. After discharge, 36.6% had nausea and 11.9% had vomiting. The incidence of severe nausea was 13.3%, and 5% had severe vomiting.[34] Efforts to address this problem must continue.[35]

The Fourth Consensus Guidelines for the Management of Postoperative Nausea and Vomiting have been issued.[31] Multiple PONV risk factors have been identified (Box 14.4). Strategies to reduce the risk of PONV and PDNV are noted in Box 14.5.[31,34,36,37]

Multimodal Antiemetic Therapy

Since the causes of postoperative nausea and vomiting are multifactorial, a multimodal approach using drugs with different mechanisms of action is the most effective prophylaxis and therapy.[31,38] Several classes of drugs are used for therapy (Box 14.6).

Glucocorticoids

Dexamethasone is a popular drug for the prevention of PONV. A dose of 4 mg IV is recommended after anesthesia induction rather than at the end of surgery. The efficacy of dexamethasone 4 mg IV is similar to ondansetron 4 mg IV and droperidol 1.25 mg IV. Some clinicians prefer a higher dose of 8 mg IV. The mechanism of action is unclear although several theories have been proposed. Data from animal studies suggest that it exerts its antiemetic effects through central inhibition of the nucleus tractus solitarii.[39] A reduction of serotonin in the central nervous system (CNS) via a reduction of tryptophan, decreased release of GI serotonin, a decrease in 5-HT$_3$ turnover in the CNS, and inhibition of prostaglandin synthesis have all been proposed.[39–41] Although corticosteroids are associated with numerous side effects with repeated use, a single dose for an antiemetic effect is generally safe.[31,32] The effect on wound healing and infection has been reported, and a single dose of dexamethasone does not increase wound complications.[42–43] An increase in blood glucose may occur 6 to 12 hours postoperatively in patients with impaired glucose tolerance, type 2 diabetes, or obesity. The increase in blood glucose after administration of IV dexamethasone either 4 or 8 mg in patients with type 2 diabetes was approximately 40 mg/dL.[44] Since the onset of action of dexamethasone is 1 hour, it is most effective in decreasing PONV when administered prior to the induction of anesthesia. Since the duration of action is approximately 72 hours, it complements the significantly shorter duration of action of ondansetron to produce a prolonged PONV effect.

TABLE 14.6   Recommended Prophylaxis for High-Risk Dental Procedures in High-Risk Patients

		SINGLE DOSE 30–60 MIN BEFORE PROCEDURE	
Situation	Antibiotic	Adults	Children
No allergy to penicillin or ampicillin	Amoxicillin or ampicillin*	2 g orally or IV	50 mg/kg orally or IV
Allergy to penicillin or ampicillin	Clindamycin	600 mg orally or IV	20 mg/kg orally or IV

*Alternatively, cephalexin 2 g IV for adults or 50 mg/kg IV for children, cefazolin or ceftriaxone 1 g IV for adults or 50 mg/kg IV for children.
Murphy DJ, Din M, Hage FG, et al. Guidelines in review: comparison of ESC and AHA guidance for the diagnosis and management of infective endocarditis in adults. *J Nucl Cardiol.* 2019;26(1):303–308.
Cephalosporins should not be used in patients with anaphylaxis, angioedema, or urticaria after intake of penicillin or ampicillin due to cross-sensitivity.

BOX 14.4   Risk Factors for PONV in Adults

Risk Factors
- Female gender
- History of PONV or motion sickness
- Nonsmoking
- Younger age
- General vs regional anesthesia
- Use of inhalation anesthetics and nitrous oxide
- Postoperative opioids
- Duration of anesthesia
- Type of surgery (cholecystectomy, laparoscopic surgery, gynecologic)
- ASA physical status

Conflicting Evidence
- Menstrual cycle
- Provider experience
- Perioperative fasting
- Body mass index
- Anxiety

Disproven
- Nasogastric tube
- Migraine
- Supplemental oxygen

ASA, American Society of Anesthesiologists; *PONV,* postoperative nausea and vomiting.
From Gan TJ, Belani KG, Bergese S, et al. Fourth consensus guidelines for the management of postoperative nausea and vomiting. *Anesth Analg.* 2020;131(2):411–448.

BOX 14.5   Strategies to Reduce the Risk of Postoperative Nausea and Vomiting

- Avoid general anesthesia by the use of regional techniques
- Use propofol for induction and maintenance
- Avoid nitrous oxide in procedures lasting over 1 hr
- Avoid inhalation anesthetics
- Minimize intra- and postoperative opioids
- Adequate hydration
- Use sugammadex instead of neostigmine for neuromuscular blockade reversal
- Minimize fasting
- Use at least two different antiemetics

Adapted from Gan TJ, Belani KG, Bergese S, et al. Fourth consensus guidelines for the management of postoperative nausea and vomiting. *Anesth Analg.* 2020;131(2):411–448; Nathan N. Management of postoperative nausea and vomiting: the 4th consensus guidelines. *Anesth Analg.* 2020;131(2):410.

BOX 14.6   Current Antiemetic Medications by Drug Classes

Corticosteroids
Dexamethasone, methylprednisolone

Phenothiazines
Chlorpromazine, prochlorperazine

Butyrophenones
Droperidol, haloperidol

Benzamides
Metoclopramide

Anticholinergics
Scopolamine

Antihistamines
Hydroxyzine, dimenhydrinate, meclizine

5-HT₃ Antagonists
Ondansetron, dolasetron, granisetron, tropisetron, palonosetron, ramosetron

NK-1 Antagonists
Aprepitant, vestipitant, fosaprepitant, netupitant, rolapitant, casopitant

Benzodiazepines
Midazolam, lorazepam

5-HT₃, 5-hydroxytryptamine-3; *NK-1,* neurokinin 1.

Methylprednisolone 40 mg IV is also effective for prophylaxis of nausea and vomiting.[31,32]

5-HT₃ Receptor Antagonists

Ondansetron is the most widely used antiemetic, and it is the gold standard for comparison of other agents. It is generally thought to have a greater inhibitory effect on vomiting as compared to nausea, although some data note a similar efficacy for both.[31,34] The standard dose is 4 mg administered at the end of the procedure. Its popularity arises in part due to the relative lack of significant side effects. At higher doses, QT interval changes may occur. A single 32-mg IV dose of ondansetron used for prevention of chemotherapy-induced nausea and vomiting (CINV) has been withdrawn from the market because it can prolong the QT interval and could possibly cause a torsades de pointes cardiac arrhythmia. The relatively short duration of action (4–6 hours) makes it unlikely to be effective for PDNV. The efficacy of the 5-HT₃ antagonists increases when combined with dexamethasone.[31,32,34] Other first-generation serotonin antagonists are granisetron (Kytril) and dolasetron (Anzemet). Palonosetron (Aloxi) is a second-generation serotonin antagonist with a long half-life of 44 hours, which makes it preferable for PDNV. It is typically administered at the beginning of surgery. It is also marketed as a combination product with netupitant (Akynzeo) for prevention of acute and delayed CINV.[45]

All first-generation 5-HT$_3$ antagonists may adversely prolong the QTc interval. IV dolasetron is no longer available for that reason. Some medical conditions that may lead to susceptibility to prolonged QT interval are noted in Box 14.7. Serotonin syndrome has been reported with concurrent use of 5-HT$_3$ receptor antagonists and other serotonergic drugs, including selective serotonin reuptake inhibitors (SSRIs) and serotonin and norepinephrine reuptake inhibitors (SNRIs).[46]

Neurokinin 1 Receptor Antagonists

Aprepitant (Emend) and its IV prodrug fosaprepitant (Emend), netupitant/palonosetron (Akynzeo), and rolapitant (Varubi) are substance P/neurokinin 1 (NK-1) receptor antagonists. Neurokinin receptors are found in the nucleus of the solitary tract (NST), where they are involved in the central regulation of visceral function. NK-1 receptor antagonists are believed to provide antiemetic activity by suppressing activity at the NST, where vagal afferents from the GI tract converge with inputs from the area postrema and other regions of the brain that initiate emesis. Aprepitant has been approved by the Food and Drug Administration (FDA) for PONV, while netupitant/palonosetron and rolapitant have been approved for CINV. Rolapitant is characterized by a long half-life of 180 hours and an active metabolite with a half-life of 158 hours. It is marketed for delayed CINV but may also be effective for prevention of PDNV.[47,48]

Butyrophenones

Droperidol in small doses of 0.625 to 1.25 mg has been used for decades to prevent and treat PONV. It is generally administered at the end of surgery, and it acts as a dopamine receptor blocking agent in the CNS. Like any dopamine blocking drug, it may cause extrapyramidal side effects and is contraindicated in patients with Parkinson disease. In 2001 the FDA issued a black box warning restricting its use due to potential prolongation of the QT interval. The anesthesia community objected that, at the low clinical doses used, this effect was unlikely. The warning suggested an electrocardiogram (ECG) be performed before droperidol is used. As that is impractical, its routine use has decreased dramatically in the United States. Haloperidol also has antiemetic properties when used in low doses of 1 to 2 mg. Administration at the beginning or end of surgery is equally efficacious.[49] Even though it has similar effects to droperidol on the QT interval, it does not contain a black box warning. Some clinicians use it as an alternative to droperidol.[31,30]

Transdermal Scopolamine

The scopolamine patch is an effective antiemetic when applied the evening before surgery. It has an onset time of approximately 4 hours and a minimum duration of 24 hours. Its effect is to prevent nausea and vomiting by blocking transmission of cholinergic impulses from vestibular nuclei to higher centers in the CNS and from the reticular formation to the vomiting center. Common side effects are reflective of its central anticholinergic effects: sedation, blurred vision, dizziness, and dry mouth. It appears most effective for prevention of nausea when a patient-controlled analgesia device is used for postoperative pain.[50,51]

Benzodiazepines

Whether the benzodiazepines have antiemetic action has been a long-standing area of controversy. Lorazepam has been used as an adjunct for CINV; however, newer drugs are currently used. Two recent meta-analyses (2016) suggest that midazolam may have a clinically significant antiemetic effect. They note that administration of preoperative or intraoperative IV midazolam is associated with a significant decrease in overall PONV, nausea, vomiting, and rescue antiemetic use.[52,53] It appears to decrease dopamine's emetic effect in the chemoreceptor trigger zone and decreases the release of serotonin by binding to the γ-aminobutyric acid (GABA) receptor complex.[50] Concerns that administering a sedative near the end of surgery may prolong recovery limit the dose.[54]

Metoclopramide

Metoclopramide is a weak antiemetic that exerts a mild dopamine receptor blocking effect. Minimal effects are seen unless doses greater than 20 mg are used. It has a short half-life of 30 to 45 minutes, which may explain why many reports note little effect if it is given at the beginning of surgery. Dyskinesia or extrapyramidal effects can be seen with higher doses.[33,55] Like droperidol it is contraindicated in patients with Parkinson disease. Since metoclopramide has potent gastrokinetic effects, its use is also contraindicated for patients with intestinal obstructions.

Clinical Use of Antiemetics

Clinicians have established guides for the use of antiemetics based on common risk factors. Multimodal PONV and PDNV prophylaxis should be considered for patients at moderate to high risk for PONV. All prophylaxis in children at moderate or high risk for PONV should include combination therapy using a 5-HT$_3$ antagonist and a second drug. Because the effects of interventions from different drug classes are additive, combining interventions has an additive effect in risk reduction.[31–33]

When rescue therapy is required, the antiemetic should be chosen from a different therapeutic class than the drugs used for prophylaxis and potentially one with a different mode of administration. If PONV occurs within 6 hours postoperatively, patients should not receive a repeat dose of the prophylactic antiemetic. An emetic episode more than 6 hours postoperatively can be treated with any of the drugs used for prophylaxis except dexamethasone, transdermal scopolamine, aprepitant, and palonosetron.[31–33] Agents with a rapid onset are preferred. Doses for select antiemetics are listed in Table 14.7.

PSYCHIATRIC DRUGS AND ANESTHESIA

The incidence of psychiatric illness is increasing, with an estimated 9.6 million individual adults (4.1% of adults in the United States)

TABLE 14.7   Drugs for Postoperative and Postdischarge Nausea and Vomiting

Drug	Usual Adult Dose	Optimal Timing	Comment
5-HT₃ Antagonists			
Ondansetron (Zofran)	Adult 4–8 mg IV Child 50–100 mcg/kg (max 4 mg)	End of surgery	Effective for prevention of both nausea and vomiting; more effective for PONV than PDNV; administer at end of procedure
Granisetron (Kytril)	Adult 1 mg IV Child 40 mcg/kg up to 0.6 mg	End of surgery	Administer at end of procedure
Palonosetron (Aloxi)	0.075 mg IV	Induction	Long duration may make it effective for PDNV
Dopamine Antagonists			
Droperidol (Inapsine)	0.625–1.25 mg IV	End of surgery	See text for discussion of black box warning
Amisulpride (Barhemsys)	5–10 mg	Induction	Selective dopamine D₂/D₃-antagonist; no sedation, extrapyramidal effects, or QTc prolongation in antiemetic doses
Metoclopramide (Reglan)	10–20 mg IV	End of surgery	Contraindicated in patients with gastric obstruction due to prokinetic effects
Antihistamines			
Diphenhydramine (Benadryl)	25 mg IV or IM	Induction	Sedation prominent
Glucocorticoid			
Dexamethasone (Decadron)	Adult 4–8 mg IV Child 150 mcg/kg up to 8 mg	1 hr prior to induction	May produce hyperglycemia postoperatively in diabetics
Anticholinergic			
Scopolamine transdermal (Transderm-Scop)	2.5 cm² patch contains 1.5 mg scopolamine	Prior evening or 2 hr prior to surgery	Long duration may make it effective for PDNV
Neurokinin 1 Antagonist			
Aprepitant (Emend)	40 mg PO	Induction	Long duration may make it effective for PDNV
Rolapitant (Varubi)	90 mg PO	Induction	Good for PDNV due to long duration

5-HT₃, Serotonin; *IM*, intramuscular; *IV*, intravenous; *PDNV*, postdischarge nausea and vomiting; *PO*, oral; *PONV*, postoperative nausea and vomiting.

suffering from serious mental illness as defined by the National Survey on Drug Use and Health.[56] The National Surgical Quality Improvement Program reported that anxiolytic medication (AXM) was used by 16% of patients undergoing a noncardiac operation. Use of AXMs was an independent risk factor for poorer short-term outcome after surgery. Antidepressant medications were used by 21% of patients, but they were not an independent risk factor for poor outcome.[57] The prevalence of depression and anxiety has been shown to be substantially greater among cardiac surgery patients compared to the general population. Depression and anxiety after cardiac surgery are associated with longer durations of stay, greater rates of hospital readmission, reoperation, and short- and long-term mortality.[58,59]

Most psychiatric drug therapy should be continued into the preoperative period. Maintaining antidepressants, anxiolytics, antipsychotics, and other psychotropic agents will ensure the patient's disease is better controlled during surgery. In the past, discontinuation of the monoamine oxidase inhibitors (MAOIs) was recommended 2 to 3 weeks prior to surgery. This practice is no longer used as it is logistically and medically impractical. Withdrawal requires titration of replacement therapy, which is frequently unsuccessful. Modern anesthetic techniques can be successfully adapted to the patient's condition and drug therapy. Important perioperative considerations for patients taking select psychiatric medications are reviewed in the following sections.

Antidepressants

Depression is treated with antidepressive medications, psychotherapy, electroconvulsive therapy (ECT), or a combination of these approaches. Several drug classes are useful for the treatment of depression, and they are listed in Table 14.8. The goal of antidepressant treatment is complete remission of symptoms because partial response is associated with an increased risk of relapse. Antidepressant treatment is usually given for 6 to 9 months following remission to consolidate recovery. For patients with recurrent depressive episodes, long-term maintenance therapy is indicated.[60,61]

Select Serotonin Reuptake Inhibitors

SSRIs are the first-line therapy for major depression and the most widely prescribed class of antidepressants.[62,63] They are generally well tolerated and safe. Common side effects include restlessness, insomnia, nausea, diarrhea, headache, dizziness, fatigue, and sexual dysfunction. SSRIs can cause hyponatremia, particularly in elderly patients. They can also increase the risk of bleeding by inhibiting serotonin uptake by platelets. In surgical patients, a small evidence base suggests that SSRI use is associated with bleeding and adverse outcomes in cardiac and orthopedic surgery due to the antiplatelet effects of SSRIs.[64–66] Recent studies indicate there is no bleeding risk in patients undergoing coronary artery bypass grafting (CABG).[65] When SSRIs are stopped abruptly, discontinuation symptoms (including nervousness, anxiety, irritability, electric-shock sensations, bouts of crying, dizziness,

TABLE 14.8 Antidepressant Drugs

Drug Class	Generic Name	Trade Name	Comment
SSRIs	Fluoxetine	Prozac	First-line treatment for depression. May increase the risk of bleeding due to inhibition of serotonin uptake by platelets. Significant effects on CYP450 isoenzymes may lead to various drug interactions. Abrupt discontinuation may lead to discontinuation syndrome. May lead to serotonin syndrome when combined with other serotonergic drugs.
	Paroxetine	Paxil	
	Sertraline	Zoloft	
	Fluvoxamine	Luvox	
	Citalopram	Celexa	
	Escitalopram	Lexapro	
SNRIs	Desvenlafaxine	Pristiq	May produce dose-dependent increase in blood pressure. Can precipitate serotonin syndrome or neuroleptic malignant syndrome. Abrupt withdrawal may lead to severe discontinuation syndrome. Used for analgesic effect in diabetic neuropathy.
	Duloxetine	Cymbalta	
	Venlafaxine	Effexor	
	Levomilnacipran	Fetzima	
TCAs	Amitriptyline	Elavil	Anticholinergic side effects such as urinary retention, dry mouth, blurred vision, and confusion are common. Orthostatic hypotension and cardiac conduction abnormalities may occur. A preoperative ECG should be obtained to rule out conduction changes. Direct-acting vasopressors such as phenylephrine are preferred over indirect drugs such as ephedrine.
	Desipramine	Norpramin	
	Imipramine	Tofranil	
	Nortriptyline	Pamelor	
	Protriptyline	Vivactil	
	Doxepin	Sinequan	
MAOIs	Isocarboxazid	Marplan	Enzyme inhibiting effects can persist for up to 2 wk after disconsolation. Interaction with serotonergic drugs, bupropion and sympathomimetics, can lead to serotonin syndrome. Avoid meperidine due to severe excitatory drug interaction.
	Selegiline	Ensam	
	Phenelzine	Nardil	
	Tranylcypromine	Parnate	
Atypical	Bupropion	Wellbutrin	Bupropion produces dose-related seizures. It is prescribed for smoking cessation. It blocks reuptake of both norepinephrine and dopamine.
	Mirtazapine	Remeron	
	Trazodone	Desyrel	
	Nefazodone	Serzone	
	Vilazodone	Viibryd	

MAOIs, Monoamine oxidase inhibitors; *SNRIs,* selective norepinephrine reuptake inhibitors; *SSRIs,* selective serotonin reuptake inhibitors; *TCAs,* tricyclic antidepressants.

insomnia, confusion, nausea, and vomiting) can occur. Withdrawal effects are most severe with paroxetine because of its short half-life and least likely to occur with fluoxetine because of its long half-life. The SSRIs have an inhibitory effect on CYP450 isoenzymes and may interact with many other drugs that rely on hepatic metabolism, including β-blockers, benzodiazepines, and antiarrhythmics. Interactions with other serotonergic drugs may lead to serotonin syndrome.[60,61] Citalopram and escitalopram may prolong the QT interval, although a recent study (2016) found no increased risk of cardiovascular outcomes in patients treated for depression.[67,68] Unless a patient-specific concern develops, the SSRI should be continued throughout the perioperative period.[69]

Serotonin Syndrome

Serotonin syndrome is a rare but potentially life-threatening condition associated with increased serotonergic activity in the central and peripheral nervous systems. It can be caused by individual drugs, an overdose, or, most commonly, a drug interaction. The mechanism is thought to be overstimulation of 5-HT_{1A} and possibly also 5-HT_2 receptors through an excess of serotonin precursors or agonists, increased serotonin release, reduced serotonin uptake, and decreased serotonin metabolism. Drugs that are associated with serotonin syndrome are listed in Table 14.9.[70–73] The syndrome is characterized by mental status changes, autonomic instability, neuromuscular hyperactivity, and hyperthermia (Table 14.10).[74,75] Symptoms may appear within minutes or up to 24 hours after the initial use of medication, a change in dose,

or the addition of a new serotonergic drug. Mortality may result from rhabdomyolysis with renal failure, hyperkalemia, disseminated intravascular coagulation, and/or acute respiratory distress syndrome.

Diagnosis is made using the Hunter Serotonin Toxicity Criteria, which require the presence of one or more of a group of symptoms (Box 14.8). Clonus (spontaneous, inducible, and ocular) is the most important sign in the Hunter Criteria. This neuromuscular feature has been strongly associated with serotonin toxicity.[76]

Most cases of serotonin syndrome are mild and may be treated by cessation of the drugs and supportive care. Benzodiazepines may be used to treat agitation and tremor. Patients with moderate or severe cases of serotonin syndrome require hospitalization. Critically ill patients may require neuromuscular paralysis, sedation, and intubation. If serotonin syndrome is recognized and complications are managed appropriately, the prognosis is favorable.[77]

First-line therapy includes cyproheptadine, an H_1-receptor antagonist with antiserotonergic and anticholinergic properties. Cyproheptadine should be started at a dose of 12 mg orally or through a nasogastric tube. An additional 2-mg dose is given every 2 hours until symptoms improve or the maximal dose of 32 mg has been reached. The usual maintenance dose of cyproheptadine is 8 mg three times daily.[78]

Tricyclic Antidepressants

Tricyclic antidepressants (TCAs) and MAOIs remain valuable alternatives to the SSRIs and SNRIs for patients with moderate to severe treatment-resistant depression. TCAs are probably the most commonly

TABLE 14.9 Drugs Implicated in Serotonin Syndrome

Drug Class	Agents
Monoamine oxidase inhibitors	Phenelzine, moclobemide, isocarboxazid, selegiline, tranylcypromine
SSRIs	Sertraline, fluoxetine, fluvoxamine, paroxetine, citalopram, escitalopram
SNRIs	Duloxetine, venlafaxine, desvenlafaxine
Tricyclic antidepressants	Amitriptyline, doxepin, clomipramine, nortriptyline, imipramine, desipramine
Antibiotics	Linezolid
Opiate analgesics and pain medications	Meperidine, fentanyl, tramadol, pentazocine
OTC cough/cold medications	Dextromethorphan
Antimigraine agents	Almotriptan, sumatriptan
Drugs of abuse	Amphetamine, cocaine, methylenedioxymethamphetamine (MDMA or Ecstasy), lysergic acid diethylamide (LSD)
Antiemetics	Metoclopramide, ondansetron
Anticonvulsants	Carbamazepine, valproic acid
Herbal products	Ginseng, nutmeg, St. John's wort
Other	Lithium, methylene blue, buspirone, tryptophan

OTC, Over the counter; *SNRIs,* selective norepinephrine reuptake inhibitors; *SSRIs,* selective serotonin reuptake inhibitors.

TABLE 14.10 The Triad of Neuromuscular, Autonomic, and Mental Status Effects Seen in Serotonin Syndrome

Neuromuscular Effects	Autonomic Effects	Mental Status Effects
• Hyperreflexia	• Hyperthermia	• Anxiety
• Tremor	• Tachycardia	• Agitation
• Myoclonus	• Tachypnea	• Confusion
• Ocular clonus	• Abdominal pain	• Hallucinations
• Hypertonia	• Diarrhea	• Delirium
• Rigidity	• Diaphoresis	• Hyperreactivity
	• Flushing	• Disorientation
	• Mydriasis	
	• Hyper- or hypotension	

BOX 14.8 Hunter Serotonin Toxicity Criteria: Decisions Rules

In the presence of serotonergic agent:
1. IF (spontaneous clonus = yes) THEN serotonin toxicity = YES
2. OR ELSE IF (inducible clonus = yes) AND {(agitation = yes) OR (diaphoresis = yes)} THEN serotonin toxicity = YES
3. OR ELSE IF (ocular clonus = yes) AND {(agitation = yes) OR (diaphoresis = yes)} THEN serotonin toxicity = YES
4. OR ELSE IF (tremor = yes) AND (hyperreflexia = yes) THEN serotonin toxicity = YES
5. OR ELSE IF (hypertonic = yes) AND (temperature > 38°C) AND {(ocular clonus=yes) OR (inducible clonus = yes)} THEN serotonin toxicity = YES
6. OR ELSE serotonin toxicity = NO

From Dunkley EJ, et al. The Hunter serotonin toxicity criteria: simple and accurate diagnostic decision rules for serotonin toxicity. *QJM.* 2003;96(9):635–642.

increase the minimum alveolar concentration (MAC) of the inhalation anesthetics. Increased peripheral catecholamines may produce exaggerated responses to indirect acting pressors such as ephedrine. This exaggerated response is prevalent upon initial TCA administration and lasts for 4 to 6 weeks. After the initial catecholamine increase, receptor down-regulation and depleted catecholamine stores result in a lesser response. If a vasopressor is administered, a direct-acting drug such as phenylephrine is preferred.[79,80]

Monoamine Oxidase Inhibitors

The MAOIs were widely used as antidepressants prior to the introduction of SSRIs, which have a greater safety profile. They are now used only when other first-line treatments are ineffective due to risk of drug and food interactions eliciting a hypertensive crisis, the risk of serotonin syndrome, and difficulty with proper dosing. The inhibition of monoamine oxidase leads to central and peripheral increases in norepinephrine, serotonin, and dopamine, producing a sympathomimetic action in nerve terminals. Monoamine oxidase has two subtypes: MAO-A and MAO-B. MAO-A preferentially metabolizes serotonin, norepinephrine, and epinephrine. MAO-B preferentially metabolizes phenylethylamine. Platelets contain exclusively MAO-A and the placenta exclusively MAO-B. Approximately 60% of human brain MAO activity is of the A subtype.[79]

Severe cases of serotonin syndrome have been reported in patients treated with MAOIs who took over-the-counter dextromethorphan, the illegal methylenedioxymethamphetamine (Ecstasy), or who started treatment with serotonin reuptake inhibitors, meperidine, or atypical antipsychotics such as aripiprazole.

Due to the risk of serotonin syndrome, serotonergic drugs and MAOIs should not be used together or within 2 weeks of each other. Some drugs with MAOI activity, such as the antimicrobial agent linezolid (Zyvox), and some serotonergic drugs, such as the cough suppressant dextromethorphan, sumatriptan (Imitrex, and generics), tramadol (Ultram, and generics), methadone, and St. John's wort, may not be recognized as serotonergic but can cause serotonin syndrome when taken concurrently with an SSRI or SNRI.[60,61]

The use of meperidine in a patient treated with MAOIs may result in a long-recognized drug interaction, which may produce agitation, headache, skeletal muscle rigidity, hyperpyrexia, and death.[71] An increase in serotonin activity in the brain is presumed to be responsible for excitatory reactions evoked by meperidine. Meperidine and other phenylpiperidines are inhibitors of neuronal serotonin uptake. Slowed breakdown of meperidine due to N-demethylase inhibition by

used adjunct analgesics in the management of both neuropathic and somatic chronic pain. Amitriptyline is the prototype antidepressant used in this context. In general, pain relief may be expected in 7 to 14 days. The TCAs commonly cause anticholinergic effects (urinary retention, constipation, dry mouth, blurred vision, and confusion), orthostatic hypotension, weight gain, sedation, and sexual dysfunction. They can cause cardiac conduction delay, which can lead to arrhythmias. Amitriptyline should be avoided in patients with a history of heart disease (conduction disorders, arrhythmias, or heart failure) and closed-angle glaucoma. Many clinicians routinely get a baseline ECG for patients taking TCAs to screen for long QT syndrome prior to surgery.

Patients treated with TCAs may have altered responses to anesthesia-related drugs. An increase in CNS catecholamine levels may

MAOIs is the presumed explanation for hypotension and depression of ventilation. There is evidence that meperidine toxicity is increased only when both MAO-A and MAO-B are inhibited. Derivatives of meperidine (fentanyl, sufentanil, alfentanil) have been associated with adverse reactions in patients treated with MAOIs, although the incidence seems to be less than with meperidine. Morphine does not inhibit uptake of serotonin, but its opioid effects may be potentiated in the presence of MAOIs.[71,79]

In the past, these drugs were discontinued prior to surgery; however, the safest approach is to continue these drugs and adjust the anesthetic plan to make changes such as avoiding meperidine and indirect-acting vasopressors. An exaggerated hypertensive response to administration of an indirect-acting vasopressor such as ephedrine may occur. If needed, the use of a low-dose direct-acting agent such as phenylephrine is preferred. Details regarding a patient's MAOI use must be clearly communicated to health care providers on the day of the surgical procedure.[60,61]

Serotonin Norepinephrine Reuptake Inhibitors

The SNRIs are given for major depression, anxiety, and other mood disorders, as well as chronic neuropathic pain, particularly pain associated with diabetic peripheral neuropathy. The effects of SNRIs are mediated via increases in levels of serotonin and norepinephrine in the brain. Side effects are similar to SSRIs but may also include increased sweating, tachycardia, and urinary retention. Severe discontinuation symptoms can occur when these drugs are stopped, especially with venlafaxine and desvenlafaxine, because of their short half-lives. SNRIs can cause a dose-dependent increase in blood pressure. Blood pressure should be under control before starting an SNRI and monitored during treatment.[60,61]

Lithium

Several drugs are used for the treatment of bipolar disorder, including antipsychotics, anticonvulsants, and lithium. Lithium is generally the drug of choice for maintenance treatment of bipolar disorder. Anticonvulsant drugs such as valproate, carbamazepine, or lamotrigine, or a second-generation antipsychotic such as risperidone, are frequently added. Common adverse effects of lithium include tremor, thirst, polyuria, edema, and weight gain. Confusion and ataxia can occur. Toxic renal effects, including tubular lesions, interstitial fibrosis, and decreased creatinine clearance, have been reported with long-term use of lithium. Nephrogenic diabetes insipidus can occur; it further increases the risk of lithium toxicity and may be irreversible. Hypothyroidism can occur with long-term lithium treatment and can contribute to exacerbations of bipolar illness. Lithium may cause mild leukocytosis, induce or exacerbate psoriasis, and cause severe acne, folliculitis, hair loss, and other skin reactions. Many commonly used drugs, including most nonsteroidal antiinflammatory drugs (but not aspirin), angiotensin-converting enzyme inhibitors, and diuretics, can increase serum lithium concentrations and should be avoided if possible. Discontinuation of lithium has also been associated with suicide.[61]

Lithium has a narrow therapeutic window and requires careful monitoring. Serum lithium concentrations should be monitored every 3 months (every 6–12 months in a stable patient) to maintain serum concentrations within the therapeutic range and avoid toxicity. Concentrations should be measured approximately 12 hours after the last dose. For acute treatment, target serum concentrations are 0.8 to 1.2 mEq/L. For maintenance, serum concentrations should be between 0.6 and 1.0 mEq/L. Thyroid and renal function should be monitored at baseline and every 6 months. Patients taking lithium require evaluation of electrolytes, blood urea nitrogen (BUN), and creatinine. In addition to laboratory monitoring, patients should be monitored for clinical signs of toxicity such as vomiting, diarrhea, tremor, lethargy, slurred speech, and weakness. Liver function and complete blood counts should be monitored in patients taking valproate. Complete blood counts should be monitored in patients taking carbamazepine.[60,61]

Due to its ability to replace sodium in the propagation of action potentials, lithium prolongs the duration of several nondepolarizing neuromuscular agents. Additionally, due to its blocking of the release of epinephrine and norepinephrine from the brainstem, lithium reduces the MAC of the inhalation agents.[60,81]

Antipsychotics

Patients with schizophrenia and other serious mental illnesses are at increased risk for perioperative complications. The increased complications are associated with comorbid physical disorders, hazardous health behaviors, impaired stress response, antipsychotic medications, and potential interactions between antipsychotics and anesthetic drugs. Studies suggest that patients with schizophrenia may have higher pain thresholds, higher rates of death, and postoperative complications such as confusion and ileus. Patients with schizophrenia experience more postoperative confusion, delirium, and agitation when psychiatric medications are discontinued preoperatively. They also have increased difficulty reestablishing their proper medication schedule postoperatively. It is suggested that patients with chronic schizophrenia continue their antipsychotics preoperatively.[82–86]

The antipsychotics include two major classes: dopamine receptor antagonists and serotonin-dopamine antagonists. The first-generation drugs are also referred to as typical antipsychotics and include the phenothiazines, thioxanthenes, and butyrophenones. They block dopamine receptors in the basal ganglia and limbic portions of the forebrain. The dopamine receptor antagonists, haloperidol and fluphenazine, tend to cause extrapyramidal symptoms or parkinsonian syndrome and induce few autonomic actions such as ileus and hypotension. Chlorpromazine and thioridazine tend to cause confusion and hypotension. All first-generation antipsychotic drugs have been associated with sexual dysfunction, hyperprolactinemia, neuroleptic malignant syndrome, and tardive dyskinesia. Their antidopamine actions make them effective antiemetics.

The second generation of atypical antipsychotics are serotonin-dopamine receptor antagonists or have other mechanisms. Second-generation antipsychotics have a relatively low risk of extrapyramidal effects and are probably less likely than first-generation antipsychotics to cause tardive dyskinesia and neuroleptic malignant syndrome. Some second-generation drugs, particularly clozapine, olanzapine, and quetiapine, cause more weight gain than others. The FDA requires the manufacturers of all second-generation antipsychotics to include product-label warnings about hyperglycemia and diabetes and about an increased risk of death among elderly patients with dementia. Second-generation antipsychotics are now used more commonly than first-generation drugs, even though controlled trials have failed to demonstrate a clear advantage in efficacy with the newer drugs, except for clozapine and possibly olanzapine. Clozapine is the most effective antipsychotic drug, but it should be reserved for refractory disease because of its potential for serious hematologic toxicity and strict monitoring requirements.

Anesthesia management consists of avoiding hypotension during induction due to additive depression of the anesthetic drugs. A baseline ECG to assess QT interval prolongation may be helpful. Other considerations include a tendency to have a history of seizure disorders, elevated liver enzymes, and abnormal temperature regulation.[61,82–86]

SUMMARY

Anesthesia providers must be aware of potent physiologic reactions that can occur with various medications that patients routinely take every day. Even though they are not anesthetic drugs, an understanding of the potential drug interactions is essential for providing a safe anesthetic. As increasing numbers of nonanesthetic drugs are developed, knowledge about their mechanism of action and effects is mandatory.

REFERENCES

For a complete list of references for this chapter, scan this QR code with any smartphone code reader app, or visit the following URL: http://booksite.elsevier.com/9780323711944/.

15

Chemistry and Physics of Anesthesia

Sarah E. Giron

The foundation of anesthesia practice is scaffolded by an elegant framework of chemical and physical science. Chemistry is the study of the composition, properties, and structure of matter at the atomic and molecular levels, and it describes how matter behaves when it reacts with other matter. Physics is a field of study that describes the motion, mechanics, force, and energy of matter, and it examines how matter behaves through space and time. Taken together, these complex fields explain such actions as pressure, flow, diffusion, expansion, contraction, and other processes that are intimately intertwined with the delivery of anesthetics. From the ancient philosophic beginnings of atomic theory and the proverbial falling apple of newtonian physics (Sir Isaac Newton, 1642–1727), to current advances in quantum mechanics and breakthroughs in anesthetic delivery systems, chemistry and physics have led to advances in and application of anesthesiology. To understand these laws and theories is to understand the how and why of anesthesia practice; it provides rationale for clinical interventions and allows for the manipulation of powerful processes to optimize patient care.

The chemistry and physics of anesthesia are detailed in this chapter primarily by atomic and kinetic molecular theories, newtonian physics, thermodynamics, and the quantum mechanics of electromagnetic radiation. This chapter describes complex theories and how the theories apply to nurse anesthesia practice. Thus this chapter provides a short, concise resource that focuses on the scientific principles guiding modern anesthesia.

GENERAL CHEMISTRY: MATTER AND ENERGY

The universe is composed of two main entities: matter and energy. Matter is the tangible composition of the universe that may be solid, liquid, gas, or plasma. Solids are defined as materials that resist changes in shape and volume. Liquids are fluids that exhibit minimal to no compressibility and may change volume with changes in pressure and temperature. Gases are also fluids but are compressible and easily change volume with changes in pressure and temperature. Energy can be defined as the exertion of force (kinetic energy) or the capacity to do work (potential energy) and will be discussed later in this chapter.

ATOMIC STRUCTURE

Atomic theory has its origins in the philosophic musings of the ancient Greek philosopher Democritus, who described indivisible building blocks of matter as "atomos."[1] The orbital theory of atomic structure was later put forth by Ernesto Rutherford (1871–1937) and improved upon by Neils Bohr (1885–1962), who described electron orbits in terms of energy levels and the ability to emit quantized energy by stimulated emission. The atomic theory describes atoms as having a central core, known as the nucleus, which contains protons and neutrons. The orbiting particles around the nucleus are called electrons (Fig. 15.1) and are negatively charged. Protons have a positive charge and are larger than electrons. Neutrons lack a charge and are similar in size to protons. The number of protons in an atom constitutes its atomic number and uniquely identifies the atom as a chemical element; atomic numbers are most commonly seen to organize and classify elements in the periodic table of elements and are denoted by the top number in each element box (Fig. 15.2).

Electron Configuration

Atoms have electrons that orbit in shells around the nucleus. Each shell can contain only a set number of electrons. Electrons must fill lower shells before occupying higher shells. Quantum physics has refined the electron shell model by designating the shells with n-values 1, 2, 3, 4, 5, 6, and 7, which correspond with increasing energy levels. Electron shells are further divided into subshells with the designations s, p, d, f, and g. These subshells may hold only 2, 6, 10, 14, and 18 electrons, respectively. Subshells are further subdivided into orbitals. Orbitals may contain only two electrons that spin in opposite directions. An s subshell has 1 orbital, a p subshell has 3 orbitals, a d subshell has 5 orbitals, and so forth. Electrons occupy lower energy level orbitals but may temporarily jump to higher level orbitals when they absorb energy. Electrons that jump to higher levels will emit their excess energy and return to their lower energy state (see "Lasers" later in this chapter). Thus for an element like nitrogen that has an atomic number of 7, an atom of nitrogen will have 7 protons and 7 electrons. The electron configuration for ground state (nonionic) nitrogen is $1s^2 2s^2 2p^3$. Notice how the superscript numbers equal the total number of electrons or the atomic number (Fig. 15.3).

Angular Momentum/Spin

Nuclei and electrons have an angular momentum known as spin. Atomic particles possess an intrinsic axis upon which they rotate (or spin), which is analogous to the axis on which the Earth rotates. The spin of an electron or proton is not directly measurable, but the uneven distribution of charge it produces is measurable. A magnetic moment is created, which is essentially a minute electric current loop (see "Magnetic Resonance Imaging" later in this chapter).

Ions

Ions are atoms that have gained or lost electrons from their natural composition. An atom that has gained one or more electrons is called an anion and is more negatively charged. An example of an anion would be a chloride anion, written as Cl^-. Conversely, an atom that has lost one or more electrons is called a cation and is more positively charged. An example of a cation would be a potassium cation, written as K^+. Ions are important in chemical bonding and aqueous solubility. The mass number (or atomic mass number) is the number of protons and neutrons in an atom and is denoted as the bottom number in the

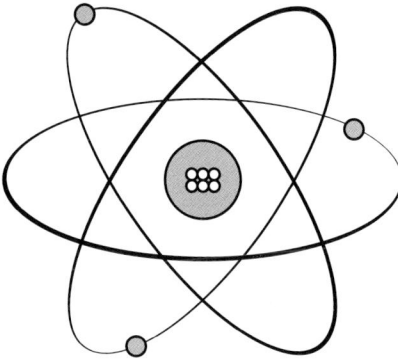

Fig. 15.1 Atomic structure showing nucleus containing protons and neutrons with orbiting electrons.

periodic table of elements (see Fig. 15.2). Isotopes of the same element have the same number of protons but different numbers of neutrons and therefore have different mass numbers.

MOLECULAR BOND TYPES

Molecules are composed of two or more bonded atoms. Electrons in the outermost shell are called valence electrons and are involved in molecular bonding. Molecular bonding may occur by direct sharing of electrons or by thermodynamic interaction due to the distribution of the electron charge. Atoms with unpaired valence electrons are reactive and tend to form bonds that will fill their outer shells. Covalent bonds and electrostatic bonds are two general types of bonds. Atoms may bond to atoms of the same element (e.g., oxygen [O_2]) or to different element atoms (e.g., water [H_2O]). When atoms of differing elements are bonded they are referred to as compounds.

Covalent Bonds

The physical sharing of electrons between atoms constitutes a covalent bond. The sharing of one pair of electrons is called a single bond, sharing two pairs of electrons is a double bond, and sharing three pairs of electrons is a triple bond. Often covalent bonds are stronger than electrostatic bonds. Covalent bonding may be between same or different atoms that share similar electronegativity.

Electrostatic Bonds

Electrostatic bonds are made by the attraction of electrons between atoms due to electron distribution. Electrostatic bonding may include ion-to-ion interactions, ion-to-dipole interactions, or dipole-to-dipole interactions and follows the general rule of "opposites attract," with negative charges attracting positive charges.

Ion-Ion Bonding

Ion-to-ion bonds are the strongest of the electrostatic bonds. These bonds are not directional and occur anywhere along the outer electron shell of an atom. Molecules with ionic bonds have high melting and boiling points. Sodium chloride (table salt) is an example of ion-to-ion bonding (Fig. 15.4).

Ion-Dipole Bonding

Ion-to-dipole bonds are weaker than ion-to-ion bonds, with only partial charges involved. Some molecules have structural arrangements that produce an uneven distribution of electrons. This uneven distribution of charges creates a dipole in which there is a more positive or more negative side to the molecule, although the molecule does not have a formal charge. An example of a molecule with an uneven charge distribution is water. The spatial arrangement of water's hydrogens toward one side of an oxygen atom causes that side to have a more positive character and the opposite side to have a more negative character. This water dipole may bond to an ion of opposite charge. Sodium and chlorine ions bond to water through ion-to-dipole interactions (Fig. 15.5).

Dipole-Dipole Bonding

Water is an example of dipole-to-dipole molecular bonding. The spatial arrangement of water's hydrogens at a 105-degree angle to each other causes this molecule to be dipolar (Fig. 15.6). The dipolar nature of water molecules allows them to form weak bonds with one another (Fig. 15.7). The polar sides of water molecules also enable them to bond to ions and other polar molecules. For this reason, water is a convenient solvent for many substances, such as drugs. The surface tension of water is a physical characteristic that is caused by water's dipole-to-dipole intermolecular attractions.

Some molecules may have induced dipoles caused by momentary uneven spatial distribution of electrons. Induced dipoles are not permanent. These temporary dipoles may lead to weak bonding between nonpolar molecules. Oils are composed of nonpolar molecules that display induced dipole bonding, often called London dispersion forces. London dispersion forces are the weakest of all molecular bonds. Despite this weakness, London dispersion forces at very low temperatures allow oxygen and nitrogen to become liquids.

Molecular Bonding Representations

There are several ways to denote bonding and electron distribution. The Lewis structure (electron dot structure) shows the valence electrons as they bond among atoms. Lewis structures may show dots or lines to represent electrons. Again, only outer shell valence electrons are represented and not lower, fully filled shells. Skeletal diagrams are another frequently used method to represent molecular bonding. In organic chemistry, skeletal diagrams use lines to show atom bonding, often omitting the letter C for carbon (Fig. 15.8).

Valence shell electron pair repulsion diagrams are more descriptive Lewis structures based on the theory of the same name. These diagrams represent electron repulsion and the resultant approximation of the geometric distribution of atoms in covalently bonded molecules (Fig. 15.9).

Molecular Modeling

Molecular models are detailed representations of molecules. Electrons are in constant orbit in an atom, and attempts have been made to graphically represent their possible space-occupying locations (Fig. 15.10). Space-filling models reflect the electron cloud of specific atoms in a molecule. These models can appear as spheric, ball and stick, or ribbonlike representations of atoms and molecules that are affixed to one another. Molecular modeling therefore expands the understanding of both molecular geometries and molecular behavior.[2]

Isomers

Isomers are molecules that have the same chemical formula but different structures. The number and type of atoms and bonds are the same in isomers, but the arrangement of the atoms is different. Isomers may be structural isomers or stereoisomers. Structural isomers have the same molecular formula, but their atoms are located in different places. Enflurane and isoflurane are examples of structural isomers. Structural isomers are truly different molecules with differing physical and chemical properties. Stereoisomers are molecules that have a similar geometric arrangement of atoms but differ in their spatial position. Stereoisomers may be enantiomers or diastereomers. Enantiomers are

PERIODIC TABLE OF THE ELEMENTS

																	2 **He** 4.002602 Helium
1 **H** 1.00794 Hydrogen																	
3 **Li** 6.941 Lithium	4 **Be** 9.012182 Beryllium											5 **B** 10.811 Boron	6 **C** 12.0107 Carbon	7 **N** 14.0067 Nitrogen	8 **O** 15.9994 Oxygen	9 **F** 18.9984032 Fluorine	10 **Ne** 20.1797 Neon
11 **Na** 22.989770 Sodium	12 **Mg** 24.3050 Magnesium											13 **Al** 26.981538 Aluminium	14 **Si** 28.0855 Silicon	15 **P** 30.973761 Phosphorus	16 **S** 32.065 Sulfur	17 **Cl** 35.453 Chlorine	18 **Ar** 39.948 Argon
19 **K** 39.0983 Potassium	20 **Ca** 40.078 Calcium	21 **Sc** 44.955910 Scandium	22 **Ti** 47.867 Titanium	23 **V** 50.9415 Vanadium	24 **Cr** 51.9961 Chromium	25 **Mn** 54.938049 Manganese	26 **Fe** 55.845 Iron	27 **Co** 58.933200 Cobalt	28 **Ni** 58.6934 Nickel	29 **Cu** 63.546 Copper	30 **Zn** 65.409 Zinc	31 **Ga** 69.723 Gallium	32 **Ge** 72.64 Germanium	33 **As** 74.92160 Arsenic	34 **Se** 78.96 Selenium	35 **Br** 79.904 Bromine	36 **Kr** 83.798 Krypton
37 **Rb** 85.4678 Rubidium	38 **Sr** 87.62 Strontium	39 **Y** 88.90585 Yttrium	40 **Zr** 91.224 Zirconium	41 **Nb** 92.90638 Niobium	42 **Mo** 95.94 Molybdenum	43 **Tc** (98) Technetium	44 **Ru** 101.07 Ruthenium	45 **Rh** 102.90550 Rhodium	46 **Pd** 106.42 Palladium	47 **Ag** 107.8682 Silver	48 **Cd** 112.411 Cadmium	49 **In** 114.818 Indium	50 **Sn** 118.710 Tin	51 **Sb** 121.760 Antimony	52 **Te** 127.60 Tellurium	53 **I** 126.90447 Iodine	54 **Xe** 131.293 Xenon
55 **Cs** 132.90545 Caesium	56 **Ba** 137.327 Barium	57* **La** 138.9055 Lanthanum	72 **Hf** 178.49 Hafnium	73 **Ta** 180.9479 Tantalum	74 **W** 183.84 Tungsten	75 **Re** 186.207 Rhenium	76 **Os** 190.23 Osmium	77 **Ir** 192.217 Iridium	78 **Pt** 195.078 Platinum	79 **Au** 196.96655 Gold	80 **Hg** 200.59 Mercury	81 **Tl** 204.3833 Thallium	82 **Pb** 207.2 Lead	83 **Bi** 208.98038 Bismuth	84 **Po** (209) Polonium	85 **At** (210) Astatine	86 **Rn** (222) Radon
87 **Fr** (223) Francium	88 **Ra** (226) Radium	89** **Ac** (227) Actinium	104 **Rf** (261) Rutherfordium	105 **Db** (262) Dubnium	106 **Sg** (266) Seaborgium	107 **Bh** (264) Bohrium	108 **Hs** (277) Hassium	109 **Mt** (268) Meitnerium	110 **Ds** (271) Darmstadtium	111 **Rg** (272) Roentgenium	112 **Cn** (285) Copernicium	113 **Nh** (286) Nihonium	114 **Fl** (289) Flerovium	115 **Mc** (289) Moscovium	116 **Lv** (293) Livermorium	117 **Ts** (294) Tennessine	118 **Og** (294) Oganesson

58 **Ce** 140.116 Cerium	59 **Pr** 140.90765 Praseodymium	60 **Nd** 144.24 Neodymium	61 **Pm** (145) Promethium	62 **Sm** 150.36 Samarium	63 **Eu** 151.964 Europium	64 **Gd** 157.25 Gadolinium	65 **Tb** 158.92534 Terbium	66 **Dy** 162.500 Dysprosium	67 **Ho** 164.93032 Holmium	68 **Er** 167.259 Erbium	69 **Tm** 168.93421 Thulium	70 **Yb** 173.04 Ytterbium	71 **Lu** 174.967 Lutetium
90 **Th** 232.0381 Thorium	91 **Pa** 231.03588 Protactinium	92 **U** 238.02891 Uranium	93 **Np** (237) Neptunium	94 **Pu** (244) Plutonium	95 **Am** (243) Americium	96 **Cm** (247) Curium	97 **Bk** (247) Berkelium	98 **Cf** (251) Californium	99 **Es** (252) Einsteinium	100 **Fm** (257) Fermium	101 **Md** (258) Mendelevium	102 **No** (259) Nobelium	103 **Lr** (262) Lawrencium

Atomic Number → 1
                 H → Symbol
                 1.00794 → Atomic Weight
                 Hydrogen → Name

Fig. 15.2 The periodic table of elements.

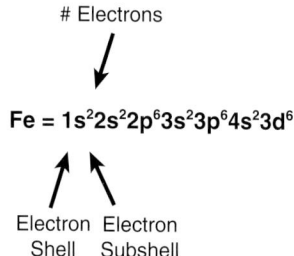

Fig. 15.3 Electron configuration of ground state (nonionic) iron (Fe).

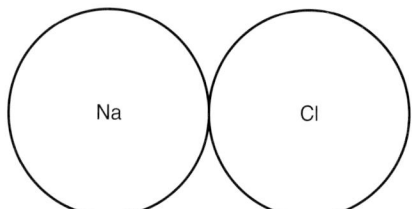

Fig. 15.4 Ion-to-ion bond representation between sodium (Na^+) and chloride (Cl^-) ions.

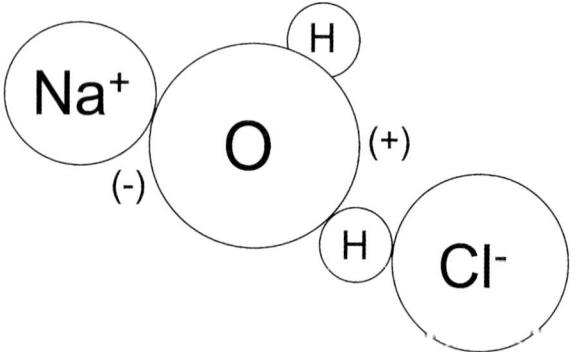

Fig. 15.5 Ion-to-dipole bond representation between a water molecule and sodium ion.

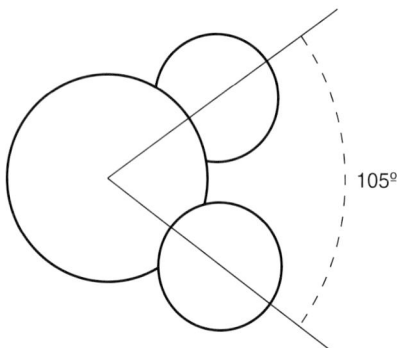

Fig. 15.6 Bond angle between two hydrogens and a water molecule.

mirror images of one another, cannot be superimposed, and possess similar chemical and physical properties. Enantiomers are optically active and can rotate polarized light in a clockwise fashion (denoted by the prefix + or *dextro*) or counterclockwise fashion (denoted by the prefix – or *levo*). Racemic chemical compositions contain 50% of the levo form of the isomer and 50% of the dextro form of the isomer. Racemic epinephrine used to treat laryngeal edema is an example of a racemic mixture. Diastereomers are not mirror images and may have differing physical and chemical properties.

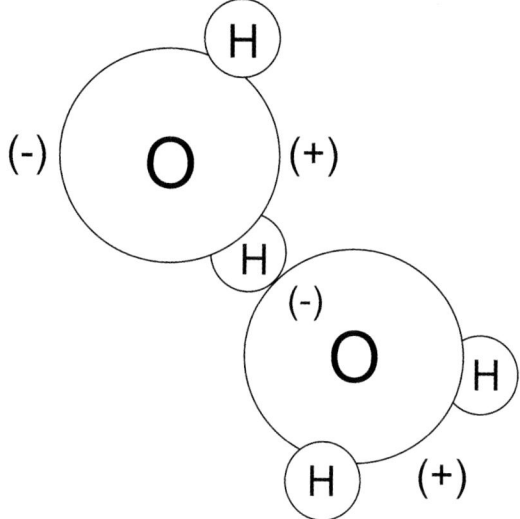

Fig. 15.7 Dipole-to-dipole bond representation between two water molecules.

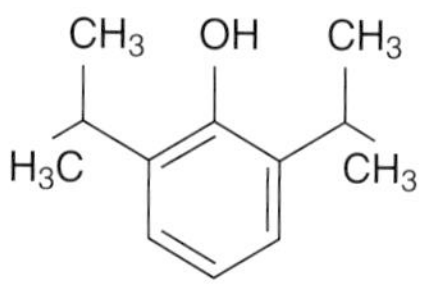

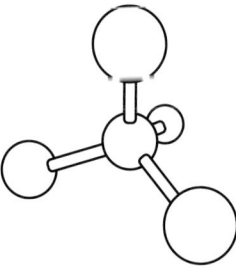

Fig. 15.8 Skeletal diagram of 2,6-diisopropylphenol molecule.

Fig. 15.9 Valence shell electron pair repulsion (VSEPR) diagram of a tetrahedral-shaped molecule.

BOND BREAKING

Bond energy is the amount of energy needed to make or break a bond. Energy is released when a bond is formed, and energy is consumed when a bond is broken. The energy released when a bond is formed is the same amount of energy required to break that same chemical bond. Short bonds, such as covalent bonds, tend to possess greater bond energies than longer, electrostatic bonds. When molecular bonds are broken, new molecular bonds are often formed, and energy is released. An example of this is adenosine triphosphate (ATP) conversion to adenosine diphosphate. Energy is consumed in the process of breaking an ATP bond. A greater amount of energy is released when the free phosphate forms new bonds with hydrogen.[3] Bond energies are measured as an enthalpy change (ΔH; see next section).

Enthalpy

Enthalpy is the total amount of energy possessed by a system. A system can be on the atomic scale or the macroscopic scale. The enthalpy of a system is the total of all kinetic and potential energy. The stored, or potential, energy includes its height in relation to the force of gravity

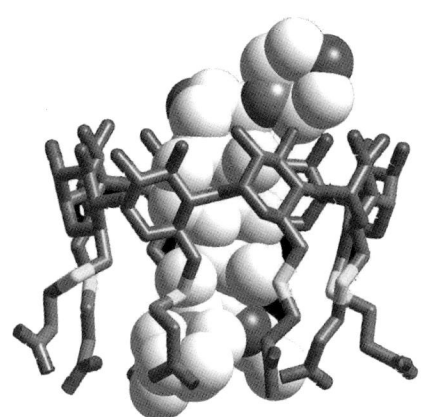

Fig. 15.10 Molecular model of sugammadex encapsulating a rocuronium molecule. (From Zhang M-Q, et al. A novel concept of reversing neuromuscular block: chemical encapsulation of rocuronium bromide by a cyclodextrin-based synthetic host. *Angew Chem Int Ed.* 2002;41(2):265. Reproduced with permission.)

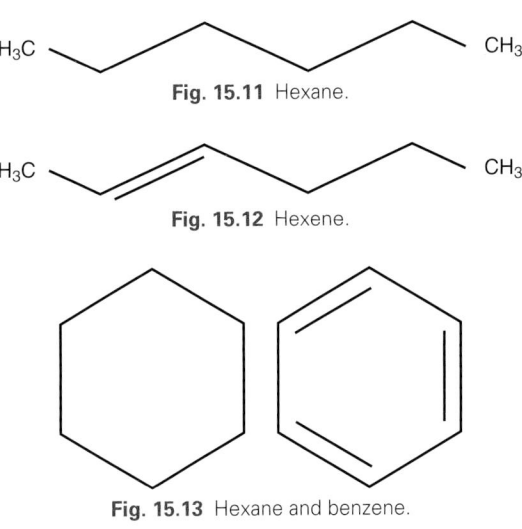

Fig. 15.11 Hexane.

Fig. 15.12 Hexene.

Fig. 15.13 Hexane and benzene.

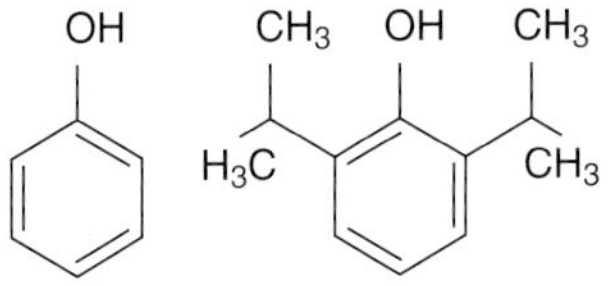

Fig. 15.14 Phenol and 2,6-disopropylphenol molecules.

and the energy stored in the bonds of its molecules, atoms, and even subatomic particles. All movement, as well as stored energy, must be accounted for and summated to know the enthalpy of a system. Thus the total amount of energy contained within a system becomes increasingly difficult to quantify, especially as the complexity of the system increases. Measuring all the energy in a particular system requires a simpler method to evaluate the energy involved in chemical reactions. Therefore, change of energy (ΔH) rather than total energy (enthalpy) of a system is measured.

ORGANIC COMPOUNDS

Organic chemistry is the study of carbon-containing molecules, and it is fitting that nurse anesthetists be familiar with this field since all biologic life on Earth is based on carbon-containing compounds. Carbon is a unique atom that combines with many atoms in multiple arrangements, owing to its four valence electrons available for bonding. Carbon may make single, double, or triple covalent bonds with other atoms or molecules.

Hydrocarbons

Hydrocarbons are molecules composed entirely of carbon and hydrogen atoms. These molecules are often found in straight chains with or without branches. Saturated hydrocarbons are single-bonded carbon chains with all available carbon bonds attached to hydrogen. Hydrocarbons containing only single-bonded carbon atoms are called alkanes. The six-carbon hydrocarbon shown in Fig. 15.11 is called a hexane. The *hex-* prefix denotes six carbons, and the *-ane* suffix denotes an alkane with all single bonds. Any other groups that are attached to the hydrocarbon are substituents or functional groups.

Unsaturated hydrocarbons have one or more double or triple bonds between carbon atoms. Hydrocarbons containing double-bonded carbons are called alkenes, and triple-bonded carbons are called alkynes. The six-carbon hydrocarbon containing a double bond is called hexene (Fig. 15.12).

Cyclic hydrocarbons are carbon chains in a ring structure. They may contain multiple carbon atoms and may have single, double, or triple bonds. Naming of cyclic hydrocarbons is done by first determining the parent chain (the cyclic hydrocarbon with the greatest number of carbons), then determining alkyl groups, and any substituent or functional groups. Next, the carbons are numbered such that the carbons with functional groups or substituents have the lowest possible

number. Then the functional groups and substituents are placed in alphabetic order with a dash (-) placed between the number and name of each substituent. The cyclic hydrocarbons hexane and benzene (1,3,5-cyclohexatriene) are shown in Fig. 15.13.

Saturated and unsaturated hydrocarbons that are missing hydrogens are known as alkyls, are very reactive, and bond to functional groups. Cyclic hydrocarbons that are missing a hydrogen on any carbon atom are called aryls, are reactive, and bind with functional groups.

Functional Groups

Functional groups impart unique characteristics to molecules. There are many functional groups in organic chemistry, and several have importance in anesthesia.

Amines are derivatives of ammonia (NH_3) and have the general formula NR_3. Only one or two of the R groups may be hydrogen. All amines have a lone pair of electrons on the nitrogen.

Alcohols have the general formula ROH, where R represents any alkyl group. The hydroxyl group (OH) of alcohols is highly polar and easily forms hydrogen bonds with other polar molecules. The polarity of the hydroxyl group allows alcohols to dissolve many other polar molecules.

Phenols are similar to alcohols in that they both have the general formula ROH. The R in phenols represents an aryl group (benzene). A simple phenol is polar due to the hydroxyl group, but more complex phenols such as propofol (2,6-diisopropylphenol) are not water soluble (Fig. 15.14).

Ethers have the general formula ROR′, where R and R′ are alkyl groups attached by oxygen. Ethers are inert and do not react with oxidizing or reducing agents, but they are highly flammable. Both alkyl groups of the outdated anesthetic agent diethyl ether are bonded to oxygen (Fig. 15.15). Halogen substitution on ethers alters anesthetic characteristics (such as blood solubility and potency) while lowering flammability.

Several functional groups contain a structural arrangement of carbon double bonded to oxygen. This is known as a carbonyl group and is structurally identified as C=O. The carbonyl group is polar, with the oxygen

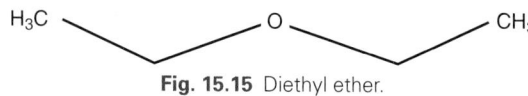

Fig. 15.15 Diethyl ether.

being more electrically negative. This polar characteristic is imparted to functional groups that contain a carbonyl group. The carbonyl group, though not a functional group by itself, is a key component of the following functional groups: aldehydes, ketones, carboxylic acids, esters, and amides.

- Aldehydes have the general formula RCHO.
- Ketones have the general formula RCOR′.
- Carboxylic acids have the general formula RCOOH.
- Esters have the general formula RCOOR.
- Amides have the general formula $RCONH_2$, RCONHR, or $RCONR_2$.

SOLUBILITY

Solubility is the maximum amount of one substance (solute) that is able to dissolve into another (solvent). Factors that may affect the solubility of solutes in solvents are the intermolecular interactions between the substances, temperature, and pressure.

Solids and Liquids

Solubility is enhanced by intermolecular interactions between substances that have similar electron configurations. "Like dissolves like" is often used to describe solubility. Salt (NaCl) solubility in water is an example. The similar polarity of water and salt's constituent parts promote dissolving. Temperature also affects solubility. Energy is required to break the bonds of dissolving substances. Most often this is an endothermic reaction, meaning it requires more energy than it produces; it consumes heat rather than produces heat. With endothermic reactions, solubility is increased with increased temperature; the additional energy (heat) drives greater dissolving. Most reactions of solids dissolving in liquids are endothermic. Occasionally the process may be exothermic, meaning energy is released in excess of the energy required to break the bonds of the solute. In this unique scenario, increases in temperature will decrease solubility. Pressure exerts little to no influence on the solubility of solids and liquids.

Gases

Gas solubility in liquids is inversely related to temperature. As temperature increases, less gas is able to dissolve into a liquid. An increased temperature represents greater kinetic energy. Greater kinetic energy allows dissolved gas molecules to escape and prevents further dissolving. Lower temperature slows the kinetic energy of gas molecules, allowing them to dissolve into liquids. A clinical example of temperature affecting solubility is seen with the slower emergence of hypothermic patients receiving volatile agent general anesthetics. The hypothermic patient retains anesthetic gases in the blood because of increased solubility related to temperature.[4] Gas solubility in a liquid is directly proportional to pressure and is described by Henry's law.[5]

Henry's Law

Henry's law (William Henry, 1775–1836) states that "at constant temperature, the amount of gas dissolved in a liquid is directly proportional to the partial pressure of that gas at equilibrium above the gas-liquid interface." The formula is as follows:

$$p = kc$$

where p is the partial pressure of the solute above the solution, k is Henry's constant, and c is the concentration of the solute in solution.

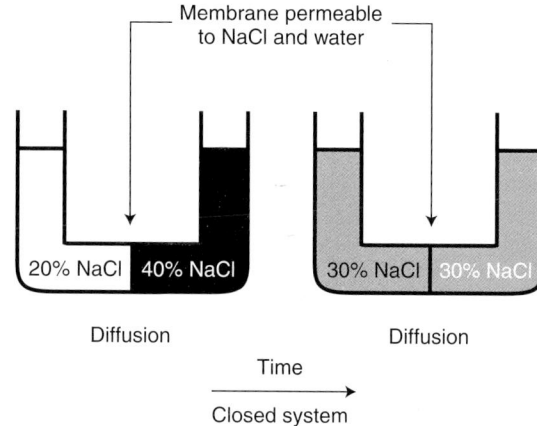

Fig. 15.16 Diffusion of water and NaCl.

Increasing the partial pressure of a gas above a liquid will increase the amount of gas that dissolves in the liquid. Increasing oxygen delivery (by raising Fio_2 %) to patients to improve arterial oxygenation (Pao_2) and overpressurizing (i.e., using high concentrations of) volatile anesthetics reflect the direct relationship of pressure and solubility described by Henry's law. With both administering high Fio_2 and in overpressurizing, the process of significantly increasing the concentration of oxygen or volatile anesthetic (measured as partial pressures) delivered to a patient increases the alveolar concentration, resulting in an increased amount dissolved in the blood and a faster uptake.

DIFFUSION

Diffusion is the net movement of one type of molecule through space as a result of random motion to minimize a concentration gradient (Fig. 15.16). This basic process occurs by brownian (Robert Brown, 1773–1858) motion, which is driven by the inherent kinetic energy of the molecules.[6] Temperature is directly proportional to kinetic energy. Kinetic energy allows molecules to move freely in a fluid, and therefore mixtures of fluids tend to evenly distribute. The velocity at which a molecule may distribute is determined by its molecular weight. Every molecule at a given temperature will have the same kinetic energy, independent of its size, but its velocity may differ. From the formula for kinetic energy, $KE = (1/2) mv^2$, it is determined that, if the mass of a molecule is changed, there must be an opposite change in velocity. Greater velocity correlates with faster diffusion. Thus molecules with smaller mass will diffuse faster.

Graham's Law

Thomas Graham (1805–1869) determined that the rate of effusion (gas diffusion through an orifice) of a gas is inversely proportional to the square root of its molecular weight. The formula for this relationship is as follows:

$$r = 1/\sqrt{mw}$$

where r is the rate of diffusion and mw is the molecular weight. Graham's law describes the faster diffusion of smaller molecules compared to larger molecules and is helpful in understanding the effect of molecular weight on diffusion. However, Graham's law is limited in fully describing all factors influencing diffusion.

Diffusion Through Permeable and Semipermeable Membranes

Diffusion may occur through open space or through permeable membranes (such as tissues). Diffusion of a fluid (gas or liquid) through a

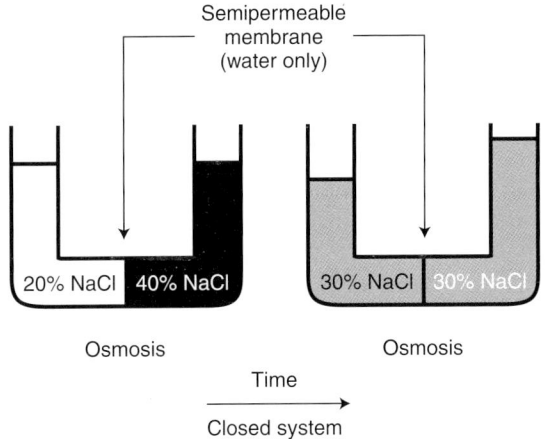

Semipermeable
membrane
(water only)

20% NaCl | 40% NaCl   30% NaCl | 30% NaCl

Osmosis   Osmosis

Time

Closed system

Fig. 15.17 Osmosis of water through a semipermeable membrane.

permeable membrane is dependent on five factors: The concentration gradient, tissue area, and fluid tissue solubility are directly proportional to diffusion; membrane thickness and molecular weight are inversely proportional to diffusion.

Osmosis

Osmosis is the movement of water across a semipermeable membrane to equilibrate a concentration gradient (Fig. 15.17). Semipermeable membranes are permeable to water only and not to solutes. Osmotic pressure is the force needed to stop osmosis from occurring. Oncotic pressure is the osmotic pressure exerted by plasma proteins and electrolytes in capillaries. Oncotic pressure balances the hydrostatic pressure tendency to push water out of capillaries and is approximately 28 mm Hg. Thus the vascular system is a semipermeable membrane that responds to intravascular delivery of colloids by sequestering fluid.[7,8]

Diffusion in Anesthesia

Diffusion is a passive process driven by entropy (discussed later in this chapter). The diffusion of oxygen and nitrous oxide represents both positive and negative consequences of this process. Nitrous oxide diffuses into air-filled cavities, therefore delivery of nitrous oxide is contraindicated in patients with pneumothorax or where air-filled cavity expansion is undesirable.[9] Nitrous oxide administration can cause expansion of endotracheal cuffs that yields tracheal mucosal damage[9–11] and distention of the bowel if administered during certain colorectal surgeries.[12,13] Apneic oxygenation is well known and exemplifies the beneficial process of diffusion.[14] An intubated patient who has previously been ventilated with 100% oxygen and remains connected to the ventilation circuit with 100% oxygen flow will maintain an acceptable PaO_2 if ventilation is ceased. The continual diffusion of oxygen into the blood is driven by a concentration gradient that continually diffuses oxygen into the alveoli via the ventilator circuit. Consequently the diffusion of gases across biologic tissues by Fick's law is discussed next.

Fick's Law

Fick's law for diffusion of a gas across a tissue plane is a law that accounts for molecular weight, concentration gradient, solubility, and membrane interactions. Fick's law states that diffusion of a gas across a semipermeable membrane is directly proportional to the partial pressure gradient, the membrane solubility of the gas, and the membrane area and is inversely proportional to the membrane thickness and the

molecular weight of the gas. Specific application of the Fick equation for diffusion of respiratory gases is as follows:

$$J = \alpha D / \Delta x (PaO_2 - PcapO_2)$$

where J is diffusion flux, α is the solubility constant for oxygen, D is diffusivity, Δx is the membrane thickness, and ($PaO_2 - PcapO_2$) is the alveolar-capillary oxygen partial pressure difference. Fick equation allows determination of pulmonary gas exchange.[15,16] The diffusion hypoxia that occurs upon anesthesia emergence (if nitrous oxide is discontinued and low inspired oxygen is administered to the patient) is explained by Fick equation.[17]

NEWTONIAN PHYSICS

GRAVITY

All life on Earth is well aware of gravity. From our first steps to our last, gravity affects every facet of our daily lives. It is a unidirectional force that pulls objects down toward Earth's center. Gravity appears to pull on heavy objects with greater force than lighter objects, but this is not necessarily true. Aristotle saw gravity this way and felt it was due to an object's desire to return to its natural position at rest on the Earth. It took 2000 years to change that perspective. Gravity pulls on all objects with a force of 9.81 m/sec per sec (32 ft/sec per sec). Sir Isaac Newton's law of gravity stated, "[e]ach particle of matter attracts every other particle with a force which is directly proportional to the product of their masses and inversely proportional to the square of the distance between them." The formula for gravity is:

$$\text{Gravitational force} = (G \times m1 \times m2) / \left(d^2\right)$$

where G is the gravitational constant ($6.67 \times 10^{-11} Nm^2/kg^2$), $m1$ and $m2$ are the masses of the two objects for which you are calculating the force, and d is the distance between the centers of gravity of the two masses. Remember that mass and weight are not the same. Mass is the total of all matter in an object—the sum of the mass of all the electrons, protons, and neutrons. Weight is the total effect of gravity pulling on all the electrons, protons, and neutrons contained in an object. For instance, average humans may weigh 70 kg on Earth due to the gravitational pull on all their atoms, but they would weigh less on the Moon, secondary to the lower gravitational pull. Conversely, the same humans would weigh 2.5 times their Earth weight on Jupiter (if they could stand there) because of a higher gravitational pull. Regardless, a human's mass or total amount of matter remains the same whether on Earth, the Moon, or Jupiter.

$$\text{Mass} \times \text{force of gravity} = \text{weight}$$

The Earth attracts all other objects around it with a force of 9.81 m/sec per sec, and those objects in turn attract the Earth in relation to their mass and distance from the planet. The formula for gravitational acceleration is:

$$g = GM_e / r_e^2$$

where g is gravitational acceleration, G is the gravitational constant, M_e is the mass of Earth, and r_e^2 is the mean radius of Earth. Earth's attraction for objects is proportional to mass for all objects at the same distance. One might want to say that objects with greater mass would accelerate or be pulled faster to Earth, but objects also resist movement proportional to their mass (Newton's second law of motion, the law of acceleration). Gravity pulls on one atom of carbon with a force of 9.81 m/sec per sec, and the mass of a carbon atom resists this pull with a force of x. Gravity pulls on two carbon atoms with a force of 9.81 m/sec per sec on each atom for a total gravitational force of 9.81 m/sec per sec × 2, or 19.62 m/sec per sec. The mass of two carbon atoms resists movement twice (2×) as much as the mass of one carbon atom, thus the net gravitational effect (falling) is the same. This is how objects with greater mass are pulled by gravity with the same force and fall at the same acceleration as objects with lesser mass.

This equal attraction on objects is often hidden in everyday life, owing to the effect of air molecules interacting with falling objects. Assuredly, all objects fall due to gravity at the same speed in a vacuum that is devoid of other molecules. Air molecules possess energy, move about, and interact with other matter. This causes friction. Greater friction equals greater force against the pull of gravity and slowing of a fall, but in a vacuum all objects fall equally at equal velocities.

NEWTON'S LAWS OF MOTION

- Newton's first law (law of inertia): A body in motion tends to stay in motion unless acted upon by another force.
- Newton's second law (law of acceleration): Acceleration of a body is in the direction of and proportional to the force (F), and that acceleration (a) is inversely proportional to the mass (m) of the body, F = ma. If multiple forces exist, the direction and acceleration are proportional to the sum of all the forces. These are called vectors.
- Newton's third law (law of reciprocal action): For every action, there is an equal and opposite reaction; objects exert equal but opposite forces on one another.[18]

FORCE

Force is the amount of energy required to move an object. From the understanding that the force of gravity pulls equally on all objects proportional to mass, a standardization of force became possible. Because we know that gravity pulls (accelerates) all objects with a force of 9.81 m/sec per sec, this force would also be 9.81 m/sec per sec if applied to any given weight. The force of gravity applied to 1 kg of weight creates a standard by which other forces may be compared, quantified, and measured. Thus the force required to accelerate a 1-kg weight 1 m/sec became known as the newton.

The newton is the standard measure of force derived from the force of gravity.

$$newton = 1\ m/sec/sec$$
$$= 1/9.81\ kg\ weight\ or\ 102\ g\ weight$$
$$gravity = 9.81\ m/sec/sec$$

One newton is equivalent to 1/9.81 kg weight or 102 g weight. Force is mass multiplied by acceleration. The formula for force is:

$$F = ma$$

where F is force, m is mass, and a is acceleration. Often the newton is too large a unit to be used to express small measures of force, therefore the dyne is used. A dyne is 1/1000 of a newton. A dyne is the force required to move 1 g of weight 1 cm/sec. Dynes are used in calculating systemic (SVR) and pulmonary vascular resistance (PVR).[19,20]

PVR is the measure of the pulmonary vascular system's resistance to flow from the right ventricle. Normal PVR is 100 to 200 dyne sec/cm^5. SVR is the measure of the peripheral vascular system's resistance to flow that must be overcome for flow to occur. The left ventricle must therefore pump blood with a force greater than the resistance of the vascular system. The formula for calculating SVR is 80 × (MAP − CVP)/CO = SVR, where MAP is mean arterial pressure, CVP is central venous pressure, and CO is cardiac output. Normal SVR is 800 to 1200 dyne sec/cm^5.

Another application of force measurement used in anesthesia is accelerometry, which is used to measure the degree of neuromuscular

blockade.[21,22] Accelerometry uses a piezoelectric disk to generate an electric current in proportion to acceleration (see "Piezoelectric Effect" later in this chapter). An accelerometer measures the acceleration caused by the contraction of a muscle after nerve stimulation. A comparison of baseline stimulated muscle twitches (forces) to twitches suppressed by neuromuscular blocking agents allows for the quantification of the degree of neuromuscular blockade.[23] Accelerometers provide objective twitch data referenced to the patient's baseline twitch response.[24] Visual or tactile assessment of twitch heights is subjective and less reliable than accelerometry.[24,25]

Force is a basic phenomenon of physics that permeates the universe. Because all matter possesses mass, and all mass has some degree of acceleration, force exists everywhere. All forces possess direction. The study of force direction is explored with vectors.

Vectors

Two basic types of values describe our physical world: scalar values and vector values. Scalar values are fully described by magnitude alone; they possess no motion, and they include mass, energy, and work. Vector values are fully described by magnitude and direction. Vectors express motion and are described by force, speed, velocity, acceleration, distance, and displacement. Vector diagrams are scaled representations of vectors, with an arrow starting at a given magnitude and pointing in the direction of the force summation.

An electrocardiogram (ECG) is an example of a type of vector diagram that allows us to calculate the predominant direction of electrical force in the myocardium. An ECG records electrical flow as an upward or downward deflection on graph paper. When the flow is toward the positive electrode, an upward deflection will record. When the flow is away from the positive electrode, a downward deflection will record. Twelve-lead ECGs are scaled graphs with multiple points of reference used to measure the force direction of the electrical conductance. As multiple points of reference are recorded, the predominant direction of electrical flow may be determined (vector summation). This is the principle behind determining axis deviation of the heart.

Axis deviation estimates the summation of forces that shift from the normal direction of electrical flow in the heart. ECG vector diagrams are scaled clockwise from 0 degrees in the east position. The normal axis of electrical flow summation in the heart is between −30 degrees and +90 degrees. The axis determination steps that follow are based on identifying the positive (upward) deflections of the 12-lead ECG, which represents electrical flow toward the positive electrode. Because the normal axis of electrical flow is between −30 and +90 degrees, positive deflections in leads I and II would represent electrical flow in the normal direction. Negative deflections in lead I or lead II would reflect a deviation of normal axis and require determination of the electrical flow vector. Vector deviations are described as left, right, or right superior. Several methods are available for quick determination of myocardial electrical axis deviation. Fig. 15.18 and Tables 15.1 and 15.2 offer help in determining axis deviation.

PRESSURE

Pressure is defined as force over area, where P is pressure, f is force, and a is area:

$$P = f/a$$

Increasing the area in which a given force is applied will result in a lower pressure. The smaller the area to which the set force is applied, the greater the pressure. The standard unit of measurement for pressure is the pascal (Pa). A pascal is the force of 1 newton (N) over 1 square meter.

$$Pa = 1N/1m^2$$

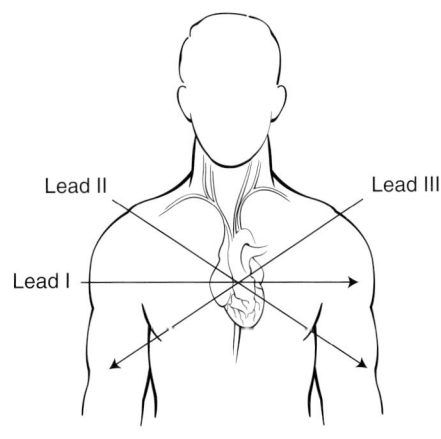

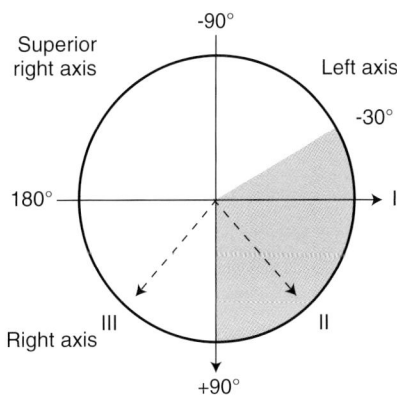

Axis deviation vectors

Fig. 15.18 Electrocardiogram lead placement with vector direction and location of normal and abnormal axes.

TABLE 15.1 Axis Deviation Determination Methods

Vector Method	Inspection Method	Grant Method
I+, aVF+ = Normal axis	I+, III+ = Normal axis	I+, II+ = Normal axis
I–, aVF– = Superior right	I– = Right axis	I+, II– = Left axis
I–, aVF+ = Right axis	III–, II– = Left axis	I–, II+ = Right axis
I+, aVF– see lead II (if II+ = Normal; if II– = Left axis)		I–, II– = Superior right

TABLE 15.2 Axis Deviations From Normal

Normal Axis	–30 to +90 degrees
Left axis deviation	–30 to –90 degrees
Right axis deviation	+90 to ±180 degrees
Superior right axis deviation	–90 to ±180 degrees

A pascal equals 102 g acting over an area of 1 m². Remember, a newton equals 102 g weight. This is a very small unit of pressure. As the newton was fractionalized to the dyne for the purpose of establishing a more convenient unit of force measurement, the pascal was increased 1000 times to create the kilopascal (kPa) unit. A kilopascal is more convenient to use for measuring pressures. A kilopascal equals 1000 N or 102 kg acting over an area of 1 m².

$$Pa = 102 \ g/m^2$$
$$kPa = 102 \ kg/m^2$$

Syringes are an example of the pressure generated by a force over a given area. Equal force (20 N) applied to the plungers of different syringes generates different pressures, depending on the area over which the force was applied. The force applied will cause greater pressure on injection with a tuberculin (TB) syringe (plunger area = 8.55×10^{-6} m²) than with a larger 10-mL syringe (plunger area 3.42×10^{-5} m²). As you increase the area to which a fixed force (20 N) is applied, the product of the equation, which is pressure (in atmospheres [atm] or millimeters of mercury [mm Hg]), becomes smaller.

$$P = f/a$$

TB syringe: 20 N/8.55×10^{-6} m² =
    2339.18 kPa, 17,543.94 mm Hg, or 23.08 atm
10 – mL syringe: 20 N/3.42×10^{-5} m² =
    584.79 kPa, 4386.28 mm Hg, or 5.77 atm
30 – mL syringe: 20 N/5.99×10^{-5} m² =
    334.16 kPa, 2506.40 mm Hg, or 3.29 atm

These calculations show the extremely high pressures that can be generated by exerting a force over a small area. The TB syringe generates more than 20 atm of pressure and can rupture catheters if used to flush or dislodge blockages. Larger syringes are recommended for flushing or unclogging enteral feeding tubes because of the potential for generating high pressures with smaller syringes.[26–28]

Atmospheric Pressure

As previously discussed, gravity pulls on all objects, including atoms and molecules in the atmosphere. Because these atoms and molecules have low mass, they have low gravitational pull, but are nonetheless pulled toward Earth. The cumulative effect of gravity on atmospheric gases gives rise to atmospheric pressure. Atmospheric gases are less concentrated at altitude and more concentrated at sea level. Atmospheric pressure is the gravitational force on gases in a given area. This can be measured and is equivalent to 100 kPa (or 14.7 lb/in², 1020 cm H_2O, or 760 mm Hg—all equivalent to one another) at sea level. Thus atmospheric pressure is lower at the top of Mount Everest (approximately 228 mm Hg) and higher at sea level (760 mm Hg). Standard pressure in the International System of Units (SI) is 100 kPa. Other units of pressure measurement include the following (shown with their equivalents). The following equivalents are pertinent in anesthesia practice:

1 torr = 1 mm Hg
1 kPa = 10.2 cm H_2O = 7.5 mm Hg
1 atm (atmosphere) = 760 mm Hg = 760 torr = 1 bar = 100 kPa
    = 1020 cm H_2O = 14.7 lb/in₂

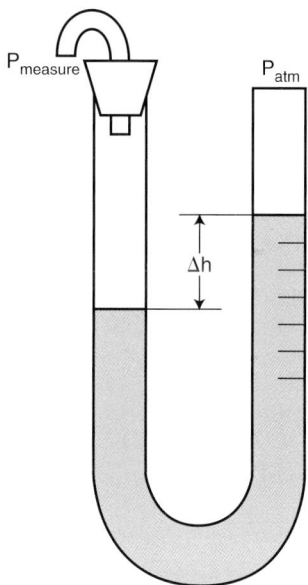

Fig. 15.19 Manometer showing change in liquid column height (Δh) related to pressure applied.

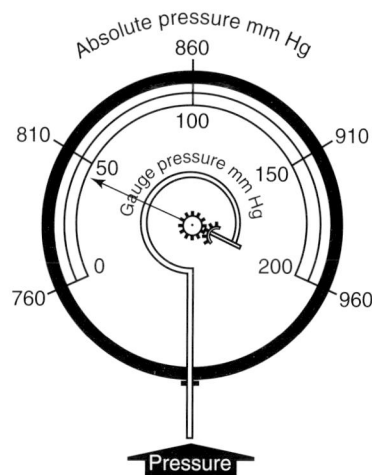

Fig. 15.20 Bourdon gauge showing gauge pressure *(inside pressures)* referenced to absolute pressure *(outside pressures)*.

Pressure Measurement

The simplest method for determining pressure is by using a manometer. A manometer is a liquid-filled tube that is open to atmospheric pressure on one end and exposed to a pressure for measurement on the other end (Fig. 15.19). A pressure greater than atmospheric pressure (760 mm Hg) will displace the column of liquid proportional to the pressure difference (Δh). Calibrating the column of liquid allows for quantification of the pressure.

A sphygmomanometer uses an inflatable cuff connected to a mercury-filled manometer to measure blood pressure. As the inflated cuff is slowly deflated, the arterial flow resumes causing a pressure wave that is transmitted to a mercury column. The mercury column is calibrated to show the measured pressure in millimeters of mercury (mm Hg). An advancement in blood pressure measurement is oscillometry. Oscillometry automates noninvasive blood pressure measurements by recording the oscillations in pressure caused by arterial pulsation.[29] As an inflated cuff is deflated, multiple measurements are made of these oscillations. Oscillations increase at systolic pressure and are maximal at MAP. Algorithmic computation of systolic and diastolic pressures is derived from the MAP. Often these noninvasive automated blood pressure monitors use the piezoelectric principle to record the pressure oscillations and a microprocessor to derive the systolic and diastolic measurements.[30] Invasive blood pressure monitors use a piezoelectric transducer that converts pressure waves into electrical signals. Blood pressure measurements are gauge pressures that are zeroed to atmospheric pressure.

Gauge and Absolute Pressure

Different pressure measurements may use different zero reference points. The zero reference point may be a complete vacuum devoid of all molecules and molecular collisions that impart pressure. This is true zero pressure and is the reference point used when measuring absolute pressure. Absolute pressure is atmospheric pressure plus gauge pressure. Gauge pressure is zero referenced at atmospheric pressure and reads zero at 760 mm Hg at sea level. Gauge pressure is absolute pressure minus atmospheric pressure.

Bourdon gauges are often used in anesthesia to measure high pressures, such as in gas cylinders, and are zero referenced to atmospheric pressure (Fig. 15.20). Bourdon gauges contain a coiled tube that expands as pressure is applied. A linkage connects the coil to a rotating

arm that records the pressure. The American Society for Testing Materials (ASTM) International mandates that the zero reading of Bourdon gauges lies between the 6 o'clock and 9 o'clock positions.

THERMODYNAMICS

The three laws of thermodynamics explain the relationship between heat and energy and their exchange during work processes:

1. *Law of conservation of energy.* Energy cannot be created or destroyed. The increase in the internal energy of a thermodynamic system is equal to the amount of heat energy added to the system minus the work done by the system on the surroundings.
2. *Energy moves toward greater entropy or randomness.* The entropy of an isolated system not in equilibrium will tend to increase over time, approaching a maximum value at equilibrium.
3. *Absolute zero (0K or −273.15°C) is void of all energy.* Absolute zero is theoretical because it has been impossible to achieve. As a system approaches absolute zero, all processes cease, and the entropy of a system approaches a minimum value.

ENERGY

Energy can be defined as the capacity to do work (potential energy) or the exertion of force (kinetic energy). Energy can be expressed as mechanical work, chemical reactions, or heat. The unit of measurement for energy is the joule. A joule is the force of 1 N that moves its point of application 1 m in the direction of that force. Two types of energy are potential energy and kinetic energy. Potential energy is energy waiting to be used; it is energy that is stored and available to be converted into power. Potential energy is defined as mass (m) times gravity (g) times height (h):

$$PE = mgh$$

Kinetic energy is the energy of movement, as even the word *kinetic* is derived from the Greek word *kinētikos*, "to move." Kinetic energy is defined as one half the product of mass times the velocity squared:

$$KE = (1/2) mv^2$$

ENTROPY

Entropy is the universal trend toward equilibration. It is the process that allows everything from ice melting to gas expansion. Sleep and the induction of general anesthesia have been proposed to be entropic processes.[31–34] All of these processes involve the equilibration of energy. Even matter is a form of energy. Entropy is unidirectional; it is the movement of energy from a higher concentration to a lower concentration, and thus energy moves because of a gradient. The difference in the gradient influences the speed of the flow. The greater the gradient difference, the greater the flow, and it is always from the higher concentration to the lower concentration. All energy and matter tend to follow this rule. An example of this unidirectional action is adding ice to lemonade. Ice does not make lemonade colder; instead, lemonade makes ice warmer. Entropy ends when all energy is equally distributed. Diffusion (see previous section in this chapter) is another process driven by entropy. Entropy is the underlying process promoting spontaneous and elicited movement in day-to-day activities and the universe in general. Essentially, entropy drives the universe. This process should be kept in mind when learning or reviewing any dynamic concepts of anesthesia.[35]

TEMPERATURE

Matter may change form with the addition of greater heat energy. An example seen every day is the melting of an ice cube into liquid water and the transformation of liquid water into water vapor with the addition of greater heat energy. Liquid water, with the addition of heat energy, expands. This is due to the water molecules moving apart with greater kinetic energy, which ultimately allows them to escape individually as a vapor (e.g., a boiling pot of water on a stove). Another liquid, mercury, also expands with the addition of heat energy. When placed in the bottom of a closed glass cylinder, the expansion is limited to one direction in relation to the energy applied. This is a simple application of heat energy (kinetic energy) interacting with matter to allow analysis of the thermal state: a thermometer.

Temperature is the measurement of the thermal state of an object. Heat is thermal energy; temperature is the quantitative measurement of that energy. Several temperature scales exist: Fahrenheit, Celsius, and Kelvin (Fig. 15.21). Gabriel Daniel Fahrenheit (1686–1736) is credited with inventing the mercury thermometer (1714) and devising the Fahrenheit temperature scale. The Celsius (Anders Celsius, 1701–1744) or centigrade scale is the primary scale used for everyday temperature measurements. The Kelvin scale (William Thompson, Lord Kelvin, 1824–1907) was developed to better reflect mathematically the temperature/pressure relationship of gases and is used when calculating their behaviors. Water freezes at 273.15K and boils at 373.15K. Conversion among temperature scales is as follows:

Celsius to Kelvin: $K = C + 273$
Celsius to Fahrenheit: $°F = 1.8(°C) + 32$
Fahrenheit to Celsius: $°C = (°F - 32)/1.8$
Standard temperature is 273.15 K (0°C).

Heat Loss

Heat and energy are the same. Heat loss (or energy loss) of a system, as discussed previously, is unidirectional from the higher concentration to the lower concentration, from hotter to less hot. Even ice possesses heat (energy). Remember absolute zero, 0K (−273.15°C or −459.67°F), is the absence of all energy and therefore the absence of all heat. The human body is a system that contains energy, and much of this energy is in the form of heat. Humans continually exchange heat with the environment from a high concentration to a lower concentration. On a very hot day or in a very hot room, one could become hyperthermic. Similarly, in a cold room, one could become hypothermic, especially if part of the body surface is exposed. Clothes, hair, skin, and fat insulate

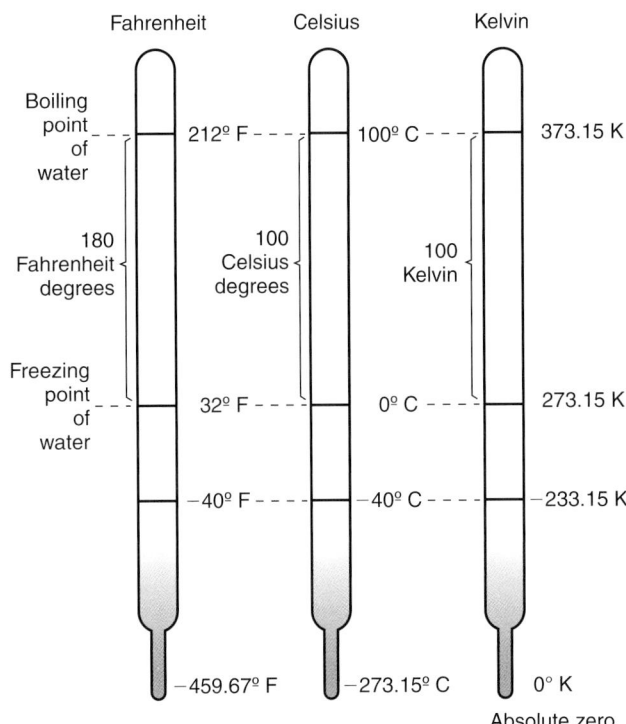

Fig. 15.21 Temperature scales referenced to Kelvin.

humans from heat loss, and protective mechanisms exist that further lessen heat loss. Here, the chapter will focus on heat loss in the cool operating room environment.

Vasoconstriction of peripheral vessels slows heat loss from the human body. An example is the vasoconstriction seen in limbs when exposed to a cold environment. The reverse thermoregulatory mechanism to promote heat loss is vasodilation when exposed to a hotter environment. Directing blood to or away from the periphery aids in the conservation or removal of a body's heat energy, respectively. This thermoregulatory mechanism is disrupted under anesthesia by vasodilating drugs, specifically volatile anesthetics. Volatile and regional anesthetics vasodilate vessels, including those in the periphery, causing greater blood flow to the surface of a body.

Core Temperature Redistribution

Core temperature redistribution is the process of increased heat loss from the body resulting from the vasodilating effects of volatile and regional anesthetics, which cause greater blood flow and therefore heat flow to the body's surface from the core.[36–38] A patient's core temperature can drop quickly due to the vasodilating actions of anesthetics, with the greatest decrease occurring in the first hour after anesthetic administration.[37] It is imperative that the anesthetist be cognizant of this heat loss mechanism and take measures to decrease it.[39–41] Covering all exposed areas of a patient minus the surgical site, using a heat and moisture exchanger (HME) on the anesthetic circuit, administering warm fluids, wrapping the head in blankets or applying a warming cap, and warming the operating room all decrease heat loss. The use of forced warm air devices is also effective at decreasing heat loss in the operating room environment.[42–44]

Blood flow to the body's surface encourages heat loss by four primary processes. In decreasing order they are:

1. Radiation
2. Convection
3. Conduction
4. Evaporation

Radiation

Radiation is the most significant mechanism by which humans lose heat, especially in patients under anesthesia. Radiation of the infrared electromagnetic wavelength transfers heat energy from warm bodies to the less warm operating room environment (walls, ceiling, equipment, etc.). Electromagnetic radiation (EMR) is pure energy (see discussion on this later in the chapter). Infrared radiation from bodies is greatest in areas of highest blood flow. Heads lose the greatest amount of heat due to the high percentage of blood flow (so perhaps your mother is correct in advising you to wear a hat on a cold day). Blood carries body heat, and the greater amount of blood and heat transported to the head, the greater the heat loss from radiation.

Convection

Convection is the process by which heat creates air currents. Bodies transfer kinetic energy to air molecules on the surface of the skin. The heated air molecules then move about with greater kinetic energy, rise, and are replaced by colder (less kinetic energy) air molecules. Bodies then transfer more kinetic energy to these molecules, which rise and are again replaced by cooler air molecules. When thinking of convection, it helps to think in terms of currents.

Conduction

Conduction is the transfer of heat via contact with a less warm object. Where two objects are in direct contact, heat exchange occurs from the higher concentration to the lower concentration (entropy). An example would be holding a cold soda can. The sensation of cold is the direct loss of heat from your hand to the can. Cold is not transferred to your hand; heat is transferred to the can. A patient on a cold operating room table will conduct body heat to the less warm table by physical contact. This is not a significant process in adult patients, but for pediatric patients who have a large body surface area compared to overall mass it is quite significant. Use of warming pads or blankets on operating room tables stops or reverses this heat transfer. Warming blankets may add heat energy to a patient, depending on the temperature and establishment of a thermal gradient.

Evaporation

Evaporation is not usually a large contributor to patient heat loss. Heat loss from evaporation includes moisture evaporation from the patient's skin as well as exhaled water vapor. The process of evaporation, which is the phase change from liquid to gas, requires energy. The source of energy needed for this process comes from the environment surrounding the evaporating substance. Latent heat of vaporization is the amount of heat energy per unit mass required to convert a liquid into the vapor phase. The energy withdrawn from the environment to convert 1 g water into vapor is 2500 joules, or approximately 600 calories. An example of this is the cooling off one feels after getting out of a swimming pool. The energy used to change the water into a vapor comes mostly from the body. Bodies lose heat energy to this process and experience a state of lower thermal energy. Patients who have areas of the body surgically prepped with liquids (e.g., isopropyl alcohol, povidone-iodine, and chlorhexidine gluconate) experience heat loss by this method. The process of breathing also causes heat loss through exhaled water vapor. This is not usually a high heat loss method in adult patients but may become significant in pediatric patients when using high fresh gas flow rates. Lower fresh gas flows, when appropriate, and use of an inline humidifying apparatus (such as HME) decrease the evaporation of pulmonary water content and limit heat loss by this mode. One should consider these interventions with all intubated general anesthetics to prevent not only heat loss but also the pulmonary drying effects of dehydrated gases.

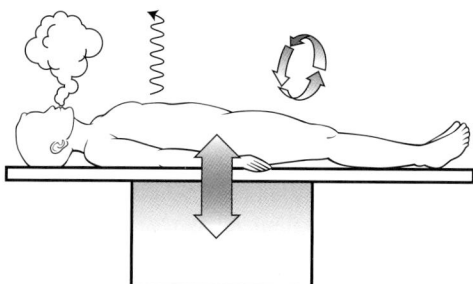

Fig. 15.22 Heat loss mechanisms of radiation, convection, conduction, and evaporation in patients under anesthesia.

Heat loss from patients is primarily due to radiation of infrared EMR.[45] Convection is the second largest method of heat loss in anesthetized patients.[45,46] Conduction and evaporation cause heat loss to lesser extents but remain a concern. Prevention of heat loss is extremely important for decreasing the higher morbidity experienced by hypothermic patients.[47–49] As Fig. 15.22 illustrates, the use of forced warm air devices, lower gas flow rates, humidification systems, warming the operating room, and covering and insulating patients are all effective methods to decrease patient heat loss.[43,50]

Vaporization. Vaporization is the process of converting liquids or solids into vapors and requires energy. Evaporation is the specific process of vaporizing liquids. As stated previously, the latent heat of vaporization is the energy needed to transform a given amount of liquid into a gas and is measured in kilojoules. The temperature at which the bulk of a liquid at a given pressure converts to a vapor is the boiling point. The temperature of a liquid will not rise above its boiling point; instead, the additional heat energy transforms the liquid into gas. Heating a liquid to its boiling point increases the kinetic energy of the liquid's molecules. Further addition of heat energy (above the boiling point) is transferred to molecules, which break away from the surface and become a gas. "The rate of vaporization depends only on the temperature, the vapor pressure of the liquid, and the partial pressure of the vapor above the evaporating liquid."[51] As gas molecules escape the liquid, they exert a pressure known as vapor pressure, measured in millimeters of mercury. Increasing heat will increase molecular kinetic energy, which will increase the rate of vaporization. In a closed container, equilibrium will be achieved between molecules in the gaseous phase and those in the liquid phase.

All liquids that have high vapor pressures at room temperatures are known as volatile liquids. Vapor pressure and boiling points are inversely related. Vapor pressures of the volatile anesthetics at standard temperature and pressure (STP) are as follows:

- Isoflurane: 238 mm Hg
- Sevoflurane: 160 mm Hg
- Desflurane: 660 mm Hg

Vapor pressures are unique characteristics of liquids that depend solely on temperature. Different liquids exert different vapor pressures at a given temperature. Because different volatile anesthetics have different vapor pressures, vaporizers must be calibrated for each specific agent. Placing the wrong agent into a vaporizer will deliver a greater or lower concentration of volatile anesthetic than what the practitioner intends to administer. If a high vapor pressure volatile anesthetic agent is placed inside a vaporizer calibrated for a lower vapor pressure volatile anesthetic, the output of that vaporizer will be higher than indicated on the control dial. If a volatile anesthetic agent with a lower vapor pressure is placed inside a vaporizer calibrated for a higher vapor pressure anesthetic, the output of that vaporizer will be lower than indicated on the control dial.[52]

Absolute Zero

The preceding discussion covered the first and second laws of thermodynamics, with examples applied to the practice of anesthesia. With a unidirectional perspective and an understanding that energy can neither be created nor destroyed, the third law becomes self-evident. Absolute zero is the theoretic state devoid of all energy. No matter how much energy is distributed, it will still be present. The lowest possible state of universal entropy would still possess energy, even though it would be very low. There is energy in the universe, and therefore it will always be present in some form and to some degree. The absolute absence of energy is therefore impossible. That does not prevent us from calculating the theoretic temperature that would be devoid of energy. The theoretic temperature of absolute zero is $-273°C$ (0K, $-460°F$).

KINETIC MOLECULAR THEORY

Thermodynamics set the foundation for explaining the overall action of a system's energy. The kinetic molecular theory builds on newtonian physics and thermodynamics, and it focuses on molecular movement (energy) and forces between these molecules. This theory explains how molecules behave as they follow the previously described laws of thermodynamics. Kinetic molecular theory was created as a conceptual framework to encompass the findings of Charles, Boyle, and Gay-Lussac, including the universal gas law that unified their studies. The following is a review of basic matter characteristics.

- Matter is composed of small particles called molecules, and molecules are composed of atoms. Matter can take the form of a solid, liquid, or gas.
- Solids: Molecules in a solid are held together closely by intermolecular forces. They may move about slightly and vibrate.
- Liquids: Molecules in a liquid are held together by intermolecular forces and may slide or flow by one another.
- Gases: Molecules in a gas move linearly, and the attractive forces between molecules are less than their kinetic energy. They move almost completely free of one another.

The kinetic molecular theory, which best describes the action of gases, makes some generalized assumptions for simplicity:

1. Molecules have no volume.
2. Gas molecules exert no force on each other unless they collide.
3. Collisions of molecules with each other or the walls of the container do not decrease the energy of the system.
4. The molecules of a gas are in constant and random motion.
5. The temperature of a gas depends entirely on its average kinetic energy. The energy of a gas is entirely kinetic.

The kinetic molecular theory was created to explain the ideal gas law. Though the ideal gas law adequately explains the general behavior of gases it does not take into account the small volume of gas molecules and their intermolecular interactions. These flaws are further addressed in the section covering van der Waals equation.

GAS LAWS

The kinetic molecular theory was based on the discoveries of three scientists: Jacques Charles (1746–1823), Robert Boyle (1627–1691), and Joseph Louis Gay-Lussac (1778–1850). They each studied isolated components of pressure, volume, and temperature to explore the relationship of these components. Charles studied the relationship of volume and temperature at constant pressure. He found that the volume-to-temperature relationship is directly proportional. This means that, at a constant pressure, volume will increase as temperature increases, and vice versa. Boyle studied the relationship of pressure and volume at constant temperature. Boyle found that the pressure-to-volume relationship is indirectly proportional. Thus, at a constant temperature, pressure will increase as volume decreases, and vice versa. Gay-Lussac studied the relationship of pressure and temperature at constant volume. Gay-Lussac found that the pressure-to-temperature relationship is directly proportional. At a constant volume, as pressure increases, temperature will increase, and vice versa. The gas laws allow one to calculate the behavior of gases when one of the three factors of pressure, volume, or temperature remains unchanged. The clinical significance of these laws is expressed by the ability to calculate the available volume of oxygen from a cylinder of any known pressure. This and other examples are available at the end of the chapter. Table 15.3 summarizes the laws and the interrelationship of pressure, volume, and temperature.

TABLE 15.3	Gas Laws: Gas Properties and Relationships		
Property Constant	Studied Properties	Property Relationship	Law
Pressure	Temperature, volume	Directly proportional	Charles
Temperature	Pressure, volume	Inversely proportional	Boyle
Volume	Pressure, temperature	Directly proportional	Gay-Lussac

Universal Gas Law

As the universal gas law unified the findings of Charles, Boyle, and Gay-Lussac, it also became known as the unified gas law or ideal gas law. The formula is as follows:

$$PV = nrT$$

where P is pressure, V is volume, n is the number of moles, r is a constant (0.0821 L atm/mol K), and T is temperature. A mole is the gram molecular weight of a gas. Atomic (or molecular) weight is the additive weight of all the atomic particles, protons, neutrons, and electrons in an atom or molecule. An example is a mole of helium. Helium has a molecular weight of 4. Placing "gram" after helium's atomic weight gives us a "mole" of helium, therefore 4 g of helium is 1 mole of helium. This amount of gas establishes a standard reference for calculations (see Fig. 15.2).

Using the universal gas law, one can calculate the volume for which 1 mole of a gas will expand at any given temperature or pressure. In the example given, the volume in liters that 1 mole of gas will expand to at 1 atm pressure at standard temperature (0°C) is calculated. Celsius is converted to Kelvin.

$$1 \text{ atm } (x) = 1 \text{ mole } (0.0821 \text{ L atm/mol K}) (273 \text{ K})$$
$$x = 22.4 \text{ L}$$

One mole of any gas at 0°C will expand to 22.4 L.

As this is a conceptual text, it is easier to view the universal gas law as PV = T to focus on the relationship between pressure, volume, and temperature. It is easy to see mathematically how increasing or decreasing any value would affect the other values, as described previously. The universal gas law can be rearranged as follows:

$$PV = T \text{ or } T/P = V \text{ or } T/V = P$$

Increasing one value will increase or decrease the other values to maintain balance in the formula. The universal gas law allows understanding and quick determination of such things as how much oxygen is available to be released from a partially full oxygen cylinder, and at what temperature a full oxygen cylinder will exceed its recommended pressure when heated.

Avogadro's Number

Amedeo Avogadro (1776–1856) was able to show that in a mole of any gas there are 6.023×10^{23} molecules. A mole of gas is equal to the molecular weight of the gas expressed in grams. A mole of helium, which weighs 4 g, contains 6.023×10^{23} atoms. Similarly, a mole of oxygen weighs 32 g and contains 6.023×10^{23} molecules. Oxygen is a molecule composed of two oxygen atoms bonded together, and therefore the molecular weight of the diatomic oxygen molecule is 32, not 16.

Van der Waals Forces

Unfortunately the simplicity of the universal gas law is not 100% accurate in fully describing the interaction of gases with their environment. The universal gas law is also called the ideal gas law because it explains the behavior of gases if they were "ideal." An ideal gas would possess molecules that occupy no volume and never interact with other molecules. Gas molecules do have volume and do occupy space, and therefore the volume they occupy must be taken into account when calculating a gas's expansion or contraction. The universal gas law does not account for gas molecule volume because Charles, Boyle, and Gay-Lussac did not account for this in their studies (remember, the universal gas law unified the work of Charles, Boyle, and Gay-Lussac). An ideal gas also assumes no intermolecular forces. However, molecules do interact with one another, and this behavior alters the net effect of kinetics as calculated by the universal gas law. Van der Waals (Johannes Diderik van der Waals, 1837–1923) equation corrects the universal gas law and accounts for molecular volume and molecular interaction in a gas. Van der Waals equation is as follows:

$$(P + n^2 a / V^2)\,(V / n - b) = RT$$

where P is the pressure of the fluid, V is the total volume of the container holding the fluid, a is a measure of the attraction between the particles, b is the volume excluded by a mole of particles, n is the number of moles, R is the gas constant, and T is the absolute temperature.

Because the deviations between the ideal gas law and the van der Waals equation are not clinically significant, the simplicity of the universal gas law and molecular kinetic theory are immensely valuable for approximating the behavior of gases used for anesthesia.

Dalton's Law of Partial Pressures

According to the kinetic molecular theory, pressure is purely the result of molecular collisions with the walls of a container. If there are more molecules in a container, there will be more collisions, and thus greater pressure. Dalton's law (John Dalton, 1766–1844) states that the total pressure of a system is the additive pressure of each individual gas in a mixture. Multiple gases in a mixture will each exert a pressure in proportion to its percentage in the mixture. The total pressure is the summation of individual molecular collisions with the walls of a container:

$$P_t = P_1 + P_2 + P_3 + P_4 + P_5 + \ldots$$

An example is the mixture of gases that compose medical air at atmospheric pressure:

79% nitrogen: 0.79×760 mm Hg = 600.4 mm Hg partial pressure of nitrogen

21% oxygen: 0.21×760 mm Hg = 159.6 mm Hg partial pressure of oxygen = 760 mm Hg total atmospheric pressure

Adiabatic Changes

Reaching a stable state of entropy in any system takes time as rapid expansion or compression of gases may exceed the speed of energy equilibration with the surrounding environment. Rapid expansion or compression of a gas without equilibration of energy with the surrounding environment is called an adiabatic process and entails no increase or decrease in a system's energy.

Remember that the energy of a gas is almost entirely kinetic. Temperature is the measurement that quantifies the energy distribution among the molecules in a system. One could think of temperature measurement as a quantification of a system's kinetic energy per area. An example would be the experience of placing your hand in sunlight. The surface area of that sunlight measured is equal to the surface area of your hand. It is warm. Now place a magnifying glass with a surface area equal to that of your hand in the sun, and focus that same amount of sunlight energy onto a pinpoint area of your hand. Ouch! The same amount of energy experienced over a smaller area is measured as a higher temperature. The temperature measurement is higher, but the system's energy total has not increased or decreased. The total sunlight energy hitting your hand is the same but is distributed over a different area.

Energy Concentration Effect

Compressing a gas quickly will intensify the kinetic energy (molecular movement) such that the thermal measurement of the gas will be higher. This quick compression of the gas's area does not allow the system's energy to dissipate into the surrounding environment. Thus the temperature will quickly rise proportional to the decreased volume. Although the temperature will be higher, the total energy of the system does not increase. A gas that is compressed quickly has little time to distribute any of its energy, so the thermal measurement becomes higher. This is the mechanism a diesel engine uses to ignite diesel fuel. Quick compression of diesel fuel vapor intensifies the kinetic energy of the gas, with a corresponding increase in temperature, until the ignition temperature is achieved and spontaneous ignition occurs. This effect, though unlikely, could happen with a compressed gas cylinder that is opened quickly. The rapid reexpansion and recompression of gas as it rushes through the outlet channels of a cylinder could increase the temperature significantly. The high temperature generated could cause a burn or ignite any grease placed on the cylinder O-ring, thus oil or grease is not recommended for use on any cylinder of compressed gas. Usually rapid recompression in the cylinder stem is not a concern, but it is possible and has occurred. It is, however, more likely that the opposite (rapid expansion of the gas as it leaves the cylinder) will occur.

Energy Dilution, Joule-Thompson Effect

The Joule-Thompson effect, named after James Prescott Joule (1818–1889) and William Thompson, Lord Kelvin, explains the cooling effect that occurs with adiabatic expansion of a gas. Rapid expansion of a gas causes the temperature measurement to decrease in exactly the opposite of the process explained previously. When we lower the pressure of a gas (i.e., increase its volume) quickly, we lower the energy per area. The temperature measurement will be lower when the volume is rapidly expanded. The total energy of the gas has not changed, but the expression (or thermal measurement) is decreased related to the increased volume. The temperature may be so low that frosting may occur at the cylinder outlet. Potentially, one could suffer a freeze injury. So why does this not always occur when anesthetists open gas cylinders? If done slowly, energy from the environment will move into the gas, and ambient temperature will equalize with the lower kinetic energy per area of expanding gas. The second law of thermodynamics (entropy) explains the maintenance of temperature when opening a gas cylinder slowly. Opening a cylinder slowly therefore would not be an adiabatic process. The slow opening of a gas cylinder allows the expanding gas to draw energy from the environment to maintain an equal distribution of energy, and one observes no changes in the temperature of the gas.

FLUID FLOW

Basic Principles of Fluid Mechanics

Fluids are defined by their response to stress. Stress is the distribution of force per unit area. The stress, or force distribution, may be tangential (i.e., a shear stress) or it may be perpendicular (i.e., a normal force). Strain is the deformation caused by stress. Fluids continuously change shape (flow) when subjected to shear stress and respond in one of two ways to perpendicular forces:

1. Resist compression (e.g., liquids)
2. Become compressible and easily expandable (e.g., gases)

Both liquids and gases are fluids. Forces associated with fluids are gravity, pressure, and friction. Friction is resistance to flow from surface interaction and is proportional to viscosity. Viscosity is the physical property of a fluid that relates shear stress to the rate of strain. Viscosity is the inherent property of a fluid that resists flow. Flow is the result of pressure forces in a fluid established by differences in pressure from one point to another, which creates a pressure gradient. All flow moves from higher pressure or resistance to lower pressure or resistance. The following laws and principles apply to both compressible (gas) and incompressible (liquid) fluids. Flow is defined as the quantity of a fluid passing a point per unit of time, where F is the mean flow, Q is quantity, and t is time.

$$F = \frac{Q}{t}$$

Types of Flow

The three types of flow that occur through tubes and orifices are laminar, turbulent, and transitional. Laminar flow is a type of flow in which all molecules of a fluid travel in a parallel path within the tube. The molecules in the center of the tube encounter the least adhesive force from the walls of the tube and therefore move at a velocity twice that of the mean flow. Flow decreases near the walls and ceases at the wall. True laminar flow predominates in the smallest airways (terminal bronchioles). Transitional flow is a mixture of laminar flow along the walls of a tube with turbulent flow in the center. Turbulent flow is described as chaotic with irregular eddies throughout. Laminar, transitional, and turbulent airflow are illustrated in Fig. 15.23.

Poiseuille's Law

Laminar flow is described mathematically by Poiseuille's law (Jean Louis Marie Poiseuille, 1797–1869). Poiseuille's law is:

$$F = (\pi r^4 \Delta P)/(8\,n\,l)$$

where F is flow, π is the constant pi, r^4 is radius to the fourth power, ΔP is the pressure gradient, n is viscosity of fluid, and l is the length of tube. According to Poiseuille's law, the radius of the tube will have the most dramatic effect on flow. Doubling the radius will result in a 16-fold increase in flow. A tripling of the radius increases flow 81-fold. Therefore flow through a 16-gauge (1.65 mm) intravenous catheter is much greater than through a 20-gauge (0.89-mm) catheter. If the viscosity of a fluid is increased, flow decreases. Patients with polycythemia have decreased blood flow due to increased blood viscosity. Increasing the length of a tube decreases the flow. If the length of a tube is decreased by 50%, there will be a corresponding doubling of the flow. If the length of a tube is doubled, flow decreases by half.

Clinical application of Poiseuille's law in anesthesia is exemplified during the process of transfusing blood. To improve flow when delivering a unit of packed red blood cells, a large-diameter intravenous catheter (18-gauge or larger) is recommended, a pressure bag may be placed on the unit of packed red blood cells to increase the driving

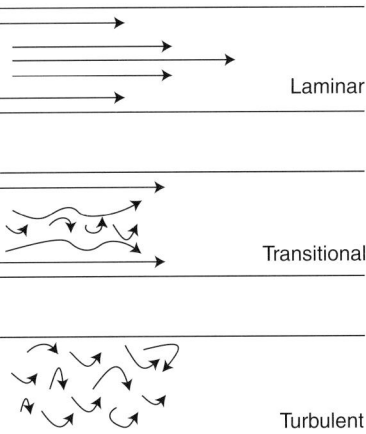

Fig. 15.23 Three types of flow: laminar, transitional, and turbulent.

pressure (pressure gradient), and the packed red blood cells may be diluted with normal saline to lower the viscosity.[53] These interventions are a direct manipulation of the factors associated with Poiseuille's law and significantly improve flow of blood to the patient. Of all the changes that may be made, increasing the diameter of the intravenous catheter will have the most dramatic effect on increasing flow. Large-bore intravenous lines, such as an introducer central line, are best for rapid, large-volume infusion.

Mechanical ventilation of patients also reflects the factors associated with Poiseuille's law. The larger the endotracheal tube (or larger diameter), the better flow of gas for ventilation. Delivery of β_2 receptor agonists such as albuterol increase the diameter of the bronchial tubes of the lungs to improve flow. Increasing the peak inspiratory pressure establishes a higher pressure gradient, which improves flow and delivered tidal volumes. Increases in the pressure gradient and flow velocity may initially improve flow but risk converting that flow to turbulent flow. Turbulent flow may also result when molecules of a fluid encounter rough, irregular walls or angles greater than 25 degrees. Turbulent flow often occurs in the medium to large airways of the lung and predominates during periods of peak flow, coughing, and phonation. Orifice constriction, such as glottic closure, causes laminar flow to become turbulent. Smaller bronchial tubes of the lung have slower velocities, and laminar flow is maintained. The presence of laminar, turbulent, or transitional flow is determined by the Reynolds number.

Reynolds Number

The Reynolds number (Osborne Reynolds, 1842–1912) is an index that incorporates the factors of Poiseuille's law with the addition of a fluid's density to determine whether a given flow will be laminar or turbulent. The Reynolds number is directly proportional to the density of the fluid, linear velocity of the flow, and tube diameter; flow is inversely proportional to fluid viscosity. The equation is as follows:

$$\text{Reynolds number} = \frac{vpd}{\eta}$$

where v is the linear velocity of fluid, p is density of fluid, d is diameter of tube, and η is viscosity. A Reynolds number greater than 2300 reflects a predominantly turbulent flow. Conversely, a Reynolds number less than 2300 reflects predominantly laminar flow. Delivery of helium-oxygen mixtures to status asthmaticus patients, who are refractory to standard treatments, is based on the understanding of density's role in reestablishing laminar flow.[54] Helium, which has a significantly lower density (0.1786 g/L at STP) than nitrogen (1.251 g/L at STP), improves flow by restoring laminar flow through the significantly narrowed airways of a severe asthma attack.

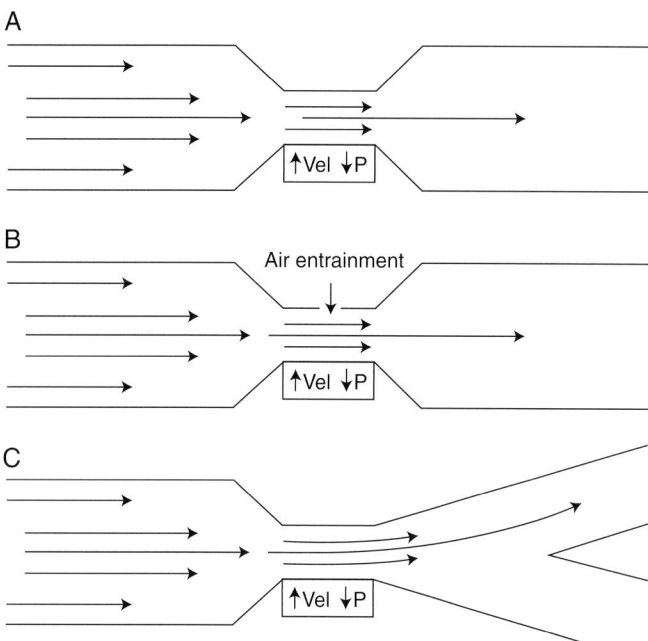

Fig. 15.24 (A) Bernoulli principle. (B) Venturi effect. (C) Coanda effect. *P*, Pressure; *Vel*, velocity.

Bernoulli Principle

Bernoulli principle (Daniel Bernoulli, 1700–1782) describes the effect of fluid flow through a tube containing a constriction. As flow passes through a narrowing in a tube, the velocity of that flow increases, and there is a corresponding decrease in pressure at the area of narrowing (Fig. 15.24A). This drop in pressure is explained by the conservation of energy law. For a steady flow of incompressible fluids, the sum of pressure, potential energy, and kinetic energy per unit of time must remain constant. The relationship of the pressure gradient to mass flow requires the pressure to decrease when the velocity increases. The Bernoulli equation is as follows:

$$P + \tfrac{1}{2}\,\Delta V^2 + pgh = constant$$

where P is pressure, Δ is density, V is velocity, g is gravitational acceleration, and h is height. Bernoulli equation is useful in determining flow through tubes that narrow, but it does not account for friction, and it assumes no changes in density or flow rate. This simple equation explains the pressure velocity relationship if fluid flows past a constriction. The velocity of a fluid is equal to the flow rate divided by the area of flow.

$$Velocity = \frac{Quantity\ of\ flow\ per\ unit\ of\ time}{area}$$

If a given quantity of flow is 4 L/min over an area (tube) with a volume of 2 L, the fluid velocity would be 2 L/min. If this flow meets a narrowing in its path that decreases the cross-sectional volume to 1 L, the fluid velocity would increase to 4 L/min.

$$V1 = \frac{4\ L/min}{2\ L/min} = 2\ L/min$$

$$V2 = \frac{4\ L/min}{1\ L/min} = 4\ L/min$$

This shows the increase in velocity associated with a narrowing in a tube for a given fluid flow (assuming no changes in density or height). The first law of thermodynamics, the law of the conservation of energy, dictates there must be a corresponding decrease in pressure. The energy of the flowing system does not change because of a constriction, rather the expression of that energy has changed. Essentially more energy is imparted toward velocity as opposed to pushing on the walls of the tube (pressure). Thus velocity increases and pressure drops to maintain conservation of energy.

Metered-dose inhalers (MDIs) use the Bernoulli principle to create a jet past a constriction that aerosolizes a drug in the expanding flow of gas. The necessity for large and sometimes cumbersome equipment is obviated by MDIs, which are able to consistently deliver aerosolized particles of medication into a fluid stream.[55] A more applicable example of the Bernoulli principle is taking advantage of the pressure drop across the narrowing in a tube of fluid flow. The Venturi effect relies on the lower pressure at a constriction to entrain air or fluid into a fluid path.

Venturi Effect

The Venturi effect (Giovanni Battista Venturi, 1746–1822) utilizes the pressure drop across a narrowing in a tube. By placing an orifice at the narrowed region of flow, air is allowed to be entrained and enter the flow (see Fig. 15.24B). Air may be entrained into a flow of liquid, or a liquid may be entrained into the flow of a gas.[56] Jet ventilation uses this entrainment of air to augment lung ventilation volumes.[57–59] Nebulizers use the Venturi effect to deliver both humidification and medications such as albuterol.[60] Nebulizers effectively deliver medications into fluid paths, such as ventilator circuits, but have been replaced to a large extent by MDIs.

Coanda Effect

The Coanda effect (Henri Coanda, 1885–1972) explains the tendency of fluid flow to follow a curved surface upon emerging from a constriction (see Fig. 15.24C). This may cause preferential flow to one tube at a bifurcation just past a narrowing in a tube.[61] Beyond a narrowing in a tube, there will be an increase in pressure corresponding with a decrease in the velocity of the fluid flow. If, at a widening in a tube, there is a division of flow with different angles, the return to a higher pressure will occur at different points along the bifurcated tube. The bifurcated tube with the delayed reestablishment of higher pressure (and corresponding lower velocity) may preferentially attract a greater percentage of the total flow toward its path. The path with the greater flow will receive a higher volume of fluid or gas at the expense of the path with lesser flow. In situations where this flow is blood in vessels or gas in the lungs, this diversion of flow could be hemodynamically consequential.[62–64]

Laplace's Law

Laplace's law (Pierre Simon Laplace, 1749–1827) describes the relationship of wall tension (T) to pressure (P) and radius (r) in cylinders and spheres:
- Cylinders: T = Pr
- Spheres: 2T = Pr

Tension is a stress force exerted over a given area. It is measured in newtons per centimeter (N/cm). In cylinders, wall tension increases with an increased radius; similarly, increasing pressure will increase wall tension.[65] Laplace's law shows why smaller diameter capillaries do not burst during periods of hypertension, whereas larger vessels or aneurysms may. An abdominal aorta maintains a mean arterial pressure along its length, including within an aneurysm, if present. Aneurysms, which have a greater radius than the rest of the aorta, have a corresponding greater tension and are more likely to rupture. Laplace formula, when rearranged, reflects the direct relationship of tension to radius in both the aorta and an aortic aneurysm at a constant pressure:

$$P = \frac{T}{r}$$

Example 1—Cylinders: If the mean aortic pressure is 100 mm Hg with a normal radius of 2 cm and an aneurysm radius of 4 cm, the tension is calculated as follows:

$$Pr = T$$

1. Normal aorta: 100 mm Hg (P) × 2.0 cm (r) = (T)
   1.33 N/cm^2 (100 mm Hg) × 2.0 cm = 2.66 N/cm
2. Aortic aneurysm: 100 mm Hg (P) × 4.0 cm (r) = (T)
   1.33 N/cm^2 (100 mm Hg) × 4.0 cm = 5.32 N/cm

The aortic aneurysm in this example has twice the wall tension of the normal aorta (mm Hg were converted to N in the formula). Any increase in blood pressure will increase the already high wall tensions of an aneurysm, and wall failure may result in dissection or rupture.[66]

In a sphere, wall tension is half that of a cylinder of the same radius. Applying Laplace's law to saccular aneurysms shows the relationship between increasing tension and an increasing radius:

Example 2—Spheres: If the mean pressures of two saccular aneurysms are 100 mm Hg, one with a radius of 0.5 cm and the other with a radius of 1 cm, the tension for each is calculated as follows:

$$Pr = 2\ T$$

1. Small saccular aneurysm:
   100 mm Hg (P) × 0.5 cm (r)/2 = T
   1.33 N/cm^2 (100 mm Hg) × 0.5 cm/2 = 0.3325 N/cm
2. Large saccular aneurysm:
   100 mm Hg (P) × 1.0 cm (r)/2 = T
   1.33 N/cm^2 (100 mm Hg) × 1 cm/2 = 0.665 N/cm

Greater wall tension would be present in a large saccular aneurysm (0.665 N/cm) than in a small saccular aneurysm (0.3325 N/cm), and any increases in pressure would risk further increases in wall tension and rupture. Decreasing pressure will decrease wall tension in both cylinders and spheres and is the rationale for controlling blood pressure in patients with aneurysms.[67]

Laplace's law, as applied to a cardiac ventricle of increasing size, explains the necessary inotropic response but eventual failure of contractility with increasing wall tension and pressure:

$Pr = 2\ T$
Increased pressure = Increased wall tension
Increased radius = Increased wall tension
Increased wall tension = Increased contractility
(Frank – Starling curve)

Laplace's law is often used to describe the dynamics of alveoli. Laplace's law directly applies to alveoli in the absence of surfactant. Without surfactant, small alveoli would collapse as they would require higher pressure to open compared to larger alveoli. This is portrayed in Fig. 15.25 by rearranging the formula for pressure.

Surfactant is a substance that lowers surface tension in the alveoli and prevents the effects observed with Laplace's law. By lowering surface tension, the pressure required to open alveoli is lowered. Surfactant lowers surface tension more in smaller alveoli than in larger alveoli, owing to the concentration effect that occurs when an alveolus contracts.[68] Greater surfactant concentration has greater surface tension, lowering ability. Surfactant therefore has the ability to equilibrate surface tension among different-sized alveoli and create stabilized alveolar pressures (Fig. 15.26).

WAVES

Waves are a very important phenomenon in everyday life as well as in anesthesia. Waves exist macroscopically, such as ocean waves and

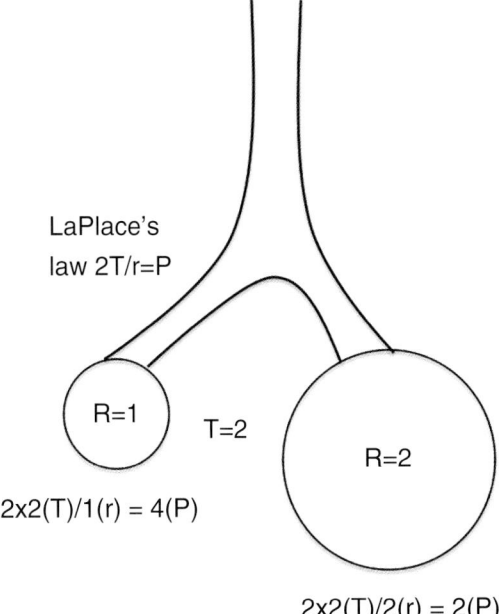

LaPlace's law 2T/r=P

R=1   T=2   R=2

2×2(T)/1(r) = 4(P)

2×2(T)/2(r) = 2(P)

Fig. 15.25 Alveoli and Laplace's law. In the absence of surfactant, the pressure needed to ventilate small alveoli would be greater than the pressure needed to ventilate large alveoli. Small alveoli would collapse (atelectasis).

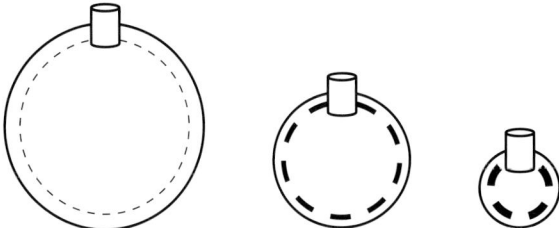

Fig. 15.26 Increased surfactant concentration *(dashed line)* with decreasing alveolar size.

sound waves. They also exist within atoms and as light energy. Waves surround us and exist within us. Understanding waves and wave action is key to understanding the basic ripple (energy) that permeates the universe. Waves are a periodic disturbance or motion and are essentially the movement of energy. The "disturbance" is energy, and energy is what is transported, or moved, along the wave front.

Wave Types

The two basic types of waves are transverse waves and longitudinal waves. Transverse waves are composed of up-and-down movement. In a transverse wave, the particles in the medium move perpendicular (up and down) to the wave direction. EMR waves are examples of transverse waves. Longitudinal waves are composed of back-and-forth movement along the direction of the wave. In a longitudinal wave, the particles in the medium move forward parallel to the direction of the wave (propagation). There is no up-and-down motion in longitudinal waves. The wave energy causes only compression and decompression (rarefaction) to occur along its path. These are pressure fluctuations. Sound waves are examples of longitudinal waves.

Wave characteristics:
- *Frequency:* Waves per second; measured in cycles per second, called hertz (Hz).
- *Wave length:* Distance from one wave top (crest) to the next.
- *Period or phase shift:* How far the wave "slides."

- *Amplitude:* Height of the wave.
- *Speed:* Measured in meters per second (m/sec).
- *Wave part:* Crest is the wave top, trough is the wave bottom.
- *Pressure waves:* Can be reflected, refracted, diffracted, or absorbed (interfered) by other waves.
- *Reflection:* Waves reflect off a medium at the same but opposite angle; the angle of incidence is the angle at which a wave strikes a medium. An example of acoustic reflection occurs anytime one hears an echo.
- *Refraction:* Redirection due to contact with a new medium. The human eye uses refraction to redirect light in the cornea to relay images in the optic nerve.
- *Diffraction:* Spreading or scattering; bending around an object. Examples of light diffraction are seen as the rainbow on compact discs or the iridescence on roast beef deli slices.
- *Absorption or interference:* Waves may interfere with other waves or be absorbed by matter. When waves interfere, amplitudes are additive. Constructive interference is when the crest of one wave passes through the crest of another wave or the trough of one wave passes through the trough of another wave, and the resultant wave is greater. Addition of two positive amplitudes or two negative amplitudes results in a greater value or wave height. Destructive interference is when the crest of one wave passes through the trough of another wave. Amplitudes from one crest are added to the negative amplitudes from the other wave's trough, and the height of the resultant wave is decreased.

Pressure Waves (Sound Waves)

Sound waves are pressure fluctuations that deviate from ambient pressure and are measured in Pa. Sound pressures are measured on a sound pressure level that uses a logarithmic decibel scale to narrow the wide range (20 Hz to 20 kHz) of amplitudes audible to the human ear. Sound waves are longitudinal waves that propagate through matter (solid, liquid, gas) at varying speeds determined by the medium's elastic modulus (stiffness), density, and temperature. The speed of sound through air at 0°C is 740 miles per hour. In the absence of matter, there are no sound waves as sound waves do not exist in a vacuum and only travel through matter.

Ultrasonography. Sound waves above the auditory limit of the human ear (20 kHz) are known as ultrasound. Ultrasonography uses ultrasound waves to construct a visual image of internal structures by examining the reflection of sound. Ultrasonography is useful for assisting simple procedures such as intravenous catheter insertion or for more invasive diagnostic assessment such as transesophageal echocardiography.[69-73] Ultrasonography uses a signal generator that transmits sound waves through tissues and a transducer to record the time delay for the returning reflected sound waves. The speed of sound waves in tissues is unique and constant to specific tissue compositions, and therefore the time delay of the returning reflected sound waves allows calculation of the location of different internal structures. Not all sound waves are reflected back to the transducer; some sound waves will have been refracted in a new direction, diffracted in multiple directions, or interfered with by tissues that cause attenuation or conversion to heat and resultant dissipation. The fraction of the original signal that is reflected back to the transducer must be amplified and processed into a visual display. The introduction of ultrasonography was made possible by the development of piezoelectric crystals that act as both signal generators and signal transducers (see "Piezoelectric Effect" next). A burst of ultrasound pressure waves is produced, followed by measurement of the reflected waves; this process is repeated many times a second, permitting real-time imaging of internal structures by computational analysis.

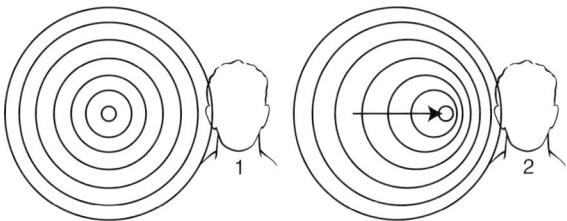

Fig. 15.27 Doppler effect.

Piezoelectric effect. Piezoelectric crystals are unique quartz, ceramic, or polymer compositions that contain a matrix of polarized molecules that respond to (1) electric current by changing shape and (2) mechanical stresses by generating an electric current. Piezoelectric crystals derive their name from the Greek prefix *piezein*, which means "to press tight or squeeze." The shape change caused by an electric current creates a pressure fluctuation around the crystal; this is a pressure wave. If a piezoelectric crystal is subjected to an alternating electric current, it will vibrate, creating many pressure waves in quick succession. The rate at which the crystal vibrates is called its resonant frequency. When not responding to an electric current, piezoelectric crystals are at rest and respond to the mechanical stress of the pressure waves by creating a small electric current.

Doppler effect. The Doppler effect (Christian Johann Doppler, 1803–1853) describes the change in frequency of a propagated wave from a moving object. The sound of a siren changes to a higher frequency as it approaches a listener and lowers in frequency as it departs. Listener 1 in the Doppler effect figure (Fig. 15.27) will hear a sound emitted from a stationary object with a fixed frequency. Listener 2 will hear a sound emitted from a moving object with increasing frequency as the sound approaches and lessening frequency when it passes. This is due to the "stacking up" of the wave fronts emitted from an approaching object and the stretching of the wave fronts when it recedes.

The Doppler effect, when applied to echocardiography, allows the determination of blood flow direction and speed. As blood cells flow to or away from an ultrasound signal, reflected waves are either compressed or expanded. This change in frequency allows calculation of blood velocity:

$$V = \frac{\Delta f}{\cos \theta} \times \frac{c}{2f_t}$$

where V is velocity of blood, Δf is the difference in transmitted frequency and received frequency, f_t is the transmitted frequency, c is the speed of sound in blood, and θ is the angle of incidence between the ultrasound beam and blood. Spectral display presents Doppler ultrasound data in a time-velocity graph that allows greater assessment of hemodynamics on a beat-to-beat basis.

Electromagnetic Waves

The term *electromagnetic* succinctly expresses the dual nature of electricity and magnetism as the two are intimately intertwined. Where there is electric current, there are also magnetic waves. Where there are changing magnetic waves, there is also an electric current. EMR is composed of two waves, electric and magnetic, oscillating in unison but perpendicular to one another. The electromagnetic wave is propagated perpendicularly to these oscillating waves. Electromagnetic waves possess both electric and magnetic potential. Electromagnetic waves (also known as EMR) are similar to pressure waves in that they both possess frequency and amplitude. Another similarity is that they may be reflected, refracted, diffracted (scattered), or absorbed. The unique wave properties of EMR include its composition, velocity, and independence of transport by matter. EMR differs from pressure waves (sound waves) in its velocity. The speed of EMR in a vacuum is

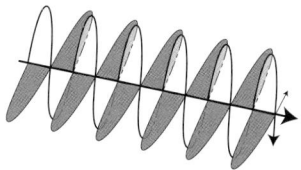

Fig. 15.28 Electromagnetic wave showing electric wave oscillating perpendicular to magnetic wave.

TABLE 15.4 Comparisons of Electromagnetic Radiation and Sound Wave Properties

	EMR	Sound Waves
Speed	300,000,000 m/sec	344 m/sec
Wave type	Transverse	Longitudinal
Energy motion	Perpendicular to propagation	Parallel to propagation

EMR, Electromagnetic radiation.

3×10^8 m/sec (186,000 miles/sec), whereas sound cannot exist in a vacuum. The speed of EMR in air closely approaches 3×10^8 m/sec. The speed of sound in air is only 331 m/sec (740 miles/hr). EMR and sound waves may travel through matter at varying speeds, but only EMR can propagate independently of matter. Sound waves only travel through matter and cannot exist in a vacuum, as shown in Fig. 15.28 and Table 15.4.

Inverse Square Law

Waves represent the propagation of energy from a source. As energy moves away from its source, its strength decreases. Newton showed that the strength of the emanating energy is inversely proportional to the square of its distance from its source, as follows:

$$I1 = \frac{(d2)^2}{I2(d1)^2}$$

where I1 equals intensity at the original distance, I2 is the lower intensity at a new distance, d1 is the distance from original source, and d2 is the new distance from the source. Newton originally calculated this for the force of gravity; however, it has applications throughout physics.[74] This relationship is represented by the inverse square law figure (Fig. 15.29), where the *y* plane is twice the distance from the source than plane *x*. The energy intensity at I2 is one-fourth the intensity at I1. The inverse square law applies to pressure waves, electricity, light, and radiation, with the intensity of each decreasing with increasing distance from its source.

Magnetism

Magnets are a unique form of matter in which the charges are aligned in an orderly fashion. There are flows of magnetic currents, or field lines, in all magnets. To observe these invisible fields, place a magnet under a piece of paper and spread iron filings on top. The filings will line up along the magnetic fields. Magnetism is a force between electric currents. Flowing charged particles not only move energy along that current but also disrupt, or alter, the surrounding environment. This altering is not apparent unless one is looking for it. Hold a compass near a wire carrying an electric current. The needle will move and align itself along the flow of magnetism. Turn the wire, and the compass needle will turn. There is a force between the electric current and the compass needle (magnet). Magnetic fields are measured with a Gauss meter in units of teslas: 10,000 gauss (G) equal one tesla (T). The Earth's magnetic field strength is 0.00005 T (0.5 G). A small magnet's strength

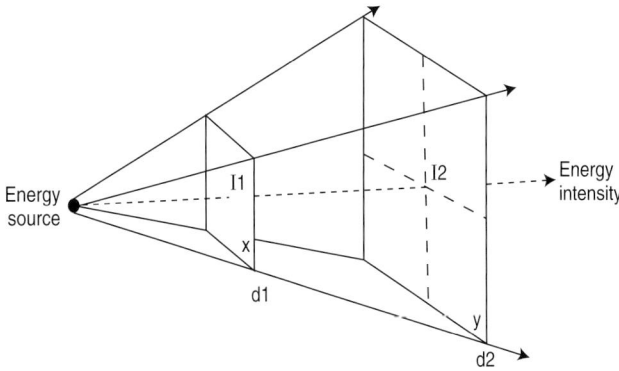

Fig. 15.29 Inverse square law representation of decreasing intensity with increasing distance.

is 0.01 T (100 G). The magnet's strength in a magnetic resonance imaging (MRI) machine is 1 to 3 T (10,000–30,000 G).

Magnetic Resonance Imaging

MRI uses a strong, continuous magnetic field to uniformly realign the spin of protons within the hydrogen atoms of water. As the proton axes are pulled into one of two possible realigned positions, a radiofrequency pulse is delivered at resonant frequency to energize the protons. The protons will then reemit this energy. The radiofrequency pulses are delivered in thin "slices" that may be made in the sagittal, coronal, or axial planes. Computer-generated analysis of these data produces detailed representations of internal tissues. The magnetic field used is very strong, and specific safety considerations need to be addressed when delivering anesthesia care in an MRI suite.

MRI safety. Because of the high strength of the magnetic field in and around an MRI scanner, special precautions must be observed. Any ferrous material will interact with the magnetic field, gaining kinetic energy and thermal heat. Movable ferrous objects will also be attracted to the MRI magnet and will be pulled into the magnetic field with great force. Patients and personnel are at potential risk for both thermal injuries from implanted ferrous objects and traumatic injury from ferrous objects violently pulled into the magnetic field. The American College of Radiology has designated four safety zones that surround an MRI scanner, with zone 4 representing the immediate area around the scanner. Zone 4 poses the greatest risk of injury and has the most stringent guidelines.[75] All ferrous materials such as pagers, phones, jewelry, identification badges, and pens must be removed before entering zone 4. Patient stretchers, oxygen tanks, IV poles, and any other ferrous objects must be kept outside zone 4. Specially designed stretchers and anesthesia machines are designated for zone 4 to prevent attraction to the magnet.

Implanted ferrous materials such as ferrous foreign bodies, prosthetics, stents, and pacemakers have been studied for MRI safety. A review of current guidelines regarding the acceptability of various devices for scanning is recommended.[75-78] Many implanted devices can be safely scanned in an MRI, and any knowledge of or concerns about potential ferrous interaction should be brought to the attention of the designated MRI personnel.[75]

Electricity

Electricity is the change in potential energy caused by the movement of electrons from an area of high concentration (high charge density) to an area of low concentration (low charge density). The fundamental unit of charge is *e*; it represents one electron's energy and is extremely small. Dealing with the energy of a single electron is difficult, so we use a quantized measurement called a coulomb (C): 1 C = 1.60222$10^{19}$ *e*.

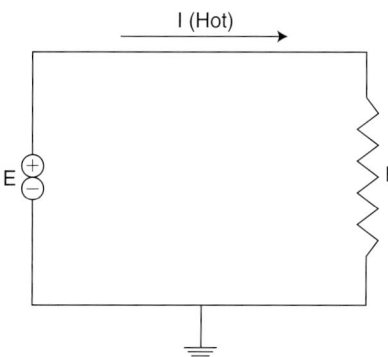

Fig. 15.30 Basic electric circuit showing a live (hot) wire (I = current), a load (R = resistance), and a grounded neutral wire (E = volts).

Coulomb's Law

Coulomb's law (Charles-Augustin de Coulomb, 1736–1806) states that like charges repel each other, and opposite charges attract each other inversely to the square of their distance. In short, opposite charges will attract more when closer together, and like charges will repel more when closer together. The electrical potential energy unit is the volt. It represents electrical "pressure" or the gradient of charges that could potentially flow. Electric current (I) is the rate of flow of an electric charge through a conductor. In operating room electrical equipment, the conductor is usually copper wire. Copper is a good conductor, and therefore the resistance to flow is low. In insulators, also known as dielectrics, electrons are not easily moved and therefore resist the flow of electricity. Current is measured in amperes (A), and 1 A = 1 C/sec. A volt is the SI unit for 1 J/C.

Ohm's Law

The potential flow of electric charge is proportional to actual current after accounting for resistance. Resistance is calculated by Ohm's law (Georg Ohm, 1789–1854):

$$E = IR$$

where E represents volts or potential energy, I is current, and R is resistance. Resistance is measured in ohms (Ω). Ohm's law measures resistance to electrical flow (Fig. 15.30).

Electrical Flow

In an electrical current, electrons flow from a surplus of electrons to a deficiency of electrons. Electricity must have a complete circuit for electrical flow to occur. A simple circuit is shown with a positive side (live, hot), a negative side (neutral), and a ground. The ground is a conductor that is connected to the earth (ground) and provides a low, resistive, alternate route for electricity to flow through in the case of an electrical surge. Electricity may be provided by direct current (DC) or alternating current (AC). In DC circuits, the flow of electrons is always in one direction. In AC circuits, the flow of electrons reverses direction (alternates) at a set frequency, usually 60 Hz (United States) or 50 Hz (Europe) (1 Hz = 1 cycle/sec). Electricity is delivered by the power company as AC because its voltage can easily be maintained while traveling long distances to customers via the power grid. Operating room equipment and most residential and institutional electrical equipment operate on AC. A simple AC circuit is the same as a simple DC circuit, except resistance is more complex with AC circuits, and the positive side alternates between both wires. In AC circuits, resistance is called impedance and is the total of all forces that impede electrical flow. In addition to the inherent characteristics of the conductive material, capacitance and inductance contribute to AC impedance. Capacitance

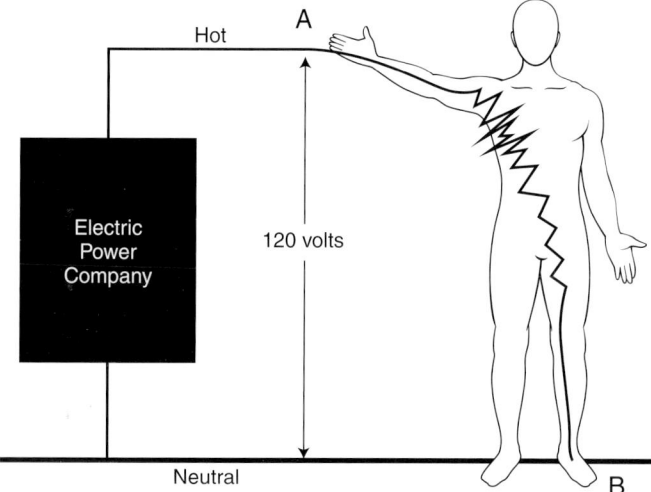

Fig. 15.31 Electric shock. *A* is point of contact and *B* is connection to ground.

is the capacity to store charge. A capacitor is composed of two parallel conductive plates separated by an insulator. When a capacitor is exposed to a voltage source in an open circuit, one plate will store a positive charge, and the other will store a negative charge. Capacitors have useful applications in electronic devices but can leak stray capacitance. There are no absolute insulators, and stray capacitance may create an unintended charge in the casing of electrical equipment. Electromagnetic inductance is the transfer of an electric current between circuits without physical contact using induced magnetic waves. Any conductors carrying an electric current will also carry a magnetic field. In AC circuits, the charge is alternating, and so the magnetic field will change, too. This changing magnetic field may induce a small electric current in nearby conductive materials such as equipment metal casings, even in the absence of physical contact between the circuit and the casing.

Electric shock. Stray capacitance and inductance may contribute a low risk of shock because they are low-current flows. Direct contact with exposed electrical wiring constitutes a high risk of electric shock because of higher voltages. Current leakage from wires to equipment casing exposes patients and operating room personnel to the risk of shock by three mechanisms:

1. Direct wire contact with metal casing due to insulation damage or faulty construction
2. Inductance due to the magnetic field of the AC, producing a small electrical flow in the surrounding metal casing despite no direct contact
3. Stray capacitance from the buildup of electrical potentials with an AC circuit despite no closed circuit electrical flow[79]

If a patient or a member of the operating room personnel makes contact with both a live wire and the ground, the individual may complete an electric circuit and receive a shock. For a shock to occur, a complete circuit must be made. This can happen if a person is standing on the earth and contacts the live wire in a circuit (Fig. 15.31). Shocks may be macroshocks or microshocks. A macroshock refers to large amounts of current conducted through the patient's skin and other tissues. Injuries may be minor or severe depending on the amount of current and the duration of exposure. Electric current seeks the path of least resistance and is often dissipated throughout the body tissues. The amount that reaches the heart is often insufficient to cause arrhythmias.

However, conductive materials in a patient's body may place that patient at greater risk by providing a low resistive path for electricity to flow to the heart. Microshock is the delivery of small amounts of

TABLE 15.5	Effects of Macroshock and Microshock
Macroshock (mA)	**Effect**
1	Perception
5	Maximal harmless current
10–20	"Let-go" current
50	Loss of consciousness
100–300	Ventricular fibrillation
6000	Complete physiologic damage
Microshock (μA)	**Effect**
20	Ventricular fibrillation in dogs
100	Ventricular fibrillation in humans[53]

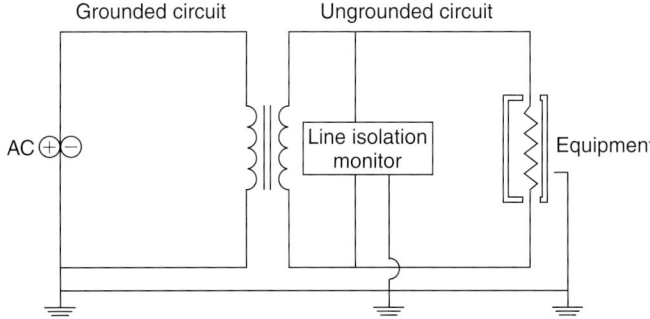

Fig. 15.32 Ungrounded operating room electric circuit isolated from grounded hospital electrical system. Note that the electrical equipment casing and line isolation monitor are connected to ground, but the electric circuit is not. *AC,* Alternating current.

current directly to the heart. The amount of current that may produce ventricular fibrillation has been found to be 50 microamperes or lower.[80,81] Table 15.5 gives a comparison of how different levels of microshock and macroshock affect the human body.

Electrical safety. To decrease the risk of shock, operating room electrical systems are isolated from the main grounded electrical supply system. A transformer is used to isolate the electrical supply systems from one another. A transformer uses the principle of magnetic inductance to transfer electricity from one system to another system without having physical contact. This allows the operating room power supply to be ungrounded, preventing a circuit from being completed when a person contacts one live wire. However, if a person contacts both wires in a circuit, shock may occur as the path of electricity flows through the person from one line to the other. Operating room equipment casing (or housing) is grounded to divert electrical flow in case of internal live wire contact with the metal housing.

If there is contact between the live wires and the ground (fault), such as when wiring touches the equipment casing, the system will become a grounded system. A second fault will enable a shock because the newly grounded system will allow a completed circuit to pass through a person in the operating room that is grounded when a live wire is contacted. To prevent a first fault from being unnoticed, a line isolation monitor is placed between the live wires and ground to measure their impedance to flow (Fig. 15.32).[82] If a live wire has contact or high capacitance to ground, the line isolation monitor will alarm. Line isolation monitors are usually set to alarm at 2 to 5 mA potential leak. If a line isolation monitor alarms, the last piece of equipment plugged in should be disconnected and inspected to verify that it is the offending piece of equipment. Equipment that activates a line isolation monitor may still be operational but increase the potential risk of shock should a second fault occur because it has converted the isolated power supply system to a grounded system. Line isolation monitor alarms may also be activated because of the cumulative effect of minor leakages of many pieces of properly functioning electrical equipment, but this does not mean a risk is present. Newer systems alarm at 5 mA to account for this normal leakage.

Electrocautery

Electrocautery devices use high-frequency electric currents to cauterize, cut, and destroy tissue. These devices may be unipolar or bipolar. Bipolar electrocautery devices have two tips: one to supply the electric current and the other to return the current. Bipolar devices do not require a return electrode and are less likely to cause burns or injuries apart from the local area of use. Unipolar devices have only one tip to

deliver an electric current, and a large surface area return electrode with good conductive contact must be placed on the patient (commonly referred to as a grounding pad). The path of current flow from the unipolar device to the return electrode (grounding pad) should not cross the patient's heart.

The high current flows used in electrocautery units may cause electromagnetic inductance, which in turn may cause artifact in other electrical equipment such as ECG monitors. Pacemakers may also sense the electromagnetic inductance as inherent electrical activity and not initiate a paced impulse. This could put the patient at risk for asystole if the patient is void of a native heart rhythm.[83] Electrocautery interference has also been documented as initiating paced tachycardic rhythms.[84,85] Placing a pacemaker magnet over the patient's pacemaker resets the pacemaker to a continuous, asynchronous mode. Not all pacemakers are reset to a continuous, asynchronous mode, and interrogation of the pacemaker is recommended to understand its settings and functions prior to surgery using electrocautery or before placing a magnet over the device.

QUANTUM PHYSICS

ELECTROMAGNETIC RADIATION

Newtonian physics is helpful in describing the wavelike properties of EMR but is incomplete in its description. Originally it was assumed that EMR, like sound waves, was propagated through a medium. A "luminiferous ether" was thought to fill the universe and was the suspected medium through which EMR traveled. The famous Michelson-Morley[86,87] experiment successfully disproved the existence of the "ether," but did not determine how EMR propagates. Max Planck (1858–1947) later theorized that EMR is quantized, meaning it is emitted only in discrete quantities of energy, and this revolutionized our perspective of the universe. Planck constant expresses the quantized nature of EMR, as defined by energy, time, and frequency:

$$E = h\nu$$

where E represents energy, h is Planck constant (6.626068×10^{-34} m^2 kg/sec), and ν is frequency.[88] Albert Einstein introduced the photon concept of Planck's discrete energy quanta, and together with others ushered in the study of quantum mechanics.[89,90] Quantum mechanics is a branch of physics that explores the subatomic dynamics of pure energy and the quasi-realm of energy/mass transition.

EMR is now thought to travel as photons or packets of energy and can be observed as both a particle and a wave, depending on how scientists study and measure it. The dual nature of behaving as both a particle and a wave is unique to EMR.[91] EMR is called a photon when

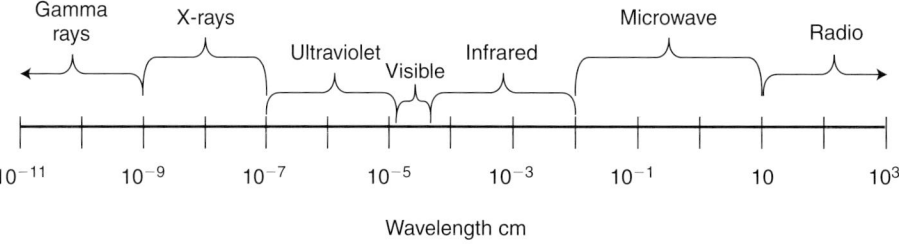

Fig. 15.33 Electromagnetic radiation spectrum. Increasing energy associated with decreasing wavelength (increasing frequency) along the electromagnetic radiation spectrum is shown. Example: X-rays possess shorter wavelengths, greater energy, and greater ability to permeate matter than microwaves, which have longer wavelengths and lower energy.

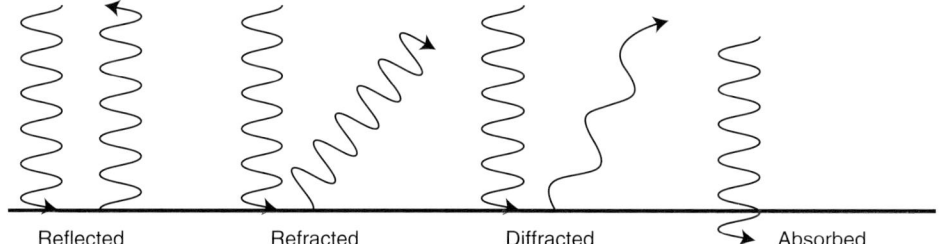

Fig. 15.34 Electromagnetic radiation interactions with matter.

it exhibits particle-like behaviors. Despite their behavior, photons have no mass. They are pure energy. The energy of EMR is directly related to its frequency. Higher frequencies correspond to higher energies, and lower frequencies correspond to lower energies. The velocity of EMR in a vacuum remains constant and does not change depending on the frequency. The understanding of energy as a quantized event promoted numerous advances in physics, which ultimately found application in anesthesia. The perspective of EMR as photons allows us to better explain many dynamic interactions of EMR and matter. Fig. 15.33 shows the EMR spectrum.

ELECTROMAGNETIC RADIATION/MATTER INTERACTION

EMR exists independently of matter. Sound (pressure) waves do not exist without matter through which their energy is transmitted. Both may be reflected, refracted (scattered), diffracted (redirected), or absorbed (interfered) by matter (Fig. 15.34). An example of the interaction of EMR with matter is visible light. Visible light is composed of a narrow band of EMR frequencies between 4.3×10^{14} and 7.5×10^{14} Hz (400–700 nm wavelengths). These frequencies of EMR are the only frequencies an eye can detect. When we see a color, we actually see the reflected frequencies that correspond to that color. Visible light is composed of the colors red, orange, yellow, green, blue, indigo, and violet, and was first described by Newton. Visualizing the color blue represents the reflected EMR frequencies between 495 and 570 nm. The other visible light frequencies are not seen because they have been absorbed and scattered by the material that appears blue. Materials that absorb EMR increase their vibration energy (kinetic energy), owing to their absorption of energy. One experiences this when wearing white or black clothing in sunlight. Black clothing absorbs many more frequencies of visible light and gains greater kinetic energy, which causes heat. White clothing appears white because of the high reflection of the visible light spectrum; it gains less kinetic energy and therefore less heat. The phenomenon of matter reflecting, scattering, and absorbing specific EMR frequencies has many applications in health care and in anesthesia specifically.

EMR may also be converted into other forms of energy such as electricity (gas discharge), heat (incandescence), and chemical energy (photoluminescence) but must obey the law of conservation of energy. When matter is exposed to EMR, it too may change form. The analysis of EMR's interaction with matter is the underlying principle of x-ray fluoroscopy, anesthetic gas measurement, pulse oximetry, and lasers.

RADIOGRAPHY

X-Rays

X-rays are able to pass through different organic materials to varying degrees and allow the "photographic" imaging of internal structures. Though x-ray and fluoroscopic imaging offer great medical benefit, they also possess potential for great harm. X-rays are ionizing radiation and lie in the higher energy frequencies of the EMR spectrum (see Fig. 15.33). They possess high energy and have the ability to ionize atoms and molecules. X-rays can cause DNA damage and be mutagenic.[92] Proper protection is imperative for health care personnel when working near or with x-rays and can be implemented by incorporating three factors of safety: (1) distance from the x-ray source, (2) barriers, and (3) exposure time to x-rays. The inverse square law explains how energy intensity significantly decreases with distance from its source.[93] X-rays obey this law, and the minimum recommended distance from an x-ray source is 6 feet. The greatest intensity of an x-ray is directly in front of the beam generator. Standing at least 6 feet away and behind or to the side of the beam direction lessens exposure. Although the energy intensity of x-rays decreases significantly with greater distance from the source, proper shielding is also important. Lead barriers are efficient absorbers of x-ray energy, and lead aprons and thyroid shields should be worn. X-ray technicians often wear dosimeter badges that measure total exposure to x-rays over a period of time. Greater exposure (both in proximity to and duration of) x-rays is associated with greater risks. Institutional policies establish guidelines for exposure limits as well as which personnel should don dosimeter badges. Unless practitioners are exposed to radiographic procedures frequently, the doses

BOX 15.1 Organic and Inorganic Anesthetic Gas Analysis Technologies

Organic and Inorganic Anesthetic Gas Analysis
- Infrared absorption analysis
- Raman scattering
- Mass spectrometry
- Piezoelectric analysis
- Interferometric refractometry
- Gas-liquid chromatography

Oxygen Analysis
- Electrogalvanic cell (fuel cell)
- Polarographic electrode (Clark electrode)
- Paramagnetic oxygen sensor
- Fluorescence quenching
- pH optode

Carbon Dioxide Analysis
- Infrared absorption analysis
- Severinghaus P_{CO_2} electrode
- Fluorescence quenching
- pH optode

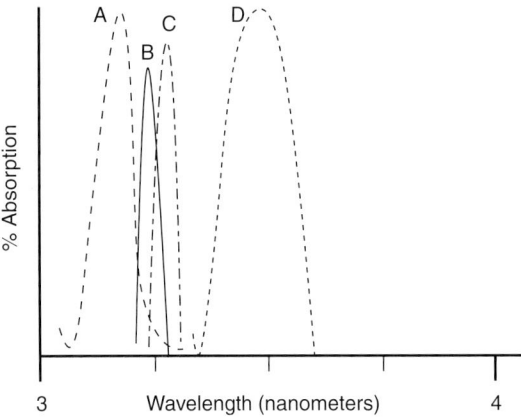

Fig. 15.35 Individual anesthetic gas infrared absorption spectra (representation only, not actual). *A, B, C,* and *D* indicate four different theoretic anesthetic gases.

received usually fall well below established limits for maximal allowable exposure. Shielding, minimizing exposure time, and increasing distance from the x-ray source remain the most important factors within the control of the practitioner.

GAS ANALYSIS

Gas analysis technologies use several methods to measure organic and inorganic gases. The methods described herein focus on the technologies that are prevalent in the field of anesthesia. The gas analysis technologies shown in Box 15.1 are the most common technologies used to analyze anesthetic gases, oxygen, and carbon dioxide.

Organic and Inorganic Anesthetic Gas Analysis

Infrared Absorption Analysis

Infrared absorption analysis uses each volatile agent's ability to absorb specific frequencies of EMR in the infrared spectrum. A sample of a gas or a mixture of gases is subjected to a known range of infrared frequencies. The frequencies lost due to absorption are measured, and the gas or gases may be identified by the specific frequencies each gas absorbs. Anesthetic agents' infrared absorption spectra are unique but close in frequency. Newer infrared absorption analysis monitors are capable of identifying specific agents without preprogramming the specific agent. Concentration is determined by the amount of infrared absorption (Fig. 15.35).

Raman Scattering Analysis

The interaction of EMR with matter is the underlying principle used with Raman scattering analysis of gases. Raman scattering passes a monochromatic laser beam through a gas mixture, causing an increased vibration frequency of the excited gas molecules (Fig. 15.36). A laser is a high-intensity beam of a known specific EMR frequency (see laser discussion in this chapter). When this laser beam interacts with an anesthetic gas molecule, it may be absorbed (as previously described with infrared absorption analysis) or scattered. Scattering is a frequency change (energy change) of the initial laser beam after

it interacts with gas molecules. The laser frequency interacting with the molecules may be scattered at higher or lower frequencies. Each anesthetic gas scatters laser frequencies uniquely. A gas or gas mixture may be analyzed and identified by comparing the gas sample scattering spectrum to that of known gas scattering spectrums. The scattered frequencies measured in this spectral analysis are represented as Stokes lines.

Raman scattering technology requires only that a gas molecule be polyatomic for identification, thus Raman scattering analysis can identify oxygen, carbon dioxide, nitrogen, nitrous oxide, and all volatile anesthetics, including mixtures of volatile anesthetics.[94] Because helium is monoatomic, helium cannot be analyzed by Raman scattering. Raman scattering analyzers return the sample to the patient circuit and therefore do not require waste gas scavenging; they are small and portable, but do require calibration. It should also be noted that they are less accurate with pediatric cases, which use high fresh gas flow rates and small tidal volumes.

Mass Spectrometry

Mass spectrometry historically has been the dominant technology for anesthetic gas analysis, though it has increasingly been replaced by more portable and efficient infrared absorption analysis and Raman scattering analysis technologies. Mass spectrometry ionizes gas molecules and passes them through a magnetic field. The gas molecules with the lowest mass-to-charge ratio are easily deflected by the magnetic field and collected by an ion detector (Fig. 15.37). Ionized gas molecules with higher mass-to-charge ratios are deflected less by the magnetic field and detected by other ion detectors. Identification of a gas is based on the amount of deflection.

Piezoelectric Gas Analysis

Piezoelectric gas analysis incorporates both the piezoelectric effect and Henry's law to determine concentrations of gases.[95–97] A piezoelectric crystal will vibrate at a set frequency when an electric current is applied to it. A vibrating piezoelectric crystal coated with a liquid solution will alter its resonant frequency when exposed to a gas. As the gas dissolves into the liquid, in proportion to its concentration above the liquid gas interphase, the resonant frequency of the crystal is altered. The degree of frequency change is proportional to the concentration of gas that dissolves into the liquid. The amount of gas that dissolves into the piezoelectric crystal's liquid coating is directly related to the partial pressure of that gas. This is explained by Henry's law. A drawback of this technology is that it does not identify the specific anesthetic agent.[98]

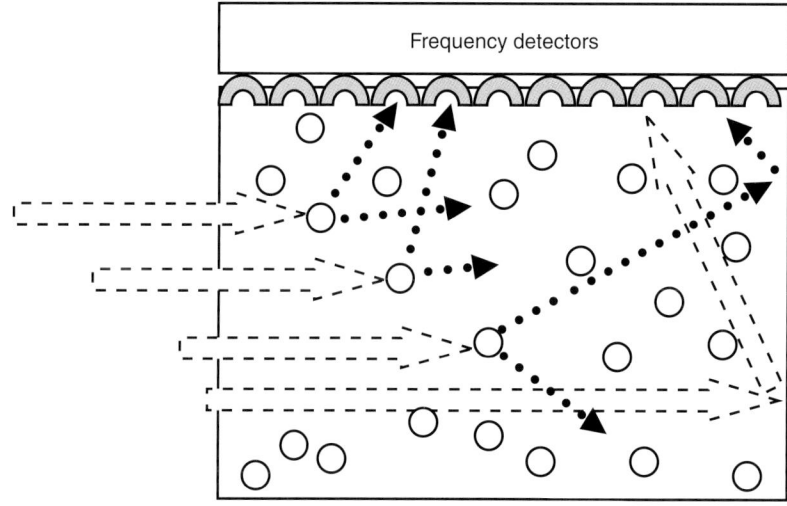

Fig. 15.36 Raman scattering gas analysis technology.

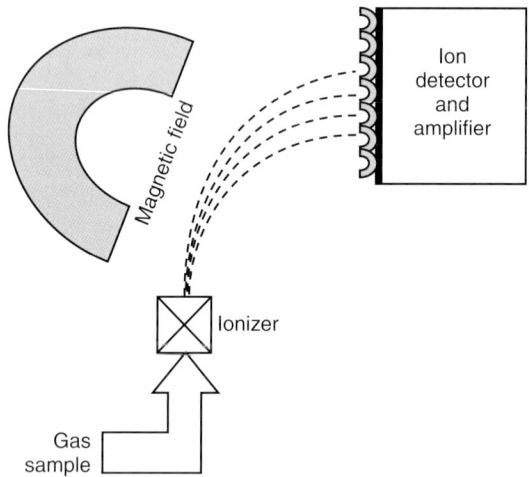

Fig. 15.37 Mass spectrometry gas analysis technology.

Photoacoustic Gas Analyzer

The photoacoustic gas analyzer subjects a gas sample to a filtered, pulsating infrared light beam in a closed chamber. The pulsating beam causes the gas molecules to increase then decrease in temperature. The increase and decrease in temperature cause the chamber pressure to increase and decrease according to Gay-Lussac's law. Microphones along the chamber measure the pressure waves. A photoacoustic gas analyzer can measure anesthetic gases, mixtures of these gases, and carbon dioxide.[99] The units are small, portable, and accurate.

Oxygen Analysis

The primary role of oxygen in biologic systems underscores the importance of identification and measurement of this gas when delivering anesthetics. Purposeful redundancy is used in oxygen measurement, and more than one technology is often used at a time. In the practice of anesthesia, oxygen content analysis is accomplished with several technologies. These technologies take advantage of oxygen's unique physicochemical properties and interaction with EMR. The most commonly used technologies pertaining to anesthesia practice are reviewed in the following section.

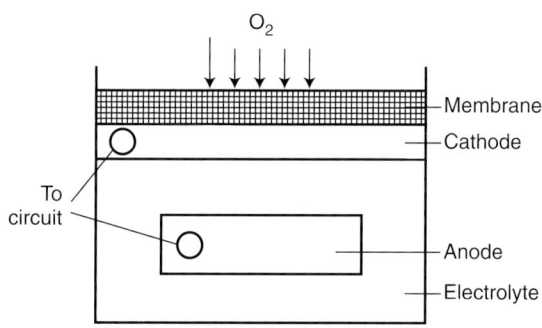

Fig. 15.38 Electrogalvanic fuel cell.

Electrogalvanic Cell (Fuel Cell) Electrochemical-Oxygen Analyzer

The electrogalvanic cell (Fig. 15.38) is also called a fuel cell because the reaction that takes place creates its own electric current by consuming its "fuel." The electrogalvanic sensor has a membrane that is permeable to gases but not liquids. At the anode of the sensor, electrons are liberated in an oxidative reaction. This is shown with a lead (Pb) anode:

$$2Pb \rightarrow (Pb^{+2}) + 4e^-$$

The meter measures the current produced by the electrons consumed in the reaction at the cathode (silver or gold):

$$O_2 + 4e^- \rightarrow 2O_2, \, 2O_2 + 2H_2O \rightarrow 4(OH)^-$$

The electron flow between the anode and cathode is directly proportional to the partial pressure of oxygen in the sample gas. Current flows in proportion to oxygen concentration.

Electrogalvanic cells have a limited life related to the concentration and duration of oxygen exposures. Because of this, some nurse anesthetists remove the oxygen sensor from the circle system if an anesthesia machine is left on and not in use for extended periods of time, such as overnight. Most anesthesia machines have minimal oxygen flow at all times, so removing the electrogalvanic cell from the flow of higher oxygen concentration will extend its duration of usefulness.

Polarographic Electrode (Clark Electrode)

The Clark polarographic oxygen electrode consists of a voltage source and a current meter connected to a platinum cathode and a silver (Ag) anode (Fig. 15.39). The electrodes are immersed in a potassium chloride (KCl) electrolyte cell. A membrane permeable to oxygen, but not electrolytes, covers one surface of the cell. A polarizing voltage is applied between the electrodes. At the anode, electrons are liberated by the oxidative reaction of silver with the chloride electrolyte:

$$4Ag \rightarrow 4Ag^+ + 4e^-, \; 4Ag^+ + Cl^- \rightarrow 4AgCl$$

The meter measures the current produced by the electrons consumed in the reaction at the cathode:

$$O_2 + 4e^- \rightarrow 2O_2, \; 2O_2 + 2H_2O \rightarrow 4(OH)^-$$

Current flows in proportion to oxygen concentration. If there is no current applied to these cells, there will be no consumption of the electrodes.[100]

Paramagnetic Oxygen Sensors: Magnetomechanical Dumbbell Principle

The paramagnetic oxygen sensor uses oxygen molecules' unique attraction into magnetic fields. Few other gases are attracted by magnetic fields. The paramagnetic oxygen sensor is constructed with two

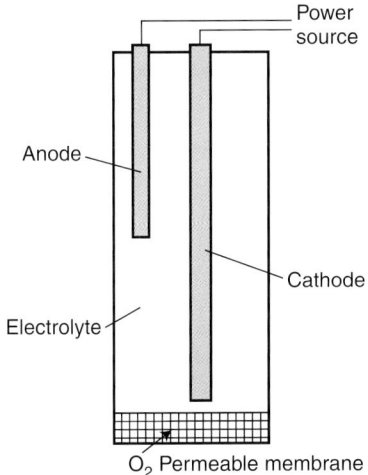

Fig. 15.39 Polarographic electrode.

nitrogen-filled bulbs attached together by a stem; this resembles a dumbbell. This dumbbell-shaped apparatus is suspended parallel to a magnetic field in its "at-rest" state. Nitrogen is not attracted or repelled by magnetic fields. The introduction of oxygen into this sensor causes the dumbbell apparatus to be displaced out of the magnetic field as oxygen is attracted into the field (Fig. 15.40). The amount of displacement of the dumbbell apparatus is directly proportional to the concentration of oxygen. Originally these sensors measured the physical displacement of the dumbbell apparatus but were prone to artifact caused by vibration and external movement. These sensors now incorporate a small optical mirror that reflects a projected light beam. The light beam is reflected onto a photocell that generates a small voltage used to counteract the displacement of the dumbbell apparatus. Increased oxygen concentration increases the displacement of the dumbbell apparatus, which in turn directs a greater amount of reflected light onto the photocell. By using a generated electric current to counteract the dumbbell apparatus, displacement proportional to the oxygen concentration, external movement, and artifact are eliminated. These sensors are highly accurate, compact, and durable.

Paramagnetic Transducer

The paramagnetic transducer type of oxygen analyzer utilizes the same unique attraction of oxygen molecules to a magnetic field (Fig. 15.41). Rather than utilizing the displacement of a mechanical apparatus, the transducer measures the pressure difference between a known gas and a sample gas. There are several variations on this principle that measure pressure or flow alterations in relation to the attraction of oxygen concentrations to a magnetic field.

Fluorescence Quenching

Fluorescence is caused by a molecule emitting light (photons) in response to being energized. Certain molecules exhibit fluorescence in response to an electric current or exposure to EMR. These molecules are sometimes said to "glow in the dark." Neon lights are an example of noble gas fluorescence initiated by an electric current. Chemical fluorescence is seen in some sea life and in glow sticks. Both electrically and chemically initiated fluorescence are caused by energizing an electron to a higher energy level. The energized (excited) electron then returns to its lower energy level (resting state) by releasing a photon (spontaneous emission). The released photon is observed as light, and its color represents the emitted photon's frequency.[100]

Fluorescence quenching is a technology that uses oxygen's ability to suppress, or quench, certain molecules from fluorescing. When a fluorescent molecule is excited to a higher energy state, it will emit a

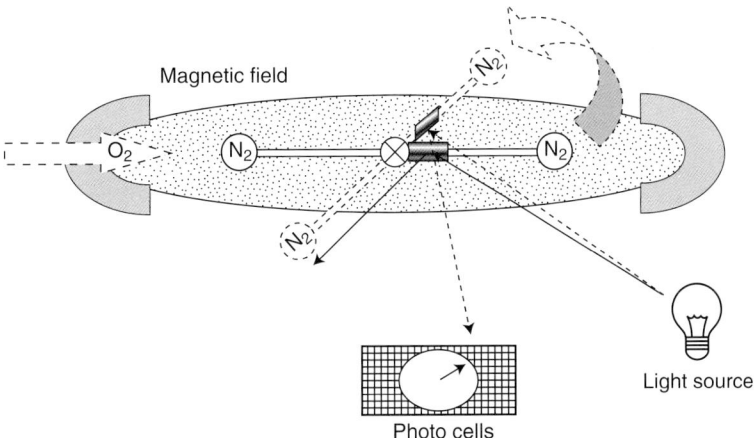

Fig. 15.40 Paramagnetic oxygen sensor.

Electromagnet

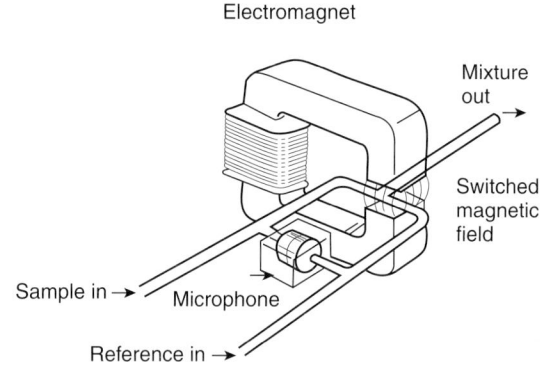

Fig. 15.41 Paramagnetic oxygen analyzer. (Courtesy Datex-Ohmeda, Madison, WI.)

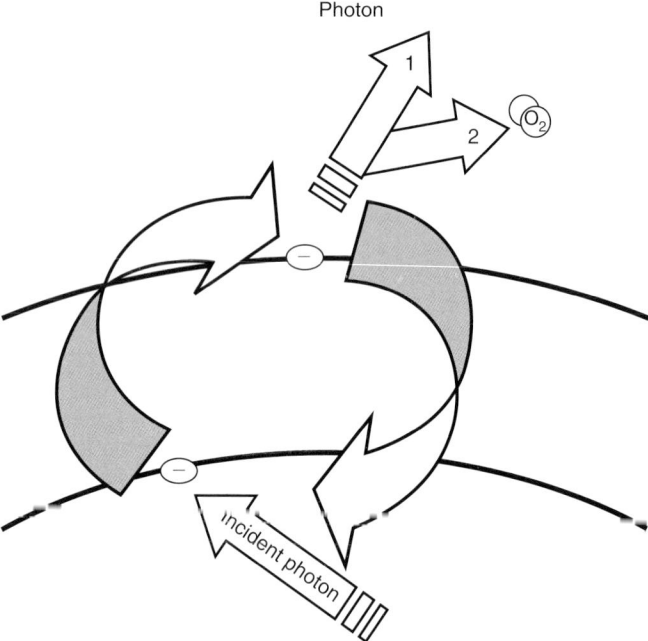

Fig. 15.42 Fluorescence-quenching principle. *1,* Photon release as fluorescence. *2,* Energy absorption by oxygen, which quenches fluorescence.

photon. Oxygen, if present, will absorb this photon and prevent its release. The amount of fluorescence that is quenched is directly proportional to the concentration of oxygen present. The oxygen concentration can be analyzed by measuring the amount of emitted photons (Fig. 15.42).

Carbon Dioxide Analysis

Fluorescence Quenching

Fluorescence quenching technology also may be used to measure carbon dioxide. Carbon dioxide is not the quencher of fluorescence; instead, it causes a change in pH, liberating hydrogen ions, which react with a quenching agent or a fluorescent dye in the sensor. Fluorescence is altered by the protonation of these chemical components. The measured change in fluorescence is proportional to the concentration of carbon dioxide.

Colorimetric Carbon Dioxide Sensor

A dry-state sensor that undergoes a color foundage in the presence of carbon dioxide is often used to differentiate endotracheal intubation from esophageal intubation. These sensors use the fluorescence principle to

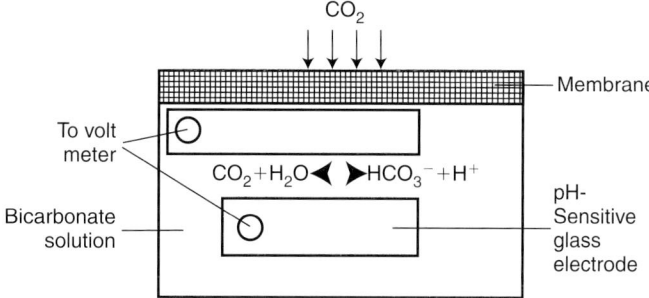

Fig. 15.43 Severinghaus partial pressure of carbon dioxide in arterial blood (Pco$_2$) electrode.

indicate carbon dioxide in the gas phase. A paper is impregnated with a fluorescent dye that, in the presence of carbon dioxide, will fluoresce or change color. A phase-transport agent facilitates the reaction to produce an immediate color change (e.g., purple to yellow), indicating carbon dioxide. Colorimetric carbon dioxide sensors indicate the presence, but not the amount, of carbon dioxide.

Severinghaus Pco$_2$ Electrode

The Severinghaus Pco$_2$ electrode (Fig. 15.43) is frequently used in anesthesia for analyzing carbon dioxide.[101] It uses a pH-sensitive electrode immersed in a bicarbonate solution with a gas-permeable membrane. Carbon dioxide diffuses into the sensor and is converted into free hydrogen ions, generating a current of electric charge. The current is proportional to the carbon dioxide concentration.

PULSE OXIMETRY

Pulse oximetry makes use of the fact that different types of matter absorb different EMR frequencies. Oxygenated and deoxygenated hemoglobin are uniquely different molecules and thus interact differently with EMR. By measuring specific frequencies that are absorbed by a pulsatile blood supply, the percentage of oxygenated and deoxygenated blood in the sample can be determined. The algorithm used to make these calculations is derived from the Beer-Lambert law (August Beer, 1825–1863; Johann Heinrich Lambert, 1728–1777). This law is based primarily on the work of Lambert. Lambert's laws state that (1) the luminance of perpendicular light on a surface is proportional to the inverse square of the distance it travels from its source, (2) the luminance intensity of angled light is proportional to the cosine of the angle with the normal, and (3) luminance intensity decreases exponentially as the light travels through a medium. The Beer-Lambert law is as follows:

$$It = Ii \times e^{-DC_\alpha}$$

where It is the transmitted light, Ii is the incident light, and e^{-DC_α} is the distance through the medium, concentration, and absorption coefficient (Fig. 15.44). Pulse oximetry applies the Beer-Lambert law to the absorption of two specific frequencies (infrared and visible red) by hemoglobin. Oxygenated hemoglobin absorbs the infrared frequency that corresponds to a wavelength of 940 nm, and deoxygenated hemoglobin absorbs the visible red wavelength of 660 nm (Fig. 15.45). Analysis of the wavelength that is most absorbed corresponds to that form of hemoglobin. If the wavelength of 940 nm is absorbed, the hemoglobin present is the oxygenated form. Pulse oximeters display a percentage measurement of saturated hemoglobin (Spo$_2$). Pulse oximeters measure the amount of absorption of these two specific wavelengths many times a second.

Pulse oximetry is inexpensive and portable, and allows early detection of hemoglobin desaturation.[102–104] Probes may be placed on the

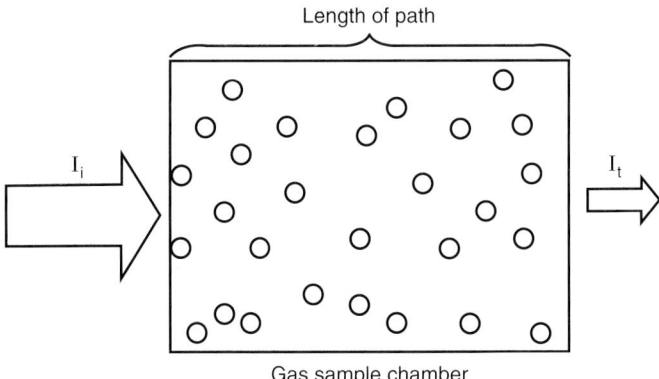

Fig. 15.44 Incident light intensity change when transmitted through a medium.

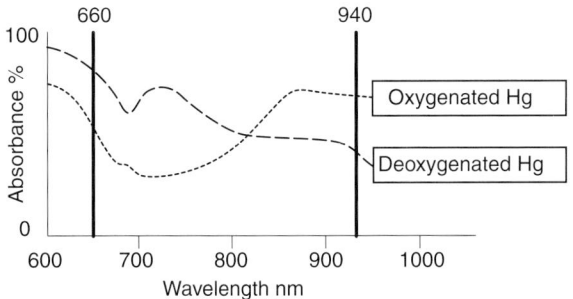

Fig. 15.45 Oxygenated hemoglobin and deoxygenated hemoglobin wavelength absorption spectra. The intersection where oxygenated and deoxygenated hemoglobin absorb the same frequency amount is the isobestic point. *Hg*, Hemoglobin.

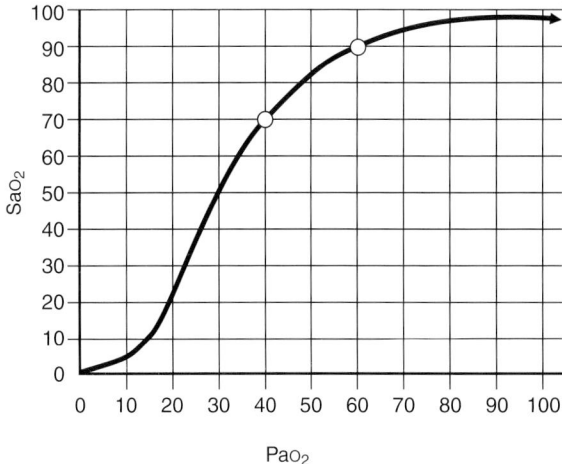

Fig. 15.46 Oxyhemoglobin dissociation curve. Pao_2, Partial pressure arterial oxygen; Sao_2, oxygen saturation as measured by blood analysis.

digits, ears, nose, tongue, or even the forehead to detect a pulsatile arterial blood flow. The oxyhemoglobin saturation curve displays the oxygen saturation (Sao_2) relationship to Pao_2. Important points along this curve include an Sao_2 of 90%, which corresponds to the critically low Pao_2 of 60 mm Hg. An Sao_2 of 70% corresponds to a Pao_2 of 40 mm Hg (Fig. 15.46) and is the saturation at which cyanosis becomes apparent.[105] Pulse oximetry is of great value and has become a standard of practice. Both a digital display and an auditory tone alert the nurse anesthetist to the patient's hemoglobin saturation.[106]

Disadvantages of pulse oximetry include the susceptibility to artifact from movement and ambient light sources, the risk of burns in poor perfusion states, and the limitation in detecting pulsatile blood flow in hypothermic or vasoconstricted patients. Additionally, some nail polish pigments and acrylics interfere with accurate estimates of oxygen saturations, while indigo carmine, indocyanine green, and methylene blue administration can yield transient false pulse oximetry readings.[107] It should also be appreciated that any state of abnormal hemoglobin (e.g., methemoglobinemia or carboxyhemoglobinemia) will also yield erroneous Spo_2 values.[108-111] During high Fio_2 delivery, ventilation-perfusion abnormalities may be masked. A Pao_2 of 100 mm Hg and a Pao_2 of 500 mm Hg will both give the same pulse oximeter reading (Spo_2) of 100%, regardless of the delivered oxygen. Lastly, pulse oximeters do not measure respiratory rate.[112-115]

LASERS

Lasers derive their name from the acronym **L**ight **A**mplification by **S**timulated **E**mission of **R**adiation. Certain atoms that have been energized by an incident photon may move an electron to a higher orbit, but that electron stays there only momentarily, releases a photon, and quickly returns to its resting energy level (see "Fluorescence

Quenching" earlier). This is called spontaneous emission. When many incident photons raise many electrons to higher energy levels, the spontaneous emission that occurs is chaotic, with photons radiating in multiple directions. However, if many atoms of a particular matter are continually energized by incident photons while their electrons are already in a higher energy state, then photons of the same frequency and direction will be emitted as the electrons are forced down to their natural resting state. This is called stimulated emission and is the basis of laser function. Continual energizing of certain atoms forces photons of the same frequency (monochromatic) and direction to be emitted in unison. Population inversion is the condition in which the majority of electrons in an atom are in a higher energy level rather than in their natural resting state; the natural balance of resting electrons to energized electrons has been inverted. Population inversion is required to allow continual production of monochromatic, coherent, and unidirectional photons used in lasers. The intensity of lasers and the ability to direct the beam have many applications in medicine, and present unique considerations for nurse anesthetists (Fig. 15.47; Table 15.6).

Laser Risks

The risk of fire is ever present with lasers and of critical importance in the operating room. Three components are needed to produce a fire: fuel, oxygen, and an ignition source. Lasers are a potent ignition source especially in the presence of oxygen, which is used intraoperatively. Drapes, dressings, and linens are a few of the combustible materials (fuel) that may ignite during surgery,[116] so to mitigate risk, operative lasers should never be kept active when not in use. The nurse anesthetist should be aware of the fire risk during laser surgeries and be prepared to take rapid action. Commonly, lasers are used for otorhinolaryngologic surgeries, and the anesthetist should monitor for endotracheal tube fires and use low inspired oxygen concentrations and a nonflammable or shielded endotracheal tube.[117] Some authors recommend placing saline with methylene dye in the endotracheal tube cuff to dissipate heat and signal cuff rupture.[118] For these procedures, or any other procedure that utilizes intraoperative lasers, the patient should have the eyes shielded with saline pads and laser goggles. Operating room personnel also should wear appropriate eye protection when intraoperative lasers are in use.[119] A source of saline to extinguish a potential fire should be immediately available. If an airway fire does occur, stop oxygen flow, stop ventilation, extubate the patient, extinguish the fire, mask ventilate, and reintubate the patient.[120] The patient should then be referred for airway assessment and medical treatment, including bronchoscopy, lavage, and steroids.

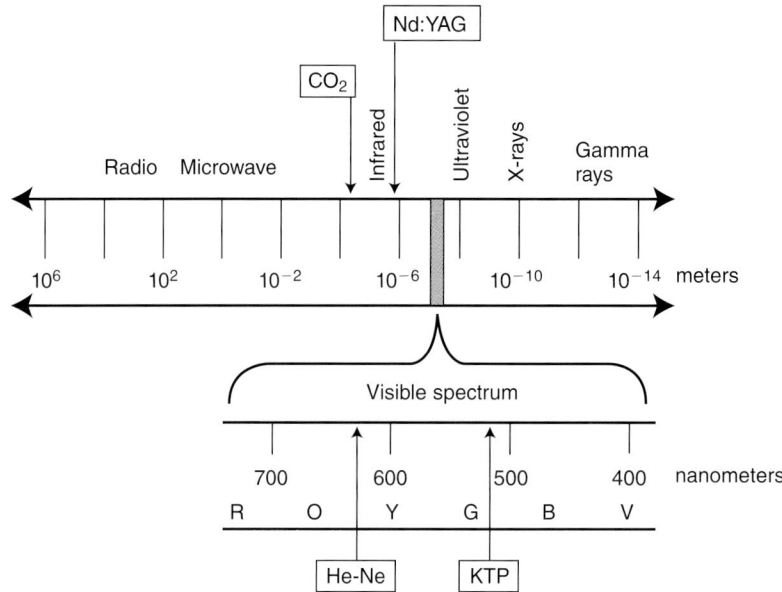

Fig. 15.47 Common medical laser frequencies. *CO₂*, Carbon dioxide; *He-Ne*, helium neon; *KTP*, potassium titanyl phosphate; *Nd:YAG*, neodymium-doped yttrium aluminum garnet; *R O Y G B V*, red, orange, yellow, green, blue, violet.

TABLE 15.6	Medical Lasers and Uses		
Laser	**Wavelength**	**Tissue Penetration**	**Characteristics/Uses**
He-Ne	633 nm	None	Aiming beam for invisible lasers
CO_2	10,600 nm	<0.5 mm	Highly absorbed by water
			Good for superficial lesions
			Used in airway surgeries
Argon	488 nm	0.5–2.0 mm	Selectively absorbed by hemoglobin
	514 nm		Good for hemangiomas, moles
			Also used in eye and ear surgery
KTP	1060 nm	0.5–2.0 mm	Highly absorbed by hemoglobin
			Multiple uses
YAG	1064–2940 nm	2–6 mm	Variable intensities
			Used to ablate and destroy tissues
			Multiple uses

CO_2, Carbon dioxide; *He-Ne*, helium neon; *KTP*, potassium titanyl phosphate; *YAG*, yttrium aluminum garnet.

■ SUMMARY

The historical view of the universe as a machine following fixed specific rules often allowed for unequivocal laws to be discovered. For a time, the actions of the universe seemed destined to be unlocked and forever understood. Unfortunately, or fortunately, this is not the case. The mechanistic view of the universe in newtonian physics loses its ability to describe certain phenomena, and this underscores a significant limitation. Advances in our knowledge of quantum events may shed light on phenomena that remain elusive.[121]

Quantum physics has brought us new insight into the subatomic world and uncovered the limitations of classical physics in fully describing the actions and reactions of the universe. What newtonian physics has done for the physical world, quantum physics promises to do for the nonphysical world: both the world of pure energy and the

quasi-world of energy/mass transition. Events in the quantum world are not determined by fixed, describable outcomes; instead, quantum events are described by probabilities. Phenomena that remain only partially understood in anesthesia may be clarified by discoveries in quantum study. Consciousness, awareness, and minimum alveolar concentrations (MACs) are all described in anesthesia as probabilities. Consciousness and awareness are not on-off phenomena, but rather fall within a spectrum. Delivery of anesthetics is sometimes measured not in fixed set doses but in ranges (or MACs) that provide a guideline for the probability of a desired outcome. Though the concept is controversial, it has been suggested that consciousness is a quantum event that can only be understood by the study of quantum mechanics.[122-125] Newtonian physics and physical chemistry will remain valued sciences that describe many processes in the field of anesthesia well, but quantum study may someday bring new advances and applications to anesthesia. Safer, more effective anesthesia techniques and technologies may evolve out of quantum understanding, or the mere search itself may stimulate new developments. Regardless, the future is exciting. Chemistry and physics have provided and will continue to provide a conceptual and analytic framework from which the nurse anesthetist can derive understanding, establish clinical rationales, and direct the practice of safe and effective anesthetic management of all patients.

REFERENCES

For a complete list of references for this chapter, scan this QR code with any smartphone code reader app, or visit the following URL: http://booksite.elsevier.com/9780323711944/.

16

Anesthesia Equipment

Darin L. Tharp, Michael P. Dosch

"To a large extent, anesthesia machines are inherently dangerous. A machine that has the power to induce anesthesia necessarily has the power to cause death and serious injury. An anesthesia department may want to institute periodic training to make sure that everyone in the department is familiar with all of the machines in the hospital."[1]

It would disturb any of us to read in the news about an adult, without driver's training, who attempted to drive a car and caused injury or death as a result. Should it not be equally disturbing to learn that, even after the introduction of electronic self-check routines, some anesthetists believe that the anesthesia workstation checks itself or that they feel they were never taught how to properly check the machine?[2,3] Since anesthesia equipment malfunction is so rare, misuse and human error are much more of a threat to patient safety than outright malfunction.[4-8] However, when errors in the use of gas delivery equipment occur, the outcome is often mortality or serious morbidity.[5] Human error can be most effectively combated by an industry commitment "to ensure that no patient is harmed by anesthesia" (the mission of the Anesthesia Patient Safety Foundation).[9] The means of accomplishing this goal are educational and motivational. We anesthetize patients who have many different kinds of problems, for many different kinds of surgical and diagnostic procedures. It is the purpose of this chapter to provide timely, accurate, and safe information about this important and ubiquitous patient-safety technology.

This edition will focus on anesthesia workstations in current practice. The main additions to this chapter are the discussion of open lung (lung-protective) ventilation strategies in the perioperative setting, the preuse checklist for the anesthesia workstation and its impact on patient safety, and new adaptive modes of ventilation (pressure control with volume guarantee, autoflow, pressure support, and continuous positive end-expiratory pressure [CPAP]). Differences between workstations are presented if understanding these differences is important to using the workstation safely. Brief descriptions of current anesthesia workstations are presented (Aisys, Aespire, and Avance [GE Healthcare, Madison, WI]; Fabius GS, Apollo, and Perseus A500 [Dräger Medical, Telford, PA]).

A major objective of this chapter is that readers will gain skill and safety in the use of the anesthesia workstation. Therefore, throughout the chapter, explicit directions on how to use the workstation safely are presented; these directions are based on manufacturers' guidelines and on reports of mishaps from the anesthesia literature. Because of the variety of workstations currently in use, no direction in this chapter can be considered universally applicable. The directions given here must be adapted to individual practice settings only after study of the operators' manuals and appropriate local peer review.

Several factors make learning about anesthesia workstations difficult. Each model has unique aspects—even those from the same manufacturer. It is not always possible for every anesthetist to be available when department in-service education is conducted. In addition, continuing education content may be too limited, or an opportunity to use new equipment soon after an educational session may not occur. New equipment constantly appears in the anesthesia work area. Although anesthesia equipment is designed to meet all legal and technical requirements, the designers of the equipment are not users. Some design limitations may be recognized only when they are used clinically.[10] Instructional materials accompanying equipment are often inadequate. For example, no matter how well written, supplying one instruction manual *per workstation* is inferior to supplying one manual *per user*. The potential lack in equipment competency caused by these factors can be a safety problem. Users may be held legally responsible for knowing and following manufacturers' instructions (checklists, operating manuals) and warnings because these may contribute to the standard of care. Some courts have defined deviation from manufacturers' instructions as prima facie negligence.[11]

This chapter views the anesthesia workstation from a systems approach, much like the 2008 PreAnesthesia Checklist.[12] For example, all workstations have systems to provide (and measure) gas composition, including life-sustaining gases (oxygen), anesthetizing gases, and metabolic by-products (carbon dioxide). When this capability of every anesthesia workstation is understood, one need only determine how a particular machine accomplishes this and how this function is checked before use to operate the machine safely (in this respect). Once all the systems, and their interplay, are understood, learning new equipment is easier. High-fidelity patient simulation is a novel approach that holds promise for both learning anesthesia equipment more efficiently and studying anesthesia workstation hazards. Simulation has allowed exploration of questions that could not be studied in the past because of risks to patients.[13-18]

ORGANIZATION OF THE ANESTHESIA WORKSTATION

Presenting the anesthesia workstation as a litany of components does not promote retention, much less aid in the development

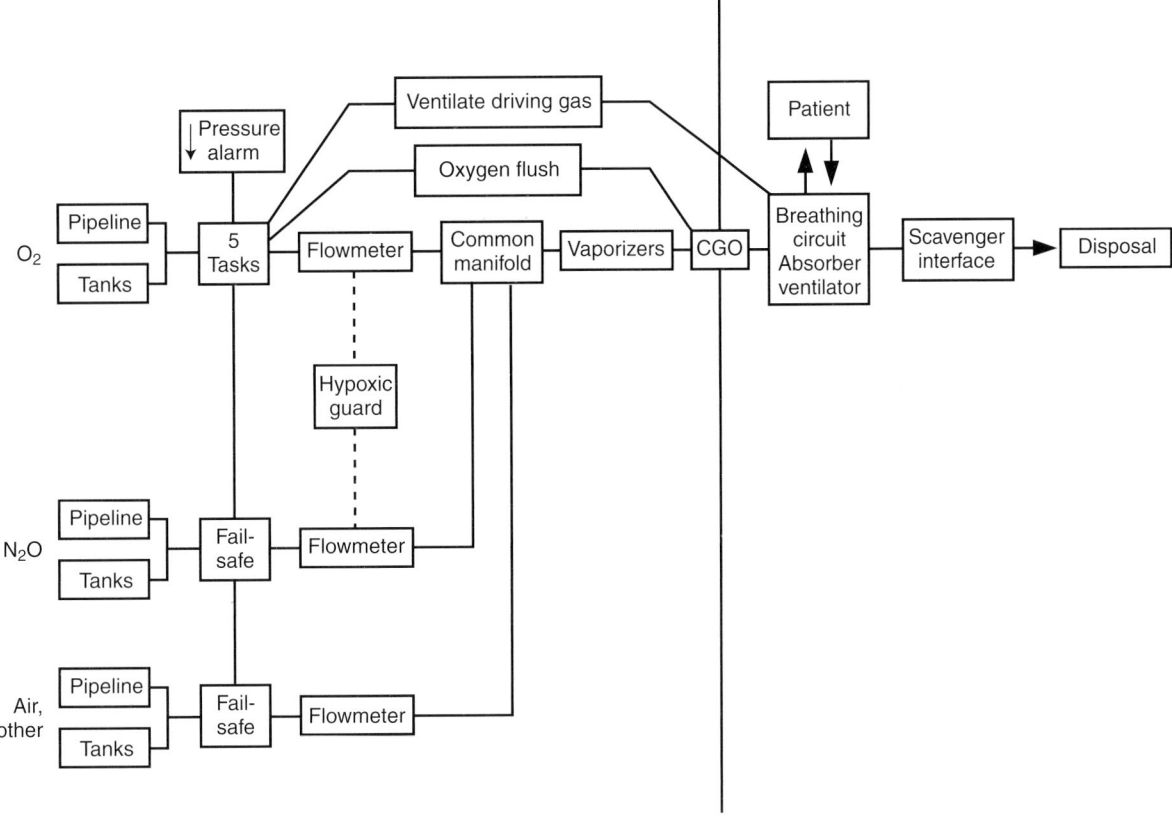

Fig. 16.1 Supply, processing, delivery, and disposal (SPDD) model. *CGO,* Common gas outlet. (Courtesy Michael P. Dosch.)

a conceptual understanding of the overall organization of the machine. An accurate concept of the overall organization should help one to understand the role of the individual components better, which should in turn promote correct use and thus patient safety. This section presents the supply, processing, delivery, and disposal (SPDD) model.

Supply, Processing, Delivery, and Disposal Model

The SPDD model is depicted in Fig. 16.1 and Box 16.1. This model is comprehensive in that the path of gases can be followed from their arrival in the operating room to their disposal from it. Most system components can be located easily within the overall scheme. Gas flows in the diagram proceed generally from left to right. The vertical bar separates components within the machine and proximal to the common gas outlet (left side), from external components downstream from the common gas outlet (right). The fact that nitrous oxide and air, unlike oxygen, have only one task in the machine is easy to appreciate. The five functions of oxygen are easy to follow. Understanding the similarities and differences between the fail-safe and hypoxic guard systems is facilitated. The model makes clear that the scavenging system, rather than the patient, is the ultimate destination of gases. Oxygen is central to the figure because it is the most essential gas delivered. The reader should note that not every component of the SPDD model in Box 16.1 is depicted graphically in Fig. 16.1. The reader should make frequent reference to the model while reading this chapter.

The model organizes the information based on how components are used rather than on the pressures to which they are exposed. From the viewpoint of pressure to which components are exposed, components

are classified as part of the high-, intermediate-, or low-pressure systems within (proximal to the common gas outlet) the anesthesia workstation (Box 16.2).

Introduction of new anesthesia workstations will invariably raise questions about the adequacy and safety of older equipment.[1,19] One way a user or department can determine whether equipment is obsolete is by considering how closely it meets current practice needs, by the availability of service, and by the presence of essential safety features.[20,21] These criteria become apparent when one becomes familiar with all four components of the SPDD model, which can be utilized as the framework upon which current and future equipment is appraised. Typical components of an anesthesia workstation can be found in Box 16.3.

SUPPLY

The concept of supply is concerned with these questions: How do gases (and electric power) come to the anesthesia workstation? What are the likely faults and hazards?

Pipeline Supply

Configuration

Oxygen is produced by the fractional distillation of liquid air. It is delivered to facilities and stored as a liquid at a temperature of −160°C.[22] The liquid oxygen is converted to a gas and supplied to hospital pipelines at a pressure of 50 psi (344 kPa). In the operating suite, main and partial-area shutoff valves are present to isolate sections with leaks, interrupt supply in case of fire, and allow repair work on subsections. Wall outlets, or hoses dropped from the operating room ceiling, are

---

BOX 16.1   Components in Supply, Processing, Delivery, and Disposal (SPDD) Model

Supply
How Do Gases Come to the Anesthesia Workstation?
(Site: Back of the Machine)
- Pipeline
  - Wall outlets
  - Connecting valves and hoses
  - Filters and check valves
  - Pressure gauges
- Cylinders
  - Hanger yokes (yoke block)
  - Filters and check valves
  - Pressure gauge
  - Pressure regulators

Processing
How Does the Anesthesia Workstation Prepare Gases
Before Delivery to the Patient? (Site: Within the Machine,
Proximal to Common Gas Outlet)
- Fail-safe (oxygen pressure-failure devices)
- Flowmeters (main, auxiliary, common gas outlet, scavenging)
- Oxygen flush
- Low oxygen pressure alarms
- Ventilator-driving gas
- Proportioning systems (hypoxic guard)
- Oxygen second-stage regulator (if present)

- Vaporizers
- Check valves distal to vaporizers (if present)
- Common gas outlet

Delivery
How Is the Interaction of Gases Controlled and Monitored?
(Site: Breathing Circuit)
- Gas delivery hose connecting common gas outlet and breathing circuit
- Breathing circuits
  - Nonrebreathing
  - Circle
- Carbon dioxide absorption
- Ventilators
- Integral monitors
  - Oxygen analysis
  - Disconnect
  - Spirometry (volumes and flows), capnography, airway pressure
- Ventilator alarms
- Addition of positive end-expiratory pressure
- Means of humidification

Disposal
How Are Gases Disposed? (Site: Scavenger)
- Scavenger systems
  - Interface—closed (active and passive) or open
  - Scavenger flowmeter

BOX 16.2   Components in the High-, Intermediate-, and Low-Pressure Pneumatic Systems

High-Pressure System (Exposed to Cylinder Pressure)
- Hanger yoke
- Yoke block with check valves
- Cylinder pressure gauge
- Cylinder pressure regulators

Intermediate-Pressure System (Exposed to Pipeline Pressure—Approximately 50 psi)
- Pipeline inlets, check valves, and pressure gauges
- Ventilator power inlet
- Oxygen pressure-failure devices
- Flowmeter valve
- Oxygen second-stage regulator (if present)
- Flush valve

Low-Pressure System (Distal to Flowmeter Needle Valve)
- Flowmeter tubes
- Vaporizers
- Check valves (if present)
- Common gas outlet

finished with quick-connect couplers. These couplers are used so the connection of the anesthesia workstation supply hoses to the wall outlets does not require tools. However, the springs and rubber gaskets (O-rings) these couplers contain provide a connection that is less secure than a wrench-tightened connection; thus they are a common source of leaks.[23-25]

Systems processing nitrous oxide are similar. Nitrous oxide is delivered to the hospital in large (size H) cylinders, which are connected to a manifold. Regulators reduce the pressure so that nitrous oxide, like oxygen and air, is supplied to the pipelines at 50 psi.[22] Consequently, 50 psi is the normal working pressure of the anesthesia workstation. Shutoff valves and wall outlets with quick-connect couplers are similar for nitrous oxide, air, and oxygen. Delivery piping for all pipeline gases uses the diameter index safety system (DISS) to prevent misconnections. In this system, gas-piping connections are sized and threaded differently so that cross-connection is difficult though not impossible (Fig. 16.2).[23,26] In spite of modern equipment that met standards, the connection of a nitrous oxide hose to a carbon dioxide wall outlet resulted in brief hypercarbia without lasting complications.[27]

Supply hoses connect the pipeline inlets on the back of the workstation to the wall outlets. At the pipeline inlet, a filter, check valve, and pressure gauge are present. The check valve ensures unidirectional forward flow so that a workstation running on cylinder supplies, with the hoses disconnected at the wall outlet, does not leak (Fig. 16.3). The filter may help prevent damage to the anesthesia workstation from particulate matter present in the pipeline gas supply.[28]

Problems With Pipeline Supply

Some of the problems associated with pipeline use can be particularly dangerous because they are occult or infrequent. Pressure loss, excess pressure, cross-connection of gas delivery pipelines, contamination, leaks, and theft of nitrous oxide (for recreational use) have been reported.[29,30] There were 45 deaths related to pipeline problems in the United States from 1972 to 1993, and this number is probably an underestimate.[31] Two patients became hypoxemic during anesthesia due to delivery to a hospital of nitrogen tanks with oxygen fittings in 1996.[26] Seven deaths related to piped medical gases were reported from 1997

BOX 16.3 Typical Components of an Anesthesia Workstation

Battery Backup for 30 Minutes

Alarms

- Grouped into high, medium, and low priority.
- High-priority alarms may not be silenced for more than 2 min.
- Certain alarms and monitors must be automatically enabled and functioning prior to use, either through turning the workstation on or by following the preuse checklist: breathing circuit pressure, oxygen concentration, exhaled volume, or carbon dioxide (or both).
- A high-priority pressure alarm must sound if user-adjustable limits are exceeded, if continuing high pressure is sensed, or for negative pressure.
- Disconnect alarms may be based on low pressure, exhaled volume, or carbon dioxide.

Monitors

- Exhaled volume
- Inspired oxygen, with a high-priority alarm within 30 sec of oxygen falling below 18% (or a user-adjustable limit)
- Oxygen supply failure alarm
- A hypoxic guard system must protect against less than 21% inspired oxygen if nitrous oxide is in use.
- Anesthetic vapor concentration must be monitored.
- Pulse oximetry, blood pressure monitoring, and electrocardiogram (ECG) are required.

Pressure in the breathing circuit is limited to 12.5 kPa (125 cm H_2O).

The electrical supply cord must be nondetachable or resistant to detachment.

Cylinder Supplies

- The workstation must have at least one oxygen cylinder attached.
- The hanger yoke must be pin-indexed, have a clamping device that resists leaks, and contain a filter. It must have a check valve to prevent transfilling and a cylinder pressure gauge.

- There must be cylinder pressure regulators. The workstation must use pipeline gas as long as pipeline pressure is >345 kPa (50 psi).

Flowmeters

- Single control for each gas
- Each flow control must be next to a flow indicator.
- There must be a uniquely shaped oxygen flow control knob (if present).
- Valve stops (or some other mechanism) are required such that excessive rotation will not damage the flowmeter.
- Oxygen flow indicator is to the right side of a flowmeter bank.
- Oxygen enters the common manifold downstream of other gases.
- An auxiliary oxygen flowmeter is strongly recommended.

An oxygen flush is present, capable of 35–75 L/min flow that does not proceed through any vaporizers.

Vaporizers

- They must be concentration calibrated.
- An interlock must be present.
- Liquid level must be indicated and designed to prevent overfilling.
- "Should" use keyed-filler devices.
- No discharge of liquid anesthetic occurs from the vaporizer, even at maximum fresh gas flow.

Pipeline Gas Supply

- Pipeline pressure gauge
- Inlets for at least oxygen and nitrous oxide
- Diameter index safety system (DISS) protected
- In-line filter
- Check valve

Checklist must be provided (it may be electronic, performed manually by the user, or have elements of both)

A digital data interface must be provided.

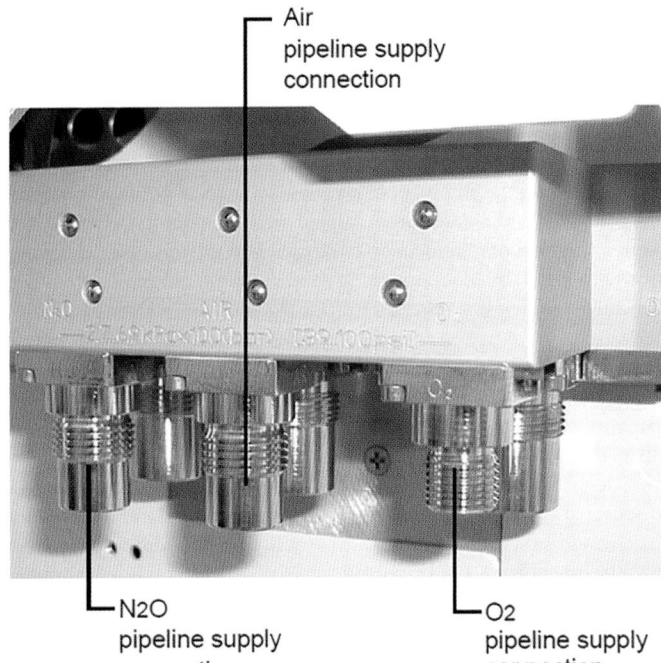

Fig. 16.2 Pipeline connections using the diameter index safety system (DISS) ensure that only the correct gas hose can be connected to each inlet on the back of the anesthesia workstation and at the wall outlet. (From *Apollo Operator's Instruction Manual*, Document No. 90 38 237, Rev. 01. Telford, PA: Dräeger Medical Inc; 2005. © Dräegerwerk AG & Co. KGaA, Lubeck. All rights reserved.)

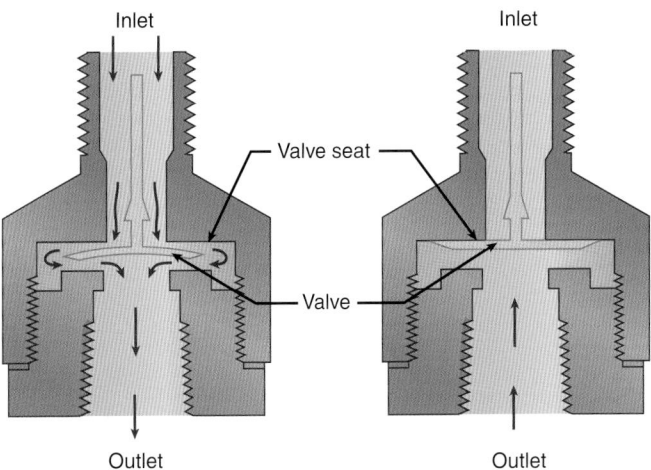

Fig. 16.3 Check valve in the pipeline gas supply inlet at the back of the anesthesia workstation. Gas enters from the supply hose at "Inlet" and proceeds *(downwards in the illustration)* into the workstation *(left)*. The right panel shows that gas cannot leak out of the workstation if the supply hose is disconnected. (From Bowie E, Huffman LM. *The Anesthesia Machine: Essentials for Understanding.* Madison, WI: Ohmeda, a Division of BOC Health Care, Ind; 1985. In Miller RD, et al., eds. *Miller's Anesthesia.* 7th ed. Philadelphia: Elsevier; 2010.)

to 2001.[32] Two patients became hypoxemic due to purging of oxygen lines with nitrogen in 2000.[33] A serious failure of the bulk liquid oxygen supply was noted in 2004, but no patients were harmed.[34] Water was reported in air flowmeters in 2013 and 2015.[35,36] In 2019, a hypoxic breathing mixture was created by nitrogen contamination of pipeline oxygen, causing hypoxemia in two patients and cardiac arrest in one.[37] Complications can arise if oxygen analyzers fail or are misused.[2,38,39] Until you can prove it wrong, always trust an oxygen analyzer that is reporting low inspired oxygen.

Pipeline supplies of gas have been reported to contain particulate, gaseous, and bacterial matter, other contaminants, and water.[28,29,35,40] The Joint Commission allows site visitors to randomly approach and question operating room staff, to ensure they are aware of the location and function of pipeline shutoff valves and alarms related to gas supplies in their area.[40]

Loss of Oxygen Pipeline Pressure

Loss of oxygen pipeline pressure is indicated by the pipeline pressure gauge. In addition, if pressure loss is profound, the oxygen low-pressure (high-priority audible and visible) alarm is engaged, and the fail-safe valves halt the delivery of all other gases. Some newer workstations are designed to switch to air to drive the ventilator bellows when oxygen pipeline pressure is lost.

Two simulation studies point to the need for change in the way we teach and respond to loss of oxygen pipeline pressure.[15,18] In a simulated loss of pipeline oxygen, most residents recognized the oxygen pressure-loss alarms. But less than half knew how to change an empty oxygen cylinder, attempted to change it (even after prompting), or recognized that bag-valve-mask (Ambu) ventilation would lead to patient awakening.[18] A group of volunteer specialist anesthetists (who had completed residency and were in practice) managed a simulated oxygen pipeline failure equally poorly.[15] In their preuse check, 70% failed to identify an empty oxygen cylinder, and only 25% checked for backup ventilation equipment (a bag-valve-mask) before induction. Most failed to conserve cylinder oxygen (by using low fresh gas flows and turning off the mechanical ventilator), and all used untested pipeline supplies of oxygen when informed that pressure had been restored.[15] These responses could be considered unwise at least, or unsafe at worst. In a third report, more than 700 anesthetics were given over a 3-week period without any checks that the emergency oxygen cylinder was full.[41]

Management of a loss of oxygen pipeline pressure has the following goals: maintenance of oxygenation, ventilation, and depth of anesthesia; and confirmation and assurance of safe oxygen supply.[15] Box 16.4 gives suggestions for management.[15,18,34,42–45] With complete loss of oxygen pipeline pressure, an immediate next step should be to fully open the E cylinder of oxygen, disconnect the pipeline, and consider the use of low fresh gas flows and manual ventilation (using the circle system). These latter actions act to conserve the emergency cylinder supply of oxygen while continuing to supply volatile anesthetic vapor. If the E cylinder of oxygen is not fully opened, flow from it may end before the cylinder is empty. Disconnecting the supply hose at the quick-connect fitting at the wall, though not strictly necessary during an oxygen pressure loss, is recommended for two reasons. First, it must be disconnected in the case of a cross-connection (which is more fully described later), otherwise the contents of the oxygen cylinder will not flow. Remembering one strategy that is effective for two reasonably similar problems is easier than remembering two different strategies. Second, if the loss of pipeline pressure is followed by the flow of contaminated contents from the oxygen pipeline, disconnecting when pipeline pressure is lost protects the patient from exposure to these contaminants.

BOX 16.4 Management of Oxygen Pipeline Supply Failure, or Crossover

Always check for the presence of a full E cylinder and an alternative means of ventilation (bag-valve-mask [Ambu] device) before using an anesthesia workstation. If pipeline pressure fails or fraction of inspired oxygen drops, follow these steps:

1. Do not attempt to fix the oxygen analyzer—it must be trusted until it can be proved wrong.
2. Turn on the backup oxygen cylinder on the workstation fully, then disconnect the pipeline. Ensure that the measured fraction of inspired oxygen (Fio_2) begins to rise. If the Fio_2 does not increase (with fresh gas flow adequate to wash in the O_2 quickly), ventilate the patient by Ambu bag with room air.
3. Use low flows of oxygen. Maintain anesthesia with a volatile agent. Ensure that Fio_2 and agent concentration are appropriate.
4. Turn off the ventilator and ventilate manually through the circle system.
5. Call for help if needed; calculate the time remaining for the current cylinder; call for additional oxygen cylinders, and install them on the workstation if needed.
6. Find out how long the problem is expected to last; participate in the hospital disaster plan, which may require prioritizing oxygen for those patients who need it most.
7. Do not reconnect patient to pipeline gas until the gas supply is tested.
8. If unable to use the circle, ventilate with an oxygen source (freestanding cylinder) or with room air via a bag-valve-mask device, and institute total intravenous anesthesia.

Although excessive pipeline pressure will not trigger alarms in the machine, it should do so in the hospital physical plant or engineering department. Excessive pressure can damage respiratory apparatus or machinery of various types connected to the pipeline, including the anesthesia workstation.

Cross-Connection of Gases

Cross-connection of gases can occur anywhere from the liquid oxygen supply and piping, to the wall outlets, hoses, and internal circuitry of the anesthesia gas workstation. Incidents of cross-connection continue to be reported (as recently as 2019).[27,37,46–48] Fatalities have been associated with the shipment in error to the hospital of liquid nitrogen instead of oxygen, liquid carbon dioxide rather than nitrous oxide, the unintentional cross-connection of oxygen and nitrous oxide pipelines during renovation of an operating room, and alteration of an oxygen flowmeter so that it would fit a nitrous oxide outlet in a cardiac catheterization laboratory. A common factor associated with patient injury has been failure to use an oxygen analyzer.

Although not all the previously mentioned incidents involved patients connected to an anesthesia workstation, cross-connections also continue to be reported in anesthetized patients. In 1997, a case was described in which the nitrogen hose from the workstation was discovered to be fitted with a quick-connect coupler for air (at the end that would be plugged into the wall outlet).[26] This did not result in patient injury but would have allowed the delivery of 100% nitrogen had the machine been set to deliver air only. The consequences of this type of error in the oxygen wall-outlet hose could be disastrous. In 1995 it was reported that two patients became hypoxemic as a result of delivery of liquid nitrogen to the hospital in a tank with oxygen fittings.[49] In 2009 a wall fitting for carbon dioxide in a lithotripsy area allowed connection of a nitrous oxide hose from the anesthesia workstation, resulting in end-tidal carbon dioxide over 105 mm Hg.[27] Cross-connections caused a death in Sydney in 2016 and caused hypoxemia in two Florida patients in 2019, with subsequent bradycardia in one and cardiac

TABLE 16.1 Characteristics of E Cylinders*

Gas	Color, US (International)	Service Pressure psi (kPa × 10⁻²)	Capacity (L)	Pin Position
Oxygen	Green (white)	1900 (131)	660	2–5
Nitrous oxide	Blue (blue)	745 (51)	1590	3–5
Air	Yellow (black and white)	1900 (131)	625	1–5

*Note that slightly different values may be found in different sources. Data from Dorsch JA, Dorsch SE. *A Practical Approach to Anesthesia Equipment*. Philadelphia: Lippincott Williams & Wilkins; 2011; Standard Specification for Particular Requirements for Anesthesia Workstations and Their Components [F1850-00]. Philadelphia: American Society for Testing and Materials; 2005; NFPA 99: Health Care Facilities [Table 5.1.11]. Quincy, MA: National Fire Protection Association; 2012:49.

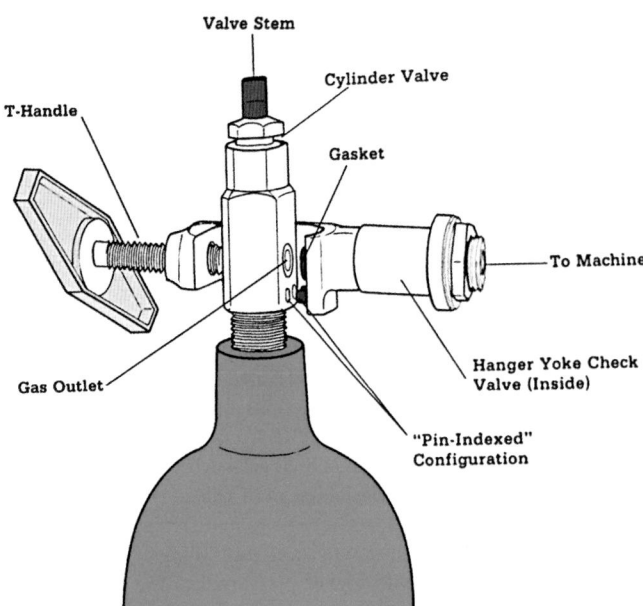

Fig. 16.4 Pin index safety system, cylinder valve, and yoke. (Modified from Bowie E, Huffman LM. *The Anesthesia Machine: Essentials for Understanding*. Madison, WI: Ohmeda, a Division of BOC Health Care, Ind; 1985.)

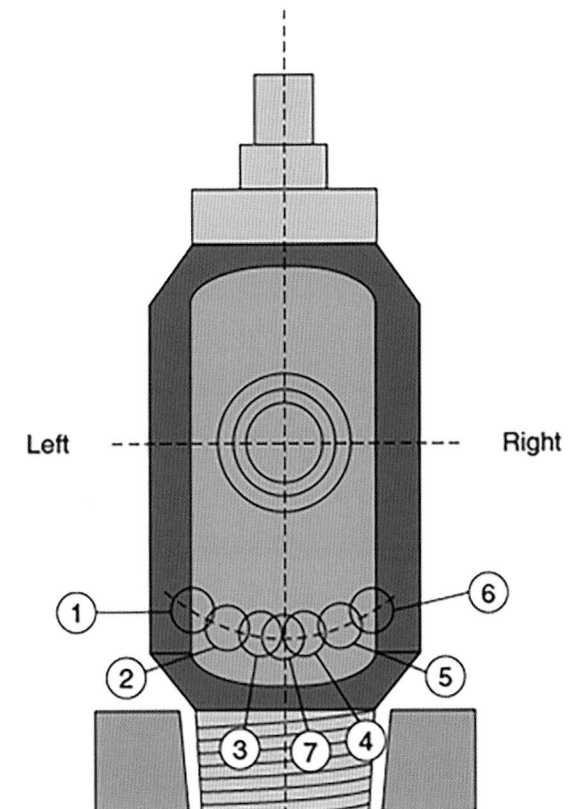

Fig. 16.5 Pin index safety system: pin positions. (Modified from Ehrenwerth J, Eisenkraft J, Berry J, eds. *Anesthesia Equipment: Principles and Applications*. 2nd ed. Philadelphia: Elsevier; 2013.)

arrest in the other.[37,50] These incidents underscore our susceptibility to the errors of ancillary personnel who install and test gas delivery apparatus. But they also highlight many patient-safety aspects under our control: properly checking oxygen analysis monitors and the anesthesia workstation before use, and proper response to oxygen-analyzer alarms.

In the event of a suspected crossover, a declining inspired oxygen concentration would be observed. The initial actions should be to open the emergency cylinder oxygen supply, disconnect the pipeline, and use low fresh gas flows and manual ventilation (see Box 16.4). If the pipeline is not disconnected, the pipeline gas will continue to flow rather than the cylinder oxygen supply because the pressure distal to the cylinder regulator is set at 45 psi (310 kPa), compared with the typical pipeline pressure of 50 psi (344 kPa). Lower pressure is intentionally set on the cylinder regulator so that flow proceeds from the higher-pressure pipeline source if a cylinder is inadvertently left open after the machine has been checked.[51] This is analogous to the situation with an intravenous main line and a piggyback line: Whichever is held higher is the one that will flow (greater hydrostatic pressure). In the case of cross-connection between oxygen and nitrous oxide pipelines, the contents of the oxygen pipeline (now nitrous oxide) continue to flow (because the pipeline pressure is 50 psi), whether or not the oxygen cylinder is open. Thus, regardless of the problem with the pipeline supply (lack of pressure or cross-connection), the cylinder must be opened; disconnecting the pipeline in any instance of problems with the pipeline is safe. If the pipeline is not disconnected and has pressure within it, the emergency supply of oxygen may not flow from the cylinder.

Cylinder Supply

Cylinders are present on the anesthesia workstation as reserves for emergency use. Thus, they should be open only when they are checked or when the pipeline supply is unavailable.[52] A fresh oxygen cylinder is obtained if the cylinder on the machine has inadequate pressure, depending on the availability of pipeline supplies and additional backup oxygen cylinders (see "Anesthesia Workstation Checklist" later). Cylinders are labeled, marked, and color coded (Table 16.1).[53] Anesthetists who practice outside the United States must be aware that the color scheme differs from country to country. Service pressure and cylinder contents are reported slightly differently in various sources.[54]

Pin position refers to the pin index safety system (PISS) illustrated in Figs. 16.4 and 16.5. In this system each cylinder valve has a unique arrangement of holes that correspond to its intended contents. The holes mate with pins in the yoke, which is the point where cylinders are attached to the anesthesia workstation. The PISS is thus another means of preventing misconnections. The system can be defeated if the pins are missing, are removed, or if more than one washer is used. Anesthetists should check both pins and washers whenever cylinders are replaced. Furthermore, they should be aware that not all E cylinders are of precisely the right size to fit properly on the machine. Installation of a longer aluminum cylinder has interfered with the casters and prevented an anesthesia workstation from being moved.[55]

The cylinder valve is the most fragile part of the cylinder so it must be protected during transport. The cylinder valve consists of a body, the port where gas exits, a conical depression (opposite the port) for the securing screw, the holes where the pins on the yoke fit, and safety relief devices. If a fire causes the temperature and pressure within the cylinder to increase, safety relief devices release cylinder contents in a controlled fashion rather than explosively. Manufacturers use one or more of the following on cylinder valves: a frangible disk that bursts under pressure, a valve that opens at extreme pressure, or a fusible plug made of Wood metal (which melts at elevated temperatures).

The hanger yoke serves three functions: It orients cylinders, provides a gas-tight seal, and ensures unidirectional flow into the machine. It also contains a filter. A unidirectional valve within the hanger yoke minimizes the likelihood of transfilling, or of leakage to the atmosphere (if a yoke is empty). It also allows cylinders to be replaced during use. If two cylinders of the same gas are open, transfilling occurs when gas flows from the cylinder with higher pressure into the cylinder with lower pressure, rather than proceeding toward the flowmeters. Transfilling is a potential fire hazard because filling a cylinder generates heat. The cylinder pressure gauge is a Bourdon-type gauge (Fig. 16.6).

Immediately distal to the hanger yoke for each gas is a regulator (Fig. 16.7). Two diaphragms move together, connected by a rod. The smaller of the two diaphragms opens or closes the high-pressure inlet (from the cylinder). Gas entering the regulator exerts pressure on the larger diaphragm, whose movement tends to close the inlet. Thus, gas can enter the regulator only at a rate controlled by a feedback loop. The outlet pressure is adjustable by a screw and spring that bear on the inlet diaphragm. The high (but variable) cylinder pressure is converted

to a constant downstream pressure (45 psi [310 kPa]), set intentionally at slightly less than pipeline pressure to prevent silent depletion of cylinder contents.[40] Pipeline pressure varies depending on the load that is placed on it throughout the facility. If a cylinder is left open and pipeline pressure drops below 45 psi, then gas will flow preferentially from an open cylinder. No alarm will sound to warn the user of this condition.[29] Furthermore, if the cylinder is left open after checking and the pipeline fails, the operator will not be alerted to the failure at the

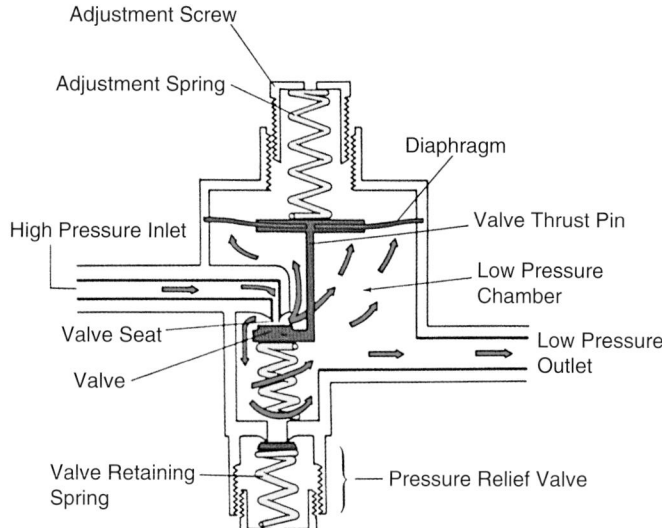

Fig. 16.7 A schematic view of a cylinder regulator. (From Bowie E, Huffman LM. *The Anesthesia Machine: Essentials for Understanding.* Madison, WI: Datex-Ohmeda; 1985.)

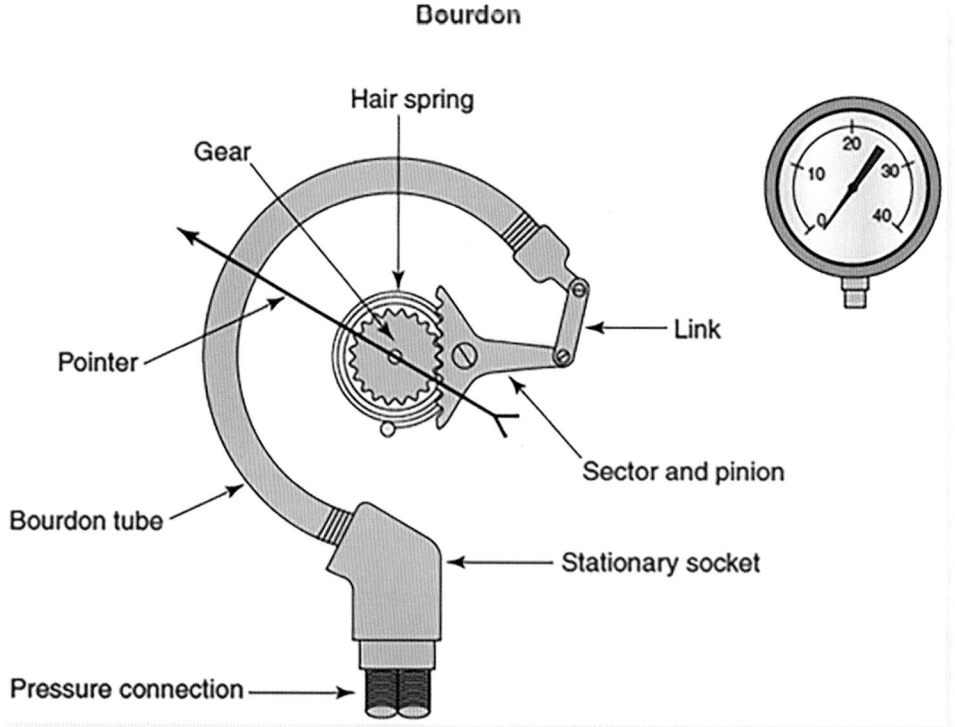

Fig. 16.6 Bourdon-type pressure gauges are aneroid gauges used for measuring cylinder (and pipeline) pressure. (Modified from Ehrenwerth J, Eisenkraft J, Berry J, eds. *Anesthesia Equipment: Principles and Applications.* 2nd ed. Philadelphia: Elsevier; 2013.)

time it occurs because gas will simply begin to flow from the cylinder without alarms. If the mechanical ventilator is in use, a full E cylinder of oxygen may be depleted in as little as 1 hour because the driving gas in a bellows ventilator is usually oxygen.[42,56] The low oxygen supply failure alarm that rings subsequently announces the end of the emergency supply instead of its beginning. This is the rationale for keeping cylinders closed after their pressure has been checked.

The US Department of Transportation issues regulations for the manufacture, handling, transport, storage, and disposal of cylinders. These regulations have binding legal force. Industry advisory groups such as the Compressed Gas Association (CGA) and the National Fire Protection Association also have a role in setting cylinder standards. Cylinders are constructed of steel approximately 0.24 inch in thickness. Only nonferrous (aluminum) cylinders may be used in the magnetic resonance imaging (MRI) environment.[54] Fatalities have occurred when steel cylinders have impacted patients in the MRI scanner.[57]

An awareness of the rules for the safe handling and use of cylinders is important for proper utilization.[29,58] Gas under pressure in cylinders has enormous potential energy, which may be lethal if it is released in a rapid, uncontrolled fashion following damage to the cylinder valve. Selected rules for safe handling of cylinders are presented in Box 16.5.

When installing a cylinder, check the labels, crack the valve, check that both PISS pins are present, check that only one washer is present, place the cylinder in the hanger yoke, observe for the absence of an audible leak, and check for proper gauge pressure. The valve is "cracked" to remove dirt from the port. This is done by opening the valve briefly and carefully before the cylinder is placed on the machine. While cracking the valve, hold the cylinder securely, and do not point the port toward oneself or other personnel.

When relying on cylinder supplies in an emergency, one must be able to calculate how long an oxygen cylinder will last. The following relationship should be used:

$$\frac{Capacity\ (L)}{Service\ pressure\ (psi)} = \frac{Contents\ remaining\ (L)}{Gauge\ pressure\ (psi)}$$

That is, the cylinder capacity when full is related to the gauge pressure when full (the service pressure), in the same proportion as the (unknown) contents remaining are related to the current gauge pressure. Remember to consider the oxygen flow rate set on the flowmeter when deciding how long the available liters will last. As an example, if

the oxygen flow is 2 L/min, and the cylinder's oxygen gauge pressure is 500 psi, how long will the cylinder last? From Table 16.1, we know that the service pressure is 1900 psi and the capacity is 660 L. Substituting these values into the previous relationship, we obtain the following:

$$\frac{660\ L}{1900\ psi} = \frac{x\ L}{500\ psi}\ and\ x = 174\ L$$

Since 2 L of oxygen flow each minute, the cylinder will last approximately 87 minutes (174 L ÷ 2 L/min). This type of calculation is not applicable to compressed gases stored as liquids (nitrous oxide or carbon dioxide). It should be remembered that this calculation refers only to requirements at the flowmeters and assumes manual ventilation. Use of a mechanical ventilator consumes approximately a minute volume of driving gas each minute and thus should be avoided in situations in which oxygen supply is limited to cylinders only.[56]

Cylinder contents must meet the purity requirements for medical gases established by the *US Pharmacopeia* (USP). The contents are also regulated by the US Food and Drug Administration (FDA). Oxygen is used to power ventilators throughout the hospital because it is dry, readily available, and relatively inexpensive.

Nitrous oxide is stored as a liquid, therefore the cylinder pressure of 745 psi (5136 kPa) represents the vapor pressure of liquid nitrous oxide at room temperature. The nitrous oxide cylinder pressure gauge remains at 745 psi until the liquid is gone; at this point, the cylinder is more than three-quarters empty. After this point, the nitrous oxide cylinder pressure swiftly declines with further use. Thus nitrous oxide cylinders should be changed if their pressure is less than 745 psi. Rapid removal (>4 L/min) from a nitrous oxide cylinder may cause the formation of frost on its wall or freezing of the valve, owing to rapid cooling as the liquid nitrous oxide evaporates. Nitrous oxide is non-flammable, but it does support combustion.[29,54] Anesthesia personnel must be alert to the possibility of nitrous oxide abuse.[59]

Atmospheric air is not dry. Hospitals that use compressors to create their own medical air actively dry it because liquid water condensed in the air pipelines can cause serious damage to equipment such as anesthesia workstations.[35,36] Medical air is composed of nitrogen (78%), oxygen (21%), and argon (nearly 1%). Carbon dioxide (0.03%) and other gases are present in trace amounts.

Electric Power Supply

Electric power is supplied to the anesthesia workstation through a single power cord, which can become dislodged. Because of this possibility, as well as the possibility of loss of main electrical power, new anesthesia workstations are generally equipped with battery backup sufficient for at least 30 minutes of limited operation.[60] Which systems remain powered during this period is specific to each model, thus users must read the operator manuals. Patient monitors (e.g., electrocardiogram [ECG], noninvasive blood pressure, gas analysis, pulse oximetry), fresh gas flowmeters, vaporizers, and ventilators may or may not continue to function during the period that battery backup is used.

Electrical receptacles are usually found on the back of the workstation so that monitors or other equipment can be plugged in. These convenience receptacles are protected by circuit breakers or fuses. It is a mistake to plug devices that convert electric power into heat into these receptacles (air or water warming blankets, intravenous fluid warmers) for two reasons. First, these devices draw a lot of amperage (relative to other electric devices) so they are more likely to cause a circuit breaker to open. Second, the circuit breakers are in nonstandard locations (so check for their location before your first case). If a circuit breaker opens, all devices that receive power there (such as monitors and, in some configurations, the mechanical ventilator) may cease to function. If one is not familiar with the circuit breaker location, valuable time may be lost while a search is conducted.

BOX 16.5 Rules for Safe Handling of Compressed Gas Cylinders

Always
- Protect the cylinder valve when carrying a cylinder; it is the most fragile part.

Never
- Stand a cylinder upright without support; if a rack or stand is not available, lay it on its side.
- Leave empty cylinders on the workstation.
- Leave the plastic cover on the port while installing the cylinder.
- Use more than one washer between a cylinder port and the yoke.
- Rely only on a cylinder's color for identification of its contents; read its labeling.
- Oil valves.
- Remove a cylinder from a yoke without filling the space with a yoke plug if available, which is a backup strategy for guarding against check valve failure.

Loss of Main Electric Power

Devices that typically require wall-outlet electric power include mechanical ventilators, physiologic monitors, room and surgical-field illumination, digital displays for electronic flowmeters, cardiopulmonary bypass pump/oxygenators, air warming blankets, gas/vapor blenders (Tec 6 [GE Healthcare]), and vaporizers with electronic controls (Aladin cassettes in the Aisys).

Devices that typically do not rely on wall-outlet electric power include spontaneous or manually assisted ventilation, mechanical flowmeters, scavenging, laryngoscope, flashlights, manual intravenous bolus or gravity-controlled infusions, battery-operated peripheral nerve stimulators or intravenous infusion pumps, monitoring by the anesthetist using the five senses, manual blood pressure cuffs, and variable bypass vaporizers (e.g., Tec 7 [GE Healthcare]; Vapor 2000 [Dräger Medical]).

Generally, hospitals have emergency generators that will supply operating room electrical outlets in the event power is lost. But these backup generators are not completely reliable. A 90-minute interruption in power during cardiopulmonary bypass, complicated by almost immediate failure of the hospital generators, has been described.[61,62] Injury to personnel as they hurried in the dark to fetch lights and equipment was an unanticipated hazard.

With power failure in older anesthesia workstations, the principal problems were loss of room illumination, failure of mechanical ventilators, and failure of electronic patient monitoring.[63] In general, new anesthesia workstations have battery backup sufficient for 30 minutes of operation; however, they are typically without patient monitors (e.g., ECG, pulse oximetry, gas analysis). Mechanical ventilation may or may not be powered by the backup battery (depending on the model). New flowmeters that are entirely electronic (Aisys and Avance [GE Healthcare]) require a backup pneumatic/mechanical (needle valve and flowtube) flowmeter.[64–67] Mechanical flowmeters with digital display of flows have a backup glass flow tube that indicates total fresh gas flow (Fabius GS[68] and Apollo [Dräger Medical]).

New anesthesia workstations with mechanical needle valve flowmeters and variable bypass vaporizers (e.g., Apollo [Dräger Medical] and Aespire [GE Healthcare]) allow for the delivery of gases and agents indefinitely during electrical power failure.[53,68] However, in the event of generator failure, anesthesia monitoring would be limited to flashlight illumination and assessment using the five senses. The Apollo (Dräger Medical) provides gas and vapor delivery, mechanical ventilation, and integrated monitoring (e.g., oxygen, breathing circuit volume and pressure, gas analysis) for 30 minutes or more if main electrical power is lost.[69,70] Patient monitors will not function on battery power. Pneumatic functions remain even after the battery is exhausted: vaporizers, sensitive oxygen ratio controller (S-ORC) (fail-safe and hypoxic guard), adjustable pressure-limiting (APL) valve, flowmeters, breathing pressure gauge, cylinder and pipeline pressure gauges, and total fresh gas flowmeter.

Due to the differences between models, it remains important to understand and anticipate how each particular anesthesia workstation responds when main electrical power is lost. This information may be reviewed in the operator manual.

PROCESSING

In this section the various aspects of the anesthesia workstation's preparation of gases before their delivery to the patient are discussed.

Manufacturers and Models

Manufacturers of anesthesia workstations common in the United States include Dräger Medical and GE Healthcare. There are some imported models in the market as well. Dräger Medical, Inc. (Telford, PA) is the manufacturer of the Narkomed series (6000 and 6400, GS, MRI, Mobile models), the Apollo, Perseus, and Fabius GS. GE Healthcare (Madison, WI) is the manufacturer of the Aisys, Avance, Aespire, Aestiva, and Aestiva MRI.

Anesthesia workstations that are not currently produced remain in widespread use because their service life is long, often 10 to 15 years or more. The differences among new anesthesia workstations are significant, thus what one learns on one model may not transfer very well to a different model. This is particularly true of preanesthesia checkout (see later). The differences are pointed out in this chapter when they are relevant to clinical practice or to demonstrate by comparison how systems function. This section continues with an overview of several current anesthesia workstations, which are summarized in Table 16.2.

Apollo

The Dräger Apollo (Fig. 16.8) features a quiet piston ventilator, which corrects tidal volume for leaks, compliance, and fresh gas flow (by fresh gas decoupling).[64,69,70] Mechanical ventilation is activated in two steps (the mode is chosen and then confirmed by a second key press). Autoflow is a dual-control mode similar to pressure control with volume guarantee [PCV-VG]). Synchronized intermittent mandatory ventilation (SIMV) may be used in either volume or pressure modes. Volume-controlled ventilation (VCV) is accurate over a wide range of tidal volumes (20–1400 mL).[70,71] Mechanical needle valves govern fresh gas flow, which is electronically measured and displayed on screen. A backup total fresh gas flowmeter tube is present.

Fabius GS

The Dräger Fabius GS (Fig. 16.9) does not include physiologic monitors. The thermal anemometry (hot wire) flow sensor in the breathing circuit is available in this machine and other Dräger models.[68] Ventilator gas flow is piston driven and corrects tidal volume for compliance and leaks. The machine uses a manual checklist with several electronic self-tests (e.g., system, leaks and compliance, flow sensor, oxygen sensor). With the Fabius GS (as with all the new models), users must review the operator manual to check the machine correctly. Sample preanesthesia checkout procedures are available.[72]

The Fabius GS breathing circuit is lower volume than older anesthesia workstations (2.8 L plus bag, of which 1.2 L is absorbent volume).[69,73] The absorber head is not warmed. As with the Apollo, fresh gas decoupling causes the manual breathing bag to fluctuate during the mechanical ventilator cycle, which serves as a disconnect alarm.

In case of electric power failure, there is a 45-minute battery reserve with fresh gas, vaporizers, integrated monitors, and ventilator operational. Because they are not part of the anesthesia workstations, patient monitors will not function. Several pneumatic functions remain after the battery is exhausted: vaporizers, hypoxic guard, APL or popoff valve, flowmeters, breathing pressure gauge, cylinder and pipeline pressure gauges, and common gas outlet flowmeter.

Perseus A500

The Perseus A500 is the most recent anesthesia workstation developed by Dräger. It is the first anesthesia workstation to include a turbine ventilator.[60] The Perseus utilizes a unidirectional impeller, which draws and compresses gas from the reservoir bag before releasing it into the external circuit.[60] During mechanical ventilation, the impeller spins continually to create a small circular flow in the breathing circuit. This allows for good gas mixing and for spontaneous breathing.[74] Visually the reservoir bag will compress with ventilator inspiration and expand with ventilator exhalation, which is opposite of other Dräger models that utilize a fresh gas decoupler.[74] The Perseus also compensates the tidal volume for leaks, fresh gas flow, as well as patient and breathing circuit

TABLE 16.2 Features of Current Anesthesia Workstations

Feature	Dräger *Apollo, Fabius, Perseus*	GE *Aisys, Aespire, Avance, ADU*
Breathing circuit monitors	All	All
Pressure transducer	Hot-wire anemometer	Variable-orifice flow sensor (D-Lite sensor in ADU)
Volume and flow		
Oxygen paramagnetic	All	All
Infrared gas analysis (N_2O, CO_2, agents)	All	All
Breathing circuit suitable for low fresh gas flow (low volume, low leaks), easy disassembly and disinfection	All	All
Control of humidity in breathing circuit	Heated breathing circuit (except Fabius)	Condenser
CO_2 absorbent—canisters or loose fill	All	All
Interfaces with physiologic monitors and electronic medical record	All	All
Electronic self-check with manual aspects (differs in each model)	All	All
Flowmeter control	Needle valve (Fabius, Apollo) Electronic gas mixer (Perseus)	Needle valve (ADU, Aespire) Electronic gas mixer (Aisys)
Fresh gas flow display	Electronic (all) All	Glass tube (Aespire) Electronic (ADU, Aisys)
Vaporizers—variable bypass	Pneumatic control (Fabius, Apollo, Perseus)	Pneumatic control (Avance, Aespire)
Blender (e.g., Tec 6)	Any model	Electronic controls (Aisys) Avance, Aespire
Ventilator flow generated by	Piston (Apollo, Fabius) Turbine (Perseus)	Bellows (all)
Ventilator modes	**Apollo** Manual/ spontaneous, VCV, PCV. Optional: PSV, Autoflow. **Perseus** Standard manual/spontaneous, PCV, PC-BiPAP, VCV, Autoflow, SIMV. Optional: CPAP, PC-BiPAP (all + PSV); PC-APRV.	**Aisys** Manual/ spontaneous, VCV. Optional: PCV, PCV-VG, SIMV, CPAP, PSV.
Scavenging	Open interface typical (closed interface available)	Open interface typical (closed interface available)
Battery backup, at least 30 min	All	All

APRV, Airway pressure release ventilation; *BiPAP,* bilevel positive airway pressure; *CPAP,* continuous positive airway pressure; *PC* or *PCV,* pressure control ventilation; *PCV-VG,* pressure control ventilation with volume guarantee; *PSV,* pressure support ventilation; *SIMV,* synchronized intermittent mandatory ventilation; *VCV,* volume control ventilation.

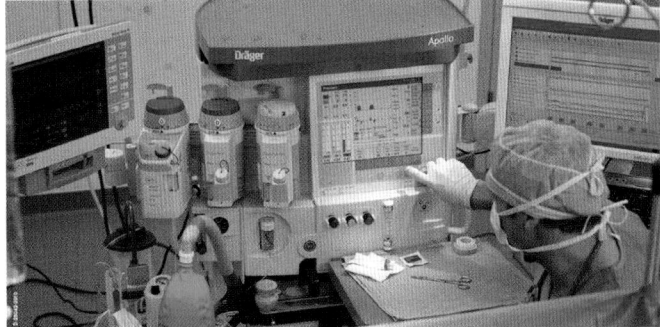

Fig. 16.8 Dräger Apollo. (Courtesy Dräger Medical, Inc, Telford, PA.)

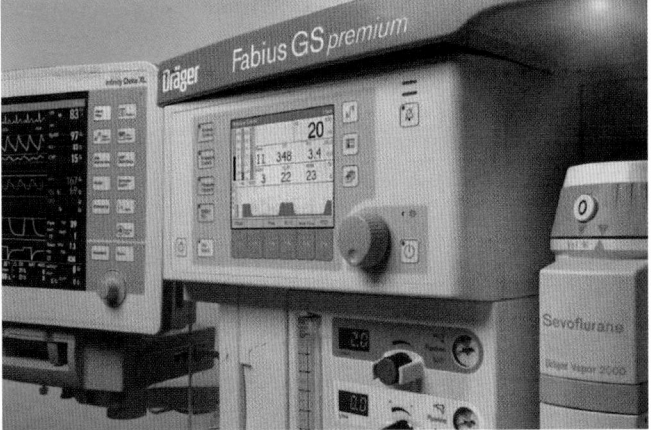

Fig. 16.9 Fabius GS. (Courtesy Dräger Medical, Inc, Telford, PA.)

compliance.[60] Together with its turbine design it has been shown to enable faster changes in gas concentration during low-flow anesthesia than Fabius.[60,75] Perseus offers an optional "econometer" to alert the clinician when fresh gas flow is in excess of that required by the patient.[60]

Aisys

The Aisys CS2 (GE Healthcare), like Avance, includes physiologic monitors (e.g., ECG, blood pressure, pulse oximetry).[67,76,77] The Aisys

(Fig. 16.10), introduced in 2005, uses the oxygen-driven standing bellows Smartvent 7900 (like Aestiva) but offers more modes.[78] PCV-VG, which is only available in Aisys and Avance, is a dual control mode. Autoflow, a ventilation mode found on Dräger anesthesia workstations, is similar. Spirometry is included to help monitor and control

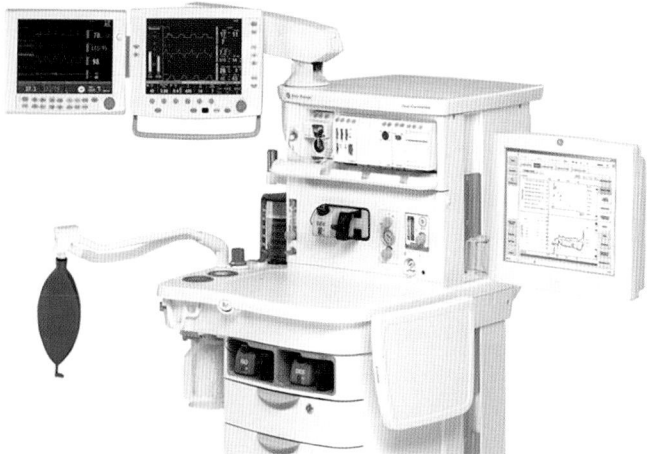

Fig. 16.10 GE Healthcare Aisys. (Courtesy GE Healthcare, Madison, WI.)

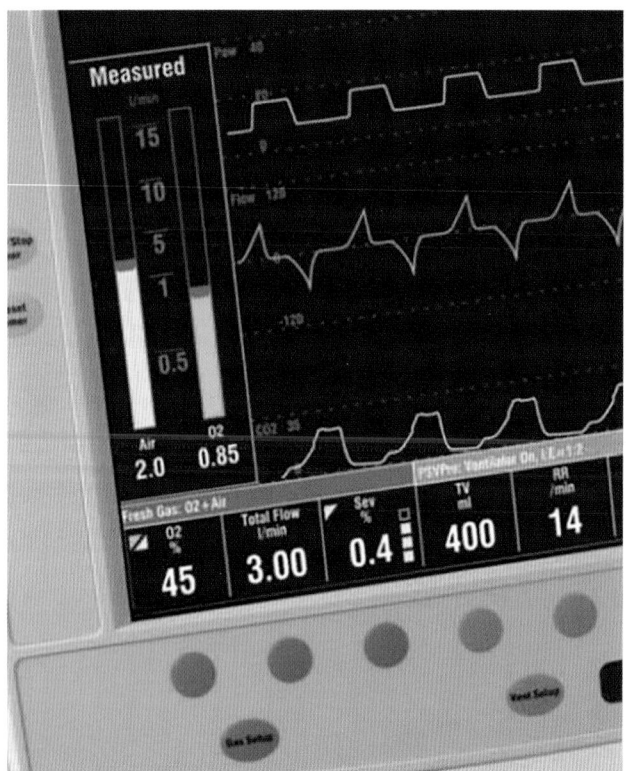

Fig. 16.11 Electronic control of inspired oxygen, carrier gas, and total fresh gas flow, Aisys. (Courtesy GE Healthcare, Madison, WI.)

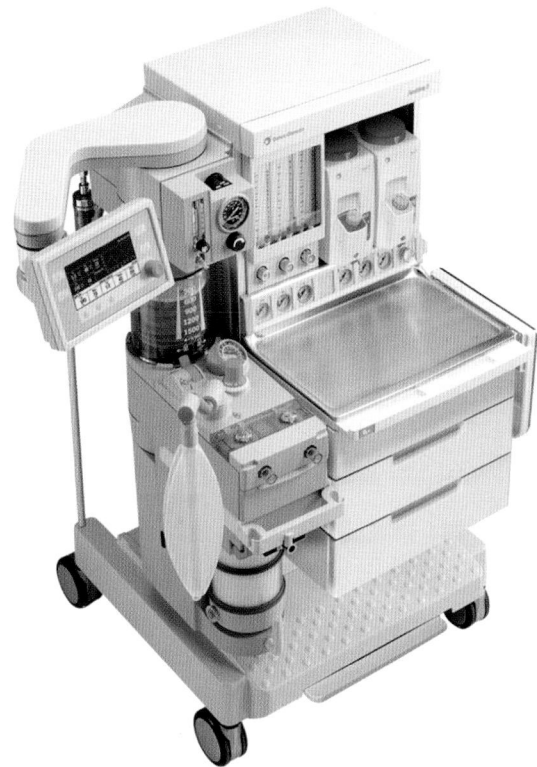

Fig. 16.12 GE Healthcare Aestiva. (Courtesy GE Healthcare, Madison, WI.)

ventilation. Like most modern ventilators, the low circuit volume, freedom from leaks, and microprocessor control support the use of low-flow anesthesia. The fresh gas inlet enters the circle system proximal to the inspiratory valve (like Aestiva).[79]

Aisys uses Aladin cassette vaporizers, which are electronically controlled. Aisys is similar to Avance and unique in the North American market in that it uses an electronic mixer to control, measure, and display fresh gas flow (Fig. 16.11). The user no longer controls the flow of each gas directly but instead selects the desired carrier gas (nitrous oxide or air), total fresh gas flow, and inspired oxygen concentration. There are no needle valves or glass flow-meter tubes to control individual flows of oxygen, nitrous oxide,

or air. In case of electronic failure there is a backup needle valve and glass flowmeter tube for control and display of total fresh gas flow.[64,66,76]

Aestiva

The Aestiva (GE Healthcare) (Fig. 16.12) has many traditional (i.e., mechanical/pneumatic) systems but with a modern and capable 7900 ventilator. Gas analysis and patient physiologic monitors must be added (like Fabius).[64,80] The 7900 ventilator uses an oxygen-driven standing bellows capable of manual, spontaneous, VCV, PCV, pressure support ventilation (PSV)–Pro (which includes apnea backup),[80] and SIMV.

The flow sensors compensate tidal volume for compliance losses and leaks in the absorber head and bellows, therefore the ventilator is accurate to very low tidal volume (range 20–1500 mL).[80] These variable orifice flow sensors (like most flow sensors) have shown some sensitivity to moisture in the breathing circuit.[81] The Aestiva uses a checklist that relies on the user to perform more manual procedures than the checklist for the Apollo, Fabius, or Aisys.[72]

Flowmeters are traditional mechanical needle valves with glass flowmeter tubes. Thus there is no electronic capture of fresh gas flow, as in machines with digital flow display. The oxygen sensor is the galvanic fuel cell type, and the hypoxic guard is mechanical (Link-25).[80] The breathing circuit is relatively high volume (5.5 L, including dual canisters of 1.35 kg absorbent each).[73,82,83] The Aestiva is also available in a version compatible with the MRI suite.

Aespire

The Aespire (GE Healthcare) (Fig. 16.13) is similar to the Aestiva in most of its systems but more compact. The standing bellows, oxygen-driven ventilator offers tidal volume compensation. Volume control and pressure control are the two modes of ventilation available.[84]

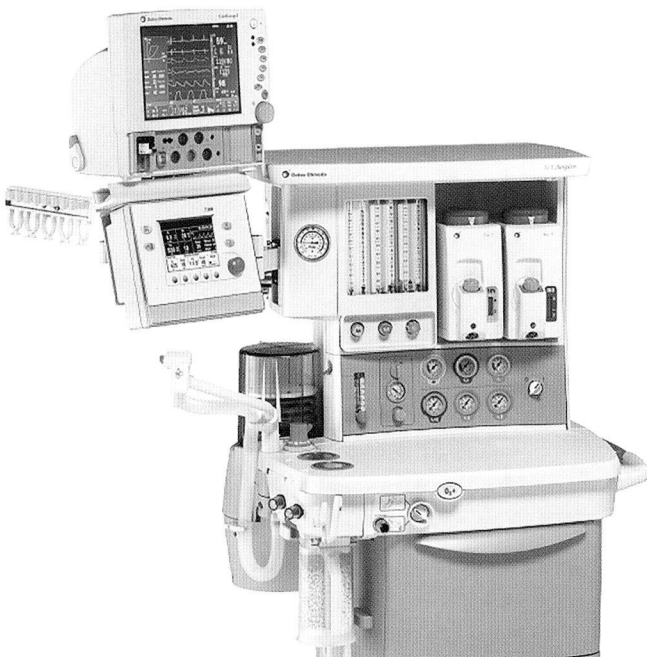

Fig. 16.13 GE Healthcare Aespire. (Courtesy GE Healthcare, Madison, WI.)

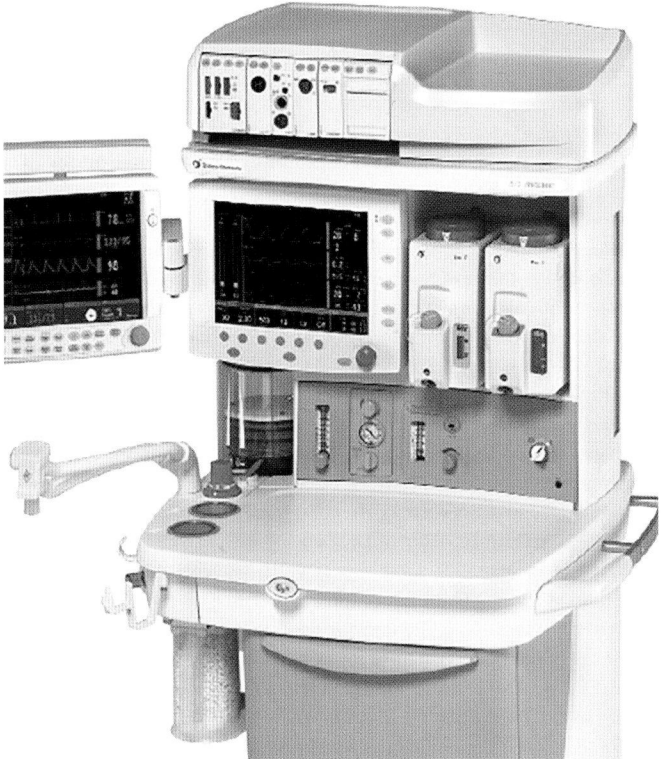

Fig. 16.14 GE Healthcare Avance. (Courtesy GE Healthcare, Madison, WI.)

Avance

The Avance (GE Healthcare) (Fig. 16.14) is similar to the Aisys in most respects: electronic fresh gas flow controls with backup pneumatic control, modern and capable multimode ventilator, spirometry, and integrated physiologic monitoring. The pneumatic/mechanical Tec 6 and Tec 7 vaporizers included in the Avance are the primary difference between it and the Aisys.

> ### BOX 16.6 Components of Flowmeters
>
> - Knob
> - Needle valve
> - Valve stops (not present on all workstations)
> - Flowtube
> - Indicator float

ADU

The ADU (GE Healthcare) and other older designs are discussed on a companion website.[85]

Path of Gases Through the Anesthesia Workstation

Oxygen, nitrous oxide, and air follow similar paths through the anesthesia workstation (see Fig. 16.1). Each passes from its supply point to a flowmeter. All gases (except oxygen and, in newer models, air) pass through a fail-safe valve before proceeding to their flowmeters. This valve is held open by pressure in the oxygen circuitry within the anesthesia workstation. After passing through their respective flowmeters, the gases are joined for the first time in a common manifold. Oxygen is always added to the common manifold downstream of other gases so that the chance of hypoxic breathing mixtures is lessened (e.g., in the event that a flowmeter tube has cracked).[86] The combined gases enter any vaporizer that is turned on and then pass through the common gas outlet. Formerly, a delivery hose with a locking connection conducted gases from the common gas outlet to the breathing circuit. Currently the connection from flowmeters to the breathing circuit is often internal and thus free of any chance of disconnection or misconnection.

The breathing circuit and ventilator (or manual breathing bag in the circle) transport gases to and from the patient. An amount equal to the fresh gas flow per minute (minus patient uptake, plus gases excreted) leaves the breathing circuit and is conducted to the scavenger interface. From there it is disposed of in the hospital ventilation or suction systems.

Five Tasks of Oxygen

Oxygen has five tasks in the anesthesia workstation: It (1) proceeds to the fresh gas flowmeter, (2) powers the oxygen flush, (3) activates fail-safe mechanisms, (4) activates oxygen low-pressure alarms, and (5) compresses the bellows of mechanical ventilators (see Fig. 16.1). The other gases supplied by the machine have only one pathway; they are transported via flowmeter and breathing circuit to anesthetize the patient (nitrous oxide) or sustain life (oxygen and air). Some newer machines can switch to air as a driving gas for the ventilator bellows if oxygen pressure is lost.

Flowmeter

The first task of oxygen is proceeding through the flowmeter and on to the patient as a life-sustaining gas. Flowmeters have several components (Box 16.6). Control knobs are color and touch coded; thus oxygen flow control knobs are distinct, in both visual appearance and tactile form, from the control knobs for the other gases (Fig. 16.15).[87]

It is not necessary to use more than fingertip force to shut off gas flow. The needle valve, which controls gas flow through the flowmeter, can be damaged if excessive force is used. Valve stops (Fig. 16.16) are usually incorporated to prevent damage, though some workstations lack them (e.g., ADU). Flow increases when the knob is turned counterclockwise. Most current anesthesia workstations use mechanical needle valves; Avance, Aisys, and Perseus A500 use electronic controls for flow. On these machines, backup oxygen controls using mechanical/pneumatic needle valves are present in case of electronic or electrical failure.

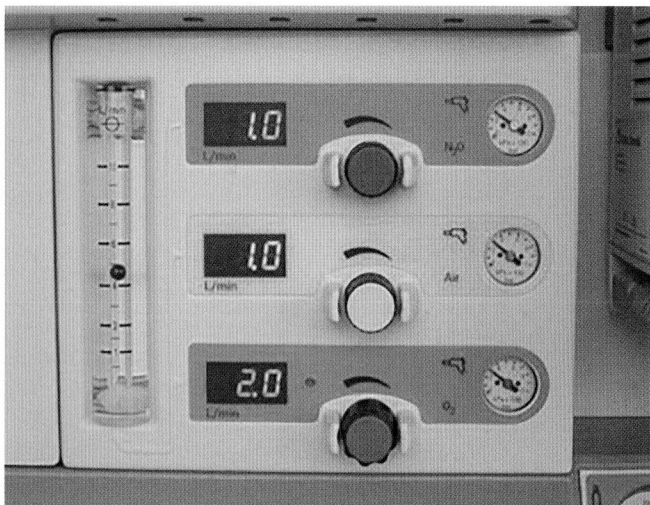

Fig. 16.15 Flowmeters on the Fabius GS are arranged vertically. The oxygen knob *(at the bottom)* is different visually, and to touch, from control knobs for air and nitrous oxide. To the left of each flow-control knob is a digital display of flow and the common gas outlet flowmeter (glass tube); to the right is the pipeline pressure gauge for each gas. (Copyright Drägerwerk AG & Co. KGaA, Lubeck. All rights reserved.)

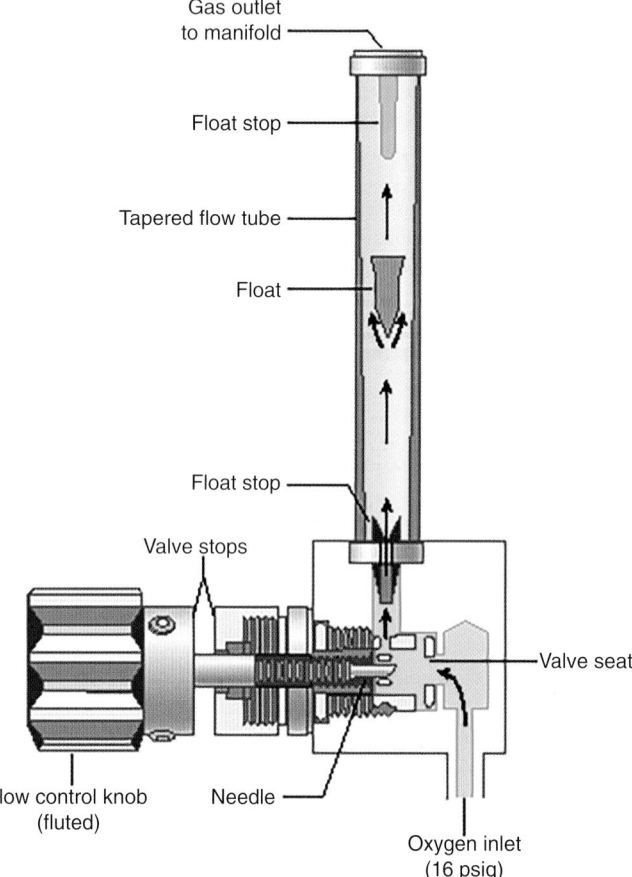

Fig. 16.16 Flowmeter components. (From Bowie E, Huffman LM. *The Anesthesia Machine: Essentials for Understanding.* Madison, WI: Datex-Ohmeda; 1985. In Miller RD, et al., eds. *Miller's Anesthesia.* 8th ed. Philadelphia: Elsevier; 2015.)

Display of fresh gas flow. An indicator float in a glass tube (Thorpe tube) is the classic way to capture and display fresh gas flow. Oxygen is calibrated to ±5% concentration (or ±20 mL/min flow) at room temperature and sea level.[65] Flowmeter tubes are specific for each gas

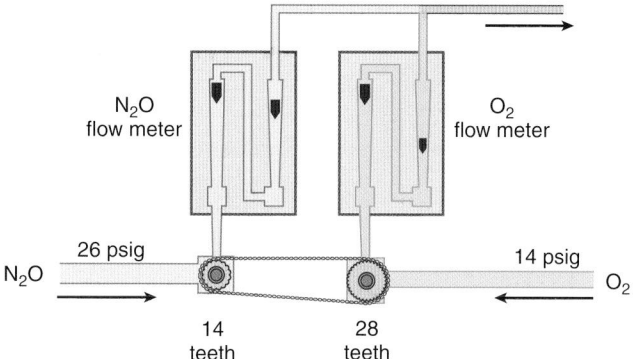

Fig. 16.17 When two flowmeters are present for one gas, they are arranged in series (gas flows first through fine [calibrated in mL] then coarse [calibrated in liters] flow tubes). The figure also depicts the Link-25 proportioning system. (From Miller RD, et al., eds. *Miller's Anesthesia.* 7th ed. Philadelphia: Elsevier; 2010.)

and cannot be interchanged. The flowtube is tapered to be narrower at its bottom. Thus it may be referred to as a variable orifice flowmeter because the annular opening around the float is larger at higher flows. If a gas has two tubes, they are connected in series with a single control valve (Fig. 16.17). It is standard in the United States (but not in the United Kingdom) for the oxygen flowtube to be placed to the right of other flowtubes. Flowmeters on the Fabius GS are unique in that they are arranged vertically rather than side by side (see Fig. 16.15).[68,73] Glass flowtubes are the most fragile part of the machine. They are susceptible to breakage, leaks at their seals, and inaccuracy due to the presence of dirt or static electricity.[29]

Rather than using glass flowtubes, many newer anesthesia workstations capture flows electronically by means of an anemometer or by a transducer and chamber of known volume. The chamber fills to a set pressure, and then the gas is allowed to proceed. The number of times this cycle occurs per minute can be converted to gas flow, which can be saved and sent to the automated medical record. These newer machines dispense with glass flowtubes, instead displaying fresh gas flows as numbers with or without colored bar graphs on a computer screen (e.g., Fabius GS, Aisys, Apollo, Perseus). Machines with electronic gas mixers and flow displays have a backup needle valve and glass flowmeter to control and measure total fresh gas flow in the event of power failure. Setting fresh gas flow on the Aisys, Avance, or Perseus is unique since the flowmeter controls and display are all electronic. The user sets the inspired oxygen concentration desired, the total fresh gas flow, and what carrier gas is desired (nitrous oxide or air) (see Fig. 16.11).[66,74,77,88]

Care of flowmeters. Flowmeters with conventional needle valves and glass flowtubes should be turned off before pipelines are connected, cylinders are opened, or the machine is turned on. If a flowtube is left open, the float will shoot to the top of a glass tube and may damage it. Flowmeters should be included in visual monitoring sweeps. Never adjust a flowmeter without looking at it. Read ball-type indicator floats in their center (Dräger) and plumb bob–type floats at the top (older Datex-Ohmeda). Remember to turn off flowmeters after each case, particularly at the end of the day. Failure to do so may contribute to premature drying of the carbon dioxide absorbent, which not only hastens its exhaustion but has been implicated in an increased degradation of volatile agents, the generation of carbon monoxide in canisters, and canister fires.[89–91]

Other flowmeters

Auxiliary oxygen flowmeters. Auxiliary oxygen flowmeters are an accessory currently offered on most models of anesthesia workstations. They are useful for attaching a nasal cannula or simple face mask. In the past it was common to attach a nasal cannula to an adapter at the common gas outlet. The auxiliary oxygen flowmeter is advantageous because the breathing circuit and gas delivery hose (if present, between the common gas outlet and breathing circuit) remain intact while supplemental oxygen is delivered to a spontaneously breathing patient. Thus, if the need arises to switch from a nasal cannula to the circle breathing system during a case, it can occur rapidly without the possibility of forgetting to reconfigure the breathing circuit properly. Another advantage is that an oxygen source is readily available for the Ambu bag if the patient needs to be ventilated manually for any reason during a case (e.g., breathing circuit failure). One disadvantage is that the auxiliary flowmeter is unusable if the pipeline supply has lost pressure or been contaminated; this is because the auxiliary flowmeter is supplied by the same wall outlet and hose connection that supplies the main oxygen flowmeter. If users do not realize this, time could be wasted while they attempt to use this potential oxygen source.[16,92] Another disadvantage is that the fraction of inspired oxygen (Fio$_2$) supplied cannot be varied with the auxiliary flowmeter. The chance of fire in sedated patients undergoing head and neck surgery can be lessened by using reduced FiO$_2$ concentrations, scavenging the oxygen to prevent pooling, and tenting the drapes.[93–95]

Emergency oxygen flowmeters. Emergency oxygen flowmeters (Fig. 16.18) are used as a backup on anesthesia workstations with electronic gas mixers. If the computer display, electronics, or electric power fails, the emergency oxygen flowmeter can still supply wall oxygen to the breathing circuit and vaporizers.

Scavenging flowmeters. Scavenging flowmeters are used on most new machines, which use open scavenging interfaces. An indication

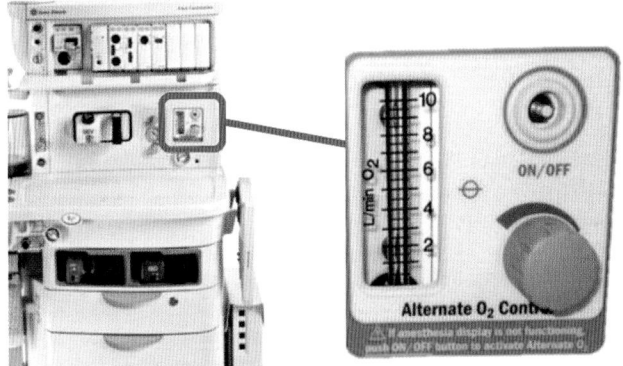

Fig. 16.18 Emergency oxygen flowmeter on Aisys. (Courtesy GE Healthcare.)

that suction is adequate is mandatory with these systems to avoid exposure to waste anesthesia gases (see "Disposal" later). Unfortunately the suction indicator is usually not visible from the operator's normal position.[96] On the Apollo, for example, it is on the left side of the machine under the breathing circuit.[84] On the Aisys, the scavenger suction flowmeter (marked "AGSS") is behind the bellows on the left side of the machine.

Oxygen Flush

The second task of oxygen in the processing area of the machine is to supply the oxygen flush valve. The flush valve delivers a very high flow of oxygen to the breathing circuit (>25–35 L/min).[77,97,98]

The purpose of the flush valve is to quickly fill the breathing circuit with oxygen. The flush valve is often protected by a rim that lessens the chance of accidental activation. Should this occur, barotrauma can result. Users should avoid activating the flush while the mechanical ventilator is in the inspiratory phase; during this phase, the ventilator relief valve closes, preventing gas from exiting to the scavenger, and resulting in increased pressure on the lungs.[96] If flushing is necessary for filling the ventilator bellows, it should be done in short pulses during the expiratory phase. Alternatively, increasing the fresh gas flow to 8 to 10 L/min for a few breaths will fill the bellows promptly and without the risk of barotrauma.

The oxygen flush line proceeds directly from the gas supply source to the common gas outlet (see Fig. 16.1). Activating the flush bypasses the vaporizers and adds 100% oxygen to the breathing circuit. If partial pressures of nitrous oxide or volatile agent have already been established in the breathing circuit (during maintenance), excessive use of the oxygen flush tends to dilute these inhaled agents and may lessen the depth of anesthesia.

Fail-Safe Systems

If pipeline oxygen pressure fails, and other gases such as nitrous oxide keep flowing, the patient might receive a hypoxic gas mixture (<21% oxygen). Therefore anesthesia workstations incorporate devices that halt the supply of all other gases in the event of oxygen supply pressure failure. These are called fail-safe systems. They are designed so that the set concentration of oxygen at the common gas outlet does not decline if the oxygen pipeline pressure decreases.[99] This requirement is satisfied by the presence of gatelike valves in the internal supply line for nonoxygen gases. The gate in each is held open by pressure in the oxygen line (Fig. 16.19). Flow of nitrous oxide may be shut off with oxygen pressure below a set limit (e.g., Avance, Aisys, Fabius GS) or proportionally decreased (e.g., Aestiva).[65,68,76,77,80] It is important to note that

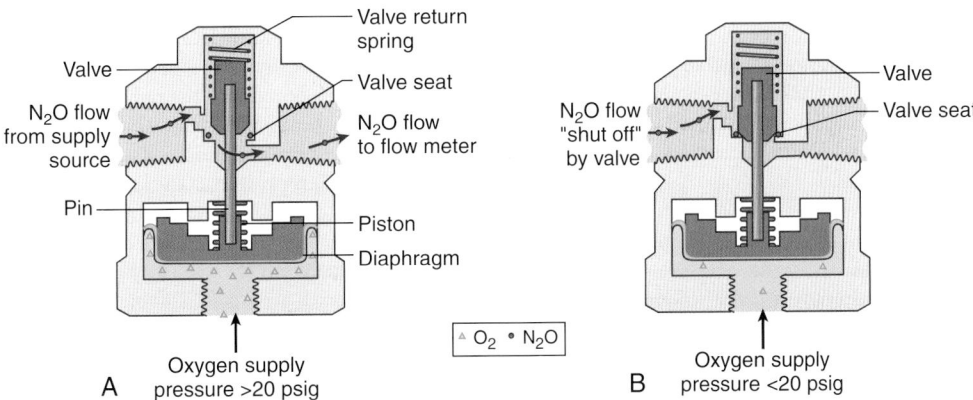

Fig. 16.19 Fail-safe valve in the nitrous oxide line. (A) Open. (B) Closed. (From Bowie E, Huffman LM. *The Anesthesia Machine: Essentials for Understanding.* Madison, WI: Datex-Ohmeda; 1985. In Miller RD, et al., eds: *Miller's Anesthesia,* 7th ed, Philadelphia, 2010, Elsevier.)

fail-safe systems do not analyze oxygen pipeline contents, so they are activated only if oxygen pipeline pressure falls. They do not protect the patient from a crossover, in which oxygen pipeline pressure is intact but the line does not contain oxygen.

Fail-safe devices were once placed in air lines as well, with the rationale of leaving oxygen (however briefly) as the last gas flowing, even if oxygen pipeline pressure is lost. However, it is not possible to deliver a hypoxic mixture of air (as long as the fresh gas flow rate is sufficient), and leaving air flowing is useful to drive the ventilator bellows in case of oxygen pipeline pressure failure.[100]

Newer equipment places the fail-safe valves in the nitrous oxide line only, and rely on electronic proportioning systems to prevent hypoxic gas mixtures if oxygen pipeline pressure fails. This is accomplished by shutting off nitrous oxide and leaving agent and air flowing, with air available to drive the ventilator bellows.

Low-Pressure Alarms

The fourth task of oxygen is powering the low-pressure alarms, which signal the operator when pressure is lost in the oxygen circuitry. The older oxygen supply failure alarm was a container with a whistle at its outlet that was pressurized by oxygen when the anesthesia workstation was turned on. When pipeline pressure decreased to 28 psi, or when the machine was shut off, a characteristic loud whistle was heard as the container released its contents. Newer models lack this distinctive alarm, substituting a variety of high-priority visual and auditory alarms.[23,39,41] The proper response to loss of pipeline pressure is discussed earlier in this chapter (see "Supply").

Ventilator Driving Gas

The fifth task of oxygen in many anesthesia workstations is compression of the ventilator bellows. The Aestiva ventilator uses 100% oxygen as its driving gas.[82] The Aisys may use either air or oxygen and will switch automatically from oxygen to the secondary drive gas (air) if oxygen pressure is lost.[64]

Piston ventilators use electric motors to compress the bellows and deliver tidal volume (e.g., Fabius GS, Apollo).[19,68] The Perseus uses an electrically powered, spinning turbine to generate positive pressure ventilation.[60]

Thus, piston or turbine ventilator delivery of tidal volume is unaffected by variation in, or even the absence of, oxygen pipeline pressure. Piston or turbine ventilators may operate for prolonged periods with only cylinder supplies of gases because they do not consume oxygen to drive the bellows. This is an advantage in office-based anesthesia, in other settings where pipelines are not available, and in emergency loss of pipeline pressure.[101]

Proportioning Systems (Hypoxic Guard)

All current anesthesia workstations incorporate nitrous oxide–oxygen proportioning (hypoxic guard) systems designed to prevent the delivery of hypoxic breathing mixtures. All link oxygen and nitrous oxide flows so that final breathing mixtures at the common gas outlet are at least 23% to 25% oxygen. The ratio of nitrous oxide to oxygen is thus kept at no more than a 3 to 1 ratio.

An example of a pneumatic-mechanical proportioning system is the Link-25 (used on Aestiva and Aespire). In this system, the flowmeter control knobs for nitrous oxide and oxygen are linked by a chain; oxygen flow is increased automatically when nitrous oxide flow is increased. The Link-25 system (Fig. 16.20) also incorporates secondary regulators, so it has both pneumatic and mechanical components.

On contemporary machines, these hypoxic guard systems are electronically controlled. Dräger Medical calls their system a "sensitive

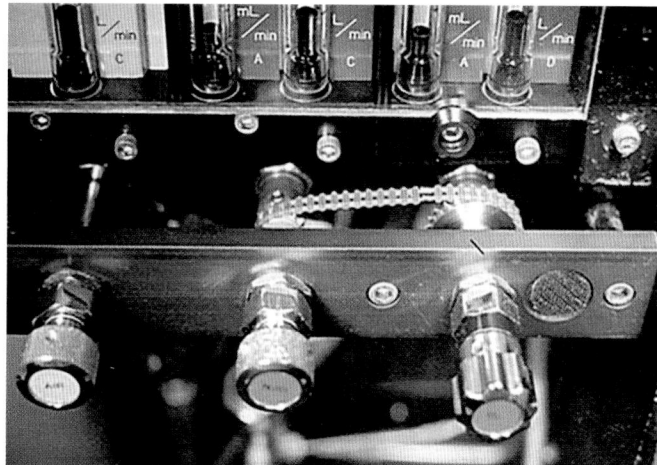

Fig. 16.20 A chain connects oxygen and nitrous oxide flow controls in the Link-25 proportioning system. Either may be adjusted separately, but the chain enforces at most a 3:1 ratio of nitrous oxide to oxygen. The chain is not normally visible. (Courtesy Datex-Ohmeda, Madison, WI.)

> **BOX 16.7 Circumstances Under Which Hypoxic Guard Systems Can Permit Formation of a Hypoxic Breathing Mixture**
>
> - Wrong supply of gas in oxygen pipeline or cylinder
> - Defective pneumatics or mechanics
> - Leaks downstream of flow control valves
> - Inert gas administration (e.g., a third gas such as helium)
> - Administration of air (or Fio$_2$ <0.30) at very low fresh gas flow

---

oxygen ratio controller (S ORC)," and uses it in the Apollo, Fabius, and Perseus models.[60,70]

This system maintains at least 23% oxygen but does so by limiting nitrous oxide flow. Electronic alarms are incorporated, and the system includes a nitrous shutoff (so a fail-safe system is also incorporated).

Hypoxic guard systems are not foolproof. With fresh gas flow set to deliver 25% oxygen, the S-ORC hypoxic guard was unable to maintain Fio$_2$ of at least 21% in almost all patients when fresh gas flow was less than 1.5 L/min.[100,102,103]

Box 16.7 lists situations in which a hypoxic breathing mixture can be delivered despite the use of these systems. Lack of oxygen in the oxygen pipeline may be detected with an oxygen analyzer. A system that is broken or defective should be detected in the preuse checklist, as should leaks downstream of the flowmeters.[104] It is not widely appreciated that the hypoxic guard systems link only nitrous oxide and oxygen. Perhaps because of the name, the faulty assumption is made that all hypoxic breathing mixtures are prevented. These systems would not prevent the administration of a hypoxic mixture if a third inert gas (such as helium) is present on the anesthesia workstation. Nor do they prevent hypoxic mixtures if low Fio$_2$ and low fresh gas flows are used simultaneously. The proper use of a calibrated oxygen analyzer in each general anesthetic will always be of vital importance.

Oxygen Analysis

Systems that warn of trouble with oxygen supply (low pressure alarms, fail-safe system) or that lessen the chances of hypoxemia when nitrous oxide is used (hypoxic guard system) are based on pressure within the oxygen circuitry of the anesthesia workstation. They do not sample the oxygen lines to determine that oxygen is present. There is only one system that ensures that oxygen is actually present in the pipeline or cylinder (and, ultimately, in the breathing circuit): inspired oxygen analysis. Monitoring inspired oxygen is mandatory in every anesthetic, and the function of the oxygen monitor must be checked before initiating care because general anesthesia may need to be induced as a backup plan in any anesthetic.[12,105]

Two types of sensors are in current use: the electrochemical or galvanic fuel cell (Aestiva, Aespire, Fabius) and the paramagnetic analyzer (in most other models). The paramagnetic analyzer is widely used because of its fast response, low cost, and extremely low maintenance requirements.[106] A paramagnetic analyzer is often incorporated in airway gas monitors (which use infrared absorption to detect anesthetic agents, nitrous oxide, and carbon dioxide).

Vaporizers

Underlying Physical Principles

A vapor is composed of molecules (in the gaseous phase) of a substance that is a liquid at room temperature and 1 atmosphere of pressure. Vaporization proceeds at a rate that depends on the physical characteristics of the vaporizing liquid and the temperature. Different liquids evaporate at different rates, quantified by their vapor pressure. Elevated temperature increases the rate of evaporation of any liquid, whereas decreased temperature slows the rate. As evaporation proceeds, the remaining liquid and its container cool because heat energy is carried from the liquid with the energetic, mobile, evaporating molecules. An example would be the cooling effect of stepping out of the shower or the chilling effect of evaporating gasoline or ether on the hand. In both cases, the evaporating molecules acquire the latent heat of vaporization from their surroundings. Thus one would expect an anesthetic vaporizer to cool as vaporization proceeds. This cooling slows the rate of further vaporization. To prevent this, materials such as copper are chosen for containing liquid anesthetics in current vaporizers. Copper has high thermal conductivity (transferring environmental heat easily to the liquid anesthetic) and high thermal capacity (acting as a thermal reservoir to help stabilize liquid anesthetic temperature).[29,107]

The rate of vaporization depends only on the temperature, the vapor pressure of the liquid, and the partial pressure of the vapor above the evaporating liquid—not on the ambient pressure of the remaining gases present. For example, water at a constant temperature evaporates at the same rate into completely dry air regardless of whether it is at sea level, in a hyperbaric chamber, or at elevations far above sea level.

Classification and Design

Variable bypass. Table 16.3 compares current variable-bypass vaporizers with heated-vapor (Tec 6) types.[29,108–112] All vaporizers blend the combined flow of fresh gases from the flowmeters with sufficient vapor to form clinically useful concentrations. The problem is ensuring that the vapor concentration is appropriately limited. For example, a fully saturated isoflurane vapor consists of nearly 31% isoflurane (238 mm Hg [31 kPa], the saturated vapor pressure of isoflurane at 20°C divided by the barometric pressure of 760 mm Hg [101 kPa]).[113] To limit vapor output to a clinically useful concentration, only a small portion of the fresh gas flow is allowed to come into contact with the liquid and pick up anesthetic vapor.

The splitting ratio (gas entering the vaporizing chamber, divided by total fresh gas flow) is automatically determined in a variable-bypass vaporizer by the resistance to flow in its internal channels; the operator merely has to set the control dial to the desired concentration (Fig. 16.21). Setting the dial to a higher percentage increases the amount of flow sent through the vaporizing chamber. The small portion of the gas flow entering the vaporizing chamber (carrier gas or

Characteristic	Variable Bypass	Injector
Example	Datex-Ohmeda Tec 4, 5, 7 Aisys Aladin Dräger Vapor 19, 2000	Datex-Ohmeda Tec 6 (Desflurane)
Splitting ratio (carrier gas flow)	Variable bypass (vaporizer determines carrier gas split)	Dual circuit (carrier gas is not split)
Method of vaporization	Flowover	Gas/vapor blender (heat produces vapor, which is injected into fresh gas flow)
Temperature compensation	Automatic temperature compensation mechanism	Electrically heated to a constant temperature (39°C, thermostatically controlled)
Calibration	Calibrated, agent specific	Calibrated, agent specific
Position	Out of circuit	Out of circuit
Capacity	Tec 5, 300 mL; Tec 7, 225 mL; Vapor 19, 200 mL; Aladin, 250 mL	390 mL

TABLE 16.3   **Classification of Vaporizers**

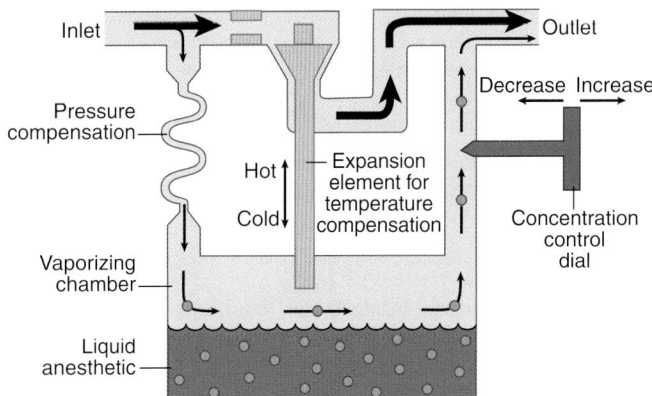

Fig. 16.21 The Dräger Vapor 19 vaporizer. (From Miller RD, et al., eds. *Miller's Anesthesia*, 7th ed, Philadelphia: Elsevier; 2010.)

chamber flow) flows over the liquid and picks up anesthetic vapor. Full saturation of the carrier gas is ensured by means of a series of wicks and baffles. This fully saturated (and thus known) concentration of carrier gas at the vaporizing chamber outlet is then diluted with the balance of the fresh gas that bypassed the vaporizing chamber (bypass flow) to produce the desired final concentration at the vaporizer outlet.

A temperature-compensation device is built into variable-bypass vaporizers so that more gas is directed into the vaporizing chamber if the vaporizer cools. Variable-bypass vaporizers are calibrated for concentration and are agent specific. Like the Tec 6, variable-bypass vaporizers are out of circuit, meaning out of the breathing circuit. Their capacities for liquid agent are listed in Table 16.2. Variable-bypass vaporizers in the Aisys are electronically controlled and based on inputs from pressure, flow, and temperature sensors at various sites in the vaporizer (Fig. 16.22).

Measured flow (Vernitrol). Anesthetists who practice in the military, or who use older equipment on mission trips outside of North America, may encounter measured-flow vaporizers. In a measured-flow vaporizer, the operator determines how much gas should be bubbled through the anesthetic liquid by means of a formula; this amount is then set on a second oxygen flowmeter, marked "Oxygen for Vernitrol." If the vaporizer cools, the operator must recalculate

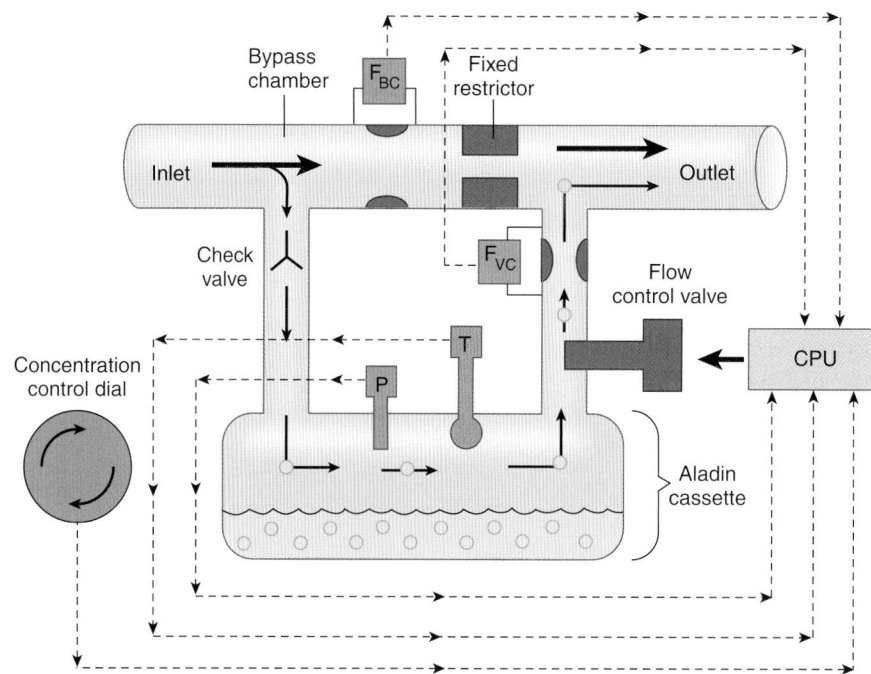

Fig. 16.22 The Aladin vaporizer found on the Aisys workstation. A microprocessor controls output by monitoring F_{BC} (bypass chamber flow), F_{VC} (vaporizing chamber flow), P (pressure), and T (temperature) in the vaporizing chamber. (From Miller RD, et al, eds. *Miller's Anesthesia*. 8th ed. Philadelphia: Elsevier; 2015.)

and set a new chamber gas flow; this is called manual temperature compensation. These devices can be used with multiple agents and are out of the breathing circuit. It is possible to use them safely, but their design is not as inherently safe as that of more modern types.[114] Measured-flow vaporizers are no longer manufactured in the United States, and factory service for them is no longer available. The military still trains anesthetists on the use of these vaporizers, and they may be seen overseas.

Tec 6 injector. The Tec 6 vaporizer uses a completely different principle of operation as compared with variable-bypass types (Fig. 16.23); it is a heated, dual-circuit injector (blender) vaporizer.[110,115,116] Fresh gas flow from the common manifold passes through the vaporizer in one circuit. This fresh gas never flows over or comes into contact with the liquid agent (as it would in a variable-bypass vaporizer). Instead, an appropriate amount of vapor is added to the fresh gas as it flows through the vaporizer. The vapor output has two control points. One is the setting on the concentration control dial, and the other is linked to a transducer that is responsive to the amount of fresh gas flow. Thus more vapor is delivered from the vapor circuit if either the dial setting or the fresh gas flow is increased. To maintain a known vapor pressure in the second circuit, the Tec 6 is heated to 39°C; this produces a vapor pressure of approximately 1500 mm Hg (200 kPa). Desflurane is near boiling at room temperature; if it were placed in a conventional variable-bypass vaporizer it would constitute nearly 100% of the output at first, and a hypoxic breathing mixture would result.[117] Modern variable-bypass vaporizers like Aladin are able to deliver desflurane accurately and safely because they incorporate a variety of sensors and electronic controls.[112]

The output of any modern vaporizer may be influenced by extremes of fresh gas flow, extremes of temperature, or backpressure from the breathing circuit and ventilator. Current vaporizers function accurately over a wide range of settings, at various ambient temperatures and fresh gas flows (Table 16.4).[110–112,118] Furthermore, they are more resistant than previous models to the effects of intermittent backpressure (the so-called pumping effect) that increases vaporizer output. This is

accomplished by incorporating unidirectional valves at the vaporizing chamber inlet or outlet, or distal to the vaporizer.

Using Vaporizers

Contemporary vaporizers are secured to the anesthesia workstation in manifolds that hold two or three units. The operator is prevented from delivering more than one agent simultaneously by an interlock system. The interlock ensures that only one vaporizer is on, that gas enters only the one that is on, that all vaporizers are locked in so that leaks are decreased, and that trace vapor output is minimal when a vaporizer is off.[29]

Variable-bypass and Tec 6 vaporizers are all filled in a similar fashion. Funnel-type (Fig. 16.24) and keyed-filler–type (Fig. 16.25) systems are still found. Keyed-filler types are preferred because their use lessens the chance that filling with the wrong agent will occur (although it is still possible).[113,117,119–125] Overfilling is unlikely when the vaporizer is filled in its normal operating position, and the liquid level indicators are visible to the operator. These indicators usually take the form of a sight glass with two etched lines, corresponding to low and maximum liquid levels within the vaporizer. To fill the vaporizer, the anesthetist should turn the vaporizer off, check the anesthetic liquid (to ensure that the agent and the vaporizer match), and then pour it in until the liquid level indicator shows that the vaporizer is full (when the liquid level reaches the maximum line on the sight glass).[113,118,126] It is a misconception that while using the keyed-filler vaporizer, one should hold the bottle up until it stops bubbling. If the vaporizer is turned on, is not horizontal, or the keyed-filler device is not perfectly tight on the bottle, overfilling may result.[122] Overfilling may result in discharge of liquid anesthetic from the vaporizer outlet, which has caused patient injuries.[29] The Tec 6 uses a similar system, but the desflurane bottle has a permanently attached, noninterchangeable spout. The sight glass on the Tec 6 is a liquid crystal display that indicates when the level of liquid is low enough to allow the addition of a full bottle, and it shows when the sump is full. Although the Tec 6 vaporizer is unique in that it

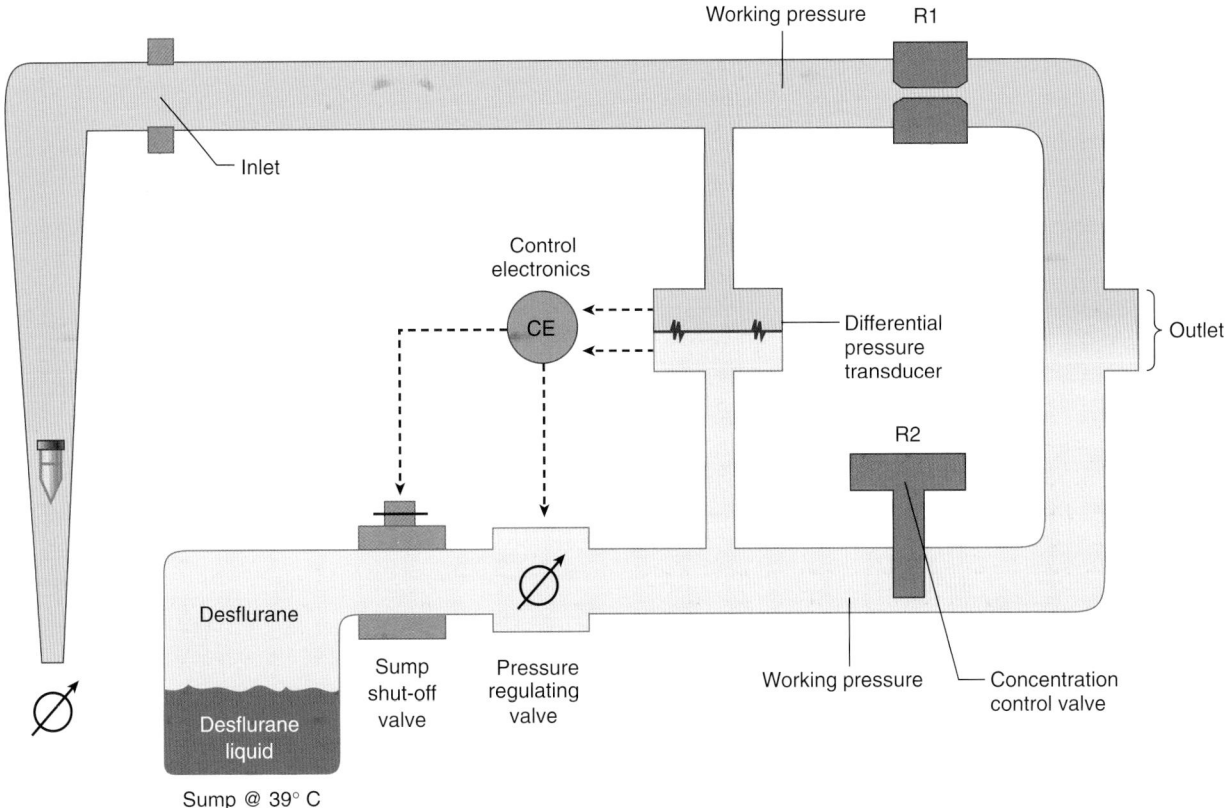

Fig. 16.23 Principle of operation of the Tec 6 vaporizer. (From Miller RD, et al, eds. *Miller's Anesthesia*. 7th ed. Philadelphia: Elsevier; 2010.)

TABLE 16.4 Accuracy of Current Vaporizers*				
Characteristic	GE Tec 6	GE Tec 7	Dräger Vapor 2000	GE Aladin (Aisys)
Fresh gas flow (L/min)	0.2–10	0.2–15	0.25–15	0.2–8
Temperature (°C)	18–30	18–35	10–40	18–25

*The vaporizers listed function accurately within the ranges specified.

can be filled while in operation,[110] it is safer to turn it off momentarily to do so. All variable-bypass vaporizers must be shut off while they are being filled.[67,118,122]

Models

The Dräger Vapor 19 fits in a manifold with an interlock system. If a vaporizer is removed from the machine, a short-circuit block must be added for leaks to be prevented. The interlock protects against simultaneous inhaled agent administration regardless of which vaporizer is removed. There is no check valve between the vaporizer outlets and the common gas outlet in Dräger anesthesia workstations. The Vapor 19 has a button that must be depressed before the control dial can be turned on. All contemporary vaporizers are designed to increase agent concentration as the dial is turned counterclockwise (as viewed from above).

The Dräger Vapor 2000 (Fig. 16.26) is similar to the Vapor 19 except that it is removable by hand. It has a unique T (transport) setting that

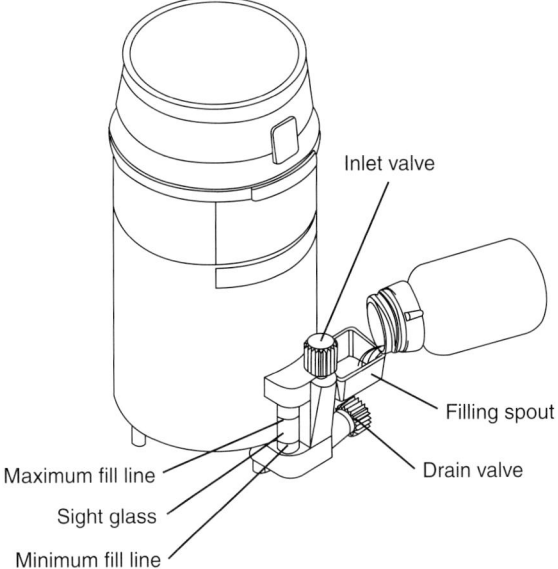

Fig. 16.24 Filling a vaporizer with a funnel-type filling system. (From Dräger Medical Inc. *Narkomed 2C Anesthesia System—Setup and Installation Manual*. Telford, PA: Drägerwerk AG & Co., and Lubeck, Germany: KGaA; 1994.)

allows the vaporizer to be tipped or transported without liquid anesthetic fouling the control mechanisms.

The GE Tec 7 is a variable-bypass vaporizer similar to the older Tec 4 and Tec 5 models. It is designed to require less frequent service.

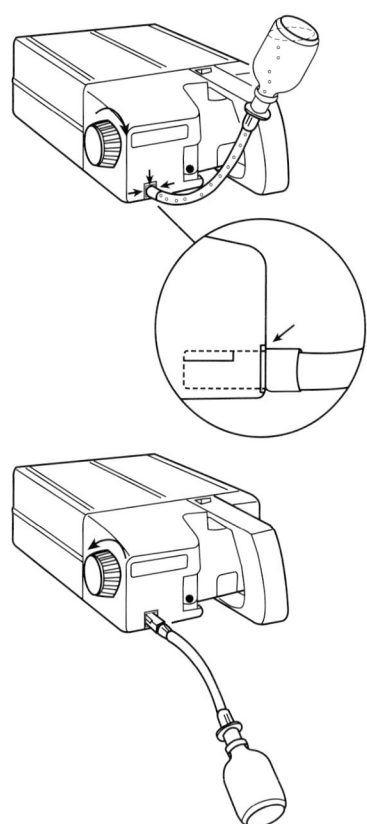

Fig. 16.25 Filling a vaporizer with a keyed-filler system. (From *S/5 Anesthesia Delivery Unit User's Reference Manual,* Catalog No. 8502304. Madison, WI: Datex-Ohmeda; 2000.)

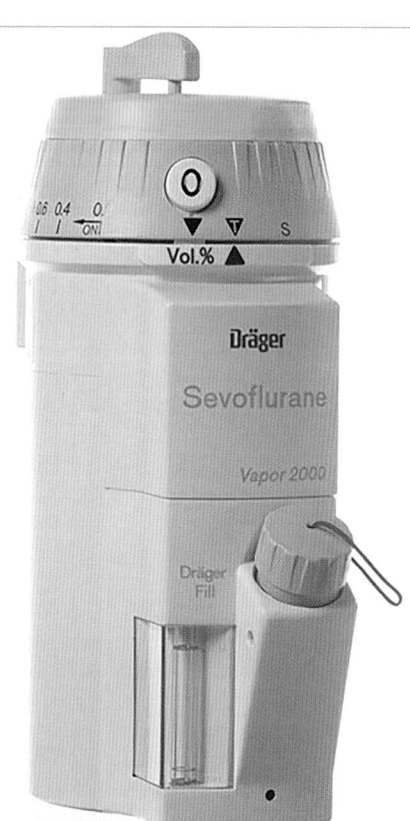

Fig. 16.26 The Dräger Vapor 2000. Note the "T" (transport) setting to the right of "0." (© Dräger. Image reprinted with permission.)

Use of the GE Tec 6 desflurane vaporizer is unique, as could be suspected from its unique principle of operation. However, it is not difficult to use. To fill the Tec 6, check the desflurane bottle to ensure that it is the right agent, push it into the vaporizer firmly, and rotate it upward until the display indicates that the vaporizer is full. The operator then rotates the bottle downward and holds it for an instant (to allow any drops to drain back into it). Finally, the operator supports the bottle while withdrawing it from the vaporizer (Fig. 16.27).[110] If the Tec 6 leaks as it is being filled, check for the lack of an O-ring on the bottle spout.[124]

The operator turns the Tec 6 vaporizer on by turning the concentration control dial to the on position while depressing the dial release (on the back of the dial, opposite the zero indicator). The vaporizer requires electric power and a warm-up period of approximately 10 minutes before it can be used from a cold start.[110]

The Tec 6 has several visual indicators that are grouped in a status display (Fig. 16.28).[110] These include a light that indicates "Operational" status, a "No Output" indicator light (and audible alarm), a

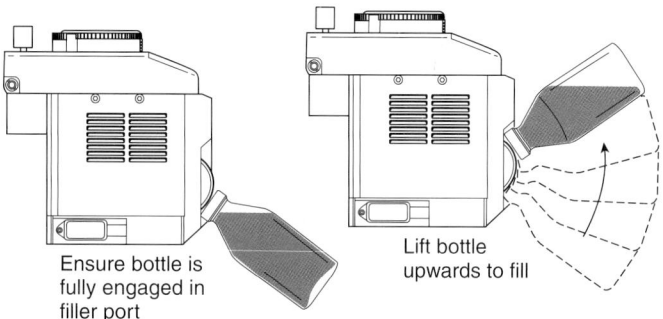

Ensure bottle is fully engaged in filler port

Lift bottle upwards to fill

Fig. 16.27 Filling the Datex-Ohmeda Tec 6 vaporizer. (From Tec 6 Vaporizer: Operation and Maintenance Manual. Madison, WI: Datex-Ohmeda; 1993.)

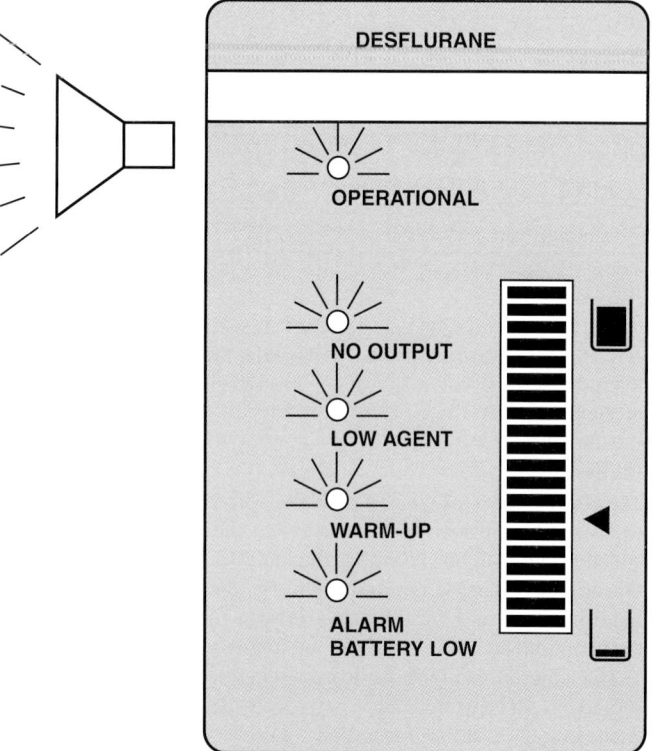

Fig. 16.28 Display panel of the Datex-Ohmeda Tec 6 vaporizer. (From Tec 6 Vaporizer: Operation and Maintenance Manual. Madison, WI: Datex-Ohmeda; 1993.)

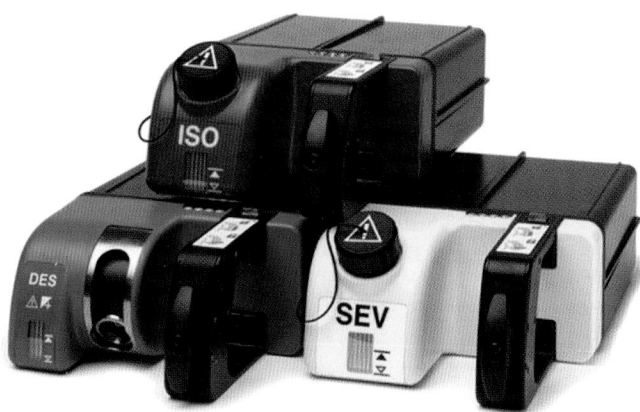

Fig. 16.29 GE Aladin vaporizer cassettes. The sevoflurane cassette is plugged into the vaporizer port. (Courtesy Datex-Ohmeda, Tewksbury, MA.)

"Low Agent" light (and audible alarm), a "Warm-Up" status light, and an "Alarm Battery Low" light. The No Output alarms are activated if the agent level is less than 20 mL, if the vaporizer is tilted more than 10 degrees from the vertical, if there is a power failure lasting longer than 10 seconds, or if an internal malfunction occurs. The cause of a No Output alarm may be sought if it occurs during a case; however, considering the rapid emergence that is characteristic with desflurane, the operator should ensure continued depth of anesthesia by switching to a different agent without undue delay.

Preoperative checkout for variable-bypass vaporizers is relatively straightforward. Proper checkout and functionality should include (1) confirmation the vaporizer is in the off position, (2) level of fullness, (3) verification that the filling cap is tightly closed, and (4) assessment of a functioning interlock. Depending on the machine, they may need to be checked for leaks as well.[53] The Tec 6 requires a more extensive checkout. After performing the appropriate leak test of the machine low-pressure system, the operator checks the amber Alarm Battery Low indicator and replaces the battery if necessary. Next, the operator should turn the Tec 6 on to at least 1%, while disconnecting its electrical plug. Within 15 seconds of disconnection, the No Output light and alarm should activate. If they do not, the battery must be replaced and the vaporizer retested before use. If everything is functioning correctly, the operator reconnects the power and turns the dial to the off position, then presses the mute button for 4 seconds to test all alarms and the display. When the mute button is pressed, all lights and the alarm should activate.[110]

The Aladin (Aisys) vaporizer uses one central electronic control mechanism for all agents.[112,127] Cassettes containing the liquid anesthetic are inserted into a port connected to these control mechanisms, which recognizes the contents of the cassette and dispenses agent into the stream of fresh gas flow (Fig. 16.29). The cassette inserted into the control mechanisms is checked as part of the electronic checklist daily. The Aisys will not deliver volatile agent or nitrous oxide without main power or battery backup and adequate oxygen pressure.

Hazards of Contemporary Vaporizers

Many of the hazards historically associated with the use of vaporizers have been corrected by advances in design, but a few hazards remain (Box 16.8). Vaporizer contamination with incorrect agents continues to be noted.[117,119,120] Diligence during filling is not enough to prevent contamination. Departments should strongly consider replacing funnel-type with keyed-filler vaporizers in equipment purchases.

Aladin vaporizers found on Aisys are not sensitive to tipping. If any other vaporizer is tipped by more than 45 degrees from the vertical, the operator manual or a field service technician must be consulted. Tipping is hazardous because the entry of liquid agent into the control assembly at the top of the vaporizer can have unpredictable effects on its function, including potential overdose to the patient. The vaporizer sump can be drained and gas run through it for a specified time and at a specified concentration before the vaporizer is returned to use. For the recommended corrective action for a particular make and model, the operator manual must be consulted.

Overfilling may be prevented by following the manufacturer's guidelines for filling (e.g., fill only to the top etched line on the liquid level indicator glass, fill only when the vaporizer is off).[113] Regular preventive maintenance of vaporizers is important since vaporizers go out of calibration and may then deliver too-high or too-low concentrations of an agent.[128] Leaks are relatively common and are often due to malposition of vaporizers on its mount, accidental dislodgement, loss of gaskets, or mechanical damage.[123,129–131] These leaks may not be detected with the standard checklist. Tec 6 vaporizers can also leak liquid while being filled if the desflurane bottle is missing the rubber O-ring near its tip.[124] This can be mistaken for a defective vaporizer. As vaporizers incorporate electronics, they are susceptible to electronic failure or unanticipated interactions of new designs with each other.[129,132,133] Case reports detail Aladin vaporizers failing due to fresh gas mixer failure and from copious emesis soaking the machine.[134,135]

New Agents and Low Flows

Low fresh gas flows should not be instituted too early after induction when desflurane or sevoflurane is used. Induction at low flows would be extremely prolonged, creating the risk of awareness in the time interval between offset of intravenous induction agents and onset of action of the volatile agent. Overpressure can be combined with low flows, but 18% of 2 L contains far fewer desflurane molecules than 18% of 6 L, and it is the number of molecules presented to the brain per unit time that causes an increase in anesthetic tension within the brain.

Imagine a 1000-mL sink filled with water, with 100 mL/min inflow (of which 1 mL is methylene blue) and 100 mL/min outflow. The goal is turning the initially colorless water in the sink as blue as the inflow solution. Now imagine the effect of increasing the inflow and outflow to 500 mL/min (of which 5 mL is methylene blue). Would the 1000 mL in the sink turn blue any faster in the second case? Of course, but not because the concentrations are different (both inflows are 1% methylene blue), but because the rate of inflow in the second example is a greater proportion of the capacity of the sink.

Wash-in is based on the concept of a time constant. One time constant (equal to capacity divided by flow) brings a system 63% of the way to equilibrium, two time constants to 86%, and three time constants to 95%. Thus the first sink will reach 63% of equilibrium in 10 minutes (1000 mL ÷ 100 mL flow), whereas the second sink reaches this same degree of equilibrium in only 2 minutes (1000 mL ÷ 500 mL flow). In the same way, the volume (capacity) of the functional residual capacity and breathing circuit can be brought to equilibrium with the inflow more quickly by using a higher rate of inflow (fresh gas flow). A rational approach for ensuring anesthesia that conserves volatile agents would include a nonrebreathing (semiopen) induction (fresh gas flow, 5–8 L/min), followed by low fresh gas flow during maintenance (fresh gas flow, 1–2 L/min). This approach helps conserve tracheal heat and humidity, gases, and agent. Emergence, like induction, must occur at higher, non-rebreathing flows; otherwise it will be unacceptably prolonged.

DELIVERY

This section discusses how the flow of gases to and from the patient is controlled and monitored.

Breathing Circuits

Fundamental Considerations

The **purpose** of all types of anesthesia breathing circuits is the delivery of oxygen and anesthetic and the elimination of carbon dioxide. Carbon dioxide is eliminated from the breathing circuit by washout with adequate fresh gas flow or by absorption in carbon dioxide–absorbent granules.

Any breathing circuit creates some **resistance** to gas flow. Resistance in a circuit may be minimized by reducing the circuit's length and increasing its diameter, avoiding the use of sharp bends, eliminating valves, and maintaining laminar flow. It is important to decrease resistance to flow because added airway resistance is uncomfortable for the conscious patient. Furthermore, the unconscious or anesthetized patient, challenged by increased work of breathing, may not be able to increase respiratory effort, and hypoventilation may occur. The resistance of the anesthesia breathing circuit is low, typically less than that of an endotracheal tube.

Rebreathing of exhaled gases occurs with the use of anesthesia breathing circuits (as it does in space or submarine environments). Rebreathing does not normally occur in other breathing circuits, such as those in the ventilators used in intensive care units. Rebreathing may be useful. Its advantages include cost reduction, an increase in tracheal warmth and humidity, and a decrease in the potential for exposure of operating room personnel to trace and waste gases (because of decreased rate of release of anesthetic gases into the environment). The degree of rebreathing in an anesthesia breathing circuit is increased as the fresh gas flow is decreased because there is relatively less fresh gas added to the circuit, and more of the next inhalation will be exhaled gas. Higher fresh gas flow is associated with less rebreathing in both circle- and Mapleson-type circuits. The higher the fresh gas flow, the more quickly the composition of gas in the breathing circuit will resemble that at the common gas outlet (the dialed-in concentrations of agent, nitrous oxide, and oxygen).

Patients under anesthesia may rebreathe any component of their exhalations—nitrogen, O_2, CO_2, N_2O, and volatile agent. The effects of rebreathing each of these components differ. Rebreathing of exhaled oxygen has no ill effects. Rebreathing of exhaled nitrogen slows induction. Nitrogen that is not eliminated from the breathing circuit delays the establishment of the desired agent concentration, thus high fresh gas flows are appropriate during induction. In contrast, rebreathing of exhaled agent during maintenance is highly desirable for cost and environmental considerations. Rebreathing of CO_2 has the undesirable effect of producing respiratory acidosis, so it is best avoided. Because higher flows reduce the discrepancy between desired concentrations and the concentrations actually inspired, they are appropriate during emergence as well. At the end of an anesthetic, as the flow of volatile agent and N_2O is turned off, it would be undesirable for exhaled agent and N_2O to be rebreathed because this would delay emergence. So gas that is free of agent (and nitrous oxide) is supplied at high flow during emergence to create a favorable concentration gradient that speeds elimination of agents from the body.

Dead space is increased to some degree with the use of any respiratory apparatus. The effect of an increase in mechanical (apparatus) dead space is that rebreathing of exhaled CO_2 is more likely. This is one reason that ventilator tidal volumes are set much larger than the volume of a spontaneous breath. To avoid hypercarbia in the face of an acute increase in dead space, a patient must increase minute ventilation (V_E). Conversely, because alveolar ventilation is the minute ventilation minus dead space ventilation ($V_A = V_E - V_D$), if the patient's minute ventilation is fixed (such as by respiratory depression), increasing dead space decreases alveolar ventilation and increases arterial CO_2 tension.[136] Dead space ends where the inspiratory and expiratory gas streams diverge. In a circle system, dead space ends at the Y-piece. It is not increased by longer inspiratory and expiratory corrugated plastic hoses (although, with longer limbs in the breathing circuit, there may be compliance losses that decrease tidal volume). Use of a face mask is associated with greater dead space than is the use of an endotracheal tube.

The anesthesia workstation uses **dry gases** so that the problems of internal corrosion and bacterial colonization are minimized. However, provision of completely dry gases to the patient's airway can cause various problems. It is common for anesthesia providers to use various means of passively humidifying and heating inspired gases (with a heat and moisture exchanger or by using low fresh gas flows). Active humidification has become less common because it is less effective at preventing hypothermia than heated-air surface warming blankets and because the added moisture can clog gas-analysis lines and soda lime granules, interfere with inspiratory and expiratory flow sensors, or obstruct unidirectional valves.[81]

Anesthesia breathing circuits are unique among respiratory equipment in the degree to which they allow manipulation of the inspired concentration of a variety of components for therapeutic benefit. Each component of the breathing mixture follows its own concentration gradient because it is made to wash into the breathing system, and then from the breathing system into the patient's lungs. In the lungs, gases flow down their concentration gradients, interchanging with pulmonary and blood gases. Understanding the pharmacokinetics of inhaled agent administration involves not only knowledge of respiratory physiology but also familiarity with the physiology of the patient-machine system. For example, the concentration set on the dial differs from the concentrations in the breathing circuit, in the lungs, in the blood, and in the brain. Furthermore, these concentration differences are not constant but vary over time, depending on a number of patient- and machine-related factors. The inspired concentration most closely resembles that delivered from the common gas outlet when rebreathing is minimal or absent (this is typical at high fresh gas flow). Of course, it is desirable that the alveolar concentration differs from the inspired concentration at times. At the start of the emergence phase, the inspired concentration of anesthetic is decreased so that anesthetic gas is washed out while ventilation is continued. Thus, emergence is very different from passively "waking up," and is as much an active process as induction.

Classification of Breathing Circuits

Table 16.5 gives a classification of breathing circuits that is based on whether a reservoir (breathing bag) is present and on the degree to which rebreathing occurs.[137] Patients have access to the atmosphere only in open systems; this is not true in semiopen, semiclosed, or closed systems. A reservoir is present in these three types to provide for the moments during the inspiratory phase when flow in the trachea is greater than fresh gas flow. Both nonrebreathing (Mapleson, Bain) systems and the circle system, at fresh gas flows greater than minute ventilation, are semiopen.[138] If the fresh gas flow to the circle system is less than minute ventilation, some rebreathing must be occurring. If the APL (pop off) valve is closed and very low fresh gas flows are used, the supply of O_2, N_2O, and agent just matches the patient's uptake.[139] In such a closed-circuit system, rebreathing is total.

Nonrebreathing circuits. Mapleson published a classification of nonrebreathing circuits in 1954; this classification is still used today.[140] Rebreathing is prevented in systems like the Mapleson D (Fig. 16.30) because during the pause between expiration and the next inspiration, fresh gas fills the corrugated limb, forcing the previously exhaled gas distally (toward the reservoir). If fresh gas flow is sufficient, no alveolar

gas is rebreathed. The common features of nonrebreathing systems are listed in Box 16.9. These circuits offer very low resistance to breathing and can be used for patients of almost any age, from premature infants to adults. The fresh gas flow required to prevent rebreathing is two to three times minute ventilation.[87] This number can be calculated; however, in practice, many use a minimum fresh gas flow of 5 L/min. Rather than a formula, one may choose a sufficient fresh gas flow to avoid inspired CO_2 on the capnogram, bearing in mind that this minimum fresh gas flow may vary during the course of the anesthetic.[141]

The Bain system is a modified Mapleson D circuit because the arrangement of its components (entry point of fresh gas, reservoir bag, and APL valve) is similar to that of the Mapleson D. However, in the Bain system, the fresh gas hose is directed coaxially within the corrugated limb, and this configuration gives the inhaled gases greater heat and humidity. Unfortunately, unrecognized kinking or disconnection of this relatively hidden fresh gas hose converts the entire corrugated limb into dead space.[142-144] The resulting respiratory acidosis can be severe enough to cause arrhythmias.[144] Users of Bain systems must test the circuit for these problems before they use the system. The Pethick test or a similar one should be used to test for air leaks.[87]

The use of nonrebreathing circuits has declined for several reasons. Many modern anesthesia workstations are not designed to

TABLE 16.5 Classification of Breathing Circuits

Type	Reservoir	Rebreathing	Example
Open	No	No	Open drop Insufflation Nasal cannula or simple face mask
Semiopen	Yes	No	Circle at high fresh gas flow (more than minute ventilation); or a nonrebreathing circuit
Semiclosed	Yes	Yes (partial)	Circle at low fresh gas flow (less than minute ventilation)
Closed	Yes	Yes (complete)	Circle at extremely low fresh gas flow, with adjustable pressure-limiting valve closed

BOX 16.9 Common Features of Nonrebreathing Systems

- All lack unidirectional valves.
- All lack soda lime carbon dioxide absorption.
- Fresh gas flow determines the amount of rebreathing in all.
- Resistance and work of breathing are low in all (no unidirectional valves; no absorbent granules).

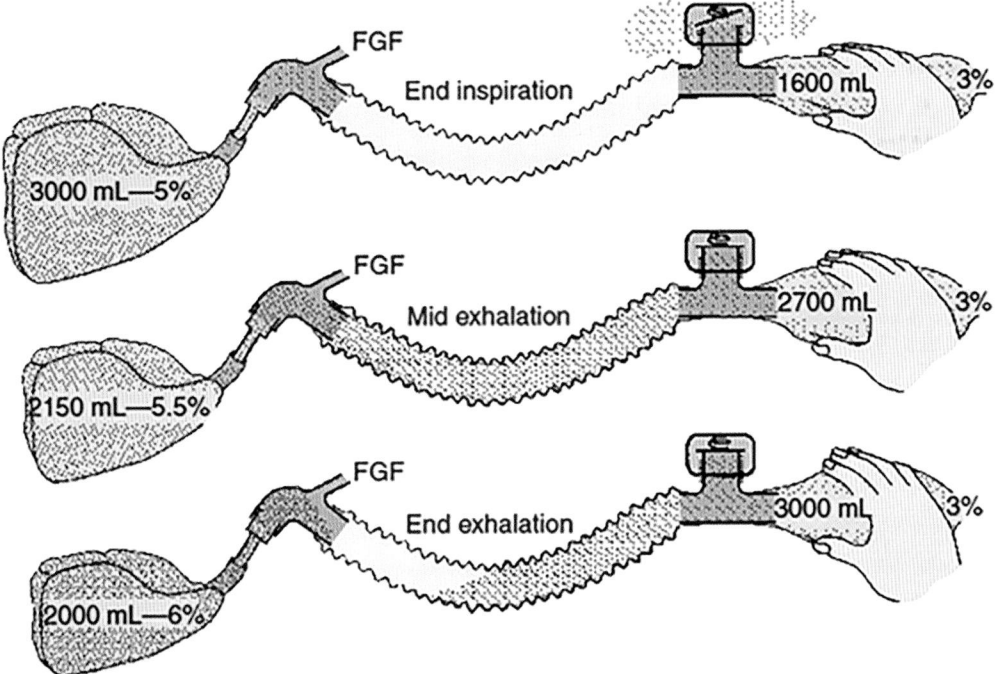

Fig. 16.30 Mapleson D system. Between the end of an expiration and the start of the next inspiration, fresh gas flow (FGF) pushes exhaled gases (containing CO_2) toward the reservoir bag. Thus the patient's inspired gas will come from the corrugated limb and be free of CO_2, as long as fresh gas flow is sufficient. (Modified from Ehrenwerth J, Eisenkraft J, Berry J, eds. *Anesthesia Equipment: Principles and Applications.* 2nd ed. Philadelphia: Elsevier; 2013.)

accommodate them (e.g., Fabius GS). It is more common to see a pediatric circle system used, which is characterized by smaller and less compliant corrugated limbs, as compared with the adult circle system. The minimum weight of a child for which a pediatric circle would be suitable has been stated as 10 to 20 kg; however, when infants of mean weight as low as 6 kg were studied, the pediatric circle was equal to a nonrebreathing circuit in preserving blood gas values and end-tidal CO_2, whether assisted or spontaneous breathing was used.[145] No one guideline applies to all situations because the decision on whether to use a pediatric circle system in any given child depends on familiarity, clinical judgment, and the anticipated duration of unassisted respiration.

Pediatric circle systems do not place undue burdens (in terms of work of breathing) on spontaneously ventilating patients.[146] The pediatric circle system is low compliance, the work of breathing associated with it is reasonable, it requires less reconfiguration to set up, and it allows the use of lower fresh gas flows (the high fresh gas flow required in nonrebreathing circuits cools children and is more costly).[147] Modern monitoring such as capnography and spirometry allows a high degree of confidence that a child is being ventilated adequately with the pediatric circle.

If a nonrebreathing circuit is used in the middle of a schedule of adult cases using the circle system, some disassembly and reassembly are required, accompanied by the possibility of error or misconnection. The small amount of resistance offered by the soda lime canisters and unidirectional valves of the circle system is deleterious only during spontaneous respiration, which is limited in duration in most general anesthesia for children. The advantages and disadvantages of nonrebreathing circuits are summarized in Box 16.10. Although they are useful, nonrebreathing circuits are associated with loss of heat from the patient and with greater use of inhalation agents, owing to their requirement for relatively high fresh gas flow.

Circle system. The circle system is the breathing circuit most commonly used in the United States because it prevents rebreathing of carbon dioxide while allowing rebreathing of all other gases. Gas flow during mechanical ventilation is shown in Fig. 16.31. The circle system has separate inspiratory and expiratory limbs. Gas in the inspiratory limb only goes toward the patient; gas in the expiratory limb only proceeds away from the patient. The inspiratory and expiratory unidirectional valves enforce this flow pattern, which ensures that all exhaled gas is directed through the absorbent granules, cleansing

it of carbon dioxide. Rebreathing takes place at low fresh gas flows; however, if the valves are functioning and the granules are unexpired, no rebreathing of carbon dioxide can occur.

A single-limb, coaxial circle system is also available in which, like the Bain, the inspiratory limb is contained within the expiratory (Fig. 16.32). It is checked and used like any circle system. Like the Bain, the coaxial circle is less bulky and is thought to provide greater heat and humidity to inhaled gases. Disadvantages include the potential for obstruction or lack of patency of either limb, which may cause respiratory acidosis or even mimic esophageal intubation.[142,143] This respiratory acidosis does not respond to increased minute ventilation; if exhaled gases are not forced through the absorbent granules, no amount of ventilation will cleanse carbon dioxide from the exhaled gases. The tests for inner tube patency that can be used for a Bain circuit are not readily adaptable to the coaxial circle system.

Gas enters the circle system from the common gas outlet, and it exits the circle to the scavenger via the APL valve (or the ventilator relief valve if mechanical ventilation is used). The APL valve creates an adjustable leak during manual ventilation. If it is completely open and the bag is squeezed, all gas exits to the scavenger because it is the path of least resistance. If the valve is completely closed, all gas ventilates the lungs, and the pressure within the circle increases because the fresh gas flowing in has no means of escape. The setting of the APL valve is constantly adjusted during manual ventilation of the lungs so that a resistance sufficient to force gas to inflate the lungs is maintained. If gas cannot exit through the APL valve or ventilator relief valve, pressure will build within the system.[148]

Unidirectional valves create a pattern of gas flow that forces exhaled gases through the CO_2 absorbent granules (Fig. 16.33). The valve leaflet (disk) is subject to damage, occlusion, foreign body contamination, and sticking with collected moisture or absorbent dust, particularly on the expiratory valve disk.[51,149–151] Daily performance of a preanesthesia checklist, as well as regular maintenance, should enable the operator to detect or prevent most of these problems. Thus there are only two common reasons for an increase in inspired CO_2: The absorbent granules have been exhausted or the unidirectional valves are faulty. Fig. 16.34 shows that incompetence of an inspiratory or expiratory valve turns the entire corrugated limb into dead space.[87,152] This usually results in an increase in inspired and expired CO_2.

If inspired CO_2 of more than 3 mm Hg is detected on the capnograph (Figs. 16.35 and 16.36), the fresh gas flow should be increased to 5 to 8 L/min; this converts the system to a semiopen configuration, in which rebreathing of exhaled gases is minimized. Similar to the principle in the Mapleson nonrebreathing circuit, a high fresh gas flow in the circle dilutes exhalations and sends them to the scavenger. If substantially increasing the fresh gas flow causes the inspired CO_2 to decrease, the absorbent granules are exhausted and should be replaced at the end of the case. Some workstations (e.g., Aisys, Apollo) with prepackaged granules or canisters allow granules to be changed during the case, although they are not meant to function for more than very brief periods without a canister attached. Furthermore, it is safest to change between cases, as problems with changing granules leading to hypoventilation continue to be reported.[153–159] If elevated inspired CO_2 persists in spite of the higher fresh gas flow, the unidirectional valves are likely to be incompetent. The operator should remove the expiratory valve (if possible), inspect and dry it, and then reassemble it (while ventilating the patient with an Ambu bag).[29] Note that this may be more difficult in newer absorber heads (e.g., Aisys) and will always be more difficult when the user has never performed it before. This argues for reading the operator manual and practicing without a patient attached before the maneuver is attempted because failure to reassemble the valve quickly will result in hypoventilation and interruption in volatile

---

BOX 16.10 Nonrebreathing Systems: Advantages and Disadvantages

Advantages
- Lightweight
- Convenient
- Easily sterilized and scavenged
- Exhaled gases in corrugated limb may give heat and humidity to inhaled gas (Bain)

Disadvantages
- Unrecognized disconnection or kinking of fresh gas hose in the Bain circuit (use Pethick test)
- Pollution and increased costs of agents and gases, owing to need for higher flows
- Loss of heat from patient
- May require disconnection of circle fresh gas supply hose and scavenger connections for assembly; can be reassembled improperly

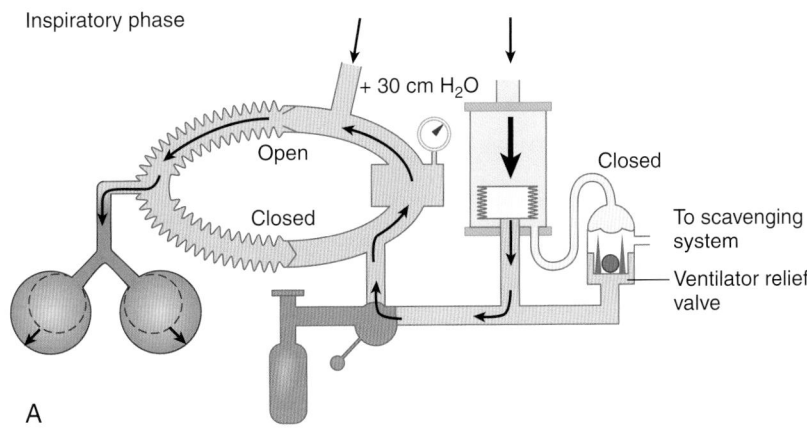

Inspiratory phase

+ 30 cm H$_2$O

Open

Closed

Closed

To scavenging system

Ventilator relief valve

A

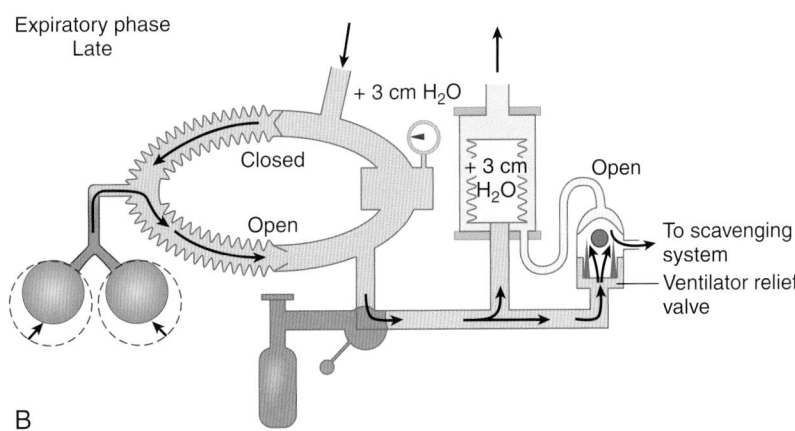

Expiratory phase
Late

+ 3 cm H$_2$O

Closed

+ 3 cm H$_2$O

Open

Open

To scavenging system

Ventilator relief valve

B

Fig. 16.31 Gas flow in a circle system during mechanical ventilator inspiration. (A) Shows inspiration. As driving gas compresses the bellows, it propels gas into the inspiratory limb past the inspiratory unidirectional valve, inflating the lungs. Driving gas pressure also closes the ventilator relief valve, which is the route to the scavenger. (B) Shows expiration. Lung deflation propels gas into the expiratory limb past the expiratory unidirectional valve. The exhaled gases fill the bellows to a small pressure first, then excess gas proceeds to the scavenger via the ventilator relief valve. A small weight within the ventilator relief valve makes filling the bellows the path of least resistance, until a small positive end-expiratory pressure (PEEP) builds up, lifting the weight, and opening the valve. NOTE: (1) Fresh gas flows into the circle continuously, and (2) flow in the circle is unidirectional, which forces all exhaled gas through the carbon dioxide absorbent granules. (From Miller RD, et al., eds. *Miller's Anesthesia.* 7th ed. Philadelphia: Elsevier; 2010.)

anesthetic delivery. Perhaps the best recommendation is to bring a new anesthesia workstation into the room; any valve adjustment can take place outside the pressure of the clinical situation and will not distract the anesthetist from patient care.

It is mandatory to check unidirectional valves before use. There are a multitude of means proposed to check the unidirectional valves, which vary in ease of performance and complexity.[29,150,160] One suggested method with applicability to a variety of workstations is as follows: A spare breathing bag is placed on the elbow fitting at the patient's end of the Y-piece, and mechanical ventilation of this "artificial lung" is begun. The user carefully observes that the valves lift and fall, and that gas flows back and forth in a tidal fashion between the mechanical ventilator bellows and the artificial lung expected during inspiration and expiration.[12,161] Breathing through the elbow or mask of a clean circuit (with a paper mask on) is an alternative method, but it presents problems of cross contamination. Dräger suggests a similar test but also breathing through each limb individually as follows.[68] If the

inspiratory limb is detached and occluded with one's palm, the operator should be able to exhale, but not inhale, through the expiratory limb, provided that the expiratory unidirectional valve is competent. Similarly, if the inspiratory limb is replaced and the expiratory limb detached and occluded, the operator should be able to inspire, but not expire, through the inspiratory limb. This test may be more sensitive than the first test mentioned. If a preanesthesia check is performed daily, the capnograph is used properly, and the operator is aware of the steps that should be taken in the event of an increase in inspired CO$_2$, perhaps this more rigorous test need be performed only if unidirectional valve function is in doubt, particularly because it is problematic to perform this more rigorous test in a hygienic fashion.[29]

Simulating manual or ventilator breathing checks not only for unidirectional valve function, but also for obstruction to expiration secondary to mold flash or plastic wrap emboli, creates problems that have resulted in mortality.[5,151,162–169] Checking for breathing circuit obstruction is critical because an obstructed circuit can prevent positive

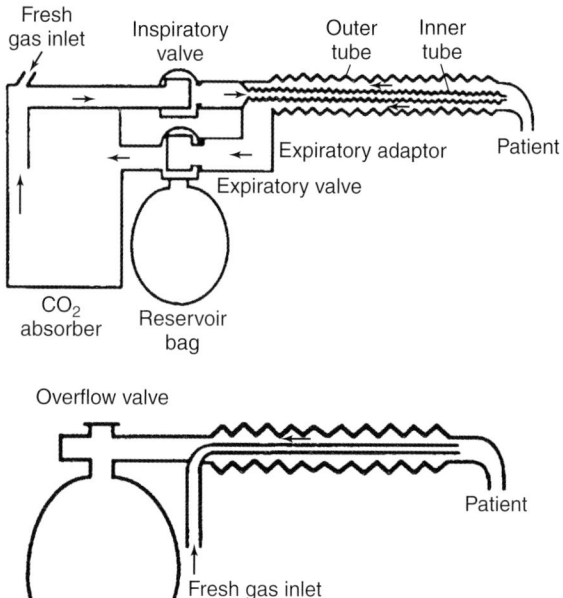

Fig. 16.32 In the coaxial circle system *(top)*, the inspiratory limb is contained within the expiratory limb, like the Bain *(bottom)*.

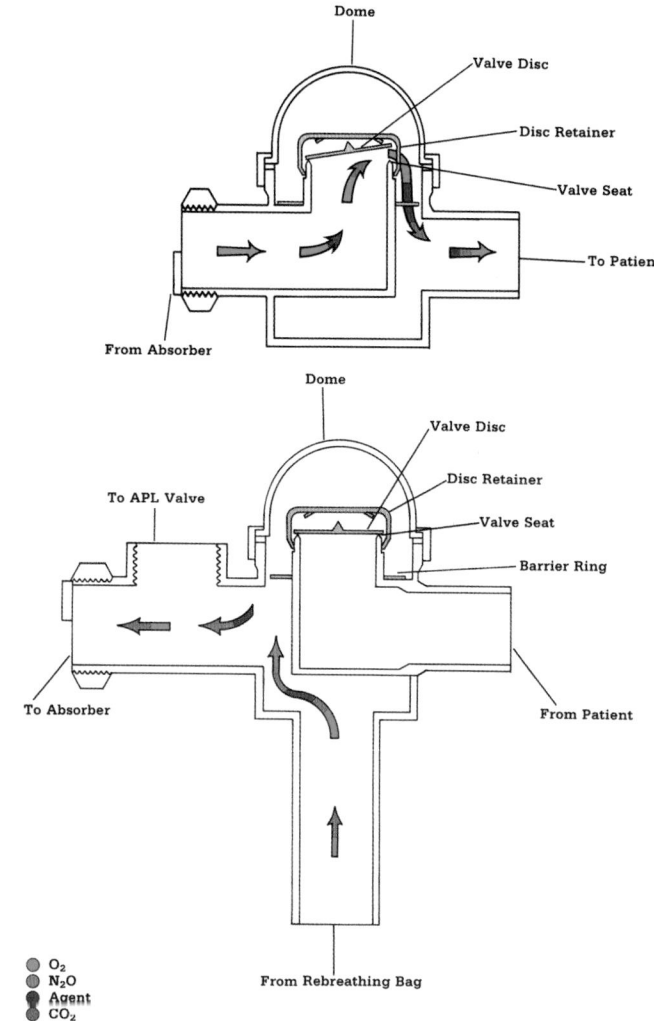

Fig. 16.33 Gas flows in inspiratory *(top)* and expiratory *(bottom)* unidirectional valves during inspiration. (From Bowie E, Huffman LM. *The Anesthesia Machine: Essentials for Understanding.* Madison, WI: Datex-Ohmeda; 1985.)

pressure ventilation, simulating bronchospasm at induction.[5] Newer workstations have electronic routines to check for leaks and compliance. This helps the ventilator accurately deliver the set tidal volume. These checks must be repeated when the type of circuit is changed, for example, from adult to pediatric. With any newer workstation, the corrugated plastic breathing circuit hoses should be expanded before the electronic leak and compliance test is initiated. These automated checks do not reliably detect breathing circuit obstruction due to foreign bodies or stuck valves.[10]

The advantages and disadvantages of the circle system are listed in Box 16.11. One advantage of at least partial rebreathing is relative constancy of inspired concentrations. In a completely nonrebreathing circuit, each breath is fresh gas, so depth can vary much more quickly. The use of lower flows also reduces the cost of volatile agents and the rate of release of anesthetic agents into the environment.[170,171] Not only can low flows reduce cost, but they reduce the environmental and greenhouse effects of anesthetic agents, which are appealing goals.[171,172] The global warming potential of 1 hour of anesthesia maintenance at 1 minimum alveolar concentration (MAC) and fresh gas flow of 2 L/min with sevoflurane is like driving a car of average fuel efficiency 8 miles. One hour of isoflurane is like driving 15 miles; 1 hour of nitrous oxide (0.6 MAC) is like driving 112 miles; and 1 hour of desflurane is like driving 387 miles.[173]

The circle conserves respiratory tract humidity. Misconnections occur much less frequently now than in the past because the diameter of breathing hoses (22 mm) has been standardized to be different from the diameter of scavenger hoses (19 or 30 mm). Nevertheless, misconnections continue to be reported.[174–178] Maintenance of the circle system is detailed in operator manuals, and these must be consulted before one disassembles and cleans the absorber head.

Several design changes in newer circle systems facilitate low-flow anesthesia. Low fresh gas flow is desirable to reduce pollution and the cost of using volatile agents and nitrous oxide, preserve tracheal heat and moisture, delay the drying of carbon dioxide–absorbent granules, and preserve patient body temperature. Factors that enhance the safety

and efficiency of low flows in modern circle breathing systems and ventilators are shown in Box 16.12.

A dual-canister absorber head like the Aestiva has a larger volume than many of the newer designs.[73,75,78,80,179,180] Circles with smaller volume will have shorter time constants. The time constant equals capacity divided by flow, and measures how quickly a breathing system reaches equilibrium with a change in the inflow. In a circle system with lower volume, changes in dialed concentration of agent will be reflected more quickly in the inspired concentration, at any flow rate, as compared to a higher volume circle system. In a nonrebreathing circuit, or a circle system at flows substantially higher than minute ventilation, each breath reflects the dialed concentration of the agent because there is no rebreathing of exhaled gases in either. Thus, a circle system with higher flows is suitable when rapid changes are desired, such as at induction and emergence.

There are, however, circumstances in which to avoid low fresh gas flows (e.g., <1 L/min). Absolute contraindications include patients with smoke inhalation injury, malignant hyperthermia, or other conditions in which washout of potentially dangerous gases or a high oxygen uptake is expected. If equipment breakdown occurs midcase that would affect the safety of low flows (i.e., failure of inspired oxygen

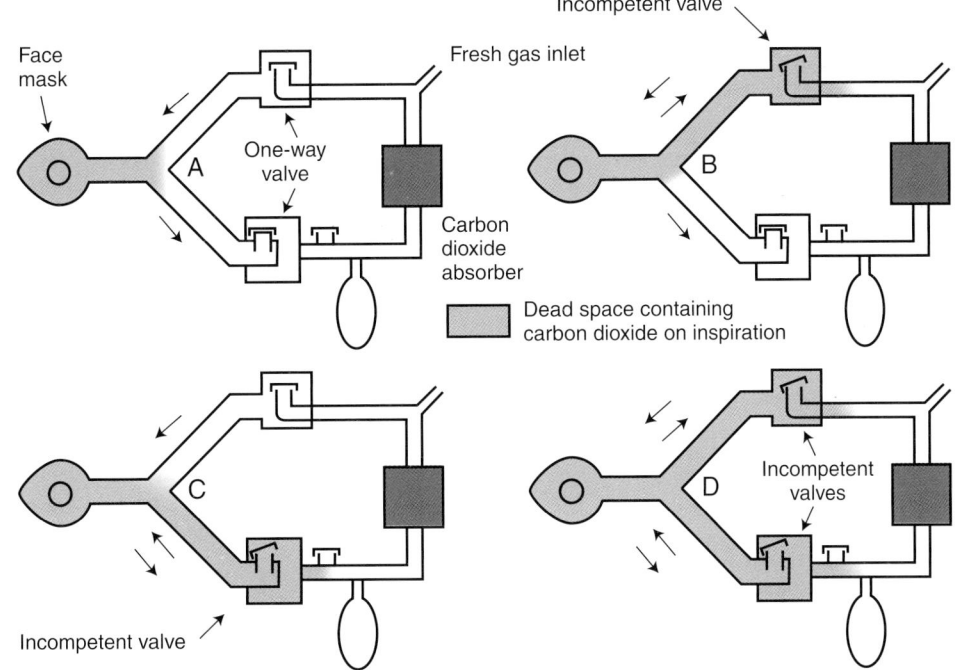

Fig. 16.34 Incompetence of a unidirectional valve. (A) Normal function. Incompetence of an inspiratory valve (B), an expiratory valve (C), or of both unidirectional valves (D) creates dead space *(stippled area)* that extends through the entire ipsilateral corrugated breathing hose. (Modified from Gravenstein JS, et al. *Capnography in Clinical Practice.* Boston: Butterworth; 1989.)

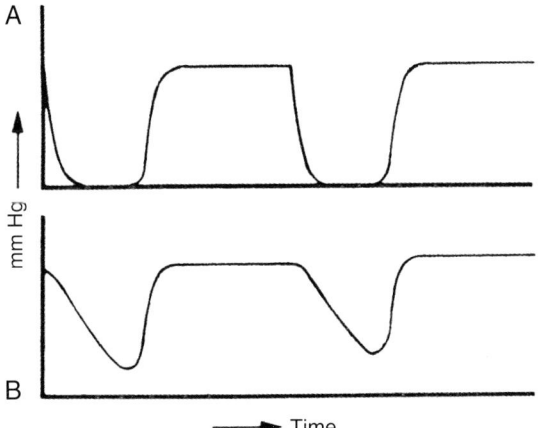

Fig. 16.35 Compared with a normal capnogram (A), a capnogram recorded when the inspiratory unidirectional valve is incompetent (B) shows increases in inhaled and exhaled carbon dioxide pressure and an abnormally prolonged downstroke. The prolonged downstroke during the inspiratory phase occurs because the patient inspires mixed alveolar and fresh gas from the inspiratory limb rather than fresh gas alone. (Modified from Gravenstein JS, et al. *Capnography in Clinical Practice.* Boston: Butterworth; 1989.)

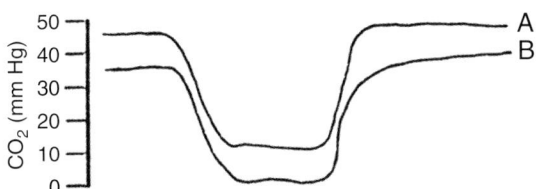

Fig. 16.36 Compared with a normal capnogram (B), a capnogram recorded with an incompetent expiratory unidirectional valve (A) shows increases in inspired and expired carbon dioxide concentration but no changes in morphology. (Modified from Gravenstein JS, et al. *Capnography in Clinical Practice.* Boston: Butterworth; 1989.)

BOX 16.11 Circle System: Advantages and Disadvantages

Advantages
- Constant inspired concentrations
- Conservation of respiratory tract heat and humidity
- Minimal operating room and environmental pollution
- Useful for closed-system, low-flow, and semiopen configurations
- Low resistance (less than the endotracheal tube; not as low as in nonrebreathing circuits)

Disadvantages
- Relatively complex
- Opportunities for misconnection or disconnection
- Malfunctioning unidirectional valves cause serious problems
  - *Open:* Rebreathing
  - *Closed:* Occlusion
- Less portable than nonrebreathing circuits
- Increased dead space (true of all respiratory apparatus; extends to the point where inspired and expired gas streams diverge [i.e., at Y-piece])

---

or anesthetic agent monitors, or failure of soda lime granules), higher flows should be used. Relative contraindications to low fresh gas flows include the use of older equipment that is less leakproof, face mask anesthesia, during rigid bronchoscopy, and ventilation using uncuffed endotracheal tubes.[181]

Humidification and prevention of nosocomial infection are desirable with the use of any respiratory apparatus. Both of these goals may be addressed with breathing circuit filters that incorporate heat and moisture exchange with filtration (HMEF).[182] The use of low flows during maintenance results in an increase in circuit humidity and a lower rate of use of volatile agents. Heat- and moisture-exchanging filters precipitate exhaled water vapor on their filter media. The next inhalation returns this moisture to the patient. HMEF filters may slow

BOX 16.12 Breathing System and Ventilator Design Features That Support Low-Flow Anesthesia

- Compliance and leak testing, automatic leak detection
- Fresh gas compensation or decoupling
- Warmed absorber heads (in some models)
- Low-volume and less-leaky absorber heads (allow faster equilibration of dialed and delivered agent concentration)
  - Fabius GS 1500-mL canister (Fabius GS volume is 2800 mL, including bag for entire breathing system)
  - Aestiva 2700 mL (canisters alone)
  - Aisys 2.7 L (vent mode), 1.2 L (bag mode)
  - Apollo and Perseus have heated breathing circuits that are low volume.
- No mandatory minimum oxygen flows (there are exceptions; Aespire and Aestiva, at 50 mL/min)

BOX 16.13 Carbon Dioxide Absorption in Soda Lime

1. $CO_2 + H_2O \leftrightarrow H_2CO_3$
2. $H_2CO_3 + NaOH \leftrightarrow Na_2CO_3 + H_2O +$ energy
3. $Na_2CO_3 + Ca(OH)_2 \rightarrow CaCO_3\downarrow + NaOH$

For soda lime, reaction 1 is also called the first neutralization reaction; reaction 3 is also called the second neutralization reaction. Note that activator is regenerated in step 3. KOH may take the place of NaOH, and K_2CO_3 may take the place of Na_2CO_3 in steps 2 and 3.

the rate of heat loss from the patient because they decrease the rate of evaporation of water from the tracheal mucosa. They may also confer the benefit of bacterial and viral filtration. Even if HMEF are used, cleaning the bellows is necessary after anesthesia has been provided to a patient with a disease transmitted by airborne particles or oral secretions. To limit contamination of the workstation, consider avoiding the mechanical ventilator, using bacterial/viral filters on the Y-piece or on each limb, ensuring the filter is connected proximal to the gas sampling lines, and changing the soda lime after the case.

The American Association of Nurse Anesthetists (AANA) Standards for Nurse Anesthesia Practice and infection control guidelines call on anesthetists to use safety precautions to minimize the risk of infection for the patient, the anesthetist, and other staff.[183,184] It is certain that anesthesia equipment, as well as providers, are contaminated with potential pathogens.[185] Furthermore, many of the surfaces of the anesthesia workstation and monitors have been shown to be contaminated with blood, both visible and occult.[186] It is therefore mandatory for patient safety to ensure that departmental cleaning and sterilization programs are adequate, that good housekeeping during administration of anesthesia is practiced, and that universal precautions are observed. For equipment, the AANA advocates a classification system and specific equipment recommendations that are published in their *Infection Control Guide*.[183] In addition, manufacturers include directions for cleaning and sterilizing equipment in their operation and maintenance manuals.

Carbon Dioxide Absorption

Carbon dioxide absorption makes rebreathing of exhalations possible. Thus it conserves agent, oxygen, nitrous oxide, and tracheal humidity, while preventing the respiratory acidosis that would result from the rebreathing of CO_2.

Fresh gas flow determines the amount of rebreathing in the circle system. A circle system with fresh gas flows of 0.3 to 0.5 L/min (closed circuit) provides near-total rebreathing and full reliance on absorbent for prevention of rebreathing of CO_2. At the other extreme, use of a circle system with fresh gas flows above minute ventilation (>5–8 L/min) is associated with little if any reliance on absorbent granules because exhaled carbon dioxide is rapidly diluted and sent to the scavenger with such high fresh gas inflows.[87,181] This relationship can be confusing. When faced with exhausted granules, which cause an increase in expired (and inspired) CO_2, one may be tempted to increase minute ventilation (V_E) by increasing tidal volume, respiratory rate, or both. This approach is ineffective with exhausted absorbent (even though it is the obvious response for controlling hypercarbia from other causes)

because the patient simply inspires more of a gas mixture from which CO_2 has been inadequately absorbed. The correct response to hypercarbia associated with exhausted absorbent is increasing fresh gas flow (and then changing the absorbent at the end of the case). Whereas this can be accomplished midcase with the newer absorbent canister designs, it is safest to wait until the case is over, controlling CO_2 with high fresh gas flow in the interim.

Chemistry

The chemistry of soda lime CO_2 absorption is shown in Box 16.13. The ionic reactions take place on the surface of the granules in an aqueous medium. An appropriate water content (10%–20% depending on formulation) is important for the speed and efficiency of the reactions. Dry granules become exhausted much more quickly than moist granules. Activators (NaOH, KOH) are added to increase the speed of the reaction. Potassium hydroxide is used much less frequently because it has been implicated in reactions that produce carbon monoxide and compound A from degradation of inhaled anesthetic agents.[187,188] The activator combines with carbonate ions in a reversible reaction that produces water and energy. The absorption of 1 mole of CO_2 produces 13,000 kcal of heat energy.[136] Absorbents contain ethyl violet as an indicator of absorbent pH. Fresh CO_2 absorbent has a caustic alkaline pH because of the sodium hydroxide. As the reactions proceed, the pH becomes less alkaline. At a critical pH of 10.3, the ethyl violet changes from colorless to blue-purple.

Soda lime does not regenerate to any extent; in other words, it does not regain capacity to absorb CO_2 during periods when it is not in use. Its capacity is similar whether it is used continuously or intermittently. However, it does exhibit some color reversion (a change in appearance from blue-purple back to white) during a rest period. The color of the absorbent at the beginning of the day may not reflect its remaining capacity because of this color reversion.[136] When a subsequent anesthetic is begun, the color of absorbent that had not seemed exhausted initially may quickly change to blue-purple. Therefore it is recommended that the user judge the degree of color change at the end of each case, and change the canister before the next case if necessary.

Soda Lime

The characteristics of soda lime and other selected absorbents are listed in Table 16.6.[90,189–198] The main constituent of most absorbents is calcium hydroxide. Hardeners (silica and kieselguhr) may be added to soda lime. Absorbents are manufactured to have a water content between 13% and 20% by weight. The size of the granules is 4 to 8 mesh, meaning they will pass through screens with four to eight holes per inch. The selection of granule size involves a compromise between resistance to flow and absorption efficiency. Larger granules have less resistance to gas flow; however, they are also less efficient because their surface area is relatively small with respect to their mass. Fine granules or soda lime dust would have a great deal of resistance to gas flow, but their efficiency would be high because of their increased surface area.

TABLE 16.6 Characteristics of Absorbents

Component	Sodasorb (WR Grace)	Medisorb (GE)	Drägersorb 800 Plus (Dräger)	Amsorb Plus (Armstrong Medical)*	Litholyme (Allied Health Care)	Spiralith (Medipore)
Ca(OH)$_2$ %	50–100	70–80	75–83	>80	>75	—
NaOH %	3.7	< 3.5	1–3	0	0	—
KOH %	0	0	0	0	0	—
LiOH %	—	—	—	—	—	95
Li$_2$CO$_3$ %	—	—	—	—	—	3
LiCl %	—	—	—	—	< 3%	—
Water content %	15–17	16–20	~16	13–18	12–19	Unknown**
Size (mesh)	4–8	4–8	4–8	4–8	4–8	—
Indicator	Yes	Yes	Yes	Yes	Yes	No

*Amsorb also contains CaCl2 1% (as humectant) and CaSO4 and polyvinylpyrrolidine 1% (as hardeners).
**The water content in Spirolith is chemically bound, so it does not desiccate.
Data from Olympio MA. *APSF Newsl.* 2005;2:25–29; Higuchi H, et al. *Anesth Analg.* 2001;93:221–225; Wissing H, et al. *Anesthesiology.* 2001;95:1205–1212; Yamakage M, et al. *Anesth Analg.* 2000;91:220–224; http://www.spiralith.com; http://www.litholyme.com/images/Litholyme_MSDS.pdf; and https://microporeusa.com/wp-content/uploads/2020/11/SAFETY-DATA-SHEET-Dry-LiOH.pdf.
Numbers are approximations that may not sum to 100%.
CaCl2, Calcium chloride; *Ca(OH)2,* calcium hydroxide; *CaSO4,* calcium sulfate; *KOH,* potassium hydroxide; *LiCl,* lithium chloride; *Li2CO3,* lithium carbonate; *LiOH,* lithium hydroxide; *NaOH,* sodium hydroxide.

Soda lime degrades most current inhalation agents, with sevoflurane degraded most and desflurane least. Degradation may produce compound A (sevoflurane), carbon monoxide (the ethyl methyl ethers isoflurane and desflurane), and other compounds. Degradation is favored by dry absorbent and the presence and quantity of strong bases (potassium hydroxide more than sodium hydroxide).[187,199-201]

Sevoflurane is unstable in soda lime, producing compound A. Compound A is lethal in rats at 130 to 340 ppm and may cause renal injury at 25 to 50 ppm. Compound A concentrations of 25 to 50 ppm are achievable in normal clinical practice if extremely low fresh gas flows are used. The incidence of toxic (hepatic or renal) or lethal effects from sevoflurane, used in millions of humans, is comparable to desflurane.[202] The product insert does not recommend sevoflurane at total fresh gas flows less than 1 to 2 L/min for more than 2 MAC hours.[203] The production of compound A may be affected by the particular workstation used. At a constant fresh gas flow, it was produced least in the workstation with the lowest circuit and absorbent volume.[192] This thinking may be changing. Because some modern absorbents are free of strong bases (Amsorb, Litholyme, Spiralith), they produce no or negligible Compound A under any fresh gas flow, whether they are desiccated or normally hydrated.[171,190,194,195,198] While Compound A is nephrotoxic in rats, it has not been shown to be so in humans, after more than 120 million sevoflurane anesthetics have been administered (as of 2003).[171]

Carbon monoxide is produced by desflurane, much more than isoflurane, when these agents are in contact with absorbent granules. Sevoflurane produces little, if any, carbon monoxide. Production of carbon monoxide is greatest in dry absorbent. It is recommended that oxygen be turned off at the end of each case, absorbents changed regularly (particularly if fresh gas flow is left on over the weekend or overnight), and low flows used (this will tend to keep granules moist). Current recommendations for safe use of absorbent are summarized in Box 16.14.

Absorbents Lacking Strong Bases

The strongly basic activators (NaOH and particularly KOH) have been convincingly implicated in the carbon monoxide problem with the methyl ethyl ethers (especially desflurane) and the generation

BOX 16.14 Recommendations on the Safe Use of Carbon Dioxide Absorbents

1. Use carbon dioxide absorbents with lower (or no) amounts of strong bases (particularly potassium hydroxide [KOH]).
2. Create institutional, hospital, and/or departmental policies regarding steps to prevent desiccation of the carbon dioxide absorbent.
3. Turn off all gas flow when the workstation is not in use.
4. Change the absorbent regularly, on Monday morning for instance.
5. Change absorbent whenever inspired CO$_2$ reaches 3 mm Hg (alternatively, use color change).
6. Change all absorbent, not just one canister in a two-canister system.
7. Change absorbent when uncertain of the state of hydration, such as when the fresh gas flow has been left on for an extensive or indeterminate time period.
8. If compact canisters are used, consider changing them more frequently.

Low flows also have a role in preserving humidity in absorbent granules. Use relatively low fresh gas flows for the majority of procedures, changing flows from high to low as soon as practical in any given case (after the patient has attained maintenance levels of volatile anesthetic).

of compound A by sevoflurane. Many absorbents available in North America lack KOH and may have reduced amounts of NaOH (see Table 16.6). Because of the potential lower efficiency of absorbents that lack all strong bases, many traditional soda lime–based absorbents have been modified to include less NaOH and no KOH (see Table 16.6).[196] The goal is to maintain efficiency while lessening the production of byproducts. Dräger Medical makes an absorbent with decreased amounts of NaOH and no KOH: Drägersorb 800 Plus. GE Medical supplies Medisorb, which lacks KOH, in the prefilled canisters for all their anesthesia workstations (i.e., Aestiva, Aisys). Eliminating both activators entirely produces an absorbent that has similar physical characteristics and carbon dioxide absorption efficiency as compared with soda lime, while avoiding the problems of Compound A or carbon monoxide generation (Amsorb Plus [Armstrong Medical Ltd., Coleraine, Northern Ireland]).[90,193,204,205]

Lithium may also be used as a catalyst for soda lime absorbents. Litholyme (Allied Healthcare Products Inc, St Louis, MO) is a $Ca(OH)_2$-based absorbent, which contains lithium chloride as a catalyst (see Table 16.6).[206,207] Litholyme does not degrade inhaled agents to carbon monoxide or Compound A even if desiccated, does not undergo color reversion, and is efficient in absorbing carbon dioxide.[207]

Lithium hydroxide is the main constituent of Spirolith, a unique absorbent that is efficient and does not degrade volatile agents. It does not desiccate since its water content is chemically bound.[197,208] Spirolith is a powder enclosed in a polymer sheet, making the absorbent recyclable, and also limiting the danger to eyes and skin posed by caustic dust in traditional absorbents. Because it lacks a color indicator, it may only be used with inspired CO_2 ($Fico_2$) monitoring.[195]

Using Carbon Dioxide Absorbents

Certain similarities are apparent with all absorbents. The resistance of filled canisters in a circle system is low. Resistance of other breathing circuit components, particularly the endotracheal tube, is greater. Inhaled dust from absorbents containing strong bases is caustic and a respiratory irritant (it may lead to laryngospasm, bronchospasm, and pneumonia).[136] A trap for water, which also prevents the passage of dust toward the patient, may be incorporated distal to the granules in circle systems; if present, it must be emptied periodically. In addition, when the breathing circuit is pressurized for checkout, consider releasing the pressure through the APL valve rather than through the elbow at the patient's end. This technique not only prevents the propulsion of dust toward the patient but is also useful for checking APL valve function.

Absorbent efficiency is decreased by channeling and the wall effect.[205,209] The amount of CO_2 absorbed varies throughout the canister. The inside edge of the canister wall is a low-resistance pathway. Exhaled gas follows this pathway, or other low-resistance pathways, through the canister, forming channels whose capacity to absorb CO_2 is exhausted before the capacity of the bulk of the absorbent is used. Thus the wall effect and channeling produce exhaustion of absorbent before its theoretic capacity has been reached. To help prevent these two effects, shake the canister before installation in the circle system to promote uniform packing throughout.[136] Finally, ensure that the canister is without cracks and, if loose-fill granules are used, the lid is in the locked position after refilling. Cracks, even in new canisters, are not an uncommon source of circuit leaks. Because absorber mounts allow a change of canisters during a case, a leaking, cracked, malpositioned, or even absent canister may pass automated checkout procedures.[210-212] There is at least one case report of a canister exploding open, spreading granules on the floor when the circuit pressure went above 30 cm H_2O while bag-masking a patient after induction. This caused a rather large leak, and upon further testing it was shown that the soda lime canister was not properly locked after it was refilled.[213]

Exhaustion and Replacement of Canisters

The clinical signs of absorbent exhaustion are shown in Box 16.15. Some of these signs (e.g., hyperventilation) may be masked in the anesthetized patient. In practice, increased $Fico_2$ and absorbent color change are primary indications of exhaustion. It is unwise to rely on color change or canister temperature alone as a measure of exhaustion.[214] The process of canister replacement for Aestiva-style dual-canister absorbers is illustrated in Fig. 16.37, and the steps for replacement are shown in Box 16.16. Canister replacement for the Aisys is shown in Fig. 16.38.

Do not change Aestiva-style dual canisters or loose fill in the middle of a case, and be hesitant to change absorbent midcase on any machine. If the new canister is placed in its clear plastic holder upside down,

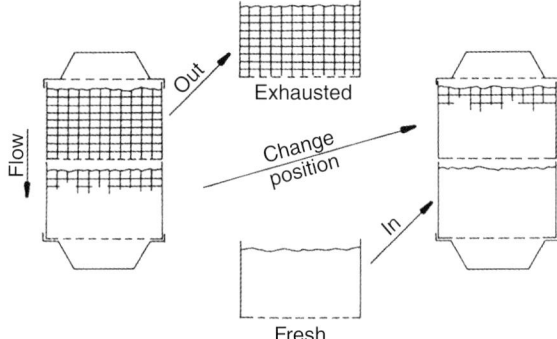

Fig. 16.37 Changing dual-canister carbon dioxide absorbers. (From Schreiber P. *Safety Guidelines for Anesthesia Systems*. Telford, PA: Drägerwerk AG & Co., and Lubeck, Germany: KGaA; 1985.)

Note: Be hesitant to change any canister in midcase, as they do not always go back together smoothly. Do not change a dual canister in the middle of a case; convert to a semiopen breathing circuit by using 5–8 L/min fresh gas flow.

or if for any other reason the circuit cannot be reassembled promptly, resumption of ventilation might be delayed.[153-155] If granules do become exhausted, a safer alternative strategy is to change fresh gas flow to one to two times the minute ventilation; this approach should ensure that expired CO_2 is reduced to acceptable levels. The granules can then be replaced after the case.

Each canister (top or bottom) in an Aestiva-style dual absorber contains 1.1 kg of granules in a volume of 1400 to 1500 mL.[80,82,215] This compares to 0.8 kg per canister in the Aisys. Each 100 g of

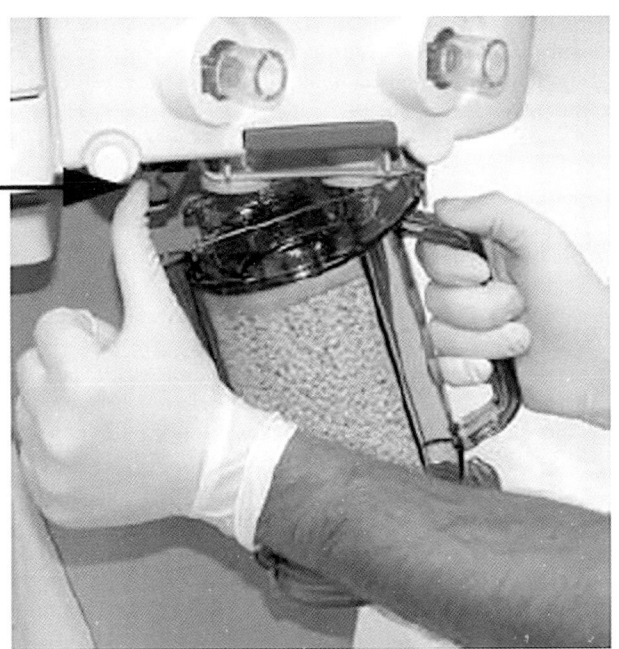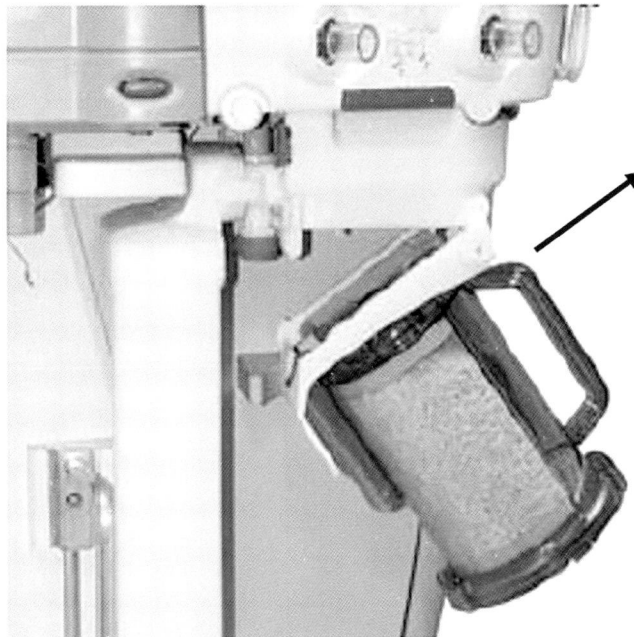

Fig. 16.38 Changing carbon dioxide granules in the Aisys, viewed from the left side of the workstation. First release the latch *(at thumb in left panel),* and the canister will pivot downwards on its hinge *(right).* Pull the old canister out, slide the new canister in on the bracket rails, then rotate upwards until the latch clicks. (From Datex-Ohmeda, Inc. *Aisys User's Reference Manual—Part 2 of 2,* Document No. M1122365 10 07 01 04 23. Tewksbury, MA: Datex-Ohmeda, Inc.; 2008.)

granules has a theoretical capacity to absorb as much as 15 L of CO_2 before the outlet concentration is 1% (7.6 mm Hg), assuming that no channeling occurs. The average to maximum production of CO_2 by the anesthetized adult is 12 to 18 L/hr.[136] Therefore, when total rebreathing is occurring during closed circuit anesthesia, the top canister in an Aestiva might be expected to last for 8 to 10 hours of continuous use. A much longer life is observed clinically for these large canisters, principally because higher flows are used (typically in many clinical settings, 2–4 L/min of fresh gas flow). These higher flows cause increases in both the dilution of exhaled CO_2 and the rate of washout of exhalations from the breathing circuit to the scavenger. In one study in which fresh gas flows of 4 L/min were used, two canisters were used for 67 and 79 hours (anesthesia time) over 2.5 weeks without exhaustion, with a final minimum water content in some segments of 4% to 8.5%.[216] Proper monitoring of an anesthesia workstation during the administration of anesthesia is to remain vigilant for the signs of absorbent exhaustion, and change it when indicated.[217]

The manufacturer of Sodasorb recommends that the absorbent be changed if it is left in the machine for longer than 48 hours.[136] Dräger recommends that absorbent in the Fabius be changed if the machine has been idle for 48 hours, or at least each week on Monday.[68] These extremely cautious guidelines are based on two problems that could arise with extended use. First, the ethyl violet indicator present along the wall of the canister may be inactivated by drying or intense light. Second, dehydration of the granules occurs over time, particularly if higher gas flows or an excessive amount of oxygen flush is used. It is not uncommon for gases to be left flowing accidentally overnight or over the weekend. The resultant dehydration of the granules reduces their efficiency and makes production of carbon monoxide and compound A more likely.[90] Since a change in color is not entirely reliable, an $FiCO_2$ of 3 mm Hg (~0.5%) has been proposed as a threshold for changing canisters due to exhaustion.[197]

Ventilators
Classification and Theory of Operation

Gas-driven bellows ventilators. Modern ventilators using compressible bellows are multimode, double-circuit, electronically controlled, volume- or pressure-limited ventilators. Because they are electronically controlled, these ventilators cannot operate without main electrical power or a backup battery. Ventilators in current use may be classified with respect to a number of parameters (Box 16.17). See Fig. 16.31, which shows gas flow in the breathing circuit with mechanical ventilation. The bellows generate inspiratory flow similar to the anesthetist's hand squeezing a breathing bag, in that both force gas into the patient's lungs by compressing a gas reservoir. The mechanical ventilator is a "bag in a bottle"; it uses the force of compressed gas (O_2 or air) as the driving mechanism to compress the bellows. Gases inspired and expired by the patient are within the bellows, which separates patient gases from the surrounding driving gas. Leaks in the bellows may cause dilution of gas within the bellows (from the driving gas) or loss of agent and oxygen from within it.[218]

Without a means of escape, the continual addition of fresh gas flow into the breathing circuit would cause increased volume and pressure within it (and in the patient's lungs). A ventilator relief valve (also known as the spill valve or overflow valve) maintains circuit volume and pressure by releasing gas to the scavenger in an amount equal to the fresh gas flow per minute. The ventilator relief valve opens only during the expiratory phase (see Fig. 16.31). Driving gas closes this relief valve during inspiration by preventing gas within the bellows from exiting to the scavenger as the bellows are compressed. During early expiration, a weight within the ventilator relief valve holds the pathway to the scavenger closed until the bellows have filled. This creates 2 to 3 cm H_2O of positive end-expiratory pressure (PEEP) within the breathing circuit. This small amount of PEEP is inherent to the design when a standing bellows mechanical ventilator is used.[53,219]

Note that the "Bag/Vent" switch set to "Vent" or "Auto" removes the reservoir bag and APL valve from the breathing circuit (not true for ventilators with fresh gas decoupling). Therefore, in a standing bellows ventilator, the APL valve can be open during mechanical ventilation without causing a leak.

Hanging bellows. A few ventilators with gas-driven bellows have hanging bellows. To distinguish between ascending (standing) and descending (hanging) bellows, use the mnemonic, "Asc*e*nd and desc*e*nd contain *e*'s, so look at the bellows during *e*xpiration to distinguish them." Both standing and hanging bellows are safe; both are capable of alerting the user to a disconnection, as long as appropriate monitoring is used.[220] Standing bellows have an advantage in that they will not fill in the event of a disconnect, whereas hanging bellows may fill with room air even when completely disconnected from the patient. Water may gather in hanging bellows (lessening tidal volume and creating an infection risk), but this should be lessened if the absorber head is heated.

Piston-driven ventilators. Piston ventilators use an electric motor to compress the gas in a rigid piston during inspiration. They use no driving gas, and thus will not deplete the oxygen cylinder in case of oxygen pipeline failure.[221] Piston ventilators, like gas-driven bellows, are safe and effective.

In the Apollo ventilator, the piston is out of view, and its motion is not normally visible during mechanical ventilation. The Fabius GS also has a piston ventilator, but the bellows travel vertically and their movement is continuously visible through a window to the left of the flowmeter bank.

Low pressure alarms, pressure and capnography waveforms, and the movement of the manual breathing bag (which remains in the breathing circuit during mechanical ventilation) are used to discover circuit disconnects. The manual breathing bag increases in size during inspiration due to diversion of fresh gas flow to it by the decoupling valve. The piston ventilator has positive and negative pressure relief valves built in. If the pressure within the piston reaches 75 ± 5 cm H_2O, the positive pressure relief valve opens. If the pressure within the piston declines to -8 cm H_2O, the negative pressure relief valve opens, and room air is drawn into the piston, protecting the patient from negative end-expiratory pressure (NEEP).[68,70]

There are several advantages to a piston ventilator.[221] It is quiet. There is no PEEP (2–3 cm H_2O is mandatory on standing bellows ventilators because of the design of the ventilator spill valve). There is great precision in delivered tidal volume in volume control mode, owing to compliance and leak compensation, fresh gas decoupling, and the rigid piston design. There are fewer compliance losses with a piston, as compared with a flexible standing bellows compressed by driving gas. Electricity is the driving force for the piston, so if oxygen pipeline pressure fails, or pipeline supplies are unavailable (as in office-based settings), mechanical ventilation may continue without exhausting the cylinder oxygen simply to drive the bellows. Piston ventilators (like gas-driven bellows) are capable of all modern ventilation modes.

The piston design also has some disadvantages.[29] It does not display the characteristic motions of a standing bellows during disconnects or when the patient is breathing over and above the ventilator settings. But disconnects can be seen in a piston ventilator with fresh gas decoupling (see later) because the manual breathing bag remains in the breathing circuit during mechanical ventilation with a piston. The piston is quiet, so that it may be harder to hear its regular cycling. The piston ventilator design cannot easily accommodate nonrebreathing circuits, although this is also true of newer ascending bellows ventilators like the Aisys. The piston has the potential for NEEP and dilution of the patient's inspired gas with room air.

Turbine ventilators. Inspiratory flow is generated in the turbine ventilator of the Perseus A500 by a spinning impeller. Delivered tidal volume or inspiratory pressure is sensed by inspiratory and expiratory flow and pressure sensors, controlled electronically, and established by the P_{Max}/PEEP valve and turbine speed. The impeller spins at a slow speed continually, which facilitates spontaneous respirations if present, and promotes efficient mixing of gases throughout the breathing circuit. There is no decoupling valve. The manual breathing bag remains in circuit during mechanical ventilation, decreasing in size during inspiration.[74,75] Patients recover from desflurane anesthesia slightly faster using a Perseus, as compared to a Fabius.[75]

Typical Ventilator Alarms

Modern ventilators have safety alarms to protect the patient from a number of conditions (Box 16.18). One important safety feature of modern equipment is that apnea (disconnect) alarms are enabled with the first breath sensed. Alarm fatigue and improperly set ventilator alarms were identified within the top 10 health hazards related to the use of technology.[222] Audible alarms should not be silenced permanently in routine circumstances.

Ventilator Modes and Settings

Besides increased tidal volume accuracy (because of compliance and leak compensation), the most notable advance in current ventilators is

BOX 16.18 Typical Ventilator Alarms

Pressure Alarms
- High (isolated or continuing)
- Subatmospheric
- Volume—low tidal or minute volume
- Rate—high respiratory rate
- Reverse flow (may indicate incompetence of expiratory unidirectional valve in the breathing circuit)

Apnea/Disconnect Alarms
- These may be based on the following:
  - Chemical monitoring (lack of end-tidal carbon dioxide)
  - Mechanical monitoring
  - Failure to reach normal inspiratory peak pressure, or failure to sense return of tidal volume
  - Spirometry
  - Failure of standing bellows to fill during exhalation
  - Failure of manual breathing bag to move and fill during mechanical ventilation (workstations with fresh gas decoupling—Apollo, Fabius, Narkomed 6000)
  - Other—lack of breath sounds or visible chest movement.

TABLE 16.7 Lung Protection Strategies

Goals: Avoid or Limit	Actions
Volutrauma	Tidal volume (V_T) 5–7 mL/kg predicted body weight
Barotrauma, stress and strain on lung tissue	Peak inspiratory pressure (PIP) <35 cm H_2O Plateau pressure (P_{plat}) <28 cm H_2O Driving pressure (= P_{plat}-PEEP) <16 cm H_2O
Atelectasis	Position head-up when possible Alveolar recruitment maneuvers PEEP 5–8 cm H_2O (higher if abdominal hypertension, or adverse positioning) Avoid Fi_{O_2} >0.8 Use lowest Fi_{O_2} that will keep Sp_{O_2} 88–95%

Data from Hess D, Kacmarek R. *Essentials of Mechanical Ventilation.* 4th ed. New York: McGraw-Hill Education; 2019.

their expanded modes of ventilation, most of which are pressure control. PCV allows more efficient and safe ventilation for certain types of patients. PCV-VG (or Autoflow) helps to maintain tidal volume in the face of changing lung compliance (e.g., when pneumoperitoneum is applied or released). PSV and CPAP are important recent additions to assist patients who are spontaneously breathing, which is seen with much greater frequency since the adoption of the laryngeal mask airway. The improvement in accuracy afforded by modern ventilators at small tidal volumes means that switching of circuits (e.g., to a nonrebreather for small children) is not used as often. This helps avoid potential misconnects. Finally, the proliferation of ventilation modes and monitors (spirometry, flow-time waveforms) has been matched by additional controls available (e.g., inspiratory flow and time, trigger window and sensitivity, Pmax, Tpause). Whereas the additional controls allow ventilation to be optimized for a wide variety of patients and situations, they add complexity and learning burdens for the workstation operator. The reader should consult discussions of individual controls and how the various controls interact.[87,219]

Protective (open lung) ventilation. Two trends have forced a reexamination of how intraoperative ventilation is managed. One is the growing recognition that our ventilator settings may contribute to lung injury, atelectasis, and postoperative pulmonary complications.[223–227] The second was spurred in 2020 when, during the Covid-19 pandemic, anesthesia workstations were widely used to chronically ventilate intensive care unit patients.[228] The need to adapt our normal practices and the various functions of the workstation for this population amplified the focus on preventing ventilation-associated lung injury (VALI) through protective lung (or open lung) ventilation.

The goals of protective lung injury include preventing volutrauma, barotrauma, and lung inflammation due to alveolar wall stress; minimizing atelectasis; and avoiding hyperoxemia (Table 16.7). These goals may be served in different ways depending on patient needs.

Volume-controlled ventilation. All ventilators offer VCV. In this mode, the desired V_T is delivered at a constant flow. The ventilator is volume limited, time cycled, and constant flow in VCV. Inspiration is terminated when the desired V_T is delivered or if an excessive pressure is reached (60–100 cm H_2O).[68,70,76] Patients under general anesthesia often have decreased functional residual capacity and compliance.[229]

Because volume is controlled, alveolar ventilation and arterial carbon dioxide can be maintained despite changes in pulmonary function.[230] However, with VCV, the peak inspiratory pressure is uncontrolled and rises as the patient's compliance decreases or airway resistance increases.

V_T is adjusted to prevent atelectasis, and respiratory rate (RR) is adjusted to keep end-tidal carbon dioxide at the desired value. Tidal volumes in the range of 5 to 7 mL/kg ideal (predicted) body weight, with PEEP and alveolar recruitment maneuvers, are currently advocated to avoid the dangers of atelectasis and ventilator-induced lung injury.[225,231] Peak inspiratory pressure (PIP) is monitored but not controlled. Typical initial settings for VCV in an adult are V_T 5 to 7 mL/kg ideal body weight, RR 6 to 12 breaths per minute titrated to end-tidal CO_2, and inspiratory:expiratory (I:E) ratio 1:2. PEEP of 5 to 10 cm H_2O may be added to prevent atelectasis.[230] In any mode, if the flow-time waveform shows that expiratory flow is incomplete before the next inspiration (resulting in auto-PEEP), RR should be decreased, or the I:E ratio prolonged (e.g., 1:3 instead of 1:2).[219,230]

Pressure-controlled ventilation. In PCV mode, PIP (Pmax) is limited, and the cycle is controlled by time, with a decelerating flow pattern. In a decelerating flow pattern, inspiratory flow is strongest early in inspiration (to reach the set pressure quickly) and declines to flow just sufficient to maintain the set pressure later in inspiration. This flow pattern increases lung inflation and oxygenation at the lowest PIP. However, the increase in mean airway pressure may decrease venous return and cardiac output.[232] Inspiratory pressure is controlled rather than volume (as with VCV).[230,233] Tidal volume is uncontrolled and increases if compliance increases or airway resistance falls. If the desired tidal volume is not obtained, either Pmax or inspiratory rise (the rate of inspiratory flow) can be increased. Target pressure is adjusted for the desired V_T; RR is adjusted to maintain a reasonable end-tidal carbon dioxide. In patients with low compliance (e.g., morbidly obese), PCV may result in an increased tidal volume at a lower PIP compared to VCV, especially if PIP had been high when using VCV (e.g., in laparoscopic abdominal or pelvic surgery). V_T must be monitored closely in PCV. During PCV, if pulmonary compliance drops (e.g., application of pneumoperitoneum) or airway resistance increases (e.g., bronchospasm, kinked endotracheal tube), delivered V_T may drop substantially. Conversely, if pulmonary compliance improves (e.g., release of pneumoperitoneum, return to supine from steep Trendelenburg position) or airway resistance decreases, V_T may increase substantially.

There are several indications for PCV. Patients for whom high inspiratory pressure is particularly dangerous may benefit (e.g., laryngeal

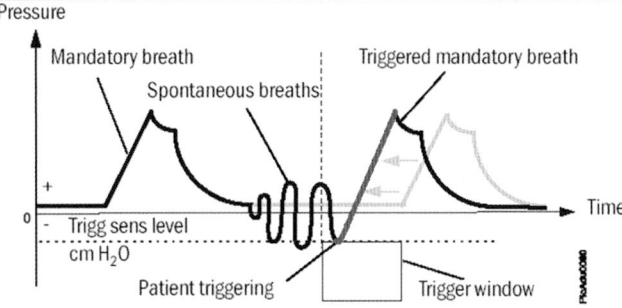

Trigger window and sensitivity level for SIMV

Fig. 16.39 Trigger window and sensitivity may be set when choosing synchronized intermittent mandatory ventilation (SIMV). (From *S/5 Anesthesia Delivery Unit User's Reference Manual*, Catalog No. 8502304. Madison, WI: Datex-Ohmeda; 2000.)

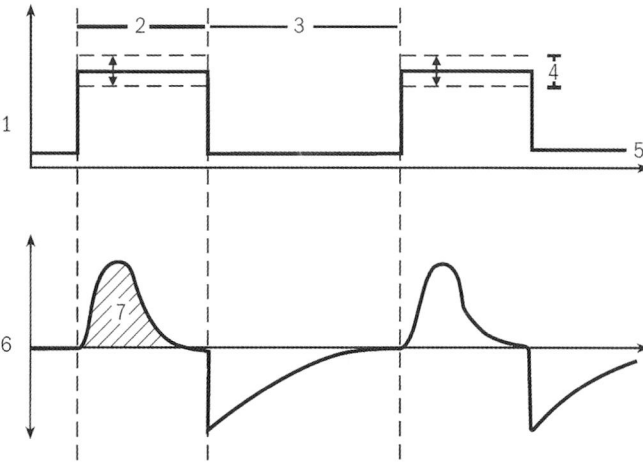

Fig. 16.40 Pressure-controlled ventilation with volume guarantee. The pressure waveform at top shows that peak inspiratory pressure is adjusted up and down (4) to deliver the set tidal volume. The bottom is a flow-time waveform. *1*, Paw waveform; *2*, Tinsp; *3*, Texp; *4*, Variable pressure to deliver desired TV; *5*, PEEP; *6*, Flow waveform; *7*, TV. *Paw*, Airway pressure; *PEEP*, positive end-expiratory pressure; *Texp*, time for expiration; *Tinsp*, time for inspiration; *TV*, tidal volume. (From *Aisys User's Reference Manual—Part 2 of 2*, Document No. M1122365 10 07 01 04 23. Tewksbury, MA: Datex-Ohmeda, Inc; 2008.)

mask airway, emphysema, neonates).[234] In patients with low compliance, PCV can often produce higher tidal volumes than VCV (e.g., pregnancy, laparoscopic surgery, morbid obesity, or adult respiratory distress syndrome). PCV can compensate for leaks (e.g., infants with uncuffed endotracheal tubes, laryngeal mask airway). PCV may provide effective ventilation and lower airway pressure during one-lung ventilation.[233,235]

Typical initial settings for PCV in an adult include pressure limit 12 to 20 cm H_2O, RR 6 to 12 breaths per minute, and I:E ratio 1:2. PEEP 5 to 10 cm H_2O may be added to help prevent atelectasis.[219] Pressure control is the basis of other modes, such as PCV-VG (which adjusts inspiratory pressure to lessen variation in delivered V_T; see hereafter) and as SIMV with pressure control breaths.

Synchronized intermittent mandatory ventilation. With the advent of the laryngeal mask airway (LMA) and the prevalence of short, ambulatory, or office-based surgical procedures, spontaneous breathing has become much more common during general anesthesia. But it may be difficult to maintain a light enough plane of anesthesia to permit spontaneous ventilation, while still retaining sufficient depth for surgery to proceed. If the spontaneously breathing patient is maintained in a plane of anesthesia that is too deep, respiratory acidosis will occur as a result of hypercarbia. Indeed, it is difficult to see how anesthetized patients breathing without pressure assistance could ever have normal blood gas tensions, given the influence of respiratory depressant volatile agents and intravenous drugs, as well as the effects of positioning. Yet if the patient is kept under a lighter plane of anesthesia, then ventilator dyssynchrony, bucking, and awareness are risks that can occur. The traditional solution was to assist ventilation manually because unsynchronized volume control ventilation was all the mechanical ventilator could provide. Ventilation modes that can support a spontaneously breathing patient (i.e., provide normocapnia without ventilator dyssynchrony) include SIMV, PSV, CPAP, and airway pressure release ventilation (APRV).[219,230,236,237] On newer anesthesia workstations, SIMV may be selected based on either pressure- or volume-controlled breaths. SIMV can be used for anything from full to partial support of ventilation. Typical settings for SIMV mirror those used for VCV (or PCV if a pressure-controlled mode is chosen).

In SIMV the intermittent mandatory breaths are delivered in synchrony with the patient's spontaneous efforts. Trigger window (percent) and sensitivity may need to be adjusted (Fig. 16.39). Any spontaneous breaths occurring outside the trigger window for the next large mandatory breath may also be pressure supported (SIMV-PS).[68,77]

Trigger window controls the percent of time during expiration that the ventilator is sensitive to spontaneous breaths (the negative pressure generated by the patient's diaphragm). Sensitivity controls how much negative pressure the patient needs to generate before a breath is triggered. If spontaneous breaths are triggered too often (e.g., by motion in the surgical field), the trigger window should be reduced or the sensitivity made more negative.[238]

Pressure-controlled ventilation with volume guarantee. PCV-VG (on GE machines; Autoflow on Dräger models) was created to address the problem that V_T in pressure control mode varies, sometimes strikingly, when the patient's compliance changes. Like PCV, the basic controls are maximum pressure and rate; in PCV-VG, however, a target V_T is also set. Like PCV, the ventilator delivers breaths using a decelerating flow pattern at a pressure that is less than Pmax; in PCV-VG, the inspiratory pressure is adjusted to deliver the target V_T, using the lowest possible pressure, and staying within the maximum pressure limit. PCV-VG begins by delivering a volume breath at the set V_T. The patient's compliance is determined from this volume breath, and the inspiratory pressure level is then adjusted for the next breath. PCV-VG combines the advantages of pressure-controlled ventilation with an assured volume delivery, yet dynamically compensates for changes in the patient's lung characteristics (Fig. 16.40).[77,219]

Pressure support ventilation. PSV is similar PCV in that it is a pressure-controlled ventilation mode, but with an RR of zero. It is like SIMV in that it is responsive to the patient's efforts, delivering pressure to the airway (which causes inspiratory flow), provided the effort occurs within a trigger window and enough negative inspiratory pressure is generated. Thus it is only useful for patients who are breathing spontaneously. There is no minimum minute ventilation, although some ventilators allow setting an apnea backup rate or delay (PSVPro on Aisys).[219,230]

PSV is useful to augment the V_T of a spontaneously ventilating patient during maintenance or emergence. It may also be useful during denitrogenation, in part because PEEP may be added in patients at high risk for atelectasis.[225] The primary setting is the pressure-support level, which is typically set at 10 cm H_2O for adults, and adjusted based on tidal volume and end-tidal carbon dioxide levels. Trigger window, sensitivity, maximum inspiratory flow, and apnea backup rate may also be set, depending on the particular ventilator (Fig. 16.41).

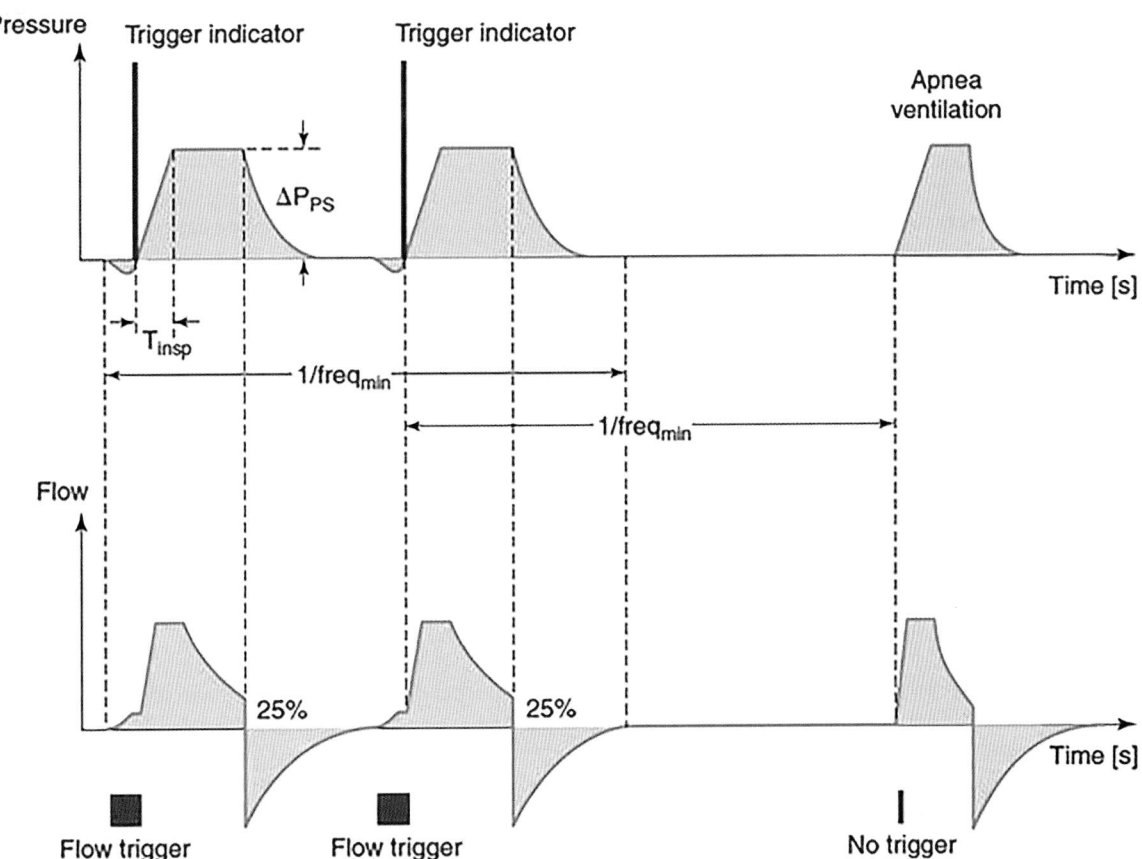

Fig. 16.41 Trigger window and sensitivity settings interact with the patient's spontaneous breaths in pressure-support ventilation. The two breaths at the left are triggered by patient efforts; the breath at the right comes only after a period of apnea. (Modified from Ehrenwerth J, Eisenkraft J, Berry J, eds. *Anesthesia Equipment: Principles and Applications.* 2nd ed. Philadelphia: Elsevier; 2013.)

Continuous positive airway pressure, bilevel positive airway pressure, and positive end-expiratory pressure. CPAP may be available as a mode on some newer workstations. If not, manipulation of ventilator settings can be done to achieve both CPAP and bilevel positive airway pressure (BiPAP) assistance. Whether using an endotracheal tube, LMA, or face mask, one can use these modes if there is a proper seal and connection to the ventilator. CPAP may be useful during denitrogenation and immediately postextubation, in particular for patients at risk for postoperative atelectasis.[225] One may engage CPAP by selecting PSV mode, adjusting the pressure support to zero, and adding PEEP to the desired CPAP level. For instance, setting the pressure support to 0 cm H_2O and PEEP to 5 cm H_2O will maintain a continuous airway pressure of 5 cm H_2O. CPAP increases intrathoracic pressure, prevents airway and alveolar collapse, prevents atelectasis, and maintains functional residual capacity. However, CPAP does not assist the bellows function of the chest and thus cannot ensure alveolar ventilation. Also, as CPAP delivery pressure (PEEP) is increased, conscious patients may find the resistance to exhalation troublesome.[239]

BiPAP settings include Pmax greater than PEEP, PEEP greater than zero, and times at High and Low pressure.[239] The patient may breathe spontaneously throughout the respiratory cycle. The periodic drop to the low pressure may be better tolerated by patients and can (unlike CPAP alone) maintain adequate minute ventilation (even without patient effort) as well as provide the benefits of CPAP mentioned earlier. Typical BiPAP settings on an anesthesia ventilator are time at High and Low pressure, Pmax, and PEEP.[219,230,239]

Safety Features of Modern Ventilators

Flexibility. The availability of pressure control modes is a major advantage, allowing more challenging patients to be ventilated efficiently, such as patients with acute respiratory distress syndrome or morbid obesity who are difficult with VCV mode. PCV also increases safety for patients in whom excessive pressure must be strictly avoided, such as neonates and infants, and patients with emphysema. PSV and SIMV are quite valuable in supporting the patient with spontaneous respirations.

Accuracy at lower tidal volumes. Factors contributing to a discrepancy between set and delivered tidal volumes are especially acute in pediatrics. They include the large compression volume of the circle system relative to the infant's lung volume, leaks around uncuffed endotracheal tubes, the augmentation of delivered V_T produced by fresh gas flow, and the difficulty of setting a small V_T using an adult bellows assembly.[64]

Modern ventilators in VCV mode have an unprecedented V_T range for two reasons: (1) greatly increased accuracy in V_T delivery achieved through electronic compliance and leak testing, and (2) V_T that is compensated for these factors and for changes in fresh gas flow. They are able to ventilate smaller patients much more accurately than any previous anesthesia ventilator could. This has significantly lessened the need for nonrebreathing (Mapleson) circuits and made care safer because anesthetists no longer have to disassemble and reconfigure a nonrebreathing circuit for a child in the middle of several adult cases. However, it is mandatory to substitute pediatric circle disposable hoses for small tidal volumes (<200 mL with the Fabius).[240] The lower limit of accuracy for V_T in VCV mode is 20 mL (for Fabius,[68] Aestiva, Apollo,[70] Avance,[65] and Aisys[78]). When sensors or disposable breathing circuit types are changed for a pediatric case, users must repeat the leak and compliance tests of the preanesthesia check so that maximum V_T accuracy is ensured. Likewise, these must be repeated when returning to the adult configuration.

Compliance and leak testing. Accuracy in delivered V_T comes with a price. An electronic leak and compliance test is part of the morning checklist, and it must be repeated every time the circuit is changed to a circuit with a different configuration (adult circle to pediatric circle, or adult to long circuit). Users must familiarize themselves with whether vaporizers and other components are included in the leak and compliance test because what is actually checked varies between different models.

The placement of the sensor used to compensate tidal volumes for compliance losses and leaks has some interesting consequences. The Aestiva flow sensors are placed between the disposable corrugated breathing circuit limbs and the absorber head. Here they are able to compensate tidal volumes for fresh gas flow, compliance losses, and leaks internal to the workstation and absorber head, but not for any of these that occur distally (in the breathing hoses). The Apollo, Aisys, and Fabius test compliance and leaks of all components to the Y-piece via a pressure transducer within the internal circuitry near the bellows. Here the sensor is relatively protected from moisture.

Fresh gas decoupling vs tidal volume compensation. Another factor adding to modern ventilator accuracy is that they correct delivered tidal volume in VCV mode for changes in fresh gas flow. In older ventilators, the delivered V_T is the sum of the volume delivered from the ventilator and the fresh gas flowing during the inspiratory phase, so the actual delivered V_T changes as fresh gas flow is changed. For example, consider a patient with a fresh gas flow of 4 L/min, an RR of 10, an I:E ratio of 1:2, and a V_T of 700 mL. During each minute, the ventilator spends a total of 20 seconds in inspiratory time and 40 seconds in expiratory time (as a result of the 1:2 ratio). During these 20 seconds, the fresh gas flow is 1320 mL (one-third of 4000 mL/min fresh gas flow). So each of the 10 breaths of 700 mL is augmented by 132 mL of fresh gas flowing while the breath is being delivered, and the actual delivered V_T is 832 mL/breath (a 19% increase).

What happens when we decrease the fresh gas flow to 1000 mL/min? During each minute, the ventilator spends 20 seconds in inspiratory time and 40 seconds in expiratory time (1:2 ratio). During 20 seconds, the fresh gas flow is 330 mL (one-third of 1000 mL/min fresh gas flow). So each of the 10 breaths of 700 mL is augmented by 33 mL of fresh gas flowing while the breath is being delivered, making the total delivered tidal volume 733 mL/breath. This means that decreasing fresh gas flow from 4000 to 1000 mL/min, without changing ventilator settings, has resulted in a 12% decrease in delivered V_T (832 mL to 733 mL). It would not be surprising if the end-tidal carbon dioxide rose slightly as a result.

The situation is more acute with a child ventilated in VCV mode without fresh gas flow compensation. Assume a 10-kg patient with a fresh gas flow of 4 L/min, an RR of 20, I:E ratio of 1:2, and a V_T of 60 mL. During each minute, the ventilator spends 20 seconds in inspiratory time and 40 seconds in expiratory time (1:2 ratio). During these 20 seconds, the fresh gas flow is 1320 mL (one-third of 4000 mL/min fresh gas flow). So each of the 20 breaths of 60 mL is augmented by 66 mL of fresh gas flowing while the breath is being delivered, making the total delivered V_T 126 mL/breath. This is a 110% increase above what is set on the ventilator. Decreasing fresh gas flow from 4 to 1 L/min, again without changing ventilator settings, decreases tidal volume (by the same calculation) from 126 to 76 mL (a 40% reduction).

There are two approaches to dealing with the problem. The Apollo and Fabius use fresh gas decoupling (Fig. 16.42). Fresh gas flow during inspiration is not added to the delivered V_T because it is diverted (by the closed decoupling valve) to the manual breathing bag, which remains in circuit during mechanical ventilation. The same fresh gas decoupled circuit is shown during expiration in the bottom panel of Fig. 16.42. The piston refills with the patient's exhaled gas and fresh gas contained in the manual breathing bag (through the open decoupling valve). The ventilator relief valve is now open, allowing excess gas to exit to the scavenger.

Fresh gas decoupling helps ensure that the set and delivered tidal volumes are equal in spite of changes in fresh gas flow. The visual appearance of the circuit during mechanical ventilation is unusual in that the manual breathing bag (normally quiescent in bellows ventilators) moves with each breath. Further, this manual breathing bag movement is opposite to the movement seen in a mechanical ventilator bellows, which empties during inspiration and fills during expiration. With fresh gas decoupling, the manual breathing bag inflates during inspiration (due to fresh gas flow) and deflates during expiration as the contents empty into the piston. With fresh gas decoupling, if there is a disconnect, the manual breathing bag rapidly deflates because the piston retraction draws gas from it.

The second approach to preventing augmentation of delivered V_T by fresh gas flow is called tidal volume compensation, which is used in the Aestiva and Aisys (among others). The volume and flow sensors provide feedback that allows the ventilator to adjust the delivered V_T so that it matches the set V_T in spite of changes in fresh gas flow.

V_T accuracy is not an issue if PCV mode is chosen. In PCV, pressure is controlled, and tidal volume is allowed to vary with change in lung compliance and airway resistance. Monitoring delivered V_T and end-tidal CO_2 allows adjustment of inspired pressure to create V_T within the desired range. Or one may choose Autoflow or PCV-VG, which adjust inspired pressure to maintain target V_T automatically.

Suitability for low flows. Low fresh gas flow during maintenance is desirable to reduce pollution, enhance environmental sustainability, reduce the cost of volatile agents and nitrous oxide, preserve tracheal heat and moisture, prevent soda lime granules from drying, and help preserve patient body temperature. Factors that enhance the safety and efficiency of low-flow anesthesia in modern ventilators are shown in Box 16.12. As can be seen, a traditional-sized absorber head like the Aestiva is roughly twice the volume of some of the newer designs. All newer, nondisposable portions of the breathing circuit are designed to be more leakproof than earlier designs.

Electronic selection of positive end-expiratory pressure. Electronic selection of PEEP is safer than previous approaches, which involved adding adapters to the expiratory limb of the breathing circuit. Add-on adapters came in different varieties, depending on how much PEEP was desired (e.g., 5 or 10 cm H_2O), and were intended to be placed between the expiratory limb of the breathing hoses and the expiratory unidirectional valve. Case studies have identified the accidental placement of these add-on PEEP adapters onto the inspiratory limb, where they cause complete obstruction to flow in the breathing circuit.[241] Newer ventilators have the ability to generate PEEP in the correct location by simply inputting the desired PEEP level as part of the ventilation mode selected.

Current Ventilator Designs

GE Healthcare 7900 "SmartVent." The 7900 was designed to provide consistent delivered V_T in spite of changes in fresh gas flow, small leaks, and absorber or bellows compliance losses. It uses variable-orifice flow sensors (proximal to the inspiratory and expiratory limbs) and pressure sensors to accomplish this.[219,242] The ventilator can use

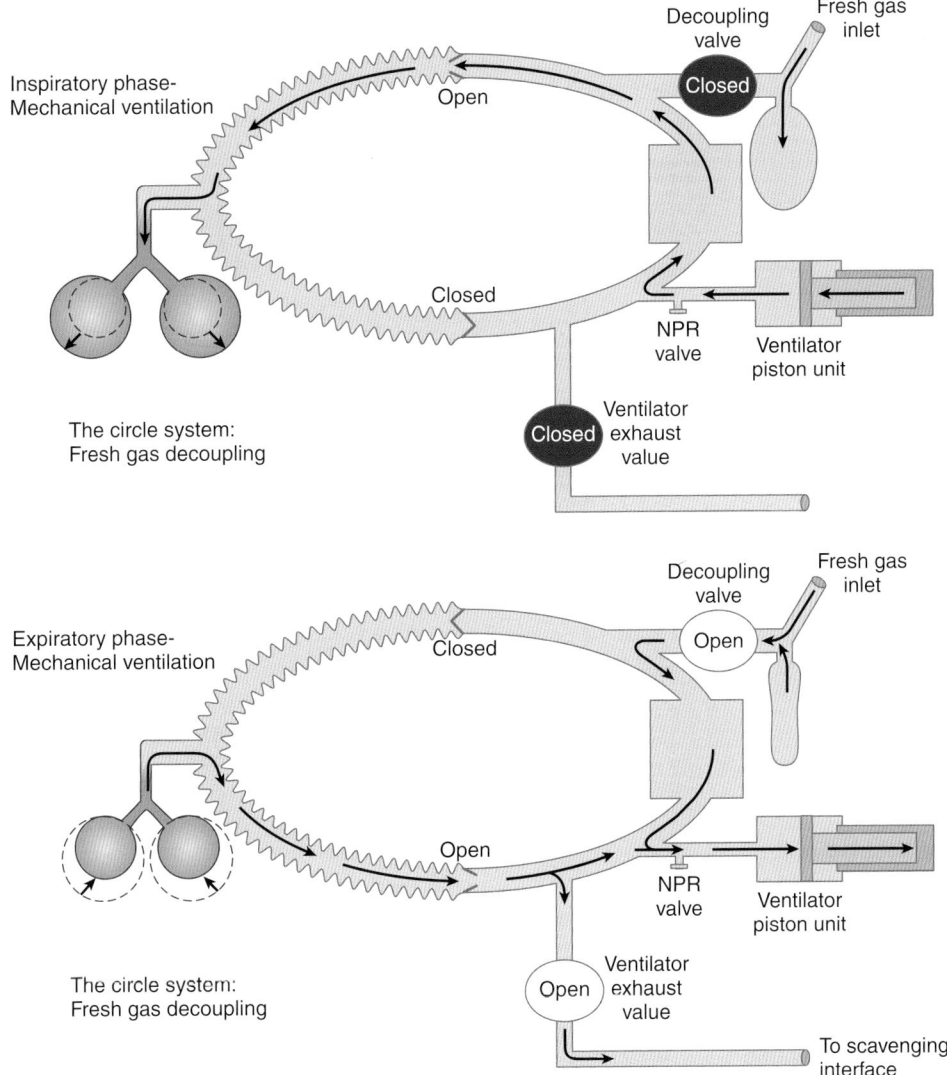

Fig. 16.42 Circle breathing system with fresh gas decoupling. (See text for explanation.) *NPR*, Negative pressure relief valve. (From Miller RD, et al., eds. *Miller's Anesthesia.* 7th ed. Philadelphia: Elsevier; 2010.)

either oxygen or air as a driving gas and will switch automatically to air if oxygen pipeline pressure is lost. Available modes include manual/spontaneous, VCV, PCV, and SIMV (in either volume or pressure mode with pressure support). PSV is available as PSV-Pro, the "Pro" indicating protection against apnea, because the ventilator will revert to the backup (PCV) settings if no spontaneous breaths are detected. PCV-VG is available on the Aisys and Avance. PEEP is integrated and electronically controlled. Spirometry loops are available. It is found on a variety of workstations, including Aestiva, Aisys, and Avance.

GE Healthcare 7100. The 7100 is similar to the 7900 except that the selection of modes is not as extensive. The 7100, like the 7900, features tidal volume compensation. It is found on the Aespire.

Fabius GS ventilator. The Fabius GS ventilator is a piston ventilator.[68,221] It offers pressure control, volume control, pressure support, SIMV-volume with PSV, and manual/spontaneous modes. There is no mechanical "Bag/Vent" switch. Switching between modes is accomplished by electronic keypad. It corrects delivered V_T for compliance losses by measuring circuit compliance, and for fresh gas flow changes by fresh gas decoupling. Electronic PEEP is integrated. One can view measured respiratory parameters or ventilator settings (but not both

simultaneously) on the monitor screen. VCV and SIMV-volume are accurate to very low tidal volumes (range 20–1400 mL). Pediatric circle system (low compliance) hoses are used for tidal volumes less than 200 mL, and the ventilator self-test should be repeated when changing circuits.

The piston movement is visible in a window to the left of the flowmeter bank. Like the Apollo, it provides a visible indication of lung inflation and potential disconnects in that fresh gas is diverted to the manual breathing bag, which inflates during mechanical ventilator inspiration and deflates during expiration. The piston design avoids NEEP by entraining room air if pressure within the bellows is less than atmospheric pressure. The "fresh gas low" error message warns of this condition.

Apollo ventilator. The Apollo ventilator is a piston similar to the Fabius except that spirometry is displayed. The absorber head is heated. Modes are manual/spontaneous, volume and pressure control, pressure support, and SIMV in either volume or pressure mode. Autoflow is available as an option.[70,219]

Perseus A500 turbine ventilator. The Perseus is unique in that an impeller spins to generate inspiratory flow (Fig 16.43). The ventilator

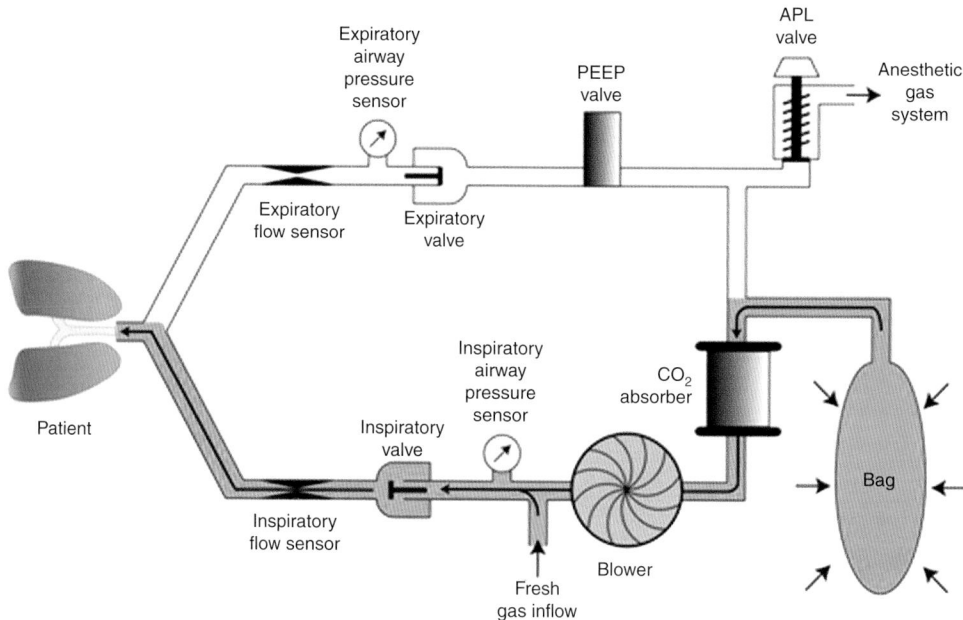

Fig. 16.43 Breathing circuit of Perseus. (© Drägerwerk AG & Co. KGaA, Lubeck (depending upon the company possessing the rights). All rights reserved.)

features a full suite of modes, including manual/spontaneous, PCV, VCV, autoflow, SIMV, CPAP, and PSV. Unique to this ventilator, BiPAP and APRV are available.

Traditional Anesthesia Ventilators

The Datex-Ohmeda 7000, 7800, and ADU and the Dräger AV-2, AV-E, and Narkomed 6000 Divan ventilators were covered in previous editions of this text. Departments that still retain or use older ventilators should ensure that all personnel are familiar with them and can use them safely in an emergency.[1]

Critical Incidents Related to Ventilation

Disconnects and other causes of low pressure in the breathing circuit. Clinical experience with anesthesia ventilators and breathing circuits has identified several situations that have led to critical incidents. Vigilance directed toward situations that have the potential to cause patient injury may contribute to the prevention of future occurrences (Box 16.19). Failure to ventilate caused by disconnection has been called the most common preventable equipment-related cause of mishaps.[29] The most common site for disconnection is between the breathing circuit and the endotracheal tube (at the Y-piece).[220] Disconnects can be partial or complete. Recent reported causes of low pressure (leak) conditions are many: absorbent granules changed between cases by ancillary personnel but improperly reassembled or even left open,[213,243,244] defective absorber canister,[158,245] failure of the "Bag/Vent" switch,[246,247] leaks in corrugated hoses,[248] incompetent ventilator relief valve,[249] leaks from a hot wire anemometer sensor,[250] the gas sampling line preventing manual ventilation by preventing closure of an APL,[251–255] and ventilator failure due to moisture in flow sensors.[81] The variety of faults leading to low pressure accidents emphasizes proper performance of preanesthesia equipment checklists (though not all of these faults were detected, most were detectable). It also emphasizes being prepared to manage low pressure in the breathing circuit regardless of its cause.

Protocols for managing leaks and other causes of low pressure in the breathing circuit have been published.[45,256] Prevention of disconnects involves a thorough preanesthesia check of equipment, including a high pressure leak check of the breathing circuit before use on every patient.

BOX 16.19   Causes of Critical Incidents

Underlying Causes of All Critical Incidents
- Improper or infrequent maintenance
- Inadequate in-service education
- Substandard equipment monitoring
- Failure to check equipment before use
- Lack of familiarity with equipment standards

Causes of Critical Incidents
Failure to Ventilate
- Disconnection
- Failure to initiate ventilation or resume it after an interruption
- Misconnections of breathing circuit
- Occlusion or obstruction of breathing circuit
- Kinking or plugging of endotracheal tube
- Kinking of fresh gas delivery hose
- Mold flash or plastic emboli from wrapping material
- Leaks
- Failure or improper reassembly of bellows after cleaning
- Damage to or disconnection of pressure monitoring or other hoses
- Failure of pipeline and tank oxygen supply
- Driving a vent with cylinders (when pipeline is unavailable) causes rapid tank depletion
- Inadvertent application of suction to the breathing circuit
- Failure of scavenger interface negative-pressure relief valve
- Intubation of trachea with nasogastric tube, which is then connected to suction

Barotrauma
- Excess inflow to breathing circuit (flushing during ventilator inspiration)
- Ventilator relief valve may stick closed
- Control assembly problems

A primary monitor for disconnection is continuous auscultation of breath sounds with a precordial or esophageal stethoscope, as well as direct visual observation of chest movement (both are recommended by standards).[12,184] Electronic monitors for disconnection include capnography and pressure- and volume-based alarms (see Box 16.18).[45,220]

Because electronic monitors may have alarms disabled, either inadvertently or intentionally (because of artifacts, monitor failure, or alarm fatigue), there is no substitute for the anesthetist's vigilance through remaining in touch with the patient with the five senses.

To manage inability to ventilate due to low pressure in the breathing circuit, first ensure ventilation is occurring by checking breath sounds. If not, and the circuit has obviously lost volume (emptied bellows), check for disconnects quickly, then try to ventilate manually using the anesthesia breathing circuit. Using the breathing circuit is superior to immediately using a bag-valve-mask because volatile agents can continue to be administered. If no volume loss is apparent, check settings of fresh gas flow, scavenger, and ventilator, as well as monitor artifact.[45] Do not interrupt ventilation for diagnosis of machine problems. If initial assessments of low pressure are not identified quickly, proceed to manual ventilation with backup ventilation equipment (Ambu bag) without undue delay.[256]

Failure to initiate or resume ventilation. Failure to initiate or resume ventilation may be less likely in the future because of the incorporation of modern monitoring in current anesthesia workstations, all of which possess common features that add to patient safety. They have a centralized data and alarm display, as well as alarms prioritized to warnings, cautions, and advisories. They provide electronic preuse checklists.[257] Furthermore, the apnea and disconnect alarms are typically enabled once a breath is sensed. Therefore the anesthesia workstation should alert the operator to a failure to turn on a mechanical ventilator after intubation or to a failure to resume ventilation after the ventilator is shut off either temporarily (in the middle of a case for radiography) or permanently (during emergence). If turning off a mechanical ventilator temporarily midcase, it is safest to leave one's finger on the switch until it is time to resume ventilation.

The number of different alarm conditions programmed into a modern anesthesia workstation with integrated monitoring is staggering, consisting of a six-page list in the Aisys operator manual.[67] It is absolutely necessary to read the manuals and participate in training for workstations of such complexity.[77,258] Although equipment has improved dramatically, some of the underlying causes of failure to ventilate and of barotrauma will likely remain problems for the foreseeable future (e.g., lack of knowledge or training, failure to use checklists).

Barotrauma and high pressure in the breathing circuit. Although such problems as misconnections are less likely now than in the past because of improvements in design, other possible causes of failure to ventilate, or barotrauma, are still hazards: occlusion, bellows leaks, failure of gas supply, failure of the ventilator relief valve, and inadvertent application of suction or positive pressure to the airway.[143,148,152,259,260]

Unlike disconnects and other low-pressure breathing circuit problems, high pressure in the breathing circuit can evolve quickly and produce devastating consequences, allowing little time for diagnosis or correction. Sustained high intrathoracic pressure rapidly and severely impedes venous return and cardiac output. The causes of sustained high pressure in the breathing circuit are diverse. Obstruction to exhalation (but not inhalation) has been caused by direct connection of wall oxygen to a tracheal tube,[259] improper manufacture of a scavenger assembly,[261] failure to remove plastic wrap around a soda lime canister before installing it in the workstation,[153,262] malfunctioning ventilator relief valve,[148] occlusion of the lumen of a breathing circuit extender adaptor by mold flash or other plastic debris,[162–165,167,263] insertion of an occluded disposable PEEP valve into the breathing circuit,[162] and an occluded expiratory unidirectional valve.[51] Most of these obstructions would have been easily detected by a preinduction high-pressure check of the breathing circuit (leak test), with release of pressure through the APL valve, and by checking for obstructions in the breathing circuit (i.e., using a flow test, using a second breathing bag as an artificial lung during checkout to ensure gas flows properly in the breathing circuit, or simply by breathing through the circuit). Consequences of obstructed breathing circuits

included high PEEP, decreased venous return, cardiovascular collapse, pneumothorax, massive subcutaneous emphysema, or death.

The algorithm for responding to sustained high pressure in the breathing circuit is as follows[45]: (1) Assess patient-related causes such as bronchospasm, (2) try manual ventilation with the breathing circuit (in "Bag" mode), and (3) consider disconnecting the patient from the breathing circuit and resuming ventilation with bag-valve-mask (Ambu bag) while assuring anesthesia depth via total intravenous anesthesia (TIVA). If the high pressure is relieved during manual ventilation with the anesthesia circuit, it is likely that the ventilator relief valve is at fault. The ventilator is unusable until this valve is serviced. If circuit pressure is sustained during manual ventilation with the circuit, it is likely that the APL valve or scavenger is obstructed.

The anesthesia workstation and malignant hyperthermia. When an unexpected malignant hyperthermia (MH) crisis arises during a case, one follows a protocol, including (as far as equipment is concerned) withdrawal of triggering agents (volatile agents and succinylcholine), hyperventilating with oxygen 100%, increasing fresh gas flow, and (if time and help are available and can be spared from other more important tasks such as mixing dantrolene) changing the disposable breathing circuit components and granules.[264,265] Activated charcoal filters are easily applied between the inspiratory and expiratory ports and the corrugated limbs of the breathing circuit. They quickly and reliably reduce the concentration of volatile agent in the breathing circuit and are recommended by the Malignant Hyperthermia Association of the United States (MHAUS).[265,266]

When preparing the anesthesia workstation for a patient who is known to be susceptible, change the breathing circuit and carbon dioxide absorbent granules, disable or remove the vaporizers, and flush all traces of volatile agent from its internal circuitry. The old guideline was flushing with a fresh gas flow rate of 10 L/min for 20 minutes. New evidence indicates that this may be very inadequate for some workstations, with the Fabius requiring as much as 104 minutes.[83,264,267–273] MHAUS recommends a 90-second flush, adding charcoal filters to both limbs, and high fresh gas flow (10 L/min) throughout maintenance, in addition to other recommendations.[274]

DISPOSAL

The final D of the SPDD model addresses the concern of gas disposal.

Scavenging Systems and Disposal of Waste Anesthesia Gases

Scavenging is the collection of waste anesthetic gases from the breathing circuit and ventilator and their removal from the operating room. An amount equal to the fresh gas flow must be scavenged each minute.[275,276] Otherwise, the breathing circuit and the patient's lungs will either gain or lose pressure, resulting in barotrauma or failure to ventilate. The components of the scavenger are listed in Box 16.20 and shown in Fig. 16.44.

Advisory recommendations for exposure to waste anesthetic gases are published by the Occupational Safety and Health Administration (OSHA).[276] OSHA advises that no worker should be exposed to more than 2 ppm halogenated agents (0.5 ppm if used with nitrous oxide), and no more than 25 ppm nitrous oxide, based on a time-weighted 8-hour average concentration. Levels in unscavenged anesthetizing locations may be as high as 7000 ppm (0.7%) N_2O and 85 ppm (0.008%) halothane.[23] The highest levels are found in the anesthetist's workstation and between the anesthesia workstation and the wall.[22] Operating room personnel working in ear, nose, and throat suites had measurable levels of exhaled sevoflurane higher than controls up to 18 hours after being on duty, although this study did not report what type of scavenging, if any, was used.[277] The health effects of chronic exposure to inhalation agents are unproved, though it is clear that occupational exposure to nitrous oxide should be avoided.[202]

Several variables determine the attainable reduction in waste anesthetic gases in the operating room, including the degree of room ventilation, the condition of anesthesia equipment, the effectiveness of the scavenger, and the anesthetic techniques of the user. However, with appropriate attention to these areas, trace gas levels within the operating room can meet OSHA requirements.[24,278]

The most important component of the scavenger system is the interface (between the breathing circuit and wall suction) because it protects the patient's airway from excessive buildup of positive pressure and from exposure to suction. There are two types of interfaces: closed and open (Fig. 16.45; also see Fig. 16.44). The closed interface is found on older workstations.[279,280] A closed interface is useful where passive scavenging

is used (no dedicated suction line for the scavenger). Note that hospital accreditors currently require active scavenging in the United States.[278] A closed interface communicates with the atmosphere only through valves. A means for relief of positive pressure is mandatory for all closed

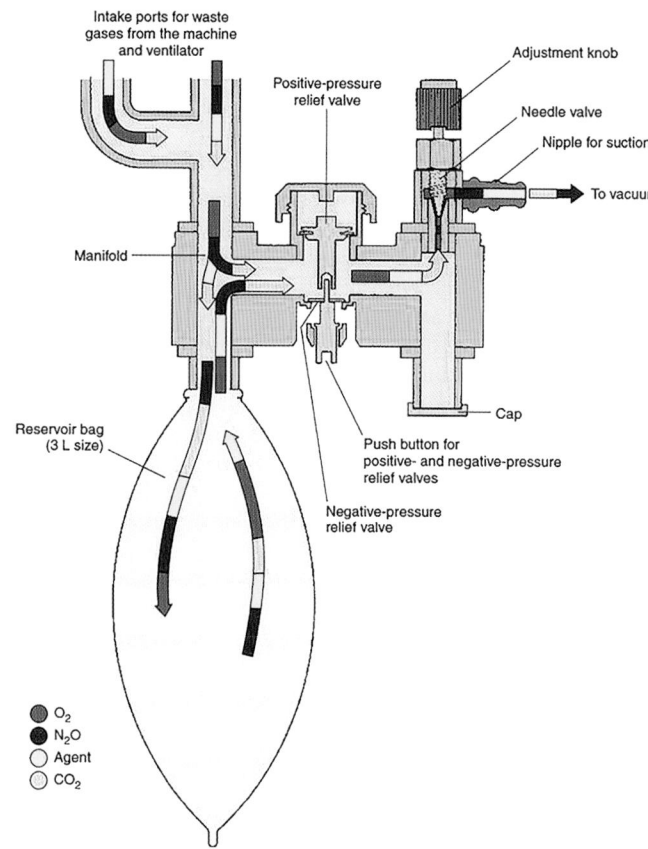

Fig. 16.45 Closed scavenger interface attached to suction. Note the reservoir, the positive and negative pressure relief valves, and the capped extra port. (Modified from Ehrenwerth J, Eisenkraft J, Berry J, eds. *Anesthesia Equipment: Principles and Applications.* 2nd ed. Philadelphia: Elsevier; 2013.)

BOX 16.20   Components of the Scavenging System

Gas collection assembly—at adjustable pressure-limiting (APL) valve and ventilator relief valve
Transfer tubing—19 or 30 mm, sometimes color-coded yellow
Scavenging interface (most important part)
- Closed interface (all older models)
  - Communicates to atmosphere only through valves
  - If used with passive disposal system, must have positive pressure relief
  - Used with active (suction) disposal system; must have positive *and* negative pressure relief
- Open interface (most new models)
  - No valves; open to atmosphere (both negative and positive pressure relief "built in")
  - Must be used *only* with active systems
  - Reservoir required
    Safety:
  - Safer than closed interface for the patient; no barotrauma
  - Less safe than closed interface for the caregiver (if used improperly)
Gas disposal tubing
Gas disposal assembly—active disposal (common) or passive disposal

---

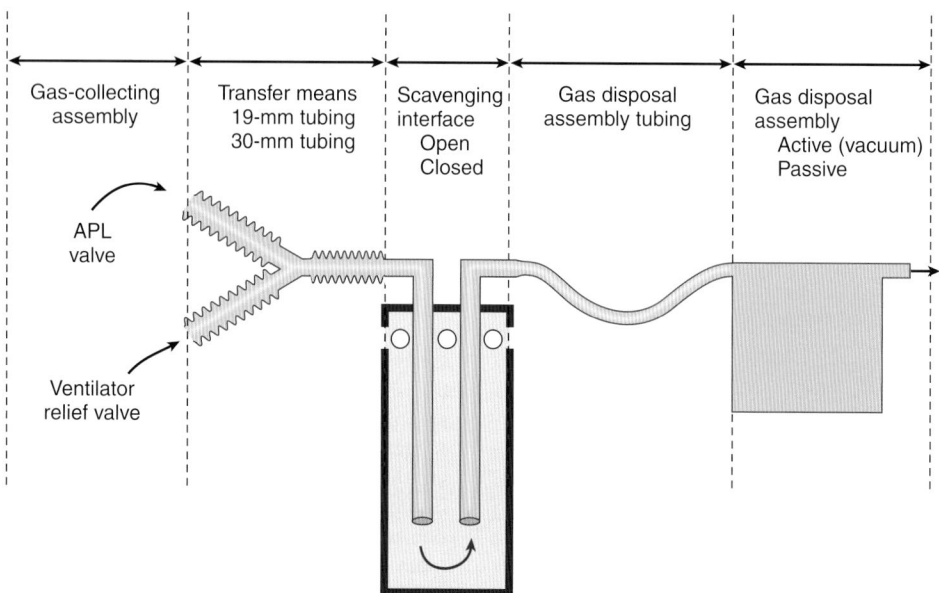

Fig. 16.44 Components of the scavenging system. *APL,* Adjustable pressure-limiting valve. (From Miller RD, et al., eds. *Miller's Anesthesia.* 7th ed. Philadelphia: Elsevier; 2010.)

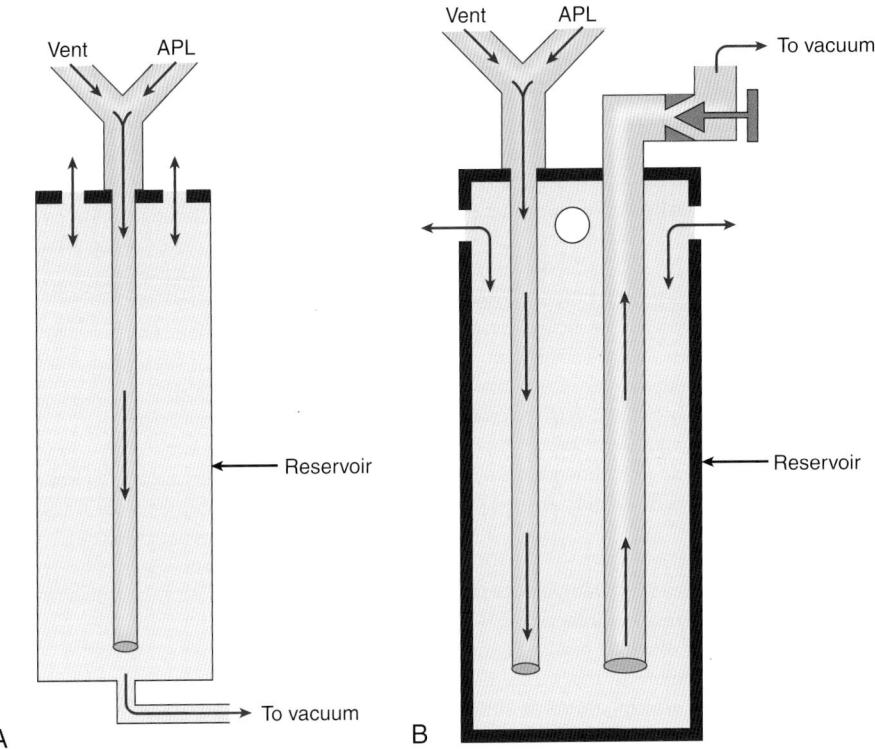

Fig. 16.46 The open scavenger interface. (A, B) Two open scavenging interfaces. Each requires an active disposal system. The open interface shown in A differs somewhat from the one shown in B. The operator can regulate the vacuum by adjusting the vacuum control valve shown in B. *APL*, Adjustable pressure-limiting valve; *Vent*, ventilator relief valve. (From Miller RD, et al., eds. *Miller's Anesthesia.* 7th ed. Philadelphia: Elsevier; 2010.)

interfaces. If the suction attached to the scavenger fails or if a hose distal to it becomes kinked, positive pressure relief valves operate before the pressure buildup within the scavenger is transmitted to the breathing circuit and the lungs. In this case, the positive pressure relief valve opens and releases waste gases into the operating room air. If the closed interface is attached to suction, a negative pressure relief valve is also mandatory. The negative pressure relief valve on the closed interface opens to draw in room air when suction is excessive, preventing the emptying of gas from the patient and breathing circuit. Suction should be adjusted in a closed interface as fresh gas flows change, so that the scavenger reservoir bag is neither flat nor overdistended.[280]

Since the closed interface relief valves can fail,[281] an open scavenger interface is supplied by the manufacturer on all new workstations (Fig. 16.46). The open interface is open to the atmosphere. There are no valves, such as those found in closed interface systems, to impede the flow of gases into, or out of, the reservoir. Each patient exhalation is led to the bottom of the open interface reservoir, where a second tube withdraws it by suction before the next exhalation arrives. Use of the device with appropriate suction is critical to its proper function.[279] If scavenger suction is inadequate, all patient exhalations and waste gases will be released into the operating room.[281] The open interface affords patient safety advantages. Though rare failures of open interface scavenging have been reported, at least there is no chance of relief valve failure (as with the closed interface), which can cause barotrauma or the application of suction to the breathing circuit.[282,283] The device is perhaps less safe for the operator who is unfamiliar with its use, since the operator may be exposed to increased concentrations of waste anesthetic gases. The smell of volatile agents during a case is abnormal, and its cause must be investigated. The threshold for smelling volatile

agents is variously stated as 5 to 300 ppm.[24,275] Thus, if any agent is smelled, the concentration is excessive (i.e., well above that described in the OSHA advisory).[278]

Many factors, in addition to the scavenger, affect exposure to waste anesthetic gases. Alterations in technique can greatly lessen occupational exposure. Guidelines for limiting exposure are listed in Box 16.21.[24,275, 284-286] Policy consideration for management of waste anesthetic gases and occupational exposure were published by AANA in 2018.[275]

RISK MANAGEMENT

Department-Level Aspects

Risk management is defined as a detection system designed to predict failures and ensure that precautions to prevent patient harm are taken.[138] Typical anesthesia risk management activities include preoperative and postoperative rounds, avoiding indifferent treatment of patients, maintaining vigilance and high standards of care, peer review, continuing education, and the commitment to delivery of high-quality and humane patient care. In terms of equipment, risk management includes cleanliness, daily performance of equipment checklists, familiarity with equipment manuals, and appropriate equipment maintenance.[138,287]

The Safe Medical Device Act of 1990 requires hospitals to report instances in which medical devices cause or contribute to death, serious illness, or serious injury.[288] All health care personnel who become aware of a problem with a device must remove the equipment from contact with patients and report the problem to their supervisors. The hospital risk manager then conducts an investigation and reports the results to the FDA within 10 working days. The most common barrier to investigation of a critical incident, and the degree to which anesthesia equipment may have contributed to it, is alteration of the equipment (i.e., it has been cleaned, disassembled, or tested).[289] In the case of patient injury in which equipment may be at fault, it is most helpful if equipment (including wastebaskets and syringes in the anesthesia work area) is sequestered "as is," pending a forensic evaluation conducted by the representatives of the hospital, the manufacturer, and perhaps the patient. Equipment logs should be kept for each anesthesia workstation and include reports of maintenance, critical incidents, additions or alterations, pollution control, and vaporizer calibration. Preventive maintenance should be done at intervals specified by the manufacturer (usually two to four times per year) by qualified, factory-trained technicians.[138]

Individual Risk Management

The department-level risk management plan requires the active involvement of all department members. In addition to participation in the department-level activities noted earlier, individuals play a vital role in three further aspects of risk management for equipment: performance of the workstation checklist before use, limiting equipment-related disease transmission, and reducing trace and waste gas exposure through alteration of work practices (the latter two were discussed earlier in this chapter).

Anesthesia Workstation Checklist

Reports of equipment problems surfacing in the 1980s prompted the professional societies to develop a recommended anesthesia checklist.[290–293] Although equipment failures are rare, they are often the result of human error in the use of the equipment.[4,5,290,293] Failure to check anesthesia equipment adequately has been reported as a factor in up to 30% of critical incidents.[294,295] Users reported that they often did not perform the preanesthesia checklist, and many did not feel competent in their ability to perform it correctly.[3] When a checklist was performed, 30% of the anesthesia workstations in one study had serious faults discovered.[2] Checklists have been the focus of several studies of fault-detection ability and much comment.[257,293,296–302] It is possible that proper and consistent use of checklists will not only prevent critical incidents but also help teach users to learn how anesthesia workstations function.[14] Performance of the preanesthesia checklist is required by various standards.[12,302] Performing and documenting the equipment check has been associated with decreased mortality.[303] One-third of recent closed claims (and six of eight breathing circuit claims) were judged to be preventable if an adequate preanesthesia checklist had been performed.[5]

In order to improve this process, a new preanesthesia checkout (PAC) was published in 2008 (Boxes 16.22 and 16.23).[12] It became necessary to abandon the 1990s FDA checklist because it recommended procedures that no longer worked for different model workstations. Considering the significant differences between models, and variations in their self-test routines, no one set of procedures can cover all anesthesia workstations. This new checklist is a statement of principles of what should be checked, how often, and who should check it, rather than a procedures list. For example, the availability of backup ventilation equipment and backup oxygen supplies, and the calibration of the oxygen analyzer, must be checked regardless of which workstation is used. But how these actions are performed varies from workstation to workstation. If they have not done so already, anesthesia departments need to develop specific procedures and training for the workstations they use, in consultation with manufacturers and the operator instruction manuals. User training is also vital, and departments should ensure that all department members are trained on all workstation types in use.[178]

The Aestiva is a system that must be manually checked; there are no electronic aspects to the checklist.[53] At the other extreme, some anesthesia workstation checkout procedures rely primarily on electronic checklists. These electronic self-check routines (like that in the Aisys, Fabius, Perseus, and Apollo) may help prevent errors and omissions in the preanesthesia checklist.[304] Electronic checklists of this type are not all identical, but

---

BOX 16.21   Means of Limiting Exposure to Waste Anesthetic Gases

- Check the scavenger (for correct level of suction) before use.
- Perform regular preventive maintenance of room ventilation systems.
- Perform regular preventive maintenance of all anesthesia equipment.
- Conduct personnel monitoring and ambient trace gas monitoring.
- Seek the source of the smell of anesthetics noted during a case.
- Keep a good mask fit.
- Avoid unscavengeable techniques (open drop, insufflation).
- Prevent flow from breathing system into room air (e.g., pause fresh gas flow during intubation of the trachea).
- Turn on anesthetic gases only after the mask is on the patient.
- Turn off anesthetic gases before suctioning.
- Wash out anesthetics into the scavenger at the end of the case.
- Do not spill liquid agent.
- Use cuffed endotracheal tubes.
- Use low fresh gas flows.
- Check the workstation regularly for leaks.
- Disconnect nitrous oxide at the wall outlet at the end of the day.
- Use total intravenous anesthesia.
- Avoid use of nitrous oxide.

BOX 16.22   Summary of Preanesthesia Checkout Recommendations

To Be Completed Daily	To Be Repeated Before Each Case
1. Verify that auxiliary oxygen cylinder and self-inflating manual ventilation device are available and functioning.	
2. Verify that patient suction is adequate to clear the airway.	*
3. Turn on anesthesia delivery system and confirm that AC power is available.	
4. Verify availability of required monitors, including alarms.	*
5. Verify that pressure is adequate on the spare oxygen cylinder mounted on the anesthesia workstation.	
6. Verify that the piped gas pressures are 50 or greater psi.	
7. Verify that vaporizers are adequately filled, and, if applicable, that the filler ports are tightly closed.	*
8. Verify that there are no leaks in the gas supply lines between the flowmeters and the common gas outlet.	
9. Test scavenging system function.	
10. Calibrate, or verify calibration of, the oxygen monitor and check the low oxygen alarm.	
11. Verify that carbon dioxide absorbent is not exhausted.	*
12. Conduct breathing system pressure and leak testing.	*
13. Verify that gas flows properly through the breathing circuit during both inspiration and exhalation.	*
14. Document completion of checkout procedures.	*
15. Confirm ventilator settings and evaluate readiness to deliver anesthesia care. (ANESTHESIA TIME OUT)	*

psi, Pounds per square inch.
From Sub-Committee of the American Society of Anesthesiologists (ASA) Committee on Equipment and Facilities: Recommendations for PreAnesthesia Checkout Procedures, 2008. Available at http://www.asahq.org/resources/clinical-information/2008-asa-recommendations-for-pre-anesthesia-checkout.

BOX 16.23   Recommendations for Preanesthesia Checkout Procedures

General Considerations

The following document is intended to serve not as a preanesthesia checkout (PAC) itself, but rather as a template for developing checkout procedures that are appropriate for each individual anesthesia workstation design and practice setting. When using this template to develop a checkout procedure for systems that incorporate automated checkout features, items that are not evaluated by the automated checkout need to be identified, and supplemental manual checkout procedures included as needed.

Simply because an automated checkout procedure exists does not mean it can completely replace a manual checkout procedure or that it can be performed safely without adequate training and a thorough understanding of what the automated checkout accomplishes. An automated checkout procedure can be incomplete and/or misleading. For example, the leak test performed by some current automated checkouts does not test for leaks at the vaporizers. As a result, a loose vaporizer filler cap, or a leak at the vaporizer mount, could easily be missed.

Ideally, an automated checkout procedure should clearly reveal to the user the functions that are being checked, any deficient function that is found, and recommendations for correcting the problem. Documentation of the automated checkout process should preferably be done in a manner that can be recorded on the anesthesia record.

Operator's manuals, which accompany anesthesia delivery systems, include extensive recommendations for equipment checkout. Although these recommendations are quite extensive and typically not used by anesthesia providers, they are nevertheless important references for developing workstation-specific and institution-specific checkout procedures.

Personnel Performing the PAC

The previously accepted *Anesthesia Apparatus Checkout Recommendation* placed all of the responsibility for pre-use checkout on the anesthesia provider. This guideline identifies those aspects of the PAC that could be completed by a qualified anesthesia and/or biomedical technician. Critical checkout steps (e.g., availability of backup ventilation equipment) will benefit from intentional redundancy (i.e., having more than one individual responsible for checking the equipment). *Regardless of the level of training and support by technicians, the anesthesia care provider is ultimately responsible for proper function of all equipment used to provide anesthesia care.*

Adaptation of the PAC to local needs, assignment of responsibility for the checkout procedures, and training are the responsibilities of the individual anesthesia department. Training procedures should be documented. Proper documentation should include records of completed coursework (e.g., a manufacturer course) or, for in-house training, a listing of the competency items taught and records of successful completion by trainees.

Objectives for a New PAC

1. Outline the essential items that need to be available and functioning properly prior to delivering every anesthetic.
2. Identify the frequency with which each of the items needs to be checked.
3. Suggest which items may be checked by a qualified anesthesia technician, biomedical technician, or a manufacturer-certified service technician.

Basic Principles

The anesthesia care provider is ultimately responsible for ensuring that the anesthesia equipment is safe and ready for use. This responsibility includes adequate familiarity with the equipment, following relevant local policies for performing and documenting the PAC, and being knowledgeable about those procedures.

Depending on the staffing resources in a particular institution, anesthesia technicians and/or biomedical technicians can participate in the PAC. Each department should decide whether or not the available technicians can or should be trained to assist with checkout procedures.

- Critical items will benefit from redundant checks to avoid errors and omissions.
- When more than one person is responsible for checking an item, all parties should perform the check if intentional redundancy is deemed important, or either party may be acceptable, depending on the available resources.
- Whoever conducts the PAC should provide documentation of successful performance. The anesthesia provider should include this documentation on the patient chart.
- Whenever an anesthesia workstation is moved to a new location, a complete beginning-of-the-day checkout should be performed.
- Automated checks should clearly distinguish the components of the delivery system that are checked automatically from those that require manual checkout.
- Ideally, the date, time, and outcome of the most recent check(s) should be recorded and the information made accessible to the user.
- Specific procedures for preuse checkout cannot be prescribed in this document because they vary with the delivery systems. Clinicians must learn how to effectively perform the necessary preuse check for each piece of equipment they use.
- Each department or health care facility should work with the manufacturer(s) of their equipment to develop preuse checkout procedures that satisfy both the following guidelines and the needs of the local department.
- Default settings for ventilators, monitors, and alarms should be checked to determine whether they are appropriate.
- These checkout recommendations are intended to replace the pre-existing FDA-approved *Anesthesia Apparatus Checkout Recommendations*. They are not intended to be a replacement for required preventive maintenance.
- The PAC is essential to safe care but should not delay initiating care if the patient needs are so urgent that time taken to complete the PAC could worsen the patient's outcome.

Guidelines for Developing Institution-Specific Checkout Procedures Prior to Anesthesia Delivery

These guidelines describe a basic approach to checkout procedures and rationale that will ensure that these priorities are satisfied. They should be used to develop institution-specific checkout procedures designed for the equipment and resources available. (Examples of institution-specific procedures for current anesthesia delivery systems are published on the same website as this document.)

Requirements for Safe Delivery of Anesthesia Care

- Reliable delivery of oxygen at any appropriate concentration up to 100%
- Reliable means of positive pressure ventilation
- Backup ventilation equipment available and functioning
- Controlled release of positive pressure from the breathing circuit
- Anesthesia vapor delivery (if intended as part of the anesthetic plan)
- Adequate suction
- Means to conform to standards for patient monitoring

Specific Items

The following fifteen items need to be checked as part of a complete PAC. The intent is to identify what to check, the recommended frequency of checking and the individual(s) who could be responsible for the item. For these guidelines, the responsible party would fall into one of four categories: Provider, Technician, Technician or Provider, or Technician and Provider. The designation "Technician and Provider" means that the provider must perform the check whether or not it has been completed by a technician. It is not intended to make the use of technician checks mandatory. The intent is not to specify how an item needs to be checked, because the specific checkout procedure will depend upon the equipment being used.

Continued

BOX 16.23   Recommendations for Preanesthesia Checkout Procedures—cont'd

1. Verify auxiliary oxygen cylinder and self-inflating manual ventilation device are available and functioning.

   Frequency: Daily.

   Responsible Parties: Provider and technician.

   Rationale: Failure to be able to ventilate is a major cause of morbidity and mortality related to anesthesia care. Because equipment failure with resulting inability to ventilate the patient can occur at any time, a self-inflating manual ventilation device (e.g., Ambu bag) should be present at every anesthetizing location for every case and should be checked for proper function. In addition, a source of oxygen separate from the anesthesia workstation and pipeline supply, specifically an oxygen cylinder with regulator and a means to open the cylinder valve, should be immediately available and checked. After checking the cylinder pressure, it is recommended that the main cylinder valve be closed to avoid inadvertent emptying of the cylinder through a leaky or open regulator.

2. Verify that patient suction is adequate to clear the airway.

   Frequency: Prior to each use.

   Responsible Parties: Provider and technician.

   Rationale: Safe anesthetic care requires the immediate availability of suction to clear the airway if needed.

3. Turn on anesthesia delivery system and confirm that AC power is available.

   Frequency: Daily.

   Responsible Parties: Provider or technician.

   Rationale: Anesthesia delivery systems typically function with backup battery power if AC power fails. Unless the presence of AC power is confirmed, the first obvious sign of power failure can be a complete system shutdown when the batteries can no longer power the system. Many anesthesia delivery systems have visual indicators of the power source showing the presence of both AC and battery power. These indicators should be checked, and connection of the power cord to a functional AC power source should be confirmed. Desflurane vaporizers require electrical power and recommendations for checking power to these vaporizers should also be followed.

4. Verify availability of required monitors, including alarms.

   Frequency: Prior to each use.

   Responsible Parties: Provider or technician.

   Rationale: Standards for patient monitoring during anesthesia are clearly defined. The ability to conform to these standards should be confirmed for every anesthetic. The first step is to visually verify that the appropriate monitoring supplies (blood pressure cuffs, oximetry probes, etc.) are available. All monitors should be turned on and proper completion of power-up self-tests confirmed. Given the importance of pulse oximetry and capnography to patient safety, verifying proper function of these devices before anesthetizing the patient is essential. Capnometer function can be verified by exhaling through the breathing circuit or gas sensor to generate a capnogram, or verifying that the patient's breathing efforts generate a capnogram before the patient is anesthetized. Visual and audible alarm signals should be generated when this is discontinued. Pulse oximeter function, including an audible alarm, can be verified by placing the sensor on a finger and observing for a proper recording. The pulse oximeter alarm can be tested by introducing motion artifact or removing the sensor.

   Audible alarms have also been reconfirmed as essential to patient safety by American Society of Anesthesiologists (ASA), American Association of Nurse Anesthetists (AANA), Anesthesia Patient Safety Foundation (APSF), and The Joint Commission. Proper monitor functioning includes visual and audible alarm signals that function as designed.

5. Verify that pressure is adequate on the spare oxygen cylinder mounted on the anesthesia workstation.

   Frequency: Daily.

   Responsible Parties: Provider 'end technician.

   Rationale: Anesthesia delivery systems rely on a supply of oxygen for various workstation functions. At a minimum, the oxygen supply is used to provide oxygen to the patient. Pneumatically powered ventilators also rely on a gas supply. Oxygen cylinder(s) should be mounted on the anesthesia delivery system and determined to have an acceptable minimum pressure. The acceptable pressure depends on the intended use, the design of the anesthesia delivery system, and the availability of piped oxygen.

   Typically, an oxygen cylinder will be used if the central oxygen supply fails.

   If the cylinder is intended to be the primary source of oxygen (e.g., remote site anesthesia), then a cylinder supply sufficient to last for the entire anesthetic is required. If a pneumatically powered ventilator that uses oxygen as its driving gas will be used, a full "E" oxygen cylinder may provide only 30 minutes of oxygen. In that case, the maximum duration of oxygen supply can be obtained from an oxygen cylinder if it is used only to provide fresh gas to the patient in conjunction with manual or spontaneous ventilation. Mechanical ventilators will consume the oxygen supply if pneumatically powered ventilators that require oxygen to power the ventilator are used. Electrically powered ventilators do not consume oxygen, so the duration of a cylinder supply will depend only on total fresh gas flow. The oxygen cylinder valve should be closed after it has been verified that adequate pressure is present, unless the cylinder is to be the primary source of oxygen (i.e., piped oxygen is not available). If the valve remains open and the pipeline supply should fail, the oxygen cylinder can become depleted while the anesthesia provider is unaware of the oxygen supply problem.

   Other gas supply cylinders (e.g., Heliox, CO_2, Air, N_2O) need to be checked only if that gas is required to provide anesthetic care.

6. Verify that piped gas pressures are 50 or greater psi/g.

   Frequency: Daily.

   Responsible Parties: Provider and technician.

   Rationale: A minimum gas supply pressure is required for proper function of the anesthesia delivery system. Gas supplied from a central source can fail for a variety of reasons. Therefore, the pressure in the piped gas supply should be checked at least once daily.

7. Verify that vaporizers are adequately filled and, if applicable, that the filler ports are tightly closed.

   Frequency: Prior to each use.

   Responsible Parties: Provider. Technician if redundancy desired.

   Rationale: If anesthetic vapor delivery is planned, an adequate supply is essential to reduce the risk of light anesthesia or recall. This is especially true if an anesthetic agent monitor with a low agent alarm is not being used. Partially open filler ports are a common cause of leaks that may not be detected if the vaporizer control dial is not open when a leak test is performed. This leak source can be minimized by tightly closing filler ports. Newer vaporizer designs have filling systems that automatically close the filler port when filling is completed. High and low anesthetic agent alarms are useful to help prevent over- or under-dosage of anesthetic vapor. Use of these alarms is encouraged, and they should be set to the appropriate limits and enabled.

8. Verify that there are no leaks in the gas supply lines between the flowmeters and the common gas outlet.

   Frequency: Daily and whenever a vaporizer is changed.

   Responsible Parties: Provider or technician.

   Rationale: The gas supply in this part of the anesthesia delivery system passes through the anesthetic vaporizer(s) on most anesthesia delivery systems. In order to perform a thorough leak test, each vaporizer must be turned on individually to check for leaks at the vaporizer mount(s) or inside the vaporizer. Furthermore, some workstations have a check valve between the flowmeters and the common gas outlet, requiring a negative pressure test to adequately check for leaks. Automated checkout procedures typically include a leak test but may not evaluate leaks at the vaporizer especially if the vaporizer is not turned on during the leak test. When relying upon automated testing to evaluate the system for leaks, the automated leak test would need to be repeated for each vaporizer in place. This test

BOX 16.23 Recommendations for Preanesthesia Checkout Procedures—cont'd

should also be completed whenever a vaporizer is changed. The risk of a leak at the vaporizer depends upon the vaporizer design. Vaporizer designs where the filler port closes automatically after filling can reduce the risk of leaks. Technicians can provide useful assistance with this aspect of the workstation checkout because it can be time consuming.

9. Test scavenging system function.

Frequency: Daily.

Responsible Parties: Provider or technician.

Rationale: A properly functioning scavenging system prevents room contamination by anesthetic gases. Proper function depends upon correct connections between the scavenging system and the anesthesia delivery system. These connections should be checked daily by a provider or technician. Depending upon the scavenging system design, proper function may also require that the vacuum level is adequate, which should also be confirmed daily. Some scavenging systems have mechanical positive and negative pressure relief valves. Positive and negative pressure relief is important to protect the patient circuit from pressure fluctuations related to the scavenging system. Proper checkout of the scavenging system should ensure that positive and negative pressure relief is functioning properly. Due to the complexity of checking for effective positive and negative pressure relief, and the variations in scavenging system design, a properly trained technician can facilitate this aspect of the checkout process.

10. Calibrate, or verify calibration of, the oxygen monitor and check the low oxygen alarm.

Frequency: Daily.

Responsible Parties: Provider or technician.

Rationale: Continuous monitoring of the inspired oxygen concentration is the last line of defense against delivering hypoxic gas concentrations to the patient. The oxygen monitor is essential for detecting adulteration of the oxygen supply. Most oxygen monitors require calibration once daily, although some are self-calibrating. For self-calibrating oxygen monitors, they should be verified to read 21% when sampling room air. This is a step that is easily completed by a trained technician. When more than one oxygen monitor is present, the primary sensor that will be relied upon for oxygen monitoring should be checked.

The low oxygen concentration alarm should also be checked at this time by setting the alarm above the measured oxygen concentration and confirming that an audible alarm signal is generated.

11. Verify that carbon dioxide absorbent is not exhausted.

Frequency: Prior to each use.

Responsible Parties: Provider or technician.

Rationale: Proper function of a circle anesthesia system relies on the absorbent to remove carbon dioxide from rebreathed gas. Exhausted absorbent as indicated by the characteristic color change should be replaced. It is possible for absorbent material to lose the ability to absorb CO_2, yet the characteristic color change may be absent or difficult to see. Some newer absorbents do change color when desiccated. Capnography should be used for every anesthetic, and when using a circle anesthesia system, rebreathing carbon dioxide as indicated by an inspired CO_2 concentration greater than 0 can also indicate exhausted absorbent.

12. Conduct breathing system pressure and leak testing.

Frequency: Prior to each use.

Responsible Parties: Provider and technician.

Rationale: The breathing system pressure and leak test should be performed with the circuit configuration to be used during anesthetic delivery. If any components of the circuit are changed after this test is completed, the test should be performed again. Although the anesthesia provider should perform this test before each use, anesthesia technicians who replace and assemble circuits can also perform this check and add redundancy to this important checkout procedure. Proper testing will demonstrate that pressure can be developed in the breathing system during both manual and mechanical ventilation and that pressure can be relieved during manual ventilation by opening the adjustable pressure-limiting (APL) valve.

Automated testing is often implemented in the newer anesthesia delivery systems to evaluate the system for leaks and also to determine the compliance of the breathing system. The compliance value determined during this testing will be used to automatically adjust the volume delivered by the ventilator to maintain a constant volume delivery to the patient. It is important that the circuit configuration that is to be used be in place during the test.

13. Verify that gas flows properly through the breathing circuit during both inspiration and exhalation.

Frequency: Prior to each use.

Responsible Parties: Provider and technician.

Rationale: Pressure and leak testing does not identify all obstructions in the breathing circuit or confirm proper function of the inspiratory and expiratory unidirectional valves. A test lung or second reservoir bag can be used to confirm that flow through the circuit is unimpeded. Complete testing includes both manual and mechanical ventilation. The presence of the unidirectional valves can be assessed visually during the PAC. Proper function of these valves cannot be visually assessed because subtle valve incompetence may not be detected. Checkout procedures to identify valve incompetence that may not be visually obvious can be implemented but are typically too complex for daily testing. A trained technician can perform regular valve competence tests. Capnography should be used during every anesthetic and the presence of carbon dioxide in the inspired gases can help to detect an incompetent valve.

14. Document completion of checkout procedures.

Frequency: Prior to each use.

Responsible Parties: Provider and technician.

Rationale: Each individual responsible for checkout procedures should document completion of these procedures. Documentation gives credit for completing the job and can be helpful if an adverse event should occur. Some automated checkout systems maintain an audit trail of completed checkout procedures that are dated and timed.

15. Confirm ventilator settings and evaluate readiness to deliver anesthesia care. (ANESTHESIA TIME OUT)

Frequency: Immediately prior to initiating the anesthetic.

Responsible Parties: Provider.

Rationale: This step is intended to avoid errors due to production pressure or other sources of haste. The goal is to confirm that appropriate checks have been completed and that essential equipment is indeed available. The concept is analogous to the "time out" used to confirm patient identity and surgical site prior to incision. Improper ventilator settings can be harmful, especially if a small patient is following a much larger patient or vice versa. Pressure limit settings (when available) should be used to prevent excessive volume delivery from improper ventilator settings.

Items to Check
- Monitors functional?
- Capnogram present?
- Oxygen saturation by pulse oximetry measured?
- Flowmeter and ventilator settings proper?
- Manual/ventilator switch set to manual?
- Vaporizer(s) adequately filled?

they do cover most essential functions, can detect leaks, and can measure breathing circuit compliance. All of these new workstations require that the circuit be occluded for the electronic self-tests, then reconfigured to be ready for use. The Aisys and Apollo warn if leaks greater than 150 to 250 mL/min are detected.[67,70] If leaks are detected, users should check that all breathing circuit connections are tight, as well as the bellows and ventilator relief valve if these are accessible. Ensure that the Y-piece is properly occluded, gas flows are closed, and the gas sampling lines are not connected to the circuit (in the Apollo, these must be connected).

The user performs a few manual tests at the end (e.g., suction, cylinder pressure, high-pressure leak check of the reassembled breathing circuit, flow test of the unidirectional valves, and oxygen analysis). The great advantage of electronic self-tests is that, unlike checks performed by humans, the workstation cannot forget steps or perform steps incorrectly. The disadvantages include the lack of knowledge of what is being checked in the electronic self-tests, even after consulting the operator manual. For example, the negative-pressure leak test has been found to be most sensitive in detecting low pressure system leaks.[304] However, it is impossible to determine from the operator manuals for Apollo or Aisys whether their electronic self-test uses this method. Furthermore, some steps over and above the electronic self-test must always be performed by the user. Models differ in their clarity in prompting users to perform these checks, and users may make the assumption that the electronic self-test "does it all," and no further checks on their part are required.[3] For example, there are many recent reports of obstructions in the breathing circuit or other problems that prevented ventilation, yet the workstations were most often reported to have passed some attempt at a preuse checklist.[168,177,212,263,282,283,305–310] One current model's self-test allows users to accept an intentionally created and complete obstruction of the expiratory limb and initiate patient care, whereas two other workstations failed the self-test and prevented the user from proceeding.[10] A vaporizer with a leak significant enough to prevent positive pressure ventilation was reported to have passed the self-test.[311] A workstation whose CO_2 absorbent granules were missing was reported to pass the self-test.[211,312] A misconfigured workstation passed all self-tests, and yet, after induction, could not deliver a single positive pressure breath. Delay in establishing effective ventilation resulted in asystole, requiring atropine and chest compressions.[176] These recent and numerous reports of breathing circuit problems leading to inability to ventilate, not caught by attempts at daily checkout, are particularly ominous considering that one of the most frequently missed steps in the checkout is failure to check for a bag-valve-mask (Ambu bag).[5,15,18,313]

There is no substitute or shortcut for the recommended anesthesia workstation assessment of function. A properly performed checkout will answer the following questions: Is there oxygen in the oxygen line? Can the patient breathe unobstructed through the circuit? Can the patient be given a positive pressure breath? Are there leaks in the breathing circuit once reassembled? Is backup ventilation equipment present in the room? Users can and should incorporate simple checks that are easy to perform at the end of any model workstation self-test that ensure these basic safety requirements are met: (1) checking the oxygen analyzer, (2) checking that the circuit is unobstructed and that the unidirectional valves are functioning properly, (3) checking the reassembled breathing circuit for leaks with high pressure, and (4) checking for the presence of a bag-valve-mask (Ambu bag).[10,12,177,293,310] Adding these four steps at the end of any workstation self-test will increase safety. Check that the oxygen analyzer reads 21% when exposed to room air, and the reading increases when the sensor is exposed to gas from the oxygen pipeline (step 10 of the 2008 PAC). Check for a bag-valve-mask (step 1). While checking for backup ventilation equipment (e.g., Ambu bag), walk around the workstation, checking for cylinder oxygen pressure, suction, and an extra circuit; the location of circuit breakers; the presence of a cylinder wrench and head strap; and whether gas analysis monitors are scavenged.

Two user-performed breathing circuit checks are vital and are not done by any model's electronic self-test. Step 12 of the PAC is a breathing circuit leak check, and step 13 (flow test) checks that the breathing circuit is unobstructed. To ensure that all breathing circuit connections are gas tight, always perform a high-pressure check of the reassembled breathing circuit after the checklist is complete. Gas should be released from the pressurized circuit by opening the APL valve. This checks its function, as well as propelling any absorbent dust toward the scavenger, and not the elbow. Perform a flow test to ensure that the unidirectional valves are working properly and that the circuit is not obstructed by mold flash, foreign objects, or plastic wrapping.[10,12,29,162,165] The flow test uses a second breathing bag as a test lung, observing for inward and outward movement between bellows (or manual breathing bag) and test lung. Alternatively, one may breathe through the circuit.[29]

There is no minimum test other than that suggested by the operator instruction manuals and the PAC. In administering an anesthetic for an emergency surgical procedure, the PAC guideline recognizes that patient needs can be so urgent that harm might come to the patient with even a few minutes delay to check the workstation thoroughly. There are, however, a few steps that can be taken to increase safety even when time is limited. One should always check suction, expected data on all monitors (ECG, Non invasive blood pressure (NIBP), SpO_2, FiO_2, capnography), backup means of ventilation (e.g., Ambu bag), and perform a high-pressure leak test of the breathing circuit before the mask is placed on the patient's face. During preoxygenation (whether in emergencies or as a matter of routine in every case), take a brief moment to check the breathing bag for fluctuations. Respiratory effort that is visible in the breathing bag before induction ensures that the patient is breathing, the mask fit is good, and oxygen is flowing. A situation in which any of these conditions is absent requires immediate attention.

SUMMARY

Current anesthesia workstations are a result of design improvements as well as better integration of electronic controls, physiologic monitors, and machine function monitors. Anesthesia workstations have undergone significant developments over the years, necessitating continued review to maintain competence. Equipment proficiency must be a part of every anesthesia clinician's toolkit.[314] Hopefully, through study of this chapter, current equipment will be more widely understood. In this manner, our future patients may "sleep" in safety, afforded the level of care that we all wish for ourselves and our loved ones.

REFERENCES

For a complete list of references for this chapter, scan this QR code with any smartphone code reader app, or visit the following URL: http://booksite.elsevier.com/9780323711944/.

17

Clinical Monitoring I: Cardiovascular System

Mark A. Kossick, Bethany K. Seale

Monitoring of anatomic and physiologic variables during an anesthetic allows anesthetists to enhance patient safety and meet established standards for professional practice.[1] Many different monitors are commonly used to assist in the delivery of an anesthetic, and it is the responsibility of the anesthetist to assimilate data provided by monitors to make appropriate clinical judgments. Consequently, the application of critical thinking skills, thorough physical assessment, vigilance, and the appropriate selection and application of monitors (including configuration) are key requirements in the process of monitoring.

Fundamental monitoring and assessment techniques include inspection (visual examination), auscultation, and palpation. They provide essential objective and subjective data not available from advanced monitoring modalities and can alert the anesthetist to occult problems in select patients. Inspection of the patient can provide information regarding the adequacy of oxygen delivery and carbon dioxide elimination, fluid requirements, as well as positioning and alignment of body structures. Auscultation is used to verify correct placement of airway devices such as the endotracheal tube and laryngeal mask airway, to assess arterial blood pressure (BP), and to continually monitor heart sounds and air exchange through the pulmonary system. Palpation can aid the anesthetist in assessing the quality of the pulse and degree of skeletal muscle relaxation, as well as locating major vascular structures when placing central venous lines or performing regional anesthesia techniques.

Critical thinking skills are cardinal prerequisites for successful monitoring of a patient's anesthetic. In addition, it is well known that errors in anesthesia care are minimized when anesthetists remain alert and vigilant. This chapter reviews the more commonly used noninvasive and invasive cardiovascular monitors in anesthesia practice.

ELECTROCARDIOGRAM MONITORING

The continuous monitoring of the cardiovascular status via the electrocardiogram (ECG) is a requirement for any patient receiving an anesthetic. This includes assessment of heart rate, rhythm, ectopy, and in particular for some patients ST segments and T waves. Computerized real-time ST segment analysis continues to be incorporated in many operating rooms (ORs), intensive care units (ICUs), and postanesthesia care units (PACUs) across the country. Many factors support this trend, including the development of practice guidelines by professional societies that advocate such monitoring techniques in select patient populations[2,3] and the demographics of the general surgical population. Approximately one-third of patients scheduled for noncardiac surgery have risk factors for coronary artery disease (CAD), and postoperative myocardial infarction (MI) is three times as frequent in patients with ischemia.[4] Research has shown prolonged stress-induced ischemia (i.e., ST segment depression) to be the major cause for cardiac morbidity (MI) after significant vascular surgery[5]; a meta-analysis involving 995 patients has also shown a direct relationship between recurrent ischemia detected by computer-assisted ST segment analysis in patients with acute coronary syndromes and the occurrence of MI and death.[6] The overall incidence of perioperative ischemia in patients with CAD scheduled for cardiac or noncardiac surgery ranges from 20% to 80%.[7,8]

As a result of its low cost, noninvasiveness, widespread availability, and designation as a standard of care for monitoring of all anesthetized patients,[1] the ECG remains a common and required diagnostic tool in the OR. Compared with Holter monitors, ST segment trending monitors have on average a sensitivity of 74% and specificity of 73% in detecting myocardial ischemia.[9] When used to guide treatment in patients with silent ischemic episodes or patients considered high risk, they may reduce morbidity.[5,6,10]

Current recommendations for ST segment deviation thresholds account for the influence of gender, ECG lead, age, and race on position of the ST segment.[11-14] In particular, two chest leads (V_2 and V_3) have been shown to exhibit the greatest shift of the ST junction (i.e., J point) and as such must be accounted for in applying diagnostic criteria for myocardial injury. Otherwise the proportion of false positives would increase.

The degree of elevation (or depression) is relative to an isoelectric line, which is commonly referenced as the PR segment. The PR segment extends from the end of the P wave to the start of ventricular depolarization (e.g., appearance of a Q wave) (Fig. 17.1). The ST junction is defined as where the QRS complex ends and the ST segment begins. It is also synonymous with the J point. In the clinical setting some biomedical engineers have eliminated the J point in their computerized ST segment analysis software algorithms (Fig. 17.2). Recommended threshold values for ST segment elevation are listed in Table 17.1.[11] For ST segment depression the threshold values are -0.5 mm (-0.05 mV) for males and females of all ages in ECG leads V_2 and V_3 and -1.0 mm (-0.1 mV) in all other ECG leads.[12] When these threshold values are met, an imbalance between oxygen supply and demand may exist (e.g., myocardial ischemia/injury).

It should be appreciated when critiquing the literature that researchers may use the J point in combination with the ST point as a means to determine the degree of ST segment deviation. Examples would include assessing the extent of ST segment shift by measuring 60 ms (1.5 mm) or 80 ms (2 mm) from the J point. Fig. 17.2 contrasts these two means of calculating ST segment deviation. Measuring the degree of ST segment depression or elevation at the J point represents the most current recommendations by the American College of Cardiology, American Heart Association, and Heart Rhythm Society to accurately determine the extent of ST segment deviation.[11,15]

For anesthesia providers who use ST segment analysis software that incorporates a J point in combination with an ST point, caution should be exercised in blindly accepting numerical ST segment deviation

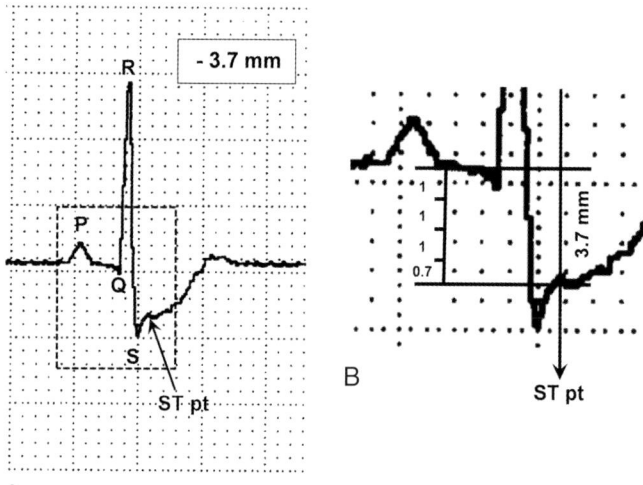

A

Fig. 17.1 A single cardiac cycle (ST snippet) and enlarged section of the snippet providing greater details. The PR segment is measured from the end of the P wave to the beginning of the QRS complex. (A) A depressed ST segment that is upsloping. The junction between the S wave and ST segment defines the ST point. (B) The PR segment is extended out via a horizontal line. This serves as an isoelectric reference (no deviation of the electrocardiogram stylus upward or downward) to determine the degree of ST segment shift. The distance from the extended PR segment to the ST point demonstrates that the ST segment is 3.7 mm depressed (i.e., J point depression of 3.7 mm). (Reprinted with permission from Kossick MA. *EKG Interpretation: Simple, Thorough, Practical.* 3rd ed. Park Ridge, IL: AANA Publishing.)

TABLE 17.1   Threshold Values for ST Segment Elevation

Gender and Age	ECG Leads	J Point Elevation
Male >40 yr of age	I, II, III, aVR, aVL, aVF V$_1$, V$_4$, V$_5$, V$_6$	1 mm (0.1 mV)
	V$_2$, V$_3$	2 mm (0.2 mV)
Male <40 yr of age	V$_2$, V$_3$	2.5 mm (0.25 mV)
Females	I, II, III, aVR, aVL, aVF V$_1$, V$_4$, V$_5$, V$_6$	>1 mm (0.1 mV)
	V$_2$, V$_3$	1.5 mm (0.15 mV)
Male and females	[†]V$_3$R, V$_4$R	0.5 mm (0.05 mV)
Males <30 yr of age	[†]V$_3$R, V$_4$R	1 mm (0.1 mV)
Male and females	[‡]V$_7$, V$_8$, V$_9$	0.5 mm (0.05 mV)

[†], right ventricular ECG leads; [‡], posterior chest leads; *ECG*, electrocardiogram; *mV*, millivolt.
Data from Galen SW, et al. AHA/ACCF/HRS expert consensus document: AHA/ACCF/HRS recommendations for the standardization and interpretation of the electrocardiogram. Part VI: acute ischemia/infarction a scientific statement from the American Heart Association Electrocardiography and Arrhythmias Committee, Council on Clinical Cardiology; the American College of Cardiology Foundation; and the Heart Rhythm Society endorsed by the International Society for Computerized Electrocardiology. *J Am Coll Cardiol.* 2009;53:1003-1011.

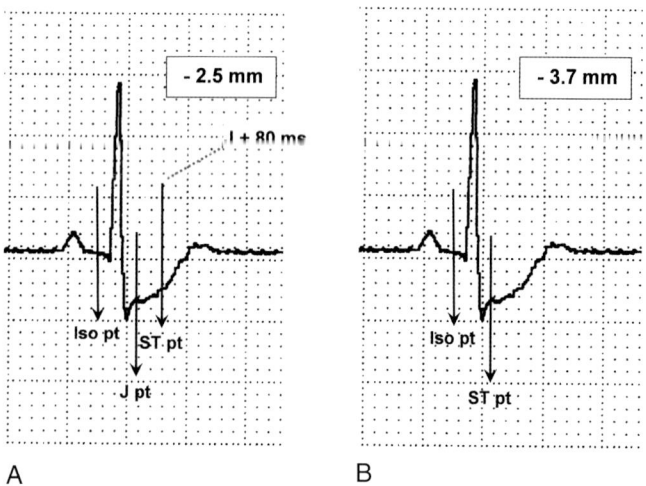

A   **B**

Fig. 17.2 Two ST snippets illustrating two different techniques to calculate ST segment depression values. ST snippet (A) measures ST segment deviation 80 ms (2 mm) from the J point. ST snippet (B) measures ST segment depression at the J point. The most recent American Heart Association/American College of Cardiology Foundation/Heart Rhythm Society recommendations for standardizing and interpreting the electrocardiogram advocate measuring ST segment changes at the J point (i.e., B). (Reprinted with permission from Kossick MA. *EKG Interpretation: Simple, Thorough, Practical.* 3rd ed. Park Ridge, IL: AANA Publishing.)

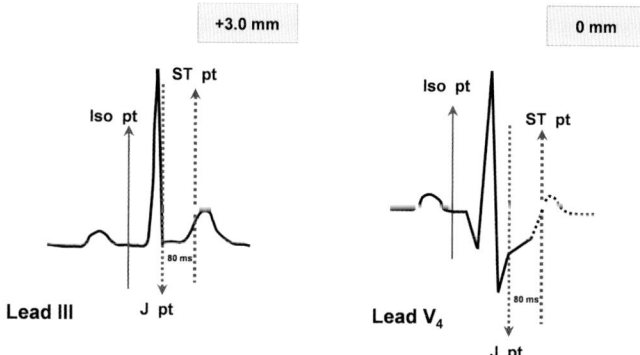

Fig. 17.3 Two cardiac cycles from leads III and V$_4$ illustrating a shortened ST segment. Use of a J + 80 ms value to measure ST segment deviation in each lead results in the ST point intersecting the T wave, thus producing inaccurate ST segment deviation values. For lead III the misplaced ST point produces a false positive and for lead V$_4$ a false negative. (Reprinted with permission from Kossick MA. *EKG Interpretation: Simple, Thorough, Practical.* 3rd ed. Park Ridge, IL: AANA Publishing.)

values. Shortened ST segments are predictably associated with tachyarrhythmias, which can result in T waves encroaching on ST segments. Should this occur, the use of older software designed by biomedical engineers in determining ST segment deviation values (e.g., J + 80 ms or even J + 60 ms) could lead to an ST point intersecting a T wave instead of the ST segment. In this circumstance, the computer-derived ST segment deviation value would reflect either a falsely elevated ST segment, suggesting myocardial injury (false positive), or the masking of a significant ST segment depression (false negative) (Fig. 17.3). Thus, it is apparent that critical assessment of computer-generated ST segment deviation values is vital to avoid making errors in management of patients.

Regarding the significance of the various forms of ST segment depression, it is important to recall that a horizontal or downsloping depressed ST segment has greater specificity (fewer false positives) than an upsloping depressed ST segment. Adding upsloping ST segment changes to myocardial injury diagnostic criteria does improve overall sensitivity but at a sacrifice to specificity and positive predictive value.[16,17] Also, it is noteworthy to recall that it is more challenging to

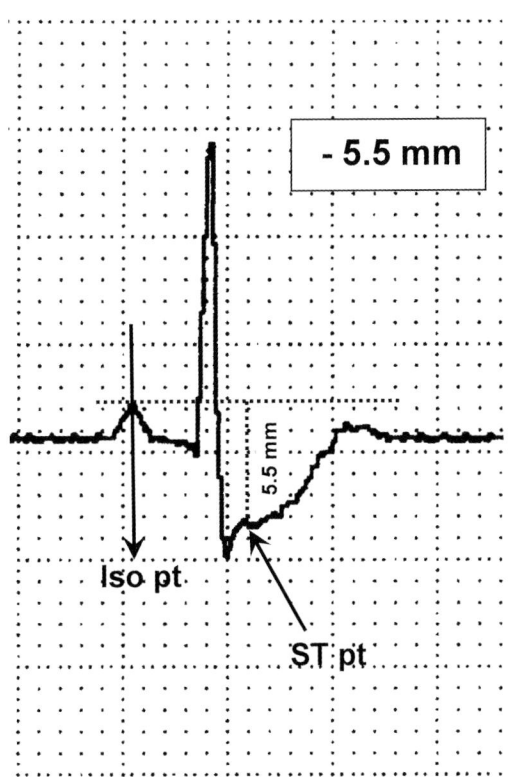

Fig. 17.4 Iso point incorrectly placed on top of the P wave by an electro-cardiogram monitor, producing an exaggerated ST segment deviation value. (Reprinted with permission from Kossick MA. *EKG Interpretation: Simple, Thorough, Practical*. 3rd ed. Park Ridge, IL: AANA Publishing.)

identify the regions of the myocardium impacted with the appearance of ST segment depression versus elevation.[11]

Setting the ST Segment Parameters

Most manufacturers of computerized ST segment analysis monitors have sophisticated algorithms that allow fairly consistent and accurate placement of ST measurement points. Nevertheless, anesthetists should periodically assess these parameters and change them as needed; responding to false trends secondary to incorrectly placed ST measurement points could lead to iatrogenic injury. In fact, manufacturers have incorporated software that permits health care providers to override the monitor's placement of ST measurement points. A common technique for setting ST measurement points involves adjustment of two (Iso point and ST point) or three (Iso point, J point, and ST point) variables. Manipulation of a keypad or touchscreen device on the ECG monitor permits the operator to scroll each of these points along a horizontal axis. The points are depicted as vertical lines that intersect various components of a single cardiac cycle (see Fig. 17.2). Fig. 17.4 illustrates the consequences when real-time ST segment analysis software incorrectly places the Iso point on the apex of the P wave. The application of an ST segment deviation algorithm can reduce the occurrence of such mishaps and improve overall management of patients at risk for ischemic changes (Fig. 17.5).

Other significant variables to account for when monitoring patients at risk for ischemic events include ECG electrode placement, ECG lead selection, gain setting, and frequency bandwidth. Each of these is briefly reviewed here.

Electrocardiograph Electrode Placement

It is fairly common to see ECG electrodes placed incorrectly on a patient in an attempt to "move an operating room schedule along." Many times

with a physical status (PS) I or II patient, accurate ECG electrode placement is not a significant issue. However, in patients with risk factors for CAD, such inattentiveness can lead to iatrogenic injury by producing deviated ST segments, inverted T waves, or pathologic Q waves that can be viewed as real problems. Proper placement of the limb lead and chest lead electrodes is described in Table 17.2. For emphasis, the precordial leads should be placed via palpation of the costae, not by gross visual estimation of an intercostal space (Fig. 17.6). Understandably, some surgical procedures do not permit the use of optimal ECG lead selection and placement; ECG electrode(s) can interfere with skin preparation and surgical incision. Under these circumstances, a less than optimal ECG lead placement may be required with the sacrificing of a preferred chest lead and/or limb lead. When this occurs the reason for not monitoring in the desired ECG lead should be documented on the anesthetic record to provide evidence of still meeting established AANA practice standards (III, V, VII, and IX).[1] Similarly, when feasible, anesthesia providers should observe ECG technicians' placement of resting 12 lead ECG electrodes. Correct placement of electrodes can be inconsistent (even grossly misplaced), which will mitigate accurate ECG interpretation for evidence of ischemia, some types of arrhythmias, and ectopy.

Electrocardiographic Lead Selection

The decision regarding which ECG leads to monitor during the course of an anesthetic can be extremely important relative to the medical history of the patient. Improper selection can result in unrecognized myocardial ischemia, injury, or infarction. Research has validated that use of a single ECG lead for ischemic monitoring in patients with documented CAD is inadequate; monitoring with multiple leads enhances patient safety. In patients at risk for ischemic events, this author recommends the maximum number of ECG leads be displayed (e.g., 3, 7, 12 [derived 12 lead]) during the perioperative period to enhance continuous and comprehensive assessment of ST segment and T-wave changes (Figs. 17.7 and 17.8). Which leads are optimal to use for detecting significant ST segment changes should be based on the preanesthetic assessment. First and foremost, if a preoperative 12-lead ECG has been done, "fingerprinting" of this tracing should serve as the primary guide for lead selection during the perioperative period. For example, if the baseline 12-lead shows significant primary ST segment changes in limb leads III and aVF, then this lead set should be prioritized for continuous display in the respective anesthetizing location. The ECG monitoring system software will dictate what lead display options can be configured. For example, with Philips software and a five-cable ECG lead system, a derived 12-lead (EASI) can be continuously displayed (see Fig. 17.8). With other manufacturers and a five-cable ECG lead system, a true V lead (e.g., V_3), a modified chest lead V_5 (e.g., central subclavicular 5 [CS_5]), and a limb lead II can be configured for ECG monitoring (Fig. 17.9). The potential value of a preoperative 12-lead ECG is relative to it being correctly recorded by the ECG technician (each ECG electrode was properly placed, ECG lead wires were correctly attached, the patient was in a supine position while it was recorded,[18] and the low-frequency cutoff was set with a lower limit not exceeding 0.67Hz[18,19]).

In patients without a preoperative 12-lead or who have a baseline 12-lead that is unremarkable (unknown ST fingerprint), the literature suggests leads V_3, V_4, V_5, limb lead III, and aVF (in this order of preference) be selected for continuous monitoring for ST segment elevation or depression.[20-25] Limb lead II is recommended for assessment of narrow QRS complex rhythms, particularly if the P wave is significant for diagnostic criteria (e.g., atrial flutter, atrial fibrillation, junctional rhythms).

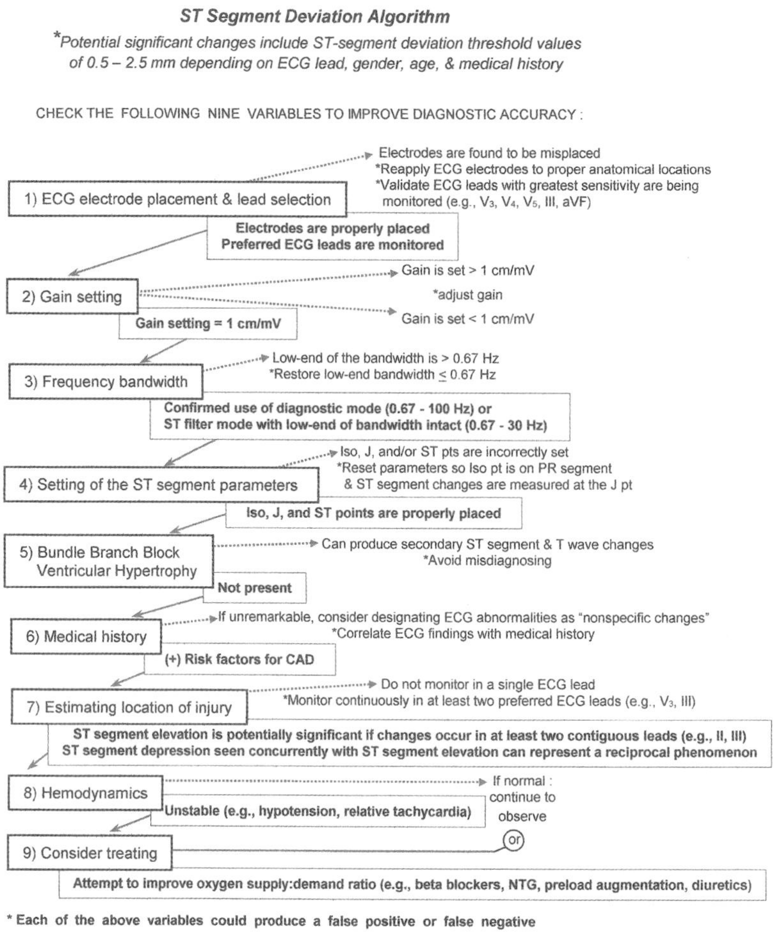

ST Segment Deviation Algorithm
*Potential significant changes include ST-segment deviation threshold values
of 0.5 – 2.5 mm depending on ECG lead, gender, age, & medical history*

CHECK THE FOLLOWING NINE VARIABLES TO IMPROVE DIAGNOSTIC ACCURACY :

1) ECG electrode placement & lead selection
→ Electrodes are found to be misplaced
*Reapply ECG electrodes to proper anatomical locations
*Validate ECG leads with greatest sensitivity are being monitored (e.g., V_3, V_4, V_5, III, aVF)

**Electrodes are properly placed
Preferred ECG leads are monitored**

2) Gain setting
→ Gain is set > 1 cm/mV
*adjust gain
Gain is set < 1 cm/mV

Gain setting = 1 cm/mV

3) Frequency bandwidth
→ Low-end of the bandwidth is > 0.67 Hz
*Restore low-end bandwidth ≤ 0.67 Hz

**Confirmed use of diagnostic mode (0.67 - 100 Hz) or
ST filter mode with low-end of bandwidth intact (0.67 - 30 Hz)**

4) Setting of the ST segment parameters
→ Iso, J, and/or ST pts are incorrectly set
*Reset parameters so Iso pt is on PR segment & ST segment changes are measured at the J pt

Iso, J, and ST points are properly placed

5) Bundle Branch Block Ventricular Hypertrophy
→ Can produce secondary ST segment & T wave changes
*Avoid misdiagnosing

Not present

6) Medical history
→ If unremarkable, consider designating ECG abnormalities as "nonspecific changes"
*Correlate ECG findings with medical history

(+) Risk factors for CAD

7) Estimating location of injury
→ Do not monitor in a single ECG lead
*Monitor continuously in at least two preferred ECG leads (e.g., V_3, III)

**ST segment elevation is potentially significant if changes occur in at least two contiguous leads (e.g., II, III)
ST segment depression seen concurrently with ST segment elevation can represent a reciprocal phenomenon**

8) Hemodynamics
→ If normal : continue to observe

Unstable (e.g., hypotension, relative tachycardia)

(or)

9) Consider treating

Attempt to improve oxygen supply:demand ratio (e.g., beta blockers, NTG, preload augmentation, diuretics)

* Each of the above variables could produce a false positive or false negative

Fig. 17.5 An ST segment deviation assessment and treatment algorithm. (Reprinted with permission from Kossick MA. *EKG Interpretation: Simple, Thorough, Practical.* 3rd ed. Park Ridge, IL: AANA Publishing.)

The 1988 recommendation for V_5 and limb lead II as preferred ECG leads[26] in patients where ST segment monitoring is desired has been mitigated by other researchers, critical care task forces, and major publications.[2,21,23,27,28] Landesberg et al. studied 185 consecutive patients undergoing vascular surgery who were monitored by continuous 12-lead ST trend analysis during the perioperative period and up to 72 hours postoperatively. Chest lead V_3 was found to detect ischemia earliest and most frequently (86.8%). Lead V_4 was the second most diagnostic lead (78.9%), and V_5 was third (65.8%). With those patients sustaining MI, V_4 was the most sensitive lead (83.3%), with V_3 and V_5 being the second most sensitive (75%).[23] In this study, MI was diagnosed if cardiac troponin I levels were greater than 3.1 ng/mL and were accompanied by symptoms of ischemia or the presence of ECG criteria (i.e., ST segment elevation, ST segment depression, or large Q waves). Of interest was the observation that 97% of ischemic events were expressed as ST segment depression—not elevation—and ST shifts were considered significant if their duration of change exceeded 10 minutes. As reported elsewhere in the literature, monitoring in multiple leads was advocated as a means to improve sensitivity for detecting ST segment changes.[5,23,24,26]

Given this information, it is prudent for anesthesia providers to monitor and assess multiple ECG leads in the operating room. In the absence of an ST segment fingerprint, this author advocates the following ECG lead combinations (for ST segment elevation or depression)

in patients with documented or identified significant risk factors for ischemic heart disease:

1. For a five-cable ECG recording system, the three-lead set of V_3, MCL_5, and aVF (the use of MCL_5 precludes the use of limb lead III) or V_3 combined with limb lead III and aVF.
2. For a three-cable ECG recording system, a two-lead set comprised of MCL_5 is combined with limb lead aVF. To date, an MCL_2, MCL_3, and MCL_4 have not been established/validated in the literature. Although not validated through research, a theoretical configuration of each of these modified chest leads is possible.

Extended monitoring capabilities help to optimize detection of regionalized myocardial ischemia. Many times this entails nothing more than changing the lead selector switch to another ECG lead (e.g., III changed to aVF) or displaying a multilead ECG when indicated or continuously during an anesthetic (Fig. 17.10). The latter produces an ECG recording of all six limb leads and a single chest lead, permitting the anesthetist to more comprehensively assess available ECG data, including arrhythmias, the mean QRS axis (limb leads I and aVF), T-wave morphology, ST segment changes, QT intervals, and the presence of right or left bundle branch block.

With the introduction into clinical practice of the derived 12-lead system (EASI), nurses and physicians have a convenient method to globally assess the overall well-being of the myocardium (see Fig. 17.8). The 12-lead is derived from modified vectorcardiographic leads and requires the use of a five-cable ECG lead system.[29] To monitor with this

TABLE 17.2   Proper Placement of Electrocardiographic Electrodes for Monitoring Chest Leads and Limb Leads via the Mason-Likar Lead Position

RA	†Over the outer right clavicle
LA	†Over the outer left clavicle
LL	†Near the left iliac crest or midway between the costal margin and left iliac crest, anterior axillary line
RL	At any convenient location on the body (e.g., upper right shoulder)
V_1	Fourth intercostal space right of the sternal border
V_2	Fourth intercostal space left of the sternal border
V_3	Equal distance between V_2 and V_4
V_4	Midclavicular line at the fifth intercostal space
V_5	Horizontal to V_4 on the anterior axillary line or if difficult to identify (anterior axillary line), then midway between V_4 and V_6
V_6	Horizontal to V_5 on the midaxillary line
V_7	Horizontal to V_6 on the posterior axillary line
V_8	Horizontal to V_7 below the left scapula
V_9	Horizontal to V_8 at the left paravertebral border
V_3R	Placed right side of chest wall in mirror image to chest lead V_3
V_4R	Placed right side of chest wall in mirror image to chest lead V_4

†, Mason-Likar ECG electrode placement; *LA*, left arm electrocardiographic (ECG) electrode; *LL*, left leg ECG electrode; *RA*, right arm ECG electrode; *RL*, right leg ECG electrode.
Data from Paul K, et al. AHA/ACC/HRS scientific statement: recommendations for the standardization and interpretation of the electrocardiogram. Part I: the electrocardiogram and its technology: a scientific statement from the American Heart Association Electrocardiography and Arrhythmias Committee, Council on Clinical Cardiology; the American College of Cardiology Foundation; and the Heart Rhythm Society. Endorsed by the International Society for Computerized Electrocardiology. *JACC.* 2007;49(10): 1109-1127.

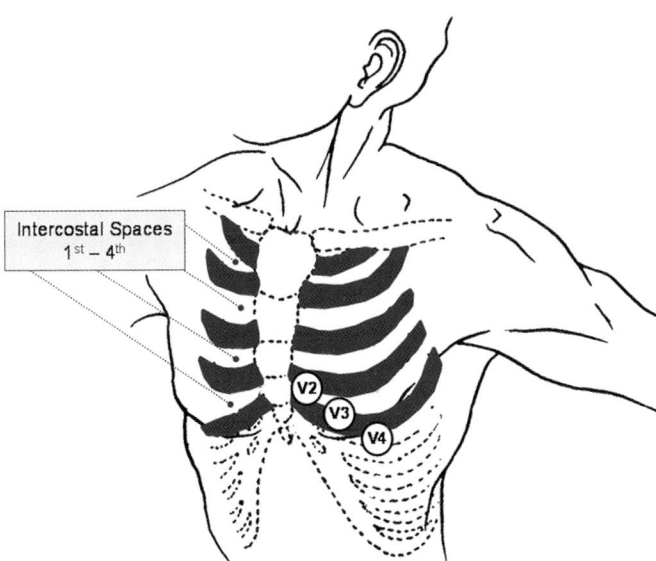

Fig. 17.6 Precordial electrodes V_2, V_3, V_4 positioned across the ventrolateral aspect of the thorax. V_2 placement: 4th intercostal space (ICS) left of the sternum; V_3: equal distance between V_2 and V_4; V_4: left midclavicular line at the 5th ICS. (Reprinted with permission from Kossick MA. *EKG Interpretation: Simple, Thorough, Practical.* 3rd ed. Park Ridge, IL: AANA Publishing.)

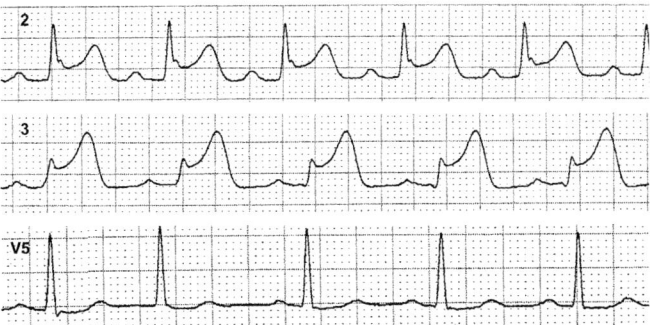

Fig. 17.7 Monitoring in three electrocardiogram leads during anesthetic administration captured significant ST segment elevation. The greatest change in ST segments occurred in limb lead III, followed by limb lead II. Noteworthy was the failure of lead V_5 to demonstrate any appreciable change in the ST segment. Postoperatively a cardiology consultation resulted in a diagnosis of Prinzmetal angina.

system, the five ECG electrodes are placed in unconventional locations: LA electrode over the manubrium; chest (V) electrode lower body of the sternum; LL electrode left midaxillary, horizontal to the chest electrode; RA electrode right midaxillary, also horizontal to the chest electrode; and the RL electrode in any convenient location. Current and past research suggests the derived 12-lead is comparable (but not equivalent)[19] to the standard 12-lead for multiple cardiac diagnosis in adults and children (e.g., ST segment changes, MI, wide QRS complex tachycardia, QT interval measurements).[30-34] It is possible that patients at substantial risk for CAD would benefit from global ischemic monitoring via a derived 12-lead. This software option also eliminates any need to consider "preferred" ECG leads because all six limb leads and six chest leads can be viewed during an anesthetic.

In contrast to a derived 12-lead or five-cable ECG electrode system, a three-cable system offers challenges to anesthesia providers concerning potential errors with ECG lead configuration. The literature documents that health care providers consistently struggle with modified chest lead configuration—even those who routinely monitor the ECG.[35] Modified chest leads offer an alternative to true chest leads when only a three-cable ECG recording system is available. Introduced into clinical practice in 2003 was the modified chest lead $MAC_{1(L)}$ (modified augmented chest lead V_1). This modified chest lead is configured using augmented limb lead aVL and has been shown to have a diagnostic accuracy similar to true chest lead V_1. The internal validity of this finding was based on His bundle recordings, used as the gold standard for distinguishing between premature ventricular ectopy and premature aberrantly conducted beats.[36] The simplicity of this unique ECG lead has the potential to reduce modified chest lead configuration errors. Additional research is needed to substantiate this theoretical advantage (e.g., ease of configuration of $MAC_{1(L)}$ versus modified chest lead V_1 [MCL_1]). Fig. 17.11 illustrates the ECG configuration of $MAC_{1(L)}$, as well as the similarities in morphologic characteristics of single cardiac cycles recorded in V_1 and $MAC_{1(L)}$.

In summary, practitioners who limit ECG monitoring and assessment to a single lead or pair of leads in patients with documented or recognized risk factors for ischemic heart disease are potentially compromising patient safety by not using (when available) multiple-ECG-lead display configuration options.[2] In such patients, the continuous display of three ECG leads, a multilead ECG (six limb leads and one true chest lead), or a derived 12-lead could be of clinical benefit. The literature substantiates that myocardial ischemia (T-wave and/or ST segment changes) can be regionalized and completely missed when viewing two or fewer ECG leads. Similar concerns exists when three-cable ECG lead

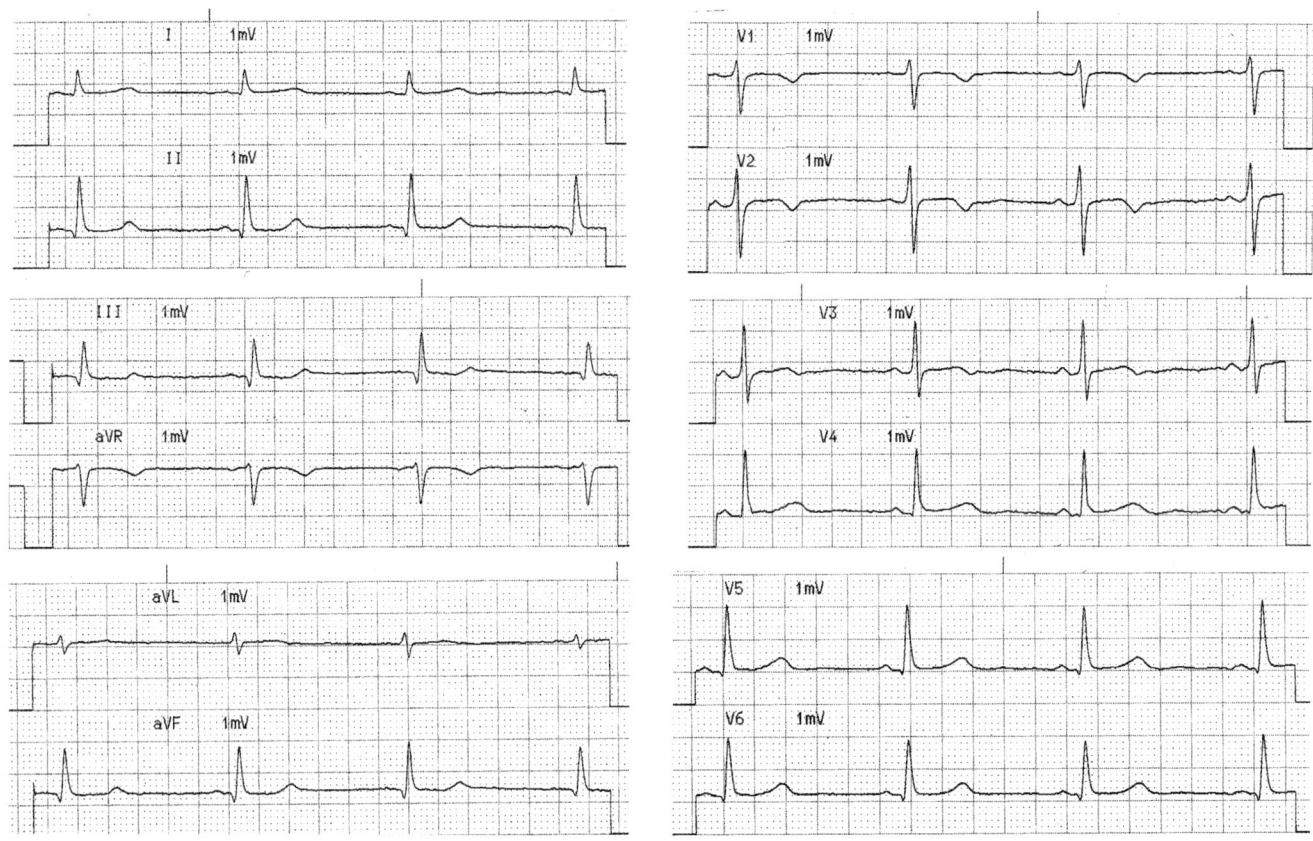

Fig. 17.8 Derived 12-lead electrocardiogram (ECG [EASI]) recorded just prior to anesthetic induction in the operating room. The ECG monitor can be configured to continuously display all 12 leads for comprehensive assessment of ST segments and rhythm changes.

systems are used in place of available five-cable ECG lead systems. The latter permits the viewing of a true chest lead, which is always preferable over a modified chest. Unarguably, critical assessment of all available patient data will help anesthetists exercise better judgment during an anesthetic and potentially improve anesthetic outcome.

Gain Setting and Frequency Bandwidth

Two other potential problems with continuous ST segment monitoring relate to the amplitude at which the ECG monitor has been set and whether filtering of the electrical signal is excessive. When accurate visual assessment of ST segments is a priority during an anesthetic, the gain of the ECG monitor should be set at standardization (i.e., a 1-mV signal delivered by the ECG monitor produces a 10-mm calibration pulse). This gain setting fixes the ratio of the ST segment and QRS complex size so that a 1-mm ST segment change is accurately assessed (e.g., potential myocardial injury). Failure to recognize the use of other gain settings can lead to overdiagnosis or underdiagnosis of myocardial injuries (ST segment changes). Fig. 17.12 illustrates how changes in gain settings, incorrect ECG electrode, and/or lead wire placement can confound ST segment assessment.[19,37,38]

The filtering capacity of the ECG monitor is yet another potential source of artifact. Research has demonstrated that filtering out the low end of the frequency bandwidth (e.g., 0.05 to 0.5 to produce a new bandwidth range of 0.5–40 Hz) of the monitor's electrical signal can lead to distortion of the ST segment (elevation or depression) and T wave (inverted).[39,40] For this reason in many (but not all) cases, the diagnostic mode of an ECG monitor should be used when ST segment analysis is a priority during an anesthetic. However, as noted earlier, the low-frequency cutoff has been amended by the American National Standards Institute (ANSI) and the Association for the Advancement of Medical Instrumentation (AAMI) to a value not to exceed 0.67 mV for routine filters.[18] This recommendation has also been endorsed by the International Society for Computerized Electrocardiology.[19]

Clearly, the sensitivity and specificity of computerized real-time ST segment analysis software is dependent on the ability of the anesthetist to critically analyze the large number of factors that influence displayed ST segment values. Attentiveness to such variables as the patient's physical status, ECG lead placement and selection, verification of proper placement of the Iso point, ST point, type of electronic filtering used by the ECG monitor, and gain setting may affect anesthetic outcome in patients at risk for myocardial ischemia or injury. In essence, overreading of ECG data is not optional but is an essential part of anesthesia care.

CENTRAL VENOUS AND ARTERIAL HEMODYNAMIC MEASUREMENTS

Central venous and pulmonary artery catheters (PACs) are not commonly used in the general surgical population. In fact, since the introduction of the PAC in 1970, the frequency of its use as a monitoring tool for significant surgical procedures has significantly diminished. Even during cardiac or large invasive vascular surgical procedures, many surgeons and anesthesia providers have opted for less invasive means to assess hemodynamic measurements (e.g., FloTrac sensor). Part of the rationale for this change in practice relates to insufficient evidence demonstrating mortality benefit from use of the PAC[41] as well as published cardiovascular management guidelines that advise against the use of PACs in patients who undergo noncardiac surgery.[42]

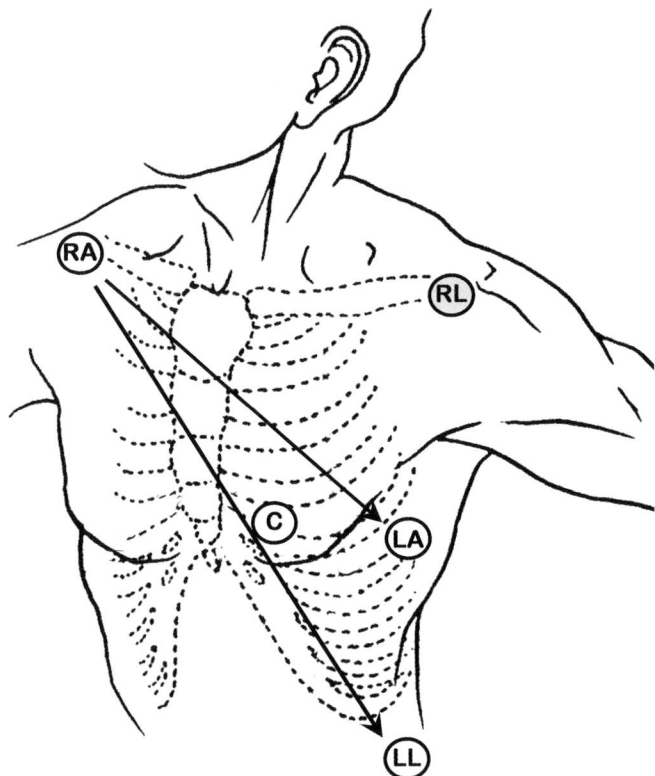

Fig. 17.9 Preoperative electrocardiogram (ECG) configured with a five-cable ECG system to continuously display limb lead II (right arm [RA] negative and left leg [LL] positive), true V_3 chest lead (C), and modified chest lead 5 (MCL$_5$, i.e., central subclavicular 5 [CS$_5$]). V_3 electrode placement (C): equal distance between V_2 and V_4. Lead selector switch set to display lead I causes the RA electrode to become negative and the left arm (LA) electrode (placed in the V_5 position) to become positive (CS$_5$). (Reprinted with permission from Kossick MA. *EKG Interpretation: Simple, Thorough, Practical.* 3rd ed. Park Ridge, IL: AANA Publishing.)

The literature is clear in regard to numerous challenges health care providers face in accurately interpreting data derived from PACs and central venous lines.[43] Cardinal concepts that relate to critical assessment of hemodynamic data will be reviewed in this section of the clinical monitoring chapter.

Practice guidelines for PAC use have been recommended and established by various professional societies.[44] It is also recognized that the competency of health care providers to manage central venous and arterial hemodynamic parameters can vary significantly. In one study, attending physicians from the departments of medicine, surgery, and anesthesia were unable to demonstrate the basic skill of correctly determining the pulmonary artery occlusive pressure (PAOP) from a clear tracing and applying PAC data for proper patient treatment.[45] Research with anesthesiologists who specialize in cardiovascular anesthesia care also demonstrated cognitive deficits with the use of the PAC (e.g., 39% of cardiovascular anesthesiologists could not correctly interpret a PAOP waveform).[46] Results from these two studies suggest that the understanding of PAC data among health care providers is extremely variable, and misinterpretation of PAC data may result in increased morbidity and mortality. It is likely that similar deficiencies in the application and interpretation of PAC data exist for advanced practice nurses (including certified registered nurse anesthetists [CRNAs]), knowing failing scores were noted on competency tests used to assess other areas of critical care.[35] Such research findings have caused several groups to develop guidelines for the indications of a PAC, along with competency requirements for interpretation of data.[44,47]

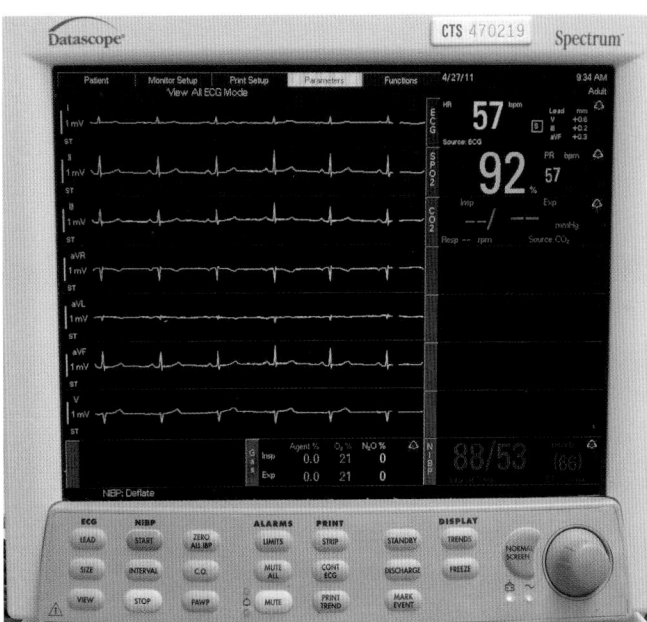

Fig. 17.10 Multilead electrocardiogram (ECG) displayed in the operating room. ECG leads displayed include limb leads I, II, III, aVR, aVL, aVF, and true chest lead V_3. This configuration permits a more comprehensive view of cardiac anatomy. (Reprinted with permission from Kossick MA. *EKG Interpretation: Simple, Thorough, Practical.* 3rd ed. Park Ridge, IL: AANA Publishing.)

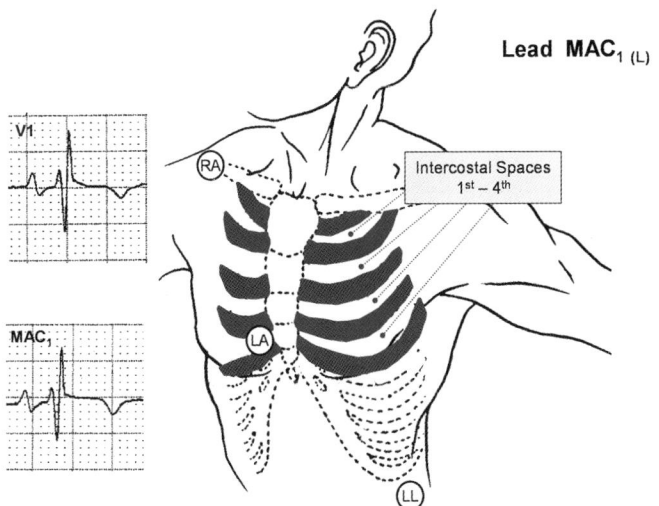

Fig. 17.11 Modified augmented chest lead V_1 (MAC$_{1 [L]}$). It is configured by (1) using limb lead aVL, which causes the left arm (LA) electrode to become positive, and (2) placing the LA electrode in the V_1 position. The remaining electrocardiogram electrodes are placed in their normal positions. The two single cardiac cycles shown above illustrate great similarity in cardiac cycle morphology (rSR$_1$) between V_1 and MAC$_{1(L)}$. (Modified and reprinted with permission from Kossick MA. *Evaluation of a New Modified Chest Lead in Diagnosing Wide Complex Beats of Unknown Origin.* Dissertation. Memphis, TN: The University of Tennessee Health Science Center; 2003:2, 9.)

Physiology and Morphology of Hemodynamic Waveforms

Essential to accurate interpretation of hemodynamic data derived from central venous lines is a solid foundation in what constitutes "normal" distances, pressures, and waveform morphology for central venous pressure (CVP), right ventricular (RV), PA, and PAOP recordings.

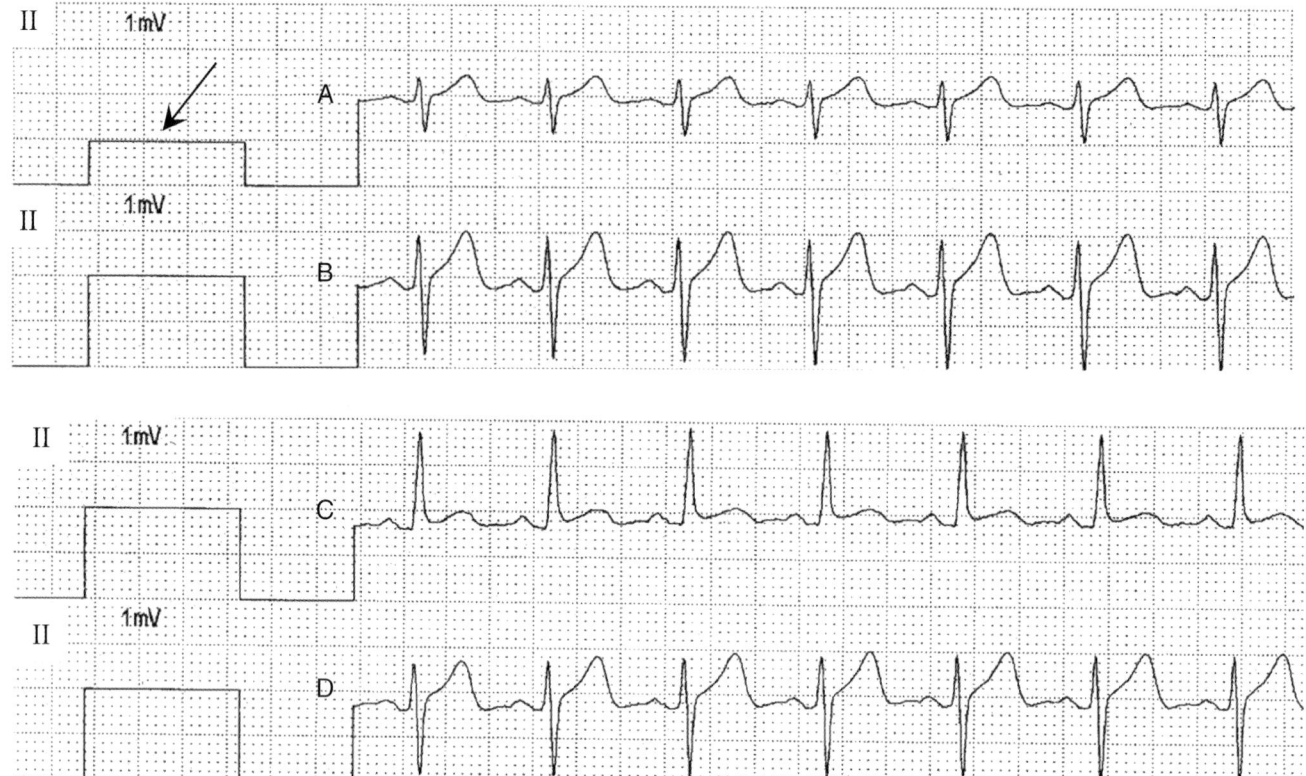

Fig. 17.12 Series of electrocardiographic (ECG) recordings illustrating how the gain setting and incorrect ECG electrode placement can lead to misinterpretation of ST segment changes. In strip *A*, the gain setting *(arrow)* on the ECG monitor has been set at half standardization (1 mV = 5 mm); it grossly gives the appearance of a minor ST segment change. When concurrent strip *B* is compared with strip *A*, it becomes apparent that use of smaller gain settings can mask ST segment deviation. Therefore, if a 0.5-mm ST-segment deviation in ECG strip *A* were to occur, it would equate with a 1-mm change. A similar error in assessment of ST segment changes can occur secondary to misplaced ECG electrodes. ECG strip recording *C* has all limb lead electrodes properly placed and displays an ST segment elevation of approximately 0.75 mm. In contrast, ECG rhythm strip *D* mistakenly has the left leg electrode placed in the second intercostal space, midclavicular line, and therefore is not representative of a lead II. The end result is an ST segment that is falsely elevated (approximately 1.5 mm), suggesting inferior transmural myocardial injury. (Reprinted with permission from Kossick MA. *EKG Interpretation: Simple, Thorough, Practical.* 2nd ed. Park Ridge, IL: AANA Publishing; 1999:26-27.)

TABLE 17.3   Distance to the Junction of the Venae Cavae and Right Atrium From Various Distal Anatomic Sites

Location	Distance (cm)
Subclavian	10
Right internal jugular vein	15
Left internal jugular vein	20
Femoral vein	40
Right median basilic vein	40
Left median basilic vein	50

TABLE 17.4   Distance From the Right Internal Jugular Vein to Distal Cardiac and Pulmonary Structures

Location or Structure	Distance (cm)
Junction venae cavae and right atrium	15
Right atrium	15–25
Right ventricle	25–35
Pulmonary artery	35–45
Pulmonary artery wedge position	40–50

Table 17.3 illustrates the approximate distances for reaching the junction of the venae cavae and the right atrium (RA) from various distal anatomic sites. Table 17.4 lists the anticipated distances for reaching various cardiac and pulmonary structures from the right internal jugular vein. Advancement of a catheter 10 cm beyond these distances without the production of a characteristic waveform could indicate coiling of the central line. If this problem arises with a PAC, the balloon should be deflated and the catheter withdrawn. If any resistance is met during

withdrawal, a chest radiograph should be taken to rule out knotting or entanglement with the chordae tendineae.

Right Atrial Pressure Waveform

Familiarity with the anticipated distances of relevant hemodynamic anatomy, normal intracardiac pressures, pulmonary pressures (Table 17.5), and waveform morphology facilitates accurate interpretation of PAC data and placement of central lines. For example, under normal circumstances, a CVP tracing will generate mean RA pressures in the range of 1 to 10 mm Hg. The fidelity of the transducing system determines if discernible *a*, *c*, and *v* waves will be displayed once the distal tip of a central line lies just above the junction of the venae cavae and the RA (Fig. 17.13). The *a* wave is produced by contraction of the RA, the *c* wave by closure of the tricuspid valve, and the *v* wave by passive filling of the RA (which encompasses a portion of RV systole). The reason the *a* wave is commonly larger than the *c* wave is based on the position of the catheter relative to the physiologic event responsible for the pressure change. In essence, RA systole and the subsequent increase in atrial pressure is detected by a catheter positioned just above (or inappropriately within) the RA, whereas RV systole (a more distal physiologic event relative to the position of a CVP catheter) indirectly increases RA pressure by closure of the tricuspid valve.

TABLE 17.5 Normal Intracardiac and Pulmonary Pressures

Location	Absolute Value (mm Hg)	Range (mm Hg)
MRAP	5	1–10
RV	25/5*	15–30/0–8
PA S/D	25/10*	15–30/5–15
MPAP	15	10–20
PAOP	10	5–15
MLAP	8	4–12
LVEDP	8	4–12

LVEDP, Left ventricular end-diastolic pressure; *MLAP*, mean left atrial pressure; *MPAP*, mean pulmonary artery pressure; *MRAP*, mean right atrial pressure; *PA*, pulmonary artery; *PAOP*, pulmonary artery occlusive pressure; *RV*, right ventricular; *S/D*, systolic/diastolic.
*Values are systolic pressure/diastolic pressure.

Right Ventricular Pressure Waveform

Further advancement of a PAC (~10 cm) produces dramatic changes in the morphology of the hemodynamic waveform. As shown in Fig. 17.14, a brisk upstroke (isovolumetric contraction and rapid ejection [RV systole]) and steep downslope (reduced ejection and isovolumetric relaxation [RV systole and diastole]) are viewed on an oscilloscope when a PAC is advanced through the right intraventricular cavity. A PAC with the distal balloon inflated should remain in the RV for as short a time as possible to reduce the incidence of ventricular ectopy or the development of a conduction defect such as right bundle branch block. Because it is undesirable to leave the tip of a central line in the RV, pressures generated during RV systole and RV diastole are assessed indirectly via the CVP port of a PAC and distal tip of the PAC. The former is used to estimate RV end-diastolic pressure (EDP) and the latter RV systolic pressure via the PA systolic recording. Thus RVEDP is used to estimate RVED volume (RVEDV), which approximates RV preload (and, less accurately, LV preload).

Pulmonary Artery Pressure Waveform

When a catheter enters the PA, the diastolic pressure is acutely increased with little change in systolic pressure. The upstroke of the PA tracing is produced by opening of the pulmonic valve, followed by RV ejection. The downstroke contains the dicrotic notch, which is produced by sudden closure of the pulmonic valve leaflets (the beginning of diastole).

Pulmonary Artery Occlusive Pressure Waveform

Final advancement of a PAC by 5 to 10 cm should produce a PAOP tracing. This waveform is similar to a CVP (the *a* wave is produced by left atrial [LA] systole, the *c* wave by closure of the mitral valve, and the *v* wave by filling of the LA, as well as upward displacement of the mitral valve during left ventricular [LV] systole), except that the

1st Cardiac Cycle   3rd Cardiac Cycle

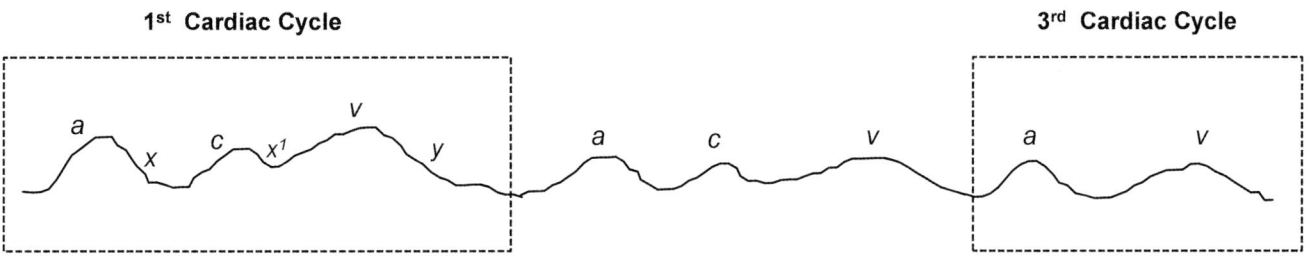

Fig. 17.13 Positive and negative waveforms of a central venous pressure tracing. The third cardiac cycle in this figure does not produce a *c* wave.

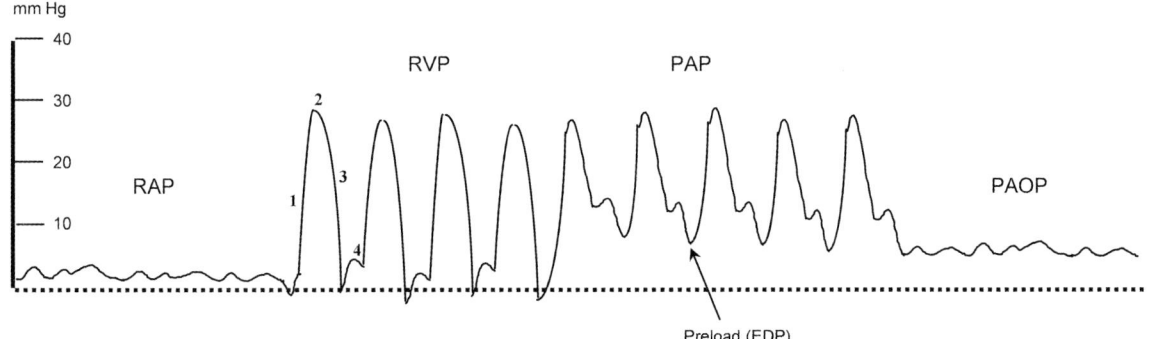

Fig. 17.14 Pressure waveforms during positioning of a pulmonary artery catheter (PAC). *EDP*, End-diastolic pressure; *PAOP*, pulmonary artery occlusive pressure; *PAP*, pulmonary artery pressure; *RAP*, right atrial pressure; *RVP*, right ventricular pressure. *1*, Isovolumetric contraction (ascent of pressure waveform); *2*, rapid ejection; *3*, isovolumetric relaxation (mid-descent of pressure waveform); *4*, atrial systole (slight increase in pressure).

pressure values are somewhat greater. In addition, it is less common to detect a *c* wave on a PAOP tracing because retrograde transmission of LA pressure (produced by closure of the mitral valve) is significantly attenuated within the pulmonary circulation. The characteristic waveform morphologies of a PAOP tracing are shown in Fig. 17.14.

Negative Waveforms

The descents that follow the *a*, *c*, and *v* waves of a CVP or PAOP tracing are labeled as *x*, x^1, and *y* (see Fig. 17.13). The *x* descent corresponds to the start of atrial diastole (its terminal component [just before the upstroke of the *c* wave (or in its absence, the *v* wave)] with RVEDP and LVEDP), the x^1 descent is produced by downward pulling of the septum during ventricular systole, and the *y* descent corresponds to opening of the tricuspid valve.

Correlation of Pressure Waveforms and the Electrocardiogram

The interpretation of hemodynamic waveforms can be facilitated by correlating their morphology and timeline with the ECG. The *a* wave of a CVP tracing, which is produced by atrial contraction, will follow depolarization of the atria (P wave on the ECG). The *c* and *v* waves occur after the beginning of ventricular depolarization (QRS complex), or the *v* wave may not appear until shortly after the T wave (Figs. 17.15 and 17.16). When compared with the CVP tracing, the PAOP recording shows greater hysteresis between the waveforms of the ECG and the display of *a*, *c*, and *v* waves—meaning there is a greater distance between ECG activity and the subsequent pressure waveform. Identification of abnormal waveforms is greatly facilitated by the use of the ECG; for example, without an ECG recording, large positive waveforms on a PAOP tracing can be diagnosed as either cannon *a* waves or large *v* waves.

Distortion of Pressure Waveforms

Arrhythmias can produce significant alterations in hemodynamic waveforms. Atrial fibrillation, junctional rhythms, and premature ventricular contractions (PVCs) can alter the shape of *a* waves. With atrial fibrillation, no synchronized atrial contraction occurs. In the CVP or PAOP tracing, this can lead to the loss of *a* waves or the appearance of small fibrillatory *a* waves. Complete atrioventricular block and some forms of junctional arrhythmias cause the atria to contract against a closed tricuspid valve, which can produce large cannon *a* waves (Fig. 17.17). Ventricular pacing can be associated with both the presence of cannon *a* waves and loss of *a* waves. The former occurs if a patient does not have an atrioventricular sequential pacemaker; the latter when ventricular pacing is used in the setting of asystole (neither atrial nor ventricular depolarization is occurring). Valvular defects can also produce dramatic changes in the CVP and PAOP tracings, causing an increase in the amplitude of the *v* wave secondary to regurgitation (e.g., with mitral regurgitation a portion of the stroke volume (SV) is ejected retrograde into the pulmonary circuit, owing to an incompetent mitral valve). Recognition of such abnormalities is critical for accurate recording of pressure measurements and proper placement of central lines. Significant tricuspid regurgitation can cause a CVP recording to mimic an RV tracing, and mitral regurgitation can lead to a PAOP recording to appear as a PA tracing. Specifically, large *v* waves become superimposed on *a* waves. For the indistinguishable PA and PAOP recording, analysis of an SvO$_2$ blood sample can assist in making a differential diagnosis. The saturation will be elevated (>77%) if the catheter is in a wedged position, assuming the distal tip is not in a region of the lung that is atelectatic, which in contrast would produce a false-negative result (normal or low SvO$_2$). As a precautionary measure, a catheter suspected of being in a wedged position should not be

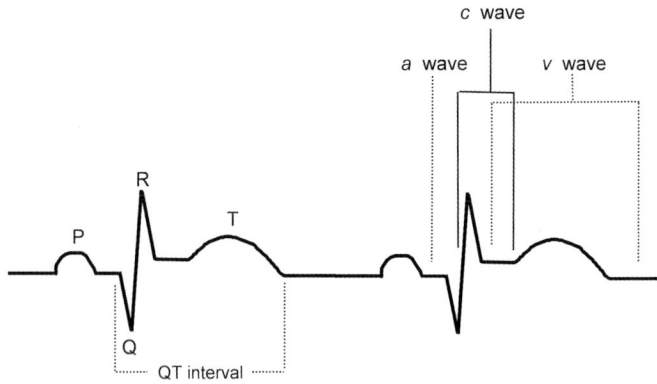

Fig. 17.15 Temporal relationship between the electrocardiogram and hemodynamic waveforms.

flushed with the fluid contained in the pressurized transducing system. Although the overall incidence of PA rupture is low (0.064%),[48] flushing of a wedged catheter (as well as balloon overinflation) can result in vascular damage ranging from minor endobronchial hemorrhage to massive hemoptysis.

Significant tricuspid regurgitation and mitral regurgitation may also be associated with normal CVP and PAOP tracings.[49] These occur in patients with a low volume status and compliant atria. In addition, a poor correlation has been found between the size of the *v* wave and the degree of regurgitation. Also of interest is the finding that large *v* waves can be observed in the absence of significant regurgitation. This phenomenon can occur whenever an acute increase in preload occurs, which dynamically reduces atrial and pulmonary vascular compliance.[49]

Whenever large *v* waves are detected on a CVP or PAOP tracing, estimates of preload should be measured just before the upstroke of the *v* wave (or *c* wave when present). This point on the pressure recording equates with the EDP, the moment just before ventricular systole that ultimately produces the large *v* waves. Box 17.1 indicates how various rhythm disturbances, pacing, and valvular defects can distort the CVP tracing.

Implications of Hemodynamic Values

Prior to implementing clinical interventions based on hemodynamic data, it is important for anesthesia providers to assess a patient's clinical condition relative to both current and past medical and surgical histories. This assessment process will assist in establishing "personalized hemodynamic values," which allows the hemodynamic data to be interpreted and managed relative to known pathophysiologic conditions that can skew normal hemodynamic parameters.[50,51] For example, a patient with acute LV myocardial ischemia will have a reduction in LV compliance. This change will result in an overestimation of left ventricular end-diastolic volume (LVEDV [suggesting volume overload]) via a recorded pulmonary artery diastolic pressure (PADP). This illustrates the importance of a comprehensive assessment process to avoid a one-size-fits-all paradigm in the management of "abnormal" hemodynamic values, which could lead to patient harm.

In addition, it is understandable that appropriate interventions can at times be implemented secondary to isolated/individual PAC values. However, the literature also recognizes that trends in hemodynamic values may be of greater significance in determining the best clinical interventions when correlated with other clinical markers.[52] It is also essential that anesthesia providers ensure that monitoring equipment used to measure hemodynamic values is correctly calibrated and positioned. For example, transducers should be zeroed and positioned

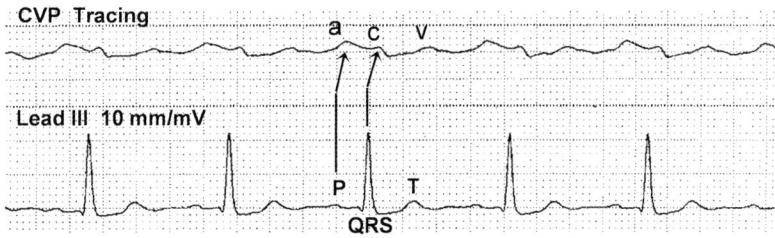

Fig. 17.16 Electrocardiographic recording with a concurrent central venous pressure tracing that demonstrates hysteresis between atrial depolarization (P wave) and the production of an *a* wave, as well as the QRS complex and the associated *c* and *v* waves.

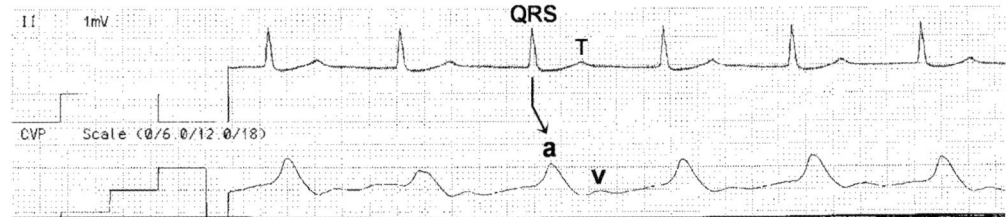

Fig. 17.17 Electrocardiographic recording of a junctional rhythm *(top)* in which there is simultaneous retrograde atrial and antegrade ventricular depolarization (as evidenced by the lack of a P wave in each cardiac cycle). This results in the right atrium contracting against a closed tricuspid valve. As a consequence, the central venous pressure *(CVP)* tracing *(bottom)* has cannon *a* waves.

BOX 17.1   Factors That Can Distort Central Venous Pressure and Pulmonary Artery Occlusive Pressure Tracings

Loss of *a* Waves or Only *v* Waves
- Atrial fibrillation
- Ventricular pacing in the setting of asystole

Giant *a* Waves—"Cannon" *a* Waves
- Junctional rhythms
- Complete AV block
- PVCs (simultaneous atrial and ventricular contraction)
- Ventricular pacing (asynchronous)
- Tricuspid or mitral stenosis
- Diastolic dysfunction
- Myocardial ischemia
- Ventricular hypertrophy

Large *v* Waves
- Tricuspid or mitral regurgitation
- Acute ↑ in intravascular volume

↑, Increase; *AV*, atrioventricular; *PVCs*, premature ventricular contractions.

---

appropriately to the respective anatomy (phlebostatic axis), and the recording of PAC pressure values should be taken at end expiration. This section will discuss potential causes and implications of different hemodynamic values.

PRELOAD ASSESSMENT: STATIC AND DYNAMIC INDICES

Central Venous Pressure

The CVP serves as a measurement of pressure in the superior vena cava and may provide an indirect estimate of preload, RA pressure and

RVEDV, and overall RV function.[53,54] The numeric value of the CVP is influenced by multiple factors, including total blood volume, central venous vascular compliance/tone, intrathoracic and intraabdominal pressures, V/Q abnormalities of the lung, ventilator settings (e.g., application of positive end-expiratory pressure [PEEP]), orthostasis, changes in cardiac compliance, cardiac output (CO), and valvular deficiencies.[55-57] Table 17.6 lists the causes of elevated and depressed CVP.

The CVP has long been used to assess and manage a patient's intravascular volume status. It is regarded as a method to determine preload; however, its ability to accurately predict fluid responsiveness (an increase in CO or SV following a preload challenge) has been questioned by many researchers.[53,54,58] Marik et al. compiled a comprehensive, landmark meta-analysis that reviewed 43 studies and a total of 1802 patients who received fluid responsiveness maneuvers. Their meta-analysis found CVP measurements are unable to accurately measure fluid responsiveness due to the curvilinear shape of the ventricular pressure-volume curve. The curve not only shows a poor relationship between ventricular filling pressure and ventricular volume but also that the curve is disrupted by diastolic dysfunction or diminished ventricular compliance.[53] Nevertheless, the CVP is an especially important tool in certain clinical situations. For example, a high CVP value is associated with acute kidney injury and increased mortality rates. It is also a requirement to calculate systemic vascular resistance (SVR), an invaluable estimate of the pressure gradient for organ perfusion.[55,59]

Stroke Volume Variation and Pulse Pressure Variation

As a replacement for static measurements of preload responsiveness, some studies have recommended intravascular fluid management be based on dynamic preload indices such as stroke volume variation (SVV) and pulse pressure variation (PPV) via minimally invasive monitoring devices.[52,60,61] Static preload indices such as CVP, PAOP, and global end-diastolic volume (GEDV) are dependent on the individual shape of a patient's Frank-Starling curve as well as a ventricular compliance curve (Fig. 17.18).[59] Therefore, at any given time, these indices may or may not reflect a patient's true preload value and/or

TABLE 17.6   Potential Causes of Elevated Central Venous Pressure, Pulmonary Artery Pressure, and Pulmonary Artery Occlusive Pressure

CVP	PAP	PAOP
• RV failure	• LV failure	• LV failure
• Tricuspid stenosis or regurgitation	• Mitral stenosis or regurgitation	• Mitral stenosis or regurgitation
• Cardiac tamponade	• L-to-R shunt	• Cardiac tamponade
• Constrictive pericarditis	• ASD or VSD	• Constrictive pericarditis
• Volume overload	• Volume overload	• Volume overload
• Pulmonary HTN	• Pulmonary HTN	• Ischemia
• LV failure (chronic)	• "Catheter whip"	

ASD, Atrial septal defect; *CVP*, central venous pressure; *HTN*, hypertension; *L*, left; *LV*, left ventricular; *PAOP*, pulmonary artery occlusive pressure; *PAP*, pulmonary artery pressure; *R*, right; *RV*, right ventricular; *VSD*, ventricular septal defect.

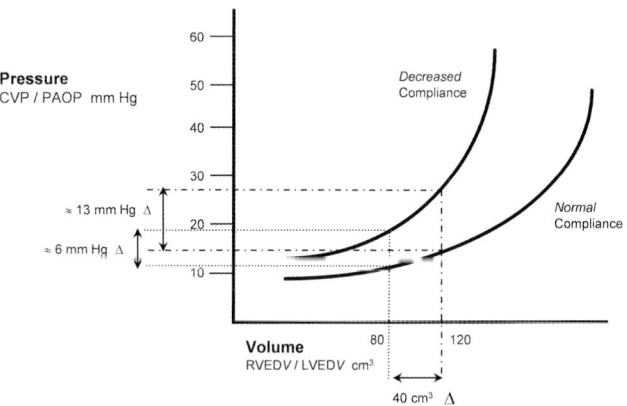

Fig. 17.18 Effect of changes in ventricular compliance on CVP (which estimates RVEDP) and PAOP (which estimates LVEDP). The curve with *decreased compliance* distorts the relationship between pressure values and estimated ventricular volume. A preload of 80 cm^3 in a compliant versus noncompliant ventricle generates a pressure difference of ≈ 6 mm Hg *(flat portion of each curve)*. On the steeper portion of both curves, the relationship between volume and pressure is skewed even more dramatically. A preload of 120 cm^3 generates a pressure difference of ≈ 13 mm Hg, which can ultimately lead to a gross overestimation of ventricular preload. Δ, Change; *CVP*, central venous pressure; *LVEDP*, left ventricular end-diastolic pressure; *LVEDV*, left ventricular end-diastolic volume; *PAOP*, pulmonary artery occlusive pressure; *RVEDP*, right ventricular end-diastolic pressure; *RVEDV*, right ventricular end-diastolic volume.

responsiveness; changes in either Frank-Starling curves or ventricular compliance curves can occur secondary to numerous variables such as pharmacologic interventions and/or pathophysiology.[59] Therefore it is recommended that dynamic preload values be used instead of static preload values when evaluating and assessing a patient's fluid responsiveness.[59]

Foundational to these recommendations is recognition of cardinal physiologic concepts; changes in SV[62] and PP (PP = Systolic blood pressure [SBP] – Diastolic blood pressure [DBP])[63] are affected by the relationship shared between the cardiovascular and respiratory

systems. With respirations, cardiac output dynamically changes.[60,64] Dynamic indices (e.g., SVV, PPV, inferior vena cava diameter variations, response to passive leg raising [PLR], end-expiratory occlusion tests) can be used to evaluate a patient's response to changes in preload. For example, a provider can assess preload responsiveness by monitoring the SVV after infusing a small bolus of fluid; if less SVV occurs after the infusion is complete (e.g., a change from 17% to 15%), then the reduction in SVV can represent a patient who will respond/require further preload augmentation.[59]

Current methods of evaluating SVV and PPV were developed after a 1987 study that evaluated the relationship between systolic pressure variation (SPV) and hypovolemia in dogs.[65] Due to the dynamic variations that occur within the cardiopulmonary system during respiration, certain criteria must be met for SVV and PPV measurements to be accurate: Patients must be mechanically ventilated with at least a 7- to 8-mL/kg tidal volume with no spontaneous respiratory effort, and patients must be in normal sinus rhythm. Other variables that can affect SVV and PVV values (and must be taken into consideration before applying such hemodynamic data) include fluctuations in exogenous catecholamine dependence/administration, abnormal intraabdominal pressures (e.g., ascites, laparoscopic insufflation, open abdomen), and decreased chest wall compliance.[59,61,64,66-73] SVV variability and/or PPV can be monitored using several Food and Drug Administration–approved minimally invasive devices. These devices include PiCCO Plus (Pulsion Medical Systems), LiDCO Plus and LiDCO Rapid (LiDCO Group Plc), and FloTrac [Edwards Lifesciences].[61]

Research has revealed that preanesthetic SVV is significantly correlated with a decrease in cardiac output during anesthesia induction; studies have found that patients with lower preanesthetic SVV had a lower incidence and significantly slower onset of decreased CO than those with higher SVV values[60] and that SVV is a reliable diagnostic tool when evaluating patients' fluid responsiveness in both the operating room and intensive care settings.[71-76] In mechanically ventilated patients, the range for normal SVV is 10% to 13%.[77] Values higher than 12% to 13% imply patients will respond positively to an increase in preload.[59,72]

Multiple studies have shown PPV has high specificity and sensitivity when determining fluid responsiveness; patients who exhibit PPV values of greater than 12% are likely to be responsive to fluid resuscitation.[67,70] A PPV range of 10% to 15% has been recommended as a goal to avoid excessive as well as insufficient fluid administration, as both can be associated with deleterious patient outcomes.[77] Furthermore, the 2016 Surviving Sepsis Campaign now recommends using dynamic preload indices such as PPV to guide fluid administration.[77,78] Some research states that PPV is associated with greater accuracy for predicting fluid responsiveness than SVV and to be more cost effective since it requires only an arterial catheter.[67,79,80] The use of hemodynamic indices such as SVV and PPV for predicting fluid responsiveness are an evolving trend in patient care[77]; further studies will be needed to better understand the application of these indices in the management of differing patient populations and conditions.[52,77,81-83]

Pulmonary Artery/Pulmonary Artery Occlusion Pressures

Like the RV waveform, the PA tracing occurs within the QT interval of the ECG. LVEDP can be estimated by measuring the pressure value that exists just prior to the upstroke of the PA waveform (see Fig. 17.14). When properly used, the PAOP recording has the potential to improve the clinician's ability to make a differential diagnosis in critically ill patients. Like the CVP, LVEDP and PAOP indirectly assesses ventricular function and therefore have distinct limitations. To ensure that accurate pressure recordings are documented, the mean or diastolic pressure should always be determined at end expiration (whether the patient is spontaneously breathing or receiving PPV). This is the time when pleural pressures are approximately equal to atmospheric pressures (except when PEEP is being used). The rationale for this timing relates to the fact that vascular pressure recordings are calibrated relative to atmospheric pressure. As stated previously, the correct area on the pressure recording to determine preload (e.g., LVEDP) is just before the upstroke of the *v* wave (or *c* wave, if present). Causes of an elevated PAOP are listed in Table 17.6. A false high value can also be produced by a phenomenon called catheter whip, which is exaggerated oscillation of the PA tracing. This can occur with excessive catheter coiling if the tip of the PA catheter is near the pulmonic valve; it also occurs in patients with dilated pulmonary arteries and/or pulmonary hypertension.

Variables That Influence Hemodynamic Measurements

Recognizing how numerous variables can skew displayed pressure values is essential for proper management of hemodynamic parameters. Most of the data obtained from a PAC allows only for indirect assessment of cardiovascular function and pulmonary indices. For example, PADP approximates PAOP, which approximates LA pressure, which approximates LVEDP, which provides an estimate of LVEDV. Table 17.7 lists clinical factors that can skew these pressure and volume relationships. Obviously, reliance on indirect pressure measurements mandates that the anesthetist understand how to interpret these data in light of such limitations. For most patients who require a PAC or CVP, it should be assumed that several, if not numerous, pathophysiologic states exist (e.g., cardiovascular disease, pulmonary dysfunction) that will potentially skew the pressure-to-pressure and pressure-to-volume relationships. Of the variables listed in Table 17.7, several require further discussion. Many of the factors listed can be viewed as disruptions or obstructions of the continuous column of blood that exists between the right atrium and left ventricle. This is the case for valvular defects and pulmonary factors.

The goal for placement of a PAC is to have it reside in a West zone III[84] of the lung; this usually does occur because the bulk of pulmonary blood flow lies within this physiologically defined region of the lung. In this position, the pulmonary artery pressure (PAP) is greater than the pulmonary venous pressure (PVP), which is greater than the AP. This zone corresponds to a complete circuit or conduit that allows for direct communication between right-sided heart and pulmonary pressures with left-sided intraventricular pressures (Fig. 17.19). It is important to recall that each of the lung zones is physiologically—not anatomically—defined; thus a zone III can change into a zone II (PAP > AP > PVP) or a zone I (AP > PAP > PVP), which is also known as a no-flow zone.

Factors that contribute to the dynamic state of zone III include the application of PEEP (see Fig. 17.19), significant diuresis, acute respiratory distress syndrome (ARDS),[85] hemorrhage, and a change in patient position (e.g., supine to sitting or lateral decubitus, dependent lung status). The influence of PEEP is contingent on the quantity applied, intravascular volume status, and pulmonary compliance. Normally, less than 50% of PEEP is transmitted to the microvasculature—even less if pulmonary compliance is poor (e.g., patients with ARDS).[86] In contrast, patients with decreased volume status (e.g., left atrial pressure [LAP] <5 mm Hg) who receive PEEP as low as 7.5 cm H_2O can have collapse of the pulmonary capillaries, which distorts the PAOP.[87] A PAC located in zone I or II will produce marked variations in the PAOP waveform recording during the ventilatory cycle. In addition, *a* and *v* waves (cardiac influences) are lost, and the PAOP exceeds the PADP. This is in contrast to a PAOP recording produced by a catheter located in a true wedge position in a zone III. The distinguishing

TABLE 17.7	Factors That Alter the Relationships Among Central Cardiovascular Pressures and Volumes
CVP ≠ PADP	• Change in RV compliance (e.g., PS) • Tricuspid valve disease
PADP ≠ PAOP	• Pulmonary HTN • MR or AR • Lung zone I or II • Tachycardia • ARDS • RBBB
PAOP ≠ MLAP	• Juxtacardiac pressure (e.g., PEEP) • Lung zone I or II • Mediastinal fibrosis • RBBB
MLAP ≠ LVEDP	• Juxtacardiac pressure (e.g., PEEP) • Mitral valve disease • Change in LV compliance (e.g., AS)
LVEDP ≠ LVEDV	• Juxtacardiac pressure (PEEP) • Ventricular interdependence • Change in LV compliance (e.g., ischemia)

AR, Aortic regurgitation; *ARDS,* acute respiratory distress syndrome; *AS,* aortic stenosis; *CVP,* central venous pressure; *HTN,* hypertension; *LVEDP,* left ventricular end-diastolic pressure; *LVEDV,* left ventricular end-diastolic volume; *MLAP,* mean left atrial pressure; *MR,* mitral regurgitation; *PADP,* pulmonary artery diastolic pressure; *PAOP,* pulmonary artery occlusive pressure; *PEEP,* positive end-expiratory pressure; *PS,* pulmonic stenosis; *PVR,* pulmonary artery vascular resistance; *RBBB,* right bundle branch block; *RV,* right ventricular.

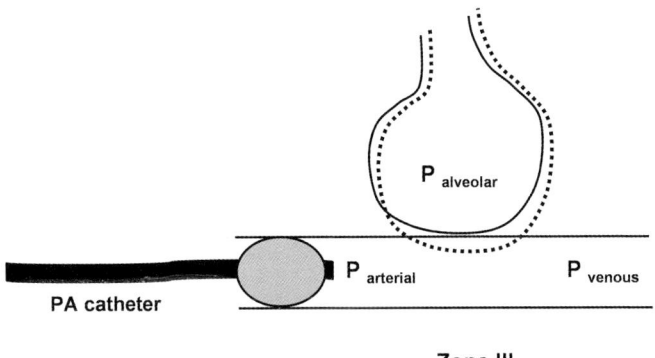

Zone III

$$P_a > P_v > P_A$$

Fig. 17.19 Pulmonary artery catheter with balloon inflated (wedging) in a West lung zone III. In this zone, pulmonary pressures equilibrate during diastole because both arterial and venous pulmonary pressures are greater than alveolar pressures. The addition of positive end-expiratory pressure *(dashed-line alveolus)* or hypovolemia can convert a zone III to a zone I or II and lead to distended alveoli and inaccurate estimates of pressures distal to the invagination. P_a, Arterial pressure; P_A, alveolar pressure; P_v, venous pressure; *PA,* pulmonary artery.

criteria include the development of a characteristic waveform with balloon inflation and a PAOP reading less than or equal to the PADP. The latter criterion assumes that no valvular defect is present, which could also cause the mean PAOP to exceed the PADP.

A rapid heart rate (HR) can also skew the relationship between PADP and the PAOP. Research has demonstrated that LA-paced induced tachycardia (increased HR from 74 to 124 beats per minute)

TABLE 17.8   Potential Clinical Diagnosis via the Use of Hemodynamic Values: Interpretation of Pulmonary Artery Catheter Data

CVP	PADP	PAOP	Interpretation
Low	Low	Low	Hypovolemia, transducer not at phlebostatic axis*
Normal or high	High	High	LV failure
High	Normal or low	Normal or low	RV failure, TR, or TS
High	High	Normal or low	Pulmonary embolism
High	High	Normal	Pulmonary HTN
High	High	High	Cardiac tamponade, ventricular interdependence, transducer not at phlebostatic axis*
Normal	Normal or high	High	LV myocardial ischemia or MR
Low	High	Normal	ARDS†

*Phlebostatic axis is the fourth intercostal space, midanteroposterior level (not midaxillary line); for the right lateral decubitus position, fourth intercostal space midsternum; for the left lateral decubitus position, fourth intercostal space at the left parasternal border.
†ARDS patients commonly require initial fluid administration for hemodynamic stability.
ARDS, Acute respiratory distress syndrome; *CVP*, central venous pressure; *HTN*, hypertension; *LV*, left ventricular; *MR*, mitral regurgitation; *PADP*, pulmonary artery diastolic pressure; *PAOP*, pulmonary artery occlusive pressure; *RV*, right ventricular; *TR*, tricuspid regurgitation; *TS*, tricuspid stenosis.

can produce an 11 mm Hg gradient between the PADP and LVEDP.[88] The increase in PADP and decrease in LVEDP result from the shortening of diastole, which reduces the amount of blood being transported from the pulmonary circulation to the left ventricle.[89] Also, as HR increases, the left atrium begins to contract against a partially closed mitral valve.[90]

Another variable that significantly influences PAC data is a change in ventricular compliance. To illustrate this point, consider the fact that a high PAOP (or LVEDP) can exist in patients with an elevated preload with normal ventricular compliance, as well as in patients with a low preload with poor ventricular compliance. A patient with reduced ventricular compliance (e.g., myocardial ischemia, LV hypertrophy, cardiac tamponade, or ventricular interdependence) has a high PAOP or PADP that results in overestimation of LVEDV (see Fig. 17.19) and underestimation of LVEDP. In the setting of poor compliance, PAOP is not a reliable index for LVEDV.[90] In fact, it has been shown that during myocardial revascularization procedures, high PAOP values exist more than 50% of the time in conjunction with a low volume status (as determined by echocardiography), with patients responding favorably (despite a high PAOP) to an increase in intravascular volume.[91]

To summarize, the PADP correlates poorly (by ≥5 mm Hg) with the PAOP under the following circumstances: when pulmonary vascular resistance (PVR) is elevated (e.g., chronic obstructive pulmonary disease, human papillomavirus, pulmonary embolus, ARDS, hypercarbia), when HRs exceed 130 beats per minute, when severe mitral or aortic regurgitation is present, or when a lung zone III has changed to a zone II or I (e.g., in the presence of hypovolemia, PEEP). Increases in PVR and HR cause the PADP to exceed PAOP. Severe regurgitation and lung zone changes produce the opposite effect, with PADP being less than the PAOP; this may also hold true for right bundle branch block, as one research group found that this conduction defect caused the PADP (in the setting of normal PVR) to be up to 7 mm Hg less than the mean LAP.[92] A review of the gross interpretation of CVP and PAOP values is presented in Table 17.8.

Assessment of Cardiac Output With Advanced Hemodynamic Monitoring

Determination of CO assists health care personnel to provide rational hemodynamic therapy, evaluate the response to such therapy, and determine the adequacy of tissue perfusion, which is linked to maintenance of arterial BP, delivery of oxygen, and removal of wastes. It also permits for the calculation of other hemodynamic indices (e.g., PVR and SVR).

Cardiac index (CI) is another hemodynamic parameter used by some practitioners as an alternative to CO; the premise for its use is to adjust CO values to accommodate for the patient's height and weight. Although this value is individualized by its indexing to the patient's body surface area (BSA), it should be understood that CI does not account for the lack of uniformity of predicted basal oxygen consumption and metabolic rates resulting from differences in sex, age, or changes in clinical status (e.g., declines with anesthesia and increases with hyperthermia). In addition, the relationship between BSA and blood flow is indistinct.[93] CI is calculated by dividing CO by BSA. The plotting of height and weight on a body surface chart estimates the BSA in square meters (Fig. 17.20). Commonly quoted normal values are 5 to 6 L/min for CO and 2.8 to 3.6 L/min • m² for CI.

There are several techniques for evaluation of CO, including both invasive and noninvasive methods. Invasive methods include PAC thermodilution, transpulmonary thermodilution (with or without arterial waveform analysis), and esophageal Doppler monitoring. Noninvasive methods are a newer trend in estimating CO and managing patient care; these methods include noninvasive cardiac output (NICO) via carbon dioxide measurement, magnetic resonance imaging, transesophageal echocardiography, and thoracic impedance.

Thermodilution Cardiac Output Measurement Techniques

The most commonly used technique for determining CO is thermodilution, whereby an analog computer calculates the CO using the modified Stewart-Hamilton equation. This method was first used by Fegler in 1954.[94] The traditional PAC thermodilution technique is still considered a gold standard. It achieves CO measurements through the injection of a known quantity of an indicator solution (most commonly 5% dextrose in water, although 0.9% normal saline has a similar density factor) through the proximal port of a thermodilution PAC.[95]

The injected solution is considered a thermal indicator because it is cold relative to body temperature. It rapidly mixes with the incoming blood and is carried through the RV until it is detected by the thermistor near the end of the catheter in the PA. The computer plots a time-temperature curve, with the area under the curve being inversely

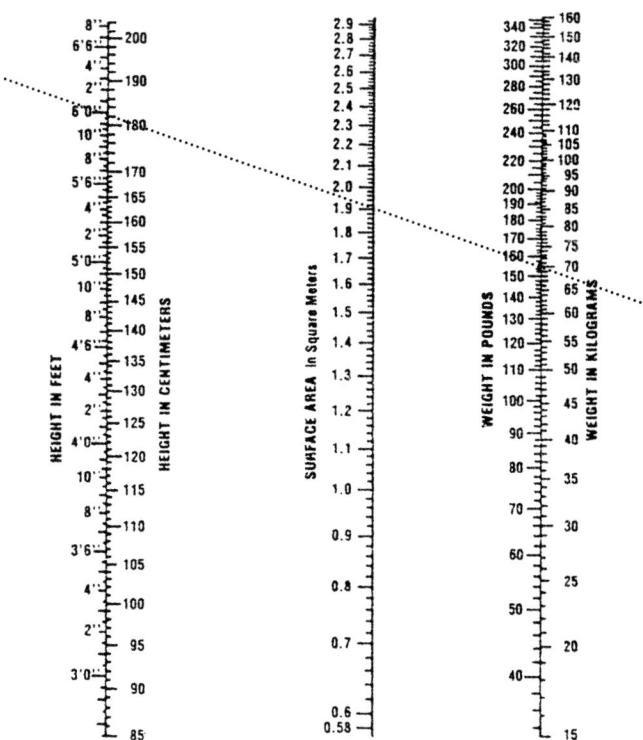

Fig. 17.20 Chart used to calculate body surface area. In this example, a height of 6 feet and a weight of 155 lb translates into a surface area of approximately 1.9 m².

proportional to the CO; therefore larger curves are not desired. Variables that can influence recorded values include the computation constant (which varies with catheter size, injectate volume, and temperature), temperature of the injectate (desired range of 0°–24°C),[96] volume of injection,[96] speed of injection (which should take ≤4 sec),[97] and the timing of injection (it should be consistent [i.e., administered at the same time during each respiratory cycle]).[98] Iced injectates have not been shown to offer any significant advantage over room temperature injectates.[96] In fact, cold indicator solutions injected rapidly into the RA have been shown to produce arrhythmias,[99] including sinus bradycardia.[100] The volume of injectate can significantly affect the CO estimate: too much injectate underestimates CO and too little can cause overestimation of CO.[101] Research that has examined the impact of valvular or septal defects on thermodilution CO (TDCO) values has produced conflicting results, but some studies show tricuspid regurgitation can result in retrograde ejection of injectate back past the valve.[101-104] A list of variables that can skew CO measurements is provided in Table 17.9.

The accuracy for TDCO (including when performed in patients in the lateral position) is ±10%, and the reliability is ±5%.[105] These values are lower in the pediatric population,[106] in patients who have low CO,[107] and for measurements taken in the OR.[108] Anesthetists should be careful not to overinterpret small changes (e.g., 5%–10%) and should never express values beyond one decimal point. The common practice of averaging three CO values has also been shown to improve accuracy and should be taken at end expiration.[109]

A further advancement in CO technology has been achieved via the placement of thermal filaments within the RV portion of the PAC and near the tip of the thermistor (e.g., the Vigilance system [Edwards Lifesciences Corporation] and the OptiQue system [Abbott Labs]). A sophisticated computer algorithm permits for analysis of a thermal signal created by small quantities of heat being emitted from the PAC—a

pulsed warm thermodilution continuous cardiac output (TDCCO) technique. This heat signal is eventually transmitted by the blood to the distal thermistor, which permits for continuous cardiac output (CCO) assessment.[110] An adequate signal-to-noise ratio is necessary to produce accurate and reliable CCO measurements. Research has shown a low ratio (derived from a core body temperature >38.5°C) can result in inaccurate CCO values.[111] One advantage of a CCO catheter is the elimination of the time-consuming administration of a thermal injectate through the proximal port of the PAC. It also reduces the number of discrepancies in thermodilution CO values that can occur with inconsistent injectate administration relative to the respiratory cycle.

A drawback to the CCO device is the hysteresis in recording hemodynamic information. Although the monitor displays updated CO figures every 30 seconds, they nonetheless do not represent real-time data. Instead, the CCO values depict the average CO from the prior 3 to 6 minutes.[112] This can be a significant limitation in patients who develop acute hemodynamic changes occurring in response to hemorrhage and resuscitation.[113] In this setting, a standard bolus thermodilution technique is preferable.

Manufacturers of TDCCO monitors have attempted to circumvent this limitation by developing "Fast-Filter" and "Urgent" modes to supplement the "Normal" mode of data processing. One investigation found a significant decline in the precision of CO measurements when the Fast-Filter and Urgent modes were used.[114] The reliability and accuracy of the device in intensive care and surgical patients have been established with recordings taken in the supine position[111,115] and with the backrest elevated to 45 degrees.[116] Nevertheless, some investigators have found the TDCCO technique to be less precise than bolus thermodilution.[117-120]

In spite of reports in the literature of a positive clinical outcome based on the use of TDCCO,[121,122] future studies will be required to establish whether CCO measurements reduce the length of hospitalization and improve morbidity and mortality rates.[123]

Transpulmonary Thermodilution Cardiac Output Measurement Techniques

Transpulmonary thermodilution (TPTD) is a relatively new, less invasive method of analyzing CO through the tip of a femoral arterial thermistor catheter after an injectate has been administered in the superior vena cava. This measurement, if calibrated with pulse contour analysis, can allow for continuous CO monitoring. Available devices include PiCCO and VolumeView. Like traditional PACs, TPTD also uses the Stewart-Hamilton principle. According to the manufacturer, 15 mL saline below 8°C must be injected through the injection port; a larger volume and cooler temperature are required since the injectate must travel farther than the distance seen with traditional TDCO to reach the thermistor tip (femoral artery).[124]

In addition to CO measurements, TPTD devices are capable of estimating SV, SVR, and SVV along with global end-diastolic volume index (GEDVI), systolic function, and extravascular lung water index (EVLWI).[125,126] GEDV is calculated by combining the end-diastolic volumes of all four heart chambers. A volumetric marker of preload, GEDV is the difference between intrathoracic thermal volume (ITTV) and pulmonary thermal volume (PTV).[127-129] Once the GEDV is calculated, it can be indexed to the patient's BSA, resulting in GEDVI. Although the normal range for GEDVI is 680 to 800 mL/m², it is stressed that GEDV is age and gender dependent, and to use this value to guide fluid resuscitation without recognizing these factors would be unacceptable.[130] Research has been mixed as to whether GEDVI should be indexed to the patient's actual BSA or predicted BSA, as GEDVI values indexed to actual BSA resulted in significantly lower values than those indexed to predicted BSA. One study found that each

TABLE 17.9	Variables That May Influence Thermodilution CO Values	
Overestimates	**Underestimates**	**Unpredictable**
• Low injectate volume	• Excessive injectate volume	• Right-to-left ventricular septal defect
• Injectate that is too warm	• Injectate solutions that are too cold	• Left-to-right ventricular septal defect
• Thrombus on the thermistor of the PAC		• Tricuspid regurgitation
• Partially wedged PAC		

CO, Cardiac output; *PAC,* pulmonary artery catheter.

year in age increased GEDVI by 9 mL, and each centimeter of height increased GEDVI by 15 mL.[131]

Extravascular lung water estimates the amount of water inside the lungs that exists outside the pulmonary vasculature, including interstitial, intracellular, alveolar, and lymphatic fluids.[132,133] An increase in EVLWI (normal value 3–7 mL/kg) is consistent with pulmonary edema, ARDS, and potential acute lung injury (ALI).[125,134] Because these devices are able to estimate EVLWI, they are especially helpful for patients with significant cardiovascular and/or pulmonary failures as they can guide clinicians' decisions regarding fluid administration.[125,126,131] One study revealed that TPTD EVLWI measurements evaluated over several days predicted mortality in ALI and ARDS patients better than consecutive chest radiographs.[134]

Although TPTD is comparable in its accuracy to the PAC thermodilution method of estimating CO,[124,135,136] it has several drawbacks. A major concern is its level of accuracy if the patient has significantly diminished CO. If the patient's CO reaches less than 2 L/min, the device is unable to provide any measurement data due to lack of reliability.[137] User error can potentially impact any thermodilution CO estimation, including both traditional PAC and TPTD methods (e.g., required number of injectate boluses to calculate an average value for CO, volume and temperature of injectate, speed of injectate administration).[125] With TPTD, if room temperature injectate boluses (vs iced injectates) are used, a slight but statistically significant overestimation of CO,[138,139] GEDVI, and EVLWI[139] can occur. Monitoring of CO via TPTD is contraindicated in any patients with femoral vascular prostheses.[125]

Unless combined with arterial pressure waveform analysis (i.e., pulse contour analysis [PCA],[140] pulse power analysis [PPA][141]), TPTD devices are unable to determine rapid changes in hemodynamically unstable patients as they can provide only intermittent CO measurements.[125] However, after initial calibration, PCA monitoring devices allow TPTD to provide real-time measurements of CO.[126] Pulse contour analysis is based on the principle that the area under the systolic portion of the arterial pressure curve is related to SV.[125,142] LiDCO, a proprietary device, utilizes PPA, and according to its manufacturer it uses clinically insignificant doses of lithium chloride as an indicator instead of requiring a saline bolus for its CO measurements.[141] Cardiac output is calculated from the area under the curve of lithium level changes in relation to time since injection.[124] Some TPTD devices analyze the arterial waveform without the need for external calibration; these devices include Vigileo/FloTrac [Edwards Life Sciences] and MostCare [Vytech, Padova Italy].[125,141] Calibration of PCA devices is recommended more frequently in several clinical settings: when arterial resistance changes over time (e.g., vascular leak syndrome),[125] after acute hemodynamic changes or any intervention that alters vascular impedance,[141] and is encouraged on an hourly basis if cardiac output measurements are mandatory for understanding changes in hemodynamic status.[125]

It is recommended in the setting of prolonged major surgery or cardiac surgery, where hemodynamic instability is likely, that patient care could be optimized with advanced hemodynamic monitoring;

techniques that do not require frequent calibration (such as the PAC) are preferred to allow for earlier treatment of hypovolemia and/or hypoxemia.[51] For this reason, TPTD methods that depend on recurring calibration may be undesirable in this setting due to the likelihood of frequent and/or acute hemodynamic changes.[125] Transpulmonary thermodilution monitors that use pulse waveform analysis (PWA) as a component of their hemodynamic calculations can be disrupted by several factors: severe vasoconstriction, continuous renal replacement therapy (dialysis done over 24 hours each day for hemodynamically unstable patients), severe aortic valve disease, and intraaortic balloon pump therapy.[124] Although TPTD CO monitors are able to provide estimates of global cardiac function through calculation of GEDVI, unlike PAC CO monitors, they are unable to estimate right and left cardiac pressures and volumes[125] or measure mixed venous oxygen saturation.

A Cochrane review of 13 studies including 5686 ICU patients revealed that when the PAC is used alone, without a correctly designed treatment strategy based on hemodynamic data, it did not change hospital mortality rates, hospital length of stay (LOS), or cost of ICU care. These researchers did find the PAC to be a useful diagnostic tool when used by health care providers who are well trained in hemodynamic assessment and the numerous variables that can skew PAC data. The authors recommended additional research of less invasive CO monitoring methods (such as TPTD) be done before clinicians consider replacing PAC monitoring with less invasive monitoring methods as a new gold standard.[143] The 2017 Canadian Cardiovascular Society (CCS) published guidelines on perioperative cardiac risk assessment and management of patients undergoing noncardiac surgery; their guidelines did not recommend the use of a PAC in this patient population.[42] One of the studies used to support this recommendation was a 2005 meta-analysis. It included 13 randomized control trials (RCTs) involving 5051 patients; the results showed that PAC use offered no benefit to patient outcomes.[144]

The European Society of Intensive Care Medicine published in 2014 a consensus statement on shock and hemodynamic monitoring. Recommendations included a preference for dynamic over static hemodynamic variables to evaluate patients' fluid responsiveness, but not to routinely use dynamic measures in shock patients. The consensus also recommended against the use of routine PAC insertion in shock patients.[145] In 2016 the Surviving Sepsis Campaign also recommended the use of dynamic measurements over static measurements when evaluating septic patients' fluid responsiveness. The authors found that dynamic methods had improved diagnostic accuracy over static methods when assessing potential fluid responsiveness.[78] Their recommendations included both noninvasive methods, such as passive leg raises and fluid challenges, and more invasive methods, such as monitoring PPV under mechanical ventilation (Fig. 17.21).[78]

Other Hemodynamic Indices

Some authors encourage the use of calculated indices to optimize the care of critical care patients. These indices include PVR, pulmonary

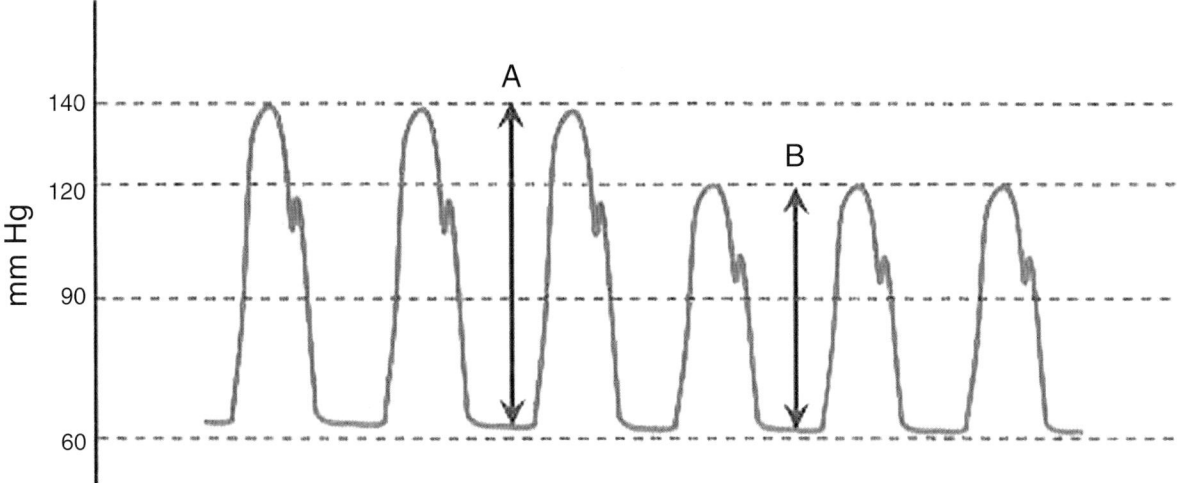

Fig. 17.21 A series of radial arterial pressure waveforms depicting variability in pulse pressure (PP). Pulse pressure variability (PPV) can be calculated as the PP max – PP min / mean PP. Multiply the calculated value x 100 allows PPV to be expressed as a percentage. PP (A) = 140 – 60 = 80; PP (B) = 120 – 60 = 60; PPV% = 80 – 60 = 20 / 70 = 0.285 x 100 = 28.6%.

vascular resistance index (PVRI), SVR, systemic vascular resistance index (SVRI), and CI. The potential advantages and limitations of each index will be reviewed.

The PVRI (PVR calculated with the CI instead of the CO) is equal to the difference in pressure across the pulmonary circuit (mean PAP – PAOP) divided by flow (CI) times 80. This formula is taken from Ohm's law (with the variables mathematically manipulated) for electric currents (R [Resistance] = V [Voltage] = I [Current]). A normal value is considered to be 45 to 225 dynes • sec/cm^5 • m^2. Two limitations of extrapolating physiologic resistance from Ohm's law are (1) blood flow is pulsatile and not flowing continuously through a set of rigid pipes, and (2) resistance is not uniform throughout the pulmonary circuit. The electrical counterpart describes resistance not in alternating currents but in direct currents.[146]

When PVR is used clinically, it should be viewed as a gross estimate of RV afterload; similarly, SVR is associated with LV afterload. In the intact heart, afterload is defined as systolic wall stress or the impedance the ventricles must overcome to eject their SV. It is important to understand that vascular resistance is not synonymous with afterload but is used as an extension of the concept. PVR, like SVR, can affect afterload, but neither formula accounts for changes in ventricular wall thickness or radius, which are components of afterload.

SVRI is calculated as the difference between systemic input pressure (mean arterial pressure [MAP]) minus the output pressure (right atrial pressure [RAP] or CVP), divided by the CI times 80. The normal range is 1760 to 2600 dynes • sec/cm^5 • m^2. SVRI is commonly used to offer some guidance in the use of vasoconstrictors (e.g., phenylephrine infusion) or afterload reduction (e.g., intravenous nitroglycerin or sodium nitroprusside). The limitations described previously for PVR also hold true for SVR, although perhaps to a lesser extent, because the systemic vasculature has lower compliance. In general, supporting afterload via vasoconstrictors should be deferred until maximization of preload or the use of positive inotropes has proven to be ineffective.

Mixed Venous and Central Venous Oxygen Saturation

Since its introduction in 1981, measuring mixed venous oxygen saturation (SvO$_2$) has been described as a means to indirectly monitor oxygen delivery. This is based on the fact that SvO$_2$ is determined by pulmonary function, cardiac function, oxygen delivery, tissue perfusion, oxygen consumption (VO$_2$), and hemoglobin concentration. During the

course of an anesthetic (excluding cases of major trauma or hemorrhagic shock), it is not unusual for pulmonary function, hemoglobin content, and oxygen consumption to remain relatively stable. Therefore proponents of SvO$_2$ monitoring state that it is reasonable to assume that a decrease in SvO$_2$ reflects a change in global oxygen delivery, presumably via a reduction in CO.[147,148] In contrast, some researchers have found a poor correlation between SvO$_2$ and CO, which can occur with cyanide toxicity, and sepsis.[124,149,150] This may be explained by the dependence of SvO$_2$ upon CO as well as other variables such as hemoglobin levels, VO$_2$, and arterial oxygen hemoglobin saturation (SaO$_2$); fluctuations in SvO$_2$ values are common and may explain why some studies show variability in SvO$_2$ and CO correlation.[151] However, some researchers have found SvO$_2$ to be a major determinant of serum lactate levels; lactate levels are related to levels of circulation, perfusion, and metabolic activity and are strongly associated with CI values.[152]

Continuous mixed venous oximetry is measured by fiberoptic reflectance spectrophotometry through two fiberoptics housed in the PAC. One fiberoptic transmits narrow wavelengths of light to the distal catheter. The extent of light absorption and reflection is a function of the quantity of oxyhemoglobin and deoxyhemoglobin present in the PA.[153] The receiving fiberoptic transports the reflected light to a microprocessor that interprets the signal and displays an SvO$_2$ value; the normal range of SvO$_2$ is 65% to 77%. Factors that increase SvO$_2$ values include left-to-right shunts, hypothermia, sepsis, cyanide toxicity, a wedged PAC, and an increase in CO. SvO$_2$ decreases with hyperthermia, shivering, seizures, reduced pulmonary transport of oxygen, hemorrhage, and decreased CO. Sustained low values (e.g., 50%) merit investigation followed by appropriate intervention(s). It has also been demonstrated that some SvO$_2$ monitoring systems adapt well to acute changes in hematocrit.[154] In addition, research with two-wavelength and three-wavelength SvO$_2$ oximetry catheters has shown the systems to be comparable in accuracy.[155]

Central venous oxygen saturation (ScvO$_2$) monitoring has been advocated as a surrogate for SvO$_2$ when a less invasive form of hemodynamic monitoring is indicated. Modified central venous catheters (CVCs) that contain a fiberoptic lumen can measure ScvO$_2$ when positioned at the junction of the superior vena cava and right atrium. A major difference between SvO$_2$ and ScvO$_2$ measurements is that the latter is considered a regional indicator of venous oxygen saturation; it measures venous O$_2$ saturation from the upper body and head. In contrast, SvO_2 measurements depend on blood flow from the superior vena cava, inferior vena cava, and coronary sinus (which has an O_2 content of ~7 mL/dL [venous O_2 saturation of 35%]). Also, the mixed venous O_2 content is greater in the inferior vena cava than in the superior vena cava.[156,157] The net effect of these differences is that, under normal conditions (e.g., in unanesthetized subjects),[157] the $ScvO_2$ is approximately 2% to 3% less than the SvO_2.[156-159] However, the literature also reports the opposite relationship. From a monitoring perspective, research indicates that the use of $ScvO_2$ as a substitute for SvO_2 is both advocated[149,160-166] and discouraged.[51,158,162-164,167] Numerous clinical investigations in different practice settings with patients having diverse pathologic states have been conducted. A 2005 meta-analysis shows that SvO_2 and $ScvO_2$ are clinically equivalent and that the differences found between values can be due to differing study approaches and methods; these authors state that it is important for the anesthesia provider to evaluate the patient's trends when applying SvO_2 and/or $ScvO_2$ data.[168]

The use of SvO2 and/or $ScvO_2$ in management of septic patients is a continued area of interest and research. Three landmark studies (ProCESS,[165] ARISE,[169] ProMISe[170]) found that early goal-directed therapy (EGDT) did not improve mortality outcomes for severely septic or septic shock patients. Published in 2017, the 2016 Surviving Sepsis Campaign: International Guidelines for Management of Severe Sepsis now reflect that research. They no longer suggest using an $ScvO_2$ goal of 70% or greater (or SvO_2 ≥65%) or a CVP of 8 to 12 mm Hg during the first 6 hours of resuscitation. The guidelines now state that within the first hour of recognizing severe sepsis and septic shock, clinicians should measure a lactate level (and remeasure if the initial lactate level is >2 mmol/L), acquire blood cultures before administering broad-spectrum intravenous antibiotics, administer 30 mL/kg crystalloid for hypotension or a serum lactate level of 4 mmol/L and greater, followed by the use of vasopressors if the patient is hypotensive during or after fluid resuscitation to maintain a MAP of 65 mm Hg or greater.[78] Researchers studying the use of $ScvO_2$ or SvO_2 measurements to guide patient care in the ICU recommend an individualized approach[168] and for the clinician to evaluate the patient's VO_2, SaO_2, hemoglobin, and CO requirements instead of using a systematic or standardized SvO_2 goal.[151] Other studies have stated the importance of evaluating lactate levels in septic patients,[78,171] and one meta-analysis study found lactate clearance levels to be superior to $ScvO_2$ alone when used during standard resuscitation protocols. Those authors suggested measuring lactate levels every 2 hours until the patient has attained a lactate clearance level greater than 10%.[172] An example of obtaining a lactate clearance measurement would be to draw an initial serum lactate level at the time that septic shock is diagnosed or strongly suspected, then obtain a second measurement 6 hours later; thus the formula would be ([lactate $_{initial}$ – lactate $_{delayed}$] / lactate $_{initial}$) × 100%; e.g., ([5 mmol/L – 2.5 mmol/L{6 hr later}] / 5.0 mmol/L) × 100% = 50%.

In conclusion, the cost-benefit ratio of using PACs that provide TDCO, TDCCO, or SvO_2 measurements, or even CVC with $ScvO_2$-monitoring capabilities, remains controversial. As with any physiologic monitor, the potential to promote health or cause harm is determined by the clinician's ability to interpret and apply data.[173] A similar analogy can be made for computerized ST segment analysis, whereby failing to account for numerous variables when interpreting ST segment shifts can potentially lead to iatrogenic injury. Therapeutic strategies should be guided by knowledge of the patient's underlying pathophysiology, individualizing hemodynamic parameters to meet the patient's current clinical scenario and understanding the limitations of the respective hemodynamic monitoring device.

ARTERIAL PRESSURE MONITORING

As with ECG monitoring, professional societies have designated the routine assessment of arterial BP to be essential for the safe conduct of any anesthetic; at minimum, BP should be recorded at least once every 5 minutes.[1] This frequency of assessment should be increased for patients noted to have any systemic disease that limits physiologic reserve, such as CAD or valvular heart defects (e.g., aortic stenosis). The coauthors advocate a BP assessment at 1-minute intervals during the induction period of most anesthetics, the rationale being that many commonly administered induction agents are associated with cardiac depressant and/or vasodilatory effects. The concomitant disruption or gross activation of homeostatic reflexes can lead to substantive changes in hemodynamics, even in relatively healthy patients. It is also known that the hemodynamic response to many drugs used during induction of anesthesia can be unpredictable, owing to differences in pharmacokinetics and pharmacodynamics among patients.

Blood pressure monitoring can be accomplished through both noninvasive and invasive techniques. Each recording modality will be reviewed, with an emphasis on clinical relevance. Other resources provide a comprehensive description of the theoretical underpinnings for the calculation of noninvasive and invasive arterial BP data. In today's modern OR environment, noninvasive blood pressure (NIBP) monitoring is most often recorded by automated BP cuffs that can be configured to measure SBP, DBP, and MAP in a standard mode, stat mode, at varied frequencies of assessment, and adjusted for patient age and habitus. The literature recommends that BP cuffs have a bladder dimension of approximately 40% the circumference of the extremity.[174] Bladders that are not properly sized and cuffs that are not applied firmly to the extremity can lead to inaccurate recordings. For example, cuffs that are applied loosely to the extremity, positioned below the level of the heart, or are too small can produce arterial BP values that are falsely elevated.[175]

In general, the benefits outweigh the risks of taking frequent NIBP recordings during an anesthetic. Nevertheless, injury and harm can occur with automatic NIBP measurements and may include damage to peripheral nerves (e.g., ulnar), development of a compartment syndrome, or interference with delivery of drugs through an intravenous line. For example, propofol sequestered in a forearm during BP cuff inflation can cause intense pain. This can be avoided by routinely placing the BP cuff on the extremity without the peripheral intravenous line. In circumstances in which the scheduled surgery involves an upper extremity, the BP cuff and intravenous line can be placed on the contralateral arm (brachium or antebrachium), with the caveat that the NIBP must be configured so BP measurements are recorded in the manual mode to prevent unexpected disruption of the delivery of intravenous induction drugs. Alternatively, a lower extremity (thigh or calf) can be used for BP measurements.

In morbidly obese patients, it is not unusual to have to relocate a BP cuff from the upper arm because of the cone shape of the extremity. An alternative BP monitoring site is the forearm. However, NIBP measurements taken in the forearm with the patient in supine or sitting position, or with the head of the bed elevated 45 degrees, can overestimate the more proximal brachial BP.[176,177] Formulas have been proposed to correct for such discrepancies. For example, in an obese patient with a diastolic forearm pressure of 80 mm Hg and an arm circumference between 32 and 44 cm, the adjusted DBP would equal 72.4 mm Hg. This is derived from the following equation:

$$\text{Brachial DBP} = (0.59 \times \text{Forearm DBP}) + 25.2$$

This formula was proposed based on a study of 129 subjects with an average body mass index of 40 ± 7 kg/m².[176] Discrepancies in BP measurements have also been noted between upper and lower extremities and between arms. In study participants up to 16 years of age, SBP has been shown to be greater in the thigh and calf than in the arm. In contrast, DBP and MAP are lower in the calf and thigh than in the arm.[178] Patients most likely to exhibit interarm BP differences are those who are obese and who have a higher HR and SBP.[179] Concerns about accuracy also arise when measuring BP noninvasively versus invasively. One group of investigators found NIBP taken in the upper arm in patients with septic shock to correlate poorly with arterial line pressure measurements, specifically causing an overestimation of MAP with the noninvasive technique.[180]

It is apparent that a substantive change has occurred in recent years in the number of adults and children in the United States who are classified as obese. Consistent with this change are the findings that mean midarm circumference has increased across the country, with the greatest increase occurring in 20- to 39-year-olds. This change should cause anesthesia providers to be more attentive to the daily task of selecting properly sized BP cuffs. In fact, research has shown that up to 39% of all hypertensive patients and 47% of self-reported diabetic patients should not have their BP measured with the standard adult-size cuff.[181] Inattentiveness to this basic and essential monitoring need could cause the anesthetist to process inaccurate hemodynamic data (e.g., overestimated BP recordings) and ultimately contribute to a poor surgical outcome.

Direct measurement of arterial BP is considered by many to be the gold standard for recording BP. Many anatomic locations can be used for direct BP measurement, with the most common being the radial artery. Other, less commonly used arteries are the ulnar, brachial, axillary, femoral, and dorsalis pedis arteries. Risks associated with placement of an intraarterial catheter include infection (localized and systemic), thrombus formation, hematoma, vasospasm, embolization, injury to adjacent nerves and veins, ischemia to extremities or digits, loss of a limb secondary to poor collateral circulation, iatrogenic injuries (air embolization, intraarterial injection of drugs meant to be administered intravenously), and acute blood loss due to an unexpected disruption of the transducing system (e.g., cracked or disconnected stopcock). A displaced transducer (no longer level with the phlebostatic axis) can show a false increase in arterial BP if positioned substantially below the level of the heart. Assessment of an abnormal BP recording should include an understanding of problems inherent to a fluid-pressure monitoring system. To mitigate the ongoing risks of direct arterial BP monitoring, constant vigilance on the part of the anesthetist is paramount.

Monitoring BP directly offers several distinct advantages, including beat-to-beat assessment of BP, limited hysteresis in measured values, and easy access for arterial sampling of blood for any number of laboratory tests (e.g., arterial blood gases, serum electrolytes, glucose, hemoglobin levels). Indications for direct arterial BP monitoring include surgical procedures in which there is potential for acute and/or gross changes in hemodynamics. This would include operations such as repair of aortic aneurysms, carotid endarterectomy, and craniotomies. Even with lower risk surgical procedures, direct arterial BP monitoring may be indicated, particularly if preoperative BP is poorly controlled (labile), or when intraoperative monitoring of somatosensory-evoked potentials produces frequent gross movement of the upper extremities, which can mitigate the effectiveness of providing noninvasive BP recordings. Patients with comorbidities may be at substantial risk for a stroke or heart attack during periods of acute stress (e.g., laryngoscopy or emergence from an anesthetic) if BP is not directly monitored.

Risks associated with placement of a radial artery catheter can be minimized if precautionary measures are taken. This would include positioning the hand and wrist on an arm board. A roll should be placed beneath the wrist, and the fingers and thumb should be taped

securely across the board. This position keeps the hand from interfering with manipulation and placement of the needle-catheter system; it also facilitates palpation of the radial artery. Commonly, a 20-gauge nontapered catheter is used (a 22 gauge is optional) to penetrate an area of skin that has been prepped with antiseptic solution and infiltrated with local anesthetic. The needle, bevel pointing upward, is directed at a 45-degree angle toward the palpated pulse. If bone is encountered with the tip of the needle during advancement, the complete catheter system (catheter and needle) is slowly withdrawn while observing for the free flow of arterial blood; sometimes the artery can be pierced without a "flash back" (unintentional transfixion-withdrawal method). If no blood is seen during catheter withdrawal, the needle system is directed slightly laterally (in either direction) and readvanced. Once arterial blood is seen in the lumen of the catheter, the angle of the needle is reduced to approximately 30 degrees, then advanced slightly (a few millimeters). The catheter is subsequently threaded off the needle. "Fatigue" at a puncture site may occur, at which time a new artery may be chosen to cannulate, or a "fresh set of hands" (perhaps another anesthesia provider or member of the surgical team) may be used to repeat the attempt at arterial puncture. After verifying correct placement of the catheter within the lumen of the artery (free flow of blood through the rigid tubing when vented to air), it is important to securely fasten the arterial catheter to the skin and apply a sterile dressing on top of the puncture site.

The transducing system should be zeroed to atmospheric pressure (with the stopcock vented to air) and referenced at the level of the left atrium. In patients with poor vascular compliance, the arterial tracing can produce an "overshoot" or "ringing" phenomenon. If not recognized, BP recordings will overestimate SBP and MAP values. In contrast, a dampened waveform, which can develop with a flexed wrist or low pressure in the continuous-flush device, can lead to an underestimation of BP recordings (Fig. 17.22). Direct arterial pressure measurements, although very accurate in many clinical circumstances, can still produce BP recordings that are significantly skewed and lead to inappropriate interventions (e.g., preload augmentation, indiscriminate use of vasoactive drugs).

TRANSESOPHAGEAL ECHOCARDIOGRAPHY MONITORING

Transesophageal echocardiography (TEE) has been established as a safe, noninvasive diagnostic tool for monitoring numerous cardiac parameters to guide medical, surgical, and nursing care. Identification of systolic wall motion abnormalities (SWMA) and vascular aneurysms, calculation of ejection fraction and ventricular preload, and measurement of blood flow within heart chambers and across valves are a few ultrasound imaging utilities that are applied during TEE. Guidelines for indications and training proficiency have been advocated by medical professional societies.[182]

The use of sound waves to define anatomic structures in the human body was first described by Dussik et al. in 1947. These investigators attempted to outline the cerebral ventricles by driving sound waves across the skull.[183] In 1971, C.D. Side and R.G. Gosling were the first to report the assessment of cardiac function via transesophageal techniques.[184] Nearly 50 years later, substantial advancements in the medical application of ultrasound have occurred, leading, in some circumstances, to an improvement in surgical outcomes.[185] Fundamental to the interpretation of data obtained by TEE is an understanding of the physics of ultrasound. Ultrasound waves are inaudible to the human ear, having a frequency greater than 20,000 Hz. The transducers use elements of silicone or piezoelectric crystals to translate sound waves into electric signals. Piezoelectric crystals are known to produce

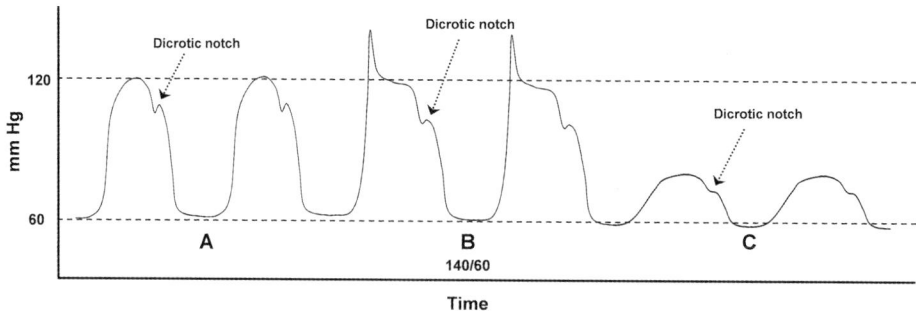

Fig. 17.22 Radial arterial pressure waveforms. (A) Normal morphology, (B) overshoot, (C) dampened. With waveform B, the overshoot should be ignored regarding the displayed systolic blood pressure.

ultrasound waves by vibrating when exposed to an electric current. The opposite also occurs, in that they produce voltage in response to an ultrasound echo or when pressed (i.e., subjected to mechanical stress) or released. The electric current produced has been shown to be of sufficient magnitude to temporarily illuminate a small bulb. Thus piezoelectric crystals function as both generators and receivers of ultrasound waves and electric currents.

The process of how an ultrasound image is produced depends on the object undergoing imaging. For example, within the esophagus, ultrasound waves emitted by piezoelectric elements are absorbed, reflected, or scattered. When reflected by an organ (e.g., heart), the ultrasound echo produced is received by the piezoelectric elements housed within the TEE probe. These elements then generate an electrical impulse that is processed, amplified, and subsequently displayed as an image on the echograph machine.

The number of piezoelectric elements manufacturers can place within a probe ranges from single elements to hundreds; the arrangement of the elements and the dimensional output of the probe (one-, two-, three-dimensional) determine the number required in certain probes.[186] One-dimensional (1D) arrangement options include linear array (LA), annular array (AA), and curved array (CA) transducers. Linear array transducers consist of elements placed in a linear fashion. In AA transducers, the elements are placed in concentric circles; CA transducers employ elements that are arranged in fan or curved shapes. Two-dimensional (2D) arrangements include matrix arrays (MA) and segmented annular arrays[186] (Fig. 17.23). The frequency of the piezoelectric crystals in TEE probes ranges from 3.5 to 7.5 MHZ.[186,187] This frequency range allows for greater detail in displayed images. Unfortunately, the tradeoff for clearer images is lower tissue penetration. Thus smaller frequency values (e.g., 2.5 MHz) are required in transthoracic echocardiographic probes due to the greater distances between the elements and distal anatomic structures.

Clinically, three primary ultrasound imaging techniques are used: the M-mode, 2D imaging, and the Doppler exam. The M-mode provides high picture resolution, with 1000 images per second. It is commonly described as unidimensional and produces a well-focused, narrow ultrasound beam. It is sometimes referred to as an ice-pick view. With the 2D scan, the ultrasound beam is electronically steered across a target field. The intermittent ultrasound pulses are produced by varying the firing sequence (phasing) of individual piezoelectric crystals. The monitor subsequently displays an image that is somewhat triangular or appears as a "slice" of pie. This produces excellent spatial orientation; however, at 30 images per second, the pictures are less well defined. The Doppler exam incorporates the concept of frequency shift, which was first described in 1842 by Austrian physicist Christian Doppler. The clinical application of this concept involves viewing red blood cells (RBCs) as moving reflectors of ultrasound. As ultrasound reflects

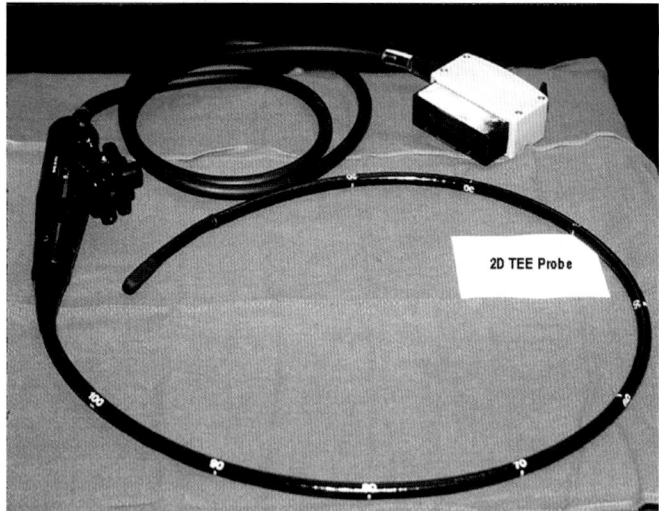

Fig. 17.23 A 170-cm transesophageal echocardiography probe with centimeter markings is displayed. Examination depth is approximately 35 to 40 cm from teeth. The positioning-holding mechanisms are located on control knobs, allowing for manipulation of the probe in the anterior, posterior, and lateral planes. *2D TEE,* Two-dimensional transesophageal echocardiography.

off the moving RBCs, echoes are produced, which are then recorded by the TEE transducer. With the flow of RBCs toward the TEE probe, the distance between the sound source and its reception changes. This phenomenon is referred to as a frequency shift. It is analogous to the change in pitch of a train whistle as the locomotive approaches the station: Sound waves are compressed, and the pitch increases (i.e., the frequency shifts). In contrast to RBCs, body fluids (in this case, plasma) only minimally reflect ultrasound. Spectral and color-flow Doppler exams performed with echographs incorporate this concept by assigning different colors to RBCs that move toward and away from the source of ultrasound. This permits easy visualization of retrograde flow of blood across incompetent heart valves, as may occur with MR. For example, the retrograde flow of blood from the LV into the left atria during MR is seen distinctly as a mosaic pattern of color.

Doppler exams are recognized as being beneficial in determining the etiology of regurgitation and the adequacy of valve repair, as well as influencing surgical management, such as the use or nonuse of cardiopulmonary bypass.[185,188-190] However, the research regarding esophageal Doppler monitoring and its role in goal-directed hemodynamic/fluid therapy during noncardiac surgery is mixed. A 2018 FEDORA trial studying 450 low- to moderate-risk patients over multiple health care centers found esophageal Doppler monitor–guided goal-directed hemodynamic therapy reduced postoperative complications in

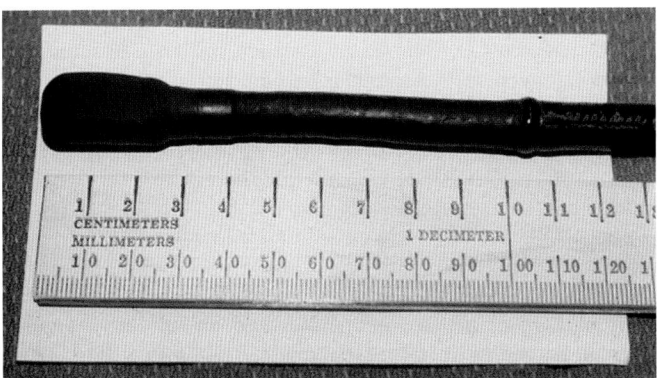

Fig. 17.24 Transesophageal echocardiography probe. Distal tip contains thermistor and piezoelectric elements.

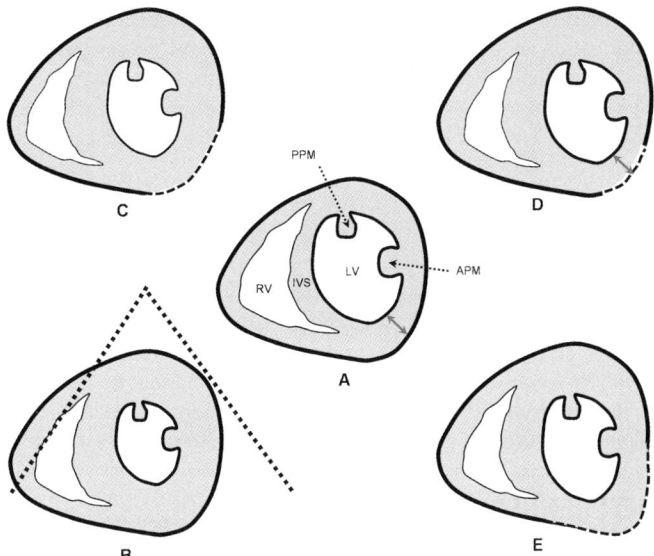

Fig. 17.25 Midpapillary muscle level short-axis view of the heart (A) during diastole, (B) during systole with normal wall thickening and inward movement of endocardial surface, (C) systole with area of hypokinesia (decreased wall thickening), (D) systole with an area of akinesia (no change in wall thickness), and (E) systole with an area of dyskinesia (paradoxical movement). *APM,* Anterior papillary muscle; *IVS,* interventricular septum; *LV,* left ventricle; *PPM,* posterior papillary muscle; *RV,* right ventricle.

intermediate-risk surgery, while 180-day postoperative mortality was unaffected.[191] A 2019 meta-analysis reviewing 11 studies encompassing 1113 patients did not support the use of intraoperative transesophageal Doppler monitoring during colorectal surgery.[192]

Fundamental elements of the TEE exam include positioning the TEE probe (Fig. 17.24) in the esophagus, either under sedation or after induction of the anesthetic. During the examination, cardiac anatomy can be assessed, myocardial ischemia can be diagnosed via the presence of SWMA, and blood flow through heart chambers and across valves can be seen. By convention, the posterior structures are displayed at the top of the screen (apex of the sector) and anterior structures at the bottom. The first image displayed in a standard exam is the short-axis view of the aortic valve. At a depth of approximately 35 to 40 cm from the teeth, the aortic valve leaflets and coronary arteries are seen. Rotation and angulation of the probe can allow a long-axis view of the right and left atria, tricuspid and mitral valves, pulmonic and aortic valves, and right and left ventricles. This view is useful for assessing stenotic valves, identifying masses within the atria or ventricles, and observing the overall size of each heart chamber. A short-axis view of the LV can be obtained with further advancement of the probe and angling of the tip. This position is also referred to as the standard monitoring view, which allows the echocardiographer to assess for SWMA. Normal ventricular wall motion (which is not entirely uniform) increases during systole, and the endocardial surface moves inward. Approximately 87% of the normal SV is derived from shortening in the short axis of the ventricle, with little contribution from the long axis.

Abnormal wall motion can be described by three terms: hypokinesia, akinesia, and dyskinesia. Hypokinesia represents contraction that is less vigorous than normal; wall thickening is decreased. Akinesia depicts the absence of wall motion and can be associated with MI. Dyskinesia correlates with paradoxic movement (i.e., outward motion during systole) and is a hallmark of MI and ventricular aneurysm (Fig. 17.25). Not all wall motion abnormalities are diagnostic of an imbalance between myocardial oxygen supply and demand. Abnormal loading conditions, asynchronous ventricular depolarization (e.g., left bundle branch block), echo dropout due to haphazard reflection of ultrasound off myocardial walls in lateral fields of the sector arc, or improper use of the gain controls of the TEE probe can lead to an erroneous diagnosis of SWMA. In addition, the duration of SWMA can persist well after coronary reperfusion has been restored (e.g., 6 hours), indicating a stunned myocardium.[193] In canine research, a 50% decline in coronary blood flow has been shown to serve as a threshold for hypokinesia. In contrast, a 75% reduction in coronary blood flow commonly produces ST segment deviation. Thus there is greater hysteresis and less sensitivity with ischemia-induced ECG changes than

with ischemia-induced SWMA.[194,195] This finding is consistent with classic research done by Tennant and Wiggers in 1935.[196]

To summarize, the best single view for routine monitoring for SWMA (myocardial ischemia) is the short axis at the midpapillary muscle level (see Fig. 17.25), followed by the apical segment in the same axis. The midpapillary muscle level includes segments of the myocardium that are perfused by all three coronary arteries. This level is created by dividing the long axis of the LV into three parts (i.e., the basal, mid-, and apical regions). The midregion extends from the tips to the bases of the papillary muscles. Interestingly, the skill required to identify gross SWMA by anesthesiologists, residents, and CRNAs (compared with those trained in echocardiography) can be acquired with limited experience; one study group successfully identified 95% of regional wall motion abnormalities.[197]

Newer imaging techniques introduced with TEE include contrast echocardiography, selected three-dimensional (3D) techniques, parametric imaging modes, speckle tracking approaches,[198,199] tissue Doppler imaging, strain/strain rate, smaller sized indwelling TEE probes,[200] and harmonic imaging modalities. Continued research with these echocardiographic diagnostic tools will help elucidate what patient populations may benefit most from their application, although many current ultrasonography machines do not have the ability to allow 3D or speckle tracking and some upgrades are cost prohibitive to most medical centers. Recent investigations have shown that live/real-time 3D echocardiography is a feasible way to estimate the area of the aortic valve orifice in patients with stenotic lesions to evaluate patients with suspected CAD for myocardial wall motion and perfusion abnormalities and to better visualize/detect cardiac lymphomas.[201-203] The valuable role of echocardiography in the management of critically ill patients is a developing area of research; the European Society of Intensive Care Medicine recommends critical care echocardiography (CCE) as a first-line evaluation of hemodynamic status when determining the type and degree of shock instead of more invasive methods.[145,190,204,205] The Surviving Sepsis Campaign reinforces the value of

CCE in its recommendations and its ability to provide more in-depth information about the patient's hemodynamic status.[78] Some research has found that clinicians can evaluate the prognosis of shock via echocardiographic monitoring of the left ventricle with speckle tracking.[200] The use of CCE is especially useful in clinical situations that can cause inaccurate measurements or missed diagnoses in TPTD CO methods, such as the presence of severe aortic or mitral regurgitation,[206] significantly decreased CO,[207] intracardiac shunts, moderate to severe tricuspid regurgitation,[208] regurgitant volume increases with increased PEEP,[209] and dynamic LV outflow tract obstruction.[210] Echocardiography can be used to identify and evaluate MI and cardiac trauma.[211-213]

SUMMARY

With continued advancements in technology and improved clinical databases derived from research, future monitoring techniques offer promise for continued improvement in anesthesia care. The development of specialized task forces[214] comprising multiple professional societies also contributes substantively to professional practice. Understandably, anesthesia providers should continue to maintain a healthy skepticism of reported advancements in monitoring modalities. The decision to change practice routines should occur only after critiquing the reported merits of any research findings. Ultimately, this clinical paradigm will allow patients to benefit from medical and nursing care derived from evidence-based practice.

REFERENCES

 For a complete list of references for this chapter, scan this QR code with any smartphone code reader app, or visit the following URL: http://booksite.elsevier.com/9780323711944/.

18

Clinical Monitoring II: Respiratory and Metabolic Systems

Greg Bozimowski, Andrea J. Teitel

"Every breath you take, and every move you make…I'll be watching you."

Sting, 1983[1]

The lyrics to the song "Every Breath You Take" were written decades ago and refer to an obsession-based relationship, but when considered in the context of monitoring respiratory status during anesthesia they succinctly define the contract between the nurse anesthetist and the patient undergoing anesthesia care. Clinical monitoring in the perioperative setting or remote locations is the process of observing physiologic responses to surgery, procedure, and anesthesia and is the essence of what the Certified Registered Nurse Anesthetist (CRNA) does to ensure an optimal, safe anesthetic outcome. CRNAs need to embrace this part of their role with an obsessive, nearly compulsive approach.

It is important to consider the monitoring modalities utilized for their value in reducing patient morbidity and mortality. Research provides rationale to support the standardization of minimal monitoring modalities. Standards are available to the anesthesia provider from both the American Association of Nurse Anesthetists (AANA) and the American Society of Anesthesiologists (ASA). It is a matter of clinical judgment by the anesthetist that determines what modalities beyond those minimally required will provide useful information when added to the anesthetic plan of care. It is through this evidence-based approach that best practices are developed.

Above all, human vigilance must be maintained and considered primary in assessing patient responses to anesthesia and surgical procedures. Human error is always possible and may be associated with adverse outcomes. Monitoring alone cannot prevent adverse outcomes, but a timely response to warnings can have a positive impact. It cannot be emphasized enough that reliance on technology must never be allowed to lull the clinician into complacency. Although accuracy and reliability of monitors continue to improve, the potential for machine malfunction and artifact is ever present. The patient is always the primary source of information. Timely human response to intraoperative events remains the key to predicting, avoiding, and managing untoward responses to anesthesia and surgery. As such, the use of technology in combination with provider vigilance remains the patients' best defense against preventable respiratory critical events. The basic human senses of sight, hearing, touch, and even smell remain crucial tools in clinical monitoring because the patient is the primary source of assessment data.

This chapter reviews the relevant standards for respiratory and temperature monitoring outlined by the AANA. Because systematic processes can provide consistency, a practical systems approach to monitoring is presented. Respiratory monitoring is reviewed as it relates to the ongoing assessment of airway and breathing using not only the human senses but also technologic tools used by nurse anesthetists. The modalities to be discussed in this chapter include the precordial stethoscope, carbon dioxide detection devices, and pulse oximetry. Thermoregulation is significantly altered under anesthesia, therefore temperature monitoring modalities are also reviewed in this chapter. Finally, implications for the education of nurse anesthetists and the future of clinical monitoring are visited.

MONITORING STANDARDS

Monitoring standards are published and reviewed by anesthesia professional associations so that minimal standards in the provision and monitoring of care can be recommended. Such standards are intended to lend guidance to anesthesia providers and health care facilities in evaluating quality of care and developing and improving the safety of practice while educating the public regarding patient rights and expectations. The AANA *Scope of Anesthesia Practice* states, "CRNAs are accountable and responsible for their services and actions, and for maintaining their individual clinical competence." In this regard, CRNAs are accountable for their practice and responsible for an understanding of and adherence to the standards of care set forth. Standard 9 of the AANA *Standards for Nurse Anesthesia Practice* outlines specific monitoring requirements necessary for compliance (Table 18.1).[2]

The AANA *Scope of Anesthesia Practice* states, "The practice of anesthesiology is a recognized nursing and medical specialty unified by the same standards of care." As it applies to monitoring, this is reflected in the published practice standards of both organizations. The ASA *Standards for Basic Anesthetic Monitoring, Standard 2,* states, "During all anesthetics, the patient's oxygenation, ventilation, circulation, and temperature shall be continually evaluated." Throughout the course of care, these standards emphasize continuous monitoring by the anesthesia provider and, additionally, it is specifically written that during moderate or deep sedation, continuous monitoring of end tidal carbon dioxide ($ETco_2$) shall be utilized to evaluate the adequacy of ventilation. The ASA standards also explicitly state that the use of $ETco_2$ monitoring should be utilized when propofol is administered during endoscopy procedures.[3]

These standards acknowledge and emphasize the importance of vigilant monitoring as the basis of safety in anesthesia practice. In addition, the standards point out that the CRNA must constantly be in attendance of the patient until the responsibility for care can be safely transferred to another qualified health care provider. They further point out that these are intended to be minimum requirements and should be exceeded as deemed necessary in the judgment of the anesthetist. In most cases, when certain monitoring modalities are not used, they must be at least immediately available. Whereas it may seem obvious that standards should be followed, a closed-claims study revealed that nearly half of the time anesthesia standards were not followed and, in particular, monitoring standards were among those most often breached.[3]

TABLE 18.1　Standards for Nurse Anesthesia Practice

Standard 9

Monitor, evaluate, and document the patient's physiologic condition as appropriate for the procedure and anesthetic technique. When a physiologic monitoring device is used, variable pitch and threshold alarms are turned on and audible. Document blood pressure, heart rate, and respiration at least every 5 minutes for all anesthetics.

Parameter	Modifier
a. Oxygenation	Continuously monitor oxygenation by clinical observation and pulse oximetry. The surgical or procedural team communicates and collaborates to mitigate the risk of fire.
b. Ventilation	Continuously monitor ventilation by clinical observation and confirmation of continuous expired carbon dioxide during moderate sedation, deep sedation, or general anesthesia. Verify intubation of the trachea or placement of other artificial airway device by auscultation, chest excursion, and confirmation of expired carbon dioxide. Use ventilatory monitors as indicated.
c. Cardiovascular	Monitor and evaluate circulation to maintain patient's hemodynamic status. Continuously monitor heart rate and cardiovascular status. Use invasive monitoring as appropriate.
d. Thermoregulation	When clinically significant changes in body temperature are intended, anticipated, or suspected, monitor body temperature. Use active measures to facilitate normothermia. When malignant hyperthermia (MH) triggering agents are used, monitor temperature and recognize signs and symptoms to immediately initiate appropriate treatment and management of MH.
e. Neuromuscular	When neuromuscular blocking agents are administered, monitor neuromuscular response to assess depth of blockade and degree of recovery.

Adapted from the American Association of Nurse Anesthetists. *Scope and Standards for Nurse Anesthesia Practice*; 2019. Available at http://www.aana.com.

CLOSED-CLAIMS ANALYSES

Closed-claims studies can provide valuable insight into monitoring techniques and habits that could be useful in preventing future anesthesia mishaps. Mortality rates have improved in recent years due to advances in respiratory monitoring modalities, implementation of evidence-based practice, utilization of surgical checklists, preoperative patient optimization, and the use of effective communication, teamwork, and education.[4] When there is deviation from these practices, the potential for adverse patient outcomes exists. The AANA Foundation closed-claims research team (CCRT) was established in 1995 to identify the role of contributing factors associated with damaging events and adverse outcomes resulting in malpractice claims involving CRNAs.[5] In an AANA CCRT evaluation of preventable closed-claims review of 123 cases, errors in judgment occurred in more than 65% of the cases (n = 82). These errors included failure to recognize, diagnose, and treat serious problems, inappropriate anesthesia care, inappropriate preparations and/or planning, cognitive biases, production pressure, lack of

vigilance, normalization of deviance, and lack of situational awareness.[5] Closed-claims studies indicate that preventable respiratory-related events commonly cause damage resulting in malpractice claims and payouts. A retroactive closed claims analysis of adverse respiratory outcomes found, "In every hypoventilation claim, regardless of the type of anesthetic technique, a failure to optimally monitor the patient's ventilation was identified as a sentinel, contributory practice pattern."[6] Therefore, it remains critically important that anesthesia providers remain attuned to the respiratory status of their patients at all times, while also maintaining attention to all other physiologic parameters. The incidence of esophageal intubation was drastically reduced with the advent of $ETco_2$ monitoring, demonstrating the value of technological advances.[7]

Incident monitoring systems and practices can be used to collect data for practitioners to use to develop safer processes, as is the case in the often-referenced analogies made to the aviation industry.[8] The vigilance needed for effective clinical monitoring can be thought of as a means to avoid critical incidents. A multitude of external factors can have an impact on the human capability to be vigilant. Anyone entering an operating room or other location where anesthesia is provided could easily identify several distractors. Environmental factors such as noise, music, temperature, and human interaction can be disruptive. Factors such as fatigue, boredom, sleep deprivation, and circadian disruption from extended work hours have been implicated in human error at one time or another, as well as self-initiated distractions such as the use of handheld devices.[9-11]

Review of critical incidents and closed-claims analyses has provided insight into how clinicians can enhance safety and prevent mishaps through their use of monitors with alarms. Equipment malfunctions, as well as a lack of familiarity with equipment or user error, have all been shown to contribute to incidents.[9,12] As monitoring technology becomes more computerized with a dependency on electronics, electricity, and electrical components, there exists a greater potential for malfunction and failure; making it is essential to have backup methods for monitoring and ventilating patients.[13] The increasing practice of providing anesthesia care in areas outside of the operating room, has been implicated in an increased number and severity of liability claims likely due unfamiliarity and/or scarcity of available monitors.[14] It behooves the anesthetist to be aware of the differences in equipment and availability of all resources when providing care away from more familiar settings.

ALARM FATIGUE

The AANA Practice Standard 9 specifically indicates that alarm limit parameters and audible warning systems should be used, and a specific statement is made recommending the use of variable pitch alarms and that threshold alarms should be activated.[2] The value of variable pitch commonly used in pulse oximetry equipment has been widely appreciated for its ability to provide information regarding subtle changes in oxygen saturation using the sense of hearing, prior to visualizing the monitor. Alarms are designed to protect the patient by alerting the practitioner that the individual is at increased risk and needs immediate assistance.

An area of concern related to electronic monitoring devices is a phenomenon referred to as alarm fatigue. Alarm fatigue is a form of human error occurring when a practitioner is desensitized to alarms or alerts.[15] The ideal alarm would be easy to localize and recognize. It would be evident despite other noises and alarms yet would allow for effective communication between care providers. The ideal monitoring device would also elicit a minimal number of false alarms. Alarms in many medical devices fall short of the ideal and as a result are subject to being ignored or even disabled by the practitioner. It has been demonstrated that many alarms generated during the course of an anesthetic are clinically irrelevant, with only a small incidence indicating a critical event.[16] As a result, it is not surprising that little progress has been made in combating alarm fatigue.

It is also necessary that when a monitor alarms, the practitioner evaluates and investigates the cause of the alarm, rather than simply dismissing the data provided as erroneous. Cognitive error occurs when the practitioner does not believe the information provided, often as a result of unconsciously held biases made in conjunction with failed analysis of the clinical situation. An example of this is when a pulse oximeter continuously alarms and the anesthesia provider focuses on reapplying the monitor to several extremities instead of recognizing that the alarm is a result of hypoxia and hypoventilation.

SYSTEMATIC APPROACH TO MONITORING

A systematic process shown to be effective in reducing anesthetic morbidity and mortality should be the goal when planning appropriate monitoring to be used. As monitoring standards guide practice by prescribing minimums of adherence, other processes can be helpful in defining how monitoring should occur and which modalities should be used. In addition, a systematic approach to problem solving for the cause of alarms or adverse patient responses can speed the anesthetist to provide remedy. As stated, monitoring alone cannot prevent adverse outcomes; the CRNA must also interpret the information correctly and then timely intervene to maintain patient safety. The use of a systematic approach to this leads to a more consistent practice.

The act of administering anesthesia results in a physiologic response to the pharmacodynamics and pharmacokinetics of each substance given. The insult of the surgical or diagnostic procedure performed also results in a physiologic response. As such, observation of the human system's response is the monitoring of the pharmacology of the agents used and the physiology of the human system. As the science and process for quality assurance and improvement have evolved, much has been learned and written about the value of a systematic approach to the analysis of critical incidents and crisis management. The concepts used in quality assurance management can be applied to anesthesia monitoring because a primary function of the nurse anesthetist is to prevent or respond to critical incidents to assure a quality anesthetic in terms of safety and efficacy.

A proactive approach to clinical monitoring involves an obsession-like commitment to vigilance in observation utilizing all the human senses and technological aids, and the development of a habit of systematic monitoring may reduce the likelihood of an unnoticed response. Many algorithms, cognitive aids, and protocols have been written to guide the practitioner through crisis management such as cardiac emergencies, anaphylaxis, or malignant hyperthermia; however, there is a scarcity of literature regarding its application to routine monitoring. While cognitive aids and the use of mnemonics have not been equivocally shown to improve outcomes, it is intuitive that such aids may be useful in the development of an inclusive, vigilant approach to routine monitoring during the education of anesthesia providers, as well as more appropriate responses to critical incidents that result from airway or other respiratory events. The habit sometimes referred to as "sweeping" the anesthesia field, to visualize the patient with the eyes following a path to the anesthesia machine via the airway and breathing circuit and progressing to the monitoring modalities used, has long been taught as a means of increasing vigilance and attention to detail. The well-known mantra of the ABCs—observing the **a**irway, **b**reathing (respiration), and **c**irculation—remains foremost and critical in anesthesia clinical monitoring. The addition of D for evaluating **d**rug effects completes the basic monitoring approach in anesthesia. Some evidence

TABLE 18.2	Crisis Management Algorithm
Algorithm	**Descriptor**
C—Circulation, Color	Determine adequacy of circulation, check pulse, blood pressure; ECG notes oxygenation through assessment and oximetry
O—Oxygen, Oxygen analyzer	Check oxygen delivery system, hypoxic guard
V—Ventilation, Vaporizer	Ventilate by hand to assess breathing circuit and airway patency, assess chest excursion and auscultation; assess $ETco_2$; check vaporizer function
E—Endotracheal tube	Thorough assessment of ETT function if used, including patency, seal, etc.
R—Review monitors, Review equipment	Review all monitors in use, ensure appropriate calibration and maintenance, review any and all equipment in contact with the patient
A—Airway	Check patency of the entire airway including the nonintubated airway. Assess for laryngospasm, foreign body, obstruction, bronchospasm, etc.
B—Breathing	Assess pattern, rate, and depth of respirations; examine, auscultate, and review $ETco_2$ and pulse oximeter monitors
C—Circulation	Repeat assessment of circulation
D—Drugs	Review drugs given; consider needed pharmacologic intervention; consider possibility of medication administration error

ECG, Electrocardiogram; *$ETco_2$*, end tidal carbon dioxide concentration; *ETT*, endotracheal tube.

suggests that checklists provide an effective means of identifying causes of failure and incidents.[17] In an anesthesia context, additional foci for monitoring can include (1) **c**olor (i.e., cyanosis); (2) **o**xygen and oxygen analyzers; (3) **v**entilation, vaporizer, or pump settings and status; (4) **e**ndotracheal tube (ETT) patency and placement, including other alternative airway devices; and (5) **r**eview of monitors, equipment, and drug effects. This expanded the crises response algorithm can be remembered as COVERABCD (Table 18.2).[18-20]

AIRWAY MONITORING

Monitoring the airway includes the observance of gas exchange from the upper to lower airways. Assessment of airway patency is performed continuously throughout the perioperative period. Ventilatory movement of the chest must be observed, and the presence of any sign of airway obstruction such as retractions or seesaw motion of the chest and abdomen is noted. Seeing the presence of condensation in an airway device or clear mask can serve to indicate the presence, although not adequacy, of gas exchange. The sense of touch can also be helpful to perceive subtle movement of air exchange, which can be felt on the hand of the anesthetist. The sense of smell can be the first aid in detecting a disconnected circuit or airway device when volatile agents are being used. Listening for the presence of abnormal airway sounds such as stridor is crucial in noting airway obstruction. While many practitioners tend to rely on electronic means of monitoring respirations, the precordial stethoscope is a valuable tool in auscultating the presence or absence of airway exchange during all phases of the anesthetic, regardless of the type administered.[21,22] Ensuring adequacy of ventilation, when using an ETT or laryngeal mask airway (LMA), must include verification of placement by assessing breath sounds and chest expansion, as well as verification of the presence of carbon dioxide (CO_2) in the expired gas ($ETco_2$).[2,3] Whereas failure to successfully intubate is problematic, failure to recognize misplacement is catastrophic.

Respiratory Monitoring: Ventilation

Merely ensuring the presence of airway movement does not ensure adequate gas exchange. Monitoring respiratory parameters is aimed at evaluating both ventilation and oxygenation. The patient must be observed for adequate minute ventilation throughout the anesthetic course. A difficult airway and/or inadequate ventilation can be encountered at any point in the perioperative period.[4]

Skin and nail bed color should be observed as part of the whole patient assessment picture; however, skin color changes alone are not a reliable measure of whether ventilation and oxygenation are adequate. Cyanosis is a late sign of anemia or hypoxia and can be difficult to assess accurately, given such variables as differences in lighting during certain procedures and lack of controls in comparisons of patients' coloring throughout the perioperative period. In addition to physical assessment skills, monitoring the adequacy of ventilation must be done throughout the perioperative period, using multiple parameters. Several themes are evident that relate to safety and vigilance in monitoring when reviewing closed-claims studies for anesthesia incidents. The most prominent of these is the value of certain specific monitors and their alarms. These include pulse oximetry, $ETco_2$ measurement, oxygen analyzers, and disconnect alarms. Of equal importance is the users' ability to ensure the proper function of these prior to administering an anesthetic.[14]

Assessing the respiratory rate and tidal volume is crucial to ensuring adequacy of minute ventilation, as well as interpreting patient response to pharmacologic agents and surgical stimuli. At the most basic level, assessment of ventilation is accomplished through visualization of chest excursion and auscultation of breath sounds. The value of the precordial or esophageal stethoscope is twofold: It provides continuous assurance that ventilation is occurring and it can be used to detect changes in breath sounds.[22] With the reliance on electronic devices, the use of a simple monaural stethoscope has diminished, and its use may at times represent a divide between anesthetists educated during a simpler time and those who were initiated since the use of electronic ventilation monitoring became standard; however, many nurse anesthesia educators believe that the use of a precordial stethoscope by students in clinical helps to encourage the habit of close respiratory monitoring. An electronic device that has been shown to accurately measure respiratory rate using acoustic monitoring transducers may serve to supplement other means of respiratory monitoring.[23] This device senses turbulent air flow through a sensor placed on the upper airway. The monitor provides a readout of respiratory rate and has been shown to be well tolerated by patients. Whereas acoustic respiratory monitoring does not identify stridor or other adventitious sounds, it can alert the anesthetist to apnea. In addition, it offers the added benefits of being effective despite the presence of large body habitus or extraneous room noises, which limit the value of a traditional precordial stethoscope. This method of detecting apnea has shown promise in the postanesthesia care unit (PACU) and was shown to be more reliable than the more frequently used thoracic impedance technology, which relies on movement of electrocardiographic electrode leads.[22,24] The use of noninvasive respiratory volume monitors (RVM) during sedation and in the postanesthesia recovery period has gained some notice in the literature. Through electrodes placed on the thorax, the RVM can measure respiratory rate (RR), tidal volume (TV), and therefore minute ventilation (MV). These devices can record measurements and trends and have been shown to be more sensitive than capnometry measurements of $ETco_2$ in detecting hypoventilation in sedated patients and may become

a more commonly marketed and used tool for the purpose of monitoring intraoperative and postoperative spontaneous ventilation.[25,26]

Carbon Dioxide Monitoring

The measurement of arterial blood gases (ABGs) to determine the level of CO_2 provides direct measurement of ventilation and metabolic status, and the necessity of this action may be indicated at times. The means of measuring the CO_2 tension in the blood ($Paco_2$) is based on hydrogen ion concentration because CO_2 reacts with water to produce hydrogen ions through a reversible reaction. This reaction yields carbonic acid, which dissociates to yield hydrogen and bicarbonate ions,[27-29] as shown in the following equation:

$$CO_2 + H_2O \leftrightarrow H_2CO_3^- \leftrightarrow H^+ + HCO_3^-$$

The production of carbonic acid also allows for the qualitative—and to a limited extent, quantitative—detection of the presence of CO_2 through the use of disposable $ETco_2$ detector devices. These colorimetric devices react to changes in pH and display it as a color change. They are widely used in emergency settings to verify proper placement of an ETT.[30,31] These devices are sensitive enough to detect carbon dioxide quickly; however, in most cases a minimum of six breaths has been suggested to avoid misinterpretation. With advances in newer technologies, colorimetric devices may become even more rapid and reliable.[32,33] It is important to be aware that false positives may result from the detection of CO_2 from air forced into the stomach during mask ventilation or the presence of carbonated beverages or antacids in the stomach.[34]

The means used to measure CO_2 level must be based on the patient's condition, the type of anesthetic administered, and the complexity of the surgical procedure. The continuous measurement of CO_2 in expired gas provides a practical, noninvasive, and accurate reflection of arterial blood carbon dioxide and is the most common means of monitoring carbon dioxide levels in the anesthesia setting. As previously mentioned, it is also a monitoring standard of care during general anesthesia for the patient being ventilated or whose ventilations are being assisted, as well as during moderate or deep sedation, unless precluded or invalidated by the nature of the patient, procedure, or equipment.[2,3]

Accuracy of $ETco_2$ as a correlation with arterial carbon dioxide has been well documented. $ETco_2$ is said to be approximately 2 to 5 torr lower than arterial CO_2 in patients who have no cardiac or pulmonary abnormalities.[35,36] Pathologies that result in an increased dead space, as well as significant alterations in hemodynamic stability, will increase the variance seen between $ETco_2$ and arterial measurements.[36] An in-depth discussion of CO_2 dissociation and O_2–CO_2 exchange is presented in chapter 29.

Capnometry measures only carbon dioxide in respiratory gas, whereas *capnography* refers to the continuous analysis and recording of the measurement. The term *capnogram* is used to describe a continuous display of CO_2 during the phases of ventilation. The continuous measurement of $ETco_2$ is accomplished through the use of infrared analysis. When a gas mixture containing more than one substance (e.g., an exhaled gas sample) is analyzed, a quantitative measurement can be made to determine the proportional contents. Each gas in the mixture absorbs infrared radiation at a different wavelength. The amount of CO_2 is measured by detecting its absorbance at specific wavelengths and filtering the absorbance related to other component gases.

Sampling of $ETco_2$ can be accomplished through either a nondiverting (mainstream) or diverting (side stream) monitor. A nondiverting monitor measures gas directly within the breathing system. Gas passes through a wide-chambered sensor that fits over a connector between the anesthesia circuit and mask adapter. The sensor is connected to the monitor by a cable. Nondiverting monitors offer several advantages. They have minimal sampling-time delays, use few disposable items, and do not require scavenging because gas is not removed from the system. Disadvantages include the inability to measure gases other than CO_2 and nitrous oxide, an increase in circuit dead space by the adapter, and greater risk of interference by condensation and secretions. In addition, because the sensor and cable are attached in proximity to the patient, the added weight may cause traction on the tube, increase the risk of circuit disconnect, and make sampling in a nonintubated patient difficult.[35]

The other, more commonly used, CO_2 monitor type is the diverting monitor. The diverting monitor extracts gas from sample tubing attached near the patient end of the circuit and pumps it to the monitor. Disadvantages include the need for scavenging of sampled gases because they are removed from the circuit, and some risk of contamination by condensation or secretions also exists. Advantages of the diverting system include minimal increase in dead space and versatility in gas analysis because the sample can also be sent to anesthetic agent monitors. In addition, the small, lightweight tubing can be adapted to sample awake, spontaneously breathing patients through the mouth, nares, or simple mask.[35]

It has become common to adapt the sampling line of a diverting $ETco_2$ monitor to trace a capnogram in awake or sedated, spontaneously breathing patients receiving O_2 via simple mask or nasal cannula. Whereas there is a possibility of air or oxygen entering the sample line and resulting in a lowered $ETco_2$ value due to dilution, the use of $ETco_2$ monitoring as a warning of hypoventilation or excess sedation has gained attention outside of the anesthesia setting. For example, $ETco_2$ monitoring has been shown to be a more sensitive indicator of hypoventilation than clinical observation or pulse oximetry when used during sedation in the emergency department setting.[31,37] Other studies note the value of $ETco_2$ monitoring during sedation, as well, and note the advantage over pulse oximetry alone in detecting hypoventilation in patients receiving supplemental O_2. It has been suggested that, like pulse oximetry, $ETco_2$ monitoring should be considered a standard of care for patients receiving sedation outside the operating room.[31,38]

End tidal carbon dioxide capnography. Capnography can record CO_2 as a component of expired lung volume or as a measure of CO_2 alone throughout the phases of respiration plotted against time. Time capnography is most commonly used in the perioperative setting. Basic interpretation of the $ETco_2$ capnogram is a necessary skill. The capnogram can differentiate between normal and abnormal patterns of ventilation that result from patient pathologies, anesthesia system problems, or unexpected patient responses during anesthesia.

The normal time capnogram can be recorded at varying speeds. A fast speed setting of approximately 12.5 mm/second allows interpretation of individual respiratory components and short-term changes, whereas a slow speed of approximately 25 mm/minute displays long-term changes.[39] Although no standard descriptions exist for the components of the capnogram, it is typically described as encompassing four basic phases (Fig. 18.1). These phases are often displayed in a classic waveform shape best recorded during mechanical ventilation in an intubated patient. It is important to note that the basic shape of the wave form will vary depending on the mode of airway management used (e.g., ETT, LMA, simple mask, nasal cannula) as well as in comparison to the spontaneously breathing patient.

Although the shapes may vary, the represented phases apply universally. The first phase is the end of inspiration and very beginning of expiration. Gas sampled at this point identifies the baseline. This sample comes from the anatomic dead space and contains no CO_2. This portion in a normal capnogram should approximate zero. The second phase is the expiratory upstroke. Gas sampled represents a mix of dead

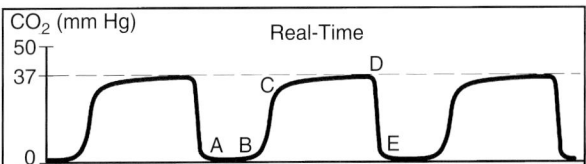

Fig. 18.1 The four phases of a normal capnogram. *A-B* represents baseline; *B-C* represents expiratory upstroke; *C-D* represents expiratory plateau; *D* represents end tidal concentration; and *D-E* represents descent to original baseline. (Courtesy Repironics, Inc., Murrysville, PA.)

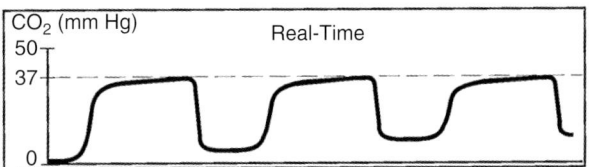

Fig. 18.2 Elevation of the baseline indicates CO_2 rebreathing. (Courtesy Repironics, Inc., Murrysville, PA.)

space and alveolar gas and thus records measurable CO_2. This phase represents the rapid passing of initial expired gas through the upper airways. The third phase represents the plateau and records alveolar emptying of CO_2. In the normal pulmonary measurement, the plateau is very nearly flat. This phase represents the longest duration of the measurement. $ETco_2$ is measured at the end of the plateau just prior to the beginning of the fourth phase, which is displayed as the rapid decrease in CO_2 concentration of sampled gas as a result of inspiration of air or O_2. This downstroke returns the recorded CO_2 measurement to or very near to zero. Variations in the capnography tracing can be very subtle and represent specific alterations in the ventilatory process. Some common deviations are worth noting. In the process of evaluating the capnogram, the anesthetist should note the respiratory rate, whether ventilation is spontaneous or mechanical, the value of measured end-expired CO_2, the shape of the recorded waveform, and the presence of additional respiratory efforts. Deviations from what is normally a close approximation of arterial CO_2 can occur. $ETco_2$ measurements may be inaccurate in the presence of significant ventilation and perfusion mismatching. When ventilation-to-perfusion ratio is large, the resultant increase in dead space causes a low concentration of $ETco_2$ overall.[40–42] In addition, small tidal volumes, reflecting inadequate alveolar ventilation, may produce $ETco_2$ recordings that significantly underestimate arterial CO_2 levels.

After esophageal intubation, an initial, slight upstroke of carbon dioxide may be seen in those rare circumstances when carbon dioxide may be sampled from the stomach, as mentioned previously in reference to disposable $ETco_2$ detector devices. These CO_2 measurements are the result of excess air blown into the stomach, possibly during overzealous ventilation or a partially obstructed airway. Such a waveform will display for a very brief period and be followed by a measurement of zero.

A waveform that fails to return to baseline during the first and fourth phases indicates that rebreathing of carbon dioxide is occurring. This can be the result of inadequate fresh gas flow in the nonrebreathing system or a depleted or ineffective carbon dioxide absorber (Fig. 18.2). Although this may be detected over time, it can be difficult to distinguish.

Sloping of the plateau phase represents a progressive prolongation of expiration. It is typically the result of either an obstruction of expired gas flow at some point along the airway or ventilation-perfusion mismatch (Fig. 18.3). It also can be indicative of chronic obstructive lung disease because CO_2 is exhaled more slowly from diseased portions of

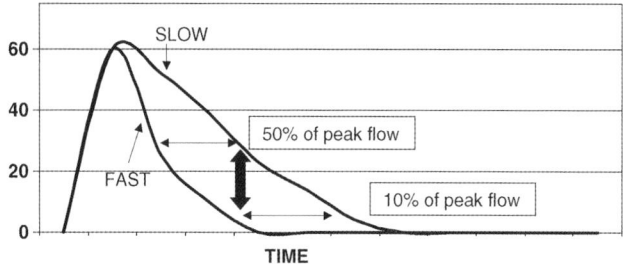

Fig. 18.3 Inspiratory flow waveform demonstrating the effect of impedance on decay of flow. In a patient with stiff lungs (e.g., acute respiratory distress syndrome) and a fast time constant, flow decay is rapid. In the patient with normal compliance and high airway resistance (e.g., chronic obstructive pulmonary disease), the flow decay is prolonged. In these two breaths with the same peak flow, 10% of the fast-time constant is equivalent to 50% of the slow-time constant. (From Branson RD. Functional principles of positive pressure ventilators: implications for patient-ventilator interaction. *Respir Care Clin N Am.* 2005;11(2):119–145.)

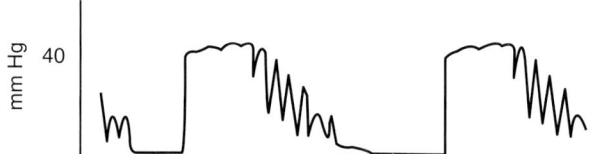

Fig. 18.4 Cardiac oscillations occur as a result of contractions of the heart and great vessels. (From Miller RD. *Miller's Anesthesia.* 8th ed. Philadelphia: Elsevier; 2015.)

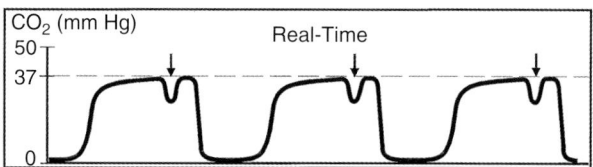

Fig. 18.5 Clefts displayed as a spontaneous inspiration asynchronous with controlled ventilation. (Courtesy Repironics, Inc., Murrysville, PA.)

the lungs (with more significant airway narrowing) than from areas with less severe narrowing. Plateau-phase sloping can also occur with kinking of the ETT or any aspect of the circuit tubing. Changes in the waveform from baseline normal should always be evaluated to determine the cause and necessary interventions.

Regular, sawtooth waves within the expiratory phase at a rate equal to the heart are likely the result of cardiac oscillations (Fig. 18.4). This is the result of the contraction of the heart and great vessels forcing gas in and out of the lungs. This is a common occurrence in pediatric patients owing to the relative size of the heart to the thorax.

During mechanical ventilation in an anesthetized and/or paralyzed patient, spontaneous respiratory effort may be seen if the anesthetic depth is insufficient to prevent respiration or when inadequate muscle relaxation is present. The resultant capnogram is often referred to as curare cleft (Fig. 18.5). This irregular asynchronous waveform may occur within the mechanically ventilated wave or separate from it. Causes of increased or decreased ETCO$_2$ levels are noted in Box 18.1.

Transcutaneous carbon dioxide monitoring. Accurate analysis of ETCO$_2$ reflects adequacy of ventilation. Transcutaneous CO$_2$ monitoring does not provide immediate, breath-by-breath verification of ETT placement nor the presence of respirations, therefore its use is not common in the anesthesia care realm. Nonetheless it is a reliable, noninvasive means of CO$_2$ measurement and can be useful in detecting hypoventilation. Transcutaneous CO$_2$ measurement is a noninvasive measure of Paco$_2$. It can either estimate Paco$_2$ or determine trends in the measurement. Transcutaneous CO$_2$ monitoring can be accomplished using the same technology that is commonly used for measurement of oxygen saturation through pulse oximetry. The electrode used provides a measurement of CO$_2$ through measurement of H$^+$ ion change. Transcutaneous CO$_2$ monitors have gained notice for their value in analyzing analysis during circumstances in which ETCO$_2$ measurement may be inaccurate, as in the case of ventilation-perfusion mismatching.[43] In such cases as severe obesity, which may affect ventilation-perfusion ratios as a result of reduced functional residual capacity, transcutaneous CO$_2$ monitoring may provide a more accurate estimate of arterial carbon dioxide than ETCO$_2$. In addition, transcutaneous CO$_2$ monitoring has been shown to accurately approximate ABG analysis in critical care patients.[44,45] An added benefit of transcutaneous CO$_2$ measurement may be seen in monitoring the awake patient at risk of hypoventilation in whom ETCO$_2$ monitoring is impractical.

BOX 18.1   Causes of High and Low End Tidal Carbon Dioxide

Increased ETCO$_2$
Increased CO$_2$ Delivery/Production
Malignant hyperthermia, fever, sepsis, seizures, increased metabolic rate or skeletal muscle activity, bicarbonate administration/medication side effect, laparoscopic surgery, clamp/tourniquet release

Hypoventilation
COPD, neuromuscular paralysis or dysfunction, CNS depression, metabolic alkalosis (if spontaneously breathing), medication side effect

Equipment Problems
CO$_2$ absorbent exhaustion, ventilator leak, rebreathing, malfunctioning inspiratory or expiratory valve

Decreased ETCO$_2$
Decreased CO$_2$ Delivery/Production
Hypothermia, hypometabolism, pulmonary hypoperfusion, low cardiac output or arrest, pulmonary artery embolism, hemorrhage, hypotension, hypovolemia, V/Q mismatch or shunt, auto-PEEP, medication side effect

Hyperventilation
Pain/anxiety, awareness/"light" anesthesia, metabolic acidosis (if spontaneously breathing), medication side effect

Equipment Problems
Ventilator disconnection, esophageal intubation, bronchial intubation, complete airway obstruction or apnea, sample line problems (kinks), ETT or LMA leaks

CNS, Central nervous system; *CO$_2$,* carbon dioxide; *COPD,* chronic obstructive pulmonary disease; *ETT,* endotracheal tube; *LMA,* laryngeal mask airway; *PEEP,* positive end-expiratory pressure; *ETCO$_2$,* end tidal carbon dioxide; *V/Q,* ventilation perfusion.
Adapted from Newmark JL, Sandberg WS. Noninvasive physiologic monitors. In Sandberg WS, et al., eds. *The MGH Textbook of Anesthetic Equipment.* Philadelphia: Elsevier; 2011:137.

Flow, Volume, and Pressure Monitoring of Ventilation

Many modern anesthesia machines offer the ability to monitor spirometry loops. Observation of spirometry loops can provide rapid evaluation of changes in lung compliance and resistance. A spirometry loop is a graphic representation of a dynamic relationship between two respiratory variables: flow and volume or pressure and volume. Pressure-volume loops provide insight into lung compliance and show volume on a vertical axis and airway pressure on the horizontal axis (Fig. 18.6). Flow-volume loops provide information on pulmonary resistance and show flow on the vertical axis and volume on the horizontal axis (Fig. 18.7). The goal of mechanical ventilation is to mimic natural breathing patterns.[46]

The forces that oppose lung expansion determine compliance of the lung. Ideal distending pressures, V/Q matching, alveolar recruitment, homogeneity, and prevention of ventilator-induced lung injury results in optimal compliance.[46] In states of high compliance, minimal force is needed for expansion; conversely, when compliance is low, higher force (pressure) is needed for lung expansion. Compliance is shown by a pressure-volume loop in Fig. 18.6. Decreases in compliance will be apparent on a flow-volume loop as a loop that requires an increase in pressure to achieve a similar volume as a normal loop. Furthermore, an

increase in flow during exhalation will have a higher peak and a steeper slope.[35] Decreases in compliance can occur as a result of pulmonary embolism, bronchoconstriction, pneumothorax, insufflation of the abdomen for laparoscopic surgery, or even inadequate muscle relaxation, to name a few causes. Compliance may be increased in emphysema, positive end-expiratory pressure (PEEP), or simply by resolving those factors that decrease compliance.[47]

Changes in resistance can also be detected by loop spirometry. An increase in resistance may occur when an ETT is kinked or blocked, when there is an airway obstruction, and when bronchoconstriction is seen. Mild bronchospasm may cause slight changes in the flow-volume loop, but, as the spasm progresses, a decreased flow throughout exhalation can be seen. In a pressure-volume loop, increased resistance manifests as an increased pressure needed to deliver the same volume as that prior to the added resistance.[47]

Respiratory Monitoring: Oxygenation

It is obvious that ensuring adequate oxygen delivery to the tissues is of paramount importance in the safe delivery of anesthesia. Monitoring of oxygenation follows the course of oxygen delivery from the source to the patient until distribution within the body. The anesthetist must evaluate the adequacy of the gas machine's delivery of O_2 and the efficiency of its delivery to the alveoli during ventilation. Oxygenation monitoring by itself constitutes only a part of the whole picture when considering the respiratory process. Hypoventilation, hypercapnia, and impending respiratory arrest can occur despite adequate oxygenation, particularly during the administration of supplemental O_2.[48]

Like ventilation monitoring, the means to ensure oxygenation uses multiple senses and technologies. Monitoring oxygenation starts with O_2 delivery analysis and is covered in depth elsewhere in the text. It is crucial to note that ensuring delivery of O_2 from the source does not ensure adequate uptake and distribution of O_2 on the part of the patient.

To assess the major aspects of acid-base balance and respiratory function, including oxygenation, ABG analysis is most helpful. Although the need for frequent sampling and analysis of ABG is dictated by the patient's physiologic status or surgical procedure, noninvasive, continuous monitoring of oxygenation through clinical observation and pulse oximetry is the standard of care[2] (see Table 18.1). Clinical observation parameters also include an assessment of skin color and temperature, nail bed perfusion signs, assessment of depth and rate of respirations, auscultation of breath sounds, and assessment of upper airway patency.

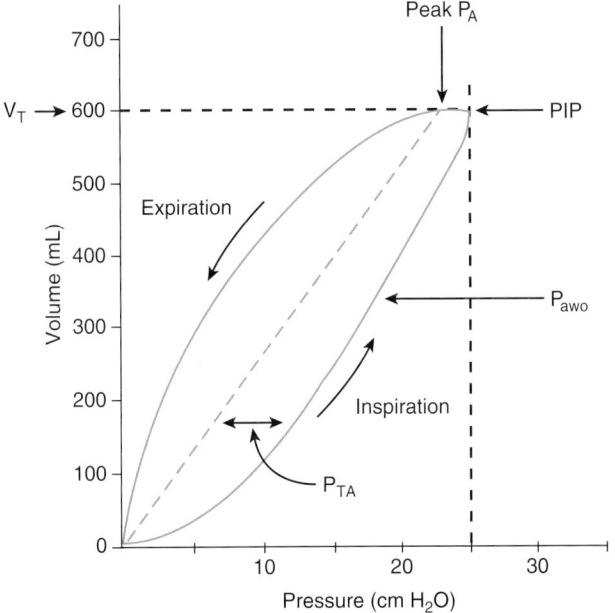

Fig. 18.6 Pressure-volume loop showing the peak inspiratory pressure *(PIP)*, pressure at the airway opening *(P_{awo})*, alveolar pressure *(P_A)*, and transairway pressure *(P_{TA})*. (From Cairo JM. *Pilbeam's Mechanical Ventilation: Physiological and Clinical Applications*. 6th ed. St. Louis: Elsevier; 2016.)

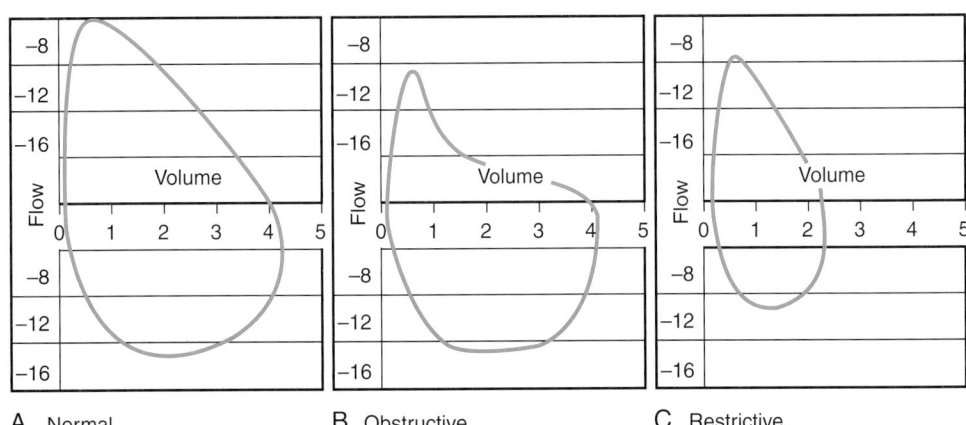

Fig. 18.7 Flow-volume loop showing curves for normal (A), obstructive (B), and restrictive (C) lung disease. (From Rakel RE, Rakel DP. *Textbook of Family Medicine*. 9th ed. Philadelphia: Elsevier; 2016.)

Pulse Oximetry

The use of pulse oximetry is commonplace in many health care settings and has proven valuable in detecting hypoxemia. Pulse oximetry measures heart rate and percent of oxygen saturation (Sao_2) of hemoglobin (Hgb) continuously and noninvasively. The technology involved in providing the transcutaneous measurement uses a spectrophotometer to determine Sao_2. Oxygenated Hgb absorbs light at a different wavelength than nonoxygenated Hgb. At a red wavelength between 650 and 750 nm, reduced oxygen hemoglobin absorbs more light than oxyhemoglobin does. In the infrared wavelengths of 900 to 1000 nm, the opposite occurs.[48,49] A light signal is emitted from one diode and transmitted through tissue, most commonly a finger, to an oppositely placed photosensitive diode that measures the amount of unabsorbed red light. This method is sometimes referred to as transmittance technology. Pulse oximeters can distinguish arterial from venous blood by measuring the change in transmitted light during pulsatile flow. The pulse oximeter converts the detected light to a plethysmograph signal that measures the drop in light intensity with each beat.[50]

Oxygen saturation physiology. To understand the measurement and significance of monitoring oxygen saturation via pulse oximetry, it is important to understand the physiology of oxygen transport and the factors that influence the binding to, and release from, Hgb. This is expressed in the following equation:

$$Hgb + O_2 \leftrightarrow HgbO_2$$

The reversibility of the reaction allows for the release of O_2 to the tissues. Oxygen is transported throughout the body and is either physically dissolved in the blood or chemically combined with Hgb. The vast majority is carried bound to Hgb. As a result, the oxygen-carrying capacity is mainly dependent on the amount of Hgb. If varying concentrations of O_2 are added to a volume of blood, after allowing the mixture to equilibrate, the oxygen tension (Po_2) of the gas can be measured. Because it is known that 0.003 mL of O_2 will dissolve in 100 mL of blood (at a Po_2 of 100 mm Hg), the remaining O_2 bound to Hgb can be determined. In short, the Po_2 of the plasma determines the amount of O_2 that binds to Hgb. Like oxygen carrying capacity, this is expressed in milliliters per 100 mL of blood.[51,52]

The proportion of Hgb bound to O_2 is expressed as percent saturation and excludes that amount dissolved in the blood. The relationship between oxygen tension and percent of oxygen saturation is illustrated in the oxyhemoglobin dissociation curve (Fig. 18.8). It shows how the availability of O_2 (Po_2 in plasma) can affect the reversible reaction between O_2 and Hgb. The curve demonstrates that the amount of O_2 carried by Hgb (percent saturated) increases rapidly to a Po_2 of approximately 60 mm Hg and slows thereafter, as displayed by a flattening of the curve. As blood travels to the systemic capillaries, the oxygenated Hgb releases O_2 to tissue with lower oxygen tension. In the 10 to 40 mm Hg range, the curve is very steep. This demonstrates that small decreases in Po_2 can result in significant dissociation of O_2 for use by the tissue. For example, at a Po_2 of 40 mm Hg, Hgb is approximately 75% saturated with O_2, whereas at 20 mm Hg, only 32% is saturated. This relationship can be altered by a variety of physiologic changes. The result is a shift in the curve either to the right, indicating a more readily release of O_2 from Hgb at the tissue level, or to the left, indicating a greater attachment of O_2 to Hgb, thereby decreasing release to tissues (Table 18.3).[51,52]

Clinical use of pulse oximetry. Although many studies regarding the use of pulse oximetry show conflicting impact on outcome, it should be intuitive that early detection and warning of hypoxemia, followed by appropriate interventions, will improve care. Pedersen et al.[53,54] reviewed more than 21,000 perioperative patients and reported that the incidence of hypoxemia ranged from 1.5 to 3 times less in patients

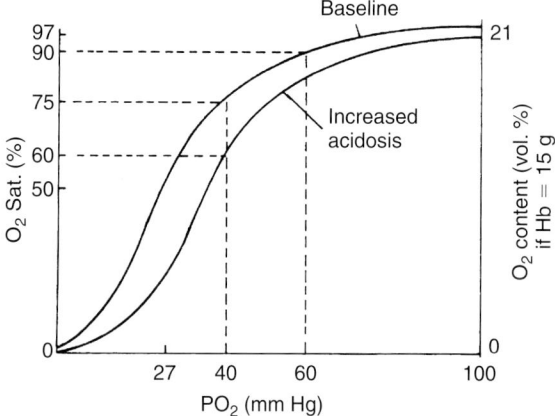

Fig. 18.8 Oxyhemoglobin dissociation curve. (From Roberts JR, et al., eds. *Roberts and Hedges' Clinical Procedures in Emergency Medicine.* 7th ed. Philadelphia: Elsevier; 2019:26.)

TABLE 18.3 Factors Influencing the Oxyhemoglobin Dissociation Curve	
Curve Shift to the Right	**Curve Shift to the Left**
Elevated CO_2	Decreased CO_2
Elevated temperature	Decreased temperature
Elevated levels of 2,3-DPG	Decreased levels of 2,3-DPG
Decreased pH, acidosis (elevated H^+ ions)	Elevated pH, alkalosis (decreased H^+ ions)

CO_2, carbon dioxide; *2,3-DPG,* 2,3-Diphosphoglycerate; *H^+,* hydrogen. Adapted from Levitzky MG, ed. *Pulmonary Physiology.* 9th ed. New York: McGraw-Hill; 2018.

monitored with pulse oximetry. Perhaps one of the greatest benefits of pulse oximetry is in its simplicity. The pulse oximeter is calibrated by the manufacturer and needs little or no further maintenance. It is basic to apply, and ongoing product development has made the device quite portable and durable. Its efficiency in measuring O_2 saturation has been shown to be accurate within 2% when oxygen saturation is between 80% and 100% and approximately 5% when saturation falls below 80%.[48]

Despite the qualities of pulse oximetry, it is essential to understand the optimal use and limitations. Pulse oximeters can use a variety of sensor types applied to the body. The finger probe is the most commonly used and is available as a reusable clip-on device or disposable stick-on probe. The finger probe is often used successfully on the toe as well, particularly in the pediatric population. Although monitors continually improve, motion artifact can still be problematic. Using alternative sites can be helpful. Forehead, ear, or nose probes can be used with comparable accuracy and reliability.[34,55] The site of application of the pulse oximeter probe should be assessed at reasonable intervals during particularly long periods of use and changed as needed to avoid skin irritation or ischemia because prolonged application of a clip-on probe could potentially compromise perfusion. Another common problem associated with inaccurate measurement or sensor difficulties with pulse oximeter monitoring is the vasoconstriction state that results from cold temperatures or inadequate circulation. During such circumstances, measurement may be improved by using oximeter sites closer to the central circulation and away from the periphery, such as the forehead, nose, or ear.[56,57]

Pulse oximeters utilizing reflectance technology have shown promise in reducing inaccuracies in pulse oximetry related to vasoconstriction or other limiting factors associated with transmittance technology. In reflectance pulse oximetry the light emitter is adjacent to the detector, rather than across from it, and thus measures the backscatter of light. The sensor is typically placed on a forehead but could be placed elsewhere. These oximeters have been shown to provide accurate and in some cases more reliable measurement of perfusion than typical sensors and have even been used to monitor tissue perfusion of surgical flaps.[58-60]

Discussion surrounding the impact of the presence of nail polish on pulse oximeter measurement is not as common as when the technology was in its infancy, and studies suggest that improved monitor sensitivity has virtually eliminated any effect nail polish might once have had on pulse oximetry readings.[61,62] A less commonly occurring but still problematic issue is the presence of abnormal hemoglobin. For example, methemoglobin absorbs light equally to oxyhemoglobin. As a result, pulse oximeter measurements are falsely underestimated when oxygen saturation is above 85% and overestimated when oxygen saturation is below 85%. Likewise, abnormally high levels of carboxyhemoglobin can cause the oximeter to overestimate oxygen saturation. Sickle cell anemia and other rarer forms of anemia may also impact the accuracy of pulse oximeter measurements. Injectable dyes for diagnostic use, such as methylene blue or indigo carmine, will result in a significant, but transient, decrease in the measured oxygen saturation by pulse oximetry. This is because the presence of the dye alters the absorption of infrared light. Technology available on some pulse oximeters enables the monitor to distinguish between normal Hgb and carboxyhemoglobin or methemoglobin and quantitatively measure amounts of these variant forms of hemoglobin.[63]

Cerebral oximetry. Monitoring for adequacy of oxygenation specific to the brain has been demonstrated through the use of near infrared spectroscopy (NIRS) in monitoring, which is referred to as cerebral oximetry. Cerebral oximeters utilize emitter/sensor pads similar to reflectance pads applied to the forehead, which measure light attenuation from the emitting light source. As opposed to pulse oximetry, which utilizes plethysmography to differentiate pulsatile flow, cerebral oximeters provide measurements of oxygen supply versus demand within a region. Nonquantitative cerebral oximeters use wavelengths of 730 and 810 nm and measure the ratio of oxygenated Hgb to total Hgb within a region. The ratio is expressed as a percentage value and may be abbreviated as rSO_2. Quantitative cerebral oximeters utilize wavelengths of 775, 825, 850, and 904 nm. They also measure tissue oxygen index as a ratio of oxygenated Hgb to total Hgb.[64]

This technology has been used during cardiac bypass surgery but is also being implemented for other procedures and situations when cerebral perfusion may be compromised, as well as in research to determine best practices to maintain cerebral perfusion.[65,66]

Temperature Monitoring

The standards of care from both the AANA and the ASA support the notion that the ability to monitor patient body temperature is essential.[2,3] Temperature monitoring alerts the anesthetist to hyperthermia, and, as is more commonly the case, hypothermia. The American Society of PeriAnesthesia Nurses (ASPAN) defines hypothermia as a core temperature of less than 36°C (<96.8°F). It has been reported that approximately 70% of postoperative patients experience some degree of hypothermia, whereas other estimates indicate as much as 90% of surgical patients experience some adverse effect of hypothermia.[67,68] Risks of hypothermia include wound infection and delayed healing, increased O_2 consumption through shivering, increased risk of cardiovascular incidents and myocardial infarction, interference with blood coagulation, and increased rate of sickling in sickle cell

patients.[68,69] Hypothermia has also been shown to result in a prolonged stay in PACU, thus increasing the cost of care during the perioperative period.[67]

Appropriate and aggressive means of maintaining normothermia intraoperatively should be instituted, and key to this is temperature monitoring. National quality improvement initiatives supported by the Centers for Medicare and Medicaid Services (CMS) have partnered with health care organizations and accrediting bodies to promote best practices aimed at improving surgical care. These initiatives have identified essential factors in preventing postoperative complications. Not the least of these identified areas of care is centered on maintenance of normothermia. An understanding of the potential causes of variations in core body temperature is valuable in appreciating the importance of temperature monitoring.[69]

Thermoregulation

Body temperature is tightly regulated through the process of thermoregulation, which occurs in a three-phase process: afferent thermal sensing, central regulation or control, and efferent responses. Peripheral sensors send thermal information via tracts in the anterior spinal cord, such as the spinothalamic tract, to various regions of the brain, including the hypothalamus. Behavioral responses to changes in temperature (i.e., layering clothing, seeking warmth) are the most important aspect of thermoregulation in persons who are awake; however, anesthesia prevents patients from responding accordingly. As a result, they must rely on autonomic efferent responses such as shivering, vasoconstriction, and sweating. General anesthetics do not have significant effects on sweating but do reduce shivering and vasoconstriction thresholds. Neuraxial anesthesia also affects thermoregulatory control, resulting in hypothermia.[70,71]

Normothermia can be defined as a body temperature of 37°C. It is important to note that there is typically a variance between core and peripheral temperatures. This is key to appreciating the value of core versus peripheral temperature measurement. Hyperthermia, or core temperatures exceeding 38°C, can be seen intraoperatively. The genetic predisposition to drug-induced malignant hyperthermia is one well-known if not common cause, and the possibility alone warrants the use of intraoperative temperature monitoring during general anesthesia.[72] Other causes of fever may include infection or hypermetabolic states. Certain recreational drugs such as amphetamines, ecstasy, or cocaine can raise the body temperature through an increased rate of metabolism.[73] Drugs such as atropine can inhibit the sweating response, resulting in impaired regulatory response and a rise in the core temperature. In the anesthesia setting, these effects are typically overshadowed by the multiple factors in place that serve to lower core temperature.

Hypothermia, or core temperature below 36°C, occurs for multiple reasons. The ambient room temperature is one obvious cause of hypothermia. Reports suggest that the greatest amount of heat loss occurs during the first hour in the perioperative setting and that patients in rooms at a temperature of 21°C will all develop hypothermia. Radiant heat loss, or that transfer of body heat into a cooler environment, accounts for the majority of heat loss in the patient undergoing surgery. This is followed by evaporative loss from liquids on the skin, such as from cleansing or perspiration or through the expiration of warm, moist air. In addition, convective heat loss (through moving cool air) and conductive heat loss (through contact with a cooler object such as an operating room table) contribute. Redistribution of lower-temperature blood from the vasodilated, anesthetized periphery to the central compartment also accounts for significant heat loss.[68,74] General and regional anesthesia inhibit thermoregulation and cause significant vasodilation such that temperature monitoring is warranted. During local anesthesia or sedation, temperature monitoring should be considered under circumstances in which the patient is at risk of hypothermia and should always be immediately available. It is important to note that normal core body temperature can vary between individuals, as well as within individuals at different points within their circadian rhythms. As a result, monitoring patient temperature is most beneficial when done continuously rather than intermittently and is most valuable when evaluated for trends.[74]

Temperature monitoring modalities. Temperature is an important parameter in the complete monitoring of homeostasis in the perioperative period. The AANA and ASA practice standards allow for some discretion on the part of the anesthesia provider in deciding under what circumstances temperature monitoring should occur. The ASA states that body temperature monitoring should occur whenever significant changes in temperature are "intended, anticipated, or suspected." The AANA states, "When clinically significant changes in body temperature are intended, anticipated, or suspected, monitor body temperature. Use active measures to facilitate normothermia. When malignant hyperthermia (MH) triggering agents are used, monitor temperature and recognize signs and symptoms to immediately initiate appropriate treatment and management of MH."[2,3]

To ensure monitoring is done and active warming strategies used, it is essential that the anesthetist be well aware of the factors that place patients at risk for perioperative hypothermia. Some of these risk factors include high ASA status, lengthy or involved surgical procedures, combined epidural and general anesthesia, surgery of long duration, elderly patients, and those with lean body mass. Interestingly, another identified risk factor for hypothermia is failure to monitor temperature. Protective factors of increased body weight, higher preoperative temperature, and warmer rooms were noted to help maintain normothermia.[74,75]

Technology used for temperature monitoring varies often by site measured. Thermistor, thermocouple, and platinum wire devices are frequently used with electronic monitors and have been shown to be accurate and reliable. Liquid crystal temperature monitors have been used for skin temperature monitoring; however, although these are noninvasive and convenient, they lack specific accuracy both in measurement and in interpretation between readings by separate observers.[34]

There has been some debate as far as how best to measure temperature; indeed, each site has certain advantages and disadvantages (Table 18.4). Skin temperature measurement is convenient and noninvasive; however, its accuracy as a reflection of core body temperature is unreliable. Temporal artery temperature measurements use infrared technology to measure blood temperature close to the surface with a device swiped across the forehead and down along the temporal artery. Some studies suggest this approximates oral and axillary temperatures to a reasonably close degree; however, others question their accuracy.[70,76]

Core temperature monitoring is believed to be the most reflective of thermal status in humans. This includes temperature monitoring at the tympanic membrane, distal esophagus, bladder, nasopharynx, or pulmonary artery.[70] The type of surgery may play an important role in determining the optimal location for temperature monitoring. For example, in liver transplantation, bladder temperature has been shown to closely approximate pulmonary artery temperature measurements. Esophageal monitoring may be less reflective of core temperature during open heart surgery because of the exposed thoracic cavity. For many surgeries, the tympanic membrane may be considered an ideal site, particularly because of its close proximity to the brain, therefore providing an accurate reflection of brain temperature. It should be noted, however, that tympanic membrane temperature measurement using aural probes with thermocouples provides this reliable assessment as opposed to the popular but less accurate use of infrared technology.[76,77]

ANESTHESIA EDUCATION AND PATIENT MONITORING

Teaching clinical monitoring begins in the classroom and is reinforced and emphasized in the clinical learning environment. As with all aspects of anesthesia education, teaching the art and science of clinical monitoring of the patient must be well thought out. Many educational programs and anesthesia departments use some form of simulation-based education as a supplement to clinical experience. Simulation learning is designed to give additional interactive practice and can also serve to review critical incidents and adverse events.[78] The use of

TABLE 18.4 Comparisons of Body Temperature Monitoring Sites

Monitoring Site	Advantages	Disadvantages
Bladder	Reflects core temperature Correlates accurately with other core sites	Invasive—requires urinary catheter placement Risk of UTI
Pulmonary artery	Reflects core temperature Correlates accurately with other core sites	Invasive—requires PA catheter Not reliable during open chest procedures
Esophageal	Considered by most authors to reflect core temperature Ease of insertion	Slight potential for oral or esophageal trauma, bleeding Not useful in awake patients Inaccurate if placed too close to the stomach
Nasopharynx	Considered by most authors to reflect core temperature Ease of insertion	Potential for nasopharyngeal trauma, bleeding Less useful in awake patients Inaccurate if breathing through nares
Tympanic	Considered by most authors to reflect core temperature Accurate if contact probe is used Ease of insertion Possible for awake patients	Slight potential for tympanic membrane trauma Possible to push ear wax from canal to membrane Infrared device less accurate
Axillary	Safe, noninvasive, ease of placement Reasonable correlation with core in adducted arm when placed close to axillary artery	Not a direct measurement of core temperature Influenced by IV fluids Easily dislodged

IV, Intravenous; *PA*, pulmonary artery; *UTI*, urinary tract infection.

simulated clinical experience can assist in developing critical decision-making skills through repetition.

A part of vigilance in monitoring lies in developing habits that promote frequent, almost ritualistic, patterns of assessment and visualization. Many students have a tendency to first focus on the electronic devices while forgetting the ongoing physical assessment of the patient. It is the role of the instructor to promote effective routines by explaining the underlying rationale, as well as by example. Another important part of learning to closely monitor the patient is training the senses to notice changes in the clinical picture. Every anesthetist should be able to discern when the changing audible tones of the pulsatile measurement of the pulse oximeter monitor indicate decreasing oxygen saturation. One should rapidly recognize the subtle development of abnormal airway sounds heard through a precordial stethoscope. These are only several of the basic clinical skills essential to anesthesia practice, and the anesthesia student requires time, experience, and appropriate habits to fully develop them.

Beyond learning the use and interpretation of monitoring methods, the student must also learn to appreciate the potential artifacts that can occur during electronic measurement. Because artifacts can result in false alarms, there exists the potential to ignore important alarms if their validity is uncertain. The student and experienced provider must learn to assimilate all data to make the right interpretation.[79]

SUMMARY

Whereas technology advances the anesthetist's ability to monitor important physiologic functions in ways previously unheard of, the importance of the human factor in anesthesia delivery and monitoring does not appear to be replaceable any time soon. Clinical monitoring is a human skill that uses all of the senses. The importance of maintaining adequate ventilation and oxygenation has been underscored in reviews of closed-claim studies, thereby emphasizing the need for vigilant, continuous monitoring of these parameters in the patient receiving anesthesia. A systematic approach to monitoring can be useful in keeping the anesthetist vigilant. Of all monitoring modalities, $ETco_2$ and pulse oximetry have been shown to be of particular value, and improvements in technology have brought more accurate and dependable means of evaluation. Hypothermia is an all too common occurrence under anesthesia, and management must center on prudent temperature monitoring. Clinical standards of care, as developed by the recognized professional anesthesia organization, must be adhered to continuously and reevaluated frequently. Outcome studies are warranted to justify the use of monitoring modalities, and the potential benefits must outweigh the potential risks.

REFERENCES

For a complete list of references for this chapter, scan this QR code with any smartphone code reader app, or visit the following URL: http://booksite.elsevier.com/9780323711944/.

19

Clinical Monitoring III: Neurologic System

Vincent E. Ford, Virginia C. Simmons

Early anesthetists John Snow and Arthur Guedel proposed the use of clinical and neurologic signs to evaluate and determine the depth of anesthesia. Snow described the "five stages of narcotism" in response to anesthesia using chloroform.[1] Guedel further refined these signs by developing a set of physical criteria for the "clinical signs and stages of anesthesia" that are based on the autonomic nervous system responses to anesthesia.[2] Neurologic signs, such as respiratory rate and rhythm, ocular movement, pupillary size, and reflexes were used to evaluate the depth of ether anesthesia.[1,2]

Today, the practice of anesthesia incorporates sophisticated technology for neurologic monitoring in addition to the classic neurologic signs as determined by Guedel and Snow. Due to the significant pharmacodynamic effects of anesthetic medications on the cardiovascular system, it is impractical to depend solely on clinical signs for assessing anesthetic levels or neurologic function. Furthermore, the adult brain comprises approximately 2% to 3% of body weight but requires 15% to 20% of cardiac output. The enormous metabolic activity of neurologic tissue substantiates this fact. Monitoring the neurologic status of a patient demands a thorough knowledge of the modern devices used and the skills needed to navigate a rapidly changing clinical environment. The most important goal of intraoperative monitoring (IOM) of the central nervous system (CNS) is to identify and rapidly treat possible neurologic injuries such as CNS ischemia prior to onset of permanent deficits.[3] Tenets of quality neurologic monitoring during anesthesia include[4]:

1. Possessing thorough knowledge of the monitors and modalities available for neurologic monitoring
2. Selecting appropriate neurologic monitor(s) with high sensitivity and specificity (i.e., low false positive and false negative) for data acquisition and guiding patient management[5]
3. Understanding the various pathologic disease states that increase the potential for cerebral ischemia during a period of increased or decreased blood flow
4. Choosing anesthetic medications and doses that best preserve cerebral blood flow (CBF)
5. Identifying and intervening promptly if deleterious neurologic changes occur during the perioperative period to prevent irreversible neurologic damage[5]

The neurophysiologic parameters that can be monitored during anesthesia and surgery include cerebral electrical activity, CBF, cerebral oxygen content, intracranial pressure (ICP), and cerebral metabolic rate of oxygen consumption ($CMRO_2$). Monitoring of the CNS electrical activity is performed by means of electroencephalography (EEG) and brainstem auditory-, sensory-, and motor-evoked potentials (EPs). Monitoring CBF velocity is achieved by transcranial Doppler (TCD) ultrasonography. ICP can be determined by the use of intraventricular catheters and fiberoptic intraparenchymal microtransducers. Near infrared spectrometry (NIRS) is a measure of cerebral oxygen content.

Lastly, $CMRO_2$ can be measured through invasive techniques such as placement of intracerebral partial pressure of oxygen (Po_2) electrodes and jugular venous oximetry.[6] Select methods for monitoring neurologic functions are presented in Box 19.1.

This chapter examines monitors currently used in clinical practice, the effects that anesthetic medications exert on CNS monitoring modalities, and preservation of neurologic function during the perianesthetic period. A thorough discussion of neurophysiology and the principles that regulate cerebral vascular autoregulation, CBF, and cerebral perfusion pressure are presented in Chapter 31. Methods that can be used to assess CNS integrity and their indications, advantages, and disadvantages are noted in Table 19.1.

ELECTROENCEPHALOGRAM

EEG Fundamentals

The brain is an electrochemical organ that generates electrical impulses in specific patterns. The voltage from the ionic current generated between neurons in the brain can be recorded. The electrical activity from the surface of the brain that can be observed through an EEG is called electrical brainwaves. The brain does not emit electrical waves; rather, the EEG is a sensitive monitor that measures the differences in electrical potentials in groups of neurons between brain regions.[7] Electrodes used to produce the EEG are placed on the patient in a standardized sequential configuration, these examine the electrical signals produced by the CNS in response to external stimuli. These responses are known as evoked potentials, or EPs. Auditory, visual, and tactile stimuli cause the neurologic EP response to occur. Sensory-evoked responses are elicited by somatosensory-evoked potentials (SSEPs), visual-evoked potentials (VEPs), and brainstem auditory–evoked potentials (BAEPs). Motor responses are measured by motor-evoked potentials (MEPs). Specific alterations in the EP signal can help diagnose a host of conditions, including systemic hypoxia, brain trauma, and ischemic and hemorrhagic stroke. The information gained from an EEG can also be used to assess and guide the depth of anesthesia during neurosurgical procedures.[8]

The basic components of the EEG waveform include frequency, amplitude, and the overall morphology (shape). Frequency refers to the rate of or duration between impulses. Amplitude is defined as the peak-to-peak measurements in a vertical plane and is measured in microvolts. The morphology or shape is comprised of the wave amplitude and the frequency at which the waves occur. The ability to detect significant changes in EEG waveforms is a complex process that requires specialized training. There are four common types of brainwaves that comprise the EEG: alpha, beta, delta, and theta waves (Table 19.2). There are also several variants or subgroups of waves noted during specific activities. Some of these waveform variants are gamma and mu waves. Gamma waves are typically seen with high-order activity such

BOX 19.1 Specialized Methods of Neurologic Monitoring

- EEG—electroencephalogram
- SSEP—somatosensory-evoked potential
- MEP—motor-evoked potential
- VEP—visual-evoked potential
- BAEP—brainstem auditory–evoked potential
- BIS—bispectral index
- NIRS—near infrared spectroscopy
- TCD—transcranial Doppler ultrasonography
- ICP—intracranial pressure

as problem solving and analytic thinking; they represent the activity of groups of neurons. Mu waves represent synchronous firing of neurons during rest.[9-11] Depending on the situation, it can be difficult to distinguish artifact from normal variations of EEG patterns, especially as the majority of anesthetic agents inhibit neuronal activity.[12-14] An example of an EEG recording is presented in Fig. 19.1.

The head and much of the scalp may be inaccessible during intracranial surgical procedures, so the standard 21-channel EEG used to detect generalized neuronal activity is rarely used. IOM during craniotomy is usually accomplished with a 2- to 4-channel recording with computer processing to simplify the interpretation. Depression of and characteristic changes in EEG activity can be seen with reductions in CBF, oxygen, or glucose delivery. During an awake state, the

TABLE 19.1 Brain Monitoring Methods

Method	Spacial Resolution	Temporal Resolution	Purpose	Advantages	Disadvantages
ICP	Global	Continuous	Measure ICP	Reliable Quantitative Allows monitoring of CPP and calculation of secondary indices	Invasive Risk of infection Risk of hemorrhage
Jugular oximetry (SjvO$_2$)	Global	Continuous	Measure adequacy of hemispheric oxygenation	Quantitative Allows monitoring of AVDO$_2$ and O$_2$ER	Susceptible to artifacts Local complications (e.g., infection, thrombosis)
EEG	Global	Continuous	Monitoring electrical brain activity Detection of seizures	Technique well standardized Only method to diagnose nonconvulsive seizures	Qualitative Relatively insensitive to secondary insults
SSEP	Global	Continuous	Monitoring integrity of sensory pathways	Technique well standardized Simple	Qualitative Fairly insensitive to secondary insults
Bedside Xe-133 CBF	Regional	Discontinuous	Measure hemispheric CBF	Quantitative	Only accurate if radiotracer injected into carotid artery Radioactivity
Laser Doppler flowmetry	Local	Continuous	Measure cortical CBF	Accurate Dynamic information	Qualitative Invasive Susceptible to artifacts Only monitors 1–2 mm^3 of tissue
Thermal diffusion flowmetry	Local	Continuous	Measure cortical CBF	Simple Dynamic information	Qualitative Invasive Monitors small volume of tissue
TCD	Regional	Continuous	Measure CBF velocities	Simple Noninvasive Allows measuring PI, VMR	Qualitative and indirect assessment of CBF Difficult to keep probes in place
Brain tissue P$_{O_2}$	Local	Continuous	Measure cerebral oxygenation	Quantitative Sensitive Probes also measure brain temperature	Invasive Susceptible to artifacts Monitors small volume of tissue
NIRS	Local	Continuous	Measure cerebral oxygenation	Noninvasive	Measures only relative changes Susceptible to artifacts
Microdialysis	Local	Discontinuous	Measure cerebral metabolism	Sensitive Quantitative	Invasive Complicated technique Labor intensive Unclear which is the best parameter to monitor

AVDO$_2$, Arteriovenous oxygen difference; *CBF*, cerebral blood flow; *CPP*, cerebral perfusion pressure; *EEG*, electroencephalogram; *ICP*, intracranial pressure; *NIRS*, near infrared spectroscopy; *O$_2$ER*, oxygen extraction rate; *PI*, pulsatility index; *P$_{O_2}$*, partial pressure of oxygen; *TCD*, transcranial Doppler; *SSEP*, somatosensory-evoked potentials; *VMR*, vasomotor reactivity.

From Rabinstein AA. Principles of neurointensive care. In Daroff RB, Jandovic J, eds. *Bradley's Neurology in Clinical Practice.* 7th ed. London: Elsevier; 2016.

TABLE 19.2 **Comparison of Electroencephalography Waveform Types**

Waveform and Frequency (Hz)	Characteristics
Alpha (7.5–14)	Occurs with eyes closed during deep relaxation
Beta (14–40)	Normal awake consciousness, alertness, logic, and critical thinking
Theta (4–7.5)	Light sleep
Gamma (>40)	High-level information processing
Delta (0.5–4)	High amplitude, associated with deep sleep

high-frequency and low-amplitude beta waves are most prominent. There is a transient increase in beta waves with the onset of ischemia or hypoxia, with eventual development of increased-amplitude theta and delta waves. As ischemia or hypoxia increase, beta waves begin to disappear, and there is an appearance of low-amplitude delta waves. This progresses to electrical activity suppression with occasional bursts of activity. The onset of irreversible damage can be determined when there is complete electrical silence, as seen with an isoelectric or flat EEG pattern.

Monitoring the EEG intraoperatively for the development of delta waves allows for the recognition of an increased risk of ischemic damage to the brain. After the induction of anesthesia and prior to the start of surgery, an EEG tracing will be established to determine a baseline pattern. To allow for reliable EEG interpretation during the

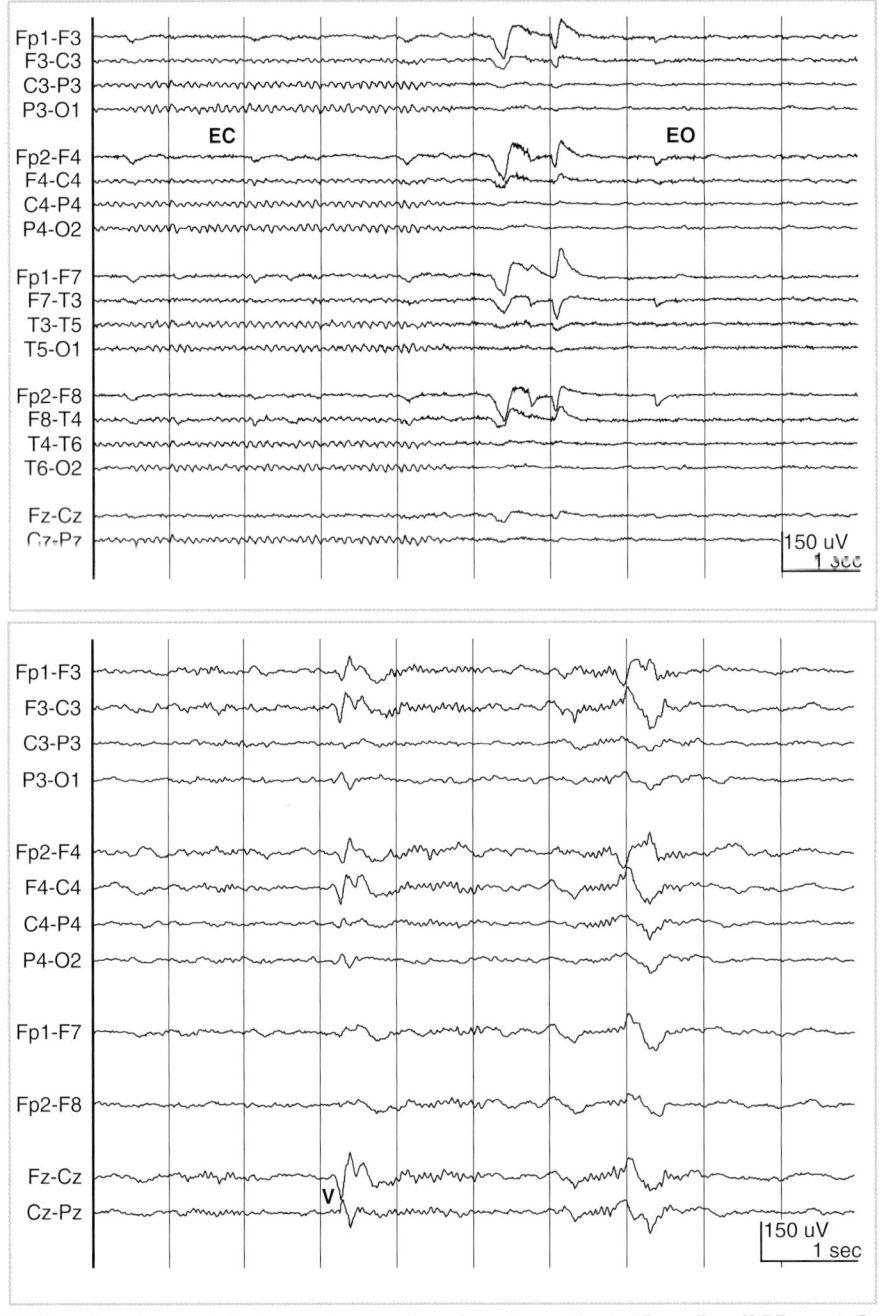

Fig. 19.1 Samples of normal electrographic recordings from two patients. (From Daroff RB, et al. *Bradley's Neurology in Clinical Practice.* 7th ed. St. Louis: Elsevier; 2016.)

TABLE 19.3 Effects of Inhalation Anesthetics on EEG

Inhalation Agent	Low-Dose Inhalation Anesthesia	Moderate-Dose Inhalation Anesthesia	High-Dose Inhalation Anesthesia	EEG Amplitude	Dose for Burst Suppression
Desflurane	< Alpha waves > Beta waves	> Beta waves	Diffuse delta and theta	↑ Low dose ↑ Anesthetic dose ↑ or 0 High dose	>1.2 MAC
Isoflurane	< Alpha waves > Beta waves	> Beta waves	Diffuse delta and theta	↑ Low dose ↑ Anesthetic dose ↑ or 0 High dose	>1.5 MAC
Sevoflurane	< Alpha waves > Beta waves	> Beta waves	Diffuse delta and theta	↑ Low dose ↑ Anesthetic dose ↑ or 0 High dose	>1.2 MAC
Nitrous oxide (alone)	> Beta waves	> Beta waves	> Beta waves	↑ Low dose ↑ Anesthetic dose ↑ High dose	Not seen in clinical concentrations

↑, Increase; 0, no effect; *EEG,* electroencephalogram; *MAC,* minimum alveolar concentration.
Adapted from Seubert CN, McCauliffe JJ, Mahla ME. Neurologic monitoring. In: Gropper MA, et al., eds. *Miller's Anesthesia.* Philadelphia: Elsevier; 2020:1267.

administration of anesthesia, the type and amount of medication given should be titrated to inhibit the sympathetic nervous system without obliterating the EEG waveform. Changes in the depth of anesthesia should be immediately communicated to the EEG technician such that false-positive ECG patterns suggestive of ischemia can be disregarded. The EEG can only provide information about the integrity of the brain's cerebral cortical structures; therefore neuronal ischemia and infarction are possible in the subcortical regions, spinal cord, or cranial and peripheral nerves.[15]

Anesthetic Effects on EEG

Considerations for Inhalation Anesthetics and EEG Interpretation

Interpreting the EEG in the presence of anesthetic medication administration can be confounding because the majority of anesthetic agents inhibit neuronal activity and depress EEG waveforms. Instead, generalized assumptions are made that brain function is adequate or inadequate during anesthetic management based on trends. There are two major reasons why the EEG tracing is difficult to correlate with patient outcomes. First, dose-related cerebral inhibition occurs with inhalation and intravenous agents, as they increase frequency and decrease amplitude of the EEG waveforms (Tables 19.3 and 19.4).[16-21] The second variable involves environmental factors (e.g., artifact) and manipulation of the brain, which add to the complexity of interpretation.

Inhalation agents depress $CMRO_2$ in a dose-dependent manner, resulting in decreased regional tissue oxygen consumption and vascular constriction. As a result, these medications have a global effect of decreasing CBF. However, the net effect of a volatile agent's influence on CBF is dependent on the direct vasodilatory properties of the individual drug and the vasoconstricting effects associated with catecholamine release. Older adults and those patients with baseline slowing of the EEG are more sensitive to the effects associated with isoflurane and desflurane.[22] When administered in "approximate" doses, inhalation agents induce a significantly greater depression of EEG activity as compared to intravenous anesthetic agents.[23]

Induction Agents

Induction doses of etomidate and propofol have similar effects on the EEG by increasing the frequency and decreasing the amplitude of beta waves. This beta-rhythm EEG activity correlates with the patient losing consciousness after drug administration; time- and dose-related neuronal depression is seen with anesthetic drugs.[24,25] One difference between these two drugs is that myoclonus, which can occur with the use of etomidate, is not reflected on EEG signals.[26] Coincidently, the EEG frequency decreases as the serum levels of etomidate rise, thereby leading to burst suppression. Burst suppression can be achieved with both of these induction agents in higher dosage ranges. Burst suppression is a term used to describe an EEG pattern associated with alternating high-voltage, mixed frequency, slow-wave activity, along with periods of electrical suppression that last several seconds (Fig. 19.2). This type of electrical activity is unpredictable, and the duration is variable. Burst suppression is also typically seen with a decrease in cerebral circulation and oxygenation, as well as with hypothermia, particularly during cardiopulmonary bypass surgery. Burst suppression may be desirable during manipulation of brain tissues as it decreases $CMRO_2$, which is neuroprotective.[23-25] Burst suppression can be achieved during anesthesia using a variety of anesthetic agents. These agents include etomidate, propofol, dexmedetomidine, and inhalation agents, which all provide varying levels of suppression of electrical activity in a dose-dependent manner.[24,26,27] Propofol enables a deeper state of unconsciousness as compared to dexmedetomidine by inducing large-amplitude slow oscillations that produce prolonged burst suppression states.[28-31] Unilateral burst suppression is indicative of ischemia or injury to the brain. Forethought should be given to the use of sevoflurane in patients with known epileptiform EEG activity; the activity may be accentuated by these inhalation agents in lower concentrations.[25,32,33]

Opioids can produce EEG slowing in the delta range, especially at moderate and higher doses. Initial excitation with faster frequencies, burst suppression, or an isoelectric pattern usually does not occur with narcotics. Muscle relaxants have no direct effect on the EEG.[11]

A summary of the effects of intravenous anesthetic medications on EEG recordings is shown in Table 19.4. There is a synergistic depressant effect on EEG sensory-evoked responses when various intravenous agents are administered concomitantly.

PROCESSED EEG WAVEFORMS

The interpretation of a raw EEG is often difficult and can depend on the waveform quality, lead placement, artifact or electrical interference, and skill level of the clinicians in interpreting the waveforms. To

TABLE 19.4   Intravenous Anesthetic Medications and Their Effect on the EEG

Medication	Effect: EEG Frequency	Effect: EEG Amplitude	Burst Suppression
Etomidate			
Low dose	Fast frontal beta activity		Yes, with high doses
Moderate dose	Fast frontal frequency spindles		
High dose	Diffuse delta → burst suppression → silence	↓, 0	
Propofol			
Low dose	Loss of alpha; frontal beta		Yes with high doses
Moderate dose	Frontal delta; waxing/waning alpha		
High dose	Diffuse delta → burst suppression → silence	↓, 0	
Ketamine			
Low dose	Loss of alpha, variability	↓	No
Moderate dose	Frontal rhythmic delta		
High dose	Polymorphic delta; some beta	Low amplitude beta	
Benzodiazepines			
Low dose	Loss of alpha; increased frontal beta activity	0	No
High dose	Frontally dominant delta and theta		
Opioids			
Low dose	Loss of beta; alpha slowing	None	No
Moderate dose	Diffuse theta; some delta		
High dose	Delta, often synchronized		
Dexmedeto-midine	Moderate slowing, prominent spindles	↓, 0	No

Alpha = 8–13 Hz frequency; beta ≥13 Hz frequency; delta ≤4 Hz frequency; theta = 4–7 Hz frequency.
↓, Decrease; 0, no effect; *EEG*, electroencephalogram.
Adapted from Seubert CN, McCauliffe JJ, Mahla ME. Neurologic monitoring. In: Gropper MA, et al., eds. *Miller's Anesthesia*. Philadelphia: Elsevier; 2020:1267.

further analyze the EEG, multiple methods are used, including compressed spectral array (CSA) and density spectral array (DSA). The CSA and DSA are obtained, calculated, and displayed by collecting, assessing, and providing a summary of each of the waves (alpha, beta, theta, delta) over a period of time. A mathematical description for the timeframe, using the amplitude and frequency of the waves, is accomplished by using a fast Fourier transform (FFT) algorithm. Applying an FFT algorithm is typically thought of as breaking down a signal into a

variety of components and then reconstructing the useful information into an analysis of the complex signals. The Fourier analysis also results in a compressed view of EEG waveforms. The compressed data are presented in a two- or three-dimensional graph. Depending on the display used, these data appear as either a CSA or a dot matrix DSA.

The processed information collected and displayed for the CSA and DSA is analyzed for the waveform relationships using the amplitude and frequency and illustrated in two- or three-dimensional graphs. These relationships are expressed as the spectral edge frequency (SEF), median frequency, and relative delta power. Most commonly, the SEF is used and represented by the EEG frequency and power activity, which falls below 90% (SEF90).[30,31] As frequency declines below a predetermined power, the spectral edge changes. In the presence of general anesthesia or cerebral injury, frequency and power decline, thereby causing a change in the spectral edge. The modern EEG calculates the computerized spectral array, which is then used during anesthesia to determine the depth of anesthesia or unilateral injury, based on the processed results.[34,35] General anesthesia produces a reduction in high-frequency waves and an increase in low-frequency amplitudes.

MONITORS FOR ASSESSING CNS BLOOD FLOW AND OXYGENATION

Cerebral Oximetry via Near Infrared Spectroscopy

Cerebral oximetry uses NIRS to assess cerebral oxygen saturation. This noninvasive monitor allows the practitioner to detect decreases in CBF in relation to $CMRO_2$. Regional oxygen saturation is determined by the difference in intensity between transmitted and received light delivered at specific wavelengths (as described by the Beer-Lambert law), as with pulse oximetry. The light source is applied to the patient's forehead, and it is then transmitted through tissue and bone. NIRS can better penetrate deep into thick tissues, allowing physiologic interpretation of oxygenation by evaluating, in real time, the transmission and absorption of infrared light by hemoglobin in brain tissue. The NIRS of electromagnetic waves ranges from approximately 750 to 2500 nm. The localized volume of cerebral blood (of which 70% is venous) is analyzed. The near infrared wavelengths used in commercial devices are between 700 and 950 nm, where the absorption spectra of oxygenated and deoxygenated hemoglobin are maximally distinguishable.

As in any monitoring modality there are conditions that can decrease the accuracy of the information obtained. Changes in blood pressure, partial pressure of carbon dioxide in arterial blood ($Paco_2$), regional blood volume, hemoglobin concentration, and individual variability (e.g., differences in extracranial tissue) all effect NIRS readings. Contamination of the signal occurs with increased levels of hypoxia in the tissues on the scalp, leading to distorted signals and brain oxygenation readings. When using the NIRS monitor, the anesthetist must be careful to consider peripheral oxygenation of the scalp, as the NIRS value may not be fully reflective of cerebral oxygenation.[36,37] For these reasons, definitive values that would be suggestive of cerebral ischemia do not exist. However, measuring NIRS values prior to induction allows for its use as a trend monitor throughout the intraoperative course.

Currently the most frequent uses of NIRS are in neonatology, during cardiac surgery, and during carotid endarterectomy. The goal of supportive intervention is to maintain the NIRS value at a minimum of 75% of the baseline reading. Avoiding cerebral desaturation during these procedures is believed to reduce complications relating to cerebral ischemia. A systematic review of patients undergoing shoulder arthroscopy in the beach chair position or internal carotid artery cross-clamping during carotid endarterectomy showed that the majority of these patients experienced periods of significant cerebral desaturation. A greater than 20% reduction in cerebral oxygen saturation

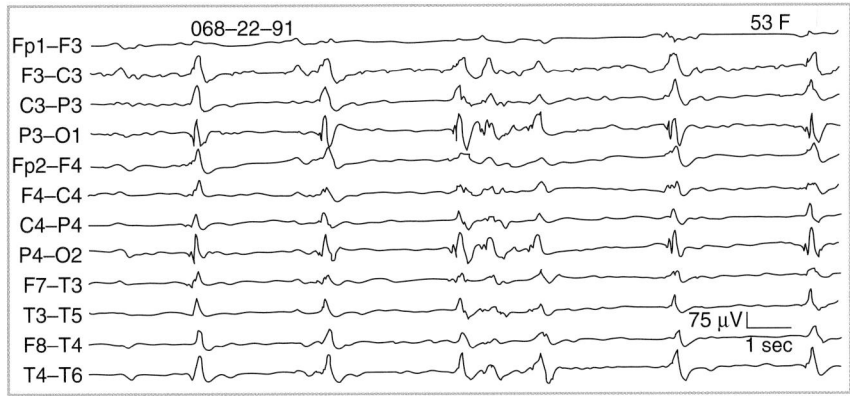

Fig. 19.2 Burst suppression pattern on the electroencephalogram of a 53-year-old woman with anoxic encephalopathy following cardiorespiratory arrest. The patient died several days later. (From Daroff RB, et al. *Bradley's Neurology in Clinical Practice.* 7th ed. St. Louis: Elsevier; 2016.)

is correlated with regional and global ischemia during carotid endarterectomy. Following thoracic surgery, major orthopedic surgery, and abdominal surgery, the occurrence of postoperative cognitive dysfunction might be related to intraoperative cerebral desaturation.[38] Currently there is a lack of evidence to define what specific cerebral oxygen saturation value, as assessed by NIRS, correlates with an "abnormal" level suggestive of cerebral ischemia. In addition, scientific data do not indicate that patients monitored via NIRS have a lower rate of mortality as compared to those who are not monitored.[39]

Transcranial Doppler Ultrasonography

TCD ultrasonography is accomplished by the use of a probe positioned on the temporal bone that emits ultrasound waves. This noninvasive monitoring modality allows for the anesthetist to monitor blood flow velocity within the large arteries of the brain, most commonly the middle cerebral artery, and detect instances of hyperperfusion and hypoperfusion.[40] Continuous pulsed Doppler waves are transmitted and received to produce acoustic information. Specific parameters that can be ascertained by TCD monitoring include flow direction, peak systolic and end-diastolic flow velocity, flow acceleration time, and intensity of pulsatile flow. Microemboli can be detected by TCD, and monitoring of cerebral integrity during specific surgical cases such as carotid endarterectomy may be beneficial.[40-42] A specific limitation associated with TCD monitoring is that, in individuals with greater thickness of the temporal bone, the Doppler waves can be impeded, which hinders accurate analysis.

Jugular Bulb Oxygen Venous Saturation

Measurement of a mixed venous blood sample from the jugular bulb ($SjvO_2$) provides an estimation of the degree of global oxygen delivery (supply) and extraction (demand) by the brain. The internal jugular vein has a dilated region known as the jugular bulb, which is the portion of internal jugular vein that enters the jugular fossa. Located at the base of the skull, the jugular bulb receives blood drainage from both left and right cerebral hemispheres—approximately 70% from the ipsilateral hemisphere and 30% from the contralateral hemisphere. The jugular bulb can be accessed from 1 cm below and 1 cm anterior to the mastoid process. A fiberoptic catheter can be inserted through the internal jugular vein and into the jugular bulb under fluoroscopy. The $SjvO_2$ catheter has two optical fibers. The first emits light, and the second absorbs the light and transmits it to a photosensor. The absorption of the reflected light from oxygenated and deoxygenated hemoglobin is then expressed as a percentage.

Indications for $SjvO_2$ monitoring include cerebral hypoxia detection, ischemia evaluation among patients with increased ICP or traumatic brain injury, hyperventilation management, and optimization of cerebral perfusion pressure. $SjvO_2$ values between 55% and 75% have been found to be a reasonable predictor of positive outcomes after traumatic brain injury if the ICP is also maintained within a normal range. A value < 55% indicates inadequate CBF (from hyperventilation, reduced cerebral perfusion pressure, or vasospasm) or an increased $CMRO_2$. A value > 75% can result from a hyperemic condition, a reduced cerebral metabolism requirement (from neuro-cell death or mitochondrial dysfunction) or damaged brain tissue resulting in poor oxygen extraction and diffusion problems. Those patients with a $SjvO_2$ less than 55% or greater than 75% and an elevated ICP had poor outcomes.[43,44] Contraindications for $SjvO_2$ monitoring include neck or cervical spine injury or trauma, coagulopathy, and impaired venous drainage.[45]

EVOKED POTENTIALS

Evoked potentials are electrical potentials that are measured in response to a particular type of stimulus. As anesthetic medications have an inhibitory effect on cerebral activity, the ability to determine a neurologic response may be altered. Intraoperatively, EPs are used to guide the surgical strategy and to act as a warning of neurologic deficits to prevent irreversible damage. Auditory, visual, motor, and somatosensory stimuli are commonly used for clinical EP studies during surgical procedures. Injuries to neural structures can arise from heat (electrocautery), mechanical stress (retraction), ischemia (ligation, edema, and vessel damage), and loss of functional integrity (transection). Many nervous system structures encountered during surgical procedures lack perineurium, which protects against longitudinal retraction, and epineurium, which protects against retraction. The "elastic limit" of such nerves is approximately 20%, suggesting that stretching the nerve farther may produce irreversible damage.[46] EPs also can be affected by hypothermia, hypotension, positioning, and anemia. These systemic effects may develop slowly, and they are potentially reversible if prompt intervention occurs.

Early detection is the key to reducing serious complications. Early detection must then be paired with continuous communication among the anesthesia provider, surgeon, and neurophysiologist. There is variability in the amount of change in latency or amplitude that necessitates intervention in different patients. For instance, stimulation of a peripheral nerve evokes a neurologic response. This response is recorded as voltage over time. The general appearance of an SSEP waveform is presented in Fig. 19.3. Acute changes or trends in waveform patterns as compared to the patient's baseline tracing are monitored. The morphology of the EP tracing varies depending on the peripheral nerve that is stimulated (Fig. 19.4). Three components of the waveform that are examined are the general appearance, amplitude, and latency. Amplitude represents the intensity of the evoked response, and latency is indicative of the time necessary for the evoked response to be measured in the brain. A 50% decrease in amplitude or a 10% increase in latency is suggestive of the possibility of cerebral ischemia, and the surgical team should be made aware of this change.[37] The threshold or stimulating current that is used also aids in assessment of neurologic integrity.

What are the best anesthetic agents to use for surgical procedures when using EPs? A balance must be established between providing an adequate depth of anesthesia while optimizing conditions that allow monitoring of neurologic structures. Each specific type of EP has a unique interaction with the anesthetic delivered. Lipophilic agents that interfere with neuronal membrane conduction also interfere with subcortical conduction, therefore these agents cause an increase in both interpeak latencies and control conduction time. Anesthetic agents that interfere with EEG also interfere with EP. Changes occur because the component frequencies of the EP are the same as that of the EEG. Lastly, inhalation and intravenous anesthetic agents depress EP waveforms in

a dose-dependent manner. Generally, inhalation agents have a greater depressant effect of EP waveforms as compared to intravenous agents. The combination of inhalation and intravenous anesthetic agents has a synergistic depressant effect on SSEP waveforms (Fig. 19.5).

Somatosensory-Evoked Potentials

SSEPs are used to monitor the integrity of the neural structures along both the peripheral and central somatosensory pathways of the brain and spinal cord. SSEPs are usually induced by stimulation of a peripheral nerve, which contains both a sensory and motor component that combine to provide a mixed signal. These stimulations can be induced through mechanical devices, but electrical stimulation gives a more robust response. A maximal electrical stimulation is not required to elicit a response from the nerve. There are several types of electrodes that can be used for stimulating peripheral nerves, including subdermal needles and conductive solid gel disk electrodes. Typically, the lower extremities can be monitored by stimulating the posterior tibial nerve, located midway between the medial border of the Achilles tendon and posterior border of the medial malleolus in the ankle. The upper extremities are monitored by placing the stimulus at the median nerve, located between the tendons of the flexor carpi radialis and the palmaris longus. If these common sites cannot be accessed, two alternate sites are the common peroneal nerve in the popliteal fossa (which may be used for the lower extremity) and the ulnar nerve (either at the wrist or ulnar notch) for the upper extremities.

A multichannel montage is recommended for recording a combination of cortical and subcortical SSEPs. Corkscrews (head), subdermal needles, and disk EEG electrodes are instruments commonly used for recording. For upper limb SSEP studies, electrodes are placed over Erb point both ipsilateral and contralateral to the stimulus. Erb point is located on the side of the neck, 2 to 3 cm above the clavicle and in front of the transverse process of the sixth cervical vertebra. Pressure over this point elicits Erb-Duchenne paralysis, and electrical stimulation over this area elicits various potentials measured in the arm. For lower limb studies, the electrode is placed at the ipsilateral popliteal fossa. Several different characteristics of SSEPs can be measured. Peak latencies are the easiest to measure and standardize, but like other characteristics they can vary with age, tissue mass, electrical stimulus, and

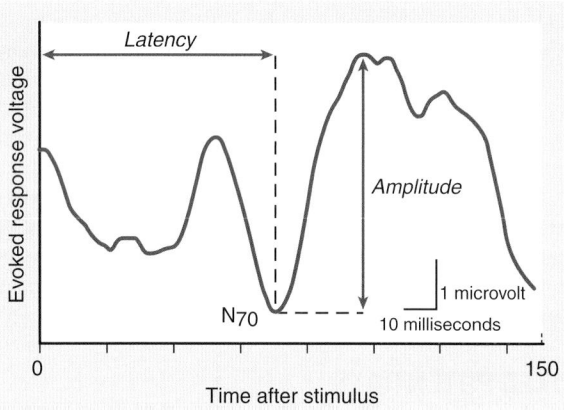

Fig. 19.3 Visual-evoked response tracing of amplitude versus time after stimulus. The measurement of latency and amplitude for the negative peak at 70 msec (N_{70}) is shown. (From Cottrell JE, Patel P. *Cottrell and Patel's Neuroanesthesia*. 6th ed. Edinburgh: Elsevier; 2017:114.)

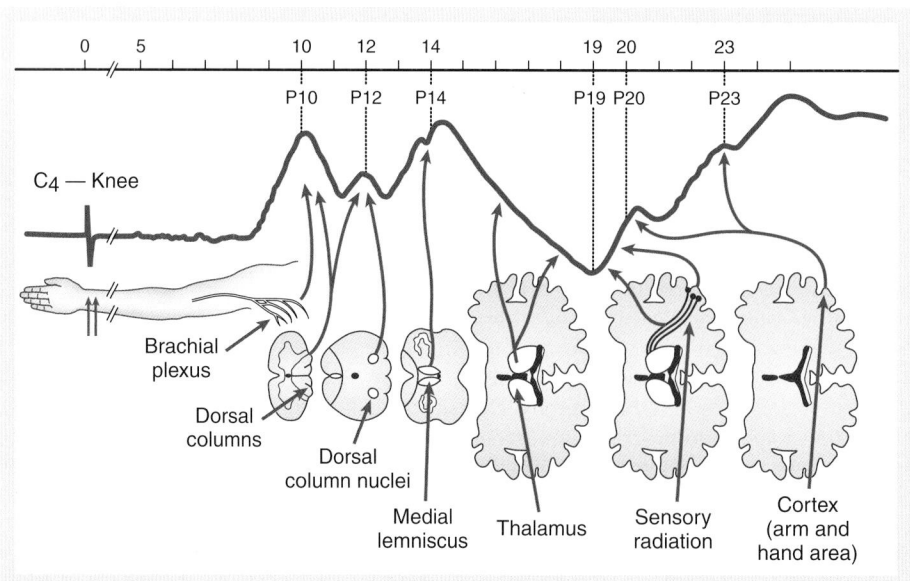

Fig. 19.4 Example of somatosensory-evoked potential peaks. (From Wiederholt WC, et al. Stimulating and recording methods used in obtaining short-latency somatosensory evoked potentials [SEPs] in patients with central and peripheral neurologic disorders. *Ann N Y Acad Sci.* 1982;18[6]:388:349.)

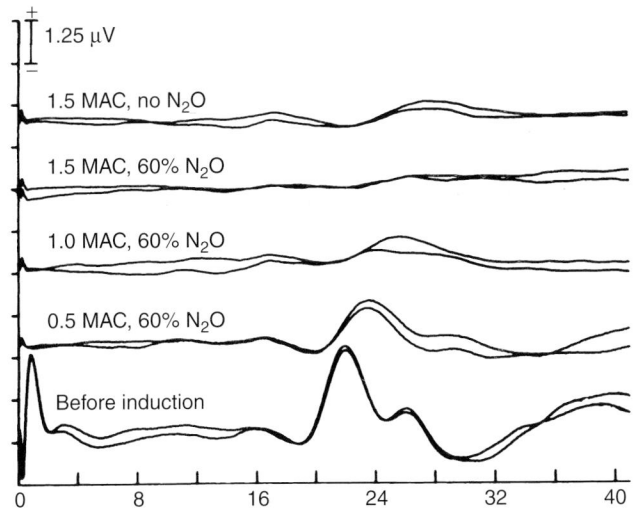

Fig. 19.5 Representative somatosensory-evoked potential-isoflurane. *MAC,* Minimum alveolar concentration; *N₂O,* nitrous oxide. (From Peterson DO, et al. Effects of halothane, enflurane, isoflurane, and nitrous oxide on somatosensory evoked potentials in humans. *Anesthesiology.* 1986;65:35-40.)

limb length. Spinal SSEP electrodes are placed over the spinal cord. SSEPs are usually processed signals, meaning they are processed as an average, with electrical filters to remove background noise, instead of providing real-time electrical waveforms. Interpretation of the compound action potential depends on the site of stimulus and distance to the recording electrodes.

Almost all anesthetic agents produce a dose-related increase in latency and decrease amplitude, with the exception of ketamine, etomidate, and opiates. However, it has been noted in other studies that ketamine and etomidate may cause changes in latency and amplitude.[47] Monitoring conditions for SSEPs are obtained with narcotic-based anesthetics, total intravenous anesthetics, a 0.5 or less minimum alveolar concentration (MAC) per total end tidal inhaled concentration of an inhalation agent, or a combination of these.[48,49] The use of nitrous oxide potentiates the depressant effects on the inhalation agents.[50] Administration of paralytic agents does not affect SSEP monitoring; however, paralytic agents can improve SSEP quality by reducing the amount of electromyographic noise or interference from muscle groups near SSEP recording electrodes.[51] Accordingly, if neuromuscular blockade is not administered, motor responses can be elicited.

Although sometimes limited in their evaluation of neurologic diseases, the value of SSEPs in the operative setting is high.[43] SSEPs can be utilized in an effort to prevent neurologic damage, follow up induced physiologic changes, and locate the central sulcus.[52] SSEP monitoring is used for a variety of surgical procedures. For instance, alterations in the SSEP waveform can indicate high-risk or neurologic injury during aortic cross-clamping. During cerebral aneurysm surgery, changes in SSEPs can indicate the possible occlusion of parental vessels, directing the positioning of important aneurismal vascular clips. In addition, monitoring SSEP waveforms allows surgeons to selectively shunt the operative carotid artery during endarterectomy.

Motor-Evoked Potentials and Electromyography

MEPs are used to monitor the functional integrity of motor tracts, particularly in the corticospinal tract. Whereas SSEPs can be used to assess the dorsal column (fasciculus cuneatus and gracilis) and the lateral sensory tract of the spinal cord, the data provided by SSEPs can also lead clinicians to make assumptions on changes in anterior motor tracts because the stimulation is a mixed nerve (motor and sensory) signal. However, because they are not directly measured, motor deficits can occur despite the presence of normal SSEP waveforms. MEPs can provide critical information about the status of the anterior spinal cord and internal capsule.

The motor cortex or spinal cord can be used as a site for stimulation. Stimuli used to produce MEPs can be either electrical or magnetic. Current techniques in IOM almost exclusively use electrical stimulation. Direct stimulation of the motor cortex is commonly elicited by straight cutaneous or corkscrew needles on the scalp or electrodes placed directly on the brain after surgical exposure. Cortical pyramidal cells are activated directly (producing descending D waves) or indirectly (producing descending I waves).[53] Evoked potentials are recorded as neurogenic potentials in the distal spinal cord or peripheral nerve. They also can be recorded as myogenic potentials of innervated muscle. The IOM technician and surgeon coordinate to identify the optimal moments during the surgery prior to MEP stimulation.

Advances in technology and the refinement of methodologies are significantly changing intraoperative neurophysiologic monitoring of the spinal cord. The clinical application of spinal D-wave and muscle MEP recordings is becoming standard in many procedures. D-wave changes have proven to be the strongest predictors of maintained corticospinal tract integrity, and therefore, of motor function/recovery. Combining the use of muscle MEPs with D-wave recordings provides the most comprehensive approach for assessing the functional integrity of the spinal cord motor tracts during select surgeries. MEPs are considered the gold standard for monitoring the motor pathways, whereas SSEPs continue to be valuable for assessing the integrity of the dorsal (sensory) column. Thus, multimodal monitoring combining SSEP and MEP monitoring is the standard for spinal surgery.[49] The use of MEPs in intracranial surgery can be divided into two categories, vascular lesions and parenchymal lesions. Direct motor cortex stimulation has been used to define the edge of motor cortex tumors.[53] Safety concerns regarding the use of MEP include bite/tongue injuries, thermal injury, cardiovascular arrythmias, and seizures. Bite injuries due to jaw muscle contraction during transcranial electric stimulation are the most common but still infrequent complication, having an estimated incidence of about 0.2%.[54] Soft bite blocks are recommended to protect tongue and lips during stimulation due to the contraction of jaw muscles or trigeminal nerve stimulation.

Stimulation and monitoring of motor components of nerves are important in the operating room, but they require an active stimulus to produce an action potential. Electromyography (EMG) can be both passive and active. EMG has the capability to stimulate a motor nerve and monitor the known innervated muscle groups. EMG can also passively "listen" to all muscle groups as continuous activity is observed and recorded. The ability to passively monitor nerves allows the surgeon to be more aware of what nerve is being stimulated with surgical manipulation. EMG monitoring is also remarkably effective in detecting nerves that may be encapsulated by scar tissue or tumors.

EMG analysis of the facial nerve, cranial nerve VII, for related surgeries has been used and researched extensively. Monitoring needle electrodes are typically placed in the orbicularis oculi and the orbicularis oris muscles. To assess the cervicofacial and temporofacial divisions of the facial nerve as it divides from the posterior aspect of the parotid gland, both of these muscles require monitoring. Other cranial nerves such as IX, X, XI, and XII can and have been used for monitoring purposes as well. Furthermore, EMG inspection of the right and left recurrent laryngeal nerves during thyroidectomy, as well as other head and neck surgical procedures, can be performed with use of a nerve integrity–monitoring endotracheal tube.[55] The choice of

TABLE 19.5 Monitoring of Cranial Nerves

Cranial Nerve		Monitoring Site or Method*
I	Olfactory	No monitoring technique
II	Optic	Visual-evoked potentials
III	Oculomotor	Inferior rectus muscle
IV	Trochlear	Superior oblique muscle
V	Trigeminal	Masseter muscle and/or temporalis muscle (sensory responses can also be monitored)
VI	Abducens	Lateral rectus muscle
VII	Facial	Orbicularis oculi and/or orbicularis oris muscles
VIII	Auditory	Auditory brainstem responses
IX	Glossopharyngeal	Stylopharyngeus muscle (posterior soft palate)
X	Vagus	
	Superior laryngeal branch (motor)	Cricothyroid muscle
	Recurrent laryngeal branch (motor)	Posterior cricoarytenoid Lateral cricoarytenoid Thyroarytenoid Transverse arytenoid Oblique arytenoid Thyroepiglottic Aryepiglottic
XI	Spinal accessory	Sternocleidomastoid and/or trapezius muscles
XII	Hypoglossal	Genioglossus muscle (tongue)

*Unless otherwise specified, monitoring is performed via electromyographic activity of the muscle(s) listed.
Adapted from Sloan TB, et al. Evoked potentials. In: Cottrell JE, Patel P. *Cottrell and Patel's Neuroanesthesia.* 6th ed. Edinburgh: Elsevier; 2017:118.

TABLE 19.6 Spinal Nerve Roots and Muscles Most Commonly Monitored

Spinal Cord Nerve(s)		Muscle(s)
Cervical	C2–C4	Trapezoids, sternocleidomastoid
	C5, C6	Biceps, deltoids
	C6, C7	Flexor carpi radialis
Thoracic	C8–T1	Adductor pollicis brevis, abductor digiti minimi
	T5–T6	Upper rectus abdominis
	T7–T8	Middle rectus abdominis
	T9–T11	Lower rectus abdominis
	T12	Inferior rectus abdominis
Lumbar	L2	Adductor longus
	L2–L4	Vastus medialis
Lumbosacral	L4–S1	Tibialis anterior
	L5–S1	Peroneus longus
Sacral	S1–S2	Gastrocnemius
	S2–S4	Anal sphincter

From Sloan TB, et al. Evoked potentials. In: Cottrell JE, Patel P. *Cottrell and Patel's Neuroanesthesia.* 6th ed. Edinburgh: Elsevier; 2017:119.

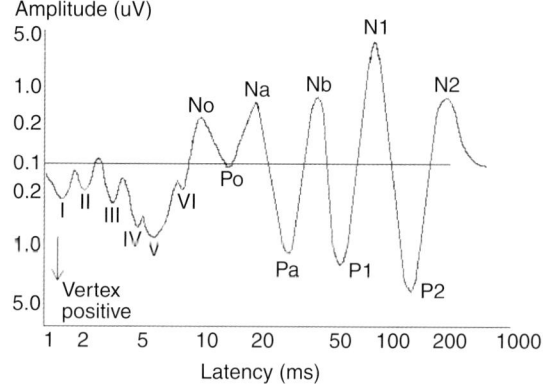

Fig. 19.6 Auditory-evoked potentials—common potentials *(labeled with Roman numerals)* that can be measured to assess different areas of the auditory and brainstem pathways. Peak I relates to the peripheral portion of the cochlear nerve inside the internal auditory canal. Peak II relates to the cochlear nucleus and the area where the eighth cranial nerve enters the brainstem. Peak III correlates to the area of the brainstem at the level of the cochlear nucleus, and potentially the ipsilateral superior olivary nucleus. Peaks IV and V relate to the brainstem along the ascending auditory pathway between the cochlear nucleus and the inferior colliculi. Peak VI relates to the medial geniculate body. Peak VII *(not shown)* relates to auditory radiations. (Modified from Barlow HB, Mollon JD. *The Senses.* Cambridge, England: Cambridge University Press; 1982.)

anesthesia is essentially unrestricted, with the exception of avoiding paralytic agents. Moreover, the efficacy of partial paralysis has not been studied extensively. Monitoring methods for cranial and spinal nerves are shown in Tables 19.5 and 19.6.

The frequency and density of discharges elucidate the type of damage to the actual nerve. Simple benign contact with the nerve causes few random discharges. A response train is associated with more significant nerve irritation. Neurotonic discharges are associated with nerve irritation as well as impending nerve damage. Elimination of environmental factors should be considered prior to diagnosing nerve damage. Trains of stimulation can also be caused by thermal changes (electrocautery or cold irrigation), drilling, traction, and/or nerve ischemia.

Brainstem Auditory–Evoked Potentials

BAEPs are used to monitor the entire auditory pathway from the distal auditory nerve to the midbrain, inadvertently allowing monitoring of basic brainstem function. The acoustic stimulus used is typically a standard broadband repeating click. Generally, repetition is approximately 10 Hz, and the intensity is approximately 65 to 70 dB above the click-perception threshold. The stimulus is delivered via an earphone placed in the auditory canal. For best results, care must be taken to (1) place the transducer after the head is positioned, so as not to cause abrasive injury to the ear canal, and (2) ensure that the internal auditory canal is free of any built-up cerumen or fluid. Fluid, saline, cerebrospinal fluid, and

soap can dampen or change the sound and delay responses. Recording electrodes are determined by the type of BAEPs stimulated in the patient.

BAEPs have five main peaks, which are represented by roman numerals (Fig. 19.6). Peak I relates to the peripheral portion of the cochlear nerve inside the internal auditory canal. Peak II relates to the cochlear nucleus and the area where the eighth cranial nerve enters the brainstem. Peak III correlates to the area of the brainstem at the level of the cochlear nucleus, and potentially the ipsilateral superior olivary nucleus. Peaks IV and V relate to the brainstem along the ascending auditory pathway between the cochlear nucleus and the inferior colliculi. Measured peaks must be compared with relative norms for age, sex, intensity, polarity, and repetition rate.

BAEPs are clinically useful as they are very resistant to interference (other than structural pathology within the brainstem). As such, BAEPs are not significantly affected by narcotics, benzodiazepines, ketamine, nitrous oxide, propofol, or muscle relaxants. However, the use of a lidocaine infusion has been known to affect BAEPs.[56,57] Additionally, inhalation agents can affect BAEPs, and their effect is proportional to the dose of inhalation agent administered.[56]

A common effect on BAEPs during anesthesia and surgery is hypothermia. Even mild hypothermia (patient temperature <35°C) has been associated with increased latency and prolonged interpeak intervals during BAEP analysis.[58] BAEPs can also be exaggerated, as demonstrated by an increase in latency with low partial pressure of carbon dioxide ($Paco_2$) seen during hyperventilation.

The auditory nerve can be directly monitored by the surgeon during the surgical procedure. The monitoring electrode is placed on the nerve itself after surgical exposure, and its response is measured as an auditory nerve compound action potential (AN-CAP). When the eighth nerve is involved, the AN-CAP is referred to as the eighth nerve potential. The AN-CAP, like the BAEP, can be used to determine auditory nerve insult or injury. For auditory brainstem responses, the noninverting (positive) electrode is placed at C2 or high on the forehead. The inverting (negative) electrode is typically placed on the mastoid or earlobe. However, if neither of these sites is practical (owing to surgical exposure), then the tragus of the ear may be used as an alternate site.

Electrocochleography (ECochG) is a specific test used to provide information about the cochlea and the distal section of the auditory nerve. Components of the ECochG include the cochlear microphonic, cochlear summating potential, and the eighth nerve CAP. The clinical utility of this modality can be found in estimating hearing thresholds in patients in whom behavioral audiometry cannot be performed, evaluating auditory neuropathy, and diagnosing Meniere disease.[59]

Otoacoustic emissions (OAEs) testing records the sounds that the ear produces itself. This test is used to detect hearing disorders due to cochlear dysfunction or indicate irregularities to the inner ear pathway.[60] OAEs are sometimes used, but this test is not an EP. Because a stimulus is not used, there is only a recording device. No stimulus is required because the normal cochlea does not just receive sound but also emits OAEs, which are produced specifically by the cochlea and most probably by the cochlear outer hair cells as they expand and contract. These sound transmissions can be recorded; they are typically used to assess auditory hair cell function and not the internal structure of the ear.

Visual-Evoked Potentials

VEPs are used to monitor the function of the visual pathway, which comprises the retina to the occipital cortex and everything in between, including the optic nerve and the optic chiasm. A series of visual stimuli are produced, and the cerebral responses are amplified, averaged by a computer, and displayed. The two major classes of VEP stimulation are patterned and unpatterned (luminance). VEPs can be obtained during procedures with patients either awake or anesthetized. Typically, awake tests consist of a pattern stimulus. The two most common pattern stimuli are pattern reversal and pattern onset/offset stimuli. Pattern reversal stimulus consists of black-and-white checks (checkerboard) that change phase (but maintain the same luminescence) at a predetermined number of reversals per second. Pattern onset/offset stimulus consists of a black-and-white checkerboard that exchanges with a diffuse background with the same luminescence.

Because such stimulation cannot be used in conjunction with anesthesia or even sedation, a stroboscopic or light-emitting diode (LED) flash (luminescence) stimulus must be used in such cases. Intraoperative flash stimulation is delivered through closed eyelids via fiberoptic light sources with attached reflective shields.[61] The flash VEP is created from a flash that has a predetermined strength

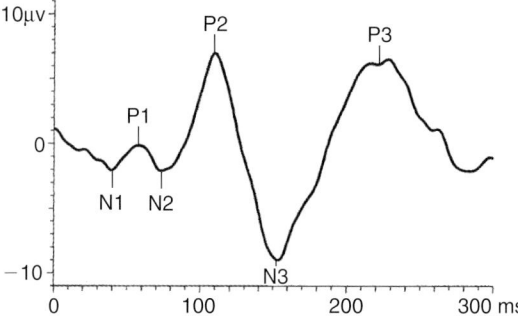

Fig. 19.7 Flash visual-evoked potential. The three positive deflections that characterize the potential and are subsequently measured are denoted as *P1, P2,* and *P3.* The three negative deflections that characterize the potential and are subsequently measured are denoted as *N1, N2,* and *N3.* (Adapted from Odom J, et al. Visual evoked potentials standard. *Doc Ophthalmol.* 2004;108:115–123.)

against a dim background of certain luminance. Recording electrodes are fixed to the scalp and, as always, placed relative to bony landmarks. The active electrode is placed on the scalp over the visual cortex. The ground electrode can be placed at the forehead, mastoid, earlobe, or both earlobes.

Monocular stimulation is typically used to avoid masking of unilateral conduction abnormality. Care should be taken to ensure that no light enters the eye not being stimulated. Closure with a patch and tape is usually sufficient to block light. Preoperatively, a comprehensive ocular physical assessment should be made to use as a comparison to the postoperative result. For example, extreme pupillary size or anisocoria (inequality of pupil diameter) can be compared to the preoperative pupillary size. Pupils do not need to be dilated for flash VEPs, and the cornea should be carefully moistened to prevent drying. Mydriatics and miotics should not be used with awake tests. It is also important to compare VEPs with appropriate age- and sex-related normal values.

The action potential of VEPs varies depending on the type of stimulus used. Flash VEPs consist of a series of negative and positive waves, with the earliest detectable response occurring approximately 30 ms poststimulus. For flash VEP, the N2 and P2 peaks are the most robust components, peaking at approximately 90 and 120 ms, respectively (Fig. 19.7). Unfortunately, flash VEPs are more variable between subjects than between pattern responses. Some question the usefulness of intraoperative VEPs because, in anesthetized patients, stable recording was either not obtainable or not consistent among study participants.[62,63] Indications for monitoring EPs are noted in Table 19.7 (also see Table 8.4 for the effects of various anesthetic agents on neurophysiologic monitoring of evoked potentials).

Multifocal VEP (mfVEP) monitoring is an important development in evaluating the functionality of the visual pathway. Traditional VEP monitoring evaluates the overall function of the visual pathway. In comparison, the mfVEP is designed to detect minor abnormalities in optic nerve transmission and provides the ability to localize and map the defect. To assess local defects in the visual field, the mfVEP responses must be compared with normal controls. Current applications of mfVEP include diagnosis and treatment of optic neuritis/multiple sclerosis, ruling out nonorganic visual loss and evaluating asymmetry of visual function caused by optic nerve dysfunction.[64]

BISPECTRAL INDEX

Extensive research with bispectral index (BIS) monitoring has allowed for the analysis and processing of EEG electrical signals; the result is then displayed as a numeric value between 0 and 100, which is representative of the patient's level of consciousness. This technology relies on a combination of frequency domain analysis and time domain

TABLE 19.7   Recommended Monitoring Modalities and Anesthetic Regimens for Surgical Procedures

| | MONITORING MODALITIES | | | | | ANESTHETIC RECOMMENDATION | |
| | | | ELECTROMYOGRAPHY | | | | |
Type of Procedure	Somatosensory-Evoked Potentials	Transcranial Motor–Evoked Potentials	Free Run	Stimulated	Auditory Brainstem Responses	Volatile (Inhalational Anesthetics)	Total Intravenous Anesthesia
Spine Skeletal							
Cervical	•	•	•				•
Thoracic	•	•	•	•			•
Lumbar instrumentation	•		•	•		•	
Lumbar disc			•	•		•	
Head and Neck							
Parotid			•	•		•	
Radical neck			•	•		•	
Thyroid			•	•		•	
Cochlear implant			•	•		•	
Mastoid			•	•		•	
Neurosurgery							
Spine							
Vascular	•	•					
Tumor	•	•					
Posterior fossa							
Acoustic neuroma			•	•	•	•	
Cerebellopontine	•	±	•	•	±		•
Vascular	•		•		±		•
Supratentorial							
Middle cerebral artery aneurysm		•					
Tumor in motor cortex	•	•					•

• Recommended for most surgeries; ± recommended for some procedures (depending on specific location of pathology).
Adapted from Jameson LC, et al. Monitoring of the brain and spinal cord. *Anesthesiol Clin.* 2006;74(4):777-791.

analysis in combination with a proprietary mathematic algorithm that produces an index of the anesthetic depth of the patient. BIS measurement is functional in determining the level of anesthesia produced with inhalation agents, but remains less predictable with pediatric patients and during regional and intravenous anesthesia.[65]

Several devices on the market today use a combination of processed EEG signals to determine the depth of anesthesia, including BIS monitoring (Medtronic), Entropy Module (GE Healthcare), Cerebral State Monitor (Danmeter), SNAP II monitor (Stryker), AEP Monitor/2 (Danmeter), and SEDLine Patient State Analyzer (Hospira).

The BIS monitor uses a proprietary algorithm to process a single frontal EEG signal, which calculates a dimensionless number that provides a measure of the patient's level of consciousness. The algorithm is also thought to consider the electricity produced by skeletal muscle known as electromyography (EMG). The monitor also offers a bilateral sensor for assessment of symmetry. BIS values range from 100 (awake) to 0 (absence of brain activity). BIS values between 40 and 60 suggest adequate general anesthesia for surgery. Values below 40 indicate a deep hypnotic state. Targeting a range of BIS values between 40 and 60 is advocated to prevent anesthesia awareness while still allowing a reduction in the administration of anesthetic agents (Fig. 19.8).[66] The ability of

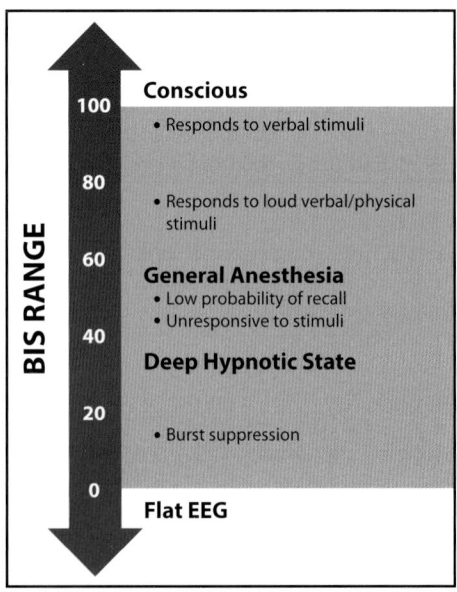

Fig. 19.8 Bispectral index ranges with various anesthetic depths.

the BIS monitor to successfully prevent awareness remains controversial. BIS-guided anesthesia reduces the incidence of awareness with recall in high-risk patients.[67] A study comparing BIS-guided anesthesia to measurement of the end tidal anesthetic concentration (ETAC) found that ETAC, which is routinely monitored, was superior in preventing recall.[68] Another study demonstrated a reduction in the incidence of awareness, while at the same time suggested that deep anesthesia, as defined by a sustained BIS value of less than 40 for more than 5 minutes, is associated with increased postoperative mortality (the B-Aware trial).[69] The concern was that adverse outcomes are increased with additional risk factors such as hypotension, high concentrations of anesthetic gases, and patient comorbidities. Other studies do not support the notion that BIS is no more effective than evaluating ETAC.[70] The BIS has also been used to assess the depth of anesthesia prior to and during emergence, to potentially decrease the time between termination of the surgical procedure and extubation. However, as compared with anesthetic management guided by ETAC, BIS guidance does not increase the incidence of earlier tracheal extubation in patients undergoing fast-track cardiac surgery.[71] The BIS may be most advantageous when used as a trend monitor that can be interpreted with other objective data (e.g., vital signs, end tidal concentration of an inhalation agent, intravenous agents used) to help guide anesthetic depth.

SUMMARY

The use of neurologic monitoring does not guarantee prevention of neurologic injury. However, technologic advances in neurologic monitoring promote patient safety. Several factors contribute to intraoperative EEG and EP changes, making interpretation of the monitoring device more challenging. Some of these factors include hypothermia, hyperthermia, volatile and intravenous anesthetic agents, surgical intervention, previous neurologic injury, and excessive auditory and visual stimulation. Providing anesthesia for neurologic surgical procedures requires knowledge of both basic and advanced anesthesia techniques. The anesthesia provider must combine the data and trends from clinical monitoring devices with clinical signs and symptoms to best assess patient neurologic function and well-being. Postoperative neurologic changes may also occur, so continued monitoring is essential to reduce the incidence of preventable permanent neurologic changes. Cooperation and communication among the surgeon, IOM staff, the neurobiologist, and the anesthetist remain vital to safe neurologic monitoring and improved surgical outcomes.

REFERENCES

For a complete list of references for this chapter, scan this QR code with any smartphone code reader app, or visit the following URL: http://booksite.elsevier.com/9780323711944/

20

Preoperative Evaluation and Preparation of the Patient

Sarah A. Sheets

A crucial element of the perioperative care of the surgical patient includes a timely and thorough preoperative assessment. A fine-tuned approach to patient evaluation then enables appropriate interventions when required to properly prepare the patient for the upcoming anesthesia and surgery. For any patient scheduled to undergo anesthesia, preoperative evaluation is compulsory to help identify factors that increase the risk associated with anesthesia and the status of the patient relative to the proposed surgery. Essential goals of preoperative assessment and preparation of the patient include the following:

- Optimize patient care, satisfaction, comfort, and convenience.
- Minimize perioperative morbidity and mortality by accurately assessing factors that influence the risk of anesthesia or might alter the planned anesthetic technique.
- Minimize surgical delays or preventable cancellations on the day of surgery.
- Determine appropriate postoperative disposition of the patient (i.e., given the patient's status, whether the procedure is best performed on an ambulatory, inpatient, or intensive care basis).
- Evaluate the patient's overall health status, determining which if any preoperative investigations and specialty consultations are required.
- Optimize preexisting medical conditions by encouraging requisite lifestyle changes (i.e., weight reduction, smoking termination, minimizing alcohol ingestion, access to ongoing health care monitoring).
- Formulate a plan for the most appropriate perianesthetic care and postoperative supportive patient care.
- Communicate patient management issues effectively among care providers.
- Communicate and provide specific instruction to patients in regard to preoperative preparation (i.e., fasting and *nil per os* [NPO] guidelines, blood glucose management, home medication administration).
- Educate patient regarding surgery, anesthesia, and expected intra- and postoperative care, including postoperative pain treatments, to reduce patient anxiety and increase patient satisfaction.
- Ensure time-efficient and cost-effective patient evaluation.

The preoperative visit begins with a thorough review of the patient's medical records and patient interview, followed by the physical examination. A comprehensive medical history and physical examination are the cornerstones of a systematic approach to continued patient preparation. Information gathered from this evaluative process guides further individualized assessment (e.g., obtaining diagnostic tests, specialist consultation). The extent of this preoperative workup depends on the existing medical condition of the patient, the proposed surgical procedure, and the type of anesthesia. Significant findings from this initial evaluation enable the anesthesia provider to make adjustments in the patient's care (i.e., initiate specific treatment modalities to optimize the patient's condition for the proposed surgery and anesthesia). A thoughtfully executed preoperative history and physical have been found to be more predictive of surgical complications than objective preoperative testing.[1]

Important strategies for achieving high-quality, cost-effective patient evaluation include the following:

- Educating the practitioner (e.g., regarding the cost of diagnostic tests) and thereby modifying practice patterns
- Developing and implementing evidence-based best practice guidelines
- Using clinical pathways (interdepartmental teamwork required)
- Disseminating information regarding protocols, thereby avoiding duplication of services
- Performing economic analyses of services, including cost-effectiveness and cost-benefit studies
- Rendering efficient resource management
- Providing for outcomes measurement

PREANESTHESIA ASSESSMENT CLINIC

The preanesthesia assessment clinic has emerged as the most effective means of providing convenient "one-stop shopping" designed to (1) permit patient registration, (2) obtain a medical history and perform a physical examination, (3) promote patient teaching, (4) meet or schedule appointments with medical consultants, (5) complete any required preoperative diagnostic testing, and (6) improve regulatory compliance and operating room efficiency. Successful preanesthesia assessment clinics have realized a reduction in patient anxiety, direct cost, last-minute surgical cancellations, overall length of hospitalization after surgery, and diagnostic testing, in addition to improvement in patient education and a shift from inpatient to outpatient surgery status. The preanesthesia assessment clinic allows patients scheduled for elective surgery to be evaluated and their condition optimized sufficiently in advance of the surgery.[2]

Timing of Patient Assessment

To allow ample time for necessary risk assessment, preoperative testing, and specialty consultations, ideal preoperative assessment for surgery

BOX 20.1   Conditions That Would Benefit From Early Preoperative Evaluation

General
- Medical conditions inhibiting ability to engage in normal daily activity
- Medical conditions necessitating continual assistance or monitoring at home within the past 6 mo
- Admission within the past 2 mo for acute episodes or exacerbation of chronic condition
- Use of medications (e.g., anticoagulants or monoamine oxidase inhibitors) for which modification of schedule or dosage might be required

Cardiocirculatory
- History of angina, coronary artery disease, myocardial infarction, symptomatic arrhythmias
- History of cardiac rhythm device in case device interrogation or reprogramming by appropriate personnel will be necessary
- Poorly controlled hypertension (diastolic >110 mm Hg, systolic >160 mm Hg)
- History of congestive heart failure

Respiratory
- Asthma or chronic obstructive pulmonary disease that requires chronic medication; acute exacerbation and progression of these diseases within the past 6 mo
- History of major airway surgery, unusual airway anatomy, or upper or lower airway tumor or obstruction
- History of chronic respiratory distress requiring home ventilatory assistance or monitoring

Endocrinologic
- Diabetes treated with insulin or oral hypoglycemic agents (unable to control with diet alone)
- Adrenal disorders
- Active thyroid disease

Hepatic
- Active hepatobiliary disease or compromise

Musculoskeletal
- Kyphosis or scoliosis causing functional compromise
- Temporomandibular joint disorder with restricted mobility
- Cervical or thoracic spine injury

Oncologic
- Patients receiving chemotherapy
- Other oncological processes with significant physiologic compromise

Gastrointestinal
- Obesity (BMI of 35 or greater)
- Hiatal hernia
- Symptomatic gastroesophageal reflux

Modified from Barash PG, ed. *ASA Refresher Courses in Anesthesiology.* Philadelphia: Lippincott Williams & Wilkins; 1996 [vol 24].

and anesthesia should take place well in advance of the proposed surgery. Patients with complex medical conditions should be evaluated at least 1 week before the scheduled procedure. Because of present economic realities, patients undergoing more complex procedures, and those who have complicated medical conditions (see Box 20.1),[3] are frequently not admitted to the hospital before the day of surgery. Preoperative evaluation on the day of surgery can result in last-minute discoveries (e.g., of inappropriate fasting, suspected difficult airway,

preexisting medical condition) that may result in surgical delay or cancellation. The timing of the preanesthesia assessment does not appear to influence outcome of anesthesia.[4] In one study, no difference in the cancellation rate for ambulatory patients was observed between groups seen within 24 hours and groups seen within 1 to 30 days of the scheduled surgery.[5] Regardless of when performed, this focused evaluation must be performed by a practitioner qualified to administer anesthesia.

CHART REVIEW

To provide the basis for and direction of the patient interview and physical assessment, the patient's past and current medical records should be reviewed preoperatively. Ideally the anesthesia provider will have the opportunity to review the patient's medical records before the interview with the patient or caregiver.

Past Medical Records

For a patient who has undergone surgery at the same institution in the past, previous anesthesia records should be retrieved and reviewed, especially if complications are suspected. If past medical records are not available, the patient must provide details of significant anesthetic experiences. If this information suggests that the patient has an unusual condition (e.g., atypical plasma cholinesterase, susceptibility to malignant hyperthermia), surgery may be delayed so that medical records can be obtained for review to provide further information that might affect patient care, or measures should be taken (e.g., avoidance of succinylcholine, provision of trigger-free anesthetic technique) to avoid consequences associated with the condition.

Patient Chart or Electronic Medical Record

A review of the current medical record includes verifying that the surgical and anesthesia consents are accurate and complete. The names of the patient and surgeon, the date, and the proposed procedure should be matched with those on the operating room schedule. Demographic or baseline data, such as the age, height, and weight of the patient, can often be obtained from the admitting record. Vital-sign trends and input-output totals are transcribed from graphic flow sheets, which may also contain pertinent data (e.g., daily blood glucose values for the diabetic patient).

Progress notes and consultation reports provide a valuable overview of the health history and physical status of the patient. Medical treatments, such as drug dosages and schedules, may be derived from these materials, but diagnostic test results should be obtained directly from their original sources. This retrieval of primary data prevents the possible misinterpretation of data that were transcribed incorrectly. Knowledge gleaned from a review of progress notes and consultative reports enables the anesthesia provider to formulate supplementary questioning, seek further specialist consultations, or obtain additional diagnostic testing as needed.

Baseline data concerning the patient, such as cultural diversity, coping mechanisms, or patient limitations (e.g., hearing impairment), can often be derived from nursing notes and can effectively guide the anesthesia provider in conducting a thorough preoperative interview. Increasingly the anesthetist must be able to appropriately interact with culturally diverse populations to properly evaluate and educate patients.

A preanesthesia questionnaire is included on the patient's chart and should be part of the admission paperwork to be completed by the patient or the patient's caregiver and consists of a concise checklist regarding the patient's health history and medical care. When properly completed and readily available on the chart, the preanesthesia questionnaire enables the anesthesia provider's visit with the patient to be accomplished more efficiently. Interview questions and physical assessment are appropriately directed toward abnormal findings and areas of concern.

PATIENT INTERVIEW

The preoperative interview may be conducted in person or by telephone. The in-person patient interview is preferred, but for patients who are unable to visit the hospital setting (e.g., who live far from the hospital, have transportation constraints, or because of infectious diseases such as Covid 19), an opportunity to participate in a telephone interview should be made available. Regardless of the location or approach used, the interview promotes a trusting relationship between the patient and anesthesia provider.

When the interview is performed in a caring and unhurried manner, the patient's degree of trust and confidence in anesthesia care is enhanced. The manner with which the provider addresses the patient and the family facilitates this trust and confidence in the care they are about to receive. In settings where the interview is happening the day of the procedure, the anesthesia provider has a small window of time to establish this relationship. For example, when the interview occurs in the setting of the hospital preoperative preparation area on the day of the procedure, the encounter the anesthesia provider has with the patient may be only 30 minutes prior to the start of the case. In less desirable circumstances it also may be the first conversation they are having regarding the topic of anesthesia.

Thoughtful methods of approach can help the anesthesia provider efficiently establish an open line of communication with the patient. For instance, patients' perception of time spent with a provider is greater when the provider sits, rather than stands, during the interview. Simply by having the provider sit during the interview, patients report a more positive exchange and more comprehensive understanding of their circumstances.[6]

In the manner of introduction, the anesthesia provider can extend respect by using the patient's surname (Mr. Smith, Mrs. Jones) unless instructed differently. The anesthesia provider can introduce oneself to the patient in this manner: "Hello, I am [name and role of provider]. How would you like to be addressed?"[7] During introductions, the title of the anesthesia provider and the provider's specific role in the patient's perioperative care should also be defined. The patient is entitled to know what role the interviewer plays in the perioperative process. Many times a nurse practitioner or physician assistant may conduct the assessment. The professional appearance and attitude of the anesthesia provider can also create a positive impression during the preoperative visit.

If not done the day of the procedure, the environment of the preoperative interview should be staged to maximize the quality and effectiveness of the interaction. Adequate lighting enhances effective communication. Distractions such as an operating television set or smartphone should be mitigated. The interviewer should ensure that the time and location of the interview are convenient and private for the patient.

Because the preoperative interview is a private interaction between the patient and the clinician, a tactful request that visitors remain outside the interview area, unless the patient wishes family members to be present, will be necessary. Otherwise the patient may not volunteer confidential health information, such as a history of substance abuse or sexual history. In certain situations, however, assistance from a family member or caregiver is required. The health history may be provided, for example, by the parent of a pediatric patient or by an interpreter for a patient with cognitive or language barriers.

The patient interview is designed to achieve specific objectives (Box 20.2).[8] A valuable step in preparing the patient or responsible

BOX 20.2 Objectives of the Preoperative Interview

- Ensure that the goals of preoperative assessment are met.
- Provide preoperative education to the patient and family.
- Obtain written documentation of informed and witnessed consent.
- Acquaint the patient and family with the surgical process (to reduce stress and increase familiarity).
- Evaluate the patient's social situation with respect to surgery (e.g., support network).
- Motivate the patient to comply with preventive care strategies (e.g., smoking cessation, improvement of cardiovascular fitness).

Modified from Cassidy J, Marley RA. Preoperative assessment of the ambulatory patient. *J Perianesth Nurs.* 1996;11(5):334–343.

BOX 20.3 Patient Education Objectives

- Promote interactive communication between patient and care provider.
- Encourage patient participation in making decisions about perioperative care.
- Maximize and enhance patient self-care skills and participation in continuing care during the postoperative phase.
- Increase the patient's ability to cope with own health status.
- Increase patient compliance with perioperative care.
- Provide individualized preoperative instructions regarding the following:
  1. Where and when laboratory tests, consultations, and diagnostic procedures will be completed
  2. Appropriate time at which the patient should cease ingestion of food and drink
  3. Personal considerations (e.g., comfortable clothes to wear; no jewelry or makeup; what personal items to bring; leave valuables at home; bring favorite toy, comforter, or book)
  4. Postoperative considerations and instructions (e.g., anticipated recovery course, discharge instructions, how to deal with complications)
  5. Person to contact if the patient's physical condition changes (e.g., upper respiratory tract infection, cancellation)
- Detail the process of arrival and registration on arrival to the surgical facility (i.e., time and location of arrival).
- Review advance directive information as required by law in some states.
- Explain the surgical facility policies to the patient and family.

Modified from Cassidy J, Marley RA. Preoperative assessment of the ambulatory patient. *J Perianesth Nurs.* 1996;11(5):334–343.

caregivers (e.g., family members, legal guardian) for the scheduled surgery includes an educational process during which the staff counsels the patient concerning fundamental perioperative issues (Box 20.3).[8] Reinforcing information to the patient verbally and in writing is essential to gaining patient compliance. Coordinating the patient's visit to the preanesthesia assessment clinic to include educational time is ideal for the patient.

The interview process, along with patient education, yields beneficial consequences of reduced patient anxiety and increased patient satisfaction. Positive interactions between the patient and the anesthesia provider have an impact that extends far past the perioperative environment. Compliance with perioperative instructions increases when the patient is treated with respect. Patient satisfaction and compliance with perioperative instructions result in decreased length of stay, decreased costs, and overall improved clinical outcomes.[6]

Medical History

The extent of a patient's health history depends partly on the amount of information available in the chart before surgery. If the surgeon has already documented a thorough medical history and physical examination, the interview can focus on confirming major findings and obtaining information that directly relates to the anesthetic management of the patient. The anesthesia provider must obtain and document a detailed health history, however, if the history is unavailable in the chart during the preoperative visit.

The health history should be obtained in an organized and systematic way, as with the preanesthesia questionnaire, to minimize possible omission of important data. Open-ended and direct questions targeting each category of the checklist can be posed. With this approach, more detailed and graded responses are elicited from the patient. To avoid overwhelming or confusing a patient, questions are asked separately and formulated in comprehensible or layperson's terms.

Surgical History

The surgical history of a patient may be learned from the chart or preoperative interview. Most patients only vaguely recall surgical experiences, even from childhood operations. Information regarding complications related to previous operations such as a peripheral nerve injury or uncontrolled blood loss should be elicited to determine the need for further investigation.

Anesthetic History

Past anesthetic experiences are often not as easily defined as the surgical history. It is vitally important to determine the reaction of a patient to previously administered anesthetics. Adverse reactions to anesthetic agents and techniques (e.g., prolonged vomiting, difficult airway, malignant hyperthermia, postoperative delirium, anaphylaxis, and cardiopulmonary collapse) may have simply been an annoyance to the patient or could have been life threatening. Preoperative knowledge of these complications allows the anesthetic approach to be modified and the recurrence of the complication thereby prevented. Causative factors are also thoroughly investigated in patients who note that a previous operation was aborted. Difficulties with airway management can alter the approach to endotracheal intubation, if indicated. Vague reports of fever and convulsions merit further investigation to rule out an episode of malignant hyperthermia.

Familial Anesthetic History

Numerous inherited diseases involving metabolic derangements may affect a patient's reaction to stress and certain drugs, including anesthetic agents. The patient is specifically asked whether any family member ever experienced an adverse reaction to anesthesia during surgery. Familial tendencies for diseases such as atypical plasma cholinesterase, malignant hyperthermia, porphyria, or glycogen storage diseases (e.g., glucose-6-phosphate dehydrogenase deficiency) are then investigated. A diagnosis should be established before the surgery proceeds because adjustments in the anesthetic management of the patient may be required.

Drug History

A preoperative drug history provides an excellent guide for the direction and depth of the patient interview and assessment. Drug dosages, schedules, and durations of treatment are reviewed and the patient questioned about the purpose and effectiveness of these medications. For example, an interview with a patient receiving β-adrenergic blockers can focus in greater detail on the cardiovascular system. Patients on medications for hypertension or angina pectoris require further investigation and possibly specialty consultation if they have not been recently evaluated.

Adverse Drug Effects and Interactions

During the preoperative evaluation, current drug therapy must be carefully reviewed for side effects and potential interactions with anesthetic agents. One drug-management strategy is to discontinue nonessential medications preoperatively in the hope of reducing the potential for adverse interactions. The therapeutic benefits of these drugs are weighed against the risks of abrupt discontinuation. Abrupt discontinuation of long-standing medication may lead to the development of undesirable withdrawal symptoms. With occasional exceptions the majority of medications are continued preoperatively. Should a decision be made to withhold a particular drug before surgery, sufficient time should be allowed for metabolic clearance (ideally 3–5 half-lives).[8,9]

Drug Allergies

A patient's drug history should include information regarding allergic reactions to certain foods and medications. The most common cause of drug hypersensitivity reactions during anesthesia are neuromuscular blocking agents and antibiotics.[9] Prior allergic responses are investigated so they can be differentiated from adverse drug reactions. Use of certain antibiotics and opioids may be avoided because of gastrointestinal side effects. However, these do not represent a true allergic response. A distinction between allergic reactions and adverse effects is crucial because an allergy to a drug is an absolute contraindication to its use. Medications within the same classification of a drug allergy should be avoided, and heightened awareness of a potential allergic reaction is required during the perioperative period.

Latex Sensitivity

Patient sensitivity to latex products may be the basis of an allergic reaction. The incidence of intraoperative reaction to latex is on the decline secondary to heightened awareness, preventative measures, and manufacture of nonlatex hospital supplies. Up to 20% of intraoperative anaphylactic reactions have been attributed to latex sensitivity.[10] The preoperative questioning of patients should include inquiry regarding specific latex sensitivity or allergy. Patients at increased risk for latex sensitivity should be cared for in a no-latex setting and scheduled as the first case of the day to reduce the likelihood of aeroallergen latex exposure. The diagnosis of latex allergy is based on the findings of the history and physical examination and if necessary in vivo (skin-prick test is the most sensitive) and in vitro testing. Preoperative testing is indicated only when there is a family history of reactions or when patients report experiencing symptoms such as a rash, swelling, or wheezing when exposed to latex. Patients at high risk for latex sensitivity include those with a history of the following:[11-14]

- Chronic exposure to latex-based products (e.g., industrial workers using protective gear, occupational exposure to latex)
- Spina bifida, urologic reconstructive surgery
- Repeated surgical procedures (more than nine)
- Intolerance to latex-based products (e.g., balloons, rubber gloves, condoms, dental dams, rubber urethral catheters)
- Allergy to food and tropical fruits (e.g., avocado, banana, buckwheat, celery, chestnut, kiwi, mango, papaya, passion fruit, peach)
- Intraoperative anaphylaxis of uncertain cause
- Health care professionals, especially with a history of atopy or severe dermatitis, hand eczema

Social History

The addictive nature of tobacco and alcohol, in addition to illegal drugs, exerts a detrimental influence on several aspects of life in the United States.

- Approximately 31.9 million Americans aged 12 years or older (11.7%) were classified as illicit drug users in 2021.

- Nearly one-quarter of all deaths (75,000 annually) in the United States are caused by addictive substances.
- The economic burden of addiction (e.g., health care expenditures, missed work, crime) is estimated at more than $400 billion annually.

Certain drugs, despite their social or recreational application, may be associated with adverse and life-threatening consequences with long- or short-term use or overdose. The social history provides an excellent opportunity to explore the extent of self-medication. Open-ended questions, posed in a professional and nonjudgmental manner, are most likely to elicit detailed information from the patient. At this time, the patient can also be educated about the adverse consequences of substance abuse, especially as such substances affect anesthetic care.[15]

Smoking

Many patients arrive for anesthesia and surgery with a history of smoking either tobacco or electronic cigarettes (e-cigarettes, vapes). In the United States some disturbing statistics are associated with this form of substance abuse:[16-22]

- One in five deaths in the United States is related to smoking. Cigarette smoking is the leading cause of preventable premature death in the United States (approximately 480,000 premature deaths annually). Smokers are 12 to 13 times more likely to die than nonsmokers.
- Cigarette smoking has declined in youth (9.3% in US high schools); however, the use of e-cigarettes and hookahs has increased.
- In 2013, use of e-cigarettes among young adults (18–24 years of age) was higher than adults in all age groups.[27]
- As of 2013, 32.5% of e-cigarette users were never or former smokers.[27]
- Smoking causes nearly 90% of all lung cancer and 80% of all deaths from chronic obstructive pulmonary disease (COPD).
- Smoking increases the risk of coronary heart disease and stroke two to four times.
- Exposure to secondhand smoke causes 7300 deaths a year from lung cancer and 34,000 deaths from coronary heart disease in adult nonsmokers in the United States.
- Use of e-cigarettes in and around children has caused an increase in poison control center calls from 1 per month in 2010 to 215 per month in 2014.
- Children can suffer from acute nicotine intoxication from exposure or direct ingestion of e-liquid resulting in seizures, coma, respiratory arrest, and death.

The inhaled components of tobacco and e-cigarette smoke lead to multiple pathophysiologic changes within the body. Nicotine and carbon monoxide are just two of the more than 6000 noxious components that have been identified in tobacco and e-cigarette smoke.[23] Nicotine, a toxic alkaloid, produces ganglionic stimulant effects and is the tobacco component that affects the cardiovascular system.[24] The overall adverse impact tobacco and e-cigarette smoking has on health is vast (Tables 20.1 and 20.2).[19,20] Carbon monoxide readily occupies the oxygen-binding sites of hemoglobin (approximately 250–300 times greater affinity for hemoglobin than oxygen).[20] Oxygen transport to the tissues and resultant oxygen use is thereby drastically reduced. In the heavy smoker carboxyhemoglobin may be as high as 15%, which effectively reduces the patient's oxyhemoglobin percentage accordingly. The adverse effects of nicotine on the cardiovascular system and carbon monoxide on oxygen-carrying capacity are short lived (half-life of nicotine is 40–60 minutes[21]; half-life of carbon monoxide if room air is breathed is 130–190 minutes).[22] Constituents of liquids and aerosols in e-cigarettes are noted in Table 20.2.

Patients should be instructed to stop smoking at least 12 to 48 hours before surgery. Short-term (e.g., 12 hours) preoperative abstinence

from tobacco smoke reduces the deleterious effects of nicotine and carbon monoxide on cardiopulmonary function.[23] Smoking cessation for even one night before surgery reduces heart rate, blood pressure (BP), and circulating catecholamine levels and allows carboxyhemoglobin values to return to normal levels.[25]

Patients who smoke have a higher incidence (a nearly sixfold increase) of postoperative pulmonary complications (pneumonia and atelectasis).[26] A smoking history of more than 20 pack-years equates to an increased risk of perioperative complications. Smoking cessation of less than 4 weeks does not reduce the risk of postoperative respiratory complication.[27] Longer periods of smoking cessation (≥8 weeks) result in a marked improvement in pulmonary mechanics (e.g., enhanced ciliary function, decreased mucous secretion and small airway obstruction, and enhanced immune function). Patients who stopped smoking less than 2 months before surgery had nearly four times the pulmonary complications (e.g., purulent sputum, secretion retention, bronchospasm, pleural effusion, pneumothorax, segmental pulmonary collapse, pneumonia) of those who abstained from smoking for longer than 2 months. However, even short-term smoking cessation is effective in reducing postoperative complications when compared with patients who continued to smoke up until the time of surgery. A reduction in postoperative wound-related complications occurs in patients who stop smoking preoperatively. Patients who smoke should be advised to quit, even immediately prior to surgery, without fear of worsening pulmonary outcomes or increasing psychological stress as a result of acute abstinence. Effective interventions, including behavioral support and nicotine replacement therapy, should be made available to smokers considering abstinence at this time.

The influence of environmental tobacco smoke (also known as secondhand or passive smoke) on children has been found to produce disturbing respiratory consequences, including increased reactive airway disease, abnormal results of pulmonary function tests, and increased respiratory tract infections.[28,29] The perioperative complications in children exposed to smoke include laryngospasm, coughing on induction or emergence, breath holding, postoperative oxyhemoglobin desaturation, and hypersecretion.[30-36]

Alcohol Intake

Alcohol-attributable deaths equal approximately 95,000 each year, 261 per day, and shorten the lives of those who die by an average of 29 years.[37,38] Perioperative complications, such as arrhythmias, infection, and alcohol withdrawal syndrome, are increased two- to fivefold in chronic excessive alcohol users.[39] Postoperative complications can be reduced with 4 or more weeks of abstinence prior to surgery.[40] Information regarding the type and amount of alcohol regularly consumed and the frequency of consumption is important in the evaluation for anesthesia and surgery. Often an accurate assessment of a patient's alcohol intake may be difficult to obtain. The Alcohol Use Disorders Identification Test (AUDIT), a self-reporting questionnaire designed to identify problem drinkers, can be incorporated into the preoperative interview of suspected problem drinkers.[41] A less confrontational and a reliable approach to evaluating a patient's potential for an alcohol problem uses the mnemonic *CAGE*, which refers to the following four questions:[42-44]

1. Do you feel you should *c*ut down on your alcohol consumption?
2. Have people *a*nnoyed you by criticizing your drinking habits?
3. Have you felt *g*uilty about your drinking?
4. Have you ever had a drink first thing in the morning to steady your nerves or get rid of a hangover (*e*ye-opener)?

A patient reporting more than two positive responses is at high risk for alcoholism and an increased likelihood of experiencing withdrawal

TABLE 20.1	Effects of Tobacco Smoking	
System	**Pathophysiologic Effects**	**Perioperative Effects**
Respiratory	Recurrent cough Mucous hypersecretion Mucociliary dysfunction Loss of integrity of airway epithelium Increased upper and lower airway reactivity Recurrent chest infections Loss of elasticity of airways Increased closing volume COPD	Laryngospasm and bronchospasm Sputum retention Hypoxemia Baro/volutrauma Need for reintubation Postoperative atelectasis Postoperative chest infection
Cardiovascular	Tachycardia Hypertension Raised carbon monoxide levels Reduced oxygen-carrying capacity Left shift of oxyhemoglobin dissociation curve Reduced oxygen delivery Increased blood viscosity Atheroma and clot formation Risk of myocardial, cerebral, and peripheral vascular ischemia/infarction Venous thromboembolism risk	Tachycardia Hypertension Perioperative risk of myocardial ischemia Venous thromboembolism risk
Hematology	Hypercoagulability Increased blood viscosity High white blood cell count Impaired humoral activity and cell-mediated immunity Increased risk of infection Vulnerable to autoimmune diseases Reduced ability to attack malignant cells	Risk of perioperative sepsis Risk of perioperative arterial/venous clot formation
Wound healing	Prolonged wound healing because of long-term immunosuppression and poor tissue perfusion	Wound breakdown Perioperative wound infection
Bones	Reduced bone density and osteoporosis Increased fracture risk	
Cancer associations	Lung Gastrointestinal (esophageal, stomach, liver, pancreas, bowel) Head and neck Genitourinary (bladder, ovarian, cervical) Leukemia	

COPD, Chronic obstructive pulmonary disease.
From Shorrock P, Bakerly N. Effects of smoking on health and anaesthesia. *Anaesth Int Care Med.* 2015;17:141–143.

TABLE 20.2	Constituents of Liquids and Aerosols in E-cigarettes	
Chemical	**Description**	**Physiologic Impact**
Nicotine	Common nicotine concentrations are 0–24 mg	Sympathomimetic, cardiac, vascular, endocrine, and immunologic toxicity Drug-to-drug interactions
Propylene glycol	Artificial flavoring	Carcinogenic
Glycerol	Artificial flavoring	Cardiotoxic, carcinogenic
Diacetyl	Artificial flavoring	Pulmonary toxicity
Acrolein, formaldehyde, and acetaldehyde	Toxic compound generated in aerosol	Pulmonary and vascular toxicity, carcinogenic
Heavy metals	Contained in e-liquid and aerosol	Pulmonary, vascular, and nephrotoxicity
Toluene	Volatile compound generated in aerosol	Central nervous system depressant

symptoms.[43] Both AUDIT and CAGE have been shown to be effective in identifying the abusive alcohol consumer.[44]

In the heavy drinker, it is important to determine whether the patient has experienced seizures, abrupt withdrawal syndrome, or delirium tremens as a consequence of alcohol abuse. Clinical signs suggestive of alcohol withdrawal include increased hand tremors, autonomic hyperactivity (e.g., sweating, tachycardia, systolic hypertension), insomnia, anxiety, restlessness, nausea or vomiting, transient hallucinations (visual, tactile, or auditory), psychomotor agitation, and grand mal seizures.[43]

Chronic alcohol abuse results in the development of tolerance, physical dependence, and multisystem organ dysfunction. Tolerance to alcohol is evidenced by a resistance or cross-tolerance to other central nervous system (CNS) depressants. For example, the anesthetic requirement of hypnotics, opioids, and inhalation agents is increased in the chronic alcoholic; however, exaggerated responses to anesthetic agents are likely during periods of acute intoxication or advanced alcoholism. This effect is attributed to the additive depressant effects of alcohol and anesthetic agents. Enzymatic function and plasma albumin concentrations may also be reduced in patients with alcoholic hepatic insufficiency. As a result, greater circulating concentrations of unbound intravenous agents may result in an exaggerated and prolonged drug effect. This enhanced drug response has not been shown to occur with propofol in patients with moderate liver cirrhosis.[44,45]

An insidious progression of multisystem organ dysfunction is also characteristic of long-term alcohol abuse. Numerous illnesses are attributable to the toxic adverse effects of advanced alcoholism on overall health and nutrition. Predictably, postoperative morbidity and mortality rates are increased in alcoholic patients as a result of poor wound healing, infection, bleeding, pneumonia, and further hepatic deterioration.[46]

Illicit Drug Use

Use of illicit drugs (e.g., cocaine, cannabis, "crack," lysergic acid diethylamide-25 [LSD], amphetamines, heroin, hallucinogens, inhalants, prescription-type psychotherapeutics or opioids used nonmedically) is a significant health care issue in the United States. The 2016 data from the Centers for Disease Control and Prevention (CDC) have shown continued escalation of prescription opioid use with opioid overdose deaths topping all previous estimations.[47] The use of these substances increases the risk for adverse consequences and drug interactions during anesthesia. In addition, patients receiving medically assisted treatment for abstinence of opioids present pain management challenges that need to be addressed prior to provision of anesthesia.

An accurate illicit drug history is often difficult to obtain because of the patient's fear of legal reprisal or refusal to believe a drug problem exists. During the physical examination, the anesthesia provider should look for signs that indicate illicit drug use by the patient. A diagnosis of recent or continuing drug abuse should be suspected in patients exhibiting the following on physical examination:[44]

- Evidence of drug injection (e.g., track marks or scarring), thrombotic veins, phlebitis, tattoos (may be used to mask the sites), ablation of venous return leading to unilateral edema of the nondominant hand, subcutaneous skin abscesses
- Ophthalmologic changes, such as pupillary constriction from opioid use, pupillary dilation with amphetamine use, nystagmus from phencyclidine (PCP) use
- Lymphadenopathy secondary to nonspecific activation of the immune system as a result of repeated injections of impurities
- Malnourishment as a result of amphetamine abuse (opioid users tend to be well nourished)
- Poor dental care and bruxism (involuntary grinding and clenching of teeth) from amphetamine use
- Nasal perforation from cocaine abuse

Primary concerns for the anesthesia provider are the likelihood of the patient exhibiting acute abuse or possible withdrawal syndrome.[45] Signs and symptoms of acute abuse of the more common substances are listed in Box 20.4.[48-51] Elective surgery should be delayed or canceled in patients suspected of being under the influence of an illicit drug until further patient evaluation can be

---

BOX 20.4 Signs and Symptoms of Acute Substance Abuse

Cannabis (Marijuana or Hashish)
- Tachycardia, labile blood pressure, headache
- Euphoria, dysphoria, depression, occasional anxiety and panic reactions, psychosis (rare)
- Poor memory and decreased motivation with chronic use

Cocaine and Amphetamines
- Tachycardia, labile blood pressure, hypertension, myocardial ischemia, arrhythmias, pulmonary edema
- Excitement, delirium, hallucinations to psychosis
- Euphoria: feeling of excitation, well-being, and enhanced physical strength and mental capacity
- Hyperreflexia, tremors, convulsions, mydriasis, sweating, hyperpyrexia, exhaustion, coma with overdose

Hallucinogens: LSD, PCP
- Sympathomimetic and weak analgesic effects
- Altered perception and judgment; high doses may progress to toxic psychosis
- PCP produces dissociative anesthesia with increasing doses

Opioids
- Respiratory depression, hypotension, bradycardia, constipation
- Euphoria (most marked with heroin)
- Pinpoint pupils with overdose; decreased level of consciousness to coma

LSD, Lysergic acid diethylamide-25; *PCP*, phencyclidine.
From Cheng DCH. The drug addicted patient. *Can J Anaesth.* 1997;44(5 Pt2):R101–R111; Cavaliere F, et al. Anesthesiologic preoperative evaluation of drug addicted patient. *Minerva Anestesiol.* 2005;71(6):367–371.

---

performed. Suspicion of acute substance abuse should be followed up with a urine screen for drug identification. Abstinence syndrome typically exhibits increased sympathetic and parasympathetic responses resulting in hypertension, tachycardia, abdominal cramping and diarrhea, tremors, anxiety, irritability, lacrimation, mydriasis, algid sweat, and yawning.[52]

A patient-specific pain management plan should be considered with patients receiving medically assisted treatment (MAT) for abstinence of opioids. The patient may present with a delineated plan from their pain management provider indicating current medications and suggestions for pain management in the perioperative period. Drug therapies for opioid abstinence include antagonists that directly compete with opiates typically used in anesthesia. These include methadone (for opioid de-addiction), suboxone (for maintenance of opioid abstinence), and naltrexone (for maintenance of abstinence with opioids or management of cravings in alcohol abuse). If an opioid-based anesthetic is planned, the scheduled withdrawal of MAT with opiate bridging should be considered. In this case, the anesthesia provider should be prepared by greater than normal opioid analgesic requirements, hyperalgesia, and other sequelae related to opioid tolerance.[53] Often a multimodal pain management plan using a combination of regional anesthesia, local infiltration of the surgical site, with long-acting local anesthetics, ketamine, gabapentin, intravenous lidocaine, clonidine, and/or cyclooxygenase-2 (COX2) inhibitors will allow for the continuation of the patient's current MAT.[54,55] Regardless of the anesthetic plan, an empathetic and understanding approach by the anesthesia provider can help gain the patient's trust and prepare the patient to have realistic expectations around perioperative pain management.

Synthetic Androgens

Anabolic steroids are self-administered in an attempt to increase muscle mass, strength, and growth, and improve athletic performance, but such actions can result in hepatic and endocrine system dysfunction. Risks associated with long-term androgen steroid supplementation include impaired liver function, cholestatic jaundice, hepatic adenocarcinoma, peliosis hepatis, myocardial infarction (MI), atherosclerosis, hypercoagulopathy, stroke, hypertension, dyslipidemia, and psychiatric and behavioral disturbances in susceptible patients.[56-60] The hepatotoxic effects have important implications for the anesthetic management of a chronic steroid abuser, particularly with agents metabolized by the liver, and such patients should undergo preoperative liver function testing.

Herbal Dietary Supplements

Patients should be questioned regarding their use of nonprescription herbal medications to determine the herb's name, the duration of herbal therapy, and the dose taken. If patients are in doubt as to the herbal medications they are taking, they should be encouraged to bring the herbal products with them to their preoperative workup. Certain herbal products are known to influence blood clotting, affect blood glucose levels, produce CNS stimulation or depression, or interact with psychotropic drugs (Table 20.3).[61,62] When practical, discontinuation of dietary supplements should be encouraged 2 to 3 weeks prior to anesthesia.[63]

PATIENT EVALUATION: OVERVIEW OF SYSTEMS

Upper Airway

Assessment of the airway should be performed preoperatively in every patient regardless of the plan of anesthetic management. It is important to evaluate the patient before anesthesia to identify those patients at risk for difficult airway management (e.g., difficult bag

TABLE 20.3 Clinically Important Effects and Perioperative Concerns of Selected Herbal Medicines and Recommendations for Discontinuation of Use Before Surgery

Herb: Common Name(s)	Relevant Pharmacologic Effects	Perioperative Concerns	Preoperative Discontinuation
Echinacea: purple coneflower root	Activation of cell-mediated immunity	Allergic reactions; decreased effectiveness of immunosuppressive actions of corticosteroids and cyclosporine; potential for immunosuppression with long-term use; inhibition of hepatic microsomal enzymes may precipitate toxicity of drugs metabolized by the liver (e.g., phenytoin, rifampin, phenobarbital)	No data
Ephedra: ma huang	Increased heart rate and blood pressure through direct and indirect sympathomimetic effects	Risk of myocardial ischemia and stroke from tachycardia and hypertension; ventricular arrhythmias with halothane; long-term use depletes endogenous catecholamines and may cause intraoperative hemodynamic instability (control hypotension with direct vasoconstrictor, e.g., phenylephrine); life-threatening interaction with monoamine oxidase inhibitors	At least 24 hr before surgery
Ginger: *Zingiber officinale*	Food flavoring, upper gastrointestinal tract discomfort, nausea, motion sickness, rheumatoid arthritis	Antiplatelet properties; potential to increase risk of bleeding	At least 7 days before surgery
Garlic: *Allium sativum*	Inhibition of platelet aggregation (may be irreversible); increased fibrinolysis; equivocal antihypertensive activity	Potential to increase risk of bleeding, especially when combined with other medications that inhibit platelet aggregation	At least 7 days before surgery
Ginkgo: duck foot tree, maidenhair tree, silver apricot	Inhibition of platelet-activating factor	Potential to increase risk of bleeding, especially when combined with other medications that inhibit platelet aggregation	At least 36 hr before surgery
Ginseng: American ginseng, Asian ginseng, Chinese ginseng, Korean ginseng	Lowers blood glucose; inhibition of platelet aggregation (may be irreversible); increased PT-PTT in animals; many other diverse effects	Hypoglycemia; potential to increase risk of bleeding; potential to decrease anticoagulation effect of warfarin	At least 7 days before surgery
Kava: awa, intoxicating pepper, kawa	Sedation, anxiolysis	Potential to increase sedative effect of anesthetics; potential for addiction, tolerance, and withdrawal after abstinence unstudied	At least 24 hr before surgery
St John's wort: amber, goat week, hardhay, *Hypericum*, klamatheweed	Inhibition of neurotransmitter reuptake, monoamine oxidase inhibition is unlikely	Induction of cytochrome P-450 enzymes, affecting cyclosporine, warfarin, steroids, protease inhibitors, and possibly benzodiazepines, calcium channel blockers, and many other drugs; decreased serum digoxin levels	At least 5 days before surgery
Valerian: all heal, garden heliotrope, vandal root	Sedation	Potential to increase sedative effect of anesthetics; benzodiazepine-like acute withdrawal; potential to increase anesthetic requirements with long-term use	No data

PT-PTT, Prothrombin time–partial thromboplastin time.

Donoghue TJ. Herbal medications and anesthesia case management. *AANA J.* 2018;86(3):242–248; Kaye AD, et al. Perioperative anesthesia clinical considerations of alternative medicines. *Anesthesiol Clin North America.* 2004;22:125–139; Chadha RM, Egan BJ. Perioperative considerations of herbal medications. *Curr Clin Pharmacol.* 2017;12(3):194–200.

TABLE 20.4   Components of the Preoperative Airway Physical Examination

Airway Examination Component	Nonreassuring Findings
Length of upper incisors	Relatively long
Relation of maxillary and mandibular incisors during normal jaw closure	Prominent "overbite" (maxillary incisors anterior to mandibular incisors)
Relationship of maxillary and mandibular incisors during voluntary protrusion of the jaw	Patient cannot bring mandibular incisors anterior to (in front of) maxillary incisors
Interincisor distance	<3 cm
Visibility of uvula	Not visible when tongue is protruded with patient in sitting position (e.g., Mallampati class >II)
Shape of palate	Highly arched or very narrow
Compliance of mandibular space	Stiff, indurated, occupied by mass, or nonresilient
Thyromental distance	<3 ordinary fingerbreadths
Length of neck	Short
Thickness of neck	Thick
Range of motion of head and neck	Patient cannot touch tip of chin to chest or cannot extend neck

From Apfelbaum JL, et al. Practice guidelines for management of the difficult airway: an updated report by the American Society of Anesthesiologists Task Force on Management of the Difficult Airway. *Anesthesiology.* 2013;118:251–270.

mask ventilation or endotracheal intubation). The initial physical examination of the patient includes careful inspection of the teeth, inside of the mouth, mandibular space, and neck in a sequential fashion to determine predictors of airway management difficulties (Table 20.4).[64] Certain body structural features, metabolic disease states, and congenital or acquired structural anomalies are associated with difficult airway management (Box 20.5).[65,66] The combination of subtle or minor physical anomalies may result in a difficult tracheal intubation even when each factor individually is not expected to pose a problem. A thorough exam allows the anesthesia provider to plan and prepare equipment for potential difficulty. Examples include video-assisted laryngoscope, positioning pillows, and/or difficult airway cart. For a complete review of airway examinations see chapter 24.

Tests for Prediction of Difficult Intubation

Several screening tests for predicting difficult endotracheal intubation are recommended as part of the preoperative patient evaluation. No single test should be relied on exclusively when the airway is evaluated; a combination of evaluative criteria should be used to increase the predictive value for difficult intubation.

Mallampati classification. A popular technique for airway assessment is the modified Mallampati airway classification, which entails examination of tongue size relative to the oral cavity.[67] During the assessment for the Mallampati classification, the patient is seated upright with the head in neutral alignment, while the examiner sits opposite the patient at eye level. The patient is asked to open the mouth as wide as possible and maximally extrude the tongue. The patient is encouraged not to phonate during this maneuver because phonation may inappropriately elevate the soft palate. The airway is then classified based on the structures visible on direct examination of the oropharynx (Fig. 20.1).[67] Endotracheal intubation is generally easy in a patient with a Mallampati class I airway and can be expected to be difficult in a patient with a Mallampati class III or IV airway. Mallampati airway classification has been criticized as not being a reliable or sensitive predictor of difficult intubating conditions. Because of the unusually high incidence of false-positive and false-negative findings associated with the system, it should not be used as the only means of screening for the difficult airway.

Thyromental distance. Thyromental distance can be quantified to enable prediction of difficulties with laryngoscopy. Thyromental distance represents the straight distance, with the neck fully extended and the mouth closed, between the prominence of the thyroid cartilage and the bony point of the lower mandibular border. In adults, a thyromental distance of less than 6-7 cm, which is approximately three adult fingerbreadths, is associated with difficult endotracheal intubation because the pharyngeal and laryngeal axes may not properly align, and difficult laryngoscopy can be anticipated.[68]

Interincisor distance. The degree of mouth opening, largely a function of the temporomandibular joint, is a vital component of airway assessment. Limited temporomandibular joint movement is a well-recognized contributor to difficult endotracheal intubation. An adult should be able to open the mouth at least 4 cm, allowing two to three fingers to be placed between the upper and lower incisors. An interincisor gap of less than two fingerbreadths is associated with difficulty in endotracheal intubation.[69] Some patients who are able to open their mouths sufficiently while awake experience limitations in temporomandibular joint mobility after anesthesia is induced. This limited movement renders the visualization of laryngeal structures difficult. In this situation, forward protrusion of the mandible can be attempted for opening the mouth adequately to allow direct laryngoscopy.[70]

Head and neck movement (atlantooccipital function). Moderate flexion of the neck on the chest and full extension of the atlantooccipital joint aligns the oral, pharyngeal, and laryngeal axes into the McGill or "sniff" position. In this position, less tongue obscures the laryngeal view during laryngoscopy. Limitations to atlantooccipital joint extension, which are frequently attributed to cervical arthritis or a small C1 gap, enhance the convexity of the neck and push the larynx anteriorly. This situation can impair laryngoscopy and render endotracheal intubation difficult.

Mandibular mobility. Have the patient demonstrate the ability to move the jaw forward and bite the upper lip. Being able to protrude the mandible in front of the central incisors indicates relative ease for maneuvering the laryngoscope.

Dentition

The incidence of perianesthetic dental injury in patients undergoing general anesthesia involving endotracheal intubation ranges from 0.02% to 0.07% and is associated with patients who have preexisting poor dentition and characteristics linked with difficult laryngoscopy and intubation (e.g., limited neck motion, previous head and neck surgery, craniofacial abnormalities, history of previous difficult tracheal intubation). Because dental injuries are the most common reason for anesthesia-related medicolegal claims (accounting for one-third of all claims in the United States),[71] a preanesthesia inspection of the teeth should be performed and documented for each patient. Otherwise fractured or missing teeth may be falsely attributed to damage occurring during airway instrumentation. The patient with protuberant or loose maxillary incisors should be informed of the increased risk of tooth injury or loss with laryngoscopy. An informed consent to proceed with the anesthetic plan, despite this dental risk, must then be

BOX 20.5 Conditions Associated With Difficult Airway Management

Head
- Mass defects (e.g., encephalocele, soft tissue sarcoma)
- Macrocephaly (e.g., severe hydrocephaly, Dandy Walker syndrome, mucopolysaccharidoses [Hurler syndrome])
- Interference with airway access (e.g., thoracopagus conjoined twins, stereotactic frame)

Facial Anomalies
- Maxillary and mandibular deformities
- Maxillary hypoplasia (e.g., Apert syndrome, Crouzon disease)
- Mandibular hypoplasia, microgenia, micrognathia (e.g., Pierre Robin syndrome, Treacher Collins syndrome, Goldenhar syndrome, cri du chat syndrome, Nager syndrome)
- Mandibular hyperplasia (e.g., cherubism)
- Temporomandibular joint anomalies
- Reduced mobility (e.g., arthrogryposis multiplex congenita, diabetes, Dutch-Kentucky syndrome, Hecht-Beals syndrome), ankylosis (inflammatory, congenital, traumatic, infectious)

Thoracoabdominal
- Morbid obesity, sleep apnea syndrome, Prader-Willi syndrome
- Kyphoscoliosis
- Prominent chest or large breasts
- Full-term or near-term pregnancy

Mouth and Tongue Anomalies
- Microstomia
- Congenital anomalies (e.g., Freeman-Sheldon [whistling face] syndrome)
- Acquired anomalies (e.g., burn)
- Stomatitis (e.g., noma)
- Tongue disease
- Macroglossia
- Congenital (e.g., Beckwith-Wiedemann syndrome, Down syndrome, congenital hypothyroidism, Pompe disease)
- Swelling (e.g., burns, trauma, Ludwig angina)
- Tumors (e.g., hemangiomas, lymphangioma)
- Protruding upper incisors (e.g., Cockayne syndrome)
- Foreign body

Nasal Pathology
- Choanal atresia
- Tumors (e.g., encephaloceles, gliomas, foreign body)

Palate Pathology
- Arch and cleft defects
- Soft-palate swelling and hematomas

Pharynx
- Adenoid and tonsillar disease

- Hypertrophy
- Tumors and abscesses
- Lingual tonsils
- Pharyngeal wall pathology
- Retropharyngeal and parapharyngeal abscesses
- Inflammatory disease (e.g., epidermolysis bullosa, erythema multiforme bullosum)
- Scarring (e.g., Behçet syndrome)

Laryngeal Pathology
- Supraglottic
- Laryngomalacia
- Supraglottis (epiglottitis)
- Glottic
- Congenital lesions (vocal cord paralysis, laryngeal web, cyst, laryngocele)
- Papillomatosis
- Granuloma formation
- Foreign body
- Subglottic
- Congenital stenosis
- Infectious (croup)
- Inflammatory (edema, traumatic stenosis)

Tracheal and Bronchial Tree Pathology
- Tracheomalacia (e.g., Larsen syndrome)
- Croup
- Bacterial tracheitis
- Mediastinal masses
- Vascular malformation
- Foreign body aspiration
- Other (e.g., tracheal stenosis, webbing, fistula, diverticulum)

Neck
- Mass lesions
- Lymphatic malformation, hemangioma, teratoma, goiter, abscess
- Skin contracture (postburn, inflammatory [scleroderma, epidermolysis bullosa, erythema multiforme bullosum])
- Webbed (e.g., Turner syndrome)

Spine
- Limited cervical spine mobility
- Congenital (e.g., Klippel-Feil syndrome)
- Acquired (e.g., surgical [fusion], trauma [vertebral fracture], inflammatory [ankylosing spondylitis])
- Cervical spine instability
- Congenital (e.g., Down syndrome, Larsen syndrome, Möbius syndrome, Morquio syndrome)
- Acquired (e.g., trauma [subluxation, fracture], inflammatory [rheumatoid arthritis])

Modified from Holzman RS. Airway management. In Davis PJ, Cladis FP, eds. *Smith's Anesthesia for Infants and Children.* 9th ed. Philadelphia: Elsevier; 2017; Fiadjoe JE, et al. The pediatric airway. In: Cote CJ, Lerman J, Anderson BJ, eds. *A Practice of Anesthesia for Infants and Children.* 6th ed. Philadelphia: Elsevier; 2019.

documented. If the patient is properly informed of the likelihood of dental damage, the anesthesia provider may not be held liable should dental injury occur.[72] For this reason, it is important that the time of the charted assessment be before the charted time of laryngoscopy or airway intervention.

The location and condition of crowns, braces, and other significant dental work are also noted. Prosthetic devices such as partial plates and dentures are removed before surgery unless they significantly improve the mask fit. An extremely loose tooth may be extracted before laryngoscopy to prevent its aspiration during anesthesia.

Class I   Class II   Class III   Class IV

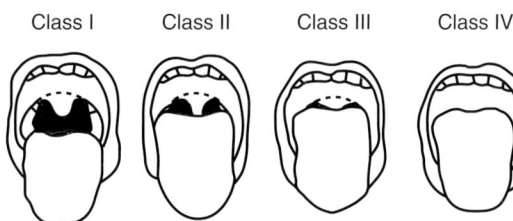

Fig. 20.1 Modified Mallampati classification of pharyngeal structures. *Class I*, Soft palate, tonsillar fauces, tonsillar pillars, and uvula visualized. *Class II*, Soft palate, tonsillar fauces, and uvula visualized. *Class III*, Soft palate and base of uvula visualized. *Class IV*, Soft palate not visualized. (From Samsoon GL, Young JR. Difficult tracheal intubation: a retrospective study. *Anaesthesia.* 1987;42:487–490.)

Musculoskeletal System

Obesity

Evaluation of the musculoskeletal system usually begins with a general assessment of the size and stature of the patient. Baseline height and weight information can be obtained from the admission data or by direct questioning of the patient during the health history interview. Body weight is then compared with normal values for a given height in relation to the patient's age and gender. Ideal body weight, for example, can be determined for men and women (Box 20.6). The actual weight of the patient is compared with the calculated ideal body weight. Body weight that is 20% in excess of the ideal body weight at a particular height constitutes obesity. A body weight that is twice the ideal body weight is deemed morbidly obese.

A more scientific approach to describing weight in relation to height uses the measure of body mass index (BMI). Box 20.6 presents the formula for calculating BMI and incorporates it into examples for an average and an overweight individual of the same height. The adult patient weight classification based on BMI is as follows: overweight, 25 to 29.9 kg/m²; Class 1 obesity, 30 to 34.9 kg/m²; Class 2 obesity, 35 to 39.9 kg/m²; and Class 3 obesity (sometimes referred to as "severe" obesity), greater than or equal to 40 kg/m². Two-thirds of the adult population in the United States are overweight or obese.[73] Obese patients are at risk of illness from a multitude of pathologic conditions that require detailed workup. Anesthesia management of the obese patient is discussed in detail in Chapter 48.

The Class 3 obese patient is at greater risk for cardiopulmonary aberrations, sleep-disordered breathing, and abnormal airway issues. Preoperative assessment scheduled in advance of the surgery should reflect careful attention to these concerns.[72] Appropriate diagnostic testing prior to bariatric surgery has been proposed (Box 20.7).[74,75] Much of this testing centers around the likelihood of patients presenting for bariatric surgery with preexisting metabolic complications or nutritional deficiencies. The extent of preexisting comorbid medical conditions needs to be thoroughly evaluated preoperatively, typically by internal medicine physicians. Serious or life-threatening comorbid conditions associated with obesity are noted in Box 20.8.[74] Patients should receive cardiac assessment in accordance with the American Heart Association guidelines.[76] Asymptomatic patients should be screened for coronary disease if they have an abnormal baseline electrocardiogram (ECG), a history of coronary artery disease/valvular disease, or are more than 50 years of age with at least two of the following: metabolic syndrome, diabetes, hypertension, smoking, dyslipidemia, or family history of coronary disease.[77] Patients without comorbid conditions may not require further preoperative workup because diagnostic testing should be individualized based on identified needs.[78]

Obstructive sleep apnea is a breathing disorder, prevalent in the obese population, distinguished by periodic, partial, or complete

---

BOX 20.6 Calculation of Ideal Body Weight and Body Mass Index

Ideal Body Weight (IBW)
IBW (male) = 105 lb + 6 lb for each inch >5 ft
IBW (female) = 100 lb + 5 lb for each inch >5 ft

To Calculate Body Mass Index (BMI):
BMI = Weight in kg/(height in meters)²

Example 1
70 kg/1.7 m² = 70 kg/2.89 m = 24 kg/m²

Example 2
125 kg/1.7 m² = 125 kg/2.89 m = 43 kg/m²

BOX 20.7 Recommended Diagnostic Testing of Candidates for Bariatric Surgery

- 12-lead electrocardiogram—if at least one risk factor for coronary heart disease, poor functional capacity, or both
- Chest radiograph (posteroanterior and lateral)—if BMI ≥40 kg/m²
- Complete blood cell count
- Glycosylated hemoglobin
- Serum chemistries with parameters for liver and kidney function
- Fasting blood glucose
- Lipid profile (total cholesterol, triglycerides, high-density lipoprotein cholesterol, low-density lipoprotein cholesterol)
- Thyroid function (thyrotropin)
- Coagulation studies
- Ferritin
- Vitamins (B₁₂, 25-hydroxyvitamin D, other fat-soluble vitamins if considering a malabsorptive procedure)
- Minerals and trace elements (e.g., zinc, selenium, calcium, magnesium)

Adapted from Eldar S, et al. A focus on surgical preoperative evaluation of the bariatric patient—the Cleveland Clinic protocol and review of the literature. *The Surgeon.* 2011;9(5):273–277; Poirier P, et al. Cardiovascular evaluation and management of severely obese patients undergoing surgery: a science advisory from the American Heart Association. *Circulation.* 2009;120(1):86–95; Thompson J, et al. Anesthesia case management for bariatric surgery, *AANA J.* 2011;79(2):147–160.

---

obstruction of the upper airway during sleep.[79] More than 70% of patients presenting for bariatric surgery have obstructive sleep apnea.[78] Particular attention is given to a history of snoring, apneic episodes, frequent arousals during sleep (vocalization, shifting position, extremity movements), morning headaches, and daytime somnolence. The physical examination would include airway evaluation, nasopharyngeal characteristics, neck circumference, tonsil size, and tongue volume.[80,81] A concise, easy to use screening questionnaire for undiagnosed obstructive sleep apnea known as STOP-Bang (Box 20.9) has been shown to be highly sensitive for categorizing obstructive sleep apnea severity.[82]

Polysomnography is the current gold standard test for establishing a clinical diagnosis of obstructive sleep apnea. If the findings of the history and physical examination are suggestive of obstructive sleep apnea, a decision in consultation with the surgeon should be made regarding obtaining a preoperative sleep study. If the diagnosis of obstructive sleep apnea is confirmed, the patient will be evaluated to determine optimal levels of continuous positive airway pressure

BOX 20.8 Comorbid Conditions Associated With Obesity

- Known sleep apnea in which patient is noncompliant with continuous positive airway pressure (CPAP)
- HbA$_{1C}$ (glycosylated hemoglobin) >8% (average blood sugar >200 mg/dL)
- Diabetic nephropathy, retinopathy, or neuropathy
- Cirrhosis
- Pulmonary hypertension
- Pseudotumor cerebri (with severe headaches or impending vision loss)
- Significant coagulopathy (including history of pulmonary embolus, bleeding diathesis, hypercoagulable syndrome, excessive bleeding, more than one deep venous thrombosis, taking Coumadin or clopidogrel medication)
- Chronic steroid therapy
- Oxygen dependent (does not necessarily have to be constant)
- Wheelchair-bound most of the time
- Systemic disease and poor functional capacity (including multiple sclerosis, inflammatory bowel disease, scleroderma, lupus, cancer)
- Severe venous stasis ulcers
- Recent complaint of chest pain (undiagnosed)

Adapted from Eldar S, et al. A focus on surgical preoperative evaluation of the bariatric patient—the Cleveland Clinic protocol and review of the literature. *The Surgeon.* 2011;9(5):273–277.

BOX 20.9 STOP-Bang Questionnaire for Obstructive Sleep Apnea Screening

STOP

1. **S**noring: Do you *snore* loudly (loud enough to be heard through closed doors)?	Yes	No
2. **T**ired: Do you often feel *tired*, fatigued, or sleepy during daytime?	Yes	No
3. **O**bserved: Has anyone *observed* you stop breathing during your sleep?	Yes	No
4. Blood **P**ressure: Do you have or are you being treated for high blood *pressure*?	Yes	No

Bang

BMI: BMI >35 kg/m^2?	Yes	No
Age: Age >50 yr?	Yes	No
Neck circumference: Neck circumference >40 cm?	Yes	No
Gender: Male?	Yes	No

High risk of OSA: Yes to ≥3 questions
Low risk of OSA: Yes to <3 questions
From Chung F, et al. High STOP-Bang score indicates a high probability of obstructive sleep apnoea. *Br J of Anaesth.* 2012;108:768–775.

TABLE 20.5 Recommendations for Perioperative Glucocorticoid Coverage

Degree of Surgical Stress	Recommended Dose
Minor (inguinal hernia repair)	Preoperative corticosteroid dose + hydrocortisone 25 mg or equivalent
Moderate (lower extremity revascularization, total joint replacement)	Preoperative corticosteroid dose + hydrocortisone 50–75 mg or equivalent
Major (cardiac surgery, aortic aneurysm repair)	Preoperative corticosteroid dose + hydrocortisone* 100–150 mg or equivalent every 8 hr for 48–72 hr

*Hydrocortisone has mineralocorticoid activity at doses above approximately 100 mg/day. The mineralocorticoid activity of hydrocortisone may produce undesirable side effects, including fluid retention, edema, and hypokalemia. It is preferable to use a glucocorticoid without mineralocorticoid activity, such as methylprednisolone, when the total dose of hydrocortisone exceeds 100 mg/day. Methylprednisolone 4 mg is equivalent to hydrocortisone 20 mg.
From Nagelhout J, Elisha S, Waters E. Should I continue or discontinue that medication? *AANA J.* 2009;77(1):59–73.

includes a drying agent and proper upper airway anesthesia, should be instituted.

The patient should be questioned about the use of antiobesity drugs such as amphetamines, nonamphetamine Schedule IV appetite suppressants, and antidepressants (e.g., fluoxetine, sertraline).[84]

Ankylosing Spondylitis and Rheumatoid Arthritis

Disorders of the musculoskeletal system include degenerative disk disease (osteoarthritis), ankylosing spondylitis, and rheumatoid arthritis (RA). The chronic pain and inflammation of spinal or extraspinal joints associated with these diseases limit the degree of patient mobility. Tolerance for positions required during surgery and regional anesthesia techniques should therefore be ascertained preoperatively. Traditional ankylosing spondylitis multimodal approach of treatments (nonsteroidal antiinflammatory drugs [NSAIDs], sulfasalazine, glucocorticoids, and local corticosteroid injections), and biologic therapies (tumor necrosis factor-α [TNF-α] antagonists) may be included in pharmacologic regimens for such patients.[84]

If the dosage and duration of corticosteroid therapy are considerable in patients with rheumatoid arthritis, perioperative supplementation also may be necessary to avoid hemodynamic instability. Patients considered at risk for adrenal insufficiency include those who received the hydrocortisone equivalent of more than 20 mg daily for longer than 3 weeks during the previous year and those who are receiving replacement corticosteroid treatment for adrenal insufficiency.[86] Patients with proven or suspected adrenal insufficiency or suppression should be evaluated for perioperative steroid coverage (Table 20.5).[87] The least amount of steroid supplement perioperatively should be used to minimize the risk of surgical site infection and postoperative wound complications.[88]

Although less common than osteoarthritis, ankylosing spondylitis and rheumatoid arthritis have greater implications for anesthetic management. Systemic manifestations are extensive during the advanced stages of both disorders. Patients frequently have pain, inflammation, and limited mobility in affected joints, such as those in the back and hands. Extreme ankylosis and joint deformity often make peripheral venous access and intraoperative positioning a challenge. On physical examination, limited range of motion of the

(CPAP) therapy. Patients already receiving CPAP therapy will be asked to bring their cleaned home CPAP units to the hospital for postoperative application as needed. If the hospital is to provide the CPAP device, the patient needs to be queried as to the type of interface device the patient uses, pressure settings, and whether supplemental oxygen is required.

Particular attention is given to airway evaluation to determine the likelihood of difficult endotracheal intubation. Patients who are obese, have short, thick necks, or have obstructive sleep apnea have a higher incidence of difficult or failed endotracheal intubation (8%)[83] than the general population (1:2200).[73] If a problem is anticipated and an awake tracheal intubation is planned, then proper patient preparation, which

TABLE 20.6 Biological Agents—Half-Life, Mechanism of Action, Management During Perioperative Period, and Major Side Effects

Drug	Half-Life	Mechanism of Action	Management	Side Effects
Etanercept	3.5–5.5 days	Anti-TNF	Withdraw 10 days before surgery	Increased risk of infection
Adalimumab	10–20 days		Withdraw 30 days before surgery	
Infliximab	9.5 days		Withdraw 19 days before surgery	
Certolizumab	14 days		Withdraw 28 days before surgery	
Golimumab	14 days		Withdraw 28 days before surgery	
Abatacept	12.6 days	T-cell inhibitor	Withdraw 25 days before surgery	Increased risk of infection, headache, gastrointestinal disorders
Rituximab	18–22 days (effects can last for months)	B-cell inhibitor	Withdraw 100 days before surgery	Increased risk of infection, Stevens-Johnson syndrome, hypotension, arrhythmias
Tocilizumab	11–13 days	IL-6 receptor antagonist	Withdraw 26 days before surgery	Increased risk of infection, hepatotoxicity
Anakinra	4–6 hr	IL-1 receptor antagonist	Withdraw 1–2 days before surgery	Increased risk of infection, hepatotoxicity

IL, Interleukin; *TNF,* tumor necrosis factor.
From Franco AS, Iuamoto LR, Pereira RMR. Perioperative management of drugs commonly used in patients with rheumatic diseases: a review. *Clinics (São Paulo).* 2017;72(6):386–390.

temporomandibular joint and cervical spine, and reduced mouth opening, can make tracheal intubation more difficult. In rheumatoid arthritis, this limitation is compounded by restrictions in vocal cord movement or tracheal stenosis caused by cricoarytenoid arthritis. These changes may be evidenced by preoperative hoarseness, stridor, painful speech, or dysphagia. Restrictive lung disease, polychondritis, pleural and pericardial effusions, and cardiac conduction abnormalities may be present during advanced stages of ankylosing spondylitis or rheumatoid arthritis.[85]

Pharmacologic considerations when caring for a patient with rheumatoid arthritis include side effects of disease-modifying anti-rheumatic drugs (DMARDs) and other biologic agents used in the treatment of rheumatoid arthritis. The method of action of these pharmacologic interventions causes immune deficiency resulting in delayed wound healing, wound dehiscence, and surgical site infection.[89] Because of these adverse effects, some DMARDs and biologic agents should be held in the perioperative period. Select biologic agents and their important pharmacologic properties are noted in Table 20.6.

Neurologic System

Preoperative evaluation of the neurologic system includes the determination of CNS or peripheral nervous system dysfunction. An initial neurologic examination consisting of the following should be performed:[90]

- *Musculoskeletal (motor) system:* Observe the patient's gait, ability to perform toe-and-heel walk, ability to maintain the arms held forward; evaluate the patient's grip strength
- *Sensory system:* Physical distinction of vibration, pain, and light touch on the patient's hands, feet, and limbs
- *Muscle reflexes:* Deep, superficial, and pathologic
- *Cranial nerve abnormalities:* Obtained by patient medical history and observation
- *Mental status and speech pattern:* Appearance, mood, thought processes, cognitive function

Knowledge of clinical manifestations of neurologic disease is essential for the preoperative evaluation of patients with CNS or peripheral nervous system disorders. Signs and symptoms of increasing intracranial pressure and cerebral ischemia are important to note, so the

BOX 20.10 Signs and Symptoms of Increased Intracranial Pressure and Ischemia

- Papilledema
- Unilateral or bilateral mydriasis
- Headaches, postural, worse in morning, made worse by coughing
- Nausea and vomiting
- Slurred speech
- Disorientation and altered levels of consciousness
- Flaccid hemiplegia or hemiparesis
- Abducens or oculomotor palsy
- Neck rigidity
- Respiratory disturbances
- Arterial hypertension, with corresponding decreases in heart rate (represents a physiologic attempt to enhance cerebral perfusion when intracranial pressure is high)
- The appearance of Q waves, deep and inverted T waves, prolonged QT intervals, and ST segment elevations on the electrocardiogram (ECG) may reflect hypothalamic ischemia and sympathetic overactivity.

clinician should document a detailed account of preexisting neurologic impairment (Box 20.10). These abnormalities are most often attributed to vasospasm after a subarachnoid hemorrhage, but myocardial ischemia should be ruled out before surgery.[91] Fever and leukocytosis can also follow a subarachnoid hemorrhage as a result of meningeal irritation by subarachnoid blood. The progression of neurologic dysfunction to coma, obtundation, and decerebrate rigidity worsens the overall prognosis of the patient with an intracranial mass or hemorrhage. This prognosis mirrors that of a patient who has sustained an acute head injury. The patient with an initial Glasgow Coma Scale (Table 20.7)[92] score of less than 8 is considered comatose. Patients with a score of 8 or less usually require tracheal intubation and mechanical hyperventilation.[93]

Diagnostic reports should be reviewed so that the extent of neurologic and coexisting disease can be determined. These reports include the results of electromyography, conduction velocity studies, electroencephalography, computed tomography (CT), magnetic resonance

TABLE 20.7   Glasgow Coma Scale

Response	Score
Eyes Open	
Spontaneously	4
To speech	3
To pain	2
Never	1
Best Motor Response	
Obeys commands	6
Localizes pain	5
Withdraws (flexion)	4
Abnormal flexion (decortication)	3
Extensor response (decerebration)	2
None	1
Best Verbal Response	
Oriented	5
Confused conversation	4
Inappropriate words	3
Incomprehensible sounds	2
None	1
Range of Scores	3–15

Modified from Teasdale G, Jennett B. Assessment of coma and impaired consciousness: a practical scale. *Lancet.* 1974; 2(7872):81–84.

imaging (MRI), and cerebral arteriography studies. Consultation with a neurologist and obtaining preoperative electromyography, for example, are recommended for patients with complaints of extremity weakness, pain, or paresthesia. This screening is especially important in patients at greater risk for peripheral neuropathy (e.g., patients with long-standing diabetes, patients with uremia, and chronic alcoholics with nutritional deficits).

Documentation of symptoms and reports of abnormal preoperative neurologic findings is important in these patients. Preoperative CT or MRI that reveals a 0.5-cm midline shift of the brain is significant and can confirm suspicions of intracranial hypertension. Additional radiologic signs of raised intracranial pressure include mass, hydrocephalus, cerebral edema, obliteration of cerebral fluid cisterns around the brainstem, and effacement of ventricles and cortical sulci.[93]

The size and location of an intracerebral aneurysm are represented on cerebral arteriography. This information can facilitate the prediction of the surgical approach and guide the evaluation of neurologic involvement. The degree of collateral circulation in the patient with cerebrovascular occlusive disease can be determined from arteriographic films. In a patient with vertebral artery involvement, for example, extremes in head flexion, extension, and rotation are avoided. Because of the associated risks of perioperative myocardial ischemia and infarction in patients undergoing a carotid endarterectomy procedure, a thorough cardiac evaluation by a cardiologist, including 12-lead ECG and stress testing, is advised.[94]

Information gained from the preoperative evaluation of neurologic function can enlighten the management of a patient with a CNS or peripheral nervous system disorder. For example, sedatives are avoided in patients with intracranial hypertension, especially when an altered level of consciousness accompanies the hypertension. Affected patients may be extremely sensitive to the CNS-depressant effects of such drugs as opioids.

Doses, schedules, and adverse effects of therapeutic regimens should also be considered before surgery. Serum concentrations of anticonvulsants such as phenytoin and phenobarbital do not need to be documented unless drug withdrawal or significant changes are expected.[95] A complete blood cell count is obtained for patients receiving prolonged phenytoin therapy because of the risk of agranulocytosis associated with this drug. As with anticonvulsant therapy, corticosteroid therapy is continued perioperatively in patients with a CNS tumor. Although the exact mechanism of the beneficial effects of corticosteroids is unknown, it is theorized to involve the reduction of cerebrospinal fluid production or cerebral edema as a result of capillary membrane stabilization. Blood glucose levels are also determined for the patient treated with either dexamethasone or methylprednisolone because hyperglycemia frequently accompanies the use of these drugs. Heightened risks of pulmonary infection and gastrointestinal irritation are unlikely in the patient undergoing perioperative therapy.[96]

Cardiovascular System

Preanesthesia patient evaluation for cardiovascular risk includes the determination of the following: (1) preexisting cardiac disease (e.g., hypertension, ischemic heart disease, valvular dysfunction, cardiac arrhythmias, and cardiac conduction abnormalities, with or without evidence of ventricular failure); (2) disease severity, stability, and prior treatment; (3) comorbidity (e.g., diabetes mellitus, peripheral vascular disease, chronic pulmonary disease, obesity); and (4) surgical procedure. The type of surgery for which the patient is scheduled impacts on the likelihood of developing perioperative adverse cardiac events (cardiac death, MI) within 30 days following surgery (Box 20.11).[4] The prevalence and adverse consequences of cardiovascular disease make it a prime consideration in the overview of systems.

Major cardiac conditions that correlate with increased perioperative morbidity and mortality have been described by the European Society of Anaesthesiology (Box 20.12).[4] In addition, risk indices are available to establish where the patient exists on the continuum of risk. Table 20.8 demonstrates three tools recommended by the American College of Cardiology Foundation/American Heart Association (ACC/AHA) that serve as predictors for perioperative morbidity and mortality based on cardiac risk factors.[99] A Revised Cardiac Risk Index (RCRI), which offers an improved predictive risk index for major postoperative cardiac complications, is noted in Box 20.13. The RCRI is the simplest and most prevalently used, but like the other indices has its limitations on its ability to predict morbidity and mortality in certain subsets of patients.[98] Whenever a patient has signs of significant cardiovascular disease, referral to a cardiologist is indicated for assessment and possible intervention.[4]

The patient's functional capacity, measured in metabolic equivalents (METs), can be simply and accurately assessed preoperatively by asking a set of questions (see Table 20.9),[77,99] and is recommended as part of cardiac risk assessment.[100] Patients with good functional capacity (>4 METs) may proceed for surgery provided patients with cardiac risk factors are properly managed with statin and β-blocker therapy as described later in this section. Good functional capacity (>4 METs) may be determined by an affirmative answer to two simple questions: (1) Are you able to walk four blocks without stopping regardless of limiting symptoms? (2) Are you able to climb two flights of stairs without stopping regardless of limiting symptoms?[101] The inability to climb two flights of stairs or walk a short distance is indicative of poor functional capacity and is associated with an increased incidence of postoperative cardiac complications in noncardiac surgery.[102,103] Patients with

BOX 20.11   Surgical Risk Estimates

High Risk (Cardiac Risk >5%)
- Aortic surgery
- Major vascular surgery
- Peripheral vascular surgery

Intermediate Risk (Cardiac Risk 1%–5%)
- Intraperitoneal
- Transplant (e.g., renal, liver, pulmonary)
- Carotid
- Peripheral arterial angioplasty
- Endovascular aneurysm repair
- Head and neck surgery
- Major neurologic/orthopedic (e.g., spine, hip)
- Intrathoracic
- Major urologic

Low Risk (Cardiac Risk <1%)
- Breast
- Dental
- Endoscopic
- Superficial
- Endocrine
- Cataract
- Gynecologic
- Reconstructive
- Minor orthopedic (e.g., knee surgery)
- Minor urologic

From De Hert S, et al. Preoperative evaluation of the adult patient undergoing noncardiac surgery: guidelines from the European Society of Anaesthesiology. *Eur J Anaesthesiol.* 2011;28(10):684–722.

BOX 20.12   Active Cardiac Conditions for Which the Patient Should Undergo Evaluation and Treatment Before Noncardiac Surgery

Unstable Coronary Syndromes
- Unstable or severe angina
- Recent myocardial infarction (MI) within 30 days

Decompensated Heart Failure
Significant Arrhythmias
- High-grade atrioventricular block
- Symptomatic ventricular arrhythmias
- Supraventricular arrhythmias with uncontrolled ventricular rate (>100 beats/min at rest)
- Symptomatic bradycardia
- Newly recognized ventricular tachycardia

Severe Valvular Disease
- Severe aortic stenosis (mean pressure gradient >40 mm Hg, area <1 cm^2 or symptomatic)
- Symptomatic mitral stenosis

Clinical Risk Factors
- History of ischemic myocardial disease
- Currently stable but history of heart disease
- History of cerebrovascular disease
- Diabetes (insulin dependent)
- Renal failure (serum creatinine [SCr] >2 mg/dL)

From De Hert S, et al. Preoperative evaluation of the adult patient undergoing noncardiac surgery: guidelines from the European Society of Anaesthesiology. *Eur J Anaesthesiol.* 2011;28(10):684–722.

moderate to poor functional capacity (<4 METs) should be further assessed to identify cardiac risk factors.[104]

A standard means of categorizing the degree of cardiovascular disability is the New York Heart Association classification tool (see Table 20.10).[105,106] When the patient interview is conducted, specific inquiry should be made regarding the presence of dyspnea, chest pain, fatigability, syncope, palpitation, and the factors that predispose to angina.

Hypertension

The updated classification of hypertension is defined as normal BP: 120/80 mm Hg systolic/diastolic; elevated BP: 120 to 129/<80; stage 1: 130 to 139/80 to 89; and stage 2: >140/>90.[107] Hypertension is the most common circulatory derangement to affect humans and is a major risk factor for coronary artery disease[102] and increased perioperative mortality.[108] In 2018, nearly 0.5 million deaths in the United States included hypertension as a primary or contributing cause.[109] Increasingly, patients undergoing surgery have stage 2 hypertension and accompanying target-organ damage, or uncontrolled stage 3 hypertension (systolic BP >180 mm Hg, diastolic BP >110 mm Hg, or both). This problem can be attributed to the lack of or inadequacy of medical treatment, or to patient noncompliance. In such a situation, elective surgery may be postponed for further patient assessment and normalization of the preoperative blood pressure.[110,111] Consultation with an internist can be pursued for the medical evaluation and treatment of the patient with uncontrolled or newly diagnosed hypertension. These recommendations are aimed at reducing the occurrence of perioperative hemodynamic instability and consequently the incidence of myocardial ischemia. Both complications are more likely to

occur when hypertension is not effectively treated before surgery.[112] With the goal of reducing perioperative risk, delaying surgery is justified in hypertensive patients with target-organ damage (or suspected damage) such as ischemic heart disease, heart failure, renal damage, and cerebrovascular diseases if either of the following scenarios is probable:[113]

- Conditions can be improved by such postponement to the extent that the perioperative risk would be considerably decreased.
- Care may be influenced by further preoperative examination.

Delaying elective surgery in patients with mild to moderate hypertension only for the purpose of blood pressure control may not reduce perioperative risk.[113] A systolic BP below 180 mm Hg and diastolic BP below 110 mm Hg is not an independent risk factor for perioperative cardiovascular complications.[77]

The practitioner taking the medical history should focus on identifying comorbid diseases, such as diabetes mellitus, and social risk factors (i.e., tobacco use, alcohol or caffeine consumption, illicit drug use [especially cocaine or amphetamines]). What medications the patient takes to manage hypertension should be established. In general, the substances used affect the central and peripheral components of the sympathetic nervous system by altering the synthesis, release, biotransformation, or end-organ action of norepinephrine. Because the circulatory-depressant effects of general anesthesia may be additive, the combination of antihypertensive drugs and anesthetics is of concern. Complaints of syncope and dizziness also are investigated. These symptoms may be the clinical manifestations of cerebrovascular insufficiency, although a diagnosis of drug-induced orthostatic hypotension should be considered preoperatively. This diagnosis can be confirmed

TABLE 20.8 **Comparison of the RCRI, the American College of Surgeons NSQIP MICA, and the American College of Surgeons NSQIP Surgical Risk Calculator**

	RCRI	American College of Surgeons NSQIP MICA	American College of Surgeons NSQIP Surgical Risk Calculator
Criteria	...	Increasing age	Age
	Creatinine ≥2 mg/dL	Creatinine >1.5 mg/dL	Acute renal failure
	HF	...	HF
	...	Partially or completely dependent functional status	Functional status
	Insulin-dependent diabetes mellitus	...	Diabetes mellitus
	Intrathoracic, intraabdominal, or suprainguinal vascular surgery	Surgery type: • Anorectal • Aortic • Bariatric • Brain • Breast • Cardiac • ENT • Foregut/hepatopancreatobiliary • Gallbladder/adrenal/appendix/spleen • Intestinal • Neck • Obstetric/gynecologic • Orthopedic • Other abdomen • Peripheral vascular • Skin • Spine • Thoracic • Vein • Urologic	Procedure (CPT code)
	History of cerebrovascular accident or TIA	...	...
	...	...	ASA physical status class
	...	...	Wound class
	...	...	Ascites
	...	...	Systemic sepsis
	...	...	Ventilator dependent
	...	...	Disseminated cancer
	...	...	Steroid use
	...	...	Hypertension
	Ischemic heart disease	...	Previous cardiac event
	...	...	Sex
	...	...	Dyspnea
	...	...	Smoker
	...	...	COPD
	...	...	Dialysis
	...	...	Acute kidney injury
	...	...	BMI
	...	...	Emergency case
Use outside original cohort	Yes	No	No
Sites	Most often single-site studies, but findings consistent in multicenter studies	Multicenter	Multicenter

Continued

TABLE 20.8   Comparison of the RCRI, the American College of Surgeons NSQIP MICA, and the American College of Surgeons NSQIP Surgical Risk Calculator—cont'd

	RCRI	American College of Surgeons NSQIP MICA	American College of Surgeons NSQIP Surgical Risk Calculator
Outcome and risk factor ascertainment	Original: research staff, multiple subsequent studies using variety of data collection strategies	Trained nurses, no prospective cardiac outcome ascertainment	Trained nurses, no prospective cardiac outcome ascertainment
Calculation method	Single point per risk factor	Web-based or open-source spreadsheet for calculation (http://www.surgicalriskcalculator.com/miorcardiacarrest)	Web-based calculator (www.riskcalculator.facs.org)

ASA, American Society of Anesthesiologists; *BMI;* body mass index; *COPD,* chronic obstructive pulmonary disease; *CPT,* Current Procedural Terminology; *ENT,* ear, nose, and throat; *HF,* heart failure; *NSQIP,* National Surgical Quality Improvement Program; *NSQIP MICA,* National Surgical Quality Improvement Program Myocardial Infarction Cardiac Arrest; *RCRI,* Revised Cardiac Risk Index; *TIA,* transient ischemic attack.

BOX 20.13   Revised Cardiac Risk Index

Risk Categories
- High-risk surgery (aortic, major vascular, peripheral vascular)
- Ischemic heart disease (previous myocardial infarction; previous positive result on stress test, use of nitroglycerin; typical angina; ECG Q waves; previous PCI or CABG)
- History of compensated previous congestive heart failure (history of heart failure; previous pulmonary edema; third heart sound; bilateral rales; evidence of heart failure on chest radiograph)
- History of cerebrovascular disease (previous TIA; previous stroke)
- Diabetes mellitus (with or without preoperative insulin)
- Renal insufficiency (creatinine >2.0 mg/dL)

Estimated Rates for Postoperative Major Cardiac Complications Per Number of Risks
- 0 risk factors: 0.4%
- 1 risk factor: 0.9%
- 2 risk factors: 7%
- ≥3 risk factors: 11%

CABG, Coronary artery bypass grafting; *ECG,* electrocardiogram; *PCI,* percutaneous coronary intervention; *TIA,* transient ischemic attack. From Lee TH, et al. Derivation and prospective validation of a simple index for prediction of cardiac risk of major noncardiac surgery. *Circulation.* 1999;100(10):1043–1049; Freeman WK, Gibbons RJ. Perioperative cardiovascular assessment of patients undergoing noncardiac surgery. *Mayo Clin Proc.* 2009;84(1):79–90.

TABLE 20.9   Exercise Tolerance in Metabolic Equivalents (METs) for Various Activities

Estimated Energy Expenditure	Physical Activity
1 MET*	*Poor functional capacity*
	Self-care; eating, dressing, or using the toilet; walking indoors and around the house; walking 1–2 blocks on level ground at 2–3 mph[2]
4 METs	*Good functional capacity*
	Light housework (e.g., dusting, washing dishes); climbing a flight of stairs without stopping, or walking up a hill longer than 1–2 blocks; walking on level ground at 4 mph; running a short distance; heavy housework (e.g., scrubbing floors, moving heavy furniture); moderate recreational activities (e.g., golf, dancing, doubles tennis, throwing a baseball or football)
>10 METs	*Excellent functional capacity*
	Strenuous sports (e.g., basketball, cross-country skiing [>8 km/hr],[3] rope skipping, running, soccer, swimming [>3.5 km/hr], weight training)

*MET is defined as the amount of oxygen consumed while sitting at rest and is equal to 3.5 mL oxygen/kg/min.
mph, Miles per hour; *km/hr,* kilometer per hour.
Modified from Jetté M, et al. Metabolic equivalents (METS) in exercise testing, exercise prescription, and evaluation of functional capacity. *Clin Cardiol.* 1990;13(8):555–565; Fleisher LA, et al. 2014 ACC/AHA guideline on perioperative cardiovascular evaluation and management of patients undergoing noncardiac surgery. *J Am Coll Cardiol.* 2014;64:e77–e137.

---

by measuring a significant decrease in the blood pressure as the patient rises from the supine position. The lack of hemodynamic compensatory responses that normally accompany positional changes may then predict their absence during anesthesia and surgery.

The physical examination of the patient includes the following:[114,115]
- *Overall appearance:* Truncal obesity with purpura and striae suggestive of Cushing disease
- *Vital signs:* Measurement of blood pressure in both arms
- *Funduscopic examination:* Hypertensive retinopathy
- *Neck:* Carotid bruits, distended veins, or enlarged thyroid gland
- *Heart:* Abnormal rhythm or size, murmurs, or heart sounds
- *Lungs:* Rales or bronchospasm
- *Abdomen:* Bruits, masses, enlarged kidneys, or abnormal aortic pulsation

- *Extremities:* Delayed or absent femoral pulses secondary to aortic coarctation; evidence of atherosclerosis, peripheral edema
- *Neurologic evaluation:* See "Neurologic System" earlier.

Ischemic Heart Disease

Myocardial ischemia occurs secondary to insufficient oxygen and nutrient supply (increased demand, reduced blood supply, or both) to meet the metabolic requirements of the myocardial cells. Nearly one-third of the estimated 30 million patients undergoing surgery annually in the United States is at high risk for coronary artery disease or

TABLE 20.10 New York Heart Association Functional Classification of Cardiovascular Disability

Classification	Cardiovascular Status
Class I	*Patients with cardiac disease*
	No functional limitations to physical activity, such as walking or climbing stairs; ordinary physical activity not associated with undue fatigue, palpitations, dyspnea, or anginal pain
Class II	*Patients with cardiac disease who are comfortable at rest*
	Slight functional limitations to physical activity, such as walking or climbing stairs rapidly, or during emotional stress; patients are comfortable at rest; ordinary physical activity results in fatigue, palpitation, dyspnea, or anginal pain
Class III	*Patients with cardiac disease resulting in marked limitations to physical activity*
	Patients are comfortable at rest; less than ordinary physical activity causes fatigue, palpitations, dyspnea, or anginal pain
Class IV	*Patients with cardiac disease resulting in inability to carry on any physical activity without discomfort*
	Symptoms of cardiac insufficiency or anginal syndrome may be present even at rest; if any physical activity is undertaken, discomfort is increased

Modified from Bansal M., et al. Assessment of cardiac risk and the cardiology consultation. In Kaplan JA, et al. *Kaplan's Cardiac Anesthesia for Cardiac and Noncardiac Surgery,* 7th ed. Philadelphia: Elsevier; 2017.

factors for cardiovascular disease.[115] Risk factors for ischemic heart disease include advanced age, smoking, diabetes mellitus, hypertension, pulmonary disease, previous MI, left ventricular wall motion dysfunction, and peripheral vascular disease.[116] The preoperative evaluation of a patient with known or suspected ischemic heart disease is aimed at determining the severity, progression, and functional limitations imposed by cardiovascular disease. Myocardial ischemia, cardiac arrhythmias, and left ventricular dysfunction are usually precipitating factors for patient symptomatology. Complaints of undue fatigue, angina pectoris, palpitations, syncope, or dyspnea should be thoroughly investigated. A 12-lead ECG can be reviewed for evidence of myocardial ischemia or infarction, cardiac arrhythmias or conduction abnormalities, and ventricular hypertrophy. Routine testing with a 12-lead ECG is not recommended for low-risk surgeries. Testing with a 12-lead ECG is recommended only for patients with known coronary heart disease or other significant structural heart disease.[77] However, signs and symptoms of myocardial ischemia may not be apparent at rest. Therefore, the response of the patient to various activities such as walking a certain distance or climbing several stairs must be determined (see Tables 20.9 and 20.10).[77,100,106]

Anginal symptoms can also be classified according to the stability of precipitating factors, the frequency of the events, and the duration of pain. Stable angina (characterized as substernal discomfort brought on by exertion, relieved by rest or nitroglycerin, or both in <15 minutes, and having a typical radiation to the shoulder, jaw, or the inner aspect of the arm) is unlikely to pose a significantly greater threat of MI perioperatively than those who have the absence of anginal symptoms.[117] Unstable angina is defined as: (1) newly developed angina

occurring within the past 2 months; (2) angina that has progressively worsened with an increased frequency, intensity, or duration, is less responsive to medicine, or that occurs when the patient is at rest; or (3) angina that lasts longer than 30 minutes, exhibiting transient ST- or T-wave changes without development of Q waves or diagnostic elevation of enzymes.[106] *Unstable angina is associated with the highest risk for perioperative MI.*[118] In the patient with unstable angina, elective surgery is canceled until the cardiovascular status of the patient has been thoroughly evaluated and optimized. Advanced diagnostic techniques such as coronary angiography and exercise ECG may be used for determination of the extent and functional impairment of ischemic heart disease.

The overall risk of MI after general anesthesia is approximately 0.3% in the population at large.[119] In patients known to have had an MI between 3 and 6 months of surgery, the risk of perioperative reinfarction increases to approximately 6%. If the MI occurred 1 to 2 months prior to surgery, the risk of reinfarction is approximately 19%. The reinfarction rate is 33% if surgery is performed within less than 30 days of the MI.[77] If reinfarction occurs, the mortality rate is approximately 50%. The highest at-risk period appears to be within 30 days after an acute MI; therefore the ACC/AHA guidelines recommend waiting at least 60 days after an MI before a patient undergoes elective surgery. Patients who have survived coronary revascularization and are asymptomatic are at lower risk of reinfarction when undergoing noncardiac surgery.[77] The universal definitions of myocardial injury and MI are noted in Table 20.11.[120]

Coronary stents. Approximately 528,000 coronary stents are placed annually in US patients to open clogged coronary arteries.[121] Coronary stents (either bare metal or drug-eluting) were designed to prevent arterial restenosis after percutaneous coronary intervention (PCI) with balloon angioplasty. Bare metal stents (BMSs), although beneficial over balloon angioplasty in reducing the incidence of restenosis, experience a restenosis rate of 20%.[122] Drug-eluting stents (DESs) were developed to further reduce the incidence of stent thrombosis, and restenosis rates approaching 5% after 2 years are reported.[123] Postprocedure pharmacotherapy involves long-term oral dual antiplatelet therapy (DAPT) consisting of aspirin (continued almost always indefinitely) and a P2Y$_{12}$ inhibitor (clopidogrel, prasugrel, or ticagrelor), which is continued for a minimum of 6 months to prevent in-stent coronary artery restenosis.[124] Approximately 5% of these patients will require noncardiac surgery within 1 year after placement of coronary stents.[125] There is an increased risk of coronary stent thrombosis, perioperative MI, hemorrhagic complications, and death in patients having noncardiac surgery performed early after stent placement.[126,127] Fig. 20.2[124] describes preoperative assessment and management considerations for patients presenting for surgery in which coronary artery stents have been placed. Management of patients with coronary stents is discussed in detail in Chapter 26.

Left Ventricular Dysfunction

Active left ventricular failure is the prominent cardiovascular risk factor for patients undergoing noncardiac surgery.[128] Heart failure can be broken down into two subsets of patients: those with preserved ejection fraction (EF ≥50%) and those with reduced ejection fraction (EF <49%).[129] Although patients with heart failure with preserved EF (HFpEF) have better perioperative outcomes than do patients with reduced EF (HFrEF), a diagnosis of heart failure places patients at significantly higher risk of perioperative mortality than other disease processes.[77] Patients with ischemic cardiomyopathy are at even greater risk for perioperative MI and ventricular dysfunction.[130] Heart failure is defined by the presence of any of the following: history of congestive

TABLE 20.11   **Universal Definitions of Myocardial Injury and Myocardial Infarction**

Criteria for Myocardial Injury

The term *myocardial injury* should be used when there is evidence of elevated cardiac troponin values (cTn) with at least 1 value above the 99th percentile upper
   reference limit (URL). The myocardial injury is considered acute if there is a rise and/or fall of cTn values.

Criteria for Acute Myocardial Infarction (MI) (Types 1, 2, and 3 MI)

The term *acute myocardial infarction* should be used when there is acute myocardial injury with clinical evidence of acute myocardial ischemia and with detection of
   a rise and/or fall of cTn values with at least 1 value above the 99th percentile URL and at least one of the following:
- Symptoms of myocardial ischemia
- New ischemic ECG changes
- Development of pathologic Q waves
- Imaging evidence of new loss of viable myocardium or new regional wall motion abnormality in a pattern consistent with an ischemic etiology
- Identification of a coronary thrombus by angiography or autopsy (not for types 2 or 3 MI)

Postmortem demonstration of acute atherothrombosis in the artery supplying the infarcted myocardium meets criteria for type 1 MI. Evidence of an imbalance
   between myocardial oxygen supply and demand unrelated to acute atherothrombosis meets criteria for type 2 MI. Cardiac death in patients with symptoms
   suggestive of myocardial ischemia and presumed new ischemic ECG changes before cTn values become available or abnormal meets criteria for type 3 MI.

Criteria for Coronary Procedure–Related Myocardial Infarction (Types 4 and 5 MI)

Percutaneous coronary intervention (PCI)–related MI is termed type 4a MI.

Coronary artery bypass grafting (CABG)–related MI is termed type 5 MI.

Coronary procedure–related MI ≤48 hr after the index procedure is arbitrarily defined by an elevation of cTn values >5 times for type 4a MI and >10 times for type 5
   MI of the 99th percentile URL in patients with normal baseline values. Patients with elevated preprocedural cTn values, in whom the preprocedural cTn levels are
   stable (≤20% variation) or falling, must meet the criteria for a >5- or >10-fold increase and manifest a change from the baseline value of >20%. In addition, with at
   least one of the following:
- New ischemic ECG changes (this criterion is related to type 4a MI only)
- Development of new pathologic Q waves
- Imaging evidence of loss of viable myocardium that is presumed to be new and in a pattern consistent with an ischemic etiology
- Angiographic findings consistent with a procedural flow-limiting complication such as coronary dissection, occlusion of a major epicardial artery or graft, side-
    branch occlusion-thrombus, disruption of collateral flow or distal embolization

Isolated development of new pathologic Q waves meets the type 4a MI or type 5 MI criteria with either revascularization procedure if cTn values are elevated and
   rising but less than the prespecified thresholds for PCI and CABG.

Other types of 4 MI include type 4b MI stent thrombosis and type 4c MI restenosis that both meet type 1 MI criteria.

Postmortem demonstration of a procedure-related thrombus meets the type 4a MI criteria or type 4b MI criteria if associated with a stent.

Criteria for Prior or Silent/Unrecognized Myocardial Infarction

Any one of the following criteria meets the diagnosis for prior or silent/unrecognized MI:
- Abnormal Q waves with or without symptoms in the absence of nonischemic causes
- Imaging evidence of loss of viable myocardium in a pattern consistent with ischemic etiology
- Pathoanatomic findings of a prior MI

ECG, Electrocardiogram.

From Thygesen K, Alpert JS, Jaffe AS, et al. Fourth universal definition of myocardial infarction. *Circulation.* 2018;138(20):e618–e651.

heart failure, pulmonary edema, or paroxysmal nocturnal dyspnea; physical examination showing bilateral rales or S₃ gallop; or chest x-ray showing pulmonary vascular redistribution.[77] Prominent signs include moist rales in the lungs often associated with tachypnea. These extraneous sounds may be confined to the bases, with mild degrees of left ventricular failure, or they may be generalized throughout the lungs with acute pulmonary edema. As a result of sympathetic nervous system stimulation, resting tachycardia may also be present. A third heart sound (S_3) or ventricular gallop, jugular vein distention, and peripheral edema are significant. In the presence of congestive heart failure as confirmed by a chest radiograph, elective surgery should be postponed until optimal ventricular performance can be achieved.

Patients exhibiting dyspnea of unknown origin, current or prior heart failure with worsening dyspnea, or other relevant change in clinical status should undergo preoperative evaluation of left ventricular function if an assessment has not been performed within the previous 12 months.[77] Tests of resting left ventricular function include cardiac magnetic resonance,[131] radionuclide angiography, two-dimensional echocardiography, and contrast ventriculography. Systolic left ventricular dysfunction is defined as a left ventricular EF

of less than 50% with and without accompanying diastolic dysfunction.[132] A left ventricular EF of less than 35% as determined by echocardiography is associated with greater incidence of postoperative heart failure and death.[133]

Valvular Heart Disease

Basic lesions of valvular heart disease may involve stenosis, incompetence, or both. In adults aortic and mitral valve lesions are more common than those involving the tricuspid or pulmonic valve. Despite decreasing incidence, rheumatic heart disease is still the most common cause of adult valvular disease. Degenerative disorders (sclerosis, fibrosis) and congenital diseases are less common causes. Stenotic valves cause the chamber proximal to the obstruction to increase the work of maintaining a stroke volume; this eventually results in hypertrophy. Normal valves can episodically accommodate up to seven times the normal cardiac output (e.g., in intense physical exercise in the normally active patient). Valvular stenosis is usually chronic and severe before cardiac output decreases. In valvular incompetence, the chambers both proximal and distal to the lesions are involved because regurgitant flow during one phase of the cardiac cycle is added to forward flow during

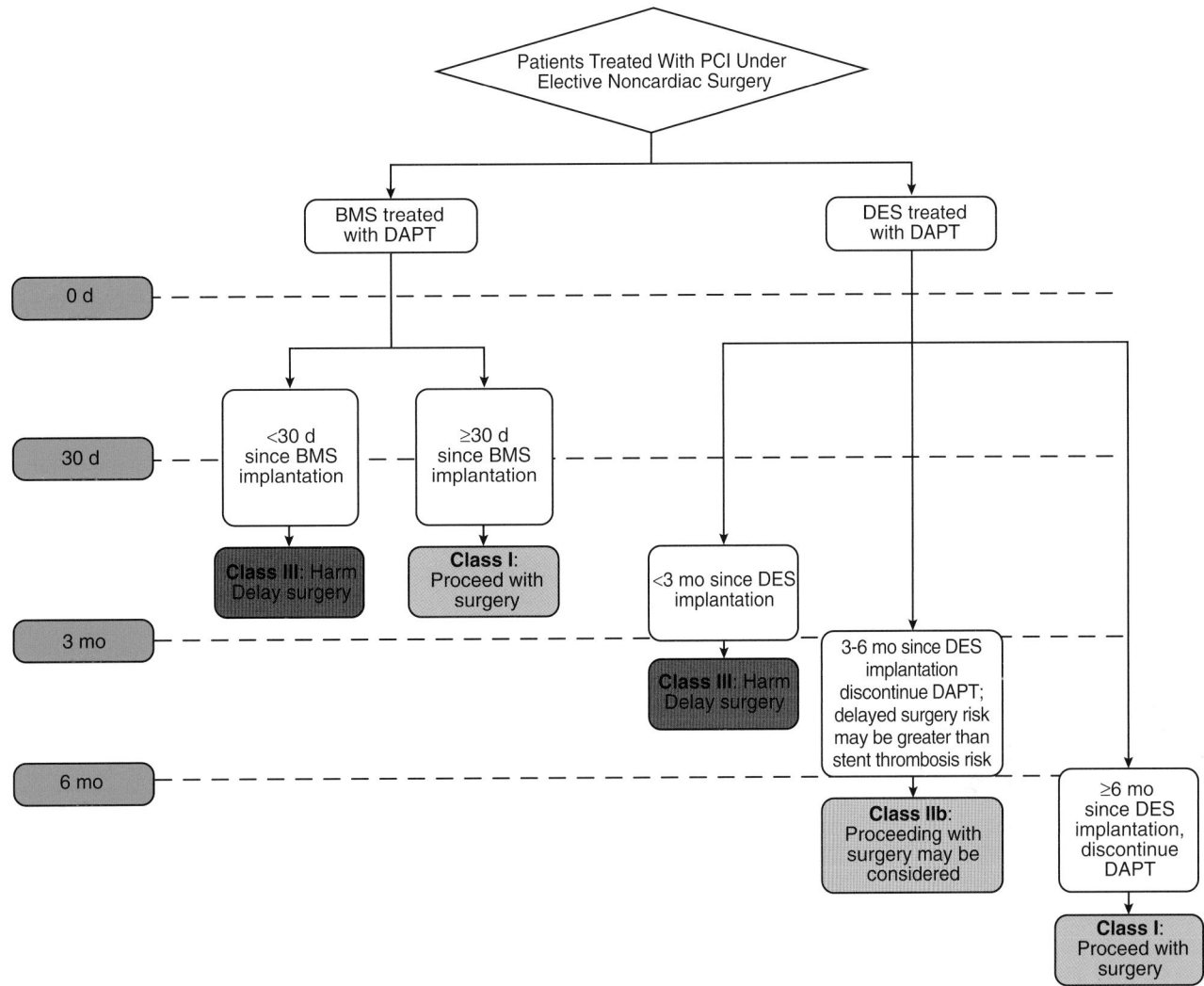

Fig. 20.2 Treatment algorithm for the timing of elective noncardiac surgery in patients with coronary stents. *BMS,* Bare metal stent; *DAPT,* dual antiplatelet therapy; *DES,* drug-eluting stent; *PCI,* percutaneous coronary intervention. (From Levine GN, et al. 2016 ACC/AHA guideline focused update on duration of dual antiplatelet therapy in patients with coronary artery disease: a report of the American College of Cardiology/American Heart Association Task Force on Clinical Practice Guidelines. *J Am Coll Cardiol.* 2016;68:1082–115.)

subsequent systole. Because lesions are almost never entirely unitary, in stenosis some regurgitation is common and vice versa. It is important to identify the type of valvular lesion before surgery. Evaluation of the clinical symptoms and cardiac catheterization data regarding valve area and gradients, combined with assessment of data from any surgical history (e.g., correction of congenital heart lesions), is an important component of the preoperative evaluation of patients with valvular heart disease.

Severe aortic stenosis poses the greatest patient risk for noncardiac surgery,[77] especially when the cross-sectional area of the aortic valve is less than 1 cm^2. Severe aortic stenosis is associated with a 14-fold greater incidence of perioperative sudden death.[134] When moderate to severe valvular stenosis or regurgitation is suspected, an echocardiogram should be obtained if one has not been performed within the previous year, or if significant change in clinical status is present. For patients in whom aortic stenosis is symptomatic, elective noncardiac surgery should be postponed until after cardiac surgical consultation.[77] Chapter 25 describes the perioperative care of patients with valvular heart disease.

Arrhythmias

Patients with cardiac arrhythmias must have an adequate preoperative evaluation to ascertain the nature of the arrhythmia, associated underlying heart disease, and type of antiarrhythmic therapy. Whether symptoms of palpitations or dizziness have been relieved may be a sign of successful therapy or continuing problems. Other cardiac symptoms such as dyspnea, angina, or syncope may suggest worsening of associated cardiac disease. Treatment of the underlying disease preoperatively may aid in control of arrhythmia in the perioperative period. All patients with a history of symptomatic arrhythmias should undergo electrocardiography with rhythm strip before surgery. Other preoperative laboratory evaluations should include measurement of potassium and magnesium levels, determination of antiarrhythmic drug levels (if possible), and chest radiography (in the presence of structural cardiac disease).

Ventricular arrhythmias are classified into three categories: benign ventricular arrhythmias (unifocal premature ventricular contractions), potentially malignant ventricular arrhythmias (patient has known organic heart disease and is on antiarrhythmic therapy), and malignant ventricular arrhythmias (patient has organic heart disease, hemodynamic compromise, and possibly a family history of sudden death).[135] Few data are available to help correlate the risk of arrhythmias and perioperative risk.[106] In the absence of cardiac disease, benign ventricular arrhythmias do not carry a significantly increased surgical risk.[136] In patients with severe coronary artery disease, recent MI, or peripheral vascular disease, arrhythmias may increase perioperative risk.[137,138]

Cardiovascular Implantable Electronic Devices (Pacemaker, Implantable Defibrillators)

When a patient presents for surgery with an implanted cardiac device, preprocedural planning can help minimize risk to both the patient and the device. This planning includes knowledge of the device, its indication for use, and functional assessment (Box 20.14).[139-142] Because of the evolving complexity of these devices, direct interrogation by a qualified member of the cardiovascular implantable electronic device (CIED) management team remains the only trustworthy method for evaluating battery status, lead performance, and adequacy of current settings.[143] Pacemakers can mask the toxicity of antiarrhythmic drugs, electrolyte disorders, and myocardial ischemia and irritability. In general, the ECG should be examined for pacemaker malfunction as evidenced by unexpected pauses. If the patient's heart rate is slower than the pacing rate, pacing spikes should appear on the ECG. To determine whether these pacing impulses are associated with myocardial contractions, the clinician should palpate a peripheral pulse. Evaluation of a pacemaker becomes more difficult when the patient's heart rate is faster than the pacing rate. A Valsalva maneuver slows the patient's rate so that pacing impulses appear on the ECG. Generally, because sensing is lost before pacing, the pacemaker is probably functioning normally if (1) it has been in place for fewer than 2 years, (2) chest radiography demonstrates that leads are intact, and (3) impulses do not appear on the ECG.[144] Chest radiography should provide information on electrode placement, the presence of electrode fracture, and even battery depletion.[145]

If each pacing impulse is not associated with a pulse, or if the symptoms that led to pacemaker implantation have returned, cardiology consultation should be considered.[144] Anesthesia providers sometimes must decide whether a transvenous, temporary pacing wire should be inserted preoperatively. Persistent bradycardia not responsive to intravenous administration of atropine or exercise is one indication. Bifascicular block in a patient with a history of syncope suggests underlying, unrecognized complete heart block. Such patients can benefit from the availability of transvenous pacing.

BOX 20.14 Perioperative Guidelines for the Patient With a Cardiovascular Implantable Electronic Device

Preoperative Key Points

- Establish the indication for the permanent pacemaker, for example, symptomatic third-degree heart block, type II second-degree heart block, sinus node dysfunction, recurrent neurally mediated syncope, some forms of cardiomyopathy.
- Establish the indication for the implantable defibrillator, for example, history of cardiac arrest not secondary to a temporary condition.
- Identify device and manufacturer (available from manufacturer's identification card).
- Notify the cardiovascular implantable electronic device (CIED) management team of the planned procedure, including anatomic location of surgery, whether monopolar electrosurgery will be used, and whether other sources of electromechanical interference (EMI) will be present. Have the pacemaker or defibrillator interrogated by a qualified member of the CIED management team (physicians or staff) who monitors the device function shortly before the anesthetic. Pacemakers should be routinely interrogated annually and implantable cardioverter devices (ICDs) every 3–4 months. Pacemakers should be assessed within 12 mo of elective surgery. ICD function should be assessed within 6 mo of surgery.
- Obtain a copy of this interrogation, including current settings. Ensure that the device will pace the heart with appropriate safety margins.
- A prescription for the perioperative management of the patient with the CIED should be communicated to the procedure team from the CIED team.
- Consider replacing any device near the end of its elective replacement period in a patient scheduled to undergo either a major surgery or surgery within 25 cm of the generator.
- Is the patient device dependent for antibradycardia? Determine the patient's underlying rhythm/rate to evaluate the need for backup pacing support.
- Evaluate effect of magnet on pacemaker function. Identify the magnet rate and rhythm if a magnet mode is present and magnet use is planned. Will device automatically reset to preoperative settings when a magnet is removed?
- Program minute ventilation rate responsiveness to "Off," if present.
- Program all rate enhancements to "Off."
- Consider increasing the pacing rate to optimize oxygen delivery to tissues for major cases.
- Inactivation of ICD tachyarrhythmia detection is recommended for all procedures using monopolar electrosurgery or radiofrequency ablation above the umbilicus. ICD arrhythmia detection can be suspended by placement of a magnet over the pulse generator.

Intraoperative Key Points

- Is electromagnetic interference (EMI) likely during the procedure? Interference is unlikely if the device is <10 yr old and bipolar cautery is >15 cm (below the umbilicus) from device lead or generator.
- Have a magnet immediately available for patients with CIEDs who are undergoing a procedure that may involve EMI.
- Monitor cardiac rhythm/peripheral pulse with pulse oximeter or arterial waveform.
- Disable the "artifact filter" on the electrocardiogram (ECG) monitor.
- Avoid use of monopolar electrosurgery.
- Use bipolar electrocautery system or ultrasonic (harmonic) scalpel if possible; if not possible, then pure cut (monopolar electrosurgery) with short bursts of ≤5 sec is better than "blend" or "coag."
- Position the electrosurgical unit (ESU) current return pad in such a way that it will prevent electricity from crossing the generator-heart circuit, even if the pad must be placed on the distal forearm and the wire covered with sterile drape.
- If the ESU causes ventricular oversensing, pacer quiescence, or tachycardia, limit the period(s) of asystole or reprogram the device.

Postoperative Key Points

- Have the device interrogated by a qualified member of the team (physician or staff) who monitors the device function postoperatively. Some rate enhancements can be reinitiated, and optimum heart rate and pacing parameters should be determined. The ICD patient must be monitored until the antitachycardia therapy is restored.

It also must be determined whether exercising the muscles adjacent to the generator causes dizziness. The presence of this symptom, indicating that myopotentials may be inhibiting the pacemaker, implies that muscle fasciculations caused by succinylcholine and shivering should be avoided. A complete discussion of anesthetic management of patients with cardiac devices can be found in Chapter 27.

Diagnostic Testing to Assess Cardiovascular Disease

Multiple tests are available to define the presence of cardiac disease. Preoperative cardiac testing should not be performed unless the results are likely to influence patient management. The ACC/AHA guidelines include an algorithm for determining the appropriateness of preoperative testing.[77]

Several noninvasive tests are available for preoperative assessment of the high-risk patient (i.e., three or more risk factors and poor functional capacity). A 12-lead ECG alone is not a predictor of perioperative major adverse cardiac events, therefore it is often useful to use this test as an adjunct to other noninvasive testing regimens.[146] The exercise stress ECG is preferred.[131] Stress testing with exercise or pharmacologic stress agents is designed to increase myocardial work and permit measurement of myocardial response to the increased workload. The exercise stress test not only is a standardized means of obtaining a functional history of angina but also provides excellent documentation of how ischemia manifests its effects on the cardiovascular system. By examining the stress test report one can learn the extremes of blood pressure and heart rate the patient can tolerate while awake (although exactly how these correlate with the anesthetized state is a matter of debate), the location of ischemic leads, and whether arrhythmias are associated with ischemia. Significant coronary disease is likely if ST segment depression is greater than 0.2 mV, if ST depression occurs early in the test, if little increase in blood pressure or heart rate occurs at the time of ST depression, or if hypotension occurs. Hypotension is considered an ominous finding and usually prompts cardiac catheterization.

Patients with good exercise tolerance rarely benefit from more than the exercise stress test.[147] Perioperative risk is considered low if exercise stress testing does not produce signs of myocardial ischemia at a reasonable workload (>85% of predicted maximum heart rate).[148] Although it is useful in diagnosing coronary artery disease, its value as a preoperative test has been questioned,[97] even in patients undergoing major vascular surgery.[149] Stress testing is not indicated in patients with intermediate risk factors (i.e., fewer than three risk factors), even if major vascular surgery is planned, provided the patient has complete heart rate control with β-blocker therapy.[108] Patients who are able to tolerate a good exercise stress workload, even those with stable angina, are unlikely to have myocardial dysfunction.[150]

Pharmacologic stress testing can be performed in patients unable to exercise or in those who take digoxin. Two pharmacologic techniques, which incorporate either echocardiography or radionuclide scintigraphy, are used: (1) dipyridamole or adenosine, both of which cause a coronary steal phenomenon by redistributing coronary blood flow without direct negative inotropic effects, and (2) dobutamine for inotropic stress testing.[151]

Additional noninvasive studies are available for preoperative testing such as stress myocardial perfusion imaging (MPI), stress echocardiography, resting transthoracic echocardiography, pharmacologic stress echocardiography, cardiac CT, cardiac magnetic resonance (CMR), and adenosine stress CMR.[131,152] The discovery of any defect is highly predictive of an increased likelihood of a postoperative cardiac event.[77] There is insufficient evidence to support the clinical utility and development of appropriate guidelines for these tests at this time.[137]

Cardiac catheterization provides definitive information about the distribution and severity of coronary artery disease and may be indicated for patients with New York Heart Association class III or IV criteria who are undergoing high-risk surgical procedures.[148] Significant stenosis means narrowing of a major coronary artery by more than 70% or narrowing of the left main coronary artery by more than 50%. However, it is important to look beyond the coronary anatomy and concentrate on other findings that can guide perioperative decision making.

Three readily identifiable findings that indicate poor ventricular function are a cardiac index of less than 2.2 L/m², a left ventricular end-diastolic pressure of greater than 18 mm Hg, and an EF of less than 40%.[153] Taking note of ischemia-induced dysfunction of the papillary muscles can help in avoiding later confusion about the configuration of the pulmonary wedge pressure waveform and the significance of intraoperative changes in wedge pressure. Wall motion abnormalities should be noted. Areas of akinesis (no movement during systole) usually represent nonviable regions of myocardium and are relatively fixed deficits. In contrast, areas of hypokinesis (reduced contraction during systole) may represent ischemic but nonetheless viable regions of myocardium. This should alert anesthesia providers to a potentially dynamic situation in which alterations in the balance of myocardial oxygen supply and demand can either improve or worsen regional ischemia and associated contractility.

Cardioprotective Pharmacotherapy

Appropriate pharmacologic therapy should be instituted preoperatively in patients exhibiting clinical risk factors (e.g., angina pectoris, prior MI, heart failure, stroke/transient ischemic attack, renal dysfunction, and diabetes mellitus requiring insulin therapy) and moderate to poor functional capacity. Patients having up to two clinical risk factors should be managed with statin and β-blocker therapy preoperatively.[154] If stable left ventricular dysfunction is present, angiotensin-converting enzyme (ACE) inhibitor therapy is recommended.

Statins. In addition to their lipid-lowering benefit, statins are valuable for enhancing endothelial function, improving atherosclerotic plaque stability, decreasing oxidative stress, and reducing vascular inflammation. Common statins used perioperatively include atorvastatin, fluvastatin, lovastatin, pravastatin, rosuvastatin, and simvastatin.[155] Recommendations are as follows[156]:

- Institute therapy between 30 days and at least 1 week before high-risk surgery.
- Continue statin therapy perioperatively.

β-blockers. Low-dose titration of β-blockers restores the oxygen supply/demand mismatch, reduces perioperative ischemia, redistributes coronary blood flow to the subendocardium, stabilizes plaques, increases ventricular fibrillation threshold, and may reduce the risk of MI and death in high-risk patients undergoing cardiac surgery.[155] The routine use of β-blockers in low-risk patients or patients having noncardiac surgery has been associated with increased rates of mortality and morbidity from hypotension, bradycardia, and stroke.[77,156,157] Recommendations are as follows:

- Continue β-blockers in patients previously treated with β-blockers for ischemic heart disease, symptomatic arrhythmia, or hypertension.
- Indicated for patients with high cardiac risk, known ischemic heart disease, or stress-induced myocardial ischemia who present for high-risk cardiovascular surgery.
- Initiation of β-blocker therapy should occur long enough in advance of the procedure (>45 days) to assess patient tolerance to therapy.

ACE inhibitors. ACE inhibitors are beneficial in reducing heart failure, MI, and death when administered in the perioperative period in patients with left ventricular dysfunction.[158] Common ACE inhibitors used perioperatively include captopril, enalapril, lisinopril, benazepril, and ramipril. Recommendations are as follows:[154]

- Recommended in cardiac stable patients with left ventricular dysfunction for intermediate- to high-risk surgery and considered for those scheduled for low-risk surgery.

Antiplatelet agents. DAPT is prescribed for patients who have undergone PCI with coronary artery stent placement. The regimen includes aspirin and a $P2Y_{12}$ inhibitor (clopidogrel, prasugrel, ticagrelor, cangrelor). Recommendations regarding the perioperative continuation or discontinuation of these agents take into account the risks of stent restenosis, the risks of intraoperative bleeding, and the type of stent the patient has implanted. If the implantation of the stent occurred prior to the year 2003, it is safe to assume that it is a BMS. Further useful information includes the type of DES, given that different agents are used to prevent stent restenosis and may have differing DAPT requirements. Fig. 20.2 outlines the new algorithm introduced by the ACC/AHA for decision making regarding this regimen. The guidelines recommend the following:[126]

1. Elective noncardiac surgery should be delayed 30 days after BMS implantation and optimally 6 months after DES implantation.
2. In patients treated with DAPT after coronary stent implantation who must undergo surgical procedures that mandate the discontinuation of $P2Y_{12}$ inhibitor therapy, it is recommended that aspirin be continued if possible and the $P2Y_{12}$ platelet receptor inhibitor be restarted as soon as possible after surgery.
3. When noncardiac surgery is required in patients currently taking a $P2Y_{12}$ inhibitor, a consensus decision among treating clinicians as to the relative risks of surgery and discontinuation or continuation of antiplatelet therapy can be useful.
4. Elective noncardiac surgery after DES implantation in patients for whom $P2Y_{12}$ inhibitor therapy will need to be discontinued may be considered after 3 months if the risk of further delay of surgery is greater than the expected risks of stent thrombosis.
5. Elective noncardiac surgery should not be performed within 30 days after BMS implantation or within 3 months after DES implantation in patients in whom DAPT will need to be discontinued perioperatively.

Novel oral anticoagulants. New oral anticoagulant agents (Table 20.12)[159] are prescribed for management of patients with a history of atrial fibrillation, deep venous thrombosis, pulmonary embolism, and at times prosthetic heart valves. These agents can either be Factor Xa inhibitors (rivaroxaban, apixaban) or thrombin inhibitors (dabigatran). As with antiplatelet agents, the risks of surgical bleeding versus recurrent thrombosis need to be considered. New reversal agents such as idarucizumab (Praxbind) are becoming available for emergency situations that require rapid reversal of anticoagulant effects. Recommendations for the perioperative management of these agents are as follows:

- Cessation for patients with atrial fibrillation depends on their $CHADS_2$ score ($CHADS_2$: *c*ongestive heart failure, *h*ypertension, *a*ge >75, *d*iabetes, previous *s*troke. All criteria get 1 point except the stroke, which gets 2 points. CHADS score >4 = high risk, 3–4 = intermediate risk, <3 = low risk).[159]
- For agents without a reversal, it is recommended that the drug be stopped 3 elimination half-lives prior to the procedure.[7]
- Agents should be resumed 24 to 48 hours after a surgical procedure provided that surgical bleeding is controlled.[160,161]
- Bridging therapies should be considered for high-risk patients.

Respiratory System

A detailed evaluation of the respiratory system is crucial because of the relative frequency of complications associated with respiratory disease. From an epidemiologic perspective some form of lung disease is

TABLE 20.12   Anticoagulant Medications

Agent		Indication	Mechanism of Action	Recommended Interval Between Last Dose and Procedure
Antiplatelet Agents				
Aspirin		Dual antiplatelet therapy (DAPT)	Cyclooxygenase inhibitor	7–10 days
Cilostazol (Pletal)		Claudication associated with peripheral vascular disease	Phosphodiesterase inhibitor	2 days
Thienopyridine agents	Clopidogrel (Plavix)	DAPT	$P2Y_{12}$ ADP receptor antagonist	5 days
	Prasugrel (Effient)	DAPT	$P2Y_{12}$ ADP receptor antagonist	7 days
	Ticagrelor (Brilinta)	DAPT	$P2Y_{12}$ ADP receptor antagonist	5 days
Novel Oral Anticoagulants				
Dabigatran (Pradaxa)		Atrial fibrillation, DVT, PE	Direct thrombin inhibitor	1–2 days (CrCl ≥50 mL/min), 3–4 days (CrCl <50 mL/min)
Rivaroxaban (Xarelto)		Atrial fibrillation, DVT, PE	Direct factor Xa inhibitor	1 day for normal renal function, 2 days (CrCl 60–90 mL/min), 3 days (CrCl 30–59 mL/min), 4 days (CrCl 15–29 mL/min)*
Apixaban (Eliquis)		Atrial fibrillation, DVT, PE	Direct factor Xa inhibitor	1–2 days (CrCl >60 mL/min); 3 days CrCl 50–59 mL/min), 5 days (CrCl ≤30–49 mL/min)

ADP, Adenosine diphosphate; *CrCl,* creatinine clearance; *DVT,* deep venous thrombosis; *PE,* pulmonary embolism.
From Baron TH, et al. Current concepts: management of antithrombotic therapy in patients undergoing invasive procedures. *N Engl J Med.* 2013;368:2113–2124.
*Hart RG, et al. Anticoagulants in atrial fibrillation patients with chronic kidney disease. *Nature Reviews Nephrology.* 2012;8:569.

present in nearly 25% of the adult population. The most common problems are COPDs, such as chronic bronchitis, emphysema, and asthma, which are major predictors for postoperative pulmonary disorders.[162] In their acute or chronic forms, the lung diseases are second only to coronary artery disease as a cause of death. Patients with COPD are twice as likely to have postoperative pulmonary complications.[163] Risk factors associated with increased postoperative respiratory morbidity and mortality rates include preoperative sepsis, emergency operations, age (begins at age 50 and increases with each additional decade), history of smoking, comorbid diseases (e.g., cardiovascular disease, congestive heart failure, diabetes, chronic kidney disease, neurologic impairment, American Society of Anesthesiologists [ASA] physical status class III or greater), preoperative weight loss, functional dependence for activities of daily living, chronic bronchitis, asthma, interstitial lung disease, upper respiratory infection, obstructive sleep apnea, obesity (as little as 20% overweight), type of surgery (abdominal, thoracic), prolonged duration of anesthesia (3–4 hours or longer), elevated creatinine, and pulmonary hypertension.[164-166] The surgical site (major abdominal, aortic, and thoracic surgeries) has been found to be the most important risk factor for the development of postoperative pulmonary complications.[166,167]

Emphysema and Chronic Bronchitis

The preparation of a patient with two forms of COPD—emphysema and chronic bronchitis—depends largely on the severity of the respiratory disease as reflected by the preoperative history, physical examination, and diagnostic testing. Elective surgery is postponed when severe dyspnea, wheezing, pulmonary congestion, or hypercarbia (partial pressure of arterial carbon dioxide [$Paco_2$] >50 mm Hg) is evident. The risk of postoperative respiratory failure in such circumstances is drastically increased. Consultation with a pulmonologist may be necessary for further evaluation and optimization of the respiratory status of the patient before anesthesia and surgery. Interventions to improve the pulmonary status of the patient with chronic bronchitis are the primary focus before surgery. Prophylactic measures that may reduce pulmonary risk are cited in Box 20.15.[165,168-170] Specific antibiotic therapy is initiated in patients with thick, purulent sputum and pulmonary infiltrates on the chest radiograph. Administration of prophylactic antibiotics to "sterilize" the sputum is not recommended because secondary resistant infections may develop and complicate the perioperative management of the patient. To enhance the mobilization and clearance of pulmonary secretions, chest physiotherapy and adequate hydration can be instituted. There is a lack of quality studies demonstrating the benefit of chest physiotherapy for noncardiothoracic surgery. Incentive spirometry may be beneficial in reducing postoperative pulmonary complications after upper abdominal surgery.[4]

The most reliable way to reduce the incidence of perioperative pulmonary complications is to have patients stop smoking cigarettes. Eight weeks after smoking cessation the pulmonary complication rate correlates with that of nonsmokers.[42] This intervention may not be feasible when initial meetings with the patient occur within days or hours of the scheduled procedure.

Several diagnostic tests are used for clinically differentiating bronchitis and emphysema in patients in the advanced stages of COPD. Arterial blood gases, for example, may document the presence of preoperative hypoxemia or hypercarbia. An abnormally low partial pressure of arterial oxygen (Pao_2) value (<60 mm Hg) with or without $Paco_2$ retention, often reflects a state of chronic bronchitis. A $Paco_2$ of greater than 45 mm Hg and an arterial oxygen saturation (Spo_2) of less than 90% is associated with an increased incidence of postoperative pulmonary complications; however, it is not predictive of whether the patient is fit for surgery.[171] Over time the patient can develop cor

---

BOX 20.15 Therapeutic Maneuvers to Decrease Risk of Pulmonary Complications

Preoperative
- Instruction in and application of respiratory maneuvers
- Smoking cessation
- Antibiotic treatment of pulmonary infection
- Antibiotic treatment of chronic bronchitis
- Expectorants
- Psychologic preparation
- Bronchodilator therapy for asthmatics
- Maintenance of good nutrition
- Chest physiotherapy
- Weight reduction

Postoperative
- Adequate pain control with minimization of postoperative opioid analgesia with epidural analgesia, when appropriate, and PCA administration of opioids (rather than intravenous boluses as needed), opioid sparing techniques with ERAS pathways
- Avoid nasogastric intubation when possible
- Maximal inspiration maneuvers, incentive spirometry, chest physiotherapy
- Mobilization of secretions
- Early mobilization of elderly patients
- Cough encouragement
- Heparin prophylaxis in selected cases

PCA, Postconceptual age; *ERAS*, enhanced recovery after surgery.
Data from Mohr DN, Lavender RC. Preoperative pulmonary evaluation. Identifying patients at increased risk for complications. *Postgrad Med.* 1996;100(5):241–244, 247–248, 251–252; Odor PM et al. Perioperative interventions for prevention of postoperative pulmonary complications: systematic review and meta-analysis. *BMJ.* 2020;368:m540. Wang JS. Pulmonary function tests in preoperative pulmonary evaluation. *Resp Med.* 2004;98(7):598–605; Pfeifer KJ, Smetana GW. Pulmonary risk assessment and optimization. *Hosp Med Clin.* 2016;5:176–188.

---

pulmonale because of the adverse effects of chronic hypoxemia on pulmonary vasculature. Neither preoperative hypoxemia nor hypercarbia has been found to be an independent predictor for the development of postoperative pulmonary complications; they are not absolute contraindications for noncardiac surgery.[166] Preoperative arterial blood gas analysis is considered routine for thoracic surgery, except in a fit patient.[172] The chest radiograph may suggest a diagnosis of COPD if slight abnormalities on the chest radiograph, including emphysemic bullae and pulmonary hyperlucency (which reflect vascular deficiencies in the lung periphery), are apparent. Diaphragmatic flattening and a vertical orientation of the cardiac silhouette also are characteristic. Chronic bronchitis, on the other hand, is rarely recognized through chest radiography unless secondary infections are present. Preoperative chest radiographs seldom change patient management and have not been shown to impact on the incidence of postoperative pulmonary complications,[4] and they may be indicated only in patients with known cardiopulmonary disease who are scheduled to undergo higher risk surgical procedures (i.e., upper abdominal, esophageal, thoracic, or aortic surgery).[166,172]

In addition to their role in categorizing patients with COPD, pulmonary function tests are occasionally used as diagnostic adjuncts for confirming the severity of airflow obstruction and its reversibility with bronchodilator therapy. In both chronic bronchitis and pulmonary emphysema, a decrease of the forced exhaled volume in 1 second (FEV_1) occurs in comparison with the forced vital capacity (FVC). FEV_1/FVC ratios of less than 80% indicate the presence of

BOX 20.16 Pertinent Asthmatic Data Obtained From the Medical History

Asthma Control and Current Therapy

- Frequency of asthmatic attacks, wheezing at exercise, or wheezing >3 three times in last 12 mo?
- Time interval since the last attack?
- Recent asthma exacerbation? How long since the patient was last hospitalized or treated in the emergency department for an asthmatic attack?
- Increased use of inhaled short-acting β-agonists? Use per week?
- Current or past use of inhaled corticosteroids?
- Most recent course of oral corticosteroids?
- What works best for treating an acute asthmatic event?

Asthma History and Complicating Conditions or Factors

- Recent upper respiratory tract infection (<2 wk) or sinus infection?
- Recent pneumonia? Was this documented on chest radiograph?
- What triggers an asthmatic attack?
- The severity of attacks: Was endotracheal intubation or intensive care unit admission required?
- History of pulmonary complications with prior surgical procedures?
- History of long-term corticosteroid use or corticosteroid-dependent asthma?
- Nocturnal dry cough
- Hay fever
- Exposure to passive smoke
- Obesity
- Obstructive sleep apnea

Modified from Karlet M, Nagelhout J. Asthma: an anesthetic update. *AANA J.* 2001;69(4):317–324; Tirumalasetty J, Grammer LC. Asthma, surgery, and general anesthesia: a review. *J Asthma.* 2006;43(4):251–254; Regli A, von Ungern-Sternberg BS. Anesthesia and ventilation strategies in children with asthma: part I–preoperative assessment. *Curr Opin Anaesthesiol.* 2014;1:288–294.

an obstructive process. Individual values of pulmonary function test results may be misleading. The FEV_1, for example, may already be low if the vital capacity is also decreased or the patient is uncooperative with the spirometric tests.

Numerous studies have found routine preoperative pulmonary function studies to be poor indicators of postoperative pulmonary complications and are not recommended.[4,173] All patients scheduled to undergo lung resection should have spirometric assessment preoperatively to estimate postoperative FEV_1 and suitability for resection.[163,174] It is not necessary to routinely obtain spirometric data prior to high-risk noncardiothoracic surgery. The value of pulmonary function testing prior to noncardiothoracic surgery is unproven and should be reserved for symptomatic patients with chronic debilitating conditions (i.e., myasthenia gravis).[166,175]

Asthma

Unlike other COPDs, asthma is characterized by reversible airflow obstruction. Inflammation of the airways is the hallmark of asthma. Distal bronchoconstriction results from airway hyperreactivity to stimuli that have little or no effect on normal airways. Precipitating factors include allergens, exercise, upper respiratory tract infections (URI), emotional stressors, and unidentified triggers.[174] Pertinent asthmatic data obtained from the medical history are detailed in Box 20.16.[176-178]

Information gleaned from these questions will help establish the nature and stability of the disease process. Patients with a history of coexistent cardiovascular disease, copious sputum production,

previous perioperative complications from asthma, recurrent nocturnal awakenings from asthma, frequent or continuous systemic corticosteroid requirement, or a recent hospitalization or emergency visit for asthma are considered to be at greater risk for perioperative aggravation of their asthma. Asthma should be under optimal medical management before a patient undergoes elective surgery and anesthesia. If the patient has a persistent cough, dyspnea, wheezing, or tachypnea on the day surgery is scheduled, it is best to reschedule surgery to allow for additional treatment of the asthma.[178]

The need for diagnostic testing is based on the clinician's assessment of the severity of the disease and magnitude of the operative procedure. An ECG is indicated if right ventricular hypertrophy is presumed, typically implying long-standing insufficient therapy. A chest radiograph is considered only if the patient is suspected of having an acute infiltrative process (e.g., pneumonia, pneumothorax in an acute exacerbation), or if a recent change in the patient's physical status is suggestive of a worsening pulmonary condition.[179] Arterial blood gases are usually indicated only when signs of debilitating chronic respiratory insufficiency (e.g., hypoxia, hypercarbia) are suspected or in patients with acute asthma who require emergency surgery. If age appropriate, spirometric evaluation consisting of a peak expiratory flow rate should be performed the morning of surgery if active disease is suspected. The results should be compared with the patient's best value in recent weeks. Findings will be as follows:

- *Normal:* 80% to 100% of baseline
- *Moderate exacerbation:* 50% to 80% of baseline
- *Severe episode indicating the need for delay of surgery and more intensive therapy:* Less than 50% of baseline

Peak expiratory flow is of limited use in assessing asthma preoperatively because other symptoms or clinical signs of poor asthma control are usually present.[179]

Early preoperative patient assessment promotes optimizing pharmacotherapy in the days prior to the scheduled surgery (Table 20.13).[178] Patient medications should be continued up to and on the day of surgery. Prophylactic β-adrenergic metered-dose inhalers should be used on the morning of surgery and accompany the patient to the operating room. Oral medications may be taken with a sip (1–2 oz) of water up to 1 to 2 hours before surgery. Therapeutic serum theophylline levels, 10 to 20 mcg/mL, should be confirmed if theophylline is used. Supplemental stress doses of corticosteroids may be appropriate if the patient has recently taken corticosteroids. Antianxiety premedication should be considered; psychologic triggers such as anxiety are common.

Ensure adequate hydration (e.g., minimize the fasting interval) to reduce airway desiccation and improve mobilization of secretions. If signs and symptoms of infection are present, surgery may be postponed until antibiotic therapy, based on sputum Gram stain and cultures, is initiated.

Upper Respiratory Tract Infection

Children with URI, particularly those younger than 1 year, have an increased risk (two- to sevenfold increase) of respiratory-related adverse events intraoperatively and postoperatively. The increased risk persists for up to 6 weeks and results in heightened airway irritability. The derangements associated with URI include decreased diffusion capacity for oxygen, decreased lung compliance, increased airway resistance, increased ventilation-perfusion mismatch, hypoxemia, and increased airway reactivity. Adverse perioperative events include laryngospasm, bronchospasm, postextubation croup, atelectasis, mucous plugging, and impaired oxygenation (e.g., bronchospasm, laryngospasm, hypoxemia, atelectasis, croup, and stridor). Signs and symptoms of URI include sore throat, inflamed and reddened nasopharyngeal and oropharyngeal mucosa, sneezing, rhinorrhea (clear

TABLE 20.13   Stepwise Treatment for Children (>5 Yr of Age) With Asthma

Using two or more canisters of β_2-agonist per month or >10–12 puffs/day, ≥3 × symptomatic per week, or waking 1 night/week indicates poorly controlled asthma and requires a step up in asthma treatment

Step 1: Mild intermittent asthma
Inhaled short-acting β_2-agonist as required

Step 2: Regular preventer therapy
Add inhaled steroids (in addition to inhaled short acting β_2-agonist)
Start with budesonide or beclomethasone 100 mcg bid, fluticasone 50 mcg bid or equivalent
<5 yr of age: consider leukotriene antagonist if inhaled steroids cannot be used

Step 3: Initial add-on therapy
Add inhaled long-acting β_2-agonist (in addition to inhaled steroids)
Consider
- Increasing inhaled steroids
- Adding leukotriene antagonists
- Theophylline
<5 yr: addition of leukotriene antagonist if already on inhaled steroid (see step 4)

Step 4: Persistent poor control
Increase inhaled steroids up to 800 mcg of budesonide equivalent per day
<5 yr: refer to a pediatric respiratory specialist

Step 5: Continuous or frequent use of oral steroids
Lowest oral dose for adequate control
Maintain high-dose inhaled steroids
Refer to a pediatric respiratory specialist
<5 yr: refer to a pediatric respiratory specialist

From Regli A, von Ungern-Sternberg BS. Anesthesia and ventilation strategies in children with asthma: part I–preoperative assessment. *Curr Opin Anaesthesiol.* 2014;1:288–294.

secretions) or mucopurulent nasal secretions, nasal congestion (including watery eyes), malaise, bulging and tender eardrums with associated inflammation, nonproductive cough, and fever of 37.5°C to 38.5°C (>38°C associated with lower respiratory tract involvement). Also present may be laryngitis or tonsillitis, viral ulcers in the oropharynx, and white blood cell count greater than 12,000 cells/mm³ with a left shift. Positive chest findings such as pulmonary congestion and rales are usually associated with lower respiratory tract involvement.

Each case should be reviewed individually. The decision to operate frequently depends on the urgency of the surgery, the duration and complexity of the surgery, and the need for instrumentation of the airway (Fig. 20.3).[180] Children with uncomplicated URIs may undergo elective procedures without significantly increasing anesthesia complications. It is important to obtain a specific history to distinguish a chronic state from an acute, superimposed symptomatic infectious process, which has predictive value for morbidity. Parents will be the best resource for establishing baseline conditions. If the parents state that the child typically has a cold or chronic runny nose (clear rhinorrhea) and is in an optimal state (afebrile, without respiratory distress), short elective procedures may be considered. If the child has a productive cough from lower respiratory tract involvement or an infectious purulent-appearing runny nose, elective surgery should be postponed for at least 2 weeks.[181] However, it may be necessary to schedule children who have chronic URIs for procedures such as myringotomy with ventilation tube placement or tonsillectomies because URIs are commonly associated with these conditions. Exercise caution with children younger than 5 years (consider postponing the

procedure for children <1 year of age) because risks are increased. If the child is older than 1 year with a resolving URI, it is reasonable to proceed with minor procedures not requiring endotracheal intubation (intubation with URI increases risk 11-fold).

Infectious nasopharyngitis (without lower respiratory tract involvement) requires postponing the surgery for 2 weeks after peak symptoms.[182] If the child exhibits signs and symptoms of lower respiratory tract involvement, it is prudent to postpone an elective surgical procedure for 4 to 6 weeks, the time necessary to minimize airway hyperactivity.

Laboratory testing may consist of a complete blood count, including differential. The value of obtaining a preoperative white blood cell count has been questioned because it is of little value and rarely is a factor in determining whether to proceed with the surgery. Nasal or throat cultures may be obtained if signs of an infectious process are observed. A chest radiograph is not warranted, especially if chest sounds are clear. Pulmonary function tests and arterial blood gas analysis rarely offer any useful information.

Recommendations for a child presenting for surgery with a mild URI include the following:[183]
- Discuss the increased risk of adverse perioperative events with parents and the surgical team.
- Try to avoid intubation if possible (laryngeal mask airway [LMA] or mask use has a lower risk).
- Preoperative albuterol treatment can be used as prophylaxis against perioperative bronchospasm.
- Humidification of inspired gases is thought to decrease airway dryness and maintain ciliary clearance.
- The febrile child presenting for an elective procedure with wheezing, rhonchi that do not clear with coughing, an abnormal chest x-ray film, elevated white count, or decreased activity level should be rescheduled.
- The well-appearing, afebrile child with a recent, uncomplicated URI and clear secretions may be able to safely undergo anesthesia.

Gastrointestinal System

Evaluation of the gastrointestinal system includes preoperative determination of the presence of nausea and vomiting, diarrhea, occult or overt gastrointestinal bleeding, abdominal or referred pain, abdominal distention, palpable masses, dysphagia, or gastric hyperacidity with or without reflux. The fluid and electrolyte status of the patient is reviewed, especially when gastrointestinal symptoms are associated with weight loss or malabsorption. Active bleeding requires preoperative hemoglobin concentration measurement. The hematocrit value may be falsely elevated as a result of hemoconcentration in patients with acute or chronic bleeding. Radiographic and CT scans of the abdomen are reviewed for evidence of obstruction or masses. The presence of peptic ulcer disease or esophageal hiatal hernia is also ascertained. For affected patients, prophylactic measures to reduce the risk of aspiration and its adverse pulmonary sequelae (e.g., aspiration pneumonitis) are instituted before surgery.

Hepatobiliary System

Preoperative evaluation of the hepatobiliary system includes screening for the presence of acute or chronic liver parenchymal disease such as hepatitis or cirrhosis, or cholestatic liver disease. Because of the tremendous reserve of the liver, progression of hepatic disease is often insidious. Signs and symptoms may be inapparent or vague until physiologic functions of the hepatobiliary system (Box 20.17) are markedly affected. Liver function tests are also limited in their ability to reflect the acuity and extent of hepatobiliary disease.[184] Considerable damage to the liver may be evident before laboratory test results are altered.

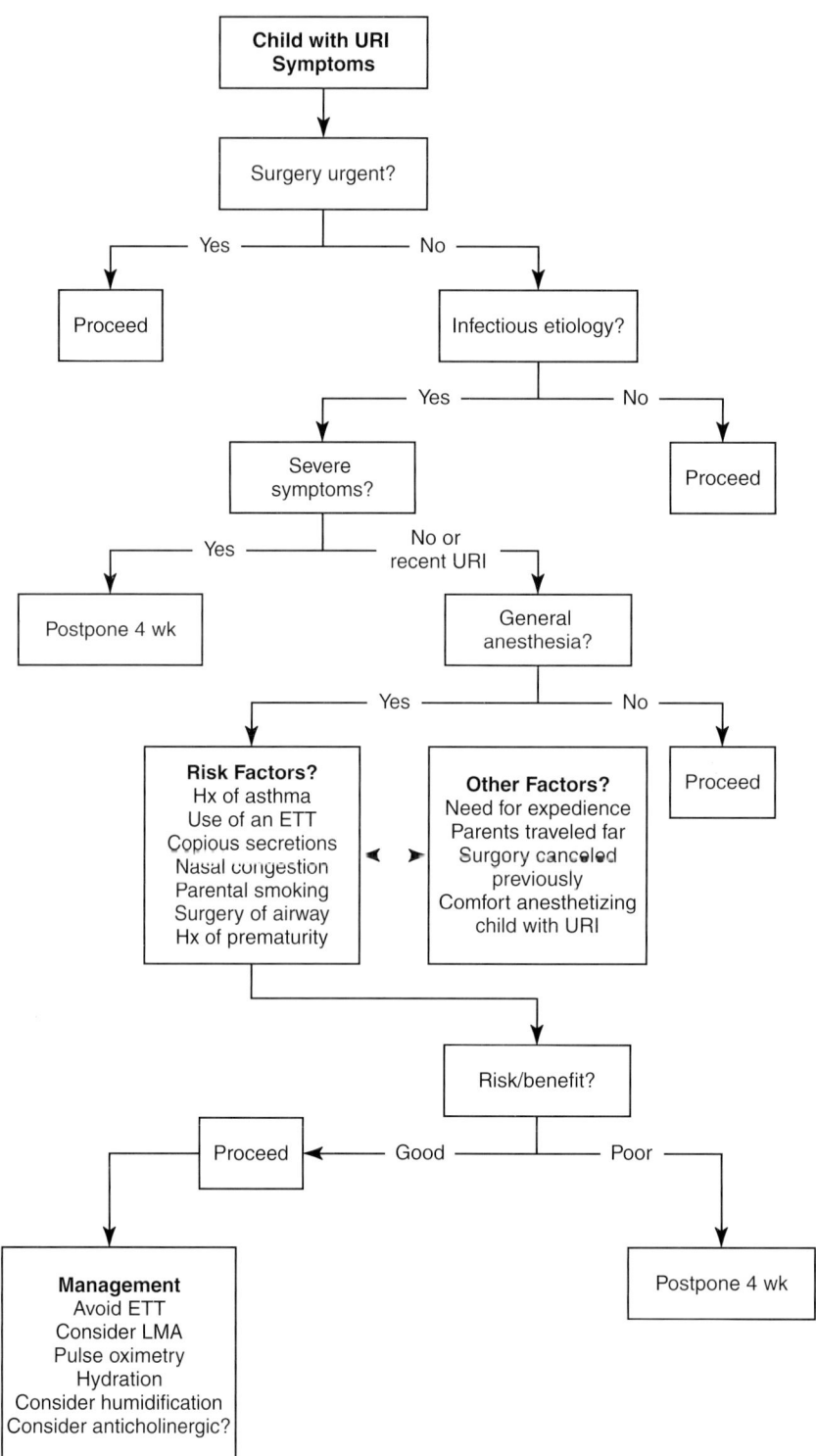

Fig. 20.3 Suggested algorithm for the assessment and anesthetic management of the child with an upper respiratory infection. *ETT*, Endotracheal tube; *Hx*, history; *LMA*, laryngeal mask airway; *URI*, upper respiratory infection. (From Tait AR, Malviya S. Anesthesia for the child with an upper respiratory tract infection: still a dilemma? *Anesth Analg.* 2005;100:59–65.)

During the early stages of hepatitis or cirrhosis, the clinical presentation ranges from one in which the patient is asymptomatic with normal liver function tests to one in which the patient has malaise, weight loss, abdominal discomfort, and mild jaundice with mild elevations in bilirubin levels. In cases of unexplained jaundice or elevated transaminase levels, suspicions of hepatobiliary dysfunction should be thoroughly investigated by a preoperative consultation with a gastroenterologist. Elective surgery is postponed until a definitive diagnosis and treatment are established and indicators of active inflammation (e.g., transaminase levels, cellular infiltration on liver biopsy) have subsided.[185] Further decompensation of hepatic function may follow anesthesia and surgery, notably after intraabdominal procedures.

Progression of hepatobiliary disease to overt hepatic failure may be evidenced by gross abnormalities of liver function test results, including coagulopathy; extreme jaundice with or without cyanosis; generalized tremors and increased deep tendon reflexes; ascites, spider nevi, and hepatosplenomegaly; hepatorenal failure; and signs of hepatic encephalopathy.[186,187] Elective surgery is avoided at this time because surgery on a patient with hepatic failure is associated with an extremely high incidence of morbidity and mortality. Anesthesia may be required, however, for a patient who requires a palliative or emergent

BOX 20.17 Physiologic Functions of the Hepatobiliary System

Bilirubin Formation and Excretion
- Conjugation of free bilirubin and secretion into bile

Carbohydrate Metabolism
- Glycogenesis
- Gluconeogenesis
- Glycogenolysis

Fat Metabolism
- Lipogenesis
- Lipolysis

Protein Metabolism
- Formation of proteins, such as albumin, prothrombin, transferrin, and glycoprotein
- Synthesis of plasma cholinesterase
- Deamination of proteins, such as hormones, into ammonia and urea

Hormone Metabolism Drug Detoxification
- Conversion of lipophilic drugs into inactive hydrophilic substances
- Hydrolysis of ester linkages by plasma cholinesterase

Vitamin Storage
- Storage of fat-soluble vitamins A, D, E, and K
- Storage of antipernicious anemia factor, vitamin B_{12}

Synthesis of Coagulation Factors and Inhibitors
- Synthesis of most clotting factors, including prothrombin, fibrinogen, factors V, VII, IX, and X
- Synthesis of antithrombin
- Mast-cell production of heparin

Phagocytosis
- Filtration and destruction of bacteria and debris in blood circulating through hepatic sinusoids by Kupffer cells

procedure. Placement of a portocaval shunt and the surgical control of hemorrhage from esophageal varices are common procedures, given the growing number of patients with advanced liver disease. Anesthetic management is supportive in such situations and is focused on minimizing the risk of further hepatobiliary deterioration. Administration of phytonadione (AquaMEPHYTON) and transfusion of fresh frozen plasma and cryoprecipitate may be required for the correction of preoperative coagulopathy. Sedative premedicants are avoided in the disoriented or somnolent patient in whom hepatic encephalopathy has been diagnosed. Because of the rapid development of hypoglycemia, the patient's blood glucose level is checked preoperatively. The acid-base balance, electrolyte status, and extent of hepatorenal reserve may be determined by arterial blood gas analysis, serum multiphasic profiles, and liver function tests.[187]

The interpretation of liver function tests should be approached cautiously. Differential diagnosis of parenchymal versus cholestatic liver disease is limited by the insensitivity and nonspecificity of current laboratory analysis, especially serum transaminase and alkaline phosphatase levels.[188] Aspartate transaminase (AST), or serum glutamic oxaloacetate transaminase (SGOT); alanine transaminase (ALT), or serum glutamic pyruvic transaminase (SGPT); and lactate dehydrogenase (LDH) are commonly measured hepatocellular enzymes also distributed throughout cells of the lungs, heart, kidneys, and skeletal muscles. Increases in their serum concentrations are therefore not always indicative of hepatobiliary disease. Greater specificity can be derived from isoenzyme-5 fractions of the enzymes such as LDH.[189]

In cases of biliary obstruction or irritation, alkaline phosphatase enzymes may be released from the cells of bile ducts. Increases in serum concentrations of these enzymes also help differentiate hepatic dysfunction caused by parenchymal disease from that caused by cholestasis. The interpretation of these results is again limited by the presence of extrahepatic stores of alkaline phosphatase. In this situation cholestatic liver disease can be confirmed by high serum levels of conjugated (direct) bilirubin.[199] Causative factors are then determined from discussions with a gastroenterologist and the results of ultrasound, CT, and endoscopic retrograde cholangiopancreatographic scans.

When acute parenchymal injury is evident, prolongation of prothrombin time offers the most rapid and reliable hallmark of liver dysfunction and is shown to have prognostic significance. It reflects the inability of the acutely damaged liver to synthesize clotting factors. Although the production of albumin is also affected, its plasma half-life exceeds that of prothrombin. Hypoalbuminemia may then be inapparent for days after an acute hepatocellular insult.[191]

Once a functional impairment of the liver has been established, the cause is investigated as part of the preoperative evaluation. Cirrhosis and hepatitis, for example, are frequently associated with long-standing alcohol abuse. The increasing consumption of alcohol in the United States parallels the rising incidence of liver disease. Exposure to hepatotoxic agents in the workplace, such as carbon tetrachloride or vinyl chloride, should be ruled out. Hepatotoxic drugs may then be discontinued or avoided before surgery. These drugs commonly include acetaminophen and other NSAIDs, aspirin, methyldopa, isoniazid, and rifampin.[192,193] Finally a diagnosis of infectious hepatitis should be pursued in patients with hepatobiliary disease of unknown cause and in patients considered to be at high risk, which includes those with a history of hemodialysis, multiple blood transfusions, or intravenous drug abuse. Because of the virulent nature of the hepatitis viruses, care of an infected patient also poses an occupational hazard for anesthesia providers.[194] Maximum precautions must be consistently exercised, and vaccination with the hepatitis B virus, as recommended by the CDC, should be performed.[195]

The Child-Pugh score was developed to predict surgical mortality in patients with cirrhosis. It assigns points for five variables: total bilirubin level, serum albumin level, international normalized ratio (INR), ascites, and hepatic encephalopathy. Patients are categorized into Child-Pugh class A, B, or C. The predicted perioperative mortality for intraabdominal surgery in these patient groups is class A (10%), class B (30%), and class C (80%). Patients in Child-Pugh classes A and B are suitable candidates for surgery with preoperative optimization. Patients in Child-Pugh class C are usually treated medically. Surgery, if necessary, is delayed until liver function improves.[190] A further discussion of anesthesia and liver disease can be found in Chapter 33.

Renal System

Evaluation of the kidneys and urinary tract includes preoperative determination of the patient's volume status and presence of polyuria; urinary incontinence or retention; microscopic or frank hematuria; recurrent infections in the form of glomerulonephritis, pyelonephritis, or cystitis; dysuria; and oliguria or anuria. Fluid balance is calculated from the patient's intake and output during the hospital stay. For example, preoperative dehydration may be evident with symptoms such as dry mucous membranes, postural hypotension, increased capillary refill time, and tachycardia in a patient receiving long-term diuretic therapy. Polyuria, when not attributed to diuretics, may reflect glycosuria or, rarely, inadequate secretion of antidiuretic hormone (diabetes insipidus). Urinary retention and other signs of neurogenic bladder may be caused by a spinal cord injury or long-standing diabetes mellitus. Frequent catheterizations are often necessary in such situations, increasing the patient's risk for developing chronic urinary tract infections. Preoperative urinalysis and culture are therefore required so that infection can be ruled out. Treatment and resolution should be accomplished before elective surgery is performed, especially for procedures involving the placement of a prosthetic graft for a mitral valve or total hip replacement. Problems with intraoperative bladder catheterization can be anticipated in patients with dysuria or voiding difficulties. In older men these problems are frequently attributed to chronic prostatism. Untreated prostatic hypertrophy, in addition to renal calculi and congenital malformations of the ureters, results in obstructed urinary outflow. Over time these conditions may lead to a state of chronic renal insufficiency or failure.

Any suspicion of renal dysfunction should be investigated before surgery. Unfortunately, clinical evidence of renal insufficiency may not be apparent until at least 70% of nephrons are nonfunctional. Accurate diagnosis of renal insufficiency is further limited by the insensitivity of laboratory tests (see Table 20.14).[196] Acute kidney injury where there is rapid deterioration in kidney function is defined by elevated creatinine of greater than 26.4 μmol/L within 48 hours; elevated serum creatinine of greater than 1.5 times baseline, which is known or presumed to have occurred within the previous 7 days; and urine output less than 0.5 mL/kg for 6 hours.[197] Blood urea nitrogen (BUN) concentrations, for example, do not accurately reflect glomerular filtration rate (GFR). Although urea is freely filtered at the glomerulus, it is reabsorbed to a large and variable extent through the tubules. BUN levels are also affected by the amount of protein ingested in the gastrointestinal tract and the amount of urea metabolized by the liver, as well as by the catabolic state of the patient. Because tubular reabsorption of creatinine does not occur, creatinine levels correlate more with the GFR than do BUN concentrations. The serum levels of creatinine, a byproduct of skeletal muscle metabolism,

can reflect the muscle mass and catabolic state of each patient. This characteristic limits its precision in determining the magnitude of nephron loss. Normal serum creatinine levels may be higher in a muscular man than in a woman. Conversely, serum creatinine levels can remain within the normal range in the elderly patient despite a progressive decline in glomerular function[198] because of the decrease in muscle mass associated with aging.

The most commonly used endogenous marker of renal reserve or GFR is creatinine clearance, which reflects the ability of glomeruli to excrete creatinine into the urine at a given blood concentration.[199] The drawbacks of this assessment lie in the cost and time required for the collection of urine samples. As a general principle, urine is collected over a 24-hour period, and the creatinine clearance rate is measured by the following equation:

$$GFR (mL/min) = UV \div P$$

Where U is the urinary concentration of creatinine (mg/dL), V is the volume of urine (mL/min), and P is the plasma concentration of creatinine (mg/dL).

Accurate measures of GFR also can be calculated from a 2-hour specimen.[200] Creatinine clearance or GFR values between 50 and 80 mL/min are indicative of mild renal dysfunction. Renal failure is otherwise evident when creatinine clearance levels decrease to less than 10 mL/min.

TABLE 20.14 Common Renal Function Tests	
Test	**Reference Range**
Urea nitrogen	5–25 mg/dL
Creatinine	0.5–1.5 mg/dL
Sodium	133–147 mmol/L
Potassium	3.2–5.2 mmol/L
Chloride	94–110 mmol/L
CO_2	22–32 mmol/L
Uric acid	2.5–7.5 mg/dL
Calcium	8.5–10.5 mg/dL
Phosphorus	2.2–4.2 mg/dL
Urinalysis, Routine	
Color	Straw-amber
Appearance	Clear-hazy
Protein	0 mg/dL
Blood	Negative
Glucose	0 mg/dL
Ketone	0 mg/dL
pH	4.5–8
Specific gravity	1.002–1.030
Bilirubin	Negative
Urinalysis, Micro	
Red blood cells	0–3/high-power field
White blood cells	0–5/high-power field
Casts	0–2/low-power field

Modified from Yu ASL, et al., eds. *Brenner and Rector's The Kidney.* 11th ed. Philadelphia: Elsevier; 2020.

Many surgical patients with chronic renal failure are undergoing dialysis, usually hemodialysis performed at the hospital or renal facility. Others undergo continuous ambulatory peritoneal dialysis. The goal of dialysis therapy is to maintain a reasonable degree of homeostasis, although BUN and creatinine concentrations remain abnormal. The preoperative evaluation and preparation of the patient with chronic renal failure should therefore focus on fluid and electrolyte balance, and on the extent of concomitant diseases.[201] Estimates of volume status are derived from the amount of weight gained between periods of dialysis. Fluid overload may also be evidenced by jugular vein distention, peripheral and periorbital edema, and bibasilar rales.

Preoperative measurement of serum potassium concentration is recommended within 6 to 8 hours of surgery regardless of whether dialysis is performed, because unexpected hyperkalemia with its adverse cardiac effects is known to occur rapidly. In cases in which the serum potassium level exceeds 5.5 mEq/L and congestive heart failure is apparent, elective surgery should be delayed until after dialysis. When postponement is not feasible, as with emergency surgery to relieve a pericardial effusion or procedures to revise a hemodialysis shunt, measures to reduce the serum potassium concentration are then instituted.

Although hemoglobin ranges from 5 to 8 mg/dL are not unusual in patients with chronic renal failure, a hemoglobin level should also be obtained as part of the preoperative evaluation. Chronic anemia is predominantly caused by decreases in renal erythropoietin production and enhanced fragility of red blood cells in the presence of uremia. It is further exacerbated by blood loss experienced with hemodialysis and chronic gastrointestinal bleeding. When extreme fatigue and pallor, limited exercise tolerance, and persistent tachycardia are evident before major surgery, the transfusion of packed red blood cells may be necessary. Because repeat transfusion and immunosuppression therapy are often required during the course of chronic renal failure, the patient is at greater risk for being infected with the hepatitis virus, human immunodeficiency virus (HIV), or both. Coagulopathies are also suspected. The most likely cause is a decrease in platelet adhesiveness secondary to the chronic state of metabolic acidemia. Hemodialysis can be effectively used for the correction of prolonged bleeding times before surgery in this situation.

Throughout the perioperative period most therapeutic regimens for patients with chronic renal failure can be continued, including the administration of antihypertensives, digitalis preparations, corticosteroids, and insulin.[202] Requirements for preoperative sedation may be less than anticipated, and medications with prolonged durations such as diazepam are avoided.[203] Peripheral arteriovenous shunts should be assessed for patency and infection. Measurement of noninvasive blood pressures and application of intravenous lines are avoided in the limb of the graft. Administration of gastrointestinal preparations (e.g., antacids and gastrokinetic agents) and drainage of peritoneal dialysate aimed at reducing the risks of regurgitation and pulmonary aspiration are instituted when preparing the patient with chronic renal failure for anesthesia and surgery.

Endocrine System

Endocrine diseases of concern in the preoperative evaluation include diabetes mellitus, thyroid gland disorders, and adrenocortical dysfunctions. End-organ effects of each of these diseases increase perioperative risk substantially. For example, morbidity and mortality rates are 5 to 10 times greater in diabetic patients with renal and autonomic nervous system involvement.[204]

Diabetes

Diabetes mellitus is the most common endocrine disorder, affecting more than 34 million people in the United States, with 1 in 4 people

TABLE 20.15 Distinguishing Features of Diabetes Mellitus

	Type 1	Type 2
Previous name	Insulin-dependent diabetes	Noninsulin-dependent diabetes
Age of onset	Childhood	Middle age or elderly
Timing of onset	Abrupt	Gradual
Predisposing factors	Genetic	Obesity, pregnancy, drugs
Prevalence	0.2%–0.3%	2%–4%
Insulin requirement	Always	Infrequent
Ketoacidosis	Common	Rare
Systemic complications	Frequent	Frequent

Modified from Crandell J, Shamoon H. Diabetes mellitus. In Goldman L, Schafer AI, eds. *Goldman's Cecil Medicine*. 26th ed. Philadelphia: Elsevier; 2020:1527–1547.

unaware that they have it. Over 88 million people have prediabetes, where blood sugar levels are higher than normal but not high enough for a diabetes diagnosis.[205] It represents a dysfunction in glucose metabolism caused by impaired synthesis, secretion, or use of insulin.

Most patients with diabetes (90%–95%) are not dependent on exogenous insulin for the regulation of blood glucose levels. As shown in Table 20.15, the patient with noninsulin-dependent (also known as adult onset or type 2) diabetes often benefits from diet modification, weight control, and exercise alone. An oral or injectable hypoglycemic agent (Table 20.16) may also be added to the patient's therapeutic regimen.[206] The remaining 5% to 10% of patients with diabetes are dependent on insulin preparations listed in Table 20.17 and are therefore classified as having insulin-dependent, or type 1, diabetes mellitus.[207,208] These patients are susceptible to periods of hyperglycemia and ketoacidosis. As a result of microvascular changes, they are also prone to the development of severe end-organ complications, including diabetic retinopathy and cataract formation, somatic and autonomic insufficiency (orthostatic hypotension, bradycardia, gastroparesis), and nephropathy. Because of acquired abnormalities in the macrovasculature, patients with type 2 diabetes are more likely to have hypertension, coronary artery disease (which frequently is asymptomatic), and peripheral vascular disease. Death in the majority of patients with diabetes is secondary to complications of atherosclerosis (e.g., MI, stroke).[209]

Proper perioperative glucose management reduces postoperative morbidity and mortality; therefore, an evaluation of a patient with diabetes, notably one with type 1 diabetes mellitus, is ascertaining the degree of preoperative blood glucose control and the presence of major organ system dysfunction. Renal and cardiovascular complications of diabetes substantially heighten perioperative risk. Particular attention should be paid to the following:

- Diabetes—type of disease, method of home monitoring, and usual metabolic control
- Drugs—antidiabetic medication, medication for associated diseases
- Cardiovascular disease—including an assessment of exercise tolerance
- Renal disease—electrolyte assessment, hemodialysis regime if applicable
- Neuropathy—peripheral and autonomic, in particular gastric paresis
- Airway—diabetics with stiff joint syndrome (due to glycosylation) often have limited mobility of the upper cervical spine. Thus, they

TABLE 20.16 Oral and Noninsulin Injectable Hypoglycemic Therapy

Class	Mechanism of Action	Generic Name	Trade Name	Route of Administration	Frequency of Administration
α-glucosidase inhibitors	• Delay carbohydrate absorption from intestine	Acarbose Miglitol	Precose Glyset	Oral Oral	tid tid
Amylin analogue	• Decrease glucagon secretion • Slow gastric emptying • Increase satiety	Pramlintide	Symlin	Injection	Prior to every meal
Biguanide	• Decrease HGP • Increase glucose uptake in muscle	Metformin	Glucophage	Oral	daily or bid
Bile acid sequestrant	• Decrease HGP • Increase in creatinine levels	Colesevelam	Welchol	Oral	daily or bid
DPP-4 Inhibitors	• Increase glucose-dependent insulin secretion • Decrease glucagon secretion	Alogliptin Linagliptin Saxagliptin Sitagliptin	Nesina Tradjenta Onglyza Januvia	Oral Oral Oral Oral	daily daily daily daily
Dopamine-2 agonist	• Activates dopaminergic receptors	Bromocriptine	Cycloset	Oral	daily
Glinides	• Increase insulin secretion	Nateglinide Repaglinide	Starlix Prandin	Oral Oral	tid with meals tid with meals
GLP-1 receptor agonists	• Increase glucose-dependent insulin secretion • Decrease glucagon secretion • Slow gastric emptying • Increase satiety	Albiglutide Dulaglutide Exenatide Exenatide XR Liraglutide Semaglutide	Tanzeum Trulicity Byetta Bydureon Victoza Ozempic	Injection Injection Injection Injection Injection Injection, Subcut, oral	Once weekly Once weekly bid Once weekly daily Once weekly, once weekly, daily
SGLT2 Inhibitors	• Increase urinary excretion of glucose	Canagliflozin Dapagliflozin Empagliflozin	Invokana Farxiga Jardiance	Oral Oral Oral	daily daily daily
Sulfonylureas	• Increase insulin secretion	Glimepiride Glipizide Glyburide	Amaryl Glucotrol Diabeta Glynase Micronase	Oral Oral Oral Oral Oral	daily AM daily AM daily AM daily AM daily AM
Thiazolidinediones	• Increase glucose uptake in muscle and fat • Decrease HGP	Pioglitazone Rosiglitazone	Actos Avandia	Oral Oral	daily daily

TID, three times daily; *HGP,* hepatic glucose production; *daily,* once daily; bid, twice daily; *DPP-4,* dipeptidyl peptidase 4; *GLP-1,* glucagon-like peptide 1; *Subcut,* subcutaneous; *SGLT2,* sodium glucose co-transporter 2; From Cavaiola TS, Pettus JH. Management of type 2 diabetes: selecting amongst available pharmacological agents. In: Feingold KR, Anawalt B, Boyce A, et al., eds. *Endotext.* South Dartmouth, MA: Endotext. org; 2000. https://www.ncbi.nlm.nih.gov/books/NBK425702/; Drugs for type 2 diabetes. *Med Lett Drugs Ther.* 2019;61(1584):169–178.

may be more likely to have a poor view on direct laryngoscopy and have difficulties with tracheal intubation.[210] Patients with a long-standing history of diabetes require a close look at the airway to assess for potential difficulties.[4]

Both early preoperative evaluation and workup of diabetic patients are important. This is especially true in patients who are noncompliant, whose blood glucose level is poorly controlled, and with newly diagnosed diabetes because modifications in their care may be necessary before surgery. Early assessment allows for consultation with a medical internist to optimize the patient's preoperative condition before anesthesia and surgery. An internist can begin monitoring of hemoglobin A_{1C} (HbA_{1C}) values and determine what interventions, if any, are indicated. Efforts to reduce the HbA_{1C} to as close to normal as possible are desirable. Levels less than 5.7% are normal, 5.7% to 6.4% are high risk, and 6.5% or more are diabetic. These values can give a good indication of glycemic control perioperatively and

should be considered in the perioperative period regarding glucose management.[211]

Patients with preoperative hyperglycemia (≥216 mg/dL), who do not have an official diagnosis of diabetes and thus are untreated, may be at risk of higher mortality at 1-year postsurgery.[212]

For this reason, elective surgery is postponed in cases of extreme hyperglycemia and ketoacidosis until such time that corrective measures may be instituted.

Consultation with a cardiologist may also help a practitioner evaluate and improve the preoperative cardiac status of a patient with diabetes, especially if the patient is undergoing a procedure associated with a greater risk of perioperative myocardial ischemia, such as a carotid endarterectomy or an abdominal aortic aneurysm resection. Because of the high incidence of ischemic heart disease in this population, exercise stress testing and a 12-lead ECG may be performed. Orthostatic hypotension, resting tachycardia, and lack of respiratory variability in

TABLE 20.17	Insulin Preparations and Guidelines			
Insulin Type	**Onset**	**Peak (hr)**	**Duration (hr)**	**Comments**
Very Rapid				
Lispro; Aspart	IV immediate; Subcut 5–15 min	Subcut 0.5–1.5	Subcut 3–4	Usually administered immediately prior to a meal; use Subcut or via an insulin pump, but not recommended for continuous infusion
Short Acting				
Regular	IV immediate; Subcut 30–60 min	Subcut 2–3	Subcut 3–6	Usually administered 30–60 min before meals; most common in continuous IV infusions
Intermediate Acting				
NPH	Subcut 2–4 hr	Subcut 6–10	Subcut 10–16	Often combined with regular insulin
Lente	Subcut 3–4 hr	Subcut 6–12	Subcut 12–18	
Long Acting				
Ultralente	Subcut 6–10 hr	Subcut 10–16	Subcut 18–20	Perioperative use uncommon
Glargine	Subcut 4 hr	Minimal peak activity	Subcut 24	May be administered as usual to provide basal insulin levels during surgery
Combinations				
75/25 (75% protamine lispro, 25% insulin lispro)	Subcut 30–60 min	Dual	10–14	
70/30 (70% NPH, 30% regular)	Subcut 30–60 min	Dual	10–16	Usually given before breakfast
50/50 (50% NPH, 50% regular)	Subcut 30–60 min	Dual	10–16	Usually given before dinner

IV, Intravenous; *NPH*, neutral protamine Hagedorn; *Subcut,* subcutaneous.

cardiac rhythm may reflect autonomic neuropathy (present in 20%–40% of diabetic patients). Abnormalities in autonomic function may also result in bladder atrophy and delayed gastric emptying times in nearly 50% of diabetic patients.[213] Administration of a gastrokinetic agent such as metoclopramide should be considered before surgery to reduce the incidence of regurgitation and pulmonary aspiration during general anesthesia.

It is best to schedule surgery as early in the day as possible to minimize the fasting period. Just before surgery, diabetic patients who require insulin or oral hypoglycemic agents should have blood glucose checked. Depending on the type and length of surgery and the lability of diabetes, blood glucose levels are checked intraoperatively and in the postanesthesia care unit at 1- to 4-hour intervals. There continues to be discussion as to optimal levels; however, a safe goal of perioperative insulin therapy is to maintain the serum glucose level at less than 180 mg/dL, while avoiding hypoglycemia.[214] Several different regimens are available for the treatment of diabetic patients undergoing surgery and anesthesia. Consultation with the physician responsible for managing the diabetes is helpful in determining an acceptable range of serum glucose and when and what type of insulin therapy may be appropriate. Considerations for managing the diabetic patient are as follows:

Mild hyperglycemia is preferable to hypoglycemia.

- For patients with either insulin-dependent or noninsulin-dependent diabetes, the most important goal of perioperative management is the prevention of hyperglycemia and especially hypoglycemia, in addition to their adverse consequences, during surgical stress.

Night before the procedure:

- Continue usual dose of PM (afternoon/evening) glargine/NPH (neutral protamine Hagedorn) or mixture (can recommend

two-thirds usual dose if tightly controlled) as long as the patient is allowed a usual diet.

Morning of procedure:

- Patients undergoing short, simple procedures early in the morning where preoperative fasting is required can be managed by delaying the patient's normal diabetes treatments until the patient is ingesting food in the early postoperative period. It should be noted that procedures requiring a patient with diabetes to fast are customarily scheduled early in the morning to minimize disruption of routine diabetic treatments.
- Patients taking oral hypoglycemic agents should withhold the short half-life agents (e.g., repaglinide) on the day of surgery and withhold the longer-lasting agents (e.g., chlorpropamide and glimepiride) for up to 48 hours.
- Fasting patients who are receiving insulin should have intravenous access established. A crystalloid solution containing 5% glucose should be available to infuse for maintenance of optimal blood glucose levels. The intravenous route still has the risk of making the patient hyperglycemic or hypoglycemic if the glucose or insulin infusions become unbalanced. The tighter the control of glucose levels, the more frequent the glucose monitoring. The subcutaneous route of insulin administration has been criticized as being too unpredictable in its absorption, especially perioperatively, with alterations in blood pressure and cutaneous blood flow.[215]
- Patients should not take a short-acting insulin bolus the morning of the procedure unless the blood glucose level is greater than 200 mg/dL, and more than 3 hours preoperatively.
- In the patient with type 1 diabetes a common approach, especially for brief procedures, is to subcutaneously administer a

TABLE 20.18   Perioperative Management of the Patient With an Insulin Pump

Preoperative preparation: topics to discuss with patient	Choice to continue the pump during surgery
	Ensure adequate supply of pump consumables for entire surgical stay
	Resite the infusion set the day before surgery and monitor blood glucose
	Position of infusion site away from operative field and cautery and accessible to anesthetist
	Overnight basal assessment prior to surgery
	Consultation with the management team and patient to confirm self-management competency
Perioperative management	Assess glucose hourly
	If glucose is not controlled switch to an intravenous infusion
	Disconnect the pump in emergency surgery and switch to intravenous insulin
	Do not use in radiology procedures
Postoperative management	Check capillary glucose hourly until patient is able to self-manage
	Increase frequency of testing for 48 hr postoperatively

Adapted from Partridge H, et al. Clinical recommendations in the management of the patient with type 1 diabetes on insulin pump therapy in the perioperative period: a primer for the anaesthetist. *Br. J Anaesth.* 2016;116(1):18–26.

fraction (50% of usual dose) of the patient's usual morning dose of intermediate- or long-acting insulin and institute continuous 5% glucose infusion.

Insulin pumps.[216]

- Determine the type of insulin in the pump, basal pump rate, and the insulin sensitivity factor (an estimate of magnitude of reduction in the blood glucose level when 1 unit of the pump insulin is administered). Table 20.18 outlines the suggested perioperative management of the patient with an insulin pump.
- Prior to any sedation ascertain whether the patient is able to recognize symptoms of hypoglycemia, and whether the patient plans to properly manage the pump.
- Examine the pump for signs of irritation or leakage.
- Considerations regarding the type of procedure include:
  - Positioning requirements (i.e., prone). For this position in particular, the pump should be padded or relocated depending on the duration of surgery and encroachment by position.
  - Discontinuation of the pump may need to be considered for lengthy noncardiac surgery, and in procedures involving x-ray, MRI, or defibrillation exposure regardless of duration or procedure.

Thyroid Gland Disorders

Although disorders of the thyroid gland are relatively uncommon, the anesthesia provider may still encounter patients with hyperthyroidism or hypothyroidism who require surgery. Most have undergone adequate medical therapy before anesthesia and surgery are performed. Nevertheless, the anesthesia provider should be aware of the clinical manifestations of thyroid gland dysfunctions (Table 20.19).[217,218]

Hyperthyroidism. Hyperthyroidism is caused by an excess secretion of thyroid hormones 3,5,3′-triiodothyronine (T_3) and tetraiodothyronine (thyroxine or T_4). It is evident in such conditions as Graves disease, toxic goiter (multinodular, single), thyroid carcinoma, and pituitary tumors that oversecrete thyroid-stimulating hormone (TSH). Signs and symptoms reflect a hypermetabolic state with sympathetic overactivity (e.g., tachycardia, atrial fibrillation, fever, tremor) resulting from the primary effects of thyroid hormones on the adenylate cyclase system.[219]

The preoperative preparation of the hyperthyroid patient is aimed at attaining a euthyroid state. This may be accomplished through administration of antithyroid drugs such as methimazole or propylthiouracil for 6 to 8 weeks, followed by iodine for 7 to 14 days. Not only does propylthiouracil decrease the overall synthesis of thyroxine, but it also lessens its conversion into the more potent T_3. Reversible agranulocytosis is infrequently seen with long-term therapy. A complete blood cell and platelet count should be determined preoperatively. β-antagonist drugs such as propranolol and atenolol daily are also useful adjuncts in the management of hyperthyroidism. The goal of oral beta blocker therapy should be to maintain a heart rate of less than 80.[217] These drugs ameliorate signs of sympathetic nervous system overstimulation such as tachycardia, diaphoresis, and tremors.

All drugs used to manage hyperthyroidism, including propylthiouracil and propranolol, should be continued perioperatively, including the morning of surgery, and elective surgery is postponed until the patient is rendered euthyroid. If emergency surgery cannot be delayed for a patient with symptomatic hyperthyroidism, a continuous infusion of esmolol (100–300 μg/kg/min) may be initiated to control unwanted tachycardia (goal heart rate <90 beats/min).[220] Higher doses of preoperative anxiolytics and sedatives such as benzodiazepines may also be required. Anticholinergics are avoided because of their interference with normal heat-regulating mechanisms and their potentiation of tachyarrhythmias.

Hypothyroidism. Hypothyroidism represents several conditions, such as chronic thyroiditis or Hashimoto disease, in which tissues are exposed to decreased circulating concentrations of T_3 and T_4. The cause of hypothyroidism may be primary, resulting from the destruction or hypofunction of the thyroid gland, or secondary, resulting from insufficient TSH production. The diagnosis of hypothyroidism is confirmed by decreased serum concentrations of T_3 and T_4, with or without secondary increases in TSH levels.[220,221]

The treatment of hypothyroidism consists of administration of T_4, levothyroxine sodium (Synthroid) replacement therapy, with the restoration of intravascular volume and electrolyte status. Elective surgery need not be delayed for patients with mild to moderate hypothyroidism. No difference in perioperative outcome has been noted between untreated hypothyroid patients and patients who are euthyroid.[222]

Adrenocortical disorders. Disorders of the adrenal cortex, ranging from hyperadrenocorticism to hypoadrenocorticism, are the result of primary disease of the adrenal cortex or pituitary gland, ectopic production of adrenocortical hormones by malignant tissue, or most commonly treatment with exogenous corticosteroids. Steroids are commonly used to treat bronchial asthma, autoimmune diseases, and connective tissue disorders such as rheumatoid arthritis. Their high-dose administration for prolonged periods or their excess levels in circulating glucocorticoid hormones characteristically result in Cushing syndrome. This syndrome is clinically manifested as hypertension and hypovolemia, truncal obesity with an accumulation of interscapular fat ("buffalo hump"), abdominal and gluteal striae, plethoric facial appearance (moon facies), easy bruising, osteoporosis, personality changes, menstrual irregularities, and hirsutism. Hyperaldosteronism—an excess of mineralocorticoid hormones—may be manifested as hypertension in association with marked hypokalemia (plasma

TABLE 20.19 Clinical Features of Thyroid Gland Disorders

	Hyperthyroidism	Hypothyroidism
General	Heat intolerance; weight loss; tremor; excessive sweating; warm, moist skin	Cold intolerance, thinning or coarsened hair, alopecia, arthralgia, "strawberries and cream" complexion, dry skin, gruff voice
Metabolic	Pyrexia, hyperglycemia, hypercalcemia	Hypothermia, hypoglycemia, hyponatremia
Cardiovascular	Sinus tachycardia, premature ventricular contractions, wide pulse pressure, elevated systolic blood pressure, decreased diastolic blood pressure, peripheral edema, increased left ventricular contractility, cardiac output and ejection fraction, atrial fibrillation, ischemic heart disease, congestive heart failure	Bradycardia, heart block, QT prolongation, reduced contractility, diastolic hypertension, cardiomegaly, ischemic heart disease, congestive heart failure, increased peripheral resistance, pericardial effusions
Respiratory	Dyspnea, increased minute volume, respiratory muscle weakness, reduced vital capacity, reduced compliance	Hypoventilation, attenuated response to hypoxia/hypercapnia, reduced diffusion capacity, myxedematous infiltration of respiratory muscles, sleep apnea
Gastrointestinal and liver	Diarrhea, nausea, vomiting, abdominal pain, elevated liver function tests	Decreased gastrointestinal motility, constipation
Neurologic	Anxiety, irritability, hyperactive reflexes, tremor, insomnia; depression, psychosis, withdrawal, and apathy in elderly	Fatigue, lethargy, slow mental function, hypoactive reflexes, depression, psychosis, myxedema coma
Musculoskeletal	Goiter, weight loss, proximal myopathy, bone resorption	Goiter, lethargy, large tongue, amyloidosis, peripheral neuropathy, muscle stiffness
Ophthalmic	Exophthalmos, lid lag, upper lid retraction, reduced blinking, corneal ulceration	Periorbital edema
Renal		Impaired free water clearance
Hematologic	Thrombocytopenia, neutropenia, mild anemia	Anemia, reduced plasma volume, coagulopathy
Neuromuscular	Peripheral myopathy, generalized muscle weakness, familial periodic paralysis, myasthenia gravis	
Goiter	Airway compromise, stridor, positional dyspnea, dysphagia, altered voice	Airway compromise, stridor, positional dyspnea, dysphagia, altered voice

potassium [K] <3 mmol/L). Its major alterations involve sodium and water retention, potassium depletion, and metabolic alkalosis.

Adrenocortical insufficiency may be of a primary origin (Addison disease) or caused by the secondary inhibition of adrenocortical function by prolonged exogenous steroid therapy. Clinical signs are less obvious than those of Cushing disease and include skin hyperpigmentation, weight loss, muscle wasting, hypotension, intravascular volume depletion, hypoglycemia, hyponatremia, and hyperkalemia.[223]

The preoperative preparation of a patient with adrenocortical dysfunction includes the correction of fluid and electrolyte disturbances and the treatment of coexisting disorders such as hypertension and diabetes mellitus. Glucocorticoid or mineralocorticoid replacement therapy is also continued perioperatively. Patients are at risk for depression of the hypothalamic-pituitary-adrenal (HPA) axis if they have (1) received 20 mg or more of prednisone, or equivalent, for 5 or more days, or (2) been treated for 1 month or more. HPA axis suppression may persist for 6 to 12 months after discontinuation of treatment.[224] A reliable test to assess adrenocortical function, the short adrenocorticotropic hormone (ACTH) stimulation test, may be performed to evaluate the need for a supplemental steroid.[225] If the patient presenting for surgery is at risk for HPA axis depression, or if findings (i.e., hyponatremia, hyperkalemia, hypotension, eosinophilia) are consistent with adrenal insufficiency, then need for exogenous corticosteroid supplementation should be assessed (see Table 20.5). For patients currently receiving high-dose steroid therapy, such as those with chronic hypoadrenocorticism or Addison disease, further supplementation of the daily maintenance doses may be required based on the surgical stress. This recommendation, although controversial regarding the need for additional supplementation,[226,227] is based on

concerns that additional cortisol may not be released from the adrenal cortex as a result of its primary hypofunction or secondary suppression in response to surgical stress. Unexplained hypotension in spite of intravenous fluid repletion or cardiovascular collapse may then ensue during major surgical procedures.

DIAGNOSTIC TESTING

Appropriate laboratory evaluations and diagnostic procedures should be obtained and the results considered to determine the patient's surgical and anesthetic risk, in addition to the need for appropriate health care modifications. The controversy lies in which tests are necessary and appropriate for specific settings. The rationale for performing "routine" tests has been under intense scrutiny, primarily because of recent and ongoing changes in health care economics. A protocol that delineates the indications for testing should be established by each surgical facility and approved by the medical staff. When protocols are followed for ordering preoperative laboratory tests, the total number of tests performed has been reduced 50% to 60%, and the appropriateness of the tests has improved.[229] A necessary step in the implementation process for preoperative testing guidelines is the education of the medical staff. Centralizing the test-ordering process such as in the preoperative assessment clinic makes standardization and compliance more attainable.

Routine Diagnostic Testing

It has been traditional practice, even within the past decade, to order a battery of routine evaluative tests before a patient undergoes surgery and anesthesia. Routine ordering of preoperative diagnostic tests remains a common practice in many institutions. Until the early 1990s, the rationale for obtaining preoperative diagnostic tests was rarely questioned. Tests were frequently ordered for a variety of reasons but were often unrelated to findings based specifically on the patient's history and physical examination. Reasons cited for ordering the standard battery of preoperative tests include the following:[230-232]

- To follow customary practice at an institution
- To adhere to institutional or legislative mandates that dictate the tests be performed
- To further evaluate and determine the progress of a known disease or condition because preexisting medical conditions have a greater risk for intraoperative and postoperative complications
- To detect asymptomatic yet modifiable conditions that could alter anesthetic and surgical care
- To detect asymptomatic but unmodifiable conditions that could alter anesthetic and surgical risk
- To screen for conditions unrelated to the planned surgery
- To acquire baseline results that might be useful in the perioperative period
- To protect against medicolegal involvement

When considering the value of preoperative tests, the following must be considered:

1. The diagnostic procedure should be cost effective—that is, the costs saved from knowing the results exceed the expense of performing the test.
2. The diagnostic procedure should have a positive benefit-risk ratio—that is, the benefit derived from conducting the test outweighs the harm that might ensue from a false-positive result.
3. Test results are available for interpretation and recuperative intervention before surgery.
4. Test results will yield information that could not be obtained from the history and physical examination.
5. Abnormal test results in an asymptomatic patient would influence the patient care, the surgery, or the anesthesia management.

Without any clinical sign the likelihood of observing a significant anomaly is very small for diagnostic procedures such as ECG,[230] chest radiography,[230-233] or laboratory tests.[230,234] Asymptomatic disease is rarely of clinical concern in perioperative surgical care. In addition, unexpected abnormal findings from preoperative testing tend not to affect the upcoming surgery.[235] When a battery of routine preoperative tests is conducted, abnormal test results potentially alter patient care only 0.22% to 0.56% of the time.[230,234] A consistent conclusion of most studies is that routine preoperative laboratory screening is not cost effective or predictive of postoperative complications,[229,236] and is unnecessary when an extensive history and physical examination do not suggest any patient abnormalities.[1,237-241] However, the tendency remains, on the part of the preoperative physician, to continue ordering the battery of routine tests in spite of professional society recommendations to the contrary.[241]

Limitations to Routine Preoperative Diagnostic Testing

Studies estimate that at least 10% of the more than $30 billion spent on laboratory testing annually in the United States goes to preparing patients for surgery.[242] Although added health care costs are the most apparent limitation to performing the routine battery of preoperative tests, additional factors can negatively affect the patient and care providers. The indiscriminate ordering of tests for diagnostic evaluation increases the likelihood that at least one test will be abnormal in a healthy patient.[230] False-positive, or even false-negative, test results can lead to additional medical evaluation and the potential for increased morbidity. Abnormal laboratory tests for continuous data are defined in probabilistic terms and assume a normal patient

population distribution.[230,231] Approximately 5% of test results in normal patients are reported as abnormal. False-positive test results may lead to additional follow-up tests, which can place the patient at risk of increased morbidity.[243] Abnormal test results that were not further pursued and lack of documentation of the rationale for not investigating abnormal test results have increased the medicolegal risk for physicians.[244]

Timing of Diagnostic Testing

In general, diagnostic testing results are deemed current within 6 months of the scheduled surgery if the test results are normal and if the patient's current health status indicates no change has occurred since the test was performed.[246] However, specific tests require more current data analysis. A serum potassium level should be obtained within 7 days of surgery for patients receiving diuretics or digitalis, and blood glucose level determinations should be obtained on the day of surgery for patients with diabetes controlled by medication. An ECG, when indicated, is considered adequate within 30 days prior to elective surgery for patients with stable disease.[77] Chest radiographs taken within 6 months are generally acceptable if the patient's pulmonary condition is stable.[247]

Indications for Diagnostic Testing

A continuing point of controversy relates to disagreement about which tests are appropriate for specific patients, surgeries, and conditions. Difference of opinion exists among and within medical specialties regarding which tests are appropriate. Suggested guidelines for ordering various diagnostic tests, based on results of the patient's history and physical examination, have been offered for diagnostic procedures (Box 20.18) and laboratory tests (Box 20.19).

Pregnancy Testing

Routine preoperative pregnancy testing in women of childbearing age remains controversial. If a patient is concerned about possible pregnancy, uncertain of her pregnancy status, or if the physical examination or medical history suggests the possibility of pregnancy (e.g., because of information regarding sexually active status, time of last menstrual period, presence or absence of birth control methods), a preoperative pregnancy test should be offered with the patient's consent on the evening prior to or morning of the surgery.[1,248] A serum human chorionic gonadotropin (hCG) measurement performed either the day prior to surgery or on the morning of surgery (realizing the potential for delay while awaiting the hCG result) should be considered for patients less than 1 month past the expected date for their initial missed period.

Currently available urine pregnancy tests may yield false-negative or false-positive results until week 5 of the pregnancy.[249] Depending on the test used, the test may not detect certain variants of hCG or may only have a window of detection for very early pregnancy. In addition, factors such as the hydration status of the patient being tested may skew results.[250]

Issues to address when deciding whether to test include the following:

- Policies of the hospital or health care facility based on medical staff bylaws. The medical facility should have established guidelines, supported on ethical, legal, financial, and scientific relevance, that delineate when testing for pregnancy is appropriate.[251]
- All women should be advised of the potential fetal risk (e.g., premature labor, spontaneous abortion) secondary to the underlying surgical condition and surgical uterine stimulation that is unrelated to anesthesia.[248] The incidence of congenital abnormalities is no greater in pregnant women who undergo surgery than it is in those with a surgery-free pregnancy.[249,250] There is not enough evidence

to support or deny the risk of anesthesia on the parturient in early pregnancy.[251]

Despite this finding, patients are sometimes advised to postpone elective surgery until postpartum or at least well after the first trimester when fetal organogenesis is complete.

- Patients should be privately questioned about the possibility of pregnancy. When adolescent patients present for surgery, consider using female staff for the interview in the absence of family members.
- Patients should be offered pregnancy testing despite history, except in patients with a history of hysterectomy or bilateral salpingo-oophorectomy.[252]

Chest Radiography

A preoperative chest radiograph is of minimal predictive importance and is not cost effective as a screening test for postoperative respiratory problems. Therefore it is not to be recommended without specific indications from the medical history and physical examination, that is, new or unstable cardiopulmonary disease.[1,4,253,254] The risk of performing a routine preoperative chest radiograph in asymptomatic patients less than 75 years of age is greater than the benefit.[244]

Electrocardiography

A routine preoperative ECG is not necessary unless a specific indication is present.[1,240,242] Many medical facilities continue to use an age-specific criterion for acquiring a preoperative ECG, regardless of indications—or lack of indications—based on the patient's medical history and physical examination. The recommended minimum age for routinely conducting a baseline ECG, if deemed necessary by the facility, has gradually increased to 65 years or older and is considered current if tested within 1 year of the procedure, provided no changes in the patient's condition have occurred.[77,255]

The value of obtaining a routine preoperative 12-lead ECG in asymptomatic, low-risk patients who are having cataract surgery[256] has been questioned.[257,258] This rethinking of indications for when to order a preoperative ECG has been challenged for the following reasons:

- It has not been shown to be cost effective.[259,260]
- It is a poor predictor of perioperative complications.[258,260,261]
- It is of limited value in detection of ischemia in asymptomatic individuals.[262,263]
- Abnormal preoperative ECGs rarely lead to alteration in patient care.[264]
- No evidence supports the value of a baseline ECG.[257,258,265]

FASTING CONSIDERATIONS

Part of the anesthesia provider's role in patient preparation involves establishing an appropriate fasting interval for the patient. This requires knowledge of risk factors for pulmonary aspiration of gastric contents weighed against the consequences of prolonged fasting. The risk of perioperative pulmonary aspiration of gastric contents that results in morbidity or mortality is relatively low, so the recommendations for withholding oral feeding before elective surgery have recently become much more liberal. When studies were conducted challenging the traditional fasting times (≥7 hours) for clear liquids, the results appeared to show that a reduced fasting interval does not increase the risk of pulmonary aspiration in normal, healthy individuals.[266] In fact, preoperative ingestion of carbohydrate supplements up to 2 hours before elective colorectal surgery has been shown to result in shorter hospital stay, faster return of bowel function, and less muscle mass loss. Therefore this practice has become part of the Enhanced Recovery After Surgery (ERAS) protocols for many facilities.[267]

> **BOX 20.18 Indications for Diagnostic Procedures**
>
> **Chest Radiograph**
> - Previous abnormal results on chest radiography
> - History of malignancy in which pulmonary metastasis might alter the surgical therapy
> - History of tuberculosis (TB) or a positive skin test result for TB and no history of treatment
> - History suggestive of pulmonary infection (e.g., new or chronic productive cough or blood-tinged or purulent-appearing sputum)
> - Suspected intrathoracic pathologic condition (e.g., tumors, vascular ring)
> - History of congenital heart disease
> - History of prematurity associated with residual bronchopulmonary dysplasia
> - Severe obstructive sleep apnea (patient may have cardiomegaly)
> - Down syndrome (patient may have asymptomatic subluxation of the atlantoaxial junction)
> - Symptomatic or debilitating asthma, chronic obstructive pulmonary disease, or cardiovascular disease
>
> **Electrocardiogram**
> - Patients at risk for cardiovascular disease (e.g., because of cocaine abuse, hypertension, chest pain, renal insufficiency, peripheral vascular disease, thyroid disease, diabetes mellitus [age ≥40 yr], inability to exercise, significant pulmonary disease, smoking [>40 pack-years], history of ischemic heart disease, history of compensated or prior heart failure, history of cerebrovascular disease)
> - History of previously unevaluated pathologic-sounding murmur or palpitation
> - Family history reveals possibility of inherited prolonged QT syndrome
> - Patients with history of morbid obesity, moderate to severe sleep apnea, or chronic anatomic airway obstruction (e.g., Pierre Robin syndrome) may be at risk for right-sided heart strain
>
> Adapted from Zaglaniczny K, Aker J, eds. *Clinical Guide to Pediatric Anesthesia*. Philadelphia: Saunders; 1999; Institute for Clinical Systems Improvement. *Health Care Guidelines: Preoperative Evaluation*. 9th ed. ICSI; June 2010. http://www.icsi.org/preoperative_evaluation/preoperative_evaluation_2328.html.

The traditional policy of fasting after midnight fails to address three variables that influence gastric emptying for surgery: (1) time of the scheduled surgery, (2) time at which the patient retired for the night, and (3) variability in gastric emptying for solids and fluids among individuals. Prolonged fasting, especially in children, can be highly distressing in addition to causing physiologic alterations. Periods of long preoperative fasting have been shown to contribute to the following:

- Dehydration[267]
- Hypoglycemia (in smaller children)[268]
- Hypovolemia
- Increased irritability[268]
- Enhanced preoperative anxiety[269]
- Reduced compliance with preoperative fasting orders[267]
- Thirst and related discomforts (e.g., hunger, headache, unhappiness)[270]

Pulmonary Aspiration Risk

Recent ingestion of food and liquid before surgery contributes to an increased risk of pulmonary aspiration. Solid foods must be digested to a bolus diameter of less than 2 mm before the food can pass through the pylorus.[271] This process normally takes several hours for solids, whereas liquids pass through the pylorus in 1 to 2 hours.

BOX 20.19   Indications for Laboratory Testing

Complete Blood Count
- Hematologic disorder
- Vascular procedure
- Chemotherapy
- Unknown sickle cell syndrome status

Hemoglobin and Hematocrit
- Age <6 mo (<1 yr if born prematurely)
- Hematologic malignancy
- Recent radiation or chemotherapy
- Renal disease
- Anticoagulant therapy
- Procedure with moderate to high blood loss potential
- Coexisting systemic disorders (e.g., cystic fibrosis, prematurity, severe malnutrition, renal failure, liver disease, congenital heart disease)

White Blood Cell Count
- Leukemia and lymphomas
- Recent radiation or chemotherapy
- Suspected infection that would lead to cancellation of surgery
- Aplastic anemia
- Hypersplenism
- Autoimmune collagen vascular disease

Blood Glucose Level
- Diabetes mellitus
- Current corticosteroid use
- History of hypoglycemia
- Adrenal disease
- Cystic fibrosis

Serum Chemistry
- Renal disease
- Adrenal or thyroid disease
- Chemotherapy
- Pituitary or hypothalamic disease
- Body fluid loss or shifts (e.g., dehydration, bowel prep)
- Central nervous system disease

Potassium
- Digoxin therapy
- Diuretic therapy
- ACE inhibitors or angiotensin receptor blockers

Creatinine and Blood Urea Nitrogen
- Cardiovascular disease (e.g., hypertension)
- Renal disease
- Adrenal disease
- Diabetes mellitus
- Diuretic therapy
- Digoxin therapy
- Body fluid loss or shifts (e.g., dehydration, bowel prep)
- Procedure requiring radiocontrast

Liver Function Tests
- Hepatic disease
- Exposure to hepatitis
- Therapy with hepatotoxic agents

Coagulation Studies
INR, Prothrombin Time, and Partial Thromboplastin Time
- Leukemia
- Hepatic disease
- Bleeding disorder
- Anticoagulant therapy
- Severe malnutrition or malabsorption
- Postoperative anticoagulation to establish a baseline

Platelet Count and Bleeding Time
- Bleeding disorder
- Abnormal hemorrhage, purpura, history of easy bruising

Urinalysis
- Not indicated as a routine screening test

Pregnancy Test
- Possibility of pregnancy

Medication Levels
- Monitor for medications (e.g., theophylline, phenytoin, digoxin, carbamazepine) if patient exhibits signs of ineffective therapy, potential drug side effects, or poor drug compliance or has recently changed medication therapy without documentation of the drug level

ACE, Angiotensin-converting enzyme; *INR*, international normalized ratio (prothrombin time).

Historically, patients have been required to fast for extended periods in an attempt to ensure an empty stomach. However, sustained fasting does not guarantee that the stomach will be empty at the time of surgery.[272]

Part of the preoperative evaluation process identifies patients who are at risk for aspirating gastric contents into the lungs and developing aspiration pneumonitis. Factors associated with an increased risk of pulmonary aspiration of gastric contents are listed in Box 20.20.[273–276]

Fasting Interval

When the fasting interval is minimized, patients (especially children) are reported to be less irritable, less thirsty, and less hungry; to have fewer headaches; to be more comfortable; and generally to tolerate the preoperative phase better than patients who have fasted for longer periods of time. Modest amounts of clear liquids taken orally 2 to 3 hours[277-283] preoperatively, when compared with a conventional fasting interval of "7 to 8 hours" or "after midnight," are acceptable and have been shown to lower residual gastric volume (stimulation of the gastric emptying reflex) and raise gastric pH in a majority of patients. Acceptable clear fluids (e.g., water, apple juice, black coffee, black tea, clear juice drinks, clear Jell-O, clear broth, ice, popsicles, Pedialyte) may be given to healthy, unpremedicated patients. A 2016 study found no, or only a minimal, increase in gastric volume at 2 hours post-ingestion in patients allowed to add reduced-fat milk in their coffee.[284] Chewing gum or sucking on candy does not warrant delay or cancellation of the operation[285] and should be avoided once fasting from clear liquids has commenced.[286] In light of these findings, recommended fasting guidelines for otherwise healthy individuals have been liberalized (Box 20.21).[285,287]

BOX 20.20 Conditions That Increase the Risk of Regurgitation and Pulmonary Aspiration During Anesthesia

- Age extremes (<1 yr or >70 yr)
- Anxiety
- Ascites
- Collagen vascular disease (e.g., scleroderma)
- Depression
- Esophageal surgery
- Exogenous medications (e.g., opioids, premedication)
- Failed intubation or difficult airway history
- Gastroesophageal junction dysfunction (e.g., hiatal hernia)
- Mechanical obstruction (e.g., pyloric stenosis, duodenal ulcer)
- Metabolic disorders (e.g., hypothyroidism, chronic diabetes, hepatic failure, hyperglycemia, obesity, renal failure, uremia)
- Neurologic sequelae (e.g., those of developmental delays, head injury, hypotonia, seizures)
- Pain
- Pregnancy
- Prematurity with respiratory problems
- Smoking
- Type and composition of gastric contents (e.g., solid foods and milk products)

BOX 20.21 Fasting Guidelines for Healthy Patients (All Ages) Undergoing Elective Surgery

- No chewing gum (nicotine gum allowed with patient counseling) or candy after midnight (foreign body aspiration concern)
- Clear liquids up to 2 hr before surgery*
- Breast milk until 4 hr before surgery
- No infant formula, nonhuman milk,[†] or light meal[‡] for at least 6 hr before surgery
- Prescribed medications (e.g., premedication) administered with a sip of water or prescribed liquid mixture (up to 150 mL for adult; up to 75 mL for children) up to 1 hr before anesthesia

* Consider the possibility that the case may proceed earlier than scheduled.

[†] Because nonhuman milk is similar to solids in gastric emptying time, the amount ingested must be considered when determining an appropriate fasting period.

[‡] A light meal typically consists of toast and clear liquids. Meals that include fried or fatty foods or meat may prolong gastric emptying time. Both the amount and type of foods ingested must be considered when determining an appropriate fasting period.

From American Society of Anesthesiologists. Practice guidelines for preoperative fasting and the use of pharmacologic agents to reduce the risk of pulmonary aspiration: application to healthy patients undergoing elective procedures: an updated report by the American Society of Anesthesiologists Task Force on Preoperative Fasting and the Use of Pharmacologic Agents to Reduce the Risk of Pulmonary Aspiration. *Anesthesiology.* 2017;126:376–393.

Premedication

In instances when the anesthesia provider feels that aspiration risk is high even when standard fasting intervals have been followed (i.e., diabetic patients, patients with abnormal physiology), premedication may be required. Pharmacologic interventions may help mitigate aspiration risk in high-risk categories. Gastrointestinal stimulants (metoclopramide), blockade of gastric acid secretion (famotidine), and antiemetics (ondansetron, aprepitant), or a combination of some of these modalities, may be helpful.[287]

AMERICAN SOCIETY OF ANESTHESIOLOGISTS PHYSICAL STATUS CLASSIFICATION SYSTEM

With the conclusion of the preanesthesia assessment, assignment of an ASA physical status classification is made for each patient. The classification ideally represents a reflection of the patient's preoperative status and is not an estimate of anesthetic risk. For greater accuracy to be attained from its interpretation, the ASA status should also remain independent of the proposed surgical procedure.[288-291]

Advent and Purpose

In 1941 the ASA developed a system "to classify the physical condition of a patient requiring anesthesia and surgery." In 1961 the system was revised into five categories, and in 1980 a sixth category was added to include brain dead organ donors. The last revision occurred in 2014 and can be reviewed in Table 20.20.[292] The purpose of the ASA classification, then and now, is to provide a consistent means of communication to anesthesia staff, within and among institutions, about the physical status of a patient. Furthermore, it allows for a standardized interpretation of anesthesia outcome based on one criterion.

Despite rough correlations between patient physical status and postoperative outcome, *the ASA classification system does not represent an estimate of anesthesia risk.*[288-291] Although a patient in poor physical health is known to be at greater risk for negative outcome, this does not account for other factors that influence perioperative morbidity and mortality. These factors include the duration and involvement of the surgical procedure, the degree of perioperative monitoring, and unfortunate circumstances such as human error or equipment failure.

Definition

The current ASA classification system ranges from class I through VI, with E denoting an emergent procedure. By definition a patient classified as ASA status I is a healthy individual except for the condition that has necessitated surgery. A healthy young woman about to undergo an emergency dilation and curettage for vaginal bleeding, for example, is classified as ASA status IE. At the other end of the spectrum, a 74-year-old man with hypertension, uncontrolled diabetes, and unstable angina who is scheduled for a coronary artery bypass graft procedure is classified as ASA status IV.[292]

Limitations of the Current System

Despite the numerous benefits of the ASA classification system, it has its shortcomings. Namely the current system is not explicit enough in its categorization to account for every patient, and this can result in patient misclassification. If the physical status classification system is used for statistical or reimbursement purposes within a department, overclassification is often the consequence. Overclassification of a patient also occurs when the proposed surgical procedure is incorporated into the assignment of ASA physical status. This improper classification, or overclassification, of patient status thereby limits the degree of accuracy attained from its original interpretation. As a result, correlations between preoperative status and postoperative outcome are skewed. Despite the shortcomings of the system, ASA physical status continues to be assigned to each patient as a summary of the preoperative evaluation.

PREVENTING OPERATIVE ERRORS

The Joint Commission has endorsed a universal protocol for eliminating wrong site, wrong procedure, and wrong patient surgeries. It has been endorsed by more than 40 of the leading medical, nursing, and health care leadership organizations. The guidelines are to be used in all hospitals, ambulatory care surgery centers, and office-based surgery sites (Box 20.22).

TABLE 20.20 ASA Physical Status Classification System

ASA PS Classification	Definition	Examples, Including, but Not Limited to:
ASA I	A normal healthy patient	Healthy, nonsmoking, no or minimal alcohol use
ASA II	A patient with mild systemic disease	Mild diseases only without substantive functional limitations. Examples include (but not limited to): current smoker, social alcohol drinker, pregnancy, obesity (30 < BMI < 40), well-controlled DM/HTN, mild lung disease
ASA III	A patient with severe systemic disease	Substantive functional limitations; one or more moderate to severe diseases. Examples include (but not limited to): poorly controlled DM or HTN, COPD, morbid obesity (BMI ≥40), active hepatitis, alcohol dependence or abuse, implanted pacemaker, moderate reduction of ejection fraction, ESRD undergoing regularly scheduled dialysis, premature infant PCA <60 wk, history (>3 mo) of MI, CVA, TIA, or CAD/stents
ASA IV	A patient with severe systemic disease that is a constant threat to life	Examples include (but not limited to): recent (<3 mo) MI, CVA, TIA, or CAD/stents, ongoing cardiac ischemia or severe valve dysfunction, severe reduction of ejection fraction, sepsis, DIC, ARD, or ESRD not undergoing regularly scheduled dialysis
ASA V	A moribund patient who is not expected to survive without the operation	Examples include (but not limited to): ruptured abdominal/thoracic aneurysm, massive trauma, intracranial bleed with mass effect, ischemic bowel in the face of significant cardiac pathology or multiple organ/system dysfunction
ASA VI	A declared brain-dead patient whose organs are being removed for donor purposes	

- The addition of "E" denotes emergency surgery: An emergency is defined as existing when delay in treatment of the patient would lead to a significant increase in the threat to life or body part.

ARD, Acute renal disease; *ASA*, American Society of Anesthesiologists; *BMI*, body mass index; *CAD*, coronary artery disease; *COPD*, chronic obstructive pulmonary disease; *CVA*, cerebral vascular accident; *DIC*, disseminated intravascular coagulation; *DM*, diabetes mellitus; *ESRD*, end-stage renal disease; *HTN*, hypertension; *MI*, myocardial infarction; *PCA*, postconceptual age; *TIA*, transient ischemic attack.
From http://www.asahq.org/~/media/sites/asahq/files/public/resources/standards-guidelines/asa-physical-status-classification-system.pdf

BOX 20.22 Guidelines for Implementing the Universal Protocol for Preventing Wrong Site, Wrong Procedure, and Wrong Person Surgery

Conduct a Preprocedure Verification Process

Address missing information or discrepancies before starting the procedure.

- Verify the correct procedure, for the correct patient, at the correct site.
- When possible, involve the patient in the verification process.
- Identify the items that must be available for the procedure.
- Use a standardized list to verify the availability of items for the procedure. (It is not necessary to document that the list was used for each patient.) At a minimum, these items include:
  1. Relevant documentation. Examples: History and physical, signed consent form, preanesthesia assessment
  2. Labeled diagnostic and radiology test results that are properly displayed. Examples: Radiology images and scans, pathology reports, biopsy reports
  3. Any required blood products, implants, devices, special equipment
- Match the items that are to be available in the procedure area to the patient.

Mark the Procedure Site

At a minimum, mark the site when there is more than one possible location for the procedure and when performing the procedure in a different location could harm the patient.

- The site does not need to be marked for bilateral structures. Examples: tonsils, ovaries
- For spinal procedures: Mark the general spinal region on the skin. Special intraoperative imaging techniques may be used to locate and mark the exact vertebral level.
- Mark the site before the procedure is performed.
- If possible, involve the patient in the site marking process.
- The site is marked by a licensed independent practitioner who is ultimately accountable for the procedure and will be present when the procedure is performed.*
- Ultimately, the licensed independent practitioner is accountable for the procedure—even when delegating site marking.
- The mark is unambiguous and is used consistently throughout the organization.
- The mark is made at or near the procedure site.
- The mark is sufficiently permanent to be visible after skin preparation and draping.

- Adhesive markers are not the sole means of marking the site.
- For patients who refuse site marking or when it is technically or anatomically impossible or impractical to mark the site (see examples below): Use your organization's written, alternative process to ensure that the correct site is operated on. Examples of situations that involve alternative processes:
  1. Mucosal surfaces or perineum
  2. Minimal access procedures treating a lateralized internal organ, whether percutaneous or through a natural orifice
  3. Teeth
  4. Premature infants, for whom the mark may cause a permanent tattoo

Perform a Time-Out

The procedure is not started until all questions or concerns are resolved.

- Conduct a time-out immediately before starting the invasive procedure or making the incision.
- A designated member of the team starts the time-out.
- The time-out is standardized.
- The time-out involves the immediate members of the procedure team: the individual performing the procedure, anesthesia providers, circulating nurse, operating room technician, and other active participants who will be participating in the procedure from the beginning.
- All relevant members of the procedure team actively communicate during the time-out.
- During the time-out, the team members agree, at a minimum, on the following:
  1. Correct patient identity
  2. Correct site
  3. Procedure to be done
- When the same patient has two or more procedures: If the person performing the procedure changes, another time-out needs to be performed before starting each procedure.
- Document the completion of the time-out. The organization determines the amount and type of documentation.

*In limited circumstances, site marking may be delegated to some medical residents, physician assistants (PAs), or advanced practice registered nurses (APRNs).

SUMMARY

An important feature of patient care is a timely and thorough preoperative assessment to identify factors that increase the risk of anesthesia and surgery. The preoperative evaluation and preparation of the patient involve integration of information obtained from the patient interview, chart review, physical examination, and interpretation of the results of necessary diagnostic tests. The anesthesia provider can then assimilate the assessment data and devise and implement the most appropriate anesthetic plan for the patient.

REFERENCES

For a complete list of references for this chapter, scan this QR code with any smartphone code reader app, or visit the following URL: http://booksite.elsevier.com/9780323711944/.

21

Fluids, Electrolytes, and Goal-Directed Therapy

Crystal Trinooson, Nilu G. Patel

FLUID VOLUME, TYPES OF FLUIDS, AND OVERVIEW OF FLUID MANAGEMENT

Perioperative fluid management is an integral component of anesthetic practice, which involves maintaining intravascular volume, augmenting cardiac output (CO), maintaining tissue perfusion, promoting oxygen delivery, correcting and maintaining electrolyte balance, enhancing microcirculatory flow, and facilitating the delivery of nutrients and clearance of metabolic waste.[1,2] Targeted fluid administration is vital to compensate for acute volume alterations intraoperatively and to mitigate increased oxygen demands associated with metabolic derangements and surgical trauma.

The impacts of perioperative fluid handling are seen acutely in the intraoperative and immediate postoperative periods, but recently there has been a tremendous focus on the relationship between perioperative fluid administration and long-term outcomes in surgical patients. A growing body of evidence suggests that fluid balance and the complications associated with inappropriate fluid administration impact not only acute postsurgical recovery but also long-term morbidity.[3-9]

NORMAL PHYSIOLOGIC DISTRIBUTION AND REGULATION OF FLUIDS

An understanding of body fluid distribution and regulation is essential for anesthesia practice. Total body water (TBW) in an average adult represents roughly 60% of lean body mass.[10] Fluid is physiologically distributed as intracellular volume (ICV), which represents roughly two-thirds of TBW, and extracellular volume (ECV), which represents one-third of TBW.[11] The normal electrolyte composition of ICV differs greatly from that of ECV.[12] The primary cation of the ECV is sodium, and the primary anion is chloride. Potassium is the primary cation of the ICV and phosphate the primary anion.[10,12] The resting membrane gradient for these electrolytes is maintained by the sodium-potassium adenosine triphosphate enzyme (Na + K + ATPase) in the cell membrane that uses cellular energy to actively transport sodium ions into the ECV.[12,13] The cell membrane is permeable to water, and as a result the ICV and ECV maintain a state of osmotic equilibrium despite their varied solute composition.[12,13] The daily fluid volume required to maintain TBW homeostasis in a healthy adult who is normothermic with standard metabolic function is approximately 25 to 35 mL/kg per day (~2–3 L/day).[10,14,15] Extracellular volume is further subdivided by the vascular endothelium into two additional compartments. The

intravascular compartment contains plasma volume and represents roughly one-fourth of ECV. The interstitial compartment is composed of extravascular fluid in the tissue spaces, and represents roughly three-fourths of ECV (Fig. 21.1).[12,13,15,16] ECV is also composed of a small amount of transcellular fluids, including cerebrospinal fluid, synovial fluid, gastrointestinal secretions, and intraocular fluid.[10,12,17] Transcellular fluids are anatomically isolated from the fluid dynamics that impact the remaining ECV, and therefore they are considered nonfunctional.[17,18] Each of these volumes can be corroborated in laboratory testing with the use of radioactive water, isotope-tagged red blood cells, and selectively permeable protein-bound radioactive tracers.[10,19]

Fluid exchange between the extracellular compartments is largely dependent on Starling forces, four transcapillary pressures whose gradients dictate direction of fluid movement across the capillary epithelium.[19] Capillary hydrostatic pressure (Pc) is the intravascular blood pressure, driven by the force of the CO and impacted by vascular tone. Interstitial fluid pressure (Pif) is the hydrostatic pressure of the interstitial space. Relative to atmospheric pressure, Pif of most tissues is slightly negative; this is thought to be due to the contraction of lymphatic vessels in the interstitium.[19-21] Rigid or encapsulated tissues of the kidneys, brain, bone marrow, and skeletal muscle have a slightly positive Pif.[19,21] Plasma oncotic pressure (πp) is the osmotic force of colloidal proteins within the vascular space. Interstitial oncotic pressure (πif) is the osmotic force of colloidal proteins within the interstitial space (Fig. 21.2).[19] Due to a smaller molecular weight and higher concentration relative to other plasma proteins, albumin is the primary determinant of both capillary and interstitial oncotic pressures.[19,20] Increases in Pc and πif favor filtration of fluid into the interstitial space; increases in Pif and πp favor absorption of fluid into the intravascular space.[10,12] The relationship between these forces is described by the Starling equation as noted[10,19,21]:

$$\text{Net Filtration (Jv)} = Kf \,([Pc - Pif] - \sigma[\pi p - \pi if])$$

where Jv is the net fluid movement between compartments; Kf is a filtration coefficient that accounts for capillary surface area and endothelial permeability to water (capillary hydraulic conductivity); and [Pc − Pif] − σ[πp − πif] is the net driving force.

Increased Kf favors filtration.[20,22] σ is a reflection coefficient that ranges from 0 to 1 and accounts for the varying degree of endothelial permeability to substances such as albumin and large polar molecules. A σ of 0 indicates that the endothelium is freely permeable to the substance; a σ of 1 indicates that endothelium is completely impermeable

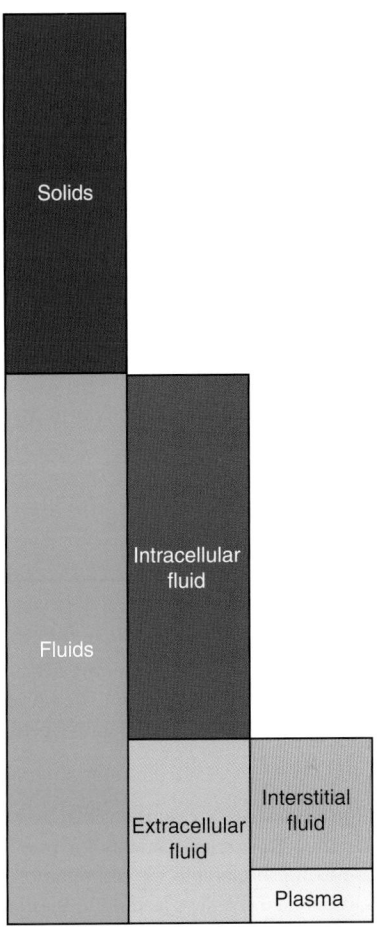

Fig. 21.1 Fluid compartments. Fluids comprise approximately 60% of the body weight. Two-thirds of the fluid is intracellular, and one-third is extracellular, which includes interstitial fluid and plasma. (Adapted from Applegate E. *The Anatomy and Physiology Learning System.* 4th ed. St. Louis: Elsevier; 2011:408.)

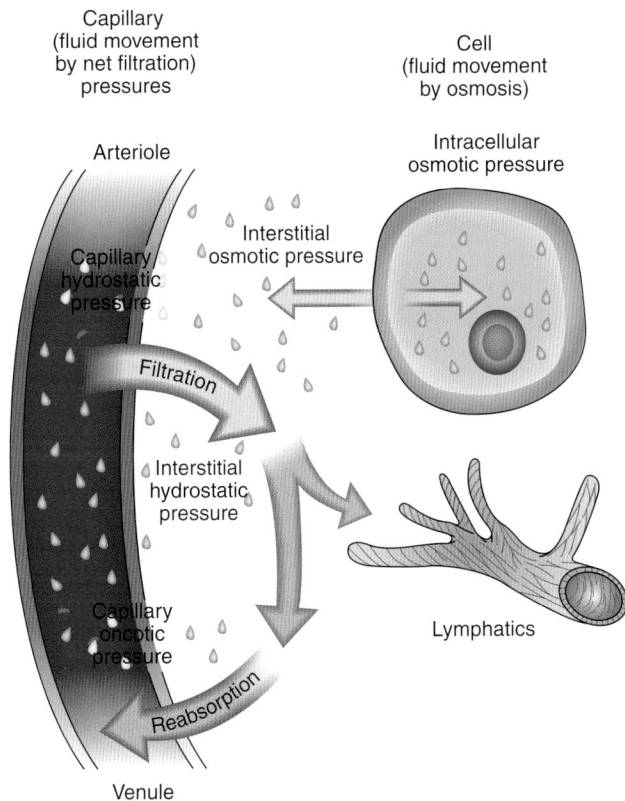

Fig. 21.2 Capillary filtration forces. Water, electrolytes, and small molecules exchange freely between the vascular compartment and the interstitial space at the site of capillaries and small venules. The rate and amount of exchange are driven by the physical forces of hydrostatic and oncotic pressures and the permeability and surface area of the capillary membranes. The two opposing hydrostatic pressures are capillary hydrostatic pressure and interstitial hydrostatic pressure. The two opposing oncotic pressures are capillary oncotic pressure and interstitial oncotic pressure. The forces that favor filtration from the capillary are capillary hydrostatic pressure and interstitial oncotic pressure, and the forces that oppose filtration are capillary oncotic pressure and interstitial hydrostatic pressure. The sum of their effects is known as net filtration pressure (NFP). In the example of normal exchange illustrated here, a small amount of fluid moves to the lymph vessels, which accounts for the net filtration difference between the arterial and venous ends of the capillary. (Adapted from McCance KL, et al. *Pathophysiology.* 7th ed. St. Louis: Elsevier; 2014:106.)

to the substance (during capillary filtration, 100% of the substance is reflected back into the vascular lumen).[20-23]

Positive net filtration favors fluid exudation into the tissues; negative net filtration favors fluid absorption into the vasculature.[10,19] Net filtration tends to be slightly positive at the arterial end of capillaries and slightly negative at the venous end.[19,20] The overall balance of filtration pressures within the capillaries of the entire body is slightly positive such that a small percentage of intravascular volume is constantly filtered into the interstitial space at a rate of approximately 2 mL/min under normal physiologic conditions.[19,20] This volume is returned to the intravascular space via the lymphatic system. Under euvolemic conditions, net fluid filtration is roughly equal to lymphatic flow.[19-22]

Starling's description of transcapillary forces has helped form the basis for our understanding of microcirculatory fluid dynamics over the past century, but recent evidence examines the importance of the capillary epithelium specifically, the endothelial glycocalyx in maintaining fluid homeostasis.[24-26] The glycocalyx is a gel layer on the luminal surface of the vascular endothelium that plays an important protective role in transcapillary fluid exchange, microcirculatory flow, blood component rheology, plasma oncotic pressure, signal transduction, immune modulation, and vascular tone.[25,26]

Ranging from 0.1 to 1.2 μM in diameter, the glycocalyx is composed of a matrix of glycoproteins, polysaccharides, and hyaluronic acid that bind to ionic side chains and plasma proteins to create a physiologically active barrier within the vascular space.[11,25] This dynamic barrier ionically repels negatively charged polar compounds in addition to

blood components, to create a zone of exclusion between the surface of the glycocalyx and the center of the vessel, aiding in the prevention of blood component adhesion to the vascular wall and augmenting laminar blood flow.[25] By binding to circulating plasma albumin, the glycocalyx also helps to preserve capillary oncotic pressure and decrease capillary permeability to water, thus modulating the impact of plasma hydrostatic pressure on net filtration.[24,25] This regulating function has been described as the double barrier effect,[11,13] and it has led to the development of a revised Starling equation as follows[25]:

$$\text{Net Filtration } (J_v) = K_f ([P_c - P_{if}] - \sigma[\pi_p - \pi_{sg}])$$

where π_{sg} is the oncotic pressure in the subglycocalyx space between the endothelium and the glycocalyx. Furthermore, the glycocalyx plays an important role in modulating inflammatory processes. This space is thought to contain inflammatory mediators whose binding sites are enclosed by the matrix, thus helping prevent leukocyte adhesion except in circumstances of acute inflammation or endothelial damage.[25] Other functions of the glycocalyx include scavenging of free radicals, binding and activation of anticoagulation factors, and signal transduction that helps regulate local vasoactive responses to mechanical stress.[25,27]

In addition to the microcirculatory dynamics that govern transcapillary fluid volume distribution, there are a series of neurohormonal influences and feedback mechanisms that help to finely regulate electrolyte and fluid balance.[12] Normal daily alterations in TBW are minute and intricately regulated by the renin-angiotensin-aldosterone system (RAAS), antidiuretic hormone (ADH), and atrial natriuretic peptide (ANP) pathways.[10,12,15,27-29] Sodium is one of the primary determinants of serum osmolality and water transport, thus the regulation of ECV is largely dependent on sodium homeostasis.[12] This concept is important when discussing perioperative sodium loading and appropriate selection of intravenous fluids.

The RAAS is an important regulator of physiologic sodium homeostasis.[12,29] In response to hypotension (as detected by intracardiac and renal afferent arteriole baroreceptors) and systemic sympathetic stimulation, the juxtaglomerular cells of the kidney release the enzyme renin. The interaction of circulating renin with the precursor angiotensinogen causes cleaving of angiotensinogen to the active substance angiotensin I. Angiotensin I exerts local vasoconstrictor activity, but its primary role is as a precursor for the more potent angiotensin II. This change occurs in the lungs as a result of angiotensin-converting enzyme (ACE) acting as a catalyst for the conversion of angiotensin I to angiotensin II. Angiotensin II is a potent vasoconstrictor and directly stimulates the renal tubules to reabsorb sodium and water. It also causes the adrenal cortex to release aldosterone, which further stimulates sodium and water retention by the kidneys.[12,29]

The ADH pathway functions primarily to regulate water balance. In response to even minute increases in serum osmolality (as detected by osmoreceptors in the hypothalamus), the posterior pituitary gland releases ADH, which causes aquaporin channels within the kidney to transiently reabsorb large quantities of water. This helps preserve circulating volume and contributes to a tremendous increase in urine concentration and osmolality.[12,19] ADH also plays an important role in preserving blood pressure by acting as a potent arterial vasoconstrictor. Decreases in circulating blood volume (as detected by baroreceptors in the atria, carotid body, and aorta) stimulate this hormone's release, although the mechanism is much less sensitive than osmolality-mediated secretion.[30,31] The detection of increased serum osmolality also causes the hypothalamus to stimulate thirst.[12]

Stretch receptors within the cardiac atrial walls stimulate the release of ANP from cardiac myocytes as a result of increased-preload or hypervolemic states. This stimulates the kidney to release sodium and water, thus reducing circulating blood volume and offloading the heart. ANP also produces specific vasoactive responses in the afferent and efferent renal arterioles to increase the glomerular filtration rate, and it inhibits the release of renin and ADH.[29] Conversely, during periods of decreased preload, atrial receptors inhibit the release of ANP.[15]

These mechanisms combine with many other complex renal, hormonal, vascular, and metabolic processes to carefully maintain fluid and electrolyte balance.[15] In the healthy adult, inputs such as water and electrolyte intake (nutrition and free water intake) are closely balanced by outputs (sweat, respiratory losses, gastrointestinal losses, and urine output) to such a degree that daily water fluctuation represents only approximately 0.2% of TBW.[10,15]

COMPOSITION AND RELATIVE ADVANTAGES OF VARIOUS INTRAVENOUS FLUIDS

The selection of intravenous fluids for perioperative management continues to be a controversial decision in modern anesthetic practice. Despite a general consensus regarding the overall goals of fluid resuscitation to restore intravascular volume, microvascular flow, and tissue

TABLE 21.1 Composition of Crystalloid Solutions

Concentration	Plasma	Plasmalyte-A/ Normosol-R/ Isolyte-S	Lactated Ringer	0.9% Sodium Chloride
Sodium (mEq/L)	142	140–141	130	154
Potassium (mEq/L)	4	5	4	
Chloride (mEq/L)	103	98	110	154
Phosphate (mEq/L)	1.4	1*		
Magnesium (mEq/L)	2	3		
Calcium (mEq/L)	5		3	
Lactate (mEq/L)			28	
Acetate (mEq/L)		27		
Gluconate (mEq/L)		23		
pH	7.4	7.4	6.2	5.6
Osmolality (mOsm/L)	291	294–295	275	310

*Isolyte-S only.

perfusion, there continues to be a longstanding debate over the safety and efficacy of crystalloid solutions as compared to colloid solutions for volume resuscitation during the perioperative period.[32]

Crystalloids

Crystalloids are aqueous electrolyte solutions that have been a mainstay of volume resuscitation in surgical patients for over a century.[17,33,34] Crystalloid infusions are preferable for resuscitation of dehydration conditions (conditions of TBW loss leading to plasma hypertonicity) such as prolonged fasting states, active gastrointestinal losses, polyuria, and hypermetabolic conditions.[17] The administration of isotonic crystalloid solutions under these circumstances contributes to the hydration of the entire ECV, restoring water and electrolyte homeostasis to both intravascular and interstitial spaces for normal cellular processes. The use of crystalloids to replace active intravascular losses in the perioperative setting is beneficial for providing immediate restoration of circulating vascular volume, preservation of microcirculatory flow, decrease in hormone-mediated vasoconstriction, and correction of plasma hyperviscosity associated with acute hemorrhage. Crystalloids are also preferred for their lack of allergenic potential, their ease of metabolism and renal clearance (compared to colloids) when infused in appropriate volumes, and their preservation of electrolyte balance despite active intraoperative plasma losses.[1,7,13,14] However, because isotonic crystalloids are distributed evenly throughout the extracellular space, their ability to expand plasma volume is transient. Due to low molecular weight, crystalloid solutions contribute to hemodilution of plasma proteins and loss of capillary oncotic pressure. This favors filtration of approximately 75% to 80% of administered volumes into the interstitial space.[1,35] The composition of common isotonic crystalloid solutions varies (Table 21.1). Their relative advantages and disadvantages are discussed later.

Sodium chloride 0.9% is the original crystalloid solution; it is known as normal saline (NS) and is presently the most commonly administered intravenous fluid worldwide.[1,13,14,33] NS was determined to be a physiologic solution over a century ago based on in vitro erythrocyte studies comparing the effects of a 0.9% saline infusion with those of a 0.6% solution; the term NS persists today.[33] However, of all the isotonic crystalloid preparations available for fluid resuscitation, 0.9% saline is the least physiologic.[15]

NS contains roughly equal concentrations of sodium and chloride, although the normal physiologic concentration of sodium in plasma is higher than that of chloride.[33,36] The presence of an extraordinarily high chloride load contributes to acid-base imbalances, and there is a potential for 0.9% saline to contribute to dose-dependent hyperchloremic metabolic acidosis.[14,36] Even if compensatory mechanisms preserve a normal plasma pH, the use of 0.9% saline for volume resuscitation in acute losses is associated with marked alterations in base excess secondary to chloride load. This effect may exacerbate volume overload if negative base excess is used as an infusion trigger.[1,17,36]

Hyperchloremia has a substantial impact on renal function. This is thought to be due, in part, to the impact of excess renal reabsorption of chloride on renal arteriolar vascular resistance, leading to a decrease in glomerular filtration rates.[36,37] Hyperchloremia may also impair renal handling of bicarbonate. The increased sodium load introduced by large volumes of 0.9% saline has been shown to cause increased salt and water retention, hemodilution, and interstitial edema well into the postoperative period. It has been determined that the administration of 2 L NS to healthy volunteers contributes to a positive sodium and water balance that takes up to 2 days to excrete.[11] This duration may be significantly prolonged in surgical patients.[7,11,15]

The long-term clinical significance of these effects and the relationship between NS administration and renal impairment have been the subject of multiple studies. In 2015, the 0.9% Saline vs Plasma-Lyte 148 for Intensive Care Unit Fluid Therapy (SPLIT) trial evaluated 2278 patients across four intensive care units (ICUs) and found that the use of a buffered crystalloid did not reduce the risk of acute kidney injury (AKI) compared to the use of saline.[38] Limitations included the relatively small volume of crystalloid administered (median volume = 2 L) and the exclusion of patients with Acute Physiology and Chronic Health Evaluation (APACHE)-II scores of 25 or greater, limiting the generalizability of the findings to higher risk patients.[38]

A 2018 systematic review of 15 studies with 4067 patients found that low-chloride solutions had no impact on mortality or renal replacement therapy (RRT) requirements compared to high-chloride solutions. However, investigators acknowledged that the overall quality of available evidence was low and that a variety of component study factors (e.g., low volume of study fluids) contributed to a low statistical power.[39]

The Saline against Lactated Ringer's or Plasma-Lyte in the Emergency Department (SALT-ED) trial compared the impact of balanced crystalloid administration against that of saline among 13,347 patients in a single-center emergency department and found no difference in hospital-free days (days alive after discharge before day 28).[40] The secondary outcome demonstrated lower incidence (P = 0.01) of major adverse kidney events within 30 days (MAKE30) in the balanced crystalloids group.[40]

Concurrently, the Isotonic Solutions and Major Adverse Renal Events Trial (SMART) examined 7942 patients in five ICUs and found that, compared to saline, balanced crystalloids significantly reduced MAKE30 among critically ill patients.[41]

To address the question of outcomes among the critically ill, in 2019 the Cochrane Collaboration published a review of 21 randomized controlled trials (RCTs) with 20,213 critically ill adult and child participants. The data showed, with a high degree of certainty, no advantage of balanced crystalloids over saline in preventing in-hospital mortality. Though balanced crystalloids conferred benefit for reducing metabolic derangements in many of the component RCTs, the evidence demonstrated no difference in the incidence of AKI compared to saline. However, the degree of certainty for this outcome was lower, suggesting that additional trials may alter this conclusion.[42]

A meta-analysis of nine studies (32,777 patients) revealed no significant difference between balanced crystalloids and saline in the incidence of mortality, moderate-to-severe AKI, or RRT. However, as with

other studies, the results revealed low-quality existing evidence with a need for larger ongoing trials.[43]

Despite these findings, current publications of the Enhanced Recovery After Surgery (ERAS) Society and others continue to strongly recommend the use of balanced crystalloid solutions for perioperative fluid management and in the setting of high-volume fluid resuscitation due to the abundance of observational data on the reduction of metabolic derangements.[44,45] A series of ongoing trials may help provide more conclusive evidence in the future.[46,47]

A decided role of NS in modern anesthetic practice is in the administration of small volumes to neurosurgical patients. As a result of its mild hyperosmolality, 0.9% saline is the preferred fluid for patients at risk for cerebral edema.[36] NS may also be indicated in fluid management of patients with anuria and end-stage renal disease who cannot excrete the potassium content of more balanced crystalloid solutions.[14] Hypertonic saline solutions of 3% or greater are sometimes used in low-dose infusions in trauma and head-injured patients. These solutions promote volume expansion that mobilizes intracellular and interstitial fluids into the intravascular space. This may confer some protection for patients with intracranial hypertension, but there are significant risks associated with its infusion, including vascular irritation, a sudden and pronounced fluid shift into the intravascular space, and the potential for dehydration of neural cells leading to osmotic demyelination syndrome.[14,36,48]

Lactated Ringer (LR) is an electrolyte solution that contains sodium lactate as a bicarbonate substrate, or buffering agent.[48,49] This helps to maintain the electrochemical balance and neutral pH of the solution while decreasing the anionic requirement for chloride.[14,48] LR is a relatively low-cost solution compared to other balanced salt solutions, and its use as a resuscitative fluid has also been shown to be more effective in preserving intravascular volume than the use of 0.9% saline. LR is not recommended for large-volume administration in diabetic patients because the byproducts of hepatic metabolism of lactate can result in gluconeogenesis.[48] The infusion of LR may also contribute to a mild metabolic alkalosis because of the alkalinizing effect of lactate metabolism. LR is mildly hypotonic and may cause transient serum hypoosmolality and associated cerebral edema. As a result, LR is contraindicated in patients with traumatic brain injury or other neurovascular insults.[7,14,50] LR contains calcium, and it is contraindicated for infusion with citrated, the preservative used in blood and blood products due to the risk of coagulation.[36]

Plasmalyte-A, Normosol-R, and Isolyte S are the most isotonic of the balanced salt solutions.[36,51] These solutions have the most favorable acid-base profile compared to plasma; they preserve physiologic pH and renal perfusion better than 0.9% saline.[36] They also utilize sodium gluconate and sodium acetate as alkalinizing buffers rather than lactate. Furthermore, because they do not contain calcium, these solutions are compatible with blood products.[11,36,51]

Colloids

Colloids are suspensions of high-molecular-weight molecules in electrolyte solutions that produce intravascular volume expansion by directly increasing πp and interacting with the endothelial glycocalyx to decrease transcapillary filtration.[11,22,25] This preparation is effective for plasma volume expansion, and colloid solutions are often used perioperatively for their fluid-sparing effects compared to crystalloids.[35,36] Aside from packed red blood cells, albumin is the only naturally occurring colloid solution available for infusion; a variety of synthetic colloids are also available worldwide.[35] Colloid solutions are classified by molecular weight, concentration, and half-life.[15]

Dextrans are among the oldest artificial colloids, and they possess high-molecular-weight polymers (40–70 kDa) derived from bacterial metabolism of sucrose. They were first manufactured in the 1940s.[33,48] They are markedly hyperosmolar and have a half-life of roughly 6 to 12 hours.[36,46] These compounds are known to cause acute renal failure by multiple mechanisms, including indirect hyperosmotic renal injury and direct renal tubular damage as a result of accumulation.[15,36,48] Dextran use is associated with a variety of coagulopathic effects due to impairment of von Willebrand factor, activation of plasminogen, and interference with platelet aggregation.[48,52] Dextrans may also adhere to the surface of platelets and red blood cells and interfere with cross-matching of blood products.[48,52] Dextrans are no longer used in clinical practice due to the propensity to cause acute renal failure and induce anaphylaxis and coagulopathy.[15,17,36,52,53]

Gelatins are synthetic colloids derived from bovine components.[15] They have a molecular weight of 30 to 35 kDa; this is lower than most other colloids and contributes to a shorter half-life (roughly 2–4 hours) and limited duration of plasma expansion.[17,36,48] Gelatins, like dextrans, interfere with platelet function, cause nephrotoxicity, and have a high propensity for causing anaphylaxis, particularly if urea-linked formulations are used.[11,17,36,48,50,52] There are concerns regarding the potential of gelatins to transmit bovine spongiform encephalitis (BSE). The actual risk of this transmission is unknown.[13] A 2016 meta-analysis examined adverse effects of gelatin-containing plasma expanders compared to crystalloids and albumin. Though the available data was limited, the results indicated an increased risk of anaphylaxis, renal injury, acquired coagulopathy, and mortality.[54] Due to ongoing safety concerns and in light of insufficient evidence suggesting any benefit from their use, the use of gelatins in clinical practice has been cautioned.[17,52,54]

Hydroxyethyl starches (HES) are synthetic macromolecules derived from starchy plants, including potatoes, maize, and sorghum. Consequently, they can cause allergic reactions in patients with reactivity to these and other components.[11] HES are synthesized by substituting hydroxyl groups at the second, third, and sixth carbon atoms of the macromolecule and are classified according to their molecular weight and substitution ratios. The C2/C6 ratio compares the degree of substitution at the second carbon to that at the sixth. A high C2/C6 ratio indicates that HES will be difficult to metabolize and will thus provide prolonged plasma volume expansion.[48] The use of HES in clinical practice has been controversial. Many of the landmark initial studies on the safety and efficacy of HES were later retracted as a result of the discovery that the supporting evidence was fabricated.[53] Despite this, HES have been widely used, particularly in the European Union.[56] The clinical impact of HES has been studied extensively because of the prevalence of their use in perioperative and critical care settings.[11,55] First-generation HES (hetastarches and hexastarches) are the highest molecular-weight solutions (>450 kDa) and often have the greatest substitution ratios (0.6–0.7).[48] These solutions are associated with dose-dependent coagulopathy because of hemodilution and binding of clotting factors, interference with platelet adhesion, inhibition of fibrin polymerization, and alterations in plasma viscosity.[11,56] HES can also accumulate to form interstitial colloid deposits in subcutaneous and other organ tissues leading to severe pruritus and nephrotoxicity.[10,11,56] This effect was originally thought to be associated with the prolonged metabolic profile of first-generation HES, but studies have demonstrated that this effect occurs across all generations of HES.[11,53] Second-generation solutions, pentastarches, are medium-weight solutions (200–260 kDa) with a substitution ratio of 0.5. Third-generation HES are low-molecular-weight tetrastarches (70–130 kDa) with a substitution ratio of 0.4.[48] RCTs have demonstrated the risk of kidney injury, dialysis requirements, coagulopathy, sepsis, and even increased mortality associated with HES.[11,57]

Furthermore, these adverse impacts have been shown to persist up to 90 days after HES administration.[58,59] Based on these and other findings, the US Food and Drug Administration (FDA) issued a black box warning for HES solutions in 2013 to notify the public of the risks of renal injury and increased mortality.[56,59,60]

There continued to be some ongoing interest in the use of HES for resuscitation of acute blood loss in trauma patients and as a component of perioperative fluid management. A 2016 systematic review evaluated the relative risk of HES compared to crystalloids in patients having elective noncardiac surgery. The investigators determined that there was insufficient evidence to identify a significant difference in outcomes (mortality, AKI, length of stay, and infection).[61] A meta-analysis of RCTs of colloids versus crystalloids examined over 16,000 patients, including critically ill patients, surgical patients, and those with traumatic injuries. Their analysis found that the risks of renal injury and increased mortality were significant only in the critically ill subgroup.[62] This may be the result of a loss of endothelial glycocalyx integrity causing alterations in transcapillary fluid dynamics in the critically ill.[26]

The Pharmacovigilance Risk Assessment Committee (PRAC) of the European Medicines Agency (EMA) issued a sudden recommendation in January 2018 to fully suspend all HES solutions from the market in the wake of two drug utilization studies indicating that HES were being used in critically ill and septic populations in defiance of the EMA's 2013 recommendation.[63]

Pushback to this decision from a group, including one of the original authors of the 2013 Colloids Versus Crystalloids for the Resuscitation of the Critically Ill (CRISTAL) trial, cited their earlier evidence showing no difference in 28-day mortality or RRT among 2857 critically ill patients. However, 90-day mortality was reduced in the colloid group, as were vasopressor use and mechanical ventilation days by day 28.[64,65,66]

Following this decision, a study of 1057 patients undergoing abdominal surgery was published to evaluate the hypothesis that HES reduced major postoperative complications compared to balanced crystalloids. The study found no difference in outcomes between the groups.[67]

Albumin is a fractionated blood product produced from pooled human plasma. It has a molecular weight of 65 to 69 kDa and is heat treated to inactivate pathogens and eliminate the risk of disease transmission.[15,25,48] Commercially prepared albumin solutions were developed in the mid-1940s as plasma volume expanders for use in military trauma settings.[33] The use of albumin in these settings was preferred for rapid restoration of circulating volume in active loss situations where transfusion was not readily available. Albumin is often utilized in modern-day anesthetic practice as a volume expander in circumstances of active loss not requiring transfusion.[7,35,68] Small volumes of albumin provide a greater degree of intravascular resuscitation as compared to equal or greater volumes of crystalloid. However, albumin preparations are significantly more costly than crystalloid solutions.[1] Albumin is often utilized in goal-directed approaches to reduce complications associated with tissue edema, but it does carry a risk for anaphylaxis or other immune-mediated reaction.[11,13,23]

Albumin is a carrier for a number of protein-bound ionic substances, including drugs and their metabolites, electrolytes, enzymes, and hormones. In the presence of hypoalbuminemia, the administration of albumin may be advised.[20] Albumin has a negative electrostatic charge. Albumin molecules bind ions, which increase plasma osmolality and intravascular volume; this phenomenon is called the Donnan effect.[19] One of the more commonly cited outcome assessments associated with albumin is the Saline Versus Albumin Fluid Evaluation (SAFE) study, a trial of nearly 7000 critically ill patients who were randomized to receive 0.9% saline or 4% albumin solutions. The study demonstrated that no difference in clinical outcomes existed, except in cases of neurotrauma, where patients in the albumin cohort had a higher incidence of mortality.[69]

As a result of the targeted expansion of the intravascular space, colloids may be the preferred solution for replacement of circulating blood volume in patients with intact endothelial glycocalyx undergoing acute volume losses.[25,26] However, the use of albumin and other colloids in patients with endothelial injuries may lead to pulmonary edema and other end-organ complications.[23] Furthermore, the administration of colloid solutions to patients who are euvolemic has been known to contribute to ANP-mediated hypervolemic endothelial disruption.[25,26,69] Therefore practitioners are cautioned to avoid colloids in patients with clinical conditions likely to precipitate endothelial injury such as hyperglycemia.[26]

The risks and benefits of crystalloids and colloids in critically ill patients concluded that there is no benefit to the administration of colloids as compared to crystalloids, and that their cost does not justify their use in critically ill patients.[70] Since albumin is less likely to cause nephrotoxicity and to disrupt the vascular endothelium, it has the potential to preserve renal perfusion in patients with septic shock.[71] Later evidence suggested albumin administration may help preserve the integrity of the glycocalyx in early sepsis.[7,35] The Surviving Sepsis Campaign issued updated guidelines in 2017, including a recommendation for albumin as a component of early resuscitation for septic patients requiring large-volume crystalloid infusion. However, the evidence for this recommendation was weak.[72] The National Institute for Health and Care Excellence (NICE) in the United Kingdom also issued a clinical guideline recommending that albumin be considered for use in septic patients.[1,36,73] The Cochrane Collaboration published an updated 2018 review comparing colloids to crystalloids in critically ill patients and found that albumin produced no difference in 30- or 90-day mortality, RRT requirement, or allergic reactions.[32]

Evidence suggests an acceptable safety profile for albumin, and the administration of small allotments to volume-responsive patients is still advocated in the context of some goal-directed approaches.[32,74,75] However, in light of insufficient high-quality evidence demonstrating clear benefit, the cost of albumin may not justify its use except in certain circumstances.[35,36] Further studies on volume-responsive surgical patients and the critically ill will help to define the role of colloid administration in anesthetic practice.

IMPACT OF SURGERY AND ANESTHESIA ON VASCULAR FLOW AND ORGAN PERFUSION

Surgery and anesthesia exert complex physiologic responses that impact vascular flow and organ perfusion. Stimulation of somatic and autonomic afferent nerves in the area of surgical incision triggers the activation of the hypothalamic-pituitary axis (HPA).[76,77] As a result of this central nervous activation, the hypothalamus releases corticotropin-releasing hormone, prompting the anterior pituitary gland to secrete adrenocorticotropic hormone (ACTH), which then elicits the creation and release of cortisol from the adrenal cortex.[76-78] Cortisol stimulates protein catabolism, hepatic gluconeogenesis and glycogenolysis, and increased hepatic production and release of plasma proteins.[77] These processes maintain energy substrate levels and contribute to increased πp to help preserve intravascular volume. Such evolutionary mechanisms provide cellular energy and circulating volume for the body in times of increased metabolic demand but may be maladaptive in the setting of hyperglycemia or vascular overload. Hyperglycemia is a major risk factor for damage or destruction of the endothelial glycocalyx. It also impairs wound healing, contributes to osmotic diuresis, and interferes with immune responses.[25,78,79]

The physiologic stimulation associated with surgery also causes the release of catecholamines. Surgical trauma causes direct stimulation of sympathetic nerves, which triggers a substantial release of catecholamines from the adrenal medulla, causing sympathetic nervous system effects such as increased heart rate, increased systemic vascular resistance (SVR), microcirculatory vasoconstriction, which results in increased basal metabolic rate, and increased oxygen demand.[77] Sympathetic stimulation, in combination with hyperosmolar conditions, triggers the release of ADH and causes vasoconstriction, reabsorption of water, and potassium excretion.[19,78] Depending on the magnitude of the surgical trauma and the resulting hemodynamic changes, this release may continue for hours postoperatively.[80]

Surgical trauma and tissue injury stimulate local endothelial release of cytokines and other inflammatory mediators that contribute to hyperthermia, increased oxygen demands, and regional alterations in microcirculatory flow.[78,79,81] Low-level cytokine release is beneficial by promoting local hemostasis and migration of neutrophils to the site of injury; unrestricted or prolonged release can contribute to vasodilation, endothelial damage, increased filtration, tissue edema, insulin resistance, intravascular loss, hypotension, and decreased organ perfusion.[78,79,82] Severe tissue damage associated with prolonged surgery or traumatic injury, particularly in open abdominal cases, may promote inflammatory loss of gastrointestinal endothelial integrity leading to translocation of bacteria and systemic inflammatory responses.[78,83] One of the most beneficial effects of cortisol is the profound antiinflammatory effect it exerts by inhibiting the production, release, and vascular aggregation of inflammatory mediators.[82,84]

During periods that result in hypovolemia or hemorrhage, decreased Pc favors absorption and supplies an autotransfusion of fluid volume from the interstitial space into the intravascular space. Conversely, hypervolemia or vascular overload may cause a marked increase in Pc and a dilutional decrease in πp that favor filtration, overfilling the interstitial space, and overwhelming the lymphatic system. The development of interstitial edema is a primary cause of tissue congestion, capillary collapse, loss of waste removal and nutrient exchange capabilities, decreased microcirculatory flow, and tissue ischemia.[20,22]

Laparoscopic surgery is often preferred because its minimally invasive approach contributes to a reduction in tissue damage, blood loss, and inflammatory release (particularly of cytokines). However, laparoscopy carries risks of its own.[78,85] Increased intraabdominal pressure, secondary to pneumoperitoneum, causes direct mechanical suppression of splanchnic blood flow leading to transient splanchnic ischemia and microcirculatory changes.[85,86] Sympathetically mediated vasoconstriction of the splanchnic circulation also sacrifices gut mucosal tissue perfusion and predisposes the gastrointestinal epithelium to ischemia-reperfusion injury when vascular flow is restored.[85] During insufflation of the abdomen, particularly if done rapidly or to high pressures (>12–15 mm Hg), peritoneal and mesenteric afferent receptors may stimulate a vagal response.[86] Abdominal insufflation contributes to a significant increase in central venous pressure (CVP) as a result of the shunting of blood from the splanchnic circulation into the thorax. This elevation in right ventricular preload also stimulates the release of ANP.[86] Increased intraabdominal pressures may contribute to a decrease in cardiac preload by decreasing venous return. Furthermore, insufflation in hypovolemic patients may cause cardiac collapse if insufflation pressures are high enough to compress the inferior vena cava.[85,86]

Afterload is markedly increased because of elevated intrathoracic pressure and compensatory increases in SVR; this contributes to a reduction in stroke volume (SV). Although vascular flow may be decreased, mean arterial pressure (MAP) is often elevated because of increased SVR. A study on the impact of pneumoperitoneum on patients who were classified as American Society of Anesthesiologists (ASA) I and II found that insufflation to pressures of 10 to 15 mm Hg significantly decreased both right and left ventricular ejection fractions.[87] Patients with normal myocardial function are able to compensate for these hemodynamic alterations with tachycardia and increased left ventricular stroke work to preserve CO at the expense of increased oxygen demand. However, patients with volume overload or who have decreased ventricular function may develop cardiac failure as a result of their inability to compensate.[86,87]

Anesthetic interventions may help mitigate many of these responses. Opioids and dexmedetomidine are known to be very effective at reducing HPA-mediated stress responses; however, enhanced recovery strategies discourage the administration of large doses of opioids.[75,78] Neuraxial anesthesia helps to mitigate spinal cord transmission of autonomic afferent impulses, which would otherwise stimulate HPA. This effect is most pronounced in procedures of the lower extremities and pelvis.[78,87] Dexmedetomidine can be used as an anesthetic adjunct or premedication to provide opioid-sparing analgesic effects and to attenuate the hemodynamic stress of laparoscopy.[88,89]

The concept of goal-directed fluid management is intricately connected to physiologic changes during surgery. Judicious and timely administration of fluids and vasoactive support to meet defined perfusion targets has been shown to support oxygen balance and mitigate the body's neuroendocrine response to surgical stress.[3,5,31] Furthermore, maintenance of euvolemia throughout the perioperative period helps to preserve the glycocalyx and its associated microvascular functions.[25]

HISTORICAL APPROACH TO FLUID MANAGEMENT

For much of the past 60 years, fluid management has relied on formulaic fixed-volume approaches to standardize fluid administration for all surgical patients, regardless of volume status at onset of surgery, myocardial and renal function, and vascular tone. These traditional methods often involved uniform calculations used to assess the fluid requirement of a given patient. Perhaps the most common of these was the 4-2-1 calculation; this was used in combination with estimates of fasting deficit, formulaic assessments of surgical insensible losses, and calculated ratios for replacement of blood loss (Box 21.1).[90] The driving concept behind many of these approaches was the theory that fasting patients incurred a preoperative "fluid debt" and required volume preloading to help maintain physiologic stability and homeostasis.[13] Scientific evidence challenges this assessment because it does not account for cardiovascular and renal function in individual patients, nor does it consider the true impact of fasting in elective surgical patients.[91,92] The routine use of preemptive fluid administration to correct perceived fasting deficits often contributed to overload-associated perioperative complications.[3,7,25] Furthermore, current knowledge indicates that prophylactic volume administration in euvolemic patients creates substantial risk of disrupting the endothelial glycocalyx and contributing to pathologic fluid overload.[10,26]

Such data do not discount the possibility of hypovolemia in the preoperative period. Given the substantial risks of arbitrary fluid administration, current evidence encourages the utilization of hemodynamic measures to evaluate fluid responsiveness in patients with active preoperative volume losses.[17] It is important to note that the use of bowel preparations may cause excessive fluid losses. As a result of the impact of these mechanisms on perioperative outcome, enhanced recovery strategies focus on reducing fasting times and evaluating the necessity of hypertonic bowel preparations. The practice of prophylactic bowel preparation prior to colorectal surgery does not decrease postoperative complications.[93] In addition to hypovolemia, routine prophylactic bowel preparation is being eliminated from enhanced recovery from anesthesia protocols.

More recent data from the American College of Surgeons National Surgical Quality Improvement Program (ACS-NSQIP) review of 27,804 elective colorectal surgical patients showed that while bowel

BOX 21.1   Historical Fluid Management Calculations

4-2-1 Calculation for Determining Maintenance Fluid Requirement
- 0–10 kg: 4 mL/kg/hr
- 11–20 kg: 4 mL/kg/hr for the first 10 kg; 2 mL/kg/hr for every kg >10
- >20 kg: 4 mL/kg/hr for the first 10 kg; 2 mL/kg/hr for the next 10 kg; 1 mL/kg/hr for every kg >20

Estimated Fluid Deficit
- Estimated Fluid Deficit = Maintenance Fluid Requirement × Fasting Hours

Guidelines for Replacement of Surgical Losses
- Superficial trauma (orofacial): 1–2 mL/kg/hr
- Minimal trauma (herniorrhaphy): 2–4 mL/kg/hr
- Moderate trauma (major nonabdominal or laparoscopic abdominal surgery): 4–6 mL/kg/hr
- Severe trauma (major open abdominal surgery): 6–8 mL/kg/hr

Recommendation for Replacement of Blood Loss
- Crystalloid—3:1 (3 mL for every 1 mL estimated blood loss)
- Colloid or blood—1:1 (1 mL for every 1 mL estimated blood loss)

preparation alone conferred no benefit against infection, the combined use of bowel preparation and prophylactic oral antibiotic therapy reduced the incidence of surgical site infection better than antibiotic preparation alone.[94] A recent review with consideration of enhanced recovery principles supports this conclusion.[95] The 2019 practice guidelines of the American Society of Colon and Rectal Surgeons strongly support the continued use of bowel preparation in conjunction with oral antibiotic prophylaxis for patients undergoing elective colorectal surgery.[96] The adoption of more isotonic bowel preparation solutions in clinical practice may help mitigate some of the excessive fluid losses and electrolyte derangements associated with hypertonic agents, and ongoing adherence to enhanced recovery principles can help optimize patient status despite mechanical bowel preparation.[75]

Animal studies that were conducted as early as the 1970s measured evaporative abdominal losses in closed chambers and demonstrated that evaporative losses from fully exteriorized bowel surfaces plateaued at 1 mL/kg per hour.[97] The tendency for traditional calculations to overestimate fluid requirements in open abdominal cases was the impetus for a multitude of studies in the early 2000s on the impact of restrictive and goal-directed fluid therapies in improving outcomes of colorectal patients.[98-100] Many of these helped form the basis for contemporary goal-directed fluid management approaches.

The concept of the "third space" was introduced in the 1960s as a nonfunctional component of the ECV. Prior to understanding the role of neuroendocrine mechanisms in the stress response, the original study hypothesized that redistribution of extracellular fluids (ECFs) contributed to the tendency of postoperative patients to retain sodium and water.[101] By excluding fluid administration and utilizing isotope tracers to tag plasma components, the investigators hoped to identify the mechanisms of fluid redistribution. They measured suction contents, specimens, sponges, and laparotomy packs for isotopes and hemoglobin. They ultimately concluded that there was a measurable deficit in functional ECV (volume subject to transcapillary fluid dynamics) not attributable to blood loss, hence the third space.[101] The third space concept became a justification for the use of liberal perioperative fluid administration to compensate for redistribution of

BOX 21.2 Consequences of Inappropriate Fluid Administration

Underresuscitation	Overresuscitation
• Hypovolemia; decreased circulating volume • Decreased microvascular perfusion leading to decreased oxygen delivery • Reduced tissue perfusion • End-organ complications • PONV • Renal dysfunction • Myocardial ischemia • Hemoconcentration leading to increased blood viscosity, thrombotic events	• Vascular overload; acute CHF • Microvascular congestion leading to decreased oxygen delivery • Endothelial glycocalyx disruption • Decreased tissue oxygenation • Altered coagulation and potential hemorrhage • Hemodilution leading to anemia, thrombocytopenia, altered viscosity, coagulopathy, decreased oxygen carrying capacity • Decreased gut motility (ileus, delayed gastric emptying, anastomotic leak) • Increased infection rates; poor wound healing • Decreased organ perfusion • Increased EVLWI and prolonged postoperative mechanical ventilation • Increased incidence of ventilator-associated pneumonia • Hepatic congestion and dysfunction • Abdominal compartment syndrome

CHF, Congestive heart failure; *EVLWI*, extravascular lung water index; *PONV*, postoperative nausea and vomiting.

ECV into this nonfunctional space.[17,18] Nonetheless, the practice of replacing third space deficits became a doctrine of historical anesthetic practice.[102] Fluid management techniques that continue to account for the third space have been shown to result in poor clinical outcomes and gross fluid accumulation of up to 10 kg of perioperative weight gain.[10,17,18]

The tendency of historical approaches to support liberal fluid administration continues in the recommendations for managing acute blood loss. The 3:1 ratio of crystalloid solutions to estimated blood loss (EBL) was introduced to preserve intravascular volume while accounting for the interstitial filtration of crystalloids; however, evidence demonstrates that the actual observed ratio is less than 2:1.[10,24]

A significant limitation of historical methods that are associated with fluid administration is the reliance on static and nonspecific indices of fluid balance such as MAP, CVP, and urine output. Despite the value of these measures in the context of standard monitoring and basic vital support, they are not predictive of volume responsiveness.[2] MAP is an unreliable index of volume status; hypotensive patients may have a "relative hypovolemia" associated with altered vascular tone or impaired cardiac function despite adequate or excessive intravascular volume. Conversely, patients who are dependent on adequate preload may have intact compensatory mechanisms that preserve normotension.[103] Historic approaches often rely on fluid volume to treat hypotension, regardless of the cause (e.g., volume preloading to treat or prevent hypotension related to neuraxial sympathectomy, bolus fluids on induction of anesthesia to compensate for myocardial depression and vasodilation).[25,90] CVP is largely dependent on venous return; baseline values may also be altered in patients with right heart impairment, severe pulmonary disease, valvular disease, and portal hypertension.[103,104] Studies involving critically ill patients, including those with sepsis, demonstrated that only half of patients with low CVP values are fluid responsive.[105] Therefore CVP has limited value as a fluid

administration target and may lead to an extraordinarily high incidence of fluid overload in patients who may not be able to compensate for the increased vascular volume.[103,104]

Reliance on urine output as a measurement of volume status is not an accurate target for fluid administration because it can be impacted by a myriad of factors, including enhanced neuroendocrine responses.[106] Furthermore, volume administration in anesthetized oliguric patients with high levels of circulating ADH may preferentially expand the interstitial space.[23,80] ADH secretion can continue in the postoperative period, and patients who receive excessive intraoperative fluid volume may have difficulty excreting their salt and water overload postoperatively.[68,80]

A systematic review comparing restrictive perioperative fluid management with conventional techniques aimed at reversing oliguria, and the result indicated there was no difference in the incidence of oliguria or postoperative renal failure.[106] This and other studies challenge the classic concepts that (1) excess perioperative fluid is easily filtered by the kidneys, and (2) large fluid volumes are nephroprotective.[37]

Historical perspectives associated with fluid management have taught us that the administration of intravenous fluid is associated with advantages but also unintended physiologic consequences that can impair homeostasis. Much like other pharmaceutic interventions, intravenous fluids have clear indications, benefits, and (dose-dependent) side effects.[7,26,103] Despite the controversy related to the amount, strategy, and type of fluids to be administered perioperatively, there is widespread recognition among anesthetists and critical care providers of the consequences associated with intravenous fluid administration (Box 21.2).[7,17,103,104]

PERIOPERATIVE GOAL-DIRECTED FLUID THERAPY

The impact of perioperative goal-directed fluid therapy (GDFT) on the clinical outcomes of surgical patients has made the approach of fluid management a crucial component of anesthetic practice, particularly within the milieu of outcome-driven care. Achieving optimal fluid balance during the perioperative period is challenging, particularly if relying on standard monitoring parameters such as heart rate, blood pressure, urine output, and CVPs. These parameters, as discussed previously, often provide erroneous estimates of volume status. Research has demonstrated that perioperative GDFT is beneficial in reducing complications, supporting the timely recovery of bowel function in major abdominal surgery, and improving overall survival rates.

The foundational outcomes assessment of early GDFT was the 1980s trial by Shoemaker et al. evaluating the impact of targeting supernormal hemodynamic and oxygen transport values in patients undergoing high-risk surgical procedures. The study was based on the observation that survivors of high-risk surgical procedures had greater oxygen delivery (Do_2), arterial oxygen content (Cao_2), and cardiac index (CI) than nonsurvivors. By placing pulmonary artery catheters (PACs) in subjects preoperatively and utilizing the hemodynamic data to help augment CI and oxygen delivery index (Do_2I) throughout the perioperative period, the investigators were able to significantly impact overall survival. Patients in the PA catheter protocol group had reduced mortality, reduced ICU stays, and reduced perioperative complications compared to those in the control.[107] Shoemaker furthered his findings by publishing a large body of work on the impact of hemodynamic monitoring and measures of oxygen transport on survival among surgical and critically ill patients in septic shock.[108-110] Although supernormal hemodynamic targets are no longer advocated, Shoemaker's work continues to be valued for its fundamental contribution to the advancement of goal-directed therapy.[111]

As a result of concerns regarding supernormal hemodynamic end points, Research conducted by the mixed venous oxygen (Svo_2)

Collaborative Group studied over 10,000 patients across 56 ICUs in 1995 to determine if targeting supernormal hemodynamic values improved survival in critically ill patients. They concluded that normal values of CI and Do_2 yielded the same results as supernormal values. Thus there was little to no benefit in attempting to "force feed" oxygen to the tissues during periods of increased oxygen consumption.[112]

As a result of the impact of these and other studies, GDFT became a subject of broad interest and the focus of multiple research efforts.[2,8,9,111,113] The utility of GDFT in the intraoperative setting and a growing body of evidence to support its role in yielding positive patient outcomes catalyzed ongoing collaborative efforts between intraoperative and postoperative care providers in the provision of integrated perioperative fluid management. However, there were concerns about the necessity of placing an invasive monitoring device such as the PAC to obtain hemodynamic values. Cannesson published a study on the relationship between arterial blood pressure and respiratory variation in plethysmography during positive pressure ventilation.[114] This relationship and the concept of pulse contour analysis are the basis for many of the minimally invasive and noninvasive technologies used to determine volume responsiveness in modern practice.[4-6,103,104] GDFT has now been widely adopted as a standard of care in Europe and readily accepted as a guideline for clinical practice in the United States.[115,116]

More recent studies have sought to provide ongoing evaluation of the efficacy of GDFT in patients with sepsis. A meta-analysis of large RCTs evaluated 3723 patients with early septic shock at 138 hospitals around the world.[117] The findings showed that GDFT yielded no difference in outcomes or mortality and produced higher costs compared to standard care. A possible explanation of these results posited by the authors is the improvement in contemporary standard care.[111,117]

Recognition of the significance of oxygen transport balance and widespread adoption of hemodynamic parameters as both triggers and end points for fluid administration in emergency and perioperative medicine and critical care have narrowed the gap between GDFT and standard care of the septic patient.[8,35,50] The guidelines of the Surviving Sepsis Campaign also reflect some of these trends. MAP and CVP are recommended as dynamic variables to determine fluid responsiveness.[72,118]

Multiple early trials of GDFT revealed that goal-directed approaches yielded better outcomes and often delivered less total fluid volumes than those administered according to the liberal standards of care at that time.[35,75,98-100,113,115] Studies over the past decade have further examined the role of fluid restriction in uniquely promoting best patient outcomes. However, analysis of restrictive fluid management techniques has often been limited by a high degree of inconsistency in defining "restrictive" approaches. One study found that a "liberal" approach, as defined by one author, was only 10 mL different than a "restrictive" approach, as defined by another.[119] The contemporary solution to this challenge is to define a fluid management approach using perioperative weight gain as a surrogate indicator for hypervolemia.

The "zero balance" approach aims to avoid surplus fluid administration to achieve normovolemia as measured by strict maintenance of preoperative body weight throughout the perioperative period. Most zero-balance techniques involve a basal fluid infusion along with 1:1 fluid or blood product replacement of measurable blood and fluid losses as indicated.[75,120] Early studies on restrictive approaches showed that the zero balance approach decreased the incidence of postoperative morbidity compared to standard care.[121] Another trial evaluated 85 patients presenting for elective colectomy and compared GDFT within a fluid-restricting ERAS protocol to management with the ERAS protocol alone. Patients in the GDFT group received more intraoperative fluid and had better aortic flow, but there was no difference in patient-reported standard recovery scores (SRS), postoperative complication rate, or length of hospital stay.[122]

A series of meta-analyses examined the effects of GDFT on perioperative outcomes in major surgeries and found that GDFT significantly reduced perioperative complications (including AKI) and hospital length of stay.[9,124-126] Three of the studies showed that GDFT reduced mortality[123-125]; one of these demonstrated mortality benefit without decrease in morbidity.[123] Another review of 41 RCTs showed that GDFT yielded a significant decrease in morbidity with no effect on mortality.[126]

The Restrictive Versus Liberal Fluid Therapy (RELIEF) trial evaluated 3000 patients undergoing major abdominal surgery and receiving restrictive versus liberal fluid therapy. Restrictive fluid management was associated with increased risk of AKI and was not shown to confer any benefit for 1-year disability-free survival.[127] Subsequently, Cochrane analysis compared restrictive fluid therapy to GDFT to determine if restrictive approaches are more beneficial in terms of patient outcomes and cost. The review concluded that existing data are insufficient to determine superiority of either approach and that further high-quality research is needed.[128]

A single-center hospital registry study evaluated data on 92,094 noncardiac surgery patients to assess the relationship between intraoperative fluid management and postoperative outcomes. The results yielded a U-shaped distribution, whereby both liberal and restrictive fluid therapy produced greater morbidity, mortality, hospital length of stay, and cost than did fluid optimization.[129]

Some sources advocate for GDFT in high-risk surgical patients, with a zero-balance approach in low-risk cases.[8] The FEDORA trial examined the impact of perioperative GDFT in 420 low- to moderate-risk patients and demonstrated a significant reduction in complications and hospital length of stay.[130] This is noteworthy because it is the first outcomes assessment of its kind in a non–high-risk patient population.

A review of ERAS protocols in *JAMA Surgery* illustrated a combined fluid management strategy using elements of zero-balance fluid therapy (weight gain avoidance) with those of GDFT (targeted hemodynamic interventions and oxygen delivery optimization).[131] This has also been referred to as "goal-directed fluid restriction."[35]

A joint consensus statement on perioperative fluid therapy in colorectal surgery by the American Society for Enhanced Recovery (ASER) and Perioperative Quality Institute (POQI) recommends GDFT as the fluid strategy of choice in reducing perioperative complications but concedes that the zero-balance approach may be an acceptable alternative.[132] The ultimate aim of GDFT is to utilize individualized hemodynamic end points to support oxygen transport balance by minimizing oxygen demand and optimizing CO, tissue oxygenation, capillary and macrovascular flow, oxygen and nutrient delivery, and end-organ perfusion.[5,133] This augments the ability of surgical patients to tolerate the metabolic and hemodynamic disturbances associated with surgery, thus improving clinical outcomes (Box 21.3).

Perioperative Goal-Directed Therapy Protocols

The success of GDFT in improving clinical outcomes is largely the result of its algorithmic approach evaluating fluid responsiveness, identifying appropriate support measures when fluid is not indicated, and optimizing oxygen transport balance.[111,131] GDFT protocols often begin with a baseline assessment of target hemodynamic measures, followed by the administration of a small volume fluid bolus (200–250 mL) to assess the patient's position along the Frank-Starling curve.[111] By integrating fluid administration triggers, small volume boluses, and defined targets for cessation of fluid therapy, GDFT protocols provide important clinical end points for assessing response to fluid intervention and preventing vascular overload. These guidelines also provide prompts for consideration of vasoactive or inotropic support. Most protocols promote constant reassessment of factors such as preload

BOX 21.3 Measured Outcomes of GDFT as Compared to Standard Fluid Management Approaches in High-Risk Surgical Patients

- ↓Infection rate
- ↓Duration of mechanical ventilation
- ↓Bowel motility
- ↓PONV
- ↓Coagulopathy
- ↓Hemorrhage
- ↓Cardiovascular complications
- ↓Respiratory complications
- ↓Anemia
- ↓Hypotension
- ↓Length of hospital stay
- ↓30-day organ complication rate
- ↓ICU length of stay in high-risk patients
- ↓Urinary tract infections
- ↓Incidence of postoperative renal impairment
- ↓Perioperative mortality rates among patients at very high risk for perioperative death

GDFT, Goal-directed fluid therapy; *ICU*, intensive care unit; *PONV*, postoperative nausea and vomiting.

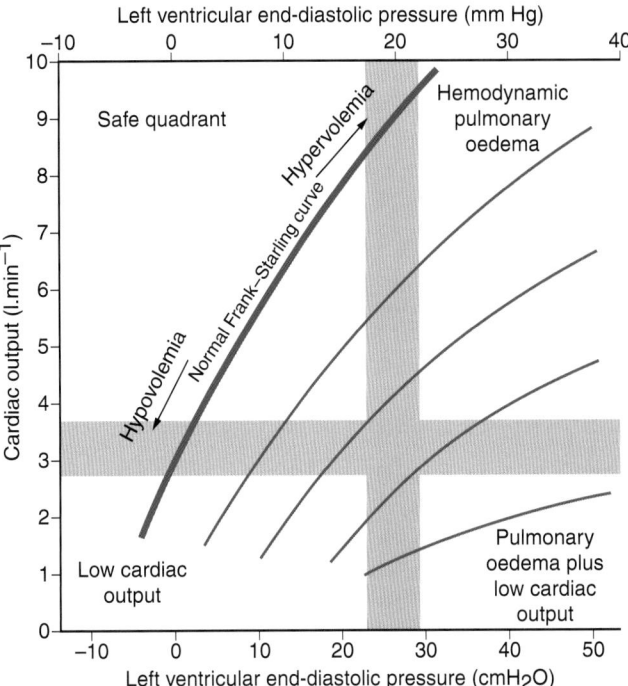

Fig. 21.4 Quadrant diagram relating cardiac output to left ventricular end-diastolic pressure. The thick blue curve is a typical normal Frank-Starling curve. To the right are curves representing progressive left ventricular failure. *(Top left)* The safe quadrant, which contains a substantial part of the normal curve, but much less of the curves representing ventricular failure. *(Top right)* The quadrant representing normal cardiac output but raised left atrial pressure, attained at the upper end of relatively normal Frank-Starling curves (e.g., hypervolemia). There is a danger of hemodynamic pulmonary edema. *(Bottom left)* The quadrant representing normal or low left atrial pressure but low cardiac output, attained at the lower end of all curves (e.g., hypovolemia). The patient is in shock. *(Bottom right)* The quadrant representing both low cardiac output and raised left atrial pressure. There is simultaneous danger of pulmonary edema and shock, and the worst Frank-Starling curves hardly leave this quadrant. (From Lumb AB. *Nunn's Applied Respiratory Physiology*. 8th ed. Philadelphia: Elsevier; 2017:413.)

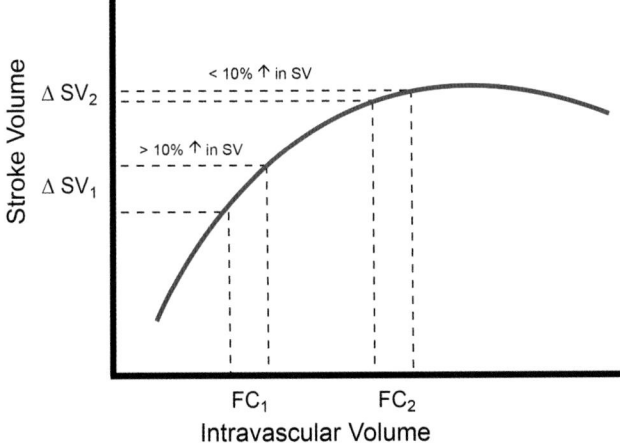

Fig. 21.3 Optimal fluid administration. *FC,* Flow cell; *SV,* stroke volume. (From Miller TE, et al. State-of-the-art fluid management in the operating room. *Best Pract Res Clin Anaesthesiol.* 2014;28[3]:262.)

responsiveness and oxygen delivery (every 5–10 minutes). This aids in the timely administration of fluid and other interventions, such as vasoactive medications, that have been shown to have a tremendous impact on preserving both endothelial and global perfusion.[2,4,5,26]

Hemodynamic Monitoring and Patient Goal-Directed Therapy

Perioperative goal-directed therapy relies on modern hemodynamic modalities to provide measurable clinical end points as a guide for both initiation and cessation of fluid administration. The ability to recognize relevant clinical end points and manipulate real-time physiologic targets to optimize regional and global perfusion during surgery allows the anesthetists to focus on definitive interventions involving fluid replacement, vasoactive support, inotropy, and/or blood transfusion. Measures of fluid responsiveness, oxygen transport, and microvascular flow help focus fluid delivery to ensure optimal volume and to mitigate the significant consequences associated with fluid mismanagement (Fig. 21.3).

The Frank-Starling Mechanism

The basis of the Frank-Starling mechanism is the relationship between left ventricular end-diastolic volume (LVEDV) and myocardial contractility (as measured by SV). An increase in left ventricular preload will, to an extent, increase myocardial contractility by stretching cardiac sarcomeres and optimizing the overlap of actin and myosin filaments to generate greater myocardial force.[19,111] This allows the myocardium to compensate for increases in ventricular preload. The Frank-Starling mechanism is highly effective until the point at which the sarcomere cannot generate additional force. Further increases in preload after this threshold will generate no further increases in SV.[134]

This relationship is depicted as a classic left ventricular pressure-volume curve, with volume (LVEDV) appearing on the x-axis and pressure (SV) appearing on the y-axis (Fig. 21.4).[11] The ascending portion of this curve represents preload dependence. Patients whose cardiac profile correspond to this curve will respond to fluid volume by increasing SV. The plateau portion of the curve represents preload independence, and patients along this portion of the curve are unable to generate any additional myocardial force in response to fluid volume. Knowledge of individual patient physiology is important in assessing a patient's position along the curve. Patients with normal left ventricular function are on the physiologic curve. The long ascent of this curve suggests that the heart will continue to increase contractility in response to greater volumes of fluid. Patients with heart failure or ventricular dysfunction are on the pathophysiologic curve. The long plateau of this curve indicates that the heart can tolerate only small volumes of fluid before it is unable to increase contractility. Patients with poor ventricular compliance may proceed from a state of preload dependence to one of volume overload with the addition of very small volumes of fluid.

This underscores the importance of small fixed-volume fluid boluses as part of GDFT protocols.[111] The differentiation between preload dependence and preload independence is perhaps one of the most vital components of GDFT in tailoring interventions to individual cardiovascular status and preventing complications associated with fluid overload. Failure to recognize preload independence in hypotensive patients is often the mechanism for inappropriate fluid administration.

Dilution Technique and Devices

Dilutional techniques involve the introduction of a fixed volume of injectate into the vascular system and the consequent measure of CO and other hemodynamic variables based on the area under a time-temperature or concentration-time curve.[135] The thermodilution PAC is the classic dilutional monitoring device. A fixed volume of chilled injectate is introduced into the right atrium (RA), and blood temperature is measured with a thermistor in the pulmonary artery. CO is calculated according to the area under the time-temperature curve.[135] Low CO coincides with a larger area under the curve because of the time required for the chilled fluid to transit through the heart. The PAC is the most invasive of the hemodynamic monitors used in GDFT, and it can be very useful in the comprehensive assessment of cardiac function, pulmonary artery occlusion pressure (PAOP), and measures of pulmonary edema, but it also carries significant risks (including bleeding, pulmonary artery rupture, thrombus, infection, and arrhythmias).[135,136]

The PiCCO hemodynamic system (Pulsion Medical Systems, Feldkirchen, Germany) involves calibrated pulse waveform analysis to provide measures of fluid responsiveness, contractility, preload, afterload, and extravascular lung water with separate central venous and central arterial (often femoral) lines.[137] Calibration is performed with traditional transpulmonary thermodilution; the chilled injectate is introduced into the venous line, and blood temperature is measured in the artery. The PulsioFlex monitoring platform (Pulsion Medical Systems, Feldkirchen, Germany) can also incorporate data from other inputs to provide central venous oxygen saturation (Scvo$_2$) and noninvasive measures of organ function.[137,138]

The VolumeView set (Edwards Lifesciences, Irvine, CA, USA) utilizes a femoral arterial catheter with an integrated thermistor in conjunction with a central venous line to provide hemodynamic data as well as transpulmonary thermodilution-based measurements.[139] The EV1000 monitoring component (Edwards Lifesciences, Irvine, CA, USA) provides integration of both noninvasive and invasive data, including central venous, arterial, and noninvasive inputs to provide dynamic measures of fluid responsiveness in addition to global hemodynamic values and measures of tissue oxygenation.[139,140]

The LiDCOplus/PulseCO hemodynamic monitoring system (LiDCO, London, UK) is a calibrated pulse waveform analysis device that utilizes a chemical dilution technique. A fixed volume of lithium chloride is administered intravascularly via peripheral or central venous access, and lithium ion concentration is measured with a sensor in the artery. The software component of the system evaluates preload responsiveness and can be used to calculate measures of oxygenation with the input of blood gas values. The accompanying LiDCOunity monitoring platform integrates additional data, including depth of anesthesia.[141]

Pulse Contour Analysis

Pulse contour analysis provides dynamic measures of preload responsiveness by quantifying the degree of change of arterial, capnography, or pulse oximetry waveforms associated with cyclic respiratory variations and the resulting pleural pressure. Measures of fluid responsiveness include plethysmography variability index, stroke volume variation (SVV), systolic pressure variation, and pulse pressure variation (PPV). These dynamic indices are particularly valuable in assessing real-time response to fluids and vasoactive interventions and are often utilized as part of minimally invasive or noninvasive technologies. The utility of noninvasive monitoring platforms lies in their favorable low-risk profile, and also offers the additional advantage of continued monitoring during the immediate postoperative period. The ability to evaluate hemodynamic measures throughout the perioperative period helps ensure continuity of GDFT and promotes enhanced recovery strategies. The use of noninvasive technology to measure dynamic parameters is based on the physiology of cyclic intracardiac pressure changes during ventilation.[5,6,104,114]

The increase in pleural pressure of mechanically ventilated patients during inspiration augments left ventricle (LV) filling as a result of compression of pulmonary veins and pleural restriction of right ventricle (RV) filling (leading to enhanced LV compliance); this contributes to an increase in SV. During expiration, SV falls when the reduced RV preload has had time to transit through the heart.[6,104] The degree of variation in SV is more prominent during hypovolemia due to the following: (a) increased intrathoracic pressure from PPV decreases RV filling, (b) greater inspiratory impact on RV afterload if alveolar pressure exceeds pulmonary arterial and venous pressures impeding RV ejection, and (c) greater ventricular contractility in response to the LV preload "bolus" if the patient is on the ascending portion of the Frank-Starling curve.[6]

Dynamic measures derived from pulse contour analysis are considered to be predictive of fluid responsiveness if the calculated value is greater than 13%.[6,101] However, there is a well-documented gray zone in which values of 9% to 13% fail to accurately predict fluid responsiveness in up to 25% of patients; correlation with additional hemodynamic measures is recommended.[2,6,142] Despite the utility of these parameters for predicting fluid responsiveness and providing real-time measures of cardiovascular response to interventions, there are some known limitations with their use (Table 21.2).[6,24]

Arterial waveform analysis is used for assessment of cardiac output and fluid responsiveness. Some current applications involve the integration of a specialized sensor-containing pressure transducer with a monitoring platform that utilizes proprietary algorithms to compute hemodynamic values.[143] Examples include the FloTrac sensor with the EV1000 or Hemosphere platforms (Edwards Lifesciences, Irvine, CA, USA)[140,144] and the ProAQT with the PulsioFlex platform (Pulsion Medical Systems, Feldkirchen, Germany).[138] The LiDCOrapid/PulseCO system (LiDCO, London, UK) uses a platform-based sensor that interfaces with a standard arterial pressure transducer to provide hemodynamic data.[141]

Evolution of hemodynamic monitoring capability and widespread interest in the use of dynamic measures to guide fluid management and clinical care has led to the development of noninvasive monitors. The ClearSight system (Edwards Lifesciences, Irvine, CA, USA) is a noninvasive inflatable finger cuff that utilizes the volume clamp method to apply continuous uniform pressure to the artery; recording of the cuff pressure yields a finger arterial pressure waveform.[145] The data undergo algorithmic reconstruction with the EV1000 platform to produce a brachial arterial pressure waveform, and a complex physiologic model integrates real-time arterial waveform analysis data with individual patient parameters and digital feedback to produce cardiac

TABLE 21.2 Limitations of Dynamic Measures

Limitation	Cause
Spontaneous ventilation	Spontaneous ventilation produces a dissimilar waveform variation as a result of negative intrathoracic pressure. Furthermore, the degree of variance produced by spontaneous ventilation is small, and respiratory rate and tidal volume may be irregular.
Small tidal volumes	The dynamic variables measured by pulse contour analyses have been tested using tidal volumes of 8 mL/kg. Smaller tidal volumes may be insufficient to produce significant intrathoracic pressure changes to predict fluid responsiveness. In the setting of low-tidal volume ventilation, small values may not be predictive, but values >13%–15% will still indicate fluid responsiveness.
Open chest	Measurements based on intrathoracic pressure variations lose their reliability in open thorax conditions; echocardiography is recommended.
Sustained arrhythmias	Variations in stroke volume are likely to be caused by beat-to-beat variability in SV secondary to decreased cardiac filling times or loss of atrial kick, rather than fluid responsiveness.
PEEP	High levels of PEEP may elevate intrathoracic pressure such that hemodynamic variables will be falsely elevated.
Right heart dysfunction	Elevation of dynamic variables in patients with severe right heart disease may reflect ventilation-associated alterations in RV afterload rather than volume responsiveness.

PEEP, Positive end-expiratory pressure; *RV,* right ventricle; *SV,* stroke volume.

output measures.[140,145] This methodology also forms the basis for the CNAP (Continuous Noninvasive Arterial Pressure) double finger sensor (CNSystems Medizintechnik AG, Graz, Austria).[146] A summary of hemodynamic measures can be found in Table 21.3.

Esophageal Doppler and Echocardiography

Esophageal Doppler monitoring applies Doppler ultrasound technology to assess thoracic aortic blood velocity and provide real-time measures of LV function and aortic compliance in addition to dynamic measures of preload responsiveness such as corrected flow time (FTc), SV, and change in peak aortic pulse wave velocity (ΔP).[8,75,133,143,147,148] It offers a less invasive means for direct measurement of hemodynamic parameters, and esophageal Doppler monitoring has become a standard of care in the United Kingdom.[133] Transesophageal echocardiography is a gold standard for direct evaluation of cardiac function and volume status, although its use is limited to those who have been board certified by the National Board of Echocardiography.[149] Perioperative echocardiography can provide invaluable data by providing real-time visualization of ventricular size, systolic and diastolic functional status, valvular abnormalities, volume status, wall motion abnormalities, and cardiac handling of fluid administration.[150,151]

Measures of Transthoracic Impedance

Thoracic impedance cardiography (ICG), or thoracic electrical bioimpedance (TEB), is based on known distinctions in measurable electrical conductance between various biologic structures and their relationship to hemodynamics throughout the cardiac cycle.[75,143] TEB devices utilize paired surface electrodes around the thoracic margins at the level of the neck and the diaphragm. Low level alternating electrical current

is transmitted through the chest from the outside sensors and seeks the path of least resistance through the chest cavity in accordance with Ohm's law.[8,143] Electrocardiography and electrical impedance (resistance) are measured by the inside sensors. The timing and amplitude of variations in impedance associated with fluctuations in blood flow during the cardiac cycle are mapped as a continuous waveform and integrated with software data to produce measurements of cardiac output and other hemodynamic parameters.[5,8,75,143] Limitations of this modality, particularly in devices that rely on change-of-phase measurements, include interference from pleural and pericardial effusions, arrythmias, aortic valve insufficiency, aortic aneurysm, morbid obesity, and movement artifacts.[75,143,152]

There are multiple TEB devices available for clinical use. These include the Aesculon (Osypka Medical, Berlin, Germany),[153] the BioZ Cardio Profile (SonoSite, Inc, Bothell, WA, USA),[154] the NICaS (NI Medical, Petah Tikva, Israel),[155] the Starling SV (Cheetah Medical, Vancouver, WA, USA),[156] and the Task Force (CNSystems Medizintechnik AG, Graz, Austria).[157]

Measures of Tissue Oxygenation

The use of oxygen transport measures as targets for GDFT has long been known to impact survival rates in high-risk and critically ill patients.[5] Measures of tissue oxygenation evaluate global tissue oxygen balance with measurement of arterial, mixed venous, and central venous blood gases, and calculation of oxygen consumption (Vo_2) and delivery (Do_2). Integrated invasive technologies combine invasive lines (PAC, central venous catheter, arterial line) with software inputs of blood gas data to calculate tissue oxygenation measures. The primary goal for GDFT is to maintain oxygen transport balance by optimizing Do_2 (fluid optimization, preservation of CO and microcirculatory flow, transfusion) and to minimize Vo_2 (opioids, β-blockers, maintenance of normothermia).[5,76,78,111,158] Active blood loss during surgery causes an imbalance in oxygen transport through loss of both circulating volume and oxygen carrying capacity. The judicious administration of packed red blood cells to optimize Do_2 is an important and often controversial consideration in perioperative fluid management. This topic is discussed in detail in Chapter 22.

Perioperative Goal-Directed Therapy and Enhanced Recovery

Optimal perioperative fluid replacement and management is a fundamental component of fast-track programs such as ERAS, which is a proactive, multimodal, patient management pathway aimed at improving surgical outcomes. Protocols for ERAS incorporate best practices that are designed to provide optimal fluid therapy, reduce the profound stress response attributed to surgery, promote nonopioid postoperative pain modalities, and maintain baseline organ function postprocedure. Ultimately, goals for the ERAS pathway for major surgical procedures are to decrease postoperative complications, to accelerate recovery after surgery, and to promote early mobilization and discharge from hospitalization.[159] A growing body of evidence supports the ERAS pathway based on documented improvements with postoperative outcomes and the overall decrease in health care costs associated with surgery.[160]

A colorectal surgeon from Denmark, Henrik Kehlet was the first to coin the concept of enhanced recovery in the 1990s when he asked the simple question, "Why is the patient still in the hospital after surgery?" He determined the causes were multifactorial, yet he concluded that the common issues faced by postoperative patients were ultimately caused by delays in both gut function and physical mobility after surgery.[161] Based on these observations, protocols were developed aimed at addressing the issues that contribute to prolonged postoperative convalescence and promote interventions that facilitate an improved state of health.

TABLE 21.3 Common Hemodynamic Measures

Abbreviation	Parameter	Normal Values	Measures
CO/CI	Cardiac output/cardiac index	CO: 4–8 L/min CI: 2.5–4 L/min/m²	Measures volume of blood pumped by the left ventricle in 1 min; CI is normalized for body surface area (BSA)
Do_2I	Oxygen delivery index	Do_2I: 450–650 mL/min/m²	Calculated value, which combines hemoglobin concentration, hemoglobin carrying capacity, CI, and arterial oxygen saturation to provide an indicator of tissue perfusion
EVLWI	Extravascular lung water index	3–7 mL/kg	Measure of fluid filtration into the interstitial space of the lung; index of pulmonary edema
FTc	Corrected flow time	330–360 ms	Measures the forward flow of blood through the aorta during systole (flow time) and corrects it to a heart rate of 60 beats/min; surrogate index of left ventricular ejection time
GEDI	Global end-diastolic index	680–800 mL/m²	Preload (end-diastolic) measurement of all cardiac chambers; measure of volume status normalized for BSA
O_2ER/O_2ERe	Oxygen extraction ratio/oxygen extraction ratio estimate	Values are organ-dependent; normal range from 22%–30%	O_2ER is a direct measure of the difference between arterial and venous oxygen saturation at a given tissue; O_2ERe is calculated based on the difference between arterial and mixed or central venous oxygen saturation
ΔPV	Change in peak velocity	>12% predicts preload responsiveness	Change in peak aortic pulse wave velocity
PPV/ΔPP	Pulse pressure variation/Δ pulse pressure	>13% predicts preload responsiveness	Variation in arterial pulse pressure
PVI	Plethysmography variability index	>14% predicts preload responsiveness	Calculated variability in amplitude of pulse oximetry plethysmography
$Scvo_2$	Central venous oxygen saturation	Normal value 70% (~2%–8% lower than Svo_2 values caused by cerebral oxygen consumption)	Venous oxygen saturation of blood in the superior vena cava as measured by a central venous catheter
SPV	Systolic pressure variation	>14% predicts preload responsiveness	Variation in systolic pressure based on pulse contour analysis
SV/SVI	Stroke volume/stroke volume index	SV: 60–100 mL/beat SVI: 33–47 mL/m²/beat	SV measures volume of blood pumped by the left ventricle in one heartbeat; SVI is normalized for BSA
SVR/SVRI	Systemic vascular resistance/systemic vascular resistance index	SVR: 800–1200 dynes-sec/cm⁻⁵/m² SVRI: 1970-2390 dynes-sec/cm⁻⁵/m²	Measure of resistance of peripheral circulation; index of afterload; SVRI is normalized for BSA
Svo_2	Mixed venous oxygen saturation	Normal value 60–80% (~2%–8% higher than $Scvo_2$ values due to mixed venous blood from both the IVC and SVC)	Venous oxygen saturation of blood in the pulmonary artery as measured by a PAC
SVV	Stroke volume variation	>13% predicts preload responsiveness	Variation in stroke volume calculated by esophageal Doppler monitoring measurements or based on pulse-contour analysis

Enhanced Recovery After Surgery

ERAS was initially developed for colon resection surgery. Enhanced recovery principles are now being used for various surgical procedures, including abdominal vascular surgeries, esophagectomy, pancreatectomy, gastric resection, cystectomy, colorectal surgeries, gynecologic surgeries, orthopedic, and bariatric procedures.[160-162] ERAS programs, specifically for abdominal surgical procedures, have been implemented in many countries around the world and are well established in 17 countries to date.[160] The ERAS Society has developed 22 treatment items under the ERAS Protocol (Fig. 21.5).

Lassen et al.[163] developed a consensus review of clinical studies demonstrating optimal perioperative care utilizing ERAS protocols for patients undergoing colorectal surgery. The authors determined that 15 of the 20 treatment items reviewed suggested that the evidence demonstrated a strong indication that the ERAS protocols are beneficial and improve postsurgical outcomes. Implementation of the various ERAS

protocols requires a multidisciplinary team committed to consistently integrating the treatment items for each surgical patient during the perioperative continuum, which include the preoperative, intraoperative, and postoperative time periods.

Preoperative Fluid Management in ERAS Protocol

Optimal perioperative fluid management is an essential component of the ERAS pathway and important for improving postsurgical outcomes. The long-standing practice standard for preoperative surgical patients was nil per os (NPO) for at least 6 to 8 hours. This practice contributed to a state of relative dehydration and metabolic demand prior to surgery.[164,165] The goal of ERAS during the preoperative period is for the patient to arrive in the operating room in a euvolemic state.[166,167] A Cochrane review of research articles demonstrated substantial evidence that allowing clear fluids up to 2 hours prior to surgery during the preoperative fasting period does not increase complications.[168,169]

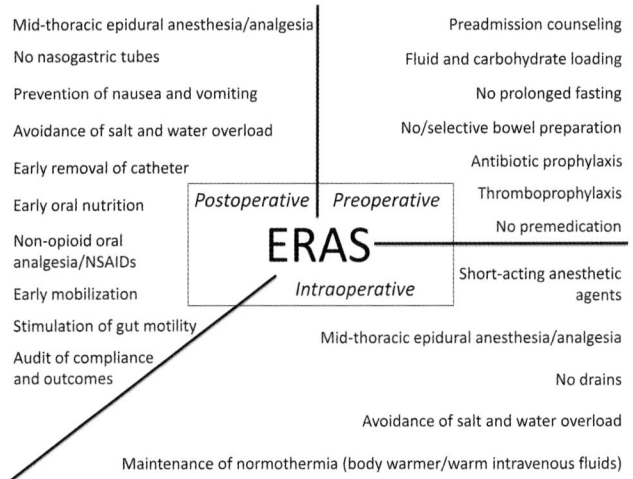

Fig. 21.5 Components of Enhanced Recovery After Surgery (ERAS). (From Varadhan KK, et al. Enhanced recovery after surgery: the future of improving surgical care. *Crit Care Clin.* 2010;26[3]:527-547.)

Furthermore, the practice standard for prolonged 8-hour fasting demonstrated neither a reduction in gastric contents nor an increase in gastric fluid pH.[169] Based on this and other evidence, in 2017 the ASA updated its practice guidelines for preoperative fasting. The new guidelines recommend the following fasting intervals[170]:
Clear liquids: 2 hours
Breast milk: 4 hours
Infant formula/nonhuman milk/light meal: 6 hours
Heavy meal (fried foods, fatty foods, meats): 8 hours

Miller et al.[166] recommend avoiding the routine use of mechanical bowel preparation (MBP) prior to colorectal surgery as an additional means of preventing dehydration on the day of surgery. The administration of hypertonic MBP for colorectal surgical patients can vary based on the surgeon's preference. The existing evidence indicates that MBP results in fluid shifts and increases postoperative morbidity.[169,171,172] Implementing two ERAS interventions of supplying a carbohydrate drink up to 2 hours prior to surgery and eliminating MBP when possible are proven methods that have contributed to improved optimization of the patient during the preoperative phase.[171,172] Supplying a carbohydrate drink 2 hours prior to surgery has the added benefit of maintaining adequate preoperative glucose and insulin levels, thereby reducing preoperative thirst, hunger, and anxiety levels experienced by the patient.[169] Decreasing NPO time results in a reduced state of relative dehydration prior to surgery. Thus the patient is subsequently less likely to develop hypotension caused by hypovolemia during the intraoperative phase. Patients are also less likely to be fluid responsive after the induction of anesthesia when compared to patients undergoing traditional preoperative fasting protocols.[172,173]

Intraoperative Fluid Management in ERAS Protocol

Traditional intraoperative fluid management consisted of replacement of perceived fasting-related volume deficits according to the 4-2-1 calculation and accounted for insensible or third space losses ranging from 1 to 15 mL/kg per hour. This estimate was highly subjective, and the volume infused varied among anesthesia providers. The concept of third space loss continues to be considered controversial because the initial trials studying ECV were flawed.[174] Standard fluid replacement during surgery also incorporates the EBL during the procedure, thus an additional 3 mL of crystalloid solution is administered for each milliliter of blood loss that is estimated by the practitioner.

Cumulatively, the surgical patient can receive intravenous fluid replacement based upon four concepts of fluid deficit: NPO fluid deficit, maintenance fluid requirements, third space fluid shifts or losses, and EBL. The standard fluid replacement paradigm is subjective, and it can vary based on the anesthetist's estimates and preferences. Liberal fluid administration can result in net weight gain experienced by the patient. Even a modest weight gain of approximately 3 kg as a result of intravenous fluid administration after elective colonic resection is associated with delayed recovery of gastrointestinal function, increased rate of complications, and prolonged hospital length of stay.[122,167] Overall, there is definitive scientific evidence suggesting that excessive fluid administration during the intraoperative phase contributes to detrimental side effects such as edema of the gut wall and prolonged ileus.[167,175] Lobo et al.[167] determined that a "change in fluid management alone on the day of surgery has been shown to reduce postoperative complications by 50%."

Perioperative Goal-Directed Therapy and ERAS

Incorporating an ERAS protocol such as GDFT reduces variations in practice. For example, a provider may treat intraoperative hypotension with a fluid challenge, ranging from a bolus of crystalloid or colloid solution of 250 to 500 mL, whereas another provider may opt to support hypotension pharmacologically with vasopressor therapy. Surgical outcomes can be improved by reducing treatment variability by using GDFT during intraoperative anesthetic management.

Postoperative Phase and ERAS

Fluid management within the ERAS protocol is continued when the patient transitions to the postoperative phase. Early discontinuation of intravenous fluid therapy and initiation of oral intake are encouraged. The authors conclude that the several liters of crystalloid fluid administered on postoperative day 1 to treat reduced urine output can cause postoperative ileus and delay hospital discharge.[166,175]

New Paradigm in Perioperative Fluid Management

Fluid therapy utilizing an ERAS pathway is largely based on the goal of maintaining euvolemia.[131,132,166,167] Fluid replacement during surgery is necessary and is often the first line of treatment for hemodynamic support and a conduit for medication administration. The traditional approach to perioperative volume therapy has been standardized and simplistic based on a fixed-volume approach. However, the subjective factors such as evaporative losses, third space loss, and ambiguous EBL amounts result in variations in fluid management and oftentimes excessive perioperative fluid administration.[101,162]

Another component of ERAS is to mitigate the physiologic changes the body experiences in response to surgery and to avoid fluid shifts. The body releases catabolic hormones and inflammatory mediators to facilitate salt and water retention in an effort to preserve intravascular volume and maintain blood pressure.[122] The physiologic response to surgery results in indirect and direct cellular injury. Direct surgical trauma from incision, heating elements such as cautery, retraction of internal organs, and so on, can lead to primary cellular injury. Primary cellular injury can impair oxygen and nutrient delivery to vital organs resulting from global and local perfusion changes. Secondary cellular injury is a process caused by the stress response associated with surgery that results in the release of local inflammatory mediators or the systemic effects of cytokines, inflammatory mediators, or hormones. The combination of both primary and secondary injury at the cellular level has been attributed to delayed wound healing and gut dysfunction, and may lead to postsurgical complications.[122,175,176] The two fundamental elements that affect postsurgical outcomes are attributed to fluid therapy and effective pain management.

ELECTROLYTE BALANCE

Disorders of Sodium Balance

Sodium and water balance within the various fluid compartments are in a dynamic state of change, and they are a vitally important component in determining the intravascular fluid volume. Sodium is the most abundant electrolyte in the ECV and, along with chloride, is responsible for the majority of osmotic activity of the ECV. A key physiologic action of sodium relates to its effect on increasing or decreasing ECV and ICV osmolality or tonicity. Water moves between ECV and ICV across cell membranes from an area of low solute concentration to high solute concentration to achieve equilibrium. These changes in water concentration are largely determined by sodium. The concentration of sodium is significantly higher in the ECV as compared to the ICV (ECV = 140 mEq/L, ICV = 25 mEq/L). The action of the Na-K-ATPase pump, which is located within cellular membranes, utilizes cellular energy to maintain cation ionic neutrality between the ECV and ICV.

An example of the physiologic effect associated with sodium disorders concerns the influence of sodium on the water content within neurons in the brain. The blood-brain barrier (BBB), unlike peripheral capillary beds, has only limited permeability to ionic solutes. The result of this limited permeability in the BBB prevents equilibration of osmotically active ionic solutes between ECV and ICV. This lack of permeability to sodium (and consequent failure to equilibrate osmotically active solutes between the intravascular and interstitial spaces) changes the osmotic gradients between fluid compartments, leading to the precedence of sodium over plasma proteins as the most important osmotically active substance influencing the water content of the brain tissues.[177]

Sodium imbalances reflect an impaired concentration between water and sodium. Evaluation of sodium imbalance should take into consideration both the volume of the solvent (water) and the amount of solute sodium (NA^+) present in the solution. Likewise, treatment of sodium imbalances can involve restriction or expansion of water volume and enhanced elimination or supplementation of sodium. One example involves the development of dilutional hyponatremia that can occur during various surgeries, including endometrial ablation and transurethral resection of the prostate. The absorption of large quantities of hypotonic fluid, which is used as irrigation, enters the ECV and causes NA^+ to become diluted. The hyponatremia that ensues can have deleterious effects on the brain and the heart. Thus there is no actual loss of sodium, but a dilution effect has occurred. This syndrome is commonly treated by decreasing ECV with fluid restriction or by administering diuretics to decrease intravascular volume. As the ECV contracts, NA^+ moves from the interstitial space back into the intravascular space. The result of normalizing ECV NA^+ concentrations allows for typical physiologic functioning.

The causative factors and manifestations associated with hyponatremia are listed in Box 21.4. The rapidity and extent by which significant hyponatremia occurs will determine the severity of clinical manifestations (Table 21.4). Of particular interest to anesthetists is hyponatremia resulting from the syndrome of inappropriate secretion of ADH (SIADH), which is further discussed in Chapter 37. Water intoxication and SIADH can also lead to hyponatremia from an excess of water, not loss of sodium.

Hyponatremia

Hyponatremia results in a condition in which the intracellular environment is hyperosmolar relative to the ECV leading to an influx of water into the ICV. One of the most significant consequences of hyponatremia is cerebral edema. As the brain is contained within the fixed confines of the cranium, cerebral edema is poorly tolerated. Compensatory mechanisms can delay the development of symptomatic cerebral

---

BOX 21.4 Hyponatremia: Classification, Causative Factors, and Manifestations*

Isotonic Hyponatremia (Pseudohyponatremia)
Serum osmolality 270–300 mOsm/kg
Causes: Hyperlipidemia, hyperproteinemia, multiple myeloma, infusion of isotonic nonelectrolytic substances (e.g., glucose, mannitol glycine)

Hypertonic Hyponatremia
Serum osmolality >300 mOsm/kg
Causes: Hyperglycemia, mannitol excess glycerol therapy

Hypotonic Hyponatremia
Serum osmolality <270 mOsm/kg

Hypovolemic hypotonic hyponatremia
Causes: Diuretics, salt-losing nephropathy, ketonuria, Addison disease, vomiting, diarrhea, third spacing of fluids, excessive sweating

Isovolemic hypotonic hyponatremia
Causes: SIADH, renal failure, hypothyroidism, drugs, water intoxication, porphyria, pain, stress, positive pressure ventilation

Hypervolemic hypotonic hyponatremia
Causes: Nephrotic syndrome, cirrhosis, congestive heart failure, renal failure

Clinical Manifestations
- Nausea and vomiting
- Cramps
- Weakness
- Agitation
- Confusion
- Headache
- Anorexia
- Cerebral edema
- Seizures
- Coma

*Serum sodium <135 mEq/L.
SIADH, Syndrome of inappropriate secretion of antidiuretic hormone.

TABLE 21.4 Sodium Levels and Physiologic Manifestations

Plasma NA+ Concentration mEq/L Levels	Signs/Symptoms
135–130	No signs/symptoms, mild neurologic signs/symptoms possible
129–125	Nausea, malaise
124–115	Headache, lethargy, altered level of consciousness
<115 and/or rapid onset	Seizures, coma, respiratory arrest, cerebral herniation

---

edema. Brain cells can maintain osmotic equilibrium by extruding intracellular solutes, thereby reducing intracellular osmolality. However, if the extrusion of solute by brain cells is inadequate to compensate for the hypoosmolar influence of the ECF, an intracellular influx of water may lead to symptomatic cerebral edema neuronal cell death.[178]

Clinical studies have demonstrated that when compared with men or postmenopausal women, menstruating women are at increased risk

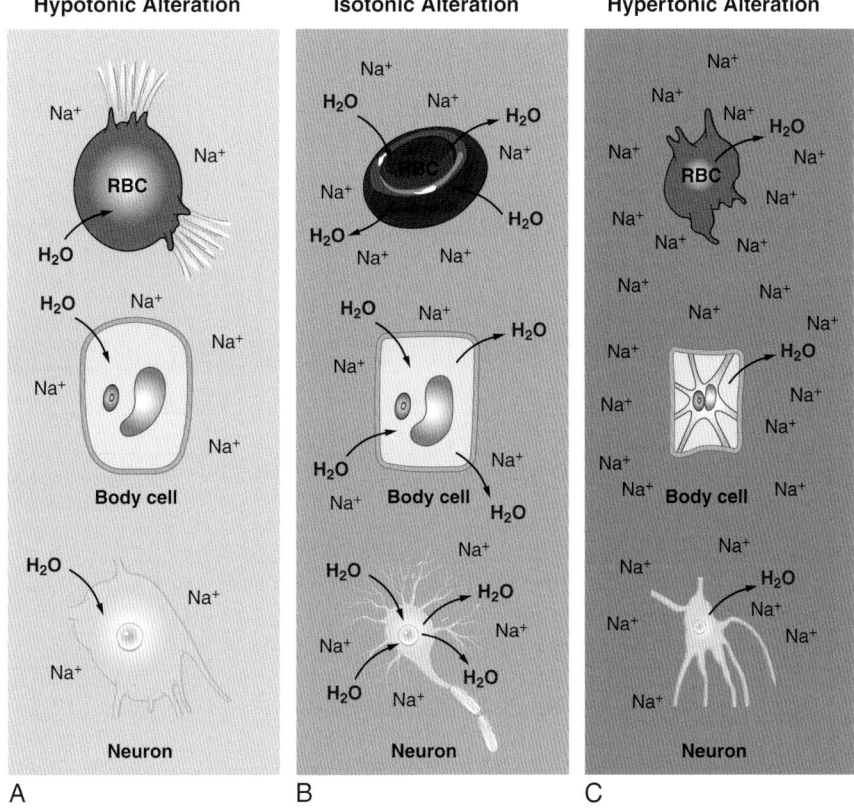

Fig. 21.6 Effects of alterations in extracellular sodium concentration in RBC, body cell, and neuron. (A) *Hypotonic alteration:* Decrease in ECF sodium *(Na)* concentration (hyponatremia) results in ICF osmotic attraction of water with swelling and potential busting of cells. (B) *Isotonic alteration:* Normal concentration of sodium in the ECF and no change in shifts of fluid in or out of cells. (C) *Hypertonic alteration:* An increase in ECF sodium concentration (hypernatremia) results in osmotic attraction of water out of cells with cell shrinkage. *ECF,* Extracellular fluid; *ICF,* intracellular fluid; *RBC,* red blood cell. (From McCance KL, et al. *Pathophysiology.* 7th ed. St. Louis: Elsevier; 2014:110.)

of brain damage resulting from hyponatremia. It is believed that estrogen and progesterone inhibit the efficiency of the Na-K-ATPase pump, which is essential to the extrusion of intracellular solutes to maintain osmotic equilibrium in hyponatremia; female sex hormones may facilitate movement of water into the brain through the mediation of ADH.[179]

Hyponatremia is the most common electrolyte abnormality in hospitalized patients. The development of hypervolemic hyponatremia in patients with congestive heart failure (CHF) or cirrhosis is associated with an increased risk of death.[180,181] Even mild stable euvolemic hyponatremia caused by SIADH has been associated with cognitive defects and gait disturbances. Overly rapid correction of serum sodium, particularly in patients with chronic hyponatremia, can cause neurologic complications such as seizures, spastic quadriparesis, and coma because of osmotic demyelination.[15] Vasopressin receptor antagonists, the vaptan drug class, which includes tolvaptan (Samsca) and conivaptan (Vaprisol), are available to treat hypervolemic or euvolemic hyponatremia that is caused by CHF, cirrhosis, and polycystic kidney disease. These medications antagonize arginine vasopressin by inhibition of renal V1a, V1RA, V2, and V3RA receptors. The result is increased free water excretion by the kidneys.[182]

Initial treatment of hyponatremia typically includes fluid restriction and diuresis. Intravenous conivaptan has been used for short-term treatment of euvolemic hyponatremia. Oral treatment with tolvaptan can increase serum sodium concentrations in patients with hypervolemic or euvolemic hyponatremia caused by cirrhosis, heart failure, or SIADH, but has not been shown to reduce mortality. Overly rapid correction of serum sodium can cause osmotic demyelination, but this

side effect has not been reported after administration of tolvaptan.[183] Fig. 21.6 depicts differences in ECV sodium concentration and the effect on various cells.

Aggressive treatment of acute hyponatremia can be associated with severe neurologic effects. Fig. 21.7 contains guidelines that highlight the treatment of hyponatremia. In instances when chronic hyponatremia occurs, rapid correction of serum sodium can lead to the neurologic disorder known as myelinolysis. Myelinolysis, originally known as central pontine myelinolysis, can lead to disorders of the upper neurons, spastic quadriparesis, pseudobulbar palsy, mental disorders, and (in some cases) death. Patients at particular risk for myelinolysis are those who have been hyponatremic for more than 48 hours and individuals who have had orthotopic liver transplantation or a history of alcohol abuse. Optimal treatment of hyponatremia must balance the risks of cerebral edema against the risks of myelinolysis.[184]

The risk of myelinolysis can be reduced by correcting serum NA^+ levels in a deliberate manner. It has been suggested that serum NA^+ concentrations should be increased by no more than 1 to 2 mEq/L per hour. In symptomatic patients, this is accomplished by infusing 3% saline at a rate of 1 to 2 mL/kg per hour. Once the patient is clinically stable, NA^+ administration should be slowed to raise serum NA^+ not more than 10 to 15 mmol/L in 24 hours.[184]

Hypernatremia

Hypernatremia can result from several causes (Fig. 21.8, Box 21.5, and Table 21.5) but is usually the result of impaired water intake.[185] Inadequate administration of free water to hospitalized patients can lead

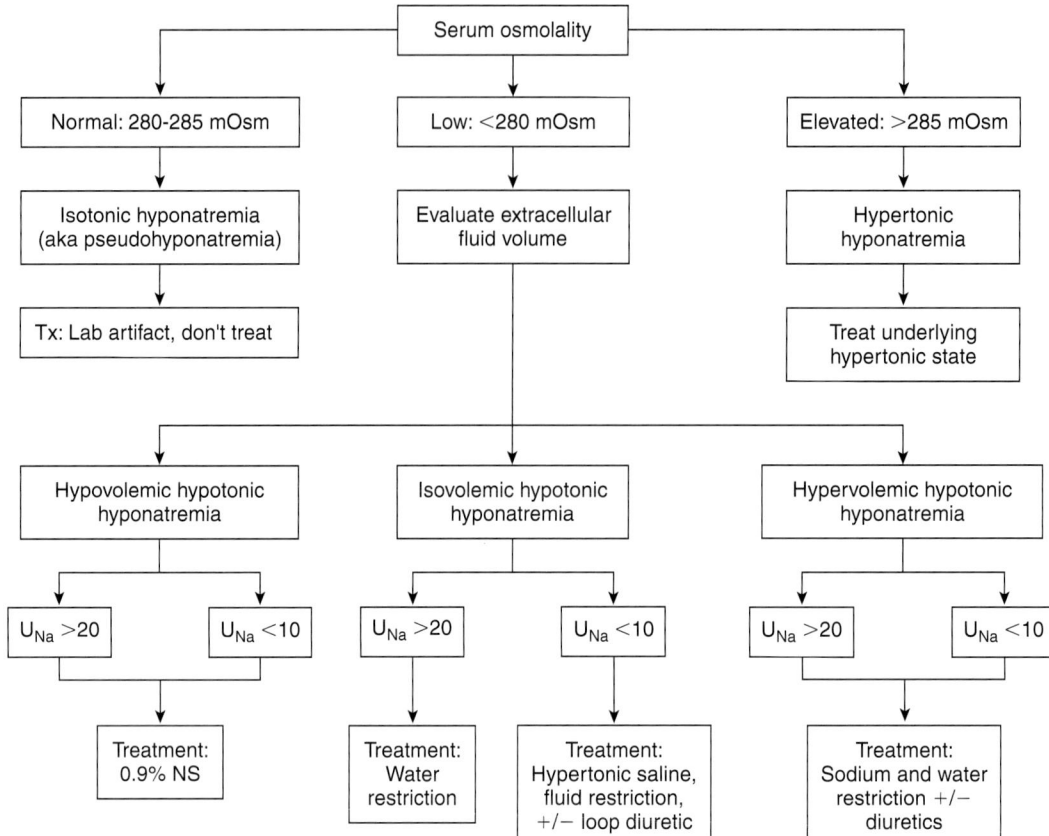

Fig. 21.7 Treatment of hyponatremia. *NS,* Normal saline; *Tx,* treatment; U_{Na}, urinary sodium. (Modified from Ferri FF. *Practical Guide to the Care of the Medical Patient.* 8th ed. Philadelphia: Elsevier; 2011.)

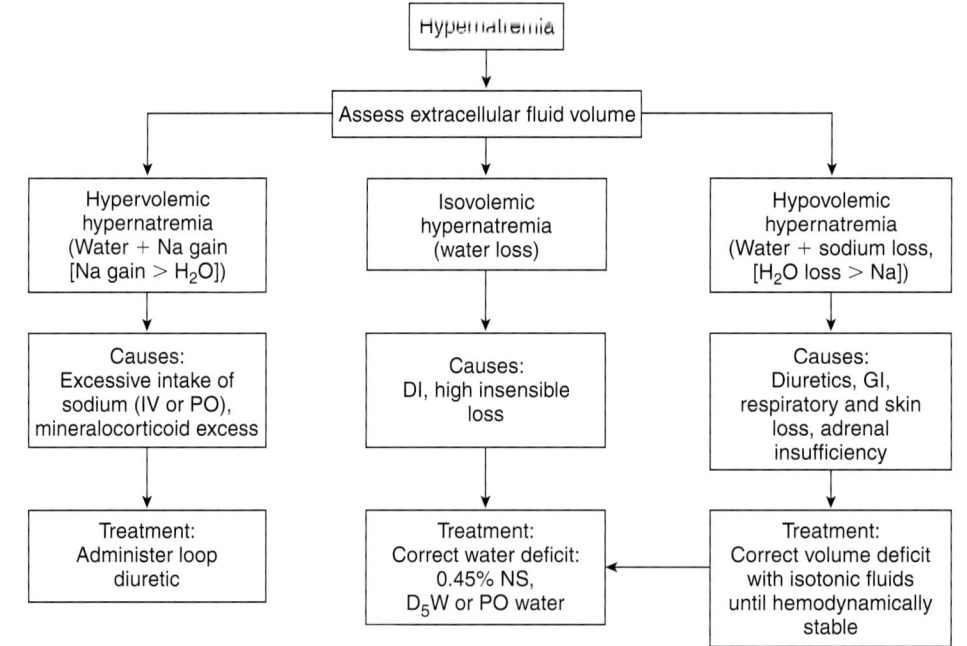

Fig. 21.8 Hypernatremia (serum sodium *[Na]* >145 mEq/L). *DI,* Diabetes insipidus; *GI,* gastrointestinal; *NS,* normal saline; *PO,* oral. (Modified from Ferri FF. *Practical Guide to the Care of the Medical Patient.* 8th ed. Philadelphia: Elsevier; 2011.)

BOX 21.5 Hypernatremia: Classification, Causative Factors, and Manifestations*

Hypernatremia With Dehydration and Low Total Body Sodium
Causes: Vomiting, diarrhea, continuous gastrointestinal suctioning, osmotic diuresis (e.g., mannitol)

Hypernatremia With Low Total Body Water and Normal Total Body Sodium
Causes: Diabetes, neurogenic, renal disease, sickle cell disease, medications (e.g., aminoglycosides)

Hypernatremia With Increased Total Body Sodium
Causes: Hypertonic saline infusion, Cushing syndrome, Conn syndrome, hemodialysis

Physiologic Manifestations
Neurologic
- Thirst
- Weakness
- Seizure
- Coma
- Intracranial bleeding
- Disorientation
- Hallucinations
- Irritability
- Muscle twitching
- Cerebral edema

Cardiovascular
- Increased NA$^+$-hypervolemia-tachycardia, increased preload, increased myocardial oxygen consumption
- Decreased NA$^+$-hypovolemia-tachycardia, decreased preload

Respiratory
- Increased NA$^+$-pulmonary edema

Renal
- Polyuria or oliguria
- Renal insufficiency

*Serum sodium >145 mEq/L.

TABLE 21.5 Clinical Signs of Hypernatremia With Increasing Serum Osmolality

Osmolality (mOsm/kg)	Neurologic Signs and Symptoms
350–375	Confusion, restlessness, agitation, headache
376–400	Ataxia, tremors, weakness
401–430	Hyperreflexia, muscle twitching/spasm
>430	Coma, seizures, death

BOX 21.6 Sodium Equations for Clinical Use

Sodium Deficit
Sodium deficit (mEq) = ([Na$^+$] goal – [Na$^+$] plasma) × TBW
TBW = total body water = body weight × 60%

Free Water Deficit
Free water deficit = ([Na$^+$]/140) –1) × TBW

Corrected Sodium
Corrected sodium = ([Na$^+$] + 0.016) × (glucose – 100)

Serum Osmolality (Calculated)
(2 × [Na$^+$]) + (BUN/2.8) + (glucose/18)

Fractional Excretion of Sodium (Fr$_{exc}$ Na$^+$)
Fr$_{exc}$ Na = ([Na$^+$] urine) + (creatinine plasma/[Na$^+$] plasma) + (creatinine urine)
<1% = prerenal (hypovolemia)
>2% = intrinsic renal disorder

BUN, Blood urea nitrogen.
From Rhee P, Bellal J. Shock fluids and electrolytes. In Townsend CM, et al., eds. *Sabiston Textbook of Surgery.* 20th ed. Philadelphia: Elsevier; 2017:86.

Box 21.6. If the hypernatremia is acute (i.e., <24-hour duration), water deficits can be replaced relatively rapidly with hypotonic solutions. If chronic hypernatremia accompanied by volume depletion is present, the volume disorder is corrected first with isotonic crystalloids. Once the circulating volume has been restored, hypotonic solutions are used to correct the water deficit. Plasma sodium should be decreased by 1 to 2 mEq per hour until the patient is clinically stable, and correction of serum sodium to normal levels should gradually progress over the subsequent 24 hours.[187]

Disorders of Potassium Balance

Potassium (K$^+$) is the principle intracellular electrolyte within the ICV, which accounts for 98% of the body's supply. The difference between intracellular K$^+$ (150–160 mEq/L) and extracellular K$^+$ (3.5–5.0 mEq/L) concentrations and the dynamic balance between K$^+$ within these compartments are in large part responsible for the resting membrane potential of the cell.[188] Homeostasis is maintained by absorption of K$^+$ from the gastrointestinal tract and by renal excretion or reabsorption into the peritubular capillary network. Renal regulation of K$^+$ is dependent on (1) the concentration gradient between the distal tubules and collecting duct relative to the peritubular capillary network, (2) the distal convoluted tubular flow rate and NA$^+$ concentration, (3) the concentration of aldosterone, and (4) changes in pH (acidosis/alkalosis). Aldosterone has a potent effect on K$^+$ levels. Hyperkalemia causes adrenal cortical synthesis and release of aldosterone, which promotes potassium excretion from the distal renal tubules. Disturbances in serum K$^+$ result from an imbalance between intracellular and extracellular distribution of K$^+$ or an abnormality in the total body stores of K$^+$. The symptoms associated with hyperkalemia and hypokalemia result in altered resting membrane potential.

Hypokalemia

Hypokalemia (defined as serum K$^+$ <3.5 mEq/L) can result from an absolute deficiency caused by gastrointestinal loss, renal loss, intracellular shift, increased nonrenal losses, endocrinopathies, and poor intake (Box 21.7). It is the most common electrolyte abnormality encountered during clinical practice. Redistribution of K$^+$ from the ECV to the ICV

to an iatrogenic hypernatremia. In cases of slow-onset hypernatremia, the brain can adapt by conserving intracellular solutes, which allows maintenance of normal ICV. Rapidly occurring hypernatremia can be accompanied by rapid shrinking of the brain and concomitant traction on intracranial veins and venous sinuses, leading to intracranial hemorrhage.[186] As with hyponatremia, rapid treatment used to correct chronic hypernatremia can lead to negative physiologic effects, as large volumes of free water may lead to cerebral edema.

Correction of hypernatremia is accomplished by replacement of the water deficit, which can be calculated using the formulas provided in

BOX 21.7 Five Most Common Causes of Hypokalemia

1. Renal losses	Diuretic use, drugs, steroid use, metabolic acidosis, hyperaldosteronism, renal tubular acidosis, diabetic ketoacidosis, alcohol consumption
2. Increased nonrenal losses	Sweating, diarrhea, vomiting, laxative use
3. Decreased intake	Ethanol, malnutrition
4. Intracellular shift	Hyperventilation, metabolic alkalosis, drugs
5. Endocrinopathy	Cushing disease, Bartter syndrome, insulin therapy

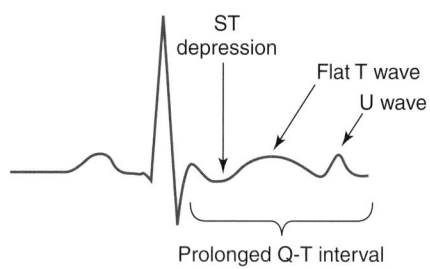

Hypokalemia

Fig. 21.9 Electrographic changes in hypokalemia. (From Marx JA, et al. *Rosen's Emergency Medicine*. 8th ed. Philadelphia: Elsevier; 2014:1640.)

can also lead to hypokalemia. β-adrenergic stimulation, insulin, and alkalosis all promote the movement of K^+ into the ICV.[189]

Hypokalemia is 11 times more likely to occur with patients routinely treated with thiazide diuretics and twice as high for men as compared to women.[190] Mild decreases in serum K^+ are often well tolerated, but symptoms that may occur include palpitations, skeletal muscle weakness, and muscle pain. With a serum K^+ value of less than 2.5 mEq/L, signs and symptoms include paresthesia, depressed deep tendon reflexes, fasciculations, muscle weakness, and altered level of consciousness. In patients with cardiac disease, including ischemia and CHF, mild to moderate hypokalemia increases the potential for dysrhythmias. Common cardiac dysrhythmias associated with hypokalemia are first- and second-degree heart block, atrial or ventricular fibrillation, and asystole. The electrocardiographic (ECG) abnormalities associated with hypokalemia include ST segment depression, flattened T wave, and the presence of a U wave (Fig. 21.9).

Treatment of hypokalemia depends on the severity of the symptoms accompanying the K+ deficit. In the face of hemodynamically compromising cardiac dysrhythmias, aggressive IV administration of K^+ is warranted. IV replacement of K^+ should be accomplished with the patient under continuous ECG monitoring. Rates of IV administration as rapid as 40 mEq per hour can be given if K^+ levels are less than 2.0 mEq/L, although a maximum rate of 10 to 20 mEq per hour is recommended to avoid an iatrogenic hyperkalemia.[191]

Once serious symptoms associated with hypokalemia (e.g., respiratory muscle weakness or dysrhythmias) have been reversed, IV replacement can be discontinued, and oral supplementation is appropriate. It is recommended that IV potassium be replaced along with chloride because the hypochloremia makes it difficult for the kidney to conserve K^+.[189] Furthermore, potassium chloride should be mixed in a dextrose-free solution to prevent stimulation of insulin, leading to increased redistribution of K^+ to the intracellular space.[192]

The association between preoperative potassium with a 30-day mortality and adverse cardiovascular event (MACE) has been long debated. Recently it has been determined that patients with preoperative hyperkalemia (K^+ >5.5 mEq/L) and hypokalemia (K^+ <4.0 mEq/L) undergoing noncardiac surgery are at increased risk of developing MACE with 30 days postoperatively.[193]

Hyperkalemia

Hyperkalemia is defined as a serum K^+ greater than 5.0 mEq/L and occurs less commonly as compared to hypokalemia if renal causes are excluded.[192] In addition to impaired renal excretion of potassium, causes of hyperkalemia include a high intake of potassium and a shift of potassium from ICV to ECV. This can lead to increased lactic acid production and apoptosis. Medications such as digoxin, ACE inhibitors (ACEIs), angiotensin receptor blockers (ARBs), and β-blockers can all increase ECV potassium. By decreasing angiotensin, ACEIs/ARBs can cause hyponatremia and hyperkalemia. Similarly, β-blockade (and specifically $β_1$-receptor antagonism of the macula densa) inhibits renin release, thus decreasing the release of aldosterone, potentially causing hyponatremia and hyperkalemia. Specific causes of hyperkalemia are listed in Box 21.8. Due to the inward and outward flux of K^+ that consistently occurs during myocardial cell depolarization and repolarization, hyperkalemia that occurs rapidly can have dramatic effects on cardiac rhythm. ECG changes that are associated with increased levels of K^+ are outlined in Table 21.6.

Treatment of hyperkalemia should be preceded by exclusion of pseudohyperkalemia, which is a laboratory artifact. Pseudohyperkalemia results from hemolysis of the blood sample, leukocytosis, thrombosis, or prolonged fist clenching during blood drawing. The treatment strategy accomplishes three physiologic events: (1) stabilization of cardiac membrane, (2) driving K from ECV to ICV, and (3) removal of K^+ from the body. For patients who are predisposed to developing chronic hyperkalemia (e.g., renal failure), an oral K^+ binding medication patiromer (Veltassa) can be used. This oral agent is an unabsorbed anion polymer that exchanges a calcium-sorbitol compound for K^+ within the gastrointestinal lumen and leads to decreased serum K^+. Treatment of hyperkalemia is based on the severity of the patient's presenting signs and symptoms (Table 21.7).

It has been customary to administer 10 units regular insulin intravenously with one ampule of D50 for patients with hyperkalemia. A complication of this therapy is the frequent occurrence of clinically significant hypoglycemia. To minimize this possibility and still adequately treat hyperkalemia, the use of 5 units regular insulin intravenously or 0.1 units/kg intravenously has been suggested.[194]

Disorders of Calcium Balance

Calcium is a divalent cation, and 99% is found in bones as hydroxyapatite (inorganic compound, which contributes to bone rigidity). The remaining 1% of calcium exists in the plasma and body cells. Calcium is vitally important for structural integrity of bone, but perhaps most important to anesthetists is its role as a second messenger that couples cell membrane receptors to cellular responses. The action of calcium as a second messenger is critical to functions such as muscle contractions and release of hormones and neurotransmitters.[195] In addition to the second messenger function, calcium plays an important role in blood coagulation and muscle function, including myocardial contractility.[196]

Although most of the body's calcium is found in the bones, a small percentage is freely exchangeable with the ECV. Calcium in the ECV is found in three distinct fractions. Ionized calcium accounts for 50% of the calcium in the ECV and is the physiologically active portion of circulating calcium. The remainder of the circulating calcium is bound either to anions (10%) or plasma proteins, primarily albumin (40%).[196]

BOX 21.8 Causes of Hyperkalemia*

Pseudohyperkalemia
- Hemolysis of sample
- Thrombocytosis
- Leukocytosis
- Laboratory error

Increased Potassium Intake and Absorption
- Potassium supplements (oral and parenteral)
- Dietary (salt substitutes)
- Stored blood
- Potassium-containing medications

Impaired Renal Excretion
- Acute renal failure
- Chronic renal failure
- Tubular defect in potassium secretion
- Renal allograft
- Analgesic nephropathy
- Obstructive uropathy
- Interstitial nephritis
- Chronic pyelonephritis
- Potassium-sparing diuretics
- Miscellaneous (e.g., lead, systemic lupus erythematosus, pseudohypoaldosteronism)

- Hypoaldosteronism
- Primary (Addison disease)
- Hyporeninemic hypoaldosteronism (renal tubular acidosis type 4)
- Congenital adrenal hyperplasia
- Drug-induced (e.g., nonsteroidal antiinflammatory drugs; angiotensin-converting enzyme; heparin; cyclosporine)

Transcellular Shifts
- Acidosis
- Hypertonicity
- Insulin deficiency
- Drugs
- β-blockers
- Digitalis toxicity
- Succinylcholine
- Exercise
- Hyperkalemic periodic paralysis

Cellular Injury
- Rhabdomyolysis
- Severe intravascular hemolysis
- Acute tumor lysis syndrome
- Burns and crush injuries

* Serum potassium >5 mEq/L.
From Marx JA, et al. *Rosen's Emergency Medicine: Concepts and Clinical Practice.* 9th ed. Philadelphia: Elsevier; 2018:1621.

TABLE 21.6 Electrocardiographic (ECG) Changes Associated With Hyperkalemia

Potassium mEq/L	ECG Change
>5.5–6.5	Peaked T waves
>6.5–7.5	P wave flattening or disappearance, PR prolongation
>7.0–8.0	QRS prolongation
>8.5	QRS complex degrades to sine wave pattern, ventricular fibrillation and cardiac arrest

Changes in pH alter the extracellular distribution of calcium, with acidemia decreasing the protein-bound fraction and increasing the ionized fraction.[23] The total fraction of calcium circulating within the blood is 9.0 to 10.5 mg/dL.

It is the ionized fraction of calcium that is most clinically significant because this form is available for physiologic reactions. Total serum calcium levels are largely dependent on the albumin concentration. Direct measurement of ionized calcium is the preferred method in critically ill patients.[197] Serum calcium levels are maintained primarily by the release or inhibition of parathyroid hormone (PTH), but also by vitamin D and calcitonin. During periods of hypercalcemia or hypocalcemia, the levels of PTH decrease or increase, respectively, and cause a series of biologic events in an attempt to normalize serum calcium (Fig. 21.10).

Hypocalcemia

The specific causes and clinical features associated with hypocalcemia are listed in Box 21.9. In the intraoperative period, the most likely causes of hypocalcemia are hyperventilation and massive rapid transfusion. Hyperventilation leads to an increased pH, which facilitates increased protein binding of calcium, thus decreasing serum ionized calcium. Citrate is a preservative added to packed red blood cells. This chemical chelates or binds calcium, decreasing serum calcium available for physiologic reactions. Massive rapid transfusion of packed red blood cells can cause acute hypocalcemia (this topic is further discussed in Chapter 22).

Treatment of acute hypocalcemia involves the infusion of calcium salts. Calcium chloride is the most bioavailable parenteral preparation of calcium (272 mg of elemental calcium). It results in the most rapid correction of hypocalcemia. However, it can cause significant venous irritation and tissue necrosis as compared to calcium gluconate. If a central line is present, then administration via the central route can decrease the incidence of complications. One regimen used to treat hypocalcemia includes administration of 10 mL of 10% calcium gluconate (93 mg of elemental calcium) over 10 minutes, followed by an infusion of 0.3 to 2 mg/kg per hour of elemental calcium.[23] Correction of serum calcium should be guided by ionized calcium levels.

Hypercalcemia

Hypercalcemia typically results from the movement of calcium from bone to the ECV, which exceeds the ability of the kidney to excrete calcium (Box 21.10). Primary hyperparathyroidism accounts for more than half of all cases of hypercalcemia, with malignancy being the second most common cause. Treatment of hypercalcemia involves volume expansion with NS, which increases renal excretion of calcium. The addition of a loop diuretic further enhances renal excretion. Bisphosphonates, mithramycin, calcitonin, glucocorticoids, and phosphate salts have also been used to treat hypercalcemia.[198] For patients who rapidly develop hypercalcemia, which results in life-threatening

TABLE 21.7   **Guidelines for Treatment of Hyperkalemia**

Clinical Feature	Therapy	Onset	Duration	Mechanism of Action
Electrocardiographic Evidence of Pending Arrest				
Loss of P wave and widening QRS; immediate effective therapy indicated	1. Intravenous (IV) infusion of calcium salts*: 10 mL of 10% calcium chloride over 10-min period *or*	1–3 min	30–60 min	Membrane stabilization
	10 mL of 10% calcium gluconate over 3–5 min	1–3 min	30–60 min	Membrane stabilization
	2. IV infusion of sodium bicarbonate: 50–100 mEq over 10–20-min period	5–10 min	1–2 hr	Shifts potassium intracellularly
Electrocardiographic Evidence of Potassium Effect				
Peaked T waves; prompt therapy needed	1. Glucose and insulin infusion: IV infusion of 50 mL of $D_{50}W$ and 5 units of regular insulin; monitor glucose	30 min	4–6 hr	Shifts potassium intracellularly
	2. Immediate hemodialysis			
Biochemical Evidence of Hyperkalemia and No Electrocardiographic Changes				
Effective therapy needed within hours	1. Potassium-binding resins in the gastrointestinal (GI) tract	1–2 hr	4–6 hr	Gastrointestinal excretion
	2. Promotion of renal potassium excretion: diuretic—Furosemide 40 mg IV	15–30 min	2–3 hr	Renal excretion

*Calcium chloride yields three times the ionized calcium as calcium gluconate; calcium chloride = 27 mg/mL; calcium gluconate = 9 mg/mL.

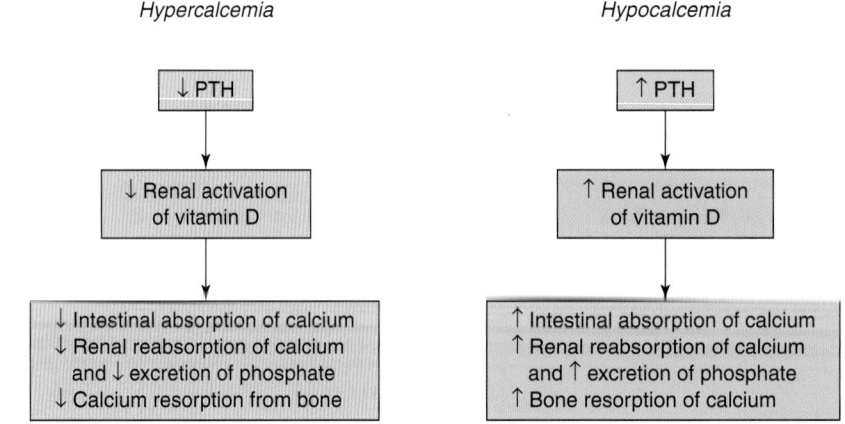

Fig. 21.10 Hormone regulation of calcium balance. *PTH*, Parathyroid hormone. (From McCance KL, et al. *Pathophysiology*. 7th ed. St. Louis: Elsevier; 2014:119.)

dysrhythmias, hemodialysis is an acute treatment to rapidly lower serum calcium.

Disorders of Magnesium Balance

Magnesium is the second most abundant intracellular cation, second only to potassium. Approximately 40% to 60% is stored in muscle and bone, 30% within cells, and 1% in serum. Regulation of magnesium metabolism occurs in the intestines and kidneys. The physiologic importance of magnesium includes its role as a cofactor in numerous enzymatic reactions, including those involving energy metabolism, protein synthesis, neuromuscular excitability, and the function of the Na-K-ATPase pump. Chronic hypomagnesemia increases cardiovascular death in both men and women by 8% and 16%, respectively.[199]

An intravenous infusion of magnesium may relieve severe bronchospasm, and it can decrease postoperative pain.[200,201] Normal magnesium plasma concentrations range from 1.5 to 3.0 mEq/L.

Hypomagnesemia

Hypomagnesemia is common in hospitalized patients, especially critically ill patients. Magnesium deficiency can be the result of increased renal or gastrointestinal loss or poor magnesium intake and/or medications[202] (Box 21.11). Hypomagnesemia has an inhibitory effect on the Na-K-ATPase dependent pump resulting in decreased ICV potassium. This can alter the cardiac resting membrane potential, specifically phase 4 (resting membrane potential) of the cardiac action potential. ECG changes seen with hypomagnesemia include flat T waves, presence of U waves, prolonged QT interval, widened QRS complexes, and atrial and ventricular arrhythmias. Thirty percent of patients who consume excessive amounts of alcohol are admitted to the hospital with hypomagnesemia caused by poor dietary intake and the associated diuretic effect.[203] Severe hypomagnesemia can be treated with IV administration of 1 to 2 g of magnesium sulfate over 5 minutes while the ECG is monitored, followed by administration of 1 to 2 g per hour.[204]

Hypermagnesemia

Hypermagnesemia is most commonly the result of iatrogenic causes (e.g., intravenous administration) (Box 21.12). Hypermagnesemia can result from the treatment of preeclampsia, preterm labor, ischemic heart disease, and cardiac dysrhythmias. The symptoms of

BOX 21.9 Causes and Clinical Features of Hypocalcemia*

Causes

Parathyroid Hormone Insufficiency

Primary hypoparathyroidism
- Congenital syndromes
- Maternal hyperparathyroidism

Secondary hypoparathyroidism
- Neck surgery
- Metastatic carcinoma
- Infiltrative disorders
- Hypomagnesemia, hypermagnesemia
- Sepsis
- Pancreatitis
- Burns
- Drugs (chemotherapeutics, ethanol, cimetidine)

Vitamin D Insufficiency

Congenital rickets
Malnutrition
Malabsorption
Liver disease
Renal disease
- Acute and chronic renal failure
- Nephrotic syndrome

Hypomagnesemia
Sepsis
Anticonvulsants (phenytoin, primidone)

Parathyroid Hormone Resistance States (Pseudohypoparathyroidism)/Calcium Chelation

Hyperphosphatemia
Citrate
Free fatty acids
Alkalosis
Fluoride poisoning

Clinical Features

Neuromuscular
- Paresthesias
- Muscle weakness
- Muscle spasm
- Tetany
- Chvostek sign (facial/eye muscle twitching)
- Trousseau sign (carpopedal spasm)
- Hyperreflexia
- Seizures

Cardiovascular
- Bradycardia
- Angina
- Hypotension
- Congestive heart failure
- Cardiac arrest
- Digitalis insensitivity
- QT prolongation

Pulmonary
- Bronchospasm
- Laryngospasm

Psychiatric
- Anxiety
- Depression
- Irritability
- Confusion
- Psychosis
- Dementia

*Serum calcium <8.5 mg/dL; ionized calcium <4.0 mg/dL.
From Marx JA, et al. *Rosen's Emergency Medicine: Concepts and Clinical Practice.* 9th ed. Philadelphia: Elsevier; 2018:1623-1624.

hypermagnesemia include depression of the peripheral and central nervous system, hypotension, QRS segment widening, PR and QT segment prolongation, heart block, and cardiac arrest. The symptoms are dependent on the rapidity and degree of increased magnesium levels. Magnesium potentiates the action of nondepolarizing neuromuscular relaxants, and their use should be carefully monitored in patients with hypermagnesemia.[205] Treatment of hypermagnesemia involves discontinuing the administration of magnesium; in urgent situations, such as bradycardia, heart block, and respiratory depression, calcium chloride should be used as an antagonist.

Disorders of Phosphate Balance

The majority of phosphate is located in bone (85%). The small amount that is present within the plasma exists as (1) phospholipids, (2) phosphate esters, and (3) inorganic phosphate, which is the ionized form. Intracellular phosphate has numerous metabolic effects, such as being a component part of ATP and 2,3-diphosphoglycerate (2,3-DPG). It also acts as a buffer in the regulation of acid-base balance. The concentration of phosphate in plasma is inversely proportional to that of calcium. Phosphate levels are tightly controlled by the same mechanism that governs calcium levels, PTH, vitamin D, and calcitonin (see Fig. 21.10).

Hypophosphatemia

Hypophosphatemia is defined as a serum phosphate concentration of less than 2.0 mg/dL. The most likely causes of hypophosphatemia are increased renal excretion and intestinal malabsorption. Respiratory alkalosis can cause low phosphate levels because of the accelerated use of ATP by cells. With hypophosphatemia, decreased 2,3-DPG is available in red blood cells. This causes a leftward shift of the oxyhemoglobin dissociation curve and increases the affinity between hemoglobin and oxygen (decreased oxygen unloading to the tissues). The result of decreased oxygen delivery to cells results in anaerobic metabolism, decreased ATP formation, and acidosis. The consequences of decreased ATP include hypoxia, heart block, bradycardia, and asystole.

Hyperphosphatemia

Hyperphosphatemia is defined as a serum phosphate level greater than 4.7 mg/dL. The majority of phosphate exists within the ECV, and cellular destruction (e.g., metastatic disease) is a leading cause. Increased phosphate levels can produce clinically significant hypocalcemia as calcium and phosphate are further deposited within bone. Therefore signs and symptoms associated with low serum phosphate are synonymous with hypocalcemia, as previously described.

BOX 21.10 Causes and Clinical Features of Hypercalcemia

Definition
- *Mild hypercalcemia:* Serum Ca^{2+} 10.5–11.9 mg/dL (2.5–3 mmol/L) or Ionized Ca^{2+} 5.6–8 mg/dL (1.4–2 mmol/L)
- *Moderate hypercalcemia:* Serum Ca^{2+} 12–13.9 mg/dL (3–3.5 mmol/L) or Ionized Ca^{2+} 8–10 mg/dL (2–2.5 mmol/L)
- *Hypercalcemic crisis:* Serum Ca^{2+} 14–16 mg/dL (3.5–4 mmol/L) or Ionized Ca^{2+} 10–12 mg/dL (2.5–3 mmol/L)

Causes
Primary Hyperparathyroidism

Malignant Disease
- Parathyroid hormone–related protein
- Ectopic production of 1,25-dihydroxyvitamin D
- Other bone-resorbing substances
- Osteolytic bone metastasis

Medications
- Thiazide diuretics
- Lithium
- Estrogens
- Vitamin D toxicity
- Vitamin A toxicity
- Calcium ingestion

Granulomatous Disorders
- Sarcoidosis
- Tuberculosis
- Coccidioidomycosis
- Berylliosis
- Histoplasmosis
- Leprosy

Nonparathyroid Endocrine Disorders
- Hyperthyroidism
- Adrenal insufficiency
- Pheochromocytoma
- Acromegaly
- Vasoactive intestinal polypeptide–producing tumor

Miscellaneous
- Milk-alkali syndrome
- Immobilization
- Idiopathic hypocalcemia of infancy
- Physiologic (in the newborn)

Clinical Features
Neurologic
- Fatigue, weakness
- Confusion, lethargy
- Seizures
- Coma
- Hypotonia, diminished deep tendon reflexes

Cardiovascular
- Hypertension
- ST segment elevation
- Sinus bradycardia/arrest, atrioventricular block
- Electrocardiographic abnormalities (short QT interval, bundle branch block)
- Ventricular dysrhythmias
- Potentiation of digoxin toxicity

Renal
- Polyuria, polydipsia
- Dehydration
- Loss of electrolyte
- Prerenal azotemia
- Nephrolithiasis
- Nephrocalcinosis

Gastrointestinal
- Nausea, vomiting
- Anorexia
- Peptic ulcer disease
- Pancreatitis
- Constipation, ileus

Adapted from Marx JA, et al. *Rosen's Emergency Medicine: Concepts and Clinical Practice.* 9th ed. Philadelphia: Elsevier; 2018:1624-1625.

BOX 21.11 Causes of Hypomagnesemia*

Excessive alcohol intake
Pregnancy
Renal losses
- Acute and chronic renal failure
- Postobstructive diuresis
- Acute tubular necrosis
- Chronic glomerulonephritis
- Chronic pyelonephritis
- Interstitial nephropathy
- Renal transplantation

Gastrointestinal losses
- Chronic diarrhea
- Nasogastric suctioning
- Short-bowel syndrome
- Protein-calorie malnutrition
- Bowel fistula
- Total parenteral nutrition
- Acute pancreatitis

Endocrine disorders
- Diabetes mellitus
- Hyperaldosteronism
- Hyperthyroidism
- Hyperparathyroidism
- Acute intermittent porphyria

Medications
- Aminoglycosides
- Amphotericin
- β-agonists
- Cisplatin
- Cyclosporine
- Diuretics
- Pentamidine
- Proton-pump inhibitors
- Theophylline

Congenital disorders
- Familial hypomagnesemia
- Maternal diabetes
- Maternal hypothyroidism
- Maternal hyperparathyroidism

*Serum Mg^{2+} <1.5 mEq/L.
From Marx JA, et al. *Rosen's Emergency Medicine: Concepts and Clinical Practice.* 9th ed. Philadelphia: Elsevier; 2018:1627.

BOX 21.12 Hypermagnesemia*

Causative Factors
- Renal failure
- Excessive magnesium administration
- Adrenal insufficiency

Clinical Manifestations
Serum Magnesium Levels (mg/dL)
4–5 = Decreased deep tendon reflexes
5–7 = Hypotension
10 = Respiratory paralysis, coma
10–15 = Heart block
10–24 = Cardiac arrest

*Serum Mg^{2+} >3 mEq/L.
From Marx JA, et al. *Rosen's Emergency Medicine: Concepts and Clinical Practice.* 9th ed. Philadelphia: Elsevier; 2018:1648.

Aluminum hydroxide, which is contained in antacids, decreases serum phosphate by binding within the gastrointestinal tract. Dialysis can also be used to treat severely elevated phosphate levels. Table 21.8 includes causes and manifestations associated with phosphate imbalances.

TABLE 21.8   Alterations in Phosphate Balance

	Causes	Manifestations
Hypophosphatemia (<2.0 mg/dL)	Intestinal malabsorption related to vitamin D deficiency	Conditions related to decreased oxygen transport and ATP creation
	Magnesium/aluminum containing antacids	Platelet dysfunction
	Chronic alcohol misuse	Bone reabsorption
		Altered nerve and muscle function
	Malabsorption syndromes	Confusion
	Respiratory alkalosis	Coma
	Increased renal excretion associated with hyperparathyroidism	Seizures
		Muscle weakness
		Respiratory failure
		Cardiomyopathy
Hyperphosphatemia (>4.7 mg/dL)	Acute/chronic renal failure	Symptoms related to hypocalcemia
	Treatment of metastatic tumor	Chronic calcification of soft tissues (e.g., joints, lungs, kidneys)
	Long-term use of laxatives/enemas containing phosphates	
	Hypoparathyroidism	

Adapted from Doig AK, Huether SE. Cellar environment fluids and electrolyte acids and bases. In: McCance KL, ed. *Pathophysiology.* 7th ed. St. Louis: Elsevier; 2014:121.

SUMMARY

As updated scientific information refutes commonly accepted beliefs regarding fluid administration, anesthetists will need to modify their practice to help ensure optimal patient outcomes. Goal-directed fluid therapy allows for a measured approach to intravenous fluid administration based on real-time physiologic data. This will result in improved perfusion to vital organs, as well as minimize the possibility of edema formation and damage to the endothelial glycocalyx. Additionally, electrolyte disorders can dramatically complicate an anesthetic course and result in morbidity and mortality. A thorough knowledge of the physiologic effects, signs and symptoms, and treatment of electrolyte abnormalities is essential for competent anesthesia practice.

REFERENCES

For a complete list of references for this chapter, scan this QR code with any smartphone code reader app, or visit the following URL: http://booksite.elsevier.com/9780323711944/.

22

Blood and Blood Component Therapy

Richard P. Wilson

A number of different factors affect patient's hemodynamic stability and ability to coagulate. Infectious disease, tissue and vascular injury, along with fluid shifts and blood loss can contribute to hemodynamic disturbances. Blood component therapy is one method utilized by anesthesia providers to treat hemodynamic disturbances and involves multiple steps. The ability to manage patients using proper component therapy is important in the effort to ensure patient safety and promote optimal physiologic outcomes. Blood component therapy includes the ability to recognize the need for treatment, proper compatibility testing, identifying and obtaining the correct product, and safe transfusion of the products. Transfusion of blood products primarily focuses on red blood cell (RBC) components to restore intravascular volume along with increasing oxygen-carrying capacity in those who need it. Transfusions can also improve hemostasis and hemodynamic stability. Anticipation of the need for blood component therapy due to fluid shifts or blood loss can be identified early in the perioperative process with a detailed preoperative assessment, understanding of the proposed procedure, and proper communication with the surgical care team. The American Society of Anesthesiologists (ASA) released its practice guidelines for perioperative blood management (Box 22.1).[1]

ESTIMATED BLOOD VOLUME AND LOSS

When considering blood component therapy, two factors to consider are estimated total blood volume and estimated allowable blood loss. To calculate estimated blood volume (EBV), the age and kilogram body weight of the patient are utilized (Table 22.1).[2,3]

Once blood volume is estimated, the next step is to calculate the amount of allowable blood loss based on the lowest acceptable hematocrit (Hct) concentration that considers the patient's condition and comorbidities. The formula for calculating the maximal allowable blood loss (MABL) is[4]

$$MABL = \frac{EBV \times (Initial\ Hct - Lowest\ Acceptable\ Hct)}{Initial\ Hct}$$

Estimation of blood loss during the intraoperative setting is based on both objective and subjective measures making it difficult to obtain an exact number. Traditionally, surgical blood loss has been estimated by viewing the amount of blood on surgical sponges, laparotomy sponges, surgical drapes, surgical gowns, and blood volume in suction canisters. The exact numbers can vary significantly between practitioners. When visually estimating blood loss, it is anticipated that a fully soaked surgical sponge holds 10 mL of blood, and a fully soaked laparotomy sponge holds 100 to 150 mL of blood.[5-11] In a prospective study of 85 patients undergoing laparoscopic urologic surgery, blood loss was estimated using direct visual measurement along with several different accepted formulas. Results from the study varied. Estimation

of blood loss from direct visual measurements ranged from 200 mL to 2200 mL. According to the study, blood loss formulas both underestimated and overestimated the actual amount of blood loss. The study concluded the formulas showed poor agreement with direct visual measurement and therefore may not be reliable measurements for blood loss.[6] A prospective study by Adkins et al. looked at simulated blood loss and the variation between different practitioners' measurements. Their results showed no significant differences in the measurement of blood loss using direct visual measurements no matter the provider, level of education, or years of experience. In this study, the confidence in blood loss estimation decreased as the simulated amount of blood loss increased.[5]

Due to the difficulties of accurately quantifying blood loss intraoperatively, the patient's hemodynamic response should also be monitored closely. Symptoms of increased blood loss include tachycardia, decreased blood pressure, and eventually decreased oxygen saturation (Spo_2) in the peripheral capillaries. According to the ASA guidelines mentioned earlier, monitoring vital organ perfusion can be accomplished with additional techniques such as echocardiography, urine output, cerebral oximetry, near infrared spectroscopy (NIRS), arterial blood gas analysis, and mixed venous oxygen saturations. Laboratory values that assess hemoglobin (Hgb), Hct, platelets, fibrinogen, thromboelastography (TEG), activated partial thromboplastin time (aPTT), and international normalized ratio (INR) should be evaluated if there is either a belief or actual signs of anemia or coagulopathy.[1]

TRANSFUSION INDICATORS

The traditional hemoglobin (10 g/dL) and hematocrit (30%) transfusion trigger is now believed to have potentially caused unnecessary transfusions and even transfusion-related deaths.[12-14] The determination to transfuse blood products should be based on multiple factors such as hemoglobin and hematocrit levels along with the anesthetist's clinical judgment of the patient's condition, vital organ perfusion, and anticipated course of the clinical case. The ASA organized task forces in 1996 and 2006 to develop guidelines on blood component therapy to help assist clinicians with best practices for transfusion therapy.[15,16]

In 2016, the American Association of Blood Banks (AABB) reviewed randomized controlled trials (RCTs) regarding transfusions of packed red blood cells (PRBCs) and compared results between "liberal" and "restrictive" thresholds. The data from 12,587 participants suggested that "restrictive" thresholds did not show an increase in myocardial infarction, 30-day mortality rates, rebleeding, cardiovascular events, and other deleterious patient outcomes. They concluded that a more restrictive transfusing threshold (7–8 g/dL) was safe and should be considered for most hemodynamically stable patients in the intensive care unit (ICU).[17]

BOX 22.1 ASA Practice Guidelines for Perioperative Blood Management—Summary

Preoperative Patient Evaluation
- Early preoperative evaluation
- Review of medical records, specifically:
  - Previous blood transfusion
  - History of drug-induced coagulopathy (anticoagulants, vitamins, herbal supplements)
  - Congenital coagulopathy
  - History of thrombotic events
  - Risk factors for organ ischemia (cardiorespiratory disease may lower trigger for red blood cell [RBC] transfusion)
- Discuss risks vs benefits of blood transfusion with patients, and confirm their preference.
- Review available labs, ordering additional tests as indicated: hemoglobin (Hgb), hematocrit (Hct), and coagulation profile.
- Conduct patient physical exam: ecchymosis, petechiae, pallor.

Preadmission Patient Preparation
- Administer erythropoietin, with or without iron, in select patient populations to reduce allogeneic blood transfusion.
- If time permits, administer iron to patients with iron-deficiency anemia.
- Discontinue anticoagulants, in consultation with appropriate specialists, and transition to shorter acting drugs.
- If possible, discontinue nonaspirin, antiplatelet agents in advance of surgery.
  - Continue aspirin on a case-by-case basis.
- Weigh risks of thrombosis vs increased bleeding.
- Confirm that blood and components are available if significant blood loss or transfusion anticipated.
- Prior to admission, offer patient opportunity to donate autologous blood, if preferred, and time allows for erythropoietin reconstitution.

Preprocedure Preparation
- Blood management protocols utilize:
  - Algorithmic strategies to reduce usage of blood products.
  - Restrictive RBC transfusion strategy to reduce transfusions.
    - Evaluate potential for ongoing bleeding, intravascular volume status, organ ischemia, and cardiovascular reserve.
    - Administer RBC unit by unit with interval reevaluations.
  - Transfusion avoidance strategy in patients refusing transfusion or is not possible.
  - Massive transfusion protocol strategy when indicated.
  - Institution's maximal surgical blood order schedule.
- Reversal of anticoagulants
  - For urgent reversal administer prothrombin complex concentrate (PCC) in consultation with a specialist, or fresh frozen plasma (FFP).
  - Administer vitamin K for select patients with nonurgent reversal and restoration of warfarin.
- Antifibrinolytics for prophylaxis of excessive blood loss
  - Employ prophylactic antifibrinolytics with use of allogeneic blood transfusion in patients undergoing cardiopulmonary bypass.

- Consider prophylactic antifibrinolytics in certain orthopedic, liver surgery, and procedures at high risk for excessive bleeding.
- Acute normovolemic hemodilution (ANH)
  - Consider ANH to reduce allogeneic transfusions in patients at risk for excessive bleeding.

Intraoperative and Postoperative Management of Blood Loss
- Allogeneic RBC transfusion
  - Administer blood without consideration of duration and storage.
  - Utilize leukocyte-reduced blood to reduce complications associated with allogeneic blood transfusion.
- Reinfuse recovered RBCs, when appropriate, as a blood-sparing intervention intraoperatively
- Intraoperative and postoperative patient monitoring
  - Periodically visual assessment of surgical field, communicate with surgeon to assess presence of coagulopathy or surgical bleeding.
  - Utilize standard methods to quantify blood loss, including drains, suction canisters, and sponges.
  - Monitor for perfusion of vital organs using standard monitoring along with clinical and physical exam.
    - Additional monitoring as indicated: renal ultrasound, cerebral oximetry, arterial blood gases (ABGs), and mixed venous oxygen support.
  - Monitor Hgb and Hct for suspected anemia.
  - Monitor standard coagulation tests such as international normalized ratio (INR), activated partial thromboplastin time (aPTT), fibrinogen, viscoelastic assay such as thromboelastography, and platelet count if coagulopathy suspected.
  - During and after transfusion, assess for sign of transfusion reaction, including hyperthermia, hemoglobinuria, microvascular bleeding, hypoxemia, respiratory distress, increased peak airway pressure, urticaria, hypotension, and signs of hypocalcemia.
    - For suspected transfusion reaction: (1) immediately stop transfusion, (2) initiate supportive care, and (3) notify the blood bank.
- Treatment of excessive bleeding
  - Before platelet transfusion, obtain platelet count and function (if drug-induced dysfunction is suspected).
  - Obtain coagulation tests before transfusion of FFP.
  - Assess fibrinogen levels before administration of cryoprecipitate.
  - Utilize desmopressin in patients with excessive bleeding and platelet dysfunction.
  - Consider topical hemostatics such as fibrin glue or thrombin gel.
  - Documented fibrinolysis, consider antifibrinolytics such as e-aminocaproic acid.
  - PCCs may be indicated in patients with excessive bleeding and increased INR.
  - Consider recombinant activated factor VII for excessive bleeding caused by coagulopathy, as a last resort; also consider fibrinogen concentrate.

Adapted from American Society of Anesthesiologists Task Force on Perioperative Blood Management. Practice Guidelines for Perioperative Blood Management. *Anesthesiology*. 2015;122:241–275.

Transfusion triggers have been the topic of many studies especially in the context of blood conservation strategies. According to a study released in 2020, many of the guidelines for RBC transfusion recommend never transfusing at a Hgb greater than or equal to 10 g/dL (except in special circumstances), and almost always transfuse at a Hgb less than 6 g/dL.[12] Several clinical trials in the 1990s retrospectively compared a "restrictive" versus "liberal" transfusion threshold, and

RCTs followed on this topic. The overall outcomes showed that in most patients, except those with myocardial ischemia, a. Hgb as low as 7 g/dL was a safe transfusion threshold. Newer guidelines address other clinically useful transfusion triggers, including arterial oxygen delivery, mixed venous oxygen saturation, central venous oxygen saturation, lactate levels, and signs of myocardial ischemia such as hypotension and/or tachycardia. They identify how an optimal transfusion trigger

TABLE 22.1 Average Blood Volumes

Age	Blood Volume (mL/kg)
Premature infant at birth	90–105 mL/kg
Term newborn infant	80–90 mL/kg
Infants (<3 mo)	70–75 mL/kg
Childhood to Adult	
Male	70 mL/kg
Female	65 mL/kg
Obese	Lean body weight plus 20%

should avoid both premature and delayed infusions, while taking into consideration anemia tolerance of the various organs.[12-14] The AABB recommended that transfusion-based decisions be driven by evidence from multiple critical elements instead of a single transfusion trigger (Box 22.2).[18]

PATIENT BLOOD MANAGEMENT

The AABB developed a strategy (patient blood management [PBM]) geared toward caring for patients who may need a blood transfusion (Box 22.3). Blood management should consider every facet of the decision-making process, from the initial patient evaluation through the clinical management of the transfusion. PBM is a multidisciplinary and multimodal approach designed to optimize patient outcomes while also helping to guarantee blood components are available for those in need.

Key aspects of PBM in the perioperative period include (1) optimization of the patient's RBC production, (2) minimization of blood loss, and (3) treatment of anemia. Strategies have been developed to enable clinicians to minimize allogenic blood transfusions and maintain safe and effective care for their patients. Table 22.2 lists the PBM performance measures and principles The Joint Commission recognizes as vital to patient safety.[19,20]

The ASA practice guidelines encourage clinicians to evaluate patients throughout the entire perioperative period for risk of bleeding. The guidelines and recommendations that encompass the periods of patient evaluation are found in Box 22.1. Addressing PBM issues during different perioperative time periods gives the practitioner the ability to recognize and properly treat conditions that put the patient at increased risk of bleeding or hemorrhage. Blood conservation strategies are an important concept that can help lead to a decrease in intraoperative blood loss, especially with the increased emphasis placed on both cost and availability of specific blood products as well as the possibility of transfusion-related complications.

CONSERVATION STRATEGIES

RBC Alternatives

Erythropoietin is an essential hormone for the production of RBCs. It is excreted by the kidneys in response to anemia and hypoxia. However, it has been shown that in critically ill patients, endogenous production of erythropoietin can be diminished in response to these conditions.[21] In 2019 Cho et al. performed a meta-analysis of RCTs looking at erythropoietin use and the incidence of allogenic RBC transfusions during hospital stays. The results included 4750 patients and showed that administration of erythropoietin preoperatively was associated with a significant reduction in allogenic blood transfusions for all patients across a variety of surgical procedures.[22]

BOX 22.2 The American Association of Blood Banks (AABB) Red Blood Cell Transfusion Recommendations

1. Restrictive transfusion strategy for hemoglobin (7–8 mg/dL) in hospitalized, stable patients. *Grade: High*
2. Restrictive transfusion strategy for hemoglobin (≤8 mg/dL) in hospitalized patients with preexisting cardiovascular disease with symptoms. *Grade: Moderate*
3. No recommendation for liberal or restrictive transfusion threshold in stable hospitalized patients with acute coronary syndrome. *Grade: Very low*
4. Transfusion decision should be influenced by symptoms in addition to hemoglobin concentration. *Grade: Low*

From Carson JL, et al. Red blood cell transfusion: a clinical practice guideline from the AABB. *Ann Intern Med.* 2012;157(1):49–58.

BOX 22.3 Patient Blood Management Strategies—Summary

Preoperative Suggestions
- Screen for and treat anemia. Manage any underlying disorders that may lead to anemia.
- Treat iron deficiency and administer erythropoiesis-stimulating agents as indicated.
- Identify and manage any bleeding risks such as medications or chronic diseases.
- Assess patient reserve and optimize patient-specific tolerable blood loss.
- Formulate management plan with evidence-based transfusion strategy.
- Preoperative autologous blood donation in select situations.
- May require preoperative visit up to 30 days prior to elective surgery to accommodate therapy.

Intraoperative Suggestions
- Perform elective surgery when hematologic status is medically optimized.
- Use meticulous blood-sparing surgical techniques.
- Continually measure and assess hemoglobin and hematocrit.
- Plan and optimize fluid management of nonblood products.
- Optimize cardiac output, oxygen delivery, and ventilation.
- Use blood salvage and autologous transfusion when possible.

Postoperative Suggestions
- Treat anemia with erythropoiesis-stimulating agents and iron deficiency as indicated.
- Vigilant monitoring and management of postoperative bleeding.
- Maintain normothermia to minimize oxygen consumption.
- Avoid and/or treat infections promptly.
- Carefully manage anticoagulant medications.

Adapted from Goodnough LT, Shander A. Patient blood management. *Anesthesiology.* 2012;116(6):1367–1376; Shander A, et al. Patient blood management in Europe. *Br J Anaesth.* 2012;109(1):55–68.

Preoperative Guidelines

Proper preoperative evaluation that focuses on a patient's hematology includes a review of previous medical records, laboratory test results, and a patient or family interview. Studies show that characteristics of congenital or acquired disease processes such as sickle cell anemia, factor VIII deficiency, liver disease, and idiopathic thrombocytopenia purpura may be associated with increased complications from blood transfusions. Specific laboratory tests such as Hgb, Hct, and coagulation studies may give the clinician a better idea of

TABLE 22.2 Patient Blood Management

TJC* Performance Measures	Principles
Transfusion Consent	Formulate plan of proactive management for avoiding and controlling blood loss tailored to clinical management of individual patient, including anticipated procedures.
RBC Transfusion Indication	Employ multidisciplinary treatment approach to blood management using a combination of interventions (e.g., pharmacologic therapy, point-of-care testing).
Plasma Transfusion Indication	Promptly investigate and treat anemia.
Platelet Transfusion Indication	Exercise clinical judgment; be prepared to modify routine practices (e.g., transfusion triggers) when appropriate.
Blood Administration Documentation	Restrict blood drawing for unnecessary laboratory tests.
Preoperative Anemia Screening	Decrease or avoid the perioperative use of anticoagulants and antiplatelet agents.
Preoperative Blood Type Screening and Antibody Testing	

*TJC, The Joint Commission.
Adapted from Goodnough LT, Shander A. Patient blood management. *Anesthesiology.* 2012;116(6):1367–1376; The Joint Commission. *Implementation Guide for the Joint Commission Blood Management Implementation Measures.* (Library of Other Measures). https://www.jointcommission.org/assets/1/6/PBM_Implementation_Guide_20110624.pdf. Accessed 2016.

the potential need for blood products or risk of excessive bleeding during the intraoperative and postoperative periods. Discontinuation of anticoagulation medications (e.g., warfarin, clopidogrel, aspirin) when clinically safe is recommended, and administration of reversal agents (e.g., vitamin K, prothrombin-complex concentrate, fresh frozen plasma [FFP]) may be indicated if urgent anticoagulation reversal is necessary. In addition, certain procedures that anticipate significant amounts of blood loss may benefit from the administration of tranexamic acid.[1,16,23]

Autologous Transfusions

Autologous transfusions by definition are the reinfusion of a patient's native blood or blood components that were salvaged during a surgical procedure or donated prior to a surgical procedure that is expected to lose a significant amount of blood. Benefits of autologous transfusion include reduced risk of transmission infection and the ability to preserve anonymous blood supplies. A 2014 study of 2251 patients undergoing total hip arthroplasty demonstrated that targeted autologous donations reduced the need for allogenic blood transfusions.[24] The three types of autologous donations are preoperative autologous donation (PAD), acute normovolemic hemodilution (ANH), and cell salvage.[25]

Preoperative Autologous Donation

This process involves blood collection in advance of an elective procedure. The PAD is then available for transfusion back into the patient when needed during the surgical procedure. Ideally, the PAD should take place 48 to 72 hours prior to the procedure to allow for equilibration of the patient's blood volume. Oral or intravenous iron

BOX 22.4 Autologous Blood Donation

Advantages
- Prevents transfusion-transmitted disease
- Prevents red cell alloimmunization
- Supplements the blood supply
- Provides compatible blood for patients with alloantibodies
- Prevents some adverse transfusion reactions
- Provides reassurance to patients concerned about blood risks

Disadvantages
- Does not affect risk of bacterial contamination
- Does not affect risk of ABO incompatibility error
- Costlier than allogeneic blood
- Results in wastage of blood not transfused
- Increased incidence of adverse reactions to autologous donation
- Subjects patient to perioperative anemia and increased likelihood of transfusion

Adapted from Goodnough LT, Shander A. Patient blood management. *Anesthesiology.* 2012;116(6):1367–1376; Goodnough LT. Autologous blood donation. *Anesthesiol Clin North America.* 2005;23:263–270; Silvergleid AJ. Surgical blood conservation: preoperative autologous blood donation. UpToDate. http://www.uptodate.com/contents/surgical-blood-conservation-preoperative-autologous-blood-donation. Accessed 2021.

supplements may be given to maintain proper erythropoiesis. Advantages and disadvantages of this technique are listed in Box 22.4. The patient may have to undergo multiple phlebotomy attempts and must be able to tolerate the hematologic and cardiovascular changes of a reduced blood volume. Complications can include bacterial contamination due to improper collection, handling, and storage. Increased costs have been associated with PAD, and up to 50% of predonated blood goes unused and must be wasted.[26] Conditions where PAD should not be used include any preexisting anemia, cyanotic heart disease, ischemic heart disease, aortic stenosis, and/or uncontrolled hypertension.[25,27]

Acute Normovolemic Hemodilution

This technique takes place in the operating room and involves the withdrawal of whole blood from the patient prior to surgery with subsequent crystalloid or colloid replacement. The whole blood that is collected is labeled and stored in the operating room and returned to the patient once surgery is ended or hemostasis is achieved. The goal for hemodilution is to achieve a hematocrit of 20%. Advantages of this technique are reduced costs and a decreased amount of actual blood loss during surgery because of the diluted blood compared to whole blood. The blood extracted from the patient also contains platelets and clotting factors, which are ideal for reinfusion either during or at the end of the surgical case when increased amounts of blood loss are happening. A significant potential complication is hemodynamic instability due to the significant decrease in Hct associated with ANH. This type of blood conservative strategy is not suggested for patients at risk for myocardial ischemia or with any significant organ dysfunction that relies on a stable Hgb and Hct. Finally, data are inconclusive as to the actual effectiveness of this technique because of the lack of quality published research.[25]

Cell Salvage

Cell salvage involves collection of blood from the surgical field from suction or surgical drains that is either filtered or washed and then reinfused into the patient. Cell salvage is commonly used during cardiothoracic, orthopedic, vascular, and neurologic surgeries. Blood cells collected are first separated, filtered, and washed before being reinfused into the patient. The safety record for this technique is favorable, and one of the advantages is it provides a supply of RBCs in proportion to the amount being lost. With point of care testing, cell salvage can provide a cost-effective way of reducing requirements for allogenic blood when large volume losses occur. It is also an acceptable means of therapy for some Jehovah's Witnesses. The 2018 Association of Anaesthetists guidelines for cell salvage recommend (1) cell salvage be used to help reduce the amount of allogenic (donor) red cell transfusion and postoperative anemia, (2) trained personnel and equipment be available 24 hours a day, (3) it be used if the surgical blood loss is anticipated to be more than 500 mL (the only exception is parturients who are having a cesarean section), (4) a full explanation of the risks and benefits be provided to the patient, and (5) using leucodepletion filters during the reinfusion of salvaged blood during cancer surgery.[28]

Cell salvage is contraindicated in those patients with sepsis or in some cancerous surgical procedures. Other complications that may occur during the reinfusion of cell salvaged blood include electrolyte disturbances, dilutional coagulopathy, and disseminated intravascular coagulation (DIC). Studies have shown that using cell salvage techniques can reduce allogenic blood transfusion up to 40%.[25,29-31] A summary of indicated surgical procedures that may benefit from cell salvage use as well as the relative contraindications are listed in Table 22.3.[32-36]

Directed Donor Transfusions

Directed donor transfusions occur when blood is donated from a relative or friend for transfusion into a preestablished matched patient. It was developed in an effort to reduce patient risk associated with anonymous donor transfusions, including transmission of diseases. In a directed donation, the patient chooses the donor, and the physician submits an order for the donor to give blood 5 days in advance of the patient's surgical procedure. Some limitations include the fact that facilities cannot guarantee the units will be available and even transfused if the blood is needed. In addition, the lack of high-quality evidence to support this process has led to selected facilities not accepting directed donations.

COMPATIBILITY OF TRANSFUSION

Before transfusion therapy can be initiated, blood compatibility must be established. Prior to the administration of blood products, the clinician must ensure that proper testing has occurred regarding the patient's specific blood type, circulating plasma antibodies, and antibodies to RBC antigens. Table 22.4 lists the blood types and blood group compatibility.

ABO blood type and Rhesus (Rh) antigen testing are a prerequisite prior to any blood transfusion, and compatibility must be matched in an effort to reduce the potential for a hemolytic blood reaction. ABO blood type is determined by the presence or absence of antigens on the RBC. For example, the A blood type has only the A antigen, the B blood type has only the B antigen, and the AB blood type has both the A and B antigens. The O blood type does not have either antigen. The Rh antigen is a transmembrane protein that can be found on the surface of the RBC, and if the blood has this protein it is considered Rh positive.[37] If the patient has blood type A and is positive for the Rh antigen, then it is common to say that the individual has type A positive blood. There are many different types of Rh antigens; however, the most common one tested is the Rh D antigen since it is the most immunogenic.

TABLE 22.3 Cell Salvage Summary

General Indications for Cell Salvage

Specialty	Surgical Procedure
Cardiac	Valve replacement Redo bypass grafting
Orthopedics	Major spine surgery Knee replacement Hip replacement
Urology	Radical retropubic prostatectomy Cystectomy Nephrectomy
Neurosurgery	Giant basilar aneurysm
Vascular	Thoracoabdominal aortic Aneurysm repair Abdominal aortic aneurysm repair
Hepatic	Liver transplant
Other	Jehovah's Witnesses Unexpected massive blood loss Red cell antibodies

Relative Contraindications to Cell Salvage

Pharmacologic Agents
- Clotting agents (e.g., Avitene, Surgicel, Gelfoam)
- Disinfectant irrigating solutions for topical use (e.g., oxygenated water, betadine, distilled water, alcohol, antibiotics meant for topical use)
- Anticoagulant drugs
- Synthetic resins such as methyl methacrylate
- Catecholamines (pheochromocytoma)
- Oxymetazoline (Afrin)
- Papaverine

Contaminants in the Operating Field
- Urine
- Bone chips
- Fat
- Bowel contents
- Infection
- Amniotic fluid

Other Conditions
- Malignant tumors or neoplastic cells
- Hematologic disorders
- Thalassemia
- Sickle cell disease
- Miscellaneous
- Carbon monoxide (electrocautery smoke)

From Esper SA, Waters JH. Intra-operative cells salvage: a fresh look at the indications and contraindications. *Blood Transfusion*. 2011;9(2):139–147.

A blood type and screen and crossmatch are two common laboratory tests that are utilized when matching a patient's blood to donor blood in the blood bank. A type and screen determines the patient's ABO type, presence of the Rh D antigen, and the existence of any other commonly known antibodies. A crossmatch tests the patient's blood against the prospective donor's blood to determine if any adverse reaction occurs. It is essentially a trial transfusion.[21]

Those with type O negative blood are considered universal donors, and their blood may be used for transfusion in all blood types. Those with type AB positive blood are termed universal recipients and may

TABLE 22.4 Relationship Among Blood Groups, Antigens, Antibodies, and Blood Compatibility

Blood Group	Antigen on Red Blood Cell	Antibodies in Serum	Blood Group Compatibility
A	A	Anti-B	A, O
B	B	Anti-A	B, O
AB	A and B		AB, A, B, O
O		Anti-A and Anti-B	O only
Rh positive	D		Rh positive and Rh negative
Rh negative		Anti-D if sensitized	Rh negative

receive a transfusion of any blood type. All other blood types must be safely matched before receiving a RBC transfusion.[37] A donor's blood must be identical or compatible to the recipient for transfusion.

EMERGENCY TRANSFUSIONS

During emergency situations, the patient's specific blood type may not be immediately available before transfusion, or the blood type may be unknown due to multiple factors. In these circumstances uncross-matched type O blood that is Rh positive may be given to persons of childbearing age that have never received a type O, Rh-positive blood transfusion in the past. When a clinician is unaware of the patient's previous history of transfusions or needs to emergently administer to a female of childbearing years, type O Rh-negative blood is indicated to decrease the likelihood of a hemolytic reaction. In the case of receiving type O blood, the patient may be switched back to the original ABO blood type only when inventory permits, bleeding has slowed or stopped, and (most importantly) a recent crossmatch using a sample of the patient's serum/plasma indicates compatibility.

MASSIVE TRANSFUSION PROTOCOLS

One of the leading causes of preventable death after trauma is hemorrhage. Traumatic hemorrhage may account for up to 50% of deaths within the first 24 hours after the injury. The early and rapid delivery of blood products during traumatic hemorrhage, with a primary goal of treating acute coagulopathy, has improved mortality in this patient population.[38] Massive transfusions are defined in several different ways such as transfusion of 10 units of PRBCs in 24 hours, loss of one blood volume, or transfusion of greater than 5 units of PRBCs within 4 hours with continued hemorrhage. Massive transfusion protocols (MTPs) were developed in the mid to late 2000s with the goal of establishing a process for coordinated and timely delivery of blood products and adjunctive therapies throughout the hospital. They were developed in response to blood product delays and concerns of improper administration during massive transfusions.[39]

Goals of MTPs include rapid provision of blood and blood products that represent whole blood. This includes PRBCs to maintain tissue oxygenation and other fractionated products (i.e., FFP and platelets) to address coagulopathy in the early stages of trauma. Triggering MTPs early in the resuscitation phase is crucial for improving patient outcomes. Activating MTPs too early can lead to inappropriate utilization of blood products along with the risks associated with blood

transfusions. Late activation of MTPs could lead to a delay in a time-sensitive lifesaving intervention.[38] Several studies have recommended a prediction scoring system to assess timely initiation of MTPs. The Assessment of Blood Consumption (ABC) and Trauma-Associated Severe Hemorrhage scores have both shown to perform similarly in predicting timely initiation of MTPs.[39]

The exact ratios of blood products (e.g., PRBCs, FFP, cryoprecipitate, platelets) may vary between institutions. Initial recommendations from 2014 included transfusing plasma and universal RBC in a plasma to RBC ratio of 1:1 or 1:2 and a single donor platelet apheresis unit or donor platelet pool for each 6 units of RBCs.[40] More recent studies have led MTPs to also include administration of calcium chloride, cryoprecipitate, and tranexamic acid because of the effect they have on the coagulation cascade and ability to promote blood clot formation.[39-42] Potential complications that can occur during resuscitation using MTPs can include coagulation abnormalities, complications related to blood storage, immunosuppression and infection, hypothermia, and lung injuries associated with transfusions.[42] The decision to initiate and discontinue a MTP should be interdisciplinary and involve communication between the anesthesia and surgical teams along with the blood bank.[43]

BLOOD COMPONENTS

Fractionation of whole blood is the process of separating it into its component parts (e.g., RBCs, platelets, plasma, and factor concentrates). The ability to administer individual blood components allows the practitioner to target patient-specific needs (Table 22.5). For example, minor hemorrhage with signs of decreased tissue oxygenation may require only the transfusion of RBCs, whereas the urgent reversal of anticoagulation would necessitate the need for FFP. For patients with platelet dysfunction or thrombocytopenia, a platelet transfusion may be the only blood product needed, and those with hypofibrinogenemia associated with massive bleeding or consumptive coagulopathy may require cryoprecipitate in addition to other blood products. Table 22.6 lists Food and Drug Administration (FDA)–approved coagulation protein deficiencies and therapies available in the United States.[44]

TRANSFUSION PRACTICE GUIDELINES
Packed Red Blood Cells

PRBCs are the component of choice for improving hemoglobin concentrations and oxygen-carrying capacity. Patients undergoing surgery may experience adverse outcomes, including myocardial and cerebral ischemia, with significant blood loss and decreased oxygen delivery to the tissues. Banked blood may be good for up to 42 days and usually contains approximately 300 mL of total volume at an Hct of 65%. A common assumption is that 1 unit of PRBCs will increase the Hgb 1 g/dL and the Hct 2% to 3% depending on the unit volume. A study of 60 patients with pelvic fractures showed only a 1.9% increase in Hct for each unit of 300 mL of PRBCs transfused.[45] Recommendations for PRBC infusion in adult patients is usually 1 mL for each 2 mL of blood loss. The recommendation for pediatric patients is higher, at 10 to 15 mL/kg. Infants have a larger volume of blood per kilogram, so the recommendation for this patient population is 15 mL/kg for PRBC transfusions.[46]

Platelets

Platelets are essential for adequate hemostasis and are transfused for platelet dysfunction or thrombocytopenia. Platelets are available as platelet concentrates, separated from 1 unit of whole blood by

TABLE 22.5   Characteristics of Blood Components

Blood Component	Content	Volume (mL)	Plasma (mL)	Shelf Life
Red Cell Products				
Whole blood	RBCs (Hct 40%–45%), WBCs, plasma, platelets (nonviable)	500–515	~300	21–35 days at 1–6°C (depending on anticoagulant) 24 hr if unrefrigerated
Packed RBCs	RBCs (Hct 60%–80%), WBCs, plasma, platelets (nonviable)	250–300	~25–50 mL	21–42 days at 1–6°C (depending on anticoagulant)
Leukocyte-reduced RBCs (filtered)	RBCs (Hct 90%), minimal plasma	200	Minimal	21–42 days at 1–6°C (depending on anticoagulant)
Washed RBCs	RBCs (Hct 60%), some WBCs	340	0	24 hours
Frozen RBCs	RBCs (Hct 90%, minimal WBC and platelets (nonviable)	170–190	0	10 years at –80°C
Platelets	Platelets, some WBCs, some RBCs, plasma			Open, 24 hr at 20–24°C with continuous agitation Closed, 5 days at 20–24°C with continuous agitation
Single donor (apheresis)	$\geq 3 \times 10^{11}$ platelets/unit	~300 (200–400)	~250	
Random donor	$\geq 5.5 \times 10^{10}$ platelets/unit	50	50	
Plasma-Derived Products				
Fresh frozen plasma (frozen within 6–8 hr of phlebotomy)	Plasma with all coagulation factors and inhibitors, complement, fibrinogen, albumin, globulins	*Whole blood donor:* 200–250 *Apheresis donor:* 400–600	200–250 400–600	1 year at –18°C; 24 hours at 1–6°C once thawed
Plasma frozen within 24 hr (separated from whole blood stored at 4–6°C within 24 hr of collection)	Plasma with all coagulation factors and inhibitors, but with lower levels of V and VIII; complement, fibrinogen, albumin, globulins	200–250	200–250	1 yr at –18°C; 24 hr at 1–6°C once thawed
Cryoprecipitate-reduced plasma (fresh frozen plasma with cold-induced precipitate removed)	Similar to fresh frozen plasma but deficient in XIII, VIII, fibrinogen, and von Willebrand factor	200–225	200–225	1 yr at –18°C; 24 hr at 1–6°C once thawed
Cryoprecipitate	Factor VIII (minimum 80 IU), XIII, fibrinogen (minimum 150 mg), von Willebrand factor, plasma, fibronectin	5–20	5–20	1 yr at –18°C; 4–6 hr at room temperature once thawed

Hct, Hematocrit; *RBCs,* red blood cells; *WBCs,* white blood cells.
From Shen MC, Zimmerman JL. Use of blood components in the intensive care unit. In Parillo JE, Dellinger JEZ, eds. *Critical Care Medicine.* Philadelphia: Elsevier; 2014:1377.

centrifuge from 6 to 10 donors. Alternatively, single-donor apheresis platelets are available for patients with alloantibodies, but at an increased expense. Treatment for bleeding caused by thrombocytopenia or abnormal platelet function includes a platelet transfusion (Box 22.5). In an average adult it is expected that transfusion of one platelet concentrate will increase the platelet count (by approximately 5–10 × 10³/µL). One platelet concentrate per 10 kg of body weight is the recommended therapeutic dose.[15] ABO incompatibility may lead to shortened survival of platelets and a small degree of hemolysis, therefore ABO matching is preferred but it is not essential for transfusion. Indications for treatment with platelets include individuals with a platelet count less than 10 × 10³ platelets/µL who are stable and not bleeding to prevent spontaneous bleeding. For those actively bleeding, the recommendation is to transfuse platelets if the level is less than 50 × 10³ platelets/µL (Box 22.6).[21,47-49]

Fresh Frozen Plasma

FFP contains all coagulation factors. A unit of FFP usually contains 200 to 250 mL of volume, which can replenish inadequate factors as a result of dilution or coagulation dysfunction. FFP is prepared from whole blood or apheresis, and, if frozen at –18°C to –30°C within 8 hours, may be stored for up to 1 year. The majority of FFP is transfused for the management of acquired bleeding disorders. Evidence suggests that a patient may still have adequate coagulation factors with as little as 20% to 30% of normal values.[41,50] FFP is the most commonly used plasma product, and if not transfused within 24 hours after being thawed concentrations of factors V and VIII will begin to decline.[21]

Reversal of warfarin therapy, correction of known factor deficiency, elevated prothrombin time (PT) and PTT (>1.5 normal time) with evidence of microvascular bleeding, and correcting microvascular bleeding due to factor deficiency in massive transfusion are all indications for FFP (Table 22.7). Urgent reversal of warfarin therapy should be treated with 5 to 8 mL/kg of FFP. Factor deficiencies require 10 to 20 mL/kg of transfused FFP to elevate coagulation levels by 20% to 30%.[50]

Cryoprecipitate

Cryoprecipitate contains 100 units of factor VIII, 200 mg of fibrinogen, and both fibronectin and von Willebrand factor (vWF). Thus it is

TABLE 22.6 FDA-Approved Coagulation Proteins and Replacement Therapies Available in the United States

Coagulation Protein Deficiency	Inheritance Pattern	Prevalence	Minimum Hemostatic Level	Replacement Sources
Factor I (fibrinogen)			50–100 mg/dL	Cryoprecipitate, FFP, fibrinogen concentrate
Afibrinogenemia	Autosomal recessive	Rare (<300 families)		
Dysfibrinogenemia	Autosomal dominant or recessive	Rare (>300 variants)		
Factor II (prothrombin)	Autosomal dominant or recessive	1 in 2 million births	30% of normal	FFP, factor IX complex concentrates
Factor V (labile factor)	Autosomal recessive	1 in 1 million births	25% of normal	FFP
Factor VII	Autosomal recessive	1 in 500,000 births	25% of normal	Recombinant factor VIIa (15–20 µg/kg), FFP, factor IX complex concentrates
Factor VIII (antihemophilic factor)	X-linked recessive	1 in 5000 male births	80%–100% for surgery/life-threatening bleeds, 50% for serious bleeds, 25%–30% for minor bleeds	Factor VIII concentrates (recombinant preferred)
von Willebrand disease Type 1 and 2 variants Type 3	Usually autosomal dominant Autosomal recessive	1% prevalence 1 in 1 million births	>50% VWF antigen and ristocetin cofactor activity	DDAVP for mild to moderate disease (except type 2B; variable response to 2A); cryoprecipitate and FFP (not preferred, except in emergencies); factor VIII/VWF concentrates, viral attenuated, intermediate purity (preferred for surgery, for disease unresponsive to DDAVP, and for type 3)
Factor IX (Christmas factor)	X-linked recessive	1 in 30,000 male births	25%–50% of normal, depending on extent of bleeding, surgery	Factor IX concentrates (recombinant preferred); FFP not preferred except in dire emergencies
Factor X (Stuart-Prower factor)	Autosomal recessive	1 in 500,000 births	10%–25% of normal	FFP or factor IX complex concentrates
Factor XI (hemophilia C)	Autosomal dominant; severe type is recessive	4% of Ashkenazi Jews; 1 in 1 million general population	20%–40% of normal	FFP or factor XI concentrate
Factor XII (Hageman factor), prekallikrein, high-molecular-weight kininogen	Autosomal recessive	Not available	No treatment necessary	—
Factor XIII (fibrin stabilizing factor)	Autosomal recessive	1 in 3 million births	5% of normal	FFP, cryoprecipitate, or viral-attenuated factor XIII concentrate

DDAVP, Desmopressin; *FDA*, US Food and Drug Administration; *FFP*, fresh frozen plasma; *VWF*, von Willebrand factor.
From Ragni MV. Hemorrhagic disorders coagulation factor deficiencies. In Goldman L, Schafer AI, eds. *Goldman's Cecil Medicine*. 25th ed. Philadelphia: Elsevier; 2016:1174.

frequently used to correct inherited or acquired coagulopathies. It can be used in the intraoperative setting for patients at risk of hemorrhage due to factor deficiencies; however, there are currently no observational studies that indicate a patient with an inherited or acquired factor deficiency is at increased risk of bleeding. Cryoprecipitate is collected by thawing FFP to 4°C and collecting the precipitate by centrifuge, which is rich in the factors mentioned earlier.[21] Studies show that 1 unit of cryoprecipitate per 10 kg of body weight can lead to a 50-mg/dL increase in the patient's plasma fibrinogen concentration. It is believed that cryoprecipitate should be used only in specific indications such as patients actively bleeding who have von Willebrand disease, those undergoing massive transfusion who have microvascular bleeding with fibrinogen levels less than 80 to 100 mg/dL, and prophylactically in patients with congenital fibrinogen deficiencies or von Willebrand disease who are unresponsive to DDAVP (desmopressin).[52,53]

STORAGE OF BLOOD

Two of the benefits related to blood transfusions are increased oxygen-carrying capacity and improved coagulopathy. During storage, banked blood has been shown to undergo structural and functional changes over time (Box 22.7).[54-56] These changes may cause deficient blood components and potential increases in morbidity and mortality. As time passes, RBC energy stores, 2,3-diphosphoglycerate, and adenosine triphosphate levels are depleted while potassium levels increase.[54-56] The membrane losses and RBC changes that occur over time are known as a blood storage lesion. An observational study of over 6000 patients undergoing cardiac surgery demonstrated that patients who received RBCs stored for more than 2 weeks had an increase in risk of postoperative complications. In addition, those patients who received blood stored for more than 2 weeks also experienced a reduction in short-term and long-term survival.[57]

RINGER LACTATE AND BLOOD TRANSFUSIONS

Previous guidelines recommended normal saline (NS) solution over Ringer lactate (LR) as the carrier fluid for blood transfusions. When blood is stored, citrate-phosphatase-dextrose (CPD) is added to prevent blood from coagulating. The reasoning for this recommendation was the belief that the amount of calcium in the blood would increase

BOX 22.5 American Association of Blood Banks Summary of 2015 Platelet Transfusion Guidelines

Recommendations include evidence grade

1. Transfuse hospitalized patients with therapy-induced lymphoproliferative thrombocytopenia prophylactically, at risk for spontaneous bleeding, and a platelet count 10×10^9 cells/L or less. *Grade: Strong*
2. Prophylactic transfusion prior to elective central line placement with platelet count less than 20×10^9 cells/L. *Grade: Weak*
3. Prophylactic transfusion for patients with elective lumbar puncture with a platelet count less than 50×10^9 cells/L. *Grade: Weak*
4. Prophylactic transfusion for patients having major elective neuraxial surgery with a platelet count less than 50×10^9 cells/L. *Grade: Weak*
5. Prophylactic transfusion for patients who exhibit perioperative bleeding, are thrombocytopenic, and having cardiopulmonary bypass. *Grade: Weak*
6. No recommendation for transfusion in patients receiving antiplatelet therapy who have an intracranial hemorrhage. *Grade: Uncertain*

From Kaufman RM, et al. Platelet transfusion: a clinical practice guideline from the AABB. *Ann Intern Med.* 2015;162:205–213.

BOX 22.6 Suggested Minimum Platelet Counts Before Invasive Procedures

Very-High-Risk Procedures—75,000/µL to 100,000/µL
- Neurosurgery
- Ocular surgery (except cataract extraction)
- Thyroid surgery
- Prostatectomy

Moderate-Risk Procedures—50,000/µL
- Liver biopsy
- Dental extraction
- Most surgical procedures

Low-Risk Procedures—30,000/µL
- Endoscopy
- Bronchoscopy
- Lumbar puncture (with scrupulous technique)

Very-Low-Risk Procedures—No Platelet Transfusions Necessary
- Bone marrow biopsy
- Cataract extraction

From Abrams CS. Thrombocytopenia. In Goldman L, Schafer AI, eds. *Goldman's Cecil Medicine.* 25th ed. Philadelphia: Elsevier; 2016:1160.

when using LR to levels greater than the chelating capabilities of the CPD resulting in clot formation. Initial studies showed, when using LR in blood transfusions, that smaller clots may form in intravenous tubing if blood was administered at slower rates.[58,59] However, newer evidence highlights that at rapid infusion rates of 540 mL/hour (such as those used in trauma cases or massive transfusions), or if the blood unit is infused within 60 minutes of initiation, there was no difference in clot formation when using LR versus NS.[59-61]

BLOOD TRANSFUSION COMPLICATIONS

Allogenic RBC transfusions are associated with significant risks to the patient (Table 22.8). Although complications after blood transfusions are rare, according to the Centers for Disease Control and Prevention (CDC),

TABLE 22.7 Suggested Indications for the Transfusion of Fresh Frozen Plasma

Indication	Recommendation
Disseminated intravascular coagulopathy	Consider transfusion with FFP, platelets, and cryoprecipitate if clinical evidence of bleeding. There is no supporting evidence for prophylactic transfusion in absence of bleeding despite abnormal coagulation tests.
Reversal of warfarin effect	FFP should only be used for the reversal of warfarin anticoagulation in the presence of *major* bleeding if prothrombin complex concentrate is not available. In the absence of bleeding, overanticoagulation should be managed by withholding warfarin therapy and initiating oral/intravenous vitamin K.
Perioperative transfusions	Majority of FFP use in this setting is in cardiac surgery. Meta-analysis does not suggest reduction in perioperative blood loss with prophylactic FFP use.
Before invasive procedures	*Regional/Neuraxial Blockade* For elective surgery, relevant anticoagulants and antiplatelets should be stopped according to local/national guidelines. With regard to warfarin reversal: Urgent procedures: consider 2.5–5 mg of oral/intravenous vitamin K. Immediate reversal: consider FFP, although no high-level evidence exists to support this. *Intensive Care* Minor derangements in PT/INR are common in ICU patients and often caused by vitamin K deficiency. As mentioned, patients with an elevated INR can still have adequate levels of coagulation factors. Systematic reviews have not shown any clear benefit of prophylactic FFP use to reduce bleeding related to planned procedures.

FFP, Fresh frozen plasma; *ICU,* intensive care unit; *INR,* international normalized ratio; *PT,* prothrombin time.
From Shah A, et al. Evidence and triggers for the transfusion of blood and blood products. *Anaesthesia.* 2015;70:10–9, e3–e5.

BOX 22.7 Changes in Banked Blood

- Depletion of 2,3-diphosphoglycerate (DPG)
- Depletion of adenosine triphosphate (ATP)
- Oxidative damage
- Increased adhesion to human vascular endothelium
- Acidosis
- Altered morphology of red blood cells (change in shape, decreased flexibility, membrane loss)
- Accumulation of microaggregates
- Hyperkalemia (as high as 17.2 mEq/L)
- Absence of viable platelets (after 2 days of refrigerated storage)
- Absence of factors V and VIII
- Hemolysis
- Accumulation of proinflammatory metabolic and breakdown products such as lysophospholipids

From Corazza ML, Hranchook AM. Massive blood transfusion. *AANA J.* 2000;68(4):311–314; Tinmouth A, et al. ABLE Investigators Canadian Critical Care Trials Group: clinical consequences of red cell storage in the critically ill. *Transfusion.* 2006;46(11):2014–2027; Shander A, et al. Patient blood management in Europe. *Br J Anaesth.* 2012;109(1):55–68.

TABLE 22.8 Summary of Risks and Side Effects of Allogeneic RBC Transfusion

Type of Risk	Incidence (Per Unit Transfused)
Infections	
Viruses	
Zika	United States: None
Human immunodeficiency virus (HIV)	1:1,500,000–1:2,000,000
Hepatitis B virus (HBV)	1:200,000–1:360,000
Hepatitis C virus (HCV)	1:1,000,000–1:2,000,000
Bacteria	
All	1:28,000–1:143,000
Parasites	
Malaria	1:4,000,000
Prions	
New variant Creutzfeldt-Jakob disease	No reported cases in the United States
Immunologic Reactions	
Hemolytic transfusion reactions (TR)	
Acute hemolytic TR	1:625,000
Delayed hemolytic TR	1:400,000
Alloimmunization	1:1600
Immunosuppression	1:1
Anaphylaxis	1:20,000–1:50,000
Transfusion-related acute lung injury	1:8000
Mistransfusion	
All RBC mistransfusions	1:14,000–1:18,000
Anaphylactoid reactions	1:150,000
Fatalities	1:600,000

RBC, Red blood cell; *TR*, transfusion reaction.
Adapted from Spahn DR, et al. More on transfusion and adverse outcome: it's time to change. *Anesthesiology*. 2011;114(2):234–236; Glance LG, et al. Association between intraoperative blood transfusion and mortality and morbidity in patients undergoing noncardiac surgery. *Anesthesiology*. 2011;114(2):283–292; Goodnough LT. Transfusion medicine. In Goldman L, Schafer AI, eds. *Goldman's Cecil Medicine*. Philadelphia: Elsevier; 2016:1191–1198.

the most common reactions are febrile and allergic reactions. Complications that occur within the first 24 hours are labeled acute, while delayed complications may develop days, months, or even years after a transfusion.[62] Serious complications are usually caused by the incompatibility of transfused products, and the severity and/or frequency of complications increases according to the amount of volume transfused. Acute lung injury, immunomodulation, allergic reactions, febrile reactions, and acute and delayed hemolytic reactions are a few of the immune-mediated complications associated with blood transfusions.[21,63,64]

Viral and Bacterial Risks

The current rate of viral and bacterial transfusion transmission is extremely low (see Table 22.8). However, even with improved testing and blood management, and despite enhanced safety of the blood supply, infectious complications can still occur. Bacterial contamination of blood remains a risk and increases with the length of time blood is

stored. Contamination of platelets is of particular concern. Platelets are stored for a maximum of 5 days at room temperature and carry a very small risk of bacterial contamination.

Hemolytic Reactions

An acute hemolytic transfusion reaction can happen when a transfusion occurs in an incompatible recipient. The hemolysis that occurs is mediated by a complement-mediated immune mechanism that causes destruction of the donor's RBCs by the recipient's antibodies. Although these reactions are very rare, they can have deleterious consequences such as shock and DIC.[65,66] Errors leading to hemolytic transfusion reactions usually involve clerical errors or an improperly performed type and crossmatch. Presenting symptoms may include pain at the infusion site, fever, chills, back pain, substernal pain, mental status changes, dyspnea, hypotension, hemoglobinuria, or tendency to bleed. A number of these symptoms may be masked under general anesthesia, making the diagnosis more complicated. Therefore unexplained hypotension, hemoglobinuria, or a hemorrhagic episode shortly after the start of a transfusion should lead the anesthetist to consider a hemolytic reaction as a differential diagnosis.[21,65] Initial treatment consists of discontinuing the transfusion and providing hemodynamic supportive measures and fluid management with NS. In severe reactions, a transfusion of FFP, platelets, and cryoprecipitate may help to counteract potential or actual coagulopathies.[65,67]

A delayed hemolytic transfusion reaction is more common and most often results in mild symptoms. The breakdown of RBCs is gradual and less severe in a delayed reaction and includes symptoms such as jaundice, decreased hemoglobin concentrations, and hemoglobinuria. Slightly more than one-third of patients are asymptomatic and usually require no therapy. Both obstetric patients and those who have received a prior blood transfusion are at the greatest risk of developing a delayed reaction.[21,65,67]

Transfusion-Related Acute Lung Injury

According to the FDA, prior to the year 2016 the leading cause of death due to transfusions was transfusion-related acute lung injuries (TRALI). It is estimated that TRALI occurs in up to 0.1% of patients receiving transfusions or 1 in every 5000 transfused blood components. The incidence may be higher (up to 5%–8% of the time) in the critically ill population.[68] However, due to strategies initiated in the early 2000s that were designed to mitigating this complication, the incidence has dropped dramatically.[69] TRALI occurs when the alloreactive plasma antibodies within blood products lead to clumping and activation of leukocytes, resulting in acute lung injury and noncardiogenic pulmonary edema.[21] TRALI is defined as a new acute lung injury within 6 hours after blood product administration in the absence of other known risk factors or causes for acute lung injury.[70]

The symptomatology is similar to transfusion-associated circulatory overload (TACO) and includes hypoxemia, acute respiratory distress, and increased peak airways. The major distinguishing symptom between TRALI and TACO is that the prior will exhibit hypotension and fever.[71] Classifications for transfusion-related acute lung injury are listed in Table 22.9. The transfusion of RBCs leads to a larger number of deaths when compared to plasma and platelet transfusions because RBC transfusions occur more often. The treatment of TRALI includes discontinuation of the transfusion along with ventilatory and hemodynamic support.[69-72]

Transfusion-Associated Circulatory Overload

Since 2016, TACO has been the leading cause of death in transfusion complications.[68] It is associated with an increase in morbidity, length of stay, and hospital cost.[72,73] Pulmonary edema can occur as a result of TACO due to circulatory overload, which typically results when patients receive large volumes of transfused products over short periods of time.

TABLE 22.9 Transfusion-Related Acute Lung Injury Classifications

Classification	Risk Factors	Conditions That Must Be Met
Type I	None	1. Acute onset 2. Hypoxemia 3. Bilateral pulmonary edema on imaging 4. No left atrial hypertrophy noted 5. Symptom onset during or within 6 hr of transfusion 6. No temporal relationship to an alternative risk factor for acute respiratory distress syndrome (ARDS)
Type 2	1. Same as ARDS 2. Mild baseline ARDS with deterioration of respiratory status due to the transfusion	1. Acute onset 2. Hypoxemia 3. Bilateral pulmonary edema on imaging 4. No left atrial hypertrophy noted 5. Symptom onset during or within 6 hr of transfusion 6. 12 hr of stable respiratory condition preceding the infusion

Adapted from Kleinman S, Kor DJ, et al. Transfusion-related acute lung injury (TRALI). UpToDate. https://www.uptodate.com/contents/transfusion-related-acute-lung-injury-trali?topicRef=1615&source=see_link. 2020. Accessed August 2021.

Those with underlying cardiovascular or renal disease may be at a higher risk. TACO is estimated to occur in 1% to 4% of patients receiving a transfusion and occurs higher in those who are critically ill and in ICUs. It should be suspected in any patient experiencing respiratory distress or hypertension 6 to 12 hours after completion of a transfusion. Although hypertension is a distinguishing feature between TRALI and TACO, hypotension and shock can also occur with TACO.[71] Other findings may include hypoxia, tachycardia, widened pulse pressure, jugular vein distension, or rales/wheezing within the lungs. Immediate treatment for TACO should include discontinuation of the transfusion and supportive care for both the respiratory and cardiovascular systems. Supplemental oxygen and fluid mobilization with diuresis are two of the primary treatments along with ventilatory support.[74]

Allergic Reactions

Allergic reactions can occur between donor plasma proteins and the immunoglobulin E (IgE) antibodies within the host patient. Only a very small amount of allergic protein is needed to elicit a reaction, which does not require previous blood exposure. Symptoms of an IgE-mediated reaction are usually minor and limited to urticaria and erythema, which can be treated with diphenhydramine.[1]

If IgA deficient, the patient may be at an increased risk for a more severe allergic reaction, especially if the patient has received blood products previously. IgA-deficient patients may develop IgE antibodies to IgA after initial exposure to blood products. Upon a second exposure to IgA-containing blood products, the patient may develop anaphylaxis characterized by bronchospasm, dyspnea, and hypotension. Anaphylaxis can occur with only a few milliliters of the donor blood transfusion. If the patient has a history of anaphylactic reaction to blood transfusion, then washed blood, which removes any residual IgA, should be given.[21]

SUMMARY

Blood component therapy is an important strategy for managing patient deficits in intravascular volume, oxygen carrying capacity, and hemostasis. To effectively utilize this strategy, the anesthetist must be educated in many different aspects of blood component therapy, including assessment of need and treatment of complications. Being able to anticipate and identify changes in the patient's condition, intelligently communicate the patient condition as it relates to hemodynamic changes, and provide the specific blood component needed will help lead to better patient outcomes.

REFERENCES

For a complete list of references for this chapter, scan this QR code with any smartphone code reader app, or visit the following URL: http://booksite.elsevier.com/9780323711944/

23

Positioning for Anesthesia and Surgery

Jennifer Lynn Thompson

The act of positioning a patient for surgery is a group endeavor that requires knowledge, teamwork, timing, and communication to protect against injury. The goal of patient positioning is to allow optimal surgical access while minimizing potential risk to the patient. Every surgical position carries some degree of risk that is magnified once an anesthetic is administered, which renders the patient unable to make necessary changes in positioning as needed. To prevent patient injury, clinicians must be knowledgeable about possible hazards associated with various surgical positions.

PHYSIOLOGIC EFFECTS OF SURGICAL POSITIONS

Anesthesia providers are intimately involved in coordinating and directing patient positioning and are continually monitoring and assessing the subsequent changes in the patient's physiologic status. Numerous factors have an effect on these changes: the surgical position, the length of time, the padding and positioning devices used, the type of anesthesia given, and the operative procedure. These changes most frequently involve (1) the cardiovascular system, (2) the respiratory system, (3) the nervous system, and (4) other vulnerable areas such as the skin, eyes, breasts, and genitalia.

Cardiovascular System

Cardiac output and blood pressure are generally decreased under general anesthesia in response to myocardial depression and vasodilation induced by anesthetic medications. As a result, blood pools in dependent body areas, reducing preload and decreasing stroke volume. Administration of neuromuscular blocking agents also contributes to decreased venous return because normal muscle tone is abolished. Additionally, opioids have the potential to slow the heart rate, further decreasing cardiac output and blood pressure. In healthy patients, mean arterial pressure (MAP) is maintained by compensatory increases in heart rate and systemic vascular resistance (SVR), but elderly patients and those with preexisting diseases are less adaptive to these hemodynamic changes. Compensatory mechanisms to increase heart rate when hypotension occurs are blunted by general anesthetics, rendering cardiac output and blood pressure more susceptible to gravitational forces.

With the patient under anesthesia, hemodynamic changes are usually minimal in the supine and lateral positions.[1,2] However, cardiac output and blood pressure are often decreased in the sitting, prone, and flexed lateral positions, where the lower extremities are dependent.[1,3] Although central venous pressure (CVP) is increased in the prone position, left ventricular volume is reduced, probably due to decreased venous return and increased intrathoracic pressure.[4] Cardiac index (CI) may be decreased[5,6] or unchanged[5] in the prone position compared with the supine; the effect may be frame dependent.[6] In the lateral decubitus position with the kidney rest elevated, hypotension is likely because the legs are dependent, venous return is reduced

by extreme flexion, and the kidney rest may compress the great vessels.[1,3] Conversely, blood pressure may appear normal or higher in the lithotomy position, in which elevation of the legs above the trunk provides a gravity-dependent central redistribution of blood volume or autotransfusion.[3]

Mean arterial pressure increases or decreases by approximately 2 mm Hg per inch for each change in height between the heart and a body region.[7] Therefore regions elevated above the heart in the head-up, sitting, and lithotomy positions may be at risk for hypoperfusion and ischemia, particularly if hypotension occurs. The decrease in hemodynamic parameters depends on the degree of elevation of the torso. Hemodynamic changes are minimal if the patient is placed in a 45-degree, head-up sitting position, but cardiac output decreases 20% if the patient is raised to 90 degrees because venous blood pools in the extremities. When the patient is in the seated position, as compared with supine, CI, CVP, and pulmonary capillary wedge pressure (PCWP) decrease significantly and SVR increases.[8] In procedures in which the head is elevated and cerebral perfusion is a concern, invasive arterial blood pressure monitoring should be instituted, with the transducer placed at the level of the circle of Willis.[9] Additionally, measuring cerebral oxygen saturation trends may be useful.[10]

Positioning devices and mechanical ventilation may contribute to decreased cardiac output and hypotension. In the lateral decubitus position, elevation of the kidney rest under the flank may cause vena cava compression. When the patient is in the lateral decubitus position, the kidney rest should lie under the dependent iliac crest.[1] Extreme flexion of the hips in some variations of the prone or lithotomy positions may occlude the femoral vessels and contribute to decreased venous return.[11] Large tidal volumes and positive end-expiratory pressure (PEEP) may generate high intrathoracic pressures, with a subsequent reduction in venous return, right atrial filling, and cardiac output.[12]

A variety of methods have been suggested for attenuating the hemodynamic changes associated with surgical positioning. Slow assumption of the surgical position allows the cardiovascular system time to compensate for position-induced hemodynamic alterations. Because hemodynamic changes may be influenced by anesthetic technique, using a nitrous-narcotic technique or a lighter level of anesthesia (<0.5 minimum alveolar concentration) or gradually attaining a deeper level of anesthesia may attenuate position-induced hypotension.[3] Intravascular volume loading before positioning can reduce or eliminate hypotension.[1,6] However, volume replacement must be done judiciously because excessive fluid administration can lead to volume overload in susceptible individuals when the patient is returned to the supine position or when the vasodilatory effects of general anesthetics are terminated.[3]

The Trendelenburg position is often used to treat hypotension because it is assumed to increase venous return and MAP. When placed in a head-down position, normotensive individuals compensate for increases in CVP and pulmonary artery pressure (PAP) with vasodilation and a decrease in heart rate from stimulation of barore-ceptor reflexes. However, hypotensive individuals may not respond in the same manner. Investigators have demonstrated variable effects of the Trendelenburg position on cardiovascular parameters. Changes in intrathoracic blood volume of 2% to 3% in unanesthetized normovole-mic individuals are reported with the Trendelenburg position.[13] CVP, mean PAP, and pulmonary artery occlusion pressure can be increased in the head-down position, but this increase may not reflect changes in CI, stroke volume, or MAP.[13,14] Others have shown no increase in MAP, an increase in SVR, and a decrease in CI in hypotensive patients placed in the Trendelenburg position.[15]

Hypovolemia can be unrecognized in the lithotomy and Trendelen-burg positions because MAP can appear normal despite volume deficit. Volume replacement can be assessed as adequate until acute hypoten-sion occurs when the patient is returned to the horizontal position. An additive effect can occur if the Trendelenburg position is used to supplement the lithotomy position.[15]

Patients with comorbidities may be susceptible to the detrimental effects of various positions. The combination of the lithotomy posi-tion and a head-down tilt can have a detrimental effect on myocardial function in patients with coronary artery disease, because CVP, PAP, and PCWP are increased, whereas cardiac output is decreased. The Trendelenburg position may increase myocardial work by increasing central blood volume, cardiac output, and stroke volume. Individuals with very poor cardiac function can have decreased cardiac output if the increased central blood volume moves them to a worse position on the Frank-Starling curve.[16] The lower extremities of individuals with peripheral vascular disease may be at risk of ischemia in the lithotomy and Trendelenburg positions because a relative state of hypoperfusion exists when the lower extremities are elevated above the heart. Addi-tionally, when the extremities are elevated above the level of the heart, the patient may be at higher risk for compartment syndrome.[17]

The prone and Trendelenburg positions may increase venous pres-sure in the head, with resultant swelling of facial, pharyngeal, and orbital structures. Intracranial pressure can be elevated when the head is dependent because venous pressures are transmitted to the head and intracranial structures through the valveless jugular system. Cerebral blood flow can be decreased when inflow is limited by venous conges-tion in intracranial structures.[16] Postoperative visual loss (POVL) may result from an increase in ocular venous pressures and concomitant decrease in ocular perfusion pressure. Facial edema, macroglossia, and airway edema are reported following the prone and head-down posi-tions.[18] When the patient is prone, positioning the head level or higher than the heart to minimize venous outflow obstruction may prevent the development of facial edema.[19]

Respiratory System

During spontaneous respiration in awake patients, contraction of the diaphragm and intercostal muscles causes expansion of the thoracic cavity in both an anterior-posterior and a lateral direction. Downward displacement of the diaphragm generates a negative intrathoracic pres-sure and allows lung expansion as gas flows inward. Lung elastance and chest-wall compliance affect the amount of pressure necessary to expand the alveoli for a given change in volume. Gravitational factors affect the distribution of ventilation and perfusion within the lung, as well as the shape of the thoracic cavity and movement of the diaphragm and abdominal contents.

Postural changes may significantly alter compliance, lung volumes, and the distribution of ventilation and pulmonary blood flow. Posi-tioning devices may cause mechanical interference with movement of the belly wall and abdominal contents, the chest wall, or the dia-phragm.[20] Therefore anesthetic-induced depression of ventilation may

be worsened by the majority of surgical positions. Individuals with pre-existing diseases that alter respiratory function may be more suscepti-ble to the deleterious ventilatory effects of surgical positions.

Effective respiratory gas exchange depends on a balance of ventila-tion and perfusion throughout the lungs. Gravitational effects on gas and blood flow are thought to result in differences in ventilation and perfusion in different lung segments. In both awake and anesthetized patients, gravitational forces are theorized to create a gradient that favors perfusion in dependent portions of the lungs and ventilation in nondependent regions.[21,22] However, new imaging techniques have identified a concentric pattern of blood flow in the lungs, with central regions receiving a greater proportion of flow than the periphery.[23,24] The mechanism for this gradient has not been identified, but the diam-eters and branching patterns of pulmonary vessels and the distance blood must flow to reach a site are possible factors. Nongravitational factors such as cardiac output, pleural pressures, and lung volumes are also thought to play a factor in regional lung perfusion.[21,24]

Positional changes may result in redistribution of ventilation and perfusion. These changes are evident less in the sitting position and more so in the prone and lateral positions. In the prone position, changes in ventilation-perfusion ($\dot{V}/\dot{Q}$) ratios have been postulated as the cause of improved oxygenation.[21] More lung volume is pres-ent posteriorly than anteriorly, where anterior mediastinal structures occupy significant space; as a consequence, posterior lung segments are better ventilated. Ventilation is more uniform, and $\dot{V}/\dot{Q}$ matching is better in the prone position than in the supine position due to the alleviation of pressure from the anterior structures on the posterior lung tissue.[22]

In the lateral decubitus position, both ventilation and perfusion are greater in the dependent lung than in the nondependent lung in awake, spontaneously breathing patients. With the addition of anes-thesia, positive pressure ventilation, and paralysis, the upper lung becomes easier to ventilate than the dependent lung, thereby creating a $\dot{V}/\dot{Q}$ mismatch. $\dot{V}/\dot{Q}$ mismatching in the lateral decubitus position may affect oxygenation, especially with procedures requiring one-lung ventilation. Hypoxic pulmonary vasoconstriction in the unventilated lung further redistributes blood flow to the dependent lung to improve oxygenation.[24]

Changes in the elastance and resistance of the diaphragm and abdo-men occur when shifting between positions. These changes have little effect on movement of the chest wall in healthy individuals but may have an effect in persons with conditions that predispose to abnormal-ities of lung function.[25] In the prone position, diaphragmatic excursion can be limited by the abdominal viscera if the abdomen is compressed by the weight of the body or positioning devices. If the abdomen hangs free, gravity allows the abdominal contents to shift, reducing interfer-ence with diaphragmatic movement.[26,27] In the anesthetized patient in the lateral position, abdominal contents shift cephalad, moving the hemidiaphragm of the dependent lung upward, thereby decreasing ventilation in the dependent lung and reducing its compliance.[28] In the nondependent lung of the anesthetized patient, ventilation is greater and compliance is increased due to the caudal shift of the upper hemi-diaphragm allowing unrestricted lung excursion (see Chapter 30).

Lung capacities are decreased with most position changes. In the supine position, functional residual capacity (FRC) and total lung capacity are significantly decreased compared with the sitting position due to the cephalad shift of the diaphragm caused by pressure of the abdominal viscera.[20,25] Some investigators have found an increase in FRC with patients in the prone position, when the abdomen hangs free.[21,29] Theories pose that better matching of ventilation and perfu-sion, rather than changes in lung volumes or capacities, cause improve-ments in oxygenation in the prone position.[20]

The lithotomy position has little effect on the compliance of the respiratory system in healthy, conscious volunteers.[20] However, extreme flexion of the thighs in the exaggerated lithotomy position compresses the abdomen, shifts the abdominal viscera cephalad, and limits diaphragmatic movement. As a result, compliance and tidal volume are reduced, and airway pressures and dead space/tidal volume ratios are increased.[30] This effect may be amplified in obese individuals.[29,31]

The sitting position is more favorable for ventilation and has less effect on lung volumes than other positions. The more the torso is elevated, the smaller the effect on lung mechanics. Forced vital capacity and FRC are within normal parameters in the seated position.[26] The abdominal contents shift caudally and anteriorly, causing less interference with diaphragmatic movement and allowing greater expansion of dependent lung regions.[20] Compared with the supine position, in which the abdominal muscles are used for spontaneous breathing, in the sitting position, the rib cage contributes more to ventilation.[26] However, respiratory benefits of the sitting position can be attenuated when the sitting position is modified to minimize cardiovascular effects. Flexion of the lower extremities at the hip and elevation of the legs can cause abdominal contents to shift cephalad against the diaphragm limiting diaphragmatic excursion and decreasing FRC and closing volumes.[9]

The Trendelenburg position exacerbates the deleterious ventilatory effects of the various positions. The diaphragm is displaced cephalad, and its excursion is limited by shifting of the abdominal contents, decreasing the FRC progressively as the degree of Trendelenburg position increases. Movement of the mediastinum toward the head may result in the tip of the endotracheal tube migrating into the right mainstem bronchus.[32,33] This complication may also occur upon establishment of the pneumoperitoneum, in which the diaphragm is displaced in a cephalad direction by pressurized gas.[33,34]

PATHOPHYSIOLOGY OF NERVE INJURY

Transection, compression, and stretch are the primary mechanisms responsible for nerve injuries.[35,36] Nerves may be transected by surgical maneuvers or by trauma. Compression can happen when a nerve is forced against a bony prominence or a hard surface such as an armboard or operating table. In the lateral position, for example, the weight of the superior leg pushes against the dependent extremity and may compress the common peroneal nerve of the dependent leg against the operating table. Stretch injuries occur where nerves such as the sciatic nerve or brachial plexus have a long course across many structures. Peripheral nerves have some laxity that allows a limited amount of elongation. However, excessive elongation or stretch may cause conduction changes, axonal disruption, or interruption of the nerve's vascular supply.[37,38] Traction injuries can occur when a peripheral nerve is pulled over or under immovable structures.[38] For example, the femoral nerve can be kinked under the inguinal ligament when the thighs are flexed on the abdomen, as in the exaggerated lithotomy position.

A common component of all peripheral nerve injuries is ischemia. Intraneural blood flow may be compromised by stretch, compression, or disruption of the nerve tissue itself. Other causes include occlusion of major vessels, emboli, tissue edema, or inhibition of perfusion at the capillary level.[38] For example, pressure applied over a body surface may limit venous capillary outflow, causing a rise in venous capillary pressure and a decrease in the hydrostatic pressure gradient between interstitial tissues and the capillary.[39] Ultimately, tissue edema occurs as fluid is sequestered in the cells and interstitial space. As venous capillary pressure rises, the arterial-venous pressure gradient is reduced, decreasing flow to tissues along the capillary. As venous and tissue pressures continue to rise, arterial inflow is eventually obstructed and

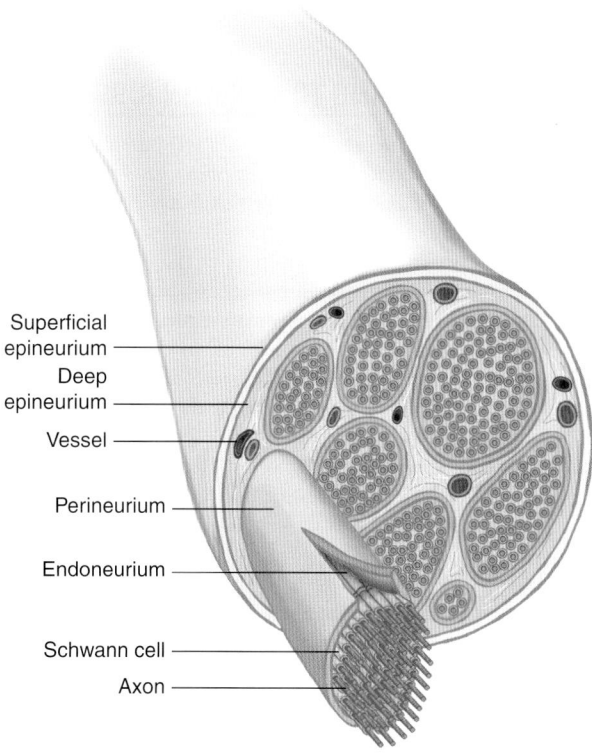

Fig. 23.1 Cross section of a peripheral nerve trunk showing its components. (From Patton KT. *Anatomy & Physiology*. 10th ed. St Louis: Elsevier; 2019:476.)

Labels in figure: Superficial epineurium; Deep epineurium; Vessel; Perineurium; Endoneurium; Schwann cell; Axon

ischemia results. Low mean arterial blood pressure may augment the development of ischemic conditions.[35]

Tissue metabolism continues even in the absence of blood flow. When ischemia ensues, adenosine triphosphate (ATP) production is decreased, causing failure of the transmembrane sodium-potassium pump and accumulation of sodium within the cell. The resulting osmotic pressure gradient favors the movement of water into the cells. Intracellular volume is increased, and tissue edema occurs.[40] A vicious cycle of ischemia results as tissue pressures increase, preventing the movement of fluid and nutrients from the capillaries into the cells.

The susceptibility of peripheral nerves to developing ischemia may be partially due to their anatomic structure (Fig. 23.1). Peripheral nerves are composed of bundles of nerve fibers (fascicles), and their vascular supply is encased in protective connective-tissue coverings. Each nerve fiber is composed of one or more axons sheathed by Schwann cells (neurolemma) that are either myelinated or unmyelinated. The axons and neurolemma are covered by a loose connective tissue called the endoneurium. The perineurium is a tough connective tissue that binds the fascicles into identifiable structures. The epineurium consists of two layers: an inner epineurium that supports the fascicles and an outer epineurium that covers the external surface of the nerve.[41] The quantity of these protective tissues varies between nerves and even along the same nerve. The entire nerve trunk is covered by a loose layer of connective tissue that allows it to slide across joints and other tissues.[38,41]

Peripheral nerves have an extensive microvascular supply. Blood vessels in the epineurium run parallel to the nerve and form numerous anastomoses with the perineurium. Collateral connections between the perineurium and the endoneurial capillaries run obliquely between the layers and thus may be more susceptible to compression by increases in tissue pressure. In addition, the endoneurial space lacks lymphatic vessels, so edema and fluid accumulation in this region may obstruct the microcirculation.[37]

FACTORS CONTRIBUTING TO NERVE INJURIES

Perioperative peripheral nerve injuries (PPNI) are frequently attributed to incorrect surgical positioning; however, current evidence indicates that the etiology of PPNI is multifactorial and involves patient predisposition, precipitating physiologic and mechanical factors.[42,43] Perioperative factors that contribute to the development of nerve injuries include ancillary positioning devices, prolonged surgical procedures, and anesthetic technique. Patient-related factors include gender, advanced age, extremes in body habitus, and preexisting medical conditions such as diabetes mellitus, tobacco use, and hypertension. Intraoperative occurrences such as hypovolemia, hypotension, induced hypothermia, hypoxia, and electrolyte disturbances have also been associated with nerve injury.[44] However, the precise mechanism of nerve injury is often unclear, suggesting that further investigation is needed to identify causative factors.[42,45]

Positioning Devices

Controlled studies of complications related to specific positioning devices are largely nonexistent. Isolated case reports provide much of the evidence that is known about nerve injuries attributable to improper use of positioning devices. Ancillary positioning devices, such as tight padding or straps used to restrain the patient or an extremity, can cause skin breakdown or nerve injury if excessively tightened.[46,47] For example, the lateral femoral cutaneous nerve in the thigh is susceptible to injury by tight table straps. Common peroneal nerve injury has been attributed to the improper use of stirrups. Brachial plexus injury has been caused by an armboard falling off the operating room (OR) table[48] or the improper use of shoulder braces with steep Trendelenburg position.[47] Compression injury of the radial nerve has been reported after the intraoperative use of tourniquets and blood pressure cuffs and by compression between the humerus and a firm surface, such as a positioning device.[49,50] Improper placement of an axillary roll may cause compression of neural and vascular structures of the brachial plexus.[51]

Length of Procedure

Prolonged surgical procedures contribute to postoperative positioning complications. POVL, nerve injuries, and compartment syndrome have been associated with a variety of procedures and positions in which the common denominator was a duration of more than 4 hours.[52-55] Rhabdomyolysis and acute renal failure also have been reported after lengthy procedures.[56,57] One possible explanation is that during long procedures the weight of the body causes external compression of dependent tissues and states of low perfusion.[57] The longer this situation persists, the higher the potential for development of edema and ischemic injury.

Anesthetic Techniques

Anesthetic techniques may contribute to the development of position-related injuries.[58] Patients receiving general anesthesia cannot move in response to painful stimuli generated by uncomfortable body positions. The constraints of the procedure or surgeon may limit movement even when patients are sedated. Muscle relaxation due to neuromuscular blocking drugs or volatile anesthetics may contribute to stretch injuries by allowing increased mobility of joints.[43] For example, limited elbow extension from tight biceps muscles can be overcome by neuromuscular blockade, allowing the arms to be extended flat and

subsequently stretching the median nerve.[35] The hypotensive effects of general anesthetics may lower perfusion pressures below acceptable levels in patients who are hypertensive or have other comorbidities. The use of hypotensive techniques to reduce blood loss should be balanced against the risk of possible complications resulting from decreased perfusion pressures, particularly during prolonged procedures and in the sitting, lithotomy, and Trendelenburg positions, in which gravity affects blood flow.

Although neuraxial and peripheral nerve blocks are associated with both permanent and temporary nerve injuries, the majority of injuries are not related to positioning but to poor block technique, hematoma formation, and direct needle trauma.[59] However, recognition of nerve injury may be delayed when providers attribute the patient's symptoms to the residual effects of regional blocks and local anesthetics.[60,61] Anesthetists must have a high index of suspicion when return of function is delayed beyond what is expected for a particular technique or local anesthetic and when patients complain of severe pain in the presence of a seemingly adequate block.

PATIENT-RELATED FACTORS CONTRIBUTING TO NERVE INJURIES

Body Habitus

Extremes of body habitus correlate with an increased incidence of positioning complications.[54,56,57] Individuals who are underweight may develop decubiti or nerve damage due to lack of adequate adipose tissue over bony prominences.[54,62] For example, thin patients may be at higher risk for sciatic nerve damage when the opposite buttock is elevated,[35] and thinner women (body mass index [BMI] <22) are more likely to develop ulnar neuropathy.[59,62] Individuals with a muscular physique may also be at increased risk for compartment syndrome and ulnar nerve injury.[36,63]

Obesity increases morbidity from positioning because large tissue masses place increased pressure on dependent body parts. Extreme abduction of the arms may cause stretch injuries to the lower roots of the brachial plexus, whereas the upper roots may be damaged by excessive rotation of the head to the opposite side. Ulnar neuropathy has been associated with an increased BMI.[64] Adipose tissue is poorly perfused and may contribute to this problem. For example, in the lateral position, a heavy superior extremity may interfere with perfusion by exerting substantial pressure on the inferior extremity.

Preexisting Conditions

Preexisting conditions appear to be associated with an increased risk of developing postoperative position-related injuries. Hypertension, diabetes mellitus, peripheral vascular disease, peripheral neuropathies, and alcoholism can exacerbate the physiologic effects of various positions.[38] Nerve injury and preexisting neuropathies are more common in patients with diabetes,[35] and diabetes is the most common metabolic cause of spontaneous isolated femoral neuropathy.[65] A history of smoking within 1 month of the surgical procedure has been identified as a risk factor for nerve injury, as well as for delayed healing.[54,66] Individuals with subclinical ulnar nerve entrapment, which may not be apparent to the patient or anesthetist, are also at risk for nerve injuries.[67,68]

Box 23.1 highlights factors associated with position-related injuries.

PERIOPERATIVE NEUROPATHIES

In the awake patient, pain or discomfort from extreme body positioning would prompt optimization of position for the relief of symptoms. The induction of anesthesia renders a patient unable to make these changes

BOX 23.1   **Factors Associated With Position-Related Injuries**

Positioning Devices
- Table straps
- Leg holders and stirrups
- Axillary roll
- Bolsters
- Fracture table post
- Shoulder braces
- Positioning frames
- Headrests
- Ether screen

Length of Procedure
- >4–5 hr

Body Habitus
- Obesity
- Malnutrition
- Bulky musculature

Preexisting Pathophysiology
- Anemia
- Diabetes mellitus
- Peripheral vascular disease
- Liver disease
- Peripheral neuropathies
- Alcoholism
- Limited joint mobility
- Smoking

Anesthetic Technique
- General anesthesia
- Hypotensive techniques
- Neuromuscular blockade

and therefore susceptible to injury. The addition of muscle relaxants may allow body or extremity positioning that the awake patient would not otherwise tolerate, making the patient even more vulnerable to injury.[38] Table 23.1 and Box 23.2 identify specific nerve injuries associated with positioning and recommendations for prevention.

Ulnar Neuropathy

Ulnar neuropathy is one of the most frequently reported injuries after surgery and anesthesia, yet its causation is not completely understood.[3,36,67] Damage to the ulnar nerve results in the inability to oppose the fifth finger and diminished sensation to the fourth and fifth finger and, if prolonged, can result in atrophy of the intrinsic muscles of the hand, creating a clawlike contracture.[69]

The ulnar nerve traverses the length of the upper extremity from its origins as a branch of the medial cord of the brachial plexus to its terminal branches in the hand. In the upper arm, the ulnar nerve passes along the anterior aspect of the medial head of the triceps muscle and posterior into the groove between the medial epicondyle of the humerus and the olecranon (Fig. 23.2).[70] In this region, the nerve is sheathed in the cubital tunnel before exiting and passing between the two heads of the flexor carpi ulnaris. The cubital tunnel retinaculum (CTR) forms the roof of the cubital tunnel (see Fig. 23.2), a potential area for nerve compression because fibrous tissue and the elbow capsule form a semirigid canal that changes shape with flexion and extension of the forearm.[54] Direct pressure on the cubital tunnel from contact on an unpadded armboard or surgical table may cause nerve compression.[70,71] When the elbow is flexed, the distance between the olecranon and medial epicondyle increases, stretching the CTR and decreasing the size of the tunnel, and it can increase pressure on the nerve.[36,72]

Although excessive flexing of the elbow and direct compression of the ulnar nerve at the condylar groove may contribute to ulnar neuropathy, current consensus is that the cause is multifactorial and not always preventable.[71] Ulnar neuropathy is more frequently associated with male gender,[38,62,67] the presence of a preexisting asymptomatic neuropathy,[67] prolonged hospital stays,[38,62] and extremes of body habitus.[38,59] Anatomic variations, such as a larger coronoid process and less subcutaneous tissue over the ulnar region, are hypothesized to explain the gender difference findings.[62] Although often blamed on

intraoperative positioning, the prevalence of ulnar neuropathy is similar in medical and surgical patients and most often has a delayed onset (median of 3 days).[73]

Recommendations for positioning to prevent ulnar nerve injury in anesthetized patients include the use of padding, placing the arms in either a supinated or neutral forearm position, and abducting the arms less than 90 degrees if armboards are used.[71,74] If the arms are secured on armboards, the forearm should be supinated (palm up) or neutral, because pronation (palm down) may increase pressure over the ulnar nerve.[75] When the patient's arms are tucked at the side of the body, they should be in a neutral position with the palms facing inward (Fig. 23.3). Anatomic changes in the cubital tunnel with flexion and extension suggest that excessive flexion of the elbow should be avoided when the patient is in the lateral position or if the arms are secured across the chest. Evidence supports the conclusion that ulnar nerve palsy is not always a preventable complication despite the best efforts at careful positioning and padding.[71,74,75]

BRACHIAL PLEXUS INJURIES

The brachial plexus is vulnerable to injuries in almost every surgical position, particularly if the arms are abducted or the head is rotated (Fig. 23.4). When the patient is supine, abduction of the arms greater than 90 degrees stretches the plexus around the humeral head. Turning the head to the side with the arms abducted can cause stretching and compression of the contralateral brachial plexus beneath the clavicle.[76] Even tucking the arms next to the body is not without risk if the head is turned laterally and the shoulders are depressed. When the patient is prone, inadequate support of the shoulders allows them to sag anteriorly, causing traction on the plexus. Also in the prone position, extending the arms over the head may compress the plexus between the clavicle and first rib.[76]

In the lateral decubitus position, brachial plexus injury is most commonly the result of excessive stretching, usually because of arm abduction greater than 90 degrees, external rotation, extension and lateral flexion of the head, and posterior shoulder displacement.[35] In the lateral position, the weight of the chest can compress the lower shoulder and axilla, putting pressure on the axillary neurovascular bundle. An "axillary roll" can be placed just caudal to the dependent axilla to relieve this pressure.[71,72]

Brachial plexus injuries are also associated with positioning devices. Injuries can be caused by an unsecured arm slipping off an armboard or an armboard falling off the OR table, causing excessive stretch of the plexus. Sometimes used during steep Trendelenburg position, shoulder braces placed too close to the base of the neck can compress neurovascular structures and cause brachial plexus neuropathy. Although best avoided, shoulder braces, if used, are properly placed at the distal end of the clavicle over the acromioclavicular joint.[48,77,78]

Spreading of the sternal retractor during cardiac surgery causes the clavicle to move posteriorly and the first rib to rotate upward, pinching the plexus between the two.[77] Dissection of the internal mammary artery requires wider, asymmetric chest retraction to allow adequate visualization and may predispose to brachial plexus neuropathy. To prevent brachial plexus injury during cardiac surgical procedures, caudad placement of the sternal retractor and avoidance of excessive and prolonged asymmetric chest wall retraction are recommended.[79,80]

SPINAL CORD INJURY

Cheney et al.[42] compared claims documented since 1990 to the outcome claims in the pre-1990 American Society of Anesthesiologists (ASA) closed-claims database and found that spinal cord injury claims

TABLE 23.1	Common Nerve Injuries: Etiology and Prevention	
Nerve/Nerve Group Injured	**Potential Cause**	**Positioning Recommendation**
Brachial plexus	*Supine, Trendelenburg, Lithotomy*	
	Arm abducted >90 degrees on armboard	Do not abduct arm >90 degrees
	Arm falls off table edge and is abducted and externally rotated	Ensure arms are adequately secured
	Arm abduction and lateral flexion of the head to the opposite side	Support head to maintain neutral alignment
	Trendelenburg	
	Shoulder braces placed too medial or lateral	Place well-padded shoulder brace over the acromioclavicular joint
		Avoid use if possible
	Lateral	
	Thorax pressure exertion on dependent shoulder and axilla	Place roll caudad to the axilla supporting the upper part of the thorax
	Prone	
	Arms abducted >90 degrees	Abduct arms minimally
Ulnar nerve	Arm pronated on armboard	Supinate forearm on padded armboard
	Arms folded across abdomen or chest with elbows flexed >90 degrees	Do not flex elbows >90 degrees
	Arms secured at side with inadequate padding at the elbow	Place sufficient padding around elbow
	Arms inadequately secured at side, elbows extend over table edge	Draw sheet should extend above the elbow and be tucked between the patient and the mattress
Radial nerve or circumflex nerve	Arm pressed against vertical positioning or retractor post or pole securing ether screen	Place adequate padding between or ensure arm is not pressing against vertical posts or pole
Suprascapular nerve	Patient in lateral position rolls semiprone onto dependent arm with shoulder circumduction	Stabilize patient in lateral position
Sciatic nerve	Malnourished/emaciated patient supine or sitting on inadequately padded table	Generous soft padding under buttock
	Legs straight in sitting position	Flex table at knees
	Lithotomy	
	Legs externally rotated with knees extended	Minimal external rotation of legs; knees should be flexed
Common peroneal nerve	*Lithotomy*	
	Fibular neck rests against vertical bar of lithotomy stirrup	Adequate padding between leg and stirrup
	Knees extended, legs externally rotated	Knees flexed with minimal external rotation
	Lateral	
	Undue pressure on downside leg	Padding under the fibular head
Posterior tibial nerve	*Lithotomy*	
	"Knee crutch" stirrups supporting posterior aspect of knees	Generous padding under knees
		Avoid use of this stirrup for prolonged procedures
Saphenous nerve	*Lithotomy*	
	Foot suspended outside vertical bar, leg rests on bar	Sufficient padding between legs and vertical bar
	Excessive pressure on medial aspect of leg from "knee crutch" stirrups	Sufficient padding between stirrup and leg
Obturator nerve	*Lithotomy*	
	Excessive flexion of the thigh at hip	Minimal hip flexion
Pudendal nerve	Traction of legs against perineal post or orthopedic fracture table	Generous padding between perineum and post

Modified from American Society of Anesthesiologists. Practice advisory for the prevention of perioperative peripheral neuropathies 2018: an updated report by the American Society of Anesthesiologists Task Force on Prevention of Perioperative Peripheral Neuropathies. *Anesthesiology.* 2018;128(1):11–26; Phillips N. *Berry & Kohn's Operating Room Technique.* 14th ed. St. Louis: Elsevier; 2017:479–528; Heizenroth PA. Positioning the patient for surgery. In Rothrock JC. *Alexander's Care of the Patient in Surgery.* 15th ed. St. Louis: Elsevier; 2015:155–185.

had surpassed ulnar nerve injury claims. However, spinal cord injury claims were primarily associated with neuraxial blocks in anticoagulated patients and with blocks for acute and chronic pain management. Although rare, hemiparesis and quadriplegia are associated with surgical procedures performed in the sitting and prone positions.[81-83]

Midcervical flexion myelopathy with temporary or permanent quadriplegia may occur when the head is flexed on the neck in the sitting or prone positions. When the head is flexed, the spinal cord moves anteriorly and may be compressed against the posterior vertebral body. Ischemia may result from a combination of compression and stretch

BOX 23.2 An Updated Report by the American Society of Anesthesiologists Task Force on Prevention of Perioperative Peripheral Neuropathies

Preoperative History and Physical Assessment

- Review a patient's preoperative history and perform a physical examination to identify body habitus, preexisting neurologic symptoms, diabetes mellitus, peripheral vascular disease, alcohol dependency, arthritis, and sex (e.g., male sex and its association with ulnar neuropathy).
- When judged appropriate, ascertain whether patients can comfortably tolerate the anticipated operative position.

Positioning Strategies for the Upper Extremities
Positioning Strategies to Reduce Perioperative Brachial Plexus Neuropathy

- When possible, limit arm abduction in a supine patient to 90 degrees.
  - The prone position may allow patients to comfortably tolerate abduction of their arms to >90 degrees.

Positioning Strategies to Reduce Perioperative Ulnar Neuropathy

- Supine patient with arm on an armboard: Position the upper extremity to decrease pressure on the postcondylar groove of the humerus (ulnar groove).
  - Use of either supination or the neutral forearm positions may be used to facilitate this action.
- Supine patient with arms tucked at side: Place the forearm in a neutral position.
- Flexion of the elbow: When possible, avoid flexion of the elbow to decrease the risk of ulnar neuropathy.

Positioning Strategies to Reduce Perioperative Radial Neuropathy

- Avoid prolonged pressure on the radial nerve in the spiral groove of the humerus.

Positioning Strategies to Reduce Perioperative Median Neuropathy

- Avoid extension of the elbow beyond the range that is comfortable during the preoperative assessment to prevent stretching of the median nerve.

Periodic Assessment of Upper Extremity Position During Procedures

- Periodic perioperative assessments may be performed to ensure maintenance of the desired position.

Positioning Strategies for the Lower Extremities
Positioning Strategies to Reduce Perioperative Sciatic Neuropathy

- Stretching of the hamstring muscle group: Positions that stretch the hamstring muscle group beyond the range that is comfortable during the preoperative assessment may be avoided to prevent stretching of the sciatic nerve.
- Limiting hip flexion: Since the sciatic nerve or its branches cross both the hip and the knee joints, assess extension and flexion of these joints when determining the degree of hip flexion.

Positioning Strategies to Reduce Perioperative Femoral Neuropathy

- When possible, avoid extension or flexion of the hip to decrease the risk of femoral neuropathy.

Positioning Strategies to Reduce Perioperative Peroneal Neuropathy

- Avoid prolonged pressure on the peroneal nerve at the fibular head.

Protective Padding

- Padded armboards may be used to decrease the risk of upper extremity neuropathy.
- Chest rolls in the laterally positioned patient may be used to decrease the risk of upper extremity neuropathy.
- Padding at the elbow may be used to decrease the risk of upper extremity neuropathy.
- Specific padding to prevent pressure of a hard surface against the peroneal nerve at the fibular head may be used to decrease the risk of peroneal neuropathy.
- Avoid the inappropriate use of padding (e.g., padding too tight) to decrease the risk of perioperative neuropathy.

Equipment

- When possible, avoid the improper use of automated blood pressure cuffs on the arm (i.e., placed below the antecubital fossa) to reduce the risk of upper extremity neuropathy.
- When possible, avoid the use of shoulder braces in a steep head-down position to decrease the risk of perioperative neuropathies.

Postoperative Physical Assessment

- Perform a simple postoperative assessment of extremity nerve function for early recognition of peripheral neuropathies.

Documentation

- Document specific perioperative positioning actions that may be useful for continuous improvement processes.

From Practice Advisory for the Prevention of Perioperative Peripheral Neuropathies: an updated report by the American Society of Anesthesiologists Task Force on prevention of perioperative peripheral neuropathies. *Anesthesiology.* 2018;128(1):11–26.

because the spinal cord lengthens with flexion. Like a rubber band, the cord becomes thinner as it stretches, and the caliber of the vessels supplying the cord can be reduced.[83] Increased vertebral venous pressure is also proposed as leading to postoperative spinal cord injury. The absence of valves between the central venous and epidural venous systems allows direct transmission of increased abdominal or intrathoracic pressure to the vertebral venous systems.[84] Congestion in the veins draining the spinal cord, coupled with hypotension, may result in decreased spinal cord perfusion and the onset of new neurologic deficits.[83] Hyperflexion of the head on the neck in any position may be avoided by allowing a minimum of two fingerbreadths between the sternum and mandible.[3]

Somatosensory evoked potentials (SSEPs) have been suggested as being useful in identifying position-related changes in spinal cord function.[85] However, neurologic defects have emerged postoperatively despite normal intraoperative SSEP readings.[3,86,87] A study by Schwartz et al.[86] evaluated the role of transcranial electric motor-evoked potential (tce-MEP) and its recommended use for the detection of not only spinal cord injury but also brachial plexus and ulnar nerve injury due to positioning.

POSTOPERATIVE VISUAL LOSS

POVL is a rare but devastating complication of nonophthalmic surgery. It may occur in one or both eyes and refers to a variety of visual

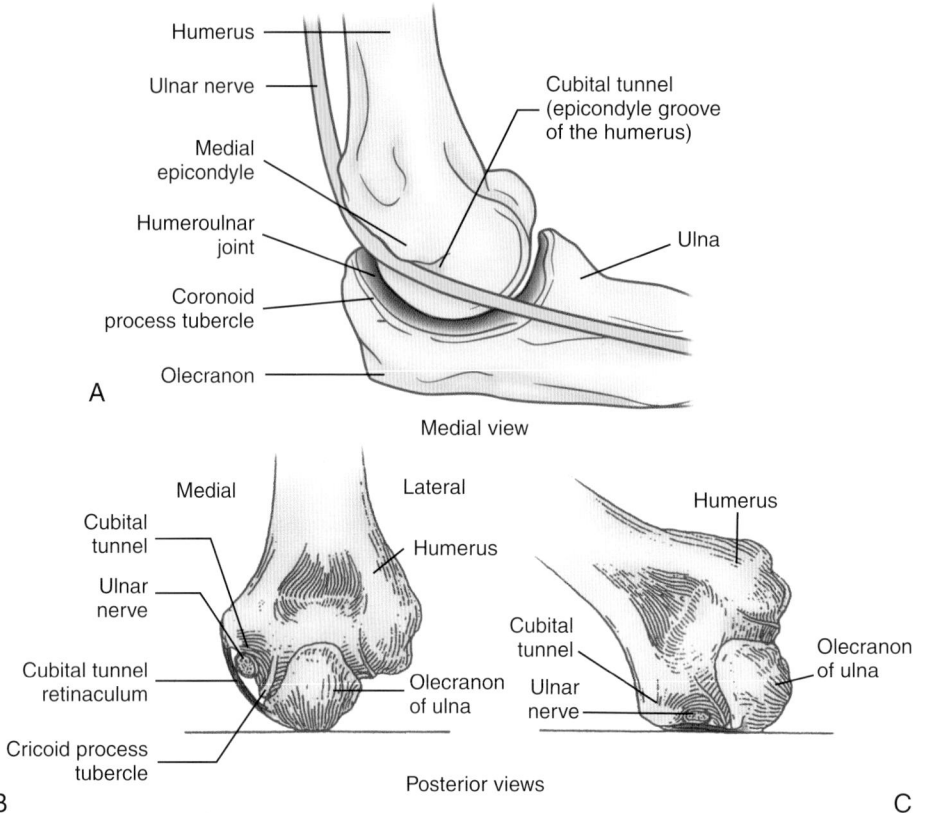

Fig. 23.2 The ulnar nerve at the cubital tunnel. (A) Medial view. (B) Posterior view. Note cubital tunnel retinaculum over the ulnar nerve in the cubital tunnel. (C) Posterior view with elbow tilted on medial side. Note the ulnar nerve compressed. (From Rothrock JC. *Alexander's Care of the Patient in Surgery.* 15th ed. St. Louis: Elsevier; 2015:162.)

defects ranging from decreased visual acuity to total blindness.[88] Visual loss after nonophthalmic surgery is generally attributable to five causes: ischemic optic neuropathy (ION), central retinal artery occlusion (CRAO), central retinal vein occlusion, cortical blindness, and glycine toxicity.[89] Of these causes, patient positioning may be a contributing factor in the development of ION and CRAO. In the ASA POVL registry, ION and CRAO accounted for 81% of all cases, with ION accounting for 89% of POVL after prone spinal procedures.[19,90]

As the name implies, ION is the result of ischemia in a portion of the optic nerve. The optic nerves may be susceptible to hypoperfusion. The central retinal and posterior ciliary arteries are end arteries and lack anastomoses with other arteries[91] (Fig. 23.5). Thus the structures supplied by these vessels are in a "watershed" region, meaning that the region receives a dual blood supply from the most distal branches of two arteries. Watershed areas are reportedly vulnerable to ischemia if a portion of the blood supply is interrupted.[88,92] Although the ocular circulation lacks autonomic innervation, autoregulation still occurs in the ophthalmic and central retinal arteries.[91] The limits of autoregulation in the ocular circulation are unknown. Preexisting diseases such as diabetes and hypertension that disrupt autoregulatory mechanisms may contribute to ischemic episodes during periods of hypotension.[93] ION is divided into two types: anterior ION (AION) and posterior ION (PION). AION is characterized by optic nerve injury occurring anterior to the lamina cribrosa, whereas PION results from optic nerve injury posterior to the lamina cribrosa.[94]

A large case-control study on ION associated with spine surgery identified six independent and significant risk factors, including male sex, obesity, Wilson frame use, longer operative times, greater blood loss, and a lower colloid to crystalloid ratio in the nonblood fluid administration.[44,95,96] Significant risk factors found by other researchers include male sex, anemia from blood loss greater than 1 L, surgery lasting over 5 hours, diabetes, hypertension, vascular disease, smoking, and intraoperative hypotension.[44,95] Despite the association of various risk factors, ION has occurred in healthy patients and in the absence of these perioperative factors.[44,95,97]

Whereas the exact cause of ION is still unclear, risk reduction strategies are aimed at avoiding both increased intraocular pressure and decreased optic nerve perfusion.[44,88] Just as cerebral perfusion pressure equals MAP minus intracranial pressure, ocular perfusion pressure (OPP) is the difference between MAP and intraocular pressure (IOP).[98,99] Intraoperative and anesthetic events that decrease MAP and thus reduce OPP include general anesthetics, hypotension, hemorrhage, and hypovolemia. Venous pressure and the ratio of aqueous humor production to absorption affect IOP. An increase in venous pressure may impede aqueous humor outflow into the venous system, causing a rise in IOP.[99] As IOP approaches MAP, OPP will decrease. During surgery, ocular venous pressure can be increased by a head-down tilt, increased abdominal and right atrial pressure, and obstruction of jugular venous return.[92] Both steep Trendelenburg position and beds such as the Wilson frame, where the head is positioned much lower than the heart, may exacerbate venous congestion and increase IOP. Unlike CRAO, ION does not seem to be associated with pressure on the globe, because ION has occurred in patients whose heads were secured with pin-type headrests.[19]

CRAO is a less common cause of POVL than ION and is caused by decreased blood supply to the entire retina. In 93 cases of POVL

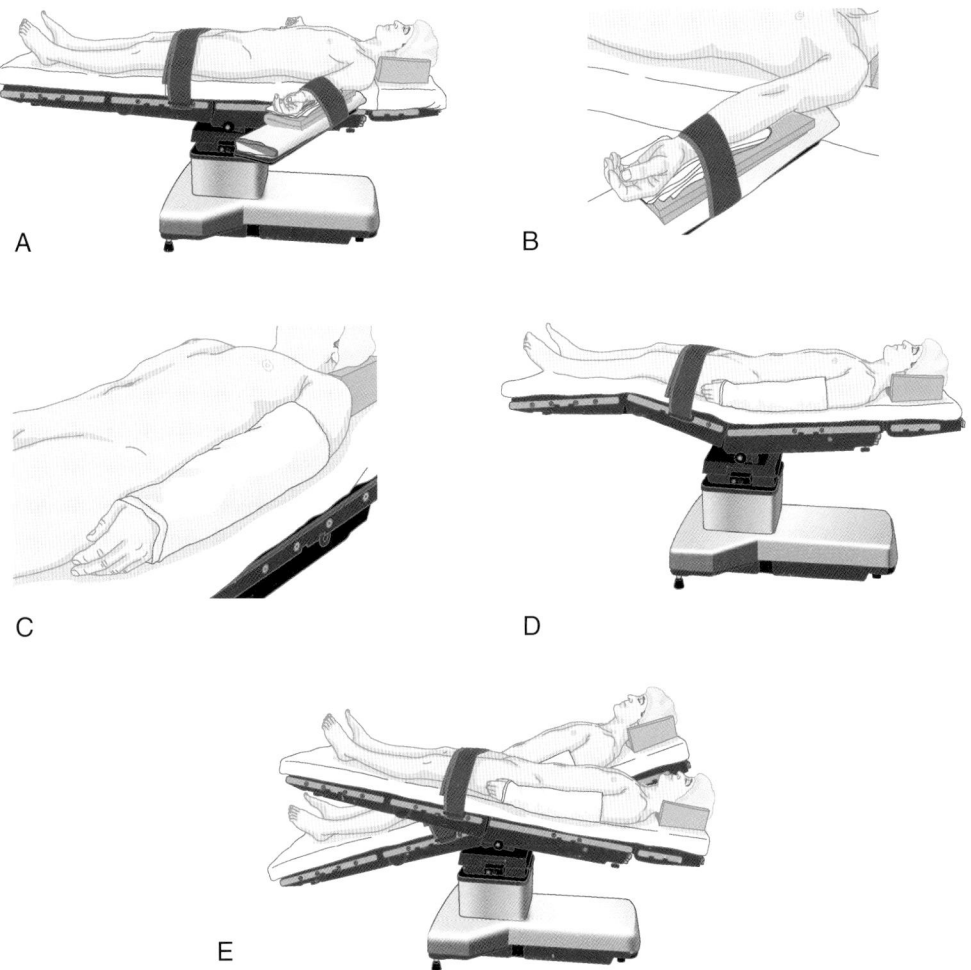

Fig. 23.3 (A) Supine. Note the asymmetry of the base of the table, placing the patient's center of gravity over the base if positioned in the usual direction. (B) Arm position on the armboard. Abduction of the arm should be limited to less than 90 degrees whenever possible. The arm is supinated, and the elbow is padded. (C) Arm tucked at patient's side. Arm in neutral position with palm to hip. The elbow is padded, and one needs to ensure that the arm is supported. (D) Lawn-chair position. Flexion of the hips and knees decreases tension on the back. (E) Trendelenburg position (head tilted down) and reverse Trendelenburg position (head tilted up). Shoulder braces should be avoided to prevent brachial plexus compression injuries. (From Miller RD, Pardo Jr MC. *Basics of Anesthesia*. 7th ed. Philadelphia: Elsevier; 2017.)

following prone spinal surgery, only 10 cases were attributed to CRAO.[90] The central retinal artery is one of the first branches of the internal carotid artery and nourishes the internal layer of the retina. The most common cause of CRAO is improper head positioning that results in external pressure on the eye.[44,95] Other causes can include emboli, due to a hypercoagulable state, that migrates to the central retinal artery and causes unilateral blindness. Perioperative factors associated with CRAO are prone spine operations, cardiopulmonary bypass surgery, and head and neck procedures where injections are performed around the nose and eyes.[95] CRAO typically presents as severe unilateral vision loss immediately following surgery. Although many treatments are recommended for CRAO, few have proven efficacy, and prognosis is poor.[99]

General risk factors for central retinal vein obstruction syndrome include hypertension, cardiovascular disease, increased BMI, open angle glaucoma, and sickle cell anemia. Because external pressure on the globe may cause central retinal vein obstruction, when the patient is placed prone for procedures on the head and neck, some suggest the use of three-pin headrests that securely immobilize the head rather

than the horseshoe headrest.[100] Although the three-pin headrest avoids the potential for external ocular compression, POVL from ION has occurred despite its use.[90]

A practice advisory for perioperative visual loss associated with spine surgery was developed in 2006 and updated in 2012, based on the synthesis and analysis of opinions of spine surgeons, neuroophthalmologists, and anesthesiologists. A summary of practice points, including major considerations from the ASA practice advisory for the prevention of POVL, can be found in Box 23.3.

Much remains to be learned about POVL. Although factors such as hypertension, vascular disease, obesity, and smoking have been associated with POVL, specific methods for identifying at-risk patients are not available, and reasons that POVL occurs in patients without obvious risk factors are unknown. Patients at high risk of developing POVL include those undergoing lengthy procedures in the prone or steep Trendelenburg position, especially if surgery is accompanied by significant blood loss. During the preoperative interview, high-risk patients should be informed of the risk of POVL. Although periodic intraoperative monitoring of hemoglobin or hematocrit is suggested,

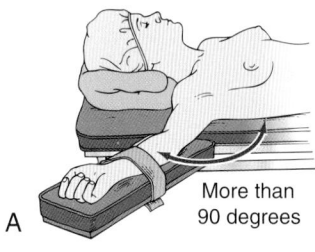

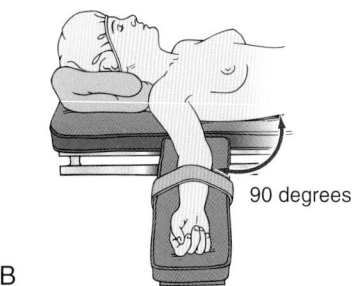

Fig. 23.4 Position of arm on armboard should not exceed 90 degrees because otherwise injury to the brachial plexus may result. (A) Incorrect positioning. (B) Correct positioning. (From Phillips N. *Berry & Kohn's Operating Room Technique.* 14th ed. St. Louis: Elsevier; 2022.)

safe lower limits for hematocrit are unknown. Deliberate hypotensive techniques to prevent blood loss during spine surgery should be avoided in individuals with chronic hypertension or other factors that place them at risk for POVL.[19] Avoidance of direct pressure over the eye is recommended to avoid CRAO. The prone patient's head should be placed in a neutral position (avoid excessive flexion) and level with or slightly elevated above the heart (10-degree head-up tilt) when possible[96] (Fig. 23.6). This prone position with the horseshoe adapter is the least preferred head support technique because of pressure on the eye and POVL (see Fig. 23.6C and D).[19] If necessary, it should be used only for short procedures. The foam head pillows with cutouts are preferred (see Fig. 23.6A). A complete discussion of POVL associated with prone positioning for orthopedic procedures can be found in Chapter 45.

OTHER POSITION-RELATED INJURIES

Position-related injuries range from minor skin abrasions and backache to events with serious morbidity (Table 23.2). Complications of these injuries can lead to tissue necrosis, infection, renal failure, paralysis, loss of limbs, and even loss of life. Although most individuals recover from minor position-related injuries without sequelae, more serious injuries may prolong a patient's hospital stay and recovery, cause psychological trauma, and perhaps even result in permanent disability. Anesthetists must not minimize the physical, psychological, social, and financial impact of transient injuries that resolve over hours, days, or months. Permanent, disabling injuries are even more devastating to patients and providers.

Compartment Syndrome

Compartment syndrome is a rare but potentially life-threatening complication that causes damage to neural and vascular structures from tissue swelling as a result of increased pressures and decreased tissue perfusion in muscles with tight, fascial borders. Because tissue swelling typically occurs when blood flow returns to a region after a period of ischemia, the syndrome has also been called a reperfusion injury. Increased compartmental pressure compromises arteriolar supply

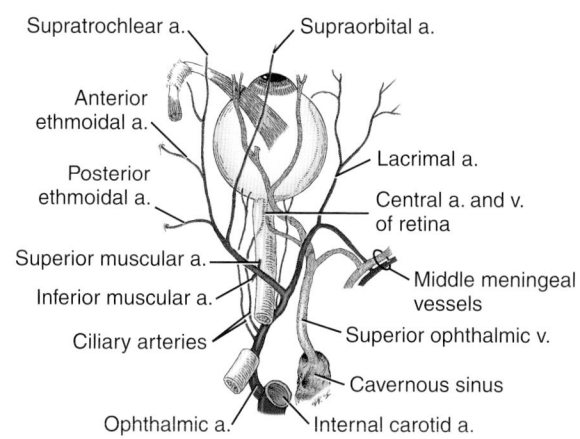

Fig. 23.5 Superior view of the orbital arteries and veins. *a*, Artery; *v*, vein.

and results in ischemia with subsequent muscle and nerve infarction.[51,101-104] Although compartment syndrome occurs most often in the lower extremities, it may also occur in the upper extremities or in the abdomen as a result of tight wound closures.[51] Compartment syndrome can be precipitated by intraoperative hypotension in conjunction with leg elevation that causes low-flow states. Because local arterial pressure decreases by 0.75 mm Hg per centimeter change in height above the right atrium, elevation of the legs puts the patient at greater risk.[101]

Long surgical duration with the patient in lithotomy position is the distinguishing characteristic of surgeries where patients develop lower extremity compartment syndrome.[104,105] Compartment pressures increase over time in the lithotomy position, and the legs should be periodically lowered to the level of the body if the procedure lasts beyond 2 to 3 hours. Other risk factors that might contribute to the development of compartment syndrome include Trendelenburg position, advanced age, extremes of body habitus, patient history of nerve ischemia or neuropathy, connective tissue disease, anemia, hypotension, and the use of vasoconstrictive drugs.[51,102,103] Although anesthetic technique has not been implicated as causing compartment syndrome, general and regional anesthesia can contribute to intraoperative hypotension and impaired blood flow.[51,105,106]

Unless the syndrome is promptly diagnosed and treated, permanent neuromuscular damage will occur. Fasciotomy is generally considered the definitive treatment because less-aggressive therapies will not release the constricted compartments. If untreated, the syndrome progresses to tissue necrosis with rhabdomyolysis and acute renal failure (crush syndrome). The need for amputation or even death can occur.[51]

Venous Air Embolism

Venous air embolism (VAE) is a well-known consequence of surgery performed in the sitting position. However, VAE may occur in any position where a negative pressure gradient exists between the right atrium and the veins at the operative site.[108-111] The precise incidence of VAE is unknown, but there is an increased incidence in surgeries performed in the sitting position.[112-114] Air that enters the right side of the heart can limit gas exchange in the lungs as it displaces blood in the pulmonary vasculature. Complications of VAE are dependent on both the rapidity and volume of air entrainment. Physiologic effects range from no effect for minimal amounts of air to hypotension, arrhythmias, cardiac arrest, and death with larger volumes.[111-114] Another potential complication is that if air emerges through the left ventricle, disruption of blood flow to the heart or brain from micro-air emboli can result in a myocardial infarction or cerebrovascular accident.

BOX 23.3 Perioperative Blindness

- Providers should consider informing patients who are having spine surgery in the prone position with prolonged duration and/or substantial blood loss that they have a small but unpredictable risk of perioperative visual loss (POVL).
- POVL can be caused by direct pressure on the globe resulting in central retinal artery occlusion (CRAO).
- Ischemic optic neuropathy (ION) is the most common cause of POVL associated with prone spine surgery in adult patients.
- Factors that significantly and independently increase the risk of ION associated with spine surgery in the prone position include male sex, obesity, use of Wilson frame, longer surgical duration, larger blood loss, and a lower percentage of colloid in the nonblood fluid administration.
- Risk reduction strategies include:
  - Avoid direct pressure on the eye.
    - Avoid the horseshoe headrest, which has a small margin of error, or any headrest that does not allow adequate assessment of the eyes during the procedure.
  - Perform and document periodic eye checks throughout the perioperative period.
    - Assess patient vision when the patient becomes alert.
    - An urgent ophthalmologic consultation should be obtained if there is concern for postoperative visual loss.
  - Minimize venous pressure and congestion in the head.
    - Keep the head in a neutral position at or above the heart level.
    - Avoid using the Wilson frame if possible.

- Minimize bleeding.
  - Avoid coagulopathy.
  - Modify surgical technique.
- Decrease the duration of the prone position.
  - Stage prolonged procedures if possible.
- Avoid significant hemodynamic changes as much as possible.
  - Closely monitor blood pressure.
  - Monitor hemoglobin and hematocrit periodically throughout surgery.
  - Use colloid along with crystalloid for nonblood fluid resuscitation.
  - Resume normotension and normotension after turning patient supine unless medically contraindicated.
- Prognosis is poor for POVL due to ION and CRAO and usually results in permanent visual loss.
- Consider magnetic resonance imaging to rule out intracranial causes of visual loss.
- Antiplatelet agents, steroids, or intraocular-lowering agents have not been shown to be effective for treatment of perioperative ION.
- Hyperbaric oxygen therapy treatment has been proposed for CRAO with the highest chance of significant improvement in visual acuity resulting when treatment is started within 6 hr of the onset of symptoms.

Adapted from Practice Advisory for Perioperative Visual Loss Associated with Spine Surgery 2019: an updated report by the American Society of Anesthesiologists Task Force on Perioperative Visual Loss, the North American Neuro-Ophthalmology Society, and the Society for Neuroscience in Anesthesiology and Critical Care. *Anesthesiology.* 2019;130(1):12–30; Kla KM, Lee LA. Perioperative visual loss. *Best Pract Res Clin Anaesthesiol.* 2016;30(1):69–77.

Paradoxic air embolism (PAE) can occur in the patient with a patent foramen ovale (PFO). Studies in vivo and in cadavers indicate that the incidence of PFO can be as high as 35% in the general population.[108,111,112] In the patient with PFO, air can enter the systemic circulation when right atrial pressure is greater than left atrial pressure, a reversal of the normal pressure gradient. Very small amounts of air in the arterial system can result in severe cardiovascular and neurologic complications.

Because VAE and PAE carry the potential for serious consequences, identifying individuals at risk for these complications is important. Preoperative transesophageal echocardiograph (TEE) with contrast is the gold standard for detection of PFO in patients scheduled for surgery in the sitting position.[109,113,114] The cost of TEE is thought to be justified because it is a low-risk, semiinvasive procedure, and the sequelae of PAE are severe. However, PFO can be present, and PAE can occur despite negative preoperative TEE.[113] Because TEE is costly and has rare but serious complications, transcranial Doppler studies are recommended as an alternative, noninvasive approach with excellent diagnostic capability in detection of right-to-left shunting.[113,115]

In addition to the use of standard anesthetic monitoring techniques, selection of appropriate monitoring for the detection of air embolism is based on the sensitivity of each modality. TEE, precordial Doppler ultrasonography, capnography ($ETco_2$), end-tidal nitrogen (ETN_2), and pulmonary artery catheterization vary in their ability to detect intraoperative VAE. TEE is the gold standard as it is the most sensitive, having the ability to identify emboli less than 0.2 mL/kg, and can be used to position right atrial catheters.[112,116] Disadvantages to the use of TEE are it requires specialized training, requires considerable time, comes with risk to the patient, and may not provide a continuous monitor of cardiovascular events.

The precordial Doppler is often used to monitor for VAE when patients are in the sitting position. The probe is placed over the third to sixth intercostal spaces to the right of the sternum. The precordial Doppler is the most sensitive noninvasive monitor and is less expensive and cumbersome than TEE.[110,113] However, it does not have the advantage of localizing entrained air within the cardiac chambers, it is sensitive to electrical interference from OR equipment, and its effectiveness can be reduced by auditory fatigue in the anesthetist.[110,112,116] Most frequently used for sitting cases, Doppler devices have not traditionally been advocated for management of VAE during procedures performed in the prone position because of the excessive pressure that it may exert on the chest wall.

VAE increases dead space and contains nitrogen; monitoring capnography will reveal a drop in end-tidal CO_2 and the presence of end-tidal nitrogen. A "mill-wheel murmur" is a characteristic of VAE that can be heard through the esophageal or precordial stethoscope.[116] Air in the coronary arteries can cause ischemic electrocardiographic changes, and air in the pulmonary vessels can result in an increase in PAP and hypoxia. These signs occur later than changes detected by TEE, Doppler, or capnography and are indicative of PAE or large emboli.[110,112]

Entrained air emboli can be removed from the circulation by aspiration through a multiorifice central venous catheter, although success rates of appreciable air aspiration are far from ideal.[117] For patients undergoing surgery in the sitting position, the catheter is placed in the right atrium at the junction of the superior vena cava.[109,116] Patients who are prone should have the CVP catheter positioned at the junction of the inferior vena cava (IVC) and right atrium because air emboli from spinal surgery enter the venous circulation through the lumbar epidural veins and IVC.[117] The risks of central venous catheter placement, the potential for VAE, and the cardiopulmonary risks of the position must be weighed against the benefits of fluid volume management and air recovery with a CVP catheter. See Chapter 31 for further discussion on detection and treatment of VAE.

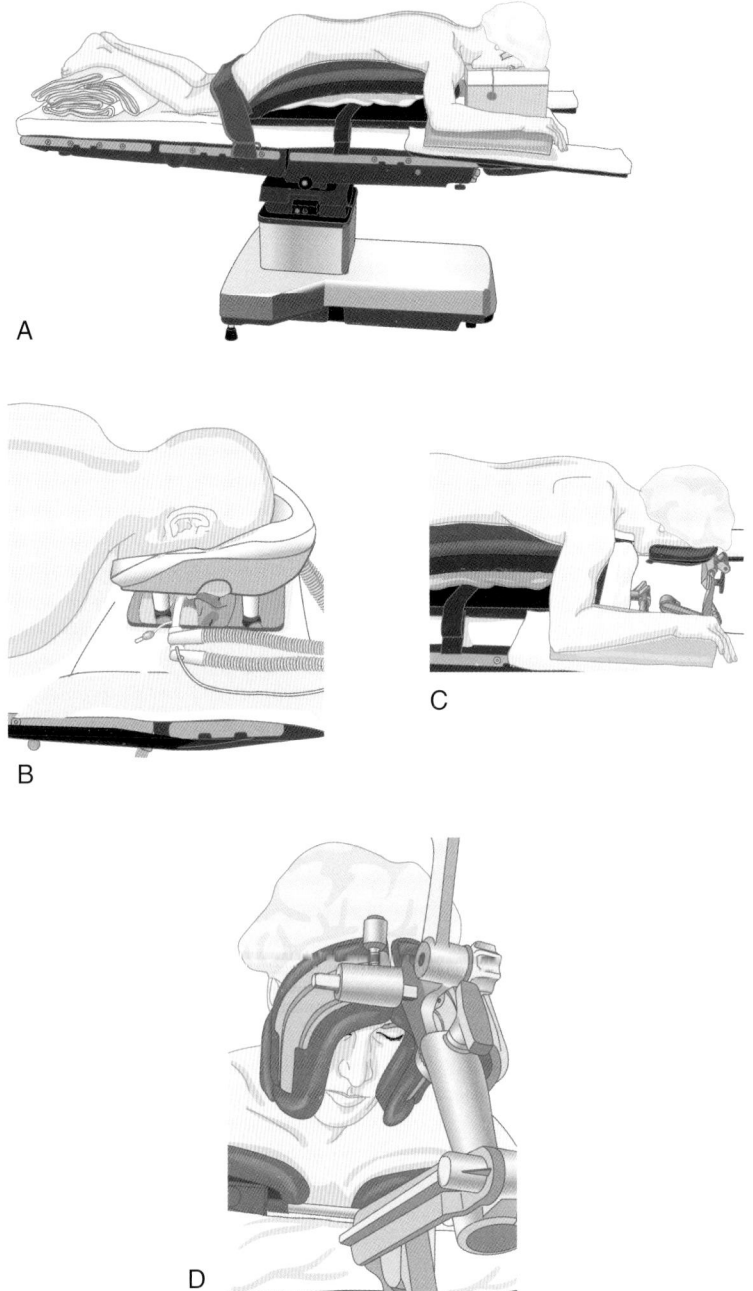

Fig. 23.6 (A) Prone position with Wilson frame. Arms are abducted less than 90 degrees whenever possible. Pressure points are padded, and chest and abdomen are supported away from the bed to minimize abdominal pressure and preserve pulmonary compliance. Foam head pillow has cutouts for eyes and nose and a slot to permit the endotracheal tube to exit. Eyes must be checked frequently. (B) Mirror system for prone position. Bony structures of the head and face are supported, and monitoring of eyes and airway is facilitated with a plastic mirror. (C) Prone position with horseshoe adapter. Head height is adjusted to position neck in a neutral position. (D) Prone position, face seen from below. Horseshoe adapter permits superior access to airway and visualization of eyes. Width may be adjusted to ensure proper support by facial bones. (From Miller RD, Pardo Jr MC. *Basics of Anesthesia*. 7th ed. Philadelphia: Elsevier; 2017.)

Airway Complications of Surgical Positions

Anesthetized patients in various surgical postures are vulnerable to endotracheal tube displacement, airway edema, and passive regurgitation. The endotracheal tube may become dislodged, kinked, or disconnected when the patient is moved or upon position change. A right mainstem intubation may occur as a result of flexion of the neck or when the patient is placed in steep Trendelenburg position. With neck flexion, the endotracheal tube moves downward and may inadvertently enter the right mainstem bronchus.[118,119] In the Trendelenburg position, pressure of the abdominal contents forces the diaphragm cephalad and may cause a similar occurrence.[34]

Extensive edema of the face, tongue, and oropharyngeal structures has been reported after procedures in the prone, head-down, and sitting positions.[120,121] In the prone and head-down positions, gravitational forces or increases in hydrostatic pressures may restrict venous return

TABLE 23.2 Positioning Related Injuries

Body System or Anatomic Location	Potential Injury
Head, eyes, ears, nose, and throat	Postoperative vision loss Corneal abrasion Facial edema Vocal cord edema
Cardiovascular	Vascular occlusion Deep vein thrombosis Ischemic injuries
Respiratory	Atelectasis Endobronchial intubation
Neurologic	Peripheral neuropathy Quadriplegia Decreased cerebral blood flow Increased intracranial pressure
Genitourinary	Myoglobinuria Acute renal failure
Musculoskeletal	Amputation Backache Compartment syndrome Rhabdomyolysis
Integumentary	Abrasion Alopecia Decubiti

from the head and neck. Excessive flexion of the head on the neck with patients in the sitting position may obstruct jugular venous return, resulting in macroglossia and airway edema. Oral airways, endotracheal tubes, and esophageal stethoscopes may compress the base of the tongue and limit lymphatic drainage. The endotracheal tube can become kinked with extreme degrees of flexion or may compress the arytenoids and epiglottis, resulting in postoperative supraglottic edema. Macroglossia or upper airway edema may necessitate leaving the patient intubated after surgery until the edema subsides.[121] It may be prudent to verify an air leak around the endotracheal tube or examine the larynx via direct laryngoscopy before extubation in suspected patients.

SURGICAL POSITIONING

The Supine Position (Dorsal Decubitus)

The supine position is most frequently used for surgical procedures on the abdomen, head, neck, extremities, and chest, owing to the favorable exposure it allows. When positioning the patient supine, the head should be maintained in a neutral position on a small pillow or donut. The arms should be either comfortably positioned and secured alongside the trunk or positioned on padded armboards.[3,37,119] If the patient has severe arthritis, decreased mobility of the head and neck, or neuropathy of the upper extremities, it is best to position using patient preference prior to the induction of anesthesia. During prolonged procedures, the head should be repositioned at intervals and the occiput massaged to prevent alopecia due to prolonged pressure. Gel-type donuts may more evenly distribute pressure.[43]

The ligaments of the vertebral column relax with anesthesia and can result in postoperative backache. Placing a pillow under the patient's knees or placing the table in a slight "lounge chair" position, with the

patient's hips and knees flexed and the trunk slightly elevated, increases patient comfort.[3,119] The legs must remain uncrossed to avoid pressure from the superior extremity damaging the superficial peroneal nerve in the dependent leg and the sural nerve in the superior leg. If prolonged surgery is anticipated, the heels should be elevated off the mattress to prevent pressure sores; however, using too large a support to elevate the heels can cause hyperextension of the knees and pain postoperatively. Gel pads or mattresses more evenly distribute the patient's body weight and prevent reddened areas after lengthy procedures.[3]

If the arms are tucked, the elbow must not be allowed to hang over the edge of the operating table because ulnar nerve damage may occur. When tucked, the hands should be placed in a neutral position, the elbow padded, with the palms facing the hip[73,75,76] (see Fig. 23.3). If the arms are secured on armboards, the forearm should be supinated; pronation may result in compression of the ulnar nerve against the armboard. The arms should be abducted less than 90 degrees, and the head should be maintained in a neutral position to avoid brachial plexus stretch injuries.[73,75,76]

Trendelenburg/Reverse Trendelenburg Positions

Trendelenburg position (head-down position) is often used temporarily to increase venous return during episodes of hypotension and is used to supplement the primary surgical position and improve surgical exposure. Physiologic alterations vary greatly depending on the degree of tilt and the primary position. An increase in central venous, intracranial, and intraocular pressures is observed with the Trendelenburg position and may contribute to edema of the face, tongue, oropharynx, and eyes.[13-16]

The increasing use of robotic-assisted surgery often requires the use of steep Trendelenburg and presents challenges in positioning. Increased injury following robotic-assisted surgery has been attributed partially to robotic arms obscuring the provider's view of the patient, putting patients at risk for injuries due to sliding on the OR table or from unrecognized compression from equipment.[122] The risk of sliding can be partially mitigated by the use of antiskid bedding, lithotomy positioning, or padded cross-torso straps. Regardless of safety equipment use, using the least degree of Trendelenburg possible for adequate equipment placement and for the shortest duration of time is the best defense against injury.

Various complications have been observed due to the Trendelenburg position, and many are the result of positioning devices. Improperly positioned shoulder braces designed to prevent the patient from sliding when in a steep Trendelenburg position can injure the brachial plexus and should not be used when the arm is extended on an armboard. Placement of the shoulder brace in a position that is placed too medial can result in depression of underlying bony structures and compression of the plexus. Braces placed too lateral may result in a stretch injury of the brachial plexus. The brace should be placed over the acromioclavicular joint and should be avoided if at all possible because nerve injury can still occur despite proper placement.[14-16,75,122] The arms are vulnerable to injury in the Trendelenburg position particularly if they are positioned on armboards and inadequately restrained. The arms can slip off, hyperextend, and abduct above the level of the shoulder, stretching the plexus.[3,14,75]

The reverse Trendelenburg position (head-up position), often used in laparoscopic surgeries, can also predispose patients to injury. The positioning of the head higher than the heart reduces perfusion pressure to the brain and should be monitored closely. When too tight, table straps used to prevent the patient from sliding in the reverse Trendelenburg position have resulted in lower-extremity neuropathies and pressure ulcers[14] (see Fig. 23.3). The use of a footboard is preferable to the overzealous tightening of the table strap if a steep reverse Trendelenburg position is necessary.

The Lithotomy Position

The lithotomy position is used for surgical procedures that require access to any perineal structure. In the typical lithotomy position, the legs are held in flexion and abduction above the level of the torso by a leg-holding device[43] (Fig. 23.7). The level of lithotomy position needed is dependent on the type of surgery and surgical access (Fig. 23.8). In low lithotomy position, the legs are almost level with the torso, whereas in exaggerated lithotomy position, the legs are suspended with boots or stirrups so that the feet are well above the body. A hemilithotomy position, with one leg elevated, is also used for some orthopedic procedures.[14,43,119]

The arms are usually positioned either tucked at the sides or abducted on armboards. In the hemilithotomy position, one arm may be secured across the chest. The same cautions for positioning the upper extremity apply as in the supine position. Strict attention must be paid to the fingers, if the arms are tucked at the sides, to avoid a potentially disastrous crush injury or amputation if they become trapped when the foot section is raised[3,75,119] (see Fig. 23.7D). Many neurovascular complications can occur in the lithotomy position because of the position of the leg and hip.[43,75] Both legs should be elevated and lowered simultaneously when they are placed in a leg-holding device; raising and lowering the legs separately can cause hip dislocation, spinal torsion, or postoperative back pain. Acute abduction and external rotation of the hips can also cause femoral nerve or lumbosacral plexus stretch injuries. Flexion of the hips more than 90 degrees in the lithotomy position

can cause neural damage by stretching the sciatic and obturator nerves or by direct pressure of femoral neurovascular structures under the inguinal ligament, with subsequent arterial or venous occlusion and nerve palsy. Leg holders that support the leg under the knee can compromise vascular structures in the popliteal space.[43,75]

Peroneal nerve injury is frequently associated with the lithotomy position because of its anatomic course.[35] The nerve crosses the knee joint laterally and wraps around the fibular head before traveling down the lower leg. Depending on the type of leg holder used, the nerve can be injured by compression against the upright bar or against the supporting cradle of the leg holder. The saphenous nerve courses down the medial aspect of the lower leg and is also at risk for compression in the leg holder. Care must be taken to adequately pad any points of potential compression.[75]

The Lateral Decubitus Position

The lateral decubitus position is often used for surgeries involving the thorax and kidneys when the supine position cannot provide sufficient exposure. Orthopedic procedures involving the hips, shoulders, or extremities can also require this position for better access to the surgical site. When a nephrectomy is performed using a lateral approach, exposure of the kidney can be facilitated by elevating the kidney rest beneath the dependent iliac crest and flexing the operating table so that the operative flank is higher than the upper torso or legs[3,43,75] (Fig. 23.9).

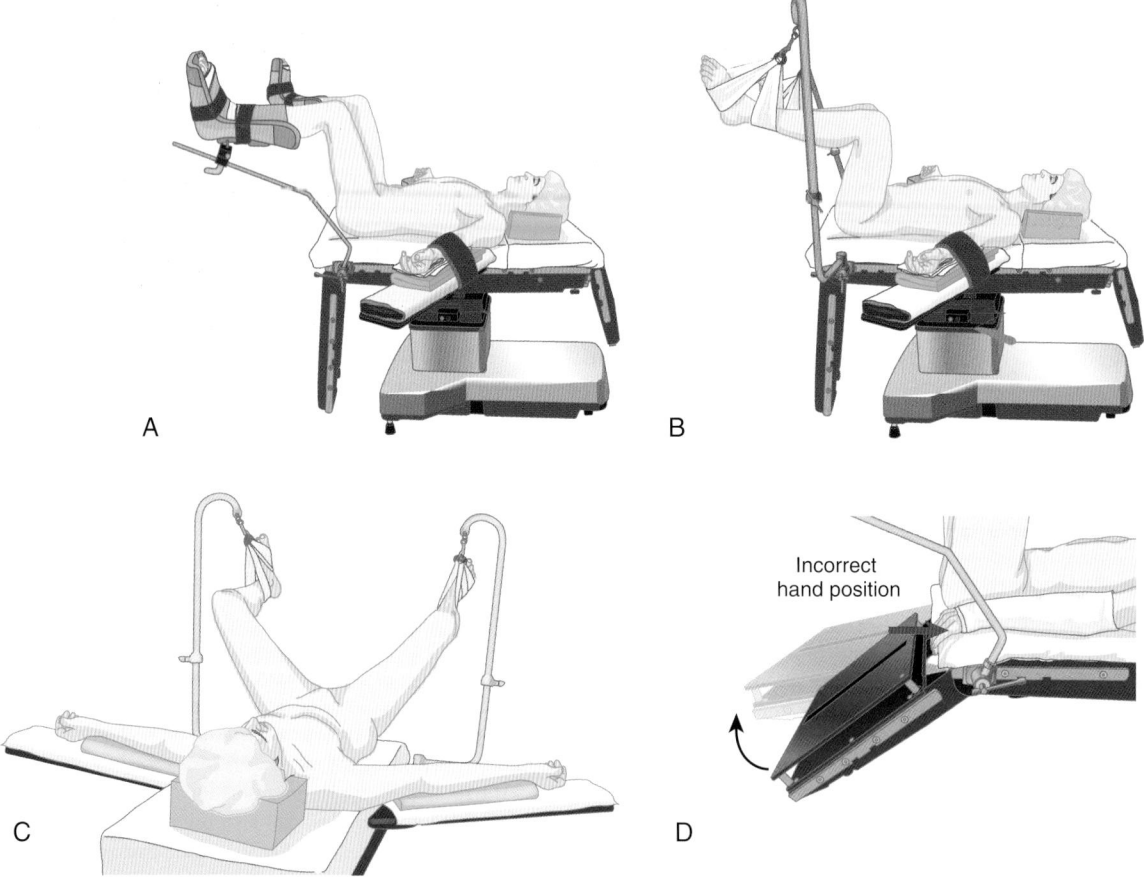

Fig. 23.7 (A) Lithotomy position. Hips are flexed 80 to 100 degrees with the lower leg parallel to the body. Arms are on armrests away from the hinge point of the foot section. (B) Lithotomy position with "candy cane" supports. (C) Lithotomy position with correct position of "candy cane" stirrups away from lateral fibular head. (D) Improper position of arms in lithotomy position with fingers at risk for compression when the lower section of the bed is raised. (From Miller RD, Pardo Jr MC. *Basics of Anesthesia.* 7th ed. Philadelphia: Elsevier; 2017.)

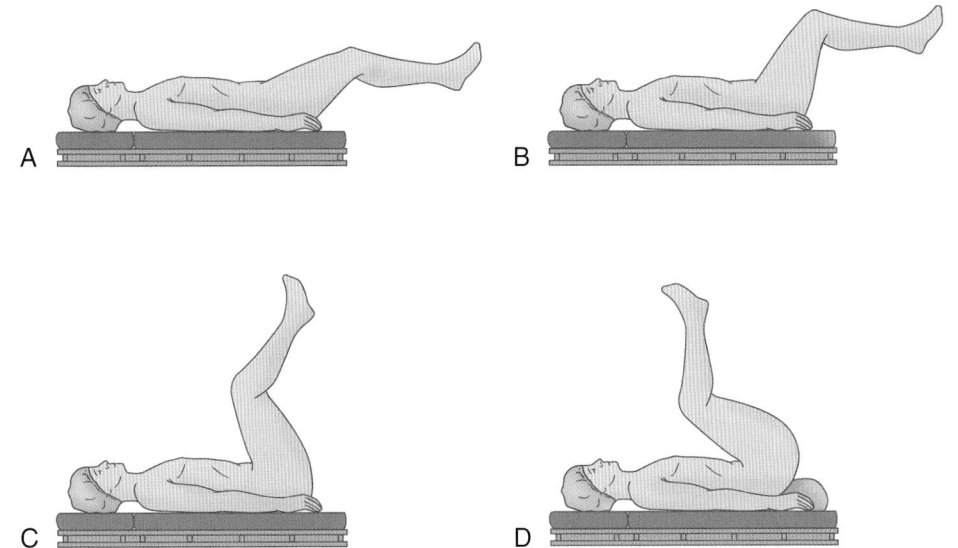

Fig. 23.8 Four basic types of lithotomy position with progressively increasing leg elevation. (A) Low. (B) Standard. (C) High. (D) Exaggerated. (From Rothrock JC. *Alexander's Care of the Patient in Surgery*. 15th ed. St. Louis: Elsevier; 2015:177.)

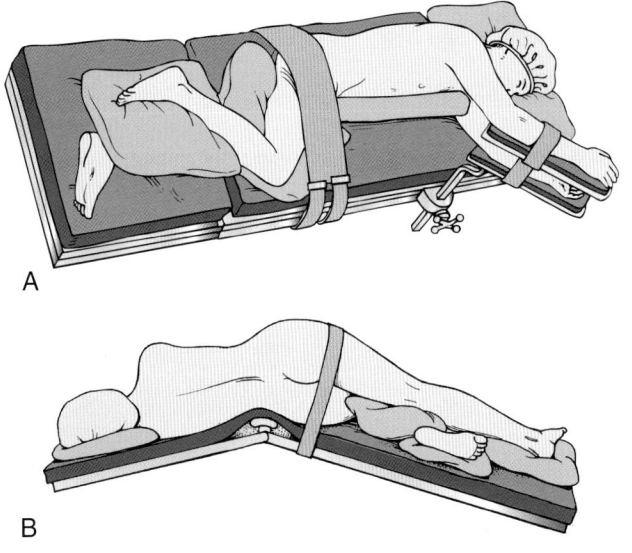

Fig. 23.9 (A) Standard left lateral decubitus position. (B) Flexed lateral position with the kidney rest properly elevated under the iliac crest. (From Phillips N. *Berry & Kohn's Operating Room Technique*. 13th ed. St Louis: Elsevier; 2017:496–497.)

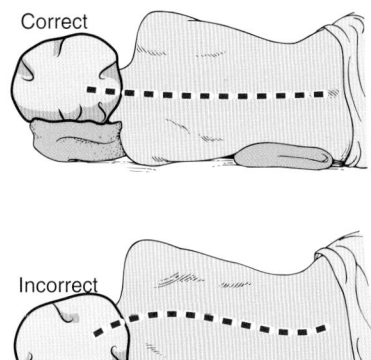

Fig. 23.10 Proper alignment of spinal column in lateral position. (From Phillips N. *Berry & Kohn's Operating Room Technique*. 13th ed. St Louis: Elsevier; 2017:497.)

Initially the patient is placed supine for induction of anesthesia and intubation. If a beanbag is used to support the torso, it is placed flat on the operating table prior to the patient's arrival in the OR. Before the patient is positioned, the endotracheal tube, breathing circuit, intravenous and monitoring lines, and any other devices should be secured so that none are beneath the body after the turn. The anesthetist should control the airway, head, and neck, as well as coordinate the turn.

Particular attention should be paid to body alignment in the lateral position. The shoulders, hips, head, and legs are maintained in the same plane and turned simultaneously to avoid stress and twisting of the torso and spine (Fig. 23.10). The head and neck remain aligned with the spine in a neutral position. The head should be supported on pillows or a donut and not allowed to hang, tilt laterally, hyperflex, or hyperextend. The dependent eye and ear must be free of pressure. A gel donut is useful for keeping the dependent ear suspended and pressure free.

Once the patient is in the lateral position, flexing the knee and hip of the dependent leg stabilizes the patient. The nondependent leg remains straight and is supported by a pillow placed between the lower extremities. Positioning the legs in this manner prevents bony prominences of the legs from resting on each other and reduces compression of the inferior leg by the superior extremity (see Fig. 23.9A). Padding should be placed along the lateral aspect of the dependent leg, extending from the knee to the heel to protect the peroneal nerve from external pressure against the table or beanbag.

The dependent arm is positioned on a padded armboard perpendicular to the torso and flexed less than 90 degrees at the elbow.[35,71] The nondependent arm is placed to avoid interference with surgical exposure—usually parallel to the dependent arm and level with the shoulder on a well-padded arm-holding device. Alternatively, both arms may be positioned on a single armboard with adequate padding between them. Perfusion to the upper extremities, especially the dependent arm, should be periodically assessed by palpating the radial artery and checking capillary refill.[3,35]

The dependent shoulder and upper extremity are susceptible to compression in the lateral position. A small (axillary) roll is placed under the dependent thorax, slightly caudad to but not directly in the axilla, to lift the thorax and relieve pressure exerted on the shoulder, axillary vessels, and brachial plexus of the dependent arm.[3,124] It is useful to obtain blood pressures in the nondependent arm because of potential for neurovascular compression in the dependent arm from the blood pressure cuff.[3] It is important to recognize the potential for inaccuracy in blood pressure readings if the arm is not level with the right atrium.[125]

Ancillary positioning devices such as beanbags, pillows, sandbags, braces, and adhesive tape aid in securing the patient and preventing rotation of the trunk. If tape or straps are used to stabilize the torso, they should be placed just caudal to the axilla to reduce the risk of brachial plexus injury.[43] Placement across the ribs can impair ventilation. Soft tissue injury may occur if straps or tape is overly tight.

Rhabdomyolysis has been reported after use of the lateral decubitus position.[126,127] Prolonged operating time, hypotension, and pressure of the operating table against gluteal and flank muscles have been described as contributory factors. The anesthetist, as well as the entire operating team, should ensure that the operating table is well padded and that positioning devices are properly placed. Furthermore, prolonged or excessive hypotension should be avoided to ensure adequate tissue perfusion.

The Sitting Position

The term *sitting position* commonly refers to any position in which the torso is elevated from the supine position and is higher than the legs. A true sitting position in which the torso is elevated at 90 degrees to the legs is rarely used. The modified sitting position, in which the torso is elevated 45 degrees, the head is flexed, and the legs are elevated and flexed, is more commonly used. This position is variously described as the lounging, lawn chair, or beach chair position.[43] Although its use is reportedly decreasing in popularity, some neurosurgeons favor the sitting position for posterior fossa and cervical spine procedures because it allows excellent visualization of intracranial structures and facilitates drainage of blood and cerebral spinal fluid from the wound. During shoulder arthroplasty and arthroscopy, the sitting position reduces brachial plexus stretch and aids surgical exposure and manipulation of the arm and shoulder.[7]

Placement of the patient in the sitting position involves flexion of the OR table, elevation of the backrest and legs, and sometimes head-down rotation. For neurosurgical procedures, a three-pin head holder is generally used to secure the head. The device provides better head stabilization compared with other headrests, but jugular venous obstruction can occur if the head is excessively flexed on the neck. At least two fingerbreadths of space should be allowed between the neck and mandible (Fig. 23.11).[8,9,109,110]

A horseshoe headrest is often used to support the head for shoulder procedures performed in the sitting position. Straps or adhesive tape secures the head to the headrest. Vigorous surgical manipulation of the arm and shoulder can move the patient's body toward the operative side of the table. If the head is firmly secured to the headrest, excessive traction or stretch can be placed on the neck and brachial plexus. If the restraining straps are loose, the head can become partially or completely dislodged from the headrest, introducing the potential for cervical spine injury. Accidental extubation can occur if the endotracheal tube is secured by a supporting device and the head is displaced.

Serious complications associated with the sitting position are among the reasons that the position is falling out of favor. VAE is the most feared complication, but pneumocephalus, quadriplegia, and peripheral nerve injuries are also possible. Profound hypotension and bradycardia from activation of the Bezold-Jarisch reflex may occur when shoulder surgery is performed in the sitting position under an interscalene block.[7,118]

The Prone Position

The prone position provides optimal exposure for a variety of procedures performed on the spine, certain orthopedic procedures, and some rectal procedures. The prone position has also been advocated for intracranial procedures, owing to the decreased risk of VAE compared with the sitting position.[109] Many modifications of the prone position exist (Fig. 23.12). Anesthetists must become familiar with the various methods of securing the patient in the prone position and recognize the potential hazards of each variation or device.

In the prone position, the torso is typically supported on a frame or with rolls that extend from the shoulders to the iliac crests. Alternatively,

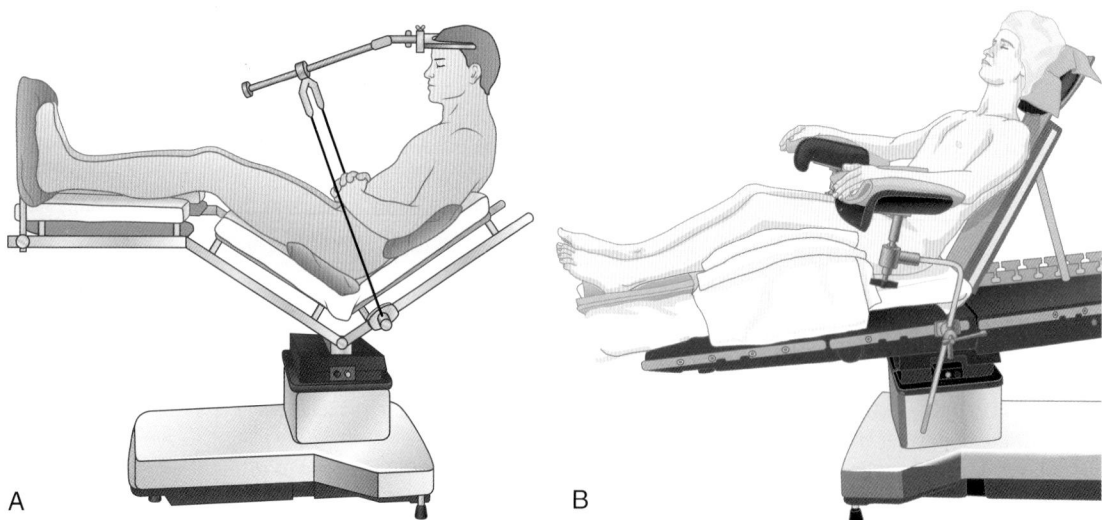

A   B

Fig. 23.11 (A) Sitting position with Mayfield head pins. The patient is typically semirecumbent rather than sitting because the legs are kept as high as possible to promote venous return. Arms must be supported to prevent shoulder traction. Note that the head holder support is preferably attached to the back section rather than the thigh section of the table so that the patient's back may be adjusted or lowered emergently without first detaching the head holder. (B) Sitting position adapted for shoulder surgery. Note the absence of pressure over the ulnar area of the elbow. (From Miller RD, Pardo Jr MC. *Basics of Anesthesia*. 7th ed. Philadelphia: Elsevier; 2017.)

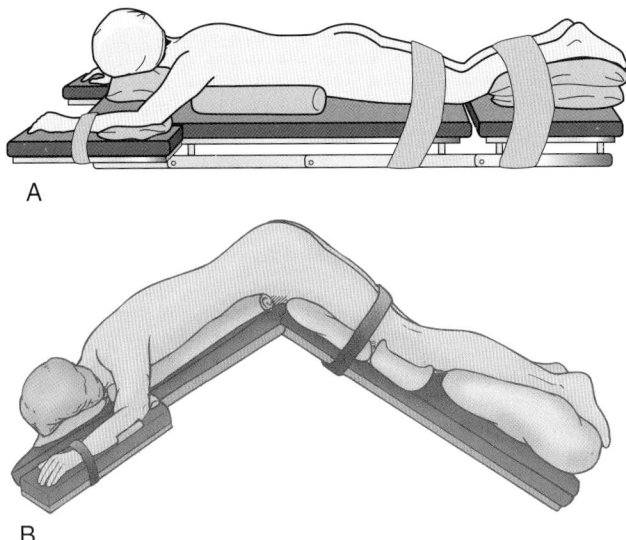

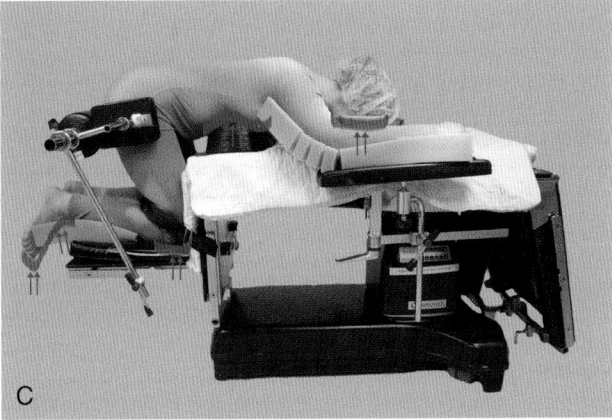

Fig. 23.12 Variations of the prone position. (A) Classic prone position with the torso supported on chest rolls. (B) Jackknife position. (C) Knee-chest position. (A, From Phillips N. *Berry & Kohn's Operating Room Technique.* 13th ed. St. Louis: Elsevier; 2017:495; B, From Rothrock JC. *Alexander's Care of the Patient in Surgery.* 15th ed. St. Louis: Elsevier; 2015:182; C, From St-Arnaud D. Safe positioning for neurosurgical patients. *AORN J.* 2008;87[6]:1167.)

supports can be placed crosswise at the pelvis and shoulders. The lower legs are supported with pillows, and the upper extremities may be tucked at the sides or supported on armboards with the arms flexed at the shoulders and elbows. Care must be taken to pad pressure points at elbows, knees, and ankles. Breasts and genitalia must be positioned to limit pressure on them.[71,75]

When a posterior approach is planned and the prone position is necessary, the patient is anesthetized on the gurney and then log-rolled onto the bed, frame, or rolls with good body alignment maintained. Thoughtful planning of monitor placement allows turning without removal of monitors during this critical period and avoids delays. Typically, the patient is disconnected from the breathing circuit to avoid accidental extubation. The anesthetist should control the airway, head, and neck, as well as coordinate the turn.

Head, neck, shoulder, and arm mobility must be assessed preoperatively; arm placement can be limited by ankylosis of shoulder or elbow joints. Depending on the surgeon's preference, the arms may be tucked parallel to the sides with a draw sheet or supported on armboards. If tucked, the arms should be secured in a natural position with the palms facing the thighs. Plastic or metal arm "sleds," with sufficient padding, can be used to protect the arms and vascular access sites

from compression by the bodies of the surgical team. If the arms are not tucked at the sides, they should be carefully rotated into position. The preferred arm placement is flexed, slightly abducted, and with the forearms and hands lower than the shoulders and adequately supported.[38,71] The arms should rest at a comfortable height on the armboards and should not support the weight of the shoulders. Padding should be placed under the shoulders to prevent sagging of the shoulders and stretching of the brachial plexus.[38,71,75]

Particular care must be taken to maintain alignment of the head and neck in the prone position. The head should be supported in a neutral position with a head-holding device. Hyperextension or lateral rotation of the neck should be avoided because either may compromise spinal cord blood flow, especially in elderly individuals with narrowing of the spinal canal due to osteoarthritis.[71] Stretch injuries of the brachial plexus may also occur with lateral head rotation.[43,71,86]

A primary goal of positioning a patient prone is to avoid pressure on the abdomen, which can impede venous return, increase venous pressures, and interfere with ventilation by inhibiting movement of the diaphragm.[3,38] Furthermore, increased venous pressure will contribute to a greater blood loss from the surgical site. Valves are not present in the intervertebral veins that drain the vertebral and spinal cord venous plexuses into the lumbar veins. External abdominal pressure is transmitted to the vena cava and communicated to the lumbar epidural veins.[38,43] Positioning devices that allow the abdomen to hang freely are associated with greater decreases in inferior vena cava pressures than those that compress the abdomen and therefore prevent engorgement of spinal venous plexuses.[43] Engorged epidural veins are fragile and easily traumatized, and the ensuing blood loss will decrease surgical exposure and contribute to hypotension. Studies suggest that in the prone position, the degree to which pulmonary mechanics are altered depends on the positioning device used, not on body habitus.[3,38] The Jackson table resulted in the smallest change in pulmonary compliance and peak airway pressures when compared with the Wilson frame and chest rolls. The investigators hypothesized that the Jackson table allows the abdomen to hang freely, permitting better diaphragmatic excursion and lower intraabdominal and intrathoracic pressures.[3]

Meticulous attention must be paid to protection of the eyes because corneal abrasions and POVL are complications associated with prone position. Several devices, including three-point skull fixation, the horseshoe headrest, and foam cushions, allow the head to be placed in a neutral position while the eyes are kept free of pressure. However, the head may slip or rotate on the horseshoe headrest, allowing pressure to be applied over the globe and placing the patient at risk of POVL. Although three-point skull fixation is often recommended for securing the head and protecting the eyes in the prone position, POVL has occurred despite the use of this device.[90]

CLOSED-CLAIMS STUDIES

Surgical positions are associated with numerous potential complications that can be detrimental to a patient's short- and long-term outcomes. Although the potential for various complications is generally well known, the precise incidence and cause of position-related injuries are often difficult to determine. Because the frequency of these events is low, contributing causes are frequently multifactorial, and uniform reporting does not exist. Position-related injuries are thought to be underreported in the scientific literature.[42,58] Fear of litigation or damage to one's professional reputation may prevent anesthesia providers from reporting such events. However, case reports, closed-claims studies, and retrospective analyses of databases can provide insight into position-related injuries and shed light on precipitating causes and outcomes.

Both the American Association of Nurse Anesthetists Foundation (AANA-F) and the ASA have conducted studies of closed malpractice claims from professional liability insurance companies. These studies provide a rich source of data about position-related complications. The ASA Closed Claims Project (ASA-CCP) was initiated in 1985.[128,129] Because the ASA-CCP involves primarily anesthesiologists, the AANA-F conducted a similar study to examine outcomes of care provided by Certified Registered Nurse Anesthetists (CRNAs). Dental claims are excluded from both the AANA-F and ASA-CCP studies.[128,130]

An analysis of the ASA-CCP revealed that death (26%), nerve injuries (22%), and permanent brain damage (9%) were the major causes of liability.[58] Nerve damage included injuries to both the peripheral nervous system and spinal cord but not to the brain. Nerves most commonly affected were the ulnar (28%), brachial plexus (20%), lumbosacral nerve root (16%), and spinal cord (13%). Injuries to all other nerves accounted for only 8% of the nerve damage claims. Although claims for nerve injury have remained constant over time, claims for ulnar nerve injury have decreased whereas those from spinal cord injury have increased.[42,58]

Specific causative factors could not be identified in the majority of claims in the ASA-CCP. When the association of anesthetic technique with nerve injury was examined, regional anesthesia was more frequently associated with nerve-injury claims—particularly of the spinal cord and lumbosacral nerve root—than general anesthesia. However, 85% of ulnar nerve injuries were associated with general anesthesia. The quality of anesthesia care was judged as appropriate in 66% of all nerve injury claims, as compared with 42% of non–nerve-damage cases. However, care was deemed appropriate in only 46% of spinal cord damage claims. Other factors associated with nerve damage included positioning and positioning devices, intraoperative trauma, and paresthesias during regional block performance.[42]

The AANA-F closed-claims study compared 151 claims (68%) in which a CRNA was judged to have contributed to the adverse outcome (CRNA related) with 72 claims (32%) in which the CRNA was judged not to have contributed to the adverse event (non–CRNA related).[131] Death (32%), nerve injury (12%), brain injury (12%), and eye injury (10%) were the primary outcomes of CRNA-related claims. No significant difference in the type of outcome was found between CRNA-related claims and non–CRNA-related claims. Reviewers evaluated the appropriateness of care and found care to be inappropriate in 52% of CRNA-related cases, appropriate for 30%, and impossible to assess in the remaining cases.[132]

The AANA-F and ASA-CCP studies highlight the importance of following standards of care and properly documenting perioperative activities. Standards for nurse anesthesia practice identify thorough, complete, and accurate documentation as an expectation of nurse anesthesia practice.[133] In the event of a malpractice claim, thorough documentation assists reviewers in determining the quality of care provided.

Several limitations are inherent in closed-claims studies. First, the purpose of data collected by professional liability insurance companies is to investigate malpractice claims, not to improve patient safety. Not all anesthesia-related injuries result in a liability claim. Therefore data from closed-claims studies are not a random or even representative sample because only those cases in which a claim was filed and subsequently closed are included. Second, the incidence of various outcomes cannot be described because the total number of cases performed by insured providers is unknown.[131] For these two reasons, closed-claims data are not suitable for calculation of risk. However, analysis of closed-claims data can identify issues confronting practitioners and suggest methods for improving practice or making changes in systems.[131,134]

Other factors limit the conclusions that can be drawn from closed-claims data. Many cases that might be included in the database are eliminated because of inadequate documentation. In addition, closed-claim studies and quality assurance data categorize claims by type of injury rather than cause. Inadequate documentation and inability to determine the role played by various factors can limit the ability of reviewers to determine the cause of injury.[58] Finally, reviewers' knowledge of patient outcomes may bias their opinions on the quality of care provided.[130]

In both studies, monetary awards were higher in those cases resulting in more severe outcomes and when anesthesia care was determined to be less than appropriate. Although some suggest that position-related nerve injuries are largely preventable,[38] the ASA analysis of nerve injury claims revealed that payouts were frequently made even when anesthesia care was judged appropriate.[42] This suggests that current knowledge of methods for preventing nerve injury is inadequate and that further research into mechanisms of nerve injury is needed.

SUMMARY

Surgical positioning alters normal cardiovascular and respiratory physiology. These positional changes can be augmented by anesthetic techniques, patient pathophysiology, and body habitus. The implications of physiologic changes associated with each position should be considered when the procedure is planned, when positioning is initiated, and when the patient is returned to the supine posture. Anesthetists must recognize and anticipate both the publicized complications and the potential for damage inherent in each surgical position. Prevention is the best method for decreasing both the incidence of position-related injuries and the associated physical, psychological, and economic costs to the patient.

REFERENCES

For a complete list of references for this chapter, scan this QR code with any smartphone code reader app, or visit the following URL: http://booksite.elsevier.com/9780323711944/

24

Airway Management

Jeremy S. Heiner

Effective airway management is a cornerstone of safe anesthesia practice, and an essential skill for all anesthesia providers. In addition to the managing the operating room (OR), nurse anesthetists are also responsible for managing the airway in many other health care settings. Maintenance of oxygenation and ventilation are primary goals during airway management for both difficult and routine (nondifficult) airways. Proper management of a difficult airway occurs as a result of experience and regular management of normal airways, thoughtful planning, and effective preparation. Therefore it is important that anesthesia providers become familiar with appropriate decision-making strategies and methods for providing adequate ventilation during airway management. These strategies and methods pertain not only to routine airways but also to anticipated difficult airways, unanticipated difficulty with intubation and/or ventilation, failed airways, patients at risk for aspiration of gastric contents, and patients who present with any other type of airway compromise.

An understanding of airway anatomy and appropriate airway assessment techniques facilitates the development of a comprehensive airway management plan. Complete and thorough assessment of the airway guides management plans, which may involve placing an airway while the patient is awake or after the induction of anesthesia, using any one of a variety of airway adjuncts. Familiarization with the different airway adjuncts is important so that anesthesia providers may become comfortable with their use in a variety of airway management situations and changing airway dynamics, in order to facilitate safe practices for the establishment of a protected airway.

Removal of an airway management device should be part of the overall airway management plan. Consideration should be given to patient, surgical, and anesthetic risk factors before removing any airway adjunct. Ultimately, the removal of an airway is determined by the patient's ability to meet extubation criteria and maintain adequate spontaneous ventilation and oxygenation. Finally, it is important to understand the risk factors and complications of airway management in order to develop the most appropriate and safe airway management plan for the patient.

ANATOMY AND PHYSIOLOGY OF THE AIRWAY

The airway is divided into upper and lower sections. The cricoid cartilage separates the upper and lower airways. Thus anatomic structures included in the upper airway are the nose, mouth, pharynx, hypopharynx, larynx, and cricoid cartilage. Anatomic structures that constitute the lower airway include trachea, bronchi, bronchioles, terminal bronchioles, respiratory bronchioles, and alveoli. This section reviews primary structures, innervation, blood supply, and normal and abnormal functions of the upper airway structures.

Developmental Anatomy

Upper Respiratory Tract

Unlike the structures of the lower respiratory tract, the upper respiratory tract arises from bony structures of the head. Endochondral

bone is preformed in cartilage. The bones form initially from the optic, olfactory, and otic capsules. These capsules merge with the midline cartilaginous structures to form the embryologic vestiges of the ethmoid, the sphenoid, the petrous portion of the temporal bone, and the base of the occipital bone. Direct ossification of membranous tissue known as the mesenchyme occurs during early embryologic development to form membranous bone. The membranous bones include the temporal bone, the parietal bone, the frontal bone, and portions of the occipital bones and the pharyngeal arches. The pharyngeal arches are complex structures also known as the branchial arches that extend anterior to posterior. Development of these structures begins at day 22 (week 4 after fertilization).[1]

Embryologically, there are six arches that develop from five structures. The first through fourth arches and the sixth arch go on to develop the airway structures, and the fifth arch disappears with fetal development. The arches all contain a covering of tissue that will eventually become the nerves, muscles, and cartilage of the airway. These will become the tissues of the oropharynx, the middle ear, the hyoid bone, and the laryngeal cartilages. The first arch becomes the jaws, the second arch becomes the facial structures and the ears, the third arch becomes the hyoid bone and structures of the upper pharynx, the fourth and sixth arches become the structures of the larynx and the lower pharynx, and the fifth (as mentioned) disappears. The tongue is formed from the mesoderm of multiple arches. The anterior two-thirds of the tongue is developed from the first arch. The mesoderm of the third and fourth arches comprises the posterior third of the tongue. Spaces found between the arches are known externally as clefts and internally as pouches. The cleft between the first two arches becomes the external auditory meatus. The internal pouch between the first and second arches forms the majority of the tympanic cavity and the eustachian tubes. The other clefts disappear as the fetus develops. The pouches contribute to the development of the glandular structures of the head and neck. The palatine tonsils arise from the second pouch, the inferior parathyroid glands and the thymus arise from the third pouch, the superior parathyroid glands arise from the fourth pouch, and the ultimobranchial structures arise from the inferior portion of the fourth pouch as well.[1]

Nose. The nose and mouth are the external openings to the respiratory tree. The large surface area of the nasal mucosa warms and humidifies inspired air while causing significant resistance to breathing. The nose is the primary passage by which air enters the lungs. Because of the surface area over the turbinates and the sinuses, the nasal passages are well suited for the humidification of air and primary filtration. As air passes through the nose, it meets the turbinates, which cause directional changes in the airflow. Branches of three arteries (e.g., the maxillary [sphenopalatine], ophthalmic, and facial [septal]) provide a rich supply of blood to the nasal mucosa. The innervation of the nose is from the maxillary and opthalmic branches of the Trigeminal nerve. These nerves also supply the nasopharynx, nasal septum, and palate.

Parasympathetic innervation arises from the seventh cranial nerve and the pterygopalatine ganglion. Sympathetic innervation is derived from the superior cervical ganglion. Sympathetic stimulation results in vasoconstriction and shrinkage of the nasal tissue. Depression of the sympathetic nervous system, as occurs with general anesthesia, may cause engorgement of the nasal tissues, resulting in a potential increase in bleeding during manipulation of nasal airways.

Mouth. The oral cavity is separated from the nasal passages by the hard and soft palates. The hard palate is stationary and remains in the same position. The soft palate covers the posterior third to half of the oral cavity. The soft palate rises during eating to prevent food and liquids from passing from the mouth into the nose, and thereby decreases the chance of aspiration. With age, obesity, and other conditions, this structure may stretch and become more movable. When an individual is asleep or paralyzed, as with general anesthesia, this structure can fall back against the nasal passages, blocking air movement and causing symptoms similar to sleep apnea. The tongue is a large muscular organ that fills most of the oral cavity and is involved in the tasting and ingestion of food. It relaxes when the individual is either asleep or paralyzed, which increases the potential for airway obstruction. The uvula protects the passageway from the oral cavity into the oropharynx. This pendulous piece of tissue extends from the posterior edge of the middle of the soft palate into the oral cavity. If swollen, enlarged, or injured, it can be a cause of airway obstruction. The palatine tonsils are walnut-shaped structures that sit on both sides of the posterior opening of the oral cavity. They are partially buried in the soft tissue at the base of the tongue and are protected by the anterior and posterior tonsillar pillars. Underdevelopment of the tongue, maxilla, and/or mandible can result in upper airway obstructive disorders such as Pierre Robin sequence, Apert syndrome, and Treacher Collins syndrome. Other disorders, such as Beckwith-Wiedemann syndrome and Down syndrome, can result in airway obstruction as a result of macroglossia.[2]

Pharynx. The pharynx is divided into three compartments: nasopharynx, oropharynx, and hypopharynx (laryngopharynx). The pharynx extends from the base of the skull to the level of the cricoid cartilage. The nasopharynx lies anterior to C1 and is bound superiorly by the base of the skull and inferiorly by the soft palate. The openings to the auditory (eustachian) tubes and the adenoids are found in the nasopharynx. Sensory innervation of the mucosa is derived from the maxillary division of the trigeminal nerve. The oropharynx lies at the C2 to C3 vertebral level, and it is bound superiorly by the soft palate and inferiorly by the epiglottis. It opens, from the oral cavity, through the anterior tonsillar pillar (i.e., the palatoglossus muscle) and posterior tonsillar pillar (i.e., palatopharyngeus muscle). This opening into the oropharynx is also known as the fauces. The fauces is located directly posterior to the oral cavity, with its borders including the soft palate superiorly, the palatoglossal and palatopharyngeal arches (i.e., anterior and posterior tonsillar pillars) laterally, and the tongue inferiorly. Identification of the fauces is a part of the Mallampati classification during airway assessment. The hypopharynx lies posterior to the larynx, and it is bound by the superior border of the epiglottis and the inferior border of the cricoid cartilage at the C5 to C6 level. The upper esophageal sphincter lies at the lower edge of the hypopharynx and arises from the cricopharyngeus muscle. This muscle acts as a barrier (within the upper esophagus) to prevent regurgitation in a conscious patient.

Numerous nerves supply motor and sensory fibers to the airway. The glossopharyngeal, vagus, and spinal accessory nerves share nuclei in the medulla and innervate all the muscles of the pharynx, larynx, and soft palate. Branches of the trigeminal nerve innervate the nasal

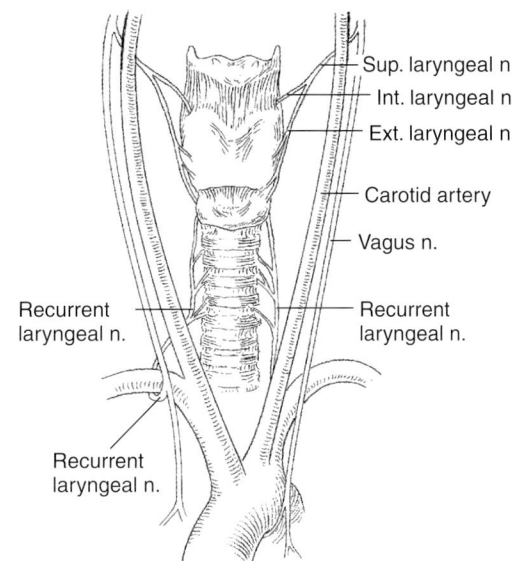

Fig. 24.1 Anatomy of the right and left, superior and recurrent laryngeal nerves. *ext,* External; *int,* internal; *n,* nerve; *sup,* superior.

cavity. Afferent (sensory) stimuli elicited when the posterior wall of the pharynx is touched are carried by the glossopharyngeal nerve to the medulla, where they synapse with nuclei of the vagus nerve and the cranial portion of the spinal accessory nerve. The efferent response returns primarily through the vagus nerve, resulting in the gag reflex as the muscles of the pharynx elevate and constrict.

Two branches of the vagus nerve innervate the hypopharynx: the superior laryngeal nerve (SLN) and the recurrent laryngeal nerve (RLN) (Fig. 24.1). The superior laryngeal nerve divides into the internal and external branches. The internal branch of the SLN provides sensory input to the hypopharynx above the vocal cords, which includes the base of tongue, epiglottis, aryepiglottic folds, and arytenoids. The external branch provides motor function to the cricothyroid muscle of the larynx.

The RLN provides sensory innervation to the subglottic area and the trachea. The RLN is so named because it recurs (loops) around other structures. The right RLN branches from the vagus nerve and recurs (loops) around the right subclavian artery, and the left RLN branches from the vagus nerve and recurs (loops) around the aortic arch. Traction on either of these structures during thoracic surgery can cause injury to the RLN, causing hoarseness, stridor, or possibly respiratory distress. The motor component of the RLN provides motor function to all the muscles of the larynx except the cricothyroid muscle.

The SLN and RLN may be damaged by surgery, neoplasms, and neck trauma. Dissecting aortic arch aneurysms and mitral stenosis can place pressure on the left RLN, causing hoarseness. Unilateral RLN injury usually results in hoarseness but does not compromise respiratory status. The vocal cords compensate by shifting the midline toward the uninjured side. In the acute phase of bilateral injury to the RLN, unopposed tension and adduction of the vocal cords result in stridor, which may deteriorate into severe respiratory distress and possibly death. Patients with chronic injury develop compensatory mechanisms that allow for normal respiration and gruff or husky speech. Injury to the superior laryngeal nerve is not associated with respiratory distress.

Larynx. The larynx begins with the epiglottis and extends to the cricoid cartilage. The larynx is composed of (1) three single cartilages (e.g., thyroid, cricoid, and epiglottis), (2) three paired cartilages (e.g.,

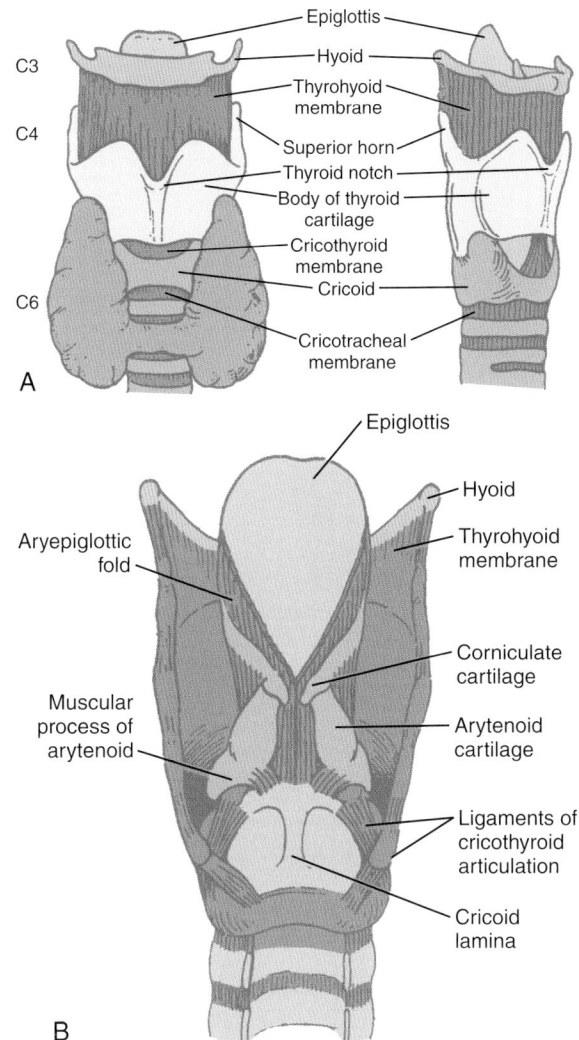

C3

C4

C6

A

- Epiglottis
- Hyoid
- Thyrohyoid membrane
- Superior horn
- Thyroid notch
- Body of thyroid cartilage
- Cricothyroid membrane
- Cricoid
- Cricotracheal membrane

B

- Epiglottis
- Hyoid
- Thyrohyoid membrane
- Aryepiglottic fold
- Corniculate cartilage
- Arytenoid cartilage
- Muscular process of arytenoid
- Ligaments of cricothyroid articulation
- Cricoid lamina

Fig. 24.2 (A) Anterior view of the laryngeal cartilages. External frontal *(left)* and anterolateral *(right)* views of the larynx. Notice the location of the cricothyroid membrane and thyroid gland in relation to the thyroid and cricoid cartilages in the frontal view. The horn of the thyroid cartilage is also known as the cornu. In the anterolateral view, the shape of the cricoid cartilage and its relation to the thyroid cartilage are shown. (B) Posterior view of laryngeal cartilages. Cartilages and ligaments of the larynx are seen posteriorly. Notice the location of the corniculate cartilage within the aryepiglottic fold. (Modified from Ellis H, Feldman S. *Anatomy for Anaesthetists.* 6th ed. Oxford, UK; Blackwell Scientific; 1993; Hagberg CA. *Hagberg and Benumof's Airway Management.* 4th ed. Philadelphia: Elsevier; 2018.)

arytenoid, corniculate, and cuneiform), and (3) intrinsic and extrinsic muscles (Figs. 24.2 and 24.3). These structures function in an intricate manner to provide (1) protection to the lower airway against aspiration, (2) patency between the hypopharynx and trachea, (3) protective gag and cough reflexes, and (4) phonation. In the adult, the larynx begins between the third and fourth cervical vertebrae and ends at the level of the sixth cervical vertebra (e.g., cricothyroid muscle). The anterior and lateral aspects of the larynx are formed by the thyroid and cricoid cartilages. Anteriorly, the thyroid cartilage fuses and forms the thyroid notch, which connects to the hyoid bone superiorly by the thyrohyoid membrane. The thyroid cartilage connects to the cricoid cartilage anteriorly and inferiorly by the cricothyroid membrane. Posteriorly, the thyroid cartilage rises toward the hyoid bone at the base of the

tongue to the posterior cornu. The thyroid cartilage is connected to the hyoid bone by the thyrohyoid fascia and muscles of the larynx.

The posterior portion of the thyroid and cricoid cartilages forms the posterior border of the larynx. Internal to the larynx are the epiglottis and three paired cartilages. The epiglottis exists as a single leaflike cartilage. The epiglottis rests above the glottic opening, where it closes the glottic aperture during swallowing. The superior vallecula is formed by the space between the epiglottis and the base of the tongue. The inferior vallecula is formed by the space between the inferior edge of the epiglottis and the true vocal cords.

The intrinsic muscles of the larynx control the tension of the vocal cords, as well as the opening and closing of the glottis (Table 24.1). In contrast, the extrinsic muscles of the larynx connect the larynx, hyoid bone, and neighboring anatomic structures (Box 24.1). The primary function of the extrinsic muscles is to adjust the position of the larynx during phonation, breathing, and swallowing.

Blood supply to the larynx originates from the external carotid, which branches into the superior thyroid artery. The superior thyroid artery eventually gives rise to the superior laryngeal artery, which supplies blood to the supraglottic region of the larynx. The inferior laryngeal artery, a terminal branch of the inferior thyroid artery, supplies the infraglottic region of the larynx.

Lower Respiratory Tract

As the fetus develops, the respiratory system evolves into complex developmental interactions between the endodermal-derived epithelium and the mesoderm. Both contribute to lung development. The lungs and airways develop through a five-stage process. These include the embryonic, pseudoglandular, canalicular, and terminal sac phases, and maturation.[3]

During the embryonic phase, the endodermal respiratory diverticulum (laryngotracheal groove) develops. This occurs during weeks 4 through 7. The laryngotracheal groove develops from the ventral surface of the foregut. During this period, fibroblast growth factor (FGF-10) causes stimulation and proliferation of cells that will eventually express fibroblast homologous factor (FHF). As the laryngotracheal groove grows and develops, it becomes the primitive lung bud. By day 28, it has grown caudally to the splanchnic mesoderm. It divides into the right and left bronchial buds. This then progresses through the development and expression of the epithelial lining of the lower respiratory system. Cartilage, muscle, and connective tissue arise from the same tissues that form the smooth muscle of the blood vessels. The bronchopulmonary segments appear by day 42 of fetal development.

During the pseudoglandular stage, there is rapid growth and proliferation of the peripheral airways. This occurs during weeks 6 through 16. Repeated branching of the distal ends of the epithelial tubes results in 16 or more generations of the bronchial tubes and the development of the terminal bronchioles. The airways are filled with liquid at this time. The cellular structure is characterized by tall columnar epithelium.

The next phase of development is known as the canalicular stage. This occurs most often during weeks 16 through 26, when the airways widen and lengthen. This space will eventually become the large volume of air space in the expanded lung after birth. Terminal and respiratory bronchioles along with terminal saccules develop. Cuboidal cells of the terminal sacs differentiate into alveolar type II cells. Secretion of surfactant begins at this time. Type II alveolar cells that are adjacent to a vessel flatten and differentiate into type I cells. As the type II and type I cells develop, vascularization appears. The vascularization is associated with the development of the respiratory bronchioles and the alveoli necessary for air exchange after birth. Along with other growth factors, vascular endothelial growth factor participates in the

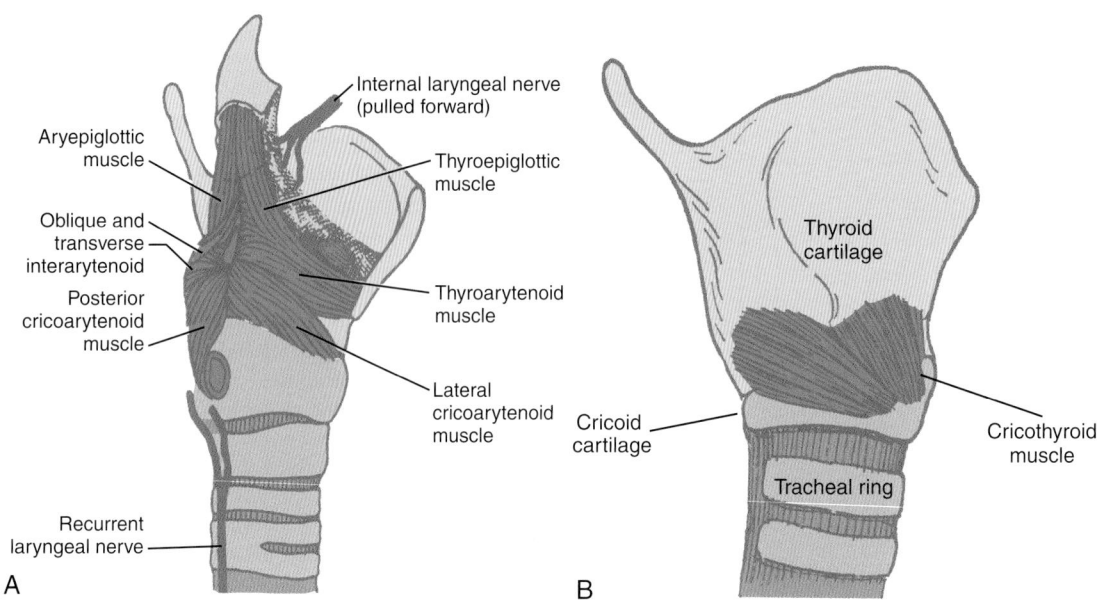

Fig. 24.3 Posterior view of the larynx showing the laryngeal cartilages and muscles. (A) Intrinsic muscles of the larynx and their nerve supply. (B) The cricothyroid muscle and its attachments. (Modified from Ellis H, Feldman S. *Anatomy for Anaesthetists.* 6th ed. Oxford, UK: Blackwell Scientific; 1993; Hagberg CA. *Hagberg and Benumof's Airway Management.* 4th ed. Philadelphia: Elsevier; 2018.)

TABLE 24.1   Intrinsic Muscles of the Larynx

Muscles Involved	Nervous Innervation	Main Function
Posterior cricoarytenoids	Recurrent laryngeal nerve	Abduction of vocal cords
Lateral cricoarytenoids	Recurrent laryngeal nerve	Adduction and lengthening of arytenoids causing glottis closure
Interarytenoid (transverse and oblique arytenoids)	Recurrent laryngeal nerve	Closing of posterior commissure of the glottis causing vocal cord narrowing
Thyroarytenoids and vocalis	Recurrent laryngeal nerve	Shortening (reduced tension) and adduction of vocal cords
Aryepiglottic	Recurrent laryngeal nerve	Constriction of laryngeal vestibule
Cricothyroids	Superior laryngeal nerve (external branch)	Adduction and increasing tension of vocal cords

From Tarrazona V, Deslauriers J. Glottis and subglottis: a thoracic surgeon's perspective. *Thorac Surg Clin.* 2007;17:561–570.

BOX 24.1   Extrinsic Muscles of the Larynx

Muscles That Elevate the Larynx
Suprahyoid Muscles
- Stylohyoid
- Digastric
- Mylohyoid
- Geniohyoid

Pharyngeal Muscle
- Stylopharyngeus

Infrahyoid Muscle
- Thyrohyoid: depresses hyoid, causing laryngeal elevation

Muscles That Depress the Larynx
Infrahyoid Muscles
- Omohyoid
- Sternohyoid
- Sternothyroid

From Tarrazona V, Deslauriers J. Glottis and subglottis: a thoracic surgeon's perspective. *Thorac Surg Clin.* 2007;17:561–570.

formation of blood vessels that will surround the alveoli. At the end of this phase, air exchange is possible, though inefficient.

The terminal sac phase occurs during weeks 24 through 36. Branching of the respiratory bud continues, and further development of the terminal buds is expressed as primitive alveoli. Capillaries begin to develop around the terminal buds and proliferate at the same time as the primitive alveoli develop. Cells further differentiate throughout this period, and by week 26 a primitive blood-gas barrier has developed.

By week 36, mature alveoli can be seen. This requires FGF and platelet-derived growth factor. Development of alveoli will continue for approximately 3 years after birth. A change in the relative relationship of parenchyma to total lung volume contributes to lung growth until the second year of life. From the third year of life until adulthood, lung growth continues.[3]

Trachea. The trachea originates at the inferior border of the cricoid cartilage and extends to the carina (Fig. 24.4). It is approximately 10 to 20 cm long in adults. The cricoid cartilage is the only cartilage of the trachea that is a complete cartilaginous ring. The remainder of the trachea is composed of 16 to 20 C-shaped cartilaginous rings. The

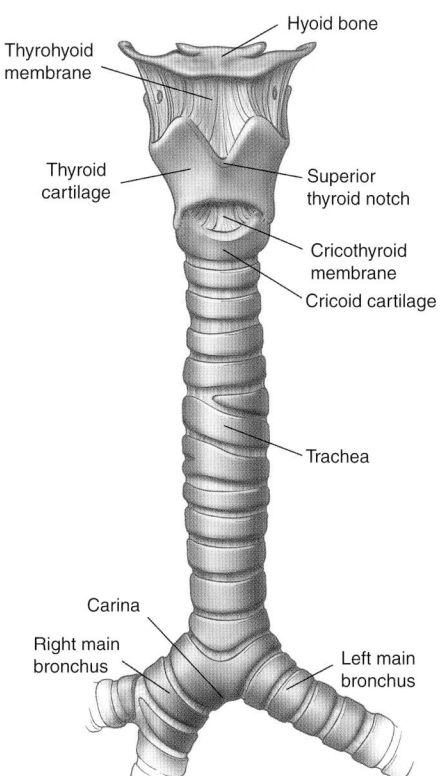

Fig. 24.4 Principal features of the larynx and trachea *(anterior view)*. Tracheobronchial angles vary widely. The angle of the right mainstem bronchus is approximately 25 to 30 degrees, whereas the angle of the left mainstem bronchus is 45 degrees. (From Minnich DJ, Mathisen DJ. Anatomy of the trachea, carina, and bronchi. *Thorac Surg Clin.* 2007;17:571–585.)

posterior side of the trachea is formed by the trachealis muscle. It lacks cartilage and instead it connects the free ends of the tracheal cartilages with smooth muscle, which helps to accommodate the esophagus during the act of swallowing. The primary function of the trachealis muscle is to constrict the trachea causing air to more forcibly exit the trachea (i.e., during coughing). The cartilaginous rings and plates continue deeper into the tracheal bronchial tree until the bronchi reach 0.6 to 0.8 mm in size. At this point, the cartilage disappears, and the bronchi are termed bronchioles. The function of the bronchi is to provide humidification and warming of inspired air as it passes to the alveoli.

The angle of bifurcation of the right mainstem bronchus is approximately 25 to 30 degrees. The bifurcation to the right upper lobe is approximately 2.5 cm from the carina. The angle of the left mainstem bronchus is 45 degrees. The left mainstem bronchus is approximately 5 cm long, before it bifurcates into the left superior and inferior lobe bronchi.

The tracheobronchial tree receives sympathetic innervation from the first through fifth thoracic ganglia. Parasympathetic innervation is derived from branches of the vagus nerve. The carina is richly innervated, making it extremely sensitive to sensory stimulation.

Diaphragm

The diaphragm arises from four structures: (1) the septum transversum, (2) the dorsal esophageal mesentery, (3) the pleuroperitoneal folds, and (4) the body wall mesoderm. The diaphragm develops in the cephalic region and descends into position between the abdominal and pleural cavity contents as the embryo develops. The nerve supply for the diaphragm arises from the cords of the third, fourth, and fifth

cervical nerves, and travels with the descending diaphragmatic structure as the phrenic nerve. The phrenic nerves lie within the pericardium as the fetus matures and after birth. Because of the development of the diaphragm in the cephalic position and the merging of four structures, drugs that impair fetal development can result in potential congenital deformities, including diaphragmatic hernia.[3]

AIRWAY EVALUATION

Evaluation of the airway is central to any airway management plan. A proper airway evaluation should be conducted in a thorough and systematic fashion to determine potential problems. A substantial amount of research over the past 20 years has identified how individual airway examinations can be poor and unreliable predictors of difficulty. Currently, no single examination consistently demonstrates high sensitivity and specificity with minimal false-positive or false-negative reports.[4,5] Instead, many researchers have advocated for a more comprehensive airway management plan that involves the use of multiple airway assessments to identify a difficult airway.[6-8] One area of airway management that may now render some airway examinations obsolete is the advent of videolaryngoscopy (VL). Ultimately, an appropriate airway management plan considers multiple airway examinations, time constraints, the availability of equipment, and presence of experienced personnel.

Current recommendations concerning evaluation of the airway are to employ several preoperative assessments (Table 24.2).[8-11] To recognize possible difficult airway conditions, and to make "sensible airway management decisions," airway assessments should be tailored to the patient, the operative procedure, and the situation to formulate a comprehensive airway management plan.[11,12]

There is no system that reliably and consistently predicts airway difficulty with 100% certainty.[13] Instead of focusing on conditions that affect the ability to intubate only, a more all-encompassing assessment of the airway has been described.[14] The following four areas of airway management focus the airway assessment on conditions that could lead to difficulty with:

1. Bag-mask ventilation (BMV)
2. Direct laryngoscopy (DL) and VL, including endotracheal tube (ETT) delivery and tracheal intubation (TI)
3. Supraglottic airway ventilation
4. Cricothyrotomy airway placement (e.g., needle, percutaneous or surgical)

A series of acronyms was developed to facilitate a thorough and systematic assessment of airway features (Box 24.2) that may lead to difficulty with hand mask, supraglottic device, ETT, and cricothyrotomy airway ventilation and placement.[14]

In addition to an airway examination, a history of a difficult airway is a strong indication for current airway difficulties. Therefore an evaluation of the patient's anesthetic history should be included in the airway assessment.[15] A careful review of prior anesthetic records and information obtained directly from the patient or family members can reveal past difficulties and offer insight concerning specific techniques used to previously manage the patient's airway. Clues that may indicate a history of difficult airway management may include chipped or broken teeth, bruised lips, previous sore throat after general surgery, past postoperative dysphonia, a memory of TI, an unexpected admission to an intensive care unit (ICU), or a pharyngeal, esophageal, or tracheal perforation.[15,16] Weight gain or loss can influence airway anatomy, and the patient may not necessarily present with the same airway conditions as in the past. Furthermore, pathologies or conditions such as an airway tumor or hematoma, which may have previously caused difficulty but have since been treated or removed, may not influence the current airway to the same degree as in the past.

TABLE 24.2   Components of the Preoperative Airway Physical Examination*

Airway Examination Component	Indication of Airway Difficulty
Length of upper incisors	Relatively long
Relation of maxillary and mandibular incisors during normal jaw closure	Prominent "overbite" (maxillary incisors anterior to mandibular incisors)
Relation of maxillary and mandibular incisors during voluntary protrusion (ULBT)	Inability to protrude mandibular incisors anterior to maxillary incisors
Interincisor distance	<3 cm
Visibility of uvula	Not visible when tongue is protruded with patient in sitting position (e.g., Mallampati class III or greater)
Shape of palate	Highly arched or very narrow
Compliance of mandibular space	Stiff, indurated, occupied by mass, or nonresilient
Thyromental distance	Less than three ordinary fingerbreadths
Length of neck	Short
Thickness of neck	Thick (>43 cm in circumference)
Range of motion of head and neck	Patient cannot touch tip of chin to chest or patient cannot extend neck

*This table displays some findings of the airway physical examination that may suggest difficulty with laryngoscopy and intubation. The decision to examine some or all of the airway components shown in this table depends on the clinical context and judgment of the practitioner. The table is not intended as a mandatory or exhaustive list of the components of an airway examination. The order of presentation in this table follows the "line of sight" that occurs during conventional oral laryngoscopy.

ULBT, Upper lip bite test.

From Berkow LC. Strategies for airway management. *Best Pract Res Clin Anaesthesiol.* 2004;18(4):531–548.

BOX 24.2   Four Areas of Airway Management With Factors Associated With Difficulty

Indication of Difficulty With Bag Mask Ventilation
- Mask seal impeded by beards, altered anatomy, or nasogastric tubes
- Obstruction of the upper or lower airway
- Obesity with redundant upper airway soft tissue and greater chest and abdominal mass compressing the lungs
- Age >55 related to loss of upper airway tissue elasticity
- No teeth, leading to improper facial structure for the bag mask
- Stiff lungs (e.g., increases in airway resistance and decreases in pulmonary compliance)
- Sleep apnea or snoring

Indication of Difficulty With Direct Laryngoscopy and Videolaryngoscopy With Tracheal Intubation
- Look externally (if it looks difficult it probably is)
- Evaluate the 3-3-2 rule*
- Mallampati score (classes III and IV indicating increased difficulty)
- Obstruction of the upper airway
- Obesity with increased neck circumference and redundant soft tissue
- Scarring, radiation, or masses on the neck
- Neck mobility that is impaired by disease of immobilization (direct laryngoscopy)
- Operator experience

Indication of Difficulty With Supraglottic Airway Device Placement and Ventilation
- Restricted mouth opening
- Obstruction of the upper airway
- Distortion of airway anatomy preventing an adequate seal
- Stiff lungs (e.g., increases in airway resistance or decreases in pulmonary compliance)

Indication of Difficulty With Cricothyrotomy Airway Placement
- Distortion of neck anatomy (e.g., hematoma, infection, abscess, tumor, scarring from radiation)
- Obesity or a short neck limiting cricothyroid identification
- Trauma in or around the cricothyroid area
- Impediments causing limited access to the neck (e.g., halo device, fixed flexion abnormality)
- Surgery causing limited access to anatomic landmarks

* 3-3-2 rule = three fingerbreadths between incisors; three fingerbreadths between tip of the chin (mentum) and chin-neck junction (hyoid bone); two fingerbreadths between chin-neck junction (hyoid bone) and thyroid notch.

Adapted from Walls RM, Murphy MF, eds. *Manual of Emergency Airway Management.* 4th ed. Philadelphia: Lippincott Williams & Wilkins; 2012:8–21.

Multiple airway assessments exist that help the anesthetist predict difficulty with BMV, DL and VL with TI, supraglottic airway ventilation, and cricothyrotomy airway placement (see Box 24.2). The following sections consider airway evaluations specific to each of the four areas of airway management.

Bag-Mask Ventilation Assessment

Adequate BMV skills are important for effective airway management. A sufficient seal between the facemask and the patient's face is imperative. Proper BMV can be achieved by placing the left thumb and index finger around the collar of the facemask at both the mask bridge and chin curve, while compressing the left side of the mask onto the face with the palm of the left hand (Fig. 24.5). The middle and ring fingers can then be placed on the bony part of the mandible to help compress the mask to the patient's face and to raise the chin. The fifth finger can be placed at the angle of the mandible to provide an anterior jaw-thrusting maneuver. Mask-retaining straps can be placed behind the patient's head and then be connected to the collar of the mask to apply pressure at various angles and promote a better mask seal.

If BMV is believed to be inadequate, then a series of steps can be performed (Box 24.3) to facilitate ventilation. First, the patient's head and neck can be repositioned into a sniffing position. Second, if the tongue or airway soft tissue is thought to be the cause of obstruction,

then the placement of an oropharyngeal airway (OPA) may help bypass the obstruction. However, the placement of an OPA can be considered prior to any attempt at BMV. Third, if BMV continues to remain inadequate, then place both thumbs on either side of the facemask bridge with both index fingers on either side of the mask chin curve on the body of the mask. The middle fingers can then be placed on either side of the mandible at the chin, the ring fingers on the bony part of the mandible, and the fifth fingers on each angle of the mandible to provide a jaw thrust while a second provider inflates and depresses the anesthesia bag. Alternatively, a second provider may stand at the side

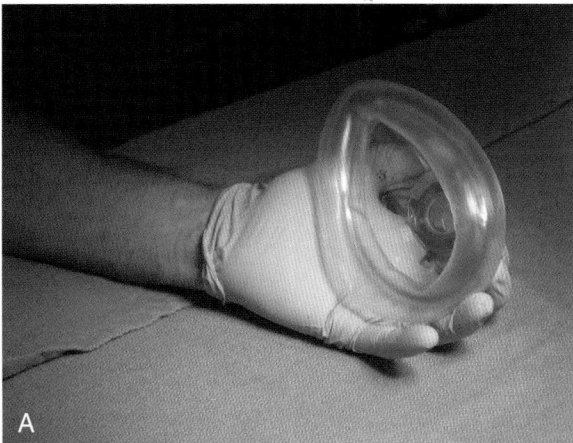

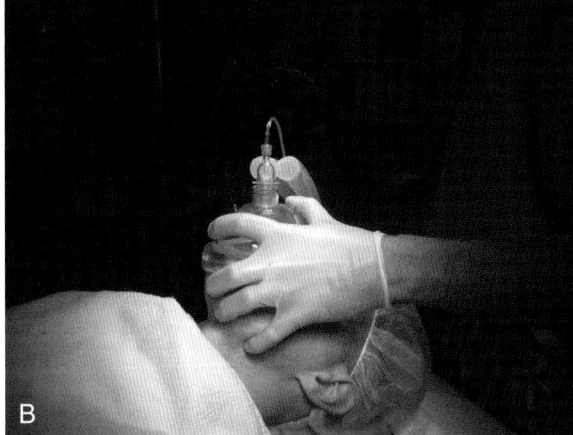 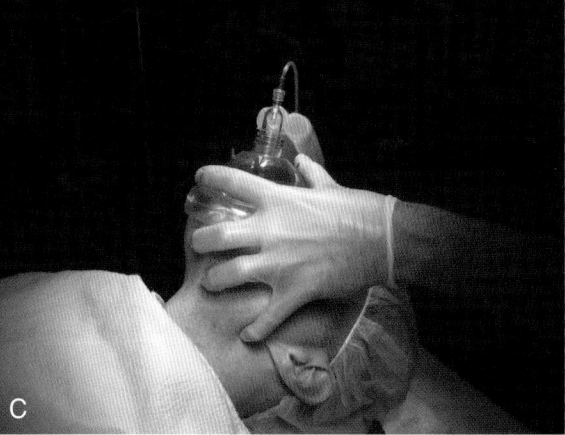

Fig. 24.5 Suggested hand technique for facemask ventilation. (A) The thumb, index finger, and thenar eminence of the palm encircle the collar, while the hypothenar eminence extends below the mask. (B) One-handed mask technique. The thumb and index finger encircle the collar of the mask, while the middle finger grasps the mental protuberance (chin), and the ring and little fingers grip the body of the mandible to pull the mask securely onto the face while gently extending the head. (C) Jaw thrust with one-handed mask technique. Middle and ring fingers grasp the mandible and pull upward into the mask, while the little finger is moved to the angle of the jaw and pulls backward and upward to maintain subluxation (jaw thrust). (From Hagberg CA. *Benumof and Hagberg's Airway Management*. 3rd ed. Philadelphia: Elsevier; 2013:335.)

BOX 24.3 Proper Sequence for Bag-Mask Ventilation When Difficulty Is Encountered

1. Assure proper positioning of the patient that avoids compression of the airway.
2. Attempt ventilation with one (left) hand (can consider use of mask strap on opposite side of mask [right] to improve mask seal).
3. Reposition the head into a sniffing position.
4. Place oropharyngeal airway (may consider earlier placement).
5. Proceed with two-handed mask ventilation while assistant compresses ventilation bag.
6. Consider placement of a supraglottic device and consider awakening the patient.
7. Consider laryngoscopy and tracheal intubation if no previous attempts.
8. Proceed with cricothyrotomy if ventilation and intubation become impossible.

---

of the bed to provide the mask seal while the provider at the head of the bed inflates the anesthesia bag in preparation for intubation (Fig. 24.6). Fig. 24.7 depicts the placement of a two-provider orientation for airway management. If ventilation continues to remain inadequate, then a supraglottic airway device (SAD) may be placed while the decision to

awaken the patient is considered. Consider laryngoscopy, using either direct or video technique, and tracheal intubation if it has not previously been attempted. In the event that all these maneuvers fail, then a cricothyrotomy should be considered.

The incidence of difficult BMV has been described as being between 0.9% and 7.8%, and the incidence of impossible BMV as 0.15%.[17-21] Difficulty with BMV can occur because of an inappropriate mask seal (such as with the presence of a beard). Inadequate ventilation during BMV is evidenced by (1) minimal or no chest movement, (2) inadequate or deficient exhaled carbon dioxide (e.g., lack of condensation and spirometric reading), (3) reduced or absent breath sounds, and (4) a decreasing oxygen saturation (e.g., <92%).[11,18] Improving the patient's position can improve BVM by elevating the shoulders, neck, and head, which is known as ramping (Fig. 24.8). Multiple factors have been identified as predictors for difficulty with BMV (see Box 24.2); these include mask seal impediments, upper airway obstructions, obesity, elderly patients, Mallampati scores of III or IV, a short thyromental distance, snoring, and poor lung compliance.[17,18,20,21]

Mask seal impediments such as facial hair, altered facial anatomy, lack of teeth causing the face to cave inward, or a nasogastric tube can cause air leakage out of the mask and prevent adequate positive pressure ventilation. Some of these factors can be modified, such as shaving

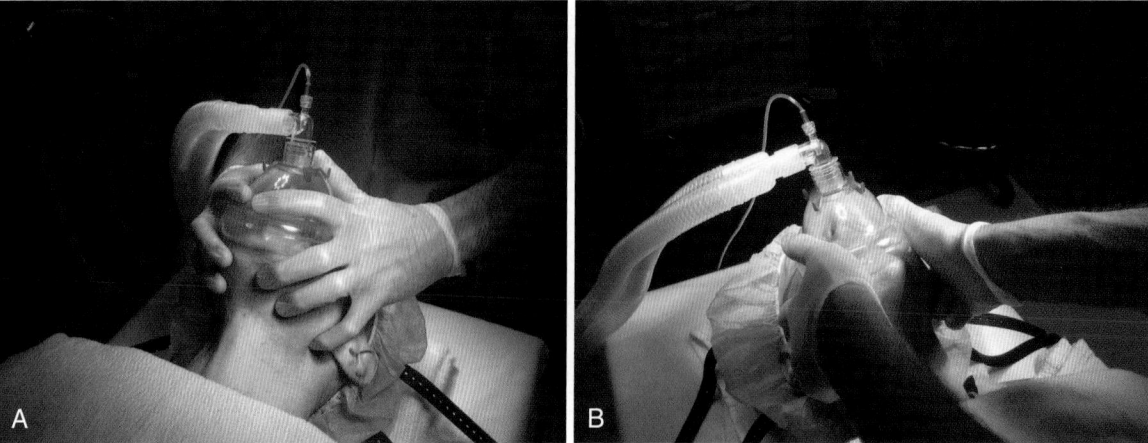

Fig. 24.6 Two-handed mask technique. (A) Provider above patient. The thumb and index finger of both hands encircle the collar of the mask to create a seal to the face, while the middle and ring fingers grasp the mandible, pulling from below and assisting with the jaw thrust maneuver. The little fingers of both hands grip the angles of the mandible to complete the jaw thrust. (B) Provider holding mask below and to the side of patient. The thumbs hold the rim of facemask to create a seal to the face, while the index fingers grip the angles of the mandible to perform a jaw thrust. This technique allows the provider above the patient to prepare for airway manipulation (e.g., laryngoscopy, fiberoptic intubation). (From Hagberg CA, ed. *Benumof and Hagberg's Airway Management*. 3rd ed. Philadelphia: Elsevier; 2013:336.)

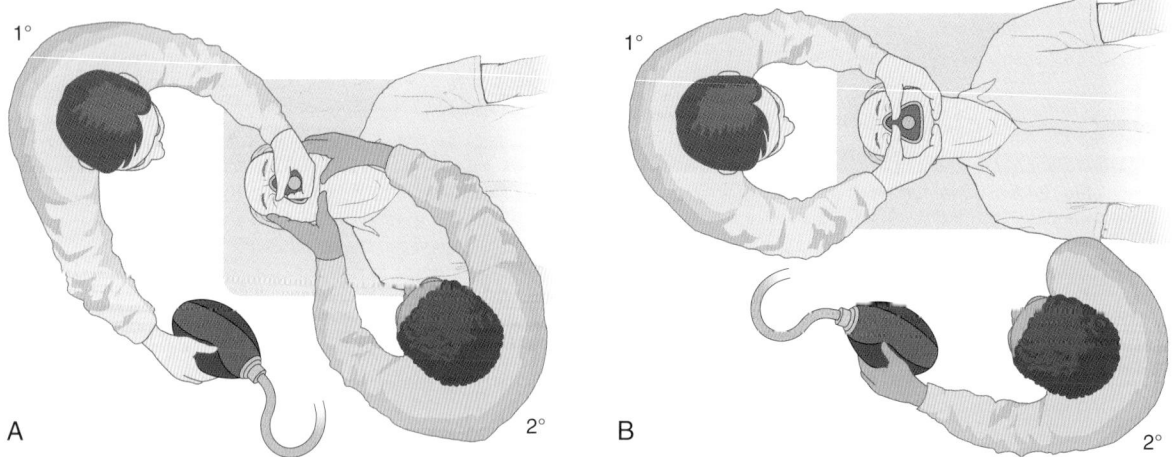

Fig. 24.7 (A) Two-person mask ventilation effort with second provider providing a jaw thrust. (B) Two-person mask ventilation effort with primary provider maintaining a mask seal and performing a jaw thrust while second provider squeezes the anesthesia bag. (Redrawn in Miller RD, Pardo M, eds. *Basics of Anesthesia*. 6th ed. Philadelphia: Saunders; 2011; originally from Benumof JL, ed. *Airway Management: Principles and Practice*. St. Louis: Mosby; 1996.)

the patient's beard, delaying removal of dentures, and removing the nasogastric tube. The decision to shave a patient's beard or remove an existing gastric tube should be individualized to the patient's condition and situation, especially since removal of a gastric tube may cause a buildup of gastric secretions in the stomach.

Obstruction may occur in the upper or lower airway and can severely limit the effectiveness of BMV. Upper airway obstructions should be considered an emergency, recognized early, and managed with extreme care because of the potential to become total airway obstructions. The hallmark signs of an upper airway obstruction in the unanesthetized patient include a hoarse or muffled voice, difficulty swallowing secretions, stridor, and dyspnea. Stridor and dyspnea are ominous signs of severe respiratory obstruction in the hypopharyngeal and/or laryngeal area.[14] There are several potential causes of an upper airway obstruction (Boxes 24.4 and 24.5). The relative management of

these conditions is discussed later in this chapter (see "Management of the Difficult and Failed Airway"). It is important to treat the airway with care because these conditions have the potential to severely impair ventilation and oxygenation, as well as cause difficulty with laryngoscopy and TI.

Lower airway obstructions typically manifest with high peak airway pressures, low tidal volumes, and impaired ventilation. These conditions can be caused by pathologic, congenital, or acquired causes (see Boxes 24.4 and 24.5) and should be managed in a way that provides optimal ventilation and oxygenation for the patient.

Obstructive sleep apnea (OSA) and snoring were recognized as predictors of difficult mask ventilation.[17,18,20] Studies have revealed that patients with a history of snoring and sleep apnea are more likely to have obstruction and difficulty with BMV.[17,18,22] An obstructive tongue and collapse of posterior oropharyngeal soft tissue are thought to be

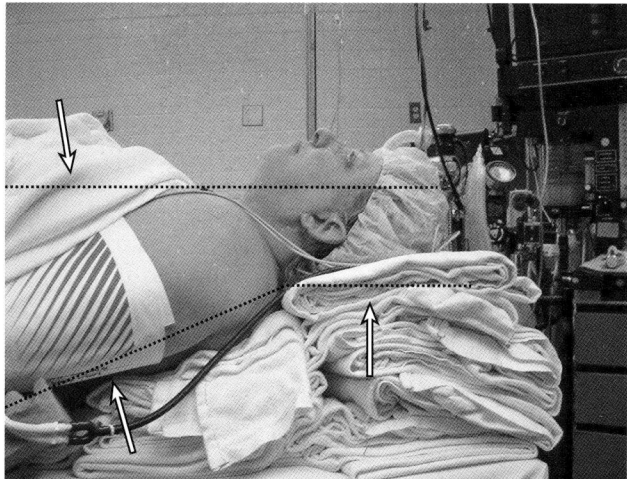

Fig. 24.8 Example of a ramp created using blankets to improve positioning. Optimal positioning is observed when an imaginary horizontal line can be drawn from the sternal notch and extending just anterior to the ear on the face or to the tragus of the ear. Arrows pointing up indicate blanket ramp; arrow pointing down indicates imaginary line between the ear and sternal notch. (From Chestnut DH, et al., eds. *Chestnut's Obstetric Anesthesia: Principles and Practice.* 5th ed. Philadelphia: Elsevier; 2014:693.)

BOX 24.4 Causes of Upper and Lower Airway Obstruction

Upper Airway Obstruction
Facial
- Burns
- Congenital abnormalities
- Trauma

Oropharyngeal
- Abscesses (e.g., peritonsillar)
- Ludwig angina
- Sleep apnea
- Tongue

Pharyngeal and Laryngeal
- Angioedema
- Foreign bodies
- Epiglottitis
- Hematomas
- Hemorrhage
- Laryngospasm
- Laryngotracheobronchitis (croup)
- Subglottic stenosis
- Tumors or lesions

Lower Airway Obstruction
Trachea
- Angioedema
- Aspirated foreign bodies
- Hematoma
- Hemorrhage
- Tumors or lesions

Bronchial and Alveolar
- Acute respiratory distress syndrome (ARDS)
- Aspiration pneumonia
- Asthma
- Bronchospasm
- Chronic obstructive pulmonary disease (COPD)
- Pulmonary edema

Extrapulmonary
- Morbid obesity (body mass index >30 kg/m^2)
- Pregnancy
- Trauma

From Berkow LC. Strategies for airway management. *Best Pract Res Clin Anaesthesiol.* 2004;18(4):531–548.

BOX 24.5 Congenital and Acquired Conditions Associated With Difficult Airway Management

Conditions With Associated Pathology Relating to Airway Difficulty
Congenital
- *Pierre Robin syndrome:* Retrognathia, micrognathia, glossoptosis, cleft palate
- *Treacher Collins syndrome:* Mandibular hypoplasia, micrognathia, facial bone hypoplasia, choanal atresia, cleft palate
- *Goldenhar syndrome:* Hemifacial microsomia, mandibular hypoplasia; vertebrae may be incomplete, fused, or missing
- *Mucopolysaccharidosis:* Macroglossia, odontoid hypoplasia, dental anomalies, sleep apnea
- *Klippel-Feil syndrome:* Short neck, fusion of two or more cervical vertebrae, limited range of neck motion
- *Down syndrome:* Macroglossia, flattened nose, cervical spine abnormalities, obstructive sleep apnea, dental anomalies

Acquired
- *Morbid obesity:* Thick neck with redundant airway tissue, obstructive sleep apnea
- *Acromegaly:* Macroglossia, prognathism, vocal cord swelling
- *Ludwig angina:* Infection at the floor of the mouth, trismus
- *Abscesses (oral, retropharyngeal):* Distortion or stenosis of the airway tissues, trismus
- *Laryngeal papillomatosis:* Viral infection causing tumors or papillomas within the larynx
- *Epiglottis:* infection causing swelling of the epiglottis, laryngeal edema
- *Croup:* infection causing laryngeal edema and subglottic edema
- *Rheumatoid arthritis:* Limited cervical spine range of motion, temporomandibular joint ankylosis, cricoarytenoid arthritis
- *Ankylosing spondylitis:* Cervical spine ankylosis, decreased chest expansion
- *Tumors involving the airway:* Distortion or stenosis of the airway, fibrosis with fixation from irradiation
- *Trauma (airway, cervical spine):* Distortion, edema, hemorrhage of the airway

may be the result of excessive weight from both chest and abdominal tissues causing compression on the lungs, especially in the supine and head-down positions. Pregnant patients in the third trimester may also be difficult to ventilate because the gravid uterus can compress the lungs, creating elevated airway resistance. Furthermore, obese patients tend to have decreased functional residual capacities (FRCs), which predispose them to desaturate more quickly, even after appropriate preoxygenation periods. One study reported that the time to reach a preoxygenation end-tidal oxygen value of 85% or greater was similar in both obese and lean patients. However, the authors observed that apnea-induced desaturation occurred more quickly, and hypoxemia was more profound, in the obese population.[23] Time to desaturation should be considered in the overall airway management plan because any time delay after the induction of anesthesia in the obese population may result in significant hypoxemia.

Redundant tissue of the upper airway may be another factor that leads to difficulty with BMV because excessive soft tissue in the oropharyngeal and pharyngeal cavities can cause resistance to airflow during positive pressure ventilation.[14,24] Therefore ideal positioning (e.g., ramping the patient), adequate preoxygenation, a secondary airway management plan with alternative airway adjuncts readily available, and assistance from other anesthesia professionals should be considered prior to the induction of anesthesia in the obese patient.

the cause of difficulty and obstruction. Patients with a history of OSA should be encouraged to bring their positive pressure device (e.g., continuous positive airway pressure [CPAP] or biphasic positive airway pressure [BiPAP] machine) from home to the hospital for use in the postanesthesia care unit.[22]

Significant obesity (body mass index >30 kg/m^2) has been identified as a potential risk factor for difficult BMV.[17,18,21] Difficulty with BMV

Obesity is a risk factor for both effective ventilation and laryngoscopy because excessive upper airway soft tissue may inhibit direct visualization of the glottis. Morbid obesity, now known as class 3 obesity or "severe obesity", is generally associated with a body mass index greater than 40 kg/m^2.[25,26]

Apneic Oxygenation

Apneic oxygenation is a strategy used to provide a patient with oxygen during times of apnea, and more specifically during intubation of the trachea. Even without lung expansion and diaphragmatic movements, alveoli will continue to receive oxygen if a higher concentration gradient exists in the upper respiratory areas. Approximately 250 mL/min of oxygen diffuses from the alveoli into the bloodstream during apnea, whereas only 8 to 20 mL/min of carbon dioxide is transferred into the alveoli. This difference is the result of blood gas solubility and hemoglobin's affinity for oxygen which causes the alveoli's net pressure to become slightly subatmospheric, facilitating gas to flow from the pharynx into the alveoli. Apneic oxygenation can sustain a patient's partial pressure of arterial oxygen (PaO_2) for significant amounts of time without ventilation. However, hypercapnia and acidosis are probable if either spontaneous or assisted breaths are not administered within a reasonable amount of time. The process of providing apneic oxygenation during an intubation procedure requires a patent upper airway and a nasal cannula. Initially the nasal cannula can be placed under an anesthesia facemask during preoxygenation and is then set to a high flow rate (15 L/min) during apnea to drive oxygen into the hypopharynx and become entrained within the trachea. The effects of such high nasal cannula oxygen flows on airway tissues can be minimized as long as this technique is utilized for short-term apneic episodes. Apneic oxygenation may be considered for use in obese patients who require intubation or in other patients who are at risk for rapid desaturation during apnea.[27]

Advanced age (>55 years) is associated with difficult BMV.[17,18] Older patients may have decreased upper airway muscle tone as a result of inelastic or aged tissue. In addition, elderly patients commonly have loose or missing teeth, or are edentulous, which can cause the airway soft tissue to sink inward. These factors contribute to a poor mask seal and an inability to perform adequate BMV. Anesthesia practitioners may consider leaving dentures in place (as long as they are easily removable) in the edentulous patient prior to instrumentation of the airway. This may be done to conserve the facial structure and facilitate a better mask seal.

Decreases in lung compliance can contribute to ineffective BMV because of the inability to effectively move ventilated gases into the alveoli. Conditions such as bronchospasm, pulmonary edema, acute respiratory distress syndrome, or pneumonia (see Box 24.4) can cause peak airway pressures to rise and compliance to decrease, resulting in ineffective BMV and poor oxygenation of the patient. The ability of the anesthetist to recognize potential and actual upper and lower airway problems early is essential when managing the airway.

Direct Laryngoscopy and Videolaryngoscopy With Tracheal Intubation Assessment

DL, VL, and TI are different procedures. DL is the process of airway instrumentation with a laryngoscope to acquire a direct line of sight with the laryngeal opening and supporting structures. VL is an indirect procedure for viewing the laryngeal opening using a camera that is embedded on the tip of the laryngoscope which is then linked to a video monitor. TI is the process of placing an ETT into the trachea proximal to the carina and can be done utilizing either direct or indirect laryngoscopy. Usually when anesthesia professionals perform a DL or VL it is with the intent of completing TI, and as a result laryngoscopy and intubation are generally performed together in sequence. Airway assessments specific to DL, VL, and TI are therefore discussed together in this section.

A primary goal during airway evaluation is to determine factors that predispose a patient to difficulty with DL, VL, and TI. The distinction among these procedures has not always been clear in the literature, and the definition of difficulty can vary. However, the incidence of difficult TI has been described to be between 1.5% and 8.5%, and the incidence of failed TI has been estimated to be between 0.3% and 0.5%.[6,28-30] The actual incidence of failure will vary depending on patient characteristics and the current situation (i.e., obstetric emergency, airway trauma, airway pathology). As described earlier, individual airway assessments have not demonstrated an ability to reliably and consistently predict difficulty. Therefore, multiple airway assessments should be used when evaluating for potential difficulty with DL, VL, and TI.

Combinations of difficult airway assessments have been used with varying degrees of predictive success.[8,28,31-33] A significant concern when performing the different airway assessments is the variation in measurements.[6] The variability among practitioners when performing airway evaluation techniques alters the validity of findings between studies. This highlights the importance of conducting airway evaluations the way they were intended every time. The most commonly cited airway assessments used to evaluate for DL, VL, and TI include (1) the modified Mallampati classification, (2) thyromental distance (TMD), (3) interincisor gap distance, (4) atlantooccipital joint mobility and cervical range of motion, (5) mandibular protrusion test, (6) evaluation for obstruction of the upper airway, and (7) measurement of neck circumference (specifically for obese patients).

Mallampati Classification

The Mallampati classification is a commonly used technique of assessing the mouth opening, size of the tongue, size of the oral pharynx, and posterior oropharyngeal structures. First developed by Rao Mallampati, this classification originally described three classes.[34] Later, Samsoon and Young[35] added a fourth class, which is now often referred to as the modified Mallampati test (MMT) (Fig. 24.9; Table 24.3). When performing the assessment, the patient is instructed to sit upright, extend the neck, open the mouth as much as possible, protrude the tongue, and avoid phonation. The MMT uses a classification system to evaluate tongue size relative to the oropharyngeal space and is categorized as follows:

- *Class I:* Full visualization of the entire oropharynx, including soft palate, uvula, fauces (created by two tonsillar pillars known as the palatoglossal and palatopharyngeal arches), and possibly the palatine tonsils located between the tonsillar pillars (not always identified)
- *Class II:* Visualization of the soft palate, fauces, and uvula
- *Class III:* Visualization of the soft palate and base of the uvula
- *Class IV:* Visualization of the hard palate only

Ezri et al.[36] suggested adding a class "zero" to the MMT, which is the ability to see any part of the epiglottis on mouth opening and tongue protrusion, and found a 1.2% incidence. However, most researchers and clinical practitioners use the Samsoon and Young I to IV modification of the Mallampati classification.

Evaluations of the MMT have shown some correlations with difficulty when either class III or IV is measured.[35,36] However, by itself, the MMT has been unreliable at consistently predicting the presence or absence of a difficult airway.[37,38] Variability in the administration of the MMT and practitioner subjectivity of assessment can result in the assessment of different classifications between similar patients. Nevertheless, when used in combination with other airway assessments, the MMT can help increase the predictive ability of both laryngoscopic and intubation difficulties. For

Mallampati Classification

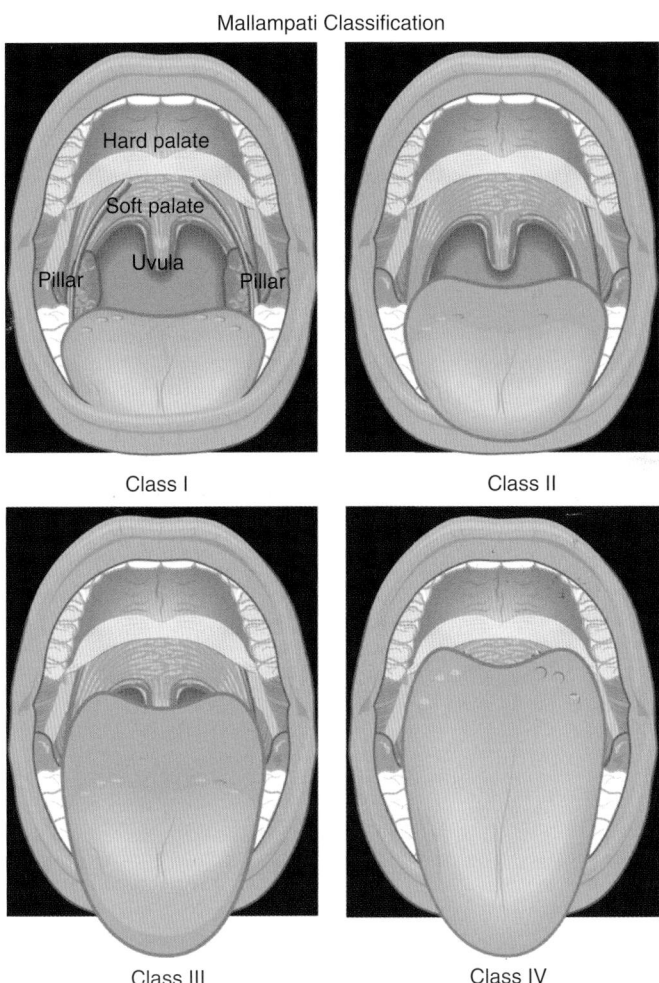

Fig. 24.9 Modified Mallampati classification. Performed with the patient sitting up and maximally protruding the tongue; visibility of the soft palate, fauces, tonsillar pillars, and uvula are noted. Class I describes full visualization of all structures. Class II allows visualization of the soft palate, fauces, and uvula. Class III allows visualization of the soft palate and the base of the uvula. With class IV, only the hard palate is visible. (Courtesy Cleveland Clinic.)

TABLE 24.3	**Mallampati Airway Classification**
Classification	**Description of Visualized Structures**
I	Soft palate, fauces, uvula, pillars visible
II	Soft palate, fauces, uvula visible
III	Soft palate, base of uvula visible
IV	Hard palate visible only

From Berkow LC. Strategies for airway management. *Best Pract Res Clin Anaesthesiol.* 2004;18(4):531–548.

example, the combination of high Mallampati classification levels of III or IV and a large neck circumference (>43 cm, as measured at the thyroid cartilage) were predictors of intubation problems.[12,25] Other researchers identified the combination of high Mallampati classifications, decreased TMDs, and limited interincisor openings as strong predictors of both laryngoscopic and intubation difficulties.[6,28,33]

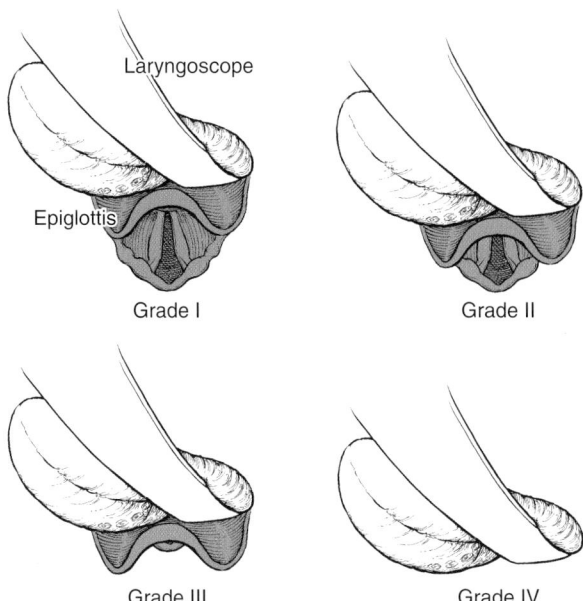

Fig. 24.10 Cormack and Lehane grading system. Grade I is visualization of the entire glottic opening. Grade II is visualization of only the posterior portion of the glottic opening. Grade III is visualization of the epiglottis only. Grade IV is visualization of the soft palate only. (From Cormack RS, Lehane J. Difficult tracheal intubation in obstetrics. *Anaesthesia.* 1984;39[11]:1105–1111.)

Cormack and Lehane Grading System

An objective scoring system frequently used by researchers and clinicians to describe laryngoscopic difficulty is the Cormack and Lehane grading scale (Fig. 24.10). This scale was originally described in 1984 and updated in 1998 to better define the grade II views.[39,40] It offers an objective assessment of the pharyngeal structures, glottic structures, and glottic opening during laryngoscopy and is rated as follows:

- *Grade I:* Full view of the glottic opening, including the anterior commissure and posterior laryngeal cartilages
- *Grade IIa:* Partial view of the vocal cords (anterior commissure not seen) and full view of posterior laryngeal cartilages
- *Grade IIb:* Only the posterior portion of the glottic opening can be visualized (posterior laryngeal cartilages)
- *Grade III:* Only the epiglottis can be visualized; no portion of the glottic opening can be seen
- *Grade IV:* Epiglottis cannot be seen; only view is of the soft palate

Cormack and Lehane grades I and IIa and IIb are generally associated with easier intubations, although a grade IIb is likely more difficult than the IIa view. Grades III and IV correspond with higher degrees of intubation difficulty.[39] Other authors have focused on an assessment to quantify the percentage of glottic visualization in an effort to limit the ambiguity that exists between Cormack and Lehane grades I and II. The percentage of glottic opening (POGO) is the percentage of the vocal cords visualized. It is defined as the linear span from the anterior commissure to the interarytenoid notch. A 100% POGO score is a full view of the glottis and includes the anterior commissure to the interarytenoid notch. A POGO score of 0% signals that no portion of the glottic opening is seen (including the interarytenoid notch). Objective scoring between 0% and 100% is dependent on the judgment of the individual performing the laryngoscopy, and POGO scoring has been shown to provide good intra- and interobserver reliability.[41]

Thyromental Distance

The TMD is a measurement of the thyromental space. This space is an available pliable compartment, directly anterior to the larynx, where the tongue can be displaced during laryngoscopy to improve direct line of site with the glottic opening. The tongue is a malleable structure that can be displaced within the oropharyngeal and pharyngeal compartments. The thyromental space is bordered laterally by the neck, superiorly by the mentum, and inferiorly by the semifixed hyoid bone. The TMD is measured from the thyroid notch to the lower border of the mentum (at the chin) when the patient's head is extended and the mouth is closed (Fig. 24.11B). A TMD less than 6 cm, or three ordinary fingerbreadths, is associated with a higher incidence of difficult intubation. Research has indicated that the thyromental space should accommodate most tongue sizes but that a small space would only facilitate a relatively small tongue.[32,42] Some conditions, such as radiation or pathologic factors (e.g., tumors), may render the thyromental space noncompliant, hindering tongue placement and causing it to protrude into the pharyngeal space. A malplaced tongue that does not fit into the thyromental space can obstruct the line of site to the glottic opening during DL.

Another condition affecting tongue placement into the thyromental space is known as mandibular hypoplasia. This condition results in a TMD of less than three fingerbreadths and may cause difficulty with DL and TI because the tongue cannot be displaced into the small submandibular space. Furthermore, the larynx may be tucked underneath the tongue or be positioned relatively anterior to the base of the tongue in the pharyngeal space, causing difficulty with laryngoscopic views. This condition is commonly called an anterior larynx, and unless the tongue can be detracted anteriorly away from the pharyngeal space, little can be done to improve the direct line of site view. In contrast, VL has shown to provide improved laryngeal visualization in patients with difficult direct line of site views.[43,44]

The assessment of a long TMD (>9 cm) may also indicate a potentially difficult laryngoscopy and intubation. The indication for difficulty is due to a large hypopharyngeal tongue, caudal larynx, and longer mandibulohyoid distance (MHD). The MHD measures the vertical distance from the angle of the mandible to the hyoid bone and is usually assessed by radiograph. A long TMD and MHD may position the glottic opening caudally in the neck and beyond the visual horizon. If the larynx is more caudally situated in the pharyngeal compartment, then the tongue is also likely to be positioned lower because the tongue muscle is hinged to the hyoid bone.[45,46] This can lead to both a greater distance to the glottic opening during laryngoscopy and an obstructed view caused by a greater amount of tongue mass in the hypopharyngeal space. In addition, a history of sleep apnea and snoring can provide further evidence of a possible hypopharyngeal tongue, which has been shown to cause difficulty with both mask ventilation and intubation.[46,47] Similar to other airway assessment tests, researchers have found limited predictability when the TMD test was used by itself and therefore recommend that it be used as part of a multivariable airway assessment.[25,30]

The 3-3-2 rule has been described by some authors as a nonscientifically based test to ensure that upper airway geometry is adequately assessed.[48] The 3-3-2 rule is an assessment that evaluates various airway proportions using fingerbreadths as a measurement (see Fig. 24.11). It is a combination of different geometric dimensions that relate mouth opening and the size of the mandibular space to the position of the larynx in the neck.[14] The first "3" estimates oral access (the interincisor gap distance), which should accommodate at least three fingerbreadths. The second "3" assesses the mandibular length (TMD) from the tip of the mentum to the mandible-neck junction and gauges the ability of the tongue to displace within the submandibular space during

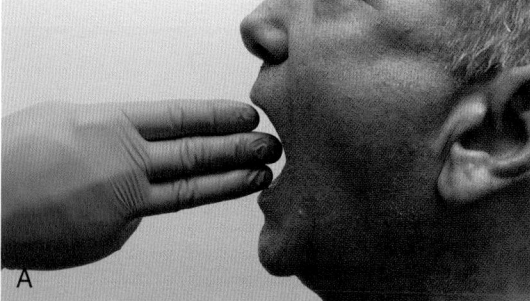
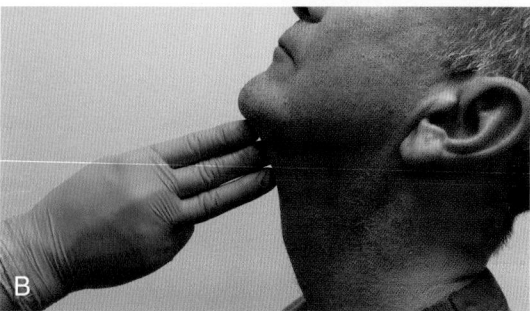
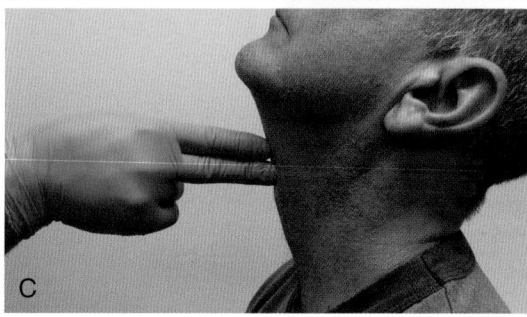

Fig. 24.11 The 3-3-2 assessment. (A) Mouth opening (distance between upper and lower incisors) at least three fingerbreadths. (B) Mentum (protruding part of chin) to thyroid notch, as known as thyromental distance, at least three fingerbreadths. (C) Thyroid notch to hyoid bone at least two fingerbreadths. (From Elisha S, Nagelhout JJ, Heiner JS. *Current Anesthesia Practice*. St. Louis: Elsevier; 2021:48.)

laryngoscopy. The "2" is a modification of the MHD, which is a nonradiographic measurement from the mandible-neck junction to the tip of the thyroid notch and assesses the position of the larynx (glottic opening) in relation to the base of the tongue. More than two fingerbreadths indicates that the larynx may be positioned too far down the neck and could be difficult to visualize. Less than two fingerbreadths indicates that the larynx may be tucked under the base of the tongue, which would be indicative of an anterior larynx. This combination of airway assessments allows the anesthetist to perform multiple airway measurements in a rapid and sequential manner.

The sternomental distance (SMD) is measured from the sternal notch to the lower border of the mentum at the chin with the mouth closed. There is some debate regarding a normal SMD length with the number ranging from greater than 12.5 cm to 15 cm. However, most researchers will agree that a SMD of less than 12.5 cm is a predictor for a difficult laryngoscopy and intubation.[49] The SMD is helpful when determining the length of head and neck extension. This can be assessed by first measuring the SMD with the head and neck in the neutral position and then again with the head and neck extended. The measurements are then used to calculate the difference. Extensions of less than 5 cm have been reported as an indicator for difficult laryngoscopy.[49] Similar to other preoperative airway exams, the SMD in

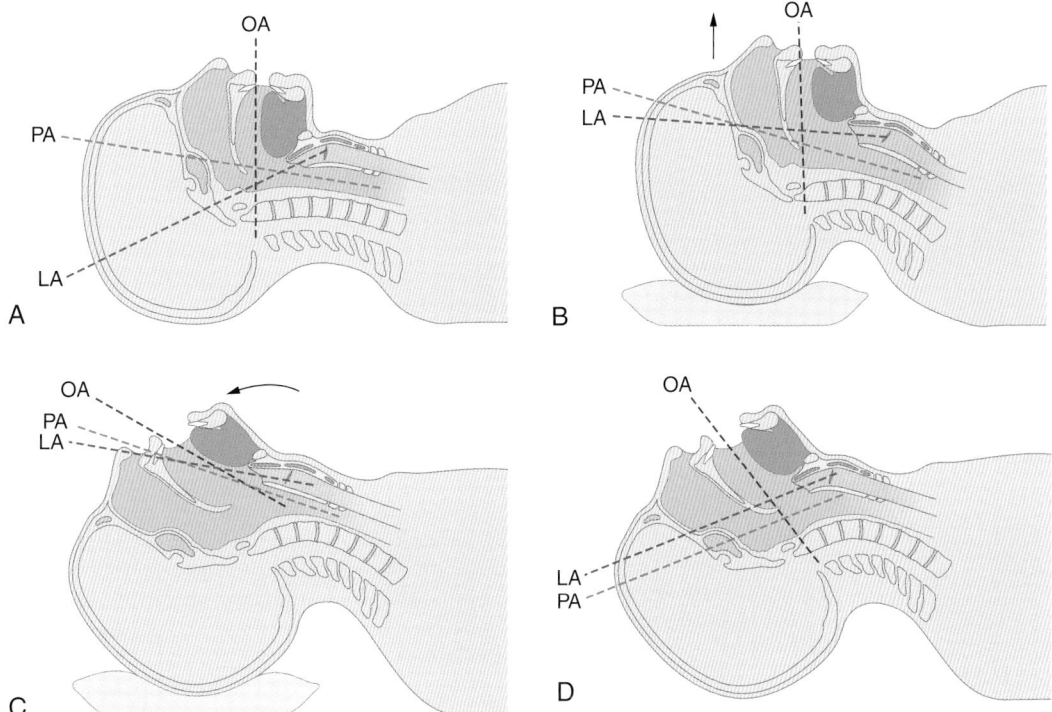

Fig. 24.12 Oral axis (*OA*), pharyngeal axis (*PA*), and laryngeal axis (*LA*) for intubation. (A) Nonaligned position. (B) Head resting on a pad causes flexion of the neck and aligns the PA and LA. (C) Head resting on pad causes flexion of the neck, and neck extension into the sniffing position aligns the OA, PA, and LA. (D) Extension of the neck without head elevation aligns PA and LA, but not the OA. (From Miller RD, Pardo MC, eds. *Basics of Anesthesia*. 6th ed. Philadelphia: Elsevier; 2011:226.)

isolation is not an adequate predictor of difficult laryngoscopy and/or intubation, and instead should be used in combination with several other preoperative airway exams in an effort to effectively predict difficulty with airway management.

Interincisor Gap

As discussed previously, the interincisor gap is important to assess when performing a DL or VL because the size of the mouth opening can affect the ability to introduce a laryngoscope device and to create a direct line of sight with the laryngeal opening.[15] The challenge with a narrow mouth opening is placing both the laryngoscope blade's 2-cm flange and the ETT into the mouth while maintaining good visualization of the vocal cords. Thus a predictor of difficult intubation is an interincisor opening of less than 3 cm. An increase in maxillary incisor length can reduce the interincisor gap and create a sharper angle between the oral and glottic openings. Furthermore, prominent incisors or "buck teeth" increase the risk of dental damage from any hard device used to manipulate the airway. Finally, loose or awkwardly sized teeth can either impede the placement of a laryngoscope blade, VL device, and ETT or create an obstruction if a tooth is dislodged and falls posteriorly into the laryngeal opening or trachea.

Atlantooccipital Joint Mobility

The full range of neck flexion and extension varies from 90 to 165 degrees and decreases approximately 20% between ages 16 and 75. The atlantooccipital joint provides the highest degree of mobility in the neck, with a normal head extension of up to 35 degrees. Proper atlantooccipital joint mobility is required for an adequate sniffing position. The sniffing position is important because it helps to improve DL views by promoting displacement of the tongue by better aligning

the oral, pharyngeal, and laryngeal axes (Fig. 24.12). Evaluation of atlantooccipital joint extension is conducted with the patient seated upright in a neutral face-forward position; the patient is then asked to lift the head back with the chin up as far as possible. When extension is reduced to 23 degrees, visualization may become difficult.[50] If the patient demonstrates substantial or complete immobility of the atlantooccipital joint, then significant compromise with DL should be anticipated. Furthermore, cervical spine diseases such as cervical pathology (e.g., degenerative disease, rheumatic disease, neurologic pathology, trauma, or previous surgical intervention) or spinal abnormalities (e.g., Down syndrome) may lead to difficult laryngoscopy and difficult airway management in general. VL has been shown to be an effective method for placing an ETT in patients with limited cervical spine mobility or in patients where the cervical spine requires minimal or no movement.[43] Either VL or flexible endoscopy (i.e., fiberoptic scope) has shown to be effective when managing the airway with patients who have limited cervical spine mobility or those who require cervical spine immobilization.[51]

Mandibular Protrusion Test

The mandibular protrusion test, also known as the upper lip bite test (ULBT), is an evaluation technique that demonstrates the patient's ability to extend the mandibular incisors anterior past the maxillary incisors. The purpose of this airway test is to first assess the patient's maxillary incisor length (e.g., presence of buck teeth), and then to assess the mobility of the patient's temporomandibular joint function and forward subluxation of the jaw. The presence of these indicators can lead to problematic oral airway placement, noneffective relief of soft tissue obstruction from poor mandibular movement, difficulty introducing the laryngoscope blade into the mouth, and an obstructive view of the glottic opening caused by

MANDIBULAR
PROTRUSION TEST

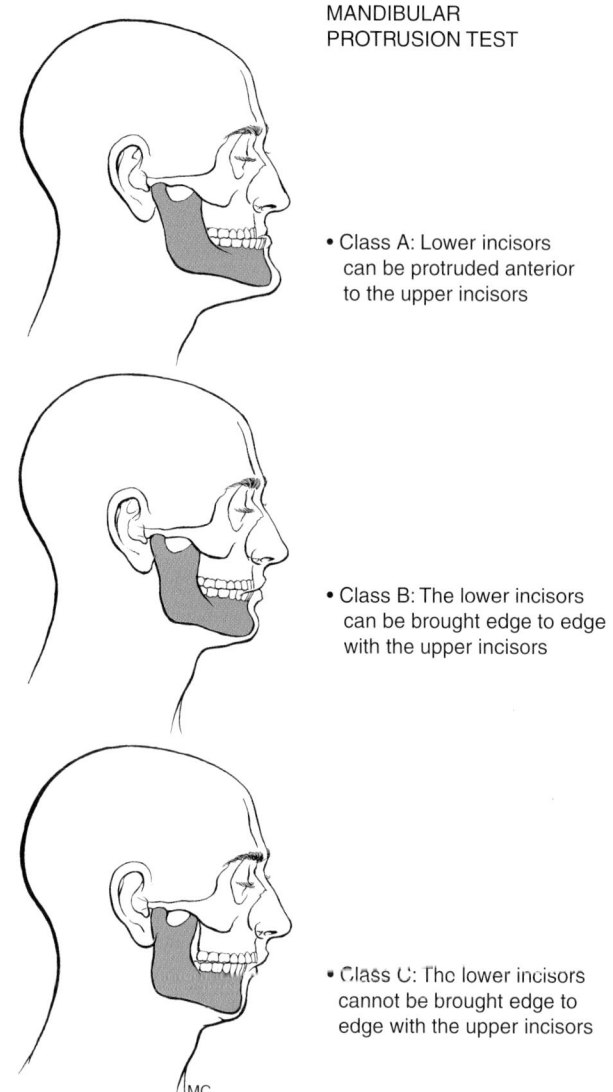

- Class A: Lower incisors
  can be protruded anterior
  to the upper incisors

- Class B: The lower incisors
  can be brought edge to edge
  with the upper incisors

- Class C: The lower incisors
  cannot be brought edge to
  edge with the upper incisors

MC

Fig. 24.13 Mandibular protrusion test classes A, B, and C (also known as the upper lip bite test). (Redrawn from Munnur U, et al. Airway problems in pregnancy. *Crit Care Med.* 2005;33:S259 2S60.)

malplacement of the tongue. Difficulty with laryngoscopy arises when the patient is unable to protrude the mandibular incisors anterior past the maxillary incisors (Fig. 24.13). The test has three classifications:

- *Class A:* Patient can protrude the lower incisors anteriorly past the upper incisors and can bite the upper lip above the vermilion border (line where the lip meets the facial skin).
- *Class B:* Patient can move the lower incisors in line with the upper incisors and bite the upper lip below the vermilion border but cannot protrude lower incisors beyond.
- *Class C:* Lower incisors cannot be moved in line with the upper incisors and cannot bite the upper lip.

Assessment of an ULBT class C indicates a potential difficult laryngoscopic view, whereas class A indicates a good view using conventional laryngoscopy.[52]

The ULBT was found to be a valuable assessment tool for the prediction of difficult ventilation when used in combination with other assessment techniques such as increased neck circumference and a history of snoring.[53] Furthermore, the ULBT has been shown to be useful in the assessment of temporomandibular joint function and the prediction of

difficult laryngoscopies when used in combination with the modified Mallampati classification.[52,54] However, the ULBT has been shown to be an unreliable assessment technique when used in the edentulous population and has demonstrated poor predictability when used as a single screening test for the assessment of laryngoscopic difficulty.[55]

Supraglottic Airway Assessment

Supraglottic airway ventilation may be the primary means of managing an airway or it can be used for rescue ventilation in the event that face-mask ventilation is difficult or fails. Similar predictors related to difficulty with mask ventilation, laryngoscopy, and intubation can also be used to indicate difficulty in placing and ventilating with a supraglottic airway device (SAD). These predictors include a restrictive mouth opening, a distortion in the upper airway anatomy, and both upper and lower airway obstruction (see Box 24.2).

The interincisor gap is an important assessment to consider when introducing any airway adjuncts into the mouth. As identified earlier, an assessment of less than 3 cm indicates a restricted oral access causing difficult SAD placement.[15] Furthermore, some researchers have indicated that reductions in atlantooccipital joint movement due to conditions such as ankylosing spondylitis and rheumatoid arthritis may cause difficulty with some SAD placements, such as the laryngeal mask airway (LMA).[56,57]

Obstruction at the level of the larynx, trachea, or below can reduce or completely block ventilation from a SAD (see Box 24.4). In addition, fixed upper airway lesions, such as oropharyngeal tumors or a disruption or distortion in the upper airway anatomy, may make SAD placement difficult and lead to ineffective ventilation from a compromised "seat and seal."[48,58]

Finally, conditions affecting the lower airways resulting in decreases in pulmonary compliance or increases in airway resistance can cause peak airway pressures to rise, which may also make supraglottic airway ventilation difficult. For example, bronchospasm or acute respiratory distress syndrome require higher ventilatory pressures to facilitate adequate gas exchange within the lungs. Severe obstruction or restriction as a result of lung pathophysiology may limit the amount of ventilation that can be accomplished with a SAD and even allow for the possible risk of vomiting and pulmonary aspiration.[58,59]

Cricothyrotomy Airway Assessment

An assessment of the neck is part of any comprehensive airway examination and should be conducted with the intent of identifying factors that may indicate difficulty with cricothyrotomy placement. The need for an invasive airway usually occurs on an emergency basis. Invasive airway management consists of a needle cricothyrotomy, percutaneous (wire guided) cricothyrotomy, surgical cricothyrotomy, or a tracheotomy. Since surgeons are more likely to perform a tracheotomy, the primary focus will be on assessments aimed at identifying factors that lead to difficulty with cricothyrotomy procedures.

Even though there is no absolute contraindication for the placement of an emergency cricothyrotomy, there are conditions that make performing this procedure difficult or even impossible (see Box 24.2). Murphy and Walls[14] described using the mnemonic *SHORT* as a means for remembering *surgery, hematoma, obesity, radiation,* and *tumor*s, which are conditions associated with difficult cricothyrotomy placement. Any condition that causes a distortion of the airway, such as trauma, surgery, infection, tumors, or physical impediments in or around the cricothyroid area, may cause difficulty with invasive airway access. A hematoma from surgery (e.g., carotid endarterectomy), an infection of the soft tissue around the airway (e.g., Ludwig angina), an oral or pharyngeal abscess, a tumor in or around the neck, or radiation causing scarring of the neck tissue can distort the neck anatomy, making a cricothyrotomy neck incision and tube placement into the trachea challenging. However, none of these factors should be considered a contraindication when emergency airway access is required. In addition, recent or past neck trauma or surgery can alter neck anatomy and cause scarring or acute bleeding, again making cricothyrotomy procedures difficult. Finally, neck impediments such as a halo device or a rigid cervical collar may impede emergency access or make the procedure technically difficult and should be removed when possible.

A short neck, obesity, scarring, or fixed flexion abnormality are all indications for a difficult cricothyrotomy placement. Both a short neck and excessive soft tissue around the neck can make finding the cricothyroid membrane and surrounding anatomic landmarks challenging. When performing the preoperative airway assessment on patients who exhibit any of these characteristics, mark the cricothyroid membrane prior to airway manipulation so it can be located rapidly in the event of an emergency. Furthermore, make readily available the appropriate equipment and personnel to save time when and if emergency airway access is indicated.

Radiologic and Ultrasonographic Imaging

Imaging technologies such as magnetic resonance imaging (MRI) and computed tomography (CT) can identify pathologies and alterations in airway anatomy and increase the predictive value of anticipated difficulty. These technologies can help anesthetists formulate appropriate airway management plans. Advantages of the CT scan include the ability to accurately depict pathology involving bones and soft tissues and the ability to view images in the sagittal, coronal, axial, and three-dimensional views. Furthermore, CT scans have become the gold standard for ruling out fractures of the cervical spine.[60]

Whereas CT scans can image both bone and soft tissue, an MRI offers detailed information on soft tissues only. An MRI can help assess the impact that pathologic processes have on soft tissue, such as the altered patency of an airway caused by a tumor in the neck. However, CT and MRI tests are not currently used on a routine basis because of the economic costs and time-delaying factors associated with their use, especially if there is no indication to perform them.

Ultrasonography has been shown to be useful as a predictor for difficult laryngoscopy. Excessive pretracheal soft tissue, as assessed by ultrasound, in combination with a large neck circumference and a history of sleep apnea, were all positive predictors for difficult laryngoscopy in an obese population.[61] Furthermore, point of care ultrasound (POCUS) provides bedside imaging of airway anatomy, including the cricoid cartilage and vocal cords.[62] As such, ultrasonography may be a useful technique for the identification of the cricoid cartilage and cricothyroid membrane in an obese individual (Figs. 24.14 and 24.15).[63] The effectiveness of POCUS as an airway assessment tool has yet to be determined. However, as it is being used with more frequency, it is likely to emerge as a useful adjunct in the assessment of the difficult airway.

When assessing the airway and preparing for manipulation, the anesthetist should perform a multivariable assessment. This assessment is based on patient, surgical, and situational requirements and is crucial for the identification of factors that are associated with difficult mask ventilation, laryngoscopy and intubation, supraglottic device, and cricothyrotomy placement.

TRACHEAL INTUBATION

Tracheal intubation remains a cornerstone of traditional airway management and may be performed by various methods (e.g., DL, flexible intubating scope, intubating LMA, VL). The technique chosen for TI is dependent on the patient's history, physical examination (including airway assessment), and previous anesthetic history (e.g., difficult intubation). Indications for TI can be found in Table 24.4.

The TI procedure is preceded by careful attention to optimal head and neck positioning for laryngoscopy. Flexion of the neck and extension of the atlantooccipital joint, or sniffing position, allows for proper alignment of the oral, pharyngeal, and tracheal axis (see Fig. 24.12). This can be accomplished using pillows, towels, blankets, or the OR table's positioning functions (Fig. 24.16). Furthermore, elevation of the shoulders, head, and neck (ramping; see Fig. 24.8) in an effort to align the tragus of the ear with the sternum may help in patients identified as potentially difficult to intubate. Manipulation of the head and neck must be used with caution in patients with decreased cervical range of motion caused by degenerative disease, rheumatic disease, neurologic pathology, trauma, or previous surgical intervention (Fig. 24.17).

Sufficient preoxygenation may help to delay arterial desaturation prior to the induction of anesthesia and during subsequent apneic situations. Effective preoxygenation increases pulmonary oxygen content and eliminates much of the nitrogen (~79% of room air) from the FRC. A functional FRC can theoretically oxygenate a healthy individual for up to 8 minutes. However, without preoxygenation, the oxygen reserve in the FRC is limited, leading to a decrease in the time an anesthetist has to secure the airway. Preoxygenation should include 100% inspired oxygen, a tight mask seal, instructing the patient to breathe at normal tidal volumes for 3 to 5 minutes, and providing a minimum fresh gas flow of at least 5 L/min. Signs of adequate preoxygenation are a respiratory bag that moves with each inspiration/expiration, a well-defined end-tidal CO_2 waveform, and a fraction of expired oxygen that increases to 90% or greater. If time is limited, there is some evidence that supports a patient taking eight vital capacity breaths within 60 seconds, before the induction of anesthesia, with equivalent results to 3 minutes of tidal volume breathing.[64] Finally, as discussed earlier, the concept of apneic oxygenation using a nasal cannula with flows reaching 15 L/min to insufflate oxygen into the pharyngeal airway may help to delay desaturation during apnea in a patient with a patent airway.

The technique for DL is dependent on the type of laryngoscope blade used for the procedure, but the premise of control/displacement of the tongue from right to left and elevation of the epiglottis remains the same for both techniques. The use of the curved (e.g., Macintosh) laryngoscope blade requires the anesthetist to (1) place the tip of the laryngoscope in the vallecula and (2) apply tension to the hyoepiglottic ligament using a gentle lifting force, which (3) promotes indirect elevation of the epiglottis. In contrast, the use of the straight (e.g., Miller) laryngoscope blade requires the anesthetist to (1) place the tip of the laryngoscope posterior to the epiglottis and (2) apply gentle force to directly lift the epiglottis. Levering action should never be applied to the patient's dentition. Such action risks dental damage and diminishes the quality of the laryngoscopic view. The technique backwards-upwards-rightwards-pressure (BURP) has been demonstrated to improve visualization of the vocal cords and can be achieved by the clinician manipulating the larynx at the neck with the right hand during laryngoscopy.[65]

If an adequate laryngoscopic view cannot be achieved after DL, then strategies and algorithms for the difficult or failed airway should be followed. Maintenance of adequate oxygenation and ventilation is of the utmost priority during TI and can be facilitated by the use of various adjunctive airway equipment and techniques.

MANAGEMENT OF THE DIFFICULT AND FAILED AIRWAY

Management of the difficult airway is a multifaceted process that begins with the airway assessment, considers decision-making strategies suggested by the various difficult airway algorithms, continues with a primary airway management plan, and is then flexible with an

Thyroid Cartilage   Cricothyroid Membrane   Cricoid Cartilage

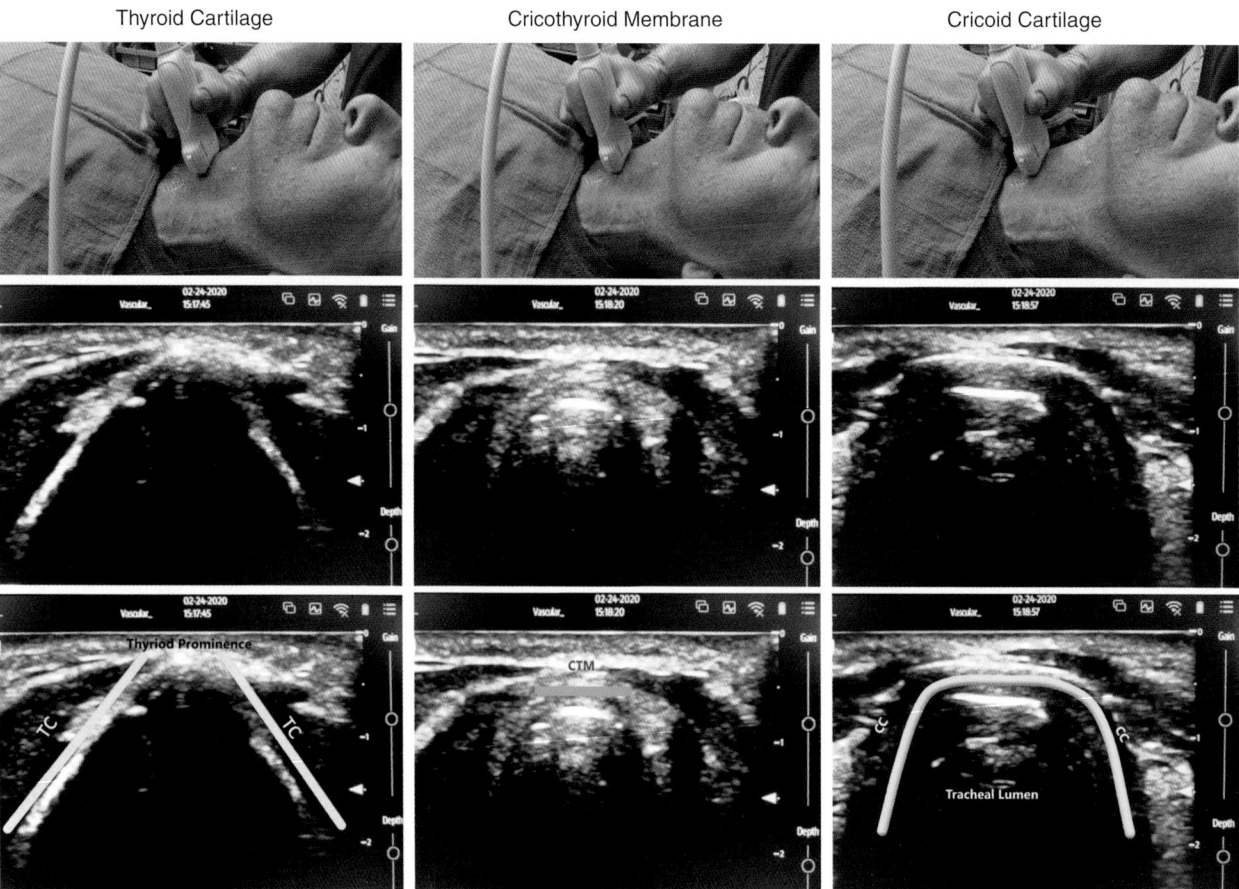

Fig. 24.14 Thyroid-Airline-Cricoid-Airline (TACA) ultrasound technique with the ultrasound probe positioned in the transverse (lateral) plane on the neck at the level of the thyroid cartilage. **T** (thyroid cartilage)—identify the thyroid cartilage as an inverted V or triangular structure *(outlined in yellow lines in left lower image)*. **A** (airline or air-tissue border)—move caudad until the hyperechoic white line is visualized *(middle images)*. The air within the tracheal lumen can be seen as a white cloud mass at the center of the screens. **C** (cricoid cartilage)—move further caudad until a hypoechoic structure resembling a horseshoe or arch or upside-down U is seen *(outlined with yellow lines in right lower image)*. Posterior to the cartilage is a white lining representing the air-tissue border. **A** (airline)—return cephalad back to the air-tissue border and mark this site *(the green line in the middle lower image)*. *CC*, Cricoid cartilage; *CTM*, cricothyroid membrane; *TC*, thyroid cartilage. (Technique from Kristensen MS, Teoh WH, Rudolph SS, et al. A randomised cross-over comparison of the transverse and longitudinal techniques for ultrasound-guided identification of the cricothyroid membrane in morbidly obese subjects. *Anaesthesia.* 2016;71[6]:675–683. Images courtesy APEX Live.)

understanding of how to proceed when initial airway management plans fail. Part of a thorough airway management plan is the consideration of patient characteristics and conditions that predispose the patient to difficulty with facemask ventilation, supraglottic airway use, laryngoscopy, TI, and cricothyrotomy. As discussed in previous sections, multiple patient characteristics and conditions are associated with difficult airway management. Therefore, an important aspect of airway management is obtaining the competency and knowledge to deal with the identified difficult airway and the less common unexpected failed airway.

The unexpected failed airway (also known as the unanticipated difficult airway) consists of an airway that has previously been evaluated as having no external identifiers indicating difficulty. In other words, the anesthesia provider does not expect or anticipate difficulty with facemask ventilation, laryngoscopy, intubation, or other airway management techniques. However, after the patient is anesthetized, difficulty then occurs with ventilation, intubation, or both. Although rare, a common cause of an unanticipated difficult intubation has been shown to be enlarged lymphoid tissue at the base of the tongue (i.e., lingual tonsil hyperplasia), which cannot be evaluated externally.[66,67] Instead,

this condition is discovered during laryngoscopy by a failure to visualize the glottic opening and a description of a grade III or IV airway. In one case series, lingual tonsil hyperplasia was found to be the most common cause of unanticipated difficulty with the airway. Although lingual tonsil hyperplasia is often asymptomatic, there are indicators that may alert the anesthetist to the presence of this potential obstruction, which include sore throat, dysphagia, globus sensation, snoring, palpation of a lump in the throat, and OSA.[67]

Definition of a Difficult and Failed Airway

The definition of a difficult airway varies within the existing literature, making it challenging to identify the true incidence. However, in broad terms, a difficult airway has been described as a clinical situation in which a trained anesthetist experiences difficulty with facemask ventilation, laryngoscopy, intubation, or all of these.[11] A significant amount of subjectivity is possible among observers when performing the different airway assessments, leading to various interpretations of predicted airway difficulty. Ultimately, it is not enough to simply identify a difficult airway; instead, it is important to possess the knowledge and skills that guide intervention after difficulty has been identified or when

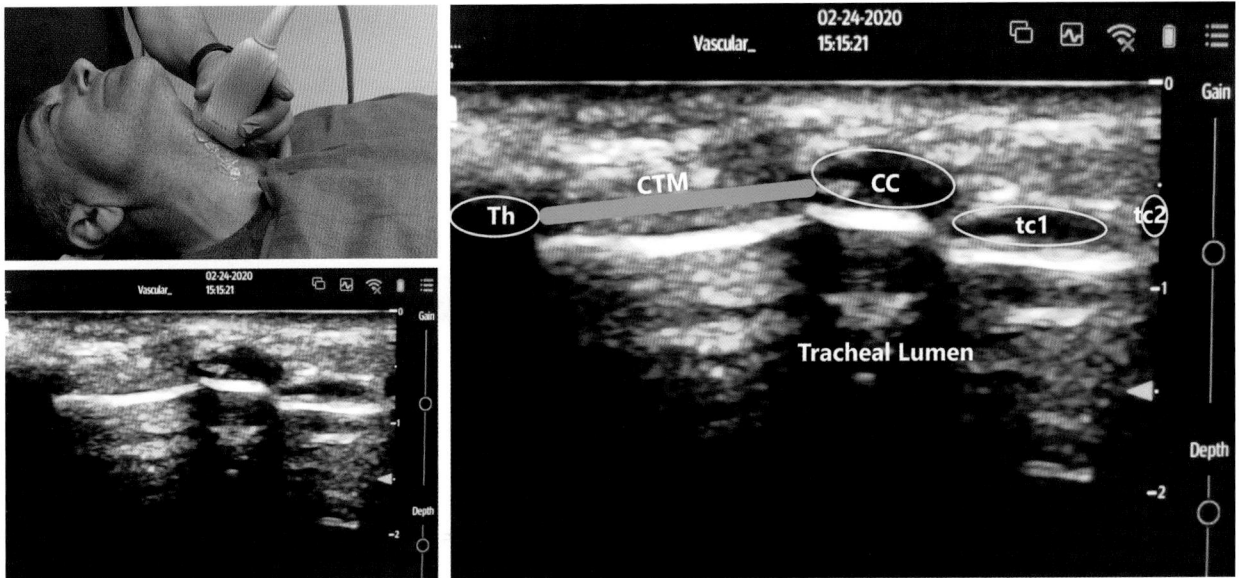

Fig. 24.15 String of pearls technique with the ultrasound probe positioned in the sagittal (vertical) place at the center of the neck at the level of the thyroid cartilage. Visualize the thyroid cartilage, cricothyroid membrane, cricoid cartilage, and tracheal rings in one image (i.e., string of pearls). The cartilage rings appear as a string of hypoechoic beads *(outlined with yellow)* sitting on a prominent white line that is the air-tissue interface *(solid white lines)*. The cricoid cartilage is the most cephalad and prominent of these beads. The cricothyroid membrane is the hyperechoic structure linking the cricoid cartilage to the thyroid cartilage *(outlined with green line)*. *CC*, Cricoid cartilage; *CTM,* cricothyroid membrane; *tc1*, first tracheal cartilage; *tc2*, second tracheal cartilage; *Th*, thyroid cartilage. (Technique from Kristensen MS, Teoh WH, Rudolph SS, et al. A randomised cross-over comparison of the transverse and longitudinal techniques for ultrasound-guided identification of the cricothyroid membrane in morbidly obese subjects. *Anaesthesia*. 2016;71[6]:675–683. Images courtesy APEX Live.)

TABLE 24.4 Indications for Tracheal Intubation

Condition	Indication
Anesthesia and surgical	High risk of aspiration of blood (e.g., head and neck trauma, bleeding into respiratory tract) or gastric contents (e.g., severe gastroesophageal reflux disease, inadequate gastric emptying, gastrointestinal obstruction) Predicted difficult airway Intraoperative patient positioning that may impede access to the airway (e.g., prone, lateral decubitus) Ineffective oxygenation or ventilation with supraglottic devices (e.g., mask ventilation, laryngeal mask airway)
Surgical	Airway access shared with surgeon (e.g., otolaryngologic and head-neck surgery) Surgery requiring paralysis using neuromuscular blocking medications (e.g., intraabdominal surgery) Surgical procedures affecting ventilation and perfusion (e.g., cardiothoracic surgery) Prolonged surgical time
Medical	Inadequate airway protection or suppressed airway reflexes (e.g., Glasgow Coma Scale <10) Ineffective oxygenation or ventilation (e.g., noninvasive positive pressure respiratory assist device, mask ventilation, laryngeal mask airway) Critical illness (e.g., inadequate respiratory function, acute respiratory distress syndrome, sepsis) Controlled management of arterial carbon dioxide content (e.g., prevention of hypercapnia for increased intracranial pressure)

Modified from Henderson J. Airway management in the adult. In Miller RD, et al., eds. *Miller's Anesthesia*. 7th ed. Philadelphia: Elsevier; 2009:1573–1610.

unanticipated difficulty is encountered. Knowing what to do when an airway proves difficult will ensure that proper ventilation is provided in a timely manner.

As discussed earlier, there are four strategic areas of airway management that affect ventilation and thus oxygenation of the tissues. The methods of providing ventilation are as follows:

1. Mask ventilation with an appropriate mask seal with or without a jaw thrust maneuver
2. Placement of a SAD such as an LMA
3. Placement of an ETT into the trachea
4. Placement of an invasive airway such as a cricothyrotomy tube

Problems or indications of complexity with one or more of these four methods would suggest a difficult airway. Additionally, there are several situations when an airway provider could experience difficulty with one or more of the four strategic areas of airway management. These situations include airway difficulty as a result of (1) anatomic challenges (i.e., mandibular hypoplasia, Mallampati III or IV airway), (2) pathophysiologic challenges (i.e., laryngeal mass, expanding neck hematoma, subcutaneous emphysema), (3) traumatic challenges (i.e., face or neck trauma), and/or (4) physiologic challenges (i.e., severe hypoxemia, severe hypotension, or acidosis).

When managing an airway, the signs that indicate difficulty must be recognized in a timely manner. Indications of difficult facemask ventilation include (1) gas flow leaks out of the facemask and increasing use of the oxygen flush valve, (2) poor chest rise, (3) absent or inadequate breath sounds, (4) gastric air entry, (5) poor carbon dioxide return and an altered capnography waveform, (6) a decreasing oxygen saturation of less than 92% as measured by pulse oximetry using a 100% inspired oxygen concentration, and (7) necessity of using an oral or nasal airway and performing a two-handed mask ventilation technique.[18,68] Difficult laryngoscopy and TI have been consistently identified in the literature as the inability to visualize any

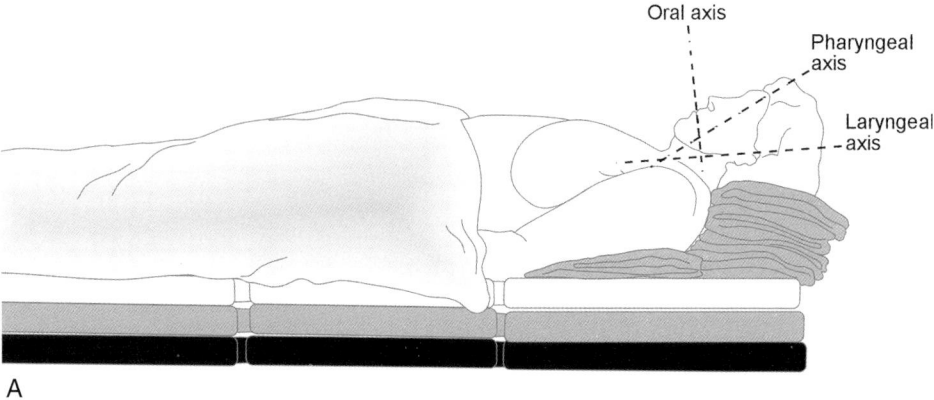

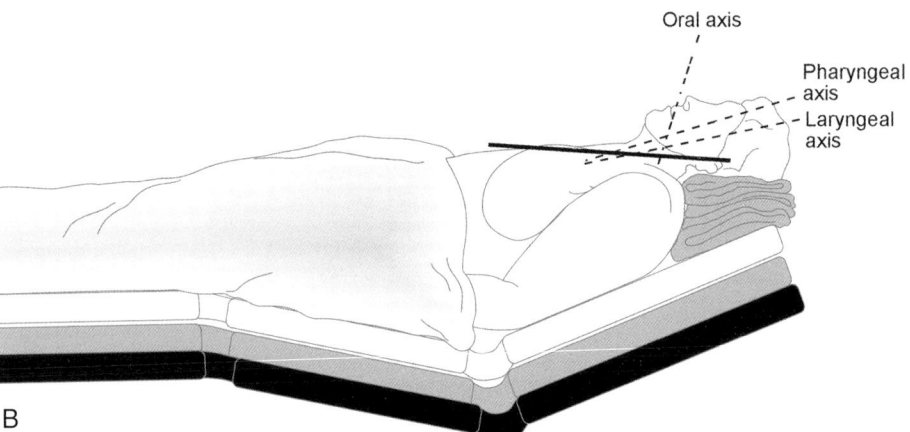

Fig. 24.16 Improving oral, pharyngeal, and laryngeal axis alignment by raising the head of the operating room table. (A) Supine position. (B) Head-up position. (From Thompson J, et al. Anesthesia case management for bariatric surgery. *AANA J.* 2011;79[2]:147–160.)

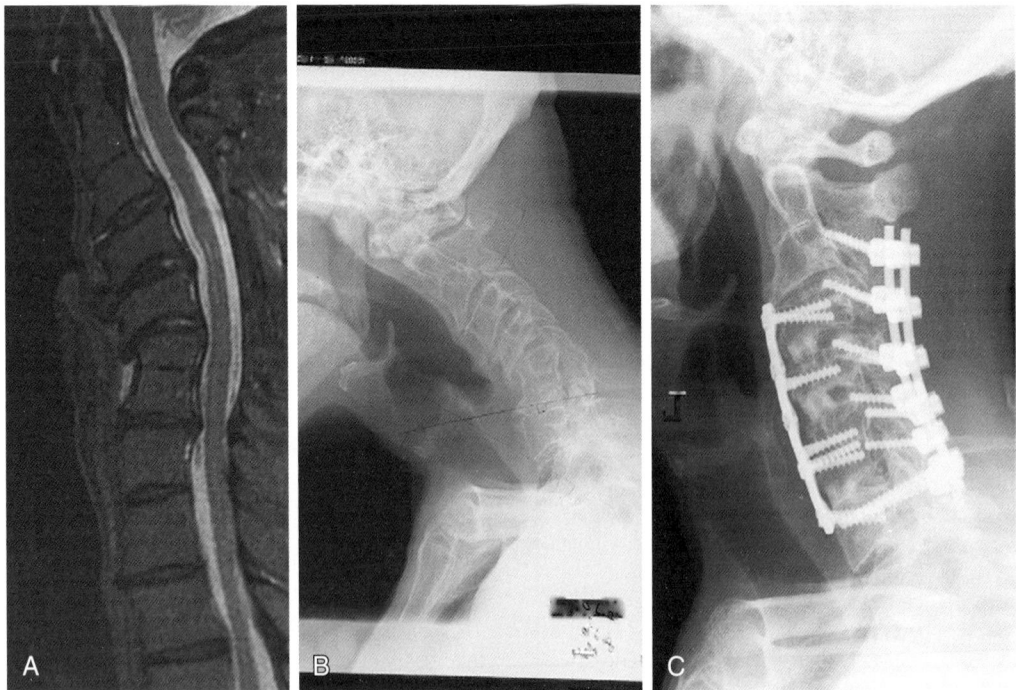

Fig. 24.17 Sagittal magnetic resonance image (A) and lateral radiograph (B) of a 60-year-old man with a prior laminectomy and Klippel-Feil malformation at C2-C3 show progressive fixed kyphotic deformity. (C) Lateral postoperative radiograph after a three-staged procedure, including posterior release, C3-T1 posterior spinal fusion, and C3-T1 correction to anterior cervical discectomy and fusion, shows marked reduction of fixed deformity. (From Chi JH, et al. Complex deformities of the cervical spine. *Neurosurg Clin N Am.* 2007;18[2]:295–304.)

portion of the vocal cords (e.g., Cormack and Lehane grade III or IV) after multiple attempts using a standard laryngoscope. In addition, difficulty with laryngoscopy and intubation has been described as requiring multiple operators in the presence or absence of tracheal pathology. Furthermore, evidence of a failed intubation was identified as an inability to place an ETT after multiple laryngoscopic attempts.[11] Difficulty with a supraglottic device may also be apparent when placement requires multiple attempts or more than one airway practitioner. Furthermore, objective indications of difficulty with supraglottic ventilation are similar to those described for facemask ventilation earlier, as well as a leak pressure less than 10 to 15 cm H_2O and a poor expired tidal volume.[16] Finally, difficulties with invasive airway placement, such as a cricothyrotomy, are apparent with bleeding at the site of insertion, an inability to identify the correct anatomic structures, or trouble accessing the cricothyroid membrane and puncturing through into the trachea.

Incidence of a Difficult and Failed Airway

Adverse events related to difficulty with airway management continue to occur both the OR and throughout the hospital, and researchers agree there is continued room for improvement.[69] In 2008, the Royal College of Anaesthetists in the United Kingdom and the Difficult Airway Society (DAS) gathered information from the administration of 2.9 million general anesthetics in an attempt to identify the incidence of major complications related to airway management. The major complications identified were death, brain damage, emergency surgical airway placement, and unanticipated ICU admission. They found that a major complication occurred at a ratio of 1:22,000 general anesthetics, with a mortality rate of 1:180,000.[69] Other researchers have focused strictly on the occurrence of a difficult airway, such as a laryngoscopic view grade II or III, and have reported a 1% to 18% incidence. The incidence of failed TI is relatively uncommon (reported as 0.045%–0.35%), with the high end of this range relating to obstetric patients and other surgical patients with known difficulties.[68,70] As previously mentioned, the incidence of difficult facemask ventilation has been described between 0.9% and 7.8%, with the variation in results occurring as a result of different study parameters.

Finally, researchers have reported a SAD failure rate of 0.19% to 1.1%, mostly caused by an inadequate seal from improper placement, surgical table rotation, poor dentition, male gender, and increased body mass index.[71,72]

The incidence of difficult intubation and ventilation is much higher in patients with neck or mediastinal pathology, previous surgery, or radiation. For example, one study evaluated 181 patients with pharyngolaryngeal disease and found that 50 (28%) were difficult to intubate, and 4 (2.8%) were impossible to intubate.[73] Other researchers performed a retrospective analysis on patients with deep neck infections, such as Ludwig angina, and found a 3.8% incidence of failure to intubate, necessitating a tracheostomy.[74] The true incidence of situations in which practitioners cannot intubate and subsequently cannot ventilate or oxygenate is difficult to assess because of the failure to consistently and accurately report these occurrences. However, some authors have reported an incidence of 1:2250 in nonparturients and as high as 1:300 in parturients, whereas another researcher reported four cases of impossible mask ventilation and intubation in 53,041 cases involving induction of anesthesia.

When assessing the frequency of emergency cricothyrotomy placement, the Fourth National Audit Project from the United Kingdom reported an occurrence of 1:2500 to 50,000 general anesthetic cases.[69] Other researchers explained that the incidence of emergency cricothyrotomy placement is strongly influenced by the clinical situation and contributing patient factors.[76] For example, the incidence of emergency cricothyrotomy placement resulting from failed TI in the emergency department (ED) has been reported as 0.3% to 0.8%, increasing to 1.4% in trauma patients, and was reported to be as high as 11% in

the prehospital setting. Other research also concluded that difficult airways may be encountered more frequently outside of the OR.[77-79] The Fourth National Audit Project reported that airway-related adverse events, which led to death or brain damage, were 30 to 60 times more likely to occur in the ED or ICU.[80]

Difficult Airway Algorithms

When considering an approach to airway management, the anesthetist must address certain issues prior to the induction of anesthesia. The following are five questions, termed "the airway approach algorithm," which may initially help in the development of an airway management plan:

1. Is airway management necessary?
2. Is DL or VL and TI be suspected to be difficult?
3. Can supralaryngeal ventilation be used or is it potentially difficult?
4. Has the risk for aspiration been minimized, or is there a significant risk of aspiration?
5. Is the patient at risk of rapid desaturation?

If the answer to each of these questions is yes, then the airway is deemed manageable by conventional means, and the anesthetist may proceed with the induction of anesthesia followed by muscle relaxation to provide optimal conditions for laryngoscopy and intubation. If, however, the answer to any question is no, then the anesthetist should either abandon airway management altogether and proceed with an alternative anesthetic option (e.g., monitored anesthesia care, regional anesthesia) or follow the guidelines set forth by various professional associations for the management of anticipated airway difficulty. The questions asked by the airway approach algorithm are being recommended as a primary part of the ASA Difficulty Airway Algorithm by the ASA task force in charge of updating the the ASA Difficult Airway Algorithm, which will be released after the publication of this text.

Difficult airway management is multifactorial and necessitates an awareness of the interactions between the patient's condition, the clinical setting, and the anesthesia provider's experience and skill level. Each of these factors alone or in combination can contribute to poor outcomes during airway manipulation and must be considered when developing airway management strategies. Tools that help the anesthetist formulate plans for safe airway care in the face of both known and unanticipated difficulties are called difficult airway algorithms. Multiple difficult airway algorithms exist, such as the American Society of Anesthesiologist (ASA) difficult airway algorithm (Fig. 24.18) and the DAS difficult intubation guidelines (Fig. 24.19). Importantly, having many guidelines suggest that difficult airway algorithms are based on the opinions of experts in the field of airway management but lack empirical evidence. Reasons given have included the significant challenges with the design of randomized controlled trials, the infrequency of certain difficult airway events (e.g., failed airway or cricothyrotomy), and an inability to account for confounding variables such as individual practitioner experience.[81] However, the widespread distribution of the different guidelines has resulted in a reduction in airway-related critical accidents.[81,82] Overall, it is important to remember that difficult airway algorithms are simply guidelines that provide structure for decision making and tools for use when managing difficult airways, but they do not preclude personal responsibility and sound clinical judgment.

ASA Difficult Airway Algorithm

The difficult airway algorithm, established in 1991 by the ASA, gave anesthesia practitioners the first standardized approach for the management of the anticipated or unanticipated difficult airway. The practice guidelines were updated in 2003, and again in 2013, and is currently under review for an update to be released after the publication of this text. The algorithm provides guidelines for dealing with difficult facemask ventilation, difficult laryngoscopy, difficult TI, and failed intubation. Assessment of the airway and use of the difficult airway algorithm provide the

1. Assess the likelihood and clinical impact of basic management problems:
   A. Difficult ventilation
   B. Difficult intubation
   C. Difficulty with patient cooperation or consent
   D. Difficult tracheostomy

2. Actively pursue opportunities to deliver supplemental oxygen throughout the process of difficult airway management

3. Consider the relative merits and feasibility of basic management choices:

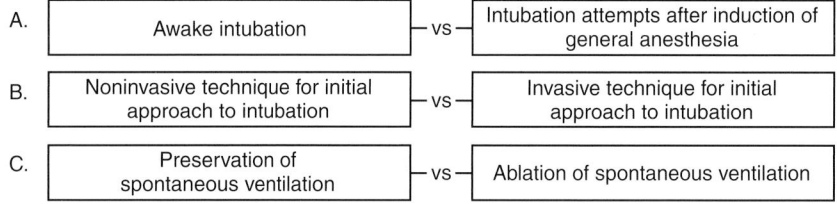

A.	Awake intubation	– vs –	Intubation attempts after induction of general anesthesia
B.	Noninvasive technique for initial approach to intubation	– vs –	Invasive technique for initial approach to intubation
C.	Preservation of spontaneous ventilation	– vs –	Ablation of spontaneous ventilation

4. Develop primary and alternative stategies:

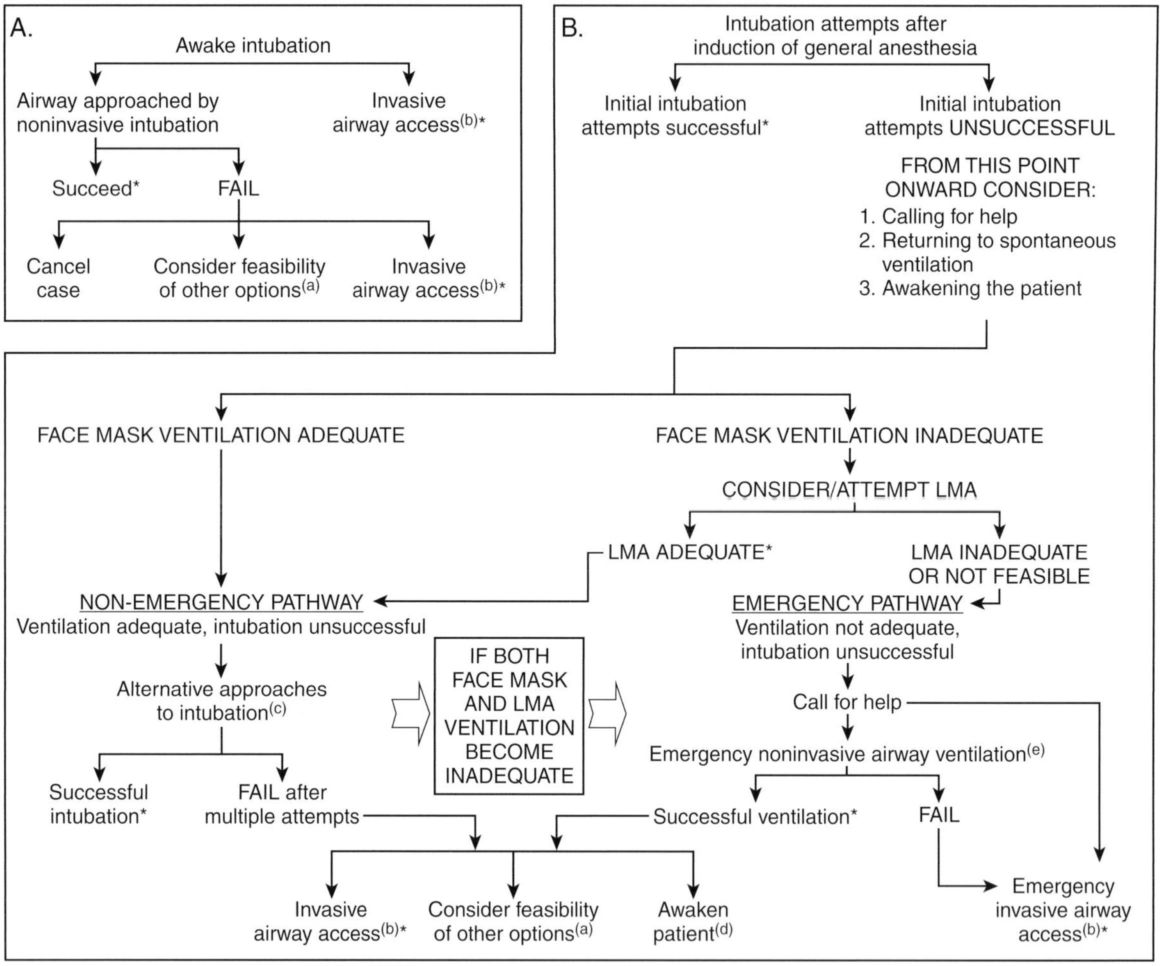

A. Awake intubation

- Airway approached by noninvasive intubation
- Invasive airway access[(b)]*

From noninvasive intubation:
- Succeed*
- FAIL

From FAIL:
- Cancel case
- Consider feasibility of other options[(a)]
- Invasive airway access[(b)]*

B. Intubation attempts after induction of general anesthesia

- Initial intubation attempts successful*
- Initial intubation attempts UNSUCCESSFUL

FROM THIS POINT ONWARD CONSIDER:
1. Calling for help
2. Returning to spontaneous ventilation
3. Awakening the patient

FACE MASK VENTILATION ADEQUATE

FACE MASK VENTILATION INADEQUATE
↓
CONSIDER/ATTEMPT LMA

- LMA ADEQUATE*
- LMA INADEQUATE OR NOT FEASIBLE

NON-EMERGENCY PATHWAY
Ventilation adequate, intubation unsuccessful

EMERGENCY PATHWAY
Ventilation not adequate, intubation unsuccessful

Alternative approaches to intubation[(c)]

IF BOTH FACE MASK AND LMA VENTILATION BECOME INADEQUATE

Call for help

Emergency noninvasive airway ventilation[(e)]

- Successful intubation*
- FAIL after multiple attempts
- Successful ventilation*
- FAIL

- Invasive airway access[(b)]*
- Consider feasibility of other options[(a)]
- Awaken patient[(d)]
- Emergency invasive airway access[(b)]*

*Confirm ventilation, tracheal intubation, or LMA placement with exhaled CO_2.

a. Other options include (but are not limited to) surgery utilizing face mask or LMA anesthesia, local anesthesia infiltration, or regional nerve blockade. Pursuit of these options usually implies that mask ventilation will not be problematic. Therefore, these options may be of limited value if this step in the algorithm has been reached via the emergency pathway.

b. Invasive airway access includes surgical or percutaneous tracheostomy or cricothyrotomy.

c. Alternative noninvasive approaches to difficult intubation include (but are not limited to) use of different laryngoscope blades, LMA as an intubation conduit (with or without fiberoptic guidance), fiberoptic intubation, intubating stylet or tube changer, light wand, retrograde intubation, and blind oral or nasal intubation.

d. Consider re-preparation of the patient for awake intubation or canceling surgery.

e. Options for emergency noninvasive airway ventilation include (but are not limited to) rigid bronchoscope, esophageal-tracheal Combitube ventilation, or transtracheal jet ventilation.

Fig. 24.18 The American Society of Anesthesiologists Difficult Airway Algorithm. (From Apfelbaum JL, Hagberg CA, Caplan RA, et al. Practice guidelines for management of the difficult airway: an updated report by the American Society of Anesthesiologists Task Force on Management of the Difficult Airway. *Anesthesiology.* 2013;118[2]:251–270.)

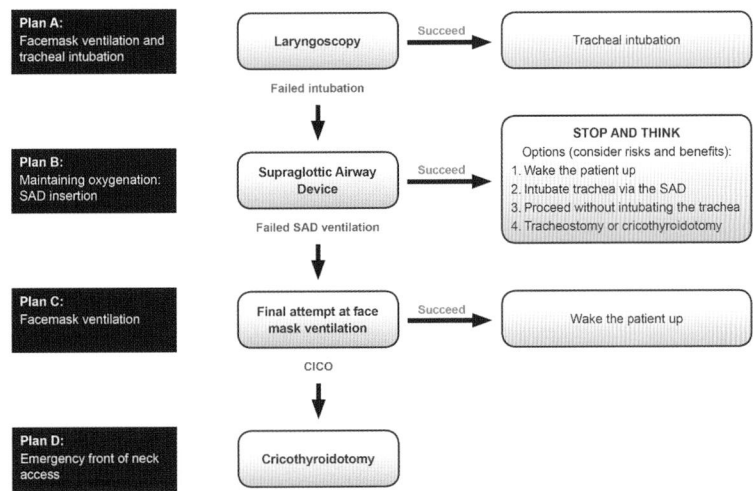

Fig. 24.19 The Difficult Airway Society (DAS) Difficult Intubation Guidelines. (From Frerk C, et al. Difficult Airway Society 2015 guidelines for management of unanticipated difficult intubation in adults. *Br J Anaesth.* 2015;115[6]:827–848.)

TABLE 24.5 **Airway Adjuncts and Alternative Airway Techniques***				
Supraglottic Airways	**Videolaryngoscopes**	**Stylets**	**Fiberoptic Scopes**	**Cricothyrotomy**
LMA Classic	GlideScope	Eschmann stylet (bougie)	Fiberoptic bronchoscope	Melker
LMA Proseal or Supreme,	McGrath Laryngoscope	Lighted stylet (e.g., Trachlite)	Fiberoptic laryngoscope with	Fastrach
Intubating LMA Fastrach,	C-MAC (Karl Storz)	Tube exchangers	various blade sizes	Commercial retrograde wire
LMA C-Trach			Fiberoptic flex tip laryngoscope	intubation kit
Cobra PLA	Airtrach		blades	Bougie assisted surgical
Streamlined liner of the	Shikani Optical Stylet		Ambu aScope disposable flexible	technique
pharynx airway (SLIPA)	Bonfils		intubating endoscopes	
i-gel	Pentax-AWS (Airway Scope)			
Combitube	Bullard Laryngoscope			
King LT/LTS-D				

*This table is not all-inclusive as many new airway adjuncts continue to be released.
LMA, Laryngeal mask airway; *LT,* laryngeal tube; *LTS-D,* disposable laryngeal tube with gastric access; *PLA,* perilaryngeal airway.

practitioner with four end points: (1) intubation awake or asleep, (2) adequate or inadequate facemask ventilation or LMA ventilation, (3) approach to intubation by special means, and (4) surgical or nonsurgical emergency airway access. Each of these end points entails using specific airway equipment and techniques to facilitate ventilation (Table 24.5). According to the algorithm, an organized plan should be initiated when a difficult airway is encountered. In essence, the philosophy of the ASA difficult airway algorithm has been explained by the following:

1. Plan ahead and be prepared for failed attempts at intubation.
2. If you are suspicious of airway trouble, then intubate awake.
3. If you get into trouble and can still ventilate the patient, then awaken the patient.
4. When making intubation choices, do what you do best.

DAS Difficult and Failed Intubation Guidelines

Proposed updates to the 2013 difficult airway algorithm include: (1) placing the airway approach algorithm questions at the beginning of the algorithm; (2) removing the consideration of returning to spontaneous ventilation or awakening the patient after initial unsuccessful intubation attempts; (3) limiting intubation and other airway management attempts to 3 or less; (4) focusing on confirmation of ETCO2 during ventilation attempts; (5) remaining aware of time during airway management; (6) removing emergency noninvasive airway ventilation from the "emergency pathway"; and (7) removal of the exhaustive list of airway adjuncts at the bottom of the algorithm. Blind intubation techniques (i.e., lighted stylet,

blind oral or nasal intubation) are no longer listed or recommended. In addition, a new infographic is being considered that depicts both the awake intubation pathway as well as the airway management pathway after induction of anesthesia. At the time of this text release, these updates are currently under revision by the ASA task force in charge of updating the the ASA Difficult Airway Algorithm.

The primary focus of the DAS difficult intubation guidelines is the unanticipated difficulty and failure of TI (see Fig. 24.17). These guidelines promote a simplified plan ("A, B, C, and D") within a single-page algorithm. Emphasis is placed on airway assessment, preparation, positioning, preoxygenation, prioritizing oxygenation, and limiting the number of airway interventions in an effort to limit the amount of trauma and complications during management.[83] Communication failures with the various airway plans occur, and the algorithm stresses the need for clarity when requesting assistance. The developers of the guidelines highly recommend that each time an airway plan fails, the airway manager verbalizes the failure to the team and then immediately verbalizes moving to the next airway plan in an effort to inform the entire perioperative team of the situation. The guidelines also highlight the importance of planning for failure during the preinduction briefing. Other pertinent suggestions about each airway plan contained within the guidelines include the following[83]:

- *Plan A*: Maximize success of TI on the first attempt (e.g., preparation, preoxygenation, positioning). Limit laryngoscopy attempts to no more than three. Declare failed intubation and verbalize implementation of plan B.

- *Plan B*: Emphasis is maintenance of oxygenation using a SAD. Second-generation SADs are recommended because of their reliability for first-time placement, high seal pressure capabilities, separation of the gastrointestinal and respiratory tracts, and compatibility with fiberoptic video devices. Video- or fiberoptic-guided TI is recommended instead of blind techniques using bougie stylets or through SADs because blind techniques may cause significant trauma. Cricoid pressure should be removed during SAD placement. There should be a maximum of three attempts. Declare failed SAD placement and verbalize implementation of plan C.
- *Plan C*: Attempt to oxygenate using a facemask. If facemask ventilation is possible, awaken the patient. Provide complete paralysis if facemask ventilation fails. Declare failed mask ventilation and verbalize implementation of plan D.
- *Plan D*: Declare cannot intubate and cannot ventilate/oxygenate, proceed with cricothyrotomy. Attempts to oxygenate the patient should continue (e.g., facemask, SAD, and nasal cannula). Surgical cricothyrotomy using a scalpel for access is the preferred rescue technique. DAS guidelines recommend regular practice with this technique.

There are similarities between the ASA difficult airway algorithm and other airway algorithms. For example, in the event of failed intubation, the ASA difficult airway algorithm reverts to facemask ventilation, and if that proves inadequate it moves to ventilation with an LMA. The DAS algorithm suggests using the LMA as means for ventilation and oxygenation immediately after a failed intubation, and then if the LMA fails it suggests reverting back to facemask ventilation. Both the ASA and DAS algorithms advocate for awakening the patient if initial attempts at intubation fail but subsequent ventilation attempts succeed. Furthermore, both recommend the placement of a cricothyrotomy if intubation has failed and both facemask and LMA ventilation have proven to be inadequate, although the DAS guidelines promote the surgical cricothyrotomy approach.[11,83]

It is worth noting the important role of the SADs within the difficult airway algorithms. SADs are used for rescue ventilation at two points in the ASA difficult airway algorithm: first, in the anesthetized patient whose trachea cannot be intubated but who can be ventilated with a facemask (anesthetized nonemergency limb); second, in the anesthetized patient whose trachea cannot be intubated and whose lungs cannot be conventionally ventilated (anesthetized emergency limb). The DAS algorithm recommends using a SAD device if initial TI fails. Comparable uses can also be found in national recommendations from Germany and Italy.[84-86]

The number of laryngoscopic attempts and the total procedural duration for intubation are quantifiable objective measurements used by multiple airway management guidelines as indications of airway difficulty. Most airway management guidelines allow three or less laryngoscopic attempts and 5 to 10 minutes of total procedural time before they classify the airway as a failed laryngoscopic intubation.[75,81,87] The number of laryngoscopic attempts is limited to prevent excessive airway instrumentation potentially leading to airway trauma, bleeding and increased difficulty. In an anticipated difficult airway, the first attempt at intubation should be the best attempt and should be associated with optimal preparation. When an unanticipated difficult intubation is encountered, the first attempt is usually the "awareness" look or view, and the second attempt should be performed under the best possible conditions (e.g., proper head and neck extension, head and shoulders elevated, experienced practitioner). If subsequent attempts are performed, alternative approaches should be considered (e.g., blade change, bougie stylet assist VL) as well as potentially changing providers.[88]

Many of the airway algorithms advocate for the use of different difficult airway adjuncts and strategies, including awake intubation, as long as ventilation is adequate and time permits. The choice of which adjunct to use is based on clinical judgment, which again should consider the patient's condition, the clinical setting, and the anesthesia provider's experience and skill level.

Frequent training in the clinical setting, at workshops, or during simulation scenarios can help increase familiarity with difficult airway management strategies and the use of different airway adjuncts and may play a role in decreasing complications associated with difficult airway management.[89,90] Ultimately, the primary goal of difficult airway management is to maintain ventilation and oxygenation, and each airway algorithm has been developed to assist in achieving this objective.

Difficult Airway Cart

A dedicated difficult airway cart or box is very useful during management of difficult airway situations. There is no definitive list of equipment, and the contents of the difficult airway cart should be decided on by the anesthesia department personnel based on the likely caseload and department budgets. The recommended basic components of the difficult airway cart are devices for (1) standard laryngoscopy, (2) intubation by alternative means, and (3) tube position control; and (4) equipment for anesthetizing the airway (Box 24.6).[81] Some difficult airway carts may also contain video and flexible intubating (i.e., fiberoptic) laryngoscopy devices.

Awake Intubation

When airway management is anticipated to be difficult, and the clinical scenario is such that the patient should remain spontaneously breathing, many airway guidelines suggest awake intubation using either a video-laryngoscope or a flexible intubating (fiberoptic) endoscope. There are several benefits to awake intubation, the first being that patients will maintain their own ventilation. In addition, the size of the pharynx may be improved because, due to the patient's inherent muscle tone, the tongue will move forward in the pharyngeal area, and sufficient lower esophageal sphincter tone should persist. Awake intubation allows the patient to maintain spontaneous ventilation and will preserve pharyngeal/laryngeal muscle tone. Regional anesthesia (e.g., airway blocks) provides an increased margin of safety and can help to facilitate both the viewing of airway structures and the placement of an ETT.[29] Anesthetizing an airway can be a time-consuming endeavor and may need to be abandoned if the patient is unwilling or unable to cooperate in an elective situation. However, in an emergency there is no absolute contraindication to awake intubation if it is considered the safest option for TI.

Sedative medications can be used to help the patient better tolerate an awake intubation. Agents that have been used include midazolam, propofol, etomidate, ketamine, fentanyl, remifentanil, and dexmedetomidine.[91] Dexmedetomidine has been shown to be effective as the sole sedative agent for awake TI in patients with local anesthetic allergies.[92] However, sedative mediations are not always required for an awake intubation. Agent selection depends on the clinical situation (e.g., an emergency that requires immediate airway access versus an anticipated difficult airway for a scheduled surgery), availability of the medication, and the provider's familiarity with the sedative agent. In addition, combinations of these medications are frequently used in clinical practice to reduce the total amount of any one drug given, especially as most cause respiratory depression in a dose-dependent fashion.

Caution should be exercised in patients with any degree of respiratory compromise or who are at risk for developing respiratory failure because even small doses of sedative medications may induce apnea. Furthermore, sedative and opioid analgesic agents decrease both pharyngeal and laryngeal muscle tone, which can lead to a total obstruction of the airway. Finally, deep sedation, or sedation levels that approach general anesthesia, defeat the purpose of performing an awake intubation and increase the risk for loss of airway reflexes, upper airway obstruction, and airway failure.[91]

Awake Intubation Techniques

An awake intubation is the placement of an ETT into the trachea while the patient is "awake" or not under the influence of general anesthesia.

BOX 24.6 Suggested Components of the Difficult Airway Cart

Standard Airway Equipment
- Oral and nasal airways of various sizes
- Tongue blades
- Flexible stylets
- Endotracheal tubes (cuffed and uncuffed) from size 2.5–8.0
- Miller laryngoscope blades sizes 0, 1, 2, 3, and 4
- Macintosh laryngoscope blades sizes 2, 3, and 4
- Extra laryngoscope batteries and bulbs
- Magill forceps
- Salem sump—16 and 18 French
- Suction catheters—10, 12, and 14 French
- Oxygen mask
- Nasal cannula
- Oxygen with 15 L/min regulator
- Ambu bag

Alternative Airway Equipment Options
- Supraglottic airway devices of different sizes (e.g., laryngeal mask airways—sizes 3, 4, and 5)
- Intubating supraglottic airway device
- Combitube or King laryngeal tube
- Lighted stylet (e.g., Trachlite)
- Eschmann stylet (e.g., gum elastic bougie)
- Tube exchanger—small, medium, and large
- Ventilating stylet
- Needle cricothyrotomy set
- Retrograde intubation set
- Melker percutaneous cricothyrotomy set
- Transtracheal jet ventilator

Tube Position Control
- Stethoscopes
- CO_2 detectors
- Esophageal detector device

Topical or Infiltration Anesthesia
- Syringes—3, 5, 10, and 20 mL (three or four of each size)
- Angiocatheters—14, 16, 18, and 20 gauge (three each)
- Xylocaine jelly (2%)
- Lidocaine—4% topical, 2% for injection
- Surgilube
- Nebulizer
- Atomizer
- 4×4 gauze pads

Video Laryngoscope Options
- Airtraq
- C-MAC
- GlideScope
- McGrath Mac or Series 5

Fiberoptic Bronchoscopy Equipment
- Tongue clamp
- Light source
- Endoscopy mask
- Flexible fiberoptic compatible oral airway (e.g., Ovassapian intubating airway)

intubation is an essential component of difficult airway management and should be a primary option any time abolishment of spontaneous ventilation is contraindicated. There are two awake techniques that can be considered after the patient has been prepared and the airway has been anesthetized:

1. Perform laryngoscopy with a standard or videolaryngoscope to (a) facilitate TI or (b) diagnostically determine whether the patient is truly difficult to intubate.
2. Perform intubation using a flexible intubating endoscope with a preloaded ETT that can be passed into the trachea.

The use of awake laryngoscopy to diagnostically determine difficulty with TI may help with the decision to (1) proceed with video or a flexible (fiberoptic) intubating scope (FIS) guided techniques (while the patient is awake) or (2) proceed with anesthesia induction and neuromuscular blockade to optimize airway conditions. Another option to determine airway difficulty is the use of a preoperative endoscopic airway examination. The purpose of this technique is to view the airway anatomy and determine airway difficulty through an endoscope using minimal sedation and local anesthesia topicalization prior to entering the OR. It has been shown to reduce the need for awake intubation and can help identify airway lesions that would otherwise not be seen in traditional external airway assessments.[93]

When performing an awake FIS intubation, either an oral or a nasal ETT can be used. The nasopharyngeal space often provides a direct line of sight to the laryngeal opening; however, this route may carry an increased risk of hemorrhage or soft tissue damage. Situations where an awake intubation would be necessary include patients with previous airway difficulty, unstable neck fractures, halo devices, small or limited oral openings, upper airway impingement by a mass, facial or neck trauma, severe burns of the face and/or neck, physiologic compromised patients (i.e., severe hypoxemia and/or hypotension), and patients in the critical care setting.

Patient Preparation

For maximum patient cooperation, the awake procedure must be clearly explained, and consent must be obtained. It is difficult, if not impossible, to proceed if the patient is uncooperative or unwilling to participate. Depending on the situation and the patient's condition, judicious use of anxiolytics or sedatives may be considered, as previously discussed. Examples of medications that may be considered when anesthetizing the airway are shown in Table 24.6. Administration of an antisialagogue (such as atropine 0.5–1 mg intravenous [IV] or intramuscular [IM] or glycopyrrolate 0.2–0.4 mg IV or IM) can help dry secretions and maximize the view of the laryngeal structures. Furthermore, an antisialagogue will decrease the secretion of saliva, allowing topical local anesthetics to penetrate the mucosa to a greater degree and enhancing anesthesia of the oral cavity, tongue, oropharynx, and hypopharynx. However, 20 minutes is usually required to effectively decrease secretions.

The risk of aspiration must always be considered when the airway reflexes have been anesthetized. Therefore medications that decrease stomach acid production and promote gastric emptying should be considered. Vasoconstriction of the nasal passages reduces the risk of mucosal damage and hemorrhage. Solutions containing 0.05% oxymetazoline (Afrin) or phenylephrine (Neo-Synephrine) can be sprayed into the nose 2 to 3 minutes prior to application of the local anesthetic. Cocaine (4%) has the benefit of local anesthetic action as well as promoting vasoconstriction.

The most widely used local anesthetic for anesthetizing the airway is lidocaine in various forms (liquid, gel, and ointment) and concentrations. Cocaine (4%), benzocaine (20%), and tetracaine are also effective anesthetics. Peak serum lidocaine levels are highest 30 minutes after instillation. Use of lidocaine within the recommended dosage keeps

"Awake" is somewhat of a misnomer, because, owing to inherent airway reflexes, it is very challenging to place an ETT without the use of local anesthesia, sedation, or both. However, patients are awake in the sense that they are cooperative and ventilating spontaneously. Awake

TABLE 24.6 Medication Considerations for Awake Intubation

	Medication	Indication
Intravenous Medications	Antisialagogue (glycopyrrolate or atropine)	Dry secretions in the airway
	Propofol	Provides sedation and anxiolysis, and assists with patient cooperation
	Midazolam	
	Ketamine	
	Etomidate	*Caution with respiratory depression and decreased muscle tone*
	Dexmedetomidine	
	Fentanyl	
	Remifentanil	
	Nonparticulate antacid (e.g., bicitra)	Aspiration prophylaxis
	Gastrokinetic (e.g., metoclopramide)	
	Histamine 2 antagonist (e.g., famotidine, ranitidine, cimetidine)	
Topical or Infiltration Medications	Phenylephrine (1%)	Vasoconstrictors for nasal intubation
	Lidocaine (2%, 4%, 5%)	Topical local anesthesia
	Cetacaine	Topical local anesthesia
	Benzocaine (20%)	Topical local anesthesia
	Cocaine (4%)	Topical local anesthesia and vasoconstrictor
	Lidocaine (2%)	Infiltration nerve block

serum lidocaine levels below toxic levels.[94,95] The evidence regarding the maximum safe dose for the topical administration of local anesthetics is controversial. However, an estimate of the maximum safe dose of local anesthesia should be calculated prior to any administration (e.g., lidocaine 4–5 mg/kg IV). Finally, clinical judgment of the situation is required, and the anesthetist should continually assess for signs and symptoms of toxicity.

AIRWAY BLOCKS

Anesthetizing the airway can be accomplished using topical anesthesia, by infiltration, or a combination of these two methods. The anesthetic requirements for the airway include sensory inhibition of the nasal, oral, pharyngeal, laryngeal, and tracheal mucosa. Specific branches of three cranial nerves need to be anesthetized to effectively perform an awake oral or nasal intubation. The three cranial nerves include the trigeminal, glossopharyngeal, and vagus nerves (Fig. 24.20). Both the ophthalmic and maxillary divisions of the trigeminal nerve provide sensory innervation to the nasal septum and lateral wall. In addition, the mandibular division of the trigeminal nerve forms the lingual nerve, which provides sensation to the anterior two-thirds of the tongue. The glossopharyngeal nerve provides sensory innervation to the posterior third of the tongue, the upper larynx, and the inner surface of the tympanic membrane via its lingual branches and other branches that connect to the tongue. Finally, the vagus nerve provides sensory innervation to the hypopharynx, larynx, and trachea via the SLN and RLN. The internal laryngeal branch of the SLN provides sensation above the vocal cords, and the RLN provides sensation below the vocal cords (Fig. 24.21).

Topical Anesthesia

Anesthesia applied to the nasal septum, nasal wall, and nasopharynx blocks the anterior ethmoidal, nasopalatine, and sphenopalatine nerves that originate from the ophthalmic and maxillary divisions of the trigeminal nerve. As discussed earlier, a topical vasoconstrictor should be applied to decrease the chance of bleeding during nasal instrumentation. These areas can be anesthetized using either viscous lidocaine or 4% lidocaine solution sprayed down each naris. The nasal and oral cavities, as well as the nasopharynx and oropharynx, may also be anesthetized by adding 4 to 10 mL of 4% lidocaine with 1 mL of 1% phenylephrine to either a handheld nebulizer or a nebulizer attached to a facemask.[91] As the patient breathes through the nose and mouth, small droplets of local anesthetic are deposited on the mucous membranes. This method is also used for anesthetization of subglottic tissue. Nebulization requires a minimum of 10 to 20 minutes and may necessitate additional topical anesthesia during the awake procedure.

An alternative approach to nebulization is providing topical anesthesia by atomization using a mucosal atomization device. Atomization produces larger droplets than nebulization, resulting in more medication coating the upper airway mucosa and producing a denser block. The provider also has the ability to direct where the atomized lidocaine is placed within the oropharynx and hypopharynx. Adequate atomization of the oral cavity and pharyngeal cavities can be performed with 10 mL or less of 4% lidocaine and a small amount of 5% lidocaine paste.

Anesthetizing the mouth and oropharynx decreases the gag and coughing reflexes associated with awake intubations. Some providers apply topical sprays to the anterior portion of the tongue and mouth. Benzocaine 20% (Hurricaine) spray is a topical anesthetic with a quick onset and short duration. A half-second spray delivers approximately 0.15 mL (30 mg), which is estimated to be approximately one-third of the toxic dose (100 mg). Cetacaine spray contains benzocaine (14%), tetracaine (2%), butyl aminobenzoate (2%), benzalkonium chloride, and cetyl dimethyl ethyl ammonium bromide. The combination of these medications shortens the onset time and increases the duration of action.[96] Methemoglobinemia is associated with the use of benzocaine, and it has been reported after the use of these topical sprays. If benzocaine is used, only conservative amounts of these sprays should be applied.

Topical anesthesia applied to the posterior tongue, vallecula, and anterior epiglottis can be enhanced with 5% lidocaine paste. The application of a "lidocaine lollipop," which can be made by coating the tip of a tongue blade with 5% lidocaine paste, to the back of the tongue allows the paste to melt and coat the base of the tongue, the vallecula, the anterior epiglottis, and at times even the vocal cords. The tongue blade should be held in place for 1 to 2 minutes to allow the lidocaine paste to liquefy and coat the tongue and lower structures. Additionally, atomization using 4% lidocaine solution can provide effective topical anesthesia of these areas if the lidocaine paste is unavailable.

Topical anesthetization of the vocal cords is best accomplished by spraying local anesthetic directly onto the cords.[97] This can be accomplished by depositing local anesthetic down the endotracheal tube when it is in close approximation to the vocal cords, and then instructing the patient to take a deep breath. This causes the patient to cough, indicating that local anesthetic was deposited on the vocal cords. Another option is using the atomizer to spray the cords with local anesthesia while viewing with a flexible intubating endoscope or videolaryngoscope. After visualization of the vocal cords is achieved, 4% lidocaine solution can be visually deposited directly onto the vocal. An alternative option for deposition of local anesthetic using the fiberoptic scope is to place an 18-gauge epidural catheter through the suction channel. This allows precise topical injection of local anesthesia onto visualized airway structures.

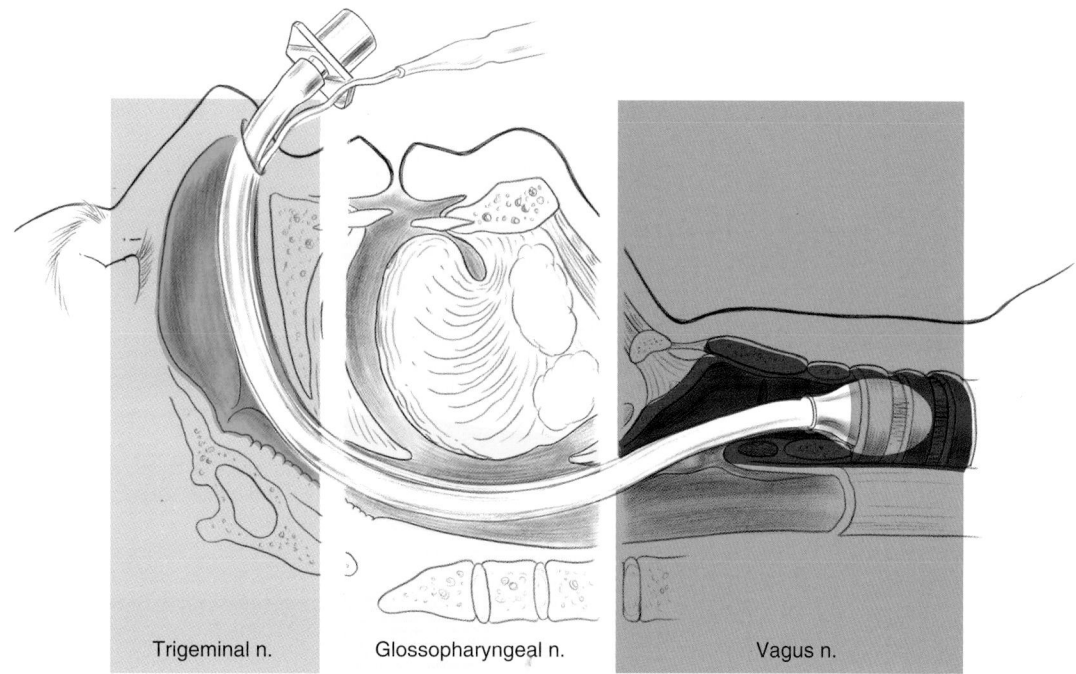

Fig. 24.20 Cranial nerve innervation of the upper airway. *n,* Nerve. (From Brown DL, et al., eds. *Atlas of Regional Anesthesia*. 5th ed. Philadelphia: Elsevier; 2017:204.)

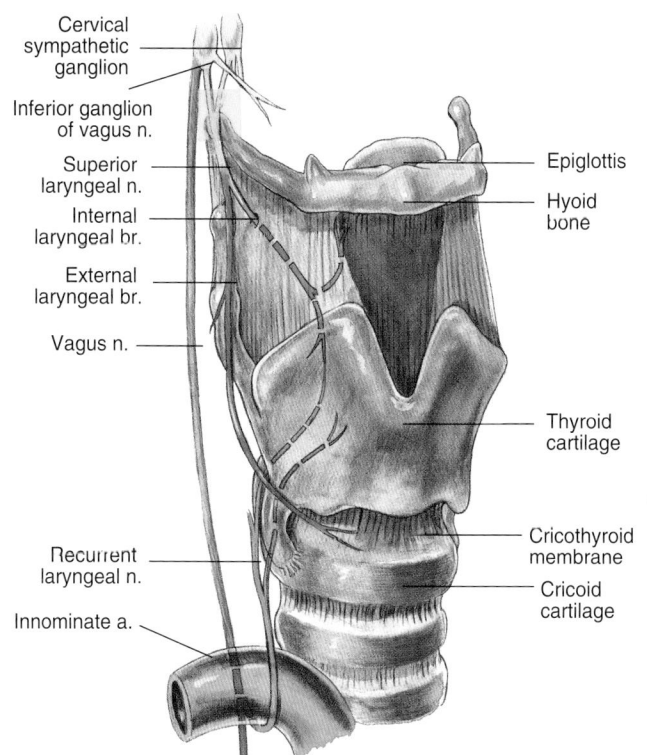

Fig. 24.21 Laryngeal anatomy and nerve innervation. *a,* Artery; *br,* branch; *n,* nerve. (From Brown DL, et al., eds. *Atlas of Regional Anesthesia*. 5th ed. Philadelphia: Elsevier; 2017:205.)

Topical anesthetization of the upper airway can be achieved quickly and safely, provided the anesthetist prepares the patient, calculates the appropriate toxic dose of local anesthetic to be used, and becomes familiar with these and other topical anesthesia techniques. Alternative upper airway anesthesia approaches, which can be used alone or in combination with topical anesthesia techniques, are infiltration nerve blocks. Both topical and infiltration techniques have demonstrated acceptable conditions for awake TI.[98,99]

Glossopharyngeal Nerve Block

The lingual branches of the glossopharyngeal nerve along with other nerve branches supply sensory innervation to the posterior third of the tongue, the upper larynx, and the inner surface of the tympanic membrane. To block the lingual branch with infiltration anesthesia, the practitioner first anesthetizes the tongue with topical anesthesia and then has the patient open the mouth and protrude the tongue forward. The anesthetist then displaces the tongue to the opposite side with a tongue blade, resulting in the formation of a gutter (Figs. 24.22 and 24.23). Where the lingual gutter meets the base of the palatoglossal arch, a 23- or 25-gauge spinal needle is inserted approximately 0.25 to 0.5 cm and aspirated for air. If air is obtained on aspiration, the needle has been placed too deeply and should be withdrawn until no air is aspirated. If blood is obtained, the needle must be withdrawn and repositioned more medially to avoid possible intracarotid injection. After correct positioning, 1 to 2 mL of 2% lidocaine is injected, and the block is then repeated on the opposite side.[91,96]

Superior Laryngeal Nerve Block

The superior laryngeal nerve block provides a dense block of the supraglottic region. To perform the block, the practitioner locates the greater cornu of the hyoid bone, which lies beneath the angle of the mandible and can be palpated with the thumb and index finger on either side of the neck as a rounded structure (Fig. 24.24). The hyoid bone is then displaced toward the side that is being injected to help stabilize the bone and facilitate identification of structures for the injection of the local anesthetic. The needle is inserted perpendicular to the skin, and advanced to contact the inferior border of the greater cornu (Fig. 24.25). The needle is then "walked off" the caudal edge of the hyoid bone where it then meets the thyrohyoid membrane. Resistance may

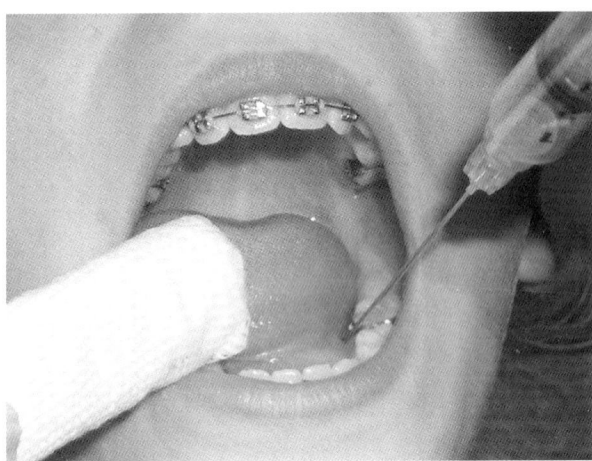

Fig. 24.22 Glossopharyngeal nerve block.

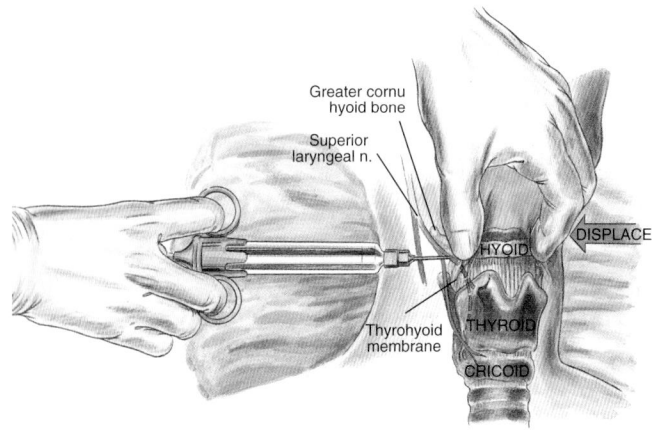

Fig. 24.24 Superior laryngeal nerve block anatomy and technique. *n,* Nerve. (From Brown DL, et al., eds. *Atlas of Regional Anesthesia.* 5th ed. Philadelphia: Elsevier; 2017:14.)

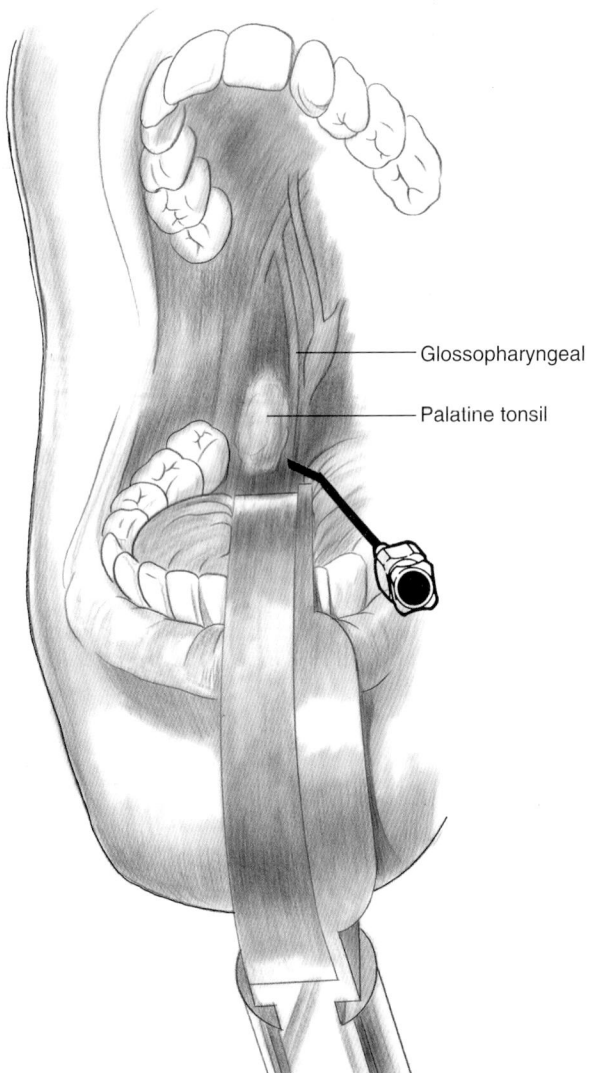

- Glossopharyngeal n.

- Palatine tonsil

Fig. 24.23 Glossopharyngeal nerve block anatomy and technique. *n,* Nerve. (From Brown DL, et al., eds. *Atlas of Regional Anesthesia.* 5th ed. Philadelphia: Elsevier; 2017.)

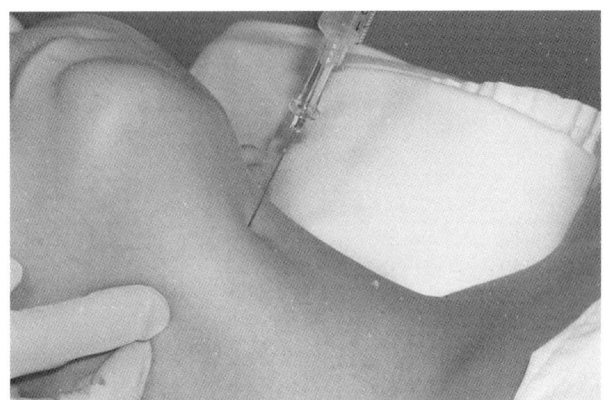

Fig 24.25 Superior laryngeal nerve block.

be appreciated as the tip of the needle may be felt to "bounce" on the thyrohyoid membrane.[100] This site approximates the area where the superior laryngeal nerve pierces the thyrohyoid membrane. Aspiration should confirm there is no air or blood, and 1 mL of local anesthetic (e.g., 2% lidocaine) is deposited above this membrane. The needle is then advanced an additional 2 to 3 mm through the membrane, and 2 mL of local anesthetic is deposited. The block is then repeated on the other side. Again, aspiration is performed before the injection of the local anesthetic. If air is aspirated, the needle has been placed too deep and is in the pharynx, and the tip of the needle should be withdrawn and repositioned. The same type of needle redirection should occur if blood is aspirated.

Transtracheal Block

A transtracheal block is accomplished by injecting local anesthetic through the cricothyroid membrane (Fig. 24.26). To administer the block, first palpate the cricothyroid membrane with the index and middle fingers (Fig. 24.27) and localize the skin. Then attach a 22-gauge needle or a 24-gauge angiocatheter to a syringe containing 3 to 5 mL of 2% lidocaine. Place the needle midline and puncture in a caudad direction through the cricothyroid membrane while aspirating continuously. When air bubbles are aspirated through the solution, the tip of the needle is in the tracheal lumen. If using an angiocatheter, the catheter is advanced into the tracheal lumen and the needle withdrawn, which may produce coughing.[100] The patient is then instructed to take

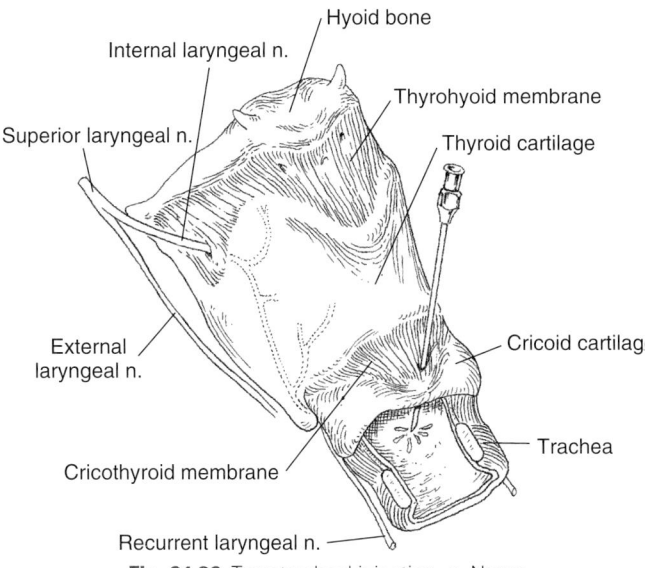

Fig. 24.26 Transtracheal injection. *n*, Nerve.

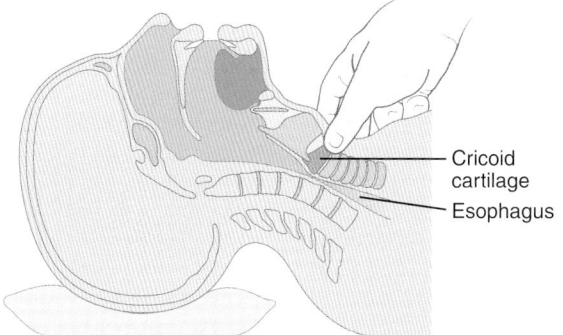

Fig. 24.28 Application of cricoid pressure. (From Miller RD, Pardo MC, eds. *Basics of Anesthesia*. 6th ed. Philadelphia: Elsevier; 2011:229.)

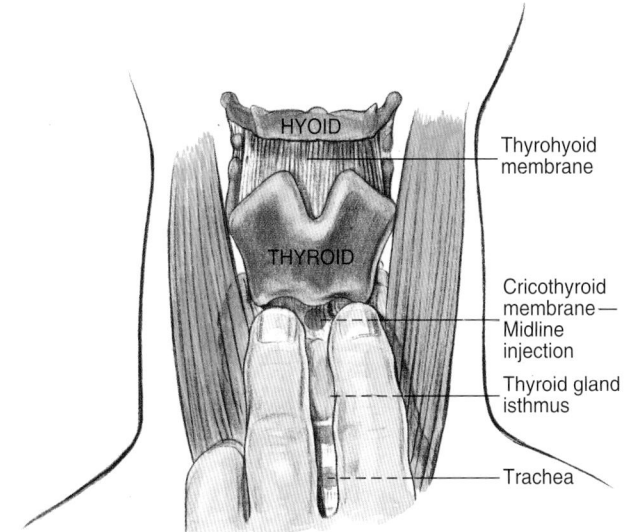

Fig. 24.27 Transtracheal nerve block anatomy and placement. (From Brown DL, et al., eds. *Atlas of Regional Anesthesia*. 5th ed. Philadelphia: Elsevier; 2017:216.)

a deep breath. On inspiration, the local anesthetic is injected into the tracheal lumen. This will cause the patient to cough, spraying the local anesthetic onto the vocal cords. Care must be taken to stabilize the needle so as not to tear the tracheal mucosa when the patient coughs. Use of the softer angiocatheter may decrease trauma.

CRICOID PRESSURE

British anesthetist Brian Arthur Sellick first described cricoid pressure in 1961 as the posterior displacement of the cricoid cartilage against the cervical vertebrae with the patient in a 20-degree head-up position to prevent regurgitation and possible aspiration of stomach contents during the induction of general anesthesia. As such, cricoid pressure, which is also known as the Sellick maneuver, has remained a mainstay of anesthetic practice, particularly in patients at risk for

aspiration who receive rapid-sequence induction for general anesthesia. The optimal amount of force necessary to effectively occlude the esophagus without obstruction of the trachea is between 30 and 40 Newtons (N). It is recommended that 10 to 20 N (e.g., 1–2 kg-force) cricoid pressure be applied prior to loss of consciousness and that the pressure be increased to 30 to 40 N (e.g., 3–4 kg-force) after loss of consciousness (Fig. 24.28).[101] This pressure is equivalent to a firm pressure or a pressure that would cause discomfort if applied to the bridge of the nose.

The efficacy of cricoid pressure as an intervention to decrease the incidence of gastric aspiration and occlude the esophagus has been questioned on the grounds that initial studies researching cricoid pressure's effectiveness to prevent aspiration were conducted using cadavers.[102,103] The application of cricoid pressure can interfere with visualization of the patient's airway during laryngoscopy and induce relaxation of the lower esophageal sphincter.[103,104] Furthermore, MRI has demonstrated that the esophagus can be found lateral to the cricoid ring in more than 50% of patients. This proportion may increase to 90% after the application of cricoid pressure, theoretically hampering esophageal occlusion during posterior displacement of the cartilaginous cricothyroid ring.[105] However, there continues to be debate, claiming that the anatomic location and movement of the esophagus during the application of cricoid pressure is irrelevant to the efficiency of the Sellick maneuver because it is the hypopharynx that is compressed. In a cohort of nonsedated volunteers, MRI showed that compression of the alimentary tract occurs with both midline and lateral displacement of the cricoid cartilage relative to the underlying vertebral body.[106]

The application of cricoid pressure is not a benign procedure. Cricoid pressure of more than 40 N applied to the awake individual has been associated with laryngeal discomfort and retching. Furthermore, holding cricoid pressure during active vomiting may result in rupture of the esophagus and should be released immediately if vomiting occurs.[107] Another contraindication to the use of cricoid pressure is a cervical spine injury, since pressure from the applied force of the cricoid cartilage against the cervical spine could exacerbate the injury.[108] The application of pressure during rapid-sequence induction has been shown to decrease upper and lower esophageal sphincter tone.[101] Other complications attributed to the use of cricoid pressure include (1) airway obstruction (e.g., partial or complete), (2) cervical spine compression, (3) glottic visualization impediments during laryngoscopy, (4) difficulty with facemask and SAD ventilation, and (5) trouble with TI.[102,103,108] However, the use of cricoid pressure is widespread and has value in the right circumstances.[109] The decision to use cricoid pressure should consider the potential benefits against the potential complications and should be made based on the clinical situation.

ADJUNCT AIRWAY EQUIPMENT AND TECHNIQUES

Over the past 2 decades, multiple adjunctive airway devices have been developed for use in both routine and difficult airway management situations. Airway adjuncts include ETT guides, lighted stylets, rigid laryngoscopes, indirect rigid fiberoptic laryngoscopes, FIS, SAD, VL, and any device or piece of equipment that supports airway management. Techniques used for difficult intubation and ventilation may include any one or a combination of airway adjuncts. To improve proficiency, frequent use of adjunctive airway equipment should be considered in nonemergent or simulated practice situations.[89,90] Ultimately, the selection of an airway adjunct for airway management is based on familiarity and skill with the device, as well as (1) the need for airway control, (2) the ease of laryngoscopy, (3) the ability to use supralaryngeal ventilation, (4) aspiration risk, and (5) the patient's tolerance for apnea.[15] It is beyond the scope of this chapter to review all adjunctive equipment related to airway management as many airway tools and management devices exist. What follows is a review of the more common airway devices and equipment.

Supraglottic Airway Devices

Supraglottic airway devices are airway adjuncts that provide ventilation above the glottic opening. Different terminology has been used to describe these devices depending on where they are placed. For example, devices that sit above or surround the glottis (e.g., LMA, facemask) are truly supraglottic. In contrast, those devices that pass behind the larynx and enter the upper esophagus (e.g., Combitube, King LT [laryngeal tube] airway) are known as retroglottic or infraglottic devices. However, because ventilation with all these devices is performed superior to the glottic opening, SAD is the preferred terminology. The choice of any SAD is dependent on the clinical situation and preference of the provider. Indications for these devices include (1) rescue ventilation for difficult mask ventilation and failed intubation; (2) an alternative to endotracheal intubation, in appropriately selected patients, for elective surgery in the OR; and (3) as a conduit to facilitate endotracheal intubation.[110] SADs have proven to be valuable tools for airway management, especially in the patient who is difficult to ventilate and/or intubate. These devices are well tolerated by patients because they follow the same inherent pathway as the airway, and unlike laryngoscopy they require minimal tissue distention in the hypopharyngeal space.

Laryngeal Mask Airway

Since its introduction into clinical practice in 1981, the LMA has been used extensively in airway management. Its development has been hailed as one of the most significant advances in airway management since the ETT.[111] The LMA can be used as the primary airway device during appropriate surgical procedures and is considered a valuable airway tool when managing a difficult airway. A great deal of literature exists that reports the successful use of the LMA as a primary airway device and as a conduit for intubation of the trachea.[111-113]

The LMA Classic (Fig. 24.29) was used extensively in Europe, primarily in England, before its introduction in the United States in 1989. Today the LMA Unique (Fig. 24.30) is more ubiquitous in everyday practice because it is single use only. Several variations of the LMA exist, including the Flexible, ProSeal, Supreme, and Fastrach models (all from Teleflex, Wayne, PA). In daily clinical use, the LMA can be used in place of BMV during general anesthesia. An appropriately sized LMA is generally based on patient kilogram weight (Table 24.7). Laryngeal mask insertion is usually accomplished using the classic technique, which is fully deflating the cuff and placing a water-soluble lubricant on its posterior surface. The practitioner inserts the LMA

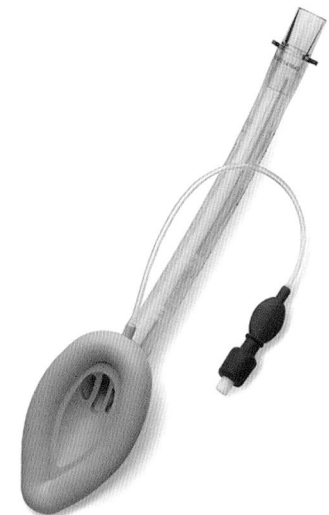

Fig. 24.29 LMA Classic. (Courtesy Teleflex Inc.)

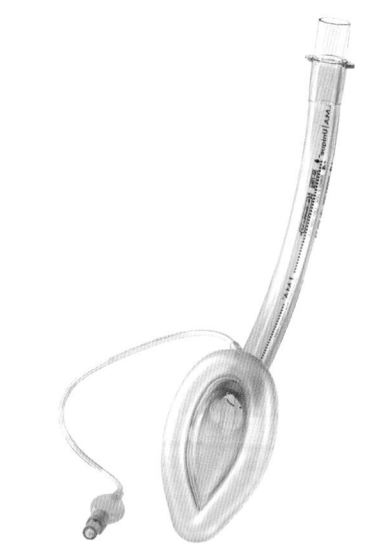

Fig. 24.30 LMA Unique. (Courtesy Teleflex Inc.)

midline into the mouth with the posterior surface pressed flat against the palate of the mouth and then advances with the index finger along the palatopharyngeal curve. Reports have indicated between an 88% and 95% success rate on the first attempt with an experienced provider.[114] If initial attempts at LMA placement are difficult, then the LMA should be removed and intubation should attempted with the patient in a proper sniffing position. In addition, if the LMA encounters resistance when it reaches the posterior pharyngeal wall, it is many times due to the distal tip having folded back as a result of aggressive posterior pressure, and the airway simply needs to be retracted and advanced again, applying a more upward pressure toward the top of the patient's head. If continued resistance occurs, then the operator can place the right index finger between the superior portion of the LMA and the palate and "flip the tip" back into normal position while advancing the device with the opposite hand. When properly placed, final resistance denotes placement of the LMA's tip in the hypopharynx, and the black line on the tubing will be even with the upper lip. The cuff is then inflated, sealing the airway over the larynx. Intracuff pressures should not exceed 60 cm H_2O. The esophageal opening at the base of the hypopharynx has no seal. If the LMA cuff is overinflated, it

TABLE 24.7 Appropriate LMA Sizing Based on Patient Weight With Maximum Cuff Inflation Volumes

LMA Size	Patient Weight* (kg)	Maximum Cuff Inflation (Air) LMA Classic, Unique, Proseal, Flexible, and Fastrach	Maximum Cuff Inflation (Air)—Maximum OG Size LMA Supreme
1	<5	Up to 4 mL	Up to 5 mL 6-French OGT
1.5	5–10	Up to 7 mL	Up to 8 mL 6-French OGT
2	10–20	Up to 10 mL	Up to 12 mL 10-French OGT
2.5	20–30	Up to 14 mL	Up to 20 mL 10-French OGT
3	30–50	Up to 20 mL	Up to 30 mL 14-French OGT
4	50–70	Up to 30 mL	Up to 45 mL 14-French OGT
5	70–100	Up to 40 mL	Up to 45 mL 14-French OGT
6 (LMA Classic only)	>100	Up to 50 mL	

*The Classic, Unique, Proseal, Supreme, Flexible, and Fastrach model sizes are based on similar patient weights.
From Teleflex, Wayne, PA.
LMA, Laryngeal mask airway; *OG,* orogastric; *OGT,* orogastric tube.

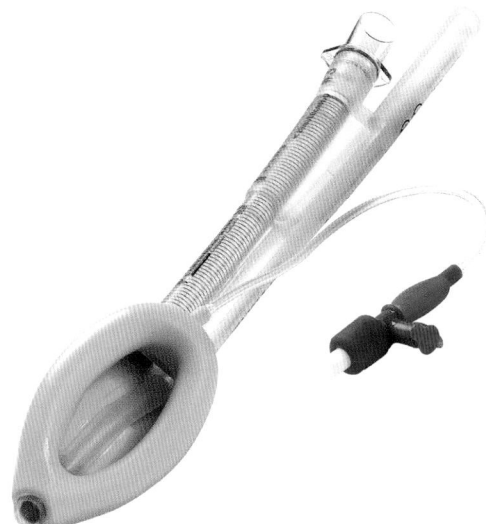

Fig. 24.31 ProSeal LMA. (Courtesy Teleflex Inc.)

can open the upper esophageal sphincter or potentially cause posterior cricoarytenoid muscle fatigue.[115]

Alternative techniques and maneuvers can be used for LMA placement. A tongue blade can be used (similar to placement of an oral airway) to reposition the tongue into the thyromental space allowing a larger opening within the oral cavity and easier placement. The LMA can also be introduced into the mouth with the opening initially facing the palate. It is then advanced until the LMA reaches the oropharynx, when it is rotated 180 degrees counterclockwise and advanced into its final position. Another technique is to partially or fully inflate the LMA cuff with air before insertion. Finally, guided techniques using an Eschmann stylet (bougie) or a laryngoscope to facilitate placement have been reported.[116] The LMA Flexible is a variation of the LMA Classic that utilizes a smaller diameter wire-reinforced barrel. Indications for use include surgeries on the mouth, pharynx, face, or jaw, or any other procedure in which the head may be moved, when heavy drapes cover the patient's face and head, or if the barrel cannot be secured at the midline.

Second-Generation Supraglottic Devices

Compared to original SAD designs, second-generation SDAs (1) attempt to reduce the risk of aspiration by incorporating a channel for gastric decompression and suctioning of secretions, (2) have reinforced tips that prevent folding, (3) incorporate improved cuff designs to help create a better cuff seal allowing for higher ventilation pressures, and (4) are more rigid in their design to prevent rotation and to facilitate easier insertion.[59,117] Indeed, current difficult airway algorithms support the use of these second-generation SADs for the previously

mentioned reasons.[83] Several different types of second-generation devices exist, including but not limited to the LMA ProSeal (PLMA) and LMA Supreme (Teleflex, Wayne, PA), i-gel (Intersurgical, Wokingham, UK), and the AuraGain (Ambu, Glen Burnie, MD). A significant amount of research and discussion is available describing the use of and comparing second-generation SADs.[118-123] The King LTS-D (Ambu, Glen Burnie, MD) is considered a second-generation SAD; however, its use is primarily in the prehospital setting, and it is not suitable as a conduit for TI. Ultimately, because these devices have all been proven to be effective for ventilation, the selection of any SAD will most likely be a result of the clinical situation and the airway provider's experience and comfort level.

The PLMA was introduced in 2000 as an alternative SAD to the LMA Classic, and it comes in the same sizes (Fig. 24.31). Modifications compared to the LMA Classic include (1) a larger and deeper bowl with no grille, (2) posterior extension of the mask cuff, (3) a gastric drainage tube running parallel to the airway tube and existing at the mask tip, (4) a silicone bite block, and (5) an anterior pocket for seating an introducer or finger during insertion.[123,124] The PLMA was designed with a second posterior cuff, which when inflated helps to separate the respiratory and gastrointestinal tracts, and a second tube developed for the insertion of a gastric tube into the esophagus without passing through the hypopharynx. The addition of this esophageal gastric drain tube allows the practitioner to identify misplacement and decompress the patient's stomach of air or solid contents and may vent regurgitated stomach contents.

Compared to the LMA Classic, insertion of the PLMA takes an additional few seconds, but the overall success is equivalent. In addition, the airway seal is improved by 50%, allowing a peak ventilation pressure of up to 28 to 30 cm H_2O (vs the 20 cm H_2O with the LMA Classic).[117,119] The PLMA has been used in laparoscopic surgery (though this is controversial), as well as in the obese, intensive care, trauma, and difficult airway populations.[125] A disposable version of the PLMA, named the LMA Supreme (Fig. 24.32), has a fixed curve design for easier insertion, a gastric access port superior to the ventilation channel, and an integrated bite block. Peak ventilation pressures were slightly lower when compared to the PLMA (e.g., 26–28 cm H_2O), although first-time insertion success rates were slightly higher with the LMA Supreme. Finally, the LMA Supreme has demonstrated similar capabilities as a ventilation and oxygenation device in challenging cases.[120,122,126]

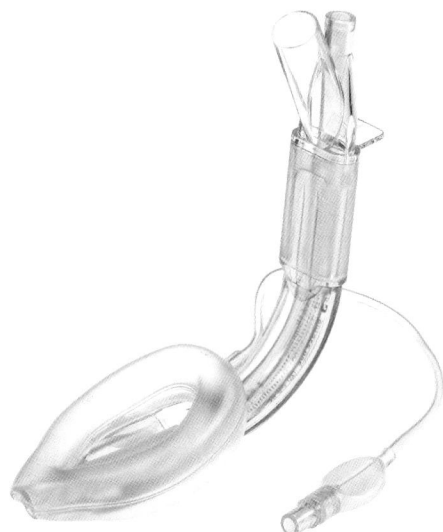

Fig. 24.32 LMA Supreme. (Courtesy Teleflex Inc.)

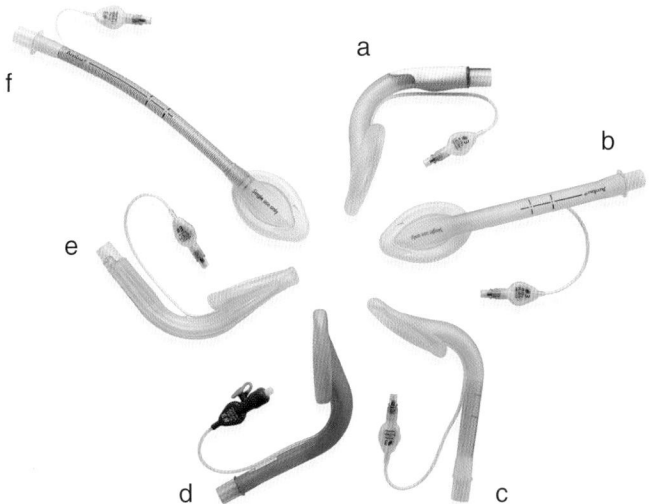

Fig. 24.34 Ambu product family. Beginning at the top and rotating clockwise: *(a)* Aura-I; *(b)* AuraStraight; *(c)* AuraOnce; *(d)* Aura40; *(e)* AuraGain; *(f)* AuraFlex. (Courtesy Ambu.)

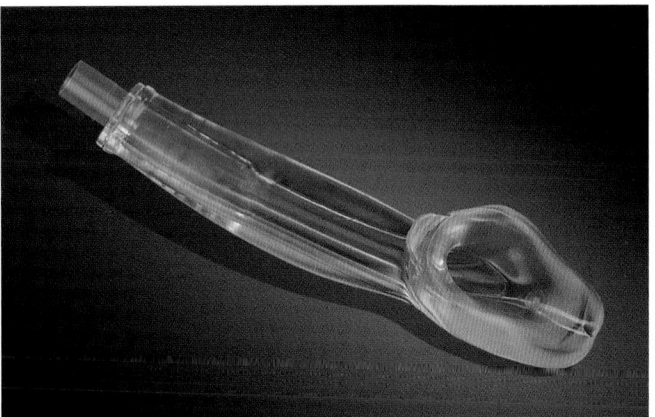

Fig. 24.33 i-gel. (From Hagberg CA, ed. *Benumof and Hagberg's Airway Management*. 3rd ed. Philadelphia: Elsevier; 2013:495.)

The i-gel is a single-use second-generation SAD designed for anesthesia and airway rescue (Fig. 24.33). Instead of an inflatable cuff, the i-gel mask is made of a medical grade thermoplastic elastomer, which is soft, gel-like, and transparent. The device occupies the entire hypopharynx and laryngopharynx, is designed to create a noninflatable anatomic seal of the perilaryngeal structures while avoiding compression trauma, and relies on contact with these anatomic structures to create an effective seal for ventilation. The channel of the device can be used as a conduit for intubation under fiberoptic guidance. The i-gel incorporates a gastric channel to provide an early warning of regurgitation, allow for the passing of a nasogastric tube to empty the stomach contents, and facilitate venting. It also has an integral bite block to reduce the possibility of airway occlusion and a buccal cavity stabilizer to aid with insertion and reduce the potential for rotation. The tip of the i-gel mask is blunt to prevent it from flexing either forward or backward. Recent evidence suggests that proper placement of the device provides both a good seal and effective ventilation.[127] Clinical trials focused on the i-gel have demonstrated relative ease of insertion, high seal pressures, and a lower incidence of sore throat when compared with other SADs.[121,123]

The Ambu AuraGain is another preformed anatomically curved single-use SAD that includes a gastric access port as well as intubating capabilities (Fig. 24.34). The device includes an integrated bite block and comes in both pediatric and adult sizes. Limited data exist regarding use of the AuraGain, however, when compared to other SADs. It appears to have similar capabilities with respect to airway leak pressures, ease of insertion, and successful insertion when used in children.[128]

The King LT differs from other SADs in that it does not have a mask that covers the laryngeal opening. Instead, this device is a one-time use, double lumen tube with a large oropharyngeal balloon and a smaller esophageal balloon. Ventilation ports are situated anteriorly between both balloons. A single pilot balloon is used to inflate both balloons when the device is situated in the airway. The larger oropharyngeal balloon isolates both the oropharynx and nasopharynx from above, and when inflated lifts the base of the tongue anteriorly while providing stabilization of the device. The distal esophageal balloon sits at the esophageal inlet and isolates the esophagus from below, providing a high-pressure esophageal seal. The newer King LTS-D model (Fig. 24.35) is disposable and includes a gastric vent posterior to the airway tube that accommodates an 18-French nasogastric suction tube for suctioning air and gastric secretions. The LTS-D is designed for blind insertion during emergency airway management but is not suitable as a conduit for intubation. The King LT model has the capacity to achieve a ventilatory seal of 30 cm H_2O or higher. Scant data are available regarding the use of the LTS-D model when compared to other SADs; however, evidence suggests it is popular in the prehospital environment because of its ease of insertion.[112,129] Several other SADs have been introduced for single airway use. Examples include the Cobra perilaryngeal airway, which is a single lumen tube with a circumferential distal cuff just proximal to a distal adaptor that looks like a cobra head and is intended to expand hypopharyngeal tissue. Similar to the i-gel, the streamlined liner of the pharyngeal airway does not have an inflatable cuff, but it does have the capacity to ventilate, and it contains a reservoir to capture regurgitated material.

Intubating Supraglottic Airway Devices

Intubating SADs offer the ability to ventilate and then to attempt either a blind or flexible endoscopic-guided tracheal intubation (with an ETT) through a barreled channel. There are several types of intubating SADs, including the LMA Fastrach (Teleflex Inc., Wayne, PA), the air-Q (Mercury Medical, Clearwater, FL), and the Aura-I (Ambu, Glen

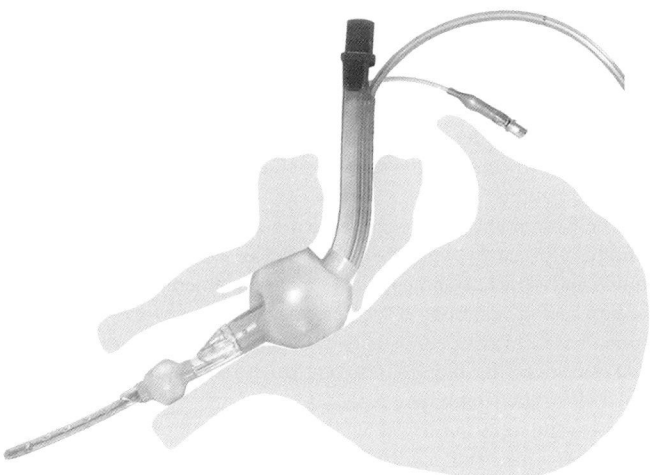

Fig. 24.35 King LTS-D tube correctly inserted. (Courtesy King Systems.)

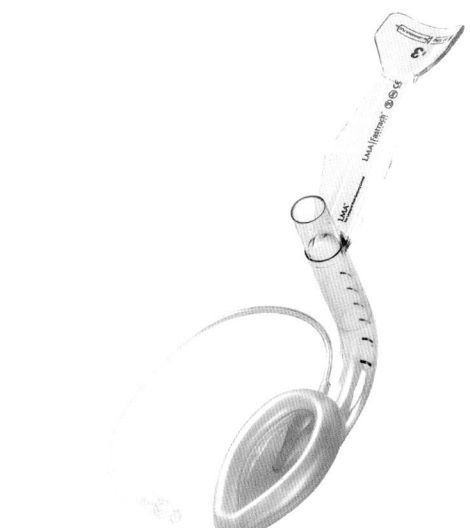

Fig. 24.36 Fastrach LMA. (Courtesy Teleflex Inc.)

Burnie, MD). A common indication is when difficulty with facemask ventilation or with TI occurs. Intubating SADs allow for continued ventilation and provision of anesthesia until TI is accomplished.

Perhaps the most well-known intubating SAD is the LMA Fastrach (Fig. 24.36), also known as the intubating LMA, which was released in 1997 and was specifically designed for use in anticipated and unanticipated difficult airway situations.[130] The LMA Fastrach has been used successfully in the "cannot intubate and cannot ventilate" scenario, in situations where a difficult intubation is anticipated, and in prehospital emergency airway situations where intubation is not possible by DL.[131,132]

The rigid curved design of the LMA Fastrach allows the mask aperture to align with the glottis vestibule. The primary distinguishing features, as described by the Fastrach inventor, Dr. Archie Brain, include (1) an anatomically curved 13-mm internal diameter rigid airway tube that can accommodate an 8.5-mm ETT, (2) an integrated guiding handle at the proximal end to facilitate insertion, (3) a vertically oriented semirigid epiglottic elevating bar, and (4) a guiding ramp built into the floor of the mask aperture.[133] The device comes in sizes 3, 4, and 5. A description of the steps required for placing an LMA Fastrach can be found in Box 24.7. After successful ETT placement, the rigid LMA Fastrach should be removed to avoid sustained pressure on the hypopharyngeal tissues. An

---

BOX 24.7   LMA Fastrach and Endotracheal Tube Placement

Initial Preparation

1. Confirm integrity of LMA and ETT cuffs (consider using prewarmed polyvinylchloride ETT) and then deflate cuffs.
2. Lubricate ETT with water-soluble lubricant at distal end and pass through to Fastrach lumen to lubricate inside the channel.
3. Lubricate anterior and posterior surfaces of LMA Fastrach cuff with water-soluble lubricant.
4. If using flexible endoscopic guided approach, prepare the flexible scope device and lubricate channel.

LMA Fastrach Placement for Supraglottic Ventilation

1. Hold device by the metal handle in dominant hand and open the airway.
2. Insert cuff into mouth with mask tip in contact with the palate (rigid handle portion will be near the chin).
3. Maintain firm upward pressure with the palate and posterior pharynx while advancing the LMA Fastrach into place until resistance is felt or handle meets face (only rigid handle and end of tube will protrude from mouth).
4. Inflate the cuff.
5. Confirm adequate ventilation (ventilation confirmation should indicate consistent end-tidal CO_2 waveform, positive change in color on CO_2-detecting devices, and equal bilateral breath sounds).
6. May manipulate device gently using handle until ventilation is optimized.

ETT Placement Through LMA Fastrach

1. Remove 15-mm connector from ETT and set aside (may place on ventilator circuit for easy placement back onto ETT postintubation).
2. Place ETT through Fastrach LMA lumen until it reaches the 15-cm marking. At this position the ETT is about to push the epiglottic elevating bar up, moving the epiglottis out of the way.
3. *Blind Approach:* Use the Fastrach handle to lift anteriorly, blindly insert ETT into trachea (should not encounter resistance) and inflate ETT cuff balloon.
   a. *Flexible Endoscopic-Guided Approach:* is the preferred approach Insert flexible scope though ETT channel and visualize glottis opening. Advance flexible scope into trachea and then advance ETT over scope channel. Can confirm placement by visualization of carina and tracheal rings.
4. Finish by placing ETT connector back on ETT and attempt ventilation (ventilation confirmation should indicate consistent end-tidal CO_2 waveform and equal bilateral breath sounds).

Remove Fastrach LMA

1. Remove ETT connector and set aside (may place on ventilator circuit for easy placement back onto ETT postintubation).
2. Deflate ETT balloon and Fastrach LMA balloon.
3. Place Fastrach stylet on the end of the ETT and provide countertraction caudally as the LMA Fastrach is removed.
4. When the ETT is visualized below the Fastrach cuff at the level of the mouth, hold ETT, remove stylet so that the ETT balloon cuff can pass through the LMA Fastrach barrel, and then remove the LMA Fastrach completely.
5. Replace ETT connector and reconfirm correct ETT placement in trachea (ventilation confirmation should indicate consistent end tidal CO_2 waveform and equal bilateral breath sounds).

ETT, Endotracheal tube; *LMA,* laryngeal mask airway.

---

adaptation of the Fastrach is the C-Trach intubation device. This device was introduced in 2004 and added a fiberoptic cable and monitor screen (magnetically mounted) to the handle. However, this device has not been widely accepted because of the cumbersome viewing monitor.

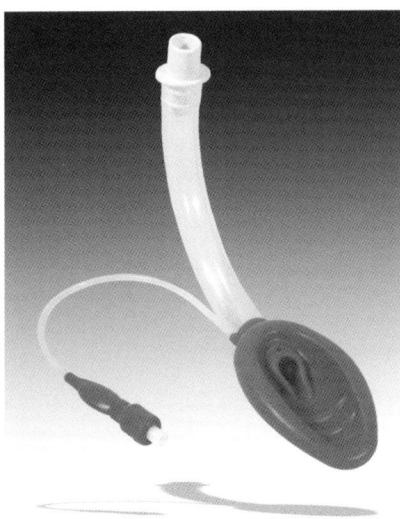

Fig. 24.37 Intubating laryngeal airway or air-Q. (Courtesy Mercury Medical.)

Physician-inventor Daniel Cook developed an oval-shaped laryngeal mask that allows ventilation through the device and intubation with a standard ETT. This masked laryngeal airway known as the air-Q (Fig. 24.37) comes in reusable and disposable forms. The air-Q device is nonrigid and does not contain an epiglottic elevating bar; it does come with a removal stylet, though, which provides stabilization of the ETT while the device is being removed. The air-Q was primarily designed as a routine SAD with intubating capabilities using standard ETTs, and unlike the LMA Fastrach it provides pediatric sizes. The device has proven to be a safe and effective conduit for intubation in the pediatric population, utilizing the fiberoptic-guided technique.[134] The Ambu Aura-i (see Fig. 24.34) is a disposable SAD primarily suited for conditions where intubation is not needed, but it has the capability to facilitate standard ETT passage for TI. The device has a built-in anatomically correct curve, incorporates a bite-resistant connector block, and comes in pediatric and adult sizes that are each color coded. As with all adjunctive airway equipment, intubating SADs should be used in routine cases to gain experience and ensure familiarity with the device and technique before its use is attempted in an emergent situation.

Several new LMAs have recently been developed that have intubating capabilities. The LMA Unique EVO (Teleflex, Wayne, PA) is a single-use SAD with a preformed curve to facilitate placement. It has an integrated bite block, a silicone cuff, and an integrated color-coded cuff pressure monitoring system. The Unique EVO comes in adult sizes only, and it can accommodate a 7- to 8-mm ETT. The LMA Protector (Teleflex, Wayne, PA) is a single-use SAD with a preformed rigid curve design that incorporates a dual gastric channel. The Protector is designed to channel high-volume, high-pressure gastric contents away from the airway, and it allows for the ability to suction secretions or gastric contents out of the airway upon removal of the device. The cuff and airway tube are made of silicone. The Protector also contains an integrated color-coded cuff pressure monitoring system and an elongated cuff purported to create a more secure esophageal seal. This SAD comes in adult sizes and allows a 6.5- to 7.5-mm ETT and a 16- to 18-French gastric tube.

Supraglottic Tubes

Several supraglottic tubes (also known as retroglottic or infraglottic tubes) have been developed over the past several years. Devices in this class include the Combitube, King LT airway, Rusch Easy Tube, and LaryVent. These devices are placed blindly through the mouth and positioned into the esophagus. These tubes have a distal balloon to occlude the esophagus and a larger proximal balloon to occlude the posterior oropharynx. Between the two balloons is a ventilation port at approximately the level of the trachea. These devices can be used for both rescue and routine management, and for prehospital difficult airway situations.

The Combitube is a double-lumen airway device that is inserted blindly into the hypopharynx. This device contains an esophageal lumen and a tracheal lumen. The esophageal lumen has a blocked distal port and perforations at the pharyngeal level, whereas the tracheal lumen has only an open distal end. Regardless of tracheal or esophageal placement, the lungs may be ventilated. The most important factor when using the Combitube is to determine which ventilation port is actually ventilating the airway, which can be difficult. The availability of newer SADs has led to a decrease in the use of the Combitube.

Supraglottic Device Considerations

Familiarity with the different SAD models, their ease and speed of insertion, and their high likelihood of success in difficult airway situations make them an extremely valuable airway rescue device. A significant concern with the use of SADs is the possibility of aspiration during insertion and ventilation. Inflation of the stomach with air, regurgitation, and aspiration of gastric contents are all possible complications associated with SAD use; however, the incidence of aspiration has proven to be small, at 1 to 2 per 10,000 cases.[135] Furthermore, with the use of second-generation SADs, the risk of aspiration may be further reduced.

These devices can also be malpositioned or cuffs overinflated, resulting in failure to ventilate the patient. Malpositioning of the LMA and overinflation of the cuff may result in a disruption of the seal over the glottis, could disrupt the function of the gastric drainage port, or may create additional pressure to the sidewalls of the pharynx and posterior wall of the larynx. If this occurs, the epiglottis can be pushed back against the glottic opening, obstructing the airway.

Pathology at or below the laryngeal level may render SADs ineffective as a ventilation device. Indeed, LMA failures have been reported with both obstructions within the hypopharynx and obstructions below the hypopharynx, such as subglottic obstructions (e.g., tracheal thrombosis, tracheal stenosis, tumors), obstetric patients, aspiration, or severe rheumatoid arthritis.[15,136]

In obstetric anesthesia, the LMA is used when TI has failed and ventilation with a facemask is difficult or impossible. In the "cannot intubate and cannot oxygenate" scenario, the LMA (or another SAD of choice) should be attempted prior to a cricothyroidotomy. Finally, SAD use in nonsupine positions should be used with caution and evaluated on a case-by-case basis according to the situation. Insertion of a SAD can be challenging in the lateral and prone positions, and may lead to failed placement or failed ventilation.

Intubation Stylets

Trachlite Lighted Stylet

The Trachlite (Laerdal Medical, Wappingers Falls, NY) (Fig. 24.38) is a lighted stylet that uses transillumination of the neck to accomplish endotracheal intubation. As the light source enters the glottis opening, a well-defined circumscribed glow is noticed below the thyroid prominence and can be readily seen on the anterior neck. Placement of the Trachlite in the esophagus results in a much more diffuse transillumination of the neck without this circumscribed glow. The Trachlite utilizes a bright light source that does not require low ambient light for optimum performance. In addition, a retractable stylet helps to increase intubation success.

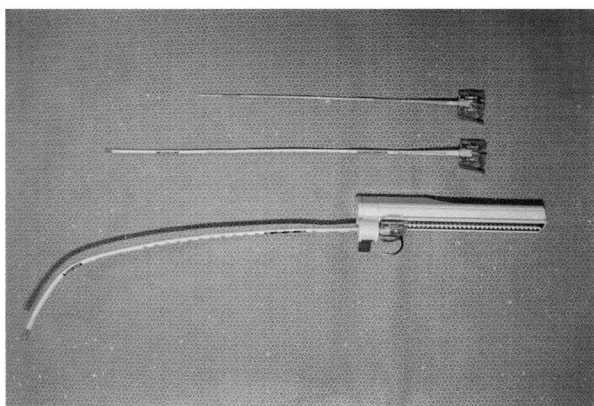

Fig. 24.38 Trachlite lighted stylet.

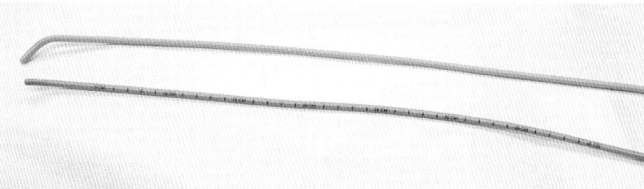

Fig. 24.39 Eschmann stylet or gum elastic bougie.

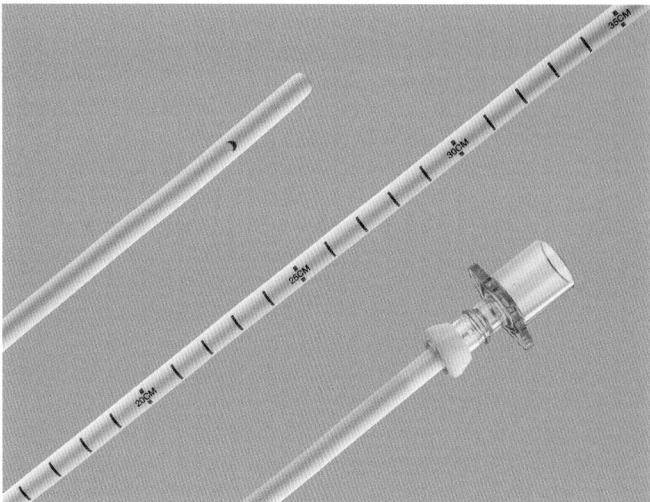

Fig. 24.40 Cook airway exchange catheter. (From Cook Medical Incorporated, Bloomington, IN.)

The device is less affected by anterior placement of the larynx, is less stimulating than conventional laryngoscopy, and may be associated with a lower incidence of sore throat. The Trachlite may be used in patients with a small oral opening or minimal neck manipulation, and it can be used in both the anticipated and the unanticipated difficult airway when conventional laryngoscopy has failed.

The risk of pharyngeal injury or failure is increased, and the Trachlite is not recommended, with any upper airway anomaly such as foreign body, tumor, polyps, or soft tissue injuries. Furthermore, it may be more difficult to accurately place and see the Trachlite in patients with short, thick necks or redundant soft tissue. Since the advent of fiberoptic stylets, videolaryngoscopes, and disposable FIS the use of transillumination to facilitate intubation has declined. Furthermore, several difficult and failed airway algorithms do not recommend blind intubation techniques because of the risk of oro- and hypo-pharyngeal mucosal injury. In 2009, Laerdal decided to cease production of the Trachlite stylet and tracheal lightwand.

Eschmann Stylet (Gum Elastic Bougie)

The Eschmann stylet (Fig. 24.39) is a 15-French flexible stylet that is 60 cm in length with a 40-degree bent distal tip. The stylet is used when the glottic opening is difficult to visualize (e.g., Cormack and Lehane grade IIb or III). Placement first involves visualization of the epiglottis or posterior arytenoid cartilages. The stylet is advanced behind the epiglottis and placed into the glottic opening. Feeling the stylet "bounce" along the tracheal rings as it is advanced into the trachea helps to confirm placement, but it is not always felt. The stylet should be advanced until the 25-cm marking is at the lip, where the stylet is then held in place. An ETT is inserted over the stylet and slid into the trachea. If resistance is felt, the ETT can be rotated 90 degrees to the left and then advanced. An alternative technique is to advance the ETT over the tracheal-placed Eschmann stylet until the ETT is in the oropharynx. DL or VL is then performed while an assistant holds the stylet in place. The ETT is then advanced through the glottic opening and into the trachea. Care should be taken not to advance the Eschmann stylet further into the trachea and risk bronchial or distal tracheal puncture. The Eschmann stylet or "bougie stylet" may be utilized during several potential clinical scenarios, including (but not limited to) (1) aiding advancement of an ETT during VL, (2) guiding ETT placement during difficult TI, (3) during tracheal extubation when it can be left in situ, and (4) during open surgical cricothyrotomy when it can facilitate tracheal tube placement.

Airway Exchange Catheters

Airway exchange catheters (AECs) facilitate the interchanging of an existing ETT and/or extubating the trachea. These catheters are capable of gas exchange using either jet ventilation or oxygen insufflation from an adapter and bag mask (Fig. 24.40). The AEC is introduced through the existing ETT with the distal tip placed proximal to the carina.[137] The ETT can then be removed and the new ETT placed over the AEC, which acts as a stylet guide into the trachea. If the new ETT encounters resistance or a "hang-up" during advancement, withdrawing the ETT 2 to 3 cm and rotating it 90 degrees may facilitate passage. If ETT placement was initially difficult, the AEC can be left in the trachea after the extubation of a difficult airway in the event that the patient requires reintubation. Care should be taken not to advance the AEC distally into either of the mainstem bronchi or to exert excessive force, which could result in a tracheal or bronchial perforation. If jet insufflation is used with the AEC, then muscle paralysis should be considered to prevent glottic closure. An oral airway device (or other airway device that promotes airway opening) can assist with maintenance of an open airway and gas egress.

Flexible Scopes and Fiberoptic Stylets

Scopes can be either flexible or rigid and assist with the placement of ETTs through visual confirmation. These devices can be used during routine airway management but are more frequently employed when the airway is expected to be difficult or during management of an unanticipated difficult airway.

Flexible (Fiberoptic) Intubating Scopes (FIS)

Flexible intubating scopes (FIS) were once known as fiberoptic bronchoscopes because they originally consisted of multiple strands of tiny glass fibers that transmit light. These fibers were bound together inside a rubberized coating that allowed for flexibility. Today these flexible scopes have a camera at the distal end of the flexible tip that transmits images to an external screen for viewing. Flexible intubating scopes can be used to evaluate the airway, facilitate awake intubation in a patient with an identified difficult airway, check ETT placement, change an existing ETT, and perform postextubation evaluations. Within the FIS are working channels that can carry oxygen, act as suction ports, or be used to instill local anesthetic. The handle contains a lever for controlling the distal end of the scope through one plane (either up or down). The second plane is navigated using side-to-side rotation of the scope by the operator's hand and wrist. Light is supplied by an external light source or by the viewing monitor.

The limitations of intubation using FIS should be considered prior to performing this procedure, but ultimately the decision to proceed is based on the anesthetist's clinical judgment and experience with these devices. Limitations of FIS include the following:

- Impaired viewing due to fogging, especially if the flexible scope is cold. Soaking the scope in warm saline, using an antifog liquid, or placing the scope in the buccal mucosa below the patient's lip for 5 seconds before use may help prevent fogging.
- Copious secretions or blood can obstruct the operator's view. This may be prevented with the instillation of oxygen at 10 to 15 L/min through one of the side channels or with effective suctioning.
- The FIS should be used with extreme caution in patients with epiglottitis, laryngotracheitis, or bacterial tracheitis because aggressive contact with inflamed tissue may cause a partial obstruction to convert into a total airway obstruction.
- Caution should be used in patients with airway burns because of the hyperirritability of the airway.
- The use of the FIS is very limited in airway trauma since the presence of blood, tissue, and mucus in the airway may obscure the lens and make visualization impossible. Adequate visualization of the larynx and trachea may also be difficult if significant soft tissue trauma is present resulting in tissue edema.
- Lack of patient cooperation may make awake flexible intubation difficult, if not impossible.
- In hypoxic situations where both intubation and ventilation have failed and immediate airway access is required, it may be prudent to attempt a different airway technique because of time constraints.

Indications for use of the FIS include the following:

- *An anticipated difficult airway.* These patients usually have a history of intubation difficulty and upper airway obstructions such as angioedema, tumors, abscesses, hematomas, Ludwig angina, or lingual hyperplasia.
- *Cervical spine immobilization.* For example, patients with traumatic cervical injuries, an unstable cervical spine, or a cervical spine with a severely decreased range of motion.
- *Anatomic abnormalities of the upper airway.* Patients with a restricted mouth opening or hypoplastic mandible or who are morbidly obese may fall into this category.
- *Failed intubation attempt, but ventilation possible with a mask or SAD.* In these unanticipated difficult airway situations, the operator has time to set up and perform the flexible intubation technique using either an endoscopy mask or SAD as a conduit for the flexible scope.

The FIS can be used for oral or nasal intubation, with the patient either awake or asleep. An awake flexible intubation is most commonly performed for an anticipated difficult airway. Preparation for an awake flexible intubation includes educating the patient regarding what to expect, removing or drying up secretions, anesthetizing the patient's airway, and providing adequate sedation.

Topical anesthesia, nerve blocks, or a combination of the two can be used to anesthetize a patient's airway. Several drying agents and sedation options exist. Radiation can cause fibrosis and loss of mucus-producing glands, so drying of the airway can be extensive with the use of an antisialagogue in this patient population. Either atropine or

glycopyrrolate may be administered 5 to 20 minutes before the procedure. Another option is to use suction and gauze to dry up existing secretions immediately prior to anesthetizing the airway. Administration of light sedation may help reduce the patient's stress and provide for a calmer environment. Several options exist, including midazolam, ketamine, propofol, dexmedetomidine, fentanyl, or remifentanil.[138] However, carefully titrated amounts, using small bolus doses, should be considered to avoid hypoventilation and oversedation.

Preparation for flexible intubation is important. Appropriate suction devices, equipment, and medications should be readily available. Success with a FIS is dependent on familiarity and experience with the device. This may be accomplished with continued training using intubation manikins, or high-fidelity patient simulators, or during routine airway management in the clinical setting.[139] With oral intubations, FIS guide (such as the Williams, Berman, or Ovassapian airway) facilitates placement of the scope into the pharyngeal area and can help prevent damage to the shaft of the scope if the patient were to bite down (Fig. 24.41). The operator can perform the technique either at the head of the bed with the patient in the supine position or from the side of the bed using a frontal approach with the patient in a sitting position (Fig. 24.42). The sitting technique may help prevent tissues from falling against the posterior pharynx (impeding flexible endoscopic views), may help decrease anxiety in an awake patient, and has been used in patients with upper airway masses that compress the airway.[140]

An ETT is first loaded onto the FIS and is then inserted through either the mouth or nose and advanced to the posterior pharynx. The larger the ratio between the flexible scope shaft and the internal diameter size of the ETT, the more the potential for hang-up of the ETT on airway structures. The scope can be manipulated in two planes by adjusting the lever on the handle up or down and by rotating the scope laterally with the wrist. The dominant hand holds the handle with the arm bent and resting on the operator's shoulder or positioned to look through the eyepiece on the handle while the other hand holds the distal portion of the scope to keep it taut (see Fig. 24.42). Care must be taken to keep the FIS in the midline while the tip is advanced toward the epiglottis. The operator should be able to visualize the different airway structures (if not using a flexible scope guide) as the scope is advanced through the oropharyngeal, pharyngeal, and laryngeal spaces. If at any point the view is lost and the operator is unsure of the scope's location in the airway, it should be retracted until identifiable airway anatomy is visualized. Insufflation of oxygen through the suction port not only aids in the oxygenation of the patient but also helps keep the optics clear. The tip of the FIS is delivered through the glottic opening and advanced until the tracheal rings come into view. The ETT is then advanced downward through the cords into the trachea, with the FIS used as a stylet. If hang-up is encountered, the ETT should be slightly retracted, rotated 90 degrees, and then advanced. The ETT should never be forced into the airway because this may cause vocal cord trauma. After the ETT is advanced into the trachea, the operator can verify placement by visualization of the carina.

Suctioning is difficult through the suction port. A more advantageous use of this channel is to provide the patient with supplemental oxygen. A 2- to 4-L flow through this port can provide additional oxygen to the patient and keeps debris from collecting on or near the port and lens. The administration of local anesthesia through the port or through an epidural catheter threaded down the port is another use of this channel.

Newer FIS, such as the Ambu aScope, are single patient use. For those FIS that are not single patient use, follow the manufacturers' recommended instructions for cleaning and disinfecting.

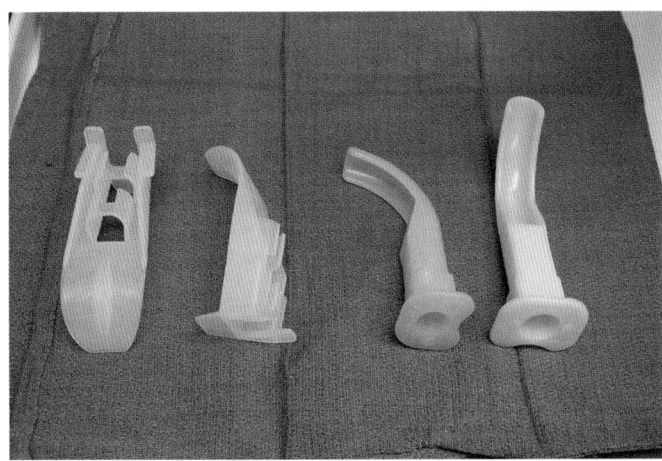

Fig. 24.41 Ovassapian (*left*) and Williams (*right*) airways.

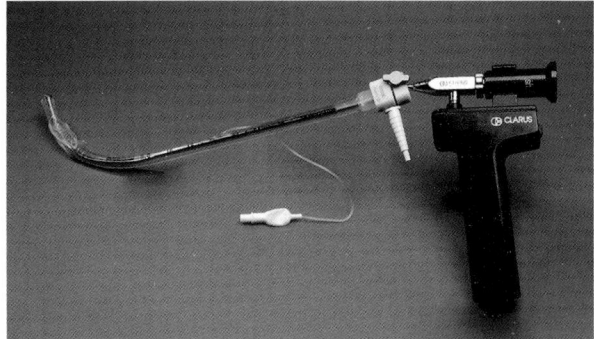

Fig. 24.43 Shikani optical stylet. (From Marx JA, et al., eds. *Rosen's Emergency Medicine*. 8th ed. St Louis: Elsevier; 2014:19.)

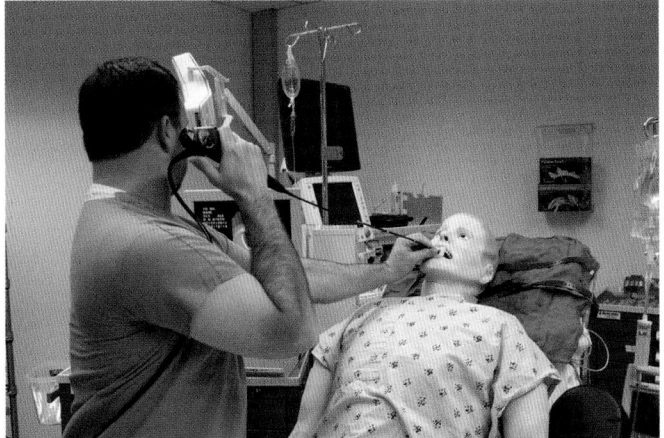

Fig. 24.42 FIS intubation technique (frontal approach).

Instructions regarding solution, dilution, soak times, and rinsing must be closely followed to ensure the integrity and longevity of the equipment.

Rigid and Semirigid Fiberoptic Stylets and Laryngoscopes

Rigid and semirigid fiberoptic stylets and laryngoscope devices can be used in difficult airway situations, when intubation has failed, or during routine airway management.[141],[142] These devices provide the operator with an indirect view of the glottic opening through a transmitted image via a fiberoptic bundle that is enclosed in a preformed design. The use of both rigid and semirigid fiberoptic stylets allows the operator to see around the tongue, which makes them suitable for patients with limited cervical spine mobility. Trauma to the airway and a limited mouth opening are other indications for these devices. Examples of semirigid fiberoptic stylets include the Shikani optical stylet (SOS) and the Levitan First Pass Success (LFPS) scope. Rigid stylets include the Bonfils Retromolar Intubation Fiberscope (Karl Storz Endoscopy, Tuttlingen, Germany), the airway rigid intubation fiberscope laryngoscope (RIFL), and the Bullard laryngoscope. Indications and limitations with the use of these devices are similar to those described for the flexible intubating endoscope.

Shikani optical stylet and Levitan FPS. The SOS (Fig. 24.43) is a malleable, semirigid, intubating fiberoptic stylet that is useful in both adult and pediatric populations. It features a battery-operated light source with a high-resolution eyepiece on the handle that is then attached to a stylet. The SOS also has the ability to insufflate oxygen into the pharynx via an oxygen port connector. The malleable distal end allows configuration for varying intubation angles; this can be particularly useful for patients with a rigid or unstable cervical spine. The SOS can be used alone or in conjunction with DL.[143]

The LFPS is similar to the SOS but is intended to be used with a standard laryngoscope. Laryngoscopy is first performed with a standard laryngoscope. If the glottis opening is visualized, the LFPS can be used as a stylet to directly intubate the trachea. However, if only the epiglottis is visualized, the LFPS is placed into the airway below and posterior to the epiglottic edge. The operator then looks through the eyepiece to visualize airway structures and advance the stylet through the vocal cords. This semirigid scope has a malleable stylet to facilitate passage into the trachea. The stylet is 30 cm in length with a 5-mm diameter. Similar to the SOS, the LFPS has an oxygen port for insufflation.

Bonfils Retromolar Intubation Fiberscope and RIFL. These devices have a rigid anatomic shape with a fiberoptic bundle that affords an indirect view of the vocal cords. The rigid anatomic shape allows for visualization and intubation of the airway without aligning the oral, pharyngeal, and tracheal axes. These devices can be used on either an awake or an anesthetized patient. Because they do not require the sniffing position, they are ideal for patients with limited range of motion of the neck, such as those in cervical collars. Most have a channel for insufflation of oxygen while performing intubation and a small combination battery pack that permits portability.

The Bonfils fiberoptic stylet has a rigid shaft that is 40 cm long, has an anterior bend of approximately 45 degrees, and is meant to be advanced in the airway using a retromolar approach. Advancement of the ETT occurs after the stylet has passed through the vocal cords.

The RIFL is a hybrid design incorporating a rigid stylet that ends with a flexible tip. This scope can be adjusted up to 135 degrees with the use of a trigger on the handle as the device is advanced into the airway. The distal tip is manipulated as the operator slowly advances the stylet until it passes through the vocal cords, where the ETT is then advanced over the RIFL and placed into the trachea.

Videolaryngoscopy

VL has been described as the most significant advancement for intubation of the trachea since the development of the laryngoscope in the 1940s.[144] VL devices include illumination and a micro video camera on the laryngoscope blade, which enables the transmission of video images to an external viewing screen. Glottic visualization is indirectly accomplished, and TI is performed while the operator views the external monitor. VL is a popular choice for anticipated difficult airways and as a rescue for unexpected difficulty. Indeed, some researchers have found that video-assisted laryngoscopy provides improved visualization of the larynx over standard laryngoscopy.[75,145] VL can be learned quickly and has several advantages:

- Magnification of the airway allows the operator to visualize airway structures in greater detail.
- Blade design and anterior angulation, along with placement of the video camera on the distal portion of the blade, permit the operator to visualize structures that would otherwise be difficult or impossible to see under DL.
- The external monitor allows other practitioners to visualize airway anatomy and understand current airway conditions.
- The recording capabilities allow for education, documentation, and research.

Disadvantages of VL include cost, which can be significant, or the unavailability of the VL device. As with other optic devices, blood and secretions can obscure the viewing of airway structures. Pharyngeal injuries, such as anterior tonsil pillar, soft palate, or palatopharyngeal arch perforation, can occur from indirect ETT advancement and stylets.[147,148] In addition, indirect placement of the ETT into the glottic opening while viewing an external monitor can prove difficult. No specific VL device is recommended over another; however, speed, simplicity, reliability, and efficiency are desirable characteristics to be considered.[149] Finally, with the advent of this new technology, a debate exists regarding whether DL or VL (indirect) is better. Ultimately this is dependent on the provider's experience and competency, and many researchers recommend maintaining proficiency with both DL and VL techniques since either can act as a rescue if the other fails.[150]

GlideScope Videolaryngoscope

The GlideScope (Fig. 24.44) is perhaps the most widely used VL and has been shown to provide a laryngoscopic view equal to or better than DL without manipulation of the head into a sniffing position.[151,152] The GlideScope system provides standard geometry blades as well as hyperangulated blades with a distal 60-degree anterior bend. A camera is located in the middle part of the blade and transmits a signal via a video cable to a separate external liquid crystal display (LCD) monitor. In addition, the newest GlideScope system provides flexible intubating endoscope capabilities along with VL. The GlideScope features an antifog system that heats the lens around the video camera, preventing fogging of the device during laryngoscopy. Multiple models have been developed, such as the portable GlideScope Ranger intended for prehospital and military field use and the GlideScope Cobalt, which incorporates a disposable one-time use blade over a lighted video baton.

When performing video-assisted laryngoscopy with this device, the blade should be inserted midline; as soon as the tip of the blade is past the teeth, the operator should begin viewing the LCD monitor to identify the different airway structures and navigate to the glottic aperture. The blade should ultimately be placed into the vallecula, followed by a gentle tilt of the handle to allow visualization of the vocal cords. An accompanying rigid stylet is recommended with the use of the GlideScope to facilitate ETT delivery into the trachea. An alternative method is to bend the ETT and regular stylet at a right angle just proximal to the cuff. The ETT is inserted into the right side of the mouth by direct visualization and is advanced to the oropharynx. The operator should then view the monitor and slowly introduce the ETT using gentle forward semicircular rotation to align the tip of the ETT with the glottic opening. Once aligned, the ETT should be advanced through the vocal cords under video visualization.[146] At this point, the stylet may be withdrawn to help assist with the advancement of the ETT. The GlideScope should be cleaned before each use following the manufacturer's recommendations.

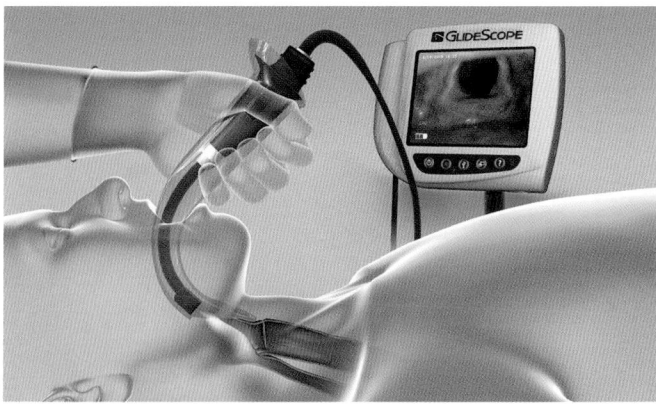

Fig. 24.44 GlideScope AVL Single Use in airway. (Used with permission, Verathon. Inc.)

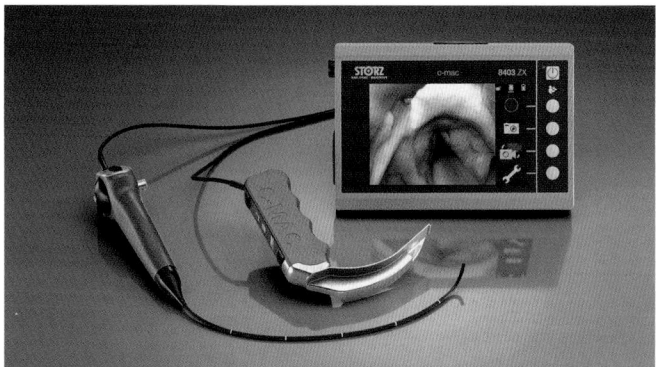

Fig. 24.45 The C-MAC videolaryngoscope with option for fiberoptic bronchoscope addition. (© KARL STORZ SE & Co. KG, Germany.)

Karl Storz C MAC Videolaryngoscope

The C-MAC videolaryngoscope system provides blade designs similar to both the standard Macintosh and Miller blades (i.e., standard geometry) as well as hyperangulated blades (Fig. 24.45). The insertion and technique using the standard blade designs is similar to DL, with the added benefit of VL, if needed. The VL handle device includes illumination and a distally placed micro video camera that resists fogging and provides an enhanced field of view. In addition, the C-MAC system incorporates videorecording that can be used for education and documentation as well as flexible endoscopy if desired. The C-MAC system has proven to be useful in patients with predicted difficult airways.[153]

McGrath Videolaryngoscope

The McGrath VL is a portable device that was initially released into clinical practice in 2007. The McGrath Series 5 VL (Fig. 24.46) requires one AA battery, whereas the newer McGrath Mac requires a proprietary 3.6-V lithium battery pack for self-contained power. Both include a rotational color LCD screen attached to the handle. A single-use disposable laryngoscope blade sleeve fits over the light source, and the Series 5 sleeve is adjustable to three different positions. The McGrath Mac blade design is similar to standard geometry blades, whereas the Series 5 is a modification of the Macintosh blade and has a similar distal hyperangulated angle. In addition, similar to the GlideScope, a semirigid or rigid stylet is recommended to assist with the placement of an ETT when using the Series 5 hyperangulated blade. The McGrath does not have an antifog mechanism but does incorporate a hydrophilic optical surface coating to minimize condensation on the light.

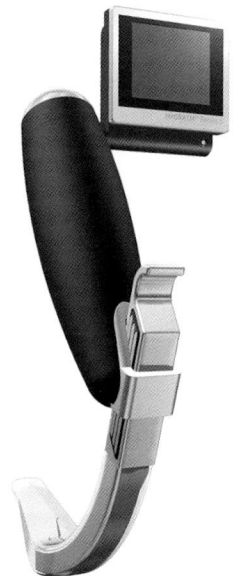

Fig. 24.46 McGrath Series 5 scope. (Courtesy LMA North America.)

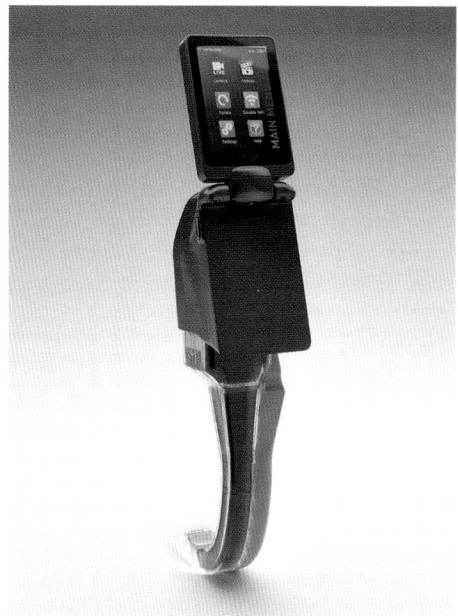

Fig. 24.48 Airtraq visualization. (Courtesy Prodol Meditec.)

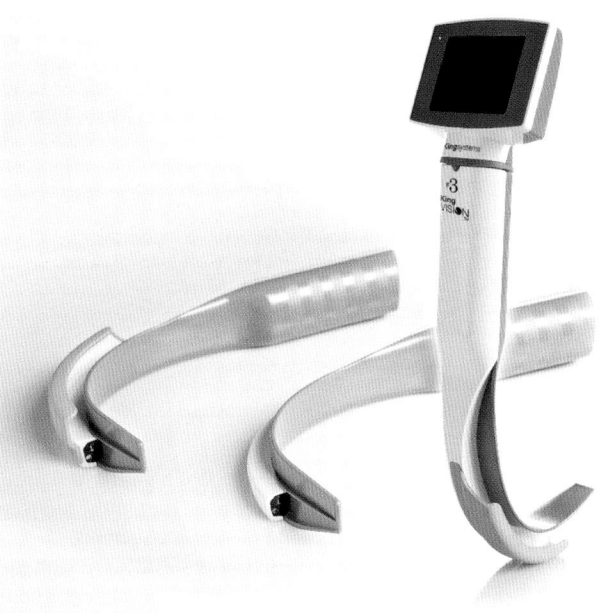

Fig. 24.47 King Vision. (Courtesy Ambu.)

The device is extremely portable and can be transported out of the OR easily as both the camera and monitor are built into the device.

Channel Scope Devices

The Pentax Airway Scope, the Res-Q-Scope II, and the King Vision (Fig. 24.47) incorporate a small video screen into the handle of each device. All use disposable blades with a near 90-degree distal bend. All allow for the preloading of an ETT into an integrated channel within the blade prior to airway manipulation. These devices can be used in patients with limited or no cervical spine mobility, in prehospital situations where space around the patient is limited, or during difficult airway management. None incorporate antifog capabilities, although the plastic material is purported to limit (but not eliminate) fogging. These devices are less-expensive alternatives than the previously mentioned VLs; however, lens contamination by fogging and blood or secretions

severely limits their viewing capabilities. Several reports support their use in difficult airway situations.[154,155]

The Airtraq (Fig. 24.48) is an optically enhanced laryngoscope that uses a series of mirrors, prisms, and lenses to magnify and enhance the laryngeal view. Like other channel and VL devices, the Airtraq is designed to provide a view of the glottic opening without manipulating the neck into a sniffing position. The blade of the Airtraq has two channels. The first channel has a lighted, heated lens; the second channel is for passage of an ETT up to a diameter of 8.5 mm. The Airtraq has a unique system that provides antifogging when the light-emitting diode (LED) is on for at least 30 seconds. There is an optional video camera that clips onto the viewfinder. When compared to standard laryngoscopy, the Airtraq was successful in achieving faster TI times, a reduced number of intubation attempts, and fewer hemodynamic changes.[156]

Subglottic Interventions and Emergency Front-of-Neck Access

With the advent of SADs, VL, and other effective airway rescue devices, the need for invasive airway access, such as a cricothyrotomy, has decreased. However, regular training and practice in emergency front-of-neck access and subglottic airway techniques continues to be important.[69,83] This is particularly true with failed intubation and subsequent failed oxygenation situations. When this occurs, the anesthesia provider must be familiar with, and avoid any delay in, the steps required for emergency subglottic airway access such as surgical cricothyrotomy or needle cricothyrotomy with transtracheal jet ventilation (TTJV). An elective cricothyrotomy can be considered in situations such as trauma or obstructive pathology, where access to the upper airway is limited.

Indications for cricothyrotomy include but are not limited to (1) failed airway (e.g., cannot intubate and subsequently cannot oxygenate); (2) traumatic injuries of maxillofacial, cervical spine, head, or neck structures that make intubation through the nose or mouth difficult to impossible or too time consuming; (3) immediate relief of an upper airway obstruction; and (4) the need for a definitive airway for neck or facial surgery, assuming intubation is not possible. There is no absolute contraindication for a cricothyrotomy in an emergency. Relative contraindications include preexisting laryngeal or tracheal diseases such as tumors, infections, or abscesses in the location of the cricothyroid membrane, distortion of neck anatomy (e.g., hematoma), bleeding diathesis, and history of coagulopathy.[158] Cricothyrotomy techniques are performed by perforating the cricothyroid membrane using either a needle or scalpel and establishing airflow into the trachea. The cricothyroid membrane is a fibroelastic membrane located inferior to the thyroid cartilage and superior to the cricoid cartilage. The three types of cricothyrotomy procedures are (1) needle cricothyrotomy with TTJV, (2) percutaneous (or wire guided) cricothyrotomy, and (3) the open surgical cricothyrotomy.

Identification of the cricothyroid membrane can be difficult in some patients, resulting in misplacement (e.g., inferior or superior to the cricothyroid membrane). The use of ultrasound as a means to correctly locate the cricothyroid membrane has shown promise (see Figs. 24.14 and 24.15) and may be considered in those patients with anticipated difficult airways prior to any airway manipulation.[159,160]

Needle Cricothyrotomy With Transtracheal Jet Ventilation

TTJV is the ventilation technique that should be attempted after the placement of a needle cricothyrotomy through the cricothyroid membrane. The procedure is performed using a large bore needle (such as a large bore angiocatheter [18 guage or larger], Ravussin needle, or Cook Emergency Transtracheal Airway Catheter) or a venous or arterial angiocatheter. Caution should be taken when using IV angiocatheters because these devices are at risk of kinking and obstruction. Consideration should be given to the use of catheters made specifically for needle cricothyrotomy that are more kink resistant. Ventilation through a catheter requires a jet injector powered by an oxygen source (Fig. 24.49). Needle cricothyrotomy with TTJV may be considered in "cannot intubate cannot oxygenate" situations. Evidence has demonstrated a significant failure rate with needle cricothyrotomy and TTJV in the emergency "cannot intubate cannot oxygenate" situation, and instead favors other cricothyrotomy techniques since these can be performed quickly and provides a larger, more secure airway.[69,157] Instead, needle cricothyrotomy and TTJV should be reserved for those airways where the anatomy is less favorable for placement of other cricothyrotomy techniques (e.g., small children age <12 years) or as a temporary means of ventilation.[158]

The needle cricothyrotomy procedure can be accomplished quickly using a large-bore catheter (≥18 gauge) inserted through the cricothyroid membrane (Fig. 24.50; see also Fig. 24.27). Once the catheter is in the airway, the lungs are ventilated using a high-pressure oxygen source with a regulating valve to control oxygen flow, but at low frequencies to avoid air trapping and barotrauma. A common frequency is between 8 and 10 breaths per minute allowing enough time for air to escape, which is confirmed with visual chest recoil prior to delivering a new breath. This requires I:E ratios of 1:3 or 1:4, with special attention focused on limiting the inspiratory time to 0.5 to 1 second to avoid high intrathoracic pressures.

Barotrauma is a significant concern because high-pressure oxygen is delivered through central wall outlets and high-flow (50–100 psi) tank regulators. Therefore, vigilant monitoring of psi pressures and a focus on longer expiratory times should occur during TTJV.[161] Most jet ventilators have a regulator that allows for changes in applied inspiratory pressures. To avoid barotrauma, inspiratory pressures should not exceed 50 psi on the regulator, and in most instances 25 to 50 psi is sufficient. A 1-second inspiration at 25 psi with a rate of 10 breaths per minute delivers between 0.5 and 1 L/sec of volume. Exhalation occurs passively through the upper airway. Obstructions to passive exhalation or excessively large tidal volumes result in hyperinflation and incomplete exhalation of CO_2 and have been shown to be a common occurrence with needle cricothyrotomies.[161] Placement of bilateral nasal airways, an oral airway, or even a SAD may facilitate exhalation and the

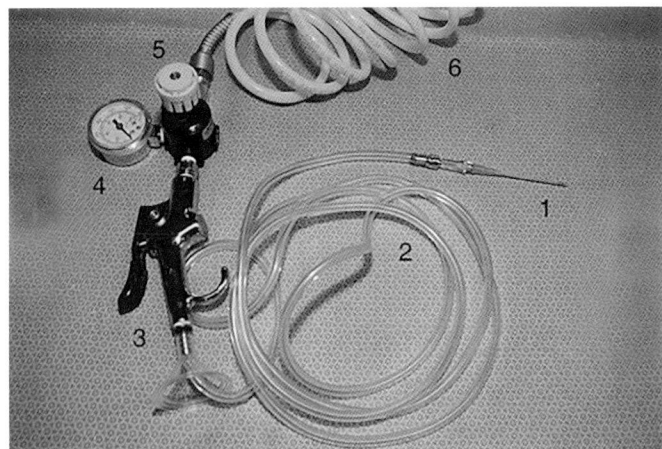

Fig. 24.49 Transtracheal jet ventilation system assembly: *(1)* intravenous angiocatheter, *(2)* small-bore tubing assembly with Luer-lock fitting, *(3)* manual on/off valve, *(4)* pressure gauge (e.g., psi), *(5)* adjustable pressure regulator, and *(6)* high-pressure hose assembly, with Diameter Index Safety System oxygen fitting *(not shown)*.

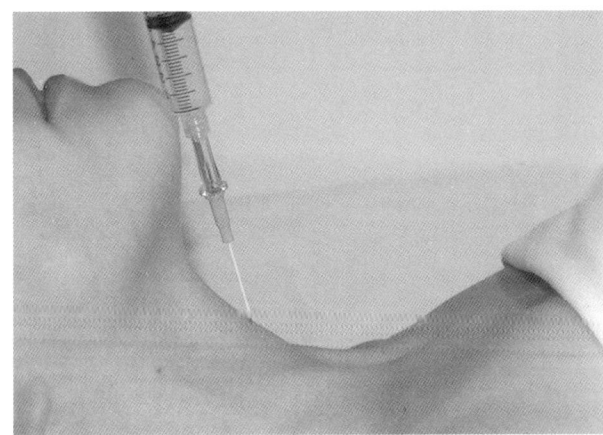

Fig. 24.50 Insertion of needle for transtracheal jet ventilation.

egress of ventilated gases. Finally, it is possible that high tracheal pressures created from TTJV can potentially stent open the glottis, allowing for improved laryngoscopic identification of airway structures.

In addition to barotrauma, other complications associated with the use of TTJV include subcutaneous emphysema, pneumothorax, pneumomediastinum, hypercarbia, esophageal puncture, drying and damage of airway mucosa, blood or mucous obstruction, catheter kinking, and inadvertent removal.[82,158] Bilateral breath sounds and bilateral chest rise should be confirmed frequently to rule out pneumothorax or dislodgement of the catheter.

Percutaneous (Wire-Guided) Cricothyrotomy

This type of cricothyrotomy uses either a needle or sharp trocar to puncture the cricothyroid membrane and gain access to the trachea. Once in place a tracheal cannula is positioned within the trachea over a wire or trocar device. The percutaneous cricothyrotomy procedure will likely be performed using a cricothyrotomy kit.[162]

Absolute contraindications are rare; however, the anesthetist should consider avoiding both the percutaneous and open surgical cricothyrotomy procedures in favor of needle cricothyrotomy and TTJV in infants and small children younger than 12 years of age. The child's larynx is small, pliable, and movable, which can make cricothyrotomy very difficult in this population.

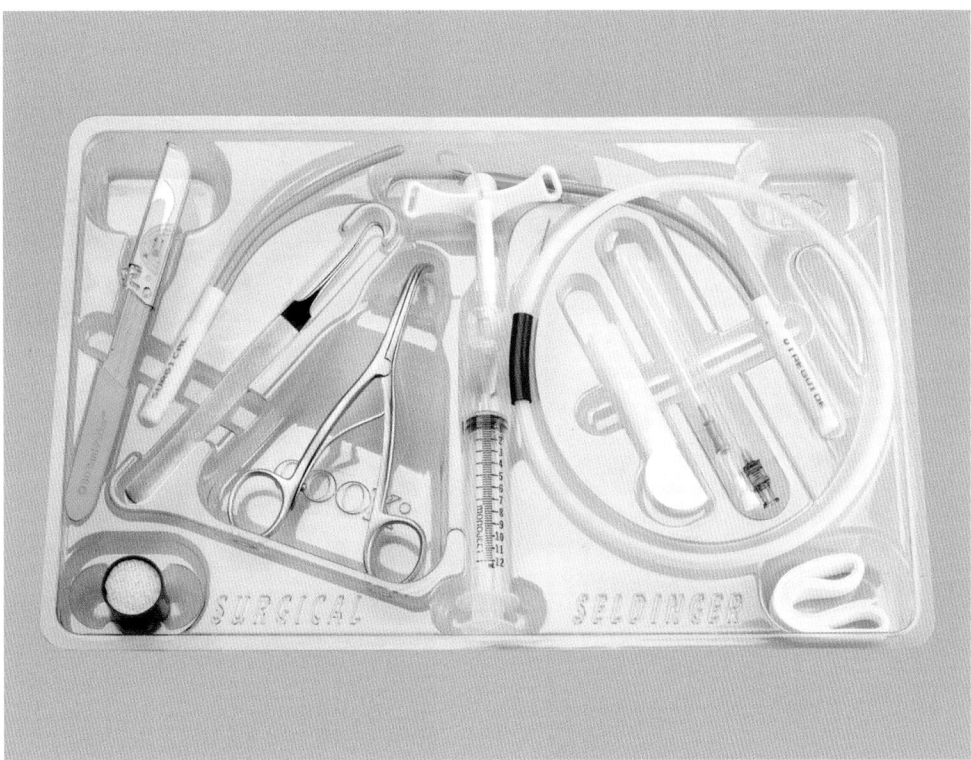

Fig. 24.51 Melker cricothyrotomy set. (From Cook Medical Incorporated.)

Complications related to the placement of a percutaneous cricothyrotomy are similar to those listed under the placement of a needle cricothyrotomy. Several cricothyrotomy kits are available, such as the Melker, the Quicktrach II, the Pertrach, and the Portex cricothyrotomy kit (PCK). The tracheal cannula is placed percutaneously using these kits either over a trocar or wire-guided using the Seldinger method. Both the Quicktrach II and PCK devices have a tracheostomy tube loaded over a trocar. The sequence of placing these devices over the trocar is as follows: (1) Check the tube cuff for air leaks, (2) palpate the cricothyroid membrane and stabilize it between the first two fingers (see Fig. 24.27 for palpation of the cricothyroid membrane), (3) insert the trocar/tube through the cricothyroid membrane at a 90-degree angle, (4) aspirate air and then advance the tracheostomy tube into the trachea, (5) remove the trocar and inflate the tube cuff, (6) confirm ventilation, and (7) secure the tube with a tracheostomy tie.

The Melker Universal Emergency Cricothyrotomy Catheter Set (Cook Critical Care, Bloomington, IN) is a commonly used percutaneous wire-guided cricothyrotomy kit. Fig. 24.51 shows a Melker cricothyrotomy kit that includes equipment for both open surgical and wire-guided techniques. The Melker kit comes in 3.5-, 4.0-, and 6.0-mm internal diameter (ID) cuffed and uncuffed tube sets. Each kit has a tracheal cannula that is fitted internally with a curved dilator. A 15-mm circuit adaptor is located at the end of the cannula and allows attachment to a bag-valve-mask or anesthesia circuit. A scalpel, syringe, introducer needle with and without a catheter, stiff guide wire, tracheal hook, and forceps are included if the kit provides the option for an open surgical technique. Tie tapes for securing the cricothyrotomy tube complete each kit.

The sequence of steps for placing a percutaneous wire-guided cricothyrotomy using the Seldinger technique is as follows:
1. Place the patient's head in a neutral position.
2. Open the proper tray and place it in a position that is comfortable and within reach for the person inserting the device. First, prepare the kit by inserting the dilator into the cricothyrotomy tube.

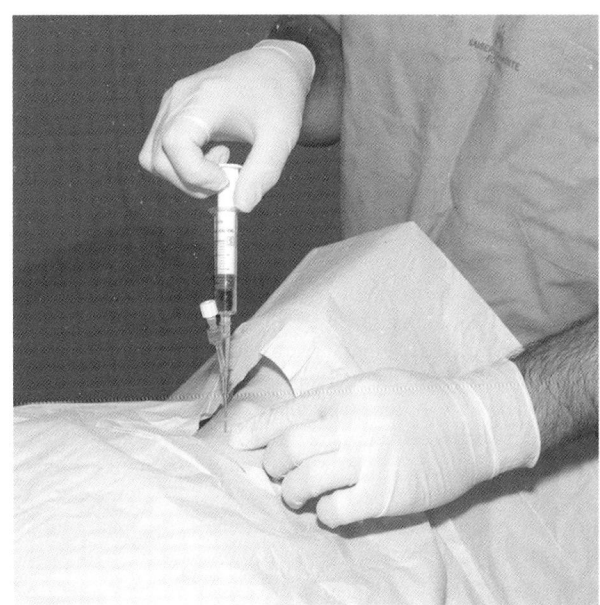

Fig. 24.52 Needle inserted through cricothyroid membrane in caudad direction with aspiration of air for confirmation of proper placement.

3. Palpate the cricothyroid membrane and then, using the introducer needle with the syringe attached, puncture the cricothyroid membrane at a 90-degree angle while aspirating with the syringe. Once air is aspirated, stop advancing the needle, and thread the catheter fully into the trachea. Attach the syringe to the catheter and again aspirate air (Fig. 24.52).
4. Insert the flexible end of the guide wire through the catheter until it is approximately 2 inches beyond the tip of the catheter (Fig. 24.53).

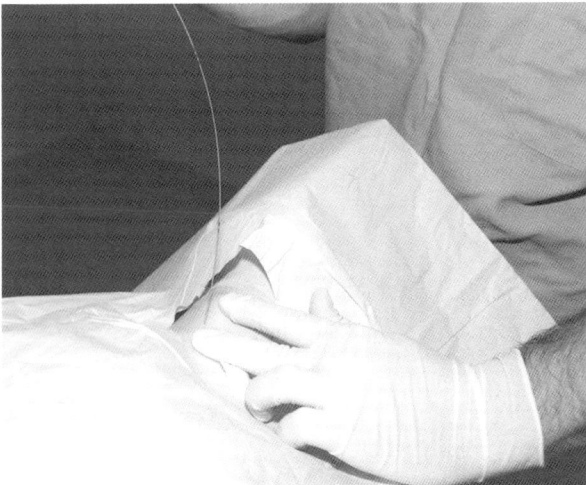

Fig. 24.53 Guide wire threaded through catheter in neck.

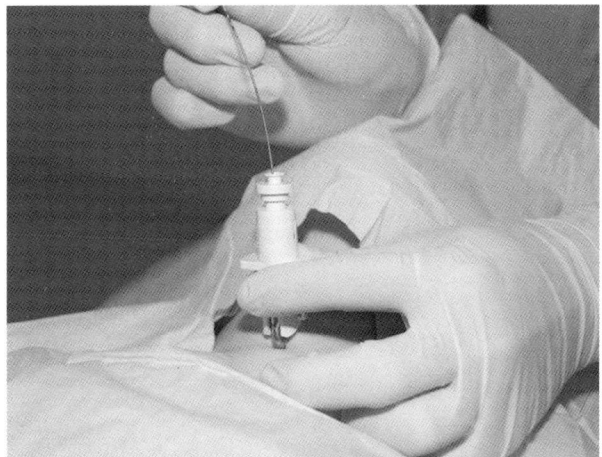

Fig. 24.55 Airway catheter/dilator threaded over guide wire, through cricothyroid membrane, and into the trachea.

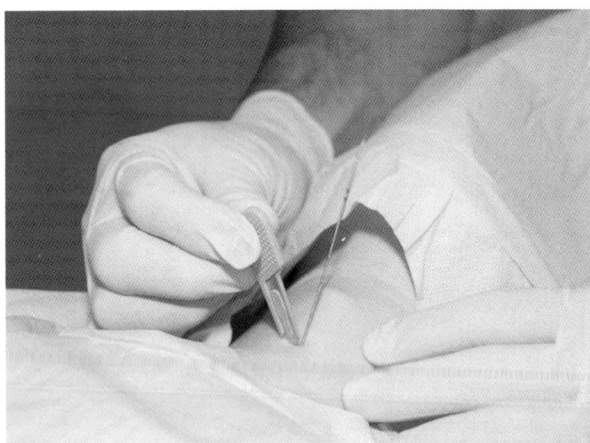

Fig. 24.54 Neck incised with scalpel along guide wire.

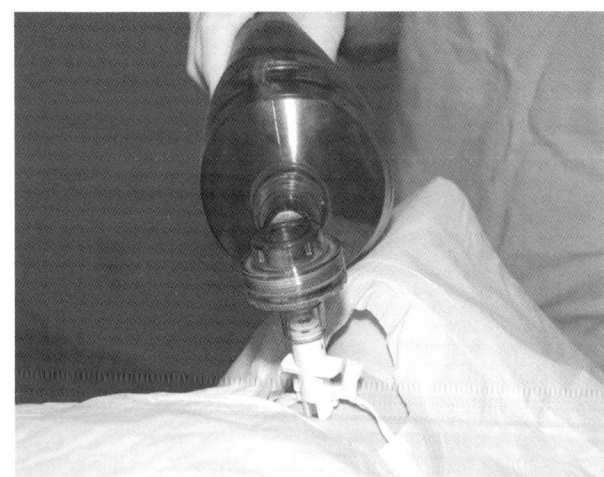

Fig. 24.56 Dilator and guide wire removed, allowing connection to a ventilation device.

5. Using the enclosed scalpel, incise the neck with a single insertion along the guide wire, with the sharp end of the blade away from the guide wire (Fig. 24.54).
6. Thread the cricothyrotomy dilator/tube over the exposed guide wire and advance to the incision. Apply steady pressure by pushing on the dilator. A loss of resistance may be felt, usually preceded by a "pop" as the catheter penetrates the cricothyroid membrane. Advance the cricothyrotomy tube off the dilator until the phalange rests firmly against the neck.
7. Remove the dilator and wire and assess for appropriate ventilation (Fig. 24.55).
8. Using sutures or the tape ties, secure the tube onto the neck while continuously ventilating the patient (Fig. 24.56).

Surgical Cricothyrotomy

A surgical cricothyrotomy is accomplished by cutting through the cricothyroid membrane with a scalpel and placing a cuffed tracheostomy tube or an ETT. Most airway algorithms and strategies recommend this procedure as a means of providing ventilation for patients who cannot be intubated or oxygenated with a facemask or SAD.[83,163]

An alternative surgical cricothyrotomy technique, known as the bougie-assisted cricothyrotomy or simply the scalpel-finger-bougie[164] technique, uses equipment found in most ORs (i.e., scalpel, bougie stylet, 6.0 Shiley tracheal tube, or a 6.0–6.5-mm ETT). The procedure is depicted in Fig. 24.57. If the cricothyroid membrane is difficult to palpate, then a vertical cut-down incision from the thyroid cartilage extending caudad several centimeters to the cricoid cartilage should allow palpation of the cricothyroid membrane within the incision. Once found with digital palpation, a transverse incision through the membrane is performed, and the inside of the cricothyroid cartilage is palpated with the nondominate index finger. At no point should the scalpel ever exist in the same plane as the operator's finger. A bougie is then advanced into the trachea over the pad of the operator's nondominant index finger while still in the incision, which verifies actual placement of the bougie within the trachea. The tube is then passed over the bougie and into the trachea.[164] A potential serious complication with this technique is false passage of the bougie and/or tube through a dissected pretracheal fascial layer of tissue. Verification of correct placement is essential and can be accomplished with visual bilateral chest rise and auscultation, but it is best verified with sustained positive end-tidal CO_2 capnography and/or with visual confirmation through the tube of the tracheal rings and carina using a flexible scope or another optical device (i.e., LFPS).

The decision to place a cricothyrotomy should never be delayed when indications are present.[76] Indeed, a review of closed-claims data for injuries related to invasive airway access suggested that failure to apply the technique early enough, before significant hypoxia developed, resulted in death or brain damage in two-thirds of the claims

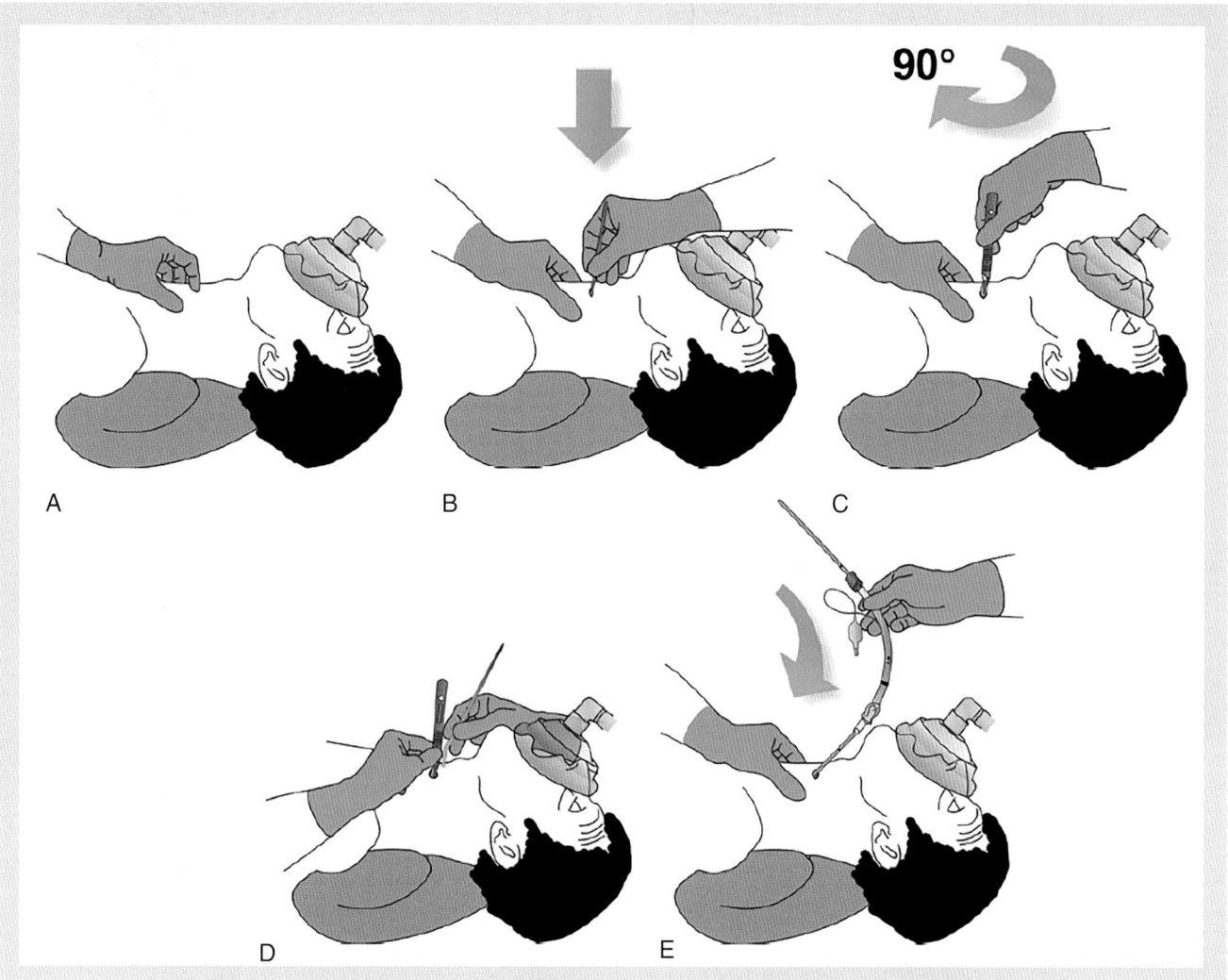

Fig. 24.57 Surgical cricothyrotomy technique with cricothyroid membrane palpable: Scalpel technique; "stab, twist, bougie, tube." (A) Identify cricothyroid membrane. (B) Make transverse stab incision through cricothyroid membrane. (C) Rotate scalpel so that sharp edge points caudally. (D) Pulling scalpel caudally to open up incision, slide coude tip of bougie down the scalpel blade into trachea. (E) Railroad 6.0-mm Shiley tracheal tube or 6.0- to 6.5-mm endotracheal tube over bougie into trachea. (From Frerk C, et al. Difficult Airway Society 2015 guidelines for management of unanticipated difficult intubation in adults. *Br J Anaesth.* 2015;115[6]:827–848. Used with permission.)

reviewed.[82] Furthermore, current airway algorithms suggest preparing for the possibility of cricothyrotomy early and promote verbalization of the failed airway and transition from one airway plan to the next in an effort to promote team situational awareness.[83] Most researchers advocate for regular training and practice in an effort to maintain proficiency with this critical skill.[83,165,166]

Retrograde Intubation

A retrograde wire-guided intubation is a front-of-neck access technique that can be considered in situations where intubation has failed but ventilation is possible. Indications can include impaired visualization of the vocal cords from blood, secretions, or anatomic anomalies; airway tumors; an unstable cervical spine; or upper airway trauma. A commercial kit is available for retrograde intubation, or the practitioner can choose to insert either a J-wire or #2 Mersilene suture thread via a cricothyrotomy and pass the device cephalad into the oropharynx. This procedure is performed by inserting a 14- to 18-gauge IV catheter or a Cook needle through the cricothyroid membrane and directing it cephalad.

After aspiration of air is confirmed, a wire or suture is then inserted through the needle and passed cephalad until it can be visualized in the posterior pharynx. It is then either advanced through the mouth or retrieved using Magill forceps. The distal end of the wire is secured with a clamp at the neck to prevent the wire from being pulled into the trachea prematurely. An ETT is then directed over the wire and passed into the trachea. As the tube enters the larynx, tension is increased on the wire or suture. Once the ETT is through the laryngeal opening and cannot pass further, the distal wire is removed at the level of the skin, and the ETT is advanced further into the trachea. Placement should be confirmed and the tube secured in place. The increased time required for completion, the potential difficulty of wire or suture retrieval, and the possibility of failure to pass the ETT limit the usefulness of this technique.

Tracheotomy

An additional surgical airway technique is the surgical tracheotomy. However, this surgical intervention has limited use in an emergency and is generally performed by a surgeon. Potential complications with

BOX 24.8   Complications of Tracheal Extubation

Respiratory
- Airway obstruction
- Breath holding
- Coughing and straining
- Hypercarbia
- Hypoxemia
- Inadequate clearance of secretions
- Laryngeal cartilage damage
- Laryngospasm
- Negative-pressure pulmonary edema
- Postextubation laryngeal edema
- Pulmonary aspiration
- Stridor
- Subglottic or supraglottic edema
- Tracheomalacia
- Vocal cord damage (e.g., edema, paralysis, or dysfunction)

Cardiovascular
- Cardiac dysrhythmias
- Hypertension
- Left ventricular failure
- Myocardial infarction
- Myocardial ischemia
- Tachycardia

Neurologic
- Cervical spine injury
- Increased intracranial pressure
- Increased intraocular pressure

Other Considerations
- Damage to dentition or other airway structures
- Inadvertent removal of equipment (e.g., nasogastric tube)
- Self-extubation
- Unintentional extubation

BOX 24.9   Standard Extubation Criteria

Global Criteria
- Acceptable hemodynamic status
- Normothermia
- Ability to maintain patent airway
  1. Return of laryngeal and cough reflexes
  2. Appropriate level of consciousness
- Adequate muscular strength
  1. Reversal of neuromuscular blockade as indicated by train-of-four ratio >0.9, tetanic response to 100 Hz for 5 sec, and double-burst stimulation without fade
  2. Head lift for >5 sec with constant strong hand grip
- Acceptable metabolic indicators
  1. Electrolytes within acceptable limits
  2. Acid-base balance within acceptable limits
- Acceptable hematologic indicators
  1. Hemoglobin level consistent with adequate oxygen delivery
- Adequate analgesia for optimal respiratory effort

Respiratory Criteria
- Adequate respiratory mechanics
  1. Vital capacity >15 mL/kg
  2. Maximal negative inspiratory force >−20 cm H_2O
  3. Adequate tidal volume of at least 4–5 mL/kg
- Ability to maintain adequate oxygenation (with Fio_2 <50%)
  1. Spo_2 >90%
  2. Pao_2 >60 mm Hg
- Ability to maintain adequate alveolar ventilation
  1. $Paco_2$ >50 mm Hg
- Acceptable spontaneous respiratory rate (breaths/min)

Fio_2, Fraction of inspired oxygen; *Pao_2,* partial pressure of oxygen in arterial blood; *$Paco_2$,* partial pressure of carbon dioxide in arterial blood; *Spo_2,* blood oxygen level.

this procedure include RLN trauma, damage to large vessels in the neck, and posterior tracheal wall perforation with esophageal trauma. In emergency situations with significant airway compromise, a surgical cricothyrotomy should be the invasive airway technique of choice. The standard tracheotomy is performed at the level of the fourth to sixth tracheal ring and below the isthmus of the thyroid gland. This procedure can take up to 30 minutes.

TRACHEAL EXTUBATION

Tracheal extubation and continued control of the airway during recovery are cornerstones of perioperative airway management. Tracheal extubation remains a logical corollary of TI, in that almost all intubations are performed with the prospect of tracheal extubation at some point during the course of a hospitalization.[11] During the perioperative period, the plan for tracheal extubation should be considered to (1) minimize alterations in cardiopulmonary physiology, (2) decrease the risk of respiratory infection and complications, and (3) reduce the postoperative length of stay while decreasing cost and resource utilization.

Tracheal extubation is not a benign procedure; it is associated with significant complications (Box 24.8).[167] Every tracheal extubation is a trial to determine whether a patient's spontaneous ventilation effort is adequate to support cardiopulmonary function. There is no guarantee that tracheal extubation will be tolerated, especially in patients with marginal cardiopulmonary reserve. Standard criteria for tracheal extubation can be divided into two categories: global and respiratory (Box 24.9). It is often impossible and impractical to fulfill the criteria in their entirety. However, the decision to extubate a patient should be based on a methodical and comprehensive evaluation of patient-, surgical-, and anesthetic-related risk factors for extubation failure (Box 24.10). Patients who require postoperative mechanical respiratory support should remain intubated until standard extubation criteria are met and risk factors for extubation failure are minimized.

Tracheal Extubation Techniques

The same vigilant care taken to initially secure the airway should be exercised when control of the airway is returned to the patient. Complications of tracheal extubation (e.g., laryngospasm) are increased when extubation is performed during Guedel stage II of anesthesia (e.g., the excitatory plane). Tracheal extubation should be performed with the patient in a surgical plane of anesthesia (e.g., deeply anesthetized or Guedel stage III) or fully awake. Advantages and disadvantages of deeply anesthetized versus fully awake extubation can be found in Table 24.8. Patients with a history of difficult intubation or who are at high risk of aspiration should be extubated when airway reflexes return, and the patient can ventilate spontaneously without difficulty. Increased cardiovascular stimulation during awake tracheal extubation can be minimized

BOX 24.10 Risk Factors for Difficult Tracheal Extubation

Patient Risk Factors
- Comprehensive airway evaluation indicating possible difficult reintubation or extubation
- Current and past medical illnesses that affect extubation tolerance (e.g., cardiopulmonary disease)
- Difficult intubation or ventilation (e.g., vocal cord paralysis or dysfunction, morbid obesity, obstructive sleep apnea)
- Generalized airway edema (e.g., tissue trauma, drug or systemic reactions, angioedema, anaphylactic or anaphylactoid reactions, sepsis, inhalation injury, burns, SIRS)
- Limited cervical spine mobility injury (e.g., hard cervical collar or halo fixation, ankylosing spondylitis)
- Tracheomalacia

Surgical Risk Factors
- Airway surgery (e.g., uvulopalatopharyngoplasty, laryngeal or tracheal surgery, tracheal resection, or reconstruction)
- Head and neck surgery (e.g., maxillofacial surgery, carotid surgery, thyroid surgery, facial and deep neck infections)
- Neurosurgical (e.g., cranial surgery, posterior fossa surgery, stereotactic brain procedures, and cervical fusion)
- Orthopedic surgery (e.g., close proximity to airway)
- Impingement of head and neck venous drainage
- Postsurgical injury (e.g., hematoma, hemorrhage, nerve injury)
- Prolonged surgical duration and intubation
- Prone or Trendelenburg position

Anesthesia Risk Factors
- Depressed neurologic status, muscular strength, or respiratory effort
- Difficult or traumatic intubation (e.g., failure to visualize glottis, intubation requiring multiple attempts or alternative techniques)
- Excessive head and neck movement during procedure
- Excessive volume resuscitation
- Intubation injury causing laryngeal incompetence or arytenoid dislocation
- Lack of cuff leak
- Laryngotracheal edema (e.g., caused by oversized endotracheal tube or dual-lumen tube, excessive cuff pressure, traumatic suctioning)

SIRS, Systemic inflammatory response syndrome.

TABLE 24.8 Tracheal Extubation Techniques

	Anesthetized	Awake
Advantages	Decreased cardiovascular stimulation Decreased coughing and straining	Return of airway reflexes Decreased risk of aspiration Airway reflex return Spontaneous ventilation
Disadvantages	Absent or obtunded airway reflexes Increased risk of aspiration Airway obstruction Hypoventilation	Increased cardiovascular stimulation Increased coughing and straining

Effective strategies for tracheal extubation in high-risk patients include (1) extubation over a flexible intubating endoscope, (2) extubation followed by placement of a supraglottic airway (e.g., LMA), (3) use of an AEC, or (4) simply leaving an ETT in place until extubation criteria are met and it is safe to remove. The placement of these short-term devices serves as a guide for expedited reintubation in the event that oxygenation or ventilation proves inadequate after extubation (e.g., reversible extubation). Advantages, disadvantages, and methods for both extubation and reintubation using these devices are discussed in Table 24.9. An antisialagogue (e.g., glycopyrrolate) and/or sedative analgesics (e.g., dexmedetomidine) may help facilitate the placement and management of these devices. Prior to extubation of a difficult airway, a discussion with the OR team regarding subsequent airway plans (in the event of initial extubation failure) should occur, just as it should when initially managing a difficult airway. These plans can include the use of SADs, VL, and cricothyrotomy.[83]

The AEC offers several benefits over the Eschmann stylet or gum elastic bougie (Box 24.11). There are three AECs currently available on the market: (1) the Endotracheal Ventilation Catheter (CardioMed Industries), (2) the Sheridan Tracheal Tube Exchanger (Hudson Respiratory Care), and (3) the Cook Airway Exchange Catheter (Cook Medical) (see Fig. 24.40). For adult patients, 11-French (external diameter: 3.7 mm) and 14-French (external diameter: 4.7 mm) AECs are generally well tolerated and allow spontaneous breathing, phonation, and the clearance of secretions. After confirmation of placement and depth, the AEC may be secured in place until it is determined that reintubation will not be required. It is important to verify that the internal diameter of the reintubation ETT approximates that of the external diameter of the AEC as much as possible to prevent the leading edge of the ETT from catching and impinging on airway structures, causing trauma, and preventing passage through the glottis. A laryngoscope can be used to lift and move supraglottic tissue; this minimizes the angle of approach and facilitates ETT passage through the glottis. If the ETT encounters an obstruction at the glottic opening, slight retraction and manual rotation 90 degrees counterclockwise can be used prior to advancement to avoid arytenoid or vocal cord impingement.

using β-blockers, α-blockers, calcium channel blockers, and vasodilators. Furthermore, coughing and straining can be attenuated by the judicious use of local anesthetics (e.g., IV, topical, intracuff lidocaine) and opioids (caution with hypoventilation).

Tracheal Extubation of the Difficult Airway

The American Association of Nurse Anesthetists and the ASA's closed-claims analysis of perioperative difficult airway management revealed that claims for death or brain damage have decreased from initial closed-claims reviews.[82,167] The development of difficult airway guidelines and new airway adjuncts (e.g., SADs and VL) has greatly improved the safety of airway management during anesthesia induction. Of particular interest is the fact that a significant portion of airway emergencies (up to one-third) happen upon extubation and recovery from anesthesia.[69] This may be attributed to the paucity of literature and guidelines regarding techniques for tracheal extubation of the difficult airway. Therefore, a preformulated airway management plan, based on extubation strategies or algorithms (Fig. 24.58), may be helpful in decreasing complications during or after extubation.[82,167]

Complications After Tracheal Extubation

Residual Neuromuscular Blockade

Residual neuromuscular blockade is a potential problem in the postoperative period and can affect tracheal extubation. Complications of residual neuromuscular blockade include (1) upper airway obstruction from pharyngeal muscle weakness, (2) hypoxemia, (3) increased risk of aspiration, (4) decreased ventilatory response to hypoxia, (5) unpleasant muscle weakness, and (6) delay in tracheal extubation.[168] Vigilant

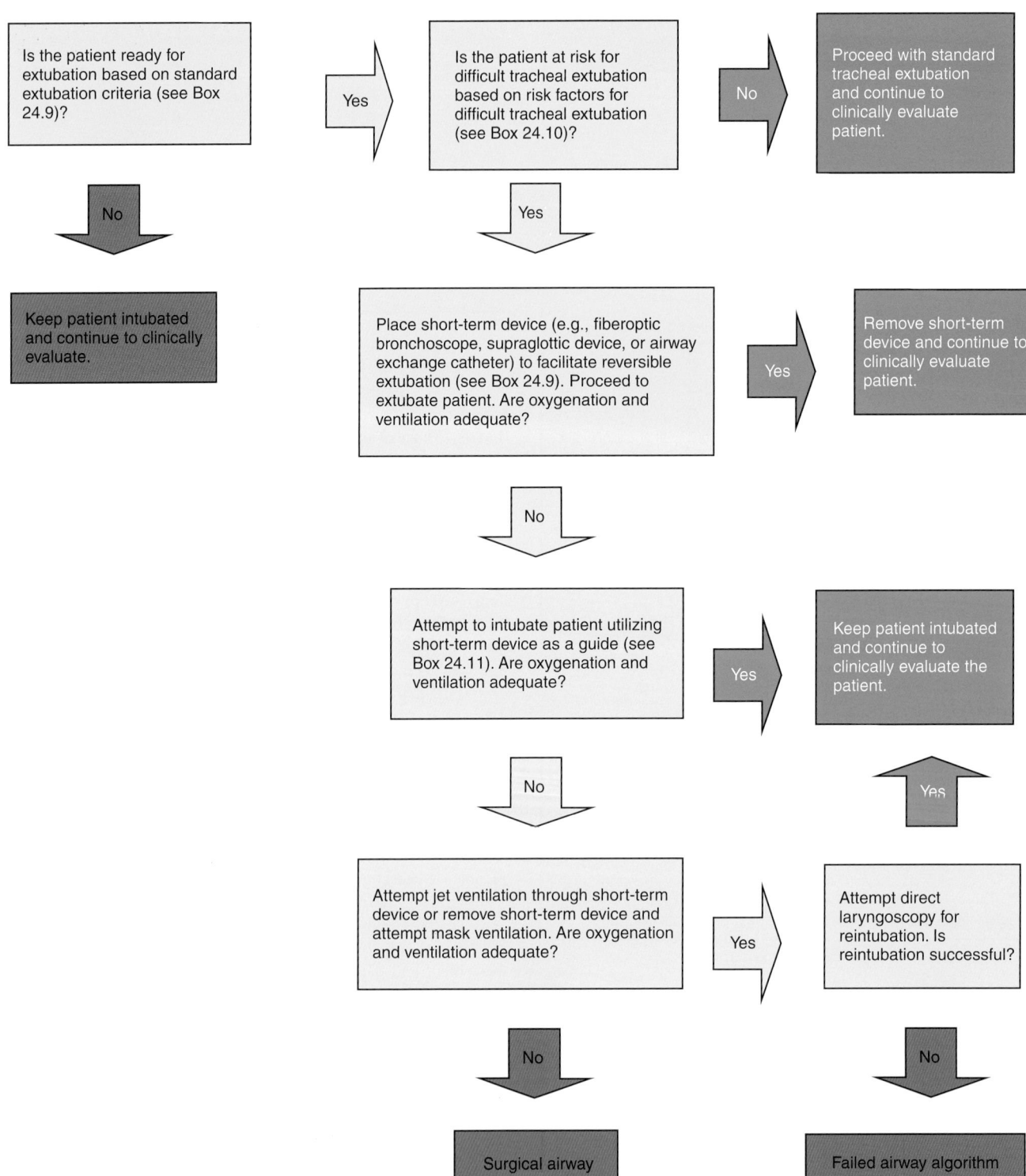

Fig. 24.58 Extubation algorithm for the difficult airway, using an airway exchange catheter. Note: "Short-term device" refers to fiberoptic bronchoscope, supraglottic airway device, or airway exchange catheter.

monitoring of neuromuscular function and correct administration of neuromuscular blocker reversal and binding agents can help to mitigate complications. Sugammadex is a cyclodextrin-based binding agent that contains a hydrophilic periphery and a lipophilic core. This agent is able to trap either rocuronium or vecuronium in a very strong cyclodextrin-target bond, effectively removing the blocking agent from the synaptic gap and rendering it inert.

Laryngospasm

Laryngospasm is the involuntary protective reflex that causes contraction of the laryngeal musculature (see Table 24.1). Bradycardia, pulmonary edema, pulmonary aspiration, and desaturation with accompanying hypoxemia are potential problems when a laryngospasm occurs, with a desaturation rate reported in up to 60% of patients. Laryngospasm is believed to occur as a result of sensory stimulation of

TABLE 24.9   Tracheal Extubation of the Difficult Airway

	Flexible Intubating Endoscope	Supraglottic Airway	Airway Exchange Catheter (AEC)
Advantages	Useful method to evaluate pharyngeal and laryngeal function, injury, pathology, and obstruction	Facilitates flexible intubating endoscopic passage and evaluation of airway through mask orifice Associated with decreased cardiovascular stimulation, coughing, and straining	Maintains continual access to the airway Lumen allows for ventilation, oxygenation, tracheal suctioning, administration of medication, and carbon dioxide monitoring
Disadvantages	Requires experience and skill to properly manipulate device May offer only a brief evaluation of the airway May cause carinal irritation	Restricted evaluation of supraglottic and pharyngeal structures if flexible scope used Periglottic obstruction will impair gas exchange through supraglottic airway	Dislodgement of AEC can occur any time during procedure Complications include trauma from deep placement, barotrauma or pneumothorax with jet ventilation, and carinal irritation Ventilation and oxygenation may not be effective
Method for extubation	Placement of flexible scope-guided oral airway (e.g., Williams or Ovassapian airway) over existing endotracheal tube Tracheal extubation Insertion of flexible scope with prefitted endotracheal tube Flexible endoscopic evaluation of airway Flexible scope is left in place within the trachea and removed when deemed appropriate	Tracheal extubation Insertion of laryngeal mask airway (LMA) LMA is left in place and removed when deemed appropriate	Placement of AEC through endotracheal tube to predetermined depth (e.g., not to exceed 25–26 cm) Tracheal extubation over AEC Confirm depth and tracheal placement of AEC by standard methods, secure with tape AEC is left in place and removed when deemed appropriate
Method for reintubation	Visual confirmation from flexible scope within trachea Appropriately sized endotracheal tube is passed over flexible scope Flexible scope is removed Placement of endotracheal tube confirmed by standard methods	Appropriately sized endotracheal tube passed through supraglottic airway tube, blindly or aided by fiberoptic bronchoscope Placement of endotracheal tube confirmed by standard methods	Remove tape and maintain depth of AEC Perform laryngoscopy to aid endotracheal tube advancement Appropriately sized endotracheal tube passed over AEC AEC removed Placement of endotracheal tube confirmed by standard methods

BOX 24.11   Benefits of the Airway Exchange Catheter

- Exchangeable 15-mm external diameter connector for manual ventilation and Luer-lock adaptor for jet ventilation
- Facilitates removal of endotracheal tube while still maintaining continual access to the airway
- Lumen allows for ventilation, oxygenation, tracheal suctioning, administration of medication (e.g., local anesthetic), and carbon dioxide monitoring
- Lumen and side ports ensure adequate airflow, while blunt tip decreases trauma to airway (see Fig. 24.40)
- Radiopaque and depth (cm) markers
- Sufficient length and rigidity guides replacement endotracheal tube into position (e.g., Seldinger technique)

the vagus nerve via the internal branch of the SLN. Afferent responses result in spasm, and closing of the vocal cords occurs from the external branch of the SLNs and the RLN. The manner in which a laryngospasm occurs includes both the tensing of the cords by the cricothyroid muscles (stimulated by the SLN) and the adduction of the cords by the thyroarytenoid and lateral cricoarytenoid muscles (stimulated by the RLN).

Laryngospasm can be caused by a number of factors, such as airway manipulation, noxious stimuli (e.g., water, blood, or mucus) within the pharynx, or stimulation of the larynx during inadequate anesthetic

depth. Tracheal extubation should therefore be performed with the patient in a surgical plane of anesthesia (e.g., deeply anesthetized or Guedel stage III) or fully awake to minimize the risk of laryngospasm. (See Box 24.9 for standard extubation criteria.)

Laryngospasm has been described as having two mechanisms. During "glottis shutter closure," intrinsic laryngeal muscles mediate vocal cord adduction, causing partial airway obstruction. In contrast, during "ball valve closure," extrinsic laryngeal muscles cause contraction of the false vocal cords and supraglottic soft tissue, resulting in complete airway obstruction. If left untreated, laryngospasm can result in hypoxia, negative-pressure pulmonary edema, and cardiovascular derangements (e.g., cardiac arrhythmias, tachycardia, bradycardia, and cardiac arrest). Treatment of laryngospasm is discussed in Box 24.12. The Larson maneuver, also termed stimulation of the laryngospasm notch, can be applied while performing a vigorous jaw thrust using bilateral firm pressure on the styloid process behind the posterior ramus of the mandible and anterior to the mastoid process. This technique has not been studied, but instead has shown anecdotal evidence for breaking a laryngospasm. Finally, when a laryngospasm occurs and rapid desaturation is observed, then paralysis with succinylcholine should not be delayed.[169]

Laryngotracheobronchitis

Laryngotracheobronchitis, or croup, involves inflammation and edema of the airway below the level of the vocal cords. Subglottic edema may manifest as stridor, which is the high-pitched inspiratory

BOX 24.12   Treatment for Laryngospasm

1. Remove stimulus (e.g., suction the pharyngeal space)
2. Administration of 100% oxygen
3. Provide an open and clear airway (e.g., placement of an oral airway)
4. Perform a jaw thrust (e.g., Larson maneuver or pressure on the laryngo-spasm notch)
5. Apply positive pressure ventilation (e.g., 10–30 cm H₂O pressure—beware of gastric insufflation)
6. Consider deepening the anesthesia with propofol (e.g., 0.5 mg/kg IV)
7. Administer succinylcholine (e.g., 0.2–2 mg/kg IV or 4–5 mg/kg IM)

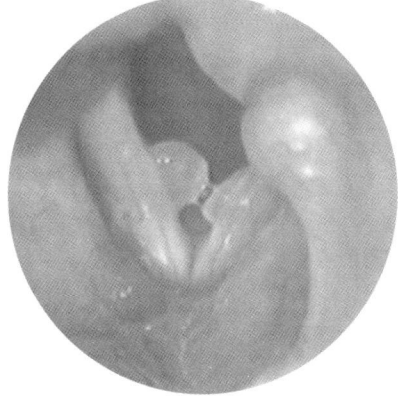

Fig. 24.59 Fiberoptic view of vocal cord polyps.

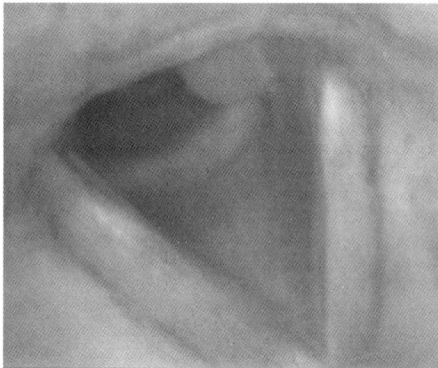

Fig. 24.60 Fiberoptic view of granuloma.

and expiratory sound caused by turbulent airflow through a partially obstructed upper airway. A "barking" cough is another distinctive symptom of croup. Croup can occur in adult and pediatric patients. However, pediatric patients are more vulnerable because of the narrow caliber of their airways. Because inflammation greatly increases airway resistance, respiratory failure can occur rapidly. Croup can be caused by (1) postintubation edema around the glottic and subglottic regions, (2) multiple intubation attempts, (3) an inappropriately large ETT causing laryngeal and tracheal capillary compression, or (4) excessive head and neck movement. Croup can occur any time during the postoperative period, but typically occurs within 3 hours of extubation. Treatment of croup is aimed at decreasing inflammation and edema using (1) humidified supplemental oxygen, (2) racemic epinephrine (e.g., 0.5 mL of a 2.25% solution in 2.5 mL of normal saline), and (3) dexamethasone (e.g., 0.1–0.5 mg/kg). Other treatment modalities include the use of a helium-oxygen mixture to facilitate oxygen delivery through narrowed airways.

COMPLICATIONS OF AIRWAY MANAGEMENT

Complications related to TI include (1) airway trauma, (2) aspiration, (3) esophageal intubation, (4) endobronchial intubation, and (5) ETT complications. Whereas individual treatments may vary, vigilant care and recognition of problems remain primary interventions if an airway complication occurs.

Airway Trauma

Iatrogenic trauma to the airway is a well-recognized complication related to airway management.[170-172] Structures damaged and sites of injury noted in the analysis include the dentition, pharynx, larynx, esophagus, and trachea.[170] Of the anesthesia-related malpractice claims, dental injury is the most common.[82,167,170] The majority of dental injuries occur during laryngoscopy and intubation, with the maxillary central incisors most at risk. However, dental injury can also occur after emergence and extubation. Risk factors for dental trauma include: (1) preexisting dental pathology (e.g., carious teeth, periodontitis, paradentosis, or fixed dental work) and (2) one or more indicators of difficult laryngoscopy and intubation (e.g., upper incisor protrusion).

Pharyngeal injury to the airway includes: (1) pharyngeal perforation, laceration, or contusion; (2) localized infection; (3) macroglossia; and (4) edema and necrosis of the uvula.[168,169] The cause of pharyngeal injury is often the result of (1) direct trauma (e.g., laryngoscopy, videolaryngoscopy, or blind pharyngeal suctioning), (2) prolonged mechanical compression and ischemia by an ETT or oral pharyngeal airway, or (3) pressure-induced nerve injury (e.g., lingual, recurrent laryngeal, or hypoglossal nerve). A malpositioned, oversized, or over-inflated LMA may also cause trauma to delicate mucosa.[168,169] Lastly, obstruction of the submandibular duct by extreme head flexion, surgical manipulation/trauma, or impingement via an ETT or bite block

can cause massive tongue swelling in extreme cases. The incidence of sore throat after intubation is approximately 40% to 65% when blood is observed on the instruments (e.g., laryngoscope) after airway manipulation. Fortunately, pain on swallowing usually lasts no more than 24 to 48 hours.

Trauma to the larynx can be subcategorized into (1) vocal cord paralysis, (2) granuloma formation, and (3) arytenoid dislocation and subluxation. Most susceptible to mechanical injury are the posterior half of the vocal cords, the arytenoids, and the posterior tracheal wall. Unilateral or bilateral vocal cord paralysis can most often be attributed to nerve or mechanical injury and may manifest as partial or complete airway obstruction. Hoarseness or airway obstruction noted in the immediate postoperative period should be evaluated for possible emergent reintubation or tracheotomy. Granuloma or polyp formation can occur at the vocal process of the arytenoids, as well as the posterior wall of the trachea (Figs. 24.59 and 24.60), both of which come into intimate contact with the ETT. The degree of injury and granuloma formation increases with increasing ETT diameter and duration of intubation. Arytenoid dislocation (e.g., complete disruption of the cricoarytenoid joint, or malpositioning of the arytenoid cartilages) can be caused by the mechanical force of an ETT against the arytenoids or by forceful ETT placement.

Esophageal laceration or perforation can occur with any attempt at intubation, especially in patients with a difficult airway or after multiple attempts. Esophageal laceration or perforation may manifest as neck erythema, edema, pneumothorax, and subcutaneous emphysema. Mediastinitis associated with esophageal injury correlates with a high degree of morbidity and mortality despite aggressive treatment with surgical drainage and antibiotics.

Tracheal laceration or perforation may be caused by overinflation of the ETT cuff, overdistention of the ETT cuff by nitrous oxide, multiple

BOX 24.13   Risk Factors for Gastric Aspiration

Patient-Related Risk Factors
- Ascites
- Cardiac arrest
- Emergency surgery
- Full stomach
- Nausea and vomiting
- Obesity
- Scleroderma
- Severe hypotension
- Trauma or stress

Anesthesia-Related Risk Factors
- Cricoid pressure
- Difficult airway management
- Inadequate depth of anesthesia
- Opioids

Gastrointestinal Pathology
- Decreased esophageal sphincter tone
- Diabetic gastroparesis
- Gastroesophageal reflux disease (GERD)
- Gastrointestinal obstruction
- Hiatal hernia
- Increased gastric pressure
- Peptic ulcer disease

Neurologic Pathology
- Decreased airway reflexes
- Decreased level of consciousness
- Head injury
- Seizures

From Nagelhout JJ. Aspiration prophylaxis: is it time for changes in our practice? *AANA J.* 2003;71(4):299–303.

intubation attempts, the use of an intubating stylet, repositioning of the ETT without cuff deflation, or the use of an inappropriately large ETT. The risk of tracheal injury is increased with tracheal distortion (e.g., neoplasm or enlarged lymph nodes), membranous trachea weakness, corticosteroid therapy, and chronic obstructive lung disease.

Aspiration

Pulmonary aspiration has two components: the movement of gastric contents from the stomach to the pharynx, followed by the movement of gastric contents from the pharynx into the lungs. Clinically significant aspiration is an uncommon complication of general anesthesia, with a reported incidence of 1 per 35,000 anesthetics.[102] Less than half of all aspirations lead to pneumonia. An analysis of the ASA Closed Claims Project (CCP), and a review of complications from several million anesthetics administered over the course of a year's time in the United Kingdom, have indicated that aspiration pneumonitis is a significant cause of morbidity and mortality.[69,82] Patient, anesthetic, and pathologic risk factors for gastric aspiration are reviewed in Box 24.13. The development of pneumonia, with subsequent ventilation perfusion abnormalities, is dependent on: (1) the type of aspirate (e.g., contaminated, acidic, particulate, or nonparticulate), (2) the volume of aspirate, and (3) the patient's comorbid conditions. Aspiration pneumonitis can be divided into two phases: phase 1 (direct chemical injury) and phase 2 (inflammatory mediator release).[102] Acute gastric aspiration can occur whenever the patient's laryngeal reflexes are inhibited. Gastric aspirate contamination into the lungs causes: (1) chemical destruction of pulmonary tissue, (2) alveolar capillary membrane edema and degeneration, (3) alveolar type II pneumocyte destruction, and (4) microhemorrhage, leading to hypoxia. Management of this condition includes positive pressure ventilation and intensive physiologic support.

A number of mechanical and pharmacologic measures can be taken to minimize the risk of gastric aspiration. During airway management and mask ventilation, limiting peak airway pressures to less than 15 to 20 cm H_2O helps minimize gastric insufflation. If higher peak airway pressures (e.g., >25 cm H_2O) are necessary for ventilation, then gastric insufflation may occur. Realistic adherence to fasting guidelines should

be instituted, and these guidelines should include consideration of the type of liquid or food consumed, patient age and characteristics, type of anesthesia and surgical procedure planned, and the presence of risk factors for gastric aspiration.

The application of cricoid pressure during rapid-sequence induction may be beneficial in preventing gastric aspiration provided that it is performed properly and does not interfere with airway management. However, the use of cricoid pressure and its efficacy have been questioned, as primary studies were done on cadavers and have not been reproduced. Furthermore, it has been demonstrated that the esophagus is not directly posterior to the trachea in a significant portion of the population, causing it to move laterally during cricoid pressure application. Finally, lateral displacement and compression of the airway can occur during cricoid pressure, artificially causing difficulty with visualization of the glottic opening.[173,174] There is evidence that esophageal occlusion does occur during correct application of cricoid pressure with 30 N of force, and it continues to be used for patients at risk for aspiration.[175]

Pharmacologic methods that decrease the acidity and volume of gastric contents may reduce the risk of gastric aspiration. The administration of nonparticulate antacids (e.g., 30 mL of sodium citrate) 10 to 20 minutes before the induction of anesthesia effectively raises the gastric pH. A histamine-blocking agent (e.g., famotidine [20 mg IV], cimetidine [300 mg IV], or ranitidine [50 mg IV]) administered at least 45 to 60 minutes preoperatively is also effective in reducing stomach acid production and raising the gastric pH. Proton pump inhibitors, such as omeprazole, may also be administered the night before surgery to help reduce acid production. The administration of a gastroprokinetic agent (e.g., metoclopramide [10 mg IV]) 20 to 30 minutes before the induction of anesthesia accelerates gastric emptying. Metoclopramide administration is contraindicated in patients with a bowel obstruction and those who have any type of dopamine deficiency such as Parkinson disease.

Esophageal Intubation

Esophageal intubation may occur during any intubation procedure. However, during difficult intubation where inadequate visualization of the glottis occurs, the possibility of inadvertently placing the ETT into the esophagus increases significantly. Unrecognized esophageal intubation can lead to severe hypoxia and catastrophic complications, up to and including death. An analysis of the ASA-CCP indicated that a significant portion of respiratory-related claims involved esophageal intubation.[82] Indeed, the results of the Fourth National Audit Project demonstrated that esophageal intubation and the lack of appropriate recognition of this complication still occur.[69] It is imperative that confirmation of ETT placement within the trachea is verified with end-tidal capnographic CO_2 monitoring. Fiberoptic bronchoscopy is another sensitive method for confirming ETT placement, although its use may not be practical after every intubation. It is important to recognize that other traditional methods of confirming ETT placement, such as equal bilateral breath sounds, symmetric chest wall movement, epigastric auscultation, and observation of tube condensation, lack specificity and can be misleading. Esophageal perforation, retropharyngeal abscess formation, subcutaneous emphysema, and pneumothorax have been documented after esophageal intubation. Mediastinitis is a potentially lethal consequence after esophageal intubation, with a mortality rate of 50%.[170]

Endobronchial Intubation

Endobronchial intubation may occur during any intubation procedure and is sometimes difficult to identify. This type of postintubation problem can contribute to high peak airway pressures, atelectasis, and inadequate ventilation. Endobronchial intubation occurs most commonly within the right mainstem bronchus. It occurs more commonly in infants and children because of the relatively short distance between the glottis and the carina. Signs and symptoms of endobronchial intubation include: (1) increased peak inspiratory pressures, (2) asymmetric chest expansion, (3) unilateral breath sounds, (4) contralateral lung deflation, and (5) hypoxemia. Endobronchial intubation may occur after initial placement of an ETT that is too deep or following extreme flexion of the neck. The tip of the ETT can move an average of 3.8 cm (up to 6 cm) toward the carina when the neck is moved from full extension to full flexion. When endobronchial intubation is discovered, the ETT cuff should be deflated and the tube carefully withdrawn into the trachea. The cuff should then be reinflated, after which the lungs should be hyperinflated sufficiently to expand any atelectatic areas.

Endotracheal Tube Complications

Complications regarding the ETT can occur any time during the administration of general anesthesia. In particular, partial or complete obstruction of the ETT may occur during a surgery of prolonged duration or in a patient with anatomic abnormalities of the airway. ETT obstruction may be caused by: (1) mechanical factors (e.g., sharp bend, kinking, or biting), (2) foreign material (e.g., mucus, blood, tissue, foreign bodies, or lubricant), or (3) the ETT cuff. The expansion of gas bubbles within the ETT cuff by nitrous oxide or overinflation of the cuff may cause partial or complete airway obstruction. Wire-reinforced ETTs may be used to decrease the risk of mechanical obstruction in patients or during surgeries at risk for this complication.

To clear a partially obstructed ETT, a suction catheter or a flexible scope can be placed down the lumen of the ETT in an attempt to dislodge and suction out the obstruction. A total obstruction that cannot be relieved quickly requires removal of the ETT, followed by reintubation.

SUMMARY

Airway management is a critical component of anesthesia practice. Knowledge of airway anatomy, physiology, and pathophysiology will aid in the formulation of appropriate airway management plans. In addition, the recognition of patient signs or symptoms and situations that indicate airway difficulty may help with the development of effective airway management strategies. Adherence to established standards and protocols, including difficult airway algorithms, can minimize complications and assist the airway provider during both anticipated and unanticipated airway difficulty. Familiarization with airway equipment and competence in a variety of airway management skills and techniques will facilitate appropriate management when a situation involving a difficult airway occurs.

REFERENCES

For a complete list of references for this chapter, scan this QR code with any smartphone code reader app, or visit the following URL: http://booksite.elsevier.com/9780323711944/.

25

Cardiovascular Anatomy, Physiology, Pathophysiology, and Anesthesia Management

Sass Elisha

CARDIOVASCULAR SYSTEM

A thorough knowledge of anatomy and physiology of the cardiovascular system is essential to anesthesia practice. Every anesthetic agent has either a direct or an indirect effect on the cardiovascular system. There are near-instantaneous and continuous changes in the cardiovascular response to surgical stimulation, physiologic alterations during surgery (e.g., blood loss), and variations in anesthetic depth. Therefore, whether the clinical concern includes decreased blood pressure during neuraxial blockade or myocardial depression during administration of an inhalation anesthetic agent, a thorough understanding of these effects and their implications to human physiology is critical.

The cardiovascular system is composed of the heart and the vasculature that carries blood, providing oxygen and cellular substrate to all cells in the body. The heart pumps deoxygenated blood to the lungs and then supplies oxygenated blood to all parts of the body. This chapter describes the anatomic and physiologic characteristics, as well as pathophysiologic changes, associated with the cardiovascular system.

Heart

Gross Anatomy

The heart is bound anteriorly by the sternum and the costal cartilages of the third, fourth, and fifth ribs and inferiorly by the diaphragm. It is positioned with the apex of the heart projecting anteriorly and inferiorly toward the left fifth intercostal space at the midclavicular line. At this location, the pulsation from the cardiac apex may be palpated. This is known as the point of maximal impulse. The first heart sound (S_1) is best auscultated in this area. A third (S_3) or fourth (S_4) heart sound, if present, can also be heard in this location. Heart sounds are generated from the vibrations caused by the closure of the atrioventricular (AV) (e.g., S_1) and semilunar (e.g., S_2) valves.[1]

Cardiac Silhouette

The superior aspect of the cardiac silhouette is formed by the transverse and ascending aorta. The right lateral border is composed of the right atrium (RA), and the mass of the right ventricle (RV) constitutes most of the inferior border of the heart. The left ventricle (LV) comprises most of the apex and the lower left lateral border of the heart. The left atrial appendage lies superior to the LV and to one side of the pulmonary artery. On x-ray it is located between the LV and the pulmonary outflow tract. The heart is rotated on its base such that the anterior surface is almost entirely composed of the RV. The base of the heart is the most superior portion of the cardiac silhouette.

Pericardium

The heart is situated within the mediastinum and surrounded by a fibrous, double-walled sac called the pericardium, which envelops the heart and the roots of the great vessels. It consists of a visceral portion, which is in intimate contact with the outer surface of the heart (epicardium), and an outer parietal portion that adheres to the fibrous pericardium (Fig. 25.1).

The fibrous pericardium is pierced superiorly by the aorta, the pulmonary trunk, and the superior vena cava. The base of the fibrous pericardium is fused with the central tendon of the diaphragm. The visceral pericardium and parietal pericardium are separated by a thin potential space known as the pericardial cavity. This space normally contains approximately 10 to 25 mL of serous fluid, which provides lubrication for the free movement of the heart within the mediastinum. In disease states, the pericardial space can fill with blood and or serosanguinous fluid, compress the heart, and decrease cardiac output (CO). In acute cardiac tamponade, the volume rapidly increases, producing myocardial dysfunction. In contrast, in chronic cardiac tamponade, the degree of pressure exerted on the heart increases slowly because the pericardial sac stretches over time to accommodate the blood that accumulates.[2] However, the pressure may eventually increase as much as 10-fold before symptoms associated with cardiac tamponade occur.[3]

The pericardium receives its arterial blood supply from the branches of the internal thoracic arteries and through the bronchial, esophageal, and superior phrenic arteries. Venous drainage from the pericardium occurs through the azygos system and the pericardiophrenic veins, which anastomose with the internal thoracic veins. Nervous innervation to the pericardium is derived from the vagus nerve, the phrenic nerves, and the sympathetic trunks.

Surface Anatomy

The atria are separated from the ventricles by the coronary sulcus (AV sulcus) (Fig. 25.2A). The right coronary artery (RCA) travels within this sulcus. The circumflex artery arises from the left coronary artery (LCA), and it travels in the coronary sulcus until it branches posteriorly. The RV and LV are separated by the interventricular sulci, which descend from the coronary sulcus to the apex. The interventricular sulci are composed of an anterior interventricular sulcus and a posterior interventricular sulcus. The anterior interventricular sulcus contains the left anterior descending (LAD) artery, which courses over the interventricular septum and continues into the posterior interventricular sulcus.

The crux of the heart is the place at which the coronary and the posterior interventricular sulci meet. Internally, it is where the atrial and ventricular septa converge (see Fig. 25.2B). This anatomic crux determines coronary artery dominance.

Cardiac Skeleton

Essential to a discussion of the chambers of the heart is a description of the fibrous skeleton, the annulus fibrosus (Fig. 25.3). Tough fibrous rings surround the AV valves and act as points of attachment for the valves. Two additional fibrous annuli develop in relation to the bases of the aorta and the pulmonary trunk. The aortic fibrous annulus is connected to the pulmonary annulus by a fibrous band called the tendon of the conus. The aortic annulus is connected to the AV annuli by the small left fibrous trigone, and the larger right fibrous trigone is called the central fibrous body. The four annuli and their interconnections constitute the fibrous cardiac skeleton.

The annulus fibrosus is the fixation point for the cardiac musculature, and it plays an important role in the structure, function, and efficiency of the heart. The annulus acts as an insulator to prevent aberrant electrical conduction from the atria to the ventricles so that AV conduction moves through one pathway only: the AV node to the AV bundle, which is also known as the bundle of His. This element increases the electromechanical efficiency of the heart and helps to prevent dysrhythmias.

Chambers of the Heart

Right atrium. The atria act as the priming chambers for the ventricles. As such, the RA acts as a reservoir for the RV and has unique anatomic

characteristics. It has a muscle wall thickness of approximately 2 mm. The RA receives blood from several sources: the superior vena cava, the inferior vena cava, and the coronary sinus (Fig. 25.4). The RA consists of two parts: an anterior, thin-walled trabeculated portion and a posterior, smooth-walled portion called the sinus venarum. The sinus venarum receives blood from the vena cava and the coronary sinus.

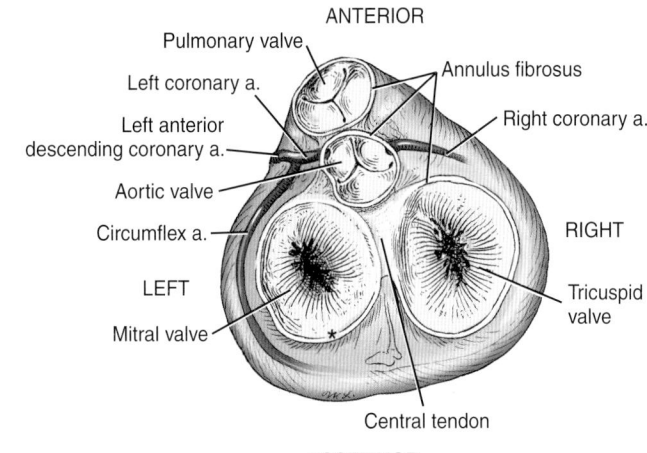

Fig. 25.3 The annulus fibrosus. *a.,* Artery.

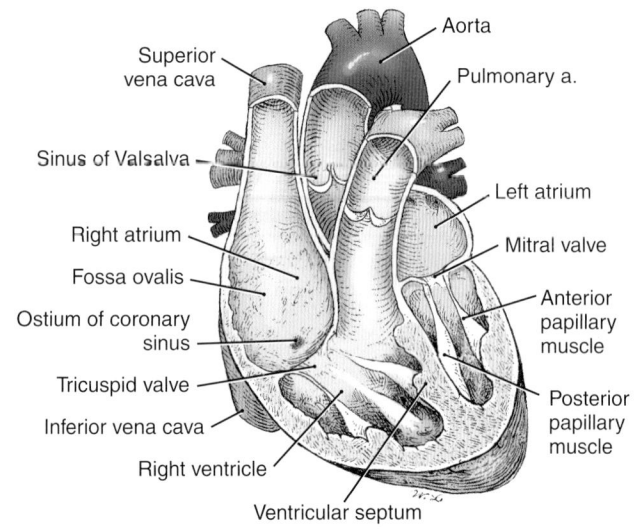

Fig. 25.4 Internal anatomy of the heart chambers. *a.,* Artery.

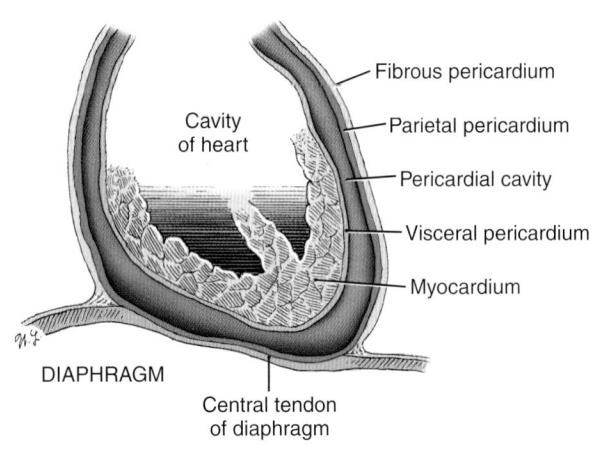

Fig. 25.1 The pericardium.

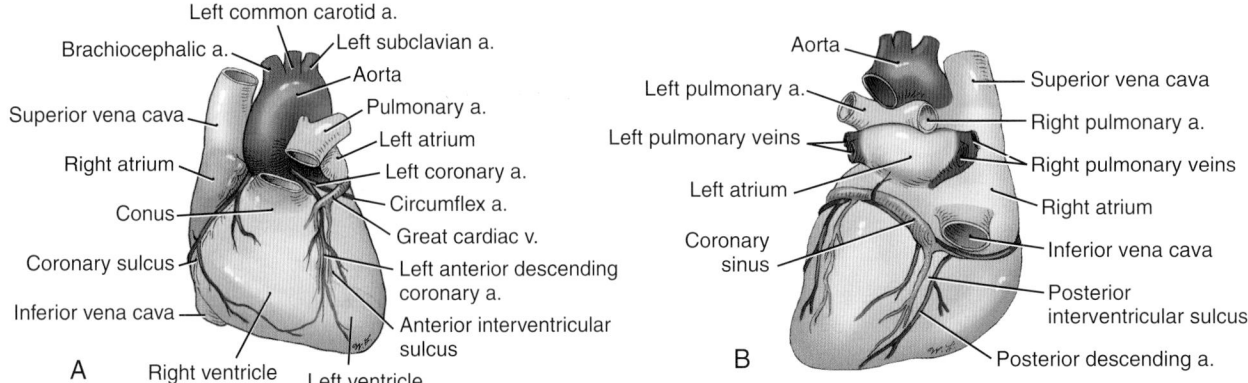

Fig. 25.2 (A) Surface anatomy of the heart *(anterior view)*. (B) Surface anatomy of the heart *(posterior view)*. *a.,* Artery; *v.,* vein.

The auricle projects to the left from the root of the superior vena cava and overlaps the root of the ascending aorta.

The superior vena cava returns blood to the RA from the upper body. The inferior vena cava returns blood to the RA from the lower body. The entrance of the inferior vena cava into the RA is protected by a rudimentary valve called the eustachian valve.[4]

The entrance from the coronary sinus into the RA is located between the AV orifice and the valve of the inferior vena cava. This opening is protected in part by a rudimentary valve of the coronary sinus called the *thebesian valve*.[5] Other distinguishing structures within the RA include the interatrial septum and the fossa ovalis cordis, which is the remnant of the fetal foramen ovale located within the septum.

Right ventricle. The RV ejects blood into the pulmonary arterial system for oxygenation and removal of carbon dioxide by the lungs. The RV communicates with the RA through the AV orifice, which is separated by the tricuspid valve. The RV also communicates with the pulmonary outflow tract through the pulmonary orifice, which is shielded by the pulmonic valve (see Fig. 25.4).

The walls of the RV are much thicker (4–5 mm) than those of the RA because of the increased pressures required to generate forward blood flow into the pulmonary artery. The superior portion of the RV as it approaches the pulmonary orifice has a conical appearance and is called the conus arteriosus or infundibulum.[6]

The inner wall of the conus is smooth, but the remainder of the right ventricular wall has a rough appearance because of the presence of several irregular muscular bundles called the papillary muscles and the trabeculae carneae. One of the trabeculae carneae (the moderator band) crosses the cavity of the ventricles and carries the right branch of the AV bundle. The papillary muscles have attachments to the ventricular walls and to the chordae tendineae. The chordae tendineae are attached to the cusps of the tricuspid valve; together with the papillary muscles, they help prevent eversion of the tricuspid valve into the RA during ventricular systole.[7]

Left atrium. The left atrium (LA) acts as a reservoir for the oxygenated blood it receives from the four pulmonary veins and serves as a pump during atrial systole. It provides a 20% to 30% increase in left ventricular end-diastolic volume (LVEDV), which is known as the atrial kick. A person who has normal myocardial performance does not rely on this increase in ventricular filling to achieve adequate CO. However, in certain cardiovascular or respiratory pathologic conditions, compromised patients do rely on this atrial kick to maintain an adequate CO. The LA is located superiorly and posteriorly to the other cardiac chambers. The walls of the LA are slightly thicker (3 mm) as compared to the RA. The LA connects to the LV through the left AV orifice, which contains the mitral valve. The atrial septum is smooth but may contain a central depression that corresponds to the location of the fossa ovalis cordis.

Left ventricle. The apex of the LV is positioned within the mediastinum in an anterior and inferior orientation. The LV receives blood from the LA and ejects it into the aorta. Left ventricular wall thickness is approximately 8 to 15 mm, or two to three times the thickness of the RV. This additional muscle mass is required to overcome the systemic vascular resistance (SVR), or afterload, and to maintain stroke volume (SV).

The ventricular septum separates the right and left ventricular cavities.[8] The upper third of the septum is smooth endocardium. The remaining two-thirds of the septum and the rest of the ventricular wall are covered with trabeculae carneae.

Two large papillary muscles are present within the LV. The anterior papillary muscle attaches to the anterior part of the left ventricular wall, and the posterior papillary muscle arises from the posterior aspect of the inferior wall. The chordae tendineae of each muscle is attached to the cusps of the mitral valve and prevents eversion of the valve during LV systole.

Myocardium

The cardiac musculature is arranged in three distinct layers: an outer epicardium, a middle muscular myocardium, and an inner endocardium. The epicardium is composed of mesothelium, connective tissue, and fat. The middle muscular myocardium consists of two muscle layers, a superficial and a deep layer. These layers are arranged in a spiral fashion and appear on cross section to run at right angles to each other. It has been postulated that the superficial and deep layers of the myocardium are not two separate layers but one tortuous and continuous layer. The arrangement of the muscle layers provides strength during contraction of the myocardium and efficient propulsion of blood toward the semilunar valves. The endocardium consists of endothelium and a layer of connective tissue.

Heart Valves

The cardiac valves increase the heart's efficiency by ensuring unidirectional flow of blood through the circuit. They open and close in response to pressure gradients that exist above (atrium) or below (ventricles) the valves. These valves may be categorized as AV, which exist between the atria and ventricle, or semilunar (pulmonary artery or aorta).

One of the most accurate ways to determine the presence of valvular pathology is by calculating the valvular area. The standard method for determining valvular area is during cardiac catheterization. Echocardiography is a noninvasive method of determining valvular area and it is used to estimate the presence and degree of valvular heart disease. The use of echocardiography is discussed later in this chapter. A cardiologist can determine valvular gradients using the Gorlin formula or its correction, which can provide information regarding the degree of pathology that exists:

$$\text{Valve Area (cm}^2) = \frac{\text{Cardiac Output (liters/min)} \times 1000}{(K)(HR)(SEP)\sqrt{\text{Mean valve gradient}}}$$

where K is a hydraulic pressure constant, heart rate (HR) (beats per minute), systolic ejection period (SEP) expressed in seconds, and square root of mean valve gradient expressed in mm Hg.[9]

Atrioventricular valves

Tricuspid valve. The tricuspid valve is positioned inferiorly to the right AV annulus, which lies between the RA and the RV. The tricuspid leaflets are well defined, thinner, and more translucent than those of the mitral valve. Three leaflets of unequal size exist: the anterior, septal, and posterior leaflets. The leaflets are attached to the chordae tendineae, which are anchored to the papillary muscles. This structure prevents eversion of the valve leaflets into the RA during ventricular systole.[10] The normal tricuspid valve area is approximately 7 cm². Symptoms associated with tricuspid valve stenosis typically occur when the valve area is less than 1.5 cm².

Mitral valve. The mitral valve is situated inferiorly to the left AV annulus between the LA and the LV. Two major leaflets, the anteromedial leaflet and the posterolateral leaflet, are connected by commissural tissue. The normal mitral valve area is 4 to 6 cm². When the surface area of the valve is decreased by half, clinical symptoms may appear. Like the tricuspid valve, the mitral valve has papillary muscles and chordae tendineae attached to the leaflets to prevent eversion of the valve during ventricular systole.[11]

Semilunar valves. The configuration of the aortic and pulmonary valves is similar. The cusps of the aortic valve are slightly thicker because it is subjected to greater pressures, which are created by left ventricular ejection. The semilunar valves are situated within the outflow tracts of their corresponding ventricles. Each valve is composed of three cusps. Above the aortic valve is a dilation known as the sinus of Valsalva, which allows the valve to open efficiently without occluding the coronary ostia or openings that communicate with the coronary arteries. Eddy currents form behind the valve leaflets and prevent contact between the valve leaflets and the walls of the aorta. Normal aortic valve area is 2.5 to 3.5 cm^2. Reduction of the valve area by one-third to one-half is associated with an increase in the symptoms caused by aortic stenosis.

Coronary Circulation

The heart is a highly aerobic organ that depends on a constant supply of oxygen to meet its high metabolic demand. It requires an elaborate arterial and venous network to ensure that myocytes are adequately supplied with oxygen and substrate to create cellular energy. The arterial system consists of epicardial and subendocardial vessels. The epicardial vessels are located superficially and most commonly become obstructed at areas of bifurcation where the blood flow is turbulent rather than laminar. Significant obstruction (50%–70% reduction in luminal diameter) can result in myocardial ischemia or infarction because of increased resistance to flow across the stenotic areas.

Coronary arteries. The left and right coronary arteries originate from the ascending aorta within the anterior and left posterior sinuses. The coronary ostia are the entrance points by which blood flows through the coronary circulation, and they are located behind the aortic cusps near the superior part of the sinus of Valsalva. The ostium of the LCA is superior and posterior to the right coronary ostium. The coronary arteries act as end arteries, and each supplies blood to its respective capillary bed[12] (Fig. 25.5).

Left main coronary artery. The left main coronary artery travels anteriorly, inferiorly, and leftward from the left coronary sinus to emerge from behind the pulmonary trunk. The caliber of this artery is greater than the right main coronary artery reflecting the increased metabolic needs of the myocardium in the left ventricle. Within 2 to 10 mm of its emergence, the left main coronary artery divides into two or more branches of near-equal diameter. The branches include the LAD artery, the left circumflex coronary artery, anterior interventricular (descending) artery, and possibly the diagonal artery.

Left anterior descending coronary artery. The LAD is a continuation of the left main coronary artery. The branches of this vessel include the first diagonal branch, the first septal perforator, the right ventricular branches (not always observed), other septal perforators, and other diagonal branches. The LAD provides blood flow to the anterior two-thirds of the interventricular septum, the right and left bundle branches, the anterior and posterior papillary muscles of the mitral valve, and the anterior lateral and apical walls of the LV. The LAD also provides collateral circulation to the anterior wall of the RV.

Left circumflex coronary artery. The left circumflex artery arises from the left main coronary artery at an obtuse angle, and it is directed posteriorly as it travels around the left side of the heart within the left AV sulcus. Branches are variable and may include the sinus node artery (40%–50% of the population), the left atrial circumflex artery, the anterolateral marginal artery, the distal circumflex artery, one or more posterolateral marginal arteries, and the posterior descending artery (10%–15% of the population). The circumflex artery supplies blood to the left atrial wall, the posterior and lateral LV, the anterolateral papillary muscle, the AV node in 10% of the population, and the sinoatrial (SA) node in 40% to 45% of the population.

Right coronary artery. The RCA supplies blood to the SA and AV nodes, the RA and RV, the posterior third of the interventricular septum, the posterior fascicle of the left bundle branch, and the interatrial septum. In approximately 90% of the population, the RCA

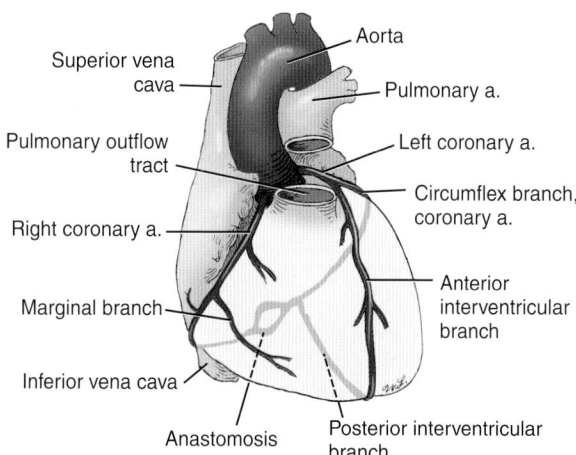

Fig. 25.5 The coronary arterial circulation. *a.*, Artery.

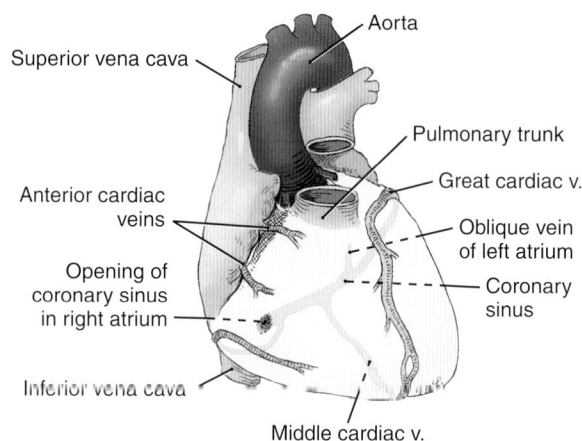

Fig. 25.6 The coronary venous system. *v.*, Vein.

leaves the right coronary sinus and descends in the right AV groove. At the crux, the RCA courses inferiorly in the posterior AV groove and terminates as a left ventricular branch.

The branches of the RCA include the conus artery, the sinus node artery (50%–60% of the population), several anterior right ventricular branches, the right atrial branches, the acute marginal branch, the AV node artery (90% of the population), the proximal bundle branches, the posterior descending artery, and the terminal branches to the LA and LV.

Coronary artery dominance. Dominance of one coronary artery is determined by the location of the coronary artery that crosses the crux and provides blood flow to the posterior descending artery. The dominant coronary artery in 50% of the general population is the right coronary. In addition, 10% to 15% of the general population are left coronary dominant, and 35% to 40% of the general population have mixed right and left dominance.

Venous drainage. An extensive venous system exists within the heart. The three major systems include the coronary sinus, the anterior cardiac veins, and the thebesian veins (Fig. 25.6).

The coronary sinus is located in the posterior AV groove near the crux. It collects approximately 85% of the blood from the LV, and for this reason it is catheterized when metabolic studies of the LV are performed. It may also be cannulated during cardiopulmonary bypass to deliver cardioplegia. The coronary sinus receives blood from the great, middle, and small cardiac veins; the posterior left ventricular veins; and the left atrial vein of Marshall.

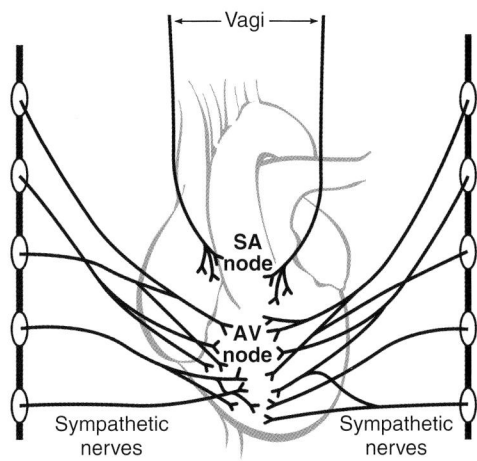

Fig. 25.7 Distribution of sympathetic and parasympathetic innervation to the heart. *AV,* Atrioventricular; *SA,* sinoatrial.

Cardiac Innervation

The autonomic nervous system is divided into the sympathetic and the parasympathetic nervous systems. Efferent impulses are transmitted from the brainstem and hypothalamus to numerous body systems, including the heart. The neurologic innervation to the heart originates from the autonomic nervous system, as well as from sensory fibers. The myocardium also has a specialized conduction system that is further discussed in this chapter.

Increased sympathetic nervous system activity increases heart rate (chronotropic), force of myocardial contraction (inotropic), and rate of AV node discharge (dromotropic). Sympathetic nervous system activation results in the mobilization of myocardial fat-free acids and glycogen for energy use by the myocardial cells. The preganglionic sympathetic nervous system fibers originate from the cells in the intermediolateral columns of the higher thoracic segments of the spinal cord and synapse at the first through the fourth or fifth thoracic paravertebral ganglia. These spinal cord segments are known as the cardioaccelerator fibers. The postganglionic fibers then travel as the superior, middle, and inferior cardiac nerves and the thoracic visceral nerves. These fibers form an epicardial plexus and are distributed over the entire ventricular myocardium. There is greater distribution of sympathetic nerves that innervate the ventricles, resulting in increased ventricular contractility (Fig. 25.7). Catecholamines released during sympathetic stimulation bind with adrenergic receptors on the heart (primarily β_1) and change the biochemical properties within the myocyte. This process is further discussed in this chapter.

Some of these postganglionic sympathetic fibers also join with the postganglionic parasympathetic fibers from the cardiac plexus and primarily innervate the SA and AV nodes and the atrial myocardium. Suppression or blockade of this thoracic portion of the spinal cord by regional anesthesia causes bradycardia and hypotension caused by inhibition of the sympathetic ganglia resulting in parasympathetic nervous system predominance.

The preganglionic parasympathetic fibers originate in the dorsal motor nucleus of the medulla. Short postganglionic fibers primarily innervate the SA and AV nodes and the atrial muscle fibers (see Fig. 25.7). For this reason, increased parasympathetic tone decreases HR. The function of the parasympathetic nervous system is primarily to slow the HR and secondarily to decrease contractility. In fact, maximal vagal nerve (parasympathetic) stimulation reduces contractility by only 30%, whereas maximal sympathetic stimulation increases contractility by 100%. Acetylcholine is the neurotransmitter of the parasympathetic nervous system. Acetylcholine binds to muscarinic receptors on the heart and decreases the rate of sinus node discharge slowing conduction velocity through the AV node. The physiologic effects of parasympathetic nervous system stimulation occur because of increased permeability of cardiac muscle cell membranes to potassium, resulting in hyperpolarization. As a result, SA and AV node cells are less excitable.

Sensory innervation to the heart originates in the nerve endings in the walls of the heart, the coronary artery adventitia, and the pericardium. These nerve endings synapse with ascending fibers in the posterior gray columns of the spinal cord, where the fibers synapse with second-order neurons. From these neurons, the fibers ascend in the ventral spinothalamic tract and terminate in the posteroventral nucleus of the thalamus.

Cardiac Conduction System

Within the myocardium lies the specialized conduction system whose purpose is to automatically initiate and coordinate the cardiac rhythm. The cells of this system differ from the other myocardial cells because they are more variable in shape, contain fewer myofibrils, and have a characteristic pale staining of the cytoplasm. The conductive system consists of the following components: the SA node, the internodal tracts, the AV node, the AV bundle, and the Purkinje system (Fig. 25.8).

Sinoatrial node. The SA node (the Keith-Flack node) is a small collection of specialized cells and collagenous tissue located along the epicardial surface at the junction of the superior vena cava and the RA. It has a prominent central artery that is a branch of the RCA. The SA node is derived from the junction of the right horn of the sinus venosus and the primitive atrium. The SA node consists of two cell types: P cells (pacemaker cells), which are pale and ovoid with large round nuclei, and intermediate or transitional cells, which are elongated. These transitional cells are intermediate between ovoid and ordinary cells. They conduct impulses within and away from the SA node. Intrinsic rate of the SA node is 60 to 100 beats/min. The speed of conduction to adjacent cells within the SA node is 0.5 m/sec.

Internodal tracts. The internodal tracts are located within the atria and are the preferential conduction pathways between the SA and the AV nodes. They are composed of a combination of closely packed parallel myocardial fibers and large pale-staining cells with a perinuclear clear zone. They have large nuclei and sparse myofibrils that resemble the Purkinje cells. Like the SA node, the internodal tracts contain P cells and transitional cells.

Three major internodal tracts exist: the anterior, middle, and posterior internodal tracts. The anterior internodal tract, or Bachmann bundle, extends into the LA and then travels downward through the atrial septum to the AV node. The middle internodal tract, or Wenckebach tract, curves behind the superior vena cava before descending to the AV node. Finally, the posterior internodal tract, or Thorel pathway, continues along the terminal crest to enter the atrial septum and then passes to the AV node.

Atrioventricular node. The AV node is located beneath the endocardium on the right side of the atrial septum, anterior to the opening of the coronary sinus. The AV node is supplied by an abundance of nerve endings as well as vagal (ganglionic) cells. The AV node causes a delay in the transmission of action potentials. This

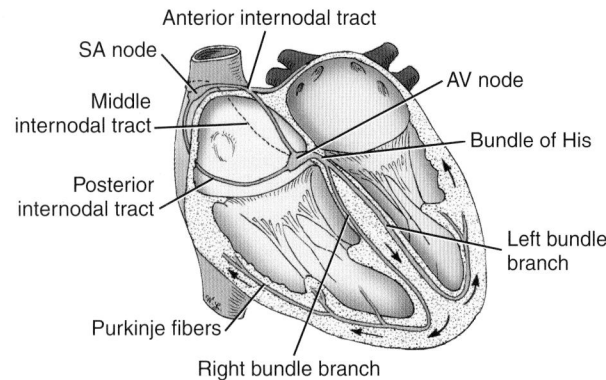

Fig. 25.8 The cardiac conduction system. *AV*, Atrioventricular; *SA*, sinoatrial.

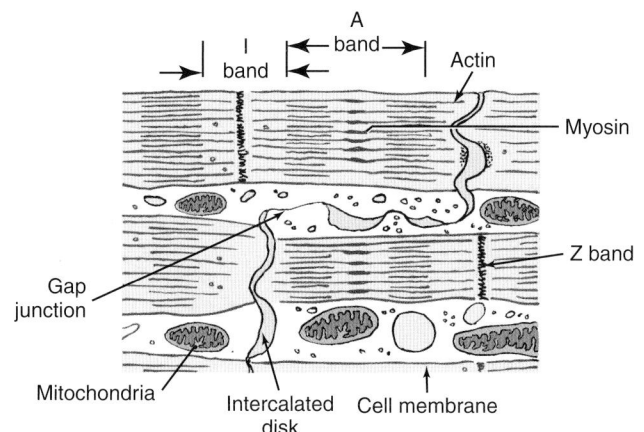

Fig. 25.9 The myocardial sarcomere.

delay may be attributed to several factors, such as the size of the AV nodal cells (smaller than the surrounding atrial cells), a decreased distribution of gap junctions between cells, a resting membrane potential that is more negative than the normal resting membrane potentials of the surrounding cells, and thus the paucity of gap junctions. Greater resistance to the transmission of an action potential exists within the AV node. Impulse conduction is considerably slower as compared to any other region within the normal cardiac conduction system (0.05 m/sec). This delayed speed allows for sufficient time for atrial depolarization and contraction (systole) prior to ventricular depolarization and contraction.

Atrioventricular bundle. The AV node is a group of cells located on the posterior aspect of the right atrium behind the tricuspid valve and near the opening of the coronary sinus. There are three functional regions that are divided according to the action potentials generated and the tissue response to electrical and chemical stimulation: atrionodal (upper region), nodal (middle region), and the nodal-His (lower region). The nodal-His is where the inferior portion of the AV node merges with the AV bundle (bundle of His). The intrinsic pacemaker cells in the AV node are capable of depolarization at a rate of 40 to 60 beats/min. The AV bundle extends from the lower end of the AV node and enters the posterior aspect of the ventricle and the Purkinje system. This AV bundle is the preferential channel for conduction of the action potential from the atria to the ventricles. Conduction velocity from the bundle of His into the left and right bundle branches along the interventricular septum is rapid (2 m/sec).

Purkinje system. The Purkinje system consists of the bundle branch system and its terminal branches. The left bundle branch extends outward under the endocardium and forms several fascicles, which innervate various parts of the LV. The anterior fascicle innervates the anterolateral wall of the LV and the anterior papillary muscle. The posterior fascicle innervates the lateral and posterior ventricular wall and the posterior papillary muscle. The anterior and posterior fascicles join to form the septal fascicle, which innervates the lower ventricular septum and the apical wall of the LV. The right bundle branch travels under the endocardium along the right side of the ventricular septum to the base of the anterior papillary muscle. The Purkinje fibers have pacemaker cells capable of firing at a rate of 20 to 40 beats/min. There is rapid velocity of impulse conduction (4 m/sec) through the Purkinje fibers, which allows for rapid depolarization of ventricular myocytes.

Structural and regulatory proteins. The myocardium has characteristics of both skeletal and smooth muscle. Like smooth muscle, cardiac muscle fibers are interconnected (syncytium), which allows for an action potential to rapidly spread to adjacent cells. Due to this

characteristic of cardiac muscle fibers, action potential propagation and muscle contraction occur as an "all-or-none" response.

The myocardial cell is similar to skeletal muscle in that it is composed of sarcomeres (Fig. 25.9). These sarcomeres contain all the microfilaments and structures that are consistent with the skeletal muscle sarcomere. The sarcomere stretches from Z line to Z line. The A bands consist of the actin filaments, which contain a bilayer filament of F-actin and tropomyosin. Along the actin filament, many active sites are available that can attach to the head of the myosin molecule. A troponin complex is necessary to inhibit actin and myosin from interacting and initiating muscle contraction. The other microfilament in the cardiac muscle is the myosin molecule. This molecule is composed of two major parts: a light meromyosin chain and a heavy meromyosin chain. The heavy meromyosin chain consists of two hinged ends and a head that plays a role in the "ratchet theory" of muscle contraction (Fig. 25.10).[1]

During sympathetic nervous system stimulation, catecholamines (primarily epinephrine and norepinephrine) are released from the central nervous system (CNS) and the adrenal medulla. Increased cardiac conduction velocity, increased force of contraction, and increased heart rate are mediated by β_1-adrenergic receptors. When catecholamines interact with β_1 receptors, they stimulate intracellular G protein activation. Adenyl cyclase activity increases and catalyzes the formation of cyclic adenosine monophosphate. A specific protein kinase is formed, and phosphorylation occurs, increasing myocardial cell permeability to calcium and sodium. Threshold potential is reached, and depolarization occurs, which increases the concentration of calcium from the sarcoplasmic reticulum and the transverse tubular system. Calcium interacts with the troponin tropomyosin complex to initiate cardiac contraction. The force of myocardial contraction is dependent on the quantity of calcium present within the cardiac cell.

The troponin-tropomyosin complex inhibits the binding of the heads of the myosin filaments with the active sites on the actin molecule (Fig. 25.11). During the initiation of contraction, calcium is released from the sarcoplasmic reticulum. Calcium binds to the troponin-tropomyosin complex and causes a conformational change so that the active binding sites on the actin filaments become exposed. The myosin cross bridges bind to the active filament and move along the actin filament by alternately attaching and detaching from the active sites, thereby causing shortening of the Z lines (Fig. 25.12). This is known as the sliding filament theory. When the actin filaments and myosin cross bridges intermingle, muscle contraction occurs. Inhibition of calcium influx into cardiac muscle cells is the proposed mechanism whereby the inhaled anesthetic agents cause depression of myocardial contractility.

Cellular energy or adenosine triphosphate (ATP) is required for this process, known as excitation-contraction coupling, to occur (Fig. 25.13). For muscle contraction to conclude, calcium reuptake into the sarcoplasmic reticulum occurs as a result of active transport. As intracellular calcium concentrations decrease, the troponin-tropomyosin complex again inhibits the interaction between actin and myosin. The process of myocardial excitation-contraction coupling reoccurs within milliseconds and throughout the myocardium. This is the primary reason for the heart's high metabolic demands (see Fig. 25.13). With a limited supply of oxygen and substrate (primarily fatty acids), such as with patients with coronary artery disease or an increased energy demand caused by tachycardia from sympathetic nervous system stimulation, myocardial ischemia and infarction can occur.

Similar length-force relationships exist within the myocardium and in skeletal muscle. The resting sarcomere length at which the muscle cell is most efficient is 2 to 2.4 μm. At greater lengths, the interdigitation of the actin and myosin is compromised, and at shorter lengths the sarcomere is unable to generate an efficient contraction.

Clinically, this concept is demonstrated by having the ideal filling pressure of the LV necessary to achieve adequate CO. Filling pressures are used to reflect the filling volumes of the ventricles and (indirectly) the amount of stretch on the ventricular muscle at rest. Filling pressures are measured by pulmonary capillary wedge pressure (PCWP) or the pulmonary artery diastolic pressure. It has been demonstrated

that at excessively high filling pressures (as in congestive heart failure) and at excessively low filling pressures (as in hypovolemia), the CO can be compromised as a result of either excessive or inadequate stretch of the left ventricular myocardium. The greater the degree of stretch of myocardial muscle fibers, the greater the number of actin filaments and myosin cross bridges that are more completely approximated. This will result in an increase in the force of cardiac contraction (Fig. 25.14). This concept is the basis for the Frank-Starling law of the heart, which is discussed later in this chapter.

Comparison—skeletal and cardiac muscle cells. Several differences exist between myocardial muscle cells and skeletal muscle cells (see Fig. 25.9). At the junctions between the fibers in the myocardial muscle mass, many branching, interconnected fibers are intercalated disks and gap junctions, or nexi. Areas of low resistance facilitate the conduction of the action potential from one myocardial cell to another.

The myocardial sarcomeres also contain increased concentrations of mitochondria due to the heart's high metabolic rate. Skeletal muscles can function both aerobically and anaerobically.

The myocardial sarcomere system has a rich capillary blood supply (one capillary per fiber) that allows for efficient diffusion and perfusion. The T-tubular system and the sarcoplasmic reticulum are extensive within the cardiac sarcomere. This situation allows for the rapid release and reabsorption of calcium from the cells. It also serves to highlight the important role extracellular calcium plays in the contractile process of the myocardial cell.

Generation of Membrane Potentials

Resting membrane potentials. The myocardial sarcomere is not merely a contractile entity. It also possesses properties common to neural tissue, such as the generation of a resting membrane potential, the ability to generate an action potential, and the conduction of the action potential from one sarcomere to the next.

The resting cell membrane is relatively permeable to potassium and relatively impermeable to both sodium and calcium. The resting membrane potential is caused by a chemical force, an electrostatic counterforce, and the sodium-potassium active transport pump.

The chemical force relies on the potential difference in ion concentration between the intracellular and extracellular environment. The ions primarily responsible for this force are sodium, potassium, and calcium.[13] The electrostatic counterforce results from the negative potential generated by the ion difference of the interior of the cell and can pull ions into the cell, especially potassium.

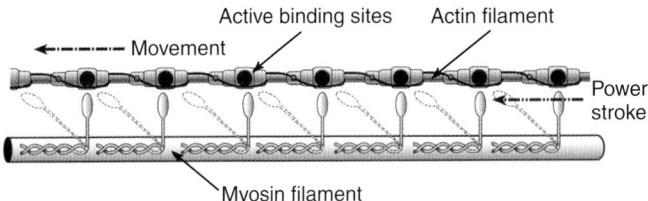

Fig. 25.10 Interaction between actin and myosin that initiates cardiac muscle contraction.

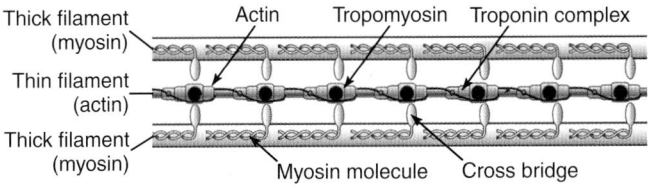

Fig. 25.11 Arrangement of actin and myosin in cardiac muscle.

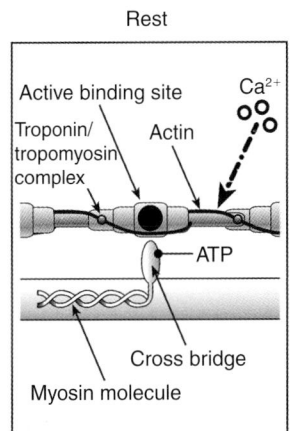
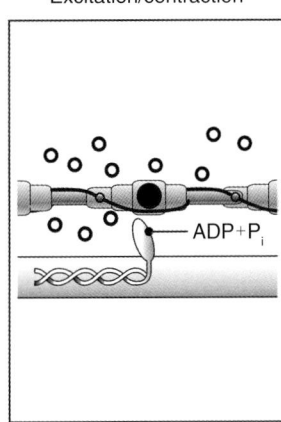
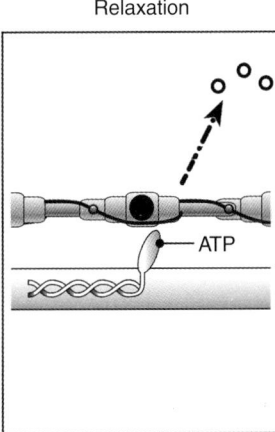

Fig. 25.12 Phases of cardiac muscle contraction. *ADP,* Adenosine diphosphate; *ATP,* adenosine triphosphate.

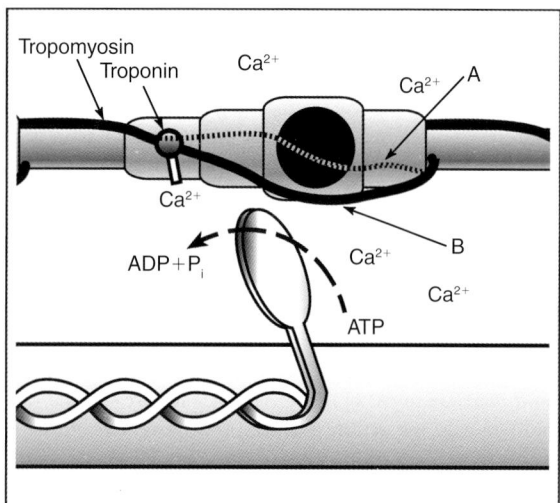

Fig. 25.13 Letter A *(dotted line)* indicates that the troponin tropomyosin complex blocks the active binding site and inhibits contraction. Letter B *(solid line)* indicates that when calcium interacts with troponin, there is a conformational change. The troponin tropomyosin complex is displaced, and interaction between actin and myosin initiates muscle contraction. Note that ATP is used during the binding, the power stroke, and the unbinding process. *ADP,* Adenosine diphosphate; *ATP,* adenosine triphosphate.

The sodium-potassium pump requires an energy source (active transport) and involves the magnesium-dependent enzyme adenosine triphosphatase located in the cell membrane. Three molecules of sodium are pumped out of the cell into the extracellular fluid for every two molecules of potassium pumped into the intracellular fluid.

Calculation of the equilibrium potential (E_m, measured in millivolts [mV]) has been accomplished by examining the concentration of an ion inside the cell versus outside the cell (see the Nernst equation that follows). Table 25.1 lists the equilibrium potentials of the most physiologically important ions. The ion most responsible for the resting membrane potential is potassium.

$$E_m = (-RT/zF) \times \log[K]_i/[K]_o$$

R is a gas constant, T is temperature in Kelvin, F is Faraday's constant, $[K]_i$ is the intracellular concentration of potassium, and $[K]_o$ is the extracellular concentration of potassium.

If a temperature of 310°K is assumed for a living human, the Nernst equation is as follows:

$$E_m = (-61.5/zF) \times \log[K]_i/[K]_o$$

The Nernst potential is useful only in discussions of a single ion. The membrane potentials are generated because the cell membrane is permeable to several different ions. Three factors affect the calculation of the effect of these different ions on the resting membrane potential: the electric charge of each ion, the permeability of the membrane to each ion, and the concentration gradient across the membrane. The following equation, the Goldman-Hodgkin-Katz equation, is a modification of the Nernst equation that accounts for these factors.

$$EMF = 61.5 \times \log([Na]_i P_{Na} + [K]_i P_K + [Cl]_o P_{Cl})/([Na]_o P_{Na} [K]_o P_K [Cl]_i P_{Cl})$$

$[K]_i$ is the intracellular ion concentration of potassium, $[K]_o$ is the extracellular ion concentration of potassium, P_{Na} is the membrane permeability of sodium, P_{Cl} is the membrane permeability of chlorine, and P_K (when calculated) is the membrane permeability of potassium.

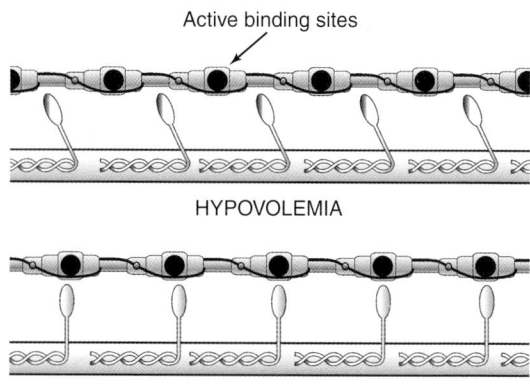

Fig. 25.14 Greater alignment of actin binding sites and myosin cross bridges causes increased myocardial contractility.

TABLE 25.1 Equilibrium Potential of Various Ions			
Ion	Intracellular Concentration (mmol)	Extracellular Plasma Concentration (mmol)	Equilibrium Potential E_m (mV)
Na+	10	145	60
K+	135	4	−94
Cl−	4	114	−97
Ca2+	10^{-4}	2	132

Ventricular Muscle Fiber Action Potential

Gate theory. The functioning of electrostatic gates has been determined for the various ions. These gates open (activated) and close (inactivated), depending on the electrical potential of the cell membrane. An electrostatic gate exists for each of the major cardiac ions (sodium, potassium, calcium, and chloride).

Phases of the action potential. The action potentials of the various parts of the conduction system vary according to their locations and functions.[14] The action potential of ventricular muscle fibers is separated into five phases (Fig. 25.15).

Phase 0, or upstroke, is represented by depolarization and involves the fast sodium channels. The fast sodium channel activation gates (M gates) open between −70 and −65 mV (threshold potential). At 0 mV, both the activation and the inactivation gates (H gates) are open. The rapid upstroke velocity of phase 0 gives a relative indication of the conductivity of the myocardial cell. Local anesthetics such as lidocaine have an inhibitory effect on phase 0 by decreasing the influx of sodium. Table 25.2 describes the phases and events of a cardiac action potential.

During *phase 1* (early rapid repolarization, +2 mV to +30 mV), the sodium gates close, the rapid influx of sodium stops, and the slower influx of calcium begins. In addition, potassium gates open and potassium moves out of the interior of the cell into the extracellular fluid.

Phase 2 (plateau phase) represents one of the characteristics of the action potential that is unique to ventricular muscle. The plateau phase exists because the slow calcium channels open at −30 to −40 mV and allow an influx of calcium. This inward calcium flux delays repolarization and prolongs the absolute refractory period. Toward the end of phase 2, a decreased permeability to potassium occurs that accounts for a small outward leakage of potassium, balanced by the calcium and sodium influx, which maintains a membrane potential near 0 mV. Calcium channel blockers exert their pharmacologic effect during phase 2.

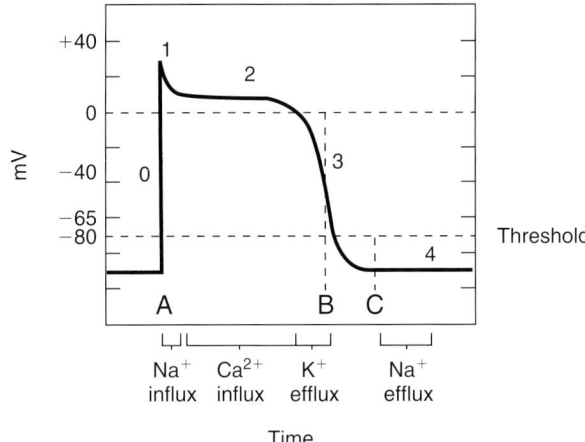

Fig. 25.15 The ventricular muscle action potential. *A* to *B*, Absolute refractory period; *B* to *C*, relative refractory period; *0*, depolarization; *1*, overshoot; *2*, plateau; *3*, repolarization (rapid); *4*, repolarization (complete).

Phase	Name	Cation Movement	Effect
0	Upstroke	Na⁺, ECF to ICF	Sodium channels open Potassium permeability decreased
1	Initial repolarization	K⁺, ICF to ECF	Sodium channels close Potassium channels open
2	Plateau	Ca²⁺, ECF to ICF	Calcium channels open
3	Final repolarization	K⁺, ICF to ECF	Calcium channels close Potassium channels open
4	Resting potential	K⁺, ICF to ECF Na⁺/Ca²⁺ ECF to ICF	Resting membrane permeability restored, sodium and potassium leak to ICF to increase threshold potential

TABLE 25.2 Cardiac Action Potential

ECF, Extracellular fluid; *ICF*, intracellular fluid.

The physiologic effects include decreased contractility, decreased heart rate, and decreased cardiac conduction velocity.[15]

Phase 3 (terminal repolarization phase) is initiated as the slow calcium channels become inactivated. This phenomenon is sustained by an accelerated potassium efflux. These events return the transmembrane potential to its resting membrane value.

During *phase 4* (diastolic repolarization phase), the sodium-potassium pump, which is dependent of ATP, reestablishes the proper intracellular-to-extracellular ionic concentrations. Phase 4 lasts from the completion of repolarization to the next action potential. Lidocaine lengthens the duration of phase 4 by decreasing the cardiac cell membrane's permeability to potassium ion, thereby decreasing the efflux of potassium and delaying the onset of the resting membrane potential.[15]

The cardiac glycoside digoxin inhibits the sodium-potassium ATP-dependent pump, decreasing sodium efflux into the extracellular fluid. As intracellular sodium concentrations increase, the exchange between sodium and calcium is decreased. The result is a higher concentration of calcium remains within the cardiac cell, and this effect is believed to be responsible for the increased inotropic effect.[15]

Refractory periods. The extended duration of the action potential of the myocardial cell protects it against premature excitation. This period of quiescence is known as the refractory period, and it can be divided into effective or absolute and relative refractory periods. The refractory periods are a result of the properties of the sodium channels during the action potential.

The term *effective* or *absolute refractory period* is used to describe the time during which a conducted action potential may not be evoked, even if an active response is elicited by a stimulus at the cellular level. This period lasts from phase 0 to the middle of phase 3, when the membrane potential drops below −60 mV. The relative refractory period is the time during the action potential when a second stimulus can result only in an action potential with decreased amplitude, upstroke velocity, and conduction velocity. The relative refractory period extends from this middle part of the phase 3 range to the beginning of phase 4, when the membrane potential ranges from −60 to −90 mV. This information can be clinically related to synchronized cardioversion. When in a synchronized mode, a shock will not be delivered during the T wave on the electrocardiogram (ECG), which represents ventricular repolarization. The relative refractory period occurs during the T wave, and electricity delivered to the chest during this time can cause electrical disorganization in cardiac cells, resulting in ventricular tachycardia or ventricular fibrillation.

Sinoatrial node action potential. Properties associated with the myocardium include contractility, automaticity, and conductivity. Various portions of the myocardium have their own intrinsic automaticity and rate of action-potential initiation. The SA node is the primary pacemaker of the heart and has several unique characteristics (Fig. 25.16). As a result of its higher resting membrane potentials, the SA node membrane is more permeable to sodium than other atrial myocardial cells. This "leakiness" gradually raises the membrane potential closer to threshold potential (−55 to −60 mV), at which time an action potential may be initiated. Therefore the action potential originating within the SA node differs from the action potential generated within the ventricular muscle mass. For this reason, the SA node is the primary pacemaker of the heart. The intrinsic rate of the SA node is 60 to 100 beats/min. The SA node and the other automatic cells exhibit only phase 4, phase 0, and phase 3 of the action potential. As rapid depolarization is absent, phase 1 or phase 2 (plateau phase) does not occur.

If the SA node fails, the area of the heart with the next highest intrinsic rate, the AV node, replaces the SA node as the pacemaker of the heart. The intrinsic firing rate of the AV node is 40 to 60 beats/min. If both the SA and the AV nodes fail, the Purkinje fibers within the ventricle have pacemaker cells capable of firing at a rate of 20 to 40 beats/min. Cardiac conduction velocity is influenced by the autonomic nervous system (sympathetic-increase, parasympathetic-decrease), myocardial ischemia (decreased within the affected cells), and medications (adrenergic-increase, cholinergic-decrease).

Physiology of the Heart

Cardiac cycle. To fully appreciate the complexities of the cardiac cycle, an understanding of the basics of heart anatomy, as well as the pressures and volumes generated within the various chambers over time, is necessary. An appreciation for the valves and their positions during the phases of the cycle is essential (Fig. 25.17). Additionally, notice that the ECG impulse generation precedes the mechanical action of the heart. This delay between the electrical impulse and the mechanical event occurs because time is needed for the wave of depolarization to spread across the myocardium before contraction can begin. In relation to the ECG, the P wave represents atrial systole, the QRS complex signifies ventricular systole, and the T wave represents ventricular repolarization.

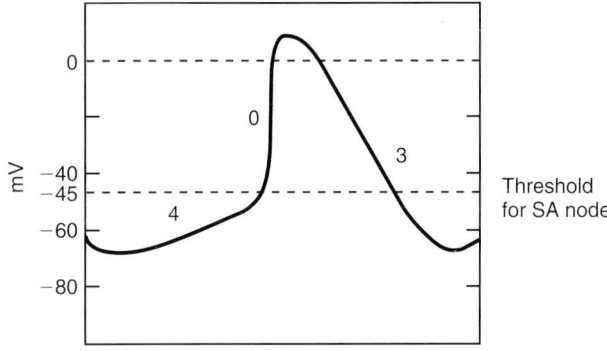

Fig. 25.16 The sinoatrial *(SA)* nodal action potential.

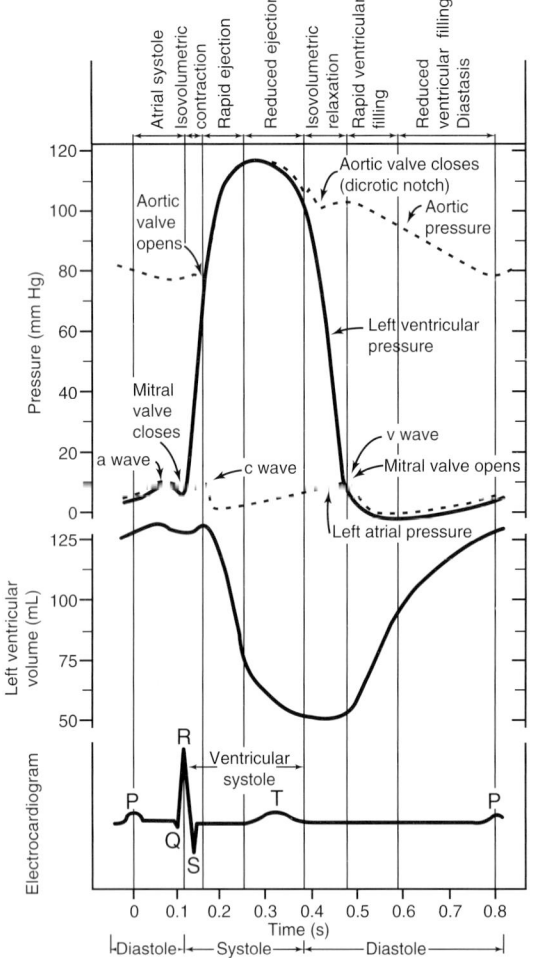

Fig. 25.17 The cardiac cycle.

The cardiac cycle extends from one ventricular contraction to the next. It may be divided into two main phases, systole and diastole. The cardiac cycle is most often described in relation to the left side of the heart. However, similar conclusions about the function of the right side of the heart may be inferred in the absence of cardiopulmonary pathology.

Diastole. During ventricular systole, the atria fill from blood returning from the venous system to the right side of the heart, and from the pulmonary circulation into the left side of the heart. The first phase of diastole is the period of isovolumetric relaxation. The ventricular muscle mass relaxes, and the tricuspid and mitral valves are closed if the ventricular pressure remains higher than the atrial

pressure. The true filling phase is divided into three periods: (1) rapid inflow, (2) reduced inflow (also known as diastasis), and (3) atrial systole. Once the left ventricular pressure drops below atrial pressure, the mitral valve opens, and the period of rapid, passive filling begins. The second period of diastole is diastasis, in which minimal changes occur in volume and in pressure as passive ventricular filling is nearly complete.

Atrial systole provides the final period of rapid filling and is commonly referred to as the atrial kick. This active process increases ventricular volume by approximately 20% immediately before ventricular systole. In patients who have severe mitral stenosis, the atrial kick may be responsible for up to 40% of the ventricular filling. Once left atrial systole and closure of the mitral valve occurs, this volume is known as LVEDV. During periods of strenuous exercise or in patients with many pathologic conditions such as shock or congestive heart failure, the additional ventricular filling is critical to maintaining SV.

Systole. After left atrial systole and closure of the mitral valve, the isovolumetric phase, or isovolumetric contraction, begins, and this period is associated with the beginning of left ventricular contraction. The ventricular myocardial fibers shorten, and pressure is increased within the ventricle. As the pressure in the left ventricle exceeds the pressure in the left atrium, the mitral valve closes. During this period, an increase in left ventricular pressure occurs without a change in ventricular diastolic volume. Isovolumetric contraction begins with closure of the mitral valve and lasts until opening of the aortic valve.

Systolic ejection begins with the opening of the aortic valve and occurs when the left ventricular pressure exceeds the aortic pressure. This phase of the cardiac cycle is divided into two periods, with the period of rapid ejection accounting for the first third of systole and the period of reduced ejection comprising the remaining two-thirds of systole. During rapid ejection, left ventricular systolic pressure peaks, and the largest amount of volume is ejected. Therefore systole is composed of isovolumetric contraction, rapid ejection, and reduced ejection. The dicrotic notch or incisura on the arterial pressure tracing occurs within the period of isovolumetric relaxation. This segment represents retrograde blood flow back into the LV before aortic valve closure. Three waveform segments are present on the left atrial pressure tracing: *a* wave, *c* wave, and *v* wave. The specific waveforms correspond to their position within the cardiac cycle: The *a* wave represents the end of atrial systole just before mitral valve closure, the *c* wave represents ventricular contraction and is produced by bulging of the mitral valve caused by increasing left ventricular pressure, and the *v* wave represents increased pressure in the LA caused by blood return from the pulmonary veins before mitral valve opening.

Physiology of coronary circulation. The anatomy of the coronary circulation has already been discussed. A description of the physiologic determinants of coronary blood flow follows.

Coronary blood flow. The rate of blood flow is determined by a change in the pressure within the vessel divided by resistance of the system. Alterations of the radius of a vessel change the flow to the fourth power of the radius. This phenomenon is an extension of Poiseuille's law, which determines the flow of a fluid through a tube.

At rest, approximately 4% to 5% of the CO, or approximately 225 mL/min of blood, passes through the coronary vasculature. Phasic changes have been documented during coronary blood flow. A greater amount of LV coronary blood flow occurs during diastole. During systole, LCA blood flow ceases to the subendocardium from compression of the subendocardial vessels due to increased myocardial muscle fiber tension; flow through the epicardial vessels is not affected during systole to this extent. The flow to the LCA is greatest during diastole as a result of the decreased resistance to flow from decreased myofibril tension that occurs as the intracavity pressure decreases (Fig. 25.18).

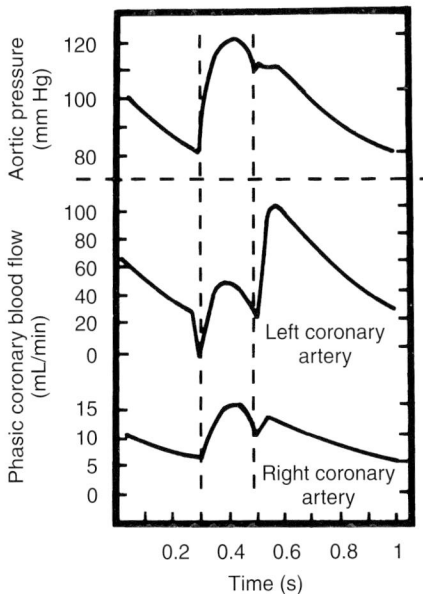

Fig. 25.18 Blood flow in the left and right coronary arteries. The right ventricle is perfused throughout the cardiac cycle. Flow to the left ventricle is largely confined to diastole. (From Hibbert B, et al. Coronary physiology and atherosclerosis. In Kaplan JA, et al., eds. *Kaplan's Cardiac Anesthesia: For Cardiac and Noncardiac Surgery.* 7th ed. Philadelphia: Elsevier; 2017:185.)

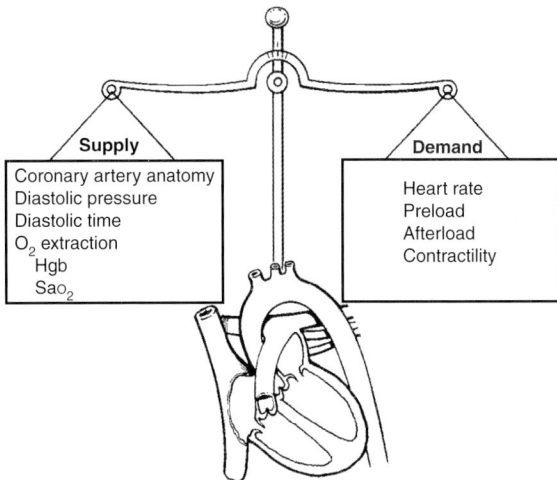

Fig. 25.19 The heart's oxygen supply and demand must be balanced by the anesthetist, who should increase the former and reduce the latter. *Hgb,* Hemoglobin; *Sao₂,* arterial oxygen saturation.

Control of coronary circulation and oxygen supply and demand. Coronary artery blood flow is regulated by intrinsic and extrinsic factors that affect coronary artery tone. Intrinsic factors include the anatomic arrangement of the coronary arteries and perfusion pressure within the coronary vessels. Extrinsic factors include compression within the myocardium, as well as metabolic, neural, and humoral factors. Blood flow through the coronary circulation is primarily controlled by the factors that determine oxygen supply and demand. Myocardial oxygen supply is determined by arterial blood content, diastolic blood pressure (DBP), diastolic time as determined by HR, oxygen extraction, and coronary blood flow. Myocardial oxygen demand is determined by preload, afterload, contractility, and HR (Fig. 25.19).

The factors that increase myocardial oxygen consumption ($M\dot{V}O_2$) are listed in Table 25.3. Notice in Fig. 25.19 that HR appears in the balance of both the supply side (as diastolic time) and demand side of the scale. Increasing HR not only increases demand but also decreases diastolic time, which is when 80% to 90% of coronary filling and myocardial perfusion occur. Increased HR is the most important factor that negatively affects $M\dot{V}O_2$. Doubling the HR doubles $M\dot{V}O_2$.[16] This phenomenon most dramatically affects patients with coronary artery disease because the supply of blood is compromised and may not be able to meet the oxygen demands caused by tachycardia. As a result, myocardial dysfunction or infarction can occur. By slowing HR and decreasing contractility, β-blocking medications increase supply and decrease demand, protecting the heart from ischemia.[17]

Due to the high metabolic demand, the myocardium extracts 65% to 70% of the available oxygen from hemoglobin. Therefore the only way to increase oxygen delivery to the myocardium is by increasing blood flow. During periods of increased myocardial oxygen demands, coronary artery vasodilation occurs and blood flow through the coronary arteries can increase by three to four times. Several vasodilator substances have been identified and are released from the myocardium in response to decreased oxygen delivery or concentration. Among these substances are adenosine, adenosine phosphate compounds,

TABLE 25.3 Components and Effects on Myocardial Oxygen Consumption

A 50% Increase in	Resultant Increase in $M\dot{V}O_2$
Heart rate	50%
Pressure work	50%
Contractility	45%
Wall stress	25%
Volume work	4%

$M\dot{V}O_2$, Myocardial oxygen consumption.

potassium ions, hydrogen ions, carbon dioxide, bradykinin, and prostaglandin. Experts believe that adenosine is one of the primary substances responsible for coronary vasodilation.

The normal physiologic parameters of the heart are presented in Table 25.4. The determinants of $M\dot{V}O_2$ include myocardial contractility, myocardial wall tension (preload), HR, and mean arterial pressure (MAP; afterload). Oxygen extraction is determined by measurement of the difference between the oxygen tension in the pulmonary arterial blood and that in the coronary sinus.

Oxygen supply relies on the blood oxygen content (see following equation), which is affected by both the oxygen carried on the hemoglobin (Hgb) molecule (constant = 1.34 mL of oxygen per gram of Hgb, exact value 1.24–1.39) and to a lesser extent the oxygen dissolved in the plasma (0.003 mL of oxygen per milliliter of plasma).

$$\text{Arterial oxygen content equation (CaO}_2) \\ = (SaO_2 \times Hgb \times 1.34) + (0.003 \times PaO_2)$$

where SaO_2 is the % of hemoglobin saturated with oxygen (normal range 93%–100%); Hgb is hemoglobin (normal range adult female 12–16 g/dL, adult male 13–18 g/dL); PaO_2 is arterial oxygen partial pressure (normal range, 80–100 mm Hg); and CaO_2 is arterial oxygen concentration, a reflection of total number of oxygen molecules in arterial blood (both bound and unbound to hemoglobin).

Other factors that have an influence on coronary circulation include the direct and indirect effects of the sympathetic nervous system and the effect of certain substrates of cardiac metabolism.

Coronary artery autoregulation. Under normal physiologic conditions, the coronary circulation, like other tissue beds in the body, exhibits autoregulation, which is the ability to maintain coronary blood

TABLE 25.4	**Normal Physiologic Parameters**
Heart size	230–280 g (female)
	280–340 g (male)
Coronary blood flow	225–250 mL/min or 4%–7% total cardiac output
Myocardial O_2 consumption	65%–70% extraction
	8–10 mL O_2/100 g/min
Normal autoregulation	60–140 mm Hg (MAP)
Coronary filling	80%–90% during diastole

MAP, Mean arterial pressure.

flow across a range of MAPs by dilating or constricting. Coronary blood flow is maintained at a constant flow rate through a MAP range of 60 to 140 mm Hg. When arterial blood pressure is less than or exceeds these pressure limits, coronary blood flow becomes pressure dependent. Therefore, during hypotension, when the coronary arteries are maximally dilated, coronary blood flow is determined by the MAP minus the right atrial pressure. Cardiac pathology (including untreated hypertension), coronary artery disease, and cardiomyopathies cause the normal autoregulatory curve to shift to the right necessitating a MAP greater than 60 mm Hg to maintain adequate myocardial perfusion.

A method for directly estimating coronary perfusion pressure (CPP) can be calculated by subtracting LVEDP from DBP (i.e., CPP = DBP – LVEDP). Under normal conditions, LVEDP (10 mm Hg) is significantly less than DBP (80 mm Hg). Therefore the major determinant of CPP is DBP.

Coronary vascular reserve is the difference between the maximal flow and the autoregulated flow. The closer these two values are, the lower the coronary reserve of the patient. Factors that increase myocardial oxygen demand and limit supply decrease coronary reserve flow and can result in myocardial dysfunction.

The concept of "coronary steal" can be used in reference to vasodilation associated with the use of medications such as adenosine, nitroglycerin, and isoflurane. When stenosis of a coronary artery exists (e.g., atherosclerotic plaque), this region of the coronary artery is maximally dilated to meet the metabolic demands of the myocardium. If vasodilator treatment is administered to a patient who has both an ischemic area of the heart that is supplied by a stenotic vessel with collateral flow and another area that has an intact autoregulated vessel, only the autoregulated vessel dilates further and has the ability to increase its flow. Therefore only the areas of the heart with intact autoregulation respond to vasodilators and receive preferential flow over the stenotic area. Lastly, by dilating the coronary arterial system, flow in the region of stenosis can decrease causing myocardial ischemia. The existence of this phenomenon is questionable. As long as adequate CPP is maintained, coronary steal and myocardial ischemia caused by isoflurane do not occur.[18,19] A second factor that could result in this phenomenon is coronary steal–prone anatomy. This has been defined as complete occlusion of one coronary artery and at least 50% occlusion of a second coronary artery that supplies collateral blood flow to the area in which the complete occlusion exists.[18] In addition, evidence suggests that the inhaled anesthetics isoflurane, desflurane, and sevoflurane produce myocardial protection during periods of ischemia in humans by decreasing the formation of free radicals, preserving myocardial ATP stores, and inhibiting intracellular calcium.[19,20] This phenomena is referred to as anesthetic preconditioning.

Cardiac output. Cardiac output is the amount of blood ejected from the LV for 1 minute. Comparing various CO values among humans requires a method for calculating output in relation to the size of the patient. The CO is measured in liters per minute. Cardiac output is indexed because a CO

of 3.5 L/min may be adequate for a woman who is 5 feet tall and weighs 95 pounds, but it is less than optimal for a man who is 6 feet 5 inches tall and weighs 250 pounds. The average CO is 5 L/min, and the average cardiac index (CI) is 2.5 L/min or more per square meter of body surface area (BSA). The formula for this relationship is CI = CO/BSA.

The primary determinants of CO are HR and SV. CO is derived by using the equation CO = HR × SV. The SV is the amount of blood ejected from the LV with each beat. The average SV is approximately 70 mL. If the average HR is 70 to 80 beats/min, a CO of 5 L/min results.

Several key factors affect SV, including preload, afterload, and myocardial contractility. When increased, all these factors increase myocardial oxygen demand. Preload is the effective tension of the blood on the ventricle or the wall tension at the end of diastole. Preload can either be passive (the flow of blood from the atria to the ventricles during diastole) or active (the volume contributed by the atrial kick). With increased preload, there is an associated increase in contractility during contraction. This phenomenon is called the Frank-Starling law of the heart, which states that the greater the wall tension (preload), the greater the compensatory increase in myocardial contractility. This mechanism allows the heart to immediately compensate for increased preload and avoid overdistention of the ventricular chambers by increasing SV, which facilitates chamber emptying. However, there is a point at which progressive increases in preload no longer increase contractility but instead can contribute to decreased myocardial performance. Increased preload increases myocardial oxygen demand. Clinically, preload can be estimated by using the PCWP and the pulmonary artery diastolic pressure. In patients with a normal mitral valve orifice and ventricular muscle function, either of these measures provides an estimate of the preload or LVEDP and volume.

Cardiac output can be calculated by applying this equation, known as the Fick principle:

$$CO\ (L/min) = \frac{O_2\ absorbed\ per\ minute\ by\ the\ lungs\ (mL/min)}{Arteriovenous\ O_2\ difference\ (mL/L\ of\ blood)}$$

This can also be expressed as:

$$CO\ (L/min) = VO_2/(C_a - C_v)O_2$$

where CO is cardiac output (Fick) (L/min), VO_2 is oxygen consumption (mL/min), and $(C_a - C_v)O_2$ is arterial venous oxygen content difference: (mL/dL) ($(C_a - C_v)O_2$ is multiplied by 10 to convert to mL/dL to mL/L).

Afterload is the wall tension the myocardium needs to generate to eject the SV against SVR. It is the pressure within the LV during peak systole. Factors affecting LV afterload include the state of the ventricular chamber and the compliance of the arterial vasculature. The shape, size, and wall thickness of the ventricle play an important role in afterload. The vascular component of the afterload includes SVR and MAP because these variables relate to the vascular compliance of the aorta. Thus increases in blood pressure increase afterload.

Afterload is most often estimated clinically by determining the SVR. The SVR may be calculated once the CO and the difference between the MAP and the central venous pressure (CVP) are known (see the following equation). The normal SVR is 800 to 1500 dynes/sec/cm[5.]

$$SVR = (MAP - CVP) \times 80/CO$$

The problem with equating afterload with SVR is that ventricular wall tension, which is an integral part of the afterload, is not considered.

Contractility of the myocardium is the state of inotropy that is independent of either preload or afterload. It may be altered by many cardiovascular disease states. Factors such as rate of pressure changes over time (dP/dt [first derivative of pressure measured over time]), force-velocity or Starling ventricular function curves, pressure-volume loops,

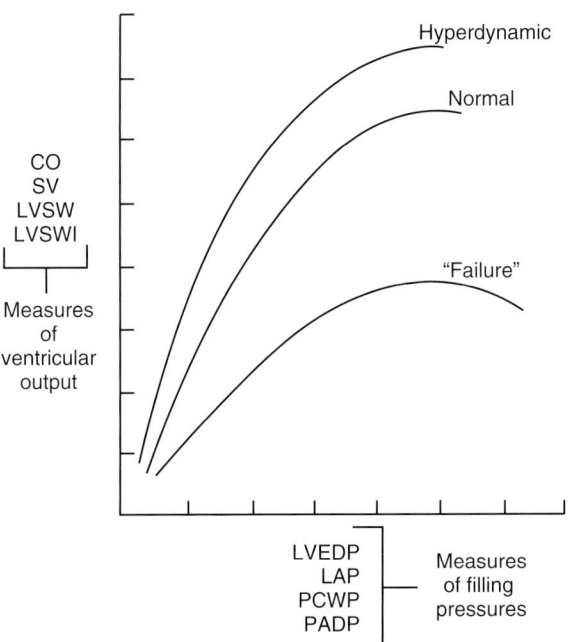

Fig. 25.20 The ventricular function curve. *CO,* Cardiac output; *LAP,* left atrial pressure; *LVEDP,* left ventricular end-diastolic pressure; *LVSW,* left ventricular stroke work; *LVSWI,* left ventricular stroke work index; *PADP,* pulmonary artery diastolic pressure; *PCWP,* pulmonary capillary wedge pressure; *SV,* stroke volume.

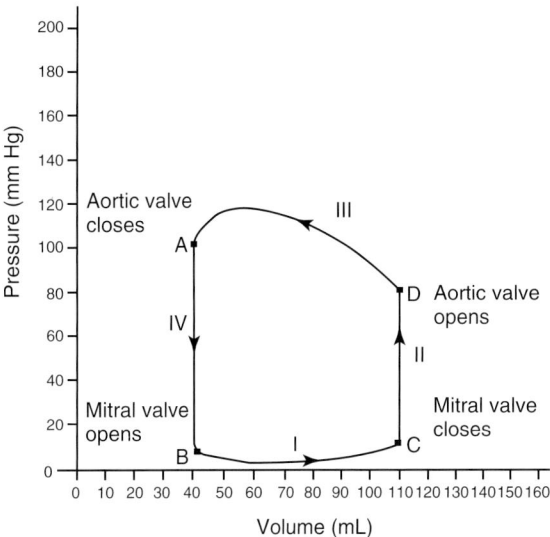

Fig. 25.21 Phases of the left ventricular (LV) pressure-volume loop, which is a continuous cycle divided into four phases. Phase I represents diastolic filling. LV filling begins at point *B* and ends at point *C*. Note the increase in volume of 70 mL from point *B* to point *C* and the upward movement of the curve at point *C*, representing a slightly increased pressure in response to the increased volume. Point *C* or mitral valve closure represents end-diastolic volume (EDV). Phase II represents isovolumetric contraction. Note there is a significant increase in pressure but no change in volume. Cardiac muscle fibers are shortening and increasing the pressure on the LV volume until point *D*, where the LV pressure exceeds aortic pressure. Phase III represents systolic ejection. Note the decrease in LV volume throughout LV systolic ejection. Phase IV represents isovolumetric relaxation. At point *A* the aortic pressure exceeds LV pressure, and the aortic valve closes. Point *A* represents end-systolic volume (ESV). The LV relaxes, and the pressure decreases significantly. At maximal LV relaxation, the mitral valve opens, and the process restarts.

ejection fraction (EF), and velocity of circumferential fiber shortening have all been used to estimate contractility.

Left ventricular dP/dt measurements require a high-fidelity recording system, and for this reason these measures are not readily available in the clinical setting. A wide range of normal values exists (800–1700 mm Hg/sec), making patient-to-patient comparisons difficult.

Ventricular function curves (Fig. 25.20) define the relationship between the left ventricular filling pressure (left ventricular diastolic pressure, left atrial pressure, PCWP) and the left ventricular stroke work index (LVSWI), which is calculated by use of the following equation:

$$LVSWI \text{ (in g/m}^2 \text{ per beat)} = 0.0136 \times SVI \times (MAP - PCWP)$$

where SVI = CI/HR and SVI is stroke volume index.

Each left ventricular function curve has a steep upstroke that has a plateau at higher filling pressures. To apply the Frank-Starling mechanism to Fig. 25.20, notice in the "normal" and "hyperdynamic" curves that as pressure (horizontal axis) increases, so does LV output (vertical axis). However, at the top of these curves there is a plateau where increasing the filling pressures no longer increases performance and can then decrease ventricular output. Symptoms may be elicited by either high or low filling pressures. On the "failure" curve, with compromised cardiac function, increases in filling pressures do not dramatically increase myocardial performance and can lead to cardiogenic shock. The clinical determination of LVSWI is an indication of the factors that contribute to CO, and it gives measures of both systolic and diastolic performance.

Left ventricular pressure-volume loops have been mentioned before as conceptual models depicting phases of the cardiac cycle. They may also be used as tools to determine myocardial performance and the presence of cardiac pathology. Left ventricular pressure-volume loops simultaneously measure chamber pressures and the resultant volumes (Fig. 25.21). Movement from left to right on the horizontal axis represents increased volume. Movement from right to left on the

horizontal axis represents decreased volume. Movement up and down on the vertical axis represents increases and decreases in pressure, respectively. The distinct phases of the left ventricular pressure-volume loop are represented in Fig. 25.22.

The interior of the curve (distance between the two vertical lines of the LV pressure-volume loop) is representative of SV. In this diagram, SV is calculated by subtracting end-systolic volume (ESV) from end-diastolic volume (EDV), or EDV (110 mL) – ESV (40 mL). Thus, in this example, SV is 70 mL. EF can then be estimated using the following equations:

$$EF = (EDV - ESV)/EDV \times 100$$

or

$$EF = (SV/EDV) \times 100$$

The EF is the percentage of the EDV ejected during systole (Fig. 25.23). The normal EF is 60% to 65%. An EF of less than 40% is associated with significant left ventricular impairment.

Deviations from the normal left ventricular pressure-volume loops occur for a variety of reasons. Factors that alter the normal loop include increases and decreases in LV preload, LV afterload, and LV contractility. These factors can be acute and transient, such as during the administration of vasoactive medications, or chronic because of myocardial compensation caused by valvular heart disease (stenosis vs regurgitation). In Fig. 25.24, these changes are consistent with valvular heart disease. As stated, many factors contribute to variations in pressure and

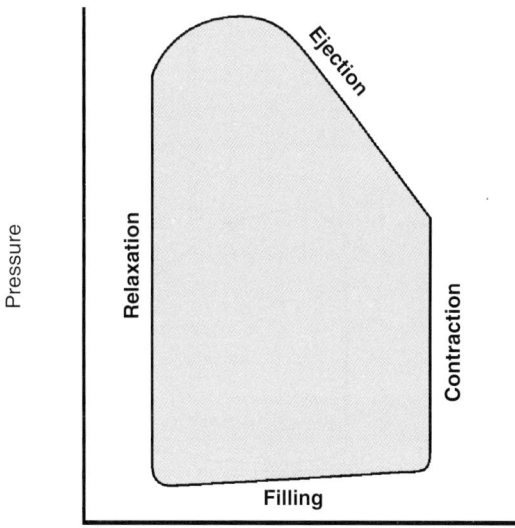

Volume
Left Ventricular Pressure-Volume Loop

Fig. 25.22 Phases of the cardiac cycle represented by a left ventricular pressure-volume loop.

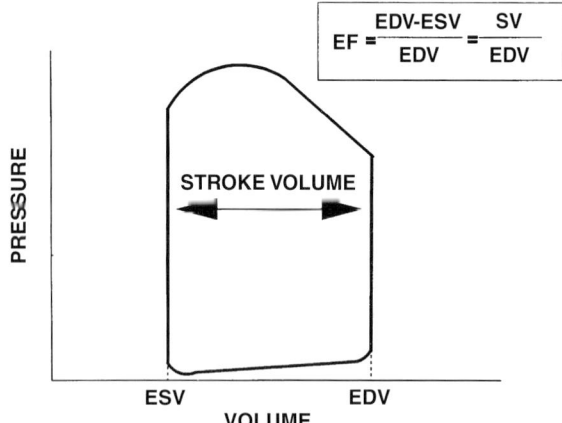

Fig. 25.23 Pressure-volume diagram indicating end-diastolic volume *(EDV)*, end-systolic volume *(ESV)*, stroke volume *(SV)*, and the equation for ejection fraction *(EF)*. (From Johnson B, et al. Cardiac physiology. In Kaplan JA, et al., eds. Kaplan's *Cardiac Anesthesia: The Echo Era.* 7th ed. Philadelphia: Elsevier; 2011:84.)

volume from beat to beat within the LV; each pressure volume loop is distinct, represents one LV systolic ejection, and is different for each contraction. A discussion of these pathologic curves is presented later in this chapter.

A clinically useful tool to determine a beat-by-beat assessment of myocardial performance is transesophageal echocardiography (TEE). When this technology is appropriately used, real-time movement of all four chambers of the heart, as well as that of the valves, may be visualized.

TEE can be used to detect valvular function and blood flows in both regurgitant and stenotic lesions. It is also useful in determining areas of hypokinesis, dyskinesis, or akinesis caused by myocardial infarction (MI), ischemia, or injury. It can be useful in determining myocardial contractility, and it is a more direct measure of intraventricular volume status than pulmonary artery catheter pressure measures. TEE has also proven useful in directing fluid and pharmacologic therapy in patients

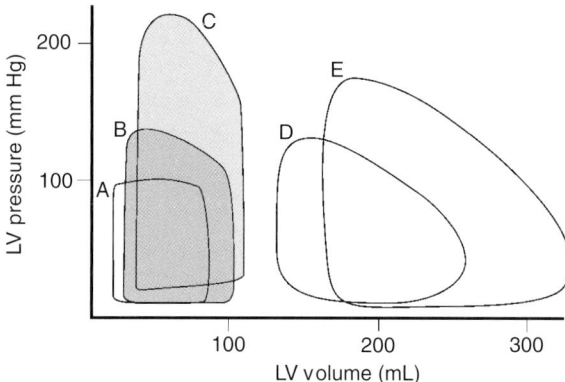

Fig. 25.24 Pathologic left ventricular pressure-volume loops. *A,* Mitral stenosis; *B,* normal curve; *C,* aortic stenosis; *D,* mitral regurgitation; *E,* aortic regurgitation.

who have undergone coronary bypass and other surgical procedures. Ventricular dysfunction or reperfusion injury, as well as the presence of intraventricular air, can be determined with TEE. This diagnostic tool is the gold standard for assessing intraoperative myocardial performance.[21] The practical problems associated with the clinical use of TEE entail acquiring the skills necessary for accurate interpretation of the visual data, the possibility of esophageal rupture, and the cost associated with its use.

Cardiovascular Reflexes

Cardiac output regulation. A direct interplay exists between CO and venous return. If either contractility or HR is not compromised, maintenance of a constant return of blood flow to the heart ensures an adequate CO. The body's regulation of CO depends on its ability to regulate HR and contractility of the myocardium, as well as constriction and distention of the vascular tree.

Many of the factors that affect CO also affect the MAP and are addressed later in this chapter in the section on regulation of MAP. Cardiovascular reflexes that can alter the CO are described in this section or in the section on regulation of MAP.

Valsalva maneuver. The Valsalva maneuver occurs as a result of forced expiration against a closed glottis. The reflex is mediated through the baroreceptors located near the bifurcation of the internal and external carotid arteries (carotid sinus) and the aortic arch. The afferent pathway is directed via Hering nerve, which is a branch of the glossopharyngeal nerve, from the carotid sinus or the vagus nerve from the aortic arch (Fig. 25.25). Stimulation of either of these areas inhibits the vasomotor center in the medulla. The response inhibits the sympathetic nervous system and stimulates the parasympathetic nervous system, producing a decrease in HR, myocardial contractility, and a rate of cardiac impulse conduction, and induces vasodilation, resulting in a decrease in blood pressure. The Valsalva maneuver also increases intrathoracic pressure, which decreases venous return and ultimately CO.

Baroreceptor reflex. The baroreceptors respond to fluctuations in arterial blood pressure. Afferent and efferent impulse transmission travels along the same pathway as previously described for the Valsalva maneuver (see Fig. 25.25). Decreases in arterial blood pressure are sensed by the baroreceptors causing increased sympathetic tone, which results in increased myocardial performance and vasoconstriction. Acute hypertension causes the opposite cardiovascular response to occur. A more in-depth explanation of the baroreceptor response and its role in short- and long-term blood pressure control is presented later in this chapter. The baroreceptor response is inhibited

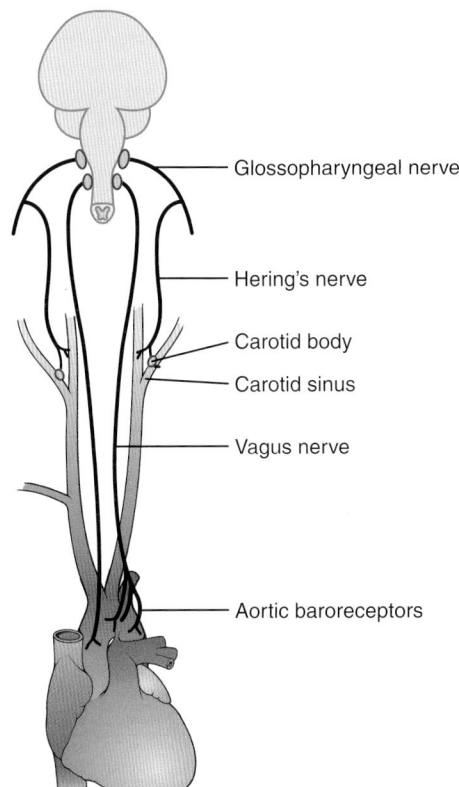

- Glossopharyngeal nerve
- Hering's nerve
- Carotid body
- Carotid sinus
- Vagus nerve
- Aortic baroreceptors

Fig. 25.25 Afferent and efferent neural pathways from carotid and aortic baroreceptors. (From Hall JE. *Guyton and Hall Textbook of Medical Physiology.* 13th ed. Philadelphia: Elsevier; 2017:220.)

by inhalation anesthetic agents in a dose-dependent manner and results in a decreased ability of the baroreceptors to respond to blood pressure changes when these agents are used. The responsiveness of the baroreceptor reflex also decreases as part of the normal aging process.

Oculocardiac reflex. Traction on the extraocular muscles (especially the medial rectus), conjunctiva, or orbital structures can cause hypotension and a reflex bradycardia, as well as dysrhythmias. The oculocardiac reflex, also known as Aschner phenomenon, may be elicited during retrobulbar block, ocular trauma, or pressure on the tissue that remains after enucleation. The afferent path of this reflex is mediated by the long and short ciliary nerves to the ciliary ganglion of the oculomotor nerve and then to the ophthalmic division of the trigeminal nerve (cranial nerve V) and finally to the gasserian ganglion. The efferent branch of the reflex is mediated by the vagus nerve (cranial nerve X). Due to the nervous system pathway, it can also be referred to as a trigeminovagal reflex. This reflex may be blunted by administering a retrobulbar block or releasing pressure on the eye or extraocular muscles. The resulting vagal response to the heart can be inhibited by an anticholinergic agent (atropine or glycopyrrolate).

Celiac reflex. The celiac reflex is elicited by traction on the mesentery or the gallbladder or stimulation of the vagus nerve in other areas of the body, such as the thorax and abdominal cavity. Stimulation of this reflex causes bradycardia, apnea, and hypotension. Clinically, the celiac reflex can be initiated indirectly as a result of a pneumoperitoneum. As with the oculocardiac reflex, the celiac reflex is frequently resolved by stopping the initiating stimulus. This vagal response to the heart can be antagonized by administration of an anticholinergic agent (atropine or glycopyrrolate).

Bainbridge reflex (atrial stretch reflex). The Bainbridge reflex is elicited as a result of an increased volume of blood in the heart, which causes sympathetic nervous system stimulation. Stretch receptors are located in the right atrium, junction of the vena cava, and pulmonary veins. The SA node is also involved in this process and can increase heart rate by 10% to 15%. This reflex helps to prevent sequestration of blood in veins, atria, and pulmonary circulation. Antidiuretic hormone secretion from the posterior pituitary gland is decreased, resulting in decreased circulating blood volume. Atrial natriuretic peptide is increased, which also promotes diuresis.

Cushing reflex. This physiologic response to CNS ischemia caused by increased intracranial pressure is called the Cushing reflex. It is triggered as a result of an elevation of intracranial pressure to a value greater than the MAP, thereby decreasing cerebral perfusion and potentially causing cerebral ischemia. An intense sympathetic nervous system response is initiated by the vasomotor center, resulting in intense vasoconstriction. These compensatory physiologic changes attempt to restore adequate cerebral perfusion. However, if cerebral ischemia is not relieved, cerebral infarction results. When the vasomotor area becomes ischemic as a result of hypotension (MAP <50 mm Hg), maximal stimulation of the vasomotor center occurs. Cushing triad is a late sign of high and sustained intracranial pressure prior to cerebral herniation. The triad of signs includes hypertension, bradycardia, and respiratory rhythm irregularity.

Chemoreceptor reflex. The central chemoreceptors are located beneath the ventrolateral surface of the medulla oblongata and are primarily stimulated by (1) decreased cerebral spinal fluid pH and (2) increased $Paco_2$. The peripheral chemoreceptors are located at the bifurcation of the internal and external carotid arteries (carotid body) and within the aortic arch (aortic body) and are primarily stimulated by (1) decreased Pao_2 and to a lesser extent (2) increased $Paco_2$ and decreased blood pH. The degree of physiologic stimulation is greater from the central chemoreceptors as compared to the peripheral chemoreceptors. The response elicited from hypoxia, hypercarbia, and acidosis stimulates the sympathetic nervous system resulting in an increased minute ventilation, blood pressure, and heart rate. Like the baroreceptor reflex, the chemoreceptor response is inhibited by the inhalation anesthetic agents in a dose-dependent manner. Thus, if residual inhalation agent is present during the emergence from anesthesia, the carbon dioxide threshold will be increased, necessitating a higher partial pressure of carbon dioxide in arterial blood ($Paco_2$) prior to the beginning of spontaneous respirations. Table 25.5 provides a summary of the cardiovascular reflexes.

Bezold-Jarisch reflex. Intense parasympathetic nervous system predominance in rare instances can lead to cardiovascular collapse. A rapid decrease in venous return to the heart activates mechanoreceptors within the LV that sense LV volume. An afferent sensory response is relayed to the medulla, which results in profound vasodilation, bradycardia, and possibly asystole. This cardiovascular response is known as the Bezold-Jarisch reflex, which can occur from a variety of causes such as neuraxial anesthesia, MI, coronary artery thrombolysis, histamine release, or nitrovasodilators. Since this response is theorized to be mediated in part by serotonin, 5-HT₃ receptor antagonists are believed to mitigate the effects. Ondansetron, a 5-HT₃ antagonist, has been shown to decrease the incidence of hypotension and possibly bradycardia following spinal anesthesia.[22]

VASCULAR SYSTEM

Anatomy

Vascular Anatomy

The vascular circulation is divided into the pulmonary circulation and the peripheral systemic circulation (Fig. 25.26). This system is composed of several functional parts.

TABLE 25.5   Cardiac Reflexes

Reflex	Stimulus	Response
Baroreceptor reflex	Hypertension resulting in baroreceptor stimulation; carotid baroreceptors send afferent response via Hering and glossopharyngeal nerves (CN IX); aortic baroreceptors send afferent response via the vagus nerve (CN X)*	Decreased heart rate, decreased contractility, peripheral vasodilation from efferent response via the vagus nerve (CN X)
Valsalva maneuver	Forced expiration against a closed glottis mediated via baroreceptors; see baroreceptor reflex for neural pathways	Decreased heart rate, decreased contractility, peripheral vasodilation from efferent response via the vagus nerve (CN X)
Cushing reflex	Increased intracranial pressure resulting in cerebral ischemia	Sympathetic nervous stimulation resulting in increased blood pressure
Chemoreceptor reflex	Decreased oxygen saturation, increased carbon dioxide, increased hydrogen ion concentration; peripheral chemoreceptors located in the carotid body and aortic arch; see baroreceptor reflex for neural pathways	Increased respiratory drive, increased blood pressure
Atrial stretch reflex (Bainbridge reflex)	Hypervolemia, increased venous return causes stimulation of atrial stretch receptors	Increased heart rate, decreased blood pressure, decreased systemic vascular resistance, diuresis
Oculocardiac reflex	Traction on the extraocular muscles (especially medial rectus) or pressure on the globe causes an afferent response via the trigeminal nerve (CN V) and results in an efferent vagal response via the vagus nerve (CN X)	Bradycardia, hypotension, and arrhythmias
Celiac reflex	Traction or pressure on structures within abdominal and thoracic cavities causes vagal nerve stimulation	Bradycardia, hypotension, and apnea
Bezold-Jarisch reflex	Decreased preload causes activation of mechanoreceptors in the LV causing parasympathetic nervous system predominance	Bradycardia, hypotension, apnea, asystole

*Efferent response increases parasympathetic tone via the vagus and sympathetic nerves.
CN, Cranial nerve; LV, left ventricle.

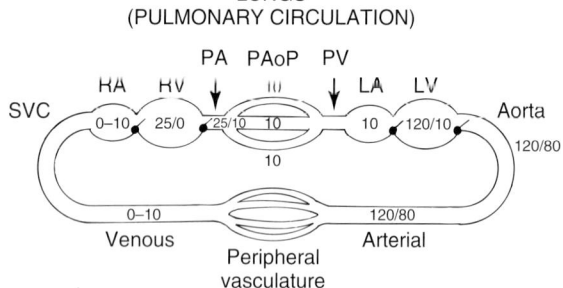

Fig. 25.26 The vascular circuit. *LA,* Left atrium; *LV,* left ventricle; *PA,* pulmonary artery; *PAOP,* pulmonary artery occlusion pressure; *RA,* right atrium; *RV,* right ventricle; *SVC,* superior vena cava.

Arteries. Arteries transport blood from the heart to peripheral tissues under high pressure. Arteries have an average diameter of 4 mm and a wall thickness of 1 mm. They have a thick layer of elastic tissue, smooth muscle, and fibrous tissue. Arteries maintain the flow of blood because of their large internal diameter. Due to the muscular layer within arterial walls, arterial constriction or dilation has a significant effect on SVR.

Arterioles. Arterioles are the last small branches of the arterial system, and they act as control valves for the release of blood into the capillary beds. Arterioles have an average diameter of 30 μm and a wall thickness of 20 μm. Like arteries, arterioles have a thick layer of elastic tissue, smooth muscle, and fibrous tissue. Constriction of the arterioles, as compared with that of other structures within the vascular system, causes the greatest increase in SVR. For this reason, arterioles exhibit the greatest pressure drop in the vascular system across the length of their vessels.

Capillaries. The exchange of fluids, nutrients, electrolytes, hormones, and other substances occurs between the blood and the interstitial fluids in the capillaries. Capillaries have an average diameter of 8 μm and a wall thickness of 1 μm. The walls of capillaries are only one cell thick and have no elastic tissue, smooth muscle, or fibrous tissue. The capillary cell membrane is semipermeable to water and other small molecules.

Venules. Venules collect blood from capillaries and gradually coalesce into progressively larger veins. Venules have an average diameter of 20 μm and a wall thickness of approximately 0.5 mm. They do not have an elastic or smooth muscle layer but have a thin fibrous layer.

Veins. Veins act as conduits for the transport of blood back to the heart (Fig. 25.27). The venous system acts as a large reservoir because veins are very distensible. They contain approximately 60% to 70% of the blood volume. They have an average diameter of 30 mm and a wall thickness of 1.5 mm. The elastic tissue and the fibrous tissue layers are similar in size to those of the arterioles, but the smooth muscle layer in the veins is smaller than that of other large vessels.

Arterial Circulation

Knowledge of the anatomy of the arterial circulation is an important part of anesthesia practice. Such information is essential for obtaining intraarterial access, assessing HR and pulse quality, understanding the anatomic relationships for the purpose of regional blocks, and understanding the physiologic implications of decreased blood flow during shock states.

Microscopic anatomy of the arterial circulation. Arteries are classically divided into two types: conducting (elastic) arteries and distributing (muscular) arteries. Conducting arteries include the major arteries, such as the aorta, and their major branches, such as the brachial, radial, and ulnar arteries. The walls of arteries are thicker than the walls of veins and consist of three major layers: the tunica intima, the tunica media, and the tunica adventitia.

Thoracic aorta. The thoracic aorta is divided into three sections: the ascending aorta is the portion that leaves the LV; the transverse

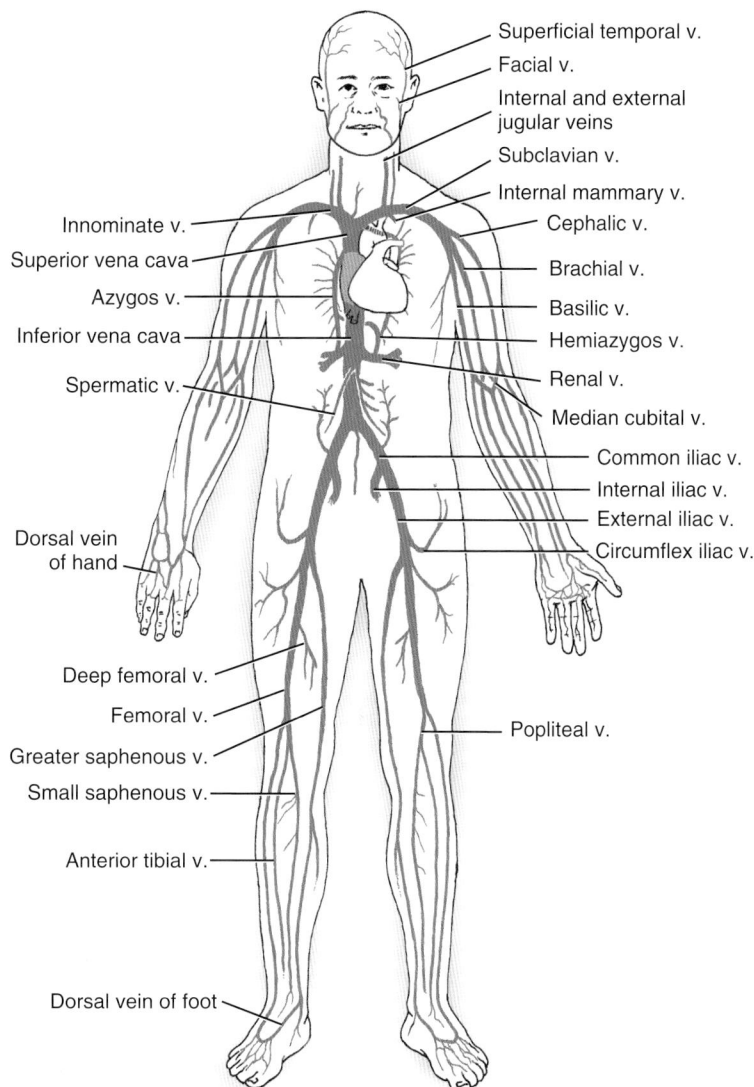

Fig. 25.27 The venous system. *v.*, Vein.

aorta, or arch, is the portion that levels off; and the descending aorta is the portion that descends into the thorax. After the thoracic aorta penetrates the diaphragm, the vessel is then referred to as the abdominal aorta (Fig. 25.28).

The first branches of the ascending aorta are the right and left coronary arteries, which are located immediately superior to the aortic valve. From this point, three major branches of the thoracic aorta exist: the brachiocephalic (innominate) artery, the left common carotid artery, and the left subclavian artery.

The brachiocephalic artery divides into the right common carotid artery and the right subclavian artery. The left and right common carotid arteries then branch into internal and external carotid arteries. The external carotid arteries supply blood to the face and neck, and the major branches are the superior thyroid artery, the lingual artery, the facial artery, the posterior auricular artery, the maxillary artery, the transverse facial artery, the middle temporal artery, and the superficial temporal artery (Fig. 25.29).

The internal carotid arteries supply 80% of blood to the brain, via the circle of Willis, and to the eyes, via the ophthalmic arteries (Fig. 25.30). The circle of Willis also receives a significant amount of blood supply from the vertebral branches of the subclavian artery.

Upper extremity arteries. The subclavian arteries branch before entering the upper arm. These branches include the vertebral arteries (as noted earlier), the thyrocervical trunk (which supplies blood to the thyroid gland as well as other structures in the neck), the internal thoracic artery (which supplies blood to the anterior chest), and the costocervical trunk (which supplies blood to the first two intercostal spaces and the muscles of the neck).

The subclavian artery continues at the border of the first rib as the axillary artery (Fig. 25.31). Branches from the axillary artery supply blood to the axillary region and include the highest thoracic artery, the thoracoacromial artery, the lateral thoracic artery, the subscapular artery, and the anterior and posterior circumflex humoral arteries.

The brachial artery begins at the terminal end of the axillary artery at the inferior border of the teres major muscle. The artery continues until the neck of the radius, where it ends by dividing into the radial and ulnar arteries. The radial artery forms the deep palmar arch, and the ulnar artery supplies blood to the superficial palmar arch.

Descending thoracic aorta. The descending thoracic aorta courses inferiorly through the posterior mediastinum on the left side of the thorax. At the level of the 12th thoracic vertebra, the aorta passes through the aortic hiatus and becomes the abdominal aorta. Branches

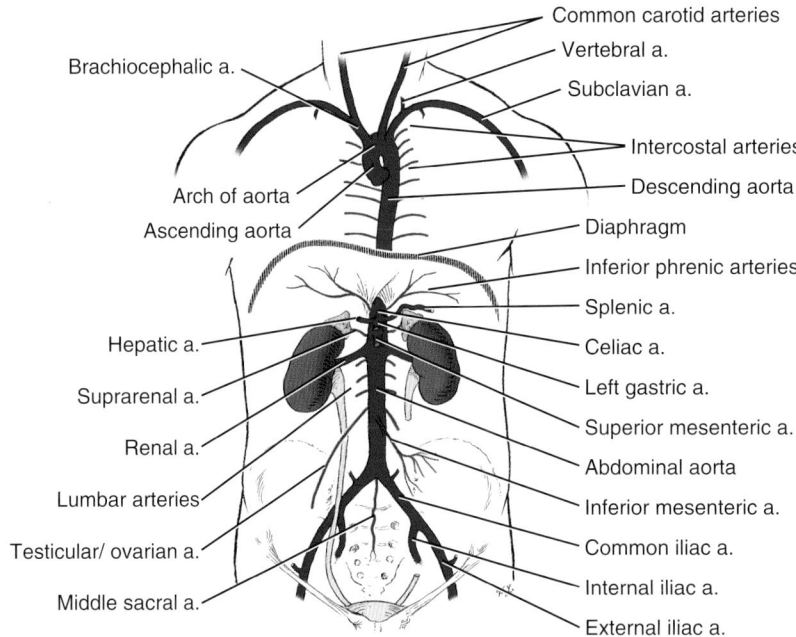

Fig. 25.28 Thoracic aorta and abdominal aorta and their branches. *a.,* Artery.

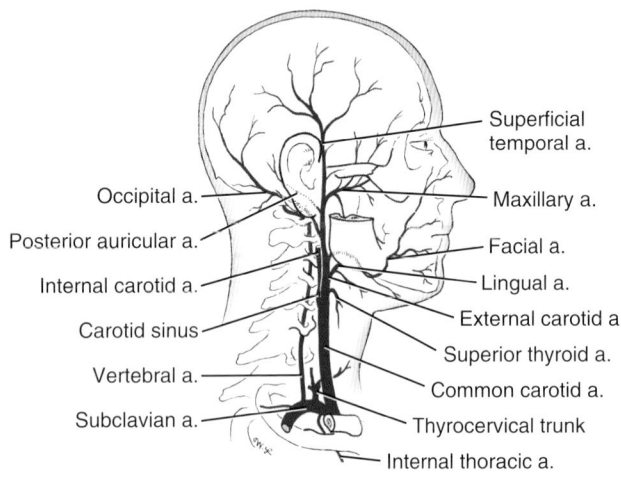

Fig. 25.29 Arterial supply to the face. *a.,* Artery.

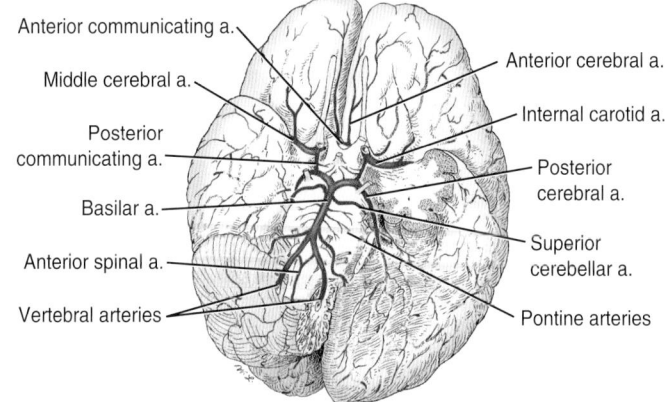

Fig. 25.30 The circle of Willis. *a.,* Artery.

of the descending thoracic aorta include the lower nine posterior intercostal arteries, the subcostal arteries, the pericardial arteries, the esophageal arteries, and the bronchial arteries.

Longitudinal blood flow to the spinal cord includes (1) two posterior and two posterolateral arteries supplying blood to the dorsal or sensory portion of the spinal cord (20% of spinal cord blood flow) and (2) one anterior spinal artery supplying blood to the anterior or motor portion of the spinal cord (80% of spinal cord blood flow). Transverse blood flow originating from the thoracic aorta is via the greater radicular artery (artery of Adamkiewicz). The exact location of this artery is variable and dependent on an individual's specific anatomic characteristics. However, the artery most often originates between spinal segments T8-T12 but it can be as low as L2 in a small segment of the population. Interruption of blood flow to the greater radicular artery in the absence of collateral blood flow has been identified as a factor that can cause paraplegia.

Abdominal aorta. As the thoracic aorta passes through the aortic hiatus of the diaphragm, it becomes the abdominal aorta. The first branches of the abdominal aorta are the inferior phrenic arteries,

which supply blood to the underside of the diaphragm and the adrenal glands (see Fig. 25.28).

The next major branch of the abdominal aorta is the celiac trunk, which supplies blood to many of the organs in the upper abdomen. Its branches include the splenic artery, the left gastric artery, the gastroduodenal artery, and the hepatic artery. The cystic artery, which supplies blood to the gallbladder, is a branch of the hepatic artery.

Below the celiac trunk of the aorta lies the superior mesenteric artery, which arises at the level of L1. This artery supplies blood to the jejunum, the ileum, and the transverse colon by means of an anastomosis with the middle colic artery. The jejunum and iliac branches unite to form the arterial arcades of the colon.

Below the superior mesenteric artery are the right and left renal arteries. The right renal artery branches to the right adrenal gland, where it is called the middle suprarenal artery. Below the renal arteries are the testicular or ovarian arteries. Inferior to the renal arteries lies the inferior mesenteric artery. This artery has branches to the transverse colon, the descending colon, the sigmoid colon, and the rectum.

Iliac arteries. The abdominal aorta terminates at the common iliac arteries in the pelvis. These arteries divide into internal and external iliac arteries. The internal iliac arteries supply blood to structures

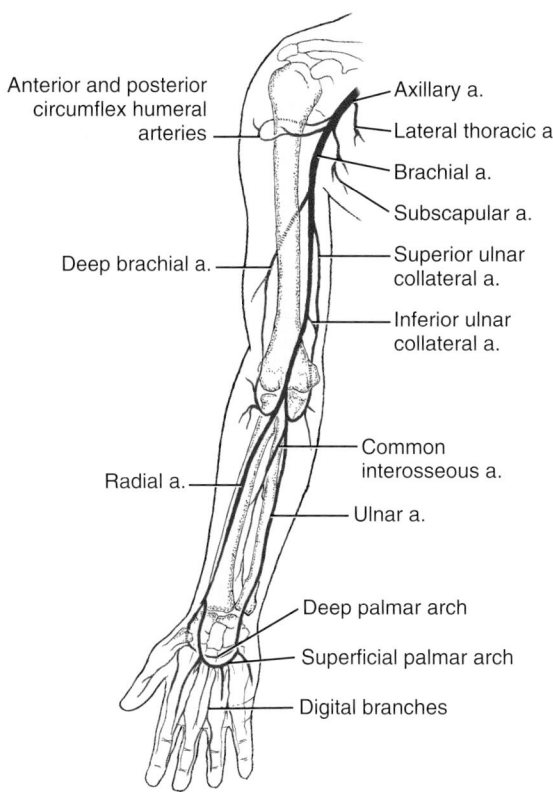

Fig. 25.31 Arterial supply to the upper extremity. *a.,* Artery.

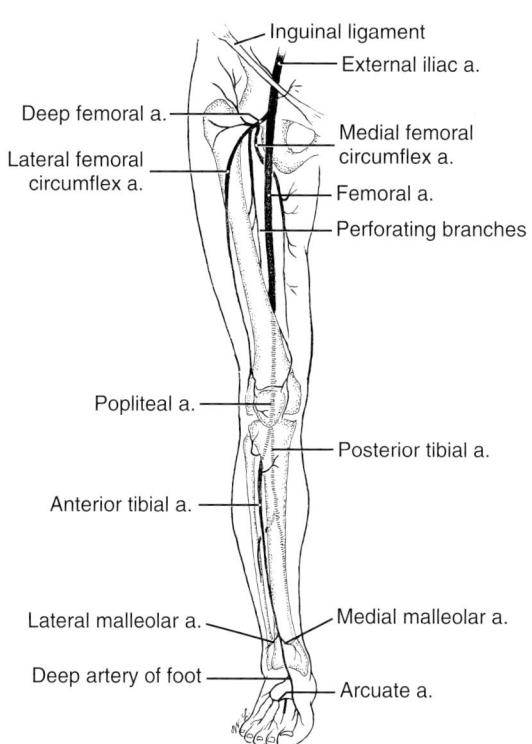

Fig. 25.32 Arterial supply to the lower extremity. *a.,* Artery.

within the pelvis, whereas the external iliac arteries supply blood to the legs. The right and left femoral arteries are branches of the external iliac arteries.

Lower extremities. The external iliac artery continues as the femoral artery and the deep femoral artery (Fig. 25.32). The femoral artery becomes the popliteal artery behind the knee and then divides into the anterior and posterior tibial arteries. The anterior tibial artery continues as the dorsal artery of the foot. The posterior tibial artery continues and supplies blood to the plantar arches. Clinically, the dorsal artery of the foot is not only an important landmark for the assessment of lower extremity circulation but also can be used for arterial cannulation if the radial artery catheter insertion is not possible.

Venous Circulation

An understanding of the anatomy of the venous system is essential for obtaining vascular access as well as for identifying significant landmarks to help locate nerve bundles when performing nerve blocks. Evaluation of venous distention is an important assessment tool to determine the presence of fluid overload and cardiovascular dynamics.

Head and neck. In the head and neck, venous drainage returns to the heart via the internal and external jugular veins. The drainage from the brain originates from the sagittal, transverse, and sigmoid sinuses. These sinuses drain into the internal jugular vein, whereas the more superficial structures of the face and head drain into the external jugular vein. Clinically, jugular venous distention can be a sign of fluid overload, cardiogenic shock, and/or cardiac compressive shock (cardiac tamponade).

Upper extremities. Superficial veins of the upper extremities include those that drain into the axillary vein, the cephalic vein laterally, and the basilica vein medially. The axillary vein drains into the subclavian vein on the right and then into the right brachiocephalic vein. The left subclavian vein drains into the left brachiocephalic vein.

The right and left brachiocephalic veins empty into the superior vena cava and account for the venous drainage that occurs from the upper extremities. Pressure and occlusion of the superior vena cava from a mass can result in a decrease in venous drainage, causing superior vena cava syndrome.

Thorax. Venous drainage of the thorax originates from the branches of the superior and inferior vena cava, as well as the azygos and hemiazygos systems. These venous networks are an important route of alternative blood return if a major obstruction of the inferior vena cava occurs. These vessels include intercostal vessels, bronchial veins, and pericardial veins.

Abdomen, pelvis, and lower extremities. The deep and superficial femoral veins receive venous drainage from the legs and join to form the external iliac veins. The internal iliac veins drain blood from the pelvis. The common iliac vessels receive blood from the internal and external iliac veins and drain into the inferior vena cava. In this region, the common iliac vessels are joined by branches from the abdomen and the hepatic portal system.

Microcirculation

Microcirculation refers to blood flow that occurs through microvessels that are present within the vasculature of tissues. The microcirculation system is composed of arterioles, capillaries, and venules. The function of the microcirculation is to control the delivery of nutrients to the capillary tissue beds, remove waste products, maintain ionic concentrations, and transport hormones to the tissues.

Anatomy. In general, a main nutrient artery enters an organ, where it branches six to eight times until the vessels are small enough to be called arterioles (<20 μm in diameter). Arterioles then branch two to five times until reaching diameters of 5 to 9 μm. Arterioles at this size are small enough to supply blood to the capillary bed.

In the capillary bed, the blood enters through an arteriole that has a muscular coat. Arterioles are connected to metarterioles, which have many interconnections to the true capillaries and whose branches are protected by precapillary sphincters. These sphincters can control blood flow through the capillary bed.

The capillary wall is a unicellular layer of endothelium surrounded by a basement membrane. The total wall thickness is 0.5 μm, and the diameter of the capillaries is 4 to 9 μm. In the capillary membrane, intercellular clefts allow the diffusion of water-soluble ions and small solutes. Plasmalemmal vesicles form channels in the cell membrane. The diffusion of substances through the cell membrane is determined by several factors: lipid solubility, water solubility, size of the molecule, and concentration difference from one side of the membrane to the other.[1]

Movement of fluid volume from the plasma and the interstitial fluid is determined by four factors: capillary pressure, interstitial fluid pressure, plasma colloid osmotic pressure, and interstitial fluid colloid osmotic pressure. Excess fluid from the interstitial space is transported through the lymphatic system, which plays an important role in the prevention of pulmonary edema formation when pulmonary artery pressures are elevated.

Local control of capillary blood flow. Blood flow to the various capillary beds is regulated by local tissue metabolic requirements. Therefore capillary blood flow may be controlled by the delivery of oxygen and other nutrients, the removal of end products of metabolism, or the maintenance of ionic balance of pH in the tissues.

Two major theories regarding regulation of capillary blood flow include the vasodilator theory and the oxygen-demand theory. According to these theories, the vessels dilate to increase the blood flow as a result of either hypoxemia or release of a vasodilator substance in response to hypoxemia. Some of the vasodilator substances that have been suggested are adenosine, carbon dioxide, nitric oxide, lactic acid, adenosine phosphate compounds, histamine, potassium ions, and hydrogen ions. These theories assume an active microcirculatory process exists that responds to tissue metabolic needs.

Certain tissue capillary beds do not function as explained by the vasodilator and the oxygen-demand theories of microcirculatory blood flow. Blood flow to the skin is dependent on external temperature and dissipation of body heat, whereas blood flow to the kidneys is dependent on the amount of fluid and sodium that needs to be excreted.

Autoregulation is another process demonstrated by certain organ tissues; it keeps blood flow through the capillary bed constant, despite the normal changes in MAP. Autoregulation has been demonstrated in such tissues as the brain, the kidney, and the coronary circulation. Autoregulation keeps the blood flow to an organ constant by way of vasodilation or vasoconstriction in response to fluctuations in MAP. When MAP is above or below autoregulatory pressures for an organ system, blood flow becomes pressure dependent.

A substance that causes secondary vasodilation of the large arteries in response to increased flow has been isolated and was once called the endothelium-derived relaxing factor.[23] Currently, it is referred to as nitric oxide. This factor is synthesized by the endothelial lining of the arterioles and the small arteries. Shear stress on the walls of the vessels accelerates the release of this substance and allows larger vessels to dilate when blood flow to the tissues increases.

Angiogenesis—Growth of Collateral Circulation

Microcirculation is a good example of vascular growth that can occur to provide collateral circulation. The growth of new vessels results in part from angiogenesis and the release of angiogenic factors. These substances are released from ischemic tissues, rapidly growing tissues, and tissues with high metabolic rates.

Several angiogenic factors have been identified, including endothelial cell growth factor,[24] fibroblast growth factor,[25] and angiogen.[26] These factors act by the dissolution of the basement membrane of the

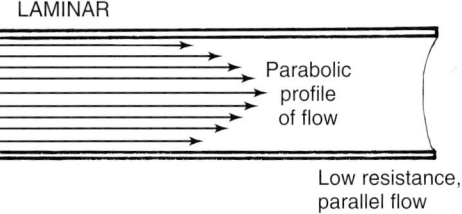
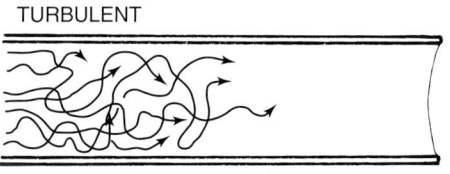

Fig. 25.33 Laminar and turbulent flow.

endothelial cells, followed by the rapid dissolution of new endothelial cells that stream out of the vessels into cords. The cells in these cords divide and then gradually fold over into a tube. The tubes then connect with other tubes to form an intricate vascular network.

Vascular flow is dependent on neurologic as well as hormonal regulation. Examples of vasoconstrictor hormones include epinephrine and norepinephrine from the CNS and the adrenal medulla, angiotensin from the lungs, cortisol from the adrenal cortex, and vasopressin from the posterior pituitary. Several vasodilator substances include bradykinin, serotonin, histamine, and prostaglandins. Various other ionic and chemical factors can also produce vasoconstriction and vasodilation and influence the flow of blood that is delivered to tissues.

Blood Pressure

Pressure, Flow, and Resistance Interrelationships

Ohm's law. Ohm's law correlates the flow of electricity (current), the applied electrical pressure (voltage), and the resistance to this flow (resistance). A modification of this law is used in medicine to describe the flow of a fluid (blood) through a tube (blood vessel), even though the vessels are dynamic rather than static. Ohm's law and fluid flow are described by the following equation:

$$Q = (P_1 - P_2)/R$$

where flow through a cylinder (Q) is equal to the change in pressure from one end of the tube to the other ($P_1 - P_2$) divided by the resistance (R) of the tube. Therefore either a decrease in resistance or an increase in pressure change across the tube increases the flow of fluid through the tube.

Blood flow. Blood flow is the quantity of blood that passes a given point in a given amount of time. Clinically, CO may be inserted into the equation as blood flow. Two types of flow exist: laminar and turbulent (Fig. 25.33).

Laminar flow has a parabolic profile that illustrates the parallel movement of molecules. Conversely, turbulent flow is described as a whirlpool and does not move as easily, thereby increasing resistance to flow. Reynolds number (Re) is a means of determining the type of flow in a tube and uses the diameter of the blood vessel (d) and the velocity (v), density (ϱ), and viscosity (n) of the fluid to determine whether turbulence occurs.

The formula for calculating Reynolds number includes the velocity of blood flow in centimeters per second multiplied by the diameter of the tube in centimeters, multiplied by the density of the fluid in grams per cubic centimeter, divided by the viscosity (see the following equation). A Reynolds number greater than 2300 reflects predominately turbulent flow. Conversely, a Reynolds number less than 2300 reflects predominately laminar flow.

$$Re = (v \times d \times \rho)/n$$

Reynolds number demonstrates that in large vessels with high velocities, such as the aorta and large arteries, turbulent flow occurs even in the straight portions of these vessels.

Poiseuille's law. Poiseuille's law (see the following equation) describes the amount of fluid flowing through a tube (Q) in relation to the pressure drop across the tube ($P_1 - P_2$), the radius of the tube (r), the viscosity of the fluid (n), and the length of the tube (l):

$$Q = ([P_1 - P_2]\,r^4)/(8 \times n \times l)$$

One of the most important factors in determining fluid flow is the radius of the vessel.

Clinical applications of Poiseuille's law include selection of intravenous (IV) catheter size, endotracheal tube size, and determination of vascular dilation or constriction in response to pharmacologic agents.

Resistance. Resistance is the impediment to blood flow in a blood vessel. Clinically it cannot be measured directly but is calculated from measures of blood flow (CO) and pressure differences in the vessels.

The units of measure most commonly used in the clinical area are centimeter-gram-second units. The normal SVR is 800 to 1500 dyne/sec/cm^{-5}, and the normal pulmonary vascular resistance is approximately one-tenth of that number, or between 50 and 150 dyne/sec/cm^{-5}.

Resistance of systems. Resistance is calculated for two major systems (Fig. 25.34). In a series system, such as the systemic vasculature, the total resistance (R_T) is equal to the sum of the collective resistance for the individual tissue beds within the system and can be expressed as:

$$R_T = R_1 + R_2 + R_3 + \ldots R_n$$

In a parallel system, such as a capillary bed, the total resistance is less than any of the individual resistances (see the following equation). Therefore the blood flow through a capillary bed such as the pulmonary capillaries is less than the resistance through any of the individual capillaries of the pulmonary system.

$$1/R_T = 1/R_1 + 1/R_2 + 1/R_3 + \ldots 1/R_n$$

Regulation of Mean Arterial Blood Pressure

Regulation of arterial blood pressure is an important function in maintaining homeostasis for patients receiving anesthesia. MAP is an important indicator of perfusion of the tissue beds. Blood pressure regulation can be categorized as either short term or long term. The choice of category depends on the onset of action, the duration of action, and the intensity of the physiologic reaction to return the MAP to normal values.

Short-term regulation. The short-term blood pressure regulators are those that respond to rapid changes in MAP and attempt to rapidly (within 30 minutes) return the MAP back to normal range. These reflexes rely on an intact autonomic nervous system, and this interaction is responsible for the rapid onset of action of these blood pressure regulators. The reflexes include baroreceptor response, chemoreceptor response, atrial stretch reflex, and CNS ischemic reflex. All these homeostatic reflexes are initiated rapidly in response to acute changes in MAP.

The cardiovascular (vasomotor) center is located in the medulla and pons. This center regulates four basic actions: vasoconstriction, vasodilation, cardiac excitation, and cardiac inhibition. These areas activate

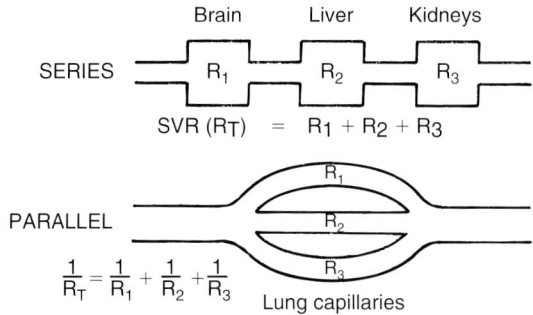

Fig. 25.34 Resistance in series and parallel systems. *R*, Resistance; *R$_T$*, total resistance; *SVR*, systemic vascular resistance.

the sympathetic and parasympathetic nervous systems in response to various stimuli. Under normal conditions, the vasomotor center maintains peripheral vascular tone.

Baroreceptors are located in the internal carotid arteries and the aortic arch and are called the carotid and aortic sinuses. They are spray-type nerve endings that increase impulse production when they are stretched. Impulses from the baroreceptors affect the inhibitory centers of the vasomotor center. At MAP of less than 60 mm Hg, the baroreceptors do not transmit impulses. However, as the MAP increases to between 60 and 180 mm Hg, impulses sent to the inhibitory area of the vasomotor center incrementally increase. The baroreceptors are most efficient in responding to rapid changes in blood pressure. They are not as efficient in long-term blood pressure regulation because they adapt to the higher pressures, in effect by being reset. Therefore the baroreceptors act as a buffer system to prevent extreme short-term swings in blood pressure. Two clinically significant examples of stimulation of the baroreceptor reflex during surgery include carotid sinus manipulation during carotid endarterectomy and aortic baroreceptor stimulation from pressure exerted on the aortic arch during mediastinoscopy.

Chemoreceptors are chemosensitive cells located within the carotid and aortic bodies. These are known as the peripheral chemoreceptors. Each area is supplied by a small nutrient artery and thereby maintains constant contact with the cardiorespiratory environment. Chemoreceptors send afferent impulses to excite the vasomotor center within the brainstem, primarily in response to decreases in Pao$_2$. Chemoreceptors play a greater role in respiratory system regulation than in blood pressure regulation.

Low-pressure receptors, or stretch receptors, are located in many areas of the vasculature, especially within the atria and pulmonary arterial tree. They act in conjunction with the baroreceptors to buffer changes in the blood pressure caused by changes in volume status.

The atrial stretch reflex is initiated by input from low-pressure receptors. Stretching of the atria caused by an increase in volume results in a dilation of the peripheral arterioles, which decreases SVR, MAP, and CO. Furthermore, hypervolemia causes the release of the atrial natriuretic factor (i.e., peptide) by the atria as a result of increased stretch.[27] This factor causes a reflex dilation of afferent arterioles in the kidney, a phenomenon that increases the glomerular filtration rate and decreases the secretion of antidiuretic hormone via signals to the hypothalamus. The combination of these events causes an increase in urine formation and an attempt to change the MAP by decreasing vascular volume.

The CNS ischemic mechanism exerts a powerful effect on the blood pressure control system. When hypotension exists, this reflex is initiated in an attempt to restore the MAP to adequate levels for CNS perfusion and especially for perfusion to the vasomotor center. The reflex is most intensely initiated when MAP is less than 20 mm

Hg, and the result is one of the most powerful sympathetic vasoconstrictor responses within the human body.[1] The stimulation persists for approximately 10 minutes, by which time either the ischemia has been relieved or the vasomotor center becomes severely ischemic and infarcts, and the stimulation ceases.

Several hormones are instrumental in the short-term regulation of MAP. The onset of action is not as rapid as that of neural control mechanisms, but activation occurs within a short time of stimulation. Norepinephrine and epinephrine are released from the CNS and the adrenal medulla during times of sympathetic stimulation and cause vasoconstriction.

Angiotensin I is converted to angiotensin II in the lungs by angiotensin-converting enzyme (ACE). This substance is one of the most potent vasoconstrictors secreted by the body. It takes approximately 20 minutes to become fully activated. Angiotensin II also plays a role in the secretion of aldosterone from the adrenal cortex. Aldosterone has a role in the long-term regulation of MAP.

The antidiuretic hormone vasopressin has both short- and long-term effects on blood pressure control. The short-term effect of antidiuretic hormone causes potent and direct vasoconstriction. The long-term control effects of antidiuretic hormone decrease urine output from the kidneys.

Two short-term systems for maintenance of blood pressure that could be classified as intermediate mechanisms are the capillary fluid shift and the stress-relaxation mechanism. Both of these mechanisms depend on an intact vascular system.

The capillary fluid shift is a simple mechanism. As the hydrostatic pressure (MAP) increases within the capillaries, a larger movement of fluid occurs across the capillary membrane. This phenomenon lowers the fluid volume within the vasculature and results in a decreased MAP.

The stress-relaxation mechanism is an example of the ability of the vasculature to compensate for hypervolemia and hypovolemia as a result of alterations of smooth muscle tone within the vasculature. As intravascular fluid volume increases, tension on the blood vessels results in dilation of the vasculature to compensate for increased volume. Conversely, as the blood volume decreases, the vessels constrict to compensate for the decreased volume to maintain MAP.

Long-term regulation. Long-term regulation of MAP includes mechanisms that eventually regulate blood volume to within normal range. The renal body fluid system is one of the major long-term regulators of MAP. Renal homeostasis of blood pressure occurs as the kidneys preferentially excrete sodium and water to maintain a normal fluid balance.

Intravascular fluid status has a direct effect on arterial blood pressure. A chronic increase in blood volume leads to increases in mean filling pressure, venous return, CO, and SVR. The combination of an increased CO and an increased SVR can increase the arterial blood pressure by more than 30%. This causes an increase in myocardial oxygen demand.

Several factors govern the effectiveness of the renal body fluid system, including the renin-angiotensin system, aldosterone secretion, and the nervous system. As fluid intake and blood pressure increase, the secretion of renin by the kidneys decreases. This decreased renin secretion causes a reduced secretion of aldosterone as a result of the decreased production of angiotensin II, which is a potent vasoconstrictor. A decrease in sympathetic nervous system response to the kidney also occurs. The net effect is an increased renal output of sodium and water.

Physiology of the Venous System

In the past, the venous system has been described as simply the return conduit for the arterial system, and it was not thought to play a very active role in the maintenance of circulation and CO. It has been determined that the venous system serves an integral role in support of the circulation.[28]

The venous system's ability to accommodate large volume changes helps to buffer the intravascular volume during periods of hypervolemia or hypovolemia and thereby helps to maintain CO. In addition, the venous system is well innervated by the autonomic nervous system and therefore has the ability to respond to the wide variations in intravascular volume that occur over the course of long surgical procedures and during intensive fluid resuscitation.

HYPERTENSION

Extent, Definition, and Etiology

The pathophysiologic cardiovascular condition that is most commonly encountered in patients who require surgery is hypertension. Hypertension affects one of every three or approximately 70 million people in the United States, and the frequency increases with age. It is vital for the anesthesia provider to understand the pathophysiology of the condition and its relation to the cardiovascular system and other body systems. Only then can a comprehensive anesthesia plan be constructed.

Patients frequently do not exhibit signs or symptoms associated with hypertension. Chronic uncontrolled hypertension affects specific target organs, including the heart, brain, and kidney. Hypertension accelerates and exacerbates the onset of atherosclerotic changes in the arterial vessels of the target organs. It is a primary risk factor for the development of coronary artery disease. Hypertension is a significant cause of congestive heart failure and cardiomyopathy because it causes increased afterload from chronic vasoconstriction. Hypertension increases the likelihood of the development of atherosclerosis, and thus chronic untreated hypertension increases the incidence of MI, stroke, and chronic kidney injury.[29]

Hypertension is classified based on its causes. Essential hypertension, also referred to as primary and idiopathic, has no identifiable cause and accounts for 95% of all cases of the disease, and its diagnosis is determined on the basis of exclusion. The relationship between an individual's genetic predisposition and environmental (modifiable) risk factors most probably influences the potential development and severity of essential hypertension. Theoretical physiologic causes of essential hypertension include sympathetic nervous system hyperactivity and/or increased activity of the renin-angiotensin-aldosterone system. Remedial (secondary) hypertension has an identifiable and potentially curable cause. Examples of pathophysiologic conditions that cause remedial hypertension include pheochromocytoma, coarctation of the aorta, renal artery stenosis, primary renal diseases (e.g., pyelonephritis, glomerulonephritis), primary aldosteronism (Conn syndrome), and hyperadrenocorticism (Cushing disease).

Guidelines regarding blood pressure values that constitute hypertension have been published by the National Institutes of Health.[30] Evidence-based guidelines for the management of hypertension in adults are given in Box 25.1. To determine accurate blood pressure measurements, two readings taken 5 minutes apart with the patient in the sitting position are necessary. It is estimated that the implementation of antihypertensive therapy is associated with a 25% decrease in cardiovascular complications and a decreased incidence of stroke of up to 38%.[31] If lifestyle modifications are unsuccessful in decreasing blood pressure to acceptable levels, then antihypertensive therapy should be prescribed.[32] In many instances, patients may have developed advanced atherosclerotic vascular disease or target-organ dysfunction before the start of treatment for hypertension.[33,34]

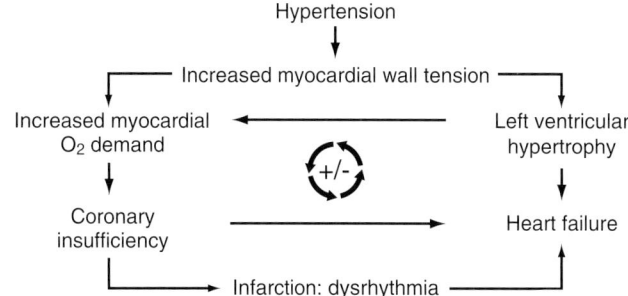

Fig. 25.35 Schematic representation of the relationship between hypertension and heart failure. (Modified from Matei VA, Haddadin AS. Systemic and pulmonary arterial hypertension. In Hines RL, Marschall KE, eds. *Stoelting's Anesthesia and Co-Existing Disease*. 6th ed. Philadelphia: Elsevier; 2012:106.)

Pathophysiology

Systemic blood pressure is regulated by interactive feedback mechanisms involving the sympathoadrenal axis and baroreceptors in the heart and great vessels. It is accepted that some degree of sympathetic hyperactivity is responsible for essential hypertension. Dysfunction of the sympathetic nervous system leads to a state of chronic vasoconstriction. In an attempt to maintain normal intravascular volume, the renal juxtaglomerular apparatus secretes renin. All the vascular and hormonal effects of renin are caused by its conversion of angiotensin I to angiotensin II. Angiotensin II is the major stimulus for the secretion of aldosterone by the adrenal cortex.

Deposition of collagen and metalloproteinases within the intima of arteries leads to vascular stiffness, and this occurs normally as part of the aging process. Narrowing of the vascular lumen and endothelial dysfunction decreases vascular dilation, and thus blood flow is decreased especially within the microvasculature. Furthermore, vascular stiffness increases afterload and myocardial oxygen demand potentially resulting in LV hypertrophy, myocardial ischemia/infarction, and/or congestive heart failure.

Anesthesia Management for the Patient With Hypertension

Preoperative Evaluation

The most important issues to address during the preoperative evaluation of a patient with hypertension is the identification and the adequacy of treatment. The goal of antihypertensive therapy is to maintain normotension on a consistent basis. Effective antihypertensive therapy that renders the patient normotensive on a routine basis may not necessarily prevent episodes of perioperative hypertension. However, patients whose conditions are well assessed and optimized before surgery have a more stable perioperative course and a lower incidence of cardiovascular system–related morbidity. Although not ideal, if perioperative DBP is maintained below 110 mm Hg, the risk of perioperative cardiac morbidity does not increase significantly.[29,35]

An adequate understanding of the pharmacology and side effects of the medications used for treating hypertension is necessary for proper management. For a complete discussion of antihypertensive drugs, see Chapter 13. Antihypertensive medications that block or depress the sympathetic nervous system response decrease the body's compensatory reflexes. These effects may be even more pronounced during anesthesia. For instance, during acute hemorrhage, the tachycardia and vasoconstriction associated with blood loss may be diminished (or may not occur) if the patient is receiving a combination β-blocker and vasodilator promoting antihypertensive drug. Patients treated with antihypertensive medications do not lose their responsiveness to vasoactive drugs but instead may respond to these substances in an exaggerated manner.

To prepare and properly manage a patient during the perioperative period, a thorough history of the cardiovascular system should be obtained in an effort to elicit any symptoms of ischemic cardiovascular disease. Hypertension is a major risk factor for coronary artery disease. Any symptoms related to coronary artery disease should be further investigated. In addition to being a risk factor for coronary artery disease, hypertension directly affects myocardial function. The chronic increase in myocardial wall tension caused by prolonged and untreated hypertension can result in left ventricular hypertrophy (LVH) (Fig. 25.35). Ventricular diastolic dysfunction occurs before the development of hypertrophy. This diastolic dysfunction is not clinically apparent, and the patient may appear to have normal cardiac function except under stressful physiologic conditions. A delayed rate of passive ventricular filling is evidence of ventricular diastolic dysfunction. The rate of ventricular filling from atrial contraction becomes predominant in hypertensive patients. This represents the inverse of normal ventricular filling patterns. Other information and results from preoperative tests that will help the nurse anesthetist evaluate and create an individualized anesthetic plan for patients with cardiac dysfunction include determining exercise tolerance, ECG, Doppler ultrasound, stress test, and cardiac catheterization results.

LVH is a consequence of chronic hypertension and increased afterload that results in an enlargement of myocardial mass. This compensatory process increases myocardial oxygen demand. Hypertrophy that occurs in response to chronic increases in intracardiac pressure is termed concentric hypertrophy. Ventricular hypertrophy also may produce subendocardial ischemia at perfusion pressures that would normally be adequate in a healthy ventricle. Concomitant development of coronary artery disease coupled with increased myocardial oxygen demand hastens and exacerbates the development of ischemic symptoms. As a rule, all patients with chronic hypertension should be suspected of having some degree of coronary artery disease.

Hypertensive cardiomyopathy and systolic ventricular dysfunction are the direct result of the pathophysiologic changes associated with chronic hypertension. This hypertensive cardiomyopathy manifests as a decrease in both EF and SV. Increasing diastolic dysfunction results in ventricular dilation in conjunction with systolic dysfunction. The subsequent replacement of myocardial cells with fibrous tissue results in a cardiomyopathy.[4]

Chronic hypertension that has remained either untreated or inadequately controlled has adverse consequences on brain, kidney, and ocular function. Patients with long-standing disease have a higher incidence of strokes than do patients whose blood pressure has been controlled.[29] The concurrent preoperative use of a β-blocker, ACE inhibitor/angiotensin receptor blocker (ARB), and statins decrease the occurrence of nonfatal MI and mortality in patients with stable coronary heart disease.[35] ACE inhibitors and ARBs can cause hypotension during anesthesia that is refractory to vasopressor administration. Vasopressin and methylene blue have been found to be effective treatments for ACE inhibitor–associated refractory hypotension (vasoplegic syndrome).[36] Discontinuing ACE inhibitors and ARBs 24 hours prior to anesthesia is associated with a decreased incidence of hypotension during anesthesia. There is no evidence that withholding these medications the day prior to surgery increases major adverse cardiac events or mortality.[37,38] Patients should be restarted on these medications the following day unless a contraindication exists.

Inadequate control of hypertension can lead to alterations in cerebrovascular and coronary artery autoregulation. For example, normal physiologic coronary artery autoregulation occurs at a MAP between 60 and 140 mm Hg. However, a patient with chronic hypertension and coronary artery disease may develop ischemic changes at a MAP of 60 mm Hg or greater. The cerebral and coronary autoregulation curves are shifted to the right in patients with chronic hypertension, necessitating higher perfusion pressures to ensure adequate organ blood flow. Therefore cerebral and myocardial ischemia may occur with significant decreases in MAP in patients with hypertension and coronary artery disease. This phenomenon makes patients with uncontrolled hypertension more susceptible to cardiac and cerebral ischemia, compared with normotensive individuals.[34] Chronic untreated hypertension can cause nephrosclerosis, which can impair renal function. Nephrosclerosis can produce proteinuria and a gradual decrease in renal function. Early treatment of hypertension results in the preservation of renal function.

Anesthesia Management

An individualized anesthetic plan must be created by determining the type and extent of cardiac pathophysiology, other disease states, and the surgical procedure. To maintain a stable intraoperative course, administration of antihypertensive medications should be continued on schedule until the time of surgery. All oral medications can be given with one or two sips of water without increased risk of aspiration.[33] It should be noted that acute hypertensive rebound can occur with abrupt cessation of antihypertensive medications. Tachycardia, hypertension, angina, and MI can result from interruption of therapy with β-blockers and other antihypertensive agents. As a general rule, preoperative antihypertensive medications should be continued up to and including the day of surgery.

Determining whether to proceed with elective surgery in a patient in whom hypertension is untreated and poorly controlled remains controversial. However, evidence suggests that patients with DBPs greater than 110 mm Hg have a significantly increased risk of perioperative cardiac morbidity.[39] This caveat may be modified in patients with hypertension in whom DBPs greater than 110 mm Hg occur frequently, despite aggressive antihypertensive drug therapy (e.g., patients with end-stage renal disease).

To attenuate sympathetic responsiveness, preoperative sedation may be indicated for patients with hypertension. Establishing control

of the blood pressure before induction should result in a more stable hemodynamic course during the induction, maintenance, and emergence from anesthesia. A fluid bolus and incremental titration of anesthetic induction agents may help decrease the degree and duration of hypotension. β-blockade therapy should be instituted days to weeks before surgery and titrated to a target HR between 50 and 60 beats per minute (bpm).[40] However, perioperative β-blockade started within 1 day or less before noncardiac surgery prevents nonfatal MIs but increases risks of hypotension, bradycardia, stroke, and death. Initiating β-blockade between 2 and 7 days may be preferable, but there is a lack of scientific data to support a benefit of beginning therapy greater than 1 month in advance.[41]

Induction of Anesthesia

Patients with hypertension may react in an exaggerated manner to induction agents and the stimulation associated with laryngoscopy and tracheal intubation. This response is highly variable and may result in hypertension or hypotension. It is dependent on the individual's physiology, degree of stimulation, adequacy of preoperative antihypertensive therapy, and amount and type of induction agents administered. Hypertensive patients are hypovolemic, as a result of renal-compensatory mechanisms, extreme vasoconstriction, or pharmacologic therapy (diuretics). Increased vasoconstriction as a consequence of hypertension results in volume contraction and a greater susceptibility to hypotension from the vasodilating and cardiac-depressant effects of anesthetic agents. Of the anesthetic induction agents, etomidate, propofol, or dexmedetomidine can be used in patients with hypertension. Etomidate offers an advantage in patients with cardiac pathology, as compared to propofol, because it preserves SV and cardiac output.[15] Due to the sympathomimetic response that occurs with the administration of induction doses of ketamine, this drug should be used with caution in patients with cardiovascular disease.

The stimuli of laryngoscopy and tracheal intubation can result in an exaggerated hypertensive response, despite postinduction hypotension. An existing hypertensive state is further compounded by intense stimulation caused by airway manipulation. Suppressing the exaggerated hypertensive response to intubation requires that a greater depth of anesthesia be achieved. However, the depth of anesthesia at induction necessary to suppress this response may produce a more profound hypotensive state. Administration of adjunct medications before induction (e.g., β-blockers or arterial dilators) can reduce the hyperdynamic sympathetic response to tracheal intubation. Hypotensive episodes can be treated with fluid administration, decreasing anesthetic depth, and administration of vasopressors. Numerous strategies have been suggested for the management of this hyperdynamic response. The sympathetic stimulatory response caused by laryngoscopy and intubation could be significantly reduced by laryngotracheal or IV administration of lidocaine.[42] Reducing the duration of airway manipulation to 15 seconds or less may be helpful. Use of a β-blocker before induction has been shown to reduce the hyperdynamic sympathetic responses.[33] Administration of fentanyl prior to induction also helps attenuate the sympathetic response.

With regard to suppression of marked hemodynamic responses, a controlled induction followed by a rapid and atraumatic intubation is imperative. Producing an adequate depth of anesthesia at induction that produces extreme hypotension may be more detrimental to both coronary and cerebral perfusion than the hypertensive response it was intended to prevent. Due to vasoconstriction, patients with untreated hypertension are frequently hypovolemic as compared with those who are normotensive. Thus adequate hydration before induction may help prevent postinduction hypotension.[29,33] A combination of low doses of more than one agent in addition to titration of medications may

TABLE 25.6	**Hemodynamic Goals for Management of Coronary Artery Disease**
Parameter	**Goal**
Preload	Decrease/maintain
Afterload	Maintain
Contractility	Decrease/maintain
Heart rate	Slow
Heart rhythm	Normal sinus rhythm

prove a better choice than a full dose of a single agent. In emergency cases in which rapidly securing the airway is of paramount importance, the choice of agents may be limited, and hyperdynamic response then becomes a secondary issue.

Maintenance of Anesthesia

A general hemodynamic goal, during anesthetic management for the hypertensive patient undergoing general anesthesia, is to maintain blood pressure within 20% of the patient's normal MAP. Intraoperative events that cause wide fluctuations in blood pressure should be anticipated and treated immediately. The most common event that precipitates intraoperative hypertension is surgical stimulation. This induces increased sympathetic stimulation resulting in the release of catecholamines, cortisol, and aldosterone, which is representative of the physiologic stress-induced response. Inhalation and narcotics administered alone and in combination have the ability to attenuate this response.[2,33,34] Altering the depth of anesthesia to suppress maximal surgical stimulation may not be adequate for achieving rapid and complete control of hypertensive responses. The adjunct use of drugs such as β-blockers and vasodilators may be necessary to achieve hemodynamic control. These drugs offer the advantage of continued control of hypertensive response in the immediate postanesthesia recovery period. Table 25.6 lists hemodynamic goals for patients with coronary artery disease.

The onset of profound hypotension during anesthesia maintenance should be immediately recognized, diagnosed, and treated. Prolonged severe hypotension has predictive significance in perioperative cardiac morbidity.[39] Treatment of hypotension may require reduction of the amount of inhalation agent used and infusion of IV fluid. Should these measures prove inadequate or untimely, a rapid-acting vasopressor such as phenylephrine or ephedrine may be administered as a temporizing measure until the cause of the hypotension can be diagnosed. It is important to realize that hypertensive patients may have exaggerated responses to vasopressor agents. The goal of intraoperative anesthesia management is maintenance of hemodynamic stability, which includes anticipation of intraoperative events that may affect cardiovascular stability, and thereby prevent extreme fluctuations in blood pressure.

Postoperative Considerations in the Hypertensive Patient

Termination of anesthesia allows for sympathetic nervous system predominance and frequently results in hyperdynamic, hypertensive responses even in patients with well-controlled hypertension. Intraoperative control of blood pressure should continue into the immediate postoperative period. Initiation of adjunct administration of antihypertensive medications should be anticipated at the end of surgery and early in the postoperative period. Adequate control of pain represents a primary antihypertensive consideration. Patients with hypertension are more susceptible to perioperative cardiac morbidity than the normotensive patient during the postoperative period. Adequate control of blood pressure in the postoperative period reduces the incidence of cardiovascular complications.[29] Maintenance of normothermia is imperative because postoperative shivering significantly increases myocardial oxygen consumption.

Pericardial Disease

In reviewing the anesthetic management of patients with pericardial disease, this section focuses on the pathophysiology, clinical presentation, and anesthetic implications of three primary disease processes: acute pericarditis, constrictive pericarditis, and cardiac tamponade.

The pericardium surrounds the heart, effectively anchoring it in a stable anatomic position while concomitantly reducing contact between it and surrounding structures. It consists of an inner visceral layer, which envelops the surface of the heart, and an outer parietal layer. The pericardial space between these layers usually contains 20 to 25 mL of clear fluid that under normal circumstances can accommodate gradual volume fluctuations. Rapid accumulation of pericardial fluid in the pericardial space can result in cardiac tamponade and cardiovascular collapse.[43]

Acute Pericarditis

Acute inflammation of the pericardium is caused by a number of disorders. The most common cause of acute pericarditis is viral infection. Post-MI syndrome (Dressler syndrome), cardiac injury (trauma, surgery), metastatic disease, irradiation, uremia, tuberculosis, and autoimmune (rheumatoid arthritis) represent the remaining primary predisposing conditions that contribute to the development of this process.[44]

Pathophysiology. It is common for a serofibrinous inflammatory reaction associated with a small intrapericardial exudative effusion to evolve. This may result in adherence of the two layers of the pericardium. The sequelae are largely dependent on the severity of the reaction, as well as on the specific cause. Most often when the condition is left untreated or undiagnosed, complete resolution is the end result. Infrequently, however, extended organization of fibrinous exudate within the pericardial sac may lead to encasement of the heart by dense fibrous connective tissue (chronic constrictive pericarditis) or to the accumulation of a large amount of pericardial fluid over time with consequent cardiac tamponade (usually fluid levels >1 L). Constrictive pericarditis and cardiac tamponade result in impaired diastolic filling, which results in decreased CO.[44]

Clinical presentation. The principal symptom associated with acute pericarditis is sudden onset chest pain. Although similar in nature to that experienced during MI, this pain is differentiated by the inclusion of a pleural component, which includes increased discomfort associated with postural changes and relief on sitting or leaning forward. Other signs that are characteristic of acute pericarditis include fever with a pericardial friction rub, absence of elevation of cardiac enzymes levels, and diffuse ST segment elevation in two or three limb leads and in most of the precordial leads. Echocardiography is another reliable method for diagnosing pericarditis and pericardial effusion.

Anesthetic management. Acute pericarditis in the absence of an associated pericardial effusion or scarring does not alter cardiac function. Specific considerations for anesthetic management are directed toward the underlying illness.

Chronic Constrictive Pericarditis

Chronic constrictive pericarditis results from pericardial thickening and fibrosis. In the past, tuberculosis was the most common cause of pericardial constriction. Currently the most common cause is idiopathic in nature and can occur following cardiac surgery, neoplasia, uremia, radiation therapy, and rheumatoid arthritis.[44,45]

Pathophysiology. Stiff, fibrous tissue encircles the heart and limits its ability to expand during diastole. The fundamental hemodynamic abnormality in chronic constrictive pericarditis is abnormal diastolic filling. Reduced myocardial compliance impairs filling of both ventricles. Consequently, filling pressures increase, and as a result pulmonary and peripheral congestion occurs. SV and CO can also be decreased. Equilibration of pulmonary artery diastolic pressure, PCWP, and right atrial pressure commonly occurs. Initially, ventricular systolic function is normal; however, over time the underlying myocardial tissue may atrophy, and systolic function decreases.

Clinical presentation. Clinical features representative of chronic constrictive pericarditis include gradually increasing fatigue and dyspnea. Typical signs of increasing venous pressure and congestion are engorgement of neck veins, hepatomegaly, ascites, and peripheral edema. In approximately 50% of patients, the fibrous enclosure becomes calcified and is visible on a chest radiograph.[33] The ECG may reveal diffuse low-voltage QRS complexes, T-wave inversion, and notched P waves. As many as 25% of patients have atrial dysrhythmias because of the involvement of atrial conduction pathways. Diagnosis is confirmed by demonstration of pericardial thickening with echocardiography or computed tomography.

The treatment used for patients with hemodynamically significant constrictive pericarditis is a pericardiotomy. Unfortunately, the surgical removal of adherent pericardium may precipitate malignant cardiac dysrhythmias and massive bleeding. Consequently, pericardiotomy is associated with relatively high perioperative morbidity and mortality rates, ranging from 6% to 19%.[46,47]

Anesthetic management. Large-bore IV lines must be established preoperatively because of the potential for sudden, rapid hemorrhage. A cardiopulmonary bypass circuit should be readily available. Invasive hemodynamic monitoring is essential. Arterial catheterization allows beat-to-beat blood pressure monitoring and assists in the evaluation of significant cardiac dysrhythmias or acute hemorrhage.

The anesthetic agents chosen for management of patients with constrictive pericarditis should preserve myocardial contractility, HR, preload, and afterload. Among these parameters, HR is of greatest concern. Cardiac output is dependent on HR in patients with constrictive pericarditis. As a consequence of limited ventricular diastolic filling, bradycardia is poorly tolerated and reflects a decrease in SV that can lead to hypotension. Using anesthetic medications that preserve HR and myocardial contractility, such as ketamine, is hemodynamically advantageous. Inhalation agents cause myocardial depression and vasodilation in a dose-dependent fashion, and therefore the concentration should be carefully titrated to avoid excessive myocardial depression and hypotension. Vigorous positive-pressure ventilation may result in a sustained increase in intrathoracic pressure, causing a decrease in venous return to the heart and consequently further reducing CO.[48]

Immediate hemodynamic improvement may not occur after removal of the constricting tissue. Consistently low CO after pericardiotomy may be secondary to diffuse atrophy of myocardial muscle fibers or myocardial damage from the underlying disease. Intensive postoperative care with inotropic support and awareness for the potential of dysrhythmias and/or hemorrhage are essential components for creating a comprehensive anesthetic plan.

Cardiac Tamponade

Cardiac tamponade is a syndrome caused by the impairment of diastolic filling of the heart because of continual increases in intrapericardial pressure.[49] Slow accumulation of fluid in the pericardial space initially causes minute increases in intrapericardial pressure. This occurs as a result of the pericardium's ability to stretch to accommodate an increased volume. If the pericardial fluid accumulates rapidly, the presence of a few hundred milliliters may cause a significant increase in intrapericardial pressure that may result in cardiovascular collapse. Cardiac tamponade that results in shock is also known as cardiac compressive shock (or obstructive shock) and can result in inadequate peripheral perfusion, acidosis, and death (Fig. 25.36).

The causes of cardiac tamponade include (1) trauma, including sharp or blunt trauma to the chest and dissecting aortic aneurysms; (2) complications associated with cardiac surgery; (3) malignancy within the mediastinum; and (4) expansion of pericardial effusions after any form of pericarditis.[50]

Pathophysiology. Normal intrapericardial pressure is subatmospheric. Accumulation of pericardial fluid leads to an increase in intrapericardial pressure. As a result, diastolic expansion of the ventricles decreases. As in constrictive pericarditis, poor ventricular filling develops and leads to peripheral congestion and a decrease in SV and CO. The decrease in SV decreases peripheral perfusion causing catecholamine release manifested as tachycardia, vasoconstriction, and increased venous pressure, which helps maintain CO. If these mechanisms fail, cardiac collapse can occur.[51] The left ventricular pressure-volume loop associated with cardiac tamponade represents decreased LV volume and decreased SV due to compression (Fig. 25.37).

Clinical presentation. In addition to obvious indications of cardiac distress, specific signs of cardiac tamponade include Beck triad: hypotension, jugular venous distention, and muffled heart sounds.[52] Another specific finding associated with cardiac tamponade is pulsus paradoxus, which is an exaggerated decrease in systolic blood pressure (i.e., >10 mm Hg) that normally occurs with inspiration. Other conditions that may result in pulsus paradoxus are chronic obstructive pulmonary disease, obesity, and congestive heart failure. Jugular venous distention occurs because of a decrease in forward blood flow through the heart.

In cardiac tamponade, chest radiography may show an enlarged cardiac silhouette. The ECG usually demonstrates a decrease in voltage across all leads or electrical alterations of either the P wave or the QRS complex.[53] Echocardiography is the most sensitive, noninvasive method for detection of pericardial effusion and exclusion of tamponade. Use of a pulmonary artery catheter may reveal equilibration of right and left atrial pressures and right ventricular end-diastolic filling pressures at approximately 20 mm Hg.[54]

The definitive treatment for cardiac tamponade is pericardiocentesis, performed percutaneously by needle decompression, through a subxiphoid incision, or via thoracotomy or video-assisted thorascopic surgery to create a pericardial window. In contrast to patients with constrictive pericarditis, immediate hemodynamic improvement occurs once the pericardium is opened and direct pressure exerted on the heart is relieved. However, despite this fact, pulmonary edema, acute right and left ventricular dysfunction, and circulatory collapse can occur.[55]

Anesthetic management. Preoperatively the patient's clinical status should be optimized. This includes expansion of intravascular fluid volume, use of positive inotropic agents, and correction of acidosis. Volume expansion can augment preload and improve SV during cardiac tamponade.[56,57] The degree to which these measures are instituted depends on the hemodynamic state of the patient. Severely compromised patients require immediate intervention, which may include an emergency pericardiocentesis. Invasive hemodynamic monitoring should be established before the procedure. Intraarterial and CVP catheters are required for frequent sampling of blood, continuous blood pressure monitoring, and assessment of intravascular fluid status.

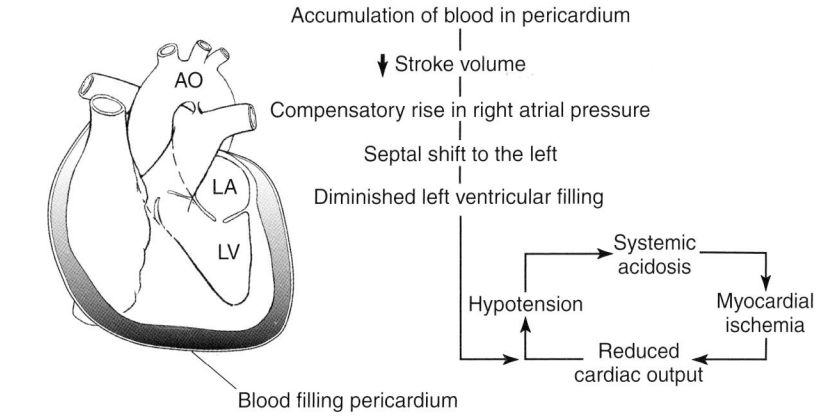

Fig. 25.36 Pathophysiology associated with cardiac tamponade. *AO*, Aorta; *LA*, left atrium; *LV*, left ventricle.

CARDIAC TAMPONADE

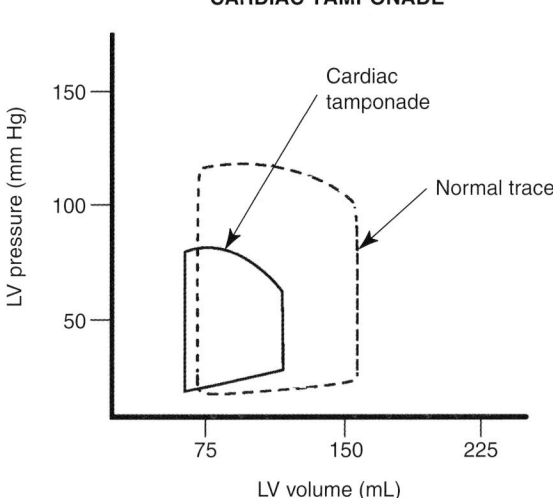

Fig. 25.37 Left ventricular pressure-volume loop associated with cardiac tamponade.

TABLE 25.7 Hemodynamic Goals for Management of Cardiac Tamponade

Parameter	Goal
Preload	Maintain or increase
Afterload	Maintain
Contractility	Maintain or increase
Heart rate	Maintain
Heart rhythm	Normal sinus rhythm
Treatment	Pericardiocentesis, pericardial window

Local infiltration anesthesia can be accomplished for emergency operative correction of cardiac tamponade.[57] Severe hypotension and cardiac arrest after induction of general anesthesia in patients with tamponade can occur.[58,59] The potential for decompensation associated with the use of general anesthetics is attributed to direct myocardial depression and vasodilation in patients with established impairment of cardiac filling. The use of positive-pressure ventilation in such patients may result in a decrease of venous return to the heart and can further decrease CO.[60] Intubation should be delayed until definitive management of the cardiac tamponade has occurred. If intubation is necessary prior to cardiac intervention, an awake approach utilizing local anesthetics to anesthetize the airway may help to (1) preserve spontaneous ventilation and (2) avoid the administration of cardiac depressive medications used for the induction of anesthesia. After percutaneous pericardiocentesis and the improvement of hemodynamic status, induction of general anesthesia and initiation of positive pressure ventilation are sufficient for further surgical exploration.

When it is not possible to relieve intrapericardial pressure that causes cardiac tamponade before the induction of anesthesia, the same anesthetic principles that are applied to the anesthetic management of patients with constrictive pericarditis should be used, including the use of anesthetic agents that preserve myocardial contractility, HR, preload, and afterload. Due to the sympathomimetic effects of ketamine, this drug has been advocated for the induction and maintenance of anesthesia.[4,57] However, many combinations of anesthetic agents that preserve the previously mentioned determinants of CO have been used safely.[48,57,59]

Continuous postoperative monitoring of blood pressure, CVP, and chest tube drainage is necessary. Possible complications after pericardiocentesis include reaccumulation of pericardial fluid, coronary laceration, cardiac puncture, and pneumothorax. Table 25.7 lists hemodynamic goals for patients with cardiac tamponade.

Acquired Valvular Heart Disease

The cardiac valves are membranous leaflets that separate the chambers of the heart. When open, they allow blood flow between the chambers and great vessels, and when closed, they prevent regurgitant blood flow between the chambers or backflow from the great vessels. A valve orifice of normal size presents a small degree of flow obstruction and thereby creates a hemodynamically insignificant gradient. Primary dysfunction of the mitral and aortic valves represents the most common and most severe hemodynamic derangement. Acquired primary dysfunction of the tricuspid or pulmonic valves is rare and therefore is not addressed in this chapter.

Valvular disease is classified according to the type of lesion that exists, stenosis, insufficiency, or mixed lesions. Valvular stenosis is a narrowing of the valvular orifice, which restricts flow through the orifice when the valve is open. This situation creates an increase in flow resistance and increases turbulent blood flow. Valvular insufficiency results in regurgitation secondary to incomplete or partial valve closure, which allows blood to flow back through the valve into the previous chamber. In patients with mixed lesions (stenosis with insufficiency or insufficiency with stenosis), one type of dysfunction is considered dominant over the other based on the severity of clinical symptoms.

Valvular dysfunction is classified as either primary or secondary. In primary valvular dysfunction, the valve leaflets or the anchoring and supporting structures are damaged or do not function properly. In secondary valvular dysfunction, the valve is not directly damaged. However, normal valve function is altered secondary to another pathophysiologic entity. Causes of secondary valvular dysfunction include ventricular dilation, which produces mitral valve insufficiency; retrograde aortic dissection, which creates aortic valve insufficiency; and papillary muscle infarction, which causes acute mitral valve insufficiency.[61]

Cardiac output. The primary components of CO are preload, afterload, contractility, LV compliance, and HR.[61-63] Blood flow may increase due to an increase in HR or an increase in SV. As blood viscosity decreases with decreasing hematocrit and increasing flow rate, normovolemic anemia reduces cardiac afterload, thereby facilitating the augmentation of CO. This sequence of events occurs so long as intravascular volume is maintained and cardiac reserve is ample. The amount of afterload present determines the degree of tension that cardiac fibers must develop before systolic ejection can occur.[64]

Evaluation of the patient. Evaluation of the patient with valvular heart disease should focus on the pathophysiologic derangements and their effects on cardiac function and hemodynamic status. The systematic evaluation of primary valvular dysfunction should include the following:

1. *Category of valvular dysfunction*
   - Stenosis (progressive narrowing of the valve orifice)
   - Insufficiency (incomplete valve closure that causes backflow through the valve)
   - Mixed (regurgitant and stenotic dysfunction)
2. *Status of left ventricular loading*
   - LV overload from mitral or aortic regurgitation
   - Pressure overload from aortic stenosis
   - Volume under load from mitral stenosis
3. *Acute vs chronic evolution of the dysfunction*
   - Acute valvular pathology has severe and precipitous hemodynamic consequences (e.g., regurgitant valvular disease).
   - Chronic valvular pathology occurs over time, and the heart compensates for stenotic and regurgitant valvular dysfunction.
4. *Cardiac rhythm and its effects on ventricular diastolic filling time*
5. *Left ventricular function*
   - Poor LV function places the patient at higher risk for perioperative cardiac morbidity.
6. *Secondary effects on the pulmonary vasculature and right ventricular function*
   - Secondary pulmonary hypertension from valvular lesions can significantly affect RV function.
7. *Heart rate*
   - Changes in HR (either bradycardia or tachycardia) can significantly alter the hemodynamic manifestations of a specific valvular lesion.
   - Bradycardia occurring with regurgitant lesions can result in a significant increase in the regurgitant fraction and decreased SV.
   - Tachycardia is detrimental in patients with stenotic lesions because it shortens the time period for ejection, which decreases SV and increases myocardial oxygen demand.[27-30,33,34]
8. *Perioperative anticoagulation* (see Chapter 38)

Clinical symptoms. The most frequent clinical signs and symptoms associated with valvular dysfunction are congestive heart failure, dysrhythmias, syncope, and angina pectoris. Symptoms commonly associated with congestive heart failure include dyspnea, orthopnea, and fatigue. The severity of valvular and left ventricular dysfunction can be related to the patient's activity level before the onset of cardiac symptoms.[39]

Patient evaluation: compensatory mechanisms. To maintain cardiac function despite progressive valvular dysfunction, increased sympathetic activity increases to compensate for decreased peripheral perfusion. A decrease in sympathetic tone that occurs during anesthesia can cause severe hemodynamic compromise. Evaluation of the patient should include recognition of sympathetic compensatory mechanisms and strategies that can be used to maintain hemodynamic stability. Despite maximum medical therapy, patients with severe valvular dysfunction may remain in congestive heart failure.

The evaluation should also focus on associated organ dysfunction. Chronic myocardial failure that causes a decrease in cardiac output may result in significant major organ dysfunction such as renal and hepatic insufficiency, as well as poor cerebral perfusion. Symptoms of decreased cerebral perfusion include an altered level of consciousness, restlessness, agitation, lethargy, and stroke.

Diagnostic modalities. The most valuable diagnostic modalities used to evaluate valvular heart disease include electrocardiography, chest radiography, color flow Doppler imaging, echocardiography, and cardiac catheterization of both the right and left chambers of the heart. Electrocardiography can be used for evaluation of ventricular hypertrophy, atrial enlargement, axis deviation, and—most important—determining cardiac rhythm. Chest radiography demonstrates the size of the cardiac silhouette and signs of pulmonary vascular congestion. Color flow Doppler imaging can be used to determine the valvular area, transvalvular gradients, degree of regurgitation, and flow velocity and direction, and can measure cardiac function. Cardiac catheterization can be used directly to measure transvalvular gradients, estimate the degree of regurgitation, visualize the coronary arteries, and determine intracardiac pressures.[65-69]

MITRAL STENOSIS

Pathophysiology

In mitral stenosis, the mitral valve orifice becomes progressively narrowed. The normal mitral valve area is 4 to 6 cm[2]. This narrowing reduces flow from the LA into the LV during diastole. The narrowing of the mitral valve orifice has two significant hemodynamic consequences. First, a gradient develops across the valve orifice. This change represents a compensatory response directed at maintaining adequate flow. Second, as the cross-sectional area of the orifice decreases and the gradient increases, flow is restricted and left ventricular volume is decreased. The clinical symptomatology associated with severe mitral stenosis results in pulmonary congestion, decreased CO, and potential RV overload/failure. Pulmonary congestion occurs as a result of increases in left atrial pressure. Decreased SV is caused by decreased left ventricular volume. Left ventricular filling is dependent on the length of diastole, the gradient between the LA and LV, and the surface area of the mitral valve. As the valve area narrows to 1.5 to 2.5 cm[2], patients frequently develop increased HR and CO.[70] When the mitral valve area becomes less than 1 cm[2], the prolonged diastolic filling time and elevated mean left atrial pressure are incapable of maintaining normal LVEDV, and decreases in left ventricular preload occur resulting in symptoms that occur at rest.[61] Atrial systole accounts for 20% to 30% of LVEDV. Because mitral stenosis presents a fixed resistance to ventricular inflow, most of the pressure generated during atrial systole is used to overcome the resistance caused by the stenotic valve rather than used for producing forward flow. As the HR increases to greater than 90 bpm and diastolic time intervals are shortened, LVEDV is decreased. Blood flow through the mitral valve can be calculated by using the Gorlin formula, which has been described earlier.

Any subsequent increase in flow rate or decrease in diastolic filling time reflects an increase in the pressure gradient between the LA

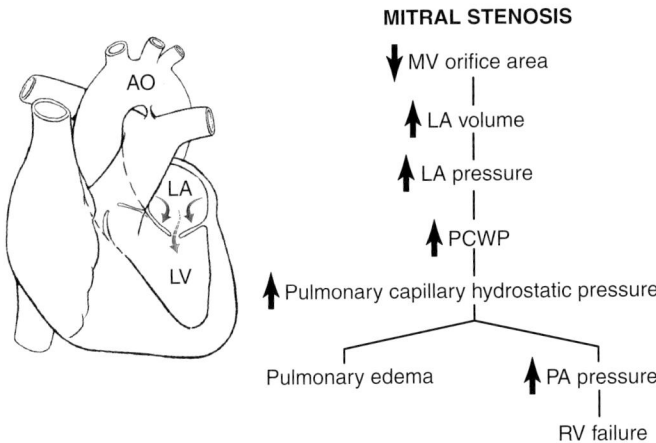

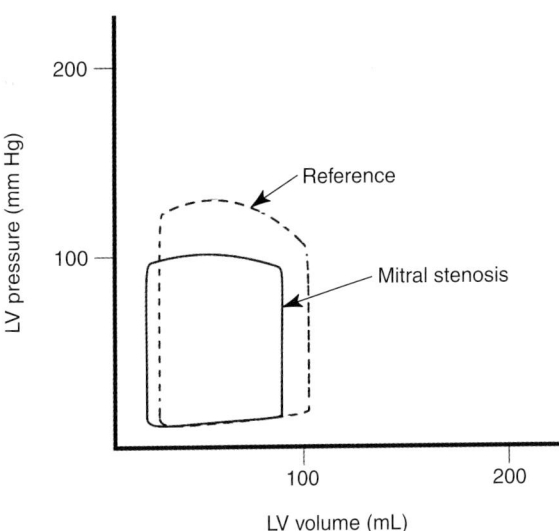

Fig. 25.38 Pathophysiology associated with mitral stenosis.

Fig. 25.39 Left ventricular pressure-volume loop associated with mitral stenosis. *LV,* Left ventricle.

and the LV. As the diastolic time interval shortens, the pressure gradient increases by the square of the increase in flow rate. Therefore any marked increase in HR can result in an increase in left atrial pressure, which can precipitate a rise in pulmonary artery pressures, potential fluid backup, and pulmonary edema.[71]

Left atrial hypertrophy and distention are consequences of elevated left atrial pressures. As a result of the increased left atrial pressure caused by mitral stenosis, the PCWP is artificially high. That is, PCWP overestimates the actual LVEDP and LVEDV. This distention of the LA can lead to atrial dysrhythmias, most commonly atrial fibrillation. The atrial systolic "kick" is lost during atrial fibrillation; this implies that diastolic filling can be maintained only by a further increase in left atrial pressure. Mean left atrial pressure is limited by the development of pulmonary congestion at pressures greater than 25 mm Hg. Elevation of left atrial pressures to greater than 25 mm Hg leads to pulmonary congestion and eventually pulmonary edema. In patients with chronic mitral stenosis, pulmonary hypertension develops because of continuous elevations in left atrial pressure (Fig. 25.38).

Pulmonary Vascular Changes in Right Ventricular Function

The pulmonary vasculature and eventually the RV are adversely affected by the chronic elevation of left atrial pressure that occurs with mitral stenosis. As mitral stenosis progresses, chronic elevation of left atrial pressure causes increased blood volume in the pulmonary vascular circuit. This can cause perivascular edema, and changes in pulmonary vascular resistance may ensue. These changes in pulmonary vascular resistance result in an increase in right ventricular afterload. As a compensatory response, right ventricular hypertrophy occurs; however, because the RV is incapable of generating high pressures, it eventually begins to fail.[61-63] As the disease progresses, overt signs of biventricular failure such as low CO with poor systemic perfusion become evident. Peripheral edema, hepatic congestion, and marked venous distention are signs of right ventricular failure. The deterioration of right ventricular function decreases adequate left ventricular filling and therefore causes further deterioration in CO (Fig. 25.39).

Anesthetic Considerations

Any anesthetic technique should be based on a thorough understanding of the pathophysiology of mitral stenosis, as well as the cardiovascular effects of the anesthetic agents administered. The following goals should be achieved in the anesthetic management of the patient with mitral stenosis:

- Maintenance of sinus rhythm at low normal heart

- Administering IV fluid to maintain LVEDV (LV preload) and thus SV without causing pulmonary congestion
- Avoid significant degree of myocardial depression
- Avoid significant increases in afterload, which can decrease SV
- Cardioversion as treatment for atrial tachyarrhythmias that cause hemodynamic instability
- Hypotension treated with phenylephrine (50–100 mcg)

The LVEDV is normal in approximately 85% of patients with mitral stenosis. An increased LVEDV in patients with mitral stenosis should alert the anesthetist to the presence of mitral or aortic insufficiency or primary coronary artery disease. Most patients with moderate mitral stenosis also have low to normal SV and therefore may have a normal EF. Approximately 33% of patients with mitral stenosis have an EF below normal (normal, 0.67 ± 0.08).[62] When the mitral valve is narrowed to less than 1 cm² (severe mitral stenosis), a mean left atrial pressure of 25 mm Hg is necessary for maintaining even an adequate resting CO. Owing to the abnormal transvalvular gradient, the PCWP overestimates LVEDP. On the PCWP, a prominent *a* wave and a decreased *y* descent are associated with mitral stenosis.

MITRAL REGURGITATION AND INSUFFICIENCY

Pathophysiology

During ventricular systole, the mitral valve is closed, preventing blood flow from the LV back into the LA. However, if for any reason the two leaflets of the mitral valve are not in opposition to each other, a portion of systolic ventricular flow regurgitates back through this incompetent (insufficient) valve. Therefore the LV has a double outlet (aorta and LA) during systolic ejection. Ejection into the aorta is a high-impedance outlet, and regurgitation through the mitral valve back into the LA is a low-impedance outlet. This condition is termed mitral regurgitation (MR) or mitral insufficiency. The degree of regurgitation (quantitatively), called the regurgitant fraction, is determined by four factors:

1. Size of the regurgitant valve orifice (surface area measured in cm²)
2. The pressure gradient between the LA and the LV
   - Inotropic state of the LV (peak systolic pressure)
   - Compliance of the LA and pulmonary veins
3. Time available for regurgitation (systole); systolic interval determines length of time during which regurgitation can occur; length of systolic time interval is inversely proportional to HR.

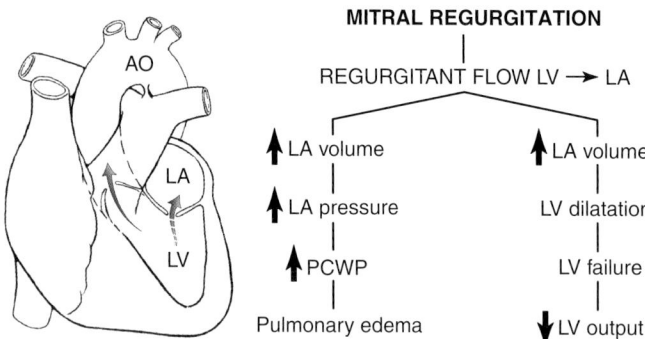

MITRAL REGURGITATION

REGURGITANT FLOW LV ⟶ LA

↑ LA volume   ↑ LA volume

↑ LA pressure   LV dilatation

↑ PCWP   LV failure

Pulmonary edema   ↓ LV output

Fig. 25.40 Pathophysiology associated with mitral regurgitation. *LA,* left atrium; *LV,* left ventricle; *PCWP,* pulmonary capillary wedge pressure.

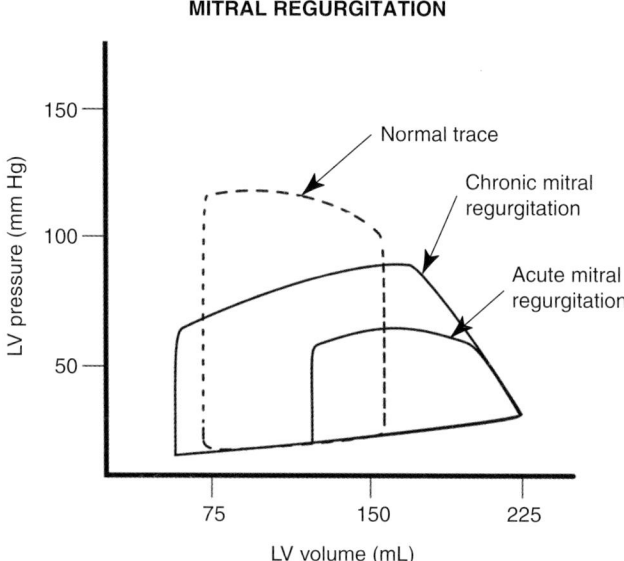

Fig. 25.41 Left ventricular (*LV*) pressure-volume loop associated with mitral regurgitation. The large volume and stroke volume associated with chronic mitral regurgitation occur because of LV hypertrophy. Notice that during the isovolumetric contraction phase, LV volume decreases as a result of the incompetent mitral valve.

4. Aortic outflow impedance SVR; regurgitant fraction can be significantly influenced by changes in impedance to aortic blood flow. Increased afterload will decrease SV.

The major pathophysiologic derangement associated with MR is volume overload of the LA and LV. This occurs because the regurgitant fraction (retrograde blood flow ejected into the LA during ventricular systole) delivers an increased diastolic volume to the LV. This increase in LVEDV results in ventricular dilation.[49,61,71] Acute MR and chronic MR have substantially different pathophysiologic manifestations. The primary determinant of these pathophysiologic adaptations is left atrial compliance. If acute MR is caused by papillary muscle rupture, which can occur after an acute MI, the mortality rate approaches 75% within 24 hours and 95% within 48 hours.[72] Chronic MR produces long-standing and gradual elevation of left atrial pressure results in remodeling of LA architecture causing LA dilation. This consequently facilitates containment of relatively large EDV while reflecting relatively low increases in LA pressures (Fig. 25.40). With chronic MR, compensatory hypertrophic changes occur in response to a continual increased left ventricular volume by increasing the left ventricular chamber size. This type of hypertrophic change is called eccentric hypertrophy.

In contrast to acute MR, the LA is small and noncompliant, but over time eccentric hypertrophic changes occur to compensate for progressive increases in volume (Fig. 25.41). In this situation, a small regurgitant volume bolus can generate deflections or *v* waves that appear in the PCWP tracing. This *v* wave appears as a result of a systolic jet (ejection) back through the incompetent mitral valve. The pressure wave produced by this jet is transmitted upstream into the pulmonary artery and designated as a pathologic *v* wave. The time delay for this pressure wave to be transmitted results in its appearance at the time interval in which the normal *v* wave (passive atrial filling) occurs.[61] The height of the *v* wave in MR does not represent a measurement of regurgitant volume but rather of left atrial compliance in relationship to the regurgitated volume. The hypertrophic LA accommodates a larger regurgitant volume, which results in small increases in pressure. The dilated and compliant LA allows the pulmonary vascular circuit to be buffered from the excessive left atrial volume. However, chronic MR causes pulmonary venous congestion, which creates pulmonary vascular reactive changes that eventually result in pulmonary artery hypertension. Distention of the LA may lead to atrial fibrillation, a common arrhythmia associated with MR. A nonhemodynamic symptom associated with MR is hoarseness. Compression of the left branch of the recurrent laryngeal nerve, which circumscribes the aortic arch, can be compressed by the enlarged LA in chronic MR. Because the recurrent laryngeal nerve provides the majority of the motor function to the vocal cords, partial paralysis of the left vocal cord could result in respiratory distress in those patients with respiratory disease.

Pulmonary Vasculature and Right Ventricular Function

In acute MR, the pulmonary vasculature is exposed to immediate and marked elevation of left atrial pressure because of a small and noncompliant LA. Pulmonary vascular congestion is precipitous and results in almost immediate development of pulmonary edema. An acute rise in left atrial pressure and congestion of the pulmonary circuit creates an increased right ventricular workload. This immediate increase in right ventricular afterload results in ventricular dilation and consequently may lead to right ventricular failure. In chronic MR, elevation of baseline pulmonary pressures is much more gradual, occurring over a prolonged period. This allows secondary pulmonary artery hypertension via intimal fibroelastosis generated by chronic perivascular edema. If the patient has coexisting mitral stenosis, pulmonary vascular resistance and right ventricular pressures may be excessively elevated.[49,61,71]

Effects of Afterload Reductions

The path of least resistance for blood flow during left ventricular systole is retrograde into the LA. Reduction of SVR via arterial vasodilation reduces impedance to systolic outflow into the aorta and increases forward flow. Conversely, increases in SVR have marked effects on the reduction in forward flow and the increase in the regurgitant fraction. A 20% increase in MAP raises LA pressure by 50% and reflects a 120% increase in regurgitant flow concurrent with a 16% decrease in forward flow.[61]

Anesthetic Considerations

An otherwise healthy patient with stable and controlled MR undergoing an ambulatory or uncomplicated surgical procedure has a minimal increase in risk of adverse hemodynamic fluctuations. Patients with cardiovascular disease who undergo major vascular, intrathoracic, intraabdominal, neurosurgical, orthopedic, or emergency procedures may have a 25% to 50% higher mortality risk than patients without the disease process. Controversy exists regarding whether the duration of surgery correlates with perioperative cardiac morbidity.[39,61]

Preoperative assessment is essential for evaluating the degree of cardiac compensation (Table 20.8; see also Table 20.7). Anesthetic

TABLE 25.8 Hemodynamic Goals for Management of Mitral Valve Lesions

Parameter	Mitral Regurgitation (Insufficiency) Goal	Mitral Stenosis Goal
Heart rate	Increase, avoid bradycardia	Low normal
Rhythm	Maintain normal sinus rhythm	Maintain normal sinus rhythm
Afterload	Decrease	Maintain normal
Pulmonary vascular resistance	Avoid increases	Avoid increases
Preload	Normal to increased	Normal to increased

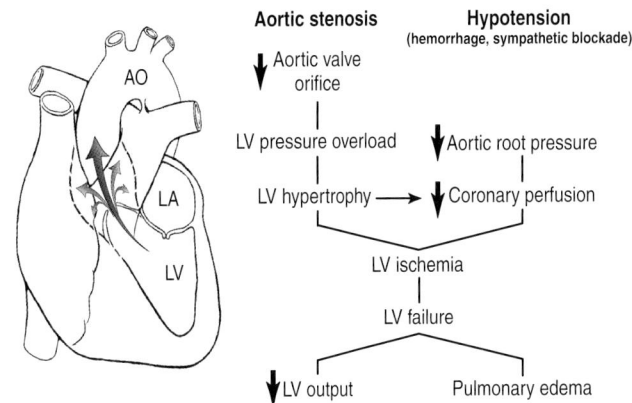

AORTIC STENOSIS

Fig. 25.42 Pathophysiology associated with aortic stenosis. *AO,* Aorta; *LA,* left atrium; *LV,* left ventricle.

management of the patient with MR should focus on these hemodynamic goals: decreasing regurgitant blood flow to enhance CO by decreasing afterload, maintaining or increasing preload, and maintaining cardiac contractility. Bradycardia or dysrhythmias that cause a loss of atrial kick can result in pulmonary congestion, left atrial and left ventricular overload, and a significant decrease in CO.[61,62]

Another anesthetic consideration for MR includes decreasing SVR or afterload. Cautiously lowering SVR via an arterial vasodilator such as sodium nitroprusside improves forward flow. However, extreme reductions in blood pressure, and especially diastolic pressure, can lead to decreased coronary artery blood flow and decreased CO.

Selection of an anesthetic technique should take into consideration the adverse effects associated with changes in HR and SVR. General anesthesia is the technique of choice in patients with MR. Regional anesthesia (spinal or epidural) is not contraindicated; however, the potential for profound and precipitous decreases in blood pressure via sympathetic blockade should be considered. Induction of general anesthesia can be safely achieved with any of the presently available agents. Hemodynamic goals include avoiding bradycardia and significant variations in afterload (both increases and dramatic decreases). The use of muscle relaxants is appropriate depending on the surgical need and so long as the resulting changes in HR do not cause bradycardia. Maintenance of anesthesia can be accomplished with narcotics and an inhalation agent. There is no definitive evidence to support that a particular inhalation agent yields superior outcomes for patients with MR. However, because all inhalation agents cause a dose-dependent decrease in myocardial contractility, their use may be detrimental in patients with severe ventricular dysfunction. In this instance, the use of opioids in combination with an infusion of dexmedetomidine and/or ketamine may provide for a more effective hemodynamic profile. Care should be given to avoid boluses of dexmedetomidine (if used) since this could result in bradycardia. Anesthetic management should primarily focus on the utilization of agents and techniques that avoid bradycardia or increases in SVR.[61] See Table 25.8 for anesthetic goals most appropriate for the management of mitral lesions.

AORTIC STENOSIS

Etiology and Pathophysiology

The most common causes of aortic stenosis include a congenital defect resulting in a bicuspid aortic valve (especially in males) and as sequelae of rheumatic valvular heart disease. Isolated aortic valvular dysfunction in patients with rheumatic heart disease is rare. Commonly, rheumatic valvular disease is associated with mitral valve involvement. Whatever

the cause, the pathophysiology remains the same and results in the need for increased left ventricular systolic pressure to overcome the left ventricular outflow tract obstruction caused by a narrowed aortic valve orifice (Fig. 25.42). During auscultation, a low-frequency systolic ejection murmur is characteristic of aortic stenosis.[42]

A normal aortic valve area of 2.5 to 3.5 cm² and SV of approximately 80 mL result in a flow rate of 250 mL/min during the interval of ventricular systole (80 mL/sec × 0.32 sec – systolic time interval). The flow rate through a normal orifice results in a minimal gradient (2–4 mm Hg). The normal left ventricular systolic pressure of 100 to 130 mm Hg is sufficient to generate flow rates of 250 to 300 mL/sec. To ensure normal flow rates and CO through the narrowed orifice, the velocity of systolic ejection must increase. For systolic ejection to increase, ventricular systolic pressure increases dramatically, depending on the degree of valvular pathology. The LV must compensate for gradually increasing mechanical impedance to ejection. This results in LVH, which allows the heart to generate high ventricular systolic pressure and overcome impedance to ejection. The elevation of systolic ejection pressure produces a gradient between the left ventricular cavity and the aorta. The valve area must be constricted by at least 50% before the gradient becomes significant to the point that symptoms occur at rest. An aortic valve area of less than 1 cm² produces a clinical triad of symptoms that includes angina (even in the absence of significant coronary artery disease), syncope, and congestive heart failure.[73] An aortic valve area less than 1 cm² represents severe aortic stenosis and should be a cause of concern during anesthetic management because of the associated increase in perioperative cardiac morbidity. The prognosis is poor if the flow velocity is greater than 4 m/sec, which corresponds to a mean aortic valve gradient greater than 40 mm Hg.[74] An aortic valve area less than 0.7 cm² is associated with sudden death.[75] For adequate assessment of the degree of valvular stenosis, both the flow rate across the valve and the pressure gradient should be evaluated either by cardiac catheterization or echocardiography.[68,69]

Left Ventricular Function

Left ventricular concentric hypertrophy is the compensatory change associated with aortic stenosis. It results in several hemodynamic adaptations that are unique to aortic stenosis and present a challenge and a dilemma with regard to anesthesia management. The consequence of LVH in aortic stenosis is a decrease in ventricular compliance, hypertrophic remodeling, and an eventual decrease in the intrinsic contractility of the myocardium.[76] The reduction in ventricular compliance affects normal hemodynamics as follows:

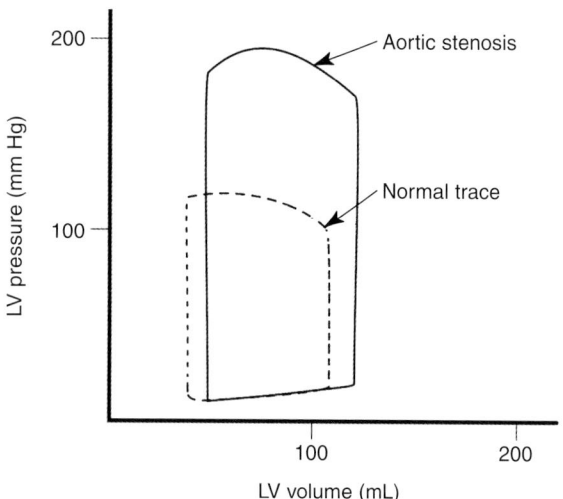

Fig. 25.43 Left ventricular (*LV*) pressure-volume loop associated with aortic stenosis.

I. Higher filling pressures are needed to produce the same amount of ventricular work.

II. To achieve adequate left ventricular filling, normal sinus rhythm must be maintained to ensure adequate LVEDV from the atrial kick.

III. Concentric ventricular hypertrophy increases myocardial oxygen demand.

   A. Myocardial oxygen consumption is increased.

      1. Myocardial mass is increased.

      2. Pressure generation (isovolumetric contraction) uses more energy than left ventricular ejection; a high intracavitary pressure must be generated to maintain CO.

      3. The ejection phase is prolonged.

   B. Myocardial oxygen supply is decreased.

      1. CPP is decreased as a result of an increase in LVEDP.

      2. Systolic coronary flow is absent because left ventricular systolic pressure exceeds aortic systolic pressure.

      3. Prolonged systolic ejection reduces the coronary perfusion interval.

      4. Subendocardial capillaries are compressed due to myocardial hypertrophy.[49,61]

Pulmonary Circuit and Right Ventricular Responses

To maintain CO in the presence of a noncompliant and hypertrophic LV, left atrial pressures increase to accommodate left ventricular filling (Fig. 25.43). Left atrial pressures greater than 18 mm Hg can cause an increase in pulmonary artery pressure, resulting in passive pulmonary venous congestion. Eventually, pulmonary fibroelastosis occurs, causing pulmonary artery hypertension. If left ventricular EF is decreased to less than 40% in association with aortic stenosis, CO can be maintained only with increases in left atrial pressures. These pressures increase to 25 to 30 mm Hg, which results in increased mean pulmonary artery pressure. Elevated mean pulmonary artery pressure increases pulmonary vascular resistance, which can cause right ventricular failure. Decreasing left ventricular preload in association with significant aortic stenosis can result in decreases in CO.

Anesthetic Considerations

The goals of anesthesia management include maintaining hemodynamic stability without causing significant alterations in compensatory mechanisms. Anesthetic management of patients with aortic stenosis should focus on the following hemodynamic factors:

- Maintain normal sinus rhythm and HR 70 to 80 bpm
- Ensure sufficient preload (LVEDV) to maintain CO
- Ensure adequate coronary perfusion by maintaining appropriate DBP values
- Avoid myocardial depression, especially with poor LV function
- Maintain or allow slight increase in afterload

General anesthesia is the preferred technique for major surgical procedures involving patients with aortic stenosis because of the ability to manipulate hemodynamic parameters, especially DBP. Neuraxial blockade (spinal or epidural) must be used with extreme caution because precipitous reductions in blood pressure associated with a sympathectomy decrease SVR.[42] Epidural anesthesia offers the advantage of a slower onset of vasodilation. Depending on the degree of compromise, the heart may not be able to compensate for moderate to severe systemic vasodilation. Therefore lower dermatome level blocks decrease the degree of systemic vasodilation and maintain afterload. Successful cardiopulmonary resuscitation is virtually impossible because of the mechanical left ventricular outflow obstruction associated with aortic stenosis. The pressure necessary to overcome outflow obstruction and produce adequate coronary artery perfusion and CO cannot be generated with closed-chest compressions. Furthermore, short periods of hypotension may lead to a decrease in coronary perfusion and should be treated with IV fluid and phenylephrine.[77] Due to the increased oxygen demands of the LV, irreversible myocardial ischemia and cardiovascular collapse can occur if hypotension is not promptly and aggressively treated.

Intraoperative control of HR and rhythm is a major goal of the anesthetic management of patients with aortic stenosis. Tachycardia can be detrimental because it decreases diastolic filling time, resulting in a reduction of left ventricular preload. The reduced time interval for coronary artery perfusion reduces oxygen supply to the myocardium. In patients with HRs greater than 110 bpm, systolic ejection time and CO are decreased.[61,62] Bradycardia (<60 bpm) is detrimental in aortic stenosis. Prolonged diastolic filling time, which occurs as a result of bradycardia, causes ventricular distention, which can further decrease CPP especially to the subendocardium.[49,61]

Monitoring and Premedication

It is prudent to titrate preoperative sedatives while vital signs can be continuously monitored. In addition to standard intraoperative monitoring, complete invasive monitoring may be required for patients with aortic stenosis, even for routine procedures. Any significant change in basic hemodynamic variables (i.e., HR, heart rhythm, LVEDV, CPP) can rapidly cause irreversible myocardial deterioration. It is imperative that these variables be monitored closely, and appropriate interventions be promptly provided to prevent adverse hemodynamic consequences. The complexity of hemodynamic monitoring modalities is dependent on the physical status of the patient, the severity of aortic stenosis, the extent of the surgical procedure, and the ability of the anesthesia provider to use and interpret hemodynamic values.

The use of intraarterial monitoring for direct beat-to-beat blood pressure assessment allows the anesthesia provider to rapidly treat undesirable hemodynamic changes. The use of intraoperative TEE provides real-time quantitative and qualitative information regarding valvular function, and changes in anesthetic management can be accomplished to maximize hemodynamic status.[78] Absolute criteria for intraoperative invasive monitoring for patients with aortic stenosis remain controversial. However, clinical judgment, experience, and the ability to appropriately use the pulmonary artery catheter should be considered before implementation.[76,79]

Maintenance of Anesthesia

Commonly used induction agents can be administered cautiously since a primary goal is to avoid profound hypotension. Tracheal intubation can be performed with any of the available muscle relaxants; however, histamine release should be avoided since it can dramatically increase HR and decrease blood pressure. Anesthetic maintenance can be accomplished with the use of an inhalation agent in conjunction with opiates. The adverse cardiovascular effects of the inhalation agents must be considered before these drugs are used. Higher concentrations of an inhaled agent result in greater degrees of myocardial depression and vasodilation. Inhalation agents must be used with caution because the myocardial depressant effect can be deleterious in patients with impaired ventricular function. The use of higher dose opioids alone, or in combination with an infusion of dexmedetomidine and/or ketamine, are alternative approaches that may help achieve cardiovascular stability without causing significant myocardial depression. Whichever combination of anesthetic medications is chosen for patients with aortic stenosis, immediate and aggressive treatment of adverse changes that occur in HR and rhythm, SVR, blood pressure, and LVEDV is paramount if successful anesthetic outcomes are to be achieved.[75,79]

AORTIC INSUFFICIENCY

Aortic insufficiency (AI), also known as aortic regurgitation, can be classified as acute or chronic and as primary or secondary, depending on the cause. Primary chronic AI is caused by rheumatic valvular disease and almost always involves the mitral valve to some degree. Primary acute AI is most commonly caused by infective endocarditis, which results in direct damage to the aortic valve cusps. Acute secondary (functional) AI results from aortic root dissection caused either by trauma or aneurysm and results in a mechanical and functional impairment of functional aortic valve closure.

Pathophysiology

The major hemodynamic aberration related to AI occurs during diastole. A portion of the blood volume ejected from the LV into the aorta regurgitates back into the ventricle because of incomplete closure of the aortic valve. AI causes volume overload of the LV. Chronic ventricular overload causes eccentric ventricular hypertrophy and chamber dilation (Fig. 25.44). The degree of regurgitation depends on three factors: the diastolic time available for regurgitation to occur, the diastolic pressure gradient between the aorta and the LV, and the degree of incompetence of the aortic valve.[71,75]

Diastolic time and diastolic pressure can be manipulated during the course of anesthesia so that the amount of regurgitant flow is decreased and the amount of forward flow is increased. An HR of 90 to 100 bpm decreases the diastolic time period, which reduces the time available for regurgitation. Reducing SVR reduces aortic diastolic pressure and decreases the gradient between the aorta and the LV. Unique pathophysiologic adaptations differentiate chronic AI from the acute form. In chronic AI, the LV has had time to compensate for the increased volume. In time, LV hypertrophy allows the LV to tolerate significant increases in volume without dramatic decreases in EF.[49,61] In situations of acute onset AI, the LV has inadequate time to adapt to volume overload, which renders compensatory mechanisms ineffective (Fig. 25.45). Frequently, left ventricular failure, pulmonary edema, and cardiovascular collapse occur. LVEDP rises precipitously in acute AI because of the inability of the LV to alter its compliance.

Patients with chronic AI can remain asymptomatic for long periods. Except during times of stress, the clinical symptoms associated with chronic AI are usually not incapacitating. End-stage AI is characterized by myocardial failure with decreased CO and precipitous elevation of

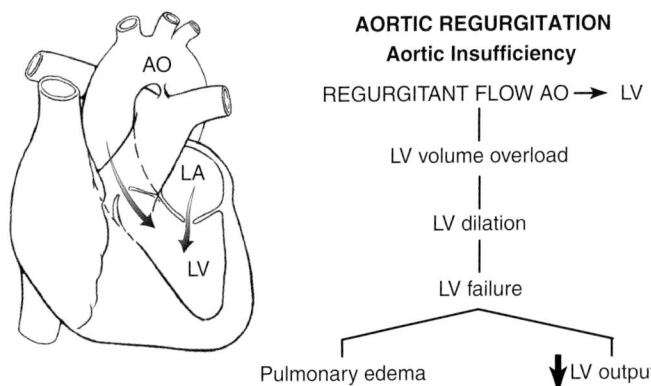

Fig. 25.44 Pathophysiology associated with aortic regurgitation. *AO*, Aorta; *LA*, left atrium; *LV*, left ventricle.

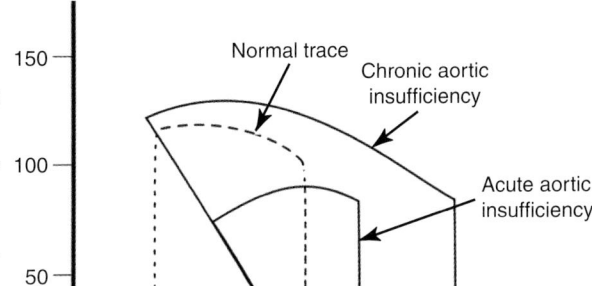

Fig. 25.45 Left ventricular (*LV*) pressure-volume loop associated with aortic insufficiency. Increased LV pressure, volume, and stroke volume are associated with chronic aortic insufficiency and are reflective of LV hypertrophy. Notice that during the relaxation phase, as isovolumetric relaxation occurs, LV volume increases as a result of the incompetent aortic valve.

LVEDV with evidence of pulmonary congestion. As long as ventricular hypertrophy and dilation do not affect the mitral valve, the pulmonary circulation is not affected by the pathophysiologic changes associated with AI. Increased myocardial oxygen consumption occurs partly because of the development of eccentric hypertrophy. The decrease in aortic diastolic pressure that results from AI reduces coronary flow and can cause subendocardial ischemia. In acute AI, a precipitous increase in LVEDP with a decrease in aortic diastolic pressure can severely compromise coronary blood flow and result in acute myocardial ischemia. The RV and pulmonary vascular circuit are usually spared in chronic AI until secondary (functional) MR occurs. This results in dilation of the mitral valve annulus. A gradual increase in LA pressure and pulmonary artery pressure caused by functional MR eventually causes pulmonary hypertension; right ventricular failure can occur if pulmonary hypertension becomes severe. In acute AI, functional MR is poorly tolerated, owing to a noncompliant LA. This situation leads to immediate pulmonary vascular congestion and pulmonary edema. Patients with asymptomatic AI have a 0.2% annual mortality rate as compared with symptomatic patients, who have a greater than 10% mortality rate per year.[74] Therefore, when evidence suggests that increases in left ventricular volume result in left ventricular dysfunction, aortic valve replacement is recommended.

TABLE 25.9　Hemodynamic Goals for Management of Aortic Valve Lesions

Parameter	Aortic Regurgitation (Insufficiency) Goal	Aortic Stenosis Goal
Heart rate	Moderate increase	Low normal
Heart rhythm	Normal sinus rhythm	Normal sinus rhythm
Afterload	Decrease	Maintain to slight increase
Pulmonary vascular resistance	Maintain	Maintain
Preload	Normal to increased	Increased

TABLE 25.10　Hemodynamic Goals for Management of Mitral Valve Prolapse

Parameter	Goal
Preload	Maintain or increase
Afterload	Maintain
Contractility	Maintain
Heart rate	Maintain
Heart rhythm	Normal sinus rhythm

Anesthesia Management

The goals for anesthesia management include increasing forward flow and decreasing the degree of regurgitation. Therefore efforts should focus on the following hemodynamic factors:

- HR should be maintained between 80 and 100 bpm
- Afterload (especially diastolic pressure) should be decreased
- Avoid myocardial depression
- Maintain normal sinus rhythm
- Maintain/increase preload

Neuraxial blockade is an appropriate anesthetic choice, depending on the invasiveness of the surgical procedure. Reduction in SVR resulting from sympathetic blockade may reduce the degree of regurgitation. The potential for immediate and uncontrolled hypotension during spinal anesthesia is a concern. However, spinal and epidural anesthesias have been used successfully for patients with AI. Induction of general anesthesia can be accomplished with any of the available IV agents. Tracheal intubation can be achieved with the use of available nondepolarizing muscle relaxants. Succinylcholine may be used, but its potential to cause bradycardia (although rarely) must be considered. Maintenance of anesthesia can be achieved with an inhalation agent. If significant ventricular dysfunction exists, an opioid-based anesthetic in combination with dexmedetomidine and/or ketamine infusion may be preferable.[59,61,62]

Monitoring and Premedication

Unless end-stage AR or significant preoperative ventricular dysfunction exists, aggressive invasive monitoring is not warranted. However, if the surgical procedure is extensive or if vasodilators or inotropes are being used, then an arterial line and a pulmonary artery catheter should be used for assessing the results and efficacy of these therapeutic agents. Premedication should be tailored to the patient's clinical condition. In elderly or debilitated patients, a conservative amount of premedication in a monitored environment should be titrated until effective.

Appropriate anesthetic management of the patient with valvular heart disease requires a basic knowledge of cardiac physiology and the pathophysiologic changes that occur with valvular dysfunction. The cardiovascular effects of all the agents, techniques, and adjunct pharmacologic agents used during anesthesia must be integrated into the anesthetic plan. A thorough understanding of the use of invasive monitoring along with other sophisticated diagnostic modalities enables the clinician to continuously monitor hemodynamic parameters. Contemporary anesthesia practice has allowed patients with severe valvular dysfunction to undergo surgical procedures that would not have been performed a decade ago.[75] Table 25.9 lists anesthetic goals for management of aortic lesions.

MITRAL VALVE PROLAPSE

Description and Etiology

The incidence of mitral valve prolapse (MVP), which was thought to be present in 5% to 15% of the US population, is presently estimated at 1.6% to 2.4% of adults.[74] A familial predisposition exists, and women are three times more likely than men to develop MVP. Other conditions frequently associated with MVP include pectus excavatum and kyphoscoliosis. Symptoms are general and include weakness, dizziness, syncope, atypical chest pain, and palpitations. Atrial and ventricular dysrhythmias are common findings in asymptomatic patients. A diagnosis of MVP is confirmed through echocardiography. Most patients with this condition remain undiagnosed. Despite infrequent signs and symptoms, MVP can produce potentially life-threatening complications. Premature ventricular contractions are the most common dysrhythmia associated with MVP. Prolonged periods of ventricular tachycardia occur in approximately 21% of patients with MVP. It is also the most common cause of isolated MR. Supraventricular tachyarrhythmias and bradycardia associated with AV block may occur. Medical therapy for MVP consists primarily of the use of β-blocking drugs, which are thought to inhibit an autonomic imbalance that exists in women who have it. Additionally, β-blocking drugs may increase end-diastolic volume and thereby decrease the degree of prolapse. Most patients with MVP do not require medical or pharmacologic management, which reflects the asymptomatic nature of this relatively common valvular abnormality (Table 25.10).[33,79]

Pathophysiology and Considerations

The pathophysiologic changes that occur in MVP primarily affect the cusps and the chordae tendineae. Involved is a myxomatous degeneration of the valve cusps that replace normal fibrous tissue. In addition, this myxomatous degeneration affects the chordae tendineae and causes them to become pliable and elongated. The valve leaflets become supple and redundant, as the valve can evert into the LA during systole.[80]

Mitral valve prolapse is undiagnosed in the majority of patients. A manifestation that commonly occurs in healthy patients who are receiving anesthesia is an unexpected dysrhythmia (e.g., premature ventricular contractions), many of which resolve spontaneously. β-blockers are the best choice for control of dysrhythmias in patients with MVP. Hemodynamic events and certain positions tend to exacerbate the degree of MVP and dysrhythmias. Hemodynamic changes that cause a decrease in ventricular preload and increase the incidence of eversion of the mitral valve are caused by increased myocardial contractility, decreased SVR, head-up or sitting positions, use of drugs that decrease ventricular preload (e.g., nitroglycerin and sodium nitroprusside), and hypovolemia.

Pharmacology

Preoperative anxiety stimulates the sympathetic nervous system, potentially increasing the degree of MVP and concomitant dysrhythmias.

Thus appropriately managing anxiety may help improve the hemodynamic profile characteristic of MVP. Anticholinergics can cause tachycardia and should therefore be omitted from the preoperative regimen.

Anesthetic Management

Regional anesthesia is acceptable for patients with MVP. SVR should be maintained slightly above normal, even in the presence of sympathetic blockade. General anesthesia is an appropriate choice and may be preferred in many instances. Whichever technique is chosen, it is important that preload be maintained. Induction of anesthesia can be accomplished with any of the available IV agents. Ketamine, with its ability to stimulate the sympathetic nervous system, should not be used in patients with MVP. Use of an inhalation agent alone or in combination with opioids is appropriate for maintenance of anesthesia. Muscle relaxants that have a stable cardiovascular profile can be used. Antibiotic prophylaxis is recommended for patients with MVP because of the potential for endocarditis. Currently, only patients with prosthetic valves, patients with prior endocarditis, heart transplant patients with a valvulopathy, and certain congenital heart disease patients now require endocarditis prophylaxis.[81]

CARDIOMYOPATHY

Cardiomyopathy is defined as heart muscle disease involving the myocardium that is chronic and frequently progressive in nature. The term is used to describe distinct cardiac pathologic conditions that can ultimately result in fatal dysrhythmias, progressive cardiac disability, and sudden cardiac death. All forms of cardiomyopathy can result in congestive heart failure and death. Cardiomyopathies can be categorically differentiated by a general pathologic cause as either extrinsic or intrinsic. Intrinsic cardiomyopathy is described as decreased contractile state of the heart muscle that cannot be attributed to a specific external causative factor. In contrast, the cause of extrinsic cardiomyopathy can be directly attributed to a disease process or toxin that adversely damages cardiac muscle. Factors that can cause extrinsic cardiomyopathy include but are not limited to ischemia, chronic inflammation, congenital heart disease, metabolic diseases (e.g., hemochromatosis), and toxins (e.g., chronic alcohol intake, chemotherapeutic agents). Frequently, histologic findings consistent with cardiomyopathies include myocyte hypertrophy, degradation of the cardiac cytoskeleton, and cellular fibrosis. The four major types of progressive cardiomyopathies include dilated cardiomyopathy (DCM), hypertrophic cardiomyopathy (HCM), restrictive cardiomyopathy (RCM), and arrhythmogenic right ventricular cardiomyopathy (ARVC). Takotsubo cardiomyopathy (TCM) most often resolves within 4 to 8 weeks after diagnosis, but the long-term prognosis has not definitively been determined.

Frequently the discovery of significant cardiomyopathy is accomplished postmortem because sudden cardiac death commonly occurs in those with this disease. A discussion of various types of cardiomyopathies, signs and symptoms, and anesthetic implications are included in the following sections.

Patients with a severe cardiomyopathy frequently present for cardiac procedures such as pacemaker implantation or heart transplantation. A thorough preoperative evaluation is essential to create a comprehensive anesthetic plan that is individualized. In addition to physical examination, an evaluation of the patient's preoperative medication regimen and assessment of the degree of compliance with medications are important parts of medical optimization. A detailed analysis of the invasive and noninvasive cardiac studies, including TEE and the cardiologist's impression of the patient's cardiac status, is vital.

Hypertrophic Cardiomyopathy

HCM, a genetically transmitted disorder, is a form of myocardial dysfunction that can cause coronary artery disease, valvular dysfunction, ventricular remodeling, and hypertension. The incidence in the adult population is approximately 1 in 500 persons.[82] Obstructive HCM has previously been referred to as idiopathic hypertrophic subaortic stenosis. Currently, the preferred term used to describe this pathologic state is HCM with or without left ventricular outflow obstruction.[83]

A summary of the pathophysiology, signs and symptoms, and anesthetic considerations is listed in Table 25.11.

Pathophysiology

Hypertrophic cardiomyopathy is the most common cause of sudden death in the pediatric and young adult populations.[84] The major cardiac changes associated with HCM include (1) ventricular hypertrophy, (2) decreased ventricular chamber size, (3) increased ventricular wall thickness, and (4) impaired ventricular relaxation. The myocardial defect associated with HCM is related to the contractile mechanism. An increase in the density of calcium channels is one abnormality that appears to lead to myocardial hypertrophy. Asymmetric hypertrophy of the interventricular septum of the LV occurs. It has been determined that there is a genetic predisposition to developing HCM.[85] Patients with HCM and sarcomere myofilament mutations have a greater degree of microvascular impairment, an increased incidence of myocardial fibrosis, and impaired myocardial remodeling.[86] The asymmetric hypertrophy of the intraventricular septum causes a left outflow tract obstruction, and the hemodynamic consequences are similar to those that are characteristic of aortic stenosis. The coronary arterial walls become narrowed because of the presence of collagen. If the entire myocardium is involved, a disproportionate hypertrophy of the intraventricular septum exists. The contraction of the hypertrophic septum bulging into the subaortic area of the left ventricular outflow tract creates a dynamic gradient. The left ventricular outflow tract is bound anteriorly by the intraventricular septum and posteriorly by the anterior leaflet of the mitral valve. The rapid acceleration of blood traveling through the narrowed outflow tract creates a Venturi effect, which pulls the anterior mitral valve leaflet into the outflow tract. An LV outflow tract obstruction is present in approximately two-thirds of patients with HCM.[87] The systolic anterior motion of the anterior mitral valve leaflet further obstructs left ventricular outflow. The valve leaflet may even contact the septum and further compromise left ventricular outflow.

The pathophysiologic abnormalities related to HCM include the presence of systolic and diastolic dysfunction. A loss of diastolic compliance results in an abnormally elevated LVEDP in the presence of low-normal end-diastolic volume. Loss of left ventricular diastolic compliance requires a greater contribution of volume from atrial contraction. As a result, congestive heart failure may ensue as left atrial pressures continue to increase.[75] Since approximately 75% of LV preload comes from the LA, maintenance of normal sinus rhythm is critical for adequate SV. The increase in LVEDP, which results from a noncompliant LV, decreases CPP to the hypertrophic LV. Altered coronary perfusion decreases myocardial blood supply, and the presence of left ventricular hypertrophy increases myocardial oxygen demand. Thickening of the internal lumen of the coronary arteries decreases myocardial perfusion, leading to ischemia.[87]

Hypertrophic cardiomyopathy with obstruction is characterized by its dynamic nature. Three basic hemodynamic parameters can affect the degree of left ventricular outflow tract obstruction. Manipulation of these parameters can exacerbate or ameliorate the hemodynamic consequences of outflow obstruction. These three parameters include preload, afterload, and contractility.[33] Increasing myocardial contractility in patients with HCM exacerbates the obstruction by increasing

TABLE 25.11	Pathology and Anesthetic Considerations for Various Cardiomyopathies		
Cardiomyopathy	**Distinctive Features**	**Signs and Symptoms**	**Anesthetic Considerations**
Dilated	Eccentric left and right ventricular hypertrophy causing systolic and diastolic dysfunction	Chest pain Jugular venous distention Weakness Exercise intolerance Rales Tachycardia Pulsus alternans Atrial fibrillation Atrial and ventricular dysrhythmias Atrioventricular valve regurgitation X-ray—pulmonary venous congestion/ spherical appearance of LV/cardiomegaly	Promote afterload reduction Avoid large fluid bolus Choose anesthetic techniques, agents that minimize myocardial depression
Restrictive	Stiff and noncompliant ventricles decrease ventricular end-diastolic volume despite near-normal systolic function	Dyspnea Fatigue Cardiomegaly Atrioventricular valve regurgitation JVD Pulmonary hypertension Rales	TEE and invasive hemodynamic monitoring IV inotropic support may be necessary Choose anesthetic techniques, agents that minimize myocardial depression
Hypertrophic	Left ventricular hypertrophy resulting in decreased LV chamber size and LV outflow tract obstruction	Chest pain Shortness of breath Palpitations Rales Systolic murmur (S_3 and S_4) Ventricular dysrhythmias Syncope	Ensure adequate preload Myocardial depression is desirable Maintenance of normal sinus rhythm Avoid tachycardia Ensure adequate depth of anesthesia
Arrhythmogenic right ventricular	Fatty tissue infiltrates; dilation and outflow tract obstruction of the right ventricle	Tachycardia Ventricular dysrhythmias (ventricular tachycardia, ventricular fibrillation) T wave inversion (leads V_1 and V_3) Bundle branch block Hypokinetic right ventricle Decreased right ventricular ejection Jugular venous distention Syncope Peripheral edema	Treat events that cause moderate to severe sympathetic nervous system predominance Monitor and treat hemodynamically compromising ventricular dysrhythmias with amiodarone

JVD, Jugular venous distention; *LV*, left ventricle; *TEE*, transesophageal echocardiography.

septal wall contraction and decreasing CO. Increased blood flow velocity causes a greater degree of systolic anterior motion of the mitral valve's anterior leaflet, creating further obstruction. Decreased preload changes left ventricular geometry and thereby brings the anterior leaflet of the mitral valve into closer proximity to the hypertrophic septum. Increases in left ventricular contractility cause the LV to empty more completely and increase the degree of septal contractility, which results in a greater degree of obstruction.[83] A summary of the signs and symptoms are included in Table 25.11.

In HCM with RV and/or LV outflow tract obstruction, conditions that impair ventricular function under normal physiologic conditions improve cardiac function. This implies that factors that normally impair contractility (e.g., myocardial depression, increased end-diastolic volume, and increased SVR) improve forward flow and diminish the degree of obstruction. Fig. 25.46 illustrates the pathology related to HCM.

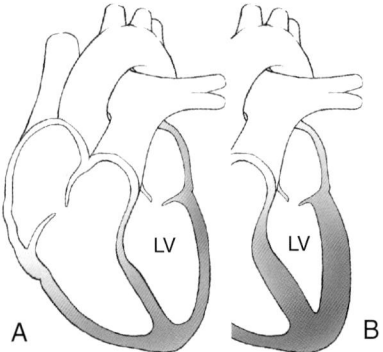

Fig. 25.46 (A) Normal LV outflow tract. (B) Hypertrophic cardiomyopathy with an enlarged interventricular septum and LV wall, a decreased LV chamber size. A further decrease of LV outflow is caused by migration of the anterior mitral leaflet toward the septum. *LV*, Left ventricle.

Anesthetic Considerations

Anesthetic management should focus on strategies that alleviate and avoid increases in LV outflow obstruction. It is imperative that adequate or slightly elevated LV volume be maintained. Measures that decrease venous return and interfere with adequate ventricular preload should be avoided. Factors that increase myocardial contractility should also be avoided. Inadequate depth of anesthesia that causes sympathetic nervous system stimulation may be detrimental. If hypotension occurs, adequate perfusion pressure should be maintained by increasing preload with fluid administration and increasing SVR with phenylephrine.

Pharmacologic therapy used to treat HCM (including β-blockers and calcium channel blockers) should be continued until the time of surgery.[15] β-blockers may be administered intraoperatively to reduce HR and contractility. Dysrhythmias must be avoided and immediately treated if they occur; the atrial contribution to left ventricular volume is necessary to maintain CO.[79,83] Table 25.12 lists hemodynamic goals for patients with HCM.

Anesthetic management must focus on increasing left ventricular preload, decreasing myocardial contractility, controlling HR, and maintaining or increasing afterload. Regional anesthesia is not contraindicated in patients with HCM. Decreases in blood pressure must be treated immediately. Hypovolemia must be avoided and expeditiously treated if it occurs. Deep general anesthesia with an inhalation agent is preferred in patients with HCM.

The potential for hemodynamic deterioration because of increasing subaortic obstruction along with secondary MR necessitates aggressive hemodynamic monitoring. Invasive monitoring via a pulmonary artery catheter allows for maintenance of adequate LVEDV. HCM is associated with reduced diastolic compliance, and therefore PCWP does not accurately correlate directly with LVEDV. The PCWP should be maintained at approximately 18 to 25 mm Hg. If the hemodynamic status deteriorates and exacerbation of outflow obstruction is suspected, β-blocking drugs (propranolol, metoprolol, or esmolol) should be administered. In addition, vasoconstrictors such as phenylephrine should be used to increase SVR.[33]

Dilated Cardiomyopathy

DCM is the most common form of cardiomyopathy, and it most often occurs in adults. As with HCM, there is believed to be a genetic link for those people who develop this cardiac pathology. Between 20% and 30% of DCM cases are caused by an autosomal dominant mutation resulting in abnormal cardiac cytoskeleton protein generation.[88] DCM can also occur in patients as a result of autosomal recessive traits, such as in patients with Duchenne muscular dystrophy. When genetic predisposition is not the cause, the specific etiology has not been definitively determined but is not limited to a viral illness, increased inflammation from metabolic abnormalities, autoimmune mechanism, or toxins. It occurs more often in men than in women and is attributed to being a significant risk factor for developing congestive heart failure. A summary of the pathophysiology, signs and symptoms, and anesthetic considerations is listed in Table 25.11.

Pathophysiology

In DCM, eccentric hypertrophy affects both left and right ventricles. As cardiac cytoskeleton uncoupling occurs, caused by interstitial fibrosis and myocardial cell death, the ventricular chambers increase in size without an associated increase in the diameter of the ventricular walls or interventricular septum. The law of Laplace, as shown in the following equation, helps to describe why the heart becomes an inefficient pump for patients with DCM. Tension on the ventricular walls is increased due to the decreased size and increased diameter of the ventricular walls. When increased ventricular volumes induce

TABLE 25.12 **Hemodynamic Goals for Management of Hypertrophic Cardiomyopathy**

Parameter	Goal
Preload	Increase
Afterload	Increase
Contractility	Decrease
Heart rate	Maintain
Heart rhythm	Normal sinus rhythm

compensatory eccentric hypertrophic changes, impaired systolic function (decreased SV) occurs because of the loss of myocardium causing decreased contractility. Myocardial oxygen consumption is increased as ventricular end-diastolic volume and pressure are increased.

$$T = (P \times R)/M$$

where T is tension, P is pressure, R is radius, and M is wall thickness. This pathologic process does not cause direct damage to the atrioventricular valves. However, as ventricular dilation occurs, changes in ventricular dimensions can cause mitral valve and/or tricuspid valve regurgitation potentially intensifying volume overload, decreased SV, and increased pulmonary congestion.

As the EF decreases, decreased peripheral perfusion causes increased circulating catecholamines, cortisol excretion, and activation of the renin-angiotensin-aldosterone system, which causes vasoconstriction and increased renal absorption of fluid. Left-sided heart failure resulting in pulmonary venous congestion or biventricular failure leads to fulminant congestive heart failure. These patients are at increased risk of thromboembolism as a result of stasis of blood from inadequate ventricular emptying.[89]

Anesthetic Considerations

Pharmacologic medical treatment for patients with DCM includes diuretics, ACE inhibitors, and digoxin. Other interventions for moderate to severe DCM include dual chamber pacing, cardiomyoplasty, or use of a left ventricular assist device. Because of the potential for severely compromised ventricular performance, minimizing myocardial depression is essential. Afterload reduction is important to promote forward blood flow through the heart. As a result, neuraxial anesthesia is an acceptable anesthetic technique for patients with DCM.[90] Narcotics and dexmedetomidine are common choices for patients with cardiomyopathy because these medications do not have a direct effect on myocardial contractility. However, patients with DCM who have a severely compromised EF depend on sympathetic nervous system innervation to augment their cardiac output. Therefore incremental titration of narcotics is warranted. Etomidate is an appropriate choice of induction agent because of the lesser amount of myocardial depression as compared to propofol. All inhalation agents cause myocardial depression in a dose-dependent fashion, thus titration of inhalation agents based on blood pressure, CVP, and PCWP is indicated.[86] Sevoflurane has been safely used in infants with DCM.[91]

Restrictive Cardiomyopathy

RCM represents several types of pathologic conditions depending on whether the myocardium or endomyocardial muscle layer is affected. Causes of myocardial RCM include genetic predisposition (e.g., familial cardiomyopathy), infiltrative disease (e.g., sarcoidosis), storage diseases (e.g., hemochromatosis), and endomyocardial dysfunction (e.g., endomyocardial fibrosis). RCM can occur in the pediatric population; however, it is one of the rarest forms of cardiomyopathy that occurs in children. It is associated with a high mortality rate once symptoms begin to develop.[92] A summary of the pathophysiology, signs and symptoms, and anesthetic considerations is listed in Table 25.11.

Pathophysiology

Infiltration of fibrous tissue and deposition into the myocardium and/or endomyocardium are the pathologic mechanisms by which RCM develops. As a result, one or both ventricles become stiff and noncompliant, which inhibits normal diastolic filling. Because of reduced end-diastolic volume (reduce ventricular preload) caused by restricted ventricular filling, SV is decreased. An increase in the sensitivity of the troponin and tropomyosin complex of calcium-mediated myofilament is thought to be the cause of genetically derived RCM.[93] Systolic ejection remains relatively normal. The atria become dilated as a compensatory response to volume overload, and left- and/or right-sided heart failure can occur. Significantly elevated RA pressures (15–20 mm Hg) and pulmonary artery systolic pressure (as high as 50 mm Hg) can occur as the disease progresses.[94]

Anesthetic Considerations

Medical management for RCM is similar to DCM and includes use of diuretics, sodium and water restriction, anticoagulation agents, and treatment of dysrhythmias. Maintenance of normal sinus rhythm, adequate preload, and minimal myocardial depression are essential to anesthetic management. As with DCM, an anesthetic technique that minimizes myocardial depression, which is accomplished using higher doses of narcotic and/or dexmedetomidine as compared to inhalation agents, may be prudent. Results from studies are often conflicting regarding the degree of myocardial depressant effects of modern inhalation agents (isoflurane, sevoflurane, desflurane) in relation to cardiomyopathy and impaired systolic ejection and diastolic relaxation.[94,95] Patients with moderate to severe cardiomyopathy depend on sympathetic nervous system activity to augment myocardial performance. Despite the minimal direct myocardial depressant effects of narcotics, their inhibition of the sympathetic nervous system has an indirect depressant effect on the heart. Thus titration of narcotics and assessment of the patient's hemodynamic status are important.

Arrhythmogenic Right Ventricular Cardiomyopathy

ARVC, also known as arrhythmogenic right ventricular dysplasia, is an autosomal dominant genetically inherited disorder. Diagnosis is often made postmortem in patients with ARVC because sudden cardiac death is a common occurrence with this cardiomyopathy. Signs and symptoms can occur during childhood, but more often manifest during adolescence. During sports-related exercise, severe intolerance caused by increasing myocardial oxygen demand can result in lightheadedness, syncope, and/or sudden death. A summary of the pathophysiology, signs and symptoms, and anesthetic considerations is listed in Table 25.11.

Pathophysiology

Fibrous fatty infiltrates invade the right ventricular myocardium and cause myocyte dysfunction and death. As a result, right ventricular cardiac output is decreased. The left ventricle undergoes this type of pathologic change in approximately half of patients with ARVC, and congestive heart failure is a sign of disease progression. Ventricular dysrhythmias are common and range from premature ventricular contractions to ventricular fibrillation. Patients with ARVC may be exquisitely sensitive to increased catecholamine levels, which may further provoke these dysrhythmias.[96]

Anesthetic Considerations

Anesthetic management for patients with ARVC should focus on identification and treatment of fatal dysrhythmias. Patients with known ARVC will have an automated implantable cardioverter defibrillator (AICD). Anesthetic concerns for pacemaker and AICD management are discussed in Chapter 27. Also, the preoperative medication regimen will include a combination of antiarrhythmics, β-blockers, and/or calcium channel blockers. Many events increase sympathetic nervous system predominance. Examples include hypoxia, hypotension, hypercarbia, and surgical stimulation. Excessive catecholamine release can induce fatal dysrhythmias. Amiodarone has been used successfully to treat dysrhythmias in these patients. Prophylactic preoperative administration of antiarrhythmic agents has not been shown to be effective at suppressing ventricular dysrhythmias intraoperatively.[80]

Takotsubo Cardiomyopathy

TCM has been described as a transient cardiac syndrome that involves left ventricular apical akinesis. The signs and symptoms mimic acute coronary syndrome. This cardiac phenomenon has also been referred to as stress cardiomyopathy, transient LV ballooning syndrome, apical ballooning syndrome, and broken heart syndrome. It is most likely to occur in postmenopausal women (~90%, mean age 66 years).[97] A patient with TCM often complains of chest pain, develops ST segment elevation on ECG, and has elevated cardiac troponin levels consistent with an acute MI. However, a cardiac angiogram will reveal an absence of significant coronary artery disease and severe left ventricular apical enlargement or ballooning. The Mayo Clinic criteria are the most widely adopted diagnostic guidelines for TCM and include (1) akinesis or dyskinesis of LV wall motion abnormalities (ballooning), (2) chest pain, (3) electrocardiographic changes (ST segment elevation or T wave inversion), (4) absence of obstructive epicardial coronary artery disease, and (5) absence of pheochromocytoma or myocarditis.

The exact mechanism by which TCM occurs has not been determined. Coronary artery vasospasm, altered myocardial fatty acid metabolism, and LV outflow tract obstruction have all been postulated. There has also been discussion of a possible genetic link. However, the leading theory is that elevated endogenous catecholamine concentrations cause myocardial toxicity leading to myocardial inflammation and dysfunction. Myocardial stunning, increased LV afterload, and decreased SV occur. Physiologic or psychological stress appears to be the trigger for the development of TCM.[98] The onset of TCM has occurred during general anesthesia. The causes are multifactorial and involve eliciting physiologic stress and catecholamine release. Some examples include anaphylaxis, local administration of cocaine, and spine surgery.[99-101] Signs can include rapidly occurring LV failure with or without pulmonary edema, MR, ventricular dysrhythmias, thromboembolism, cardiogenic shock, LV wall rupture, and cardiovascular collapse. Echocardiographic characteristics show LV wall motion abnormalities, including hypokinesia, akinesia, and dyskinesia. Systolic function is significantly reduced, with the reported EF ranging from 20% to 49%.[102]

Currently, the treatment for TCM is supportive. The majority of patients who develop TCM regain normal cardiac function within 4 to 8 weeks after onset of symptoms. However, mortality rates for TCM are higher than previously estimated, and long-term mortality exceeds that of patients with ST elevation MI.[103]

SUMMARY

As the population continues to age and the incidence of obesity rises, the prevalence of cardiovascular disease will increase to reflect the progressive nature of its pathology. Anesthesia providers are nonetheless able to safely manage these extremely critical patients with respect to the full spectrum of surgical needs. A thorough knowledge of cardiac physiology and function is imperative to maintaining administration of high-quality anesthesia care. Improved patient outcomes are consistently being achieved as better assessment, monitoring, and anesthesia management techniques are developed.

REFERENCES

For a complete list of references for this chapter, scan this QR code with any smartphone code reader app, or visit the following URL: http://booksite.elsevier.com/9780323711944/.

26

Anesthesia for Cardiac Surgery

Margaret A. Contrera, Jenna Applebee, Lindsay Shockley

Despite advances in prevention and treatment, cardiovascular disease (CVD) remains the leading cause of death globally, accounting for 31% of mortality. The World Health Organization estimates that CVD will remain the predominant cause of mortality, resulting in 23.6 million deaths by 2030, mostly from coronary artery disease (CAD).[1] In the United States, CVD causes 1 of every 3 deaths and 43% are attributed to CAD.[2] Due to the aging population, degenerative valvular heart disease (VHD) is on the rise.[3] There are currently more than 290,000 heart valve operations performed annually worldwide. This number is expected to triple by 2050, reaching 850,000 annually.[4] Both CAD and VHD lead to heart failure, which impacts more than 6.5 million Americans[5] and over 64 million worldwide.[6] The mortality rate for symptomatic patients with heart failure is a staggering 45%, worse than that of most cancers.[7] The Centers for Disease Control and Prevention estimates that $351.2 billion, or $1 of every $7 in health care costs, is spent on treatment for CVD.[2]

Scientific and medical communities, together with governmental agencies, have worked tirelessly to improve this public health burden. Consequently, new knowledge and technologic advancements have led to the development of cardiac procedures that were once inconceivable. Minimally invasive techniques, robotics, hybrid operating rooms (ORs), and mechanical circulatory-assist devices now play significant roles in the practice of cardiothoracic anesthesia. The field has become more diverse, exciting, challenging, and rewarding than ever before.

Caring for these high-risk patients undergoing complicated surgical procedures with complex technology may seem intimidating; however, as Richard Morris, a pioneer in the field of cardiothoracic nurse anesthesia advised, "It's simple really; just take care of the pump, pipes, and volume." Accordingly, the first half of this chapter covers general cardiac surgery beginning with a brief overview of the key physiologic principles that form the foundation of evidence-based anesthetic management strategies. Next, cardiopulmonary bypass (CPB) is discussed, including a description of the circuit components and their physiologic implications. Then, each phase of the perioperative period is examined, and the anesthetic implications are detailed. The second half of the chapter covers anesthetic considerations for specific CVDs and procedures. The pathophysiology of CAD and VHD is briefly reviewed, and the anesthetic management of traditional myocardial revascularization and valvular surgery is described. Next, innovative procedures for the management of atrial fibrillation (AF), the most common irregular heart rhythm, are discussed. New technologic advancements have changed the landscape of cardiac anesthesia. Consequently, the next section is devoted to the management of patients undergoing innovative, minimally invasive cardiac surgery (MICS), including valvular interventions and myocardial revascularization. This is followed by a discussion of the devices and procedures that bring new hope to the management of end-stage heart failure. The

chapter concludes with the anesthetic management of procedures on the ascending aorta and aortic arch, including considerations for deep hypothermic circulatory arrest (DHCA).

ANESTHETIC MANAGEMENT OF GENERAL CARDIAC SURGERY

Key Physiologic Principles

Appropriate management of the cardiac surgical patient begins with a comprehensive understanding of normal cardiac anatomy, physiology, pharmacology, monitoring, and the pathophysiologic response to disease. The reader is advised to review the excellent discussions of these topics found in Chapters 13, 17, 20, and 25 as background for the information presented in this chapter. Certain key physiologic principles apply to most cardiac surgical patients. An imbalance in myocardial oxygen (O_2) supply and demand, often due to CAD, leads to ischemia or infarction. The abnormal pressure and volume loads caused by stenotic and regurgitant valves cause the ventricle to compensate by altering its structure, function, and neurohormonal balance. As a result of these imbalances, the left ventricle (LV) hypertrophies by thickening or dilating. Although each disease starts with a different etiology and pathophysiologic process, with disease progression, the limits of compensation are reached, and severe decompensated heart failure ensues.

Myocardial Oxygen Supply and Demand

Myocardial injury, or infarction, is the most frequent complication following cardiac and major vascular surgery, as well as the primary cause of hospital morbidity and mortality.[8] Undoubtedly, optimizing the balance between myocardial O_2 supply and demand is of paramount importance (Fig. 26.1). Coronary perfusion pressure (CPP) is equal to the aortic diastolic blood pressure (DBP) minus the left ventricular end-diastolic pressure (LVEDP). Actual coronary blood flow is dependent on the CPP divided by the coronary vascular resistance.[9] In a healthy heart, coronary vascular resistance is autoregulated to maintain a constant coronary flow between a mean arterial pressure (MAP) of 60 to 140 mm Hg.[10] The heart alters the coronary vascular resistance based on the local metabolic need of the myocardium. MAP is therefore the most useful measure of coronary perfusion in the clinical setting.[11] However, in patients with CAD, flow is no longer autoregulated beyond partial, calcified obstruction. Instead, coronary perfusion becomes pressure dependent, especially when the MAP drops below 70 mm Hg (Fig. 26.2).[12,13] Total coronary blood flow is determined by the perfusion pressure gradient, the time allotted for flow, coronary anatomy, and coronary vascular resistance. Eighty percent of blood flow to the LV occurs during diastole when the LVEDP is low (Fig. 26.3).[14] Diastolic time progressively shortens as the heart rate increases, resulting in decreased time for coronary

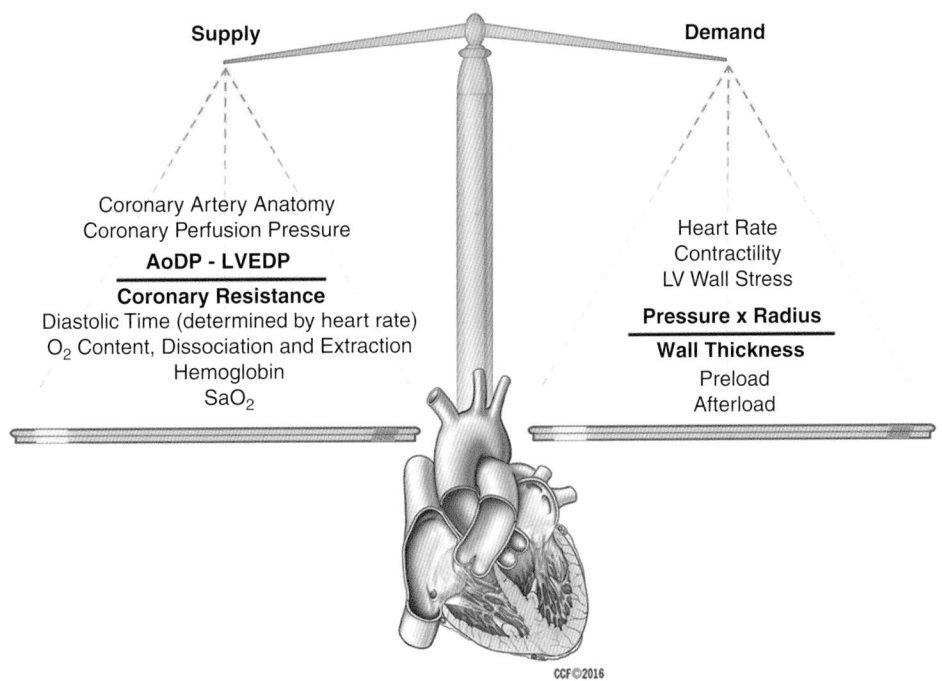

Fig. 26.1 Myocardial oxygen supply and demand balance. Note heart rate and left ventricular pressure affect both supply and demand. *AoDP,* Aortic diastolic pressure; *LV,* left ventricular; *LVEDP,* left ventricular end-diastolic pressure; *O₂,* oxygen; *SaO₂,* arterial oxygen saturation. (Reprinted with permission from Cleveland Clinic Center for Medical Art & Photography ©2020. All rights reserved.)

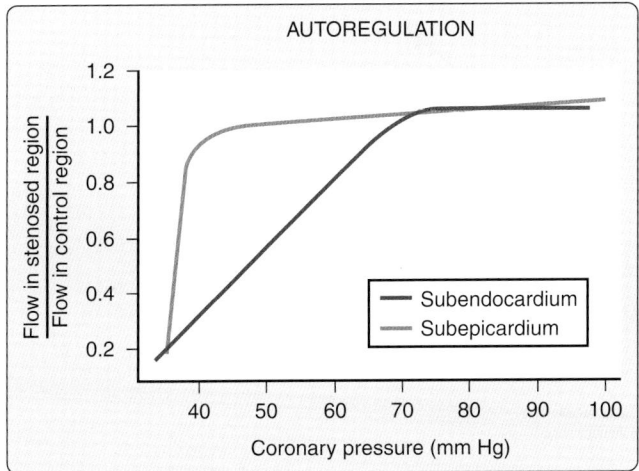

Fig. 26.2 Pressure-flow relations of the subepicardial and subendocardial thirds of the left ventricle in anesthetized dogs. In the subendocardium, autoregulation is exhausted, and flow becomes pressure dependent when pressure distal to a stenosis declines to less than 70 mm Hg. In the subepicardium, autoregulation persists until perfusion pressure declines to less than 40 mm Hg. Autoregulatory coronary reserve is less in the subendocardium. (Redrawn from Guyton RA, et al. Significance of subendocardial ST segment elevation caused by coronary stenosis in the dog. *Am J Cardiol.* 1977;40:373.)

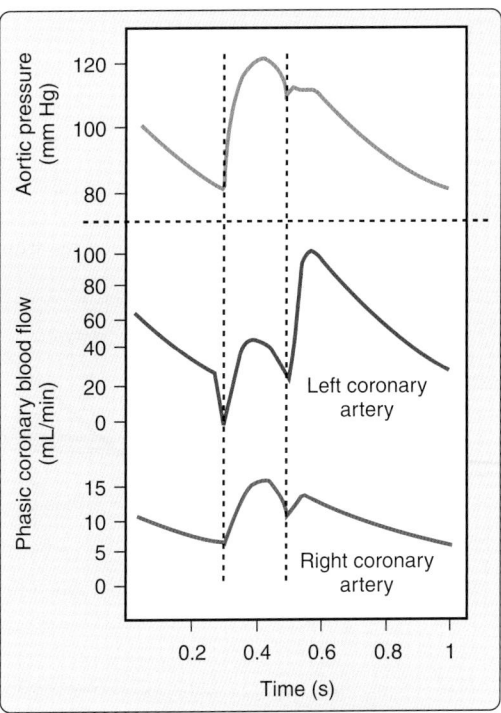

Fig. 26.3 Blood flow in the left and right coronary arteries. The right ventricle is perfused throughout the cardiac cycle. Flow to the left ventricle is largely confined to diastole. (From Pappano AJ. Properties of the vasculature. In Koeppen BM, Stanton BA, eds. *Berne & Levy Physiology.* 7th ed. Philadelphia: Elsevier 2018:369.)

perfusion at higher heart rates. The subendocardium or inner third of the heart muscle is at greatest risk for ischemia because it is exposed to the highest LVEDP, especially at peak systole.[12] Note that elevations in heart rate and LVEDP not only decrease myocardial blood supply but also increase myocardial O₂ demand. An increase in heart rate proportionally increases myocardial O₂ demand and decreases diastolic time.[9] Large epidemiologic studies show that a high heart rate is an independent predictor for cardiac and all-cause morbidity and mortality in men and women with and without CVD.[15] More

recently, intraoperative hypotension has been strongly correlated with myocardial injury after noncardiac surgery.[16-19] Therefore maintaining an adequate MAP and a low heart rate is critical, particularly in patients who have CAD or an elevated LVEDP. The ideal heart rate and BP must be individually determined, but less than 70 beats per

TABLE 26.1 Perioperative Management of Alterations in Myocardial O₂ Balance

Causes of Decreased O₂ Supply	Perioperative Management Strategy
Tachycardia (↓ diastolic time)	Keep heart rate relatively low (<70 bpm); consider β-blockers Deepen anesthesia during stimulating periods
Hypotension	Maintain high normal MAP; consider phenylephrine ↓ anesthetic depth during less stimulating periods and surgical manipulation that causes ↓ MAP
↑ PaEDP	Consider nitroglycerin or diuretic Evaluate LV volume with TEE (PaEDP is increased in patients with concentric LVH and may not reflect LVEDV)
↓ O₂ Content	Maintain SaO₂ at >95%
Anemia	Maintain adequate hemoglobin

Causes of Increased O₂ Demand	Perioperative Management Strategy
SNS stimulation	Maintain adequate depth of anesthesia Anticipate stimulating events and treat preemptively
Tachycardia	Keep heart rate relatively low (<70 bpm); consider β-blockers Deepen anesthesia during stimulating periods
↑ Preload	Consider nitroglycerin or diuretic
↑ Contractility	Consider agents that depress contractility (β-blockers/volatile anesthetics)
↑ Afterload	Avoid hypertension Consider vasodilator

↓, Decrease; ↑, increase; *bpm,* beats per minute; *LV,* left ventricular; *LVEDV,* left ventricular end-diastolic volume; *LVH,* left ventricular hypertrophy; *MAP,* mean arterial pressure; *O₂,* oxygen; *PaEDP,* pulmonary artery end-diastolic pressure; *SaO₂,* saturation of arterial oxygen; *SNS,* sympathetic nervous system; *TEE,* transesophageal echocardiography.

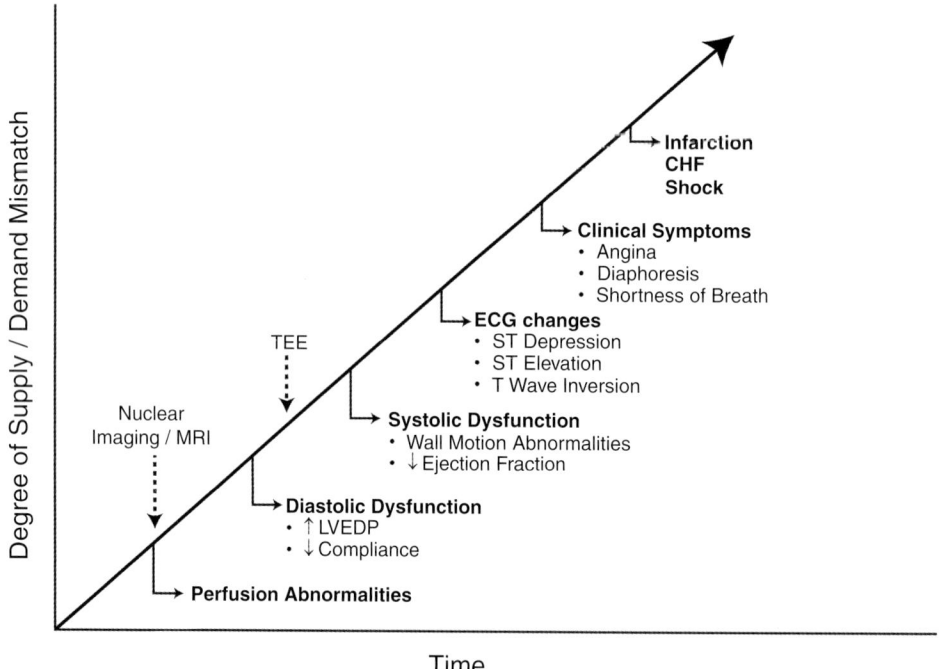

Fig. 26.4 The ischemia cascade. Pathophysiologic sequence of developing myocardial ischemia correlated with timing of detection using various cardiovascular examinations. *CHF,* Congestive heart failure; *ECG,* electrocardiogram; *LVEDP,* left ventricular end-diastolic pressure; *MRI,* magnetic resonance imaging; *TEE,* transesophageal echocardiography. (Reprinted with permission from Cleveland Clinic Center for Medical Art & Photography ©2020. All rights reserved.)

minute (bpm) and a MAP greater than 70 mm Hg are reasonable guides.[20] Patients with a thickened LV, known as concentric left ventricular hypertrophy (LVH), have an elevated LVEDP and are best managed with a higher MAP and lower heart rate. Table 26.1 outlines some of the causes of and treatments for alterations in myocardial O₂ supply and demand.

Ischemia Cascade

Myocardial ischemia leads to a cascade of events (Fig. 26.4).[21,22] It is important to emphasize that diastolic dysfunction precedes systolic dysfunction and that regional wall motion abnormalities occur on echocardiography before changes on the electrocardiogram (ECG). Transesophageal echocardiography (TEE) is the most sensitive intraoperative monitor for detecting myocardial ischemia.[23,24] An imbalance between myocardial O_2 supply and demand will initially induce diastolic dysfunction, making the ventricle stiff and less compliant.[21] Although pulmonary artery end-diastolic pressure (PAEDP) increases, it is not specific for ischemia.[23] Systolic dysfunction causes regional wall motion abnormalities that can be readily detected on TEE. Traditionally, V_5 has been considered the single best ECG lead for detecting myocardial ischemia.[22] More recently Landesberg showed that V_4 and V_3 were more sensitive than V_5 in detecting perioperative ischemia (87%, 79%, and 66%, respectively).[25] Therefore it is important to ensure that the V lead (brown) of the ECG is correctly placed at the fourth intercostal space (ICS) midclavicular line. Automated ST segment analysis is also recommended due to its high sensitivity and specificity for detecting intraoperative ischemia. Three-lead ECG systems are not recommended for monitoring perioperative ischemia.[26]

Stunning, Preconditioning, and Hibernation

When the heart muscle experiences brief periods of ischemia lasting less than 20 minutes, necrosis (cell death) does not occur, but reversible contractile dysfunction, known as stunning, can develop and last for several hours.[27-29] Many cardiac surgery patients require 12 to 24 hours of inotropic support after CPB, often due to stunning.[30,31] Ischemic preconditioning refers to a short period of ischemia improving the heart's ability to tolerate subsequently longer periods of ischemia.[27,32] Multiple animal and clinical studies have demonstrated that all inhalation agents except nitrous oxide produce a preconditioning effect, thereby protecting the myocardium from ischemia and reperfusion injury and reducing infarct size.[33-36] Internationally, there is expert consensus support for the use of inhalation agents except nitrous oxide in hemodynamically stable cardiac surgery patients as a means of reducing myocardial damage and death.[34] Consequently there has been a resurgence of inhalation anesthesia as a primary technique for cardiac surgery, especially in patients with near-normal ventricular function. The role of inhalation agents in unstable patients and those with significant LV dysfunction is less clear, and large, randomized controlled trials in cardiac surgery patients are still needed.

When stable coronary plaques cause chronic reductions in coronary perfusion, steady-state ischemia occurs, which results in left ventricular perfusion-contraction matching, or hibernation. This phenomenon is considered a self-preservation mechanism whereby left ventricular contractile function is reduced to match the amount of O_2 available.[37] Hibernation may also develop following multiple episodes of stunning.[27-29] Patients with hibernating LVs often have significantly improved function following reperfusion with coronary stents or coronary artery bypass grafting.[38-40] Differentiation of ischemic myocardium that is considered "viable or hibernating" (vs necrosed) is important because approximately 20% to 40% of patients with chronically ischemic LV dysfunction will have significant improvement after revascularization.[37,39,41] Nuclear imaging tests (single-photon emission computerized tomography [SPECT]), positron emission tomography (PET), dobutamine stress echocardiography, and cardiac magnetic resonance imaging (CMRI) are used to help determine the presence of stunning and hibernating myocardium to help determine viability.[37] Viability testing is unnecessary in patients with ischemic cardiomyopathy, as ischemia, by definition, indicates viable myocardium.[37] Common cardiovascular tests are outlined in Table 26.2.

Heart Failure

Heart failure is a complex pathophysiologic process that causes a clinical syndrome characterized by pulmonary congestion resulting from the heart's inability to fill with or eject blood in a sufficient quantity to meet tissue requirements.[42] The heart was once thought of as simply the pump of the circulatory system, but it is now known that it evolves into an "endocrine organ" under stress, actively secreting neurohormonal factors to meet the needs of the body. For example, atrial natriuretic peptide (ANP) is released from the atria in response to volume overload. B-type natriuretic peptide (BNP) is released primarily from the ventricles in response to increased wall stress. These peptides help protect the myocardium by inducing physiologic effects such as diuresis, natriuresis, and vasodilation.[43] In fact, BNP has been recognized as a powerful biomarker for diagnosis, determination of severity, and prognostication of heart failure.[44,45] Heart failure is caused by an insult that alters perfusion and leads to a state of neurohumoral imbalance. Activation of the sympathetic nervous system (SNS) and the renin-angiotensin-aldosterone system induce a host of pathologic responses. Many patients with heart failure will receive multimodal drug therapy aimed at interrupting these responses and slowing disease progression (Fig. 26.5).[43,46] The New York Heart Association (NYHA) functional classes of heart failure have prognostic significance and predict quality of life, whereas the American Heart Association (AHA) and American College of Cardiology (ACC) stages of heart failure emphasize disease progression (Table 26.3).

Left ventricular failure and remodeling. Sympathetic activation, coupled with alterations in perfusion, pressure, and volume, cause the heart to change its size, shape, and function; remodeling itself is an attempt to maintain cardiac output (CO). When the coronary flow is reduced to the point that the supply is no longer adequate to meet the metabolic demands of the myocardium, supply ischemia occurs causing an increase in ventricular compliance (dilation) and a decrease in contractility. When the metabolic demands of myocardial muscle exceed supply, demand ischemia occurs causing reduced compliance (stiffening) without initially impacting contractility.[47,48] The primary characteristics of remodeling are hypertrophy (dilation or thickening), myocyte death, and increased interstitial fibrosis. The clinical impact manifests as a change in systolic and diastolic function. Figs. 26.6 and 26.7 help summarize and visualize the process.

Systolic dysfunction. As demonstrated in Fig. 26.7C, supply ischemia resulting from MI or chronic volume overload of the LV causes eccentric hypertrophy or dilation. The chamber size increases in an attempt to preserve stroke volume (SV). In the dilated state, the heart loses its normal elliptic football shape and becomes more spheric, resembling a basketball.[49] In this shape, the heart cannot contract effectively (systolic dysfunction), and the mitral apparatus is stretched potentially to the point that results in mitral regurgitation (MR). Of patients with heart failure, 39% to 74% will experience MR.[50] The degree of systolic dysfunction is commonly expressed as an ejection fraction (EF). The EF is calculated as SV divided by end-diastolic volume (EDV). According to the American Society of Echocardiography guidelines, a normal EF is 52% to 72% in males and 54% to 74% in females. Dysfunction is graded as mild (41%–51% in males and 41%–53% in females), moderate (30%–40% in both genders), or severe (<30% in both genders).[51] When SV is reduced, the body compensates by activating the SNS to raise the resting heart rate to maintain CO.[52] Systolic heart failure (SHF) is caused by CAD, dilated cardiomyopathy, chronic volume overload (regurgitant valves, high output failure), and advanced stages associated with chronic pressure overload (AS, chronic hypertension). Myocardial infarction (MI) causes regional defects that can eventually encompass the entire myocardium, whereas other causes of heart failure typically reduce global function from the onset.[43] As shown in Fig. 26.6, SHF is associated with a volume overload of the LV that is managed using multiple drug therapies (see Fig. 26.5).

Diastolic dysfunction. Pulmonary congestion and the symptoms of heart failure can develop with a normal or near-normal EF. Diastolic

TABLE 26.2   Significant Findings on Cardiac Preoperative Testing

Diagnostic Tool	Significant Findings/Test Descriptions
Electrocardiogram or Ambulatory Electrocardiogram	ST-T wave changes, significant Q waves, new BBB If recent ACS: STEMI vs NSTEMI vs unstable angina Significant arrhythmia or conduction block BBB (concern if placing PAC) Ventricular hypertrophy Axis deviation Presence of pacemaker
Chest X-ray	Cardiomegaly Pulmonary vascular congestion/pulmonary edema Pleural effusion Presence of pacemaker or ICD
Exercise Stress Test	Level and severity of ischemic changes, leads involved Patient symptoms Maximum heart rate ≤85% of predicted
Pharmacologic Stress Test	Identification of viable vs nonviable myocardium Adenosine and dipyridamole cause vasodilation in normal coronaries leading to steal or supply ischemia in areas with CAD Dobutamine (β_1-agonist) ↑ HR and contractility inducing demand ischemia; also used for stress echocardiogram
Nuclear Imaging	Radionuclides with varying tracer actions and kinetics are used to evaluate myocardial perfusion and function
SPECT	Viable myocardium vs fixed defects (scar) Two sets of images are obtained: after stress and after rest Defects that are initially seen (ischemic area) and fill later indicate viable myocardium, whereas fixed defects indicate scar
PET	Ischemic areas of viable myocardium Ischemia shifts metabolism from fatty acids to glucose An isotope is given that attaches to glucose The scan can show flow as well as identify areas of uptake; uptake indicates ischemic areas and viable myocardium
Stress Echo (Exercise or Dobutamine)	New wall motion abnormalities Segments with new wall motion abnormalities during stress are considered ischemic and therefore viable myocardium
Cardiac Magnetic Resonance Imaging (CMR)	Global LV dysfunction and regional wall motion abnormalities Viability assessed using LV end-diastolic wall thickness or response to dobutamine as with dobutamine stress-echo
Coronary Computed Tomography Angiogram (CTA)	Identification of plaques in coronaries and aorta
Cardiac Catheterization	LVEDP Cardiac index Presence of left main, triple vessel disease, or equivalent Quality of targets Type and timing of PCI Type, location, and timing of coronary stents Presence of pulmonary hypertension

↑, Increase; *ACS*, acute coronary syndrome; *BBB*, bundle branch block; *CAD*, coronary artery disease; *CT*, computed tomography; *HR*, heart rate; *ICD*, implantable cardioverter defibrillator; *LV*, left ventricle; *LVEDP*, left ventricular end-diastolic pressure; *LVH*, left ventricular hypertrophy; *NSTEMI*, non-ST elevation myocardial infarction; *PAC*, pulmonary artery catheter; *PCI*, percutaneous coronary intervention; *PET*, positron emission tomography; *RV*, right ventricle; *SPECT*, single-photon emission computed tomography; *STEMI*, ST elevation myocardial infarction.

heart failure (DHF), which is more appropriately termed heart failure with preserved EF, is the most common type of heart failure in women and the elderly (see Fig. 26.6).[53] Demand ischemia, resulting from chronic pressure overload secondary to stenotic heart valves, obstructive cardiomyopathy, chronic hypertension, pulmonary disease, obstructive sleep apnea, or obesity, causes the myocardium to thicken (concentric hypertrophy) and compliance to decrease (see Fig. 26.7B).[43] In response to a fibrotic and noncompliant LV, filling is inadequate and LVEDP is increased, leading to pulmonary congestion despite near-normal systolic function. Diastolic failure is graded from class I to

IV based on echocardiographic examination findings.[51] The LV with concentric hypertrophy is prone to ischemia; therefore maintaining a high MAP and slow normal heart rate is crucial.[54] Hypotension should be treated promptly, usually with phenylephrine, to avoid rapid decompensation, potentially leading to cardiac arrest. If the patient arrests, chest compressions rarely generate enough pressure to perfuse the hypertrophied, noncompliant LV. The mortality and hospitalization rates are similar in both systolic and diastolic failure.[43,54] Table 26.4 compares the characteristics of patients with systolic and diastolic failure, and Table 26.5 outlines the anesthetic management strategies

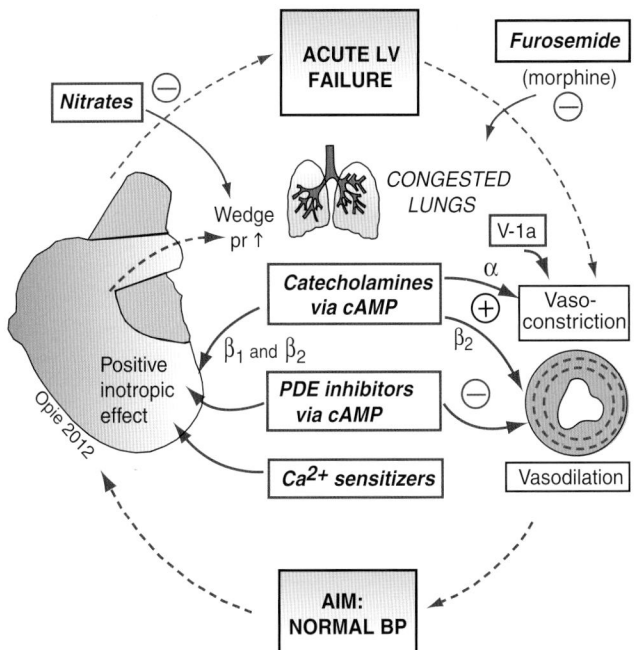

Fig. 26.5 Sites of action of drugs used for acute left ventricular *(LV)* failure. Note opposing effects of (1) vasoconstriction resulting from α-adrenergic effects (norepinephrine, high doses of epinephrine or dopamine), and (2) vasodilation resulting from vascular cyclic adenosine monophosphate *(cAMP)* elevation from β_2 effects or phosphodiesterase *(PDE)* inhibition. *alpha,* α-adrenergic; *BP,* blood pressure; *pr,* pressure; *V-1a,* vasopressin agonist action on receptor subtype 1a. (Figure © L.H. Opie, 2012. In Opie LH, Gersh BJ. *Drugs for the Heart.* 8th ed. Philadelphia: Elsevier; 2013:172.)

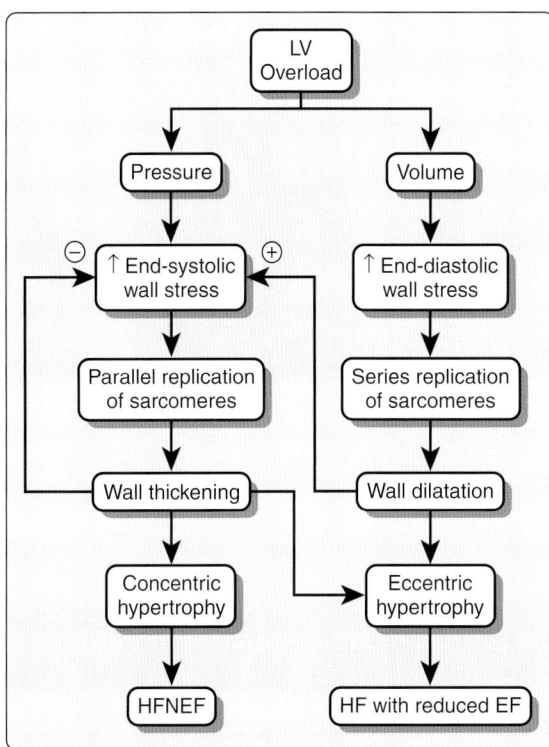

Fig. 26.6 Left ventricular *(LV)* pressure and volume overload produce compensatory responses based on the nature of the inciting stress. Wall thickening reduces (−) and chamber dilation increases (+) end-systolic wall stress, as predicted by Laplace's law. LV pressure-overload hypertrophy has been linked to heart failure with normal ejection fraction *(HFNEF),* but LV volume overload most often causes heart failure *(HF)* with reduced ejection fraction *(EF).* (From Pagel PS, Freed JK. Cardiac physiology. In Kaplan JA, et al., eds. *Kaplan's Cardiac Anesthesia: For Cardiac and Noncardiac Surgery.* 7th ed. Philadelphia: Elsevier; 2017:160.)

TABLE 26.3 Comparison of the Primary Heart Failure Classifications

ACC/AHA HF Stage	NYHA Functional Class
A—At high risk for HF but without structural heart disease or symptoms	None
B—Structural heart disease without symptoms	I—Asymptomatic
C—Structural heart disease with prior or current symptoms	II—Symptoms with moderate exertion III—Symptoms with minimal exertion
D—Refractory heart failure requiring specialized interventions	IV—Symptoms at rest

ACC, American College of Cardiology; *AHA,* American Heart Association; *HF,* heart failure; *NYHA,* New York Heart Association.
Adapted from Popescue WM. Heart failure and cardiomyopathies. In Hines RL, Marschall KE, eds. *Anesthesia and Co-Existing Diseases.* 6th ed. Philadelphia: Elsevier; 2012.

for systolic and diastolic dysfunction. Often, as DHF progresses, SHF will develop, resulting in a further decrease in SV.[43]

Right ventricular failure. Right heart failure (RHF) is most often the result of left heart failure, but it can also be caused by pulmonary hypertension (PHTN) or a right-sided MI. RHF causes systemic venous congestion, hepatomegaly, and peripheral edema.[43] Management of RHF can be more difficult than left-sided failure because fewer options exist for unloading and supporting the right ventricle (RV). The goal of managing RHF is to improve perfusion and contractility

while reducing the right heart afterload. Therefore conditions or medications that increase right heart afterload, decrease right heart contractility, increase pulmonary pressures, or exacerbate preexisting PHTN should be avoided. Typically, management includes avoiding hypercarbia, hypoxemia, acidosis, nitrous oxide (N_2O), desflurane, and the Trendelenburg position.[43] Perioperative management of RHF and PHTN requires careful titration of perioperative fluids and possibly administration of diuretics or venodilators such as nitroglycerin. Normally, the right heart is perfused throughout the cardiac cycle (see Fig. 26.3); however, when the RV is distended, coronary perfusion occurs primarily during diastole, as it does in the LV.[47] It is therefore critical to maintain the mean and diastolic perfusion pressures. In cases of hypotension, a drug with combined inotropic and vasopressor properties such as ephedrine or epinephrine is preferred.[55] Arginine vasopressin causes peripheral vasoconstriction with less increase in pulmonary vascular resistance. Milrinone, an inotrope and vasodilator, is also useful in the management of RHF and PHTN. In severe acute cases, pulmonary vasodilators, including inhaled epoprostenol (Flolan or Veletri), may prove beneficial.[56,57] Mechanical support in heart failure will be discussed later in the chapter.

Cardiopulmonary Bypass

Principles

Most cardiac surgeries must be accomplished with the aid of CPB. The machine is operated by a perfusionist, but it is imperative that

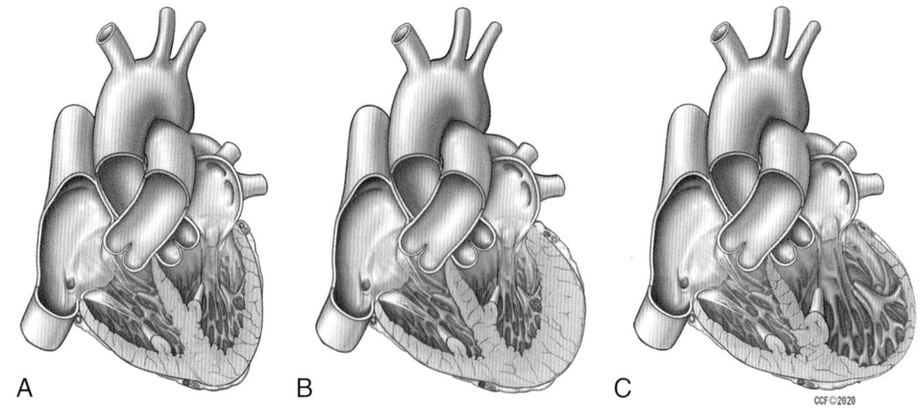

Fig. 26.7 Ventricular remodeling is a compensatory mechanism in response to abnormal pressure and volume loads. (A) Normal heart. (B) Concentric left ventricular hypertropy (LVH) in response to a pressure overload leads to diastolic failure. (C) Eccentric LVH in response to a volume overload or myocardial infarction leads to systolic failure. (Reprinted with permission from Cleveland Clinic Center for Medical Art & Photography ©2020. All rights reserved.)

TABLE 26.4 Characteristics of Patients With Diastolic and Systolic Heart Failure

Characteristic	Diastolic HF	Systolic HF
Age	Often in the elderly	Usually 50–70 yr
Gender	Often in females	Often in males
LV EF	Preserved, ≥40%	Depressed, ≤40%
LV cavity size	Normal with concentric LVH	Dilated with eccentric LVH
Chest x-ray	Congestion and/or cardiomegaly	Congestion and cardiomegaly
HTN	+++	++
DM	+++	++
Previous MI	+	+++
Obesity	+++	+
COPD	++	0
Sleep apnea	++	++
Dialysis	++	0
Atrial fibrillation	+ Usually paroxysmal	+ Usually persistent
Gallop rhythm	Fourth heart sound	Third heart sound

+, Occasionally associated with; ++, often associated with; +++, usually associated with; 0, no association; *COPD,* chronic obstructive pulmonary disease; *DM,* diabetes mellitus; *EF,* ejection fraction; *HF,* heart failure; *HTN,* hypertension; *LV,* left ventricle; *LVH,* left ventricular hypertrophy; *MI,* myocardial infarction.
Adapted from Popescue WM. Heart failure and cardiomyopathies. In Hines RA, Marschall KE, eds. *Stoelting's Anesthesia and Co-Existing Diseases.* 6th ed. Philadelphia: Elsevier; 2012.

TABLE 26.5 Anesthetic Considerations for Systolic and Diastolic Dysfunction

	Systolic Dysfunction	Diastolic Dysfunction
Preload	Already ↑, avoid overload, especially coming off pump NTG helps reduce preload and ↑ subendocardial perfusion	Volume will be needed to stretch noncompliant LV Evaluate with TEE as PaEDP ↑ and may not reflect LVEDV
Contractility	Reduced, avoid agents that cause further reductions May need inotropic support	Usually good, but caution with agents that depress function
Compliance	Increased in an effort to preserve SV	Reduced, NTG may help stiff LV relax
Afterload	Reductions will enhance forward flow as long as coronary perfusion pressure maintained SNP works well if volume is adequate	Already ↑ Higher MAP needed to perfuse thick myocardium Treat hypotension aggressively with phenylephrine
Heart rate	Usually high normal due to sympathetic activation	Slow normal to maximize diastolic time for coronary perfusion and ↓ MVO₂ Prone to ischemia Maintain SR; dependent on atrial kick (cardiovert early)
CPB	Expect large pump volumes Consider ultrafiltration, diuretic	Pump volume normal

↓, Decreased; ↑, increased; *CPB,* cardiopulmonary bypass; *LV,* left ventricle; *LVEDV,* left ventricular end-diastolic volume; *MAP,* mean arterial pressure; *MVO₂,* myocardial oxygen consumption; *NTG,* nitroglycerin; *PaEDP,* pulmonary artery end-diastolic pressure; *SNP,* sodium nitroprusside; *SR,* sinus rhythm; *SV,* stroke volume; *TEE,* transesophageal echocardiography.

the anesthetist have a clear understanding of the components and physiologic impact of CPB. The purpose of CPB is to provide a motionless, bloodless heart for the surgical procedure. This goal is achieved by temporarily diverting nearly all venous blood away from the heart and lungs to an extracorporeal circulation apparatus that adds oxygen (O_2), removes carbon dioxide (CO_2), and then filters the blood before returning it to the body.[58] The CPB circuit is continuous with the systemic circulation and provides artificial ventilation, perfusion, and temperature regulation. The heart is intermittently perfused and cooled with a chemical solution, called cardioplegia, to halt electrical activity and protect myocardial

tissue. Although the goal is to provide near-physiologic hemodynamics and acid-base balance, the technique is nonphysiologic; it incites a host of inflammatory responses, as well as platelet dysfunction and coagulopathy when the patient's blood is exposed to nonendothelial surfaces.[59]

Basic Circuit

The CPB machine consists of five basic components: a venous reservoir, the main pump, an oxygenator, a heat exchanger, and an arterial filter (Fig. 26.8). A simplified explanation of CPB is as follows: Venous (deoxygenated) blood is drained from the right side of the heart via a cannula in the atrium and vena cava, then carried by tubing to a reservoir; the main pump (centrifugal or roller) then propels the blood to an oxygenator and a heat exchanger; finally, the oxygenated blood passes through an arterial line filter before returning to the arterial circulation via a cannula in the ascending aorta to perfuse the rest of the body.[60] The modern bypass machine also performs several other functions, including delivering cardioplegia using accessory roller pumps. Suction devices are also used to vent the heart and aorta and salvage blood from the surgical field.[61]

Venous cannulas. The CPB circuit includes cannulas and tubing made of medical-grade polyvinyl chloride with a biocompatible coating to decrease the inflammatory response associated with CPB and to preserve blood components.[60] One-, two-, or multistage (meaning more than one hole to drain the blood) venous cannulas are used to remove the deoxygenated blood from the heart. A large-bore two-stage or multistage venous cannula that drains blood from both the right atrium (RA) and the inferior vena cava (IVC) is most often used for coronary artery bypass graft (CABG), aortic valve (AV), and septal myectomy procedures in which the heart remains closed and small amounts of retained blood will not interfere with the surgery (Fig. 26.9A). Open-cavity procedures such as mitral, pulmonic, and tricuspid valve surgery, or procedures that repair defects such as atrial septal defects (ASDs), patent foramen ovale (PFO) defects, or ventricular septal defects require a bloodless field. For such procedures, a technique known as bicaval or two-vessel cannulation is used: Two separate single-stage venous cannulas are individually inserted into the superior and inferior vena cava, and the vessels are snared with elastic loops to prevent systemic venous blood from entering the heart (see Fig. 26.9B).[55,61] A venous cannula may also be placed in the femoral vein for MICS, or in reoperations where the patient may need to go on bypass while the chest is opened before central access can be obtained.[62,63]

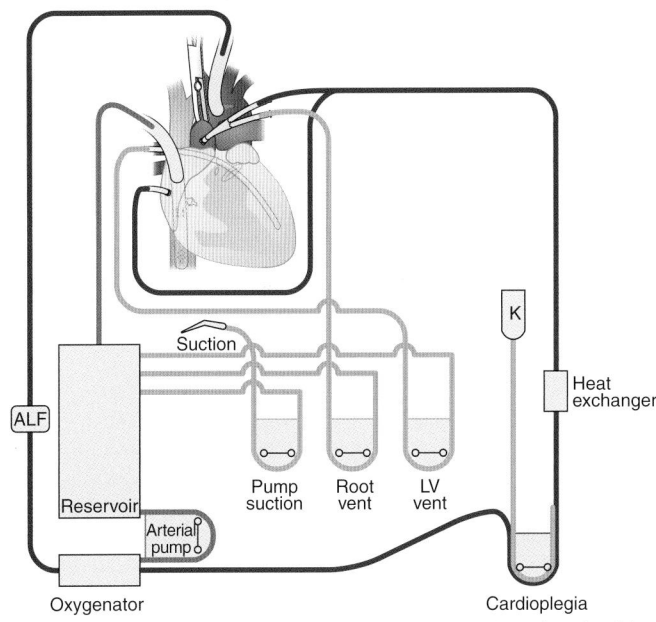

Fig. 26.8 A typical cardiopulmonary bypass circuit interfaced with a patient. *ALF,* Arterial line filter; *K,* potassium; *LV,* left ventricular. (From Miller RD. *Miller's Anesthesia.* 8th ed. Philadelphia: Elsevier; 2015:2032.)

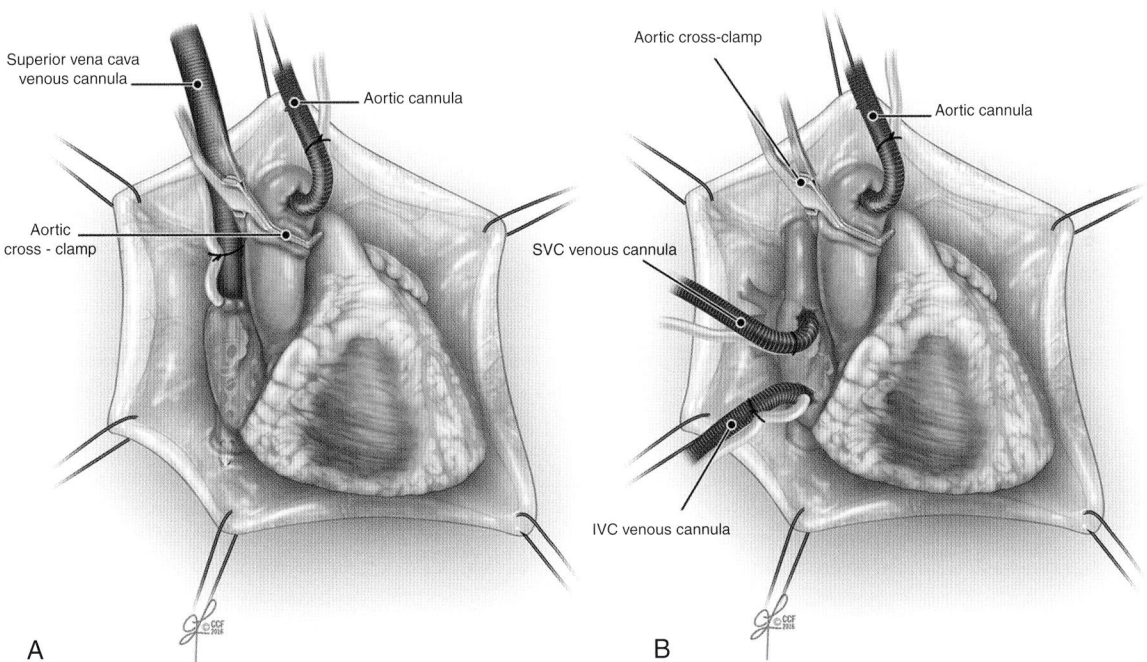

Fig. 26.9 (A) Aortic arterial cannula and single, multistaged, right atrial venous cannula. Notice the drainage holes of the venous cannula in the right atrium and inferior vena cava. Note the position of the aortic cross-clamp. (B) Aortic arterial cannulation and bicaval venous cannulas. Two separate single-stage venous cannulas are individually inserted into both the superior and inferior vena cava for most open cavity procedures. (Reprinted with permission, Cleveland Clinic Center for Medical Art & Photography ©2021. All rights reserved.)

Prime. Prime is the fluid used to fill the CPB circuit and components. It is composed of an isotonic electrolyte solution, such as lactated Ringer, Plasmalyte-A, or Normosol-R, that closely matches the principal ionic composition of blood.[64] Traditionally, the volume of the prime used to fill the CPB circuit is 1 to 2 L. Medications and other solutions are often added to the prime for a variety of purposes: colloid to decrease postoperative edema, blood to treat anemia, mannitol to promote diuresis, heparin to ensure adequate anticoagulation, and bicarbonate to treat acidosis.[65,66] Upon instituting CPB, the prime added to the circulating blood volume causes dilutional anemia, often resulting in decreased hematocrit (22%–25%).[67] The dilution is beneficial to offset some of the increase in blood viscosity that occurs when blood cools during CPB.[61]

Venous reservoir. The venous reservoir is hard or soft shelled and divided into two compartments: one for the venous drainage from the heart and the other for the blood suctioned or vented directly from the surgical field. This portion of the reservoir, referred to as the cardiotomy, is discussed in detail later.[61] Traditionally, blood drains from the patient to the reservoir by gravity; the rate is determined by the size and placement of the cannulas, the height of the bed, and the patient's intravascular volume status. With the introduction of minimally invasive techniques, gravity drainage proved inadequate due to the small size of the cannulas and tubing. Subsequently, the practice of vacuum-assisted venous drainage (VAVD) was established and is now used in both traditional surgery and MICS.[68] A vacuum regulator is added to the venous reservoir with a piece of Y tubing, and a pressure of approximately −40 mm Hg is applied. This Y tubing is used to turn on the suction or open the system to atmospheric pressure. Improved drainage can facilitate surgical exposure and decrease the necessity of adding more crystalloid and/or blood to the CPB circuit. The inherent risks include hemolysis of blood cells and air embolism. VAVD at a suction of −40 mm Hg causes less hemolysis than when the suction is increased to −80 mm Hg.[68] It is critical that the fluid level in the venous reservoir be kept sufficiently high to prevent air entrainment from the main pump, which can result in an air embolism. An alarm is incorporated into the venous reservoir to alert the perfusionist if the fluid level drops below a specified level.

Main pump. Blood is propelled through the CPB circuit by an electric pump (see Fig. 26.8). Two types of pumps are available. (1) A roller pump produces flow by subtotally compressing large-bore tubing against a tract and propelling the blood forward. Constant nonpulsatile flow is produced that is directly proportional to the number of revolutions per minute of the roller heads, regardless of arterial resistance in the circuit.[60] (2) A centrifugal pump uses a magnetically controlled impeller that rotates rapidly, creating a pressure drop that causes blood to be sucked into the housing and ejected. A major difference between the two pumps is that the flow from the centrifugal pump will vary with changes in preload and afterload. For this reason, a flowmeter must be attached to the arterial side of the pump. While the roller pump is economical and simple to use, it has the disadvantage of increased destruction of blood elements. As a result, centrifugal pumps are replacing roller head pumps in contemporary practice.[60] In the event of a power failure, a hand crank can be used to manually operate either pump.

Oxygenator. The oxygenator performs the functions of oxygenating venous blood and removing CO_2 (see Fig. 26.8). Historically, bubble oxygenators were used, but today only membrane oxygenators are in use.[60] The membrane oxygenator is a coated bundle of hollow microporous polypropylene fibers that are tightly wound to create a large surface area. Blood flows around the tightly packed fibers, and gas flows through the fibers. The gas, consisting of O_2 or a mixture of O_2 and medical-grade air, diffuses passively across the membrane and into

the blood. The O_2 level in the blood can be controlled by changing the O_2 concentration, and the amount of CO_2 removed from the blood is controlled by changing the liter gas flow rate or "sweep" of gas through the oxygenator. An inhalation anesthetic agent can also be added to the fresh gas inlet that enters the oxygenator to maintain appropriate blood concentration and depth of anesthesia while on CPB.[61]

Heat exchanger. The blood enters a heat exchanger either separately or in combination with the oxygenator (see Fig. 26.8). The heat exchanger is usually made of stainless-steel tubes with heated or cooled water flowing through them. Blood flows around the tubes, and the temperature is adjusted to the desired level.[61] Traditionally, patients were cooled to protect the heart and other vital organs during CPB. Today, active cooling is less common, and the patient's temperature is allowed to naturally drop or drift while the surgery is performed. The patient is then actively rewarmed in preparation for the termination of CPB. For some procedures, the patient is actively cooled to decrease the metabolic rate and thus oxygen consumption. This process is discussed later in the chapter (see "Surgery on the Ascending Aorta and Aortic Arch"). As the patient is rewarmed, gas solubility decreases, and air bubbles can form in the CPB circuit. Consequently, the oxygenated blood passes through a filter before it is returned to the patient.[58]

Arterial filter. The final phase of the CPB circuit requires the blood to pass through an arterial filter before returning to the arterial cannula and the rest of the body (see Fig. 26.8). The arterial filter acts as an air bubble trap and particulate filter, ideally preventing thrombi, fat globules, calcium, and tissue debris from entering the circulation. While the arterial filter used to be a separate feature, it is now commonly integrated into the oxygenator to prevent microbubbles from continuing in the circuit.[64,69] The blood is then returned to the body via the arterial cannula, which is most often placed in the ascending aorta, but alternate sites include the femoral, subclavian, or axillary artery often with a side graft.

Accessory pumps and devices

Cardiotomy and basket suction. As illustrated in Fig. 26.8, the perfusionist also operates several accessory roller pumps used to control suction devices and deliver cardioplegia. A common suction device is a Yankauer, or handheld suction tip, used to aspirate blood from the surgical field. Another type of suction device is the basket, which consists of a metal tip cylindric device with multiple holes for suctioning that can be placed in an open cardiac cavity to help drain accumulating blood (see Fig. 26.8). This shed blood can be returned to the patient in one of two ways. First, the blood can be returned to a portion of the venous reservoir (cardiotomy), which has a separate integrated filter that defoams the blood and removes air and debris that are picked up by the suction tip (pump sucker) used in the surgical field or by the vents used to drain the heart.[70] Blood returned via the cardiotomy may contain fat, bone, and other debris. Some surgeons believe that the blood suctioned by the Yankauer cannot be adequately filtered, so they choose to send this shed blood to a cell-saver device that will centrifuge and wash the blood. When the Yankauer suction is used to return blood to the cardiotomy, it is commonly referred to as the pump sucker. The disadvantage of diverting blood to the cell-saver device is that the volume of blood available for CPB is reduced, especially if there is significant bleeding. If this occurs, the cell-saver blood can be washed and the red cells returned to the venous reservoir, but plasma and platelets are removed; the process requires time. Research shows that systemic inflammatory markers are lower when no shed blood is returned to the patient undergoing CPB, and blood returned from cell-saver suction generates less inflammatory mediators than that of the pump sucker.[70] It is important to note that the pump sucker cannot be used until the patient is heparinized, therefore blood suctioned by the Yankauer is returned to the cell-saver in the beginning of the case before the patient is heparinized.

Left ventricular vent. The LV vent, if used, is a catheter placed in the left ventricle through the right superior pulmonary vein to drain blood that has accumulated in the cavity (see Fig. 26.8). Although the majority of blood is diverted from the heart during CPB, small amounts of blood may enter the LV from the bronchial arteries (which arise directly from the aorta or the intercostal arteries) or the thebesian vessels (coronary veins that drain directly into the heart). Blood and cardioplegia can also fill the LV if the patient has aortic valve insufficiency (AI; also known as aortic regurgitation [AR]). This volume can cause the LV to distend, raise LVEDP, and compromise preservation by opposing the cardioplegia flow into the coronary arteries.[59] The vented blood returns to the cardiotomy portion of the venous reservoir.

Cardioplegia pump. The perfusionist controls the infusion of cardioplegia using an accessory roller pump (see Fig. 26.8). A separate heat exchanger is utilized to regulate temperature, rate, and the pressure of cardioplegia administration.[61] Cardioplegia is further discussed under myocardial preservation.

Anticoagulation

Systemic anticoagulation is essential before cannulation and initiation of CPB. The absence of proper anticoagulation causes blood clots to form in the pump, leading to serious neurologic injury or death. Heparin is the preferred anticoagulant for cardiac surgery. Heparin binds to antithrombin III (AT III) and increases its action by 1000-fold. AT III inhibits the procoagulant thrombin and activated factor X (factor Xa).[71] The standard cardiac dosage of heparin is 400 units/kg, preferably administered through a central venous line.[72] Adequate anticoagulation is measured with point-of-care (POC) testing that includes activated clotting times (ACT) or heparin concentration assays (Hepcon). A baseline ACT is obtained before heparin administration; a normal value is approximately 80 to 120 seconds. The ACT is then measured 3 to 5 minutes after heparin administration. Historically, ACTs as low as 300 to 400 seconds were considered satisfactory, but current guidelines recommend an ACT of at least 480 seconds before CPB initiation to ensure proper anticoagulation.[61,72] A heparin concentration monitor, such as Hepcon HMS Plus (Medtronic, Inc., Minneapolis, MN, USA), can be used in place of, or in addition to, the ACT measure. The Hepcon generates a heparin dose-response (HDR) curve that is then used to calculate the most appropriate dose of heparin, maintain an adequate level of anticoagulation during bypass, and determine the amount of protamine needed to reverse the heparin after bypass. The level of anticoagulation should be checked every 20 to 30 minutes during bypass so that more heparin can be administered as needed.[73]

Patients who have been recently exposed to heparin may become "heparin resistant" and require higher doses of heparin to obtain therapeutic anticoagulation. Heparin resistance is defined as an ACT less than 480 seconds despite administration of 600 units/kg of intravenous (IV) heparin. AT III deficiency should be suspected if the patient does not become anticoagulated with additional heparin administration. AT III deficiency can be treated empirically with two units of fresh frozen plasma (FFP), AT III concentrate, or recombinant AT III. Recombinant AT III is effective in reducing heparin resistance by increasing circulating AT III without exposing patients to FFP.[74]

Heparin-induced thrombocytopenia (HIT) is an immune reaction that occurs as a direct consequence of exposure to heparin. A comprehensive review of this disorder is found in Chapter 38. For patients with a history of HIT, but a negative HIT antibody screen at the time of cardiac surgery, the American College of Chest Surgeons guidelines recommend the use of heparin only during CPB.[74] There is a decreased risk of a patient receiving a second diagnosis with HIT if the prior diagnosis occurred more than 3 months before the scheduled cardiac surgery. In patients with a positive HIT antibody screen, the use of an anticoagulant other than heparin is recommended in the preoperative and postoperative periods. In all cases, there should be no heparin added to the flush solution or heparin lock IV ports, and heparin-bonded catheters are avoided. Surgery should be postponed, if feasible, in patients with acute HIT and those who are antibody positive (subacute HIT). If urgent surgery is required, the use of bivalirudin is suggested over other nonheparin anticoagulants.[71,75]

Myocardial Preservation

Mild to moderate systemic hypothermia and cold cardioplegia are used for myocardial preservation. The patient can be actively cooled by the CPB circuit, or the patient's temperature can be allowed to drift toward the ambient room temperature. Some surgeons cool the heart topically by packing icy slush around it. The goal is to achieve hypothermic, diastolic cardiac arrest to decrease the metabolic rate, O_2 consumption, and excitatory neurotransmitter release, and to preserve high-energy phosphate substrates.[59]

A hyperkalemic crystalloid solution mixed with blood is the most commonly used cardioplegia solution today. The ratio of the mix varies but is most often a 4:1 blood to crystalloid solution (e.g., Buckberg solution). The exact composition of the cardioplegia solution is institution driven, but the first dose (induction dose) is cold (2°C–5°C) and contains 20 to 30 mEq/L of potassium. Maintenance doses are also cold and contain 12 to 16 mEq/L of potassium. The goal is to maintain a myocardial temperature between 8°C and 10°C.[58] An alternative, del Nido cardioplegia solution, originally used in pediatric heart surgery, has gained popularity in adult cardiac surgery. It consists of a 1:4 blood to a nonglucose-based crystalloid solution that is delivered as a single dose lasting up to 180 minutes. It has been used effectively and safely in adult isolated valve surgery and is associated with lower insulin requirements as well as potential time and cost savings.[76] Whole blood microplegia is a third option, which uses concentrated additives, similar to those used in del Nido, mixed with blood to cause asystole. This whole blood formulation provides adequate myocardial protection with the benefit of decreased hemodilution, due to the removal of the crystalloid component. It also provides better caloric support for ischemic myocardium without inducing hyperglycemia.[77] Microplegia is less costly than del Nido and allows for longer redosing intervals, leading to improved financial savings.[78]

The amount of cardioplegia given in any single dose can be based on time, volume, or myocardial temperature, according to the surgeon's preference. Maintenance whole blood cardioplegia is generally readministered every 15 to 20 minutes while the aorta is clamped to ensure diastolic cardiac arrest.[77] ECG activity and/or an increase in myocardial temperature indicate that cardioplegia may need to be redosed at shorter intervals.

There are two possible approaches to delivering cardioplegia: (1) antegrade, delivered down the coronary arteries, or (2) retrograde, via the coronary sinus and cardiac veins. The first dose of cardioplegia is usually antegrade, and it is given just after placement of the aortic cross-clamp. After antegrade cardioplegia is given, the perfusionist will switch to retrograde cardioplegia if being used. For administration of antegrade cardioplegia, a catheter is inserted into the aortic root, just proximal to the aortic cross-clamp, and cardioplegia is administered into the root and flows antegrade down the coronary arteries.[58] Hypothermic diastolic circulatory arrest usually follows within 1 to 2 minutes, depending on the adequacy of coronary artery perfusion. Antegrade cardioplegia can also be given directly down the coronary ostia with a special catheter when the aorta is opened for surgeries that involve the aorta or AV. In CABG surgery, it is also infused directly into the new vein or arterial bypass grafts once the distal anastomosis is completed. Myocardial preservation is occasionally incomplete if the cardioplegia does not reach the entire myocardium; therefore there may be difficulty achieving diastolic arrest, and electric activity may reappear on the ECG between doses of cardioplegia. This may occur if the coronary arteries are blocked by atherosclerotic disease or the solution has leaked into the LV due to an incompetent AV.[58,65] In these cases, retrograde cardioplegia can significantly improve myocardial preservation. Many surgeons choose to maximize myocardial protection by routinely giving both antegrade and retrograde cardioplegia.[61]

For retrograde cardioplegia, a catheter is blindly or directly inserted into the RA and advanced into the coronary sinus, the largest venous drainage vessel of the heart. To place the catheter blindly, the surgeon must often lift the heart to help locate the sinus and then advance the catheter into position by feel.[65] Lifting and manipulation of the heart frequently results in dysrhythmias and hypotension. AF is not unusual, and synchronized cardioversion may be required if the patient becomes hemodynamically unstable. If the patient is unable to tolerate the placement of the coronary sinus catheter, the surgeon may opt to place the catheter after initiation of CPB. Once on pump, the catheter can either be placed blindly or under direct visualization via an incision in the RA.[65]

Just before releasing the aortic cross-clamp, many surgeons administer a single terminal dose of warm blood (37°C) cardioplegia, frequently referred to as "the hot shot." This final cardioplegia dose contains metabolic substrates (i.e., glucose, glutamine, and aspartate), which have been found to accelerate myocardial recovery from global ischemia.[79]

Blood Conservation

A review of over 4 million cardiac surgery patients between 1999 and 2010 showed that blood product utilization was increasing and peaked at 34% in 2010, despite the publication of blood conservation guidelines by the Society of Thoracic Surgeons (STS) in 2007.[80] Currently, 10% to 15% of the nation's blood supply is used during cardiac surgery. The risks of transfusion are well documented (see Chapter 22). Blood transfusions during cardiac surgery are associated with worse short-term and long-term survival, including a dose-related increase in the number of postoperative infections with the number of red blood cell (RBC) transfusion units.[81] The donor blood supply is either stable or decreasing, thus blood is considered a finite, scarce, and expensive resource, and there is an international effort to limit its use.[82,83] Three preoperative risk factors have been linked to bleeding and blood transfusion: (1) advanced age (≥70 years), (2) low red cell volume from either preoperative anemia and/or small body size, and (3) urgent or complex surgery involving prolonged CPB times.[67]

The most critical questions are what to transfuse and when transfusion should occur. Even the 2011 STS/Society of Cardiovascular Anesthesiologists (SCA) blood conservation guidelines do not provide clear answers to these complicated questions. Oxygen-carrying capacity is extremely important in cardiac surgical patients, but research has not been able to elucidate what hemoglobin (Hgb) level correlates with organ failure or long-term adverse outcomes. The guidelines suggest transfusion for patients on CPB with a Hgb level of 6 g/dL or less, but transfusion may be justified in patients with a higher Hgb level who are at risk of decreased cerebral O_2 delivery. If the patient's Hgb level is greater than 6 g/dL and the patient's clinical situation (including comorbidities, clinical setting, and laboratory or clinical data) warrants transfusion, it is reasonable to transfuse earlier.[67] Based on the increased age and comorbidities of the typical cardiac surgical population, it is generally accepted to keep a patient's hematocrit in the 22% to 25% range.[67]

In 2011, the STS/SCA published instructions for blood conservation in clinical practice guidelines. Practitioners of cardiac anesthesia are encouraged to review this important document as this chapter discusses only the highlights. The recommended techniques that promote the conservation of blood and blood products include the administration of antifibrinolytics, blood salvage, limiting the quantity of pump prime, ultrafiltration, acute normovolemic hemodilution (ANH) when appropriate, and the development of multidisciplinary blood management teams.[67]

Antifibrinolytics. Antifibrinolytics are commonly administered to cardiac surgical patients requiring CPB to reduce surgical bleeding and the incidence of blood transfusion.[67] Aminocaproic acid (Amicar) and tranexamic acid (Cyklokapron) are both lysine analogs that inhibit plasmin, the key enzyme in the fibrinolytic cascade. Both drugs form a reversible complex with plasmin that inhibits fibrinolysis or the natural breakdown of clots.[72,84] Dosing regimens vary among institutions, but a common recommendation for aminocaproic acid is a 50 mg/kg bolus over 20 to 30 minutes followed by an infusion of 25 mg/kg per hour continued into the immediate postoperative period.[61] A standard dosing regimen of tranexamic acid is 10 mg/kg over 20 minutes, followed by 1 mg/kg per hour maintenance infusion continued into the immediate postoperative period. Tranexamic acid carries a 5% to 7% risk of seizure associated with its use, and decreased dosing is suggested in renal impairment.[61,72] Tranexamic acid is 5 to 10 times more potent than aminocaproic acid and more expensive.

Blood salvage. Blood that is suctioned from the surgical field while the patient is not on CPB, as well as the residual blood that remains in the CPB circuit at the end of bypass, should be directed into a centrifugal red cell salvage device. Blood shed from mediastinal chest tubes can also be salvaged, washed, and reinfused. As previously discussed, the blood aspirated from the field during CPB can return to the pump cardiotomy or the cell-salvage reservoir, depending on surgeon's preference.[70] The shed blood is stored in a reservoir until it reaches a quantity or weight specified by the device manufacturer. The blood is then "washed," a process that removes the serum, coagulation factors, and platelets. The red cells are preserved and placed in a bag that can then be infused into the patient. Cell-salvaged blood has a hematocrit of approximately 55% to 70%. Although the heparin is washed out of the salvaged cells, infusing large quantities of salvaged blood can contribute to a dilutional coagulopathy because this blood is devoid of coagulation factors and platelets.[70] Contraindications to the use of salvaged blood include infection and the use of topical hemostasis agents. Malignancy was previously considered a contraindication to cell-salvage administration; however, the new guidelines state, "In high-risk patients with known malignancy who require CPB, blood salvage using centrifugation of salvaged blood from the operative field may be considered because substantial data support the benefit in patients without malignancy and new evidence suggests worsened outcome when allogeneic transfusion is required in patients with malignancy."[67]

Limiting pump prime. Traditionally, the addition of pump prime to the patient's blood volume at the initiation of CPB resulted in significant hemodilution. Several mechanisms have been devised that help limit the volume of pump prime. Minicircuits that require a smaller volume of pump prime are available and should be considered for patients at high risk for anemia. VAVD in conjunction with these minicircuits has also proved helpful.[60,61,65] Retrograde autologous priming (RAP) is a technique in which the CPB prime is displaced by passive exsanguination (backbleeding) through the arterial line before initiating CPB. This can significantly reduce allogeneic blood transfusion for adult cardiac surgery patients who require CPB.[85] The patient's BP often drops during RAP, so closed-loop communication between the perfusionist and the anesthetist is key. Hypotension usually responds to small bolus doses of phenylephrine.

Ultrafiltration. Ultrafiltration is a process in which the perfusionist diverts the patient's blood to an ultrafilter made of hollow capillary fibers that act as a membrane to separate the aqueous portion of blood from the cellular and proteinaceous elements. The aqueous portion is discarded, while the RBCs and coagulation factors are hemoconcentrated.[61] Ultrafiltration raises the hematocrit and is most often performed to prevent transfusion. An adequate pump volume is needed for ultrafiltration and may be most appropriate in those patients who are volume overloaded preoperatively.[59,72]

Acute normovolemic hemodilution. ANH involves removing the patient's whole blood after placement of central venous access and ideally before surgical incision. Removing the blood before incision ensures that optimum clotting factors are present and that the clotting cascade has not been initiated.[86] The blood is stored in a citrated bag and preferably administered post-CPB; however, it may also be transfused during CPB. ANH may be considered for patients with a hematocrit greater than 38% undergoing a surgery where the need for blood products is anticipated. It is important to be aware of the minimal and maximal fill of the storage bags; if there is too little blood, the patient is at risk for citrate toxicity with transfusion, and too much blood may result in clot formation in the bag. ANH RBCs and platelets are protected from the mechanical trauma and inflammatory effects of CPB. When the blood is removed, the volume is commonly replaced with a 3:1 crystalloid to blood ratio; however, 1:1 colloid can also be used. The dilution of the blood has an added benefit of decreasing blood viscosity on pump and reducing red cells lost during bleeding.[86]

Physiologic Effects of Cardiopulmonary Bypass

Despite improvements in perfusion, anesthesia, and cardiac surgery, patients are still at risk for developing organ dysfunction after CPB. CPB provokes a systemic inflammatory response syndrome (SIRS) that may impact every organ system. SIRS and ischemia related to emboli or hypoperfusion within an organ seem to be the common pathophysiologic mechanisms. In addition to SIRS, hemostasis is also impaired as a result of CPB.[58]

SIRS is thought to be activated as a result of blood exposure to the foreign surfaces of the CPB machine. The inflammatory response to CPB can be mild, patients may be asymptomatic, or it may result in multiple organ dysfunction syndrome (MODS).[87] Ischemia-reperfusion injury or embolization may occur and cause the release of endotoxins, primarily from splanchnic hypoperfusion. Endothelial damage occurs, and the cellular immune response is activated, as are the complement and coagulation cascades. When CPB is initiated, the body exhibits a marked stress response with the elevation of cortisol, catecholamines, arginine vasopressin, and angiotensin. Large amounts of O_2-free radicals are also produced.[87] Further research is necessary to identify protective strategies as no single intervention has been found to limit the adverse outcomes related to SIRS and CPB. The most promising interventions are those that target multiple inflammatory pathways, including surgical/perioperative techniques, perfusion-related strategies, and pharmacologic measures. The use of steroids is the most widely studied intervention but has shown no improvement in clinical outcomes related to mortality, cardiac compromise, or pulmonary complications.[87,88]

Myocardial injury can occur even when protection strategies seem adequate. The degree of injury varies from asymptomatic with an elevation of cardiac enzymes postoperatively to severe with a marked decrease in cardiac function causing failure to separate from CPB. Substantial increases in cardiac enzymes may also result from the activation of SIRS and/or ischemic injury causing embolization and hypoperfusion during CPB. Myocardial injury manifesting as increased cardiac enzymes after CABG has been shown to increase the risk of both early and late death.[89]

Injury to the central nervous system (CNS) after cardiac surgery is a devastating outcome for both the patient and the family. Mild early cognitive deficits have been shown to improve in the first 3 months after surgery.[90] Late cognitive decline in CABG patients, which was originally attributed to CPB, has been shown to occur to the same degree in patients of similar age with CAD who have not undergone CPB.[91] A review of literature regarding neurocognitive outcomes and cardiac surgery revealed there is no evidence to suggest that cardiac surgery, CPB in particular, has a causal role in progression to dementia or long-term neurologic deficit.[72,92,93] Atherosclerotic disease of the ascending aorta is the biggest predictor for injury, but increased age is also a determining factor. Minimizing manipulation of the aorta when atheroma is present may decrease the risk of this neurologic insult; diagnosis can typically be made with TEE and epiaortic echocardiography. Filters on the CPB circuit decrease embolic debris, and flooding the operative field with CO_2 is thought to decrease gaseous emboli. A wide array of neuroprotective and CNS monitoring strategies have been introduced into practice; however, hypothermia is the only intervention that has proven effective. For this reason, it is imperative that the patient does not become hyperthermic and is not rewarmed rapidly after CPB.[92]

Pulmonary complications after CPB can range from mild atelectasis that develops because the lungs are not ventilated on bypass to severe pulmonary dysfunction, known as acute lung injury (ALI) or acute respiratory distress syndrome (ARDS), depending on the severity. Atelectasis and pleural effusions, which occur in 60% of cardiac surgery patients, are the most common injuries, but hemothorax, pneumothorax, and pulmonary edema may also occur.[58] Patients with preexisting respiratory disease are at increased risk for exacerbation of their existing pulmonary illness after CPB. Embolic insults, prolonged CPB, and the CPB-induced SIRS, which causes an increase in pulmonary endothelial permeability, pose the biggest risk to the development of ALI and ARDS.[72] Strategies that may help decrease these complications are low tidal volume (Vt) ventilation during CPB, giving a vital capacity breath before separation from CPB, and maintaining reduced Fio_2 and tidal volume after CPB.[58] Low Vt ventilation on CPB has been shown to reduce pulmonary edema and lung inflammation, and shorten time to extubation, especially in complex cases with prolonged CPB time. The addition of inhaled epoprostenol, a pulmonary vasodilator, during bypass reduces pulmonary artery pressure, decreases RV workload, and improves CO after separating from CPB.[94]

Renal dysfunction manifesting as acute kidney injury (AKI) is one of the major complications of cardiac surgery and serves as a major predictor of morbidity and mortality for postoperative cardiac surgical patients.[95] In 2019, Hessel[72] conducted a review of 32 studies and found that 22% of patients who underwent cardiac surgery with CPB developed acute renal failure (ARF) and 3% required renal replacement therapy. Hospital mortality was over 40% for patients with ARF and increased to over 60% in patients who required renal replacement therapy. Optimizing cardiovascular volume status and CO as well as limiting CPB time are suggested to decrease the incidence of ARF.[58,96]

Gastrointestinal (GI) system dysfunction is a relatively rare occurrence, but significantly increases the incidence of perioperative MI, renal failure, stroke, and even death. GI dysfunction seems to also be affected by hypoperfusion and/or embolic events related to CPB. Splanchnic hypoperfusion causes the release of endotoxins that can initiate SIRS.[97] The most effective strategy for avoiding intestinal ischemia is minimizing CPB time and possibly limiting the use of vasopressin.[58]

Even with adequate heparinization, CPB activates extrinsic and intrinsic hemostatic pathways as well as fibrinolysis. Contact of the blood with the internal surface of the CPB circuit results in the activation of complement, the coagulation cascade, platelets, plasminogen, and kallikrein. During CPB, platelets and clotting factors are first diluted and then denatured by mechanical trauma from the CPB circuit and suction devices.[82,83] Platelets and leukocytes are also activated by mechanical trauma. The end result is the development of coagulopathies that manifest as increased perioperative bleeding. This coagulopathy may be attenuated by the use of antifibrinolytics and ANH, which preserves some of the patient's blood and protects it from these detrimental changes.[86]

Anesthetic Considerations in the Preoperative Period

Preoperative Evaluation

Due to the serious nature of the primary disease and the high prevalence of comorbidities, all patients undergoing cardiac surgery should have a thorough preoperative evaluation, including a history of the patient's medical condition and a complete physical exam. The preoperative assessment should primarily focus on the cardiovascular system, but a thorough airway assessment must also be performed and information gathered about the pulmonary, neurologic, endocrine, renal, hepatic, and hematologic systems.

Cardiovascular system. The medical record should be examined and results of cardiovascular tests noted. Table 26.2 summarizes many of the common cardiovascular tests and findings that are used to identify cardiac pathology. Ventricular function and a history of heart failure are important considerations that affect anesthetic choice, hemodynamic management, and requirements for intraoperative pharmacologic support. Patients with a history of severe systolic heart failure and an interventricular conduction delay are likely to have a cardiac electronic implantable device (CEID), including a pacemaker alone or in combination with an implantable cardioverter-defibrillator (ICD).[98] Many patients will have a biventricular pacemaker for cardiac resynchronization therapy (CRT), which improves CO, hemodynamics, heart failure symptoms, and quality of life.[98,99] All implantable devices should be evaluated before cardiac surgery and may need to be reprogrammed just before surgery to prevent electrocautery-induced discharge.[99,100] Usually, the antitachyarrhythmia functions on an automatic ICD and the rate response (if present) on a pacemaker are suspended.[99] Patients with an ICD should have defibrillation pads placed before reprogramming so that a means for pacing and defibrillation are immediately available. The pads are positioned away from the generator to prevent damage to the device should defibrillation be necessary. A magnet must be available and the magnet response identified. In emergency situations, the magnet will usually deactivate ICD devices and place most modern pacemakers in an asynchronous mode.[99] If the programmed backup asynchronous pacing rate is less than 70, it is often advisable to have the pacemaker reprogrammed to a higher rate.

Patients with CAD or aortic stenosis (AS) often have carotid artery disease and/or peripheral vascular disease (PVD). The MAP is kept within a relatively higher range in patients with carotid disease to ensure adequate cerebral perfusion pressure.[101] The presence of PVD may limit the locations available for invasive monitoring, and the presence of aortic disease can impact the surgeon's ability to cannulate or clamp the aorta. If alternate cannulation sites are selected, this too can impact invasive line placement.

Comorbidities. For elective surgery, patient comorbidities should be optimized before the time of the operation. Multiple studies have correlated the following conditions with increased risk in the cardiac surgical population: systolic or diastolic heart failure, chronic obstructive pulmonary disease (COPD), diabetes mellitus, compromised renal function, CVD or PVD, and thyroid dysfunction.[102,103] Diabetes mellitus and perioperative hyperglycemia are associated with increases in

---

BOX 26.1   Highlights of STS Perioperative Glucose Management Recommendations

Preoperative
- Hold oral hypoglycemic for 24 hr prior to surgery.
- Hold nutritional insulin after dinner the night before surgery.
- Continue basal insulin dose (NPH dose may be cut by 1/3–1/2).
- Check glucose level frequently the day of surgery.
- Maintaining glucose at ≤180 mg/dL is reasonable.

Intraoperative
- Intermittent bolus acceptable if nondiabetic and glucose <180 mg/dL.
- Continuous infusion preferred if glucose ≥180 mg/dL.
- Continuous infusion preferred for diabetics, maintain postoperatively.
- Adjust infusion per institutional protocol with a goal of maintaining glucose at ≤180 mg/dL.
- Check glucose level every 30–60 min or more frequently.

Postoperative in ICU
- Consult endocrinology for diabetic patients.
- If glucose is persistently >180 mg/dL, continue infusion.
- If patient in ICU >3 days, target should be ≤150 mg/dL.
- Before stopping infusion, transition to subcutaneous insulin.

In Step-Down or Floor
- Endocrinology to adjust basal and nutritional insulin doses.
- General goal is ≤180 mg/dL after meals and ≤110 mg/dL fasting.
- Restart oral hypoglycemic if target achieved and no contraindications.

ICU, intensive care unit; *NPH,* neutral protamine Hagedorn; *STS,* Society of Thoracic Surgeons.
Data from The Society of Thoracic Surgeons (STS) guidelines on blood glucose management during adult cardiac surgery. *Ann Thorac Surg.* 2009;87:663–669.

---

sternal wound infections, extended length of stay, recurrence of angina, postoperative mortality, and decreased long-term survival.[104-107] The STS developed evidence-based practice guidelines for blood glucose management in the perioperative period (Box 26.1).[108] In addition, perioperative renal impairment is strongly correlated with increases in morbidity and mortality.[109] International consensus recommendations covering cardiac and vascular surgery–associated AKI were published in 2018.[110] Strategies to prevent AKI that the anesthesia provider can influence include optimizing of volume status, maintaining the MAP above 75 mmHg, using a inhalation anesthetic agent (vs propofol), and preventing hyperthermia.[110]

Laboratory studies. Laboratory studies that will assist in the perioperative period include a room-air arterial blood gas (ABG), electrolytes, serum blood urea nitrogen (BUN) and creatinine, fasting lipid profile, complete blood count, coagulation profile, hemoglobin A_{1C}, and fasting blood glucose. Any serum biomarkers drawn to evaluate ischemia, infarction (troponin), or failure (ANP/BNP) should be noted. Methicillin-resistant *Staphylococcus aureus* (MRSA) infection has a low prevalence but high mortality associated with cardiac surgery. Preoperatively, nasal swab cultures are taken, and those patients colonized with MRSA (~3.9%) have vancomycin added to their antibiotic routine.[111,112]

Airway assessment and pulmonary function. A plan must be developed to safely secure the airway and ventilate the patient while maintaining hemodynamic stability. It can be especially challenging to maintain hemodynamic stability in the face of a difficult airway, severe PHTN, lung disease, or compromised ventricular function. A double-lumen tube and a pediatric fiberoptic bronchoscope are required for procedures performed through a thoracotomy incision. If prolonged postoperative ventilation is anticipated, a slightly larger endotracheal tube (ETT) aids mechanical ventilation and pulmonary toileting.[55,113]

Surgical risk. The STS maintains a robust national database that estimates the risk of operative morbidity and mortality after adult cardiac surgery based on patient demographics and preoperative clinical variables. The risk calculator was updated last in November 2018 and is accessible on the internet.[114] Risk can be calculated for primary procedures as well as combined CABG and single valve surgeries. The risk calculation includes overall morbidity and mortality, length of stay, risk of reoperation, and several other quality measures. The AHA/ACC[115,116] recommend and current evidence supports that patients who are considered high risk because of complex pathology or significant comorbidities be cared for by a heart team at a center of excellence.[117,118] In tertiary/quaternary care centers specializing in cardiac care there are likely to be many patients and procedures that exceed any risk model's ability to accurately calculate risk. Procedures such as reoperations for multiple valve replacements in a patient with endocarditis or placement of an assist device are not included in these models.

Management of preoperative medications. Cardiac surgical patients are likely to be on multiple medications to manage their primary disease and comorbidities. As a general rule, patients should receive medicines that are used to manage their medical conditions on the morning of surgery with a sip of water.[119] However, a few medications merit further discussion.

The AHA/ACC consider the continuation of statin therapy in cardiac surgery a class I recommendation, which has the most reliable level of evidence support.[120] Clinical research has also demonstrated the benefit of perioperative β-blocker therapy to improve hemodynamic stability, decrease dysrhythmias, and reduce morbidity and mortality.[119,121,122] Unless there is a contraindication, patients having coronary surgery should receive β-blockers preoperatively, and patients who are on β-blockers for any reason preoperatively should have them continued in the perioperative period. The continuation of β-blockers has become a national quality measure. However, β-blockers should not first be initiated on the day of surgery because of the increased risk of hypotension.[115,116,123]

Medical management of hypertension, heart failure, and diabetic nephropathy includes the use of renin-angiotensin-aldosterone system blockers (RAASB) and angiotensin-converting enzyme inhibitors (ACEIs) (see Fig. 26.5). Perioperative management of these medications remains controversial. Current AHA/ACC guidelines for CABG (2011) state that "the safety of preoperative ACEIs or ARBs [angiotensin receptor blockers] in patients on chronic therapy is uncertain."[116] The updated (2017) European Association for Cardio-Thoracic Surgery (EACTS) recommends the discontinuation of ACEIs and ARBs (class I, level C) in cardiac surgery because their use is associated with an increased need for vasoactive medications postoperatively and an increase in AKI.[124] ACEIs and ARBs have also been implicated as a cause of postoperative vasoplegic syndrome.[125-127] Yet, a meta-analysis suggests that perioperative administration of RAASBs improves outcomes of patients undergoing CABG and/or valve surgery.[128] It is generally agreed that ACEIs and ARBs in patients on chronic therapy should be reinstituted in the postoperative period if the patients are stable.[116,119,124,129]

The STS guidelines recommend that medications that affect coagulation be managed on an individual basis by a multidisciplinary heart team.[67,119,124,130] A complete review of these recommendations is beyond the scope of this chapter, but a few important points will be addressed. Many patients with AF are maintained on antithrombotics, including warfarin (Coumadin), and nonvitamin K oral anticoagulants

(NOACs) that include thrombin inhibitors (dabigatran) and factor Xa inhibitors (rivaroxaban, apixaban, and edoxaban). Warfarin is usually discontinued 5 days before surgery until the international normalized ratio (INR) is less than 1.5.[124] If surgery must proceed before the INR is normalized, prothrombin complex concentrate and vitamin K can be used to reverse the anticoagulation effects of warfarin.[124] When compared to warfarin, NOACs have fewer bleeding complications with a similar thromboprophylaxis efficacy and a more predictable pharmacodynamic profile making routine monitoring less necessary.[131,132] NOACs are potent and long acting, and cannot be reversed; therefore it is expected that the risk of bleeding is increased in cardiac surgical patients on these drugs. The INR and partial thromboplastin time (PTT) do not accurately assess the anticoagulant activity of NOACs, so a thrombin time (TT), a direct measure of anti-Xa activity or plasma levels, will be used by the multidisciplinary heart team to make decisions about the timing of surgery.[124,133,134]

Aspirin (acetylsalicylic acid [ASA]) and heparin are vital in the treatment of CAD, especially in patients with acute coronary syndrome (ACS). Heparin and ASA are administered to patients requiring emergency surgery for ACS, and heparin is continued until shortly before skin incision.[116] ASA is also recommended postoperatively for patients having CABG because it increases graft patency and reduces mortality.[116] Recent guidelines state that perioperative continuation of ASA should be considered for CABG.[124] Preoperative ASA increases the risk of bleeding in more complex cardiac surgery, so an STS consensus statement recommends that ASA should be discontinued before elective cardiac surgery in patients without ACS.[119,130] However, a recent meta-analysis demonstrated ASA at any dose is associated with decreased mortality and AKI. Low-dose aspirin (≤160 mg) decreases the incidence of perioperative MI. Although low-dose ASA preoperatively increases the risk of bleeding, it did not increase the need for chest reexploration or the rate of packed red blood cell (PRBC) transfusion.[135,136]

The decision to bridge a patient who is on oral anticoagulants preoperatively is made by the multidisciplinary heart team based on the thrombotic risk and the surgical procedure. Unfractionated heparin (UFH) is the only approved drug for bridging, but low molecular weight heparin (LMWH) is sometimes used for outpatients. Bridging is initiated when INR values are no longer therapeutic. LMWH should be stopped at least 12 hours before surgery, and UFH should be stopped 6 hours before surgery.[124]

Following a percutaneous coronary intervention (PCI), patients are most often placed on ASA and a thienopyridine (ticlopidine, clopidogrel, prasugrel), which blocks adenosine diphosphate (ADP)–mediated platelet activation by binding with the $P2Y_{12}$ receptor. Initially, the ACC/AHA guidelines recommended that patients receive dual antiplatelet therapy (DAPT) for 1 year or more following placement of a drug-eluting stent (DES) and 3 months after placement of a bare-metal stent (BMS) to prevent stent thrombosis.[137] However, in 2016 the guidelines were revised because contemporary evidence showed that 6 months of DAPT is equally effective for second-generation DES.[138] Recommendations for individual patients are best made by a multidisciplinary heart team based on multiple factors, including risk of thrombosis and bleeding along with patient drug responsiveness.[138] Mini thoracotomy, transapical transcatheter aortic valve replacement (TAVR), off-pump coronary artery bypass (OPCAB), CABG, and valve replacement are considered intermediate hemorrhagic risk. Reinterventions, endocarditis, CABG for PCI failure, and aortic dissections are considered high hemorrhagic risk.[139] In general, it is recommended that elective surgery be postponed a minimum of 6 months following a DES and 1 month following BMS. If surgery is not deferrable, recommendations are to continue ASA, discontinue the $P2Y_{12}$ receptor inhibitor, and resume within 24 to 72 hours with a loading dose.[139] The interval between discontinuation of antiplatelet drugs and surgery is dependent on the medication. Traditionally, clopidogrel and ticagrelor are held for 5 days while prasugrel is held for 7 days. Newer evidence suggests that discontinuing clopidogrel and ticagrelor for 3 days may be sufficient.[124,140] Patients who are considered to be a high thrombotic risk and who require urgent surgery while on DAPT may benefit from bridging strategies using short-acting antiplatelet agents.[139] Decisions regarding the management of DAPT are individual and complex, so a multidisciplinary heart team approach is recommended.

Preparation for possible blood loss. Since cardiac surgical procedures are associated with significant blood loss, the anesthesia provider must confirm with all patients their willingness to accept blood products. In patients with specific religious beliefs or personal preferences, the permissibility of specific products and/or cell-saver devices should be discussed and documented.[67] Before induction, the anesthetist should confirm the validity of the patient's type and crossmatch as well as the anticipated blood product availability. This is particularly important in patients who have a positive antibody screen because it can sometimes take multiple hours to secure crossmatched units. Patients having "redo" sternotomy or a history of radiation to the chest should have blood immediately available before sternotomy. The section on CPB discusses blood conservation measures.

Psychological preparation and preoperative sedation. The cardiac surgical environment is a fast-paced, high-intensity area, and it is easy for team members to become task oriented and inadvertently overlook the emotional needs of the patient. Patients facing major surgery are acutely aware of their mortality and are often apprehensive about the procedure and postoperative pain. Concerns about the future of loved ones, especially those who are dependent upon them for support, are common. The preoperative interview provides a unique opportunity to gather needed data and share information about what the patient can expect. Ideally, the provider caring for the patient during the surgery should conduct the preoperative interview to establish rapport and address the patient's and family's concerns. Mentally prepared patients will be more calm, confident, and cooperative in the OR and the intensive care unit (ICU).[55]

Preoperative sedation is selected on an individual basis taking into consideration the patient's functional status and anxiety level. Generally, patients with normal LV function and few comorbidities can tolerate heavier sedation, whereas the frail require only minimal sedation. Sedation should not be so heavy as to prevent coherent patients from participating in the identification and interview process. When in doubt, sedation is withheld preoperatively and then administered in the OR while the patient is monitored during line placement.

Preparation for Surgery

Operating room preparation. The surgical suite should be readied in preparation for the planned surgical procedure before the patient's arrival. Communication with the surgical, nursing, and perfusion teams is essential to ensure that all parties are ready to act appropriately if the patient should rapidly deteriorate, requiring emergent surgical intervention and/or institution of CPB. The basic setup and monitoring are similar to most major cases, with a few additions, as outlined in Table 26.6.

Monitoring. Standard and extended monitors for cardiac surgery are listed in Table 26.6. ECG monitoring should include lead II for the detection of dysrhythmias and lead V_4 or V_5 with automated ST analysis for the detection of ischemia. In practice, the V lead may need to be placed at the fourth to fifth ICS, posterior to the axillary line, rather than at the midclavicular line, to avoid the surgical field. TEE is almost always indicated for cardiac surgery and is more

sensitive than the ECG for the detection of ischemia.[24] The 2015 STS guidelines recommend that core temperature be measured using a nasopharyngeal probe or the pulmonary artery catheter (PAC).[141] To avoid excessive nasopharyngeal bleeding, the probe should be placed at the beginning of the surgical procedure, before heparinization. It is recommended that the oxygenator arterial outlet blood temperature is used as a surrogate for cerebral temperature measurement during CPB.[141] Many centers find a peripheral temperature monitor (bladder or rectal) is useful to compare core and shell temperatures during cooling and rewarming.

Arterial line. The arterial line (A line) is placed before induction using sedation as tolerated and local anesthesia for patient comfort. Continuous monitoring of hemodynamics during induction of anesthesia is crucial when the patient has life-threatening cardiac pathology, including severe AS, left main CAD, severe PHTN, or moderate to severely decreased left or right ventricular function.

The A line is most commonly placed in the radial or brachial arteries, based on personal or institutional preference. The dominant hand artery may be selected if the surgeon plans to harvest the radial artery in the nondominate arm as a CABG conduit. Left-sided placement is preferred if the surgeon plans to use the right subclavian artery for placement of the aortic cannula.[113] Radial artery cannulation is safer than brachial artery cannulation as most of the blood flow to the hand is from the ulnar artery.[142] However, the radial pressure waveform may dampen during chest wall retraction as a consequence of subclavian artery compression between the clavicle and first rib, especially during dissection of the internal thoracic artery (ITA).[143] Some providers prefer the brachial artery because it is a more reliable measure of central aortic pressure before and after CPB.[144,145] Although concerns for thrombosis persist, the safety of brachial A line use in heparinized patients has been well documented.[145,146] A baseline ABG and ACT are obtained after A line placement.

Central venous access. Central venous access is mandatory in adult cardiac surgery for volume resuscitation and administration of vasoactive medications. In most cases, central access is obtained after the induction of anesthesia. However, it may be prudent to place the central line before induction if the patient is hemodynamically unstable or likely to decompensate on induction. Occasionally, preinduction central access is obtained because of inadequate peripheral access. The right internal jugular (IJ) vein is the preferred cannulation site because it is relatively easy to access and provides a straight, short path to the RA. If the left IJ vein is used, the anesthetist must use caution to avoid the thoracic duct and left brachiocephalic vein, which courses the IJ vein at a right angle.[146] For this reason, some providers prefer to use a short introducer on the left. Catheters placed in the IJ or subclavian vein, especially on the left, are prone to kinking during chest-wall retraction. It is now standard of care to use an ultrasound to guide central line placement since the evidence has shown increased speed, reduced infections, and decreased complications.[146]

A PAC is frequently placed instead of a central venous pressure (CVP) monitor alone, to measure intracardiac pressures (Table 26.7) and CO. The information obtained can be used to derive other hemodynamic parameters to assist patient management (Table 26.8). Generally, a PAC is preferred in complex surgical procedures and in patients with left or right ventricular failure, PHTN, or reduced LV compliance.[55] In these situations, the PAC may be the most valuable postoperatively in the ICU when TEE is no longer available. During CPB, the PAC can advance, potentially injuring the pulmonary artery (PA).[147] It is therefore recommended that the catheter be retracted 2 to 3 cm during this time, and the balloon inflated slowly (if used to wedge) after weaning from CPB.[55,147] Many providers avoid wedging completely to decrease the risk of PA damage or rupture. Defibrillation pads should

TABLE 26.6   Typical Anesthesia Preparation of the Cardiac Operating Room

Anesthesia Machine	Routine Check	
Airway	Nasal cannula, simple face mask, anesthesia facemask, oral airways	
	Laryngoscope handle, blades, endotracheal tubes	
	Suction (Yankauer and endotracheal)	
	Ambu bag and any anticipated difficult airway equipment	
Vascular Access	1–2 Large-bore PIV catheters (14 or 16 gauge preferred)	
	Blood tubing on a warmer for complex cases or expected blood loss	
	Arterial line (radial or brachial based on institutional preference)	
	R may be preferred for LITA conduit	
	L may be preferred for "redos" requiring R subclavian cannulation	
	Avoid side of radial artery conduit and sites distal to prior brachial cut-down for cardiac catheterization	
	Central venous access	
	CVP for normal LVF and primary, uncomplicated, cases in relatively healthy patients	
	PAC for poor LVF, complex surgery, and patients with multiple comorbidities	
Monitors	**Standard Monitors**	**Extended Monitors**
	ECG (II, V_5 + automated ST analysis)	PAC
	BP (noninvasive + invasive)	Specialized PACs (pacing, etc.)
	Intermittent ABGs	Cardiac output measurement
	Pulse oximetry	Mixed venous saturation
	Capnography	TEE
	Temperature (core ± peripheral)	Left atrial pressure
	CVP	BIS
	Foley catheter +/- temperature monitor	Cerebral oximetry
	Neuromuscular blockade monitor	Retrograde coronary sinus cardioplegia perfusion
	Machine with cassettes for monitoring anticoagulation (ACT or Hepcon)	pressure
	Electronic medical record	
Medications	Anesthetic sedation	
	Line placement (midazolam)	
	Transport to ICU (propofol or dexmedetomidine)	
	Anesthetic induction	
	Induction (propofol or etomidate)	
	Muscle relaxant (succinylcholine for difficult airway + nondepolarizing)	
	Narcotic (fentanyl, sufentanil, remifentanil, or hydromorphone)	
	Inhalation anesthetic	
	Heparin (400 units/kg in a syringe)	
	Antibiotic (cephalosporin +/- vancomycin and aminoglycoside)	
	Vasoactive bolus medications: nitroglycerine, phenylephrine, norepinephrine, ephedrine, epinephrine, ± glycopyrrolate, ± atropine, ± calcium	
	Infusions as needed on pumps:	
	Antifibrinolytic (aminocaproic acid or tranexamic acid)	
	Nitroglycerin (NTG) for patients with CAD or volume overload	
	Sodium nitroprusside (SNP), nicardipine, or clevidipine for patients with HTN, regurgitant valve lesions, or systolic heart failure	
	Inotrope (epinephrine or dobutamine) for patients with poor left or right ventricular function	
	Vasopressin for septic or vasoplegic individuals	
	Insulin	
Miscellaneous	Pacemaker with battery	
	Warm water mattress or forced-air warming device	

ACT, Activated clotting time; *BIS,* bispectral index; *BP,* blood pressure; *CAD,* coronary artery disease; *CVP,* central venous pressure; *ECG,* electrocardiogram; *Hepcon,* machine for determining circulating heparin concentration; *HTN,* hypertension; *ICU,* intensive care unit; *L,* left; *LITA,* left internal thoracic artery; *LVF,* left ventricular function; *PAC,* pulmonary artery catheter; *PIV,* peripheral intravenous; *R,* right; *TEE,* transesophageal echocardiography.

be placed prophylactically before PAC insertion in a patient with a preexisting left bundle branch block (LBBB) because about 3% will develop a right bundle branch block (RBBB) leading to complete heart block (CHB).[148] Alternatively, the PAC can be left in the superior vena cava (SVC) until the chest is open and then advanced. If CHB does develop, rapid CPB is an option.[149] PACs should generally be avoided in patients who have had pacemaker leads placed in the past 6 weeks because of the possibility of lead displacement.[150] Occasionally, in cardiac surgery, specialized PACs are useful, including those that can pace or continuously measure mixed venous saturation and CO. In surgical

TABLE 26.7 Normal Intracardiac Pressures

Location	Mean (mm Hg)	Range (mm Hg)
Right atrium	5	1–10
Right ventricle	25/5	15–30/0–8
Pulmonary arterial systolic/diastolic	23/9	15–30/5–15
Mean pulmonary arterial	15	10–20
Pulmonary capillary wedge pressure	10	5–15
Left atrial pressure	8	4–12
Left ventricular end-diastolic pressure	8	4–12
Left ventricular systolic pressure	130	90–140

From Mittnacht AJC, et al. Monitoring the heart and vascular system. In Kaplan JA, et al. eds. *Kaplan's Cardiac Anesthesia: For Cardiac and Noncardiac Surgery.* 7th ed. Philadelphia: Elsevier; 2017:406.

TABLE 26.8 Derived Hemodynamic Parameters

Formula	Normal Values
Cardiac Index $CI = CO/BSA$	2.8–4.2 L/min/m^2
Stroke Volume $SV = CO \times 1000/HR$	50–110 mL (per beat)
Stroke Index $SI = SV/BSA$	30–65 mL/beat/m^2
Left Ventricular Stroke Work Index $LVSWI = 1.36 \times (MAP - PCWP) \times SI/100$	45–60 kg/m/m^2
Right Ventricular Stroke Work Index $RVSWI = 1.36 \times (MPAP - CVP) \times SI/100$	5–10 kg/m/m^2
Systemic Vascular Resistance $SVR = (MAP - CVP) \times 80/CO$	900–1400 dynes/sec/cm^{-5}
Systemic Vascular Resistance Index $SVRI = (MAP - CVP) \times 80/CI$	1500–2400 dynes/sec/cm^{-5}/m^2
Pulmonary Vascular Resistance $PVR = (MPAP - PCWP) \times 80/CO$	150–250 dynes/sec/cm^{-5}
Pulmonary Vascular Resistance Index $PVRI = (MPAP - PCWP) \times 80/CI$	250–400 dynes/sec/cm^{-5}/m^2

BSA, Body surface area; *CI,* cardiac index; *CO,* cardiac output; *CVP,* central venous pressure; *HR,* heart rate; *LVSWI,* left ventricular stroke work index; *MAP,* mean arterial pressure; *MPAP,* mean pulmonary arterial pressure; *PCWP,* pulmonary capillary wedge pressure; *PVR,* pulmonary vascular resistance; *PVRI,* pulmonary vascular resistance index; *RVSWI,* right ventricular stroke work index; *SI,* stroke index; *SV,* stroke volume; *SVR,* systemic vascular resistance; *SVRI,* systemic vascular resistance index.

From Mittnacht AJC, et al. Monitoring the heart and vascular system. In Kaplan JA, et al. eds. *Kaplan's Cardiac Anesthesia: For Cardiac and Noncardiac Surgery.* 7th ed. Philadelphia: Elsevier; 2017:407.

procedures where large blood loss is anticipated, or when peripheral access is limited, a 9-French two-lumen introducer or a large-bore double-lumen central venous line is useful.

Transesophageal echocardiography. TEE is an invaluable source of information about cardiovascular anatomy and function during cardiac surgery. It is the most sensitive clinical monitor for detecting wall motion abnormalities caused by myocardial ischemia. Additional uses include evaluation of right and left systolic and diastolic ventricular function, valvular function and pathology, intravascular volume status, intracardiac air or pulmonary embolism, aortic atheroma and dissection, pericardial effusion or tamponade, and cannula or catheter placement. Unless there is a contraindication, multiple guidelines recommend intraoperative TEE in cardiac surgery for all open chamber (i.e., valvular), thoracic aortic, and transcatheter procedures, and in the setting of unexplained hemodynamic instability. TEE should also be considered (and is most often used) for CABG procedures when there is a question of concurrent valvular pathology and to detect wall motion abnormalities. Transthoracic echocardiography (TTE) is substituted for TEE in transcatheter procedures performed under monitored anesthesia care (MAC).[51,151-155] Absolute contraindications to TEE include perforated viscus and pathologic conditions of the esophagus, including strictures, diverticula, tumors, traumatic interruption, or recent suture lines.[156]

A comprehensive exam initially encompassed 20 two-dimensional (2D) views but was expanded to 28 views in 2013 when three-dimensional (3D) imaging became available.[157] A targeted perioperative TEE exam can be performed using 11 selected views.[156] M mode, 2D, and 3D imaging are all important in the evaluation of cardiac pathology. The TEE exam should be performed before CPB by a credentialed provider to identify baseline pathology and function. This information is communicated to the surgical and anesthesia teams and used for comparison after CPB to immediately evaluate the surgical repair(s) and identify new pathology or dysfunction.

The American Society of Echocardiography (ASE) and the SCA recognize TEE as a physician privilege and adhere to strict training, certification, and recertification guidelines for basic and advanced certification.[151] The American Association of Nurse Anesthetists (AANA) recognized placement of the TEE probe as a core privilege and recommends monitoring and interpretation of TEE as a special privilege for Certified Registered Nurse Anesthetists (CRNAs).[158] Although even an introductory discussion of TEE is beyond the scope of this chapter, a basic understanding of TEE is valuable for nurse anesthetists to help monitor ventricular function and intravascular volume status and to identify situations where interpretation by a credentialed provider is

advisable. Therefore a few key points and views will be discussed as they relate to cardiac anesthesia. The reader is referred to the chapters on monitoring the cardiovascular system (Chapter 17) and regional anesthesia (Chapter 50) for a discussion on the physics and practical use of ultrasound. The virtual TEE website sponsored by the Toronto General Hospital Department of Anesthesia Perioperative Interactive Education Group is highly recommended.[159]

TEE placement is accomplished after the airway is secured and the patient is fully anesthetized and relaxed since probe placement is stimulating and carries potential risk. A bite-block is inserted before or after probe placement (depending on the type) for the dual purpose of protecting the patient's teeth and probe integrity. The stomach is decompressed of air and gastric contents prior to TEE insertion with an orogastric (OG) tube that is subsequently removed to prevent interference with image quality. A generous amount of water-soluble jelly placed in the oropharynx facilitates the advancement of the probe and enhances image quality. It is important to confirm that the TEE probe handle control is in the unlocked position and moves freely before insertion (Fig. 26.10). The probe is initially placed in the posterior pharynx with the transducer facing anteriorly. This is best accomplished by flexing the probe anteriorly using the large wheel on the handle, then

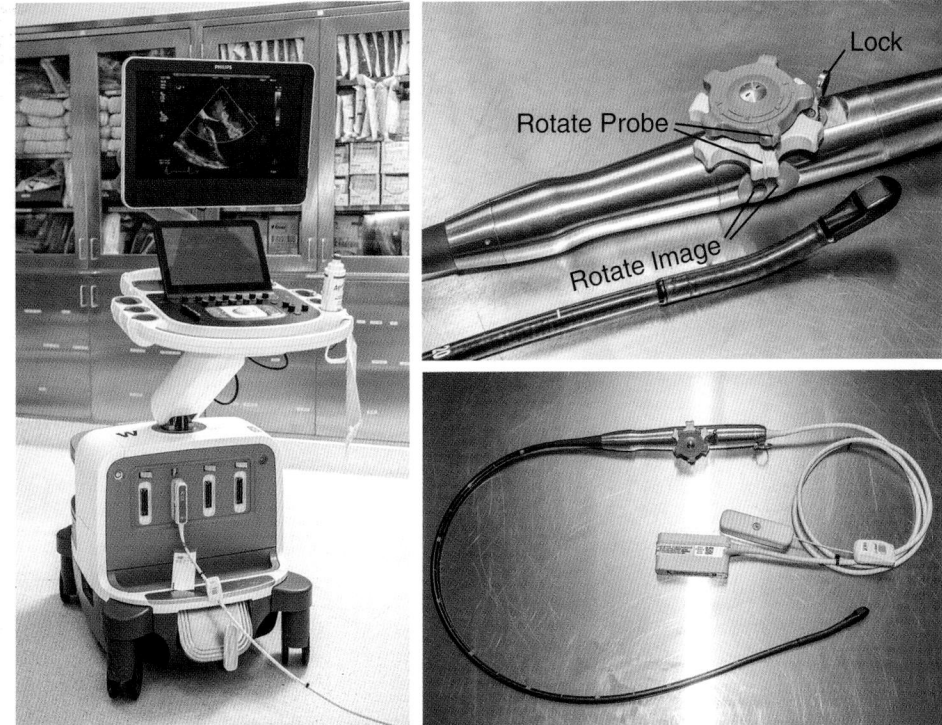

Fig. 26.10 Transesophageal echocardiography machine and probe. The probe is marked in 10-cm increments. The large wheel flexes the transducer anterior and posterior, and the small wheel flexes left and right. The lock lever stiffens the probe locking the transducer in a fixed position. The button control rotates the multiplane transducer forward from 0 to 180 degrees and back. (Reprinted with permission, Cleveland Clinic Center for Medical Art & Photography ©2021. All Rights Reserved.)

displacing the tongue using a manual tongue and jaw lift, or with the aid of a laryngoscope, and applying gentle pressure to advance the probe into the posterior pharynx. Finally, the probe is advanced gently into the esophagus. Occasionally, the tip of the probe may lodge in one of the piriform sinuses during insertion. This parapharyngeal area is vulnerable to injury, so withdrawing the probe slightly and turning the patient's head to the right before advancing helps to avoid this tissue pocket. To prevent trauma to the mouth, pharynx, or esophagus, force is never applied when placing the TEE probe.[160] TEE probe placement fails in approximately 2% of patients.[160] In this situation, a pediatric probe can be considered for small patients, or the surgeon can perform epicardial echocardiography to attain the necessary images.

All practitioners who manipulate the probe should be trained and familiar with the system controls and techniques for image optimization. As illustrated in Figs. 26.10 and 26.11, standardized terms are used for probe manipulation. The probe itself can be advanced deeper into the esophagus or stomach or withdrawn. Manually turning the probe clockwise is referred to as "turning to the right" and counterclockwise as "turning to the left." Wheels on the probe are used to flex the probe transducer. The large wheel is used to flex the transducer anteriorly toward the sternum, referred to as "anteflexing," or posteriorly toward the spine, referred to as "retroflexing." With the probe facing anteriorly, the small wheel flexes the transducer toward the patient's left or right, referred to as "flexing left" or "flexing right." A button control on the handle is used to electronically rotate the multiplane transducer from 0 degrees through 180 degrees, referred to as "rotating forward," and from 180 degrees through 0 degrees, referred to as "rotating back." The position of the multiplane transducer is shown on the image in the upper right corner of the screen. The probe is 170 cm in length and marked in 10-cm increments. There are four general areas where the transducer may be positioned within the esophagus and stomach that

Probe Manipulations

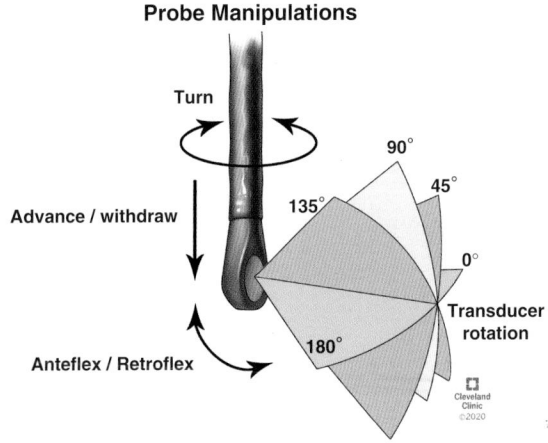

Fig. 26.11 Terminology used to describe manipulation of the transesophageal echocardiography probe during image acquisition. (Reprinted with permission, Cleveland Clinic Center for Medical Art & Photography ©2021. All Rights Reserved.)

have associated imaging planes: upper esophageal (UE), midesophageal (ME), transgastric (TG), and deep transgastric (DTG) (Fig. 26.12). The probe depth is determined on an individual basis, but UE structures usually come into view at about 25 cm and ME structures at 30 to 35 cm. TG images require anteflexion of the probe and advancing to 40 cm or more.[157,160]

The mainstay of TEE is a 2D echo. The transducer sequentially directs an ultrasound beam across a sector of the heart, and structures can be viewed moving in real time. The image will appear cone or pie shaped, with structures closest to the probe in the near field at the top of the screen and those farthest from the probe in the far field at the

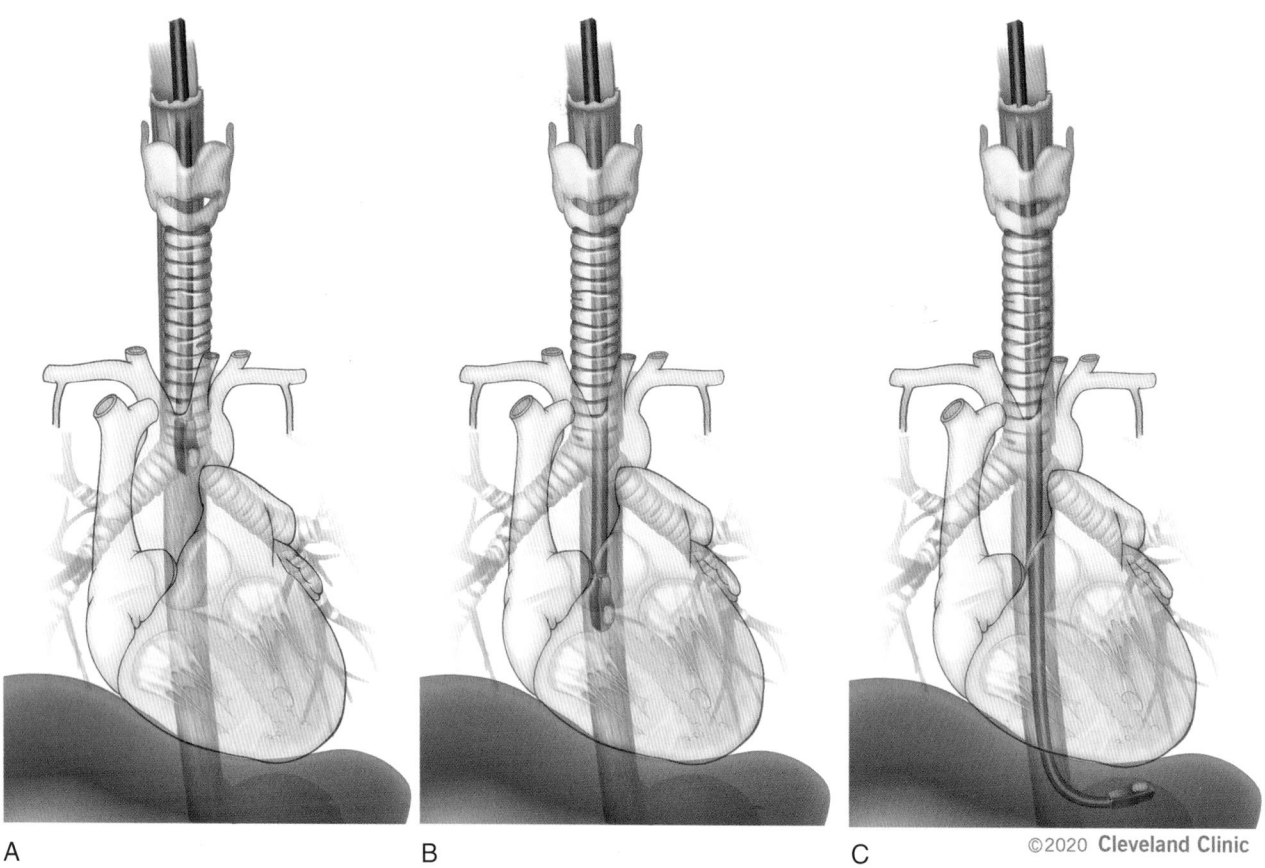

Fig. 26.12 Three standard transducer positions within the esophagus and stomach that are associated with imaging planes. (A) Upper esophageal. (B) Midesophageal. (C) Transgastric. (Reprinted with permission, Cleveland Clinic Center for Medical Art & Photography ©2021. All Rights Reserved.)

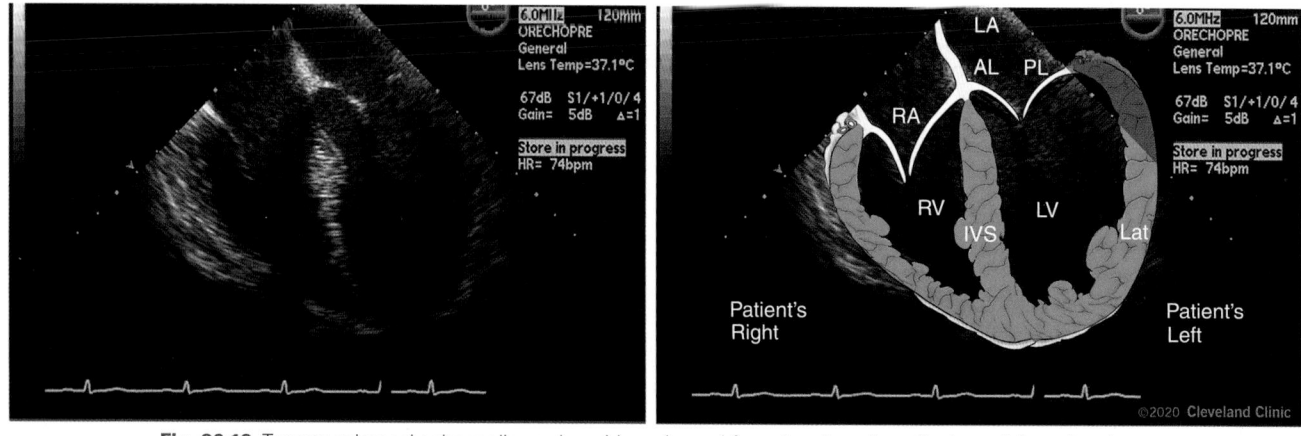

Fig. 26.13 Transesophageal echocardiography midesophageal four-chamber view displays all four chambers and the tricuspid and mitral valves. The septal and lateral left ventricular walls are monitored. *AL,* Anterior leaflet; *IVS,* interventricular septum; *LA,* left atria; *Lat,* lateral; *LV,* left ventricle; *PL,* posterior leaflet; *RA,* right atria; *RV,* right ventricle. (Reprinted with permission, Cleveland Clinic Center for Medical Art & Photography ©2021. All Rights Reserved.)

bottom. When looking at left-sided structures in ME views, the posterior left atrium (LA) is at the top of the screen and the anterior LV apex is at the bottom. Special attention should be given to the rotational position of the multiplane transducer that is displayed in the upper right corner. As shown in Fig. 26.13, in the ME view at 0 degrees, the patient's right side will be on screen left and the patient's left side on screen right. When the imaging plane is rotated to 90 degrees (Fig. 26.14), the inferior wall of the LV is on screen left, while the anterior

wall is on screen right. At 180 degrees, the mirror image of 0 degrees imaging will be displayed.[157,161]

Three Doppler techniques are used in addition to 2D echo: pulse-wave Doppler (PWD), continuous-wave Doppler (CWD), and color-flow Doppler (CFD). CFD is particularly useful in identifying valvular stenosis or regurgitation and intracardiac shunts by imaging blood flow in the heart. CFD is a form of PWD that uses the velocity and direction of blood flow to superimpose a color pattern known as *BART*

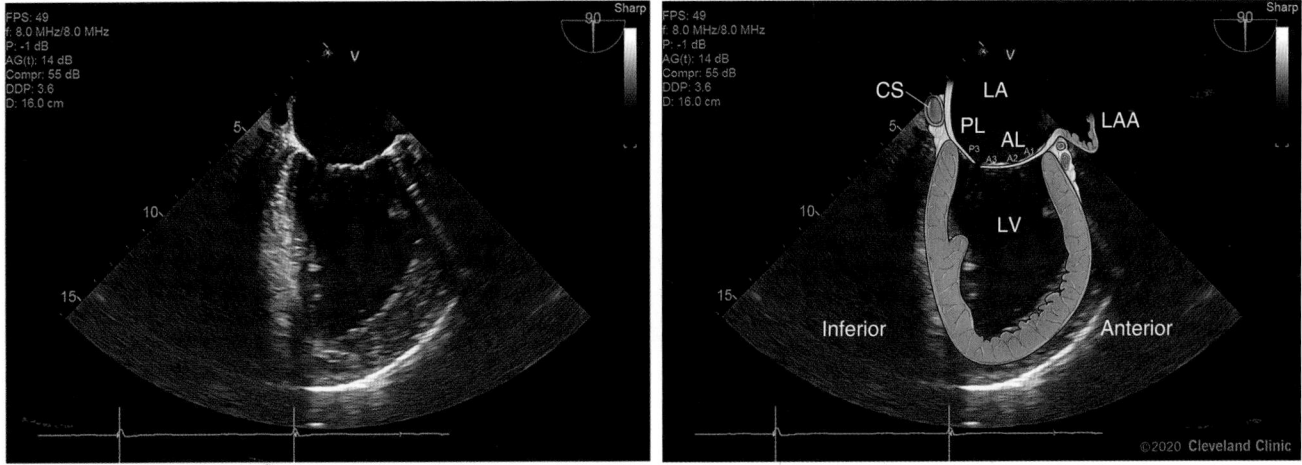

Fig. 26.14 Transesophageal echocardiography midesophageal two-chamber view displays the left atrium and ventricle with the mitral valve. The anterior and inferior walls of the left ventricle *(LV)* are monitored. *AL,* Anterior leaflet; *CS,* coronary sinus; *LA,* left atria; *LAA,* left atrial appendage; *PL,* posterior leaflet. (Reprinted with permission, Cleveland Clinic Center for Medical Art & Photography ©2021. All Rights Reserved.)

(*blue-away*; *red-toward*) technology, where blue indicates blood flow away from the transducer, and red indicates blood flow toward the transducer. There is a threshold velocity called the Nyquist limit above which the color changes to a mosaic pattern to detect turbulence or opposite color from the typical directional color pattern. This is especially useful for identifying valvular regurgitation.[154,161]

Although a comprehensive exam including 28 views is needed to accurately assess and diagnose cardiac pathology, there are views that are particularly useful for monitoring function and volume status, and these will be described in more detail. The ME four-chamber view is one of the most comprehensive and easiest to image (see Fig. 26.13). In this view, the multiplane transducer is at 0 to 20 degrees, and the probe is advanced to about 30 to 35 cm until all four chambers of the heart are imaged, along with the mitral valve and tricuspid valve. The intraatrial and intraventricular septae are imaged with the lateral wall of the LV and the free wall of the RV. The anterior leaflet of the mitral valve is adjacent to the septum, and the posterior leaflet is adjacent to the lateral wall of the LV. Turning the probe counterclockwise to the left allows imaging primarily of the left heart structures, while turning it clockwise to the right allows imaging of right heart structures. Diagnostic information can be obtained about the movement and function of the mitral valve, tricuspid valve, LV inferoseptal and anterolateral walls, and RV free wall. CFD is applied to assess valvular regurgitation. The anterior interventricular septum is perfused by the left anterior descending (LAD) artery and the posterior interventricular septum by the right coronary artery (RCA). The anterolateral wall receives a combination of blood flow from the left circumflex (LCX) artery and LAD artery.[156,157]

Turning the probe counterclockwise and focusing on the left side of the heart while rotating the multiplane transducer to between 80 and 100 degrees will generate the ME two-chamber view (see Fig. 26.14). Structures visualized in this view include the LA and left atrial appendage (LAA) at the top of the screen with the mitral valve and LV below. The LV anterior wall, whose blood supply is provided by the LAD artery, is on screen right, and the inferior wall, whose blood supply is provided by the RCA, is on screen left. The anterior leaflet of the mitral valve is adjacent to the anterior wall, and the posterior leaflet is adjacent to the inferior wall. The coronary sinus is imaged just above the posterior leaflet of the mitral valve. Diagnostic information can be obtained about LA and LV pathology, including size, wall function, or the presence of thrombus or masses. CFD is used to assess mitral stenosis and regurgitation.[156,157,161]

Rotating the multiplane transducer forward to approximately 120 to 140 degrees will image the ME long-axis (LAX) view (Fig. 26.15). In this view, the LV outflow tract (LVOT), AV, and ascending aorta can be imaged. The LA is positioned at the top of the screen with the mitral valve and LV below. The right ventricular outflow tract (RVOT) appears on the right side of the screen next to the LV. In this view, the anteroseptal LV wall, whose blood supply is provided by the LAD artery, is located on the right screen, and the inferolateral wall of the LV, whose blood supply is provided by either the LCX artery or RCA, is on the left screen. The anterior leaflet of the mitral valve is adjacent to the aorta, and the posterior leaflet is adjacent to the inferolateral wall. The ME LAX view is used to assess LA and LV size and function (including LV anteroseptal and/or inferolateral wall function), mitral valve and AV anatomy and function, and LVOT and aortic root pathology. This view is frequently used when separating from CPB to assess for air before discontinuation of the aortic root vent.[156,157,161]

The three views described earlier are useful for examining different walls of the LV and volume status. The most useful view for examining all the walls of the LV simultaneously as well as ventricular volume status is the transgastric midpapillary short-axis (TG mid-SAX) view (Fig. 26.16). With the multiplane transducer at 0 degrees, the probe is advanced into the stomach until the posterior medial papillary muscle comes into view at the top of the display. Next, the large wheel control on the handle is used to anteflex the tip so the transducer comes in contact with the gastric wall. The view is optimized by locating the anterior papillary muscle. Visualization of both the anterolateral and posteromedial papillary muscle protruding from the circular LV demonstrates that the probe is in the midventricular cross section. In this view, the RV appears like a pocket wrapped around the LV. This view, sometimes referred to as the donut view, is the only view that enables simultaneous assessment of myocardial perfusion of all LV walls supplied by all three coronary arteries. The LV inferior wall appears at the top of the screen, closest to the probe, and its blood supply is primarily the RCA. The LV anterior wall, perfused by the LAD artery, is opposite from the inferior wall and appears at the bottom of the screen. The RV appears on the left side of the screen and is perfused by the RCA and bordered by the intraventricular septum whose blood supply is the LAD artery anteriorly and the RCA posteriorly. The LV anterolateral wall, perfused by the LCX artery, appears on the right lower aspect, and the LV inferolateral (posterior) wall, perfused by a combination of RCA and LCX artery, appears on the right upper aspect. The TG

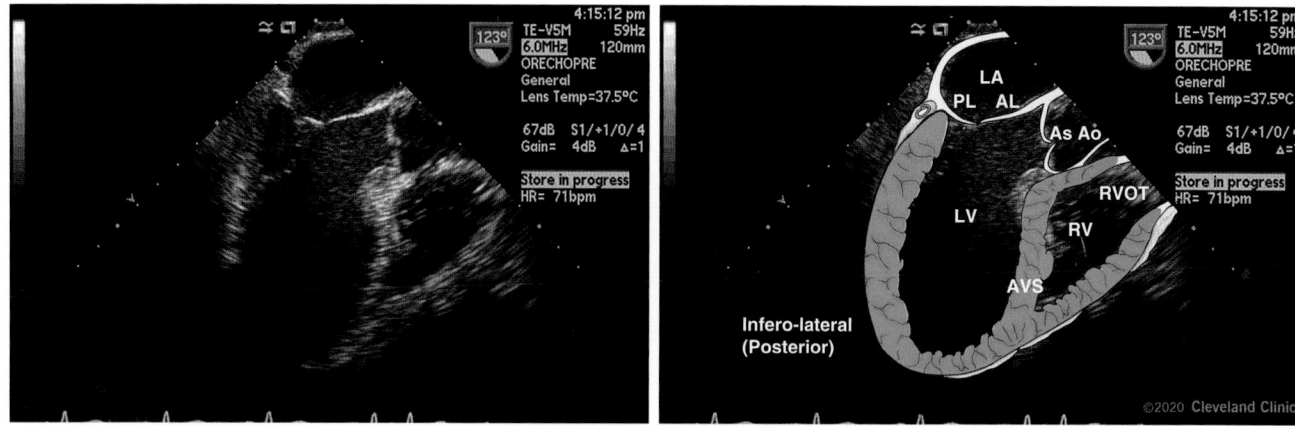

Fig. 26.15 Transesophageal echocardiography midesophageal long axis view displays the left atrium and ventricle, with the mitral and aortic valves. The anteroseptal and inferolateral left ventricular walls are monitored. *AL*, Anterior leaflet; *As Ao*, ascending aorta; *AVS*, anterior ventricular septum; *LA*, left atria; *LV*, left ventricle; *PL*, posterior leaflet; *RV*, right ventricle; *RVOT*, right ventricular outflow tract. (Reprinted with permission, Cleveland Clinic Center for Medical Art & Photography ©2021. All Rights Reserved.)

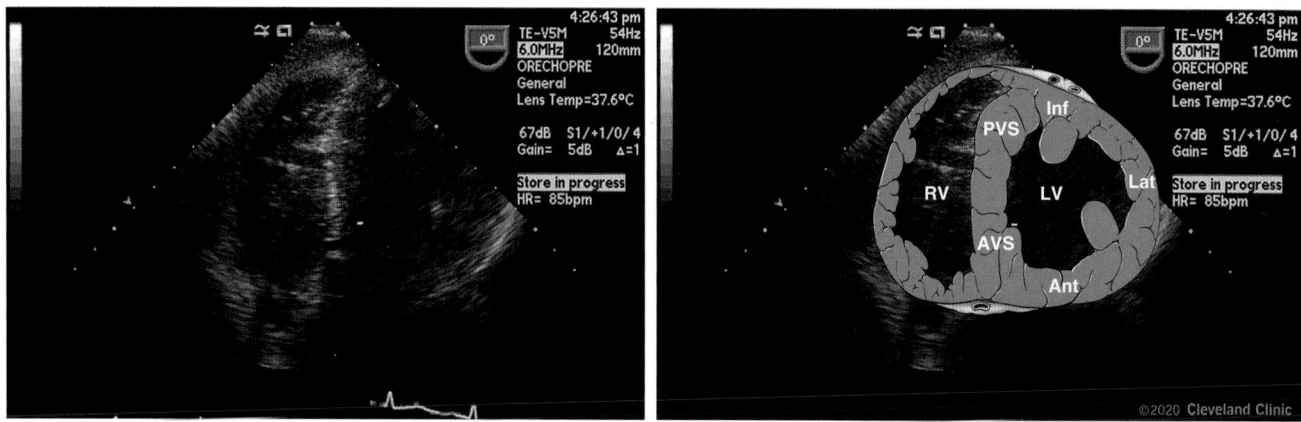

Fig. 26.16 Transesophageal echocardiography midpapillary muscle transgastric view displays the right ventricle *(RV)* and all left ventricle *(LV)* walls simultaneously. *Ant*, Anterior; *AVS*, anterior ventricular septum; *Inf*, inferior; *Lat*, lateral; *PVS*, posterior ventricular septum. (Reprinted with permission, Cleveland Clinic Center for Medical Art & Photography ©2021. All Rights Reserved.)

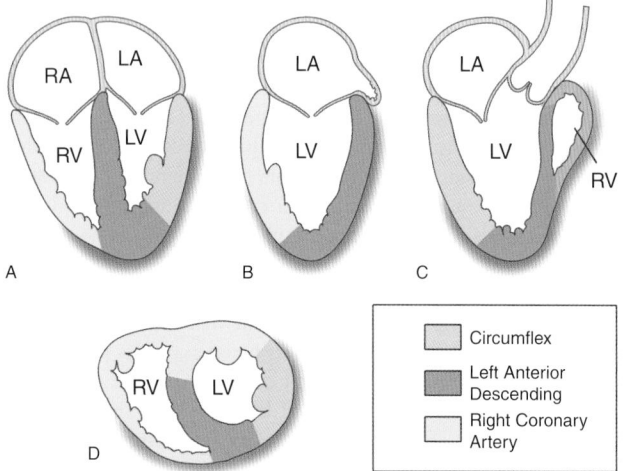

Fig. 26.17 Typical coronary flow distribution. *LA*, Left atria; *LV*, left ventricle; *RA*, right atria; *RV*, right ventricle. (Reprinted with permission, Cleveland Clinic Center for Medical Art & Photography ©2021. All Rights Reserved.)

mid-SAX view is used to examine regional wall motion. A wall that does not thicken or move toward the center of the LV is described as akinetic. A wall that moves less vigorously than normal with reduced muscle thickening is described as hypokinetic. A wall that moves outward during systole while the rest of the heart is contracting inward is described as dyskinetic and indicates infarction and the formation of a ventricular aneurysm.[162] When the patient is severely hypovolemic, the papillary muscles will touch during systole. This view enables an assessment of the patient's response to a fluid challenge. Optimization of preload will improve LV systolic function. The RV, however, should also be assessed carefully since it is more susceptible to volume. This view also enables the detection of ventricular septal defects and pericardial effusions.[156,157,161] Fig. 26.17 shows these four views along with the distribution of coronary blood flow.

Although the LV is often the focus of greatest concern during cardiac surgery, the aortic, mitral, tricuspid, and pulmonic valves, and the atria, are also of interest. The ME AV SAX view (Fig. 26.18) provides imaging of the AV in the short axis. This view is developed from the TG or ME position by withdrawing the probe into the UE and rotating the multiplane transducer to 30 to 60 degrees. Slight anteflexion may be helpful. The LA will appear at the top of the screen. The interatrial

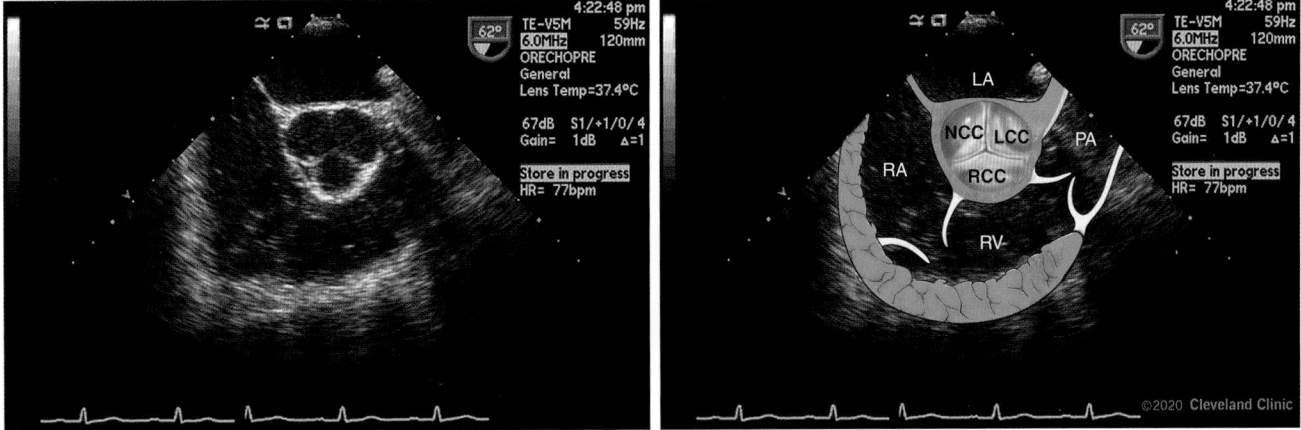

Fig. 26.18 Transesophageal echocardiography midesophageal aortic valve short axis view displays the three aortic valve leaflets with the noncoronary cusp adjacent to the intraatrial septum. *LA*, left atria; *LCC*, left coronary cusp; *NCC*, noncoronary cusp; *PA*, pulmonary artery; *RA*, right atria; *RCC*, right coronary cusp; *RV*, right ventricle. (Reprinted with permission, Cleveland Clinic Center for Medical Art & Photography ©2021. All Rights Reserved.)

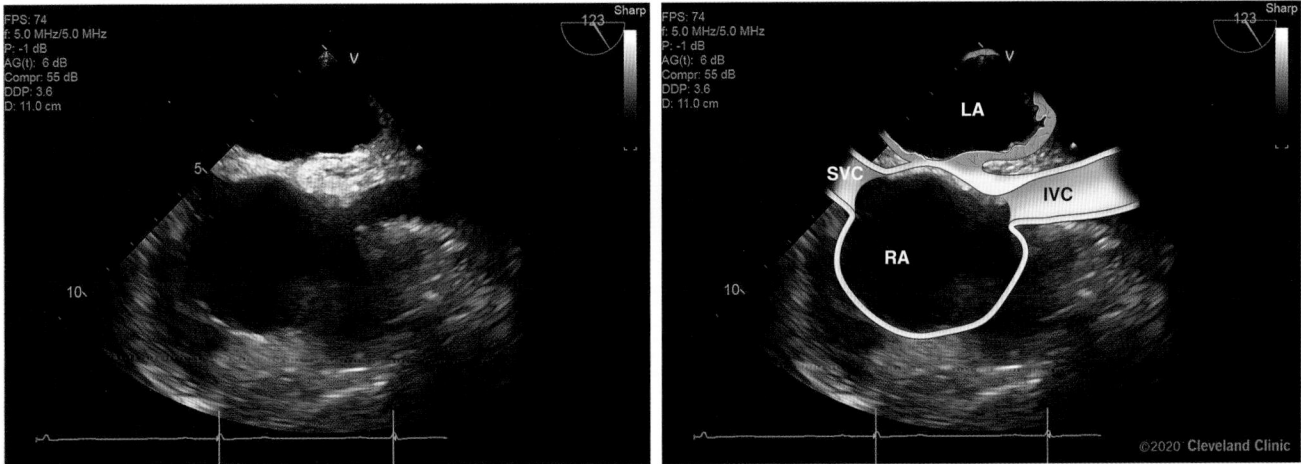

Fig. 26.19 Transesophageal echocardiography midesophageal bicaval view displays the left atrium *(LA)* and right atrium *(RA)* with the superior *(SVC)* and inferior vena cava *(IVC)*. (Reprinted with permission, Cleveland Clinic Center for Medical Art & Photography ©2021. All Rights Reserved.)

septum and RA appear on the left of the screen. The AV appears in the middle of the screen. The noncoronary cusp of a tricuspid AV is adjacent to the interatrial septum. The left coronary cusp appears on the right side below the LA. The right coronary cusp is most anterior (lower part of the screen) and adjacent the RVOT, and the pulmonary valve appears at the bottom and right side of the screen. CFD is useful for assessing shunts across a PFO or assessing for AR.[156,157,161]

Another useful view is the ME bicaval view (Fig. 26.19), which is developed by turning the probe clockwise to the right and rotating the transducer angle to 90 to 110 degrees. In this view, the LA is again at the top of the screen with the intraatrial septum appearing in the lower part of the screen. The IVC and eustachian valve appear on the left, while the RA appears in the lower middle with the right atrial appendage and the SVC appearing on the right. This view is particularly useful for guiding the placement of SVC or IVC catheters, wires, and cannulas. The intraatrial septum can be assessed using CFD to detect PFOs or ASDs. Often, a saline-contrast study is conducted using this view to assess for a smaller (probe patent) foramen ovale. Blood and saline are mixed and agitated between two 10-mL syringes (barbotage) for the test. The mixture is then injected quickly through a central line into the RA in conjunction with a Valsalva maneuver. The RA will appear to be filled with white contrast due to the gas-fluid interface from microbubbles and turbulent flow. The test is considered positive when three or more bubbles cross the interatrial septum within five heartbeats.[156,157,161]

Other extended monitors. The use of other extended monitors is related to personal preference (e.g., bispectral index [BIS] monitor) or case requirement (e.g., cerebral oximetry in surgery on the aortic arch). The BIS monitor has not been shown to reliably prevent recall,[163] but the trend is useful in detecting changes in anesthetic depth. The BIS monitor can serve as a reminder to the practitioner to administer medication to prevent recall when the inhalation agent is titrated down during periods of hemodynamic instability or when ventilation is held frequently at the surgeon's request.

Cerebral oximetry uses near-infrared regional spectroscopy (NIRS) technology, which is similar to that used in pulse oximetry. It has proven beneficial in both cardiac and major vascular surgery, especially when the procedure requires DHCA. A relative decrease in regional saturation to less than 70% of baseline or an absolute level of less than 50% is associated with an increase in adverse outcomes such as stroke, postoperative cognitive dysfunction, organ dysfunction, and mortality. NIRS has been used to extend the "safe time" of DHCA and to identify

SVC cannula malposition. NIRS helps the practitioner assess the adequacy of cerebral oxygenation and the effectiveness of interventions such as increasing BP, administering volume, or adjusting ventilation to improve oxygenation.[164,165]

Selection of medications. An enormous body of information has accumulated regarding the cardiovascular effects of various anesthetic agents. The most significant considerations are highlighted. Traditionally, the choice of anesthetic has been based primarily on preexisting ventricular function and comorbidities, coupled with the desired length of action. However, the same anesthetic combinations may cause different responses in patients with similar histories and hemodynamic profiles. Therefore the combination of medications selected for the anesthetic is far less important than the skill and judgment with which they are administered.

Inhalation anesthetics. Inhalation anesthetic agents cause myocardial depression, vasodilation, and hypotension in a dose-dependent manner. They lower the arrhythmogenic threshold to catecholamines and do not provide pain relief in the postoperative period. Newer evidence shows that the myocardial depression caused by inhalation agents is dose dependent and that they reduce myocardial infarct size by protecting the myocardium from ischemia (preconditioning effect) and reperfusion injury (postconditioning effect).[33,166,167] Other advantages include the ability to produce amnesia and blunt the sympathetic response to surgical stress and CPB. Several meta-analyses demonstrate improved outcomes when inhalation anesthetics are included as part of the anesthetic plan. Benefits include reduced troponin release, inotropic requirements, time to extubation, length of stay in the ICU and hospital, and mortality.[34,36,168-170] Desflurane is a potential concern because sudden increases in inspired concentration can lead to tachycardia and hypertension, which can be detrimental in patients who have CAD, hypertrophic cardiomyopathy (HCM), or stenotic valvular lesions. Desflurane and nitrous oxide (N_2O) raise pulmonary vascular resistance, PA pressure, and wedge pressure.[168] N_2O should be avoided just before, during, and after CPB because of the potential for expansion of air introduced into the circulation during bypass. N_2O also may cause catecholamine release and LV dysfunction.[171]

Opioids. Opioids do not cause direct myocardial depression and maintain stable hemodynamics.[172] Therefore a high-dose narcotic technique (fentanyl 100–200 mcg/kg) became popular in past decades.[55] Problems with the technique included significant bradycardia, recall, chest-wall rigidity, and prolonged intubation. Today, a primary narcotic technique is reserved for hemodynamically unstable patients. Currently, inhalation agents are often combined with modest doses of narcotics (fentanyl 5–20 mcg/kg or sufentanil 2–10 mcg/kg) in a balanced technique. The fentanyl derivatives are most popular, but morphine, hydromorphone, and other narcotics can also be used effectively. This trend favors fast-track (early) extubation in cardiac surgery since the decreased length of stay translates into reduced cost without increasing adverse outcomes.[173-175] Thus the goal of early extubation, generally within several hours, is now a major consideration in the selection of medications. The opioid crisis has also impacted cardiac surgery. Guidelines for enhanced recovery after cardiac surgery were recently published that give the use of acetaminophen, tramadol, gabapentin, and dexmedetomidine a class I recommendation to reduce postoperative pain.[175]

Sedation. Sedation before induction can be accomplished with low doses (1–4 mg) of midazolam. Caution is advised because the combination of a benzodiazepine and fentanyl-type drugs reduces systemic vascular resistance (SVR) and causes myocardial depression leading to hypotension. Sedation for transport to the ICU is often facilitated with infusions of propofol or dexmedetomidine.[55,113]

Induction agents. Induction of anesthesia can be accomplished with any of the agents alone or in combination with narcotics, volatile agents, or benzodiazepines. Etomidate causes less myocardial depression than propofol, therefore it may be preferable for use in patients who have reduced left ventricular function.[172] The significance of the adrenal suppression caused by etomidate has been the subject of much debate. A large review of studies involving single-dose etomidate induction versus other standard induction agents showed an increased incidence of adrenal insufficiency in critically ill patients.[176] However, a 2015 study of patients having cardiac surgery concluded that the adrenal suppression caused by etomidate lasted less than 24 hours and had no significant impact on outcome. Furthermore, etomidate provided more stable hemodynamic parameters when used for induction of anesthesia as compared to propofol in patients with poor LV function.[177] If adrenal insufficiency is suspected, a dose of a steroid such as hydrocortisone (100 mg IV) may be administered. Etomidate and propofol may cause pain with injection, but this can be blunted by diluting the drug and giving it slowly and/or by administering IV lidocaine or narcotic prophylactically.

Muscle relaxants. Muscle relaxants are needed to facilitate tracheal intubation, prevent movement during cannulation, and attenuate skeletal muscle contraction from shivering or defibrillation. Most nondepolarizing muscle relaxants used today lack significant cardiac effects. The choice of relaxant is based on the airway examination, patient history, and procedure length. Succinylcholine is often preferred for management of a difficult airway.[55]

Antibiotic prophylaxis. The STS has published guidelines for antibiotic prophylaxis in cardiac surgery that were reaffirmed in 2019.[175,178] A β-lactam antibiotic (cephalosporin) is the prophylactic antibiotic of choice (class IA) for cardiac surgical patients who are not at increased risk for MRSA. Cefazolin is administered within an hour of skin incision with a weight-based dose (1 g if ≤60 kg, 2 g if >60 kg, or 3 g if >120 kg). The dose should be repeated every 3 to 4 hours while the surgical incision is open. Cefuroxime 1.5 g IV is an alternative to cefazolin. Patients at increased risk for MRSA (known or presumed), including those undergoing an operation using prosthetic valvular or vascular material, should have vancomycin 1 to 1.5 g (or 15 mg/kg weight-adjusted dose) added. Vancomycin should be administered slowly over 60 to 90 minutes depending on the dose. Patients with a known β-lactam allergy should receive vancomycin and an antimicrobial with gram-negative coverage. The guidelines suggest an aminoglycoside such as gentamicin at 4 mg/kg, but a nonnephrotoxic antimicrobial like aztreonam is also acceptable. Redosing of vancomycin and the aminoglycoside is not recommended. The Surgical Care Improvement Project (SCIP) guidelines recommend that the antibiotic be administered within 1 hour of incision or 2 hours for vancomycin.[111,175,179]

Intraoperative Management

This section focuses on the management of general cardiac surgery from the time patients enter the OR until their care is safely transitioned to the ICU team. A sequential description of events that occur during most cases requiring CPB is described, so that the reader can gain an understanding of important perioperative milestones. The rationale for pharmacologic and hemodynamic management as well as patient monitoring was previously discussed. A discussion of the management of specific cases and specialized equipment follows.

The cardiothoracic OR is a fast-paced, high-intensity environment where up to a dozen practitioners must focus for extended periods. The patient population is high risk because of the prevalence of multiple comorbidities in addition to their primary cardiac pathology. The surgical procedures can be complex, and manipulation of the heart and vasculature can profoundly impact hemodynamic function. The anesthetist is required to intently focus on both the surgical procedure and the patient's response to widely varying levels of stimulation. Problems must be anticipated, and interventions must be prompt. Throughout the process, communication among the anesthesia, surgical, nursing, and perfusion teams is critical. Failure to communicate can have devastating consequences. Closed-loop communication, the practice of clearly repeating back information when one team member makes a request of another, is imperative for safety.[180]

Precardiopulmonary bypass period. The precardiopulmonary bypass period begins when the patient arrives at the operating suite and ends when the patient is on CPB. A review of the patient's preoperative vital signs and cardiac function will help the anesthetist determine the "normal" range for that individual. The general goal is to maintain hemodynamic stability. Individual hemodynamic perturbations must be considered within the context of the patient's baseline status. For example, a patient with an acceptable heart rate, MAP, O_2 saturation, and arterial pH does not need an inotropic agent if the cardiac index (CI) is below the normal range. In this particular instance, general anesthesia reduces O_2 demand, and the decreased CO is frequently adequate to meet demand. Starting an infusion of an inotrope to increase the CI within the normal range (>2.2 L/min/m^2) might paradoxically lead to ischemia by increasing myocardial O_2 demand.[181]

The prebypass period is marked by periods of widely variable stimulation. The most intense stimulation occurs at intubation, incision, sternal split and spread, sympathetic nerve dissection, pericardial incision, and aortic cannulation. Hypertension and tachycardia that occur as a result of inadequate analgesia or sympathetic activation can lead to ischemia, dysrhythmias, or heart failure. The anesthetist must anticipate these events and consider a preemptive dose of a narcotic and/or an increase in the concentration of the volatile agent. Hyperdynamic individuals may also need the addition of a short-acting β-antagonist such as esmolol (0.1–0.5 mg/kg) or an IV infusion of a titratable vasodilator such as nitroglycerin to treat the adrenergic response to these events. During the remainder of the prebypass period, including preincision and the harvesting of conduit, there is little stimulation, and the BP and heart rate tend to decrease. Hypotension and significant bradycardia may decrease the CPP and lead to ischemia. Oftentimes, intermittent boluses of phenylephrine or ephedrine may be required to support coronary perfusion.[55,162]

Preinduction period. During the preinduction period, the patient is identified and interviewed before entering the OR. The information from the preoperative assessment is reviewed, and the anesthetist confirms that there have been no significant changes in the patient's medical condition, with a particular focus on worsening symptoms and recent infectious illness. The airway is examined, and the lungs and heart are auscultated. Medications taken within the last 24 hours are recorded. The patient's willingness to accept blood products is confirmed. The interview also allows the anesthesia provider to assess patient anxiety, communicate expectations, and provide emotional support.

Once in the OR, areas prone to pressure ischemia such as the sacrum and heels may be protected by the application of foam pads. The perioperative management of ICDs and pacemakers, if present, was discussed earlier. External adhesive defibrillator pads are usually placed for patients with deactivated ICDs or a history of recent serious ventricular ectopy, as well as those having minimally invasive surgery or a repeat sternotomy. A "huddle" is performed where the surgeon and patient, together with the nursing, anesthesia, and perfusion teams, review the operative plan, needed equipment, and safety checklists. Next, the patient is moved to the OR table and standard monitors are applied (see Table 26.6). Pulse oximetry volume is adjusted to a level

that is loud enough to provide an audible warning to the clinician in case of decreasing O_2 saturation while attention is focused on another task. Some centers routinely administer supplemental O_2 during the preinduction phase, whereas others use O_2 as needed. A large-bore peripheral IV catheter (14 or 16 gauge) is placed using local anesthesia for patient comfort. Patients with normal ventricular function will often benefit from supplemental sedation, especially during invasive monitor placement. The location and timing of invasive lines were discussed in the monitoring section of the chapter. A baseline ABG and ACT are drawn from the A line. Central venous access is most often deferred until after induction, but regardless of the timing, baseline measurements are recorded after placement. When the patient and all teams (nursing, perfusion, surgery, and anesthesia) are prepared, induction can begin.[113,181]

Induction and intubation. The plan for induction is based on the length and complexity of the proposed procedure, as well as multiple patient-specific considerations, including cardiac pathology, comorbidities, ventricular function, and the airway examination. No combination of induction medications has proven superior in cardiac anesthesia. Rather, the artful skill each practitioner uses to administer preferred drugs to achieve hemodynamic stability throughout induction and intubation is most important. Generally, a combination of a sedative, hypnotic, opioid, volatile agent, and muscle relaxant, with or without lidocaine and/or a β-blocker, is used. Achieving hemodynamic stability can be especially challenging when a difficult airway must be secured. After intubation and confirmation of correct ETT placement, the fresh gas flows are adjusted; 100% O_2 has been advocated for cardiac surgery to maximize O_2 tensions, but a lower inspired concentration may prevent absorption atelectasis and reduce the risk of O_2 toxicity.[182,183] Inhalation anesthetics have been correlated with improved outcomes in cardiac anesthesia most likely because of the pre- and postconditioning effects.[35,170,184] Patients with severe LV dysfunction may require a primary narcotic technique because all inhalational agents cause some degree of myocardial depression and afterload reduction. Enhanced recovery after surgery (ERAS) protocols should also be given consideration.[175]

Preincision period. The preincision period is generally not very stimulating, so the anesthetic level can often be reduced. Occasional boluses of phenylephrine may be required for hemodynamic support. A second peripheral intravenous (PIV) line is inserted if needed, and central access is obtained. The stomach is decompressed with an OG tube before the placement of the TEE probe. Considerations for TEE probe placement can be found in the monitoring section of the chapter. The urinary catheter (which often includes a temperature sensor) is inserted, and a nasopharyngeal temperature probe may be placed.

Next, the patient is carefully positioned, and pressure points are padded. All routine positioning precautions apply along with some areas of special concern. Brachial plexus injury can occur if the arms are hyperextended or if the chest wall retraction is excessive.[113] Brachial and radial artery or nerve compression can occur if the upper arm is compressed by the ether screen or the post that is sometimes used to support the chest wall retractor during dissection of the internal mammary artery (IMA), also referred to as the ITA.[113] Occipital alopecia is a problem that develops in the weeks after surgery. The head should be placed on a well-padded surface and repositioned frequently during the operation. Nothing that can cause pressure, such as the ECG cable, should be placed under the patient's head.[181]

After final positioning, the anesthetist reconfirms the ETT position. The antibiotic infusion is completed (vancomycin may take longer), and the antifibrinolytic agent, if used, is initiated. Proper placement of monitors and lines is verified. Transducers are placed at heart level and zeroed to atmospheric pressure. All lines and access ports are labeled and neatly secured for easy access. Hemodynamic parameters, ABGs, and blood chemistry are all rechecked as needed and abnormalities are treated. Mild hypokalemia is not typically treated during the pre-CPB period since the cardioplegia solution contains significant amounts of potassium.[181] Insulin infusions may be required to lower the serum glucose level, especially in those with diabetes mellitus. The STS guidelines recommend that blood glucose levels greater than 180 mg/dL be treated with an insulin infusion in both diabetic and nondiabetic patients.[108] Insulin is titrated cautiously to avoid dramatic changes in serum glucose levels.

Incision to bypass. The incision-to-bypass period begins with intensely stimulating events: incision, sternotomy, and sternal spread. The anesthetist should prepare for these events by deepening the anesthetic and administering additional muscle relaxant if needed. The highest rate of recall in cardiac surgery has been recorded during this period, therefore an amnestic can be given if not previously administered.[185] The lungs are deflated during sternotomy to decrease the risk of cardiac or pulmonary laceration.

Repeat or redo sternotomy requires greater preparation and vigilance. Patients who have had a prior CABG may have an arterial or venous bypass graft lying directly beneath the sternum. Patients who have had prior cardiac surgery or chest radiation (often for breast cancer or lymphoma) can also have adherent scar tissue that is difficult to dissect. In these situations, the surgical team will examine the patient's lateral radiograph and possibly a MRI or computed tomography (CT) scan to determine the proximity of the cardiac structures to the sternum. If the heart appears to be adherent to the sternum, there are several management options for sternotomy and dissection. Some surgeons may expose the femoral vessels so they can quickly cannulate and institute CPB if arterial or cardiac trauma occurs during sternotomy. Other surgeons will cannulate the femoral vessels before sternotomy and institute CPB during dissection (the heart is not arrested and continues beating). Still others will sew a graft onto the right subclavian artery for arterial cannulation and use the femoral vein for venous access. An oscillating saw is often selected to perform a slow, cautious sternotomy. Communication between the surgeon and anesthetist is crucial because the lungs may need to be deflated several times for short periods. In the rare event that a cardiac structure or great vessel is damaged and bleeding becomes uncontrollable, it may become necessary to "crash on pump." IV heparin (400 units/kg) is promptly administered through the central line. If the patient is not already cannulated, the surgeon will emergently place the arterial cannula in the femoral artery or aorta, and the cardiotomy suckers will be used for venous return in what is sometimes referred to as "sucker bypass." BP is kept high enough to maintain adequate coronary perfusion, yet hypertension must be avoided to minimize excess bleeding. Crystalloid or colloid can be administered if necessary, but hemodilution will exacerbate preexisting anemia. PRBCs should be readily available in all redo or postradiation sternotomies because the potential for inadvertent vascular injury is significantly increased.[55,181]

After sternotomy, the conduit will be harvested if the procedure involves a CABG. The anesthetic considerations related to conduit harvesting are reviewed later in the chapter during the discussion of CABG. If no conduit is required, the heart and vascular structures are dissected as individual exposure requirements of the surgical procedure dictate. The period of harvesting and dissection is generally less stimulating, so anesthetic levels may be reduced. Vigilance is required so the surgeon can be alerted when excessive manipulation results in hypotension and/or dysrhythmias. Hypotension frequently responds to placing the patient in the Trendelenburg position (head down) and administering small doses of phenylephrine. The surgeon may

ask for ventilation to be held and the lungs deflated to improve the surgical view. The anesthetist is cautioned against silencing the apnea alarm when ventilation is held as the alarm serves as a reminder to the entire team that ventilation must be resumed. Inadvertent failure to ventilate is a hazard in cardiac anesthesia that can have devastating consequences. Both sympathetic nerve dissection and opening of the pericardium are additional stimulating events that may require an increased depth of anesthesia. Lifting the pericardium, on the other hand, is associated with bradycardia and hypotension because changing the position of the heart impedes venous return and may activate the parasympathetic nervous system. Most patients respond to small doses of phenylephrine or ephedrine, but occasionally the anesthetist must ask the surgeon to decrease tension on the pericardial sutures. After the pericardium is opened, surgical preparation for cannulation begins.[55,113,181]

Cannulation. Cannulation is the next major event in the prebypass period (Fig. 26.20). Full heparinization is essential before cannulation. Heparin (400 units/kg) is administered through a central line, after aspiration of blood confirms line patency and ensures intravascular administration. The ACT or heparin concentration assay is checked 3 to 5 minutes after the heparin is administered.[61] Muscle relaxants are given if needed because movement during cannulation could prove disastrous. The aortic cannula is placed first, followed by the single venous cannula or double venous cannulas (see Fig. 26.9). The retrograde cardioplegia cannula may then be inserted, or the surgeon may wait until after CPB is initiated. Once on CPB, the antegrade cannula is inserted proximal to the aortic cannula; this cannula will also be used at the end of bypass to suction air bubbles coming from the heart and will then be referred to as the aortic root vent.[61]

Surgical manipulation of the heart and great vessels during cannulation often leads to hypotension and dysrhythmias; therefore careful attention and clear communication among the anesthetist, surgeon, and perfusionist are critical. The process should not begin until 3 minutes after heparin administration. Before the aortic cannula is placed, BP is decreased to a systolic blood pressure (SBP) of 90 to 100 mm Hg or a MAP of 60 to 70 mm Hg to decrease the risk of aortic dissection.[58,61] Strategies to lower the BP include deepening the anesthetic, raising the head of the bed, or cautiously titrating vasodilators. The aortic cannula and aortic line from the CPB machine are connected and inspected, and all air bubbles are purged. Complications of aortic cannulation include arterial dissection, hemorrhage, plaque or air embolization, and inadvertent placement of the distal tip of the cannula in an aortic arch vessel. Once aortic cannulation is completed, the perfusionist will confirm intraarterial placement by verifying pressure variation in the manometer connected to the aortic line, referred to as "checking the swing." A test transfusion is then administered to confirm normal flow and pressure into the aortic cannula. Following aortic cannulation, BP is allowed to increase. Vasodilators, if used, are discontinued, the anesthetic level is returned to normal, and the head of the bed is leveled. The perfusionist can give volume through the aortic line to augment MAP as needed.[55]

Next, the venous cannulas are placed. Again, the anesthetist should watch for hypotension, dysrhythmias, or hemorrhage. When placement is completed, the perfusionist may initiate the RAP process and hypotension may occur.[186] Finally, the surgeon may choose to place the retrograde cardioplegia cannula.[65] The retrograde cannula is sometimes connected to a pressure transducer to monitor the mean pressure. The baseline retrograde pressure is generally reflective of venous pressure and should increase approximately 20 mm Hg when retrograde cardioplegia is infused. If the retrograde pressure is low, it could indicate that the cannula has fallen into the atria; if it is too high

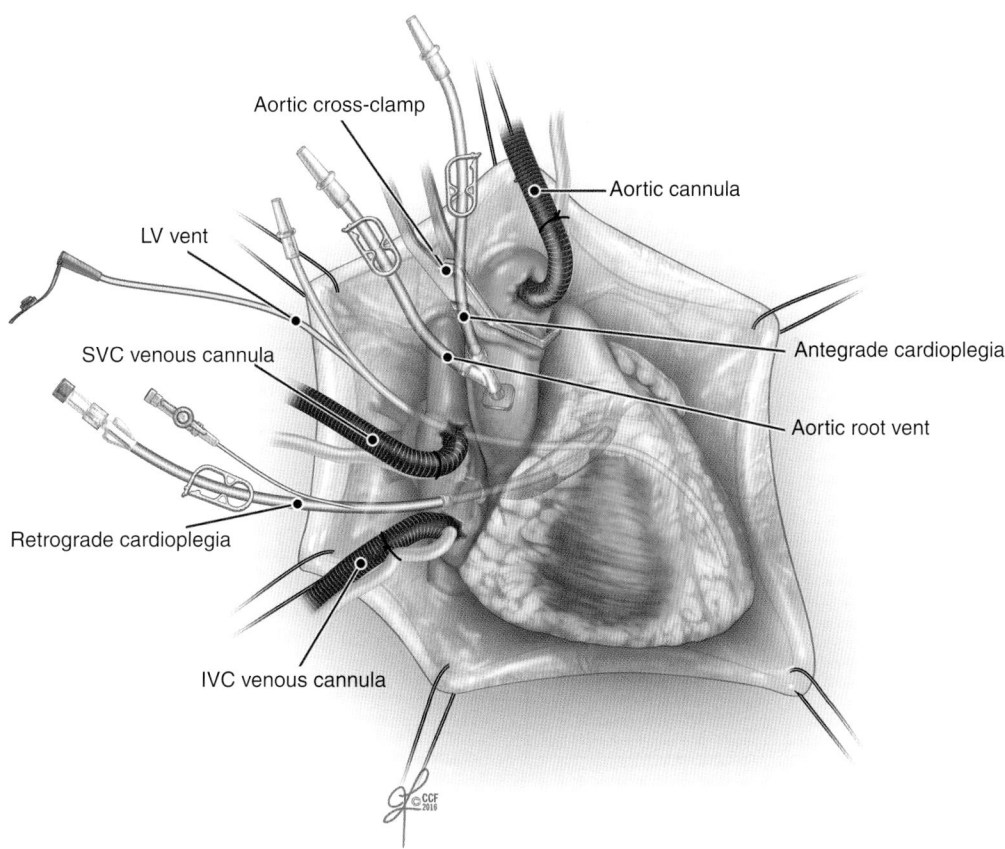

Fig. 26.20 Full cannulation for cardiopulmonary bypass (CPB). Deoxygenated venous blood is drained from the patient to the CPB machine via two separate venous cannulas (bicaval cannulation). One cannula is placed into the superior vena cava *(SVC)* and the other into the inferior vena cava *(IVC)*. Oxygenated and filtered blood from the CPB machine returns to the patient via the aortic cannula that is located distal to the aortic cross-clamp and proximal to the innominate. Cardioplegia may be administered antegrade down the coronary arteries via a cannula placed in the aorta just proximal to the cross-clamp. Cardioplegia is sometimes administered retrograde into the venous system via a balloon-tipped cannula placed in the coronary sinus. Vents are used to decompress the left ventricle *(LV vent)* and to remove air from the ascending aorta *(root vent)*. Note that the aortic vent is the same cannula that is used for antegrade cardioplegia. A Y-connector and clamps are used to control flow. (Reprinted with permission, Cleveland Clinic Center for Medical Art & Photography ©2021. All rights reserved.)

(>40 mm Hg), the catheter could be positioned too distally, increasing the risk of coronary sinus rupture. Box 26.2 contains a preparation-for-bypass checklist.[55]

Cardiopulmonary bypass period

Initiation. CPB can be initiated after the ACT is greater than 480 seconds. The venous clamp is first released, allowing blood to fill the venous reservoir; then the arterial clamp is removed, initiating CPB. Adequate venous drainage is necessary so the pump flow can be gradually increased to reach a calculated CI of 2.0 to 2.5 L/min/m². Acceptable venous drainage usually correlates with a CVP of less than 5 mm Hg and possibly a negative pressure if VAVD is used.[61] The heart should appear empty and not distended. Hypotension is common at the initiation of CPB and is most likely related to reduction in SVR due to instantaneous hemodilution and reduced blood viscosity. Phenylephrine boluses administered by the perfusionist are frequently required to augment the MAP during the initial phase of CPB. The most ominous reason for significant persistent hypotension (MAP <30 mm Hg) is an aortic dissection.[61] The diagnosis can be confirmed by TEE, and/or the surgeon may note a hematoma on the wall of the aorta. If a dissection is suspected, CPB must be discontinued until the aorta can be recannulated distal to the dissection. Other causes of persistent hypotension while on CPB include vasoplegia and sepsis.

When the CPB machine reaches full flow there will no longer be a pulsatile trace visible on the PA or A line, indicating that blood is now bypassing the lungs. Consequently, mechanical ventilation is discontinued, but the low flow oxygen (0.2 L/min) is maintained. Some surgeons choose to maintain ventilation on CPB using low tidal volumes with slow respiratory rates since newer evidence suggests that postbypass oxygenation and lung mechanics are improved.[187] During CPB, the anesthetist must ensure that adequate levels of anesthetic and muscle relaxant are maintained.[61] Confirmation that the perfusionist has turned on the vaporizer that administers the volatile anesthetic via the pump oxygenator is crucial. The perfusionist can also give IV medications via a stopcock sampling manifold attached to both the arterial and venous lines of the CPB pump. The infusion of all IV fluids and most medications are stopped. Insulin and antifibrinolytics, if used, are continued. Hyperglycemia usually manifests during CPB, especially with the use of Buckberg cardioplegia, which has high glucose content, necessitating the use of insulin. The PAC, if present, should be pulled back 2 to 3 cm to prevent pulmonary rupture.[58] Sometimes the surgeon will complete the dissection of the heart while it is still beating on CPB before applying the aortic cross-clamp. The vent for the LV is most often inserted through the right superior pulmonary vein at this time.

BOX 26.2 Preparation for Bypass: Prebypass Checklist

1. Anticoagulation
   a. Heparin administered
   b. Desired level of anticoagulation achieved
2. Arterial cannulation
   a. Absence of bubbles in arterial line
   b. Evidence of dissection or malposition?
3. Venous cannulation
   a. Evidence of superior vena cava obstruction?
   b. Evidence of inferior vena cava obstruction?
4. Pulmonary artery catheter (if used) pulled back
5. Are all monitoring/access catheters functional?
6. Transesophageal echocardiograph (if used)
   a. In "freeze" mode
   b. Scope in neutral/unlocked position
7. Supplemental medications
   a. Neuromuscular blockers
   b. Anesthetics, analgesics, amnestic
8. Inspection of head and neck
   a. Color
   b. Symmetry
   c. Venous drainage
   d. Pupils

From Grocott HP, et al. Cardiopulmonary bypass management and organ protection. In Kaplan JA, et al., eds. *Kaplan's Cardiac Anesthesia: For Cardiac and Noncardiac Surgery.* 7th ed. Philadelphia: Elsevier; 2017:1139.

BOX 26.3 Anesthesia Checklist at the Initiation of CPB

Face	Examine for color, temperature, plethora, edema, and symmetry
Eyes	Examine pupils for size and symmetry and conjunctiva for edema
CPB lines	Arteriovenous color difference should be visible
PAC	If present, pull back 3–4 cm. Mean pressure should be <15 mm Hg
CVP	<5 mm Hg, possibly negative with VAVD
Heart	Avoid distension
Ventilation	Stop when PA ejection and/or aortic ejection ceases

CPB, Cardiopulmonary bypass; *CVP,* central venous pressure; *PA,* pulmonary artery; *PAC,* pulmonary artery catheter; *VAVD,* vacuum-assisted venous drainage.

Next, the surgeon will ask the perfusionist to temporarily decrease the CPB flow while the aortic cross-clamp is applied. The clamp time is noted, and full CPB flow is then resumed. Antegrade cardioplegia is infused through a catheter placed in the aorta between the cross-clamp and the AV (see Fig. 26.9). As the infusion of the high-potassium solution reaches the myocardium via the coronary arteries, the QRS progressively widens until the heart arrests in diastole, and electrical and mechanical asystole should ensue quickly. Any heart rhythm besides asystole indicates incomplete myocardial protection and the need for additional cardioplegia. Retrograde cardioplegia through the coronary sinus may also be administered, or cardioplegia may be given directly into the coronary ostia if the aorta is opened.[65] At this time, active cooling may begin, if indicated, or the patient's temperature can drift down gradually.[58] Box 26.3 contains a checklist of items the anesthetist should check after bypass is initiated.

Maintenance. The flow rate on CPB is maintained at 50 to 60 mL/kg/min to reach a calculated CI of 2.0 to 2.5 L/min/m². An acceptable MAP on CPB is no less than 50 to 60 mm Hg. Older patients or those with known carotid disease should have a higher MAP, closer to 60 to 70 mm Hg, to ensure adequate cerebral perfusion pressure.[58,72] The mixed venous O_2 saturation should be monitored and maintained above 70%. A light anesthetic level may manifest as hypertension, which can be treated by increasing the inhalational agent on the pump or by administering a supplemental dose of IV narcotic or benzodiazepine. If hypertension persists, a vasodilator may be added. Hypotension is usually treated with bolus doses of phenylephrine by the perfusionist, but occasionally an infusion of a vasopressor may be needed. The train-of-four should be completely suppressed to prevent movement or shivering during CPB as it greatly increases O_2 consumption, which may manifest as low O_2 on the venous gas sensor.[58]

ABGs and ACTs are monitored every 30 minutes by the perfusionist, and acid-base imbalances are corrected as needed.[61] Depending on the patient's hematocrit and comorbidities, as well as the complexity of the surgical procedure, blood may be needed. Blood glucose may increase to a level that requires treatment with an insulin infusion. Patients often develop some level of hyperkalemia related to the potassium in the cardioplegia solution; however, an insulin infusion can counter this problem by driving potassium into the cell.[65,72,77] Urine output is monitored and 1 mL/kg/hr is considered satisfactory. If urine output is low and the pump volume is adequate, the addition of a diuretic can be considered, especially if the patient was taking a diuretic preoperatively.[58] If the hematocrit is low, hemoconcentration (ultrafiltration) through the CPB circuit can be considered as a blood conservation technique.

Preparation for separation from CPB. Box 26.4 outlines many of the factors that must be considered in preparation for separation from CPB. The need for possible inotropic or vasopressor support is anticipated, and infusions are prepared. Rewarming begins as the surgeon is completing the repair. The process is begun early enough to facilitate slow, gradual warming to a nasopharyngeal or bladder temperature of 36°C to 37°C.[188] A slower rate of warming is associated with better cognitive function 6 weeks post CABG.[189] During rewarming, the bladder temperature may lag 2°C to 4°C behind the nasopharyngeal or esophageal temperatures.[190]

Arterial and venous blood gases are normalized before termination of CPB. Potassium levels are addressed if greater than 5.5 mEq/L or less than 4.0 mEq/L, to decrease the incidence of dysrhythmias. If the patient is hyperkalemic, calcium may also be given to counteract the potassium and stabilize the membrane to prevent dysrhythmias. The administration of calcium is controversial. Some clinicians have a low threshold for treating low ionized calcium, given its beneficial positive inotropic effects and its essential role in the coagulation cascade.[191] Other clinicians avoid calcium because it contributes to coronary vasospasm and may exacerbate reperfusion injury.[192] Magnesium (2–4 g IV) is frequently administered prophylactically to minimize dysrhythmias, including AF.[193] In a recent meta-analysis, CABG patients who received IV magnesium intraoperatively experienced a significant reduction in postoperative AF.[194] Treatment for high glucose levels should continue, but the rate of insulin infusion often can be lowered significantly, especially in a nondiabetic patient after separation from CPB.

An adequate circulating blood volume is necessary for separation from CPB. The amount needed varies with the patient's weight, prebypass volume status, ventricular function, and comorbidities. As

BOX 26.4   Preparation for Separation-From-Bypass Checklist

1. Air clearance maneuvers completed
2. Rewarming completed
    a. Nasopharyngeal temperature 36°C–37°C
    b. Rectal/bladder temperature ≥35°C, but ≤37°C
3. Address issue of adequacy of anesthesia and muscle relaxation
4. Obtain stable cardiac rate and rhythm (use pacing if necessary)
5. Pump flow and systemic arterial pressure
    a. Pump flow to maintain mixed venous saturation ≥70%
    b. Systemic pressure restored to normothermic levels
6. Metabolic parameters
    a. Arterial pH, Po_2, Pco_2 within normal limits
    b. Hematocrit: 20%–25%
    c. K+: 4–5 mEq/L
    d. Ionized calcium
7. Ensuring all monitoring/access catheters functional?
    a. Transducers rezeroed
    b. TEE (if used) out of freeze mode
8. Respiratory management
    a. Atelectasis cleared/lungs reexpanded
    b. Evidence of pneumothorax?
    c. Residual fluid in thoracic cavities drained
    d. Ventilation reinstituted
9. Intravenous fluids restarted
10. Inotropes/vasopressors/vasodilators prepared

K^+, potassium; Pco_2, partial pressure of carbon dioxide; Po_2, partial pressure of oxygen; *TEE*, transesophageal echocardiography.
From Grocott HP, et al. Cardiopulmonary bypass management and organ protection. In Kaplan JA, et al., eds. *Kaplan's Cardiac Anesthesia: For Cardiac and Noncardiac Surgery.* 7th ed. Philadelphia: Elsevier; 2017:1141.

previously indicated, the ideal hematocrit is controversial, but most cardiac surgical patients require a hematocrit of 22% to 25% to ensure adequate tissue perfusion.[67]

As the cardiac chambers are surgically closed, the lungs are inflated to push air from the heart and pulmonary veins and to assist in filling the heart. Terminal warm reperfusion cardioplegia solution (the hot shot) is administered, and the perfusionist lowers the pump flow temporarily as the surgeon removes the aortic cross-clamp. The time of clamp removal is noted. It is not uncommon for the heart to fibrillate, especially if the myocardial preservation is suboptimal or there are electrolyte imbalances during CPB. Magnesium (1–2 g IV) and lidocaine (100 mg IV) may be given prophylactically, most often by the perfusionist, to prevent or to treat ventricular tachycardia or fibrillation. If there is a full sternotomy, the heart can be defibrillated with internal cardiac paddles placed directly on the myocardium, using 5 to 10 joules. In minimally invasive procedures, external defibrillator pads are used with 120 to 200 joules. Antidysrhythmic agents such as amiodarone may also be administered. The TEE ME LAX view is useful in monitoring for air and determining when all air pockets have been removed.[157] Intracardiac air can migrate into the coronary arteries, most commonly the RCA, because it is anatomically superior and air rises. If ischemic changes manifest on the ECG and TEE, the MAP should be increased using phenylephrine boluses to improve coronary blood flow and ensure optimal ventricular function.[55,193] The surgeon may shake the heart or insert a needle through the muscle into the ventricle in an attempt to displace residual air. Valsalva breaths can help expel residual air from the pulmonary vascular system. Many surgeons prefer the patient to be in the Trendelenburg position during de-airing to prevent cerebral embolization.[55,113,193]

Sinus rhythm is optimal, and a rate between 70 and 90 bpm represents a balance between adequate cardiac performance and myocardial O_2 demand. Temporary ventricular pacing wires are routinely placed because the intrinsic conduction system of the heart may be temporarily or permanently altered. Atrioventricular pacing is preferred for bradycardia since it preserves the atrial contribution to the CO. Unfortunately, atrial tissue is more prone to disruption or damage when the pacing wires are removed in the postoperative period, so they are placed less commonly. Patients with chronic AF are generally unable to conduct with atrial pacing. After separation from CPB when electrocautery is used, a pacemaker in a synchronous mode may sense discharge from the electrocautery as intrinsic cardiac activity causing discharge to be inhibited. This can be prevented by switching to an asynchronous pacing mode (VOO [ventricular asynchronous] or DOO [atrial ventricular sequential asynchronous]); however, this places the patient at risk for developing ventricular fibrillation as a result of the R-on-T phenomenon. The pacer should therefore be converted to a synchronous mode as soon as electrocautery use becomes limited.[55,113,193]

Once the heart begins ejecting, the lungs are gently reinflated manually, limiting the positive pressure to 30 cm H_2O, and mechanical ventilation is resumed. The anesthetist will visually inspect the lungs as they reinflate, to detect atelectasis and adequacy of reinflation. Positive end-expiratory pressure (PEEP) and/or recruitment maneuvers, such as manual sighs, can be used to treat significant atelectasis. However, overinflation of the lungs must be avoided, especially in CABG patients, because an in situ ITA bypass graft may be stretched or even disrupted during hyperinflation of the lungs. Delivery of an inhalation or IV anesthetic is resumed. Monitors and transducers are zeroed to atmospheric pressure and recalibrated. Ventricular function is assessed using TEE and direct visual inspection of the heart in the surgical field. The surgeon is notified of any concerning echocardiographic findings. Valvular integrity and ventricular wall motion are carefully examined. If left ventricular function is marginal, an inotrope such as epinephrine, dopamine, or dobutamine is initiated. Right ventricular function can be supported with epinephrine or milrinone. If hypotension persists, a vasoconstrictor such as norepinephrine may be initiated. Once the volume, hemodynamic function, and ventilation are satisfactory, weaning from CPB can begin.[55,113,193]

Separation from CPB. The perfusionist uses a clamp to gradually occlude the venous return to facilitate filling of the RV. The RV pumps the blood volume through the pulmonary system and into the LV. As the beating heart continues to fill, ejection resumes, and arterial pressure rises. The perfusionist gradually decreases CPB flow. Volume (preload) can be added through the arterial pump line until loading conditions are optimized. Once adequate volume has been supplied through the in situ arterial cannula, the line is clamped, and the time of separation from CPB is recorded. The immediate postbypass period demands close attention because hemodynamic instability and cardiovascular collapse may occur.[55,193] If a radial A line is present, the practitioner must be aware of the potential discrepancy between the radial and aortic pressures.[144] If a PAC was pulled back during the procedure and is now in the RV, it can be repositioned into the PA.[55]

Rising pulmonary pressures with falling arterial pressure may indicate severely decreased ventricular function and an inability to separate from CPB. If the patient fails separation despite significant pharmacologic support, CPB can be reinstituted and the situation reevaluated, focusing on potentially reversible causes of failure. TEE is an invaluable tool to assist in diagnosis and guide management. Visual inspection of the operative field may reveal a surgically correctable problem, such as a kinked bypass graft. Residual air can also enter the coronary circulation, causing temporary decompensation. A MAP between 75 and

95 mm Hg will improve perfusion to the right heart. If, however, no obvious anatomic problem is identified, a period of resting perfusion on CPB will help resolve the cardiac stunning that commonly occurs after cardiac surgery. Pharmacologic inotropic or vasopressor support is initiated or increased as needed. If pharmacologic support is insufficient for separation from CPB, an intraaortic balloon pump (IABP) may be placed. As a last resort, extracorporeal membrane oxygenation (ECMO) or a ventricular assist device (VAD) may be used for ventricular support.[55,113,193] The indications for and use of these devices are discussed in the section on mechanical circulatory support of heart failure.

Postbypass period

Decannulation. Blood from the pump is transfused to the patient either at a slow, continuous rate or in 100-mL increments. Caution is taken to prevent overdistention and volume overload of either ventricle. The heart should be directly visualized, and global and regional ventricular function assessed on the TEE. The TEE is used to assess for the presence of remaining intracardiac air. If present, the perfusionist will continue to drain blood from the aortic root vent to remove the air. This blood is reinfused via the aortic cannula (aka "keeping up with the vent"), and the root vent is not discontinued until all air is removed from the heart. Once the heart is de-aired, the patient is warm, major surgical bleeding is controlled, and hemodynamic stability is satisfactory, preparation for decannulation can begin. The retrograde cardioplegia cannula and LV vent, if used, are removed first. Next, the venous cannula(s) are removed. Venous decannulation gives the perfusionist volume that can then be reinfused via the aortic cannula. Then, the aortic root vent is removed. Finally, when volume and ventricular function are optimized, preparation for aortic decannulation begins. The BP is lowered to SBP of 90 mm Hg or a MAP of 70 mm Hg or less to reduce tension on the aortic wall and bleeding. Some surgeons give only a 10-mg test dose of protamine before aortic decannulation, while others prefer that half the protamine dose be administered. The time of aortic decannulation should be noted. TEE is used to evaluate the presence of aortic dissection. The remaining dose of protamine is administered as the surgeon checks for bleeding. Some surgeons prefer to pack the heart for 15 minutes following protamine administration to allow natural coagulation. Once the surgeon is satisfied with coagulation and the patient is hemodynamically stable, all lines to the CPB circuit will be handed back to the perfusionist. Any blood remaining in the CPB venous reservoir and pump tubing can be sent to the cell-saver device so that it can be washed and reinfused.[55,113,193]

Protamine administration. Protamine is used to reverse the anticoagulation caused by heparin. The positively charged protamine neutralizes the negatively charged heparin through electrostatic interaction, forming a heparin-protamine complex that renders heparin inactive. One mg of protamine reverses 100 units of heparin, but this does not consider heparin elimination. Excess protamine causes decreased platelet number and function in dogs, and protamine to heparin ratios above 1.3:1 are associated with platelet aggregation and ACT prolongation.[195,196] In clinical practice, many administer the "unit dose" of 250 mg of protamine and use the ACT together with an assessment of surgical bleeding to determine the need for more protamine.[197] Since protamine can cause blood in the pump to clot, clear, closed-loop communication among the surgeon, anesthetist, and perfusionist is essential.

Protamine reactions range from mild hypotension from histamine release to catastrophic with refractory systemic hypotension, PHTN, and RHF from either an anaphylactic (immunologic) or anaphylactoid (nonimmunologic) reaction.[197] Protamine is prepared from the sperm of salmon or a related species, and risk factors for a serious reaction

include a true vertebrate fish allergy, neutral protamine Hagedorn (NPH) insulin use, and multiple medication allergies.[198] A test dose of 10 mg of protamine should be administered at least 1 minute before giving the full dose to check for a serious reaction. The test dose of protamine should be administered before decannulation of the aortic cannulas so that the patient can be placed back on the pump should anaphylaxis develop. All pump suction should be discontinued once the protamine administration begins since clot formation in the CPB pump can have devastating consequences. Slow drug administration is the most effective strategy for avoiding hypotension, which is common when protamine is delivered rapidly. The manufacturer recommends an infusion rate of 5 mg/min, which could take up to 1 hour, but clinical studies have shown that patients adequately tolerate protamine when administered over 5 to 15 minutes.[199-201] Some practitioners give small bolus doses, while others dilute the remaining dose in 100 to 150 mL of saline for slow IV infusion. An ACT is obtained at least 3 to 5 minutes after the entire protamine dose is given to confirm the return to baseline. Alternatively, a heparin dose-response assay (Hepcon) can be used to determine the optimal protamine dose and check for residual heparin after protamine administration. Additional protamine doses of 50 to 100 mg are administered to cover residual anticoagulation if the ACT is higher than baseline or inadequate hemostasis is visualized in the surgical field.[55,113]

Hemodynamic management during separation and post bypass. During separation from CPB, and in the immediate postbypass period, it is clinically useful to think of hemodynamic management in categories or groups. Fortunately, most patients separate from CPB relatively easily (group 1), but others experience diastolic failure (group 2), systolic failure (group 3), or vasoplegia (group 4).[162] Of course, some patients will experience more than one complication, and others will begin in one group and then progress to another. Successful separation requires combining the art and science of anesthesia to manage the pump, the pipes, and the volume.

The first group includes patients with good LV function preoperatively and few comorbidities, having relatively straightforward surgical procedures that do not require more than 1 to 2 hours on CPB. These patients usually separate from CPB easily and require little support. Patients with good ventricular function usually have a BP, heart rate and rhythm, and CO within the normal range. Hyperdynamic patients usually fall into this category as well. This group of patients may need some occasional adjustments of their volume or BP, but they are generally stable during the post-CPB period.[55,162]

The second group consists of patients with significant concentric LVH and diastolic dysfunction.[162] This group tends to be volume dependent. The intravascular volume status should be continually reassessed using TEE. Reduced ventricular compliance can cause the LVEDP to be elevated despite low ventricular volume. As volume is added from the pump, these patients may become hypertensive, even though their CO is still low due to hypovolemia. In other words, this group of patients is prone to diastolic heart failure. Judicious boluses of nitroglycerin will help the LV to relax and accept volume, as well as aid in controlling hypertension. As discussed at the beginning of the chapter, patients with concentric LVH require a high MAP and adequate diastolic time to fill the noncompliant ventricle (see Table 26.4). If the MAP decreases, they are prone to ischemia; therefore they may benefit from a low-dose vasoconstrictor such as norepinephrine if the BP is low after volume has been optimized. These patients are also very reliant on their atrial kick, which can contribute up to 40% of left ventricular end-diastolic volume.[202] If the patient's heart rate is slow or nodal, atrial or atrioventricular pacing can significantly improve hemodynamic function. LVOT obstruction with possible systolic anterior motion (SAM) of the mitral valve can also occur, particularly in patients with septal hypertrophy. This problem is best assessed using TEE and treated by keeping the heart full, heart rate in the slow-normal range, and BP up (see the section on hypertrophic obstructive cardiomyopathy [HOCM]).[193] Once the diastolic filling volume, heart rate, and BP are optimized, the patients usually separate from CPB easily.[162]

The third group of patients comprises those who develop systolic failure after CPB. This group can be further subdivided into left, right, or biventricular failure.[162] As volume is added from the pump, the heart chamber(s) begin to dilate, and contractility is poor. Patients with poor preoperative left or right ventricular function, long CPB runs, complex procedures, uncorrected structural defects, or inadequate myocardial protection on CPB are at high risk for failure.[203] The pathophysiology of heart failure was discussed earlier in the chapter (see Tables 26.3 and 26.4). Many times, CPB must be reinitiated while the beating heart is given a chance to rest, and pharmacologic support is optimized. LV systolic failure is managed with an inotrope, such as epinephrine or dobutamine, combined with gentle afterload reduction using a vasodilator, such as nitroprusside, if the SVR is high.[55,193] An inotrope and vasodilator, such as milrinone, will provide inotropic support and reduce afterload. Milrinone has the added benefit of significantly increasing the flow in anastomosed saphenous vein grafts (SVGs) after CPB.[204] It may be used alone or in conjunction with other inotropes and vasopressors. Right heart failure can be initially managed with a combination of epinephrine, to support contractility, and nitroglycerin, titrated to reduce preload, while maintaining BP to support coronary perfusion. If the right heart function continues to be inadequate, a bolus and/or infusion of milrinone will reduce pulmonary vascular resistance and right ventricular afterload. Unfortunately, milrinone may decrease SVR excessively, leading to hypotension. A norepinephrine infusion may be initiated to augment the BP to a level sufficient for coronary perfusion.[205] A recent meta-analysis confirmed that inhaled pulmonary vasodilators, including epoprostenol sodium (Veletri or Flolan) or rarely (due to cost) nitric oxide, may be added to selectively dilate the pulmonary vasculature, increasing both MAP and right ventricular EF.[206] If maximal pharmacologic support fails, then mechanical support of the ventricle is considered, including the use of an IABP, ECMO, or VAD. Management of these devices is complex and specialized, thus anesthetic considerations are discussed separately (see the section on the treatment of heart failure).

The fourth and final group of patients present with persistent hypotension in the post-CPB period, despite a normal to high CO.[162] Patients in this group may be septic due to preexisting endocarditis or may develop vasoplegic syndrome. Vasoplegic syndrome is a well-described type of vasodilatory shock that occurs after CPB. The reported incidence (5%–25%) varies widely, as do the purported causes. Preoperative administration of ACEIs, ARBs, calcium channel blockers, amiodarone, and IV heparin have been implicated as potential causative agents. Diabetes and moderate-to-poor LV dysfunction are also correlated with this syndrome.[207,208] Unfortunately, no particular medical history consistently predicts manifestation of this syndrome; however, hypotension early in the pump run is predictive of its development after CPB.[209] Patients with this syndrome often require large doses of phenylephrine, or even norepinephrine, while on CPB. Post-CPB, they develop resistance to phenylephrine and respond much better to boluses of norepinephrine (16–32 mcg) or vasopressin (1–2 units). A norepinephrine and/or vasopressin infusion is often needed to support the BP. Vasopressin has been demonstrated to be more effective in the management of vasoplegic syndrome than norepinephrine.[162,210,211] Although a patient's CO may fall into the normal or even the hyperdynamic range, the heart may still benefit from low to moderate doses of inotropic support to sustain contractility in this state of vasodilatory shock. Maintaining a relatively high hematocrit level

augments preload and also improves BP.[212] Nonvasopressor agents that may also be used in the treatment of vasoplegia include corticosteroids, methylene blue, ascorbic acid, and hydroxocobalamin.[211]

Bleeding and other considerations. After the patient is decannulated, the surgeon may pack the chest to encourage hemostasis. During this period, the surgeon may need to lift the heart to inspect surgical anastomosis for bleeding on the posterior surface. Lifting and manipulating the heart and vasculature can cause significant dysrhythmias and hypotension. The surgeon should be informed if hypotension is severe or excessive in duration. Electrocautery is used routinely and may cause suppression of the pacemaker. It is recommended that the pacemaker be placed in an asynchronous mode at this time, with synchronous pacing resumed as soon as the surgeon finishes using electrocautery. Most patients require volume supplementation post bypass. Often, a combination of crystalloid, colloid, and cell-saver blood is used, generally resulting in a hematocrit of 25% to 30%.[55,193]

Persistent bleeding occasionally develops after CPB, especially if the surgery was complex and required a long pump run. The causes are multifactorial, but readily treatable problems should be addressed. Adequate reversal of heparin is confirmed via ACT or a heparin concentration assay, and additional doses of protamine are given if needed. Hypothermia accentuates hemostatic defects, so the patient and the room are warmed to promote normothermia.[193] Surgical causes of persistent bleeding are identified, as inadequate surgical hemostasis may develop and progress insidiously. Multiple studies have confirmed that transfusion may increase the rate of death as much as 70%, and it is associated with both early and late mortality even when confounders are excluded.[213-215] If bleeding persists, laboratory coagulation studies may reveal a deficiency in the coagulation cascade. Tests of whole blood viscoelasticity, including thromboelastography (TEG), Sonoclot, and rotational thromboelastometry (ROTEM), measure the platelet strength and integrity of the fibrin-platelet bond. These tests provide a more accurate and evidenced-based method of deciding which products to administer rather than traditional tests of coagulation such as the prothrombin time (PT) or PTT. A recent meta-analysis demonstrated that in adult cardiac surgery, the use of a viscoelastic blood test is associated with reduced allogeneic blood product exposure, postoperative bleeding at 12 and 24 hours, and the need for redo surgery unrelated to bleeding.[216] When postoperative bleeding is anticipated, viscoelastic tests of coagulation can be used while on CPB by adding heparinase to the sample. The STS and SCA advocate for the implementation of their transfusion guidelines supported with viscoelastic POC testing.[67,217] Any units removed as part of ANH can be reinfused any time after the protamine is administered. Platelet, plasma, cryoprecipitate, and red cell transfusions may be required depending on the underlying deficiency. Factor concentrates, including prothrombin complex, have been incorporated into many transfusion algorithms as a substitute for FFP because they are easy to use and have a lower volume and viral load. If the patient has platelet dysfunction due to preexisting pathology (e.g., uremia, liver disease), medications (e.g., ASA, thienopyridines), or even CPB, then desmopressin (DDAVP) should be considered.[217,218]

As discussed in the section on the physiologic effects of CPB, a host of other complications can arise, including ARDS, renal failure, and neurologic injury. Problems with adequate ventilation may occur in the OR, although these are most evident in the postoperative period. Most patients will respond to the addition of PEEP and other recruitment measures. If ALI is significant, an ICU ventilator with advanced ventilation modes is requested for use in the OR.[193]

Chest closure. When hemostasis has been achieved and the patient is hemodynamically stable, preparations are made for chest closure and transport to the ICU. Before closure, pacemaker capture and the ability to move the PAC freely should be assessed and documented because it is possible for the PAC to accidentally be sutured or the pacemaker wire to become dislodged. While checking is no guarantee that either complication will be avoided, identifying the problem early has the potential to prevent patient harm. The lungs are deflated temporarily when the sternum is pulled together to facilitate chest closure and prevent the kinking of bypass grafts, if present. Chest closure causes a decrease in preload and an increase in afterload, which can sometimes lead to hemodynamic deterioration. Therefore CO and TEE should be assessed before and after the chest is closed. If the patient becomes unstable, the wires are released, and the situation is reevaluated. Patients who have received massive transfusions or require high-dose pharmacologic and/or mechanical support may not tolerate the hemodynamic consequences of chest closure. In this situation, closure of the chest will be delayed, and negative pressure wound dressing (V.A.C., KCI, San Antonio, TX, USA) is applied. The patient is maintained in the ICU for the next 24 to 48 hours until hemostasis and hemodynamic stability are achieved. The patient may then return to the OR for subsequent chest washout and closure.[193]

Once the chest is closed, preparations for safe transport to the ICU are initiated. Emergency medications and airway equipment are gathered for transport because the transfer to the ICU represents a particularly vulnerable time outside of the OR. The TEE probe is removed at the end of the procedure, and an OG tube is inserted to decompress the stomach. Although stable patients may be extubated at the end of the procedure, most surgeons prefer that fast-tracking occur in the ICU.

Transport. With the numerous monitors, invasive lines, chest tubes, pharmacologic infusions, and requisite airway equipment, moving a patient safely to the ICU can be complex and hazardous. Most patients are sedated with propofol or dexmedetomidine infusions during transport and initially in the ICU. A thorough patient handoff to ICU personnel is vital for patient safety. A handoff checklist helps to ensure that all critical information is communicated to the ICU team.[180] Once the patient is hemodynamically stable and chest tube output is adequate, then weaning from mechanical ventilation usually begins.

Postoperative Bleeding and Cardiac Tamponade

Bleeding is a significant complication in cardiac surgery that is associated with an increased ICU and hospital length of stay, morbidity, mortality, and cost. In approximately 4% to 9% of cases, patients must return to the OR to have their chest reexplored for persistent bleeding, tamponade, or unexplained hemodynamic instability that is presumed to be tamponade.[219,220] Any single hour chest tube output measures above 500 mL or more than 200 mL/hr of sustained drainage is considered an indication for exploration.[221] Coagulopathy, postoperative bleeding, and/or localized compression from the blood that is in contact with the heart may all contribute to tamponade that occurs in the period immediately following cardiac surgery, even though the pericardium is left open. The compression limits diastolic filling of the heart, thus reducing SV and CO. Cardiac tamponade should also be suspected after cardiac surgery if there is a sudden dramatic decrease in chest tube drainage with concomitant hypotension, tachycardia, increased and equalizing filling pressures, and decreased cardiac indices, despite increased inotropic and vasopressor support. Severe hypotension, myocardial ischemia, and eventually cardiac arrest can ensue once venous pressures fall below pericardial pressures, causing ventricular collapse.[222,223] Pulsus paradoxus, electrical alternans, and Beck triad (hypotension, muffled heart sounds, and jugular venous distention [JVD]) are considered classic clinical indicators of cardiac

tamponade.[224] These and other symptoms of cardiac tamponade are described fully in Chapter 25.

Pericardiocentesis, subxiphoid drainage, or mediastinal exploration must occur without delay once decompensated cardiac tamponade occurs to prevent complete cardiac collapse. Crystalloid, colloid, and/or blood should be administered to optimize preload until pericardiocentesis or mediastinal exploration can be undertaken in the ICU or operating suite.[113] If the postoperative cardiac surgical patient is brought to the operative room for reexploration because of cardiac tamponade, medications such as anesthetics, sedatives, and narcotics should be either carefully titrated or avoided to prevent further myocardial depression until the tamponade is relieved. Ketamine, because of its sympathomimetic effects, may be selected for the induction of anesthesia to support heart rate, BP, and myocardial function.[55,113] Since SV is fixed, bradycardia should be avoided, and tachycardia must be recognized as an important compensatory mechanism that serves to maintain CO. If cardiac arrest seems likely to occur with induction, a temporary improvement in cardiac function can be achieved by performing a pericardiocentesis under local anesthesia before induction, to create enough drainage to provide some relief. For postoperative cardiac surgical patients returning to the OR for bleeding and cardiac tamponade who no longer have invasive monitoring in place, reinsertion of an A line and CVP will be necessary. However, surgical drainage should not be delayed for placement of central access. TEE is useful for monitoring ventricular function and as an aid in guiding the surgeon in removing trapped fluid. The patient is sometimes kept spontaneously breathing until the pericardial sac is opened to prevent further decreases in ventricular filling caused by positive pressure ventilation. If positive pressure ventilation is used, tidal volumes should be reduced to prevent further decrease in preload and CO. Once the cardiac tamponade is surgically relieved, an immediate improvement in hemodynamics is usually noted. At this time, hypertension and tachycardia from endogenous catecholamine release should be anticipated and treated accordingly.[113,225,226]

ANESTHETIC CONSIDERATIONS FOR SPECIFIC CARDIAC DISEASES AND SURGICAL PROCEDURES

Coronary Artery Disease and Myocardial Revascularization
Pathophysiology
On-pump CABG surgery is the most frequently performed cardiac surgical procedure. The 2020 STS adult cardiac surgery database shows that isolated CABG accounts for 55% of cardiac surgical procedures, and CABG in combination with one or more valve procedures accounts for another 9%.[227] This section focuses on the anesthetic considerations that pertain to patients with CAD presenting for CABG surgery. Anesthetic management for these patients requires an understanding of coronary anatomy and physiology, discussed in Chapter 25, as well as an understanding of the key physiologic principles covered at the beginning of this chapter.

CAD is a complex disease state that involves the narrowing of the coronary arteries. Coronary O_2 extraction is maximal at rest, and the only way to increase O_2 delivery to the tissues is to increase coronary flow. In normal coronaries, flow can increase 3 to 5 times over baseline when demand increases, known as coronary reserve. This protective reserve is limited with CAD; thus, when these patients increase demand by exercise or stress, they develop demand ischemia. This is symptomatically experienced as predictable, stable angina. General anesthetic medications decrease MVO_2 and thus help to protect against demand ischemia.[228]

ACS and perioperative ischemia are usually caused by supply ischemia. Ischemia occurs when a piece of plaque ruptures, causing a thrombus to form that significantly, or totally, occludes a segment of a coronary artery, leading to ischemia, dysrhythmias, and/or MI. The problem can be exacerbated by spasm, which can develop even in normal adjacent vessels.[59] The development and evolution of coronary stents have revolutionized cardiac care; in fact, most patients presenting for CABG surgery with CAD and/or ACS will have been referred for some type of PCI. Much research has been conducted comparing the risk-benefit ratio of surgical intervention to optimal medical management. The Coronary Revascularization Writing Group states that surgical intervention (CABG) is appropriate for patients with three-vessel disease with or without proximal LAD disease, two-vessel disease with proximal LAD disease, severe ischemia in two-vessel disease without proximal LAD disease, and proximal LAD disease if the left internal thoracic artery (LITA) will be used as the graft. Additionally, patients who have failed PCI or who have coronary lesions not amenable to PCI will benefit from surgery.[229] In these situations, CABG has been found to have a lower mortality risk as well as a lower risk of major cardiovascular complications or cerebral events than optimal medical management.[229-231]

Anesthetic Considerations and Surgical Options for On-Pump CABG

The anesthetist should carefully review preoperative cardiac tests to determine the location and extent of the lesions, to assess ventricular function, and to detect the possible presence of concurrent cardiac abnormalities such as AS. Table 26.2 reviews significant findings on cardiovascular preoperative testing. Preoperative ventricular function correlates with the risk of developing postoperative low cardiac output syndrome (LCOS). Patients with ACS or NYHA class IV heart failure (see Table 26.5) are at high risk of LCOS. If the patient develops cardiogenic shock, possibly requiring an IABP to maintain stable hemodynamics, the patient is in the highest risk category.[228] Patients who have had a BMS implanted within 1 month of surgery and/or DES within 6 months of surgery will have special considerations because of their antiplatelet therapy.[138] The general management of drugs affecting coagulation has already been discussed; however, in patients with recent coronary stents, the cardiologist and surgeon collaborate to determine the best management for the individual patient. For emergency procedures, both aspirin and GPIIb/IIIa inhibitors may be continued, despite the increased risk of bleeding.[228]

Optimizing myocardial O_2 supply and minimizing myocardial O_2 demand are key anesthetic considerations in CABG surgery (see Fig. 26.1). The patient must be monitored carefully for ischemia throughout the procedure using a combination of ECG and TEE findings, together with direct inspection of the heart.[72,228] Table 26.1 outlines the causes of and treatments for myocardial ischemia. Anesthetic considerations for CABG are summarized in Table 26.9. It is most important to maintain MAP at or greater than perioperative values to maintain coronary perfusion, while keeping the heart rate and LVEDP low. Patients with left-main and triple-vessel disease should have an A line and a large-bore peripheral IV in place before induction so that hypotension can be treated promptly with phenylephrine and volume. β-blockers are used to control heart rate and prevent tachycardia during intubation or during stimulating surgical events.[228] Preoperative β-blockade is a quality metric for both the National Quality Forum and the STS database, which is used for quality report cards in conjunction with Consumer Reports.[232] If the patient becomes too hypertensive, the preferred vasodilator for CABG is nitroglycerin. In low doses, nitroglycerin acts immediately to reduce preload by decreasing vascular tone; in higher doses, it also decreases coronary artery resistance. Kaplan et al.

TABLE 26.9 Anesthetic Considerations in the Management of CABG

Factor	Hemodynamic Goals	Anesthetic Considerations
Preload	Low normal	↓ LVEDP will ↑ myocardial O_2 supply and ↓ demand Nitroglycerin selectively dilates coronary vessels
Heart rate	Slow normal	Too fast → ischemia; consider β-blockade Too slow → not enough CO for coronary perfusion
Rhythm	Maintain sinus	Maintains atrial contribution to CO
Compliance	Improve	Concentric LVH (common with history of HTN) → ↓ compliance
Contractility	Depress if normal LVF Support if ↓ LVF	↓ Contractility → ↓MVO₂ If poor LVF, may not tolerate myocardial depression
SVR	Maintain	Hypertension better tolerated than hypotension Treat hypotension promptly with phenylephrine
PVR	Maintain	Usually not a problem

↓, Decreased; ↑, increased; →, leads to; *CABG*, coronary artery bypass graft; *CO*, cardiac output; *HTN*, hypertension; *LVEDP*, left ventricular end-diastolic pressure; *LVF*, left ventricular function; *LVH*, left ventricular hypertrophy; *MVO₂*, myocardial oxygen consumption; *O₂*, oxygen; *PVR*, pulmonary vascular resistance; *SVR*, systemic vascular resistance.

showed that nitroglycerin is superior to nitroprusside in patients having a CABG.[233,234]

Inhalation anesthetics should also comprise part of the anesthetic plan because of their pre- and postconditioning effect. Nitrous oxide should be avoided due to the possibility of expanding gaseous spaces. Patients considered for fast-track protocols (generally those with EFs >35%) should receive a limited dose of narcotics to allow for early extubation. High-risk patients may still require a primary narcotic technique to maintain hemodynamic stability.[228]

Conventional CABG surgery is performed through a median sternotomy with CPB. Different types of conduit can be used to bypass occluded areas of the patient's native coronary arteries to revascularize the myocardium distal to the occlusions (Fig. 26.21). The surgeon must take into consideration the viability of the myocardium, the quality of the target vessel, and the type and length of conduit needed to reach a point distal to the occlusions. The most commonly used conduits are the ITAs (formerly IMAs, as mentioned) and greater saphenous veins. The free radial artery graft is the second-choice arterial conduit after the LITA.[235] Arterial grafts have superior long-term patency, but they must be reserved for high-grade lesions.[236] Flow in the native coronary artery can compete with the flow in the arterial bypass graft. If there is not enough flow in the muscular artery, it will spasm, and blood flow will be compromised. Topical (papaverine) and IV antispasmodic drugs such as calcium channel blockers or low-dose nitroglycerin infused intraoperatively are used to treat spasm.[235,237]

The LITA is usually left in situ at its proximal origin from the left subclavian artery, dissected from the chest wall, and anastomosed to the LAD artery. A LITA graft to the LAD artery has a 10-year patency rate of 90%.[235,236] The right ITA (RITA) may be left in situ, but is more

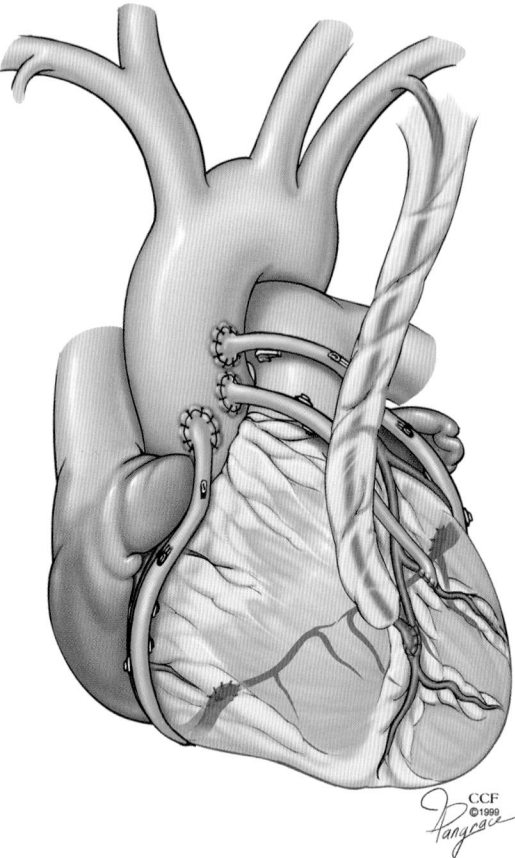

Fig. 26.21 Coronary artery bypass graft surgery. The in situ left internal thoracic artery is most often grafted to the left anterior descending native coronary. Free grafts (saphenous vein grafts, free radial artery, or right internal thoracic artery) are anastomosed proximally to the aorta (or branched from another bypass—*not shown*) and distally to a target area of the native coronary vessel that is beyond the obstruction. (Reprinted with permission from Cleveland Clinic Center for Medical Art & Photography ©2020. All rights reserved.)

frequently transected from its proximal origin to become a free graft with a proximal anastomosis originating from the aorta or another conduit. The surgical table is elevated and turned while the ITA is dissected. Lung volumes are reduced to improve the surgical view. The patient's arm should be well padded since the axillary artery can be compressed by the chest wall retractor, lowering radial A line pressures. A noninvasive cuff on the contralateral arm helps confirm the diagnosis. Brachial plexus injury may occur if the ITA retractor lifts the patient's shoulder and head off the surgical table. To prevent this, padding can be added to support the patient's head and shoulder to ensure they are not free hanging, and the surgeon should be made aware so that the retraction can be lessened.[238] Heparin is usually administered before the LITA pedicle is clamped.[228]

The radial artery is harvested endoscopically or by open surgical dissection from the forearm of the nondominant hand and is used in the same manner as the RITA. A low-dose nitroglycerin drip may be initiated to decrease the chance of radial conduit spasm. Studies have found that while there is a greater risk of spasm compared to a SVG, there is improved 5-year patency and flow.[235,239]

The SVG can also be harvested endoscopically or by open surgical dissection. As with any endoscopic procedure, the respiratory rate may have to be increased to compensate for the addition of carbon dioxide. Most vein grafts are now removed endoscopically, but there are concerns that endovascular vein harvest (EVH) might decrease long-term

graft patency.[240,241] Some surgeons request that low-dose heparin (2500 units) be given IV during EVH to decrease these issues. The vein graft is reversed for implantation so that the valves do not impede blood flow. The distal anastomosis to the native coronary artery is usually completed first, and then the proximal portion is sewn to the aorta or bridged off another graft.

Several surgical and technical complications can result in ischemia. In addition to the previously mentioned concerns about reoperations, patients who have undergone prior CABG surgery may have a patent LITA or other grafts lying directly under the sternum. Sternotomy can lead to marked ischemia and blood loss if flow in the vessel is accidentally disrupted.[63] The surgeon must take care to make bypass grafts the perfect length. LITA grafts that are too short can be overstretched with vigorous lung inflation, and free radial artery or SVGs can be overstretched when the heart is filled. On the other hand, grafts that are too long can kink when the chest is closed. Other causes of ischemia include coronary embolization of air or debris and coronary spasm.[228]

Anesthetic Considerations and Surgical Options for Off-Pump CABG

The first OPCAB procedures were attempted in the 1950s, but there has been a resurgence in popularity since retractors and epicardial stabilizing devices, such as the Octopus (Medtronic Inc., Minneapolis, MN, USA), were developed in the 1990s. Off-pump surgery is also called beating heart bypass surgery.[228,242] Although the procedure is typically performed through a full median sternotomy without the aid of CPB, a perfusionist and a primed or dry pump (based on surgical preference) should be in the OR on standby throughout the case. Occasionally, a limited anterior thoracotomy (minimally invasive direct coronary artery bypass [MIDCAB]) approach is used. The implications of the MIDCAB incision are detailed in the section on minimally invasive surgery. It is estimated that OPCAB procedures peaked in 2002 at 25% of all CABG procedures and have since declined.[243] OPCAB is performed to avoid the risks and complications associated with conventional CABG and CPB, but further research is needed to determine its relative safety. Aortic cross-clamping is avoided, theoretically decreasing the risk of debris embolization. Studies comparing the techniques showed that patients from both groups had equivalent rises in inflammatory biomarkers and similar neuropsychologic outcomes.[243] Additionally, incomplete revascularization was slightly more common in the OPCAB patients, and 1-year patency was significantly worse.[242] The STS recommends OPCAB as a blood conservation technique.[67]

Anesthetic implications and monitoring are similar to those of on-pump CABG, with a few additional concerns. The procedure is usually limited to patients with adequate LV function, and bleeding is less of a concern, so patients are even more likely to be candidates for a fast-track anesthetic plan.[228,243] In contrast to on-pump cases, in which patients' blood volumes are diluted by priming volume, OPCAB patients require crystalloid and/or colloid solutions to correct the fluid deficit and the hemodynamic changes inherent to the procedure. Patient temperature cannot be corrected on-pump, therefore hypothermia occurs. Normothermia is maintained by warming the room and using fluid warmers, warm water mattresses, or forced-air warming devices. Anticoagulation is necessary, but the decision to partially heparinize (100–200 units/kg with an intended ACT >300 sec) or fully heparinize (400 units/kg with an intended ACT >480 sec) depends on the surgeon's preference.[228] ACTs should be monitored at least every 30 minutes and heparin administered as needed to maintain adequate anticoagulation. Antifibrinolytics are not routinely used because the blood is not exposed to CPB. ABGs, electrolytes, and blood glucose should be monitored and treated every 30 to 60 minutes.

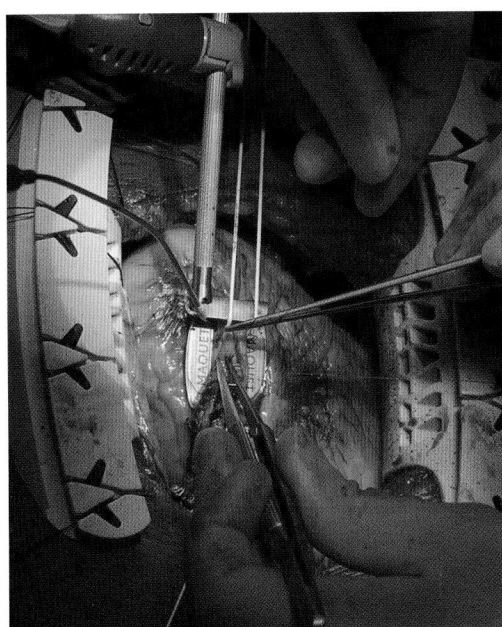

Fig. 26.22 Left anterior descending (LAD) artery anastomosis during off-pump coronary artery bypass grafting using a left internal thoracic artery (LITA) graft. The view is from the head of the patient. The Maquet mechanical stabilizer (MAQUET, Wayne, NJ) is in place together with vascular snare sutures used to transiently occlude the artery. The LITA is being anastomosed to the LAD, assisted by use of pressurized and heavily humidified carbon dioxide ("mister blower" metal cannula) to facilitate visualization of the vessel lumen. (Courtesy Alexander Mittnacht, MD, Mount Sinai School of Medicine, New York, NY.)

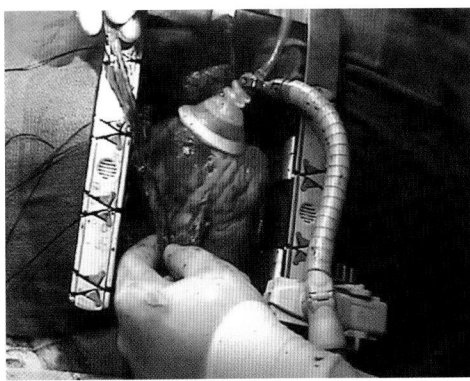

Fig. 26.23 Verticalization of the cardiac apex in an off-pump coronary artery bypass operation. (From Miller RD, et al. *Miller's Anesthesia*. 7th ed. Philadelphia: Elsevier; 2009:1925.)

To perform a bypass on a beating heart, the surgeon employs specialized compressive footplate stabilizers (Fig. 26.22) and retractors that use suction to lift and suspend the heart, verticalizing the apex (Fig. 26.23). These maneuvers compress cardiac chambers and distort valvular apparatuses, resulting in well-documented hemodynamic compromise and acute ischemia.[228,243,244] Every team member needs to be prepared for the possibility of converting to an on-pump procedure in the event of hemodynamic deterioration. Less myocardial manipulation is needed to bypass the LAD or diagonal coronary artery lesions (see Fig. 26.22), but as shown in Fig. 26.23, near verticalization of the apex is necessary to expose the posterior lateral wall for posterior descending artery (PDA) and circumflex lesions to be grafted. Some surgeons routinely shunt the coronary lesion being grafted, whereas others shunt the lesion only if regional ischemia develops.

Close communication between the anesthesia providers and the surgical team is critical. The CPP is maintained by keeping a relatively high MAP (90–100 mm Hg) during distal anastomosis. Hypotension is initially treated with volume and vasopressors (by bolus or infusion) as needed to maintain BP. The steep Trendelenburg position will facilitate surgical exposure and help restore MAP and CO.[228] Occasionally, patients will also require an inotrope to maintain hemodynamic stability. Dramatic hemodynamic changes can occur when the heart returns to a physiologic position, necessitating the abrupt withdrawal of pharmacologic support. Later, when the surgeon uses a side clamp to perform the anastomoses of the proximal graft to the aorta, the MAP is routinely lowered to approximately 60 to 70 mm Hg. Surgical drying and closure are often more rapid in off-pump procedures compared to on-pump procedures because bleeding is minimized.[228,243]

Valvular Heart Disease and Valve Surgery

VHD affects 2.5% of the population globally. Rheumatic heart disease (RHD) is still the primary cause of valvular disease in underdeveloped countries; however, in industrialized, developed countries like the United States, degenerative heart disease predominates. The prevalence of VHD rises dramatically with increasing age, reaching 13.2% after the age of 75.[245,246] These statistics are based on historical data, and large-scale echocardiographic screening suggests that the prevalence may be as high as one in two in the elderly.[247] Infective endocarditis is on the rise due to the increased prevalence of medical devices and IV substance misuse.[73,245,246,248] The proportion of cardiac surgeries that include valvular procedures has doubled over the past 2 decades. In 2020, the STS reported that 35% of cardiac surgeries involved valve repair or replacement, and a significant number of these cases involved multiple lesions or concurrent myocardial revascularization. AS is the most common valvular disease requiring surgical intervention, followed by MR, aortic insufficiency, and mitral stenosis. Right-sided valvular disease occurs much less frequently.[227,247] Often, multiple lesions are present, and a valve may exhibit both stenosis and regurgitation. In this situation, usually one problem predominates, and management is dictated by the pathology causing the majority of the patient's symptoms.[249] The ACC/AHA perioperative guidelines recommend that patients with clinically suspected moderate or severe stenosis or regurgitation undergo echocardiographic evaluation if there is a significant change in the clinical status or physical exam since their last evaluation, or if greater than 1 year has elapsed since their last evaluation. If valve replacement or repair is indicated, it should be done before elective noncardiac surgery.[123]

VHD causes abnormalities in the pressure and volume loading conditions of the heart that result in structural and functional changes. Management requires a clear understanding of the anatomy, pathophysiology, and natural history of each lesion, as discussed in Chapter 25. Echocardiography is an invaluable tool in the diagnosis and management of VHD. Three factors determine valvular flow: valve area, the pressure gradient across the valve, and duration of flow in systole and diastole. Hemodynamic management of VHD requires manipulation of heart rate and rhythm, preload, afterload, and contractility to enhance forward flow in stenotic lesions and to minimize retrograde flow in regurgitant lesions.[115,250,251] Although HOCM is not a valvular defect, its hemodynamic management is similar to that required for AS, so it is addressed in this section of the chapter.

Aortic Stenosis

AS is the most common valvular lesion among older patients in industrialized countries. Symptomatic, severe AS has a staggering mortality of up to 50% at 1 year when treated medically.[252,253] The development of the minimally invasive transcatheter approach has revolutionized valve replacement and given hope to millions. Consequently, the volume of aortic valve replacements (AVRs) has increased substantially in the past decade, particularly in older, high-risk patients.[254,255] Approximately 1% to 2% of the population has a congenital bicuspid valve.[256,257] A bicuspid valve has a smaller orifice and tends to open and close abnormally, which subjects the valve apparatus to increased shear stress and degeneration.[256,257] Hence the majority of younger patients (30–60 years of age) undergoing AVR have bicuspid valves.[246] The prevalence of degenerative AS increases markedly with age, and there is often concomitant AR.[245] Risk factors for the development of acquired AS are the same as those for atherosclerosis and CAD: increased age, male gender, smoking, hypertension, and hyperlipidemia.[41,245] Consequently, AVR is often performed in combination with CABG. Rheumatic disease accounts for up to 30% of AV pathology and usually results in mixed AS and AI, and frequently coexists with mitral valve dysfunction.[249,258] According to the STS database, in 2018 there were 25,274 isolated AVRs and 15,855 combined AVR and CABG procedures.[227]

Pathophysiology. The normal AV area measures 3 cm² ± 1 cm². Per the ACC/AHA guidelines, stenosis is considered severe when the valve area decreases to 1 cm² or less.[115,153] The stenotic orifice obstructs the LV outflow. In an attempt to generate enough pressure to push the blood forward past the stenosis, the LV muscle thickens with the parallel addition of new myofibrils (concentric hypertrophy). This forward motion causes a jet of accelerated, turbulent blood flow as it crosses the valve, similar to water flow through a partially occluded garden hose. The increased flow results in a pressure drop across the valve, secondary to the Venturi effect, with pressure in the aorta significantly less than the pressure in the LV. The 2014 AHA/ACC guidelines describe four stages of AS (A [at risk] through D [severe]) based on patient symptoms, valve anatomy, and hemodynamics. The reader should refer to these guidelines for details, but in general, a jet velocity of 4 m/sec or more and a mean pressure gradient drop of 40 mm Hg or more suggests severe AS. A jet velocity of 6 m/sec with a mean pressure gradient of 60 mm Hg or more is considered very severe or critical AS.[115,153] The pressure drop results in a characteristic slow upstroke and a high dicrotic notch on the arterial waveform, with a classic narrow pulse pressure (SBP – DBP). The patient with AS is very prone to ischemia for three reasons: (1) thick, hypertrophied muscle mass has a high O_2 requirement, (2) increased ventricular pressure inhibits coronary perfusion, and (3) a high prevalence (>50%) of coexisting CAD.[55,251] The fibrosed ventricle is noncompliant; consequently, diastolic filling becomes compromised despite preserved LV systolic function. LVEDP is elevated, despite a low left ventricular end-diastolic volume (LVEDV). Patients with AS are dependent on atrial augmentation of their CO, with atrial kick contributing up to 40% of LVEDV. The classic triad of AS symptoms (angina, syncope, and congestion causing dyspnea) correlate closely with 5-, 3-, and 2-year survival, respectively.[251] The ventricular systolic function remains normal until late in the course of the disease when the LV dilates and systolic function deteriorates.[259-262]

Anesthetic considerations and surgical options. Valve replacement is a class I recommendation for symptomatic patients with severe AS, as well as for asymptomatic patients with a LVEF less than 50%, or those having cardiac surgery for another indication.[115,250] Surgical aortic valve replacement (SAVR) is a class I recommendation for low-, medium-, and high-risk patients. TAVR is a class I recommendation for patients with prohibitive or high surgical risk and a class IIa recommendation for patients with intermediate surgical risk.[115,263] TAVR is covered in the minimally invasive section of this chapter.

Anesthetic management follows directly from an understanding of cardiovascular pathophysiology. Table 26.10 outlines the anesthetic

TABLE 26.10 Anesthetic Considerations in the Management of Aortic Stenosis

Factor	Hemodynamic Goals	Anesthetic Considerations
Preload	High normal	Need volume to stretch noncompliant LV ↑ preload reduces the gradient across LVOT LVEDP > LVEDV (use TEE to evaluate)
Heart rate	Slow normal	Too fast → ischemia Too slow → not enough CO for coronary perfusion
Rhythm	Maintain sinus	Atrial kick can contribute up to 40% of LVEDV Cardiovert early
Compliance	Improve	Thick, sclerotic LV prone to diastolic failure ↑ LVEDP reduces coronary perfusion Cautiously treat with NTG maintaining LVEDV and MAP
Contractility	Maintain	Concentric hypertrophy with normal chamber size Normal or ↑ EF initially Late dilation and falling EF
SVR	Maintain coronary perfusion gradient	Hypertension better tolerated than hypotension Treat hypotension promptly with phenylephrine Vasodilate cautiously for significant hypertension
PVR	Maintain	Diastolic failure can lead to dyspnea

↑, Increase; →, leads to; *CO*, cardiac output; *EF*, ejection fraction; *LV*, left ventricle; *LVEDP*, left ventricular end-diastolic pressure; *LVEDV*, left ventricular end-diastolic volume; *LVOT*, left ventricular outflow tract; *MAP*, mean arterial pressure; *NTG*, nitroglycerin; *PVR*, pulmonary vascular resistance; *SVR*, systemic vascular resistance; *TEE*, transesophageal echocardiography.

considerations. Preoperatively, extreme caution is required when treating angina with nitrates as hypotension can decrease coronary perfusion causing ischemia and ultimately cardiac arrest and sudden death. Cardiac compressions rarely generate enough pressure to provide adequate coronary perfusion to permit resuscitation. In patients with AS, hypotension should therefore be treated promptly with a vasoconstrictor like phenylephrine to prevent hemodynamic decompensation.[55,251,264] The anesthesia provider must be prepared for hemodynamic instability on induction and choose the medications and speed of administration accordingly. Patients often present with a significant degree of hypertension preoperatively, and BP may rise or fall abruptly during the procedure depending on the level of stimulation. Hypertension is better tolerated than hypotension, but it must be kept in mind that hypertension can also be a source of increased myocardial O_2 demand. Patients with severe AS have at least a 40 mm Hg mean (80 mm Hg systolic) pressure gradient between the LV and the aorta. Consequently, a systolic pressure of 180 mm Hg in the aorta correlates with a systolic pressure in the LV of at least 260 mm Hg.[250,265] Tachycardia decreases the diastolic time needed for adequate coronary perfusion and ventricular filling while simultaneously increasing myocardial O_2 demand. Hypotension or tachycardia must be treated promptly to avoid increased myocardial O_2 consumption, which can provoke ischemia. Vasodilators should be titrated cautiously. AF, with loss of atrial augmentation of CO, can lead to rapid hemodynamic deterioration, so prompt cardioversion is indicated.[55,113,115,266]

Stenotic AVs rarely lend themselves to repair.[266] The choice of the valve depends on patient preference, age, and comorbidities, but approximately 60% to 80% are currently replaced with a bioprosthetic (tissue) valve, and that number is increasing.[267] Other options include a mechanical valve, aortic homograft (cadaver valve), or a Ross procedure, which uses the native pulmonic valve. Table 26.11 shows various surgical options and key points about each alternative. Mechanical valves last approximately 25 to 50 years, but they are highly thrombogenic. Therefore lifelong anticoagulation is required with a vitamin K antagonist such as warfarin and occasionally endocarditis prophylaxis. NOACs are not approved for patients with mechanical heart valves.[268] Although tissue valves do not require anticoagulation, they degenerate over 10 to 20 years with durability being inversely proportional to the age at implantation. Guidelines recommend a bioprosthetic valve for patients of any age who cannot reliably take warfarin and for those older than 70 years. A mechanical valve is reasonable for patients under 60 years without contraindications to warfarin. Between age 60 and 70 years, the decision is individualized.[268] The STS mortality risk benchmark for an isolated AVR is 1.9% in an otherwise healthy patient but can increase to over 15% if the patient has multiple comorbidities and the surgery is combined with other procedures.[227] In these high-risk populations, percutaneous TAVR has revolutionized treatment.

Hypertrophic Cardiomyopathy

HCM is the preferred contemporary nomenclature for this pathophysiologic state. However, it was formerly known as idiopathic hypertrophic subaortic stenosis (IHSS). If HCM causes a LVOT obstruction, then it is often referred to as HOCM. HCM is an inherited disease that affects approximately 1 in 500 persons of all ages globally.[269] It is a heterogeneous genetic disorder with clinical presentations that range from asymptomatic to life threatening. When complications of HCM develop, they are described in three nonmutually exclusive categories: ventricular tachydysrhythmias that can lead to sudden cardiac death (SCD), especially in young athletes; progressive diastolic heart failure despite preserved LV systolic function; and AF, with a predisposition to stroke.[269,270] Before the opioid crisis, HCM was the leading cause of sudden death in young people. However, HCM can cause morbidity and death at any age.[113] The ACC and AHA recommend that the diagnosis and treatment of HCM take place in a clinical center that specializes in this disease state.[270]

Pathophysiology. Concentric LVH is the primary pathology in HCM, as opposed to AS, in which LVH is secondary to stenosis. The pathophysiology of HCM is complex and can include LVOT obstruction, MR, diastolic dysfunction, ischemia, and dysrhythmias.[269,271] HCM is categorized as either obstructive or nonobstructive, based on the degree of outflow tract obstruction and mitral valve involvement. Echocardiography is used to determine the presence of obstruction and to document the pressure gradient across the obstruction. A gradient of more than 30 mm Hg is considered significant, and a gradient of more than 50 mm Hg is the conventional threshold for surgical or percutaneous intervention if symptoms persist despite optimal medical management.[269,270] Approximately one-third of patients manifest as nonobstructive HCM, one-third manifest as obstruction even at rest, and one-third have variable obstruction based on volume-loading conditions. Approximately 25% of patients exhibit autonomic dysfunction that causes their BP to decrease or increase only slightly in response to exercise, which increases the degree of obstruction.[270,271]

Due to LVH, patients can have angina and ischemia even without significant CAD. Some patients will present with dyspnea, angina, and

syncope, but in more than half of cases sudden death or cardiac arrest is the initial finding. Patients with HCM must be evaluated for the risk of SCD.[266,269] In the subset of patients in whom basal septal hypertrophy obstructs the LVOT, ventricular contraction becomes hyperdynamic, forcing the blood to eject at high velocity to pass the obstruction. This rapid blood flow can lead to a Venturi effect that causes the anterior leaflet of the mitral valve or the chordal structures to be pulled into contact with the basal septal wall during systole (i.e., SAM) of the mitral valve. SAM increases LVOT obstruction and causes MR.[55,269] Any reduction in ventricular volume, directly or reflexively, will increase the degree of SAM-septal wall contact and exacerbate LVOT obstruction and MR. Therefore increases in heart rate and contractility and/or decreases in preload and afterload must be avoided. The atrial contribution to ventricular filling can be as much as 75%, so maintenance of sinus rhythm is essential, and synchronized cardioversion should occur promptly in patients who develop AF with hemodynamic instability.[266,270,272]

Medical management of HCM includes treatment of comorbidities and administration of β-blockers to prevent sympathetically induced tachycardia and AF, calcium channel blockers to improve diastolic relaxation, and disopyramide or other antidysrhythmic to reduce contractility and treat dysrhythmias. Sinus rhythm preserves the atrial contribution to CO. Patients with a history of cardiac arrest or symptomatic ventricular dysrhythmias will likely have an ICD.[269,271] ICDs should have their antitachyarrhythmia function suspended in the OR before surgery to prevent electrocautery-induced discharge. Means for external defibrillation must be available while the ICD is deactivated, and reactivation should occur as early as possible postoperatively. Alcohol septal ablation is the primary nonsurgical invasive therapy for HOCM.[270,271]

Anesthetic considerations and surgical options. Patients who remain symptomatic with gradients of 50 mm Hg, despite optimal medical management, are candidates for septal reduction therapy. Surgical septal myotomy via the aortic approach at an experienced surgery center is preferred over alcohol septal ablation.[269,270] Approximately two-thirds of patients will also have structural malformations of the mitral valve. It is not uncommon to find that the mitral valve will need repair or replacement at the time of myectomy.[266]

Anesthetic management (Table 26.12) is directed at optimizing preload, avoiding increases in the septal wall–anterior mitral valve leaflet contact caused by increases in heart rate or contractility, and preventing sudden reductions in afterload. Excision of the hypertrophic basal septum may result in disruption of the conduction system of the heart, with new-onset heart block requiring cardiac pacing.[55,266] After CPB is terminated, the outflow tract and mitral valve are examined using TEE. To determine the adequacy of surgical repair, the patient's heart rate and contractility are deliberately increased while the BP is simultaneously decreased, to mimic a physiologic hyperdynamic state such as exercise. An infusion of isoproterenol is ideal for achieving this goal. Dobutamine or rapid ventricular pacing (at a rate of 120 bpm), combined with an infusion of nitroglycerin, can also be used. TEE examination will reveal whether obstruction, SAM, or MR develops. If more muscle needs to be excised, or the valve needs repair or replacement to prevent SAM, CPB will be resumed so the surgeon can make the necessary adjustments.

Aortic Insufficiency or Regurgitation

AI (or AR) occurs when maladaptation of the AV leaflet or annular dilation allows a portion of the ejected SV to be regurgitated or flow retrograde from the aorta into the LV during diastole. The regurgitant blood flow causes the LV to be volume overloaded, initially causing LV pressure overload. AI can develop acutely or chronically and can be caused by a primary disease affecting the valve itself or can be

TABLE 26.11 Surgical Options for the Aortic Valve

Surgical Option	Surgical Considerations
Repair 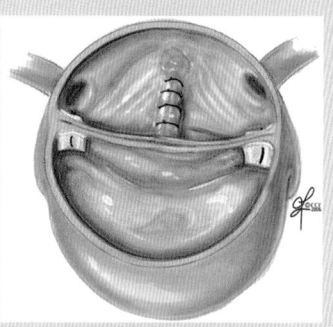 (Reprinted with permission from Cleveland Clinic Center for Medical Art & Photography © 2006-2012. All rights reserved.)	Used for aortic regurgitation, usually due to bicuspid valve Technically more difficult than mitral repair Can last a lifetime, but 20%–25% need to be replaced in 10 yr Preserves heart muscle strength and natural heart anatomy Decreased risk of infection Decreased requirement for lifelong anticoagulation
Replacement With a Mechanical Valve 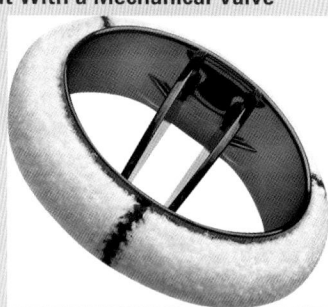 (Courtesy Medtronic Inc., Minneapolis, MN.)	Designed to last a lifetime (25–50 yr) Requires the use of lifetime warfarin so lifestyle, childbearing, and compliance must be considered Some antibiotic prophylaxis Some produce a clicking noise
Replacement With a Bioprosthetic (Tissue) Valve 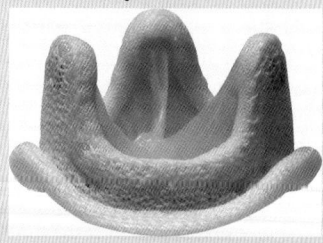 (Courtesy Medtronic Inc., Minneapolis, MN.)	Made of cow (bovine) pericardium or pig (porcine) aortic valve sewn on a frame Warfarin not usually required unless the patient is in atrial fibrillation Valve degenerates over 10–20 yr Generally, less durable if younger and more durable if older at age of implantation Straightforward, relatively low risk
Replacement With a Homograft (Also Called Allograft) 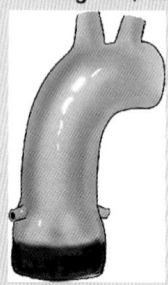 (From Otto CM, Bonow RO. *Valvular Heart Disease: A Companion to Braunwald's Heart Disease.* 4th ed. Philadelphia: Elsevier; 2014.)	Human aortic or pulmonic valve Ideal for endocarditis because the valve is less prone to infection May be a good choice for athletes because of excellent flow characteristics and no need to take warfarin Technically challenging and limited availability Last only approximately 15 yr; durability varies with age
Ross Procedure (Also Called Switch Procedure) 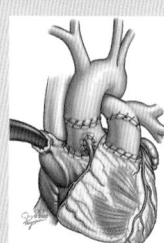 (Reprinted with permission from Cleveland Clinic Center for Medical Art & Photography © 2006-2012. All rights reserved.)	Patient's pulmonary valve is removed and used to replace the aortic valve; coronaries are reimplanted. Pulmonary valve is replaced with a pulmonary homograft. Main advantage is that the valves can grow, so a good choice for teens. Lifetime anticoagulation is not required. Pulmonary autograft (in aortic position) has approximately a 50% chance of lasting a lifetime. Pulmonary homograft has a 10% chance of needing replacement in 10 yr. Technically difficult and reoperation is challenging.

TABLE 26.12 **Anesthetic Considerations in the Management of HOCM**		
Factor	**Hemodynamic Goals**	**Anesthetic Considerations**
Preload	High normal	Volume is key; the first treatment for hypotension Optimize preload to stretch the noncompliant LV Reduces the gradient across LVOT Prevents SAM and MR PaEDP > LVEDV (evaluate with TEE)
Heart rate	Low normal	Too fast → ischemia and not enough time for ventricular filling
Rhythm	Maintain sinus	Atrial kick contributes to LVEDV Cardiovert early
Compliance	Improve	↓ due to concentric hypertrophy
Contractility	Reduce	Usually hyperdynamic Inhalation agents and/or β-blockers are used to depress
SVR	Avoid reductions	Hypertension better tolerated than hypotension Treat hypotension with volume and phenylephrine
PVR	Maintain	Not usually a problem

↓, Decrease(d); →, leads to; *EF*, ejection fraction; *HOCM*, hypertrophic obstructive cardiomyopathy; *LV*, left ventricle; *LVEDV*, left ventricular end-diastolic volume; *LVOT*, left ventricular outflow tract; *MR*, mitral regurgitation; *PaEDP*, pulmonary artery end-diastolic pressure; *PVR*, pulmonary vascular resistance; *SAM*, systolic anterior motion of the mitral valve; *SVR*, systemic vascular resistance; *TEE*, transesophageal echocardiography.

TABLE 26.13 **Anesthetic Considerations in the Management of Aortic Insufficiency Fast, Full, and Forward**		
Factor	**Hemodynamic Goals**	**Anesthetic Considerations**
Preload	High normal	Need increased volume to maintain forward flow
Heart rate	High normal	Decreased diastolic time minimizes regurgitation Avoid bradycardia
Rhythm	Usually sinus	Not usually a concern
Compliance	Maintain	Eccentric hypertrophy can lead to an LVEDV three to four times normal Return large pump volume judiciously after bypass to prevent failure
Contractility	Maintain	Normal LVF till late Surgery indicated when EF <50% May need inotropes after pump
SVR	↓	Judicious vasodilation enhances forward flow
PVR	Maintain or ↓	PVR ↑ rapidly with acute AI → acute failure
CPB	↓ LV distention	Can develop due to slow HR or nonbeating heart Consider LV vent; retrograde or ostial cardioplegia

↑, Increase(d); ↓, decrease(d); →, leads to; *AI*, aortic insufficiency; *CPB*, cardiopulmonary bypass; *EF*, ejection fraction; *HR*, heart rate; *LV*, left ventricle; *LVEDV*, left ventricular end-diastolic volume; *LVF*, left ventricular function; *PVR*, pulmonary vascular resistance; *SVR*, systemic vascular resistance.

secondary to aortic root dilation. Acute AI results in rapid deterioration and is most frequently caused by trauma, endocarditis, or aortic dissection. Chronic AI can be tolerated for decades and is caused by bicuspid or tricuspid valve degeneration in 67% of patients.[273] There are multiple other etiologies, including rheumatic fever, inflammatory or connective tissue disease (Marfan, Loeys-Dietz, or Ehlers-Danlos syndrome), idiopathic aortic root or valve dilation, hypertension-induced aortoannular ectasia, syphilis, and rheumatoid arthritis.[251]

Pathophysiology. The increased LVEDV causes increased diastolic wall tension that leads to a pattern of LV chamber enlargement known as eccentric hypertrophy, whereby the sarcomeres replicate in series. By virtue of the Frank-Starling mechanism, the increased preload results in a large SV that in turn rapidly raises aortic systolic pressure. Diastolic runoff is rapid as blood can flow antegrade through the aorta or retrograde through an incompetent AV back into the LV. The period of isovolumetric relaxation is lost as the ventricle fills throughout diastole. The period of isovolumetric contraction is shortened because the low aortic diastolic pressure affords minimal resistance to ventricular ejection. The rapid systolic ejection and diastolic runoff cause a bounding pulse, a widened pulse pressure (SBP – DBP), and an arterial waveform with a rapid rise in systolic pressure and a low dicrotic notch. Sometimes a double systolic peak called pulsus bisferiens can be seen on the arterial pressure trace. The magnitude of the regurgitant volume is directly proportional to regurgitant orifice size, diastolic time, and SVR. Ventricular compliance is increased, and the LVEDV can be three to four times greater than normal.[55,251,266] The regurgitation is graded as mild (1+ [< 30%]) to severe (4+ [≥

50%]), based on echocardiographic findings.[115] As volume overload progresses, wall tension also increases, resulting in LV pressure overload and some degree of concentric hypertrophy. The hypertrophy increases O_2 demand, and angina can develop in patients with normal coronaries. However, the O_2 debt incurred for muscle shortening is relatively low, so ischemia occurs less often than in AS.[55,274] The natural history of chronic AI is such that dilation occurs slowly over years. Ventricular compensation allows the patient to remain asymptomatic until the AI is severe, causing permanent LV dysfunction.[266] Surgery is an AHA/ACC class I recommendation for all symptomatic patients and asymptomatic patients when ventricular function falls below 50% or if the patient is undergoing cardiac surgery for other indications.[115]

Acute AI can cause rapid deterioration because the normal ventricle is unable to compensate for the sudden increase in volume. Ventricular distension leads to increased LVEDV and LVEDP. As the LVEDP approaches the aortic diastolic pressure, coronary perfusion decreases, causing ischemia and systolic dysfunction. Pulmonary congestion is likely since the forward blood flow from the LA is reduced due to higher LV diastolic volume and pressure. MR can develop as the LV dilates further.[274,275] TEE is invaluable in the etiologic diagnosis and treatment of acute AI and can help determine the need for urgent or emergent surgery.

Anesthetic considerations and surgical options. Hemodynamic management of AI (Table 26.13) is focused on enhancing forward flow and minimizing regurgitant volume. Regurgitation occurs during diastole, so a relatively high heart rate minimizes diastolic time. The patient's volume should be kept in the "high normal" range because the heart is dilated and compliance is increased. Judicious vasodilation lowers the SVR to enhance forward flow and reduce regurgitant volume, while still maintaining adequate pressure to support coronary perfusion. "Fast, full, and forward" is the frequently quoted mnemonic that reflects this hemodynamic management of AI.

During CPB, AI can lead to ventricular distention and pressure overload that directly opposes coronary perfusion and myocardial preservation. When CPB is initiated, a slow heart rate or ventricular fibrillation can result in distension. After the aortic cross-clamp is applied, cardioplegia is usually infused into the aortic root. While cardioplegia normally flows antegrade down the coronary ostia, in the presence of an incompetent valve, it can fill and dilate the LV. Even mild to moderate AI can cause LV distention; consequently, the presence of AI increases the risk of other cardiac surgical procedures. Achieving diastolic standstill in these situations often requires that cardioplegia be delivered directly into the coronary ostia and/or retrograde cardioplegia delivered through the coronary sinus. An LV vent is sometimes placed to suction away blood and fluid, thereby alleviating or preventing distension. A positive inotrope is often useful after CPB, especially if there was LV dysfunction prebypass or questionable preservation during bypass.[55,113,251]

Current guidelines suggest that aortic valve repair (AVr) and valve-sparing aortic surgery be considered over AVR, ideally performed at an experienced heart valve replacement medical center.[115,263,273,276] Traditional replacement options are the same as for AS (see Table 26.11). Percutaneous TAVR was pioneered for AS but is now also showing promise for patients with AR. TAVR is discussed in the minimally invasive section of the chapter.[277]

Mitral Stenosis

In the developed world, atherosclerotic-associated annular calcification and endocarditis are now the main etiologies of mitral stenosis, whereas RHD still prevails in underdeveloped countries.[55,278] Although RHD affects men and women equally, mitral stenosis is two to three times more prevalent in women.[278] Less common etiologies include carcinoid syndrome, left atrial myxoma, collagen diseases, and radiation heart disease.[251] Clinically, significant stenosis takes decades to develop, and symptoms do not usually appear until the valve area, which is normally 4 to 5 cm², is reduced to 2.5 cm². Many patients remain asymptomatic until the valve area is 1 cm².[115,278]

Pathophysiology. Diastolic filling of the LV is limited by the narrowed orifice, and a pressure gradient develops across the mitral valve. Left atrial volume and pressure increase, leading to atrial dilation and elevated pulmonary pressures. Right ventricular failure can eventually develop if PHTN is uncorrected. Stenosis is considered severe when the valve area is 1.5 cm² or less and very severe when it is 1 cm² or less. In severe mitral stenosis, the mean gradient across the valve generally exceeds 5 to 10 mm Hg, and PA systolic pressures are greater than 30 mm Hg.[115] The risk of surgery is 3% to 8% in most studies, but the presence of PHTN increases the risk to 12%.[278] Flow across the valve will decrease in response to an increase in CO or a decrease in diastolic time. Hence symptoms are usually first experienced during exercise or stress. Conditions such as pregnancy and sepsis may provoke AF in a previously asymptomatic patient, leading to decompensation. Approximately 33% of patients develop AF. The rapid heart rate is the primary cause of hemodynamic instability rather than the loss of atrial kick.[251] Patients with mitral stenosis and AF have an embolic stroke rate of 7% to 15% per year. Long-term anticoagulation and heart rate control are important in the management of mitral stenosis.[278]

Anesthetic considerations and surgical options. Mitral stenosis mechanically obstructs LV filling. The three procedures used to relieve this obstruction are mitral balloon valvotomy, open commissurotomy

TABLE 26.14 Anesthetic Considerations in the Management of Mitral Stenosis

Factor	Hemodynamic Goals	Anesthetic Considerations
Preload	High normal	LV chronically underloaded Adequate preload needed to maintain flow across the valve, but overloading leads to pulmonary congestion
Heart rate	Low normal	Need adequate diastolic time to fill LV Too fast→↑ gradient across valve
Rhythm	Sinus If AF, control ventricular rate	AF occurs in 33% of patients May decompensate if rapid ventricular response, otherwise reasonably well tolerated
Compliance	Maintain	Usually normal
Contractility	Maintain LV RV often needs support	LV may need inotropic support after pump Administer volume cautiously after pump, watching for RV dysfunction and volume overload RV may need support with epinephrine or milrinone
SVR	Maintain	Treat ↓ BP with volume or mixed alpha and beta drug (ephedrine) Pure alpha→ ↑ pulmonary pressures May need vasoconstrictor to offset vasodilation from milrinone but watch for pulmonary vasoconstriction
PVR	Reduce	PHTN can be mild to severe Avoid hypercarbia, hypoxia, acidosis, Trendelenburg position, nitrous oxide, and desflurane Severe cases may benefit from inhaled epoprostenol (Veletri or Flolan)

↑, Increase; ↓, decrease; →, leads to; *AF*, atrial fibrillation; *BP*, blood pressure; *LV*, left ventricle; *NTG*, nitroglycerin; *PHTN*, pulmonary hypertension; *PVR*, pulmonary vascular resistance; *RV*, right ventricle; *SVR*, systemic vascular resistance.

of the mitral valve, and replacement with a mechanical or biologic valve. Closed commissurotomy is no longer recommended. Valvotomy or repair is generally preferred to a replacement, but a left atrial thrombus, concurrent MR, or annular calcification may make replacement the treatment of choice.[115] If the patient has a history of AF and the valve is approached through a full sternotomy, the surgeon will often elect to add a MAZE procedure or pulmonary vein isolation (PVI) to treat AF. Anesthetic considerations for the MAZE procedure and other options for atrial ablation are discussed after the valve section of this chapter. The LAA may also be excised or clipped to decrease the risk of emboli.

Anesthetic considerations for mitral stenosis are outlined in Table 26.14. Maintaining a low-normal heart rate is a priority to ensure adequate LV filling during diastole. If AF is present or develops, the ventricular rate must be controlled. Conditions or medications that can exacerbate PHTN should be avoided. These include hypercarbia, hypoxemia, nitrous oxide, desflurane, and the Trendelenburg position.[251,278] Mitral stenosis is the only valve defect that causes the LV to be chronically underloaded. Volume management can be challenging because an adequate preload is needed to maintain flow across the stenotic valve, but too much volume can lead to pulmonary congestion.

The majority of patients have normal left ventricular function; however, the increase in ventricular volume that occurs after valve replacement can cause the chronically underloaded LV to dilate. If failure occurs, it is generally responsive to inotropic support.[279] PHTN with resultant RV failure can be more problematic. Patients may benefit from mild hypocapnia, judicious vasodilator therapy, and inotropic support with epinephrine or milrinone. In extreme cases, inhaled epoprostenol (Veletri or Flolan) or nitric oxide may be used to dilate the pulmonary vasculature and reduce RV afterload. Routine use of nitric oxide is limited by cost.[55,113]

Mitral Regurgitation or Insufficiency

MR (or mitral insufficiency) occurs during systole when blood is ejected retrograde into the LA due to an incompetent mitral valve. MR is present in about 2% of the US population making it the most common valve disorder across the lifespan.[245,266] The causes of MR are considered primary/organic or structural, when the regurgitation is due to a problem with the valve leaflets or chordae. Secondary or functional insufficiency results from a dilated LV stretching a structurally normal valve. In developed countries, chronic MR is usually caused by myxomatous degenerative processes that lead to leaflet prolapse, sometimes with chordal rupture. MR can also arise secondary to inflammatory diseases like RHD, lupus erythematosus, or rheumatoid arthritis; or collagen diseases and connective tissue disorders such as Marfan or Ehlers-Danlos syndrome. Functional MR is most often caused by ischemic heart disease, but it can also develop in patients who have idiopathic cardiomyopathy. The presentation of the patient with MR varies depending on the etiology or acuity of the condition. Acute MR is most often the result of papillary muscle or chordae tendineae rupture or dysfunction due to ischemia, infarction, or infective endocarditis.[251,263,266]

Pathophysiology. In MR, both the LA and the LV experience volume overload. This occurs because the total SV is equivalent to the volume of blood that is ejected antegrade into the aorta, plus the amount of blood that is ejected retrograde into the LA. The isovolumetric contraction phase of systole is minimized because the LA acts as a low-resistance vent for ventricular ejection.[278] Consequently, the EF that is calculated by TEE overestimates the actual forward flow. Pressure and volume overload lead to LA dilation. AF develops in approximately 50% of patients who undergo surgery.[113] The amount of regurgitation is dynamic and based on the size of the mitral orifice, the pressure gradient between the LA and LV, the time available for regurgitant flow, and the compliance of the receiving chamber.[251] The LA and LV compensate for the chronic volume overload by dilating in an eccentric pattern (series replication of sarcomeres) and increasing compliance to accommodate the volume load. Patients with chronic MR may be asymptomatic for years because large increases in volume can occur with minimal increases in LA pressure or PAEDP. Systolic work is not initially increased, making myocardial ischemia unlikely. Increases in heart rate and decreases in preload and/or afterload help minimize the regurgitation and enhance forward flow.[55] CO is an afterload-dependent measurement. Often TEE evaluation of MR requires pharmacologic manipulation of the BP to evaluate the regurgitant volume at various systolic driving pressures.[113,251] It is important to note that volume overload eventually induces pressure overload, leading to LV dysfunction; however, CO may be normal or only mildly reduced, even in the face of significantly compromised ventricular function. An EF of less than 60% in a patient with severe MR represents significant LV dysfunction and is predictive of a worsening outcome. This problem is often first unmasked during the attempt to separate from CPB after valve repair or replacement.[113] Pharmacologic support with epinephrine, dobutamine, or milrinone should be considered if LV dysfunction occurs.[115,250,251,266,280]

TABLE 26.15 Anesthetic Considerations in the Management of Mitral Regurgitation

Factor	Hemodynamic Goals	Anesthetic Considerations
Preload	High normal	Cautiously ↓ or ↑ to enhance forward flow
Heart rate	High normal	Decreased diastolic time minimizes regurgitation. Avoid bradycardia
Rhythm	Sinus AF, control ventricular rate	Not usually a concern as long as the rate is adequate
Compliance	Maintain	Eccentric hypertrophy of LA and LV
Contractility	Maintain	May have LV dysfunction even with mildly ↓ EF. May need inotropes after pump
SVR	↓	Cautious vasodilation enhances forward flow
PVR	↓	PHTN can be mild to severe, acute, or chronic. Avoid hypercarbia, hypoxia, acidosis, Trendelenburg position, and nitrous oxide. Severe cases may benefit from inhaled epoprostenol (Veletri or Flolan)
CPB		LV dysfunction can be unmasked after surgery

↑, Increase; ↓, decrease; *AF*, atrial fibrillation; *CPB*, cardiopulmonary bypass; *EF*, ejection fraction; *IABP*, intraaortic balloon pump; *LA*, left atrium; *LV*, left ventricle; *MR*, mitral regurgitation; *MV*, mitral valve; *PHTN*, pulmonary hypertension; *PVR*, pulmonary vascular resistance; *RV*, right ventricle; *SVR*, systemic vascular resistance.

Patients with acute MR often deteriorate rapidly. The LA cannot compensate for the abrupt increase in volume, resulting in pulmonary congestion, edema, and RHF. The pulmonary capillary wedge pressure (PCWP) will classically show an enlarged V wave, but the size does not reliably correlate with the degree of MR.[266] Acute MR must often be treated on an urgent or emergent basis with mitral repair or replacement. Oftentimes, an IABP will be used to increase coronary perfusion, decrease afterload, and support the patient during the perioperative period.[113]

Anesthetic considerations and surgical options. The preload is elevated and must be judiciously maintained or manipulated to enhance forward flow and minimize regurgitation. Inhalation agents and vasodilators are generally effective in reducing afterload and maintaining heart rate in the high-normal range (Table 26.15). Valve repair or replacement increases afterload and may unmask previously compensated LV dysfunction. An inotrope or inotrope/vasodilator may be needed after CPB. Occasionally, SAM develops after the repair, especially if the anterior leaflet is long or has redundant tissue. TEE is used to diagnose this problem.[55]

According to AHA/ACC guidelines, MR is graded as severe when the regurgitant volume is 60 mL or more or the regurgitant fraction is 50% or more. In patients with severe MR, surgery is a class I recommendation for all symptomatic patients with a LVEF greater than 30%, and asymptomatic patients with LVEF from 30% to 60% and/or left ventricular end-systolic diameter (LVESD) of 40 mm or more.[250] Mitral valve repair is recommended over replacement whenever possible, depending on the native valve pathology and on surgical expertise. The advantages of repair include improved postoperative LV function,

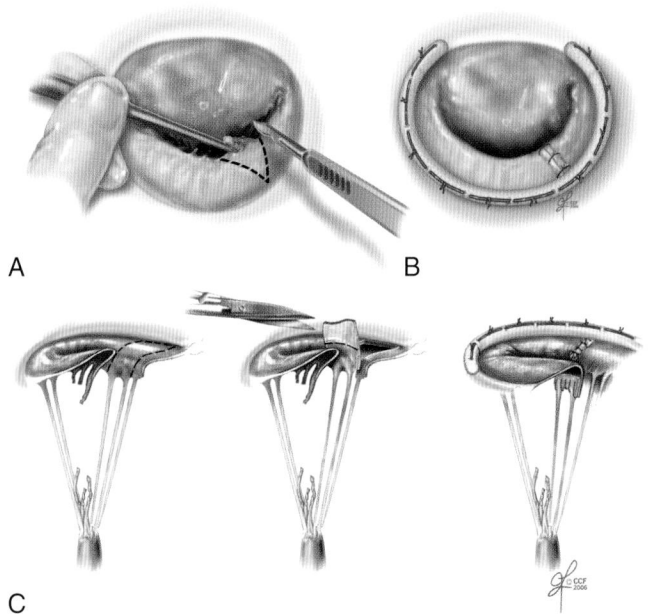

C

Fig. 26.24 Mitral valve repair. (A) Triangular resection is the technique used most often for posterior leaflet prolapse. Region to be resected is indicated. (B) Abnormal segment has been removed. Leaflet edges are sewn together. An annuloplasty ring completes the repair. (C) Chordal transfer to correct anterior leaflet prolapse. Posterior leaflet chordae are transferred to the unsupported free edge of the anterior leaflet. The posterior leaflet is repaired with a quadrangular resection. An annu-loplasty ring completes the repair. (Reprinted with permission from Cleveland Clinic Center for Medical Art & Photography © 2006-2012. All rights reserved.)

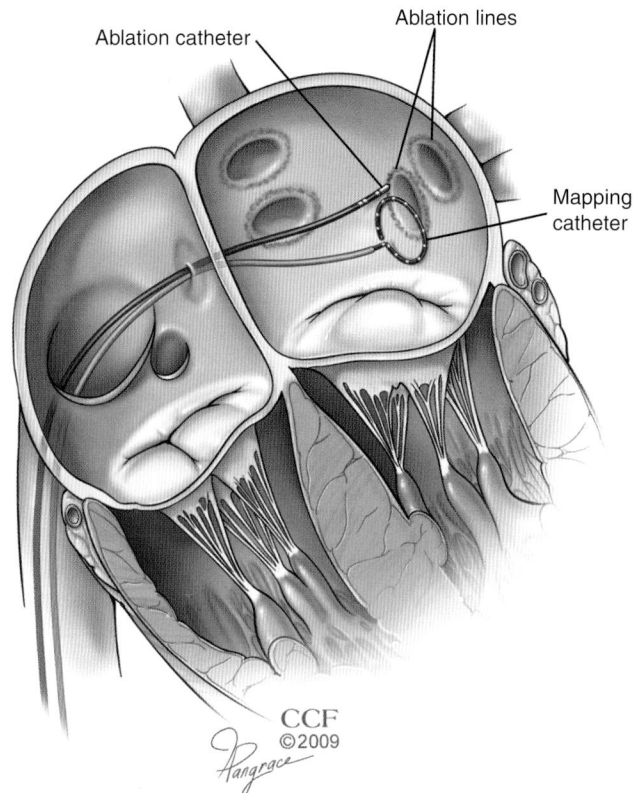

Fig. 26.25 Pulmonary vein isolation procedure. Energy is applied to the tip of the catheter to target the upper and lower pulmonary veins at the point where they connect with the left atrium. (Reprinted with permission, Cleveland Clinic Center for Medical Art & Photography ©2021. All rights reserved.)

increased long-term and short-term survival, improved quality of life, lower risk of complications, and less need for long-term anticoagula-tion. The benefits of repair or replacement are less well established in patients with an LVEF less than 30% (class IIb).[250]

Over the past decade, as surgeons have gained experience with valve repair techniques, the number of mitral valve repairs performed and the variety of approaches have risen dramatically. The mitral valve can be accessed through traditional sternotomy, partial upper sternotomy, right mini-thoracotomy, and robotic-assisted endoscopy. Posterior leaf-let abnormalities are often repaired using a triangular or quadrangu-lar resection, with a complete or partial annuloplasty ring (Fig. 26.24). Involvement of the anterior leaflet increases the complexity of the repair and requires greater surgical expertise because the chords must often be shortened, transferred, or replaced. If the patient has AF, a MAZE procedure or ablation may be performed. Severe mitral annular calcifi-cation or rheumatic disease may make repair impossible, in which case the valve can be replaced with a tissue or mechanical device.[115,263,266] When a patient has severe heart failure and is a poor surgical candidate, another US Food and Drug Administration (FDA)–approved advance-ment involves endovascular placement of a clip (MitraClip, Abbott Vascular, Abbott Park, IL) that grasps and coapts the mitral valve leaf-lets, resulting in fixed approximation of the mitral leaflets throughout the cardiac cycle. Transcatheter mitral valve replacement is currently in development with several devices already approved in Europe.[281] These alternative approaches are discussed later in the chapter.

Management of AF

Research over the past few decades has largely focused on medical and surgical therapies to treat AF. Class I recommended treatments for AF include the prescription of antiarrhythmic, rate-control, and/or

anticoagulation medications.[282] In cases when medications fail to con-trol the ventricular rate and hemodynamic instability ensues, electrical or pharmacologic cardioversion is also considered a class I recommen-dation.[283] When the aforementioned therapies are contraindicated or proven ineffective, catheter-based procedures or surgical interventions may be effective.

Catheter ablation

Procedural approaches. The abnormal electrical impulses that provoke AF often originate where the four pulmonary veins enter the LA. Therefore PVI utilizes radiofrequency energy or cryoablation to encircle and isolate each pulmonary vein and prevent the propagation of abnormal electric signals (Fig. 26.25).[284] Currently, catheter ablation is a class IIb recommendation for patients with symptomatic AF and heart failure.[282]

Anesthetic considerations. Catheter ablation procedures utilize fluoroscopy and are usually performed in electrophysiology (EP) laboratories at remote locations from the OR. Standard ASA monitoring with frequent BP measurements is sufficient. However, patients at high risk for intraoperative decompensation may require arterial and central venous access. Due to the potential for critical arrhythmias during the procedure, external defibrillation pads are placed.[285]

Catheter ablation may be performed with general endotracheal anesthesia (GETA) or MAC. Benefits to MAC include the patient's ability to report pain as an early sign of complication, the prompt iden-tification of a neurologic event, and the avoidance of risks associated with GETA. However, precise localization and ablation of abnormal foci is required, and GETA is beneficial to minimize patient movement and improve comfort during long or complex procedures. GETA also provides greater patient comfort when TEE is used to guide transseptal puncture; however, the use of intracardiac echocardiography (ICE) may be equally as effective and more suitable in patients undergoing MAC. If respiratory movement interferes with catheter-tissue contact, high-frequency jet ventilation may be useful.[285]

Antiarrhythmic medications must be discontinued prior to the procedure to properly identify the origin of arrhythmia. In addition, the administration of isoproterenol or adenosine during the procedure helps to identify areas of abnormal electrical activity.[285] Ketamine may also be useful for induction of cardiac arrhythmias since it shortens atrial conduction and stimulates the SNS.[286] Notably, remifentanil and dexmedetomidine may interfere with the identification of abnormal foci and should be avoided.[285] According to a literature review, sevoflurane, midazolam, fentanyl, and propofol do not affect cardiac conduction and are appropriate for use in these cases.[286] In patients with chronic AF, the origin of arrhythmia is easier to identify, and anesthetic agents should not interfere.

Due to the high risk of stroke associated with cardiac ablation procedures performed on the left side of the heart, chronic anticoagulation medications are continued throughout the perioperative period. Heparin is administered prior to transseptal puncture at a dose of 130 units/kg in patients on NOAC therapy and 100 units/kg in patients receiving warfarin.[285] This is followed by an infusion at a rate of 2000 to 2500 units/hour in patients receiving NOACs, and 10 units/kg/hour in patients receiving warfarin to achieve and maintain an ACT of 300 to 400 seconds.[285] Protamine reversal may or may not be administered at the conclusion of the procedure depending on the amount of bleeding present. Alternatively, for epicardial ablation, anticoagulants must be discontinued at the appropriate time prior to the procedure to decrease the risk of severe bleeding.

A major risk of cardiac ablation procedures is thermal injury leading to esophageal perforation or the formation of an atrioesophageal fistula. Therefore an esophageal temperature probe is placed following endotracheal intubation, and the interventional cardiologist performs each phase of ablation based on temperature rise within the esophagus. Another risk related to cardiac ablation is injury to the right phrenic nerve, which lies close in proximity to the right superior pulmonary vein. During intervention on the right superior pulmonary vein, high-frequency phrenic nerve pacing is utilized, and the anesthesia provider must ensure complete recovery from neuromuscular blockade at this time. The movement of catheters within the heart and the use of radiofrequency is associated with the risk of perforation, which may require immediate intervention and management. In the most severe cases, cardiac surgery must intervene, and the patient may require immediate transportation to the OR.[285]

Left atrial appendage occlusion (LAAO)

Procedural approaches. The LAA is a common site of clot formation in patients with AF. LAA closure devices may be effective in decreasing the risk of stroke in patients unable to take anticoagulation medications.[282,287] The WATCHMAN device, specifically, utilizes an endovascular approach via the femoral vein, is advanced across the interatrial septum into the LA, and self-expands once in the LAA (Fig. 26.26).[288] In March 2015 the first-generation WATCHMAN device gained FDA approval for use in patients with nonvalvular AF and at high risk for stroke.[289] Based on clinical trials and FDA approval, the AHA/ACC/Heart Rhythm Society (HRS) guideline offers a class IIb recommendation for LAAO.[282] Since this recommendation, the second-generation WATCHMAN FLX device gained FDA approval in July 2020 for patients with nonvalvular AF appropriately seeking nondrug therapy.[290]

Notably, when a patient with AF is scheduled to have an open-heart procedure, the LAA may be excised completely or surgically separated

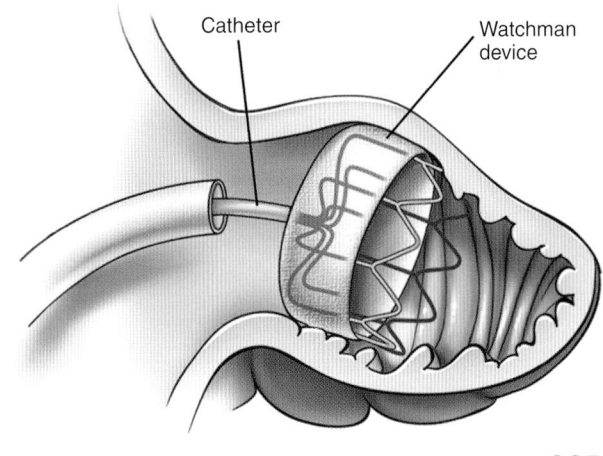

Fig. 26.26 Watchman device. The device is guided through a catheter sheath into the left atrial appendage (LAA). Once in the correct position, it self-expands and occludes the LAA from the rest of the heart, preventing the release of clots. (Reprinted with permission, Cleveland Clinic Center for Medical Art & Photography ©2021. All Rights Reserved.)

from the rest of the LA with a clip.[291] This procedure is currently a class IIb recommendation in the AHA/ACC/HRS guideline for patients with symptomatic AF who are already scheduled for open-heart surgery and are at risk for a postoperative thromboembolic event.[282]

Anesthetic considerations. Similar to cardiac ablation procedures, LAAO may be performed at remote locations from the OR. A preoperative CT scan determines the size and location of the LAA, while a preoperative echocardiogram assesses cardiac function, valvular abnormalities, and the presence of intracardiac thrombus. Fluoroscopy and TEE guide intervention throughout the procedure. In addition to standard ASA monitors, defibrillation pads should be placed to combat prolonged arrhythmia in conjunction with hemodynamic instability. Large-bore peripheral IVs and an A line are placed to quickly recognize and treat hemodynamic compromise or bleeding.[288] Many interventional cardiologists gain central venous access via the femoral vein for use by the anesthesia team if necessary.

Most patients undergoing LAAO receive GETA due to the need for continuous intraoperative TEE; however, there have been reports of the procedure being performed under MAC.[292] To perform MAC, the patient must be able to tolerate the insertion of the TEE probe and have the capacity to lie flat and still for the full duration of the procedure. In some institutions, ICE has been used in place of TEE, which better accommodates a patient undergoing MAC.[292] If GETA is used, the patient is extubated at the end of the procedure to allow for a thorough neurologic exam and to rule out a procedure-related stroke.

Due to the risk of severe bleeding, chronic anticoagulation medications are discontinued preoperatively. Prior to transseptal puncture, however, heparin is administered at a dose of 100 units/kg with a goal ACT of at least 250 seconds. The ACT may be allowed to drift back to baseline at the conclusion of the procedure or a small dose of protamine may be administered for reversal.[288]

Risks specific to the WATCHMAN procedure include severe bleeding, pericardial effusion, stroke, air embolism, and device embolization. Upon advancement of the device and deployment in the LAA, the patient may experience arrhythmias and is at risk for LAA rupture.[288] Blood products and a cardiothoracic surgical team should be readily available in the case of an emergency. The risks related to the device itself include device failure, device-related thrombus, and inadequate closure of the LAA.[293]

MAZE procedure

Surgical approaches. The most common and reliable surgical technique used to treat AF is the MAZE procedure, founded by Cox and colleagues approximately three decades ago.[294] When performed with the use of CPB, the Cox-MAZE procedure is reported to be more successful than any single, catheter-based approach and results in a greater reduction in stroke.[294] When the MAZE procedure was first pioneered, the surgeon created a series of small incisions that formed a "maze" of scar tissue throughout the atria. This scar tissue prevented the abnormal electrical impulses that caused AF, but still allowed electrical conduction from the sinoatrial (SA) node to the atrioventricular (AV) node, negating the need for insertion of a permanent pacemaker (PPM). Currently, the fourth version of the MAZE procedure is performed (MAZE IV), which reflects the many updates to the procedure over the past 30 years. Now, instead of small incisions, both radiofrequency and cryoablation energy are used to create the essential scar tissue. As mentioned previously, with the heart in direct view, techniques to surgically remove or isolate the LAA are often performed together with the MAZE procedure.

Anesthetic considerations. In most cases, the MAZE procedure is carried out in conjunction with another open-heart surgery, so the surgical approach is often dependent on the exposure required for the primary surgery. However, it is possible to perform the MAZE procedure with a traditional median sternotomy or a right mini-thoracotomy. In the case of a right mini-thoracotomy, right lung isolation is achieved with either a double-lumen endotracheal tube (DLT) or single-lumen endotracheal tube (SLT) and bronchial blocker.[295]

Convergent procedure

Surgical approaches. The convergent procedure is a hybrid approach to treat persistent, nonparoxysmal AF with the combination of epicardial and endocardial techniques. The epicardial approach is preferably performed with a subxiphoid incision, as it is a more direct route to the pericardium compared with a transdiaphragmatic approach. The posterior LA is then targeted, and ablation lines are created from the right to left inferior pulmonary veins. This portion of the procedure is generally followed by a left, video-assisted thoracotomy (VATS) for occlusion of the LAA. For the endocardial portion of the procedure, femoral access is achieved, and endocardial ablation is performed on the pulmonary veins and other areas of the heart not accessible with epicardial access. The epicardial and endocardial procedures may be performed on the same day in either a hybrid OR or an EP laboratory with OR capabilities, or a staged procedure may be performed at separate times.[296]

Anesthetic considerations. Epicardial access requires GETA with muscle relaxation, and a VATS requires a DLT for lung isolation. A TEE is inserted, and the absence of intracardiac thrombus is confirmed prior to the procedure. An esophageal temperature probe is positioned in the esophagus near the LA to monitor temperature rise throughout the operation, and central venous and arterial access are often obtained. Contraindications to the procedure include previous cardiac surgery, mediastinal radiation, or the current presence of an intracardiac thrombus.[296]

Minimally Invasive Cardiac Surgery

General Considerations

Minimally invasive surgical approaches have been performed since the 1950s, but MICS was not established until 4 decades later. Since then, the specific approaches to safely and successfully accomplish these operations have evolved considerably. Most patients desire a less invasive approach assuming it amounts to less risk. Unfortunately, the

literature does not support this perception, and there are many factors to consider to ensure optimal surgical exposure and patient safety.[297]

According to recent studies, survival rates are similar when comparing traditional median sternotomy with MICS.[297] Reasons to execute MICS include decreased bleeding, lower rates of transfusion, earlier extubation, faster mobilization, expedited discharge from the hospital, lower rates of wound infection, a lower incidence of pain, and a more cosmetic appearance. However, there are also reported complications with MICS, including increased rates of hemorrhage, complications associated with the femoral vessels following cannulation, unilateral pulmonary edema, and high rates of conversion to a conventional technique. There is controversy over whether femoral cannulation and the retrograde direction of blood flow in the descending aorta lead to increased risk of stroke. Contraindications to MICS include diffuse CAD with severe calcifications at the site of anastomoses, presence of calcification around the mitral annulus, abscesses in the setting of endocarditis, abnormal cardiac anatomy, a porcelain aorta, or a very narrow aorta.[297,298]

Surgical Approaches

What constitutes a minimally invasive approach is quite variable as there are many ways to gain exposure to the heart's valves, vessels, and surfaces. In current practice, a partial sternotomy may be performed at either the upper or lower end of the sternum (i.e., hemisternotomy). Otherwise, a sternotomy may be avoided altogether with small incisions made on either side of the chest between ICSs (i.e., mini-thoracotomy). Whenever possible, surgeons may need only port incisions to perform a total endoscopic procedure with video assistance or execute a complete robotic approach.[298] Fig. 26.27 illustrates the many unique surgical incisions used to accomplish a successful MICS.

Minimally invasive aortic valve surgery. Minimally invasive aortic valve surgery has been performed since the first reported cases of MICS in the early 1990s.[298] Due to the aging population and the growing prevalence of AS, techniques for a minimally invasive approach to the aortic valve have been perfected and are performed commonly and safely in many heart centers. Most commonly, an upper hemisternotomy is performed beginning at the sternal notch and extending inferiorly into a "hockey stick" shape around the fourth ICS. A benefit to this approach is the number of different cannulation possibilities, whether central, peripheral, or a combination of the two. Alternatively, a right mini-thoracotomy approach may be used for exposure of the aortic valve, which involves a small incision at the medial end of the third ICS. However, the view of the aortic valve with this right mini-thoracotomy may not be ideal, and although the sternum remains intact, the third or fourth rib may need to be separated from the sternum, leading to a higher degree of postoperative pain.[298]

Minimally invasive mitral valve surgery. Surgeons Cohn, Navia, and Cosgrove led the way in establishing a minimally invasive approach to the mitral valve with the use of a parasternal incision. In current practice, a right mini-thoracotomy incision at the midaxillary line is most common and has many reported advantages, including better view of the valve, a lower incidence of infection attributed to the highly perfused pectoralis muscle, lower rates of bleeding, less postoperative pain, and decreased length of hospital stay. Smaller incisions are made inferior to the initial incision for the use of supporting instruments, a port for carbon dioxide insufflation, and a videoscope if necessary. Mitral valve repair with the use of the robot was established in 1998 by Carpentier and Mohr. Using a right mini-thoracotomy incision at the fourth ICS, the robot allows total 3D vision, even smaller incisions, and better operator control (Figs. 26.28 and 26.29).[298]

Minimally invasive coronary revascularization. In current practice, a majority of CABG procedures are still performed with a traditional

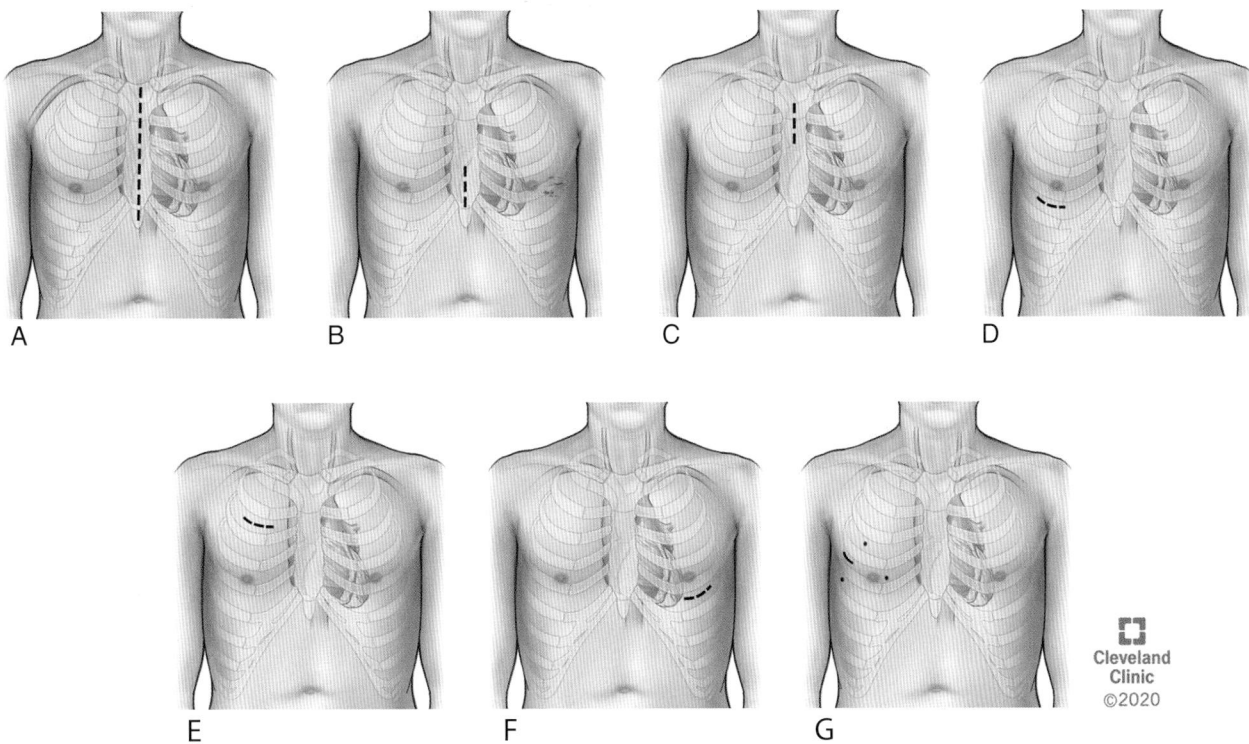

Fig. 26.27 Minimally invasive incisions. (A) Full median sternotomy. (B) Lower hemisternotomy. (C) Upper hemisternotomy. (D) Right mini-thoracotomy fifth intercostal space (ICS). (E) Right mini-thoracotomy second ICS. (F) Left mini-thoracotomy fifth ICS. (G) Robotic port incisions. (Reprinted with permission, Cleveland Clinic Center for Medical Art & Photography ©2021. All rights reserved.)

median sternotomy, but MICS is becoming more common as surgeons become increasingly comfortable with the technologies to perform a safe operation. Initially, minimally invasive coronary revascularization procedures were limited to the surgical technique MIDCAB, which involves dissection of the left internal mammary (thoracic) artery and connection to the LAD artery. When the procedure was first conducted, PCIs were often completed in conjunction with the primary procedure in the setting of multivessel CAD; however, multivessel CABG can now be performed using this minimally invasive technique.[297]

To gain access to the heart, the surgeon makes a left mini-thoracotomy incision at the fifth ICS (see Fig. 26.27). Smaller incisions are also made to allow for instruments that adequately position and stabilize the heart, as this procedure is typically performed without CPB on a beating heart. If the patient's hemodynamics become unstable due to positioning of the heart, the femoral artery and vein may be cannulated and CPB used. One limitation to the use of a MIDCAB procedure is that the right mammary artery cannot be harvested without the use of video assistance or an additional right mini-thoracotomy incision.[298]

Owing to the evolution of MICS, coronary revascularization of multiple vessels may now also be performed via a total endoscopic approach. Total endoscopic coronary artery bypass (TECAB) for multivessel CAD utilizes a robotic system, CO_2 insufflation, and single-lung ventilation. The cannulation strategy for TECAB is a total peripheral approach, and the aorta is occluded via an endoaortic balloon occlusion (EAO); both of these techniques require specific training and skill and may be a reason for avoidance of TECAB in many cardiac surgery centers.[298]

Minimally invasive septal myectomy. Transaortic septal myectomy via traditional median sternotomy has been performed to treat HOCM since its introduction in 1961.[299] One less invasive approach,

most similar to traditional median sternotomy, is transaortic access to the interventricular septum through a midline mini-sternotomy incision from the second to fourth ICS.[300] Another approach to septal myectomy is the transatrial, transmitral approach, which typically involves a 5- to 8-cm right mini-thoracotomy incision in the fourth ICS as well as additional smaller incisions for the insertion of the aortic cross-clamp, a port for CO_2 insufflation, and an atrial retractor.[301] This minimally invasive approach is convenient for mitral valve repair in conjunction with septal myectomy, and surgeons with experience in traditional septal myectomy and minimally invasive mitral valve surgery combine their techniques from each individual procedure to achieve a successful MICS.[302]

Cannulation strategies. Arterial cannulation is usually achieved via the femoral artery using a percutaneous or cutdown approach (Fig. 26.30). A preoperative computed tomographic angiography (CTA) is helpful to assess for disease and determine femoral vessel size. In the case of severe femoral atherosclerosis, arterial cannulation is achieved via the axillary or subclavian arteries. Before the advancement of the cannula through either of these vessels, TEE or fluoroscopy confirms guidewire position. If severe atherosclerosis is also present in these vessels, central aortic cannulation may be pursued; however, it is not ideal due to further limitations of the already small surgical field (see Fig. 26.9). Complications associated with arterial cannulation include loss of perfusion to a lower extremity, embolization of plaque leading to stroke, retrograde aortic dissection, femoral nerve injury, hematoma, compartment syndrome, and arterial stenosis.[303]

Similar to arterial cannulation, the most common site for peripheral venous cannulation is the femoral vein, which may also be accessed percutaneously or via open cutdown (see Fig. 26.30). TEE guidance or fluoroscopy is utilized to pass a wire from the IVC, through the RA, and into the SVC. Then a three-stage cannula is passed over the wire

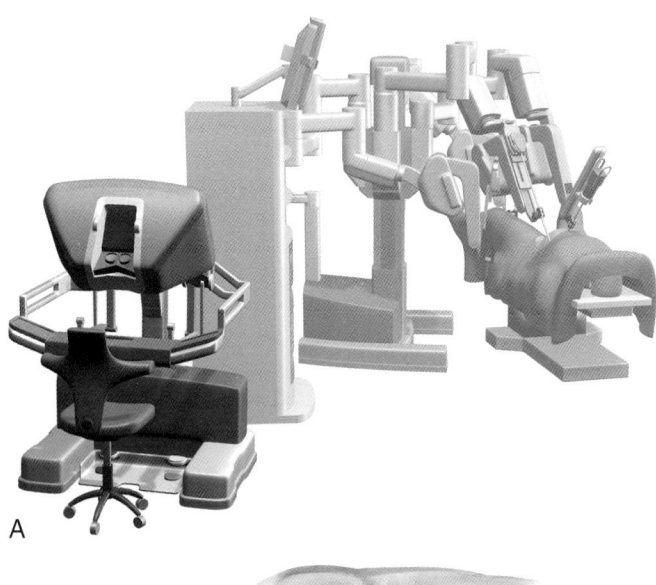

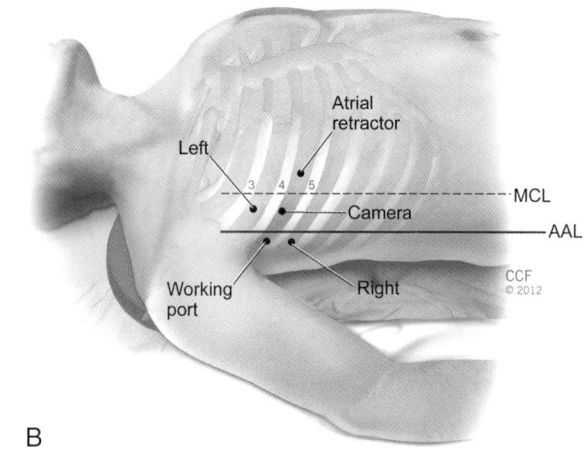

Fig. 26.28 (A) Robot used to assist cardiac surgery. The surgeon sits at the remote console and controls the two robotic arms. (B) Port placement for lateral endoscopic approach. *AAL,* Anterior axillary line; *MCL,* midclavicular line. (Reprinted with permission from Cleveland Clinic Center for Medical Art & Photography ©2020. All rights reserved.)

and into the correct position. If venous drainage is not sufficient with a single femoral cannula, the IJ vein, the subclavian vein, or the contralateral femoral vein may also be used. After induction of anesthesia, the anesthetist often places additional central venous access in the IJ vein to provide an alternative site for venous drainage during CPB. As a last resort, central venous cannulation may be used for venous drainage (see Fig. 26.9). Venous cannulation with a percutaneous approach is often associated with greater risk compared to an open cutdown as the femoral artery lies in close proximity to the femoral vein.[303]

Cannulation of the coronary sinus is required if retrograde cardioplegia administration is needed for adequate myocardial protection (see Fig. 26.30). In MICS, direct cannulation of the coronary sinus is more difficult, so the anesthesia provider typically inserts the cannula indirectly via the right IJ vein. TEE helps to guide the catheter into the coronary sinus ostium, while fluoroscopy helps determine the distance of the catheter into the coronary sinus.[304] After confirmation of adequate placement, the anesthesia provider inflates the balloon at the distal tip of the catheter with less than 1 mL of dilute contrast agent.[305] Serious risks associated with cannulation of the coronary sinus include rupture of the vessel and right ventricular perforation.[304] The use of TEE and fluoroscopy with all cannulation strategies helps decrease the risk of perforation to cardiac and vascular structures.

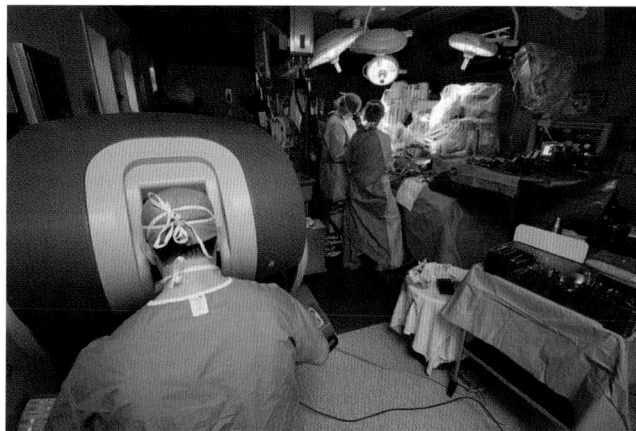

Fig. 26.29 Robotic-assisted mitral valve repair. The surgeon *(lower left)* controls the robotic arms while seated at a console remote from the patient. (From Ramakrishna H, et al. Valvular heart disease: replacement and repair. In Kaplan JA, et al., eds. *Kaplan's Cardiac Anesthesia: For Cardiac and Noncardiac Surgery.* 7th ed. Philadelphia: Elsevier; 2017:798.)

Endoaortic balloon. There are two methods of aortic occlusion for MICS, including an external transthoracic aortic cross-clamp (TCC) or a percutaneous EAO (see Fig. 26.30). The decision between aortic occlusion techniques is often based on provider experience and institutional preference. Additionally, the surgeon evaluates the preoperative CT scan to determine if the patient's ascending aorta is of appropriate size for occlusion with the EAO. A benefit to the EAO is its ability to administer cardioplegia through its proximal end, negating the need for an additional cardioplegia cannula in the ascending aorta.[306]

Proper position of the balloon is confirmed with TEE throughout the procedure, especially during its advancement from the femoral artery and during initial balloon inflation. A major risk associated with an EAO is distal migration and occlusion of the innominate artery. Some institutions monitor for this with bilateral A lines, where loss of the right arterial waveform indicates occlusion of the innominate artery. NIRS may also be used to assess for decreased cerebral oxygen concentration. It is also possible for the balloon to migrate proximally and occlude the coronary arteries; therefore, careful attention must be paid to balloon position when administering cardioplegia. Another risk associated with aortic occlusion, especially with the EAO, is aortic dissection; however, with careful monitoring of perfusion pressures in the femoral artery, this risk is not observed as frequently in current practice.[306]

Anesthetic considerations for MICS. MICS often requires specific patient positioning, one-lung ventilation, and expert knowledge of TEE. Due to less surgical exposure, greater manipulation of the heart may be required leading to more difficult hemodynamic management. External defibrillation pads must be placed because the use of internal defibrillation paddles is not possible due to limited surgical access. In addition, TEE is crucial to ensure intracardiac air removal that may become particularly challenging with limited surgical access. To promote a faster recovery with MICS, the anesthesia provider should administer narcotics judiciously, utilize alternative pain management strategies, maintain normothermia, and ensure the adequate reversal of muscle relaxant to allow prompt return of spontaneous breathing and adequate respiratory muscle strength.

Transcatheter Interventions

General considerations. With the evolution of transcatheter approaches, therapeutic options have been extended to patients at

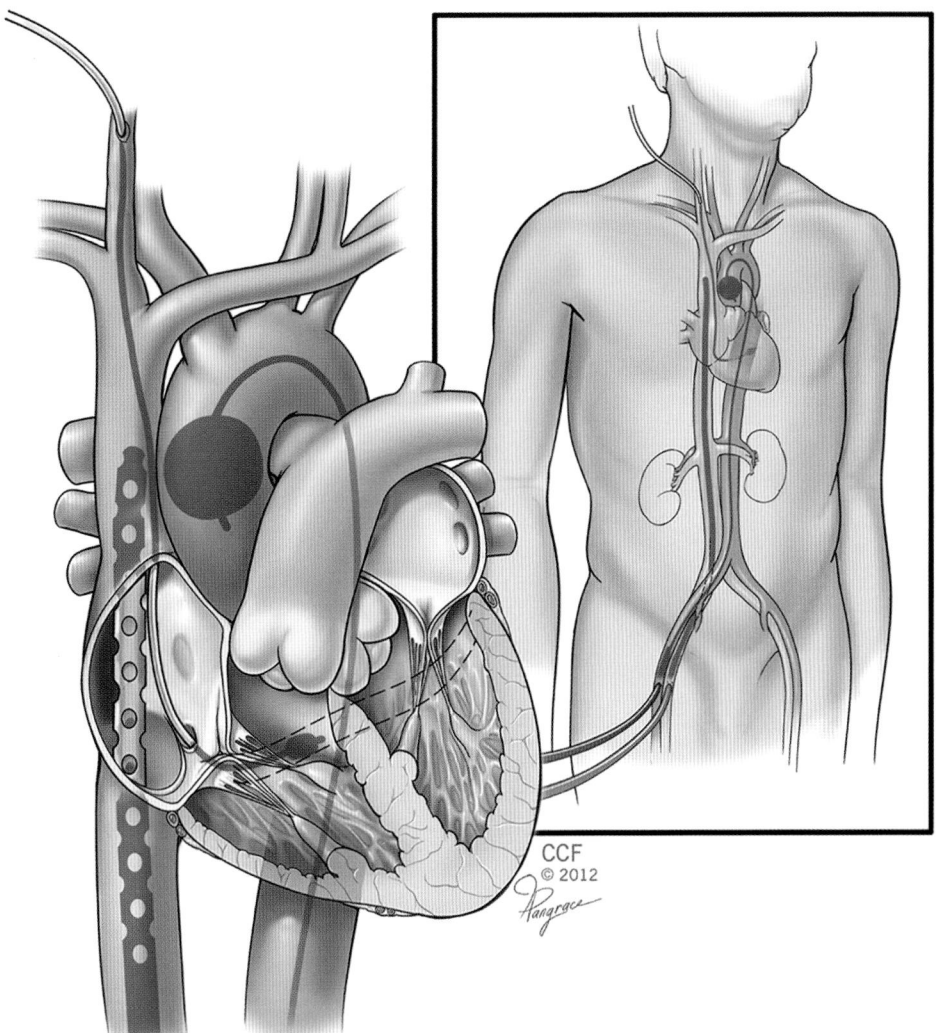

Fig. 26.30 Overview of cannulation for minimally invasive cardiac surgery showing femoral venous and arterial cannulas, a retrograde coronary sinus catheter, and an endoaortic balloon. (Reprinted with permission from Cleveland Clinic Center for Medical Art & Photography ©2020. All rights reserved.)

very high or prohibitive surgical risk. In patients considered for transcatheter valve repair or replacement, a multidisciplinary team, including a cardiothoracic surgeon and an interventional cardiologist, collaborate to determine the appropriate timing for valve intervention, whether the valve is best suited for repair or replacement, and if a surgical or percutaneous technique will be most beneficial.[263,307]

Procedural approaches

Transcatheter aortic valve replacement. In current practice, the retrograde approach to TAVR via the femoral artery is most common and preferred. In the case of iliofemoral disease, other surgical approaches to TAVR exist, including the transapical, transaxillary, subclavian, transcarotid, transaortic, and transcaval techniques (Fig. 26.31).[308,309] TAVR is an AHA/ACC class I recommendation for patients with prohibitive and high surgical risk, and a class IIa recommendation in patients with intermediate surgical risk.[263] For patients at low to intermediate surgical risk who present with asymptomatic or symptomatic severe AS, SAVR remains the class I recommendation.[263] However, surgeons are beginning to assess the feasibility of TAVR in low-risk surgical patients.[310,311]

The prosthetic valves utilized for TAVR are either balloon expandable (BE) or self-expanding (SE). The current valves in use are the bovine pericardial BE Edwards SAPIEN 3 and the porcine pericardial SE CoreValve Evolut R/Pro.[312] In addition to the advancements in prosthetic valves and delivery systems used for TAVR, vascular closure devices have been created to avoid open femoral cutdown.[310]

Balloon predilation was once considered a mandatory procedural step in TAVR to expand a native calcified valve and allow proper positioning of the new prosthetic valve.[313] However, a recent study concluded there was no difference in adverse short-term outcomes between procedures performed with balloon predilation versus without.[314] Balloon postdilation is also commonly performed following valve deployment with the goal of diminishing the degree of perivalvular AI.[315] Risks associated with balloon dilation include embolization of debris resulting in stroke, severe aortic insufficiency, and conduction disturbances requiring the implantation of a PPM device.[314]

Brief cardiac immobility is required during balloon dilation and BE valve deployment to temporarily decrease CO and ensure proper positioning. Low flow is achieved by rapidly pacing the ventricle at a rate of approximately 200 bpm to mimic a state of pulseless ventricular tachycardia. Unless the patient has a PPM device, additional venous access is achieved, and a transvenous pacemaker is advanced into the RV under fluoroscopic guidance. To decrease procedure time and avoid potential

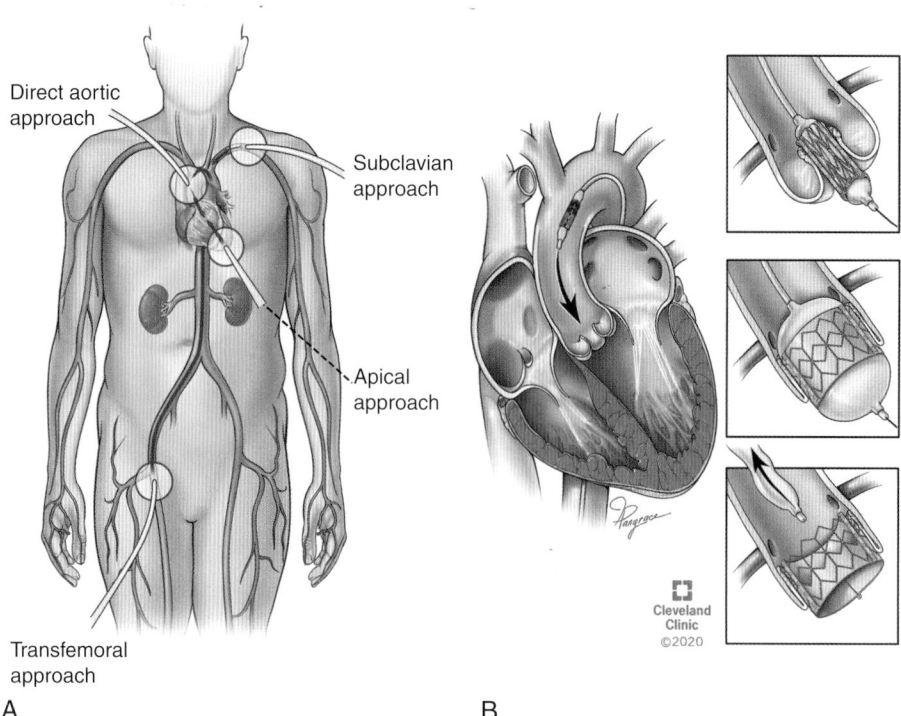

Fig. 26.31 Transcatheter aortic valve replacement. (A) Various approaches for percutaneous access to the aortic valve. (B) Retrograde, transfemoral approach using a balloon-expanding valve. (Reprinted with permission, Cleveland Clinic Center for Medical Art & Photography ©2021. All rights reserved.)

complications associated with additional vascular access, the valve delivery guidewire has recently been used for the delivery of the transvenous pacemaker as well.[316] Rapid pacing for balloon valvuloplasty or BE valve implantation may result in hemodynamic instability requiring bolus doses of phenylephrine, norepinephrine, or epinephrine. A distinct advantage of the SE CorValve is that rapid pacing is not required for valve implantation, and the device can be repositioned by the proceduralist.

One of the most common complications following TAVR is AV block requiring the need for a PPM. This risk is significantly more common with the Medtronic CoreValve (33% at 30 days) compared to the Edwards SAPIEN valve (6% at 30 days).[317,318] The new generation Edwards SAPIEN 3 valve presents slightly higher rates of AV block as compared to its predecessor.[319] In addition, paravalvular leak (PVL) is a significant risk due to varying annular sizes, valve undersizing, and/or calcification.[310] If a PVL is observed postdeployment, balloon dilation may first be tried, followed by percutaneous closure, with a high rate of success.[310,320] Cerebrovascular events occur more frequently in the early phase postprocedure (0–90 days) versus the late phase (90 days–5 years) and may be avoided with the use of cerebral protection devices (CPDs).[321] The risk of vascular complications is especially common in cases of small vessel diameter or failure of the vascular closure device. Aortic root rupture is a devastating complication of TAVR that is more likely with LVOT calcification and extensive valve oversizing.[322] BE valves present a higher risk for aortic root rupture and coronary obstruction by the native valve leaflets compared to SE valves.[309,322] Lastly, transcatheter valve embolization and migration is a critical event leading to increased morbidity and mortality and occurring in 0.92% of TAVR cases.[323]

Transcatheter mitral valve repair. MR is the most prevalent VHD across the lifespan, and the incidence increases with age.[324] The AHA/ACC guideline offers a class IIb recommendation for transcatheter repair of the

mitral valve for patients with symptomatic and severe MR at prohibitive surgical risk.[263] In current practice there are many devices available for transcatheter mitral valve repair, and each one is specific to the mitral valve leaflets, the chordae tendineae, or the valvular annulus. The MitraClip system is the leading technology for repair of the mitral valve leaflets and is currently the only FDA-approved device for mitral valve leaflet repair.[307] In the United States, the MitraClip system is only presently approved for use in high-risk surgical patients with degenerative MR.[307] The Cardiovascular Outcomes Assessment of the MitraClip Percutaneous Therapy (COAPT) trial is currently assessing the feasibility of the MitraClip system for use in patients with functional MR.[307] The concept of the MitraClip system is based on a surgical technique proposed by Alfieri in the 1990s, where an edge-to-edge strategy is used to suture the middle segments of the anterior and posterior mitral valve leaflets together to create a double-orifice valve.[307] Fluoroscopy and TEE guidance are crucial both prior to and during the procedure to thoroughly assess the mitral valve anatomy, guide transseptal puncture through the interatrial septum, and ensure proper MitraClip placement. Since MitraClip requires TEE guidance, GETA is administered.

Cerebral protection devices. Cerebrovascular accident (CVA) occurs in 9.1% of patients following TAVR and 3.9% of patients after mitral valve clipping.[325] The most reputable CPD is the Sentinel Cerebral Protection System; the third-generation device gained CE approval in 2013 and FDA approval in 2017.[326] This CPD is introduced via the right radial or brachial artery and advanced to the brachiocephalic and left common carotid arteries. For complete cerebral protection, an additional device may be inserted into the left vertebral artery in conjunction with the Sentinel device.[326] Overall, the implementation of a CPD takes less than 10 minutes in most cases and can successfully prevent an embolic CVA.

Anesthetic considerations for transcatheter interventions. All transcatheter cardiovascular procedures are performed in a hybrid

OR with fluoroscopic imaging capabilities or an EP laboratory with the means to convert urgently to an open cardiac surgery if necessary. Peripheral access is often adequate, but if central access is required the anesthesia provider may utilize a central venous sheath placed by the interventional cardiologist.[325] The anesthetist often transduces an arterial pressure from one of the A lines placed by the proceduralist. Due to the insertion of large, vascular sheaths, 70 to 100 units/kg of IV heparin are administered with a goal ACT of approximately 250 to 300 seconds.[325,327] When the procedure is complete, protamine may be administered to reverse heparin and return the ACT to baseline.[324,325]

Most percutaneous procedures are accomplished under GETA due to the need for TEE guidance. However, fluoroscopy with the addition of TTE in transfemoral TAVR allows the use of MAC. Occasionally, ICE is used to help guide specific devices into position.[326] For transfemoral TAVR, the choice of GETA versus MAC is patient and provider specific. Some patients are unable to tolerate the discomfort associated with catheter insertion or are uncomfortable lying flat for a prolonged period and may require GETA. However, patients who are ineligible for open cardiac surgery often have multiple comorbidities, and it is beneficial to maintain spontaneous respirations and avoid endotracheal intubation and ventilation. MAC is often accomplished in this frail population using small doses of midazolam and fentanyl in combination with a low-dose dexmedetomidine infusion. With MAC, the patient's neurologic function may be continuously assessed, and length of stay in the hospital is potentially reduced.[308] Managing a patient under MAC may prove challenging for the anesthesia provider as it requires great skill to balance patient comfort with respiratory protection and hemodynamic support.

Devices and Procedures Developed to Manage Heart Failure

Mechanical Circulatory Assist Devices

A mechanical circulatory assist device (MCAD) is inserted in patients with severe heart failure to maintain circulation and oxygenation to the organs and tissues of the body. The demand for MCADs has increased as the population ages and the prevalence of heart failure rises. Selecting the appropriate device for each patient is based on the ease of insertion, the degree of circulatory support required, and the length of time needed for support. Both short- and long-term devices are getting smaller, easier to implant, and last longer, with fewer complications and dramatically improved outcomes. Today, VADs are used to assume the function of the failing ventricle as a bridge to survival, recovery, decision, or transplant, and as destination therapy (DT). Many short-term MCADs have been developed that can be placed percutaneously or surgically to rescue the decompensating patient, or support the marginal patient, undergoing an interventional cardiology procedure or cardiac surgery. Similarly, technologic advancements in long-term VADs have improved markedly, so that 1-year outcomes now rival heart transplantation, and over 70% are placed as DT.[328,329] Although a comprehensive discussion of MCADs is beyond the scope of this chapter, the key features of the most commonly employed devices will be highlighted, and the general principles of anesthetic management discussed. The reader is referred to current guidelines[330-332] and excellent reviews for a more in-depth discussion on the topic.[329,333-336]

Short-term devices for acute mechanical circulatory support. For many years, acute support was limited to the IABP and ECMO. Today, multiple percutaneous and surgical devices provide temporary support for the left and/or right ventricle. Indications for short-term mechanical circulatory support include rescue from acute myocardial infarction (AMI), heart failure in the setting of nonischemic cardiomyopathy, posttransplant allograft or right ventricular failure, failure to wean from CPB, and refractory arrhythmias. In these settings, the MCAD is

used as a bridge to recovery, decision, transplant, or long-term durable device placement. Short-term devices are also placed prophylactically for high-risk PCI, ventricular tachycardia ablations, and percutaneous valve interventions.[330,335,337]

Intraaortic balloon pump. The IABP is the simplest and most commonly employed MCAD, allowing intrinsic cardiac ejection, assisted with synchronized counterpulsation. The IABP consists of a flexible, cylindric, balloon-tipped catheter positioned in the descending aorta. The catheter is attached to a drive console containing computerized circuitry to determine proper timing for balloon inflation and deflation. Helium is used to inflate the balloon at the onset of diastole, displacing blood proximally toward the coronary arteries (counterpulse), thereby increasing aortic diastolic pressure (diastolic augmentation) and coronary perfusion. At the onset of systole, the balloon deflates, creating a vacuum that reduces afterload and myocardial oxygen demand while modestly enhancing CO. In the perioperative setting it is most commonly used to stabilize a patient preoperatively and/or to help wean a patient who is having difficulty separating from CPB. Occasionally it is used to support coronary perfusion during OPCAB procedures. Sepsis, descending aortic disease, severe PVD, severe AR, and uncontrolled bleeding are contraindications to IABP placement.[55,330,333]

IABPs come in sizes between 20 and 50 mL based on the patient's height. Most commonly, the IABP is placed percutaneously through the femoral artery using a Seldinger technique; however, alternative routes of access include the abdominal aorta and the axillary, subclavian, and iliac arteries.[338,339] The catheter is then advanced retrograde through the descending aorta so that the tip of the balloon is positioned 1 to 2 cm distal to the origin of the left subclavian artery, with the lower margin well above the renal arteries. Proper sizing and positioning are important considerations to prevent complications such as vascular damage or vessel occlusion. Fluoroscopy, echocardiography, or radiography are used to confirm proper position at the time of placement, and a chest radiograph should be examined daily to assess for catheter migration. Distal pulses and urine output are evaluated regularly to rule out vascular occlusion.[55,333,334,340]

Circuitry in the drive console analyzes the aortic and ECG waveforms to ensure appropriate timing of balloon inflation and deflation, which is key to maximizing the hemodynamic benefits and avoiding unnecessary complications. Balloon inflation should be timed with the dicrotic notch of the arterial waveform, or the peak of the T wave on the ECG, so that inflation begins once the AV closes and is maintained throughout diastole. The augmented diastolic pressure should exceed the nonaugmented systolic pressure. Deflation of the balloon is timed to occur immediately before the onset of systole, at the beginning of the R wave of the ECG. Assisted systolic and aortic end-diastolic pressures should be less than the unassisted values.[334,340] Proper timing of the IABP is essential to prevent further strain on the myocardium and achieve the maximal benefit of counter pulsation. Fig. 26.32 shows arterial waveforms with correct timing and placement, and Fig. 26.33 demonstrates arterial waveforms associated with inappropriate IABP timing.[334]

Most modern consoles are unaffected by electrocautery and can accurately differentiate pacer spikes from the QRS complex when pacing is used. Timing can be difficult with irregular rhythms such as AF and faster heart rates. IABP is usually timed to inflate with each heartbeat (1:1) or every other beat (1:2) until ventricular function improves. The counterpulsation ratio can be gradually weaned to as low as 1:4 as the ventricle recovers, before it is safely discontinued. The only time it is acceptable for an IABP to be abruptly discontinued or turned off is when the patient is fully heparinized during CPB.[334] There is no definitive data to support a recommendation regarding anticoagulation for IABP. Many centers do use anticoagulation, while others do not,

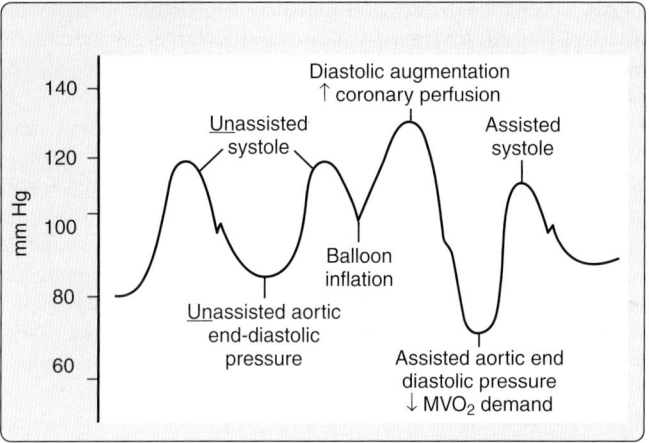

Fig. 26.32 Arterial waveforms seen during intraaortic balloon pump (IABP) assist. The first two waveforms are unassisted, and the last is assisted. Notice the decreased end-systolic and end-diastolic pressures and augmented diastolic pressures caused by IABP augmentation and the (correct) point at which balloon inflation occurs. These are waveforms generated by a correctly positioned and timed balloon. *MVO₂*, mixed venous oxygen saturation. (Courtesy Datascope Corporation.)

especially if assisting 1:1.[330] Vascular injuries, including ischemia distal to the site of the balloon, are the most common complications associated with IABP use. Other complications of IABP use include infection or bleeding at the insertion site and thrombocytopenia.[330,331,333,334]

Extracorporeal membrane oxygenation. ECMO is a temporary, closed-circuit mechanism of circulatory support that allows the heart and/or lungs to rest and recover from injury or trauma for days to weeks, while maintaining oxygenation and perfusion. Much like CPB, the ECMO circuit includes a centrifugal, nonpulsatile pump for blood propulsion, a membrane oxygenator for gas exchange, a heat exchanger for warming, an oxygen blender, and a control console.[341] There are two types of ECMO, venovenous and venoarterial, with differing indications, characteristics, and cannula configurations to achieve the desired support.

Venovenous (V-V) ECMO is indicated when respiratory failure is the principal issue, and the heart can provide adequate CO to meet circulatory needs. In patients with poor gas exchange, despite medical therapy and advanced modes of ventilation, V-V ECMO supports the lungs by improving gas exchange and allowing lung-protective ventilation.[334,342,343] Lung-protective ventilation strategies used in conjunction with V-V ECMO include the use of lower tidal volumes (3–5 mL/kg), lower oxygen concentrations (30%–50%), lower peak inspiratory

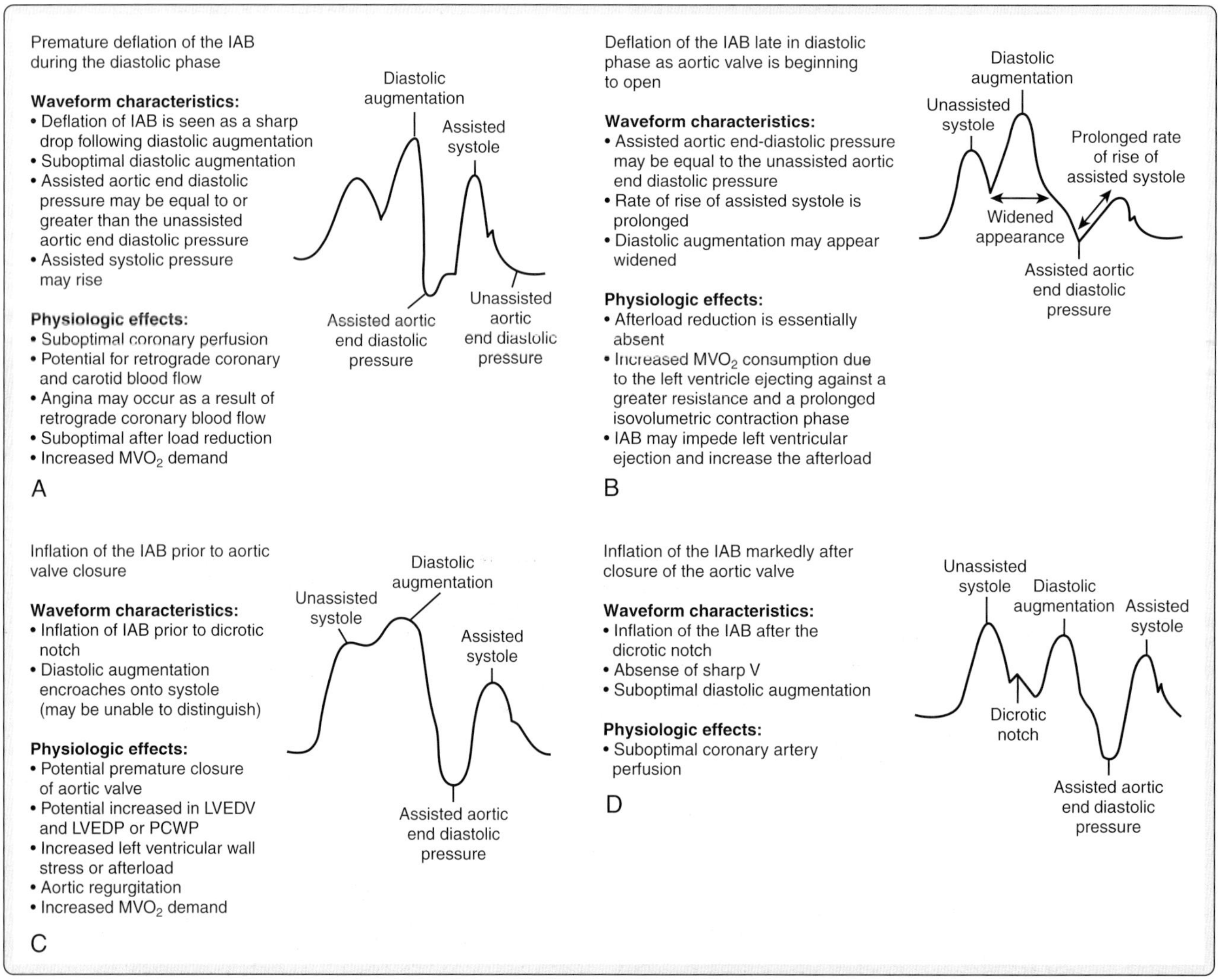

Premature deflation of the IAB during the diastolic phase

Waveform characteristics:
• Deflation of IAB is seen as a sharp drop following diastolic augmentation
• Suboptimal diastolic augmentation
• Assisted aortic end diastolic pressure may be equal to or greater than the unassisted aortic end diastolic pressure
• Assisted systolic pressure may rise

Physiologic effects:
• Suboptimal coronary perfusion
• Potential for retrograde coronary and carotid blood flow
• Angina may occur as a result of retrograde coronary blood flow
• Suboptimal after load reduction
• Increased MVO₂ demand

A

Deflation of the IAB late in diastolic phase as aortic valve is beginning to open

Waveform characteristics:
• Assisted aortic end-diastolic pressure may be equal to the unassisted aortic end diastolic pressure
• Rate of rise of assisted systole is prolonged
• Diastolic augmentation may appear widened

Physiologic effects:
• Afterload reduction is essentially absent
• Increased MVO₂ consumption due to the left ventricle ejecting against a greater resistance and a prolonged isovolumetric contraction phase
• IAB may impede left ventricular ejection and increase the afterload

B

Inflation of the IAB prior to aortic valve closure

Waveform characteristics:
• Inflation of IAB prior to dicrotic notch
• Diastolic augmentation encroaches onto systole (may be unable to distinguish)

Physiologic effects:
• Potential premature closure of aortic valve
• Potential increased in LVEDV and LVEDP or PCWP
• Increased left ventricular wall stress or afterload
• Aortic regurgitation
• Increased MVO₂ demand

C

Inflation of the IAB markedly after closure of the aortic valve

Waveform characteristics:
• Inflation of the IAB after the dicrotic notch
• Absense of sharp V
• Suboptimal diastolic augmentation

Physiologic effects:
• Suboptimal coronary artery perfusion

D

Fig. 26.33 Alterations in waveform tracings caused by errors in timing of the intraaortic balloon pump. (A) The balloon was deflated too early. (B) The balloon was deflated too late. (C) The balloon was inflated too early. (D) The balloon was inflated too late. *IAB*, intraaortic balloon; *LVEDP*, left ventricular end-diastolic pressure; *LVEDV*, left ventricular end-diastolic volume; *MVO₂*, mixed venous oxygen saturation; *PCWP*, pulmonary capillary wedge pressure. (Courtesy Datascope Corporation.)

pressures (PIPs <30 mm Hg), lower respiratory rates (8–10 breaths/min), and lower PEEPs (≤15 cm H_2O). Some patients on V-V ECMO can be extubated because gas exchange occurs via the ECMO oxygenator. V-V ECMO has become an invaluable tool to manage ARDS, including patients with Covid-19 and other respiratory illnesses.[344-346]

In V-V ECMO blood is often drained via a femoral cannula advanced in the IVC so that the tip is near the junction with the RA. A centrifugal pump propels the blood to a membrane oxygenator where O_2 diffuses in and CO_2 diffuses out. The blood, with a saturation of 75% to 85%, returns to the body via a catheter in the opposite femoral vessel, or the right IJ vein, and advances to the RA. Alternatively, a double lumen cannula (Crescent), placed in the right IJ vein and advanced into the RA and IVC, can be used. Drainage occurs via the lumen with openings in the SVC and IVC, and infusion occurs via the lumen in the RA.[333,341,346]

If left ventricular support is required in addition to pulmonary support, venoarterial (V-A) ECMO can provide complete cardiopulmonary support with flow rates of 3 to 6 L/min.[347,348] V-A ECMO is used in cardiogenic shock resulting from MI, failure to wean from CPB, allograft failure after heart or lung transplantation, pulmonary embolism or trauma, and septic or peripartum cardiomyopathy.[349] In contrast to V-V ECMO, V-A ECMO partially bypasses pulmonary circulation so a higher arterial oxygenation is achieved with lower flow rates. When used to assist in separation from CPB, cannulation for V-A ECMO is usually central where deoxygenated blood is directly drained from a cannula in the RA, and oxygenated blood is directly returned through a cannula inserted into the ascending aorta. Cannulation for V-A ECMO may also be peripheral, where deoxygenated blood is drained from a cannula in the right IJ and/or the femoral vein, and oxygen-rich blood is returned to the circulation via the femoral artery. In either case, blood drains through the venous cannula to a centrifugal pump that then circulates the blood through a membrane oxygenator for gas exchange and a heat exchanger for warming before it is returned to the patient via the arterial cannula.[273,330,347,350] V-A ECMO increases SVR, which can potentially depress native CO; increase LVEDP, LVEDV, and MVO_2; and cause pulmonary edema. This complication, generally referred to as LV distention or ECMO lung, must be closely monitored. Treatment strategies for LV distention include adding medications (e.g., inotrope) or devices (e.g., Impella) that enhance forward flow, reduce afterload (e.g., IABP), or mechanically (e.g., LV vent) or pharmacologically (e.g., diuretic) decompress the LV.[335,351]

Anticoagulation with heparin is necessary before insertion of the ECMO cannulas to prevent thrombus formation. ACTs are typically maintained between 180 and 250 seconds.[330] Since both heparin and ECMO can cause thrombocytopenia, bleeding and vascular injury are major risk factors for patients supported with ECMO. Anticoagulation is not needed for V-V ECMO if the flow rates are kept above 3 L/min. If limb perfusion is compromised, a second sheath can be inserted into the superficial femoral artery to provide antegrade perfusion.[330] Other complications associated with ECMO include stroke, infection, and multiorgan dysfunction.[341,347,348]

Ventricular assist devices

General considerations. A VAD is an MCAD that supports a failing left or right ventricle by ensuring adequate ejection of blood into either the pulmonic or systemic circulation. Both a left ventricular assist device (LVAD) and a right ventricular assist device (RVAD) consist of the same components, including an inflow cannula, a pump, and an outflow cannula. An LVAD collects oxygenated blood via an inflow cannula in the LA or LV and pumps it to an outflow cannula most often attached to the aorta but sometimes to the femoral artery. Similarly, an RVAD collects deoxygenated blood from an inflow cannula in the RA or RV and pumps blood to an outflow cannula attached to the PA. VADs are categorized according to the type of blood flow (continuous or pulsatile), length of time the device can be used for support (short, intermediate, or long term), location of the device (intra-, extra-, or paracorporeal), and the source of driving power (pneumatic or electric).[334]

Specific short-term devices. The Impella (Abiomed) propels blood continuously from the LV to the aorta using a microaxial flow device called the Archimedes screw. The Impella unloads the ventricle, reduces ventricular end-diastolic pressure, increases MAP, and decreases MVO_2. There are five systems approved for use in the United States that can be placed percutaneously or surgically (Fig. 26.34). To support the LV, the Impella 2.5 (2.5 L/min flow) and the Impella CP (4 L/min flow) can be placed percutaneously via the femoral artery and advanced retrograde across the AV under fluoroscopic guidance. The Impella 5.0 (5 L/min flow) and 5.5 (>6 L/min flow) require a surgical cutdown incision and insertion of a vascular graft to the axillary artery or direct arteriotomy of the ascending aorta. Abiomed's newest pump, the Impella 5.5, incorporates a SmartAssist fiberoptic pressure sensor that facilitates proper positioning and integrates data informatics to optimize native heart recovery and support weaning algorithms. Contraindications to an LV Impella include severe AS, mechanical AV, and severe PVD if femoral access is used.[335,336]

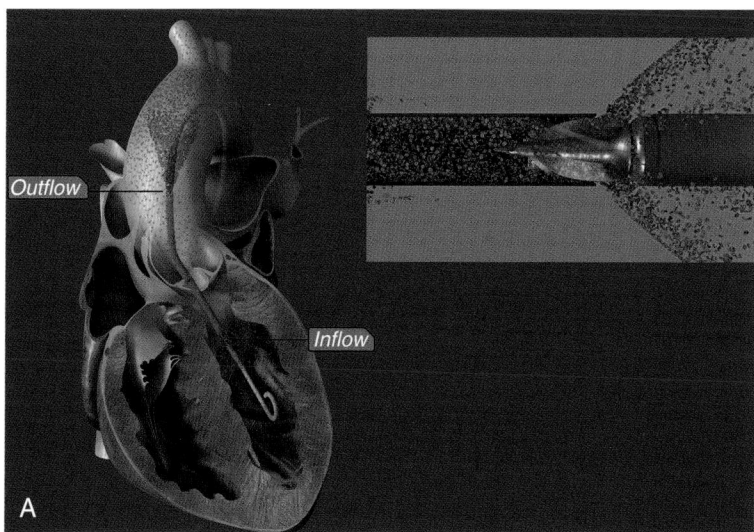
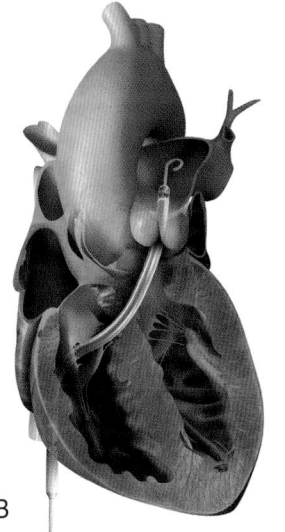
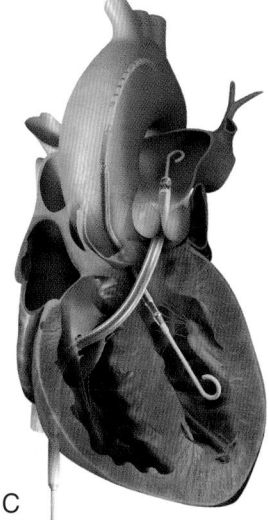

Fig. 26.34 (A–C) The Impella family of support devices. (Courtesy Abiomed Inc., Danvers, MA.)

There is also an Impella (RP) designed to provide up to 4 L/min RV support. It is placed in the femoral vein and advanced antegrade through the venous system crossing into the PA. Inflow is then in the IVC, and outflow is in the PA. Contraindications include right-sided mechanical or stenotic valves as well as prior placement of an IVC filter. Complications of percutaneous VADs, in general, include vascular injury, cardiac tamponade/perforation, ventricular arrhythmias, acute valve regurgitation, hemolysis, and thrombosis.[334,341]

The TandemHeart system (Cardiac Assist, Inc.) is a percutaneously deployed, LA to femoral artery bypass system, with an external centrifugal pump (Fig. 26.35). A cannula is inserted into the femoral vein and advanced across the atrial septum into the LA. Oxygenated blood from the LA is pumped into the femoral artery at a rate up to 5 L/min. Because of its parallel configuration, both the native LV and the TandemHeart device can contribute to forward flow. Although not FDA approved for RV support, there are reports of the TandemHeart being used to provide RA to PA support.[334,335]

CentriMag (Abbott) is a small paracorporeal centrifugal pump with a magnetically levitated impeller connected to cannulas in the heart and great vessels so it can be used for left-sided (RA-aorta), right-sided (RA-PA), or biventricular support. The system is especially practical when weaning from CPB fails because the existing cannula may be used by simply changing the adaptors. Additionally, the device can provide up to 10 L/min flow and can accommodate a membrane oxygenator if ECMO is desired to allow use on a variety of patients.[334,335,337]

The PROTEK Duo system (CardiacAssist, Inc.) is an RV assist cannula, inserted into the right IJ vein and advanced to the PA. Blood is drained from the RA and reinfused into the PA with the help of a centrifugal pump such as the TandemHeart or CentriMag.[335]

Durable devices for intermediate to long-term mechanical circulatory support

General considerations. VADs were originally conceived as a bridge to heart transplantation (BTT), and evidence clearly supports that VADs are effective in stabilizing multiorgan failure in end-stage heart failure patients who are awaiting transplant.[352,353] In 2001, the Randomized Evaluation of Mechanical Assistance for the Treatment of Congestive Heart Failure (REMATCH) trial demonstrated that compared to optimal medical management, patients who received an LVAD have a 48% reduction in the risk of death, fewer adverse events, shorter hospital stays, lower prescription cost, and improved quality of life.[354] Today the evidence is even stronger that VADs substantially improve functional capacity and quality of life, as approximately 80% of patients are NYHA functional class I or II at 24 months postimplantation.[329,355] Rapid advances in technology have significantly improved patient outcomes so that LVADs are now considered a cost-effective, durable, and safe option for the management of end-stage heart failure. The survival rate following durable MCAD implantation (82% at 1 year) is now equivalent to heart transplantation. However, following the first year, transplant survival is superior to a VAD regardless of the indication.[328,356] Nevertheless, the trajectory of modern devices suggests that this may change over time due to the reduced complications reported with newer centrifugal-flow devices.[328] More than 70% of LVADs implanted from 2017 to 2018 were placed as DT in patients who were not eligible for a heart transplant, and less than 10% were placed as BTT.[328] Additionally, a major restructuring of the United Network for Organ Sharing (UNOS) in 2018 prioritized patients who are unstable on ECMO or temporary MCAD for heart transplantation. Consequently, stable outpatients on durable long-term MCADs are at a lower urgency status, and those with complications from MCADs are required to meet more stringent requirements.

According to the most current AHA recommendations, indications for LVAD include NYHA class IIIb or IV with functional limitations despite maximal medical therapy. The Interagency Registry for Mechanically Assisted Circulatory Support (INTERMACS) system divides heart failure into seven different risk levels. Risk level 1 represents the most unstable patient, while risk level 7 denotes a hemodynamically stable patient with minimal symptoms.[329] When compared to a cohort that received a durable LVAD between 2014 and 2018, patients that received a durable LVAD in 2019 were more likely to be INTERMACS level 1 (17.1% vs 14.3%) and to have a temporary MCAD (34.8% vs 29.3%).[328] Contraindications to VAD insertion include active infection or sepsis; irreversible renal, hepatic, or neurologic dysfunction; severe PHTN unrelated to cardiac disease; metastatic cancer; and major coagulation disorders such as hemophilia and von Willebrand disease. Patients must also be able to adhere to the strict care regimen and be free of severe psychosocial disease.[330,332]

Types of durable MCAD. The three commonly implanted continuous-flow LVADs for DT are the HeartMate II (HM II, Abbot Laboratories), the HeartWare HVAD System (HVAD, Medtronic), and the HeartMate 3 (HM 3, Abbott Laboratories) (Fig. 26.36). All three devices were initially approved for BTT and then later approved for DT in 2010, 2017, and 2018, respectively. Each device unloads the LV from the apex and augments up to 10 L/min flow to the ascending aorta. They are connected to an external power source (electric or portable battery packs) via a subcutaneously tunneled driveline that exits at the level of the abdomen. For biventricular support, SynCardia's pulsatile temporary Total Artificial Heart (TAH-t) was approved in 2014 for BTT.[329,333,357]

Long-term LVADs have two distinct types of continuous-flow design: axial or centrifugal. Axial flow consists of second-generation technology where the flow is generated by a propeller in a pipe, whereas centrifugal flow is third-generation technology where the flow is generated by a bladed disc spinning in a cavity. HM II is an axial flow pump, and HVAD and HM 3 are centrifugal flow pumps. Key engineering

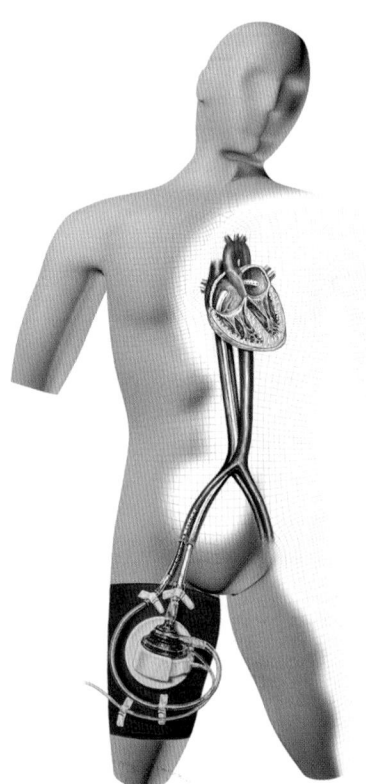

Fig. 26.35 TandemHeart. (Courtesy CardiacAssist Inc., Pittsburgh, PA.)

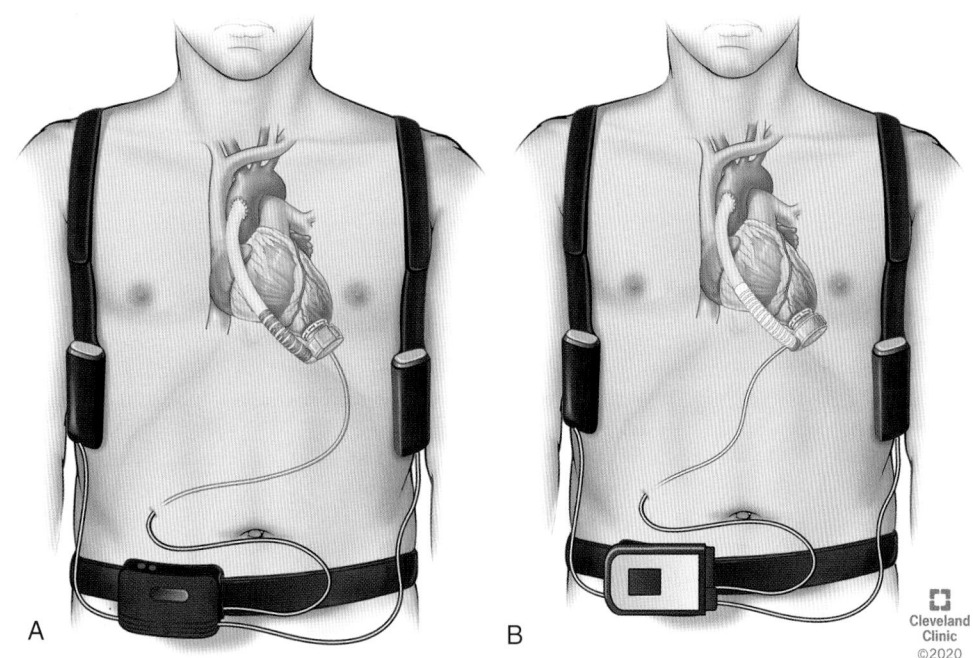

Fig. 26.36 (A) HeartWare HVAD and (B) HeartMate 3 are intracorporeal electrically powered centrifugal-flow pumps. Blood is drawn from the apex and pumped continuously to the ascending aorta. (Reprinted with permission, Cleveland Clinic Center for Medical Art & Photography ©2021. All rights reserved.)

features make the older device, HM II, less desirable. The rotor spins in blood, generating heat that can contribute to hemolysis and thrombosis.[358-360] HVAD and HM 3 have magnetically levitated, frictionless rotors. Axial pumps continue to flow even in low volume states, making them more likely to have life-threatening "suck-down" events. When preload is low, the negative pressure generated by the axial pump can cause the ventricular cavity or septum to be sucked against the pump inflow cannula, potentially triggering ventricular tachycardia. On the other hand, centrifugal output is exquisitely sensitive to loading conditions, making suck-down less likely. HM II is larger and sits in an upper abdominal pocket increasing the risk of infection. Newer generation devices are smaller so they can remain in the thoracic cavity and potentially be placed via a minimally invasive thoracotomy.[329,333,334,355] The rotor on the HM 3 has a programmed artificial pulsatility setting that causes it to accelerate and decelerate by 2000 RPMs from the set speed every 2 seconds to wash out the device and eliminate areas of stasis, reducing the risk of thrombosis.[329]

Evidence confirms that all centrifugal devices are superior to axial flow in that there is dramatically less pump thrombosis, disabling stroke, and reoperations.[355] An STS INTERMACS report confirms that only 2.1% of devices implanted in 2019 were axial flow as compared to 70.1% in 2014.[361] When comparing HVAD to HM 3, the most recent STS INTERMACS report found that HM 3 had fewer adverse events and improved survival at 1 year (87% vs 79%).[328]

The SynCardia temporary total artificial heart (TAH-t) is an option for patients with biventricular failure as a BTT. The native ventricles and valves are removed and replaced with a pneumatically driven, biventricular pump weighing less than 0.5 pound and producing pulsatile flow. The pumping chambers come in two sizes, 50 mL and 70 mL, that can generate 7.5 and 9.5 L/min flow, respectively. Survival to heart transplant is 74% to 80%. The TAH-t is initially powered and controlled by a large control console. Later, there is a smaller portable driver that allows patients to ambulate and be discharged from the hospital.[357,362]

Anesthetic management. Anesthetic management of the LVAD candidate begins with a thorough preoperative assessment of the

end-stage heart failure patient. Hepatic congestion from RHF, preoperative use of anticoagulation drugs, and exposure of the patient's blood to nonbiologic surfaces of the LVAD device can all contribute to potentially substantial blood loss and coagulopathy after placement.[357] Blood products should be available, and large-bore central and peripheral IV access secured before incision, in case rapid transfusion becomes necessary. Antifibrinolytic agents such as aminocaproic acid or tranexamic acid may be administered perioperatively to minimize blood loss. In addition to standard ASA monitors, a radial or brachial arterial catheter and CVP or PAC should be placed before induction to assist the anesthesia provider in achieving hemodynamic stability during induction. Decreases in preload and increases in afterload are poorly tolerated in patients with end-stage heart failure.[55] These patients are extremely dependent on heart rate and are considered to have a relatively fixed CO with an inability to increase SV. Rapid deterioration and cardiovascular collapse can occur on induction if the patient becomes bradycardic or loses sympathetic tone. Judicious use of etomidate with moderate-dose narcotic, a low-dose inhalation anesthetic, and a neuromuscular blocker may minimize hemodynamic instability. Ketamine with a small dose of midazolam is a useful alternative for patients that present with hemodynamic instability, but also consider that ketamine can cause myocardial depression in patients who are catecholamine depleted.[150] Sepsis is the leading cause of postoperative rehospitalization and mortality, so attention should be given to the antibiotic regimen and strict sterile technique maintained.[328,329,363]

A complete TEE examination assists with the placement and detection of anatomic problems that can potentially complicate the proper functioning of the device. AI, the presence of intracardiac shunts (PFO), mitral stenosis, tricuspid insufficiency, the presence of thrombus, RV function, and the adequacy of VAD inflow and outflow function can all be assessed using TEE.[333,364] Many concerns, such as AI, tricuspid regurgitation, or a PFO, will require surgical correction before LVAD placement for the device to function properly.[363] TEE also serves as a monitor of right and left ventricular function, thereby helping to guide fluid and hemodynamic management.[154]

Before separation from CPB, ventilation is reestablished, the device is de-aired, and its function is evaluated to confirm that it will provide adequate circulatory support. Unfortunately, 30% of LVAD recipients develop RV dysfunction after implantation so filling pressures and function are monitored closely with TEE to avoid overload. Causes of RV failure are multifactorial; these include left ventricular decompression, myocardial stunning from CPB, fixed PHTN, and right ventricular overload from LVAD activation.[55,334,357] Inotropes such as epinephrine, or a phosphodiesterase III inhibitor such as milrinone, help support function and decrease right ventricular afterload. Inhaled epoprostenol sodium (Veletri or Flolan) and (rarely, due to cost) nitric oxide may be used to dilate the pulmonary vasculature. If RV dysfunction ensues despite pharmacologic support, biventricular support should be considered.[55,333,334]

LVAD flow is very sensitive to preload and afterload. Volume is administered rapidly (mainly blood and blood products) if massive bleeding and coagulopathy develop. Patients who are potential future transplant recipients should receive blood that has been leukocyte reduced. As mentioned previously, hypovolemia can lead to a very dangerous suck-down event, which occurs more frequently with axial flow devices. The negative pressure of the pump can cause the empty ventricular septum or wall to be pulled against the LVAD inlet, potentially causing ventricular tachycardia. TEE is an invaluable tool in assessing volume status and the position of the inflow cannula, which should be in the center of the LV pointing toward the mitral valve. Both are important in preventing suck-down events.[329,334] Vasoplegic syndrome can also develop and is best managed with vasopressin because it causes less pulmonary vasoconstriction than norepinephrine or phenylephrine and will help prevent increases in right heart afterload.[55] Hypertension should be treated with a vasodilator, such as sodium nitroprusside, to avoid causing stress and malfunction of the LVAD.[363]

Rehospitalization is common for LVAD recipients, with 80% readmitted in the first year following placement.[365] Postimplant complications include infection (especially driveline, 15%–24%), bleeding (especially GI, 15%–30%), RHF (15%–25%), pump thrombosis (1.1%–12.2%), AI (30% at 2 years), and stroke (13%–30%).[329] Any of these complications can result in the need for surgical intervention, and anesthetic management will need to be individually tailored based on the cause and the patient's condition.

Cardiac Transplantation

General considerations. On December 3, 1967, in Cape Town, South Africa, Dr. Christiaan Barnard performed the first human-to-human cardiac transplantation. Today cardiac transplantation is the gold standard treatment for end-stage heart failure regardless of an ischemic or nonischemic etiology. In 1980 cyclosporines were introduced for use in cardiac transplantation recipients, drastically improving patient outcomes by effectively suppressing the immune system and avoiding rejection.[366] Due to further advancements, the rate of survival after surgery at 1, 3, and 5 years is 90.3%, 84.7%, and 79.6%, respectively.[367] The most common early complications following cardiac transplantation include AKI, early graft dysfunction, hemodynamic changes and vasoplegia, pericardial effusions, arrhythmias, and mediastinal bleeding.[368] Due to advancements in treatment options for patients with end-stage heart failure, the recipient demand greatly outweighs the donor supply.[369] Due to the increased demand for cardiac donors, the specific donor criteria has been extended to include imperfect hearts, and this poses greater challenges in the intraoperative and postoperative management of these patients.

Donor heart allocation and recipient criteria. Following the initial diagnosis of end-stage heart failure, the prognosis for survival is 50% within 5 years.[370] To optimally distribute donor hearts and increase waitlist survival, UNOS, which operates the Organ Procurement and Transplantation Network (OPTN), was established in 1984. The OPTN organizes an allocation system that distributes donor hearts to recipients based on specific policy and criteria.[369]

To address the growing recipient pool, a new set of revisions gained approval by the OPTN/UNOS board and were introduced in October 2018. The current allocation system is made up of six tiers and better distinguishes those candidates requiring the most urgent need. Status 1 patients represent those with the highest priority for transplantation, while status 6 patients are temporarily listed as lowest priority. Other factors considered when matching a donor heart with a recipient is blood type, height, weight, and geographic distance.[369]

Communication is of utmost importance to minimize graft ischemic time and limit the duration of CPB for the recipient. The ideal ischemic time is less than 4 hours but should be no longer than 5 hours to ensure optimal cardiac reserve after transplantation.[368] The time of anesthetic induction for the recipient depends on a number of factors, including surgical team expertise and patient-specific characteristics, including the need for redo sternotomy.

Surgical approaches. The two most common surgical techniques utilized for cardiac transplantation are the biatrial and bicaval approaches (Fig. 26.37). The biatrial technique was employed in the initial stages of cardiac transplantation, and the bicaval technique is the most common approach utilized today. The biatrial technique requires only four anastomoses, while the bicaval technique requires five. The order of anastomoses for the bicaval technique is based on surgical exposure and is performed in the following order: LA, IVC, PA, aorta, and SVC.[368]

Anesthetic considerations. The goal of anesthetic induction is to achieve unconsciousness and necessary paralysis for endotracheal intubation without causing cardiovascular collapse. The slow administration of induction medication is necessary, as the patient's low CO state will produce a delayed response. Because the recipient is notified of the surgery with little time in advance, the recipient is typically considered to have a full stomach so a rapid sequence intubation is performed.[368]

A critical balance must be achieved between preventing infection with antibiotic prophylaxis and avoiding rejection with immunosuppressive therapy; however, there is currently no consensus on best practice, and different routines exist among various institutions. At many facilities, high-dose steroid is administered at the start of the procedure and just prior to the removal of the aortic cross-clamp to prevent an acute immune response.[368]

After successful induction of anesthesia, a TEE probe is placed to dictate patient management prior to CPB. TEE is also effective for the assessment of intracardiac emboli caused by the low flow rates through the heart, which will prompt more careful manipulation by the surgeon to prevent dislodgement. TEE may also help to identify pleural effusions necessitating drainage to allow easier ventilation and avoidance of right ventricular dysfunction in the post-CPB period. Prior to CPB, the main ventilatory goal is to prevent an increase in pulmonary vascular resistance, which can be achieved by preventing hypoxia, hypercarbia, and hypothermia, and avoiding increased sympathetic activity.[368]

Heparin administration is required prior to aortic cannulation at the full dose of 400 units/kg with the goal of achieving an ACT of greater than 480 seconds.[368] Recent evidence promotes the usage of heparin-level guided administration compared to ACT because end-stage heart failure patients often have AT III deficiency due to long-term heparin administration.[371] Long-term exposure to heparin also increases the incidence of HIT, which is prevalent in 3.6% to 24% of heart transplant patients.[368]

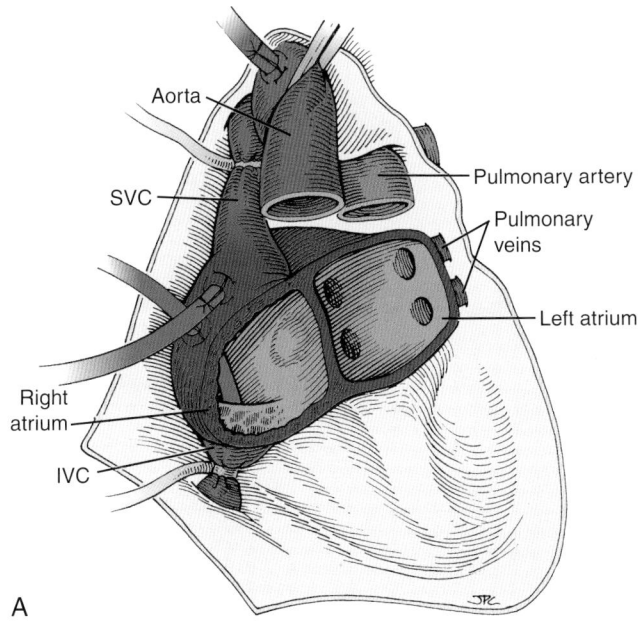

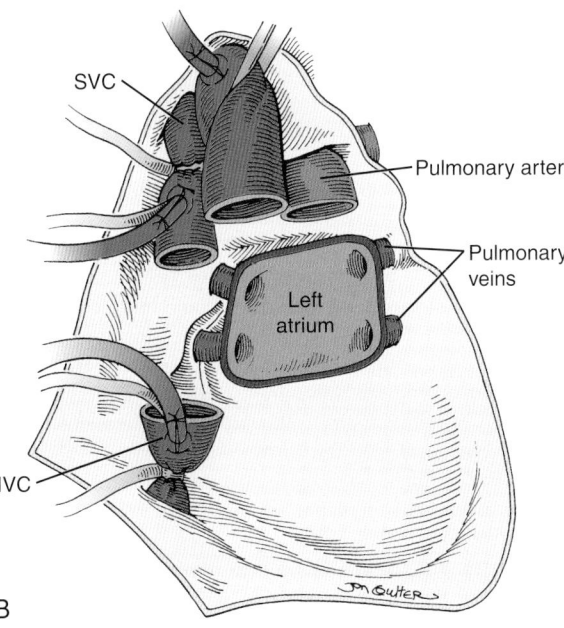

Fig. 26.37 Mediastinum after excision of the heart but before allograft placement. Venous cannulas are present in the superior *(SVC)* and inferior vena cava *(IVC)*, and the arterial cannula is present in the ascending aorta. (A) Classic orthotopic (biatrial) technique. (B) Bicaval anastomotic technique. (From Murray AW, et al. Anesthesia for heart, lung, and heart-lung transplantation. In Kaplan JA, et al., eds. *Kaplan's Cardiac Anesthesia: For Cardiac and Noncardiac Surgery.* 7th ed. Philadelphia: Elsevier; 2017:976.)

There are many factors to consider prior to separation from CPB, and guidance with TEE during this time is crucial. One of the most critical uses for TEE prior to aortic cross-clamp removal is the evaluation of intracardiac air, which is most often located near the sites of anastomoses or at the apex of the left ventricle. A steep Trendelenburg position may help prevent migration of air to the cerebral vessels at the time of aortic cross-clamp removal.[368]

As mentioned previously, the lungs should be ventilated using strategies to maintain or decrease pulmonary vascular resistance.

Temporary pacemaker leads are placed in the donor atrium and ventricle, as prolonged ischemic times often contribute to slower restoration of the heart's electrical conduction pathway. If the donor heart recovers spontaneously, this is a promising indication of minimal injury after ischemia and reperfusion. Because the donor heart is denervated, it will not respond to indirect-acting agents, including parasympatholytics, and the intrinsic heart rate will be higher at a rate of 90 to 110 bpm. Therefore, after the removal of the aortic cross-clamp, direct-acting inotropic agents are initiated, and TEE guidance helps to direct the titration of these inotropic infusions. Although the donor heart no longer responds to indirect-acting agents, the Frank-Starling mechanism is still intact, and the heart is critically dependent on adequate preload.[368]

One of the most devastating complications associated with heart transplantation, with a mortality rate as high as 86%, is right ventricular failure with or without the presence of PHTN.[368] In addition to preventing an increase in pulmonary vascular resistance, other strategies to avoid strain on the RV include maintaining adequate coronary perfusion with optimal aortic pressure and preventing overdistention. Epinephrine, milrinone, and dopamine are all options for inotropic support, although milrinone may also cause systemic vasodilation. If systemic vasoconstriction is required, vasopressin may be a better choice than norepinephrine because norepinephrine increases resistance in the pulmonary and coronary vasculature.[368]

When PHTN is present, inhaled vasodilators are preferred over systemic vasodilators, which include epoprostenol, iloprost, and nitric oxide.[368] Epoprostenol may be the most beneficial as it not only decreases pulmonary vascular resistance but also increases function of the RV.[368] If intravenous or inhaled medication does not adequately support the function of the RV, temporary support with a RVAD or ECMO may be required.[368]

Protamine should be given slowly over 10 to 15 minutes because hypotension associated with rapid administration may decrease perfusion to the RV and increase pulmonary vascular resistance. Blood transfusion places the patient at significant risk for allosensitization in the posttransplant period. Specific blood conservation techniques include ANH, RAP of the CPB circuit by the perfusionist, and administration of antifibrinolytic therapies, including tranexamic acid and aminocaproic acid.[368]

Surgery on the Ascending Aorta and Aortic Arch
General Considerations
Thoracic aortic disease consists of two subtypes: aneurysm and dissection. An aneurysm refers to a greater than 50% dilation of all three layers of the aortic wall. A dissection involves disruption of the aortic intimal layer allowing blood to track within the media layer creating a false lumen. Aneurysm and dissection are not always clinically distinct, and there are many similarities between the two regarding surgical and anesthetic management.[55,372] The cause of aortic disease is usually genetic (e.g., Marfan, Loeys-Dietz, Ehlers-Danlos, and Turner syndromes; bicuspid AV disease) in patients who present at younger ages for surgery, but acquired (e.g., hypertension, atherosclerosis, and inflammation) in older patients.[55,372,373] A discussion of aortic disease can be found in Chapter 25. This chapter focuses on anesthetic management for surgeries on the ascending aorta and arch that require CPB. Management will vary markedly, depending on what segment(s) of the aorta is (are) involved and whether the AV is preserved, repaired, or replaced. A multidisciplinary discussion regarding the plan for cannulation, invasive monitoring, and cerebral protection is critical before surgery to determine the appropriate management.

Most thoracic aneurysms (TAs) are asymptomatic and often found coincidentally following an x-ray or other test performed for an unrelated problem. Large TAs can cause a mass effect that can lead to cough, dysphasia, or hoarseness due to compression on the trachea, esophagus, or recurrent laryngeal nerve. Sometimes SVC syndrome develops.[374] Patients with a bicuspid AV or genetic mutation associated with aortic disease should be imaged and followed at regular intervals. Aortic diameter is related to wall tension and risk of dissection or rupture. Surgery is indicated for all symptomatic aneurysms and is generally indicated for asymptomatic ascending TAs that are dilated to 4.5 cm for congenital lesions (especially if there is a family history of dissection) or 5.5 cm for acquired lesions. TAs usually grow slowly over years, but an aneurysm that is growing at a rate exceeding 0.5 cm/year should also undergo surgical repair.[372] TAs and dissections of the ascending aorta and aortic arch are usually repaired using an upper hemi or full median sternotomy, depending on the size and surgeon's preference. The type of procedure will vary depending on the extent of the aneurysm or dissection, and the competency of the AV. TEE is an invaluable assessment tool for determining whether the valve can be spared or repaired and for measuring the aorta.

Aortic Dissection

A devastating complication of an aneurysm is dissection, but dissections can also occur in a normal size aorta. The dissection begins from an intimal tear that most often spreads antegrade, but can also dissect retrograde throughout the aorta, possibly encompassing the great vessels and/or the AV.[55] Acute ascending or aortic arch dissections (Crawford type A) are highly lethal, and timely surgical intervention correlates with survival. Descending dissections, distal to the left subclavian (Crawford type B), can usually be repaired on an elective basis unless there are signs of rupture or organ ischemia. The most catastrophic and lethal complication of aneurysms is rupture.

Patients with ascending or arch dissections usually present with sudden severe neck and chest pain, but symptoms mimicking a stroke, MI, or arterial embolization can also occur. Syncope is an ominous sign that cerebral or cardiac circulation is compromised. Diagnosis can be made with TEE, contrast-enhanced spiral CT scan, or MRI. Acute AI, tamponade, or limb ischemia can develop at any time.[55,373,375,376] The initial priority is to obtain adequate vascular access for both monitoring BP and transfusing the patient. The A line site should be carefully selected, avoiding ischemic limbs and locations that will be impacted by surgical cannulation.

The aim of hemodynamic management is to control the aortic shear stress, including BP, contractility, and heart rate, which can cause further dissection or rupture. The heart rate and BP are most often controlled using a β-blocker first to achieve a heart rate of approximately 60 bpm, followed by cautious vasodilation with nicardipine, nitroglycerin, or nitroprusside to achieve a MAP of 60 to 70 mm Hg.[372,373] Vasodilator therapy should not be initiated before rate control because the reflex tachycardia that may develop can increase LV ejection velocity and aortic wall stress, causing harmful expansion of the dissection.[373,377] Coexisting myocardial depression can make medication titration challenging. Some institutions have the patient prepped and draped before induction in preparation for the possibility of rupture and the need to urgently initiate CPB.

Ascending aortic aneurysm and dissection. When the aortic aneurysm or dissection involves only the root and proximal aorta, standard aortic arterial cannulation and CPB can be used since the distal aorta can be cannulated and an aortic cross-clamp placed between the cannula and the aneurysm. Alternative approaches include cannulation of the right axillary artery or the innominate artery, most often with a graft to the vessel. The femoral artery may also be used for arterial cannulation, but in this case arterial flow is retrograde from

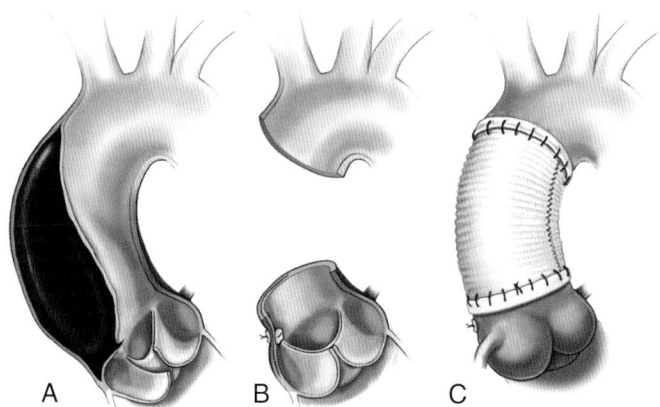

Fig. 26.38 Ascending aortic dissection repair. (A) The dissecting hematoma is seen and usually extends all the way to the iliac arteries. (B) The compromised commissure of the valve is resuspended by a full-thickness pledgeted suture. (C) The ascending aorta is replaced with a vascular graft, usually using strips of felt to reinforce the delicate adventitial tissues. (From Otto CM, Bonow RO. *Valvular Heart Disease: A Companion to Braunwald's Heart Disease.* 3rd ed. Philadelphia: Elsevier; 2009.)

the femoral artery to the cerebral vessels. Usually a single, two-stage venous cannula suffices. A simple tube graft can be used to replace the aorta when the aortic root and valve are normal (Fig. 26.38).[373] In the setting of significant AI, but a normal diameter within sinuses of Valsalva (aortic root), a simple supracoronary graft can be used, which does not necessitate coronary arteries being reimplanted. The valve is repaired or replaced, the sinuses are spared, and a Dacron tube graft is used to repair the aneurysm or dissection.[373]

If the aortic annulus or sinuses of Valsalva (where the coronary arteries attach) are involved, the options become more complicated, and the selected technique will depend on the surgeon's expertise and preferences. Four options exist, including a valve-sparing aortic root replacement, a composite valve graft with either a mechanical or biologic valve, or a homograph or allograph root replacement from a human cadaveric aorta.[378] If the aortic root (sinuses of Valsalva) is dilated, a technically difficult valve-sparing operation known as a modified David or Svensson reimplantation procedure can be used (Fig. 26.39). The aneurysm, including the root, is resected along with the sinuses of Valsalva. The coronaries are then removed with a button of native aortic tissue. The native AV (repaired if necessary) is sewn inside the Dacron graft used to repair the aneurysm. The coronary arteries are then reimplanted into the graft. When the valve cannot be spared, an alternative procedure known as the Bentall (or modified Bentall) is performed. A biologic or mechanical AV (or pulmonary homograft) is sewn into one end of the conduit, and the resulting composite valve-graft is used to replace both the AV and ascending aorta. Again, the coronaries must be reimplanted, or an aortocoronary bypass graft can be used (Cabrol technique).[372,377,379]

Aortic arch aneurysm or dissection. Aortic pathology of the arch is much more complex (Fig. 26.40A). The involvement of the cerebral vessels increases the risk of neurologic injury from both the threat of global ischemia and the embolization of atherosclerotic debris. Since cannulas and aortic cross-clamps cannot be used to divert blood flow away from the surgical field, DHCA is used to protect the cerebral tissue and other organs while the arch is replaced. If only the proximal aortic arch is involved, a hemiarch or partial arch replacement can be done. The origins of the arch vessels may be dissected en bloc so that the three vessels lie on an island of native aortic tissue that can be

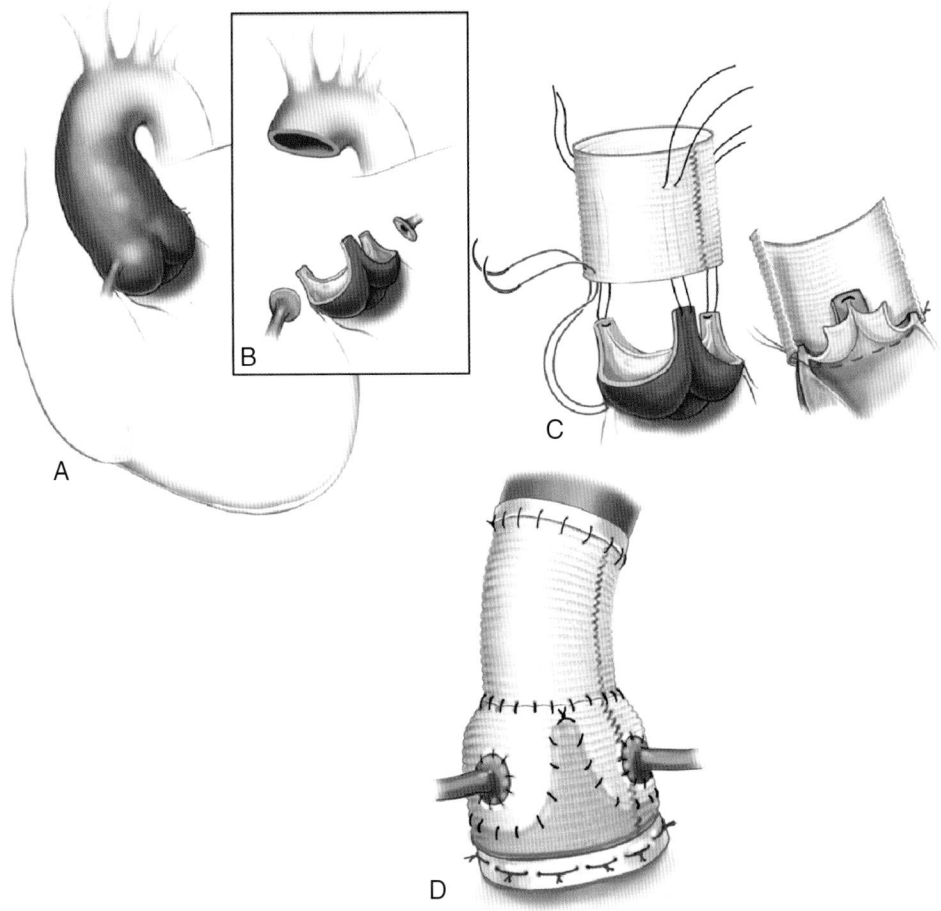

Fig. 26.39 David procedure. Aneurysmal root (A) is resected (B), including sinuses of Valsalva with coronary "buttons" mobilized away. (C) Subannular sutures (six to eight) are placed. Commissural posts are drawn up inside the valve, and the annular sutures are passed through the proximal end of the graft. (D) Annular sutures are tied gently. Then the valve is reimplanted with continuous 5-0 polypropylene suture inside the graft. Aortic continuity is reestablished with another graft of a size appropriate to the desired sinotubular junction and proximal arch. (From Otto CM, Bonow RO. *Valvular Heart Disease: A Companion to Braunwald's Heart Disease.* 4th ed. Philadelphia: Elsevier; 2014:210.)

anastomosed to the synthetic graft. Debranching procedures, in which each of the great vessels are individually anastomosed to a multibranch aortic graft, are also common. In either case, the surgeon completes the distal anastomosis to the descending aorta first, and then anastomoses either the previous aortic island containing the aortic arch vessels or the individual vessels (see Fig. 26.40B). Next, assuming axillary artery cannulation, the aortic clamp is moved proximal to the arch vessels so that CPB flow can be reestablished and the cerebral vessels perfused. Finally, the proximal aortic graft anastomosis is completed.

Aneurysms that involve the entire thoracic aorta are extremely complicated and are often repaired in stages, combining both open and endovascular techniques. As shown in Fig. 26.40B, the distal graft is sutured circumferentially to the aorta just beyond the left subclavian artery, and the free end of the graft ("elephant trunk") is placed within the descending aneurysm. The aneurysm repair is completed (often in a second procedure as shown in Fig. 26.40C) using an endovascular stent graft attached proximally to the elephant trunk, and the distal end is secured to a Dacron graft cuff.[373,375,380]

Anesthetic Management

Anesthesia implications are similar to those of other cardiac surgeries involving a median sternotomy with CPB but with several additional concerns. As discussed earlier, securing the airway may be difficult in large aneurysms that cause compression on the trachea or other airway structures.[55] Occasionally, a reinforced ETT must be used and advanced beyond the point of compression. Resistance to passing the TEE probe or OG tube may indicate the aneurysm is compressing the esophagus, which may necessitate epiaortic echocardiographic examination.

Nasopharyngeal or tympanic temperature is monitored as a reflection of cerebral temperature if DHCA is planned. The nasal probe should be placed before heparin is administered to prevent bleeding in this fragile area. Bladder and PA temperatures are measured to reflect core and shell temperatures that are used to monitor the rate of rewarming. During rewarming, nasopharyngeal and tympanic temperatures correlate much more closely with cerebral temperatures than core temperature measurements, so monitoring at the nasopharyngeal and tympanic locations decreases the risk of cerebral overwarming.[375,381,382]

A strategic approach to A line placement should consider the plan for placement of the aortic cannula and aortic cross-clamp, and the use of antegrade cerebral perfusion (ACP). For ascending aortic pathology, there is no consensus in the literature as to the best location for the A line. When the arch is involved and DHCA is planned, brachial artery hemodynamic monitoring may be preferred to the radial artery since

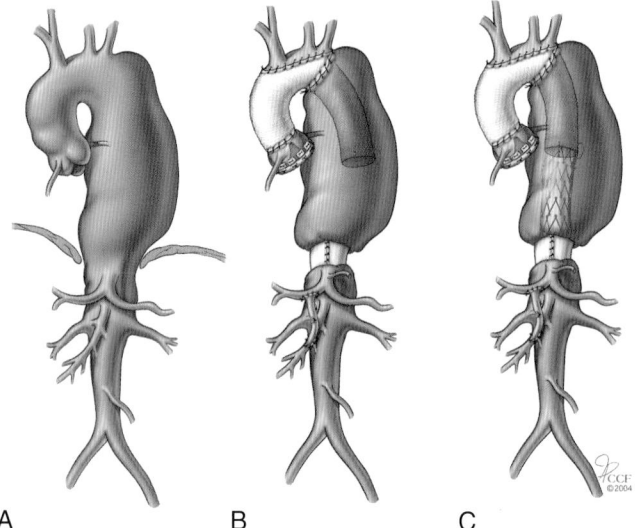

Fig. 26.40 Repair of an ascending aorta, aortic arch, and descending thoracic aneurysm. (A) Preoperative disease. (B) Stage 1 of the repair is an open procedure. The ascending aorta and arch are replaced with a Dacron graft that is sutured circumferentially to the aorta distal to the left subclavian artery. Note that the great vessels to the head are usually resected as an island of tissue that is anastomosed to the graft. The free end of the graft ("elephant trunk") is placed within the descending aneurysm. (C) Completion of the procedure using an endovascular stent graft attached proximally to the elephant trunk and the distal end secured to a Dacron graft cuff. (Reprinted with permission from Cleveland Clinic Center for Medical Art & Photography ©2020. All rights reserved.)

the brachial artery correlates more closely with aortic pressures during rewarming.[375,383] If the distal arch is involved, temporary occlusion of the left subclavian may make the placement of the A line in the right preferable. If the right axillary artery is to be cannulated for CPB or ACP, then the left radial or brachial is preferred since increased flow will cause the pressure on the right to be falsely elevated.[373,381] If a proximal descending aortic graft is anticipated, two A lines are placed: one in the upper extremity and one in a femoral artery. If occlusion of the stent-graft occurs following deployment, the lower extremity A line will have lower pressures than the upper extremity.[378]

PACs are usually indicated because large shifts in volume can be reasonably anticipated, especially if the arch is involved, along with the possibility of myocardial ischemia during the DHCA period. A large-bore, multilumen central venous introducer allows volume to be rapidly infused. Alternatively, several large-bore PIVs can be used with a standard central venous introducer. Blood loss can be significant when involving a high-pressure system such as the aorta, so RBCs should be available for transfusion. Additionally, coagulation factors may adhere to the aortic graft material creating a systemic coagulopathy. FFP and platelets are transfused (usually after the protamine is administered) as needed, based on coagulation studies and nonsurgical bleeding. Fluid warmers and airway heat and humidifiers are used following DHCA to prevent redistribution hypothermia. Consideration should be given to the use of a rapid-infusion device if large amounts of RBCs and FFP can be reasonably anticipated. Use of antifibrinolytic therapy is considered reasonable, but the infusion is generally held during the period of DHCA or initiated following DHCA.[377]

Management of AI generally includes maintenance of a relatively high heart rate and a low SVR to enhance forward flow. However, in this situation, sheer stress must be considered, so the heart rate and contractility are controlled with β-blockers, and the systolic BP is kept

below 120 mm Hg using vasodilators to minimize the risk of dissection or rupture.[372,373,377,379]

Deep Hypothermic Circulatory Arrest

Cerebral perfusion must be temporarily interrupted during repair of aneurysms and dissections involving the aortic arch. Hypothermia is the most important therapeutic intervention to prevent cerebral ischemia. The patient is cooled using CPB to maximally decrease the cerebral metabolic rate and O_2 consumption ($CMRO_2$), thereby extending the period that the brain and other organs can tolerate circulatory arrest. As cooling on CPB is initiated, most institutions cool the brain topically by placing ice bags around the head to further reduce metabolic function.[381] The target temperature for DHCA depends on the clinical setting and whether ACP or retrograde cerebral perfusion (RCP) will be used. $CMRO_2$ decreases by a factor of 2.3 for every 10°C decrease in body temperature.[384] The traditional goal is to have an isoelectric electroencephalogram (EEG), with the BIS monitor considered an easily accessible and acceptable substitute for an EEG.[113]

Once the patient is cooled to the desired temperature and the EEG shows burst suppression, or the BIS monitor reads 0, most of the blood volume is drained into the venous reservoir, and the CPB is turned off. General anesthesia is not needed once burst suppression has been achieved, but it must be reinstituted when rewarming begins. A circulatory arrest period of 20 to 30 minutes is generally tolerated when deep hypothermia, defined as a temperature of 14.1°C to 20°C, is used.[382] It is recommended that the oxygenator arterial outlet blood temperature be utilized as a surrogate for cerebral temperature measurement during CPB.[141] Combining DHCA with cold ACP may prolong the safe period to as long as 80 minutes.[375,381,385] Cerebral oximetry uses NIRS to measure the oxygen saturation of cerebral tissue. Cerebral oxygen saturation will increase with cooling and then decrease during the DHCA period. Monitoring the decrease in oxygen saturation provides insight when the acceptable length of DHCA has been reached, potentially preventing cerebral ischemia.[386] Since the viscosity of blood increases with cooling, hemodilution may be advantageous in that a lower hematocrit may allow for smaller capillaries to be perfused during the cooling process, promoting homogenous cooling of cerebral tissue and greater protection. Pharmacologic attempts at neuroprotection include the administration of propofol to decrease $CMRO_2$. Steroids, lidocaine, and mannitol have also been used. However, because no pharmacologic intervention has proved effective, these medications are not considered a substitute for achieving adequate hypothermia.[375,377]

Antegrade cerebral perfusion. If DHCA is anticipated to last more than 30 minutes, selective ACP is often used to extend safe operative time. The cerebral vessel(s) used for ACP depends on the patient's anatomy and surgeon's preference and may include the axillary, innominate, subclavian, or internal carotid arteries. The perfusionist administers blood cooled to 6°C to 12°C directly into one or more of the cerebral vessels at rates of 5 to 7 mL/kg/min at a pressure of 60 to 70 mm Hg. Many surgeons prefer to use right subclavian arterial cannulation if ACP is planned. The BP is monitored using a right radial A line during ACP to maintain the MAP between 30 and 70 mm Hg; however, the right A line should not be used to control perfusion pressure during the cooling and rewarming period, as the pressure may be falsely elevated if the right subclavian is used for CPB arterial flow.[375,381,385] Many institutions use cerebral oximetry with NIRS during ACP to ensure bilateral cerebral perfusion. Significant unilateral decrease in cerebral oxygen saturations may indicate an incomplete circle of Willis. In this situation, ACP via the left carotid artery often restores the values.[387,388]

Retrograde cerebral perfusion. RCP was popularized in past decades as a cerebral protection adjunct; however, ACP has been shown to provide superior protection. Clinical use of RCP is on the decline but is still practiced.[375,381,385] RCP requires the use of individual SVC and IVC venous cannulation. During the period of arrest, the arterial component of the CPB circuit is connected to the SVC cannula, and cold oxygenated blood (between 8°C and 14°C) is infused in a retrograde fashion at a rate of 150 to 250 mL/min. During RCP, the patient is kept in a slight Trendelenburg position to prevent air embolism. Ideally, cerebral tissue is constantly cooled at a low pressure (<20 mm Hg) to prevent venous engorgement of cerebral tissue. During RCP, the pressure within the venous system is measured during the period of circulatory arrest from the most proximal port of the central venous introducer (the side port). Advantages of RCP include relative simplicity, uniform cerebral cooling, efficient de-airing of the cerebral vessels reducing the risk of embolism, and provision of O_2 and energy substrates.[375,376]

Rewarming. Once systemic perfusion is reestablished using CPB, a period of hypothermic reperfusion is recommended. General anesthesia is resumed and antifibrinolytic therapy is initiated or also resumed. Rewarming should be done gradually, maintaining a maximal temperature gradient of 10°C between the arterial outlet and venous inflow on the oxygenator/heat exchanger. The STS recommendation

is to limit arterial outlet blood temperature to less than 37°C to avoid cerebral hyperthermia.[141] Even slight hyperthermia in patients with cerebral ischemia or infarction may exacerbate any damage.[377] The optimal temperature for CPB separation remains debatable. Some surgeons prefer a bladder temperature of 36.5°C before CPB separation to decrease bleeding, whereas others prioritize cerebral protection and separate at 35°C. Separation at lower temperatures may intensify post-CPB coagulopathy.[141]

The postbypass period includes all the considerations discussed in the section on general cardiac surgery. Coagulopathy is often significant because deep hypothermia decreases platelet count, slows enzymatic reactions in the coagulation cascade, impairs tissue factor activity, and enhances fibrinolysis. Platelets, FFP, and cryoprecipitate are often administered after surgical bleeding is controlled. Tests of viscoelasticity are useful in guiding therapy.[389,390] Hemodynamic management can be challenging as both hypertension and hypotension can be problematic. Intravascular fluid shifts are common, and the TEE is invaluable in assessing volume status. Patients are transported to the ICU intubated and sedated. The weaning process is delayed until hemodynamic stability is achieved and coagulopathy is corrected.[375,376]

SUMMARY

As the population ages, CAD, VHD, and heart failure will continue to be major health concerns. The risk profile of the average cardiac surgical patient and the complexity of the procedures continue to rise. Technology and innovative surgical approaches to managing CVD have improved the landscape of cardiac anesthesia. A clear understanding of the core physiologic and pathophysiologic principles that impact coronary blood flow and myocardial function will enable the anesthetist to adapt anesthetic management in this ever-evolving field. Each clinician is encouraged to stay abreast of the evidence-based outcome studies that have so greatly impacted our clinical practice.

REFERENCES

For a complete list of references for this chapter, scan this QR code with any smartphone code reader app, or visit the following URL: http://booksite.elsevier.com/9780323711944/

27

Perioperative Management for Patients With Cardiac Devices

Becky J. Ashlock, Judith A. Franco

The mean age in the US population is increasing. Many of these older patients have associated cardiac pathology that warrants placement of a cardiac implantable electronic device (CIED). Many patients undergoing surgical procedures or presenting to the procedural environment will have a preexisting CIED. The CIED may be a pacemaker (PM), an implantable cardioverter defibrillator (ICD; older model), a combination of both PM and ICD (modern device), or a cardiac resynchronization device (also referred to as a biventricular cardiac device). With increasing advances in technology there is greater device variability and expanded clinical application. The indications for the use of each CIED differ, including the programmability and the management in the perioperative setting may be different depending on the device. Intraoperative electromagnetic interference (EMI) can alter, disrupt, or damage these devices. Furthermore, rapid changes in technology are responsible for the lack of evidence-based practice guidelines and troubleshooting methodologies.[1,2] Therefore, it is important to avoid generalizations regarding these devices.[1,3] Instead, knowledge regarding the type of device, indications for placement, manufacturer, basic functions, programmability, battery life, response to a magnet, and device limitations should be ascertained to ensure patient safety.[4]

The key objectives that will be addressed in this chapter include:

- A generalized review of CIEDs
- The multidisciplinary team's responsibility regarding management of CIEDs
- The CIED's potential response to EMI
- Intraoperative management strategies for various CIEDs

REVIEW OF PACEMAKERS

PMs emerged approximately 70 years ago in an effort to save the lives of patients with sinus node and atrioventricular node dysfunction. Pacemakers were initially placed via thoracotomy.[5] These early devices were limited to ventricular pacing at a constant rate as sensing capabilities were unavailable. The first PMs were associated with a multitude of problems such as lead fractures, randomly changing thresholds, competition between the intrinsic heart rate and the PM rate, and EMI.

The creation of a reed switch enabled the PM to convert from synchronous to asynchronous pacing with the application of a magnet. A reed switch is composed of two magnetic metal strips located within the pulse generator. In the presence of a magnetic field or with the placement of a magnet directly over the PM, the two metal strips make contact and close the reed switch inactivating the sensing circuit. It is this change in voltage that causes the PM to asynchronously pace the myocardium.[6] The creation of a reed switch revolutionized PM technology and secured the use of PMs' place as a safe and reliable intervention for sinus and atrioventricular node dysfunction.

Today's PMs are approximately the size of a quarter (Fig. 27.1). They consist of two main components: (1) a pulse generator that houses the battery, circuitry, and connectors, and (2) the insulated lead wires that conduct energy to and from the myocardium. The pulse generator is usually implanted in the pectoral pocket on either the right or left side of the chest. Implantation is accomplished while the patient receives a general anesthetic or local anesthetic with sedation (Fig. 27.2). A sensing circuit, located within the pulse generator, picks up signals transferred from the myocardium via the leads. High amplitude is seen by the PM as intrinsic activity, and low amplitude is seen as interference commonly referred to as noise. The low amplitude signals are filtered, and native cardiac signals are sensed. The PM can interpret intrinsic activity correctly, and pacing is initiated appropriately. However, in the presence of EMI, this noise causes the PM to inaccurately sense intrinsic cardiac activity resulting in PM inhibition.[5]

A PM may contain up to three lead wires. The wires are imbedded into the right atrium, the right ventricle, both the right atrium and ventricle, or the right atrium and both ventricles. The lead systems are unipolar, bipolar, or multipolar. In a unipolar configuration, the pulse generator acts as an anode (positive electrode) and the distal end of the lead wire is the cathode (negative electrode). With a unipolar lead system there is a greater distance between the anode and cathode. With a unipolar lead, the spikes (vertical lines that represent electrical activity) on the surface electrocardiogram (ECG) are frequently larger, and the distance between the anode and the cathode places the PM at an increased risk for EMI.

Bipolar leads contain two electrodes. In a bipolar configuration, the anode and cathode are located at the distal end of the bipolar lead. As a result, there is less distance between the two poles, decreasing the chance of EMI and the potential for disruption to the PM function. Bipolar electrodes are visualized on a chest x-ray by identification of a distal ring located 1 to 3 cm from the tip of the bipolar lead (Fig. 27.3).[7] Most modern PM leads are bipolar, and their lead configuration exhibits smaller spikes on the surface ECG.

PMs have sensing and capturing responses that may be identifiable by the presence of spikes on the ECG. When the PM lead wire is placed in the right atrium there is a spike followed by a P wave on the ECG, representing atrial depolarization (Fig. 27.4). When the lead is inserted in the right ventricle, a spike followed by a QRS complex on the ECG indicates ventricular depolarization (Fig. 27.5). If the device is a dual-chamber PM (a lead is inserted in both the right atrium and ventricle), there is a spike before the P wave and before the QRS complex followed by both atrial and ventricular depolarization (Fig. 27.6). If the pacing device is sensing the patient's intrinsic rhythm and not providing a paced response due to inherent cardiac activity, only a sensing marker is visualized on the surface ECG. There are a multitude of indications for PM placement,[8] and the most common examples are listed in Box 27.1.

Types of Pacemakers

Although the focus of this chapter is on the perioperative management of implantable PMs and ICDs, there are various types of external PMs available. These external devices can be manipulated manually when a disruption in pacing occurs. The implantable PM requires reprogramming or, in some cases, magnet application to remedy unreliable or disrupted pacing behavior.

With external pacing, transcutaneous pacing pads are applied (a) anteriorly on the right upper chest and anteriorly on the left lower chest, or (b) anteriorly midchest and posteriorly between the scapulae. In either case, the transcutaneous pacing pads are plugged into a defibrillator/pacing machine and programmed accordingly (Fig. 27.7). In transvenous pacing, the pacing catheter is passed into the central circulation (usually via an introducer sheath) and into the appropriate cardiac chamber(s). The pacing lead is connected to an external pacemaker generator and is programmed as needed. Epicardial pacing leads are often inserted at the completion of cardiac surgery. These pacing wires are directly sewn, by the cardiac surgeon, onto the epicardium, passed through the skin, attached to an external pacing device, and programmed as dictated by the clinical situation.

Although different PMs are available, the language, terminology, and programming are similar (Table 27.1). With the nonimplantable devices (external, transcutaneous, or transvenous), a practitioner can diagnose a PM problem (e.g., failure to capture or sense) and immediately intervene by manipulating the programming. For example, providers can manually change the heart rate programmed on the nonimplanted pacemaker to increase the electrical output and improve capture. With an implantable PM, intervening in this manner is not an option without access to a device-specific programmer. Troubleshooting an implantable PM requires recognition of the problem, knowledge of whether the device is magnet sensitive, and access to a programmer.

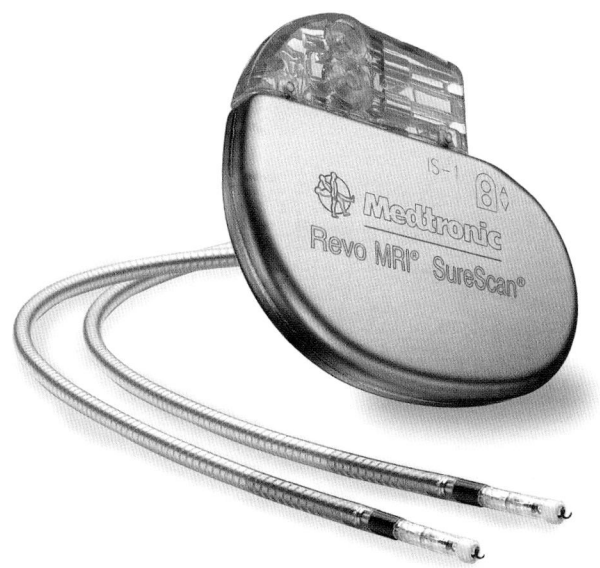

Fig. 27.1 Pacemaker. (Reproduced with permission of Medtronic, Inc.)

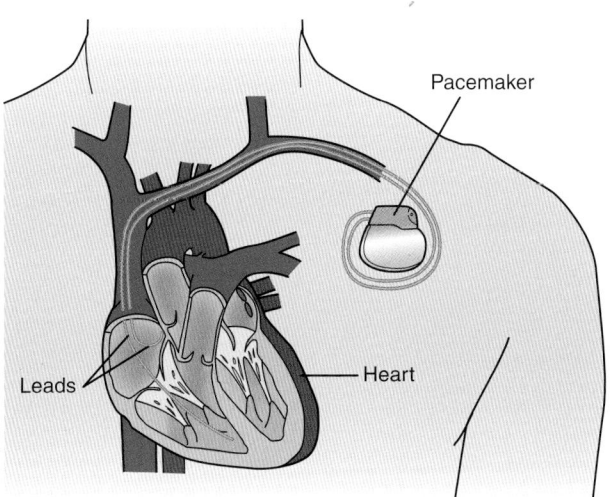

Fig. 27.2 A pacemaker is positioned in the pectoral pocket. (From Sorrentino SA, Remmert LN. *Mosby's Textbook for Nursing Assistants*. 9th ed. St. Louis: Elsevier; 2017:730.)

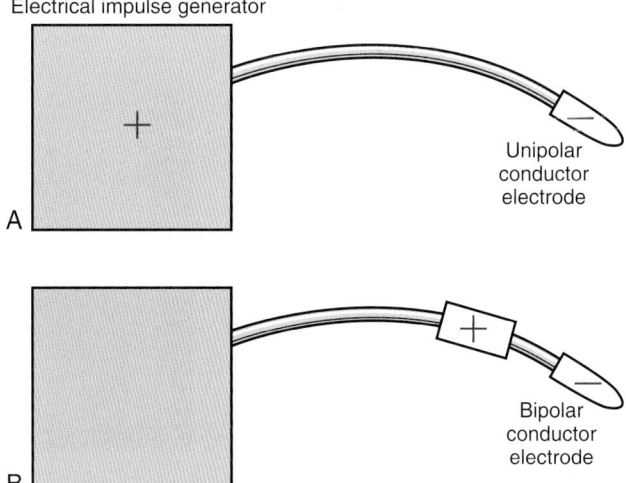

Fig. 27.3 Pacemaker electrode configurations. (A) Unipolar electrode. (B) Bipolar electrode. (From Hillegass E. *Essentials of Cardiopulmonary Physical Therapy*. 3rd ed. St. Louis: Elsevier; 2011:389.)

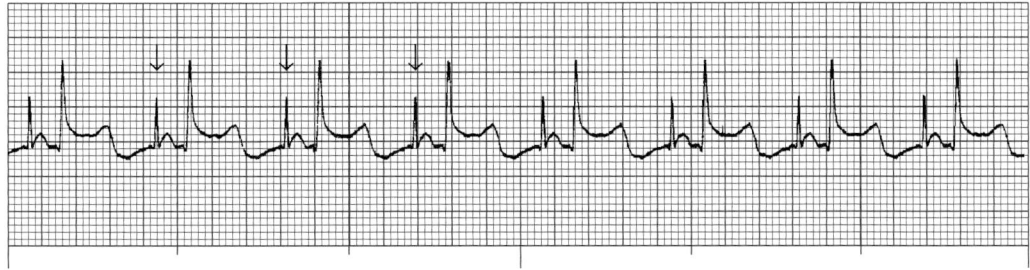

Fig. 27.4 Electrocardiogram of a single-chamber pacemaker with atrial pacing spikes *(arrows)*. (From Aehlert B. *ECGs Made Easy*. 5th ed. St. Louis: Elsevier; 2013:243.)

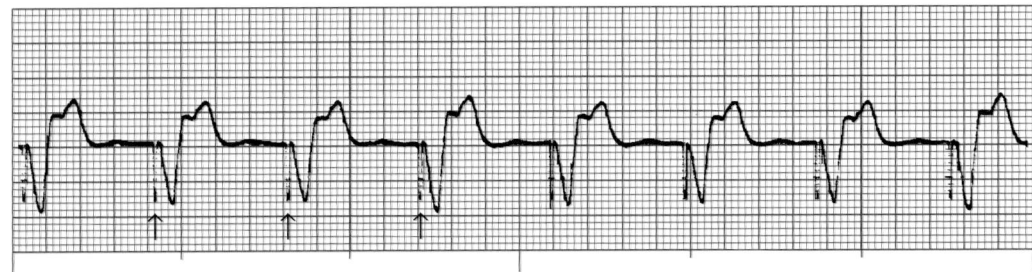

Fig. 27.5 Electrocardiogram of a single-chamber pacemaker with ventricular pacing spikes *(arrows)*. (From Aehlert B. *ECGs Made Easy*. 5th ed. St. Louis: Elsevier; 2013:244.)

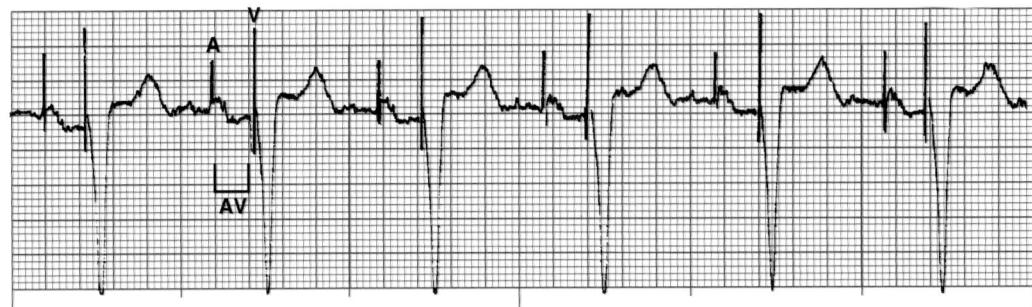

Fig. 27.6 Dual pacing: atrial and ventricular. Electrocardiogram of a dual-chamber pacemaker with atrial pacing spikes *(A)*, ventricular pacing spikes *(V)*. *AV*, Atrioventricular interval. (From Aehlert B. *ECGs Made Easy*. 5th ed. St. Louis: Elsevier; 2013:244.)

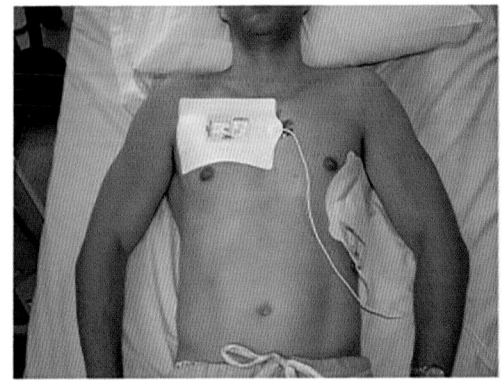

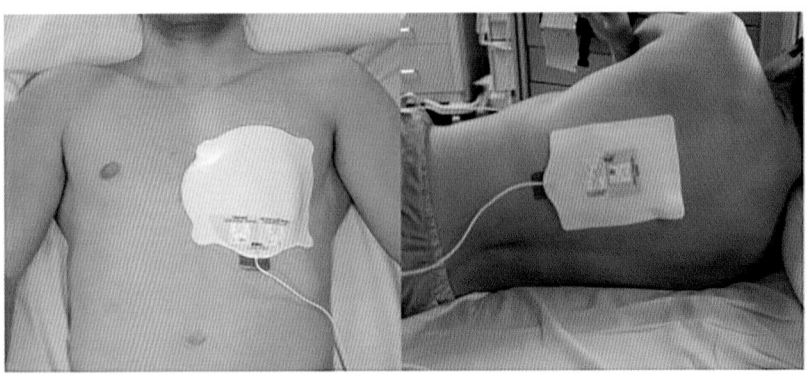

Fig. 27.7 (A) Pad placement for transcutaneous pacing. (B) Alternate anteroposterior placement. (From L'Italien AJ. Critical cardiovascular skills and procedures in the emergency department. *Emerg Med Clin North Am*. 2013;31(1):151–206.)

BOX 27.1 Indications for the Use of Pacemakers

- Sinus node dysfunction
- Atrioventricular node disease
- Chronic bifascicular block
- Long QT syndrome
- Hypertrophic obstructive cardiomyopathy
- Dilated cardiomyopathy
- Postacute phase of myocardial infarction
- Carotid sinus syndrome

From Santucci PA, Wilber DJ. Electrophysiologic interventional procedures and surgery. In Goldman L, Schafer AI, et al., eds. *Goldman-Cecil Medicine.* 26th ed. Philadelphia: Elsevier 2020: 351–357.

TABLE 27.1 Pacemaker Terminology

Heart rate	Programmed upper and lower heart rate.
Electrical output	Electrical output, measured in milliamps (mA), is the electrical output the pacemaker delivers with each charge.
Synchronous mode	Paced rate matching the underlying rate of one of the heart chambers.
Asynchronous mode	Cardiac pacing mode set independent of the heart's intrinsic rate.
Inhibited	When the patient demonstrates an intrinsic heartbeat, the pacemaker will not deliver a paced beat.
Threshold	The minimum output that will cause the myocardial chamber (atrium or ventricle) to consistently contract or capture.
Sensitivity	The lowest amplitude P or R wave that the pacemaker will recognize as an electrical signal.
AV interval	The time between the beginning of atrial systole (paced or intrinsic) and the beginning of ventricular systole (equivalent to the PR interval on the electrocardiogram).
Capture	Depolarization of a heart chamber in response to pacemaker electrical output.
Failure to capture	When the pacemaker's electrical output fails to cause myocardial depolarization.
Failure to sense	The pacemaker fails to recognize intrinsic cardiac electrical activity.

Pacemaker Codes

A three- or five-letter Heart Rhythm Society (HRS) code identifies the key functions of implantable PMs (Table 27.2). It is imperative that the anesthetist is familiar with the HRS codes and understands the functionality and result on the PM. The first letter in the code identifies the chamber where the pacing electrode is placed. If the first letter is A, the pacing lead is in the right atrium. If the first letter is V, the pacing lead is located in the right ventricle. If the first letter is D, then there is dual-chamber pacing with wire pacing located in both the right atrium and the right ventricle.

The second letter of the code identifies the chamber where the sensing electrode is placed. If the second letter is A, the sensing wire is located in the right atrium. If the second letter is V, the sensing lead is located in the right ventricle. If the second letter is D, there is a sensing wire located in both the right atrium and the right ventricle. If the second letter is O, then there is no sensing, and the PM will pace at an asynchronous rate.

The third letter of the code identifies the PM's response to the detection of a spontaneous cardiac depolarization and its effect on subsequent pacing stimuli. The device will either inhibit or trigger a pacing stimulus. If the third letter is I (inhibit), then the PM response is withheld when intrinsic sensed activity is faster than the programmed lower rate limit. If the third letter is T (trigger) in a single chamber mode, the PM will deliver a scheduled output pulse in response to sensed intrinsic activity. This programmed response is used for troubleshooting and electrophysiology studies. If the third letter is D, the PM will either inhibit or trigger in response to sensed intrinsic activity. For example, a sensed intrinsic atrial beat will inhibit atrial pacing output and trigger ventricular pacing.[9] If the third letter is O, then there is no sensing, and the PM will asynchronously provide pacing.

The fourth letter of the code represents rate modulation. A rate-adaptive sensor, located within the generator, is programmed to respond to physiologic stimuli (compensation for physical needs, illness, or stress) and allows the pacemaker to increase its lower rate limit. For example, if a patient exercises, the PM will increase the heart rate to augment the increased need in myocardial oxygen demand. Activity-based sensors are the most prevalent and use piezoelectric (material that generates a charge in response to applied mechanical stress) crystals to detect vibration and/or accelerometers, which detect acceleration and deceleration forces. Sensors that detect minute ventilation sensors, located within the PM circuitry, measure changes in transthoracic impedance during chest expansion and deflation that are associated with respiration. These measurements provide respiratory rate and tidal volume information and allow for calculation of minute ventilation. Changes in minute ventilation are an excellent reflection of changes in myocardial oxygen consumption and metabolic demand.[10] An R indicates the presence of rate modulation capability, and O indicates its absence.

TABLE 27.2 Heart Rhythm Society (HRS) Pacemaker Codes

NASPE/BPEG GENERIC PACEMAKER CODES (REVISED 2002)				
Position 1	**Position 2**	**Position 3**	**Position 4**	**Position 5**
Chamber Paced	*Chamber Sensed*	*Response to Sensing*	*Programmability*	*Multisite Pacing*
0 = None	0 = None	0 = None	0 = None	0 = None
A = Atrium	A = Atrium	I = Inhibited	R = Rate Modulation	A = Atrium
V = Ventricle	V = Ventricle	T = Triggered		V = Ventricle
D = Dual (A + V)	D = Dual (A + V)	D = Dual (T + I)		D = Dual (A + V)

The fifth and final letter in the HRS code identifies multisite pacing. The letter A indicates one or both atria are paced. The letter V indicates that one or both ventricles are paced. The letter D indicates that there is a combination of both atrial and ventricular pacing. The letter O indicates the absence of multisite pacing.[11]

Preoperative interrogation is recommended so that CIED indications, basic functions, programmability, response to magnet, battery life, and device limitations are known. The anesthetist must be able to recognize when the PM is not functioning or when the PM is responding inappropriately during the intraoperative period.

REVIEW OF IMPLANTABLE CARDIOVERTER DEFIBRILLATORS

Symptomatic bradyarrhythmias are treated with a PM, and tachyarrhythmias are often managed with an ICD. An ICD is a reliable method to restore a regular and coordinated rhythm from a lethal tachyarrhythmia.[1]

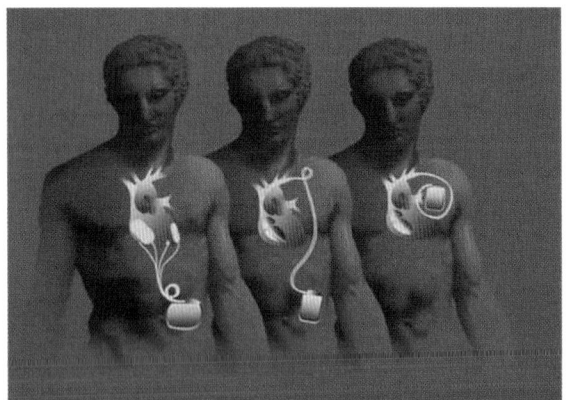

Fig. 27.8 Transformation of implantable cardioverter defibrillators. (Reproduced with permission of Medtronic, Inc.)

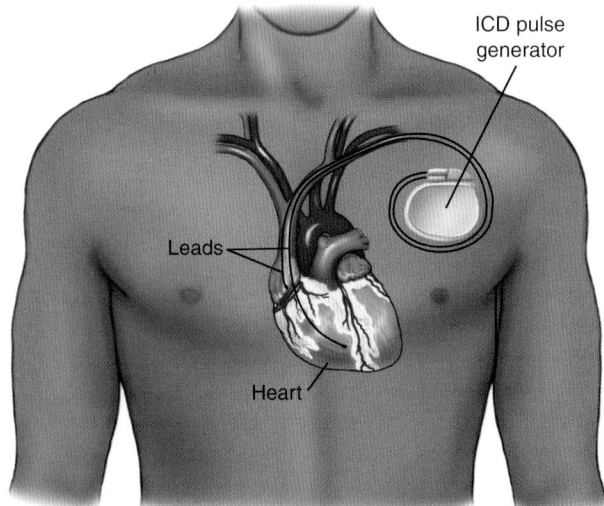

Fig. 27.9 An implanted cardioverter defibrillator *(ICD)*. (Modified from Goldberger AL. *Clinical Electrocardiography: A Simplified Approach*. 8th ed. St. Louis: Elsevier; 2013.)

Significant technologic advancements in recent years have improved the efficacy of ICDs (Fig. 27.8). The first ICD, developed in the 1980s, was primitive and was energized by simple batteries.[12] This original ICD was placed through a thoracotomy or sternotomy incision, and defibrillation patches were positioned directly on the epicardium. The lead wires were tunneled to the abdomen, which housed the defibrillator generator, and only limited programming was available. When a charge was needed, the battery sent energy to the capacitor, and once the capacitor was fully charged the energy traveled through the wire to the myocardium and delivered a shock. By the 1990s, although the ICD generator still remained implanted in the abdomen, the ICD lead/shock coils (no longer an epicardial patch) were inserted via transvenous access and implanted into the right ventricle.

Today's ICDs consist of a pulse generator, a large capacity battery, a voltage capacitor, a lead wire, and a shock coil as one unit[13] (Fig. 27.9). The generator is most often implanted in the pectoral pocket on either the right or left side of the chest while the patient receives either a general anesthetic or local anesthetic with sedation. The ICD lead/shock coil is attached to a pulse generator and positioned in the right atrium and ventricle. The capacitor delivers the current for defibrillation by receiving energy transferred from the generator's battery and discharging this energy as an electrical impulse. This impulse travels through the lead/shock coil to the myocardium and cardioverts or defibrillates the heart to treat the tachyarrhythmia. The original ICDs delivered antitachycardia therapy only. Modern ICDs are dual-function devices that contain backup pacing capabilities. This chapter will focus on ICDs with dual function (ICD + PM) unless otherwise specified.

ICDs are programmed to accomplish multiple interventions. A lead/shock coil placed in the right atrium can (a) treat bradycardia through pacing and sensing, (b) provide rate modulation, (c) initiate antitachycardia pacing, and (d) cardiovert. A lead/shock coil placed in the right ventricle can (a) treat ventricular arrhythmias, (b) initiate anticardiac pacing, (c) cardiovert and defibrillate, and (d) treat bradycardia through pacing and sensing.[14] If the device is a cardiac resynchronization device, a lead wire is threaded retrograde through the coronary sinus to the left side of the myocardium.

Indications and Terminology

The indications for ICDs include coronary artery disease, heart failure, arrhythmia, structural abnormalities, or conduction disturbances (Box 27.2).[13] As with PMs, ICDs have specific codes that

---

BOX 27.2   Indications for Implantable Cardiac Devices

- Ventricular tachycardia (VT)
- Ventricular fibrillation (VF)
- Postmyocardial infarction with an ejection fraction (EF) <35%, ≥40 days
- Cardiomyopathy from any cause with an EF <35%
- Hypertrophic cardiomyopathy and one or more risk factors for sudden death
- Awaiting heart transplant
- Long QT syndrome
- Arrhythmogenic right ventricular dysplasia
- Brugada syndrome and syncope or ventricular tachycardia
- Catecholaminergic polymorphic VT and syncope or VT on β-blocker therapy
- Cardiac sarcoidosis, giant cell myocarditis, or Chagas disease

From Santucci PA, Wilber DJ. Electrophysiologic interventional procedures and surgery. In Goldman L, Schafer AI, et al., eds. *Goldman-Cecil Medicine.* 26th ed. Philadelphia: Elsevier 2020: 351–357.

TABLE 27.3 Heart Rhythm Society (HRS) Implantable Cardiovascular Device (ICD) Codes

NASPE/BPG GENERIC DEFIBRILLATOR CODES			
Position I	Position II	Position III	Position IV
Shock Chambers	Anti-tachycardia Pacing Chambers	Tachycardia Detection	Anti-bradycardia Pacing Chambers (for Pacemaker)
O = None	O = None	E = Electrocardiogram	O = None
A = Atrium	A = Atrium	H = Hemodynamic	A = Atrium
V = Ventricle	V = Ventricle		V = Ventricle
D = Dual (A + V)	D = Dual (A + D)		D = Dual (A + D)

From Fleisher LE. *Evidence-Based Practice of Anesthesiology.* 3rd ed. St. Louis: Elsevier; 2013.

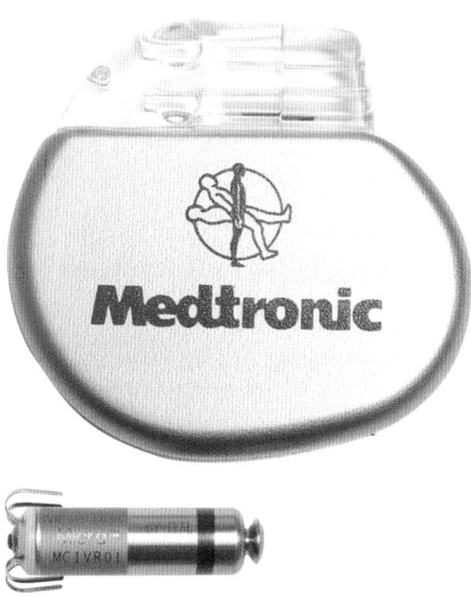
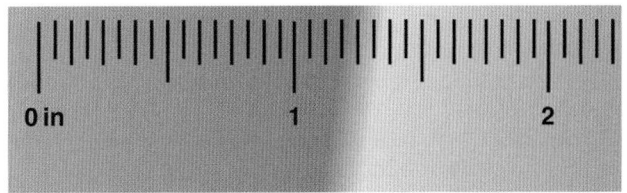

Fig. 27.10 Leadless pacemaker. (Reproduced with permission of Medtronic, Inc.)

determine individual device functionality (Table 27.3). The first letter in the HRS code describes the chamber that will be shocked, the second letter indicates the chamber where antitachycardia pacing occurs, the third letter denotes the device's method of rhythm detection, and the fourth letter identifies which chamber will deliver backup pacing. The ICD pacemaker function follows the HRS pacing coding system.

ICDs can be programmed to recognize a magnet, which will disable shock therapy, although not all devices are programmed to do so.[15] The magnet placed on an ICD will not initiate asynchronous pacing. This is a very important distinction, and the specifics will be addressed in the following section. Anesthetists must be familiar with the device codes, terminology, and capabilities to properly manage and manipulate the ICD during the perioperative period.

Implantable Cardioverter Defibrillators Therapy

Sophisticated and complicated algorithms programmed in the ICD generator activate the tachyarrhythmia features when a malignant rhythm occurs. The algorithms are programmed to sense the R-to-R wave and evaluate the rate, the abruptness of the malignant pattern, and the sustainability of the rhythm.[1] The antitachycardia pacing feature will initiate short rapid pacing bursts at a rate that exceeds the intrinsic tachycardic rate and will terminate the rhythm. The ICD cardioverts ventricular tachycardia (VT) with 1 to 30j and defibrillates ventricular fibrillation (VF) with 10 to 30j.[5] If the ICD acknowledges that the rhythm requires defibrillation, it will deliver six shocks. Once a shock is delivered, the ICD will disable any further antitachycardia pacing activity.[1]

Advancements in Technology

Over the last decade, there has been tremendous forward progress in the design and engineering of both PMs and ICDs. Advances in battery and miniaturization technology have led to the development of a leadless single-chamber intracardiac PM. These leadless PMs, approximately one-tenth the size of the traditional single-chamber PMs, are implanted directly into the right ventricle via a femoral vein catheter (Fig. 27.10). The miniaturized devices are engineered with functionality and features that match their larger predecessors. Elimination of the complications associated with traditional PM implantation (e.g., infection of the subcutaneous pocket, lead fracture and dislodgment, hematoma) may decrease hospitalizations and ultimately lower health

care costs.[16-18] Intracardiac devices do not require removal at the end of service, and they are engineered to convert to OOO mode when the battery voltage reaches the end of service.[18]

In 2012, the Food and Drug Administration (FDA) approved the use of a subcutaneous ICD (S-ICD) for the termination of life-threatening VTs in patients with structural or congenital heart disease, compromised venous access, or those at high risk of infection. The S-ICD pulse generator is implanted subcutaneously along the left lateral chest wall, and the lead/shock coil is positioned along the left sternal border.[19,20] Unlike the traditional ICD with intracardiac leads, the S-ICD delivers higher energy defibrillation shocks from outside the chest wall. The S-ICD is not indicated for patients who require pacing for bradyarrhythmias as the device will deliver only 30 seconds of immediate postshock pacing for bradycardia.[19] This device is not sensitive to manipulation with a magnet.

PERIOPERATIVE PERIOD

Preoperative

Patients who are scheduled for surgical procedures should be medically optimized and undergo a thorough history and physical, indicated laboratory testing, and an assessment of comorbidities.[6] The surgical patient with a CIED will require special attention. A multidisciplinary team approach (cardiologist or electrophysiologist, anesthetist, programmer, and surgeon) that considers the type of device, the location of the pulse generator, the type and length of procedure, the anticipated use of electrosurgical cautery (EC), and the patient's surgical position is warranted (Box 27.3).[3,21] A device-specific programmer and/or manufacturer contact number should be known as well (Table 27.4).

BOX 27.3 Preoperative Assessment of Cardiac Implantable Electronic Devices (CIEDs)

CIED Inquiry
- What is the device?
- How is the CIED programmed?
- What is the indication for device implantation?
- Is the patient pacemaker dependent, and if so what are the underlying rate and rhythm?
- Has the device been interrogated recently?
- Is the device functioning properly?
- If the device is an implantable cardioverter defibrillator (ICD), what is the recent number of shocks delivered? Is it safe to disable preoperatively or to use a magnet?
- Is the device able to recognize the magnet, and if so what is the response?
- If electromagnetic interference (EMI) is likely such as in monopolar electrosurgery [Bovie] use, or radiofrequency ablation is planned superior to the umbilicus, should I alter the pacing function to an asynchronous pacing mode or suspend the antitachycardia function, if present?
- Is the surgical site near the pulse generator?
- Is EMI likely to occur?
- Does the device need to be reprogrammed?
- Do I know what to do should the CIED become inhibited or malfunction as a result of EMI?
- Have I ensured that temporary pacing and defibrillation equipment are immediately available before, during, and after the procedure?

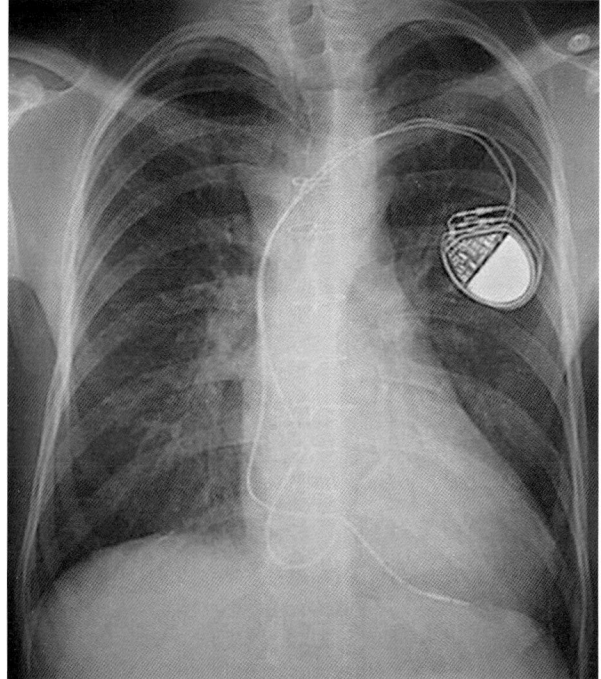

Fig. 27.11 A cardiac pacemaker battery implanted under the skin on the left chest wall is visible in this chest radiograph. The leads from the battery extend down to the right atrium and the apex of the right ventricle. (From Klatt E. *Robbins and Cotran Atlas of Pathology*. 3rd ed. St. Louis: Elsevier; 2015:51.)

TABLE 27.4 Manufacturer Contact Numbers

Biotronik	800-547-0394 www.biotronic.com
Guidant (Boston Scientific CRM) • AM Pacemaker Corporation • Arco Medical • Intermedics	800-227-3422 www.guidant.com
Medtronic • Edwards Pacemaker Systems • Viatron	800-678-2500 www.medtronic.com
St. Jude • Teletronics • Cordis • Ventritex • Siemens • Diag	800-722-3774 www.sjm.com

Some pertinent information may be found on the manufacturer-generated wallet card. This identification card lists the (a) type of device, (b) model number and serial number, (c) date of implantation, (d) name of the implanting physician or clinic, and (e) contact information for the manufacturer.[6] The information card will not include the date when the CIED was last interrogated or if the CIED has been functioning properly.

The HRS recommends routine assessment of the PM on a yearly basis and assessment of the ICD every 6 months.[22] Device interrogation will include the (a) date of last interrogation, (b) type of device,

(c) manufacturer, (d) model, (e) indications, (f) battery life, (g) lead integrity, (h) PM function and underlying rhythm or ICD therapy, (i) magnet response, and (j) any alerts.[6] Any recently initiated antitachycardia therapy should be considered when planning the perioperative management of these patients. This information may directly determine if disabling shock therapy intraoperatively constitutes a safe plan of care.[23] An incomplete preoperative assessment or failure to investigate a CIED's programmability can lead to poor patient outcomes.[24]

In an emergency, if the CIED function is unknown, assessing the ECG and obtaining a chest x-ray can be of use when there is insufficient time to interrogate. Evaluation of a 12-lead ECG may reveal a paced rhythm only if heart is currently pacing. The 12-lead ECG will not, however, inform the provider of the underlying rate, PM dependence, type of device, or response to magnet. The 12-lead ECG merely provides a real-time visualization of cardiac activity. The patient's chest x-ray is another source of information. Each CIED has a manufacturer identifier on its pulse generator. This identifier can be used to determine the manufacturer and possibly the model of the device. The chest x-ray can also alert the provider to whether the device is a PM (the presence of lead wires) (Fig. 27.11) or a defibrillator (the presence of one to two radiopaque lead/shock coils) or both (Fig. 27.12). Additional information may be obtained by placing a magnet over a CIED. If the device is a PM, asynchronous pacing may be evident. If the device is an ICD, there may be an audible tone indicating that antitachycardia therapy has been disabled. It is important to note that not all CIEDs respond in this manner. For example, at the time of publishing, ICDs manufactured by Boston Scientific and Medtronic elicit a tone when a magnet is placed; however, St. Jude, Biotronik, and Sorin ICDs do not elicit a tone with magnet placement. Some clinical factors affecting CIED functions are listed in Table 27.5.

Intraoperative

Both general anesthetics and local anesthetics with sedation are acceptable techniques and should be tailored to the patient's underlying pathology.[24] The American Society of Anesthesiologists (ASA) standard monitoring recommendations should be employed during all anesthetics. Attention to intraoperative physiologic alterations such as electrolyte and/or acid-base imbalances, ischemia, medication levels, and hypothermia can alter device thresholds and as such should be corrected.[1]

Electromagnetic Interference

EMI is defined as any external or nonphysiologic signal that interferes with PM or ICD function. Sources of EMI are present both within and outside the hospital environment. However, the intraoperative period may increase exposure to sources of potential EMI that may interfere with the function of a CIED. The degree to which EMI may interfere with the function of the CIED is variable. Inhibition of PM function, inappropriate triggering, electrical reset, damage at the lead-tissue

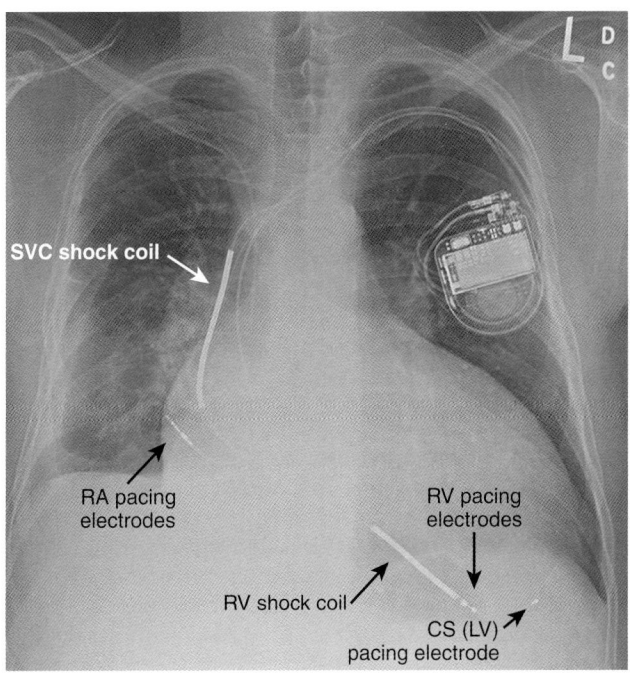

Fig. 27.12 Chest x-ray of an implanted cardioverter defibrillator. *CS,* Coronary sinus; *LV,* left ventricle; *RA,* right atrium; *RV,* right ventricle; *SVC,* superior vena cava. (From Fleisher LA. *Evidence-Based Practice of Anesthesiology.* 3rd ed. Philadelphia: Elsevier; 2013:90.)

interface, and tracking of electrical noise are all possible responses.[22] In an effort to eliminate the potential clinical consequences of EMI, modern CIEDs have been engineered to allow for filtering of noncardiac signals.[26] However, the potential for altering CIED function persists and requires both a vigilant and informed approach to managing patients who present to the surgical or procedural environment with an implantable device.

The most prevalent source of EMI in the operating room is the EC that is used to stop bleeding via cutting or coagulation of tissues. Two main types of EC are frequently employed during surgery: monopolar and bipolar. Monopolar cautery (Bovie) produces more energy than bipolar, and therefore, requires the placement of a grounding pad. The distance between the electrocautery tip and the grounding pad will determine the area in which stray current can be sensed by a CIED and misinterpreted (this is similar to the unipolar pacing lead). For this reason, the grounding pad should be positioned near the site of surgery, and a far away from the CIED generator as possible.

Bipolar electrocautery devices have the anode and cathode at the tip of the device. Due to the close proximity there is less area for stray interference to be misread by the CIED. A grounding pad is not necessary with bipolar cautery and less energy is exerted. However, if it becomes necessary to convert bipolar cautery to monopolar cautery a grounding pad must be placed on the patient.[5] Although there are no controlled studies evaluating the efficacy of using short bursts (<5 sec at a time) of energy or decreased energy, in practice it is a frequently employed technique for reducing the incidence of device interference.[6,25]

Electromagnetic interference and cardiac implantable electronic devices. EMI can be interpreted as a serious cardiac dysrhythmia that can affect the activity of PMs and ICDs. A PM may interpret EMI as intrinsic electric activity and will inhibit pacing if it is programmed to do so. In this instance, the PM oversenses electrical activity, and it will not pace the myocardium.[23] If the patient is dependent on the PM, inhibition of pacing results in loss of mechanical cardiac activity. This can be dangerous and even life threatening unless an escape rhythm emerges.[27] There are additional instances where EMI may negatively affect PM function and programmability. EMI may:

- Be viewed as noise and initiate asynchronous pacing at a rate that may cause R-on-T phenomena
- Be conducted down the lead and damage the myocardium via an endocardial burn
- Decrease battery life
- Reset the device to an alternate rate
- Be interpreted as a P wave, causing the device to pace only the ventricle, thus losing atrial kick

TABLE 27.5   Factors Affecting Implantable Cardiovascular Device Function

Factor	Effect	Reason
Shivering	Inhibits pacing	Sensed as cardiac contraction
Fasciculations (succinylcholine)	Inhibits pacing	Sensed as cardiac contraction
Electrolyte changes	Affects capture	Alters myopotential threshold
Temperature	Affects capture	Alters myopotential threshold
	Hypothermia	Increases arrhythmogenicity of myocardium
pH	Affects capture	Alters myopotential threshold
Blood transfusions	Alters pH, temperature, or electrolytes	Alters myopotential threshold
Chemotherapy	Loss of capture	Elevation of capture threshold

From Costa A, Richman DC. Implantable devices: assessment and perioperative management. *Anesthesiol Clin.* 2016;34(1):185–199.

- Result in severe bradycardia or asystole
- Reprogram and alter device settings
- Alter thresholds eliminating proper capture[1,6,10,23,27]

The effect of EMI on an ICD differs from that of a PM. When EMI is present, the ICD generator may interpret the signal as a potential tachyarrhythmia (VT or VF).[27] If the interference (e.g., cautery) lasts long enough, the device will analyze the noise and determine if antitachycardia therapy is warranted. If the ICD analysis concludes the noise as a lethal arrhythmia, the device will deliver an unnecessary shock. ECG interference can be differentiated from VT/VF on by analyzing the pulse oximeter or, if present, the arterial waveform (Fig. 27.13). Both pulse oximeter and arterial waveforms on the monitor will remain intact when the EMI noise is not a malignant rhythm. The device, however, may not make a correct determination in the presence of EMI despite sophisticated algorithms and may initiate an unwarranted shock. Information regarding what the device is programmed to do is crucial, and will aid in the anesthesia practitioner's decision of whether preoperative reprogramming is warranted or if magnet placement is a viable alternative. EMI can initiate negative effects on an ICD which may:

- Inhibit antitachycardia therapy
- Be conducted down the lead and damage the myocardium via an endocardial burn
- Permanently deactivate the device, causing it to enter a magnet mode and fail to detect lethal rhythms
- Change the programming and thresholds
- Affect the rate adaptive mode and inappropriately increase the heart rate[1,22,23]

In the hospital environment there are other potential sources of EMI that can equally disrupt device function and/or programmability. Transcutaneous electrical nerve stimulators, spinal cord stimulators, extracorporeal shock wave lithotripsy, radiation therapy, electroconvulsive therapy (ECT), radiofrequency ablation, and magnetic resonance imaging (MRI) on CIED function vary. The anesthesia provider should be aware of the potential sources and appropriate options for minimizing and managing the consequences of CIED malfunction in these areas. Box 27.4 lists recommendations for CIED management in selected nonoperative procedures.

Extracorporeal shockwave lithotripsy rarely produces EMI sufficient to interfere with CIED function; however, some inappropriate sensing and pacing inhibition have been documented.[22] During ECT, which is used to treat severe depression, electrical current is administered to the brain. The initial cardiovascular response to ECT is bradycardia followed immediately by tachycardia, which may result in the administration of inappropriate ICD shocks. According to the HRS/ASA, if the CIED is

programmed to respond to magnet application, use of a magnet is a reasonable management option, and reprogramming the device prior to ECT is not required.

Transcutaneous electrical nerve stimulation, used for the treatment of both chronic and acute pain, should be used in patients with PMs only (a) after extensive testing to ensure safety, (b) when

---

Adapted from Practice advisory for the perioperative management of patients with cardiac implantable electronic devices: pacemakers and implantable cardioverter-defibrillators 2020: an updated report by the American Society of Anesthesiologists Task Force on Perioperative Management of Patients with Cardiac Implantable Electronic Devices. *Anesthesiology.* 2020;132(2):225–252.

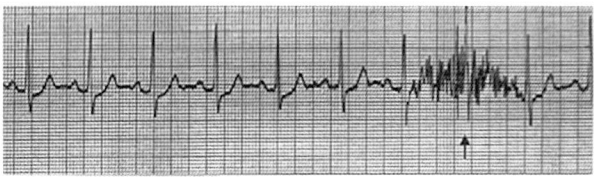

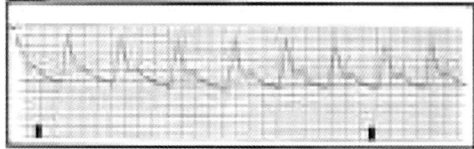

Fig. 27.13 Electrocardiogram and arterial line with electromagnetic interference.

TABLE 27.6 Preoperative Reprogramming Recommendations

Reprogramming Recommendations	Rationale
Reprogramming to an asynchronous mode on a pacemaker (PM)–dependent patient	• Expected use of monopolar cautery • Expected increase in electromagnetic interference (EMI) • Surgical site located near the pulse generator
Disable shock therapy	• If monopolar cautery used and anticipating increased EMI
Disable rate modulation	• Prohibit increases in rate due to EMI
Consider a higher asynchronous rate	• Anticipated need for increased oxygen demand
Older models may not be dual devices	• Reprogramming is suggested

BOX 27.5 Intraoperative Planning and Interventions for Patients With Cardiac Devices

- Continuously monitor and display a patient's electrocardiogram and oxygen saturation (Spo_2) as required by American Society of Anesthesiologists standards from the beginning of anesthesia until the patient is transferred out of the anesthetizing location.
- Perform continuous peripheral pulse monitoring for all CIED patients.
- If unanticipated CIED interactions occur, temporarily suspend the procedure until the source of interference can be identified and eliminated or managed.
- Visualization of the pulse waveform, consider arterial line
- Magnet placed or in the operating room (if the device is magnet sensitive)
- Placement of grounding pad away from pulse generator
- Bipolar cautery with short bursts
- Chronotropic pharmacologic support as needed
- Interrogator and manufacturer phone number available
- Emergency equipment readily available
- Position transcutaneous patches anterior and posterior if antiarrhythmic therapy is disabled
- Reprogram the device

exceptional improvement of quality of life is demonstrated, and (c) intermittently. Similarly, individual testing should be performed on patients prior to initiation of spinal cord stimulator therapy to ensure that no inhibition of pacemaker function or inappropriate triggering of antitachycardia therapy is observed.[22] Radiation, both therapeutic and diagnostic, can be safely performed for patients with CIEDs. With therapeutic radiation there is an increased risk of CIED dysfunction. Additionally, the radiation beam may have a direct effect on the pulse generator, which may result in permanent changes to the device.[21] Diagnostic radiation frequently does not have a clinically significant impact on CIED function. However, there have been documented cases of oversensing and electrical reset with computed tomography (CT) scanning.[28,29]

At present, medical devices are categorized into one of three groups by the American Society for Testing and Materials: (1) magnetic resonance (MR)–safe: an item that poses no known hazards in an MR environment; (2) MR-conditional: an item that has been demonstrated to pose no known hazards in a specified MR environment with specified conditions of use; and (3) MR-unsafe: an item that is known to pose hazards in all MR environments. MRI examinations can also interfere with CIED function. Possible adverse events specific to MRI include reed switch closure with subsequent asynchronous pacing, thermal injury at the electrode-myocardial tissue interface, and development of rapid pacing. Some manufacturers have developed an FDA-approved MR-conditional device. These MR-conditional devices require reprogramming prior to an MRI scan, and the manufacturers require that a facility undergo special training prior to administering patient scans. All major device companies are in the process of refining their technology. Continued monitoring of MR-conditional leads is needed to ensure that complication rates remain reasonable in comparison with the benefit attained.[30,31]

Reprogramming and Magnet Application

The potential for intraoperative EMI necessitates an appropriate plan to mitigate the potentially harmful effects (Table 27.6).[27] Reprogramming is recommended when there is an expectation of increased EMI, when monopolar cautery is used, or when the surgical site is in close proximity to the device generator.[6,22,27] Although the influence of EMI cannot be eliminated, the environment can be manipulated to identify EMI and control its impact. A device-specific programmer can temporarily modify the device settings. A PM can be programmed to an asynchronous mode, and an ICD can be programmed to disable antitachycardia therapy.

Intraoperative planning and interventions that can be used to decrease EMI and to limit its effects on cardiac devices are listed in Box 27.5.

The rate modulation mode is not intended to increase the heart rate indiscriminately but might do so intraoperatively in the presence of EMI. Hyperventilation, coughing or bucking, and mechanical ventilation may result in inappropriate increases in the rate of pacing.[10] Therefore, disabling rate modulation is recommended during a surgical procedure.[3,27]

Another strategy to offset the effects of intraoperative EMI is the placement of a 3-inch, round, horseshoe or rectangle magnet directly over the CIED (Fig. 27.14). Preoperative interrogation of the device manufacturer will inform the practitioner if the CIED is magnet sensitive. Most modern PMs are programmed to acknowledge the magnet, resulting in asynchronous pacing at a magnet rate. The magnet rate is frequently more rapid than the patient's intrinsic heart rate (85–100 beats per minute) to decrease the potential for R-on-T phenomenon. Magnet application will also suspend rate modulation on some PM devices.[15] Unfortunately, each PM is programmed differently and may or may not respond to magnet application. Some magnet responses may be disabled, and the magnet rate may not be the same as the programmed pacer rate.[1] Older devices may exhibit asynchronous paced rates at a lower than expected rate with magnet application, indicating a low or depleted battery.[25,32]

Magnet application on an ICD closes the reed switch, suspending antitachycardia therapy (if the ICD is programmed to do so).[11] The ICD cannot shock VT or VF unless the magnet is removed. Magnet application will not suspend rate modulation on an ICD, therefore a programmer must turn off the mode.[32] Older ICDs with a backup pacing function will not convert to asynchronous pacing with magnet application.[15] However, with newer generation ICDs (PM + ICD), the magnet will only suspend shock therapy, not asynchronously pace the heart (Table 27.7).

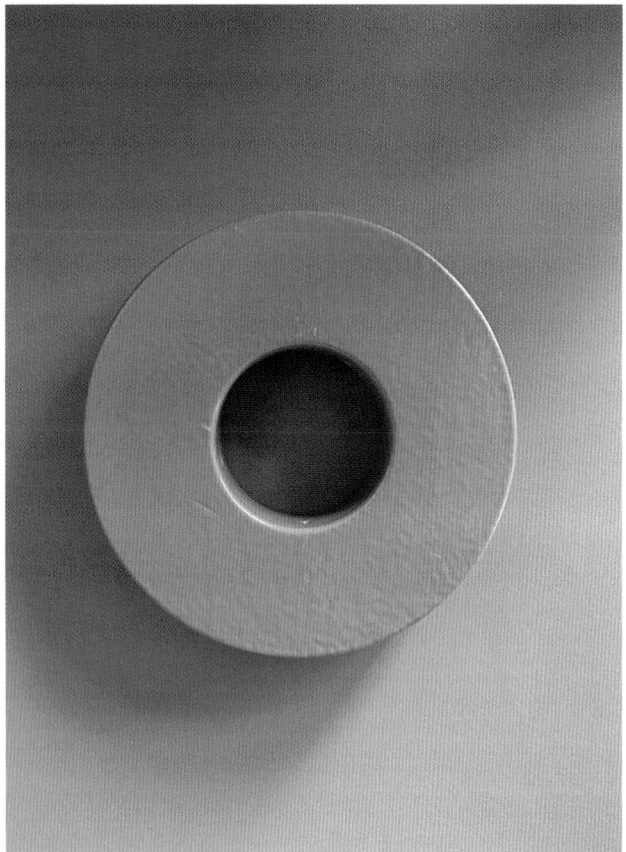

Fig. 27.14 Device magnet.

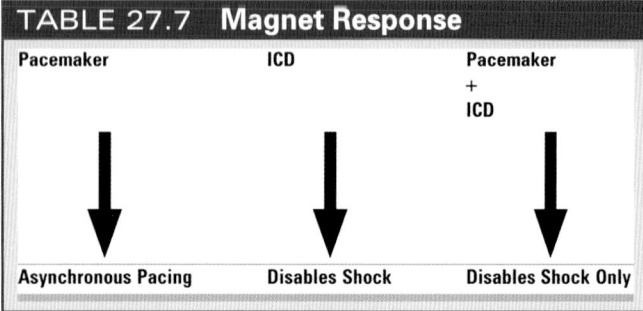

TABLE 27.7	**Magnet Response**	
Pacemaker	**ICD**	**Pacemaker + ICD**
↓	↓	↓
Asynchronous Pacing	**Disables Shock**	**Disables Shock Only**

ICD, Implantable cardiovascular device.

Three intraoperative clinical scenarios illustrate this important distinction when CIEDs are programmed to recognize magnet application:

1. Example A: EMI is inhibiting PM function (PM only). Placing the magnet directly on the PM device should initiate asynchronous pacing.

2. Example B: A surgical patient has a magnet positioned over the ICD (ICD + PM), temporarily disabling antitachycardia therapy. The patient suddenly converts to VF. Removing the magnet will allow the device to analyze the rhythm and intervene appropriately.

3. Example C: A surgical patient does not have a magnet placed over the ICD (ICD + PM). The patient develops a lethal rhythm. The ICD recognizes the rhythm as VF, analyzes that rhythm, determines shock therapy is warranted, and shocks the patient. The postshock rhythm is a bradyarrhythmia, and ICD pacing is not present. Placing a magnet to treat this bradyarrhythmia will not asynchronously pace the heart. This intervention merely results in disabling shock therapy, which can be hazardous to the patient who has just experienced VF.

Placement of a magnet on a CIED should not replace a thorough interrogation of the device.[32] Blind magnet placement can compromise safety, especially when generalizations are made regarding device function and its response to magnet placement.[1] It is important to note (a) not all CIEDs have similar programming, (b) CIED proper function should never be assumed, and (c) placement of a magnet or reprogramming the CIED does not eliminate the potential effects of EMI.[4] Direct interrogation remains the only reliable method of CIED assessment.[7] Furthermore, intraoperative magnet placement has disadvantages; the position of the patient may not be optimal to accommodate the magnet, or the magnet may not be effectively secured on the CIED.

Emergency Intervention

In the event of CIED malfunction during a hemodynamically unstable cardiac rhythm, transthoracic defibrillation paddles should be placed anteriorly and posteriorly but never directly over the device. The lowest possible energy setting required to achieve cardioversion or defibrillation should be used. Transient increases in myocardial stimulation thresholds associated with external cardioversion have been documented.[33,34] Interrogation of the device is advised following any external cardioversion or defibrillation.[2]

Postoperative Care

Patients with a CIED and EMI exposure must be monitored postoperatively. If the magnet was used to disable shock therapy, it should be removed and a complete evaluation of the device's integrity performed. A CIED is reassessed if any settings were changed and then reprogrammed to appropriate preoperative settings.[6] If rate modulation was disabled, then this mode must be restored. Recommendations for postoperative interrogation are also suggested for any surgical procedure where monopolar cautery was used, for any large and invasive surgery, for any intraoperative adverse event, and for any emergent surgery when device interrogation did not occur.[3] Consultation with a cardiologist should occur as necessary.[6] All interventions should be recorded in the patient's medical record.

■ SUMMARY

Rapidly evolving technology, expanding indications for implantation, and an aging population increase the likelihood that the anesthetist will be responsible for the care of a patient with a CIED. Complex devices, lack of standardization among manufacturers, variable programmability and response to magnet therapy, and the lack of evidence-based management guidelines caused by rapid innovation and improvements in CIEDs all complicate perioperative management. A basic understanding of the indications for CIED implantation and device function is essential. Furthermore, a systematic approach for providing a safe, efficient, and individualized plan of perioperative care is vital for optimum patient outcomes.

REFERENCES

For a complete list of references for this chapter, scan this QR code with any smartphone code reader app, or visit the following URL: http://booksite.elsevier.com/9780323711944/

28

Anesthesia for Vascular Surgery

Sass Elisha

PERIPHERAL VASCULAR DISEASE

Atherosclerosis is the most common cause of peripheral vascular occlusive disease. This degenerative process involves the formation of atheromatous plaques that may obstruct the vessel lumen resulting in a reduction in distal blood flow. The pathophysiologic process is systemic, progressive, and primarily affects the arteries due to plaque formation, which can lead to stenosis and potentially occlusion of the vascular lumen; thrombosis from hypercoagulability, resulting in acute organ ischemia; embolism from microthrombi or atheromatous debris; and weakening of the arterial wall, resulting in aneurysm formation. Atherosclerosis is an inflammatory condition that is partially caused by cholesterol plaques, which occur within arteries. In response to cholesterol plaques, immune cells such as macrophages and monocytes liberate proinflammatory cytokines, which leads to a progressive increase in the size of plaques. The lipid cap that envelopes the plaque can rupture, resulting in intraluminal thrombosis or plaque emboli. The most common risk factors associated with atherosclerosis are shown in Box 28.1. Endothelial dysfunction is a potential cause of increased hemodynamic variability during anesthesia. Smoking, elevated proinflammatory mediators, and diabetes mellitus are major risk factors in the pathogenesis of atherosclerosis in the arterial tree. Typical symptoms associated with peripheral occlusive disease include claudication, skin ulcerations, gangrene, and impotence.[1] The extent of disability is primarily influenced by the development of collateral blood flow. The mortality rate in patients with vascular disease is two- to sixfold higher than in the general population.[2] Hypercoagulability resulting from platelet interaction with leukocytes and other cells that modulate the immune response plays a major role in the development of atherosclerosis.[3,4] Researchers have discovered heritable genetic factors that predispose patients to developing vascular disease.[5]

Treatment for peripheral occlusive disease may range from pharmacologic therapy to surgery. Surgical therapy includes transluminal angioplasty, endarterectomy, thrombectomy, endovascular stenting, and arterial bypass. Some common surgical maneuvers used to bypass occlusive lesions are aortofemoral, axillofemoral, femorofemoral, and femoropopliteal procedures. Bypass techniques may be classified as inflow or outflow procedures depending on the level of the obstruction, with the dividing axis occurring at the level of the groin. Temporary occlusion of the operative artery is mandatory during surgical bypass, as this temporarily further reduces blood flow and oxygen delivery. The development of collateral circulation provides alternative vascular blood flow in patients with occlusive disease.[6,7] Initially, angiogenesis or the development of new vessels supplies collateral blood flow that is sufficient to meet tissue oxygen demands. As the disease progresses, the blood flow is decreased, and the oxygen supply is unable to meet the tissues' demand, which could result in myocardial dysfunction, neurologic dysfunction, renal dysfunction, and/or limb ischemia.

Preoperative Evaluation

The atherosclerotic process in occlusive disease is not limited to peripheral arteries and should be expected to be present in the coronary, cerebral, and renal arteries. More than half of the mortality associated with peripheral vascular disease results from adverse cardiac events.[8] There is a clear association between the development of aortic aneurysms and coronary artery disease (CAD).[9] It has been estimated that 42% of patients presenting for abdominal aortic aneurysm (AAA) repair have significant CAD.[10] Preoperative cardiovascular evaluation and treatment are beneficial for reducing not only perioperative risk but also late cardiovascular events. After elective AAA repair, the 5-year survival rate and incidence of major adverse cardiovascular events is 86%.[11] Cardiac pathology, which often occurs in this patient population, must be managed aggressively to optimize cardiac functioning and decrease morbidity and mortality from cardiac causes.

Preoperative Pharmacologic Management

β-blockade. The advantages of β-blockade, as it relates to factors that affect myocardial oxygen supply and demand, have been extensively studied in patients with peripheral vascular disease. The use of β-blockers is recommended in patients at high risk for myocardial ischemia and infarction.[12] For patients having an AAA repair, there is a 10-fold decrease in cardiac morbidity associated with adequate preoperative β-blockade.[13] β-blockade therapy should be instituted days to weeks before surgery and titrated to a target heart rate between 50 and 60 beats per minute (bpm).[14] Perioperative β-blockade started within 1 day or less before noncardiac surgery prevents nonfatal myocardial infarctions (MIs) but increases the risk of hypotension, bradycardia, stroke, and death. Initiating β-blockade between 2 and 7 days before surgery may be preferable, but there is a lack of scientific data to support the benefit of beginning therapy more than a month in advance.[15] Vascular surgery patients with limited heart rate variability after receiving β-blockers exhibit less cardiac ischemia and decreased postoperative troponin values and have a decreased mortality from all causes 2 years postoperatively.[16] For patients taking β-blockers, these medications should be continued up to the day of surgery and during the postoperative period.[17]

Statins. It is suggested that statins decrease perioperative mortality in patients with vascular disease by decreasing adverse cardiovascular and cerebrovascular events and death.[18] These drugs have cardioprotective effects, as they reduce vascular inflammation, decrease the incidence of thrombogenesis, enhance nitric oxide bioavailability, stabilize atherosclerotic plaques, and lower lipid concentrations. It is reasonable to start a statin drug in this patient population. If prescribed, a statin should be instituted 30 days prior to the surgical procedure and continued throughout the postoperative period.[15] Statin therapy that is started preoperatively and continued through discharge has been associated with reduced 30-day mortality and an absolute 18% improvement in

BOX 28.1 Risk Factors Related to the Development of Atherosclerotic Lesions

- Advanced age
- Smoking
- Hypertension
- Diabetes mellitus
- Insulin resistance
- Obesity
- Family history and genetic predisposition
- Physical inactivity
- Gender (males at greater risk than females)
- Hyper/hypohomocysteinemia
- Elevated C-reactive protein
- Elevated lipoprotein
- Hypertriglyceridemia
- Hyperlipidemia

5-year survival after vascular surgery.[18,19] Specifically, patients who were prescribed statins and then underwent endovascular aortic aneurysm repair (EVAR) had greater residual aneurysm sac regression within the first years postoperatively.[20]

Antiplatelet medications. It has been unclear whether patients having noncardiac surgery who are at increased risk for MI should receive aspirin throughout the perioperative period. The results of current evidence and the Perioperative Ischemic Evaluation 2 (POISE-2) research trial indicate that perioperative aspirin does not prevent MI and does not alter the risk of a perioperative cardiovascular event.[21] The outcomes were unchanged for those subjects who took aspirin for a prolonged period compared to those who started aspirin prior to surgery. Aspirin did, however, increase the risk of major bleeding. In patients who have been on a long-term aspirin regimen and have aspirin withheld during the perioperative period, it is important to ensure that aspirin is restarted after the increased risk period for bleeding has passed (i.e., 8–10 days after surgery). On the basis of currently available literature, aspirin should not be administered to patients undergoing surgery unless there is a definitive guideline-based primary or secondary prevention indicated.[22,23]

The presence of concurrent pulmonary, renal, neurologic, and endocrine dysfunction should be identified, and measures should be taken to improve organ function before surgery. Acute kidney injury (AKI) is common during the perioperative period in patients undergoing vascular surgery, and this condition is associated with a high risk for cardiovascular-specific mortality comparable to that seen with chronic kidney disease.[24] Strategies used to help prevent perioperative AKI are discussed later in this chapter. Preoperatively, the greater the number of comorbidities that exist, the greater the risk of morbidity and mortality during the perioperative period.

Monitoring

The extent of perioperative monitoring should be based on the presence of coexisting disease and the type of surgery. The detection of myocardial ischemia should be a primary objective in patients with vascular disease. Methods for assessing cardiac function include electrocardiography (ECG), pulmonary artery pressure, and transesophageal echocardiography (TEE) monitoring. The effectiveness of pulmonary artery catheters (PACs) in improving patient outcomes remains controversial. Many randomized controlled trials have been performed to assess whether they offer any benefit. It was determined that PAC monitoring had no effect on mortality or length of hospital stay. Additionally, there were higher rates of pulmonary embolism, pulmonary infarction, and

hemorrhage in the PAC group.[25-27] Furthermore, PACs have not been associated with decreased intraoperative mortality or morbidity, and they are associated with increases in the duration of ventilation and length of stay (LOS) in the intensive care unit (ICU) following cardiac surgical procedures.[26] Specific indications for the use of PAC may be indicated (e.g., complex cardiac surgery).[28]

Due to the global nature of atherosclerotic disease, some degree of systemic cardiovascular disease in patients with peripheral vascular disease should be assumed.[10] Patients with hypertension and/or angiopathology rely on increased mean arterial pressures (MAPs) to perfuse their vital organs. Thus cerebral and coronary autoregulation occur within a higher range compared to patients without peripheral occlusive vascular disease (60–140 mm Hg). Short, sustained periods of hypotension can result in cardiac or neurologic ischemia. Direct intraarterial blood pressure monitoring allows for near–real-time determination of blood pressure values. Information ascertained from an arterial line, such as fluid volume status, acute fluctuations in blood pressure caused by surgical intervention, and titration of vasopressor/vasodilator medications, helps to guide treatment decisions.

In the future, the use of noninvasive hemodynamic monitoring modalities may prove to decrease morbidity and mortality during anesthesia care by allowing the anesthetist to make pharmacologic choices based on cardiac output and myocardial oxygen supply and demand. Guided titration of vasoactive medications along with patient-specific, goal-directed intravenous fluid therapy could improve survivability in this patient population. More scientific evidence will be needed on these interventions prior to making practice guideline recommendations.

Anesthetic Selection

The anesthetic technique chosen for patients having vascular surgery depends on the type of surgical procedure to be performed and the presence of coexisting disease. Maintaining consistent hemodynamic control and avoiding significant episodes of intraoperative hypertension and hypotension are vital to (1) maintaining oxygen delivery to vital organs, (2) decreasing the possibility of increased myocardial oxygen consumption, and (3) decreasing the potential for hemorrhagic stroke. In certain instances, infiltration of local anesthetic and intravenous sedation may be sufficient, whereas more invasive surgical procedures require the use of general anesthesia. Regional anesthesia for surgery on the lower extremities may decrease the overall morbidity and mortality associated with this patient population. Numerous studies have failed to yield demonstrative evidence that any single anesthetic technique decreases morbidity and mortality following vascular surgery. A comprehensive meta-analysis combining data from 141 studies involving 9559 patients suggested a 30% reduction in mortality for those patients who received a combined general anesthetic (GA) and epidural combination. A reduction in the rate of MI, stroke, and respiratory failure was found when epidural anesthesia was used in patients undergoing aortic surgery.[29] A major study has been conducted to evaluate various end points associated with major vascular surgery.[30] None of these studies have definitively concluded that superior outcomes depend on the anesthetic technique used.[31] A positive consideration for administering inhalation and intravenous anesthetic agents is that anesthetic medications decrease the rate of oxygen demand and help to protect neurologic and cardiac tissue in patients having noncardiac surgery.[32] In addition, a meta-analysis reviewing epidural analgesia versus opioids for postoperative pain relief in patients undergoing abdominal aortic surgery showed an overall decreased rate of MI in those patients who received epidural analgesia.[33] Epidural analgesia provided during the postoperative period has significant physiologic advantages. Specific benefits of using an epidural for major abdominal vascular surgery are summarized in Box 28.2. In addition, many patients having vascular surgery are

Patients having vascular surgery are at increased risk for developing a venous thromboembolism (VTE) during the postoperative period. In one study, VTE was detected in 18.1% of patients with aortoiliac obstruction and 21% of patients after AAA repair.[36] The incidence of VTE continued to be elevated after discharge. All methods intended to prevent the formation of deep vein thrombosis (DVT), including pharmacologic management, should be employed throughout the postoperative period. Low-molecular-weight heparin is frequently used to bridge the time between withholding oral anticoagulants and surgery. It is important to restart oral anticoagulant medications postoperatively after the risk of bleeding is decreased to minimize DVT and VTE. Increased postoperative hematocrit concentration is associated with an increased risk of 30-day mortality from DVT and pulmonary embolism.[37]

ABDOMINAL AORTIC ANEURYSMS

Incidence

The incidence of AAA is estimated to be between 3% and 10% for patients over 50 years of age in the Western world.[38] Improved detection of AAAs is the result of increased screening of asymptomatic aneurysms by noninvasive diagnostic modalities such as computed tomography (CT), magnetic resonance imaging (MRI), and ultrasonography. The occurrence of AAAs has increased because of the increased age of the general population and the vascular changes that occur as a result of aging.[39] AAAs are two to six times more common in men than in women, and are two to three times more common in white men than in black men.[38] Women with AAAs are being treated at older ages and typically have AAAs that are smaller in diameter, as compared to men.[40] In men, AAAs most frequently begin to occur at 50 years of age and peak at 80 years of age.[41]

Risk Factors

The incidence of AAAs in a given population depends on the presence of risk factors (Box 28.3). Independent risk factors thought to be causes rather than markers for the development of an AAA include age, gender, and smoking. Smoking is the risk factor that is most highly correlated with AAA. In cigarette smokers, the incidence of AAAs increases fivefold.[38] There is an association between chronic inflammation and angiopathy. The specific mechanism that links inflammation and vascular disease has not been definitively established, but elevated cytokine levels appear to play a central role.[42]

Mortality

Elective AAA repair is one of the most frequent vascular surgical procedures, with approximately 40,000 operations performed in the

receiving anticoagulant therapy and will receive heparin intraoperatively; therefore there is a remote risk that neuraxial anesthesia could lead to epidural hematoma formation.[34]

Postoperative Considerations

Postoperative pain management is important to consider after peripheral vascular surgery. Most clinicians agree that postoperative administration of narcotics not only provides patient comfort but also contributes to cardiac stability. The perioperative use of dexmedetomidine is also advantageous due to its sympatholytic effects, analgesic properties, and minimal effects on respiration. The use of epidural opioids and local anesthetics in patients recovering from vascular surgery is an important component of postoperative care because pain can greatly enhance sympathetic nervous system stimulation. Despite a decrease in discomfort during the postoperative course, these patients must be monitored for possible adverse events, such as MI, hypotension, or respiratory depression, which could be attributed to the administration of epidural opioids and local anesthetics. Acute pain increases inflammatory mediators such as creatinine kinase, C-reactive protein, interleukin-6 (IL-6), and tumor necrosis factor, which can lead to regional blood flow alterations, organ dysfunction, and cell death.[35]

United States annually.[43] Mortality rates for elective abdominal aortic aneurysmectomies have decreased since the 1970s. The present mortality rate ranges from 1% to 11%, although it is most commonly estimated at 5%. This is compared with mortality rates of 18% to 30% in the 1950s.[38,44-47] Even with the advent and increased frequency of EVAR, long-term mortality rates are similar, at approximately 15% to 17%.[48] Advanced detection, earlier surgical intervention, extensive preoperative preparation, refined surgical techniques, higher quality hemodynamic monitoring, and improved anesthetic techniques have all contributed to this improvement in surgical outcomes. Data suggest a low risk of rupture for AAAs less than 4 cm in diameter; however, the risk dramatically increases for AAAs with a 5-cm diameter or greater. Surgical intervention is recommended for AAAs 5.5 cm or greater in diameter.[49] Unfortunately, mortality rates for patients with undetected or untreated ruptured aortic aneurysms have not followed the trend of those who have surgical intervention. Estimates of mortality resulting from ruptured AAAs vary from 35% to 94%.[43,50-52] Combining prehospital mortality with operative mortality, the overall mortality for AAA rupture is 80% to 90%. The 5-year mortality rate for individuals with untreated AAAs is 81%, and the 10-year mortality rate is 100%.[53] Other criteria for surgical intervention for AAA include ruptured AAA, a 4- to 5-cm AAA with greater than 0.5-cm enlargement in less than 6 months, patients who are symptomatic for AAA, and a 5-cm AAA or greater for elective repair for patients with a reasonable life expectancy. Early detection and elective surgical intervention can be lifesaving because elective surgical mortality is less than 5% in most studies.[54]

Diagnosis

Physical Examination

Asymptomatic aneurysms may be detected during routine examination as a pulsatile abdominal mass. Smaller aneurysms are often undetected on routine physical examination. AAA screening rates remain below 50%. AAAs are frequently discovered incidentally by primary practitioners, and some patients undergo unnecessary ultrasound screening.[55] It has been estimated that less than 30% of AAAs are identified during routine physical examination. A more extensive scoring system that includes additional risk factors such as the presence of carotid artery or peripheral arterial disease, obesity, hypertension, smoking, diabetes, and advanced age may increase the rate of detection to almost 90% of AAAs.[56]

Imaging

A minimally invasive method used to initially diagnose the presence of AAA is by ultrasound. Ultrasound is helpful to determine if an AAA is present, but it is not highly accurate in determining the extent of the AAA or if rupture has occurred.[57] CT angiography (CTA) allows for a more precise view of the aneurysm morphology, including aneurysm size, vessel wall integrity, and adjacent anatomic definition such as the iliac arteries. CTA has become the imaging test of choice for AAA because of its high-quality resolution, rapid image acquisition, and wide availability.[58] The information gained from CTA is valuable to the surgeon and interventional radiologist for initial determination of the surgical intervention (e.g., open or EVAR) and the extent of the distal and proximal aneurysm if an endovascular stent graft is to be implanted.

ABDOMINAL AORTIC RECONSTRUCTION

Patient Selection

As a result of recent advances in surgical and anesthetic techniques, the 30-day perioperative mortality rate associated with elective open repair of AAAs is estimated to be 3% to 4.5%.[59] Most patients with

TABLE 28.1 Criteria for High Risk in Abdominal Aortic Aneurysm Repair

Parameter	Criterion
Age	>70 yr
Gender	Female
Cardiac	History of myocardial infarction Angina pectoris Myocardial disease Q waves on ECG ST/T wave changes on ECG Ventricular ectopy Hypertension with left ventricular hypertrophy Congestive heart failure
Endocrine	Diabetes
Neurologic	Stroke
Renal	Chronic or acute renal failure
Pulmonary	Chronic obstructive pulmonary disease Emphysema Dyspnea Previous pulmonary surgery

ECG, Electrocardiogram.
Modified from Pairolero PC. Repair of abdominal aortic aneurysms in high-risk patients. *Surg Clin North Am.* 1989;69:765–774; Holt PJE, Thompson MM. Abdominal aortic aneurysms: evaluation and decision making. In Cronenwett JL, Johnston W, eds. *Rutherford's Vascular Surgery.* 8th ed. Vol. 2. Philadelphia: Elsevier; 2014; Woo EY, Damraur SM. Abdominal aortic aneurysms: open surgical treatment. In Cronenwett JL, Johnston W, eds. *Rutherford's Vascular Surgery.* 8th ed. Vol. 2. Philadelphia: Elsevier; 2014.

abdominal aneurysms, including the elderly, are considered surgical candidates. Although advanced age contributes to an increased incidence of morbidity and mortality, age alone is not a contraindication to elective aneurysmectomy.[60] However, physiologic age is more indicative of increased surgical risk than chronologic age. Contraindications to elective repair include intractable angina pectoris, recent MI, severe pulmonary dysfunction, and chronic renal insufficiency.[61] Patients with stable CAD and coronary artery stenosis of greater than 70% who require nonemergent AAA repair do not benefit from revascularization if β-blockade has been established.[44] Table 28.1 lists characteristics that define high-risk patients; however, in most cases, the presence of an AAA warrants surgical intervention.[53]

The dimensions of an aneurysm can change over time. AAAs expand by approximately 4 mm/yr.[62] Aneurysmal vessel dimensions correspond to the law of Laplace:

$$T = P \times r$$

where T = wall tension, P = transmural pressure, and r = vessel radius.

As the radius of a vessel increases, the wall tension increases. Wall tension is directly proportional to the vessel radius and intraluminal pressure and inversely proportional to wall thickness. Therefore the larger the aneurysm, the higher the likelihood of spontaneous rupture.

As previously stated, aneurysms measuring more than 5 cm in diameter generally require surgical intervention, but aneurysms measuring less than 5 cm should not be considered benign, and monitoring of the condition is indicated.[44] An aneurysm has the potential to rupture regardless of its size. As the diameter of the aneurysm increases in size, the risk of rupture increases (Table 28.2).[1] In contradiction to the current thought that increased wall shear stress increases the risk of

TABLE 28.2 Range of Potential Rupture Rates for a Given Size of Abdominal Aortic Aneurysm

AAA Diameter (cm)	Rupture Risk (%/yr)
<4	0
4–5	0.5–5
5–6	3–15
6–7	10–20
7–8	20–40
>8	30–50

AAA, Abdominal aortic aneurysm.
From Brewster DC, et al. Guidelines for the treatment of abdominal aortic aneurysms: report of a subcommittee of the Joint Council of the American Association for Vascular Surgery and Society for Vascular Surgery. *J Vasc Surg.* 2003;37:1106–1117.

aortic rupture, it has been shown that aortic rupture may occur more often at sites with low wall shear stress due to blood flow recirculation resulting in thrombus deposition, aortic wall degeneration, and eventual rupture.[63] Due to increased wall stress at the bifurcation of the aorta and the iliac arteries, AAAs most frequently develop in the infrarenal aorta, although approximately 5% to 15% involve the suprarenal aorta. It is estimated that approximately 40% of AAAs also involve the iliac arteries.[1]

Patient Preparation

Perioperative MI is the most common reason for poor outcomes in noncardiac surgery for patients with vascular disease. Optimization of myocardial oxygen supply and demand and modification of cardiac risk factors are the major goals of preoperative risk reduction. β-blockers and statins are the important preoperative pharmacologic treatments for medical management.[17,19] Prophylactic coronary revascularization does not reduce the incidence of perioperative cardiac events.[64] Preoperative cardiac testing is recommended only if interpretation of the results will change anesthetic management.[15,65,66]

Preoperative fluid loading and restoration of intravascular volume are perhaps the most important techniques used to enhance cardiac function during abdominal aortic aneurysmectomies. Reliable venous access must be secured if volume replacement is to be accomplished. Large-bore intravenous lines and central lines can be used to infuse fluids or blood. Massive hemorrhage is an ever-present threat, therefore the availability of blood and blood products should be ensured. Provisions for rapid transfusion and intraoperative blood salvage should be confirmed.

Routine Monitoring

Standard monitoring methods include ECG (with display of lead II for detection of dysrhythmias and the precordial V_5 lead for analysis of ischemic ST segment changes), pulse oximetry, and capnography. An esophageal stethoscope allows for continuous auscultation of heart and breath sounds, as well as temperature monitoring. Placement of an indwelling urinary catheter is necessary for continuous measurement of urinary output and renal function. Neuromuscular function should be routinely monitored.

Invasive Monitoring

Maintaining cardiac function is crucial for a successful surgical outcome. Cardiac function should be closely monitored during abdominal aortic reconstruction. Invasive blood pressure monitoring permits

beat-to-beat analysis of the blood pressure, immediate identification of hemodynamic alterations related to aortic clamping, and access for blood sampling. However, information obtained from PACs has been shown to have low sensitivity and low specificity in detecting myocardial ischemia when compared with ECG and TEE. As previously discussed, PACs are not routinely indicated unless a specific purpose warrants their use.[26]

By detecting changes in ventricular wall motion, TEE provides a sensitive method for assessing ventricular wall motion abnormalities. TEE is a primary method of intraoperative cardiac assessment in patients undergoing surgery on the heart and the aorta.[65,67] Wall motion abnormalities also occur much sooner than electrocardiographic changes during periods of reduced coronary blood flow.[52] When TEE is used to guide intraoperative hemodynamic management, patients with left ventricular diastolic dysfunction have a decreased incidence of developing congestive heart failure and atrial fibrillation.[68,69] The most common abnormalities detected by intraoperative TEE include hypovolemia, low ejection fraction, right ventricular failure, segmental wall motion abnormalities, and pulmonary embolus.[70] Myocardial ischemia poses the greatest risk of mortality after abdominal aortic reconstruction. Intraoperative monitoring may enable earlier detection and intervention during ischemic cardiac events.

Aortic Cross-Clamping

Abdominal aortic reconstruction is one of the most challenging situations for the anesthetist due to the frequency and degree of hemodynamic variability during cross-clamping and unclamping of the aorta. This is further complicated by the fact that most patients having an aortic aneurysm repair are elderly and have varying degrees of coexisting disease. Perhaps the most dramatic physiologic change occurs with the application of an aortic cross-clamp. Temporary aortic occlusion produces various hemodynamic and metabolic alterations.

Hemodynamic Alterations

The hemodynamic effects of aortic cross-clamping are affected by the clamp application site along the aorta, the patient's preoperative cardiac reserve, and the patient's intravascular volume. The most common site for cross-clamping is infrarenal because most aneurysms appear below the level of the renal arteries. Less common sites of aneurysm development are the juxtarenal and suprarenal areas.

During aortic cross-clamping, hypertension occurs above the cross-clamp, and hypotension occurs below the cross-clamp. Aortic cross-clamping increases plasma levels of catecholamines, aldosterone, cortisol, prostaglandins, and other stress hormones that are associated with a sympathetic nervous system response. There is an absence of blood flow distal to the cross-clamp in the pelvis and lower extremities.[6] An increase in afterload causes the left ventricular myocardial wall tension to increase, which in turn increases myocardial oxygen demand. Patients with poor left ventricular function are at risk for developing congestive heart failure during this period. MAP and systemic vascular resistance (SVR) also increase. Cardiac output may decrease or remain unchanged. Pulmonary artery occlusion pressure (PAOP) may increase or remain unchanged. Table 28.3 summarizes the physiologic changes associated with aortic cross-clamping.

Patients with adequate cardiac reserve commonly adjust to sudden increases in afterload without the occurrence of adverse cardiac events. However, patients with ischemic heart disease or ventricular dysfunction are unable to fully compensate as a result of the hemodynamic alterations. The increased left ventricular wall stress attributed to aortic cross-clamp application may contribute to decreased global ventricular function and myocardial ischemia. Clinically, these patients experience increases in PAOP in response to aortic cross-clamping. Aggressive

TABLE 28.3   The Physiologic Changes Associated With Aortic Cross-Clamping

Hemodynamic Changes	Metabolic Changes	Intraoperative Interventions
Increased arterial blood pressure above the clamp	Decreased total body oxygen consumption	*Reduce Afterload* Sodium nitroprusside Inhalation anesthetics Milrinone Shunts and aorta to femoral bypass
Decreased arterial blood pressure below the clamp	Decreased total body carbon dioxide production	*Reduce Preload* Nitroglycerin Atrial to femoral bypass
Increased wall motion abnormalities and left ventricular wall tension	Increased mixed venous oxygen saturation	*Renal Protection* Fluid administration Mannitol Furosemide Dopamine N-acetylcysteine Renal cold perfusion
Decreased ejection fraction and cardiac output	Decreased total body oxygen extraction	*Miscellaneous* Hypothermia Decrease minute ventilation Sodium bicarbonate
Decreased renal blood flow	Increased catecholamine release	
Increased pulmonary occlusion pressure	Respiratory alkalosis	
Increased central venous pressure	Metabolic acidosis	
Increased coronary blood flow		

Adapted from Norris EJ. Anesthesia for vascular surgery. In Miller RD, et al., eds. *Miller's Anesthesia*. 9th ed. Philadelphia: Elsevier; 2020; Holt PJE, Thompson MM. Abdominal aortic aneurysms: evaluation and decision making. In Cronenwett JL, Johnston W, eds. *Rutherford's Vascular Surgery*. 9th ed. Vol. 2. Philadelphia: Elsevier; 2019.

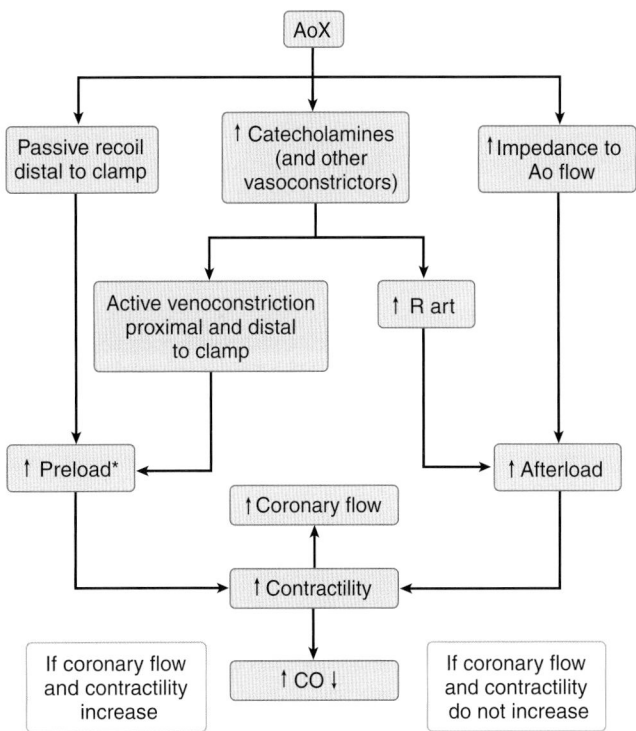

Fig. 28.1 Systemic hemodynamic response to aortic cross-clamping. Preload *(asterisk)* does not necessarily increase with infrarenal clamping. Depending on splanchnic vascular tone, blood volume can be shifted into the splanchnic circulation, and preload will not increase. *Ao,* Aortic; *AoX,* aortic cross-clamping; *R art,* arterial resistance. (Adapted from Gelman S. The pathophysiology of aortic cross-clamping. *Anesthesiology.* 1995;82:1026-1060.)

pharmacologic intervention is required for restoration of cardiac function during this time. An algorithm that depicts the systemic hemodynamic responses to aortic cross-clamping is shown in Fig. 28.1.

Metabolic Alterations

After application of an aortic cross-clamp, the lack of blood flow to distal structures results in a hypoxic and ischemic environment. In response to tissue ischemia, metabolites such as cytokines, prostaglandins, nitric oxide, and arachidonic acid are formed and released into circulation. Furthermore, anaerobic metabolism leads to the accumulation of serum lactate. The release of arachidonic acid derivatives may be a contributing factor leading to cardiac instability and myocardial depression during aortic cross-clamping.[38] Thromboxane A_2 synthesis, which is accelerated by the application of an aortic cross-clamp, may be responsible for the decrease in myocardial contractility and cardiac output that occurs.

Traction on the mesentery is a surgical maneuver used for exposing the aorta. Mesenteric traction syndrome is associated with this procedure. Decreases in blood pressure and SVR, tachycardia, increased cardiac output, and facial flushing are common responses to mesenteric

traction. Although the cause of this syndrome is unknown, it has been associated with high concentrations of 6-keto-prostaglandin F1α, a stable metabolite of prostacyclin, at the time of mesenteric traction.[71] The 6-keto-prostaglandin F1α levels and hemodynamic stability return to preclamp values as reperfusion occurs.

The neuroendocrine response to major surgical stress is believed to be mediated by cytokines such as IL-1B, IL-6, and tumor necrosis factor, as well as plasma catecholamines and cortisol.[72] These mediators are thought to be responsible for triggering the inflammatory response that results in increased body temperature, leukocytosis, tachycardia, tachypnea, and fluid sequestration. Patients who have an exaggerated plasma stress mediator release have longer operative and cross-clamp times and require a greater number of blood transfusions.

Effects on Regional Circulation

Acute kidney injury. Hypoperfusion to tissues that are distal to the aortic clamp occurs. Renal insufficiency and acute renal failure are severe complications associated with abdominal aortic reconstruction. Suprarenal and juxtarenal cross-clamping are associated with a higher incidence of altered renal dynamics and can decrease renal blood flow by as much as 80%. However, significant reductions in renal blood flow occur even when aortic cross-clamping is performed below the renal arteries. Infrarenal aortic cross-clamping is associated with a 40% decrease in renal blood flow.[38] Thus renal insufficiency more commonly occurs with suprarenal as compared to infrarenal cross-clamping. AKI may occur in as many as 18% of patients undergoing aortic aneurysm repair. Preoperative evaluation of renal function is the best method of assessing and anticipating which patients may develop postoperative renal dysfunction. Preexisting renal impairment appears to be the main factor associated with AKI. A complete evaluation of renal function is required during the preoperative period, and patients with a low glomerular filtration rate should be managed with more aggressive renal protection interventions.[73]

Suprarenal cross-clamp times longer than 30 minutes increase the risk of postoperative renal failure. Even though renal blood flow is restored after unclamping, prolonged effects associated with ischemic reperfusion injury (IRI) occur. The injury caused to the renal tubular epithelium decreases the glomerular filtration rate. This effect may lead to acute renal failure, which is fatal in 50% to 90% of patients who have undergone aneurysmectomy.[74] Clamp positioning above the renal arteries is predictive of severe AKI in patients treated with open surgical repair (OSR).[75] AKI is a common problem after elective infrarenal EVAR, and preoperative renal dysfunction appears to be the main factor associated with AKI. AKI is associated with higher mortality rates and long-term cardiovascular events after surgery.[75,76] The administration of renal-dose dopamine, mannitol, sodium bicarbonate, and/or loop diuretics has not been scientifically proven to preserve or improve renal function postoperatively. The use of balanced crystalloid solutions decreases the incidence of AKI.[77] Minimizing the use of nephrotoxic medications such as nonsteroidal antiinflammatory drugs and aminoglycoside antibiotics preoperatively is prudent. Intraoperative renal perfusion with cold solution appears to have a renal protective effect and decrease the incidence of AKI.[78] Atrial natriuretic peptide (ANP) causes vasodilatation of the preglomerular artery, inhibition of the angiotensin axis, and prostaglandin release, which promotes renal vascular dilation. During the AKI reflow period, the natriuretic effect of ANP could be useful in preventing tubular obstruction in patients undergoing major surgery such as cardiovascular surgery.[77] The most important interventions to protect from AKI are aggressive hemodynamic stabilization and minimization of aortic clamp times, which have proven efficacy.[79]

Spinal cord ischemia. Spinal cord damage causing paraplegia can occur during aortic occlusion. The incidence of paraplegia during thoracic and thoracoabdominal aneurysm repair is estimated to be between 1% and 13%.[80] Longitudinal blood flow to the spinal cord includes (1) two posterior and two posterolateral arteries supplying blood to the dorsal or sensory portion of the spinal cord (20% of spinal cord blood flow) and (2) one anterior spinal artery supplying blood to the anterior or motor portion of the spinal cord (80% of spinal cord blood flow). Transverse blood flow originating from the aorta is via the greater radicular artery (artery of Adamkiewicz). The exact location of this artery is variable and depends on an individual's specific anatomic characteristics. The artery most often originates between spinal segments T8 and T12, but it can originate as low as L2 in a small segment of the population. This explains why the presence of paraplegia with aortic cross-clamping is unpredictable. Interruption of blood flow to the greater radicular artery in the absence of collateral blood flow has been identified as a factor that can cause paraplegia in patients having AAA repair. The incidence of neurologic complications increases as the aortic cross-clamp is positioned higher or more proximal to the heart. Somatosensory-evoked potential (SSEP) monitoring has been advocated as a method of identifying spinal cord ischemia. However, SSEP monitoring reflects dorsal (sensory) spinal cord function and does not provide information regarding the integrity of the anterior (motor) spinal cord.[6] Motor-evoked potential (MEP) monitoring is capable of determining anterior cord function. This monitoring modality relies on intact neuromuscular functioning for analysis, which limits its use in abdominal aortic aneurysmectomies because neuromuscular blocking drugs are routinely used. Alternative methods for reliable evaluation of spinal cord ischemia are still under investigation.[81]

Spinal cord protection strategies include distal aortic perfusion, cerebrospinal fluid drainage, and mild hypothermia. Maintenance of

TABLE 28.4 Hemodynamic Responses to Aortic Unclamping and Therapeutic Interventions

Hemodynamic Changes	Metabolic Changes	Intraoperative Interventions
Decreased arterial blood pressure	Increased lactate	Decrease anesthetic depth
Decreased myocardial contractility	Increased total body oxygen consumption	Decrease vasodilators
Decreased systemic vascular resistance	Decreased mixed venous oxygen saturation	Increase fluids
Decreased central venous pressure	Increased prostaglandins	Increase vasoconstrictor drugs
Decreased preload	Increased activated complement	Reapply cross-clamp for severe hypotension
Decreased cardiac output	Increased myocardial depressant factors	Consider administration of mannitol and sodium bicarbonate
Increased pulmonary artery pressure	Decreased temperature	
	Metabolic acidosis	

Adapted from Norris EJ. Anesthesia for vascular surgery. In Miller RD, et al., eds. *Miller's Anesthesia.* 9th ed. Philadelphia: Elsevier; 2020; Holt PJE, Thompson MM. Abdominal aortic aneurysms: evaluation and decision making. In Cronenwett JL, Johnston W, eds. *Rutherford's Vascular Surgery.* 9th ed. Vol. 2. Philadelphia: Elsevier; 2019.

normotension (systolic blood pressure ≥120 mm Hg) through the second postoperative day decreased the incidence of paraplegia during thoracic aortic reconstruction.[82,83]

Ischemic colon injury is a well-documented complication associated with abdominal aortic resections. Ischemia of the colon is most often attributed to manipulation of the inferior mesenteric artery, which supplies the primary blood supply to the left colon. This vessel is often sacrificed during surgery, and blood flow to the descending and sigmoid colon depends on the presence and adequacy of the collateral vessels. Increased intraabdominal pressure has also been implicated in ischemic colon injury. Mucosal ischemia occurs in 10% of patients who undergo AAA repair. In less than 1% of these patients, infarction of the left colon necessitates surgical intervention.[74]

Aortic Cross-Clamp Release

While the aorta is occluded, metabolites that are liberated as a result of anaerobic metabolism (such as serum lactate) accumulate below the aortic cross-clamp and induce vasodilation. As the cross-clamp is released, SVR decreases, and blood is sequestered into previously dilated veins, decreasing venous return. Reactive hyperemia causes transient vasodilation secondary to the presence of tissue hypoxia, release of adenine, and liberation of an unknown vasodepressor substance that may act as a myocardial depressant and peripheral vasodilator.[74] This combination of events results in decreased preload and afterload. The hemodynamic instability that may ensue after the release of an aortic cross-clamp is called declamping shock syndrome.[84] Evidence demonstrates that venous endothelin (ET), and specifically ET-1, may be partially responsible for the hemodynamic alterations that accompany declamping shock syndrome. Venous ET-1 has a positive inotropic effect on the heart and a vasoconstricting effect on blood vessels. Table 28.4 summarizes the most commonly observed hemodynamic responses to aortic unclamping and therapeutic interventions.

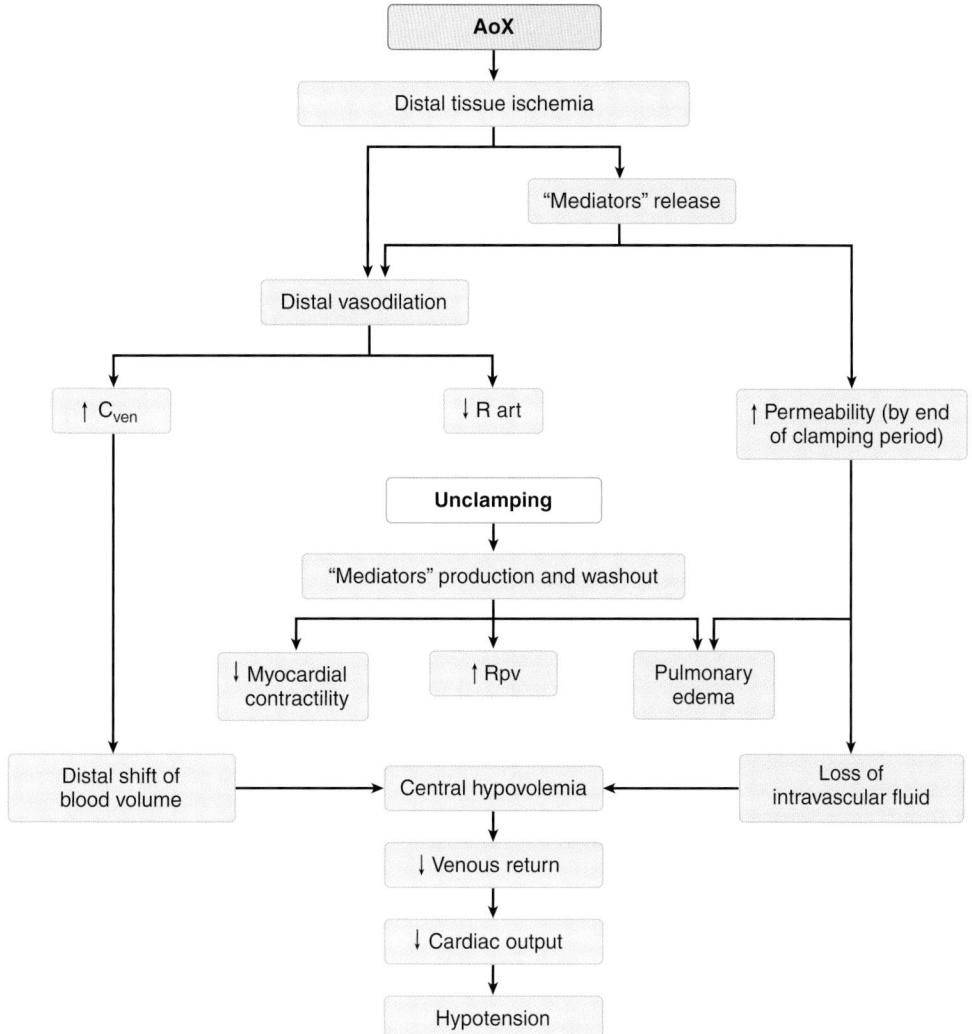

Fig. 28.2 Systemic hemodynamic response to aortic unclamping. *AoX,* Aortic cross-clamping; C_{ven}, venous capacitance; *R art,* arterial resistance; *Rpv,* pulmonary vascular resistance. (From Gelman S. The pathophysiology of aortic cross-clamping and unclamping. *Anesthesiology.* 1995;82:1026-1060.)

The magnitude of the response to unclamping the aorta may be manipulated. Although SVR and MAP decrease, intravascular volume may influence the direction and magnitude of the change in cardiac output. Restoration of circulating blood volume is paramount in providing circulatory stability before release of the aortic clamp.[64,74,85] The site and duration of cross-clamp application, as well as the gradual release of the clamp, influence the magnitude of circulatory instability. Thus effective communication between the anesthetist and the surgical team is vital during the operative procedure. Partial release of the aortic cross-clamp over time often results in less severe hypotension. Vasopressors and/or inotropic agents are administered to help minimize hypotension. An algorithm depicting the systemic hemodynamic response to aortic unclamping is shown in Fig. 28.2.

IRI is a complex metabolic process that occurs during application of the cross-clamp (ischemia) and subsequent unclamping of the aorta (reperfusion). IRI is characterized by metabolic, thrombotic, and inflammatory components. Cells that comprise tissues remain metabolic despite low blood flow, and they liberate cytotoxic mediators during anaerobic metabolism. During cellular ischemia, reactive oxygen species and increased intracellular calcium further inhibit mitochondrial activity and adenosine triphosphate generation. Specific body tissues vary in terms of the time it takes for their cells to

become necrotic. The degree of cellular necrosis is primarily determined by the duration of ischemia. The no-reflow phenomenon occurs when the microvasculature is occluded by platelets, neutrophils, and thrombi, causing inadequate perfusion and further increasing cellular necrosis.[1] Reinstituting blood flow increases inflammatory cell influx and cytotoxic substance washout into the central circulation.[82] Myocardial stunning and dysrhythmias can occur due to decreased cellular energy, increased reactive oxygen metabolites, and increased intracellular calcium, necessitating inotropic support.[86] Other manifestations associated with IRI include tissue edema, acute respiratory distress syndrome, compartment syndrome, bacterial translocation, renal failure, and multisystem organ failure.[1]

Surgical Approach

The standard surgical approach for elective abdominal aortic reconstruction is a transperitoneal incision. The advantages of this route include exposure of infrarenal and iliac vessels, ability to inspect intraabdominal organs, and rapid closure.[87] Unfavorable consequences associated with the transperitoneal approach include increased fluid losses, prolonged ileus, postoperative incisional pain, and pulmonary complications.

The retroperitoneal approach is an alternative to the standard route. Its advantages include excellent exposure (especially for both

TABLE 28.5 Comparison of Transperitoneal and Retroperitoneal Approaches

Transperitoneal	Retroperitoneal
Advantages	
Familiarity	Exposure for juxtarenal and suprarenal aneurysms
Access to infrarenal aorta and iliac vessels	Decreased fluid loss
Visualization of intraabdominal viscera	Improved postoperative respiratory function
Rapid opening and closure	Better-tolerated incisional pain
	Avoids formation of intraabdominal adhesions
Versatility	Does not elicit mesenteric traction syndrome
Disadvantages	
Increased fluid losses	Inaccessibility to distal right renal artery
Less postoperative ileus	
More frequent postoperative respiratory complications	
Increased postoperative incisional pain	

Modified from Sicard GA, et al. Retroperitoneal versus transperitoneal approach of repair of abdominal aortic aneurysms. *Surg Clin North Am.* 1989;69:795–806; Woo EY, Damraur SM. Abdominal aortic aneurysms: open surgical treatment. In Cronenwett JL, Johnston W, eds. *Rutherford's Vascular Surgery.* 9th ed. Vol. 2. Philadelphia: Elsevier; 2019.

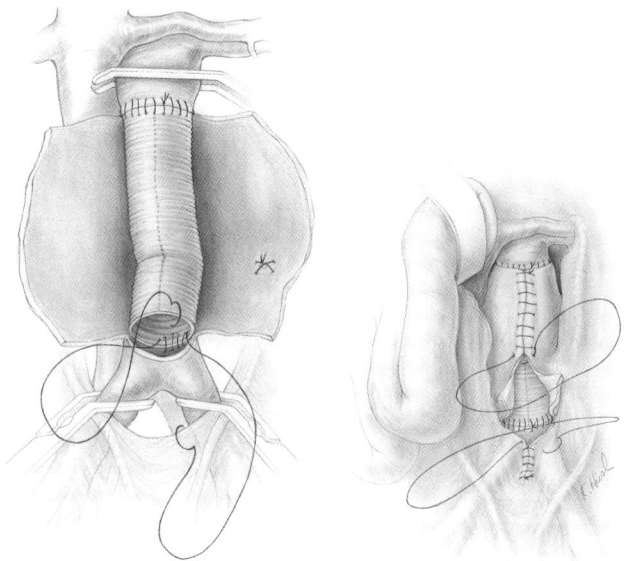

Fig. 28.3 Dacron graft used to repair an aneurysm. (From Zarins CK, Gewertz BL. *Atlas of Vascular Surgery.* 2nd ed. Philadelphia: Churchill Livingstone; 2009.)

juxtarenal and suprarenal aneurysms and in obese patients), decreased fluid losses, less incisional pain, and fewer postoperative pulmonary and intestinal complications. In addition, the retroperitoneal approach does not elicit mesenteric traction syndrome.[87] The reported limitations of this approach are the unfamiliarity of surgeons with this technique, poor right distal renal artery exposure, and the inability to inspect the integrity of the abdominal contents. Table 28.5 compares the standard and retroperitoneal surgical approaches. After cross-clamping, the aneurysm is incised, and a synthetic graft is sewn distally and proximally to the aneurysm. The aortic adventitia is then resewn over the synthetic graft (Fig. 28.3).

Management of Fluid and Blood Loss

Extreme loss of extracellular fluid and blood should be expected during repair of AAAs. The degree of surgical and evaporative losses and third spacing will determine the magnitude of the patient's fluid volume deficit. Furthermore, the surgical approach, the duration of the surgery, and the experience of the surgeon affect the total blood loss. Most blood loss occurs because of backbleeding from the lumbar and inferior mesenteric arteries after the vessels have been clamped and the aneurysm is opened.[88] Anticoagulation with the use of heparin also contributes to blood loss. Excessive bleeding, however, can occur at any point during surgery, and blood replacement is often necessary during open abdominal aortic resections.

Owing to the heightened awareness of transfusion-related morbidity, the use of autologous blood via a cell-saver system is a standard procedure. Presently, three options are available for administering autologous transfusions: preoperative deposit, intraoperative phlebotomy

and hemodilution, and intraoperative blood salvage. Ideally, patients donate their own blood to minimize the intraoperative use of homologous blood products and the subsequent risk of transfusion-related viruses. With anemia and decreased hemoglobin, oxygen transport is decreased, thus placing the patient with systemic vascular disease at increased risk for MI and stroke. Autotransfusion blood-salvaging systems may be used for replacing intraoperative blood loss. A study at the Mayo Clinic demonstrated a 75% reduction in transfused banked blood when intraoperative autologous red cell salvage was used. It was a prospective study of 100 patients who underwent elective abdominal aortic resections, and 80% of patients received only their own blood.[88] An increased number of banked red blood cell units infused is an independent risk factor for poor outcome after cardiac surgery.[89] Evidence suggests that there is no difference with respect to 30-day mortality between a hematocrit of 24% and a hematocrit of 30% in patients having cardiac surgery.[90]

Presence of Concurrent Disease

Preoperative Management

The presence of underlying CAD in patients with vascular disease has been well documented. Reports suggest that CAD exists in more than 50% of patients who require abdominal aortic reconstruction and is the single most significant risk factor influencing long-term survivability.[8,91,92] MIs are responsible for 40% to 70% of all fatalities that occur after aneurysm reconstruction.[6,46] Preoperative cardiac evaluation begins with the identification of risk factors that may contribute to adverse cardiac events and subsequent death. When preoperative CAD exists, an increased incidence of postoperative adverse cardiac complications has been demonstrated.[93]

The end point of any method of preoperative cardiac evaluation for aneurysmectomies is identification of functional cardiac limitations. Depending on the degree of cardiac dysfunction, preoperative optimization of cardiac function may range from simple pharmacologic manipulation to surgical intervention. The American College of Cardiology and the American Hospital Association guidelines on perioperative cardiovascular evaluation and care for noncardiac surgery are generally followed when preparing patients for these procedures. Optimizing patient preoperative pathophysiologic states (Box 28.4) minimizes the overall rate of morbidity and mortality.

Intraoperative Management

Anesthetic Selection

Several anesthetic techniques are available for abdominal aortic resections. Although each technique has its advantages and disadvantages, no single technique has been proven to be definitively superior. Anesthetic selection should be based on the following objectives: providing optimum analgesia and amnesia, facilitating relaxation, maintaining hemodynamic stability, preserving renal blood flow, and minimizing morbidity and mortality.

General anesthesia. Circulatory stability is especially desirable for patients undergoing AAA reconstruction, especially for those with CAD. All inhalation anesthetics may depress the myocardium and cause hemodynamic instability. Therefore high concentrations of inhalation agents should not be used in patients with a moderate to severe decreased ejection fraction. The degree of myocardial depression is dose dependent, and it is acceptable to administer inhalation agents at lower inhaled concentrations. Beneficial effects attributed to inhalation agents include the ability to alter autonomic responses, reversibility, rapid emergence, potentially earlier extubation, neurologic protection, and cardioprotection.[33] Cardiovascular stability provided by opioids has been well documented, and this feature is especially attractive for patients with ischemic heart disease and ventricular dysfunction. Provision of intense analgesia for the initial postoperative period after major abdominal vascular surgery (i.e., administration of neuraxial opioid) does not alter the combined incidence of major cardiovascular, respiratory, and renal complications.[94] Despite the absence of direct myocardial depression, the sympathetic nervous system inhibition that ensues may decrease SVR and heart rate. Therefore, especially in an individual with a moderate to severely decreased ejection fraction, narcotics should be carefully titrated to the patient's hemodynamic response. Dexmedetomidine is an option since it functions to inhibit the sympathetic nervous system by decreasing central catecholamine release, does not inhibit respiration, and provides postoperative analgesia.

Regional anesthesia. The use of epidural anesthesia for abdominal aneurysmectomies is commonly considered. The benefits of epidural use include (1) decreased preload and afterload, (2) preserved myocardial oxygenation, (3) reduced stress response, (4) excellent muscle relaxation, (5) decreased incidence of postoperative thromboembolism, (6) increased graft flow to the lower extremities, (7) decreased pulmonary complications, and (8) improved postoperative analgesia. Potential disadvantages include the possibility of an epidural hematoma (risk increases with anticoagulation) and severe hypotension during blood loss or unclamping.[34,95]

The use of thoracic epidural analgesia (TEA) in patients having coronary artery bypass surgery decreases the incidence of postoperative supraventricular arrhythmias and respiratory complications. General anesthesia with TEA does not increase the risk of mortality, MI, or neurologic complications compared to GA alone.[96]

Combination techniques. The use of a combined general anesthesia and epidural anesthesia provides the benefits of epidural anesthesia with the ability to provide amnesia and controlled ventilation. Due to neuraxial blockade, a "light" GA can be administered. Postoperative epidural analgesia improves postoperative respiratory function and blood flow to distal tissues. Furthermore, postoperative epidural analgesia reduces postoperative pain and pulmonary complications in patients with chronic obstructive pulmonary disease (COPD), as compared to general anesthesia alone after open aneurysm repair.[97] However, the major risks associated with neuraxial anesthesia are subarachnoid or epidural hemorrhage (resulting in hematoma after heparinization) and hypotension, which may be difficult to treat especially during an episode of acute blood loss.

In summary, all the aforementioned anesthetic techniques can be used safely and can demonstrate positive outcomes. Even more important than anesthetic selection is the clinical management of each patient. Observation, accurate interpretation, and immediate intervention to minimize dramatic hemodynamic variability during the anesthetic process reduce morbidity and mortality to a much greater extent than selection of a superior anesthetic technique.

Fluid Management

Maintaining intravascular volume may be an extreme challenge during abdominal aortic resections. Controversy exists regarding whether the

---

BOX 28.5   Postoperative Considerations for Patients Having Abdominal Aortic Aneurysm Repair

- Continue invasive hemodynamic monitoring
- Treat acute blood pressure extremes, arrhythmias (atrial fibrillation)
- Assess for postoperative myocardial infarction
- Provide ventilatory management with weaning and extubation
- Assess for abdominal compartment syndrome
- Evaluate hemoglobin, hematocrit, coagulation status, and adequacy of volume replacement
- Assess blood urea nitrogen/creatinine and urine output
- Institute deep vein thrombosis prophylaxis per protocol

BOX 28.6   Potential Complications of Juxtarenal or Suprarenal Aortic Occlusion

- Renal failure
- Hemorrhage
- Distal arterial occlusion
- Infarction
- Pulmonary or cardiac dysfunction
- Impotence
- Paraplegia
- Thrombosis
- Pseudoaneurysm formation
- Aortoenteric fistula

---

administration of crystalloids or colloids affects the overall incidence of morbidity and mortality. Blood losses initially can be replaced with crystalloids at a ratio of 3:1. The combination of crystalloid and colloid administration is also acceptable. Regardless of the choice of fluid, volume replacement must be dictated by physiologic parameters. Fluid replacement should be sufficient to maintain normal cardiac filling pressures and cardiac output, and a urine output of at least 1 mL/kg/hr. Patients with limited cardiac reserve can develop congestive heart failure if hypervolemia occurs. As mentioned previously, cell-saver blood retrieval can be used, and vascular access should include two large-bore intravenous lines and a central venous catheter. Goal-directed fluid therapy may help to optimize a patient's intravascular volume and hemodynamic status.

Hemodynamic Alterations

Hemodynamic changes are likely to occur throughout the procedure. Adequate preoperative sedation should be given before the placement of invasive monitoring equipment. Fluctuations in heart rate and blood pressure should be anticipated during induction and intubation. Preoperative replacement of fluid deficits prevents exaggerated responses to vasodilating induction agents. For patients with adequate left ventricular function, hemodynamic stability can be preserved with a "slow" and controlled induction using higher doses of opioids and sympathomimetic agents if hypotension develops. The response to mesenteric traction (discussed previously) is also associated with stimulation of the celiac reflex, which results in bradycardia and hypotension.

Postoperative Considerations

Cardiac, respiratory, and renal failure are the most common complications observed postoperatively in patients recovering from abdominal aortic reconstruction. Cardiovascular function must be closely monitored in the ICU for at least 24 hours after surgery. Maintaining adequate blood pressure, intravascular fluid volume, and myocardial oxygenation is paramount during this period. MI frequently contributes to postoperative morbidity and mortality; serial cardiac enzyme analysis may be justified. Pharmacologic agents used in the treatment of hypertension or hypotension must also be available.

Most patients require ventilatory assistance during the postoperative period. Vigilant monitoring of respiratory function is mandatory, especially when epidural catheters are used for postoperative analgesia. To address the significant number of serious postoperative complications (Box 28.5), intensive and continuous assessment of the patient condition is vital. Patients are admitted to the ICU for high-acuity monitoring and care.

Juxtarenal and Suprarenal Aortic Aneurysms

Although most AAAs occur below the level of the renal arteries, 2% extend proximally and involve the renal or visceral arteries.[98] Juxtarenal

aneurysms are located at the level of the renal arteries, but they spare the renal artery orifice. More proximal suprarenal aneurysms include at least one of the renal arteries and may involve visceral vessels. The effects of aortic cross-clamping for juxtarenal or suprarenal aneurysms are similar to those for infrarenal aortic occlusions; however, the magnitude of hemodynamic alterations increases as the aorta is clamped more proximally.

Renal failure, although possible during infrarenal aortic cross-clamping, occurs more often because of suprarenal aortic occlusion. Maintaining adequate intravascular volume and administering osmotic and loop diuretics may minimize renal ischemia and dysfunction.

Paraplegia is possible when the blood supply to the spinal cord is interrupted by aortic cross-clamping at or above the level of the diaphragm. Increasing the MAP or decreasing cerebrospinal fluid (CSF) pressure by placing a catheter in the subarachnoid space to drain CSF may be used as a means to increase spinal cord perfusion pressure.[98] Total body hypothermia and neurologic monitoring (i.e., SSEPs and MEPs) can be used to decrease the incidence of paraplegia. Early detection and intervention for spinal cord ischemia can decrease the incidence of permanent paraplegia after endovascular stent grafting (EVSG) of the descending thoracic aorta. Neurologic deficits can become evident weeks after surgery. Routine SSEP monitoring, serial neurologic assessment, arterial pressure augmentation, and CSF drainage may benefit patients at risk for paraplegia.[99] Box 28.6 summarizes the complications that may result from juxtarenal or suprarenal aortic occlusion.

Ruptured Abdominal Aortic Aneurysm

A high mortality rate of 80% to 90% is associated with a ruptured AAA, whereas postoperative mortality is estimated to range from 40% to 50%.[100] The mortality after surgery to repair a ruptured AAA does not vary based on the type of surgical repair (open vs endovascular).[101] The most common symptoms of ruptured AAAs include a triad of severe abdominal discomfort or back pain, altered level of consciousness caused by hypotension, and a pulsatile abdominal mass.[102] Other common symptoms include syncope, groin or flank pain, hematuria, and groin hernia. Risk factors associated with an increase in mortality in patients with a ruptured AAA are noted in Box 28.7.

Hypotension and a history of cardiac disease are two factors associated with the poorest prognosis.[51] Patients with these symptoms should be immediately transferred to the operating room for surgical exploration. When hypotension is absent, more time is available for comprehensive preoperative assessment and testing; however, decompensation and cardiovascular collapse can occur rapidly.

Once the patient arrives in the operating suite, performing a brief preoperative evaluation to establish peripheral and central venous access is a priority. Provisions for fluid, blood, and blood product

BOX 28.7 Risk Factors Associated With an Increased Risk of Mortality in Abdominal Aortic Aneurysm Rupture

- Increased age
- Women
- Nonwhite race
- Insurance status (higher for those who self-pay or are on Medicaid in the United States)
- Comorbid conditions
- Congestive heart failure
- Renal failure
- Valvular heart disease

From Cronenwett JL, Johnston W. *Rutherford's Vascular Surgery*. 9th ed. Vol. 2. Philadelphia: Elsevier; 2019.

TABLE 28.6 Classification Schemes of Acute Aortic Dissection

Classification	Site of Origin and Extent of Aortic Involvement
DeBakey	
Type I	Originates in the ascending aorta and extends at least to the aortic arch and often to the descending aorta (and beyond)
Type II	Originates in the ascending aorta; confined to this segment
Type III	Originates in the descending aorta, usually just distal to the left subclavian artery, and extends distally
Stanford	
Type A	Dissections that involve the ascending aorta (with or without extension into the descending aorta)
Type B	Dissections that do not involve the ascending aorta

From Braverman AC, et al. Diseases of the aorta. In Bonow RO, et al., eds. *Braunwald's Heart Disease: A Textbook of Cardiovascular Medicine*. 9th ed. Vol. 2. Philadelphia: Elsevier; 2012:1320.

administration is necessary, as rapid massive hemorrhage is a distinct possibility. The use of blood salvaging techniques and the ability to rapidly infuse blood and fluids are indicated. Insertion of an arterial line is essential, as significant fluctuations in blood pressure should be expected. Vasopressors such as phenylephrine and epinephrine given as a bolus and by infusion should be available. Hemodynamic stability must be the primary objective, and anesthetic induction and maintenance agents must be selected on a case-by-case basis.

Cardiovascular stability is the primary focus until blood loss from the proximal aorta is controlled by surgical intervention. Fluid resuscitation can begin with crystalloids; colloids and blood products can be administered as they become available. Intraoperative blood salvage provisions should be available. Coagulation studies and other laboratory tests, including hemoglobin, hematocrit, and ionized calcium values, should be obtained. Calcium is a positive inotrope, which is necessary for myocardial contractility. Large amounts of citrate used as a preservative in banked blood bind calcium ions and result in relative hypocalcemia. Decreased myocardial contractility—as evidenced by hypotension, increased left ventricular end-diastolic pressure, and increased central venous pressure—can be caused by hypocalcemia. Increased bleeding can also be caused by intraoperative hypocalcemia. If hypocalcemia occurs, calcium chloride can be administered, as guided by ionized calcium levels. Dilutional thrombocytopenia is the most common reason for coagulopathy to develop after massive intravenous fluid and blood administration. The use of fresh frozen plasma has been shown to decrease the total transfusion requirement and the incidence of coagulopathies.[37]

The hemodynamic effects of aortic cross-clamping and release are similar to those for elective surgery; however, responses may be extreme especially if hypotension exists when the clamp is released. Most patients require large amounts of fluid and blood replacement, and therefore postoperative mechanical ventilation is recommended. Patients experiencing hypovolemic shock are exquisitely sensitive to the myocardial depressant and vasodilatory effects of anesthetic agents. Titration of anesthetic agents and the use of vasopressors and/or positive inotropes are warranted. Additionally, ventilation may be difficult due to surgical displacement of the diaphragm cephalad. This will decrease lung expansion and functional residual capacity and increase peak pressures. Because positive pressure ventilation decreases venous return, hypotension can occur. Minimizing peak inspiratory pressures and administering higher concentrations of oxygen will help maximize venous return and maintain oxygen saturation. Manual initiation of a positive pressure breath will improve alveolar recruitment and distention.

THORACIC AORTIC ANEURYSMS

The mortality associated with elective thoracic aneurysm repair is 22%, and if rupture occurs, it increases to 54%.[103] Patients with aortic dissections have a predicted survival of only 3 months if they do not undergo surgical repair because the incidence of rupture is high.[104] Aneurysms have been described for hundreds of years; however, the development of the arterial prosthesis that led to successful bypass options did not occur until 1951.[105] The refinement of endovascular stent grafts, surgical and perfusion techniques, and intraoperative management have contributed to improved surgical outcomes.

Classification

Aneurysms of the thoracic aorta may be classified with respect to type, shape, and location. Typically, aneurysms involving all three layers of the arterial wall—tunica adventitia, tunica media, and tunica intima—are considered to be true aneurysms. In comparison, aneurysms that solely involve the adventitia are termed false aneurysms. The shape of the lesion also can serve as a means of characterizing aneurysms. Fusiform aneurysms have a spindle shape and result in dilation of the aorta. Saccular aneurysms are spherical dilations and are generally limited to only one segment of the vessel wall. Aortic dissection is the result of a spontaneous tear within the intima that permits the flow of blood through a false passage along the longitudinal axis of the aorta. If an aortic dissection is extensive, it is difficult for the surgeon to isolate the aneurysm and secure a graft, due to the weakened aortic wall. There are two major classification schemes for aortic dissections, based on the location. These are the DeBakey and Stanford classifications (Table 28.6). Thoracoabdominal aortic aneurysms (TAAAs) are classified using the Crawford classification (Fig. 28.4).

Etiology

Atherosclerosis is the most common cause of aneurysmal pathology. Atherosclerotic lesions occur most often in the descending and distal thoracic aorta and are most often classified as fusiform. Less common causes include aortic dissection and various mechanical, inflammatory, and infectious processes. The various causes of aortic aneurysms are classified in Box 28.8.

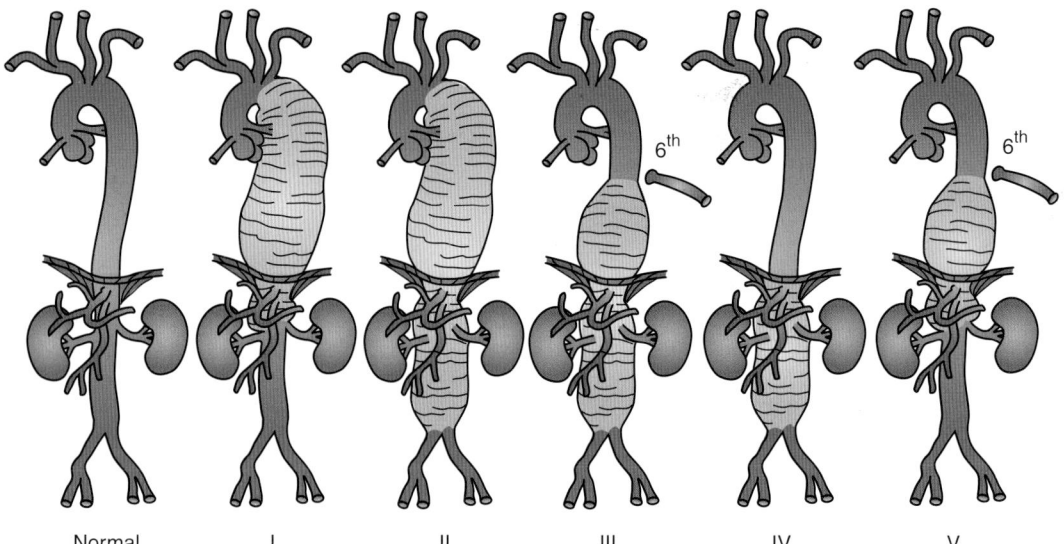

Normal   I   II   III   IV   V

Fig. 28.4 Crawford classification of thoracoabdominal aortic aneurysms. Type I, distal to the left subclavian artery to above the renal arteries. Type II, distal to the left subclavian artery to below the renal arteries. Type III, from the sixth intercostal space to the renal arteries. Type IV, from the 13th intercostal space to the iliac bifurcation (entire abdominal aorta). Type V, below the sixth intercostal space to just above the renal arteries. (From Cronenwett JL, Johnston KW. *Rutherford's Vascular Surgery*. 9th ed. Vol. 2. Philadelphia: Elsevier; 2019:2096.)

BOX 28.8 Etiology of Thoracoabdominal Aortic Aneurysms

Degenerative
- Nonspecific (commonly considered arteriosclerotic), dysplastic (80%)

Mechanical (Hemodynamic)
- Dissections (15%–20%)
- Poststenotic
- Arteriovenous fistula
- Blunt or penetrating trauma

Connective Tissue
- Ehlers-Danlos syndrome
- Marfan syndrome

Inflammatory (Noninfectious)
- Takayasu disease
- Behçet syndrome
- Reiter syndrome
- Kawasaki disease
- Microvascular disorder (e.g., polyarteritis)
- Ankylosing spondylitis
- Rheumatoid aortitis
- Periarterial inflammatory disease (e.g., pancreatitis)

Infectious
- Tuberculosis
- Bacterial
- Fungal
- Spirochetal (syphilis)

Anastomosis
- Postarteriotomy
- Postoperative pseudoaneurysm

Diagnosis

The symptomatology of thoracic aneurysms is often related to the site of the lesion and its compression of adjacent structures. Pain, stridor, and cough may result from compression of thoracic structures. A change in the quality of one's voice, resulting in hoarseness, can occur from impingement by the aneurysm on the left recurrent laryngeal nerve. This can occur because the left recurrent larynx nerve bifurcates from the vagus nerve at the level of the aortic arch. Symptoms related to aortic insufficiency may be observed in aneurysms of the ascending aorta. An upper mediastinal mass may be an incidental finding on conventional chest radiography in an asymptomatic patient. Further investigation with noninvasive methods such as CT scan and MRI can describe the specific anatomic characteristics and location of the aneurysm.

Treatment

As previously described, a high mortality rate is associated with the rupture of thoracic aneurysms, therefore early detection and surgical intervention make a significant contribution to long-term survival. Hemodynamic compromise and increased complexity of the aneurysm are associated with increased postoperative mortality. The surgical approach and the method of aneurysm resection vary according to the location of the lesion within the thoracic aorta. Resection of the ascending aorta and graft replacement necessitate the use of complete cardiopulmonary bypass or partial cardiopulmonary bypass (atrial-femoral: left atrial cannulation to a centrifugal pump, and reinfusion to a femoral artery cannula). If extracorporeal circulation is not indicated, heparin (50–100 units/kg) is required prior to aortic cross-clamping. For complete cardiac bypass, total systemic heparinization with 400 units/kg is necessary, and monitoring of activated clotting time is needed.[106] Depending on the proximity of the aneurysm to the aortic arch, the aortic valve may require replacement. Surgical resection of lesions in the transverse arch compromises cerebral perfusion. For these higher aneurysms various bypass techniques, combined with profound hypothermia and circulatory arrest, have been used.[107]

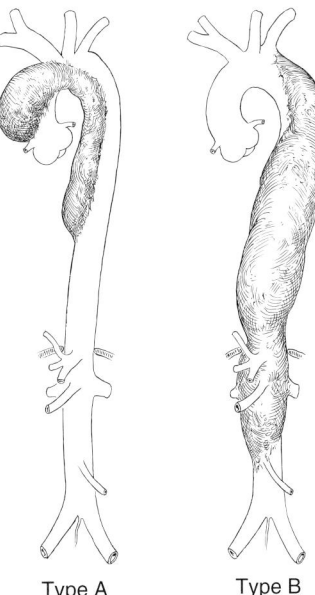

Type A   Type B

Fig. 28.5 Types of aortic dissection. Type A involves the ascending aorta and may extend into the aortic arch. Type B starts at the proximal descending aorta and extends distally.

Aneurysms of the descending aorta may be resected after application of an aortic cross-clamp; however, perfusion to distal organs can be compromised during this procedure. Arterial line and pulse oximetry monitoring should occur on the right side because impingement of the left subclavian artery, which provides blood flow to the left hand, is possible. A double lumen tube is placed, and deflation of the left lung is necessary to avoid left lung contusion and improve the surgical operating conditions. The patient is positioned in the left lateral decubitus position, and a left-sided thoracotomy is accomplished. The extent of the thoracotomy is determined by the extent of the aneurysm. A lower thoracic incision is associated with a decreased incidence of postoperative pulmonary dysfunction.[108]

AORTIC DISSECTION

Aortic dissection is characterized by a spontaneous tear of the vessel wall intima, permitting the passage of blood along a false lumen. Although the cause of dissections is unclear, lesions that were thought to be related to cystic necrotic processes may actually be caused by variations in wall integrity. Hypertension is the most common factor that contributes to the progression of the lesion. Manipulation of the ascending aorta during cardiac surgery may be associated with aortic dissection.[109] The symptoms of aortic dissection are the result of interruption of blood supply to vital organs. The most serious complication is aneurysm rupture. Diagnosis can be accomplished by the previously mentioned noninvasive techniques.

Treatment of dissecting aortic lesions depends on their location within the thoracic aorta (Fig. 28.5). Type A lesions have the highest incidence of rupture and require immediate surgical intervention. Type B lesions may initially be managed medically, with the administration of arterial dilating and β-adrenergic blocking agents.

In summary, surgical resection of thoracic aortic lesions enhances long-term survival. Refinement of surgical techniques and improvements in perfusion technology have reduced the overall mortality rate. The surgical method used is dependent on the location of the aortic lesion. Anesthesia for aneurysms of the ascending and transverse aorta requires cardiopulmonary bypass.

DESCENDING THORACIC AND THORACOABDOMINAL ANEURYSMS

Preoperative Assessment

Patients who undergo major vascular surgery are often elderly and have varying degrees of concurrent disease. Most patients who develop a descending thoracic aortic aneurysm (DTAA) are asymptomatic. Operative surgical decisions are based on the size, extent, and rate of expansion of the aneurysm. For patients with degenerative aortic disease, surgical repair is advised for aneurysms 6 cm or larger. Independent risk factors for DTAA include pain, increased age, COPD, renal insufficiency, aneurysm size, and aneurysm expansion rate.[110]

The importance of a thorough preoperative evaluation cannot be overemphasized. Special attention should be directed toward cardiac, renal, and neurologic function. Although most fatalities related to thoracic aortic surgery are cardiac in origin, renal and neurologic dysfunction contribute to poor surgical outcomes.[111] Preoperative renal dysfunction is directly related to postoperative renal failure and is thought to be one of the strongest contributors to renal deterioration after surgery.[83,111] Neurologic function should be carefully assessed in the preoperative phase. Paraplegia is one of the most devastating consequences of thoracic aortic surgery, and any alteration in lower extremity function should be noted. Hoarseness related to compression of the recurrent laryngeal nerve should be assessed and documented. The left recurrent laryngeal nerve is most susceptible due to its close proximity to the aortic arch. Bilateral recurrent laryngeal nerve compression or damage can result in respiratory compromise.

Intraoperative Management
Monitoring

Intraoperative monitoring devices used for thoracoabdominal aneurysm resection are the same as those used for abdominal aneurysmectomies. Direct intraarterial blood pressure and pulmonary artery pressure monitoring is standard during extracorporeal circulation. If the aneurysm involves the thoracic region or the distal aortic arch, right radial arterial line monitoring is preferred because left subclavian arterial blood flow may be compromised during surgery. The use of TEE is suggested for cardiac monitoring in patients with myocardial dysfunction. An indwelling urinary catheter is used for assessing renal function. To facilitate exposing the descending thoracic aorta, a double-lumen endotracheal tube is inserted to allow for one-lung ventilation. As a result, careful monitoring of oxygenation is mandatory. Routine use of pulse oximetry may be limited if the left subclavian artery is manipulated; therefore the right hand, the ear, or the nose should be used for monitoring oxygen saturation. Finally, a lumbar intrathecal catheter is inserted to access CSF pressure. SSEPs and/or MEPs are often used to monitor and detect neurologic dysfunction.

Spinal Cord Ischemia

Neurologic dysfunction is a serious complication associated with thoracic aortic aneurysm (TAA) reconstruction. Spinal cord injury is categorized into immediate and delayed paraplegia. The incidence of immediate paraplegia with DTAA ranges from 0% to 3% if surgery is performed with adjunctive procedures or clamp times are less than 10 minutes. However, the incidence of paraplegia and/or paresis for patients having TAA repair is 7.1% ± 6.1% (range 0%–32%).[112] Impending spinal cord injury depends on the type of aneurysm, surgical technique, cross-clamp time, and use of spinal cord protection interventions.[113] The exact incidence of delayed paraplegia is unknown, but it is believed that as many as 25% of all spinal cord injuries are delayed. The primary preoperative risk factors for delayed paraplegia include type 2 aneurysms, emergency procedures, number of sacrificed segmental segments, and renal failure. The main postoperative factors include hemodynamic instability caused by atrial fibrillation, bleeding, multiorgan failure, and sepsis.[110]

Several techniques have been successfully applied in an effort to decrease the incidence of neurologic dysfunction after thoracic aortic surgery. These include SSEP and MEP monitoring, CSF drainage, hypothermia, reattachment of intercostal arteries, and distal aortic perfusion. Systemic hypothermia and selective cooling of the spinal cord may lengthen ischemic time intervals; however, the clinical benefits are unclear.[114] The use of various bypass mechanisms and distal shunts may minimize the length of aortic occlusion time.

Spinal cord perfusion pressure can be estimated by calculating the arterial blood pressure minus the CSF pressure. During aortic clamping, CSF pressure increases whereas arterial pressure decreases distal to the clamp. The spinal cord perfusion pressure can therefore be manipulated by altering arterial blood pressure and draining CSF through an intrathecal catheter.[114,115] The most influential interventions used to protect the spinal cord during thoracic aortic cross-clamping include (1) routine CSF drainage (CSF pressure <10 mm Hg), (2) endorphin receptor blockade (naloxone infusion), (3) moderate intraoperative hypothermia (<35°C), (4) avoiding hypotension (MAP >90 mm Hg), and (5) optimizing cardiac function.[116] It is postulated that increased levels of excitatory amino acid neurotransmitters bind to opioid receptors in the spinal cord and induce spinal cord edema. Therefore administration of naloxone may inhibit edema formation. Avoiding the use of sodium nitroprusside is indicated, as arterial dilation may cause a "steal phenomenon," further decreasing spinal cord blood flow.

Methods for detecting spinal cord ischemia were discussed previously. The intraoperative use of SSEPs and MEPs can provide early identification of neurologic dysfunction, but these monitoring modalities do not ensure spinal cord integrity. Factors that contribute to the development of neurologic deficits include the level of aortic clamp application, ischemic time, embolization or thrombosis of a critical intercostal artery, failure to revascularize intercostal arteries, and the urgency of surgical intervention.[114,115] Delayed paraplegia may also be the result of IRI, although the exact mechanism of injury has not been proven.[110,117,118] Additional complications of thoracoabdominal aortic reconstruction are listed in Box 28.9.

Anesthetic Management

The principles of perioperative management of TAAs and DTAAs are similar to those previously discussed for abdominal aortic aneurysmectomies. Anesthetic selection should be based on the presence of concomitant disease processes, with the objective of maintaining cardiovascular stability and minimizing morbidity and mortality. Intraoperative monitoring should focus on detection of myocardial, neurologic, and renal ischemia. The hemodynamic consequences of aortic cross-clamping should be attenuated by the use of pharmacologic adjuncts. Restoration of circulating blood volume minimizes the hemodynamic alterations caused by the release of the aortic clamp.

Postoperative Considerations

After surgery is completed, if a double-lumen endotracheal tube was used, it should be replaced with a standard endotracheal tube since postoperative ventilatory assistance is usually required. Airway anatomy may become edematous during surgery, causing difficulty with ventilation and reintubation. Under these circumstances, the double-lumen endotracheal tube may be left in place. Replacement of the endotracheal tube can proceed in the postoperative period after the airway edema has dissipated. Recurrent laryngeal nerve dysfunction can contribute to breathing difficulties after extubation.

BOX 28.9 Complications Following Thoracoabdominal Aortic Aneurysm Repair

Early Complications
- Respiratory failure (most common complication)
- Hemorrhage
- Myocardial infarction
- Congestive heart failure
- Early paraplegia
- Embolization/thrombosis
- Distal artery occlusion
- Bowel ischemia
- Sexual dysfunction
- Infection
- Renal failure
- Cerebrovascular accident

Late Complications
- Delayed paraplegia
- Graft thrombosis
- Fistula formation
- False aneurysm
- Graft infection

Close observation of neurologic, circulatory, pulmonary, and renal status is warranted in the postoperative phase. Hemodynamic control is vital to maintaining perfusion to vital organs without creating excessive demands on the heart or the aortic graft. Careful monitoring of respiratory status aided by arterial blood gas analysis is indicated. Epidural analgesia with the use of local anesthetics, narcotics, or both can be administered for pain relief.

ENDOVASCULAR AORTIC ANEURYSM REPAIR

In 1991 the first EVSG procedure was performed to repair an infrarenal aortic aneurysm. The development of this technique allows surgeons to repair an AAA in a less invasive manner. Due to severe cardiac and respiratory pathology, as many as 30% of patients with aortic aneurysms are poor surgical candidates.[119] Thus EVAR was initially developed to help patients with severe coexisting disease who were not considered viable surgical candidates. Presently, EVAR is the treatment of choice for the majority of patients with an AAA.[120] In high-risk patients having elective AAA repair, the 30-day and 1-year mortality rates are significantly decreased with EVAR as compared to OSR.[121] Researchers suggest that the patient population that may benefit most from EVAR are high-risk patients.[122] Furthermore, patients who are prone to aortic aneurysm development commonly have significant coexisting diseases (Box 28.10).

Endovascular aortic repair is associated with improved 30-day outcomes (all-cause mortality, readmission, surgical site infection, pneumonia, and sepsis) as compared to OSR.[122-124] In one study, the 30-day mortality rate was 1.7% in the EVAR group vs 4.7% in the OSR group. Secondary interventions most often caused by endoleak were more common in the EVAR group (9.8% vs 5.8%).[125] However, there was no significant difference between the groups with respect to 2-year survival. A comparison of EVAR vs OSR showed that mortality was 0.6% and mean LOS was 5.8 days for EVAR, whereas in-hospital mortality for OSR was 4.6%, and the average LOS was 11.9 days.[126] EVAR is associated with decreased procedure duration, a decreased need for transfusion of blood and blood products, a shorter duration of hospitalization, and decreased morbidity compared to OSR.[127] Perioperative

BOX 28.10 Predisposing Factors for Patients Who Are Prone to Aortic Aneurysm Development

- Hypertension
- Male gender
- Heart disease
- Smoking
- Chronic obstructive pulmonary disease
- Diabetes mellitus
- Renal impairment
- Carotid artery disease
- Peripheral arterial disease
- Family history

Data from Townsend CM, et al. *Sabiston Textbook of Surgery.* 20th ed. Philadelphia: Elsevier; 2017.

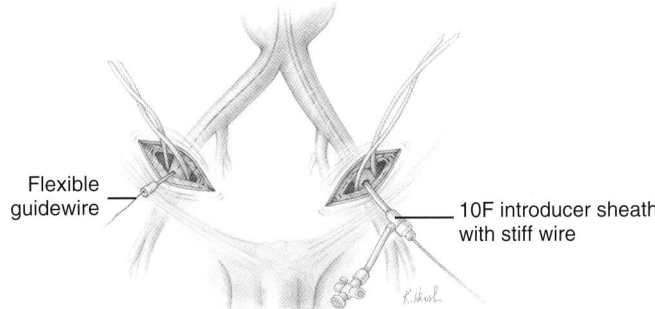

Fig. 28.6 Femoral cutdown and insertion of introducer sheath. (From Zarins CK, Gewertz BL. *Atlas of Vascular Surgery.* 2nd ed. Philadelphia: Churchill Livingstone; 2009.)

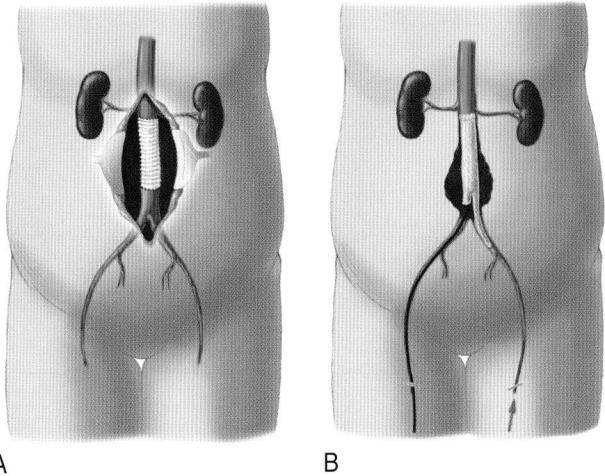

Fig. 28.7 Comparison of (A) open surgical repair and (B) endovascular aortic aneurysm repair.

mortality after EVAR has remained similar in recent years despite improvements in techniques, devices, and proficiency. Randomized trials such as the Endovascular Aneurysm Repair 1 (EVAR 1), Dutch Randomized Endovascular Aneurysm Management (DREAM), and Open versus Endovascular Repair (OVER) trials showed lower 30-day mortality rates for EVAR as compared to OSR. However, late mortality rates (24–36 months postoperatively) are similar for EVAR and OSR.[128]

Reinterventions occur more frequently after EVAR than after OSR.[129] The primary reason for a secondary corrective procedure is due to endoleak. Endoleak is a term that is used to describe the inability of the EVSG to isolate blood flow into the aneurysm sac. Endoleak has been determined to be a significant risk factor for late open conversion. The overall risk of late failure is approximately 3% per year.[124]

EVAR is also being used to treat patients with TAAs. The mortality rate for EVAR for elective DTAA repairs range from 3.5% to 12.5%, as compared with an open approach, where mortality is approximately 10%.[130] Reports also show that EVAR has a low incidence (0%–6%) of spinal cord ischemia and paraplegia.[131] Potential explanations for the decreased incidence of spinal cord trauma as compared to OSR are (1) no thoracic aortic cross-clamping and (2) no prolonged periods of extreme hypotension. Perioperative hypotension (MAP <70 mm Hg) was a significant predictor of spinal cord ischemia in patients undergoing EVAR for TAA.[132]

The overall mortality rate for patients with a ruptured AAA who are alive when diagnosed in emergency departments is 40% to 70%.[133] Since the 1950s, mortality from ruptured AAAs has decreased only 3.5% per decade.[134] Patient survival after emergency repair with EVAR has increased from 2005 to 2011. A significant improvement is noted particularly in those patients who survive the first 24 hours postoperatively.[135] The 30-day mortality rate after AAA rupture is estimated to be 10% to 45%.[136] Even though secondary interventions and EVSG surveillance are required, the use of EVAR for both ruptured AAAs and TAAs in patients with suitable anatomy is a lifesaving option.[137] Medical centers that consider EVAR for ruptured AAA repair have immediate CT imaging capabilities, trained endovascular teams, adequate endovascular supplies, and a specially arranged surgical suite.

Procedure

The most significant intraoperative advantages with EVAR as compared to OSR are the absence of aortic cross-clamping and the absence of an incision that extends from the xiphoid process to the pubis. EVAR involves deployment of an EVSG within the aortic lumen. The graft restricts blood flow to the portion of the aorta where the aneurysm exists. This procedure is also performed for patients who have TAAs or

TAAAs. Cannulation of both femoral arteries is performed. As seen in Fig. 28.6, a guide wire is threaded through the iliac artery to the level of the aneurysm. Next, a sheath is inserted over the guide wire and positioned at the aneurysm location through the use of fluoroscopy. The proximal end of the sheath must extend beyond the aneurysm, and care must be taken to avoid occlusion of the renal arteries. Once the sheath is deployed, radial force or fixation mechanisms such as hooks or barbs on the stent become embedded into the aortic wall to prevent stent migration (Fig. 28.7).

The surgical procedure may take place in a traditional operating room or an interventional radiology suite. Compared with the conventional surgical method, advantages of the endovascular approach include the absence of aortic cross-clamping, improved hemodynamic stability, decreased incidence of embolic events, decreased blood loss, a reduced stress response, decreased incidence of renal dysfunction, and decreased postoperative discomfort.[138,139] Systemic anticoagulation with heparin (50–100 units/kg) is administered prior to catheter manipulation.[140] Administration of a broad-spectrum antibiotic is recommended prior to surgery. The anesthetic techniques that can be used for EVAR include general anesthesia, neuraxial blockade, or local anesthesia with sedation.[141]

Local anesthesia with sedation, as compared to general anesthesia, is associated with decreases in nonfatal cardiac morbidity, respiratory complications, renal failure, and overall mortality.[142,143] There is also decreased pulmonary morbidity as compared with general anesthesia, and local anesthesia with sedation is associated with a shorter LOS as compared with general and neuraxial anesthesia.[144] The goals for intraoperative management for EVAR include maintaining hemodynamic stability, providing analgesia and anxiolysis, and being prepared to rapidly convert to an open procedure. Local or neuraxial anesthesia is associated with fewer ICU admissions, decreased length of hospitalization, and fewer systemic complications, as compared to general anesthesia.[145] In an alternative analysis there was no difference in 30-day mortality associated with either local anesthesia or general anesthesia

provided for EVAR. However, shorter operative times, shorter length of hospitalization, and fewer postoperative complications were associated with a local anesthetic technique.[146]

With infrarenal or suprarenal EVAR, creatinine clearance values can decrease by 10% in the first year.[147] However, proximal endovascular graft migration can occur, causing renal artery occlusion and postoperative renal failure.[148] Fenestrated EVSGs that are constructed to allow blood to flow to the renal arteries can be used safely for those patients who have juxtarenal or suprarenal aortic aneurysms.[149] Plasma catecholamine concentrations and mediators of the systemic immune response are decreased in patients who undergo the endovascular approach as compared with patients who undergo conventional repair.[150,151] Furthermore, there is evidence suggesting that patients who undergo EVAR release less plasma cortisol, develop significantly less sepsis, and may encounter a reduced incidence of systemic immune response syndrome as compared to those having traditional open AAA repair.[152] Some of the complications that can arise from the EVAR approach include (1) endograft thrombosis, migration, or rupture; (2) graft infection; (3) iliac artery rupture; and (4) lower extremity ischemia.[153] Fatal cerebral embolism resulting in sudden respiratory arrest has occurred during EVAR.[154] Box 28.11 lists potential complications associated with EVAR.

Endovascular graft design and durability continue to improve. Graft devices are either unibody (come in one piece) or modular (come in multiple pieces). The endograft fabric is either woven polyester (Dacron) or polytetrafluoroethylene. There is no significant difference in biologic response when comparing these two materials.[155] The graft skeleton is constructed of stainless steel, Nitinol, or Elgiloy (Fig. 28.8). Nitinol stents are popular because they exhibit minimal shortening after deployment when exposed to body temperature. There is considerable interest and research involving drug-eluting stents. In initial clinical trials, researchers have shown that restenosis rates are improved with the newer generation endovascular stents.[156,157] EVSGs have undergone modifications to meet anatomic challenges and improve patient outcomes. In the past, endovascular repair has been limited to infrarenal AAAs and isolated TAAs. The advent of fenestrated and branched endografts have made endovascular repair of thoracoabdominal and juxtarenal aneurysms possible. Fenestrated EVSGs are safe and effective in short- and midterm postoperative follow-up.[158] Continued evolution of endograft technology

BOX 28.11 Potential Complications Associated With EVAR

Graft and Deployment Complications
- Failed deployment
- Microembolization
- Migration/occlusion of major branch arteries (i.e., renal, mesenteric)
- Aortic perforation/aneurysm rupture
- Aortic dissection
- Hematoma formation
- Endoleak
- Stenosis/kink/thrombosis
- Graft tear
- Damage to access arteries (femoral → iliac)
- Infection

Radiologic Implications
- Radiation exposure
- Allergy to contrast dye
- Renal insufficiency from contrast dye

Systemic Complications
- Neurologic (CVA, paraplegia)
- Cardiac morbidity/mortality
- Pulmonary insufficiency
- Renal insufficiency
- Postimplantation syndrome

CVA, Cardiovascular accident; *EVAR,* endovascular aneurysm repair.

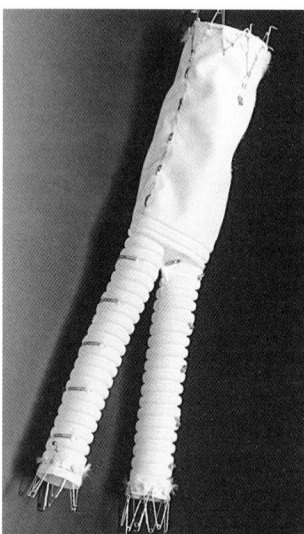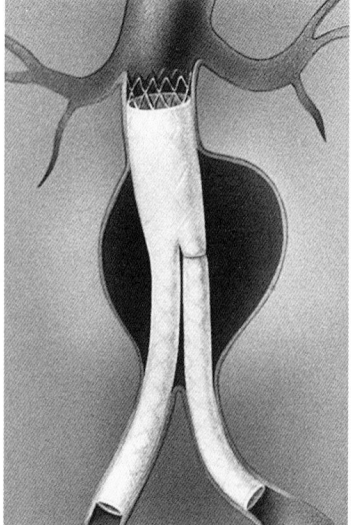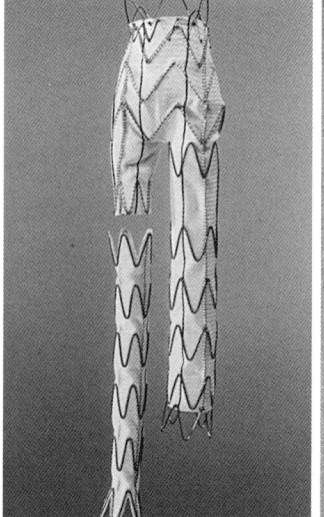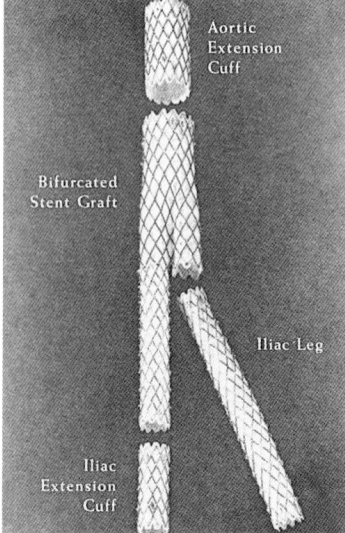

Fig. 28.8 Various types of endovascular grafts. (Adapted from Cronenwett JL, Johnston KW. *Rutherford's Vascular Surgery.* 7th ed. Vol. 2. Philadelphia: Saunders; 2010:1363-1383.)

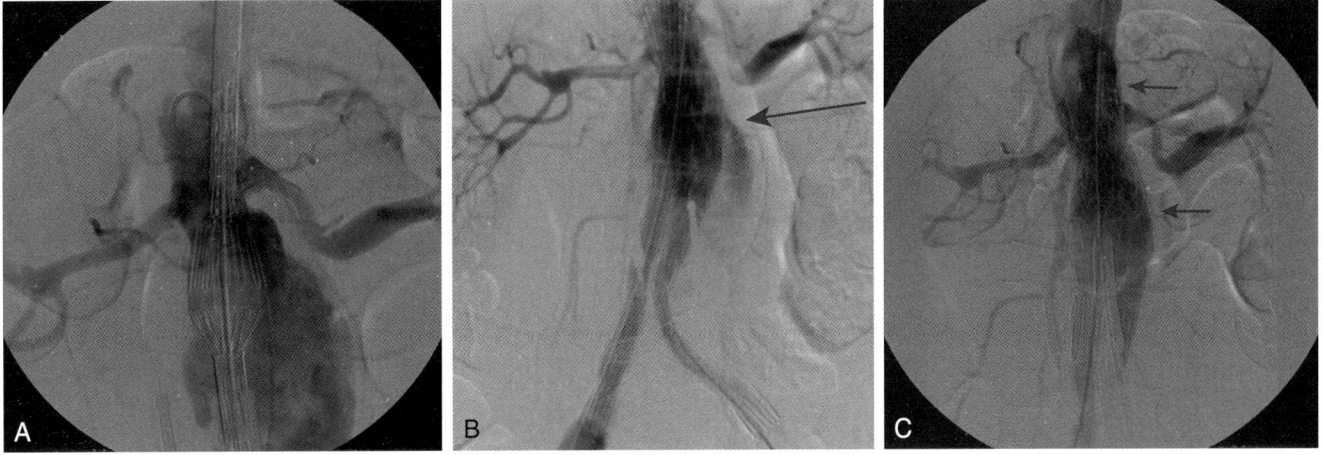

Fig. 28.9 (A) Short aortic neck immediately before endovascular aneurysm repair. (B) Type IA endoleak *(arrow)* after initial endograft placement and molding balloon angioplasty. (C) Resolution of the type IA endoleak after placement of a 5010 giant Palmaz stent (*arrows* show proximal and distal extent). (From Cronenwett JL, Johnston W. *Rutherford's Vascular Surgery.* 8th ed. Vol. 2. Philadelphia: Elsevier; 2014:1348.)

TABLE 28.7   Classification of Types of Endoleak

Classification	Description	Treatment
Type I endoleak	Attachment site leaks	Proximal or distal graft extension Secondary endograft Open repair
Type II endoleak	Branch leaks (i.e., lumbar artery, renal artery, internal iliac artery, inferior mesenteric artery)	Monitoring for enlargement Laparoscopic clip application Embolization
Type III endoleak	Graft defect (fabric tear, modular disconnection)	Secondary endograft Open repair
Type IV endoleak	Graft wall fabric porosity/suture holes	Observation Open repair
Endotension	Systemic pressure in aneurysm sac despite no evidence of endoleaks	Secondary endograft Open repair

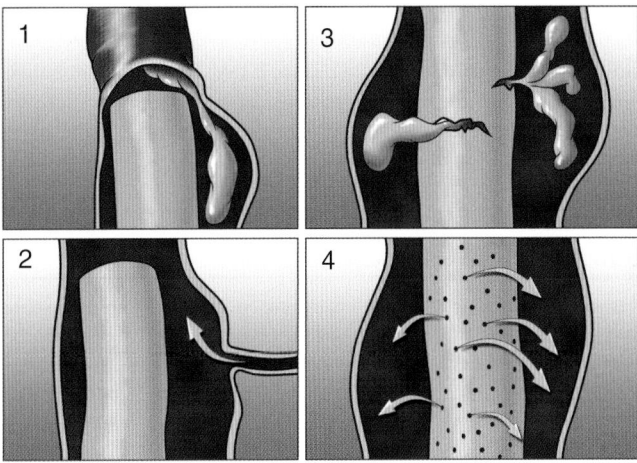

Fig. 28.10 *1,* Type I endoleak; *2,* type II endoleak; *3,* type III endoleak; *4,* type IV endoleak.

will maximize the benefit and minimize complications in patients with a range of aneurysmal disease.

Endoleak (Fig. 28.9), which was noted earlier as persistent blood flow and pressure (endotension) between the endovascular graft and the aortic aneurysm, is a serious complication of this procedure. Types of endoleaks are listed in Table 28.7 and shown in Fig. 28.10. Endoleak diagnosed by postoperative CT scan has been reported to occur in 15% to 52% of patients.[159] The majority of endoleaks are type II, and 70% close spontaneously within the first month after implantation.[160] Type II endoleaks are caused by collateral retrograde perfusion and are associated with long-term complications. Types I and III endoleaks are caused by device-related problems and most often occur soon after EVSG implantation.[161] The most frequent interventions used to correct these complications include implantation of a second endograft or open repair.[162] One long-term study has demonstrated that EVAR yields good results as compared to an open repair, but the overall durability of the open surgical procedure is superior.[163]

As described in the EVAR 1 study, reinterventions due to endoleak were required in three times as many patients who had EVAR as compared to an open procedure. Of these endoleaks requiring reintervention, 7% were discovered within 1 month of implantation, and another 13% occurred within 4 years postoperatively.[148] A comparison of the outcomes comparatively evaluating EVAR and open AAA repair (in nearly 40,000 patients) has been reported. Perioperative mortality (≤30 days postoperative) and the risk of mortality 3 years postoperatively were lower after EVAR compared with OSR. At 3 years postoperatively, the risk of mortality was similar to patients having an OSR. Follow-up interventions were more common after EVAR, most often due to the EVSG. Lastly, the risk of rupture was greater with EVAR within an 8-year postoperative period.[122]

As EVSG-related endoleaks are the most likely causes of late aneurysm rupture, post-EVAR surveillance is an important factor in avoiding the risk of late aneurysm rupture.[164] A large proportion of late ruptures are amenable to endovascular treatment. Postoperative follow-up care for patients who have undergone EVAR is vital because long-term outcomes have not been quantitatively established. Physical examination and contrast-enhanced CT scans are recommended at 1, 6, 12, and 18 months postoperatively, and then annually.[165] Additionally, abdominal x-rays should be obtained on a regular basis. Lifelong

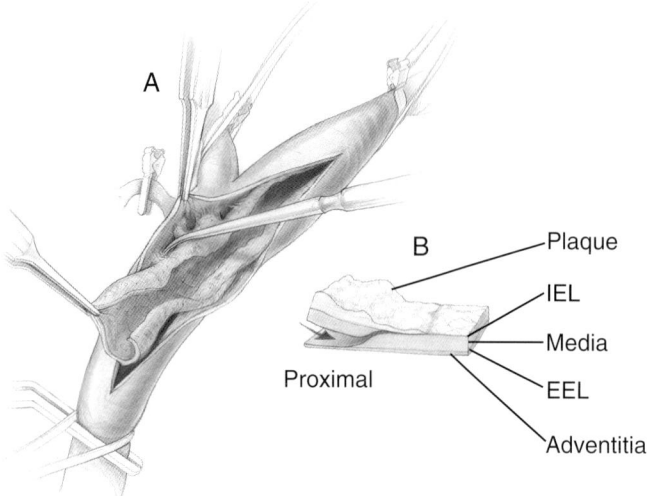

Fig. 28.11 (A) Removal of plaque from carotid artery. (B) Formulation of plaque on the intima of the carotid artery. *EEL,* External elastic lamina; *IEL,* internal elastic lamina. (From Zarins CK, Gewertz BL. *Atlas of Vascular Surgery.* 2nd ed. Philadelphia: Churchill Livingstone; 2009.)

radiographic evaluation and surveillance is necessary to monitor aneurysm size, graft migration, and endoleak. Intensive follow-up care, the need for reinterventions, and the cost of the endograft make EVAR more expensive than open repair.[166]

CEREBROVASCULAR INSUFFICIENCY AND CAROTID ENDARTERECTOMY

Carotid endarterectomy (CEA) is the second most common vascular operation performed in the United States every year (the first being coronary revascularization). Cerebrovascular accidents (CVAs, strokes) are the third leading cause of death in the United States.[167] More strokes are caused by cerebral ischemia than by intracranial hemorrhage. In carotid atherosclerotic disease, subintimal fatty plaques can increase in size over time and incrementally occlude the vascular lumen, which results in decreased cerebral blood flow (CBF). The plaque may rupture and release fibrin, calcium, cholesterol, and inflammatory cells. This phenomenon can lead to abrupt occlusion of the lumen from thrombosis due to platelet activation, or an embolus may form and decrease CBF distal to the carotid artery. In each scenario, an abrupt decrease in CBF leads to transient ischemic attacks (TIAs) or strokes. Note the anatomic details associated with the removal of plaque and the involvement within the layers of the carotid artery in Fig. 28.11.

More than half of all strokes are preceded by a TIA. The Framingham study reported that the risk of a stroke was 30% 2 years after a TIA had occurred and approximately 55% 12 years after a TIA had occurred.[168] It is this increased risk of stroke associated with TIA that provides the rationale for the use of CEA, the surgical procedure in which the internal carotid artery is incised and the plaque within the carotid arterial lumen is removed to improve CBF.

Indications

Since 1954, specific indications for and expected outcomes of CEA have been the subject of heated debate. Ischemic stroke accounts for approximately 80% of first-time strokes and is primarily caused by atheromatous plaques. The initial indication for CEA was symptomatic stenosis but not complete occlusive carotid disease. This presentation occurs in most patients who undergo carotid surgery. Some centers have extended the indications to include evolved (nondense),

nonhemorrhagic strokes and asymptomatic severe stenosis or lesser stenosis associated with contralateral occlusive disease. The North American Symptomatic CEA Trial concluded that CEA for patients with recent hemispheric TIAs and high-grade stenosis (70%–99%) had a risk reduction of 65% for the development of an ipsilateral stroke 2 years after surgery, compared with patients whose conditions were medically managed.[169] The Executive Committee for the Asymptomatic Carotid Atherosclerosis Study demonstrated that asymptomatic patients with at least 60% carotid artery stenosis who underwent CEA had a 53% lower 5-year risk of ipsilateral stroke than patients who were treated medically.[170] Other widely reported large-scale studies, including the Asymptomatic Carotid Atherosclerosis Study (ACAS) and the European Asymptomatic Carotid Surgery Trial (EACST), demonstrated a benefit of CEA with medical therapy (aspirin and atherosclerotic risk factor reduction) over medical therapy alone for patients with carotid stenosis in the 60% to 99% range.[171,172] These trials showed a similar absolute and relative reduction in risk for stroke of approximately 5% and 50%, respectively, at 5 years for CEA over medical therapy. Symptomatic patients are at a higher risk than asymptomatic patients for perioperative adverse events. However, the benefit of CEA in patients with recent ipsilateral carotid territory symptoms and moderate to severe carotid stenosis is much greater than the benefit of CEA in asymptomatic patients.[173]

Morbidity and Mortality

The surgical outcomes reported for CEA vary due to differences in patient populations and varying degrees of surgical expertise. Other variables that cannot be stratified in studies but may affect patient outcomes include the state of collateral flow through the circle of Willis, the presence of concurrent atherosclerotic disease in the cerebral vasculature, the size and morphology of the offending plaque, the specific presenting symptoms, and the presence of concurrent cardiovascular disease.[174] Carotid artery stenosis is the primary cause of approximately 20% of all strokes.[175] The recommended acceptable perioperative stroke rates are less than 3% in asymptomatic patients, less than 5% in symptomatic patients, and 10% or less in patients with recurrent disease or existing strokes.[176] Morbidity rates related to CEA have been reported to be at or below these recommended limits.[176,177] The perioperative MI rate of 2% to 5% illustrates the global nature of atherosclerotic disease and represents the greatest contribution to overall morbidity. The perioperative mortality rate for CEA is approximately 0.5% to 2.5%,[178,179] and the long-term postoperative stroke incidence ranges from 1% to 3% per year.[180] In a multicenter cohort of black and white adults in the United States, the incidence and mortality rates associated with a stroke decreased from 1987 to 2011. The decreases varied across age groups but were similar across sex and race.[181]

Patient Selection

The risks associated with CEA and stroke must be measured against the risks associated with undergoing medical management. The patients who benefit most from CEA are those with stenosis of greater than 70%; it is less beneficial in symptomatic patients with 50% to 69% stenosis.[175] Surgical intervention is most beneficial in men who are older than 75 years and are within 2 weeks of their last ischemic event.[182] As mentioned previously, the Framingham study identified the incidence of stroke after TIAs and demonstrated an increased risk of stroke in patients with untreated disease. Preoperative neurologic dysfunction was found to be the most significant factor for predicting postoperative stroke incidence (4%). Several conditions that can increase the risk of perioperative complications include severe preoperative hypertension, CEA performed in preparation for coronary artery bypass, angina, internal carotid artery stenosis near the carotid siphon, age older than

BOX 28.12   Factors Contributing to Morbidity During Carotid Endarterectomy

- History of stroke
- Operative timing
- Hyperglycemia
- Multiple comorbidities
- Age
- Contralateral carotid artery disease
- Progressing stroke
- Ulcerative lesion
- Intraoperative hemodynamic instability
- Surgery with shunt
- Surgery without shunt

BOX 28.13   Preoperative Risk Factors for Patients Scheduled for CEA

- Neurologic (cerebrovascular accident)
- Coronary artery disease
- Hypertension
- Diabetes
- Renal disease
- Thromboembolism

CEA, Carotid endarterectomy.

Heart Association (AHA) recommendations for perioperative cardiac assessment are in Table 28.8.

75 years, and diabetes mellitus.[183] Box 28.12 identifies various factors that contribute to morbidity during CEA.

In the past, emergent CEA or carotid artery stenting (CAS) after acute CVA was not considered safe. However, more evidence suggests that these surgical interventions, after an acute neurologic ischemic episode, are performed to reduce the risk of neurologic damage and recurrent stroke. Even within 72 hours after tissue plasminogen activator administration for thrombolysis, patients were not at risk for increased complications associated with the surgical procedure.[184]

Diagnosis

The neurologic symptoms associated with cerebral vascular dysfunctions such as TIAs and strokes are often related to decreased CBF. Whereas there are multiple causes for symptoms such as lightheadedness, altered levels of consciousness, aphasia, and acute motor deficits, these deficits warrant testing to determine if carotid stenosis is present. Asymptomatic carotid bruits may be a sign of carotid artery disease. However, not all carotid bruits indicate the presence of significant carotid artery disease. Amaurosis fugax manifests as monocular blindness and occurs in 25% of patients with high-grade carotid artery stenosis. This syndrome is believed to be caused by microthrombi that migrate into the internal carotid artery and decrease the blood supply of the optic nerve via the ophthalmic artery. Standard diagnostic imaging techniques used to assess the extent of carotid disease include duplex ultrasonography, digital subtraction angiography, CTA, and magnetic resonance angiography.[185]

Preoperative Assessment

The presence of concurrent CAD and carotid stenosis is well documented. Although stroke is a devastating consequence of CEA, MI contributes more often to poor surgical outcomes than stroke. Although coronary angiography may not be justified in all patients undergoing CEA, a systematic approach for identifying CAD and its subsequent risks should be performed before elective surgery.

Patients with no significant medical history, normal physical examination, and normal ECG should proceed directly to surgery; these patients have low surgical risks. If abnormal cardiac function is discovered during the preoperative assessment, further evaluation and testing should be performed. The presence of significant comorbidities will determine the extent to which further preoperative testing is appropriate. Box 28.13 lists preoperative risk factors in patients having CEA. Preoperative pharmacologic optimization for patients with vascular and cardiac disease was discussed earlier in this chapter. Vascular surgery is associated with an increased risk of major adverse cardiac events.[186] For a complete discussion of cardiac optimization, see Chapter 20. The American College of Cardiology Foundation (ACCF) and American

Intraoperative Considerations

Cerebral Physiology

CBF can remain relatively constant at different cerebral perfusion pressures as a result of cerebrovascular autoregulation. Cerebral perfusion pressure can be expressed as the difference between MAP and intracranial pressure (ICP). During CEA, ICP is usually not elevated, therefore MAP plays the predominant role in determining cerebral perfusion pressure. When MAP is maintained between 60 and 160 mm Hg, CBF remains constant. However, the adverse effects of chronic systemic hypertension shift the patient's cerebral autoregulatory curve to the right, and therefore a higher than normal MAP may be required to ensure adequate cerebral perfusion. CBF is also influenced by arterial carbon dioxide and oxygen concentrations, as well as anesthetic agents. Profound hypocarbia causes cerebral vascular constriction by decreasing CBF. Cerebral steal can occur with hypercarbia as it leads to cerebral vascular dilation in cerebral vessels. However, in those areas of the brain that are at risk of developing ischemia caused by atherosclerotic plaques, the cerebral vessels are maximally dilated. Therefore causing profound cerebral vascular dilation decreases CBF and increases the potential for regional ischemia. Inhalation agents increase CBF due to cerebral vascular dilation in a dose-dependent fashion. Anesthetic agents, with the exception of ketamine, decrease the cerebral metabolic rate of oxygen consumption ($CMRO_2$).

Normal CBF is approximately 50 mL/100 g per min. Neuronal function is generally maintained at levels greater than 25 mL/100 g per min. Blood flow that is less than this critical value jeopardizes cellular function. Decreased perfusion and ischemia can be reflected in changes in consciousness. Cellular death occurs at levels less than 6 mL/100 g per min, as evidenced by the flattening seen on an electroencephalogram (EEG).

Carotid occlusive disease jeopardizes the cerebral perfusion pressure in the ipsilateral artery. Ischemia leads to the disruption of autoregulation and compensatory vasodilation, causing blood flow to become pressure dependent. During CEA, a primary goal is to ensure adequate CBF by maintaining and, if necessary, augmenting MAP.

Cerebral Monitoring

In addition to standard monitoring, direct intraarterial pressure must be continuously assessed via arterial line placement. During CEA, hemodynamic variability frequently occurs. Owing to the high incidence of CAD and neurovascular disease in patients having a CEA, prompt and tight control of blood pressure is imperative.

During repair, the carotid artery cross-clamp is applied distally and proximally to the carotid incision. Various monitoring techniques have been proposed for assessing the adequacy of CBF during this maneuver. A summary of select cerebral monitoring techniques is presented

TABLE 28.8 ACCF/AHA Recommendations for Perioperative Cardiac Assessment

	Scenario	Recommendation
Class I	Patients in need of emergency noncardiac surgery	Proceed directly to the operating room.
	Patients with active cardiac conditions, unstable or severe angina (not stable angina), decompensated heart failure, significant dysrhythmia (high-grade AV block, Mobitz type II block, third-degree AV block, symptomatic ventricular arrhythmias, symptomatic bradycardia, and supraventricular arrhythmias including atrial fibrillation with HR >100 beats/min), and severe valvular disease	Provide perioperative surveillance, risk stratification, and risk factor management.
	Patients undergoing low-risk procedures	Proceed with planned surgery.
	Patients with poor (<4 METs) or unknown functional capacity and no clinical risk factors	
Class IIa	Patients with functional capacity ≥4 METs without symptoms	Proceed with planned surgery.
	Patients with poor (<4 METs) or unknown functional capacity and three or more clinical risk factors* who are undergoing intermediate-risk surgery	Proceed with planned surgery with heart rate control.
	Patients with poor (<4 METs) or unknown functional capacity and one or two clinical risk factors* who are undergoing vascular surgery or intermediate-risk surgery	
	Patients with poor (<4 METs) or unknown functional capacity and three or more clinical risk factors* who are undergoing vascular surgery	Consider further testing if it will change management.
Class IIb	Patients with poor (<4 METs) or unknown functional capacity and three or more clinical risk factors* who are scheduled for intermediate-risk surgery	Consider noninvasive testing if it will change patient management.
	Patients with poor (<4 METs) or unknown functional capacity and one or two clinical risk factors* who are scheduled for vascular surgery or intermediate-risk surgery	

*Clinical risk factors include ischemic heart disease, compensated or prior heart failure, diabetes mellitus, renal insufficiency, and cerebrovascular disease.
Class I recommendations suggest that procedures/treatments should be performed; class IIa recommendations suggest that it is reasonable to perform the procedure/treatment; class IIb recommendations imply that the procedure/treatment should be considered; and in class III the intervention should not be performed because it may not be helpful and may potentially be harmful to the patient.
ACCF/AHA, American College of Cardiology Foundation/American Heart Association; *AV,* atrioventricular; *HR,* heart rate; *METs,* metabolic equivalents.
From Cronenwett JL, Johnston KW. *Rutherford's Vascular Surgery.* 9th ed. Philadelphia: Elsevier; 2019: 507.

BOX 28.14 Cerebral Monitoring Modalities During General Anesthesia for CEA

- Electroencephalogram: assesses cortical electrical function
- Somatosensory-evoked potential: assesses sensory-evoked potentials
- Carotid stump pressure: assesses perfusion pressure in the operative carotid artery
- Transcranial Doppler: assesses blood flow velocity in the middle cerebral artery
- Cerebral oximetry: assesses cerebral regional oxygen saturation (near infrared spectroscopy)

CEA, Carotid endarterectomy.

in Box 28.14. Each of these monitoring modalities has limitations. The most sensitive and specific measure of adequate CBF is responsiveness in an awake patient.

EEG monitoring constitutes the gold standard in identifying neurologic deficits related to carotid artery cross-clamping.[175,187] EEG has demonstrated reliability in monitoring cortical electrical function.[188] Loss of β-wave activity, loss of amplitude, and emergence of slow-wave activity are all indicative of neurologic dysfunction. Limitations surrounding EEG monitoring include (1) the effect of blood pressure, temperature, and anesthetic agents on monitoring; and (2) the fact that this modality detects EEG changes only on the superficial layers of the brain and not in deep cortical structures such as the brainstem.

Carotid stump pressure has been used as a means of assessing collateral flow.[189] After the carotid cross-clamp is placed, blood flow from the nonoperative carotid artery and the basilar artery provides blood flow

to the circle of Willis. A catheter is placed into the distal portion (above the cross clamp) of the operative internal carotid artery, and the pressure can be monitored. Carotid stump pressure is a gross measurement of the pressure within the circle of Willis. A carotid stump pressure of less than 40 to 50 mm Hg reflects neurologic hypoperfusion and is a criterion for shunt placement. However, there is no correlation between stump pressures and EEG changes.[177] In one study, a carotid stump pressure of less than 50 mm Hg had a positive predictive value for only 36% of patients who exhibited ischemic changes on EEG during carotid artery cross-clamping.[190] A combination of stump pressure and either transcranial Doppler (TCD) or EEG appears to improve the detection of cerebral ischemia during carotid artery cross-clamping.[191]

SSEP monitoring can be used to identify inadequate CBF during cross-clamping; however, false-positive results can occur. In addition, SSEPs reflect the sensory integrity of the spinal cord and the brain, therefore a motor deficit can occur despite a normal SSEP waveform. Additionally, there are no values for decreased amplitude and increased latency that definitively correlate with cerebral ischemia. Monitoring both SSEP and EEG is more sensitive for predicting perioperative deficits as compared to using either monitoring modality in isolation. Patients who experience perioperative strokes are 17 times more likely to have a change in either EEG or SSEP than other patients.[192]

TCD velocity monitoring has been used to detect adverse cerebral events during CEA. TCD is noninvasive and measures cerebrovascular dynamics through the CBF velocity. The use of TCD during CEA to determine if carotid shunt placement is necessary is a reliable method to decrease adverse neurologic outcomes.[193] TCD can also be used during the postoperative period to detect ischemia and the presence of cerebral hyperperfusion syndrome (CHS).

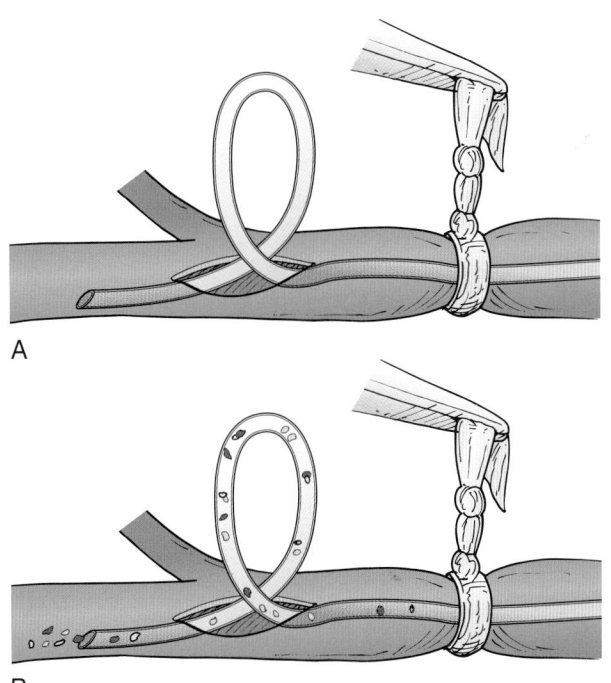

Fig. 28.12 Pitfalls of carotid shunt placement. (A) Potential traumatic injury to the distal internal carotid artery intima. (B) Potential for embolization of atherosclerotic debris or air. (From Cronenwett JL, Johnston W. *Rutherford's Vascular Surgery*. 7th ed. Vol. 2. Philadelphia: Saunders; 2010:1452.)

Near infrared spectroscopy (NIRS) measures cerebral oxygenation. A greater than 20% reduction in regional cerebral oxygenation coincides with regional and global cerebral ischemia during CEA.[194] Despite the established advantages of using NIRS monitoring in cardiac surgery, its routine use is less established during noncardiac procedures. Both NIRS and TCD monitoring are independently accurate in predicting the need for selective shunting by detecting cerebral ischemia during CEA and general anesthesia.[195] As compared with stump pressure monitoring, cerebral oximetry more accurately predicts cerebral oxygenation.[196] Box 28.14 outlines the cerebral monitoring modalities that can be used during general anesthesia for CEA.

Cerebral Protection

The major objective during carotid artery revascularization is to maintain cerebral CBF and oxygenation. Prevention of cerebral ischemia can be accomplished in one of two ways: by increasing collateral flow (placement of intraluminal shunt) or by decreasing cerebral metabolic requirements (anesthetic medications). Multiple interventions are available for cerebral protection, including avoiding hyperglycemia, hemodilution, maintenance of normocarbia, and tight control of arterial blood pressure. Anesthetics, except for etomidate, have cerebral protective properties and may be used to minimize the degree of cerebral ischemia. Shunt placement is commonly used to allow blood to flow proximally and distally to the carotid cross-clamp during intimal plaque dissection. Potential complications associated with carotid shunt placement are depicted in Fig. 28.12.

Cerebral ischemic events are most often the result of embolic complications and frequently occur during the postoperative period. The need for shunt placement is based on surgeon preference and information obtained using intraoperative monitoring techniques to determine CBF. Furthermore, propofol decreases $CMRO_2$ to 40%

below normal values.[114] Dexmedetomidine also decreases cerebral oxygen consumption and CBF in animal models.[197] During transient focal ischemia, propofol decreases the $CMRO_2$, which results in cerebral protection. The disadvantages of administering propofol during CEA surgery include myocardial depression and hypotension. The inhalation agents also decrease $CMRO_2$ in a dose-dependent fashion. Nitrous oxide should be avoided due to the potential for pneumocephalus from microbubble expansion after carotid artery unclamping.[175,182]

Blood Pressure Control

The presence of hypertension in patients with cerebrovascular disease is well known, and therefore one of the most challenging aspects of care associated with anesthesia for CEA is blood pressure control. Patients with cerebral insufficiency are vulnerable to perioperative blood pressure instability. Hypotension occurs in 10% to 50% of patients who undergo CEA and is believed to be the result of carotid sinus baroreceptor stimulation. Conversely, 10% to 66% of patients experience hypertension, which is attributed to surgical manipulation of the carotid sinus.[198] Preoperative blood pressure control, volume status, and depth of anesthesia can also contribute to intraoperative hemodynamic instability. During carotid artery cross-clamping, maintaining the MAP at 20% or greater of the patient's preoperative mean pressure decreases postoperative cognitive dysfunction.[199]

Blood pressure control must begin in the preoperative phase. All patients should continue taking their antihypertensive medications until the time of surgery. Patients with systolic blood pressure greater than 180 mm Hg may be at increased risk of stroke and death.[182] Additional pharmacologic agents may be required in the preoperative period, especially during the insertion of intravenous and intraarterial catheters, to reduce increases in heart rate and blood pressure. The induction of anesthesia, the initial incision, dissection, manipulation of the carotid sinus, and emergence from anesthesia are all events that precipitate blood pressure fluctuations. The use of pharmacologic adjuncts, such as short-acting β-adrenergic blockers, may stabilize blood pressure during induction and emergence. Continuous intravenous use of nitroglycerin or sodium nitroprusside should be available to treat hypertension. Patients with chronic hypertension are predisposed to dramatic decreases in blood pressure after the induction of general anesthesia. This condition must be treated promptly and can be successfully managed by providing intravenous fluids or administering appropriate vasopressors. Hypotension and bradycardia, which result from carotid sinus baroreceptor manipulation, may be inhibited by stopping surgical stimulation, infiltrating the region with local anesthesia, and administering an anticholinergic (as necessary).

Anesthetic Management

The anesthetic objectives for vascular surgery are similar to those for any type of elective procedure: to provide analgesia and amnesia, to facilitate surgical intervention, and to minimize operative morbidity and mortality. Goals that are specific to CEA include maintaining cerebral and myocardial perfusion and oxygenation, minimizing the stress response, and facilitating a smooth and rapid emergence. However, it may be difficult to maintain the integrity of one system without adversely affecting the other. For example, raising the arterial blood pressure to augment cerebral perfusion can increase myocardial oxygen demand, which may lead to ischemia. In addition, significantly decreasing blood pressure can lead to cerebral hypoperfusion. Therefore the anesthetic goal is to optimize perfusion to the brain, minimize myocardial workload, ensure cardiovascular stability, and

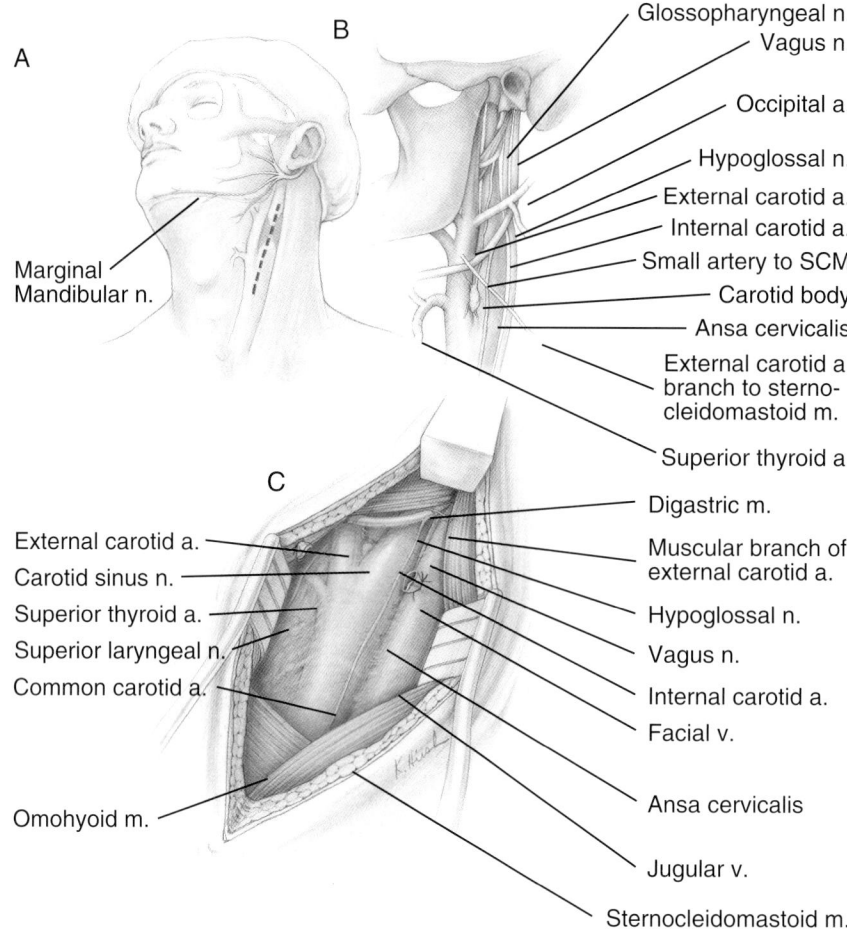

Fig. 28.13 Carotid endarterectomy. (A) Incision site. (B, C) Anatomic structures presented at the carotid surgical site. *a*, Artery; *m*, muscle; *n*, nerve; *SCM*, sternocleidomastoid; *v*, vein. (From Zarins CK, Gewertz BL. *Atlas of Vascular Surgery.* 2nd ed. Philadelphia. Churchill Livingstone; 2009.)

allow for rapid emergence. Anticoagulation is achieved via administration of heparin (50–100 units/kg) prior to carotid artery cross-clamping. The decision to administer protamine upon completion of the surgical procedure is based on the surgeon's impression. Protamine administration is associated with a reduction in bleeding complications without increasing major thrombotic outcomes, including stroke, MI, or death after CEA.[200] Protamine administration is associated with hypotension. Anaphylaxis is a rare but life-threatening side effect. An understanding of the physiology of the cerebrovascular system is important for optimal anesthetic management. Fig. 28.13 illustrates the anatomy of structures in this region. This knowledge enables the selection of appropriate monitoring and anesthetic techniques that will protect and improve cerebral and myocardial perfusion.

Anesthetic Selection

The long-standing question has been whether there is an advantage of regional vs general anesthesia for CEA. The General Anesthetic versus Local Anesthetic for Carotid Surgery Trial (GALA), as well as a Cochrane meta-analysis, indicate no significant difference between the two anesthetic techniques.[201,202] The anesthetic selection is based on the surgeon's preference, the patient's condition, and the preoperative evaluation. Advantages of a regional technique are that an awake patient can respond to commands and allow for continuous assessment of neurologic function. If the patient's level of consciousness decreases as a result of cerebral hypoperfusion,

surgeons can then place a shunt. Other potential benefits include improved patient satisfaction, decreased cost, and minimization of potential postoperative cognitive effects associated with general anesthesia.[203-205] Disadvantages include patient agitation and inability to remain still, minimal airway control, seizure or stroke during carotid artery clamping, and limited ability to give anesthetic medications. Advantages of general anesthesia include the ability to perform more extensive and difficult surgical procedures, better airway control, the ability to administer cerebral protectants, and improved blood pressure control.[175,182]

Regional anesthesia. A regional anesthetic (RA) technique during CEA requires a deep and superficial cervical plexus block, which is accomplished by anesthetizing cervical nerves II to IV.[175] Superficial cervical blocks do not anesthetize the region at the angle of the mandible, which is innervated by the trigeminal nerve. Local infiltration may be required. As noted previously, the greatest advantage of RA is the ability to directly assess neurologic function in an awake individual. Assessing level of consciousness is the most effective method of assessing the adequacy of CBF and detecting cerebral ischemia. In fact, assessment of consciousness in the awake patient may be more sensitive than conventional EEG in detecting cerebral ischemia. Researchers reviewed data from 399 patients who underwent CEA while receiving either GA or RA. The authors concluded that perioperative strokes occurred less often when RA was administered, especially in high-risk patients.[206] Another study compared middle cerebral artery blood flow velocity using TCD monitoring in patients undergoing CEA with either local or GA.[207] There is significant evidence to support that the preservation of cerebral circulation is better maintained in patients who receive local anesthesia.[208-211] In addition, further evidence suggests that patients who receive GA are more likely to receive a shunt compared with those who receive RA.[212] RA resulted in fewer hemodynamic fluctuations and fewer intraoperative vasoactive medication requirements as compared with GA during perioperative management of CEA.[213] However, despite these seemingly physiologic advantages, no differences were observed in outcomes between the RA and GA groups. The use of RA has been associated with shorter operative times, fewer cardiopulmonary complications, and a shorter duration of postoperative hospitalization.

One limiting factor for the use of RA is patient tolerance. The individual is mildly sedated; therefore preoperative education is essential, and patient cooperation during surgery is vital. Anxiety, fear, and apprehension can initiate sympathetic stimulation, and as a result extreme hemodynamic responses can occur. Deep sedation, which is sometimes necessary in an apprehensive patient, may confound the neurologic assessment, subsequently negating the advantages of a regional technique. Additionally, hypercarbia can result from hypoventilation, and dysphoria is more likely to occur. Furthermore, converting to a GA technique once surgery has begun can be problematic. Symptoms indicating that adequate cerebral perfusion has been compromised include dizziness, contralateral weakness, decreased mentation, and loss of consciousness. In the event that this scenario occurs, immediate shunt placement is warranted. If symptoms associated with cerebral hypoperfusion do not resolve rapidly with shunt placement, emergent airway management is necessary.

General anesthesia. Although the use of RA has numerous advantages, GA is also used during CEA. Perhaps the greatest benefit of this technique is that it counters the most cited disadvantage of regional anesthesia: lack of patient tolerance during the procedure. GA promotes a motionless field during surgery. In addition, inhalation agents may provide hemodynamic stability and may have beneficial effects on cerebral circulation.[214] By decreasing cerebral and cardiac metabolism, the inhalation agents provide a degree of protection against ischemia, an effect called anesthetic preconditioning.[215-217]

There is no scientific evidence to suggest that patient outcome is improved when inhaled agents are used compared to narcotic-based techniques. In studies of inhalation agents, the critical regional CBF (the blood flow measurement for which EEG signs of ischemia occur) during isoflurane anesthesia was less than when other volatile anesthetics were used.[214,218] The effects of sufentanil on cerebral hemodynamics were similar to those of isoflurane.[219] Remifentanil can be used, and its rapid metabolism improves neurologic recovery. The inhalation agents may alter the monitoring methods used for detecting cerebral ischemia, such as EEG and SSEP monitoring. In these cases, GA may require modification, and direct communication between the anesthesia and surgical teams is vital. When carotid artery cross-clamping without shunting occurs, MAP values must be 20% or greater of the patient's preoperative MAP to help ensure adequate cerebral perfusion through the contralateral carotid artery and decrease the possibility of postoperative cognitive dysfunction.[199] The use of nitrous oxide during CEA can potentially increase the incidence of a clinically significant pneumocephalus. During shunt placement and carotid artery cross-clamp release, microbubbles can be entrained into the carotid artery blood flow. Nitrous oxide is also known to cause hyperhomocysteinemia. Increased homocysteine can increase the postoperative cardiac risk and long-term mortality and

increase the potential for carotid artery restenosis.[220,221] If nitrous oxide is used, it should be discontinued before removal of the carotid artery cross-clamp.[175,182]

In summary, there is no scientific consensus supporting the notion that a specific anesthetic technique is superior in decreasing perioperative morbidity and mortality post-CEA. Ensuring adequate cerebral and cardiac perfusion by treating hypertensive and hypotensive episodes aggressively is important. An anesthetic plan that allows for a rapid assessment of neurologic function at the completion of surgery should be selected.

Postoperative Considerations

Perhaps the most common problem experienced in the postoperative period is hypertension. Although the specific cause remains unclear, postoperative hypertension is likely related to changes in sensitivity of the carotid baroreceptor reflex. A systolic blood pressure greater than 180 mm Hg is associated with an increased incidence of TIA, stroke, or MI.[183] Patients with a systolic blood pressure of 145 mm Hg or less tend to have fewer postoperative complications.[169] A postoperative blood pressure of 140/80 mm Hg or less is recommended.[222] Chronic hypertension during the postoperative period can lead to the development of CHS as described later. Postoperative hypertension often resolves within 24 hours after surgery. Postoperative hypotension is less common but can be more difficult to treat because raising the blood pressure increases myocardial oxygen demand. Reestablishing normal pressures can be accomplished by careful titration of fluids and vasopressors.

Although an uncommon complication, carotid artery hemorrhage can occur in the postoperative phase. Hemorrhage is a devastating event that requires immediate surgical intervention. One of the initial manifestations of hemorrhage may be upper airway obstruction, which may make reintubation difficult due to tracheal deviation. Emergency management of a patient with airway compromise as a result of carotid artery hemorrhage and hematoma includes immediate evacuation of the hematoma. In addition, recurrent laryngeal nerve damage can occur, which routinely manifests as inspiratory stridor. Respiratory insufficiency can be problematic for patients who have preexisting respiratory conditions. Tension pneumothorax also can occur because the apices of the lungs extend above the clavicles toward the surgical site. Treatment includes immediate lung reexpansion via chest tube insertion or needle decompression. Damage to the carotid body can lead to blunting of the chemoreceptor reflex, necessitating the administration of supplemental oxygen. Lastly, CHS may result from increased blood flow to the brain as a result of a loss of cerebral vascular autoregulation. The mechanism of action that causes this phenomenon is unclear; however, it is hypothesized that CHS may occur as a result of chronic cerebral ischemia or altered cerebrovascular autoregulation. Signs and symptoms of CHS include severe headache, visual disturbances, altered level of consciousness, and seizures. CHS may occur more often in patients who have had a contralateral CEA within the last 3 months and undergo a second CEA for occlusion on the ipsilateral side.[223]

The incidence of postoperative stroke after CEA was discussed previously. Unfortunately, even after successful revascularization of the carotid artery, occlusion can recur at a rate of 3% per year.[179] Although symptoms are present in only a small percentage of patients (3%–5%), the incidence of recurrent carotid stenosis may be much larger than that reported because asymptomatic cases may be overlooked.[223] As many as 25% of patients experience a neurocognitive decline up to 1 month after surgery. Patients who are predisposed to this decline are those with diabetes and advanced age.[224] The exact mechanism responsible for postoperative cognitive dysfunction has not been scientifically identified. Postoperative complications associated with CEA are listed in Box 28.15.

Owing to the anatomic location of and potential neurologic complications after CEA, postemergence neurologic integrity should be assessed. In addition to neurocognitive functioning, clinical assessment of cranial nerve function should be performed (Table 28.9). The anatomic locations of the cranial nerves in relation to the internal, external, and common carotid arteries are shown in Fig. 28.14.

CAROTID ARTERY ANGIOPLASTY STENTING

A less invasive surgical approach for the treatment of carotid artery stenosis is carotid artery angioplasty and stenting (i.e., CAS). Controversy exists regarding the degree of success that this procedure affords as an alternative to CEA. The best application of CAS is still evolving, and many studies comparing stenting with endarterectomy are ongoing. Best practices regarding proper patient selection, technique, and timing of the procedure are still being explored.[225,226] The current incidence of stroke after CEA is approximately 2%. A meta-analysis noted that, compared to CAS, CEA decreases the risk of stroke at 30 days, increases the risk of MI, and has no effect on the risk of death.[227]

The first large multicenter randomized controlled trial comparing CEA vs CAS was the Stenting and Angioplasty with Protection Patients at High Risk for Endarterectomy (SAPPHIRE) trial.[228] The rate of event-free survival at 1-year postsurgery was 88% for the CAS group and 79.9% for the CEA group. The stroke rate after 1 year was lower in the CAS group as compared with the CEA group (6.2% vs 7.9%, respectively). As for cardiac morbidity, the rate of MI for CAS vs CEA was 1.9% vs 6.6% at 30 days postoperatively. Overall, cardiac morbidity was 3% for CAS and 6.2% for CEA. The conclusion drawn from the SAPPHIRE trial was that CAS does not yield inferior outcomes as compared with CEA. However, the study methodology was criticized, and some experts questioned whether the results could be replicated.[229] A new 3-year follow-up report of the SAPPHIRE study group indicates that in patients with severe carotid artery stenosis and increased surgical risk, no significant difference could be shown in long-term outcomes between patients who underwent CAS with an emboliprotection device and those who underwent endarterectomy.[230]

The Endarterectomy versus Angioplasty with Symptomatic Severe Carotid Stenosis (EVA-3S) trial was designed to compare the outcomes from CAS vs CEA. The study population included patients with symptomatic carotid stenosis of at least 60%. The study was stopped early because of a high incidence of stroke and death (9.6% compared with 3.9% for CEA at 30 days after surgery). The conclusion was that CEA was superior to CAS for this patient population when considering risk of stroke at 30 days and 6 months postoperatively.[231] Another randomized controlled trial, the Stent-Protected Angioplasty versus Carotid Endarterectomy (SPACE) trial, yielded high but similar statistics for 30-day stroke death rates (6.8% for CAS and 6.3% for CEA).[232]

The goal of the Carotid Revascularization Endarterectomy versus Stenting Trial (CREST), a randomized controlled trial, was to determine which procedure (CAS or CEA) was more effective in preventing stroke and death. Inclusion criteria were patients who were symptomatic and had greater than 50% carotid artery stenosis and those who were asymptomatic with greater than 60% carotid artery stenosis. The preliminary results from the first stage of the trial, which included 1000 patients, are encouraging and compare favorably with CEA. The rate of death or stroke from any cause during the 30 days after the procedure was 3% for asymptomatic patients under 80 years of age and 2.7% for symptomatic patients under 80 years of age.[233] Initial indications were that CAS was associated with an increased incidence of stroke in octogenarians. However, it has now been determined that the incidence of stroke resulting from CAS is similar to the CEA results for all age groups.[234] The CREST data show that the health-related quality of life in patients who underwent CAS is superior to those who underwent CEA for up to 1 year postoperatively.[235] The CREST study was conducted over a 10-year period. It was determined that there were no significant differences between patients who had CEA vs CAS with respect to stroke, MI, and death.[236]

> ### BOX 28.15 Postoperative Complications of Carotid Endarterectomy
>
> - Hemodynamic instability
> - Myocardial ischemia/Infarction
> - Cerebral hyperperfusion syndrome
> - Stroke
> - Respiratory insufficiency
> - Recurrent/superior laryngeal nerve damage
> - Hematoma
> - Carotid body dysfunction
> - Tension pneumothorax
> - Acute carotid occlusion

TABLE 28.9 Cranial Nerve Assessment for the Patient Scheduled for CEA

Cranial Nerve	Function	Abnormal Response
VII (facial)	Muscles of facial expression, saliva secretion	Inability to smile symmetrically; contralateral asymmetry indicates possible stroke; nerve injury on ipsilateral side
IX (glossopharyngeal)	Swallowing, pharyngeal muscle	Difficulty swallowing with ipsilateral Horner syndrome (i.e., ptosis, miosis, exophthalmos, reduced sweating)
X (vagus) → superior and recurrent laryngeal nerves	Laryngeal muscle movement	Minor swallowing problems, fatigued voice; vocal cord paralysis, hoarseness, inadequate gag reflex; may test speech by having the patient say "EEE"
XI spinal accessory	Shoulder muscles	Ipsilateral weakness in neck and shoulder with shrugging
XII (hypoglossal)*	Muscles of tongue	Tongue sticks out and moves side to side; tongue droops to ipsilateral side; difficulty with speech and chewing, high-pitched sounds, hoarseness

*This nerve traverses the internal carotid artery.
CEA, Carotid endarterectomy.
From Heffine MS. Care of the vascular surgical patient. In Odom-Forren J, ed. *Drain's Perianesthesia Nursing: A Critical Care Approach*. 6th ed. St Louis: Elsevier; 2013.

Case selection guidelines for CAS are listed in Table 28.10. Prior to CAS, a high-resolution MRI is taken of the patient's aortic arch and carotid arteries, as well as a cerebral angiogram. This allows evaluation of the individual anatomy and angiopathology of the aortic arch, brachiocephalic artery (for right carotid artery stent), or left common carotid artery. The type of sheaths, stents, and cerebral embolic protection device needed can then be determined. Femoral artery access is obtained, and a sheath is then threaded through the aortic arch and into the operative carotid artery. The guide wire/embolic protection device is advanced through the sheath and positioned across the stenotic region. An embolic protection device sequesters emboli during angioplasty and stenting to avoid distal occlusion in cerebral arteries (Fig. 28.15). A distal embolic protection device lowers the risk of intraoperative and postoperative adverse events.[237] This filterlike device is inserted distal to the area of stenosis prior to the angioplasty and stent deployment to catch microthrombi and pieces of plaque that could lodge within the brain. Angioplasty with a 5-mm balloon dilates the carotid artery, and then the stent is deployed. The guide wire/device wire is removed after angiographic confirmation that carotid artery dissection or occlusion has not occurred. Fig. 28.16 shows carotid artery patency after angioplasty and stent placement.

Anesthetic Considerations

The anesthetic technique used most often for patients having CAS is local anesthesia at the femoral insertion site, minimal sedation, antithrombotic therapy, and observation for hypotension and bradycardia.[238] Anticoagulation is initiated with a heparin bolus (50–100 units/kg) to maintain an activated clotting time greater than 250 seconds.[239] Balloon inflation in the internal carotid artery can stimulate the baroreceptor response, resulting in prolonged bradycardia and hypotension. Glycopyrrolate or atropine can be given prior to inflation to offset this vagal response. Fluoroscopy will be used throughout the surgery

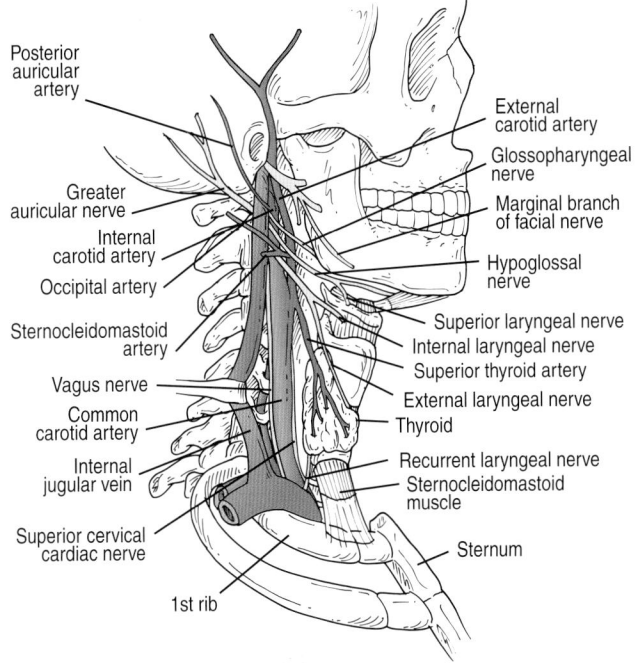

Fig. 28.14 Relationship of the cranial nerves and their major branches to the common, internal, and external carotids in the neck. (From Eisele DW, Smith RV, eds. *Complications in Head and Neck Surgery*. Philadelphia: Elsevier; 2009.)

TABLE 28.10	Case Selection for Carotid Artery Stenting	
CAS Worse	**CAS Better**
Clinical Features	
Advanced age (≥80 yr)	COPD
Intolerance of antiplatelet agents	CHD with an abnormal cardiac stress test, unstable angina, or myocardial infarction
Severe renal dysfunction	<1 mo ago
	Valvular heart disease
	Congestive heart failure (EF <30%)
	Contralateral recurrent laryngeal nerve dysfunction
	Severe obesity
Anatomic Features	
Access related	Previous neck irradiation
Shaggy aorta	Previous radical neck surgery
Eggshell aorta	Tracheostomy
Severely angulated type III aortic arch	Neck immobility
Aortoiliac occlusive disease	Recurrent stenosis
Target vessel related	High lesions (>C2)
Heavy calcification	Contralateral carotid occlusion
Severe tortuosity	
String sign	
Fresh thrombus	
Unstable plaque	

CAS, Carotid artery stenting; *CHD,* coronary heart disease; *COPD,* chronic obstructive pulmonary disease; *EF,* ejection fraction.
Adapted from Cronenwett JL, Johnston W. *Rutherford's Vascular Surgery.* 9th ed. Vol. 2 Philadelphia: Elsevier; 2019.

so it is important that all operating room personnel are protected with lead shielding.

Complications associated with CAS are listed in Box 28.16. The most common complication associated with this procedure is stroke caused by thromboembolism.[240] Interventions for a patient with an acute stroke include airway and hemodynamic management. Immediate CT scan and identification of the presence of an embolus is

critical. Neurologic deficits are significantly reversible if CBF is restored within 2 hours. Treatment with catheter-directed recombinant tissue plasminogen activator is approved for acute ischemic stroke that is believed to be caused by an embolus. Catheter-based thrombectomy using snares or balloon angioplasty to restore blood flow and remove the thromboembolic material has also been used successfully. In general, the incidence of CVA is greater with CAS,

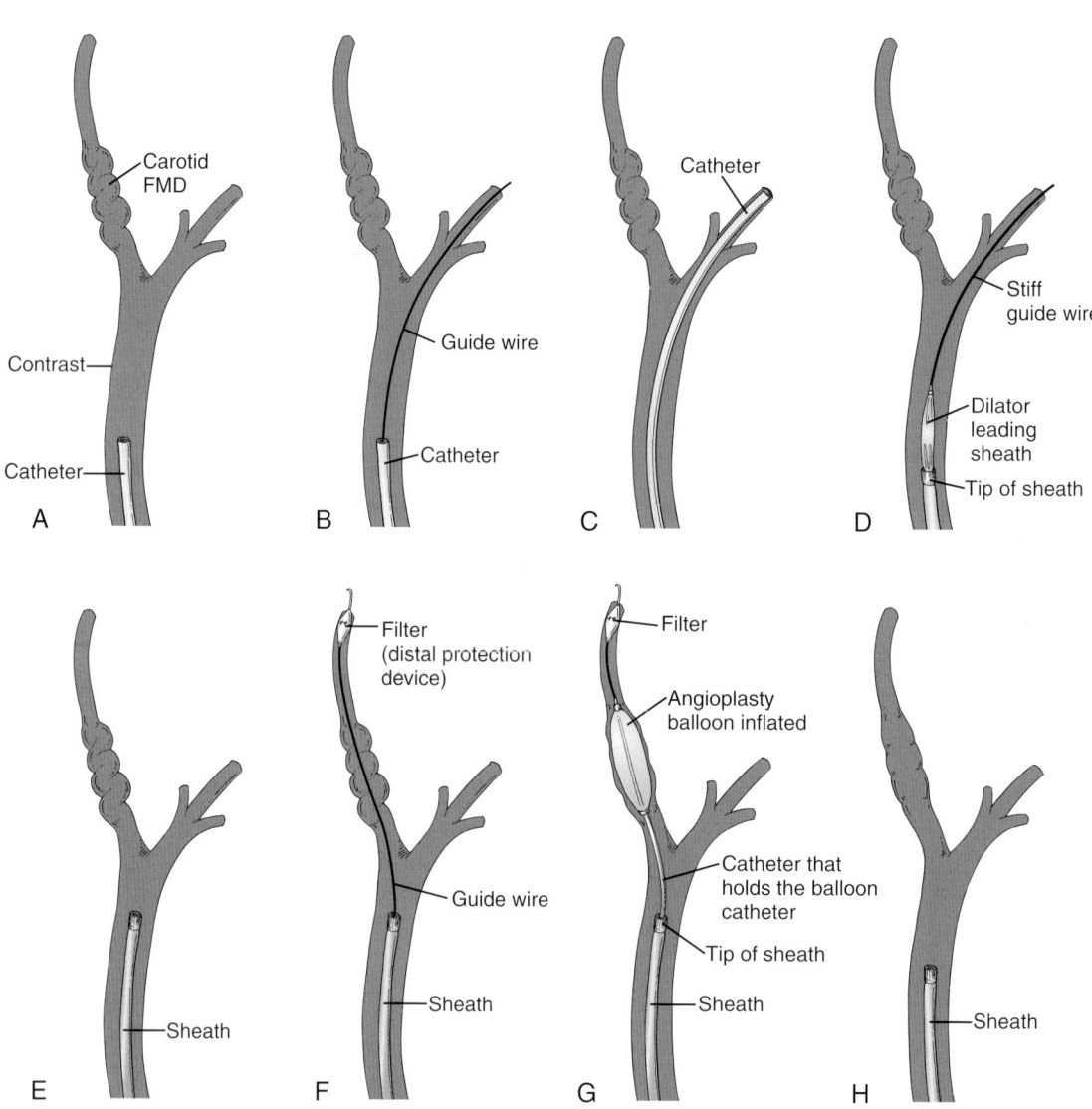

Fig. 28.15 Endovascular technique. (A) Internal carotid artery narrowed by fibromuscular dysplasia. An arteriogram was performed through a carotid catheter. (B) Guide wire placed in the external carotid artery by using a roadmap of the carotid bifurcation. (C) Cerebral catheter advanced into the external carotid artery. (D) Stiff guide wire advanced into the external carotid artery. The carotid access sheath is advanced over the exchange guide wire. (E) Carotid sheath in place with the tip of the sheath in the distal common carotid artery. (F) Cerebral protection device in place in the distal internal carotid artery. (G) Balloon angioplasty of the fibromuscular lesion in the internal carotid artery. (H) After balloon angioplasty, the patency of the lumen has improved significantly. *FMD,* Fibromuscular dysplasia. (From Cronenwett JL, Johnston W. *Rutherford's Vascular Surgery.* 9th ed. Vol. 2. Philadelphia: Elsevier; 2019:1528.)

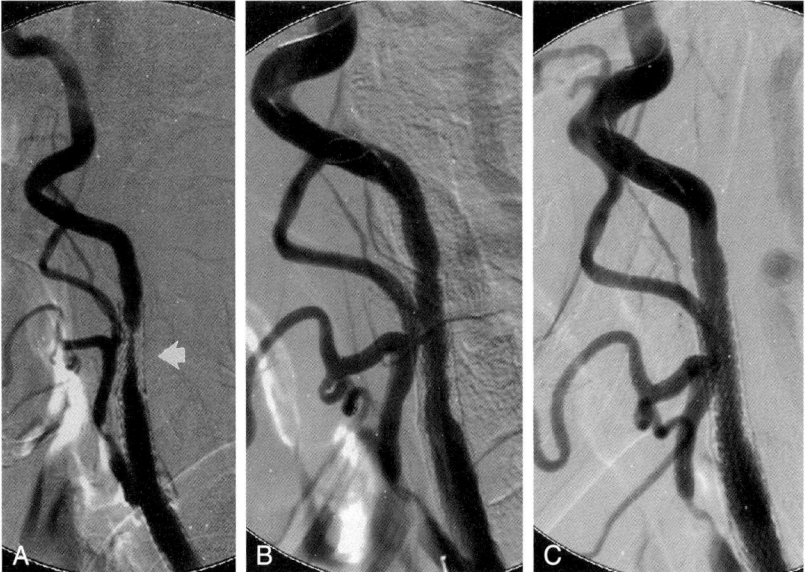

Fig. 28.16 (A) High-grade restenosis of internal carotid artery *(arrowhead)* 11 months after carotid angioplasty/stenting with a wall stent. (B) After angioplasty alone. (C) After placement of a nitinol stent. Note filter protection device in distal internal carotid artery. (From Rutherford RB. *Vascular Surgery.* 8th ed. Vol. 2. Philadelphia: Elsevier; 2014.)

and the incidence of MI is greater with CEA. The long-term morbidity and mortality comparing the two surgical interventions are presently inconclusive. Due to the increased risks of periprocedural stroke, CEA is thought to be the preferred method for the management of asymptomatic carotid stenosis.[241]

Patients typically remain in the postanesthesia care unit for 30 minutes after carotid stent placement and are then transferred to a monitored floor. A carotid duplex scan is performed prior to discharge and then routinely obtained at 6 weeks, 6 months, 1 year, and yearly thereafter. Patients remain on aspirin therapy for anticoagulation for life.[242]

BOX 28.16 Complications Associated With Carotid Artery Stenting

- Stroke
- Myocardial ischemia/infarction
- Bradycardia
- Hypotension
- Deformation of expandable stent
- Stent thrombosis
- Horner syndrome
- Cerebral hyperperfusion syndrome
- Carotid artery dissection
- Carotid artery rupture
- Hemorrhage resulting from anticoagulation

SUMMARY

As the mean age of people in the United States increases, treatment of vascular disease is one of the fastest changing areas of medicine. Minimally invasive vascular surgical techniques are being introduced that are revolutionizing the options available for treatment. Many highly invasive surgical techniques are now being performed as interventional radiologic procedures. Anesthetic management for vascular procedures is far different from just a few years ago and requires that we adapt to ever-new treatment strategies. As technology practice evolves, we will be better able to assess growing evidence that suggests the superiority of these procedures in decreasing patient morbidity, mortality, and convalescence.

REFERENCES

For a complete list of references for this chapter, scan this QR code with any smartphone code reader app, or visit the following URL: http://booksite.elsevier.com/9780323711944/.

29

Respiratory Anatomy, Physiology, Pathophysiology, and Anesthesia Management

Jeremy S. Heiner

Knowledge of the respiratory system is essential to the practice of anesthesia. A thorough understanding and command of the entire respiratory system is necessary because anesthetists give oxygen to the majority of patients, administer inhaled anesthetics down a cascade of concentration gradients through the lungs, provide artificial ventilation for many patients under general anesthesia, and monitor and interpret blood gas analysis, capnography, and oximetry.

The respiratory system provides the essential basic functions of extracting oxygen (O_2) from the atmosphere and delivering it to the blood while excreting carbon dioxide (CO_2). In addition, the respiratory system is involved in the functions and processes of maintaining acid-base balance, phonation, pulmonary defense, and metabolism (synthesis and breakdown of bioactive materials). The general components of the respiratory system are the conducting airways, the lungs and their blood supply, the portions of the central nervous system responsible for control of the muscles of ventilation, the chest wall, and the thoracic muscles responsible for ventilation. These anatomic and physiologic functions are all discussed in this chapter.

ANATOMY AND PHYSIOLOGY OF THE RESPIRATORY SYSTEM

Knowledge of airway anatomy is not only necessary for understanding respiratory physiology but also essential for the practice of anesthesia. The upper airway consists of the nose, mouth, nasopharynx, oropharynx, hypopharynx, and larynx. The lower airway consists of the trachea; main, lobar, and segmental bronchi; conducting, terminal, and respiratory bronchioles; alveoli ducts; and alveolar sacs.

ANATOMIC STRUCTURES OF THE RESPIRATORY SYSTEM

Nose

Inhaled air enters the body through the nose or mouth. Air passing through the nose is filtered, heated to body temperature, and humidified. The external nose is only a small part of the nasal air passageway; the major portion lies inside the nostrils and includes three scroll-shaped turbinate bones called the nasal conchae.

The cartilage around the entrance to the nostrils that can flare during heavy breathing is called the alar cartilage or ala nasae ("nasal wings"). Each nostril opening (anterior naris) leads directly into the vestibule, which is the anterior expanded portion of the nasal cavity. The vestibule is lined with cutaneous epithelium. Its initial lower half contains sebaceous glands and coarse hairs, which serve to filter incoming air. The base of the nasal cavity is at a level higher than the opening of the nostril. This has implications during nasal intubation, necessitating that the apex of the nose be elevated superiorly with gentle pressure while the tube is inserted parallel to the roof of the mouth. The endotracheal tube (ETT) should be directed not upward into the turbinates but rather along the floor of the nose formed by the superior aspect of the palatine bone, which forms the hard palate of the mouth directly below the nose. Prolonged nasotracheal intubation is associated with obstruction of the nasal sinuses, sinus infection, and fever. Intranasal infections can produce an intracranial infection via vascular connections.

The anterior portion of the external nose, the vestibule, expands above and behind into triangular spaces, or fossae. The fossae are separated from each other by the nasal septum, which also separates the two nostrils. The septum is formed by the ethmoid and vomer bones superiorly and the vomeronasal and nasal septal cartilages inferiorly. The nasal fossae usually communicate freely with the paranasal air sinuses (frontal, ethmoid, maxillary, and sphenoid). They open into the nasopharynx by the posterior nares (also known as choanae) and are bordered medially by the nasal septum and laterally by three turbinates arranged one above the other. Choanal atresia is a birth defect characterized by obstruction of the posterior nasal airway. This obstruction may be life threatening in the obligate nose-breathing newborn.

The conchae are scroll-shaped prominences projecting from the lateral walls and have their free margins directed downward and inward. The conchae overlie the superior, middle, and inferior meatus, which contain the openings to the paranasal sinuses. The superior concha is the smallest of the three, and the middle concha extends forward much farther than the superior concha. The inferior concha, which lies along the inferior part of the lateral wall of the nasal cavity, is in the pathway of airflow in the nose, and it is the one most commonly injured during nasal intubation or nasal intrumentation. It extends to within approximately 2 cm of the middle of the anterior naris, and its posterior tip lies approximately 1 cm in front of the pharyngeal orifice of the eustachian tube. Eustachian drainage can become obstructed when the inferior concha or adenoid tonsils become inflamed. Such obstruction can lead to middle ear pathology.

The nasal cavities are lined with mucous membranes that are continuous with those of the pharynx. The mucosa can be divided into respiratory and olfactory areas because it not only lines the tracts followed by respired air but also covers the cells that act as the receptors for smell. The olfactory epithelium occupies the apical third of the nasal cavity. This epithelium contains afferent fibers from the olfactory nerves (cranial nerve I) that communicate through the cribriform plate of the ethmoid bone to the adjacent olfactory bulb. Signals then progress to the other parts of the rhinencephalon. The respiratory mucosa lines the lower two-thirds of the nose and consists of pseudostratified ciliated columnar epithelium interspersed with goblet cells that produce mucus. Although the morphology of cells changes progressively toward the terminal bronchioles, this general arrangement of stratified ciliated epithelium with goblet cells persists throughout the majority of air passages within the respiratory system. The directed motion of the cilia within the respiratory tract is toward the exterior of the nasal cavity or toward the pharyngeal areas for swallowing.[1-5]

The principal arterial supply of the nasal fossae arises from the ophthalmic arteries through the anterior and posterior ethmoid branches, and from the internal maxillary artery through the sphenopalatine arteries. Because of the location of the interior maxillary artery, it is sometimes ligated for the treatment of persistent nosebleed. The veins accompany the arteries; the ethmoid veins open into the superior sagittal sinus, and the nasal veins drain into the ophthalmic veins and then into the cavernous sinuses. Nasal infections can result in meningitis because of this venous communication between the intracranial and intranasal circulation. The sensory nerves from the upper respiratory tract come from the ophthalmic nerve and the maxillary nerve (both are branches of cranial nerve V). Lymphatic drainage from the cavities of the nose is via the deep cervical lymph nodes adjacent to the internal jugular vein.

Through the functioning of the nasal hairs, the mucus-producing epithelium, and the rich arterial supply, the nose has important functions that include filtration, humidification, and heating of inspired air. As long as the incoming air is not extremely cold, the nose can warm the inspired air to nearly body temperature and moisten it to nearly 100% relative humidity. The heating and humidifying functions of the nose are affected by general anesthesia. The inspiration of cold, dry gas often dries the nasal and pharyngeal mucosa and passageways, causing a sore throat even if no instrumentation of the airway occurs.

The hairs at the entrance to the nostrils are of minor importance to filtration because they remove only large particles. More important is the removal of particles by turbulent precipitation. Air passing through the nasal passageways hits many obstructions, including the septum, the turbinates, and the pharyngeal wall. When the inspired air is forced to change direction, the inhaled particles cannot change course as rapidly, and they become embedded in the mucus-covered surfaces of these processes. The particles trapped in the mucus are moved by the cilia either to the naris or posteriorly to the pharynx to be expectorated or swallowed. The trapping and removal of particles is important because it does not allow entry of infectious, carcinogenic, or irritating substances. Nasal filtration is extremely effective for particles above 10 mcm and less than 1 nm, but filtration efficiency is inverse to particle size for particles that are between 10 nm and 1 mcm.[1-5]

Pharynx

The pharynx is a wide, muscular tube that is a part of both the respiratory tract and the alimentary canal. Its upper border is the base of the skull, and it extends to the level of the C6 vertebra where it becomes continuous with the esophagus. If a foreign body is ingested, such as a coin, it can be frequently lodged at this level. The pharynx is lined by a musculomembranous coat and divided into three parts: the nasopharynx, which extends from the posterior nares (choanae) to the end of the soft palate; the oropharynx, which is bounded superiorly by the soft palate and anteriorly by the tonsillar pillars and oral cavity, and extends inferiorly to the tip of the epiglottis; and the hypopharynx (laryngopharynx), which extends from the tip of the epiglottis to the level of C6, or the beginning of the esophagus.

The pharyngeal region includes the tonsils, which are composed of four aggregations of lymphoid tissue: the palatine tonsils (major

TABLE 29.1 The Nine Cartilages of the Larynx

UNPAIRED CARTILAGES		PAIRED CARTILAGES	
Number	Name	Number	Name
1	Epiglottic	4 and 5	Arytenoids
2	Thyroid	6 and 7	Corniculates
3	Cricoid	8 and 9	Cuneiforms

tonsils), which lie in the tonsillar fossae at the boundary of the oral cavity and oropharynx (these are the tonsils that can be visualized in back of the mouth); the lingual tonsils, which extend across the tongue from the base of each palatine tonsil; the tubal tonsils, which are positioned on the roof of the nasopharynx inferior and lateral to the pharyngeal tonsils; and the pharyngeal tonsils (adenoids), which are located in the center part of the nasopharyngeal roof. The lymphoid tissue of the tonsils forms the Waldeyer tonsillar ring, which acts as a first line of defense against bacterial invasion of the nasal, oral, and buccal passages. If inflamed, the pharyngeal tonsils may obstruct airflow through the choanae and are sometimes removed by an adenoidectomy. Likewise, chronic tonsillitis is an indication for removal of the palatine tonsils via tonsillectomy.[1-5]

Larynx

The adult larynx extends from vertebrae C3 to C6 and is primarily a protective structure to prevent aspiration during swallowing. Its use for vocalization evolved secondarily. The larynx consists of one bone, nine cartilages (Table 29.1), ligaments, muscles, and membranes.

The hyoid bone is the chief support for the larynx, and it is the only bone that does not form a joint with another bone. Its anterior aspect can be easily palpated, and its location is sometimes used as a measure of airway assessment for laryngoscopy. The thyroid cartilage and the cricoid cartilage make up the principal part of the framework of the larynx, whereas internally the epiglottis protects the vocal cords and the entrance to the trachea against aspiration of foreign material such as food or fluids.

Laryngeal Cartilages

There are three paired and three single laryngeal cartilages. The epiglottis resides in close proximity to the root of the tongue and is vertical to the opening of the larynx. It is attached inferiorly to the body of the thyroid cartilage by the thyroepiglottic ligament just above the vocal cords, to the base of the tongue by mucosal membrane tissue known as the median and lateral glossoepiglottic folds, and to the back of the hyoid bone by the hyoepiglottic ligament. The furrow between the glossoepiglottic folds and the base of the tongue is called the vallecula epiglottica and serves as the situation point for the tip of a curved laryngoscope blade. Pressure by the laryngoscope blade within the vallecula on the hyoepiglottic ligament serves to move the epiglottis closer to the base of the tongue and better expose the laryngeal opening. The epiglottis serves to protect the larynx from foreign body entry. During swallowing or laryngospasm, elevation of the larynx closes the epiglottis, effectively sealing off the trachea.

The thyroid cartilage is the largest cartilage of the larynx, formed by two quadrangular plates or laminae fused near the midline anteriorly. Its strength affords a great deal of protection to the larynx. The thyroid cartilage halves meet at a peak that form the laryngeal prominence or Adam's apple. The thyroid cartilage is larger and more prominent in adult males, is a primary external landmark on the neck, and functions to protect the vocal cords.

The cricoid cartilage is palpable just below the thyroid gland, and its level corresponds to the beginning of the trachea and the esophagus. It is the only true ring of cartilage encircling the airway. Anteriorly, the cricoid cartilage lies below the thyroid cartilage, with the cricothyroid membrane intervening. The cricoid is the most inferior of the nine laryngeal cartilages. The arytenoid cartilages articulate on the superior posterior aspect of the cricoid cartilage, which is slanted forward. The paired arytenoid cartilages are attached to the posterior ends of the vocal cords. The paired corniculate (median) and cuneiform (more lateral) cartilages are embedded in the aryepiglottic folds, and they provide support to these structures. These cartilages cause the two bumps seen in the aryepiglottic folds, which are often (but incorrectly) called the arytenoids when visualized during laryngoscopy.

In adults, the narrowest portion of the larynx is the opening between the true vocal cords (aka cricoid opening or rima glottidis) during relaxation. However, in children younger than 8 years of age, the narrowest portion of the larynx is the cricoid cartilage and possibly the subcricoid region. This anatomic difference is of clinical significance: A tube with adequate clearance through the vocal cords may create mucosal pressure at the level of the cricoid ring in children less than 8 years of age. For this reason, uncuffed ETTs were traditionally used in children less than 8 years of age. However, it is more commonplace to use a cuffed tube in pediatric patients for the added assurance of tidal volume delivery, to reduce the amount of pressure on the cricoid and subcricoid regions and to decrease the need for an ETT change because of incorrect sizing.[3]

Laryngeal Membranes

The thyrohyoid membrane suspends the larynx from the hyoid bone. The cricothyroid membrane lies between the cricoid and the thyroid cartilages. The easiest and most rapid laryngotomy can be performed through this membrane. Cricothyrotomy is recommended for the emergency establishment of an airway when both endotracheal intubation and mask ventilation are unsuccessful. A transtracheal block can be performed by puncturing the cricothyroid membrane with a needle and injecting a local anesthetic into the trachea.

Interior of Larynx

The larynx is divided into three compartments by the false vocal cords and the true vocal cords. The false vocal cords are also known as the vestibular folds. They are narrow bands of fibrous tissue covered by mucous membranes and are located to either side and superiorly to the true vocal cords. The false vocal cords are involved with respiration, aspiration prevention, and phonation. The first compartment within the larynx is the supraglottic area, also called the vestibule, which extends from above the false cords to the tip of the epiglottis. On each side of the vestibule is located a pharyngeal sinus (the pyriform sinus). This recess is a potential location for lodging of foreign bodies that enter the pharynx or for noncentered ETTs. The second compartment of the larynx is the area between the false cords and the true cords known as the laryngeal ventricles. The third area is the infraglottic region below the true cords and above the beginning of the trachea. The rima glottidis (cricoid opening) is the space between the true vocal cords.[1-5]

Movements of the Vocal Cords

The true vocal cords are fibromembranous folds attached anteriorly to the thyroid cartilage and posteriorly to the arytenoids. The focal points of movement are the arytenoid cartilages, which rotate and slide up and down on the sloping cricoid cartilage. Several of the muscles controlling laryngeal movement (Box 29.1) act as pairs and have opposing actions, though some work in tandem. The laryngeal vestibule (i.e., laryngeal

---

> ### BOX 29.1   Intrinsic Muscles of the Larynx
>
> **Laryngeal Inlet**
> - Closed by the aryepiglottic and oblique arytenoid muscles
> - Opened by the thyroepiglottic muscle
>
> **Glottic Opening**
> - Opened by the posterior cricoarytenoid muscles
> - Closed by the transverse arytenoid and the lateral cricoarytenoid muscles
>
> **True Vocal Cords**
> - Lengthened by the cricothyroid muscles
> - Shortened by thyroarytenoid muscles

inlet) is closed, and the epiglottis pulled inferiorly to cover the laryngeal vestibule, by the aryepiglottic muscle, oblique arytenoid muscles, and thyroepiglottic muscle. The glottic opening is dilated (abducted) by the posterior cricoarytenoid muscles and closed (adducted) by the interarytenoid and lateral cricoarytenoid muscles. The cricothyroid muscles increase tension on (lengthen) the true vocal cords, and the thyroarytenoid muscles decrease tension on (shorten) them. The cricothyroid and thyroarytenoid muscle sets can alter the tension on the vocal cords and are important for determining the pitch of the voice.[4]

Nerve Supply to the Larynx

Both the superior and inferior laryngeal nerves are branches of cranial nerve X, the vagus nerve. The superior laryngeal nerve arises from the ganglion nodosum of the vagus and divides into two branches, the internal and external. The external branch of the superior laryngeal nerve is smaller and extends to the inferior constrictor muscle of the pharynx and to the cricothyroid muscles. These muscles change the position of the cricoid and thyroid cartilages resulting in a lengthening or increase in tension of the vocal cords. If these muscles are paralyzed, the voice becomes weak, rough, and easily fatigued. Voice hoarseness, particularly of recent onset, should be investigated in the preoperative evaluation as a potential indicator of vocal cord palsy or airway obstruction. The internal branch of the superior laryngeal nerve enters the larynx through the thyrohyoid membrane and is distributed to the mucous membranes of the larynx and epiglottis. It provides sensation from the inferior side of the epiglottis down to the true cords (the superior side of the epiglottis is innervated by the glossopharyngeal nerve). The internal branch also innervates the interarytenoid muscles, which are important in phonation.

The inferior (or recurrent) laryngeal nerves arise from the bilateral vagus nerves at different levels. The left nerve descends with the vagus, loops around the arch of the aorta, and then courses superiorly to the trachea. The right recurrent laryngeal nerve travels with the vagus nerve as far as the right subclavian artery; it loops around this artery and then comes back up the neck. The recurrent laryngeal nerve supplies sensation to the larynx below the level of the vocal cords and innervates all the intrinsic muscles of the larynx except the cricothyroid muscles and part of the interarytenoid muscles. Damage to the recurrent laryngeal nerve(s) during trauma, surgery on the neck, or from airway devices or anesthetic blocks can lead to unilateral or bilateral vocal cord paralysis with hoarseness or dyspnea.[5,6] Blood supply to the larynx is provided by the superior thyroid artery (a branch of the external carotid artery) and the inferior thyroid artery (a branch of the thyrocervical trunk, which arises from the subclavian artery).[1-5]

Trachea

The trachea is lined by pseudostratified ciliated columnar epithelium, and extends from the inferior larynx to the carina, where it bifurcates

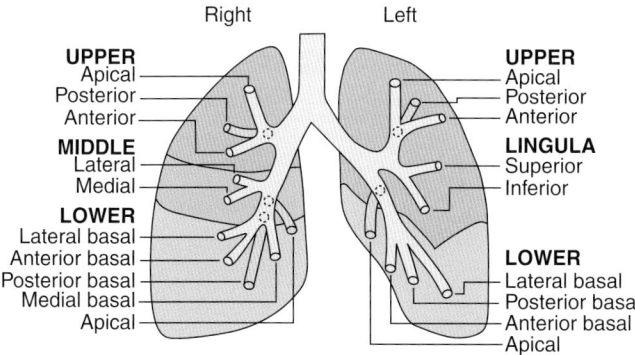

Right   Left

UPPER
Apical
Posterior
Anterior
MIDDLE
Lateral
Medial
LOWER
Lateral basal
Anterior basal
Posterior basal
Medial basal
Apical

UPPER
Apical
Posterior
Anterior
LINGULA
Superior
Inferior
LOWER
Lateral basal
Posterior basal
Anterior basal
Apical

Fig. 29.1 Lobes and bronchopulmonary segments of the lungs. *Red,* upper lobes; *blue,* lower lobes; *green,* right middle lobe. The 19 major lung segments are labeled. Some sources will combine the apical and posterior segments (i.e., apical posterior) demonstrating only 18 lung segments. (From Lumb AB. *Nunn's Applied Respiratory Physiology.* 8th ed. Philadelphia: Elsevier; 2017:6.)

BOX 29.2   Lung Lobes and Segments

I. Right lung
  A. Right upper lobe (three segments)
    1. Apical
    2. Anterior
    3. Posterior
  B. Right middle lobe (two segments)
    1. Medial
    2. Lateral
  C. Right lower lobe (five segments)
    1. Superior (apical)
    2. Anterior basal
    3. Posterior basal
    4. Lateral basal
    5. Medial basal

II. Left lung
  A. Left upper lobe (four segments)
    1. Apical posterior
    2. Anterior
    3. Superior lingular
    4. Inferior lingular
  B. Left lower lobe (four segments)
    1. Superior (apical)
    2. Anteromedial basal
    3. Posterior basal
    4. Lateral basal

---

into the two mainstem bronchi. In adults of normal size, the distances are fairly constant: The distance from the incisors to the larynx is approximately 13 cm, as is that from the larynx to the carina. Therefore the distance from the incisors to the carina is approximately 26 cm (note the length markings on ETTs). The blood supply to the trachea is through the inferior thyroid artery, which comes from the thyrocervical branch of the subclavian artery. Some perfusion is also received from the superior thyroid, bronchial, and internal thoracic arteries. Blood is drained by the inferior thyroid veins. Sensory innervation of the trachea is via the vagus nerve for both parasympathetic and nociceptive stimuli.

The trachea has a diameter of approximately 2.5 cm, and it is supported by incomplete rings of cartilage that open posteriorly and prevent tracheal collapse under the negative pressure generated during spontaneous respiration. The trachea extends down to the level of T4-T5, where the carina is located. This level corresponds anteriorly to the angle of Louis on the sternum, which is the articulation of the second rib. The trachea is not a rigid structure; it expands and contracts to accommodate head and neck movement. In an intubated patient, flexion of the neck causes a fixed ETT to move downward, and endobronchial intubation may result. During extension of the head and neck a fixed ETT at the mouth causes upward movement that can result in extubation. In pediatric patients, the range of this movement was demonstrated to increase with patient age and height.[7] The apparent movement of the ETT in relation to head flexion may seem paradoxic; the mnemonic "the hose follows the nose" can be used as a memory aid. Neck rotation to the left or right tends to cause tracheal elevation and risk of endobronchial intubation.[1-5]

Bronchi

At the carina, the trachea divides into the right and left bronchi (Fig. 29.1). The cellular structure begins to change at this point from columnar to cuboidal epithelium, and the cartilaginous rings thin into plates once the bronchi penetrate the lungs. From the carina, the bronchi branch off at slightly different angles. The right bronchus takes a less acute angle from the trachea, approximately 25 degrees, whereas the left bronchus branches off at 45 degrees. In addition, the right mainstem bronchus is wider and shorter (2 cm) than the left one (4 cm). Because the right bronchus is more nearly vertical than the left, the tendency is much greater for ETTs, suction catheters, or aspirated foreign materials to enter the right side after passing the carina. Additionally, the beveled tip of an ETT makes right-sided intubation more likely. The

side opening (Murphy eye) located at the distal end of the ETT allows the delivery of gas if the beveled tip of the tube is closely opposed to the similarly angled right main bronchus.

Each mainstem bronchus divides into lobar bronchi (three on the right; two on the left) that lead to the major lung lobes. The right mainstem bronchus divides at 2 to 2.5 cm from the carina into the right upper lobe (RUL) bronchus. It can branch off sooner in some individuals. The right main bronchus then continues for 3 cm as the bronchus intermedius before giving rise to the right middle lobe bronchus and the right lower lobe bronchus. The left main bronchus is 4 to 5 cm long before bifurcating into the left upper lobe bronchus and the left lower lobe bronchus.

Each successive division of the airways is referred to as a generation, with the mainstem bronchi representing the first generation, the lobar bronchi representing the second, and so on. The lobar bronchi divide into the third generation of airways, called segmental bronchi, which deliver ventilation to the various bronchopulmonary segments of the lung. There are 10 bronchopulmonary segments in each lung, but on the left, the apical and posterior segments and the anterior basal and medial basal segment pairs each arise from a single bronchial branch (Box 29.2). Therefore only eight third-generation bronchi are found on the left. Segments whose names contain the word *basal* are located adjacent to the diaphragm. The bronchopulmonary segments create distinct anatomic and functional units. The segments are separated by connective tissue, so gas-exchange properties or pathology tend to be isolated to a segment. A bronchopulmonary segment can also be excised as a unit.

Each subsegmental bronchus divides several times, giving rise to numerous bronchioles. With succeeding generations and multiplication of the number of airways, the total cross-sectional area becomes very large, and the airflow velocity decreases. There are 20 to 25 total generations before the alveoli. By the seventh generation, the diameter of bronchioles is approximately 2 mm, beyond which they are referred to as small airways. When the diameter has decreased to 1 mm they are referred to as terminal bronchioles. The terminal bronchioles are the last structures perfused by the bronchial circulation and are the end of the conducting airways (anatomic dead space, as discussed later). In the latter generations, the cross-sectional area of the airway has expanded so much that the velocity of airflow becomes very slow, and gas moves largely by diffusion as compared to bulk flow.

BOX 29.3 Characteristics of Progressive Airway Divisions

With each succeeding generation:
- Number of airways ↑
- Cross-sectional area ↑
- Airflow velocity ↓
- Muscular layer ↑
- Cartilage ↓

- Mucous glands ↓ (absent in bronchioles)
- Goblet cells ↓
- Ciliated cells ↓
- Cuboidal, then squamous cells ↑

TABLE 29.2 Conditions That Affect the Pleural Space

Material in Pleural Space	Medical Name
Air	Pneumothorax
Air under pressure	Tension pneumothorax
Blood	Hemothorax
Serous fluid	Pleural effusion
Pus	Empyema or pyothorax
Organized blood clot	Fibrothorax
Lymph	Chylothorax

With succeeding generations the histology of the airways changes, in a progression characterized by thinning of the walls, to transition to the gas-exchanging morphology of the respiratory zone (Box 29.3). The terminal bronchioles divide into the respiratory bronchioles and are the first location where gas exchange occurs with the blood. The respiratory bronchioles are perfused by the pulmonary circulation. These airways are characterized by occasional outpouching of alveoli (air sacs). The respiratory bronchioles divide into several alveolar ducts that lead to circular spaces called atria. Each atrium opens into two to five alveolar sacs, which are spaces lined by alveoli. The terminal airways are very small and lack cartilage for supportive opening; instead they rely on the connections with the adjacent matrix of pulmonary parenchyma in which they are situated and airflow within to remain open. For this reason they are prone to closure from compression of the pulmonary tissue during respiration or if emphysema, for example, expands the volume of adjacent air spaces and compresses the airways. The lung volume at which small airways tend to close during exhalation is called the closing volume. Conditions such as obesity or chronic obstructive pulmonary disease (COPD) can cause an increase in closing volume into the range of normal tidal breathing. Closing volume encroachment within tidal volume results in the closure of some small airways before the intended tidal volume has been fully expired. Small pores in the alveoli, known as the pores of Kohn, serve to allow collateral gas flow between alveoli and provide a mechanism of relief from gas stagnation from airway closure.[8]

Respiratory Zone

The respiratory bronchioles along with the alveolar ducts, sacs, and alveoli comprise the respiratory zone, which is the area where gas exchange takes place. All parts of the airway prior to this (nose to terminal bronchioles) are referred to as the conducting zone. These areas conduct gas without exchanging gas with the blood. Some refer to the respiratory bronchioles and alveolar ducts where limited gas exchange takes place as the transitional zone because structures here function both to conduct gas and to participate in some gas exchange. The alveoli are the air sacs that are tightly packed and closely approximated with pulmonary capillaries. The typical maximum number (~300 million) alveoli is reached by age 9 years. The alveoli are characterized by very thin walls composed of squamous epithelium. There are three types of cells that form the alveoli: type I pneumocytes, which are the structural cells; type II pneumocytes, which produce surfactant to reduce alveolar collapse from surface tension; and type III pneumocytes, which are macrophages. The average alveolar diameter is approximately 250 mcm, therefore the total surface area available for gas exchange is 60 to 80 m^2.[9] The respiratory zone also contains nonciliated bronchiolar cells known as club cells (or Clara cells), which serve a number of metabolic and antiinflammatory processes, and serve as progenitor cells (i.e., similar to stem cells) for themselves and the other pneumocytes. Club cells have a distinctive dome-shaped luminal surface with short microvilli and secrete components that make up the extracellular substance lining the respiratory bronchioles. These cells produce and secrete proteins and cytochrome P450 enzymes that are involved in the biotransformation of many inhaled harmful and toxic substances (i.e., tobacco smoke, ozone, hydrocarbons, and numerous other substances). The primary protein secreted by club cells is uteroglobin (because it is also found in the pregnant uterus), also known as club cell secretory protein (CCSP). Uteroglobin (or CCSP), along with other proteins, lipids, and glycoproteins secreted by club cells, binds with and helps to protect pulmonary surfactant, essentially stabilizing the lipoprotein secreted by type II alveolar cells. Club cells may play a role in the development of adenocarcinoma and other chronic lung diseases.[10]

Pulmonary Hilum and Contents

The nerve supply to the bronchi and lungs arises chiefly from the sympathetic nerves and the vagus nerve (which supplies sensory and parasympathetic innervation). All conduits to the lung pass through the hilum (pleural form is *hila*), which is the connection of the mediastinum to the pedicle of each lung. The structures included in each hilum include the mainstem bronchus, pulmonary artery and vein, bronchial arteries and veins (which drain into the azygos system), lymphatics, lymph nodes, pulmonary nerve plexuses, and pulmonary ligament. All of this is surrounded by connective tissue. The serous membrane covering the lung is called the pleura.

Pleura

The pleura is a serous membrane that lines the thoracic wall and lungs. The parietal pleura lines the chest wall, mediastinum, and diaphragm. When it reaches the hilum it is then reflected back to cover the lungs as the visceral pleura. Between these two layers is a potential space called the pleural cavity. The touching surfaces of the two layers of pleura remain slippery by a small amount of serous fluid. Certain conditions can result in occupation of liquids or gas within the pleural space (Table 29.2), which may affect ventilation and lung expansion. Infected intrapleural blood can clot and organize to form a fibrothorax, which must be peeled from the surface of the lung (in a procedure called lung decortication) so the lung can reexpand.

The two pleural layers are closely opposed, with only a capillary-thin layer of pleural fluid between them in a potential space called the pleural space. The parietal pleura is very sensitive to pain, and conditions that cause accumulation of pleural fluid or friction between the layers can cause discomfort. Different areas of the pleura may produce characteristic pain patterns: The costal pleura creates localized pain, the diaphragmatic pleura creates diffuse pain, and areas supplied by the phrenic nerve may radiate pain to the neck or back. Posterior to the mediastinum, the pleura doubles up and descends downward as the pulmonary ligament.

If communication is created across the pleura, accumulation of air in the pleural space is referred to as pneumothorax. In a closed chest (e.g., a pulmonary bleb ruptures, creating a communication to the pleural space), a tension pneumothorax develops as inspired air accumulates in the pleural space and is not expelled. With an opening through both pleura (such as with open chest trauma), the external wound may create a simple pneumothorax, which does not tend to cause high intrathoracic pressures. In either type of pneumothorax, the elastic recoil of the lung tends to favor lung collapse once the negative pressure of the pleural space is disrupted by the breach.[1-5]

Mediastinum

The mediastinum is the region located between the two pleural sacs. It exists in the center of the thoracic cavity but is slightly displaced to the left by the presence of the heart. Therefore the left lung represents 45% of the total lung capacity (TLC), whereas the right lung represents 55%. Perforation of the larynx, trachea, pharynx, or esophagus, which sometimes occurs during esophagoscopy, bronchoscopy, or traumatic intubation, can produce mediastinitis, a life-threatening infection of an area containing the trachea, esophagus, and major blood vessels and heart. The mediastinum is divided into four divisions separated by the pericardium (Table 29.3). Common procedures involving the mediastinum include coronary artery bypass, cardiac valve replacement, aortic aneurysm repair, thymectomy for myasthenia gravis, resection of tumors, and mediastinoscopy for diagnosis and staging of cancer.

MECHANICS OF BREATHING

Inspiratory muscle contraction lowers intrathoracic pressure and causes the volume of the thoracic cavity to increase. Boyle's law explains that the increase in volume creates a reduction in pressure (i.e., negative pressure), which causes air to be drawn into the lungs from the atmosphere. Spontaneous respiration involves the movement of gas caused by negative pressure forces (or vacuum) created by contraction of the diaphragm (and other inspiratory muscles). In contrast to negative pressure ventilation, positive pressure ventilation requires the generation of positive forces from within the upper airway to overcome intrathoracic pressure and expand the lungs.

The respiratory muscles are listed in Fig. 29.2. The diaphragm and external intercostal muscles contract during normal breathing (eupnea). Whereas the diaphragm increases the superior-inferior dimension of the chest, the external intercostals increase the anterior-posterior diameter by elevating the ribs and sternum. Each half of the diaphragm is innervated by a branch of the phrenic nerve, which arises from the third, fourth, and fifth cervical spinal nerve roots. This anatomy gives rise to the mnemonic "C3, 4, and 5 keep the diaphragm alive." The diaphragm is almost solely responsible for quiet respiration. Loss of external intercostal muscle function from a thoracic spinal cord injury, high spinal or epidural block, or an increased concentration of volatile agents usually does not impair respiration in individuals without pulmonary disease. However, if coupled with paralysis of the phrenic nerve and resulting paralysis of a hemidiaphragm (such as may occur with interscalene blocks), then dyspnea may result. Spinal cord injuries above the level of C5 usually lead to dependence on mechanical ventilation.

Normally, eupneic expiration results from passive recoil of the chest wall and does not require muscular contraction, although the internal intercostal muscles may be used to augment exhalation. During forced exhalation (e.g., with coughing and the clearing of secretions), the abdominal muscles, particularly the rectus abdominis, the transversus abdominis, and the external and internal oblique muscles, are used. For forced inhalation, the external intercostal muscles play a more prominent role, along with accessory breathing muscles in the neck and

TABLE 29.3 Divisions of the Mediastinum

Subdivision	Location	Contents
Superior	Above level of the sternal angle, extending superior to the thoracic inlet	Thymus, esophagus, trachea, great vessels
Anterior	Between sternum and pericardium	Thymus
Posterior	Between vertebral column and posterior pericardium	Esophagus, thoracic aorta, thoracic duct
Middle	Between anterior and posterior divisions, bounded laterally by the parietal pleura	Heart, distal trachea, mainstem bronchi, and great vessel trunks

Muscles of inspiration

Core muscles

- External intercostals
  (contract to elevate ribs)

- Diaphragm
  (contracts to expand thoracic cavity)

Accessory muscles

- Scalene
  (helps to elevate clavicle and sternum)

- Sternocleidomastoid
  (contracts to elevate sternum)

- Pectoralis minor
  (contracts to pull ribs outwards)

Muscles of expiration

Core muscles

- Internal intercostals
  (contract to pull ribs down)

- Diaphragm
  (relaxes to reduce thoracic cavity)

Accessory muscles

- Abdominals
  (contract to compress abdomen)

- External and internal obliques
  (contract to compress abdomen)

- Rectus abdominis
  (contracts to compress abdomen)

- Transverse abdominis
  (contracts to compress abdomen)

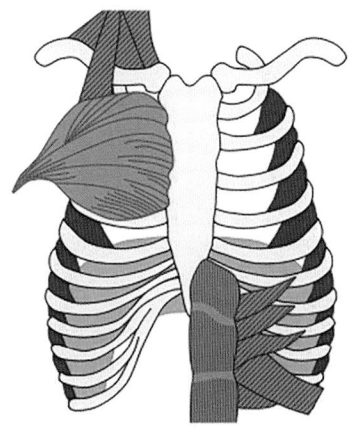

Fig. 29.2 Inspiratory and expiratory muscles.

chest (i.e., pectoralis minor). The diaphragm descends approximately 1 to 2 cm during eupneic breathing, but this excursion can increase to as much as 10 cm during forceful breathing. For air to move into the alveoli, alveolar pressure must be less than atmospheric pressure. This can be achieved through either an increase in atmospheric pressure (as in positive pressure ventilation) or a reduction in alveolar pressure, as during spontaneous breathing (negative pressure ventilation). During forceful inspiration, the sternocleidomastoid, scalene muscles, and pectoralis minor contract in conjunction with the diaphragm and intercostals.

The muscles of ventilation are attached to the cartilaginous and bony components (ribs, sternum, and vertebrae) of the chest. Conditions that impede chest excursion, such as thoracic kyphosis, may require reduction to further increase the chest diameter. The two domes of the diaphragm separate the thoracic and abdominal cavities and function separately, such that injury to a phrenic nerve results in paralysis in the diaphragm only on that side. The central tendon on the underside of the diaphragm provides a site of rigidity, allowing the diaphragm to tense and flatten without pulling against an external insertion point, as do other muscles. The central tendon includes an orifice for passage of the inferior vena cava. The two other prominent openings through the diaphragm include the esophageal and aortic hiatus. The esophagus passes through the esophageal hiatus, and the aorta, azygous vein, and thoracic duct pass through the aortic hiatus. When the diaphragm contracts during spontaneous inspiration, it flattens and moves the abdominal contents downward, raising intraabdominal pressure while lowering intrathoracic pressure. Pressure within the alveoli becomes slightly negative with respect to atmospheric pressure, and gas flows inward through the conducting airways to expand the lungs. When half of the diaphragm is paralyzed it cannot contract and moves upward from its normal position as a result of intraabdominal pressure and negative intrapleural pressure. When the nonaffected diaphragm contracts (moving downward), the paralyzed diaphragm moves upward, and when the nonaffected diaphragm relaxes (moving upward), the paralyzed diaphragm moves downward, resulting in paradoxic movements.[1-5]

Lung Compliance

Lung compliance is defined as the change in volume divided by the change in pressure (V/P). For a given change in pressure, a more compliant lung has a greater change in volume than a less compliant one. Fig. 29.3 shows pressure-volume relationships for a lung. As with many respiratory physiology concepts, it is easier to consider the application to a single alveolus (which aids in understanding) than to conceptualize the overall pulmonary system that involves many regions existing along a continuum of conditions. In considering lung compliance, the curve in Fig. 29.3 represents the collective contribution of alveoli that are almost collapsed at the beginning of inspiration, alveoli that are distended, and alveoli that exist at various intermediate volumes.

Static lung compliance is defined as a change in lung volume per unit of pressure change within the lung when air is not moving. It is the pressure required to maintain pulmonary volume with the lungs at rest. Static compliance reflects the compliance of the lung tissue and chest wall alone. Static compliance is decreased by conditions that make the lung difficult to inflate, such as fibrosis, obesity, vascular engorgement, edema, acute respiratory distress syndrome (ARDS), and external compression (e.g., that caused by tight dressings or a surgeon leaning on the patient's chest). Static compliance is increased by emphysema, which destroys the elastic tissue of the lung. This makes the emphysematous lung easier to inflate, but without the needed elastic recoil. The problem with emphysema is not inflation but rather deflation. The

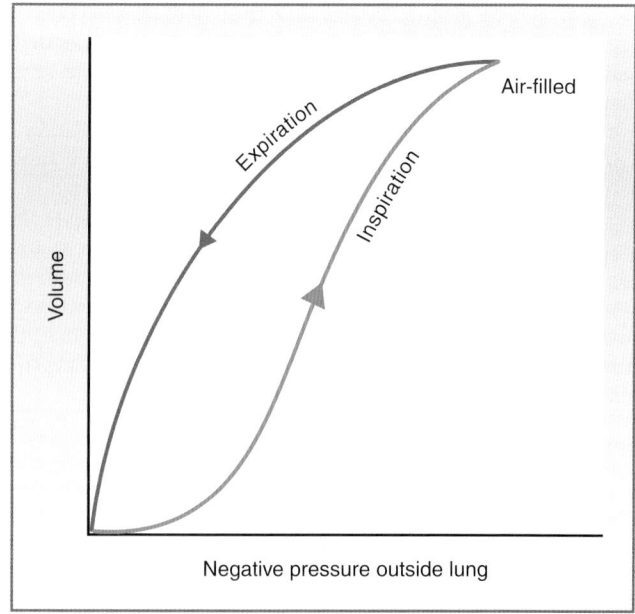

Fig. 29.3 Compliance of the lung during negative pressure ventilation. The relationship between lung volume and lung pressure is obtained by inflating and deflating an isolated lung. The slope of each curve is the compliance. In the air-filled lung, inspiration (inflation) and expiration (deflation) follow different curves, which is known as hysteresis. (From Costanzo LS. *Physiology*. 5th ed. Philadelphia: Elsevier; 2014:195.)

loss of elastic tissue results in small airway collapse as the lung deflates and gas trapping occurs. It is important to note that compliance changes as lung volume changes. In other words, compliance is volume dependent. Fig. 29.3 shows that the lung is less compliant at both very low and very high lung volumes. Alveoli require greater pressure to be inflated when they are almost empty or almost full. When an alveolus is collapsed, a significant increase in pressure is necessary for inflation to begin. Observe in Fig. 29.3 that the slope of the inspiratory curve is less at both low volumes and very high volumes, signaling a decrease in lung compliance at both of these points. At low volumes, more energy is required (i.e., more negative pressure) to begin to expand the lungs. At high volumes, the alveoli are almost at capacity, and further changes in pressure result in less changes in volume. During the expiratory curve there is a less negative (more positive) pressure as the chest wall relaxes back to the resting level and the volume of air within the lung is expelled.

Lung compliance is a measure of lung stiffness. Compliance is the amount of force required to cause elastic deformation, with the described measurement being opposite elastance. For example, high elasticity results in low compliance, and low elasticity results in high compliance. Lung compliance results from the interplay of various factors that tend to either promote or restrict lung expansion. Much of the energy required to expand the lungs, particularly at low volumes, is created by surface tension in the fluid lining of the alveoli that cause the alveoli to contract inward. Although not a high-fidelity measurement, static effective compliance can be calculated easily using the following equation:

$$\text{Statice compliance (Cstat)} = \frac{\text{tidal volume (Vt)}}{\text{(plateau pressure [Pplat]} - \text{PEEP)}}$$

Plateau pressure is the pressure observed during the momentary exhalation delay when the lungs are at end inspiration. An inspiratory pause on the ventilator is an easy way to observe the plateau pressure.

After subtracting the added positive end-expiratory pressure (PEEP), the plateau pressure is then divided into the measured tidal volume of that breath, producing a measure of lung compliance. A static compliance of 60 to 100 mL/cm H_2O is considered normal. However, the most useful clinical application of compliance measurement is in monitoring trends to evaluate changing physical status or the effectiveness of PEEP and other treatment modalities. Because the plateau pressure may be affected by both lung elastance and pressure external to the lung (such as abdominal insufflation), static compliance may not be the most accurate way to measure lung compliance in the clinical setting (refer to section that describes transpulmonary pressure).

Dynamic lung compliance refers to the change in lung volume per unit of pressure change within the lung during air movement. It is the measured pressure during gas flow (i.e., inspiratory flow). The components of dynamic compliance include chest wall and lung tissue compliance in combination with the effects of airway resistance. Airway obstruction (e.g., such as bronchospasm or the presence of foreign bodies in the airway) can greatly decrease dynamic compliance.[11] The equation for dynamic compliance is calculated as:

$$\text{Dynamic compliance (Cdyn)} = \frac{\text{tidal volume (Vt)}}{\text{(peak inspiratory pressure} - \text{PEEP)}}$$

Modern anesthesia ventilators can calculate and trend compliance through tracing of pressure-volume curves.

Lung Elastic Recoil

The forces that cause elastic recoil of the lung are responsible for emptying the lung during exhalation and have a significant influence on lung compliance. In addition to actual elastic fibers, the surface tension of the liquid film that lines the alveoli contributes to elastic recoil by inherently causing a contracting force. The surface tension occurs as a gas-liquid interface is generated by the cohesive forces among the molecules of the liquid. Surface tension is what causes water to bead and form droplets.

Surface tension at the gas-fluid interface between the alveolar walls and the gas inside them contributes to reducing the size of alveoli, particularly when the alveoli are at low volumes. At end expiration, surface tension increases the pressure required to inflate the alveoli, contributing to the flat portion of the lung compliance curve. This concept is often attributed to the law of Laplace ($P = T/r$), which states that if surface tension (T) is constant, pressure (P) would increase as radius (r) decreases. Pulmonary surfactant secreted by alveolar type II cells counteracts the influence of surface tension on the lungs. With surfactant present, as alveolar radius decreases, surface tension also decreases, so that pressure remains more constant. Surfactant consists of proteins and phospholipids, primarily dipalmitoylphosphatidylcholine. The surface-active agent serves to lower the surface tension of the fluid lining the alveoli and decrease the work of breathing.

Although the law of Laplace has traditionally been applied to understanding alveolar pressure-tension relationships, there is controversy as to whether alveoli should be treated as spherical (and thus subject to the law) or not. Geometricians postulate that closely packed alveoli would not maintain the shape of spheres, but rather that of polyhedrons because their sides would be flattened against each other. The classical application of Laplace described the concept of alveoli as distinct balloonlike structures wherein pressure differentials can cause small alveoli to collapse and expel their gas into larger ones. The fact that alveoli are not individually suspended, but rather part of a connective tissue mesh, argues against this concept. The presence of pores of Kohn also argues against this theory because the pores allow pressure equalization between adjacent alveoli.

Connective tissue and elastic forces certainly play an important role in preventing alveolar closure.[12]

It is clear that surfactant is crucial for reducing surface tension and preventing collapse of alveoli as well as small airways. Surfactant is a lipoprotein that coats the inner surface of the alveoli, alveolar ducts, and distal respiratory bronchioles causing a reduction in surface tension at end expiration; prevents lung collapse; and facilitates lung expansion. The cylindric shape of distal airways (i.e., respiratory bronchioles that connect to alveolar ducts) lends to the application of the law of Laplace to the role of surfactant in these structures. Surfactant probably also helps prevent fluid bridging (connection of fluid lining from opposite sides of an airway at low volumes), which could impair gas flow.[13]

In the fetus, surfactant is not produced until approximately 28 to 32 weeks of gestation and does not reach mature levels until approximately 35 weeks of gestation. The lack of surfactant is the predominant cause of respiratory distress syndrome (RDS) in premature infants. Formation of surfactant can be hastened by the administration of glucocorticoids (particularly a steroid that crosses the placenta, such as betamethasone) to the parturient mother when premature delivery is threatened or imminent. The direct administration of synthetic surfactant to the airways of premature newborns has also greatly reduced the incidence of RDS. Amniocentesis is sometimes performed to determine whether mature surfactant levels are present in the premature fetus. The ratio of lecithin to sphingomyelin (the L:S ratio) indicates the amount of mature surfactant (dipalmitoyl lecithin) in proportion to the amount of surfactant precursor (sphingomyelin).

Pleural, Intraalveolar, and Transpulmonary Pressures

Pleural pressure is the pressure that exists within the pleural space outside the lung between the visceral pleura of the lung and the parietal pleura of the inner chest wall. Although the elastic forces of the lung tend to favor lung collapse, the chest wall is constantly under tension to expand. This is why normal inspiration requires very little energy. At the end of exhalation, the outward recoil of the chest wall is balanced by the inward elastic recoil of the lung tissue and surface tension of the alveoli (when surfactant is not present). At this resting end-expiratory point, the opposing forces of the lungs and chest wall produce negative pressure in the pleural space. In addition to the balance of these inward and outward recoil forces, pleural pressure is influenced secondarily by an extensive lymphatic network that is continuously pulling fluid and proteins out of the lungs and thus augmenting the negative pressure within the intrapleural space. Essentially, the negative pressure within the pleural space acts like a suction cup to keep the lungs inflated. In the upright position intrapleural pressure is more negative at the apex of the lung as compared to the base. This is because the weight of the lung tissue, blood, lymph drainage, and other intrapulmonary and chest contents pushes on the pleural space with a positive pressure, making the pressure within the intrapleural space less negative as it travels toward the lung base. During inspiration the chest wall expands, creating a greater outward force and resulting in a decreased (more negative) intrapleural pressure. Conversely, during expiration, the chest wall forces retract inward, resulting in an increased (less negative) intrapleural pressure. It is important to note that the pressure within the intrapleural space during the respiratory cycle is always negative (subatmospheric) but can become zero (atmospheric) if the chest wall and parietal pleura are breached such as in a pneumothorax.

Intraalveolar pressure (also known as intrapulmonary pressure) is the pressure applied to the inside of the alveoli. Between each inspiratory and expiratory cycle there is no air movement, and as long as the airways are open the intraalveolar pressure is the same as atmospheric pressure (760 mm Hg). This resting (i.e., no gas flow) intraalveolar pressure is referred to as zero. Since atmospheric pressure is relatively constant, pressure in the lungs must be higher or lower than atmospheric pressure for air to flow between the atmosphere and the alveoli. As the diaphragm contracts during inspiration, intraalveolar pressure decreases (i.e., falls below atmospheric pressure) causing air to flow from an area of high pressure (atmosphere) to an area of lower pressure (alveoli), resulting in an increased intrapulmonary volume. At the end of inspiration, when intraalveolar pressure again equals atmospheric pressure, the airflow stops. During expiration, the diaphragm and other respiratory muscles relax causing a slight increase in intraalveolar pressure, resulting in a net movement of gases out of the alveoli toward the atmosphere and producing a decrease in intrapulmonary volume. Airflow stops at the end of expiration when again intraalveolar pressure is equal to atmospheric pressure. The positive and negative changes in pressure refer to the movement of air. As long as gases (i.e., air, oxygen, etc.) are present inside the alveoli, a constant pressure will exist within to help keep them open.

The difference between intraalveolar pressure and intrapleural pressure is called the transpulmonary pressure. It is the pressure that is delivered to the lung tissue itself independent of chest wall and abdominal forces. In essence, transpulmonary pressure is the net pressure that distends the lungs during contraction of the inspiratory muscles or during positive pressure ventilation. The higher the transpulmonary pressure is, the more distended the lung is (i.e., bronchioles, alveoli). The transpulmonary pressure is always positive in a normal spontaneously breathing individual whose physiology is unaltered. This is a due to the negative intrapleural pressure in the following equation:

Transpulmonary pressure (P_L) = Intraalveolar pressure (P_{alv})
$-$ Intrapleural pressure (P_{pl})

If the transpulmonary pressure were to equal zero (e.g., intraalveolar pressure = intrapleural pressure), such as occurs in a pneumothorax, the lung would collapse due to the lack of negative force outside the lung and the resulting elastic recoil of lung parenchymal tissues.

Transpulmonary pressure fluctuates as both the intraalveolar and pleural pressures alternate between inspiration and expiration (Fig. 29.4). During normal inspiration, intraalveolar pressure can fluctuate by as little

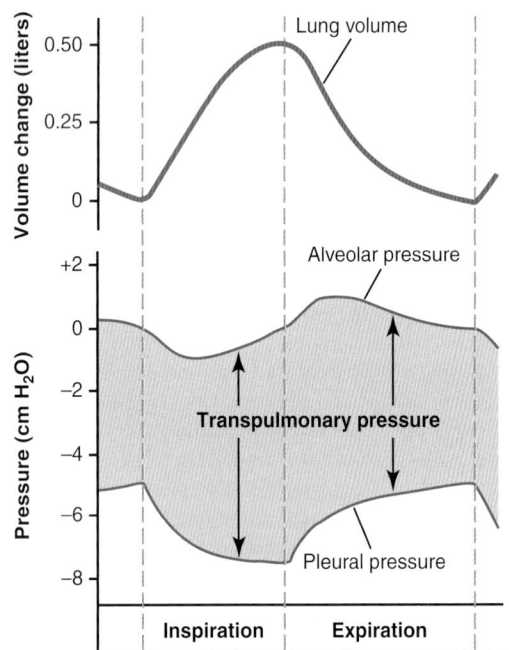

Fig. 29.4 Alveolar, pleural, and transpulmonary pressures. (From Hall JE, Hall ME. In *Guyton and Hall Textbook of Medical Physiology.* 14th ed. Philadelphia: Elsevier; 2021:492)

as 1 to 2 mm Hg. Consequently, very little pressure is required during eupneic ventilation. If lung compliance is reduced (i.e., increase in elastance or resistance to inflation) during spontaneous respiration, the generation of a more negative intrapleural pressure will be required to effect the same change in intraalveolar pressure to inflate the lung. As a result there is a greater difference between intrapleural and intraalveolar pressure, and therefore a greater transpulmonary pressure.

During positive pressure ventilation, the lungs' resistance to inflation is not the only contributor to dynamic or static pressures generated as a result of volume inflation. Stiffness of the chest wall, abdominal insufflation during laparoscopic surgery, obesity, Trendelenburg position, pathology exterior to the lungs, and other factors can increase the pressure required to inflate the lungs. Traditional measures of lung compliance, based on peak or plateau pressure, cannot differentiate these factors from lung parenchymal stiffness. High insufflating pressures or high PEEP are frequently necessary in these circumstances and can cause barotrauma or volutrauma to the lung. However, when conditions outside of the lung parenchyma (e.g., abdominal insufflation, pleural effusion, massive ascites) impede lung expansion, higher ventilating pressures may not represent actual high intrapulmonary pressures, but instead the high pressures may be required simply to overcome extraneous pressure from outside the lung and would not be as harmful to the lung.

This differentiation provides the clinical application of transpulmonary pressure. In a patient with increased extraneous pressure such as an increase in chest wall compliance or an increase in extraneous forces applied to the thorax (e.g., abdominal gas insufflation, obesity, positioning), the increase in airway pressures caused by these factors is not a true indication of actual lung stress (i.e., pressure on parenchymal lung tissue). Therefore, although the peak inspiratory pressure may be elevated, the difference between them (i.e., the transpulmonary pressure) will be normal. The esophageal pressure is an accurate representation of the adjacent intrapleural pressure, and it can be measured using an esophageal measurement device, which appears similar to an esophageal stethoscope. This allows calculation of the transpulmonary pressure, which can guide an appropriate ventilation strategy that avoids undue stress on the lung.[14]

Transpulmonary pressure has been found to be an effective measure of compliance, which discounts extrapulmonary effects. The esophageal calculation of transpulmonary pressures can guide the selection of appropriate tidal volume and PEEP settings to achieve open lung status while avoiding overdistention and mechanisms associated with ventilator-induced lung injury.[14] Patients with acute lung injury (ALI) have demonstrated significantly improved oxygenation when ventilation was guided by maintaining a transpulmonary pressure at 0 to 10 cm H_2O at end expiration and less than 25 cm H_2O at end inspiration.

Resistance to Breathing

Several factors oppose the inflation of the lungs, including the static elastic recoil of the lung, frictional resistance of lung tissues, and resistance to airflow. Rheologic characteristics of airflow affect its ability to pass through conducting airways. Laminar flow is an orderly movement, where molecules are moving along a generally straight path. In laminar flow, the gas in the center of the stream moves faster than that closer to the wall because frictional resistance slows molecules near the vessel wall. Compared to turbulent flow, laminar flow is characterized by lower pressures. During turbulent flow, resistance greatly increases because molecules move in various directions. The rheologic calculation of Reynolds number (Re) predicts when flow of a fluid (or gas) will be laminar or turbulent. Re is calculated as follows:

$$Re = \rho v d / \eta$$

where v = velocity of fluid flow, d = diameter of the vessel, p = density of the fluid, and η = viscosity of the fluid. This version of the formula would apply to flow through a tube (such as the airways). In open systems, length is substituted for diameter. When the inertial forces of density, velocity of flow, and diameter increase, Re increases. Increasing viscosity of the fluid reduces the product. A Reynolds number greater than 2300 reflects predominately turbulent flow. Conversely, a Reynolds number less than 2300 reflects predominately laminar flow.

Throughout the airways, both laminar and turbulent flows occur. True laminar flow occurs in smaller airways, where the diameter is small and linear velocity is very low. Linear velocity is inversely proportional to cross-sectional area for any flow rate. Turbulence is greatest in large airways, and turbulence caused by branching of the airways produces the breath sounds heard on auscultation. Resistance to laminar flow follows Poiseuille's law (R = 8çl/r⁴, where ç equals viscosity). Resistance (R) to laminar airflow is directly proportional to the length (l) of the tube and inversely proportional to the fourth power of the radius (r). Therefore doubling the radius of the tube decreases resistance 16 (2⁴) times. Normally, approximately 40% of the total airway resistance resides in the upper airways (nasal cavity, pharynx, and larynx).

Although resistance to airflow is greatest in individual small airways, the net total resistance to airflow of the small airways is very low because they represent a massive number of parallel pathways. Under normal circumstances, the greatest resistance to airflow resides in medium-sized bronchi, whose smooth muscle tone greatly affects airway resistance. During lung inflation, increasing lung volumes exert retractive forces on the airways, resulting in a reduction in airway resistance. During forced expiration, dynamic compression of the airways increases airway resistance and may promote airway collapse (most likely in small airways with no cartilaginous support).

The clinical application of these concepts resides in strategies to reduce airflow resistance. Bronchodilators will reduce resistance to airflow by increasing the radius of the pathway, as predicted by Poiseuille. The size of an ETT may confer greater or lesser resistance, based on the length and (much more significantly) the internal diameter of the tube. Clinical application of Re suggests that lower velocity (lower inspiratory flow or lower inspiratory:expiratory ratio) and lower density would promote laminar flow and create lower ventilating pressures. The reduction in density is the conceptual basis for combining helium with oxygen (heliox) to improve pulmonary gas distribution in obstructive lung disease.

Other influences on airflow include the autonomic nervous system and pathologic conditions. The autonomic nervous system affects the tone of the bronchial smooth muscle. The sympathetic nervous system and sympathomimetic drugs (e.g., norepinephrine, epinephrine, and isoproterenol) produce bronchodilation facilitating airflow. The parasympathetic nerves and parasympathomimetic drugs (e.g., acetylcholine) cause bronchoconstriction, increasing resistance to airflow. Parasympatholytic drugs (e.g., atropine and ipratropium) therefore cause bronchodilation (though mildly). Irritation of the airway by foreign bodies or inhaled irritants causes reflex bronchoconstriction, which causes reduced airflow.

Lung Volumes and Capacities

There are multiple lung volumes and capacities. Table 29.4 gives an overview of related terms and values related to lung volumes and capacities for a normal-size adult male. The amount of gas that enters and leaves the body with each breath is approximately 350 to 500 mL and represents the tidal volume (Vt). The minute volume (MV) equals Vt multiplied by the respiratory rate. However, because some ventilation occupies the conducting zone, only a portion of the minute ventilation (V̇e) participates in gas exchange. The amount of alveolar ventilation in a minute equals Vt minus anatomic dead space (the volume of the conducting airways, which is approximately 2 mL/kg of body weight) multiplied by the ventilatory rate. The rate of alveolar ventilation will be indirectly proportional to the arterial CO_2 tension. The residual volume (RV) is the volume of gas left in the lung after a maximal exhalation (approximately 1.2–1.5 L). The RV cannot be removed from the lungs voluntarily and is important because it is a component of the functional residual capacity (FRC), which represents alveolar gas used for oxygenation of the blood between breaths or in periods of apnea. The expiratory reserve volume is the volume of gas expelled from the lungs during a maximal forced exhalation, starting at the end of a normal tidal exhalation. The inspiratory reserve volume is the volume of gas inhaled into the lungs during a maximal forced inhalation, starting at the end of a normal tidal inspiration (2.5–3 L).

The sum of the four basic lung volumes is the TLC. Several types of lung capacity measures exist, each of which is the sum of two or more lung volumes. TLC is the volume of air in the lungs after a maximal inspiratory effort (~6 L in a 70-kg adult). The vital capacity is the amount of air that can be forcibly exhaled from the lungs after a maximal inspiratory effort (~4.5–5 L). The FRC is the volume of gas contained in the lungs after normal quiet expiration. It is the sum of the RV

TABLE 29.4 Glossary for Static Lung Volumes and Capacities

Measurement	Symbol	Definition	Capacity (mL)
Volumes			
Residual volume	RV	Volume of air remaining in the lungs after maximum expiration	1200
Expiratory reserve volume	ERV	Maximum volume of air expired from the resting end-expiratory level	1100
Tidal volume	Vt	Volume of air inspired or expired with each breath during quiet breathing	500
Inspiratory reserve volume	IRV	Maximum volume of air inspired from the resting end-inspiratory level	3000
Capacities			
Inspiratory capacity	IC = IRV + Vt	Maximum volume of air inspired from the end-expiratory level (the sum of IRV and Vt)	3500
Vital capacity	VC = IRV + Vt + ERV	Maximum volume of air expired from the maximum inspiratory level	4500
Functional residual capacity	FRC = RV + ERV	Volume of air remaining in the lungs at the end-expiratory level (the sum of RV and ERV)	2300
Total lung capacity	TLC = IRV + Vt + ERV + RV	Volume of air in the lungs after maximum inspiration (the sum of all volume compartments)	5800

and expiratory reserve volume (~2.2–2.4 L). The inspiratory capacity is the volume of air inhaled into the lungs during a maximal inspiratory effort that begins at FRC (~3.5–3.8 L). Fig. 29.5 gives a graphic representation of lung volumes and normal flow measurements.

Closing volume describes the phenomenon during exhalation when small airways collapse, hindering further emptying of distal lung units. Closing volume is defined as the volume above residual volume where small airways close, whereas closing capacity describes the absolute volume of gas in the lung when small airways close (the closing capacity is the sum of the closing volume plus the residual volume). The closing volume is normally below residual volume in an individual but increases from approximately 30% of the TLC at age 20 years to approximately 55% at age 70 years. Certain conditions increase the closing volume, such as supine positioning, pregnancy, obesity, COPD, congestive heart failure (CHF), aging, or anything that decreases residual volume.[15] In abnormal conditions, if the closing volume exceeds the FRC, airway closure occurs during tidal breathing, resulting in

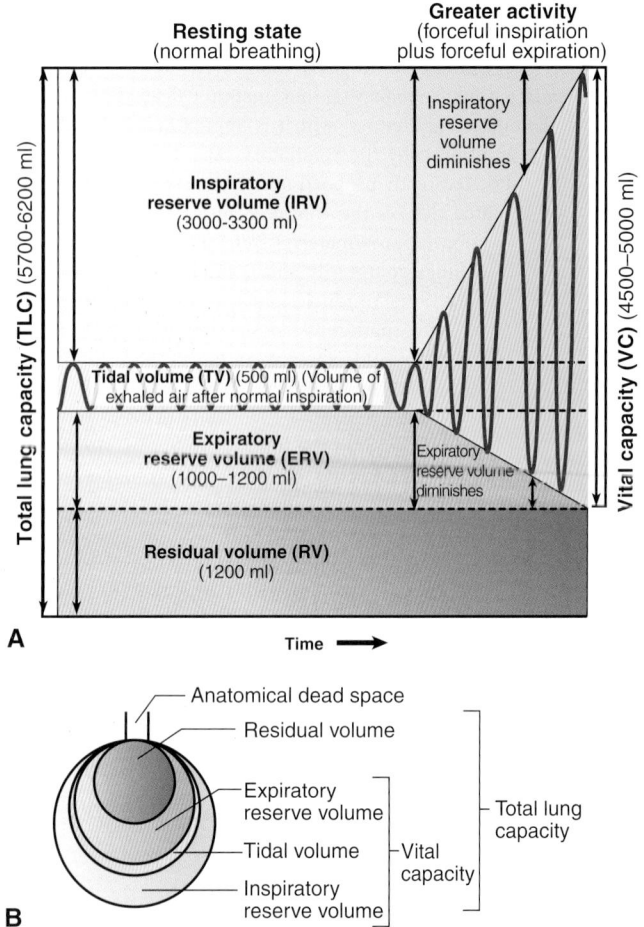

A Time →

B

Fig. 29.5 Pulmonary ventilation volumes. (A) The chart shows a tracing like that produced with a spirometer. (B) The diagram shows the pulmonary volumes as relative proportions of an inflated balloon. During normal, quiet breathing, approximately 500 mL of air is moved into and out of the respiratory tract, an amount called the tidal volume. During forceful breathing (like that during and after heavy exercise), an extra 3300 mL can be inspired (the inspiratory reserve volume), and an extra 1000 mL or so can be expired (the expiratory reserve volume). The largest volume of air that can be moved in and out during ventilation is called the vital capacity. Air that remains in the respiratory tract after a forceful expiration is called the residual volume. (From Patton KT, Thibodeau GA. *The Human Body in Health and Disease.* 7th ed. St. Louis: Elsevier; 2018:476.)

poorly ventilated or unventilated alveoli and intrapulmonary shunting. The shearing forces of repetitive airway opening and closing also lead to airway injury.[16] Measurements of closing volume analyzing washout characteristics of inert gas are more sensitive indicators of small airway disease (such as from smoking) than is measurement of spirometry.[17]

GAS EXCHANGE IN THE LUNGS

Dead Space

Dead space refers to ventilation that does not participate in gas exchange. The volume of the conducting airways represents the anatomic dead space and normally equals approximately 2 mL/kg of body weight. Alveoli that are ventilated but not perfused comprise the alveolar dead space because they neither deliver oxygen nor remove CO_2 from the blood. The sum of the anatomic dead space plus the alveolar dead space is the physiologic dead space (V_D). Because perfused ventilation equilibrates with arteriolar CO_2 and nonperfused (dead space) ventilation does not, the proportion of dead space ventilation can be calculated by comparing the ratio of CO_2 in the arterial blood and in the exhaled gas. This is calculated with the Bohr equation:

$$\% V_D = (PaCO_2 - PeCO_2)/PaCO_2$$

where $PaCO_2$ is the arterial partial pressure of CO_2 as determined from arterial blood gas (ABG) measurement, and $PeCO_2$ is the PCO_2 (partial pressure of carbon dioxide) of mixed expired gas as determined by capnography. Certain pathologic conditions, such as pulmonary embolus, increase the alveolar dead space and can abruptly decrease the end tidal CO_2 ($ETCO_2$) levels monitored with capnography.[1–5]

Regional Distribution of Alveolar Ventilation

Gravity and other factors influence ventilation and perfusion such that both are unevenly distributed throughout the lungs. In the normal upright lung, the alveoli at the base are more compliant than those at the apex, meaning that those at the base exhibit a greater change in volume with each breath. This is considered to be a result of the effect of gravity on the interconnected parenchyma of the lung, whereby the greatest "pull" is exerted on the more superior portions of lung. The alveoli in the nondependent areas of the lung are held in a more open state even at rest, whereas alveoli at the base are more compressed. During inspiration, then, the alveoli at the bases are able to accept more new gas. Alterations to the resting volume or impingements on lung compliance may change this relationship. Pregnancy or obesity may hinder expansion of lower units or may cause compression that results in collapsed dependent areas. If this is the case, other lung areas become more compliant. The sigmoidal shape of the compliance curve (see Fig. 29.2) reveals that alveoli become less compliant at higher volumes (e.g., in nondependent alveoli at high lung volume) and at very low volumes (e.g., in dependent alveoli at very low resting lung volumes).

Alveolar Oxygen and Carbon Dioxide Levels

The levels of O_2 and CO_2 in alveolar gas are determined by several factors. These include (1) the amount of alveolar ventilation, (2) the inspired concentrations of O_2 and CO_2, (3) the flow of mixed venous blood to the lungs, and (4) the body's consumption of O_2 and production of CO_2. In a person spontaneously breathing room air, each breath brings approximately 350 mL of fresh air (21% of which is O_2) into the alveoli, which already contain over 2 L of gas (the FRC). Each exhalation removes approximately 350 mL of gas consisting of 5% to 6% CO_2. Every minute, approximately 250 mL of O_2 diffuse from the alveoli into the pulmonary capillary blood, whereas approximately 200 mL of CO_2 diffuse from the pulmonary capillary blood into the alveoli. The ratio of the amount of CO_2 produced to the quantity of O_2 consumed is called the respiratory quotient (RQ = 200 mL CO_2 produced divided by 250 mL O_2 consumed = 0.8). The proportion of CO_2 production and O_2 consumption varies with energy source (greater with more carbohydrates and lower with more fat), but 0.8 is the typical result from a mixed diet.

Approximately 21% of dry atmospheric air is O_2; therefore at the standard barometric pressure of 760 mm Hg, the partial pressure of O_2 in atmosphere (Po_2atm) equals 0.21×760 mm Hg, or 160 mm Hg. Only 0.04% of atmospheric air is CO_2, so Pco_2atm = 0.3 mm Hg. As the inspired air passes through the upper airways, it is heated to body temperature and humidified to a relative humidity of nearly 100%. The partial pressure of water vapor at body temperature is a fairly constant 47 mm Hg. The Po_2 of inspired air (Pio_2) saturated with water vapor at standard atmospheric pressure = $0.21 \times (760$ mm Hg $- 47$ mm Hg), or 149 mm Hg.

The inspired gas mixes with the gas already in the alveoli (FRC) and rapidly equilibrates with the pulmonary capillary blood. The alveolar Po_2 (Pao_2) can be calculated with the alveolar air equation:

$$PAO_2 = PiO_2 - (PACO_2/RQ)$$

Thus, during breathing of atmospheric air, when alveolar Pco_2 ($Paco_2$) is 40 mm Hg and the RQ is 0.8, $Pao_2 = (0.21 \times [760$ mm Hg $- 47$ mm Hg]$) - 40$ mm Hg/0.8 = 99 mm Hg. Therefore, using the alveolar air equation, one can calculate the Pao_2 if the atmospheric pressure, inspired O_2 concentration, and $Paco_2$ (which is approximately equal both to the end tidal Pco_2 and the arterial Pco_2 [$Paco_2$]) are known, because water vapor pressure and RQ are fairly constant. If the inspired O_2 concentration differs from that of room air, then that fraction replaces the 0.21. Pao_2 is less than Pio_2 because the CO_2 is delivered to the alveoli by the pulmonary blood flow at the same time that O_2 is taken up from the alveoli. Therefore $Paco_2$ divided by the RQ approximates the amount of O_2 that was removed from the alveoli by the pulmonary capillary blood flow.[1-5]

Effects of Alveolar Ventilation on Carbon Dioxide and Oxygen

Within certain limits, $Paco_2$ is inversely proportional to alveolar ventilation. If alveolar ventilation is doubled, then $Paco_2$ and $Paco_2$ are reduced by half (if CO_2 production remains unchanged).

As alveolar ventilation increases, Pao_2 also increases slightly. However, doubling alveolar ventilation does not double Pao_2; according to the alveolar air equation, reduction of the $Paco_2$ raises the Pao_2, bringing Pao_2 closer to the Pio_2.

PULMONARY BLOOD FLOW

The lungs have a dual blood supply: (1) the bronchial arteries (usually one on the right and two on the left), and (2) the pulmonary arteries, which bring unoxygenated blood to the lungs from the right ventricle. The bronchial arteries arise from the descending aorta and carry approximately 2% of the cardiac output to nourish the nonrespiratory tissues: lung parenchyma, bronchi, nerves, pulmonary vessels, and visceral pleura. Bronchial arteries do not participate in fresh gas exchange with the alveoli. The branches of the bronchial arteries accompany the bronchial divisions as far as the respiratory bronchioles. The bronchial veins return deoxygenated blood from the first part of the bronchi and drain into the azygos, hemiazygos, or posterior intercostal veins. The remainder of the deoxygenated blood is returned via the pulmonary veins.

The pulmonary circulation provides blood flow to the structures distal to the terminal bronchioles, including distal nonrespiratory tissues and the respiratory units. The pulmonary artery arises from the right ventricle and branches into the right and left pulmonary arteries, which further branch to accompany the bronchi. Although the pulmonary artery receives the entire CO of the right ventricle, its walls are less muscular and more distensible than those of the aorta, and the pulmonary artery pressure (PAP) is considerably less than the pressure in the aorta. The pulmonary arteries rapidly subdivide into terminal branches, which have thinner walls, much less smooth muscle, and greater internal diameters than corresponding branches of the systemic arterial tree. Pulmonary vessels are also much shorter than systemic vessels, and, according to Poiseuille's law, a decrease in length decreases resistance. Subsequently, pulmonary vascular resistance (PVR) is very low, approximately one-eighth of systemic vascular resistance (SVR).

PVR is fairly evenly distributed among the arteries, capillaries, and veins, whereas most of the resistance in the systemic circulation is in the muscular arteries. Although pulmonary venous resistance is very low, it can decrease further when blood flow increases. This results from passive changes in resistance caused by recruitment and distensibility of the pulmonary vessels. Recruitment is the opening to perfusion of pulmonary vessels that were previously not perfused. Distensibility is an increase in diameter of a pulmonary vessel that is already being perfused, and it results from the vessel's compliance.

The sympathetic nervous system influences PVR, as do certain substances circulating in the pulmonary blood. PVR is increased by norepinephrine, serotonin, histamine, hypoxia, endothelin, leukotriene, thromboxane, prostaglandin (e.g., $PGF_2\alpha$), and hypercapnia.[18] It is decreased by prostacyclin analogs (e.g., epoprostenol), endothelin receptor antagonists (e.g., bosentan), phosphodiesterase type 5 inhibitors (e.g., sildenafil), acetylcholine, and isoproterenol (minimal effect). Short-term or limited-use medications to reduce PVR include inhaled nitric oxide, sildenafil, tadalafil, iloprost, treprostinil, and riociguat.[18-20]

The respiratory units are the site of gas exchange between alveolar air and pulmonary capillary blood. After participating in gas exchange in the respiratory zone, blood is returned to the heart by way of the pulmonary veins. The pulmonary vessels also anastomose with the bronchial vessels at the junction of the terminal and respiratory bronchioles. Thus the pulmonary veins carry oxygenated blood from the respiratory units and deoxygenated blood from the visceral pleura and distal bronchi. The venous bronchopulmonary anastomoses are significant in their contribution to the normal anatomic shunt (the addition of unoxygenated blood to the left chambers of the heart). Evidence of this crossover is observed during complete cardiopulmonary bypass: Blood enters the left atrium, even though all blood is shunted from the right heart by the venous cannula. This occurs because blood flow continues through the bronchial vessels, which anastomose with the pulmonary veins, which in turn ultimately drain into the left atrium; this is one reason a ventricular drain may be inserted during surgery to prevent overdistention of the heart. Five pulmonary veins ultimately return blood to the left heart.

Pulmonary Blood Flow and Hypoxic Pulmonary Vasoconstriction

Although pulmonary vessels are less muscular as compared to systemic arteries, the low pressure of the system makes pulmonary blood flow very sensitive to small changes in arterial tone. Unlike the systemic circulation, where hemodynamic influences are more global, pulmonary blood flow is more readily and locally regulated by changes in oxygen and carbon dioxide tension. In contrast to the systemic circulation, high oxygen tension and hypocapnia vasodilate pulmonary vessels (which helps those vessels pick up more oxygen), whereas hypoxia, hypercarbia, and acidosis cause vasoconstriction. Hypoxic and/or atelectatic alveoli has the strongest influence on local pulmonary blood flow regulation and causes blood flow to be actively diverted at a precapillary site by a process known as hypoxic pulmonary vasoconstriction. This protective physiologic reflex acts to shunt blood away from focal hypoxic areas of the lung in an effort to improve the matching of ventilation and perfusion. See Chapter 30 for a discussion of the characteristics and significance of hypoxic pulmonary vasoconstriction during pulmonary surgery.

Relationship of Pulmonary Blood Flow and Ventilation

In the normal upright lung, a greater portion of the blood flow is distributed to the dependent regions because of the effects of hydrostatic pressure and greater distention of dependent pulmonary vessels. Likewise, differences in compliance of the ventilating tissue also result in a general increase in the proportion of ventilation from nondependent (least ventilation) to dependent (most ventilation) of the lungs. There are two caveats to these rules. Although they describe what occurs during spontaneous respiration well, the spatial distribution of these relationships is altered during positive pressure ventilation. In addition, the lung zones are commonly portrayed in textbooks in nicely demarcated lines of latitude, a model appreciated for its simple elegance.

Although there may be a general increase in perfusion from top to bottom of the lung, it should be noted that gravity alone does not determine physiologic perfusion. If it did, then it would be observed that the greatest blood flow in the body would be in the lower extremities, with the least in the head, a cogent point of explanation offered by Levitzky.[21] Gravity interacts with elastic forces to influence ventilation, and with vessel recruitment to alter distribution of perfusion. The gravitational model explaining ventilation-perfusion matching has been called into question, and there is evidence that regional perfusion zones may be situated with the greatest blood flow in the lower core areas of the lungs, with zones 2 and 1 more resembling concentric spheres radiating toward the periphery.[22] Furthermore, there is an impressive body of evidence that supports the distribution of ventilation to perfusion, at least in part, dependent on the diameter and branching patterns of both pulmonary vascular and pulmonary bronchial structures.[23]

Despite the fact that the gravitational model explaining ventilation-perfusion distribution between zones (as described by West in 1964) has not been completely confirmed by both animal and human studies, it does serve as a useful model for considering the relationships between ventilation and perfusion, and more specifically the conditions under which intraalveolar pressure may impede vascular flow.[24] In this model, regions of the lung are divided into zones according to the relative intravascular and intraalveolar pressure (Fig. 29.6).

In the parts of the lung where alveoli exist at a greater resting volume, alveolar pressure can exceed pulmonary arterial pressure so that perfusion is impeded. This is called zone 1, and it represents alveolar dead space because the region is ventilated but not perfused. Normally, zone 1 either does not exist or exists only in a very small margin of lung area around the apical border during spontaneous ventilation. However, the use of PEEP or high airway pressures during positive pressure and/or mechanical ventilation can create or expand this zone.

The intermediate zone is zone 2, which consists of a variable relationship between vascular and alveolar pressure. A point is described in zone 2 along the continuum of decreasing intraalveolar pressure where arterial pressure exceeds alveolar. Below that point, flow is solely dependent upon arterial flow and unrelated to alveolar or venous pressure. This concept is described as a waterfall zone, as when rising water finally overflows a dam. At that point, the height of the dam does not influence the flow; only the upstream inflow does. The zone 2

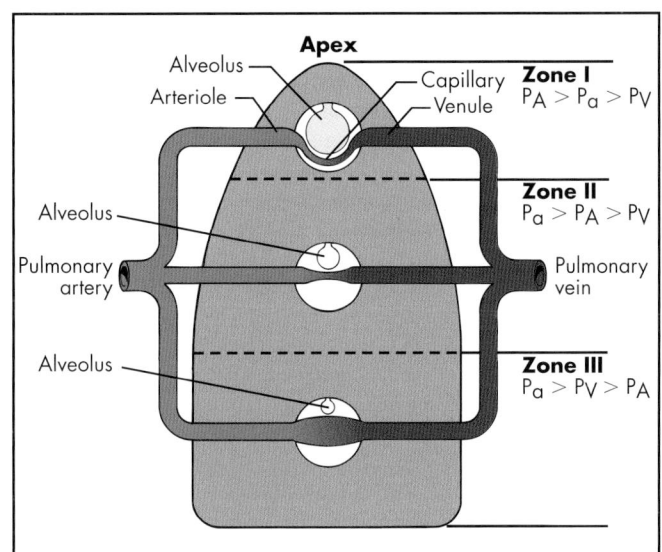

Fig. 29.6 Gravity and alveolar pressure. Effects of gravity and alveolar pressure on pulmonary blood flow in the three lung zones. In zone I, alveolar pressure *(PA)* is greater than arterial and venous pressure, and no blood flow occurs. In zone II, arterial pressure *(Pa)* exceeds alveolar pressure, but alveolar pressure exceeds venous pressure *(PV)*. Blood flow occurs in this zone, but alveolar pressure compresses the venules (venous ends of the capillaries). In zone III, both arterial and venous pressures are greater than alveolar pressure, and blood flow fluctuates depending on the difference between arterial and venous pressures. (From McCance KL, Huether SE. *Pathophysiology: The Biologic Basis for Disease in Adults and Children.* 8th ed. St. Louis: Elsevier; 2019:1240.)

relationship is not static, but fluctuation in alveolar pressure related to respiration can variably occlude capillary flow.

The dependent portion of the lung, where both pulmonary arterial and venous pressures exceed alveolar pressure, is known as zone 3. This zone represents continuous blood flow throughout the respiratory cycle. Thus there is no obstruction to blood flow. The tip of a pulmonary artery catheter should be placed within this zone to ensure continuous communication with the left heart. Alveoli in this zone rest at a lower volume than in zones 1 and 2, and so have a greater compliance with the ability to better expand to ideally match ventilation to perfusion within the lung.

West later described a fourth zone in the most dependent portions of lung, wherein extravascular pressure from mechanical compression or interstitial fluid compresses the vessels and occludes their flow.[25]

Pulmonary Edema

The normal distance for diffusion from the alveolar air space into the pulmonary capillary blood cells is less than 1 µm. The gas must traverse the surfactant layer, the flat alveolar type I cells, the interstitial space, the endothelial cells that make up the wall of the pulmonary capillary, a minute amount of plasma, and then finally the membrane of the red blood cell. The pulmonary system is designed to allow free passage of gases across this series of structures, collectively called the respiratory membrane. However, that inherent "leakiness" does predispose this area to unintended movement of fluid.

There is a fine balance between the forces that tend to hold fluid within the pulmonary capillaries (e.g., plasma colloid oncotic pressure) and the forces that tend to favor fluid movement into the interstitial space (e.g., capillary hydrostatic pressure, interstitial fluid colloid oncotic pressure, and negative interstitial fluid pressure). In normal circumstances, the net effect of these forces favors movement into the

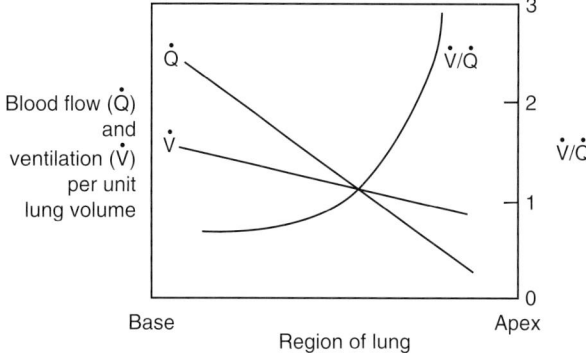

Fig. 29.7 Ventilation-perfusion relationships throughout the lung.

interstitium, helping to divert fluid from the adjacent leaky capillaries and prevent accumulation into the alveoli.[26] Although the interstitium has a large compliance for removing accumulating transudate fluid, derangements in the previously mentioned factors can lead to fluid accumulation within the interstitium or alveoli and disrupt gas exchange.

Pulmonary vascular congestion can cause an increase in capillary leakage into the interstitium, resulting in a greater distance for gas diffusion. If capillary leak overcomes the compliance and capacity of the interstitial space, then fluid may begin to pass into the alveoli. Pulmonary edema affects O_2 diffusion more than CO_2 excretion because CO_2 is 20 times more diffusible than O_2. Many conditions can result in pulmonary edema. The high capillary pressures associated with heart failure or an excessive administration of intravenous fluid volume can increase the fluid content within the lungs. Pulmonary capillary pore size can increase in sepsis, smoke inhalation, and other toxic conditions. Brain trauma can produce an intense sympathetic discharge, resulting in neurogenic pulmonary edema.

A condition that occasionally occurs during emergence from anesthesia is postobstructive pulmonary edema, also referred to as negative pressure pulmonary edema (NPPE). This can occur if the patient experiences laryngospasm or airway obstruction after extubation and then attempts forceful inhalations against the closed glottis. The result is a drastic increase in negative intrathoracic pressure that pulls fluid from the pulmonary capillaries into lung tissue and can cause alveolar-capillary membrane trauma. Common signs of NPPE are evident as upper airway obstruction with strong diaphragmatic effort, shortness of breath, pulmonary rales, decreased oxygen saturation, and/or production of pink, frothy sputum from the lower airway.

The onset of pulmonary edema can be rapid and is usually treatable. The symptoms resolve rapidly; in most cases, patients are discharged within 24 hours. Treatment includes removing the precipitating condition (e.g., relieving airway obstruction) and general supportive measures: oxygen, maintenance of a patent airway, noninvasive continuous positive airway pressure (CPAP), intubation with PEEP when needed to maintain oxygenation, diuretics, and potentially steroids. Unlike pulmonary edema related to fluid overload, treatment for NPPE does not routinely include diuretic therapy. However, many reported cases do include the use of diuretics and corticosteroids.[27] The three mainstays of treatment remain treatment of the precipitating condition, normalization of ventilation and oxygenation, and reduction of lung congestion and fluid. Treatment summary is included in Box 29.4.

Ventilation-Perfusion Relationships in the Lung

Normally, ventilation $(\dot{V})$ is approximately 4 L/min, whereas pulmonary blood flow $(\dot{Q})$ is approximately 5 L/min resulting in a ventilation-perfusion ratio $(\dot{V}/\dot{Q})$ of 0.8 for the entire lung. However, $\dot{V}$ and $\dot{Q}$ must be matched within the lung at the alveolar-capillary level for gas exchange to occur.

Dependent portions of the lung receive a greater amount of blood flow as compared to the nondependent portions because of the effects of gravity and vessel recruitment and distensibility. Additionally, ventilation is predominant to the more compliant portions of the lung. Normally at FRC, the dependent regions of the lung are more compliant, whereas alveoli in the nondependent portions can be more inflated (tented open) and less compliant in certain circumstances (e.g., positive pressure ventilation and PEEP). Consequently, more evenly matched ventilation and perfusion favor the dependent lung portions, resulting in optimal gas exchange.

During spontaneous breathing both blood flow and ventilation are greatest at the lung bases. Ventilation flow normally decreases from dependent to nondependent regions of the lung. Due to gravitational effects, there is also an accompanying decrease in perfusion (which is even greater). Therefore the $\dot{V}/\dot{Q}$ ratio increases as measured progressively from base to apical lung areas (Fig. 29.7). In addition, $\dot{V}/\dot{Q}$ varies: In alveoli that are ventilated but not perfused, $\dot{Q}$ equals 0, so $\dot{V}/\dot{Q}$ equals infinity (i.e., dead space); in alveoli that are perfused but not ventilated, $\dot{V}$ equals 0, so $\dot{V}/\dot{Q}$ equals 0 (i.e., a shunt). Similarly, alveoli that are ventilated but poorly perfused are described as dead space, whereas alveoli that are perfused but poorly ventilated are termed shuntlike; the latter contribute to the $\dot{V}/\dot{Q}$ mismatch of the lung. Shuntlike alveoli (low $\dot{V}/\dot{Q}$) have relatively low Po_2 and high Pco_2 when compared with dead space–like alveoli (high $\dot{V}/\dot{Q}$), which have relatively high Po_2 and low Pco_2.

Ventilation-perfusion mismatch can result from a number of causes. A pulmonary embolus of thrombus, air, or other material that passes through the pulmonary artery to obstruct blood flow through the pulmonary capillaries creates alveolar dead space. Likewise, very high airway pressure from aggressive ventilation or PEEP can produce alveoli that are ventilated but not perfused. Similarly, very low CO results in low pulmonary blood flow and therefore increases the $\dot{V}/\dot{Q}$ ratio. This is reflected by a low $ETco_2$ on capnography and an increased gradient between the end tidal and the arterial Pco_2.

Total pulmonary venous admixture (unoxygenated blood delivered to the left side of the heart) is the sum of the shunt and shuntlike states. Bronchopulmonary anastomoses are a cause of normal anatomic shunt, along with thebesian veins, which drain into the left side of the heart and usually account for less than 2% of the CO. Airway obstruction, alveolar collapse (atelectasis), and alveolar filling processes, such as pneumonia, also produce shunt.

Some diagnostic studies can definitively identify ventilation-perfusion abnormalities. A lung scan after a single breath of xenon 133 (^{133}Xe) gas or aerosolized technetium-99m can be used to determine the location of poorly ventilated areas in the lung, whereas intravenous injection of dissolved radioisotope reveals areas of the lung that are poorly perfused. Together these comprise a ventilation-perfusion scan. Pulmonary angiography (radiography with injection of intravenous contrast dye) of the pulmonary vasculature can be used to determine whether any pulmonary blood vessels are obstructed, such as with a pulmonary embolism.[1-5]

Effects of General Anesthesia on Respiratory Physiology

General anesthesia affects the matching of ventilation and perfusion in several ways. Changing position from upright to supine, and induction of general anesthesia, results in a significant decrease in FRC (see Chapter 23). With positive pressure ventilation, the distribution of ventilation becomes more uniform throughout the lung, so both the dependent and nondependent alveoli receive approximately the same amount of ventilation. This leads to a wider scatter of ventilation and perfusion because there is relatively more ventilation of underperfused alveoli. General anesthesia also causes a significant decrease in CO, which is exacerbated by positive pressure ventilation, especially if it is accompanied by PEEP. This may promote an extension of zone 1 areas, although this theoretic effect is probably overstated. Atelectasis is a common finding with general anesthesia and is the main cause of the 10% shunt commonly observed in patients under anesthesia.[26]

Although hypoxic pulmonary vasoconstriction is partially effective in diverting blood flow away from poorly ventilated lung regions, most inhaled anesthetics (as well as potent vasodilators, such as nitroprusside and nitroglycerin) decrease the effectiveness of hypoxic pulmonary vasoconstriction, whereas most intravenous anesthetics have minimal effects. The inhibition of hypoxic pulmonary vasoconstriction contributes to the decrease in PaO_2. The increase in the alveolar-arterial PO_2 difference usually occurs when volatile inhaled anesthetic agents are used in significant concentrations.

General anesthesia, particularly when administered in combination with muscle relaxants, increases chest-wall compliance (i.e., less elastic) Laryngoscopy and endotracheal intubation can increase airway resistance by stimulating airway irritant receptors, thereby decreasing dynamic compliance (i.e., can restrict airflow). However, most inhaled anesthetics (except for nitrous oxide [N_2O]) act as bronchodilators. In addition, medications that are used to produce general anesthesia depress the ventilatory response to CO_2, metabolic acidosis, and hypoxia (as discussed later in this chapter).[28]

Oxygen and Carbon Dioxide Exchange

As blood flows through the lungs, the mean pulmonary transit time is approximately 4 to 5 seconds, with the blood spending approximately 0.75 second in the pulmonary capillaries. However, in the normal lung, it takes only one-third of the time, or 0.25 second, for equilibration to occur between the alveolar air and the pulmonary capillary blood. During exercise, CO may be so greatly increased that the time a blood cell spends in a pulmonary capillary can be reduced to 0.25 second. This decreased time available for diffusion has a much greater effect on the exchange of O_2 than on that of CO_2 because CO_2 diffuses approximately 20 times more rapidly than O_2. Diffusivity is defined as the solubility divided by the square root of the molecular weight. Carbon dioxide is a heavier molecule than O_2 but is 24-fold more soluble in body fluids than O_2.[4]

Oxygen Transport

The blood carries O_2 in two ways: (1) physically dissolved in the plasma, and (2) bound to hemoglobin (Hgb) in the red blood cells. Normally 99.7% of the O_2 carried is bound to Hgb. Without adequate Hgb, the cardiovascular system could not transport sufficient O_2 to meet the metabolic demands of the tissues.

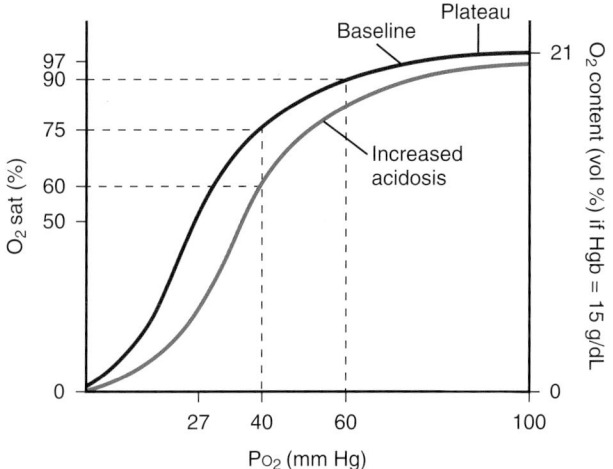

Fig. 29.8 Oxyhemoglobin dissociation curve. (From Roberts JR, et al. *Roberts and Hedges' Clinical Procedures in Emergency Medicine and Acute Care.* 7th ed. Philadelphia: Elsevier; 2019.)

The solubility coefficient of oxygen in plasma is 0.003, so there is 0.003 mL of O_2 per every 1 mm Hg partial pressure of PO_2 dissolved in 100 mL of whole blood. Therefore, with a PaO_2 of 100 mm Hg, only 0.3 mL of O_2 is transported dissolved per deciliter of plasma. Each gram of Hgb can combine with 1.39 mL of oxygen; however, because of factors that contaminate this process (such as the presence of methemoglobin), a factor of 1.36 is applied in clinical calculations. Therefore, if the level of Hgb is 10 g/100 mL, then at 100% saturation, 1.36 mL of O_2 is bound to Hgb per 100 mL of blood. Note that a Hgb level of 10 g/100 mL of blood corresponds to a hematocrit of 30% as the hematocrit is normally approximately equal to the Hgb level multiplied by 3.

The normal hematocrit for a male is approximately 45% (Hgb 15 g/dL) and for a female is approximately 39% (Hgb 13 g/dL). Centrifugation of the blood in a capillary tube separates the cells from the plasma. A thin layer called the buffy coat separates the plasma and the red blood cells (erythrocytes). This thin layer (~1% of the volume of the blood) consists of white blood cells and platelets.[4]

Oxyhemoglobin Dissociation Curve

The affinity of Hgb for oxygen fluctuates with various physiologic conditions. This unique characteristic means that Hgb changes its affinity for oxygen because of its allosteric characteristics depending on the environment. Hgb changes its conformational shape in response to high oxygen concentrations, such as in the lungs, allowing oxygen to bind more readily to the heme component of the Hgb protein. Conversely, in areas of lower oxygen concentrations (i.e., peripheral tissues), Hgb alters its shape to allow for the unloading of oxygen and delivery to peripheral cells. Hgb's affinity for oxygen is described by the relationship between the saturation of Hgb at a given PO_2 in the plasma and is represented by the oxyhemoglobin ($HgbO_2$) dissociation curve (Fig. 29.8). This relationship between PO_2 and $HgbO_2$ is described by a sigmoidal curve that is steep at lower PO_2 values and nearly flat when the PO_2 is greater than 70 mm Hg. As the PO_2 of the plasma increases, the amount of O_2 bound to the Hgb also increases, but not in a linear manner. This phenomenon occurs as each of the four Hgb subunits combines with O_2, and each combination facilitates the next. Similarly, when the O_2 is unloaded at the peripheral tissues, each dissociation facilitates the next. Therefore this S-shaped curve is extremely important physiologically. Interaction between O_2 and Hgb is also influenced by pH, PCO_2, temperature, and the concentration of 2,3-diphosphoglycerate (a metabolite of glucose hydrolysis during glycolysis).

The changing affinity of Hgb for O_2 facilitates loading at the pulmonary capillaries and unloading of the O_2 at the peripheral capillaries and cells. The S-shaped $HgbO_2$ dissociation curve is displaced to the left of the normal curve by hypocapnia, a decrease in temperature, alkalosis, and a decrease in 2,3-diphosphoglycerate levels, resulting in an increased affinity of the Hgb for O_2 (a higher saturation for a given Po_2). When exposed to increased temperature, hypercapnia, acidosis, and elevated 2,3-diphosphoglycerate levels, the affinity of Hgb for O_2 decreases. This results in a shift of the $HgbO_2$ dissociation curve to the right, and therefore O_2 more readily diffuses to the tissues. Note that the conditions that favor the release of O_2 from the Hgb to the tissues are likely to be associated with increased tissue metabolism, which would increase the O_2 demand. The influence of pH and Pco_2 on the $HgbO_2$ dissociation curve is referred as the Bohr effect. The position of the oxyhemoglobin curve can be quantified by the P_{50}, which is simply used as an indicator to identify a shift in the curve. The P_{50} corresponds to the Pao_2 at which 50% of the Hgb is saturated. Under normal conditions, adult human blood has a P_{50} of 26 to 27 mm Hg. If the $HgbO_2$ dissociation curve shifts to the right, the P_{50} increases; if it shifts to the left, the P_{50} decreases.

Other factors that affect O_2 transport include carbon monoxide poisoning and methemoglobinemia, both of which cause a left shift in the oxyhemoglobin dissociation curve. Carbon monoxide binds to Hgb (forming carboxyhemoglobin) with over 200 times the affinity of O_2.[29] Carbon monoxide binds with the heme moiety of Hgb causing a conformational change in Hgb, which prevents the off-loading of O_2 from the other three oxygen binding sites at peripheral tissues. In addition, to a small degree carbon monoxide inhibits the peripheral utilization of O_2 at the tissue level by impairing oxidative phosphorylation at the cellular mitochondrial level. Without a multiple-channel oximeter, carboxyhemoglobin provides a misleadingly high reading because it interprets the Hgb as being "saturated," without distinguishing the inability of the Hgb to unload O_2. Carbon monoxide poisoning is primarily treated by removal from the source, and with high flow and high levels of FiO_2. In severe cases hyperbaric O_2 therapy may be used.[29]

Methemoglobin is Hgb with its iron molecule in its ferric state (Fe^{3+}) instead of the normal ferrous state (Fe^{2+}). In the ferric state, the Hgb iron atoms do not combine with O_2. Methemoglobinemia can be caused by nitrate poisoning (nitroprusside overdose) or toxic reactions to oxidant drugs, such as the local anesthetic prilocaine. Methemoglobinemia is treated with O_2 therapy and methylene blue at a dose of 1 to 2 mg/kg administered intravenously over 5 minutes.[30]

Oxygen Content Calculations

Hgb saturation is continuously monitored in anesthetized patients, but the saturation provides only a relative value; 100% saturation of a Hgb level that is one-half of a normal value represents a similar amount of oxygen as a 50% saturation of the normal amount of Hgb. Absolute values for the amount of O_2 in arterial blood are yielded by the O_2 content equation:

$$CaO_2 = (1.36 \times Hgb \times \% \text{ arterial Hgb saturation}) + (PaO_2 \times 0.003)$$

where CaO_2 is the arterial O_2 content, and Pao_2 and percent of Hgb saturation are obtained from ABG analysis. CaO_2 is normally approximately 20 mL of O_2 per 100 mL of arterial blood (when Hgb is 15 g/dL and Pao_2 >90 mm Hg).

The amount of O_2 in mixed venous blood is calculated with the following equation:

$$C\overline{v}O_2 = (1.36 \times Hgb \times \% \text{ mixed venous Hgb saturation}) + (P\overline{v}O_2 \times 0.003)$$

where $C\overline{v}O_2$ is the mixed venous O_2 content, and $P\overline{v}O_2$ and percent of Hgb saturation are obtained from mixed venous blood gas analysis of blood drawn from the distal lumen of a pulmonary artery catheter (the only site in the body with truly mixed venous blood). $C\overline{v}O_2$ is normally approximately 15 mL of O_2 per 100 mL of mixed venous blood when Hgb is 15 g/dL and $P\overline{v}O_2$ is 40 mm Hg.

Subtraction of $C\overline{v}O_2$ from CaO_2 yields the arteriovenous O_2 content difference. This difference is useful in determining the relationship between O_2 delivery to the body's tissues and the O_2 demand of the tissues. Normally the difference is approximately 5 mL/dL of blood. A difference greater than 5 mL/dL of blood can be associated with a low cardiac output because the blood takes longer to traverse the capillaries in the tissues, or an increase in the metabolic state and need for more O_2 within the tissues. Both result in more O_2 being extracted. A difference of less than 5 mL/dL of blood can be associated with systemic arteriovenous shunts, which allow blood to bypass the tissue capillaries; such shunts occur during hyperdynamic sepsis.

The amount of O_2 in pulmonary capillary blood is calculated with the following equation:

$$CpCO_2 = (1.36 \times Hgb \times \% \text{ pulmonary capillary Hgb saturation}) + (PpCO_2 \times 0.003)$$

where $CpcO_2$ is the pulmonary capillary O_2 content. $PpcO_2$ (partial pressure of oxygen in the pulmonary capillary) is derived from the alveolar air equation described earlier in this chapter; the assumption is made that pulmonary capillary blood equilibrates completely with the partial pressure of oxygen in the alveolar air. The pulmonary capillary oxygen saturation cannot be measured but is estimated by plotting the $PpcO_2$ on the oxyhemoglobin dissociation curve and determining the corresponding Hgb saturation. $CpcO_2$ is normally approximately 21 mL of O_2 per 100 mL of pulmonary capillary blood (when Hgb is 15 g/dL and $PpcO_2$ is 99 mm Hg).

The CaO_2, $C\overline{v}O_2$, and $CpcO_2$ are used in the shunt equation:

$$\dot{Q}S/\dot{Q}T = (CpCO_2 - CaO_2)/(CpCO_2 - C\overline{v}O_2)$$

In this equation, $\dot{Q}S$ is the shunt blood flow, $\dot{Q}T$ is the total blood flow (CO), $CpcO_2$ is the pulmonary capillary O_2 content, CaO_2 is the arterial O_2 content, and $C\overline{v}O_2$ is the mixed venous O_2 content.[28] The shunt equation estimates the fraction of cardiac output that perfuses alveoli that are absolutely nonventilated. In actuality, the shunt calculation represents the sum effects of countless lung units of varying $(\dot{V}/\dot{Q})$ relationships throughout the lung; however, the calculation is useful to monitor trends in oxygenation, help diagnose the cause of observed hypoxemia, and guide alveolar recruitment maneuvers such as PEEP. The proof of this equation is illustrated in Fig. 29.9 and lies in the assumption that if there were no shunt (see Fig. 29.9A), all arterial blood would have been fully oxygenated in the alveolar capillaries. Therefore ($CpcO_2 = CaO_2$) and the numerator of the equation would be zero, thus so would its quotient. On the other hand, with a theoretic 100% shunt (see Fig. 29.9B), no blood would become oxygenated and thus ($C\overline{v}O_2 = CaO_2$); the difference of each from $CpcO_2$ would be the same, and the number divided by itself would equal 1.0, denoting 100% shunt. Fig. 29.9C illustrates a theoretic 50% shunt, where the CaO_2 equilibrates between the $CpcO_2$ and the $C\overline{v}O_2$, so its difference from the $CpcO_2$ is twice that from the $C\overline{v}O_2$, denoting a 0.5 shunt fraction.

One characteristic of the existence of a significant shunt proportion is hypoxemia unresponsive to supplemental oxygen administration. When blood is passing through the lungs unoxygenated, no increase in fraction of inspired oxygen (Fio_2) delivered to other regions can

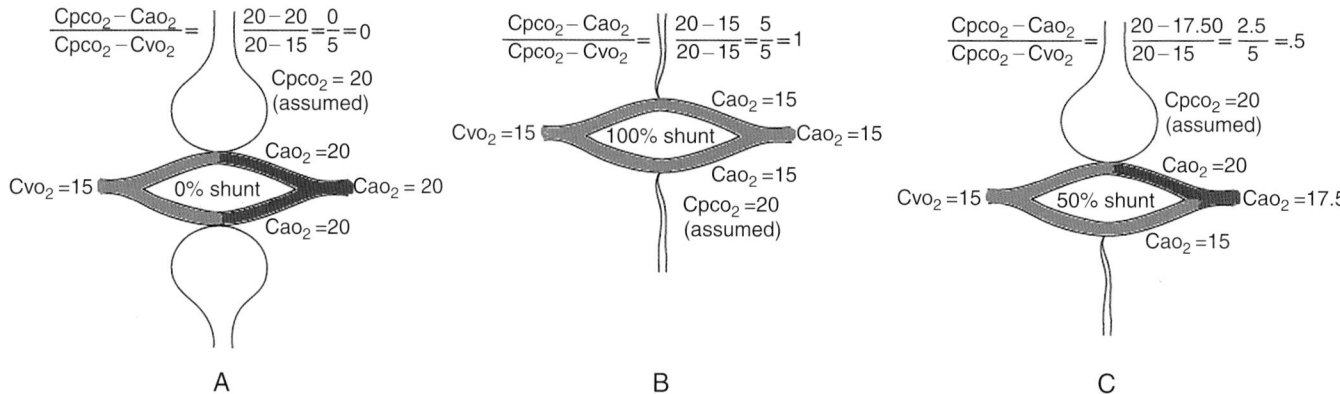

Fig. 29.9 Calculation of the shunt fraction for various theoretic conditions: (A) no shunt, (B) complete shunt, (C) 50% shunt.

overcome the hypoxemia. This is because under normal circumstances, those normal lung regions are already achieving 100% saturation of the Hgb. Therefore they cannot overcompensate for the venous admixture contributed by the shunt areas. In assessing hypoxemia, once hypoventilation and low inspired oxygen are ruled out, improvement in Pao_2 in response to supplemental oxygen favors $\dot{V}/\dot{Q}$ mismatch, as opposed to true shunt or possibly a diffusion disorder (the latter of which can be identified through a test of diffusing capacity of carbon monoxide in the lung [DLCO]).

Transport of Carbon Dioxide

The blood carries CO_2 in three forms: (1) in physical solution, (2) chemically combined with the amino acids of blood proteins, and (3) as bicarbonate ions. Approximately 5% to 10% of the total CO_2 transported in the blood is carried in physical solution. Chemical combination of CO_2 with the terminal amine groups of blood proteins forms carbamino compounds. The reaction occurs rapidly and does not require enzymes. Carbamino compounds constitute another 5% to 10% of the blood's total CO_2 content. The remaining 80% to 90% of the CO_2 in the blood is carried as bicarbonate. Within the red blood cell and in the presence of carbonic anhydrase, CO_2 combines with water to form carbonic acid. The carbonic acid can dissociate into a bicarbonate ion and hydrogen (H^+) according to the following chemical reaction:

$$CO_2 + H_2O \xrightarrow{\text{carbonic anhydrase}} H_2CO_3 \rightarrow H^+ + HCO_3^-$$

When HCO_3^- leaves the blood cells, chloride ions enter to maintain electrical neutrality. This is the so-called chloride shift or hamburger shift.[31]

Carbon Dioxide Dissociation Curve

As expected, decreases in the $Paco_2$ correspond to a decrease in the total CO_2 content in the blood. This is caused by corresponding decreases in the levels of bicarbonate and carbamino compounds. When the $Paco_2$ falls, the amount of the total CO_2 decrease is affected by the presence of O_2 in the blood. When blood contains mainly oxygenated Hgb, the CO_2 dissociation curve shifts to the right, reducing the blood's capacity to hold CO_2. When the blood contains mostly deoxyhemoglobin, the curve shifts to the left, increasing the capacity to carry CO_2. This effect is known as the Haldane effect, which explains how the blood is able to load more CO_2 at the tissue level (where more deoxyhemoglobin is present) and unload CO_2 in the pulmonary capillaries (where more oxyhemoglobin is present) (Fig. 29.10).

The Haldane effect describes how the oxygenation of Hgb affects the transport and elimination of CO_2. The fact that deoxyhemoglobin is a weaker acid than oxyhemoglobin accounts for the Haldane effect. Deoxyhemoglobin more readily accepts the H^+ produced by the dissociation of carbonic acid (which happens in the extrapulmonary capillaries). This permits more CO_2 to be carried in the form of bicarbonate ions (Haldane effect). Then at the pulmonary capillary level the increase in O_2 concentration results in an increase in oxyhemoglobin, which stimulates the dissociation of H+ from Hgb. Bicarbonate then reenters the red blood cell (in exchange for Cl-) and combines with H+ to produce CO_2 and H_2O. Carbon dioxide unbinds to hemoglobin and other plasma proteins, and together with the CO_2 dissolved in blood plasma, diffuses into the alveoli for exhalation.

The Bohr effect explains how higher CO_2 and H^+ ions levels affect O_2 delivery and transport. Excess H+ ions cause Hgb to change its conformational shape, effectively lowering its affinity for O_2. This can happen in situations of low pH (acidosis) or high $Paco_2$ (hypercapnia), which causes a rightward shift in the oxyhemoglobin dissociation curve and the need to release more O_2 to peripheral capillaries and tissues. The ability to more readily deliver and release O_2 to cellular areas and tissues that have a higher metabolism and produce more CO_2 (i.e., heart and brain) is a result of the Bohr effect. A suppressed Bohr effect is seen in lower CO_2 concentrations (i.e., hyperventilation with hypocapnia).[28]

ACID-BASE BALANCE

The respiratory system plays an important role in maintaining normal pH balance within the body. It works along with the kidneys and the buffer systems to balance the acids and bases of the blood and other body tissues, allowing them to function normally. Hydrogen ions interact with negatively charged regions of other molecules, such as proteins, altering their structural conformation and effectively altering their behavior. Besides affecting the oxyhemoglobin dissociation curve, blood pH alters the activity of various enzymes, thereby changing metabolic functions in all body tissues. Severe metabolic acidosis that results from prolonged cardiopulmonary arrest must be treated with sodium bicarbonate because protein-receptor sensitivity and other enzymatic functions must be restored before epinephrine can be effective in the resuscitation.

Metabolism of substances ingested as food produces mainly acidic metabolic waste products. Under normal conditions, a tremendous amount of the acid produced daily can be removed from the body by the respiratory system as exhaled CO_2. The acidic products are known as volatile acids because they can be converted from carbonic acid into CO_2 gas that is exhaled. Through exhalation of CO_2, the lung eliminates over 10,000 mEq/day of carbonic acid. A much smaller amount

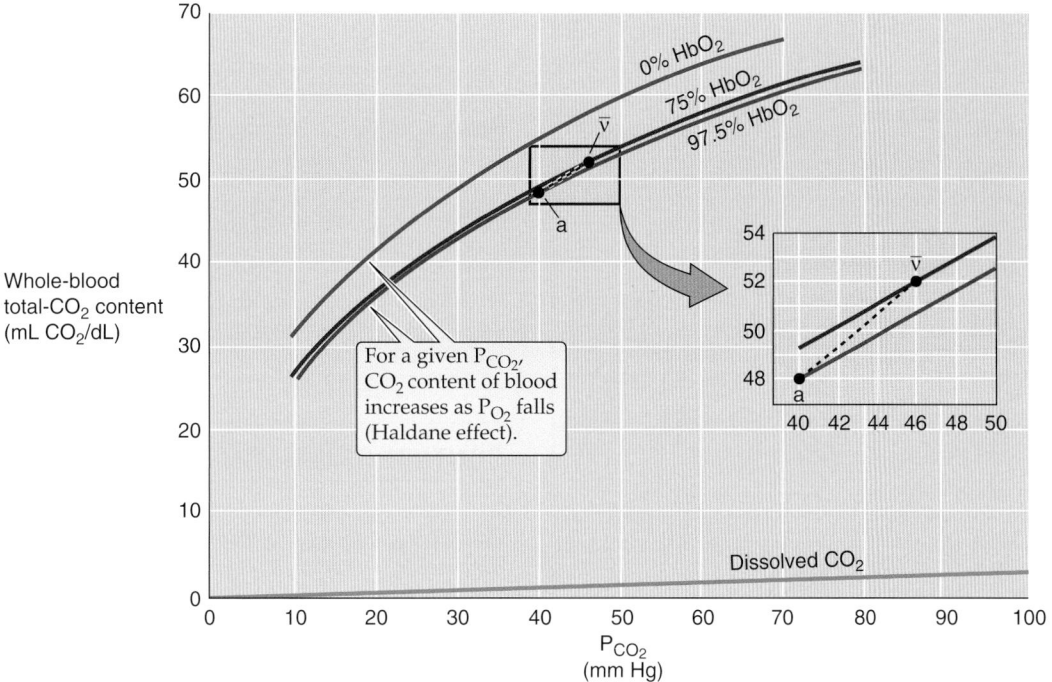

Fig. 29.10 CO_2 dissociation curves (Haldane effect). (From Boron WF, Boulpaep EL. *Medical Physiology.* 3rd ed. Philadelphia: Elsevier; 2017:657.)

of nonvolatile or fixed acids is also produced during normal metabolic breakdown of food at the rate of approximately 100 mEq/day; these acids are primarily removed by the kidneys.[28]

In addition to the efforts of the respiratory system and kidneys to regulate pH levels, buffers in the human body maintain pH within the physiologic range. The buffers consist mainly of bicarbonate, phosphate, and proteins. A buffer is a mixture of substances that usually consists of a weak acid and its conjugate base. When a strong acid or base is added to a buffer system, the changes in H^+ concentration are much smaller than those that would occur if the same amount of acid or base were added to pure water or another nonbuffered solution.

Interpretation of Arterial Blood Gases

Analysis of ABGs can provide useful information concerning the relationship of acid production and acid removal by the lungs and kidneys. Acid-base disturbances can be categorized into four major groups: respiratory acidosis, metabolic acidosis, respiratory alkalosis, and metabolic alkalosis. Each can be considered compensated under certain conditions.

Although it may seem that a great number of acid-base states are possible, only 11 conditions exist (Table 29.5). Blood gases in a normal individual have a pH in the range of 7.35 to 7.45, $Paco_2$ ranges from 35 to 45 mm Hg, and bicarbonate concentration is normally 22 to 26 mEq/L.

Acidosis

Any process that leads to an elevation in $Paco_2$ tends to lower arterial pH, resulting in respiratory acidosis. An acute change in $Paco_2$ of 10 mm Hg is associated with a change in pH of 0.08 units. An increase in $Paco_2$ with a normal bicarbonate level is termed uncompensated respiratory acidosis.

Metabolic acidosis should more properly be referred to as nonrespiratory acidosis because it does not always involve alterations in metabolism. Causes of this condition include ingestion (poisoning), infusion, production of a fixed acid (lactic acidosis), and decreased excretion of

acid by the kidneys. A base change of 10 mEq/L is associated with a pH change of 0.15 unit (in the absence of a change in $Paco_2$). Therefore, if the bicarbonate level increases by 10 mEq/L, then the pH also increases by 0.15 unit. A decrease in bicarbonate level when the Pco_2 remains at approximately 40 mm Hg is termed uncompensated metabolic acidosis. The combination of respiratory acidosis and metabolic acidosis is termed mixed acidosis and can produce a drastically decreased arterial pH.[28]

Alkalosis

When alveolar ventilation exceeds the point required to match CO_2 production, both $Paco_2$ and $Paco_2$ decrease below 35 mm Hg. As the pH rises, this hyperventilation results in respiratory alkalosis. Elevated pH accompanied by a decrease in $Paco_2$ in the presence of a normal bicarbonate level is termed uncompensated respiratory alkalosis. If alveolar ventilation is maintained at normal levels, hypocarbia can occur because of an increase in alveolar ventilation or a decrease in CO_2 production, as occurs with hypothyroidism or hypothermia.

Metabolic alkalosis occurs when fixed acid loss is increased or when the intake of bases is abnormally high. Elevated pH accompanied by above-normal increases in the bicarbonate level when the Pco_2 is maintained at approximately 40 mm Hg is termed uncompensated metabolic alkalosis. The combination of respiratory alkalosis and metabolic alkalosis produces mixed alkalosis in which the arterial pH is markedly elevated.[28]

Compensatory Mechanisms

The respiratory system can rapidly compensate for metabolic acidosis or alkalosis by altering alveolar ventilation. It normally occurs because changes in blood H^+ concentrations affect central chemoreceptors, resulting in prompt increases or decreases in alveolar ventilation and altering the $Paco_2$ within minutes. The kidneys can compensate for respiratory acidosis and metabolic acidosis of nonrenal origin by excreting fixed acid and retaining bicarbonate. Conversely, the kidneys compensate for respiratory alkalosis or metabolic alkalosis of nonrenal

TABLE 29.5   Acid-Base States

pH	CO₂	HCO₃	Clinical Examples
>7.45	↓	↑	**Mixed Alkalosis** Overresuscitation (hyperventilation and excess bicarbonate administration)
	•	↑	**Metabolic Alkalosis** Vomiting
	↓	•	**Respiratory Alkalosis** Acute hyperventilation (neurogenic, or pain)
7.45			
7.40–7.45	↑	↑	**Compensated Metabolic Alkalosis** Long-term hypokalemia or bicarbonate ingestion
	↓	↓	**Compensated Respiratory Alkalosis** Chronic hyperventilation (as in chronic ICP)
	•	•	**Normal**
7.40	•	•	**Normal**
7.35–7.40	•	•	**Normal**
	↑	↑	**Compensated Respiratory Acidosis** Chronic hypoventilation (as in COPD)
	↓	↓	**Compensated Metabolic Acidosis** Renal failure
7.35			
<7.35	↑	•	**Respiratory Acidosis** Acute hypoventilation (opioid overdose)
	•	↓	**Metabolic Acidosis** Diabetic ketoacidosis
	↑	↓	**Mixed Acidosis** Respiratory and circulatory arrest

Upward arrow = above normal range, *downward arrow* = below normal range, *circle* = within normal range. *COPD,* Chronic obstructive pulmonary disease; *ICP,* intracranial pressure.

origin by decreasing H⁺ excretion and decreasing retention of bicarbonate. Renal compensatory mechanisms act more slowly than respiratory mechanisms and may take several days. When evaluating blood gas analyses, compensated acidosis involves finding abnormalities of both the CO_2 and the HCO_3^- in the same direction, with the pH below 7.4 but above 7.35. Conversely, compensated alkalosis involves finding abnormalities of both the CO_2 and the HCO_3^- in the same direction, with a pH above 7.4 but less than 7.45. Ascribing the abnormality to respiratory or metabolic is then based upon which abnormality (CO_2 or HCO_3^-) in their present level would be responsible for the directional change in pH (toward acidosis or alkalosis). In spite of observing a compensatory change in CO_2 or bicarbonate, an acid-base disorder is considered uncompensated if that mechanism has not been able to bring the pH back into a normal range. Compensation will not "overshoot" and create a pH disorder in the opposite direction because the drive for compensatory mechanisms is diminished as the pH approaches normal. Acid-base disorders wherein the CO_2 and HCO_3^- are both abnormal in different directions (one high, the other low) are termed mixed acidosis or alkalosis.[28]

Treatment of Blood Gas Abnormalities

For the patient who is mechanically ventilated, respiratory acidosis and respiratory alkalosis can be treated with a simple increase or decrease in the amount of alveolar ventilation. Respiratory acidosis should not be treated with sodium bicarbonate because the bicarbonate dissociates into more CO_2, worsening the acidosis. To restore stable and spontaneous circulation, mild to moderate metabolic acidosis can be treated with hyperventilation and correction of shock. Certain types of severe metabolic acidosis (pH <7.20) may be treated with sodium bicarbonate. The total body bicarbonate deficit is equal to the base deficit (in mEq/L) that is obtained from the blood gas values: The patient's bicarbonate level is subtracted from the normal bicarbonate level; the difference is multiplied by the patient's weight (in kilograms) and then by 0.3 (which is equal to the extracellular fluid compartment and the volume of distribution for bicarbonate). Complete correction of the base deficit is not indicated; only half of the calculated dose of bicarbonate is initially recommended. Severe lactic acidosis is treated with bicarbonate, but the acidosis associated with renal failure is better treated with dialysis. The hyperosmolarity and high sodium content of bicarbonate are usually contraindicated for patients with renal failure.[28]

CONTROL OF BREATHING

The respiratory centers in the brainstem control breathing by automatically generating a cycle of inspiration and expiration (Fig. 29.11). This spontaneously generated sequence can be modified by reflexes or by higher centers in the brain. The respiratory centers affect the nerves of the spinal cord, which innervate the muscles of respiration. For example, the cervical branches of the spinal nerves C3, C4, and C5 form bilateral phrenic nerves, which innervate the diaphragm, and nerves originating at the thoracic spinal cord level innervate the external intercostal muscles. The spontaneous respiratory rhythm is generated by the medullary respiratory center, which is located in the reticular formation of the medulla under the floor of the fourth ventricle. The dorsal respiratory group and ventral respiratory group are dense collections of respiratory neurons located in the tractus solitarius. This region contains projections of cranial nerves IX and X and processes signals related to chemoreceptors, lung stretch receptors, gag and cough reflexes, and others. The dorsal respiratory group is considered the pacemaker of normal breathing, that is, the area that drives respiration. The ventral respiratory group contains neurons controlling inspiration and expiration but is quiescent during normal respiration. The pons contains the apneustic center (in the lower pons) and the pneumotaxic center (in the upper pons), both of which modify the output of the medullary respiratory center. The normal function of the apneustic center is unknown, but if it is severed, the result is apneustic breathing (i.e., prolonged inspiration with occasional expiration). The pneumotaxic center is thought to be the inspiratory cutoff switch, which functions to fine-tune and smooth the respiratory pattern.

The activity of the brainstem's breathing centers is modulated by information received from afferent spinal nerves and higher brain centers, as occurs in voluntary control of breathing. Additionally, a great number of sensors in the lungs, cardiovascular system, muscles, tendons, skin, and viscera can affect the control of breathing by eliciting reflex changes. Stimulation of stretch receptors in the lungs can elicit three respiratory reflexes: the Hering-Breuer inflation reflex, the Hering-Breuer deflation reflex, and the paradoxic reflex of Head. The Hering-Breuer inflation reflex helps prevent overdistention of the alveoli at high lung volumes by inhibiting large systolic tidal volume (Vts) and may decrease the frequency of the inspiratory efforts by causing a transient apnea. The Hering-Breuer deflation reflex is responsible for the increased ventilation elicited when the lungs are deflated abnormally, such as in pneumothorax, or it may have a role in the periodic spontaneous deep breaths (sighs) that help to prevent atelectasis. The paradoxic reflex of Head results during partial block of the vagus nerve, such that lung inflation results in further deep inspiration instead of the apnea expected when the nerve is fully functional. This reflex may be involved in generating the first breath of the newborn baby.[32]

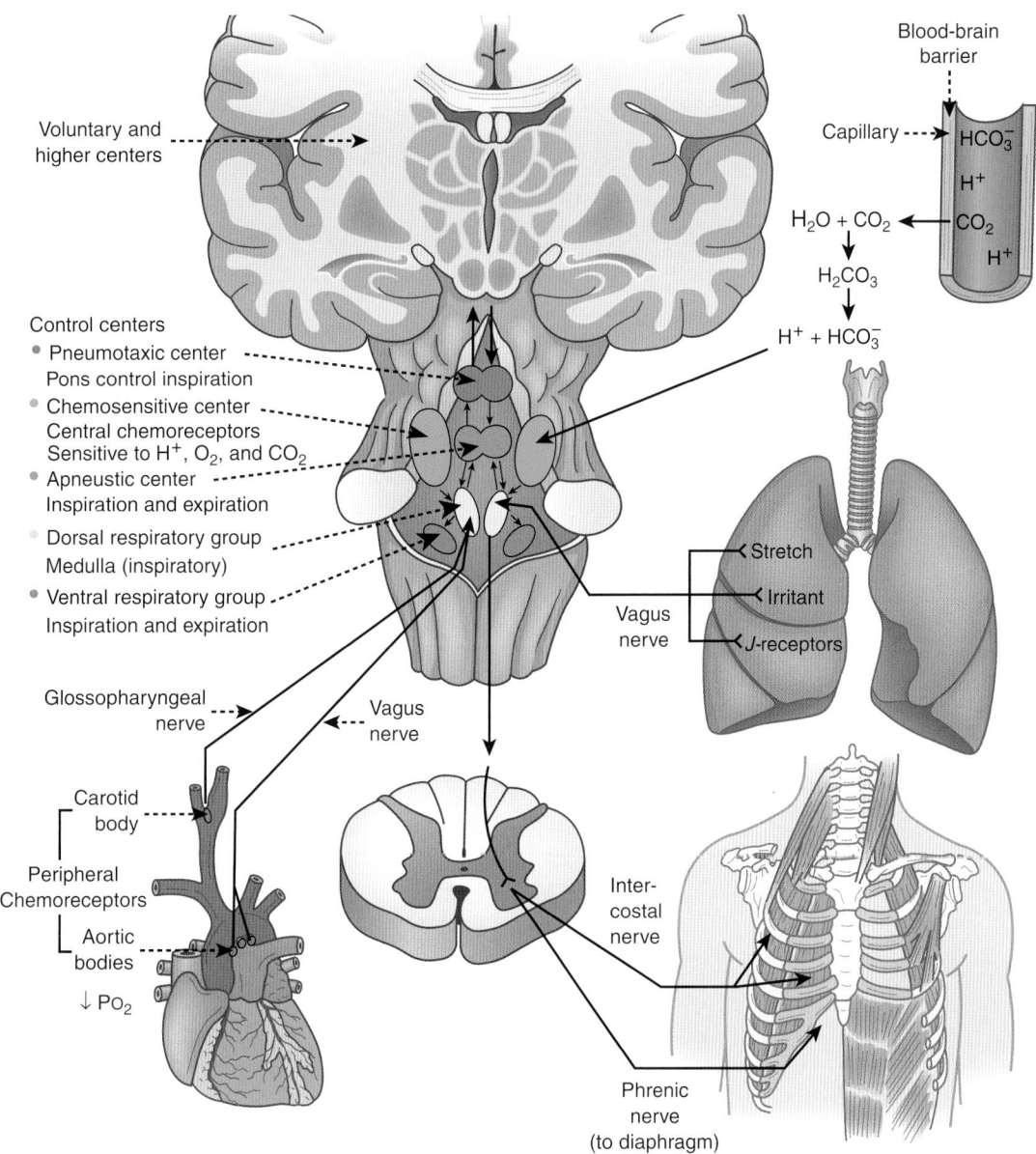

Fig. 29.11 Neurochemical respiratory control system. (From McCance KL, Huether SE. *Pathophysiology: The Biologic Basis for Disease in Adults and Children*. 8th ed. St. Louis: Elsevier; 2019:1233.)

Chemical or mechanical irritation of the airways may elicit a reflex cough or sneeze, rapid deep breathing (hyperpnea), bronchoconstriction, and increased blood pressure. The vagus nerve provides afferent pathways for all of the airway's irritant receptors, except for the nasal mucosa receptors, which send information centrally by means of the trigeminal and olfactory tracts. Pulmonary embolism typically causes rapid, shallow breathing, whereas pulmonary vascular congestion causes hyperpnea. The vascular receptors that initiate these responses are named J receptors (for juxtapulmonary capillary). Stimulation of receptors in the muscles, tendons, and joints can also increase minute ventilation during exercise. Elevated blood pressure stimulates the arterial (carotid and aortic) baroreceptors, resulting in apnea and bronchodilation. Somatic pain tends to cause hyperpnea, whereas visceral pain usually causes apnea or decreased ventilation. Stimulation of the arterial chemoreceptors by decreased Pao_2, increased $Paco_2$, or low

pH tends to increase lung inflation and cause hyperpnea, bronchoconstriction, and an increase in blood pressure. Table 29.6 summarizes the respiratory control reflexes.[1-5]

Chemical Control of Breathing

The arterial and cerebrospinal fluid partial pressures of CO_2 are probably the most important inputs to the brainstem centers for establishing the ventilatory rate and Vt. Hypoxemia potentiates the ventilatory response to CO_2. Its effect is that, for any particular $Paco_2$, ventilatory response becomes greater as the Pao_2 decreases. Opioids, anesthetics, and hypnotic drugs (Fig. 29.12) may profoundly depress the ventilatory response to CO_2. COPD also depresses the ventilatory response to hypercapnia so the hypoxic drive may be more prominently responsible for maintaining spontaneous breathing in these patients, and administering high Fio_2 may reduce their spontaneous ventilatory

TABLE 29.6   Reflex Mechanism of Respiratory Control

Stimulus	Reflex	Receptor	Afferent Pathway	Effects
Lung inflation	Hering-Breuer inflation reflex	Stretch receptors within smooth muscles of large and small airways	Vagus	Respiratory—cessation of inspiratory effort, apnea, or decreased breathing frequency; bronchodilation Cardiovascular—increased heart rate, slight vasoconstriction
Lung deflation	Hering-Breuer deflation reflex	Possibly J receptors, irritant receptors in lungs, or stretch receptors in airway	Vagus	Respiratory—hyperpnea
Lung inflation	Paradoxic reflex of head	Stretch receptors in lungs	Vagus	Respiratory—inspiration
Negative pressure in upper airway	Pharyngeal dilator reflex	Receptors in nose, mouth, upper airways		Respiratory—contraction of pharyngeal dilator muscles
Mechanical or chemical irritation of airways	Cough	Receptors in upper airways, tracheobronchial tree	Vagus	Respiratory—cough, bronchoconstriction
	Sneeze	Receptors in nasal mucosa	Trigeminal, olfactory	Respiratory—sneeze, bronchoconstriction Cardiovascular—increased blood pressure
Face immersion	Diving reflex	Receptors in nasal mucosa and face	Trigeminal	Respiratory—apnea Cardiovascular—decreased heart rate, vasoconstriction
Pulmonary embolism		J receptors in pulmonary vessels	Vagus	Respiratory—apnea or tachypnea
Pulmonary vascular congestion		J receptors in pulmonary vessels	Vagus	Respiratory—tachypnea, possible sensation of dyspnea
Specific chemicals in the pulmonary circulation	Pulmonary chemoreflex	J receptors in pulmonary vessels	Vagus	Respiratory—apnea or tachypnea, bronchoconstriction
Low Pao_2, high $Paco_2$; low pH	Arterial chemoreceptor reflex	Carotid bodies, aortic bodies	Glossopharyngeal, vagus	Respiratory—hyperpnea, bronchoconstriction, dilation of upper airway Cardiovascular—decreased heart rate, vasodilation, etc.
Increased systemic arterial blood pressure	Arterial baroreceptor reflex	Carotid and aortic arch stretch receptors	Glossopharyngeal, vagus	Respiratory—apnea, bronchodilation Cardiovascular—decreased heart rate, vasodilation
Increased systemic arterial blood pressure		Muscle spindles, tendon, organs, proprioceptors	Various spinal pathways	Respiratory—provide respiratory controller with feedback about work of breathing, stimulation of proprioceptors in joints causes hyperpnea
Somatic pain		Pain receptors	Various spinal pathways	Respiratory—hyperpnea Cardiovascular—increased heart rate, vasoconstriction

Pao_2, partial pressure of O_2 in arterial blood; $Paco_2$, partial pressure of carbon dioxide.
Modified from Levitzky MG. *Pulmonary Physiology*. 9th ed. New York: McGraw-Hill; 2018:237–238.

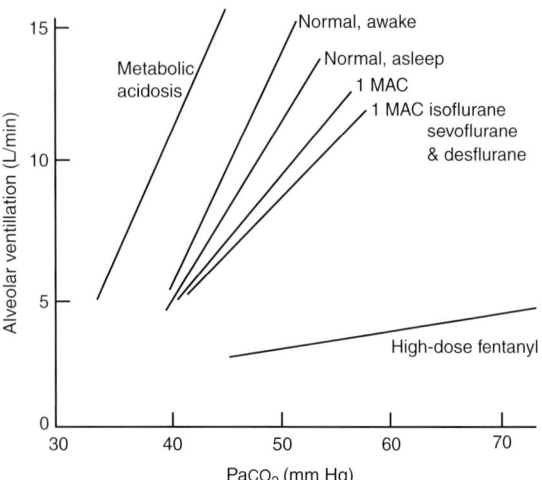

Fig. 29.12 Carbon dioxide response curve. *MAC*, Minimum alveolar concentration.

drive. Metabolic acidosis shifts the CO_2 curve to the left so that for any particular Pco_2, ventilation is increased during metabolic acidosis.

A depressed or abnormal response to CO_2 during sleep may be involved in central sleep apnea (characterized by pauses of at least 10-second duration between breaths, with cessation of respiratory effort).[33] Central sleep apnea, which possibly is caused by a defect in the chemoreceptors or brainstem respiratory control center, may be an important contributor to sudden infant death syndrome.

The arterial peripheral chemoreceptors are positioned to detect large changes in Pao_2 as arterial blood leaves the heart. They are located in the carotid and aortic bodies. In addition to detecting changes (particularly decreases) in arterial O_2, they also can detect changes in $Paco_2$ and arterial pH. The carotid bodies apparently exert a much greater influence on the medullary respiratory centers than the aortic bodies. The afferent nerve from the carotid body is Hering nerve, a branch of the glossopharyngeal nerve. The afferent pathway from the aortic body is the vagus nerve (see Fig. 29.11). If a decrease in Pao_2 is detected, the afferent response is almost instantaneous and results in an increase in respiratory rate and volume as well as an increase in cardiac output. These responses aim to improve the PaO$_2$ and blood flow (i.e., oxygen delivery) to vital organs that are most sensitive to hypoxia (i.e., brain and kidneys).

The central chemoreceptors are in contact with cerebrospinal fluid but are not directly exposed to arterial blood (because of the blood-brain barrier). Central chemoreceptors are most responsive to changes in cerebral spinal fluid pH (i.e., H$^+$ ion concentrations). However, charged ions (such as hydrogen and bicarbonate) do not easily cross the blood brain barrier (BBB), and changes in arterial pH that do not result from changes in PCO$_2$ take considerably longer to affect the cerebrospinal fluid. In contrast, if the arterial PCO$_2$ changes, CO$_2$ rapidly diffuses through the BBB; therefore changes in PaCO$_2$ are rapidly transmitted (<2 minutes) to the cerebrospinal fluid, affecting the central chemoreceptors and central respiratory drive. After diffusing through the BBB, CO$_2$ reacts with H$_2$O to form carbonic acid. Carbonic acid then dissociates into H$^+$ and bicarbonate ions within the medulla resulting in direct stimulation of chemoreceptive neurons by H$^+$ ions (see Fig. 29.11).

The central chemoreceptors are located just beneath the surface of the medulla. They are not stimulated by hypoxia. In fact, their activity may even be suppressed by it. The central chemoreceptors are majorly responsible for determining the resting ventilatory level and long-term maintenance of blood CO$_2$ levels. The central chemoreceptors contribute approximately two-thirds of the ventilatory response, whereas the peripheral chemoreceptors contribute the remaining one-third.[34]

RESPIRATORY SYSTEM PATHOLOGY

OBSTRUCTIVE SLEEP APNEA

Definition

Obstructive sleep apnea (OSA) is a mechanical obstruction to breathing caused by the relaxation of pharyngeal musculature during sleep. It is characterized by episodes of breathing cessation that last 10 or more seconds. Obesity hypoventilation syndrome is a distinct entity from OSA. It is defined as the triad of obesity, daytime hypoventilation, and sleep-disordered breathing without an alternative neuromuscular, mechanical, or metabolic cause.

Incidence and Outcome

OSA occurs in as many as 24% of males and 9% of females. Obesity is the most significant precipitating factor, with OSA being noted in 40% of obese individuals, and 80% of those presenting for bariatric surgery.[35] OSA is becoming increasingly prevalent in children and demonstrates many of the same characteristics as observed in adults. Between 7% and 10% of children are habitual snorers, and OSA is estimated to exist in 1% to 4% of preschool-age children. OSA is associated with increased postoperative complications and is an independent risk factor for increased morbidity in the hospitalized patient.[36,37]

Etiology and Pathophysiology

The primary causative factor for OSA is obesity, although it can exist in nonobese individuals. Factors in the pharyngeal musculature cause collapse during sleep under negative inspiratory pressure. Chronic hypoxemia and hypercarbia lead to an inflammatory state and a variety of secondary pathologies. OSA has been linked as a causative factor in atherosclerosis, hypertension, stroke, insulin resistance, diabetes, dyslipidemia, and other disorders (Table 29.7).[38-40] Sleep apnea is associated with a decrease in FRC of the lung, so sleep apnea patients may present with not only a more challenging airway, but also with less oxygen reserve when they become apneic.

TABLE 29.7 Comorbidities Associated With OSA

Category	Condition	Prevalence (%)
Cardiac	Treatment-resistant hypertension	63–83
	Congestive heart failure	76
	Ischemic heart disease	38
	Atrial fibrillation	49
	Dysrhythmias	58
Respiratory	Asthma	18
	Pulmonary hypertension	77
Neurologic	First-ever stroke	71–90
Metabolic	Type 2 diabetes mellitus	36
	Metabolic syndrome	50
	Hypothyroidism	45
	Morbid obesity	50–90
Surgical	Bariatric surgery	71
	Intracranial tumor surgery	64
	Epilepsy surgery	33
Others	Gastroesophageal reflux disease	60
	Nocturia	48
	Alcoholism	17
	Primary open-angle glaucoma	20
	Head and neck cancer	76

OSA, Obstructive sleep apnea.
From Seet E, Chung F. Obstructive sleep apnea: preoperative assessment. *Anesthesiol Clin*. 2010;28(2):199–215.

Clinical Features and Diagnosis

Patients with sleep apnea often present with multiple comorbidities related to their obesity or to chronic hypoxemia from the apneic disorder. Common comorbidities include systemic and pulmonary hypertension, ischemic heart disease, and CHF. A hallmark of OSA is habitual snoring and fragmented sleep, which can lead to daytime somnolence.

Polysomnography (see later) provides an objective measure of sleep apnea, but it is expensive and impractical to apply to every patient with risk factors who presents for surgery. A number of questionnaires such as the Berlin questionnaire have been developed as screening tools for OSA. These provide a low-cost, simple approach to identifying OSA. The components of the STOP questionnaire are as follows: S, snore loudly; T, daytime tiredness; O, observed cessation of breathing or choking/gasping during sleep; P, high blood pressure. The STOP questionnaire is often paired with four additional variables of the Bang questionnaire: B, body mass greater than 35 kg/m^2; A, age older than 50 years; N, neck circumference greater than 40 cm; G, male gender. Used together, the STOP-Bang questionnaire demonstrates sensitivity of nearly 100% and specificity of approximately 40%[36] (see Chapter 48, Box 48.2).

Polysomnography is used to establish the diagnosis of OSA, which is based on the number of abnormal respiratory events per hour of sleep (the apnea plus hypopnea index [AHI]). Diagnostic criteria vary among institutions, but an index of greater than 5 if associated with sleep-related symptoms, or an index of greater than 15 alone, is diagnostic for the condition. The AHI also describes severity, with AHI greater than 15 being moderate, and AHI greater than 30 being severe.[35] Investigators are identifying a variety of at-home and in-hospital diagnostic and screening tools for the identification of sleep apnea. Although polysomnography is the most definitive validation of OSA, it is usually not necessary to delay a surgical case solely for this test. Based on the STOP-Bang assessment, the anesthetic plan can be formulated around a presumptive diagnosis of OSA. Unless the preoperative workup discovers previously unrecognized cardiovascular disease (such as pulmonary hypertension, resting hypoxemia, or significant hypoventilation), there is no reliable evidence that delaying surgery or providing more detailed investigation of the degree of OSA will improve outcomes. Consideration of the interplay among baseline state of health, severity of obesity, complexity of the surgery, and anticipated requirements for postoperative opioids should inform the anesthetic plan for each individual.

Treatment

Weight loss is an important goal for the obese patient with OSA. Patients who are obese and undergo bariatric surgery demonstrate a decreased requirement for sleep apnea therapy after the weight loss. The use of CPAP devices has become the gold standard in the management of OSA. CPAP devices utilize a facemask held tightly to the face during sleep, which provides positive airway pressure. This pressure stents the airway open, relieves the obstruction, and promotes more continuous breathing and sleep. Although CPAP is a very effective treatment modality, sleeping with a bulky and sometimes noisy mask can be difficult to tolerate, and adherence to the therapy is as low as 50% among sleep apnea subjects. As a result, other emerging treatments include an implantable stimulator of the hypoglossal nerve to increase pharyngeal tone, nasal end-expiratory pressure devices, positional therapy, oral devices that move the mandible forward, procedures to shrink pharyngeal tissue, and/or pharmacologic adjuncts. Procedures to reduce tissue mass range from minor radiofrequency intervention to surgical procedures, such as uvulopalatopharyngoplasty and adenotonsillectomy in pediatric or adult patients with tonsillar hypertrophy. Adjunctive therapy includes analeptic drugs such as modafinil and armodafinil, methylxanthines, doxapram, serotonin modulators, and tricyclic antidepressants. Drug therapy is intended to reduce daytime sleepiness, reduce cardiovascular complications, strengthen pharyngeal musculature, and reduce rapid eye movement (REM) sleep, among other effects.[41-43]

Anesthetic Management

CPAP may be implemented preoperatively to improve respiratory function, and it is even more contributory postoperatively when respirations are compromised by opioids and residual anesthesia. Patients on CPAP at home may be instructed to bring their device to the hospital so that it can be used following surgery. Research is equivocal regarding whether perioperative CPAP therapy reduces complications other than the obvious reduction in airway obstruction. Considering the cost and logistics involved with the process of continuing CPAP in the perioperative period, individual institutional resources can inform the decision of the extent to which CPAP is used perioperatively.

Careful airway evaluation is an important step in anesthetic preparation and management. Redundant tissue in the neck region is common in OSA (even more so than is general obesity), and it may impede effective head positioning, mask ventilation, or laryngoscopy. The anesthetist should anticipate airway difficulty and rapid desaturation from reduced FRC. Elevation of the head and shoulders facilitates airway management and ventilation. It is prudent to have a videolaryngoscope and other airway adjuncts immediately available during airway management. Use caution with sedative medications prior to surgery. As a result of central nervous system sensitization, patients may be hypersensitive to the effects of benzodiazepines and opioids. Effective doses may be extremely small, and this effect may persist even after physical

TABLE 29.8   Suggested Management of the Patient With Obstructive Sleep Apnea

Screening	STOP-Bang questionnaire.
	Polysomnography for definitive diagnosis, but not required solely for anesthesia.
Preoperative	Preoperative sedation should be judicious, followed by continuous patient observation, ideally with oximetry.
Positioning	Ramp upper body for intubation.
Induction	Anticipate difficult airway.
	Make videolaryngoscope or other airway adjuncts readily available.
Intraoperative	Use regional anesthesia when possible.
	For general anesthesia, use short-acting agents.
	Limit long-acting opioids and minimize muscle relaxants as possible.
	Provide PEEP to reduce postoperative atelectasis.
Emergence	Confirm muscle paralysis reversal with attention to residual relaxation.
	Elevate upper body and extubate when fully awake.
Postoperative	Use multimodal and nonopioid analgesia.
	Regional techniques for analgesia.
	CPAP in recovery if recurring obstruction or history of home use.
Discharge	Minor surgery or regional anesthesia or sedation, and minimize opioid administration = same-day discharge.
	Major surgery, substantial opioid need, severe OSA, or home CPAP = monitor overnight.

CPAP, Continuous positive airway pressure; *OSA,* obstructive sleep apnea; *PEEP,* positive end-expiratory pressure.

symptoms have been surgically ameliorated (e.g., through uvulopalatopharyngoplasty). The same concerns apply postoperatively. Patients receiving preoperative sedation should be observed, and pulse oximetry is recommended. Extubation must be undertaken carefully with vigilant monitoring of the patient's respiratory status in the recovery area since the patient with OSA is at risk for airway obstruction from residual anesthetic and depressant medications. Airway obstruction occurs in 25% of pediatric patients with OSA following tonsillectomy, in contrast to 1% of those without OSA. Analgesics and general somnolence may lead to airway obstruction in the recovery area. Multimodal analgesia and regional techniques may help limit the need for systemic opioids.

It is prudent to provide additional postoperative monitoring to patients with moderate to severe OSA. This may include longer postanesthesia care unit (PACU) time, admission to a monitored bed, prolonged blood oxygen saturation (SpO_2) monitoring, and disqualification from same-day discharge, depending on the patient's condition. CPAP is helpful in the PACU, and patients who use this treatment at home should be encouraged to bring their device for use in the postanesthetic period. If the patient can receive CPAP therapy and monitoring for apneic episodes and desaturation, ICU admission is not indicated solely on the basis of the OSA unless the patient has other specific indications. See Table 29.8 for suggested management of the patient with OSA.

PULMONARY FUNCTION TESTING

An understanding of pulmonary function evaluation will be helpful before discussing pathologies that involve airflow limitations. A

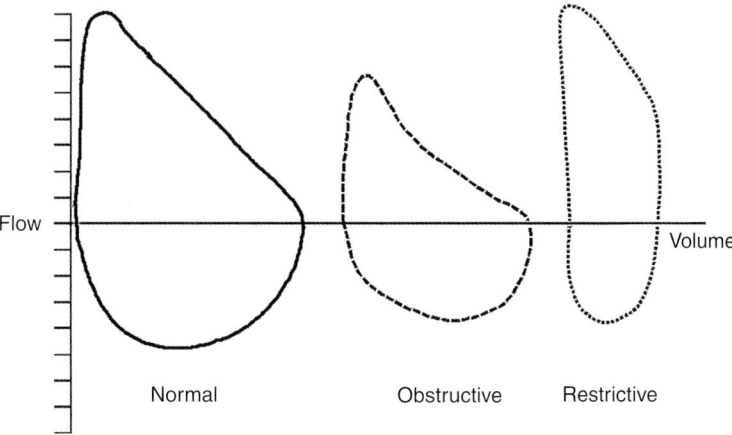

Fig. 29.13 Flow-volume loops in disease. Characteristic deformities of pulmonary flow-volume loops related to obstructive and restrictive disease.

number of examinations may be performed to evaluate lung volumes and the inspiratory and expiratory flow of gas. Many of these are derived by having the patient breathe through a closed circuit with measurement of gas flow and composition. Measurement of pulmonary volume over time is called spirometry. A glossary of static lung volumes and capacities is presented in Table 29.4. A standard flow-volume loop is drawn in a clockwise direction, with inspiratory flow below the x-axis, and expiratory flow above it. Flow rates (in liters per second) are represented on the y-axis (see Fig. 29.4). The zero point on the x-axis represents full inspiration because the lungs cannot be totally emptied due to the residual volume. In Fig. 29.4 the scale below the x-axis provides corresponding approximate absolute values of lung volume. The most important portion of the loop in most cases is the expiratory flow and volume that begins at this point and ends when the loop reaches the x-axis again as it transitions to inspiratory flow. Values for an individual's flow and volume pattern are measured in absolute terms and are compared to predicted values based on performance of healthy subjects with similar anthropometric characteristics (age, gender, and height, and sometimes other factors such as weight and race).

Spirometry is based on a forced air capacity (FVC) maneuver, which requires concerted patient effort; a lack of effort may produce erroneous results.[44] The FVC is divided into several time intervals, of which the FEV_1 (forced expired volume in 1 second) is the most reproducible. The volume of air that is exhaled in 1 second from a maximal inspiration is measured as the FEV_1. Patients with increased airway resistance exhibit decreased FEV_1 and FEV_1/FVC ratios. Normal FEV_1 varies with age, declining as age increases.[45] Normally the FEV_1 volume is at least 80% of the vital capacity. This is an important point used to differentiate low FEV_1 due to obstructive disease from low FEV_1 due to restrictive disease (where the vital capacity is also reduced, and the ratio of FEV_1/FVC is preserved).

Respiratory activity represented by the midportion of the expiratory curve is the most effort-independent and the most sensitive indicator of small airway disease. The parameter measured is the $FEF_{25\%-75\%}$ (forced expiratory flow rate between 25% and 75% of the exhaled breath). The normal $FEF_{25\%-75\%}$ of 4 to 5 L/sec may decrease markedly in those with pulmonary disease, with early changes evident sooner in patients with obstructive disease than in those with restrictive disease. Reduction in the $FEF_{25\%-75\%}$ wherein the curve begins to take a concave shape usually appears before significant change occurs in the FEV_1.[44] It is not as reproducible as the FEV_1, but it is more sensitive to airway obstruction.[46]

Flow-volume loops also provide information about disease processes through characteristic shapes (Fig. 29.13). Obstructive disease is

characterized by a reduced peak flow rate and a sloping of the expiratory limb. This occurs as small airways close during expiration, noticeably reducing the flow rate during expiration. Restrictive disease is characterized by normal or heightened peak expiratory flows, but a very narrow loop, reflecting the reduced vital capacity. Obstructions to airflow may also be variable, as in tracheomalacia, such that changes in pressure may both augment and reverse the obstruction in the course of each respiratory cycle. In this case, the location of the lesion (being intrathoracic or extrathoracic) determines whether the obstruction will be relieved or made worse by inspiration or expiration (Fig. 29.14). Airway obstructions lead to characteristic patterns on a flow-volume tracing as well (Fig. 29.15).

The diffusion capacity (DL) is another form of pulmonary function testing, which assesses the ability of gas to traverse the alveolar-capillary membrane. Factors related to Fick's law of diffusion correlate the diffusion capacity to clinical conditions (i.e., thickness of the membrane [fibrosis] or surface area for diffusion [emphysema]). Vascular or interstitial pathology, such as pulmonary hypertension, will decrease the DL, whereas polycythemia will increase it. The DL is also influenced by alterations in ventilation-perfusion matching, such as pulmonary embolism, which would cause it to decrease. The DL test is commonly performed by having the patient inhale a single breath containing a small amount of carbon monoxide. Carbon monoxide is highly diffusible and binds avidly with Hgb so that any reduction in transfer to the blood is indicative of loss of surface area of the alveolar-capillary membrane. New methods of assessing the DL now also use nitric oxide as the traced gas, as it may provide a more sensitive indicator of interstitial disease. The DLCO is reported as the uptake of carbon monoxide in milliliters per minute per mm Hg or as a percentage of predicted value. There is no specific value correlated with perioperative complications, but reductions in DLCO are associated with increased exacerbations in COPD and a significantly increased 3-year mortality in patients with pulmonary hypertension.[46]

CHRONIC OBSTRUCTIVE PULMONARY DISEASE

The American Thoracic Society and European Respiratory Society define COPD as a "preventable and treatable disease state characterized by airflow limitation that is not fully reversible. The airflow limitation is usually progressive and is associated with an abnormal inflammatory response of the lungs to noxious particles or gases...."[47] COPD should be considered in any patient with ongoing cough, sputum production, or dyspnea with history of exposure to risk factors. Diagnosis is made by spirometric demonstration of airflow obstruction that is not fully reversible (postbronchodilator FEV_1:FVC ratio <0.7).[48]

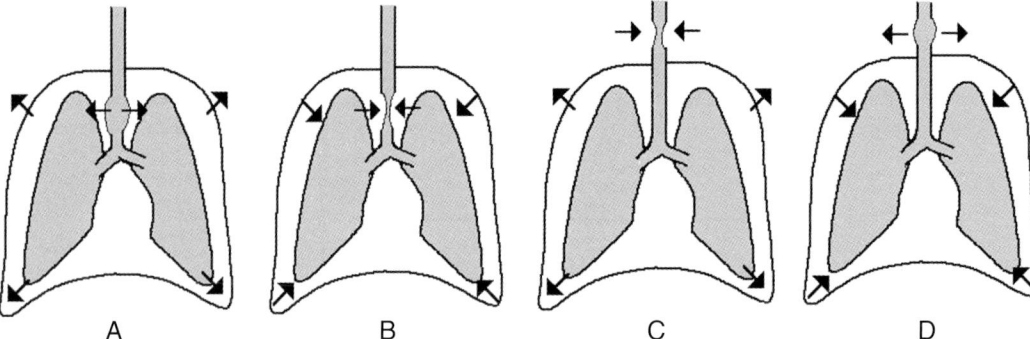

Fig. 29.14 Variable airway obstructions during spontaneous respiration. A variable intrathoracic obstruction will be subjected to negative pressure during inspiration and will be stented open (A); however, as intrathoracic pressure rises during expiration, an intrathoracic obstruction will be compressed (B). A variable extrathoracic obstruction will be subjected to negative intratracheal pressure during inspiration and will be compressed (C); however, as intratracheal pressure rises during expiration, the extrathoracic obstruction will be pushed open (D).

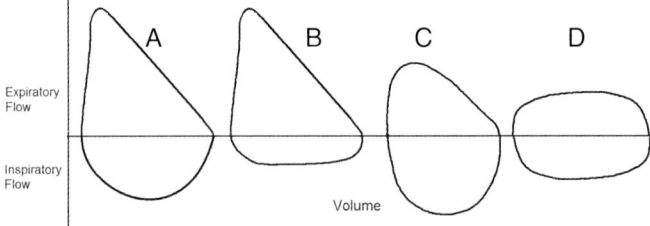

Fig. 29.15 Flow volume loops—airway obstruction. The dynamic effects of airway obstruction during inspiration and expiration are compared to the normal flow volume loop (A). (B) An extrathoracic obstruction that causes airway compression and decreased inspiratory flow results in an inspiratory flow pattern that is abnormally affected. (C) An intrathoracic obstruction that causes airway compression and decreased expiratory flow results in an expiratory flow pattern that is abnormally affected. (D) A fixed obstruction (e.g., foreign body in the airway) abnormally affects both the inspiratory and expiratory flow patterns.

The terms *chronic obstructive pulmonary disease* and *chronic obstructive lung disease* are widely used as synonyms for pathology involving airflow obstruction that does not change over months to years. COPD is caused by a mixture of small airways disease and parenchymal destruction in various combinations and proportions from one individual to the next. Two specific disorders, emphysema and chronic bronchitis, provide the prototypes of pathologic changes in COPD. Emphysema is characterized by the destruction of parenchyma that leads to loss of surface area, elastic recoil, and structural support to maintain airway patency. Bronchitis is characterized by narrowing of small airways by inflammation and mucous production. There are also numerous chronic conditions referred to collectively as peripheral airways disease or small airways disease. These entities are not mutually exclusive; peripheral airways disease often precedes onset of emphysema, and chronic bronchitis and emphysematous changes often coexist to define COPD. As a rule, COPD is observed most often in individuals with an extensive history of smoking, and the disease process takes 30 years or longer to manifest. Other chronic diseases such as cystic fibrosis, tuberculosis, and bronchiectasis are not included in the definition of COPD.[47] Restrictive diseases such as scoliosis, other forms of pulmonary fibrosis, or obesity are also not included. Differential diagnosis of COPD compared with other common lung disorders is presented in Table 29.9.

TABLE 29.9	**Differential Diagnosis of COPD**
Diagnosis	**Suggestive Features***
COPD	Onset in midlife; symptoms slowly progressive; long-term smoking history; dyspnea during exercise; largely irreversible airflow limitation
Asthma	Onset early in life (often childhood); symptoms vary from day to day; symptoms occur at night or in early morning; allergy, rhinitis, or eczema also present; family history of asthma; largely reversible airflow limitation
Congestive heart failure	Fine basilar crackles on auscultation; chest radiograph shows dilated heart, pulmonary edema; pulmonary function tests indicate volume restriction, not airflow limitation
Bronchiectasis	Large volumes of purulent sputum; commonly associated with bacterial infection; coarse crackles or clubbing on auscultation; chest radiograph or CT scan shows bronchial dilation, bronchial wall thickening
Tuberculosis	Onset at all ages; chest radiograph shows lung infiltrate or nodular lesions; microbiologic confirmation; high local prevalence of tuberculosis, or known exposure
Obliterative bronchiolitis	Onset at younger age, in nonsmokers; may have history of rheumatoid arthritis or fume exposure; CT scan taken on expiration shows hypodense areas
Diffuse panbronchiolitis	Most patients are male and nonsmokers; almost all have chronic sinusitis; chest radiograph and HRCT scan show diffuse small centrilobular nodular opacities and hyperinflation

*These features tend to be characteristic of the respective diseases but do not occur in every case. For example, a person who has never smoked can develop COPD (especially in developing countries, where other risk factors may be more important than cigarette smoking); asthma can develop in adults and even in elderly patients.
From López-Campos JL, Soler-Cataluña JJ, Miravitlles M. Global strategy for the diagnosis, management, and prevention of chronic obstructive lung disease 2019 report: future challenges. *Arch Bronconeumol.* 2020;56(2):65–67.
COPD, Chronic obstructive pulmonary disease; *HRCT,* high-resolution computed tomography.

Definition

Peripheral airways disease involves inflammation of the terminal and respiratory bronchioles, fibrosis and narrowing of the airway walls, and goblet cell metaplasia.[49] A small sampling of conditions that are characterized as small airways disease includes sarcoidosis, Wegener granulomatosis, mineral dust–associated airways disease, disease from exposure to fumes and toxins, and bronchocentric granulomatosis.[50] Chronic bronchitis refers to chronic or recurrent excess mucous secretion occurring on most days for at least 3 months of the year for at least 2 successive years. A critical element is the presence of airway obstruction of expiratory airflow. Emphysema is defined as a chronic lung condition characterized by abnormal permanent enlargement of the air spaces distal to the terminal bronchioles, which is accompanied by destruction (i.e., loss of elasticity) of alveolar walls and structures supporting alveoli without obvious fibrosis.[49] Alveolar tissue that has been destroyed is largely incapable of regeneration, and therefore the changes that occur in emphysema are irreversible. Emphysema is subclassified as centrilobular or panlobular. In centrilobular emphysema, dilation predominantly affects the respiratory bronchioles in the upper lung lobes. In panlobular emphysema, tissue destruction is widespread, affecting all areas of the acinus (the cells that define the "berry-bunch" shape of the alveoli) and distributed throughout the lung.[44] Destruction of lung tissue that is associated with emphysema leads to four primary alterations in pulmonary function: (1) Increases in size of acini cause compression of adjacent small airways and increase airflow resistance, (2) consolidation of alveoli leads to loss of alveolar surface area and impairs gas diffusion, (3) heterogeneity of disease in different parts of the lungs leads to mismatch of ventilation and perfusion, and (4) loss of alveolar walls also decreases the amount of pulmonary capillaries resulting in an increase in right ventricular workload.[4]

Incidence and Outcome

COPD affects more than 5% of adult Americans and is the third leading cause of death.[48] Chronic bronchitis and emphysema are the most common causes of COPD. The social and economic impacts of COPD are enormous. Patients who have advanced stages of obstructive lung disease are unable to work and frequently cannot participate in activities of daily living. Even in milder cases, activities are often restricted. The economic cost of COPD is estimated to be over $50 billion in the United States.[48] Death related to COPD is not only caused by respiratory failure but is also associated with related comorbidities such as lung cancer and heart disease.[51]

Etiology and Pathophysiology

In general, the development of COPD causes an exaggerated inflammatory reaction in the lungs. The principal factor that predisposes a patient to the development of COPD is cigarette smoking.[51] Environmental pollution appears to have some role, but its effects are minor compared with those of cigarette smoking, particularly as the disease occurs in the United States. COPD may develop in some patients because of an imbalance between protease and antiprotease activities in the lungs; α_1-antitrypsin deficiency is the primary genetically related cause. α_1-antitrypsin is produced in the liver and helps to protect lung tissue from damage by neutrophil elastase. Smoking can cause an immune-related release of neutrophil elastase that is inadequately regulated due to deficient levels of α_1-antitrypsin. This results in degradation of pulmonary connective tissue and a potential early development of COPD.[52] Unfortunately, α_1-antitrypsin administration is expensive and has not demonstrated good results as a treatment.[52,53]

The dominant feature of the natural history of COPD is progressive airflow obstruction, as reflected by a decrease in FEV_1. Three causes of decreases in FEV_1 are as follows: (1) a decrease in the intrinsic size

of bronchial lumina, (2) an increase in the collapsibility of bronchial walls (this cause is the most difficult to quantify), and (3) a decrease in elastic recoil of the lungs.[44] Distinct morphologic changes can be found in the airways of patients exposed to ongoing inflammatory challenges. In chronic bronchitis, a proliferation of the compound tracheobronchial mucous glands occurs in the subepithelial layers of the airway wall. Excessive airway mucus and thickened airway walls cause a narrowing of the functional airflow channel. Airway narrowing is primarily related to a thickening of the airway walls, not an increase in smooth muscle tone as is more prominently observed in asthma. Destruction of parenchyma results in a loss of elastic support, which also contributes to airway narrowing.[54] Although COPD is defined as being irreversible, contemporary science is focusing on the limited amount of reversibility that can improve patients' quality of life and slow progression of the disease. Between 25% and 50% of patients with COPD also have enhanced airway reactivity.[55] While bearing similarities to asthmatic bronchial reactivity, it appears that in COPD airway hyperresponsiveness affects small airways more so than larger ones.[56]

The defense system of a patient with COPD is disrupted by the excessive production of mucus and by paralysis of the mucociliary transport system, which leads to microbial colonization. The presence of microbial organisms in the airway secretions of patients with chronic bronchitis is common and does not necessarily imply the presence of an acute infection. Instead, chronic colonization of the airway plays a cyclic role in the ongoing pathogenesis of COPD, whereby bacteria increase mucous production, reduce ciliary motility, cause influx of neutrophils that lead to fibrosis, alter the host response to cigarette smoke, induce a chronic inflammatory response, and enhance airway reactivity.[57] General changes in lung functioning include:

1. Destruction of lung connective tissue, which normally provides elastic pull on the outsides of bronchi and bronchioles, reduces the tethering of airways of the pulmonary interstitium, leads to premature collapse of the airways from external pressure, and increases poor distribution of inspired air. Consequently, the exchange of CO_2 and O_2 between the blood and alveolar air is impeded. Compensation for lower diffusion of gases is partly achieved via collateral ventilation by diffusion across alveolar walls.[58]
2. Injury and inflammation of the bronchial tubes and alveoli increase the resistance to airflow during both inspiration and expiration. More forceful breaths or quicker breaths are needed for maintaining even normal levels of ventilation.[59]
3. Lung compliance increases with the tissue damage, and the airways' narrowing and greater collapsibility impede the ability of the ventilatory muscles to empty the lung completely. Hyperinflation results, raising the resting end-expiratory position of the lungs. Because the lung is more expanded, the inspiratory muscles operate from a shorter initial length and produce less force when shortened.
4. The more horizontally placed diaphragm is less able to lift the rib cage. The diaphragm may contract ineffectively, such that the abdomen moves inward rather than outward with each inspiration.[60]
5. Because of the increased demands for work output placed on the respiratory muscles, the energy requirement of these muscles escalates. A greater proportion of the CO goes to these muscles. If hypoxemia is present and increased ventilation is required (e.g., as in exercise), the energy supply of the muscles may become inadequate, and respiratory muscle fatigue is ultimately produced.[61]
6. The expansion of the lung and thorax also misaligns the intercostal muscles and accessory respiratory muscles. To compensate, patients may assume special postures, such as leaning forward.[62]
7. Inflammation allows noxious agents in the air to reach the more deeply located tissues in the lung and gain access to blood vessels, macrophages, mast cells, and nerves in the lung. Airway irritation

increases; as a result, asthmatic episodes occur because the introduction of noxious agents causes the release of spasmogenic agents from tissue cells and nerve endings.[62]

General Gas Exchange Characteristics

The ability of compensatory mechanisms to preserve ventilation and ABG tensions varies. The diffusion capacity of CO_2 is much greater than O_2, allowing for the preservation of relatively normal CO_2 levels until severe obstruction occurs. When chronic obstruction leads to CO_2 retention and hypercapnia, acid-base disorders can occur that shift the normal central ventilatory response to a peripheral hypoxic drive response that relies on a decrease in Pao_2 concentrations to increase ventilation.[63] Minute ventilation ($\dot{V}e$) in COPD generally is normal to above normal. Usually, $Paco_2$ does not increase beyond normal levels in COPD until FEV_1 is less than 1 L. In comparison, Pao_2 is not appreciably restored by an increase in depth of breathing, and even slight variations in $\dot{V}/\dot{Q}$ ratios in the lung adversely affect oxygenation.[49] Oxygen delivery (DO_2) to the tissues is preserved as much as possible by an increase in cardiac output a greater extraction of O_2 from the blood, polycythemia, or some combination of these three factors. Consequently, respiratory muscle work is greater than normal, and O_2 use by the muscles is increased.

Associated Conditions

Cigarette Smoking

Cigarette smoking has been firmly established as the primary environmental risk factor associated with emphysema and bronchitis.[47] Its pathogenic mechanism is not known. The unchecked protease hypothesis holds that emphysema is caused by damage to elastic fibers because of an imbalance between elastase and α_1-antitrypsin in the lung.[64] In addition, evidence that oxidants have a role in lung damage is increasing. The lungs of cigarette smokers are subject to an enhanced oxidant burden. Oxidants are highly reactive electron acceptors capable of removing electrons from a variety of molecules. The process of oxidation may reversibly or irreversibly damage compounds of all chemical classes, including nucleic acids, proteins and free amino acids, lipids and lipoproteins, and carbohydrates. In this regard, oxidants can damage cells and extracellular matrix components critical for normal lung function. Cigarette smoke and activated lung phagocytes generate an increase in the level of oxidants.[65,66] Additionally, excess sputum production and hyperplasia of the mucous glands of the trachea and large bronchi are linked to cigarette smoking.[65] The risk of COPD is not limited to cigarette smoking; smoking other types of tobacco or marijuana, exposure to secondhand smoke, and even fetal exposure to smoke during pregnancy may predispose to COPD.[67]

Chronic lung hyperinflation results in diaphragmatic flattening, and a reduction in contractile force results, attributable to the Frank-Starling mechanism. Besides this gross effect, oxidative stress leads to loss of contractile proteins (i.e., myosin), further reducing the contractile force.[68]

Peripheral Circulation in COPD

COPD can change the determinants of systemic venous return by altering the mechanical characteristics of either the heart or the lungs. When a forced expiratory breathing pattern occurs (e.g., during exercise), positive intrathoracic pressure is generated during expiration. The positive swings in pressure cyclically decrease systemic venous return, leading to an exaggeration of respiratory variation in arterial blood pressure or to pulsus paradoxus.[69] Pulsus paradoxus as a result of COPD causes a drop in both systolic and diastolic blood pressure, which worsens as the degree of airflow obstruction worsens.[70] Increases

in lung volume may directly impede systemic venous return through compression of the vena cava or heart. Normally, inspiration augments systemic venous return because of a decrease in right atrial pressure.[71]

Patients with COPD often have an increase in cardiac output mediated by an increase in catecholamine levels and by a redistribution of blood flow and volume from the high-capacitance splanchnic regions to the lower-capacitance cardiac, cerebral, and muscle regions.[71]

A characteristic enhanced heart rate response has also been identified. Four parameters of airway obstruction (FVC, the ratio of FEV_1 to FVC [% FEV_1], the ratio of RV to TLC [RV/TLC], and % RV) have been correlated with the heart rate response to hypoxia. This increased response appears to be the result of an unknown mechanism of diseased lung tissue.[72]

Fluid retention in COPD. It appears that patients with hypoxic and hypercapnic respiratory failure caused by emphysema or chronic bronchitis, or from both, have impaired renal function with reduced renal plasma flow and decreases in glomerular filtration.[73]

Note that cardiac responses to chronic and acute pressure increases are not the same. Chronic pressure overload causes right ventricular hypertrophy, whereas acute pressure changes cause right ventricular dilation.

Other Air Space Abnormalities

Bullae, a manifestation of some forms of emphysema, are air-containing spaces greater than 1 cm in diameter that result from the destruction and dilation of air spaces distal to terminal bronchioles. Bullae have an outer wall consisting of the visceral pleura and an inner wall consisting of tissue derived from confluent alveoli. Bullae can grow to sizes occupying a significant proportion of the hemithorax, in which case they are referred to as giant.[74] A bulla or bullae that become symptomatic may warrant surgical resection. Similar to bullae, blebs are collections of air within the layers of the visceral pleura. They occur when air migrates from the lung parenchyma, and they usually form near the apices. Because blebs do not involve the functional lung units (i.e., respiratory bronchioles, alveolar ducts, and alveoli), they are not a form of emphysema; however, they do pose the risk of causing pneumothorax.

Clinical Features and Diagnosis

The clinical presentation associated with COPD varies markedly. Chronic productive cough and progressive exercise limitation are the hallmarks of COPD. Other common symptoms are dyspnea and wheezing, but COPD may progress to respiratory failure or cor pulmonale. Key findings in COPD are listed in Table 29.10.

Diagnostic Testing

Pulmonary function tests. Spirometry is not recommended as a screening tool, and it has limited benefit in anesthetic risk assessment in contrast to the cost of performing the procedure.[75] Although the FEV_1 indicates the degree of airflow obstruction, it correlates poorly with symptoms and therefore may not solely indicate the severity of pulmonary disease.[44] Furthermore, severe pulmonary disease will manifest in functional limitations and characteristic physical traits, which will be evident to the anesthetist even in the absence of airflow measurement. Spirometry is most useful to primary care providers when evaluating patients with unexplained dyspnea and in those in whom COPD is suspected. Current evidence-based guidelines note that a smoking history of greater than 40 pack-years is the single best variable for predicting airflow obstruction, and the combination of greater than 55–pack-year history, wheezing on auscultation, and patient self-reported wheezing almost assures that obstruction (FEV_1:FVC ratio <0.7) is present.[48]

TABLE 29.10	**Clinical Hallmarks of COPD**
Assessment	**Typical Finding**
General appearance	Range from overweight and dusky, to thin, emaciated; pursed-lip breathing; anxious; prominent use of accessory muscles; barrel chest; jugular vein distention; rapid weight loss carries poor prognosis
Cough	Chronic, productive throughout the day (most characteristic with prominent bronchitis)
Dyspnea	Chronic, progressive increase (dyspnea precipitated by decreasing levels of activity)
Breath sounds	Rhonchi, wheezing
Heart sounds	Split S_2, pulmonary/tricuspid insufficiency
Radiographic features	Flat diaphragm; areas of increased radiolucency; rapid tapering of vascular markings
Spirometry	Elevated TLC, RV, FRC, RV:TLC ratio; reduced FEV_1, FEV_1:FVC ratio
Echocardiography	Increased pulmonary artery pressure, decreased RV contractility
Blood gas exchange	Reduced DLCO, hypoxemia (most characteristic of prominent emphysema)

COPD, Chronic obstructive pulmonary disease; *DLCO*, carbon monoxide diffusion in the lung; *FEV_1*, forced expiratory volume in 1 sec; *FRC*, functional residual capacity; *FVC*, forced vital capacity; *RV*, residual volume; *TLC*, total lung capacity.
From Mirza S, Clay RD, Koslow MA, et al. COPD guidelines: a review of the 2018 GOLD report. *Mayo Clin Proc.* 2018;93(10):1488–1502.

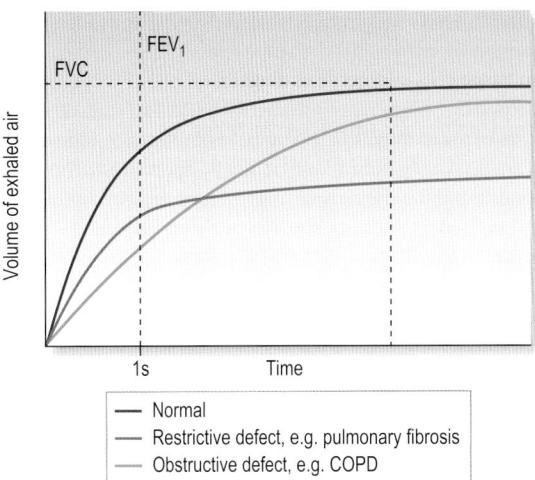

Fig. 29.16 Changes in the forced expiratory volume in 1 second (FEV_1) and the forced expiratory capacity (FVC) in obstructive and restrictive pulmonary disease. *COPD*, Chronic obstructive pulmonary disease. (From Naish J, Court DS. *Medical Sciences.* 2nd ed. Philadelphia: Elsevier; 2015:632.)

Reduction in the FEV_1 is a hallmark of obstructive disease; however, it may also characterize restrictive disease. In severe obstructive lung disease, expiratory flow rates are greatly decreased and the FEV_1:FVC ratio is reduced. The ratio is evaluated in addition to the FEV_1 alone because in restrictive disease the FEV_1 is reduced secondary to a reduction in the vital capacity so the reduction in FEV_1 alone does not indicate expiratory airflow obstruction. A low FEV_1 combined with a normal FEV_1:FVC is indicative of restrictive disease (Fig. 29.16). Measurement of lung volumes in obstructive disease demonstrates an increased RV and often an increased FRC. Slowing of expiratory flow and gas trapping associated with premature distal airway collapse is responsible for the increase in RV. When spirometry is used to grade the severity of COPD (FEV_1:FVC <0.7), the postbronchodilator FEV_1 compared to predicted levels is the primary determinant (i.e., $FEV_1 \geq 80\%$ = mild, 50%–79% = moderate, 30%–49% = severe, and <30% = very severe). The number of exacerbations and hospitalizations per year is also directly correlated with 3-year mortality and can be considered in the evaluation of severity of COPD.[67]

Arterial blood gas analysis. ABG analysis is helpful in determining the severity of gas exchange abnormality and guiding management of patients with COPD. COPD can manifest with impaired exchange of oxygen and CO_2 (Pao_2 <60 mm Hg, $Paco_2$ >45 mm Hg, and presence of cor pulmonale), generally based on the severity of the disease and the relative contributions of emphysema and chronic bronchitis. When emphysema predominates, compensatory hyperventilation can maintain oxygenation until the disease is very advanced. Although patients maintain adequate ABG values, they do so at the cost of significantly increased work of breathing, and general muscle wasting occurs. In chronic bronchitis, the alveolar capillary membrane is intact, but excess mucus in the airways impedes gas flow. Chronic hypoxia in the lung causes PVR to rise and to increase work on the right ventricle. The patients become polycythemic and hypoxemic. Cyanosis is more common in patients with chronic bronchitis.

Chest radiography and computed tomography. Radiographic abnormalities may be minimal, even in the presence of advanced COPD. Hyperlucency of the lungs (caused by arterial vascular deficiency in the lung periphery) and hyperinflation (flattening of the diaphragm with loss of the silhouette) suggest the diagnosis of emphysema.[4] If bullae are also present, the diagnosis of emphysema is virtually certain; however, only a small percentage of patients who have emphysema have bullae. Computed tomography (CT) can delineate the pulmonary parenchyma much better than standard chest radiography. CT may also be used to quantify the amount of air trapping. Although conventional radiography has 60% to 80% sensitivity to diagnose COPD, CT scanning improves sensitivity to 90%.[46]

Treatment

Treatment of COPD is focused on relieving symptoms and reducing the incidence of exacerbations. There is no treatment to reverse the course of COPD, but smoking cessation can slow the forward progression of the disease. Medical management is aimed at promoting bronchodilation using inhaled β_2-agonists, corticosteroids, or anticholinergics. Although a low baseline level of cholinergic tone normally influences bronchial caliber, cholinergic influence is found to be elevated in COPD, with fluctuations in airway diameter attributable to changes in cholinergic tone.[76] Anticholinergics that block the M_1 and M_3 receptors would be ideal because the M_2 acts in negative feedback to reduce acetylcholine release. In addition, the M_2 receptor also reduces adenylate cyclase, so blockade of the M_2 receptors confers the advantage of enhancing the response to β-agonists.[54] Tiotropium is a long-acting anticholinergic that is more selective for the M_3 receptor than ipratropium and atropine, and it dissociates more rapidly from the M_2 receptor. Given a 24-hour duration of action, tiotropium is gaining popularity as the ideal anticholinergic for reducing cholinergic tone in COPD.[77,78] The choice of agents in general is largely based on individual patient response and tolerance of different agents. A joint position statement by the American College of Physicians, American College of Chest Physicians, American Thoracic Society, and the European

Respiratory Society recommends the following approach to medical management of symptomatic patients[48]:

1. Bronchodilators *may* be used for mild COPD (FEV_1 60%–80%).
2. Bronchodilators are *recommended* for FEV_1 less than 60%. The specific drug prescribed is based on patient tolerance, side effects, and cost and may consist of a long-acting β_2-agonist, anticholinergic, or corticosteroid. Combination therapy may be used, although combination therapy does not show a consistent advantage over monotherapy.
3. Pulmonary rehabilitation may be used for patients with FEV_1 greater than 50% and is recommended for those with FEV_1 less than 50%.
4. Oxygen therapy is used to maintain Pao_2 greater than 60 mm Hg (Spo_2 >88%) for patients who have resting hypoxemia below this level.

At all stages of COPD progression, removal of offending and exacerbating factors is recommended (particularly cessation of smoking and administration of the influenza vaccine). Surgical treatments that are used to reduce symptoms in COPD include lung volume reduction surgery (LVRS), bullectomy, and lung transplantation. LVRS removes severely diseased portions of lung, leaving behind a greater proportion of better-functioning tissue. The result is improved elastic recoil, diaphragmatic function, and reduction in exacerbations. LVRS is most effective for predominantly upper lobe emphysema.[67]

Preoperative Evaluation

The surgical site and the preoperative status of the patient are critical factors in predicting the incidence of postoperative complications. The risk of respiratory complications is generally proportional to the proximity of the surgical site to the diaphragm.[47] Multiple factors are predictive of postoperative respiratory difficulties, but no preoperative pulmonary function test establishes absolute contraindications to surgery. The preoperative evaluation of patients with COPD should determine the severity of the disease and identify treatments for reducing inflammation, improving secretion clearance, treating underlying infection, and increasing airway caliber to ensure the best surgical outcome. Although the FEV_1 has previously been used as the primary indicator of disease severity, other factors such as body mass index, functional dyspnea, and exercise tolerance along with the FEV_1 provide useful assessment of prognosis in patients with COPD.[51,79] The multidimensional BODE index (*b*ody mass index, airflow *o*bstruction, *d*yspnea, and *e*xercise capacity) is one tool used to assess disease severity.[80] Despite their heterogeneity, treatment algorithms are primarily driven by a single measurement: FEV_1 as a percentage of its predicted value (FEV_1 %). In 2011, a major shift in Global Initiative for Chronic Obstructive Lung Disease (GOLD) treatment recommendations was proposed that stratifies patients with COPD on the basis of symptoms.[47,67] GOLD recommends that spirometry be required for the clinical diagnosis of COPD to avoid misdiagnosis and to ensure proper evaluation of severity of airflow limitation. The assessment of the patient with COPD should always include assessment of (1) symptoms, (2) severity of airflow limitation, (3) history of exacerbations, and (4) comorbidities. The widely used GOLD classification system is shown in Table 29.11. The recommendations were recently updated to add (1) assessment and regular evaluation of inhaler technique to improve therapeutic outcomes; (2) examination of symptoms and future risk of exacerbations to provide the map for pharmacologic management of stable COPD; (3) starting patients with persistent symptoms on a long-acting bronchodilator (a long-acting β_2-agonist [LABA] or a long-acting muscarinic antagonist [LAMA]), and if symptoms persist, then adding dual bronchodilator therapy; (4) for patients with progressive symptoms on a long-acting bronchodilator, advancing

TABLE 29.11 **Global Initiative for Chronic Obstructive Lung Disease (GOLD) Classification of Severity of Airflow Limitation in COPD, Based on Post–Bronchodilator FEV_1**

IN PATIENTS WITH FEV_1/FVC <0.70	
GOLD 1: mild	FEV_1 ≥80% predicted
GOLD 2: moderate	50% ≤ FEV_1 <80% predicted
GOLD 3: severe	30% ≤ FEV_1 <50% predicted
GOLD 4: very severe	FEV_1 <30% predicted

COPD, Chronic obstructive pulmonary disease; *FEV_1,* forced expiratory volume in 1 sec.
From Global Strategy for the Diagnosis, Management and Prevention of COPD, Global Initiative for Chronic Obstructive Lung Disease (GOLD) 2017. http://goldcopd.org. Accessed 2020.

to dual-bronchodilator therapy rather than the combination of an inhaled-corticosteroid and a long-acting bronchodilator; and (5) a shift toward a more personalized approach to treatment with strategies for escalation and deescalation of pharmacotherapy.

The causes of acute exacerbations of COPD are multifactorial and may be explained only partially by airway infection or inflammation. Multiple contributing factors may include bronchitis, underlying airway hyperresponsiveness, inhalation of noxious agents, mucous plugging, pneumonitis, cardiovascular disease, CHF, and generalized systemic inflammation. Signs of COPD may be subtle, thus clinical assessment should look for increased respiratory effort, altered breathing patterns, abnormal breath sounds, and a productive cough. A consensus statement by the American Thoracic Society defines dyspnea as "a subjective experience of breathing discomfort that is comprised of qualitatively distinct sensations that vary in intensity. The experience derives from interactions among multiple physiologic, psychologic, social, and environmental factors and may induce secondary physiologic and behavioral responses."[81,82]

A history of or the presence of atopy (predisposition to allergies), childhood respiratory impairment, high serum immunoglobulin E (IgE) levels, and eosinophilia is suggestive of asthmatic bronchitis, which is generally more responsive to treatment than is smoking-induced COPD. The value of preoperative pulmonary function tests is questionable for nonpulmonary surgery.[47] Data from resting Spo_2, dyspnea-related functional limitation, exercise capacity, and body mass index will lead to useful assessment of the patient's pulmonary reserve. If pulmonary function tests are available, spirometry should be assessed before and after bronchodilator or steroid treatment (or both) so that airway disease reversibility can be evaluated. The patient's response to bronchodilators provides important information regarding the management of COPD, with an improvement in FEV_1 of 12% to 15% from baseline indicating a significant response.[44] Other changes considered significant are improvements in FVC (of at least 10%), and $FEF_{25\%-75\%}$ (of at least 20%). A lack of significant improvement does not preclude use of bronchodilators during anesthesia.[46]

Numerous conditions predispose a patient with COPD to infectious complications, including dehydration, decreased ability to cough, immobility, and decreased mucociliary clearance. Optimal control of airway inflammation may require antimicrobial therapy preoperatively. Increasing cough, dyspnea, chest pain, fatigue, worsening blood gas values, and other signs may indicate an acute exacerbation of COPD. The patient may report a change in sputum volume, color, or consistency. Viruses are the most frequent causative

TABLE 29.12 FDA-Approved Drugs for COPD		
Drug	**Delivery Device**	**Usual Adult Dosage**
Inhaled Short-Acting Anticholinergic		
Ipratropium		
Altrovent HFA (Boehringer Ingelheim)	HFA MDI (200 inh/unit)	2 inhalations qid PRN
Generic—single-dose vials	Nebulizer	500 mcg qid PRN
Inhaled Short-Acting Beta$_2$-Agonist/Short-Acting Anticholinergic Combination		
Albuterol/Ipratropium		
Combivent (Boehringer Ingelheim)	CFC MDI (200 inh/unit)	2 inhalations qid PRN
Combivent respimat (Boehringer Ingelheim)	MDI (130 inh/unit)	1 inhalation qid PRN
DuoNeb(dey) generic	Nebulizer	2.5–9.5 mg qid PRN
Inhaled Long-Acting Beta$_2$-Agonists		
Indacterol—*Arcapta Noehaler* (Novartis)	DPI (30 inh/unit)	75 mcg once/day
Salmeterol—*Serevent Diskus* (GSK)	DPI (60 inh/unit)	50 mcg bid
Formoterol—*Foradil Aerolizer* (Merk)	DPI (60 inh/unit)	12 mcg bid
Perforomist (Dey)	Nebulizer	20 mcg bid
Arformoterol—*Brovana* (Sunovion)	Nebulizer	15 mcg bid
Inhaled Long-Acting Anticholinergics		
Tiotropium—*Spiriva HandiHaler* (Boehringer Ingelheim)	DPI (60 inh/unit) DPI (60 inh/unit)	18 mcg once/day 1 inhal. bid
Glycopyrrolate—*Seebri Neohaler* (Sunovium)		
Aclidinium—*Tudorza Pressair* (Forest)	DPI (60 inh/unit)	400 mcg bid

bid, Twice per day; *FDA,* US Food and Drug Administration; *inh,* inhalations; *qid,* four times per day; *PRN,* as needed.

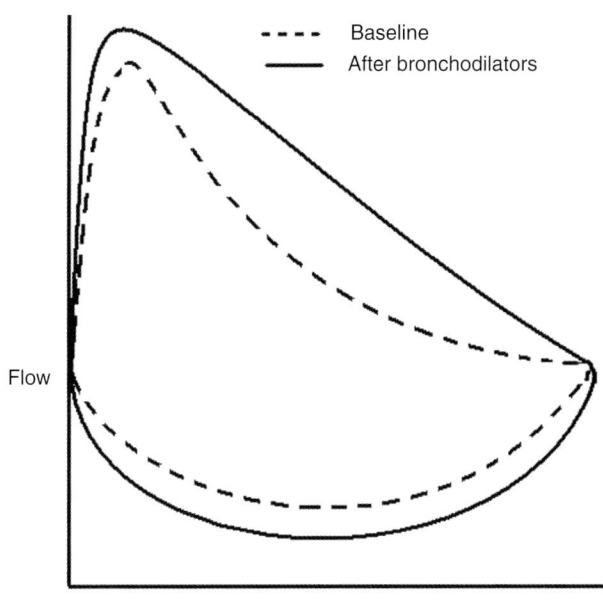

Fig. 29.17 Flow-volume loop, demonstrating expected improvement after bronchodilator therapy.

Anesthetic Management

Presently, there is a lack of scientific evidence that supports a specific anesthetic regimen for patients with COPD. However, there are general principles that can guide anesthetic planning. COPD patients are susceptible to the development of acute respiratory failure during the postoperative period. Therefore continued intubation of the trachea and mechanical ventilation of the lungs may be necessary, particularly after thoracic and upper abdominal surgery. Postoperative ventilation is more likely to be needed in those patients with low Pao$_2$ and dyspnea at rest. Assessment of respiratory function can be performed effectively and inexpensively by considering relevant factors, such as the GOLD classification or BODE score (see Table 29.11). The initial study using the BODE demonstrated a lower score among survivors than among those who died from any cause up to 52 months postoperatively (3.7 ± 2.2 vs 5.9 ± 2.6, *p* < 0.005).[80] When categorized into four quartiles (BODE indices of 0–2, 3–4, 5–6, and 7–10, respectively), there was significant correlation in the mortality rates among patients with higher BODE scores.[85]

Regional Anesthesia

Regional anesthesia is frequently recommended to avoid airway management and mechanical ventilation in patients with COPD.[67,71] Sedation should be used with caution to avoid any respiratory depression. Complications such as pneumothorax and impaired respiratory muscle function (from phrenic nerve block or high spinal block) can quickly lead to respiratory decompensation. Neuraxial anesthetic techniques that produce sensory anesthesia above T6 are not recommended since the potential for decreasing expiratory reserve volume, impairing cough effort, and creating anxiety-provoking weakness is too great.[86]

General Anesthesia

General anesthesia is often provided with a volatile anesthetic (to facilitate bronchodilation) and humidification (to prevent drying of secretions). It is often associated with an increase in the alveolar-arterial difference in Po$_2$ (Pao$_2$ − Pao$_2$). Causes include a decrease in FRC when neuromuscular blocking agents are used, as well as small airway closure and atelectasis. Atelectasis normally occurs after induction of

organisms in acute exacerbations of chronic bronchitis.[83] Acute infection is associated with epithelial desquamation and correlates with airway hyperreactivity that may persist for 3 to 6 weeks after the resolution of symptoms.[84] Measures to improve respiratory skeletal muscle strength include good nutrition and balanced fluid and electrolyte intake. Bronchodilators should be used if the patient exhibits some degree of airway obstruction, and coughing may temporarily increase in frequency as greater quantities of sputum are removed. Some commonly used bronchodilators are listed in Table 29.12. If pulmonary function tests are performed, the degree of reversibility (Fig. 29.17) will suggest the potential for and the means of improving ventilation in the perioperative period.

An increased plasma concentration of bicarbonate in the presence of a low or normal Paco$_2$ suggests chronic CO$_2$ retention compensated by acute hyperventilation. In situations where the Paco$_2$ is chronically elevated, care should be given to avoid drastic reductions. Sudden decreases in Paco$_2$ can result in alkalemia since the kidneys cannot rapidly excrete excessive amounts of bicarbonate.

general anesthesia, and it has been found to worsen with muscle paralysis and prolonged surgical duration.[87] It is interesting to note that patients with chronic hyperinflation appear to be less likely to develop atelectasis than subjects with healthy lungs, possibly because of airway closure before alveolar collapse or because of resistance to early alveolar collapse from long-standing lung hyperinflation, which prevents prompt formation of atelectasis.[88]

There is some evidence that volatile anesthetics reduce the function of cilia in the respiratory tract.[89] Opioids pose less threat to disrupting ventilation-perfusion matching and may be an appealing option. However, the residual respiratory depressant effects of opioids must be considered, particularly in the COPD population, which is frequently elderly. N_2O should be avoided since bullae may enlarge and rupture.

Ventilation Management

Ventilation strategies should focus on (1) maintaining adequate oxygenation, (2) eliminating CO_2, (3) avoiding barotrauma from excessive inspiratory pressures, (4) avoiding alveolar injury from repetitive airway closure and subsequent reopening, and (5) avoiding volutrauma from either excessive tidal volumes or from auto-PEEP. Oxygenation is managed first with increases in FiO_2; however, high FiO_2 concentrations can result in absorptive atelectasis and/or oxidative damage. Adequate hydration should be provided to prevent excessive drying of respiratory secretions. In managing CO_2 elimination, providers should avoid correction of chronic hypercapnia during mechanical ventilation. In the face of long-term renal compensation, doing so may result in an unintended alkalemia and may make ventilator weaning difficult.

Patients with COPD suffer from air trapping and have difficulty effectively moving gas into the respiratory zone. Excessive airway secretions and bronchial reactivity can impede inspiration. Intermittent vital capacity maneuvers to recruit atelectatic alveoli may help improve oxygenation during surgery,[88] and PEEP can assist with maintaining small airway patency. If the airways are noncompliant, such as with bronchitis, then slower inspiration, perhaps with an inspiratory pause, is helpful to allow time for gas to redistribute from higher compliance areas to less-ventilated lung areas. Obstructive disease commonly requires longer expiratory times (lower inspiration:expiration [I:E] ratio) to allow more time for expiration. The lower I:E ratio causes an increase in peak pressures as a result of higher inspiratory flows needed to deliver the tidal volume during a shorter inspiratory cycle. There does not seem to be any benefit when prolonging expiratory times beyond 4 seconds.[90] During expiration small airway closure and emphysematous loss of elasticity impede complete emptying of the tidal breath. As a result, inspiration begins during the respiratory system's positive recoil pressure. Thus breath stacking can occur, which builds pressure due to incomplete emptying prior to the beginning of the next inspiration. This is known as auto-PEEP or intrinsic PEEP (PEEPi).[91,92] In the past, external PEEP (PEEPe) was generally not used in patients with COPD because hypoxemia is often improved with increases in FiO_2 and because the risk of barotrauma resulting from further hyperinflation was deemed too great. The risk of PEEP exacerbating incomplete emptying is greater in patients with COPD.[93] However, cyclic closure and reopening of small airways with each breathing cycle is also detrimental, and judicious use of PEEP may avoid this low-volume tissue injury.[93] Research suggests that a PEEPe that is less than the PEEPi in the presence of expiratory flow limitation may assist patients in overcoming the inspiratory mechanical load of PEEPi, ultimately decreasing the work of breathing and eliminating or decreasing atelectatic areas and airway closure.[93-95] Patients whose peak cycling pressures remain essentially unaffected by PEEPe experience the greatest improvement with minimal untoward effects.[96] In the operating room, the clinician can best diagnose PEEPi by assessing whether exhalation is still taking

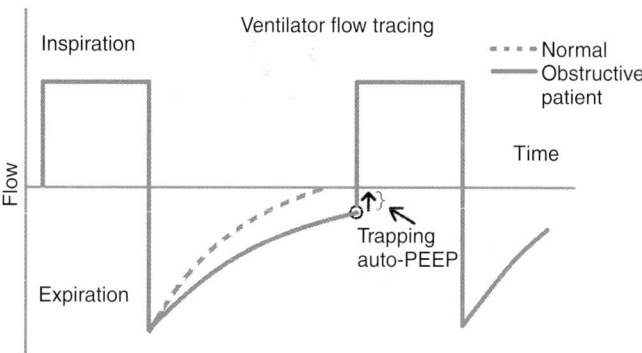

Fig. 29.18 Development of intrinsic positive end-expiratory pressure (PEEPi) is suspected when the expiratory flow tracing does not reach the zero line before the subsequent inspiration begins. (From García Vicente E, et al. Ventilación mecánica invasiva en EPOC y asma. *Med Intensiva.* 2011;35[4]:288–298.)

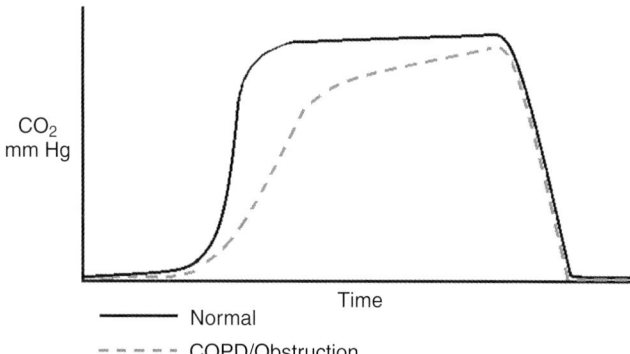

Fig. 29.19 Capnograph of a patient with expiratory airway obstruction. *COPD,* Chronic obstructive pulmonary disease.

place when the next inhalation begins.[97] Newer generation anesthesia machines, which provide dynamic flow and volume tracings of the respiratory cycle, have improved the ability to adequately ventilate patients with COPD (Fig. 29.18). Monitoring flow-volume tracings or the capnograph for expiratory airflow obstruction (Fig. 29.19) may also help guide decision making about whether incomplete emptying threatens the development of PEEPi. When PEEPe is added, it should be titrated in 2.5- to 5-cm H_2O increments while peak cycling pressures are closely monitored. Because PEEP is intended to avoid closure of small airways and alveoli that would exist at the lower (flat) portion of the compliance curve, the pressure-volume tracing can be used to determine the appropriate amount of PEEP to administer. Research demonstrates that PEEP set just above the lower inflection point of the compliance curve provides optimal oxygenation[98-101] (Fig. 29.20). This point can be clinically difficult to determine; however, it connects understanding of the physiologic concept of the compliance curve with the clinical intervention of PEEP.

Postoperative Care

Postoperative care of patients with COPD is directed at minimizing the incidence and severity of pulmonary complications because of the increased risk for developing acute respiratory failure.[102] Postoperative pulmonary complications are most often characterized by atelectasis followed by pneumonia and decreases in PaO_2.[97] These patients require close monitoring; minute ventilation may not change, but often respiratory rate increases, and Vt decreases after the termination of mechanical ventilation.[96] The choice of drugs or anesthetic techniques does not seem to predictably alter the incidence of

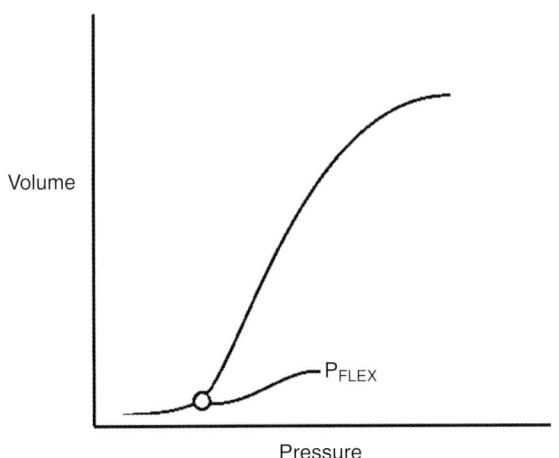

Fig. 29.20 The lower inflection point *(P_FLEX)* of the pressure-volume curve of the airway suggests an optimal pressure for setting positive end-expiratory pressure (PEEP).

postoperative pulmonary infections. Whether a relationship exists between the duration of anesthesia and the incidence of postoperative pulmonary complications is unclear. It is recommended that patients perform pulmonary toilet maneuvers and incentive spirometry in the postoperative period to help mobilize secretions and improve ventilation.[102]

ASTHMA

Definition

The National Asthma Education and Prevention Program Expert Panel Report 3 (EPR-3) defines asthma as follows:[103]

[A] chronic inflammatory disorder of the airways in which many cells and cellular elements play a role: in particular, mast cells, eosinophils, neutrophils (especially in sudden onset, fatal exacerbations, occupational asthma, and patients who smoke), T lymphocytes, macrophages, and epithelial cells. In susceptible individuals, this inflammation causes recurrent episodes of coughing (particularly at night or in the early morning), wheezing, breathlessness, and chest tightness. These episodes are usually associated with widespread but variable airflow obstruction that is often reversible either spontaneously or with treatment.

The pathogenesis of asthma involves chronic inflammation of the respiratory tract and the widespread propagation of inflammatory mediators, which is what primarily differentiates it from COPD.[67]

Various theories underlie the cause of asthma. The three overarching theories suggest that asthma may result from the following:
1. *Deficiency of acquired immunity.* Lack of exposure to immunologic challenges in early life allows a predominance of the Th2-type cytokine response and a general atopy.
2. *Genetics.*
3. *Exposure to respiratory system irritants.* These include airborne allergens (house-dust mite), irritants (tobacco smoke), and viral respiratory infections (respiratory syncytial virus).

A general approach to classification discriminates between extrinsic or intrinsic asthma. Although this system is conceptually helpful, its two groups are not mutually exclusive. Extrinsic asthma (or allergic asthma) most commonly affects children and young adults and involves exacerbation by infectious, environmental, psychological, or physical factors, whereas intrinsic asthma (or idiosyncratic asthma) usually develops in middle age without specifically identifiable

attack-provoking stimuli. It is of significance that the clinical features of idiosyncratic asthma are essentially indistinguishable from the immune-mediated response.

Incidence and Outcome

Up to 25 million persons in the United States have asthma. It is the most common chronic disease of childhood, affecting an estimated 6 million children. Asthma affects the lives of patients, their families, and society in terms of lost work and school, reduced quality of life, and avoidable emergency department (ED) visits, hospitalizations, and deaths.[103]

Pathogenesis and Pathophysiology

Our contemporary understanding of asthma is that it is not a single entity but a heterogeneous clinical syndrome characterized by episodes in which airways are hyperresponsive at times interspersed with symptom-free periods.[104] Bronchoconstriction is a factor long associated with the asthmatic symptom complex, but asthma is much more than bronchoconstriction. Airway inflammation and a nonspecific hyperirritability of the tracheobronchial tree are now recognized as being central to the pathogenesis of even mild cases of asthma. Permanent changes in airway anatomy, referred to as airway remodeling, magnify the inflammatory response.[104,105] Some manifestations of airway remodeling include fibrosis, mucous hypersecretion, smooth muscle hypertrophy, and angiogenesis.[103]

Allergic (atopic) asthma is triggered by antigens that provoke a T-lymphocyte–generated, IgE-mediated immune response.[106] It is often associated with a personal or familial history of allergic disease. In susceptible patients, exposure to even microscopic amounts of an offending agent can cause activation of lymphocytes and cytokine release, setting into motion an immune-mediated inflammatory response. Endobronchial biopsy specimens, even from asymptomatic patients, frequently show an active inflammatory process. Eosinophils, mast cells, neutrophils, and macrophages are the most common mediators of the proinflammatory cascade.

Potent biochemical mediators released from proinflammatory and airway epithelial cells promote vasoconstriction, increased smooth muscle tone, enhanced mucous secretion, submucosal edema, increased vascular permeability, and inflammatory cell chemotaxis. Leukotrienes have been identified as especially potent spasmogenic and proinflammatory substances. Released molecules that are toxic to the airway epithelium cause patchy desquamation, exposing cholinergic nerve endings and compounding the bronchoconstrictive and hyperirritable response. Asthmatic symptoms are a result of airway inflammation, edema, and hypersensitivity to irritant stimuli and proinflammatory substances. The degree of airway hyperresponsiveness and bronchoconstriction appears to parallel the extent of inflammation.[107,108] When airway reactivity is high, asthmatic symptoms are generally more severe and unrelenting, requiring additional therapeutic interventions.[104]

The mechanisms underlying nonimmunologic asthma are less clearly defined. Nonimmunologic asthma occurs in patients with no history of allergy and normal serum IgE. These patients typically develop asthmatic symptoms in response to some provocative or noxious stimulus such as cold air, airway instrumentation or irritation, climate changes, or an upper respiratory illness. Recent upper respiratory infection may precipitate bronchospasm in any patient, but the risk is higher in patients with a history of asthma. The increased bronchomotor tone associated with viral respiratory infections may persist for as long as 5 weeks.[84] Nonasthmatic children with an upper respiratory infection are two to seven times more likely to experience an adverse event perioperatively and are more prone to postoperative

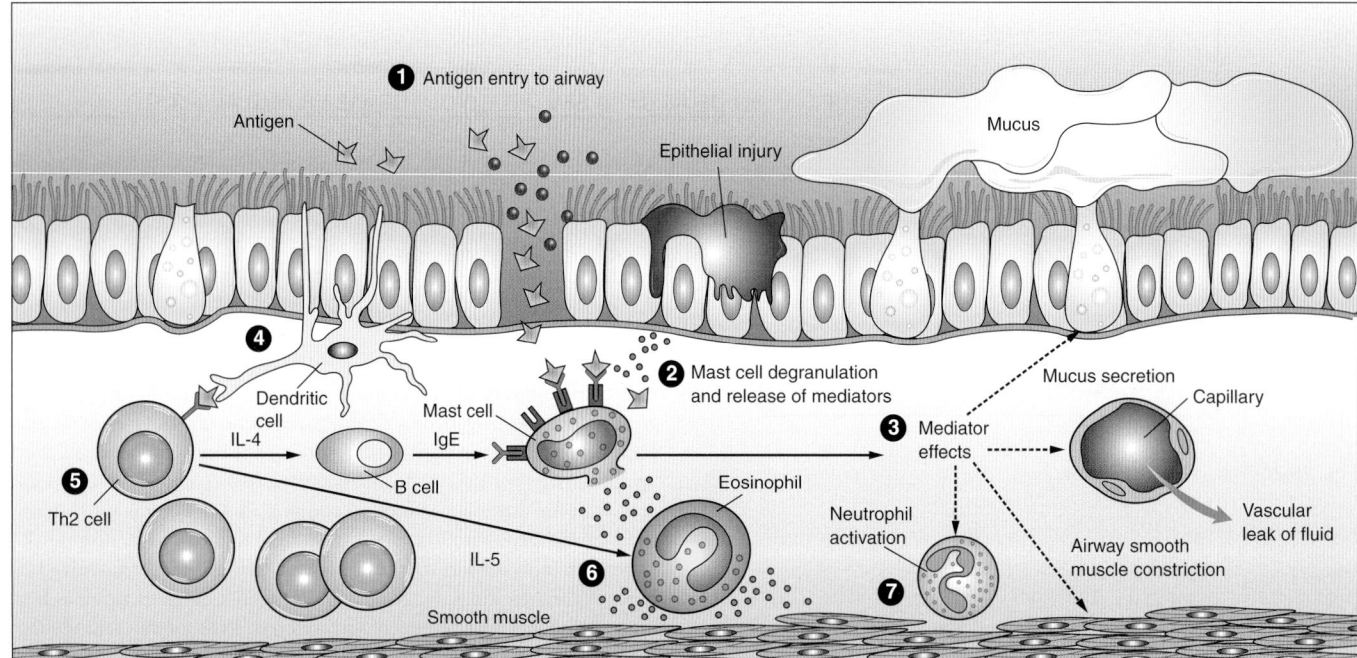

Fig. 29.21 Pathogenesis of immune response related to asthma. (1) Inhaled antigen binds to mast cells covered with preformed IgE. (2) Mast cells degranulate and release inflammatory mediators such as histamine, bradykinins, leukotrienes, prostaglandins, platelet-activating factor, and interleukins. (3) Secreted mediators induce active bronchospasm (airway smooth muscle constriction), edema from increased capillary permeability, and airway mucous secretion from goblet cells. (4) The antigen is also detected by dendritic cells that process and present it to Th2 cells at the same time as the inflammatory response is occurring. (5) Interleukin-4 (IL-4) and many other interleukins (see text) are produced. IL-4 promotes switching of B cells to favor immunoglobulin E (IgE) production. (6) IL-5 produced by Th2 cells activates eosinophils. Eosinophil products, such as major basic protein and eosinophilic cationic protein, damage the respiratory epithelium. (7) Many other inflammatory cells, including neutrophils, further contribute to the inflammatory process. *IgE,* Immunoglobulin E. (From McCance KL, Huether SE. *Pathophysiology: The Biologic Basis for Disease in Adults and Children.* 8th ed. St. Louis: Elsevier; 2019:1265.)

desaturation.[109] Controlled asthma appears to have a significantly decreased degree of risk for postoperative pulmonary complications versus noncontrolled asthma.[110] Poorly controlled asthma (defined by frequent rescue inhaler use or ED visits within 30 days) is associated with an increase in respiratory complications, which affect overall surgical risk, hospital length of stay, and in-hospital mortality.[111]

Immune mechanisms appear to be causally related or contributory to the development of asthma in more than 50% of cases, but many patients with asthma have disease mechanisms from both categories. Asthma that begins in childhood tends to have a strong allergic component, whereas asthma that occurs in adults tends to be nonallergic or to have a mixed cause.[104] As a general rule, nonallergic mechanisms of exacerbation are more prevalent in the perioperative period.[112]

IgE-mediated asthma occurs after initial antigen exposure and results in IgE antibody formation. On repeat exposure to an antigen, the IgE antibodies cause mast cells to release multiple inflammatory mediators. These mediators directly constrict small and large airways, increase capillary permeability, stimulate vasoconstriction, and increase mucous gland secretion, which contributes to mucous plugging. The pathogenesis of the immune response related to asthma is described in Fig. 29.21.

The mechanism of exercise-induced bronchospasm is unknown. One popular theory suggests that a high minute ventilation ($\dot{V}e$) and the low temperature or low H_2O content of inspired gas (which requires greater heat and water transfer from the mucosal surface to the inspired gas) generate a bronchoconstrictive response. Another theory proposes that the evaporation of water from respiratory mucosa

and the resultant increase in the osmolarity of the surface-lining fluid induce the degranulation of mast cells. A third theory suggests that reactive hyperemia of the bronchial mucosa occurs with rewarming, resulting in airway narrowing.[113] Regardless of the mechanism, most symptoms last less than 1 hour and are usually very responsive to administration of β_2-adrenergic receptor agonists.[114]

Occupational asthma develops when irritants directly stimulate vagal nerve endings in the airway epithelium. Infection-induced asthma with acute inflammation of the bronchi may be caused by viral, bacterial, or mycoplasmal infections. Aspirin-induced asthma occurs in some predisposed individuals as a result of cyclooxygenase inhibition that drives arachidonic acid metabolism toward the lipoxygenase pathway, with subsequent leukotriene production.[115] This peculiar response can also occur with the use of other nonsteroidal antiinflammatory agents. The aspirin-induced asthma variant is not IgE mediated or allergic in nature. It can be clinically associated with the presence of nasal polyps.

Clinical Features and Diagnosis

Airflow limitation is caused by a variety of changes in the airway, all influenced by airway inflammation[103]:

*   *Bronchoconstriction*—bronchial smooth muscle contraction that quickly narrows the airways in response to exposure to a variety of stimuli, including allergens or irritants.
*   *Airway hyperresponsiveness*—an exaggerated bronchoconstrictor response to stimuli.
*   *Mucous secretion*—produced by the hypersecretion of the glycoprotein mucin.

TABLE 29.13   Classification of Severity of Asthma in Adults and Children Older than 12 Not Currently Taking Long-Term Controllers

	CLASSIFICATION OF ASTHMA SEVERITY (YOUTHS ≥12 YR AND ADULTS)			
		PERSISTENT		
Components of Severity	**Intermittent**	*Mild*	*Moderate*	*Severe*
Impairment				
Symptoms	≤2 days/wk	>2 days/wk but not daily	Daily	Throughout the day
Nighttime awakenings	<2×/mo	3–4×/mo	>1×/wk but not nightly	Often 7×/wk
Short-acting β_2-agonist use for symptom control	≤2 days/wk	>2 days/wk but not daily	Daily	Several times per day
Interference with normal activity	None	Minor limitation	Some limitation	Extremely limited
Lung function	Normal FEV_1 between exacerbations • FEV_1 >80% predicted • FEV_1:FVC normal	• FEV_1 >80% predicted • FEV_1:FVC normal	• FEV_1 >60% but <80% predicted • FEV_1:FVC reduced 5%	• FEV_1 <60% predicted • FEV_1:FVC reduced >5%
Risk				
Exacerbations (consider frequency and severity)	0–2/yr	>2/yr	>2/yr	>2/yr
	Frequency and severity may fluctuate over time Relative annual risk of exacerbations may be related to FEV_1			

FEV1, Forced expiratory volume in 1 sec; *FVC,* forced vital capacity.
From Broaddus VC, et al., eds. *Murray and Nadel's Textbook of Respiratory Medicine.* 6th ed. Philadelphia: Elsevier; 2016:737; National Heart, Lung, and Blood Institute. National Asthma Education and Prevention Program 2020. https://www.nhlbi.nih.gov/health-topics/asthma. Accessed 2020.

- *Airway edema*—as the disease becomes more persistent and inflammation becomes more progressive, edema, mucous hypersecretion, and formation of inspissated mucous plugs further limit airflow. Key hallmarks of asthma include[103,107]:
- Recurrent wheezing
- Dyspnea (may parallel the severity of expiratory airflow obstruction)
- Cough (productive or nonproductive; frequently at night or early morning)
- Recurrent labored respirations with accessory muscle use
- Tachypnea (a respiratory rate >30 breaths per minute and a heart rate of 120 suggests severe bronchospasm)
- Recurrent chest tightness
- Prolonged respiratory expiratory phase
- Fatigue
- Symptoms occur or worsen with exercise, viral infection, environmental allergens or irritants, changes in weather, stress, or menstrual cycles

Clinical classification of asthma is noted in Table 29.13, and corresponding treatment protocols are shown in Fig. 29.22. Typical attacks are short lived, lasting minutes to hours. Between attacks the asthmatic patient may be entirely symptom free; however, underlying airway remodeling is still evident.[105,106] Severe obstruction that is refractory to bronchodilator therapy is known as status asthmaticus. This variant occurs in persons with a genetic predisposition[116] and requires an escalating approach to therapy for symptoms that may persist over a number of days. Status asthmaticus also can represent an emergency situation. Although rare, anesthetists may be called upon to administer ketamine or volatile anesthetics as part of the treatment for status asthmaticus.[117-119] Use of accessory muscles of respiration and the increased work of breathing associated with a

protracted asthmatic episode can result in respiratory muscle fatigue and respiratory failure.

During exacerbations, pulmonary function tests may reflect acute expiratory airflow obstruction (decreased forced expiratory flow [$FEF_{25\%-75\%}$]; decreased FEV_1:FVC). Viscid mucous secretion may compound airway obstruction and narrowing while producing airway collapse.[114] The asthmatic episode produces not only airflow obstruction but also gas exchange abnormalities. The resulting low $\dot{V}/\dot{Q}$ state produces arterial O_2 desaturation.[120] Hypoxemia is common, but in most patients with acute bronchospasm CO_2 elimination is relatively well preserved until $\dot{V}/\dot{Q}$ abnormalities are severe. An increased arterial CO_2 tension may indicate impending respiratory failure in the acutely ill asthmatic patient. Chronic asthma may eventually lead to irreversible lung destruction, loss of lung elasticity, pulmonary hypertension, and lung hyperinflation.

Diagnostic Testing

Pulmonary function tests. Lung function testing offers limited value to anesthetic risk assessment and should not be performed routinely based solely on the presence of asthma. Although spirometry is used to determine candidacy for lung resection surgery, it has limited value before extrathoracic surgery, even in patients with asthma or other lung disease. Even when spirometry is used to document the degree of airflow limitation, there is no fixed threshold that precludes surgery.[110]

When pulmonary function tests are performed, they provide information related to the degree of impairment and the reversibility of airway limitation. RV, FRC, and TLC all increase because of an increase in volume of the gas trapped beyond closed airways, and lung deflation is less because of airway obstruction. Comparison of current and prior pulmonary function test results is useful. Tolerance of activities is used for classifying the degree of dyspnea.[121] The patient in remission may

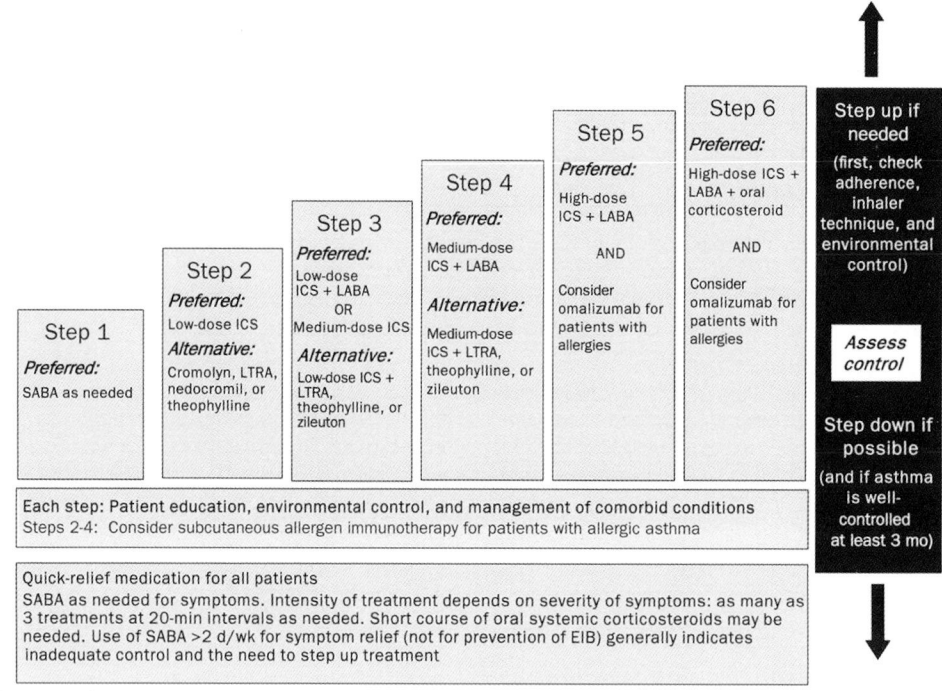

Fig. 29.22 Stepwise approach to treating asthma in adults and children older than 12. *EIB*, Exercise-induced bronchospasm; *ICS*, inhaled corticosteroid; *LABA*, long-acting β-agonist; *LTRA*, leukotriene receptor antagonist; *SABA*, short-acting β-agonist. (From National Heart Lung and Blood Institute. *National Asthma Education and Prevention Program, Expert Panel Report 3: Guidelines for the Diagnosis and Management of Asthma.* Bethesda, MD: US Department of Health and Human Services; 2007.)

have negative results on all parameters of pulmonary function and can be tested with a cholinergic agonist such as methacholine for bronchial provocation and clarification of the diagnosis of asthma.[122] The hallmark of a developing exacerbation of asthma is a reduction in the peak expiratory flow rate.[103]

Arterial blood gas analysis. An increased CO_2 diffusion capacity (compared with that of O_2) in combination with an increased respiratory rate generally produces ABG analysis results that reflect the presence of respiratory alkalosis. Even slight hypercapnia may indicate severe air trapping and potential impending respiratory failure.

Chest radiography. Because nearly 75% of asthma patients have a normal chest radiograph, chest radiography is not helpful in diagnosing or determining the severity of asthma. Hyperinflation with flattening of the diaphragm may be evident.

Electrocardiography. Changes evident on electrocardiography, such as ST segment changes, right ventricular strain, and right axis deviation, usually manifest only in severe attacks and generally are of little significance with regard to the asthmatic condition.

Sputum analysis. Eosinophilia, which is common in asthmatic patients, may be manifested as the production of grossly purulent sputum. Microscopic evaluation may reveal Curschmann spirals and Charcot-Leyden crystals, rather than polymorphic neutrophils associated with infection.

Serum values. Eosinophilia (defined as >275 eosinophils/mm³ of blood) is common in asthmatic patients with active IgE-mediated bronchial asthma, but its presence does not serve to differentiate extrinsic from intrinsic asthma. Asymptomatic patients with asthma generally have a total blood eosinophil count that is less than 50/mm³, with an increasing count often signaling the acceleration of bronchial asthma even before such patients experience symptoms. Determination of an increased eosinophil value in the absence of signs and symptoms of asthma requires that a differential analysis be undertaken. Tests for

detection of IgE antibodies are performed only if an identifiable and avoidable substance is suspected. In this instance, consultation with a physician skilled in testing for allergic disease may be indicated.

Anesthetic Management

Several important anesthetic considerations and risk-reduction strategies should be considered prior to the day of surgery. The EPR-3 recommends the following to reduce the risk of complications during surgery[103]:

- Review the level of asthma control prior to surgery. This includes medication use (especially oral systemic corticosteroids within the past 6 months) and pulmonary function.
- Prior to surgery, provide medications that improve lung function if lung function is not well controlled. A short course of oral systemic corticosteroids may be necessary.
- For patients receiving oral systemic corticosteroids during a 6-month period prior to surgery, and for selected patients on long-term high-dose inhaled corticosteroids (ICS), administer 100 mg hydrocortisone every 8 hours intravenously during the surgical period, and reduce the dose rapidly within 24 hours after surgery.

Preoperative Evaluation

A careful preoperative history, physical examination, and review of patient medications are essential to discerning the current disease status. Frequent nocturnal awakenings due to respiratory difficulty, recent increases in medication use, and signs of viral infection may signal an increased likelihood of intraoperative difficulties.[123] Elective procedures in patients who are exhibiting significant respiratory symptoms should be postponed in an effort to provide a more optimal state before surgery can occur.[124]

The predictive value of routine pulmonary function testing does not warrant screening use of this modality; rather, it should be used only when patient condition and surgical procedure cause concern for the patient's pulmonary recovery.[48] FEV and peak expiratory flow rate, which can be measured with inexpensive handheld devices, may be helpful in assessing current respiratory status. Values that fall to within 30% to 50% below expected baseline values indicate a moderate episode of bronchoconstriction. Values below 50% of normal indicate a severe episode.[123]

Medication management of asthma is similar to that of COPD. Anticholinergics are more commonly used with COPD, whereas corticosteroids are more highly effective in patients with asthma.[125] Pretreatment with systemic corticosteroids has been advocated in patients with asthma undergoing surgical procedures. However, corticosteroid pretreatment should be considered several days prior to surgery (if possible) in an effort to maximize lung function.[126] Complications of steroid therapy such as delayed wound healing, infection, or adrenocortical insufficiency are rare with these isolated doses. Patients taking either an oral or high-dose inhaled steroid prior to surgery should either continue their current therapy or receive intravenous steroids if clinically indicated depending on the anticipated degree of surgical stress.[126,127]

Anxiolytics can reduce anxiety and may help prevent a stress-induced bronchospasm. Anticholinergics such as atropine and glycopyrrolate exhibit mild bronchodilating effects and dry secretions but can increase heart rates to undesirable levels Their routine preoperative use has not been established. Use caution with opioids in patients whose respiratory difficulties are evident or when using opioids associated with histamine release, such as morphine and the other phenanthrenes. Fentanyl and the other phenylpiperidine analogs commonly used in anesthesia (with the exception of meperidine) have been widely used and are safe.[128,129] The use of histamine-2 (H_2)–receptor blocking agents such as cimetidine and ranitidine to reduce gastric volume and acidity should be avoided.[109,129] Bronchospasm can occur after the administration of H_2-receptor antagonists, possibly resulting from loss of inhibitory feedback control via presynaptic H_2-receptor blockade, resulting in increased histamine release. Commonly prescribed drug therapy for asthma is listed in Table 29.14. If airway management is anticipated, it may be sensible to administer a short-acting beta$_2$-agonist 20 to 30 minutes prior to airway manipulation.

Intraoperative Management

Despite a lack of definitive controlled clinical studies, regional anesthetic techniques are generally considered to be safer than general anesthesia. The placement of an ETT in the trachea is extremely stimulating and can result in a bronchospasm. If providing general anesthesia, and it is possible to avoid intubation, then other means of securing the airway should be considered such as a supraglottic airway.[130] Avoid spinal or epidural levels to the midthoracic area or higher since they can cause a decrease in FRC, expiratory reserve volume, and the ability to cough.

Common induction medication (such as propofol and ketamine) have been used successfully in asthmatic patients, but some differences exist. Ketamine is the only induction drug with bronchodilating properties, which makes it the agent of choice in patients with active asthmatic symptoms who require emergency surgery. Thiopental, thiamylal, methohexital, and propofol were evaluated for their effects in patients with and without asthma. None of the asthmatic patients who received propofol exhibited wheezing 2 and 5 minutes after intubation. Wheezing after intubation occurred in 26% to 45% of the patients who received one of the three barbiturates. Propofol was determined to be advantageous for routine induction in asthmatic patients.[131]

Inhalational agents produce bronchial relaxation and have all been used successfully in patients with asthma during the intraoperative period. However, isoflurane and desflurane are both mild respiratory irritants, which may be a consideration during emergence. It is common practice to blunt this effect with the administration of opiates. Sevoflurane is the agent of choice for inhalation induction in children.[132,133] Other anesthesia-related medications that should be avoided in asthmatic patients include atracurium, mivacurium, and morphine because of histamine release, and β-receptor blockers, which may produce bronchoconstriction. If a β-blocker is desired, esmolol is the preferred choice because of its relative β$_1$ selectivity and very short half-life. Prostaglandins, such as the F$_2$α subtype that is used to stop postpartum bleeding, should be avoided in asthmatic patients, as should ergonovine and related ergot derivatives, because of the risk of bronchospasm. Many practitioners avoid long-acting muscle relaxants and the associated possibility of residual muscle weakness in patients with asthma. Ketorolac and other nonsteroidal inflammatory agents should be avoided in patients with aspirin-intolerant asthma.[134]

A strategy for mechanical ventilation that avoids lung hyperinflation and barotrauma while allowing for longer expiratory times should be considered. A reduction in $\dot{V}e$, by limiting inspiratory times and prolonging expiratory times, and moderate permissive hypercapnia have been suggested.[135-137]

Intraoperative Bronchospasm

Bronchospasm may occur abruptly in surgical patients. Airway manipulation, acute exposure to allergens, or the stress of surgery can provoke wheezing in a patient who was previously asymptomatic. Wheezing often suggests potentially reversible bronchoconstriction, but the extent or degree of wheezing is a notoriously poor indicator of the degree of airway obstruction.[121] In addition, care must be taken to differentiate wheezing of asthmatic origin from other causes of wheezing, such as pneumothorax, ETT obstruction, carinal stimulation, endobronchial intubation, anaphylaxis, pulmonary edema, pulmonary embolism, or pulmonary aspiration.[138]

In anesthetized patients, prominent manifestations of the asthmatic episode are wheezing, increased mucous secretion, high inspiratory pressures, a slanted expiratory CO_2 waveform, and hypoxemia. Mechanical ventilation and positive airway pressure are associated with a higher incidence of air trapping and lung hyperinflation, and the associated inflammation can result in a pneumothorax.[120] Additionally, alveolar overdistention may lead to decreased venous return and cardiac output. The combination of impaired ventilation and hypoxemia can precipitate an increase in PVR, enhanced right ventricular afterload, and finally hemodynamic collapse.

If an episode of bronchospasm occurs during anesthesia, the following steps are recommended:

1. Deepen the level of anesthesia with a volatile agent, propofol, ketamine, lidocaine, or a combination that rapidly increases anesthetic depth.
2. Administer 100% O_2.
3. Administer a short-acting β$_2$-agonist (SABA).
4. In severe cases, administer epinephrine intravenously or subcutaneously (in doses of 10 mcg/kg).
5. Administer intravenous corticosteroids—hydrocortisone 2 to 4 mg/kg.
6. Consider intravenous aminophylline if long-term postoperative mechanical ventilation is planned.

Theophylline has little efficacy for the treatment of acute bronchoconstrictive episodes.[139] Episodes of severe airway obstruction may not respond to bronchodilator treatment, and cessation of wheezing may occur with the worsening of obstruction (i.e., the "ominously silent chest").

TABLE 29.14 FDA-Approved Drugs for Asthma

Drug	Adult Dosage	Pediatric Dosage
Inhaled Beta₂-Agonists, Short Acting		
Albuterol		
Proair	90–180 mcg q 4–6 hr PRN	≥4 yr; 90–180 mcg q 4–6 hr PRN
Proventil		
Ventolin		
Generic single-dose vials	1.25–5 mg q 4–8 hr PRN	2–4 yr; 0.63–2.5 mg q 4–6h PRN
		5–11 yr: 1.25–5 mg q 4–8 hr PRN
Acc/Nub single-dose vials	—	2–12 yr: 0.63 or 1.25 mg tid–qid PRN
Levalbuterol		
Xopenex	90 mcg q 4–6 hr PRN	≤4 yr: 90 mcg q 4–6 hr PRN
Xopenex	0.63–1.25 mg tid q 6–8 hr PRN	6–11 yr; 0.31–0.63 mg tid q 6–8h PRN
Pirbuterol—Maxair Autohaler	200–400 mcg q 4–6 hr PRN	≤12 yr: 200–400 mcg q 4–6 hr PRN
Inhaled Corticosteroids		
Beclomethasone dipropionate	40–320 mcg bid	5–11 yr: 40–80 mcg bid
QVAR	180–720 mcg bid	6–17 yr: 180–360 mcg bid
Budesonide—Pulmicort		
Flexhaler Pulmicort Respules	—	1–8 yr: 0.25 mcg bid or 0.5 mg once/day or bid or 1 mg once/day
Generic single-dose vials	80–320 mcg bid	≤12 yr: 80–320 mcg bid
Ciclesonide—*Alvesco*	160–320 mcg bid	I6–11 yr: 80–160 mcg bid
Fluticasone propionate	100–1000 mcg bid	4–11 yr: 50–100 mcg bid
Flovent Diskus	88–880 mcg bid	
Flovent HFA	222–888 mcg once/day in evening or 220 mcg bid	4–11 yr: 88 mcg bid
Mometasone furoate—*Asmanex Twisthaler*		4–11 yr:110 mcg 1×/day in evening
Oral Glucocorticoids		
Methylprednisolone—generic	7.5–60 mg once/day or every other day or 40–60 mg	0–11 yr: 0.25–2 mg/kg once/day or every other day
Medrol	once/day or divided bid × 3–10 days for an acute	(max 60 mg/day) or 1–2 mg/kg per day divided
Prednisolone—generic	exacerbation	bid ×3–10 days (max 60 mg/day) for an acute
Prelone		exacerbation
Orapred		
ODT		
Pediapred		
Prednisone—generic		
Inhaled Beta₂-Agonists, Long Acting		
Salmeterol—*Serevent Diskus* (GSK)	50 mcg bid	≤4 yr: 50 mcg bid
Formoterol—*Foradil Aerolizer*	12 mcg bid	≤5 yr: 12 mcg bid
Inhaled Corticosteroid/Long-Acting Beta₂-Agonist Combinations		
Fluticasone propionate/		
Salmeterol		
Advair Diskus	1 inhalation bid	4–11 yr: 1 inhalation (100/50 mcg) bid
Advair	2 inhalations bid	≤12 yr: 1 inhalation bid
		≤12 yr: 2 inhalations bid
Budesonide/formoterol		
Symbicort	2 inhalations bid	≤12 yr: 2 inhalations bid
Mometasone/formoterol		
Dulera	2 inhalations bid	≤12 yr: 2 inhalations bid
Leukotriene Modifiers		
Montelukast—generic *Singulair*	10 mg PO once/day	≤1 yr: 4 or 5 mg PO once day

TABLE 29.14 FDA-Approved Drugs for Asthma—cont'd

Drug	Adult Dosage	Pediatric Dosage
Zafirlukast—generic	20 mg PO bid	5–11 yr: 10 mg PO bid
Accolate		≤12 yr: 20 mg PO bid
Zileuton—*Zyflo*	600 mg PO qid	≤12 yr: 600 mg PO qid
Extended release		
Zyflo CR	1200 mg PO bid	≤12 yr: 1200 mg PO bid
Anti-IgE Antibody		
Omalizumab—*Xolair*	150–300 mc SC q 4 wk or 225–375 mg SC 2 wk	≤12 yr: 150–300 mg q 4 wk or 225–375 mg q 2 wk
Theophylline		
Generic	300–600 mg/once day or divided bid	10 mg/kg per day (max 300 mg/day)
Theo-24	300–600 mg once/day	
Theochron	300–600 mg once/day	
Anti-interleukin-5 (IL-5) Antibodies		
Mepolizumab *(Nucala)*, reslizumab *(Cinqair)*, and benralizumab *(Fasenra)*	For treatment of severe asthma in patients who have elevated eosinophil levels. Intravenous or subcutaneous injections monthly	Hypersensitivity reactions have occurred with all three drugs; the reslizumab package insert includes a boxed warning about a risk of anaphylaxis

FDA, US Food and Drug Administration.
Adapted from Drugs for asthma. *Med Lett Drugs Ther.* 2017;59(1528):139–146.

When treating bronchospasm, SABAs may be administered by metered-dose inhaler or nebulizer. Multiple doses may be necessary, but it should be noted that these drugs do exhibit a plateau in efficacy. Therefore extremely high doses or intravenous β-agonist do not confer additional advantage. Anticholinergic agents such as ipratropium bromide (0.25–0.5 mg nebulizer every 20 minutes × 3) should be used in moderate to severe cases as a second-line therapy to SABA. Because inflammation is central to asthma exacerbation, corticosteroids are becoming more acceptable for acute usage to prevent the need for longer term therapy.[140,141] In cases refractory to other bronchodilators, magnesium sulfate (2 g intravenously over 20 minutes) has been demonstrated to be safe and effective. Magnesium is effective as both a direct smooth muscle relaxant and an antiinflammatory medication.[142] Research attention is turning to traditionally chronic-acute medications, such as montelukast, for their utilization in acute therapy.[140] In severe cases, use of helium-oxygen (heliox) and noninvasive ventilation may promote gas flow and prevent intubation in cases of impending respiratory failure.[103] However, the use of heliox is associated with decreased FiO_2 levels.

Emergence

There are both advantages and disadvantages to deep or awake extubation. A deep extubation may be preferable to avoid the mechanical stimulation from the ETT upon awakening. However, residual anesthesia and/or muscle paralysis can cause hypoventilation without a secure airway. An awake patient who meets criteria for extubation confirms the return of airway reflexes and adequate tidal volumes; however, the presence of the ETT within the trachea can cause significant pulmonary stimulation potentially resulting in a bronchospasm. Either way, a judgment must be made as to when to extubate the patient, with the understanding that the earliest possible time is advantageous to avoid prolonged mechanical bronchial stimulation. Administration of opioids may help diminish airway sensitivity.

The use of anticholinesterase reversal agents has also been an area of concern. Administration of an anticholinesterase medication should consist of the minimum adequate dose. To ensure a more complete anticholinergic effect, a small increase in the coadministered dose of atropine or glycopyrrolate is suggested. Sugammadex does not have the cholinergic actions and may be preferred in patients with a reactive airway.[143]

Asthma and the Pregnant Surgical Patient

Effective control of asthma symptoms during pregnancy is important for the health and well-being of both mother and fetus, and it ensures adequate oxygen supply. Uncontrolled asthma increases the risk of perinatal mortality, preeclampsia, preterm birth, and low birthweight infants. It is safer for pregnant women to be treated with asthma medications than to suffer from asthma symptoms and exacerbations. The EPR-3 report recommends the following general strategies when caring for women during pregnancy:

- Albuterol is the preferred SABA. Most data related to safety during human pregnancy are available for albuterol.
- Inhaled corticosteroids are preferred for long-term control. Budesonide is the preferred ICS since most evidence of ICS use during pregnancy is with budesonide. However, no evidence exists precluding the use of other ICS medications during pregnancy.
- Around the time of delivery, note that β-agonists, which promote bronchodilation, also relax the uterus and may impede the progress of labor or encourage postpartum bleeding.
- Prostaglandin preparations and ergot alkaloids, which reduce uterine bleeding, can lead to bronchoconstriction.

PULMONARY HYPERTENSION

Definition

Pulmonary hypertension is defined by a mean PAP at least 25 mm Hg with a pulmonary capillary occlusion pressure of no more than 15 mm Hg. Pulmonary arterial hypertension (PAH) is a subgroup of pulmonary hypertension characterized by vascular cell proliferation and cellular changes in low-resistance pulmonary arteries that increase the PVR.[144] PAH represents an advanced stage of a large number of cardiovascular diseases.[145]

Although patients with severe PAH would not be considered candidates for nonessential surgical procedures, several other operations (i.e., lung transplant or balloon atrial septostomy) may be needed as treatment.[146,147]

Incidence and Outcome

PAH is a rare disorder, and its true incidence is unknown; however, it is estimated to affect approximately 15 million people.[145] PAH is characterized by a rapidly progressive course with a 79% mortality rate within 5 years of clinical diagnosis.[148] The degree of increase in pressure in the pulmonary circulation has an important influence on the patient's life expectancy,[149] and prognosis is largely determined by right ventricular integrity.[150] Factors that predict perioperative complications include emergency surgery, major surgery, long operative time, use of general anesthesia, and increased New York Heart Association functional class.[144] Pulmonary hypertension carries an increased risk of respiratory failure (~25%), heart failure, and death following noncardiac surgery.[151,152] The perioperative mortality rate associated with PAH is high, even in mild to moderate disease.[145] Reviews of outcomes among patients with PAH demonstrated perioperative death rates of 7%[144] and 18%.[153] The mortality rate among obstetric patients with PAH undergoing surgery was found to be near 25%.[154]

Etiology

PAH may be caused by many associated conditions, including drug effects, connective tissue disorders, COPD, sarcoidosis, and idiopathic/genetic causes. Five main categories describe the types of pulmonary hypertension: (1) PAH, (2) pulmonary hypertension due to left heart disease, (3) pulmonary hypertension due to lung diseases and/or hypoxia, (4) chronic thromboembolic pulmonary hypertension, and (5) causes with unknown mechanisms.[154]

Pathophysiology

Normally, pulmonary vasculature is highly distensible resulting in circulatory low resistance.[155] PAH is characterized by an increase in vascular tone resulting in the growth and proliferation of pulmonary vascular smooth muscle. Initial reversible vasoconstriction may progress to muscle hypertrophy and irreversible degeneration.[156] Overload of the right ventricle can lead to cor pulmonale and inhibition of coronary perfusion.

Clinical Features and Diagnosis

Pulmonary arterial hypertension may be either acute or chronic. In almost all patients with PAH, dyspnea and exercise intolerance are usually the first complaints.[150,157] Patients may also have angina. Right atrial hypertrophy, right ventricular hypertrophy, or both, may be evident on electrocardiogram (ECG). Chest radiography may demonstrate an enlarged pulmonary artery.[158] Cardiac catheterization combined with pulmonary angiography provides the greatest amount of information regarding assessment, cardiac reserve, and the effects of pulmonary vasodilator therapy in patients with PAH.[156] Vasodilator therapy is attempted when a vasoconstrictor component is identified. A vasodilator challenge may be performed during cardiac catheterization using a rapid and effective pulmonary vasodilator such as nitroglycerin, isoproterenol, nifedipine, prostaglandin E₁, prostacyclin, prostaglandin E₂, hydralazine, nitroprusside, or adenosine to determine the potential reversibility of PAH.[159] Frequently, open-lung biopsy is performed for assessment of the histopathologic composition of small pulmonary arteries.[160] Noninvasive evaluation includes Doppler echocardiography for measurement of the velocity of tricuspid regurgitation (which correlates well with invasive PAP measurements) and pulmonic peak flow velocity.[161,162] ETco₂ can also serve as an indicator of the presence of PAH, due to the underlying vascular

TABLE 29.15 Medications Used to Treat Pulmonary Arterial Hypertension

Drug	Route	Usual Adult Dosage
Soluble Guanylate Cyclase	Oral	1–2.5 mg tid
Riociguat—*Adempas*		
Endothelin Receptor Antagonists	Oral	5–10 mg once/day
Ambrisentan—*Letairis*	Oral	62.5 mg bid for 4 wk, then 125 mg bid
Bosentan—Tracleer	Oral	10 mg once/day
Macitentan—*Opsumit*	Oral	20 mg/tid
Phosphodiesterase 5 (PDE 5) Inhibitors		
Sildenafil	Oral	40 mg once/day
Revatio		
Tadalafil—*Adcirca*	IV	2–40 ng/kg per min continuous infusion
Prostacyclins		
Epoprostenol	Inhalation	2.5–5 mcg/inhalation
Veletri	Oral	6–9 times/day
Folan		0.25–21 mg bid
Iloprost—*Ventavis*	SC or IV	40–160 ng/kg per min
Treprostinil—*Orenitram*	Inhalation	continuous infusion 9 breaths (54 mcg) qid
Remodulin		
Tyvaso		

IV, Intravenous; *SC*, subcutaneous.
From Ambrisentan (Letairis) and tadalafil (Adcirca) for pulmonary arterial hypertension. *Med Lett Drugs Ther.* 2016;58:1485.

defect. ETco₂ is significantly reduced in patients with PAH, as compared with pulmonary venous hypertension or the absence of pulmonary vascular disease.

Attempts to alleviate varying degrees of pulmonary hypertensive disease have had mixed success. Medications that cause pulmonary artery vasodilation are commonly used and may be helpful in patients with reversible vasoconstriction (Table 29.15). α- and β-adrenergic antagonists have shown the least benefit, whereas prostacyclins demonstrate the best, and newer medications such as ρ-kinase inhibitors show good promise.[146] Possible beneficial effects of pulmonary arterial dilation are preservation of lung function, prevention of right ventricle deterioration, and improved survival.

Anesthetic Management

The principal objectives during anesthesia management in a patient with PAH are to (1) prevent any increases in PAH and (2) avoid major hemodynamic changes.[157] Preoperative evaluation should include ECG, echocardiogram, chest x-ray, and ABG. Underlying medical conditions (such as COPD) should be optimized. Chronic therapy for PAH should not be discontinued. Intraoperative hypotension should be treated with vasopressors.[145]

The anesthetic plan should focus on cardiovascular support, particularly related to the pulmonary vasculature. Overall, conditions that increase the PVR (hypoxemia, hypercarbia, acidosis, pain, hypothermia) should be avoided.[144] General or regional anesthesia may be used. Peripheral nerve blocks with sedation and monitored anesthesia care should be provided when possible for minor surgical procedures.

Neuraxial anesthesia may cause significant acute decreases in SVR resulting in lower preloads, cardiac outputs, and systemic perfusion pressures, which could adversely affect RV function. Furthermore, a high thoracic blockade can result in cardioaccelerator fiber blockade causing bradycardia. A thoracic epidural may be considered with careful management. There is significant risk for adverse cardiac and respiratory complications with the use of general anesthesia in patients with severe pulmonary hypertension.[144] Etomidate provides the least amount of cardiac depression and is frequently the induction medication of choice. Ketamine should be avoided since it can potentially cause an increase in PVR. An opioid-heavy technique in combination with lower concentrations of volatile agents has been used successfully. N_2O should be avoided because it can cause small increases in PVR and its use is associated with lower Fio_2 concentrations. Sympathetic stimulation from desflurane should be avoided.

Unless the surgical procedure is minor, blood pressure should be monitored with an intraarterial catheter. Central venous lines are usually placed for more invasive surgical procedures. Pulmonary artery catheters are reserved for major surgical procedures. Hypotension during surgery should be treated aggressively since it can begin a downward spiral from which it is difficult to recover. Discrimination between a drop in SVR or right ventricular failure is important since the treatments will differ. Vasopressors are indicated for acute decreases in SVR, whereas inhaled nitric oxide or iloprost are used when the right ventricle is failing.[163,164]

COR PULMONALE

Definition

The term *cor pulmonale* refers to right heart failure secondary to pulmonary pathology. Typically this results from pulmonary hypertension that leads to progressive right ventricular hypertrophy, dilation, and eventual cardiac decompensation. This situation arises from a variety of disorders that affect the structure and function of the lungs (Box 29.5). COPD is the leading cause of cor pulmonale.[165]

Incidence and Outcome

In individuals older than 50 years of age, cor pulmonale is the third most common cardiac disorder (after ischemic heart disease and hypertensive cardiac disease). The male:female ratio of incidence of the disease is 5:1, and 10% to 30% of patients admitted to the hospital with coronary heart failure exhibit cor pulmonale.[166] The incidence of pulmonary hypertension among patients with advanced COPD is estimated to be 50%.[167]

Prognosis is determined by the pulmonary disease responsible for the increased PVR. In patients with COPD in whom Pao_2 can be maintained at near-normal levels, the prognosis is favorable. However, in COPD patients with progressive hypoxemia, hypercarbia, and airflow obstruction cor pulmonale is associated with a significant increase in mortality.[168] Prognosis is poor for those patients in whom cor pulmonale is the result of gradual obstruction of pulmonary vessels by intrinsic pulmonary vascular disease or pulmonary fibrosis. These anatomic changes cause irreversible alterations in the pulmonary vasculature, resulting in fixed elevations in PVR.

Etiology

Diseases that affect the lung, vasculature, upper airway, or chest wall can lead to pulmonary hypertension and cor pulmonale. The most common cause of acute cor pulmonale is pulmonary embolism. COPD is associated with the functional loss of pulmonary capillaries and subsequent arterial hypoxemia; these events initiate pulmonary vasoconstriction, which is the leading cause of chronic cor pulmonale. The World Health Organization has proposed a classification of conditions

---

BOX 29.5   Diagnostic Classification of Pulmonary Hypertension

Group 1: Pulmonary Arterial Hypertension (PAH)
1. Idiopathic PAH
2. Heritable PAH
    1. *BMPR2*
    2. *ALK1, ENG, SMAD9, CAV1, KCNK3*
    3. Unknown genes
3. Drug and toxin induced
4. Associated with:
    1. Connective tissue diseases
    2. HIV infection
    3. Portal hypertension
    4. Congenital heart disease
    5. Schistosomiasis

Group 1′: Pulmonary Venoocclusive Disease (PVOD) and/or Pulmonary Capillary Hemangiomatosis (PCH)

Group 1″: Persistent Pulmonary Hypertension of the Newborn

Group 2: Pulmonary Hypertension due to Left Heart Disease
1. Left ventricular systolic dysfunction
2. Left ventricular diastolic dysfunction
3. Valvular disease
4. Congenital/acquired left heart inflow/outflow tract obstruction and congenital cardiomyopathies

Group 3: Pulmonary Hypertension due to Lung Diseases and/or Hypoxia
1. Chronic obstructive pulmonary disease
2. Interstitial lung disease
3. Other pulmonary diseases with mixed restrictive and obstructive pattern
4. Sleep-disordered breathing
5. Alveolar hypoventilation disorders
6. Chronic exposure to high altitude
7. Developmental lung diseases

Group 4: Chronic Thromboembolic Pulmonary Hypertension (CTEPH)

Group 5: Pulmonary Hypertension With Unclear Multifactorial Mechanisms
1. Hematologic disorders: chronic hemolytic anemia, myeloproliferative disorders, splenectomy
2. Systemic disorders: sarcoidosis, pulmonary histiocytosis, lymphangioleiomyomatosis
3. Metabolic disorders: glycogen storage disease, Gaucher disease, thyroid disorders
4. Others: tumoral obstruction, fibrosing mediastinitis, chronic renal failure, segmental PH

ALK1, Activin receptor-like kinase type 1; *BMPR2*, bone morphogenetic protein receptor type 2; *CAV1*, caveolin-1; *ENG*, endoglin; *HIV*, human immunodeficiency virus; PAH, pulmonary arterial hypertension.
From Simonneau G, et al. Updated clinical classification of pulmonary hypertension. *J Am Coll Cardiol.* 2013;62:D34–D41.

---

associated with cor pulmonale. Diseases associated with hypoxic pulmonary vasoconstriction include the following:
- COPD
- Bronchiectasis
- Chronic mountain sickness

- Cystic fibrosis
- Idiopathic alveolar hypoventilation
- Obesity-related hypoventilation syndrome
- OSA
- Neuromuscular disease
- Kyphoscoliosis
- Pleuropulmonary fibrosis
- Upper airway obstruction

Diseases that produce obstruction or obliteration of the pulmonary vasculature include the following:

- Pulmonary embolism
- Pulmonary fibrosis
- Pulmonary lymphangitic carcinomatosis
- Idiopathic PAH
- Progressive systemic sclerosis
- Sarcoidosis
- Intravenous drug abuse
- Pulmonary vasculitis
- Pulmonary venoocclusive disease

Pathophysiology

Pulmonary hypertension is always an underlying pathology of cor pulmonale. In COPD, polycythemia, hypoxic pulmonary vasoconstriction, hyperinflation, and the reduction in size of the pulmonary vascular bed lead to pulmonary hypertension.[169] Sustained pulmonary hypertension produces hypertrophy of the smooth muscle in the tunica media, and remodeling of the vascular smooth muscle leads to irreversible increases in PVR. An imbalance in nitric oxide and endothelin is also contributory, with the balance tipped toward the vasoconstrictive effects of endothelin.[169] The rate at which right ventricular dysfunction develops depends on the magnitude of pressure increase in the pulmonary circulation and on the rapidity with which this increase occurs. For example, pulmonary embolism may lead to right ventricular failure in the presence of a mean PAP as low as 30 mm Hg. By contrast, when PAH occurs gradually, as it does in COPD, right ventricular compensation occurs; CHF rarely occurs before mean PAP exceeds 50 mm Hg.

The normal pulmonary circulation can accommodate a maximal right ventricular output with minimal increase in pulmonary pressure via distention of existing vessels or recruitment of unused vessels. The compensatory mechanism for pressure overload on the right ventricle involves enhancement of contractility and an increase in preload, which result in an increase in right ventricular end-diastolic volume.[170] In response to chronic pressure overload imposed by the PAH, right ventricular hypertrophy occurs. Brain natriuretic peptide shows a positive correlation to ventricular stretch, which occurs in cor pulmonale.[169] Cor pulmonale can acutely occur from sudden increases in PVR that result in significant right ventricular strain, such as pulmonary embolism or ARDS.[171,172]

Clinical Features and Diagnosis

Clinical manifestations of cor pulmonale are often nonspecific and obscured by COPD. Echocardiography may be useful,[172] but right-sided heart catheterization is usually required for diagnosis. Cardiac catheterization combined with pulmonary angiography provides the most definitive information on the degree of PAH, cardiac reserve, and the effects of pulmonary vasodilator treatment.[156]

Symptoms associated with cor pulmonale include retrosternal pain, cough, dyspnea on exertion, weakness, fatigue, early exhaustion, and hemoptysis.[156] Occasionally, hoarseness secondary to left recurrent laryngeal nerve compression by the enlarged pulmonary artery is present.[166] Syncope on exertion may occur as a result of right ventricular stroke volume decreases in the presence of a fixed PVR elevation.

Physical signs of cor pulmonale include the following:

- Elevation of jugular venous pressure
- Cardiac heave or thrust along the left sternal border and S_3 gallop
- Presence of an S_4 heart sound secondary to significant right ventricular hypertrophy
- A widely split S_2 heart sound
- Possible murmur of pulmonic and tricuspid insufficiency
- Hepatomegaly, ascites, and lower extremity edema (late signs)

Diagnostic Testing

Electrocardiography. Right atrial displacement, right ventricular hypertrophy, right atrial hypertrophy, and right atrial enlargement may be observed. P pulmonale (tall, peaked p waves) is a characteristic sign. Patients may develop concomitant supraventricular tachydysrhythmias (i.e., tachycardic atrial fibrillation, sinus tachycardia, and paroxysmal atrial tachycardia).

Imaging studies. On chest radiography, enlargement of the pulmonary arteries is observed, followed by right ventricular hypertrophy. Meeting criteria for pulmonary artery dilation has 98% sensitivity for diagnosing pulmonary hypertension.[169] Echocardiography may be helpful to demonstrate enlargement, dilation, or thickening of the right ventricle, with or without tricuspid valve regurgitation, and elevated pulmonary artery systolic pressure. Shifting of the intraventricular septum as a result of increased right ventricular end-diastolic volume is another characteristic finding.[169] All these findings suggest the presence of acute or chronic PAH. Magnetic resonance imaging provides better evaluation of the ventricular wall thickness than echocardiography.

Treatment

The three major drug classes for treatment of PAH are prostanoids, endothelin receptor antagonists, and phosphodiesterase inhibitors. Goals of treatment include (1) right ventricular workload decreases, (2) PVR reductions, (3) prevention of PAP increases, and (4) the avoidance of major hemodynamic changes. Diuretics may be used to reduce cardiac workload but not at the expense of an inadequate preload.[169] Improvement of gas exchange is the primary focus of treatment in COPD patients with cor pulmonale.[156,173] Treatment includes supplemental administration of O_2 to maintain a PaO_2 of greater than 60 mm Hg or an arterial O_2 saturation of greater than 90%. O_2 is the only vasodilator with a selective effect on pulmonary vessels that is not associated with a risk of worsening hypoxemia.[174] Ventilation under anesthesia should focus on maintaining low airway pressures and avoiding PEEPi.[172]

Heart-Lung Transplantation

A heart-lung transplantation may ultimately be needed when cor pulmonale progresses despite the provision of maximal medical therapy.

In general, preoperative preparation of the patient with cor pulmonale includes the following:

- Elimination and control of acute or chronic pulmonary infections
- Reversal of bronchospasm
- Improvement in clearance of secretions
- Expansion of collapsed or poorly ventilated alveoli
- Hydration
- Correction of any electrolyte imbalance

Anesthetic Management

Regional anesthesia technique may be appropriate as long as a high sensory level of anesthesia is not required because any decrease in SVR in the presence of a fixed PVR may result in severe hypotension.[175]

General Anesthesia

Volatile agents decrease PVR. N_2O has been shown to increase PVR in patients with primary pulmonary hypertension. Intravenous

TABLE 29.16	Classification of Acute Pulmonary Embolism	
Category (Frequency)	Presentation	Therapy
Massive PE (5%–10%)	Systolic blood pressure <90 mm Hg or poor tissue perfusion or multisystem organ failure plus extensive thrombosis, such as "saddle" PE or right or left main pulmonary artery thrombus	Anticoagulation (usually starting with intravenous UFH), plus consider advanced therapy: systemic thrombolysis, pharmacomechanical catheter-directed therapy, surgical embolectomy, or inferior vena cava (IVC) filter
Submassive PE (20%–25%)	Hemodynamically stable but moderate or severe right ventricular dysfunction or enlargement, coupled with biomarker elevation indicative of right ventricular microinfarction and/or right ventricular pressure overload	Anticoagulation usually with intravenous UFH until decision made regarding implementation of advanced therapy; controversy centers on this group. For systemic thrombolysis, reducing the rate of cardiovascular collapse and death must be balanced against the increased rate of hemorrhagic stroke. For patients at low bleeding risk with severe right ventricular dysfunction, consider same interventions as for massive PE
Small to moderate PE (70%)	Normal hemodynamics and normal right ventricular size and function	Anticoagulation with parenteral therapy as a bridge to warfarin or, alternatively, with oral rivaroxaban regimen as monotherapy

PE, Pulmonary embolism; *UFH*, unfractionated heparin.
From Goldhaber SZ. Pulmonary embolism. In Mann DL, et al, eds. *Braunwald's Heart Disease: A Textbook of Cardiovascular Medicine*. 11th ed. Philadelphia: Elsevier; 2019.

agents, with the exception of ketamine, appear to have little effect on PVR. During all stages of anesthesia, hemodynamic manipulation that increases PAP must be avoided. Five key principles should be followed[144,156]:

- Maintain adequate oxygenation.
- Avoid acidosis.
- Avoid the use of exogenous and endogenous vasoconstrictors.
- Avoid presenting stimuli that increase sympathetic tone.
- Avoid hypothermia.

A complete discussion of heart and lung transplants can be found in Chapter 41.

PULMONARY EMBOLISM

Definition

Pulmonary embolism is caused by a dislodged thrombus that travels into the pulmonary vascular bed. A significant pulmonary embolus obstructs blood flow causing severe gas exchange and circulatory decreases. Classification of acute pulmonary embolisms is given in Table 29.16.

Incidence and Outcome

Being a major source of morbidity and mortality, pulmonary embolism affects between 300,000 and 600,000 people in the United States annually. One-third of these develop postthrombotic syndrome (long-term complications such as swelling, pain, and discoloration in the affected limb), one-third of people with pulmonary embolism die within 1 month of diagnosis, and one-fourth of them present with sudden death as the first symptom.[176] Pulmonary emboli originate from deep vein thrombosis (DVT) of the iliofemoral vessels in approximately 90% of patients, although other sites of thrombus formation include the pelvic veins, the renal and hepatic veins, the axillary veins in the upper extremities, and the right atrium.[177] Pulmonary embolism occurs in approximately 1% of surgical patients overall,[178] but the incidence is as high as 30% among high-risk orthopedic procedures.[179] Mortality from perioperative pulmonary embolism is approximately 10%.[178,180]

Etiology

Pulmonary embolism can result from a number of factors (i.e., individual patient health and comorbidities, hematologic disorders, or recent/upcoming surgery), which can either individually or combined affect its development (Box 29.6). The incidence of symptoms from DVT is greater

BOX 29.6 Thromboembolic Risk Factors

Hereditary Thrombophilias
- Protein C deficiency
- Protein S deficiency
- Antithrombin III deficiency
- Factor V Leiden mutation
- Prothrombin 20210 G → A variation
- Hyperhomocysteinemia
- Dysfibrinogenemia
- Familial plasminogen deficiency

Acquired Surgical Predispositions
- Major thoracic, abdominal, or neurosurgical procedures requiring general anesthesia and lasting >30 min
- Hip arthroplasty
- Knee arthroplasty
- Knee arthroscopy
- Hip fracture
- Major trauma
- Open prostatectomy
- Spinal cord injury

Acquired Medical Predispositions
- Prior venous thromboembolism
- Advanced age (>60 yr)
- Malignancy
- Congestive heart failure
- Cerebrovascular accident
- Nephrotic syndrome
- Estrogen therapy
- Pregnancy and the postpartum period
- Obesity
- Prolonged immobilization
- Antiphospholipid antibody syndrome
- Lupus anticoagulant
- Inflammatory bowel disease
- Paroxysmal nocturnal hemoglobinuria
- Behçet syndrome

From Morris TA, Fedullo PF. Pulmonary thromboembolism. In Broaddus VC, et al., eds. *Murray and Nadel's Textbook of Respiratory Medicine*. 6th ed. Philadelphia: Elsevier; 2016:1002.

with more proximal sites of thrombosis. Three major factors promote the formation of venous thrombi: stasis of blood flow, venous injury, and hypercoagulable states. These three components are described as the Virchow triad and underlie the risk factors for venous thrombosis. Smoking and obesity have been shown to be independent risk factors for pulmonary embolism in women,[181] and malignancies are a particularly high risk for pulmonary embolism. Cancer patients are found to have over twice the incidence of venous thromboembolism as that in the general population, and this risk is heightened further when indwelling central venous catheters are in place.[182] Other, less common causes of pulmonary embolism include air, CO_2 insufflation, tumor, bone, fat, catheter fragments, and amniotic fluid. Fillers used in illicit drug preparations by intravenous drug abusers may also cause pulmonary embolism. Of particular concern to anesthesia providers are air emboli caused by the opening of venous structures during surgery or by disconnected intravenous lines and CO_2 gas emboli caused by the insufflation of the gas into an open vein during laparoscopic surgery.

Most thrombus-causing pulmonary emboli resolve within 8 to 21 days of the initial presentation; 10% to 20% are estimated to develop into unresolved emboli; and 0.5% to 4% lead to the development of chronic PAH. Chronically unresolved emboli that lodge in major pulmonary arteries may become incorporated into the vascular walls and obstruct blood flow. Patients with such emboli are surgical candidates, representing approximately 1000 cases in the United States each year.[183]

Pathophysiology

Once a thrombus has formed, it rarely remains static. It can be dissolved through fibrinolysis, become organized into a vessel wall, or be released into the circulation. Because thrombi are most friable early in their development, it is then that the greatest risk for embolization exists.

If the fragment is released from its site of formation, it can be rapidly swept into one of the pulmonary arteries. It may pass through the vasculature completely, disintegrate, and block several smaller pulmonary vessels; or, if the thrombus is sufficiently large, it may impact against one or both pulmonary arteries and cause pulmonary collapse, massive infarction, and ultimately cardiac arrest.[184]

Within the pulmonary capillaries, hemorrhage is frequently seen distal to the site of the embolism. The alveolar structures in this area can remain viable for a period.[184] However, if the clot does not dissolve or if it is not quickly squeezed through the vasculature, the alveolar structure will be permanently damaged. Bronchial circulation limits the possibility of pulmonary infarction, and substantial damage is unusual unless an embolus completely blocks a large artery or preexisting lung disease is present.[185] In fact, less than 10% of emboli cause any type of infarction.[186]

Occlusion at any point along the pulmonary arterial tree results in reduced ventilation distal to the obstruction. Impaired gas exchange, alveolar edema, and in some cases alveolar necrosis can occur. Pulmonary embolism can lead to increased PVR, pulmonary hypertension, right heart stress, and potential right ventricular failure. Cardiac anomalies, such as patent foramen ovale or an atrial septal defect, can result in a paradoxic embolism, which increases the risk of ischemia to the brain, kidneys, and other organs.[186]

Pulmonary Function

Pulmonary circulation. Normally the pulmonary circulation has a very large reserve capacity. However, when PAPs increase, previously unfilled capillaries are recruited, and distention occurs. This allows for obstruction of at least half of the pulmonary circulation before a substantial increase in PAP becomes manifest.[184] Obstruction of

blood flow is further reduced by serotonin and platelet-activating factor from platelets of the embolus, vasoactive peptides from plasma, and histamine from mast cells.[187] Occlusion of approximately 70% of the pulmonary vascular bed results in PAH with subsequent right ventricular failure, increased end-diastolic pressures, development of dysrhythmias, and possibly of tricuspid valve incompetence.[185] Pulmonary edema may follow because blood flow is diverted to alternate areas of lung.[184,188] Acute pulmonary edema develops when hyperperfusion from intact circulation to the perfused lung results in extravasation of fluid into the alveoli. If the clot fractures and passes quickly, or if the affected area is minimal, the PAPs gradually decrease with embolus resolution by fibrinolysis or transformation onto the vessel wall as a scar.[185]

The right ventricle will initially increase stroke volume through adrenergic activation. Eventually, though, the increased ventricular volume shifts the intraventricular septum and reduces left heart output. The reduction in left ventricular output can compromise coronary filling and lead to ischemia, which further degrades contractility.[187]

Gas exchange. An embolus can have a significant effect on gas exchange. Moderate hypoxemia without CO_2 retention is often seen after pulmonary embolism as both physiologic shunt and dead space increase. In spontaneously breathing patients, $PaCO_2$ is maintained at the normal level after pulmonary embolism by increasing the respiratory rate. The resultant increase in ventilation may be substantial because of the large physiologic dead space. Anesthetized patients not spontaneously breathing cannot increase ventilation, resulting in quicker $PaCO_2$ increases and O_2 saturation decreases.[186,189]

The difference between $PaCO_2$ and end tidal PCO_2 ($PETCO_2$) is a very useful indicator in pulmonary embolism, with high sensitivity and specificity.[186] The mixed $PETCO_2$ tends to be low because of the high $\dot{V}/\dot{Q}$ ratio in the embolized region. Particularly if underlying ventilation and perfusion prior to embolization were well matched, the $PETCO_2$ is an accurate and immediate indicator of the status of pulmonary gas exchange. In anesthetized patients, the $PaCO_2$ continues to increase more quickly because of this increase in dead space without ventilatory compensation. If the embolus does not completely occlude the vessel, the discrepancy between $PETCO_2$ and $PaCO_2$ may not be as great.[184]

Clinical Features and Diagnosis

The patient's clinical presentation depends largely on the size of the embolus. Signs and symptoms of pulmonary embolism vary and are common to a number of disorders. Therefore the differential diagnosis may be difficult (Box 29.7). The Wells Clinical Model for predicting

---

BOX 29.7 **Differential Diagnosis of Acute Intraoperative Pulmonary Embolism**

- Anaphylactic reaction
- Aortic dissection
- Aortic stenosis
- ARDS
- Brainstem stroke
- Bronchospasm
- Cardiac tamponade
- COPD exacerbation
- Early sepsis
- Equipment malfunction (i.e., $ETCO_2$ line disconnection)
- Heart failure
- Hypertrophic cardiomyopathy
- Myocardial infarction
- Pneumothorax
- Pulmonary hypertension
- Tension pneumothorax

ARDS, acute respiratory distress syndrome; COPD, chronic obstructive pulmonary disease; $ETCO_2$, end tidal carbon dioxide.

TABLE 29.17 Wells Clinical Model for Predicting the Pretest Probability of Pulmonary Embolism

Variable	Points Assigned
Clinical signs and symptoms of deep venous thrombosis	3.0
An alternative diagnosis is less likely than pulmonary embolism	3.0
Heart rate >100 beats/min	1.5
Immobilization or surgery in the previous 4 wk	1.5
Previous deep venous thrombosis or pulmonary embolism	1.5
Hemoptysis	1.0
Malignancy (on treatment, treated in the past 6 mo, or palliative)	1.0

Score	Clinical Assessment Probability
<2 points	Low probability
2–6 points	Intermediate probability
>6 points	High probability

From Kearon C. Diagnosis of pulmonary embolism. *CMAJ.* 2003;168:183–194.

BOX 29.8 Most Common Symptoms and Signs of Pulmonary Embolism

Symptoms
- Otherwise unexplained dyspnea
- Chest pain, either pleuritic or "atypical"
- Anxiety
- Cough

Signs
- Tachypnea
- Tachycardia
- Hypotension
- Decreased, altered, or loss of ETco$_2$

- Hypoxemia
- Hypercarbia
- Low-grade fever
- Left parasternal lift
- Jugular venous distension
- Tricuspid regurgitant murmur
- Accentuated P2
- Hemoptysis
- Leg edema, erythema, tenderness

From Goldhaber SZ. Pulmonary embolism. In Mann DL, et al, eds. *Braunwald's Heart Disease: A Textbook of Cardiovascular Medicine.* 11th ed. Philadelphia: Elsevier; 2019.

the pretest probability of pulmonary embolism is commonly used to determine which patients may be at risk (Table 29.17). Dyspnea of sudden onset appears to be the only common historic complaint. Sudden hypotension and tachycardia, wheezing, tachypnea, and signs of right ventricular overload are common. Hypoxemia is a constant feature of pulmonary embolism, possibly owing to intrapulmonary shunting. Because pulmonary embolism often occurs without premonitory signs, and the symptoms are not highly specific in the acute setting, diagnosis is often presumptive and by exclusion. Box 29.8 outlines common clinical findings (history and symptoms) in patients who have developed a pulmonary embolism.

Small emboli often go unrecognized; however, multiple small emboli can produce extensive obstruction of the pulmonary capillary bed, possibly causing PAH and cardiac failure. Generally, however, small thromboemboli are incorporated into the arterial wall and have little effect on either parenchyma or the circulation. Patients may complain of dyspnea on exertion that may lead to syncope. At times a right ventricular "heave" or a split-second heart sound can be detected on examination. Patients with medium-sized emboli may present with pleuritic pain accompanied by dyspnea, a slight fever, and a productive cough that yields blood-streaked sputum. These patients usually are tachycardic. A small pleural effusion can develop and mimic the appearance of pneumonia.

Massive emboli can produce sudden cardiac collapse. Preceding symptoms range from pallor, shock, and central chest pain to sudden loss of consciousness. In patients with cardiac collapse, the pulse becomes rapid and weak, blood pressure decreases, neck veins become engorged, and cardiogenic shock may be present or impending. In addition, a decrease in PETco$_2$ and an increase in Paco$_2$ occur, with the difference between the values increasing as conditions worsen. If a pulmonary artery catheter is in place, rapid increases in PAPs are observed. A right ventricular strain pattern

may be seen on an ECG and/or echocardiogram. The prognosis for these patients is very poor.[184]

Diagnostic Testing

Few of the common preoperative tests indicate the presence of pulmonary embolism. A number of imaging and laboratory tests are available for diagnosis (Table 29.18). The most common electrocardiographic signs are noted in Box 29.9 and Fig. 29.23. In addition, echocardiography may demonstrate right ventricular dilation or dyskinesis, septal shift, tricuspid regurgitation, or dilation of the pulmonary artery. In the patient with pulmonary embolism, ABG analysis generally reveals hypoxemia, an increase in the alveolar-arterial oxygen tension gradient, and increased differences between Paco$_2$ and PETco$_2$, which result from ventilation of underperfused alveoli (i.e., increase in total dead space).[189] Massive pulmonary embolism is associated with severe hypoxemia and hypocapnia (caused by initial hyperventilation). An initial difference between Paco$_2$ and PETco$_2$ is common early during the embolic event.[186] Some common conditions associated with an increased risk for DVT are given in Tables 38.8 and 38.9.

There are limited laboratory analyses useful to support the diagnosis of pulmonary embolism. The D-dimer assay cannot confirm pulmonary embolism; however, an elevated (abnormal) result requires further investigation for its diagnosis. Troponin I and troponin T levels are elevated in less than one-half of cases of significant pulmonary embolism; therefore their presence is not useful for diagnosis, but elevation of troponins is associated with adverse outcomes, including death and the need for aggressive resuscitation.[190]

Prevention

Aggressive efforts at prevention have been successful in reducing the occurrence of DVT in surgical patients. Use of compression stockings, intermittent pneumatic compression devices, administration of various anticoagulants and thrombolytics, and ambulation are typical measures for preventing embolus formation. Overall efforts that help reduce the risk of pulmonary embolism in surgical patients are aimed at avoiding venous stasis, hypercoagulability, and vessel injury. These involve placing an inferior vena cava filter prior to surgery in patients at high risk for pulmonary embolism,[191] ensuring administration of lower extremity circulatory aids before anesthetic induction,

TABLE 29.18 Diagnostic Tests for Suspected Pulmonary Embolism

Test	Comments
Oxygen saturation	Nonspecific, but suspect PE if there is a sudden otherwise unexplained decrease
Electrocardiogram	May be normal, especially in younger, previously healthy individuals; may provide alternative diagnosis, such as myocardial infarction or pericarditis
Echocardiography	Best used as a prognostic test in patients with established PE, rather than as a diagnostic test; many patients with larger PE will have normal echocardiograms
Lung scanning	Usually provides ambiguous results, used in lieu of chest CT for patients with anaphylaxis to contrast agent, renal insufficiency, or pregnancy
Chest CT	Most accurate diagnostic imaging test for PE; beware if CT result and clinical likelihood are discordant
Pulmonary angiography	Invasive, costly, uncomfortable; used primarily when local catheter intervention is planned
D-dimer	An excellent "rule out" test if normal, especially if accompanied by low clinical suspicion
Venous ultrasonography	Excellent for diagnosing acute symptomatic proximal DVT, but a negative test does not rule out PE, because a recent leg DVT may have embolized completely; calf vein imaging is operator dependent
Magnetic resonance imaging	Reliable only for imaging proximal segmental pulmonary arteries; requires gadolinium but does not require iodinated contrast agents

CT, Computed tomography; *DVT,* deep vein thrombosis; *PE,* pulmonary embolism.
From Goldhaber SZ. Pulmonary embolism. In Mann DL, et al, eds. *Braunwald's Heart Disease: A Textbook of Cardiovascular Medicine.* 11th ed. Philadelphia: Elsevier; 2019.

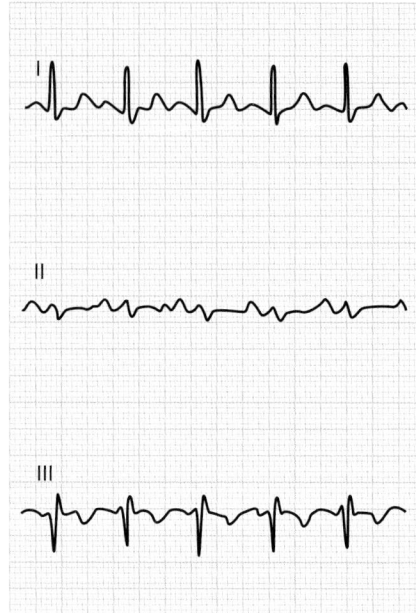

Fig. 29.23 Classic electrocardiogram of pulmonary embolus. Note the "S1, Q3, T3" pattern. (From Weitz JI, Ginsberg JS. Venous thrombus and embolism. In *Goldman's Cecil Medicine.* 26th ed. Philadelphia: Elsevier; 2020:480.)

BOX 29.9 Electrocardiographic Signs Associated With Pulmonary Embolism

- Tachycardia
- Negative T wave in V1–V5
- McGinn-White S1Q3T3
- Right axis deviation >90 degrees
- Negative T wave in II, III, aVF
- Pulmonary P wave
- R > S or Q in aVR
- Right ventricular ischemia
- Complete or incomplete RBBB

RBBB, Right bundle branch block.

BOX 29.10 Medical Management for Acute Pulmonary Embolism

- Begin UFH intravenous therapy as soon as massive PE is suspected.
- Goal of UFH infusion should be an aPTT of at least 00 sec.
- Limit volume resuscitation to 500–1000 mL as excessive volume may worsen right ventricular failure.
- Administer vasopressors and inotropes if there is evidence of hemodynamic instability.
- Determine risk of thrombolytic therapy.
- Consider placement of IVC filter, catheter embolectomy, or surgical embolectomy if thrombolytic therapy is too risky.
- Avoid the combination of thrombolytic therapy and IVC filter insertion.
- Consider immediate referral to medical institution that specializes in massive PE.

aPTT, Activated partial thromboplastin time; *IVC,* inferior vena cava; *PE,* pulmonary embolism; *UFH,* unfractionated heparin.
Adapted from Goldhaber SZ. Pulmonary embolism. In Mann DL, et al., eds. *Braunwald's Heart Disease: A Textbook of Cardiovascular Medicine.* 11th ed. Philadelphia: Elsevier; 2019.

preventing hypothermia with the use of active warming devices, and avoiding hypoxemia or any factor that could lead to acidosis. Anesthetic technique may contribute to risk reduction. For example, the use of neuraxial anesthesia, which causes vasodilation in the lower extremities, reduces the incidence of DVT by 50% in comparison to general anesthesia.[192]

Medical and Surgical Treatment

Guidelines for treatment of pulmonary embolism are summarized in Box 29.10. Anticoagulation is the most common intervention, aimed at preventing further insult. Clot removal is most often accomplished with thrombolytic agents. Surgical intervention is indicated for patients who are unresponsive to other measures; however, this represents a small number of patients.[193] Currently the most common surgical procedure for patients with pulmonary embolism is placement of an umbrella filter, which traps thromboemboli. Vena cava filters are usually indicated for patients with bleeding disorders who are not able to tolerate standard anticoagulant therapy or for those who are refractory to anticoagulant therapy. The filter is placed in the inferior vena cava under fluoroscopic guidance, usually below the renal veins at the L2-L3 level. Suprarenal placement is required when a thrombus directly involves the renal veins or has propagated above the level of the renal veins. The presence of an infrarenal filter in a pregnant woman may place the mother and fetus at risk because of the possibility that the filter will come in contact with the gravid uterus. Suprarenal placement prevents this risk.[192]

Thromboendarterectomy is the treatment of choice for chronic large vessel thromboembolic PAH.[194] Desired results include decreased PVR, improved CO, restoration of exercise tolerance, and resolution of hypoxemia. Improvements in RV function and hemodynamics may be prompt, whereas improvements in gas exchange occur over weeks to months. Although the role of pulmonary embolectomy remains controversial, in the few patients who do not benefit from optimal medical therapy, it remains an acceptable procedure.[195] Catheter-directed embolectomy techniques include (1) the administration of thrombolytic agents directly at the site of embolism; (2) rheolytic embolectomy, which injects pressurized saline into the clot causing it to break up and be aspirated; (3) rotational embolectomy, which fragments the clot using a small rotational device at the catheter tip, which continually aspirates the fragments; and (4) suction embolectomy, which aspirates a clot through a large lumen catheter.[196]

Anesthetic Management

Anesthetic management for a patient with a pulmonary embolus is primarily aimed at preventing further embolism and providing respiratory and cardiovascular support.[196] Table 29.19 outlines preventative prophylactic measures for patients at risk of pulmonary embolism. The use of a high Fio_2 supports pulmonary vasodilation. If PAP is monitored, the anesthesia provider will have additional information to optimize right-sided heart function and assess the effects of anesthetic management on PVR.[188] However, the risk-benefit ratio of a pulmonary artery catheter should consider the possibility that these catheters may dislodge clots in the right side of the heart. Induction is often performed with etomidate. Ketamine may increase PVR.[186] The use of N_2O limits the amount of Fio_2 that can be administered. The use of N_2O is contraindicated in patients with venous air embolism because of the potential for N_2O to rapidly expand the volume of the embolism.[185] Patients with moderate to severe pulmonary embolism are often experiencing acute right-sided heart failure. Medications that minimally depress cardiac function, such as opiods, should be considered.

Persistent severe hypotension, such as that accompanying a massive pulmonary embolism, may necessitate the use of a cardiotonic agent or partial or full cardiopulmonary bypass. The goal is preservation of perfusion to the brain and heart until cardiopulmonary bypass is started and surgical removal of the clot attempted.[188] Patients with pulmonary embolism are extremely sensitive to any anesthetic agent. It is critical to have heparin ready to support initiation of bypass if necessary. Although separation from bypass is beyond the scope of this chapter, the anesthetist should anticipate that difficulties may be encountered. Reports of operative mortality during pulmonary embolectomy range from 11% to 55%, with much higher rates among patients experiencing cardiac arrest.[197]

Detection of Pulmonary Embolism During Anesthesia

In the intubated patient under general anesthesia, clinical presentation is limited to objective signs. A decreasing or variable $PETCO_2$ waveform and value, as well as tachycardia, are usually the first signs of pulmonary embolism.[188,189] These can be followed by a decrease in blood-oxygen saturation (Sao_2) and ABG results, indicative of unexplained arterial hypoxemia. In the case of massive pulmonary embolism, abrupt, unexplained hypotension with loss of $PETCO_2$ and tachycardia are the classic (albeit nonspecific) signs. In some cases of massive pulmonary embolism, cardiac arrest may occur. Increased PAP and central venous pressure (CVP) are observed in combination with a decrease in systolic and diastolic blood pressures.[189] Bronchospasm may occur.[183] Finally, ECG changes that indicate right axis deviation, incomplete or complete right BBB, or peaked T waves may be observed in the presence or absence of an accompanying systolic ejection murmur[184,189] (see Fig. 29.23 and Box 29.9).

TABLE 29.19	**Prevention of Venous Thromboembolism**
Condition	**Strategy**
Total hip or knee replacement; hip or pelvis fracture	Warfarin (Coumadin) (target INR 2.5) × 4–6 wk
	LMWH/subcut (e.g., fondaparinux 2.5 mg subcut [except for total knee replacement]) or rivaroxaban 10 mg daily or dalteparin 2500–5000 units daily subcut where available
	IPC ± warfarin
Gynecologic cancer surgery	LMWH consider 1 mo of prophylaxis
Thoracic surgery	IPC *or* GCS *plus* unfractionated heparin, 5000 units bid or tid
High-risk general surgery (e.g., prior VTE, current cancer, or obesity)	IPC *or* GCS *plus* unfractionated heparin, 5000 units bid tid or LMWH
General, gynecologic, or urologic surgery (without prior VTE) for noncancerous conditions	GCS *plus* unfractionated heparin 5000 units bid or tid
	Dalteparin 2500 units subcut once daily
	Enoxaparin 40 mg subcut once daily
Neurosurgery, eye surgery, or other surgery when prophylactic anticoagulation is contraindicated	GCS ± IPC
Neurosurgery	Unfractionated heparin 5000 units bid or tid
	Enoxaparin 40 mg subcut once daily
	GPC *or* IPC
	Consider surveillance of lower extremity by ultrasonography
Orthopedic surgery	Enoxaparin 30 mg twice daily
	Enoxaparin 40 mg once daily*
	Dalteparin 5000 units once daily*
	Fondaparinux 2.5 mg subcut daily
	Warfarin (target INR = 2–3)
	GCS *plus* IPC
General surgery	Unfractionated heparin 5000 units bid or tid
	Enoxaparin 40 mg daily
	Dalteparin 2500 or 5000 units once daily
	GCS *plus* IPC
Pregnancy	Enoxaparin 40 mg daily
	Dalteparin 5000 units daily
Medical patients	Unfractionated heparin 5000 units bid or tid
	Enoxaparin 40 mg daily
	Dalteparin 5000 units once daily
	Fondaparinux 2.5 mg subcut daily in patient who cannot tolerate heparin
	Consider surveillance of lower extremity by ultrasonography
	GCS *plus* IPC
Long-distance air travel	LMWH for high-risk patients

*Approved only for total hip replacement prophylaxis.
GCS, Graduated compression stockings; *INR*, international normalized ratio; *IPC*, intermittent pneumatic compression; *LMHW*, low molecular weight heparin; *subcut,* subcutaneous; *VTE*, venous thromboembolism.
Modified from Goldhaber SZ. Deep vein thrombosis and pulmonary thromboembolism. In: Jameson JL, et al., eds. *Harrison's Principles of Internal Medicine.* 20th ed. New York: McGraw Hill; 2018:1631–1636; Goldhaber SZ. Pulmonary embolism. In Mann DL, et al., eds. *Braunwald's Heart Disease: A Textbook of Cardiovascular Medicine.* 11th ed. Philadelphia: Elsevier; 2019.

Intraoperative Management of Acute Thromboembolism

In the case of suspected pulmonary embolism in the anesthetized patient, treatment requires rapid intervention because cardiovascular decompensation can occur quickly. First and most important, an airway must be established if the patient is not already intubated, with administration of a 100% FiO_2 initiated. Second, delivery of the anesthetic agent must be discontinued.[188] Next, the circulatory system should be supported with the infusion of intravenous fluids or blood (or both) as needed, and sympathomimetics initiated if necessary. Norepinephrine may be the vasopressor of choice because of its ability to support contractility and improve brain perfusion through vasoconstriction.[187] Epinephrine, dopamine, or a combination of dobutamine and norepinephrine may also be helpful. Ventricular dysrhythmias should be treated with intravenous administration of lidocaine or amiodarone, and the patient should receive PEEP for optimization of oxygenation.[185] If symptoms are refractory to treatment, thrombolysis or pulmonary embolectomy may be necessary. Severe hemodynamic difficulty should be anticipated, and resuscitative efforts should be continued into the ICU as needed. In severe cases, cardiopulmonary bypass may be necessary until the obstruction can be relieved.

Patients with pulmonary embolism present particular management challenges during their postoperative course, which may include reperfusion edema, persistent hypoxemia, pericardial effusion, psychiatric disorders, and pulmonary blood flow steal. The areas of the lung to which pulmonary artery flow has been restored are subject to development of reperfusion pulmonary edema, presumably as a manifestation of oxidant- and protease-mediated ALI. Other possible causes are extracorporeal circulation, anticoagulation, and an increase in perfusion pressure in a previously obstructed pulmonary artery. Severe complications can ensue, including significant pulmonary hemorrhage and respiratory disturbances, or death may occur.[197] This syndrome may develop 3 to 5 days after surgery.[198] Some evidence has demonstrated that after pulmonary thromboendarterectomy for relief of chronic thromboembolic PAH, perfusion lung scans often reveal new perfusion defects in pulmonary artery segments not involved in the primary pulmonary embolism and subsequent endarterectomy.[199] This phenomenon has been labeled pulmonary blood flow steal, and it is believed to be caused by postoperative redistribution of regional PVR due to the altered (widened) architecture of the affected vessels that received the vascular intervention. However, the cause of new perfusion defects could also be a result of residual pulmonary artery disease, and future studies are posed to investigate this potential cause.[199]

RESTRICTIVE PULMONARY DISEASES

Definition

Restrictive pulmonary disease is defined as any condition that interferes with normal lung expansion during inspiration, and it is characterized by a TLC below the 5th percentile.[44] Typically it includes disorders that increase the inward elastic recoil of the lungs or chest wall (Table 29.20). Consequently, the alteration in pulmonary dynamics results in both reduced lung volumes and capacities and decreased lung or chest-wall compliance. Some restrictive diseases produce ventilation abnormalities and $\dot{V}/\dot{Q}$ mismatching, whereas others lead to impairment of diffusion. FEV_1 and FVC are both decreased, owing to a reduction in TLC or a decrease in chest-wall compliance or muscle strength. However, the FEV_1:FVC ratio is normal or elevated.

Impairment-producing restrictive pulmonary diseases can be classified as (1) acute intrinsic, (2) chronic intrinsic, or (3) chronic extrinsic. Acute intrinsic disorders are primarily caused by the abnormal movement of intravascular fluid into the interstitium of the lung and alveoli secondary to the increase in pulmonary vascular pressures

TABLE 29.20   Common Causes of Restrictive Lung Disease

Cause	Example
Interstitium	
Interstitial fibrosis, infiltration	Asbestosis
Pulmonary edema	Left ventricular failure
Pleura	
Pleural disease	Fibrothorax
Thoracic Cage and Abdomen	
Neuromuscular disease	Poliomyelitis
Skeletal abnormalities	Severe kyphoscoliosis
Marked obesity	Gross obesity
Chest trauma	Broken rib(s)

Modified from Grippi MA, et al. Approach to the patient with respiratory symptoms. In Grippi MA, et al., eds. *Fishman's Pulmonary Disease and Disorders.* New York: McGraw-Hill; 2015:382.

occurring with left ventricular failure, fluid overload, or an increase in pulmonary capillary permeability. Examples of acute intrinsic disorders include pulmonary edema, aspiration pneumonia, and ARDS. Chronic intrinsic diseases are characterized by pulmonary fibrosis. Conditions that produce fibrosis of the lung include idiopathic pulmonary fibrosis (IPF), radiation injury, cytotoxic and noncytotoxic drug exposure, O_2 toxicity, autoimmune diseases, and sarcoidosis. Chronic extrinsic diseases can be defined as disorders that inhibit the normal lung excursion. They include flail chest, pneumothorax, and pleural effusions. They also include conditions that interfere with chest-wall expansion, such as ascites, obesity, pregnancy, and skeletal and neuromuscular disorders.

The pulmonary system and its functions are directly manipulated by the administration of anesthesia. The effect of intraoperative pulmonary insult or preexisting pulmonary disease on respiratory function during anesthesia and the postoperative period is predictable: Greater degrees of pulmonary impairment lead to marked alterations in intraoperative respiratory status and higher rates of occurrence of postoperative pulmonary complications. This section illustrates the pathophysiologic changes involved in these clinical disorders and discusses their clinical presentation, diagnosis, treatment, and anesthetic implications.

Pulmonary Edema

Pulmonary edema is not an independent disease entity but the result of a variety of disease processes. Pulmonary edema is the accumulation of excess fluid in the interstitial and air-filled spaces of the lung. The mechanisms responsible for its development include an increase in hydrostatic pressure within the pulmonary capillary system, an increase in the permeability of the alveolocapillary membrane, and a decrease in intravascular colloid oncotic pressure.[200]

The etiology and pathophysiology of pulmonary edema is based on the principle of Starling's law of transcapillary fluid exchange, or simply Starling forces. The pulmonary capillary endothelium is semipermeable. Pulmonary interstitial fluid pressures, both hydrostatic (peak inspiratory flow [Pif]) and osmotic (πif), along with the hydrostatic pressure in the pulmonary capillaries (Pc) and the osmotic pressure of the plasma (πp), are the primary determinants that balance fluid exchange across this semipermeable barrier.[201] These factors, which ultimately determine the amount of fluid that leaves the pulmonary vascular space, are incorporated into what is known as the Starling equation. A simplified version of this equation is as follows:

$$\dot{Q} = k[(Pc–Pif)–(\pi p–\pi if)]$$

where $\dot{Q}$ is the total amount of fluid that traverses the endothelial membrane and k is the fluid filtration coefficient, which describes quantitatively the permeability of the membrane.[200,201] Pc represents the force favoring fluid movement out of the vessel wall and is in direct opposition to the Pif. The Pif, when positive, tends to force fluid inward through the capillary membrane; when it is negative, it tends to force fluid outward.[4] The πp and Pif also oppose each other, with the πif keeping fluid within the capillary and the Pif pulling it outward into the interstitium. Overall, the balance of forces shown in the Starling equation favors fluid filtration into the interstitial space. Fluid filtered into the alveolar interstitial space does not enter the alveoli because under normal conditions the alveolar epithelium is composed of very tight junctions that prevent fluid and protein from entering alveolar air spaces. The fluid moves to the extravascular interstitial space, where the lymphatic vessels remove all the filtered fluid and return it to the systemic circulation.[202]

Pulmonary edema can occur if any variable in the Starling equation is altered in the direction favoring increased fluid filtration. High pressure (Pc) and increased permeability (k) are the two most important components of the Starling equation that are altered in states of pulmonary edema. Because of this, pulmonary edema is classified as being either cardiogenic (high pressure, hydrostatic) or noncardiogenic (altered or increased permeability).

Cardiogenic pulmonary edema occurs whenever the Pc is increased. Increased Pc is the most common form of pulmonary edema. Cardiogenic pulmonary edema is initiated by some type of left-sided heart incompetence or failure. The term *left ventricular failure* implies that reduced functionality has occurred in left ventricular contractility, which ultimately leads to a decrease in both stroke volume and cardiac output. Incomplete left ventricular emptying elevates left ventricular end-diastolic volume, which in turn elevates left ventricular end-diastolic pressure. Increased left ventricular end-diastolic pressure is "reflected back," causing elevation of the left atrial, pulmonary venous, and pulmonary capillary pressures. When pulmonary capillary pressure reaches levels of 20 to 25 mm Hg (normal range, 10–16 mm Hg), the rate of fluid transudation often exceeds lymphatic drainage capacity, and alveolar flooding occurs.

Coronary artery disease, hypertension, cardiomyopathies, mitral regurgitation, and mitral stenosis are a few of the cardiac conditions that may increase pulmonary intravascular hydrostatic pressure (Pc) and predispose a patient to developing pulmonary edema. Although an elevated left ventricular end-diastolic pressure is the major cause of an increase in Pc, and therefore pulmonary edema, it is important to realize that several noncardiac problems also may increase Pc. These include pulmonary venoocclusive disease, fibrosing mediastinitis, head trauma, cerebrovascular accident, exposure to high altitudes, and overhydration.

Noncardiogenic pulmonary edema is associated with an increase in endothelial permeability caused by an insult that disrupts the barrier function of the blood-tissue interface. Unlike cardiogenic pulmonary edema, in which the capillary endothelium remains intact and no leakage of protein is noted, noncardiogenic pulmonary edema is associated with leakage of both fluid and protein from the vascular space.[201] Because this respiratory membrane disruption cannot be easily or directly measured, noncardiogenic pulmonary edema is said to exist when suspicious chest radiographic evidence coexists with insufficient hemodynamic basis. The presence of a pulmonary wedge pressure less than 12 mm Hg and the absence of a significant history of cardiac disease generally suffice for exclusion of a hemodynamic mechanism.

BOX 29.11 Conditions Associated With ARDS, Categorized by Possible Mechanisms of Injury

Direct Injury	Indirect Injury
Pneumonia	Sepsis
Aspiration	Major trauma
Pulmonary contusion	Multiple blood transfusions
Toxic inhalation	Pancreatitis
Near drowning	Cardiopulmonary bypass
Reperfusion injury (e.g., after lung transplantation)	Drug overdose
	Adverse effect of medication

ARDS, acute respiratory distress syndrome.
From Lee WL. Slutsky AS. Acute hypoxemic respiratory failure and ARDS. In Broaddus VC, et al., eds. *Murray and Nadel's Textbook of Respiratory Medicine.* 6th ed. Philadelphia: Elsevier; 2016:1744.

Although a multitude of disorders are associated with noncardiogenic pulmonary edema, the most commonly encountered cause is systemic sepsis that leads to ARDS. Other clinical conditions associated with ARDS and noncardiogenic pulmonary edema include the aspiration syndromes, inhalation of toxic fumes and gases, and the embolization phenomena (Box 29.11).

Pulmonary edema is nearly always associated with some type of preexisting disease state or insult. If a patient with pulmonary edema has a history of CHF, hypertension, or ischemic heart disease, the presence of cardiogenic pulmonary edema can be assumed. In addition to systemic sepsis, anaphylaxis, pancreatitis, disseminated intravascular coagulation, trauma, multiple transfusions, and near-drowning can all result in noncardiogenic pulmonary edema.

Neurogenic Pulmonary Edema

Neurogenic pulmonary edema begins with a massive outpouring of sympathetic nervous system stimulation triggered by central nervous system insult. This centrally mediated central nervous system overactivity typically occurs in the hypothalamic area. Excessive sympathetic activation induces remarkable hemodynamic alterations, primarily systemic and pulmonary vasoconstriction. The left ventricle fails because of the inordinate workload imposed by the systemic hypertension resulting in pulmonary blood volume increases and a functional imbalance between the failing left ventricle and the normal right ventricle.[201] Although this sequence seems to parallel that of cardiogenic pulmonary edema, a permeability component exists, as evidenced by the high protein concentration found in the pulmonary secretions of affected patients.

Uremic Pulmonary Edema

Uremic pulmonary edema is seen in those patients with metabolic disturbances as a result of renal insufficiency or failure. Overhydration and expansion of the circulating blood volume lead to increases in pulmonary capillary pressures. Again, a leaky component exists because of the metabolic abnormalities associated with uremia. Hemodialysis reduces the circulating blood volume of these patients and promotes resolution of this type of pulmonary edema.[201]

High-Altitude–Related Pulmonary Edema

High-altitude–related pulmonary edema can occur in the absence of left ventricular failure whenever an individual overexerts before acclimating to a high altitude. The pathogenesis of this form of pulmonary edema is unclear, but it may be the result of intense hypoxic pulmonary arterial vasoconstriction or massive sympathetic discharge triggered by cerebral hypoxia.[202]

Pulmonary Edema Due to Upper Airway Obstruction

Pulmonary edema caused by upper airway obstruction results from prolonged, forced inspiratory effort against an obstructed upper airway. The most common cause of this type of pulmonary edema in adults is laryngospasm after extubation and general anesthesia. In children, pulmonary edema after obstruction caused by croup, epiglottitis, and laryngospasm is also well documented. Vigorous inspiration against airway obstruction creates high negative intrathoracic, transpleural, and alveolar pressures, enlarging the pulmonary vascular volume and subsequently the interstitial fluid volume. The capacity of the lymphatics becomes overwhelmed, and interstitial fluid transudes into the pulmonary alveoli. Hypoxia causes a massive sympathetic discharge that results in systemic vasoconstriction and a translocation of fluid from the systemic circulation to the already expanding pulmonary vascular and interstitial spaces. Hypoxia also increases pulmonary capillary pressures. Because hypoxia alters myocardial activity, left atrial function and left ventricular function are reduced.

During obstruction, vigorous inspiratory efforts are unsuccessful because of the airway obstruction. Unsuccessful expiration produces an increase in intrathoracic and alveolar pressures. PEEPi is also produced during this stage. Relief of the obstruction results in cessation of PEEPi.

The consequence of these events is the sudden massive transudation of fluid from the pulmonary interstitium into the alveoli, which results in pulmonary edema. The malignity of pulmonary edema is determined by the extent of prior alveolar and capillary damage, and the immensity of hemodynamic and cardiovascular alterations.

Not all of those who experience an acute airway obstruction develop pulmonary edema, and no specific risk factors for its occurrence have been identified. Factors that may predispose to its formation after obstruction include youth, male gender, long periods of obstruction, overzealous perioperative fluid administration, and the presence of preexisting cardiac and pulmonary disease.

Treatment includes prompt recognition of the condition, securing a patent airway, supportive therapy with oxygenation, and administering diuretics. Although the onset of pulmonary edema after laryngospasm is usually immediate, cases have been reported of the occurrence of pulmonary edema several hours after laryngospasm. Therefore it is recommended that patients who develop laryngospasm be closely observed postoperatively.

The diagnosis of pulmonary edema and its differentiation into cardiogenic and noncardiac categories necessitates taking a detailed medical history and performing a physical examination, chest radiography, and ABG analysis.

Physical examination reveals increased respiratory effort. As water accumulates, the lungs become heavy and noncompliant, and a decrease in FRC occurs. This increase in the volume of extravascular lung fluid provides a potent stimulus for surrounding interstitial stretch receptors (J receptors), the activation of which results in tachypnea. Tachypnea is usually not relieved by the administration of O_2 or the return of Pao_2 to normal values. Intercostal retractions and use of accessory muscles are apparent on physical examination. Signs of sympathetic stress stimulation, such as hypertension, diaphoresis, and tachycardia, are often noted. The expectoration of pink, frothy sputum is indicative that alveoli have been flooded.[201]

The detection of basilar crackles on auscultation is the traditional hallmark of early pulmonary edema. In reality, by the time crackles become audible, excess water has already flooded the alveoli and overflowed into the terminal bronchioles.[199] It is in the bronchioles, not in the alveoli, that the crackles of pulmonary edema are generated. The earliest and most often disregarded clinical sign associated with pulmonary edema is rapid, shallow breathing.

In cardiogenic pulmonary edema, heart size may be increased. High CVPs, an S_3 or S_4 gallop, and jugular venous distention are often observed.[200] Chest radiography is still the most reliable and expedient tool for early detection of pulmonary edema. In cardiogenic pulmonary edema, the cardiac silhouette may appear abnormal or enlarged; in noncardiogenic pulmonary edema, it can be enlarged or remain normal. Interstitial edema can be observed before the alveoli flood and the onset of clinical signs occurs. Pleural effusions are common, and a whited-out or butterfly appearance may be noted.[201]

ABG analysis reveals hypoxemia secondary to $\dot{V}/\dot{Q}$ abnormalities. When right-to-left shunting is significant, the Pao_2 can be affected by any change in the central venous O_2 content. Increases in O_2 consumption or decreases in cardiac output further reduce the Pao_2. The $Paco_2$ may be low, normal, or elevated. The initial hypocarbia is related to tachypnea and high minute volumes; at later stages, hypercarbia is frequently secondary to muscle fatigue and exhaustion. Changes in pH usually reflect changes in $Paco_2$, but metabolic or lactic acidosis (or both) may occur from tissue O_2 deficiency, low cardiac output or sepsis.

Anesthetic Management

Pulmonary edema is considered a medical emergency, and immediate intervention is required for treatment of the underlying disease, support of other failing organ systems, and optimization of O_2 delivery.[200] O_2 administration is a primary treatment and should be administered early using either a nasal cannula or facemask. If oxygenation does not improve with the administration of high Fio_2, intubation and positive pressure ventilation with either PEEP or CPAP must be initiated. Institution of positive pressure mechanical ventilation in patients with acute pulmonary edema usually results in a prompt increase in oxygenation and, in some cases, in cardiac output. Improvement occurs because of superior inflation and $\dot{V}/\dot{Q}$ matching. Improvement in left ventricular function (i.e., cardiac output) may occur secondary to four possible mechanisms: (1) improvement in arterial oxygenation and therefore improvement of myocardial O_2 supply, (2) reduction in the extreme pleural pressure swings present with spontaneous ventilation and hence reduction in afterload on the left ventricle, (3) decrease in the workload of the failing heart because of a reduction in work of breathing (and therefore a reduction in O_2 requirement) effected by a mechanical ventilator, and (4) decrease in preload (and a subsequent reduction in venous return) occurring secondary to the use of positive pressure ventilation.

Pharmacologic therapy includes the use of vasodilators, inotropes, steroids, and diuretics. For more than 50 years, morphine sulfate has been used in the treatment of cardiogenic pulmonary edema because of its venodilatory and preload-reducing properties.[201] Nitroprusside is effective at decreasing preload and afterload. The reduction in systemic blood pressure and afterload provided by nitroprusside alleviates the impedance to left ventricular ejection. This may result in better cardiac function, with a subsequent lowering of left atrial pressures. Inotropic agents such as dopamine or dobutamine improve myocardial contractility and lower cardiac filling pressures. In patients with chronic CHF and pulmonary congestion, digitalis augments contractility and promotes decreases in left atrial and ventricular filling pressures. (The use of steroids is discussed later in this chapter in the section on ARDS.)

Fluid balance is managed with both fluid restriction and diuresis. This therapy helps achieve a negative fluid balance in hydrostatic pulmonary edema, in which Pc is high. Even in permeability pulmonary edema, in which Pc is thought to be low, any decrease in the hydrostatic pressure further reduces the net movement of pulmonary microvascular fluid outward.[200] Potent diuretics such as furosemide not only lower left atrial filling pressure by decreasing systemic venous tone but also induce diuresis of the expanded extravascular volume.

The type of fluid, whether crystalloid or colloid, that should be used in the presence of pulmonary edema remains controversial. Regardless of the type used, it is generally agreed that fluids should be restricted.

ASPIRATION PNEUMONITIS

Definition

Aspiration is a rare yet serious complication associated with general anesthesia. Much effort is expended to prevent this untoward occurrence and minimize sequelae if it does occur. It can occur at any time during the course of anesthesia administration, and if severe, a multitude of serious complications may follow.[203]

Pneumonitis caused by perioperative aspiration (Mendelson syndrome) was described by Curtis Mendelson in 1946 after he observed a number of deaths among obstetric patients.[204] Mendelson's laboratory investigations led him to the conclusion that two entirely separate clinical aspiration disorders existed. One followed the aspiration of solid food and produced a picture of laryngeal or bronchial obstruction, whereas the other resulted from direct acid injury to the lung and produced the asthmalike syndrome that now carries his name.[205] Aspiration pneumonitis in patients receiving anesthesia results from the intersection of three components: (1) Gastric contents escape from the stomach into the pharynx, (2) those contents enter the lungs, and (3) they are of a caustic nature and so result in lung tissue injury. This results from preexisting disease, airway manipulation, and the inevitable compromise in protective reflexes that accompany the anesthetized state. Aspirates may be categorized as contaminated, acidic, alkaline, particulate, and nonparticulate. Aspiration pneumonitis is a chemical injury to the lung and is different than aspiration pneumonia, which is a resulting infection within the lung. Not all aspirations lead to aspiration pneumonia, and when it does occur it is usually in individuals who have aspirated infected material or who are immunocompromised. Ingestion of highly acidic or particulate aspirate may cause severe respiratory damage without an infectious component. Patients who initially show no signs of infection, however, may develop pneumonia over time because of the severity of the lung injury and prolonged respiratory support.[206]

Incidence and Outcome

Pulmonary aspiration has been estimated to occur in approximately 1 of 3000 anesthetics.[206,207] This incidence is roughly doubled for cesarean section surgery[208] and emergency surgery.[209] Fortunately the majority of aspiration incidents require little or no treatment. Warner et al.[210] reviewed 215,488 general anesthetics and studied the outcomes of pulmonary aspiration. They noted that approximately 60% of episodes were asymptomatic, 20% were symptomatic but required only conservative treatment or short-term ventilation, 15% required mechanical ventilation for more than 6 hours, and 5% of episodes led to death (Fig. 29.24). The overall mortality was 1 in 71,829 anesthetic procedures. Several of their findings were interesting. Complications developed in equal percentages among those who received and those who did not receive pharmacologic acid aspiration prophylaxis. Patients who aspirated but did not develop symptoms within 2 hours could be discharged. If signs or symptoms did not emerge in that time frame they would not occur subsequently. Not surprisingly, the largest number of aspirations occur during induction and intubation or on emergence within 5 minutes of extubation. They found no serious morbidity from pulmonary aspiration in nearly 120,000 elective procedures in American Society of Anesthesiologists (ASA) class I or II.

In a later study, the same group reported on the incidence of aspiration in infants and children.[211] Although pediatric patients are often reported as having a higher incidence of aspiration than adults,[209] the

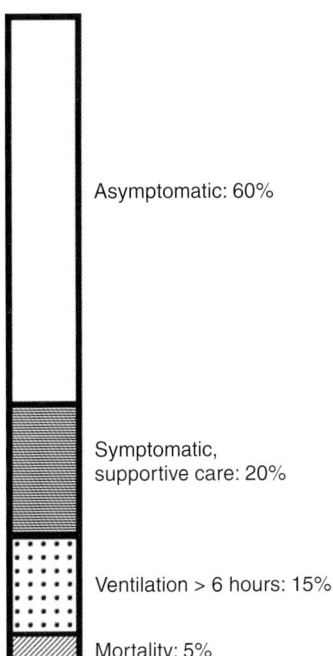

Fig. 29.24 Outcomes of patients with perioperative aspiration (percentages approximate). (Data from Warner MA, et al. Clinical significance of pulmonary aspiration during the perioperative period. *Anesthesiology.* 1993;78[1]:56–62.)

researchers found no increase in the incidence among young patients. They noted 24 aspirations in a series of 63,180 general anesthetic procedures. Fifteen of the 24 children did not develop symptoms within 2 hours, and no treatment was required. Five children required respiratory support, three for more than 48 hours. No deaths occurred. Several risk factors for aspiration are listed in Box 29.12.

The Anesthetic Incidence Monitoring Study database in New Zealand noted 133 cases of aspiration out of 5000 reported anesthesia incidents.[212] Five deaths occurred. Aspiration was confirmed by clinical signs or radiography. Predisposing factors included abdominal pathology, obesity, diabetes, neurologic deficit, lithotomy position, difficult intubation, reflux disease, hiatal hernia, and inadequate anesthesia leading to straining and bucking.

In an interesting study, researchers examined general anesthesia administered by mask in obstetric patients who required surgery immediately after vaginal delivery.[213] Procedures included placental extraction; repair of vaginal, cervical, and perineal tears; and uterine manipulation. This database in Israel involved 1705 anesthetic procedures, and only one case of mild pneumonitis occurred.

Etiology

Although vomiting and gastroesophageal reflux are common clinical events, aspiration usually occurs only when normal protective reflexes (swallowing, coughing, gagging) are inhibited.[210] Reflex responses to aspiration are automatically blunted with depression of consciousness. The most common time period for depression of protective airway reflexes, without a secure airway, is during anesthetic induction and emergence.[210]

Three aspiration syndromes have been identified: (1) chemical aspiration pneumonitis (Mendelson syndrome), (2) mechanical obstruction, and (3) bacterial infection (i.e., aspiration pneumonia). Since acute chemical pneumonitis poses the greatest difficulty to anesthesia providers, the pathophysiology, presentation, and anesthetic implications of Mendelson syndrome are discussed.

BOX 29.12 Risk Factors for Gastric Aspiration

- Emergency surgery
- Full stomach
- Obstetrics
- Gastrointestinal obstruction
- Ascites
- Diabetic gastroparesis
- Gastroesophageal reflux
- Hiatal hernia
- Peptic ulcer disease
- Difficult airway management
- High gastric pressure or reduced lower esophageal sphincter tone
- Impaired airway reflexes
- Head injury
- Depressed level of consciousness
- Seizures
- Obesity
- Scleroderma, CREST, or other connective tissue disorders affecting the esophagus
- Trauma or stress
- Nausea and vomiting
- Opioid administration
- Cricoid pressure
- Residual neuromuscular relaxation
- Cardiac arrest, severe hypotension

CREST, *C*alcinosis, *R*aynaud phenomenon, *e*sophageal dysmotility, *s*clerodactyly, and *t*elangiectasia.

The type and amount of the aspirate that causes aspiration pneumonia is often characterized according to the pH, volume, and type of gastric material aspirated. It has long been considered that gastric fluid volume (GFV) greater than 0.4 mL/kg (25 mL/70 kg) and a pH less than 2.5 are significant indicators of risk for aspiration sequelae. However, these markers were arbitrarily defined in 1974[214] and widely accepted in clinical practice without rigorous study. Efforts to reach these levels preoperatively have unnecessarily included insertion of nasogastric tubes, as well as multidrug pharmacologic intervention. Unfortunately, the experiment by Roberts and Shirley significantly lacked adequate scientific design to derive recommendations on assessing risk or administering prophylaxis to patients to reduce aspiration.[214] Questions have therefore been raised as to the validity of the data behind these recommendations, with the suggestion that a reappraisal is in order.[215]

A GFV greater than 0.4 mL/kg is more common, even in fasting individuals, than the overall incidence of aspiration would suggest if this were a major risk factor for aspiration. In one study comparing gastric content differences in healthy obese versus lean patients, a GFV greater than 25 mL and pH less than 2.5 were noted in 26.6% of obese and 42% of lean patients.[216] These data suggest that healthy obese patients do not exhibit delayed gastric emptying and that many patients routinely fall into the arbitrary range of GFV greater than 25 mL and pH less than 2.5 without experiencing aspiration. Although the volume of aspirate correlates with the severity of pulmonary damage, there is less of a correlation between the actual volume in the stomach and the risk of pneumonitis. A review of the value of routine nasogastric tube use after abdominal surgery demonstrated a slight increase in pulmonary complications among patients nonselectively treated with a nasogastric tube. The applicability of this information to short-term use under anesthesia is unknown, but it should be noted that gastric tubes not only provide evacuation but also may provide a conduit for regurgitation. Their value in patients not at risk for aspiration is unclear.[217]

Acidity plays a role in aspiration-induced lung damage; however, preoperative pharmacologic manipulation of gastric pH has not been proven to be clinically effective.[210,211] It is time to shift the focus away from GFV and pH and toward patient characteristics, patient condition, and anesthetic practices that place the patient at risk for pulmonary aspiration. Attention to the presence of factors listed in Box 29.12, and in particular to the presence of multiple factors, will likely improve the ability to predict aspiration risk better than overattention to the questionable and nonspecific factors of GFV and gastric pH. Gastrointestinal (bowel) obstruction, emergency surgery with a known full stomach, pregnancy with a gravid uterus, and acute trauma are some of the highest risk patient populations for aspiration. Point-of-care ultrasound is a technique that can assess both gastric content and volume to help determine aspiration risk. Ultrasound assessment is being used more frequently to quantify gastric content and volume.[218]

Pathophysiology

The pathophysiology of aspiration pneumonitis is typically characterized by four stages: (1) The aspirated substance causes immediate damage to the lung parenchyma, resulting in tissue damage. (2) Atelectasis results within minutes, owing to a parasympathetic response that leads to airway closure and a decrease in lung compliance. (3) One to 2 hours after the injury an intense inflammatory reaction occurs, characterized by pulmonary edema and hemorrhage. Inflammatory cytokines, including interleukin-8 (IL-8) and tumor necrosis factor-α (TNF-α) released by alveolar macrophages, play a central role. The attracted neutrophils also play a key role in this phase by releasing oxygen radicals and proteases. (4) By 24 hours after the insult, secondary injuries result from fibrin deposits and necrosis of alveolar cells.

When aspiration is severe, damage to the entire alveolar-capillary barrier, including the basement membranes and capillary endothelial cells, may occur. It is important to note that physical damage is done to the lung endothelium instantly on contact with caustic aspirate. The use of bronchoscopy or deep tracheal suctioning with the intent of halting the damage is currently not recommended.[209] Unless the patient has aspirated a particulate substance that can be retrieved, deep suctioning after aspiration will probably cause more irritation than any benefit from reversing the process. Immediate suctioning of the mouth and pharynx to prevent further aspiration is indicated.

Hypoxemia occurs secondary to a shunting effect due to atelectasis. Initially, $Paco_2$ tends to be low because of hyperventilation from hypoxic drive and because of the mechanical and irritative stimuli to the large airways and parenchyma. Hypercarbia associated with hypoventilation is a negative prognostic sign. Because atelectasis is common, PEEP is commonly used as a treatment modality for patients who require mechanical ventilation. Damage to the lung parenchyma causes an increase in the permeability of the alveolar-capillary membrane followed by a profound capillary leak syndrome. This capillary leak produces flooding of the interstitium and alveolar spaces with a protein-rich fluid. Mucus rapidly buffers the acidic fluid entering the lungs. Despite this, initial contact with highly acidic material has still been shown to increase the vascular permeability in a very predictable fashion. In addition to the inactivation of surfactant by the gastric aspirate itself, the loss of protein through the impaired capillary wall can cause changes in surfactant production, which can contribute to reduced lung compliance. Hemodynamic changes may include hypotension and reduction in CO from hypoxemia-induced myocardial ischemia and acidosis.

In the inflammatory stage, there is a release of various phagocyte-derived substances such as reactive oxygen metabolites, nitric oxide, and proteases. This stage is characterized by neutrophil infiltration, which has been found to be an important negative factor in the eventual outcome after aspiration. Research has demonstrated that inhibition of alveolar macrophages will decrease the levels of inflammatory mediators and neutrophil recruitment to the area of injury.[219] Direct inhibition of neutrophils with neutrophil aggregation inhibitors, such as pentoxifylline and lidocaine, is gaining research interest for their potential to improve outcomes of pneumonitis. Lidocaine has been demonstrated to inhibit neutrophil chemotaxis,[209] suppress superoxide production,[220] reduce reperfusion injury,[221] and improve outcomes following acid aspiration.[222]

Clinical Features and Diagnosis

Arterial hypoxemia, the hallmark sign of aspiration pneumonitis, is frequently the first sign of aspiration. Because the majority of aspiration incidents are asymptomatic or mildly symptomatic, unexplained hypoxemia occurring in otherwise healthy patients postoperatively may often be a vague sign of silent aspiration. Other signs of aspiration include tachypnea, dyspnea, tachycardia, hypertension, and cyanosis.

Diagnosis may be difficult to establish unless the aspiration is witnessed or gastric contents are visualized directly in the airway or suctioned from an ETT. ABG analysis and chest radiography are needed for evaluation. Infiltrates may not initially be seen on radiography after an acute episode. However, when seen, they are frequently located in perihilar and dependent lung regions.

Anesthetic Management

Preoperative Management

Recognizing risk factors and decreasing the overall risk (including avoidance of general anesthesia) are important steps in preventing aspiration. When the use of general anesthesia is unavoidable in at-risk patients, taking the following steps may help minimize the risk of aspiration or at least limit its consequences.

Nil per os (NPO) policy has been a mainstay of prophylaxis against aspiration by aiming to reduce patients' intragastric volume by the time they undergo anesthesia. The suggestion by Roberts and Shirley that a GFV greater than 0.4 mL/kg would predispose to aspiration gave credence to this approach. Following this concept, practitioners have instructed patients to refrain from oral intake for 8, 12, and sometimes as much as 16 hours (e.g., afternoon-scheduled surgeries, for which the patient is told to remain "NPO after midnight"). However, these NPO periods are unnecessarily long to ensure stomach emptying of most low-fat foods, and the prolonged NPO periods contribute more to patient discomfort, dehydration, and insulin resistance than to ensuring an empty stomach.[223] It has become evident that clear liquids leave the stomach within 2 hours of ingestion, but gastric acid secretion continues, even in the absence of food intake. Therefore, in the absence of prokinetic stimulation by oral intake, a fasting patient may have a higher gastric volume and acidity than one who was allowed clear fluids closer to the time of surgery. The effects of gastrin and cholecystokinin on stimulating gastric emptying in response to clear liquid ingestion are greater than the effect of the migrating motor complex in emptying the stomach in the absence of food or liquid intake. As a result, patients who are allowed liberal intake (without upper limit of volume) of clear fluids up to 2 hours before a procedure have higher gastric pH and lower volume than those who fasted for more than 4 hours.[224,225] Contemporary understanding of this concept has led to revision of blanket NPO guidelines in favor of food-specific guidelines, particularly a much more liberal approach to clear liquid ingestion preoperatively (Fig. 29.25).

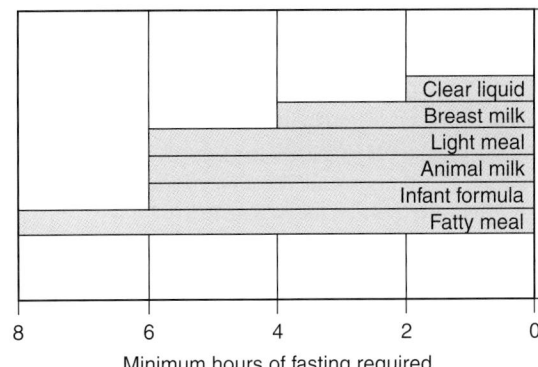

Preoperative fasting guidelines for various foods

Minimum hours of fasting required

Fig. 29.25 Preoperative fasting guidelines. (Data practice guidelines for preoperative fasting and the use of pharmacologic agents to reduce the risk of pulmonary aspiration: application to healthy patients undergoing elective procedures: an updated report by the American Society of Anesthesiologists Task Force on Preoperative Fasting and the Use of Pharmacologic Agents to Reduce the Risk of Pulmonary Aspiration. *Anesthesiology.* 2017;126[3]:376–393.)

TABLE 29.21	Medications for Aspiration Prophylaxis*
Medication Type	**Common Examples**
Gastrointestinal stimulants	Metoclopramide
Histamine-2 antagonists	Ranitidine
	Famotidine
Proton pump inhibitors	Omeprazole
	Lansoprazole
Antacids	Sodium citrate
	Sodium bicarbonate
	Magnesium trisilicate
Antiemetics	Droperidol
	Ondansetron
Anticholinergics†	Atropine
	Scopolamine
	Glycopyrrolate

*The routine preoperative use of these medications to decrease aspiration risk in patients with no apparent increased risk is not recommended.
†The use of anticholinergics to decrease aspiration risk is not recommended.
Data from American Society of Anesthesiologists Committee on Standards and Practice Parameters. Practice guidelines for preoperative fasting and the use of pharmacologic agents to reduce the risk of pulmonary aspiration: application to healthy patients undergoing elective surgery. *Anesthesiology.* 2011;114:495–511.

Pharmacologic prophylaxis for aspiration may be considered to reduce risk factors for pneumonitis. Agents such as gastrokinetics, histamine blockers, anticholinergics, antacids, proton pump inhibitors, and antiemetics are all used alone or in various combinations to raise gastric pH, lower gastric volume, and reduce the incidence of emesis (Table 29.21). Although scientific evidence does not support the routine use of prophylactic agents, practitioners may administer them when indicated for patients who are at risk. Although previously used to inhibit gastrointestinal activity, anticholinergic agents are no longer supported for prophylactic use, and they may even antagonize other useful agents. For example, metoclopramide raises barrier pressure (which opposes gastric regurgitation) by increasing the tone of the lower esophageal sphincter; however, anticholinergics inhibit this effect. Metoclopramide stimulates gastric emptying and acts as an antiemetic.

Clear, nonparticulate antacids such as sodium citrate or sodium citrate with citric acid (bicitra) have been shown to be clinically effective in increasing the pH of gastric contents. Desired onset of action occurs within 15 minutes, and duration of action is 1 to 3 hours. Although citrate preparations may last up to 6 to 7 hours, some patients will also experience a rebound increase in gastric acid production, so if surgery is delayed more than 1 hour after citrate administration it may be prudent to repeat the dose.[226]

Intravenous administration of the H_2-receptor blockers such as ranitidine or famotidine 45 to 60 minutes before surgery can raise gastric pH. Famotidine provides the best profile of duration of action and low incidence of side effects.[227] Although the H_2-blockers reduce gastrin-induced acid production, they are less effective against vagal or muscarinic influence. In contrast, proton pump inhibitors irreversibly bind to H^+/K^+ ATPase, blocking the final pathway for acid production. They are therefore more effective in reducing acid production, but for maximal effectiveness they must be administered as a dose the night before surgery and then repeated preoperatively. In emergency cases or where the prior-night dose was not performed, H_2-receptor blockers may provide a better option for single-dose therapy.

Although cricoid pressure has long been considered a foundation of management of aspiration risk, the effectiveness of this technique has been called into question.[228-231] Confounding findings include that in a significant number of patients the esophagus is not aligned directly posteriorly to the trachea,[232,233] and there are numerous reports of aspiration despite application of cricoid pressure.[234] Other suggestions are that cricoid pressure is inconsistently applied, or cricoid pressure itself will reduce lower esophageal sphincter pressure (LESP), thereby increasing the gradient for gastric regurgitation.[235,236] This LESP reduction appears to be a reflex mechanism in response to cricoid pressure and can be blunted by remifentanil.[237] Others have indicated that esophageal position is irrelevant since it is the hypopharynx that is compressed by the application of cricoid pressure.[238] Nonpharmacologic mechanisms such as head elevation may offer some benefit. Proponents of cricoid pressure believe that whereas the procedure may not exactly compress the esophagus as Sellick envisioned, it may nonetheless provide a barrier against regurgitation.[238,239,240] Although the overall benefit of cricoid pressure is questionable, it is still widely considered a standard of care.[241]

Intraoperative Management

If intubation is not expected to be difficult, a rapid-sequence induction (rather than awake endotracheal intubation) is acceptable in the patient with aspiration risk. There is little evidence that modified rapid sequence technique (which allows for gentle mask ventilation) worsens aspiration incidence. In fact, providing oxygenation and ventilation through the induction period is preferable in patients at risk for rapid oxygen desaturation.[242] Because difficult intubation itself is a risk factor for aspiration, there should be a low threshold for performing awake intubation, or at a minimum utilizing videolaryngoscopy, in a patient with aspiration risk who may also pose airway challenges. Endotracheal intubation is considered the optimal approach for airway isolation, but regurgitated material can seep around the ETT cuff, particularly if it is not lubricated.[243,244] Preventive measures in the anesthetic plan include ensuring that the patient is fully awake before extubation and manifesting protective reflexes, residual neuromuscular blockade is minimized to the extent possible, the degree of narcosis does not impair the level of consciousness postoperatively, and the stomach has been evacuated.

If vomiting or aspiration occurs during induction, immediate treatment includes tilting of the patient's head downward or to the side, rapid suctioning of the mouth and pharynx, and endotracheal intubation. It is recommended to suction the trachea prior to positive pressure ventilation, but there is no robust evidence to support the efficacy of this technique. There is little benefit in performing bronchial suctioning in most cases, and bronchoscopy should be reserved for those patients suspected of having aspirated solid material. If aspiration is severe, surgery may be postponed. ABG analysis should be performed for determination of the extent of hypoxemia. Early application of PEEP is recommended for improving pulmonary function and combating atelectasis.[215]

Oxygenation should be supported with increases in FiO_2 only to the minimum extent necessary. The damage to pulmonary parenchyma from caustic aspiration predisposes the tissue to oxygen toxicity. Indiscriminate administration of oxygen may worsen tissue damage.[245] For pharmacologic treatment of aspiration pneumonitis, the use of steroids is controversial and is usually reserved for treatment in the ICU after other therapies have been unsuccessful. Lidocaine 1.5 mg/kg is probably not harmful and may be helpful as a neutrophil aggregation for improving long-term outcome after aspiration.[222] Although most cases of aspiration are of sterile material (such as typical gastric acid), leukocytosis, fever, and infiltrate on x-ray are common findings in aspiration pneumonitis. The clinical findings resemble but do not indicate bacterial colonization (i.e., pneumonia). For this reason, the routine use of antibiotics is not recommended. Antibiotics are indicated only if the fever does not resolve within 48 hours, if there is risk for bacterial colonization (e.g., a patient on high-pH gastric tube feedings or aspiration of fecal material), or if protected-sample bronchial or blood cultures indicate infection. Box 29.13 gives the standard treatment protocol for aspiration pneumonitis.

The common time course of symptoms after aspiration has been characterized. Warner et al.[210] noted that the condition of the patient at 2 hours after the aspiration was prognostic of the patient's eventual course. Patients could be discharged if they did not manifest significant symptoms within 2 hours of the incident. Their criteria were as follows: (1) Patients did not develop symptoms that included a new cough or a wheeze, (2) no decrease in SpO_2 of greater than or equal to 10% of preoperative levels occurred when the patient was breathing room air, (3) patients did not exhibit an A-a gradient of greater than or equal to 300 mm Hg, and (4) no radiographic evidence of pulmonary aspiration was present.

ACUTE RESPIRATORY DISTRESS SYNDROME

Definition

The term *acute respiratory failure* is often used synonymously with *acute* (formerly *adult*) *respiratory distress syndrome*. Although ARDS

TABLE 29.22   Berlin Definition of ARDS

Criterion	Definition
Timing	Within 1 wk of a known precipitant, or new/worsening respiratory symptoms
Chest imaging (chest radiograph or CT scan)	Bilateral opacities—not fully explained by effusions, lobar/lung collapse, or nodules
Origin of edema	Respiratory failure not fully explained by cardiac failure or fluid overload If no risk factor for ARDS is present, need objective assessment (e.g., echocardiogram) to exclude hydrostatic edema
Oxygenation Mild	200 mm Hg < arterial Po_2/Fio_2 ≤300 mm Hg with PEEP or CPAP ≥5 cm H_2O
Moderate	100 mm Hg < arterial Po_2/Fio_2 ≤200 mm Hg with PEEP ≥5 cm H_2O
Severe	Arterial Po_2/Fio_2 ≤100 mm Hg with PEEP ≥5 cm H_2O

ARDS, Acute respiratory distress syndrome; *CPAP,* continuous positive airway pressure; *CT,* computed tomography; *Fio₂,* fraction of inspired oxygen; *PEEP,* positive end-expiratory pressure.
Adapted from Ranieri VM, et al. Acute respiratory distress syndrome: the Berlin definition. *JAMA.* 2012;307(23):2526–2533.

may be caused by or associated with a variety of clinical conditions, most patients with this disease demonstrate similar clinical and pathologic features regardless of the cause of lung injury. Common features include a history of a preceding noxious event that served as a trigger for the subsequent development of ARDS and insult to the alveolar-capillary membrane that results in increased permeability and subsequent interstitial and alveolar edema.[246] Clinical presentation is characterized by dyspnea, severe hypoxemia, diffuse bilateral pulmonary infiltration, and stiffening and noncompliance of the lungs.

In 2012, the Berlin definition of ARDS was developed (Table 29.22). The degree of hypoxemia was stratified into mild, moderate, and severe based on the arterial $Po_2{:}Fio_2$ ratio, and a requirement for PEEP of 5 cm H_2O or greater was included (whether applied by ETT or, in the setting of mild disease, by noninvasive ventilation). The term *acute lung injury* was eliminated. Given that the use of pulmonary artery catheters has decreased dramatically due to a demonstrated lack of benefit, the need for a pulmonary arterial wedge pressure measurement was eliminated. Revised recommendations focus on objective testing (e.g., echocardiography) to exclude cardiogenic edema if no risk factor for ARDS could be identified. Acute ARDS was explicitly defined as ARDS developing within 1 week of a known risk factor.[247]

Incidence and Outcome

Risk factors for the development of ARDS appear to be additive. Occurrence is 25% with the presence of one risk factor, 42% with the presence of two, and 85% with the presence of three.[248] The mortality rate for ARDS remains high, at approximately 50%.[249] However, the mortality rate often exceeds 90% when gram-negative septic shock precedes ARDS development.[250]

Etiology

The most common events and risk factors associated with the development of ARDS include (1) sepsis, (2) bacterial pneumonia, (3) trauma, and (4) aspiration pneumonitis.[251] Other causes include diseases of the

central nervous system, metabolic events (e.g., pancreatitis and uremia), disease states that result in the release of inflammatory mediators (e.g., extrapulmonary infections, disseminated intravascular coagulation, anaphylaxis, coronary bypass grafting, and transfusion reactions), and other forms of shock (cardiogenic or hypovolemic) (see Box 29.11).[247]

Pathophysiology

The pathophysiology of ARDS is centered on severe damage and inflammation to the alveolar-capillary membrane. Research has focused on the release of cytokines and membrane-bound phospholipids from the capillary endothelium and the activation of leukocytes and macrophages (via the complement system) within the lungs.[252] As in pneumonitis, neutrophils play a role in the pathology of ARDS, and IL-8 has been identified as the main chemotactic factor for neutrophils.[253]

Phospholipids, prostaglandins, and leukotrienes are all involved in the immune response during ARDS. Some of their actions include pulmonary vasoconstriction, bronchoconstriction, and alterations in vascular reactivity and permeability. One of the primary actions of prostaglandins and leukotrienes is to assist with the attraction and regulation of neutrophils. Neutrophils have a major impact in the pathogenesis of ARDS. Once neutrophils cross the alveolar-capillary membrane and enter the alveoli at the sites of inflammation, their effects within the airways can be both helpful and harmful.

Microemboli formation is a common manifestation of ARDS. Complement system activation and the release of thromboplastin from soft tissue injury can trigger the coagulation system. Damage to the alveolar-capillary membrane impairs oxygenation, and loss of lung compliance makes it difficult to effectively ventilate patients. The effect of microemboli, prolonged alveolar hypoxia and hypercapnia, and injury to the alveolar tissue leads to increases in PVR. High alveolar pressures from aggressive positive pressure ventilation further contribute to increased right ventricular afterload and ventilator induced lung injury to lung parenchyma. This afterload increase leads to cor pulmonale in 25% of cases,[254] and shunting across a patent foramen ovale occurs in 20%.[255] Associated right ventricular dysfunction increases the associated mortality from ARDS,[256] particularly when plateau pressures are high.[257]

Clinical Features and Diagnosis

The clinical presentation of ARDS resembles that of pulmonary edema and aspiration pneumonitis. Patients appear dyspneic, hypoxemic, and hypovolemic, and they often require intubation and mechanical ventilation. Noncardiogenic pulmonary edema is a hallmark finding. Findings on histologic examination are similar to those of aspiration pneumonitis, with the exception that fibrosis of lung is more pronounced. Recovery of lung function is unpredictable. Milder cases resolve quickly, whereas others progress to fibrosis and death.

Treatment

Treatment is supportive and includes correction of hypoxemia, afterload reduction, and inotropic support as indicated. Maintaining tissue oxygenation and reducing further lung damage are the main goals of therapy. Preserving end-organ perfusion is of utmost importance. Multiple therapies have been attempted to improve ventilation and reduce shunt in ARDS patients. Other than lung protective ventilation[258] and prone positioning, no other therapy is consistently utilized. Possible therapeutic options include corticosteroids, inhaled nitric oxide, exogenous surfactant, and extracorporeal gas exchange.[259]

Anesthetic Management

Anesthetic preparation includes evaluation of the patient's respiratory, cardiac, and renal status. The anesthetist should carefully manage

TABLE 29.23	Features of Pressure-Controlled Versus Volume-Controlled Ventilation			
	Set Parameters	**Variable Parameters**	**Clinical Implications**	**Clinical Conditions**
Pressure-controlled ventilation (PCV)	Peak pressure target, inspiratory time, RR, PEEP	Tidal volume, inspiratory flow	Controls airway pressure, but tidal volume becomes a function of lung compliance (no guaranteed tidal volume or minute ventilation). Allows estimation of end-inspiratory alveolar pressure based on ventilator settings. Variable inspiratory flow helpful for patients with high respiratory drive.	Severe asthma COPD Salicylate toxicity
Volume-controlled ventilation (VCV)	Tidal volume, RR, inspiratory flow pattern, inspiratory time	PIP, end-inspiratory alveolar pressure	Guaranteed delivery of tidal volume but may result in high or injurious lung pressures. End-inspiratory alveolar pressure cannot be reliably estimated and must be measured (plateau pressure).	Acute lung injury ARDS Obesity Severe burns

ARDS, Acute respiratory distress syndrome; *COPD,* chronic obstructive pulmonary disease; *PEEP,* positive-end expiratory pressure; *PIP,* peak inspiratory pressure; *RR,* respiratory rate.
From Seigel TA. Mechanical support and noninvasive ventilatory support. In Marx JA, et al., eds. *Rosen's Emergency Medicine: Concepts and Clinical Practice.* 8th ed. Philadelphia: Elsevier; 2014:24.

vascular volume to avoid transudation of water into the lungs and give meticulous attention to avoiding air in vascular lines due to the potential for right-to-left shunting. Useful monitoring should include invasive blood pressure, CVP monitoring, cardiac filling pressures, cardiac output, and a urinary catheter.

Ventilator settings should be noted, and special attention should be devoted to peak inspiratory pressures and PEEP levels. Considering the prominence of cor pulmonale, the ventilation strategy must balance the need for alveolar recruitment with the potential for overloading the right ventricle. As PEEP is added, alveoli are recruited, improving oxygenation and reducing afterload on the right ventricle. However, at a point, alveolar overdistention will tip the balance beyond benefit and into detrimental effects, as the intrapulmonary pressure provides impedance to cardiac output.[260] The concept of permissive hypercapnia limits aggressive ventilation in the interest of minimizing mean airway pressures; however, the effects of hypercapnia on increasing the PVR are varied. Some report a significant reduction (20%) in right ventricular ejection,[261] whereas others have found the hemodynamic effects temporary and nondetrimental.[262] In any case, right ventricular function should be monitored along with blood gas results as outcome goals for any ventilation strategy used in ARDS. Rising CVP as well as chamber dilation, reduced ejection fraction, and septal deviation or paradoxic motion as shown by echocardiography are means of identifying right ventricular dysfunction.[263]

A lung protective ventilation strategy is often used, aimed at minimizing airway pressures and avoiding barotrauma and volutrauma in the face of severely reduced compliance. One of the most accepted and evidence-based therapies for ARDS is a lung protective strategy for mechanical ventilation that uses 6 to 8 mL/kg predicted body weight tidal volumes and an escalating PEEP.[258] Plateau pressures are monitored and pressures of 30 mm Hg and lower are recommended. Some approaches are referred to as open lung strategies, implying a primary goal of preventing atelectasis and airway closure. Open lung approaches have tended toward use of high levels of PEEP, but there is growing evidence that more modest levels may be equally effective.[260,264] Protective ventilation strategies vary in their details. In some cases, very unconventional ventilation approaches such as high-frequency oscillation may be used. Oscillation has demonstrated mixed results, but in some studies an improvement in gas exchange has occurred.[265,266] Strategies focused on supporting right ventricular performance may include prone positioning.[263] Prone positioning improves airway pressures and gas exchange, and it reduces the

indicators of cor pulmonale.[267-269] Some common modes of ventilation are shown in Tables 29.23 and 29.24; however, Table 29.25 provides a sampling of some protective ventilation protocols that have been used in ARDS research or as guidelines.

TRANSFUSION-RELATED PULMONARY DISEASE

With increasing awareness of a host of complications related to blood transfusion, the connection to pulmonary complications has become a significant area of concern. The primary transfusion-related pulmonary complication is transfusion-related acute lung injury (TRALI).

Definition

TRALI is a form of acute lung injury associated with blood transfusion and characterized by pulmonary infiltrates and hypoxemia. TRALI is defined as acute onset hypoxemia, bilateral lung infiltrations on the chest radiograph, and no evidence of circulatory overload; all of these occur during or within 6 hours of blood transfusion in a patient with no other risk factor for ALI. TRALI resembles ARDS in clinical presentation, but unlike ARDS it has a lower mortality and is self-limiting with spontaneous resolution usually occurring within 96 hours.[270]

Incidence and Outcome

TRALI is a leading cause of transfusion-related fatalities, and it is the most common cause of major morbidity and death after transfusion[271-274]; 5% to 10% of cases are fatal, and the incidence is believed to be 1 in 5000 transfused blood units.[274-276] There is a prevailing sense that TRALI is underdiagnosed, and so the incidence may be much higher than reported. Poor recognition, passive reporting instead of active monitoring, and the inclusion of cases that do not fully meet diagnostic criteria for TRALI are all reasons for a lack of a true understanding of the incidence.[274,275]

Etiology

TRALI is thought to occur because of an interaction between transfused blood products and the recipient's white blood cells. Attention first focused on an immune mechanism, particularly surrounding the human leukocyte antigens (HLAs) and human neutrophil alloantigens (HNAs) in the recipient. The findings that some victims did not demonstrate elevated antibody titers and that TRALI could be induced in excised lungs both indicated there is at least one other mechanism. In cases of nonimmune TRALI, reactive lipid products released from

TABLE 29.24 Ventilator Strategies: Features of Potential Options

Mode	Parameters Set by Provider	Clinical Scenario
Continuous Mechanical Ventilation (CMV)		
Assist-control (A/C)	Pressure or volume control, RR	Paralyzed or deeply sedated patient, sedated patients with intermittent spontaneous respiratory effort; can lead to hyperventilation
Intermittent Mandatory Ventilation (IMV)		
Synchronized intermittent mandatory ventilation (SIMV)	Pressure or volume control, RR (backup rate)	Patients with regular but poor spontaneous respiratory effort; if used in deeply sedated patients, set RR will need to be higher
Continuous Spontaneous Ventilation (CSV)		
Pressure-support ventilation (PSV)	Level of pressure support, PEEP	Spontaneously breathing patients with good respiratory effort requiring minimal ventilatory support
Continuous positive airway pressure (CPAP)	Level of CPAP	Alert, spontaneously breathing patients with immediately reversible causes of respiratory distress; COPD and ACPE are classic indications for noninvasive ventilation
Bilevel positive airway pressure (Bi-PAP)	IPAP and EPAP	Similar to CPAP

ACPE, Acute cardiogenic pulmonary edema; *COPD*, chronic obstructive pulmonary disease; *EPAP*, expiratory positive airway pressure; *IPAP*, inspiratory positive airway pressure; *PEEP*, positive end-expiratory pressure; *RR*, respiratory rate.
From Seigel TA. Mechanical support and noninvasive ventilatory support. In Marx JA, et al., eds. *Rosen's Emergency Medicine: Concepts and Clinical Practice.* 8th ed. Philadelphia: Elsevier; 2014:25.

TABLE 29.25 Ventilation Protocol Used in the ARDS Network Study

Parameter	Protocol
Mode of ventilation	Volume assist control
Tidal volume	≤6 mL/kg predicted body weight
Plateau pressure	≤30 cm H_2O
Frequency	6–35 breaths/min, titrated for pH 7.3–7.45
I:E ratio	1:1 to 1:3
Oxygenation goal	Arterial Po_2 55–80 mm Hg, or Spo_2 88%–95%
Fio_2/PEEP (cm H_2O) combinations allowed	0.3/5, 0.4/5, 0.4/8, 0.5/8, 0.5/10, 0.6/10, 0.7/10, 0.7/12, 0.7/14, 0.8/14, 0.9/14, 0.9/16, 0.9/18, 1/18–24
Weaning	By pressure support, required when Fio_2/PEEP ≤0.4/8

ARDS, Acute respiratory distress syndrome; *I:E ratio*, inspiratory:expiratory ratio; *Fio₂*, fraction of inspired oxygen; *PEEP*, positive end-expiratory pressure.
From The Acute Respiratory Distress Syndrome Network. Ventilation with lower tidal volumes as compared with traditional tidal volumes for acute lung injury and the acute respiratory distress syndrome. *N Engl J Med.* 2000:342(18):1301–1308.

the donor blood cells may act as the trigger. In either form of TRALI, neutrophils play an important role. Theories often entertain a two-hit hypothesis, assuming that a preexisting factor is present in victims, which leads to the abnormal reaction to the allograft blood.[277,278] This hypothesis helps explain why TRALI occurs only in some individuals.

Predisposing factors for TRALI frequently surround events that may prime the immune system (e.g., recent surgery, malignancy, sepsis, alcoholism, liver disease). Increased levels of HLA and previous ALI as risk factors point to immunologic predisposition.[279] Donor risk factors also play an important role in development of TRALI. For example, pregnancy causes an elevation in HLA in many women, and a high proportion of TRALI cases arise in individuals who receive blood products donated by women with leukocyte antibodies. For this reason, the United Kingdom halted use of plasma from female donors in 2003, and a significant reduction in the incidence of TRALI ensued. Although TRALI has occurred in association with a wide variety of blood products, the greatest incidence follows platelet transfusion.[270]

Pathophysiology

Upon activation, neutrophils become trapped within the pulmonary microvasculature, causing congestion and leading to noncardiogenic pulmonary edema. Complement activation and the release of oxygen free radicals with proteases then causes damage to the capillary endothelium, which also promotes fluid leak into the alveoli. Platelets play an important role in TRALI because they are activated and then sequestered in the lungs through their interaction with neutrophils.[280]

Clinical Features and Diagnosis

TRALI, by definition, is associated with blood transfusion, so symptoms begin during or up to 6 hours after transfusion of any blood product. Acute onset and hypoxemia are key findings, with Pao_2:Fio_2 ratio less than 300. Bilateral infiltrates are found on chest radiography. Clinical symptoms include fever, chills, and dyspnea. Hypertension and hypotension occur with equal frequency.

It is important to distinguish TRALI from other causes of lung dysfunction, and diagnosis must exclude any other precipitating factor for ALI. Cardiogenic causes and acute hypersensitivity reactions or ABO incompatibility reactions must also be excluded. TRALI appears with similar symptomatology as transfusion-related circulatory overload (TACO). TACO usually presents with tachycardia, dyspnea, and pulmonary edema. The key differentiating factor is that signs of circulatory overload or predisposition to circulatory overload (e.g., CHF) exist in TACO but not in TRALI. Circulatory overload should be ruled out before presuming a diagnosis of TRALI for patients with coronary artery disease or CHF, or who are status post lung resection (particularly with peripheral edema, jugular vein distension, S_3 heart sound). Patients who develop TACO often show signs of circulatory overload prior to the blood infusion.

Treatment

Treatment is largely supportive, similar to the treatment for ARDS. A lung-protective ventilation strategy is used for patients requiring mechanical ventilation.

Anesthetic Management

Management of the patient who develops TRALI requires immediate cessation of the transfusion. Intravenous fluids are used to support blood pressure if the patient is hypotensive, and diuretics are not indicated. Because the respiratory distress is due to microvascular injury rather than fluid overload, the majority of cases require mechanical ventilation. However, resolution occurs more quickly than it does with ARDS.

Appropriate attribution of cause is important to guide the correct treatment. Finding of anti-HLA or HNA antibodies in plasma support the diagnosis of TRALI, whereas signs of fluid overload (clinical signs or elevated brain natriuretic peptide) support the diagnosis of TACO.[281,282]

DRUG-INDUCED PULMONARY DISEASE

Drug-induced pulmonary injury occurs in several hundred thousand people each year in the United States. Knowledge of doses and the potential adverse effects of the prescribed medications may prevent or minimize drug-induced damage. The rapid development of nanotechnology also lends concern for new forms of pulmonary toxicity. Nanoparticles, because of their extremely small size, can gain access to physiologic areas that traditional molecules cannot. In particular, in the respiratory tract, carbon nanotubes cause damage to alveolar cells, form granulomas, and lead to fibrosis. This damage leads to release of proinflammatory cytokines and generation of oxygen free radicals.[283-285] With the growing use of nanotubes in medications, cosmetics, disease treatment, and other applications, it is likely that new forms of pulmonary toxicity will grow in incidence.

Mechanism

The mechanism of drug-induced pulmonary injury is not well defined. It has been shown that cytotoxic drugs used in the treatment of cancer cause pulmonary insult by a combination of the direct toxic effects of a drug or its metabolite and of their indirect effects (i.e., the enhancement of inflammation or immune processes). The clinical features produced by different cytotoxic agents are similar, but chronic pneumonitis and fibrosis are the most commonly associated clinical syndromes. Box 29.14 lists various agents that may produce pulmonary toxicity. The pathogenesis of pulmonary toxicity is uncertain but has been found to include disruption of the endothelial cells and changes in calcium homeostasis that lead to toxic injury. The mechanisms of drug-induced pulmonary injury associated with noncytotoxic drugs are less well defined but may involve changes in pulmonary homeostasis. Noncytotoxic agents can induce the development of numerous clinical syndromes. Several commonly implicated agents are discussed in the following sections.

Noncytotoxic Drug-Induced Pulmonary Disease

Amiodarone

Amiodarone is one of the most frequently prescribed medications for ventricular dysrhythmias. Pulmonary disease from amiodarone occurs with 5% to 15% prevalence and takes the form of chronic interstitial pneumonitis, organizing pneumonia, ARDS, or a solitary mass of fibrosis.[286] Toxicity may be related to direct toxicity, immunologic mechanisms, or activation of the renin-angiotensin system.[287]

BOX 29.14 Classification of Drug-Induced and Related Pulmonary Diseases by Type of Medication

Chemotherapeutic

Cytotoxic
- Azathioprine
- Bleomycin
- Busulfan
- Chlorambucil
- Cyclophosphamide
- Etoposide
- Interleukin-2
- Melphalan
- Mitomycin C*
- Nitrosoureas
- Procarbazine
- Vinblastine
- Zinostatin

Noncytotoxic
- Bleomycin*
- Cytosine arabinoside*
- Gemcitabine*
- Methotrexate*
- Procarbazine*

Antibiotic
- Amphotericin B*
- Nitrofurantoin
  - Acute*
  - Chronic
- Sulfasalazine

Antiinflammatory
- Acetylsalicylic acid*
- Gold
- Interferons
- Leukotriene antagonists
- Methotrexate
- Nonsteroidal antiinflammatory agents
- Penicillamine*

Analgesic
- Placidyl*
- Propoxyphene*
- Salicylates*

Cardiovascular
- Amiodarone*
- Angiotensin-converting enzyme inhibitors
- Anticoagulants
- β-blockers*
- Dipyridamole
- Flecainide
- Protamine*
- Tocainide

Illicit
- Heroin*
- Methadone*
- Methylphenidate
- Cocaine
- Talc granulomatosis

Inhalant
- Aspirated oil
- Oxygen*

Intravenous
- Blood products*
- Sodium morrhuate*
- Ethiodized oil (lymphangiogram)

Miscellaneous
- Appetite suppressants
- Bromocriptine
- Complement-mediated leukostasis*
- Dantrolene
- Hydrochlorothiazide*
- Methysergide
- Radiation
- Systemic lupus erythematosus (drug induced)
- Tocolytic agents*
- Tricyclics*
- L-Tryptophan

* Typically present as acute and subacute respiratory insufficiency. From Dulohery MM, et al. Drug-induced pulmonary disease. In Broaddus VC, et al., eds. *Murray and Nadel's Textbook of Respiratory Medicine.* 6th ed. Philadelphia: Elsevier; 2016:1276.

Clinical diagnosis of amiodarone-induced pulmonary toxicity is based on the presence of two or more of the following signs and symptoms[288]:

1. New onset of pulmonary symptoms such as dyspnea, cough, or pleuritic chest pain
2. Detection of new chest radiographic abnormalities such as an interstitial or alveolar infiltrate

3. A decrease in DLCO of 20% from the pretreatment value; if no pretreatment values are available, then a value equal to less than 80% of the predicted value
4. Abnormal gallium-67 uptake by the lungs
5. Characteristic histologic changes of lung tissue obtained by bronchoscopic or open-lung biopsy

Amiodarone-induced pulmonary toxicity is commonly characterized by an insidious onset with nonproductive cough, hypoxemia, progressive dyspnea, weight loss, pleuritic chest pain, pleural effusion, and occasional fever.[286,289] Some patients present with a rapidly progressive dyspnea, high fever, and hypoxemia. Chest radiographs demonstrate parenchymal infiltrates with a predominant diffuse alveolar, interstitial, or mixed pattern that may progress to fibrosis.[290] Pleural thickening and effusions also have been reported. Pulmonary function tests performed at the onset of pulmonary toxicity reveal abnormalities typical of restrictive lung disease. Onset usually occurs after 2 months and is dose related, occurring most commonly if doses greater than 400 mg/day are used.[286] Toxicity is rare when given acutely. Therapeutic options are limited. In cases where drug withdrawal is not desirable, corticosteroids are helpful at ameliorating the disease.[291] When the drug is discontinued, resolution of toxic signs is gradual due to the drug's half-life of approximately 40 to 70 days. Fibrosis, when it occurs, is not irreversible.[286]

Cytotoxic Drug-Induced Pulmonary Disease

Three clinical syndromes are associated with cytotoxic drug-induced pulmonary injury and include (1) chronic pneumonitis and fibrosis, (2) acute hypersensitivity lung disease, and (3) noncardiogenic pulmonary edema.[292] These syndromes may coexist.

Chronic Pneumonitis and Fibrosis

The pattern of interstitial pneumonitis and fibrosis is the most frequently encountered in drug-induced pulmonary injury. The mechanism of injury is a direct cytotoxic effect of a drug or its metabolites on the endothelial, interstitial, or alveolar epithelial cells. The cytotoxic effect elicits an inflammatory response on lung parenchyma characterized by the proliferation of macrophages, lymphocytes, and other inflammatory cells. This inflammatory response leads to the deposition of fibrin within the alveoli, which produces interstitial inflammation and fibrosis.

Interstitial pneumonitis can be classified as acute, subacute, or chronic. The chronic form is the most common. Manifestations of these subgroups include dyspnea, dry cough, low-grade fever, fatigue, and malaise that develops over several weeks to months. Chest radiography demonstrates diffuse interstitial infiltrates. Bleomycin is the causative agent most often implicated in interstitial pneumonitis. Treatment includes discontinuation of the offending agent with or without institution of corticosteroid therapy; prognosis is variable. Other antineoplastics implicated in pneumonitis and fibrosis are trastuzumab, gemcitabine, temsirolimus, everolimus, paclitaxel, docetaxel, irinotecan, gefitinib, oxaliplatin, topotecan, and imatinib.[293]

Syndrome of Hypersensitivity Lung Disease

Hypersensitivity lung disease has been associated with the cytotoxic agents bleomycin, methotrexate, L-asparaginase, procarbazine, etoposide, teniposide, and mitoxantrone.[293] Common pulmonary manifestations include a nonproductive cough, dyspnea, and chest pain. The systemic response may show fever, urticaria, arthralgias, hypotension, and/or eosinophilia. Chest radiography may reveal pneumonitis, pleuritis, and pleural effusion. Corticosteroid use may or may not be indicated, and prognosis is generally favorable.

Drug-Induced Pulmonary Edema

The development of noncardiogenic pulmonary edema is an acute but rare phenomenon that occurs after the administration of some antineoplastic agents. Numerous pharmacologic agents used in the treatment of cancer have been implicated in the development of toxic pulmonary side effects. Cytotoxic agents most commonly implicated in pulmonary insult include bleomycin, busulfan, carmustine, methotrexate, cytosine arabinoside (cytarabine), gemcitabine, imatinib, and cyclophosphamide. Pulmonary toxicity in the use of antineoplastic agents is defined as the development of clinical signs and symptoms of pulmonary distress that were not present during the pretreatment studies. The prevalence of diffuse pulmonary infiltration occurring as a result of drug toxicity is reported to be as high as 20%.

Prototype Agents Implicated in Pulmonary Insult

Bleomycin. Bleomycin, an antitumor antibiotic, is the most common chemotherapeutically induced potentiator of pulmonary injury. Despite the benefits of bleomycin therapy, the development of pulmonary toxicity is the limiting factor of its use.[294] The most common adverse effect of bleomycin is the development of interstitial fibrosis. The incidence of pulmonary fibrosis is approximately 20%, with a 1% mortality rate. Anesthesia-related problems usually occur postoperatively and are associated with exposure to high Fio_2 concentrations. Symptoms of toxicity initially include a dry hacking cough and dyspnea on exertion. Progression of lung disease is associated with dyspnea at rest, tachypnea, fever, and cyanosis. Changes on chest radiography usually occur later and manifest as bibasilar reticular infiltrates that may progress to consolidation.

Several investigators have suggested that patients undergoing general anesthesia who have a concurrent history of bleomycin therapy should receive the lowest possible O_2 concentrations that allow maintenance of adequate Pao_2.[295,296] The use of steroids has been effective in some patients.

Anesthetic management of bleomycin-treated patients. Although universally accepted guidelines for the management of a bleomycin-treated patient undergoing general anesthesia are lacking, the following suggestions have been made:

- O_2 saturation should be monitored continuously and ABG analysis performed intermittently.
- Immediately before anesthesia, 100% O_2 should be administered for 1 to 4 minutes.
- After induction, a target Pao_2 should be chosen and the Fio_2 maintained at the lowest level that allows adequate oxygenation.
- The use of PEEP should be considered.
- Crystalloid solutions should be administered carefully and the use of colloid solutions considered if large fluid volumes are required.
- The patient should be informed of the possible need for postoperative ventilation.
- Postoperatively, the Fio_2 should be kept at the lowest possible setting that maintains the target Pao_2.

The choice of anesthetic technique varies, but as with all surgical procedures, careful evaluation and management are essential. There are no reports suggesting the superiority of regional anesthesia in patients treated with bleomycin.

Methotrexate. Methotrexate is an analog of folic acid that inhibits cellular reproduction by causing an acute intracellular deficiency of folate coenzymes. Methotrexate is used in the treatment of malignant and benign conditions, which include leukemia, osteogenic sarcoma, choriocarcinoma, polymyositis, psoriasis, and connective tissue disorders (particularly rheumatoid arthritis). Regardless of the route of administration, pulmonary toxicity has been reported to occur with all forms of delivery, with an incidence of 7.6%. Acute pulmonary dysfunction occurs most often; however, the onset of pulmonary dysfunction may also be chronic. The syndrome often develops over 7 to 14 days and is characterized by fever, dry cough, dyspnea, hypoxemia, and bilateral pulmonary infiltrates. Improvement may begin 10 to 14 days after onset.

PULMONARY OXYGEN TOXICITY

Etiology

As with all prescribed drugs, the risks of the adverse effects of O_2 administration must be considered despite its beneficial effects. The prolonged use of high concentrations of O_2 (>50% for >24 hours) is potentially toxic and may result in irreversible lung damage.[295] The rate of development of O_2 toxicity is directly related to the exposure: partial pressure of inspired O_2 and duration of administration. Deleterious effects have been reported with briefer administrations.[297]

Normobaric hyperoxia can result in four clinical syndromes: (1) acute tracheobronchitis, (2) absorption atelectasis, (3) acute alveolar lung injury (ARDS), and (4) bronchopulmonary dysplasia. When nitrogen is replaced with O_2, absorption atelectasis occurs in the alveoli that are poorly ventilated. The loss of the so-called nitrogen splint promotes alveolar collapse.

Pathophysiology

The pathogenesis of pulmonary O_2 toxicity is linked to the excessive production of free O_2 radicals.[298] Free radicals are molecules that contain one or more unpaired electrons. Free radicals are highly reactive metabolites of O_2 (e.g., superoxide anion, hydrogen peroxide, and hydroxyl radical) that overwhelm antioxidant systems, including cellular enzymatic defenses (superoxide dismutase, catalase, glutathione peroxidase) and nonenzymatic scavengers (α-tocopherol acetate). Free radicals exert their toxic effect on cell and organelle membranes; they interfere with vital cellular functions, causing inactivation of enzymes and transport proteins, membrane lipid peroxidation, and inhibition of cell growth and division. Factors predisposing to oxygen toxicity are increased exposure (concentration + duration), advanced age, and radiation therapy to the thorax and use of chemotherapeutic agents that alter antioxidant defense mechanisms or generate oxidants.

Clinical Features and Diagnosis

The earliest manifestations are related to the effects on the tracheobronchial mucosa. Symptoms may occur after 6 hours of O_2 exposure and include substernal chest pain that is prominent with inspiration, tachypnea, and a nonproductive cough. By 24 hours, paresthesia, anorexia, nausea, and headache occur. Physiologic changes include a decrease in tracheal mucous velocity, vital capacity, pulmonary compliance, and diffusing capacity and increased $Pao_2 - Pao_2$. Some individuals develop signs of mild airway obstruction. Chest radiography demonstrates an alveolar and interstitial pattern.

Management

Both hyperoxia and hypoxemia have undesirable effects. The goal is to deliver the lowest level of Fio_2 needed for maintaining adequate arterial O_2 saturation (generally, a Pao_2 >90 mm Hg). Measures such as PEEP should be used for decreasing the need for high Fio_2. In cases of oxygen toxicity, corticosteroid therapy may be useful in reducing antioxidant enzyme activity.

AUTOIMMUNE DISORDERS

Autoimmune diseases, connective tissue diseases, collagenosis, and *rheumatologic diseases* are terms used interchangeably in clinical medicine.

BOX 29.15 Pulmonary Manifestations of Collagen Vascular Diseases

Rheumatoid Arthritis
- Pleural disease (effusions)
- Diffuse interstitial pneumonitis
- Necrobiotic nodules
- Caplan syndrome
- Pulmonary hypertension (arteritis)
- Apical fibrobullous disease
- Bronchiolitis obliterans with and without organizing pneumonia
- Cricoarytenoid arthritis

Systemic Lupus Erythematosus
- Pleural disease (pleuritis, effusions)
- Atelectasis
- Acute lupus pneumonitis
- Diffuse interstitial lung disease
- Pulmonary hemorrhage
- Respiratory muscle dysfunction

Progressive Systemic Sclerosis
- Diffuse interstitial fibrosis
- Pulmonary vascular disease
- Aspiration pneumonia
- Chest-wall restrictions secondary to thoracic skin sclerosis
- Pleural disease

Polymyositis—Dermatomyositis
- Interstitial pneumonitis
- Aspiration pneumonia
- Respiratory myositis
- Pulmonary hypertension
- Bronchiolitis obliterans organizing pneumonia

Mixed Connective Tissue Disease
- Diffuse interstitial lung disease
- Pulmonary hypertension (vasculitis)
- Pleural disease
- Diaphragmatic muscle dysfunction

Sjögren Syndrome
- Respiratory mucosal dryness
- Pleurisy
- Chronic airway disease
- Lymphocytic interstitial pneumonia
- Pseudolymphoma
- Lymphoma
- Amyloid
- Pulmonary hypertension (vasculitis)

These entities are often characterized by multiple-organ involvement and inflammation. Most of these disorders have unknown causes; however, the inflammatory process is immunologically mediated, as evidenced by the presence of autoantibodies, rheumatoid factor, and immune complexes, as well as by elevation of the sedimentation rate and the observation of certain clinical characteristics. Pulmonary manifestations are common and often assume a major role in the disease process. Characteristic restrictive lung changes may result if pulmonary impairment is sufficiently severe. Box 29.15 lists pulmonary manifestations of various collagen vascular diseases.

Sarcoidosis

Sarcoidosis is a multisystemic disorder characterized by the presence of epithelioid-cell granulomata. It is described as an intense interaction of activated lymphocytes and macrophages that results in tissue injury. The disease most often involves the lungs, reticuloendothelial system, skin, eyes, and myocardium. The prevalence of disease globally is 16.5/100,000 men and 19/100,000 women. The disease predominantly occurs in those aged 20 to 40 years.[299] A preponderance of the disease among blacks and varying phenotypes among other ethnic groups points to a strong genetic influence.[300] The cause of sarcoidosis is unclear; no organic or inorganic causative agent has been consistently found. The route of transmission also is uncertain and may be related to human lymphocyte antigen polymorphisms, which lead to granuloma formation after various interactions of antigens, HLA molecules, and T-cell receptors.[301] Interferon-γ and cytokines such as TNF-α, IL-12, and IL-18 play a critical role in the formation of granulomatous lesions.[302]

Most sarcoid granulomata resolve spontaneously, leaving no scar. Others persist for a longer duration, with little or no fibrosis, and still others become hyalinized, fibrotic areas that cause tissue damage. Pulmonary involvement is primarily in regions rich in lymphatic vessels, such as the subpleural, perivascular, and peribronchial areas. Often, adjacent nonspecific inflammatory changes, as well as alveolitis with cellular infiltrates, are noted.[303]

Parenchymal infiltration and fibrosis result in a decrease in lung compliance, impairment of diffusing capacity, and a reduction in lung volumes. A restrictive pattern of ventilation is usually observed, but many patients exhibit a reduced FEV_1:FVC and increased airway resistance. $\dot{V}/\dot{Q}$ imbalance and a decrease in Pao_2 occur in response to a nonuniform decrease in lung compliance. An obstructive pattern resulting from endobronchial disease or peribronchial fibrosis may occur simultaneously. Pulmonary hypertension occurs in varying percentages but is reportedly as high as 50% to 70% in some groups (particularly lung transplant patients).[304] Cor pulmonale may develop in the presence of severe pulmonary fibrosis. Inhaled prostacyclin and sildenafil may be used to reduce pulmonary hypertension.

Clinical presentation is varied and may be categorized as asymptomatic (occurring in 20% of individuals investigated and based on the detection of abnormality of chest radiography) or symptomatic (characterized by nonspecific features ranging from fever, fatigue, anorexia, weight loss, chills, and night sweats to dyspnea and blindness). The lung is the most commonly affected organ, with pulmonary involvement occurring in more than 90% of individuals with sarcoidosis.[301] Respiratory symptoms are those typical of interstitial involvement and include dyspnea, dry cough, and retrosternal chest pain (35%–50% of patients). Less common symptoms include wheezing, hemoptysis, pleural effusion, and clubbing of the fingers. Sarcoidosis is one of the few chest diseases that concurrently involve lymph nodes in the lung (hilar region) and the mediastinum. On radiography, intrathoracic involvement has been classified into four categories. Stage I is characterized by bilateral, symmetric, hilar, and mediastinal adenopathy; stage II by hilar adenopathy and diffuse pulmonary infiltrates; stage III by diffuse pulmonary infiltrates without adenopathy; and stage IV by pulmonary fibrosis.[301] Stage I is associated with the most favorable prognosis, and stage IV with the poor outcomes.

The diagnosis of sarcoidosis requires evidence of multisystem disease (i.e., multiorgan presence of granulomas). Extrathoracic involvement typically involves lymphatics, skin, liver, eye, spleen, and bone. Salivary glands, heart, nervous system, and larynx involvement occur in small percentages. Although not a common site, laryngeal involvement should cause concern about possible difficulty with airway instrumentation, and awake intubation techniques should be considered if

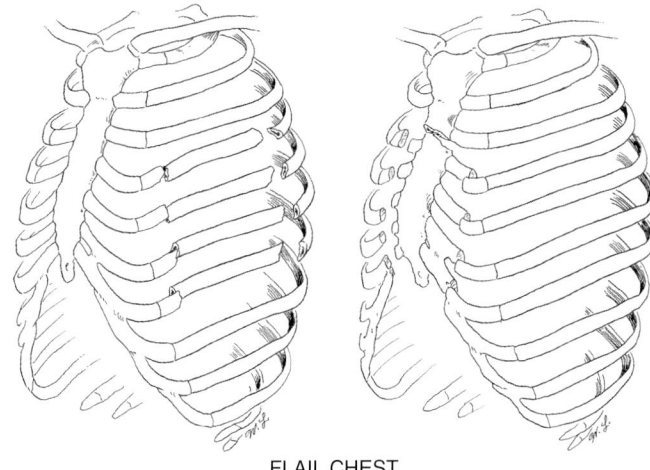

FLAIL CHEST

Fig. 29.26 Fracture of several adjacent ribs in two places with lateral flail or central flail segments. (From Marx JA, et al., eds. *Rosen's Emergency Medicine: Concepts and Clinical Practice.* 9th ed. Philadelphia: Elsevier; 2017.)

intubation is required. Laryngeal involvement is signaled by hoarseness, dyspnea, dysphagia, dysphonia, cough, or stridor. When laryngeal involvement exists, it affects the supraglottic area in 80% and the subglottic area in 20%.[299] Tracheotomy, transoral resection, corticosteroids, and laser resection may be used to treat laryngeal granulomas.

The overall prognosis in sarcoidosis is good. The acute onset is usually followed by a self-limiting course of approximately a 2-year duration with spontaneous resolution in approximately 20%. Although controversial, treatment with corticosteroids (topical, inhaled, enteral, or parenteral) is frequently used and can produce relief of symptoms, clinical remissions, and suppression of inflammation and granuloma formation. Other therapies include methotrexate, azathioprine, leflunomide, and mycophenolate.[301] Infliximab has been found to be effective in treating sarcoidosis because of its role as a monoclonal antibody to TNF, which has a prominent role in sarcoidosis.[305,306]

The mortality rate for patients with sarcoidosis after 5 years is approximately 4% to 10% and is attributed to respiratory failure, azotemia from renal injury caused by chronic hypercalciuria, cardiac arrest resulting from myocardial involvement, and/or massive hemoptysis due to colonization of bullae by *Aspergillus fumigatus*.

FLAIL CHEST

Flail chest is a condition that results from chest trauma and multiple rib fractures. It is reported to occur in 5% of patients who sustain thoracic injury (Fig. 29.26).[307] The hallmark of flail chest is paradoxic movement of the chest wall at the site of the fracture. During inspiration, the chest wall is drawn inward, owing to the negative intrathoracic pressure; it is drawn outward during expiration, when the intrathoracic pressure increases above atmospheric pressure (Fig. 29.27). Inefficient lung inflation caused by rib fracture and paradoxic breathing limits alveolar ventilation and may progress to hypoventilation, hypercapnia, and progressive alveolar collapse.[308] Treatment includes pain control with interventions that may include intercostal nerve block with a local anesthetic or insertion of an epidural catheter with a local anesthetic or opioid. In severe cases, tracheal intubation with mechanical ventilation and PEEP may be required (Box 29.16). Ventilator settings are adjusted so that wide fluctuations in pleural pressure are decreased or avoided. Surgical fixation of the rib cage may be indicated in some patients for persistent pain, severe chest-wall instability, or a progressive decline in

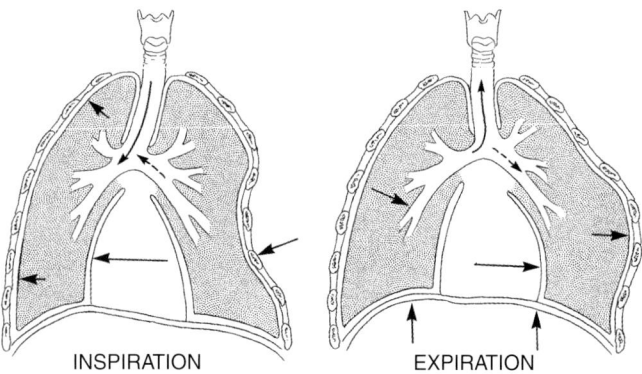

Fig. 29.27 Flail chest: paradoxic respiration. On inspiration, flail section sinks in as chest expands, impairing ability to produce negative intrapleural pressure to draw in air. Mediastinum shifts to uninjured side. On expiration, flail segment bulges outward, impairing ability to exhale. Mediastinum shifts to injured side. Air may shift uselessly from side to side in severe flail chest (broken arrows). (Redrawn from Marx JA, et al, eds. *Rosen's Emergency Medicine: Concepts and Clinical Practice.* 9th ed. Philadelphia: Elsevier; 2017.)

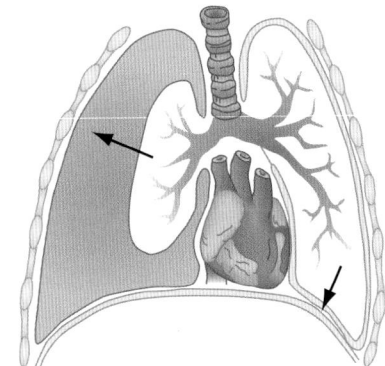

Fig. 29.28 Closed pneumothorax. Simple pneumothorax is present in the right lung, with air in the pleural cavity and collapse of right lung. *Arrow* in right lung indicates the right lungs inability to expand because of the trapped intrathoracic air. *Arrow* in the left lung indicates the left lungs limited ability to expand as intrathoracic pressure increases. (From Marx JA, et al, eds. *Rosen's Emergency Medicine: Concepts and Clinical Practice.* 9th ed. Philadelphia: Elsevier; 2017.)

> **BOX 29.16 Indications for Treatment of Flail Chest With Mechanical Ventilation**
>
> Respiratory failure manifested by one or more of the following criteria:
> - Clinical signs of respiratory fatigue
> - Respiratory rate >35/min or <8 min
> - P_{AO_2} <60 mm Hg at F_{IO_2} ≥0.5
> - Pa_{CO_2} <55 mm Hg at F_{IO_2} ≥0.5
> - Alveolar-arterial oxygen gradient >450
> - Clinical evidence of severe shock
> - Associated severe head injury with lack of airway control or need to ventilate
> - Severe associated injury necessitating surgery

pulmonary function testing in a patient with flail chest.[309] The mortality rate is directly related to the underlying and associated injuries. It has been reported to be between 8% and 35%.[308]

PNEUMOTHORAX

Pneumothorax can be subdivided into three categories, depending on whether air has direct access to the pleural cavity.

Simple Pneumothorax

In simple pneumothorax, no communication exists between the atmosphere and the pleural space (Fig. 29.28). Additionally, no shift of the mediastinum or hemidiaphragm results from the accumulation of air in the intrapleural space. The severity of pneumothorax is graded on the basis of the degree of collapse: Collapse of 15% or less is small, collapse of 15% to 60% is moderate, and collapse of greater than 60% is large. Treatment of a simple pneumothorax is determined by the size and cause of injury and may include catheter aspiration or tube thoracostomy; close observation of the patient with simple pneumothorax is essential.

Communicating Pneumothorax

With a communicating pneumothorax, air in the pleural cavity exchanges with atmospheric air through a wound or defect in the chest wall (Fig. 29.29). A communicating pneumothorax represents a severe

ventilatory disturbance because the affected lung collapses on inspiration and expands slightly on expiration. The exchange of air in and out of the wound results in a large functional dead space and a decrease in the efficacy of ventilation.

The chest wall opening should immediately be covered with an occlusive dressing. The dressing should be taped on three sides to prevent influx of air on inspiration and allow egress of air from inside the thorax on expiration to avoid the development of tension pneumothorax. Treatment measures include administration of supplemental O_2, tube thoracostomy, and intubation. Mechanical ventilation may be indicated.

Tension Pneumothorax

Tension pneumothorax develops when air progressively accumulates under pressure within the pleural cavity (Fig. 29.30). If the pressure becomes too great, the mediastinum shifts to the opposite hemithorax, and this causes compression of the contralateral lung and great vessels. Subsequently, venous return is decreased, and air enters the pleural space but cannot exit. Respiratory and cardiac disturbances commonly manifest as decreases in blood pressure and cardiac output an increase in CVP, altered $\dot{V}/\dot{Q}$ with shunting of blood to nonventilated areas, and hypoxemia. The hallmark signs associated with a tension pneumothorax are hypotension, low O_2 saturation, tachypnea, tachycardia, increased CVP, and increased airway pressure. Other findings include absence of breath sounds on the affected side, asymmetric chest-wall movement, tracheal shift, displacement of the cardiac impulse, and hyperresonance to percussion in the affected hemithorax. The patient may exhibit extreme anxiety.

Tension pneumothorax is potentially lethal, and immediate treatment is essential. Decompression of the chest can be performed with the insertion of a 14-gauge angiocatheter into the second or third rib interspace anteriorly or the fourth or fifth rib interspace laterally. A rush of air may be heard when decompression successfully occurs. Angiocatheter decompression is only an immediate temporizing measure since a chest tube, via a finger thoracostomy, is required for definitive decompression of the tension pneumothorax.

Hemothorax

A hemothorax is caused by the accumulation of blood in the pleural cavity. It is usually a result of trauma (Fig. 29.31), but other causes include the rupture of small blood vessels in the presence of inflammation, pneumonia, tuberculosis, or erosion by tumors.

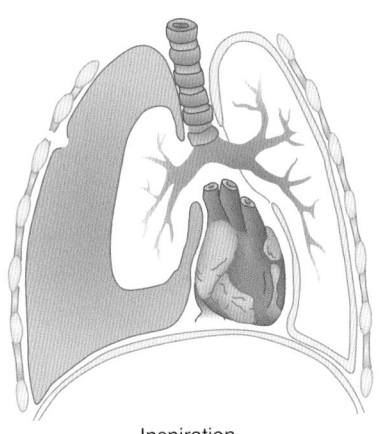
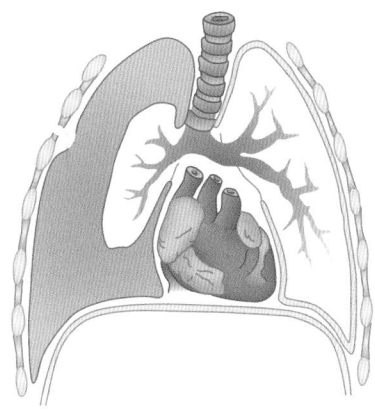

Inspiration   Expiration

Fig. 29.29 Communicating pneumothorax. The right lung has collapsed, and air is present in the pleural cavity, with communication to the outside through the defect in the chest wall. In sucking chest wounds, lung volume is greater with expiration. (From Marx JA, et al, eds. *Rosen's Emergency Medicine: Concepts and Clinical Practice.* 9th ed. Philadelphia: Elsevier; 2017.)

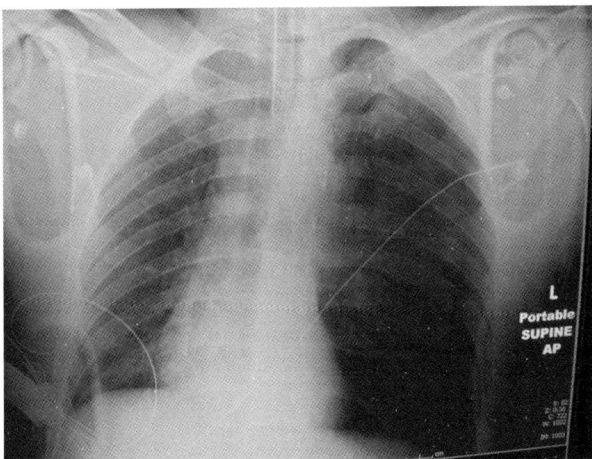

Fig. 29.30 Tension pneumothorax. Hyperlucency is noted, mostly toward the left lung base, because the x-ray is a supine exposure. Shift of the mediastinum toward the right is noted. (From Marx JA, et al, eds. *Rosen's Emergency Medicine: Concepts and Clinical Practice.* 9th ed. Philadelphia: Elsevier; 2017.)

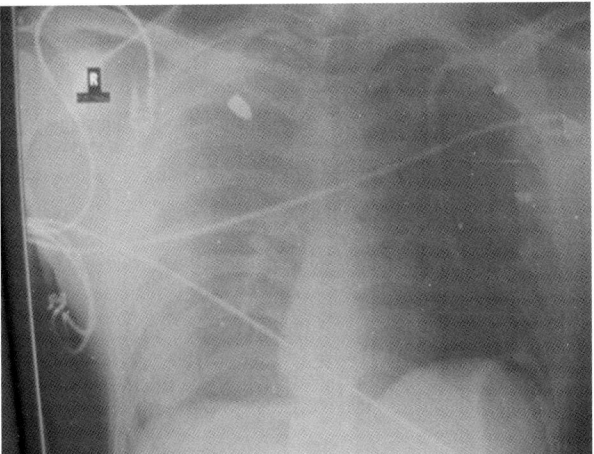

Fig. 29.31 Hemothorax secondary to gunshot wound. Note haziness over right hemithorax with bullet seen in right upper lobe. (From Marx JA, et al, eds. *Rosen's Emergency Medicine: Concepts and Clinical Practice.* 9th ed. Philadelphia: Elsevier; 2017.)

The treatment of hemothorax consists of airway management as necessary, restoration of circulating blood volume, and evacuation of the accumulated blood. Thoracostomy may be indicated if the initial bleeding rate is greater than 20 mL/kg/hr. If bleeding subsides but its rate remains greater than 7 mL/kg/hr, if chest radiograph worsens, or if hypotension persists after initial blood replacement and decompression, then a thoracostomy is indicated.

Pathogenesis

Different presentations may be distinguished, according to the mechanism of injury.

Spontaneous. Pneumothorax is usually caused by rupture of alveoli near the pleural surface of the lung after a forceful sneeze or cough. This mechanism is most common in individuals with a long, narrow chest and in those with emphysema.

Traumatic. Hemothorax, pneumothorax, tension pneumothorax, and/or flail chest may occur after blunt or penetrating chest trauma. However, these most often occur after rib fracture. Hemopneumothorax is probably more common with a penetrating injury.

Iatrogenic. Hemothorax and pneumothorax may occur after any of the following:

- Subclavian central line insertion (incidence 2%–16%)
- Supraclavicular or infraclavicular brachial plexus block (interscalene and intercostal block are possible, but less prevalent causes)
- Barotrauma (resulting from overdistention of the alveoli by PEEP or high peak pressure; abrupt deterioration of Pao_2 and cardiovascular function during mechanical ventilation should arouse suspicion of pulmonary barotrauma, especially pneumothorax)
- Other surgical procedures (e.g., mediastinoscopy, radical neck dissection, mastectomy, axillary lymph node dissection, or nephrectomy)

Nitrous Oxide and Pneumothorax

The blood-gas partition coefficient of N_2O (0.47) is 34 times greater than that of nitrogen (0.014). This differential solubility allows N_2O to leave the blood and enter an air-filled cavity 34 times more rapidly than nitrogen can leave the cavity and enter the blood. As a result, the volume or pressure with the air-filled cavity increases. An often-cited study determined that 75% N_2O doubles the volume of a pneumothorax in 10 minutes.[310] N_2O is theoretically acceptable if the chest tube, treating a pneumothorax, is patent and functioning because little pleural air should be present, and any accumulation should be evacuated by the chest tube. A closed pneumothorax is a contraindication for the administration of N_2O. There should be a high suspicion for an unrecognized pneumothorax in patients with a history of chest trauma who develop a decrease in pulmonary compliance (i.e., increased pulmonary inspiratory pressures) during administration of anesthesia.

ATELECTASIS

Definition

Atelectasis is an abnormal condition characterized by a collapse of pulmonary tissue that prevents the alveolar exchange of CO_2 and O_2. Atelectasis can involve a small, localized area or an entire lung. Atelectasis is common with all general anesthetics. It commonly develops within the first few minutes of induction of anesthesia, regardless of the mode of ventilation used, and can persist for hours to days after anesthesia, depending on the extent and location of surgery.[311] Atelectasis commonly forms adjacent to the diaphragm in dependent lung regions. Compression of lung tissue, absence of diaphragmatic-induced negative pressure, impaired surfactant, and absorption of oxygen from nitrogen-free alveoli are common causes of atelectasis. Atelectasis and airway closure are responsible for the vast majority of impaired gas exchange observed under anesthesia and can affect as much as 90% of patients who receive a general anesthetic.[312]

Etiology and Pathophysiology

Atelectasis can result from a blockage or obstruction of many small bronchi or of a major bronchus. The loss of diaphragmatic tone and function during general anesthesia is a major contributing factor to atelectasis, which characteristically develops within minutes after anesthesia induction. As small airways close due to maldistribution of ventilation under positive pressure breathing, or due to the cephalad migration of abdominal contents, the gas within the affected alveoli is absorbed, and there is no further ventilation to reopen those alveoli. Reduction in the Fio_2 can help reduce the degree of atelectasis (as measured by the shunt fraction).[313]

Incidence and Outcome

Atelectasis occurs almost universally under general anesthesia and is the most common cause of postoperative respiratory dysfunction. Postoperatively, it occurs most often after thoracic and upper abdominal procedures, with incidence rates reaching 80%. In lower risk surgeries, postoperative atelectasis is most often subclinical and resolves spontaneously within 24 to 48 hours. No evidence supports whether atelectasis predisposes one to the development of pneumonia.

Treatment

Historically, practitioners used large tidal volumes (10–15 mL/kg) to combat atelectasis intraoperatively. Although the concept of injury related to high-pressure barotraumas has been long understood, the understanding of ventilator-associated lung injury being related to high ventilating volumes, even in the presence of moderate-peak inspiratory pressures (volutrauma), has changed the approach to establishing ventilator tidal volumes.[258,273,314] To reduce the deleterious effect of high volumes, smaller tidal volumes of 6 to 8 mL/kg are more beneficial for mechanical ventilation, particularly in cases of respiratory distress syndromes. There is evidence that this reduction in tidal volume does not worsen the degree of atelectasis.[315] The use of PEEP and various maneuvers to reopen (recruit) and maintain alveoli have been proposed to reduce atelectasis.[316] A vital capacity maneuver can be used as a recruitment exercise by intermittently expanding the lung to 30 cm H_2O and holding that pressure for approximately 10 seconds.[313,317] Such recruitment maneuvers are most effective when combined with other strategies such as reduction in Fio_2 or open-lung ventilation approaches.

Open-lung ventilation describes a myriad of approaches to providing mechanical ventilation with the goal of preventing atelectasis. Pressure-control inverse ratio ventilation (PC-IRV) and airway pressure release ventilation (APRV) are approaches designed to maintain a higher mean lung volume and thereby reduce airway closure and atelectasis. APRV is analogous to CPAP, with intermittent release phases that allow the lung volume to drop briefly and permit exhalation. APRV provides several advantages over more controlled ventilation modes (such as PC-IRV) since it can be used in spontaneously breathing patients allowing a preservation of respiratory effort and airway protective reflexes. Neuromuscular blockade is not required, and it causes less patient-ventilator dyssynchrony.[318]

Standard postoperative measures for improving pulmonary function include incentive spirometry, deep breathing, intermittent positive pressure breathing, and administration of CPAP. The use of CPAP is the most effective method for increasing FRC from the interventions previously listed.

PLEURAL EFFUSION

Pleural effusion is the abnormal accumulation of fluid in the pleural space. It is usually an indication of disorders or disease complications in the surrounding structures. Possible causes of effusion are (1) blockage of lymphatic drainage from the pleural cavity; (2) cardiac failure, which causes an increase in pulmonary capillary pressures and eventual movement of fluid into the pleural cavity; (3) reductions in plasma colloid osmotic pressure; and (4) infection or any other inflammatory process of the pleural membranes that alters capillary membrane permeability.

Treatment modalities include tube thoracostomy, thoracentesis, and pleurodesis. Pleurodesis is a procedure used to prevent the reaccumulation of pleural fluid. Inflammation is produced with injection of a sclerosing agent, usually tetracycline, into the chest tube; adhesion formation and fusion of the pleural membranes result.

SKELETAL DISORDERS

The primary pathophysiology of skeletal disorders is an alteration in the structure of the thorax that diminishes chest-wall excursion. Disorders commonly producing this restriction of breathing include sternal deformities, kyphoscoliosis, and ankylosing spondylitis.

Pectus Deformities

Pectus Excavatum

Pectus excavatum, also referred to as funnel chest, is the most common chest-wall deformity, occurring in 1 in 400 children.[319] It is a congenital anomaly characterized by depression of the sternum (usually above the xiphoid-sternal junction) and symmetric or asymmetric prominence of the ribs on either side. Pectus excavatum is a genetically heritable abnormality that is associated with adolescent scoliosis.[320] If uncorrected, the disease usually worsens at adolescence. A widely used surgical procedure, the Nuss procedure, inserts a metal rod behind the sternum to reverse the concavity.[321]

Clinically, the majority of patients are asymptomatic unless pectus excavatum is extreme. Patients with pectus excavatum have reduced chest cavities and TLC compared with normal individuals. However, pulmonary function is often normal except in severe cases where vital capacity, TLC, and maximum breathing capacity may be diminished. The indications for repair of pectus excavatum are the subject of controversy. Conflicting data have been presented regarding whether the repair of pectus excavatum is performed only for cosmetic purposes or whether it improves cardiorespiratory function and exercise toler-ance.[321] Patients with Marfan syndrome have a high incidence of chest-wall deformities. They are usually seen in their most severe form and are often accompanied by scoliosis. Other musculoskeletal diseases may be present in patients with pectus excavatum. Congenital heart disease, mitral valve prolapse, and asthma also occur more frequently in patients with pectus excavatum. ECG abnormalities are common and attributable to the abnormal chest-wall configuration, as well as the displacement and rotation of the heart into the left thoracic cavity. A systolic ejection murmur of grades II to III or IV is often identified.

Pectus Carinatum

Pectus carinatum is characterized by a longitudinal protrusion of the sternum. It is the second most common chest deformity, occurring in 1 or 2 persons per 1000. A familial tendency exists, and the disorder is more frequent in males than in females (4:1). The pathogenesis is unclear, and the disorder may be congenital or acquired. The develop-ment of pectus carinatum is thought to result from the overgrowth of the costal cartilages, which results in displacement of the sternum. The development of pectus carinatum has also been associated with severe childhood asthma and rickets.[322] The physiologic effects are probably related to the restriction of thoracic excursion. Patients with pectus carinatum have an increased incidence of congenital heart disease, including ventricular septal defect, patent ductus arteriosus, atrial-septal defects, and mitral valve abnormalities.[323] Surgery is the only effective treatment for pectus carinatum, and it is performed to allevi-ate possible cardiopulmonary dysfunction and to prevent progressive postural deformities, as well as for cosmetic reasons.

Kyphoscoliosis

Definition

Kyphosis is a deformity marked by an accentuated posterior curvature of the spine. Scoliosis is a lateral curvature. Kyphoscoliosis results when kyphosis and scoliosis occur concomitantly, causing a lateral bending and rotation of the vertebral column. Scoliosis alone, despite its sever-ity, does not cause sensory or motor impairment. In contrast, kyphosis and kyphoscoliosis may cause spinal cord damage because of the sharp angulation of the spine. Respiratory dysfunction as a result of pulmo-nary restriction from an altered thoracic cage is associated with scolio-sis, significant kyphosis, and severe kyphoscoliosis.

Incidence and Outcome

Scoliosis is the most common spinal deformity, with an incidence of 4 persons per 1000.[324] The etiologic classification of scoliosis is divided into five categories: idiopathic, congenital, neuropathic (e.g., poliomy-elitis, cerebral palsy, syringomyelia, and Friedreich ataxia), myopathic (e.g., muscular dystrophy and amyotonia congenita), and traumatic. Idiopathic scoliosis is the most common deformity, accounting for 80% of all cases. The presence of cervical scoliosis should alert anesthesia personnel to potential difficulties in airway management. Any signif-icant curvature involving the thoracic spine may alter lung function. Unless the deformity is severe, patients with kyphosis are generally able to maintain normal pulmonary function. In contrast, even mild forms of scoliosis can result in impaired ventilatory function.

Although not totally consistent, vital capacity and FEV_1 less than 50% of that predicted during initial testing suggest an increased risk of pulmonary complications postoperatively.[325-327] The Cobb angle (being >100–110 degrees) is also moderately predictive of restrictive disease and potential pulmonary complications.[325,326]

Severe thoracic deformity may result in respiratory alterations during sleep. Several types of breathing abnormalities have been

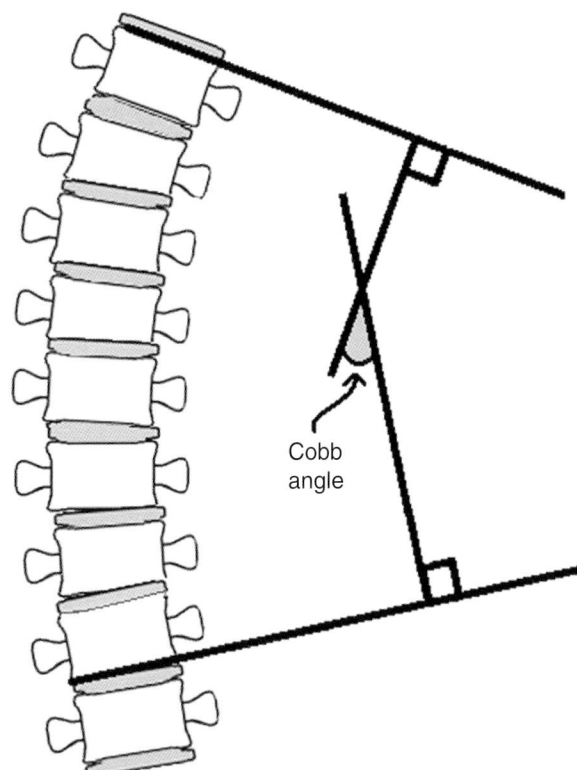

Fig. 29.32 Cobb method of measuring scoliosis curves. The most tilted vertebrae above and below the curve are identified. Horizontal lines are drawn parallel with the plane of each vertebra. Perpendicular lines inter-secting those horizontal lines intersect at the angle of curvature.

documented, including obstructive apnea and hypopnea. The lowest O_2 saturations occurred during REM sleep.[328,329] Because of chronic effects on the pulmonary system, surgical correction of these spinal abnormalities does not result in immediate improvements, and in fact abrupt and short-term deterioration of respiratory mechanics can occur during the procedure while patients are anesthetized.[330]

Clinical Features and Diagnosis

Reduced pulmonary function occurs with curvatures of greater than 60 degrees, and pulmonary symptoms can develop with curvatures greater than 70 degrees (as measured by the Cobb technique) (Fig. 29.32). Curvatures of greater than 100 degrees may be associated with significant restriction and gas exchange impairment.[331] In general, the greater the curvature, the greater the loss of pulmonary function, and the greater the risk of inefficient gas exchange.[329] At the time of diag-nosis, it is often possible to document a reduction in lung capacity. The characteristic deformity seen in scoliosis causes one hemithorax to become relatively smaller than the other.

Skeletal chest-wall deformity in kyphoscoliosis leads to a develop-mental reduction in both lung volumes and the pulmonary vascular bed.[332] Ventilatory failure associated with severe kyphoscoliosis pro-duces a lung size that is 30% to 65% of normal. As the patient ages, the chest wall becomes less compliant; this increases the work of breathing and leads to hypoventilation and respiratory muscle weakness.

The main features of lung mechanics in the patient with early-stage scoliosis are reduced lung volumes (vital capacity, TLC, FRC, and RV) and reduced chest-wall compliance. In the late stages of disease, $\dot{V}/\dot{Q}$ mismatching with hypoxemia (attributed to alveolar hypoventilation because of a decrease in Vt), increased PAP, hypercapnia, abnormal response to CO_2 stimulation, increased work of breathing, and cor pulmonale occur and eventually lead to cardiorespiratory failure.[332] Reduction in vital capacity to 60% to 80% of the predicted value is a typical finding.[331] FEV_1:FVC is normal unless other pulmonary diseases are present. Although normocarbia prevails for most of the clinical course, an elevated $PaCO_2$ signifies the onset of respiratory failure. The severity of hypercapnia most closely correlates with the patient's age and inspiratory muscle strength.

Associated Conditions

Scoliosis may be associated with several cardiovascular abnormalities, of which mitral valve prolapse is the most common. If mitral regurgitation is present, antibiotic prophylaxis is indicated before surgical manipulation. Other common changes include an increase in PVR and ensuing PAH, which leads to the development of right ventricular hypertrophy. Several contributing factors are thought to be responsible for the development of increased PVR. First, arterial hypoxemia results in pulmonary vasoconstriction. Second, changes in the pulmonary arterioles as a consequence of the increased pulmonic pressure may cause narrowing and result in irreversible PAH. Third, a compressed chest wall may increase vascular resistance in affected areas. Lastly, development of scoliosis at an early age inhibits growth of the pulmonary vascular bed.

Treatment

The management of scoliosis may include (1) observation of the problem without active medical treatment, (2) treatment by nonoperative methods that include the use of braces or electronic stimulators, and (3) operative methods such as anterior or posterior spinal fusion and instrumentation such as Harrington rod insertion.[333] Debate continues regarding the long-term effectiveness of various treatment modalities concerning short- and long-term complications that can also arise after surgery.[334]

Anesthetic Management

Preoperative evaluation. The severity of scoliosis and any underlying conditions must be noted. Any reversible pulmonary involvement such as pneumonia should be corrected before elective surgery. ABG analysis may be indicated if there is suspicion of significant pulmonary impairment. Because these procedures can potentially involve large blood losses, autologous blood can be donated by young, healthy, asymptomatic patients. Blood typing and crossmatch are also required.

When sedatives are used in the preoperative area, care must be taken to ensure that respiratory status is not depressed. The need for intraoperative monitoring is dictated by the type of surgery and the physical status of the patient. No specific anesthetic techniques have been shown to be superior in patients with scoliosis, but N_2O may increase PVR by direct vasoconstrictive effects on the pulmonary vasculature. It has been suggested that scoliosis is associated with an increased incidence of malignant hyperthermia, but concrete evidence is lacking.[335]

With significant manual distraction of the spine during the procedure, assessment of neural integrity may be required using somatosensory and motor-evoked potentials. Although increasingly less common, a "wake-up" test may be requested after placement of surgical instrumentation. This should be communicated between surgeon and anesthetist prior to the procedure. At the designated time, the anesthetic is lightened and the patient is observed to follow commands and demonstrate motor function. The anesthetic must be planned to allow the patient to become able to hear and follow commands, while still tolerating the ETT in the prone position. After successful demonstration, anesthesia is rapidly reinstituted to facilitate the conclusion of the procedure.

The use of somatosensory-evoked potentials and motor-evoked potential monitoring has reduced the requirement for the wake-up test. Neural monitoring, however, also necessitates customization of the anesthetic plan to reduce interference with the signals. High-dose volatile agent concentration or wide swings in anesthetic depth can influence sensory-evoked potential monitoring. Muscle relaxants interfere with motor-evoked response monitoring. All anesthetic agents depress somatosensory-evoked potentials to a varying degree. Administration of volatile anesthetics should not exceed a minimum alveolar concentration of 1 MAC. A technique using continuous infusions of propofol and opioid is a common approach. Communication between the monitoring technician and anesthetist is essential.

Intraoperative management. Considerable fluid and blood loss may occur during surgery. The surgeon may request the institution of deliberate hypotension. Deliberate hypotension can be produced with the use of one or more of the following: potent inhalation anesthetics, vasodilators (e.g., sodium nitroprusside, nitroglycerin), or β-adrenergic blocking agents (e.g., propranolol, esmolol). The risks and potential benefits should be weighed against the effects of deliberate hypotension. Traditional wisdom was that the mean arterial blood pressure can be safely maintained at a lower level of 60 mm Hg. However, the lower limit of cerebral autoregulation is highly variable. Discrepancies between blood pressure measurement devices and the actual perfusion pressure of the brain may be significant. The incidence of both blindness from retinal hypoperfusion in the prone position and cerebral injury from deliberate hypotension call for extreme caution when deliberately lowering the blood pressure during this procedure.[336-338] Hypothermia prevention using a forced air warming blanket, heat-moisture exchange (HME) filter, and warmed intravenous fluids should be used. Careful positioning is essential.

Postoperative care. The decision of whether to use mechanical ventilation postoperatively is based on the severity of scoliosis, the patient's preoperative physical status, and the occurrence of intraoperative events. Most patients with mild to moderate pulmonary dysfunction are able to undergo safe extubation in the operating room. Those with severe deformity should be weaned slowly.

Ankylosing Spondylitis

Definition

Ankylosing spondylitis, also known as rheumatoid spondylitis and Marie-Strumpell disease, is a chronic inflammatory disorder that primarily affects the spine and sacroiliac joints and produces fusion of the spinal vertebrae and the costovertebral joints.

Etiology and Incidence

The cause of ankylosing spondylitis remains unclear. However, it is strongly associated with the histocompatibility antigen HLA-B27, the presence of which is detected in more than 90% of whites with the disease.[339] It is a disease of adults younger than 40 years, and it demonstrates a predilection for males (male:female ratio of 9:1). The disease is rare in nonwhites.

Clinical Features and Diagnosis

Ankylosing spondylitis is diagnosed on the basis of clinical criteria that include (1) chronic low back pain with limitation of spinal motion (<4 cm as measured by the Schober test), (2) radiographic evidence of bilateral sacroiliitis, and (3) limitation of chest-wall expansion (<2.5 cm increase in chest circumference measured at the fourth intercostal space). Extraskeletal manifestations of this disease include iritis, cardiovascular involvement (cardiac conduction defects, aortitis, and aortic insufficiency in 20% of individuals), peripheral arthritis, fever, anemia, fatigue, weight loss, and fibrocavitary (fibrobullous) disease of the apexes of the lungs. The most limiting factors associated with ankylosing spondylitis are pain, stiffness, and fatigue.

Complications

Pulmonary complications are reported to occur in 2% to 70% of patients with ankylosing spondylitis. Apical fibrosis is the most common abnormality, followed by interstitial lung disease, respiratory impairment due to chest-wall restriction, sleep apnea, and spontaneous pneumothorax. A pulmonary lesion begins with apical pleural thickening and patchy consolidation of one or both apexes in apical fibrosis. This often progresses to dense bilateral fibrosis and air space enlargement. Patients with apical fibrosis usually have advanced ankylosing spondylitis. Cardiac complications associated with ankylosing spondylitis include aortic valve diseases, conduction disturbances, cardiomyopathy, and ischemic heart disease.[340]

The most common thoracic complication is fixation of the thoracic cage as a result of costovertebral ankylosis, which causes a restrictive defect and can lead to pulmonary dysfunction.[341] In patients with this complication, motion of the thoracic cage is restricted due to fusion of the costovertebral joints; this restriction leads to a decrease in thoracic excursion. Respiratory function typically demonstrates a restrictive pattern with mild reductions in TLC, vital capacity, and DLCO along with normal or slightly increased RV and FRC. Pulmonary compliance, diffusion capacity, and ABG values are usually normal.[341] Despite having abnormal pulmonary function, the majority of patients with ankylosing spondylitis are able to perform normal physical activities without exhibiting pulmonary symptoms.

Bone ankylosis may occur in the numerous joints around the thorax (i.e., the thoracic vertebrae and the costovertebral, costotransverse, sternoclavicular, and sternomanubrial joints), resulting in limitation of chest-wall movement. Patients with ankylosing spondylitis rarely complain of respiratory symptoms or functional impairment unless they have coexisting cardiovascular or respiratory disease. Progressive kyphosis is equivalent to progressive rigidity of the thorax. Increased diaphragmatic function compensates for decreased thoracic motion, allowing lung function to be well preserved. Regional lung ventilation in patients with ankylosing spondylitis is normal unless they have preexisting apical fibrosis.

Cervical spondylosis can occur in any of the cervical vertebrae. The degenerative changes may result in nerve root entrapment by foraminal encroachment. The phrenic nerve, which innervates the diaphragm, is supplied primarily by the C4 nerve root and to a lesser extent by the C3 and C5 nerve roots. Hemidiaphragmatic paralysis is a rare but potential complication secondary to C4 nerve root compression.

Cricoarytenoid involvement may exist and can lead to respiratory dysfunction and upper airway obstruction. Cricoarytenoid dysfunction can manifest as a hoarse, weak voice, and, depending on the degree of dysfunction, even stridor. Respiratory failure from cricoarytenoid dysfunction can occur requiring therapeutic tracheostomy. In all reported cases, laryngeal symptoms were present before cricoarytenoid arthritis caused airway compromise. A case of acute respiratory failure and cor pulmonale resulting from cricoarytenoid arthritis has also been reported in a patient with ankylosing spondylosis.[342]

Treatment

Medical therapy for adult patients with ankylosing spondylosis is supportive and preventive. Most patients are asymptomatic. Depending on the severity of disease involvement, management may consist of the use of corticosteroids and nonsteroidal antiinflammatory agents.

Anesthetic Management

Patients with ankylosing spondylosis have specific anesthetic requirements.[343] Management of the upper airway is the priority because of the potential for obstruction. Cervical spine involvement may result in limitation of movement. The ankylosed neck is more susceptible to hyperextension injury, and cervical fracture may occur. Awake intubation, with or without the use of a flexible intubating endoscope, is indicated. In rare situations, tracheostomy must be performed with the patient under local anesthesia before anesthesia can be induced. A regional anesthetic technique may not be feasible because of skeletal involvement that precludes access or because of neurologic complications such as spinal cord compression, cauda equina syndrome, focal epilepsy, vertebrobasilar insufficiency, and peripheral nerve lesions. Patients with cardiovascular system involvement may require antibiotic coverage, treatment of heart failure, or insertion of a temporary pacemaker before surgery. Restriction of chest expansion necessitates a thorough pulmonary assessment, and immediate postoperative mechanical ventilation is likely. Careful attention for proper positioning is essential.

▌SUMMARY

A comprehensive knowledge of respiratory anatomy and physiology is needed to conduct an accurate patient assessment and manage relevant pathophysiology. An understanding of anatomic characteristics (i.e., the shorter, straighter, right mainstem bronchus), physiologic derangements from anesthesia (i.e., atelectasis and ventilation-perfusion mismatches), perianesthetic complications (i.e., aspiration pneumonitis), preexisting illnesses (such as COPD), and iatrogenic illnesses (i.e., chemotherapeutic-induced pulmonary toxicity) will assist in the proper care of patients with these pulmonary concerns.

REFERENCES

For a complete list of references for this chapter, scan this QR code with any smartphone code reader app, or visit the following URL: http://booksite.elsevier.com/9780323711944/.

30

Anesthesia for Thoracic Surgery

Michael Rieker, Caroline Killmon

Thoracic surgery is greatly facilitated by the contribution of anesthesia care, which can isolate the movement of one lung during ventilation and create a quiet surgical field. Although this procedure requires advanced techniques related to airway management, it has been in existence almost as long as tracheal intubation itself. In 1928, Guedel, Magill, Waters, and other pioneers first achieved closed endotracheal anesthesia. The treatment of tuberculosis and empyema, however, required isolation of the infected lung, and in 1931 Joseph Gale and Ralph Waters first described "closed endobronchial anesthesia." Bronchial blockade for selective ventilation and lung isolation was reported by Magill in 1936. In 1950 Björk and Carlens were credited with the first use of a double-lumen endotracheal tube (ETT) for thoracic surgery, the bronchospirometric double-lumen tube (DLT), which Carlens described the year before.[1,2] DLTs evolved in design, and the use of the Fogarty embolectomy catheter for bronchial blockade gave way to the Univent tube invented by Inoue and colleagues.

Development of airway devices is continuously evolving, and anesthetists caring for patients undergoing thoracic surgery must be skilled at insertion, maintenance, and monitoring of these devices for proper function. However, the process of lung isolation facilitates the surgical procedure but compounds a central concern in thoracic anesthesia: maintaining effective gas exchange in the face of ventilation-perfusion (V/Q) mismatch. General anesthesia creates atelectasis, which is compounded by muscle relaxants and lateral positioning, but ventilation and perfusion are further mismatched when the thorax is opened, and ceasing ventilation of one lung is the final insult. Fortunately, physiologic processes such as hypoxic pulmonary vasoconstriction (HPV) combat the inherent shunt, and anesthetic management is geared toward supporting those processes while fostering oxygenation through various ventilation modalities. Hypoxemia during thoracic surgery is defined as a decrease in oxygen saturation (Sao_2) via pulse oximetry of less than 85% to 90%.[3] It also may be defined as an arterial oxygen tension (Pao_2) of less than 60 mm Hg when the patient is being ventilated at an inspired oxygen fraction (Fio_2) of 1%.[3] Previous reports indicated that the incidence of hypoxemia during one-lung ventilation (OLV) was 5% to 10%; however, the incidence of hypoxemia during OLV is currently less than 4% in part because of the use of flexible bronchoscopy to achieve optimal position of lung isolation devices.[3,4] Lesser degrees of hypoxemia are also attributable to the introduction of newer, volatile anesthetics that cause less inhibition of HPV in a dose-dependent manner and less venous admixture during OLV.[3]

Besides managing the complexities of a DLT or bronchial blocker, the anesthetist must also be cognizant of the effects of underlying disease as it relates to management of ventilation (bullous disease contraindicating nitrous oxide [N_2O]), interactions with anesthetic drugs (small cell carcinoma being associated with myasthenic syndrome, volatile anesthetics, and inhibition of HPV), and even concerns about oxygen toxicity (in patients treated with bleomycin and other chemotherapeutics).

PREOPERATIVE PREPARATION

Bronchogenic carcinoma is the leading cause of cancer deaths in the United States, making up almost 25% of cancer deaths.[5] Lung cancer is most often discovered only once the patients exhibit symptoms; even with aggressive multimodal treatment (surgical resection, chemotherapy, radiation, immunotherapy, and gene therapy), prognosis is poor. According to the National Cancer Institute, the 5-year survival rate for lung cancer is 20.5%.[6] However, resection of the affected lung tissue offers a better prognosis as compared to radiation and chemotherapy, so cancer is a common indication for lung surgery. There is a strong association between lung cancer and chronic obstructive pulmonary disease (COPD), such that the incidence of lung cancer is four times higher among COPD sufferers than it is in the general population, and underlying COPD almost doubles the 3-year mortality from lung cancer.[7-9] Many patients presenting for lung surgery will have complex underlying pathology. Therefore evaluating respiratory function and predicting postresection function are crucial to anticipating the patient's intraoperative and postoperative care needs.

The surgical risk assessment for patients in need of pulmonary resection surgery focuses on the risk of potential postoperative complications and whether postoperative pulmonary function will be sufficient to allow for an adequate quality of life. Between 20% and 30% of patients with lung cancer are found to be surgical candidates,[10] and almost 40% of these candidates are disqualified based on poor lung function alone.[11] The anesthetic risk assessment specific to pulmonary surgery focuses on how the underlying pathology will challenge the maintenance of adequate gas exchange and general homeostasis under OLV, and the potential for postoperative respiratory failure to make weaning and extubation difficult. However, mortality from unresected carcinomas is sufficiently high that the risks of postoperative complications would need to be extraordinarily significant before they would preclude surgery. COPD is the progressive destruction of alveoli and lung architecture that occurs over the course of multiple years. Considering the aging nature of our population and the increase in the incidence of obesity, it is not surprising that lung resection surgeries are now being performed on more patients who have end-stage COPD or morbid obesity, or who are of advanced age.[12,13] Evidence shows that these patients can be treated safely. The American College of Chest Physicians (ACCP) does not set a maximal age cutoff for pulmonary surgical candidacy.[14] Changes in surgical techniques, especially the use of video-assisted thoracoscopic surgery (VATS), have markedly decreased the incidence of postoperative pulmonary complications and will necessitate a reevaluation of the testing required for

BOX 30.1 Summary of Preoperative Factors That Predict Postoperative Complications

Factors That Characterize Average Risk
- FEV_1 >2 L or 80% of predicted
- PPO FEV_1 >80% of predicted
- PPO FEV_1 + PPO DLCO both >40%
- $\dot{V}O_2$ max >15 mL/kg/min
- Ability to climb three flights of stairs

Factors That Characterize Elevated Risk
- FEV_1 <2 L or <40% of predicted
- PPO FEV_1 <40% of predicted
- PPO DLCO <40% of predicted
- PPO product (FEV_1 × DLCO) <1650
- $\dot{V}O_2$ max <10 mL/kg/min
- Inability to climb one flight of stairs
- Oxygen desaturation >4% during exercise

DLCO, Diffusing capacity of the lungs for carbon monoxide; FEV_1, forced expiratory volume 1; PPO, predicted postoperative, $\dot{V}O_2$ max, maximum volume of oxygen.

TABLE 30.1 Anesthetic Considerations in Lung Cancer Patients: The Four Ms

Mass effects	Obstructive pneumonia, lung abscess, superior vena cava syndrome, tracheobronchial distortion, Pancoast syndrome, recurrent laryngeal nerve or phrenic nerve paresis, chest wall or mediastinal extension
Metabolic effects	Lambert-Eaton syndrome, hypercalcemia, hyponatremia, Cushing syndrome, syndrome of inappropriate antidiuretic hormone secretion (SIADH)
Metastases	Particularly to brain, bone, liver, and adrenal glands
Medications	Chemotherapy-induced lung changes (bleomycin = pulmonary toxicity, doxorubicin = cardiac toxicity, cisplatin = renal toxicity)

Modified from Slinger PP, Johnston MR. Preoperative assessment and management. In Kaplan JA, Slinger PD, eds. Thoracic Anesthesia. 3rd ed. Philadelphia: Churchill Livingstone; 2003.

preoperative assessment.[15] Given the large physiologic changes that occur after pneumonectomy, complete pulmonary function testing, as well as cardiac testing, is indicated.

Fear of creating pulmonary insufficiency by lung resection is an important concern, and numerous studies have attempted to determine the lowest limit of pulmonary function that will allow surgery to be safely performed. However, research findings are limited in their ability to predict particular complications. Studies performed to predict postoperative pulmonary complications after lung resection demonstrate that patients develop both pulmonary and cardiac complications such as dysrhythmias, myocardial infarction, pulmonary embolism, pneumonia, and empyema. These complications influence the duration of mechanical ventilation and outcome; however, none of these complications can be predicted by preoperative studies of pulmonary function. Box 30.1 presents some commonly used preoperative assessment criteria for lung resection.

History and Physical Examination

Cancer patients who undergo lung resection typically have a history of multiple risk factors and signs of respiratory disease. Risk factors include cigarette smoking, air pollution, and industrial chemical exposure. The smoking history that is so commonly associated with these patients increases the incidence of ischemic heart disease or hypertension. Therefore patients must be evaluated for exertional dyspnea, productive cough, hemoptysis, cyanosis, poor exercise tolerance, and chest pain.

The presence of ischemic cardiac disease that is severe, unstable, or associated with dysrhythmias should indicate consultation from a cardiologist to help mitigate the risk of cardiac complications. Because severe COPD may significantly limit physical activity, a pharmacologic cardiac stress test may be helpful to identify coronary insufficiency.[16] The use of perioperative β-blockade is controversial, and nonselective agents may be particularly detrimental if they inhibit bronchodilation. However, cardioselective β-blockers have been found to be beneficial in COPD patients undergoing vascular surgery.[17] β-blockade may be considered to reduce cardiac risk[18]; at the least, patients currently taking β-blockers should continue their regimen throughout the surgical encounter. The surgical plan must be carefully considered for patients

with coronary diffusion defects that show greater than 20% reversibility. In cases of high-risk cardiac disease, lung surgery may be delayed for 6 weeks to allow coronary artery bypass first.[16] With the increasing popularity of off-bypass coronary revascularization, the two procedures can more easily be performed in a single surgical encounter.[19]

Patients with lung cancer should be assessed for effects of the primary tumor, as well as effects of secondary pathologies and side effects of therapy (Table 30.1). Dyspnea while in the supine position may result from COPD, compression of the airway by a mediastinal mass, or diaphragmatic displacement due to obesity. A high index of suspicion should also be maintained for hormonal abnormalities because many lung tumors cause paraneoplastic syndromes characterized by the secretion of endocrine-like substances such as adrenocorticotropic hormone,[20] antidiuretic hormone,[21] serotonin, parathyroid-like hormone,[22] and insulin-like growth factor,[23] causing a variety of metabolic abnormalities.[24] Cushing disease may lead to metabolic alkalosis, hypokalemia, and hyperglycemia.[25,26] Hypercalcemia occurs in 10% to 25% of patients with lung cancer related to parathyroid-like hormone, increased calcitriol, or overactivity of osteoclasts. The finding of hypercalcemia carries a very poor prognosis. Clinical signs may include polyuria, polydipsia, confusion, vomiting, abdominal cramps, bradycardia, and mental status changes. Treatment of hypercalcemia includes intravenous (IV) hydration with normal saline, loop diuretics, bisphosphonates, calcitonin, or hemodialysis. Neuroendocrine tumors comprise 20% of lung cancers, and 5% of them produce carcinoid syndrome.[27] In those patients, histamine-stimulating drugs and adrenergic agonists may precipitate the flushing, hypotension, and tachyarrhythmias related to serotonin release. Paraneoplastic neurologic syndromes represent autoimmune dysfunctions associated with cancers. In total, 1% to 2% of patients with small cell lung cancer develop Lambert-Eaton myasthenic syndrome (LEMS).[28] In this syndrome, antibodies are formed that inhibit voltage-gated calcium channels. This decreases the release of acetylcholine from presynaptic nerve terminals,[29] resulting in weakness and sensitivity to nondepolarizing muscle relaxants. Usually, the initial presentation with autonomic dysfunction (80% of patients with LEMS) includes orthostatic hypotension followed by weakness that progresses upward from the legs.[30] In contrast to myasthenia gravis, LEMS involves dysfunction of the calcium channels. Repetitive stimulation or activity improves function (as more acetylcholine is mobilized), and anticholinesterase drugs are not an effective treatment. Treatment includes immunoglobulin, corticosteroids, or 3,4-diaminopyridine (3,4-DAP), which opens potassium channels and

BOX 30.2 Preoperative Evaluation of Patients for Pulmonary Surgery

1. Evaluate comorbidities:
   - Smoking-related complications
   - Cor pulmonale
   - Effects of paraneoplasms
   - Cardiovascular disease (unstable angina, MI within 6 weeks, or significant dysrhythmias = high risk of cardiac complications)
2. Treatment side effects (particularly from cytotoxic drugs and radiation)
   - ECG and chest x-ray for signs of cardiovascular dysfunction and effects of lung pathology
3. Laboratory assessment of electrolytes, blood count, albumin, and renal function indicators
4. Lung function testing: 80-40-35-15 rule:
   - FEV_1 and DLCO >80% predicted = no additional testing needed. If <80 or dyspnea present, diffusing capacity and postoperative function should be predicted
   - PPO FEV_1 and DLCO <40% predicted = increased risk; exercise testing should be evaluated
   - VE/VCO_2 slope >35 = increased risk of mortality and postoperative complications
   - $\dot{V}O_2$ max <15 mL/kg/min = increased risk
5. For COPD, consider blood gas and response to bronchodilators

COPD, Chronic obstructive pulmonary disease; *DLCO,* diffusing capacity of the lungs for carbon monoxide; *ECG,* electrocardiogram; *FEV₁,* forced expiratory volume 1; *MI,* myocardial infarction; *PPO,* predicted postoperative; *VE/VCO₂ slope,* measurement of ventilatory efficiency (minute ventilation relative to CO_2 exhalation) normally <30; *$\dot{V}O_2$ max,* maximum volume of oxygen.

increases calcium concentrations in the nerve terminal. Other autoimmune channelopathies can affect voltage-gated potassium channels and prolong acetylcholine release, causing myotonia, or affect autonomic ganglia, causing orthostatic hypotension and arrhythmias.[31]

Physical examination findings in COPD are commonly barrel chest deformity, accessory muscle use or paradoxic breathing movement, pursed-lip breathing, and tympanic percussion notes on the chest. Auscultation reveals rhonchi or wheezing. Signs of cor pulmonale include jugular vein distention or peripheral edema, split S_2 heart sound, pulmonary or tricuspid valve insufficiency murmurs, and rales auscultated over the lungs.[32] Nutritional status, commonly compromised in patients with cancer, is also important to note because hypoalbuminemia and malnutrition are associated with increased postoperative complications such as pneumonia.[33] Box 30.2 lists important elements of the preoperative evaluation.

Diagnostic Data

Chest Radiograph

A chest radiograph should be obtained to determine the presence of associated disease and COPD complications (tumor infringement on airway or vascular structures, bullous disease, congestive heart failure, or pneumothorax). The radiograph does not provide abundant information regarding the degree of COPD, but findings characteristic of COPD include hyperinflation, increased anteroposterior thoracic diameter, and diaphragm flattening. Emphysema-related bullae may be present, and infection or pleural effusions may be noted preoperatively and treated to improve the postoperative course. The locations of masses can be identified. In some patients, it can be ascertained whether lesions compress mediastinal structures, cause tracheal shift,

or invade the airway. This information is important to predict whether intubation will be difficult, whether induction of anesthesia could cause collapse of the airway, or whether surgical dissection may be difficult and potentially involve excessive bleeding. Evidence of increased pulmonary vascular resistance (PVR) resulting from compression of the vascular bed increases the likelihood of right ventricular failure and worsens the prognosis following lung resection. Relevant signs include prominent pulmonary arteries with rapid tapering of the vasculature and a widened right heart border.

Electrocardiogram

An electrocardiogram (ECG) is useful for assessing signs of right ventricular hypertrophy. In such a case, the ECG shows a tall R wave in V_1 (>6 mm), R/S ratio greater than 1 in lead V_1, and a ratio less than 1 in V_6, along with a right-axis deviation and diminished amplitude limb leads.[34-36] Right atrial hypertrophy causes the initial component of a biphasic P wave in lead V_1 to be larger than the second component. Strain characteristics such as ST segment depression and T-wave inversion, as well as incomplete or complete right bundle branch block, may be observed. The ECG has excellent specificity for identifying left ventricular hypertrophy (LVH), but less sensitivity for detecting it.[37,38] Therefore, if ECG criteria are inconclusive, echocardiography may be helpful to further elucidate the status of the right ventricle. Findings of pathologic Q waves and evidence of LVH preoperatively correlate with an increased incidence of postoperative ischemia and infarction.[39]

Echocardiogram

Echocardiographic findings that are consistent with pulmonary disease are increased thickness of the right ventricular free wall, chamber enlargement, septal shift, tricuspid regurgitation, and a decreased right ventricular ejection fraction. In response to chronic hypoxia, HPV causes elevated pulmonary artery pressures. This results in increased right ventricular afterload, which can lead to right ventricular dysfunction. Increased PVR and right ventricular strain cause concern in patients undergoing pneumonectomy or extensive partial resection because of the added resistance produced by clamping the vasculature of one lung in the surgical procedure. Echocardiography is the best initial tool for assessing pulmonary hypertension, but additional studies with pulmonary angiography, ventilation-perfusion scintigraphy, computed tomography (CT), and magnetic resonance imaging (MRI) may also be used for more in-depth evaluation.[40] In an observational study consisting of 105 patients undergoing thoracic surgery, 37% had alterations in their anesthesia management based off transthoracic echocardiography (TTE) findings, mostly reflecting right ventricular pathologies.[41]

Laboratory Assessment

Measurement of preoperative room air arterial blood gases should be considered for patients with COPD, and it is useful in guiding postoperative ventilation. Carbon dioxide (CO_2) retention with an arterial partial pressure ($PaCO_2$) greater than 45 mm Hg is an indicator of poor ventilatory function. However, hypercapnia is not a reliable predictor of increased risk of perioperative pulmonary complications.[42] Preoperative hypoxemia (SaO_2 <85%–90%) and, particularly, desaturation during exercise may be predictive of increased complications following thoracic surgery.[43,44] However, in general, blood gas analysis is not a reliable tool for predicting postoperative pulmonary complications,[45] and the correlation between desaturation during exercise and postoperative complications is not a consistent finding.[46]

Hypoalbuminemia is the most common laboratory finding and serves as an important predictor of pulmonary complications. Numerous studies have demonstrated increases in postoperative pulmonary complications among patients with low serum albumin levels (generally <3.6 g/dL).[47-50] This factor increases risk as much as 2.5 times,[49] and albumin level maintenance is a measured factor in the American College of Surgeons National Surgical Quality Improvement Program (NSQIP).[51] The blood urea nitrogen level is also identified by NSQIP data as a predictive factor for pulmonary complications when it is greater than 22 mg/dL.[49,50]

Other laboratory analyses should include renal function indicators (particularly for patients treated with nephrotoxic drugs such as methotrexate, gemcitabine, and cisplatin),[52,53] sodium (related to syndrome of inappropriate antidiuretic hormone secretion [SIADH]),[24] and calcium (due to parathyroid hormone–like protein).[22,54]

Pulmonary Function Tests

Patients presenting for lung resection should undergo pulmonary function testing to assess for airflow limitation, diffusion defect, and cardiopulmonary reserve.[55] Assessment should include the response to bronchodilators for patients who demonstrate obstructive disease (see Fig. 29.17). The American Thoracic Society considers a 12% improvement in forced expiratory volume 1 (FEV_1) post–bronchodilator therapy to be significant. Whereas this parameter has a low sensitivity to diagnose asthma,[56] the relative responsiveness of the patient to bronchodilators can suggest the utility of using bronchodilators for intraoperative management. Pulmonary assessment by spirometry should be based on values obtained post–bronchodilator therapy, as these would represent the patient's potential lung function once optimized on medications. No single pulmonary function measurement provides an overall risk assessment. For example, although the FEV_1 is the most prevalent spirometric measurement, one case series of 100 thoracic surgery patients with very low FEV_1 values (<35%) demonstrated a low rate of mortality and ventilator dependence (although the patients showed a prolonged duration of hospitalization and air leak).[57] In another series of 109 elderly patients, stair-climbing ability was better correlated (inverse relationship) with postoperative cardiopulmonary complications than was forced vital capacity (FVC) or predicted postoperative (PPO) FEV_1.[58] Therefore a multimodal approach must be taken, considering airflow (PPO FEV_1), parenchymal function (diffusing capacity of the lungs for carbon monoxide [DLCO]), and cardiopulmonary reserve (maximum volume of oxygen [$\dot{V}O_2$ max]). The general cutoff points indicating increased risk among these parameters is below 40% for PPO FEV_1 and DLCO, and 15 mL/kg/min for $\dot{V}O_2$ max. However, the surgical approach must also be considered as part of the risk evaluation. A large study involving more than 13,000 subjects validated that PPO FEV_1 and PPO DLCO estimates were inversely proportional to the rate of complications and mortality. However, the absolute rate of complications and mortality was significantly lower in patients undergoing thoracoscopic, rather than open, lobectomy, even when the PPO FEV_1 and PPO DLCO were less than 40%.[59]

It should be noted that guidelines used to assess surgical candidacy are not intended to dictate candidacy for anesthesia. If the patient is a candidate for surgery, it is less likely that there will be anesthetic-specific concerns about pulmonary function that would override the surgical decision, particularly as many of these surgeries are performed to treat cancer. Notwithstanding this, it is helpful for the anesthetist to understand the patient's risk stratification to plan for the level of ventilatory support required during and after surgery. Assessment must consider multiple functional variables. Similar to standards set by the American Thoracic Society and the European Respiratory Society, the ACCP proposes the following assessment of risk factors for patients with lung cancer undergoing lung surgery: Preoperative FEV_1 greater than 80% of the predicted value (or >2 L for pneumonectomy or >1.5 L for lobectomy) indicates average risk,

and no further assessment of lung function is required. The DLCO should be assessed if diffuse parenchymal disease or dyspnea on exertion is noted. If the FEV_1 or DLCO is less than 80% of the predicted value, then the PPO FEV_1 and DLCO are assessed.[42] This is accomplished either through radionucleotide scanning or mathematically (based on the proportion of total lung that will remain after the planned resection). The PPO FEV_1 can be calculated by multiplying the current FEV_1 by the fraction of functioning lung or the fraction of lung segments that will remain after surgery.[16] For high-risk patients, more detailed assessment via radionuclide scanning, CT scanning, or MRI is advisable. Postoperative PPO FEV_1 values greater than 40% of the predicted value for the patient indicate average risk. Values less than 30% of the predicted value indicate increased risk, and intermediate values warrant exercise testing to assess oxygen consumption ($\dot{V}O_2$ max). A $\dot{V}O_2$ max of less than 15 mL/kg/min indicates high risk, whereas a value greater than 15 mL/kg/min indicates average risk.[42] The European Respiratory Society places $\dot{V}O_2$ max more prominently in the assessment and considers high-risk cutoffs as being less than 30% for PPO FEV_1 and DLCO, and less than 10 mL/kg/min for $\dot{V}O_2$ max.[55] Regarding anesthetic planning, average-risk patients (e.g., PPO FEV_1 >40%) are likely to be extubated immediately following surgery. High-risk patients (e.g., PPO FEV_1 <30%) have a higher likelihood of requiring some degree of postoperative ventilation. Planning for intermediate-risk patients (e.g., PPO FEV_1 30%–40%) is further individualized based on other assessment parameters.

Ventilation-Perfusion Assessment

When the preoperative lung function tests indicate that the patient is at an increased risk for perioperative complications, split lung function tests of ventilation and perfusion are valuable for predicting postresection lung function.[55,60] Removal of a diseased portion of lung may not decrease overall lung function; in fact, it may improve it. The extent of pulmonary surgery has been found to correlate inversely with the intraoperative partial pressure of arterial oxygen (PaO_2), where patients undergoing pneumonectomy had higher PaO_2 than those undergoing lobectomy, which in turn were higher than those undergoing segmentectomy.[4] This paradox is related to the corresponding amount of perfusion of the diseased lung. With larger, central tumors (such as would require a pneumonectomy), perfusion, and thus shunting under OLV, is diminished in comparison to a more peripheral lesion requiring a limited resection. Likewise, the results of perfusion scanning can predict the degree of hypoxemia during OLV, as the degree of perfusion to the operative lung is proportional to the degree of potential shunt produced when ventilation to that lung ceases.[4]

Ventilation can be measured by having the patient inhale one vital capacity breath of a radioisotope and then measuring isotope counts with multiple scanners placed over the chest wall. IV injected radioisotope can be imaged to show the distribution of perfusion to all areas of the lung. After determining function in various areas of the lung, calculations can then estimate postresection function by multiplying the current function by the fraction of functioning lung that will remain postoperatively. Calculations based on segmental lung regions may help predict outcomes for patients undergoing lung volume reduction surgery. This procedure of removing emphysematous portions of lung to improve overall lung function has proved efficacious and particularly beneficial in allowing resection of cancerous lung tissue from patients in whom overall lung function studies would have contraindicated surgery.[42] Lung volume reduction surgery is most useful in patients with heterogeneous emphysema (particularly when the emphysematous lobe is also the one containing the tumor), where removal of a lung segment or lobe will result in better pulmonary function overall. Incidentally, this effect is appreciated more often with upper rather than lower lobectomy, in which patients with a low preoperative FEV_1 tend to demonstrate improvement in the FEV_1 following upper lobectomy.[61]

Dynamic MRI and quantitative CT are newer modalities used to determine postresection pulmonary function.[62,63] Dynamic MRI traces the movement of oxygen or sulfur hexafluoride to reflect diffusing capacity.[64] Quantitative CT is intended to provide more specific data than global measurements such as FEV_1. This scan can be used to quantify low-attenuation (emphysematous) areas of the lung to determine both overall proportion and regional distribution of disease. Results are comparable to FEV_1 in predicting obstruction.[65] Volumetric CT has been shown to achieve higher correlation and precision with measured postoperative lung function than with conventional procedures.[66]

Diffusion Capacity

Diffusion capacity (DLCO) tests the lungs' ability to allow transport of gas across the alveolar-capillary membrane. The capacity of the lung to exchange gas across the alveolar-capillary membrane is determined by its structural and functional properties. The structural properties include the following: lung gas volume, the path length for diffusion in the gas phase, the thickness and area of the alveolar capillary membrane, any effects of airway closure, and the volume of hemoglobin in capillaries supplying ventilated alveoli. The functional properties include the following: absolute levels of ventilation and perfusion, the uniformity of the distribution of ventilation relative to the distribution of perfusion, the composition of the alveolar gas, the diffusion characteristics of the membrane, the concentration and binding properties of hemoglobin in the alveolar capillaries, and the carbon monoxide and oxygen tensions in the alveolar capillaries in that part of the pulmonary vascular bed that exchanges gas with the alveoli.[67]

It is difficult to measure the diffusing capacity of oxygen as it is limited by cardiac uptake and total body consumption, thus carbon monoxide (CO) is used due to its high affinity for hemoglobin (200–250 times that of oxygen).[68] The patient inhales a small amount of CO, holds the breath for 10 seconds, and exhales; the amount of CO in the exhaled breath is then measured. After subtracting the amount of CO that should be expired with dead space air, the amount exhaled provides an indicator of the diffusion of gases in the lung. As cigarette smoking is the most common source of carboxyhemoglobin (COHb), patients must be asked to refrain from smoking or other sources of CO exposure on the day of the test. COHb produces an acute, reversible decrease in DLCO largely due to its effects on CO backpressure and the decreased Hb binding sites for test gas CO.[67]

A DLCO less than 40% of the predicted value has been associated with increased complications following pulmonary surgery. However, DLCO has been found to have good specificity but low sensitivity as an independent measurement. The product of the predicted values for DLCO and FEV_1 may provide better reliability than single measures. This measurement, called the PPO product, was found by Pierce to be less than 1650 in 75% of those who died.[69]

Cardiopulmonary Reserve

Maximal oxygen consumption ($\dot{V}O_2$ max) testing during exercise is also a strong predictor of patient outcome.[32,42,70] A $\dot{V}O_2$ max less than 10 mL/kg/min (or 40% of the predicted value) is associated with increased mortality, whereas a $\dot{V}O_2$ max greater than 20 mL/kg/min is a favorable finding.[71] These values may be roughly estimated by evaluating the patient's physical ability, in which the ability to climb five flights of stairs suggests a $\dot{V}O_2$ max greater than 20 mL/kg/min, and the inability to climb one flight of stairs suggests a $\dot{V}O_2$ max of less than 10 mL/kg/min.[72] Cardiopulmonary exercise testing may be applied to evaluate patients prior to pulmonary surgery. For example, the inability to walk 500 m in a 6-minute walk test was correlated with a significant

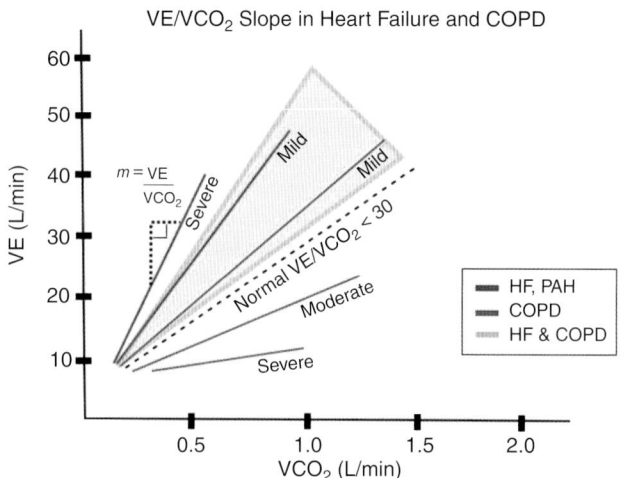

Fig. 30.1 VE/VCO$_2$ slope in heart failure and COPD. *COPD,* Chronic obstructive pulmonary disease; *HF,* heart failure; *PAH,* pulmonary artery hypertension.

increase in the duration of hospital stay, atrial fibrillation, and blood transfusion in patients undergoing pulmonary lobectomies.[73]

Additionally, current literature supports the utilization of the VE/VCO$_2$ slope in assessing the probability of postoperative pulmonary complications. The VE/VCO$_2$ slope is a measurement of ventilatory efficiency (minute ventilation relative to CO_2 exhalation), which is normally less than 30.[74] A VE/VCO$_2$ slope of more than 35 (at maximal exercise) was the single parameter most strongly associated with the probability of mortality and postoperative complications in an observational study among COPD patients compared to $\dot{V}O_2$ max measurements and is recommended in clinical practice for preoperative evaluation for lung resection.[75] As one of the most commonly used parameters of ventilatory efficiency in the clinical literature, the VE/VCO$_2$ slope increases in mild to severe heart failure and, contrarily, decreases in severe to very severe COPD compared with milder disease (Fig. 30.1).[76] In early stages of COPD, the VE/VCO$_2$ slope can actually be increased (due to an increase in dead space and/or due to concomitant pulmonary hypertension). However, in the more advanced stages of COPD, precisely because of worsening mechanical constraints and desensitization of the chemoreceptors leading to hypercapnia, the VE/VCO$_2$ slope can be lower.[76,77] Consequently, in a patient with heart failure and COPD, the VE/VCO$_2$ slope may remain stable (but still higher when compared to a healthy patient) if the value of a high slope in heart failure is markedly reduced by a lower value in severe COPD.[76]

Patient Optimization

Aggressive treatment of acute or reversible components of respiratory disease greatly decreases the risk of postoperative complications. Treatable preoperative conditions include infections, excess bronchial secretions, pleural effusions, bronchospasm, dehydration, electrolyte imbalance, cigarette smoking, alcohol abuse, and malnutrition.

Smoking is not only a major risk factor for chronic lung disease but also a strong predictor of perioperative complications. Among patients undergoing noncardiac surgery, pulmonary complications occurred in 22% of smokers, 13% of past smokers, and only 5% of nonsmokers.[78] In a study of lung cancer patients, 87% were smokers who carried a 1.5% rate of mortality, whereas nonsmokers had only a 0.4% rate of mortality. Smokers in that study demonstrated twice the rate of complications as did nonsmokers.[79] The correlation of complications with the duration of smoking history can be calculated using the pack-year index (the product of the packs per day smoked times the years of smoking at that rate).

Patients with greater than a 20 pack-year history have demonstrated increased incidence of complications compared with those who have a more modest smoking history.[80,81] The VE/VCO$_2$ slope was also increased in symptomatic, but not in asymptomatic, smokers without diagnosed COPD.[76]

Smoking cessation may reduce postoperative complications; however, the timing of this intervention is important. Most research indicates that smoking cessation for less than 4 weeks prior to surgery does not alter risk of complications at all.[78,82,83] Some data suggest that short-term smoking cessation (<1 month) may cause increases in mucous production, which may actually increase complications[78,84]; however, research findings are equivocal on the concept of increasing complications.[83,84] Carboxyhemoglobin levels have shown a significant decrease rapidly after smoking cessation, and improvement of nasal mucociliary clearance occurs within 1 to 2 weeks; however, the implications of these findings for postoperative complications are unclear.[85,86] The rates of complications are reduced in proportion to the amount of time after quitting, with a threshold of at least 4 weeks to observe improvement and even more improvement noted after 8 weeks.[82,83] Only in one very large study was a trend toward slight reduction in complications noticed with less than 1 month of smoking cessation, and complications further decreased in proportion to the total duration of cessation.[79] Smoking cessation counseling and intervention is a widely recommended strategy for medical management of COPD patients. Many anesthetists have seen or will start to see the use of electronic cigarettes (e-cigarettes). UK public health authorities have stated that e-cigarette use is likely to be at least 95% less toxic than cigarette use, yet it carries electronic (overheating, explosion), physical (e-liquid leaks, damaged components), chemical (composition, quality and impurities of e-liquid), and operational safety (complexity of modular devices) hazards.[87] Many countries have incorporated e-cigarettes in smoking cessation programs; however, the American Cancer Society does not recommend the use of e-cigarettes as a cessation method, as e-cigarettes have not been approved by the Food and Drug Administration as a safe and effective cessation product.[87,88] Owing to the urgent nature of treating pulmonary carcinoma, delaying surgery to allow for an adequate period of smoking cessation is an impractical goal.

Monitoring Plan

The purpose of monitoring during thoracic surgery is the quick recognition of sudden and severe changes in ventilation and hemodynamics that can accompany positioning, OLV, and surgical manipulation of the airway and thoracic structures. According to American Association of Nurse Anesthetists (AANA) guidelines, standard monitors should be used.[89] Airway pressure monitoring helps detect changes in airway compliance and assists in identifying the proper placement of DLTs. Capnography is useful for determining the adequacy of when one lung is deflated and for detecting abrupt changes in cardiac output, which may accompany positioning or surgical manipulation. Considering preexisting ventilation derangements and changes with lateral position, the gradient of end tidal to arterial CO$_2$ may be wider than the typical 5 mm Hg. There is evidence that, even if the gradient is determined early, it may not remain the same throughout the intraoperative course.

Electrocardiogram

All patients require continuous monitoring of the ECG. Typically, anesthetists monitor a limb lead (II) for easy rhythm recognition and a precordial lead to add sensitivity for detection of ischemia. A landmark article by London identified V$_5$ as the precordial lead, which would add the most sensitivity to ischemia detection.[90] That article noted that monitoring a combination of leads II and V$_5$ will help detect more than 85% of myocardial ischemic episodes. A more recent study (2014),

which accounted for both the changing pattern of ischemia over time (onset vs peak), as well as comparison to preoperative values, found lead V$_4$ to be the most sensitive for detecting ischemia, followed by V$_5$.[39] In practice, concerns for positioning, surgical site prep, and access to the skin electrode may result in the precordial lead not being placed in the precisely correct location. Various studies have determined that myocardial ischemia frequently occurs in leads V$_3$ through V$_6$.[39,91,92] A consistent finding is that monitoring a combination of leads is significantly more effective than monitoring a single lead.[39,90,93] A second intraoperative lead monitored in the V$_{4-5}$ position or in whatever anterolateral position provides the most isoelectric ST segment is desirable.[39]

Arterial Pressure Monitoring

Arterial blood pressure monitoring allows the anesthetist to identify acute hypotension during surgical manipulation. It also facilitates sampling of arterial blood for blood gas analysis. It is recommended to assess an arterial blood gas upon 15 minutes of instituting OLV for a baseline value and guide to augment ventilation if needed. For thoracotomies, the arterial cannula is generally placed in the dependent arm, where it is more easily stabilized. For mediastinoscopy, the arterial monitoring site (right side) is selected to provide indication of innominate artery occlusion (see section on mediastinoscopy).

Pulse pressure variation (PPV) is a value that can be obtained from an arterial waveform that aids in the estimation of cardiac preload and fluid responsiveness.[94,95] PPV is measured by identifying the maximum individual arterial waveform (during inspiration) and the minimum (during exhalation) on the undulating continuous waveform, then determine the systolic and diastolic pressure value for the largest, or maximum, inspiratory individual waveform. The difference in these two values is your pulse pressure. Repeat this assessment for the minimum individual waveform. Utilize the following formula to find your PPV value: PPV% = [(P$_{max}$ − P$_{min}$) / (mean of the pulse pressures) × 100].[95] To use PPV, a patient must be in normal sinus rhythm, intubated and mechanically ventilated making no spontaneous respiratory efforts, ventilated with at least 8 mL/kg of tidal volume, and have no significant alterations to chest-wall compliance, such as an open chest.[95] It has been proposed that the shunt through the nonventilated lung decreases the PPV value due to the absence of cyclic change of intrathoracic pressure. Thus PPV threshold values seem to be lower in OLV than two-lung ventilation. Currently few studies have addressed the reliability of PPV to assess fluid responsiveness in an open-chest setting during thoracic surgery. Current published data are heterogeneous and conflicting. Meta-analysis results indicate low-quality evidence on PPV reliability to identify responsiveness in patients with volume loading in the open-chest scenario.[96]

Central Venous Pressure Monitoring

Central venous pressure (CVP) monitoring is not required for routine thoracotomies but may be indicated if the patient's volume status is unclear, large fluid shifts are anticipated, or peripheral access cannot be obtained. In complex cases, a CVP line may help manage fluid status and provide central access for vasoactive medications. Increased filling pressures (CVP or pulmonary capillary wedge) have been associated with greater lung injury and prolonged mechanical ventilation following complex pulmonary surgery.[97] Fluid management is complex as patients are prone to developing interstitial and alveolar edema. The effects of existing pulmonary disease, prior chemoradiotherapy, OLV, direct lung manipulation by the surgeon, and ischemia-reperfusion phenomena can all damage the glycocalyx and underlying endothelial cells as well as affect epithelial alveolar cells and surfactant. This may lead to lung injury. Guidelines for enhanced recovery after lung surgery

(ERAS) recommendations have been published.[98] CVP readings are not reliable in an open-chest, laterally positioned patient. In addition, a large-bore CVP line can provide access for rapid infusion and access site should transvenous pacing or pulmonary artery pressure monitoring become necessary.

The CVP line can be inserted via the external or internal jugular veins or the subclavian veins. An external jugular line is more easily kinked in the lateral position. One should remain alert to the possibility of pneumothorax with the insertion of central lines. A pneumothorax on the ventilated (nonoperative) side can lead to severe hypoxemia during OLV. If a subclavian approach to venous cannulation is planned, the insertion site should be on the same side as the planned thoracotomy.

Cardiac Performance Monitoring

Pulmonary artery pressure monitoring is intended to provide estimation of left ventricular pressures and guide the support of cardiac performance with fluids and cardiovascular drugs. In spite of its past popularity, pulmonary artery catheterization has not been demonstrated to improve patient outcomes in either cardiac or noncardiac surgery,[99,100] nor is it helpful in predicting postoperative complications.[55,101] There have even been suggestions that right heart catheterization may promote cardiac complications.[102] If pulmonary artery monitoring is deemed useful, the anesthetist must be cautious in interpreting values when pulmonary disease is present because the normal correlation of right and left ventricular pressures may be inaccurate. The use of pulmonary artery catheters has specific limitations during OLV. Lung pathology or HPV may alter the resistance in pulmonary vessels and reduce the correlation between pulmonary artery occlusion pressure and left ventricular pressure.[103] More than 90% of pulmonary artery catheters float into the right lung.[104] During right thoracotomy, then, the catheter will likely be in the nondependent, collapsed lung and give a false low reading for cardiac output. Finally, care must be taken to ensure that a pulmonary artery catheter is not situated in a vessel that will be clamped during the course of lung resection. A better evaluation of cardiac filling, contractility, and valvular performance would come by way of echocardiography. Preoperative echocardiography is indicated when suspicion exists of valvular disease, outflow tract obstruction, ventricular dysfunction, or pulmonary hypertension.[18,55]

LATERAL DECUBITUS POSITION

The most frequent position chosen for surgical exposure during thoracotomy is the lateral decubitus position. A roll is placed beneath the torso just caudal to the axilla to prevent compression of the neurovascular bundle and forward rotation of the humeral head. It is important to note that, whereas this roll is commonly called an axillary roll, is better considered an axillary support roll because positioning it in the axilla may cause neurovascular compression. Hyperabduction of the arms is prevented to keep the brachial plexus from stretching against the humeral head. Arms can be separately padded and extended forward on arm boards. Strategies for supporting the nondependent arm may include a pillow between the arms, a padded Mayo stand (which provides good access to IV or arterial lines in the dependent arm), or specially made double arm boards. Pulse oximetry or frequent palpation of the radial pulse ensures the integrity of circulation to the hand.

The head is supported on pillows to maintain alignment of the head and neck with the spine. Lateral flexion of the neck can cause compression of the jugular veins or vertebral arteries, compromising cerebral circulation. The dependent ear can be compressed by the weight of the head. Careful padding or use of a foam doughnut relieves this pressure, but care must be taken to prevent corneal abrasion and retinal ischemia

by avoiding pressure on the eyes. Because the brachial plexus arises from the cervical vertebrae, stretching of one side of the neck can occur if the head is not maintained in a neutral position resulting in neuropathy. A complete discussion of positioning and potential nerve injuries is presented in Chapter 23. Another pressure point of concern with the lateral position is the region near the common peroneal nerve. These pressure points are located near the fibular head of the dependent leg and the femoral head of the nondependent leg if a stabilizing strap is placed over the patient.

Physiology of the Lateral Decubitus Position

Positional changes and alterations in chest wall integrity produce significant alterations in ventilation and perfusion of the lungs during thoracic surgery. Due to the critical nature of the procedure and the degree of pulmonary pathology that is frequently associated with these patients, a thorough knowledge of positioning, ventilation, perfusion, and strategies to minimize the potential for hypoxia are discussed. A thorough discussion of pulmonary anatomy and physiology is present in Chapter 29.

Upright Position

The distribution of perfusion in the lungs depends on gravity in relation to the level of the heart and on pressures transmitted through alveoli. In a spontaneously breathing, upright patient, perfusion increases from the apex to the base of the lung (Fig. 30.2). Ventilation also increases from apex to base, based on the relative compliance of alveoli. Owing to downward traction from gravity, negative pleural pressure is greatest at the apex of the lung, and this factor keeps alveoli distended (Fig. 30.3). Dependent alveoli are less distended

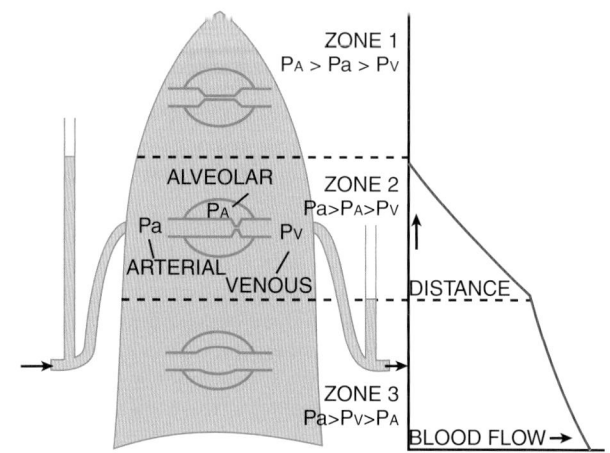

Fig. 30.2 The lung is divided into three zones according to the relative magnitudes of the pulmonary arterial, venous, and alveolar pressures (*Pa*, *Pv*, and *PA*, respectively). In zone 1, alveolar pressure exceeds arterial pressure, so the collapsible vessels are held closed and there is no blood flow. In zone 2, arterial pressure exceeds alveolar pressure, but alveolar pressure exceeds venous pressure. Under these conditions, a constriction occurs at the downstream end of each collapsible vessel, and the pressure inside the vessel at this point is equal to alveolar pressure, so the pressure gradient causing flow is arterial-alveolar. This gradient increases linearly with distance down the lung, and therefore, so does blood flow. In zone 3, venous pressure exceeds alveolar pressure, and the collapsible vessels are held open. Here, the pressure gradient causing flow is arteriovenous, and there is constant perfusion of alveoli. (From West JB. Explanation of the uneven distribution of blood flow in the lung, based on the pressures affecting capillaries. In West JB, Luks AM, eds. *Respiratory Physiology: The Essentials.* 11th ed. Philadelphia: Lippincott Williams & Wilkins; 2021:54.)

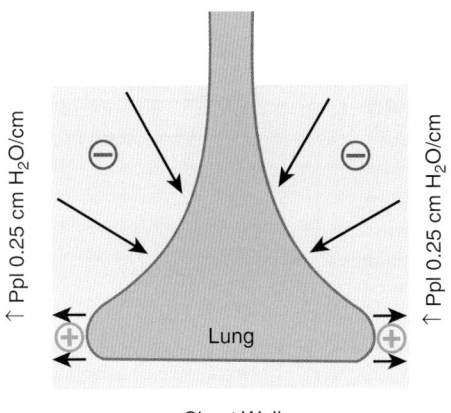

Fig. 30.3 Schematic diagram of the lung within the chest wall, showing the tendency of the lung to assume a globular shape because of its viscoelastic nature. The tendency of the top of the lung to collapse inward creates a relatively negative pressure at the apex, and the tendency of the bottom of the lung to spread outward creates a relatively positive pressure at the base. Therefore, pleural pressure *(Ppl)* increases by 0.25 cm H_2O, in a caudad direction, per centimeter of lung dependency. (From Triantafillou AN, et al. Physiology of the lateral decubitus position, the open chest, and one-lung ventilation. In Kaplan JA, Slinger PD, eds. *Thoracic Anesthesia*. 3rd ed. Philadelphia: Churchill Livingstone; 2003.)

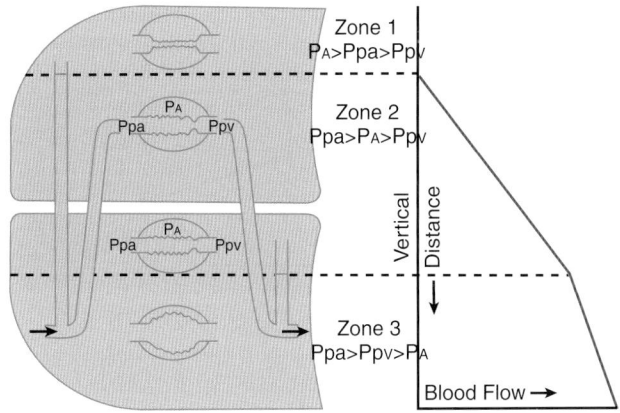

Fig. 30.5 Schematic representation of the effects of gravity on the distribution of pulmonary ventilation and blood flow in the lateral decubitus position. The vertical gradient in the lateral decubitus position is less than in the upright position; consequently, blood flow in zones 2 and 3 is less. Nevertheless, pulmonary blood flow increases with lung dependency and is greater in the dependent lung than in the nondependent lung. *PA*, Alveolar pressure; *Ppa*, pulmonary arterial pressure; *Ppv*, pulmonary venous pressure. (From Triantafillou AN, et al. Physiology of the lateral decubitus position, the open chest, and one-lung ventilation. In Kaplan JA, Slinger PD, eds. *Thoracic Anesthesia*. 3rd ed. Philadelphia: Churchill Livingstone; 2003.)

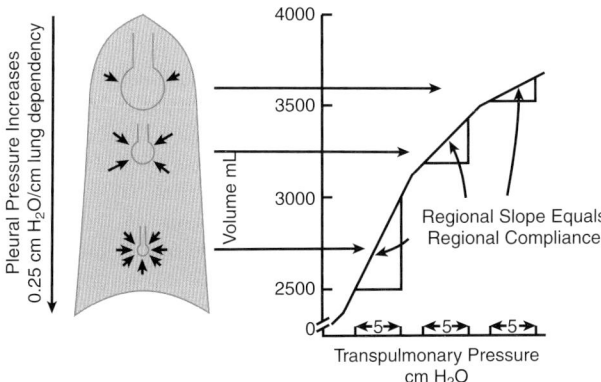

Fig. 30.4 Due to gravity, alveoli in the most dependent portions of the lung are compressed by the tissue above, whereas those in the most nondependent portions are suspended open. At end inspiration and end expiration, the pressure inside all alveoli is equalized with atmospheric pressure; however, an increasing gradient of pleural pressure toward dependent areas creates a gradient in transpulmonary pressure at rest. Whereas the change in transpulmonary pressure during inspiration is equal for all alveoli, alveoli in dependent regions are on the steep portion of the compliance curve tend to be more compliant, and therefore, receive the largest share of the tidal volume. (From Triantafillou AN, et al. Physiology of the lateral decubitus position, the open chest, and one-lung ventilation. In Kaplan JA, Slinger PD, eds. *Thoracic Anesthesia*. 3rd ed. Philadelphia: Churchill Livingstone; 2003.)

and therefore, more compliant (can expand by a greater volume for a given pressure change because they are starting at a lower resting volume). Therefore, most of a tidal volume (Vt) breath is distributed to the dependent alveoli (Fig. 30.4). The increase in both ventilation and perfusion from apex to base is not parallel and is certainly more complexly arranged than in neatly divided zones. However, the general increase in ventilation and perfusion from top to bottom results in efficient gas exchange.

Awake Lateral Position

In the lateral position, less vertical distance is present to cause differences in the intrapleural pressure and blood pressure gradients (Fig. 30.5). Abdominal contents displace the diaphragm in a cephalad direction on the dependent side. Starting from a higher position in the thorax, the dependent hemidiaphragm can contract further. During inspiration, therefore, contraction of the diaphragm causes more of the Vt to fill the dependent lung. Perfusion is dependent upon gravity, and when in the lateral position it is also greatest in the dependent lung (Fig. 30.6). Overall, the relationship of greater ventilation and perfusion in the dependent lung is unchanged, and gas exchange remains efficient.

Anesthetized Lateral Position, Chest Closed, With Spontaneous Ventilation

A change in the distribution of ventilation is seen with the induction of anesthesia, even when spontaneous respiration is maintained. Functional residual capacity (FRC) decreases almost immediately upon the induction of anesthesia. The weight of the mediastinum and the cephalad displacement of the diaphragm by abdominal contents further decrease FRC in the dependent lung and reduces the proportion of the favorable zone 3 area. Lower volumes in each lung shift their place on the compliance curve. The lungs are less compliant when they are either at a very high volume (distended alveoli) or a very low volume (atelectasis). In the anesthetized patient, the nondependent lung moves from a flat, noncompliant portion of the compliance curve to a more compliant position. Although anesthesia results in a net loss of FRC, the relative proportion of FRC in the nondependent lung increases in contrast to the dependent lung.[105] As the dependent lung loses FRC, its volume becomes so low as to decrease its compliance. It shifts to a less compliant, flatter portion of the curve (Fig. 30.7). Ventilation is therefore preferentially distributed to the nondependent lung, whereas gravity-dependent blood flow preferentially goes to the dependent lung, resulting in a V/Q mismatch.

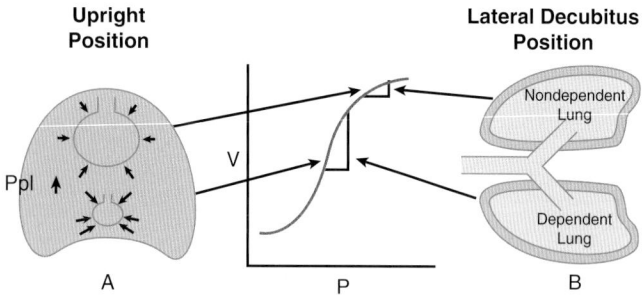

Fig. 30.6 (A) An increasing gradient of intrapleural pressure from top to bottom of lungs creates different resting volumes of alveoli and variation in regional compliance, as described in Fig. 30.5. (B) In the lateral decubitus position, gravity-related effects translate to greater compliance of the dependent lung and lesser compliance of the nondependent lung. Therefore, in the spontaneously breathing individual, more ventilation is delivered to the dependent lung. *P*, Transpulmonary pressure; *PPL*, intrapleural pressure; *V*, alveolar volume. (From Triantafillou AN, et al. Physiology of the lateral decubitus position, the open chest, and one-lung ventilation. In Kaplan JA, Slinger PD, eds. *Thoracic Anesthesia.* 3rd ed. Philadelphia: Churchill Livingstone; 2003.)

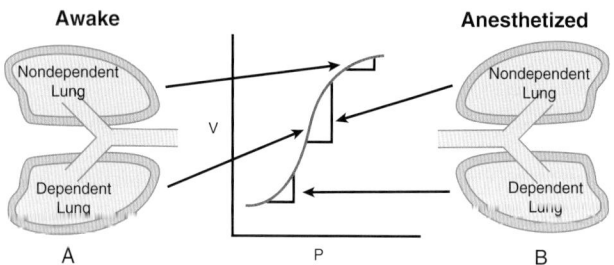

Fig. 30.7 (A) Regional compliance of lungs in the awake patient in lateral decubitus position. (B) Regional compliance of lungs in the anesthetized patient in the lateral decubitus position. Induction of anesthesia causes a loss of lung volume in both lungs, with the nondependent lung moving from a flat, noncompliant portion of the pressure-volume curve to a steep, compliant portion. The dependent lung moves from the highly compliant portion toward the lower flattening of the curve. In some areas of the dependent lung, resting alveolar volume is so low that atelectasis and airway closure impede inflation. Therefore, in the anesthetized patient in the lateral decubitus position, more tidal ventilation shifts toward the nondependent lung (where there is less perfusion), creating a ventilation-perfusion mismatch. *P*, Transpulmonary pressure; *V*, alveolar volume. (From Triantafillou AN, et al. Physiology of the lateral decubitus position, the open chest, and one-lung ventilation. In Kaplan JA, Slinger PD, eds. *Thoracic Anesthesia.* 3rd ed. Philadelphia: Churchill Livingstone; 2003.)

Anesthetized, Paralyzed, Mechanically Ventilated

Under mechanical ventilation, the diaphragm no longer contributes to ventilation of the lower lung, and FRC further declines as the compression from abdominal viscera is no longer counteracted by the force of the contracting diaphragm (Fig. 30.8). With the initiation of mechanical ventilation and the absence of diaphragmatic contraction, ventilation further shifts to follow the path of least resistance, favoring the nondependent lung. The V/Q relationship further deteriorates. The addition of positive end-expiratory pressure (PEEP) to mechanical ventilation may help restore FRC and improve the V/Q ratio.

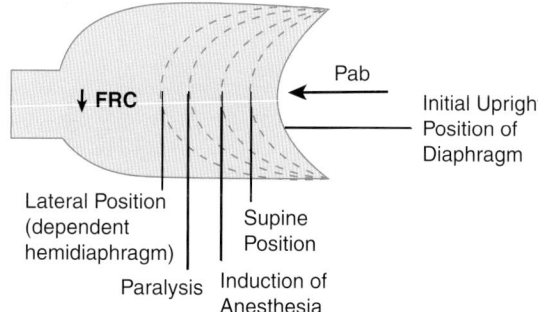

Fig. 30.8 Anesthesia and surgery may cause a progressive cephalad displacement of the diaphragm. The sequence of events involves assumption of the supine position, induction of anesthesia, causation of paralysis, and lateral decubitus positioning (wherein abdominal contents mostly press upon the dependent hemidiaphragm). This movement of the diaphragm and the downward displacement of the mediastinum result in decreased functional residual capacity *(FRC)* and contribute to pushing the dependent lung to the lower flattening of the compliance curve. *Pab*, Pressure of the abdominal contents. (Adapted from Benumof JL. *Anesthesia for Thoracic Surgery.* 2nd ed. Philadelphia: Elsevier; 1995.)

Anesthetized, Open Chest

Upon opening the thorax there is an immediate decrease in resistance to gas flow in the nondependent lung, as the lung detaches from the chest wall. This causes further loss of ventilation to the dependent lung, in preference for the nondependent lung. The mediastinum also further shifts downward (compressing the dependent lung) because of loss of negative intrapleural pressure in the nondependent lung, which helped to distend it. Ventilation to the dependent lung is decreased in proportion to the displacement of the lung by the mediastinal structures. Compression of the great vessels may cause a decrease in venous return and cardiac output causing circulatory compromise. Any spontaneous respiration becomes very inefficient as paradoxic movement of air occurs on inspiration from the open-chest lung into the dependent lung, which has greater negative intrapleural pressure. Upon expiration, gas exits the dependent lung and enters both the trachea and the open-chest lung, causing the lung to expand (Fig. 30.9). Paradoxic respiration compromises fresh gas exchange in the dependent lung as part of the Vt moves between the lungs. Positive pressure ventilation diminishes the effects of mediastinal shift and paradoxic respiration. However, during mechanical ventilation, the open chest provides no resistance, and the greatly increased compliance of that lung allows a higher proportion of ventilation to go to the nondependent lung, which is the least perfused area of the thorax. The less ventilated, better perfused, dependent lung contributes to physiologic shunt, as blood flows through atelectatic areas without acquiring oxygen. Although the prevalence of different zones is not as evenly distributed as diagrams would suggest, the lateral, anesthetized, paralyzed, open-chest patient does exhibit significant regional areas of ventilation and perfusion mismatching.

Anesthetized, Open Chest, With One-Lung Ventilation

The succeeding cascade of changes leading up to the anesthetized open chest results in significant V/Q mismatch. There is little resistance to ventilation of the nondependent lung, whereas the effects of gravity promote perfusion to the dependent lung. When ventilation to the nondependent lung is ceased, ventilation is directed to the dependent lung. The remaining perfusion to the nondependent lung creates a shunt, but HPV reduces the shunt by 50% by diverting much of that blood toward the dependent lung. The PaO_2 is higher during OLV in the lateral position than it is in the supine position, as clamping the airway to the nondependent lung reverses some of the changes that cause the V/Q disparity in the anesthetized patient.

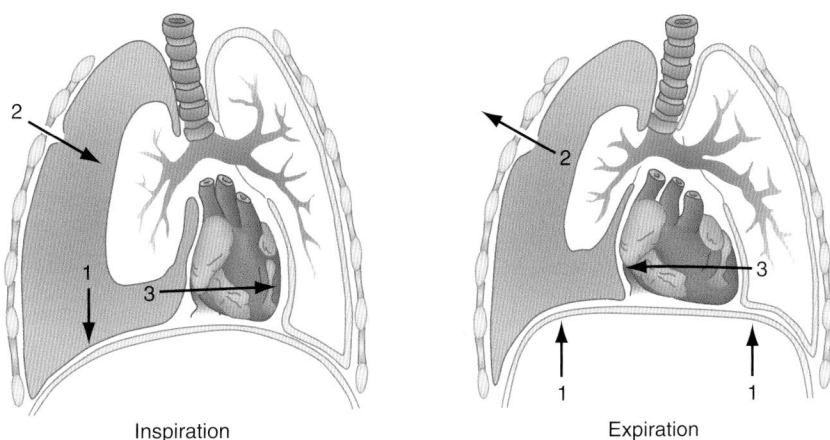

Inspiration

Expiration

Fig. 30.9 Inspiration: The diaphragm contracts causing negative intrathoracic pressure *(arrow 1)* that draws air through the sucking chest wound in the pleural cavity *(arrow 2)* and causing the mediastinal structures to shift to the patient's left *(arrow 3)*. Expiration: The diaphragm recoils *(arrow 1)* causing air to exit the chest *(arrow 2)* and allowing the mediastinum to shift back to normal position *(arrow 3)*. The collapsed lung paradoxically shrinks on inspiration and expands on expiration. (From Walls R, et al. *Rosen's Emergency Medicine.* 8th ed. Philadelphia: Elsevier; 20:387.)

ONE-LUNG VENTILATION

Indications for Lung Separation

The ability to provide distinct ventilation to the separate lungs facilitates pulmonary surgery by providing a quiet surgical field. This is particularly helpful in the case of thoracoscopic surgery, in which visualization and the ability to manipulate the operative lung are limited. Thoracic surgeons will commonly consider lung separation an absolute requirement for pulmonary surgery. However, surgery can be performed on a lung that is being ventilated, and thoracic surgery alone is not an absolute indication for OLV. In fact, in the case of pediatric patients, gentle dual-lung ventilation is indicated and appropriate in either the presence of airway concerns that preclude use of a lung-separating device or the inability to maintain oxygenation with OLV. Certain situations, such as infectious contamination of one lung, are absolute indications for OLV, but most common thoracic surgeries create relative indications for lung separation in that they can safely be accomplished without it. Indications for lung separation are noted in Box 30.3.

Methods of Lung Separation

Several devices have been developed to enable isolation of one lung and ventilation of the other. The single-lumen endobronchial tube was developed in 1931 to isolate an infected lung.[106] Mimicking this simple approach by advancing a 7.5-mm wide, 32-cm long ETT over a fiberoptic scope into one bronchus may still be used in some circumstances. A disadvantage of using a single-lumen tube for OLV is that the ability to ventilate or suction the operative lung is lost. Another disadvantage is that use of a single-lumen tube in the right lung would probably occlude the right upper lobe orifice. However, in an emergent situation, use of a single-lumen tube advanced blindly down the right bronchus or placed into the left bronchus aided by a bronchoscope can be lifesaving. A summary of lung separation devices is presented in Table 30.2. Given that each approach (DLT vs bronchial blocker) has relative merits, neither can be recommended as a superior method of lung separation for thoracic surgery.

Double-Lumen Endobronchial Tubes

DLTs consist of a single tube with two lumens. The bronchial lumen is identified by its blue cuff and is designed to be inserted into either

---

BOX 30.3 Indications for Lung Separation

Absolute

1. Isolation of one lung from the other to avoid spillage or contamination
   - Infection
   - Massive hemorrhage
2. Control of the distribution of ventilation
   - Bronchopleural fistula
   - Bronchopleural cutaneous fistula
   - Surgical opening of a major conducting airway
   - Giant unilateral lung cyst or bulla
   - Tracheobronchial tree disruption
   - Life-threatening hypoxemia related to unilateral lung disease
3. Unilateral bronchopulmonary lavage
   - Pulmonary alveolar proteinosis

Relative

1. Surgical exposure—high priority
   - Thoracic aortic aneurysm
   - Pneumonectomy
   - Thoracoscopy
   - Upper lobectomy
   - Mediastinal exposure
2. Surgical exposure—medium (lower) priority
   - Middle and lower lobectomies and subsegmental resections
   - Esophageal resection
   - Procedures on the thoracic spine
3. Postcardiopulmonary bypass pulmonary edema/hemorrhage after removal of totally occluding unilateral chronic pulmonary emboli
4. Severe hypoxemia related to unilateral lung disease

Adapted from Moise O, et al. Separation of the two lungs (double-lumen tubes, bronchial blockers, and endobronchial single-lumen tubes). In Hagberg CA, ed. *Hagberg and Benumof's Airway Management.* 4th ed. Philadelphia: Elsevier; 2018:471.

---

the left or right mainstem bronchus. The bronchial lumen will be used to initially ventilate the corresponding lung. The tracheal lumen is positioned midtrachea, and the corresponding port will ventilate the

TABLE 30.2   Types of Lung Separation Devices

Type	Examples	Notes
Endobronchial tube	Bronchocath, Carlens, Robertshaw, White	Left bronchus intubation preferable. Large size increases difficulty of transoral insertion, but facilitates emptying of surgical lung. Right-side more challenging to position, but may be preferable for descending aortic aneurism. Carlens and White: carinal hook aids placement when visualization is poor (hemorrhage/hemoptysis).
Bronchial blocker	Ardnt, Cohen, Coopdech, Univent	Easier basic tube insertion, but requires a fiberoptic bronchoscope, thus takes longer to situate. Lung deflation may require suction. More often dislodged. Preferable if postoperative intubation planned. Cohen: flexible tip can be manipulated. Arndt, Coopdech: blocker is adapted to a regular endotracheal tube.

opposite lung. The bronchial lumen does not necessarily have to be placed within the bronchus of the operative lung (Fig. 30.10).

Features

Several types of DLTs are used in thoracic surgery. DLTs are designed for insertion either in the right or the left bronchus. Right-sided tubes include features to accommodate the proximity of the upper lobe bronchus. Disposable polyvinyl chloride tubes are available in French (F) sizes 26, 28, 35, 37, 39, and 41. The F scale refers to three times the external diameter of the ETT (in millimeters). The internal lumen diameters range from 3.4 mm to 6.6 mm,[107] although there is wide size variation between manufacturers.[108,109] It would be most important for the anesthetist to ascertain the appropriate size fiberscope that will fit through the intended tube lumens. Despite the perceived smaller size of the lumens, DLTs do not increase breathing resistance significantly in comparison to single lumen tubes.[104,110] A newly integrated DLT has been utilized in the clinical environment. The VivaSight-DL (Fig. 30.11) is a DLT that has a video imaging device and light source at the distal end of the tracheal lumen, and a single use video/power cable that displays images of the airway onto a specific video monitor for as long as the device remains in place. The VivaSight-DL has an injection port leading to two lumens along the tube's wall to aid in cleaning of the imaging lens. The VivaSight-DL provides continuous, real-time observation of the carina during surgery, which may help prevent dislodgement and assist in repositioning the DLT during OLV.[111] Despite the reduced need for flexible bronchoscopy with the VivaSight-DL, a flexible intubating bronchoscope (endoscope) must be available in every case, whether or not the anesthetist is using the VivaSight-DL or a standard DLT.[112]

Advantages and Disadvantages

Although the presence of two lumens limits the internal diameter of each, the external diameter of a DLT is large. The 37F DLT has an outer diameter equivalent to that of a standard 11-mm internal diameter (ID) ETT. For this reason, DLTs are not used for small children; the external diameter of the 26F DLT, which is the smallest version, is 7.5 mm.[113] Sizing of DLTs is determined by patient height, usually leading to the

use of 35F to 37F tubes in females, and 39F to 41F tubes in males. More specifically, DLT use can include 35F for women up to 160 cm, 37F for women over 160 cm, 37/39F for men less than 175 cm, and 39/41F for men over 175 cm.[114]

The distance from the carinal bifurcation to the right upper lobe is 1.5 to 2 cm, as compared with a 4- to 5-cm left mainstem bronchus. Modifications have been made in right-sided tubes to allow ventilation through a slot in the endobronchial cuff or to use two bronchial cuffs, but even slight movement of the right DLT can lead to malpositioning. Many practitioners have resolved to use left-sided DLTs for all right and left thoracotomies unless a left-sided tube is contraindicated by internal lesions of the airway, compression of the trachea or main bronchi by an external mass, or the presence of a descending thoracic aortic aneurysm, which can compress or erode the left main bronchus. This is due to the close proximity of the right upper bronchi to the carina. The bronchial cuff of a right-sided DLT is more likely to occlude the right upper lung lobe and further decrease ventilation. Intubation with the large DLT can pose a challenge, even in patients with a normal airway; insertion in those with poor airway anatomy may be particularly challenging.

Complications Associated With Double-Lumen Tubes

The most common complication associated with a DLT is malpositioning. Fig. 30.12 demonstrates some variations of DLT positioning. Rupture of a thoracic aneurysm is possible with a left-sided DLT if the aneurysm compresses the left mainstem bronchus. Damage to the vocal cords or arytenoid cartilages is possible from a carinal hook. A carinal hook can also break off, requiring retrieval with a bronchoscope. Bronchial rupture, which was thought to be caused by overinflation of the bronchial cuff, has been reported.[115,116] Owing to the possibility of its being inserted too deeply, a DLT can also cause the entire Vt to be delivered to a single lung lobe, creating the potential for barotrauma. The larger size of the DLT is probably also responsible for the slightly increased incidence of hoarseness and vocal cord lesions observed in patients following DLT, versus using a bronchial blocker for lung separation.[117]

Insertion of Double-Lumen Endotracheal Tubes

The DLT has two curves along its length to aid in its placement. A stylet aids placement through the larynx. Some practitioners prefer the Macintosh blade for intubation because it offers greater clearance for the tube and may decrease the chance of balloon rupture from the teeth.[118] For laryngoscopy, the lubricated DLT is advanced with the distal curve concave anteriorly until the vocal cords are passed. The stylet is usually removed at this point to reduce the potential of the rigid tube causing mucosal damage. The tube is then rotated 90 degrees toward the bronchus that is to be intubated. The DLT is advanced to approximately a 27-cm depth in females or a 29-cm depth in males, or until resistance is met.[119]

The tracheal cuff requires 5 to 10 mL of air, and the bronchial cuff requires 1 to 2 mL of air. Overinflation of the bronchial cuff can cause its lumen to become narrowed or occluded and increases the risk of bronchial damage. Unlike most tracheal high-volume, low-pressure cuffs, the bronchial cuff holds a small volume and can exert high pressure on the endobronchial mucosa. For that reason, unless unilateral lung contamination exists, the bronchial cuff should be deflated during the procedure once OLV is no longer needed. After the tube is situated in the bronchus, adapters are attached to the two lumens for interface with the anesthesia circuit. Auscultation of breath sounds is a simple, though not highly reliable, method of determining the position of a DLT (Box 30.4). When properly positioned, breath sounds should be auscultated in all fields of the lung corresponding to the bronchial lumen (depending on the use of a

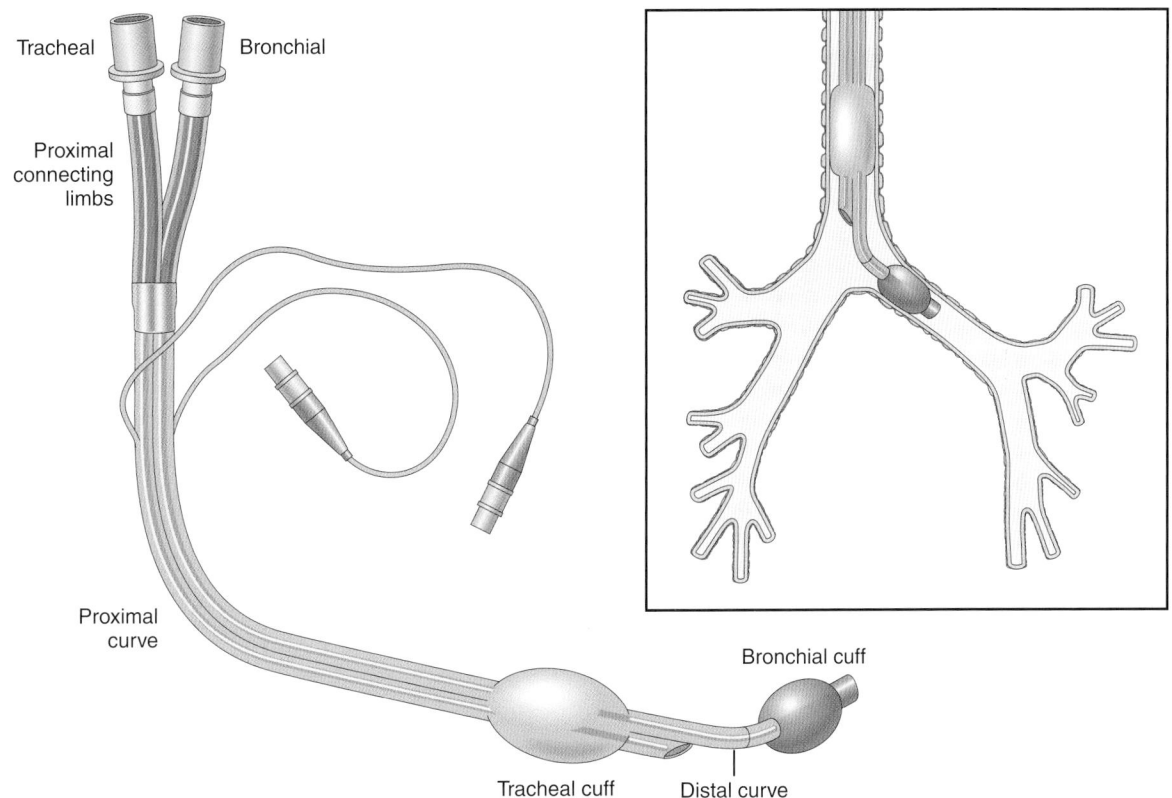

Fig. 30.10 The double-lumen endobronchial tube. Inset shows a left-sided tube correctly positioned in the bronchus. (From Pardo MC, Miller RD. *Basics of Anesthesia*. 7th ed. Philadelphia: Elsevier; 2018:471.)

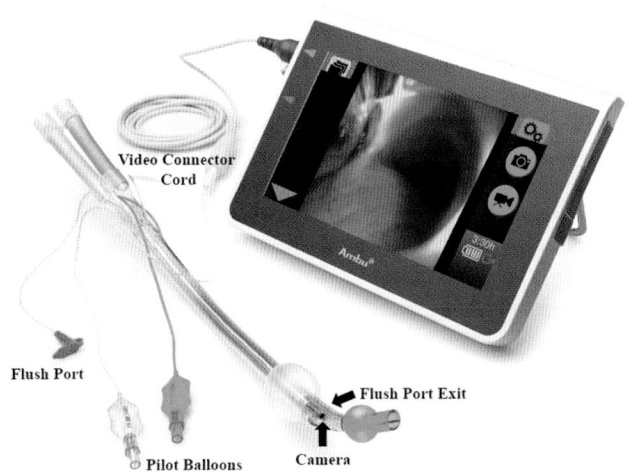

Fig. 30.11 VivaSight-DL111. Video connector cord displays images during intubation and throughout the surgical procedure to confirm double-lumen tube positioning. The flush port utilizes saline or air to clear the camera lens of secretions.

left- or right-sided tube) when that lumen alone is ventilated. Breath sounds should be heard only in the opposite lung when the tracheal lumen is ventilated. Fig. 30.13 outlines some auscultation findings expected with various tube positions.

Flexible bronchoscopy is essential to verify placement of the DLT (Box 30.5; see Fig. 30.13). Visualization using a flexible intubating bronchoscope has revealed a 38% to 83% incidence of malpositioning of DLTs that were judged by auscultation to be properly placed.[107,120] Some particular advantages of fiberoptic inspection of the DLT over auscultation are guidance during initial placement, the ability to

visualize the correct depth of the bronchial cuff, and visualization of proper positioning of the right upper lobe port (if present). Placement of the tube should again be verified by bronchoscopy after the patient is positioned laterally because the DLT will commonly withdraw from the bronchus by 1 cm.[121] When separation of the lungs is required to prevent cross-contamination, the integrity of the bronchial seal can be tested by connecting a tube from the bronchial port to a water seal and then providing ventilation through the tracheal lumen. Incompetence of the bronchial cuff will be evidenced by egress of bubbles in the water seal (Fig. 30.14).

Bronchial Blockers

A bronchial blocker consists of a catheter with an inflatable balloon that blocks the bronchus of the operative lung. Blockers can be incorporated into a side channel of an ETT (e.g., Univent tube), or they can be separate devices that are inserted either through the regular ETT lumen or outside of it (more common in pediatrics) (Fig. 30.15). Common options for stand-alone bronchial blockers include the 8F Fogarty embolectomy catheter, the Cohen Flextip blocker, the Coopdech blocker, the EZ blocker, and the Arndt bronchial blocker (formerly known as the wire-guided endobronchial blocker).

Features

Bronchial blockers are guided into the appropriate bronchus with the aid of a bronchoscope (Fig. 30.16). Wire-guided blockers have a loop on the end through which the fiberscope is passed, facilitating guidance of the blocker into the bronchus after the fiberscope. The Cohen blocker has a steerable tip to facilitate advancement into the appropriate bronchus. The Univent tube consists of an integrated ETT with a second lumen for a deployable bronchial blocker. The EZ blocker has a forked distal end that functions like the Carlens hook to rest on the

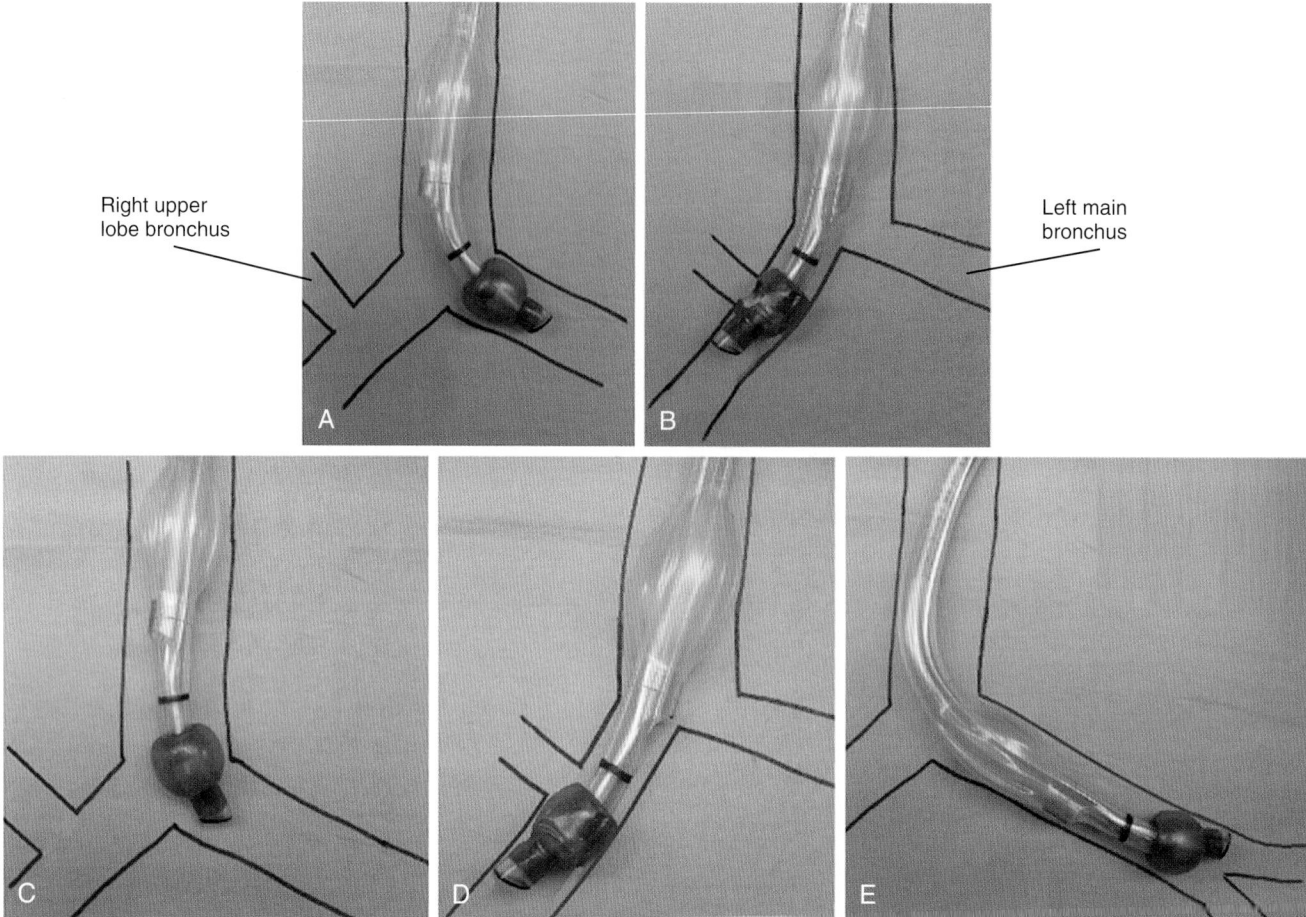

Figure	Description	Ventilating through the bronchial lumen produces breath sounds:	Ventilating through the tracheal lumen produces breath sounds:
A	Correct position of left DLT	Left lung	Right lung
B	Correct position of right DLT	Right lung	Left lung
C	DLT insertion too shallow	Both lungs	Diminished or absent if bronchial cuff obstructs trachea; otherwise, both lungs
D	DLT too deep in right bronchus	Right middle and lower lobes	Left lung or right upper lobe (depending on depth of tracheal cuff)
E	DLT too deep in left bronchus	Left lung	Left lung

Additional variations are possible, such as if a left-sided DLT is inadvertently positioned in the right bronchus, or vice versa. Auscultation provides a quick check, but fiberoptic confirmation is preferable for definitive confirmation.

Fig. 30.12 Positioning variations of the double-lumen endobronchial tube *(DLT)*.

BOX 30.4   Auscultation of Breath Sounds After Placement of a Double-Lumen Tube

1. Inflate the tracheal cuff.
2. Verify bilaterally equal breath sounds. If breath sounds are present on only one side, both lumens are in the same bronchus. Deflate the cuff and withdraw the tube 1–2 cm at a time until breath sounds are equal bilaterally.
3. Inflate the endobronchial cuff.
4. Clamp Y-piece to the endobronchial lumen and open the lumen to atmosphere.
5. Verify breath sounds in the correct lung (tracheal side) and the absence of breath sounds in the opposite lung (bronchial side).

6. *Verify the absence of air leakage through the bronchial lumen*
7. Unclamp and reconnect the endobronchial lumen and verify bilateral breath sounds.
8. Clamp Y-piece to the tracheal lumen and open the lumen to atmosphere.
9. Verify breath sounds in the correct lung (bronchial side) and the absence of breath sounds in the opposite lung (tracheal side).
10. Verify that breath sounds are equal at the apex of the lung and at the base. If the apex is diminished, withdraw the tube until upper lung sounds return.
11. *Verify the absence of air leakage through the tracheal lumen*

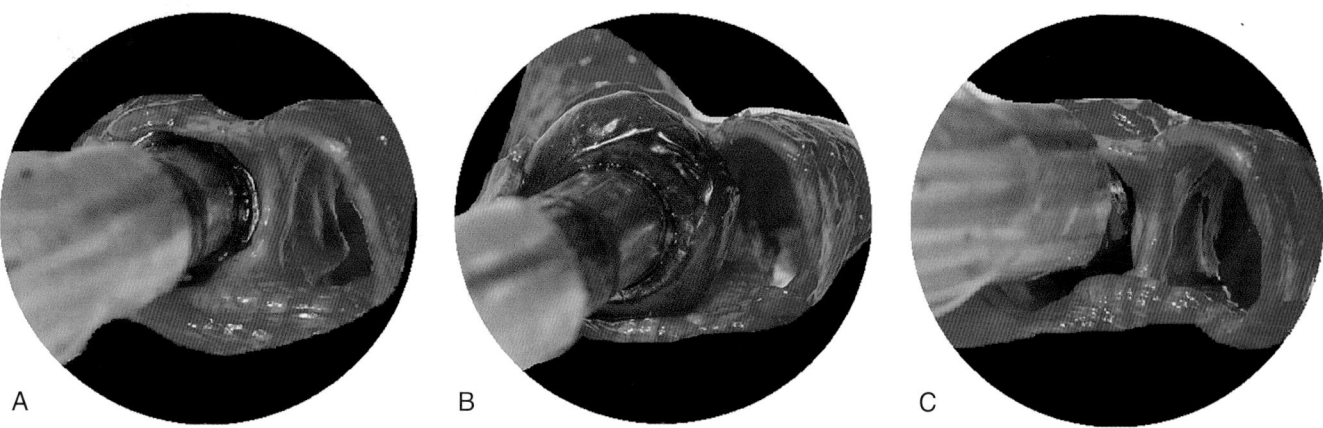

A   B   C

Fig. 30.13 Verification of double-lumen tube position with a fiberoptic bronchoscope. (A) Correct position; bronchial cuff visualized just beyond the carina. (B) Tube too shallow; bronchial cuff herniating across the carina. (C) Tube too deep. See additional description in Box 30.5.

BOX 30.5 Flexible Bronchoscopy to Verify Placement of a Double-Lumen Tube

1. Insert the scope through the tracheal lumen. Visualize the carina distally. (Confirm that the tracheal orifice is within the trachea and not a bronchus, or that the tube is not displaced proximally such that the bronchial cuff fills the trachea.)
2. Visualize the bronchial (blue) cuff 1–2 mm beyond the carina. Ensure that the cuff is not too proximal or overinflated such as to herniate across the carina and obstruct the contralateral bronchus.
3. Insert the scope through the bronchial lumen. Visually confirm that the tip of the bronchial lumen is unobstructed. For left-sided tubes, visualize the bronchial carina distal to the tube tip. For right-sided tubes with a right upper lobe (RUL) ventilation port, visualize that the RUL bronchus is aligned with the ventilation port.

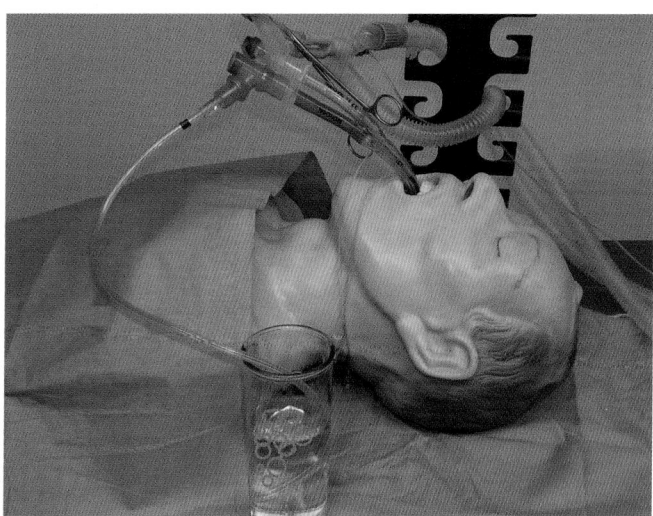

Fig. 30.14 Water seal setup to test for leaks around the bronchial cuff.

carina, while one arm of the fork has the inflatable balloon to occlude the bronchus it occupies.

Advantages and Disadvantages

Because insertion of a DLT is more complicated, bronchial blockers are more useful in patients with a difficult airway or a tracheostomy. These devices are beneficial for patients who are already intubated, when changing to another tube would compromise ventilation. They can also be used for pediatric lung separation, even in children younger than 2 years of age, with a special small-sized blocker.[122,123]

Positioning the bronchial blocker requires more time than the DLT, and placement is dependent on the use of a fiberscope. In comparison to DLT, blockers have a greater incidence of becoming malpositioned. Because a bronchial blocker affords little conduit for egress of gas, lung deflation is often less effective than with a DLT. This can be particularly troublesome in thoracoscopic surgery. Suction of the blocker port can be helpful, but excessive negative pressure or duration can cause damage. Blockers also do not allow suctioning, particularly when separation is indicated by unilateral infection or bleeding. In that case, removal must follow special procedures to avoid contaminating the opposite lung.[124] The bronchial blocker is plagued with the same challenge as the DLT in blocking the right bronchus, but the DLT has the advantage of being able to exclude either lung with a left-sided device. Therefore bronchial blockers are reserved by some exclusively for left-sided surgery.

The airway exchange catheter (AEC) is an essential piece of equipment for thoracic anesthesia, as there have been various case reports of anesthetists utilizing AECs for DLT placement. Most AECs have a small lumen that allows oxygen insufflation or jet ventilation. Many times AECs will also be utilized at the end of procedures to exchange the DLT for a standard ETT to prevent undue airway damage if long-term ventilation is needed postoperatively. When utilizing an AEC for DLT placement after intubation with a single-lumen ETT, it must be of sufficient length to ensure tracheal introduction of the DLT.[125] Considering the length of the DLT, the distance down the airway to the lower trachea, and additional length needed at its proximal end for control of the tube, the AEC must be more than 70 cm long. When a thin AEC is used, resistance to passage of the DLT at the glottis can occur. A laryngoscope should be used to lift supraglottic tissue to help the tube pass the angle between the pharynx and the larynx. A counterclockwise rotation of the tube will disengage it if it is temporarily stuck at the level of the glottis.[125]

To avoid airway perforation, the AEC should never be advanced against resistance. All AEC DLT guides have depth markings to monitor the depth of insertion. Although placement of the AEC in a more distal airway decreases the chance of the catheter slipping out of the trachea during tube exchange, it is safer for the guide to remain above

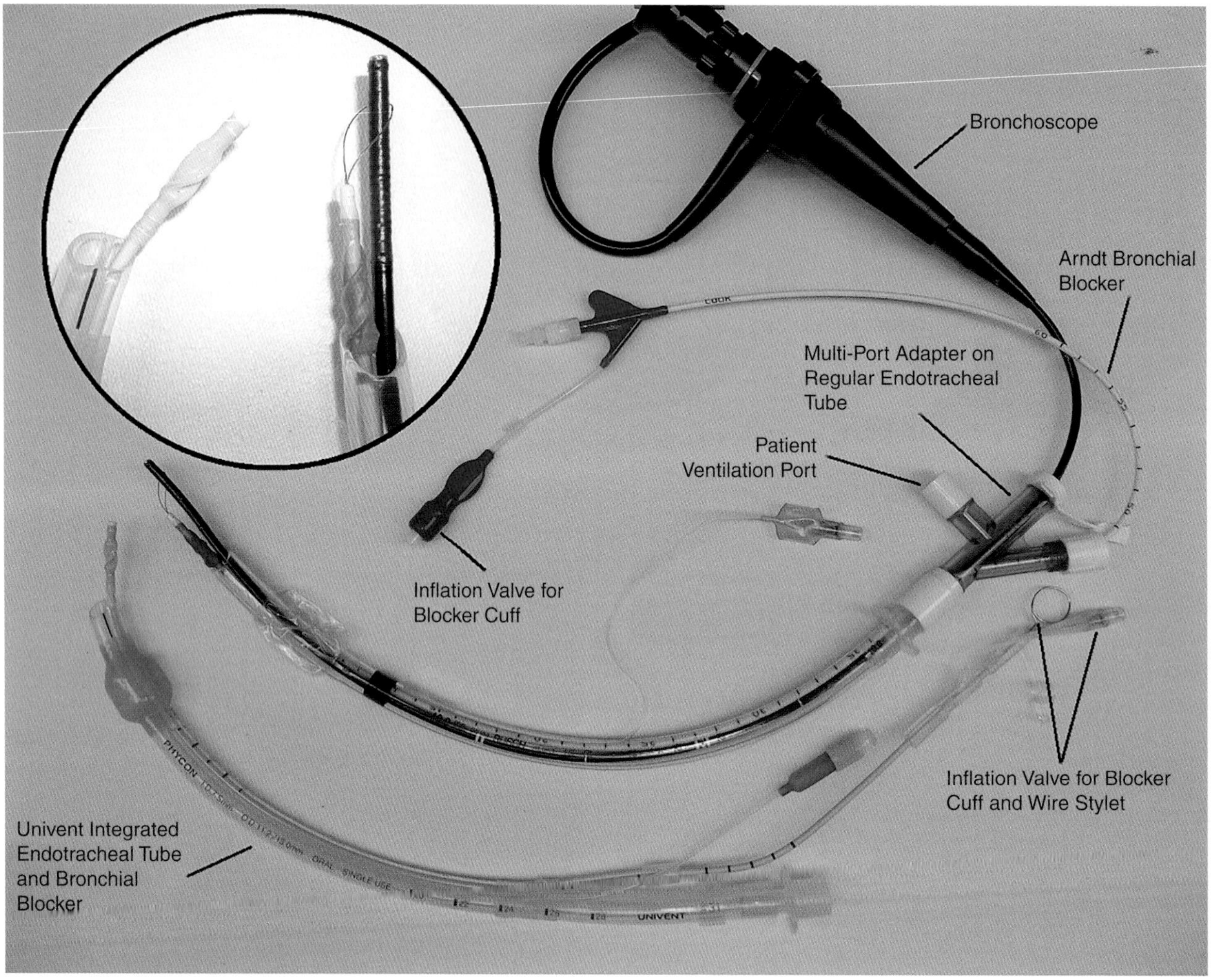

Bronchoscope

Arndt Bronchial
Blocker

Multi-Port Adapter on
Regular Endotracheal
Tube

Patient
Ventilation Port

Inflation Valve for
Blocker Cuff

Inflation Valve for Blocker
Cuff and Wire Stylet

Univent Integrated
Endotracheal Tube
and Bronchial
Blocker

Fig. 30.15 The Uninvent *(bottom)* and Arndt *(top)* bronchial blockers. Inset shows detail of Uninvent double-lumen tube design and Arndt wire guidance loop.

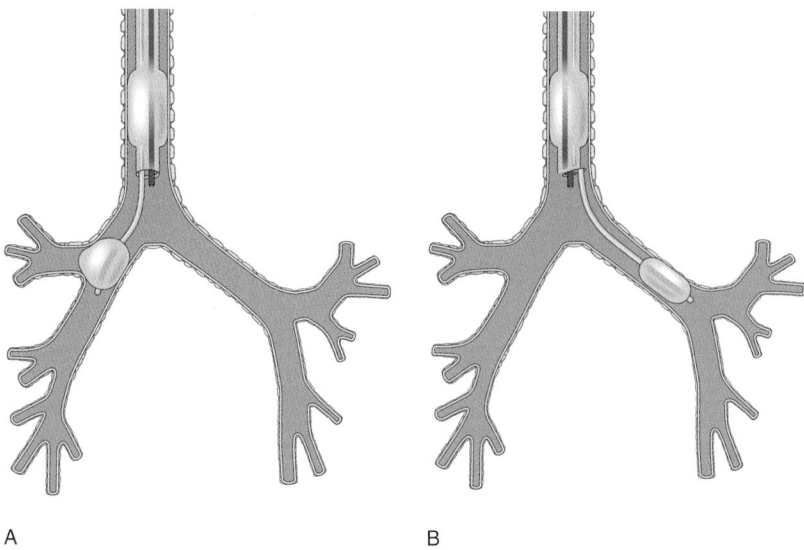

A   B

Fig. 30.16 Positioning of the bronchial blocker in the right (A) and left (B) lung. The fiberoptic bronchoscope is used to establish and verify correct position. (From Pardo MC, Miller RD. *Basics of Anesthesia.* 7th ed. Philadelphia: Elsevier; 2018:475.)

the carina in the lower trachea to avoid laceration of the bronchus. The AEC should not be inserted beyond the 25-cm mark at the teeth in adults.[125]

Insertion of Bronchial Blockers

The method used for inserting the bronchial blocker depends on the device. Typically, it involves basic tracheal intubation and insertion of the blocker through the tube, followed by the fiberscope, which is used for final positioning. Variations include wire-guided catheters, which are already mounted on the fiberscope when it is inserted, and pediatric extraluminal blockers, which are inserted in the trachea, followed by intubation, followed by fiberoptic inspection and positioning of the blocker. Of note, when utilizing a Univent tube, the fiberoptic bronchoscope is inserted into the ETT lumen while directing the bronchial blocker, preventing connection for ventilation to the anesthesia circuit. With the utilization of a bronchial blocker adapter, ventilation can be achieved via the side port as the bronchial blocker is being placed using a flexible intubating bronchoscope (see Fig. 30.15).

Physiology of One-Lung Ventilation

During two-lung ventilation, blood flow to the dependent lung averages approximately 60% (Fig. 30.17). When one lung is allowed to deflate and OLV is started, any blood flow to the deflated lung becomes shunt flow, causing the PaO_2 to decrease. Without autoregulation of pulmonary blood flow, a 40% shunt would be anticipated. The lungs have a compensatory mechanism of increasing vascular resistance in hypoxic areas of the lungs, and this diverts some blood flow to areas of better ventilation and oxygenation. This mechanism, which is present in most mammals, is termed HPV (or the von Euler–Liljestrand mechanism).[126] HPV is a reflex intrapulmonary feedback mechanism in inhomogeneous lungs that improves gas exchange and arterial oxygenation. Whereas hypoxemia causes vasodilation in the general circulation, alveolar hypoxia has the opposite effect on pulmonary arteries. HPV is a unique compensatory mechanism, suited specifically to matching pulmonary blood flow with well-oxygenated areas of the lung.

The cellular mechanism for HPV involves a redox-based oxygen sensor in smooth muscle cells of the pulmonary arteries, particularly the precapillary vessels (probably focused on the electron transport chain of the mitochondria of these cells). Hypoxia likely reduces production of activated oxygen species (AOS) such as H_2O_2; however, there are experimental discrepancies in the literature regarding whether a true increase or decrease in production of AOS occurs, as these AOS act as second messengers and lead to inhibition of voltage-dependent potassium channels.[126,127] These discrepancies may relate to variation among experimental groups in the use of freshly isolated pulmonary artery smooth muscle cells from resistance arteries, the severity of hypoxia induced, attention to pH and PcO_2, and challenges in AOS measurement.[127] The end result is an influx of extracellular calcium via the L-type calcium channels, which results in myosin light chain phosphorylation and ultimately vasoconstriction.[126-129] Box 30.6 lists the characteristics of HPV.

HPV during OLV is effective in decreasing the cardiac output to the nonventilated lung by approximately 50% (Fig. 30.18).[127] HPV can increase the PVR by 50% to 300%, and the response can persist for long periods of time in the face of chronic hypoxia.[128] In fact, the chronic increase in PVR from COPD can be responsible for pulmonary vascular remodeling that leads to cor pulmonale.[130] HPV occurs whether the lung is rendered hypoxic by atelectasis or by ventilation with a hypoxic mixture. It is initiated within seconds of hypoxia and reaches its maximum effect in approximately 15 minutes. HPV improves arterial oxygenation when the amount of hypoxic lung is between 20% and 80%, which occurs during OLV.[131] When less than 20% of the lung is

Blood Flow Distribution: Two-Lung Ventilation

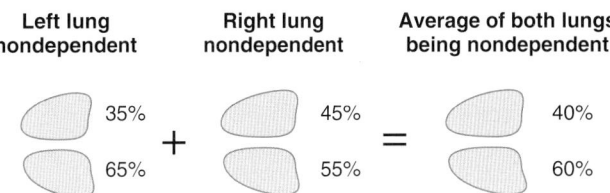

Fig. 30.17 When the left lung is the nondependent lung, the distribution of blood flow between the nondependent and dependent lungs is 35%:65%. When the right lung is the nondependent lung, blood flow distribution between the nondependent and dependent lungs is 45%:55%. Average one-lung ventilation blood flow distribution is a nondependent:dependent ratio of 40%:60%. (From Benumof JL. *Anesthesia for Thoracic Surgery.* 2nd ed. Philadelphia: Elsevier; 1995.)

BOX 30.6 Characteristics of Hypoxic Pulmonary Vasoconstriction

- A local reaction occurring in hypoxic areas of lung. May be very localized due to regional atelectasis (as in one-lung ventilation) or may affect both lungs entirely in hypoxic situations (such as those leading to high-altitude pulmonary edema).
- Opposite to systemic reaction to hypoxia, causes vasoconstriction in all but very proximal pulmonary arteries.
- Triggered by alveolar hypoxia, not arterial hypoxemia.
- Onset and resolution are within seconds following changes in partial pressure of oxygen (PO_2).
- Peak effect occurs within 15 min.
- May be inhibited by vasodilators and augmented by chemoreceptor agonists (almitrine).

Conversion of Two-Lung to One-Lung Ventilation: Blood Flow Distributions

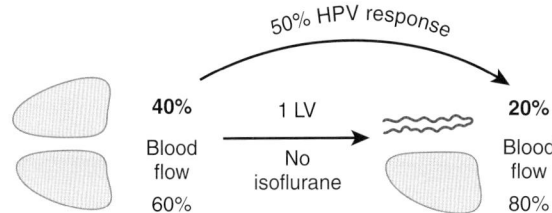

Fig. 30.18 Two-lung ventilation nondependent:dependent lung blood flow ratio is 40%:60%. When two-lung ventilation is converted to one-lung ventilation, the hypoxic pulmonary vasoconstriction *(HPV)* response decreases the blood flow to the nondependent lung by 50%, and the nondependent:dependent lung blood flow ratio becomes 20%:80%. *LV,* Lung ventilation. (From Benumof JL. *Anesthesia for Thoracic Surgery.* 2nd ed. Philadelphia: Saunders; 1995.)

hypoxic, the total amount of shunt is not significant. When more than 80% of the lung is hypoxic, HPV increases PVR, but the amount of well-perfused lung is not sufficient to accept enough diverted flow to maintain arterial oxygenation.

HPV is effective in decreasing shunt flow, and avoiding drugs or events that inhibit this mechanism is important pulmonary shunting (Box 30.7). Alveolar and intravascular volume derangements can inhibit the effects of HPV. Hypervolemia or high cardiac output may override HPV by recruiting constricted vessels.[132] Conversely, hypovolemia may trigger adrenergic vasoconstriction, reducing flow to well-ventilated portions of lung.[133] Overdistention of alveoli may also reduce perfusion to well-ventilated lung areas by creating the zone 1 V/Q scenario. For these reasons, normal fluid volume should be maintained during OLV; moderate Vt (6 mL/kg) should be used, and excessive PEEP should be avoided.[105] Hypocapnia and alkalosis decrease HPV.

Many vasodilatory drugs inhibit HPV, including nitroglycerin, nitroprusside, dobutamine, some calcium channel blockers (e.g., nifedipine, nicardipine, and verapamil), and some β2-agonists (such as isoproterenol).[105] Vasoconstrictive drugs, including dopamine, epinephrine, and phenylephrine, may preferentially constrict normally oxygenated pulmonary vessels and reestablish the shunt flow, opposing the effects of HPV.[131]

ANESTHETIC MANAGEMENT DURING ONE-LUNG VENTILATION

Choice of Anesthetic

Side effects associated with general anesthesia stem from a variety of mechanisms and can negatively impact intraoperative and postoperative pulmonary function. They include impairment of HPV, disruption of V/Q matching, neural and pain-induced hypoventilation, postoperative residual muscle relaxation, and atelectasis. Few studies have been able to demonstrate clear differences in patient outcomes based on anesthetic technique alone. However, some factors have emerged as important in the pulmonary surgical patient.

Clinical doses of potent inhalation agents do not significantly alter the mechanism of HPV. Volatile agents offer several benefits in thoracic surgery. They allow the use of a high fraction of inspired oxygen (Fio_2) to help prevent hypoxemia during OLV. They produce bronchodilatory effects and decrease airway irritability in patients who will be subjected to direct manipulation of lung tissue. In some studies, volatile agents resulted in a decreased inflammatory response compared to IV agents.[134,135] In contrast, the dose of narcotics required to obtund airway reflexes could depress ventilation and necessitate postoperative ventilation. Volatile agents are rapidly eliminated at the end of surgery and allow for early extubation. For these reasons, volatile agents are usually chosen as the primary anesthetics during thoracic surgery.

IV anesthetics do not inhibit HPV, and, whereas all volatile agents theoretically do, the volatiles act as vasodilators in a dose-dependent manner.[136] HPV can be expected to remain intact if volatile agents are administered at less than 1.5 of the minimum alveolar concentration.[137-139] Most analyses fail to demonstrate a difference in gas exchange between IV and inhaled techniques.[140] Furthermore, there is no difference in perioperative morbidity and mortality whether inhalational anesthesia or total IV anesthesia is administered.[141]

To prevent hypoxia and any significant increase in PVR, N_2O is generally avoided in favor of an air-oxygen mixture. N_2O increases PVR in healthy patients as well as in those with preexisting pulmonary hypertension.[103] This is cause for even greater concern with concurrent right ventricular dysfunction. Another indication to avoid N_2O includes patients with bullous or emphysematous lungs. Because N_2O is highly diffusible, increased air can be trapped within the lung. An air-oxygen mixture prolongs emptying of the operative lung (noting nitrogen stenting) in contrast to pure oxygen or an N_2O mixture.[142]

The choice of specific opioids or hypnotics will not influence pulmonary outcomes, but there is concern related to the choice of muscle relaxants used. Postoperative residual neuromuscular blockade can occur with both intermediate and long-acting relaxants and is present regardless of the use of neuromuscular monitoring.[143] However, the incidence of residual relaxation associated with the use of long-acting relaxants (e.g., pancuronium) is significantly higher, and complications from it are more frequent compared with the use of intermediate-acting relaxants.[144] Muscle weakness may follow long surgeries, even with adequate tests of neuromuscular recovery.[145] Therefore the use of shorter-acting muscle relaxants and conservative monitoring, dosing, and reversal practices are indicated in the pulmonary surgical patient. In one study of thoracic surgical patients necessitating OLV, the reversal of moderate neuromuscular blockade with sugammadex resulted in significantly fewer episodes of hypoxia in the early postoperative period compared with neostigmine.[146] The incorporation of sugammadex will likely become a more prominent practice due to its ability to effectively and efficiently reverse deep neuromuscular blockade by aminosteroid neuromuscular blockers. Of note, the incidence of bronchospasm has been cited within the literature as an adverse reaction of sugammadex administration and should be of particular concern when administering to patients with pathologic respiratory states.

The Role of Regional Anesthesia

When compared with general anesthesia, regional anesthesia may be beneficial in reducing atelectasis, pneumonia, respiratory failure, and other pulmonary complications.[147] Unfortunately, regional anesthesia as the sole anesthetic technique is impractical for open-lung cases; however, regional anesthesia can offer postoperative analgesia without the respiratory depressant effects of systemic opioids, which confers great benefits. Epidural anesthesia was found to reduce complications for both patients with normal FEV_1 and those with airflow obstruction.[148] The sympathectomy that is associated with neuraxial blockade causes vasodilation. Some have questioned whether epidural anesthesia would inhibit HPV, but because HPV is a locally mediated event epidural anesthesia has been found to be similar to IV or balanced techniques with regard to pulmonary gas exchange.[149]

Analgesia for Thoracic Surgery

A thoracotomy is known as one of the most painful operations, and postoperative pain can be very protracted, as in postthoracotomy pain syndrome (PTPS). PTPS is defined by the International Association for the Study of Pain (IASP) as pain that recurs or persists along a thoracotomy incision at least 2 months following the surgical procedure.[150] Most of the pain is caused by resection of thoracic tissue and bone in order for the surgeon to enter the chest cavity. This can lead to complications such as pneumonia and atelectasis.[103] Pain immediately after thoracic surgery causes splinting, decreased respiratory effort, hypoxemia, and respiratory acidosis. Aggressive management of pain is aimed at seeking a balance between comfort and respiratory depression in patients with decreased lung function. Residual pain exists in half of thoracotomy patients after 1 year and in one-third of patients after 4 years.[104]

Several options can be considered in the management of postoperative pain. Patients can titrate IV patient-controlled analgesia to obtain a more constant level of analgesia than that provided by intermittent intramuscular injections, but the benefits of avoiding systemic opioids have made regional anesthesia emerge as a superior method of pain control.

Thoracic epidural analgesia is considered one of the most effective methods for treating postoperative pain.[151] An epidural catheter is placed at the level of T6 to T8 and infused with epidural opioids or dilute solutions of local anesthetics to provide analgesia. The efficacy of epidural analgesia may be improved with adjunctive interventions, such as IV administration of ketamine, dexmedetomidine, acetaminophen, and nonsteroidal analgesics.[152]

As an alternative regional anesthesia technique, paravertebral nerve blocks can be placed at the level of the incision plus one or two intercostal interspaces above and below. A paravertebral nerve block can be performed with or without the use of a catheter and provides unilateral coverage of the chest wall by anesthetizing the nerves as they exit the intervertebral foramina, providing a somatosensory as well as sympathetic dermatomal block.[153] This technique provides good short-term pain relief and reduces opioid requirements. Paravertebral block provides quality pain control to rival epidural analgesia.[154,155] In the setting of a patient presenting for decortication for infectious pathology, it is vital to consider the close proximity of the paravertebral space to the pleural cavity likely deferring the placement of a catheter. Additionally, these catheters are challenging to place, with an incidence of pneumothorax between 1% and 10% as well as risk of epidural spread of medication.[153]

Intercostal blocks can be performed percutaneously or under direct visualization in the pleural cavity by the surgeon in the field at the end of the procedure. Specifically, intercostal blocks carry an increased risk of local anesthetic systemic toxicity (LAST) if not performed properly. Multiple-levels injections are required to ensure adequate analgesia, and risks include significant bleeding from trauma to the intercostal artery, block failure, and pneumothorax.[153]

A relatively newer regional block that offers advantages and has been gaining popularity is the erector spinae block. Like many regional techniques this block can also be performed as a single shot technique or by placing a catheter for continuous infusion. Most anesthesia providers view this as a peripheral nerve block. An erector spinae block is performed by injecting local anesthetic deep to the erector spinae fascia, superficial to the transverse process utilizing ultrasound. The local anesthetic can then spread and provide coverage from C7 to T10 dermatomes unilateral to the injection. Analgesia is believed to occur from diffusion of the anesthetic into the paravertebral space where it acts on the ventral and dorsal thoracic spinal nerves. Benefits of this technique include lack of significant sympathetic blockade, it can be performed under preoperative sedation or general anesthesia, a single injection can cover the entire chest wall, and it eliminates the risk of an epidural-related hematoma in a patient with or without anticoagulation medications.[153]

Management of One-Lung Ventilation
Ventilation Modes

The primary goal during OLV is to maintain adequate arterial oxygenation and protect the lung, while providing a surgical field favorable for visualization and manipulation of the operative lung (Table 30.3). In the past, large Vt of 10 to 15 mL/kg were recommended to prevent atelectasis in the dependent lung and maintain an adequate FRC. Contemporary understanding is that high volumes predispose to volutrauma,

which is associated with increases in cytokine inflammatory mediators, alveolar fibrin deposition, and other markers of procoagulant effect that contribute to acute lung injury (ALI).[156,157]

During OLV, patients frequently develop auto-PEEP and have an increased FRC such that large Vt is unnecessary. Understanding the detrimental effects of high Vt has led to the more contemporary approach of using more physiologic volumes (e.g., 6 mL/kg on the left and 8 mL/kg on the right), adding PEEP to those patients without auto-PEEP and limiting peak inspiratory pressures to less than 25 cm H_2O.[149,156-158] With this approach, patients will maintain adequate or even improved oxygenation (as compared with using a higher Vt) and minimal elevations in $Paco_2$.[105,159] It is preferable to allow permissive hypercapnia, rather than aggressively attempting to maintain a normal $Paco_2$, as hypercapnia supports HPV and directly reduces the cytokine response.[160,161] The $Paco_2$ should be maintained below 60 to 70 mm Hg to reduce the incidence of dysrhythmias, hypotension, and pulmonary hypertension. Although a high Fio_2 should induce vasodilation in the dependent lung and improve blood flow, hypocapnia causes vasoconstriction and should be avoided. PEEP must be employed when using a low Vt, otherwise alveolar derecruitment and atelectasis will occur, reducing Pao_2.[162] Implementation of an alveolar recruitment maneuver prior to initiating OLV can help to support better Pao_2 throughout the OLV period.[163] Recruitment maneuvers are not universally accepted. Besides opening airways, they may also translocate cytokines into the circulation,[164] impede hemodynamics, and provide only a transient effect.[165]

An appropriate air-oxygen mixture, at times as high as an Fio_2 of 1, is necessary to maximize the Pao_2. However, considering the potential for oxygen toxicity (particularly in a setting of absorptive atelectasis or history of chemotherapeutic administration),[166] Fio_2 should be maintained at the lowest level that will support adequate Spo_2.[136] This approach also leaves a reserve intervention in the case of hypoxemia. Increasing the Fio_2 in the face of declining oxygenation allows time to plan other interventions (such as checking tube placement). On 100% oxygen, by the time the Spo_2 falls, the insult will be more advanced, and the saturation will continue to decline during diagnosis and management of the issue.

Research validates the protective ventilation strategy, including end-expiratory pressures above the lower inflection point on the pressure-volume curve, a Vt less than 6 mL/kg, inspiratory pressures less than 20 cm H_2O above the PEEP value, permissive hypercapnia, and preferential use of pressure-limited ventilatory modes.[167-169] The superiority of pressure or volume modes of ventilation has not been definitively determined. It is compelling to consider that pressure-controlled ventilation limits maximal airway pressure and that the square pressure waveform provides more widespread alveolar recruitment, but research has been equivocal about demonstrating consistently better outcomes based on the ventilation mode.[170-173]

Hypoxemia During One-Lung Ventilation

The incidence of hypoxemia during OLV is currently less than 4%.[3] Although HPV attempts to normalize the relationship between ventilation and perfusion, it is not 100% effective at doing so. Certain characteristics predict the degree of hypoxemia that will be exhibited by a patient under OLV. Anatomically, the right lung is larger than the left lung, and thus proportionally there is a greater amount of perfusion to the right lung. This is the reason that there is an increased incidence of hypoxemia during right-sided surgery (see Fig. 30.17).[174] The usual detrimental effect of lateral positioning on oxygenation paradoxically benefits the patient during OLV. Lateral positioning with mechanical ventilation normally imbalances V/Q matching by distributing more ventilation to the nondependent lung, while gravity encourages more

TABLE 30.3   Recommendations for Avoiding Hypoxemia and Acute Lung Injury During One-Lung Ventilation

Setting	Rationale	Questions
Fio_2 <1.0	Fio_2 of 1.0 can facilitate atelectasis, inducing atelectotrauma and, paradoxically, hypoxemia.	Is there any cutoff point (e.g., Spo_2) to set the Fio_2?
Low Vt (e.g., 6 mL/kg) (or low pressures)	High Vt (or high pressures) can lead to volutrauma (or barotrauma).	What is the ideal Vt for one lung?
Routine use of PEEP	PEEP is beneficial for oxygenation and for lung protection.	What is the best PEEP? How can it be determined?
Recruitment maneuvers	Recruitment maneuvers improve oxygenation and acheive a better distribution of aeration.	Should it be used routinely? How should it be applied?
Routine use of CPAP to nondependent lung	CPAP is beneficial for both oxygenation and lung protection.	Are their situations during one-lung ventilation where CPAP is contraindicated?
Permissive hypercapnia	High Pco_2 can be beneficial in avoiding ALI.	In order to avoid hemodynamic instability, what is the optimal Pco_2?
Inhalational anesthetics + TEA	TEA does not inhibit HPV allowing a lower inhalational anesthetic MAC value; Inhalational anesthetics can reduce the potential for ALI.	What are the effects of TEA on ALI?

ALI, Acute lung injury; *CPAP,* continuous positive airway pressure; *Fio_2,* fraction of inspired oxygen; *HPV,* hypoxic pulmonary vasoconstriction; *Pco_2,* partial pressure of carbon dioxide; *PEEP,* positive end-expiratory pressure; *RM,* recruitment maneuvers; *Spo_2,* blood oxygen saturation; *TEA,* thoracic epidural anesthesia; *TV,* tidal volume; *VATS,* video-assisted thoracoscopic surgery.
From Şentürk M, et al. Intraoperative mechanical ventilation strategies for one-lung ventilation. *Best Pract Res Clin Anaesthesiol.* 2015;29(3):357–369.

perfusion to the dependent lung. During laterally positioned OLV, direction of all ventilation to the dependent lung creates a more beneficial match of ventilation and perfusion. In fact, Pao_2 is found to be significantly worse in procedures (such as lung transplant) where OLV is performed in supine patients.[136] Some patient data also predict the degree of hypoxemia that will be encountered during OLV. The reduction in FEV_1, paradoxically, is sometimes inverse to the degree of hypoxemia experienced. As a measure of disease progress, a lower FEV_1 indicates worse disease; but as a measure of air trapping, patients with a lower FEV_1 sometimes develop intrinsic or auto-PEEP that helps keep their airways patent and beneficially reduces hypoxemia during OLV.[174] V/Q scanning, if completed preoperatively, can help the anesthetist to predict the potential for intraoperative shunt under OLV because perfusion to the operative lung is inverse to the potential shunt.[175] A last-minute predictor is the end tidal CO_2 ($ETco_2$). Being dependent on blood flow to the lung, $ETco_2$ is a surrogate measure of perfusion.[176] The degree of decline in $ETco_2$ when switching from two-lung ventilation to OLV indicates the degree of blood perfusing the nondependent lung, and therefore a greater initial decline predicts inferior oxygenation during OLV. Alveolar recruitment maneuvers and the use of subsequent PEEP at 8 cm H_2O improve arterial oxygenation during OLV.[177]

Should hypoxemia occur during OLV, the anesthetist should assess for physiologic causes or tube malpositioning. Physiologic causes include bronchospasm, decreased cardiac output, hypoventilation, low Fio_2, or pneumothorax of the dependent lung. Tube malpositioning implies that movement of the DLT may have excluded a portion of dependent lung, usually the upper lobe. Assessing the position of the DLT should be the initial intervention, as a large proportion of hypoxemic episodes are remedied by tube repositioning.[4] If physiologic causes have been ruled out, and adequate lung separation and ventilation have been determined, one or more of the following interventions will help improve Pao_2. First, continuous positive airway pressure (CPAP) to the nondependent, nonventilated lung is almost 100% efficacious in increasing Pao_2. This can be accomplished with a compact breathing system, such as a Mapleson C with a manometer

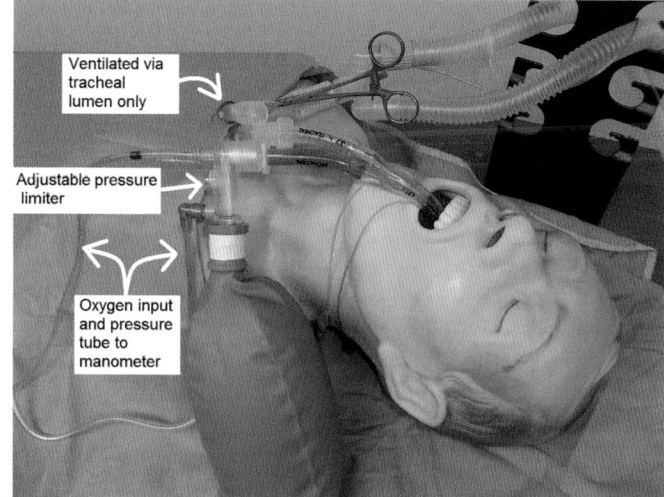

Fig. 30.19 Continuous positive airway pressure apparatus for improving oxygenation of the nonventilated lung.

for pressure determination, attached to the lumen of the deflated lung (Fig. 30.19), or with a calibrated, adjustable device made specifically for this purpose. Application of CPAP should help to oxygenate the persistent blood flow through the nondependent lung, but too much pressure will cause the lung to inflate, reducing surgical exposure. The lowest level of effective CPAP should be sought (start at 2 cm H_2O). The reservoir bag on the CPAP device can also be used to provide intermittent ventilation to the operative lung, should that intervention become necessary. Providing gentle ventilation with a separate system will minimize the diminution of surgical exposure, as opposed to ventilating the lung with the same vigor as that required for the dependent lung. As an alternative to CPAP, a small catheter can be used to deliver low-flow oxygen insufflation to the nondependent lung without generating pressure. This approach may be adequate to reduce the shunt and reverse hypoxemia in mild cases.[178]

Besides shunt flow through the operative lung, atelectasis and reduced FRC in the dependent lung may also degrade the Pao$_2$. If CPAP to the nondependent lung does not improve oxygenation, PEEP applied (or titrated upward) to the dependent, ventilated lung acts to recruit collapsed airways, increasing lung compliance and FRC. Excessive PEEP may detrimentally reduce cardiac output. Combined with a fast respiratory rate and/or high inspiratory:expiratory ratio (I:E ratio), PEEP may impair adequate exhalation, leading to a net volume increase through auto-PEEP and the potential for volutrauma to the dependent lung. The actual end-expiratory pressure should be monitored during OLV to ensure that it does not significantly exceed the intended level of PEEP.

Other methods of improving oxygenation during OLV include combining PEEP and CPAP to the respective lungs, and intermittent reinflation of the nondependent lung. Innovative ventilatory approaches such as high-frequency jet ventilation to the operative lung and selective oxygenation to nonoperative lobes of the operative lung via a bronchial blocker or bronchoscope are also used.[178-181] Jet ventilation is effective at reducing the shunt, but lung movement can be deleterious, which makes monitoring CO$_2$ levels and effective CO$_2$ removal challenging.[182]

If CPAP and PEEP fail, early ligation of the pulmonary artery in pneumonectomy patients may be used to improve oxygenation. If the pulmonary artery is planned to be ligated during the procedure, clamping it will immediately stop all significant flow through the lung contributing to the shunt. For the same reason, manual compression of the lung will also improve the Pao$_2$, but the expense of cardiac output and tissue trauma advises against this as a regular strategy.[183] If it becomes impossible to maintain adequate oxygenation with OLV in spite of CPAP and PEEP, manual two-lung ventilation can be used, with pauses in ventilation coordinated with the surgeon's activities to facilitate exposure, suturing of the lung, or other needs. Communication with the surgical team is vital throughout the procedure, especially during the evaluation and correction of hypoxia.

At the conclusion of the resection, the surgeon will commonly ask that the operative lung be reinflated using large Vt so that air leaks may be detected. At this time, the lung separator (DLT clamp or bronchial blocker) should be discontinued, and the lung inflated with slow breaths, achieving a peak inspiratory pressure of 30 to 40 cm H$_2$O.[105] Reexpansion of the lung can be observed while performing this maneuver, which also helps to reverse atelectasis in the lungs. Following lung reexpansion, the bronchial cuff should be deflated on the DLT to both reduce pressure on the bronchial mucosa and obviate any detrimental effects of slight tube malpositioning. Deflated, the cuff does not pose the threat of herniating over the carina or obstructing the lobar bronchi. Box 30.8 outlines the management of one-lung anesthesia.

Emerging techniques of OLV focus attention away from manipulating ventilation of the operative lung to manipulating perfusion of the nonoperative lung. V/Q matching can be supported by encouraging more perfusion to the ventilated lung or selectively diminishing perfusion to the nonventilated lung. Inhaled epoprostenol (prostacyclin) and NO are beneficial for increasing the perfusion of the dependent lung. The combination of inhaled epoprostenol and IV phenylephrine (for vasoconstriction of the operative lung) is an effective strategy.[184] Another experimental approach is the use of almitrine, which enhances HPV of the nonventilated lung. Studies have shown a more than 100% increase in Pao$_2$ when almitrine and NO are used on their respective lungs[185,186]; however, toxicity, cost, and challenges related to setting up and administering NO are deterrents to using these interventions as part of a routine plan except for in the most critical cases.

BOX 30.8 Management of One-Lung Anesthesia

- Ventilate:
  - Tidal volume: 6–8 mL/kg
  - Rate: 12–15 (permissive hypercapnia acceptable)
  - Fio$_2$: 0.4–0.8; maintain Spo$_2$ >90%
  - PEEP: 5–10 cm H$_2$O (2.5–5 if COPD)
  - I:E ratio: 1:2 (1:3 if COPD or intrinsic [auto-] PEEP)
- Consider alveolar recruitment maneuver prior to OLV
- Assess ABG 15 min after OLV is initiated
- Volatile anesthetics <1–1.5 MAC or IV agents
- Stepwise response to worsening hypoxemia:
  - Increase Fio$_2$
  - Confirm tube position with fiberoptic bronchoscope
  - Ensure adequacy of cardiac output
  - Remedy detrimental effects caused by anemia or vasodilators
  - Perform alveolar recruitment maneuver to DL
  - Titrate PEEP in DL
  - CPAP 5–10 cm H$_2$O to NDL
  - Intermittent or continuous two-lung ventilation
  - Low- or no-pressure oxygen insufflation to NDL or selected lobe of NDL
  - Reposition to lateral decubitus position if supine
  - Alter perfusion with almitrine to NDL; nitric oxide to DL

ABG, Arterial blood gas; *COPD,* chronic obstructive pulmonary disease; *CPAP,* continuous positive airway pressure; *DL,* dependent lung; *Fio$_2$,* fraction of inspired oxygen; *I:E,* inspiratory/expiratory ratio; *IV,* intravenous; *MAC,* minimum alveolar concentration; *NDL,* nondependent lung; *PEEP,* positive end-expiratory pressure; *Spo$_2$,* blood oxygen saturation.

THORACIC SURGICAL CONCERNS

Asthma Treatment

Asthma that is refractory to medical therapy may be treated with thermal ablation of the bronchial smooth muscle to reduce its responsiveness. Bronchial thermoplasty is performed through a fiberoptic bronchoscope. The procedure may be performed under general anesthesia or monitored anesthesia care (MAC). Either approach has positive and negative attributes. MAC provides the advantage of not needing to instrument the airway; however, suppressing the cough and irritant reflexes while preserving spontaneous ventilation can pose a challenge. Agents that provide sedation while minimizing airway compromise and bronchial irritation (such as dexmedetomidine) are beneficial.[187] General anesthesia provides control of the airway and breathing and allows a deeper state of reflex attenuation; however, weaning and extubation may pose challenges. The procedure is completed in three stages, with a few weeks between stages. Therefore the patient is not "cured" upon completion of the procedure, and postoperative complications may include bronchospasm, hypoxemia, and respiratory distress. There have been reports of reversible complete lobar collapse, asthma exacerbations, pulmonary abscess, pulmonary pseudoaneurysm, and massive hemoptysis requiring embolization postprocedure. Current literature also reflects a high incidence of acute postoperative inflammation and pulmonary consolidations extending far beyond the treated airways.[188]

Mediastinal Masses

Masses in the mediastinum can compress vital structures and cause changes in cardiac output, obstruct airflow, induce atelectasis, or produce central nervous system changes. Masses can include benign or

BOX 30.9   Common Tumors of the Anterior Mediastinum: The Four *T*s

- Thymoma
- Thyroid
- Teratoma
- Terrible lymphoma

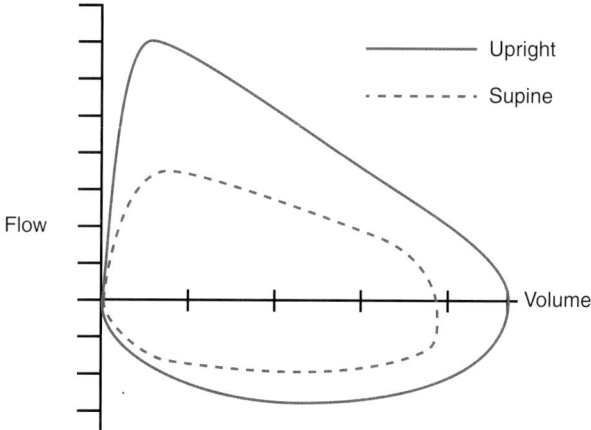

Fig. 30.20 Upright and supine flow-volume curves representative of anterior mediastinal mass. Note that an abnormality appears in the supine position when gravity causes the mass to impinge on the lower airway. The greatest decrement affects the expiratory limb of the loop, which is generally indicative of variable intrathoracic obstructions. Thoracic excursion during spontaneous inspiration relieves the pressure. This effect is lost when ventilation is changed to exclusively positive pressure input from above.

BOX 30.10   Symptoms of Mediastinal Mass

- Sweats
- Stridor
- Syncope
- Cyanosis
- Orthopnea
- Hoarseness
- Inability to lie flat
- Chest pain or fullness
- Jugular vein distention
- Superior vena cava syndrome
- Cough (especially when supine)

Data from Slinger P, Karsli C. Management of the patient with a large anterior mediastinal mass: recurring myths. *Curr Opin Anaesthesiol.* 2007;20(1):1-3; Hartigan PM, Ng JM, Gill RR. Anesthesia in a patient with a large mediastinal mass. *N Engl J Med.* 2018;379(6):587–588.

cancerous tumors, thymomas, substernal thyroid masses, vascular aneurysms, lymphomas, teratomas, germ cell tumors, metastatic lung and esophageal lesions, and neuromas (Box 30.9).[189] Surgical procedures for diagnosis or treatment of these masses may include thoracotomy, thoracoscopy, and mediastinoscopy.

Tumors within the anterior mediastinum can cause compression of the trachea or bronchi, increasing resistance to airflow. Changes in airway dynamics with supine positioning, induction of anesthesia, and positive pressure ventilation can cause collapse of the airway with total obstruction to flow. General anesthesia can therefore be very dangerous in these patients. Total airway obstruction can occur at any phase of anesthesia and through the recovery phase. Positive pressure ventilation may be impossible, even with a properly placed ETT, if the mass encroaches on the airway distal to the ETT. The airway can collapse, even when spontaneous respiration is maintained.[190] To anticipate this potential, anesthetic preparation should include the availability of a rigid bronchoscope and readiness to turn the patient lateral or prone in case of airway collapse. Cannulation for potential emergency femoral-femoral bypass should be considered if the tumor is large or if the patient becomes symptomatic.[191,192] Localization of the mass by CT or bronchoscopy may facilitate placement of the ETT distal to the mass. A major anesthetic goal is to maintain spontaneous ventilation, which retains normal airway-distending pressure gradients and can maintain airway patency when positive pressure ventilation will not.[193]

Signs and symptoms associated with respiratory tract compression should be determined preoperatively. Many patients with mediastinal masses are asymptomatic or characterized by vague signs such as dyspnea, cough, hoarseness, or chest pain. Wheezing may represent airflow past a mechanical obstruction rather than bronchospasm. Symptoms may be positional, worsening in the supine position, or other positions. A chest radiograph may show airway compression or deviation. CT, transesophageal echocardiography, and MRI may further delineate the size and effects of masses. Subclinical airway obstruction may be revealed by flow-volume loops, which demonstrate changes in flow rates at different lung volumes. A decreased maximal inspiratory or expiratory flow rate alerts the anesthetist to an increased risk of obstruction perioperatively. Comparison of flow rates obtained with the patient in the upright and supine positions can reveal whether the supine position will exacerbate the obstruction intraoperatively (Fig. 30.20; Box 30.10).[194]

Biopsy of masses should be performed with the patient under local anesthesia whenever possible. Bilevel positive airway pressure (BiPAP) has been used in this situation to support the airway and maintain spontaneous ventilation while still providing sedation.[195,196] Radiation therapy may be helpful to decrease the mass of the tumor before major surgery is attempted. For airway management, awake intubation using a flexible intubating endoscope enable the anesthetist to evaluate the large airways for obstruction and place the ETT beyond the obstruction while maintaining spontaneous ventilation. The effect of positional changes can be assessed with the bronchoscope. Spontaneous ventilation should be maintained as long as possible or throughout the procedure if feasible. The ability to effectively provide positive pressure

ventilation should be guaranteed prior to administering muscle relaxants. The use of a helium-oxygen mixture can improve airflow during partial obstruction by decreasing turbulence past the stenotic area.[197]

Mediastinal masses can cause compression of great vessels or cardiac chambers. Patients with any cardiac or great vessel involvement should receive only local anesthesia whenever possible, remain in the sitting position, and maintain spontaneous respirations. Cardiopulmonary bypass must be able to be implemented within minutes in the case of sudden cardiopulmonary collapse.

Patients with mediastinal masses may develop superior vena cava (SVC) syndrome, which is venous engorgement of the upper body caused by compression of the SVC. The following signs and symptoms are associated with SVC syndrome: dilation of collateral veins of the upper part of the thorax and neck; edema and rubor of the face, neck, upper torso, and airway; edema of the conjunctiva with or without proptosis; shortness of breath, headache, visual distortion, or altered mentation.[198] Placement of IV lines in the lower extremities is preferred; insertion in sites above the SVC could delay the drug's effect as a result of slow distribution. Fluids should be administered with caution because large volumes can worsen symptoms.

Mediastinoscopy

Mediastinoscopy involves insertion of a scope into the mediastinum via an incision made above the sternal notch. The scope is passed

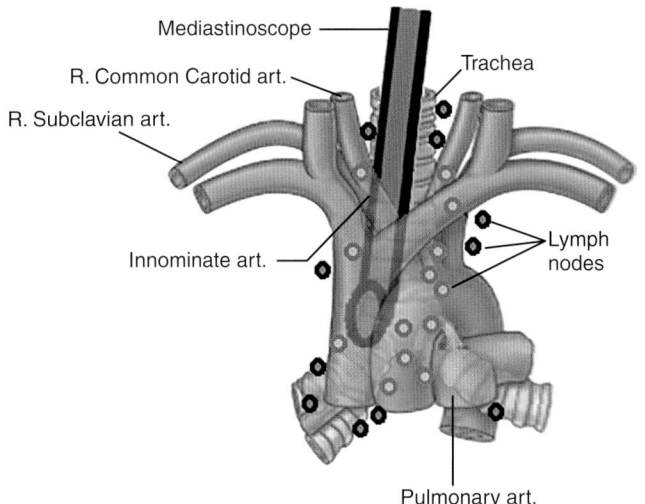

Fig. 30.21 Placement of a mediastinoscope into the superior mediastinum. The mediastinoscope passes in front of the trachea but behind the thoracic aorta. The mediastinoscope can potentially compress or damage the aorta, innominate artery, trachea, superior vena cava, and left recurrent laryngeal nerve. *Art.,* Artery; *R.,* right. (Adapted from Drake RL, et al. *Gray's Anatomy for Students.* 4th ed. Philadelphia: Elsevier; 2020.)

anterior to the trachea in close proximity to the left common carotid artery, the left subclavian artery, the innominate artery, the innominate veins, the vagus nerve, the left recurrent laryngeal nerve, the thoracic duct, the SVC, and the aortic arch.

Complications associated with mediastinoscopy include hemorrhage resulting from disruption of major vessels, pneumothorax, dysrhythmias, bronchospasm, left recurrent laryngeal nerve palsy, laceration of the trachea or esophagus, and chylothorax secondary to laceration of the thoracic duct.[199] Large-bore IV access should be in place, and banked blood should be immediately available in the event of a tear in a major blood vessel. Air embolism is also a risk if a venous tear occurs. Dysrhythmias such as bradycardia are possible with manipulation of the aorta or trachea during blunt dissection.

The mediastinoscope can place pressure on the innominate (brachiocephalic) artery prior to its division into the right common carotid artery and right subclavian artery. This can cause decreased blood flow to the right common carotid artery and right vertebral artery, and decreased right subclavian blood flow to the right arm (Fig. 30.21).[137] The decrease in cerebral flow can cause an acute ischemic stroke, especially if the patient has a history of cerebrovascular disease. Monitoring perfusion to the right arm with a pulse oximeter or radial artery catheter can detect decreased flow to the right arm and signal concurrent loss of flow to the brain via innominate artery compression. Repositioning of the mediastinoscope is required to reestablish flow to the brain. A noninvasive blood pressure cuff placed on the left arm enables continued monitoring of systemic blood pressure during periods of innominate artery compression.

Thoracoscopy

Advances in videoscopic technology have led to the increased use of thoracoscopy to replace open thoracotomy for a variety of diagnostic and therapeutic intrathoracic interventions (Table 30.4). VATS most often requires general anesthesia, and frequently requires lung isolation during ventilation. A video camera and surgical instruments are inserted via a trocar (Thoracoport) into the chest, allowing for visualization and manipulation of thoracic structures (Fig. 30.22). The surgeon has less ability to manually compress the lung during this

TABLE 30.4 **Indications for Video-Assisted Thoracoscopic Surgery**	
Diagnostic	**Therapeutic**
Pulmonary	
Identification of disease	• Lung volume reduction
Biopsy and staging of cancer	• Resection of lung tumor(s) or metastasis
Evaluation of intrapleural infection	• Lobectomy, pneumonectomy
	• Spontaneous pneumothorax
	• Blebectomy
	• Pleurodesis
	• Decortication
	• Drainage of empyema
	• Lysis of adhesions
Mediastinum	
Biopsy of tumor(s)	• Excision of cysts: bronchogenic or pericardial
Biopsy of lymph node(s)	• Resection of mediastinal tumor(s)
	• Thymectomy
	• Ligation of thoracic duct
Esophagus	
Biopsy of tumor	• Esophageal resection: vagotomy, Heller myotomy, Nissen fundoplication, transhiatal esophagectomy
Staging of cancer	• Resection of primary esophageal tumor(s)
Cardiac	
Identification of pericardial distention	• Drainage of pericardial effusion
Identification of pericardial disease	• Pericardiectomy
	• Ligation of patent ductus arteriosus
	• Minimally invasive coronary artery bypass and valve procedures
Spine	• Sympathectomy
	• Spinal surgery, discectomy, fusion
	• Spinal abscess drainage
Other	• Assessment of injury from trauma
	• Stabilization of bleeding
	• Clot evaluation

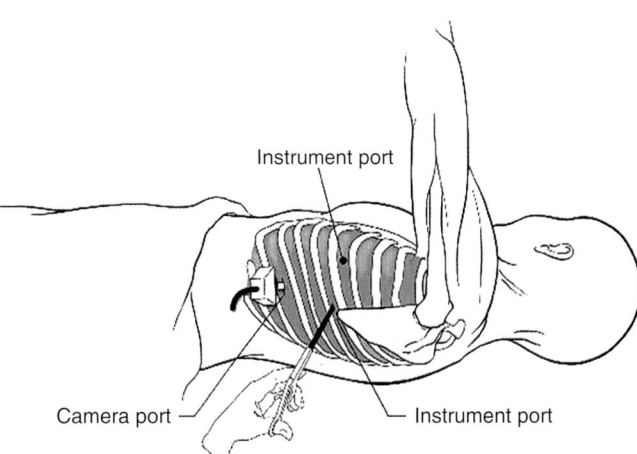

Fig. 30.22 Surgical instrument placement during video-assisted thoracoscopic surgery. (From Kitabjian L, et al. Anesthesia case management for video-assisted thoracoscopic surgery. *AANA J.* 2013;81:65–72.)

procedure as compared to during an open thoracotomy, and therefore a DLT may be preferable to a bronchial blocker to facilitate lung isolation. An arterial line is frequently inserted for VATS procedures, except with minimally invasive procedures in selected healthy patients. However, the anesthetic plan should account for the potential need for rapidly obtaining arterial blood gas samples or for possible hemorrhage, which may be difficult to control during the endoscopic procedure. In addition to the potential for rapid massive hemorrhage, other complications associated with VATS include hypoxemia, cardiac/pulmonary artery/esophageal disruption, cardiac tamponade, left recurrent laryngeal nerve damage, and pulmonary edema. In cases of severe pulmonary compromise, VATS can be performed using epidural anesthesia in the spontaneously breathing patient who is sedated with a variety of techniques.[200] The degree of postoperative pain is less with VATS as compared to an open procedure. For this reason, an epidural used solely for postoperative pain management is rarely indicated. Patients who undergo VATS have an improved quality of life for the first year postoperatively as compared to those who undergo open thoracotomy, suggesting that VATS should be the preferred surgical approach for lobectomy in stage I non–small cell lung cancer.[201] VATS is associated with greater antiangiogenic responsiveness in patients with non–small cell lung cancer as compared to open thoracotomy. The differences in antiangiogenic responsiveness may have an important effect on cancer biology and recurrence after surgery.[202]

Thoracoscopic sympathectomy for hyperhidrosis is an outpatient procedure. A DLT is preferred over a bronchial blocker because the procedure is bilateral, and the DLT can more easily switch from ventilation of one lung to the other. The procedure is performed in the supine position, and no chest tubes are inserted.

Bullectomy

Patients with bullous COPD are often treated with VATS to prevent pneumothorax or tension pneumothorax, which may result from ruptured bullae. To reduce the risk of bulla rupture, spontaneous ventilation is desirable under anesthesia until the chest is opened. Patients with severe cardiopulmonary disease may not be able to ventilate adequately under general anesthesia, however, and positive pressure ventilation may be required. Small Vt, high respiratory rates, and high FiO_2 can be delivered by gentle manual ventilation to keep airway pressures below 10 to 20 cm H_2O.[203] An alternative to positive pressure ventilation is high-frequency jet ventilation, which is used to decrease the chance of barotrauma.[204]

The use of N_2O should be avoided in bullous disease because it rapidly enlarges the air-filled spaces. The anesthetic plan can involve general or epidural anesthesia and is based on the patient's cardiopulmonary status and the anesthetist's desire to maintain spontaneous ventilation. The risk of bulla rupture persists even after surgery, so the same measures taken to avoid high airway pressure must be observed.

COMPLICATIONS AFTER THORACOTOMY

A number of complications may occur following thoracic surgery. Various factors have been correlated with an increased risk of complications. Admission to the intensive care unit or heightened surveillance should be considered for postoperative patients with the following characteristics: pulmonary fibrosis, age greater than 80 years, PPO FEV_1 or DLCO less than 40%, ASA status over 3, surgical time longer than 80 minutes, intraoperative hemorrhage, and others.[205-208] The following frequent predictors of pulmonary complications are quantified in the FLAM score (named after two of its designers: Francesco Leo and Marylene Anziani), which shows good predictive capacity for impending respiratory complications: dyspnea, chest x-ray changes, required

oxygen administration, auscultated changes, cough, and bronchial secretions.[209] Among the most common postoperative complications are respiratory failure, cardiac dysrhythmia or failure, and ALI.

Significant factors associated with ALI after pulmonary resections include right pneumonectomy, intraoperative overhydration with high vascular volume, high intraoperative airway pressure during OLV, and preoperative alcohol abuse. Other factors that have been suggested are female gender, poor postoperative predicted lung function, trauma, infection, chemotherapy, mediastinal lymphatic damage, transfusion and administration of fresh frozen plasma, oxygen toxicity, prolonged OLV (>100 min), and an increased postoperative urine output.[166,210]

OLV causes inflammatory changes in the ventilated and nonventilated lung, and some of the damage appears to occur upon reexpansion of the deflated lung.[211-215] Protective ventilation strategies should always be employed to reduce the generation of inflammatory processes.[159,216] There appears to be a lasting effect of OLV that is not reversed when reverting to two-lung ventilation. A small animal study demonstrated that after OLV has been discontinued, very low V/Q ratios in the range of 0.3 to 0.5 persist in the dependent lung.[217] This, coupled with diffuse alveolar damage in comparison to controls, suggests that anesthetists should expect hypoxemia from the resultant V/Q mismatch that may persist for an unknown period after OLV. Even in the absence of an inflammatory response there is evidence of vascular injury to lung tissue that is collapsed during OLV, which suggests that CPAP may have both short- and long-term benefits.[218]

Minimizing pulmonary intravascular pressures by intraoperative fluid restriction is advocated to decrease postoperative complications.[219] ERAS protocols recommend very restrictive fluid regimes, balanced crystalloid solutions versus 0.9% normal saline, and that IV fluids be discontinued as soon as possible and replaced with oral fluids.[98] Surgical requirements for proper hydration and tissue perfusion must be balanced with the desire to prevent high postoperative intravascular pressures that can cause acute pulmonary edema. In review of the Starling hypothesis, there is a fine balance among plasma colloid oncotic pressure (which holds fluid in the pulmonary capillaries), capillary hydrostatic pressure, interstitial fluid colloid oncotic pressure, and the negative interstitial fluid pressure that promotes fluid movement into the interstitial space away from the alveoli to foster optimal gas exchange. Any derangement of these forces, along with inflammatory mediator release and resultant vascular permeability that occurs with surgical procedures, pathology, or aggressive ventilatory methods, could ultimately lead to pulmonary edema.

Decreased cardiac output in the early postoperative period can be caused by several factors, including blood loss, herniation of the heart through a pericardial defect, right-sided heart failure, and dysrhythmias. Generally, blood entering the pleural space drains into chest tubes at a rate of less than 500 mL/day. Chest tube drainage greater than 200 mL/hour necessitates surgical exploration. An obstructed chest tube can conceal bleeding in a hemothorax. Hypotension, unexplained tachycardia, and decreasing hematocrit are other signs associated with hemorrhage.

Loss of pulmonary vasculature with lung resection can result in increased PVR and right-sided heart failure. The reduction in cardiac ejection fraction is greater following pneumonectomy than that following lobectomy. Conditions that increase the likelihood of right-sided heart failure include postoperative pneumonia, hypercarbia, and acidosis. Vasodilators are useful for decreasing the PVR. Amrinone or dobutamine can be administered for inotropic support, as needed.

Supraventricular dysrhythmias are common after thoracotomy and may herald other serious complications.[220] Morbidity and mortality rates in patients with supraventricular tachydysrhythmias are high, with 25% associated with death within 30 days postoperatively, despite institution of aggressive treatment. Administration of a β-blocking agent can help prevent atrial dysrhythmias. Metoprolol or esmolol provide rate control, and their cardioselectivity limits adverse effects on bronchial tone. Digitalis, adenosine, calcium channel blockers, and β-blockers are useful for treating supraventricular tachydysrhythmias.

Respiratory complications in the early postoperative period include atelectasis, pneumonia, respiratory failure, bronchopleural or bronchocutaneous fistula, pneumothorax, and pulmonary edema. Aggressive respiratory care to prevent deterioration and allow weaning from ventilation is vital.

Nerve injuries that may follow thoracic surgery include damage to the phrenic nerve as it passes through the mediastinum and damage to the left recurrent laryngeal nerve, which is vulnerable during dissection of aortopulmonary lymph nodes and mediastinal procedures.[221] Spinal cord injury is a possibility if an intercostal artery supplying a major radicular artery is injured or if an epidural hematoma is created by surgical dissection between the pleura and the epidural space. Nerve injuries related to surgical positioning are also possible complications.

SUMMARY

Providing anesthesia for thoracic surgery requires a comprehensive knowledge of anatomy, physiology, pharmacology, and anesthetic considerations, as this is necessary for safe patient care. The patient may have cardiac or respiratory diseases, masses, bullae, and other problems that complicate anesthetic management. Knowledge of respiratory physiology, pathophysiology, and the physiology of OLV is vital to safe and effective practice. Special equipment such as double-lumen endobronchial tubes, bronchial blockers, and fiberoptic bronchoscopes must be understood. A thorough understanding of the properties of anesthetic drugs is necessary so that the most beneficial combination of agents can be selected to manage the patient's anesthesia. Traditional ventilation concepts favoring high Fio_2 and large Vt have given way to protective ventilation strategies, considering the metabolic implications of oxygen toxicity and ALI. Protective lung strategies use lower Vt, PEEP, and modest Fio_2 levels. For pulmonary surgery, lung separation may be achieved by DLTs or bronchial blockers. Each has its own advantages, but neither is clearly preferable over the other in every case. Flexible bronchoscopy should be used to ensure proper placement of airway devices for lung separation. For hypoxemia caused by shunting during OLV, intermittent expansion of one or both lungs, CPAP applied to the operative lung, or PEEP applied to the dependent lung should be used. Judicious fluid management is an important component of reducing postoperative lung injury. Regional anesthesia is a useful adjunct for postoperative pain control. Future research and directions will include more practical methods of reducing the shunt during OLV and a better understanding of the implications of hypoxemia. More critical monitoring (such as effect-site monitoring) of oxygenation will improve the management of thoracic anesthesia.

REFERENCES

For a complete list of references for this chapter, scan this QR code with any smartphone code reader app, or visit the following URL:
http://booksite.elsevier.com/9780323711944/.

31

Neuroanatomy, Neurophysiology, and Neuroanesthesia

Laura S. Bonanno

This chapter reviews the anatomy and physiology of the central nervous system (CNS) and provides recommendations for the anesthetic management of specific neurosurgical procedures. An understanding of specific neurophysiologic concepts such as electrophysiology, cerebral blood supply, role of neurotransmitters, and the effects of anesthetic agents on cerebral physiology is important for proper management of patients undergoing neurosurgery.

ORGANIZATION OF THE CENTRAL NERVOUS SYSTEM

Cells of the Central and Peripheral Nervous Systems

The CNS includes the brain and spinal cord. The peripheral nervous system includes the cranial and spinal nerves and their receptors, and it is divided into the somatic and autonomic nervous systems. The somatic nervous system contains sensory neurons for the skin, muscles, and joints. The autonomic nervous system consists of the sympathetic, parasympathetic, and enteric subdivisions and is responsible for involuntary innervation of various organ systems.

The CNS is derived from two primary cell types: neurons and neuroglial (or glial) cells. The neuron is the basic functional cell of the CNS, and it consists of a cell body (perikaryon) and specialized cytoplasmic processes, dendrites, and a single axon (Fig. 31.1). A single axon emerges from the cell body at the axon hillock. The axon may branch to form collateral nerves at a point distal to the neuron cell body. Axon diameters range from 0.2 to 20 μm. Most of the axons in the brain are only a few millimeters long, although the axons that run from the spinal cord may be as long as 1 m. Stimulation of the dendrites produces anterograde impulse conduction (toward the neuron cell body) with subsequent conduction away from the neuron cell body by way of the axon.

Neuron cell bodies vary in size and shape and are classified as unipolar, bipolar, pseudounipolar, or multipolar. Unipolar neurons are found only in lower invertebrates. Bipolar neurons are found in the retina, ear, and olfactory mucosa. Pseudounipolar neurons have one cytoplasmic process that exits the cell and divides into two branches: one serving as the dendrite, the other as the axon. Pseudounipolar neurons are present in the dorsal root ganglia and cranial ganglion cells, enabling sensory impulses to travel from the dendrite directly to the axon without passing through the cell body. Multipolar neurons have multiple dendritic processes but only one axon and constitute the majority of the CNS neurons.

The gray matter of the CNS is composed of neuron cell bodies in the CNS, and the white matter is composed of myelinated axons. Regions of concentrated cell bodies within the peripheral nervous system form the cranial, spinal, and autonomic ganglia.

Neurons may be classified according to their specific function: motor neurons, sensory neurons, or interneurons. Motor neurons are multipolar and innervate and control effector tissues such as muscles and glands. Sensory neurons are pseudounipolar and receive exteroceptive, interoceptive, or proprioceptive input. Interneurons are pseudounipolar and connect adjacent neurons.

The neuron is bound by a bilaminar lipoprotein membrane derived from phospholipid molecules arranged with their fatty acid chains facing one another, producing an inner hydrophobic membrane. The membrane surface in contact with the extracellular fluid contains polar hydrophilic groups of phospholipid molecules. The neuronal membrane contains integral membrane proteins, which form ionic pumps, ion channels, enzymes (e.g., adenylate cyclase), receptor proteins, and structural proteins.

The neuron contains a number of common cellular organelles, including a well-developed nucleus, mitochondria (distributed throughout the cell body), and cytoplasmic processes. Ribosomes, endoplasmic reticulum, lysosomes, and Golgi complexes are also found. Neurotubules and neurofilaments extend through the cytoplasm from the dendrites to the axon terminal; they provide structural support and a pathway for intracellular transport of neurotransmitters.

The second major cell type found within the CNS is the neuroglial, or glial cell (Table 31.1). Four types of glial cells are found within the CNS: astrocytes, oligodendrocytes, microglial cells, and ependymal cells. Most neoplasms of the CNS arise from glial cells (astrocytes). Glial cells are smaller, outnumber neuronal cells, and lack dendritic and axonal processes. Although they do not participate in neuronal signaling, glial cells are essential for neuronal function. The role of neuroglia includes the maintenance of a proper ionic environment, modulation of nerve cell electrical conduction, control of reuptake of neurotransmitters, and repair after neuronal injury.

The astrocyte is the predominant glial cell. Astrocytes provide structural neuronal support, group and pair neurons and nerve terminals, regulate the metabolic environment, and are active in repair after neuronal injury.

Two distinct types of astrocytes exist: fibrous astrocytes, which are found in the white matter, and protoplasmic astrocytes, which are concentrated in the gray matter. Astrocytes have multiple processes that radiate from the cell, producing a star-shaped appearance. Some of these processes (astrocytic feet) terminate on the surfaces of blood vessels within the CNS (perivascular feet). The contact of the cerebral endothelium by astrocytes has been proposed to be essential in the development of the blood-brain barrier (BBB).[1]

Oligodendrocytes have fewer branches than astrocytes (*oligo* meaning "few"; *dendro* meaning "branches"). Oligodendrocytes form the myelin sheath of axons in the brain and spinal cord and are capable of myelinating more than one axon. However, oligodendrocytes are incapable of division and fail to regenerate after injury.

The velocity of nerve impulse conduction in an unmyelinated axon increases with the square root of the diameter of the axon. Accordingly,

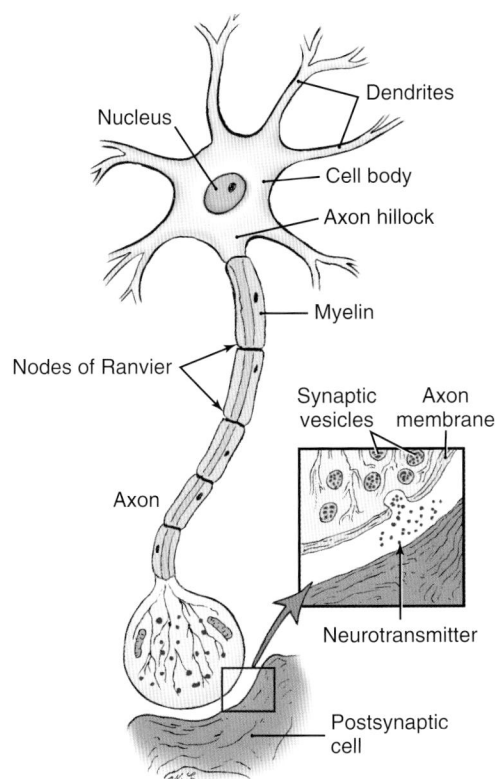

Nucleus

Dendrites

Cell body

Axon hillock

Myelin

Nodes of Ranvier

Synaptic vesicles   Axon membrane

Axon

Neurotransmitter

Postsynaptic cell

Fig. 31.1 Neuron and chemical synapse.

TABLE 31.1	Glial Cells
Type	**Major Functions**
Astrocytes	Support (for neurons)
	Metabolic and nutritive functions
Ependymal cells	Probable role in cerebrospinal fluid production
Microglia	Phagocytosis
Oligodendrocytes	Insulation (form myelin sheath in the brain and spinal cord)
Schwann cells	Insulation (form myelin sheath in the peripheral nerves)

a doubling of impulse conduction requires that the axon be doubled in size. One could only imagine the size of the peripheral nervous system without the presence of myelin. Myelin is essential to increase the velocity of impulse conduction and minimize the size of the axon. Conduction velocity is improved because myelin insulates the nerve axon and gathers voltage-gated sodium channels at distinct nodes along its projection.

Myelin is formed in the vertebral peripheral nervous system by modified glial cells termed *Schwann cells*.[2] Unlike the oligodendrocyte, the Schwann cell myelinates only one axon, surrounding the axon and forming successive layers of plasma membrane. The resultant thickness is variable in different axons. The junction between adjacent Schwann cells is devoid of myelin at 1-mm intervals along the length of the axon. This nonmyelinated portion of the axon, the node of Ranvier, is the site of electrical impulse propagation. Impulses in myelinated axons travel from one node of Ranvier to another (saltatory conduction), bypassing the area between the nodes and increasing the velocity of conduction (see Fig. 31.1). Wallerian degeneration results in the distal degeneration

of the axon after peripheral nerve injury. Proximal axon degeneration also may occur. Within 1 week of the initial injury, Schwann cells proliferate to form a tube into the area of degeneration, forming a scaffold to direct axon regeneration. Myelin regeneration precedes axon regeneration, with the myelin eventually reaching its previous thickness.

Microglial cells are the smallest neuroglial cells and are scattered throughout the CNS. They are transported throughout the CNS to sites of neuronal injury or degeneration, where they proliferate and develop into large macrophages that phagocytize neuronal debris.

Ependymal cells line the roof of the third and fourth ventricles of the brain and the central spinal canal. Ependymal cells form the cuboidal epithelium (choroid plexus), which secretes cerebrospinal fluid (CSF).

Blood-Brain Barrier

The injection of an intravenous dye causes most of the body tissues and internal organs to be stained; yet the brain and spinal cord remain unblemished. This finding led to the discovery of the BBB, which effectively isolates the brain and spinal cord extracellular compartment from the intravascular compartment.[3]

The BBB is essential for maintaining homeostasis within the CNS, and it is vital for proper neuronal function. The BBB is formed by microvascular capillary endothelial cells, pericytes (a type of mural cell), a capillary basement membrane, a neuroglial membrane, and glial podocytes (which are astrocyte projections). These structures strictly control the passage of substances into and out of the CNS. Complex and continuous tight junctions and lack of fenestrae, combined with low pinocytotic activity, make the BBB endothelium a tight barrier for water soluble molecules. In combination with its expression of specific enzymes and transport molecules, the BBB endothelium is unique and distinguishable from all other endothelial cells in the body. A number of midline brain structures receive neurosecretory products from the blood and therefore lack a BBB. These structures, known as the circumventricular organs, include the area postrema, pituitary gland (specifically the posterior lobe), pineal gland, choroid plexus, and portions of the hypothalamus.[4]

The BBB is incompletely developed in the newborn. The high vascular content of bile pigments in jaundiced newborns may enter the basal ganglia, producing kernicterus. BBB disruption can be caused by traumatic head injury, subarachnoid or intracerebral hemorrhage, or cerebral ischemia. The BBB can be disrupted in several disease processes such as multiple sclerosis, stroke, and brain tumors. Osmotically active substances may penetrate the brain or spinal cord after BBB disruption. Intentional intracarotid injection of a hyperosmolar solution crenates or shrinks the endothelial cells, opens tight junctions, and disrupts the BBB. This technique allows the delivery of chemotherapeutic drugs through the BBB for the treatment of neural malignancy.[5,6]

ANATOMY OF THE CENTRAL NERVOUS SYSTEM

Cerebral Structures

The cerebral hemispheres are the most intricately developed and largest regions of the brain (Fig. 31.2). They contain the cerebral cortex, hippocampal formation, amygdala, and basal ganglia. The cerebral cortex consists of the outer 3-mm layer of the cerebral hemispheres. The surface of the cerebral cortex is convoluted, increasing the surface area of the cerebral hemispheres. Elevated convolutions called gyri are separated by shallow grooves called sulci and by deeper grooves called fissures.

The medial longitudinal fissure divides the cerebral hemispheres into right and left halves. The lateral fissure of Sylvius and the central sulcus of Rolando divide each hemisphere into four lobes, which are

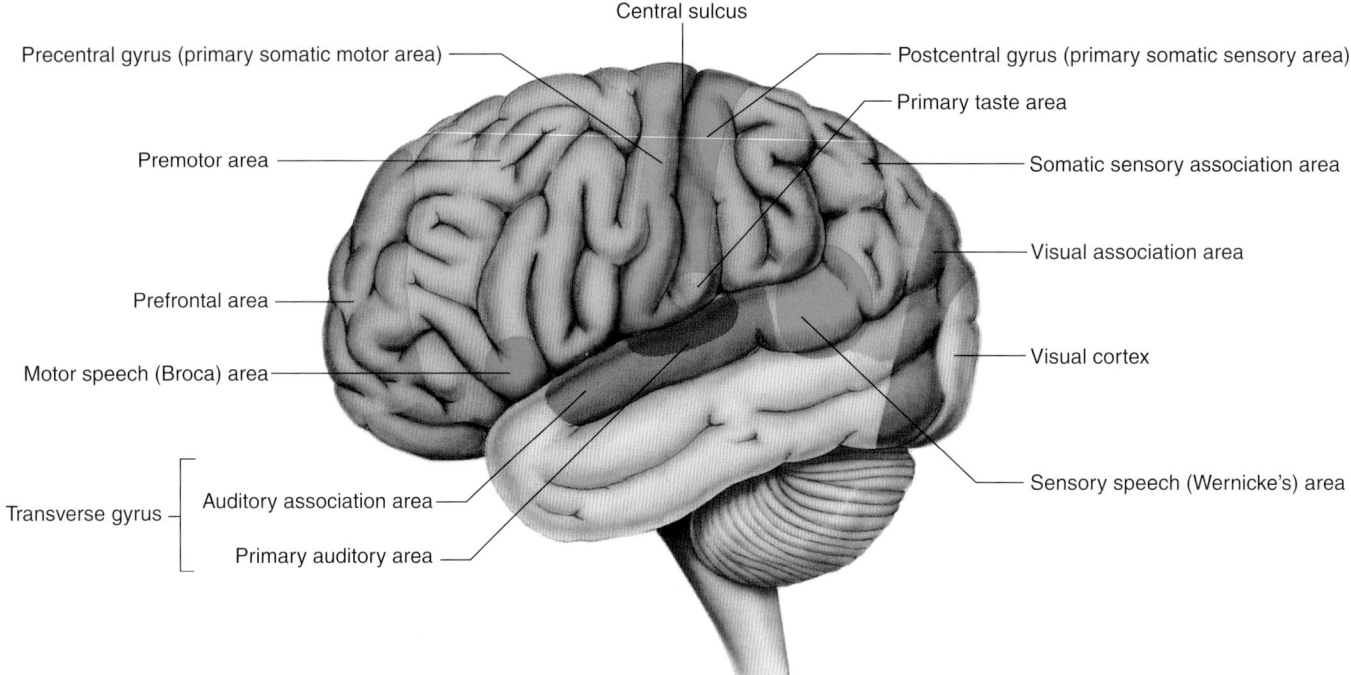

Central sulcus

Precentral gyrus (primary somatic motor area)

Postcentral gyrus (primary somatic sensory area)

Primary taste area

Premotor area

Somatic sensory association area

Visual association area

Prefrontal area

Visual cortex

Motor speech (Broca) area

Sensory speech (Wernicke's) area

Transverse gyrus

Auditory association area

Primary auditory area

Fig. 31.2 Functional areas of the cerebral cortex. (From Patton KT, Thibodeau GA. *Anatomy and Physiology.* 9th ed. St. Louis: Elsevier; 2016:458.)

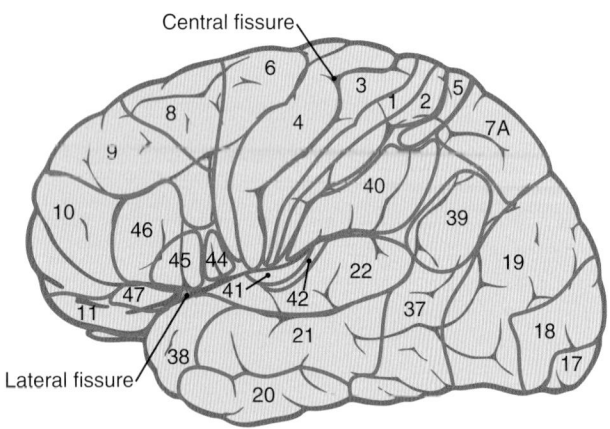

Central fissure

Lateral fissure

Fig. 31.3 Structurally distinct areas, called Brodmann areas, of the human cerebral cortex. Note specifically areas 1, 2, and 3, which constitute primary somatosensory area I, and areas 5 and 7, which constitute the somatosensory association area. (From Hall JE. *Guyton and Hall Textbook of Medical Physiology.* 13th ed. Philadelphia: Elsevier; 2016:611.)

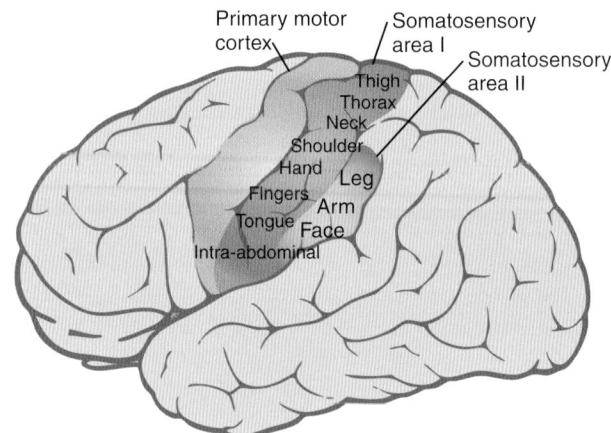

Primary motor cortex

Somatosensory area I

Somatosensory area II

Thigh
Thorax
Neck
Shoulder
Hand
Fingers Leg
Tongue Arm
Intra-abdominal Face

Fig. 31.4 Two somatosensory cortical areas, somatosensory areas I and II. (From Hall JE. *Guyton and Hall Textbook of Medical Physiology.* 13th ed. Philadelphia: Elsevier; 2016:611.)

named for the cranial bones that overlie each area. The frontal lobe, essential for motor control, and the parietal lobe, essential for the senses of pain and touch, are separated by the central sulcus. The cerebral cortex is divided into nearly 50 structurally distinct areas called Brodmann areas (Fig. 31.3). Voluntary muscle activity is controlled by the motor cortex located in the precentral gyrus, or Brodmann area 4. Brodmann areas 1, 2, and 3 make up primary somatosensory area I, also referred to as the somatosensory cortex. This area contains a high degree of localization for various body parts, whereas areas 5 and 7 function as the somatosensory association area, also known as the somatosensory association cortex (Fig. 31.4). The sensations of touch, pain, and limb position, as well as the sensory perception of grasped objects, are controlled by the somatic sensory cortex located in the postcentral gyrus of the parietal lobe. The temporal lobe, which

contains the auditory cortex, is separated from the frontal and parietal lobes by the Sylvian fissure. The occipital lobe lies posterior to the parietooccipital sulcus. Here, the visual cortex lies within the walls of the calcarine fissure on the medial brain surface.

The corpus callosum lies deep in the longitudinal fissure and contains commissural fibers that interconnect the cerebral hemispheres. These fibers arise from neurons in one hemisphere and synapse with neurons in the corresponding area of the adjacent hemisphere. The remaining major structures of the cerebral hemispheres include the basal ganglia, the amygdala, and the hippocampal formation. The basal ganglia are involved in the control of movement. The amygdala functions in the regulation of emotional behavior, response to pain and appetite, and is essential in forming the response to stressors. The hippocampal formation is essential for memory formation and learning.

The diencephalon is located in the midline between the two cerebral hemispheres and contains the thalamus, hypothalamus, epithalamus,

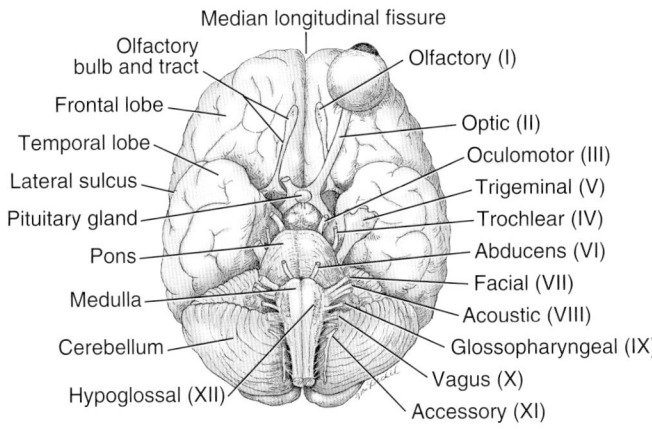

Fig. 31.5 The pons and medulla and the origin of the cranial nerves.

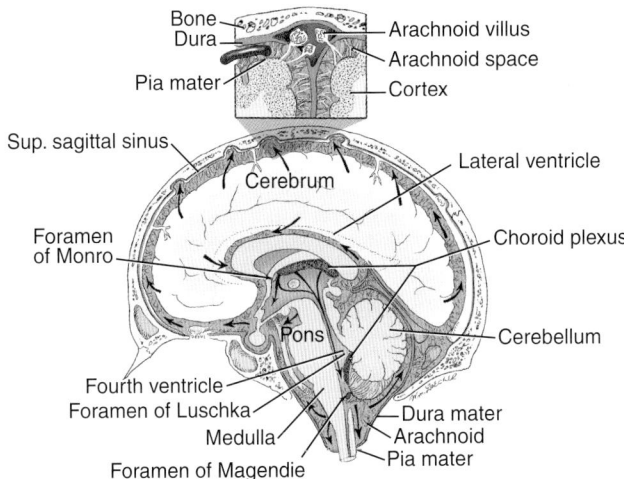

Fig. 31.6 Meninges and the flow of cerebrospinal fluid through the ventricular system.

and subthalamus. The oval-shaped thalamus integrates and transmits sensory information to various cortical areas of the cerebral hemispheres via separate thalamic nuclei. The hypothalamus is composed of several nuclei, including the mammillary bodies. The hypothalamus is the master neurohumoral organ.

The midbrain, pons, and medulla form the brainstem. The brainstem contains the reticular activating system, which functions to maintain consciousness, arousal, and alertness. The pons is anterior to the cerebellum, separated by the fourth ventricle, connecting the medulla oblongata and the midbrain (Fig. 31.5). The pons contains ascending and descending fiber tracts and the nuclei of the trigeminal nerve (cranial nerve V) and facial nerve (cranial nerve VII). The medulla extends from the pons to the foramen magnum, where it becomes continuous with the spinal cord (see Fig. 31.5). In addition to ascending and descending fiber tracts, the medulla contains respiratory and cardiovascular control centers and the vestibulocochlear nerve (cranial nerve VIII), the glossopharyngeal nerve (cranial nerve IX), the vagus nerve (cranial nerve X), the spinal accessory nerve (cranial nerve XI), and the hypoglossal nerve (cranial nerve XII) nuclei.[7]

The cerebellum appears convoluted and lies below the occipital lobe of the cerebral cortex and posterior to the pons and medulla. Structurally, it resembles the cerebral cortex, containing an outer layer of gray matter and an inner core of white matter with several nuclei embedded within. The cerebellum can be divided into three functional areas. The flocculonodular lobe (archeocerebellum) actively maintains the equilibrium, and the paleocerebellum (anterior lobe and part of vermis)

regulates muscle tone. The neocerebellum (posterior lobe plus most of the vermis) is the largest subdivision of the cerebellum and is essential in coordinating voluntary muscle activity. The cerebellum integrates information received from other areas of the CNS and the peripheral nervous system. Information from the cerebellum is transmitted to the cerebral cortex and to lower motor neurons involved in the maintenance of muscle tone, equilibrium, and voluntary muscle activity.[7]

Meninges

The brain and spinal cord are enveloped by three meningeal layers: the dura mater, the arachnoid mater, and the pia mater (Fig. 31.6). The dura mater, the thickest of the meningeal layers, overlies the cerebral hemispheres and brainstem and is functionally separated into an outer periosteal layer (adherent to the inner cranium) and an inner meningeal layer. The dura mater forms a fold, the falx cerebri, that functionally separates the cerebral hemispheres. A similar fold, the tentorium cerebelli, separates the occipital lobe and the cerebellum. The dura mater of the spinal cord is continuous with the meningeal layer of the cranial dura mater and the perineurium of the peripheral nerves. The first three cervical roots and the trigeminal nerve provide innervation of the dura mater. During awake craniotomy, the patient may complain of pain "behind the eye" when traction is applied to the dura.

The arachnoid mater is a thin, avascular membrane joining the dura mater. The subdural space, a potential space between the dura mater and the arachnoid mater, is of clinical importance. The unintentional injection of a local anesthetic during spinal anesthesia into the subdural space produces patchy, asymmetric block. In addition, injury to a blood vessel in the subdural space can create bleeding (subdural hematoma), requiring surgical intervention.

The pia mater is a thin avascular membrane adherent to the brain and spinal cord. The subarachnoid space lies between the arachnoid mater and the pia mater. In the spinal cord, the subarachnoid space extends to the S2-S3 level and is filled with CSF. In addition, the vasculature that overlies the CNS is located within the subarachnoid space. Injury to the vascular structures may produce subarachnoid hemorrhage (SAH) and hematoma.

The epidural space is located above the dura but inside the spinal canal. The epidural space contains a venous plexus and epidural fat that provides protection of the neural structures. The distance from the skin to the epidural space may be as little as 3 cm or as large as 8 cm.

Cerebrospinal Fluid

CSF is contained within the ventricles of the brain, the cisterns surrounding the brain, and the subarachnoid space of the brain and spinal cord (see Fig. 31.6). The total volume of cranial and spinal CSF in the adult is approximately 150 mL. The specific gravity varies from 1.002 to 1.009, and the pH is 7.32. CSF bathes the brain and spinal cord, cushioning these delicate structures, and controls and maintains the extracellular milieu for neurons and glial cells.

Cerebrospinal fluid is secreted by the ependymal cells of the choroid plexus within the ventricular system at a rate of approximately 30 mL/hr. Although CSF is isotonic with plasma, it is not a plasma filtrate. CSF concentrations of potassium, calcium, bicarbonate, and glucose are lower than their respective plasma concentrations, and concentrations of sodium, chloride, and magnesium are higher. The entire CSF volume is replaced every 3 to 4 hours. Normal CSF pressure is between 5 and 15 mm Hg. CSF flows from the lateral ventricles of the cerebral hemispheres through the foramen of Monro into the third ventricle, and through the aqueduct of Sylvius in the midbrain into the fourth ventricle. CSF enters the subarachnoid space through the medial foramen of Magendie and the paired lateral foramina of Luschka, opening posterior to the pons and anterior to the cerebellum.

The cisterna magna, located between the medulla and the cerebellum, is formed from the separation of the arachnoid mater from the pia mater and is filled with CSF. Two additional cisterns exist, the cisterna pontis and the cisterna basalis. CSF drains into the venous blood via the superior sagittal sinus and is absorbed by arachnoid granulations.

Spinal Cord

The spinal cord extends from the medulla at the foramen magnum to the filum terminale, a threadlike connective tissue structure that attaches to the first segment of the coccyx. Thirty-one pairs of spinal nerves carry motor and sensory information: 8 cervical, 12 thoracic, 5 lumbar, 5 sacral, and 1 coccygeal. The first pair of cervical nerves exits the spinal cord between the base of the skull and the first cervical vertebra (atlas), and the remaining 30 pairs exit between adjacent vertebrae. All the exiting spinal nerves are covered with pia mater. Because the spinal cord is approximately 25 cm shorter than the vertebral canal in adults, the lumbar and sacral nerves have relatively long roots (the cauda equina). The spinal cord fills the canal in utero, but the canal elongates at a greater rate than does the neural tissue as the child ages, forming the cauda equina.

The spinal cord is divided into dorsal, lateral, and ventral regions by the entering dorsal sensory root fibers and the outgoing ventral motor root fibers. Neuron cell bodies and unmyelinated fibers lie in the H-shaped central gray region of the cord, surrounded by fiber tracts that form the white matter. Although it does not have a uniform appearance, this general arrangement continues throughout the entire spinal cord.

The spinal gray matter is divided into the ventral and dorsal gray commissures. The ventral projections of gray matter are called the gray horns or columns; the posterior projections are called the posterior gray horns or columns. Intermediolateral gray horns or columns are found between T1 and L2. The gray matter has been subdivided into 10 (I–X) laminae of Rexed. Rexed laminae I through VI are located in the dorsal (posterior) horn and contain cell bodies that receive sensory information from the periphery. Projections from the laminae form afferent tracts. A large number of interneurons are found in laminae V, VI, and X. Laminae VII, VIII, and IX make up the ventral (anterior) horn and contain motor neurons and interneurons involved in motor functions. The gray matter is enlarged in two areas of the spinal cord, C5-C7 and L3-S2. The cervical enlargement contains neuron cell bodies that innervate the upper extremities; the lumbosacral enlargement contains neuron cell bodies that innervate the lower extremities.

The tracts or fascicles that comprise the white matter are highly organized, similar to the organization of the cerebral cortex and other areas of the brain. The dorsal white matter is composed almost exclusively of ascending sensory fiber tracts. The lateral and ventral white matter contain descending motor tracts. Commonly, fiber tracts at various levels within the spinal cord or brain decussate or cross over to the other side. As in the brain, spinal cord fiber tracts can be projection tracts connecting the spinal cord and brain, or they can be association (intersegmental, fasciculi proprii) tracts that originate and terminate entirely within the spinal cord. The association tracts play an important role in spinal reflexes.[7-10]

Shortly after emerging from the spinal cord, the meningeal coverings of the peripheral nerves merge with the connective tissue layers that cover the peripheral nerve. The outermost covering of the peripheral nerve is called the epineurium. The bundles or fascicles of axons in each nerve are covered by the perineurium, and each axon in a fascicle is surrounded by the endoneurium.

Peripheral nerves may be classified according to their diameter. Generally, the larger the diameter, the faster the conduction velocity; therefore, A alpha fibers, the fibers with the largest diameters, have the fastest conduction velocity, and C fibers, which have the smallest diameter, have the slowest conduction velocity. Between the two extremes lie A beta, A gamma, A delta, and B fibers, in decreasing order of size

and conduction velocity. A higher degree of myelination increases the conduction velocity of the nerve.

PERIPHERAL NERVOUS SYSTEM

The peripheral nervous system is divided into the somatic and autonomic nervous systems (Fig. 31.7). The somatic system contains sensory neurons for the skin, muscles, and joints. Somatic motor fibers arise from motor neurons in the ventral horn, their axons exiting the spinal cord via the ventral root. A few centimeters after emerging from the spinal cord, the somatic motor fibers join with incoming sensory fibers carrying information from afferent receptors (muscles, skin, tendons, and joints) to form a mixed nerve. As a mixed nerve approaches its site of innervation, the motor and sensory fibers separate.

Cranial nerves emerge from the cranium. Cranial nerves provide sensory and motor innervation for the head and neck. The sensory cranial nerves include the olfactory nerve (cranial nerve I), optic nerve (cranial nerve II), and vestibulocochlear nerve (cranial nerve VIII); the motor cranial nerves include the oculomotor (cranial nerve III), trochlear (cranial nerve IV), abducens (cranial nerve VI), spinal accessory (cranial nerve XI), and hypoglossal (cranial nerve XII) nerves; and the four mixed cranial nerves with both sensory and motor functions are the trigeminal nerve (cranial nerve V), facial nerve (cranial nerve VII), glossopharyngeal nerve (cranial nerve IX), and vagus nerve (cranial nerve X). Table 31.2 lists cranial and peripheral nerve fiber types, locations, and functions.

The autonomic nervous system controls involuntary visceral functions and is composed of three subdivisions: the sympathetic, parasympathetic, and enteric nervous systems. The sympathetic nervous system (SNS) and the parasympathetic nervous system (PNS) are functionally antagonistic.[8,11] The SNS and PNS originate within the CNS and require two efferent neurons: a preganglionic neuron originating within the CNS and a postganglionic neuron terminating within the effector organ (smooth muscle, cardiac muscle, or sweat gland). Autonomic fibers originating in the brain arise from cell bodies located in the brainstem. PNS fibers supplying the lower gastrointestinal tract and genitourinary systems arise from the sacral portion of the spinal cord.

TABLE 31.2	**Cranial and Peripheral Nerves**	
Fiber Type	**Location**	**Information Conveyed**
General somatic afferent	CN V, CN VII, CN IX, CN X, all spinal nerves	Pain, touch, temperature, pressure, and proprioception from muscles, tendons, and joint capsules
General visceral afferent	CN V, CN VII, CN IX, CN X, all spinal nerves	Conscious pain sensations
Special somatic afferent	CN II, CN VIII	Sight, hearing
Special visceral afferent	CN I, CN IX, CN X, CN VII (intermediate branch)	Olfaction, taste
Special visceral efferent	CN V, CN VII, CN IX, CN X, CN XI	Mastication, facial expressions
General somatic efferent	CN III, CN IV, CN VI, CN VII, all spinal nerves	Voluntary muscles (trunk and extremities), extrinsic muscles of eye, muscles of the tongue
General visceral efferent	CN III, CN VII, CN IX, CN X, spinal nerves T1 through L2 or L3, S2, S3, S4	Smooth muscle, cardiac muscle, some glands

CN, Cranial nerve.

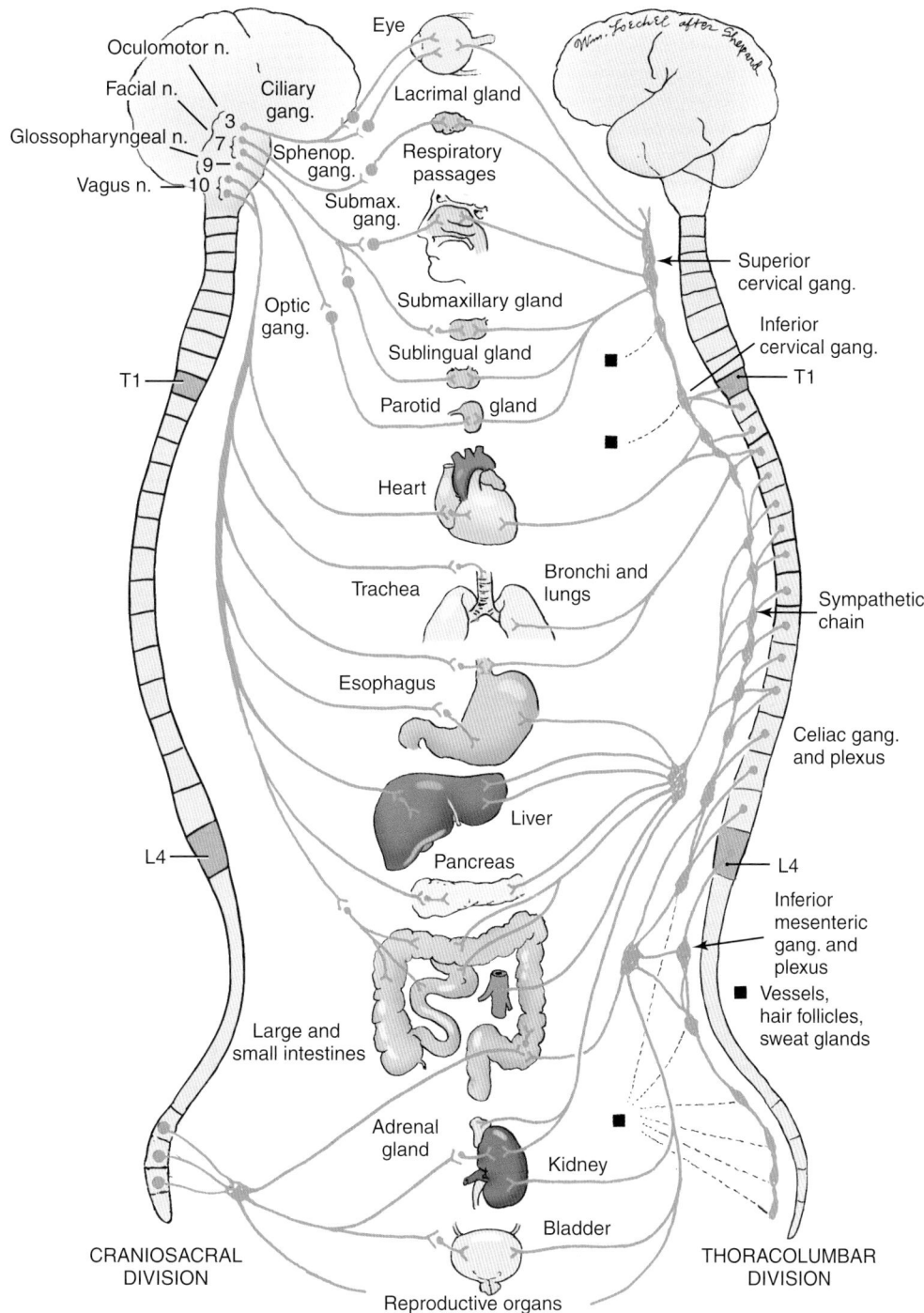

Fig. 31.7 Both divisions of the autonomic nervous system. *gang.*, Ganglion; *n*, nerve.

Sympathetic Nervous System

Preganglionic neurons of the SNS originate in the intermediolateral gray horn of the spinal cord between the first thoracic (T1) and second or third lumbar (L2 or L3) vertebra. The efferent anatomic distribution of the SNS originates from the thoracolumbar region. The myelinated preganglionic axons (i.e., preganglionic fibers of the preganglionic neurons) exit the spinal cord via the anterior (ventral) nerve root. These processes leave the spinal cord by way of a small trunk, the white rami communicantes. A series of paired paravertebral ganglia is ranged bilaterally along the spinal cord (Fig. 31.8). All the paired segmental paravertebral ganglia are connected, forming the sympathetic trunks.

These ganglia may contain the cell body of the second efferent neuron (postganglionic neuron). The preganglionic fibers of the preganglionic neuron enter the white rami communicantes and may synapse with the second efferent neuron located within the ganglion. The postganglionic fiber of the postganglionic neuron may either exit the gray ramus to enter a spinal nerve or extend through a connection between the paravertebral ganglion and one of the three (celiac, superior, or inferior) mesenteric ganglia. The postganglionic fibers then synapse with the smooth muscle of the digestive tract and other abdominal organs. SNS preganglionic axons secrete acetylcholine at their ganglionic synapses, and postganglionic fibers secrete catecholamines.[1,7,9]

Usually, one paravertebral ganglion is present for each spinal nerve, except in the cervical area, where they fuse to form two or three ganglia. On entering the sympathetic chain, the preganglionic fiber may synapse at the entry level or travel up or down the ganglionic chain before forming a synapse. Some preganglionic axons pass through the sympathetic chain without synapsing and, after leaving the chain, form a distinct nerve (e.g., splanchnic nerve) before synapsing in prevertebral ganglia, such as the superior or inferior mesenteric ganglia. Some preganglionic axons in the sympathetic trunk synapse with several postganglionic neurons located in several chain ganglia. This arrangement explains the manner in which a central SNS discharge spreads over several segments. After synapsing in the sympathetic chain, the postganglionic axons, which are unmyelinated, enter the spinal nerve through the gray ramus communicans and travel to the periphery.

The cervical ganglia are divided into superior, medial, and inferior cervical ganglia. The inferior cervical ganglion fuses with the first thoracic ganglion to form the stellate ganglion. Stimulation of SNS fibers from the superior cervical ganglion produces contraction of the radial muscle of the iris (mydriasis), relaxation of the ciliary muscle of the eye, and constriction of the blood vessels of the head. Destruction of the superior cervical ganglion, central SNS damage, or injury to other cervical paravertebral ganglia produces Horner syndrome, clinically distinguished by miosis, anhidrosis (absence of sweating), and ptosis on the affected side. Ptosis is incomplete because the primary innervation to the levator palpebrae superioris muscle of the eyelid is through the oculomotor nerve, and only a few SNS fibers innervate this muscle.[1,7,9]

Postganglionic fibers from the upper thoracic chain ganglia (stellate to T4-T5) innervate the heart and lungs. β-receptor stimulation produces an increased heart rate (positive chronotropic effect), an increase in conduction (positive dromotropic effect), and an increase in myocardial contractility (positive inotropic effect). Coronary artery α-receptor stimulation produces vasoconstriction. The resultant pulmonary effects also depend on the receptor type that is stimulated; bronchial dilation follows β_2-receptor stimulation, and mild bronchoconstriction follows α-receptor stimulation.

The SNS fibers supplying abdominal and pelvic viscera (T5 through L3) pass through the chain ganglia forming the greater and lesser splanchnic nerves, which subsequently terminate in preterminal ganglia. Postganglionic fibers from the prevertebral ganglia, such as the superior and inferior mesenteric ganglia, travel to the abdominal and pelvic viscera. Stimulation of these SNS fibers activates liver glycogenolysis and gluconeogenesis, decreases secretions from pancreatic acinar cells and β-cells, initiates lipolysis, decreases the tone and motility of the gastrointestinal tract, contracts gastrointestinal sphincters, relaxes urinary smooth muscle, and increases renin secretion from the kidney.[1,7,9]

Parasympathetic Nervous System

The efferent neurons of the parasympathetic subdivision are located in the gray matter of the midbrain and medulla. The preganglionic fibers exit the brain via cranial nerves II, VII, IX, and X. The remainder of the cell bodies of the first efferent neurons arise from the lateral horn of the sacral portion of the spinal cord (S2-S5). Therefore, due to the regions of efferent innervation, the PNS is called the craniosacral distribution. Acetylcholine is secreted by both parasympathetic preganglionic and postganglionic fibers (see Fig. 31.8).

The second efferent neuron (postganglionic neuron) of the parasympathetic subdivision may be located in a small ganglion adjacent to the innervated organ or within the organ itself. Preganglionic axons travel with the vagus to ganglia located near the organ they innervate. The postganglionic axons innervate the bronchioles, heart, coronary arteries, stomach, and large intestine up to the left colic flexure. PNS postganglionic fibers to the descending colon and the genitourinary

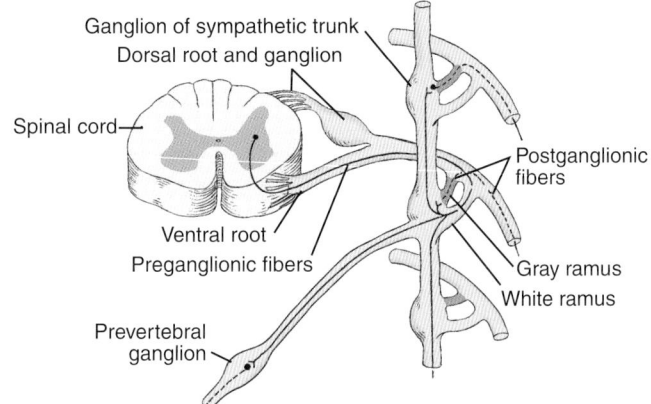

Fig. 31.8 Sympathetic ganglia.

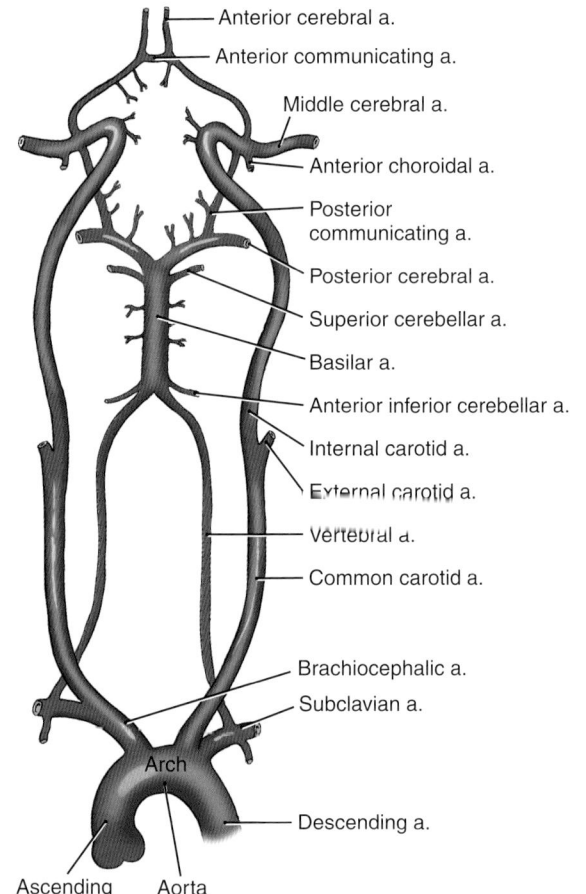

Fig. 31.9 Cerebral vasculature. *a*, Artery.

systems are supplied by parasympathetic fibers from sacral segments of the spinal cord. Most of the parasympathetic preganglionic fibers originate at the S3 and S4 segments. Shortly after exiting the spinal cord with the spinal nerves, the preganglionic fibers form the pelvic nerves (nervi erigentes), which synapse in ganglia in close proximity to the innervated organ.[1,7,9] Stimulation of the Vagus nerve accounts for approximately 75% of parasympathetic nervous system activity.

VASCULATURE OF THE CENTRAL NERVOUS SYSTEM

The brain and spinal cord are dependent on an uninterrupted blood supply to deliver essential fuels, oxygen, and glucose (Fig. 31.9). The brain receives 15% of the cardiac output, or approximately 50 mL/100 g/min. The brain's blood supply originates from two arterial circulations that receive blood from two distinct systemic arteries: The anterior circulation receives blood from the internal carotid arteries, and the posterior circulation receives blood from the vertebral arteries. These arterial systems communicate through arterial anastomoses that form the circle of Willis. The paired anterior, middle, and posterior cerebral arteries originate from the circle of Willis. Although these arterial communications exist, under normal conditions, little mixing of blood flow occurs. Intraarterial contrast studies demonstrate that the carotid artery supplies the ipsilateral cerebral hemisphere, and the vertebrobasilar system supplies the structures of the posterior fossa.

The internal carotid arteries enter the skull through the foramen lacerum and bifurcate near the lateral border of the optic chiasm, forming the anterior and middle cerebral arteries. The anterior cerebral arteries supply the medial surface of the cerebral hemispheres, and the middle cerebral arteries supply the lateral surface of the hemispheres. The striate arteries, which are branches of the middle cerebral arteries, supply the internal capsule and its motor tracts. Cerebrovascular accidents commonly involve the striate arteries. Communicating arteries provide connections between the two anterior cerebral arteries of each hemisphere (anterior communicating arteries) and between the middle and posterior cerebral arteries (posterior communicating arteries).[1,7,9]

The vertebral arteries, branches of the subclavian artery, enter the cranium through the foramen magnum and join to form the basilar artery in the vicinity of the pons. Branches of the vertebral and basilar arteries supply a wide area, including the cervical region of the spinal cord, the brainstem, the cerebellum, the vestibular apparatus and cochlea of the inner ear, parts of the diencephalon, and the occipital and temporal lobes of the cerebral hemispheres.

Venous blood exits the brain via two separate systems. The blood from the cerebral and cerebellar cortex flows through veins on the surface and empties into overlying dural venous sinuses. Venous blood from the basal portions of the brain empties into the great vein of Galen and the straight sinus. These sinuses empty into the internal jugular veins. The superficial veins of the scalp are linked to the dural sinuses by the emissary veins.[7,8]

Like the brain, the spinal cord receives blood from two arterial sources: the anterior and posterior spinal arteries, which are branches of the vertebral artery, and the radicular arteries, which are branches of segmental vessels (cervical, intercostal, and lumbar). The spinal cord blood supply is not continuous along its length, and although each spinal cord segment is perfused, blood is delivered preferentially by one of the supply sources. The cervical cord is supplied by the vertebral and radicular arteries, and the thoracic and lumbar cord is supplied by the radicular arteries arising from this respective region (intercostal and lumbar). Of particular importance is the radicular artery, the artery of Adamkiewicz, which enters the cord at approximately T7 and supplies the lumbosacral segment. Spinal cord segments that receive blood from one source are particularly prone to ischemic injury if this blood supply is interrupted. Interruption of the blood flow from the artery of Adamkiewicz results in paraplegia.[1,7,9]

ELECTROPHYSIOLOGY

The physiologic basis for the propagation of a nerve impulse lies in the structural nature of the axolemma, the differential concentration of electrolytes within the axolemma and extracellular space, and the semipermeability of the axolemma to these specific ions. The resting nerve cell has a potential difference, or voltage, created by the asymmetric distribution of sodium and potassium ions. Sodium ions are 10-fold richer in the extracellular medium, and potassium ions are 10-fold

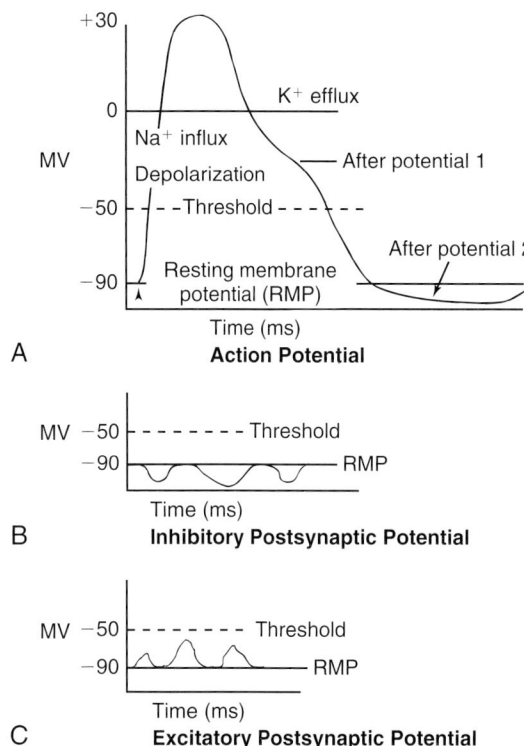

Fig. 31.10 (A) Phases of the action potential (AP) and major ionic movements during the AP. (B, C) Subthreshold changes in the resting membrane potential.

richer in the intracellular medium. The resting membrane potential is created through the excess positive charges on the extracellular surface and excess negative charges on the interior of the cell membrane. The nerve cell is said to be "polarized" in the resting state.

In the resting state, the cell membrane permeability to sodium ions is low, so little movement of extracellular sodium ions to the cell interior occurs. Although larger than sodium ions, potassium ions are freely permeable through the axolemma, and their movement creates a net deficit of positive ions within the interior of the axolemma. This ionic asymmetry is maintained by the sodium-potassium adenosine triphosphate (ATP) pump. The distribution of ions outside the cell produces a negative resting membrane potential of approximately −60 to −90 mV.

Nerve impulses are transmitted through action potentials that are generated with membrane alterations in permeability of the axolemma to sodium and potassium ions. Depolarization occurs when a stimulus of sufficient intensity (threshold potential) increases membrane permeability to sodium ions, facilitating the passage of a greater number of sodium ions into the cell interior than potassium ions to the cell exterior. The lowering of the voltage difference of the axolemma occurs as a result of gating, or the opening or closing of integral membrane proteins. Gating occurs in response to voltage differences across the axolemma (voltage-gated channel) or after the binding of a specific molecule to a receptor or channel protein (chemically gated channel [e.g., the binding of acetylcholine to the neuromuscular junction]).[1,7,9]

Sodium channels open when the threshold potential is reached, facilitating a rapid influx of sodium into the axolemma interior and producing depolarization (Fig. 31.10). The initial flow of sodium ions results in the opening of additional sodium channels. The action potential develops as the cell interior undergoes a transition from negative to positive. At the peak of depolarization, the electrical potential is 30 to 40 mV higher than the cell exterior, and sodium channels close. The action potential develops because of the change from the resting potential of −60 to −90 mV to a peak of 30 to 50 mV at the completion of depolarization. The action potential cannot occur without the delivery of a stimulus, or critical threshold potential.

For myelinated mammalian nerves, the threshold potential is 20 to 30 mV less than the resting potential. This threshold potential can be modified by a variety of factors, including pH, partial pressure of oxygen (Po_2), and partial pressure of carbon dioxide (Pco_2). Alkalosis increases neuronal excitability, and hypoxemia and acidosis depress neuronal excitability.

After depolarization, cell repolarization is initiated with the closing of sodium channels and the opening of potassium channels, allowing the flow of potassium ions to the exterior of the axolemma to return the axon to the resting potential of −60 to −90 mV. The sodium pump is active in reestablishing this ionic asymmetry. During repolarization, the axon is refractory, or unable to respond to an additional stimulus, no matter how strong. In the later phases of repolarization, the axolemma is in a state of ready refractoriness—that is, depolarization can be initiated only by a stimulus with an intensity greater than that which produced the original depolarization.

Chemical, mechanical, and electrical stimulation may elicit an action potential. Mechanical stimulation via pinching or crushing increases the membrane's permeability to sodium ions. The resulting change in ion permeability determines whether the postsynaptic neuron is either excited or inhibited.

Tissues whose sodium channels are not completely closed at rest (cardiac and smooth muscle) have a constant leak of sodium inside the cell, and excitation occurs by electrical stimulation to produce an action potential. Because these tissues repetitively discharge, they are described as having rhythmicity. The usual resting membrane potential of cells displaying rhythmicity is −60 to −70 mV. After stimulation, a wave of depolarization is transmitted to the axon terminal. At electrical synapses, the wave of depolarization crosses the 2-nm synaptic space and spreads to the postsynaptic cell (neuron or muscle cell).[1,7,9]

Synaptic Transmission

After depolarization, the flow of information is transmitted to adjacent neurons at specialized membrane sites called synapses (see Fig. 31.1). Synapses are present on dendrites and axons. Synapses may be present on axon terminals of specific neurons in contact with endocrine glands (e.g., salivary glands) or skeletal muscle. The neuron sending the information is the presynaptic neuron, and the receiving neuron is the postsynaptic neuron. Separating the presynaptic and postsynaptic neurons is a small intracellular space (the synaptic cleft). Most synaptic transmission occurs in the direction from the presynaptic to the postsynaptic neuron, but retrograde nerve impulse conduction is known to occur and modulates the strength of synaptic connections.

Synaptic transmission may be electrically or chemically mediated. Electrically mediated synapses are large compared with chemically mediated synapses. Electrical synapses have direct cytoplasmic continuity and no synaptic delay. Electrical synapses are excitatory in nature and are located in the CNS, peripherally in smooth muscle, and in cardiac muscle. Synaptic delays (delayed synaptic transmission) occur in chemically mediated transmission because of the transit time of the chemical mediator (specific neurotransmitter) from the presynaptic terminal to the postsynaptic membrane.

The majority of neurons in the CNS have chemically mediated synapses. The presynaptic neuron releases a neurotransmitter, a low molecular weight compound that diffuses across the synaptic cleft and binds to specific receptors on the postsynaptic membrane. Depolarization stimulates the uptake of calcium by the nerve terminal, fusing intracellular vesicles that contain the neurotransmitter to the presynaptic membrane. The neurotransmitters are subsequently released into the synaptic cleft. The neurotransmitter diffuses across the synaptic cleft, interacting with a specific postsynaptic receptor. Neurotransmitters that increase the permeability of the axolemma to sodium ions are excitatory (e.g., acetylcholine, glutamate); neuroinhibitory neurotransmitters (e.g., γ-aminobutyric acid [GABA], glycine) hyperpolarize the membrane by increasing the permeability to chloride ions. The neurotransmitter serotonin excites some neurons and inhibits others. The attachment of the neurotransmitter to the postsynaptic receptor can produce either an immediate (fraction of millisecond) or a delayed (from a few milliseconds up to seconds) effect on the postsynaptic membrane. The delayed transmission involves second messengers, such as cyclic adenosine monophosphate and cyclic guanosine monophosphate, which are activated when the neurotransmitter attaches to the postsynaptic membrane.[1,7,9]

NEUROTRANSMITTERS

Neurotransmitters are molecules contained within the presynaptic neuron that are discharged in a calcium-dependent manner after presynaptic depolarization and that interact with specific receptors on the postsynaptic membrane. More than 100 molecules are deposited within the synapse via this mechanism. Acetylcholine is an excitatory neurotransmitter that interacts with both nicotinic and muscarinic receptors. Additional neurotransmitters include biogenic amines (e.g., epinephrine, norepinephrine, dopamine, serotonin, histamine), amino acids (e.g., aspartate, glycine, GABA, glutamate), neuropeptides (e.g., substance P, the opioids, several hormones), and the second messenger, nitric oxide (Table 31.3).

The synthesis of neurotransmitters occurs within the presynaptic neuron terminal. The neuron regulates the synthesis, packaging, release, and degradation of the synthesized neurotransmitter. The enzymes essential for the synthesis of neurotransmitters are obtained by axonal transport and taken into the nerve terminal by transport proteins. The synthesized neurotransmitter is then packaged into synaptic vesicles by membrane transport proteins.

Acetylcholine

Acetylcholine is an excitatory neurotransmitter that is released in many areas within the body. It is the predominant neurotransmitter within the CNS, at the neuromuscular junction, within all autonomic nervous system preganglionic fibers and postganglionic parasympathetic fibers, and within postganglionic sympathetic fibers innervating sweat glands. Acetylcholine is synthesized in the presynaptic nerve terminal from acetic acid, coenzyme A, and choline in the presence of the enzymes acetyl kinase and choline acetylase. This enzyme is also referred to as choline acetyl transferase. Acetylcholine is packaged in vesicles and stored in the presynaptic terminal. Calcium uptake into the presynaptic terminal is required for acetylcholine release, and magnesium (Mg^{2+}) and manganese (Mn^{2+}) block the uptake of calcium (Ca^{2+}) and the subsequent release of acetylcholine. Acetylcholine interacts with the postsynaptic receptor for a few milliseconds before being hydrolyzed by acetylcholinesterase to acetic acid and choline. Both the acetic acid and the choline are taken up by the presynaptic nerve terminal and recycled.[1,7,9]

Cholinergic receptors are classified as either nicotinic or muscarinic. Nicotinic receptors are found in autonomic ganglia and at the neuromuscular junction. Muscarinic receptors are found on smooth muscle, cardiac muscle, and sweat glands. Acetylcholine is the neurotransmitter at cranial nerve nuclei and ventral horn motor neurons of the spinal cord, including various collateral nerves to Renshaw cells (interneurons). Acetylcholine may be interactive in neuronal circuits involved with pain reception. Acetylcholine may also act as a sensory transmitter in thermal receptors and taste bud endings.

TABLE 31.3 Common Neurotransmitters

Class	Neurotransmitter
Biogenic amines	Epinephrine
	Norepinephrine
	Dopamine
	5-hydroxytryptamine (serotonin)
	Histamine
Amino acids	γ-aminobutyric acid
	Glycine
	Glutamate
Neuropeptides	Calcitonin family
	Calcitonin
	Calcitonin gene-related peptide
	Hypothalamic hormones
	Oxytocin
	Vasopressin
	Hypothalamic releasing and inhibitory hormones
	Corticotropin-releasing factor (CRF or CRH)
	Gonadotropin-releasing hormone (GnRH)
	Growth hormone-releasing hormone (GHRH)
	Somatostatin
	Thyrotropin-releasing hormone (TRH)
	Neuropeptide Y family
	Neuropeptide Y (NPY)
	Neuropeptide YY (PYY)
	Pancreatic polypeptide (PP)
	Opioid peptides
	β-endorphin (also a pituitary hormone)
	Dynorphin peptides
	Leu-enkephalin
	Met-enkephalin
	Pituitary hormones
	Adrenocorticotropic hormone (ACTH)
	α-melanocyte-stimulating hormone (α-MSH)
	Growth hormone (GH)
	Follicle-stimulating hormone (FSH)
	Luteinizing hormone (LH)
	Tachykinins
	Neurokinin A (substance K)
	Neurokinin B
	Neuropeptide K
	Substance P
	VIP-glucagon family
	Glucagon
	Glucagon-like peptide (ARP)
	Bradykinin
	Cholecystokinin (CKK; multiple forms)
	Cocaine- and amphetamine-regulated transcript (CART)
	Galanin
	Chrelin
	Melanin-concentrating hormone (MCH)
	Neurotensin
	Orexins (or hypocretins)
	Orphanin FQ (or nociceptin)
	(also grouped with opioids)
Other	Acetylcholine
	Nitric oxide

VIP, Vasoactive intestinal peptide.

Biogenic Amines

There are five biogenic amines, which include the three catecholamines, epinephrine, norepinephrine, and dopamine, as well as serotonin and histamine. The catecholamines are synthesized in a series of hydroxylation, decarboxylation, and methylation reactions from the amino acid phenylalanine, a precursor to tyrosine. The adrenal medulla secretes both epinephrine (75%) and norepinephrine (25%). Postganglionic adrenergic neurons secrete norepinephrine; norepinephrine and dopamine are probably neurotransmitters within the CNS. Amacrine cells of the retina and some neurons of the intrinsic nervous system of the intestine secrete dopamine. As with acetylcholine, the release of norepinephrine, epinephrine, and dopamine is calcium dependent. One notable difference from acetylcholine is that norepinephrine and dopamine act by means of second messengers (slow synaptic transmission), whereas most of the actions of acetylcholine are directly on ion channels (fast synaptic transmission). The duration of effect of catecholamines is regulated by presynaptic reuptake. Enzymatic breakdown of catecholamines by monoamine oxidase and catechol-O-methyltransferase within the liver is primarily responsible for terminating their effects.

- Dopamine is an inhibitory neurotransmitter and the predominant biogenic amine within the CNS. Dopamine is concentrated within the basal ganglia. Dopamine's inhibitory effects occur through action on adenylate cyclase.
- Norepinephrine is concentrated in the reticular activating system and the hypothalamus. Norepinephrine acts as an inhibitory neurotransmitter, inhibiting impulses to the cerebral cortex.
- Serotonin is an inhibitory neurotransmitter that influences behavior and mood. Histamine is also an inhibitory neurotransmitter concentrated within the hypothalamus and the reticular activating system. Histamine requires the second messenger cyclic adenosine monophosphate to mediate its inhibitory effects.[1,7,9]

Amino Acids

Glutamate is the primary excitatory transmitter found within the cerebral cortex, the hippocampus, and the substantia gelatinosa of the spinal cord.[12] Glutamate plays a significant role in learning and memory (perhaps interactive in memory formation during awareness that occurs during anesthesia) and the appreciation of pain. Glutamate has also been implicated in excitotoxic neuronal injury after ischemic or traumatic brain injury.

Glutamate is formed from the deamination of glutamine supplied by the Krebs cycle. Glutamate may activate either an inotropic or a metabotropic amino acid receptor. N-methyl-D-aspartate (NMDA) receptors are ligand-gated inotropic receptors that produce a conformational change in the receptor, opening a sodium channel, which results in the depolarization of the postsynaptic membrane. The metabotropic receptor is an integral transmembrane receptor that regulates intracellular second messenger systems.[13]

GABA is the major inhibitory neurotransmitter found in the CNS. It is concentrated in the basal ganglia, cerebral cortex, cerebellum, and spinal cord. Activation of the GABA receptor opens neuronal membrane chloride channels, producing hyperpolarization (the hyperpolarized neuron is resistant to excitation). GABA is important in antagonizing the excitatory effects of amino acid neurotransmitters.[14]

Glycine is the primary inhibitory neurotransmitter in the spinal cord. In the past, glycine irrigation was employed during transurethral resection of the prostate. Postoperative visual impairment after the intravascular absorption of glycine suggests that glycine may act as an inhibitory neurotransmitter within the retina.

Neuropeptides

Neuropeptides have either excitatory or inhibitory physiologic effects. Common neuropeptides include the opioids, substance P, and many pituitary and pancreatic islet hormones. Substance P is an excitatory neurotransmitter found in the striatum and substantia nigra of the basal ganglia, hypothalamus, brainstem (raphe nuclei), and dorsal root ganglia of the spinal cord. Pain-fiber terminals that synapse with the substantia gelatinosa of the spinal cord release substance P.

The opioid neuropeptides include β-endorphin, enkephalins, dynorphins, and endomorphins. They act at opiate receptors distributed throughout the brain and spinal cord. Three classes of opiate receptors have been identified: delta, kappa, and mu. Dynorphin is a potent agonist at kappa receptors, and the enkephalins are agonists at delta and mu receptors. Opiate alkaloids like morphine interact with mu receptors. Morphine-like agents block slow pain pathways, raise the pain threshold, and modify the response to pain. Other effects, such as miosis and respiratory depression, result from the actions of these agents on opiate receptors located in the parts of the brain that control these functions.[2,10,15]

SENSORY PATHWAYS

Sensory or afferent pathways transmit pain, temperature, pressure, touch, vibratory sense, and proprioceptive information to the CNS. Sensory pathways also include the special senses of vision, taste, hearing, smell, and equilibrium.

Receptors for pain and temperature are located in the epidermis and the dermis; those for pressure, touch, vibratory sense, and proprioception are located in the dermis. Receptors can be classified as (1) exteroceptors, which are located near the surface of skin and oral mucosa, and (2) proprioceptors, which are located in deeper skin layers, joint capsules, ligaments, tendons, muscles, and periosteum. Several types of receptors exist. Pacinian corpuscles are receptors for vibration and pressure. Free nerve endings, Ruffini corpuscles, muscle spindles, and Golgi tendon organs are involved in movement sense. The receptors for light (or crude) touch sensations include Merkel disks, Meissner corpuscles, and the nerve plexuses surrounding some hair roots. Fibers travel from these receptors to a ganglion, where they synapse with first-order neurons, the fibers of which continue to the CNS. Fibers from receptors in the trunk and extremities travel to the dorsal root ganglion, where they synapse with first-order neurons. Most of the sensory fibers from the head, excluding those from the special sense organs (hearing, equilibrium, vision, taste, and smell), synapse in first-order neurons located in the semilunar or trigeminal ganglion.[10,11]

Pain and Temperature Pathways

Pain and temperature fibers from the head synapse in the trigeminal ganglion and enter the pons, forming the trigeminal nerve (cranial nerve V). These fibers subsequently synapse with second-order neurons in the nucleus of the descending tract of cranial nerve V. The second-order axons cross to the ventrolateral side and ascend as the ventral trigeminal tract to the ventral posteromedial nucleus of the thalamus, where they synapse with third-order neurons. From the ventral posteromedial thalamic nucleus, third-order axons ascend in the internal capsule and end in the postcentral gyrus of the cerebral cortex, which is the primary somatic sensory area of the brain.

Pain and temperature receptors in the skin of the trunk and extremities send signals to the spinal cord via the dorsal roots of the spinal nerves. The majority of these dorsal root sensory nerve fibers terminate in the dorsal horn on laminae I, IV, V, and VI (Fig. 31.11). This is the origination site of the anterolateral pathway for signal transmission up the spinal cord to the brain.[16] From this point in the dorsal horn, the anterolateral fibers decussate (cross) in the ventral commissure to the opposite anterior and lateral white columns (Fig. 31.12). The fibers then ascend cephalad via the anterior spinothalamic and lateral spinothalamic tracts to the ventral posterolateral thalamic nucleus,

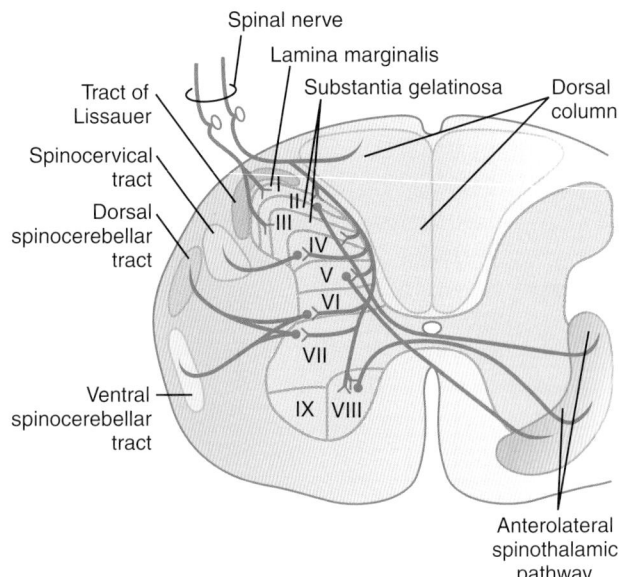

Fig. 31.11 Cross section of spinal cord, showing the anatomy of the cord gray matter and of ascending sensory tracts in the white columns of the spinal cord. (From Hall JE. *Guyton and Hall Textbook of Medical Physiology.* 13th ed. Philadelphia: Elsevier; 2016:609.)

where they synapse with third-order neurons. Axons from the third-order neurons travel in the posterior limb of the internal capsule and ultimately synapse in the postcentral gyrus, where sensations of pain, temperature, touch, and pressure are interpreted, and responses to the sensations are initiated.

Some pain and temperature fibers in the dorsal horn bifurcate into branches that synapse with internuncial (messenger) neurons. The internuncial neurons have axons that synapse with motor neurons in the ventral horn, which are not necessarily at the same level of the spinal cord. The axons can cross over and travel up or down the spinal cord before synapsing. These circuits are part of the reflex response to pain, which results in a rapid, automatic response to nociceptive stimuli.

The afferent fibers from each dorsal root ganglion come from a relatively limited area of the skin termed a cutaneous dermatome. Some overlap exists, so if a spinal nerve that supplies a certain dermatome is severed, pain and temperature sensations from that dermatome are supplied by adjacent dermatome fibers. For example, if T6 is severed, T5 and T7 sensory neurons carry pain and temperature sensations from the skin area supplied by T6. Axons entering the dorsal horn from the dorsal root ganglion send branches to one spinal segment above and one segment below in the dorsolateral column of Lissauer.[2,9,11,17]

Pressure and Crude Touch

Nerve fibers that mediate pressure and light touch from the head synapse with first-order neurons in the trigeminal ganglion. From the trigeminal ganglion, first-order axons travel to the pons, where they synapse with second-order neurons in the sensory nucleus of cranial nerve V. From the sensory nucleus of cranial nerve V, second-order axons form the dorsal trigeminal tract, which has both crossed and uncrossed fibers. The second-order fibers terminate in the ventral posteromedial nucleus of the thalamus. Third-order axons from the ventral posteromedial nucleus subsequently terminate in the postcentral gyrus of the cerebral cortex.

After leaving the dorsal root ganglion, light touch and pressure fibers from the extremities and trunk enter the dorsal white column on the ipsilateral side and bifurcate (see Fig. 31.12). One branch immediately enters the dorsal gray horn and synapses with second-order

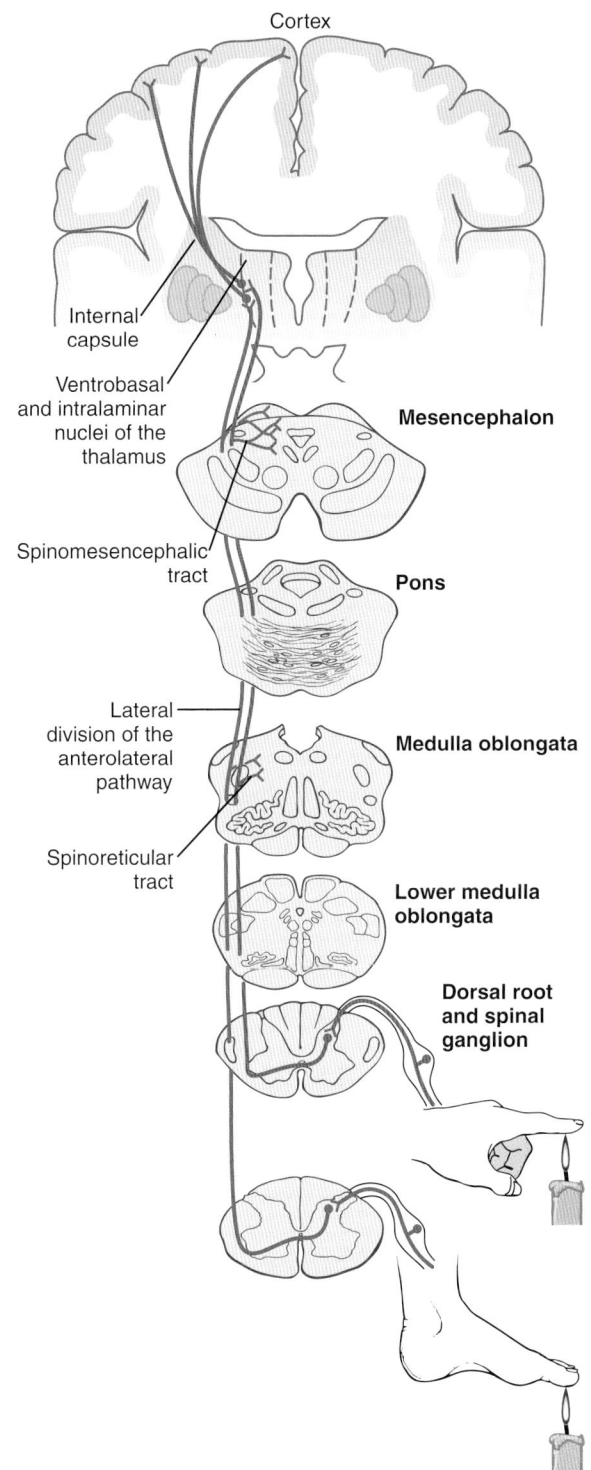

Cortex

Internal
capsule

Ventrobasal
and intralaminar
nuclei of the
thalamus

Mesencephalon

Spinomesencephalic
tract

Pons

Lateral
division of the
anterolateral
pathway

Medulla oblongata

Spinoreticular
tract

**Lower medulla
oblongata**

**Dorsal root
and spinal
ganglion**

Fig. 31.12 Pain, temperature, and crude sensations travel via the anterior spinothalamic and lateral spinothalamic tracts. (From Hall JE. *Guyton and Hall Textbook of Medical Physiology.* 13th ed. Philadelphia: Elsevier; 2016:610.)

neurons. The other branch ascends for up to 10 spinal segments before synapsing with the second-order neurons in the dorsal horn. Second-order axons from both branches cross over and enter the ventral white column, forming the ventral spinothalamic tract, which ascends to the thalamus and synapses with third-order neurons in the ventral posterolateral nucleus. Tertiary axons travel through the internal capsule to the postcentral gyrus.

Owing to the branching arrangement of the first-order fibers from the trunk and extremities, injuries to the spinal cord rarely result in the total loss of these two sensations. Each cerebral cortex receives both crossed and uncrossed pressure and light-touch fibers from the face; as a result, damage to the postcentral gyrus on one side does not result in loss of pressure and light touch sensations to the face, even though these sensations are lost on the trunk and extremities of the contralateral side.[2,10,11,17]

Vibratory Sense, Proprioception, and Discriminatory Touch

Proprioceptive fibers from muscles of the face involved in facial expression and mastication synapse in cell bodies located in the mesencephalic nucleus of the midbrain. Little is known about the complete functioning of the pathway.

Fibers from the trunk and extremities carrying proprioceptive, vibratory, and discriminatory (fine) touch sensations synapse with neuron cell bodies in the dorsal root ganglion. From the dorsal root ganglion, first-order axons enter the dorsal white column and immediately ascend to the medulla (Fig. 31.13). The fibers are somatotopically organized in the white columns. Axons from the lumbar and sacral parts of the spinal cord travel medially in the fasciculus gracilis, and fibers from the cervical and thoracic areas of the cord are located laterally in the fasciculus cuneatus of the dorsal white column of the spinal cord. Each fasciculus terminates in its respective medullary nucleus (e.g., the fasciculus gracilis terminates in the nucleus gracilis). Second-order axons decussate after leaving their medullary nucleus and form a bundle termed the medial lemniscus, which terminates in the ventral posterolateral thalamic nucleus. Third-order fibers from the ventral posterolateral nucleus terminate in the postcentral gyrus.[2,10,11,17]

There are important distinctions to be made between the dorsal column medial lemniscal system and the anterolateral system. The differences determine the types of sensory information that can be transmitted by the two systems. The dorsal column medial lemniscal system is composed of large myelinated fibers with a high degree of spatial orientation that is maintained from their origin in the dorsal root to their termination in the thalamus. Therefore, sensations that must be transmitted rapidly with a high degree of localization to the stimulus travel via the dorsal column. The anterolateral system, on the other hand, is composed of smaller myelinated nerve fibers with less spatial orientation. Hence, the anterolateral system transmits a wider variety of sensations, at a slower velocity, and with less specificity than the dorsal column system.[16] A summary of the different sensations transmitted between the two systems is shown in Box 31.1.

Pupillary light and accommodation reflexes are mediated through the Edinger-Westphal nucleus and cranial nerve III. Pupillary dilation is produced by postganglionic sympathetic fibers from the superior cervical ganglion that travel with branches of the internal carotid artery to the radial muscle of the iris.[2,10,11,17]

MOTOR PATHWAYS

Motor, or efferent, pathways transmit information from the brain to voluntary muscles of the body, smooth muscle and cardiac muscle, and some glands. The corticospinal tracts supply the voluntary muscles of the trunk and extremities; nine cranial nerves supply the voluntary muscles of the head and neck. Autonomic preganglionic fibers arise in the brain and spinal cord and transmit efferent signals to smooth muscle, cardiac muscle, and some glands (lacrimal, bronchial).[10]

Corticospinal Tract

The corticospinal tract originates in large, upper motor neurons located in the precentral gyrus of the frontal lobe (Fig. 31.14). These neurons

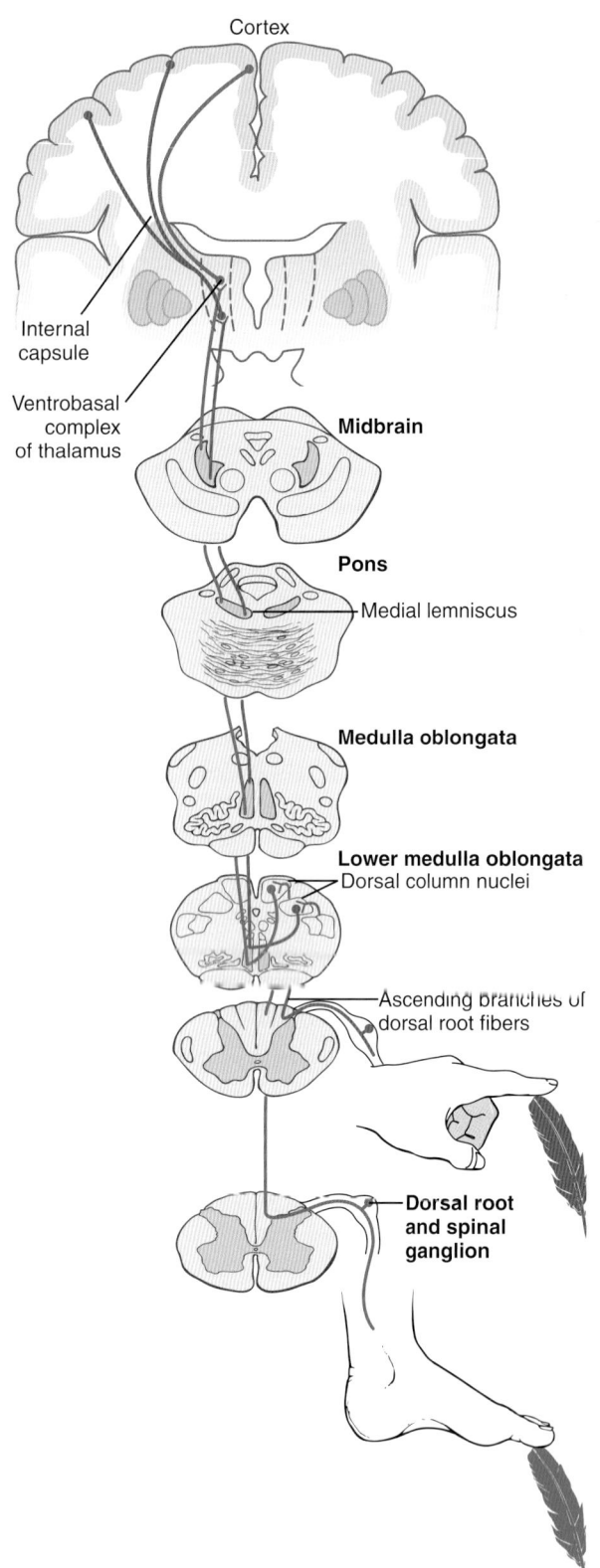

Cortex

Internal
capsule

Ventrobasal
complex
of thalamus

Midbrain

Pons

Medial lemniscus

Medulla oblongata

Lower medulla oblongata
Dorsal column nuclei

Ascending branches of
dorsal root fibers

**Dorsal root
and spinal
ganglion**

Fig. 31.13 Vibration, proprioception, and fine tactile sensations travel via the dorsal column–medial lemniscal system. (From Hall JE. *Guyton and Hall Textbook of Medical Physiology.* 13th ed. Philadelphia: Elsevier; 2016:610.)

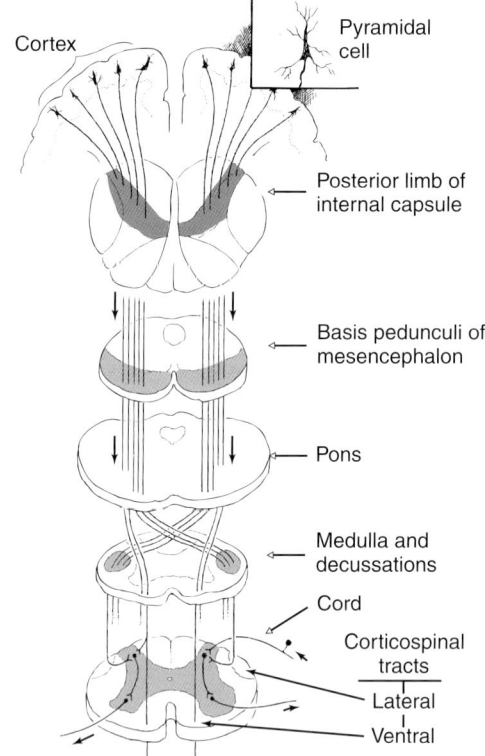

Cortex

Pyramidal
cell

Posterior limb of
internal capsule

Basis pedunculi of
mesencephalon

Pons

Medulla and
decussations

Cord

Corticospinal
tracts

Lateral

Ventral

Fig. 31.14 Corticospinal tracts. (From Hall JE. *Guyton and Hall Textbook of Medical Physiology.* 13th ed. Philadelphia: Elsevier; 2016:709.)

movements (such as the hands when writing, typing, or playing the piano) have a larger area in the gyrus than other parts of the body not involved in intricate movements. Many of the upper motor neurons are shaped in the form of a pyramid.

Axons travel from the pyramidal cells through the internal capsule, the major pathway for ascending and descending fibers between the cortex and other sites in the CNS. The internal capsule has three parts: the anterior limb, the posterior limb, and the genu, which lies between the anterior and posterior limbs. Fibers in the internal capsule are highly organized. Motor fibers to all parts of the body except the

are arranged in a specific manner. Neurons supplying voluntary muscles of the head are found in the precentral gyrus near the lateral fissure of Sylvius, and those innervating the legs and feet are found in an area of the gyrus near the median longitudinal fissure. All parts of the body are represented in the gyrus. However, areas that perform complex

face are located in the anterior limb and part of the posterior limb. Fibers supplying the face are located in the genu. From the internal capsule, the axons travel through the midbrain (basis pedunculi) to the medulla, where approximately 90% of the fibers decussate, forming the pyramids of the medulla. The corticospinal tract is frequently called the pyramidal tract, either because of the shape of the upper motor neurons or because of the site at which the fibers decussate in the medulla. The fibers that cross over form the lateral corticospinal tract. Axons from the lateral corticospinal tract continue their descent to the spinal cord. At each level of the cord, some fibers leave the lateral corticospinal tract and enter the ventral horn gray matter, where they synapse with lower motor neurons. The fibers that do not decussate (~10%) in the medulla continue to the spinal cord as the ventral corticospinal tract. The ventral corticospinal tracts cross over before synapsing with lower motor neurons in the gray matter. Axons from the lower motor neurons travel in the spinal nerves to innervate voluntary muscle.

A few corticospinal tract neurons are located anterior to the precentral gyrus. Axons from these neurons have an inhibitory effect on the lower motor neurons because they prevent them from discharging excessively. Damage to these suppressor fibers allows lower motor neurons to fire incorrect signals and either to become overexcited, resulting in hyperreflexia, or to discharge simultaneously, causing spasticity. Damage to the corticospinal tract anywhere along its route to the spinal cord can cause upper motor neuron paralysis. If the injury occurs above the decussation in the medulla, the paralysis is on the opposite side of the body. Paralysis occurs on the same side of the body if the damage occurs below the medulla. With upper motor neuron paralysis, reflexes are intact, but suppressor-fiber activity is impeded. As a result, hyperreflexia is present, and the upper motor neuron paralysis is spastic. Damage to lower motor neuron cell bodies in the ventral horn or ventral root fibers produces lower motor neuron paralysis, a flaccid type of paralysis. Cerebral palsy and amyotrophic lateral sclerosis are diseases that affect the corticospinal tracts.[2,7,9,10]

Motor Innervation to the Head

Upper motor neurons whose axons supply the voluntary muscles of the head are found in the precentral gyrus next to the lateral fissure of Sylvius. The cell bodies, whose axons supply the extrinsic muscles of the eye, are located in the middle frontal gyrus. Axons from both areas form the corticobulbar tracts, which travel through the genu of the internal capsule to the brainstem, where they synapse with neurons located in nuclei spread throughout the brainstem. Axons from these neurons form many of the cranial nerves.

Axons originating from neurons located in the midbrain form the oculomotor and trochlear nerves (Fig. 31.15). The oculomotor nerve innervates most of the external muscles of the eye (inferior oblique and the inferior, medial, and superior rectus muscles), along with the levator palpebrae superioris muscle, which raises the upper eyelid. The trochlear nerve innervates the external oblique muscle of the eye. Three other groups of nuclei have neurons whose axons form the trigeminal, abducens, and facial nerves. The trigeminal nerve innervates part of the soft palate and all the muscles of mastication. The abducens innervates the lateral rectus muscle of the eye, and the facial nerves supply all the muscles involved in facial expression.

Axons from neurons located in medullary nuclei form the glossopharyngeal, vagal, accessory, and hypoglossal nerves. Both the glossopharyngeal and vagal nerves arise from the ambiguous nucleus. The glossopharyngeal nerve supplies the stylopharyngeal muscle of the pharynx, and the vagal nerve innervates the muscles of the throat involved in swallowing and phonation. All the tongue muscles are supplied by the hypoglossal nerve. The accessory nerve innervates the trapezius and sternocleidomastoid muscles of the neck. With the

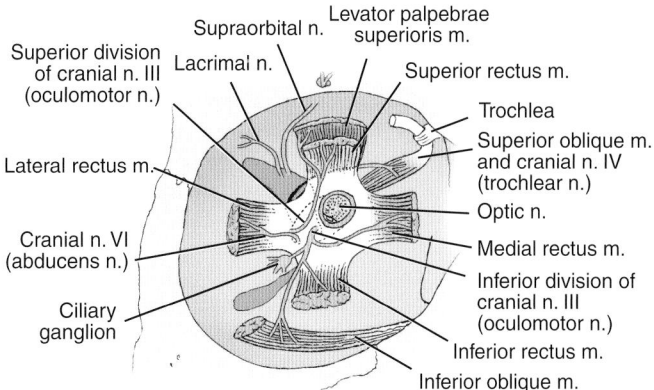

Fig. 31.15 Frontal view of the posterior orbit with its motor nerves and the extraocular muscles. *n.,* Nerve; *m.,* muscle.

exception of the facial and hypoglossal nerves, the remaining nerves receive information from both the right and the left corticobulbar tracts. The nuclei of facial nerve fibers to the upper part of the face receive axons from the left and right corticobulbar tracts; the facial nerve nuclei whose fibers supply the lower part of the face receive fibers only from the contralateral corticobulbar tract. The nuclei from the origin of the hypoglossal nerves receive innervation from only the contralateral corticobulbar tract.[2,10,11,17]

Subcortical Motor Areas

Several motor areas in the brain are outside the cerebral cortex. For the most part, these are relatively primitive motor areas that have a modulating influence on motor function. Included in the subcortical motor areas are the basal ganglia, the nucleus of Luys, the red nucleus (nucleus ruber), the substantia nigra, and the reticular formation.

The basal ganglia lie deep within the cerebral hemispheres at the level of the internal capsule. They are composed of three nuclei: the globus pallidus, the putamen, and the caudate, which are collectively termed the corpus striata. The globus pallidus and the putamen are sometimes termed the lentiform nucleus. The globus pallidus makes up the paleostriatum, and the other two nuclei are part of the neostriatum.

The globus pallidus receives input from the motor cortex and from the other basal ganglia; it sends fibers to the subcortical motor areas. The globus pallidus is connected to the thalamus by two tracts, the ansa lenticularis and the lenticular fasciculus, which merge as they enter the thalamus to form the thalamic fasciculus. The thalamus forms a feedback process by sending fibers to the caudate nucleus and motor cortex. In this way, the motor activity of the basal ganglia can be influenced by the motor cortex without the presence of direct connections between the two structures. Dopamine, an important neurotransmitter in the basal ganglia, is produced in the substantia nigra of the midbrain and then travels by axonal transport to the caudate nucleus and the putamen.

The subthalamic nucleus of Luys is located in the diencephalon and is connected to other subcortical motor areas. Lesions in this nucleus result in a suppression of motor activity.

Three motor areas are located in the midbrain: the red nucleus, the substantia nigra, and the reticular formation. The red nucleus is located at the level of the corpora quadrigemina and gives rise to the crossed rubrospinal tract. When stimulated, this tract excites alpha and gamma flexor motor neurons and inhibits extensor motor neurons. The reticular formation consists of a diffuse collection of neurons found throughout the brainstem and into the diencephalon. Two major tracts arise from the reticular formation. One tract is the uncrossed medial reticulospinal tract, which excites alpha and gamma extensor motor neurons and inhibits flexor motor neurons when stimulated. The second tract is the lateral reticulospinal tract, which contains crossed and uncrossed fibers and activates alpha and gamma flexor motor neurons and inhibits extensor motor neurons when stimulated.

Lesions contained within the subcortical motor areas produce diseases characterized by abnormal muscle tone and dyskinesia (abnormal involuntary movements). For example, in Parkinson disease, the globus pallidus and substantia nigra are affected. Huntington chorea involves atrophy of the caudate nucleus and putamen, as well as degeneration of cortical neurons. Other diseases that involve subcortical motor nuclei include athetosis, dystonia, ballismus, and Sydenham chorea.[2,10,11,17]

NEUROANESTHESIA

Creating a comprehensive plan to care for patients having neurosurgical procedures should consider the patient's condition and comorbidities, as well as specific procedural implications such as positioning, surgical approach, and surgical requirements. An overview of the effects of anesthetic agents on cerebral blood flow (CBF), cerebral metabolic rate of oxygen consumption ($CMRO_2$), and intracranial pressure (ICP) is discussed next.

The remainder of this chapter provides a general discussion of the preoperative, intraoperative, and immediate postoperative care associated with common intracranial surgical procedures.

Effects of Anesthetic Agents on Cerebral Physiology

Cerebral blood flow, cerebral blood volume (CBV), ICP, $CMRO_2$, and cerebral compliance must all be considered in concert with pharmacologic principles in the design of a neurosurgical anesthetic regimen (Table 31.4). These factors have a dramatic effect of cerebrovascular tone, blood flow, and oxygen delivery.

Inhalation Agents

The majority of anesthetic agents influence ICP by decreasing cerebrovascular resistance through cerebrovascular dilation and by dose-dependent impairment of autoregulation, producing increases in ICP and CBV and a decrease in $CMRO_2$. The changes in ICP are frequently greater in patients who have an underlying increase in ICP.[18,19] Inhalation agents decrease mean arterial pressure (MAP) and increase ICP, reducing cerebral perfusion pressure (CPP).[20-22] Isoflurane produces the greatest increases in CBF and ICP, followed by sevoflurane and desflurane.[18,23-25]

Cerebral blood flow in humans is unaltered with isoflurane-inspired concentrations of 0.6 to 1.1 minimum alveolar concentration (MAC); however, when isoflurane is increased to 1.6 MAC CBF doubles. Animal studies have shown that isoflurane may enhance the carbon dioxide (CO_2) reactivity of the cerebral vessels. Cerebral autoregulation is impaired with concentrations exceeding 1 MAC.[26,27] $CMRO_2$ is depressed with isoflurane, as with all potent inhalation anesthetics, and progressive metabolic depression occurs with concentrations of isoflurane greater than 1 MAC until the electroencephalograph (EEG) becomes isoelectric at approximately 2.5 MAC.[28,29] These properties suggest that clinically relevant doses may provide a neuroprotective effect against ischemic insults, as demonstrated in human studies of critical regional CBF during carotid clamping.[30] Although strong experimental data support a neuroprotective potential of several anesthetic agents, consistent long-term protection by either agent has not been demonstrated. Unfortunately, there is a lack of clinical studies to support the use of any one anesthetic agent over the others. Proposed mechanisms related to the neuroprotective effect

TABLE 31.4 Effects of Anesthetics on Cerebral Dynamics

Drug	Cerebral Blood Flow	$CMRO_2$	Intracranial Pressure	Cerebral Perfusion Pressure
Inhalation				
Nitrous oxide	↑	↑↑	0/↓	↓
Sevoflurane	↑	↓	↑	↓
Isoflurane	↑	↓	↑	↓
Desflurane	↑	↓	↑	↓
Intravenous				
Barbiturates	↓↓	↓↓	↓↓	0/↓
Etomidate	↓↓	↓↓	↓	0
Propofol	↓	↓	↓	↓
Ketamine	↑	↑	↑↑	↓
Benzodiazepines	↓	↓	↓	0/↓
Dexmedetomidine	↓	0/↓	0	0/↓
Morphine	0/↓	0/↓	↓	↑↓
Fentanyl	0/↓	0/↓	↓	0/↓
Alfentanil	0/↓	0/↓	↓	↓
Sufentanil	0/↓	0/↓	↓	↓
Remifentanil	0/↓	0/↓	↓	↓

$CMRO_2$, Cerebral metabolic rate of oxygen.
From Zaglaniczny KL, Aker J, eds. *Clinical Guide to Pediatric Anesthesia*. Philadelphia: Elsevier; 1999:176; Matsumoto M, Sakabe T. Effects of anesthetic agents and other drugs on cerebral blood flow, metabolism, and intracranial pressure. In Cottrell JE, Patel P, eds. *Cottrell and Patel's Neuroanesthesia*. 6th ed. Edinburgh: Elsevier; 2017:74–91.

of inhalation anesthetic agents include activation of ATP-dependent potassium channels, upregulation of nitric oxide synthase, reduction of excitotoxic stressors and cerebral metabolic rate, augmentation of periischemic CBF, and upregulation of antiapoptotic factors including mitogen-activated protein kinases.[31] Activation of intracellular signaling cascades that lead to altered expression of protective genes may also be involved.[32] The high concentrations of isoflurane necessary for abolishing cortical activity have no toxic effect on cerebral metabolic pathways.[29,33] The majority of human studies show that inspired concentrations of isoflurane of less than 1% have minimal effect on ICP and that any increase in ICP is attenuated by mild hyperventilation. An exception to this generalization is that some patients with malignant brain tumors may show increases in ICP despite hyperventilation, particularly if computed tomography (CT) shows a midline shift.[34-36]

Desflurane is unique among the potent inhalation agents in that its low blood/gas solubility facilitates a rapid emergence, which may be useful for immediate postoperative neurologic evaluation. Desflurane has effects on EEG, CBF, and $CMRO_2$ similar to those of isoflurane. Cerebral blood flow was compared using desflurane and isoflurane at two concentrations, 1 MAC and 1.5 MAC, in an air-oxygen mixture during hypocapnia without any reported difference between the two different MAC levels.[37,38] Holmström and Akeson reported that desflurane was associated with more CBF than isoflurane at the same depth of anesthesia.[39] However, the results of ICP studies are not as definitive. Muzzi et al. reported that desflurane at 1 MAC in an air-oxygen mixture with an arterial CO_2 tension ($PaCO_2$) of 26 mm Hg resulted in sustained increases in ICP until the dura was incised.[40] The physiologic effects

BOX 31.2 Neurosurgical Considerations for Omitting the Use of Nitrous Oxide

- In the presence of intracranial air (recent craniotomy, craniofacial trauma)
- When signal quality during intraoperative-evoked potential monitoring is inadequate
- When the patient has clinical evidence of moderate to severe increases in ICP
- When a "tight-brain" is clinically appreciated during the intraoperative period
- When the duration of the case is >8 hr

ICP, Intracranial pressure.

of sevoflurane are similar to those of other inhalation anesthetics, but some consider sevoflurane less vasoactive than isoflurane or desflurane.[41] In summary, all inhalational agents are known to increase CBF, CBV, and ICP. Mild hyperventilation attenuates these dose-dependent increases in ICP. Isoflurane, desflurane, and sevoflurane all preserve cerebrovascular carbon dioxide reactivity. They are all concentration-dependent cerebral vasodilators and decrease $CMRO_2$. Sevoflurane induces the least degree cerebral vasodilatation and preserves cerebral autoregulation up to 1.5 MAC, compared to isoflurane and desflurane, which impair it upon 1 MAC. In intracranial surgery, inhaled agents can be used as a maintenance anesthetic with a preference for sevoflurane.[24]

The use of nitrous oxide (N_2O) during intracranial procedures continues to be controversial. N_2O can produce increases in CBF, $CMRO_2$, and ICP. The effect of N_2O on cerebral dynamics varies widely and is influenced by what drugs are coadministered, the doses of each, and body temperature. Concomitant hyperventilation or the administration of one of several intravenous anesthetics (barbiturates, propofol, benzodiazepines, opioids) can reduce the increases in CBF and $CMRO_2$ during N_2O administration. However, the combination of N_2O and volatile anesthetics behaves much differently. Administering a volatile anesthetic in low doses (<1 MAC) may decrease CBF and $CMRO_2$. The addition of 50% N_2O with less than 1 MAC of the volatile anesthetic produces increases in both CBF and $CMRO_2$. The cerebral vasodilation produced by N_2O is greater when increasing doses of the volatile anesthetic are administered (i.e., >1 MAC). N_2O may increase CBF by 100% or more at approximately 0.5 MAC. N_2O appears to produce nonuniform changes in CBF, increasing flow in anterior regions and decreasing flow in posterior brain regions. N_2O is not thought to affect CBV or CSF dynamics.[42-46]

Many clinicians have advocated that N_2O should no longer be administered to neurosurgical patients. However, there is little scientific evidence that N_2O produces significant neurotoxicity during limited periods of exposure. Typically, only very small amounts of N_2O are broken down in the body, but when used on long cases (>12 hours), substantial accumulation of metabolic breakdown products may occur. These metabolites have been associated with megaloblastic anemia, leukopenia, impaired fetal development, and a depressed immune system. Circumstances in which the practitioner should consider eliminating the use of N_2O are listed in Box 31.2.

Another important consideration is the fact that N_2O is more soluble than nitrogen and expands closed-gas spaces. Its use should be avoided in patients with an intracranial or intravascular air compartment such as pneumocephalus.[47] Some practitioners discontinue N_2O before closure of the dura to attenuate the development of iatrogenic pneumocephalus.

Intravenous Agents

Propofol is a popular induction and maintenance agent for neurosurgical patients. It is very useful in patients with intracranial pathologic

conditions, provided that hypotension is prevented. The cerebral effects are a dose-dependent reduction in CBF and $CMRO_2$. The reductions are approximately 40% to 50%. CPP may decrease because of reductions in blood pressure after bolus induction doses; however, the reduction in CBF appears to be independent of systemic hemodynamic changes.[48,49] They are most likely due to the metabolic depressant effect and cerebral vasoconstriction.[50,51] Reductions in systemic blood pressure produce corresponding reductions in CPP.

Etomidate, like other CNS depressants, reduces $CMRO_2$ and CBF. Benefits associated with etomidate use include cerebral vasoconstriction, which results in the reduction of ICP without reducing CPP.[52-54] Major disadvantages include a high incidence of myoclonia, thrombophlebitis, nausea, vomiting, and suppression of the adrenocortical response to stress.[54,55] Many clinicians feel that etomidate should be avoided in brain-injured patients. Although it is considered an induction drug of choice in situations of hemodynamic compromise, prolonged adrenal insufficiency is a major concern. Adrenal insufficiency is of special concern in critically ill patients with sepsis and traumatic brain injury (TBI). For these reasons, it may be prudent to replace etomidate with an amnestic dose of a benzodiazepine in combination with an opioid or ketamine to facilitate endotracheal intubation. If etomidate is used, empirical adrenal replacement therapy for 24 hours should be considered.[52]

Dexmedetomidine is gaining popularity in neuroanesthesia and neurocritical care practice. This medication is a presynaptic α_2-adrenergic receptor agonist that provides "cooperative sedation," anxiolysis, and analgesia without respiratory depression.[56] Dexmedetomidine produces a dose-dependent sedation that resembles natural sleep. Sleep patterns differ from the classic GABA receptor agonists such as propofol. Patients do not experience respiratory depression and are readily arousable.[57] An advantage of this type of sedation is that procedures requiring "wake-up" tests can be more readily accomplished compared with usual anesthetic regimens.[58] Dexmedetomidine does not interfere with electrophysiologic monitoring, thereby allowing brain mapping during awake craniotomy and microelectrode recording during implantation of deep-brain stimulators. Motor- and somatosensory-evoked potentials are maintained when added to a desflurane and remifentanil technique. Dose-dependent decreases in the amplitude of motor-evoked potentials (MEPs) may occur.[59,60] Bispectral index (BIS) values are also decreased in a dose-dependent manner, to a greater extent than with propofol.[61]

Dexmedetomidine does not alter cerebral metabolism ($CMRO_2$). CBF is decreased due to cerebral vasoconstriction. This suggests uncoupling between cerebral metabolism and flow because of decreases in central catecholamine degradation. Effects on ICP are not clinically significant.[62,63]

The central sympatholytic effects also result in an antishivering action, hypothermia, and a reduction in the neuroendocrine stress response to surgery. A reduction in postoperative agitation and emergence delirium in children and adults is an increasingly used clinical action. A neuroprotective effect has been proposed, but benefits in head-injured patients remain to be clarified.[62] Analgesic- and anesthetic-sparing effects are well documented and are produced at both the brain and spinal cord levels. The greatest utilization of dexmedetomidine outside the neurosurgical intensive care environment is for awake craniotomy.

Opioid-based anesthetic techniques are popular for neurosurgical procedures because they provide a steady hemodynamic course and predictable emergence. The synthetic opioids produce dose-related reductions in CBF (decrease to 25 mL/100 g/min) and $CMRO_2$ (40%–50%).[64-67] Later investigations in patients after acute head injury or in those undergoing supratentorial craniotomy noted increases in ICP and decreases in CPP after administration of induction doses of fentanyl, sufentanil, and alfentanil.[68] These opioid-induced changes in ICP have been suggested to occur secondarily to an autoregulatory response to decreases in MAP.[64]

Fentanyl decreases the resistance to CSF absorption and results in a 10% reduction in CBV.[55,64] Sufentanil is 5 to 10 times more potent than fentanyl and has the highest therapeutic index of the clinically used opiates. Of the synthetic opiates, alfentanil produces the greatest decreases in MAP and CPP.[55,64] Remifentanil is a 4-anilidopiperidine derivative. It is characterized by an ultrashort duration of action and a metabolism independent of both hepatic and renal functions. The main drawback is a lack of residual analgesia and the risk of postoperative hyperalgesia.[69] Meperidine should be avoided in the neurosurgical patient because its metabolite, normeperidine, is known for causing seizures.

Judiciously titrated doses of naloxone reverse opioid-induced respiratory depression and normalize both CBF and $CMRO_2$. The abrupt reversal of opioid-induced respiratory depression should be avoided in neurosurgical patients. Naloxone administered is associated with hypertension, cardiac dysrhythmias, pulmonary edema, and intracranial hemorrhage.[70,71]

Newer techniques for managing craniotomies have been suggested using opioid-free or opioid-sparing techniques. There is limited evidence regarding the efficacy of avoiding opioids altogether; however, multimodal techniques are recommended in an effort to limit opioid use and improve neurologic monitoring while at the same time limiting opioid side effects.[72]

The benzodiazepines are useful for their anxiolytic, anticonvulsant, and amnestic effects. Benzodiazepines produce a dose-dependent decrease in $CMRO_2$ and reductions in CBF; however, their effects on ICP are minimal.

Flumazenil, the benzodiazepine-specific antagonist, has no effect on cerebral dynamics when administered alone. Evidence (in the canine population) suggests that a high dose midazolam anesthetic was associated with rebound increases in CBF and ICP to values greater than baseline when abrupt reversal was accomplished with flumazenil. Flumazenil may produce seizures when large doses are administered.

Ketamine has had limited popularity in neuroanesthesia. The dissociative mechanism of action may result in a stormy emergence from anesthesia, which is undesirable after neurosurgical procedures. The primary advantage associated with ketamine is the stable hemodynamic course in the presence of hypovolemia that may occur in patients with traumatic head injury and multisystem trauma. Ketamine is known to produce untoward alterations in cerebral physiology, increasing CBF by 60% to 80% and potentially elevating ICP. Ketamine also increases the resistance to CSF reabsorption in animal studies, which could lead to increases in ICP beyond that produced by increases in CBF alone. However, recent evidence demonstrates how ketamine does not increase ICP to levels previously believed and that it can be administered (as an induction agent) to patients with TBI and elevated ICP, especially in the situation of low blood pressure.[73] Cerebral metabolic rate is unchanged, but regional differences may exist.

A renewed interest in ketamine has been prompted because of its noncompetitive antagonism of the glutamine NMDA receptor. Similar compounds have been demonstrated to afford some degree of neuroprotection. Ketamine has analgesic properties as well. Analgesia occurs with subanesthetic doses, and it is widely used for sedation in combination with low doses of benzodiazepines, propofol, and other analgesics.[74] The effect on glucose utilization varies by brain region. The response of cerebral vessels to carbon dioxide is left intact.

Others suggests ketamine can be used safely in neurologically impaired patients under conditions of controlled ventilation,

coadministration of a GABA receptor agonist such as midazolam or propofol, and avoidance of N_2O.[75] Trauma patients with multiple injuries may benefit from the favorable cardiovascular effects while avoiding untoward neurologic adverse actions. Ketamine produces atypical anesthesia, thus EEG patterns also differ from standard anesthetics. On loss of consciousness and onset of analgesia, ketamine induces a transition from alpha to theta waves (slow waves with moderate to high amplitude) on the EEG. Alpha waves do not reappear until after consciousness returns and analgesia is lost. Ketamine alone does not decrease the BIS even when patients are unconscious.[76] Several researchers have, in fact, noted an increase in BIS levels when ketamine is added to a propofol, fentanyl, or sevoflurane anesthetic. Ketamine does not alter auditory-evoked potentials (AEPs), midlatency auditory-evoked potential (MLAEP), or A line autoregressive index monitors based on MLAEPs.

Nondepolarizing neuromuscular relaxants do not appear to have clinically significant direct effects on CBF or $CMRO_2$, provided MAP is not altered after administration.[77] The depolarizing agent succinylcholine in select circumstances may produce transient elevations in ICP, CBF, and $CMRO_2$.

Upper motor neuron disease may alter the peripheral nerve–stimulating response of nondepolarizing neuromuscular relaxants. Generally, the twitch response shows relative resistance to muscle relaxants on the hemiparetic or hemiplegic side, compared with the unaffected side or respiratory muscles.[78,79] Decreased sensitivity to nondepolarizing muscle relaxants is most exaggerated in the first 3 weeks of upper motor neuron disease. Therefore, monitoring neuromuscular blockade is preferentially performed on the unaffected side. Patients on chronic anticonvulsant therapy may be more resistant to long-acting nondepolarizing muscle relaxants.[80] Phenytoin causes cytochrome P450 enzyme induction, and therefore, it is possible that increased doses may be required and a decreased duration of action may occur for aminosteroid neuromuscular blockers.

Succinylcholine-induced fasciculations can cause transient increases in ICP. Thus, this medication should be used with caution for neurosurgical patents with elevated ICP. Research conducted in animals shows a small and transient rise of 10 to 15 mm Hg for 5 to 8 minutes after administration.[81] The rise is associated with an increased CBF, muscle spindle afferent activity, and electroencephalogram arousal. Fasciculation of the neck muscles causing jugular vein stasis appears to be a factor. The effects on ICP may be inhibited by pretreatment with a small dose of nondepolarizing relaxant. Furthermore, the administration of an anesthetic induction agent prior to succinylcholine may reduce the potential for ICP increases. In clinical practice, succinylcholine continues to be the medication that provides the most rapid and reliable paralysis for emergency procedures requiring airway control via rapid sequence induction. As mentioned previously, succinylcholine is contraindicated in patients with neurologic or denervated muscle because of the potential for life-threatening hyperkalemia. Succinylcholine should be avoided in patients with cerebrovascular accident, upper and lower motor neuron lesions, coma, encephalitis, closed head injury, and after severe burns and prolonged bed rest.[82]

A nondepolarizing alternative, such as rocuronium (at 1.2 mg/kg intubating dose), also facilitates endotracheal intubation within 60 to 90 seconds and avoids the known complications of succinylcholine. Rocuronium is being used with more frequency for rapid sequence induction since the availability of sugammadex, which provides rapid reversal if necessary.

Antihypertensives

β-adrenergic antagonists have great utility for the control of the inotropic and chronotropic effects of sympathetic stimulation that attend laryngoscopy, endotracheal intubation, and endotracheal extubation. Esmolol is a rapid-onset, short-acting selective β_1-adrenergic receptor antagonist. Administration of 0.5 to 1 mg/kg 1 to 2 minutes before laryngoscopy and endotracheal intubation attenuates the predictable increases in heart rate and blood pressure. Its effects on ICP are thought to be negligible. Labetalol is a selective α_1-adrenergic antagonist and nonselective β_1- and β_2-adrenergic antagonist (ratio of β-blockade to α-blockade is 7:1 for intravenous preparation). Labetalol spares presynaptic α_2-receptors; consequently, released norepinephrine produces further inhibition of catecholamine release via a negative feedback from the stimulation of β_2-receptors. Labetalol and esmolol may be preferred for the control of emergence hypertension after intracranial procedures. Some evidence demonstrated that patients treated with labetalol, as compared with esmolol, experienced a higher incidence of bradycardia in the immediate postoperative period.[83,84]

Sodium nitroprusside and nitroglycerin produce increases in CBV and ICP. Sodium nitroprusside is a direct-acting cerebrovasodilator, increasing CBV after dilation of cerebral capacitance vessels.[77,85] Deliberate hyperventilation and administration of propofol may attenuate cerebrovasodilation. Most contemporary neuroanesthetists consider nitroglycerin and sodium nitroprusside to be potent dilators of capacitance vessels and unsafe in patients with abnormal elastance. Cerebrovascular dilation increases ICP by increasing CBV. These effects can result in intracranial hypertension and potentially cerebral herniation if increased ICP already exists.[86]

INTRACRANIAL PRESSURE

Intracranial pressure refers to the supratentorial CSF pressure. The supratentorial pressure may be measured within the lateral ventricle or within the subarachnoid space over the convexity of the cerebral cortex. CSF pressure may vary markedly in different areas within the cranium, and similarly, CSF pressure in the cranial subarachnoid space may differ from that in the spinal subarachnoid space. In individuals free of neurologic pathology who are in a recumbent position, the CSF pressure measured at the lumbar cistern accurately reflects ICP. However, many factors, including the assumption of the upright position, can alter the relationship between cranial and spinal CSF pressures. In addition, in the presence of intracranial mass lesions, infratentorial CSF pressure (as measured in the cisterna magna or lumbar cistern) often decreases, whereas supratentorial pressure increases. Therefore, the measurement of supratentorial CSF pressure is a useful clinical concept.[21,87]

Determinants of Intracranial Pressure

The brain is enclosed within the cranium, and because the brain is not compressible any increase in total intracranial volume produces an accompanying increase in ICP (Monro-Kelly doctrine). Increased ICP may have a detrimental effect on neurologic function. The intracranial space is occupied by four constituent compartments: the brain (accounting for 80%–90% of the intracranial volume), the blood, intracellular water, and CSF. The intracranial contents combined have a volume of approximately 1200 to 1500 mL.[88] Under normal conditions, local CNS pressure gradients are equilibrated if the CSF circulation is patent. Because the skull is rigid, any expansion of one of these compartments must be compensated by a reduction in size of the others if ICP is to remain constant. If these compensatory mechanisms are insufficient, ICP rises. Small increases in intracranial volume can be initially accommodated with little or no effect on the ICP, but as more volume is added, intracranial compliance falls until it reaches a critical point beyond which any minimal increase in volume causes an exponential rise in ICP.[89] Intracranial hypertension may lead to global

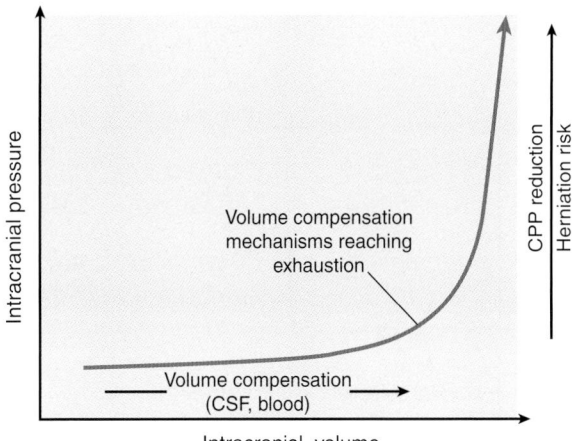

Fig. 31.16 The intracranial pressure-volume relationship. *CPP*, Cerebral perfusion pressure; *CSF*, cerebrospinal fluid. (From Miller RD, et al., eds. *Miller's Anesthesia. 9th ed.* Philadelphia: Elsevier; 2020:1870.)

reductions in CPP (CPP = MAP – ICP) from compression-induced ischemia, or may produce shifting of intracranial contents resulting in compression of the brain against the falx, the tentorium, or the foramen magnum.

Normal ICP is approximately 5 to 15 mm Hg in adults; lower values are recorded in children and infants. This pressure is determined by the relationship between the volume allowed by the structures that limit intracranial volume and the actual volume of the intracranial space. Due to the normal elastance of the intracranial contents, individuals without intracranial pathology maintain normal ICP despite transient increases that develop with coughing or during a Valsalva maneuver. Small increases in the intracranial volume do not produce abrupt increases in ICP. This normal elastance exists because the limits of the intracranial contents have not been reached. Pressures exceeding 20 to 25 mm Hg are indicative of intracranial hypertension and require monitoring and treatment.

Once intracranial volume begins to increase, dramatic increases in ICP may occur.[90] This relationship is depicted in Fig. 31.16. Although this ICP-volume curve is commonly used to explain these relationships, some suggest that the x-axis be relabeled as "volume of the growing mass" because it does not represent total intracranial volume.[91] The initial portion of the ICP curve is relatively flat because the total intracranial volume does not change with early periods of bleeding or tumor growth. This portion of the curve reflects the phenomenon of spatial compensation. As the mass (blood or tumor) increases, the volume of the intracranial compartments must decrease to maintain normal ICP. In most cases, the CSF compartment decreases in an effort to compensate for the increased intracranial volume. CSF is absorbed by the arachnoid granulations or shunted to the spinal subarachnoid space. Compensation is exhausted when the CSF compartment cannot decrease further in size and total intracranial volume increases, accounting for the increase in ICP. Once volume compensation has reached exhaustion, the subsequent increasing ICP has a direct relationship with a reduction in cerebral perfusion and an increased herniation risk (see Fig. 31.16).[92]

Measurement of Intracranial Pressure

ICP may be monitored using intraparenchymal, intraventricular, epidural, or subdural devices. The current gold standard for ICP monitoring is the intraventricular catheter because of its precision. Although it is highly invasive, it allows for drainage of CSF to lower ICP. As with any indwelling catheter, there can be insertion problems and strict sterile technique must be maintained. Infection is the most frequent

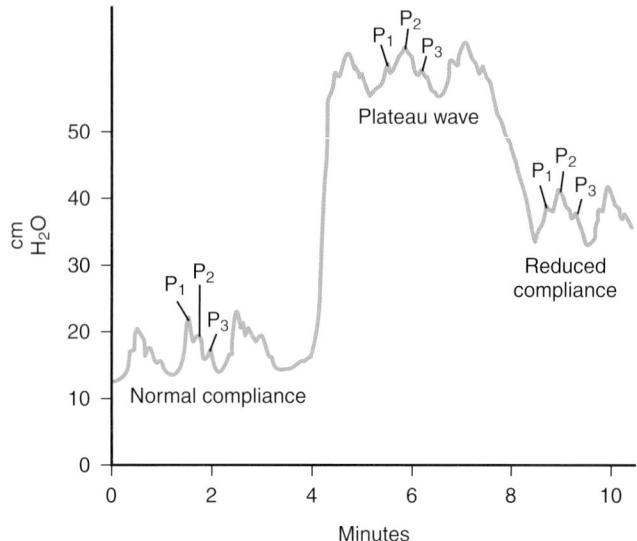

Fig. 31.17 Intracranial pressure tracings in the setting of normal and reduced compliance. Plateau wave (A wave of Lundberg) is seen in the center of the figure. (From Daroff RB, et al., eds. *Bradley's Neurology in Clinical Practice.* 7th ed. London: Elsevier; 2016:745.)

complication of ICP monitoring. Ventriculostomy carries an infection risk of up to 22%, in contrast with fiber-optic intraparenchymal monitors (1.8%). Risk factors include drainage duration greater than 5 days, CSF leak, concurrent systemic infection, craniotomy, and intraventricular hemorrhage. Neither prophylactic antibiotics nor routine catheter exchange has been shown to decrease the incidence of infection. Tract hematoma along the catheter trajectory and subdural hematoma due to ruptured bridging veins from over drainage can also occur.

Intraparenchymal probes are a popular method of measuring ICP. They are easy to use and transport and are zeroed when inserted. Infection problems are minimal. The microsensor transducer and the fiber optic transducer are the most widely available. Recommendations for ICP monitoring include patients with severe TBI and a Glasgow Coma Scale (GCS) sum score below 9 with an abnormal CT scan. If the patient has a normal CT scan but has two or more of the following criteria: age older than 40, unilateral or bilateral motor posturing, and systolic blood pressure (SBP) less than 90 mm Hg, then ICP monitoring should be provided.[93-96]

ICP is pulsatile, and the pressure waveforms provide useful information beyond numbers measured. The ICP waveforms are made of three distinct components: heart pulse waves, respiratory waves, and slow vasogenic waves (Lundberg B waves), each with a characteristic frequency. The normal ICP waveform consists of a three-peaked wave (Fig. 31.17). P1, the first and generally the tallest peak, is also known as the percussion wave and corresponds to the transmitted SBP; P2 (the tidal wave) and P3 (the dicrotic wave) are normally smaller peaks, and the notch between them corresponds to the dicrotic notch of the arterial waveform. As ICP increases, P2 and P3 rise and eventually surpass P1. Ultimately, with continued elevation of ICP, the waveform loses distinct peaks and assumes a triangular morphology. Intracranial pathology leading to sustained elevations of ICP may produce plateau waves, also known as A waves of Lundberg. These waves reflect a sudden dramatic rise in ICP to levels of 40 to 100 mm Hg, often lasting 5 to 20 minutes. Plateau waves indicate critically low intracranial compliance leading to marked changes in ICP, even with very small variations in intracranial volume. Although their pathophysiology is not fully elucidated, plateau waves are thought to be generated by brief episodes of decreased CPP (often caused by systemic hypotension),

leading to exaggerated cerebral vasodilation, increased blood volume, and increased ICP. This further decreases CPP, potentially resulting in cerebral ischemia. Cushing triad, which was originally described as systemic hypertension, bradycardia, and an irregular respiratory pattern, is a sign of a severely increased ICP indicating impending brain herniation.[95] Currently, most clinicians will include an increase in pulse pressure (the difference between the systolic and diastolic blood pressure) as part of the triad.

Intracranial Hypertension

Intracranial hypertension occurs with a sustained increase in ICP above 20 to 25 mm Hg.[97] Intracranial hypertension develops with expanding tissue or fluid mass, interference with normal CSF absorption, excessive CBF, or systemic disturbances promoting brain edema. Often, multiple factors are responsible for the development of intracranial hypertension. For example, tumors in the posterior fossa usually produce some degree of brain edema and readily obstruct CSF flow by compressing the fourth ventricle.[98]

Although many patients with intracranial hypertension are initially asymptomatic, all eventually develop characteristic signs and symptoms, including headache, nausea, vomiting, papilledema, focal neurologic deficits, altered ventilatory function, decreased consciousness, seizures, and coma. When ICP exceeds 30 mm Hg, CBF progressively decreases, and a vicious cycle is established: Ischemia produces brain edema, which, in turn, increases ICP and further precipitates ischemia. If this cycle remains unchecked, progressive neurologic damage or catastrophic herniation may result.[21,98,99] A consistent increase in ICP above 20 mm Hg requires treatment.

When intracranial hypertension is caused by hematoma, contusion, tumor, hygroma, hydrocephalus, or pneumatocephalus, surgical treatment is indicated. In the absence of a surgically treatable condition, ICP may be controlled by correcting the patient's position, temperature, ventilation, hemodynamics, and drainage of CSF. Other initial options include controlled hypocapnia (hyperventilation to a $Paco_2$ 35–40 mm Hg). On average, CBF decreases by 4% for every 1-mm Hg decrease in $Paco_2$. The effect of hyperventilation is temporary, however, as tolerance develops within hours. Hyperosmolar therapy (mannitol, hypertonic saline) and induced arterial hypertension (CPP concept) are also used. When autoregulation of CBF is compromised, hyperoncotic treatment aimed at reducing vasogenic edema and intracranial blood volume may be applied. When intracranial hypertension persists, secondary treatments may be indicated. These include forced intentional hyperventilation ($Paco_2$ <25 mm Hg), sedative induced coma, or experimental protocols such as induced hypothermia. Lastly, emergent bilateral decompressive craniectomy can be performed.[93]

Intracranial Pressure Reduction

The major interventions for treating elevated ICP are listed in Box 31.3. Selective application of these methods often results in ICP reduction, accompanied by clinical improvement. A patent airway, adequate oxygenation, and controlled ventilation provide the foundation for neuroresuscitative care in acute intracranial hypertensive states. Frequently, overlap occurs among causes of increased ICP, and this may necessitate simultaneous application of a number of different therapeutic modalities.[68]

Hyperventilation

Hyperventilation has the potential to reduce ICP via reflex vasoconstriction in the presence of hypocapnia. The vasoconstriction leads to decreases in CBF, overall cerebral fluid volume, and therefore, ICP. The potential dangers associated with inducing hypocapnia are related to the vasoconstriction and possible cerebral hypoxia that occurs,

BOX 31.3 Methods for the Treatment of Elevated Intracranial Pressure

- Insertion of intracranial pressure monitor such as a ventricular catheter or parenchymal probe; tissue oxygen partial pressure, $AVDo_2$, and CBF monitoring recommended.
- Optimize sedation and analgesia to allow for ventilatory control. Administer propofol and/or fentanyl.
- Open external ventricular drain if present for ICP >20 mm Hg for 10 minutes; repeat as needed.
- Hyperosmolar therapy:
  - 3% hypertonic saline bolus of 150–250 mL over 30 min
  - 23.4% hypertonic saline bolus of 30 mL over 10 min
  - Prior to administering 3% hypertonic saline bolus, check if Na <155 mEq/L
  - Mannitol 0.25–1 g/kg bolus once in emergency
  - Start 3% hypertonic saline drip at 30 mL/h if three or more 3% hypertonic saline boluses within 6 hr
  - Hypertonic saline can be temporarily infused in a large bore peripheral IV if central venous access is unavailable or while waiting for central venous access.
  - Check sodium and serum osmolality
- Hyperventilation:
  - Do not hyperventilate in the first 24 hr (goal $Paco_2$ of 35–40 mm Hg).
- Elevate patient's head 15–30 degrees if the surgery allows; position to improve cerebral venous return; avoid neck-vein compression; loosen cervical collar if in place.
- Avoid overhydration; target normovolemia.
- Optimize hemodynamics: mean arterial pressure, central venous pressure, pulmonary capillary wedge pressure, heart rate, and cerebral perfusion pressure; consider antihypertensive therapy as needed.
- Surgical decompression; consider decompressive craniectomy if hematoma is present.
- Consider mild hypothermia.
- Avoid corticosteroids with traumatic brain injuries.

$AVDo_2$, Arteriovenous difference in oxygen content; *CBF*, cerebral blood flow; *ICP*, intracranial pressure; *IV*, intravenous; *$Paco_2$*, partial pressure of arterial carbon dioxide.
Adapted from Stippler M. Craniocerebral trauma. In Daroff, et al., eds. *Bradley's Neurology in Clinical Practice.* 7th ed. London: Elsevier; 2016:876.

and thus, this intervention is not used initially to treat increased ICP. Excessive hypocapnia may lead to ischemia secondary to insufficient CBF. Therefore, it is not recommended in the first 24 hours after TBI or prophylactically. The reactivity of cerebral vessels to changes in $Paco_2$ is an important physiologic control system. When the physiologic control is intact, hyperventilation lowers $Paco_2$, resulting in respiratory alkalosis and subsequent vasoconstriction. When vasoconstriction is pronounced, intracranial blood volume will decrease and lower ICP. This is particularly important in known low-CBF conditions, such as severe TBI or vasospasm. To avoid cerebral ischemia, $Paco_2$ should be lowered to approximately 30 to 35 mm Hg. The vasoconstrictive effect on cerebral arterioles lasts only 11 to 20 hours because the pH of the CSF rapidly equilibrates to the new $Paco_2$ level. When hypocapnia is monitored by end tidal capnometry, the $Paco_2$ is approximately 2 to 5 mm Hg higher than end tidal carbon dioxide ($ETco_2$) readings, although many conditions can affect this gradient. Compared with autoregulation of CBF, CO_2 vascular reactivity is usually maintained even in the traumatized brain. When CO_2 vascular reactivity is lost, a poor prognosis is probable.[95,100]

Cerebrospinal Fluid Drainage

Intracranial hypertension may be reduced by a surgical CSF diversion. The long-term effectiveness of this therapeutic alternative depends on the cause of the increased ICP. Cerebral spinal fluid drainage can be cycled in 10-minute intervals when an external ventricular drain is present.[100] When brain edema produces elevation of ICP, CSF drainage may provide only transient abatement of intracranial hypertension. If external drainage is continued in this circumstance, ventricular collapse can occur and prevent further venting of CSF. Successful chronic control of increased ICP caused by hydrocephalus can be achieved with ventriculoperitoneal shunts.[68,93,100]

Surgical Decompression

Surgical decompression may be used for uncontrollable increases in ICP. Internal decompression involves the excision of brain tissue, reduction in ICP, and reduction of the potential for brainstem displacement or herniation. External decompression involves excision of the skull overlying the site of either an epidural or a subdural hematoma. Decompressive surgery is generally considered to be a last resort in patients with persistent, intractable increases in ICP.[54]

Hypothermia

Hypothermia may help to decrease ICP by decreasing $CMRO_2$ by 7% for each degree centigrade decrease in core body temperature. Temperature is lowered by convective cooling to a bladder temperature of 35°C to 36°C for 48 hours after trauma or hemorrhage. There has been considerable interest in the use of hypothermia in the management of severe TBI. However, despite promising experimental evidence, results from clinical studies have failed to demonstrate benefit. Currently, hypothermia still has a role in the management of intractable intracranial hypertension. Nevertheless, optimizing therapeutic time frames and better management of strategies for complications are required if experimental evidence for neuroprotection is to be translated into clinical benefit.[101]

Pharmacologic Manipulation of Intracranial Pressure

Diuretics

Loop diuretics (furosemide, bumetanide, ethacrynic acid) produce a general diuresis, decrease the rate of CSF production, and decrease cerebral edema. Osmotic diuretics are effective to decrease the water content of the brain. Mannitol is the most widely used osmotic diuretic for acute control of intracranial hypertension. Rapid administration of mannitol (0.25–1 g/kg) may produce vasodilation, increases in CBF, a transient rise in ICP, and a transient increase in circulating blood volume. Increases in circulating blood volume may prove to be detrimental to patients with underlying cardiac dysfunction. Prior administration of intravenous furosemide may minimize these potential complications. Decreases in ICP begin shortly after mannitol administration and may continue for up to 6 hours. Continued use of mannitol may produce hyperosmolality and electrolyte imbalance, which may be attenuated with concurrent administration of a loop diuretic.[102]

Hypertonic saline (either 3% or 23.4%) has an osmotic effect on the brain because of its high tonicity and ability to effectively remain outside the BBB. Like mannitol, hypertonic saline produces an osmolar gradient causing shrinkage of brain tissue and reduction in ICP. It also increases circulating blood volume, MAP, and CPP. The ICP reduction is seen for approximately 2 hours and may be maintained for longer periods by using a continuous infusion of hypertonic saline. The ICP reduction is thought to be caused by a decrease in water content in areas of the brain with intact BBB, such as the nonlesioned hemisphere and cerebellum. Most comparisons with mannitol suggest almost equal efficacy in reducing ICP, but there is a suggestion that mannitol may have a longer duration of action. Results from studies directly comparing hypertonic saline with standard treatment in regard to safety and efficacy are inconclusive. However, the low frequency of side effects and a definite reduction of ICP observed with use of hypertonic saline in these studies are very promising. Systemic effects include transient volume expansion, natriuresis, hemodilution, immunomodulation, and improved pulmonary gas exchange. Adverse effects include electrolyte abnormalities, cardiac failure, bleeding diathesis, and phlebitis.[103] Caution must be exhibited when administering hypertonic saline, as a rapid rise in serum sodium concentration (>9 mEq/L in 24 hours) can lead to an osmotic demyelination syndrome, also known as central pontine myelinolysis.[104] Prior to hypertonic administration, the serum sodium should be evaluated and confirmed less than 155 mEq/L since the target serum sodium levels are between 145 and 155 mEq/L.[103]

Corticosteroids

Glucocorticoids penetrate the BBB and decrease edema associated with mass lesions. Steroids have been in use for neurosurgical patients for decades. They are commonly used for primary and metastatic brain tumors to decrease vasogenic cerebral edema. Classical indications, such as perifocal edema surrounding intracranial tumors or edema associated with cerebral abscess, are other indications. Increased ICP decreases over 2 to 5 days with treatment. The most commonly used regimen is intravenous dexamethasone, 4 mg every 6 hours. Steroids may also be given in spinal cord trauma. Based on the Corticosteroid Randomization After Significant Head injury (CRASH) trial results, which showed that steroids were harmful in patients who sustained a TBI.[105]

Barbiturates

Barbiturate coma, hypothermia, or decompressive craniectomy should be considered for intracranial hypertension refractory to initial medical management. Barbiturate coma is used to reduce refractory ICP by decreasing $CMRO_2$ scavenging free radicals, preventing convulsions, and reducing the hyperthermic response to ischemia. Barbiturates induce hypotension, which at times may be very difficult to treat.[106] Volume expansion should be the first-line treatment to maintain SBP, although intravenous vasopressors may be used. The cerebral metabolic rate cannot be lowered further after burst suppression is achieved by barbiturates; theoretically, ICP will be at its lowest barbiturate-induced level when burst suppression is achieved.[107] Patients may be kept in burst suppression–induced barbiturate coma for hours to days. Although routine use of barbiturates has not been effective in reducing morbidity or mortality after severe head injury, beneficial reductions in ICP are produced. A disadvantage is the inability to perform neurologic assessments during the coma.[108]

NEUROPHYSIOLOGIC MONITORING

Neurophysiologic monitoring is discussed in detail in Chapter 19. It is important to confer with the surgeon to determine which neurophysiologic monitoring is to be used so that a comprehensive plan of care that accounts for the anesthetic considerations related to various neuromonitoring techniques can be employed.

Intraoperative monitoring (IOM) is used routinely to assess the nervous system during procedures that present significant risk of brain, spinal cord, or nerve injury. Intraoperative testing is used to identify nerves and to define brain regions and structures for resection. There is significant improvement in patient outcomes associated with neuromonitoring. The Therapeutics and Technology Subcommittee of the

---

> **BOX 31.4   Clinical Conditions Monitored During Surgery**
>
> - Epilepsy surgery
> - Cerebral tumor and vascular malformation resection
> - Intracranial aneurysm clipping
> - Movement disorders electrode placement
> - Mapping nerves, tracts, and nuclei during brainstem and cranial base surgery
> - Ear and parotid surgery near facial nerve
> - Thyroid and aortic arch surgery near laryngeal nerve
> - Carotid endarterectomy
> - Carotid balloon occlusion
> - Endovascular spinal and cerebral procedures
> - Spinal deformity correction
> - Spinal fracture stabilization
> - Spinal tumor resection
> - Cervical myelopathy decompression and fusion
> - Cervical radiculopathy decompression and fusion
> - Lumbar stenosis decompression and fusion
> - Tethered cord and cauda equina procedures
> - Dorsal root entry zone surgery
> - Brachial and lumbosacral plexus surgery
> - Peripheral nerve surgery
> - Cardiac and aortic procedures

Adapted from Nuwer MR. Clinical neurophysiology: intraoperative monitoring. In Daroff et al., eds. *Bradley's Neurology in Clinical Practice.* 7th ed. London: Elsevier; 2016:410.

American Academy of Neurology concluded that the following are useful and noninvestigational: (1) EEG, compressed spectral array, and somatosensory-evoked potentials (SSEPs) in carotid endarterectomies and brain surgeries that potentially compromise CBF; (2) brainstem auditory-evoked response and cranial-nerve monitoring in surgeries performed in the region of the brainstem or inner ear; and (3) somatosensory-evoked monitoring performed for surgical procedures potentially involving ischemia or mechanical trauma of the spinal cord.[109] MEP monitoring is commonly used during spine surgery and has a good correlation to postoperative motor outcome. The novel technique of MEP monitoring using transcranial electrical stimulation allows reliable assessment of the functional integrity of the corticospinal and corticobulbar tracts while the patient is under general anesthesia.[110]

Surgical procedures that commonly use intraoperative monitoring are shown in Box 31.4. Intracranial posterior fossa cases commonly use brain auditory-evoked potentials (BAEPs), SSEPs, and cranial nerve electromyography (EMG) monitoring. Typical applications are cerebellopontine angle and skull base tumor resection, brainstem vascular malformation and tumor resection, and microvascular decompressions. Intracranial supratentorial procedures include resections for epilepsy, tumors, and vascular malformations, as well as for aneurysm clipping. These use multimodality monitoring with a combination of EEG and SSEP monitoring together with functional cortical localization with direct cortical stimulation and electrocorticography (ECoG). Surgery of the carotid, aorta, or heart may use EEG to monitor hemispheric function or assess the need for shunting or adequacy of protective hypothermia. SSEPs are also used for these vascular cases.

Spinal surgery is the most common setting for IOM. Procedures include cervical discectomy and fusion for myelopathy, stabilization for deformities such as scoliosis, resection of spinal column or cord tumors, and stabilization of fractures. Both sensory-evoked potential

(SEP) and MEP are often used to assess the posterior columns and corticospinal tract functions. The use of MEP depends on the case because it usually requires total intravenous anesthetic and incurs some movements during surgery. As a result, some spinal cases are still carried out with SEP alone. In cases involving pedicle screw placement, EMG is monitored to detect screw misplacement. Spinal cord monitoring is also used for cardiothoracic procedures of the aorta that jeopardize spinal perfusion. Peripheral nerve monitoring is carried out for cases risking injury to the nerves, plexus, or roots. Testing can also determine which segments of a nerve are damaged when performing a nerve graft.

When SSEP monitoring is used for spinal cord surgery, the risk of paraplegia was 60% less among the monitored cases when compared with historical and contemporaneous controls. This information translates to 1 of every 200 patients that did not have paraplegia when monitoring was used. Multimodal monitoring combining SSEPs with MEPs and others is now standard for many spinal procedures. The expectation is that the rate of postoperative neurologic deficits will be reduced even further.[111]

Electroencephalography

The EEG recorded from the scalp is a summation of the excitatory and inhibitory postsynaptic potentials produced in the pyramidal layer of the cerebral cortex. EEG activity requires approximately 50% of the total oxygen consumed by the brain; the remaining 50% is needed to maintain cellular integrity. When oxygen delivery is compromised, slowing of EEG activity ensues.

Changes in EEG frequency and amplitude may be caused by administration of anesthetic drugs and changes in anesthetic depth. Low doses of potent inhalation agents with N_2O produce an active EEG. Steady-state anesthesia, regardless of the agent used, usually produces a stable EEG pattern. It is worth noting that deep levels of anesthesia and cerebral ischemia produce similar EEG changes. In both cases, fast activity is replaced by slower, larger EEG waveforms. Boluses of anesthetic drugs may produce large EEG changes indistinguishable from those seen during ischemia. The EEG provides information about the overall electrical functioning of the cerebral cortex but not much about the subcortical brain, spinal cord, or cranial and peripheral nerves.[111]

Somatosensory-Evoked Potentials

An evoked potential differs from the EEG in two main ways: (1) The EEG is a random, continuous signal that arises from the ongoing activity of the outer layers of the cortex, and an evoked potential is the brain's response to a repetitive stimulus along a specific nerve pathway, and (2) EEG signals range from 10 to 200 mV. Evoked potentials are smaller in amplitude (1, 5, 20 mV), requiring precise electrode positioning and special techniques (signal averaging) to extract the specific response from the underlying EEG "noise." The technique of signal averaging has been further developed in computer processing. The technique now used applies a stimulus repeatedly—preferably at randomized intervals—and records the evoked response over the corresponding area of the brain, averaging out mathematically the change over the number of stimuli.[112] SSEP can be used for detecting localized injury to specific areas of the neural axis by assessing cortically generated waves, or it can serve as a nonspecific indicator of the adequacy of cerebral oxygen delivery.[111]

Volatile anesthetics alter the generation and transmission of SSEP. Suppression of muscle artifact by neuromuscular blocking drugs and the ability to use much higher stimulus intensity in the anesthetized patient allow rapid production of waves that are reproducible, although they differ from those found in the awake patient. Early components of SSEP are generally resistant to anesthetic depression. Etomidate and ketamine both increase the amplitude of scalp-recorded waves by 200% to 600%. Volatile

anesthetics and N_2O depress the SSEP waveform in a dose-dependent manner. Avoiding abrupt changes in inhaled gas concentration and bolus injection of hypnotic drugs during periods of risk minimizes difficulties in determining whether waveform changes are due to surgical manipulation.[113] Furthermore, a concentration of less than 1 MAC of volatile anesthetics is recommended when monitoring SSEPs.[111,113] The effects of anesthetics on SSEP and MEP are shown in Chapter 8, Table 8.4.

Hypothermia increases SSEP latency. Latency increases approximately 3 ms with every decrease in temperature of 2°C to 3°C. This amount of change is suggestive of neural injury. Hyperthermia suppresses SSEP amplitude, with the amplitude being only 15% of that at normothermia.[113-116]

Reproducible, very short latency waves of the trigeminal system are produced by stimulation of the lip at 2 to 4 Hz (512 stimuli). This modality of evoked potential is abnormal in patients with posterior fossa masses in the region of cranial nerve V or in symptomatic hydrocephalus.[117] This modality of evoked potential monitoring may be useful in patients with large posterior fossa tumors that cause severe cranial nerve VIII dysfunction and make brainstem auditory-evoked response (BAER) monitoring impossible.[113]

BAER assesses only brainstem function, although long-latency cortical waves can be assessed to evaluate cortical function. BAER has been used extensively in patients at risk of brain injury during intracranial surgery, despite the extremely small amount of neural tissue assessed and the resistance of BAER to oxygen deprivation when compared with other neural monitors such as the EEG or SSEP waves.[113,118]

Compared with SSEPs, intraoperative factors other than surgical brain damage are relatively unlikely to alter the BAER. BAER waveforms are resistant to both intravenous and inhalational drugs.[113] Fentanyl in large doses does not alter BAER.[113,119] Propofol (2 mg/kg, followed by an infusion) increases the latency of waves I, III, and V without a change in the amplitude, but it completely suppresses middle-latency auditory waves.[113,120] N_2O produces a linear decrease in BAER amplitude from 10% to 40%[113,121]; N_2O at doses of 33% reduces the wave amplitude without altering latency.[113,122,123]

BAER waves are easily identifiable at more frequently used levels of hypothermia (29°C), although latencies are delayed by approximately 33%.[124] BAER latency is inversely related to temperature over the range of 36°C to 42°C, with a decrease in amplitude as temperature increases.[113,125]

BAER appears to be a sensitive monitor to the auditory apparatus in response to direct injury.[113] The auditory apparatus includes the cochlear hair cells, spiral ganglion, eighth cranial nerve, cochlear nuclei, superior olivary complex, lateral lemnisci, inferior colliculus, and medial geniculate thalamic nuclei.[111] Some have recommended BAER monitoring be undertaken in all patients at risk of brainstem injury, even if the primary disease causes hearing loss on the affected side.[113] BAER is also considered clinically useful for microvascular decompression procedures and acoustic tumor surgery.[111]

Aggressive intraoperative monitoring does not guarantee prevention of neurologic injury because all parts of the brain are not assessed using currently available monitoring.[113] Except when the entire brainstem is at risk, there will likely be a high incidence of cases in which BAERs are unaffected intraoperatively, yet significant impairment in motor function or consciousness occurs postoperatively.[111]

EMG monitoring is frequently used for facial nerve monitoring. Generally, two types of EMG activity are monitored. The first involves active stimulation of the nerve for localization, and the second involves spontaneous EMG activity initiated by irritation or manipulation of the nerve. It has been noted that in the presence of light anesthesia, spontaneous EMG activity caused by slight movements may become apparent and mimic neuronal irritation.[111]

TABLE 31.5 Recommended Monitoring Modalities and Anesthetic Regimens for Surgical Procedures

Type of Procedure	Somatosensory-Evoked Potentials	Transcranial Motor-Evoked Potentials	ELECTROMYOGRAPHY Free Run	Stimulated	Auditory Brainstem Responses	Volatile (Inhalational Anesthetics)	Total Intravenous Anesthesia
Spine Skeletal							
Cervical	•	•	•				•
Thoracic	•	•	•	•			•
Lumbar instrumentation	•		•	•		•	
Lumbar disc			•	•		•	
Head and Neck							
Parotid			•	•		•	
Radical neck			•	•		•	
Thyroid			•	•		•	
Cochlear implant			•	•		•	
Mastoid			•	•		•	
Neurosurgery							
Spine							
Vascular	•	•					•
Tumor	•	•					•
Posterior Fossa							
Acoustic neuroma			•	•	•	•	
Cerebellopontine	•	±	•	•	±		•
Vascular	•	•	•		±		•
Supratentorial							
Middle cerebral artery aneurysm		•					•
Tumor in motor cortex	•	•					•

• Recommended for most surgeries; ± recommended for some procedures (depending on specific location of pathology).
Adapted from Jameson LC, et al. Monitoring of the brain and spinal cord. *Anesthesiol Clin.* 2006;24:777.

The effects of muscle relaxants on EMG monitoring have not been adequately studied.[111,113] Chronically injured facial nerves may show greater sensitivity to the effects of neuromuscular blockade, suggesting lower levels of neuromuscular blockade should be used.[126] Some anesthetists do not paralyze patients during the time EMG monitoring is used. Facial nerve monitoring is considered the standard of care for acoustic tumor surgery and during other surgery that risks facial nerve function.[111]

The motor component of cranial nerves III, IV, X, XI, and XII can be monitored using EMG.[111,127,128] Recent interest in skull-base surgery has spurred EMG monitoring for lower cranial nerve preservation. The predictive value of standard neurophysiologic parameters for functional outcome, however, is limited.[129]

There is great interest in intraoperative use of MEPs because of the theoretic limitations of SSEPs in monitoring motor function.[111] MEPs assess function of the motor cortex and descending tracts. The peripheral response of the MEP is recorded by measuring the compound muscle action potential.[113] The motor cortex is stimulated by electrical or magnetic stimulation. Both volatile anesthetics and neuromuscular blocking drugs suppress these responses.[113,130,131]

Evoked potentials are affected by various anesthetics. Neuromuscular blockade resulting in a 70% or less reduction in the height of the response to ulnar nerve stimulation is compatible with MEP monitoring.[111,132] If N_2O is used, it is recommended it be kept to less than 50% or avoided if monitoring MEPs. MEPs are very sensitive to the effects of volatile anesthetics and should be avoided when this type of neuromonitoring is being utilized.[133,134] Total intravenous anesthesia using an infusion of propofol in combination with a narcotic allows for stable MEP recordings. Total intravenous anesthesia with ketamine has also been recognized as being compatible with stable MEP readings.[111,135] Recommended monitoring modalities and anesthetic techniques for various surgical procedures are shown in Table 31.5.

ANESTHETIC CONSIDERATIONS FOR SPECIFIC PROCEDURES

Supratentorial Surgery

Intracranial masses may be congenital, neoplastic (benign, malignant, or metastatic), infectious (abscess or cyst), or vascular (hematoma or malformation). Most, but not all, anesthetics can be used safely in patients with cerebral lesions. Important considerations are the effects of the anesthetic agents on ICP, CPP, CBF, $CMRO_2$, promptness of return of consciousness, drug-related protection from cerebral ischemia or edema, blood pressure control, and compatibility with neurophysiologic monitoring techniques.[136]

Most craniotomies performed within the United States today include the use of propofol for induction of anesthesia with intubation of the trachea after administration of a nondepolarizing relaxant. Maintaining anesthesia is commonly accomplished with a volatile agent and a narcotic, such as fentanyl, sufentanil, alfentanil, or remifentanil.[136]

Preoperative Evaluation

The clinical signs of a supratentorial mass include seizures, hemiplegia, and aphasia. The clinical signs of infratentorial masses include cerebellar dysfunction (ataxia, nystagmus, dysarthria) and brainstem compression (cranial nerve palsies, altered consciousness, abnormal respiration). When ICP increases, frank signs of intracranial hypertension also can develop.[98]

Preanesthetic evaluation should attempt to establish the presence or absence of intracranial hypertension. CT or magnetic resonance imaging (MRI) data should be reviewed for evidence of brain edema, midline shift greater than 0.5 cm, and ventricular size. A neurologic assessment should evaluate the current mental status and any existing deficits. Anticonvulsant therapy and medications prescribed for control of ICP (corticosteroids, diuretics) should be reviewed. Laboratory evaluation should rule out corticosteroid-induced hyperglycemia and electrolyte disturbances that may develop secondary to diuretic therapy. For anticonvulsants, amount, time of last dose, and blood levels should be noted.

The decision regarding the amount and timing of the premedication should be made only after a thorough patient evaluation. Benzodiazepines produce respiratory depression and hypercapnia. Premedication should be omitted in patients with a large mass lesion, a midline shift, and abnormal ventricular size. If premedication is desired careful titration of intravenous midazolam may begin once the patient has been delivered to the preoperative holding area. In an attempt to help control ICP in patients with mass lesions, the head of the bed should be elevated 15 to 30 degrees during transport to the preoperative holding area and the operating room. The anesthetist must be aware of existing hospital recommendations for prophylactic antibiotics to ensure proper timing and dosage.

Intraoperative Monitoring

Routine monitors for supratentorial procedures include continuous electrocardiography (ECG), cuff measurement of blood pressure, precordial stethoscope, monitoring of the fraction of inspired oxygen, pulse oximetry, temperature, peripheral nerve stimulation, $ETco_2$ monitoring, and indwelling urinary catheterization. For patients with ischemic heart disease, use of a modified V_5 ECG lead is recommended. An arterial line placed either before or immediately after anesthetic induction provides for uninterrupted blood pressure monitoring and easy access for blood sampling for laboratory analysis. SSEPs may be assessed. Methods for cerebral oxygenation monitoring are listed in Table 31.6.[137-139]

Fluid Management

Tissues within the CNS are subject to water movement governed by the BBB. The pore size in the BBB is only one-tenth that of the periphery, at 0.7 to 0.9 nm.[140] There is a fundamental difference between capillaries within the CNS and the peripheral capillaries. The BBB remains impermeable to both ions and proteins. The number of ions represents

TABLE 31.6 Cerebral Oxygenation Monitoring

Monitor	Abbreviations	Comments
Jugular bulb oximetry	$Sjvo_2$	Invasive; monitors global not focal ischemia and hypoxia; <50% desaturation suggests inadequate delivery or excessive consumption; >75% suggests hyperemia or stroke
Transcranial Doppler monitoring	rso_2	Noninvasive; monitors flow within the circle of Willis; temporal bone thickness may prevent monitoring; ratio >3 may be indicative of vasospasm; ratio <3 suggests hyperemia
Brain tissue oxygen tension	Pbo_2	Invasive; reserved for global head injuries; simultaneously estimates tissue oxygen tension and ICP; normal values 20–45 mm Hg; pathologic reading <15 mm Hg
Near infrared spectroscopy	NIRS	Noninvasive; estimates brain tissue saturation; concerns with reliability and specificity; may be best used as a trend monitor for flow

ICP, Intracranial pressure.
Adapted from Miller RD, et al., eds. *Miller's Anesthesia.* 9th ed. Philadelphia: Churchill Livingstone; 2020.

a greater magnitude in determining the net movement of water than the number of plasma proteins. There can be little doubt that osmolarity is the primary determinant of water movement across the intact BBB.[141,142]

Preoperative fluid deficits and intraoperative blood and fluid losses must be adequately replaced during neurosurgical procedures. Judicious fluid administration minimizes the occurrence of cerebral edema and increased ICP, reduced CPP, and worsened cerebral ischemia. In most neurosurgical patients, fluids that contain sodium in a concentration similar to that of serum (e.g., lactated Ringer solution or 0.9% saline) are administered in a volume sufficient for maintaining peripheral perfusion but avoiding hypervolemia (0.5–1 mL/kg/hr). Traditionally, less fluid was given than would be administered for nonneurologic surgery, although current recommendations indicate that patients should be kept isovolemic, isotonic, and isooncotic.[143-146] Glucose-containing or hypoosmolar solutions such as lactated Ringer solution should be avoided. The use of isoosmolar crystalloids is widely accepted and can be justified on a scientific basis.[142,147,148]

Hyperglycemia induces marked detrimental cerebrovascular changes during both ischemia and reperfusion.[149] An essential component in the overall management of acute brain injury, especially during the acute phase, is maintaining adequate and appropriate control of serum glucose. Intensive insulin therapy is associated with unacceptable rates of hypoglycemia and metabolic crisis and does not necessarily provide benefit. Hyperglycemia is harmful to the injured brain as it compromises microcirculatory blood flow, increases BBB permeability, and promotes inflammation. In addition, it triggers osmotic diuresis, hypovolemia, and immunosuppression.[150]

Multiple studies have demonstrated that hyperglycemia before and during an episode of global cerebral ischemia will exacerbate the neurologic injury. Hyperglycemia-enhanced ischemic injury is due to several factors, including a rise in lactate production and concomitant tissue acidosis.[151-153] Another theory suggests that hyperglycemia enhances ischemic injury by attenuating an increase in adenosine.[151,154,155] Yet another theory suggests that hyperglycemia significantly worsens the degree of acute BBB disruption that occurs during ischemia.[151,156] It is also thought that hyperglycemia is associated with a significantly reduced CBF and increased heterogeneity of regional CBF during the postischemic period.[151,157-160]

Fluid therapy is most challenging during prolonged surgical procedures or in the surgical management of multiple traumatic injuries. If tissue trauma is severe or if hemorrhage has been prolonged, patients develop a marked reduction in functional extracellular volume as a result of the internal redistribution of fluids (third-space losses). Although the extent of tissue manipulation in most routine neurosurgical procedures is small, third-space fluid losses during prolonged surgery and in patients with severe associated systemic trauma can be sufficient to decrease intravascular volume, reduce peripheral perfusion, and impair renal function. The sequestered extracellular fluid can be cautiously replaced with 0.9% saline. In the absence of diuretic therapy, a urinary output of 0.5 to 1 mL/kg/hour suggests adequate replacement, as do hemodynamic stability and cardiac filling pressures within the normal range. It is recommended that the hematocrit be kept above 28%.[136]

Anesthetic Induction and Maintenance

Although induction of anesthesia for patients undergoing craniotomy can be performed with various agents, a smooth and gentle induction of general anesthesia is more important than the drug combination used. No evidence indicates that one technique or set of drugs is better than another. A reasonable induction sequence would combine preoxygenation, propofol (1–2 mg/kg), and a nondepolarizing muscle relaxant. No evidence suggests that any of the induction agents is superior. The hemodynamic response to intubation may be blunted with the administration of fentanyl administered 3 minutes before laryngoscopy. Whatever agents are selected, the induction should be accomplished without the development of sudden and profound hypertension or hypotension.

The head is typically elevated from 15 to 30 degrees to facilitate venous and CSF drainage. The head may also be turned to the side to facilitate exposure. Excessive neck flexion may impede jugular venous drainage and increase ICP. Because of the flexion-extension-rotation of the head in combination with head fixation in a pinion headrest, the use of an armored or reinforced endotracheal tube (ETT) is recommended to avoid kinking of the tube once positioning is accomplished. The ETT follows the position of the chin. With extension of the neck, the chin and ETT move cephalad; with neck flexion, the chin and ETT move caudad. The anesthesia circuit connections must be firmly secured by simultaneously pushing and twisting to seat the plastic connectors. The risk of unrecognized disconnections may be increased because the operating table is usually turned 90 to 180 degrees away from the anesthetist, and both the patient and the breathing circuit are almost completely covered by surgical drapes.[98]

Maintenance of anesthesia may be accomplished with an oxygen-air-opioid technique, a selected potent inhalation agent, or oxygen-air and a continuous infusion of propofol. After endotracheal intubation, mechanical hyperventilation may be considered based on a discussion with the operating neurosurgeon to an $ETCO_2$ of 30 to 35 mm Hg. A baseline arterial blood gas analysis should be obtained. The patient should also be covered with blankets or a forced-air warming blanket to maintain core body temperature.

An opioid-based anesthetic technique with air in oxygen and a volatile anesthetic is a popular choice. Incremental administration of fentanyl, sufentanil, alfentanil, or an infusion of remifentanil is acceptable.

Sufentanil as a 0.5- to 1-mcg/kg loading dose, followed by either incremental boluses (not to exceed 0.5 mcg/kg/hr) or an intravenous infusion of 0.25 to 0.5 mcg/kg/hour, may be used. Sufentanil administration should be discontinued early to ensure that the patient awakens promptly. The primary advantage of remifentanil is rapid awakening. If the patient experiences hypertension or tachycardia near the end of surgery, the practitioner should consider giving either labetalol or esmolol, instead of additional opioids.[161]

A volatile agent (isoflurane, desflurane, or sevoflurane) can also be used for maintenance of anesthesia. If isoflurane is used, the concentration should remain less than 0.1%.[161] A 2016 study suggests that a Canadian Cardiovascular Society (CCS) score = 10, Mini-Mental Status Exam = 30, and GCS = 15 may be more quickly achieved postoperatively after providing a sevoflurane-based anesthetic versus propofol for maintenance during supratentorial tumor resection.[162]

N_2O may be used in an anesthetic regimen if it is deemed desirable. However, if the patient is suspected to have a pneumocephalus or if the potential for air embolism exists, N_2O use is contraindicated. N_2O expands both the pneumocephalus and the air embolus. A tension pneumocephalus acts as an expanding mass lesion. A large air embolus can cause cardiovascular collapse.[161]

Very mild hyperventilation is an important adjunct to any neuroanesthetic technique. Hypocapnia decreases ICP before opening of the dura and attenuates the vasodilation produced by the volatile anesthetic agents. Optimal hyperventilation during surgery would yield a $PaCO_2$ of 35 to 40 mm Hg. Diuretics, when indicated, may be timed just before or after the cranial vault is opened to facilitate surgical exposure.

Skeletal muscle relaxation prevents patient movement at inappropriate times. It may decrease ICP by relaxing the chest wall, decreasing intrathoracic pressure, and facilitating venous drainage. In choosing an agent for muscle relaxation, the length of the procedure and the effect of the drug on ICP should be considered.[161]

Blood pressure should remain within 10% of preoperative values. A discussion with the operating neurosurgeon should occur with an agreed upon target blood pressure value. Vasopressors may be needed to maintain the agreed-upon blood pressure.[161]

Emergence

Arguably, in no other anesthetic situation is careful attention to appropriate planning for the emergence from anesthesia as important as in neurosurgical brain tumor surgery. Sudden emergence from anesthesia can result in uncontrolled hypertension. Delirium with coughing and straining on the ETT should be avoided. In a patient with a compromised BBB, a hyperexcitable emergence can produce devastating consequences. Late emergence from anesthesia can result in a confusing diagnostic picture with possible intracranial hematoma, acute hydrocephalus, or other diagnoses masked by the residual anesthesia.[92]

A controlled emergence focuses on regulation of blood pressure, ICP, and CBF. Controlled emergence also accounts for the preexisting pathophysiology, the surgical trauma, the length of the procedure, and appropriate management of the airway.[92]

Emergence from anesthesia begins when the surgical pathology has been addressed. Collaboration with the surgeon is essential. Prior to closing the dura, the appropriate levels of postoperative blood pressure can be determined. The $PaCO_2$ should be allowed to return to a normal level. Blood pressure can then be raised to 20% above baseline prior to closing of the dura. Hypertension is considered a frequent occurrence of the postoperative period.[135,163,164] Tachycardia associated with hypertension frequently results from emergence excitement.[165] By raising the blood pressure and the $PaCO_2$ prior to dural closure, the ability of the brain to withstand systemic hypertension can be directly assessed by the surgeon.[92] Once the dura has been closed, the blood pressure is maintained at baseline levels throughout the remainder of the closure.

There is strong support for the notion that sympatholytic drugs should be used to decrease blood pressure during emergence.[166] Studies have shown that during the first hour after craniotomy for supratentorial lesions, the arteriovenous oxygen content difference is low, suggesting a state of cerebral luxury perfusion.[167,168] This event coincides with a high level of mean arterial blood pressure. Accordingly, it is supposed that this correlation is caused by changes in the mean blood pressure and impaired autoregulation. This may be deleterious because it enhances BBB leakage, provoking edema and hemorrhage.

A relationship between hypertension and postoperative hematoma formation exists.[169] The parameters for these events for each individual patient are unknown. Normal autoregulation of CBF maintains adequate perfusion at mean blood pressures ranging from 50 to 150 torr. However, the effectiveness of autoregulation during tumor resection, when combinations of anesthetic agents are used over a prolonged case, and under varying temperatures are unknown.[150,170] Labile hypertension and unstable blood pressure during the perisurgical period may contribute to intracerebral hemorrhage remote from the site of the initial neurosurgical procedure.[171] Given the evidence, and without the need to volume expand and maintain the patient in a hyperdynamic manner, it would seem prudent to institute some form of blood pressure control to provide the most controlled emergence possible.

Judicious titration of short-acting antihypertensives (esmolol, labetalol) has great clinical utility in controlling blood pressure during emergence. When access to the patient is regained, the use of anesthetic gases is discontinued, and the muscle relaxant is reversed. Intravenous lidocaine 1.0–1.5 mg/kg can be given just before suctioning for cough suppression before extubation. Rapid awakening facilitates immediate neurologic assessment and can generally be expected after a pure opioid-N$_2$O technique. Delayed awakening may result from residual opioid or remaining end tidal concentrations of potent inhalation agent. After extubation the patient is transported to the intensive care unit postoperatively for continued monitoring of neurologic function.[166]

Awake Craniotomy

In a small percentage of patients—those in whom a seizure focus may be suppressed during general anesthesia or may be adjacent to an area of eloquent cortical function—awake craniotomy may be necessary.[172] An awake craniotomy may be the most reliable method to ensure neurologic integrity in the presence of cerebral gliomas that infiltrate or come close to the especially sensitive areas of the brain. Awake craniotomy allows for localization of eloquent cortical areas by electrical stimulation and of epileptic foci through cortical recordings. Continuous monitoring of the functional integrity of the brain in awake patients is inherently protective while surgical removal of the gliomatous tissue is performed.[173] Anesthetic techniques may vary depending on whether the procedure is for tumor removal or seizure treatment.

Patient Selection

To minimize the risk of intraoperative complications, contraindications for awake craniotomy include developmental delay, lack of maturity, an exaggerated or unacceptable response to pain, a significant communication barrier, or a failure to obtain patient consent. Only those patients with the ability to clearly understand risks and benefits and who, in the opinion of the neurosurgeon and the anesthesia team, will cooperate during surgery should be considered as candidates for an awake craniotomy.[172] Seizure management should be optimized with acceptable blood levels of antiepileptic medications.

Patient Teaching

The single most important element in a successful awake craniotomy is a highly motivated, well-informed patient. Each step of the procedure is discussed with the patient and family. Special emphasis is paid to prolonged surgical procedure, positioning, head immobility, pain anxiety, monitoring, noise, seizure management, and any individual considerations.

Induction and Maintenance of Anesthesia

Upon arrival to the holding area, an intravenous line is established. Preanesthesia medications are administered; they may include antibiotics, steroids, antiemetic prophylaxis, and anticonvulsants as indicated.

In the operating room suite, application of noninvasive monitoring is completed. Last-minute questions are addressed, and the patient is induced with propofol and a laryngeal mask airway (LMA) is placed. Some sources use either dexmedetomidine singly or in combination with propofol for sedation.[174] Invasive monitoring is established (arterial line, central line, urinary catheter). The scalp is anesthetized with 0.5% bupivacaine and the head placed in a pinion head holder. The patient is carefully positioned with all bony surfaces padded and the patient carefully secured to the table to minimize a sense of falling when the table is moved during the awake phase of the surgery. Frameless stereotaxis registration is accomplished. Depending on the preoperative radiographic edema findings, hypertonic saline or mannitol is given. During draping, an area is constructed around the patient's face such that the face may be clearly seen and accessed. A light is introduced under the surgical drapes to limit darkness. During the scalp opening, spontaneous ventilation is established. Prior to the bone flap removal, the LMA is removed, and the level of anesthesia reduced until verbal communication with the patient is established.

Awake Phase

During the awake phase, all sedation must be discontinued. Any issue regarding patient comfort and concerns is addressed prior to the incision of the dura. Conversation with the patient is confined to the surgeon and one member of the anesthesia team. Stimulation of eloquent areas is carried out with results noted. Any seizures are controlled with propofol or cold saline.[175] Following the stimulation and mapping, volumetric surgical removal of the tumor or seizure focus is accomplished with interval monitoring. Upon completion of the surgical removal and requisite monitoring, intravenous sedation may be restarted and titrated to patient preference. Sedation is discontinued upon conclusion of surgery. The most common complications associated with awake craniotomy are pain, seizures, nausea, and confusion.[176,177]

Posterior Fossa Surgery

Neuropathology within the posterior fossa may impair control of the airway, respiratory function, cardiovascular function, autonomic function, and consciousness. The major motor and sensory pathways, the primary cardiovascular and respiratory centers, the reticular activating system, and the nuclei of the lower cranial nerves are all concentrated in the brainstem. All these structures are contained in a tight space with little room for edema, tumor, or blood.

Venous Air Embolus

In addition to the previously mentioned monitoring modalities, monitoring during posterior fossa surgery requires consideration of patient position and the potential for venous air embolus (VAE). Clinical situations that contribute to the occurrence of VAE are listed in Box 31.5. Air may also be entrained from the cranial pin sites of the Mayfield head holder and from improperly connected vascular lines (arterial, central, and intravenous).

BOX 31.5　Clinical Situations Contributing to Venous Air Embolism

- Patient positioning (seated, prone, steep Trendelenburg)
- Transfusion therapy
- Intravenous therapy
- Central venous catheterization
- Hepatic surgical procedures
- Urologic surgical procedures
- Posterior spinal procedures
- Epidural or caudal catheter insertion
- Bone marrow harvesting
- Laparoscopy
- Radical pelvic surgery
- Obstetric gynecologic procedures
- Thoracic procedures
- Orthopedic procedures
- Cardiac surgery
- Head and neck surgery

The occurrence of VAE depends on the development of a negative pressure gradient between the operative site and the right side of the heart. As the gradient between the cerebral veins and the right atrium increases, the potential for air entry increases. The estimated incidence of VAE during neurosurgical procedures ranges from 5% to 50%, with an increased incidence in the sitting position.[178,179] A 39% rate of VAE for posterior fossa surgery and 12% for cervical procedures has been reported.[180]

As the venous pressure at wound level may be negative, air can be entrained. This air may follow any of four pathways. Most commonly, it passes through the right heart and into the pulmonary circulation, diffuses through the alveolar-capillary membrane, and appears in expelled gas. It may also pass through a pulmonary shunt, such as a patent foramen ovale (paradoxic air embolism [PAE]). It may collect at the superior vena cava–right atrial junction. Lastly, rarely, it may traverse through lung capillaries into the systemic circulation.[181,182] Air that reaches the arterial circulation is generally associated with poor outcomes.

The physiologic consequences associated with VAE depend on both the volume and the rate of air entrainment. In the canine model, large cumulative doses of air produce sudden cardiac arrest and death; smaller cumulative doses produce less profound physiologic consequences, including increased pulmonary artery and central venous pressure, decreased cardiac output with accompanying hypotension, progressive hypotension, and dysrhythmias.[183] Despite the potentially devastating effects of VAE, a retrospective review of neurosurgery patients who had appropriate monitoring for the detection of VAE found that VAE contributed to patient morbidity or mortality in only six instances (0.4%).[184-186]

Paradoxic Air Embolism

Paradoxical air embolism develops with the entry of air into the arterial circulation. Individuals with an existing anatomic connection between the right and left sides of the heart (i.e., atrial or ventricular septal defect, probe-patent foramen ovale) are at risk. Arterial air embolism is life threatening and requires immediate identification and early management. A patent foramen ovale may exist in 30% to 35% of the population.[187] If right-sided heart pressures exceed left-sided pressures (a situation that may occur in fluid-restricted neurosurgical patients), systemic air may embolize and enter the arterial circulation through a probe-patent foramen ovale.

Patients who are placed in the sitting position should be carefully evaluated with echocardiograms if the history suggests the presence of an intracardiac defect (presence of heart murmur) or probe-patent foramen ovale. The presence of a probe-patent foramen ovale may be elicited with the injection of contrast material before, during, and after the patient produces a Valsalva maneuver. If the condition is identified, the surgical procedure should be accomplished in an alternative position.[188]

Detection of Venous Air Embolus

The entrainment of small amounts of air into the vascular system is usually of little consequence because the lungs serve as effective blood filters.[189] Small amounts of air are absorbed into the blood or enter the alveoli, where they are eliminated. However, the efficient filtering capacity of the lung may be breached by a large bolus of air. A reflexive sympathetic pulmonary vasoconstriction is produced after the release of endothelial mediators, which are ultimately responsible for the clinical manifestations (i.e., pulmonary hypertension, hypoxemia, CO_2 retention, increased dead space ventilation, and decreased $ETco_2$). The continued entry of air produces an airlock within the right ventricle, producing right ventricular failure and decreased cardiac output. Altered ventilation-perfusion relationships parallel the hemodynamic changes. Obstructed pulmonary blood flow increases dead space ventilation, resulting in decreased $ETco_2$. The entry of a large volume of air in the alveoli may be detected by the sudden appearance of end tidal nitrogen (ETN_2). Studies indicate that entrainment of small amounts of air less than 0.5 mL/kg will manifest as a decreased $ETco_2$, increased ETN_2, oxygen desaturation, altered mental status, and wheezing. Moderate amounts of entrapped air, approximately 0.5 to 2.0 mL/kg, will produce difficulty breathing, wheezing, hypotension, ST changes, peaked P waves, jugular venous distention, myocardial and cerebral ischemia, bronchoconstriction, and pulmonary vasoconstriction. Large quantities of air entrainment (>2.0 mL/kg) result in chest pain, right-sided heart failure, and cardiovascular collapse.[190]

The selection of appropriate monitoring for the detection of VAE is based on the various sensitivities of the available monitoring modalities (Table 31.7).[189] The order of sensitivity of the monitoring methods from most sensitive to least is transesophageal echocardiography (TEE) > precordial Doppler > pulmonary artery and $ETco_2$ changes > cardiac output and central venous pressure changes > blood pressure, ECG, and precordial stethoscope detection.

TEE is the most sensitive method of air embolism detection but may not be practical, especially in longer procedures. Precordial Doppler monitoring can detect air entrainment at rates as small as 0.0021 mL/kg/minute.[191] The Doppler probe is affixed over the right side of the heart along the right sternal border between the third and sixth intercostal spaces. Proper positioning over the right atrium is confirmed if a change in Doppler signal is elicited when a 10-mL bolus of saline is injected rapidly into a previously placed right central venous catheter.[191-193] Placement of a right atrial catheter affords the means for diagnosis and recovery of intravenous air and also reflects cardiac preload. When a right atrial catheter is placed, it is recommended that either radiographic confirmation or ECG confirmation of proper placement of the catheter tip be obtained.[193] Advantages and disadvantages of selected monitors for detection of VAE are noted in Table 31.7.

Capnography complements the capabilities of the Doppler device because small, hemodynamically insignificant air emboli detected with the Doppler device can be differentiated from emboli that may produce arterial hypotension. The detection of a "mill-wheel" murmur via precordial or esophageal stethoscope is a late sign of air entrainment. As noted already, TEE is the most sensitive method of air embolism detection, but it is also the most expensive. With TEE, it is possible to observe both cardiac contractility and air bubbles as

TABLE 31.7 Monitors for Detection of Venous Air Embolism

Monitor	Advantages	Disadvantages
Transesophageal echocardiography (TEE)	Most sensitive detector of air Can detect air in left side of heart, aorta	Invasive, cumbersome Expensive Must be observed continuously Not quantitative May interfere with Doppler ultrasonography
Precordial Doppler	Most sensitive *noninvasive* monitor Earliest detector (before air enters pulmonary circulation)	Not quantitative May be difficult to place in obese patients, patients with chest wall deformity, or patients in the prone/lateral positions False-negative result if air does not pass beneath ultrasonic beam (~10% of cases) Useless during electrocautery IV mannitol may mimic intravascular air
Pulmonary artery (PA) catheter	Quantitative, slightly more sensitive than ETco$_2$ Widely available Placed with minimum difficulty in experienced hands Can detect right atrial pressure greater than pulmonary capillary wedge pressure	Small lumen, less air aspirated than with right atrial catheter Placement for optimal air aspiration may not allow pulmonary capillary wedge pressure measurement Nonspecific for air
Capnography (ETco$_2$)	Noninvasive Sensitive Quantitative Widely available	Nonspecific for air Less sensitive than Doppler ultrasound, PA catheter Accuracy affected by tachypnea, low cardiac output, chronic obstructive pulmonary disease

ETco$_2$, End tidal carbon dioxide; *IV*, intravenous.
From Cottrell JE, Patel P, eds. *Cottrell and Patel's Neuroanesthesia*; 6th ed. Edinburgh: Elsevier; 2017:215.

they pass through the heart.[194] TEE is also capable of detecting PAE in the heart.

Treatment of Venous Air Embolus

Early detection and rapid treatment of VAE are important for successful outcomes (Box 31.6). The surgeon should be notified, and N$_2$O should be immediately discontinued, 100% oxygen delivered, anesthesia discontinued, and the right atrial catheter aspirated (if present).[195] The surgeon should flood the surgical field with irrigation or pack the area with saline-soaked sponges. A Valsalva maneuver or bilateral compression of the jugular veins for 5 to 10 seconds increases the cerebral venous pressure. The addition of positive end-expiratory pressure also slows air entry. However, 10 to 15 cm H$_2$O may be required to effectively elevate venous pressure when the head is elevated. The head should be lowered to decrease air entrainment. This may be accomplished by placing the operating table in Trendelenburg position. Finally, additional personnel may be required to perform the various interventions needed for proper management of a VAE.[196,197]

Supportive therapy is required for hemodynamic compromise. Administration of ephedrine, 10 to 20 mg intravenously, and an intravenous fluid bolus may improve cardiac output and blood pressure. If these measures do not restore blood pressure, additional vasopressors (such as epinephrine) may be required.

Anesthetic agents and techniques may influence the rate of air entrainment and the resulting physiologic consequences. Munson and Merrick demonstrated that the expansion of an intravascular air bubble is proportional to the delivered concentration of N$_2$O.[195] A 50% concentration doubles the initial air-bubble volume, and a 70% concentration quadruples the air-bubble volume. General endotracheal anesthesia with controlled ventilation is thought to be protective in patients experiencing VAE.

BOX 31.6 Management of Venous Air Embolus

- Notify surgeon on detection (flood surgical field with saline and wax bone edges).
- Discontinue nitrous oxide administration (if used); administer 100% oxygen.
- Perform a Valsalva maneuver or compression of jugular veins.
- Aspirate air from atrial catheter (if central venous catheter is in place).
- Support blood pressure with IV crystalloid boluses and vasopressors (i.e., epinephrine).
- Reposition patient in left lateral decubitus position with a 15-degree head-down tilt if blood pressure continues to decrease.
- Modify the anesthetic as needed to optimize hemodynamics.
- Discontinue anesthetic agents
- Postoperative follow-up should include ECG, chest x-ray, and arterial blood gases with oxygen as needed.

ECG, Electrocardiogram.

Surgical Positioning

Although many posterior fossa explorations may be performed with the patient in either the lateral or prone position, the sitting position (Fig. 31.18) is occasionally preferred because the enhanced CSF and venous drainage facilitates surgical exposure. The use of this position, however, has declined due to the potential for serious complications.[198,199] The patient is semirecumbent in the standard sitting position with the back elevated to 60 degrees and the legs elevated (with the knees flexed) to the level of the heart. The latter is important for preventing venous pooling and reducing the risk of venous thrombosis. The head is fixed in a three-point head holder with the neck in flexion, and the arms remain at the sides with the hands resting on the lap.[98]

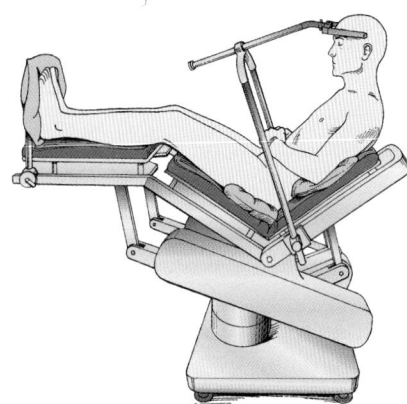

Fig. 31.18 Neurosurgical sitting position for posterior approach. Frame of head holder is attached to side rails of back section of operating room bed. Note that legs are flexed at thighs and are approximately at level of heart. Feet are padded at right angles to legs. Subgluteal padding protects sciatic nerves. (From Phillips N. *Berry and Kohn's Operating Room Technique.* 13th ed. St. Louis: Elsevier; 2017:764.)

Careful positioning is essential to prevent iatrogenic injury. Pressure points such as the elbows, ischial spines, and forehead must be protected with foam padding. Excessive neck flexion has been associated with swelling of the upper airway (venous obstruction) and, rarely, quadriplegia. This results from compression of the cervical spinal cord and decreased cervical cord perfusion when the neck is elevated above the heart. Preexisting cervical spinal stenosis probably predisposes the patient to the latter injury.[98]

Anesthetic Induction, Maintenance, and Emergence

Increased ICP, although common in patients with supratentorial lesions, is less common in patients with posterior fossa lesions. Obstructive hydrocephalus is more typical because CSF outflow is occluded at the level of the aqueduct of Sylvius or fourth ventricle. This can be readily identified preoperatively by MRI or CT and may be corrected before definitive surgical intervention with the placement of a ventricular catheter. Premedication is contraindicated in patients with obstructive hydrocephalus.

Induction should be slow and deliberate to avoid changes in cerebral perfusion and increased ICP. Because the head is generally flexed and fixed in this position, a wire-reinforced ETT may prevent intraoperative kinking. The ETT may become kinked if the patient is lightly anesthetized and bites the tube, thus a soft bit block is commonly used to prevent this potential complication. Intravenous fluid administration during posterior fossa surgery should be limited to the infusion of deficit and maintenance quantities of a balanced salt solution. Major volume resuscitation can be accomplished with the infusion of blood, colloid, or crystalloid solutions.

Emergence from anesthesia should be as smooth and gentle as possible. The intraoperative use of opioids facilitates a smooth emergence without significant coughing and bucking. The administration of lidocaine, 1.5 mg/kg intravenously, may decrease the airway irritation of the ETT.[196]

The decision to remove the ETT should be made after the anesthetic course and surgical procedure are reviewed. Intraoperative air embolism may be followed by the development of pulmonary edema. Although this condition is self-limiting, continued mechanical ventilation is the treatment of choice. Consideration must also be given to the possibility of cranial nerve damage during the operative procedure. Provided the patient is safely extubated, continued vigilant observation is essential because airway compromise may develop after injury to cranial nerves IX, X, and XI (Box 31.7).

BOX 31.7   **Postoperative Considerations for Posterior Fossa Surgery**

- Cranial nerve dysfunction
- Central apnea
- Loss of upper airway control and patency
- Altered level of consciousness
- Altered cardiomotor function
- Cardiac dysrhythmias

Adapted from Miller RD, et al., eds. *Miller's Anesthesia.* 9th ed. Philadelphia: Elsevier Saunders; 2020.

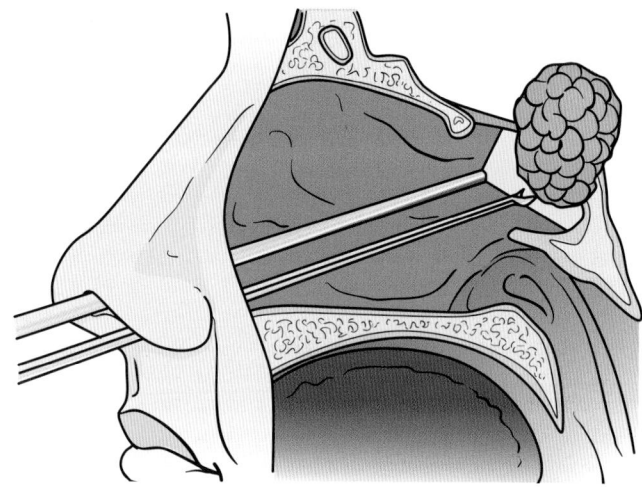

Fig. 31.19 Transnasal hypophysectomy. (From Phillips N. *Berry and Kohn's Operating Room Technique.* 13th ed. St. Louis: Elsevier; 2017:772.)

Pituitary Surgery

Approximately 10% of intracranial neoplasms are found in the pituitary gland and come to clinical attention because of their mass effects or the hypersecretion of pituitary hormones. These tumors are rarely metastatic and produce local symptoms via bone invasion, hydrocephalus, and compression of a cranial nerve (most often the optic nerve). Frontotemporal headache and bitemporal hemianopsia are the most common nonendocrine symptoms of enlarging pituitary lesions. Nonsecreting pituitary tumors account for approximately 20% to 50% of lesions in this area and are classified as chromophobe adenomas.[199,200]

Tumors that secrete excess growth hormone produce acromegaly. Increased growth hormone increases the size of the skeleton, particularly the bones and soft tissues of the hands, feet, and face. The enlarged facial structures may increase the likelihood of difficult intubation. Excess growth hormone may also contribute to the development of coronary artery disease, hypertension, and cardiomyopathy. Hyperglycemia is also a common finding, reflecting a growth hormone–induced glucose intolerance.[201]

Surgical Approach

Medical and surgical therapies exist for both functional and nonfunctional pituitary tumors. Transsphenoidal surgery (Fig. 31.19) offers several advantages over the intracranial approach. Statistically, morbidity and mortality rates are reduced because of a decrease in blood loss and less manipulation of brain tissue. In addition, the risk of inducing panhypopituitarism and the incidence of permanent diabetes insipidus are both reduced. For patients with large tumors (>10 mm), tumors of uncertain type, and tumors that have substantial extrasellar (beyond the sella turcica) extension, the transsphenoidal approach is inadequate, and a bifrontal intracranial approach is required for successful removal.[201] Current trends support the use of endoscopic approaches to pituitary tumor excision. Less invasive approaches, such as the transnasal approach combined with endoscopic resection of tumor, have been performed. The endoscopic technique is associated with less morbidity and a shorter hospital stay than the traditional approach.[202]

Preoperative Evaluation

The most common surgical approach for a hypersecreting pituitary tumor is through the nose using transsphenoidal techniques. Clinical symptoms of pituitary tumors include amenorrhea, galactorrhea, Cushing disease, and acromegaly.

Each preoperative condition has its own collection of systemic disorders and accompanying effects on intracranial dynamics that must be considered when an anesthetic technique is selected. Pituitary tumors can damage decussating optic fibers, producing blindness in the temporal half of the visual field of both eyes (bitemporal heteronymous hemianopsia). Occasionally, an aneurysm of one of the internal carotid arteries may produce nasal hemianopsia on the affected side. Patients who suffer from Cushing disease may have associated hypertension, diabetes, osteoporosis, obesity, and friability of skin and connective tissue. Patients diagnosed with acromegaly may exhibit hypertension, cardiomyopathy, diabetes, and osteoporosis, as well as cartilaginous and soft-tissue hypertrophy of the larynx and enlargement of the tongue, complicating laryngoscopy and intubation of the trachea. Patients who have panhypopituitarism may exhibit hypothyroidism, requiring preoperative thyroid supplementation.

The transsphenoidal approach usually necessitates the head and back be elevated 10 to 20 degrees. The patient's head is supported by a three-point pin head holder (known as a Mayfield head clamp) and centered within a C-arm fluoroscopy unit for radiographic control during surgery. The patient's arms are placed at the sides and padded so that injury to the ulnar nerves is avoided. The patient's airway is difficult to access during the surgical procedure; therefore, specific attention must be directed to securing of the ETT and anesthesia circuit to prevent unintended extubation and anesthesia-circuit disconnect. Hyperventilation is avoided after anesthetic induction because reductions in ICP result in retraction of the pituitary into the sella, making surgical access difficult. The anesthetist should also consider the potential for massive hemorrhage because the carotid arteries lie adjacent to the suprasellar area and may be inadvertently injured.

When the resection involves the suprasellar area, postoperative endocrine dysfunction may occur, namely, diabetes insipidus. Diabetes insipidus that occurs after most transsphenoidal procedures is usually self-limited and resolves within a week to 10 days.[200] Although the onset is usually on the first or second postoperative day, diabetes insipidus may develop during the perioperative period or in the immediate recovery period. Intraoperative diagnosis is made with the sudden onset of diuresis. The diagnosis may be confirmed with concurrent urine and serum osmolalities. If diabetes insipidus persists or if it becomes difficult to match urinary losses, then DDAVP (desmopressin) should be administered. It is available as a nasal solution, as an oral or sublingual tablet, or as a subcutaneous or intravenous solution.[203]

Anesthetic Induction, Maintenance, and Emergence

After anesthetic induction and intubation, the ETT is typically moved to the left corner of the patient's mouth and secured to the chin with adhesive and tape. A right-angled or an oral RAE ETT may be effective because such tubes are prebent and curve along the mandible when exiting the mouth. An esophageal stethoscope and temperature probe

can be inserted and secured on the lower left as well, leaving the upper lip totally exposed. An orogastric tube is placed, aspirated, and then put to gravity drainage during the procedure. The oropharynx is then packed with moist cotton gauze. The eyes are first taped closed and then covered with cotton-padded adhesive patches to prevent corneal abrasion and seepage of cleansing solution and blood into the eyes.

Anesthesia induction is typically provided using propofol, an opioid, and a neuromuscular blocking agent (either succinylcholine or a nondepolarizing neuromuscular blocking agent). Anesthesia maintenance can be provided using an inhalational combination of air and oxygen with a volatile agent (isoflurane, desflurane, or sevoflurane), or as a TIVA using any or a combination of the following: propofol, dexmedetomidine, opioids, and ketamine. Continued neuromuscular blockade will depend on the surgical need to assess for nerve function. The anesthetic plan should be discussed with the surgeon to provide the most effective operating conditions.

The topical use of vasoconstrictors and the oral and nasal submucosal injection of local anesthetic solutions containing epinephrine help constrict gingival and mucosal vessels and dissect the nasal mucosa away from the cartilaginous septum. Epinephrine use may produce hypertension or dysrhythmias or both. The use of epinephrine is relatively safe if (1) ventilation is adequate, (2) epinephrine is given in combination with lidocaine instead of saline, (3) epinephrine concentrations of 1:100,000 to 1:200,000 are used, and (4) total dose does not exceed 10 mL of 1:100,000 solution in 10 minutes for a 70-kg adult. Persistent dysrhythmias may require treatment with an antiarrhythmic drug. Hypertension may be controlled with an increased concentration of the selected inhalation agent or with labetalol or esmolol.[204]

In some cases, it may be necessary to insert a catheter into the lumbar subarachnoid space to facilitate the injection of preservative-free saline to delineate the suprasellar margins or for prevention of CSF leak postoperatively. If air is injected, N_2O must be discontinued from the anesthetic mixture because of rapid diffusion into the air present in the closed cranial vault.[204]

Emergence from anesthesia should be conducted smoothly avoiding a hyperexcitable state and coughing as described for the previously discussed procedures. Intravenous lidocaine, 1.5 mg/kg given approximately 3 minutes before suctioning and extubation, may help to decrease coughing, straining, and hypertension. Postoperatively, patients should be responsive to commands in the recovery room.

Cerebrovascular Surgery

Cerebral Aneurysms

Interventional neuroradiology is the recommended initial treatment for intracranial aneurysms. Aneurysm coiling or occlusion of the proximal arteries and obliteration of the aneurysm sac is the preferred therapy for many lesions.[205] The International Subarachnoid Aneurysm Trial and subsequent studies have shown this approach to have several advantages over craniotomy with clipping although recurrence may be higher. Endovascular treatment of ruptured aneurysms results in quicker recovery and better functional outcomes at 1 year at the expense of lower rates of complete aneurysm obliteration frequently requiring retreatment.[206]

Cerebral aneurysms are abnormal, localized dilations of the intracranial arteries. They are classified as berry (or saccular), mycotic, traumatic, fusiform, neoplastic, or atherosclerotic. Rupture of a saccular aneurysm is a leading cause of SAH.[207]

An estimated 6 million people in the United States have an unruptured brain aneurysm, or 1 in 50 people. The annual rate of rupture is approximately 8 to 10 per 100,000 people; approximately 30,000 people in the United States suffer a brain aneurysm rupture each year. Ruptured brain aneurysms are fatal in approximately 40% of cases. Of those who survive, approximately 66% suffer some permanent neurologic deficit. Brain aneurysms are most prevalent in people ages 35 to 60 but can occur in children as well. Most aneurysms develop after the age of 40, and the median age when aneurysmal hemorrhagic stroke occurs is 50 years old with typically no warning signs. Most aneurysms are small, approximately 0.125 inch to nearly 1 inch, and an estimated 50% to 80% of all aneurysms do not rupture during the course of a person's lifetime. Aneurysms larger than 1 inch are referred to as giant aneurysms and can pose a particularly high risk and be difficult to treat. Women, more than men, suffer from brain aneurysms at a ratio of 3:2.[208]

More than four of seven patients with SAH die or develop significant and lasting neurologic disabilities before they receive any treatment. A small bleed occurs in approximately 50% of patients and is often tragically ignored or misdiagnosed. Even in patients who receive prompt care, only half remain functional survivors; the remainder die or develop serious neurologic deficits.[209]

Aneurysms may arise at any point in the circle of Willis. Most aneurysms are broad based and located in the middle cerebral system. Traumatic aneurysms develop as a result of direct trauma to an artery, with injury to the wall.

Mirror aneurysms of the internal carotid system are common, and other combinations of locations occur. The site of the bleeding aneurysm is best located by CT studies, evidence of vasospasm in the immediate vicinity, and lobulation of the aneurysm wall on angiographic studies.[207]

Diagnosis of Subarachnoid Hemorrhage

Subarachnoid hemorrhage (SAH) produces an abrupt, intense headache in 85% of patients, and transient loss of consciousness may be seen in up to 45% of patients. Nausea and vomiting, photophobia, fever, meningismus, and focal neurologic deficits are not uncommon. The severity of an SAH can be graded clinically with the use of classifications such as Hunt and Hess or the World Federation of

Neurological Surgeons Scale (Table 31.8). Although surgical mortality rates vary somewhat among institutions, patients with a neurologic grade I SAH generally undergo surgical clipping with a low mortality rate (<5%), whereas grade V patients generally do not survive.[209] Unruptured cerebral aneurysms are commonly detected on brain imaging performed for reasons unrelated to the aneurysms.[210] The data on 1-year aneurysm- and procedure-related morbidity and mortality appear to support treatment over watchful waiting, as long as one avoids treating large aneurysms in those greater than 65 years of age with microsurgery.[211]

General Considerations

Hypertension often accompanies acute SAH and is believed to occur secondary to autonomic hyperactivity, which may increase transmural pressure in the aneurysmal sac. Transmural pressure is defined as the differential pressure between MAP and ICP and represents the stress applied to the aneurysm's wall (Figs. 31.20 and 31.21).[209]

Increases in blood pressure directly increase the transmural pressure and the likelihood of bleeding; conversely, reductions in blood pressure reduce transmural pressure and may compromise perfusion. Caution should be exercised when purposefully reducing transmural pressure because cerebral autoregulation may be impaired after SAH, and a reduction in blood pressure may induce or aggravate cerebral ischemia, particularly if vasospasm is present. To balance these opposing factors, many neurosurgeons attempt to maintain systolic blood pressure between 120 and 150 mm Hg before clipping the aneurysm.[205,209]

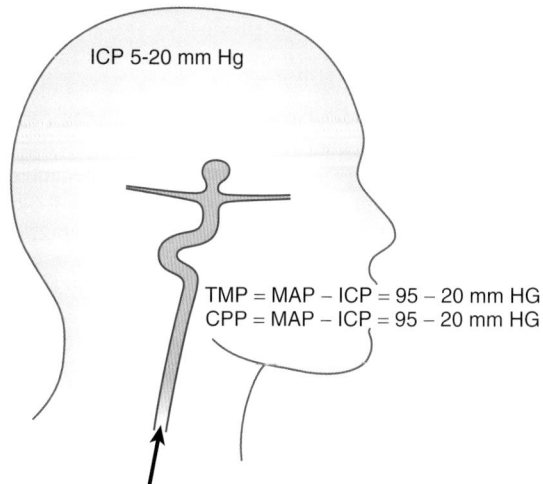

Fig. 31.20 Determinants of transmural pressure *(TMP)* and cerebral perfusion pressure *(CPP)*. Both are determined by the difference between mean arterial pressure *(MAP)* and intracranial pressure *(ICP)* and are, therefore, numerically identical. (From Cottrell JE, Patel P, eds. *Cottrell and Patel's Neuroanesthesia.* 6th ed. Edinburgh: Elsevier; 2017:229.)

TABLE 31.8 **Most Commonly Used Clinical Grading Scales for Subarachnoid Hemorrhage**
Hunt and Hess Scale
Grade 0: Asymptomatic
Grade I: Mild headache and mild nuchal rigidity, no neurologic deficit
Grade II: Moderate to severe headache but no neurologic deficit other than cranial nerve palsy
Grade III: Drowsy, confused, or mild focal deficit
Grade IV: Stupor, moderate to severe hemiparesis, and early decerebrate posturing
Grade V: Deep comatose, decerebrate posturing

World Federation of Neurological Surgeons (WFNS) Scale

	Glasgow Coma Scale	Motor Deficit
Grade I	15	Absent
Grade II	13–14	Absent
Grade III	13–14	Present
Grade IV	7–12	Present or absent
Grade V	3–6	Present or absent

From Daroff RB, et al., eds. *Bradley's Neurology in Clinical Practice.* 7th ed. London: Elsevier; 2016:990.

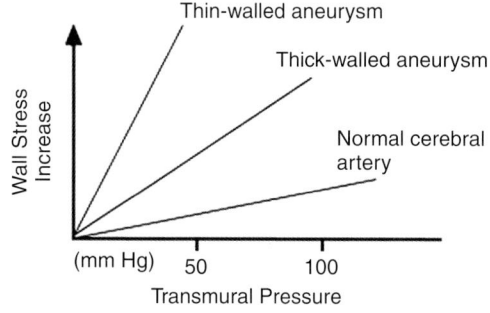

Fig. 31.21 Aneurysm wall stress.

ECG changes are common after SAH, and they have been reported to occur in 50% to 80% of patients. The most common changes involve the T wave or the ST segment, but other changes such as the presence of a U wave, QTc interval (interval corrected for heart rate) prolongation, and dysrhythmias may be present. Whether such changes in the ECG represent myocardial injury has long been debated. In the majority of patients, these changes do not appear to be associated with adverse neurologic or cardiac outcomes.[209,211]

Rebleeding from a previously ruptured aneurysm is a life-threatening complication. The incidence of rebleeding is approximately 50% in the first days after SAH, and rebleeding is associated with an 80% mortality rate.[212] The chance of rebleeding from an unsecured aneurysm declines over time; by 6 months, the risk stabilizes at approximately 3% per year. Approaches used to decrease the risk of rebleeding include early surgical clipping, the use of antifibrinolytic agents, and blood pressure control.[209,213]

Vasospasm

Cerebral artery vasospasm, a delayed and sustained contraction of cerebral arteries, continues to be a leading cause of morbidity and mortality in patients with SAH after aneurysm rupture.[207] Vasospasm is reactive narrowing of cerebral arteries after SAH. Approximately one in four patients who have an SAH will develop vasospasm. Although arterial narrowing may be detected with angiography in 60% of patients, only half of these patients develop clinical symptoms. The accompanying neurologic deterioration, arising from impaired cerebral perfusion, ischemia, and secondary infarction of the brain, peaks between the third and fourteenth day after SAH and resolves over the next 2 to 3 weeks.[213] Vasospasm causes a decrease in blood flow and a resultant lowering of CPP. Medical treatments include oral nimodipine and hypertensive therapy to enhance cerebral oxygenation in the setting of vasoconstriction. Despite maximal medical measures, 15% of patients who initially survive an SAH experience stroke or death secondary to vasospasm. For vasospasm that is refractory to medical management, endovascular therapy has emerged as an alternative or supplementary therapeutic modality. Both balloon angioplasty and intraarterial vasodilator infusion have established roles in the management of medically intractable vasospasm. The optimal method and timing of endovascular treatment, however, remains controversial. Angioplasty is ideally accomplished in patients who have already had the symptomatic aneurysm surgically clipped and for patients in the early course of symptomatic ischemia to prevent hemorrhagic transformation of an ischemia region. A balloon catheter is guided under fluoroscopy into the vasospastic segment and inflated to distend the constricted area mechanically. It is also possible to perform a pharmacologic angioplasty by direct intraarterial infusion. Papaverine is an opium alkaloid and nonspecific smooth muscle relaxant. Papaverine causes vasodilation through cyclic adenosine and guanosine monophosphate phosphodiesterase inhibition and has a half-life of nearly 2 hours. Although papaverine produced clinical improvement in 43% of treated patients, the effect was temporary, and individuals often needed multiple treatment sessions. Concerns regarding the toxicity profile and short effect of papaverine have prompted the off-label use of calcium channel antagonists such as verapamil, nimodipine, and nicardipine in the treatment of cerebral vasospasm.[205,213]

Vasospasm and the ensuing delayed ischemic deficit are thought to result from several factors. Vasospasm is initiated by the release of oxyhemoglobin, one of the blood breakdown products. However, the exact mechanism of cerebral vasospasm after SAH is not completely understood. The mechanism involves multifactorial processes and chemicals such as free radicals, lipid peroxidation, and the release of endothelin-1. Past studies on vasospasm have demonstrated prolonged smooth muscle contraction in affected arteries. Hypertrophy, fibrosis, wall degeneration, and inflammatory changes were also observed.[207,214,215]

Successful treatment of vasospasm depends on maintaining adequate CPP. This is accomplished by expanding intravascular volume (which augments blood pressure and cardiac output), avoiding hyponatremia, and preserving relative hemodilution (hematocrit ~32%).[215] Because of the risk of rebleeding, careful blood pressure control is necessary.

Nimodipine is commonly used to prevent vasospasm after neurologic trauma or hemorrhage. Nimodipine is the only calcium channel blocker shown to reduce morbidity and mortality from vasospasm. Various agents are being tested as a means to prevent or ameliorate vasospasm, including magnesium sulfate, statins, and an endothelin antagonist.[216] Cerebral vasospasm is frequently the cause of poor outcomes after successful surgical or endovascular treatment.

Currently, the most consistently effective regimen to prevent and treat ischemic neurologic deficits due to cerebral vasospasm uses hypervolemia, hypertension, and hemodilution. It is referred to as triple-H therapy. The use of nicardipine, labetalol, and esmolol can help reduce hypertension and avoid aneurysm rupture. An important goal is the prevention of hypotension so as to maintain CPP. Nimodipine is recommended for vasospasm prophylaxis in all patients with an SAH. Erythropoietin has shown to lower the incidence of vasospasm and delayed cerebral ischemia. Albumin is the preferred colloid. Induced hypervolemia and hypertension during SAH improve the impaired autoregulation within ischemic areas of the brain. This concept is important to remember since CBF is dependent on CPP in these situations, and CBF depends on intravascular volume and mean arterial blood pressure. Sufficient intravenous fluids are given to raise the CVP to 10 mm Hg. Hypervolemia is generally achieved with infusions of colloids (e.g., 5% albumin) as well as crystalloids. Hemodilution should be induced to keep the hematocrit between 27% and 30%. Hypertension often results from the fluid loading; however, vasopressors may be required at times to reach a targeted blood pressure. Hypertensive, hypervolemic therapy may induce a vagal response and profound diuresis, requiring administration of large amounts of intravenous fluids. Atropine (1 mg intramuscularly every 3–4 hours) may be given to maintain the heart rate between 80 and 120 beats/minute. Vasopressin (Pitressin), 5 units intramuscularly, may be administered to maintain the urine output at less than 200 mL/hour.

With this regimen, often only small amounts of vasopressor drugs are required. The blood pressure should be manipulated to a level necessary to reverse the signs and symptoms of vasospasm or to a maximum of 160 to 180 mm Hg systolic or a MAP up to 110 mm Hg postclipping. However, the optimal hypertensive therapy for SAH-induced vasospasm is unclear. If the aneurysm has not been clipped, the SBP is increased to only 120 to 150 mm Hg. The elevated blood pressure must be maintained until the vasospasm resolves, usually within 3 to 7 days. Response to therapy can be monitored noninvasively with transcranial Doppler. Improvement in vasospasm may be associated with a decrease in flow velocity, and angiography may be necessary.[215,217]

Timing of Surgery

Early surgery has been shown to carry higher procedural morbidity and mortality. The presence or absence of vasospasm on angiographic studies has often been a major determinant. Nevertheless, early surgery prevents devastating rebleeding and enables aggressive triple-H therapy for cerebral vasospasm. Current evidence supports that conventional open surgery or endovascular treatment should be performed as soon as possible after the onset of SAH unless contraindicated. A good outcome may be achieved with early operation (within 24–48 hours) in patients who are neurologically intact (grade I or II), regardless of whether vasospasm has been demonstrated. Such emergency intervention decreases the likelihood of rebleeding. Only 53% of grade III patients achieve a good outcome after early surgery; this indicates that the gross neurologic condition preoperatively is the best prognostic indicator of intact survival.[207] In the first few days after hemorrhage, the brain is swollen, soft, hyperemic, and prone to contusion and laceration. The International Cooperative Study on the Timing of Aneurysm Surgery guided practice for many years. This multicenter study demonstrated that SAH patients who underwent surgery on posthemorrhage days 4 to 10 had worse outcomes than patients treated on days 0 to 3 and days 11 to 14. It was concluded that patients who present with SAH on days 4 to 10 should have aneurysm surgery delayed until after day 10. Since the introduction of interventional neuroradiology techniques, practitioners have come to believe that coiling of ruptured aneurysms can be performed safely on patients who arrive on posthemorrhage days 4 to 10, and treatment need not be delayed until after day 10 as suggested.[212,218]

Impaired autoregulation may decrease cerebral tolerance to brain retraction. Although removal of a subarachnoid clot probably decreases the incidence and severity of delayed arterial narrowing, clearly operative management may be hazardous. In more severely brain injured patients (grades III–V), surgery is often delayed in anticipation of resolution of vasospasm and improvement in neurologic status.[207,212,218] Data from 2011 suggest that early surgery, in good-grade patients within 48 hours of an SAH, is associated with better outcomes than surgery performed in the 3- to 6-day posthemorrhage interval. Surgical treatment for aneurysmal SAH may be more hazardous during the 3- to 6-day interval, but this should be weighed against the risk of rebleeding.[219,220] As mentioned earlier, endovascular clipping or coiling is increasingly used to treat SAH secondary to aneurysm rupture.[206,221-223]

Preoperative Evaluation

The patient's baseline neurologic status must be ascertained. The level of consciousness may vary from perfect alertness to deep coma and is an important prognostic factor for the postoperative state. Evidence of increased ICP should be elicited preoperatively so it can be managed appropriately. Focal motor and sensory signs may indicate intracerebral extension of SAH, vasospasm, or cerebral edema.[209]

Pulmonary complications, such as pneumonia, neurogenic pulmonary edema, and atelectasis, are not uncommon. Patients often have an increased risk of aspiration because of their depressed level of consciousness, and measures should be taken to reduce gastric acidity and volume preoperatively. The use of prophylactic hypervolemia also increases the likelihood of pulmonary edema.[209]

The hemodynamic status of the patient should be assessed, with particular attention paid to the relationship between neurologic deterioration and blood pressure changes. The patient's cognitive status is a useful guide to blood pressure control. If the patient is alert, then CPP is adequate, and blood pressure goals can be established based on preoperative values. Continuous arterial blood pressure monitoring is essential. Serious dysrhythmias or evidence of ventricular dysfunction should be diagnosed preoperatively so appropriate monitoring and management can be provided.[224] The syndrome of inappropriate antidiuretic hormone and diabetes insipidus can occur in patients with SAH.

The presence of blood in the subarachnoid space may produce a 1°C to 2°C elevation of body temperature. Hyperthermia increases cerebral oxygen requirements and therefore, should be treated to prevent an increase of cerebral ischemia.[209,213,225]

Preoperative sedation is rarely necessary in these patients. Depression of ventilation associated with opioids and benzodiazepines may

result in hypercapnia, with resultant increases in CBF and ICP. Additionally, the reduced level of consciousness preoperatively and postoperatively may make clinical assessment difficult. Preoperative anxiety is not a problem in patients with a depressed level of consciousness (grades III–V), so sedation is not required. If preoperative sedation is considered necessary, a benzodiazepine (midazolam) is appropriate, and continued observation after its administration is warranted.[226-228]

Anesthetic Induction, Maintenance, and Emergence

Maintaining adequate intravascular volume requires two large-bore intravenous cannulas. Intraoperative monitoring includes continuous ECG (V_5), arterial pressure monitoring, peripheral nerve stimulator, central venous pressure monitoring, EEG, $ETco_2$ monitoring, pulse oximetry, and monitoring of temperature and fluid balance.[229]

Intraoperative neurophysiologic monitoring during intracranial aneurysm surgery is standard practice. It is an important adjunct to surgical inspection and intraoperative angiography to detect cerebral ischemia. SSEPs, particularly median and posterior tibial nerve SSEPs, are commonly monitored during anterior circulation procedures. Dural monitoring with SSEPs and BAERs are preferred for posterior circulation and aneurysm surgeries. There is a significant correlation between alterations in electrical signals and regional cerebral blood flow (rCBF), with transient electrophysiologic changes generally corresponding to good outcomes and permanent changes corresponding to postoperative deficits. EEG is also commonly used. Prior to temporary clip application, the neuroanesthesia team increases the anesthetic to achieve burst suppression on EEG. Burst suppression helps decrease metabolic demand so that the cerebral tissue can better tolerate induced ischemia during temporary clipping.[25]

The anesthetic induction should be slow and deliberate, with a depth that is sufficient to avoid the sympathetic responses that accompany laryngoscopy and endotracheal intubation. Anesthesia is frequently induced with propofol. The addition of an opioid (2–10 mcg/kg of fentanyl or 1–2 mcg/kg of sufentanil) and intravenous lidocaine (1.5 mg/kg) further blunts the patient's response to the sympathetic stimulation. An additional dose of opioid or propofol is required for the placement of the three-point pin Mayfield clamp. Injection of local anesthetic at the pin sites helps to minimize the associated sympathetic stimulation. Epinephrine should not be included with the local anesthetic because delayed absorption (up to 30 minutes after injection) may produce significant increases in blood pressure. Ventilation is controlled and the $Paco_2$ is maintained between 35 and 40 mm Hg to establish normal intracranial compliance. Mild hyperventilation ($Paco_2$ of 30–35 mm Hg) is instituted when intracranial compliance is impaired.[209]

Succinylcholine produces moderate increases in ICP; however, as noted earlier, it is commonly used since the ICP elevations have not been proven to be clinically relevant.[230-232] Alternatively, intubation can be accomplished with rocuronium.

The patient is placed in one of several positions, depending on the site of the aneurysm. Aneurysms that arise from the anterior part of the circle of Willis require that the patient be supine for a frontotemporal approach. The lateral position for a temporal approach is required for aneurysms that arise from the posterior aspect of the basilar artery. Aneurysms that arise from the vertebral artery or from the lower basilar artery require a sitting or prone position for a suboccipital approach. Aneurysms that arise from the anterior communicating artery are usually approached from the right and those from the middle cerebral and posterior communicating arteries are approached from the side on which the aneurysm is located.[233]

Anesthesia is maintained with air and oxygen or N_2O in oxygen, with incremental titrated dosages of an opioid (fentanyl, alfentanil, or sufentanil), or an infusion of remifentanil and a muscle relaxant.

Isoflurane may also be added in inspired concentrations not to exceed 1%. Patients who have intracranial aneurysms may require induced hypertension to counteract vasospasm, as discussed earlier, or therapeutic hypotension to control rebleeding.[234] However, there is a risk of cerebral infarction if the CPP decreases too much, especially in the presence of increased ICP. Thus, tight blood pressure control with cerebral monitoring is essential. In addition, controlled hypotension is commonly used intraoperatively to render aneurysms softer and more pliable at the time of clipping, as well as to minimize blood loss if aneurysmal rupture occurs during clipping.[211] Sodium nitroprusside and nitroglycerine should be used with caution or avoided since they can increase CBV and thus ICP. Propofol, labetalol, nicardipine, or enalapril can be used to induce hypotension.[203,234]

The safe limit of controlled hypotension has not been definitively established. Since the lower limit of cerebral vascular autoregulation is 60 mm Hg in cerebral arteries that are uncompromised by disease or trauma, it stands to reason that arterial reactivity may be compromised in brain tissue surrounding an aneurysm. Thus, the autoregulatory curve is likely shifted to higher pressures in these patients and those with preexisting hypertension. Therefore, decreases in MAP should be limited to no more than 20% of preoperative values.[209]

Rather than induce hypotension to facilitate clip ligation of the neck of the aneurysm, many neurosurgeons now routinely use temporary proximal occlusion of the parent vessel.[235]

The use of mild intraoperative hypothermia has been advocated for cerebral protection during periods of temporary occlusion.[236] Deliberate mild hypothermia was first used in 1955 as an intraoperative technique to ameliorate new neurologic deficits after cerebral aneurysm clipping. Subsequently, it was also used after neonatal asphyxia, head trauma, and cardiac arrest. The Intraoperative Hypothermia for Aneurysm Surgery Trial (IHAST II) was a randomized controlled trial designed to evaluate the effectiveness of mild hypothermia in decreasing neurologic deficits after aneurysm surgery. Intraoperative hypothermia did not improve the neurologic outcome after craniotomy among good-grade patients with aneurysmal SAH.[237]

At the conclusion of the anesthetic procedure, patients with good-grade aneurysms may be extubated in the operating room, although care must be exercised so that coughing, straining, hypercarbia, and hypertension are avoided. Propofol, lidocaine, or fentanyl may be used for short-term anesthesia as the procedure is being finished and for reducing the hemodynamic responses to extubation. Although the residual depressant effects of opioids may be reversed with judicious titrated dosages of naloxone, larger doses of naloxone can be hazardous in that they may cause sudden, violent awakening of the patient and marked increases in systemic blood pressure. ETTs should be retained in patients with poor-grade aneurysms and in those who have had intraoperative complications.[213]

Postoperative Care

Postoperative care is directed at the prevention of vasospasm via the maintenance of intravascular volume expansion and moderate hypertension (MAP of 80–110 mm Hg). Changes in the level of consciousness and development of focal neurologic deficits are usually early signs of vasospasm. These clinical signs should be aggressively managed with hypertension, hypervolemia, and hemodilution. Vasopressors may be used for blood pressure support. A CT scan should be used to rule out other potential causes of neurologic deterioration, including rebleeding, infarction, and hydrocephalus.[213]

Aneurysmal Rupture

Intraoperative aneurysmal rupture can be catastrophic. An abrupt increase in blood pressure during or after induction of anesthesia may

---

BOX 31.8 Management of Intracranial Catastrophes*

Initial Resuscitation
- Communicate with endovascular therapy team
- Assess need for assistance; call for assistance
- Secure the airway; ventilate with 100% O_2
- Determine whether the problem is hemorrhagic or occlusive (see text)
- *Hemorrhagic:* Immediate heparin reversal (1 mg protamine for each 100 units of heparin given) and low normal mean arterial pressure
- *Occlusive:* Deliberate hypertension, titrated to neurologic examination, angiography, or physiologic imaging studies; or to clinical context

Further Resuscitation
- Head up 15 degrees in neutral position, if possible
- $Paco_2$ manipulation consistent with clinical setting, otherwise normocapnia
- Mannitol 0.5 g/kg, rapid IV infusion
- Titrate IV agent to electroencephalogram burst suppression
- Passive cooling to 33°C–34°C
- Consider ventriculostomy for treatment or monitoring of increased ICP
- Consider anticonvulsants (e.g., phenytoin or phenobarbital)

*These are only general recommendations, and drug doses must be adapted to specific clinical situations and in accordance with a patient's preexisting medical condition(s). In some cases of asymptomatic or minor vessel puncture or occlusion, less aggressive management may be appropriate.
ICP, Intracranial pressure; *Paco2,* partial pressure of arterial carbon dioxide.
From Lee CZ, Young WL. Anesthesia for endovascular neurosurgery and interventional neuroradiology. *Anesthesiol Clin.* 2012;30(2):127–147.

---

indicate that an aneurysm has bled. The use of propofol 1 to 2 mg/kg or sodium nitroprusside 0.5 to 1 mcg/kg decreases the transmural pressure of the aneurysm. Intraoperative aneurysmal rupture necessitates maintaining the MAP between 40 and 50 mm Hg or lower to facilitate surgical control of the neck of the aneurysm or the parent vessel. Alternatively, one or both carotid arteries may be compressed for up to 3 minutes to produce a bloodless field. Rapid blood replacement and adequate intravenous access is essential. Massive transfusion using blood and blood products is necessary to maintain adequate intravascular volume.[213]

Although barbiturates have been used for protection against focal cerebral ischemia, their efficacy has not been demonstrated in this clinical situation.[238]

Interventional Neuroradiology

Treatment of aneurysms using interventional neuroradiology presents some special anesthetic considerations. These include (1) maintaining immobility during procedures to facilitate imaging, (2) rapid recovery from anesthesia, either during or at the end of procedures, to facilitate neurologic examination and monitoring, (3) managing anticoagulation, (4) treating and managing sudden hemorrhage or vascular occlusion, (5) manipulating systemic or regional blood pressures, and (6) guiding the management of the patients during transport to and from the radiology suites. Both general and intravenous sedation are used; however, general anesthesia is preferred because the procedures can be long, and manipulation of blood pressure and respiration may be necessary. The patient is prepared in a manner similar to open intracranial aneurysm clipping. Anesthesia considerations and management are also the same; however, if an intracranial emergency occurs during the procedure, several steps should be taken. Box 31.8 outlines the management of intracranial emergencies.[205] Anesthetic considerations for select interventional neuroradiology procedures are noted in Table 31.9 and in Chapter 58.

TABLE 31.9   Interventional Neuroradiologic Procedures and Primary Anesthetic Considerations

Procedure	Possible Anesthetic Considerations
Therapeutic embolization of vascular malformation	
Intracranial AVMs	Deliberate hypotension, postprocedure NPPB
Dural AVM	Existence of venous hypertension; deliberate hypercapnia
Extracranial AVMs	Deliberate hypercapnia
Carotid cavernous fistula	Deliberate hypercapnia, postprocedure NPPB
Cerebral aneurysms	Aneurysmal rupture, blood pressure control*
Ethanol sclerotherapy of AVMs or venous malformations	Brain swelling, airway swelling, hypoxemia, hypoglycemia, intoxication from ethanol, cardiorespiratory arrest
Balloon A&S of occlusive cerebrovascular disease	Cerebral ischemia, deliberate hypertension, concomitant coronary artery disease, bradycardia, hypotension
Balloon angioplasty of cerebral vasospasm secondary to aneurysmal SAH	Cerebral ischemia, blood pressure control*
Therapeutic carotid occlusion for giant aneurysms and skull base tumors	Cerebral ischemia, blood pressure control*
Thrombolysis of acute thromboembolic stroke	Postprocedure ICH (NPPB), concomitant coronary artery disease, blood pressure control*
Intraarterial chemotherapy of head and neck tumors	Airway swelling, intracranial hypertension
Embolization for epistaxis	Airway control

*Blood pressure control refers to deliberate hypo- or hypertension.
A&S, Angioplasty and stenting; *AVM,* arteriovenous malformation; *ICH,* intracerebral hemorrhage; *NPPB,* normal perfusion pressure breakthrough; *SAH,* subarachnoid hemorrhage.
From Lee CZ, Young WL. Anesthesia for endovascular neurosurgery and interventional neuroradiology. *Anesthesiol Clin.* 2012;30(2):127–147.

Arteriovenous Malformation

Arteriovenous malformations are congenital intracerebral networks in which arteries flow directly into veins. Patients with these malformations generally are younger than those with aneurysms. They may have bleeding or seizures or, less commonly, ischemia resulting from "steal" from normal areas or occurring with high-output congestive heart failure. The anesthetic concerns are similar to those associated with patients undergoing aneurysm surgery. Notably, arteriovenous malformations lack the ability to autoregulate blood flow at the site of the malformation. Surgery may be preceded with an attempt to embolize the arteriovenous malformation. The neurologic examination should be repeated after embolization to document any new deficits that otherwise might be attributed to anesthesia and surgery.

BOX 31.9   Peripheral Sequelae of Head Trauma

- Hemodynamic instability
- Abnormal breathing patterns
- Bone fractures
- Pneumothorax
- Airway obstruction
- Aspiration
- Hypoxia
- Acute respiratory distress syndrome
- Neurogenic pulmonary edema
- Electrocardiographic changes
- Hematologic
- Disseminated intravascular coagulation
- Endocrinologic
- Cervical spine injury
- Maxillofacial injuries

Adapted from Pasternack JJ, Lanier WL. Diseases affecting the brain. In Hines RL, Marshall KE, eds. *Stoelting's Anesthesia and Co-Existing Disease.* 7th ed. Philadelphia: Elsevier; 2017.

Head Trauma and Traumatic Brain Injury

Traumatic brain injury is a contributory factor in up to 50% of deaths resulting from trauma. Most patients with head trauma are young, and many (10%–40%) have associated polytraumatic injuries such as intraabdominal injuries, long-bone fractures, or both. The significance of a head injury is dependent not only on the extent of the irreversible neuronal damage caused by the injury but also on the potential for secondary injuries. These include systemic factors such as hypoxemia, hypercapnia, and hypotension; the formation and expansion of an epidural, subdural, or intracerebral hematoma; and/or sustained intracranial hypertension (Box 31.9). Sustained increases in ICP can result in irreversible brain damage. Surgical and anesthetic management is directed at treating the primary injury and preventing secondary insults.[98] Types of cerebral hematomas and mechanisms of head injuries are illustrated in Fig. 31.22.

Preoperative Management

Emergency therapy for head injury should begin before hospital admission because a large proportion of deaths occur in the prehospital environment. Therapy is based on prevention of secondary brain injury resulting from hypoxia, hypercapnia, hypotension, and expanding intracranial masses.

Airway Management

Interventions that ensure airway patency, adequacy of ventilation and oxygenation, and the correction of systemic hypotension should be conducted simultaneously with an early neurologic evaluation. Airway obstruction and hypoventilation are common. Up to 70% of patients with a head injury have concurrent hypoxemia, which may be complicated by other pulmonary insults such as pulmonary contusion, fat emboli, or neurogenic pulmonary edema. The suspicion of a cervical spine injury (10% incidence) should accompany any head injury until disproven by radiography. Manual in-line axial stabilization (MILS) that maintains the head in a neutral position should be used during airway instrumentation. Videolaryngoscopy is frequently utilized since it provides a large screen for viewing the intubation procedure. Awake intubation, with a flexible (fiberoptic) intubating scope, may be preferred for airway management if difficulty is anticipated. Patients who are hypoventilating, do not have a gag reflex, or have a GCS total score below 9 require emergent tracheal intubation and hyperventilation (Table 31.10). All other patients should be carefully observed for deterioration. Table 31.11 summarizes respiratory patterns seen with various neurologic injuries. The GCS score is a test that

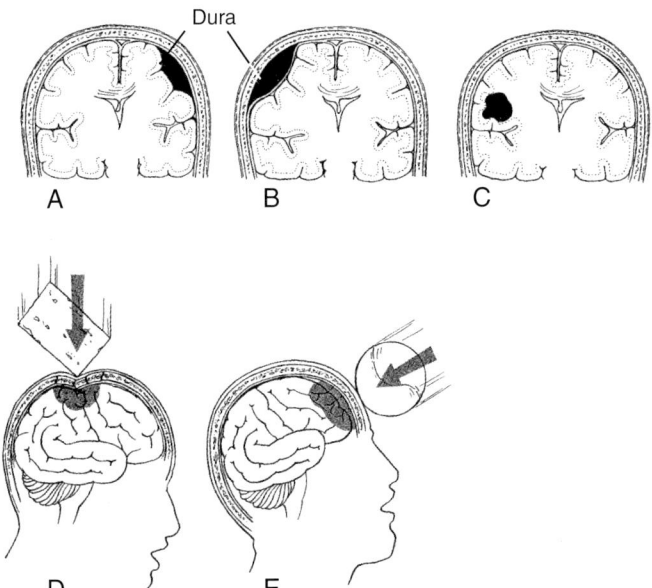

Fig. 31.22 (A) Subdural hematoma. (B) Epidural hematoma. (C) Intracerebral hematoma. (D) Direct head injury resulting in depressed skull fracture and compression injury. (E) Blow to skull resulting in tearing of blood vessels. Shaded areas on skull represent cerebral contusion. (From Black JM, Hokanson Hawks JH. *Medical-Surgical Nursing: Clinical Management for Positive Outcomes*. 8th ed. St. Louis: Saunders; 2009:1934–1936.)

TABLE 31.10 Modified Coma Scale for Infants

Response	Score
Eye Opening	
Spontaneous	4
To sound	3
To pressure	2
None	1
Verbal Response	
Oriented	5
Confused	4
Words	3
Sounds	2
None	1
Motor Response	
Obeys commands	6
Localizing	5
Normal flexion	4
Abnormal flexion	3
Extension	2
None	1

communicates the level of consciousness in patients with acute TBI, assesses neurologic trends, and can help to guide initial decision making.[239]

When intubation is indicated, the oral route provides the most efficient means of safely securing the airway. A rapid-sequence induction endotracheal intubation that avoids desaturation and hypoxemia should be performed.[240,241] Nasal intubation should be avoided in the presence of suspected basilar skull fracture, bleeding diathesis, suspected upper-airway foreign body, or severe facial fractures.[240]

Cardiovascular Assessment

Multisystem trauma often accompanies head injury, and the hypotension that results is usually from hemorrhage. These injuries must be identified and treated early in the resuscitative period. Resuscitation should be provided with either whole blood or packed red blood cells, plasma, and platelets. If blood products are not immediately available, then fluid resuscitation can be facilitated by the administration of isotonic fluid, either normal saline or lactated Ringer solution, or colloids. Glucose in water should not be used because it decreases serum osmolarity and can exacerbate cerebral edema. Because the cerebral vessels are already dilated from hypotension, rapid restoration of the normal arterial pressure precipitates brain swelling. It is extremely valuable to insert an ICP monitor during resuscitation for the monitoring of both systemic arterial pressure and ICP.[238] Dysrhythmias and ECG abnormalities in the T wave, U wave, ST segment, and QT interval are common after head injuries but are not necessarily associated with cardiac injury.[98] Blood pressure goals usually target a higher MAP after a TBI, and in the presence of increased ICP, in an effort to maintain a CPP of at least 60 mm Hg. For example, if the ICP is 20 mm Hg, then the MAP would need to be at least 80 mm Hg to preserve a CPP of 60 mm Hg. Guidelines

TABLE 31.11 Respiratory Patterns With Head Trauma

Pattern	Description	Location of Injury and Other Causes
Cheyne-Stokes respiration	Regular increase in the rate and depth of breathing that peaks and is followed by a decreasing rate and depth of breathing, which progresses to apnea; then the cycle repeats itself	Bilateral dysfunction of cerebral hemispheres; Midbrain and upper pons
Central neurogenic hyperventilation	Deep, rapid, and regular pattern of breathing	Low midbrain and upper pons; Increased intracranial pressure with head trauma
Apneusis breathing	A pause at full inspiration occurs; may see prolonged inspiratory pause alternating with prolonged expiratory pause	Mid and low pons; Hypoglycemia, anoxia, and meningitis
Cluster breathing	Periodic breathing with frequent apneic episodes	Low pons and high medulla
Ataxic breathing	Irregular breathing with shallow, deep respirations and irregular apneic episodes; usually slow	Medulla

From Drain CB, Odom-Forren J, eds. *Perianesthesia Nursing: A Critical Care Approach*. 5th ed. St. Louis: Elsevier; 2009:574.

TABLE 31.12 Guidelines for Blood Pressure Management in Common Neurologic Conditions

Diagnosis	Recommendation
Acute ischemic stroke	Keep <180/110 mm Hg if thrombolysis
	Treat only BP >220/120 if no thrombolysis
Intracerebral hemorrhage	Keep SBP <180 and MAP <130 mm Hg (ideal SBP <160 and MAP <110 mm Hg)
Subarachnoid hemorrhage from cerebral aneurysm	Keep SBP <160 mm Hg before aneurysm treated
	Caution with any reduction in BP after aneurysm treated
Traumatic brain injury	Keep MAP to maintain CPP >60 mm Hg (i.e., MAP >80 mm Hg)

BP, Blood pressure; *CPP,* cerebral perfusion pressure; *MAP,* mean arterial pressure; *SBP,* systolic blood pressure.
Adapted from Rabinstein AA, Fugate JE. Principles of neuro-intensive care. In Daroff, et al., eds. *Bradley's Neurology in Clinical Practice.* 7th ed. London: Elsevier; 2016:753.

for blood pressure management in select neurosurgical emergencies are noted in Table 31.12.

Coagulopathies

Chronic subdural hematoma. Bridging veins run between the dura and the surface of the brain. A subdural hematoma develops when these veins tear and leak blood, usually as the result of a head injury. A collection of blood then forms over the surface of the brain. In a chronic subdural collection, the problem is not discovered immediately, and blood leaks from the veins slowly over time. A subdural hematoma is more common in the elderly because normal brain shrinkage occurs with aging that stretches and weakens the bridging veins. Rarely, a subdural hematoma can occur spontaneously. Risks include head injury, old age, chronic use of aspirin or antiinflammatory drugs such as ibuprofen, anticoagulant medication, chronic heavy alcohol use, or diseases that are associated with blood-clotting problems.[242]

A 2006 study of 713 emergency referrals documented over 90 days evaluated the effect of antithrombotic therapy on neurosurgical emergency referral. Of the 713 patients, 174 (24.4%) were discovered to have intracranial or spinal hemorrhage, and 75 (43.1%) of these were on antithrombotic therapy. Seventeen of these 75 patients (22.6%) had no documented indication for antithrombotic therapy (all were on aspirin therapy), and 9 of the 29 on warfarin (31%) had an international normalized ratio (INR; prothrombin time) in excess of 3.5 on presentation.[243]

The key elements when managing coagulation abnormalities in patients presenting for emergent/urgent neurosurgery are (1) identifying the coagulopathy, (2) implementing a plan that allows for optimum coagulation status given the comorbidities of the patient, and (3) timing the period of optimum coagulation to coincide with the conclusion of surgery and the immediate postoperative period.

The relationship between coagulopathy and chronic subdural hematoma requires correction of coagulation to facilitate surgery. In one study, 42% of 114 patients presenting for drainage of chronic subdural hematoma were found to have coagulation disorders before surgery.[244] Addressing coagulopathies in the geriatric population is a situation best addressed by a multidisciplinary approach. A significant amount of blood products, or even difficult to obtain blood products, may be necessary to reverse coagulopathies. Evidence suggest that 10 to 17 mL/kg of fresh frozen plasma (FFP) is necessary to reverse Coumadin toxicity.[245]

The general principles for emergency bleeding management include discontinuing the anticoagulant; hemodynamic and hemostatic resuscitation; and obtaining coagulation tests, including platelets, fibrinogen levels, and renal function studies. In warfarin-associated bleeding, prothrombin complex concentrate (PCC) or FFP in combination with vitamin K can be administered to replace the missing functional clotting factors. Some hospitals use FFP; however, PCC is often preferred because it lowers the INR more rapidly, more completely, and without the added risks of transfusion reactions and excess volume. When reversing warfarin, concomitant vitamin K should be administered because of warfarin's long half-life. Without the use of PCC, vitamin K and FFP can take at least 12 to 24 hours to lower the INR into the reference range.[245,246]

The direct oral anticoagulants dabigatran (Pradaxa), apixaban (Eliquis), edoxaban (Savaysa), and rivaroxaban (Xarelto) are frequently being used in lieu of warfarin. Idarucizumab (Praxbind) is available for the urgent anticoagulant reversal of dabigatran.[247]

Reversal of clopidogrel (Plavix), aspirin, or aspirin plus clopidogrel may be addressed by platelet administration. Alternatively, recombinant factor VIIa has been shown to reverse the inhibitory effects of aspirin or aspirin plus clopidogrel and could be useful for bleeding complications or when acute surgery is needed during treatment with these antiplatelet drugs.[248]

Severe brain injury initiates the outpouring of tissue thromboplastin and activation of the complement system, causing disseminated intravascular coagulopathy and fibrinolysis, as well as precipitating the development of adult respiratory distress syndrome. Early recognition of abnormal prothrombin and partial thromboplastin times is crucial. Prompt therapy with FFP, cryoprecipitate, whole blood, and, if necessary, platelets may decrease the likelihood of disseminated intravascular coagulopathy.[211,212]

Increased Intracranial Pressure

The initial therapy is directed toward lowering or preventing further increases in ICP. Simple maneuvers such as using a head-up tilt of 15 to 30 degrees to keep the head in the midline position and not rotated to either side (to ensure jugular vein patency), avoiding overhydration, maintaining normovolemia, and maintaining normal (rather than increased) arterial pressure all help control ICP.[240]

In patients in whom intracranial hypertension is suspected, whether from an epidural or subdural hematoma or from diffuse brain swelling, emergency treatment directed at reducing ICP is the rational course. Treatment of an increased ICP has been described previously. Corticosteroids (dexamethasone or methylprednisolone) are of little benefit, have not been shown to help in acute TBI, and should be avoided.[105,249]

Although mannitol effectively lowers the ICP minutes after administration, its use remains controversial. The drug is indicated when either elevated ICP or a mass causes herniation with subsequent patient deterioration. The risk of increasing the size of a hematoma is negligible compared with the disastrous effects of untreated progressive uncal herniation. If decompression of transtentorial herniation is delayed, secondary hemorrhage into the brainstem can occur and cause irreversible neurologic deficit. Once mannitol is given and the ICP is reduced, the specific intracranial disorder must be identified as soon as possible if a recurrence of the patient's deterioration is to be prevented.[250,251]

Animal and human studies have demonstrated that hypertonic saline has clinically desirable physiologic effects on CBF, ICP, and inflammatory responses in models of neurotrauma.[252] Some studies suggest that 23.4% hypertonic saline is a safe and effective treatment for elevated ICP in patients after TBI.[252,253]

Mannitol therapy administered for increased ICP may have a beneficial effect on mortality when compared with pentobarbital treatment, but it may have a detrimental effect on mortality when compared with hypertonic saline in treating increased ICP in head-injury patients.[250,251]

Neurodiagnostic Evaluation

The choice between operative and medical management of head trauma is based on radiographic and clinical findings. If the patient is unconscious in the absence of a drug overdose, the ICP should be assumed to be elevated. Patients should be stabilized before any CT or angiographic studies are performed. Critically ill patients should be closely monitored during such studies. Restless or uncooperative patients may require general anesthesia or sedation if these diagnostic examinations are to be accomplished. Sedation without control of the airway should be avoided because of the risk of further increases in ICP from hypercapnia or hypoxemia. Diagnostic imaging plays an important role in the management of patients with TBI. CT is the first-line imaging technique allowing rapid detection of primary structural brain lesions that require surgical intervention. CT also detects various deleterious secondary insults, allowing for early medical and surgical management. A patient who has a CT scan that demonstrates obliteration of basal cisterns, dilation of the fourth or lateral ventricles, or a midline shift of 10 mm has an increase in ICP, which should be immediately monitored if a monitoring device is not already in place. Serial imaging is critical to identifying secondary injuries. MRI is indicated for patients with acute TBI when CT results are inconsistent with neurologic findings. However, MRI is superior in patients with subacute and chronic TBI and is also predictive of neurocognitive outcome.[254]

Intraoperative Management

Operative treatment is reserved for depressed skull fracture, depressed fractures associated with underlying brain injury, and evacuation of epidural, subdural, and some intracerebral hematomas.[255] Monitoring during anesthesia is generally similar to that for other mass lesions associated with intracranial hypertension. Intraarterial and central venous (or pulmonary artery) pressure monitoring should be established if it is not already present, but it should not delay surgical decompression in a rapidly deteriorating patient.[98,242]

Anesthetic Induction, Maintenance, and Emergence

Intubation must be accomplished as expeditiously as possible using an RSI technique with cricoid pressure. The use of cricoid pressure may need to be avoided if there is suspicion of a cervical fracture. The choice of induction agent depends on the patient's blood pressure. If hypotension is present, then either etomidate or ketamine should be considered. If hypertension is present, then propofol can be used being cautious to avoid severe reductions in blood pressure. Either succinylcholine or rocuronium can be used, as discussed earlier in this chapter.[255] Hyperkalemia may result after administration of succinylcholine in a patient with closed-head injury without paresis.[256] It is important to reduce the sympathetic response to intubation, which can be done by administering lidocaine and either fentanyl or esmolol, or a combination of both, again being cautious to avoid rapid reductions in blood pressure. Intracranial damage is usually associated with severe hypertension.

Although hyperventilation attenuates the increase in ICP when inhalation anesthetics are used in patients with head injury, early cerebral vasoconstriction in response to hypocapnia is not recommended. Hyperventilation is only recommended if there is impending uncal herniation or for brief periods during neurosurgery at the request of the neurosurgeon. The administration of inhalation anesthetics in concentrations less than 1 MAC may have a role in the treatment of intraoperative hypertension.[255]

Patients who have chronic subdural hematoma and are alert and responsive may have burr holes placed for evacuation of accumulated blood under local anesthesia with sedation. Depressed skull fractures also may be elevated while the patient is awake and under local anesthesia with sedation. This technique must be used cautiously when the patient is placed in the three-point pin head holder, is awake, and has a full stomach without a secure airway.[255]

Fluid replacement should be accomplished with glucose-free solutions. Hypovolemia results in systemic hypotension, an unstable anesthetic course, and (by decreasing cerebral oxygen delivery) increased cerebral vasodilation. An adequate hemoglobin and hematocrit, as well as electrolytes, coagulation factors, and kidney function, should be evaluated.

The decision of whether to extubate the trachea at the conclusion of the surgical procedure depends on the severity of the injury, the presence of concomitant abdominal or thoracic injuries, preexisting illnesses, and the preoperative level of consciousness. The occurrence of nausea, vomiting, and respiratory and cardiac problems are all possibilities that should be considered. Young patients who are conscious preoperatively may be extubated after the removal of a localized lesion, whereas patients with diffuse brain injury should remain intubated. Moreover, persistent intracranial hypertension requires continued paralysis, mechanical ventilation, and sedation postoperatively.[98]

■ SUMMARY

Advances in surgical approaches to tumors, vascular lesions, and TBIs necessitate constant reappraisal of the important role of anesthesia care in improving a patient's long-term outcome. Multiple intraoperative monitoring modalities are available for neurosurgical procedures. Interventional radiologic approaches are now a primary therapy for several neurologic disorders, and many new challenges exist during the anesthesia management of these patients.

REFERENCES

For a complete list of references for this chapter, scan this QR code with any smartphone code reader app, or visit the following URL: http://booksite.elsevier.com/9780323711944/.

32

Renal Anatomy, Physiology, Pathophysiology, and Anesthesia Management

Catherine Y. Morse

The kidneys are paired solid organs lying retroperitoneally on either side of the vertebral column. The main function of these organs is excreting end products of metabolism and controlling the concentration of constituents of body fluids. A rich blood supply to these vital organs, coupled with the physiologic processes of filtration, reabsorption, secretion, and excretion, maintains homeostasis of the fluid within cells. For management of anesthetized patients to be optimal, clinicians must be familiar with physiologic mechanisms utilized by the renal system to control intracellular and extracellular environments to maintain homeostasis.

This chapter addresses the effects of anesthesia and surgery on both the normal and the diseased kidney. After a discussion of the anatomic structure and physiologic mechanisms of the kidney, the effects of anesthesia on normal renal function are addressed. Pathophysiologic mechanisms associated with acute and chronic kidney injury follow. Preoperative renal assessment and anesthetic considerations for patients with impaired renal function are emphasized, and pertinent anesthetic considerations for common urologic procedures are discussed.

STRUCTURE OF THE KIDNEY

The kidneys are bean-shaped, reddish-brown organs located in the posterior part of the abdomen on both sides of the vertebral column (Fig. 32.1). These organs extend from the 12th thoracic vertebra to the 3rd lumbar vertebra; each weighs approximately 125 to 170 g in men and 115 to 155 g in women. Each kidney is approximately 11.25 cm long, 5 to 7.5 cm wide, and 2.5 cm thick. Due to hepatic displacement, the right kidney's position is slightly lower than the left kidney. The kidneys and renal vessels are embedded in fatty tissue known as perirenal fat and enclosed in renal fascia. Renal fascia and large vessels hold the kidneys in anatomic position (see Fig. 32.1).

The anterior and posterior surfaces, upper and lower poles, and lateral margin of the kidney have convex contours. The medial margin is concave because of the presence of a recessed fissure known as the hilus. Structures entering or exiting the kidney through the hilus include the renal artery and vein, nerves, lymphatics, and ureters.

A longitudinal section of the kidney reveals two distinct regions, the outer cortex and the inner medulla (Fig. 32.2). The medulla is divided into 8 to 18 triangular wedges called pyramids. The base of each pyramid is directed toward the renal cortex, and the apexes converge toward the renal pelvis. Pyramids have a striated appearance due to the presence of the loop of Henle and collecting ducts of the nephron. The apex of each pyramid, called the papilla, is composed of many collecting ducts, and those papillary ducts empty into a cup-shaped structure known as the minor calyx. Several minor calyces join to form major calyces, which come together as the renal pelvis.

The renal pelvis is the major reservoir for urine. Ureters connect the renal pelvis to the bladder.[1]

Nephron

The functional unit of the kidney is the nephron (Fig. 32.3), and approximately 1,250,000 of these units reside in each kidney. The shape of the nephron is unique, unmistakable, and admirably suited for its function. Each component of the nephron is selective with regard to its physiologic function. Filtered blood flows through the nephrons, which, in turn, retain filtered fluid known as filtrate. Through this process, end products of metabolism are excreted, and metabolically important substances such as water and electrolytes are reabsorbed as needed.

The formation of urine begins with the nephron. The nephron begins in the cortex at the glomerulus and ends where the tubule joins the collecting duct at the papilla. The glomerulus is a tuft of capillaries derived from the afferent arteriole. Blood is transported to the glomerulus by the afferent arteriole; blood that is not filtered in the nephron returns to the systemic circulation via the efferent arteriole. The filtrate from the glomeruli enters the Bowman capsule, or capsula glomeruli, then flows through a tortuous pathway in the proximal convoluted tubule, to the loop of Henle, distal convoluted tubule, and, finally, the collecting duct.

The nephron, which changes in shape and direction as it follows its course, is contained partly in the renal cortex and partly in the medulla (Fig. 32.4). The cortex contains the Bowman capsule, glomerulus, and proximal and distal tubules. The thin, descending loop of Henle comes from the proximal tubule and extends toward the pyramid. The descending loop of Henle eventually bends on itself and forms an enlarged, ascending loop of Henle. The ascending limb joins the distal convoluted tubule.[1]

The kidneys have two types of nephrons: cortical nephrons, which extend only partially into the medulla, and juxtamedullary nephrons, which lie deep in the cortex and extend deep into the medulla. Juxtamedullary nephrons comprise one-fifth to one-third of total nephrons and play an important role in concentration of urine.[2]

Renal Blood Supply

To understand how the kidneys function, it is essential to understand their blood supply. The kidneys are highly vascular, receiving 1100 to 1200 mL of blood per minute, or 20% to 25% of the cardiac output, although they represent only 0.5% of body weight. Blood reaches these organs through the renal arteries. At the hilus of the kidney, the renal artery divides into several lobar arteries and then subdivides again into interlobar arteries, which run between the pyramids. When these vessels reach the corticomedullary zone, they make well-defined arches over the bases of the pyramids. These vessels, known as arcuate arteries, divide into a series of arteries known as interlobular arteries (see Fig. 32.2). An interlobular artery may terminate as an afferent arteriole or as a nutrient artery to the tubule.

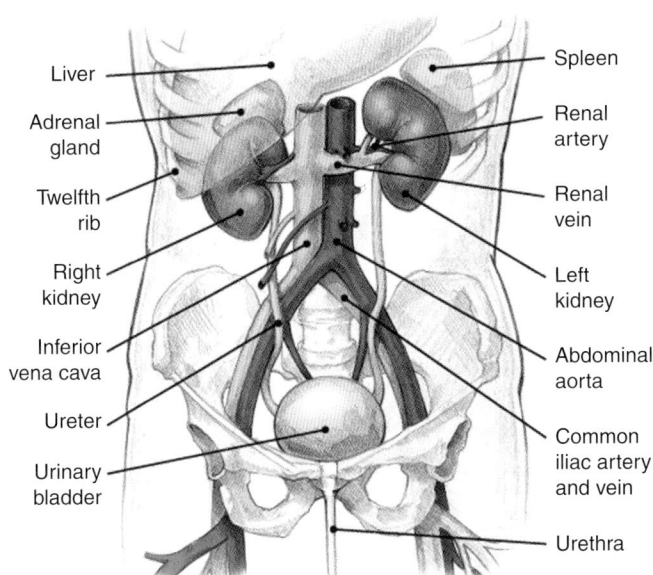

Fig. 32.1 Kidney position.

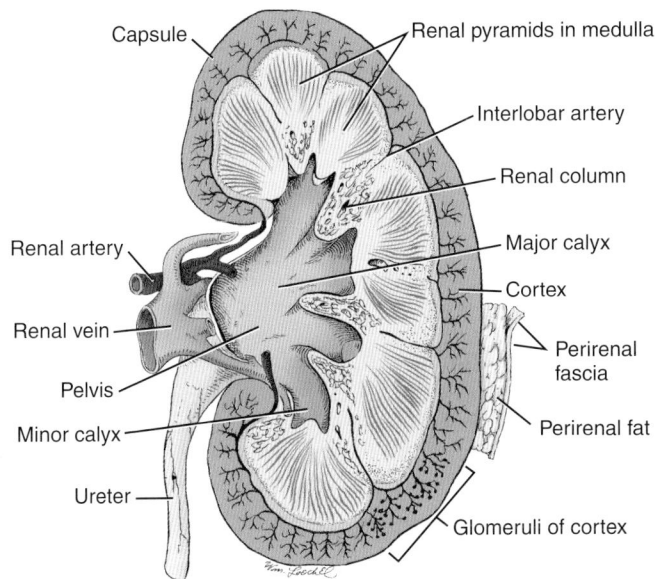

Fig. 32.2 Longitudinal section of the kidney.

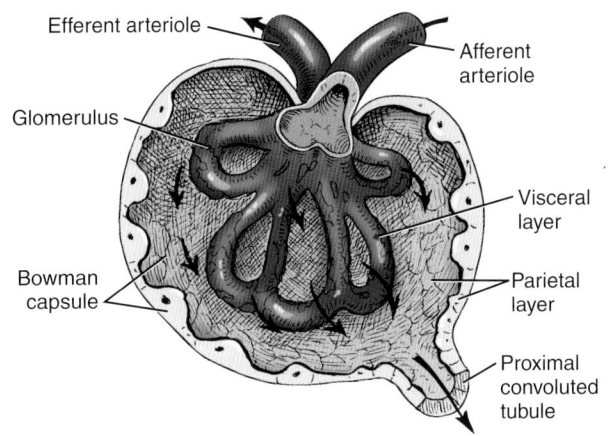

Fig. 32.3 The nephron.

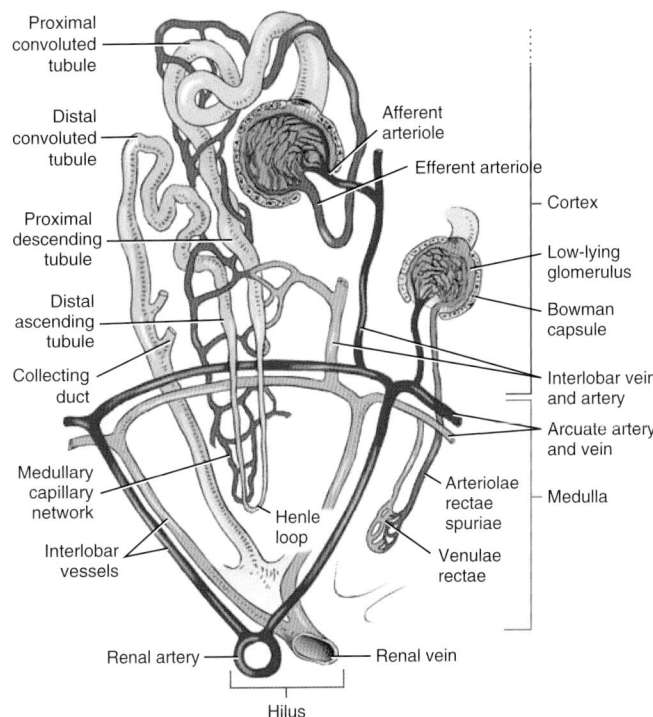

Fig. 32.4 Renal filtration.

The afferent arterioles form the high-pressure capillary bed within the Bowman capsule that is called the glomerulus. Because little or no oxygen is removed in the glomerulus, blood that is not filtered begins its passage to the venous system via the efferent arteriole. The efferent arteriole is smaller than the afferent arteriole, thereby affording some resistance to blood flow. The efferent vessel soon becomes a plexus of capillaries again, and this low-pressure bed is known as the peritubular capillary bed, which winds and twists around the proximal and distal tubule. A few hairpin loops, called vasa recta, dip down among the loops of Henle. Anatomic arrangements of these capillary beds and the renal tubules set the stage for filtration, reabsorption, and concentration of urine.

After leaving the peritubular capillary, blood returns to the central circulation via the renal veins. Renal veins are named in reverse order of the arteries, and, therefore, are the interlobular, arcuate, interlobar, lobar, and renal veins. The renal vein leaves the kidney at the hilus and empties into the inferior vena cava.

The cardiac output portion that passes through the kidney is called the renal fraction. Cardiac output in a 70-kg adult is approximately 5 - 6 L/min,

and blood flow through both kidneys is approximately 1 - 1.2 L/min, making the normal renal fraction of cardiac output between 20% and 25%. Distribution of renal blood flow is to the renal cortex and the medulla, with the cortex receiving the larger amount. Values obtained from dogs indicate that 3 to 5 mL/g/min are distributed to the cortex, 1 to 2 mL/g/min to the outer medulla, and 0.3 to 0.6 mL/g/min to the inner medulla. Only a small portion of blood (1%–2%) flows through the vasa recta in the medulla.[1]

Regulation of Renal Blood Flow

Blood flow to any organ is determined by the arteriovenous pressure difference across the vascular bed and is given by the following relationship:

$$\text{Renal blood flow (RBF)} = \text{RPF}/(1-\text{HCT})$$

where RPF is the renal plasma flow, and HCT is the hematocrit. Renal blood flow is regulated by intrinsic autoregulation and neural regulation.

Autoregulation of renal blood flow implies that blood flow remains normal despite a considerable change in pressure. With a mean arterial pressure (MAP) between 50 and 180 mmHg, renal blood flow to both kidneys remains 1000 mL/min. If mean systemic blood pressure falls below 50 mm Hg, filtration ceases. Afferent arteriole vasodilation and myogenic mechanisms are responsible for autoregulation.[1]

There is a direct relationship between renal blood flow and glomerular filtration. When renal blood flow decreases, glomerular filtration is reduced. A reduction in glomerular filtration leads to dilation of the afferent arteriole. An increase in blood flow to the glomerulus returns glomerular filtration to normal.

Myogenic mechanisms also play a role in renal autoregulation. When arterial pressure rises, the arterial wall is stretched, the vessel constricts, and blood flow remains normal. When arterial pressure decreases, the opposite effect occurs. Therefore, renal blood flow remains constant over a wide range of pressure changes.

Renal blood flow is also influenced by neural regulation. The sympathetic nervous system innervates the afferent and efferent arterioles. Autoregulation will override the adrenergic system with mild stimulation; acute sympathetic stimulation and associated vasoconstriction can decrease renal blood flow substantially. The parasympathetic nervous system is not physiologically significant in relationship to renal blood flow.[1]

RENAL PHYSIOLOGY

The kidneys maintain a steady state, which promotes homeostasis and is essential to life. This is accomplished through three major mechanisms: filtration, reabsorption, and tubular secretion. Plasma filtrate may be reabsorbed or excreted as urine depending on the physiologic needs.[2]

Filtration

Filtration, which results from pressures forcing fluids and solutes through the glomerulus, is the first step in the formation of urine. The quantity of glomerular filtrate formed each minute in all nephrons is called the glomerular filtration rate (GFR). The filtration fraction is the quantity of renal plasma flow that becomes filtrate and is defined as GFR divided by the flow to one kidney. Because the GFR is approximately 125 mL/min, and the flow to one kidney is 650 mL/min, the filtration fraction is 125/650, or 19% (approximately one-fifth) of plasma flow. Of the 125 mL/min (or 180 L/day) of this protein-free filtrate made, 99% is reabsorbed from the renal tubules, and the remaining small portion is excreted as urine.[1]

Regulation of Glomerular Filtration Rate

Glomerular filtration is also dependent on the following physiologic factors:
- The pressure inside the glomerular capillaries
- The pressure in the Bowman capsule
- The colloid osmotic pressure of the plasma proteins

The pressure inside the high-pressure glomerulus (60 mm Hg) is an outward force, whereas the colloid osmotic pressure created by proteins in the glomerulus (28 mm Hg) is an inward force that tends to hold fluid within the glomerulus. Pressure in the Bowman capsule (18 mm Hg) opposes filtration. Filtration pressure is the pressure that forces fluid through the glomerular membrane and is equal to the glomerular pressure minus the sum of the glomerular colloid osmotic pressure and the capsular pressure. With the values given, the normal filtration pressure is 10 mm Hg. Several factors can alter GFR. Increased renal blood flow, dilation of the afferent arteriole, and increased resistance in the efferent arteriole increase GFR. Afferent arteriole constriction and efferent arteriole dilation tend to decrease GFR.

A special structure called the juxtaglomerular complex regulates GFR. At the juxtaglomerular complex, the distal convoluted tubule lies between the afferent and efferent arterioles. Cells of the distal tubule

encountering the arterioles are dense, and therefore, are referred to as the macula densa. Smooth muscle cells of both the afferent and efferent arterioles consist of juxtaglomerular cells, which contain renin. Anatomically, this structure is arranged to allow fluid in the distal tubule to alter afferent or efferent arteriolar tone and thus regulate GFR.

Decreased glomerular filtration causes overabsorption of sodium ions (Na^+) and chloride ions (Cl^-) in the ascending limb of the loop of Henle resulting in a reduction in the delivery of these ions to the macula densa, which are specialized cells designed to detect small changes in osmolality. Decreases in sodium and chloride concentrations cause afferent arterioles to dilate, thus increasing renal blood flow and GFR. Sympathetic stimulation and decreased delivery of both sodium and chloride to the macula densa stimulate the juxtaglomerular cells to release renin. Renin clears angiotensinogen from the liver to form angiotensin I. In the lung, angiotensin I is changed into angiotensin II under the influence of a converting enzyme, known as angiotensin-converting enzyme (ACE). In addition to having a generalized vasoconstricting effect, angiotensin II causes efferent arteriole constriction. This causes the pressure in the glomerulus to increase and the GFR to return to normal. In this manner, the renal system autoregulates blood flow, and GFR remains relatively unchanged despite changes in systemic blood pressure.[1]

Filtrate Composition

Although permeability at the glomerulus is 100 to 500 times greater than most capillaries, glomerulus filtration is a selective process, and it is only partially understood why some substances are filtered and others are not. It is postulated that the glomerular capillary contains negatively charged pores, which are 70 to 100 nm in size, and are freely permeable to water and small molecules, as well as to some ions. Molecules with diameters up to 80 nm that do not have a negative charge are easily filtered. The glomerulus is almost impermeable to all plasma proteins but highly permeable to most other dissolved substances. Glomerular filtrate is, therefore, similar to plasma except that it lacks significant amounts of proteins.[2]

Tubular Reabsorption and Secretion

Conversion of glomerular filtrate to urine is the result of filtration at the glomerulus, tubular reabsorption, or transport from the tubular lumen to the renal cell and secretion or transport from the renal cell to the filtrate. Approximately 99% of plasma filtrate is reabsorbed in the nephron.

Tubular reabsorption permits conservation of essential substances such as water, glucose, amino acids, and electrolytes. Some substances, such as water and sodium, are reabsorbed throughout the nephron, whereas others, such as glucose, are completely reabsorbed when plasma concentrations are low. Certain substances have a reabsorption maximum value, and after that value is reached, excess filtered material is excreted, regardless of plasma concentration. This maximum value is termed maximum transport. Maximum transport occurs because of substance saturation of the carrier.

By the time the blood has reached the peritubular capillary, one-fifth of the plasma has been filtered into the Bowman capsule. The hydrostatic pressure in this low-pressure capillary bed has dropped to 13 mm Hg, whereas the osmotic pressure has increased to 30 to 32 mm Hg. The peritubular capillaries are extremely porous compared with those in other body tissues, and the proximity to the proximal and distal tubule allows movement of water and solutes from the tubule to the peritubular capillary bed. The anatomic location and colloid osmotic pressure of plasma proteins account for the rapid absorption requirements.[1]

Transport Mechanisms

Basic mechanisms of transport through the tubular membrane can be divided into active transport and passive transport. Active transport is the net movement of particles across a membrane against an electrochemical gradient, generally at the cost of metabolic energy. Passive transport involves the movement of substances across membranes and relies on either concentration gradients or chemical gradients. Active transport can be further divided into primary active transport, which requires energy, and secondary active transport, which does not require energy. Most primary active transport is for sodium. Secondary active transport is a result of the movement of sodium from the tubular lumen to the interior of the cell. For example, the active transport of sodium pulls glucose and amino acids with it. Because a carrier protein in the membrane combines with sodium and glucose, the process is termed cotransport. In addition to glucose and amino acids, chloride, phosphate, calcium, magnesium, and hydrogen ions are cotransported.

Some substances are actively secreted into the renal tubule in exchange for other molecules. Hydrogen, potassium, and urate ions are secreted in this manner. Hydrogen and potassium are generally secreted in exchange for sodium in a process termed countertransport.

When substances are actively transported from the tubule to the peritubular capillary bed, a concentration gradient that causes passive absorption of water by osmosis is established. When positive ions are actively transported, negative ions follow to maintain electrical neutrality. Chloride ions and urea are examples of substances that are passively absorbed.[1]

Proximal Tubule

At any given time, each portion of the renal nephron is selective regarding what is reabsorbed or secreted. Active transport of sodium is the primary function of the proximal tubule. Water, most electrolytes, and organic substances are cotransported with sodium. The osmotic force generated by active sodium transport promotes passive diffusion of water out of the tubules into the peritubular capillaries. Passive transport of water is further enhanced by the elevated osmotic pressure of the blood in the peritubular capillaries. Reabsorption of water leaves an increased concentration of urea within the tubular lumen, thereby creating a gradient for its passive diffusion into the peritubular plasma. As positively charged sodium ions leave the tubular lumen, negatively charged chloride ions passively follow to maintain electroneutrality. Hydrogen ions are actively secreted in exchange for sodium. Secretory transport of sodium also occurs in the proximal tubule.

As the filtrate passes along the proximal tubule, 60% to 70% of filtered sodium and water, 50% of urea, as well as potassium, calcium, phosphate, uric acid, and the bicarbonate (HCO_3) form of carbon dioxide (CO_2) have been reabsorbed. Glucose, proteins, amino acids, acetoacetate ions, and vitamins are completely or almost completely reabsorbed by active processes. Because protein molecules are too large to be reabsorbed by normal mechanisms, a special mechanism called pinocytosis is used to save proteins. In this process, the tubular membrane engulfs the protein and internalizes it. Once inside the cell, the protein is digested into amino acids that can then be absorbed into the interstitial fluid.[2]

Loop of Henle

The primary function of the loop of Henle is to establish a hyperosmotic state within the medullary area of the kidney, a function vital to conserve salt and water. Water conservation and the production of concentrated urine involve a countercurrent exchange system. The countercurrent exchange system uses a concentration gradient causing fluid to be exchanged across parallel pathways. The fluid moves up and down the parallel sides of the hairpin loop of Henle in the medulla; the longer the loop, the greater the concentration gradient. As the gradient increases from the cortex to the medulla, movement of water is enhanced. Sluggish blood flow in the vasa recta assists in maintaining the gradient. The countercurrent mechanism is described in the section Concentration and Dilution of Urine—Countercurrent Multiplication.

Late Distal Tubule

In the late distal tubule, sodium, under the influence of aldosterone, is reabsorbed. In this area, potassium is secreted into the lumen in exchange for sodium. It is mainly by this means that the potassium concentration is controlled in the extracellular fluids of the body.

The late distal tubule also secretes hydrogen against a concentration gradient. This function has a role in acid-base balance and determines the final degree of urine acidification. The late distal tubule reabsorbs 10% of filtered water. This area is permeable to water only in the presence of antidiuretic hormone (ADH).[1,2]

Collecting Duct

Collecting duct permeability to water is controlled by ADH plasma levels, which determine urine concentration. When this neurohypophyseal hormone is present, water is reabsorbed into the medullary interstitium, and the urine volume is reduced and concentrated. The collecting duct can also secrete hydrogen, and therefore, has a role in acid-base balance. Fig. 32.5 illustrates renal blood flow, filtration, reabsorption, and secretion.[1]

Renal Secretion

In addition to renin, hydrogen, and potassium, the kidneys release erythropoietin, a glycoprotein stimulating red blood cell production in the bone marrow. Any condition that causes the quantity of oxygen transported to the tissues to decrease stimulates the release of erythropoietin, production of red blood cells, and correction of hypoxia. A clinical diagnosis of anemia emerges when both kidneys are destroyed by renal disease.[1,2]

Renal Hormones

Aldosterone

Several hormones affect renal function. Aldosterone, the chief mineralocorticoid produced by the adrenal cortex, affects the distal segment of the nephron, causing the reabsorption of sodium and water. Several physiologic control systems regulate aldosterone release potassium concentration in extracellular fluid, the renin-angiotensin system, and sodium concentration in extracellular fluid. Of these, potassium is the strongest trigger, followed by renin and then sodium, respectively.[2]

Antidiuretic Hormone

ADH, a hormone synthesized in the hypothalamus but released from the neurohypophysis, also has the distal nephron as its target tissue. Because the distal tubule and collecting ducts are almost totally impermeable to water in the absence of ADH, water is not reabsorbed and is lost in the urine. In the presence of ADH, tubular permeability is increased, and water is reabsorbed. The release of ADH is controlled by the osmotic concentration of the extracellular fluids (Fig. 32.6). Osmoreceptors located near the hypothalamus sense extracellular fluid concentration and release ADH accordingly. ADH is inhibited by a stretch of atrial baroreceptors.[1,2]

Angiotensin

Angiotensin is a hormone that has a direct renal effect, as well as a general systemic effect. As previously discussed, renin is a small protein enzyme released by the kidneys. Stimuli for the release of renin include β-adrenergic stimulation, decreased perfusion to the afferent arterioles, and reduction in sodium delivery to the distal convoluted tubule. Once released, renin acts on hepatic angiotensinogen to form angiotensin I. ACE converts angiotensin I to angiotensin II in the lung. In addition to causing powerful vasoconstriction, angiotensin II stimulates aldosterone release from the adrenal cortex. Aldosterone increases salt and water retention by the kidneys. Both these actions increase arterial pressure.[1,3]

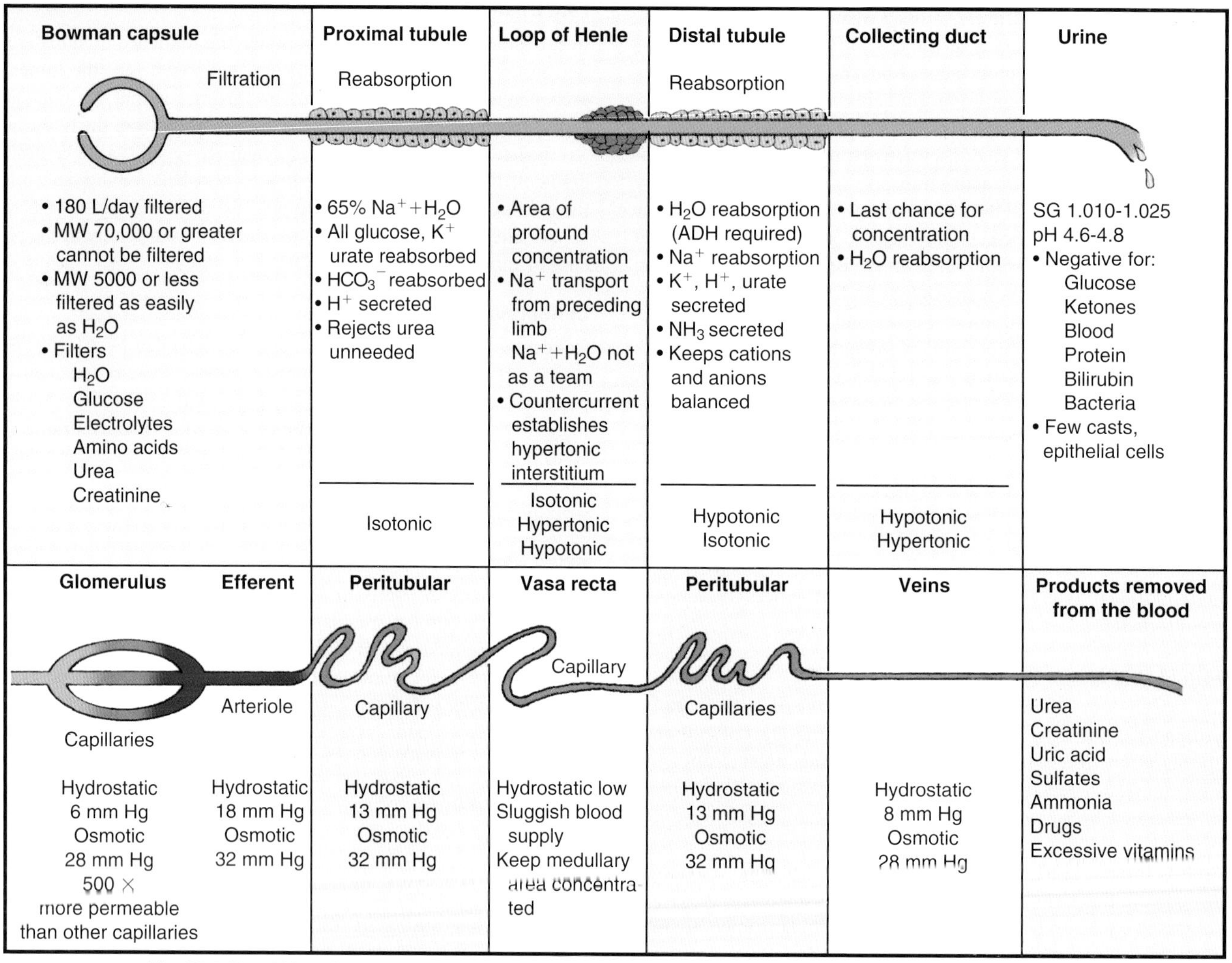

Bowman capsule		Proximal tubule	Loop of Henle	Distal tubule	Collecting duct	Urine
	Filtration	Reabsorption		Reabsorption		

• 180 L/day filtered
• MW 70,000 or greater cannot be filtered
• MW 5000 or less filtered as easily as H_2O
• Filters
  H_2O
  Glucose
  Electrolytes
  Amino acids
  Urea
  Creatinine
		• 65% Na^++H_2O
		• All glucose, K^+ urate reabsorbed
		• HCO_3^- reabsorbed
		• H^+ secreted
		• Rejects urea unneeded
			• Area of profound concentration
			• Na^+ transport from preceding limb
			  Na^++H_2O not as a team
			• Countercurrent establishes hypertonic interstitium
				• H_2O reabsorption (ADH required)
				• Na^+ reabsorption
				• K^+, H^+, urate secreted
				• NH_3 secreted
				• Keeps cations and anions balanced
					• Last chance for concentration
					• H_2O reabsorption
						SG 1.010-1.025
						pH 4.6-4.8
						• Negative for:
						  Glucose
						  Ketones
						  Blood
						  Protein
						  Bilirubin
						  Bacteria
						• Few casts, epithelial cells

		Isotonic	Isotonic Hypertonic Hypotonic	Hypotonic Isotonic	Hypotonic Hypertonic	

Glomerulus	Efferent	Peritubular	Vasa recta	Peritubular	Veins	Products removed from the blood
	Arteriole	Capillary	Capillary	Capillaries		Urea Creatinine Uric acid Sulfates Ammonia Drugs Excessive vitamins
Capillaries						
Hydrostatic 6 mm Hg Osmotic 28 mm Hg 500 × more permeable than other capillaries	Hydrostatic 18 mm Hg Osmotic 32 mm Hg	Hydrostatic 13 mm Hg Osmotic 32 mm Hg	Hydrostatic low Sluggish blood supply Keep medullary area concentrated	Hydrostatic 13 mm Hg Osmotic 32 mm Hg	Hydrostatic 8 mm Hg Osmotic 28 mm Hg	

Fig. 32.5 Renal blood flow, filtration, reabsorption, and secretion. *ADH*, Antidiuretic hormone; *SG*, specific gravity.

Atrial Natriuretic Factor

Atrial natriuretic factor (ANF) is a peptide hormone synthesized, stored, and secreted by the cardiac atria.[4] It acts on the kidney to increase urine flow and sodium excretion, and it may enhance renal blood flow and GFR. In addition, ANF antagonizes both the release and end-organ effects of renin, aldosterone, and ADH. The stimulus for ANF release is atrial distention, stretch, or pressure. ANF is one of the most potent diuretics known. Inhibition of plasma renin, angiotensin, and aldosterone can produce a dose-dependent decrease in blood pressure.[1,2]

Vitamin D

Vitamin D, along with parathyroid hormone and calcitonin, has a vital role in calcium metabolism. Vitamin D, or cholecalciferol, is obtained in the diet or synthesized by the action of ultraviolet radiation on cholesterol in the skin. To become active, cholecalciferol is first hydroxylated in the kidney to 25-hydroxycholecalciferol, then in the liver to 1,25-dihydroxycholecalciferol. Advanced renal disease is associated with abnormal serum calcium levels.[2]

Prostaglandins

Prostaglandins (PGs) such as PGE_2 and thromboxane A_2 modulate the renal effects of other hormones. PGE_2 is a vasodilator, and thromboxane A_2 produces contraction of vascular smooth muscle. Renal PGs influence renal excretion.[1,2]

Renal Regulation of Acid-Base Balance

The kidneys, along with protein buffers and the respiratory system, play a major role in regulating acid base balance. Epithelial cells of the proximal tubules, the thick portion of the loop of Henle, distal tubules, and collecting ducts secrete hydrogen into the tubular fluid. This secretory process begins with CO_2 in the epithelial cells, where, under the influence of carbonic anhydrase, CO_2 combines with water to form carbonic acid (H_2CO_3). H_2CO_3 dissociates into HCO_3 and hydrogen ions, and hydrogen ions are actively secreted into tubular fluid in exchange for sodium ions. This exchange maintains appropriate electrical balance between anions and cations in the tubular fluid.

An increase in HCO_3 in alkalosis means that the filtered amount of HCO_3 exceeds the amount of hydrogen secreted. Because excess HCO_3 must react with hydrogen ($HCO_3^- + H^+ \rightarrow H_2CO_3 \rightarrow CO_2^- + H_2O$) and be absorbed as CO_2, excess HCO_3 ions are lost in the urine along with sodium. In this way, sodium and excess HCO_3 are removed from the extracellular fluid.

In acidosis, the concentration of hydrogen ions increases to a level far greater than that of HCO_3 in the tubules. Excess hydrogen ions are lost in the urine through the phosphate or ammonia (NH_3) buffer system.

The phosphate buffer is composed of hydrogen phosphate (HPO_2^-) and dihydrogen phosphate (H_2PO_4). Both these ions become concentrated in the tubular fluid because of poor reabsorption. The quantity of HPO_2^- is normally fourfold that of H_2PO_4. Excess hydrogen ions

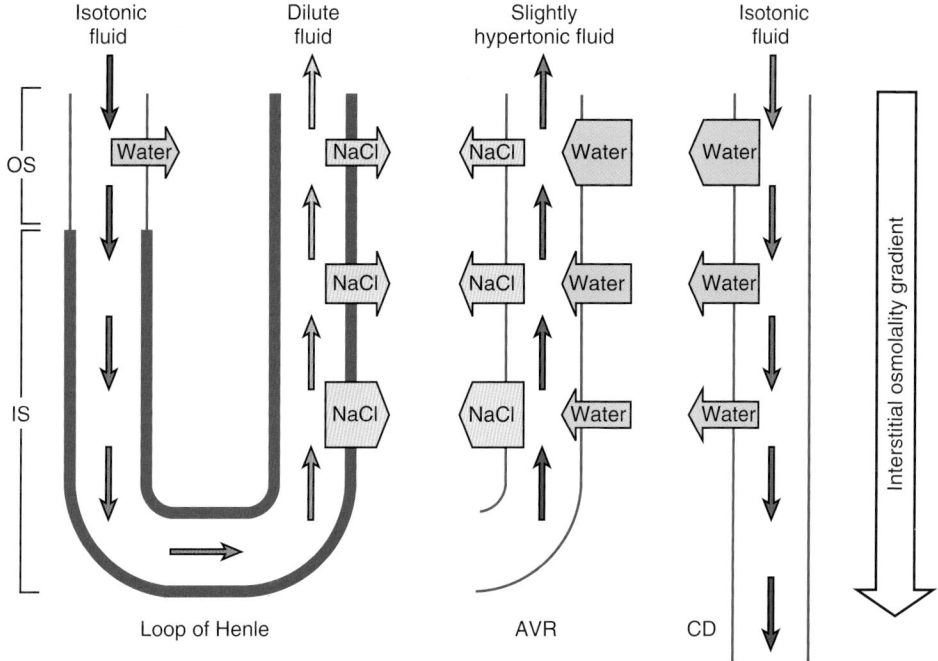

Fig. 32.6 Outer medullary concentrating mechanism based on NaCl addition to the interstitium but without water absorption from descending limbs of short loops. Arrows indicate water *(cyan)* and NaCl *(yellow)* transepithelial transport; arrow widths suggest relative transport magnitudes. Isotonic fluid is considered to have the same osmolality as blood plasma. Flow entering the ascending vas rectum *(AVR)* is assumed to arise from a descending vas rectum that is in, or near, a vascular bundle. Outflow from collecting duct *(CD)* enters the inner medullary CD. Tubule fluid flow direction is indicated by blue arrows; increasing osmolality is indicated by darkening shades of blue. Thick blue lines indicate that a tubule is impermeable to water; thin lines indicate high permeability to water. *IS,* Inner stripe; *OS,* outer stripe. (From Sands JM, et al. Urine concentration and dilution. In: Yu ASL, et al., eds. *Brenner and Rector's The Kidney.* 11th ed. St. Louis: Elsevier; 2020:274.)

entering the tubules combine with monohydrogen phosphate to form H_2PO_4, which is lost in the urine. A sodium ion is absorbed into the extracellular fluid in exchange for hydrogen. It combines with HCO_3, which was formed in the process of secretion of the hydrogen, and sodium bicarbonate is added to the extracellular fluid.

NH_3, which is synthesized by all epithelial cells except those in the thin segment of the loop of Henle, is also secreted into the tubules. NH_3 reacts with hydrogen to form the ammonium ion (NH_4). Ammonium ions are lost in the urine with chloride and other tubular anions.

The kidneys control extracellular fluid hydrogen concentration by excreting an acidic or basic urine. Excretion of acidic urine removes excess acid from the extracellular fluid, whereas loss of basic urine removes base from the extracellular fluid.[1,2]

Concentration and Dilution of Urine—Countercurrent Multiplication

Doubts have arisen about whether the classic countercurrent multiplication process, as conceptualized, provides an accurate representation of how the gradient is generated in the outer medulla. Newer theories state that the outer medullary osmolality gradient arises principally from vigorous active transport of NaCl, without accompanying water, from the thick ascending limbs of short- and long-looped nephrons. The tubule fluid of the thick limbs that enters the cortex is diluted well below plasma osmolality, and thus, the requirement of mass balance is met. This osmolality imbalance will facilitate water withdrawal from the descending limbs of long loops and from collecting ducts. Descending vasa recta are thought to be found only in the vascular bundles. Thus, the ascending vasa recta will act as the collectors of any

NaCl that is absorbed from loops of Henle and water that is absorbed from the descending limbs of long loops and from collecting ducts.

The countercurrent configuration of the ascending vasa recta, relative to the descending limbs and collecting ducts, is likely to participate in sustaining the axial gradient: As ascending vasa recta fluid ascends toward the cortex, its osmolality will exceed that in the descending limbs of long loops and in the collecting ducts. Ascending vasa recta fluid will be progressively diluted as that fluid contributes to the concentrating of fluid in descending limbs of long loops and in collecting ducts by giving up NaCl to, and absorbing water from, the interstitium (see Fig. 32.6).[5]

EFFECTS OF ANESTHESIA ON NORMAL RENAL FUNCTION

Before considering anesthetic implications for patients with renal disease, it is important to review the effects of anesthesia and surgery on normal renal function. As expected, anesthesia tends to depress normal renal function. Some differences exist among anesthetics and are discussed in the next section.

Anesthetic Effects

General anesthesia is associated with a temporary depression of renal blood flow, GFR, urinary flow, and electrolyte excretion. Although similar changes occur after spinal and epidural anesthesia, the magnitude of change tends to parallel the degree of sympathetic block and cardiovascular depression. This consistent and generalized depression of renal function has been attributed to several factors, including type and duration of surgical procedure, physical status of the patient, volume and electrolyte status, depth of anesthesia, and choice of agent.[5]

Anesthesia may alter renal function by direct or indirect effects. Indirect effects are mediated through changes in the circulatory, endocrine, or sympathetic nervous system. Anesthetic drugs alter the circulatory system by decreasing renal perfusion, increasing renal vascular resistance, or a combination of both. Drugs associated with catecholamine release lead to vasoconstriction, an increase in renal vascular resistance, a decrease in renal blood flow, and a decrease in renal function. Volatile agents such as isoflurane, desflurane, and sevoflurane cause a mild to moderate increase in renal vascular resistance as a compensatory response to decreased perfusion pressure secondary to alterations in cardiac output or systemic vascular resistance.[6-8] Desflurane has been shown to produce hemodynamic effects comparable to those produced by isoflurane.[5] It increases heart rate and decreases both MAP and systemic vascular resistance while maintaining cardiac output. In some studies, but not all, desflurane maintains arterial pressure and systemic vascular resistance to a greater degree than equianesthetic concentrations of isoflurane. Otherwise, desflurane and isoflurane have similar effects on most vascular beds, including the renal circulation.[6]

Issues regarding the renal effects of the release of free fluoride ion associated with sevoflurane metabolism have been debated. Historically, after methoxyflurane metabolism, high fluoride ion concentrations in the range of 60 to 90 μmol/L have led to nephrotoxicity characterized by polyuria. This methoxyflurane polyuria was commonly referred to as high-output renal failure. Although previously promoted to cause nephrotoxicity, sevoflurane has not produced the expected toxicity in the same way as methoxyflurane even though significant fluoride ion levels may result from prolonged administration. Methoxyflurane is not currently available in the United States. A few reasons have been theorized for the lack of nephrotoxicity of sevoflurane, even though levels of metabolically released fluoride ions can approach those of methoxyflurane. Prevailing theories are based on the fact sevoflurane metabolism is largely hepatic rather than renal. Intrarenal production of inorganic fluoride may be a more important factor than hepatic metabolism for the nephrotoxicity produced by increased serum fluoride concentration. Sevoflurane also has very low blood solubility and undergoes rapid elimination. Sevoflurane has not been associated with nephrotoxicity.[9-11]

Changes in renal function during opiate and nitrous oxide anesthesia are similar to those observed during the administration of low-dose volatile anesthesia. Preoperative hydration, lower concentrations of volatile anesthetics, and maintenance of normal blood pressure attenuate reductions in renal blood flow and GFR.[12,13] In a recent large cohort study of 138,081 noncardiac surgical patients, the incidence of acute kidney injury (AKI) was 9%. Major factors identifying patients at risk for AKI included anemia, estimated GFR, elevated risk surgery, American Society of Anesthesiologists (ASA) physical status classification, and expected anesthesia duration. The relationship between hypotension and AKI varied by underlying patient and procedural risk. Patients with low risk demonstrated no associated increased risk of AKI across all blood pressure ranges, whereas patients with the highest baseline risk demonstrated an association between even mild absolute intraoperative hypotension ranges and AKI.[14]

High levels of spinal or epidural anesthesia can impair venous return, diminish cardiac output, and reduce renal perfusion.[15-18] Epidural blocks at thoracic levels with epinephrine-containing local anesthetics cause moderate reductions in renal blood flow and GFR that parallel the decrease in mean blood pressure. Epidural blocks performed with epinephrine-free solutions generate little change in systemic hemodynamics; however, absorption of local anesthetics is enhanced in uremic patients.[18]

In summary, virtually all anesthetics have the potential to alter the physiologic state, usually depressing the cardiovascular system and affecting renal blood flow, GFR, and urinary output. Although systolic arterial blood pressure may not fall below 80 to 90 mm Hg, renal blood flow may be decreased by 30% to 40% after the administration of various anesthetics. This suggests impairment of autoregulation. In most cases, changes in renal function are transient and reversible. If they persist into the postoperative period, the cause is often a combination of factors such as preexisting renal or cardiovascular disease, significant intraoperative hypotension or severe fluid imbalance, and the importance of the direct anesthetic effects is decreased.[5,13,14]

Physiologic Responses

The renal vasculature is richly innervated by the sympathetic nervous system. Drugs or perioperative events that stimulate this system cause an increase in renal vascular resistance and a decrease in renal blood flow and glomerular filtration. Surgical stress may also alter autonomic and neuroendocrine responses. Norepinephrine from sympathetic postganglionic nerve fibers and epinephrine and norepinephrine from the adrenal medulla shift blood away from the cortical nephrons, resulting in decreases in renal blood flow, GFR, electrolyte excretion, and urinary output. Catecholamines also stimulate the release of renin, which ultimately leads to the production of angiotensin II, a potent vasoconstrictor.

Neuroendocrine changes associated with anesthesia and surgical stress involves ADH, aldosterone, and the renin-angiotensin-aldosterone system. Although the perioperative period is associated with high circulating levels of ADH and aldosterone, it is not clear whether anesthetics stimulate the release or the release is secondary to the surgical stress response. General anesthetics and opioids may cause a minor stimulus to release ADH. Laparoscopic surgical procedures have been shown to increase ADH levels. Clinical studies have specifically identified that pneumoperitoneum during laparoscopic surgery increases the level of ADH. Other studies indicate anesthetics lasting long durations had significant increases in ADH, with the greatest increase occurring at emergence.[19] Additional investigations have shown that ADH levels increase after the induction of anesthesia and are higher in subjects receiving lower concentrations of remifentanil-propofol anesthesia.[20]

ADH release is modulated by blood volume changes sensed by atrial wall stretch receptors. Hemorrhage, positive pressure ventilation, and upright positions increase ADH release.[21,22] A decrease in arterial pressure stimulates ADH release. Distention of a balloon in the atrium, negative pressure ventilation, and immersion in water up to the neck decrease ADH release.

Renin-angiotensin levels may be elevated during the perioperative period, but the role of anesthetics and stress is not clear. Some studies have reported large increases in plasma renin levels associated with the use of anesthetics, whereas others report variances dependent on type of anesthesia delivered, as well as surgical procedure. Balanced anesthesia has been found to result in higher levels of epinephrine, norepinephrine, and adrenocorticotropic hormones than total intravenous anesthesia.[23] Renin levels have been shown to increase during laparoscopic surgery, as well as levels of vasopressin, epinephrine, norepinephrine, and cortisol.[24] Hydration status prior to the start of surgery may play an important role in the intraoperative release of renin.[2]

Aldosterone, a hormone released from the adrenal gland, is responsible for the precise control of sodium excretion. It is not known whether anesthetic agents act directly on the adrenal gland to cause aldosterone release. Most likely, there is indirect influence through the neuroendocrine system and the renin-angiotensin-aldosterone system. Stimulation of the sympathetic nervous system causes renal vasoconstriction, which is a trigger for the renin-angiotensin-aldosterone system. Aldosterone leads to sodium and water reabsorption and can be associated with decreased urinary output.[2]

Nephrotoxicity of Anesthetic Agents

The kidneys are extremely vulnerable to toxicity because of their rich blood supply and the increase in concentration of excreted compounds occurring in the renal tubules during the process of reabsorption. Medullary hyperosmolality encourages concentration of all substances, including toxins. The amount of renal damage associated with nephrotoxic agents depends on (1) the concentration of the toxins, (2) the degree of toxin binding to plasma proteins and nonrenal versus renal tissue, and (3) the length of exposure of the kidneys to the toxin. Evidence indicates the release of the inorganic fluoride ions (F−) in the metabolism of the fluorinated anesthetic methoxyflurane was the causative agent in nephrotoxicity. Fortunately, none of the modern inhalation anesthetics are nephrotoxic.[5]

Fluoride Ion Toxicity

Fluoride alters renal concentration mechanisms by interfering with active transport of sodium and chloride in the medullary portions of the loop of Henle. It also acts as a potent vasodilator, resulting in increased vasa recta blood flow and washout of medullary solute. Fluoride is a potent inhibitor of many enzyme systems, including those involving ADH, which is necessary for distal nephron reabsorption of water. Proximal tubular swelling and necrosis associated with fluoride ions also contribute to nephrotoxicity. Signs and symptoms of fluoride nephrotoxicity include polyuria, hypernatremia, serum hyperosmolality, elevations in blood urea nitrogen (BUN) and serum creatinine levels, and decreased creatinine clearance. The extent of nephrotoxicity in general surgical patients has been correlated with dosage or maximum allowable concentration hours (MAC-hours), duration, and peak fluoride concentrations.[25]

Isoflurane

Isoflurane is only slightly metabolized, and defluorinated much less than other halogenated agents. In one report of nine surgical patients, mean peak serum fluoride concentration measured 6 hours after anesthesia was only 4.4 µmol.[26] Clinical experience has indicated that renal toxicity does not occur after the administration of isoflurane.

Desflurane

The metabolism of desflurane has been assessed in both animals and humans with the appearance of fluoride metabolites (fluoride ion, nonvolatile organic fluoride, trifluoroacetic acid) in blood and urine. Administration of desflurane to rats that were either pretreated or not pretreated with phenobarbital or ethanol for 3.2 MAC-hours, as well as to swine for 5.5 MAC-hours, produced fluoride levels in blood that were almost indistinguishable from values measured in control animals.[27] In human studies, desflurane administered to patients for 3.1 MAC-hours and volunteers for 7.3 MAC-hours resulted in postanesthesia serum fluoride concentrations that did not differ from background fluoride concentrations. Similarly, postanesthesia urinary excretion rates of fluoride and organic fluoride in volunteers were comparable with preanesthetic excretion rates.[28] Small but statistically significant increases in the levels of trifluoroacetic acid were found in both the serum and urine of volunteers after exposure to desflurane. Although these increases in trifluoroacetic acid were statistically significant, they were approximately one-tenth the levels seen after exposure to isoflurane. Desflurane strongly resists biodegradation, and only a small amount is metabolized in animals and humans. Desflurane does not produce nephrotoxicity.

Sevoflurane

Sevoflurane undergoes approximately 5% to 8% metabolism, and the primary metabolites are fluoride and hexafluoroisopropanol (HFIP).

The oxidative defluorination of sevoflurane in the liver with the liberation of free fluoride ions raised concerns in the past that sevoflurane, like methoxyflurane, might impair the ability of the kidneys to concentrate urine. Earlier research indicated that with methoxyflurane, renal dysfunction was likely to occur when plasma fluoride levels exceeded 50 µmol. The same does not appear to be true with sevoflurane.

Numerous published reports indicate the absence of renal toxicity after sevoflurane anesthesia. As mentioned previously, an explanation for the absence of fluoride-induced nephrotoxicity may be a lower intrarenal production of fluoride ions, which is important in the pathogenesis of this complication. The intrarenal metabolism of methoxyflurane is four times greater than that of sevoflurane.

Studies of surgical patients receiving intermediate-duration sevoflurane with high and low fresh gas flow and long-duration sevoflurane with high fresh gas flow included sensitive measures of renal function or injury. These studies also indicate the absence of renal toxicity after sevoflurane anesthesia.

In addition to the release of inorganic fluoride ions resulting from biotransformation, CO_2 absorbents degrade sevoflurane, causing the production of a type of vinyl ether called compound A. This reaction occurs in the anesthesia machine, and the resulting toxin, compound A, is then delivered to the patient via the machine breathing system. Factors associated with the generation of higher levels of compound A during administration of sevoflurane to patients include (1) higher concentration of the agent, (2) increased temperature in CO_2 absorbent, (3) low fresh gas flow rates, (4) increased states of CO_2 production, and (5) absorbents containing strong base activators such as sodium or potassium hydroxide. The potential for compound A nephrotoxicity theoretically exists although no reports of problems in clinical practice have been reported.[25]

Because the potential for renal injury exists with sevoflurane, studies in volunteers have raised the question of whether it is important to apply more sensitive measures of renal function in evaluation of this drug. Such tests have included urine concentrations or excretion of enzymes, albumin, protein, and glucose and creatinine clearance. The only proven direct toxic effect of any anesthetic agent is the fluoride-related toxicity of methoxyflurane.

Currently, the US Food and Drug Administration (FDA) recommends the use of sevoflurane for a minimum of 1 L/min of fresh gas flow and advise 2 MAC-hours at this flow rate should not be exceeded. The use of newer carbon dioxide absorbents (e.g., Litholyme, which does not react with sevoflurane) to replace soda lime–type absorbents in modern anesthesia practice has virtually eliminated any concern regarding compound A toxicity.[5,10]

ACUTE KIDNEY INJURY

AKI describes the clinical syndrome formerly called acute renal failure (ARF). AKI is defined as a renal functional or structural abnormality manifesting within 48 hours as determined by blood, urine, or tissue tests or by imaging studies. Diagnostically, the reduction in kidney function is associated with either an absolute increase in serum creatinine of 0.3 mg/dL or a percentage increase in serum creatinine of 50%. In addition, a reduction in urine output with oliguria (<0.5 mL/kg/hr) for more than 6 hours also fulfills the diagnostic criteria. Classifications are based on urine flow rates as nonoliguric (urine output >400 mL/day), oliguric (urine output <400 mL/day), or anuric (urine output <100 mL/day).

Most episodes of AKI occur in the hospital, and AKI is most common among patients in intensive care units (ICUs). After adjusting for age-related renal decline over the past 5 years, diabetic patients diagnosed with AKI increased by 139% (from 23.1 to 55.3 per 1000 persons). In the same period, nondiabetic patients' rate of increase was 230% (from 3.5 to 11.7 per 1000 persons).[29] By contrast, the incidence of community-acquired AKI is less than 1%.

BOX 32.1 Causes of Prerenal Acute Kidney Injury

Intravascular Volume Depletion
- Hemorrhage—trauma, surgery, postpartum, gastrointestinal
- Gastrointestinal losses—diarrhea, vomiting, nasogastric tube loss
- Renal losses—diuretic use, osmotic diuresis, diabetes insipidus
- Skin and mucous membrane losses—burns, hyperthermia
- Nephrotic syndrome
- Cirrhosis
- Capillary leak

Reduced Cardiac Output
- Cardiogenic shock
- Pericardial diseases—restrictive, constrictive, tamponade
- Congestive heart failure
- Valvular diseases
- Pulmonary diseases—pulmonary hypertension, pulmonary embolism
- Sepsis

Systemic Vasodilation
- Sepsis
- Cirrhosis
- Anaphylaxis
- Drugs

Renal Vasoconstriction
- Early sepsis
- Hepatorenal syndrome
- Acute hypercalcemia
- Drugs—norepinephrine, vasopressin, nonsteroidal antiinflammatory drugs, angiotensin-converting enzyme inhibitors, calcineurin inhibitors
- Iodinated contrast agents

Increased Intraabdominal Pressure
- Abdominal compartment syndrome

From Weisbord SD, Palevsky PM, et al. Prevention and management of acute kidney injury. In: Yu ASL, et al., eds. *Brenner & Rector's The Kidney.* 11th ed. Philadelphia: Elsevier; 2020:940–971.

TABLE 32.1 Major Causes of Intrinsic Acute Kidney Injury

Tubular Injury	
Ischemia due to hypoperfusion	Hypovolemia, sepsis, hemorrhage, cirrhosis, congestive heart failure
Endogenous toxins	Myoglobin, hemoglobin, paraproteinemia, uric acid
Exogenous toxins	Antibiotics, chemotherapy agents, radiocontrast, media, phosphate preparations
Tubulointerstitial Injury	
Acute allergic interstitial nephritis	Nonsteroidal antiinflammatory drugs, antibiotics
Infections	Viral, bacterial, and fungal infections
Infiltration Allograft rejection	Lymphoma, leukemia, sarcoid
Glomerular Injury	
Inflammation	Anti-glomerular basement membrane disease, antineutrophil cytoplasmic autoantibody disease, infection, cryoglobulinemia, membranoproliferative glomerulonephritis, immunoglobulin A nephropathy, systemic lupus erythematosus, Henoch-Schönlein purpura, polyarteritis nodosa
Hematologic disorders	Hemolytic uremic syndrome, thrombotic thrombocytopenic purpura, drugs
Renal Microvasculature	
	Malignant hypertension, toxemia of pregnancy, hypercalcemia, radiocontrast media, scleroderma, drugs
Large Vessels	
Arteries	Thrombosis, vasculitis, dissection, thromboembolism, atheroembolism, trauma
Veins	Thrombosis, compression, trauma

From Weisbord SD, Palevsky PM, et al. Prevention and management of acute kidney injury. In: Yu ASL, et al., eds. *Brenner & Rector's The Kidney.* 11th ed. Philadelphia: Elsevier; 2020:940.

AKI is usually divided into three broad pathophysiologic categories based on cause:

1. Prerenal AKI: diseases characterized by effective hypoperfusion of the kidneys in which there is no parenchymal damage to the kidney
2. Intrinsic AKI: diseases involving the renal parenchyma
3. Postrenal (obstructive) AKI: diseases associated with acute obstruction of the urinary tract

Each of the categories represents a unique pathophysiologic process with distinctive diagnostic parameters and prognosis. Causes of prerenal (Box 32.1), intrinsic (Table 32.1), and postrenal (Box 32.2) AKI are summarized.

Classification

Historically, AKI was classified according to urine output: oliguric, nonoliguric, or polyuric, or by its predominant cause: prerenal, renal, or postrenal. Oliguria is defined as a urinary flow rate less than 0.5 mL/kg/hour. Polyuric failure is associated with elevations of BUN and serum creatinine levels and is characterized by urine flow rates that exceed 2.5 L/day.[30] Prerenal AKI results from hemodynamic or endocrine factors impairing renal perfusion, intrinsic AKI results from tissue damage, and postrenal AKI results from urinary tract obstruction.

Current classification focuses on serum creatinine clearance and urinary output as markers for severity of injury: Acute Dialysis Quality Initiative's RIFLE (risk of renal dysfunction, injury to the kidney, failure of kidney function, loss of kidney function, and end-stage renal disease [ESRD]) or the Acute Kidney Injury Network's (AKIN) stages 1 through 3. Both classifications demonstrate that serum creatinine clearance is a sensitive marker for AKI, as opposed to urine output. Well-established classifications delineate kidney injury progression from an at-risk standpoint to complete ESRD.[29,31-33] Table 32.2 shows the RIFLE and AKIN classification systems. Additional markers, such as urine creatinine levels, angiotensinogen, or presence of proteinuria can be used in conjunction with RIFLE or AKIN classifications to aid in diagnosing the severity of AKI. However, use of diuretics must be factored in before using these additional biomarkers.[30,34,35] For these reasons, the current preferred definition for AKI diagnosis is the Kidney Disease: Improving Global Outcomes (KDIGO) definition and staging system. The main difference between the KDIGO criteria and the RIFLE classification in that the KDIGO criteria examines serum creatinine and urine output only, while the RIFLE classification also includes changes in GFR for staging in adult patients. Just like the RIFLE and AKIN classification systems that rely solely on changes

BOX 32.2 Causes of Postrenal Acute Kidney Injury

Upper Urinary Tract Extrinsic Causes
- Retroperitoneal space—lymph nodes, tumors
- Pelvic or intraabdominal tumors—cervix, uterus, ovary, prostate
- Fibrosis—radiation, drugs, inflammatory conditions
- Ureteral ligation or surgical trauma
- Granulomatous diseases
- Hematoma

Lower Urinary Tract Causes
- Prostate—benign prostatic hypertrophy, carcinoma, infection
- Bladder—neck obstruction, calculi, carcinoma, infection (schistosomiasis)
- Functional—neurogenic bladder secondary to spinal cord injury, diabetes, multiple sclerosis, stroke, pharmacologic side effects of drugs (anticholinergics, antidepressants)
- Urethral—posterior urethral valves, strictures, trauma, infections, tuberculosis, tumors

Upper Urinary Tract Intrinsic Causes
- Nephrolithiasis
- Strictures
- Edema
- Debris, blood clots, sloughed papillae, fungal ball
- Malignancy

From Weisbord SD, Palevsky PM, et al. Prevention and management of acute kidney injury. In: Yu ASL, et al., eds. *Brenner & Rectors The Kidney.* 11th ed. Philadelphia: Elsevier; 2020:940–971.

in creatinine or urine output, limitations are associated with KDIGO criteria for AKI.[34] Therefore, an examination of the patient's clinical presentation is important, in addition to using a classification system when determining the diagnosis of AKI.

Prerenal conditions leading to urine output reductions include acute reductions in GFR, excessive reabsorption of salt or water, or both. Increases in circulating levels of catecholamines, ADH, or aldosterone are physiologic factors that can decrease urinary output.[33] If not reversed, initial stages of AKI may progress to injury, tissue loss, or ESRD with progressively increasing mortality rates.[35,36]

Acute tubular necrosis may be produced by a variety of factors interfering with glomerular filtration or tubular reabsorption. Reabsorption of urea, sodium, and water are all impaired, in contrast to AKI, in which these functions are maintained.[33]

Renal hypoperfusion or a nephrotoxic insult may initiate renal failure. Surgical patients with external and internal fluid losses or sepsis may have renal hypoperfusion. The renal medulla, with its slow blood supply and active transport mechanisms, is especially susceptible to even moderate renal ischemia.

The initiating insult culminates in the development of one or more maintenance factors, such as (1) decreased tubular function, (2) tubular obstruction, (3) sustained reductions in renal blood flow, and (4) glomerular filtration. Urine flow and solute excretion are reduced. Once the maintenance period has begun, pharmacologic interventions to improve renal blood flow do not reverse the failure.

Hemodynamic optimization is crucial in preventing postoperative AKI. Decreasing the need for renal replacement therapy (RRT) decreases AKIN classification and the incidence of progression. Administering fluids and inotropes, to maintain adequate perfusion,

TABLE 32.2 RIFLE, Acute Kidney Injury Network (AKIN), and Kidney Disease: Improving Global Outcomes (KDIGO) Definitions and Staging of Acute Kidney Injury

Definitions

	RIFLE	AKIN	KDIGO
Serum creatinine level	An increase of >50% developing over <7 days	An increase of ≥0.3 mg/dL or of >50% developing over <48 hr	An increase of ≥0.3 mg/dL developing over <48 hr; or an increase of >50% developing over <7 days
Urine output*	<0.5 mL/kg per hr for >6 hr	<0.5 mL/kg per hr for >6 hr	<0.5 mL/kg/hr for >6 hr

Staging Criteria

RIFLE	Increase in Serum Creatinine Level	AKIN	Increase in Serum Creatinine Level	KDIGO	Increase in Serum Creatinine Level	Urine Output*
Risk	≥50%	Stage 1	≥0.3 mg/dL; or ≥50%	Stage 1	≥0.3 mg/dL; or ≥50%	<0.5 mL/kg per hr for >6 hr
Injury	≥100%	Stage 2	≥100%	Stage 2	≥100%	<0.5 mL/kg per hr for >12 hr
Failure	≥200%	Stage 3	≥200%	Stage 3	≥200%	<0.5 mL/kg per hr for >24 hr or anuria for >12 hr
Loss	Need for renal replacement therapy for >4 wk					
End stage	Need for renal replacement therapy for >3 mo					

*The urine output criteria for both definition and staging of acute kidney injury are the same for the RIFLE, AKIN, and KDIGO criteria.
RIFLE, Risk, injury, failure, loss, and end-stage renal disease.
From Weisbord SD, Palevsky PM, et al. Prevention and management of acute kidney injury. In: Yu ASL, et al., eds. *Brenner & Rector's The Kidney.* 11th ed. Philadelphia: Elsevier; 2020:940–971.

TABLE 32.3 Major Risk Factors for the Development of Perioperative Acute Kidney Injury

Patient	Surgery	Other
Chronic diseases of the	Emergency	Acute illness
Kidney	Nonrenal solid organ transplant	Sepsis
Heart failure	Cardiac bypass time	Multiorgan dysfunction
Hypertension	Aortic cross-clamp	
Peripheral arterial	Intraperitoneal surgery	Nephrotoxic drugs
Obstructive	Emergency surgery	ACEi
pulmonary		
Diabetes mellitus	Long-duration surgery	ARB
Alcoholism		Diuretics
Ascites		
Male		Radioopaque intravenous contrast
Obesity	Perioperative hypotension	
High ASA status		
Anemia		
Decreased glomerular filtration rate		

ACEi, Angiotensin-converting enzyme inhibitor; *ARB*, angiotensin receptor blocker; *ASA*, American Society of Anesthesiologists.
Adapted from Golden D, et al. Peri-operative renal dysfunction: prevention and management. *Anaesthesia.* 2016;71:S51–S57; Mathis MR, Naik BI, Freundlich RE, et al. Preoperative risk and the association between hypotension and postoperative acute kidney injury. *Anesthesiology.* 2020;132(3):461–475.

in the pre-, intra-, and postoperative periods, is associated with significantly decreased mortality and less risk of developing AKI.[5,37]

Patients with parenchymal disease have trouble concentrating urine, resulting in urine sodium levels that are high, and osmolality that is low. Renal damage is also associated with a progressive rise in serum urea, creatinine, uric acid, and polypeptide levels. Serum potassium levels increase, and a decrease, or dilution, occurs in the serum levels of sodium, calcium, and proteins such as albumin. Exogenous factors may alter BUN levels, and subtle changes in serum creatinine concentration are easily ignored.[5,33]

Risk Factors

Several conditions may place patients at high risk for acute renal injury. Renal reserve decreases progressively with age. Older patients are less able to cope with fluid and electrolyte imbalance and are more prone to renal damage. In the geriatric population, overall mortality rates associated with AKI increase.[13] As noted previously, in a recent large cohort study of 138,081 noncardiac surgical patients, the incidence of AKI was 9%. Major factors identifying patients at risk for AKI included anemia, estimated GFR, elevated risk surgery, ASA physical status classification, and expected anesthesia duration. The relationship between hypotension and AKI varied by underlying patient and procedural risk. Patients with low risk demonstrated no associated increased risk of AKI across all blood pressure ranges, whereas patients with the highest baseline risk demonstrated an association between even mild absolute intraoperative hypotension ranges and AKI.[14]

Patients with preexisting renal dysfunction are also at high risk. Cardiac and hepatic failure are associated with abnormal renal hemodynamics. Reduced GFR is associated with cortical redistribution of blood flow and salt and water retention. All these aberrations are increased by anesthetics, stress, and hypovolemia. Furthermore, these alterations correlate with greater incidences of postoperative AKI and mortality.[37,38] Elevated bilirubin is related to hepatitis and other liver diseases and is an independent risk factor of AKI.

Certain surgical procedures such as nonrenal solid organ transplants, prolonged cardiac bypass, or aortic cross-clamp time are associated with a higher risk of AKI. The risk increases with (1) preoperative ventricular dysfunction or bacterial endocarditis, (2) emergency or high-risk procedures, and (3) anemia or perioperative blood product administration. Postoperative bleeding with reexploration and low cardiac output requiring use of the intraaortic balloon pump also carry a higher incidence of injury.[31,39,40] Some major risk factors for the development of perioperative AKI are noted in Table 32.3.[14,41]

A ruptured abdominal aortic aneurysm commonly results in hypovolemia, shock, and the need for high aortic cross-clamping. Of these patients, 40% have renal damage, and 11% develop AKI with an associated mortality rate of 80%. Renal dysfunction after elective surgery is less profound if attention is given to adequate hydration and if a brisk diuresis is established before, and maintained during, aortic cross-clamping. The aortic clamp proximity to the renal arteries is critical. Aortic clamp placement above the renal arteries increases the risk of AKI. Aortic arteriography performed just before surgery also increases risk. Predisposing factors include preexisting renal disease with serum creatinine levels greater than 3 mg/dL, proteinuria, diabetes, and hypovolemia. Risk is reduced by (1) minimizing the amount of radiographic dye given, (2) maintaining hydration, and (3) using diuretics such as mannitol to promote diuresis. Postoperative AKI is a common complication of thoracic aorta, thoracoabdominal aorta, and aortic arch surgeries. It is observed in 6% to 18% of such surgical procedures. Predisposing factors for this complication include (1) age older than 50, (2) preoperative renal dysfunction, (3) duration of renal ischemia, and (4) amount of blood transfused.

Mechanical obstruction by calculi or prostatic disease is the most common cause of obstructive uropathy. Risk is increased by the frequent presence of hypovolemia and electrolyte imbalance and by preoperative diagnostic studies that involve the use of dye.

Hypovolemia, decreased pulmonary function, and acidosis are key factors in the development of AKI in septic patients. The use of vasoconstricting adrenergic agonists and antibiotics with nephrotoxic potential can further decrease kidney function in these patients.[35,42,43] The type of replacement fluid (crystalloids vs colloids) is important in patients at risk for developing AKI. There are several studies demonstrating colloid replacement therapy is not superior to crystalloid infusion and may increase the incidence of perioperative AKI. In patients with KDIGO, RIFLE, or AKIN scores indicating the presence of AKI, the need for replacing fluids is based on the hemodynamic parameters. Patients at low risk undergoing minor surgery should receive liberal perioperative fluid replacement (10–30 mL/kg) to reduce postoperative adverse outcomes (i.e., postoperative nausea and vomiting [PONV], pain), whereas patients at high risk undergoing major surgery will likely benefit from more stringent fluid replacement strategies or goal-directed therapy with fluid replaced to maintain urine output between 0.5 and 1.0 mL/kg/hour.[37,44]

Complications of pregnancy such as hemorrhage, amniotic fluid embolus, and toxemia carry a high risk of renal failure, although mortality in this group is reduced because patients are usually young and healthy. Proteinuria, related to or independent of pregnancy, also serves as a major risk factor for the development of AKI.[45]

In the first trimester of pregnancy, hyperemesis gravidum or septic abortion poses a risk for renal injury. Risks in the third trimester include preeclampsia, HELLP (hemolysis, elevated liver enzymes, and low platelet count) syndrome, acute fatty liver of pregnancy, or thrombosis. Diagnosis is by serum creatinine because GFR calculations are complicated due to the altered volume status of pregnant women.[5,10]

Prevention and Management

Prevention of AKI is far more successful than management after its development. Prevention can be based on the following generalizations:

- The most common cause of AKI is prolonged renal hypoperfusion.
- Prophylaxis reduces mortality more effectively dialytic therapy.
- The duration and magnitude of the initiating renal insult are critical in determining the severity of AKI.

A key strategy in reducing the incidence of AKI is limiting the magnitude and duration of renal ischemia. Prevention begins in the preoperative period.[46,47]

Preoperative Strategies

High-risk patients and procedures should be identified. Reversible renal dysfunction should be addressed, and fluid deficits and hypovolemia should be corrected using intravenous fluids and inotropes. Perioperative ADH and renin-angiotensin-aldosterone secretion can be minimized with adequate hydration before anesthetic induction and perioperative attenuation of surgical stress. Administration of saline, such as a balanced salt solution rather than solutions low in sodium, is helpful in prevention of aldosterone secretion, hyponatremia, and oliguria.[5,47]

Oliguria often signals inadequate systemic perfusion, and prevention of AKI requires its rapid recognition through appropriate monitoring and early intervention. In addition to standard monitors and a urinary catheter, monitors for patients with questionable cardiac and pulmonary function should include (1) a direct arterial line for blood pressure monitoring and (2) central venous pressure (CVP), pulmonary artery catheter, or transesophageal echocardiography as applicable for assessment of cardiac function and volume status. Noninvasive perioperative monitoring of cardiac index and other cardiac parameters may also be of value in preventing AKI. The hemodynamic end point should be adequate cardiac output and renal perfusion.[44]

Perioperative Strategies

Use of a urinary catheter is the standard means of monitoring renal function in the operating room. A fluid challenge of 500 to 1000 mL may be necessary if hourly urinary output decreases to below acceptable levels. For patients with renal compromise, 250 mL bolus is a safe alternative.

Diuretics increase urine output but do not decrease chronic renal dysfunction or mortality. The use of diuretics in the face of inadequate urinary output is common; however, it is controversial. Data suggest diuretic use to prevent AKI is not useful. Diuretic use in established AKI offers little benefit in changing outcome of mortality or need for RRT, particularly in the presence of oliguria. Given the current literature, use of diuretics for volume management when necessary in patients with AKI can be considered. However, diuretic use to prevent oliguria in the AKI setting is not indicated.[30,37,48]

High-dose diuretics have been effective in decreasing 60-day mortality rates associated with AKI. Diuretic therapy must be balanced with fluid administration to prevent hypotension and hypoperfusion. The best outcomes have been reported with furosemide and fluid balance to avoid a fluid excess or deficit. Mechanisms for protection include inhibition of sodium reabsorption and prevention of tubular obstruction through the maintenance of high renal tubule flow and pressure and reversal of intrinsic renal vasoconstriction. Prophylactic use of diuretics may be of benefit in the case of jaundice in surgical patients, excessive exposure to contrast media, hyperuricemia, or the presence of pigment in the urine.[30,46]

Fenoldopam (Corlopam) is a selective dopamine-1 (DA_1) receptor agonist. It causes both systemic and renal arteriolar vasodilation and has no effect on dopamine-2 (DA_2), α-adrenergic, or β-adrenergic receptors. Unlike dopamine, which causes renal vasoconstriction and systemic cardiovascular changes at higher doses, fenoldopam at high doses produces renal vasodilation with little systemic effects. Despite theoretically promising pharmacology, clinical benefit with fenoldopam has been limited. Attempts at developing a clinical protocol for the use of fenoldopam in AKI have so far proven unsuccessful. Currently, it is not recommended for use in AKI.[37,49] No benefit in survival or the need for RRT has been noted as compared with placebo. Other therapies under investigation include atrial natriuretic peptide (ANP), urodilatin, and nesiritide. Survival rates may be higher in patients with oliguria, who have not begun dialysis, receiving ANP for treatment of fluid overload.[37]

Treatment of Acute Kidney Injury

Therapy for AKI involves rapid recognition and correction of reversible causes, avoidance of any further renal injury, and correction and maintenance of a normal electrolyte and fluid volumes. Preventive therapy or medical interventions performed early provide the greatest chance for minimizing injury. Hyperkalemia, hyperuremia, metabolic acidosis, and fluid overload are indications for RRT, but it is uncertain what values should precipitate treatment.[43]

Key approaches include (1) administering volume (e.g., normal saline) to achieve euvolemia, (2) improving cardiac output by afterload reduction, and (3) normalizing systemic vascular resistance. Postrenal AKI secondary to prostatic hypertrophy can frequently be corrected by placement of a bladder catheter or nephrostomy tube. Intrarenal AKI can be the most complex and difficult to treat. AKI caused by glomerulonephritis or vasculitis frequently requires immunosuppressive therapy. For suspected acute interstitial nephritis, the offending medication must be determined and discontinued; a 2-week tapering course of glucocorticoids, beginning with 1 mg/kg of prednisone for 3 days, is commonly recommended despite the absence of definitive data. Serum electrolytes, creatinine, and BUN should be monitored at least daily, more frequently if the patient's renal function appears to be tenuous. Patients with AKI should also receive a low sodium, potassium, and protein diet. Early nephrology consultation will ensure that the patient receives optimal care. Some patients will require urgent hemodialysis because of marked metabolic acidosis unresponsive to sodium bicarbonate infusions; electrolyte abnormalities, such as hyperkalemia unresponsive to medical management; pulmonary edema not responding to diuretic therapy; and uremic symptoms of encephalopathy, seizures, and pericarditis. Intermittent hemodialysis and continuous RRT may be necessary.[43,44,49,50]

Prognosis. Typically, AKI secondary to prerenal causes, if diagnosed and treated early, has the best prognosis for renal recovery. Patients with prerenal AKI commonly return to baseline level of renal function and have a mortality rate of less than 10%. Similarly, patients with postrenal AKI also have a good prognosis for renal recovery if the outlet obstruction is promptly diagnosed and definitively treated.[47]

In contrast, patients with intrarenal AKI have a less predictable renal outcome, and mortality in this group varies between 30% and 80%, depending on the severity of injury. Patients who have a severe episode of AKI requiring hemodialysis may not recover renal function and may need hemodialysis indefinitely. AKI hastens progression of

BOX 32.3   Clinical Management of Perioperative Oliguria

- Oliguria is defined as a urine output <0.5 mL/kg but may be 1–2 mL/kg in a patient who has received mannitol.
- Assume oliguria is prerenal until proven otherwise. Signs of prerenal include the following:
  - Oliguria
  - High urine osmolality
  - Low urine sodium
- A common cause of postoperative oliguria is impaired perfusion and outflow obstruction. A bladder ultrasound or examination for abdominal compression may be helpful.
- Begin treatment with serial fluid boluses if assessment does not indicate overload.
- Avoid diuretic administration in the face of intravascular hypovolemia or hypotension because this may result in exacerbation of renal injury.
- Administer diuretics if there are signs of fluid overload or if oliguria persists despite fluid challenges and stabilized hemodynamics.
- If improvement is not noted with fluid challenge or diuretics, institute invasive hemodynamic monitoring (central venous pressure and arterial pressure monitoring when large fluid shifts are expected).
- Maximize renal blood flow by enhancing cardiac function: normalize preload, heart rate, and rhythm; institute afterload reduction with vasodilators or inodilator agents.
- Maintain renal perfusion pressure.
- Prophylactic pharmacologic agents may be used when renal risk is high, but there is little evidence to suggest they are better at maintaining glomerular filtration rate than volume.
- Diuretic resistance may be related to the following:
  - Acute tolerance induced by hypovolemia
  - Chronic tolerance
  - Refractory states

TABLE 32.4   Systemic Effects of Chronic Renal Disease

System	Effects
Cardiovascular	Hypertension
	Congestive heart failure
	Peripheral and pulmonary edema
	Pericarditis
	Coronary artery disease
Hematologic	Normochromic, normocystic anemia
	Platelet dysfunction
	Leukocyte, immunologic dysfunction
Neurologic	Encephalopathy
	Peripheral and autonomic neuropathy
Endocrine	Hyperparathyroidism
	Adrenal insufficiency
Respiratory	Pneumonitis
	Pulmonary edema
Gastrointestinal	Bleeding
	Nausea, vomiting
	Delayed gastric emptying
Metabolic	Acidosis
	Electrolyte imbalance

chronic kidney disease (CKD) to end-stage kidney disease and is often the major factor causing such progression.[51] Clinical management of oliguria is found in Box 32.3.

CHRONIC KIDNEY DISEASE

CKD, or chronic renal failure, is a slow, progressive, irreversible condition characterized by diminished functioning of nephrons and a decrease in renal blood flow, GFR, tubular function, and reabsorptive capacity. By definition, CKD exists when GFR is less than 60 mL/min/1.73 m² for 3 months or more.[44,51] Although many conditions may lead to renal failure, primary causes include glomerulonephritis, pyelonephritis, diabetes mellitus, hyperlipidemia, autoimmune disease, obesity, vascular or hypertensive insults, and congenital defects. A definitive link between AKI and the development of CKD is not yet established.[36] Table 32.4 outlines the systemic effects of chronic renal failure. Normal aging processes reduce nephron function by 10% for each decade of life. Therefore, renal insufficiency is common in the geriatric population.

The general course of progressive CKD can be divided into five stages.[52,53]

Stage 1: Kidney damage with normal or increased GFR
Stage 2: GFR 60 to 89 mL/min/1.73 m² with evidence of kidney damage
Stage 3: GFR 30 to 59 mL/min/1.73 m²
Stage 4: GFR 15 to 29 mL/min/1.73 m²
Stage 5: End-stage renal failure with GFR less than 15 mL/min/1.73 m²

Initial nephron injury causes adaptation in remaining nephrons, including increased glomerular size and pressure, which results in progression of renal disease. As the number of functioning nephrons declines, the signs, symptoms, and biochemical abnormalities become more severe.

Clinical signs or laboratory evidence of renal disease are absent until less than 40% of normal-functioning nephrons remain. Loss of nephron function without symptoms is known as a decrease in renal reserve. Renal insufficiency occurs when only 10% to 40% of nephrons are functioning adequately. Nocturia occurs secondary to a decrease in concentrating ability. Elimination of a large protein load or excretion of certain drugs is impaired. Preservation of remaining nephron function is a major goal in renal insufficiency.

Toxic substances such as aminoglycosides, nonsteroidal antiinflammatory drugs, and piperacillin have been implicated in causing interstitial nephritis and renal insufficiency. The administration of radiographic contrast media in at-risk patients results in renal insufficiency at the same rate as in 1979. Patients at greatest risk for developing contrast-induced renal insufficiency include those with preexisting renal insufficiency (creatinine >1.2 mg/dL) and diabetes. Strategies including the administration of N-acetylcysteine, sodium bicarbonate, and ascorbic acid have been studied.[5]

As renal function deteriorates further, end-stage renal disease develops. In this stage, concentrating and diluting properties of the kidney are severely compromised, and electrolyte, hematologic, and acid-base disturbances are common. The loss of 95% of functioning nephrons culminates in uremia, which is associated with volume overload and congestive heart failure. Uremia, which can be viewed as urine in the blood, adversely affects almost every organ system. Mortality is inevitable unless dialysis is performed for end-stage renal disease.[48]

Renal Failure and Dialysis

Greater than 600,000 Americans are diagnosed with kidney failure each year, and most of these individuals are placed on dialysis. The

BOX 32.4   Indications for Renal Replacement Therapy

Absolute Indications
- Volume overload unresponsive to diuretic therapy
- Persistent hyperkalemia despite medical treatment
- Severe metabolic acidosis
- Overt uremic symptoms
  Encephalopathy
  Pericarditis
  Uremic bleeding diathesis

Relative Indications
- Progressive azotemia without uremic manifestations
- Persistent oliguria

From Weisbord SD, Palevsky PM, et al. Prevention and management of acute kidney injury. In: Yu ASL, et al., eds. *Brenner & Rector's The Kidney.* 11th ed. Philadelphia: Elsevier; 2020:940–971.

end-stage renal failure population is projected to grow approximately 8% per year; 339 patients per 1 million receive RRT for end-stage renal disease per year, and almost half of these patients require treatment early in the postoperative period.[5,48,53] Indications for RRT are shown in Box 32.4.

Dialysis Techniques

Dialysis is a general term used to describe therapy designed to move solute from plasma through a semipermeable membrane into a chemically prescribed solution. The movement of solute (i.e., diffusive transport) depends on differences in molecular concentration between the blood compartment and the dialysate. Ultrafiltration is a technique in which a hydraulic pressure difference across a semipermeable membrane causes bulk fluid removal and solute by convective transport.

Major types of dialysis include hemodialysis and peritoneal dialysis. In hemodialysis, blood moves through a device exposing it to an individually prescribed dialysate solution across a semipermeable membrane. Hemodialysis requires systemic or regional anticoagulation. Concerns about hemodynamic stability during hemodialysis, nephron injury, and inability to adequately remove excess water and solutes have led to the development of a slower, less aggressive RRT: continuous renal replacement therapy (CRRT).

CRRT is an extracorporeal process in which blood is removed from the arterial lumen of a catheter by a peristaltic blood pump and pushed through a semipermeable membrane before being pumped back into patients via the venous lumen of the catheter. CRRT includes several treatment modalities. Pump-driven venovenous CRRT is currently the most common technique. The modalities of venovenous CRRT vary primarily by mechanism of solute removal: In continuous venovenous hemofiltration, solute transport occurs by convection; in continuous venovenous hemodialysis, it occurs by diffusion; and continuous venovenous hemodiafiltration is a combination of the two. The hybrid modalities of RRT with conventional hemodialysis equipment modified to provide extended-duration dialysis provide enhanced hemodynamic tolerability.[54]

Peritoneal dialysis. The use of peritoneal dialysis in the management of AKI has diminished as the use of continuous and hybrid therapies have improved. Peritoneal dialysis has the unique advantage of requiring minimal technology and can be performed easily at home. Access for short-term peritoneal dialysis can be obtained either by percutaneous placement of an uncuffed temporary peritoneal catheter or through surgical placement of a tunneled cuffed catheter. Peritoneal dialysis has the distinct advantage of avoiding the need for vascular access or anticoagulation. Solute clearance and control of metabolic parameters may be inferior to other modalities of RRT. Although systemic hypotension is less of an issue than with other modalities of RRT, ultrafiltration cannot be as tightly controlled. Other limitations include (1) relative contraindication in patients with acute abdominal processes or recent abdominal surgery, (2) risk of visceral organ injury during catheter placement, (3) risk of peritoneal dialysis–associated peritonitis, and (4) increased tendency toward hyperglycemia, which is associated with adverse outcomes in acute illness due to the high glucose concentrations in peritoneal dialysate.[55]

Physiologic Effects

Dialysis and ultrafiltration are associated with several physiologic effects and complications. Major systems involved include the nervous system, cardiovascular system, and respiratory system. The disequilibrium syndrome is the most severe central nervous system (CNS) effect of dialysis. This syndrome is associated with a rapid increase in brain intracellular volume because serum sodium and BUN levels are reduced. Predisposing factors include a BUN concentration greater than 150 mg/dL, hypernatremia, severe acidemia, and preexisting brain disease. The syndrome may be mild or may progress to seizures, stupor, and coma. The incidence is reduced by the avoidance of high rates of hemodialysis therapy in high-risk patients.

Hemodialysis is associated with a 30% incidence of hypotension. Contributing factors include reduced plasma volume and blunted sympathetic nervous system response associated with uremia. Acetate from the dialysate moves into the blood contributing to the hypotension by causing vasodilation and cardiac depression.

The incidence of hypotension with dialysis is less in patients who have fasted than in those who have not. Fasting prevents the contribution to systemic hypovolemia due to increased gastrointestinal blood flow and secretion of isotonic intestinal juices. Anemia should be corrected if the hematocrit is less than 20% to increase vascular resistance. Leg elevation, a decrease in dialyzer transmembrane pressure, or the use of volume expanders or vasoconstrictors usually corrects hypotension. Substitution of HCO_3 for acetate in the dialysate also decreases the incidence of hypotension.

Hypoxemia is a common side effect of hemodialysis and may be seen during peritoneal dialysis. During hemodialysis, arterial oxygen tension often decreases by 5 to 20 mm Hg. Pulmonary leukostasis and extracorporeal loss of CO_2 with a reduction in minute ventilation have been implicated. Hypoxemia is managed by increasing the inspired oxygen concentration during dialysis. The use of HCO_3 in place of acetate limits extracorporeal losses of CO_2 and reduces the incidence of hypoxemia.

Muscle cramping is the most common neuromuscular complication of dialysis. It is seen almost exclusively with hemodialysis and results from the rapid reduction of intravascular volume and serum sodium level. Intravenous administration of hypertonic saline relieves muscle cramping.

The nutritional depletion common in dialysis-dependent patients may be caused by the primary disease, dietary restrictions, or the loss of protein associated with peritoneal dialysis. Protein depletion may produce hypoalbuminemia and immune system suppression. The large quantities of hypertonic glucose solutions absorbed with peritoneal dialysis contribute to obesity, hyperglycemia, and hyperlipidemia. Administration of insulin controls hyperglycemia, and diet and exercise limit hyperlipidemia.[54,55]

PREOPERATIVE RENAL ASSESSMENT

Preoperative assessment of the patient with suspected or known renal dysfunction must include a thorough history and physical examination,

BOX 32.5 Preoperative Assessment and Preparation of the Patient With End-Stage Renal Disease

I. Clinical History
   A. Evaluate renal function.
   B. Document central nervous system deficits.
   C. Review cardiovascular history; look for significant hypertension, accelerated atherosclerosis, pericarditis, tamponade; assess extent, stability, and management of coronary artery disease.
   D. Look for history of excessive bleeding; if present consider use of desmopressin.
   E. Assess intravascular volume; correlate body weight changes with changes in blood pressure and heart rate before and after dialysis.
   F. Review pulmonary history.
   G. Dialyze ≤24 hr before surgery; ideal weight preoperatively is 1–2 kg above dry weight.
II. Physical Examination
   A. Locate and check patency of arteriovenous fistula or shunt.
   B. Evaluate vessels for venous or arterial access.
   C. Look for signs of congestive heart failure, pericarditis, or cardiac tamponade.
   D. Look for evidence of noncardiogenic pulmonary edema or aspiration.
III. Laboratory Tests
   A. Electrocardiography, chest radiography
   B. Glomerular filtration rate or creatinine clearance
   C. Blood urea nitrogen, creatinine
   D. Complete blood count with platelet count
   E. Bleeding time; prothrombin time; partial thromboplastin time
   F. Hematocrit; red blood cell index
   G. Electrolytes (especially potassium)
   H. Acid-base status
   I. Hepatitis antigen status

which includes appropriate laboratory evaluation (see Box 32.5). The medical history is the single most important source of information in establishing the presence or absence of renal disease. Poorly controlled hypertension, trauma to the urinary system, prior renal surgery, or systemic disease (e.g., diabetes) may be associated with renal impairment. A history arousing suspicion should lead to a more thorough evaluation of renal function.

Although abnormalities are commonly identified by urinalysis, the quality of urinalysis results obtained by dipstick technique varies. Abnormal urinalysis results usually fail to lead to a change in management, so the test is generally omitted. If the test is available, attention should be directed to the following:

1. *Specific gravity.* Specific gravity, a measurement of solutes in the urine, indicates the kidney's ability to excrete concentrated or dilute urine. It reflects renal tubular function and normally varies from 1.003 to 1.030, depending on fluid intake and the presence or absence of high-molecular-weight substances such as glucose or mannitol. In the absence of such substances, a specific gravity of 1.018 or greater after overnight dehydration indicates reasonable function. A low specific gravity is meaningless if the condition under which the sample was collected is not known.

2. *Urine osmolality.* Osmolality, or the number of moles of solute (measured in osmoles) per kilogram of solvent, is more unambiguous

than specific gravity. Excretion of concentrated urine (specific gravity 1.030; 1400 mOsm/kg) indicates excellent renal tubular function, whereas urinary osmolality fixed to that of plasma (serum gravity 1.010; 290 mOsm/kg) suggests renal tubular concentrating defects. Urinary diluting mechanisms are dominant after concentrating ability is lost.

3. *Proteinuria.* Proteinuria exists when more than 150 mg of protein is excreted per day. Massive proteinuria or the renal loss of more than 750 mg/day is always abnormal and usually indicative of severe glomerular damage. In addition to the association with glomerular damage, proteinuria may also be present with abnormal plasma proteins or increased concentrations of normal proteins, or when the renal tubules fail to reabsorb the small amount of filtered protein. Although proteinuria is most often associated with significant pathology, patients may present with proteinuria without renal disease under conditions of stress, fever, dehydration, exercise, or congestive heart failure. Patients who have significant proteinuria are more likely to develop AKI postoperatively than those who do not. The incidence of hypoalbuminemia and subsequent sequelae is increased in patients with severe proteinuria. In concentrated urine samples, trace or 1+ proteinuria is a nonspecific finding, whereas 3+ or 4+ proteinuria suggests glomerular disease.

The kidneys share regulation of acid-base balance with the lungs, providing the sole pathway for the excretion of the 60 mEq of hydrogen ions produced per day. Urinary pH reflects renal ability to acidify urine. Inability to excrete acid urine in the presence of systemic acidosis is indicative of renal insufficiency.[56,57]

Laboratory Tests for Renal Function

Patients with suspected or known renal disease should be tested preoperatively to evaluate GFR and renal tubular function. Urine specific gravity (1.003–1.030), urine osmolality (65–1400 mOsm/L), and urine sodium concentration (130–260 mEq/day) reflect renal tubular function, whereas BUN concentration (10–20 mg/dL), plasma creatinine level (0.7–1.5 mg/dL), and creatinine clearance (110–150 mL/min) evaluate GFR.[58-60]

Blood Urea Nitrogen

Urea, the chief end product of protein metabolism, is formed in the liver. It is excreted by glomerular filtration, but significant amounts of urea are reabsorbed along the renal tubule. Although the normal range for BUN level is 10 to 20 mg/dL, it is altered by a variety of factors, including (1) ingestion of protein, (2) anabolic and catabolic states, (3) GFR, (4) state of hydration, and (5) reabsorption of urea by the nephrons. Because of the numerous extrarenal factors influencing BUN, it is a better indicator of uremic symptoms than of GFR. Levels below 8 mg/dL suggest overhydration or underproduction of urea, whereas those between 20 and 40 mg/dL suggest dehydration, high nitrogen levels, or decreased GFR. Levels higher than 50 mg/dL almost always indicate decreased glomerular filtration. Elevations of BUN level in the presence of normal serum creatinine concentration suggest a nonrenal cause of the elevation. In general, BUN level is a late indicator of renal disease because it does not increase in most patients until the GFR is reduced by more than 50%.[46]

Serum Creatinine

Creatinine is a metabolite of creatine, a major muscle constituent. The daily rate of production of creatinine is constant and determined by skeletal muscle mass. Because creatinine is eliminated almost entirely by glomerular filtration, serum steady-state concentration is viewed as a reliable marker of glomerular function. Normal values range from 0.7 to 1.5 mg/dL, but the serum concentration can be lower in the elderly or in women who have reduced muscle mass. Patients with muscle wasting have lower levels, whereas those who are heavily muscled or those in acute catabolic states have higher values due to rapid muscle breakdown. Because the production and release of creatinine are relatively stable throughout the day and from day to day, serum levels are inversely related to GFR if a steady state exists. In other words, for every 50% reduction in GFR, creatinine level doubles. Excretion of drugs dependent on glomerular filtration may be significantly decreased despite only a slight elevation in serum creatinine level.

An elevation of both BUN and serum creatinine levels provides more information than an elevation of either level alone. The usual ratio of urea nitrogen to creatinine in the serum is 10:1. Increased ratios are seen with (1) increased urea input, (2) decreased circulatory blood volume, and (3) obstructive uropathy. Decreased ratios are seen with decreased urea input, increased creatinine production, and volume expansion.[61]

Creatinine Clearance

Creatinine clearance is a specific test of GFR and the most reliable assessment tool for renal function, which measures the glomerular ability to excrete creatinine into the urine for a given plasma creatinine concentration. Although not dependent on corrections for age or the presence of a steady state, a disadvantage of this test is the need for accurate 24-hour urine specimens. Creatinine clearance is calculated according to the following formula:

$$GFR = (Urine\ creatinine \times Urine\ volume) \times Serum\ creatinine$$

A 2-hour urine sample collected through a urinary catheter permits acceptable accuracy. In the absence of urine volume, creatinine clearance can be approximated with use of the following Cockcroft-Gault formula:

$$GFR = \frac{([140 - Age] \times Lean\ body\ weight\ [kg])}{(72 \times Serum\ creatinine\ [mg/dL])}$$

where weight is expressed in kilograms. To compensate for their smaller muscle mass, when values for women are calculated, the weight should be multiplied by 0.85.

The normal range for creatinine clearance is 95 to 150 mL/min. Mild renal dysfunction is present when creatinine clearance is 50 to 80 mL/min, and moderate dysfunction is present at values below 25 mL/min. In patients with dysfunction, the administration of drugs dependent on renal excretion should be reduced, and fluid and electrolyte balance should be carefully monitored. Patients with creatinine clearance less than 10 mL/min are anephric and require dialysis for fluid and water hemostasis.[61]

Other Tests

Advanced renal disease affects most organ systems. Additional tests that may be useful in patients with advanced renal disease include chest radiography, electrocardiography (ECG), complete blood count, serum electrolytes, and acid-base studies.

Systemic Abnormalities and Advanced Renal Disease

Renal failure is characterized by a wide variety of biochemical disturbances. Although most organ systems are involved (see Table 32.4), only those most relevant to anesthetic management are discussed in this section.

Cardiovascular Alterations

Cardiovascular disease accounts for approximately 50% of all deaths in patients on hemodialysis with 26% mortality from sudden cardiac death.[39,62] Hypertension and congestive heart failure often accompany end-stage renal disease. Ninety percent of the hypertension is volume dependent and related to sodium and water retention. The remaining 10% can be attributed to high circulatory levels of renin. The combination of hypertension, anemia, hypoalbuminemia, and circulatory overload secondary to salt and water retention contributes to peripheral and pulmonary edema and to an increased risk of developing congestive heart failure.

In nonsurgical settings, ischemic heart disease is the most common cause of death in patients with chronic renal failure. Multiple risk factors such as hypertension, hyperlipidemia, and abnormal carbohydrate metabolism contribute to this high incidence of ischemic heart disease.[39] It is a safe assumption that clinically significant coronary artery disease exists, and the prudent anesthetist should evaluate the extent and stability of the disease prior to administering anesthetic agents. Correction of coronary lesions with coronary artery bypass grafting (CABG) is associated with better outcomes than coronary angioplasty in patients on hemodialysis. Improvement of symptoms is common after the CABG procedure.[63]

Fifty percent of patients with severe uremia will present with a fibrous pericarditis. Signs and symptoms may include pain on deep inspiration or when lying down, and a friction rub over the pericardium noted during auscultation. An enlarged cardiac silhouette on chest radiography indicates pericardial effusion. Patients with uremic pericarditis occasionally develop a massive hemorrhagic effusion and cardiac tamponade, especially when anticoagulants are used for hemodialysis.[64,65]

Uremic patients exhibit a wide range of hemodynamic abnormalities when studied during hemodialysis. The striking feature of these studies is the abnormal peripheral vasculature response to dialysis-induced hypovolemia. Untreated hypovolemia decreases arterial pressure without compensatory increase in heart rate. Peripheral vascular resistance is unchanged or decreased, and cardiac output is increased.[1,5,10]

Because the potential for significant cardiovascular complications exists, patients with advanced renal disease should undergo chest radiography and ECG preoperatively. Administration of antihypertensive drugs should be continued, blood pressure should be monitored, and signs and symptoms of cerebrovascular disease should be recorded. The blood pressure should be normal or slightly elevated before induction. Because adequate intravascular volume is necessary for hemodynamic stability, the patient's weight should ideally be 1 to 2 kg greater than dry weight at the end of the last dialysis before anesthetic induction.[54,55]

Hematologic Changes

Normochromic, normocytic anemia is an inevitable finding in advanced renal disease. Hematocrit levels often decrease to the 20% to 30% range and generally parallel the degree of azotemia. The primary reason for anemia is a decrease in erythrocyte formation secondary to a decrease in production of erythropoietin by the failing kidney.[66,67] In addition, some evidence suggests uremic toxins may inactivate erythropoietin or suppress bone marrow response. A second factor contributing to anemia in uremic patients is reduction of erythrocyte life span due to an increase in hemolysis secondary to the presence of an abnormal chemical environment. Additionally, blood loss from frequent sampling for laboratory tests, loss in hemodialysis tubing, and a tendency for gastrointestinal bleeding further aggravate anemia.

Hematocrit and red blood cell indexes should be measured preoperatively, and their values should be checked against dialysis records to ensure no acute changes have occurred. Preoperative hematocrit levels are similar to those of a patient maintained on dialysis, suggesting patients can tolerate the chronic anemia; therefore, routine transfusion of blood preoperatively is not recommended for these patients. If transfusion is necessary because of acutely decreased or poorly tolerated hematocrit values, no need exists to withhold red blood cell transfusions for fear of sensitization to histocompatibility antigens.[67]

Exogenous administration of human recombinant erythropoietin corrects the anemia associated with chronic renal failure. The risks of treatment with erythropoietin include hypertension, vascular access clotting, and death. Adequate iron stores and good dialysis are essential if the response to recombinant erythropoietin or epoetin is to be maximized.[68,69] There are two erythropoiesis-stimulating agents currently available to treat anemia in patients with chronic renal disease who are on dialysis: epoetin (Procrit, Epogen) and darbepoetin (Aranesp).

Patients with chronic uremia tend to bleed excessively. Although platelet counts are only mildly reduced, a defect in platelet function appears to be responsible for prolonged bleeding time and the tendency for excessive bleeding. Dialysis partially corrects platelet dysfunction, therefore dialysis 24 hours or less before surgical intervention is recommended.

Desmopressin is known to shorten bleeding time and increase circulating levels of factor VIII, the von Willebrand antigen, in uremic patients. Desmopressin is the agent of choice because of its rapid onset and minimal side effects. Repeated doses over time may increase bleeding time between treatments. Cryoprecipitate and conjugated estrogens also shorten bleeding time and may reduce blood loss.[70]

Gastrointestinal Effects

Patients on dialysis have a high incidence of gastrointestinal mucosal inflammatory changes and are at high risk of gastrointestinal bleeding perioperatively. The use of histamine-2 (H_2) blocking drugs or antacids is recommended throughout the perioperative period for decreasing the incidence of stress ulcers.[54]

Infections

Infectious complications are common in patients with renal failure and represent a leading cause of death in dialysis-dependent patients. Protein malnutrition and abnormalities in neutrophil, monocyte, and macrophage function contribute to this problem. Mechanisms that lead to leukocyte dysfunction and increased susceptibility to infection are not known but may be related to uremia, immunosuppressive therapy, and increased exposure to invasive therapy. Frequent exposure to blood and blood products increases the risk of infection with hepatitis B and C and the human immunodeficiency viruses. Universal precautions are mandatory for the protection of both patients and health care providers.[58]

Neurologic Effects

Neurologic symptoms associated with end-stage renal disease roughly parallel the degree of azotemia. Fatigue and weakness are early complaints, and untreated patients eventually become confused and comatose. Additional early symptoms include apathy, decreased mental acuity, and lethargy. Seizures may be associated with hypertensive encephalopathy. Peripheral and autonomic nervous system neuropathy is common. Autonomic neuropathy is associated with delayed gastric emptying and places the patient at risk for aspiration pneumonitis. Preoperative assessment should include the patient's baseline awareness and mental acuity.[71]

Endocrine Abnormalities

Endocrine abnormalities in patients with end-stage renal disease include hyperparathyroidism and adrenal insufficiency. Hypocalcemia is common in patients with advanced renal disease, and hyperparathyroidism represents an appropriate compensatory increase

in parathormone in response to a reduction in serum calcium levels. Adrenal insufficiency is often secondary to exogenous steroid administration.[72]

Respiratory Effects

Respiratory complications associated with renal failure include pneumonitis and the "uremic lung." Chest radiographs of the uremic lung reveal bilateral butterfly-shaped infiltrates indicative of pulmonary edema. Pulmonary congestion and edema are usually related to volume overload. Respiratory depression may be exaggerated when sedatives or opioids accumulate in the plasma due to reduced clearance.[73]

Electrolyte Abnormalities

Abnormalities of water, electrolyte, and acid-base balance become more common as the degree of renal failure increases. With a normal diet, the kidneys typically excrete 40 to 60 mEq of hydrogen ions per day to prevent acidosis. Impaired ability of the kidney to excrete hydrogen ions with renal failure results in metabolic acidosis characterized by decreases in plasma pH and HCO_3 concentration. Acidosis is usually moderate, but symptoms of anorexia, nausea, vomiting, and lethargy, which are common in uremic patients, may be partly related to acidosis.

Sodium ion excretion by the kidney normally varies according to intake. Patients with chronic renal failure lose this flexibility and have sodium wasting or retention. In early renal insufficiency with polyuria, an increased solute load for each intact nephron results in sodium wasting. In renal failure, the patient is more likely to retain sodium. Salt and water retention leads to circulatory overload, hypertension, edema, and congestive heart failure.

Although the ability to excrete magnesium is reduced in uremic patients, hypermagnesemia is generally not a serious problem. Magnesium intake is usually reduced because of anorexia, reduced protein intake, and decreased absorption from the gastrointestinal tract.

Calcium balance is controlled by parathyroid hormone, calcitonin, and vitamin D. Vitamin D control serum calcium balance, or cholecalciferol, must undergo activation to become biologically available. Inability of the failing kidney to hydroxylate 25-hydroxycholecalciferol to 1,25-dihydroxycholecalciferol (active vitamin D) results in hypocalcemia. To maintain appropriate serum calcium levels, calcium is liberated from the bone. Patients with chronic renal failure have skeletal disorders or osteodystrophy, and defective mineralization of bone predisposes patients to fractures. Special precautions should be taken when these patients are moved and positioned.

Potassium imbalance is one of the most serious disturbances occurring in patients with renal failure. Although hypokalemia may be associated with the polyuria of renal insufficiency, end-stage renal disease invariably leads to hyperkalemia. Although the major mechanism for hyperkalemia is the inability of distal nephrons to secrete potassium in exchange for calcium, systemic acidosis also contributes to potassium imbalance. Acidosis causes potassium ions to shift from intracellular to extracellular fluid.

Fatal dysrhythmias or cardiac asystole can occur when serum potassium levels reach 7 to 8 mEq/L. Dialysis is the most effective means of managing perioperative hyperkalemia, and hemodialysis is indicated when serum potassium exceeds 6 mEq/L. Other techniques for treating hyperkalemia include insulin in glucose infusions (25–50 g of glucose with 10–20 units of regular insulin) and administration of bicarbonate (50–100 mEq intravenously slowly). These measures promote rapid translocation of extracellular potassium to the intracellular space during hyperkalemic emergencies. Hyperventilation of the lungs with respiratory alkalosis lowers serum potassium concentration by approximately 0.5 mEq/L for every 10–mm Hg change in arterial

CO_2 tension. Life-threatening cardiac dysrhythmias are treated with intravenous administration of calcium chloride. A typical dose is 1 g in adults. Although calcium does not change the serum concentration of potassium, it antagonizes the cardiotoxic effects of hyperkalemia.

Unexpected hyperkalemia can develop rapidly, so it is important to measure potassium even when dialysis has been performed within 6 to 8 hours of surgery. Hyperkalemia occurs early postoperatively and is the primary reason patients with renal failure require dialysis within the first 24 hours after surgery.[13,14,46] A complete discussion of hyperkalemia, its symptoms, and treatment can be found in Chapter 21.

Surgical procedures are becoming increasingly more common in anephric patients. The perioperative course of these patients may be complicated by a high incidence of untoward events increasing morbidity and mortality. These complications are related to the abnormal physiology of the anephric state and are predictable. Adverse outcomes are minimized by appropriate preoperative evaluation and preparation.[46] Pertinent points in the preoperative assessment and preparation of patients with end-stage renal disease are listed in Box 32.5.

ANESTHETIC MANAGEMENT OF PATIENTS WITH ADVANCED RENAL DISEASE

Preoperative preparation of patients with advanced renal disease should include an evaluation of recent laboratory measurements (i.e., electrolytes, coagulation, and creatinine), coexisting diseases, and current medications. Patients with end-stage renal disease should undergo preoperative determination of BUN and serum creatinine levels, complete blood count, bleeding-time measurement, and electrolyte studies. Special attention should be given to serum potassium, the type of and schedule for dialysis, and volume status. Additional information needed from this patient population is dry weight and "normal" preoperative concerns (e.g., nil by mouth [NPO] status, allergies).

Premedications

Discussions regarding premedication should take into consideration unexpected sensitivity to CNS depressants and delayed gastric emptying. Short-acting benzodiazepines are useful as premedication. Midazolam is preferred because it has virtually no active metabolites, and the half-life is only slightly prolonged in renal failure patients. Although this drug is useful when it is carefully titrated, patients with renal disease may be more susceptible to the sedative-hypnotic effects of benzodiazepines than those without renal dysfunction.[74,75]

Patients with renal failure should be monitored with a pulse oximetry prior to administering any sedative or CNS depressant. Reduced protein binding may be responsible for increased sensitivity to these drugs in patients with advanced renal disease. Protein binding of morphine decreases by 10% in the presence of chronic renal failure, altering free fraction only slightly because morphine is generally protein bound to such a small extent. Morphine is almost completely metabolized in the liver, resulting in two metabolites (morphine-3-glucuronide and morphine-6-glucuronide), which are both excreted by the kidney. Patients with kidney disease can develop high levels of morphine-6-glucuronide and resultant respiratory failure. Morphine is not removed by dialysis.[75]

Meperidine is more lipophilic than morphine. It is 60% protein bound and is metabolized to normeperidine, which has analgesic properties and stimulates the CNS system. Meperidine metabolites can cause convulsions when present in high concentrations and cannot be removed by dialysis. Meperidine should be avoided in patients with renal failure.

Hydromorphone does not directly cause adverse effects in renal failure; however, its metabolite, hydromorphone-3-glucuronide does accumulate. For this reason, hydromorphone should be used with caution, although it can readily be removed by dialysis.[76]

A review of publications on opioid use in patients with renal failure reveals that transdermal buprenorphine, methadone, fentanyl, and sufentanil appear to be safe in these patients. Anticholinergic drugs, such as atropine and glycopyrrolate, are partially dependent on renal elimination, although no reports of toxicity exist.

Gastric hyperacidity and gastrointestinal bleeding are common in patients with renal failure. H_2 blockers and magnesium-free antacids should be considered. Cimetidine has been used, but renal elimination accounts for 80% of total elimination, and elimination is impaired with reduced renal function. Although newer H_2 antagonists are now available, all H_2-receptor blockers are highly dependent on renal excretion. Metoclopramide is partly excreted unchanged in the urine and will accumulate in patients with renal failure.[74]

Intraoperative Monitoring

The selection of monitors for a patient with diminished or absent renal function is based on the physiologic status of the patient and the proposed surgical procedure. Frequent measurements of blood pressure and continuous recording of temperature and heart rate and rhythm are essential. ECG may allow early detection of hyperkalemia, including observation of peaked T waves, prolongation of the PR interval, and absent P waves with widened QRS complex.

Care should be taken to place ECG leads in the appropriate position on the patient to facilitate early recognition of hyperkalemia. Because these patients are often chronically anemic, a further reduction in oxygen delivery secondary to hypoxia can be extremely hazardous. Pulse oximetry is essential for the early detection of arterial desaturations. Pulse oximetry and capnography are required in all patients. Minor surgical procedures in stable patients can be monitored noninvasively.[58]

The decision to use invasive monitors depends on the patient's functional cardiac reserve and the severity and control of hypertension. Significant hypotension on induction of anesthesia is common in recently dialyzed patients. Continuous monitoring of arterial blood pressure is helpful when major surgical procedures are performed. A femoral or dorsalis pedis artery is sometimes used for cannulation because vessels in the upper extremities may be needed later for vascular shunts. Vascular volume and fluid replacement can be guided by central venous pressure monitoring. A pulmonary artery catheter is rarely indicated because sophisticated evaluation of fluid status and ventricular function can be accomplished with echocardiography.[39]

Vascular shunts and fistulas must be protected. Patency is easily monitored with Doppler imaging. Care must be taken to avoid the extremity with the shunt when placing blood pressure cuffs. Because of the immunocompromised state of these patients, strict aseptic technique is required during the placement of vascular catheters.[77,78]

Regional Anesthesia

Regional anesthesia is well tolerated by patients with advanced renal disease, provided no significant coagulation disorder is present and MAP is maintained. Regional techniques avoid most of the pharmacokinetic and pharmacodynamic problems associated with general anesthetics and sedative drugs. Major concerns regarding this type of anesthesia include (1) psychologic intolerance, (2) coagulation abnormalities, (3) presence of peripheral neuropathies, (4) difficulty in making intravascular volume adjustments, (5) risk of infection, and (6) altered drug disposition.

Arteriovenous (AV) shunts or fistulas may be surgically created with the use of local infiltration or brachial plexus block. In addition to providing analgesia, brachial plexus blocks improve surgical conditions by providing maximum vascular vasodilation and abolishing vasospasm. Studies have shown brachial plexus blocks are associated with greater brachial artery blood flow than local anesthesia, greater fistula blood flow, and decreased maturation time.[79] Brachial plexus block and local infiltration techniques are good alternatives to general anesthesia for creation of AV fistula. Age, ASA class, and cardiac status are the determining factors for choice of anesthetic technique.

Data suggest a similar duration of anesthesia with brachial plexus blocks in patients with renal failure and normal renal function.[80] High-dose mepivacaine has been used successfully for brachial plexus block in patients with end-stage chronic renal failure. Brachial plexus anesthesia with 650 mg of plain mepivacaine did not result in serious systematic toxicity in these patients despite high mepivacaine plasma concentrations.[81,82] Ropivacaine has a longer duration of action with higher plasma concentrations in renal dysfunction.[79] The use of clonidine (150 mcg) as an adjuvant for lidocaine in axillary blocks for AV fistula construction prolongs blockade, decreases heart rate and blood pressure, and provides sedative effects.[82] Creating an AV fistula 6 months prior to the first dialysis cannulation is associated with a 95% success rate.[83]

Regarding spinal or epidural anesthesia, patients with long-standing renal disease have often undergone multiple procedures and prefer general anesthetic techniques. In addition to the history, the uremic patient's bleeding time, platelet count, prothrombin time, partial thromboplastin time, and fibrinogen level should be evaluated before subarachnoid or epidural catheters are placed. Paraplegia secondary to hematoma formation with spinal anesthesia has been reported in patients with chronic renal failure and clotting abnormalities. A case of epidural hematoma in a surgical patient with chronic renal failure and epidural postoperative analgesia has been reported.[84] The only risk factor for development of epidural hematoma was a history of chronic renal failure. High-risk patients should be monitored closely for early signs of cord compression such as severe back pain and motor or sensory deficits.[5,10]

An opioid or opioid and local epidural solution rather than local solution alone allows continuous monitoring of neurologic function. If spinal hematoma is suspected, the patient should undergo immediate magnetic resonance imaging (MRI) or computed tomography (CT) scan, and decompressive laminectomy should be performed without delay.[84]

Peripheral neuropathies should be discussed with the patient and documented before regional anesthesia is undertaken. The incidence of hypotension with subarachnoid or epidural blockade may be increased because of effects of chronic hypertension or hypovolemia related to recent dialysis. Correction of hypovolemia postoperatively is hazardous. Recession of the sympathetic block in patients who cannot undergo diuresis may lead to pulmonary edema. One must weigh the advantages of fluid infusion against the effects of pressor drugs with these factors in mind.

Patients with end-stage renal disease are often acidotic, and local anesthetic toxicity may be increased with acidosis. The onset and duration of blocks have also been shown to vary in these patients, leading to "patchy blocks," which may necessitate conversion to general anesthesia. Subarachnoid blockade induced with 3 mL of 0.75% bupivacaine developed more rapidly, attained a greater level, and was of shorter duration in patients with renal failure than in control patients. The slower onset of epidural anesthesia is an advantage in these patients.

General Anesthesia

Intravenous Drugs

Intravenous anesthetics can be used in patients with advanced renal disease, but the response of these patients may be more variable than

normal. Variability arises from a complex interplay among changes in (1) volume of distribution (which is often increased), (2) protein binding (which may be decreased), (3) low pH, and (4) dependence on renal excretion for the parent drug or metabolites.

The action of many drugs is potentiated by metabolic abnormalities associated with renal failure. Highly protein-bound drugs may have a greater target-organ effect in the presence of hypoalbuminemia. The acidemia associated with renal failure may alter the proportion of the agent available to target tissue. Anemia associated with renal failure increases cardiac output and enhances delivery to the brain. Uremia alters the blood-brain barrier; this also increases sensitivity to intravenous drugs.

Ketamine and benzodiazepines are less heavily protein bound. The sympathomimetic effects of ketamine are frequently associated with an increase in blood pressure and cardiac output, which may be deleterious in hypertensive patients who are at risk for coronary artery disease or decreased left ventricular function. In addition, metabolites of ketamine depend on renal excretion and can accumulate in patients with renal failure.

The pharmacokinetic profile of narcotics can be altered in the presence of renal disease. Fentanyl is metabolized in the liver, and 85% of it appears in the urine and feces as inactive metabolites. Its slow elimination half-life is the result of a large volume of distribution. The effect is exaggerated in renal failure.[25] Chronic renal failure is associated with a decrease in alfentanil plasma protein binding, but it does not change plasma clearance of the drug. The volume of distribution at steady state is greater in patients with renal failure. Altered protein binding of alfentanil must be considered in patients with renal failure. Although the pharmacokinetics of sufentanil do not appear to be altered in patients with advanced renal disease, clearance and half-life are more variable in this group. Sufentanil should be carefully administered to these patients. Remifentanil is metabolized by nonspecific plasma esterases, and a significant reduction in clearance in patients with end-stage renal disease may be noted.[2]

Propofol has gained wide acceptance for both induction and maintenance of anesthesia and appears to be safe. Studies suggest, however, that patients with end-stage renal disease may require a higher dose to achieve hypnosis. A hyperdynamic circulation in these anemic patients may be responsible. Propofol pharmacokinetics are unaltered by established renal failure. The time interval between cessation of a propofol infusion and eye opening is significantly shorter in renal failure patients compared with controls, although blood propofol concentrations are not significantly different on emergence.[2,5,10,25]

Dexmedetomidine, an α_2-adrenergic agonist with sedative and analgesic properties, is cleared predominantly by the liver. Studies reveal minimal pharmacokinetic differences between healthy volunteers and patients with renal transplant. There were no reported differences in hemodynamics during administration of dexmedetomidine, but patients with renal failure exhibited prolonged duration of sedation.[85]

Volatile Anesthetic Agents

Inhalation agents offer some advantage in patients with renal failure. Although biotransformation of some agents may produce metabolites excreted by the kidneys, elimination of volatile agents does not rely on renal function. Volatile agents potentiate neuromuscular blocking drugs, allowing administration of reduced doses. Although the potency of these agents allows them to be administered without nitrous oxide, excessive depth of anesthesia may lead to a depression of cardiac output. Reductions in cardiac output and tissue blood flow must be avoided in these anemic patients if tissue oxygen delivery is to be maintained.

TABLE 32.5	Regional Versus General Anesthesia	
Technique	**Advantages**	**Disadvantages**

Regional	Patient responsiveness
	Minimal changes in renal hemodynamics
	May shorten hospital stays
	Allows for earlier detection of capsular tears and bladder perforation
	Lower incidence of postoperative nausea and vomiting
	Reduced amount of operative blood loss and the incidence of deep vein
	    thrombosis with transurethral resection of prostate (TURP)
		Presence of peripheral neuropathy
		Tendency for bleeding
		Patient anxiety
		Less suitable for prolonged procedures
		Hypotension with sympathetic block; may cause
		    reluctance to expand volume

Volatile anesthetics	Good airway control Blood pressure control Duration not dependent on urinary excretion Less neuromuscular blocking with drugs required Fio_2 can be increased because N_2O not necessary	Alterations in renal hemodynamics Decreased cardiac output Hypotension Increased incidence of postoperative nausea and vomiting
Intravenous anesthetics	Hemodynamic stability	Unpredictable response Hypertension Greater need for N_2O and neuromuscular blockers

Fio_2, Fraction of inspired oxygen; N_2O, nitrous oxide.

A theoretic disadvantage of inhalation agents relates to biotransformation and nephrotoxic potential, although this disadvantage is not associated with the modern inhalation anesthetics. Fluoride levels after isoflurane anesthesia increased by only 1 to 2 μmol, and desflurane is metabolized approximately one-tenth as much as isoflurane and is the least metabolized of the currently available volatile agents. In studies of patients and volunteers administered desflurane for prolonged periods, no evidence of renal, hepatic, or hematologic toxicity was observed.

Some practitioners may avoid use of sevoflurane in patients with severe renal dysfunction because of the potential for nephrotoxicity. Studies do not support this concern, and there is little evidence to support the avoidance of sevoflurane. All the current volatile anesthetics are safe in patients with renal disease.[2,5,10,25]

In summary, both regional and general anesthesia have been used successfully in patients with advanced renal disease. Advantages and disadvantages of both techniques are listed in Table 32.5.

Neuromuscular Blocking Drugs

The appropriate use of neuromuscular blocking drugs in patients with advanced renal disease has received much attention over the years. At one time, caution was advised in all cases of the use of a muscle relaxant in patients with renal disease due to concerns of prolonged duration of action. It was further theorized that, as the anticholinesterase or relaxant antagonist level decreased, the patient would be at risk of postoperative residual neuromuscular blockade. In general, the short and intermediate acting relaxants are used in patients with renal disease, but a longer duration of action may be expected. The benzoisoquinoline relaxants, cisatracurium, and atracurium are the least affected.[86] A complete discussion of the neuromuscular blocking drugs and renal disease can be found in Chapter 12.

Succinylcholine. Several problems have been associated with the use of succinylcholine in patients with renal failure. Succinylcholine is metabolized by hepatic-derived pseudocholinesterase to succinic acid and choline. A metabolic precursor of these two compounds is succinylmonocholine, which has some nondepolarizing blocking activity and is eliminated by the kidneys. Prolongation of succinylcholine has also been associated with depressed levels of pseudocholinesterase in uremic patients who require hemodialysis.

Serum potassium increases by approximately 0.5 mEq/L in both normal patients and those with renal failure. This elevation in extracellular potassium is not reliably prevented by pretreatment with a nondepolarizing muscle relaxant. The rise in serum potassium level is particularly dangerous in uremic patients who are hyperkalemic. The use of succinylcholine is inadvisable unless a patient has undergone dialysis within 24 hours before surgery and the potassium concentration is less than 5.5 mEq/L. Succinylcholine is safe in normokalemic patients who have recently undergone dialysis.[86]

Atracurium and cisatracurium. Initial reports indicated the action of neither atracurium nor vecuronium was prolonged in patients with decreased renal function; however, it now appears this is true only for atracurium. Atracurium and cisatracurium are broken down by Hoffman elimination and non-esterase-dependent hydrolysis to inactive products. Neither process is dependent on renal excretion for termination of action. Atracurium is less potent and has a shorter duration of action than cisatracurium. However, atracurium produces histamine release, which limits its desirability, and it is rarely used today. CKD does not alter pharmacokinetics or pharmacodynamics of atracurium. The pharmacodynamics of cisatracurium are not changed, but there is a slight slowing of onset. Many clinicians consider these the drugs of choice in patients with renal failure.[86]

Vecuronium. Approximately 30% of administered vecuronium is excreted via the renal system, and the duration of neuromuscular blockade is longer in patients with renal failure than in those without renal failure. Accumulation results from reduced clearance and a prolonged half-life. If vecuronium is used, a lower dose is recommended, and repeated administration should be avoided. Careful neuromuscular monitoring is essential. Vecuronium neuromuscular blockade is rapidly reversible with dialytic treatment.[87]

Rocuronium. Rocuronium is the most widely used nondepolarizing neuromuscular blocking drug. It has a rapid onset of action, producing good to excellent conditions for tracheal intubation in 60 to 90 seconds in humans. It has no clinically significant cardiovascular effects and an intermediate duration of action. A rapid onset is particularly attractive in these patients because they are subject to autonomic neuropathy and delayed gastric emptying. Rocuronium is excreted primarily in the bile, although renal excretion occurs up to 33% of the time. Renal failure reduces the clearance of rocuronium by 39%. The duration of action and recovery time are significantly prolonged in patients with renal failure.[88] In patients with renal failure, sugammadex (4 mg/kg) effectively and safely reversed profound rocuronium-induced neuromuscular block, but the recovery was slower than healthy patients.[89] Due to the prolonged sugammadex-rocuronium complex exposure in patients with severe renal impairment, researchers caution that current safety data are insufficient. A recent study in renal transplant patients, many on dialysis, found no adverse effects when sugammadex reversal was used. Patients were assessed for up to 6 months posttransplant. They concluded that sugammadex was efficacious and safe in patients who underwent renal transplantation.[90] Hemodialysis using a high-flux dialysis method is effective in removing sugammadex and the sugammadex-rocuronium complex if necessary in patients with severe renal impairment.[91]

INTRAVENOUS FLUID MANAGEMENT

Perioperative management of fluids and electrolytes in patients with renal disease is critical. The state of hydration affects renin, aldosterone, and antidiuretic levels. Dehydration and hypovolemia lead to elevations in these hormones and to a decline in urinary output. Volume overload can lead to the development of pulmonary edema. Goal-directed fluid management therapy is encouraged for patients with severe renal insufficiency and failure.

Perioperative Renal Function

Surgical patients at high risk for AKI, or those with advanced disease not requiring hemodialysis, present unique challenges. Preservation of renal function intraoperatively is dependent on the maintenance of intravascular volume and cardiovascular stability, as well as the avoidance of events causing renal vasoconstriction. Intraoperatively, urinary output is the most immediate monitor for renal function. A urinary output of 0.5 to 1 mL/kg/hour perioperatively is recommended because urinary output less than 0.5 mL/kg/hour is a risk factor for renal injury (see RIFLE and AKIN classifications in Table 32.2). Serum creatinine is a more specific assessment of renal function than urinary output.[92]

Patients with normal or mildly compromised renal function should receive balanced salt solutions at 3 to 5 mL/kg/hour. A bolus of 500 mL should improve decreased urine output related to hypovolemia. Use of mannitol or furosemide to increase urine output may further exacerbate volume depletion and should be administered cautiously. Potassium-containing solutions (lactated Ringer) are contraindicated in anuric patients.

Dialysis patients present a unique challenge to the anesthetist. This population requires a narrow window of control between hypovolemic and fluid overloaded states. Insensible losses are replaced with 5 to 10 mL/kg of 5% glucose in water (D_5W). If any urine is produced, it may be replaced with 0.45% saline.

The greater expected fluid losses of thoracic and abdominal surgery cases may require significant volume replacement. A balanced salt solution, 5% albumin, or a combination thereof is recommended for replacing these larger volumes in patients with, or at risk for, kidney disease or injury. The administration of blood products should be reserved for patients who need increased oxygen-carrying capacity. The safety of synthetic colloids in patients with preexisting renal dysfunction remains unclear, although research supports that synthetic colloids are not well tolerated by patients with ESRD.[93-95]

Renal Insufficiency

In patients with renal insufficiency, volume deficits should be replaced preoperatively, as in normal patients. Basal fluids must be carefully regulated because these patients cannot tolerate much deviation. Overall, basal fluid requirements must be related to metabolic rate and designed to provide an overall fluid balance to form isotonic urine, which will facilitate excretion of electrolytes and waste products. Intraoperative losses greater than 10% to 15% of the blood volume should be replaced with colloid solution on a 1:1 basis after red blood cell losses are corrected. Smaller losses can be replaced with the usual 3:1 ratio

of crystalloid infusion to blood loss. Third space losses are ideally replaced initially with crystalloid solution without potassium or excess chloride. Initial third space losses should be replaced with crystalloid solution at a rate of 2 to 3 mL/kg/hour. The critical goal in patients with renal insufficiency is sustaining blood volume and preventing hypotension and subsequent hypoperfusion. Monitoring of colloid osmotic pressure and hemoglobin can guide the choice between crystalloid and colloid infusions. If hemoglobin and colloid osmotic pressure are increasing, crystalloid solution is clearly indicated. If they are decreasing, crystalloid solution should be withheld in favor of colloid solution. Close monitoring of blood pressure, heart rate, CVP, pulmonary artery occlusion pressure, and cardiac output also guides fluid titration. This is especially true in patients with cardiac or respiratory compromise.[96]

End-Stage Renal Disease

Regarding perioperative fluid management, patients with end-stage renal disease who are hemodialysis dependent require special attention. Although these patients are like normal patients in terms of fluid deficit, basal, and third space requirements, they have a very narrow margin of safety. Ability to compensate for either fluid excess or fluid deficiency progressively declines as renal function is lost.

Fluid deficits must be replaced preoperatively in patients with end-stage renal disease. If deficits exceed 10% to 15% of the blood volume, invasive monitoring is justified. Dialysis is recommended on the day before anesthesia to allow time for equilibration of fluid and electrolyte shifts common with dialysis. Electrolyte levels, particularly potassium, must be checked before anesthesia. If the serum potassium is markedly elevated, attempts should be made to lower the serum level prior to administration of anesthetics. Many facilities having a large population of ESRD patients have developed clinical guidelines to manage severe potassium derangements.[37]

Basal fluids in patients with ESRD should be replaced in a manner like that for patients with renal insufficiency. Volume restriction is recommended for intraoperative losses. Third space losses should be replaced with a balanced salt solution that does not contain potassium and small amounts of chloride. Close monitoring of hemoglobin and cardiac filling pressures is indicated for all major procedures. Patients with ESRD generally require dialysis within 24 to 36 hours after major surgery.[93-95]

Uremia

Deficit replacement in patients with uremia must be guided by hemodynamic monitoring. Basal fluids should be replaced with red blood cells, fresh frozen plasma, or colloid solutions, and third space losses are best replaced with crystalloid solutions in association with frequent monitoring of hemoglobin. Cardiac filling pressures should be checked when warranted by the surgical procedure. A moderate degree of volume overload is not a grave problem. Many uremic patients require dialysis within 24 to 36 hours for the removal of mobilized fluid and the control of hypertension.

Although volume overload is most often emphasized in patients with end-stage renal disease, complications of hypovolemia are also serious. Hypotension associated with hypovolemia increases the risk of thrombosis of the arteriovenous fistula and predisposes to cardiac and cerebral ischemia. Hemodynamic goals include the avoidance of hypotension and gross fluid overload. This can be accomplished only through careful titration with the patient well monitored.[97,98]

CYSTOSCOPY

Almost all urologic surgical procedures that are not open are performed via cystoscope and in the lithotomy position. Urologic procedures performed via a cystoscope can be very quick (i.e., diagnostic cystoscopy) or last several hours (i.e., stone retrieval). A short-acting spinal anesthesia is an ideal anesthetic technique for urologic procedures performed through a cystoscope. The insertion of the cystoscope is very stimulating for the patient, so it is important to attenuate the surgical stress response by deepening the patient very early in the maintenance phase. This can be accomplished with the sympathectomy associated with spinal anesthesia or a deep anesthetic plane when using a general technique. Spinal anesthesia provides analgesia and loss of muscle movement, as well as permitting real-time assessment of mental status. When using general anesthesia technique, a laryngeal mask airway with spontaneous respirations is appropriate practice for airway management unless aspiration is a concern.

EXTRACORPOREAL SHOCK WAVE AND LASER LITHOTRIPSY

Nephrolithiasis (renal calculi) is a common condition, with a lifetime prevalence of approximately 9% in the United States. Although many renal calculi (stones) are asymptomatic, patients with symptomatic stones often require immediate treatment. Up to 2 million emergency room visits annually are for a primary diagnosis of renal colic or renal calculus with acute obstruction. The economic burden of urolithiasis is immense, and costs continue to rise. There is concerted effort to decrease direct and indirect costs of caring for patients diagnosed with nephrolithiasis with newer instrumentation and increased treatment options. Approximately 80% of upper urinary tract stones are calcium based (composed of calcium oxalate, calcium phosphate, or brushite), with the remaining 20% composed of uric acid, struvite, cystine, or (rarely) other components.[99]

CT of kidneys, ureters, and bladder (CT KUB) can identify more than 99% of stones. Ultrasound is an alternative. If a ureteric stone is less than 5 mm in diameter, it is expected it will pass without intervention. Initially medical management is attempted for stones between 5 and 10 mm in diameter, but urology input is more likely to be necessary as up to 50% of these may require intervention. Stones that are greater than 10 mm in diameter should be discussed with the urology service as they are unlikely to pass spontaneously.[100]

Extracorporeal shock wave lithotripsy (ESWL) is a very effective noninvasive treatment for urinary stones. The technique uses high-energy ultrasonic or pneumatic shock waves or lasers to fragment renal calculi into small particles. ESWL is used for stones less than 10 to 20 mm in the proximal or midureter. Stones of any size located in the distal ureters are removed using ureterorenoscopy. Success rates are highly variable, ranging from 30% to 100%. ESWL uses an external source to deliver pulses of energy into a fluid chamber, generating a shock wave. The shock wave is transmitted unimpeded through the fluid and transmitted through soft tissue (which has approximately the same density as fluid) until abrupt change in acoustic density from tissue to stone impedes the shock wave forward movement. By focusing the shock waves on a single focal point, the lithotripter concentrates energy at the stone location. Stone fragmentation by shock waves occurs because of both direct mechanical stress from the incident shock wave and indirect forces as a result of collapse of cavitation bubbles generated by the trailing negative pressure wave. For the properly selected patients, ESWL is a well-tolerated, noninvasive procedure that produces reasonable stone clearance of upper urinary tract calculi while offering low morbidity rates. Recent advances in ESWL have produced significant improvements in its safety and efficacy. A drawback to ESWL is that retreatments may be necessary.

Ureteroscopy has undergone remarkable advancements in the last 30 years. With the introduction of modern semirigid and flexible devices, stones that would have traditionally been considered for ESWL can now be managed via ureteroscopy. In fact, the application of ureteroscopic procedures for upper urinary tract calculi now surpasses that of ESWL around the world.[101]

When lithotripsy fails to resolve the stone, more invasive techniques are employed such as percutaneous nephrolithotomy.[102]

Techniques

Shock wave lithotripsy is an outpatient procedure usually performed in a hospital, ambulatory surgery center, or a mobile lithotripter. Initially, all ESWL was accomplished in water baths. Modern lithotripters create a connection with high-acoustic gel or oil or ionized water bags instead of submersion, providing for a more portable and convenient treatment regimen. Connections between the patient and the shock waves may be diminished by air pockets in the gel or oil requiring an increased number of shocks, and therefore, greater risk of tissue damage.[103,104]

Several types of lithotripters are in clinical use, and they differ in the way they generate the shock waves. Electrohydraulic (spark-gap) lithotripters rely on an underwater discharge of a high-voltage spark that rapidly vaporizes the surrounding water, generating spherically expanding shock waves. Electromagnetic lithotripters are composed of an electromagnetic coil and a closely approximated metallic plate (or membrane) inside a water-filled shock tube. Piezoelectric lithotripters produce shock waves with the use of a spheric dish containing an array of small ceramic elements.[103] Ultrasonic waves fragment stones and allow them to pass in urine. Lasers may not be as effective with larger stones (>1.5–2 cm).[105,106]

Water Immersion

The original ESWL procedure required patients to be strapped in a chair in a semireclining position, followed by submersion in water up to the clavicle. Due to patient intolerance and high risk for adverse outcomes this technique is not used today, but the principles underlying the surgical procedure are similar. The focused, reflected shock wave passes through water entering flank soft tissue. Significant effects on several systems may occur (Box 32.6).[101,107] ECG lead placement is important and should be coordinated with the surgeon. A high-quality tracing is critical because the R wave is used to trigger the shocks. Synchronization of the shock wave to the ECG has reduced the incidence of cardiac dysrhythmias, most commonly supraventricular or premature ventricular complexes, but has not eliminated them. Atropine or glycopyrrolate may be given at the request of the surgeon to increase the heart rate, and thus the shock wave rate.[107]

Contraindications and Complications

Contraindications to shock wave lithotripsy include (1) active urinary tract infection, (2) uncorrected bleeding disorder or coagulopathy, (3)

BOX 32.6 Side Effects Associated With Extracorporeal Shock Wave Lithotripsy

- Hypothermia, hyperthermia
- Cardiac arrhythmias
- Skin bruising hematomas
- Petechiae, soft tissue swelling at site
- Renal edema
- Renal hematoma
- Lung injury
- Flank pain
- Hypertension, hypotension
- Nausea, vomiting
- Respiratory difficulties

distal obstruction, and (4) pregnancy. Obesity and orthopedic or spinal deformities may make positioning difficult.[101,103] Dose-dependent hemorrhagic lesions can develop on the kidneys, secondary to vascular damage.[105-107] The colon, hepatic structure, lungs, spleen, pancreas, abdominal aorta, ileac veins, or any structure in the abdominal region may be perforated, ruptured, or otherwise damaged. Moderate to severe hemorrhage may occur but usually resolves spontaneously; patients with clotting disorders are at an increased risk. Hematuria develops in most patients, secondary to blood vessel rupture. Diabetes, new-onset hypertension, or permanently decreased renal function may result.[108]

Anesthesia

Patients will not tolerate ESWL without anesthesia. Various anesthetic techniques have been used. General anesthesia is advantageous because of its rapid onset and control of patient movement. Other techniques include spinal or epidural anesthesia, patient-controlled analgesia, monitored anesthesia care, and topical anesthesia with eutectic local anesthetics. Continuous infusions of propofol, ketamine, and alfentanil have been used alone or with midazolam. Regional anesthesia provides effective analgesia with a T4-T6 level. A short-acting spinal anesthetic using 50 mcg of sufentanil alone is popular. Epidural catheters and dressings may cause absorption of some of the shock wave, decreasing the efficacy of treatment. Akinesis is critical in reducing number and duration of treatments, determining efficacy of ESWL, and preventing potential tissue damage. General anesthesia or deep sedation techniques decrease the risk of patient movement.[101,103,108] Preoperative preparation includes the discontinuation of aspirin-containing medications, anticoagulants, platelet inhibitors, and nonsteroidal antiinflammatory agents for 7 to 10 days before the procedure and documentation of a negative urine culture to prevent postoperative urinary tract infection or sepsis. In women of childbearing age, a pregnancy test is administered if ionizing radiation is to be used during the procedure. Depending on stone composition (i.e., size, radiopacity, location) patients may be advised to drink clear liquids, take a laxative, or both the day before the procedure to enhance stone visualization. Fasting protocols are within standard guidelines for anesthesia.[103]

For lithotripsy to be most effective, the calculus must remain at the focal point. Because patient movement and patterns of respiration can change kidney and calculus position, movement must be minimized, and ventilation carefully controlled. The number and intensity of shock waves can be reduced when calculus movement is minimized.[109] An obstructed kidney or a patient exhibiting signs and symptoms of infection qualifies as an emergency case. Adequate hydration is encouraged postoperatively to promote diuresis of fragments and decrease hematuria. Proximity to lasers may cause corneal damage; strict laser protocols should be employed (i.e., eye protection).[103]

PERCUTANEOUS NEPHROLITHOTOMY

Removal of kidney stones or calculi 25 mm or smaller also can be accomplished through percutaneous nephrolithotomy. This procedure requires general anesthesia and postoperative hospitalization. Calculi are removed via a rigid operating scope inserted in the lower renal calyx under intermittent fluoroscopy. Once located, calculi are pulverized by using laser, electrohydraulic, or ultrasound probes placed directly on the stones. The procedure is performed with the patient in the prone or supine position; therefore, associated anesthetic considerations apply. The following is a list of complications of percutaneous nephrolithotomy.[110,111]

BOX 32.7 Potential complications of percutaneous nephrolithotomy

Minor	Major
Pain	Septicemia
Fever	Bleeding
Urinary tract infection	Pelvic or ureteral tears
Renal colic	Pneumothorax
	Hemothorax
	Anaphylaxis secondary to contrast dye

TRANSURETHRAL RESECTION OF THE PROSTATE

Surgical Technique

Benign prostatic hyperplasia (BPH) is the most common benign adenoma in men. Up to 40% of men will require intervention for urinary difficulty, and the frequency of those seeking medical treatment is increasing due in part to the increase in life expectancy. Medical management consists of pharmacotherapy, which may be combined with a minimally invasive technique. Drugs such as the α-blocking agents (alfuzosin [Uroxatral], tamsulosin [Flomax], doxazosin [Cardura], and terazosin [Hytrin]) or the 5-α-reductase (5AR) inhibitors (finasteride [Proscar] and dutasteride [Avodart]) are used alone or in combination such as dutasteride and tamsulosin (Jalyn). Laser therapy seems useful for selected patients with small glands. Transurethral microwave treatment and intraprostatic stents may be useful in high-risk patients. Transurethral resection of the prostate (TURP) is one of the most performed surgical procedures in men older than 60 years of age. It is being performed less frequently as medical management improves; however, it remains the gold standard in surgical treatment approaches.[112,113]

The procedure consists of opening the outlet channel from the bladder using a resectoscope in the urethra to electrically cut away the obstructing median and lateral lobes of prostate tissue. Bleeding is controlled by coagulation current. For visualization of the area, the bladder is distended, and continuous irrigation is used to wash away blood and dissected prostatic tissue. These patients are often at greater anesthetic risk because they are elderly and more likely to have cardiovascular or pulmonary problems. TURP syndrome is a rare but potentially fatal surgical complication. The incidence is reported to range from 0.78% to 1.4% of procedures. Severe TURP syndrome is extremely rare, but the mortality rate may be as high as 25%. It may occur as early as 15 minutes after the start of resection up to 24 hours postoperatively.[112] The hallmark clinical symptoms are procedure related due to a combination of water intoxication, fluid overload, and hyponatremia. The pathophysiology and clinical features of TURP syndrome are summarized in Table 32.6. Other complications of the procedure include excessive bleeding, bladder perforation, and infection. Average surgical parameters associated with a TURP are given in Table 32.7. Improved surgical techniques and knowledge of the pathophysiology, prevention, and management of TURP syndrome have minimized the risks of this procedure.[112,114-117]

There are several newer surgical techniques, including bipolar TURP (B-TURP), laser TURP (L-TURP), microwave ablation. Aquablation is new technique recently approved by the FDA for treatment of prostate glands too large to be safely removed by a traditional TURP approach. A robotic-assisted water knife works similar to a laser knife in obliterating excess prostate tissue. Due to large amounts of water, perioperative fluid management should be judicious and goal oriented.[118]

TABLE 32.6   Pathophysiology and Clinical Features of TURP Syndrome

Pathophysiology	Clinical Features
Fluid overload	Hypertension, bradycardia, arrhythmia, angina, pulmonary edema and hypoxemia, congestive heart failure and hypotension
Water intoxication or hypoosmolality	Confusion and restlessness, twitching or seizures, lethargy or coma, dilated, sluggish pupils, papilledema, low-voltage EEG, hemolysis
Hyponatremia	CNS changes as above, reduced inotropy, widened QRS complex, low-voltage ECG, T-wave inversion on ECG
Glycine toxicity	Nausea and vomiting, headache, transient blindness, loss of light and accommodation reflexes (blink reflex preserved), myocardial depression, ECG changes
Ammonia toxicity	Nausea and vomiting, CNS depression
Hemolysis	Anemia, acute renal failure, chills, clammy skin; chest tightness and bronchospasm; hyperkalemia resulting in malignant arrhythmias or brady asystole
Coagulopathy	Severe bleeding, primary fibrinolysis, disseminated intravascular coagulation

CNS, Central nervous system; *ECG,* electrocardiography; *EEG,* electroencephalography.
Adapted from Malhotra V, et al. Anesthesia and the renal and genitourinary system. In: Gropper MA, et al., eds. *Miller's Anesthesia.* 9th ed. Philadelphia: Elsevier; 2020:1945.

TABLE 32.7   Average Parameters With a Transurethral Resection of the Prostate

Parameter	Average
30-day mortality	0.2%–0.8%
Resection time	<80 min
Resected mass	20–50 g
Absorbed volume	10–30 mL of fluid per min of resection time
Blood loss	2–5 mL/min of resection time
Serum sodium nadir	132–135 mmol/L

Adapted from Malhotra V, et al. Anesthesia and the renal and genitourinary system. In: Gropper MA, et al., eds. *Miller's Anesthesia.* 9th ed. Philadelphia: Elsevier; 2020:1931–1959.

Complications

Fluid Absorption

Several complications are associated with resection of the prostate. Large amounts of irrigating solution can be absorbed through prostate venous sinuses. The amount absorbed and the rate of absorption depend on (1) glandular size to be resected, (2) congestion, (3) duration of resection, (4) irrigating solution pressure, (5) number of sinuses open at any one time, and (6) experience of the resectionist.[119-121] An average of 10 to 30 mL of fluid can be absorbed per minute of resection time, and 6 to 8 L can be absorbed in cases that last up to 2 hours.[5,114] The uptake of 1 L of irrigant into the circulation within 1 hour can decrease the serum sodium 5 to 8 mEq/L. In general, limiting resection time to 1 hour is desirable.

Complications may occur with irrigation solutions, as determined by their osmolality and solute composition. Various types of irrigating fluid have been used. Although distilled water is associated with the least optical impairment, hemolysis of red blood cells occurs due to the hypotonic composition.[122] Normal saline or lactated Ringer solution is highly ionized and promotes dispersion of high current from the resectoscope. Current irrigating solutions typically consist of Cytal (sorbitol 2.7% and mannitol 0.54%), glycine 1.2% or 1.5%, or physiologic saline.[112]

Complications specifically related to absorption of irrigating fluid include (1) volume overload with pulmonary edema, (2) dilutional hyponatremia, (3) hypoosmolality, (4) cardiac effects, (5) retinal toxic effects (with glycine), and (6) hyperglycemia. As fluid enters the vascular compartment, intravascular pressure, and myocardial work increase. The fluid dilutes plasma proteins and electrolytes, and the change in intravascular pressure favors movement of fluid from the vascular to the interstitial compartment and is poorly tolerated by patients with a cardiovascular disease. Cardiac dysrhythmias may also develop. Progressive increases in blood pressure, CVP, or pulmonary artery wedge pressure (when monitored) suggest hypervolemia. Mannitol irrigating solutions have been reported to contribute to the development of pulmonary edema and hyponatremia.[120,123,124]

Absorption of irrigating fluid also leads to dilutional hyponatremia and hypoosmolality. Sodium is a major cation of extracellular fluid and is responsible for the depolarization of excitable cells and the propagation of action potentials. The severity and speed of the drop in sodium are related to the resulting symptoms. The decrease in sodium produces an osmotic shift of fluid resulting in brain edema, increases in intracranial pressure, and neurologic symptoms. Hyponatremia usually results from water excess rather than from sodium loss. CNS symptoms associated with hyponatremia range from restlessness, headache, irritability, and confusion to blindness, coma, and seizures.

Serum sodium (Na^+) concentrations of 120 mEq/L appear to be borderline for the development of severe reactions, which are mainly ECG and CNS changes. ECG changes characterized by widening of the QRS complex and ST segment elevation are seen when the serum level decreases to 115 mEq/L. At levels less than 100 mEq/L, ventricular tachycardia and fibrillation can occur.[116,125,126] The irrigating fluid should be warmed to prevent the development of hypothermia and possible detrimental shivering.[127]

CNS symptoms associated with hyponatremia include restlessness, confusion, nausea, vomiting, coma, and convulsions. A change in mental status may be the first sign of developing hyponatremia. These symptoms can be detected more easily in patients receiving regional anesthesia. CNS symptoms are hidden under general anesthesia. Transient hyperglycemia and hypokalemia have been reported when glucose irrigation solutions have been used.[114,116,122,128]

Bladder Perforation

Perforation of the bladder is another potential complication of prostatic surgery; however, recent advances in technology have reduced its incidence. Symptoms vary, depending on whether the rupture is intraperitoneal or extraperitoneal. Pathophysiology and clinical features of bladder perforation and TURP syndrome are noted in Box 32.8.[120] These symptoms are better recognized when the patient has regional anesthesia, particularly when the regional technique does not produce a high block. With general anesthesia, only the surgeon can appreciate the inability to recover bladder fluid as a sign of perforation. The kidney may excrete small amounts of intraperitoneal fluid. However, if hemodynamic compromise occurs, suprapubic drainage is effective for removal of excess intraperitoneal fluid.

BOX 32.8   Key Points for Anesthesia Management of Transurethral Resection of Prostate (TURP)

- TURP syndrome is caused by disturbance of intravascular volume and/or serum osmolality.
- Five questions to ask prior to a TURP:
  1. What is the irrigation fluid (glycine, Cytal, or physiologic saline)?
  2. What is the bag height over the prostate?
  3. What is the size of the prostate?
  4. What is the expected duration of procedure?
  5. What is the surgical operating position (avoid Trendelenburg)?
- Techniques for detection of pending TURP syndrome include measurement of serum sodium, monitoring for fluid overload, assessment of mental status, and ethanol breath analysis.
- Treat symptomatic (mental status changes, seizures, hypotension) patients aggressively; treat asymptomatic aberrant lab values (hyponatremia, hyperglycemia) very slowly, if at all.
- CNS symptoms of headache, irritability, confusion, nausea, and vomiting are early warning signs of TURP syndrome.

CNS, Central nervous system.
Adapted from Hawary A, et al. Transurethral resection of the prostate syndrome: almost gone but not forgotten. *J Endourol.* 2009;23(12):2013–2020; Malhotra A, Malhotra V. Complications of transurethral surgery. In: Atlee JL, ed. *Complications in Anesthesia.* 3rd ed. Philadelphia: Elsevier; 2018:210–213; Gravenstein D, Hahn RG. TURP syndrome. In: Lobato EB, et al., eds. *Complications in Anesthesiology.* Philadelphia: Lippincott Williams & Wilkins; 2008:474–491.

Glycine Absorption

Absorption of glycine has been associated with toxicity. Although glycine, a normal amino acid, is a major inhibitory transmitter, particularly in the retina, toxic effects may occur from absorption during the procedure. Absorption of 1.5% glycine can cause a deterioration of vision. TURP blindness is caused by retinal dysfunction from glycine toxicity.[112,114] Clinical signs and symptoms of excess glycine absorption include nausea, vomiting, fixation and dilation of the pupils, weakness, muscle incoordination, and hypotension due to a decrease in the release of catecholamines.[114]

Glycine may also result in encephalopathy and seizure activity due to N-methyl-D-aspartate (NMDA) receptor stimulation and CNS toxicity. CNS symptoms are a consequence of its biotransformation in the liver to ammonia. Ammonia toxicity may result in encephalopathy, delayed awakening, and even coma in the postoperative period.[112] Other signs and symptoms of glycine toxicity include nausea, vomiting, headache, malaise, and weakness.

Skin Burns

The use of high voltage for cutting and coagulation during TURP may result in skin burns. Newer technology for TURP (e.g., bipolar enucleation of the prostate, laser and Aquablation therapy) reduces the risk of skin burns when compared with monopolar techniques.[118,130] ECG pads may be placed at other sites so that potential burns are avoided. Many patients who undergo TURP have pacemakers. Depending on the age of the pacemaker, these devices must be converted to a fixed rate unless they are designed to operate in the presence of applied currents.[114,129]

Blood Loss

Significant bleeding occurs in less than 1% of TURP cases. Blood loss during TURP is generally related to (1) weight of the resected tissue,

(2) resection time, and (3) skill of the surgeon.[121] Increased blood loss occurs with greater than 45 g of resected tissue and procedures lasting longer than 90 minutes. Assessment of blood loss may be difficult because of the dilution of blood in irrigating fluid. Hematocrit may be increased, decreased, or unchanged depending on the amount of fluid in the intravascular space at the time. Blood transfusion should be based on preoperative hematocrit, the duration and difficulty of resection, and a general assessment of the patient. A 2011 study of 951 robotic-assisted laparoscopic prostatectomies noted that men with larger prostates and median lobes requiring longer operative times experienced higher blood loss. Resected tissue less than 30 g generally required no transfusion. Thirty to 80 g resected possibly required up to 2 units of red blood cells, and greater than 80 g up to 4 units.[2,130]

Prevention of TURP syndrome. Prevention of TURP syndrome is, of course, the most important approach. Early identification of evolving symptoms is vital to avoid serious morbidity. Suggested preventative measures include (1) avoid the Trendelenburg position as it promotes fluid absorption, (2) limit resection time to less than 1 hour, (3) keep prostate capsule intact until the end of the resection, (4) place irrigating fluids less than 60 cm above the prostate gland, (5) measure electrolytes during and after the procedure as indicated, and (6) use a regional technique with light sedation so that mental changes can be identified.[131]

Treatment of TURP syndrome. An asymptomatic patient with mild hyponatremia only requires monitoring and observation. Mild symptoms can be managed with supportive treatment such as antiemetics, atropine, vasopressors, or diuretics, and careful observation as indicated.

If TURP syndrome is detected intraoperatively, bleeding points should be coagulated and surgery completed as soon as reasonable. Severe hyponatremia less than 120 mEq/L must be treated. The challenge is to promptly institute treatment while avoiding overtreatment. The most feared complication of rapid correction of acute hyponatremia is central pontine myelinolysis, also referred to as osmotic demyelination syndrome (ODS). The etiology is unclear; however, osmotic stress appears to cause changes in neuronal cells and the release of myelin toxins. Symptoms usually occur approximately 1 week after the osmotic stress and may include seizures, palsy, dysarthria, paralysis, mental changes, and coma. Hypertonic saline (3%–5% sodium chloride) should be given at a rate no greater than 100 mL/hour. Sodium correction should not exceed 0.5 mEq/L/hour or 8 mEq/day. Severe symptoms may require initial doses of 1 to 2 mEq/L/hour. Target levels for correction are 120 mEq/L. If 3% to 5% sodium chloride is not immediately available, 9% sodium bicarbonate can be administered to treat severe hyponatremia until 3% to 5% sodium chloride becomes available. Suggestions for the management of TURP syndrome and bladder perforations are given in Box 32.8.

Anesthesia for TURP procedures. Spinal and general anesthesia techniques are both used for TURP procedures. Spinal anesthesia is considered the anesthetic of choice because the early signs and symptoms of TURP syndrome, hypervolemia, and bladder perforation are more easily detected in a responsive patient. Under general anesthesia, cardiovascular changes must be relied on to diagnose complications.[132-134] Pain impulses from the bladder neck and prostate are propagated by afferent parasympathetic fibers originating primarily from the second and third sacral roots in concert with the pelvic splanchnic nerves. The sympathetic nerves via the hypogastric plexus, which is derived from T11-L2 nerve roots, transmit sensation from the bladder.[5] As a result, a T10 sensory level is necessary for adequate anesthesia. Intrathecal opioids are commonly included with

BOX 32.9   Management of Transurethral Resection of Prostate (TURP) Syndrome and Bladder Perforation

- Asymptomatic or mildly symptomatic patients should be observed and monitored.
- Severe TURP syndrome requires immediate aggressive therapy if the patient is to survive. The following interventions are suggested:
  - Terminate the surgery as soon as possible.
  - Administer 20 mg of intravenous (IV) furosemide.
  - Immediately obtain the following tests: hematocrit; serum electrolyte, creatinine, and glucose concentrations; serum osmolality (if available); arterial blood gas analyses; and 12-lead electrocardiography.
  - Continue or start the administration of normal saline. Hypertonic saline (3% or 5%) may be administered (at a rate <100 mL/hr) if the serum sodium concentration is <100 mEq/L, severe central nervous system side effects of hyponatremia and hypoosmolality are evident, or reduced inotropy results in cardiovascular collapse.
  - Administer IV midazolam in 1-mg incremental doses to treat twitching or seizures; a barbiturate may be added if seizures persist.
  - Auscultate chest and obtain chest radiographs to detect pulmonary edema. Intubate and mechanically ventilate the patient at the earliest evidence of pulmonary edema.
  - Transfuse packed red blood cells as necessary.
- If bleeding continues, investigate for disseminated intravascular coagulation (DIC) or primary fibrinolysis. DIC is treated with crystalloids and blood products to achieve hemodynamic stability and normal coagulation. Primary fibrinolysis responds well to aminocaproic acid (Amicar) administered as an IV infusion of 3–5 g in the first hour, followed by continuous IV infusion at 1 g/hr until the bleeding is controlled.
- Institute invasive monitoring and provide supportive therapy to maintain circulation and pulmonary function, and to prevent renal failure.

Bladder Perforation

As soon as bladder perforation is detected, undertake the following measures:
- Stop surgery and achieve hemostasis.
- Treat hypotension with IV crystalloids, vasopressors, and inotropes.
- Obtain a hematocrit. Start blood transfusion if brisk bleeding continues. Occult blood loss into the intraperitoneal or retroperitoneal space may occur.
- Perform a cystourethrogram to locate the perforation.
- For most perforations, suprapubic cystotomy, an indwelling Foley catheter, and (occasionally) ureteral stents are sufficient. In some instances, immediate exploratory laparotomy may be necessary to control bleeding and repair the perforation.

Adapted from Hawary A, et al. Transurethral resection of the prostate syndrome: almost gone but not forgotten. J Endourol. 2009;23(12):2013–2020; Malhotra V, et al. Anesthesia and the renal and genitourinary system. In: Gropper MA, et al., eds. Miller's Anesthesia. 9th ed. Philadelphia: Elsevier; 2020:1931–1959; Gravenstein D, Hahn RG. TURP syndrome. In: Lobato EB, et al., eds. Complications in Anesthesiology. Philadelphia: Lippincott Williams & Wilkins; 2008:474–491.

BOX 32.10   Advantages and Disadvantages of Laparoscopic Renal Surgery

Advantages
- More precise operative procedure due to magnification of operative site
- Reduced postoperative pain
- Improved cosmetic results
- Quicker return to normal activities
- Reduction in hospital length of stay
- Reduction of cost of care
- Less intraoperative bleeding
- Fewer postoperative pulmonary infections
- Fewer postoperative wound infections
- Reduced metabolic derangements
- Better postoperative respiratory function

Disadvantages
- Potential for extravasation of insufflated carbon dioxide to retroperitoneal space and thorax
- Potential for postoperative airway compromise secondary to subcutaneous emphysema and pharyngeal obstruction
- Increased incidence of acidosis due to absorption of carbon dioxide
- Higher incidence of intraoperative oliguria potentially due to perirenal pressure from pneumoperitoneum
- Potentially longer duration than open procedure

LAPAROSCOPIC UROLOGIC SURGERY

Laparoscopy is the process of inspecting the abdominal cavity through an endoscope. Laparoscopy started in the mid-1950s in gynecologic surgeries. Over the years, laparoscopy for general and urologic surgery has become a common procedure. Advantages and disadvantages of laparoscopic surgery are found in Box 32.10. Some examples of surgical procedures that can be done laparoscopically include varicocelectomy, percutaneous stone retrieval, nephrectomy, transplants, and radical prostatectomy.[135]

Carbon dioxide is the most universally used agent for insufflating the abdominal cavity to facilitate view during this procedure. Several pathophysiologic changes can occur after carbon dioxide pneumoperitoneum and the extremes of patient positioning. Preparation for hemorrhage and conversion to an open procedure are critical.[136] Most of the considerations for laparoscopic surgery are in Chapter 34, but two unique problems specific to urologic surgery are worth noting.

The urogenital system is a retroperitoneal system. As such, carbon dioxide insufflated in this space communicates freely with the thorax and subcutaneous tissue. Subcutaneous emphysema can occur and may extend to the head and neck. In severe cases, it may lead to submucosa swelling and airway compromise in the unprotected airway.[137]

Carbon dioxide is absorbed from the peritoneal cavity, and acidosis may develop. Because the carbon dioxide insufflation, together with steep Trendelenburg position and long procedures, may increase intraabdominal and intrathoracic pressure, controlled ventilation is mandatory. Intraperitoneal pressure greater than 10 mm Hg results in hemodynamic alterations, including decreased cardiac output and increased systemic vascular resistance. The pneumoperitoneum can cause renal cortical vasoconstriction due to activation of the sympathetic nervous system. Decreased renal perfusion activates the renin-angiotensin-aldosterone system, which causes vasoconstriction. These effects are additive to those seen with surgical

the local anesthetic. Cautious fluid loading may be used to minimize spinal anesthesia-induced hypotension. Although general anesthesia may mask early complications, it may be desirable in the patient who requires pulmonary support or who cannot tolerate a fluid load for compensation of a loss of sympathetic tone. All inhalation agents have been used successfully.[112,114,123] Some key points for anesthesia management of TURP are given in Box 32.9.

stress. Renal and hepatic perfusion may be altered.[135,136,138,139] Some suggested techniques to minimize the effect of positive pressure pneumoperitoneum include (1) employ lower insufflation pressures, (2) operate in a gasless environment, (3) substitute inert gas for carbon dioxide, (4) use drugs to antagonize the neuroendocrine response, (5) expand volume, and (6) use mechanical devices. It has been reported that the use of intermittent sequential pneumatic compression, activated over the lower limbs 15 minutes after the pneumoperitoneum, improves splanchnic and renal perfusion. This technique augments cardiac output and lowers systemic vascular resistance.[140] A complete discussion of laparoscopic surgery can be found in Chapter 34.

ROBOTIC UROLOGIC SURGERY

Robotic-assisted surgery is becoming increasing more popular for managing various urologic procedures.[141] Major urologic surgery has two main categories. The first is upper tract surgery such as simple or radical nephrectomy, radical nephroureterectomy, or nephron-sparing surgery. The second category is pelvic surgery, such as radical cystectomy, with urinary diversion and radical prostatectomy.[139]

Robotic systems consist of a surgeon's console for surgical work, a surgical cart housing video and lighting equipment, and a robotic tower supporting three or four robotic arms.

Robotic technology provides the surgeon with an enhanced and magnified three-dimensional view, a reduction in scattered ambient light, reduced surgeon fatigue, hand tremor, and improved manual dexterity. This technology also provides a predominantly bloodless field.[142,143] Pyeloplasties to correct hydronephrosis, nephrectomies, and bladder augmentation robotic procedures are being employed in the pediatric population.[144,145]

Cost savings are noted in managing adverse outcomes and decreased hospital length of stay, but these savings only offer a partial offset of the direct costs of purchasing and maintaining the robotic equipment. Competition from medical equipment companies can lower direct costs.[144] Patient outcomes are similar or improved from open and laparoscopic surgical approaches.[141,146] Wang reported decreased blood loss, decreased transfusion requirements, and shorter hospital stays.[147] Complications are commonly related to patient position, length of surgical time, and surgeon skill level.[148,149]

Robotic surgery necessitates a coordinated approach by anesthetist and surgeon because the surgery is performed using a modified laparoscopic technique and can be long in duration. The patient is placed in steep Trendelenburg position, with the addition of lithotomy positioning in prostatectomy surgery. Major complications of surgery in the Trendelenburg position include (1) neuropathies, (2) CVP elevation, (3) intraocular/intracranial pressure elevation, (4) increased pulmonary venous pressure, (5) decreased pulmonary compliance, (6) reduced functional residual capacity, and (7) swelling of the face, eyelids, conjunctivae, and tongue.[5,148,149,150,151]

Significant pulmonary alterations, such as profound hypercarbia, can develop in the perioperative environment. Although most patients with impaired gas exchange due to diaphragmatic and chest wall restriction will quickly resolve to 15% of baseline within minutes when returned to supine position, increased body mass index and smoking history significantly increase the risk of prolonged respiratory compromise.[151]

Fluid replacement should be carefully monitored. Overhydration can distort anatomic surgical landmarks and lead to profound fluid shifts in radical prostatectomy and cystectomy procedures.[147] Facial swelling requires careful airway assessment prior to extubation as reintubation may be difficult due to altered anatomic landmarks and

---

BOX 32.11 Anesthetic Considerations With Robot-Assisted Surgery

Prolonged lithotomy position predisposes to:
- Lower (and rarely upper) extremity nerve injury (particularly femoral nerve)
- Pressure areas and compartment syndrome of the lower limbs

Prolonged Trendelenburg position predisposes to:
- Ocular injury, including corneal abrasions and ischemic optic neuropathy caused by high intraocular pressures
- Laryngeal (and facial) edema and respiratory distress
- Risk of cerebral edema, as well as increased intracranial pressure, due to reduction in cerebral venous return due to the high intraabdominal pressures and head-down position
- Decreased functional residual capacity and decreased pulmonary compliance causing increased ventilatory pressures and increased atelectasis

Prolonged pneumoperitoneum predisposes to:
- Carbon dioxide subcutaneous emphysema (up to 4% of cases)
- Carbon dioxide air embolism is also possible

Adapted from Cockcroft JO, et al. Anesthesia for major urologic surgery. *Anesthesiol Clin.* 2015;33(1):165–172.

edematous soft tissue. Anesthetic considerations for robotic procedures are summarized in Box 32.11. Common management principles for urologic robot-assisted surgery are noted in Box 32.12. A complete discussion of anesthesia for robotic-assisted surgery can be found in Chapter 35.

RENAL TRANSPLANTATION

Renal transplant procedures have been a mainstream treatment for end-stage renal disease patients for years. Although brain-dead donors still comprise the largest segment of the donor pool, living related donors are rapidly increasing due to improved surgical techniques, posttransplantation management, and social media marketing efforts. Please see Chapter 41 for complete information on renal organ transplantation.

OPEN NEPHRECTOMY

Nephrectomy procedures are performed either laparoscopically or open and can be partial or total removal of the kidney, typically from tumors or polycystic disease. Laparoscopic and robotic techniques are rapidly replacing the open nephrectomy procedures due to more rapid recovery and decreased postoperative complications.[136] Open nephrectomies are typically performed in the jackknife lateral position with a raised kidney rest or other bump to displace the kidney to a more superficial location facilitating surgical access. Significant cardiopulmonary compromise may occur from the surgical position. The vena cava may be compressed by the kidney rest, decreasing venous return and blood pressure. Decreased respiratory compliance, increase in peak airway pressures, and atelectasis development in the dependent lung are common. The procedure is very stimulating, and appropriate attenuation of the stress response should be the cornerstone of the anesthetic plan, such as a combined epidural/general anesthetic.[151] Third spacing and the development of dependent edema may be significant due to surgical positioning and length of surgery. Vocal cord edema should be considered if the patient exhibits scleral edema, and it may be prudent to keep the patient intubated postoperatively. Other anesthetic concerns are related to major abdominal procedures. Postoperative pain management should be initiated perioperatively or early in the recovery phase.

BOX 32.12   Common Management Principles for Urologic Robot-Assisted Surgery

- *Duration:* approximately 3–4 hr (surgical time, 2–3 hr)
- *Incision:* multiple robotic-arm trocars with surgical instruments attached
- *Positioning:* steep head-down lithotomy (~27 degrees), arms wrapped by sides
- Warn patient about sore throat, due to the endotracheal tube, facial edema, catheter insertion, lower abdominal (and sometimes penile) pain, and the need for early mobilization
- Drugs to reduce gastric acid and increase gastric emptying (e.g., famotidine 20 mg intravenously and metoclopramide 10 mg by intravenously)
- Thromboembolic stockings (if not contraindicated)
- All invasive lines on one side (opposite side to robot assistant; usually the left) for less interference during procedure (normally a 16-gauge intravenous cannula and 20-gauge arterial cannula)
- Anesthetize patient on the surgical table, lying directly on gel pad, with gel head support
- General anesthesia, endotracheal tube (taped not tied to avoid cerebral venous congestion), positive pressure ventilation (optimal positive end-expiratory pressure)
- Orogastric tube (for gastric deflation) and oral temperature probe
- Saline-soaked ribbon gauze throat pack (to protect against gastric contents refluxing up lacrimal ducts and causing corneal burns)
- Eye protection with lubricating ointment, tape, and padding
- Padded right-angled bar placed just caudad to patient's chin to protect head from surgical instruments
- Arms wrapped by patient's sides, which limits intraoperative access: plan lines appropriately and attach patient identification to forehead after routine safety checks
- Arterial transducer on board fixed at the level of the shoulder
- Forced-air warmer to upper chest and fluid warmer
- Bolsters under knees, gel pads under ankles, and calf pumps
- Steep head-down position (try for 27 degrees, depending on patient habitus and ventilatory pressures); some centers use shoulder bolsters
- Preincision surgical antibiotic prophylaxis as per local protocol
- Intravenous dexamethasone to decrease inflammation and swelling
- Buscopan reduces bladder spasm in recovery (can increase heart rate)
- Remifentanil infusion with volatile maintenance in oxygen/air mix is used most commonly
- Avoid any patient movement during robotic instrumentation
- With careful attention to airway pressures, a second dose of muscle relaxant is rarely required
- Limit fluid therapy during procedure while lower renal tract is disrupted. For most surgery, this requires <800 mL. Then administer up to ~1200 mL of crystalloid once urethra is reconnected by the surgeon (communicate closely): total 2000 mL
- Blood loss is usually <300 mL

Surgical Conclusion

- As soon as robot is disengaged, flatten patient out and perform recruitment maneuvers to the lungs
- Consider spinal after discussion with surgeon before emergence (if bladder spasm is a problem, spinal is advised): no opiate, aim to cover 3 hr after surgery
- Sit patient up as soon as surgery is complete: slow wake up over 10–15 min while remifentanil action wears off (this period reduces cerebral edema and risk of agitation and confusion postoperatively)
- Ensure normocapnia and cuff leak before extubation
- Postoperative pain is normally only mild to moderate
- Regular multimodal analgesia, antiemetic, and venous thromboembolic prophylaxis

Adapted from Cockcroft JO, et al. Anesthesia for major urologic surgery. *Anesthesiol Clin.* 2015;33(1):165–172.

SUMMARY

Anesthetic management of the patient during the perioperative period for renal procedures depends on an understanding of both normal renal function and pathophysiologic changes in the organ system. In addition to normal anatomy and physiology, this chapter highlighted ways to assess renal function and changes in renal function secondary to anesthetics. Various stages of renal pathology were identified and management of patients with acute and chronic renal failure emphasized. Rare and common urologic procedures were identified, and pertinent anesthetic considerations discussed for each procedure.

REFERENCES

For a complete list of references for this chapter, scan this QR code with any smartphone code reader app, or visit the following URL: http://booksite.elsevier.com/9780323711944/.

33

Hepatobiliary and Gastrointestinal Disturbances and Anesthesia

Shawn B. Collins, Vanessa Jones-Oyefeso, Kurt D. Cao

An understanding of the hepatobiliary system plays an integral role in anesthetic management. Familiarity with diseases of the hepatobiliary and gastrointestinal (GI) systems can help avoid negative anesthetic outcomes. The liver is the largest internal organ and plays a critical role in maintaining the homeostasis of many other physiologic processes, most notably drug metabolism. As such, acute or chronic liver dysfunction can impair the intended response to anesthesia and result in comorbidities that must be taken into consideration.[1]

The purpose of this chapter is to give an overview of pathophysiologic processes specific to the hepatobiliary and GI system that are commonly encountered by the anesthetist. Fundamental relevant anesthetic considerations are described. More specifically, this chapter reviews the anatomy, physiology, and pathophysiology of the liver, including evaluation of liver function, anesthesia effects on liver function, and perioperative management of patients with liver disease. The chapter continues with diseases of the biliary tract, esophagus, stomach, peritoneum, intestinal tract, and spleen, and anesthetic management of patients with conditions affecting these systems. Special consideration is given to carcinoid tumors.

LIVER DISEASE

Anatomic, Physiologic, and Pathophysiologic Considerations

Located in the right upper quadrant of the abdomen, the liver is the largest internal organ. It generally extends from ribs 7 to 11 along the right midaxillary line. The liver spans an area from the right hypochondrium to a portion of the left hypochondrium and is classically divided into four lobes, which may be subdivided into multiple segments, such as the eight segments described by the Couinaud system (Fig. 33.1).[2] These subdivisions are based on the anatomic proximity of the hepatic and portal veins, though multiple classifications with different terminology are used, and no system is recognized as superior.

The liver acts as an interface between the GI tract and systemic circulation, providing numerous essential metabolic, synthetic, immunologic, and hemodynamic functions.[1] It constitutes 2.5% of total body weight but accounts for 20% of total body oxygen consumption. The liver receives approximately 25% of cardiac output via a dual arterial and venous blood supply.[3] The portal vein collects venous drainage from the spleen, stomach, small and large intestines, gallbladder, and pancreas and delivers it to the liver (Fig. 33.2). This partially deoxygenated, nutrient-rich blood represents approximately 75% of the hepatic blood supply but only half of the oxygen supply. The hepatic artery, which branches off of the abdominal aorta, provides oxygen-rich blood, representing approximately 25% of the hepatic blood supply and 50% of the oxygen supply (Fig. 33.3).[4] The hepatic artery and portal vein enter the liver and progressively branch until terminating in the hepatic sinusoids.

The basic structural unit of the liver is the hepatic lobule, which consists of plates of hepatocytes that radiate around a central vein in a hexagonal pattern with portal canals at the corners. The portal canals contain lymphatic vessels, nerves, and a portal triad, which consist of a hepatic arteriole, a portal venule, and a bile duct. Blood from the portal canal vessels flows through hepatic sinusoids located between the hepatocyte plates to the central veins, which return the blood to the inferior vena cava via the hepatic vein (Fig. 33.4). The hepatic sinusoids are composed of sinusoidal endothelial cells and function as capillaries. These cells have large fenestrations, which permit the diffusion of fluids, large plasma proteins, and other solutes into the spaces surrounding the hepatocytes known as the space of Disse.[6] Due to the nature of the sinusoidal endothelial cells, a large quantity of lymph is produced that is nearly equal in protein concentration to plasma. The hepatic sinusoids also contain Kupffer cells, which are macrophages that phagocytize 99% of the bacteria delivered from the GI tract.[5] There are between 50,000 and 100,000 hepatic lobules in a normal liver.

Hepatocytes constitute 75% to 80% of the total cellular volume of the liver and are responsible for the majority of its metabolic and synthetic functions. They are divided into three zones based on proximity to the portal tracts, with each zone being exposed to different amounts of oxygen, nutrients, and other filtered substances as blood flows from the portal tract vessels to the central veins. As a result, the hepatocytes of each zone differ enzymatically and respond differently to toxin exposure and hypoxia.[5] Bile canaliculi are located between hepatocytes and empty into terminal bile ducts. An extensive arcade of lymphatic vessels is also present within the layer of cells.[3]

The mean pressure in the hepatic artery is similar to that in the aorta, whereas portal vein pressure has been reported to range from 6 to 10 mm Hg in humans. This relatively low pressure allows the liver to function as a circulatory reservoir. The hepatic blood volume may expand considerably in patients with cardiac failure. It serves as an important blood reservoir in case of bleeding episodes, and compensates for up to 25% of the volume lost from hemorrhage by the immediate expulsion of blood from the capacitance vessels.[7] Both α- and β-receptors are present in the hepatic arterial circulation, but only α-receptors are found in the portal circulation. There is disagreement as to whether the hepatic arterial vasculature exhibits autoregulation of blood flow. Portal blood flow is dependent on the combined venous outflow from the spleen and GI tract. A decrease in either portal or arterial blood flow induces a compensatory increase in the blood flow delivered by the other system.[4]

Potent inhaled anesthetics can affect hepatic blood flow, particularly the portal blood flow, but current evidence suggests that flow is well maintained relative to oxygen demand. None of the present anesthetics adversely influence hepatic integrity by affecting hepatic blood flow.[8] The effects of volatile anesthetics on hepatic blood flow are shown in Table 33.1.

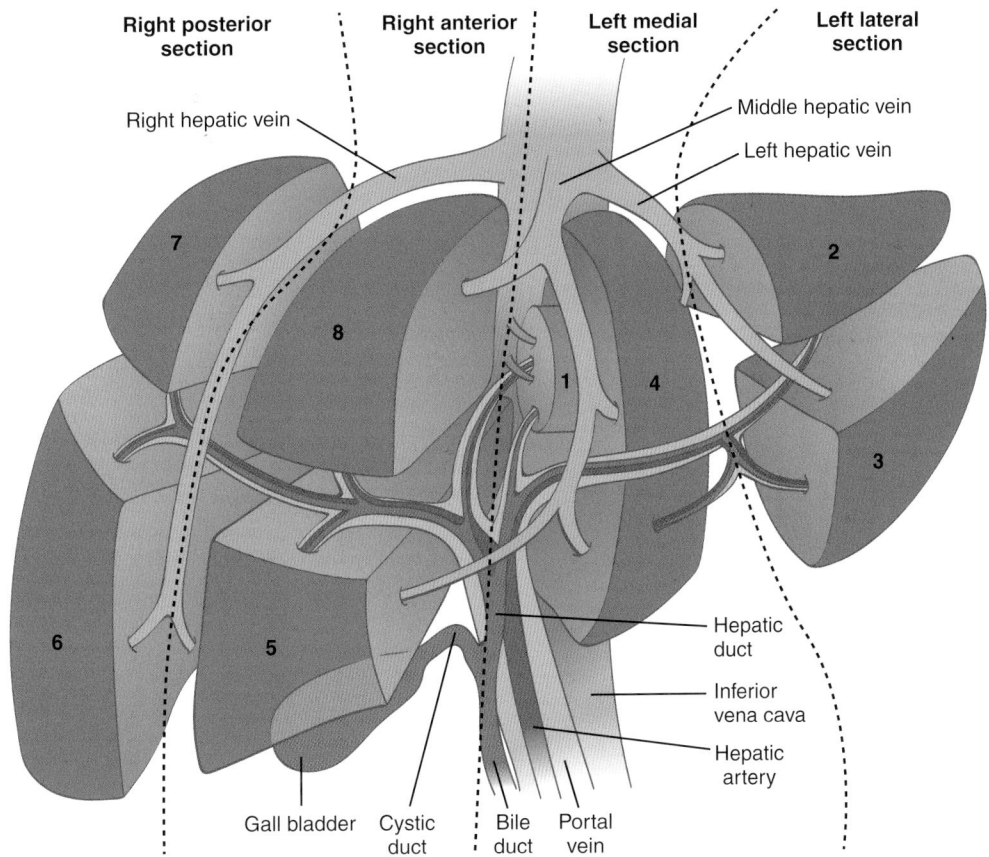

Fig. 33.1 Anatomic and functional subdivisions of the liver. The eight functional anatomic segments of the liver are demonstrated in this drawing. Each segment has its own blood supply and biliary drainage. (From Marschall MD, et al. *Stoelting's Anesthesia and Co-Existing Disease.* 7th ed. Philadelphia: Elsevier; 2018:346.)

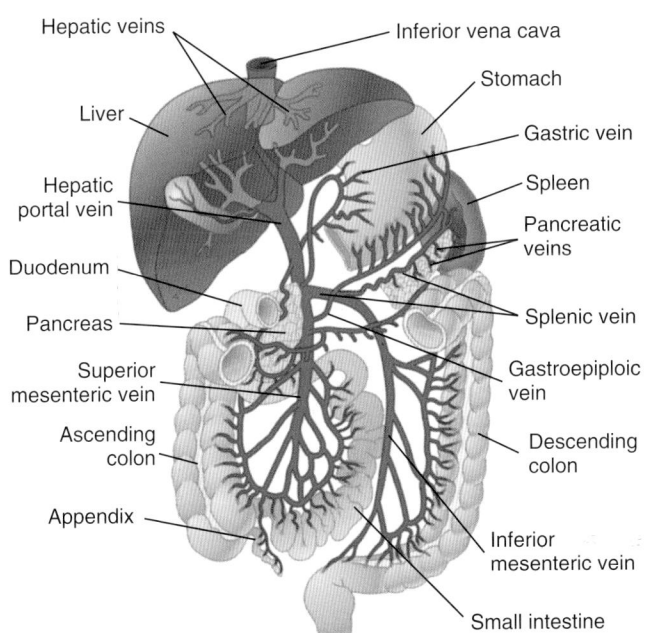

Fig. 33.2 Hepatic portal circulation. In this unusual circulatory route, a vein is located between two capillary beds. The hepatic portal vein collects blood from capillaries in visceral structures located in the abdomen and empties into the liver for distribution to the hepatic capillaries. Hepatic veins return blood to the inferior vena cava. *I,* Inferior; *L,* left; *R,* right; *S,* superior. (From Patton KT. *Anatomy & Physiology.* 10th ed. St. Louis: Elsevier; 2019:685.)

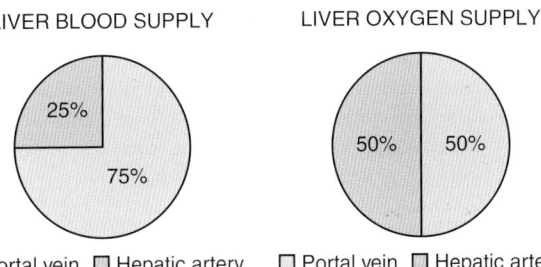

Fig. 33.3 Sources of blood and oxygen supply to the liver. (From Marschall MD, et al. *Stoelting's Anesthesia and Co-Existing Disease.* 7th ed. Philadelphia: Elsevier; 2018:346.)

Changes in hepatic artery or portal vein blood flow may not result in an overall change in total hepatic flow due to the hepatic artery buffer response (HABR). This response is a semireciprocal autoregulatory mechanism whereby changes in portal flow inversely affect hepatic arterial flow.[7] Similar rates of total hepatic flow between administration of two different anesthetic agents implies that the HABR is intact.

The liver has many physiologic functions, including synthesis and metabolism of various essential proteins, lipids, and hormones (Box 33.1). There are no artificial devices that can duplicate all functions of the liver.

Carbohydrate Metabolism

Because nutritional ingestion and energy demand may not be synchronous, the body relies on a dynamic system of energy storage and utilization. Glucose is the primary fuel source for many cells of the body

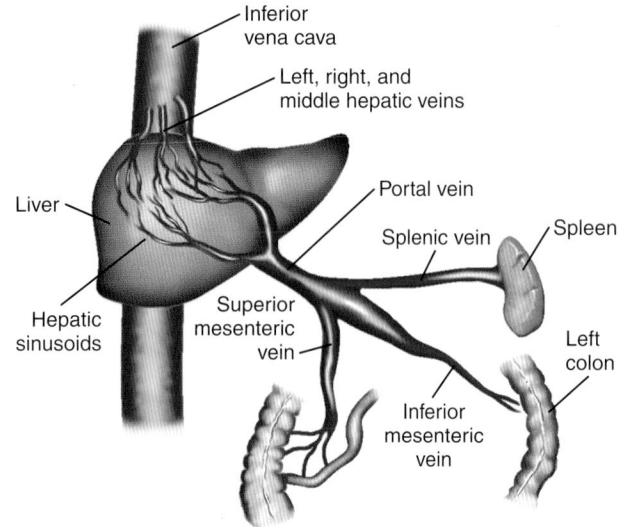

Fig. 33.4 Anatomy of the portal circulation. Blood vessels that constitute the portal circulation and hepatic outflow tracts are depicted. (From Feldman M, et al., eds. *Sleisenger and Fordtran's Gastrointestinal and Liver Disease.* 11th ed. Philadelphia: Elsevier; 2021:1443.)

TABLE 33.1 Effect of Selected Volatile Anesthetics on Hepatic Blood Flow

Volatile Anesthetic	Hepatic Artery Blood Flow	Portal Vein Blood Flow
Desflurane	Moderate dose-dependent decrease	Moderate dose-dependent decrease
Isoflurane	Minimal dose-dependent decrease	Minimal dose-dependent decrease
Sevoflurane	Minimal dose-dependent decrease	Minimal dose-dependent decrease

BOX 33.1 Selected Essential Physiologic Functions of the Liver

- Carbohydrate metabolism
- Gluconeogenesis
- Glycogenolysis
- Glycogenesis
- Protein synthesis
- Albumin (maintenance of osmolarity)
- Thrombopoietin (platelet production)
- Amino acid synthesis
- Protein metabolism
- Bile production
- Lipid metabolism
- Lipogenesis
- Cholesterol synthesis
- Coagulation factor synthesis
- Production of factors I, II, V, VII, IX, X, and XI
- Insulin clearance
- Drug metabolism/transformation
- Bilirubin metabolism

(e.g., kidney, red blood cells) and the preferred energy source for other tissues (e.g., brain). To maintain a steady blood glucose level, the liver moderates gluconeogenesis and glycogenolysis.

Gluconeogenesis is the formation of glucose from the noncarbohydrate molecules lactate and pyruvate, as well as amino acids, all of which are products of anaerobic and catabolic metabolism. It is stimulated by a decrease in glycogen stores. During periods of fasting, the liver maintains blood glucose at relatively normal levels through glycogenolysis. Initiated by epinephrine and glucagon, glycogenolysis is the process of liberating glucose from glycogen stores found in the liver (and skeletal muscle). Hypoglycemia may therefore be encountered in patients with severe liver disease due to dysfunctions in insulin clearance, a decrease in glycogen capacities, and impaired gluconeogenesis. Because these processes deplete stored nutrients, the body's energy needs can only be maintained for a limited time.

Protein Synthesis

Protein synthesis occurs primarily in the liver; this excludes immunoglobulins, which are produced by the humoral immune system. With significant liver disease, a reduction in circulating plasma protein will result in a decrease in plasma oncotic pressure. Additionally, drugs bound to proteins produced by the liver will have a greater unbound fraction if circulating proteins are reduced due to liver disease. In addition, overexpansion of the interstitial space and third spacing secondary to derangements in plasma oncotic pressure result in a large increase in the volume of distribution of clinically used medications. Clinical concerns should therefore focus on the potential for an exaggerated effect with a given dose of drug, particularly a drug that is highly protein bound. The amount of nondepolarizing muscle relaxant may also need to be increased to achieve a given level of blockade. This is secondary to an increased volume of distribution of the drug (secondary to alterations in plasma protein binding and body fluid shifts). Plasma cholinesterase, which is produced in the liver, may also be deficient. This condition may prolong the effects of succinylcholine and enhance the potential toxicity of ester local anesthetics.

Protein Metabolism

Other roles in protein metabolism performed by the liver include the synthesis of lipoproteins (important for lipid transport in the blood), the deamination of amino acids into carbohydrates and fats for production of adenosine triphosphate through citric acid cycle oxidation, and the production of urea for the removal of ammonia, which is formed by hepatic deamination processes and bacteria in the gut.

Bilirubin Metabolism

Bilirubin is a breakdown product of heme metabolism and is often classified as unconjugated or conjugated. Heme is converted to unconjugated bilirubin in the reticuloendothelial cells of the spleen. This unconjugated bilirubin is not soluble in water and is neurotoxic at sufficiently high levels. It is then bound to albumin and transported to the liver. Once in the liver, the unconjugated bilirubin is conjugated with glucuronic acid. Bilirubin is then incorporated into the bile and secreted into the intestine, where it is metabolized by bacterial enzymes and predominantly excreted in the feces.

Bile Production

The liver aids intestinal digestion by forming bile and secreting it into the common bile duct (CBD). Hepatocytes in each lobule continuously secrete fluid that contains phospholipids, cholesterol, conjugated bilirubin (the end product of hemoglobin metabolism), bile salts, and other substances. Bile is stored and concentrated in the gallbladder. In response to the intestinal hormone cholecystokinin (CCK), bile is released by the gallbladder. The presence of fat and protein in the duodenum initiates contraction of the gallbladder and movement of bile via the CBD. This duct merges with the pancreatic duct at the ampulla of Vater, which empties into the duodenum via the sphincter of Oddi (major duodenal ampulla). Obstruction of either of these ducts may result in pathologic illness that may necessitate surgical correction.

Bile secretion assists in the absorption of fat and fat-soluble vitamins (vitamins A, D, E, and K). The metabolic end products of many drugs are also removed via the bile. Liver disease may result in impaired bile production or flow, leading to steatorrhea, vitamin K deficiency, and delayed removal of active drug metabolites.

A deficiency in vitamin K results in coagulopathy due to impaired production of clotting factors II (prothrombin), VII, IX, and X.[9] The liver is responsible for producing the majority of clotting factors. Hepatocellular disease therefore results in decreased clotting factor levels and abnormal bile production. Impaired bile production ultimately manifests as altered production of vitamin K–dependent clotting factors.

Intrahepatic obstruction of blood flow (due to disease pathology) ultimately causes portal hypertension. A consequence of the resultant transmission of backward pressure is congestive splenomegaly, leading to platelet sequestration and thrombocytopenia. Therefore, severe liver disease with portal hypertension induces coagulopathy not only as a result of impairment in hepatic coagulation factor production but also as a result of a decrease in the number of circulating functional platelets. In the presence of biliary deficiency, parenteral vitamin K administration helps correct coagulopathy. However, significant hepatocellular disease may dictate the need for fresh frozen plasma (FFP) for immediate correction of coagulation factor deficits.

The use of subarachnoid and epidural blockade should be avoided in the presence of coagulopathy. Abnormalities in parameters such as prothrombin time (PT), activated partial thromboplastin time (aPTT), and platelet count are a relative contraindication to these techniques; procedures in which bleeding is a possibility are often postponed when the international normalized ratio (INR [PT]) is greater than 1.5. Nasopharyngeal instrumentation and invasive procedures must be performed cautiously and carefully in the presence of increases in PT and aPTT, a low platelet count, or other laboratory signs that arouse suspicion of coagulopathy.

Insulin Clearance

The liver is the main site for insulin clearance, removing 50% during the first portal passage, but this percentage varies widely under different conditions.[10] In patients with obesity, hyperinsulinemia, an insulin-resistant state, dyslipidemia, or type II diabetes mellitus, insulin clearance by the liver decreases. In insulin-resistant states, a reduction in hepatic insulin extraction leads to substantial peripheral hyperinsulinemia (due to insulin hypersecretion and reduced hepatic extraction of insulin).[11]

Drug Metabolism/Transformation

The enzyme systems involved in the biotransformation of drugs are primarily located in the liver. Proper hepatic function is necessary to maintain the pharmacokinetic machinery detailed in Chapter 6. Orally administered drugs may be metabolically inactivated in the liver before reaching the systemic circulation. This first-pass metabolism may limit the oral availability of highly metabolized drugs. Within the liver, phase I and II reactions are responsible for the metabolism of many exogenous substances and most drugs. The subsequent products are then excreted via excretory transporters on either the canalicular or sinusoidal membranes (Box 33.2).[12] The end products of these processes

(except in the case of a prodrug or an active metabolite) are the result of deactivation and transformation of substances into benign byproducts that are capable of being excreted in the bile or urine.

The cytochrome P450 (CYP) class of enzymes are primarily responsible for phase I reactions. More than 50 CYPs have been identified in humans, yet nearly 50% of currently manufactured drugs are metabolized by a single CYP.[13] Differences in the rate of metabolism of a drug can be due to drug interactions. When two drugs that are metabolized by the same enzyme system are coadministered, the rate of metabolism can be either decreased or increased. Enzyme induction hastens metabolism of certain coadministered medications (e.g., ethanol, barbiturates, ketamine, some benzodiazepines) and promotes tolerance to other medications metabolized by the same enzyme class. This relative tolerance can increase the clinical requirement for other drugs (e.g., sedatives, opioids, steroid muscle relaxants). Conversely, coadministration of drugs metabolized by the same CYP (e.g., cimetidine, chloramphenicol) will compete for binding to the enzyme's active site. This can result in enzyme inhibition of metabolism of one or both drugs and lead to elevated plasma levels, culminating in increased sensitivity or toxicity.

Tolerance to certain drugs results from overproduction of enzymes within hepatic enzyme systems, including the CYP system. Drugs capable of inducing this process include ethanol, benzodiazepines, ketamine, barbiturates, and phenytoin. The result is an increased clinical requirement for certain drugs such as sedatives, opioids, and muscle relaxants (e.g., vecuronium and rocuronium).

Certain drugs, such as lidocaine, morphine, meperidine, and propranolol, are highly dependent on hepatic extraction from the circulation for sufficient metabolism. Decreased blood flow to the splanchnic circulation, which occurs during hypotensive states and can even occur during an uneventful laparotomy, may decrease the metabolic clearance of these drugs. Anesthetic drug metabolism is discussed further in Chapter 6.

Laboratory Evaluation of Liver Function

No single laboratory test reliably assesses liver function. As stated previously, the huge capacity and functional reserve of the liver allow for significant disease processes to develop before evidence of liver failure is reflected in abnormal laboratory findings; abnormalities do, however, aid in differentiating parenchymal from obstructive disorders. Parenchymal disorders reflect dysfunction at the hepatocellular level, whereas obstructive disorders reflect disease processes caused by dysfunctional bile excretion.

BOX 33.2 Drug Metabolism in the Liver

Phase I Reactions
- Functionalization reactions
- Addition or exposure of a functional group (e.g., oxidation, reduction, hydrolysis)
- Typically result in the loss of pharmacologic activity (excluding prodrugs)
- Important for metabolizing many of the anesthetic drugs (e.g., midazolam, diazepam, codeine, phenobarbital, inhalation anesthetics, propofol)

Phase II Reactions
- Conjugation reactions
- Phase I product (substrate) conjugation with a second molecule
- Lead to the formation of a covalent linkage between a functional group and glucuronic acid, sulfate, glutathione, amino acid, or acetate (e.g., morphine, acetaminophen)

Ammonia is cleared by the liver and may be used to evaluate hepatic encephalopathy, but ammonia levels do not correlate well with the severity of the clinical presentation. As such, its usefulness is limited. Bilirubin levels also reflect hepatic clearance effectiveness, but it is elevated in most significant liver diseases and does not have specific diagnostic value. Albumin synthesis occurs in the liver, and hypoalbuminemia can indicate chronic liver disease once nonhepatic etiologies have been ruled out. Because albumin has a half-life of 14 to 21 days, quantitative values derived from laboratory analysis will be slow to decrease in relation to worsening liver function, making it an unreliable indicator of hepatic synthetic function in acute liver injury. The most common reason for a low albumin is chronic liver failure caused by cirrhosis. The serum albumin concentration is usually normal in chronic liver disease until cirrhosis and significant liver damage has occurred. In advanced liver disease, the serum albumin level may be less than 3.5 g/dL. Biochemical markers of liver function are identified in Table 33.2.

Serum transferases (transaminases) are the most sensitive marker for identifying acute hepatic injury. Elevations in transferase levels are common to all forms of liver injury, but the degree of elevation combined with physical examination and patient symptoms can aid in the differential diagnosis of probable types of hepatic disease.

Patients who present soon after passing CBD stones can be misdiagnosed with acute hepatitis, as aminotransferase levels often increase immediately, whereas alkaline phosphatase and γ-glutamyl transferase levels do not become elevated for several days. Asymptomatic patients with isolated, mild elevation of either unconjugated bilirubin or γ-glutamyl transferase levels usually do not have liver disease and generally do not require extensive evaluation.[14]

Overall hepatic function can be assessed by applying the values for albumin, bilirubin, and PT in the Child-Pugh classification system, which is a modified version of the earlier Child-Turcotte grading system (Table 33.3).[15]

Effects of Anesthesia on Liver Function

Patients with liver disease who require surgery are at greater risk for surgical- and anesthesia-related complications than those with a healthy liver.[16] The degree of risk is dependent on the anesthetic technique and associated sequelae, the surgery being performed, and the specific type of liver disease and its severity.

Volatile Anesthetic Selection

Given the global nature of general and regional anesthesia, administration of an anesthetic agent may reduce hepatic blood flow in a dose-dependent manner. The reduction in mean arterial pressure and cardiac output frequently seen with the use of volatile anesthetics results in a proportional reduction in hepatic blood flow. Another factor that impairs hepatic blood flow is the vasoconstrictive response of the splanchnic circulation; this response occurs as

TABLE 33.2 Clinical Significance of Liver Biochemical Tests

Test (Normal Range*)	Basis of Abnormality	Associated Liver Diseases	Extrahepatic Origin
Aminotransferases			
ALT (10–55 units/L) AST (10–40 units/L)	Leakage from damaged tissue	*Mild to moderate elevations:* Many types of liver disease. *Marked elevations:* Hepatitis (viral, toxic, autoimmune, and ischemic). AST/ALT >2 suggests alcoholic liver disease or cirrhosis of any etiology	ALT is more specific than AST for hepatic injuries. AST nonspecific: can originate from skeletal muscle, red blood cell, kidney, pancreas, brain, and myocardium
AP (45–115 units/L)	Overproduction and leakage into serum	*Moderate elevations:* Many types of liver disease. *Marked elevations:* Extrahepatic and intrahepatic cholestasis, diffuse infiltrating disease (e.g., tumor, MAC), rarely alcoholic hepatitis	Bone growth or disease (e.g., tumor, fracture, Paget disease), placenta, intestine, and tumors
GGTP (0–30 units/L)	Overproduction and leakage into serum	Same as for AP; induced by ethanol and drugs. GGTP/AP >2.5 suggests alcoholic liver disease	Kidney, spleen, pancreas, heart, lung, and brain
5' nucleotidase (0–11 units/L)	Overproduction and leakage into serum	Same as for AP	Found in many tissues, but serum elevation is relatively specific for liver disease
Bilirubin (0–1 mg/dL)	Decreased hepatic clearance	*Moderate elevations:* Many types of liver disease. *Marked elevations:* Extrahepatic and intrahepatic bile duct obstruction; viral, alcoholic, or drug-induced hepatitis; inherited hyperbilirubinemia	Increased breakdown of hemoglobin (resulting from hemolysis, disordered erythropoiesis, resorption of hematoma) or myoglobin (resulting from muscle injury)
Prothrombin time (PT) (10.9–12.5 seconds) (international normalized ratio [INR]: 0.9–1.2)	Decreased synthetic capacity	Acute or chronic liver failure (prolonged PT unresponsive to vitamin K). Biliary obstruction (prolonged PT usually responsive to vitamin K administration)	Vitamin K deficiency (secondary to malabsorption, malnutrition, antibiotics, consumptive coagulopathy)
Albumin (3.5–5 g/dL)	Decreased synthesis; increased catabolism	Chronic liver failure	Nephritic syndrome, protein-losing enteropathy, vascular leak, malnutrition, malignancy, infections, and inflammatory states

*The normal values shown in this table are for adult men and will vary with the methodology used in testing.
ALT, Alanine aminotransferase; *AP,* alkaline phosphatase; *AST,* aspartate aminotransferase; *GGTP,* γ-glutamyl transpeptidase; *INR,* international normalized ratio; *MAC,* mycobacterium avium complex; *PT,* prothrombin time.

TABLE 33.3 Grading Liver Function Using the Child-Pugh Classification System

Feature	POINTS		
	1	2	3
Albumin	>3.5 g/dL	2.8–3.5 g/dL	<2.8 g/dL
Bilirubin	<2 mg/dL	2–3 mg/dL	>3 mg/dL
Prolongation of prothrombin time (INR)	<4 sec (<1.7)	4–6 sec (1.7–2.3)	>6 sec (>2.3)
Ascites encephalopathy	None	Controlled minimal (1 and 2)	Refractory advanced (3 and 4)

The Child-Pugh class is calculated by adding the points based on the five features: class A = 5 or 6, class B = 7–9, class C = 10 and higher. The classes indicate the severity of liver dysfunction: Class A is associated with a good prognosis, and class C is associated with limited life expectancy.

INR, International normalized ratio.

a sympathetic reflex to reduced mean arterial pressure. Isoflurane increases hepatic blood flow through direct vasodilatory properties. This effect is likely offset, however, by a reduction in portal blood flow. Hypotension secondary to regional anesthetic–induced sympathectomy (e.g., epidural or subarachnoid blockade) is primarily responsible for the reduced splanchnic blood flow associated with the use of these techniques.

All of the volatile anesthetics have also been shown to reduce hepatic blood flow. Halothane causes the greatest reduction, and desflurane has slightly greater hepatic effects than sevoflurane and isoflurane. A rise in serum glutathione-S-transferase levels indicates a decrease in splanchnic circulation, which causes a transient reduction in hepatocyte oxygenation. One study has shown that liver function is well preserved after administration of desflurane.[17] Sevoflurane undergoes hepatic biotransformation, producing organic and inorganic fluoride ions. In humans, the serum levels of inorganic fluoride ion secondary to sevoflurane metabolism are generally below nephrotoxic levels. Anesthetic agents may reduce hepatic blood flow by 30% to 50% after induction. Animal data suggest, however, that isoflurane and sevoflurane cause less perturbation in hepatic arterial blood flow than other inhaled anesthetic agents; the use of these agents is therefore preferred for patients with liver disease. Studies are underway to determine the influence of sevoflurane biotransformation on renal and hepatic function, but no significant clinical toxicity has yet been reported, so it appears to be safe for clinical use.[18,19]

In developed countries, the clinical use of halothane has been superseded by the newer low-solubility agents desflurane and sevoflurane. Halothane, however, is still in use in some countries, and remains on the 2015 World Health Organization Model List of Essential Medicines, which is a list of minimum medical needs for a basic health care system. Continued awareness of the potentially deleterious effect of halothane on hepatic function is therefore justified.

Halothane administration is associated with two types of postoperative liver injury. Minor injury in 10% to 30% of patients may result in elevations in alanine aminotransferase (ALT) levels during postoperative days 1 through 10. The risk of hepatotoxicity is higher after repeat exposure to halothane. Major injury involves halothane-induced hepatotoxicity, which is a severe hepatic reaction with

elements of autoimmune allergy. Halothane-induced liver damage is also referred to as halothane hepatitis due to a similar clinical presentation. Clinical features of halothane hepatitis are listed in Box 33.3. Hepatic necrosis may be seen histologically, and the case fatality rate ranged from 14% to 71% (before liver transplant was an option). Evidence for the role of hypersensitivity is found in the increased susceptibility and shortened latency after repeat exposure, which are hallmark symptoms and signs of drug allergy. An estimated 1 in 10,000 patients develops postoperative jaundice after halothane exposure. In this population, a viral source of infection is more likely to be the cause, for instance, as a complication of intraoperative blood transfusion.

Opioid Effects

Spasm of the Oddi sphincter may cause biliary colic, or it may cause a false-positive result on intraoperative cholangiography. All opioids have been implicated in causing spasm of the Oddi sphincter, and the more potent the opioid, the greater the resultant increase in biliary pressure. The cause of the spasm is unclear, but its occurrence may be reduced with judicious titration of the anesthetic. There is a low incidence of spasm even when a fentanyl-based anesthetic is used. The treatment of suspected spasm of the Oddi sphincter involves administration of naloxone or nalbuphine. Atropine, glycopyrrolate, glucagon, and nitroglycerin also have been shown to be effective.

Anesthesia-Related Activity: Mechanical Ventilation

The sequelae of mechanical ventilation have been implicated as a contributing factor in reduced hepatic blood flow. Positive pressure ventilation can result in airway pressures that adversely affect venous delivery to the right atrium. Increased airway pressures also result in reduced CO,[20] with a consequent reduction in hepatic blood flow. Positive end-expiratory pressure further exacerbates this condition. Impairment of hepatic blood flow under these conditions may result from increased hepatic venous pressure due to increased intrathoracic pressure and from increased reflex sympathetic tone due to reduced CO. Hypercapnia and acidosis have vasodilatory effects on the hepatic circulation that result in increased blood flow, whereas hypocapnia and alkalosis exert vasoconstricting effects that result in decreased flow. The interplay of various intraoperative variables (e.g., surgical site, ventilatory mode, direct and indirect effects of the anesthetics used, physiologic responses to intraoperative events) influences the degree of variation in hepatic blood flow.

Site of Surgery

The surgical site (particularly an intraabdominal surgical site) has also been implicated as a cause of decreased hepatic blood flow (Table 33.4) in surgical patients with liver disease. Traction on the abdominal viscera may cause reflex dilation of splanchnic capacitance vessels and thereby lower hepatic blood flow.

Additional factors that may contribute to decreased hepatic blood flow intraoperatively include hypotension, hemorrhage, administration of vasoactive drugs, and pneumoperitoneum during laparoscopic surgery.[7,21]

Diseases of the Liver

Signs and symptoms indicating liver disease vary widely depending on the etiology of the underlying pathologic process. The decline in liver function may be acute, related to drug toxicity or infection, or it may follow a chronic subclinical course. The following discussion focuses

BOX 33.3 Clinicopathologic Features of Halothane Hepatitis

- Estimated incidence
  - *After first exposure:* 0.3–1.5/10,000
  - *After multiple exposures:* 10–15/10,000
- Female-to-male ratio 2:1
- Latent period to first symptom
  - *After first exposure:* 6 days (11 days to jaundice)
  - *After multiple exposures:* 3 days (6 days to jaundice)
- Risk factors
  - Older age
  - Female gender
  - Two or more exposures documented in 60%–90% of cases
  - Obesity
  - Familial predisposition
  - Induction of CYPE1 by phenobarbital, alcohol, or isoniazid
- Clinical features
  - Jaundice as presenting symptom in 25% (serum bilirubin: 3–50 mg/L)
  - Fever in 75% (precedes jaundice in 75%); chills in 30%
  - Rash in 10%
  - Myalgia in 20%
  - Ascites, renal failure, and/or gastrointestinal hemorrhage in 20%–30%

- Eosinophilia in 20%–60%
- Serum ALT and AST levels: 25–250 × ULN
- Serum alkaline phosphatase level: 1–3 × ULN
- Histopathologic features
  - Zone 3 massive hepatic necrosis in 30%; submassive necrosis in 70% (autopsy series)
  - Inflammation usually less marked than in viral hepatitis
  - Eosinophilic infiltrate in 20%
  - Granulomatous hepatitis occasionally
- Course and outcome
  - Mortality rate (pretransplantation era): 10%–80%
  - Symptoms can resolve within 5–14 days
  - Full recovery can take 12 wk or longer
  - Chronic hepatitis not well documented
- Adverse prognostic findings
  - Age >40 yr
  - Obesity
  - Short duration to the onset of jaundice
  - Serum bilirubin level >20 mg/dL
  - Coagulopathy

ALT, Alanine aminotransferase; *AST,* aspartate aminotransferase; CYPE1, cytochrome P450 2E1; *ULN,* upper limit of normal.
From Lewis JH. Liver disease caused by anesthetics, chemicals, toxins, and herbal preparations. In: Feldman M, et al., eds. *Sleisenger and Fordtran's Gastrointestinal and Liver Disease.* 11th ed. Philadelphia: Elsevier; 2021:1399.

TABLE 33.4 Reported Surgery Risk in Patients With Liver Disease

Liver Disease	Type of Surgery	Mortality	Prognostic Factors
Cirrhosis	Nonlaparoscopic biliary surgery	20%	Ascites, prothrombin time, albumin
	Peptic ulcer surgery	54%	Prothrombin time, systolic blood pressure, hemoglobin
	Umbilical herniorrhaphy	13%	Urgent surgery
	Colectomy	24%	Hepatic encephalopathy, ascites, albumin, hemoglobin
	Abdominal surgery for trauma	47%	
	Emergency abdominal surgery	57%	Child-Pugh class, urgent surgery
	Laparoscopic cholecystectomy	0.9%–6%	
	Emergency cardiac surgery	80%	Child-Pugh class
	Elective cardiac surgery	3%–46%	Child-Pugh class
	Knee replacement	0%	
	TURP	6.7%	
Chronic hepatitis	Various types	0%	
Hepatitis C	Laparoscopic cholecystectomy	0%	
Acute hepatitis	Exploratory laparotomy	Up to 100%	
Obstructive jaundice	Abdominal surgery	5%–60%	Hemoglobin, bilirubin, malignancy

TURP, Transurethral resection of the prostate.

on the more commonly encountered diseases of the liver and offers guided clinical anesthetic implications.

Acute Hepatitis

Hepatitis is a generic term that means liver inflammation. Hepatitis may be caused by several factors (e.g., toxins, alcohol, medications, viral or bacterial infections, autoimmune diseases). Acute hepatitis presents a variable clinical picture. Manifestations may extend from mild inflammatory increases in serum transaminase levels to fulminant hepatic failure. The cause of this syndrome is usually exposure to an infectious virus. Other causes include exposure to hepatotoxic substances and adverse drug reactions.

Viral Hepatitis

Although several types of hepatitis viruses are known to cause illness, typically only hepatitis A, B, and C (infections caused by the hepatitis A virus, hepatitis B virus [HBV], and hepatitis C virus, respectively) affect persons living in the United States.[22] Hepatitis D requires coinfection with HBV; hepatitis E virus diagnosis is made by exclusion after travel to an endemic area (e.g., South/Central America or Southeast

Asia). Hepatitis A and E are transmitted by the oral-fecal route, and hepatitis B, C, and D are transmitted by contact with body fluids and physical contact with disrupted cutaneous barriers.

The common clinical course of viral hepatitis begins with a 1- to 2-week prodromal period, the signs and symptoms of which include fever, malaise, nausea, and vomiting. Progression to jaundice typically occurs, with resolution within 2 to 12 weeks. However, serum transaminase levels often remain elevated for up to 4 months. If hepatitis B or C is the cause, the clinical course is often more prolonged and complicated. Cholestasis may manifest in certain cases. Fulminant hepatic necrosis in certain individuals is also possible. Table 33.5 lists the major characteristics of hepatitis types A, B, C, D, and E.

Drug-Induced Hepatitis

Drug-related injury to the liver results from an idiosyncratic reaction to a substance or an overdose resulting in toxicity. Genetic predisposition is presumed to be the most critical determinant. Important risk factors include age, gender, exposure to other substances, a history or family history of previous drug reactions, other risk factors for liver disease, and concomitant medical conditions.[23]

Alcoholic hepatitis is probably the most common form of drug-induced hepatitis and results in fatty infiltration of the liver (causing hepatomegaly), with impairment of hepatic oxidation of fatty acids, lipoprotein synthesis and secretion, and fatty acid esterification.[4]

Chronic Hepatitis

Chronic hepatitis occurs in 1% to 10% of acute hepatitis B infections and in 10% to 40% of hepatitis C infections but does not occur in hepatitis A infections.

Because chronic persistent hepatitis is limited to portal areas and is relatively benign, hepatic cellular integrity is preserved, and progression to cirrhosis is rare. Chronic lobular hepatitis involves recurrent exacerbations of acute inflammation; as in persistent hepatitis, progression to cirrhosis is rare.

Chronic active hepatitis is progressive and results in hepatocyte destruction, cirrhosis, and progressive deterioration of hepatic function. Hepatic failure and fatal chronic hepatitis are marked by clinical manifestations such as multiorgan system failure (e.g., hepatorenal syndrome [HRS]), encephalopathy, and hemorrhage from esophageal varices. Exposure to certain drugs (e.g., methyldopa, isoniazid, and nitrofurantoin) and the presence of autoimmune disorders (e.g., systemic lupus erythematosus) are potential causative factors implicated in hepatic failure, though hepatitis B or C are more typical.

Other symptoms present in chronic hepatitis include marked fatigue and jaundice; thrombocytopenia, glomerulonephritis, myocarditis, arthritis, and neuropathy may also be present. Plasma albumin levels are usually low as a result of synthetic dysfunction, and the PT is prolonged.

Nonalcoholic Fatty Liver Disease

Nonalcoholic fatty liver disease (NAFLD) is a term that encompasses a broad spectrum of liver disorders related to steatosis that is not due to alcohol consumption.[24] It can range in severity from simple benign steatosis to nonalcoholic steatohepatitis (NASH), which involves inflammation with hepatocyte injury and may progress to cirrhosis and hepatocellular carcinoma.[25] NAFLD is commonly associated with metabolic comorbidities such as obesity, diabetes mellitus, and dyslipidemia.[24] The incidence of NAFLD is increasing worldwide in parallel with the obesity and diabetes epidemics, affecting an estimated one-third of the US adult population.[26] As a result, NASH has become the most common chronic liver disease worldwide and the fastest growing indication for liver transplantation in the United States.[4,27]

Anesthetic Management for Patients With Hepatitis

Research indicates that mild chronic hepatitis confers no additional risk of surgical morbidity or mortality during laparoscopic cholecystectomy.[28] Surgical outcomes in patients with acute hepatitis are less well studied, and recommendations suggest that elective surgery should be postponed until normalization of biochemical profiles. Existing studies are many decades old, and the statistical risks associated may not reflect improvements in surgical techniques and anesthetic management. Anesthetic management recommendations for patients with hepatitis are found in Box 33.4.

Operative procedures performed in patients with alcohol intoxication are likely to be associated with increased perioperative complications, and anesthetic management must be well planned (Box 33.5). Surgery performed in those undergoing alcohol withdrawal is associated with an increased mortality rate. If surgery is of urgent or emergent nature, attention must be paid to managing comorbidities, with a focus on risk reduction and symptom management.

Cirrhosis

The term *cirrhosis* derives from the Greek word meaning "yellowish or tawny," which describes the coloration of the diseased liver. Cirrhosis is defined as the histologic development of regenerative nodules surrounded by fibrous bands in response to chronic liver injury, which leads to portal hypertension and end-stage liver disease.[29] Cirrhosis may be caused by a variety of diseases (Box 33.6), but the resultant

TABLE 33.5 Five Types of Acute Viral Hepatitis

Hepatitis Virus	Size (nm)	Genome	Route of Transmission	Incubation Period (Days)	Fatality Rate	Chronic Rate	Antibody
A	27	RNA	Fecal-oral	15–45 (mean = 25)	1%	None	Anti-HAV
B	45	DNA	Parenteral Sexual	30–180 (mean = 75)	1%	2%–7%	Anti-S Anti-HBc Anti-HBe
C	60	RNA	Parenteral	15–150 (mean = 50)	<0.1%	70%–85%	Anti-HCV
D (delta)	40	RNA	Parenteral Sexual	30–150	2%–10%	2%–7% 50%	Anti-HDV
E	32	RNA	Fecal-oral	30–60	1%	None	Anti-HEV

HAV, Hepatitis A virus; *HBc,* hepatitis B core; *HBe,* hepatitis B e-antigen; *HBs,* hepatitis B surface; *HCV,* hepatitis C virus; *HDV,* hepatitis D virus; *HEV,* hepatitis E virus.
From Goldman L, Schafer AI, eds. *Goldman's Cecil Medicine.* 24th ed. Philadelphia: Elsevier; 2012.

BOX 33.4 Anesthetic Management of the Patient With Acute Hepatitis

Preserve hepatic blood flow:
- Use isoflurane or desflurane and avoid halothane
- Maintain normocapnia
- Avoid PEEP if possible
- Provide adequate/liberal intravenous hydration
- Consider regional anesthesia if coagulation is acceptable and the procedure allows

Avoid medications with potential for hepatotoxicity or inhibition of CYP450:
- Halothane
- Acetaminophen
- Sulfonamides
- Tetracycline
- Penicillin
- Amiodarone

Thoughtful titration of neuromuscular blocking agents may be prolonged in patients with liver disease because of:
- Reduced pseudocholinesterase activity
- Decreased biliary excretion
- Larger volume of distribution

CYP450, Cytochrome P450; *PEEP,* positive end-expiratory pressure.

BOX 33.5 Management Recommendations for the Acutely Intoxicated Patient

- Anesthetic requirement is reduced
- Acute intoxication reduces MAC
- Aspiration precautions are needed
- Full stomach, alcohol-related impaired pharyngeal reflexes
- Alcohol increases GABA receptor activity
- Enhanced effects of benzodiazepines, barbiturates, propofol, other CNS depressants
- Alcohol inhibits NMDA receptors
- Reduces CNS excitability

CNS, Central nervous system; *GABA,* γ-aminobutyric acid; *MAC,* maximum allowable concentration; *NMDA,* N-methyl-D-aspartate.

BOX 33.6 Causes of Cirrhosis

Viral
- HBV
- HCV
- HDV

Autoimmune
- Autoimmune hepatitis
- PBC
- PSC

Toxic
- Alcohol
- Arsenic

Metabolic
- α_1-antitrypsin deficiency
- Galactosemia
- Glycogen storage disease
- Hemochromatosis
- Nonalcoholic fatty liver disease and steatohepatitis
- Wilson disease

Biliary
- Atresia
- Stone
- Tumor

Vascular
- Budd-Chiari syndrome
- Cardiac fibrosis

Genetic
- CF
- Lysosomal acid lipase deficiency

Iatrogenic
- Biliary injury
- Drugs: high-dose vitamin A, methotrexate

CF, Cystic fibrosis; *HBV,* hepatitis B virus; *HCV,* hepatitis C virus; *HDV,* hepatitis D (delta) virus; *PBC,* primary biliary cirrhosis; *PSC,* primary sclerosing cholangitis.
From Kamath PS, Shah VH. Overview of cirrhosis. In: Feldman M, et al., eds. *Sleisenger and Fordtran's Gastrointestinal and Liver Disease.* 11th ed. Philadelphia: Elsevier; 2021:1164.

TABLE 33.6 Laboratory Tests and Findings in Cirrhosis

Laboratory Finding	Description	Cause
AST/ALT	Normal or modest increase	Leakage from damaged hepatocytes
Bilirubin	Increased (important predictor of mortality)	Cholestasis, systemic inflammation
Albumin	Decreased in advanced cirrhosis	Decreased production; sequestered in ascites
Prothrombin time	Decreased in advanced cirrhosis	Decreased hepatic production of factor V/VII
Sodium imbalance	Hyponatremia	Inability to excrete free water (increased ADH)
Anemia	Low hemoglobin Low red blood cell count	Folate deficiency, hypersplenism, varices
Thrombocytes	Thrombocytopenia	Hypersplenism, decreased hepatic thrombopoietin production

AST/ALT, Aspartate aminotransferase/alanine aminotransferase ratio; *ADH,* antidiuretic hormone.

anatomic alterations secondary to hepatocyte necrosis are the primary cause of the deterioration in liver function. Over time, the liver parenchyma is replaced by fibrous and nodular tissue, which distorts, compresses, and obstructs normal portal venous blood flow. Portal hypertension develops and impairs the ability of the liver to perform various metabolic and synthetic processes.

Characteristics of cirrhosis are presented in Table 33.6. Obstructive engorgement of vessels within the portal system ultimately results in the transmission of increasing retrograde pressure to the splanchnic circulation. The progressive reversal of portal venous blood flow results in the formation of esophageal varices and splenomegaly. As portal hypertension persists, physical changes can be seen systemically (Fig. 33.5).

The development of esophageal varices places the patient at risk for spontaneous, severe, upper GI hemorrhage. Development of ascites (related to altered intravascular osmolarity) results in fluid retention and dysfunction of the renin-angiotensin system. The subsequent reduction in renal perfusion progresses to eventual renal failure concomitant with hepatic failure. This is referred to as hepatorenal syndrome. HRS is a severe complication of advanced liver cirrhosis that occurs in patients with ascites and marked circulatory dysfunction. HRS is functionally related to extreme renal vasoconstriction.[30] Patient

prognosis is very poor once disease has progressed to this stage. Further failure of the liver to clear nitrogenous compounds (ammonia) from the blood contributes to the development of progressive mental status changes (encephalopathy), ultimately leading to coma and death, if untreated. Recommendations for anesthetic preparation and management for patients with cirrhosis are shown in Box 33.7.

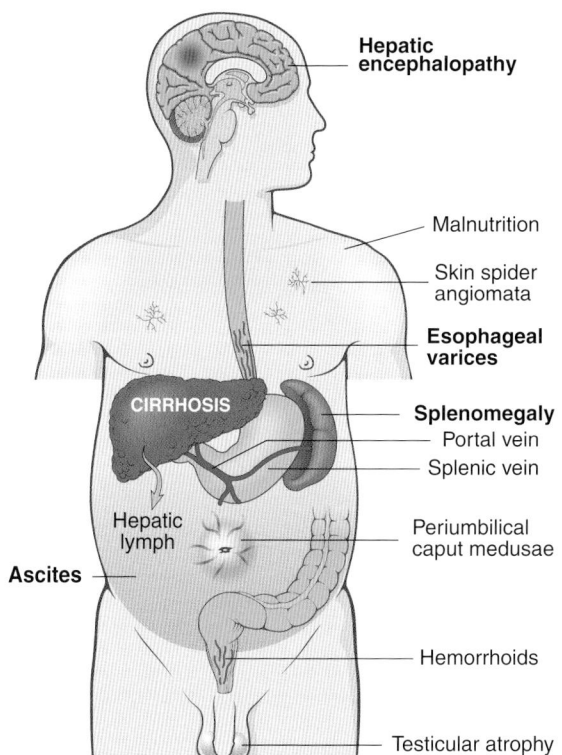

Fig. 33.5 The major clinical consequences of portal hypertension in the setting of cirrhosis, shown for men. In women, oligomenorrhea, amenorrhea, and sterility are frequent, as a result of hypogonadism. (From Kumar V, et al., eds. *Robbins Basic Pathology*. 10th ed. Philadelphia: Elsevier; 2018:637.)

Perioperative Considerations in Liver Disease

Preoperative Assessment

Preoperative assessment of patients with hepatic dysfunction necessitates the collection of diagnostic laboratory markers and physical characteristics indicative of the type and severity of liver disease present. Acute derangements in hepatic function should be identified, and the risks of surgery must be weighed against the risk of postponing the planned procedure until the physical status of the patient is improved. Urgent or emergent surgery may preclude a rigorous diagnostic workup, so it is incumbent on the anesthetist to focus on the implications of the disease process and prioritize care to minimize further physiologic insult.

The Child-Pugh score, original Model for End-stage Liver Disease (MELD) score, and the newer MELD-Sodium (MELD-Na) score have been reported to be correlated with postoperative morbidity and mortality in patients with end-stage liver disease.[31,32] The Child-Pugh score was described earlier (see Table 33.3). MELD is a scoring system that assesses the severity of chronic liver disease. It is useful in prioritizing recipients for liver transplant, as it predicts the outcome based on the calculated score. MELD uses the patient's values for serum bilirubin, serum creatinine, and the INR(PT) to predict three-month survival (interpretation of MELD score is given in Table 33.7). The original MELD score was developed to determine short-term mortality in patients receiving a transjugular intrahepatic portosystemic shunt (TIPS) procedure. It has been used by the United Network for Organ Sharing (UNOS) since the early 2000s. In 2016, UNOS updated the MELD Score to include sodium (MELD-Na) in the calculation. If the original MELD Score is 12 or greater then it is adjusted using the serum sodium value.

Hyponatremia is a reflection of the vasodilatory state in cirrhosis and is associated with several complications in patients with

TABLE 33.7 Original MELD Score Prediction of 90-Day Mortality

MELD Score	Mortality
>40	71.3%
30–39	52.6%
20–29	19.6%
10–19	6.0%
<9	1.9%

MELD, Model for end-stage liver disease.

liver disease, including severe ascites, hepatic encephalopathy, renal impairment, increased infection rate, and posttransplant problems. For every mmol decrease in serum sodium between 125 and 140 there is a small increase in mortality, and the addition of serum sodium to the MELD score can help elevate an individual's transplant priority.[33]

$$\text{Original MELD Score} = 3.78\,[\text{Ln serum bilirubin (mg/dL)}] \\ + 11.2\,[\text{Ln INR}] + 9.57\,[\text{Ln serum} \\ \text{creatinine (mg/dL)}] + 6.43$$

The MELD-Na Score can be calculated online (e.g., https://optn.transplant.hrsa.gov/resources/allocation-calculators/meld-calculator/).

Multivariate analysis of a 2007 study of 772 patients with cirrhosis undergoing major digestive, orthopedic, or cardiovascular surgery (586 patients underwent GI surgery) revealed that the MELD score, ASA physical status, and age were predictors of mortality.[31]

The existence of jaundice, prolonged PT, ascites, encephalopathy, hypoalbuminemia, portal hypertension, renal insufficiency, hyponatremia, infection, and anemia have been propped as risk factors for adverse outcomes in surgical patients.[34] In patients with cirrhosis undergoing surgery, preoperative assessment is crucial. The high risk of mortality and morbidity can be reduced by addressing coagulopathy, ascites, renal dysfunction, hyponatremia, hepatic encephalopathy, malnutrition, pulmonary conditions, cardiac conditions, and anemia, and administering antibiotic prophylaxis.[35]

Relevant information including past or current jaundice, ascites, hepatitis, blood transfusion, or substance abuse can be obtained from the patient history and by physical examination. Reviewing previous anesthetic records also may provide guidance for developing an anesthetic plan. Physical signs such as petechiae, jaundice, ascites, dependent edema, altered mental status, and asterixis (tremor of the wrist indicative of hepatic encephalopathy) suggest the presence of significant liver disease. Laboratory assessment may include the following:

- Albumin (normal values: 3.5–5 g/dL)
- Bilirubin
- PT/INR
- Creatinine
- Serum liver enzyme levels: alanine transaminase (ALT test), aspartate aminotransferase, alkaline phosphatase, lactic dehydrogenase, γ-glutamyl transpeptidase
- Complete blood count
- Serum electrolyte (especially sodium) and glucose levels
- Blood type and screen or crossmatch based on planned surgery and patient condition

Effects of Hepatic Dysfunction on Other Organ Systems

Cardiovascular Considerations

Cardiovascular complications of cirrhosis include (1) cardiac dysfunction; (2) abnormalities in the central, splanchnic, and peripheral circulation; and (3) hemodynamic changes caused by humoral and nervous dysregulation.[36] Increased levels of endogenous vasodilators such as vasoactive intestinal peptide, ferritin glucagon, and others result in a hyperdynamic circulatory state. Cardiovascular changes associated with liver disease include the following:

- Increased cardiac output
- Decreased systemic vascular resistance
- Decreased arterial blood pressure
- Systemic collateral circulation
- Arteriovenous shunting
- Portal hypertension
- Esophageal varices
- Cardiomyopathy
- Congestive heart failure

Fluid Balance and Renal Considerations

Severe hepatic disease disrupts the fluid balance, which manifests as ascites and edema. Ascites is the most common complication of cirrhosis and is associated with an increased risk of infections, renal failure, and poor long-term outcome.[37] The absolute intravascular volume is typically increased, but therapeutic paracentesis, diuretic therapy, and arteriovenous shunting create a relative hypovolemia. Severe hepatic disease (e.g., advanced cirrhosis) may result in impairment of compensatory mechanisms that initiate displacement of blood from the hepatic vascular reservoir into systemic circulation in response to sympathetic stimulation or hemorrhage.

Perioperative concerns focus on the intravascular volume and on electrolyte imbalances. Diuretic therapy should be instituted in the presence of volume overload, with special attention paid to maintaining normotension and the electrolyte balance. Perioperative preservation of adequate renal perfusion is of the utmost importance. Water restriction, controlled isotonic intravenous (IV) fluid administration, and potassium replacement may be necessary components of the preoperative plan of fluid therapy.

Fluid and electrolyte disturbances associated with liver disease include the following:

- Hypoalbuminemia
- Sodium retention
- Progressive decline in renal function
- Decreased free water clearance
- Dilutional hyponatremia
- Hypokalemia

Intraabdominal ascites exerts a profound influence on several organ systems, including the renal system. As cirrhosis progressively worsens, excessive hydrostatic pressure develops within the lymphatic and hepatic venous systems. This phenomenon, coupled with impaired albumin synthesis, produces decreased plasma oncotic pressure within the liver vasculature, and an exudative process results. Protein-rich fluid accumulates within the peritoneum, resulting in electrolyte abnormalities. The misplacement of fluids within peritoneum establishes an osmotic gradient, leading to a relative intravascular hypovolemia and sodium retention.

HRS is a clinical condition of renal failure that occurs in patients with chronic liver disease, advanced hepatic failure, and portal hypertension; it is characterized by impaired renal function and marked abnormalities in arterial circulation and in the activity of vasoactive systems. HRS may occur as a consequence of GI hemorrhage, sepsis, or surgery, or as a result of aggressive diuretic therapy, all of which place patients at risk for abnormalities in renal perfusion. Signs of HRS include progressive ascites, azotemia, oliguria, and, eventually, multisystem organ failure. Hepatic transplantation remains the only definitive treatment for HRS, and supportive therapy must be instituted until an organ match is made. The aim of most HRS therapy is to increase renal blood flow through renal vasodilation and vasoconstriction of splanchnic circulation.[38] Current treatment options for HRS are listed in Box 33.8.

Hematologic Considerations

Anemia is commonly encountered in advanced hepatic disease. The reduction in the number of red blood cells is due to hemolysis, folate deficiency, hemorrhage, and bone marrow suppression. Multiple factors can contribute to the development of thrombocytopenia, including splenic platelet sequestration, bone marrow suppression by chronic hepatitis C infection, and antiviral treatment with interferon-based therapy.[39] Reductions in the level or activity of the hematopoietic growth factor thrombopoietin may also play a role. Failure of hepatic synthetic processes results in clotting-factor deficiencies, decreased blood viscosity, and enhanced fibrinolysis resulting from decreased clearance of fibrinolytic factors.

In the context of hepatic dysfunction, excessive blood transfusion may exacerbate encephalopathy, owing to the breakdown of red blood cells and the subsequent increase of protein-rich byproducts in the plasma—byproducts that would ordinarily be metabolized by hepatocytes. When

BOX 33.8 Management of Hepatorenal Syndrome (HRS)

Prevent variceal bleeding
   Measures to prevent variceal bleeding (e.g., β-receptor blocking agent, band ligation)
   Pentoxifylline for severe alcohol-associated hepatitis
Prevention of hepatorenal syndrome (HRS)
   Avoidance of intravascular volume depletion (diuretics, lactulose, GI bleeding, large-volume paracentesis without adequate volume repletion)
   Judicious management of nephrotoxins (ACEIs, ARBs, NSAIDs, antibiotics)
   Prompt diagnosis and treatment of infections (spontaneous bacterial peritonitis [SBP], sepsis)
   SBP prophylaxis
Treatment of hepatorenal syndrome
   Discontinuation of all nephrotoxic agents (ACEIs, ARBs, NSAIDs, diuretics)
   Antibiotics for infections
   IV albumin—bolus of 1 g/kg/day on presentation (maximum dose, 100 g daily). Continue at a dose of 20–60 g daily as required to maintain the central venous pressure between 10 and 15 cm H_2O
Vasopressor therapy (in addition to albumin):
   Midodrine and octreotide—begin midodrine at 2.5–5 mg orally 3 times daily and increase to a maximum dose of 15 mg 3 times daily. Titrate to an MAP increase of at least 15 mm Hg; begin octreotide at 100 mcg subcutaneously 3 times daily and increase to a maximum dose of 200 mcg subcutaneously 3 times daily, or begin octreotide with a 25 mcg IV bolus and continue at a rate of 25 mcg/hr
   OR
   Norepinephrine—0.1–0.7 mcg/kg/min as an IV infusion. Increase by 0.05 mcg/kg/min every 4 hr and titrate to an MAP increase of at least 10 mm Hg
   The duration of vasopressor treatment is generally a maximum of 2 wk until HRS reverses or liver transplant (LT) is performed
Evaluation of patient for liver transplant

ACEIs, Angiotensin-converting enzyme inhibitors; *ARBs,* angiotensin receptor blockers; *GI,* gastrointestinal; *MAP,* mean arterial pressure; *SBP,* spontaneous bacterial peritonitis; *NSAIDs,* nonsteroidal antiinflammatory drugs.
Adapted from Feldman M, et al., eds. *Sleisenger and Fordtran's Gastrointestinal and Liver Disease*. 11th ed. Philadelphia: Elsevier, 2021:1486.

indicated, FFP, platelet, and cryoprecipitate transfusion should be undertaken to correct coagulation deficiencies before surgery.[40]

Respiratory Considerations

A decline in pulmonary function can be predicted in patients with severe hepatic disease. Arterial hypoxemia is common in the context of hepatic disease, and is often multifactorial (e.g., ascites, hepatic hydrothorax, and chronic obstructive pulmonary disease in patients with alcoholism).[41] Hepatopulmonary syndrome (HPS) is defined as the triad of liver disease, arterial deoxygenation, and widespread pulmonary vasodilation. HPS can, however, appear in patients with acute and chronic noncirrhotic portal hypertension. The exact pathogenesis of HPS is still being explored, but precapillary dilation in the lungs appears to play a central role, leading to shunting of blood into the pulmonary vasculature, ventilation-perfusion mismatch, and an increased alveolar-arterial oxygen saturation gradient. One of the characteristics of HPS is intrapulmonary vascular dilation.[41] The preoperative focus is on baseline measurement of oxygen tension or saturation and improving reversible pulmonary dysfunction (e.g., elective thoracentesis/paracentesis). Preoperative sedatives and opioids should be carefully

considered or omitted based on underlying pathology and the patient's current physical status.

Central Nervous System Considerations

Hepatic encephalopathy is a chronic, debilitating complication of hepatic cirrhosis and encompasses a wide spectrum of potentially reversible neuropsychiatric abnormalities seen in patients with liver dysfunction. Neurologic impairment stems from various metabolic abnormalities that are a direct result of the failing liver. The inability to clear neurotoxins generated in the gut (e.g., ammonia, short-chain fatty acids, mercaptans, manganese) results in a cascade of systemic disorders, including alterations in mental status that range from subtle personality change to coma. Ammonia is produced in the GI tract by bacterial degradation of amines, amino acids, purines, and urea. Once formed, ammonia is detoxified by hepatocytes in the liver. In hepatic failure, there is a decrease in functioning hepatocytes. The alterations in hepatic portal flow (shunting) that accompany cirrhosis permit ammonia to enter the systemic circulation. Ammonia causes neurotransmitter abnormalities and induces injury to astrocytes that is partially mediated by oxidative stress. These disturbances lead to astrocyte swelling and brain edema, which appear to be involved in the pathogenesis of neurologic manifestations.[42] It is noteworthy that the mechanism of encephalopathy cannot fully be attributed to ammonia; some patients with encephalopathy have normal ammonia levels, yet others with elevated ammonia levels have no encephalopathic symptoms. Research into the pathogenesis of hepatic encephalopathy is ongoing, but therapy continues to focus on pharmacologic reduction of ammonia levels with nonabsorbable disaccharides (e.g., lactulose) and antimicrobial agents (e.g., neomycin, rifaximin) that reduce the bacterial production of ammonia and other bacteria-derived toxins by suppressing proliferation of the intestinal flora.[43] When possible, the use of benzodiazepine and other sedatives should be avoided in patients with altered mental status.

Intraoperative Anesthetic Considerations

Monitoring

After thorough preoperative evaluation, anesthetic management of patients with liver disease requires consideration of the underlying pathophysiology and the attendant alterations in pharmacokinetics/pharmacodynamics for each medication administered.

Routine intraoperative monitoring may be sufficient for patients with mild hepatic dysfunction undergoing minor surgery. As previously discussed, morbidity and mortality are higher in patients with advanced liver disease. Regarding electrocardiography (ECG) monitoring, a five-cable ECG lead system is preferred over a three-cable ECG system in such patients in that it allows monitoring of a true chest lead. With the latter, only a modified chest lead can be used. Myocardial ischemia can be identified by the presence of an ST segment depression of at least 1 mm. Monitoring of ST segment trends in leads II, V_4, and V_5 can detect 96% of ST segment changes.[44]

Each of these recommendations presumes that the anesthesia provider has properly configured the computerized ST segment analysis software (e.g., verified that the ST point has been positioned over the J point and that the electrodes have been properly placed on the body). Given the potential for hemodynamic lability related to alterations in intravascular status, ascites, electrolyte irregularities, and cardiac comorbidity (e.g., cardiomyopathy), attention should be paid to ST segment analysis for signs of cardiac ischemia. In the absence of an ST segment fingerprint, leads III and V_3 are advocated for the detection of ST segment elevation or depression.[45]

Invasive hemodynamic monitoring may be indicated for patients with cirrhosis and other conditions that involve severe hepatic dysfunction. Arterial cannulation permits beat-to-beat measurement of blood pressure and provides immediate access for blood withdrawal if laboratory analysis is indicated intraoperatively. Patients with cirrhosis frequently require hemodynamic monitoring, including cardiac output assessment, particularly when admitted to the intensive care unit or when undergoing surgery.[33,46] Arterial cannulation also permits the usage of minimally invasive cardiac output monitors. Noninvasive cardiac monitors are not universally reliable and may be considered unreliable in cirrhotic patients with hyperdynamic circulation.[46] Cirrhosis is associated with a pattern of alterations in the cardiovascular system, known as cirrhotic cardiomyopathy, which is characterized by hyperdynamic circulation, elevated baseline cardiac output, reduced peripheral vascular resistance, and decreased ventricular response to physiologic, pharmacologic, and surgical stressors. Furthermore, cirrhotic patients commonly have peripheral autonomic neuropathy, which may result in pronounced hemodynamic instability.[46]

Surgeries such as liver transplant (discussed in Chapter 41) or hepatic resection require additional preparation in anticipation of extensive blood loss. As such, large-bore peripheral and central venous access is necessary for rapid fluid administration, administration of vasopressor medications, and invasive monitoring (e.g., central venous pressure [CVP], pulmonary artery catheter), especially if cardiac disease is present. Transesophageal echocardiography (TEE) monitoring also may be used in the absence of esophageal varices or significant coagulopathy.

Additional considerations for hepatic comorbidity may include blood glucose monitoring (e.g., hypoglycemia during hepatic vascular occlusion), forced air and fluid warming to prevent hypothermia (related to prolonged surgery with an open abdomen coupled with large volumes of blood loss and fluid replacement), and coagulation profile monitoring and correction with FFP, as necessary.

Anesthetic Technique and Medication Choices

In patients with severe hepatic disease, hepatic arterial blood flow does not increase when the portal blood flow and/or oxygen content in the portal venous blood decrease. This could lead to a decrease in hepatic blood and oxygen supply, with subsequent hepatic oxygen deprivation.[47] Any anesthetic plan must focus on the maintenance of arterial blood pressure and cardiac output. Often, it is not the specific anesthetic agents chosen that matter most, rather the care with which they are administered. General anesthesia can be performed safely for patients with liver disease; regional anesthesia also can be used, but coagulopathy should be considered as a contraindication to many types of nerve blockade.

Volatile anesthetic considerations were discussed earlier, with an emphasis on selecting agents that are metabolized minimally or not at all (e.g., desflurane, sevoflurane, isoflurane) by the liver.

Nitrous oxide should be avoided in open abdominal cases because of the potential for expansion of the bowel and theoretic risk of exacerbating a venous embolism resulting from positional entrainment of air. Propofol has been used safely in patients with liver disease and may be considered for use as an induction agent. The effects of benzodiazepines may be exaggerated and prolonged.[21,48]

Neuromuscular blockade selection should be based on patient physical status and the nature of the surgery (e.g., elective or urgent/emergent). Rapid sequence induction may be prudent in the cirrhotic patient with impaired gastric function and increased abdominal pressure related to ascites (Fig. 33.6). In chronic liver failure, succinylcholine may exhibit a prolonged duration of action because of decreased synthesis of plasma cholinesterase by the liver. Due to the long half-life of plasma cholinesterase (14 days), decreased plasma cholinesterase is less likely to be seen in acute liver failure. Nondepolarizing neuromuscular blocking drugs (e.g., rocuronium) used for induction or maintenance should be titrated cautiously, with the expectation that the duration of action will be extended if hepatic metabolism

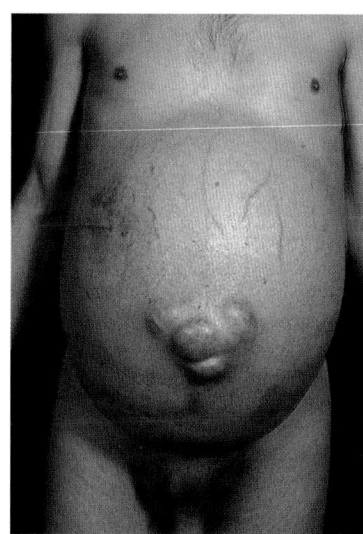

Fig. 33.6 Ascites in a patient with alcoholic cirrhosis showing distended abdomen, dilated superficial collateral veins, hemorrhagic scratch marks due to pruritus and coagulopathy, umbilical varices, and plaster in left iliac fossa indicating diagnostic paracentesis. (From Forbes A, et al., eds. *Atlas of Clinical Gastroenterology.* 3rd ed. Oxford: Mosby Ltd; 2005.)

and clearance are impaired. In patients with cirrhosis, the duration of action of vecuronium is prolonged.[21] Liver disease increases the volume of distribution and elimination half-life of rocuronium, but not its rate of clearance. The decreased elimination of rocuronium in patients with liver disease prolongs its duration of action, particularly with larger initial doses or prolonged administration. Onset time is slowed in patients with cirrhosis, most likely due to the increased volume of distribution.[21,49] A better option after intubation may be cisatracurium, which is metabolized independently of hepatic function and relies on Hoffman elimination (sensitive to temperature and pH).

Opioid activity is dependent on hepatic metabolism, and they should be administered cautiously. Coexisting pulmonary dysfunction may be worsened postoperatively by the prolonged sedative and respiratory depressant effects of opioids used perioperatively. Fentanyl is primarily metabolized by the CYP3A4 system. Administration of CYP3A4 substrates or inhibitors can increase opioid concentrations, thereby prolonging and intensifying analgesic effects and adverse opioid effects, such as respiratory depression.[50] Hepatic dysfunction has a direct impact on the CYP metabolic system.

Morphine is metabolized in a phase II reaction, undergoing glucuronidation in the liver, and should be titrated cautiously or avoided in patients with significant liver disease. Elimination of alfentanil is reduced in patients with liver disease; its volume of distribution is increased, and protein binding is reduced by the lack of α_1-acid glycoprotein.[15] Remifentanil has a very short half-life due to its metabolism by nonspecific esterases in the blood and is not reliant on hepatic or renal function. Perhaps the most compelling evidence for the lack of effect of hepatic dysfunction on the pharmacokinetics of remifentanil is that its kinetics do not change during the anhepatic phase of orthotopic liver transplantation.[51]

DISEASES OF THE BILIARY TRACT

Biliary tract disease is often characterized by a suppression or cessation of bile flow (cholestasis). The most common cause of cholestasis is obstruction of the biliary tract outside of the liver. Symptomatic presentation of obstruction and/or an inflammatory process can be attributed to gallstones, stricture, tumor, infection, or ischemia. Gallstone formation is most likely caused by physicochemical abnormalities in the formation of bile. Approximately 90% of gallstones appear as radiolucent structures composed of hydrophobic cholesterol crystals. Calcium bilirubinate generally accounts for the composition of the remaining percentage. Stones composed of calcium bilirubinate are usually seen in patients with cirrhosis and hemolytic anemia. An estimated 15 to 20 million adults in the United States have biliary tract disease, as evidenced by the presence of gallstones.[52]

Anatomic and Physiologic Overview

The biliary tract is the excretory conduit for the liver. It is composed of (1) the intrahepatic ducts, which collect bile from the liver segments; (2) the coalescence of the intrahepatic ducts and the right and left hepatic ducts; (3) the common hepatic duct, which is formed by the junction of the right and left hepatic ducts in the liver hilum; (4) the gallbladder, which serves as a bile reservoir; (5) the cystic duct, which joins the gallbladder to the CBD; and (6) the CBD, which begins at the junction of the cystic duct and the common hepatic duct and terminates in the lumen of the duodenum.[52]

The gallbladder is a pear-shaped organ capable of holding 30 to 60 mL of fluid and is attached to the liver in a shallow depression at the inferior junction of the right and left hepatic lobes. The gallbladder drains into the cystic duct, which is usually 1 to 5 cm long and arises from the narrow end, or infundibulum, of the gallbladder. The cystic duct drains into the common hepatic duct. The CBD arises from the junction of the cystic duct and the common hepatic duct and is approximately 6 mm in diameter. It passes behind the duodenum to the right of the gastroduodenal artery, traversing the head of the pancreas before entering the second part of the duodenum. The distal CBD may join with the pancreatic duct before entering the duodenum via the ampulla of Vater (Fig. 33.7). At the termination, these CBD and pancreatic ducts are enveloped in smooth muscle, the sphincter of Oddi, which provides a barrier to intestinal bacteria, maintaining the sterile environment of the biliary tract. The biliary tract can be obstructed at this termination by a pancreatic tumor.

Arterial blood supply to the gallbladder is furnished by the cystic artery, which is a branch of the right hepatic artery. The biliary ducts receive their blood supply distally from the gastroduodenal, retroduodenal, and posterosuperior pancreatoduodenal arteries and proximally from the right hepatic and cystic arteries. Venous drainage flows

into the portal vein. Lymphatic drainage flows into a cystic duct node located between the cystic duct and the common hepatic duct.

The area known as the cystohepatic triangle (Calot triangle) is bound by the common hepatic duct, the liver, and the cystic duct, and is a critical region that contains the cystic artery, the right hepatic artery, the cystic duct lymph node, and, sometimes, an aberrant right segmental bile duct. This area must be carefully dissected during cholecystectomy to avoid damaging these vital and friable structures.

The gallbladder mucosa secretes a protective mucus that prevents caustic damage by bile salts. After food is ingested, the gallbladder contracts, emptying its contents (bile) into the duodenum to assist in the digestive processes. Gallbladder contraction is primarily hormonally regulated through the action of CCK. The release of CCK from duodenal cells is mediated by the presence of intraluminal amino acids and fat. Vagal stimulation also serves a role in gallbladder contraction (secondary to the role of CCK). Indeed, vagotomy is associated with impaired gallbladder contraction and an increased prevalence of gallstones.[40]

Bile is the combined secretory product of the hepatocyte and biliary tract epithelial cells and has three main functions: (1) to emulsify and enhance absorption of ingested fats and fat-soluble vitamins; (2) to provide an excretory pathway for bilirubin, drugs, toxins, and immunoglobulin A (IgA); and (3) to maintain duodenal alkalization. The combined output of the ductal cells and hepatocytes is 500 to 1000 mL/day, which is excreted into the bile canaliculi. The bile ducts, gallbladder, and sphincter of Oddi modify, store, and regulate bile flow. The gallbladder concentrates and stores hepatic bile during the fasting state and delivers bile into the duodenum in response to a meal. Because the usual capacity of the gallbladder is only approximately 30 to 60 mL, the remarkable absorptive capacity of the gallbladder accounts for its ability to store much of the bile produced each day.[52] Absorbed bile is returned via the portal venous system to the liver.

Hepatocytes secrete bilirubin (the metabolic waste product of heme metabolism), cholesterol, bile salts, lecithin, water, and electrolytes. The epithelial cells contribute water and more electrolytes. Vagal stimulation, secretin, CCK, and gastrin stimulate ductular cell secretion and increase bile flow. In addition, bile acids serve as a positive-feedback mechanism for inducing hepatocyte and ductular secretion of bile. Gallbladder filling during fasting occurs with relaxation and contraction of the sphincter of Oddi. The sphincter of Oddi is a complex structure that is functionally independent from the duodenal musculature. It creates a high-pressure zone between the bile duct and the duodenum. The sphincter regulates the flow of bile and pancreatic juice into the duodenum, prevents the regurgitation of duodenal contents into the biliary tract, and diverts bile into the gallbladder. Vasoactive intestinal peptide induces relaxation of the sphincter of Oddi, whereas somatostatin, an inhibitory peptide, induces contraction. In states of prolonged fasting, the risk of gallstone formation increases due to the lack of CCK stimulation and consequent biliary stasis.[52]

Cholecystitis

Cholecystitis symptoms are usually the result of obstruction, infection, or both. Obstruction can be extramural (e.g., pancreatic cancer), intramural (e.g., cholangiocarcinoma), or intraluminal (e.g., choledocholithiasis). Acute cholecystitis is related to gallstones in 90% to 95% of cases. Obstruction of the cystic duct leading to biliary colic is the initial event in acute cholecystitis. If the cystic duct remains obstructed, the gallbladder distends, and the gallbladder wall becomes inflamed and edematous. Obstruction of the cystic duct by gallstones results in a triad of sudden right upper quadrant tenderness, fever, and leukocytosis.

Inspiratory effort usually accentuates the pain in the right upper quadrant (Murphy sign). Increases in plasma bilirubin, alkaline

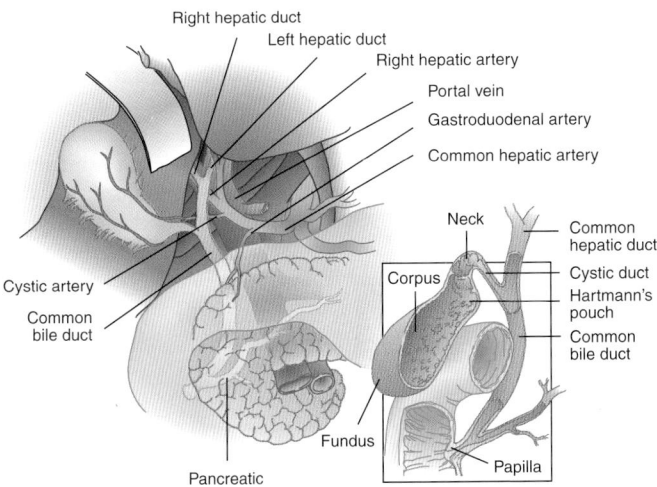

Fig. 33.7 Anatomy of the biliary tract. (From Townsend CM, et al., eds. *Sabiston Textbook of Surgery.* 18th ed. Philadelphia: Elsevier; 2008:1548.)

phosphatase, and amylase levels frequently occur. Ileus and localized tenderness may indicate perforation with peritonitis. Leukocytosis and fever are often present. Jaundice indicates complete obstruction of the cystic duct. Symptoms are frequently confused with those of myocardial infarction. Differential diagnosis is accomplished through serial ECG evaluations and laboratory analysis of serum enzymes specific to cardiac muscle. Cholescintigraphy (a contrast study that evaluates gallbladder excretion of a radiographically labeled substance) and ultrasonography are often used for clinical confirmation of the diagnosis.[40]

For most patients, the treatment for acute cholecystitis is cholecystectomy, but for those who are critically ill, the risk of general anesthesia may be greater than the benefit of a surgical procedure. An alternative, temporary treatment for these high-risk patients is decompression and drainage of the gallbladder through the insertion of a cholecystostomy tube. This minimally invasive procedure can be performed with local anesthetic infiltration and IV sedation.[53]

Patients with symptoms indicative of acute cholecystitis are often volume depleted due to oral intake intolerance, vomiting, and possible preoperative nasogastric (NG) evacuation of gastric contents. Dehydration calls for preoperative IV fluid replacement. Gastric suction may be warranted in the presence of ileus. The presence of free abdominal air, as determined by abdominal radiography or symptoms of an acute abdomen (e.g., fever, ileus, rigid and painful abdomen, vomiting, dehydration), suggests a ruptured viscus, possibly including perforation of the gallbladder. Under these circumstances, emergency exploratory laparotomy is undertaken.

Cholelithiasis and Choledocholithiasis

Acute obstruction of the CBD often produces symptoms similar to those seen in patients with cholecystitis. Recurrent bouts of acute cholecystitis induce the development of fibrotic changes in gallbladder structure, thereby impeding the ability of the gallbladder to adequately expel bile. The presence of Charcot triad (i.e., fever and chills, jaundice, right upper quadrant pain) aids in establishing the diagnosis of acute ductal obstruction. Weight loss, anorexia, and fatigue complete the symptomatology. Ductal patency may be confirmed by radiologic evaluation. Diagnostic modalities include radiography, transhepatic cholangiography, ultrasonography, cholescintigraphy, and computed tomography (CT) scan. A dilated CBD and biliary tree are typically observed in these studies. Endoscopic retrograde cholangiopancreatography (ERCP) is the usual treatment for ductal stones.

The use of ERCP in patients with suspected CBD stones not only confirms the diagnosis but also provides ductal clearance of the stones and sphincterotomy before subsequent laparoscopic cholecystectomy. It is relatively more complex than routine endoscopies, and requires adequate sedation, analgesia, and patient cooperation. ERCP is performed by passing an endoscope into the upper GI tract and into the duodenum, locating the major duodenal ampulla. The ampulla is cannulated and examined using radiographic dye to determine whether the blockage is due to a CBD stone. If a stone is present, it can typically be retrieved endoscopically. Sphincterotomy also may be performed to facilitate removal of CBD stones. Correction of ductal stenosis also may require sphincterotomy or insertion of a stent. ERCP is most commonly performed with the patient in the prone position and the head turned to the patient's right side. Patients undergoing ERCP have been found to be more anxious as compared with those undergoing a routine esophagogastroduodenoscopy (EGD). Restlessness and lack of cooperation have been reported to be one of the causative factors for post-ERCP complications such as duodenal perforation and pancreatitis. The choice of sedative is chiefly governed by the user and the patient history. Similarly, the level of sedation—up to and including general endotracheal anesthesia—is also dependent on the clinical condition of the patient and the degree of patient cooperation.[54] Patients presenting for ERCP often have comorbidities. Endoscopic clearance of stones from the CBD can prevent the need for an open operation if expertise in laparoscopic CBD exploration is not available. Patients with worsening cholangitis caused by ascending bacterial infection of the biliary system, ampullary stone impaction, biliary pancreatitis, multiple comorbidities, or cirrhosis are considered good candidates for preoperative endoscopic therapy.[52]

Anesthetic Considerations in Gallbladder and Biliary Tract Disease

Removal of gallstones is undertaken not only to relieve symptoms but also to prevent further sequelae, including cholecystitis, cholangitis, jaundice, pancreatitis, and peritonitis, all of which may result from stasis or impediment to bile flow. Contraindications to laparoscopic cholecystectomy include coagulopathy, severe chronic obstructive pulmonary disease, end-stage liver disease, and congestive heart failure.

Since the introduction of laparoscopic cholecystectomy, the number of cholecystectomies performed in the United States has increased from approximately 500,000 per year to 700,000 per year. More than 90% of cholecystectomies are performed laparoscopically. Laparoscopic cholecystectomy is now often performed in the relatively healthy patient on an outpatient basis, with discharge either later on the day of the surgery or, occasionally, after an overnight stay in the hospital. Postoperative pain management is typically less challenging with laparoscopic surgery.

A standard or rapid sequence induction with oral endotracheal intubation is required. The peritoneal cavity must be insufflated with carbon dioxide gas to provide adequate surgical exposure of anatomic structures, and mandates general endotracheal intubation to effectively seal the airway and prevent passive aspiration of gastric contents. An orogastric tube should be inserted to decompress the stomach. Maintenance requires muscle relaxation with appropriate reversal. Prophylactic antiemetics are needed due to the peritoneal irritation of insufflation, opioid use, and potential intravascular volume depletion. The peritoneal cavity must be insufflated for surgical exposure.

Insufflation of the abdomen with carbon dioxide impedes diaphragmatic excursion, causing a decrease in functional residual capacity, a decrease in closing capacity, and an increase in peak inspiratory pressure. Retroperitoneal insufflation may lead to hypotension and necessitates early recognition and repositioning of the trocar. Insufflation with carbon dioxide causes a rise in the carbon dioxide partial pressure and thus may lead to hypercarbia in the presence of inadequate ventilation. Special attention should be paid to the potential need for ventilator setting adjustment with insufflation. In the setting of intraabdominal insufflation, using pressure control ventilation rather than a volume control mode may be the best means of preventing alveolar derecruitment (measured at the bedside by a pressure-volume curve method), as it provides physiologic minute ventilation while minimizing the risk of barotrauma. The use of a reverse Trendelenburg position during laparoscopic cholecystectomy may induce a variable degree of hemodynamic compromise by impeding venous return. Occult hemorrhage is also possible and may go undetected.

Insufflation also leads to increased intraabdominal pressure (IAP). Insufflation to a pressure of approximately 15 mm Hg is routine. An IAP of 20 to 25 cm H_2O leads to increased cardiac output and CVP secondary to changes in the volume of the venous return of blood. An IAP greater than 30 to 40 cm H_2O may lead to decreased cardiac output and CVP secondary to reduced right ventricular preload. Abdominal insufflation also displaces the abdominal viscera and diaphragm in a cephalad direction, which places extra pressure on the lower esophageal sphincter (LES), thereby increasing the risk of gastric reflux.

All maintenance anesthetic drugs may be used. Some surgeons request that nitrous oxide not be used, to reduce the risk of bowel expansion, which could hinder surgical exposure. In the presence of hepatic dysfunction, isoflurane, desflurane, and sevoflurane are safe. The choice of muscle relaxant depends on the patient's ability to tolerate possible side effects of the drug, the drug's dependence on hepatic clearance, and the length of the procedure to be performed. Awake extubation is performed after the patient's airway reflexes have recovered adequately. The laparoscopic approach offers the benefit of reduced postoperative pain secondary to smaller abdominal incisions. Patients may experience shoulder pain from pneumoperitoneum, which is usually self-limiting. Evacuation of the pneumoperitoneum with a Valsalva maneuver prior to closing will assist in alleviating postoperative pain. Severe postoperative pain may be reduced by patient-controlled analgesia, intercostal nerve blocks, or neuraxial opioid administration. Abdominal pain or other symptoms originally attributed to the gallbladder may persist or recur months or years after cholecystectomy. Anesthesia for laparoscopic surgery is discussed in Chapter 34.

Open cholecystectomy may be indicated for patients who are emergently ill, patients with an existing infection, or patients in whom laparoscopy poses a particularly formidable technical challenge (e.g., in cases of morbid obesity or intraabdominal adhesions secondary to previous abdominal surgery or peritonitis). Patients who undergo open cholecystectomy often experience more complications, including a greater likelihood of severe postoperative pain and respiratory splinting (caused by the use of a right subcostal or upper abdominal midline incision), with the risk of postoperative respiratory embarrassment in the susceptible patient. Patients who have experienced severe traumatic injury or who require aggressive intensive care for multiorgan disease are at particular risk for developing acute cholecystitis secondary to the stress of severe illness. Patients with significant comorbidities, including advanced age, who undergo prolonged or complex surgical procedures (e.g., trauma surgery, cardiac surgery with cardiopulmonary bypass, abdominal aneurysm repair) that are complicated by perioperative hemodynamic lability are also at greater risk for ischemia of the abdominal viscera. The result may be the development of an acute, postoperative abdominal crisis. Under these circumstances, exploratory laparotomy for an acute abdomen may reveal necrosis and perforation of the gallbladder. This places the patient at extreme risk for developing peritonitis. The acute critical nature of the presenting illness, superimposed upon preexisting patient comorbidities, is another factor potentially complicating perianesthetic management of the patient.[40]

Full-stomach precautions should be used during the induction of and emergence from anesthesia, particularly in the presence of abdominal distention or ileus. Patients with jaundice require a more thorough preparation, owing to the likelihood of a variable degree of hepatic dysfunction. This may make for greater susceptibility to hemorrhage, exaggerated drug effects, and fluctuation in hemodynamics. Invasive hemodynamic monitoring and preparation for blood product transfusion are influenced by the patient's clinical status.

CBD exploration may be carried out in conjunction with cholecystectomy, if necessary. Glucagon may be requested by the surgeon for its spasmolytic effect in the GI system and its ability to relax the sphincter of Oddi. Note that glucagon may cause nausea at doses greater than 2 mg.

DISEASES OF THE ESOPHAGUS
Anatomic and Physiologic Overview

Esophagus is derived from the Greek words *oiso*, which is the future tense of *phero* ("to carry"), and *phagein* ("food").[55] Approximately 18 to 25 cm long, the esophagus is a hollow, muscular tube that serves to carry food or liquid to the stomach. The esophagus has three segments: cervical, thoracic, and abdominal. The cervical esophagus is bordered anteriorly by the trachea; bilaterally by the common carotid arteries, internal jugular veins, and vagal nerves; and posteriorly by the cervical muscles. Proximally, the esophagus begins where the inferior pharyngeal constrictor merges with the cricopharyngeus, an area of skeletal muscle known functionally as the upper esophageal sphincter.[56] At rest, the upper esophageal sphincter prevents entrainment of air by muscle contraction, which creates a high pressure zone.

Although collapsed when unused, the esophagus is capable of expanding to permit passage of substances; however, it remains the narrowest of the digestive tubes. Peristaltic action pushes solid matter distally toward the stomach. The LES, contracted at rest to prevent passage of gastric contents proximally into the esophagus, relaxes to permit passage of food into the stomach.

Sympathetic and parasympathetic innervation regulates esophageal muscle tone. Peristaltic activity is regulated by parasympathetic innervation via the vagus nerves. Esophageal muscular contraction and LES relaxation are regulated by stimulation of cranial nerves IX, X, and XI. Sympathetic fibers act on Auerbach (myenteric) plexus to modulate motor activity.

Esophageal Disorders

Disorders affecting esophageal motility or sphincter tone may create generalized symptoms of dysphagia, heartburn, or chest pain. Primary esophageal motility disorders include achalasia and gastroesophageal reflux disease (GERD). Achalasia is characterized by impaired relaxation of the LES and may develop secondary to systemic disease states, including diabetes, stroke, amyotrophic lateral sclerosis, and certain connective tissue diseases such as amyloidosis and scleroderma. Chronic achalasia results in dilation of the distal esophagus, and regurgitation becomes more frequent when larger amounts of food and fluid are retained. GERD is a consequence of the failure of the normal antireflux barriers to protect against frequent and abnormal amounts of gastroesophageal reflux. Symptoms range from heartburn to extraesophageal manifestations (e.g., pulmonary, ear, nose, or throat symptoms).

Chronic GERD can result in abnormal epithelial changes in the esophagus that predispose the tissue to developing a malignancy. Damage to the esophageal epithelium results in columnar epithelium replacing the normal stratified squamous cells in the distal esophagus, a condition that is referred to as Barrett esophagus. These changes create no symptoms but are a cautionary risk factor associated with adenocarcinoma of the esophagus.

In many patients, GERD may be managed conservatively with pharmacologic therapy, and surgery is withheld until medical management proves unsuccessful. Medication therapy may include antacids, mucosal protective medications, histamine (H_2) receptor blockers, proton pump inhibitors, and prokinetics designed to facilitate emptying of the stomach. Aside from failed medical therapy, other surgical indications include a mechanically defective cardiac sphincter, recurrence of symptoms after discontinuing treatment, and unacceptable side effects related to medications.

Hiatal Hernia

Hiatal hernia refers to conditions in which elements from the abdominal cavity, most commonly the stomach, herniate through the esophageal hiatus into the mediastinum.[57] Hiatal hernias are classified as type I to IV. Type I, the sliding type, is formed by the movement of the upper stomach through an enlarged hiatus. In type II, the paraesophageal type, the esophagogastric junction remains in normal position, but all or part of the stomach moves into the thorax and assumes a

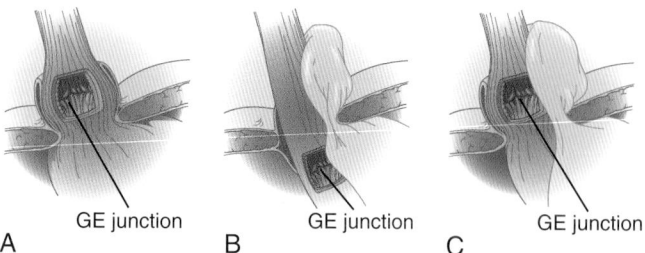

Fig. 33.8 Three types of hiatal hernia. (A) Type I, or sliding hernia. (B) Type 2, or rolling hernia. (C) Type 3, or mixed hernia. *GE,* Gastroesophageal. (From Townsend CM, et al., eds. *Sabiston Textbook of Surgery: The Biological Basis of Modern Surgical Practice.* 20th ed. Philadelphia: Elsevier; 2017:1044.)

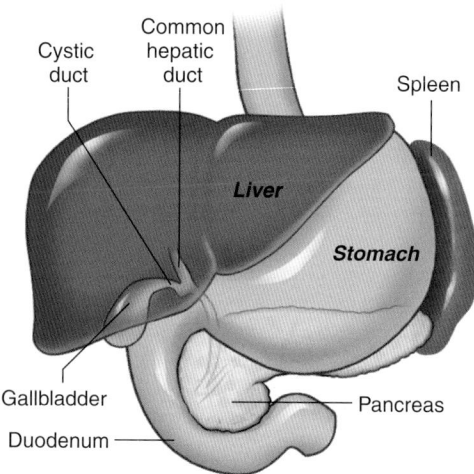

Fig. 33.9 Position of the stomach relative to the other principal organs of the upper abdomen. *I,* Inferior; *L,* left; *R,* right; *S,* superior. (From Patton KT. *Anatomy & Physiology.* 10th ed. St. Louis: Elsevier; 2019:871.)

paraesophageal position. A type III has been identified that combines the features of sliding and paraesophageal hernias (Fig. 33.8). Type IV hiatal hernias are those in which other organs, such as the colon or small bowel, are contained in the hernial sac formed by a large paraesophageal hernia.[58]

The contribution of hiatal hernia to GERD is controversial,[59] but data confirm the importance of hiatal hernia in patients with more severe esophagitis, peptic stricture, or Barrett esophagus. Several surgical approaches may be used to reduce and correct hiatal hernia, although the laparoscopic Nissen fundoplication remains common. Collis-Nissen elongation gastroplasty may be superior to Nissen fundoplication for select patients with Barrett esophagus because of the reflux-induced shortening of the esophagus, but the choice of which procedure to perform is often made intraoperatively.[60,61] Anesthetic management may include aspiration prophylaxis, as discussed previously. Application of cricoid pressure has been shown to decrease LES. However, normal gastric pressures remain; consequently, the value of cricoid cartilage pressure in rapid sequence induction has been questioned, although it remains a frequent technique in clinical practice.[62]

Anesthetic Considerations in Esophageal Disease

Special considerations may be necessary for patients with active esophageal disease. Occult disease (asymptomatic) is generally less concerning than uncontrolled disease states that manifest with reflux symptoms. A preoperative history of symptoms that indicate the presence of gastric reflux warrants aspiration prophylaxis during general anesthesia induction and emergence. Although best practice data do not support a specific regimen, modifying the acidity and/or volume of gastric contents remains a common preoperative practice. For maximum benefit, it is imperative to have an understanding of the pharmacokinetic/pharmacodynamic profile of selected preoperative medications.

Rapid sequence induction with cricoid pressure may serve to hasten protection of the airway with a cuffed endotracheal tube (ETT) and limit opportunity for aspiration of gastric contents. Usage of a laryngeal mask airway (LMA) remains controversial in patients with active reflux disease. The absence of definitive airway protection with LMA must be carefully considered, and a reasonable indication against endotracheal intubation should be present prior to implementation.

DISEASES OF THE STOMACH

Anatomic and Physiologic Overview

The principal function of the stomach is to prepare ingested food for digestion and absorption before it is moved into and through the small intestine. The initial period of digestion requires solid components of

a meal to be stored for several hours while they undergo a reduction in size and are broken down into their basic metabolic constituents.

Receptive relaxation is a process whereby the proximal portion of the stomach relaxes in anticipation of food intake. This relaxation enables liquids to pass easily from the stomach along the lesser curvature, whereas the solid food settles along the greater curvature of the fundus. In contrast to liquids, emptying of solid food is facilitated by the antrum, which pumps solid food components into and through the pylorus. The antrum and pylorus function in a coordinated fashion, allowing entry of food components into the duodenum and returning material to the proximal stomach until it has been processed appropriately for delivery into the duodenum.

In addition to storing food, the stomach participates in digestion of a meal. An example of this is the enzymatic breakdown of starch through the activity of salivary amylase. For this to work, the pH within the center of the gastric bolus needs to be greater than 5. Peptic digestion metabolizes a meal into fats, proteins, and carbohydrates by breaking down cell walls. Although the duodenum and proximal small intestine are primarily responsible for digestion of a meal, the stomach facilitates this process.[63]

The stomach is essentially composed of three sections. The thin-walled and distensible proximal portion (fundus) is located in the upper abdomen, and its function is primarily storage. The body of the stomach represents the largest portion. The body also contains most of the parietal cells and is bound on the right by the relatively straight lesser curvature and on the left by the longer greater curvature. The thick-walled distal portion of the stomach (pylorus) is responsible for mixing food and releasing it slowly through the pyloric sphincter into the duodenum. The relationship of the stomach to the other abdominal organs is noted in Fig. 33.9.

Most of the blood supply to the stomach is from the celiac artery. There are four main arteries: the left and right gastric arteries along the lesser curvature and the left and right gastroepiploic arteries along the greater curvature. In addition, a substantial quantity of blood may be supplied to the proximal stomach by the inferior phrenic arteries and by the short gastric arteries from the spleen (Fig. 33.10). Major autonomic innervation is furnished by two branches of the vagus nerve, the right posterior (celiac) branch and the left anterior (hepatic) branch.

The gastric wall consists of an external serosal layer that covers an inner oblique, a middle circular, and an outer longitudinal layer

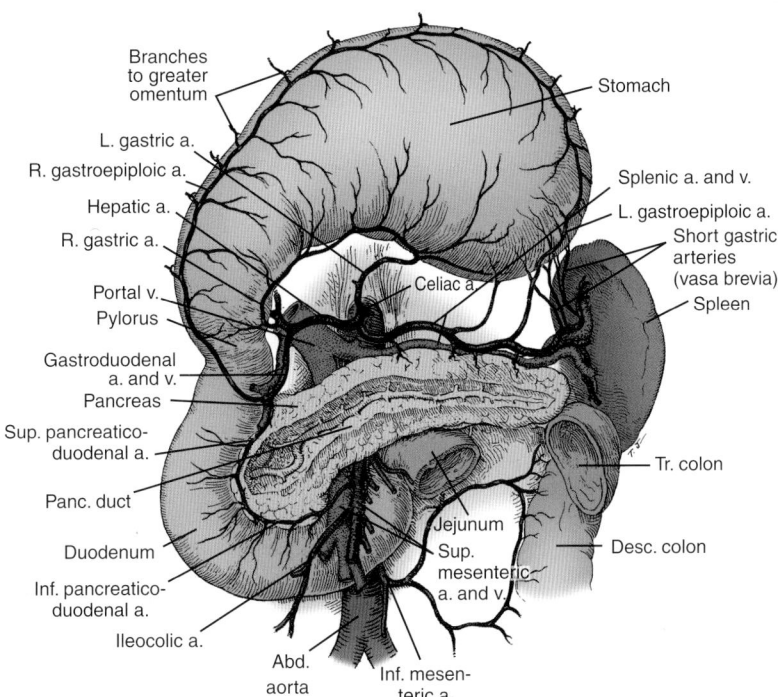

Fig. 33.10 Blood supply to the stomach and duodenum with anatomic relationships to the spleen and pancreas. *a*, Artery; *L*, left; *R*, right; *v*, vein. (From Yeo CJ, et al. *Shackelford's Surgery of the Alimentary Tract.* 8th ed. Philadelphia: Elsevier; 2019:634.)

of smooth muscle. The middle layer of smooth muscle is circular and is the only complete muscle layer of the stomach wall. At the pylorus, this middle circular muscle layer becomes progressively thicker and functions as a true anatomic sphincter between the stomach and duodenum.

The submucosa, which lies between the muscularis externa and mucosae, is a collagen-rich layer of connective tissue that is the strongest layer of the gastric wall. The submucosa contains the rich anastomotic network of blood vessels, lymphatic vessels, and Meissner plexus of autonomic nerves. The mucosa consists of surface epithelium, lamina propria, and muscularis mucosae. The latter is on the luminal side of the submucosa and is probably responsible for forming the rugae that greatly increase epithelial surface area. It also marks the histologic boundary for invasive and noninvasive gastric carcinoma.[63]

Within the gastric mucosa reside the glands that are responsible for the significant physiologic role that the stomach plays during the digestive processes. The functions of the glands and the cells lining the glands vary according to the region of the stomach in which they are found. Within the fundic mucosa lie mucus-secreting glands that provide a protective barrier against the acid outflow of the parietal cells, which are located in the same region of the stomach. The stomach has an endocrine function, as demonstrated by the secretion of pepsinogen by chief cells and serotonin by other cells. The antrum contains cells that secrete mucus (surface epithelial cells and mucous cells) and gastrin (G cells). The two important sphincters are the LES at the gastroesophageal junction and the pyloric sphincter at the gastroduodenal junction.

The stomach is very distensible, can store up to 1.5 L of fluid without any increase in gastric pressure, and normally stores food for up to 4 hours. The sight and smell of food stimulate acid and pepsinogen production. Gastrin is the major hormonal regulator of the gastric phase of acid secretion after a meal. Gastrin is released by the G cells in response to gastric distention, which stimulates parietal cell acid (hydrochloric

acid) secretion. The duodenum and upper jejunum also secrete a small amount of gastrin. Luminal acid suppresses gastrin feedback (negative feedback).

Pepsinogen and gastrin release are vagally mediated. Acid in duodenal contents induces the release of secretin, which further inhibits gastrin release and acid production. Acid in the antrum also stimulates the release of somatostatin. Somatostatin directly inhibits parietal cell acid secretion and indirectly inhibits acid secretion through inhibition of gastrin release and down-regulation of histamine release. Pancreatic bicarbonate release is also stimulated by duodenal acidity.

Gastric acid secretion by parietal cells is regulated by three local stimuli: acetylcholine, gastrin, and histamine. These three stimuli account for both basal and stimulated gastric acid secretion. Acetylcholine is the principal neurotransmitter modulating acid secretion and is released from the vagus and parasympathetic ganglion cells. Gastrin has hormonal effects on the parietal cells and stimulates histamine release. Histamine has paracrine-like effects on the parietal cells and plays a central role in the regulation of acid secretion by parietal cells after its release from enterochromaffin-like (ECL) cells. Somatostatin inhibits gastric acid secretion. Release of somatostatin from antral D cells is stimulated in the presence of intraluminal acid at a pH of 3 or less. After its release, somatostatin inhibits gastrin release and modifies histamine release from ECL cells. In some patients with peptic ulcer disease (PUD), this negative feedback response is defective. Consequently, the precise state of acid secretion by parietal cells is dependent on the overall influence of the positive and negative stimuli.[63]

Other gastric functions include providing a barrier against ingested pathogens. This goal is accomplished through the maintenance of a highly acidic environment and through a functional role in immunosurveillance. The stomach heats or cools ingested substances as needed to maintain normothermia. Parietal cells also secrete intrinsic factor (in addition to hydrochloric acid), which facilitates ileal vitamin B_{12} absorption.

Peptic Ulcer Disease

A gastric ulcer is defined by the loss of mucosa (including muscularis mucosae) due to inflammation. Ulcers may extend into the submucosa and even into the muscularis propria. All ulcers begin as erosions, but not all erosions progress to ulcers. Ulcers may be acute or chronic. Peptic ulcers are considered chronic and are most often solitary. They may occur in any portion of the GI tract that is exposed to acid-peptic juices. Approximately 98% of peptic ulcers occur in the stomach and duodenum.

It is now believed that 90% of duodenal ulcers and roughly 75% of gastric ulcers are associated with *Helicobacter pylori* infection. *H. pylori* is detected in the stomach of almost all patients with duodenal peptic ulcer and in more than 90% of gastric ulcer patients who are not nonsteroidal antiinflammatory drug (NSAID) users (after *H. pylori* infection, ingestion of NSAIDs is the most common cause of PUD). Eradication of *H. pylori* facilitates healing of peptic ulcers and essentially prevents their recurrence.[64]

The most common complications of PUD, in order of prevalence, are hemorrhage, perforation, and obstruction. Approximately one-third of patients experience at least one of these complications during the course of their PUD; pyloric channel ulcers are the ulcers that are most commonly associated with complications, particularly obstruction. Bleeding occurs when the ulcer erodes underlying blood vessels. Ulcers may perforate into adjacent organs, such as the pancreas (most common) or the liver.

Gastric outlet obstruction may develop as a result of distortion and narrowing of the pyloric area due to fibrosis, edema, or smooth muscle spasm resulting from chronic ulcer disease. It occurs almost exclusively in patients with long-standing peptic ulcers of the pyloric channel or duodenum. Surgical repair or endoscopic pyloric dilation with stents are often necessary to alleviate the symptoms of gastric outlet obstruction.[64,65]

A chronic overabundance of hydrochloric acid and pepsin (from various causes) results in erosion of the protective mucous layer of the stomach and duodenum, eventually leading to ulcerative lesions extending beyond the mucosal barrier into the submucosa and muscularis epithelial layers, and sometimes into the serosal layer. In the case of LES incompetence, ulcerative involvement of the esophagus may develop.

A chronic ulcerative lesion in the duodenum constitutes duodenal ulcer disease. This classification also includes lesions that occur before the pylorus in the lower antrum of the stomach, due to the similarity in symptoms and responses to therapy. Men 45 to 65 years of age and women older than 55 years have the highest incidence of duodenal ulcer disease. Affected patients possess twice the number of acid-secreting parietal cells.[66]

Gastritis

Stress gastritis, an inflammatory disorder of the gastric mucosa, has been referred to as stress ulcerations, stress erosive gastritis, and hemorrhagic gastritis. These lesions may lead to life-threatening gastric bleeding and by definition occur after physical trauma, shock, sepsis, hemorrhage, or respiratory failure. They are characterized by multiple superficial (nonulcerating) erosions that begin in the proximal or acid-secreting portion of the stomach and progress distally. They also may occur in the setting of central nervous system disease such as that seen with Cushing ulcer or as a result of thermal burn injury involving more than 30% of the body surface area (Curling ulcer).

Although the precise mechanisms responsible for the development of stress gastritis remain to be fully elucidated, current evidence suggests a multifactorial etiology, including drugs, chemicals, or *H. pylori* infection. These stress-induced gastric lesions appear to require

the presence of acid. Stress is considered to be present when hypoxia, sepsis, or organ failure occurs. Other factors that may predispose to the development of these lesions include impaired mucosal defense mechanisms against luminal acid such as a reduction in blood flow, a reduction in mucus, a reduction in bicarbonate secretion by mucosal cells, or a reduction in endogenous prostaglandins.[63] *H. pylori* has been identified as a major etiologic factor of gastritis-associated disease, as well as gastric and duodenal ulcers and gastric carcinoma, but it should be noted that at present *H. pylori* is not recognized as a serious occupational hazard despite the fact that anesthesia providers are frequently exposed to potential oral and ambient routes of transmission.[66] Epidemiologic findings indicate a higher prevalence of this organism in older adults, individuals of lower socioeconomic status, and those born outside the United States. Infected patients undergoing stress are at greatest risk for exacerbation of the infection, with potential development of gastric and duodenal ulceration. All these factors render the stomach more susceptible to damage from luminal acid, with resultant hemorrhagic gastritis.

Any patient with upper GI bleeding requires prompt and definitive fluid resuscitation with correction of any coagulation or platelet abnormalities. If blood is required, it should be administered without delay, and if there are specific clotting abnormalities or platelet deficiencies, FFP and platelets should also be administered. In patients being treated for sepsis, broad-spectrum antibiotic treatment and control of the source of infection need to be undertaken. Treatment of the underlying sepsis plays a major role in treating the underlying gastric erosions. Saline lavage of the stomach through an NG tube will help remove any pooled blood and prevent gastric distention, which stimulates gastrin release. NG decompression also removes noxious substances such as bile and pancreatic juice that could potentially further compromise the stomach. More than 80% of patients who present with upper GI hemorrhage stop bleeding when this approach is used. When the NG tube aspirate is clear, indicating that bleeding has ceased, intraluminal gastric pH should be maintained at greater than 5 with antisecretory agents. If the pH can be maintained above 5, more than 99.9% of acid will be neutralized, and pepsin will be inactive. Usually, this involves the use of proton pump inhibitors or, alternatively, H_2-receptor antagonists with or without combination antacid therapy. There is little evidence to suggest that endoscopy with electrocautery or heater probe coagulation has any benefit in the therapy of bleeding from acute stress gastritis.[63]

Gastric mucosal acidosis has been reported frequently in critically ill patients with respiratory failure and underlying coagulopathy, hepatic cirrhosis, hyperparathyroidism, obstructive airway disease, rheumatoid arthritis; patients undergoing prolonged, complex surgical procedures; and patients undergoing cardiopulmonary bypass. Gastritis associated with gastric mucosal acidosis is associated with increased perioperative morbidity and mortality. The splanchnic viscera is particularly vulnerable to decreased circulatory blood flow in the presence of inflammation, with the potential for breakdown of intestinal barrier function. This results in the translocation of bacteria and endotoxins into the bloodstream, leading to systemic sepsis. Ischemia and acidosis of the gut are the primary causative factors for erosion of the gut barrier function.[40]

Therapeutic Options in Peptic Ulcer Disease

The clinician has three major goals when faced with a patient with peptic ulcer disease: Symptoms need to be relieved, the ulcer needs to heal, and recurrence needs to be prevented. The major medical therapies and treatments used for the control of PUD focus on *H. pylori*. Adjuncts include oral antacids, H_2-receptor antagonists, proton pump inhibitors, sucralfate, and antibiotics. A proton pump inhibitor such as omeprazole is used in duodenal ulcer management. EGD and surgical treatment are reserved for patients who continue to experience intractable symptoms despite aggressive medical therapy, or to treat complications. These complications are often of an urgent nature and consist of GI hemorrhage, ulcerative perforation into adjacent structures such as the pancreas or jejunum, and obstruction.[67]

Antacid use for the medical treatment of PUD has potential complications that are of interest to the anesthetist. Antacids may produce an acid rebound in which gastric acid secretion increases after acid is neutralized by calcium-containing antacids. Another condition that may result from antacid therapy is the milk-alkali syndrome. In this condition, hypercalcemia, alkalosis, and an elevated blood urea nitrogen level may develop from the daily ingestion of large quantities of calcium-containing antacids and milk. Manifestations of this syndrome include skeletal muscle weakness and polyuria. Ingestion of large quantities of aluminum-containing antacids may result in acute hypophosphatemia because of increased binding of intestinal phosphorus. Skeletal muscle weakness and fatigue follow chronic overuse, resulting in pathologic fractures and osteoporosis.[40]

Hydrochloric acid secretion is blocked by H_2 antagonists, thereby promoting the healing of duodenal ulcers. All three available H_2-receptor antagonists (cimetidine, famotidine, and nizatidine) suppress basal acid output, as well as acid output stimulated by meals. After IV administration, all three agents are eliminated principally through renal excretion. For cimetidine and famotidine, it is recommended that the doses be cut in half in patients whose creatinine clearance is 15 to 30 mL/min. For nizatidine, the dose should be halved if the creatinine clearance is less than 50 mL/min.[67] A noteworthy side effect is the alteration of CYP enzyme activity in the liver, which may result in prolongation of the effects of concurrently administered drugs that rely on CYP-mediated hepatic metabolism and elimination. Famotidine is the H_2-receptor antagonist least likely to cause this effect. Other side effects of H_2-receptor antagonists include decreased hepatic blood flow, leukopenia and thrombocytopenia, mental confusion, interstitial nephritis, hepatitis, bradycardia, and hypotension.

The most effective antisecretory agents are the proton pump inhibitors (Table 33.8). Sucralfate, the aluminum salt of sulfated sucrose, not only binds to ulcers but also promotes thickening of the gastric mucous layer, thereby promoting healing processes. It has been shown to be equally efficacious when used with H_2-receptor antagonists and antacids, and it is relatively devoid of side effects.

Misoprostol is a synthetic prostaglandin that may be used as a second-line prophylactic agent to prevent ulcers in patients taking NSAIDs. H. pylori is a species of gram-negative spiral bacteria sensitive to combination therapy with a variety of antibiotics. Approximately 80% of upper GI bleeds are self-limited. Laparoscopic repair is indicated when medical therapy is unsuccessful.

Gastric Ulcer Disease

Gastric ulcers develop as a result of the degeneration of the stomach's mucosal barrier against gastric acid. Gastric ulcers can occur anywhere in the stomach and may or may not be associated with increased gastric acid secretion. Pain and anorexia predispose the patient to metabolic changes and weight loss. The most frequent complication of gastric ulceration is perforation. Most perforations occur along the anterior aspect of the lesser curvature. In general, older patients have increased rates of perforations, and larger ulcers are associated with more morbidity and higher mortality rates. Similar to duodenal ulcers, gastric outlet obstruction can also occur in patients with type II or III gastric ulcers.[63] Surgery, consisting of antrectomy with pyloroplasty and vagotomy, is undertaken if the patient's condition does not respond to medical therapy.

TABLE 33.8	Proton Pump Inhibitors	
Generic Name	**Trade Name**	**Adult Dosage Range**
Esomeprazole	Nexium	20–40 mg daily
Lansoprazole	Prevacid	15–30 mg daily
Omeprazole	Prilosec	20–40 mg daily
Pantoprazole	Protonix, Protonix IV	40 mg daily 40 mg slow infusion
Rabeprazole	Aciphex	20 mg daily
Dexlansoprazole	Dexilant	30–60 mg daily

Gastric Neoplastic Disease

Gastric cancer is the second most common type of cancer worldwide. In the United States, gastric cancer is the seventh most frequent cause of cancer-related death. Most gastric neoplasms are malignant. The incidence of these neoplasms according to type is adenocarcinoma, 95%; lymphoma, 4%; and leiomyosarcoma, 1%. The epigastric pain is similar to pain caused by benign ulcers and may mimic angina. Typically, however, the pain is constant, nonradiating, and unrelieved by food ingestion. More advanced disease may present with weight loss, anorexia, fatigue, or vomiting. Symptoms often reflect the site of origin of the tumor. Endoscopic mucosal resection has become the treatment of choice for early gastric cancer and usually is performed in association with endoscopic ultrasonography for staging. Advanced adenocarcinoma is defined as a tumor that invades the gastric wall beyond the submucosa. Most patients are men (male:female ratio of 2:1) in their fifth to seventh decades of life. Clinically, symptoms include epigastric pain, dyspepsia, anemia, and weight loss. Hematemesis and symptoms of gastric outlet obstruction are not uncommon. Female patients may develop metastatic ovarian lesions (Krukenberg tumors) composed of diffuse-type cancer cells. Unfortunately, the majority of patients with gastric cancer in the United States are diagnosed at an advanced stage.[68]

Surgical resection remains the primary curative treatment for gastric cancer and represents the best chance for long-term survival. In addition, surgical resection often provides the most effective symptom relief, particularly those of an obstructive nature. In general, total gastrectomy is performed for proximal gastric tumors and diffuse gastric cancer, and partial gastrectomy is reserved for tumors in the distal stomach. Despite increased morbidity and mortality, arguments in favor of an extended lymphadenectomy include the fact that the removal of a larger number of lymph nodes results in more accurate pathologic staging and that failure to remove these lymph nodes leaves tumor cells behind in as many as one-third of patients.[68]

Anesthetic Considerations in Gastric Disease

Despite advances in medical therapy designed to inhibit acid secretion and to eradicate H. pylori, surgery remains an important strategy for managing patients with gastric disease. Patients undergoing surgery for gastric disease are generally either acutely ill and requiring emergency surgery, as in the case of a bleeding gastric ulcer, or stable and requiring elective surgical treatment of gastric carcinoma or intractable ulcer disease. Many procedures are performed laparoscopically. Limitations to the laparoscopic approach include the risk of developing peritonitis and the risk of forming dense adhesions. Acutely ill patients are more likely to be hemodynamically unstable and dehydrated. Elective surgical patients may exhibit varying degrees of debilitation and anemia. Aspiration precautions are warranted in both groups during the anesthetic course.

Hypovolemia should be corrected with the administration of appropriate colloid, crystalloid, or blood products before the induction of anesthesia. Suggested laboratory tests include complete blood count, electrolytes, blood urea nitrogen, glucose, magnesium, calcium, phosphate, PT, and PTT. Other tests are performed based on history and physical examination. Preparations for the perioperative transfusion of blood products must be undertaken before anesthesia and surgery. Expect a moderate fluid shift with moderate to large fluid losses. Two large-bore IV catheters (14–16 gauge) are indicated.

Clinical anemia and coagulopathy should be corrected with packed red blood cells and appropriate blood products (e.g., FFP, cryoprecipitate, platelets). The use of invasive monitoring (i.e., through the use of a pulmonary artery catheter, CVP line, or arterial line) is determined by the presence of preexisting, age-related, or acquired compromise in the function of other organ systems. Potential postoperative complications include hemorrhage, hypovolemia, hypothermia, atelectasis, and ileus. A postoperative stay in the intensive care unit may be necessary, especially in the case of fluid shifts caused by peritonitis and the need for large-volume fluid resuscitation.

The anesthetic technique used in gastrectomy may include preoperative epidural catheter placement as an intraoperative adjunct and for use in postoperative analgesia. Procedures other than total and partial gastrectomy performed for gastric disease include the following:

- Billroth I (gastroduodenostomy): resection of the distal stomach with reconstruction via end-to-end gastroduodenostomy
- Billroth II (gastrojejunostomy): resection of the distal stomach with reconstruction via end-to-side gastrojejunostomy
- Laparotomy with oversewing of the ulcer and application of an omental patch

Vagotomy is usually performed for gastric ulcer surgery to decrease gastric acid secretion and to allow ulcer healing. The vagus nerve can be transected at the main vagal trunks (truncal), which interrupts transmission to the top of the stomach and other abdominal viscera, or selectively, so that only the gastric vagal nerves are interrupted. The anesthetic technique is general or laparoscopic; esophageal dilators are used to facilitate traction on the stomach. An NG tube is placed after induction.

Gastrostomy

Gastrostomy is the surgical placement of a permanent or temporary artificial opening into the stomach that exits the skin of the abdominal wall for the purpose of gastric decompression and nutritional support. Patients who require placement of a gastrostomy tube (permanent or temporary) are often neurologically incapacitated or otherwise markedly debilitated and are likely to have compromised command of their airway reflexes. This, along with the need to insufflate the stomach, places them at greater risk for aspiration.

Gastrostomy placement is performed percutaneously at the bedside, in the endoscopy suite, or in the operating room. Endoscopic guidance is used with percutaneous placement of the gastrostomy tube. Any tube feedings should be stopped at least 8 hours prior to the procedure. A bite block should be used. As a primary procedure, gastrostomy placement is commonly undertaken with sedation and local anesthesia at the incisional site and in the back of the throat. General endotracheal anesthesia is indicated in patients who require laparotomy in conjunction with endoscopic placement and in those for whom percutaneous placement under local anesthesia with sedation may be contraindicated (e.g., the comatose patient). If general anesthesia is used, the ETT may need to be held as the surgeon inserts and withdraws the gastroscope.

PANCREATIC DISEASE

Physiologic Overview

The pancreas is approximately 20 cm long; its head is tucked into the curve of the duodenum, and its tail touches the spleen. The body of the pancreas lies behind the stomach. The pancreas functions in both an exocrine digestive enzyme and endocrine hormonal capacity.

TABLE 33.9 Major Pancreatic Enzyme Groups*

Enzyme Group	Enzyme, Proenzyme, or Precursor
Proteolytic	Trypsinogen (trypsin), chymotrypsinogen (chymotrypsin), procarboxypeptidase A (carboxypeptidase A), procarboxypeptidase B (carboxypeptidase B), proaminopeptidase (aminopeptidase), proelastase (elastase)
Amylolytic	α-amylase
Lipolytic	Lipase, prophospholipase A_2 (phospholipase A_2), carboxylesterase lipase, procolipase (colipase)
Nucleolytic	Deoxyribonuclease, ribonuclease
Other	Trypsin inhibitor

*Precursor molecules are listed, with products in parentheses.

The exocrine functions of the pancreas include protein secretion and electrolyte secretion. The exocrine function of the pancreas is primarily the continuous transductal secretion of 2.5 L of clear, colorless, bicarbonate-rich (pH 8.3) pancreatic juice per day. The ionic composition consists largely of sodium, potassium, bicarbonate, and chloride, with smaller concentrations of phosphate, sulfate, zinc, and calcium. The principal function of pancreatic juice is duodenal alkalinization to promote the optimal activity of pancreatic enzymes.

The arrival of acidic chyme (partially digested gastric contents) into the duodenum and jejunum stimulates the release of the hormones cholecystokinin-pancreozymin (CCK-PZ) and secretin. Both hormones are produced in the duodenum, jejunum, and ileum. Secretin causes the pancreas to release bicarbonate and water, and CCK-PZ, released in response to the presence of fats and partially digested proteins in the duodenum, stimulates secretion of the pancreatic enzymes necessary for further intestinal digestive processes. Trypsinogen, which is produced by pancreatic cells, is converted to the active enzyme trypsin in response to the release of enterokinase by the gastric mucosa. Trypsin is responsible for the conversion of large ingested proteins into smaller peptides and amino acids in preparation for intestinal absorption.[40] The major pancreatic enzyme groups are listed in Table 33.9.

Secretion of the aqueous and enzymatic components of pancreatic juice is controlled by hormonal and parasympathetic stimuli. Administration of vagolytic agents (e.g., atropine, glycopyrrolate) or ganglionic blocking agents, along with physical interruption of the vagus nerve, may induce a decreased response to secretin. Vagotomy has also been shown to result in a decrease in the release of pancreatic bicarbonate in response to duodenal acidity.

The endocrine function of the pancreas consists primarily of regulation of plasma glucose levels through the release of glucagon and insulin. Pancreatic endocrine cells reside in the islets of Langerhans and contain multiple cell types: the A (alpha) cell secretes glucagon, the B (beta) cell secretes insulin, the D (delta) cell secretes somatostatin (growth hormone–releasing inhibitory factor, which is responsible for controlling plasma levels of insulin, glucagon, and gastrin), whereas the D_2 (delta-2) cell secretes vasoactive intestinal peptide (VIP), and the PP (or F) cell secretes pancreatic polypeptide (PP).[69] The chief physiologic function of the endocrine pancreas might be summarized as regulation of body energy (a role largely achieved by hormonal control of carbohydrate metabolism). Simply stated, insulin is the hormone responsible for energy storage, and glucagon is the hormone responsible for energy release. Insulin promotes energy storage by decreasing blood glucose levels, increasing protein synthesis, decreasing glycogenolysis, decreasing lipolysis, and increasing glucose transport into cells (except for beta cells, hepatocytes, and central nervous system cells). Glucagon promotes energy release by increasing blood glucose levels through the stimulation of glycogenolysis, gluconeogenesis, and lipolysis.

α-adrenergic sympathetic stimulation has been shown to inhibit insulin secretion. β-adrenergic sympathetic and cholinergic blockade are inhibitory to insulin secretion as well. Arterial hypoxemia, hypothermia, traumatic stress, and surgical stress all suppress insulin secretion through α-adrenergic stimulation. Insulin secretion is enhanced by parasympathetic vagal stimulation, β$_2$-adrenergic sympathetic activation, and cholinergic drug administration.

Anesthetic considerations in patients with abnormalities in pancreatic endocrine function (such as diabetes mellitus) are discussed in other chapters. The present discussion is directed toward anesthetic considerations germane to patients with inflammatory or neoplastic disease of the pancreas.

Acute Pancreatitis

The cause of pancreatitis is multifactorial. Common causes include alcohol abuse, direct or indirect trauma to the pancreas, ulcerative penetration from adjacent structures (e.g., the duodenum), infectious processes, biliary tract disease, metabolic disorders (e.g., hyperlipidemia and hypercalcemia), vascular and autoimmune causes, toxic causes, and certain drugs (e.g., corticosteroids, furosemide, estrogens, and thiazide diuretics). In industrialized nations, 80% of acute pancreatitis cases are caused by alcohol abuse or gallstones. Although 35% to 40% of attacks are induced by gallstones, only 3% to 7% of patients with gallstones develop pancreatitis. The incidence of gallstone pancreatitis is increased in white females older than 60 and is highest among patients with small gallstones (<5 mm in diameter). Severe acute pancreatitis (SAP) is associated with organ failure, local complications, prolonged intensive care stay, and mortality rates greater than 25%. In patients with SAP, multiple organ dysfunction syndrome (MODS) is the main cause of death.[70]

Patients who have undergone extensive surgery involving mobilization of the abdominal viscera are at risk of developing postoperative pancreatitis, as are patients who have undergone procedures involving cardiopulmonary bypass. Patients who have received large doses of calcium intraoperatively, particularly after cardiopulmonary bypass, have also been shown to be at risk of developing postoperative pancreatitis.[71,72] Hypothetically, the pathophysiologic mechanism for the development of postoperative pancreatitis may involve an induced autodigestion syndrome. In fact, acute pancreatitis is characterized as a severe chemical burn of the peritoneal cavity.

It is generally believed that acute pancreatitis is triggered by obstruction of the pancreatic duct, and that the injury begins within pancreatic acinar cells. That injury is believed to include, and possibly be the result of, intraacinar cell activation of digestive enzyme zymogens, including trypsinogen. The pathophysiology of acute pancreatitis can be divided into three phases. The first phase is characterized by the premature activation of trypsin in acinar cells. The second phase is the inflammatory response of the pancreas, which is disproportionate to the response of other organs to a similar insult. In the third phase, systemic activation of the immune system and remote organ dysfunctions occur.[70] Aberrant activation or release of pancreatic enzymes or injury to the acinar cells caused by one or more of the aforementioned etiologic factors results in hemorrhage, edema, and necrosis of the pancreas.

Enzymes implicated as major culprits in pancreatitis are those activated by trypsin, enterokinase, and bile acids. These enzymes are necessary for proteolysis, elastolysis, and lipolysis. The inappropriate production of these enzymes results in pancreatic inflammation, which is caused by vascular breakdown, coagulation necrosis, fat necrosis, and parenchymal necrosis. Cardiovascular complications of acute pancreatitis can lead to pericardial effusion, alterations in cardiac

rhythmicity, signs and symptoms mimicking acute myocardial infarction, thrombophlebitis, and cardiac depression. Acute pancreatitis also predisposes patients to the development of acute respiratory distress syndrome (ARDS) and disseminated intravascular coagulopathy.[73]

The pain of pancreatitis may be severe and difficult to control. Most patients require narcotic medications. Pancreatic pain may radiate from the midepigastric to the periumbilical region and may be more intense when the patient is in the supine position. Abdominal distention is often seen and is largely attributable to the accumulation of intraperitoneal fluid and paralytic ileus. Nausea, vomiting, and fever are common symptoms. Hypotension is seen in 40% to 50% of patients and is attributable to hypovolemia secondary to the loss of plasma proteins into the retroperitoneal space. Acute renal failure secondary to dehydration and hypotension may occur.

Immediate circulatory and electrolyte resuscitation restores the microcirculation and represents one of the most powerful and effective interventions, especially in patients with SAP. Fluid losses can be enormous and can lead to marked hemoconcentration and hypovolemia. Inadequate fluid resuscitation during the early stages of pancreatitis can worsen the severity of an attack and lead to subsequent complications. The fluid depletion that occurs in pancreatitis results from the additive effects of losing fluid both externally and internally. The external fluid losses are caused by repeated episodes of vomiting and are worsened by nausea, which limits fluid intake. Repeated vomiting can result in hypochloremic alkalosis. Internal fluid losses, which are usually even greater than the external losses, are caused by fluid sequestration in areas of inflammation (i.e., the peripancreatic retroperitoneum) and in the pulmonary parenchyma and soft tissues elsewhere in the body. These latter losses result from diffuse capillary leakage, which is triggered by the release of proinflammatory factors during pancreatitis. Total fluid losses may be so great that they lead to hypovolemia and hypoperfusion, and metabolic acidosis can develop as a result.[74]

In patients with SAP, the magnitude of the proinflammatory response correlates with the severity and concomitant course of disease. A simple predictive tool is C-reactive protein (CRP) levels. A CRP level exceeding 150 mg/L (an arbitrarily chosen cutoff level) within the first 72 hours correlates with the occurrence of necrotizing pancreatitis and the degree of severity.[75]

During the first several days of a severe attack, circulating levels of many proinflammatory factors, including cytokines and chemokines, are elevated. In many cases, this so-called cytokine storm triggers the systemic immune response syndrome, and as a result, the hemodynamic parameters of these patients may resemble those of patients with sepsis associated with other disease states. The heart rate, cardiac output, and cardiac index usually rise, and total peripheral resistance falls. Hypoxemia also can occur as a result of the combined effects of increased intrapulmonary shunting and pancreatitis-associated lung injury that closely resembles that seen in other forms of ARDS. Fluid management, although critical, may be particularly difficult when hypovolemia is combined with ARDS-related respiratory failure.[74]

Severely ill, malnourished patients are often given parenteral nutritional support. Pain is controlled with synthetic opioids, such as fentanyl, which are preferable to morphine. Morphine-induced spasms of the sphincter of Oddi may exacerbate bile obstruction and stasis. Normeperidine, the metabolite of meperidine, causes central nervous system activity and makes meperidine unattractive for pain management in these patients. Epidural analgesia may be appropriate in select patients.[74]

Patients with gallstone pancreatitis can be divided into two groups: those who have or have had gallbladder-derived problems (cholecystitis or biliary colic) and those whose only problems are purely related to stones in the biliary ductal system (i.e., cholangitis and pancreatitis).

Patients in the first group undergo cholecystectomy to prevent additional gallbladder attacks and eliminate the source of stones that might trigger another attack of pancreatitis. Patients in the second group, however, do not necessarily require cholecystectomy because their problem relates only to ductal stones. Theoretically, they could be treated simply by endoscopic stone clearance (ERCP) combined with endoscopic sphincterotomy, so that future stones are passed without becoming impacted in the ampulla and triggering either pancreatitis or cholangitis. Indeed, for patients with high surgical risk, the endoscopic approach is generally recommended. Patients with low surgical risk are better managed by cholecystectomy.

The choice of anesthetic technique and the extent to which monitoring modalities are used are based on an assessment of the patient's history, the severity of disease, and the degree of preexisting physical compensation. Special attention should be paid to correcting significant intravascular volume deficits. The presence of labile hemodynamics and altered hepatic function must also be discerned, and appropriate modifications made to the anesthetic plan, for example, by ensuring stable arterial pressure, using anesthetic agents and adjuvants that require minimal hepatic biotransformation, ensuring adequate oxygenation, and replacing electrolytes and blood volume.

Chronic Pancreatitis

Chronic pancreatitis is traditionally defined as having permanent and irreversible damage to the pancreas, with histologic evidence of chronic inflammation, fibrosis, and destruction of exocrine (acinar cells) and endocrine (islets of Langerhans) tissue. Chronic pancreatitis is believed to reflect repeated episodes of subclinical acute pancreatitis with unrecognized pancreatic necrosis evolving into pancreatic fibrosis.

The most common etiology of chronic pancreatitis is alcohol use (70% of cases), with the risk increasing logarithmically with increasing alcohol use. Other causes include tobacco use (increased risk of pancreatic calcifications), genetic mutation, autoimmune disease, and obstruction of the main pancreatic duct by tumors, scars, stones, or duodenal wall cysts.[76]

Chronic pancreatitis is strongly suggested by the classic diagnostic triad of steatorrhea, pancreatic calcification (evidenced radiographically), and diabetes mellitus. Steatorrhea does not occur until pancreatic lipase secretion is less than 10% of the maximum output. The most common clinical problem in chronic pancreatitis is abdominal pain causing loss of appetite that results in weight loss and malnutrition. The clinical picture may also include hepatic disease, as evidenced by jaundice, ascites, esophageal varices, and abnormalities in coagulation factor, serum albumin, and transferase levels. A disturbance in pancreatic exocrine function, with consequent enzymatic insufficiency, results in malabsorption of fats and proteins in the intestine. Patients with chronic pancreatitis also have a predisposition for pericardial and pleural effusions.[74]

Many patients with chronic pancreatitis are alcoholics who, even before the onset of pancreatitis, had hypoalbuminemia and hypomagnesemia. Those problems are exacerbated by pancreatitis. The measured values for serum albumin may decrease even further as fluid losses are treated with albumin-free crystalloid solutions. Although hypocalcemia is common, particularly during a severe attack, the low total serum calcium is usually attributable to the low levels of circulating albumin, and no treatment is needed when ionized calcium levels are normal. Occasionally, however, ionized calcium levels also may be depressed, and tetany, as well as carpopedal spasm, can occur. This necessitates monitoring the ECG for cardiac rhythm disorders (e.g., lengthened QT interval with possible reentry dysrhythmias). When cardiac rhythm disorders are present, aggressive calcium replacement is indicated.[74]

Endocrine insufficiency is another consequence of chronic pancreatitis and is especially common after pancreatic resection. Approximately half of all patients with chronic pancreatitis develop insulin-dependent diabetes. Unlike in type 1 diabetes, in patients with insulin-dependent diabetes, insulin-producing beta cells and glucagon-producing alpha cells are injured, leading to an increased risk of prolonged and severe hypoglycemia with overzealous insulin treatment.[76]

Pancreatic abscesses develop from the peripancreatic collection of fluids that become infected. Abscesses are usually secondary manifestations of chronic pancreatitis and warrant surgical drainage to prevent the spread of infectious contents to the subphrenic and pericolic spaces. Fistula formation is possible, particularly into the transverse colon. Severe intraabdominal hemorrhage is also possible as a result of erosion into major proximal arteries.

Pancreatic Pseudocysts

Most pseudocysts communicate with the pancreatic ductal system and contain a watery fluid that is rich in pancreatic digestive enzymes. Typically, patients with pseudocysts have persistent elevation of circulating pancreatic enzyme levels. Many pseudocysts eventually resolve without complications, and intervention is not mandatory in all cases unless the pseudocysts are symptomatic, enlarging, or associated with complications. The likelihood that a pseudocyst will resolve spontaneously, however, is dependent on its size. Large pseudocysts (i.e., >6 cm in diameter) are more likely to become symptomatic, either because they are tender or because of their mass effect on adjacent organs. Those that compress the stomach or duodenum may cause gastric outlet obstruction with nausea and vomiting. Those that reduce the capacity of the stomach frequently cause early satiety, whereas those impinging on the bile duct can cause obstructive jaundice. Pancreatic pseudocysts that erode into a neighboring vessel can result in formation of a pseudoaneurysm with hemosuccus pancreaticus and upper GI bleeding.

Most patients who develop symptomatic pseudocysts are best managed by pseudocyst drainage. Internal drainage can be accomplished either endoscopically (by transpapillary drainage, cystogastrostomy, or cystoduodenostomy) or surgically (by cystogastrostomy, cystoduodenostomy, or Roux-en-Y cystojejunostomy). The approach chosen depends primarily on the locally available expertise and the location of the pseudocyst, but endoscopic drainage may be preferable in patients with high surgical risk.

Surgical Therapy for Pancreatitis

Depending on the cause of the pancreatitis, several surgical approaches can be used. Endoscopic therapy is used to improve drainage of the pancreatic duct. This can be done through pancreatic duct sphincterotomy, stent placement, or pancreatic duct stone removal (including extracorporeal shock wave lithotripsy). Open surgical therapy in chronic pancreatitis is most often considered for intractable abdominal pain for which medical therapy has failed, complications involving adjacent organs, failure of endoscopic management of pseudocysts, and internal pancreatic fistulas.

Surgical drainage of a pancreatic pseudocyst is usually undertaken after a period of maturation of the cyst (usually 6 weeks with acute pancreatitis). Pseudocysts with chronic pancreatitis are generally mature at the time of diagnosis, and delay is not necessary to allow for maturation. The procedure consists of the formation of a cystogastrostomy, cystojejunostomy, cystoduodenostomy, or possibly distal pancreatectomy. The location of the pseudocyst dictates the extent and type of procedure used for providing drainage of cystic contents into the GI tract. All these approaches require general anesthesia. Percutaneous external drainage guided by CT is reserved for cases in which the pseudocyst is particularly friable.[77]

Pancreatic Tumors

Pancreatic cancer affects 25,000 to 30,000 people in the United States each year, occurs more often in men than in women, and is more common among blacks than whites. The population most commonly associated with pancreatic cancer is between 60 and 80 years of age (80%), whereas less than 2% of cases occur in people younger than 40 years. Other risk factors include a family history of pancreatic cancer or a history of either hereditary or chronic pancreatitis, cigarette smoking, and occupational exposure to carcinogens. The incidence of diabetes mellitus is increased in patients with pancreatic cancer; some studies have indicated that diabetes is a risk factor for the development of pancreatic cancer, whereas others have argued that diabetes may be a manifestation of the cancer. Coffee drinking, which was once considered a risk factor, is no longer thought to play a role in the development of pancreatic cancer.[74]

Of all pancreatic tumors, 80% to 90% can be accounted for by ductal adenocarcinomas, and an even greater percentage of the malignant tumors are ductal adenocarcinomas. Most ductal cancers (70%) arise in the pancreatic head or in the uncinate process. They are generally resected by pancreaticoduodenectomy, with or without preservation of the pylorus and proximal duodenum. Ductal cancers originating in the body or tail of the pancreas are often larger and are more likely to have spread before their presence is known.[74]

Pancreatic cancers are insidious tumors that can be present for long periods and grow extensively before they produce symptoms. Once symptoms appear, they are determined by the location of the tumor in the pancreas. Those in the head or uncinate process of the pancreas cause bile duct, duodenal, or pancreatic duct obstruction. Because the head of the pancreas is most often the locus of the tumor, biliary obstruction is likely, resulting in progressive painless jaundice. The patient may have vague and nonspecific symptoms that include dull, aching, midepigastric or back pain. Anorexia and fatigue are often present and are associated with weight loss. Other symptoms include unexplained episodes of pancreatitis, nausea, vomiting, and steatorrhea. If the tumor spreads beyond the pancreas, peripancreatic nerve plexuses may cause abdominal or back pain. In the presence of peritoneal carcinomatosis or portal vein occlusion, ascites may occur. New-onset diabetes mellitus is occasionally the first symptom of an otherwise occult pancreatic cancer. Recent studies have suggested that this form of diabetes may be mediated by a factor released from the tumor that either inhibits insulin release from islets or induces peripheral insulin resistance. Unexplained migratory thrombophlebitis (Trousseau syndrome) may be associated with pancreatic cancer and other types of malignancy. It is probably a paraneoplastic phenomenon that results from a tumor-induced hypercoagulable state.[74]

Laboratory studies usually show elevated bilirubin and alkaline phosphatase levels. Radiographic evidence is generally nonspecific; needle biopsy during CT is most helpful in making a diagnosis. Percutaneous transhepatic cholangiography and ERCP are useful diagnostic modalities. ERCP is the most useful modality for defining lesions in the body and tail of the pancreas, or in the duodenum or ampulla.[78]

Insulinoma is the most common functioning tumor of the pancreas, and affected patients have a multitude of symptoms attributable to hypoglycemia, including seizures and coma (symptoms of catecholamine release), mental confusion, and obtundation. Hypersecretion of insulin is a major manifestation of this disease and results in profound hypoglycemia. The diagnostic hallmark of the syndrome is the so-called Whipple triad: hypoglycemia (catecholamine release), low blood glucose (40–50 mg/dL), and relief of symptoms after IV administration of glucose.

Insulinoma is treated surgically, by either an open or a laparoscopic approach (except in patients with advanced metastatic disease), and

involves distal pancreatectomy, subtotal pancreatectomy, or removal of all but a small portion of pancreatic tissue around the rim of the duodenum (Child procedure).[78]

If neoplastic disease is determined to be respectable, that is, without involvement of mesenteric vessels or infiltration into the mesenteric arterial root or hepatobiliary structures, a pancreaticoduodenectomy (Whipple procedure) may be performed. This procedure involves excision of the head of the pancreas, the entire duodenum, the proximal portion of the jejunum, the distal third of the stomach, the gallbladder, and the distal half of the CBD. A Whipple procedure also can be performed for malignancies of the CBD, traumatic injury to the pancreas, or benign obstructive chronic pancreatitis.[79]

Zollinger-Ellison syndrome (ZES; gastrinoma), a neoplasm primarily arising from the duodenum, results in the release of overabundant quantities of gastrin, which leads to the secretion of massive quantities of hydrochloric acid from the parietal cells. This condition is associated with severe, intractable ulcer pain. If other endocrine neoplasias are present (i.e., thyroid or parathyroid adenoma, pituitary adenoma, insulinoma), the condition is referred to as multiple endocrine neoplasia (MEN) type I.

Gastrinoma is the second most common islet cell tumor and is the most common symptomatic, malignant endocrine tumor of the pancreas. Thus current data indicate that gastrinomas are 3 to 10 times more common in the duodenum than in the pancreas, and although up to 70% of duodenal gastrinomas have lymph node metastases, only 5% have liver metastases. Although gastrinomas have a high rate of malignancy, they are more apt to be cured than cancer of any other abdominal viscera.

Omeprazole therapy is so effective in these cases that surgery is performed only for tumor removal. Every patient with ZES is a candidate for tumor removal until proved otherwise because of systemic illness or widespread metastases. During anesthetic induction for gastrinoma excision, a rapid sequence technique is recommended because of the likelihood of a large volume of stagnant, acidic intragastric fluid. Electrolyte and intravascular volume abnormalities (e.g., from severe diarrhea) should be anticipated and corrected before surgery. Attention should also be given to intraoperative monitoring of electrolyte and fluid balances. Hypokalemia and metabolic alkalosis are likely to be present if the patient has been vomiting and is dehydrated. Furthermore, preparations for the treatment of patients with known or suspected abnormalities in endocrine function must be included in the anesthetic plan, to include blood glucose monitoring, vigilance for and timely correction of swings in vital signs and physiologic parameters, maintenance of normothermia and normocarbia, maintenance of an appropriately anesthetized state, and maintenance of renal function.[40]

Anesthetic Considerations in Pancreatic Disease

The patient undergoing surgical treatment of pancreatic disease exhibits a variable clinical picture, from jaundiced and stable with a painless pancreatic mass to severely ill with multiorgan system involvement. Patients may have severe, acute abdominal pain with possible intestinal obstruction or ileus. Aspiration precautions should be in effect during induction of anesthesia and emergence from anesthesia, and an NG tube should be placed after induction. Because these patients are likely to be diabetic (secondary to beta cell dysfunction) or hypoglycemic (as in the case of insulinoma), perioperative assessment of serum glucose and institution of appropriate control measures are warranted. Patients with pancreatitis are usually hypotensive and hypovolemic. As such, aggressive blood product and crystalloid resuscitation may be necessary throughout the perioperative period and likely will necessitate placing invasive hemodynamic lines to guide therapy and monitor central pressures.

Severe electrolyte disorders may be present, including hypocalcemia, hypomagnesemia, hypokalemia, and possibly hypochloremic metabolic alkalosis. The serum hematocrit value may be falsely increased secondary to hemoconcentration or it may be decreased secondary to the presence of a bleeding diathesis. Coagulation parameters, including platelet count, PT, aPTT, and fibrinogen levels, should be assessed at regular intervals perioperatively. Preserving renal function mandates the preoperative assessment of blood urea nitrogen, serum creatinine, and 24-hour creatinine clearance (if possible); urinalysis also should be performed. Intraoperatively, a urine output of at least 0.5 to 1 mL/kg/hour should be maintained.

A thorough assessment of preexisting pulmonary status is vital. Pleural effusions, ventilation/perfusion (V/Q) mismatching, and atelectasis may occur, and can progress to respiratory failure. A significant incidence of postoperative respiratory morbidity is associated with upper abdominal surgery, especially in association with a preoperative debilitated state and splinting secondary to pain. Pulmonary assessment includes arterial blood gas analysis, chest radiography, and pulmonary function tests, when appropriate.

Cardiovascular assessment should consider the related findings from the assessment of other organ systems so that the degree to which functional hemodynamic impairment (that may need to be corrected) is fully appreciated. Correction of preexisting hemodynamic disturbances entails restitution of plasma volume and the oxygen-carrying capacity of the blood. Ischemic changes noted on the ECG must be treated promptly. ECG changes mimicking myocardial ischemia are often seen in patients with pancreatitis.[40] ECG changes are usually in the form of T-wave inversion, ST segment depression, and rarely ST segment elevation without the presence of coronary artery disease. Potential pathophysiologic mechanisms are circulating proteolytic enzymes, a vagally mediated reflex, or systemic inflammatory response.[80]

The celiac plexus transmits visceral afferent impulses from the upper abdominal organs, including the pancreas. Celiac plexus block may be performed in patients with chronic pancreatitis, but its effects are short lived. A combination of glucocorticoid and long-acting local anesthetic such as bupivacaine is commonly used. Celiac plexus neurolysis also may be performed by injecting absolute alcohol under CT or ultrasound guidance.[76]

Pancreatectomy

Pancreatectomy is performed for a variety of reasons, including ductal obstruction, pancreatic stones or cysts, trauma, benign or malignant tumors, chronic pancreatitis, and endocrine tumors. Complete surgical excision is the only definitive treatment of ductal pancreatic cancer.

In a partial pancreatectomy, part of the pancreas, the duodenum, the gallbladder, and part of the bile duct are removed. The tail of the pancreas is joined to a portion of the small bowel. In a total pancreatectomy, the distal portion of the stomach, the gallbladder, part of the bile duct, the spleen, and the surrounding lymph nodes are removed. The remaining distal portion of the stomach is reanastomosed to a portion of the small intestine.[79]

General endotracheal anesthesia is preferred for pancreatectomy, and muscle relaxants are used. The presence of increased IAP requires a rapid sequence induction. The use of nitrous oxide should be avoided due to the expansion of air-filled spaces in the bowel. An epidural at the T9-T10 level is advised for postoperative pain control, as it seems to improve the surgical outcome.[81] An even better choice may be the use of intrathecal morphine. One study also showed that the use of intrathecal morphine for major hepatopancreatobiliary surgery is associated with a lower incidence of postoperative hypotension, reduced perioperative IV fluid requirement, and shorter hospital stays compared with thoracic epidural anesthesia.[82]

Patients undergoing extensive pancreatic surgery often require postoperative ventilatory support and intensive care unit monitoring because of the magnitude and length of the procedure, as well as their preexisting cardiopulmonary status.[40] Pancreatic transplants are discussed in detail in Chapter 41.

DISEASES OF THE INTESTINAL TRACT

Anatomic and Physiologic Overview of the Small Intestine

The overall length of the small intestine is between 5 and 7 m long; it extends from the pylorus to the ileocecal valve (ICV). The small intestine is divided into three functional anatomic and physiologic segments. The first segment, the duodenum, begins at the pylorus and has a length of approximately 20 cm. The duodenum joins the second segment, the jejunum, which has a length of approximately 100 to 110 cm, at a suspensory ligament called the ligament of Treitz. The third and longest segment of the small intestine is the ileum, which has a length of approximately 150 to 160 cm and ends at the ileocecal valve. The jejunum has a larger lumen and is thicker than the ileum, with a less extensive blood supply (one or two vascular networks versus four or five in the ileum).[83]

The mesentery, which is rich in lymphatic vessels and blood vessels, is a peritoneal membrane that tethers the ileum and jejunum to the posterior abdominal wall and facilitates intestinal motility. Branches of the superior mesenteric artery provide the primary arterial blood supply to the jejunum, the ileum, and the proximal transverse colon. Venous drainage occurs via the superior mesenteric vein. This vessel joins the splenic vein posterior to the pancreas and forms the portal vein that empties into the liver. Lymphatic drainage from the bowel wall originates from the central bowel wall lacteal, continues through the superior mesenteric nodes into the cisterna chyli, and drains into the thoracic duct and eventually into the left internal jugular and subclavian veins.[84]

The wall of the small intestine is composed of the mucosa, submucosa, muscularis propria, and serosa. The outermost serosal layer is composed of a single layer of mesoepithelial cells. These cells form the visceral peritoneum and surround the jejunum, ileum, and anterior duodenum. The muscularis propria is composed of smooth muscle—an outer longitudinal layer and an inner circular layer. The Auerbach (myenteric) plexus, which primarily controls small intestine motility and secretion and is responsible for electrical conductance within the muscle, lies between the two layers of the muscularis propria. The next layer of the small intestine is the submucosa, which is composed of fibroelastic connective tissue; the strongest component of the bowel wall is the submucosa. Within the submucosa is the Meissner plexus (submucosal plexus), which regulates local blood flow, GI motility, and glandular secretions. The innermost layer, the mucosa, has transverse folds with millions of villi. These intraluminal projections are the functional units of the intestines and greatly increase the absorptive surface.[77]

The mucosa is further subdivided into three distinct layers:
1. *Muscularis mucosae.* The deepest layer is composed of a thin muscular sheet and separates the mucosa from the submucosa.
2. *Lamina propria.* A continuous connective tissue layer between the muscularis mucosae and the epithelium. This layer serves as a support epithelium and immunogenic barrier. Constituents of this layer include plasma cells (which produce immunoglobulins), macrophages, and lymphocytes.
3. *Epithelial layer.* Covers the villi and lines the Lieberkühn crypts. The functional units of the intestines, villi, contain goblet (mucus-secreting), absorptive, and endocrine cells. The villi also secrete enzymes that are necessary for digestion and useful for nutrient absorption. Cell turnover takes 3 to 7 days.

TABLE 33.10 Gastrointestinal Hormones

Hormone	Location	Major Stimulants of Peptide Secretion	Primary Effects	Diagnostic and Therapeutic Uses
Gastrin	Antrum, duodenum (G cells)	Peptides, amino acids, antral distention, vagal and adrenergic stimulation, gastrin-releasing peptide (bombesin)	Stimulates gastric acid and pepsinogen secretion; stimulates gastric mucosal growth	Gastrin analog (pentagastrin) used to measure maximal gastric acid secretion
Cholecystokinin (CCK)	Duodenum, jejunum (I cells)	Fats, peptides, amino acids	Stimulates pancreatic enzyme secretion; stimulates gallbladder contraction; relaxes sphincter of Oddi; inhibits gastric emptying	Biliary imaging of gallbladder contraction
Secretin	Duodenum, jejunum (S cells)	Fatty acids, luminal acidity, bile salts	Stimulates release of water and bicarbonate from pancreatic ductal cells; stimulates bile flow and alkalinity; inhibits gastric acid secretion and motility and inhibits gastrin release	Provocative test for gastrinoma; measurement of maximal pancreatic secretion
Somatostatin	Pancreatic islet (D cells), antrum, duodenum	Gut: Fats, proteins, acid, other hormones (e.g., gastrin, CCK) Pancreas: Glucose, amino acids, CCK	Universal "off" switch; stimulates release of all GI secretion and motility; stimulates gastric acid secretion and release of antral gastrin; stimulates growth of intestinal mucosa and pancreas	Treatment of carcinoid diarrhea and flushing; decreases secretion from intestinal fistulas (particularly pancreatic fistulas); ameliorates symptoms associated with hormone-overproducing endocrine tumors; treatment of esophageal variceal bleeding
Gastrin-releasing peptide (mammalian equivalent of bombesin)	Small bowel	Vagal stimulation	Universal "on" switch; stimulates release of all GI hormones (except secretin); stimulates growth of intestinal mucosa and pancreas	
Gastric inhibitory polypeptide	Duodenum, jejunum (K cells)	Glucose, fats, protein adrenergic stimulation	Inhibits gastric acid and pepsin secretion; stimulates pancreatic insulin release in response to hyperglycemia	
Motilin	Duodenum, jejunum	Gastric distention, fats	Stimulates upper GI tract motility; may initiate the migrating motor complex	
Vasoactive intestinal peptide	Neurons throughout the GI tract	Vagal stimulation	Primarily functions as a neuropeptide; potent vasodilator	
Neurotensin	Small bowel (N cells)	Fats	Stimulates pancreatic and intestinal secretion; inhibits gastric acid secretion; stimulates growth of small and large bowel mucosa	
Enteroglucagon	Small bowel (L cells)	Glucose, fats	Glucagon-like peptide-1: Stimulates insulin release; inhibits pancreatic glucagon release; Glucagon-like peptide-2: Potent enterotropic factor	
Peptide YY	Distal small bowel, colon	Fatty acids, CCK	Inhibits gastric and pancreatic secretions; inhibits gallbladder contraction	

CCK, Cholecystokinin; *GI*, gastrointestinal.
Adapted from Harris JW, Evers BM. Small intestine. In: Townsend CM, et al., eds. *Sabiston Textbook of Surgery: The Biological Basis of Modern Surgical Practice*. 20th ed. Philadelphia: Elsevier; 2017:1246.

The lamina propria of the intestinal mucosa provides a barrier to pathogen entry. Within this connective tissue layer is a rich supply of immune cells that include plasma cells, lymphocytes, mast cells, and eosinophils. The plasma cells are responsible for synthesizing IgA, therefore there is a rich reservoir of IgA in the lamina propria. IgA antigen binding initiates mucous secretion, which prevents intestinal bacterial and viral uptake by disabling or facilitating neutralization of the aforementioned organisms. Lymphocytes are responsible for the

development of antibodies in response to an antigen. These antibodies are formed from precursors located in Peyer patches.[84] An additional function of the small intestinal mucosa is the production of a rich supply of hormones that regulate GI function (Table 33.10).

The small intestine is innervated by the autonomic and enteric nervous systems. These systems function independently of each other. Both divisions of the autonomic nervous system innervate the small intestine and are the extrinsic nerve supply. The parasympathetic fibers originate from the vagus nerve and travel along the path of the celiac ganglia. Parasympathetic stimulation is responsible for increased intestinal reflexes (e.g., related to the LES), intestinal motility, and secretions. Splanchnic nerves from the celiac plexus provide sympathetic innervation; activation of these nerves inhibits motility and produces vasoconstriction. Sympathetic nerve tracts are also responsible for carrying afferent pain impulses. Intrinsic motor innervation is mediated by the myenteric plexus (Auerbach plexus) and the submucosal plexus (Meissner plexus). The enteric nervous system also plays an important role in the GI tract. The enteric nervous system is comprised of intrinsic neurons, the network of neurons whose cell bodies are located within the walls of the small intestine, pancreas, and gallbladder.[85] The enteric nervous system contains as many nerve cells as the spinal cord and is unique in its extraordinary degree of local autonomy. The high degree of local autonomy allows digestion and peristalsis to continue in the event of spinal cord transection or spinal anesthesia. Spinal anesthetic inhibition of sympathetic preganglionic fibers from T8 through L3 yields a contracted small intestine that may afford superior surgical conditions.

The intestinal inhibitory reflex responds to abnormal distention by decreasing motility proximal to the locus of distention. This reflex may have significant indirect clinical implications (e.g., aspiration risk).[84] The arrival of chyme from the stomach stimulates intestinal movements that mix secretions from the liver, pancreas, and intestinal glands. A basic electrical rhythm in the longitudinal smooth muscle layer initiates action potentials in the circular muscular layers of the small intestine. This activates the muscular contractions that constitute small bowel motility. Segmental contractions mix chyme with digestive enzymes and expose it to the villi's absorptive surfaces, and peristaltic (propulsive) contractions move chyme toward the large intestine.

Malabsorption Syndromes

The small intestine is the largest endocrine gland in the body that has major immune capability and is responsible for the digestion of food and the absorption of nutrients.[84] Approximately 85% to 90% of the water entering the GI tract is absorbed in the small intestine. Malabsorption syndromes interfere with brush border processing, nutrient absorption in the small intestine through mucosal disruption, and transport of nutrients into the circulation. Numerous disorders of the small intestine manifest as abnormalities in absorption. These include diverticulosis, radiation enteritis, and gastric bypass. Primary clinical signs include unexplained weight loss, steatorrhea, and diarrhea. Other manifestations of malabsorptive disease include anemia, bone loss, and menstrual disturbance.[86] These disorders affect the absorption of the major constituents of ingested nutrients, including amino acids, carbohydrates, and fats.[73]

Fat malabsorption results in deficiencies in the uptake of fat-soluble vitamins (vitamins A, D, E, and K). Vitamin K deficiency manifests as hypoprothrombinemia. This condition is often evidenced through bleeding dyscrasias. Vitamin B_{12} deficiency results in anemia (which may also be encountered in patients with impaired iron absorption), neuropathy, and glossitis. Protein malabsorption may result in the development of peripheral edema and ascites. Tetany, osteomalacia, and pathologic fractures result from calcium deficiency caused by vitamin D malabsorption and calcium malabsorption because fatty acids bind calcium. In the setting of steatorrhea, pancreatic replacement enzymes are often effective in decreasing fat loss.[63]

The cause of malabsorption syndromes is multifactorial. The basic underlying defect is either disruption of intestinal mucosal integrity, such as from a disease processes, or loss of absorptive surface area caused by extensive surgical resection of the small intestine (i.e., short gut syndrome). The particular part of the small bowel that is resected

and the amount that is removed have a significant bearing on the degree to which deficiencies in minerals, vitamins, and electrolytes are clinically manifested and are of particular concern to the anesthetist.

Maldigestion Syndromes

Maldigestion syndromes are generally caused by failure of the chemical digestive processes to take place in the intestinal lumen or at the brush border of the intestinal mucosa.[76,86] The most common causes include pancreatic deficiency, lactase deficiency, or bile salt deficiency. Diseases that are more likely to result in malabsorption syndromes (failure to absorb and transport digested nutrients) differ from those that are responsible for maldigestion (failure of the chemical digestive process). The hallmark of maldigestion is steatorrhea. Significant pancreatic disease is usually present when a maldigestion syndrome exists because the pancreas has a large functional reserve in both normal and disease states. Chronic pancreatitis is the most common cause of pancreatic insufficiency. Other causes of maldigestion are cystic fibrosis, fistulas, gallstones (which contribute to diminished bile flow), ischemic enteritis, neoplastic disease processes, diabetes mellitus, and vitamin B_6 or B_{12} deficiency.[76]

Anatomic and Physiologic Considerations of the Large Intestine

The large intestine is approximately 3 to 5 ft long; consists of the cecum, appendix, colon, rectum, and anal canal; and may be recognized by its size, position, and the presence of haustrations (outpouchings of the colon) and the taeniae coli. The taeniae coli are three strips of longitudinal muscles that give rise to haustrations and the segmented look at the colon.[87] The arterial blood supply comprises the superior mesenteric artery (which perfuses the cecum to the splenic flexure colon), the inferior mesenteric artery (which perfuses from the splenic flexure to the superior rectum), and the internal iliac artery (which perfuses the middle and lower rectum). Venous drainage of the colon corresponds to the arterial blood supply with the middle and superior mesenteric veins contributing to the portal venous system. The superior rectal and inferior mesenteric lymph nodes receive lymph drainage from the rectum, sigmoid, and descending colon. The inguinal lymph nodes receive lymphatic drainage from the anal canal. This has implications for individuals with rectal and anal cancer.[87] The myenteric plexus regulates motor and secretory activity independently of the extrinsic system. Sympathetic innervation is derived from T10-T12 (right colon), L1-L3 (left colon), and the presacral nerves arising within the preaortic plexuses (rectum). Parasympathetic innervation is primarily from the vagus nerve (right and transverse colon) and from nerve fibers arising from S2-S4 (descending colon, sigmoid colon, and rectum). A rich endowment of lymphatics is present throughout the length of the colon and rectum.[5,88,89]

The primary function of the large colon is to store and expel waste products. Approximately 500 to 700 mL of chyme are delivered from the ileum to the cecum each day. Another function performed largely in the right colon is the absorption of sodium and water. All but 100 to 200 mL of the 1 to 2 L of ileal effluent presented to the large colon per day is reabsorbed through diffusion and active transport.

Sodium absorption occurs through active transport against a gradient and is enhanced by minerals, corticoids, glucocorticoids, and fatty acids that are produced by indigenous bacteria. Conservation of sodium is so efficient in the large colon that a normal individual may require only 5 mEq/day to maintain a sodium balance. However, a patient presenting with an ileostomy necessitates a greater intake of sodium (80–100 mEq/day) to approximate the high sodium content lost as ileal effluent. The loss of the normal colonic reabsorption of sodium chloride and water (e.g., after colectomy) may eventually exceed the small intestine's compensatory capacity to increase absorption, and clinical abnormalities in electrolyte balance follow.

Potassium is passively absorbed and secreted across the electrochemical gradient, whereas chloride is absorbed as the complementary ion to sodium and in exchange for bicarbonate. Potassium is lost through passive diffusion in the colonic mucoid secretions. Significant potassium loss is likely to occur, therefore, in the presence of colitis and villous adenoma, two disease processes notable for mucoid stools.

Inflammatory Bowel Disease

In 2015, approximately 3 million adults in the United States were diagnosed with inflammatory bowel disease. The two major types of inflammatory bowel disease are Crohn disease and ulcerative colitis (UC), which have different clinical features and manifestations (Table 33.11).

Crohn disease can involve any part of the GI tract from the mouth to the anus, but it most commonly affects the distal ileum and the proximal large colon.[90] Th1-mediated inflammation with activation of leukocytes and cytokines causes injury. The involved leukocytes release proinflammatory substances, including prostaglandins, leukotrienes, proteases, and nitric oxide, with resulting injury.[91] Progression of the disease leads to neutrophil infiltration of the crypts, with resulting abscess formation and crypt destruction.[92] Symptoms of Crohn disease may initially be described as irritable bowel. Abdominal pain and diarrhea are the most common signs (more than five stools per day), with passage of blood and mucus. If the ileum is involved, patients may have right lower quadrant tenderness, and individuals may be anemic due to decreased vitamin B_{12} absorption.[90]

The deeper layers of the intestinal mucosa are typically involved, a situation that leads to derangements in colonic absorption. Owing to the loss of functional absorptive surfaces in the large colon, patients with Crohn disease are often deficient in magnesium, phosphorus, zinc, and potassium. They also have deficiencies secondary to the loss of absorptive capability in portions of the small intestine. Protein-losing enteropathy is often encountered, as is anemia resulting from occult blood loss and deficiencies in vitamin B_{12} and folic acid. Disturbances in the enterohepatic circulation of bile in the terminal ileum are reflected in complex nutrient deficiencies, including deficiencies in proteins, zinc, magnesium, phosphorus, fat-soluble vitamins, calcium (leading to bone disease), and vitamin B_{12}.[93] This state is typical of patients with chronic Crohn disease. Folate deficiency may also be present in patients who receive sulfasalazine preparations.

Fistulas often develop between inflamed portions of the intestine and adjacent abdominal structures. There is a high incidence of abdominal and pelvic abscesses, rectocutaneous fistulas, and perirectal abscesses in these patients. Increased calcium oxalate absorption in the terminal ileum frequently occurs, resulting in a high rate of renal calculi and cholelithiasis.[94,95] Medical therapy for Crohn disease includes a variety of drugs (Box 33.9).

Surgery is performed when medical treatment fails or when complications supervene. Although effective in relieving complications, surgical resection of the diseased colon and ileum does not alter the progression of the disease. The primary goal of surgical management is to limit the operation to correcting the presenting complication, which could include bowel obstruction, fistulas, abscesses, perforation, and symptoms that indicate widespread symptomatic disease (for which total colectomy and ileal resection may be warranted). Surgical resection of small intestinal segments can lead to short bowel syndrome, with accentuated complications of malabsorption, diarrhea, and nutritional deficiencies.[96]

Most patients with Crohn disease eventually undergo surgery, and a large number require repeat or continued procedures. The recurrence rate at 10 years after surgery is 50%. A high likelihood of repeat surgery involves areas of the remaining bowel proximal to the area of a

TABLE 33.11 Diagnosis of Crohn Colitis Versus Ulcerative Colitis

Observation	Crohn Colitis	Ulcerative Colitis
Symptoms and Signs		
Diarrhea	Common	Common
Rectal bleeding	Less common	Almost always
Abdominal pain (cramps)	Moderate to severe	Mild to moderate
Palpable mass	At times	No (except for large tumors)
Anal complaints	Frequent (>50%)	Infrequent (<20%)
Radiologic Findings		
Ileal disease	Common	Rare (backwash ileitis)
Nodularity, fuzziness	No	Yes
Distribution	Skips areas	Rectum, extending upward and continuously
Ulcers	Linear, cobblestone, fissures	Collar-button
Toxic dilation	Rare	Uncommon
Proctoscopic Findings		
Anal fissure, fistula, abscess	Common	Rare
Rectal sparing	Common (50%)	Rare (5%)
Granular mucosa	No	Yes
Ulceration	Linear, deep, scattered	Superficial, universal

Adapted from Mahmoud NN, et al. Colon and rectum. In: Townsend CM, et al., eds. *Sabiston Textbook of Surgery: The Biological Basis of Modern Surgical Practice.* 20th ed. Philadelphia: Elsevier; 2017:1339.

BOX 33.9 Agents Used to Treat Crohn Disease

5-Aminosalicylate Acids (5-ASAs)
- Sulfasalazine
- Sulfa-free (mesalamine, olsalazine, balsalazide)

Antibiotics
- Metronidazole
- Ciprofloxacin

Glucocorticoids
- Classic
- Novel (controlled ileal-release budesonide)

Immune Modulators
- 6-mercaptopurine, azathioprine
- Methotrexate
- Cyclosporine/tacrolimus
- Tofacitinib

Biologic Response Modifiers
- Anti-TNF antibodies (infliximab, adalimumab, golimumab, certolizumab pegol)
- Natalizumab
- Vedolizumab
- Ustekinumab

TNF, Tumor necrosis factor.

Adapted from Ananthakrishnan AN, Regueiro MD. Management of inflammatory bowel diseases. In: Feldman M, et al., eds. *Sleisenger and Fordtran's Gastrointestinal and Liver Disease.* 11th ed. Philadelphia: Elsevier; 2021:1898–1929.

previous anastomosis. Patients with a long history of Crohn disease are also shown to have a higher risk of intestinal carcinoma.[90,97,98]

UC is a chronic inflammatory disease that causes ulceration of the colonic mucosa and extends proximally from the rectum into the colon. It is a disease characterized by remissions and exacerbations. UC is more prevalent in females and whites and has a peak incidence between ages 20 and 40. It is speculated that there is a strong genetic predisposition to the disorder, but psychological factors have also been implicated. UC lesions are limited to the mucosa and are not transmural. Inflammation begins at the crypt of Lieberkühn, with the infiltration and release of inflammatory cytokines from neutrophils, lymphocytes, plasma cells, macrophages, eosinophils, and mast cells.[99,100]

Symptoms usually include abdominal pain, fever, and bloody diarrhea. Loss of absorptive mucosal surface and decreased colonic transit time can lead to large volumes of watery diarrhea. UC is typically chronic, with periods of remission and exacerbation. UC has relatively low-grade symptoms, such as bloody stools with purulent mucus, malaise, diarrhea, and pain. In approximately 15% of patients, however, UC with acute, fulminating characteristics may occur. These patients demonstrate continuous severe abdominal pain, profuse rectal hemorrhage, and high fever. Associated symptoms include nausea and vomiting, anorexia, and profound weakness. Physical signs usually include dehydration, pallor, and weight loss. Severe blood loss may result in hypotension and shock.[101]

Associated with an acute onset of fulminating UC is toxic megacolon, which is characterized by severe colonic distention that causes shock. In patients with this condition, the distended bowel lumen (>5.5–6 cm on a supine abdominal film) provides an environment conducive to bacterial overgrowth. This condition, coupled with erosive intestinal inflammation and perforation, allows for the systemic release of bacterial toxins. Clinical signs and symptoms of toxic megacolon include fever, tachycardia, abdominal distention, pain, ileus, and dehydration. Electrolyte abnormalities, anemia, and hypoalbuminemia are also commonly present. If there is no significant improvement within a short period of medical treatment, patients arrive in the operating room for subtotal colectomy with an end ileostomy. Patients with toxic megacolon due to Crohn disease undergo surgical treatment similar to those with toxic megacolon due to UC.[101]

Patients with chronic UC are at increased risk for the development of left-sided carcinoma of the colon. An increased incidence of large-joint arthritis is seen in patients when the disease is clinically active. Concomitant liver disease, as evidenced by fatty infiltrates and pericholangitis, also may complicate the clinical picture. Other extracolonic manifestations of UC include iritis, erythema nodosum, and ankylosing spondylitis.

Therapy for UC is initially medical. As with Crohn disease, sulfasalazine preparations, antidiarrheal agents, immunosuppressive agents, and corticosteroids are the cornerstones of medical therapy. Nicotine may have a protective effect in UC but not in Crohn disease. Both Crohn disease and UC result in systemic disorders such as anemia and nutritional deficiencies, which are handled in the same supportive manner. In both diseases, surgical resection is reserved for patients with intractable complications. Whereas surgery for Crohn disease is nondefinitive and complication oriented, proctocolectomy with ileostomy is generally curative for UC and eliminates the risk of malignancy and long-term steroid use.[102]

Anesthetic Considerations in Inflammatory Bowel Disease

Anesthetic management of patients with inflammatory bowel disease begins with optimization of the patient's medical status. Correction of anemia, fluid depletion, electrolyte and acid-base disorders, and performance of a nutritional assessment are mandatory. Possible extracolonic

complications (e.g., sepsis, liver disease, coagulopathy, anemia, arthritis, hypoalbuminemia, and other metabolic abnormalities) must also be considered during planning and perioperative management.[103]

Patients on long-term steroid therapy may require prophylactic steroid coverage. Nitrous oxide should be avoided due to the possibility of bowel distention associated with its prolonged intraoperative use. Many patients require total parenteral nutrition (TPN) and bowel rest because eating may worsen symptoms. As such, the anesthetist should be aware of complications from parenteral nutritional therapy (e.g., hyperglycemia or hypoglycemia, increased carbon dioxide production, renal or hepatic dysfunction, nonketotic hyperosmolar hyperglycemic coma, and hyperchloremic metabolic acidosis). Any preexisting TPN infusion should be maintained throughout the perioperative period at the ordered infusion rate. Correction of fluid, electrolyte, and hematologic abnormalities may be necessary before surgery. Periodic laboratory assessment of metabolic status (i.e., serum glucose and electrolytes) should be performed and should guide corrective interventions. The severity of extracolonic influences on the function of other organ systems dictates appropriate technique and drug selection, as well as the extent to which invasive monitoring is used. The increased intraluminal pressure caused by the administration of anticholinesterases for neuromuscular blockade reversal has been shown to have no effect on colonic suture lines. No particular anesthetic technique is mandated; however, the use of a combined technique (epidural and general anesthesia) is attractive for both intraoperative use and postoperative analgesia requirements. A combined spinal-epidural technique may be beneficial in fast-track cases and low anterior rectal resections.[103-105]

Diverticulitis and Diverticulosis

Diverticulosis of the colon is characterized by the presence of numerous asymptomatic mucosal herniations or outpouchings in the large colon, with the highest prevalence (65%) noted in the left (sigmoid) colon. The colonic mucosa herniates through the smooth muscle layers. Structural weakness of the colonic wall (usually where arteries penetrate the tunica muscularis to nourish the mucosal layer) and intraluminar hypertension are two mechanisms theorized to be responsible for the development of diverticulosis.

Diverticulitis is inflammation of the diverticula; this syndrome manifests as abdominal pain with ileus and other symptoms that indicate an acute abdomen, such as nausea, vomiting, diarrhea, rigid abdominal distention, and dehydration. Diverticulitis occurs in only 1% of patients with diverticulosis. Inflammation of the diverticula may be localized or more widespread and may involve the mesentery and other abdominal organs. Progression of symptoms may lead to hypovolemia, hypokalemia, and shock. The presence of free intraperitoneal air, as evidenced on radiographic abdominal films, suggests perforation. Air in the retroperitoneum may be indicative of paracolic abscess. Both conditions require urgent surgical exploration. Abscess formation and visceral perforation indicate the need for urgent surgical intervention.[83]

Surgical treatment of diverticulitis is reserved for severe symptoms that are refractory to aggressive medical therapy. IV corticosteroids, antibiotics, and fluid replacement are attempted initially. Exploratory laparotomy with colectomy may be necessary under emergent conditions of acute bleeding, recurrent bleeding that fails to cease spontaneously, or sepsis. The goals of surgical exploration include fecal diversion and abscess drainage, as well as resection of the diseased colon.[40]

Complications of diverticulitis, which occur in up to 25% of patients, frequently necessitate surgical intervention. Such complications include bowel obstruction; fistulas between the sigmoid colon and the skin, bladder, vagina, or small intestine; abscesses; and peritonitis. Abscess formation after colonic obstruction and perforation is generally confined to the pelvis and may involve such structures as the abdominal wall and the subdiaphragmatic spaces. More extensive abscess formation can include the deep pelvic organs and the hip and thigh. Patients with pelvic abscesses caused by diverticulitis have significant pain, fever, and leukocytosis.

Bleeding is uncommon in patients with diverticular disease, but when present, it is often difficult to locate by endoscopy and even laparotomy. Bleeding in diverticular disease may be either occult or massive and is caused by erosion of the vessels adjacent to the diverticulum. Elective colon resection is usually considered in patients with recurrent episodes of acute diverticulitis. After a second attack of acute diverticulitis, the prevalence of complications associated with the disease approaches 50%, and the associated mortality rate is twice that of an initial attack. Diverticulitis, when present in the right colon or cecum, often mimics acute appendicitis. Surgery for appendectomy, therefore, may uncover the presence of an inflamed diverticulum or diverticulitis, necessitating extension of the procedure so that colonic resection can be performed.[40]

Abdominal Compartment Syndrome

Abdominal compartment syndrome (ACS) develops when there is abnormally high IAP (>20 mm Hg) with associated organ dysfunction. Also known as intraabdominal hypertension, ACS can be diagnosed by measuring IAP with a bladder manometer. Normal IAP is less than 10 mm Hg. At pressures greater than 10 mm Hg, hepatic arterial blood flow significantly decreases. Cardiovascular perturbations occur at 15 mm Hg. Oliguria occurs at 15 to 20 mm Hg, and anuria occurs at 40 mm Hg. Organ dysfunction develops if these increased pressures last longer than 6 hours. IAP greater than 20 to 30 mm Hg can result in organ failure and death.[106]

ACS is associated with abdominal trauma, hemoperitoneum, mesenteric arterial thrombosis, acute pancreatitis, intestinal obstruction, visceral edema (as occurs in sepsis and shock), and massive fluid volume replacement. Causes of chronic ACS include ascites, pregnancy, and intraabdominal tumors. Resuscitative efforts and exposure of the abdomen induce mesenteric edema formation and bowel dilation. Under these conditions, additional ischemic injury to the abdominal viscera is avoided by delaying closure until the gross abdominal distention is resolved.

Cardiac output is decreased secondary to decreased cardiac preload (venous return), elevated systemic vascular resistance, and elevated intrathoracic pressure. Reflex tachycardia is a baroceptor-mediated response to decreased preload, with resultant diminished diastolic filling and coronary perfusion. Intracranial filling pressures are increased. Decreased thoracic compliance and decreased lung volumes result from impaired diaphragmatic descent. The outcome is an increased pulmonary shunt fraction, atelectasis, and pulmonary edema. Impairment in renal function results from compression of the kidney and diminished glomerular perfusion. The end consequence is multiple organ failure.

ACS is treated by urgent decompressive laparotomy, which may be performed at the bedside if the patient is too unstable to move. However, surgical decompression is ideally performed in the operating room. One study showed that overall mortality after surgical decompression was 46%, with preoperative renal failure, lower preoperative IAP, and late decompression being predictive of death. This underscores the point that once the diagnosis of ACS is made, prompt intervention is needed. If medical interventions are futile or judged to be inadequate, prompt decompression is mandatory.[107]

Affected patients often have myriad medical problems that may significantly influence their outcome. The possibility of developing ACS subsequent to performing a resuscitative "damage-control" laparotomy

in a traumatically injured patient is always a consideration. Under this circumstance, immediate life-threatening injuries are addressed, and the patient is then returned to the operating room from the intensive care unit at a later date, when hemodynamic stabilization has occurred. Definitive repairs of associated, less life-threatening injuries are then undertaken, often in stages. During this time, the abdomen may be left open but packed and sealed with sterile dressings, along with a drainage appliance to resolve postresuscitation intraabdominal edema.[40] The patient may be returned repeatedly to the operating room for dressing changes until conditions are conducive for abdominal wound closure. Providing anesthesia care for these patients can be extremely challenging. Intraoperative monitoring is directed toward the maintenance of hemodynamic stability and includes knowledge of the patient's preoperative hemodynamic profile. If the patient is still receiving mechanical ventilatory support, it is of utmost importance to provide intraoperative ventilation in a mode as close as possible to that being administered in the intensive care unit. This is particularly vital in the patient with ARDS. This may require modification of the anesthesia delivery ventilator to approximate as closely as possible the minute ventilation, fraction of inspired oxygen (FiO_2), inspiratory/expiratory ratio, ventilatory rate, and level of positive end-expiratory pressure the patient has been receiving. This minimizes the potential for perioperative deterioration of previously accomplished improvement in the patient's ventilatory status. Invasive monitors brought with the patient, such as an arterial line, central venous catheter, and pulmonary artery catheter, should be used for perioperative management. Opioids and inhalation agents are used with discretion in accordance with patient tolerance. The induction of adequate muscle relaxation and amnesia with a benzodiazepine or with scopolamine assume priority in the pharmacologic anesthetic management of the physiologically labile patient. Other vasoactive agents are included as indicated for hemodynamic support. Best practice caveats for the anesthetic management of these patients are the provision of intraoperative stability and the preservation of preoperative homeostatic compensation.

One serious but rare complication of surgical decompression is the so-called reperfusion syndrome, in which the patient develops severe hypotension and acidosis immediately after the abdomen is decompressed, as a result of the release of acidotic blood from the mesenteric beds.[107] Reperfusion washout of the byproducts of anaerobic metabolism releases an array of cardiac depressants and vasodilatory mediators into the general circulation. Proper preparation is required and includes optimization of intravascular volume, acid-base status, and arterial oxygenation.[108]

The mortality rate in ACS approaches 42%, with most patients succumbing to secondary systemic inflammatory response syndrome, sepsis, and MODS. Other causes of death include respiratory failure (i.e., ARDS) and the consequences of added stress imposed on cardiac function in susceptible patients.[108]

Anesthetic Considerations in Elective Surgery of the Colon

Using either a laparoscopic or anterior open approach, the surgeon mobilizes the colon and ligates the associated blood vessels. The diseased bowel is removed, and the remaining ends of the distal and proximal colon are anastomosed together; alternatively, a colostomy or ileostomy may be created. Preoperative elimination of fecal mass and bacterial flora are critical to avoid postoperative infection. The night before admission, the patient can lavage with isotonic and isosmotic solutions orally or by way of an NG tube. Cleansing enemas also may be ordered. These techniques are often used for elective procedures in conjunction with dietary changes that emphasize the intake of fluids and low-residue foodstuffs and culminate in the intake of only clear liquids for 24 to 48 hours before surgery. IV and oral antibiotics used for bowel cleansing commonly include drugs from the aminoglycoside family (e.g., neomycin, erythromycin) and/or a combination of the cephalosporins and metronidazole.

Awareness of this preoperative preparation in patients who undergo elective bowel surgery is critical because aggressive preoperative bowel preparation predisposes a patient to water and electrolyte imbalances that may have a deleterious influence on perioperative cardiovascular function, hemodynamics, and systemic organ perfusion, particularly if the patient is elderly or debilitated. Depending on how chronic the disease process is, anemia resulting from frank or occult bleeding may be present. Malnutrition with hypoalbuminemia also may be present before surgery.

Preoperative NG drainage may be required if an adynamic colon or obstruction is present. This preoperative intervention may be superimposed on a dehydrated patient or one who is electrolyte depleted, resulting in hypochloremic hypokalemic alkalosis. The resulting fluid and electrolyte abnormalities may be of sufficient magnitude to require postponement of the procedure until volume and electrolyte resuscitation has been accomplished.

Carcinoma of the Colon

Cancer of the colon is a highly treatable and often curable disease when it is localized to the bowel. It is the second most frequently diagnosed malignancy and the third most common cause of cancer death in both men and women in the United States. Most colorectal cancers develop from adenomatous polyps. Surgery is the primary treatment and results in a cure in approximately 50% of patients. The location and amount of resection depends on the site of the cancer. If the rectum is involved, a permanent colostomy will be created. Recurrence after surgery is a major problem and is often the ultimate cause of death. The prognosis of patients with colon cancer is clearly related to the degree of penetration of the tumor through the bowel wall and the presence or absence of nodal involvement. Carcinoma of the colon accounts for approximately 50,000 deaths annually, and more than 145,000 new cases are diagnosed in the United States each years.[101] The etiology is multifactorial and includes a strong environmental correlation with diet (high red meat intake, low dietary fiber intake) and genetic predisposition. Inflammatory bowel disease is usually associated with a greater predisposition to colonic carcinoma. Stool testing for occult blood is a standard screening method. Rectal examination and colonoscopic examination with biopsy are important diagnostic modalities. Tests designed to detect genetic markers for colon cancer in stool and blood are being developed.

Right-sided colonic lesions grow along one wall of the cecum and ascending colon; they often cause symptoms, including pain, a palpable mass in the lower right quadrant, anemia, and dark-colored blood mixed with the stool. Persistent blood loss and anemia with fatigue are common, and obstruction is unlikely because the feces are more liquid. Bleeding is usually less profuse than in patients with diverticular disease. Left-sided colonic lesions grow circumferentially, and symptoms include progressive abdominal distention, pain, vomiting, constipation, cramps, and bright red blood in the stool. Obstruction is common but develops slowly.[83]

Volvulus of the Colon

Volvulus is a twisting of the bowel on its mesenteric pedicle, resulting in an occlusion of the blood supply. This condition usually affects a freely mobile colonic segment and a fixed point or set of points about which the colon twists. Approximately 75% of cases of colonic volvulus affect the sigmoid colon. Colonic volvulus is often associated with fibrous adhesions in the small intestines.[83]

Although colonic volvulus is relatively rare in the United States, it is responsible for 5% of large bowel obstruction cases. Symptoms usually

suggest the presence of acute or subacute bowel obstruction (e.g., sudden onset of acute, severe, colicky abdominal pain, vomiting, and distention). Acute strangulation of the bowel is suggested by generalized severe abdominal pain, hypovolemia, and fever. Initial therapy starts with appropriate resuscitation followed by decompression through the placement of a rectal tube through a proctoscope or the use of a colonoscope. This treatment has a high success rate (70%–80%) and allows resection as an elective procedure, which can be accomplished with reduced morbidity and mortality. If detorsion of the volvulus cannot be accomplished with either a rectal tube or a colonoscope, laparotomy with resection of the sigmoid colon and the formation of an end colostomy and mucous fistula (Hartmann operation) is required.[83]

Many patients with this condition are elderly (in their seventh to eighth decade) or debilitated and are referred from long-term care facilities. Associated disease processes include Alzheimer disease, Parkinson disease, multiple sclerosis, paralysis, pseudobulbar palsy, chronic schizophrenia, and dementia. Medications taken on a long-term basis by these institutionalized patients may include psychotropic drugs, which are known to affect intestinal motility.

Ischemic Bowel Disease

Ischemic injury to the GI tract occurs whenever the oxygen or vascular supply cannot meet the metabolic demands of the tissue. GI ischemia has many causes, including inadequate perfusion, narrowing of blood vessels from any cause, bowel obstruction and distention, drug effects, and infections that can mimic ischemic damage. Most ischemic episodes result from nonocclusive ischemic bowel disease (low-flow states), and in these cases, no vascular lesion or specific cause for ischemia can be demonstrated on pathologic examination.[109] Surgical iatrogenic causes, such as interruption of the inferior mesenteric artery as a result of aortic cross-clamping during abdominal aortic surgery, are also responsible. Prolonged hemodynamic lability in patients with significant comorbidities such as advanced age, chronic diabetes, hypertension, and atherosclerotic disease places them at even greater risk for the consequences of ischemic bowel disease. Any part or length of bowel can be affected, depending on the cause and duration of hypoxia and the state of the collateral circulation. The extent, severity, and prognosis of the syndrome of ischemic bowel disease are variable. Localized or segmental ischemia is often present. Differentiation of ischemic colitis from infectious processes, diverticulitis, or inflammatory bowel disease may be difficult. Definitive diagnosis depends on endoscopic examination with biopsy. Bowel perforation can be excluded in the differential diagnosis through radiographic or ultrasonographic examination of the abdomen for the presence of free air.

Patients with ischemic bowel disease are usually elderly. Symptoms of ischemic bowel disease typically include fever, vomiting, rectal bleeding, and abdominal cramping pain, and may be present for weeks or months. The development of sudden rectal bleeding associated with left-sided abdominal pain and peritoneal signs strongly suggests the presence of this disease process. Concomitant ischemic heart disease and peripheral vascular disease are often present in these patients.[110] Supportive measures are initially undertaken if bowel necrosis is not suspected. This includes antibiotic therapy and fluid resuscitation. In patients in whom perforation or necrosis is suspected, emergency laparotomy is indicated, with possible bowel resection and temporary or permanent colostomy. Stable patients may be candidates for vascular reconstructive procedures.[73]

Diseases of the Rectum and Anus

Diseases of the anorectal region may include neoplastic lesions. Rectal carcinomas are defined as tumors occurring up to 15 cm from the anal opening. If biopsy findings are consistent with localized adenocarcinoma, abdominal-perineal resection of the rectum and sigmoid colon with permanent colostomy may be curative. Squamous cell carcinomas of the rectum are effectively treated with chemotherapy and radiation, as well as local excision. Rectal carcinoma can spread through the rectal wall to nearby structures (the prostate and vagina), especially in the lower third of the rectum. Surgical proctectomy is another treatment option.

Other rectal diseases include rectal prolapse, which is characterized by full-thickness eversion of the rectal wall through the anus and is repaired with rectosigmoidectomy or proctopexy. Rectal prolapse is seen most often in the elderly and in females. Another rectal disease is perirectal abscess, which requires drainage; this may be performed on either an inpatient or an outpatient basis.

Perirectal fistulas typically develop secondary to infectious disease processes that cause abscess formation. Four types are generally recognized: extrasphincteric, suprasphincteric, transsphincteric, and intersphincteric. Initial therapy is incision and drainage with delayed fistulectomy to facilitate healing of the abscess.[40]

Hemorrhoids are a common affliction and have been described and treated for more than 4000 years. The refined, low-fiber diet of Western nations makes hemorrhoids extremely common in the United States, where 1 in 25 to 30 individuals is afflicted. Hemorrhoids are composed of vascular, mucosal, and muscular tissue. Although frequently attributed to varicosities, all three elements compose the hemorrhoid. There are two types of hemorrhoids: internal and external. Internal hemorrhoids originate above the dentate line, are covered with mucosa, and lack sensory innervation. Internal hemorrhoidal prolapse may be painless. Gangrenous, strangulated, extruded, or thrombosed internal hemorrhoids, however, may be extremely painful. Treatment is usually by rubber band ligation or surgical excision. External hemorrhoids originate below the dentate line and are covered with squamous epithelium that makes them easily recognizable because their covering matches the surrounding skin. The inferior rectal nerve innervates external hemorrhoids. A thrombosed external hemorrhoid appears as a bluish mass covered by epidermis. Acute thrombosis occurs suddenly and is usually very painful. Significant bleeding is uncommon but may occur in the case of spontaneous rupture. Increased pressures from straining or trauma from constipation or diarrhea may exacerbate external hemorrhoids. Distention and trauma predispose the hemorrhoidal venous plexus to stasis, with ensuing clot formation and edema.[111] Surgical excision is the treatment of choice.

Anesthesia for most perirectal and perianal procedures may be effectively provided by regional techniques such as spinal subarachnoid block or epidural blockade, as well as by local anesthesia infiltration with sedation. A particularly useful technique is a saddle block with hypobaric bupivacaine. In some cases, general endotracheal anesthesia may be necessary. Anesthetic considerations must include the effect of the patient's position (e.g., prone, jackknife, or lithotomy position) on intraoperative cardiovascular and respiratory dynamics.

Radiation Enteritis

Radiation therapy is commonly used as adjuvant therapy for various abdominal and pelvic cancers. In addition to tumor cells, however, other rapidly dividing cells in the intestinal epithelial lining may be affected by radiation. Surrounding normal tissue such as the small intestinal epithelium may sustain severe, acute, and chronic deleterious effects. The amount of radiation used appears to correlate with the probability of developing radiation enteritis. Other factors that contribute to the development of radiation enteritis are the amount of small bowel in the radiation field, previous intestinal surgery, and concurrent chemotherapy. Radiation damage tends to be acute and self-limiting, but symptoms can occur up to 25 years postradiation therapy. The most common symptoms are diarrhea, abdominal pain, and malabsorption.

The late effects of radiation injury are the result of damage to the small submucosal blood vessels and include progressive obliterative arteritis and submucosal fibrosis, eventually resulting in thrombosis and vascular insufficiency.

Operative intervention may be required in a subgroup of patients who experience chronic effects of radiation enteritis. Indications for surgical intervention include obstruction, fistula formation, perforation, and bleeding, with obstruction being the most common presentation. Operative procedures include bypass or resection with reanastomosis, sometimes under emergent conditions. The presence of adhesions and the induced increased friability of the intestinal tissues predispose affected patients to increased intraoperative bleeding and tissue third spacing. Radiation enteritis can be a relentless disease process. Almost half of patients who survive their first laparotomy for radiation-induced bowel injury require further surgery for ongoing bowel damage. Up to 25% of these patients die of radiation enteritis and complications from its management.[84,112]

Appendicitis

The appendix arises from the apex of the cecum. The length of the appendix varies from 2 to 20 cm, and the average length is 9 cm in adults. The appendiceal artery, a branch of the ileocolic artery, supplies blood to the appendix.[113] The appendix may assume any of a number of positions that influence the quality of symptoms and the site of pain when inflammation occurs.

Appendicitis occurs most often in individuals between 10 and 30 years of age and is the most common general surgical emergency. A slight prevalence for male patients over female patients exists. Obstruction of the appendiceal lumen is believed to be the major cause of appendicitis.

In the classic presentation of appendicitis, patients first note vague, poorly localized epigastric or periumbilical discomfort, which progresses to localized right lower quadrant tenderness in 80% of patients. Within 4 to 12 hours of the onset of pain, most patients also note nausea, vomiting, anorexia, or some combination of these three symptoms. If vomiting is the main symptom, the diagnosis should be questioned.[114] Patients point to localized pain at McBurney point, which is midway between the iliac crest and umbilicus; rebound tenderness, muscle rigidity, and abdominal guarding are noted. In the pregnant patient, Alder sign is used to differentiate between uterine and appendiceal pain: The pain is localized with the patient supine, and the patient then lies on her left side. If the area of pain shifts to the left, it is presumed to be uterine.

The major complication of untreated appendicitis is perforation, with resultant peritonitis, abscess, and portal pylephlebitis. The risk of perforation increases as the duration of the illness progresses, especially beyond 24 hours. Patients with perforation are more likely to have a higher fever, leukocytosis, and physical findings of peritonitis. The most severe complication of appendiceal perforation is septic thrombophlebitis of the portal vein, or portal pylephlebitis.

If the appendix perforates, abdominal pain becomes intense and more diffuse, and abdominal muscular spasm increases, producing rigidity. The heart rate rises, with an elevation of temperature above 39°C. Occasionally, pain may improve somewhat after rupture of the appendix, although a true pain-free interval is uncommon.[113]

The definitive treatment for appendicitis is appendectomy, which may be performed with general or regional anesthesia. The patient is frequently dehydrated and may require a brief period of fluid resuscitation and antibiotics for enteric anaerobic Gram-negative bacilli before the induction of anesthesia. Laparoscopic procedures are the most common techniques used for simple presentations. If an open appendectomy is performed and regional anesthesia is chosen, the analgesia level should be maintained at the T6-T8 level. If general anesthesia is selected, muscle relaxation is necessary, and aspiration precautions that include a rapid sequence induction should be considered. Local anesthesia with IV sedation may also be a useful technique.

SPLENIC DISEASE

Anatomic and Physiologic Overview

The spleen is located in the posterior left upper quadrant of the abdomen and is surrounded by the fundus of the stomach (medially), the splenic flexure of the colon (inferiorly), the left kidney and adrenal gland (posteriorly), and the diaphragm (superiorly). Attachment to these organs via suspensory ligaments, which are vascular except for the gastrosplenic ligament, protects and supports this organ.[40]

The normal spleen weighs less than 250 g, decreases in size with age, normally lies entirely within the rib cage, has a maximum cephalocaudal diameter of 13 cm by ultrasonography or maximum length of 12 cm and/or width of 7 cm by radionuclide scan, and is usually not palpable. In fact, palpability is the major physical sign of diseases affecting the spleen and suggests enlargement of the organ.

The encapsulated spleen is divided into three zones by strands of connective tissue (trabeculae) that originate from the capsule. Each compartment contains masses of lymphoid tissue called splenic pulp. Each of the three splenic compartments is surrounded by a 1- to 2-mm capsule. These compartments are (1) the white pulp, which consists of lymphatic sheaths and contains lymphocytes, plasma cells, and macrophages; (2) the red pulp, which consists of splenic cords and capillaries, and large, thin-walled, highly distensible venous sinuses, also known as the splenic sinusoids, which ultimately form the splenic vein; and (3) the marginal zone, an ill-defined vascular space that interfaces between the white pulp and the red pulp.[40,115]

Total splenic blood flow is approximately 300 mL/min and comes from the splenic artery. The splenic artery is a tortuous vessel that arises from the descending aorta. The splenic artery lies behind the posterior body of the pancreas and divides into several branches within the splenorenal ligament before entering the splenic hilum, where they branch again into the trabeculae as they enter the splenic pulp. Splenic arterial blood flow drains into the splenic vein and then contributes to portal venous blood flow.

The spleen functions in several physiologic capacities to include filtration of blood in the marginal zone, maintenance of normal erythrocyte morphology, and immune processing of blood-borne foreign antigens. The spleen is also involved in hematopoiesis in the fetus until the fifth month of gestation. Blood is filtered in the splenic sinusoids and removes nuclear remnants and excess cell membrane found in immature erythrocytes. An example of the filtration process occurs in patients with sickle cell disease, thalassemia, and spherocytosis, in which the abnormal blood cells are filtered and removed by macrophages and other cells of the reticuloendothelial system. This process can occasionally lead to worsening anemia, symptomatic splenomegaly, and, occasionally, splenic infarction. Aged red blood cells (>120 days) that have lost enzymatic activity and membrane elasticity are removed by the same processes.[40]

The spleen plays an important role in specific and nonspecific immune responses. Macrophages and specialized histiocytes engulf and remove foreign cells, particularly those that have been bound by antibodies. The production of specific antibodies (IgM) is facilitated in the white pulp through the processing of foreign antigens.[39,116] It is well established that people lacking a spleen are at a significantly higher risk for overwhelming postsplenectomy infection with fulminant bacteremia, pneumonia, or meningitis, as compared with those with normal splenic function. Asplenic subjects have defective activation

of complement by the alternative pathway, leaving them more susceptible to infection.[117] Kristinsson et al.[118] reviewed 8149 cancer-free splenectomized patients over 27 years and found these patients had a significantly increased risk of pneumococcal pneumonia, pneumonia not otherwise specified, meningitis, and septicemia. Splenectomized patients had a 1.58-fold and 3.02-fold increased risk of death from pneumonia and septicemia, respectively.

The spleen has a minor role as a reservoir of platelets. This function, however, is important in only a few pathologic conditions. The spleen is not a significant reservoir for red blood cells, but if there is a sudden decrease in blood pressure, sympathetic nervous system activation can constrict the red pulp sinuses, contributing as much as 200 mL of blood to the venous circulation and increasing the hematocrit by as much as 4%.[119]

Despite its important and myriad functions, the spleen is not essential for life. Splenectomy may be performed for benign hematologic conditions, including idiopathic thrombocytopenic purpura (ITP), thrombotic thrombocytic purpura, hereditary spherocytosis, hereditary hemolytic anemia, and hemoglobinopathies (e.g., thalassemia, sickle cell disease). Splenectomy also may be performed for malignancies such as Hodgkin or non-Hodgkin disease, lymphoma, certain leukemias, or for benign conditions such as splenic abscess, splenic cysts, the presence of an accessory spleen, wandering spleen, and splenomegaly (spleen >20 cm longitudinally). The development of primary (having no identifiable underlying cause) or secondary (having a known cause) hypersplenism may warrant splenectomy. Hypersplenism and acute splenic sequestration are life-threatening disorders in children with sickle cell anemia and thalassemia. Symptoms of hypersplenism include fatigue, malaise, recurrent infection, and easy or prolonged bleeding. These symptoms occur from a hyperfunctional spleen that removes and destroys normal blood cells.[120]

In portal hypertension, transmitted backpressure results in hypersplenism, which leads to congestive failure of splenic function. Treatment of the primary disease process usually relieves symptoms. Splenectomy, however, is often a necessary part of therapy, particularly with long-standing disorders. Splenectomy also offers a curative solution for patients with isolated splenic vein thrombosis and bleeding gastric varices.[121]

Splenic Trauma

Angiographic embolization of hemorrhaging vessels in the spleen has reduced the need for open procedures. However, the spleen is the most frequently injured abdominal organ, being involved in 25% to 60% of adults with intraabdominal trauma. Damage to the spleen is important because it is the most vascular body organ, receiving 5% of the cardiac output. Because blood loss from the spleen is mostly arterial, splenic injury can produce a lethal hemoperitoneum. Unlike the liver, hemorrhage from splenic trauma is always within the peritoneal cavity.[122] Rapid deceleration or puncture from an adjacent broken rib are common causes of spleen injuries. Any patient who has sustained blunt abdominal trauma and who has left upper quadrant pain should be suspected of having sustained splenic injury. Conservative, nonoperative treatment (with avoidance of splenectomy) may be elected for minor splenic injury. The clearest indication for urgent operation is hemodynamic instability. Because there can be no standard criteria for hemodynamic instability, a general guideline is to operate for a systolic blood pressure below 90 mm Hg or a pulse of more than 120 beats/minute if there is no immediate response to 1 to 2 L of crystalloid resuscitation and when physical examination, ultrasound, or diagnostic peritoneal lavage indicates intraabdominal blood loss.[120] Splenectomy is generally avoided in children because of the importance of splenic function (i.e., immunologic function) in growth and development.[123,124]

In hemodynamically stable patients with severe splenic damage and hemoperitoneum, the surgery can be performed laparoscopically with no related morbidity or mortality. Anesthesia concerns regarding the laparoscopic approach are related to respiratory distress, which can be exacerbated by the lateral decubitus position and by pneumoperitoneum, usually associated with multiple trauma and rib fractures. At least one study showed no negative outcomes for a laparoscopic approach, and in fact found that these patients exhibited improved postoperative respiratory compliance.[125]

In the presence of impending shock, emergency exploratory laparotomy is carried out to diagnose and treat all injuries to the abdominal viscera, including the spleen. Anesthetic management in these cases is directed by considerations for all unstable patients undergoing emergency laparotomy, particularly hemodynamic stability and renal function. A paramount consideration is maintaining physiologic hemoglobin and hematocrit levels and arterial blood pressure. Hemoglobin and hematocrit are decreased in the emergent setting not only by hemorrhagic diathesis but also from dilution secondary to aggressive volume resuscitation with crystalloid solutions. These considerations assume an integral part in the decision to implement perioperative blood product transfusion.

Anesthetic Considerations in Elective Splenectomy

Anesthetic management for splenectomy is individualized based on the patient's medical condition. Patients who have received chemotherapy must be assessed for potential organ system complications.

Minimally invasive procedures have become standard for most splenectomies, and laparoscopy is now the procedure of choice. The spleen may be removed laparoscopically if it is normal or close to normal in size. Although the operative time is significantly greater than for laparotomy, the postoperative recovery time, the risk of damage to the pancreas, the likelihood of developing subphrenic abscess and peritoneal adhesions postoperatively, and the nutritional and metabolic challenges to the patient are considerably reduced.[126]

Patients with systemic disease may be chronically ill and have decreased cardiovascular reserve. Patients who have received doxorubicin (Adriamycin) may have a dose-dependent cardiotoxicity that can be worsened by radiation therapy. Manifestations include decreased QRS amplitude, congestive heart failure, pleural effusions, and dysrhythmia. Patients may have a degree of left lower lobe atelectasis and altered ventilation. In patients treated with bleomycin, pulmonary fibrosis may occur. Methotrexate, busulfan, mitomycin, cytarabine, and other chemotherapeutic agents may cause pulmonary toxicity. Neurologically, patients may exhibit deficits after the administration of chemotherapeutic agents. Vinblastine and cisplatin can cause peripheral neuropathies. Any evidence of neurologic dysfunction should be documented. Hematologically, patients are likely to have splenomegaly secondary to hematologic disease (e.g., Hodgkin disease, leukemia). Cytopenias are common. Some chemotherapeutic agents (e.g., methotrexate, 6-mercaptopurine) may be hepatotoxic. Evaluation of liver function tests should be considered in patients considered to be at risk. Renally, some chemotherapeutic drugs (e.g., methotrexate, cisplatin) are nephrotoxic. Patients exposed to such agents may have renal insufficiency.

Laboratory tests that should be performed as indicated by the patient history and physical examination include a complete blood count, PT, PTT, bleeding time, platelet count, electrolytes, blood urea nitrogen, creatinine, and urinalysis. Consider aspiration prophylaxis and administer steroids (25–100 mg hydrocortisone) if the patient has received them as part of a chemotherapeutic or medical treatment.

Because of the potential for large blood loss, the patient should be typed and crossmatched, and the use of cell-saver recovery system is appropriate. The ability to transfuse blood products when indicated should be accommodated with the insertion of at least two large-bore IV lines if a central line is not placed. The extent of monitoring modalities is dictated by the patient's preexisting condition and anticipated perioperative course.

General endotracheal anesthesia (GETA) with or without an epidural for postoperative analgesia is used. GETA induction should include consideration of rapid sequence intubation as indicated. Intravascular volume should be restored before anesthetic induction. If the patient is hemodynamically unstable, etomidate or ketamine should be considered. Nitrous oxide should be avoided to prevent bowel distention. Appropriate measures must also be implemented intraoperatively to prevent any further deterioration in preexisting function. These measures include positioning the patient carefully, administering appropriate IV fluids, maintaining adequate urine output, monitoring hemoglobin and hematocrit levels, and avoiding anesthetics and adjuvants that place an extra metabolic burden on the renal or hepatic system. An epidural catheter may be beneficial in postoperative pain control in the absence of ITP.

CARCINOID TUMORS AND CARCINOID SYNDROME

Carcinoid tumors are slow-growing malignancies composed of enterochromaffin cells (Kulchitsky cells) and are most commonly found in the GI tract. They also may occur in the lung, pancreas, thymus, and liver.

Approximately two-thirds of carcinoids occur in the GI tract. Within the GI tract, most tumors occur in the appendix (45%), jejunoileum (28%), rectum (16%), and duodenum (4%). Carcinoid tumors are capable of metastasis and are composed of multipotent cells with the ability to secrete numerous bioactive humoral agents, the most important of which are serotonin, histamine, and kallikrein. In addition to these substances, carcinoid tumors have been found to secrete corticotropin, histamine, dopamine, neurotensin, prostaglandins, substance P, gastrin, somatostatin, pancreatic polypeptide, calcitonin, and neuron-specific enolase (Table 33.12).[113]

TABLE 33.12 Secretory Products of Carcinoid Tumors

Amines	Tachykinins	Peptides	Other
Serotonin	Kallikrein	Pancreatic polypeptide (40%)	Prostaglandins
5-HIAA (88%)	Substance P (32%)	Chromogranins (100%)	
5-HTP	Neuropeptide K (67%)	Neurotensin (19%)	
Histamine		hCGα (28%)	
Dopamine		hCGβ	
		Motilin (14%)	

hCGα, Human chorionic gonadotropin alpha subunit; *hCGβ*, human chorionic gonadotropin beta subunit; *5-HIAA*, 5-hydroxyindoleacetic acid; *5-HTP*, 5-hydroxy-L-tryptophan.
From McKenzie S, Evers BM. Small intestine. In: Townsend CM, et al., eds. *Sabiston Textbook of Surgery: The Biological Basis of Modern Surgical Practice.* 19th ed. Philadelphia: Elsevier; 2012:1259.

Adrenergic stimulation causes the release of serotonin into the circulation. Serotonin is metabolized by aldehyde dehydrogenase and monoamine oxidase to 5-hydroxyindoleacetic acid (5-HIAA), which is excreted in the urine. Elevated levels of 5-HIAA in the urine are a marker of excess serotonin production and, therefore, the presence of a carcinoid tumor. Serotonin may cause vasoconstriction or vasodilation, thus both hypertension and hypotension are possible. At normal concentrations, serotonin does not affect cardiac function; however, the elevated levels seen in carcinoid syndrome may cause both inotropic and chronotropic responses. This action is due in part to an indirect effect from the release of norepinephrine. Elevated serotonin levels also result in increased gut motility and the secretion of water, sodium, chloride, and potassium by the small intestine. Other effects attributed to elevated levels of serotonin are vomiting, bronchospasm, hyperglycemia, and prolonged drowsiness after emergence from anesthesia.[127]

Histamine release is seen predominantly in patients with gastric or foregut carcinoids and may be due to the presence of histidine decarboxylase in normal gastric mucosa. Histamine is probably responsible for the bronchospasm seen in some carcinoid patients, and it also may be the source of flushing.[127,128]

Other substances thought to be released by carcinoid tumors are the kinins, especially bradykinin. Kinins are produced by the action of proteolytic enzymes, called kallikreins, on the inactive kinin precursors.[127] Lysosomal kallikrein release is triggered mainly by sympathetic stimulation. When this occurs, the newly produced bradykinin is usually rapidly broken down and removed from the circulation by plasma aminopeptidases and kinases. When abnormally high amounts of bradykinin are released, the pathways become saturated, causing an exaggerated and prolonged effect from bradykinin. The bradykinins produce profound vasomotor relaxation, causing severe hypotension and flushing, probably via increased nitric oxide synthesis.[129,130] Bradykinin also causes bronchospasm, especially in asthmatics and frequently in patients with cardiac disease.[130]

Normally, the release of vasoactive substances causes few if any symptoms because the liver is able to rapidly inactivate these substances. If these substances reach the systemic circulation without first being metabolized by the liver, they are capable of producing carcinoid syndrome (Box 33.10).

Carcinoid syndrome may produce life-threatening perioperative hemodynamic instability. This syndrome most often occurs with primary tumors that do not drain into the portal system or with hepatic metastases (the most common site of metastasis). Although 25% of tumors actively secrete substances capable of causing symptoms, less than 10% of people with a carcinoid tumor develop the classic carcinoid syndrome.[130] Symptoms related to carcinoid syndrome include episodic cutaneous flushing (kinins, histamine), diarrhea (serotonin, prostaglandins E and F), heart disease, tricuspid regurgitation, pulmonic stenosis, supraventricular tachydysrhythmias (serotonin), bronchoconstriction (serotonin, bradykinin, substance P), hypotension (kinins, histamine), hypertension (serotonin), abdominal pain (small bowel obstruction), hepatomegaly (metastases), hyperglycemia, and hypoalbuminemia (pellagra-like skin lesions resulting from niacin deficiency).

Since the introduction of octreotide as a therapeutic option, the prognosis for patients with carcinoids has significantly improved. Nevertheless, carcinoid tumors may prove fatal for some patients. Death in these patients often results from pulmonary, cardiovascular, or hepatic involvement and dysfunction, rather than from carcinoid crisis. Overall survival is significantly worse for patients with cardiac involvement.

Carcinoid crisis, a life-threatening form of carcinoid syndrome, may be precipitated by physical manipulation of the tumor (including bedside palpation), chemical stimulation or tumor necrosis resulting from chemotherapy, and hepatic artery ligation or embolization.[131] It may occur spontaneously or during the induction of anesthesia. Clinical manifestations of carcinoid crisis include severe flushing with associated dramatic changes in blood pressure, cardiac arrhythmias, bronchoconstriction, and mental status changes. Complete surgical excision of the tumor, often with partial bowel resection and mesenteric lymphadenectomy, is generally regarded as the most effective treatment for carcinoid tumors.[130] Other procedures associated with carcinoid syndrome include cardiac valve replacement and hepatic resection for metastatic disease.

Anesthetic Management

The primary goal during the perioperative period is to prevent the release of bioactive mediators, thereby avoiding carcinoid crisis. Caution should be exercised in the anesthetic management of patients with carcinoid tumors because anesthesia may precipitate a carcinoid crisis characterized by hypotension, bronchospasm, flushing, and tachycardia predisposing to arrhythmias. Long-acting synthetic analogues of somatostatin (octreotide and lanreotide) are now the drugs of choice for symptom control. Sustained release preparations of both drugs, octreotide LAR and lanreotide autogel, are widely used, as they are effective for 4 to 6 weeks. In patients with carcinoid crises, 150 to 200 mcg of octreotide is administered every 6 to 8 hours for 24 to 48 hours prior to surgery and continued throughout the procedure.[130]

Many anesthetic techniques have been used successfully in the treatment of patients with carcinoid syndrome (Box 33.11). Most patients with carcinoid tumors undergo general anesthesia because of the need to avoid the sympathectomy associated with neuraxial anesthesia; however, both epidural and spinal anesthesia have been used successfully in these patients. Successful spinal anesthesia has been reported with the use of preoperative octreotide, fluids, and low-dose spinal anesthetic supplemented with low-dose intrathecal opioids. Laboratory tests should include the standard chemistry, blood count, liver function panel, blood glucose concentration, and ECG, as well as urinary 5-HIAA measurements.[130] The anesthetist should consider a thorough cardiac workup because the reported incidence of cardiac involvement is as high as 50% to 60%.

BOX 33.10   Signs and Symptoms of Carcinoid Syndrome

- Episodic cutaneous flushing, purple face and neck (kinins, histamine)
- Diarrhea (serotonin, prostaglandins E and F)
- Heart disease
- Tricuspid regurgitation, pulmonic stenosis
- Supraventricular tachydysrhythmias (serotonin)
- Bronchoconstriction (serotonin, bradykinin, substance P)
- Hypotension (kinins, histamine)
- Hypertension (serotonin)
- Abdominal pain (small bowel obstruction)
- Hepatomegaly (metastases)
- Hyperglycemia
- Hypoalbuminemia (pellagra-like skin lesions resulting from niacin deficiency)

Modified from Tantay H, Myslajek T. Diseases of the gastrointestinal system. In: Hines RL, Marschall KE, eds. *Stoelting's Anesthesia and Co-Existing Disease*. 6th ed. Philadelphia: Elsevier; 2012:297.

BOX 33.11 Anesthetic Considerations in Carcinoid Syndrome

- The most common clinical signs are cutaneous flushing of the head, neck, and upper thorax, wheezing, blood pressure and heart rate changes, and diarrhea.
- Preoperative assessment should include complete blood count, measurement of electrolytes, liver function tests, measurement of blood glucose, electrocardiogram, and determination of urine 5-HIAA levels. Echocardiography should be performed to determine the extent of carcinoid heart disease.
- Confirmation: >30 mg of 5-HIAA per 24-hr urine sample (normal = 3–15 mg/24 hr).
- Optimize fluid and electrolyte status and pretreat with octreotide as noted. Continue octreotide throughout the postoperative period. Aprotinin (kallikrein inhibitor) may be used to treat hypotension refractory to octreotide. Interferon-α has shown success in controlling some symptoms.
- Both histamine-1 and histamine-2 receptor blockers must be used to fully counteract histamine effects.
- Perioperative blockade of serotonin receptors.
- Anxiolytics reduce stress-related serotonin release.
- Avoid histamine-releasing agents such as morphine and atracurium. Avoid sympathomimetic agents such as ketamine and ephedrine.
- Treat hypotension with an α-receptor agonist such as phenylephrine.
- General anesthesia is preferred over regional anesthesia. Patients with high serotonin levels may exhibit prolonged recovery; therefore, desflurane and sevoflurane, which have rapid recovery profiles, may be beneficial.
- Aggressively maintain normothermia to avoid catecholamine-induced vasoactive mediator release.
- Monitor intraoperative plasma glucose because these patients are prone to hyperglycemia. Treat with insulin as is customary.
- Pay attention to procedures, treatments, and drugs that may stimulate the release of vasoactive substances from tumor cells. These include tumor-debulking surgery or hepatic artery embolization to reduce tumor size, and biotherapy (interferon for tumor shrinkage) or chemotherapy for systemic spread.
- Postoperatively, patients require careful hemodynamic monitoring. Residual tumor or metastatic disease can cause persistent release of vasoactive neuropeptides in the postoperative period and lead to hemodynamic instability.

5-HIAA, 5-hydroxyindoleacetic acid.
Adapted from Mancuso K, et al. Carcinoid syndrome and perioperative anesthetic considerations. *J Clin Anesth.* 2011;23(4):329–341; Peramunage D, Nikravan S. Anesthesia for endocrine emergencies. *Anesthesiol Clin.* 2020;38(1):149–163.

Rapid changes in blood pressure are often seen in carcinoid patients; therefore, in addition to standard monitoring, invasive monitoring is typically required.[128] Hypotension is commonly associated with induction agents, and may trigger a carcinoid crisis. Thus, the insertion of an arterial catheter is mandatory prior to the induction of anesthesia. Increased bleeding also may be encountered because abdominal carcinoids often have a rich vascular supply, and metastases may involve vessel-rich organs such as the liver. CVP monitoring may be very useful in these patients, especially during abdominal surgery for tumor resection. CVP monitoring may help exclude hypovolemia as a cause of hypotension and allow better attention to and adjustment of fluid balance.

The release of catecholamines should be avoided. Propofol and etomidate have been used to induce anesthesia; however, propofol has a more profound effect in suppressing the sympathetic response to intubation and, as long as hypotension is avoided, may be the best induction agent in patients with carcinoid syndrome. Etomidate may have less effect on heart rate and blood pressure but may not suppress laryngeal reflexes. The use of histamine-releasing agents such as morphine, thiopental, pancuronium, and atracurium should be avoided.

Succinylcholine-induced increases in IAP from fasciculations may trigger mediator release[128]; however, some researchers have not found any adverse effects with its use. Opioids that are associated with histamine release should not be used. Furthermore, only nondepolarizing neuromuscular blocking agents that do not cause histamine release should be used. Because of its cardiovascular stability, vecuronium is a good choice, and rocuronium is an effective alternative.

A balanced technique that incorporates positive pressure ventilation, an inhalation agent, a nondepolarizing neuromuscular blocking agent, and an opioid—most commonly fentanyl—may be the best choice in patients with carcinoid tumors. The use of propofol infusions has also been reported. Inhalation agents with low blood-gas solubility such as desflurane are preferred, although all available inhalation agents have been used. Nitrous oxide is also safe. High-dose opioids may be indicated because volatile anesthetics may cause myocardial depression and hypotension, resulting in the release of tumor peptides. Because these patients often have chronic right ventricular (RV) valvular lesions and heart failure, anesthetic factors that increase RV work and/or may precipitate acute RV failure should be avoided. Factors that increase RV work include hypoxemia, hypercarbia, and a light anesthetic plane.[130] Hypotension should be treated with an α-receptor agonist such as phenylephrine to avoid β-adrenergic activation.

▌ SUMMARY

Managing the anesthetic needs of patients with hepatobiliary and GI disorders requires a thorough understanding of the normal physiologic functions of the organ systems, as well as an appreciation for the systemic implications of the pathophysiologic abnormalities discussed in this chapter. Advances in anesthetic and surgical management of patients are resulting in improved outcomes, but ongoing inquiry by clinicians and researchers is still needed. The discussions in this chapter represent some of the most current evidence available in regard to providing quality anesthesia care for and management of the patient undergoing hepatobiliary and GI procedures.

REFERENCES

For a complete list of references for this chapter, scan this QR code with any smartphone code reader app, or visit the following URL: http://booksite.elsevier.com/9780323711944/.

34

Anesthesia for Laparoscopic Surgery

Nancy A. Moriber

The advent and expansion of laparoscopic surgical techniques over the past 35 years has transformed the way in which practitioners approach the care of patients during the perioperative period. Surgeons in all subspecialties, including gynecology, urology, and general surgery, are using laparoscopy to perform increasingly more complex diagnostic and therapeutic procedures (Box 34.1). In fact, in some cases laparoscopic approaches have almost entirely replaced the traditional open laparotomy. These "minimally invasive" surgical procedures offer many advantages over "open" procedures but have also created unique challenges for the anesthesia community, including those related to positioning and the creation of the pneumoperitoneum.

Although the explosion in laparoscopic surgical procedures is a relatively new phenomenon in health care, the origins of laparoscopic surgery date back over 100 years. In 1901 the first endoscopic examination of the peritoneal cavity, known at the time as celioscopy, was attempted by the German surgeon George Kelling to evaluate the effects of pneumoperitoneum on intraabdominal hemorrhage associated with such conditions as ectopic pregnancy and bleeding ulcers.[1-4] Over the next 70 years, several surgeons used laparoscopic techniques, but because of technologic limitations and a high complication rate from bowel and cautery injuries and vascular perforation, few mainstream surgeons embraced the techniques.[2] With the development of the open entry Hasson trocar in 1971 and videoscopic imagining in the mid-1980s, the safety of laparoscopy improved dramatically. Finally, in 1988 the first videolaparoscopic cholecystectomy was performed by the French surgeon Philip Mouret, and the technique soon spread worldwide as the health care community began to realize the true benefits of laparoscopy—a safer, less painful, minimally invasive alternative to open laparotomy with a faster recovery and return to normal function.[2,5,6]

After the success of laparoscopic cholecystectomy, surgeons began to apply minimally invasive approaches to a vast array of complex intraabdominal procedures, including herniorrhaphy, prostatectomy, hysterectomy, nephrectomy, splenectomy, hiatal hernia repair, among others. These techniques are now employed by many surgical specialties in patients across the life span and with significant coexisting disease. As a result, the challenges associated with laparoscopy, such as pneumoperitoneum and positioning, are coupled with increasingly critical patients, adding unique complexity to the anesthetic management for these procedures. In addition, many laparoscopic procedures are now being combined with robotic techniques, adding to the complexity of patient care (see Chapter 35). Fig. 34.1 depicts a classic approach to a laparoscopic cholecystectomy.

CREATION OF THE PNEUMOPERITONEUM

To perform laparoscopic procedures, it is necessary to create an environment in which the surgeon can clearly view all intraabdominal structures and successfully manipulate the instruments required

for surgical dissection. This is accomplished through the creation of an artificial pneumoperitoneum—the installation of air or gas into the peritoneal cavity under controlled pressure. Although complications associated with laparoscopic surgery are rare, initial entry into the abdominal cavity and establishment of the pneumoperitoneum are responsible for a significant proportion of those that do occur.[7-9] Large multicenter studies have demonstrated the risk of severe vascular injury at the time of abdominal entry, the leading cause of morbidity and mortality during laparoscopic procedures, to be between 0.1 and 6.4 injuries per 1000.[8] Risk of injury to the bowel, the second leading cause of morbidity and mortality, is approximately 0.4 cases per 1000 procedures.[9] Approximately 33% of these injuries occur with use of the Veress needle, 50% with placement of the umbilical trocar, and 17% with placement of additional trocars.[8] In addition to the risks caused by the placement of the surgical trocars, insufflation of gas into the peritoneal cavity produces significant physical stress on multiple organ systems. These physiologic effects are seen intraoperatively and can carry over into the immediate postoperative period, increasing the morbidity and mortality associated with these procedures. These effects are accentuated in the elderly and those with significant comorbidity.[10]

Two entry methods are used most commonly for the establishment of the pneumoperitoneum during laparoscopic surgery—the closed technique or the open (Hasson) procedure.[8] The closed technique may utilize blind entry with the Veress needle, blind entry with the pointed trocar, or placement of the trocar using direct vision.[8] Other techniques are available but are used less often because little evidence exists to support their superiority in respect to preventing the complications associated with needle and trocar placement. These techniques include direct entry without prior establishment of the pneumoperitoneum and the use of optical entry trocars that incorporate direct visualization during placement.[8,11-13] The choice of technique is determined by the surgeon; however, the evidence indicates that patients who are extremely thin, obese, or known to have abdominal adhesions are at increased risk for laparoscopic entry-related injuries at the umbilical entry point, and they may benefit from an alternative entry procedure such as the open (Hasson) or left upper-quadrant (Palmer point) entry technique.[8,14-16] Despite the many techniques available, there is limited evidence to support one technique over another. A Cochrane review of 57 randomized trials with 9865 participants did not demonstrate major differences in vascular or visceral injury between the two techniques. There was some evidence that an open technique did result in a lower incidence of omental perforation.[12,13]

The closed technique involves the use of a spring-loaded Veress needle to pierce the abdominal wall at its thinnest point, either in the infraumbilical or intraumbilical region. Various techniques have been used to test for proper placement of the Veress needle, including attempted saline aspiration and hanging-drop techniques. However, a review of case control and cohort studies of women undergoing

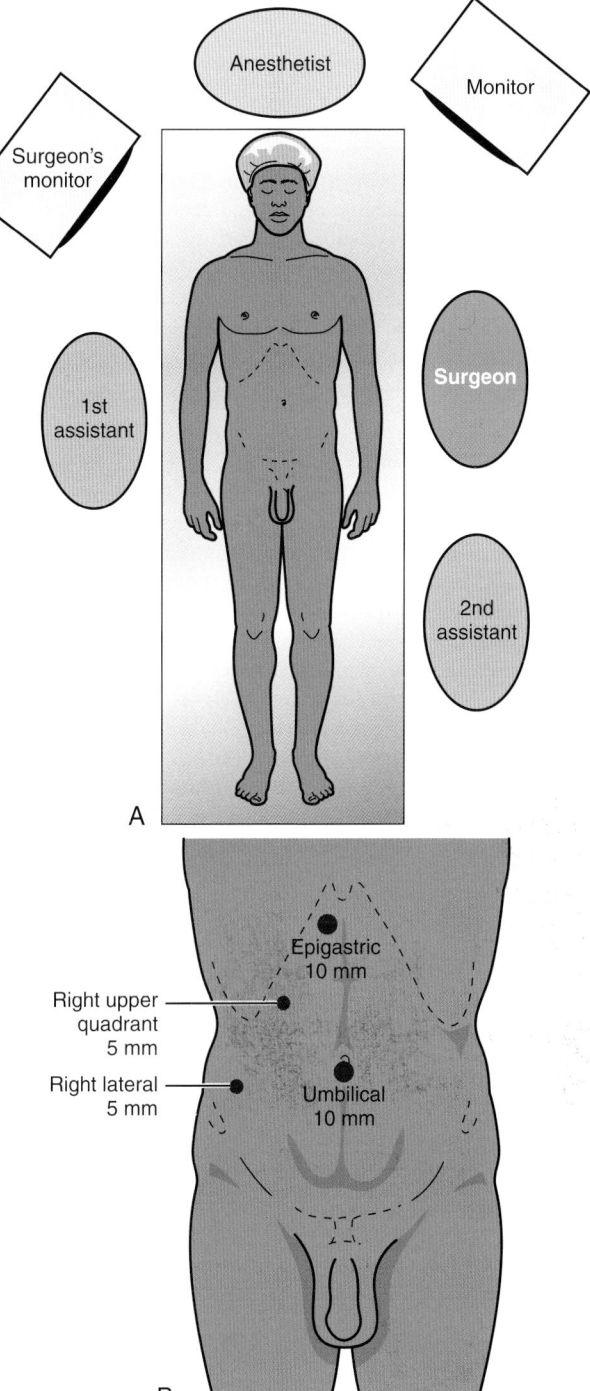

Fig. 34.1 Laparoscopic cholecystectomy. (A) Placement of personnel and monitors for gallbladder removal. (B) Trocar placement for gallbladder removal. (From Phillips N, Hornacky A. *Berry and Kohn's Operating Room Techniques*. 14th ed. St. Louis: Elsevier; 2021.)

laparoscopic procedures has shown that an intraabdominal pressure of 10 mm Hg or less reliably indicates correct placement of an umbilical Veress needle.[17,18] An appropriate nonflammable gas, usually carbon dioxide (CO_2), is then insufflated through the needle to increase the intraabdominal pressure, lift the abdominal wall, and create a space between it and the underlying organs. After insufflation of the abdomen, a trocar is inserted blindly or under direct vision to allow the surgeon to pass instruments into the abdominal cavity.[7,8] It is important to note that the rate of injury to underlying structures increases with each attempt, and an alternative site/technique should be used after two to three failed attempts.[8]

The open technique was developed by Hasson in an attempt to combine the benefits of laparoscopy with the safety of open laparotomy.[19] The technique involves the development of a 1- to 2.5-mm midline vertical incision that begins at the lower border of the umbilicus and extends through the subcutaneous tissue and underlying fascia.[20] The surgeon is then able to directly separate the abdominal wall from the underlying tissues, theoretically minimizing the risk of damage to the bowel and vasculature. Once the surgeon has entered the abdominal cavity, a blunt trocar can be placed under direct vision and sutured in place. Gas can then be insufflated directly through a side port in the Hasson trocar establishing the pneumoperitoneum.

PHYSIOLOGIC EFFECTS OF THE PNEUMOPERITONEUM

As the complexity of laparoscopic surgery and the severity of illnesses in patients undergoing these procedures continue to increase, the need to have a comprehensive understanding of the complex physiologic effects of pneumoperitoneum is essential to ensure proper care of patients. The magnitude of patient response to pneumoperitoneum is multifactorial and includes the degree of intraabdominal pressure generated during creation of the pneumoperitoneum, chemical and biophysiologic properties of the gas utilized, length of surgery, patient position, patient age, perioperative volume status, and presence of preexisting pulmonary and/or cardiovascular disease.[9,10,21,22]

The ideal gas for abdominal insufflation is one that is capable of increasing working and viewing space, while at the same time is

inexpensive, colorless, not flammable, inexplosive, easily removed by the body, and completely nontoxic to patients undergoing laparoscopic procedures. CO_2 has become the gas of choice in most instances because it possesses these properties with minimal risk of air embolization.[22,23] Other gases (including nitrous oxide, helium, argon and room air) have been utilized; however, there is currently no evidence to suggest that these produce better surgical conditions or better patient outcomes. Other studies have suggested that nitrous oxide is associated with less shoulder pain and room air with reduced hospital costs, but further research is indicated.[22,23] Whereas clinical complications have not been demonstrated following transitory elevations in intraabdominal pressure following CO_2 insufflation, prolonged periods of high intraabdominal pressure and tension, such as those required for successful laparoscopy, may be associated with significant physiologic effects.[9,10,24-26] These changes occur as a result of direct mechanical pressure and the stimulation of intrinsic neurocirculatory responses. When combined with patient and surgery-specific conditions, unique patient positioning needs (i.e., steep Trendelenburg), and variations in anesthetic technique, the net effect of increases in intraabdominal pressure on physiologic hemostasis may be unpredictable. Fortunately, long-term clinical complications of the creation of the pneumoperitoneum are rare.

Cardiovascular Effects

Multiple studies demonstrate that the creation of a pneumoperitoneum is associated with significant changes in hemodynamic and other physiologic parameters (Box 34.2). Similar hemodynamic changes have been demonstrated in the morbidly obese despite higher baseline intraabdominal pressures.[27] Consistently, increases in mean arterial pressure (MAP), systemic vascular resistance (SVR), and heart rate that are sustained over the duration of insufflation have been demonstrated.[9,21,28,29] Compression of the intraabdominal vessels and release of neuroendocrine hormones (i.e., vasopressin and renin) are implicated as causative factors in this hemodynamic response. The increases in MAP and SVR are observed regardless of whether the pneumoperitoneum is created under low pressure (12 mm Hg) or high pressure (20 mm Hg).[9,28] In some patients, the peritoneal stretch that coincides with the induction of the pneumoperitoneum may stimulate a vagally mediated bradycardia. This response can be relieved by releasing the pneumoperitoneum and then prevented by ensuring that insufflation pressures remain under 16 mm Hg.[28] If this is insufficient, treatment with anticholinergics such as glycopyrrolate or low-dose atropine may be warranted.

BOX 34.2 Pneumoperitoneum Pressure Effects: 5, 10, 20, and 40 mm Hg

Effects	5 mm Hg	10 mm Hg	20 mm Hg	40 mm Hg
Cardiovascular				
Heart rate	↑	↑	↑/↓	↓
Mean arterial pressure	↑	↑	↑	↑
Systemic vascular resistance	↑	↑	↑	↑
Venous return	→/↓	↓/↑	↓/↑	↓
Cardiac output	→/↓	→/↑	→/↓	↓
Renal				
Glomerular filtration rate	→	↓	↓↓	↓↓
Urine output	→	↓	↓↓	↓↓
Respiratory				
End-tidal CO_2	→	→/↑	→/↑	↑
Pco_2	→	↑	↑	↑
Arterial pH	→	→/↓	↓	↓

↑, increased; ↓, decreased; →, no change.
CO_2, carbon dioxide; Pco_2, partial pressure of carbon dioxide.
From Ordon M, et al. Fundamentals of laparoscopic and robotic urologic surgery. In: Partin AW, et al., eds. *Campbell Walsh Wein Urology.* 12th ed. Philadelphia: Elsevier; 2020:203–234,

Reports on the impact of abdominal insufflation on cardiac filling pressures are mixed. Several studies demonstrate increases in central pressures, whereas others show significant reductions.[21,29-31] Confounding variables, such as the use of vasodilating anesthetics and perioperative fluid restrictions, can significantly alter preload. It is known that insufflation compresses abdominal vasculature, but the extent to which this impacts venous return is not fully understood. Changes in position appear to have a greater effect on central pressures than the pneumoperitoneum itself.[21,28,29] Steep Trendelenburg produces significant increases in central venous pressure (CVP) because it facilitates venous return and increases hydrostatic pressure at the level of the external auditory meatus.[21,28] In contrast, placing the patient in the head-up or reverse Trendelenburg position reduces cardiac preload, which, in turn, will decrease cardiac index.[30]

Uniformly, studies demonstrate that the creation of the pneumoperitoneum produces significant decreases in stroke volume.[29-31] These changes appear to occur primarily as a result in decreases in venous return and not a result of changes in myocardial function. There is some evidence that compression of the aorta, production of neurohormonal factors, and activation of the renin-angiotensin-aldosterone system may not only raise SVR but have a depressant effect on myocardial function.[28]

Although it is clear that stroke volume decreases as a result of abdominal insufflation, the impact of pneumoperitoneum on cardiac output (CO) and cardiac index (CI) is variable because these parameters are influenced by a multitude of factors, including volume status, the use of positive pressure ventilation, and insufflation pressures. In several studies, CO was maintained because reductions in stroke volume were offset by increases in heart rate and increases in venous return when patients were placed in the Trendelenburg position.[28,31] Other researchers have observed significant reductions in CI after operative insufflation pressures are achieved.[32] Healthy patients undergoing laparoscopic cholecystectomy have demonstrated 30% to 40% reductions in CO using a thermodilution technique. In addition, significant reductions in left ventricular end-diastolic pressures have been demonstrated, which in turn negatively impact cardiac function if not accompanied by sufficient increases in heart rate.[32] Despite the variability in findings, patients who have been adequately fluid loaded and who have received therapies to augment venous return (e.g., compression stockings) experience significantly smaller reductions in CO as compared with control patients (20% vs 50%).[29,30]

Finally, the pneumoperitoneum appears to have an effect on the cardiac conduction system, even in healthy patients. Studies show that both low-flow and high-flow insufflation pressures significantly prolong QT dispersion (QTd) in patients undergoing laparoscopic cholecystectomy regardless of the anesthetic technique used.[33,34] The QTd reflects ventricular instability, and prolongation of this parameter is associated with an increased risk of arrhythmias and cardiac effects. Although these changes would not be expected to have clinical significance in healthy patients undergoing an elective laparoscopic procedure, they may produce significant hemodynamic effects in elderly patients with significant cardiac disease.

Hemodynamic Changes in the Elderly

Most research on the hemodynamic effects of abdominal insufflation has been conducted in young, healthy patients. Therefore, little is known about the impact of the pneumoperitoneum in the elderly population, who often present with significant comorbidities. When compared with healthy patients, patients with significant comorbidity have been shown to exhibit exaggerated hemodynamic responses to pneumoperitoneum.[10,35,36] The cumulative effects of CO_2 in the pneumoperitoneum and the reverse Trendelenburg position can result in moderate decreases in CO, as well as significant increases in filling pressures and afterload in sick patients. In one study of patients undergoing laparoscopic colorectal surgery, elderly patients exhibited greater increases in CVP and decreases in MAP, as compared with younger, healthier patients. In addition, the magnitude of these changes at different time intervals was also greater in the elderly population. These findings may reflect baseline physiologic differences in organ function and compensatory mechanisms in the elderly population.[36] In those with cardiopulmonary compromise it may be difficult to increase myocardial contractility and may be prone to the development of cardiac failure during the development of pneumoperitoneum.[10]

Respiratory Effects

Although laparoscopic surgery is associated with a significant decrease in postoperative respiratory complications, intraoperative pulmonary function is greatly impacted by both the mechanical effects of the pneumoperitoneum and introduction of CO_2 into the intraperitoneal cavity itself. Increases in intraabdominal pressure shift the end-expiratory position of the diaphragm cephalad decreasing forced vital capacity (FVC), forced expiratory volume in 1 second (FEV_1), and functional residual capacity (FRC), creating areas of atelectasis and making ventilation difficult.[37] In addition, CO_2 insufflation causes acid-base alterations that can have deleterious effects on multiple organ systems.[38]

In the presence of fixed minute ventilation, CO_2 pneumoperitoneum is associated with increases in the partial pressure of arterial CO_2 ($PaCO_2$) and end tidal CO_2 ($ETCO_2$) with or without the development of acidosis.[38] This hypercarbia been shown to induce pulmonary vasoconstriction and cause the development of cardiac dysrhythmias that may be poorly tolerated in patients with underlying pulmonary and cardiovascular disease.[39] The increases in $PaCO_2$ seen with abdominal insufflation are primarily caused by CO_2 absorption through the peritoneal serosa secondary to the increased intraabdominal pressure caused by the pneumoperitoneum. The resultant acidosis is considered to be respiratory rather than metabolic in nature. Therefore, increases in $PaCO_2$ must be offset by increases in minute ventilation, or CO_2 levels will continue to rise. Studies show that during laparoscopy, decreases in arterial pH are accompanied by a rise in partial pressure of carbon dioxide (PcO_2) but not by increases in lactate or decreases in the apparent strong ion difference.[38] These parameters return to baseline after discontinuation of CO_2 insufflation. Maximum absorption of CO_2 is noted with an intraabdominal pressure of 10 torr (mm Hg pressure). $PaCO_2$ levels are noted to reach a plateau approximately 40 minutes after the induction of the peritoneum.[38,40,41]

A major concern during the creation of the pneumoperitoneum involves the risk of subcutaneous tracking of CO_2 through misplaced trocars or rents in the peritoneum that develop during trocar placement. Compared with intraperitoneal insufflation of CO_2, extraperitoneal insufflation (subcutaneous absorption) has been associated with an unusually rapid increase in $PaCO_2$ and exceptionally high, sustained levels of CO_2.[42-44] Cases of pneumopericardium and severe emphysema of the orbit have been documented after subcutaneous absorption of CO_2.[42,43] The incidence of subcutaneous emphysema has been reported to range between 0.43% and 2.34%.[44,45] The main risk factors include an $ETCO_2$ above 50 mm Hg, operative time greater than 200 minutes, the use of six or more surgical ports, high insufflation pressures, and extraperitoneal dissections.[45] A complete list of factors that increase the incidence and degree of subcutaneous emphysema during laparoscopy are listed in Box 34.3.[42-45] The anesthesia provider should suspect the development of subcutaneous emphysema if physiologic changes such as crepitus, hypercarbia,

BOX 34.3   Factors Leading to Subcutaneous Emphysema

- Insufflator (high gas flow and high gas pressure setting)
- Intraabdominal pressure >15 mm Hg
- Multiple attempts at the abdominal entry
- Veress needle or cannula not placed in the peritoneal cavity
- Skin/fascial fit/seal around the cannulas is not snug
- Use of >5 cannulas
- Laparoscope used as a lever
- Cannula acting as a fulcrum
- Long arm of the laparoscope is a force multiplier
- Tissue integrity compromised by repetitive movements
- Structural weakness caused by repetitive movements
- Improper cannula placement, causing stressed angulation
- Soft tissue dissection and fascial extension
- Gas dissection leading to more dissection
- Procedures lasting >3.5 hr
- Positive end tidal CO_2 >50 mm Hg

From Ott DE. Subcutaneous emphysema—beyond the pneumoperitoneum. *JSLS.* 2014;18(1):1–7.

BOX 34.4   Management of Subcutaneous Emphysema

- Decrease intraabdominal pressure, if possible terminate pneumoperitoneum
- Discontinue nitrous oxide because it can increase subcutaneous emphysema volume
- Place on 100% FiO_2
- Evaluate for a pneumothorax
- Increase minute ventilation to treat hypercarbia
- Evaluate $ETCO_2$ and $PaCO_2$
- Assess chest wall and lung compliance
- Assess airway to rule out compression prior to extubation

$ETCO_2$, End tidal CO_2; FiO_2, fraction of inspired oxygen; $PaCO_2$, partial pressure of arterial CO_2.

elevated $ETCO_2$, decreased lung compliance, cardiac arrhythmias, and hypertension are observed.[44,45] Management of subcutaneous emphysema is outlined in Box 34.4.[44]

The mechanical effects of peritoneal insufflation impair ventilation. Insufflation of the peritoneum put pressure on the diaphragm and displaces it in a cephalad direction, decreasing functional residual capacity and vital capacity, and in turn inducing collapse of the dependent regions of the lungs.[37,46,47] Perfusion of these nonventilated alveoli causes the development of pulmonary shunt with impaired oxygenation and CO_2 elimination and subsequent increases in the arterial to end tidal PcO_2 difference.[37,46,47] Increases in intraabdominal pressure also affect pulmonary compliance; in supine patients, pulmonary compliance has been observed to be reduced by 43%.[21,35]

The impact of atelectasis on gas exchange has been shown to be offset by a redistribution of perfusion away from collapsed lung units when the pneumoperitoneum is established.[47] Although the exact mechanism is not known, it appears to be the result of activation of the hypoxic pulmonary vasoconstriction (HPV) reflex.[39,47] Because many anesthetics attenuate or inhibit the HPV reflex, increases in ventilation/perfusion ($\dot{V}/\dot{Q}$) mismatching and changes in oxygenation during laparoscopic surgery may reflect the physiologic effects of the anesthetics used, rather than the impact of the pneumoperitoneum itself. This

BOX 34.5   Pulmonary Function Changes Associated With Pneumoperitoneum

- Positive inspiratory pressure (PIP) ↑
- Pulmonary compliance dV/dP ↓
- Vital capacity ↓
- Functional residual capacity ↓
- Intrathoracic pressure ↑

↑, Increased; ↓, decreased; *dV/dP*, change in volume/change in pressure.

may have implications for the choice of anesthetics used during these procedures. Physiologic pulmonary changes associated with pneumoperitoneum are listed in Box 34.5.

An additive effect is observed when general anesthesia, which in and of itself reduces FRC and pulmonary compliance, is combined with pneumoperitoneum.[37,47] The surgical position employed to facilitate exposure can either aggravate or attenuate pneumoperitoneum-induced pulmonary changes. The Trendelenburg position has been shown to increase the effects of pneumoperitoneum on pulmonary mechanics. During robotic laparoscopic prostatectomy in the steep Trendelenburg position, pulmonary compliance decreased approximately 50%, and peak plateau pressures increased by 50% and remained stable over the duration of the CO_2 insufflation.[21] In contrast, the reverse Trendelenburg position partially counteracts the effects of pneumoperitoneum on the diaphragm and improves diaphragmatic function.[48]

Another impact of pneumoperitoneum is the potential for the development of endobronchial intubation as a result of a shortening of the distance from the tip of the endotracheal tube to the carina.[49,50] Because the carina is attached to the lungs, cephalad displacement of the diaphragm compresses the lungs and shifts the position of the carina upward effectively moving the endotracheal tube caudad. Studies indicate that displacement of the tube occurs within 10 minutes of creation of the pneumoperitoneum, therefore the authors recommend reconfirmation of tracheal tube position after establishment of the pneumoperitoneum.[49,50]

Controlled mechanical ventilation is necessary to maintain normocarbia in anesthetized patients undergoing laparoscopic surgery with CO_2 pneumoperitoneum. Studies of patients in the Trendelenburg position during pneumoperitoneum reveal that a 20% to 30% increase in minute ventilation is necessary to maintain prepneumoperitoneum levels and prevent respiratory acidosis.[38,51] In these studies, increasing the minute ventilation by preferentially increasing tidal volume rather than increasing respiratory rate was the preferred method. In addition, the use of the pressure control (PC) modes appears to be more effective in maintaining arterial pH when compared with the volume control (VC) modes of ventilation.[52] Patients ventilated using PC were also easier to ventilate, generating significantly lower maximum peak airway pressures and increased mean airway pressures. However, careful attention must be paid to changes in intraabdominal pressure, as significant changes in tidal volume may occur with the release of the pneumoperitoneum.

There has been a push for the use of low tidal volume ventilation strategies in patients undergoing major abdominal surgery by either the laparoscopic or open approach. It is well documented that high tidal volume ventilation is associated with the development of acute lung injury in the critically ill, ventilator-dependent patient as a result of the mechanical stress and strain placed on the lung parenchyma and the subsequent release of proinflammatory factors.[53,54] Lung protection strategies utilizing 6 to 8 mL/kg of predicted body weight, 6 to 8 cm

H_2O, plateau pressures below 16 cm H_2O, the lowest driving pressure possible, moderate positive end-expiratory pressure (PEEP), and intraoperative recruitment maneuvers every 30 minutes were associated with improved clinical outcomes, including decreased postoperative pulmonary complications and the need for postoperative intubation, and decreased length of stay.[54-57]

Patients with marginal cardiopulmonary function undergoing laparoscopic surgical procedures are at increased risk of decompensation when faced with the stress introduced by increases in intraabdominal pressure and CO_2 insufflation. Patients particularly vulnerable to the effects of exposure to prolonged CO_2 insufflation are those with increased metabolic rates (as in sepsis), large ventilatory dead space, and decreased CO.[22] Patients with chronic obstructive pulmonary disease (COPD) are at increased risk of developing postoperative complications after laparoscopic procedures.[39,58] One study demonstrated the odds ratio for postoperative complication to be 1:63 in patients with significant COPD.[58] Studies also indicate that although healthy patients experience minor changes in $PaCO_2$ and $ETCO_2$ during CO_2 insufflation, patients with COPD show significantly higher levels of CO_2 retention and subsequent respiratory acidosis.[39] Although $ETCO_2$ is standard of care for all patients, careful intraoperative monitoring of CO_2 levels during laparoscopic surgery in these patients is essential. Because of the significant arterial to end tidal PCO_2 gradient that develops during sustained pneumoperitoneum, and which is compounded in patients with chronic CO_2 retention, $ETCO_2$ may underestimate arterial CO_2. Therefore, direct measurement of $PaCO_2$ via arterial blood gases or P_TCO_2 (transcutaneous) may be warranted.[37,59] Studies show that P_TCO_2 is an accurate, noninvasive predictor of arterial carbon dioxide levels and can be used as a proxy in patients with significant cardiopulmonary disease.[59]

Mild pulmonary dysfunction after laparoscopic procedures has been shown to persist into the immediate postoperative period in patients recovering from laparoscopic surgery.[57-61] A slight restrictive breathing pattern in the postoperative period has been observed secondary to the residual effects of anesthesia, pain, and diaphragmatic dysfunction induced by stretching or reflex inhibition.[57] In addition, after laparoscopic surgery, patients may still be subjected to an elevated CO_2 load secondary to systemic absorption and subcutaneous tracking of gas during the procedure.[27] Moreover, if surgery is prolonged and exposure to pneumoperitoneum is sustained for the majority of the procedure, CO_2 may be stored in skeletal muscle and bone. It may take hours for this excess CO_2 to be excreted from the patient.[61] Despite the potential immediate negative perioperative pulmonary effects associated with laparoscopy, the procedures are associated with improved clinical outcomes.[39] Studies show that there is a substantial decrease in the incidence of postoperative pneumonia or reintubation.[39] In addition, patients demonstrate improved lung volumes with higher force-vital capacity and FEV_1.[39]

Renal Effects

The effects of pneumoperitoneum on renal physiology primarily manifest as transient increases in creatinine clearance and decreases in renal blood flow and urinary output secondary to increases in intraabdominal pressure. Oliguria has been reported but most commonly occurs only during periods of sustained high intraabdominal pressures.[27,62,63] It is proposed that the high intraabdominal pressures created during the pneumoperitoneum cause transient renal injury by reducing renal blood flow and subsequently causing hypoperfusion of the renal cortex. High intraabdominal pressures (≥15 mm Hg) create renal oxidative stress and the generation of tissue oxidases that promote tubular injury.[63] In addition, the neuroendocrine response to pneumoperitoneum results in the release of antidiuretic hormone (ADH), aldosterone, and renin.[27] Elevated hormonal levels in the presence of a pneumoperitoneum-induced respiratory acidosis induce a sympathetic response and renal vasoconstriction, which further diminishes renal blood flow.[27,62-64]

Hepatic and Splanchnic Effects

There is conflicting evidence regarding the effects of increased intraabdominal pressure on hepatic and splanchnic blood flow. Several animal studies have demonstrated that abdominal insufflation can cause marked decreases in splanchnic and liver perfusion, as well as intestinal ischemia secondary to the production of oxygen free radicals and bacterial translocation.[65,66] More recently, studies evaluating the effect of different intraabdominal pressures on oxidative stress markers in patients undergoing laparoscopic cholecystectomy have demonstrated increases in the production of lipid and protein oxidative substances that negatively impact splanchnic tissues.[67] This evidence is further supported by the fact that approximately 50% of patients undergoing laparoscopic cholecystectomy demonstrate elevated liver enzymes.[68,69] Other studies indicate that low-pressure insufflation of the abdomen either did not disrupt or improved hepatic and splanchnic perfusion, possibly secondary to the local vasodilatory effect of CO_2 on splanchnic vasculature.[70,71]

Immunologic Effects

CO_2 pneumoperitoneum also may have a negative effect on the local immune response by altering the concentrations of certain cytokine levels with the peritoneum. Several studies have demonstrated that CO_2 pneumoperitoneum influences the growth of cultured human cancer cells, and that this effect is pressure dependent.[72,73] In addition, patients receiving low insufflation pressures (6–8 mm Hg) showed statistically significant lower concentrations of C-reactive protein, interleukin-1β (IL-1β), and IL-6 and other proinflammatory factors resulting in a reduction in the postoperative inflammatory response.[74] In contrast, other studies have shown no significant differences in levels of cytokines and other proinflammatory factors between low- and high-pressure insufflation.[75] Proinflammatory cytokines and angiogenic factors have been shown to influence neoangiogenesis, adhesion formation, and normal wound healing processes. Despite the negative immunologic perturbations that follow the creation of the pneumoperitoneum, this response appears to be weaker than that induced following conventional open abdominal procedures.[76]

COMPLICATIONS OF LAPAROSCOPIC SURGERY

Although laparoscopy has revolutionized the way surgery is conducted today, it is not devoid of complications. Even though major complications are rare, when they do occur, they are usually associated with significant morbidity. More than 50% of all complications occur during entry into the abdomen and insertion of trocars. Entry-related complications involve intestinal, urinary tract, and vascular injuries, as well as carbon dioxide gas embolism.[8,77] The reported incidence of these injuries is between 0.3% and 1.0% of all laparoscopic procedures.[77,78] The most common complication, vascular injury, is reported to occur at a rate of between 0.1 and 6.4 injuries per 1000.[8] Risk of injury to the bowel, the second leading cause of morbidity and mortality, is approximately 0.4 cases per 1000 procedures.[9]

Unfortunately, approximately 30% to 50% of these injuries go undiagnosed intraoperatively, resulting in significant surgical mortality (3.5%–5%).[79] Mortality rates as high as 30% have been reported when major bowel and vascular injuries occur.[80] Delayed diagnosis may occur because initial signs and symptoms may be confused with other conditions such as anaphylaxis, gas embolism, or perioperative cardiac

events. Frequently, bleeding may be occult and confined to the retroperitoneal space, which can tamponade significant hemorrhage.

The potential for injury to intraabdominal structures during the creation of the pneumoperitoneum is easily understood when one considers the proximity of anatomic structures to the site of incision and infraumbilical puncture. The major abdominal vessels, including inferior vena cava, aorta, and iliac arteries and veins, as well as the bladder, bowel, and uterus, lie in close proximity to the entry points. Factors that increase risk of injury include body habitus, anatomic anomalies, prior surgery, surgical skill, degree of abdominal elevation during trocar placement, patient position, and the volume of gas insufflation.[8,77,78]

A prompt and coordinated response is required to prevent morbidity associated with vascular injury. Blood on aspiration of the Veress needle, free intraperitoneal blood, or unexplained hypotension and tachycardia should alert the operative team to a potential vascular injury.[77] Retroperitoneal hematomas are often difficult to visualize during laparoscopy and may become apparent only when blood loss is significant. Temporary measures to control bleeding may be possible through the abdominal trocar while resuscitative measures are instituted, but definitive treatment is usually achieved via conversion to an open laparotomy.

Visceral injuries can occur at any time during laparoscopy and are also associated with significant morbidity and mortality. Intestinal injuries occur in 0.3% to 0.5% of operative laparoscopies, and less than 50% of these are recognized at the time of surgery. Diagnosis is difficult because presenting symptoms vary significantly depending on the location of injury and degree of peritoneal contamination. Early recognition and surgical repair are essential to prevent mortality from bowel injuries. Untreated patients may develop peritonitis, sepsis, respiratory distress, and multisystem organ failure.[78] Because of the seriousness of these complications, many practitioners advocate the use of the open (Hasson) entry laparoscopic technique because it is believed to be associated with a lower incidence of unrecognized vascular and visceral injury.[8,9]

Injury to the urinary tract occurs in 0.5% to 8.3% of cases secondary to trauma from instrument manipulation, electrocautery, or laser.[81] These injuries are easily recognized by direct visualization of urine leakage from damaged structures. Therefore, urinary bladder catheterization and instillation of methylene blue dye is often employed during these procedures when significant risk of damage to urinary structures is suspected.[77]

To help decrease the incidence of major vascular and visceral injury during laparoscopic surgery, the Royal College of Obstetricians and Gynaecologists established evidence-based practice guidelines for abdominal entry in 2008.[82] These were validated by a subsequent Cochrane review that evaluated the evidence on the safety and efficacy of various abdominal entry techniques.[83] Quality randomized controlled trials and systematic reviews consistently demonstrate that placement of the primary trocar under high pressure (25 mm Hg) creates the safest distance between the anterior abdominal wall and underlying abdominal contents in order to minimize injury from trocar insertion. In addition, in healthy patients, these transitory, high intraperitoneal pressures appear to be well tolerated without significant adverse clinical effects.[9]

Another potentially life-threatening complication of laparoscopic surgery is gas embolism. Gas embolism is defined as the direct entrainment of air and/or other medical gases, such as carbon dioxide, into the arterial or venous system.[77,81] Significant gas embolism is rare, having a reported incidence of 0.001% to 0.59% and an associated mortality rate of up to 28.5%.[77,84] Massive and/or fatal gas embolisms have been reported during all types of laparoscopic procedures, including laparoscopic cholecystectomy, liver resection, and hysterectomy.[85,86] It can occur any time there are open vessels that have an intravascular pressure that is below intraabdominal pressure or with the erroneous placement of a Veress needle or trocar directly into the lumen of an intraabdominal vessel. However, studies that have evaluated methods of increasing CVP, such as the use of PEEP, to decrease the pressure gradient across vessels have not shown them to be effective in reducing the incidence of gas embolism.[85]

Both animal and human studies using transesophageal echocardiography and monitoring of pulmonary artery pressure have shown that the actual incidence of gas embolism during laparoscopic procedures is between 65% and 100%.[81,87,88] The majority of these embolisms, although minor, were still associated with respiratory and hemodynamic changes that usually resolved spontaneously. These studies raise concerns regarding best practices for appropriate monitoring during the perioperative period in patients undergoing laparoscopic procedures. Intravascular insufflation of large volumes of gas can travel to the right side of the heart where they enter the pulmonary circulation and lodge in the pulmonary outflow tract, causing increased pulmonary artery pressure, right ventricular failure, decreased pulmonary venous return with subsequent decreased left ventricular preload, decreased cardiac output, asystole, and cardiovascular collapse.[77]

Other gases such as helium have been utilized for peritoneal insufflation to avoid the negative side effects of CO_2 insufflation, including CO_2 accumulation, hypercarbia, acidosis, and sympathetic nervous system stimulation, particularly in patients with preexisting impairment in respiratory function (COPD, infancy). Although helium pneumoperitoneum is associated with a greater degree of cardiopulmonary stability, there appears to be a higher incidence of subcutaneous emphysema and life-threatening gas embolism even with entrainment of small volumes.[23,89,90]

Signs and symptoms of a significant gas embolism in the anesthetized patient include an acute decrease or loss of end tidal partial pressure of carbon dioxide (PET_{CO_2}), and an increase in end tidal nitrogen if air is entrained, which is accompanied by hypotension and/or hypoxia that cannot be explained by deep anesthesia or hypovolemia. Dysrhythmias, severe hemodynamic instability, and cardiovascular collapse can occur when large volumes of gas are entrained, especially in patients with impaired cardiovascular function and minimal cardiac reserve.[87] Large gas embolisms result in obstruction of the right ventricle or pulmonary artery resulting in a precipitous drop in cardiac output.[84]

Diagnosis of gas embolism depends on recognition of the physiologic manifestations of gas emboli and/or visual detection of gas emboli in the right side of the heart and pulmonary outflow tract. Transesophageal echocardiography is the most sensitive diagnostic technique for the detection of gas emboli and can identify emboli as small as 0.02 mL/kg.[91] However, this technology is rarely used because these volumes of air are well tolerated and usually not associated with hemodynamic changes. Changes in Doppler sounds and increases in pulmonary artery pressures will occur with volumes of 0.5 mL/kg of gas. Unfortunately, when the "classic mill wheel murmur" is audible, gas volumes of 2 mL/kg or more have been entrained, and significant hemodynamic instability is present manifesting in tachycardia, hypotension, cardiac dysrhythmias, cyanosis, and electrocardiogram (ECG) changes indicative of right-sided heart strain.[92] There have been case reports of abrupt or "seesawing" changing in $ETco_2$ that precede the occurrence of massive gas embolism in patients undergoing laparoscopic procedures.[84] These changes in CO_2 appear to be associated with small tears in vessels that intermittently entrain CO_2 prior to the development of cardiovascular collapse.

Management of gas embolism includes halting the insufflation of gas, eliminating nitrous oxide (N_2O) from the anesthetic gases if it is

---

BOX 34.6   Gas Embolism

Signs and Symptoms
- ↓ PET_{CO_2}, ↑ end tidal nitrogen
- Oxygen saturation ↓
- Chest pain, dyspnea (spinal or epidural anesthesia)
- Increased pulmonary artery pressures
- Hypotension
- Dysrhythmias
- Cyanosis
- Hypoxia
- Pulmonary edema
- Wheezing, rales
- "Mill wheel" murmur
- Detection of air in the heart by transesophageal echocardiography or precordial Doppler ultrasound

Treatment
- Discontinue gas insufflation
- Discontinue nitrous oxide
- Administer 100% oxygen
- Release pneumoperitoneum
- Flood surgical field with normal saline
- Position patient in left lateral decubitus position
- Attempt to aspirate gas via central venous catheter
- Supportive measures to maintain hemodynamics

↑, Increased; ↓, decreased; PET_{CO_2}, end tidal pressure of carbon dioxide.

---

being administered to prevent expansion of the embolism, releasing the pneumoperitoneum, flooding the field with normal saline to halt gas entrainment, placing the patient in left lateral decubitus position (Durant maneuver), aspirating the gas through a central venous catheter if in place, and supporting the hemodynamics with volume and pressors as required.[92] Low CVP increases the risk of venous gas embolism; therefore, adequate hydration should be provided for the patient undergoing laparoscopy.[93] However, the decision to obtain central venous access during laparoscopic procedures is guided by the complexity of the surgical procedure and presenting comorbidities of the patient, rather than as a means of managing perioperative gas embolism. Box 34.6 lists the signs, symptoms, and treatment of venous gas embolism.

Another set of serious but rare complications related to the creation of pneumoperitoneum occurs as a result of migration of gas into adjacent body cavities and includes unilateral or bilateral pneumothorax, pneumomediastinum, and pneumopericardium. Gas may enter the thoracic cavity via congenital defects in the diaphragm, embryonic connections between the thoracic and abdominal cavities that may open under high pressure, or through perforations in the diaphragm or pleura during upper abdominal laparoscopic procedures, most commonly during laparoscopic esophageal surgery.[44,45,94,95] The incidence of significant and grossly detectable subcutaneous emphysema during laparoscopic procedures is reported to be approximately 2.3%, while the incidence of pneumothorax/pneumomediastinum is 1.9%.[44,94-96] Another possible cause of pneumothorax is barotrauma secondary to increased airway pressures and decreased pulmonary compliance as a result of abdominal insufflation.[97] Pneumothorax caused by CO_2 insufflation may rapidly resolve spontaneously without intervention. However, pneumothorax that results from barotrauma, such as a ruptured bleb, requires surgical decompression and chest tube placement.[98] Predictors for the development of subcutaneous emphysema during laparoscopy include maximum $ETco_2$ above 50 mm Hg, operative time greater than 200 minutes, and the use of more than five entry ports.[94,95] Variables predictive of pneumothorax include all of the previously mentioned plus procedures involving laparoscopic mobilization of the esophagus and operator inexperience.[94,95]

Mild to severe localized or generalized subcutaneous emphysema is a frequent manifestation of pneumoperitoneum that occurs as a result of gas entry into the subcutaneous tissues. As previously discussed, it can be the result of trocar or Veress needle misplacement in subcutaneous tissue or the result of high intraabdominal pressure and movement of gas through defects in the peritoneum.[41-43] The incidence of extraperitoneal insufflation appears to be the same regardless of the laparoscopic entry technique utilized.[83] Most cases of subcutaneous emphysema are clinically insignificant; however, it has been associated with the development of severe hypercarbia, decreased chest compliance, and hemodynamic instability.[94] Most cases resolve spontaneously; however, severe subcutaneous emphysema of the head and neck may require that patients be left intubated in the immediate postoperative period as premature extubation prior to reabsorption of the carbon dioxide may result in loss of airway.

The ideal gas for the creation and maintenance of pneumoperitoneum would demonstrate several properties, including colorlessness, lack of flammability in the presence of electrocautery, physiologic inertness, and excretion via a pulmonary route.[89,90] Several gases have been investigated in an attempt to find an alternative to CO_2 that is devoid of hemodynamic and respiratory effects.[89,90] Both N_2O and air support combustion and could not be used in the presence of electrocautery, which is essential for successful laparoscopy.[61] Inert gases such as helium have been evaluated for use in abdominal insufflation, but helium is not highly insoluble and raises issues about safety in the presence of a significant gas embolism.[89,90,99]

Despite efforts to identify other gases suitable for the development of the pneumoperitoneum, CO_2 has proven to be the closest to an "ideal" gas for abdominal insufflation. CO_2 is readily available and inexpensive, does not support combustion, is rapidly absorbed from the vascular space, and is readily excreted by the respiratory system. However, when used in a pneumoperitoneum, prolonged CO_2 absorption can cause hypercarbia and respiratory acidosis.[89,94] It is also a known peritoneal and diaphragmatic irritant, which has been implicated as a causative factor in the development of postoperative shoulder pain.[100]

ANESTHETIC MANAGEMENT

Laparoscopic procedures have been performed using local, regional, and general anesthetic techniques. The choice of anesthetic technique is dependent upon the specifics of the surgical procedure, method of insufflation utilized, patient comorbidities, and provider/patient preference.

Local anesthesia with sedation has been used successfully in the United States for patients undergoing minor gynecologic laparoscopic surgical procedures such as diagnostic laparoscopy or extraperitoneal inguinal hernia repair since 1971.[101,102] Evidence shows there is no difference in patient outcomes when these procedures are performed under local versus general anesthesia.[102] Gasless laparoscopy has been shown to be useful in the emergency department for the diagnosis of acute abdomen and the management of hemodynamically stable patients with penetrating abdominal injury. The use of local anesthesia is facilitated by surgical techniques such as the use of single-port techniques, low-pressure pneumoperitoneum, and port and small-diameter laparoscopes.[103-105] Research indicates that compared with patients who received general anesthetics, patients who received local anesthesia had shorter hospital stays and a reduction in overall

hospital and anesthesia costs.[101,105] In addition, they demonstrated a faster recovery, decreased incidence of postoperative nausea and vomiting, and fewer hemodynamic changes.[101,105,106] However, use of this anesthetic technique requires a cooperative patient and gentle surgical manipulation. When heavy sedation is required, the combination with pneumoperitoneum can result in hypoventilation and arterial oxygen desaturation.

Regional anesthesia techniques, including spinal and epidural anesthesia, have also been used successfully for laparoscopic procedures, including cholecystectomy, without significant ventilatory compromise. Regional techniques are associated with a reduction in the stress response, early ambulation with a lower incidence of deep vein thrombosis, and effective postoperative analgesia.[107] However, significantly high sensory levels are required for these procedures, which may result in significant patient discomfort and hypotension due to sympathetic blockade. There may also be significant impact on ventilation as a result of cephalad pressure on the diaphragm that is compounded by the sensory and motor blockade. In addition, there is a high incidence of shoulder pain reported (27%–47%) secondary to diaphragmatic irritation from insufflated carbon dioxide that is not well managed by means of regional techniques.[108,109]

General anesthesia is the most common anesthetic technique used during diagnostic and surgical laparoscopy. General anesthesia allows for control of ventilation and facilitates management of patient discomfort associated with the creation of the pneumoperitoneum and changes in intraoperative position such as steep Trendelenburg. It also allows for mitigation of the hypercarbia that develops secondary to insufflation of the abdomen with carbon dioxide.

Most often, the airway is secured with a cuffed endotracheal tube to facilitate ventilation and prevent aspiration of gastric contents. Minute ventilation is increased by approximately 15% to 35% to offset CO_2 absorption and maintain $PETco_2$ between 35 and 45 mm Hg. This is most effectively performed using PC versus VC ventilation.[53] Intraoperative recruitment maneuvers, the application of individualized PEEP, and the use of innovative ventilator modes have all been successful in improving lung compliance, oxygenation, and ventilation.[55-57,110-112] PEEP requirements vary significantly among patients when protective lung strategies are employed. Therefore, PEEP settings should be individualized to maximize oxygenation, minimize driving pressures, and prevent intraoperative atelectasis.[112] Studies also show that recruitment maneuvers that use the combination of PEEP 10 cm H_2O and intermittent positive airway pressure (40 cm H_2O) for 40 seconds were most effective in improving end-expiratory lung volumes, lung compliance, and arterial oxygenation in both healthy weight and obese patients than either intervention alone.[57,111]

The use of laryngeal mask airway (LMA) and other supraglottic airway devices in patients receiving general anesthesia for laparoscopic surgery remains controversial. Several authors have expressed concerns that the increased intraabdominal and intrathoracic pressures characteristic of pneumoperitoneum place the patient at increased risk of gastroesophageal reflux and pulmonary aspiration. In addition, the classic LMA does not secure the airway, and the low seal pressures preclude the use of high airway inflation pressures without causing gastric distention.[113]

The barrier pressure (BrP) quantifies resistance to gastroesophageal reflux and is defined as the difference between the lower esophageal sphincter pressure and the gastric pressure.[114] To prevent aspiration, the gradient needs to remain positive because this will help prevent the lower esophageal sphincter from opening. A study examining the effect of induction, intubation, anesthesia, and pneumoperitoneum on barrier pressure in nonobese patients undergoing laparoscopy and obese patients undergoing laparoscopic gastric bypass showed that BrP decreased in both groups but at all times remained positive.[114] The obese patients, however, had lower BrP at all points when compared with the nonobese patients, suggesting that they may be at increased risk for aspiration.

Researchers have conducted studies to evaluate the safety and efficacy of LMAs in a variety of laparoscopic procedures. A systematic review and meta-analysis by Park et al.[115] compared the efficacies of supraglottic devices and endotracheal tubes in patients undergoing laparoscopic surgery. They found the incidence of laryngospasm, cough at devise removal, dysphagia, dysphonia, sore throat, and hoarseness to be significantly higher in those intubated with an endotracheal tube. However, there were no differences seen in oropharyngeal leak pressures, aspiration episodes, or other complications leading the authors to conclude that supraglottic airways may be an acceptable alternative to endotracheal tubes for laparoscopic procedures. A meta-analysis by Beleña et al.[116] of 704 patients undergoing laparoscopic cholecystectomy demonstrated an incidence of aspiration (0.4%). In all these studies, optimal ventilation was provided in approximately 99.5% of cases.[115,116]

Several researchers have also examined the efficacy of different types of supraglottic airway devices for the management of ventilation during laparoscopic procedures. A meta-analysis comparing the ProSeal LMA and the i-gel demonstrated that the LMA ProSeal provided higher oropharyngeal leak pressures (OLP) when compared to the i-gel with similar time to insertion and first insertion success rates.[117] Both devices did, however, allow for decompression of the stomach so that continuous gastric decompression can be accomplished.[116,117] The efficacy of the LMA Supreme versus the i-gel was also evaluated in approximately 100 patients undergoing laparoscopic surgery in the Trendelenburg position.[118] Again, both devices provided an adequate seal during controlled ventilation and allowed for decompression of the stomach throughout the procedures. Finally, the efficacy of the ProSeal LMA was also compared to the LMA Supreme in elective cholecystectomy to examine ease of insertion and OLP.[119] Whereas the LMA Supreme was easier to insert and demonstrated higher success rates for first-time insertion, the OLP was much higher with the ProSeal LMA, which allowed for the delivery of greater tidal volumes and more effective ventilation. These studies suggest that the LMA ProSeal may offer some advantages when concerns for the adequacy of ventilation exist.

The evidence suggests that under certain circumstances, the use of the LMA and other supraglottic devices may be appropriate during laparoscopy, but no general consensus exists to date.[115-117] Many clinicians feel that the risk of airway difficulties is too high to warrant their use. With the development of newer supraglottic devices that allow for decompression of the stomach and adequate high-pressure ventilation, the issue may become clearer. Recommendations for clinicians using supraglottic airways for laparoscopic procedures are presented in Box 34.7.

There is no one specific anesthetic technique that is best for laparoscopic surgery. The choice is dictated by a combination of factors, including the surgical procedure, postoperative disposition of the patient (ambulatory or in-patient), and presence of coexisting disease processes. However, the use of N_2O in laparoscopic surgery has been a source of controversy because of beliefs that N_2O contributes to bowel distention and increases the incidence of postoperative nausea and vomiting (PONV). Based on the evidence, the jury is still out.

The effect of N_2O on the incidence of PONV has been evaluated in several studies. A randomized controlled trial (2008) in three groups of patients undergoing gynecologic laparoscopy showed that N_2O increases the incidence and severity of PONV in a dose-dependent manner.[120] Patients who received 70% N_2O had a statistically significant greater incidence of nausea than patients who received no N_2O or

---

BOX 34.7 Guidelines for Use of the Laryngeal Mask Airway During Laparoscopy

- Ensure that clinician is an experienced LMA user.
- Select patients carefully (e.g., fasted, not obese).
- Use correct size of LMA.
- Use LMA that allows for gastric drainage (i.e., LMA ProSeal).
- Make surgeon aware of the use of LMA.
- Use total IV anesthetic technique or volatile agent.
- Use low-pressure insufflation.
- Avoid steep Trendelenburg position.
- Avoid inadequate anesthesia during surgery.
- Avoid disturbance of the patient during emergence.

IV, Intravenous; *LMA*, laryngeal mask airway.

50% N_2O. However, a similar study showed that the elimination of N_2O from a propofol-based anesthetic for ambulatory gynecologic surgery had no effect on readiness to discharge and did not increase the incidence of adverse postoperative events, including PONV.[121]

The effect of N_2O on bowel distention has been examined. In a randomized controlled trial involving 28 patients undergoing laparoscopic donor nephrectomy, the use of N_2O caused bowel distention in 50% of patients.[122] In 25%, the distention was severe enough to interfere with the progress of the surgery and as a result needed to be discontinued. In contrast, a randomized controlled trial examined the use of N_2O in 50 morbidly obese patients undergoing laparoscopic bariatric surgery.[123] Half of the patients received N_2O as part of the anesthetic and the other half did not. The surgeons, unaware of anesthetic technique, were unable to detect any differences in bowel distention between the groups over a 90-minute period.

There is also controversy surrounding the use of muscle relaxants for laparoscopic surgical procedures. It has been hypothesized that deep neuromuscular blockade as demonstrated by a train of four (TOF) count of zero but a posttetanic count of 1 or more, would allow for better surgical operating conditions at lower insufflation pressures.[124] However, many studies have demonstrated no differences in operating conditions or long-term benefits during laparoscopic gynecologic procedures under varying levels of neuromuscular blockade.[125,126] In addition, in these studies, deep blockade did not appear to allow for the use of lower insufflation pressures and may be associated with inadequate reversal and postoperative respiratory depression.[124,127] In contrast, in a systematic review and meta-analysis conducted by Bruintjes et al.[128] deep neuromuscular blockade was shown to improve surgical space conditions and reduce postoperative pain scores in the postanesthesia care unit. This analysis did not evaluate the incidence of intraoperative complications or patient outcomes.

There is also controversy surrounding the choice of total intravenous anesthesia (TIVA) versus inhalational anesthetics for laparoscopic surgical procedures. A Cochrane review evaluating the use of both techniques in urology, gynecology, and gastroenterology did not demonstrate the superiority of either technique.[129] There were no clinically meaningful differences in postoperative pain scores, incidence of PONV, or other adverse effects between the two groups.

POSTOPERATIVE CONCERNS

PONV is a major concern for patients undergoing laparoscopic surgical procedures. In fact, patients report that they are more worried about nausea and vomiting after surgery than they are about experiencing postoperative pain. The incidence of PONV in the laparoscopic population has been reported to be as high as 72% and is known to be associated with significant postoperative complications such as surgical wound dehiscence, aspiration, and unanticipated hospital admission.[130,131] Because the etiology of PONV is multifactorial, multimodal therapy using antiemetics that target different receptors has become standard of care.[121,132] The use of TIVA versus inhalational anesthesia does not seem to offer any advantage for reducing the incidence of PONV alone.[129] There is evidence that a combination of TIVA with multimodal antiemetic therapy has been reported to decrease the incidence of PONV. A randomized controlled trial compared TIVA and multimodal therapy with inhalation anesthesia plus multimodal therapy or propofol anesthesia alone.[133] The researchers showed that patients who received TIVA and multimodal therapy had a 90% response rate versus 63% and 66% in the other two groups. In addition, multimodal therapy was associated with a greater degree of patient satisfaction.

Although the development of laparoscopic surgical procedures has reduced the overall need for analgesia both intraoperatively and postoperatively, pain still continues to be a concern in the postoperative period. Pain after laparoscopy is comprised of three components: incisional pain (parietal pain), deep intraabdominal pain (visceral pain), and shoulder pain, which is believed to be referred visceral pain.[134] However, the majority of postoperative pain after laparoscopic surgery is typically of a visceral quality on the day of surgery, with shoulder pain predominating on the first postoperative day.[135] The creation of the pneumoperitoneum is associated with distention of the peritoneum and abdominal wall, and in conjunction with visceral dissection and/or resection activates nociceptors via the enteric nervous system.[100] The enteric nervous system is a complex system that functions to some extent independent of the central nervous system.[100] The peritoneum and viscera convey unpleasant sensations and autonomic reactions to injury via the vagus nerve giving rise to both painful and nonpainful sensations.[136,137] In addition, intraabdominal CO_2 contributes to postoperative pain by decreasing intraperitoneal pH and causing irritation of the phrenic nerve.[138]

Management of postoperative pain in laparoscopy patients is complex and involves a multimodal approach that includes opioids, nonsteroidal antiinflammatory drugs (NSAIDs), corticosteroids, and local anesthetics. The multimodal approach has been found to improve patient satisfaction, decrease opioid requirements, and decrease the incidence of postoperative complications (including PONV) and unplanned hospital admission.[100,139]

NSAIDs have proven to be of value in managing postoperative laparoscopic pain. Several types of NSAIDs have been used, including the cyclooxygenase-2 (COX-2) inhibitor celecoxib, ketorolac, and acetaminophen, and their efficacy has been repeatedly studied. Although NSAIDs are not potent enough as a sole analgesic for managing laparoscopic pain, they have been shown to act synergistically leading to decreased opioid use.[140] A double-blinded, placebo-controlled, randomized study of 80 American Society of Anesthesiologists (ASA) class I to III patients undergoing outpatient laparoscopy showed that short-term use of celecoxib decreased postoperative pain and postoperative opioid-containing analgesic requirements, while improving the quality of recovery.[141] In addition, multiple NSAIDs are being combined to optimize their effectiveness. A retrospective comparative study examining the efficacy of preemptive administration of pregabalin, acetaminophen, and celecoxib for the management of perioperative pain after robotic-assisted laparoscopic radical prostatectomy showed a decrease in both intraoperative and postoperative opioid use.[142] The efficacy and utility of celecoxib for use in the management of postoperative pain was confirmed in a 2015 Cochrane report.[143]

Glucocorticoids also have been used successfully for the management of postlaparoscopy pain. In addition to possessing antiemetic properties, glucocorticoids have antiinflammatory and analgesic properties that make them useful in the management of visceral pain. The exact mechanism is not fully understood, but it is known that glucocorticoids reduce prostaglandin synthesis by inhibiting phospholipase enzyme and COX-2. In addition, they modulate the inflammatory response by inhibiting major cytokines, including C-reactive protein, tumor necrosis factor, and several interleukins.[144] The efficacy of dexamethasone administration in decreasing perioperative opioid consumption has been evaluated in a systematic review.[145] The study showed that preoperative administration of dexamethasone decreased total opioid consumption for up to 48 hours postoperatively. In addition, it was not associated with an increase in adverse effects and was associated with the benefit of significantly decreasing the incidence of PONV. Dexamethasone in combination with NSAIDs was shown to further reduce pain scores and the need for opioids in the postoperative period.

The effectiveness of peripherally administered local anesthetics in the management of postoperative laparoscopy pain is a complicated question because research evidence remains mixed. One systematic review of postoperative pain management strategies demonstrated that infiltration of surgical incisions at the end of procedures was effective in the management of postoperative pain.[146] In addition, intravenous lidocaine infusions were shown to be useful for rescue therapy. However, neuraxial techniques were not considered necessary because of a high risk to benefit ratio. In contrast, a 2017 systematic review found little to no benefit of local infiltration of port sites or intraperitoneal instillation of local anesthetics in reducing postoperative pain scores.[140] Other techniques, such as ultrasound-guided transversus abdominus sheath block, are also being used in the management of postlaparoscopy pain by blocking the terminal branches of the lower intercostal nerves in a T8-L1 dermatomal distribution.[147-149] The evidence on the effectiveness of these techniques is mixed, and further evaluation is warranted.[140,147-149]

The prevention and management of shoulder tip pain (STP) following laparoscopic surgery has received a great deal of attention in recent years. It is estimated that up to 80% of women experience STP, which increases morbidity, delays discharge, and increases the rate of readmission.[150] While many interventions have been proposed, there is mixed evidence to support their efficacy. The choice of technique for releasing the pneumoperitoneum appears to have the greatest impact on reducing the incidence of postoperative shoulder pain.[150] The use of pulmonary recruitment maneuvers, extended assisted ventilation, and active aspiration of intraabdominal gas have been shown to reduce the severity of STP at 24 hours postoperatively. While local anesthetic instillation has not been shown to be effective in reducing incision pain, it may reduce STP for up to 8 hours.

THE FUTURE OF LAPAROSCOPIC SURGERY

Minimally invasive surgery has become the norm over the last 25 years, prompting major advances in laparoscopic techniques. Innovations in technology include the development of robotic-assisted surgical systems such as the DaVinci Surgical System, which provides for greater surgical precision, decreased postoperative pain, and shorter lengths of hospital stay[151,152] (see Chapter 35). In addition, efforts have been made to eliminate the need for pneumoperitoneum through the development of "gasless" laparoscopic systems. The gasless laparoscopy technique creates a working space for the surgeon by inserting a fan-shaped device into the abdomen to lift the abdominal wall away from the viscera, eliminating the need for CO_2 insufflation. Current research shows much promise for this technique. Compared with conventional laparoscopy, gasless laparoscopy was associated with lower intraoperative blood loss, decreased postoperative pain, and less postoperative inflammation.[153-155]

The development of robotic-assisted laparoscopic surgery has allowed surgeons to overcome some of the limitations imposed by standard laparoscopic technology.[151,152] A surgeon using robotic-assisted technology controls surgical instruments from a control console that may be immediately adjacent to the patient, within the operative suite, or at a site hundreds of miles away from the operating room. An important advantage of robotic technology is the incorporation of three-dimensional (stereoptic) imaging, which permits superior depth perception. Robotic-assisted surgery offers the surgeon improved ergonomics, superior dexterity, and the ability to use traditional open surgical skills for laparoscopic operations. Robotic-assisted surgical techniques have been used in all types of procedures—cardiac, general, gynecologic, and urologic surgical specialties. The anesthetic management of these procedures is discussed in Chapter 35.

SUMMARY

As technology advances, laparoscopic surgical techniques will be employed in increasingly more complicated procedures and patient populations. Providing safe and effective anesthetic care demands that the anesthesia care provider understand the unique challenges of laparoscopic surgery, with particular attention to the physiologic effects of carbon dioxide insufflation and pneumoperitoneum.

REFERENCES

For a complete list of references for this chapter, scan this QR code with any smartphone code reader app, or visit the following URL: http://booksite.elsevier.com/9780323711944/.

35

Anesthesia for Robotic Surgery

Nancy A. Moriber

Robotic surgical techniques originally evolved as an offshoot of the minimally invasive surgical phenomenon, and this method is rapidly becoming the preferred surgical technique in all subspecialties. Robotic systems provide surgeons with improved dexterity that translates into greater stability of surgical instruments and greater surgical precision.[1] As a result, robotic procedures have been shown to benefit both the patient and the hospital system, demonstrating improved outcomes, including decreased length of stay, decreased costs associated with hospitalization, decreased postoperative pain, decreased bleeding, decreased wound complications (including infection and incisional hernia), and improved overall patient satisfaction.[1-3] Minimally invasive robotic-assisted techniques have been utilized in a vast array of surgical specialties, including general surgery, urology, gynecology, cardiac surgery, orthopedic, and otolaryngology. However, these advances in surgical technique have created unique challenges for the anesthetic management of patients undergoing robotic procedures to ensure patient safety and hemodynamic stability.

HISTORY OF ROBOTIC SURGERY

Whereas science has seen the development of robots over the past 75 years, the first conceptualizations as an adjunct for use in surgery began in the mid- to late-1980s at the National Aeronautics and Space Administration (NASA) Ames Research Center in Palo Alto, California.[4] This work marked the beginning of the development of "virtual reality," which made it possible to interact with three-dimensional (3D) space. The NASA-Ames team took the concept of virtual reality to engineers at the Stanford Research Institute with expertise in human interface technology to develop an extremely dexterous telemanipulator that would revolutionize vascular and nerve anastomoses for hand surgery by providing surgeons with the sense that the surgical field was directly in front of them even when operating at a distance.

While the NASA-Ames group was working on its robotic system, laparoscopic surgical procedures focusing on cholecystectomy were developed in France.[4] With the widespread implementation of this type of surgical intervention, it became apparent that laparoscopy created enormous challenges for the surgeon, including degradation of the sense of touch, loss of natural 3D visualization, and impairment of dexterity as a result of the fulcrum effect, which could be resolved by the integration of robotic systems.[5,6] The fulcrum effect is a nonintuitive motion of laparoscopic instrument tips around a fixed point, which in laparoscopic procedures is considered to be the skin insertion site.

The earliest robotic surgical device was created in 1992 for use in hip replacement surgery. The RoboDoc (Integrated Surgical Systems) was developed to precisely core out the femoral shaft with 96% precision, far exceeding the 75% accuracy of manual approaches.[4] However, despite the accuracy of the instrument, it would be many years before it would be approved by the US Food and Drug Administration (FDA).

At the same time, the military became interested in developing remote surgical technologies that would enable surgeons, through telepresence, to stabilize soldiers who would otherwise die on the battlefield.[7] Although these systems have never been implemented for use on the battlefield, they provided the technology that has been integrated into many of the systems in use today.

The first robotic system approved by the FDA was the Automated Endoscopic System for Optimal Positioning (AESOP), which allowed for precise control of the camera in laparoscopic procedures and launched the era of robotic general surgery.[8] AESOP would then evolve into the Zeus Robotic Surgical System (Computer Motion, Inc.). Simultaneously, the Stanford Research Institute developed the first master-slave manipulator for medical use. This system was unique in that it was capable of offering four degrees of freedom in instrumentation motion. In 1994, the rights to this robotic system were purchased by Intuitive Surgical (Mountainview, CA), and after extensive redesign became the da Vinci surgical system, which offered greater dexterity and six degrees of freedom.[9] The da Vinci system displayed an image just above the surgeon's hands, giving the appearance that the surgical instruments operated as an extension of the hands. In April 1997, the first da Vinci robotic surgical procedure was performed in Brussels, Belgium.[10] The FDA approved the da Vinci system in 2000. Finally, in 2003, Computer Motion and Intuitive Surgical merged, combining their technology to become the da Vinci systems in use today.

Currently there are approximately 4500 da Vinci robotic systems in use worldwide, two-thirds of which are in the United States. While the da Vinci robotic systems predominate, newer systems such as the Senhance Surgical System (TransEnterix) have been introduced following FDA approval for use in both gynecologic and colorectal procedures.[11] This system integrates the latest technology and offers some advantages over the da Vinci systems, including rapid conversion to traditional laparoscopy, "haptic feedback" so that the surgeon can "feel" the pull/push of instruments, and the integration of a 3D camera with "eye-sensing control" that allows the surgeon to control the position of the camera by movement of the eyes.

Over the past 10 years, there has been a dramatic increase in the number of robotic procedures performed as a result of major advances in technology. In 2017, an estimated 644,000 robotic procedures were performed in the United States alone, more than any other country in the world.[12] Today, robotic techniques are employed in all surgical specialties, including colorectal surgery, cardiac surgery, gynecology, urology, and otolaryngology.

ROBOTIC SYSTEMS

Robotics systems are classified according to the degree of "hands on" control required from the operator. Assist devices such as AESOP are used to guide and control the location of surgical instruments but

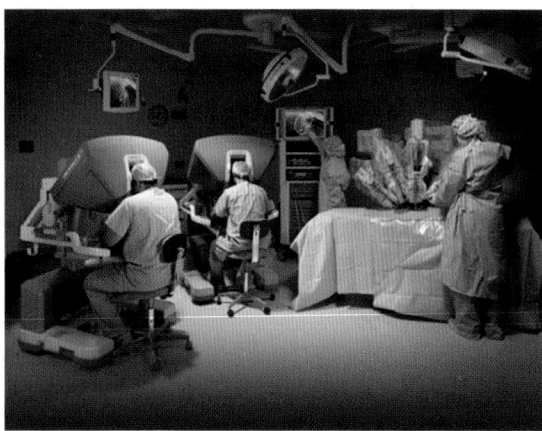

Fig. 35.1 Surgeon operates while seated at the robotic console. (Courtesy Intuitive Surgical Inc., Sunnyvale, CA.)

require the input of specific cues from the operator. They are not autonomous and cannot operate on their own. In contrast, telemanipulators, such as the da Vinci surgical system, require continuous hands-on control from the operator so that the movement of the instruments exactly replicates the motion of the operator. Currently, the da Vinci and the Senhance Surgical systems are the only FDA-approved robotic-assisted surgical systems in the United States.

The da Vinci system is the primary system in use and consists of three components: the vision cart, which includes the monitor; the surgeon console; and the patient side-cart (Fig. 35.1).[13] The vision system is comprised of the endoscope, the cameras, and all the equipment necessary to produce a 3D image of the operative field. The patient side-cart contains the robotic arms, which are designed to hold the endoscope and the surgical instruments.[13] Most systems contain three to four robotic arms; however, the FDA has recently approved the da Vinci SP (single-port) robotic platform to allow for the performance of single-site surgical procedures.[13,14] This system is currently approved for use only in the United States. The robotic arms stabilize the EndoWrist surgical instruments, which mimic the motions of the human hand and wrist in 3D space. The current EndoWrist instruments possess seven degrees of freedom, including three arm motions (in-out, up-down, side-to-side), three wrist motions (side-to-side, left, and right yaw), pitch, and rotation, allowing for greater rotation and pivoting. Once the instruments are properly positioned at the surgical field, they are docked in place by the patient side-cart.

The surgeon console stands several feet away from the operating room table and serves as an operating station from which the surgeon can manipulate the robotic arms and attached instruments within the surgical field. The surgeon's fingers are inserted into rings on the console's levers, which allows fine movement of the surgical instruments. The image displayed on the console is transmitted via two separate channels to create the virtual 3D image visualized by the operator. For safety, the surgeon's head must be placed in the viewer, or the system will lock automatically and remain motionless until it senses the presence of the surgeon's head once again. To ensure the sterility and safety of the surgical field, a second surgeon is always present to ensure that institutional protocols are followed and to adjust the camera and docked instruments as needed.

GENERAL ANESTHETIC CONSIDERATIONS

It has become clear that minimally invasive robotic surgery is associated with improved patient outcomes, especially in morbidly obese and geriatric patients, including decreased length of stay, faster recovery,

reduced perioperative blood loss, reduced postoperative pain, and a significant decrease in perioperative complications.[15-17] However, the transition to robotic surgery has created challenges for anesthetic management that are unique to patients undergoing these procedures. Additional factors must be taken into consideration, depending on the surgical specialty involved. Regardless of the procedure, however, the anesthetic plan must take into consideration the following factors: (1) prolonged surgical times, (2) spatial restrictions associated with use of the robot, (3) inability to alter patient position after docking of the robot, (4) physiologic changes associated with extreme positioning, (5) risk of postoperative visual loss (POVL), (6) physiologic consequences associated with the creation of pneumoperitoneum (see Chapter 34), and (7) implementation of enhanced recovery after surgery (ERAS) protocols.[18]

Surgical Time, Spatial Restrictions, and Mobility Issues

Robotic surgery is associated with significantly longer operative times but shorter hospital stays as compared with traditional surgical techniques.[15-18] Factors influencing surgical time are usually out of the control of the anesthesia care provider and include operator experience, surgical complexity, and the time requirements associated with patient positioning and docking/undocking of the robot. In addition, the bulkiness and proximity of the equipment in relation to the operative field limit the accessibility of the anesthesia care provider to the patient after the start of the surgical procedure. To accommodate the robot, the patient's extremities are frequently tucked at the sides and inaccessible for the remainder of the procedure. This is compounded by the fact that once the robot is docked, rapid access to the patient and emergent positional changes are difficult to achieve due to the time is takes to "undock" the patient cart. Therefore, when complications during robotic surgery occur, they may cause catastrophic implications for the patient.

There is limited access to patients for prolonged periods of time during robotic procedures, and, therefore, it is imperative the patient be adequately prepared for surgery. Additional intravenous access, the use of invasive monitoring, and blood product availability should be dictated by the patient's underlying comorbidities and the particular surgical procedure performed. It is also essential that the members of the perioperative team be trained to quickly undock the robot to allow for rapid intervention during times of crisis. Operating rooms should have established emergency undocking protocols in place to handle these situations. These protocols should clearly define the responsibilities of the surgeon at the console, the bedside assistant(s), surgical scrub nurse, circulating nurse, and anesthetists(s).[19] Operating room personnel should be provided with adequate time in a simulated environment to practice these procedures in order to improve performance and ensure positive patient outcomes. The shorter time required to undock the new Senhance Surgical System offers an advantage for institutions when making decisions to purchase new/additional robotic systems.

The proximity of the fixed robotic arms and attached surgical instruments to the patient also creates the potential for constant compression of underlying structures, including the face, nose, and chest. The anesthetist needs to ensure that adequate padding is placed between the robotic arms/instruments and the patient. Due to the extreme Trendelenburg surgical position required in most robotic surgical procedures, the risk that patients could slip on the operating room table as a result of gravitational forces is possible. Patients must be appropriately secured on the operating room table to prevent inadvertent movement and the creation of pressure points and nerve damage. Therefore, it is essential that the surgical position be assessed and documented at regular intervals (at least every 15 minutes) throughout the procedure or when changes in the position of the patient, robot, or operating room table occur.

Physiologic Changes Associated With Extreme Positioning

To facilitate surgical exposure for many robotic procedures, the steep Trendelenburg position is commonly used. Steep Trendelenburg position is defined as a 40- to 45-degree head-down tilt of the operating room table.[20,21] Patients are frequently placed in this position for several hours, resulting in significant and potentially adverse cardiovascular, respiratory, and neurophysiologic changes, which are compounded by the simultaneous creation of the pneumoperitoneum. It is difficult at times to separate the positional effects from those caused by the pneumoperitoneum, as both are frequently instituted simultaneously. The physiologic changes associated with steep Trendelenburg are summarized in Box 35.1.

Pneumoperitoneum and steep Trendelenburg create significant changes in cardiovascular parameters in both healthy patients and those with preexisting cardiovascular disease.[21-24] Mean arterial pressure (MAP), central venous pressure (CVP), and pulmonary capillary wedge pressure (PCWP) increase dramatically. Lestar et al.[21] demonstrated a threefold increase in CVP and a twofold increase in PCWP as compared to initial supine values. In addition, MAP increases by as much as 35%. The overall effect of increased filling pressure and systemic vascular resistance is a prolongation of isovolemic relaxation time. However, despite the changes in MAP and cardiac filling pressures, heart rate, stroke volume, and mixed venous oxygen saturation remain relatively unchanged.[21,23] Once the patient assumes the horizontal position and the pneumoperitoneum is released, cardiac parameters return to baseline.

The steep Trendelenburg position has significant effects on ventilation, gas exchange, and the ventilation-perfusion distribution.[23-26] Gravitational forces and the pneumoperitoneum cause a cephalad shift of the diaphragm leading to atelectasis in the dorsal parts of the lungs, alterations in lung mechanics (including increases in airway pressures), decreases in static lung and chest wall compliance, and decreases in lung volume.[26] Both peak and plateau pressures rise and continue to increase with the creation of the pneumoperitoneum.[21] As a result, end tidal carbon dioxide ($ETco_2$) levels increase, which is associated with a widening of the arterial partial pressure of carbon dioxide ($Paco_2$)–$ETco_2$ gradient.[21,23] In the presence of controlled ventilation, the arterial blood acid-base balance is relatively well maintained; however, significant abnormalities can develop in the spontaneously breathing patient without ventilatory assistance.[21] Evidence also suggests that the addition of high positive end-expiratory pressure (PEEP) (15 cm H_2O) to controlled mechanical ventilation results in higher lung dynamic compliance, better oxygenation, and more homogeneous ventilation intraoperatively.[26] The steep Trendelenburg position can also lead to the development of significant upper airway edema and increased risk of upper airway obstruction following extubation.[25,27] These changes can persist for up to 2 hours into the postoperative period and warrant vigilant monitoring for the development of airway compromise.[27] Finally, the creation of the pneumoperitoneum in the steep Trendelenburg position has been shown to shorten the distance from the vocal cords to the carina, which could potentially displace the endotracheal tube, resulting in an endobronchial intubation.[28] It is therefore imperative to reconfirm bilateral breath sounds after positioning and following abdominal insufflation.

The physiologic effects of steep Trendelenburg position on airway resistance, compliance, and lung volumes persist after emergence from anesthesia, and are magnified in patients with preexisting chronic obstructive pulmonary disease (COPD). In the steep Trendelenburg position, the ratio of maximal expiratory flow to maximal inspiratory

BOX 35.1 Physiologic Changes Associated With Steep Trendelenburg Position

Cardiovascular Changes
- Increased:
  - Mean arterial pressure (MAP)
  - Central venous pressure (CVP)
  - Pulmonary capillary wedge pressure (PCWP)
  - Systemic vascular resistance (SVR)
  - Afterload
- Unchanged:
  - Heart rate (HR)
  - Stroke volume (SV)
  - Mixed venous oxygen saturation

Respiratory Changes
- Increased:
  - Airway resistance
  - Peak airway pressure
  - Plateau pressure
  - End tidal carbon dioxide ($ETco_2$)
  - Upper airway edema
- Decreased:
  - Lung compliance
  - Vital capacity (VC)
  - Forced expiratory volume in 1 sec (FEV_1)

Cerebrovascular Changes:
- Increased:
  - Intracranial pressure
  - Hydrostatic pressure gradient
  - Cerebral vascular resistance
  - Intraocular pressure
- Decreased:
  - Cerebral venous drainage
- Unchanged:
  - Regional cerebral oxygenation
  - Cerebral perfusion pressure

flow at 50% of vital capacity (MEF_{50}/MIF_{50}) increases significantly in patients with and without COPD and returns to baseline within 24 hours. There are also significant reductions in both vital capacity and forced expiratory volume in 1 second (FEV_1), leading to lung atelectasis, which can persist for more than 5 days postoperatively in patients with COPD. Many of the prolonged changes can be attributed to the development of airway edema as a direct result of positional effects.[25]

The steep Trendelenburg position also impacts cerebral homeostasis because of its effects on cerebral perfusion and intracranial pressure (ICP). The head-down position causes a simultaneous increase in both MAP and CVP that impairs venous drainage from the head, increasing the hydrostatic pressure gradient in the cerebral vasculature.[20,29,30] The net effect is an increase in ICP, cerebral edema, and cerebral vascular resistance, which could potentially impair cerebral blood flow.[20,31] In fact, ICP rises to more than 20 mm Hg in the steep Trendelenburg position.[31] This increase is directly associated with elevations in MAP and impairments in venous drainage. In some studies, the optic nerve sheath diameter, which can be measured noninvasively with optic sonography, is a surrogate measure of elevated ICP with a measure of 6.8 mm in diameter correlating with an ICP above 20 mm Hg.[30,31] Regional cerebral oxygenation and cerebral perfusion pressures appear to be well maintained despite these physiologic changes, as a result of local cerebral autoregulation.[20,25,29] It is prudent to limit the time spent in the steep Trendelenburg position, as these hemodynamic perturbations have implications for the development of POVL.

Postoperative Visual Loss

POVL is a rare but devastating complication following surgery. It has been documented after cardiac, spine, head, and neck procedures, and, most recently, robotic surgical procedures performed in the steep Trendelenburg position.[32-35] The reported incidence of POVL is between 0.056% and 1.3%.[34] Risk factors associated with the development of POVL include gender, hypotension, prone and Trendelenburg positioning, prolonged procedures, increased blood loss, and decreased use of colloid. Prolonged surgical time in positions associated with venous congestion and rising intraocular pressures are common in robotic surgery; thus, these patients are considered to be at increased risk.[32]

The major causes of POVL include anterior ischemic optic neuropathy (AION), posterior ischemic optic neuropathy (PION), central retinal artery occlusion (CRAO), and cortical blindness.[32-35] AION is caused by occlusion or hypoperfusion of the anterior optic nerve and is most common following cardiac, major vascular, and spine procedures.[32] In contrast, PION results from infarction of the optic nerve posterior to the lamina cribrosa, usually as a result of elevated venous pressures, increased intraocular pressures, and interstitial edema, which compromise blood flow to the eye, as seen in prone and steep Trendelenburg positions.[32,33,36] While anemia and hypoperfusion are seen in patients that develop PION, the exact mechanism of injury is unknown.[34] AION and PION present with sudden onset of painless visual loss and visual field deficits and are usually discovered upon emergence from anesthesia.[34-36] CRAO and cortical blindness are usually associated with procedures in which there is a high likelihood of emboli, severe hypotension, or direct compression on the globe.[32,34]

Prevention of POVL should include risk-modification strategies that are aimed at minimizing surgical time, minimizing estimated blood loss, and decreasing venous congestion. The American Society of Anesthesiologists (ASA) and the Anesthesia Patient Safety Foundation (APSF) released recommendations for the prevention of POVL in surgical patients in 2012. These were updated in 2019 specifically for patients undergoing spine procedures but can be applied to all patients at risk for POVL.[37] The recommendations include the consideration of staged surgical procedures to reduce operative time, keeping the head at or above the level of the heart when possible, and including colloid in nonblood replacement strategies. In addition, they highly encourage the anesthetist to include a discussion of risk factors associated with POVL and the current understanding of interventions available to reduce the risk as part of the informed consent process in high-risk patients. Although the reported incidence of POVL in robotic surgery is currently low, it is recommended that efforts to reduce the degree of venous congestion and interstitial edema in the head during robotic procedures be implemented by anesthesia care providers. Recommendations for management of the patient in the steep Trendelenburg position are presented in Box 35.2. Finally, several researchers have attempted to identify pharmacologic agents that might be effective in reducing venous congestion through a reduction in intraocular pressure.[35,36,38] They examined the effect of topical β-adrenergic blockers and carbonic anhydrase inhibitors (dorzolamide-timolol, betaxolol) in patients undergoing procedures in the steep Trendelenburg position and found that these agents significantly reduce IOP and that these effects are sustained over time. Whereas a causative relationship between elevated IOP and POVL has not been found, it may be prudent to manage IOP during these procedures. A further discussion of POVL can be found in Chapter 23.

BOX 35.2 Recommendations for the Prevention of Postoperative Visual Loss

Preoperative
- Complete a thorough history and physical to identify preoperative risk factors.
- Inform patients of risk of POVL if substantial blood loss or prolonged surgical time is expected.

Intraoperative
- Assess patient's baseline blood pressure and monitor continuously. If high risk, consider invasive blood pressure monitoring.
- Treat prolonged significant decreases in blood pressure with adrenergic agonists.
- Administer crystalloids or colloids alone or in combination to maintain euvolemia.
- Avoid direct pressure on the eyes to prevent retinal artery occlusion.
- Stage procedures for high-risk patients if applicable.

Postoperative
- Assess vision when patient is awake and alert.
- If concerns over POVL arise, obtain ophthalmologic consult immediately.
- Optimize hemoglobin, hemodynamic status, and arterial oxygenation as indicated.

POVL, Postoperative visual loss.
Practice Advisory for Perioperative Visual Loss Associated with Spine Surgery 2019. An updated report by the American Society of Anesthesiologists Task Force on Perioperative Visual Loss, the North American Neuro-Ophthalmology Society and the Society of Neuroscience in Anesthesiology and Critical Care. *Anesthesiology.* 2019;130:12–30.

Enhanced Recovery After Surgery

The goal of minimally invasive robotic procedures is to improve surgical outcomes and allow patients to return to normal activity as quickly as possible. Enhanced recovery management pathways have been developed to facilitate this process. The ERAS program is an international, multimodal approach to perioperative care that aims to achieve early recovery following major surgery.[39-41] It was first designed for application in patients undergoing gastrointestinal procedures, but it has been applied across all surgical specialties, including gynecology, general surgery, cardiac, thoracic, and orthopedics procedures.

The ERAS protocol is a multidisciplinary, evidence-based list of recommendations for the care of patients during the preoperative, intraoperative, and postoperative periods in an attempt to modify the stress response to surgery and improve surgical outcomes for a faster return to function.[40,41] The protocol is comprised of approximately 20 general elements that have been shown to decrease hospitalization and perioperative complications when implemented across the perianesthesia continuum (Box 35.3).[40,42] The elements may be modified to meet the specific needs of the surgical specialty. Preoperative guidelines focus on prevention of a catabolic state associated with long periods of fasting and fluid restriction. Intraoperative and postoperative recommendations are designed to fast-track patients to promote early ambulation and feeding following surgery. An early Cochrane review of four randomized controlled trials (237 patients) demonstrated a significant decrease in length of stay, a reduction in major perioperative complications, and similar rates of readmission in patients receiving ERAS-based versus conventional care.[43] In addition, ERAS programs are associated with attenuation of the stress response, as evidenced by reduced levels of stress hormones, including cortisol, tumor necrosis

BOX 35.3 Enhanced Recovery After Surgery (ERAS) Protocol Recommendations

Preoperative
- Preadmission counseling and education, including early discharge planning
- Fluid and carbohydrate loading
- Elimination of NPO status
- No/selective bowel preparation
- Antibiotic and thromboembolism prophylaxis
- Eliminate routine use of premedication
- Prewarming

Intraoperative
- Opioid sparing anesthetic techniques
- Pain and PONV management, including nonopioid analgesics and regional techniques
- Avoidance of NG tubes and surgical drains
- Avoidance of salt/water overload (goal-directed fluid therapy)
- Active warming and maintenance of normothermia

Postoperative
- Pain and PONV management, including nonopioid analgesics and regional techniques
- Avoidance of postoperative nasogastric tubes
- Aggressive PONV prophylaxis
- Avoidance of salt/water overload (goal-directed fluid therapy)
- Early ambulation
- Early oral nutrition/stimulation gut motility
- Early catheter removal
- Audit of ERAS compliance and patient outcome

NPO, Nil per os; *PONV*, postoperative nausea and vomiting.
From Pedziwiatr M, et al. Current status of enhanced recovery after surgery (ERAS) protocol in gastrointestinal surgery. *Mod Oncol.* 2018;35(6):95.

factor, interleukins, and interferon.[40,44] This leads to faster return of gastrointestinal function and accelerated postoperative recovery. Anesthetists are in a unique position to control many aspects of care related to the successful implementation of the ERAS protocol.

Guidelines for perioperative fluid management are a main component of the ERAS protocol. Perioperative fluid overload is associated with increased morbidity, postoperative ileus, and delayed hospital discharge. In addition, hypoproteinemia associated with large crystalloid loads has been shown to cause delayed gastric emptying, increased small bowel transit time, and postoperative ileus.[45] Studies have long demonstrated that the avoidance of perioperative fluid overload, independent of the amount of fluid administered preoperatively or postoperatively, decreases the rate of postoperative complications and improves outcomes following major gastrointestinal and thoracic surgery.[46,47] Therefore, the overarching goal of fluid management during implementation of the ERAS protocol is maintenance of the euvolemic state.[40]

During the preoperative period, patients are "fed" to reduce the hemodynamic effects associated with induction of anesthesia as a result of hypovolemia.[48] Current guidelines recommend the avoidance of preoperative fasting and intentional carbohydrate loading prior to surgery.[45] Patients are permitted to consume clear fluids up to 2 hours before anesthesia to prevent dehydration. Research evidence has shown that patients who consume clear liquids up to 2 hours before surgery have lower gastric volumes as compared to patients following conventional fasting guidelines. The patients undergoing liberal clear fluid intake are at no greater risk for pulmonary aspiration. In addition, 100 g (800 mL) of a 12.5% maltodextrin carbohydrate drink (Gatorade) is administered the night before surgery, followed by an additional 50 g (400 mL) 2 to 3 hours before induction of anesthesia to reduce the catabolic state induced by preoperative fasting.[49] Overnight fasting inhibits insulin secretion and promotes the release of catabolic hormones (including cortisol and glucagon), leading to insulin resistance, glycogen depletion, and protein breakdown in the postoperative period.[49,50] It is also associated with the development of a hypovolemic state. Therefore, intraoperatively, the goal of fluid therapy is to achieve a zero fluid balance at the end of surgery.[45,49]

Intraoperative fluid requirements should be met with a basal infusion of isotonic crystalloid solutions such as lactated Ringer at a 3 ± 2 mL/kg/hour.[49] Additional volume therapy is administered by bolus based on objective measures of hypovolemia such as changes in stroke volume measured through minimally invasive techniques, as heart rate, blood pressure, urine output, and CVP are not reliable measures of volume status. Normal saline (0.9%) should be avoided because of the potential for developing hyperchloremic metabolic acidosis, which has been associated with reductions in gastric blood flow and pH, as well as changes in renal perfusion.[51] Postoperatively, resumption of oral intake should be encouraged as soon as possible to maintain a euvolemic state, reduce the risk of infection, and decrease length of stay.[40,42,52] Intravenous fluids should be discontinued unless there is a clinical indication.[40,45]

The choice of anesthetic technique for implementation of the ERAS protocol must consider the need to minimize the impact of anesthetics on organ systems and facilitate rapid awakening following surgery to speed recovery of gastrointestinal and motor function. Whereas several different techniques can be utilized to achieve this goal, short-acting agents with minimal side effects are recommended in all cases. This must include the use of an opioid-sparing technique. Aggressive postoperative nausea and vomiting (PONV) prophylaxis using a multimodal approach should also be included in all ERAS protocols.[40,42,49] This includes the use of antiemetics and total intravenous anesthesia (TIVA) with propofol rather than inhalational agents. All patients with one to two risk factors (female gender, history of motion sickness/PONV, nonsmoking status, and use of perioperative narcotics) should receive a combination of two antiemetics, whereas patients with three to four risk factors should receive two to three antiemetics in addition to TIVA and opioid-sparing strategies.[40,53] To minimize the use of perioperative opioids, pain management should be achieved with the use multimodal therapy, including nonsteroidal antiinflammatory drugs and regional anesthetic techniques. Epidural anesthesia/analgesia has been recommended for complex and open procedures. Transversus abdominis plane (TAP) blocks have also been used safely in patients undergoing gynecologic robotic procedures. Current literature demonstrates that TAP blocks are effective in reducing postoperative pain scores, decreasing overall morphine consumption, and delaying time to first opioid request.[54] Adequate recovery from neuromuscular blockade must occur to minimize the risk of postoperative respiratory depression. Finally, normothermia should be maintained throughout the perioperative period with the use of active warming devices.[49] A further discussion of ERAS techniques can be found in Chapter 21.

CONSIDERATIONS FOR SURGICAL SUBSPECIALTIES

Cardiac Procedures

Minimally invasive robotic surgical techniques have been performed successfully for many cardiac procedures. The first successful internal mammary artery harvest was performed via thoracoscopy in 1997.[55]

This was followed by the first totally endoscopic coronary artery bypass surgery (TECAB) in 1998.[56] Since then, robotic techniques have been applied in such procedures as mitral valve repair, repair of atrial septal defects, and ablation of atrial arrhythmias. The challenge for anesthesia care providers is the need for expertise in both cardiac and thoracic anesthesia, as one-lung ventilation (OLV) and creation of a capnothorax are required to successfully perform these procedures.[57] All members of the perioperative team must be ready for conversion to an open procedure should it become necessary. Preoperative preparation involves assessment of both cardiac and pulmonary function. The presence of significant pulmonary disease, including COPD and pulmonary hypertension with poor preoperative lung function may be a contraindication to the performance of robotic cardiac procedures, even in patients who are deemed suitable from a cardiac perspective.[57] Evaluation of pulmonary function should include pulmonary function testing, preoperative chest x-ray, room air arterial blood gas analysis, and assessment of functional capacity ($\geq$4 metabolic equivalent of task [METS]).[57] Patients are also evaluated for the presence of significant peripheral vascular disease and atherosclerosis, which would create excessive risk for perfusion peripheral to the site of endovascular cannulation. Contraindications to TECAB are listed in Box 35.4.

Robotically Assisted Totally Endoscopic Coronary Artery Bypass Surgery

TECAB surgical techniques are currently used in patients requiring up to quadruple-vessel bypass using either on-pump (arrested heart) or off-pump (beating heart) techniques, with results comparable to conventional techniques.[58-60] Arrested heart TECAB procedures provide more optimal conditions for performing distal arterial anastomoses. Aortic cross-clamping is accomplished through the left femoral insertion of an endoaortic occlusion balloon catheter (EAOBC), through which antegrade cardioplegia can be delivered.[57] Following induction and intubation with a double-lumen tube, patients are positioned supine with the left chest elevated 30 degrees and the left arm tucked at the side to allow access to the thoracic cavity. The da Vinci instruments and endoscope are inserted through three ports placed in third through seventh left intercostal spaces to allow harvesting of both the right and left internal mammary arteries as needed. The exact positioning of the ports depends on multiple factors, including surgeon preference, target vessels, and patient's body habitus.[59] Harvesting of the left internal mammary artery (LIMA) is completed through two working ports under endoscopic visualization via the third port.[59] Beating heart TECAB is most often performed in patients who are not candidates for endovascular balloon insertion and can be performed off-pump or with cardiopulmonary bypass (CPB) support to improve visualization.[57] CPB may be required in the presence of intraoperative hemodynamic instability, ventricular arrhythmias, or in the patient who fails to tolerate OLV strategies.

Choice of anesthetic technique for TECAB procedures is dependent on the patient's underlying comorbidities. A thorough preoperative evaluation is required to ensure that patients are optimized prior to surgery and to guide the anesthetic plan of care. General anesthesia can be accomplished with the use of intravenous induction agents, maintained with inhalational anesthetics and intravenous opioids. Adequate muscle relaxation is essential as long as da Vinci surgical instruments are in situ to prevent damage or perforation of underlying mediastinal and thoracic structures. The patient is positioned supine with elevation of the operative hemithorax at 30 degrees. Intraoperative monitoring includes the use of transesophageal echocardiography (TEE) to monitor cardiac function and determine catheter placement, bilateral arterial lines to detect migration of the EAOBC, and pulmonary artery catheter placement as indicated. Near infrared cerebral oximetry has also been used as an adjunct to monitor EAOBC position, as a decline in left-sided readings may be indicative of left common carotid artery occlusion.[57] Paravertebral nerve blocks (PVB) placed prior to induction have been shown to be an effective component of the primary anesthetic and useful for the management of postoperative pain.[61] PVB involves the injection of local anesthetic into a wedge-shaped space lateral to the spinal nerves as they emerge from the intervertebral foramina, producing unilateral somatosensory and sympathetic nerve blockade.[61] The use of PVB avoids contralateral sympathectomy, minimizes hypotension, and allows for better control of intraoperative blood pressure when compared to a thoracic epidural.

OLV is initiated once full cannulation is completed in preparation for CPB. Lung isolation can be achieved with the use of a standard double-lumen tube or bronchial blocker and managed in the traditional manner (Box 35.5). In patients unable to tolerate OLV, high-frequency jet ventilation with a single-lumen endotracheal tube has been shown to be an effective method of ventilation for TECAB procedures.[62] If this is not feasible and the procedure can be accomplished off-pump, TECAB can be successfully performed

---

BOX 35.4 Contraindications to Totally Endoscopic Coronary Artery Bypass Surgery (TECAB)

- Morbid obesity
- Small patients with insufficient thoracic space
- Presence of anatomic abnormalities
  - Pleural adhesions
  - Previous cardiac or thoracic surgery
  - Narrow intercostal spaces
  - Severe cardiomegaly
- Valvular heart disease
  - Severe aortic insufficiency
  - Severe valvular stenosis of any kind
- Severe peripheral vascular disease and atherosclerosis
- Significant preexisting pulmonary disease with poor pulmonary function tests
- Inability to tolerate one-lung ventilation

From Deshpande SP, et al. Anesthetic management of robotically assisted totally endoscopic coronary artery bypass surgery (TECAB). *J Cardiothor Vasc An.* 2013;27(3):586–599.

BOX 35.5 Management of One-Lung Ventilation for Totally Endoscopic Coronary Artery Bypass (TECAB) Surgery Procedures to Prevent Hypoxia and Hypercarbia

- 100% Fio_2
- Pressure control ventilation
  - Peak plateau pressure <30 cm H_2O
  - Respiratory rate to maintain $Paco_2$ at 35–40 mm Hg, as assessed by arterial blood gas
- CPAP to nonventilated lung
- PEEP to ventilated lung

CPAP, Continuous positive airway pressure; *Fio₂,* fraction of inspired oxygen; *Paco₂,* partial pressure of arterial carbon dioxide; *PEEP,* positive end expiratory pressure.

From Deshpande SP, et al. Anesthetic management of robotically assisted totally endoscopic coronary artery bypass surgery (TECAB). *J Cardiothor Vasc An.* 2013;27(3):586–599.

with double-lung ventilation, avoiding the need for conversion to a traditional open-chest technique.[63] Once the left lung is allowed to collapse, the chest is insufflated with 10 to 12 mm Hg carbon dioxide (CO_2) to create a capnothorax to improve surgical exposure.[57] The instruments are then inserted into the thoracic cavity, the internal mammary arteries are harvested, and CPB is instituted so that revascularization of the coronaries can be completed.

The creation of the capnothorax may be accompanied by significant hemodynamic and respiratory changes that are the result of elevated intrathoracic pressures, which cause proportional increases in CVP, pulmonary artery pressures, PCWP, and peak airway pressures.[57,64,65] These increases may be accompanied by increases in heart rate and decreases in venous return, cardiac index, and MAP.[64-66] Hypovolemic patients and patients with preexisting left ventricular dysfunction are more likely to develop hemodynamic instability, even with low insufflation pressures.[66] Hemodynamic instability may be prevented with the administration of fluid boluses to raise the CVP to approximately 10 mm Hg prior to creation of the capnothorax. The capnothorax can be created slowly with the implementation of 2–mm Hg incremental increases in intrathoracic pressure. Evidence indicates that adequate visualization of intrathoracic structures can be achieved with one-lung ventilation at a pressure of 6 mm Hg. The required intrathoracic pressure increases to 8 mm Hg if two-lung ventilation is required.[66,67] Higher insufflation pressures (>10 mm Hg) are more likely to be associated with major changes in cardiovascular and respiratory parameters.[66,67] Vasopressors and inotropic agents may be required in the presence of significant increased right and left afterload and ventricular dysfunction.

TECAB procedures also present unique challenges with respect to temperature management in the perioperative period, which is dependent on the total number of anastomoses planned and the technique employed (arrested heart vs beating heart). The closed-chest procedure is associated with a decrease in radiant heat loss, so active systemic cooling is required for myocardial protection while on bypass.[57] For one-vessel arrested heart procedures, the temperature will be allowed to drift down to 34°C to 35°C. However, for two- or more-vessel procedures, active cooling to as low at 28°C may be required. In beating heart procedures, relative maintenance of systemic temperature will be required, and the use of a forced air warming device considered.[67] Temperature should be monitored in both the bladder and a central site such as the nasopharynx or esophagus.[67] At the completion of TECAB, patients should be rewarmed to establish normothermia to prevent shivering and increased myocardial demand in the immediate postoperative period.

Mitral Valve Procedures

Minimally invasive mitral valve procedures can be performed using a variety of surgical techniques, with the ultimate goals of decreasing surgical trauma, cardiac manipulation, and length of hospital stay. Minimally invasive mitral valve repairs can be performed through either a mini-thoracotomy or closed-chest technique, whereas mitral valve replacement requires the latter to allow placement of the prosthetic valve. In the United States, the first robot-assisted mitral repair was performed at East Carolina University in 2000.[68] The current trend is toward the performance of more complex, multiple valve procedures. Robotic mitral value repair offers many advantages over traditional endoscopic techniques, including an excellent 3D view of the valvular pathology and increased maneuverability of the endoscopic instruments.[69] Patients undergoing minimally invasive robotic procedures demonstrate shorter stays in the intensive care unit, decreased blood transfusions, lower incidence of renal failure, and reduced in-hospital mortality.[70]

Robotically assisted mitral valve procedures are most often performed through a 2- to 3-cm inframammary incision in the right fourth or fifth intercostal space.[69,71] Additional trocars are inserted around the primary incision to place the robotic arms/instruments, allow insufflation of CO_2, and facilitate transthoracic aortic cross-clamping if required. The patient is positioned in a modified left lateral position with a support placed under the right upper back and shoulder so as to form a 25- to 30-degree angle with the operating table.[69,71] The pelvis is kept flat on the table. The surgeon may request a left lateral tilt to further elevate the chest, but care must be taken not to put stress on the brachial plexus. Monitoring approaches are similar to those utilized for TECAB procedures, and TEE is the standard of care to evaluate valvular function and to assess for residual mitral regurgitation before terminating CPB. Transcutaneous defibrillation/pacing pads are placed for intraoperative cardioversion and defibrillation because placement of internal paddles is not possible. OLV and thoracic insufflation are required—except in this case, the right lung is collapsed, and the right chest is insufflated. Hemodynamic instability is a concern with moderate to high insufflation pressures. Recommendations are to limit the rate of CO_2 insufflation to 2 to 3 L/minute and to maintain intrathoracic pressures within the right hemithorax at less than 10 mm Hg to avoid hemodynamic changes and prevent the development of a tension pneumothorax.[66,69,72]

The choice of anesthetic for robotic-assisted mitral valve procedures is similar to TECAB and dependent on the patient's presentation. Intraoperative and postoperative analgesia can be achieved through the use of parenteral techniques or a combination of regional and opioid-based techniques, including intercostal and paravertebral approaches.[61,71] The use of neuraxial analgesia remains controversial in light of full intraoperative anticoagulation; however, in select patients, the placement of epidural catheters in the postoperative period may be warranted.

Thoracic Procedures

Video-assisted thoracoscopic surgery (VATS) is a well-established technique for the resection of thoracic tumors because it is associated with less trauma, decreased pain, shorter duration of chest tube drainage, and decreased length of hospital stay.[73] Since 2013, robotic-assisted surgical techniques have been successfully developed for several types of resections, including lung, mediastinal, and esophageal resection, despite significant increases in cost.[73-75] When compared to traditional endoscopic thoracic procedures, minimally invasive robotic procedures are associated with similar lengths of stay and perioperative morbidity. A systematic review of minimally invasive and robotic esophagectomy by Taurchini and Cuttitta[76] found no real benefit from the robotic approach. Surgeons do, however, report that robotic procedures are easier to perform and are associated with a shorter learning curve as a result of the 3D visual field created by the da Vinci system.[73]

Robotic-assisted thoracic procedures create unique challenges for the anesthetist. Patient positioning and subsequent physiologic changes are determined by the specific surgical procedure and location of pathology. Mediastinal procedures are most commonly performed in the supine position with a slight lateral tilt (30 degrees, right-side up). Hilar or lung procedures will employ a 90-degree lateral decubitus position.[74,75] CO_2 insufflation and creation of a capnothorax is necessary to achieve adequate surgical exposure by compressing thoracic structures away from the operative field. However, as discussed in the management of robotic cardiac procedures, it is associated with significant hemodynamic instability and respiratory compromise. Hemodynamic instability may once again be prevented by the administration of fluid boluses to raise the CVP to approximately 10 mm Hg prior to creation of the capnothorax. In addition, the capnothorax

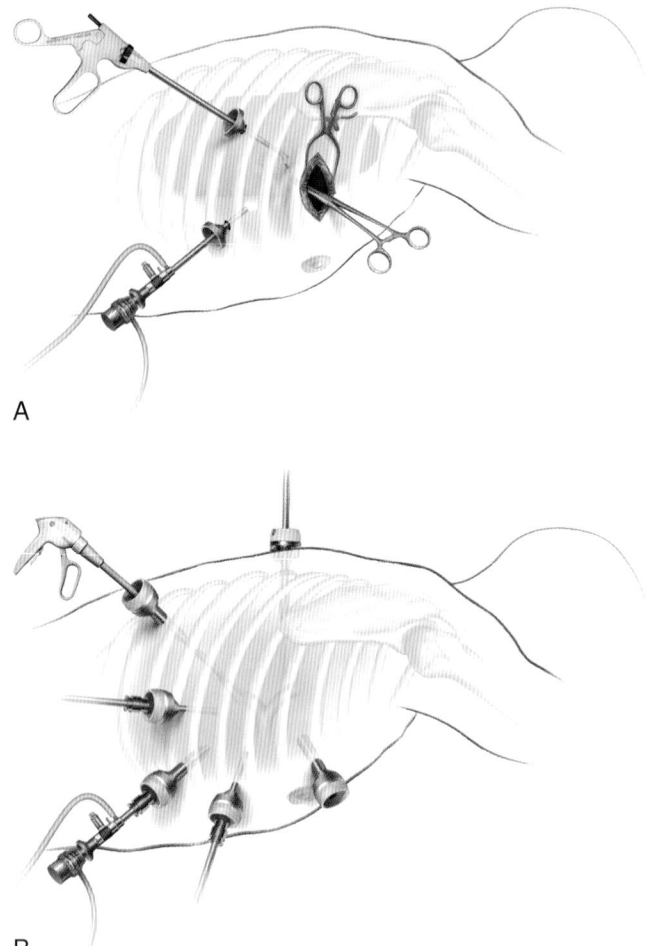

A

B

Fig. 35.2 Comparison of video-assisted thoracic surgery (VATS) lobectomy to robotic lobectomy. The two patients shown are undergoing hilar dissection. (A) VATS resection. Three incisions are shown: one for the videoscope and the other two for the right-angle clamp and stapler. The manipulation of the instrumentation and the arcs of rotation occur outside of the chest. The fulcrum of the instrumentation occurs at the chest wall, compressing and distending the intercostal nerves. (B) Robotic resection. The arcs of rotation and management of the instrumentation for dissection are within the chest, allowing surgical dissection to occur in small spaces. (From Kernstine KH, et al. Robotic lobectomy. *Op Tech Thorac Cardiovasc Surg.* 2009;13(3):204.e1–e23.)

can be established with the implementation of 2–mm Hg incremental increases in intrathoracic pressure. Vasopressors and inotropic agents may be necessary if ventricular dysfunction occurs.

Although robotic video-assisted thoracic surgery (RVATS) may offer some advantages, it is not without its potential risks. When compared with a standard VATS approach, patients undergoing RVATS procedures had increased rates of chylothorax and recurrent laryngeal nerve injury.[77] This may be due to several factors, including the use of more aggressive surgical lymph node dissection and increased use of electrocautery. Meticulous airway manipulation and assessment of vocal cord motion is necessary following these procedures. A comparison of a VATS and robotic lobectomy techniques is shown in Fig. 35.2.

General Surgical Procedures

Robotic surgical techniques have been employed in general surgery since the introduction of the earliest robotic systems. Currently, almost all gastrointestinal procedures can be successfully competed

utilizing robotic techniques, including cholecystectomy, gastrectomy, and colon resection. Advocates of general surgical robotic procedures cite improvements in 3D imaging and easier surgical manipulation, resulting in smaller surgical incisions with minimal activation of the stress response.[78] However, studies evaluating the efficacy of these procedures do not demonstrate improved patient outcomes.[79-81] When compared with traditional laparoscopic approaches, robotic general surgical techniques are not associated with a lower incidence of major or minor morbidity. However, they are associated with significantly longer operative times and significantly higher total costs.[81,82] There are also no demonstrable differences in estimated blood loss, rates of conversion to an open repair, or overall length of hospital stay. These results may be a deterrent to the long-term viability of these procedures in the general surgical population.

Anesthetic management for robotic general surgery must take into consideration the impact of patient positioning and pneumoperitoneum on hemodynamics and ventilation. Patients should have adequate intravenous access. As in most surgical cases, both arms are tucked to their respective left and right side and may restrict access. It is prudent to have a second large-bore (minimum 18G) intravenous line in place, should fluid resuscitation become necessary. The decision to use invasive hemodynamic monitoring is made on a case-by-case basis and depends on the patient's underlying comorbidities. An orogastric tube is placed to decompress the stomach, and a Foley catheter is usually inserted to monitor urinary output if the procedure will last longer than 2 hours. Maintenance of normothermia is achieved utilizing standard techniques.

Gynecologic Procedures

Robotic techniques are increasingly employed in gynecologic laparoscopic surgery because these procedures are performed in an extremely confined space (the female pelvis). With traditional laparoscopic techniques, complex surgical tasks can be difficult to perform due to limited freedom of movement and dexterity. The enhanced dexterity of the seven degrees of freedom provided by the current da Vinci system allows the surgeon to perform finer dissection, removal, and/or repair of these tissues.[18] Despite the perceived improvement in surgical technique, there is little evidence to demonstrate the superiority of robotic procedures over traditional laparoscopic techniques in this patient population.[83,84] Robotic gynecologic procedures take significantly longer at a significantly increased cost but do not demonstrate a statistically significant difference in estimated blood loss or length of hospital stay. In addition, both robotic and traditional laparoscopic techniques are associated with few major complications, similar postoperative pain scores, and similar time to resumption of normal daily activities compared to open techniques, which may not justify the increased cost associated with these procedures.[83,84] Anesthetic management of patients undergoing these procedures is similar to the general surgical population. Careful attention must be paid to the effects of steep Trendelenburg position and CO_2 insufflation on hemodynamics and ventilation. A large proportion of patients undergoing robotic gynecologic procedures are morbidly obese, and TAP blocks have been used successfully to decrease postoperative pain and minimize opioid consumption.[85]

Urologic Procedures

One of the earliest specialties to successfully employ robotic-assisted surgical techniques was urology. Wolfram et al.[86] demonstrated the safety and efficacy of this procedure in 2000. Since then, the robotic-assisted laparoscopic prostatectomy (RALP) has become one of the most common robotic procedures performed worldwide. Evidence suggests that RALP is associated with less blood loss and shorter length of stay, but a higher cost, when compared with open procedures.[87] However, the data regarding the superiority of the procedure in reducing urinary incontinence and impotency are conflicting.

The anesthetic management for patients undergoing RALP is similar to the open or laparoscopic procedures and takes into consideration the potential for significant blood loss, use of pneumoperitoneum, and hemodynamic/ventilatory changes associated with the utilization of steep Trendelenburg position. Both arms are tucked to the side and inaccessible once the robot is docked. Intravenous fluid administration should routinely be limited to less than 1 L until after the reanastomosis of the urethra is complete.

Robotic-assisted laparoscopic prostatectomy is performed in the steep Trendelenburg lithotomy position with both arms tucked to maximize surgical exposure. This position creates the potential for the patient to slide cephalad on the operating table, causing dermal injury and altering the position of the extremities, which can result in peripheral nerve damage. In addition, there is a risk of damage to abdominal wall and intraabdominal structures because the fixed robotic arms can put unintended traction on underlying tissues. The patient's position should be checked frequently and adjusted as needed. Whereas shoulder restraints or braces may appear to be a desirable option to prevent movement, their use has been associated with the development of brachial plexus injury and is not recommended.[88]

As noted earlier, the utilization of the steep Trendelenburg position in conjunction with the creation of the pneumoperitoneum also creates challenges for management of ventilation and hemodynamics. Pneumoperitoneum is associated with an increase in intraabdominal pressure, which can create significant hemodynamic changes that can be compounded if excessive perioperative bleeding occurs (see Chapter 34). Systemic absorption of CO_2 results in the development of hypercarbia, requiring compensatory increased minute ventilation. This can be accomplished successfully using either volume-controlled or pressure-controlled ventilation. The choice is dependent on the patient's underlying physiology and practitioner preference. Patients undergoing RALP are also at increased risk for the development of venous air embolism if insufflation pressures exceed venous pressures in the presence of active bleeding. Evidence of subclinical gas embolism has been reported in 17% of patients undergoing RALP.[89] Finally, prolonged steep Trendelenburg and abdominal insufflation can result in increases in ICP, placing the patient at risk for ocular complications, including visual defects and POVL.[36,90,91]

Head and Neck Procedures

As in all other surgical subspecialties, there has been a trend to employ robotic techniques in head and neck (HEENT) surgery to minimize surgical morbidity and improve cosmetic results. The first transoral robotic surgery (TORS) was performed in 2005 to resect a neoplasm at the base of the tongue.[92] Since then, robotic systems have been successfully used in transoral, transaxillary, and retroauricular approaches to head and neck pathology to perform tonsillectomy, thyroidectomy, radical neck dissection, and resection of early-stage squamous cell cancers. Several studies have shown comparable outcomes, similar rates of complications, and higher cosmetic satisfaction in patients undergoing robotic versus traditional HEENT surgical procedures.[93-95] Anesthetic management for patients undergoing these procedures is similar to the traditional approaches and is guided by the patient's underlying pathophysiology, considerations of a shared airway, and the need for perioperative nerve monitoring. Care should be taken to avoid postoperative sedation, manage severe pain, and control nausea and vomiting to minimize anesthesia recovery time and overall hospital length of stay.[96]

Orthopedic Procedures

The utilization of robotic systems in orthopedic surgery is in its infancy. Currently, the MAKO Tactile Guidance System (TGS; MAKO Surgical Corporation, Fort Lauderdale, FL) is used in many operating rooms to facilitate robotically assisted arthroplasty, including unicompartmental knee and total hip arthroplasty.[97] This system requires active participation of the surgeon and relies upon preoperative computed tomography scan imaging to create a 3D model of the knee for use by the surgeon in planning the placement of prosthetic components. These techniques have the advantage of increased surgical accuracy, optimization of component positioning, reduced complications, and improved functional outcomes.[97-99] The anesthetic management of robotic-assisted orthopedic procedures does not differ from the conventional approach.

Robotic surgical techniques have also been introduced for use in spine procedures. Early evidence of its use in the placement of pedicle screws during instrumented spinal fusions demonstrates an acceptable and consistent level of accuracy.[100] However, the impacts on radiation exposure, surgical time, and hospital length of stay are unknown. Continued use of these techniques will be needed to assess short- and long-term patient outcomes.

SUMMARY

Robotic technology continues to improve exponentially, and as a result, it can be expected to be used in an increasing number and type of surgical procedures. Whereas the outcome data to date do not demonstrate a clear advantage of robotic procedures over traditional approaches, this may change with improved accuracy, decreased operative time, and reduced costs. Providing safe and effective anesthesia care requires the anesthetist to understand the challenges associated with robotic surgical techniques and to develop a plan of care that maximizes patient outcomes.

REFERENCES

For a complete list of references for this chapter, scan this QR code with any smartphone code reader app, or visit the following URL: http://booksite.elsevier.com/9780323711944/.

36

Musculoskeletal System Anatomy, Physiology, Pathophysiology, and Anesthesia Management

Mary C. Karlet

Somatic musculature is broadly classified into three compartments—skeletal, cardiac, and smooth—based on the muscles' anatomic and functional roles. Force generated by all these muscle types depends on the transient elevation of intracellular calcium (Ca^{2+}) and activation of actin and myosin filaments. Skeletal muscle is striated in appearance. It is largely, but not always, under voluntary control. Smooth muscle is found in blood vessels and most internal organs (except the heart), is under involuntary autonomic control, and lacks striations. Cardiac muscle is striated in appearance and under control of an intrinsic pacemaker modulated by the autonomic nervous system.[1,2] The focus of this chapter is skeletal muscle, its function, and its neurologic control.

Examples of skeletal muscle tissue include muscles of the tongue, pharynx and larynx, the extrinsic eye muscles, intercostal muscles and the diaphragm in the chest, the muscles that move the scalp, and all muscles attached to the skeleton. The esophagus is unique. It is the only organ in the body that contains a mixture of smooth and skeletal muscle. The upper 2 to 4 cm of the esophagus is entirely skeletal; the middle, a mixture of skeletal and smooth muscle; and the lower 11 cm or so is entirely smooth muscle. Some skeletal muscles serve as sphincters, such as the upper esophageal sphincter, the external urethral sphincter, and the external anal sphincter. The lower esophageal sphincter is smooth muscle.[3]

Skeletal muscles of the thorax, abdomen, and extremities are innervated by myelinated efferent motor nerve fibers called alpha (α) motor neurons. These fast-conducting somatic fibers arise from cell bodies located in the ventral horn of the spinal cord gray matter (Fig. 36.1).[2]

The motor nerve axon exits through the spinal cord ventral root and travels uninterrupted to the muscle through a mixed peripheral nerve. Inputs to the ventral horn motor nerve cell body are both excitatory and inhibitory. The inputs include neurons from the brain, neurons from other spinal cord segments, and afferent neurons from various sensory receptors. A motor neuron fires an action potential when the sum of the excitatory inputs depolarizes the nerve cell body to its critical threshold potential, leading to depolarization and action potential propagation down the axon.

At the muscle, each motor nerve divides into branches that enter the muscle and end on individual muscle cells called muscle fibers. A single motor neuron and all the muscle fibers it innervates are collectively called a motor unit (Fig. 36.2). When a motor nerve fires, all the fibers within a single motor unit contract simultaneously.

Each motor unit usually contains between 100 and 200 muscle fibers; however, the motor unit may contain as few as 2 muscle fibers for fine, delicate movements or as many as 1000 for coarse movements.[1,2]

The strength of a muscle contraction is determined in large part by the number of motor units stimulated and the frequency of the stimulation. A minimal stimulus applied to a muscle may cause only a few muscle units to contract, with a weak overall response. As the stimulus is increased, more units are recruited, and a greater contraction of the muscle occurs.

OVERVIEW OF NEUROMUSCULAR TRANSMISSION

Skeletal muscles are normally relaxed and do not contract without nervous stimulation. At rest, the electrical potential difference across the muscle membrane is approximately −90 mV (inside negative). There is a high potassium ion (K^+) concentration inside the muscle cell and a high sodium ion (Na^+) concentration outside the cell.

The specialized conduction area, or synapse, where the axon of a motor neuron ends on a skeletal muscle fiber is called the neuromuscular junction (NMJ), or myoneural junction. The process of muscle contraction begins when the electrical activity of a presynaptic motor neuron communicates across this junctional cleft, or synaptic gap, to postsynaptic skeletal muscle fibers. Each skeletal muscle fiber usually has only one neuromuscular junction. The mediator substance that chemically transduces the axon's electrical message across the synaptic gap to the muscle is the neurotransmitter acetylcholine (ACh).[1,2,4]

Muscle contraction develops when the propagated action potential of the presynaptic motor neuron induces release of the chemical mediator ACh into the junctional cleft. ACh binds to specialized receptors on the postsynaptic muscle membrane. If released from the axon nerve ending in sufficient quantity, ACh-receptor (AChR) occupation induces a transient change in the electrical property of the skeletal muscle membrane, and an action potential and muscle contraction follow.[1,2,4]

In the overall process of neuromuscular transmission, a motor nerve electrical signal (action potential) is converted to a chemical signal (ACh), which generates an electrical signal (action potential) in muscle. ACh molecules bind to receptors on an area of the muscle called the motor endplate, which evokes an action potential in the muscle membrane. As described in greater detail in the following sections, the result of muscle membrane depolarization is muscle contraction.

Neuromuscular Junction

Motor nerve endings develop in intimate and precise proximity to skeletal muscle fibers forming a highly efficient communication unit.[5,6] The motor axon terminal is separated from the muscle cell it innervates by a synaptic gap of about 50 nm.[2] This anatomic alliance increases the likelihood for prompt receptor activation after transmitter release.[7-9]

The NMJ synaptic gap is contiguous with the extracellular fluid. The gap contains a structured matrix called the basal lamina, which

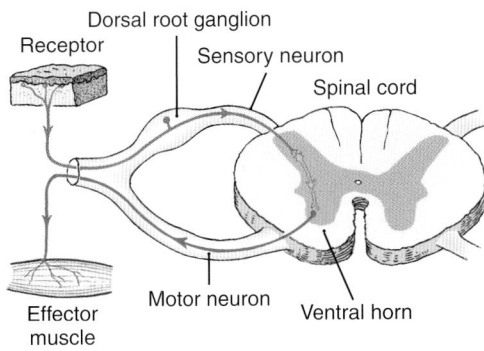

Fig. 36.1 Spinal reflex arc. Sensory information from the skin is relayed to the motor neuron in the ventral horn of the spinal cord gray matter.

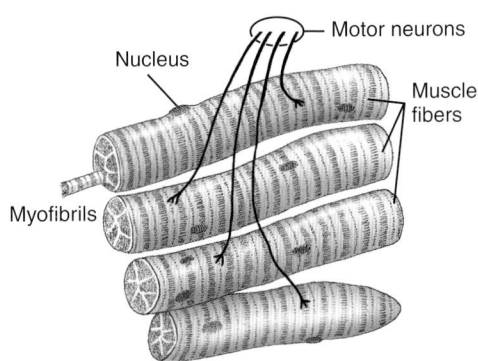

Fig. 36.2 A motor unit. One motor neuron can synapse with several muscle fibers, which contract as a unit.

facilitates robust synaptic transmission. Extracellular communication with the NMJ provides a route for drugs or toxins to gain access to the NMJ. Botulinum toxin, for example, gains access to the junction through the extracellular fluid and produces its depressive neuromuscular effects by inhibiting ACh release from the nerve ending.[2,10-13]

Both sides of the NMJ—the presynaptic motor axon and the postsynaptic muscle cell—serve specialized functions. As it nears the neuromuscular junction, the motor nerve axon loses its myelin sheath and divides into many smaller nerve fibers, which terminate as end-feet or terminal boutons.

The motor nerve end-foot is distinct from the rest of the nerve. It is rich in mitochondria and the materials and support structures necessary for the synthesis, storage, mobilization, and release of the neurotransmitter ACh. Small vesicles or quanta of concentrated ACh are particularly numerous in the part of the nerve ending closest to the junctional gap.[2] ACh is concentrated in the vesicles by an ACh-H[+] exchange pump. The ACh vesicles converge along the junctional surface of the nerve end-feet in areas called active zones.[11,14-16]

At the neuromuscular junction, each motor nerve ending closely approximates with a thickened and highly convoluted portion of the postsynaptic membrane called the motor endplate. The motor endplate is physically and functionally demarcated from the surrounding muscle membrane. The many membrane convolutions at the endplate are known as junctional folds or junctional clefts.[2,7] ACh receptors are concentrated near the shoulders of the junctional folds, lying near the ACh release sites. The close approximation of ACh release site and target receptor site ensures little transmitter waste and direct coupling of nerve signal and muscle response.[2,7] Fig. 36.3 summarizes the anatomy and dynamic function of the neuromuscular junction

The development and clustering of ACh receptors at the motor endplate near the ACh "active zones" are the result of the interaction

of synaptogenic factors such as agrin, muscle-specific tyrosine kinase (MuSK), and low-density lipoprotein receptor-related protein-4 (Lrp4).[6] As will be described later in this chapter, defects in these factors that promote healthy synapse formation are responsible for some forms of myasthenia gravis.[15]

Acetylcholine Release

Physiologic transmission of the nerve message to the muscle begins with Ca^{2+}-dependent ACh release from the nerve terminal. When a nerve impulse arrives at a motor nerve ending, the action potential causes a transient increase in Ca^{2+} conductance across the nerve membrane by activating voltage-gated Ca^{2+} channels. It is primarily the fast (P/Q-type) Ca^{2+} channels that are involved in depolarization-induced transmitter release.[2,11] Calcium enters the nerve terminal and diffuses down its electrochemical gradient. The influx of Ca^{2+} causes ACh vesicles to fuse with the nerve plasma membrane and then expel their content into the synaptic cleft.[7,11,17] The amount of ACh released is influenced by the amount of Ca^{2+} that enters the nerve terminal during nerve stimulation. The more Ca^{2+} that enters the nerve terminal, the greater the amount of ACh released. Hypocalcemia therefore can decrease ACh release from the presynaptic nerve ending.

About 150 to 300 ACh vesicles, or quanta, are released with each nerve impulse. Each individual quantum in turn contains about 10,000 ACh molecules of the neurotransmitter.[4,16] This amount of ACh and the normal abundance of postjunctional receptors at each NMJ readily ensure muscle activation. A 10-fold safety margin typically exists in normal synaptic transmission. With each nerve impulse, excess ACh is released, and excess ACh receptors are available for occupation.

Small concentrations of other divalent cations can compete with and limit Ca^{2+} influx into the nerve ending, decreasing ACh release and impairing neuromuscular transmission. When administered intravenously, magnesium sulfate, for example, can interfere with Ca^{2+} influx and produce muscle weakness by inhibiting ACh release. Aminoglycoside antibiotics also inhibit voltage-gated Ca^{2+} channels and ACh release at the NMJ and can enhance neuromuscular blockade when administered concomitant with clinical dosages of neuromuscular blocking agents.[18]

Calcium channel–blocking drugs used for the treatment of dysrhythmias and hypertension primarily block Ca^{2+} conductance through slow (L-type) channels of the heart and blood vessels. Their primary action is on the slow Ca^{2+} channels of the heart and blood vessels, but they can inhibit NMJ prejunctional Ca^{2+} influx. The large safety margin inherent in normal neuromuscular transmission obscures any clinically detectable effect these drugs may have on neuromuscular transmission. However, with disorders associated with impaired neuromuscular transmission, such as Lambert-Eaton myasthenic syndrome, the Ca^{2+} channel blocker's prejunctional attenuation of ACh release may be unmasked, and neuromuscular transmission may be further weakened.[4,17-19]

Acetylcholine Synthesis

Neurons that release the neurotransmitter ACh are called cholinergic neurons. Active cholinergic motor neurons replenish their ACh stores by continually resynthesizing the neurotransmitter. Many enzymes and other proteins needed by the nerve ending to synthesize, store, and release ACh are made in the motor nerve cell body and are transported distally to the nerve ending by a process called axonal transport.

In the axoplasm of the motor nerve ending, the enzyme choline acetyltransferase (CAT) catalyzes the reaction of two substrates, acetyl

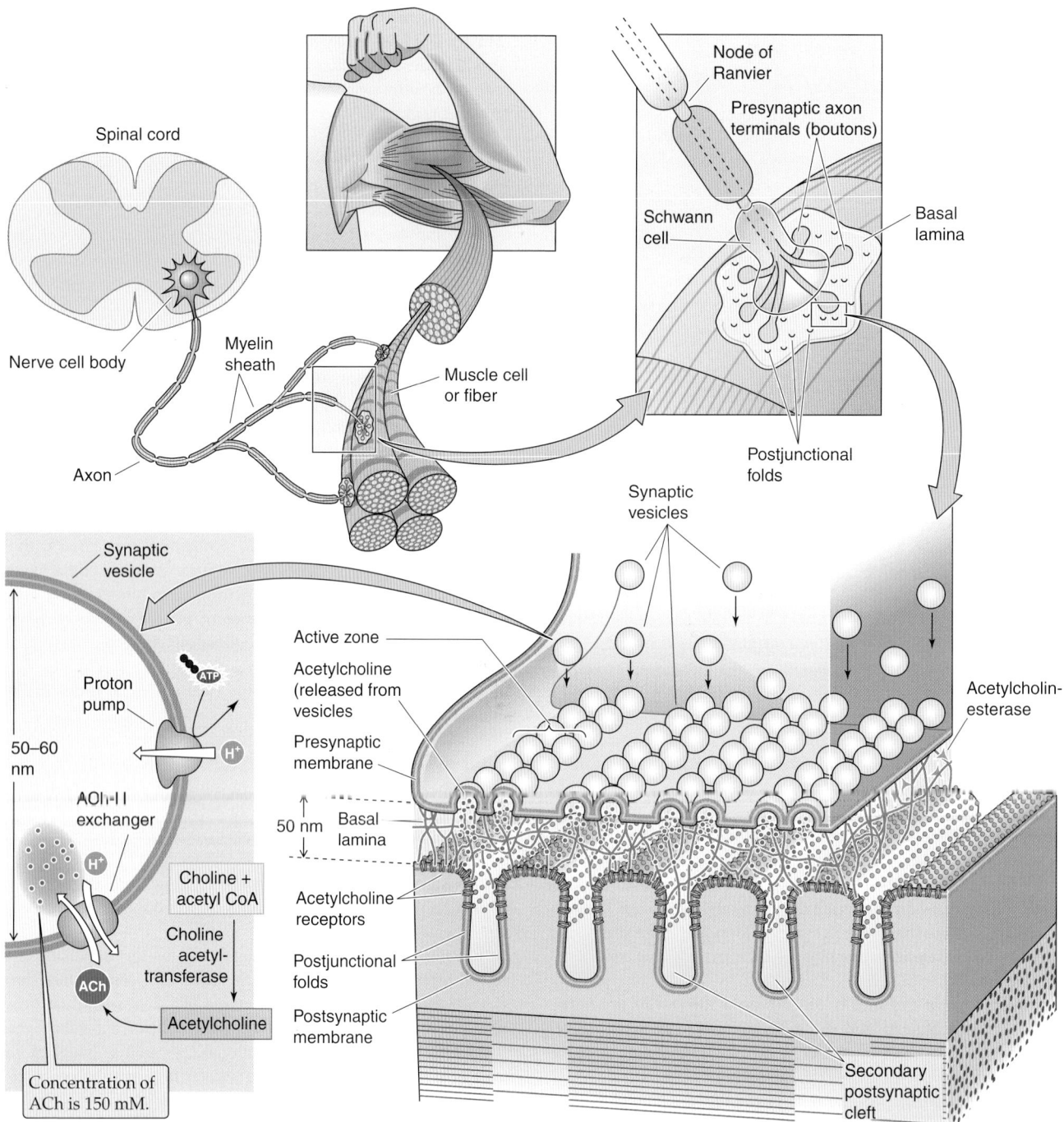

Fig. 36.3 Vertebrate neuromuscular junction or motor endplate. A motor neuron, with its cell body in the ventral horn of the spinal cord, sends out an axon that progressively bifurcates to innervate several muscle fibers (a motor unit). The neuron contacts a muscle fiber at exactly one spot, called a neuromuscular junction or motor endplate. The endplate consists of an arborization of the nerve into many presynaptic terminals, or boutons, as well as the specializations of the postsynaptic membrane. A high-magnification view of a bouton shows that the synaptic vesicles containing the neurotransmitter acetylcholine *(ACh)* cluster and line up at the active zone of the presynaptic membrane. The active zones on the presynaptic membrane are directly opposite the secondary postsynaptic clefts that are created by infoldings of the postsynaptic membrane *(postjunctional folds)*. Depolarization of the bouton causes the vesicles to fuse with the presynaptic membrane and to release their contents into the synaptic cleft. The ACh molecules must diffuse at least 50 nm before reaching nicotinic ACh receptors (AChRs). Note the high density of AChRs at the crests of the postjunctional folds. The activity of the released ACh is terminated mainly by an acetylcholinesterase. The bouton reloads its discharged synaptic vesicles by resynthesizing ACh and transporting this ACh into the vesicle via an ACh-H exchanger. *CoA,* coenzyme A. (From Boron WF, Boulpaep EL. *Concise Medical Physiology.* 1st ed. Philadelphia: Elsevier; 2022:94.)

coenzyme A (acetyl CoA) and choline, to form ACh, as seen in the following equation:

$$Choline + Acetyl\ CoA \rightarrow ACh + CoA$$

Choline is obtained locally by a Na^+-linked uptake into the cholinergic nerve ending. Acetyl CoA is synthesized from pyruvate in neuronal mitochondria. Mitochondria and other metabolic machinery used to synthesize ACh are abundant in the nerve ending (Fig. 36.4).

Each nerve ending contains more than 100,000 ACh vesicles.[2,7] A small percentage of these vesicles are positioned for rapid release "immediately available pool," while a more substantial amount is a "reserve pool" that is released more slowly. The ACh vesicles are released through exocytosis in response to action potential stimulation, but only a small fraction of the available vesicles is used to send each signal.[2,7]

Postjunctional Endplate

ACh receptors that are present at the postjuctional motor endplate are cation channels. There is a distinction between the postjunctional ACh receptor cation channels of the muscle endplate and other cation channels of nerve and muscle membranes. Motor endplate ACh channels are ligand gated—that is, they are opened or closed by the action of a chemical, ACh. Cation channels of the remaining muscle membrane, on the other hand, are voltage gated or voltage activated—that is, they open or close in response to electrical changes in the membrane.[4]

The binding of ACh molecules to postsynaptic receptors causes a transient increase in conductance in the ligand (ACh)–gated cation channels at the postjunctional motor endplate. The cation flow allows an outward current of K^+ and an inward Na^+ current. The Na^+ current predominates because it is attracted to the negative charge inside the cell. As a result, the previously polarized endplate membrane becomes transiently depolarized. The resulting postjunctional membrane voltage change is called an endplate potential (EPP).[4]

EPPs vary in strength according to the quantity of ACh released. The more ACh released, the greater the postsynaptic endplate voltage change. In other words, EPPs do not adhere to the all-or-none principle. EPPs can be summed, and their magnitude depends on the strength of the summed stimuli of ACh molecules.

The postjunctional endplate membrane does not fire action potentials. After it is depolarized by ACh-receptor occupation, the current sink created by the local EPP depolarizes the adjacent muscle membrane.[4] If the depolarizing input is great enough and reaches threshold potential, action potentials are fired from either side of the endplate in both directions along the muscle fiber (Fig. 36.5).

The transition zone where the potential developed at the endplate is converted to an action potential is called the perijunctional area. A demarcation exists between the chemically sensitive AChR channels of the endplate and the chemically insensitive but electrically sensitive Na^+ channels in the perijunctional area of the muscle membrane.

With a typical motor neuron's action potential, the EPP produced at the muscle endplate is usually sufficient to create an action potential at the muscle membrane, and muscle contraction is regularly produced.

Acetylcholine Receptor

Postjunctional neuromuscular ACh receptors have been extensively purified and their complex architecture studied in detail.[7,8,15,16,20] Approximately 30 million tightly packed nicotinic AChRs are at each neuromuscular junction.[3]

In fetal muscle, the ACh nicotinic receptor is a protein composed of five polypeptide subunits: two identical alpha (α) subunits, a beta (β) subunit, a gamma (γ) subunit, and a delta (δ) subunit, surrounding a central cation channel (Fig. 36.6). As described later in this chapter,

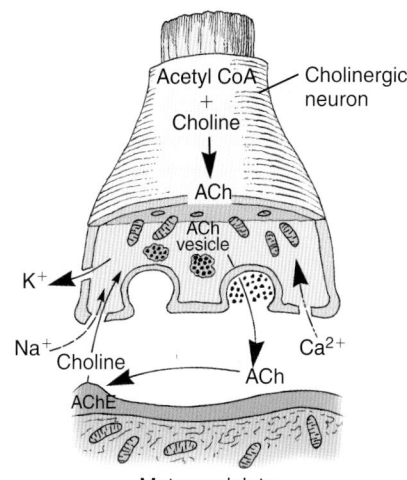

Fig. 36.4 Acetylcholine *(ACh)* synthesis from choline and acetyl coenzyme A *(acetyl CoA)* in the motor nerve ending. Calcium ion entry into the nerve ending causes the ACh vesicles to release their contents. Acetylcholinesterase *(AChE)* on the postjunctional membrane destroys ACh. Choline is recycled into the nerve ending by a sodium ion-linked transport mechanism.

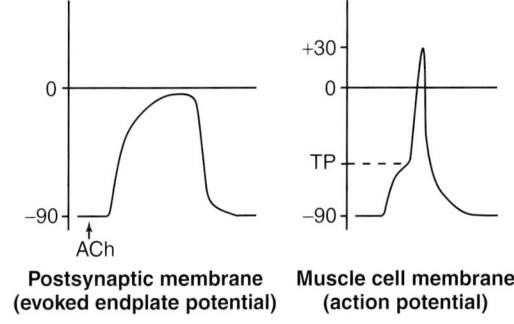

Fig. 36.5 Depiction of the depolarization characteristics (the endplate potential or generator potential) at the postsynaptic membrane in response to acetylcholine *(ACh)* occupation and the depolarization and action-potential response at the adjacent, electrically excitable muscle membrane. *TP*, Threshold potential.

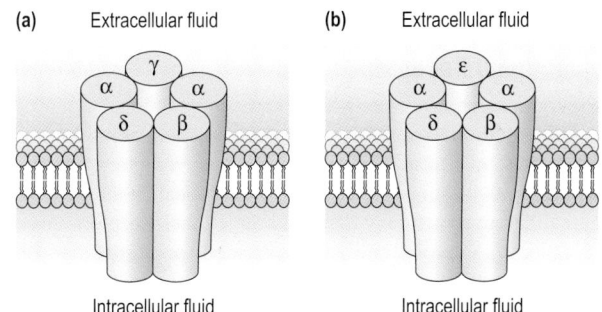

Fig. 36.6 (A) The receptor consists of (α)2, β, γ, and δ subunits in the fetal form, and (B) (α)2, β, δ, and ε subunits in the adult form. (From Shamley D. *Pathophysiology.* Philadelphia: Butterworth-Heinemann; 2005.)

the fetal subunit composition (α2βγδ) is also present at nonjunctional regions of denervated adult skeletal muscle.[7]

In adults, the AChR protein structure is similar, except that the fetal gamma subunit is replaced by an epsilon (ε) subunit.[7,8,20] The change produces an adult cholinergic postjunctional AChR (α2βεδ) that has an increased cation conductance, a shortened open time, and higher density at the NMJ.[21]

As noted earlier, the ACh receptors are clustered at the crests of the motor endplate junctional folds, which directly align with nerve terminal release sites. In active adults, only the endplate region of the muscle contains ACh receptors.[16] As little as 200 μm away from the endplate, the muscle membrane becomes practically devoid of receptors.

The ACh receptors are synthesized in the muscle cells and then incorporated into the endplate membrane as integral membrane proteins. The extracellular or junctional face of the receptor protrudes from the surface of the endplate membrane, whereas the cytoplasmic surface of the receptor is more flush to the plasma membrane surface. The proteins MuSK, Lrp4, and agrin mediate clustering of nicotinic acetylcholine receptors during NMJ formation and have critical roles in signaling between motor neurons and skeletal muscle.[22]

Activation of postjunctional AChRs and opening of AChR cation channels requires simultaneous ACh occupation at *each* of the *two* α-receptor subunits. The binding of two ACh molecules causes a conformational change in the alpha polypeptides, and the protein conformational change causes the AChR central ion channel to open.[7,8,20] If only one alpha subunit site is occupied by the agonist (ACh), the channel remains closed. As described earlier, the open channel increases the conductance to positively charged ions, particularly Na^+, an effect that produces the net depolarizing potential, the EPP. When even one ACh molecule leaves an alpha subunit, the channel snaps shut and the current stops. The opening (1 ms) and closing events are extremely fast, enabling rapid initiation and termination of the postsynaptic response.[16]

When ACh is present on the α-receptor subunit for an extended period (>20 ms), the ACh receptor may convert to a desensitized or nonconducting state.[8,16,23] Desensitization is of little consequence for normal neuromuscular transmission, but this property may contribute to the neuromuscular blocking effects of the depolarizing muscle relaxant succinylcholine, as described in Chapter 12. The alpha subunits are sites of competition between the cholinergic agonist ACh and receptor antagonists, such as nondepolarizing neuromuscular blocking agents. The outcome of the competition—neuromuscular transmission or neuromuscular blockade—depends on the concentration of ACh and the relative concentration and binding properties of the antagonist involved. Nondepolarizing muscle relaxants produce neuromuscular blockade in part because they bind to one or both alpha subunit sites and, in so doing, prevent ACh from binding to both sites and opening the channel.

Prejunctional Receptors

Cholinergic receptors are also present at the prejunctional motor nerve ending. In addition to mediating nerve transmission at postjunctional receptor sites, ACh also acts on prejunctional receptors to enhance transmitter mobilization and release. Prejunctional cholinergic receptors are different structurally than adult junctional receptors, containing 3 alpha (α) subunits, and 2 beta (β) subunits. Stimulation of the prejunctional receptors is believed to transform the motor nerve ACh pool from a reserve store to a readily releasable store so that transmitter output can keep pace with transmitter demand.[17] As a result, repeated stimulation leads to increased amount of transmitter release.

All the nondepolarizing muscle relaxants used in anesthesia practice compete with ACh for postjunctional cholinergic receptor sites to produce neuromuscular blockade. Receptor antagonist effects at prejunctional receptors may augment nondepolarizing blockade by diminishing ACh output as well. Herein also lies an explanation for the fade that is observed with neuromuscular blockade monitoring of nondepolarizing muscle relaxants. Fade of tetanic and train-of-four

stimulation may, at least in part, reflect the blockade of prejunctional ACh receptors by the muscle relaxant and failure of ACh release to keep pace with rapid stimulation.[24,25]

Acetylcholinesterase

As noted earlier, the combination of ACh with its muscle endplate receptor causes a transitory depolarization of the endplate. The EPP is short lived because soon after binding, ACh is rapidly destroyed by hydrolysis, and its depolarizing action halts.[4] Paradoxically, the rapid destruction and removal of ACh from the junctional cleft is critical for continued muscle contractile response. The ACh molecule must be off the muscle endplate receptor for the perijunctional muscle membrane to repolarize, or reset, in anticipation of further activation.

The hydrolysis of ACh to choline and acetate is rapid and efficient. Most ACh is destroyed within a few milliseconds after it is released into the junctional cleft.[2] The enzyme acetylcholinesterase (AChE), also known as true or tissue cholinesterase, catalyzes the hydrolysis. AChE is present in high concentrations on the external surface of the postjunctional muscle membranes.

$$\text{Acetylcholine} \xrightarrow{\text{Acetylcholinesterase}} \text{Choline} + \text{Acetate}$$

Much of the choline byproduct released by hydrolysis is efficiently drawn back within the prejunctional nerve terminal for use in the synthesis of new ACh.

Without AChE, the concentration of ACh would become extremely high in the junctional cleft. Under these circumstances, ACh would maintain the muscle endplate in a state of persistent depolarization, yet the muscle itself would be paralyzed.[7,23] The reason for this seemingly illogical behavior (ACh-receptor occupation, endplate depolarization, yet no muscle contraction) is that in the face of persistent endplate depolarization, the Na^+ channels of the perijunctional muscle membrane do not reactivate or reset; these voltage-gated ion channels remain closed, impeding further muscle membrane depolarization. Thus, even with persistent endplate depolarization, muscle contraction is prevented, and clinical weakness follows. A cyclic muscle membrane depolarization/repolarization sequence is necessary for normal muscle contraction to occur.

The mechanism of depolarizing muscle relaxants may, at least in part, be explained by a similar mechanism. Depolarizing muscle relaxants, such as succinylcholine, activate the muscle endplate in a manner similar to that of ACh, but they have a more protracted endplate depolarizing response because they are less rapidly metabolized. AChR occupation by a depolarizing muscle relaxant causes a prolonged depolarization of the endplate, prohibits activation of perijunctional channels, and produces a depolarizing block.[7,23]

Reversal of a nondepolarizing neuromuscular block may be accomplished by the use of cholinesterase inhibitors. Anticholinesterase agents inhibit the breakdown of ACh and, in so doing, increase the amount of ACh at the NMJ. The abundance of ACh in the synaptic gap changes the agonist:antagonist ratio and enables the agonist (ACh) to bind to the ACh receptor with greater frequency than the antagonist (nondepolarizing muscle relaxant). Hence a higher ACh concentration can overcome the receptor occupation by the muscle relaxant, and neuromuscular transmission can be restored.

Various other esterases, in addition to AChE, are present throughout the body. One that is found in the plasma is pseudocholinesterase, or nonspecific cholinesterase. Like AChE, pseudocholinesterase is capable of hydrolyzing ACh, but it also has properties separate from those of AChE. One distinction particularly relevant to anesthesia practice is the ability of pseudocholinesterase to metabolize ester local anesthetics and the depolarizing muscle relaxant succinylcholine.

Extrajunctional Receptors

In utero, before muscle innervation occurs, the muscle cells of a fetus synthesize what are termed immature, fetal, or extrajunctional receptors. These fetal receptors (γAChRs) are inserted over the entire length of the muscle cell. As the fetal NMJ develops, increasing motor nerve activity has a trophic effect in restricting the ACh receptors specifically to the NMJ.[8] As the nerve-muscle contact becomes active and matures, extrajunctional receptors disappear from the peripheral part of the muscle. If neural activity is reduced or abolished and the neural trophic influence is lost, the muscle resorts to fetal-like synthesis of γAChRs.[11,12,26]

Several situations, including stroke, spinal cord transection, thermal trauma, direct muscle damage, and prolonged immobility, have been associated with the accelerated spread of γAChRs to large areas of the skeletal muscle membrane.[11,12,26-28] These so-called denervation injuries result in an abnormal excitability of the muscle and an increase in muscle sensitivity to ACh, a condition that is called denervation hypersensitivity.[29] The extrajunctional receptors may develop within 24 to 48 hours after diminution of nerve activity. Eventually, the number of aberrant receptors per muscle fiber may increase 5- to 32-fold.[29] These receptors disappear, and muscle sensitivity returns to normal if neural input is reestablished. Extrajunctional and endplate cholinergic receptors are similar in many ways, but an important distinction pertinent to anesthesia practice is their differing response to receptor agonists and antagonists.

Clinically, extrajunctional receptors demonstrate resistance to nondepolarizing muscle relaxants. Hence larger doses of nondepolarizing relaxants may be necessary to induce neuromuscular blockade (e.g., in an immobilized limb or in parts of the body affected by a stroke).[25,26] Monitoring a nondepolarizing neuromuscular block with a peripheral nerve stimulator in a paretic limb may result in an underestimating of the magnitude of neuromuscular blockade in nonparetic muscles.[30]

Conversely, extrajunctional receptors are more easily activated by agonists (e.g., ACh, succinylcholine) than junctional receptors. Moreover, each extrajunctional channel stays open 4 to 10 times longer than junctional receptors, allowing more ions to flow (primarily Na^+ into the muscle cell and K^+ out) in response to agonist-induced depolarization.

The clinical significance of denervation injuries and the proliferation of extrajunctional receptors becomes evident with the administration of succinylcholine, which can produce alarmingly high levels of plasma K^+ in these patients.[26,28] Due to its molecular similarity to ACh, succinylcholine depolarizes both postsynaptic and extrajunctional receptors. Succinylcholine-induced hyperkalemia reflects the extensive proliferation of extrajunctional receptors along the entire muscle membrane and their prolonged and exaggerated depolarization response to agonists. Succinylcholine stimulates the aberrant cholinergic receptors and triggers a protracted opening of the cation channels, allowing excess Na^+ movement into the cell and excess K^+ movement out, down their respective gradients.

Dangerous levels of succinylcholine-induced hyperkalemia have been observed after denervation injury with doses of succinylcholine as low as 20 mg.[26] The pronounced release of K^+ in response to succinylcholine cannot be circumvented by the prior administration of nonparalyzing doses of nondepolarizing muscle relaxants.

MUSCLE PHYSIOLOGY

Skeletal muscle constitutes the greatest mass of somatic musculature. Skeletal muscle is composed of bundles of multinucleated, long cylindric cells, called muscle fibers, that typically extend the entire length of a muscle.[31] Each muscle fiber is a single cell surrounded by an electrically polarized cell membrane called the sarcolemma. The

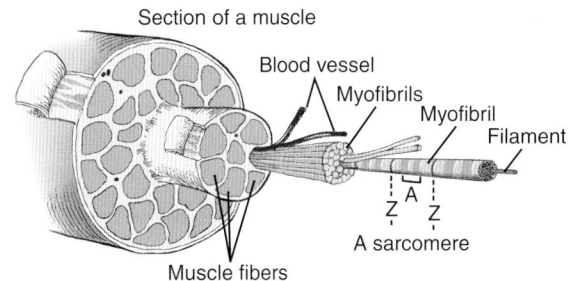

Fig. 36.7 The structural arrangement and organization at each level of the muscle assembly. The skeletal muscle is composed of muscle fibers that contain long, cylindric myofibrils. Each myofibril is made up of precisely arranged thick and thin filaments that form repeating dark and light bands called sarcomeres.

sarcolemma separates the extracellular space from the myoplasm, the muscle-fiber intracellular space. Dystrophin is a large rodlike protein that is located on the intracellular side of the sarcolemma. Dystrophin, in association with membrane glycoproteins, serves to stabilize the muscle membrane during contraction.[1] As will be discussed later in this chapter, disruption of dystrophin and its important structural features results in dystrophinopathies such as Duchenne muscular dystrophy.

Individual skeletal muscle cells are parallel to the muscle body and have no anatomic or functional bridges between them. The parallel arrangement helps maximize shortening capacity and velocity. The cells function independently so that the force of contraction of the total muscle is equal to the sum of individual fibers. This contrasts with smooth and cardiac muscle, in which the muscle cells are interdependent and are mechanically coupled to adjacent cells.[1,9]

Bundles of cylindric filaments called myofibrils run along the axis of the muscle fiber. Each skeletal muscle fiber contains several hundred to several thousand myofibrils. The myofibrils are composed of contractile proteins that impart a striking, repetitive light-and-dark banding pattern along the entire fiber length. The repeating unit, called a sarcomere, is the basic contractile unit of skeletal muscle. The alternating light-and-dark banding pattern is responsible for the classification called striated muscle. Cardiac muscle is also classified as striated muscle because it, too, has the repetitive pattern of light and dark bands.[1,9] The arrangement of the muscle fibers, myofibrils, and sarcomeres is shown in Fig. 36.7.

Most skeletal muscles bridge two skeletal attachment points and are recruited to generate force and movement in voluntary actions ranging from chewing to walking. A muscle contraction that involves shortening of the muscle length to perform work is an isotonic contraction. A muscle contraction that produces increased tension but no appreciable decrease in length is an isometric contraction.

Structure of the Contractile Apparatus

The repeating, striated arrangement of the myofibril arises from the contractile filaments that compose the sarcomere: the thick filaments and the thin filaments. The thick filaments, which are composed primarily of the protein myosin, are in the central region of the sarcomere. The thin filaments are about half the diameter of the thick filaments and are composed of the proteins actin, troponin, and tropomyosin. Myosin and actin filaments are responsible for the actual muscle contraction[9] (Fig. 36.8).

Cross sections of the myofibril reveal that each thick filament is surrounded by a hexagonal arrangement of thin filaments. The thick and thin filaments are arranged to slide over one another, overlap, and create shortening of the sarcomere.[9] With muscle contraction,

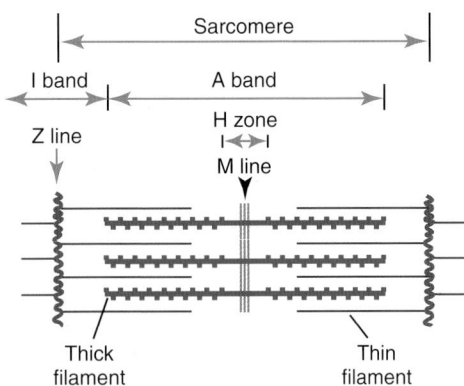

Fig. 36.8 Longitudinal diagram of a sarcomere showing the arrangement of the thick filaments (myosin) and the thin filaments (primarily actin) within the myofibril.

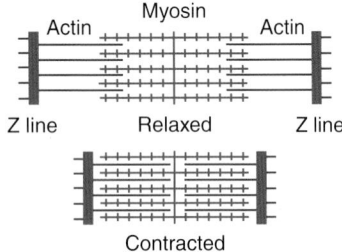

Fig. 36.9 Actin filament sliding over myosin filament during muscle contraction.

force is generated by interaction and overlap of thick and thin filaments (Fig. 36.9).

Cross-Bridge Interaction and Cycling

Sliding Filament Mechanism

Physiologic contraction of striated muscle occurs when muscle fibers are depolarized to a threshold for action potential formation. The depolarizing wave initiated by AChR occupation at the motor endplate is carried along the muscle membrane surface from one Na^+ channel to the next. Action potential depolarization of the sarcolemma spreads rapidly to the muscle cell's interior through a reticular network of intracellular tubules that are, in essence, internal extensions of the cell membrane.

This network, composed of transverse (T) tubules, forms a grid around the intracellular myofibrils and closely associates with the intracellular sarcoplasmic reticular membranes. The T tubules provide a path for the rapid transmission of the action potential from the sarcolemma to the myoplasm.[31]

The sarcoplasmic reticulum is an irregular, closed membrane structure that weaves throughout the myoplasm of the muscle cell and contains large amounts of Ca^{2+}. The sarcoplasmic reticular membrane is active in sequestering Ca^{2+} by way of numerous high-affinity Ca^{2+} active-transport carriers in its membrane. These pumps maintain a high sarcoplasmic reticular store of Ca^{2+} and a very low resting myoplasmic Ca^{2+} concentration.[9,31]

The transit of an action potential along the sarcolemma and into the T-tubule system is detected by intracellular dihydropyridine voltage sensors (DHPR). These DHPR voltage sensors are linked to calcium release channels in the sarcoplasmic reticulum. The major Ca^{2+} release channel located on the sarcoplasmic reticulum is called the ryanodine receptor (RYR). These channels are commonly called receptors because they bind the alkaloid ryanodine.[1] There is a close physical association

between DHPR and RYR. Transit of an action potential into the T-tubule system triggers a conformational change in DHPR, causing immediate opening of RYR (Fig. 36.10). When RYR opens, a favorable concentration gradient facilitates efflux of Ca2+ from the sarcoplasmic reticulum to the myoplasm.

Genetic mutations in RYR or DHPR are associated with pathologic disturbances in skeletal muscle myoplasmic Ca2+ concentrations. As we will discuss later in this chapter, defects in the RYR are a major factor contributing to malignant hyperthermia.

In response to action potential stimulation, the myoplasmic Ca^{2+} concentration rises several-fold. The overall effect is the discharge of Ca^{2+} from the terminal cisterns (rapid Ca^{2+} release sites) of the sarcoplasmic reticulum into the myoplasm by the transit of an action potential into the muscle cell.[2]

The Ca^{2+} released into the myoplasm acts as a switch to expose myosin binding sites on actin. Myosin reacts by binding to the surrounding exposed thin filament sites and forms a reversible complex with actin—the actomyosin complex. The process of myosin-actin binding in response to elevated myoplasmic Ca^{2+} is termed crossbridge formation.

When myosin binds to the actin site, it uses energy to drag the actin filaments toward the center of the sarcomere. The pull of the actin filaments accentuates the overlap of the thick and thin filaments, causing shortening of the sarcomere and culminating in muscle contraction. Cross-bridge cycling and the associated movement of actin is called the sliding filament mechanism.

If the intracellular Ca^{2+} concentration remains sufficiently high, which mainly depends on the frequency of incoming action potentials, the cycle begins again: Myosin links to actin, slides the filament, detaches, and reconnects at the next actin site.

A single sliding cycle or myosin power stroke shortens the length of the sarcomere by about 1%. The sliding cycle must be repeated about 50 times for full shortening of the muscle. The cycle continues until it is interrupted by the active removal of Ca^{2+} from the myoplasm or until adenosine triphosphate (ATP) is exhausted. Active Ca^{2+} removal from the cytoplasm back into the sarcoplasmic reticulum causes return to a configuration that prohibits myosin-actin binding, and the muscle relaxes.

The overall process by which depolarization of the muscle fiber causes Ca^{2+} release from the sarcoplasmic reticulum into the myoplasm to cause cross-bridge cycling and muscle contraction is called excitation-contraction coupling (Fig. 36.11).[2]

Box 36.1 summarizes the excitation-contraction coupling events. Box 36.2 summarizes the events leading to skeletal muscle relaxation.

Grading Contractile Force

Two major mechanisms grade skeletal muscle contractile force. One determining factor of muscle force is the number of motor units activated or recruited. With increasing voluntary effort, more and more motor units are recruited, and an increasing muscle force develops.

The other mechanism by which skeletal muscle tension is graded is by varying the frequency of the action potential discharge to the muscle. A single action potential invariably liberates sufficient Ca^{2+} ions to activate skeletal muscle contraction. The brief contraction that results from transit of a single action potential is called a twitch.[31] After a single twitch, the Ca^{2+} ions are rapidly transported back into the sarcoplasmic reticulum before the muscle has time to develop maximal tension. If a second action potential is generated before the muscle relaxes following the first action potential, the force of the second contraction is amplified. Rapidly repeated electrical impulses can cause summation of contractions and greatly increase the muscle tension. Repetitive action potentials maintain a high Ca^{2+} concentration

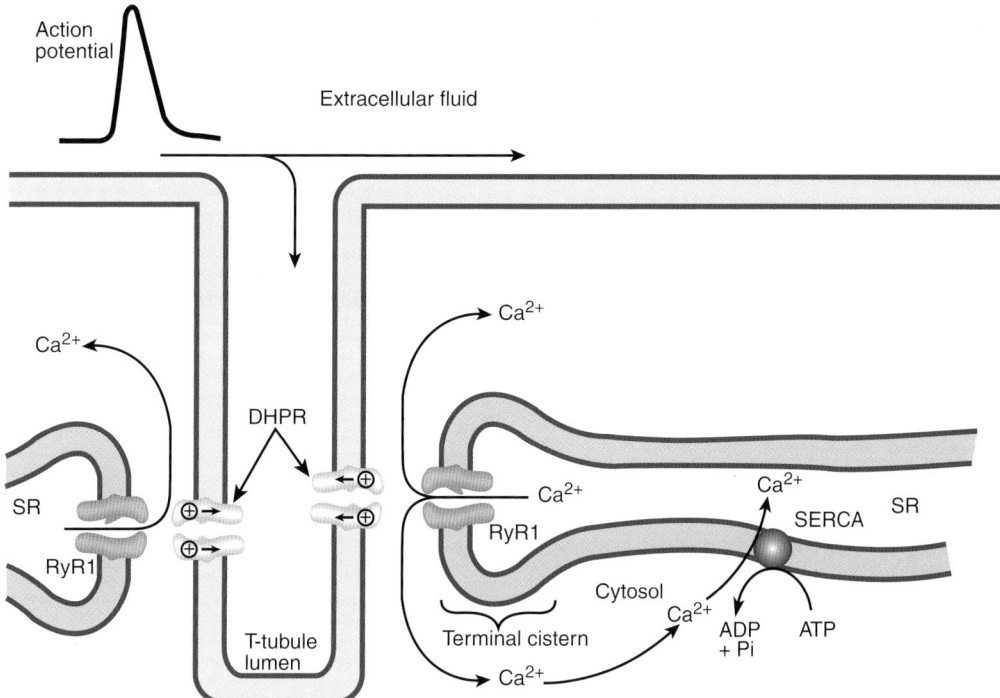

Fig. 36.10 Cellular components of excitation-contraction (E-C) coupling and relaxation in skeletal muscle. An action potential (AP) initiated at the neuromuscular junction is normally the first event in E-C coupling. The AP rapidly propagates over the sarcolemma and into the T tubules. When the T tubule is depolarized, the voltage sensors (%) in the dihydropyridine receptors *(DHPRs)* move and open the ryanodine receptors *(RyR1)*, thus permitting Ca^{2+} to flow out of the sarcoplasmic reticulum *(SR)* into the cytosol to trigger contraction. The Ca^{2+} released from the SR is subsequently returned to the SR by sarco/endoplasmic reticulum calcium-ATPase *(SERCA)* to relax the muscle. (From Blaustein MP, et al. *Cellular Physiology and Neurophysiology*. 3rd ed. Philadelphia: Elsevier; 2020:204.)

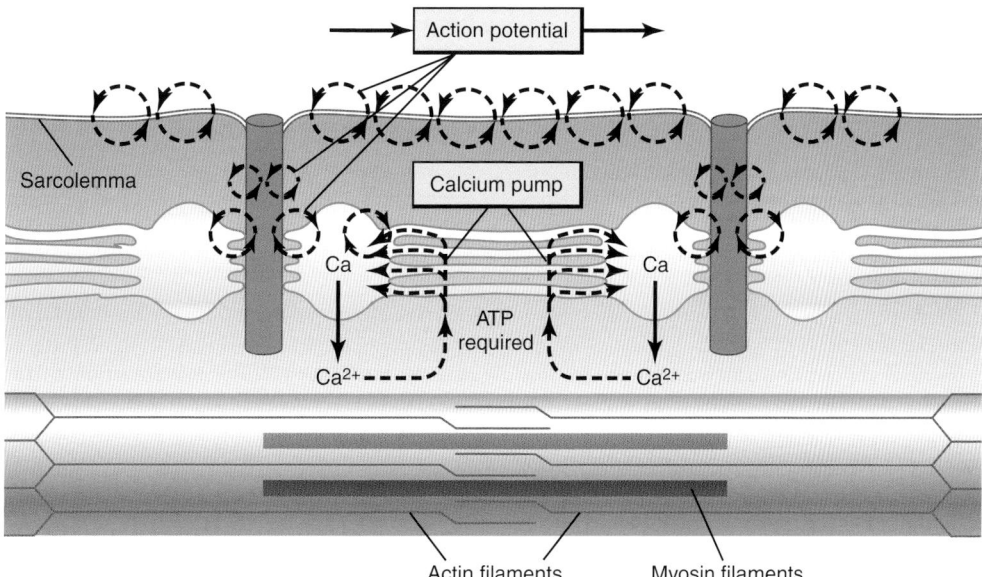

Fig. 36.11 Excitation-contraction coupling in the muscle, showing (1) an action potential that causes release of calcium ions from the sarcoplasmic reticulum and then (2) reuptake of the calcium ions by a calcium pump. *ATP,* Adenosine triphosphate. (From Hall JE, et al. *Guyton and Hall Textbook of Medical Physiology*. 14th ed. Philadelphia: Elsevier; 2021:99.)

in the myoplasm. Contractile tension increases in a sigmoidal manner as intracellular Ca^{2+} increases.[1] The greater the myoplasmic Ca^{2+} concentration, the more cross-bridge sites are exposed, and the stronger the force of the contraction. Maximal and sustained muscle tension

without relaxation—produced by the fusion and summation of successive twitch responses—is called tetanus.[2]

Fig. 36.12 shows the time course and relationship between a single action potential, the myoplasmic Ca^{2+} rise, and the resulting twitch

BOX 36.1 Steps of Neurohumoral Transmission and Excitation-Contraction Coupling

1. An action potential reaches the motor nerve ending.
2. Ca^{2+} enters the motor nerve ending; ACh is released into the synaptic cleft.
3. ACh binds to a postsynaptic cholinergic receptor at the motor endplate.
4. The motor endplate membrane depolarizes (the endplate potential [EPP]).
5. An action potential is generated at the perijunctional muscle membrane.
6. The action potential spreads along the muscle membrane and inward to the transverse tubules.
7. Depolarization of the T tubules causes Ca^{2+} release from the terminal cisterns of the sarcoplasmic reticulum.
8. Ca^{2+} triggers actomyosin complex cross-bridge formation; the sarcomere shortens; the muscle contracts.

ACh, Acetylcholine; *T,* transverse.

BOX 36.2 Steps of Skeletal Muscle Relaxation

1. ACh is hydrolyzed by AChE in the synaptic cleft.
2. The endplate and muscle membrane repolarize to their resting potentials.
3. Ca^{2+} is actively pumped back into the sarcoplasmic reticulum.
4. Myoplasmic Ca^{2+} concentration returns to a normal low level.
5. The muscle relaxes.

ACh, Acetylcholine; *AChE,* acetylcholinesterase.

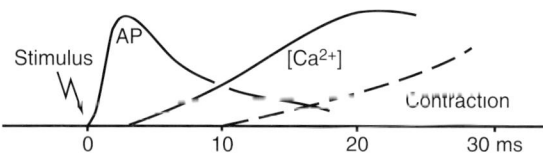

Fig. 36.12 The electrical, ionic, and mechanical responses of a skeletal muscle to a single maximal stimulus. *AP,* Action potential.

response. The action potential lasts about 2 to 4 ms. The twitch contraction begins about 2 ms after the start of the muscle membrane depolarization. The duration of the twitch varies with the type of muscle stimulated.

Slow Versus Fast Muscle

Skeletal muscle fibers are classified as type I (slow-twitch fibers) or type II (fast-twitch fibers) based on different myosin isoenzymes that distinguish the two types. The two fiber types differ in their metabolic demands, speed of contraction, and myosin ATPase activity. Muscles usually contain a mixture of both types of fibers, but one type often predominates.[1,32,33]

Slow-twitch (type I) muscle fibers are adapted for sustained movements, such as maintaining posture, and are resistant to fatigue. They have slow-twitch durations, depend on oxidative metabolism for energy, have extensive blood supplies, and have rich concentrations of mitochondria.[1,32,33] An example of a type I muscle is the soleus muscle of the leg, an important muscle used for maintaining posture and walking. Type I muscle is referred to as red muscle because its high capillary density and myoglobin content imparts a dark, rubrous color.

Fast-twitch (type II) muscle fibers usually predominate in white muscle and are primarily concerned with rapid or powerful movement of short duration. They have short-twitch durations, depend on glycolytic pathways for energy, and are easily fatigued.[1,33] Muscles

specialized for fine, skilled movement, such as extraocular muscles, and some muscles of the hand are in this category.

The diaphragm is engaged in continuous rhythmic activity to support respiratory inspiration, and so the muscle fibers must be resistant to fatigue. Infants have a greater tendency toward respiratory failure in part because at birth only 25% of their diaphragm is composed of type I fatigue-resistant fibers, compared with 55% in the adult. Before 27 weeks of gestation, type I slow fibers make up less than 10% of the total diaphragm muscle content.[32]

Energy Sources for Skeletal Muscle

Muscle contraction requires a continual supply of chemical energy (i.e., ATP) at a rate proportionate to its energy consumption. The energy consumed by skeletal muscle is used for (1) cross-bridge cycling during muscle contraction, (2) sarcoplasmic reticular resequestration of Ca^{2+} during muscle relaxation, (3) rephosphorylation of creatine to replenish creatine phosphate energy stores, (4) activation of the Na^+/K^+ pump to restore proper membrane polarization, and (5) resynthesis of muscle glycogen.[8]

The amount of ATP present in the muscles is sufficient to sustain maximal muscle power for only about 3 seconds. For this reason, actively contracting muscles must continually form new ATP. There are three metabolic systems that provide a continuous supply of ATP in muscle cells: (1) the phosphocreatine-creatine system, (2) the glycogen–lactic acid system, and (3) the aerobic system.[33]

Phosphocreatine-Creatine System

The energy-rich phosphate bonds in muscle phosphocreatine (also called creatine phosphate) supply a limited amount of energy to produce ATP in skeletal muscle. The hydrolysis of creatine phosphate to creatine and phosphate is an extremely rapid reaction that releases large amounts of energy for the conversion of adenosine diphosphate (ADP) to ATP. Creatine phosphate provides a stored source of energy that is used for short bursts of muscle power or for use at the very beginning of muscle contraction while other, more sustainable, energy-regenerating systems are being turned on.[33]

Glycogen-Lactic Acid System

Skeletal muscle stores glucose as energy-rich glycogen. With brief, intense muscle exertion, muscles meet their energy demands from the breakdown of glycogen to glucose (glycogenolysis) and the metabolism of glucose to pyruvate and lactate (glycolysis). Glycolysis occurs without the consumption of oxygen in the cytoplasm of the muscle cell. The energy released from the breakdown of glucose to pyruvate or lactate is used to convert ADP to ATP for very short periods of muscle contraction.[33] The accumulation of metabolic byproducts (e.g., lactic acid) in combination with depletion of glycogen stores are important factors contributing to muscle fatigue during prolonged exercise.[1]

Aerobic System

When oxygen is plentiful and exercise prolonged, skeletal muscle utilizes products of the glycolytic pathway, glucose, fatty acids, and other substrates, and efficiently oxidizes them to CO_2 and water in the muscle fiber mitochondria. This energy-yielding process is called oxidative metabolism. Oxidation is a slower process, but it is usually sufficient to meet the continual but more modest energy demands of more than 95% of skeletal muscle. If the energy requirements of exercise cannot be met by oxidation metabolism, an oxygen debt is incurred.[1] The aerobic system is the primary source of energy for muscle cells during prolonged exercise and for steady-state requirements.[33]

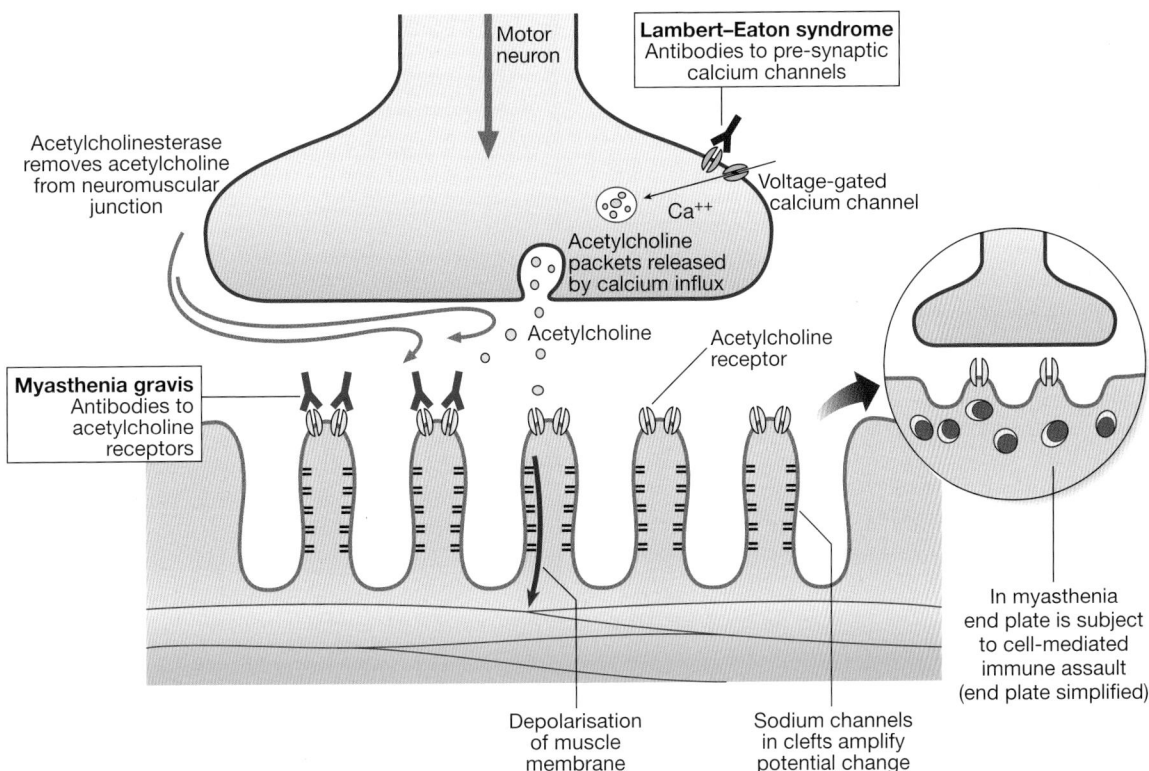

Fig. 36.13 Myasthenia gravis and Lambert-Eaton myasthenic syndrome (LEMS). In myasthenia, there are antibodies to the acetylcholine receptors on the postsynaptic membrane, which block conduction across the neuromuscular junction (NMJ). Myasthenic symptoms can be transiently improved by inhibition of acetylcholinesterase (e.g., with Tensilon [edrophonium bromide]), which normally removes the acetylcholine. A cell-mediated immune response produces simplification of the postsynaptic membrane, further impairing the safety factor of neuromuscular conduction. In LEMS, antibodies to the presynaptic voltage calcium channels impair release of acetylcholine from the motor nerve ending; calcium is required for the acetylcholine-containing vesicle to fuse with the presynaptic membrane for release into the NMJ. (From Walker BR, et al. *Davidson's Principles and Practice of Medicine.* 22nd ed. London: Elsevier; 2014:1227.)

MUSCULOSKELETAL PATHOPHYSIOLOGY AND ANESTHESIA

Musculoskeletal diseases have a wide variety of causes ranging from autoimmune destruction of tissue, to genetically determined defects in muscle membrane proteins, to pharmacologically induced alterations in Ca^{2+} metabolism. Musculoskeletal defects may reside in the NMJ, the muscle infrastructure, or the skeletal support structures.

Myasthenia Gravis

Myasthenia gravis (MG) is a chronic disease of the neuromuscular junction, manifested by skeletal muscle weakness, fatigability on effort, and at least partial restoration of function after rest.[34,35]

Epidemiology

MG is the most common disease affecting the NMJ. It occurs in 25 to 125 of every 1 million people worldwide, and studies indicate that the prevalence is increasing.[34,36-38] In individuals younger than 50 years, there is a predominance of female cases (60%–70%); in those older than 50 years, the disease is equally distributed between the sexes.[35,37] The onset may be abrupt or insidious, and the course is fluctuating, marked by periods of exacerbation and remission.[39] Spontaneous remissions that do occur sometimes persist for years.

Pathophysiology

MG is an autoimmune disease, characterized by autoantibodies directed against AChRs or receptor-related proteins at the NMJ postsynaptic membrane.[35,40-46] The complexity of MG is augmented by the presence of at least three distinct postsynaptic target proteins—NMJ dysfunction is the common feature.[34,35,40] The postsynaptic lesion appears to be caused by immune-mediated destruction or inactivation of the nicotinic AChR. The end result is a NMJ with a decreased number of functional postsynaptic AChRs (Fig. 36.13).

In the majority of patients with MG (~85%), circulating antibodies react directly with the nicotinic AChR, leading to varying degrees of dysfunction. This is the most prevalent subtype of MG and is termed AChR-MG. The alpha subunits of the AChR channel appear to be the primary immunogenic target.[35,47] Although antibodies are often detected in the sera with AChR-MG, the antibody levels do not correlate with the severity of the disease.[48-51]

Another distinct subgroup of MG involves those with antibodies against MuSK, a protein previously mentioned in this chapter as being involved in AChR clustering at the motor endplate.[34] This subgroup, termed MuSK-MG, accounts for about 10% of patients with MG. Patients with MuSK-MG have a distribution of muscle weakness typically involving the neck and respiratory muscles. Bulbar muscle involvement is common, placing these patients at increased risk for pulmonary aspiration. Often an atrophied tongue is seen.[49] Up to 50%

of these patients are likely to experience respiratory crisis requiring mechanical ventilation.[48-52] Unlike most cases of MG, serum concentrations of MuSK antibodies correlate with severity of symptoms.[48] Evidence from case series has demonstrated increased prevalence of MuSK-MG in people living closer to the equator.[49,53]

A third and small subset of patients with MG involves antibodies against Lrp4 found at the motor endplate of the NMJ. As mentioned previously in this chapter, Lrp4 works with agrin and MuSK to promote NMJ maturation and AChR clustering at the endplate.[41,42,49]

The initiating stimulus for MG producing IgE antibodies against NMJ proteins (AChR, MuSK, and Lrp4) is enigmatic.[45,46] A genetic predisposition, age, sex, and various environmental and infectious etiologies have been suggested as MG triggers.[34,47] In the majority of patients with MG, the thymus gland is a recognized trigger by producing autoantibodies against the AChR at the NMJ (the thymus seems to play a central role in the pathogenesis of AChR-MG, but not MuSK-MG).[35,40,47,50,54-56] The thymus is hyperplastic or abnormal in about 75% of patients with MG. Thymomas are present in an additional 10% to 15% of patients.[47]

The effect of pregnancy on the severity of MG is variable.[57,58] Pregnancy exacerbates symptoms of MG in about 30% of pregnant women; however, other patients with the disease experience remission or no change in symptoms during pregnancy.[58]

Anti-AChR antibodies that pass across the placenta may produce transitory symptoms of weakness in 15% to 20% of infants born to mothers with MG. Neonatal MG signs of weakness (difficulty with swallowing, sucking, and breathing; ptosis; facial weakness) in the affected infant are usually present within the first few hours after birth and may necessitate intubation and mechanical ventilation. Spontaneous remission usually occurs within 2 to 4 weeks as the maternal antibodies are cleared from the neonate's circulation.[57] Neonatal MG has been linked to both AChR and MuSK antibodies.[49]

The Myasthenia Gravis Foundation of America clinical classification scale is widely used today to categorize the severity of the disease (Table 36.1).

Clinical Manifestations

The clinical hallmarks of MG include generalized muscle weakness that improves with rest and an inability to sustain or repeat muscular contractions. Enhanced effort produces enhanced weakness. Muscle weakness can be asymmetric, confined to one muscle group, or generalized. The severity of MG can range from mild (slight ptosis only) to severe respiratory muscle weakness (myasthenic crisis). Stress, infection, and surgery seem to affect the disease process, although unpredictably.[42]

Visual symptoms (ptosis and diplopia) from extraocular muscle weakness occur in the majority of patients, especially at disease onset.[42,49,59] The disease is restricted to the ocular muscles (ocular myasthenia) in approximately 20% of patients.[34] Proximal limb and shoulder girdle musculature is often affected in patients with generalized disease. Oropharyngeal (bulbar) weakness may cause problems with articulation, chewing, swallowing, and clearing secretions. With severe disease, respiratory weakness is a critical element of focus and management.[45] Sensation and cognition are not affected by the disease process.

Other autoimmune disorders, such as hyperthyroidism, hypothyroidism, and rheumatoid arthritis, occur more often in patients with MG.[4,42]

Myocarditis may complicate MG, especially in patients with thymomas. The myocardial inflammation produces dysrhythmias, particularly atrial fibrillation and atrioventricular block.[42,60]

TABLE 36.1 Myasthenia Gravis Foundation of America Clinical Classification of Myasthenia Gravis

Class	Description
I	Eye muscle weakness, possible ptosis; no other evidence of muscle weakness
II	Eye muscle weakness of any severity, mild weakness of other muscles IIa Predominantly affecting limb or axial muscles IIb Predominantly affecting bulbar (oropharyngeal), respiratory muscles, or both
III	Eye muscle weakness of any severity, moderate weakness of other muscles IIIa Predominantly affecting limb or axial muscles IIIb Predominantly affecting bulbar (oropharyngeal), respiratory muscles, or both
IV	Eye muscle weakness of any severity, severe weakness of other muscles IVa Predominantly affecting limb or axial muscles IVb Predominantly affecting bulbar (oropharyngeal), respiratory muscles, or both
V	Intubation; with or without mechanical ventilation

Adapted from Myasthenia Gravis Foundation of America: *MGFA clinical classification.* Retrieved from https://myasthenia.org/Portals/0/MGFA%20Classification.pdf.

Treatment

Therapy for patients with MG is directed toward improving neuromuscular transmission and includes cholinesterase inhibitors, corticosteroids and other immunosuppressants, plasmapheresis, intravenous immunoglobulin (IVIG), and surgical thymectomy.[45,61,62] Additional immunomodulatory drugs are emerging.[61,63-66]

Treatment with cholinesterase inhibitors can dramatically reduce the symptoms of MG in most patients by inhibiting the hydrolysis of ACh and therefore raising the neurotransmitter's concentration at the NMJ. Increasing the synaptic concentration of ACh enhances the possibility of postsynaptic AChR occupation, which is critical for the production of a threshold-reaching EPP for muscle contraction.[41] The administration of AChE inhibitors improves muscular strength for several hours but does not affect the course of the disease.[42] Anticholinesterase treatment is particularly successful in patients with milder disease and the subtype AChR-MG.[62] The most commonly used anticholinesterase agent in the United States is oral pyridostigmine.[42,62] An oral dose of 60 mg pyridostigmine lasts 3 to 6 hours and is equivalent to an intravenous dose of 2 mg pyridostigmine (i.e., intravenous dosing is ~1/30 the oral dose). Cholinergic autonomic effects associated with anticholinesterase agents can pose problems. Increased bronchial and oral secretions, for instance, can be a serious challenge in patients with swallowing problems or respiratory insufficiency.[41]

Titration of the anticholinesterase dose can be challenging. Underdosing (poor disease control) does not sufficiently retard the muscle weakness and can result in myasthenic crisis, a severe exacerbation of myasthenic symptoms culminating in respiratory failure. About 25% of patients with MG will experience a myasthenic crisis sometime during their life. On the other hand, excessive administration of an anticholinesterase drug may precipitate cholinergic crisis by producing a surplus of ACh at the myoneural junction relative to receptor number. Cholinergic crisis manifests as a phase II–like block with paradoxic weakness. The respiratory distress of myasthenic crisis must be distinguished from

BOX 36.3   Comparison: Myasthenic Crisis versus Cholinergic Crisis

Myasthenic Crisis

May occur spontaneously or be precipitated by the stress of surgery, residual anesthetics, aminoglycoside antibiotics, infection, withholding myasthenia gravis medications

Manifestations: Severe respiratory muscle and/or bulbar muscle weakness

Treatment: Respiratory support that may include intubation or delay of extubation (if weakness occurs at the completion of surgery); urgent therapy may include plasma exchange or intravenous immune therapy

Cholinergic Crisis

May be precipitated by administration of an anticholinesterase (preoperatively or for reversal of neuromuscular blockade at the completion of a surgical procedure)

Manifestations: Muscle weakness (overstimulation at the neuromuscular junction due to an excess of acetylcholine [ACh] relative to the number of ACh receptors); cholinergic excess at muscarinic receptors (abdominal cramping, diarrhea, bradycardia, excess bronchial and oral secretions, urinary urgency, miosis)

Treatment: Respiratory system support that may include intubation or delay of extubation (if weakness occurs at the completion of surgery); anticholinergic agents (atropine, glycopyrrolate) to counteract muscarinic effects; withhold further anticholinesterase medication

the respiratory distress of cholinergic crisis as the cause and treatment of the two conditions are very different. Muscarinic manifestations predominate with cholinergic crisis (Box 36.3). An edrophonium (Tensilon) test is used to help differentiate a cholinergic from a myasthenic crisis. Increased weakness plus enhanced muscarinic effects after administration of intravenous edrophonium (1–2 mg) indicates cholinergic crisis, whereas increasing strength implies myasthenic crisis. In either crisis, treatment should be coordinated with a neurologist, and the patient should be monitored closely, often in an intensive care unit.

For patients with debilitating, widespread disease, treatment with AChE inhibitors is usually combined with immunomodulating therapy.[41] Corticosteroid therapy produces an 80% remission rate in patients with MG, in part by reducing AChR antibody levels, but therapy is limited by the side effects (e.g., osteoporosis, gastrointestinal bleeding, suppression of the hypothalamic pituitary axis, cataracts, increased susceptibility to acute infections, hypertension, and glucose intolerance) observed with long-term administration.[41,62] Other immunosuppressive drugs (azathioprine, cyclosporine, mycophenolate mofetil, tacrolimus) may be a part of treatment.[41,42,61,63] The monoclonal antibody, rituximab is promising for treatment-refractory MG resulting in safe and rapid-acting therapeutic effects.[64,65] Infection risks in the perioperative period need to be considered when patients are taking immunosuppressant agents.

Excision of the thymus gland is often recommended for adults with generalized disease and for patients with thymomas, thymus gland hyperplasia, or drug-resistant MG. Thymectomy effectively arrests or reverses the myasthenic process by removing a major source of antibody production and is generally a safe and viable treatment option.[42,54,56,67] Clinical improvement of myasthenic symptoms is seen in up to 85% of patients, but improvement may be delayed weeks to months after surgery. Postthymectomy, almost 35% of patients go into remission requiring no medications. Transsternal and endoscopic approaches have been used for surgical excision of the thymus.

Plasmapheresis (plasma exchange) arrests acute exacerbations of MG by reducing the concentration or neutralizing circulating

antibodies. Intravenous immune globulin (IVIG) may also be used as a rapid-acting, short-term treatment to improve symptoms.[42,61,66] Plasmapheresis or IVIG may be administered preoperatively to stabilize a patient before surgery or for crisis intervention to temporarily improve muscle strength.[61,62,66]

Anesthetic Implications

Several days before the operation and again immediately prior to surgery, the surgical candidate with MG should be evaluated for disease control and history, coexisting illnesses, muscle groups affected, and medical treatment. Perioperative planning should be multidisciplinary, including the patient's neurologist. Ideally, the patient with MG should be scheduled for elective surgery during a stable phase when the patient has optimal strength and respiratory function. Immunosuppressive medications should be avoided if possible in the perioperative period to decrease the risk of infection, as long as interruptions do not cause significant symptomatic effects. Premedication with sedatives or opioids may result in exaggerated respiratory depression and should be done with caution if at all.[36,68]

The continuation of the daily dose of anticholinesterase medication in the immediate preoperative period is individualized and depends to a large degree on the patient's reliance on the drug for control of symptoms.[36,68,69] Anticholinesterase therapy continued into the morning of surgery may be necessary for patients with severe disease who depend on this therapy for their well-being.[70] However, it is important to recognize that the presence of cholinesterase inhibitors may potentiate vagal responses, further modify responses to nondepolarizing muscle relaxants, and cloud the differential diagnosis and treatment of postoperative muscle weakness.[70,71] Hyperperistalsis, associated with anticholinesterase therapy, can disrupt anastomoses following bowel surgery. Discontinuing or tapering pyridostigmine before surgery may avoid complicating the anesthetic management. Patients with mild MG can usually tolerate the temporary disruption in treatment.

Electrolyte imbalance (hypokalemia, hypermagnesemia) and aminoglycoside antibiotics may aggravate muscle weakness in the patient with MG.[54] Pharyngeal and laryngeal muscle weakness, difficulty in eliminating oral secretions, respiratory weakness, and the risk of pulmonary aspiration should be considered in the anesthesia plan of care.[54,68,69,71] IVIG or plasmapheresis may be indicated to immediately improve preoperative muscle strength. Swallowing and respiratory muscle dysfunction account for much of the morbidity and potential mortality in patients with MG.[68,71,72]

Regional and local anesthesia have important utility for the surgical patient with MG in that they not only minimize or eliminate the need for intraoperative neuromuscular blockade but also provide postoperative analgesia.[36,54,73] Amide local anesthetics (ropivacaine, mepivacaine, bupivacaine, lidocaine) are preferred, as ester-type local anesthetics rely on pseudocholinesterase for metabolism, and their duration may be prolonged in patients taking cholinesterase inhibitors.

Patients with MG may be particularly vulnerable to respiratory depressant complications associated with supraclavicular and interscalene upper extremity blockade, as well as midthoracic or higher neuraxial anesthesia levels.[36,69,73,74] Sedation should be administered cautiously, if at all, to avoid respiratory depression.[73]

When general anesthesia is indicated for the surgical patient with MG, the respiratory depressant effects of sedatives, narcotics, and volatile anesthetic agents, compounded by the presence of an already weakened respiratory system, must be carefully considered.[36,71,73,75,76] Premedication should be avoided, but if necessary the smallest effective dose should be administered incrementally with continuous monitoring. Nonopioid analgesics may be suitable options for the patient with MG to avoid opioid-induced respiratory depression. The risk for pulmonary aspiration, especially for patients with bulbar involvement, should be considered in the plan of care.[36,71]

Neuromuscular blocking agents should be avoided in patients with MG if possible. In many patients, the relaxant effects of a volatile anesthetic in combination with the patient's preexisting skeletal muscle weakness are sufficient to facilitate intubation of the trachea.[75,77] Enhanced muscle relaxation occurs in a dose-dependent manner with the administration of all potent volatile anesthetics.[75,76]

Succinylcholine may be used to facilitate tracheal intubation, but the response is unpredictable.[78] Patients with MG appear to be 2.6 times more resistant to succinylcholine.[79] Normal dosages of succinylcholine may not effectively depolarize the endplate possibly because of the deficiency of viable AChRs.[78] Accordingly, for rapid-sequence induction using succinylcholine, the dose may have to be increased to 1.5 to 2 mg/kg.[79] Conversely, patients treated with cholinesterase inhibitors may exhibit a normal or prolonged response to succinylcholine. Cholinesterase inhibitors (pyridostigmine) block the effects of plasma cholinesterase (butyrylcholinesterase), as well as those of AChE at the NMJ; hence succinylcholine and other medications metabolized by plasma cholinesterase theoretically may have delayed hydrolysis and a prolonged duration of action.[36,80] Ester hydrolysis of atracurium and cisatracurium is independent of plasma cholinesterase activity.

The deficient number of functioning AChRs in patients with MG produces an extraordinary sensitivity to nondepolarizing muscle relaxants. Small doses of nondepolarizing agents, even defasciculating doses, can produce a profound block with a prolonged effect.[36,68] However, muscle relaxant requirements can be variable and unpredictable, a characteristic that makes neuromuscular blockade monitoring an essential and integral part of anesthetic management. Monitoring only one muscle group may overestimate or underestimate the degree of muscle relaxation in patients with MG.[81,82] Monitoring the neuromuscular blockade in more than one muscle group is a prudent choice to ensure safe recovery at the end of surgery.

If nondepolarizing muscle relaxants are required, a conservative and individualized approach to muscle paralysis is advised. The use of titrated smaller doses (0.1–0.2 times the ED_{95}) of shorter-acting nondepolarizing relaxants makes sense.[36,54] Patients with severe disease may require no nondepolarizing relaxants at all for surgical muscle relaxation.[76,77,83,84] Airway management with a laryngeal mask can help avoid the use of muscle relaxants for some procedures.[85]

Reversal of neuromuscular blockade with an acetylcholinesterase inhibitor is unpredictable and should be performed cautiously in patients with MG. Overtreatment with an anticholinesterase agent can precipitate a cholinergic crisis and aggravate rather than reverse the muscle weakness. If neuromuscular blockade is necessary, rocuronium has the advantage of reversal with sugammadex, thereby avoiding the need for reversal with AChE inhibitors. Several case reports have described effective use of sugammadex for reversal of rocuronium neuromuscular blockade in patients with MG.[86-89]

Complete, sustained return of muscle strength, resumption of spontaneous ventilation, and intact upper airway reflexes must be present before extubation. The patient should be informed that postoperative tracheal intubation, ventilatory support, and monitoring in an intensive care unit may be required. Several studies have attempted to determine the perioperative factors that predict a higher likelihood for myasthenic crisis and the need for postoperative ventilation, especially following thymectomy.[36] Study results have differed, but some of the factors cited for predicting the need for postoperative mechanical ventilation include body mass index greater than 28, duration of the disease longer than 6 years, pyridostigmine dose greater than 750 mg/day, positivity for ACh-receptor antibodies, the presence of coexisting

> ## BOX 36.4 Anesthesia Considerations for the Patient With Myasthenia Gravis
>
> - Carefully evaluate the patient for extent of disease, several days before surgery and again immediately prior to surgery.
> - Preoperative evaluation should focus on:
>   - Bulbar symptoms (dysphagia, dysarthria, oropharyngeal weakness, and difficulty eliminating oral secretions), which may predispose to aspiration
>   - Pulmonary function and respiratory muscle weakness to help predict the need for postoperative mechanical ventilation
>   - Myasthenia gravis (MG) therapy
>   - History of the disease
> - Search for other autoimmune diseases (diabetes mellitus, thyroid disease, systemic lupus erythematosus, rheumatoid arthritis).
> - Avoid routine premedication with sedatives or opioids.
> - If anticholinesterase medication is continued on the morning of surgery, consider muscarinic and nicotinic effects of the agent.
> - Opt for local or regional anesthesia if appropriate. In parturients with MG, neuraxial anesthesia is preferred for both cesarean and vaginal delivery.
> - For general anesthesia, avoid use of neuromuscular blocking agents (NMBAs) if possible. Volatile anesthetics alone may provide sufficient relaxation. If NMBAs are needed, titrate smaller doses of shorter-acting agents. Steroidal NMBAs allow for reversal with sugammadex. Monitor neuromuscular blockade in more than one muscle group.
> - Consider the respiratory depressant effects of sedatives, narcotics, and volatile anesthetic agents on an already weakened respiratory system.
> - Anticipate an unpredictable response to succinylcholine.
> - Ensure full return of respiratory strength prior to extubation. Closely monitor muscle strength in the postoperative period regardless of anesthesia technique.

respiratory disease, bulbar symptoms, a previous history of myasthenic crisis, a preoperative forced vital capacity less than 4 mL/kg, and severe muscle weakness.[90-94]

Skeletal muscle strength may appear to be adequate shortly after surgery but may deteriorate a few hours later. All patients, whether they receive regional anesthesia or general anesthesia, must be monitored assiduously for weakness in the postoperative period. Box 36.4 outlines important anesthesia considerations for the patient with MG.

The effects of pregnancy on MG are unpredictable. Some patients have MG symptom remission, while others have increased symptoms. Pregnant patients with MG should have antepartum anesthesia consultation with focus on the degree of respiratory and bulbar dysfunction, as well as their ability to tolerate a midthoracic level of neuraxial anesthesia. Neuraxial anesthesia is preferred in myasthenic parturients for labor analgesia and potential operative delivery. Early neuraxial analgesia for labor pain may circumvent fatigue, weakness, and stress.[57,58,73,95] As noted earlier, amide local anesthetics are preferred, as the metabolism of ester local anesthetics may theoretically be impaired if butyrylcholinesterase activity is reduced due to anticholinesterase therapy. Magnesium sulfate should be avoided in the parturient with MG because of the risk of compounding muscle weakness.[57,58,95]

Lambert-Eaton Myasthenic Syndrome

Incidence

Lambert-Eaton myasthenic syndrome (LEMS) is an autoimmune disorder affecting the NMJ that classically occurs in patients with malignant disease, particularly small cell carcinoma of the lung. LEMS often precedes the diagnosis of cancer by months to years.[17,18,96,97] LEMS is considered a paraneoplastic disease (an immune-mediated disease associated with underlying cancer), but one-third to one-half of patients have no evidence of carcinoma.[17,96,98] LEMS is a rare disease with an annual incidence about one-tenth that of MG.[82] Most patients with LEMS are men with a history of cigarette smoking, between the ages of 50 and 70 years, although cases do occur in children.[82]

Pathophysiology

The predominant defect associated with LEMS appears to be an autoantibody-mediated derangement in presynaptic P/Q-type voltage-gated Ca^{2+} channels leading to a reduction in Ca^{2+}-mediated exocytosis of ACh at neuromuscular and autonomic nerve terminals.[4,17,98-102] Calcium channel antibodies are present in 80% to 90% of patients with LEMS.[96] The decreased release of ACh from the motor nerve ending produces a reduced postjunctional response. Unlike MG, the number and quality of postjunctional AChRs remain unaltered, and the end-plate sensitivity is normal. The NMJ abnormality of LEMS is similar in location to the effects of aminoglycoside antibiotics and magnesium sulfate in which impairment of presynaptic voltage-gated channels results in attenuated ACh release.[4,96]

Clinical Manifestations and Treatment

Weak and often tender proximal muscles (hips, shoulders), fatigue, and hyporeflexia are dominant features of LEMS. Bulbar and respiratory muscles are less commonly involved. Autonomic nervous system dysfunction occurs in 75% to 80% of patients and is manifested as constipation, dry mouth, orthostatic hypotension, and urinary retention. Autonomic dysfunction is not seen with MG.[96,97]

Patients with LEMS experience a brief increase in muscle strength with voluntary contraction, distinguishing it from MG where increased effort produces increased weakness.

There is no cure for LEMS. Treatment is aimed at improving muscle strength and reversing autonomic deficits.[103] If there is evidence of an underlying malignancy, treating the cancer often improves symptoms.[96] 3,4-diaminopyridine is approved by the US Food and Drug Administration (FDA) to treat adult patients with LEMS. It improves muscle strength by prolonging activation of presynaptic voltage-gated Ca^{2+} channels, allowing more ACh to be released. Treatment should be continued preoperatively, as case reports of respiratory insufficiency have been reported when medications were held prior to surgery.[104] Immunosuppressive agents and plasmapheresis have also been used to improve muscle strength. In most patients with LEMS, pyridostigmine is of minimal therapeutic value, again differentiating it from MG.[103]

Anesthetic Implications

An index of suspicion for LEMS should be maintained in surgical patients with a history of muscle weakness and suspected or diagnosed carcinoma, especially lung cancer. Patients with LEMS are sensitive to the relaxant effects of both depolarizing and nondepolarizing muscle relaxants. Inhalational anesthetics alone may provide adequate relaxation for intubation and most surgical procedures. If muscle relaxants are required, their dosages should be reduced, and the neuromuscular blockade closely monitored.[104,105] Neuromuscular reversal with an anticholinesterase agent may be used but may produce an insufficient reversal response. Patients are at risk for postoperative respiratory failure, and close monitoring is required.[104] Prolonged ventilatory assistance may be required postoperatively. Box 36.5 summarizes anesthesia considerations for patients with LEMS.

Duchenne Muscular Dystrophy

Muscular dystrophy is a heterogeneous set of diseases that includes fascioscapulohumeral dystrophy, Emery-Dreifuss muscular dystrophy,

> ### BOX 36.5   Anesthesia Considerations for the Patient With Lambert-Eaton Myasthenic Syndrome (LEMS)
>
> - Maintain an index of suspicion for LEMS in surgical patients with a history of muscle weakness and suspected or diagnosed carcinoma of the lung.
> - Continue 3,4-diaminopyridine preoperatively.
> - Consider the possibility of autonomic nervous system disturbances.
> - Administer benzodiazepines, opioids, and other medications with sedative effects with caution, if at all.
> - Adjust muscle relaxant dose recognizing possible sensitivity to both depolarizing and nondepolarizing muscle relaxants. Assess neuromuscular blockade closely.
> - Monitor closely for postoperative respiratory failure regardless of anesthesia technique.

limb-girdle dystrophy, Becker muscular dystrophy, Duchenne muscular dystrophy (DMD), and others. Duchenne muscular dystrophy is the most common of these and has the most severe clinical course.[106]

Incidence

DMD, described by the French neurologist G.B. Duchenne in 1861, is an inherited, X-linked, recessive disease that presents in early childhood between 3 and 5 years of age. It is clinically evident almost exclusively in males and has an incidence of approximately 1 in 3500 live male births. Females are carriers of the disorder. Carriers are generally unaffected but may have variable degrees of muscle weakness and age-adjusted cardiomyopathy. Cognitive and behavioral difficulties occur in approximately 30% of patients with DMD.[107] There is no cure for the disease. Medical treatment, including corticosteroid therapy, helps preserve skeletal muscle strength, reduces the risk of scoliosis, delays cardiomyopathy onset, and stabilizes pulmonary function in many patients.[108-112] Patients with DMD are now living longer than ever before due to advances in supportive care and medical management.[113,114] However, despite improvements in survival, death often occurs in early adulthood (20–30 years of age) and is usually caused by progressive cardiomyopathy or pneumonia.[106,112]

Pathophysiology

Patients with DMD experience an infiltration of fibrous and fatty tissue into the muscle, followed by a progressive degeneration and necrosis of muscle fibers. The disease affects skeletal muscle, cardiac muscle, and smooth muscle. Muscle weakness ends with muscle destruction.

In 1987, the abnormal gene responsible for DMD was identified. This gene is located on the X chromosome and is errant in coding for the vital muscle protein dystrophin. Dystrophin is part of a large, tightly associated complex of glycoproteins that serve as structural components of the muscle fiber sarcolemma.[115,116] The dystrophin-glycoprotein complex stabilizes the sarcolemma during muscle contraction and relaxation.[117] Patients with DMD have a complete absence or a severe deficiency of the dystrophin protein, which alters sarcolemma integrity, stability, and signaling.[116,117] The dystrophin protein is present in low amounts or is structurally altered in Becker muscular dystrophy, a similar but rarer disorder that follows a milder and less progressive course than the Duchenne type.[106,117]

In the early stages of DMD, increased permeability of the sarcolemma and skeletal muscle necrosis are mirrored by elevated serum levels of the enzyme creatine kinase (CK).[106] Serum CK concentrations are greater than 50 to 100 times normal, but as muscle is lost to the destructive process, CK levels decline.[117]

Clinical Manifestations

DMD is characterized by an unremitting weakness and a steady deterioration of symmetric muscle groups. Proximal muscles of the lower extremities are usually affected first. The child exhibits a clumsy waddling gait, difficulty with climbing stairs and jumping, and frequent falls. Weakness of the pelvic girdle leads to the classic finding of Gowers sign, in which patients use their hands to climb up their legs to arise from the floor.[106] Neck flexor weakness occurs at all stages of the disease; when supine, a child with DMD has difficulty lifting the head against gravity.[106] Loss of strength is relentless, and the steady deterioration of muscle strength forces most of these boys to be wheelchair bound by age 12 years.[106,117]

Skeletal muscle atrophy is usually preceded by fat and fibrous tissue infiltration, resulting in pseudohypertrophy. The infiltrative process is most apparent in the calf muscles, which become particularly enlarged.

Degeneration of respiratory muscles (diaphragm, intercostal, accessory muscles) occurs and leads to chronic respiratory insufficiency.[118] Particularly in nonambulating patients, paraspinal muscle weakness predisposes patients to kyphoscoliosis, which further decreases the pulmonary reserve. Decreasing muscle strength leads to ineffective coughing, inability to mobilize secretions, impaired swallowing, and frequent pulmonary infections.[106,110,119,120] Chronic hypoxemia may be compounded by obstructive sleep apnea.

As the disease progresses, it affects not only skeletal muscle but also smooth muscle of the alimentary tract and cardiac muscle. Alimentary tract involvement can lead to intestinal hypomotility, delayed gastric emptying, and gastric dilation.[121]

Myocardial involvement occurs in almost all patients with progressive disease and includes dilated cardiomyopathy, supraventricular and ventricular dysrhythmias, and mitral regurgitation.[106,108,112,122-124] Preclinical cardiac involvement can be detected in up to 62% of boys between the ages of 6 and 10 years. Cardiomyopathy is present in nearly all patients by the age of 18 years.[112,123,124] The cardiomyopathy primarily involves the left ventricle (LV) and is characterized by myocyte fibrosis, thinning of the LV wall, and decreased contractility. Oral corticosteroids have been shown to slow the deterioration of cardiac function.[112] Electrocardiographic (ECG) changes occur at a young age and include sinus tachycardia, prolonged P-R interval, prominent R waves in V_1, and deep Q waves in the left precordial leads.[106]

Although often severe, compromised cardiac and respiratory conditions may be masked by the limited activity imposed by the patient's skeletal myopathy. Added stress, such as that produced by surgery, may suddenly increase cardiorespiratory demand and uncover the weakened cardiac and respiratory states.[110,125,126]

Anesthetic Implications

Children with DMD may require anesthesia for diagnostic procedures or various corrective orthopedic surgeries to prolong ambulation or improve quality of life. Surgical patients with DMD are susceptible to untoward anesthesia-related complications related to muscle weakness, muscle breakdown, and myocardial, pulmonary, and gastrointestinal involvement. Careful multidisciplinary preoperative evaluation by a cardiologist, pulmonologist, and neuromuscular specialist is suggested before any surgical procedure requiring anesthesia or sedation.[106,126-129]

For the surgical patient with DMD on long-term corticosteroid treatment, potential side effects, including peptic ulcers, glucose intolerance, and adrenal suppression, should be considered. Patients with DMD have decreased bone density due to limited mobility. Osteoporosis associated with steroid use compounds the bone fragility and increases risk for fractures. The risk of fragile bones, kyphoscoliosis, and flexion contractures can complicate surgical positioning.[106]

Consideration also needs to be given to surgical stress-dose steroid coverage for the patient on long-term glucocorticoid therapy.

Generalized muscle weakness, especially in the advanced stages of DMD, makes these patients exquisitely sensitive to the respiratory depressant properties of opioids, sedatives, and general anesthetic agents. Preoperative anxiolytics should only be administered to patients without significant risk of respiratory dysfunction and only in a setting of continuous monitoring of respiratory function. The use of regional or local anesthesia, whenever feasible, is advised.[126,129]

Aggressive preoperative respiratory therapy can help maximize the patient's pulmonary condition.[126,129] Arterial blood gas determinations help elucidate the extent of respiratory involvement and the amount of respiratory reserve. A preoperative forced vital capacity (FVC) less than 50% of predicted places the patient at increased risk for respiratory complications when undergoing general anesthesia or procedural sedation. Patients with a FVC less than 35% of predicted have a higher risk for pulmonary complications.[126,129] In one series, aggressive preoperative chest physiotherapy and incorporation of postoperative noninvasive positive pressure ventilation (NPPV) enabled patients with preoperative FVC levels of 30% and below to successfully undergo corrective spinal surgery.[130] Other reports have not shown a significant correlation between preoperative pulmonary function tests and the need for postoperative ventilatory support. Experts recommend extubation directly to NPPV for patients with baseline FVC less than 50% of predicted and strongly recommend for patients with a FVC less than 30% of predicted.[126-129] In all cases, assiduous attention to respiratory function must be continued into the postoperative period with continuous monitoring of SpO_2, and whenever possible, blood or end tidal carbon dioxide ($ETco_2$) levels. Patients at high risk of ineffective cough may benefit from postoperative mechanical insufflation-exsufflation bronchial secretion clearance devices.[126] Delayed pulmonary insufficiency, as late as 36 hours after surgery, has been reported.[121] An intensive care unit bed should be available for postprocedure care.[129] Outpatient surgery with general anesthesia of any duration is not advised.

The effects of nondepolarizing muscle relaxants must be scrupulously monitored. Some patients demonstrate enhanced muscle relaxant sensitivity, with recovery prolonged three to six times the normal duration.[131] If surgical muscle relaxation is required, a short-acting nondepolarizing muscle relaxant that is carefully titrated with the use of blockade monitoring makes sense.

Cardiomyopathy and decreased cardiac reserve makes these patients sensitive to myocardial depressant effects of general anesthetic agents, sedatives, and narcotics.[132,133] Preoperative 12-lead ECG, cardiac magnetic resonance imaging (MRI), echocardiography, and cardiology consultation is recommended to evaluate cardiac function.[108,126,134] A carefully titrated intravenous "balanced" anesthesia technique can provide a smooth cardiovascular course.[128] Ketamine and dexmedetomidine have been used successfully for anesthesia during diagnostic muscle biopsy in patients with DMD. Judicious administration of intravenous fluids is warranted. The sudden occurrence of hypotension and tachycardia during anesthesia may herald heart failure.[125]

The potential for delayed gastric emptying, plus the presence of weak laryngeal reflexes, dictates that the anesthesia plan of care includes measures for guarding against aspiration of stomach contents. Gastric decompression with a nasogastric tube should be considered for patients with gastrointestinal dysmotility. Premedication with prokinetic agents is recommended for patients with gastrointestinal dysmotility.[126]

Succinylcholine is strictly avoided in patients with DMD.[128,135,136] The altered sarcolemma can lead to rhabdomyolysis and myoglobin efflux with succinylcholine administration. The resultant massive breakdown of the diseased muscle fibers produces a profound hyperkalemia that requires extensive and tenacious treatment with calcium chloride, hyperventilation, sodium bicarbonate, and 50% dextrose and insulin. Ventricular fibrillation and intractable cardiac arrest have been associated with succinylcholine administration to patients with diagnosed and undiagnosed muscular dystrophy.[132,135,136] On the basis of succinylcholine inducing hyperkalemic cardiac arrest in patients with undiagnosed muscular dystrophy, the USFDA issued a black box warning against the administration of succinylcholine for nonemergent intubation in all pediatric patients.

Rhabdomyolysis, hyperkalemia, hyperthermia, unexplained tachycardia, and cardiac arrest have been reported after the administration of potent inhalation anesthetics to patients with DMD with and without the use of succinylcholine.[132,133,137-139] These malignant hyperthermia–like reactions may be due to the destabilizing effect of inhalational agents on an already unstable and fragile muscle membrane resulting in anesthesia-induced rhabdomyolysis.[140]

In addition to the strict contraindication of succinylcholine, some experts advocate for the strict avoidance of potent volatile inhalational agents in patients with DMD.[129,133,140,141] Given the availabilities of safe anesthesia alternatives for general anesthesia induction and maintenance, total intravenous anesthesia (e.g., propofol and short-acting opioids) can be used safely.[108,126,139,140,142]

Despite the increased risk for malignant hyperthermia–like events in patients with DMD, malignant hyperthermia and DMD are genetically distinct diseases. Current evidence indicates that DMD and Becker muscular dystrophy are not among the myopathies that are genetically associated with malignant hyperthermia.[141,142] Box 36.6 outlines important anesthesia considerations for the patient with DMD.

Malignant Hyperthermia

Malignant hyperthermia (MH) is an uncommon, life-threatening, hypermetabolic disorder of skeletal muscle, triggered in susceptible individuals by potent inhalation agents, including sevoflurane, desflurane, isoflurane, halothane, enflurane, and ether, and the depolarizing muscle relaxant succinylcholine.[143,144] There is mounting evidence that

---

BOX 36.6 Anesthesia Considerations for the Patient With Duchenne Muscular Dystrophy

- Enlist multidisciplinary preoperative consultation from pulmonologist, cardiologist, and neuromuscular specialists.
- When possible, consider local or regional anesthesia for surgical procedures.
- Implement preoperative and postoperative respiratory therapy. Extubation directly to noninvasive positive pressure ventilation is recommended for patients with forced vital capacity <50% of predicted.
- Consider the potential for delayed gastric emptying in the plan of care.
- If general anesthesia is selected, implement a trigger-free total intravenous anesthetic. Succinylcholine is contraindicated. Avoid potent volatile inhalational agents.
- Carefully position the patient considering bone fragility imposed by limited mobility and glucocorticoid use.
- Appreciate sensitivity to the respiratory depressant properties of opioids, sedatives, and general anesthetic agents. Preoperative sedation should be omitted or minimal. The smallest possible amounts of general anesthetic agents should be used.
- Monitor the cardiovascular course, considering decreased cardiac reserve and potential sensitivity to the myocardial depressant effects of general anesthetic agents, sedatives, and narcotics.
- Continue close monitoring of the patient in the postoperative period.

MH may also be triggered in some patients by stressors such as vigorous exercise and heat.[145,146]

Epidemiology/Incidence

The exact incidence of MH is unknown, but estimates are that MH complicates 1 in 100,000 surgical procedures in adults and 1 in 30,000 surgeries in children.[147] Children under 15 years of age comprise approximately 52% of all reactions.[144] A review of MH cases in New York State reported the prevalence of MH in males to be 2.5 to 4.5 times the rate for females.[148] All ethnic groups are affected in all parts of the world.[144]

The first formal case report of MH was of an Australian family, described by Denborough et al. over 50 years ago in the journal *The Lancet*.[149] Since that time, a great deal has been learned about the biochemical and physiologic components of the disease. Nonetheless, many questions remain regarding the pathophysiology, genetics, diagnosis, and significance of some clinical manifestations.

Pathophysiology

Although the cause(s) of MH are not yet known with certainty, it is agreed that MH is an inherited disorder of skeletal muscle. MH has been associated with at least 34 genetic mutations, and in many cases, the genetic defects have not been established.[150]

In most susceptible patients, a defect in calcium regulation is expressed by exposure to specific anesthetic triggers, the volatile inhalational anesthetic agents or succinylcholine. An uncontrolled rise in myoplasmic calcium results.

To date, most MH-associated genetic variants are found within the *RYR1* gene.[141,151-154] The genes *CACNA1S* and *STAC3* are involved in muscle excitation-contraction and calcium ion flow, and genetic mutations in these genes have also been linked to MH susceptibility.[144,154]

- *RYR1* encodes the ryanodine receptor, the major calcium release channel of the sarcoplasmic reticulum.
- *CACNA1S* encodes a subunit of a dihydropyridine calcium channel located in skeletal muscle T tubules.
- *STAC3* gene variants are manifested most as Native American myopathy in the Lumbee Native American tribe of North Carolina.

Mutation of *RYR1* and a defective ryanodine channel appear to underlie approximately 70% of reported cases of MH, while about 2% of cases result from mutation of *CACA1S*.[141,143,155]

MH is typically initiated in MH-susceptible (MHS) patients when specific anesthetic-triggering agents induce enhanced calcium release from myocyte sarcoplasmic reticulum. The defect involves skeletal muscle, and there is no evidence for a primary defect in cardiac or smooth muscle cells. The elevated intracellular calcium results in muscle contraction and abnormal muscle metabolism. Energy-dependent reuptake mechanisms attempt to remove excess calcium from the myoplasm, increasing muscle metabolism two- to threefold. The accelerated cellular processes increase oxygen consumption, augment carbon dioxide and heat production, deplete ATP stores, and generate lactic acid.[143] Acidosis, hyperthermia, and ATP depletion cause sarcolemma destruction, producing a marked egress of potassium, myoglobin, and CK to the extracellular fluid. Skeletal muscle constitutes 40% to 50% of our body mass, so relatively small changes in muscle metabolism may produce the dramatic systemic biochemical changes observed with MH.

Clinical Manifestations

Not all cases of MH are fulminant, but rather there is a spectrum or continuum of severity, ranging from an insidious onset with mild complications to an explosive response with pronounced rigidity, temperature rise, arrhythmias, and death.[143,156]

All anesthetic inhalational agents except nitrous oxide are triggers for MH. Succinylcholine is a trigger. No other anesthetic agents appear to trigger MH.

Although MH may present in several ways, a typical MH episode begins while the patient is under general anesthesia with a volatile anesthetic. Succinylcholine may or may not precede the MH episode. The onset of MH symptoms may occur immediately after induction of anesthesia, several hours into the surgery, or even after surgery is completed.[156] MH risk may increase up to 20 times higher when succinylcholine is used in combination with volatile anesthetics.[157] Succinylcholine also appears to accelerate the onset and increase the severity of the MH episode.[143,144] In some cases, but not all, desflurane and sevoflurane have been associated with delayed onset of MH, as long as 6 hours after induction of anesthesia.[158-160] Although an uncommon event, MH can occur in the recovery room or the intensive care unit, usually within 1 hour after general anesthesia.[161-163]

The clinical features of MH are not uniform, and the time course between onset of initial signs and fulminant MH is variable. Overall, clinical manifestations of MH reflect increased intracellular muscle Ca^{2+} concentration and greatly increased body metabolism (Box 36.7). Tachycardia and an unanticipated increase in $ETco_2$ levels >55 mm Hg (most reliable sign) out of proportion to minute ventilation are often early diagnostic clues.[143,144] Other common signs of MH include tachypnea, skin mottling, and total body or jaw muscle rigidity. Muscle rigidity is clinically apparent in most cases. Hyperthermia, which may climb at a rate of 1°C to 2°C every 5 minutes and averages 39.3°C (102.7°F), may occur early or late in the anesthetic and is a confirming sign of MH.[143,164]

Acidosis, hyperkalemia, and hyperthermia lead to cardiac irritability, a labile blood pressure, and arrhythmias that can rapidly progress to cardiac arrest. Laboratory findings mirror the muscle breakdown and include increased serum potassium, myoglobin, and CK levels. Myoglobin appears in the urine and places the patient at risk for tubular obstruction and renal failure. Arterial and venous blood gas analysis reveals mixed metabolic and respiratory acidosis. Death may result unless the individual is promptly treated.[143] Even with treatment, the individual is at risk for complications, including cerebral edema,

consumptive coagulopathy, myoglobinuric renal failure, compartment syndrome, hepatic dysfunction, and pulmonary edema.[143,144]

The variable time course and nonspecific clinical features and laboratory findings can make the diagnosis of MH difficult. Insufficient anesthetic depth, hypoxia, neuroleptic malignant syndrome, thyrotoxicosis, pheochromocytoma, and sepsis can share several characteristics with MH, making the clinical picture ambiguous and the differential diagnosis challenging to even the most experienced practitioner[143,165,166] (Box 36.8). Surgical procedures performed of necessity in a darkened operating room can further compromise the practitioner's diagnostic acumen.

Preoperative Assessment and Prevention

Patients who are MHS are usually phenotypically normal, otherwise healthy, and completely unaware of their risk until exposed to a triggering anesthetic.[143,167] Furthermore, not everyone who has the MH gene develops an MH episode upon each exposure to triggering anesthetics. An MHS patient may be anesthetized multiple times before experiencing an MH event. Although MH susceptibility cannot be ruled out by history alone, every surgical patient should be questioned about the following:

- Family history of unexpected intraoperative complications or deaths
- Family or personal history of MH, muscle rigidity/stiffness, and/or high fever under anesthesia
- Personal history of dark/cola-colored urine after surgery or exercise
- Personal or family history of high temperature or death during exercise

---

BOX 36.7 Clinical Events and Laboratory Findings During Malignant Hyperthermia (MH)

Clinical Events
- Unexplained, sudden rise in end tidal CO_2 (>55 mm Hg)
- Unexplained tachycardia
- Masseter muscle or generalized muscle rigidity
- Rising patient temperature
- Cola-colored urine (myoglobinuria)
- Mottled, cyanotic skin
- Decreased Sao_2
- Tachypnea
- Labile blood pressure
- Arrythmias

Laboratory Findings Consistent With MH
- Arterial blood gases: respiratory and metabolic acidosis
- Serum potassium >6 mEq/L
- Creatine kinase >20,000 units/L
- Serum myoglobin >170 mcg/L
- Urine myoglobin >60 mcg/L

Sao_2, % of oxygen saturation.

BOX 36.8 Signs and Symptoms Shared by Malignant Hyperthermia and Other Clinical Occurrences

Tachycardia
- Hypoxia
- Hypercarbia
- Hypovolemia
- Insufficient anesthetic depth
- Anticholinergics, sympathomimetics, cocaine, amphetamine
- Hypermetabolic states (sepsis, thyroid storm, pheochromocytoma)

Hyperpyrexia
- Heatstroke
- Blood transfusion reaction
- Infection
- Drug reaction
- Serotonin syndrome
- Iatrogenic overheating

Tachypnea, Hypercapnia
- Congestive heart failure, pulmonary edema
- Hypermetabolic states (sepsis, thyroid storm, pheochromocytoma)
- Intraperitoneal carbon dioxide insufflation
- Airway obstruction, pneumothorax
- Excess dead space, low minute volume

Masseter Muscle Rigidity
- Insufficient neuromuscular blockade
- Temporomandibular joint syndrome
- Neuroleptic malignant syndrome
- Myotonia

Since MH is an inherited disorder, all members of a family in which MH has occurred must be considered MHS unless proven otherwise. Moreover, the absence of a positive family history does not preclude MH susceptibility.

Patients with neuromuscular disease may exhibit one or more clinical features of MH in the perioperative period. There are a limited number of relatively rare diseases that have a clinical and/or genetic link to MH susceptibility. These include central core disease, King-Denborough syndrome, multiminicore myopathy, centronuclear myopathy, congenital myopathy with cores and rods, periodic paralysis, nemaline rod myopathy, idiopathic hyperCKemia, Native American myopathy, and congenital fiber type disproportion.[141,152,153,155,168-170] There appears no higher risk for MH over the general population in patients with Duchenne or Becker muscular dystrophy and myotonic dystrophy.[144,169,171]

Some otherwise healthy patients who test positive for MH on muscle biopsy have unexplained increased CK levels. Persistently elevated CK levels in an otherwise healthy patient should inform the anesthetist to the possibility of MHS and/or myopathy.[172] However, as a screening test for MH, CK levels are imprecise and nonspecific.[172,173]

Heat stroke and strenuous exercise have been implicated as causal factors of MH in some patients.[146,174] As yet, there is no clear consensus whether or how these factors cause or exacerbate MH triggering.[145,146,175,176] It may be advisable to provide a trigger-free anesthetic to patients with previously unexplained exertional heat illness or exertional rhabdomyolysis until definitive MH testing can be performed.[175]

Management of an MH Episode

Enhanced patient monitoring, earlier diagnosis and treatment, and the introduction of dantrolene are responsible for the dramatic decrease in mortality from nearly 80% 30 years ago to less than 5% today.[143]

In 1979 dantrolene sodium was introduced as a treatment for MH. Since that time, dantrolene has contributed greatly to the dramatic decline in death and disability associated with MH episodes. It remains the only drug known to specifically treat MH. Dantrolene is a unique muscle relaxant that does not work at the NMJ as do standard neuromuscular blocking drugs. Rather, it works by binding to the ryanodine calcium channel and reducing calcium efflux from the sarcoplasmic reticulum, counteracting the abnormal intracellular calcium levels accompanying MH.[144,177,178] At clinical concentrations, dantrolene does not render the muscle totally flaccid and without tone, but it may cause significant muscle weakness and respiratory insufficiency, especially in patients with preexisting muscle disease. Dantrolene may also be efficacious treating neuroleptic malignant syndrome. Calcium channel blockers should not be administered with dantrolene as they may induce life-threatening myocardial depression and hyperkalemia.[144,178]

The Malignant Hyperthermia Association of the United States (MHAUS) recommends that all patients have core temperature monitoring.[143,179] Pulmonary artery, distal esophageal, nasopharyngeal, bladder, and tympanic membrane temperature monitors are the gold standards for core temperature measurement.[179] Skin temperature does not accurately reflect core temperature during an MH event. Larach et al. showed that the risk of dying from an MH episode was 9.7 times greater when only skin temperature was being used, and the relative risk of dying was 13.8 times higher when no temperature monitors were used compared to core temperature monitoring.[164]

Early recognition of an impending MH crisis and prompt emergency response is critical for a patient's survival.[180] The incidence of MH is low, but if untreated the mortality rate is high. The earlier an MH episode is recognized and treated, the better the outcome. An increase in the time interval between the first clinical signs of MH and

the administration of dantrolene has been associated with increased complication rates.[181] Once MH is identified, it is important to discontinue triggering agents, administer dantrolene, hyperventilate with 100% O_2, cool the patient, and treat symptoms. MHAUS provides an "Emergency Therapy for MH" poster that can be hung in every surgical site. The following treatment sequence is recommended for an acute MH episode[182]:

- Call for help and alert the surgeon to conclude the procedure promptly.
- Immediately discontinue the volatile anesthetic and succinylcholine. If surgery must be continued, maintain general anesthesia with intravenous nontriggering anesthetics.
- Prepare and administer 2.5 mg/kg dantrolene intravenous bolus (based on the patient's "actual weight") and repeat as necessary every 5 to 10 minutes until symptoms abate (decreased ETco₂, decreased muscle rigidity, and/or lowered heart rate). Occasionally, a total dose greater than 10 mg/kg may be needed, but if greater than 10 mg/kg is given without reversal of symptoms, the diagnosis should be reassessed. The alkaline solution is highly irritating to vessels and should be administered through the largest vein possible.178
- Hyperventilate with 100% oxygen at high flows (at least 10 L/min) to improve tissue oxygenation and eliminate CO2.
- If available, apply activated charcoal filters (Vapor-Clean, Dynasthetics, Salt Lake City, UT) to each limb of the anesthesia circuit and replace after each hour of use. Even though the volatile anesthetic agent is discontinued when MH is first suspected, activated charcoal filters may become saturated after 1 hour.[183-185]
- If fever is present (>39°C) or if the temperature is rapidly rising, initiate cooling by lavage (orogastric, bladder, open cavities), administration of chilled intravenous normal saline, and surface cooling (e.g., hypothermia blanket; ice packs to the groin, axilla, and neck). Stop cooling measures when the core body temperature is below 38.0°C to avoid hypothermia.
- Dysrhythmias will usually respond to treatment of acidosis or hyperkalemia. Treat persistent or life-threatening arrhythmias with standard antiarrhythmic agents. Do not administer calcium channel blockers.
- Check arterial blood gases, serum electrolytes, and blood glucose until the syndrome stabilizes. Consider administration of sodium bicarbonate, 1 to 2 mEq/kg dose, for pH<7.2 and serum bicarbonate levels <10-12 meq/L (maximum dose 50 mEq).
- Treat hyperkalemia: hyperventilation; calcium chloride 10 mg/kg (maximum dose 2000 mg) or calcium gluconate 30 mg/kg (maximum dose 3000 mg) for life-threatening hyperkalemia; sodium bicarbonate, 1 to 2 mEq/kg intravenously (maximum dose 50 mEq); glucose/insulin administration (for pediatric patients: 0.1 unit regular insulin/kg intravenously and 0.5 g/kg dextrose; for adult patients: 10 units regular insulin intravenously and 50 mL 50% dextrose).
  - For refractory hyperkalemia, consider albuterol (or other sympathetic β-receptor agonist), kayexalate, dialysis, or extracorporeal membrane oxygenation if the patient is in cardiac arrest.
- Maintain urine output greater than 1 mL/kg/hour. Large losses of intravascular volume should be anticipated.
- Monitor: heart rate, core temperature, ETco₂, minute ventilation, blood gases, serum K+, serum CK, urine myoglobin, and coagulation studies as warranted by the clinical severity of the patient. Consider invasive hemodynamic monitoring.

A full complement of dantrolene, along with other drugs and equipment necessary to treat an MH crisis, must be available at all facilities, including ambulatory surgical centers and offices, where MH triggering anesthetics or depolarizing muscle relaxants are administered or stocked.[185,186] The cart should be kept in or very close to the operating room so it is available immediately if MH occurs.[144] MHAUS recommends that dantrolene be available to administer within 10 minutes of the decision to treat for MH.[186] In addition to promoting patient safety, stocking dantrolene for the treatment of MH in an ambulatory surgical setting has been shown to be cost effective.[187]

There are three preparations of dantrolene available. The original preparations of dantrolene (Dantrium, Revonto) are packaged as 20-mg vials that must be reconstituted with 60 mL of sterile water for injection. There are 3 g of mannitol in each 20-mg vial of Dantrium and Revonto. The poor water solubility of Dantrium, and to a lesser degree Revonto, requires vigorous mixing until the solution is clear.

A newer alternative formulation of dantrolene (Ryanodex) is easier to reconstitute, is available as 250-mg vials, and it requires 5 mL of sterile water diluent shaken to ensure a uniform orange, opaque suspension. With Ryanodex, the initial dantrolene treatment can be more expeditiously delivered with administration of one vial. The provider should note that there is only 0.125 g of mannitol in each 250-mg vial of Ryanodex.

Documentation of an MH episode should include patient responses, personnel involved, medications administered, interventions, and patient outcomes.

Anesthesia for Malignant Hyperthermia-Susceptible Patients

Patients known or suspected of having MH should be assessed well before their date of surgery so that anesthesia records and MH testing center reports (if available) can be collected to corroborate the history.

Standard intraoperative monitoring for the MHS surgical patients includes blood pressure, ECG, pulse oximetry, capnography, and continuous measurement of core body temperature. A cooling water mattress should be placed under the MHS patient at the start of the procedure. Dantrolene pretreatment for the MHS surgical patient is not routine.[178]

If the surgical site permits, a regional or local anesthetic technique is preferable for the MHS patient. Local anesthetics (both amide and ester) are nontriggering drugs. Preoperative administration of anxiolytics followed by a nontriggering general anesthetic can also be administered safely in concert with close monitoring of appropriate vital functions. The list of nontriggering anesthetic agents is comprehensive enough to meet most anesthetic requirements (Box 36.9). All volatile halogenated inhalation agents and succinylcholine are MH triggers and should be avoided when caring for the MHS patient.

Not all drugs have been thoroughly screened as potential MH triggers, but it is clear that the vast majority of prescription and nonprescription drugs are safe. Case reports and studies have suggested a link between statin-induced muscle toxicity and susceptibility to MH.[188]

Keys to successful perioperative outcome for the surgical patient who is MHS include the following:

- Perform preoperative care in a relaxed and quiet environment with premedication anxiolysis as appropriate.
- Avoid MH-triggering medications.
- Remove trace anesthesia gas from the anesthesia machine. Change the carbon dioxide absorbent. Ensure that anesthetic vaporizers are disabled by removing or taping in the OFF position. Flush the anesthesia machine and ventilators with oxygen set at 10 L/min or more by attaching a new breathing circuit and reservoir bag to the Y-piece of the circle system and setting the ventilator to inflate the bag periodically. Preparation of modern anesthesia workstations is complex as they have variability in their components and contain silicone parts that absorb inhalational agents and result in prolonged release of agent. The provider should review specific anesthesia machine

---

BOX 36.9 Malignant Hyperthermia: Triggering and Nontriggering Agents

Triggering (Unsafe) Agents
- All volatile inhalation anesthetics (desflurane, isoflurane, sevoflurane, enflurane, halothane)
- Succinylcholine

Nontriggering (Safe) Agents
- Local anesthetics
- Opioids
- Nitrous oxide
- Barbiturates, propofol, ketamine, etomidate
- Benzodiazepines, dexmedetomidine, droperidol
- Nondepolarizing skeletal muscle relaxants (vecuronium, atracurium, cisatracurium, pancuronium, rocuronium, mivacurium)
- Digoxin, tricyclic antidepressants, magnesium sulfate
- Anticholinesterase agents
- Anticholinergic agents
- Antibiotics
- Antihistamines
- Vasoactive drugs

---

instructions on preparation for an MH patient. Older anesthesia machines require only 20 minutes of oxygen flush for adequate preparation, while newer anesthesia machines may require longer time for the anesthesia machine to be cleaned of volatile agents with oxygen flush. During the case, fresh gas flow should be kept at 10 L/min to avoid rebound phenomenon (increased release of residual volatile anesthetic agent when fresh gas flow is reduced after a set period of flushing).[144,183,184,189-192]

- Activated charcoal filters placed on the inspiratory and expiratory proximal limbs of the anesthesia circuit decrease inhalational anesthetics to safe levels within several minutes. For both new and older machines, adding activated charcoal filters to the circuit will remove anesthetic gases and obviate the need for purging the system as described earlier. However, the anesthesia machine will still need to be flushed with high fresh gas flows (≥10 L/min) for 90 seconds prior to placing the activated charcoal filters on both the inspiratory and expiratory ports. Adding activated charcoal filters to the airway circuit is effective in keeping anesthetic agent concentration below 5 ppm for up to 12 hours with fresh gas flows of at least 3 L/min.[184,189,193,194]
- Alternatives to preparing regularly operated anesthesia machines include the use of a dedicated vapor-free machine for MHS patients or, if appropriate to the institution, the use of an intensive care unit ventilator that has never been exposed to volatile anesthetic agents.
- An MH kit or cart that contains dantrolene along with other drugs and equipment necessary to treat an MH crisis should be placed in the operating room. A full complement of Dantrium or Revonto is 36 vials, and a full complement of Ryanodex is three vials.[185]
- Ice and the ability to crush it and at least 3000 mL of cold intravenous solution should be readily available.
- The patient should be observed for signs of MH, including continuous intraoperative monitoring of the patient's ETCO$_2$, arterial oxygen saturation, and core temperature.
- All perioperative medical personnel should be informed of the preestablished treatment protocol.

Surgery in an ambulatory surgical center can be safely performed for the MHS patient with appropriate planning and if the previously mentioned safety precautions are regarded.[195] A preoperative evaluation and consultation with the surgeon will help determine the best location to perform the needed surgery.

For the MHS patient who has undergone an uneventful surgical course with a trigger-free anesthetic, assiduous monitoring should continue into the postanesthesia care unit (PACU) for at least 1 hour.[196] Patients undergoing outpatient procedures with an uneventful course may be discharged home the same day after a minimum period of 1 hour in the PACU with vital sign monitoring at least every 15 minutes and an additional 1 hour in phase 2 PACU/stepdown.[196] A myoglobin urine test can be used to document the absence of myoglobin in the urine. It is important to provide discharge instructions with clear guidance on signs, symptoms, and instructions on how to manage complications.[197]

Diagnostic Testing

The most accurate and commonly accepted test available for determining MH susceptibility is the caffeine halothane contracture test (CHCT). The CHCT is currently considered the gold standard for MH testing. This test involves taking a biopsy of skeletal muscle from the patient and measuring its contractile response to caffeine, halothane, or both. Normal muscle contracts in response to caffeine or halothane, but this is augmented in the patient with MH. The test is available at five medical centers in North America. Most muscle biopsies can be performed with local or regional anesthesia. Because the test must be completed within hours after muscle biopsy, the patient must travel to the testing site. Patients who have survived an unequivocal episode of MH are considered MHS. MHAUS recommends the CHCT for the following individuals[198]:

- The patient with an MHS family member (as determined by past suspicious MH episode, but without a known *RYR1* pathogenic genetic mutation)
- The patient with a past suspected MH event (wait 6 months postevent, depending on the degree of rhabdomyolysis)
- The patient with **severe** masseter muscle rigidity (MMR) during anesthesia with a triggering agent
- The patient with moderate to mild MMR with evidence of rhabdomyolysis
- The patient with unexplained rhabdomyolysis during or after surgery
- The patient with exercise-induced rhabdomyolysis after a negative rhabdomyolysis workup
- Signs suggestive of, but not definitive, for MH

An alternative to the CHCT for confirmation of MH susceptibility is genetic testing and DNA-based mutation analysis. Intensive investigations have focused on identifying the gene(s) responsible for MH. Most of the focus has been on searching for mutations in genes that encode the ryanodine receptor (RYR1), the dihydropyridine receptor, and associated proteins involved with muscle excitation-contraction coupling. To date, most genetic studies link MH susceptibility to *RYR1* gene variants.[199-203]

Postoperative Care After an MH Episode

The patient who has experienced an acute MH episode should be monitored in an intensive care unit for MH complications, including recrudescence, disseminated intravascular coagulation, pulmonary edema, compartment syndrome (secondary to rhabdomyolysis), and myoglobinuric renal failure. For surgery performed outside a hospital setting, a transfer protocol to a facility that has inpatient capabilities to care for a patient in an MH crisis should be in place.[204] Intravenous dantrolene should be continued at least 24 hours at approximately 1 mg/kg every 4 to 6 hours or at 0.25 mg/kg/hour by continuous

infusion.[205] Dantrolene can be stopped, or the interval between doses increased if all of the following criteria are met:

- Metabolic stability for 24 hours
- Core temp is less than 38°C
- CK is decreasing
- No evidence of myoglobinuria
- Muscular rigidity has resolved

Recrudescence of an intraoperative MH episode may occur in up to 25% of cases with a mean time from the initial reaction to recrudescence of 13 hours, underscoring the importance of continued vigilance.[143,206-208]

Masseter Muscle Rigidity

MMR, or trismus, is a sustained and forceful contracture of the masseter muscle. The contracture may be severe enough to make opening the jaw impossible ("jaws of steel"). A mild increase in masseter muscle tone or incomplete jaw relaxation after succinylcholine administration is fairly common and may be a normal response, but MMR presages MH in 20% to 30% of cases.[143] Because MMR after succinylcholine administration may be a harbinger of MH, if a patient has received succinylcholine and the jaw cannot be opened or the patient has peripheral muscle rigidity, it is advisable to discontinue the trigger anesthetic, assume it is an MH event, and immediately begin MH treatment.[143,144]

Information Resources

The MHAUS provides educational and technical information to patients and health care providers. Information is available on the online (http://www.mhaus.org). An MH hotline should be accessed for MH emergencies 24 hours a day at 1-800-MH-HYPER (1-800-644-9737). Health care providers are encouraged to report MH episodes to the North American MH Registry of MHAUS.

Myotonic Dystrophy

The myotonias are a group of inherited skeletal muscle diseases that include myotonic dystrophy, myotonia congenita, myotonia fluctuans, and paramyotonia congenita. A symptom common to all myotonias is the inability of skeletal muscles to relax after contraction or electrical stimulation. The molecular basis for the aberrant muscle contraction of myotonic dystrophy is not fully clear but appears to be due to abnormal conductance of chloride and sodium ions in the sarcolemma and other channelopathies.[209] The NMJ is not affected.

Myotonic dystrophy (dystrophia myotonica) (DM) is composed of two recognized forms, type 1 (DM1, or Steinert disease) and type 2 (DM2, or proximal myotonic myopathy [PROMM]), with overlapping phenotypes and distinct genetic defects.[210] DM1 and DM2 are characterized by skeletal muscles that are hypoplastic, dystrophic, and weak yet prone to persistent contraction.

Both disorders have multisystem features, including premature ocular cataracts, cardiac conduction problems, and endocrine disorders.[211,212] Of the two types of myotonic dystrophies, DM1 is more severe and roughly five times more common than DM2.[209,212] The discussion in this chapter will focus primarily on DM1.

Incidence

DM1 is the most common and severe inherited muscular dystrophy in adults, with an estimated prevalence of 1 in 8000 to 20,000 depending on the geographic area.[68,99,209,211] In most cases, an affected person has one affected parent. The onset of symptoms can occur at any age (infancy to old age), but most patients (~75%) develop symptoms in the second to third decade.[209,212] A slow, progressive deterioration of skeletal, cardiac, and smooth muscle occurs, resulting in death by the sixth decade in most patients. Death is due to respiratory failure, pneumonia, fatal arrhythmias, or cardiac failure.[211,213,214] Particularly with DM1, the severity of clinical symptoms increases with transmission to subsequent generations (genetic anticipation).[210]

Clinical Manifestations

The name *myotonia dystrophy* aptly identifies two prominent aspects of the disorder, myotonia and muscular dystrophy, but the disease is multisystem with involvement of almost all organ systems in the body.[209,210] Frontal balding, premature ocular cataracts, and testicular atrophy in males form a frequently recognized triad of characteristics. Endocrine abnormalities, such as insulin resistance, occur with a greater frequency than in the general population.[212]

Muscle stiffness and delayed muscle relaxation after contraction (myotonia) occurs in almost all patients with DM1 and is the most common initial symptom.[209,212] Hands, jaw, and tongue are commonly affected. Myotonic symptoms usually precede atrophy and weakness.[212]

Muscle weakness most commonly affects facial (expressionless facies), extraocular, masseter, sternocleidomastoid, and distal limb muscles. The neck flexor muscles are affected early. Dysarthria and dysphagia are frequent problems. A high arched palate limits some patients' ability to fully open their mouth. Distal limb weakness causes severe muscle debility in the later stages of the disease.[210,211,213]

Cardiac disturbances occur in most patients with myotonic dystrophy, often manifesting as intraventricular and atrioventricular conduction defects and arrhythmias.[210,211,215,216] Approximately 65% of patients with DM1 have ECG abnormalities; the most common being prolongation of the PR interval and the QRS duration.[212,215,217] Arrhythmias include sinus bradycardia, atrial tachycardia, flutter or fibrillation, and ventricular tachyarrhthmias.[209,216-218] Conduction defects are progressive and are an important cause of premature death in these patients.[215] Sudden death may result from asystole after complete heart block or from ventricular tachycardia or fibrillation.[215,217] Recommendations include a cardiac pacemaker for DM1 patients with clinically significant cardiac conduction abnormalities and an implantable cardiac defibrillator for patients with cardiac tachyarrhythmia. In a study of 406 adult patients with DM1, patients were characterized as being at risk for sudden cardiac death if the ECG had at least one of the following features: rhythm other than sinus, PR interval of 240 msec or more, QRS duration of 120 msec or more, or second- or third-degree atrioventricular block.[217] Although cardiac contractility is relatively preserved, LV systolic dysfunction and cardiomyopathy may occur at later stages.[212,219]

Weakening of the thoracic muscles, including the diaphragm and intercostal muscles, reduces the respiratory reserve and the vital capacity. In addition, central and obstructive sleep apneas and hypersomnolence are reported in nearly 90% of patients with DM1 and can coexist with decreased ventilatory response to hypoxia and hypercarbia.[209,210]

Gastrointestinal symptoms are common in patients with DM1 and may reflect involvement of smooth muscle. Gastric and intestinal dysmotility produces symptoms of bowel urgency alternating with constipation.[220,221]

Treatment

There is currently no known cure for myotonic dystrophy, and treatment is directed at symptom management.[209,210,212] Sodium channel blockers are often used therapeutic agents for targeting myotonia. These agents delay the return of skeletal muscle membrane excitability by blocking rapid Na$^+$ influx into muscle cells.[222] Other agents used to treat the myotonic contractures include a variety of antiarrhythmic drugs and anticonvulsants, which stabilize skeletal muscle membranes (phenytoin, carbamazepine, flecainide, and propafenone).[209,223] Infiltration of muscles in the operative field with a dilute local anesthetic

has been shown to alleviate refractory skeletal muscle contraction. Neuromuscular blocking agents and regional anesthetics do not consistently prevent or relieve recalcitrant contraction.[224]

Anesthetic Implications

Preoperative evaluation of the patient with myotonic dystrophy should be multidisciplinary and focus on the degree of functional muscle involvement, cardiopulmonary function, and extramuscular manifestations of the disease.[224]

Any drug that has the potential to depolarize skeletal muscle may produce an exaggerated contraction in patients with myotonic dystrophy. Succinylcholine is avoided because administration can produce intense myotonic contracture of the diaphragm, chest wall, or laryngeal muscles for several minutes, making ventilation and intubation difficult or impossible.[224] It is important to keep patients warm. Warming the operating room helps prevent postoperative shivering, which may produce myotonia in susceptible patients.

Nondepolarizing muscle relaxants may be used in these patients as long as any muscle wasting and weakness are appreciated. The response to nondepolarizing relaxants may be normal in some patients, but the initial dose of the nondepolarizer should be reduced and subsequent doses titrated in patients with muscle impairment. Neuromuscular blockade monitoring should be assessed carefully as peripheral nerve stimulation could induce myotonia that is misinterpreted as sustained tetanus even when significant neuromuscular blockade still exists.

It is difficult to predict the reaction to reversal of neuromuscular blockade with anticholinesterase agents as accumulation of ACh at the NMJ can theoretically result in aggravation of myotonia. Alternatively, sugammadex may be the more appropriate option as it has been used successfully to reverse rocuronium-induced muscle blockade in patients with myotonic dystrophy.[225,226] Reversal of neuromuscular blockade with sugammadex is indicated for these patients. Extubation should occur only after the patient is awake with full return of muscle strength.

An abnormal swallowing mechanism and ineffective cough resulting from oropharyngeal muscle involvement renders these patients vulnerable to pulmonary aspiration of gastric contents.[221,224,226,227] The temporomandibular joint (TMJ) may have a tendency to dislocate in patients with DM, therefore a gentle laryngoscopy is the aim.

The severity of respiratory compromise in patients with DM1 should not be underestimated. Pulmonary function test results may serve as useful baselines in the patient with advanced disease. The respiratory depressant effects of hypnotics, sedatives, opioids, and volatile anesthetics may compromise already weakened respiratory musculature and lead to unexpected decompensation.[224] Premedication should be avoided, especially in the patient with a history of central sleep apnea. If opioids are administered, continuous monitoring with pulse oximetry is required given the high risk for respiratory depression and aspiration.

The patient should be questioned preoperatively about syncope, dizziness, and palpitations and the ECG examined for advanced conduction blocks. It may be wise to assume that even asymptomatic patients have some degree of cardiac involvement. Diligent monitoring of cardiovascular parameters should be maintained intraoperatively and postoperatively. Conduction blocks may require access to pacemaker equipment.

When appropriate, regional anesthesia and peripheral nerve blocks using ultrasound guidance are a prudent choice for anesthesia and a successful way to provide intra- and postoperative analgesia with no or minimal doses of opioids.[224]

The ultrashort-acting opioid remifentanil may be an appropriate choice during general anesthesia to provide intraoperative analgesia. In the patient with a history of hypersomnolence, even small doses of short-acting anesthetic agents may be associated with an exaggerated and prolonged anesthetic effect. Speedy reported on a case in which a 31-year-old man with myotonic dystrophy remained unconscious and unable to maintain a patent airway for 4 hours after receiving an anesthetic that consisted of 50 mg of propofol, 0.5% sevoflurane and 50% nitrous oxide in oxygen.[228] Inhalational agents can be safely used in patients with myotonia dystrophy, but close monitoring for cardiac depression is required. The risk for MH is no greater in patients with DM1 than in the general population.[171]

Close and continuous monitoring of the patient's cardiopulmonary status (ECG and SpO_2) is required for at least 24 hours after surgery especially if the patient received sedatives or opioids.[224]

Admission to an intensive care unit for postoperative management should be considered given the significant complications that may occur in these patients. Aggressive pulmonary toilet using a mechanical cough-assist device may be needed in the postoperative period. Preoperative training can facilitate postoperative use of the cough-assist device. Completely uneventful responses to general anesthesia in myotonic patients have also been reported.

Pregnancy may exacerbate the symptoms of myotonic dystrophy. Uterine atony, postpartum hemorrhage, and retained placenta have been reported.[229] The skeletal muscle relaxant effects of magnesium sulfate can result in respiratory compromise in pregnant women with even mild DM1.[230]

Box 36.10 outlines important anesthesia considerations for the patient with DM1.

Rheumatoid Arthritis

Rheumatoid arthritis (RA) is a chronic inflammatory polyarthropathy with extraarticular involvement. The disease is multifactorial, and the clinical picture varies widely in severity, extent of involvement, and symptoms. The capricious course of the disease may be persistent and debilitating or relapsing and remitting.[231] With each successive exacerbation, new joints may become involved.

BOX 36.10 Anesthesia Considerations for the Patient With Myotonic Dystrophy Type 1 (DM1)

- Perform an extensive preoperative evaluation with a multidisciplinary medical team.
- Consider pharyngeal muscle involvement and aspiration risk in the plan of care.
- Avoid premedication (anxiolytics, sedatives, opioids) given potential exaggerated effects in patients with preexisting respiratory muscle weakness, central and obstructive sleep apneas, and hypersomnolence.
- Consider regional anesthesia and peripheral nerve blocks for anesthesia management when appropriate.
- When general anesthesia is required, avoid succinylcholine as it is potential trigger of myotonia. If needed, titrate shorter-acting nondepolarizing muscle relaxant agents judiciously based on preexisting muscle weakness.
- Monitor the electrocardiogram (ECG) closely for conduction blocks. Advanced conduction blocks may require access to pacemaker equipment.
- Keep the patient warm to prevent shivering, which can precipitate myotonia.
- Use anticholinesterase agents cautiously to reverse muscle blockade. Sugammadex has been used uneventfully in patients with DM1.
- Manage postoperative pain with nonsteroidal antiinflammatory drugs, regional techniques, and acetaminophen when appropriate. Use opioids with extreme caution.
- Anticipate slow awakening. Continue close observation and monitoring (ECG, pulse oximetry, nasal capnography) in the recovery area.

Incidence

RA is the most common form of inflammatory arthritis, affecting approximately 1% of the adult population.[231] The onset of RA can occur at any age, but most cases are diagnosed in patients between the ages of 25 and 55 years. RA is two to three times more likely to develop in women than in men.[232] The life expectancy of patients with RA may be reduced by 3 to 7 years.[233] Patients with RA are living longer, and today one-third of patients with RA are older than 60 years.[233,234]

Etiology

The exact cause of RA remains elusive, but it appears to involve a complex interplay among genetic factors, environmental triggers, and chance. Aggressive tumorlike activity in synovial tissue and impaired immunity (T-cell-mediated and T-cell-independent cytokine responses) have been implicated. Stress and other environmental factors may precipitate or aggravate the disease.[231,232]

A viral or a bacterial infection that alters the immune system in a genetically susceptible host may play a role in the etiology. The invading microbe may produce a protein similar to those in the body's own tissue, particularly joint tissue (molecular mimicry).[232] To destroy the antigen, the immune system may mount an autoimmune response and mistakenly direct its attack against its own tissue. Circulating autoantibodies, rheumatoid factors, and anticitrullinated protein antibodies (ACPA) are detectable in up to 90% of patients with RA.[232,233]

Clinical Manifestations

Joint involvement. Inflammation and destruction of synovial tissues are responsible for most of the symptoms and chronic disability associated with RA. Contributors to the inflammatory process are proinflammatory cytokines (tumor necrosis factor [TNF], interleukin-1), synovial-like fibroblasts, osteoclasts, and macrophages.[231,232,234] Joint involvement progresses in three main stages: (1) inflammation of the joint synovial membrane and infiltration by polymorphonuclear leukocytes, (2) rapid division and growth of cells in the joint (synovial proliferation and pannus formation), and (3) liberation of cytokines, osteolytic enzymes, proteases, and collagenases, which damage small blood vessels, cartilage, ligaments, tendons, and bones. Collapse of normal cortical and medullary architecture leads to erosion and dislocation of bone that is contiguous with the inflammatory cell mass.

The onset of symptoms is most often insidious, evolving over a period of weeks to months. The most common sites of onset are the hands, wrists, and feet. There is often symmetric joint involvement. Swelling, warmth, and pain in the affected joints are caused by the inflammatory process. Weight loss and fatigue are noted early in the disease course.

Dissolution of bone and disuse atrophy of bone are found in all seriously affected areas. Inflammation and erosion of bone and tissue may permanently limit the joint's full range of motion. Later stages of the disease are characterized by severe pain, joint instability, loss of physical function, and crippling deformities.

Nerve entrapment may occur at any site where peripheral nerves pass near the inflamed joint. Carpal tunnel syndrome is a common peripheral neuropathy.

Synovitis in the TMJ may limit jaw motion. An estimated 45% to 75% of patients with RA have involvement of the TMJ. As the disease progresses, flexion contractures and soft tissue swelling may lead to a marked limitation in the patient's ability to open the jaw.

Although the thoracic and lumbar spines are usually spared, involvement of the cervical spine is common and includes atlantoaxial subluxation and instability, subaxial instability, and basilar invagination.[235-239] The cervical spine is affected in up to 80% of patients with RA, and the incidence of cervical spine instability may exceed 40%.[239-241] A common site of cervical involvement is C1-C2 (Fig. 36.14). Atlantoaxial (C1-C2) instability occurs from erosion and collapse of bone and destruction of supporting cervical ligaments. Cervical vertebrae subluxation may exert pressure on the spinal cord (Fig. 36.15) or impair blood flow through the vertebral arteries[242-244] (Fig. 36.16). Cervical spine involvement may also lead to limited movement of the neck, odontoid prolapse into the foramen magnum, and severe laryngeal deviation.[236,237,243]

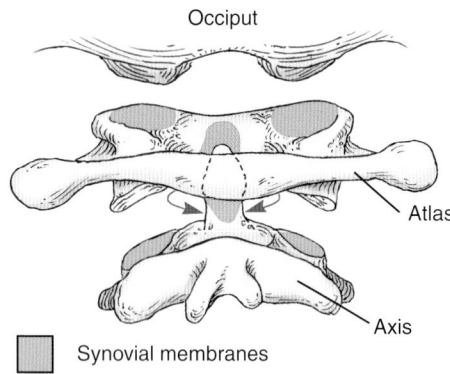

Fig. 36.14 The relationship between the occiput, the atlas (C1), and the axis (C2). The atlas supports the head and rotates about the odontoid process of the axis. The occipitoatlantoaxial articulations are lined by synovial membranes and are firmly supported by surrounding ligaments (*not shown*).

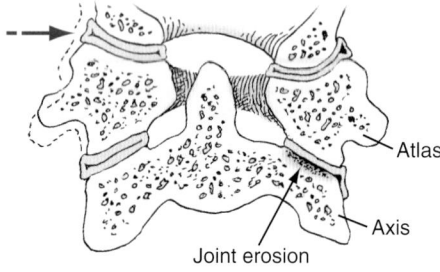

Fig. 36.15 Erosion and collapse of C1 and C2 articular surfaces can lead to a shifting of the atlas over the axis. If the subluxation is pronounced, spinal cord compression may occur.

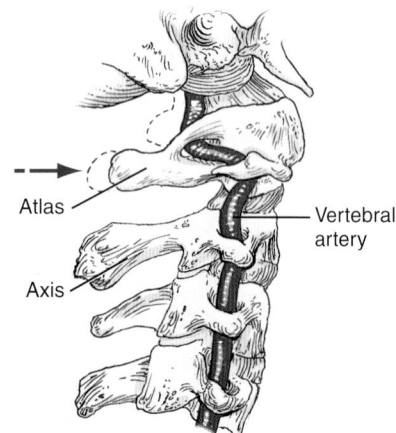

Fig. 36.16 Vertebral artery compression may result from atlantoaxial subluxation.

Arthritis extends to the cricoarytenoid joint of the larynx in 26% to 86% of patients with severe RA.[245,246] The joint may become swollen, inflamed, and fixed in a position that obstructs airflow. Vocal cord nodules and polyps also may be present. Symptoms of cricoarytenoid arthritis include tenderness over the larynx, hoarseness, pain on swallowing with radiation to the ear, and dyspnea or stridor. Patients with no overt clinical symptoms also may have significant laryngeal disease.[233]

Systemic involvement. Although the effects of RA are most clearly seen in joints, the disease is systemic. The immune-mediated inflammatory process produces extraarticular features, including cardiovascular and lung disease, anemia (anemia of chronic disease), myositis, and Sjögren syndrome.[232] The occurrence of extraarticular manifestations is usually associated with more active, erosive articular disease.

Firm, painless subcutaneous nodules occur in approximately 30% to 40% of patients with RA. The nodules usually occur over pressure points, such as the occiput, the sacrum, the ulna, or the Achilles tendon, and may be associated with pressure ulcerations.

Patients with RA have a higher risk of atherosclerosis, myocardial infarction, and stroke.[242] Pericarditis and pericardial effusion may accompany severe progressive RA and impair cardiac performance.

Pulmonary involvement manifests as pleural effusion, pneumonitis, pulmonary nodules, and interstitial fibrosis.[233,247] A restrictive type of ventilatory impairment and decreased lung volumes can produce ventilation and perfusion mismatch that can decrease arterial oxygenation.

Lacrimal duct and salivary gland destruction may result in dryness of the eyes and the mouth (Sjögren syndrome) in about 14% of patients with RA.[248]

Rheumatoid myositis, which is characterized by muscle weakness and eventual muscle necrosis and atrophy, may accompany RA. Inflamed, painful, and underused joints contribute to both osteoporosis and skeletal muscle atrophy.

Treatment

Medical therapy for RA is directed toward relief of pain, suppression of the inflammatory process, immunosuppression, prevention and correction of deformity, and control of systemic involvement.

The introduction of disease-modifying antirheumatic drugs (DMARDs) has dramatically improved long-term outcomes and quality of life for patients with RA. DMARDs used to treat RA have varied mechanisms of action and include methotrexate, sulfasalazine, and hydroxychloroquine.

The antimetabolite and antiinflammatory agent methotrexate is generally the initial DMARD of choice for patients with mild, moderate, or severe RA.[249] Oral ulcerations, bone marrow suppression, pneumonitis, and hepatic damage are potential side effects of methotrexate.[233] Due to the efficacy of methotrexate, nonsteroidal antiinflammatory drugs (NSAIDs) are now used mainly as bridge drugs for relief of acute symptoms.

Biologic response modifiers (biologics) limit joint destruction and slow the progression of the disease by blocking cytokines and cell-signaling molecules involved in the RA inflammatory and immune response. They are generally reserved for patients with moderate to severe disease.[233,234,249] Biologics, such as etanercept, adalimumab, and infliximab, work by interfering with the proinflammatory cytokine, TNF-α, and produce significant improvement in functional ability.[233,249-251]

Other biologic agents involved in various immune activation pathways (rituximab, abatacept, tocilizumab, baricitinib, tofacitinib) are used, sometimes in combination with other drugs, to treat patients who do not respond to methotrexate or TNF inhibitor treatment alone.

Glucocorticoids are potent antiinflammatory drugs that effectively suppress many aspects of the RA disease process. Because of their significant side effects (impaired wound healing, infection, hyperglycemia, osteoporosis), the risk-benefit ratio calls for limiting their use to isolated flares of the disease, low to medium dosage regimens, and adjunctive rather than primary treatment.[249,252]

Surgical interventions for relief of pain or correction or prevention of deformities include total joint replacement, synovectomy, and tenolysis.

Anesthetic Management

Complications associated with RA, as well as medications used in therapy, can impact multiple organ systems beyond the joints.[240] Preoperative examination of an individual patient's disease course, comorbidities, and medication history are likely to reveal specific features that affect the choice of anesthetic agent or mode of anesthesia.

A thorough preoperative assessment of the airway is essential. Particular attention should be directed to the TMJs, cervical spine, and cricoarytenoid joints.

Range of motion of the TMJ must be assessed before anesthesia is induced. Patients with severe TMJ involvement may be unable to open their mouth more than 1 to 2 cm. In such cases, the use of a flexible fiberoptic bronchoscope or other optically guided instruments for tracheal intubation are of proven value.

Neck pain and paresthesias are early symptoms of cervical spine instability, but history and exams alone cannot be relied upon to identify cervical spine disease.[240,253-255] Cervical myelopathy can mimic other rheumatoid complications (neuropathy, arthralgia) and make the extent of cervical involvement underappreciated.[237,256] Compression on the vertebral arteries, with interruption of vertebral artery blood flow, may cause nausea, dysphagia, blurred vision, loss of consciousness, or stroke. However, the absence of preoperative symptoms does not guarantee cervical spine stability or safety, as some patients with significant radiographic evidence of atlantoaxial or subaxial instability are entirely asymptomatic.[238,240,244,253,257] Preoperative imaging studies (radiography, CT, MRI) are essential if the degree of cervical involvement is unknown.[253-255,257]

Cervical spine instability, cricoarytenoid and TMJ involvement, and laryngeal deviation can make intubation of the trachea by direct laryngoscopy an extreme challenge. In addition to preoperative imaging studies, deviation of the larynx caused by cervical spine involvement may be detected by palpating the location of the larynx in relation to the sternal notch. Flexion, extension, and rotation of the neck must be minimized in the presence of cervical instability. Regional anesthesia is often a safe choice for the patient with RA to avoid manipulation of the neck.

Dysphonia in a patient with RA should alert the anesthetist to possible cricoarytenoid joint involvement.[258] Inflammation and narrowing of the glottic opening calls for gentle intubation with a smaller endotracheal tube. The vocal cords may be edematous and erythematous. Involvement of the laryngeal cartilages and cervical spine can predispose to difficult airway management. When intubation is required for general anesthesia, videolaryngoscopy or fiberoptic-guided intubation of the trachea are valuable tools for visualizing the airway while maintaining neutral head position and minimizing neck manipulation.[259,260] The patient should be observed closely for signs of acute airway obstruction after extubation.[237]

The anesthetist should be aware that the spread of sensory spinal anesthesia may be higher in the patient with spinal block. Epidural nodules and synovitis in the thoracolumbar spine may cause narrowing of the subarachnoid space and decrease the cerebrospinal fluid (CSF) volume. The reduced dilution of the local anesthetic may contribute to the sensory effect averaging 1.5 dermatomes higher in a RA patient.[261]

Generalized demineralization of bone increases the risk of fractures in patients with RA. Glucocorticoid therapy aggravates the osteopenia. Careful patient positioning and padding of pressure points and maintaining the natural position of the deformed joints can help prevent nerve palsies, skin ulcerations, and further structural damage to the joints.[260]

TNF inhibitors, biologics, and other immunosuppressive agents are important components of treating RA, but because of their mechanisms of action they may increase the risk for perioperative infections and delayed wound healing.[250,251,262,263] Clinical guidelines vary, but holding biologic therapy is generally advised for at least one dosage interval before major surgery (with adjustments made depending on the specific drug and pharmacokinetics of the individual agent).[235,240,242,262-267] The optimal time of stopping remains uncertain. Some experts assert that biologics may be continued preoperatively for minor operations, given the low risk of infection and impaired wound healing in these cases.[264]

Continuation of methotrexate preoperatively does not increase infection risk, and therefore most recommendations support the safety of methotrexate in the perioperative period.[235,240,242] The American College of Rheumatology recommends continuing treatment with conventional disease-modifying antirheumatic drugs through the perioperative period when RA patients undergo elective knee or hip arthroplasty.[267]

Patients receiving long-term glucocorticoid therapy may be at risk for hypophyseal-pituitary axis suppression. However, glucocorticoid use (especially dosages >10 mg of prednisone equivalents daily) are also a significant risk factor for postoperative infection and impaired wound healing in patients with RA.[240,268,269] Additional research is needed to determine how to best manage these patients, but the relationship between glucocorticoid dosage and infection risk postsurgery suggests that glucocorticoids should be tapered to minimize the risk of impaired wound healing and infection.[240,242,266,268,269]

Box 36.11 summarizes anesthesia implications for the patient with RA.

BOX 36.11 Anesthesia Considerations for the Patient With Rheumatoid Arthritis

- Perform a thorough preoperative assessment of the airway, especially assessing temporomandibular joints, cervical spine, and cricoarytenoid joints. Preoperative imagining studies (radiography, computed tomography, magnetic resonance imaging) may be indicated if the degree of cervical involvement is unknown.
- Consider local or regional anesthesia to avoid manipulation of the neck. The spread of sensory spinal anesthesia may be higher in the patient receiving subarachnoid block due to epidural nodules and synovitis in the thoracolumbar spine.
- If general anesthesia is required, airway management should minimize neck manipulation and may include use of videolaryngoscopy or fiberoptic-guided intubation of the trachea.
- Avoid flexion, extension, and rotation of the neck in the presence of cervical instability.
- Carefully position the patient considering skin and bone fragility imposed by deformed joints, limited mobility, and possible glucocorticoid use.
- Avoid antisialagogues for patients with a history of dry mouth or dry eyes (Sjögren syndrome).
- Tumor necrosis factor inhibitors and other therapy for rheumatoid arthritis suppress the immune response and increase the risk for serious infections. Holding biologic therapy is generally advised at least one dosage interval before major surgery.

SUMMARY

Understanding the pathophysiologic characteristics, clinical presentation, and supporting studies of patients with musculoskeletal abnormalities is essential for safe and effective anesthetic management. A thorough preoperative assessment helps determine overall debility, the extent of muscle strength, risk of pulmonary aspiration, and respiratory and cardiac reserve, and aids in anesthetic selection and planning for postprocedure care.

Management of cases involving musculoskeletal pathology must take into account preoperative drug therapy for the disease and the potential effect drug therapy may have on anesthetic agents and muscle relaxants. An anesthetic agent's margin of safety is often reduced in such patients; therefore fixed dosage regimens should be avoided.

REFERENCES

For a complete list of references for this chapter, scan this QR code with any smartphone code reader app, or visit the following URL: http://booksite.elsevier.com/9780323711944/.

37

The Endocrine System and Anesthesia

Mary C. Karlet

GENERAL PRINCIPLES OF ENDOCRINE PHYSIOLOGY

Body homeostasis is controlled by two major regulating systems: the nervous system and the endocrine or hormonal system.[1-3] Both of these systems communicate, integrate, and organize the body's response to a changing internal or external environment.[1-3]

Organs that secrete hormones are called endocrine glands; collectively, these glands make up the endocrine system. The purpose of the endocrine system is regulation of behavior, growth, metabolism, fluid and electrolyte status, development, and reproduction. To accomplish these complex processes, multiple hormones interact to produce precise biochemical and physiologic responses.

Endocrine glands secrete their hormone products directly into the surrounding extracellular fluid. This distinguishes them from exocrine glands, such as salivary or sweat glands, whose products are discharged through ducts. Important endocrine glands include the pituitary gland, thyroid gland, parathyroid glands, adrenal glands, pancreas, ovaries and testes, and placenta.

Hormones

Endocrine function is mediated by hormones. Hormones are the signaling molecules or chemical messengers that transport information from one set of cells (endocrine cells) to another (target cells). Hormones are released from endocrine glands into body fluids in minute quantities, but they exert powerful control over most metabolic functions.[1-4]

Transmission of a hormonal signal through the bloodstream to a distant target cell (e.g., pituitary gland to the adrenal gland) is called an endocrine function. If a hormone signal acts on a neighboring cell of a different type (e.g., pancreas α cells to pancreas β cells), the interaction is a paracrine function. If the secreted hormone acts on the producer cell itself, the interaction is an autocrine function.[4] Cytokines are peptides secreted by cells that can serve as autocrine, paracrine, or endocrine hormones.[4]

Types of Hormones

Hormones can be classified into three major categories: (1) proteins or peptides, (2) tyrosine amino acid derivatives, and (3) steroids. Table 37.1 outlines common endocrine glands, hormones, their functions, and their structures.

Peptide or protein hormones. Most hormones in the body have a water-soluble peptide or protein structure. This group of hormones includes insulin, growth hormone (GH), vasopressin (antidiuretic hormone [ADH]), angiotensin, prolactin, erythropoietin, calcitonin, somatostatin, adrenocorticotropic hormone (ACTH), oxytocin, glucagon, and parathyroid hormone (PTH). Peptide hormones are synthesized in endocrine cells as prehormones and prohormones. They are processed by the cell and stored in secretory granules within the endocrine gland until needed.[1-4] The proper stimulus to secretion causes exocytosis of the peptide or protein hormone into the extracellular fluid.

Protein hormones, such as insulin, erythropoietin, and GH, can now be synthesized for therapeutic purposes by recombinant deoxyribonucleic acid (DNA) techniques.

Tyrosine amino acid derivative hormones. Thyroid hormones (thyroxine and triiodothyronine) and catecholamine hormones (dopamine, epinephrine, and norepinephrine) are derived from the amino acid tyrosine. Thyroid hormones are stored in the thyroid gland, and catecholamine hormones are stored in the adrenal medulla, and both are released by the appropriate stimulation.[4]

Steroid hormones. All steroid hormones are lipid soluble and derived from cholesterol or have a chemical structure similar to that of cholesterol.[4] Common steroid hormones include hormones of the adrenal cortex (cortisol, aldosterone) and reproductive hormones (estrogen, progesterone, testosterone). Active metabolites of vitamin D are also steroid hormones.[1] In contrast to most other hormones, steroid hormones are not stored in discrete secretory granules but are compartmentalized within the endocrine cell and released into the extracellular fluid by simple diffusion through the cell membrane into the blood.[1]

Transport of Hormones

Once released into the circulation, steroid and thyroid hormones are bound to transport proteins. Most catecholamine and protein hormones are water soluble and circulate free, largely unbound to carriers. Plasma protein binding protects hormones from metabolism and renal clearance.[2,3] The circulating half-life of steroid and thyroid hormones is therefore typically much longer than that of peptide and catecholamine hormones. For example, the thyroid hormone thyroxine, which is over 99% protein bound, has a plasma half-life of 1 to 6 days, whereas insulin, which has essentially no plasma protein binding, has a half-life of approximately 7 minutes.[1]

The major sites of hormone degradation and elimination are the liver and the kidneys, respectively. Some hormone degradation also occurs at target cell sites.[1-4]

Hormone Receptors

Binding to a specific target cell receptor is the primary event that initiates a hormone response. The hormone receptor displays high specificity and affinity for the proper hormone ligand, and the location of the receptor directs the hormone to the specific target organ or target cell site.[2,3] Some hormones, such as insulin and GH, act on widespread target sites; others, such as thyroid-stimulating hormone (TSH), act on one target tissue. After binding, the hormone-receptor complex induces a cascade of intracellular events that produce specific physiologic responses in the target cell.[2,3]

Hormone receptor activation. Hormone receptors are located (1) on the surface of the target cell membrane, (2) in the target cell cytoplasm,

TABLE 37.1   Common Endocrine Glands, Hormones, Their Functions, and Structures

Gland/Tissue	Hormones	Major Functions	Chemical Structure
Hypothalamus	Thyrotropin-releasing hormone	Stimulates secretion of thyroid-stimulating hormone and prolactin	Peptide
	Corticotropin-releasing hormone	Causes release of adrenocorticotropic hormone	Peptide
	Growth hormone–releasing hormone	Causes release of growth hormone	Peptide
	Growth hormone inhibitory hormone (somatostatin)	Inhibits release of growth hormone	Peptide
	Gonadotropin-releasing hormone	Causes release of luteinizing hormone and follicle-stimulating hormone	Peptide
	Dopamine or prolactin-inhibiting factor	Inhibits release of prolactin	Amine
Anterior pituitary	Growth hormone	Stimulates protein synthesis and overall growth of most cells and tissues	Peptide
	Thyroid-stimulating hormone	Stimulates synthesis and secretion of thyroid hormones (thyroxine and triiodothyronine)	Peptide
	Adrenocorticotropic hormone	Stimulates synthesis and secretion of adrenocortical hormones	Peptide
	Prolactin	Promotes development of the female breasts and secretion of milk	Peptide
	Follicle-stimulating hormone	Causes growth of follicles in the ovaries and sperm maturation in Sertoli cells of testes	Peptide
	Luteinizing hormone	Stimulates testosterone synthesis in Leydig cells of testes; stimulates ovulation, formation of corpus luteum, and estrogen and progesterone synthesis in ovaries	Peptide
Posterior pituitary	Antidiuretic hormone (also called vasopressin)	Increases water reabsorption by the kidneys and causes vasoconstriction	Peptide
	Oxytocin	Stimulates milk ejection from breasts and uterine contractions	Peptide
Thyroid	Thyroxine (T_4) and triiodothyronine (T_3)	Increases the rates of chemical reactions in most cells, thus increasing body metabolic rate	Amine
	Calcitonin	Promotes deposition of calcium in the bones and decreases extracellular fluid calcium ion concentration	Peptide
Adrenal cortex	Cortisol	Has multiple metabolic functions for controlling metabolism of proteins, carbohydrates, and fats; also has antiinflammatory effects	Steroid
	Aldosterone	Increases renal sodium reabsorption, potassium secretion, and hydrogen ion secretion	Steroid
Adrenal medulla	Norepinephrine, epinephrine	Same effects as sympathetic stimulation	Amine
Pancreas	Insulin (β cells)	Promotes glucose entry in many cells, and in this way controls carbohydrate metabolism	Peptide
	Glucagon (α cells)	Increases synthesis and release of glucose from the liver into the body fluids	Peptide
Parathyroid	Parathyroid hormone	Controls serum calcium ion concentration by increasing calcium absorption by the gut and kidneys and releasing calcium from bones	Peptide
Testes	Testosterone	Promotes development of male reproductive system and male secondary sexual characteristics	Steroid
Ovaries	Estrogens	Promotes growth and development of female reproductive system, female breasts, and female secondary sexual characteristics	Steroid
	Progesterone	Stimulates secretion of "uterine milk" by the uterine endometrial glands and promotes development of secretory apparatus of breasts	Steroid
Placenta	Human chorionic gonadotropin	Promotes growth of corpus luteum and secretion of estrogens and progesterone by corpus luteum	Peptide
	Human somatomammotropin	Probably helps promote development of some fetal tissues, as well as the mother's breasts	Peptide
	Estrogens	See actions of estrogens from ovaries	Steroid
	Progesterone	See actions of progesterone from ovaries	Steroid
Kidney	Renin	Catalyzes conversion of angiotensinogen to angiotensin I (acts as an enzyme)	Peptide
	1,25-dihydroxycholecalciferol	Increases intestinal absorption of calcium and bone mineralization	Steroid
	Erythropoietin	Increases erythrocyte production	Peptide
Heart	Atrial natriuretic peptide	Increases sodium excretion by kidneys, reduces blood pressure	Peptide
Stomach	Gastrin	Stimulates hydrogen chloride secretion by parietal cells	Peptide
Small intestine	Secretin	Stimulates pancreatic acinar cells to release bicarbonate and water	Peptide
	Cholecystokinin	Stimulates gallbladder contraction and release of pancreatic enzymes	Peptide
Adipocytes	Leptin	Inhibits appetite, stimulates thermogenesis	Peptide

From Hall JE, Hall ME. *Guyton and Hall Textbook of Medical Physiology.* 14th ed. Philadelphia: Elsevier; 2021:915–927.

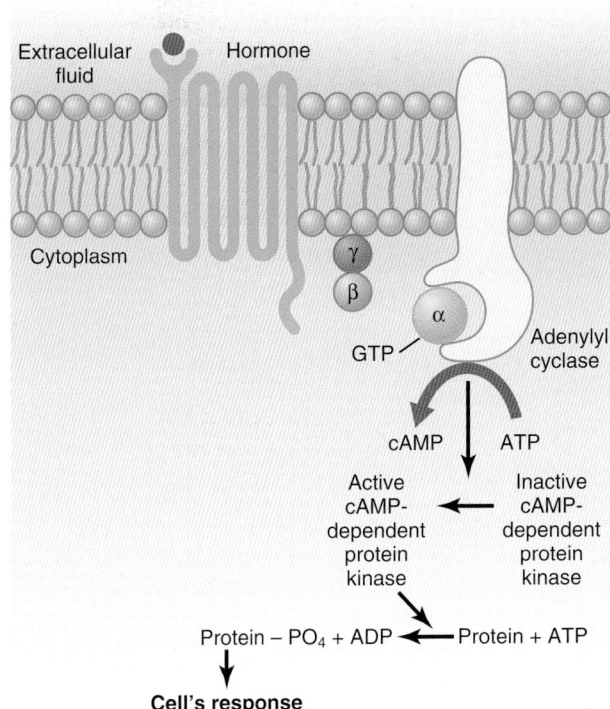

Extracellular fluid   Hormone

Cytoplasm

Fig. 37.1 The cyclic adenosine monophosphate (cAMP) mechanism by which many hormones exert their control of cell function. *ADP,* Adenosine diphosphate; *ATP,* adenosine triphosphate; *GTP,* guanosine triphosphate. (From Hall JE, Hall ME. *Guyton and Hall Textbook of Medical Physiology.* 14th ed. Philadelphia: Elsevier; 2021:924.)

or (3) in the target cell nucleus.[4] Receptors for protein, peptide, and catecholamine hormones are located in or on the surface of the target cell membrane. Hormone binding to a cell membrane receptor triggers a response by activating enzyme systems in or near the plasma membrane bilayer. The activated enzymes generate intracellular signals, called second messengers, which carry the hormone's message within the intracellular space.

Several different second-messenger systems operate in response to cell membrane receptor–hormone binding. Probably the most widely described second-messenger system is the cyclic adenosine monophosphate (cAMP) system. This transduction mechanism is initiated when a hormone occupies a G protein–associated receptor and activates the plasma membrane enzyme adenyl cyclase. The membrane-bound adenyl cyclase then catalyzes the intracellular conversion of adenosine triphosphate to cAMP; cAMP in turn becomes the hormone's intracellular messenger, activating intracellular enzymes, modifying cell membrane permeability or transport, and altering cellular gene expression[1] (Fig. 37.1). The enzyme phosphodiesterase catalyzes the hydrolysis of cAMP and terminates its intracellular actions. Hormones that use cAMP as their second messenger include TSH, vasopressin (V_2 receptor), ACTH, PTH, glucagon, catecholamines (beta receptors), follicle-stimulating hormone (FSH), and luteinizing hormone (LH).[5]

Other intracellular second messengers generated by hormones include calcium, diacylglycerol, inositol triphosphate, and cyclic guanosine monophosphate. The primary intracellular messenger has not been identified for many hormones.

In contrast to peptide and catecholamine hormones, thyroid and steroid hormones produce the desired target cell response chiefly by interacting with specific intracellular hormone receptors.[1] Thyroid and steroid hormones are small, lipophilic molecules that enter target cells by simple diffusion or by special transport mechanisms. Once within

the cell, these hormones occupy specific intracellular receptors.[2,3] Steroid hormone receptors are mainly in the cell cytoplasm. Thyroid hormone receptors are predominately in the target cell nucleus. Here, in combination with their receptors, thyroid hormones interact with DNA in the cell nucleus to enhance or suppress gene transcription or translation.[2,3] Thyroid and steroid hormones cause target cells to synthesize proteins such as enzymes or transport proteins.

Every hormone has a specific onset and duration of action. Hormones that act by binding to cell membrane receptors (peptide, protein, and catecholamine hormones) usually generate a hormonal effect in seconds to minutes. Hormones that bind to intracellular receptors and activate the transcription processes of specific genes (thyroid and steroid hormones) may require several hours or even days to generate a hormonal response.[1,4]

Hormone insensitivity accounts for some endocrine disorders such as type 2 diabetes mellitus (DM). Receptor insensitivity may occur due to impaired receptor function, the presence of antibodies that stimulate or block specific receptor binding sites, or decreased number of receptors (down-regulation).[5]

Hormone receptor regulation. Each target cell that is stimulated by a hormone has 2000 to 100,000 receptors specific to that hormone. These receptors are dynamic molecules that are constantly being destroyed and replaced, changing from day to day.[4] The receptor for insulin, for example, has a normal half-life of only approximately 7 hours.[2,3] Regulation of receptor turnover, and thus hormone receptor number, is a mechanism by which hormone activity can be precisely modulated. Hormone receptor destruction may be part of a normal endocrine response or part of an acquired or genetic disease state.

In many instances, the hormone receptor number is inversely related to the concentration of the circulating hormone. A sustained elevation of the plasma level of a given hormone may cause the target site to decrease the number of receptors per cell. This down-regulation of receptor number serves to decrease the responsiveness of a target cell to hormone excess.[1] The insulin resistance observed in obesity and type 2 DM may be partly explained by down-regulation of the insulin receptors in response to chronically high levels of circulating insulin.[2,3]

Conversely, a low circulating hormone concentration may cause the target gland to increase the number of hormone receptors per cell. This up-regulation of hormone receptor number amplifies the cell's sensitivity to hormone stimulation.[1-3]

Regulation of hormone secretion. The synthesis and secretion of hormones by endocrine glands are regulated by three general control mechanisms: neural controls, biorhythms, and feedback mechanisms.

Neural controls can evoke or suppress hormone secretion. Pain, emotion, smell, touch, injury, stress, sight, and taste can alter hormone release through neural mechanisms. Glucagon, cortisol, and catecholamines, for example, are all stimulated by the stress response to surgery and trauma. Deep general anesthesia or regional anesthesia blunts this stress response but does not eliminate it.

The secretion of other hormones is governed by genetically encoded or acquired biorhythms. These intrinsic hormonal oscillations may be circadian (e.g., the daily variability in glucocorticoid secretion), monthly (e.g., the menstrual cycle), or seasonal (e.g., thyroxine production).[6] The biorhythms also may vary at different stages of development and life (e.g., GH secretion).[7]

Feedback control is another sophisticated mechanism through which a hormonal response is controlled. Many endocrine disorders are caused by the breakdown of feedback loops.[1-3] Negative feedback acts to limit or terminate the production and secretion of a given hormone once the appropriate response has occurred. Negative feedback of a target cell product to the hormone producer (the endocrine gland) limits or prevents hormone excess. When concentrations of the

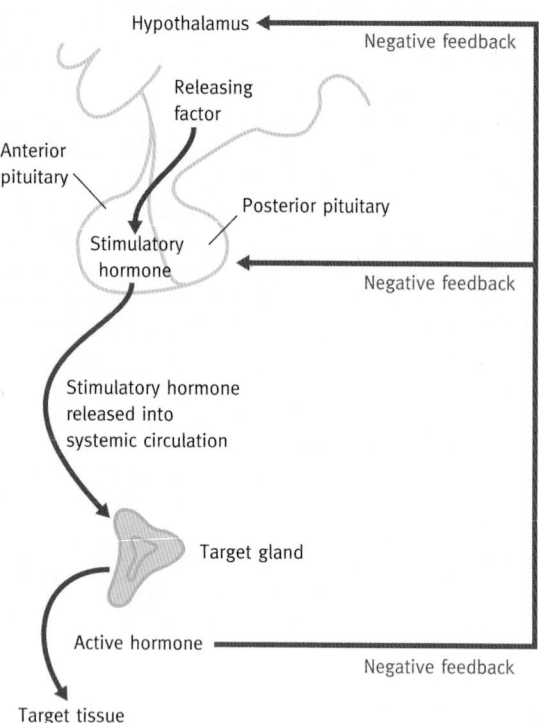

Fig. 37.2 Negative feedback control of hypothalamic-pituitary axis. (From Nicholson G, Hall GM. Hypothalamic-pituitary-adrenal function: anaesthetic implications. *Anaesth Int Care Med.* 2014;15[10]:473–476.)

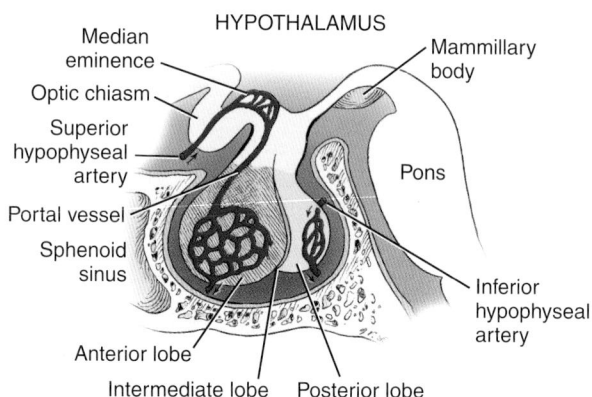

Fig. 37.3 The pituitary gland is located at the base of the brain. It is connected to the overlying hypothalamus by the pituitary or hypophyseal stalk.

product are low, feedback inhibition to the endocrine gland is lessened and hormone secretion is enhanced.

Virtually all hormones secreted from endocrine glands are controlled by some type of negative feedback mechanism.[7] For example, PTH is controlled by calcium, insulin and glucagon are controlled by glucose, and vasopressin is controlled by serum osmolarity.[6] The negative feedback mechanism is a very important system for the regulation of hormones of the hypothalamus and pituitary gland. Hypothalamic hormones stimulate the release of pituitary hormones from the pituitary gland. The pituitary hormones in turn may stimulate an output of product from peripheral target cells. Product from peripheral target tissues may then initiate feedback to the pituitary gland or the hypothalamus, or both, to inhibit pituitary and hypothalamic hormone synthesis and discharge.[2,3] Fig. 37.2 shows a typical endocrine negative feedback system.

Positive feedback is a less common hormone-regulating mechanism in which a given hormone response initiates signals amplifying hormone release. The surge in LH that precedes ovulation is stimulated by LH; this is an example of positive feedback.[2,3]

Hormones produced by nonendocrine tissues (ectopic hormones) may be abnormally elevated and without control by normal feedback systems. Ectopic hormone production is said to be autonomous.[5]

PITUITARY GLAND

Relationship Between Pituitary Gland and Hypothalamus

The pituitary gland, or hypophysis, is known as the master endocrine gland.[6,7] It secretes hormones that have far-reaching effects on various homeostatic, developmental, metabolic, and reproductive functions of the body. The pituitary is a small endocrine gland (only about 500 mg

in weight and approximately the size of a pea) centrally located at the base of the brain. It is enclosed within a bony cavity of the sphenoid bone called the sella turcica.[6,7] The pituitary gland is connected to the overlying hypothalamus by the hypophysial stalk (pituitary stalk). The hypothalamus is located below the thalamus, behind the optic chiasm, and between the optic tracts. The pituitary, hypothalamus, and some of the surrounding structures are shown in Fig. 37.3.

The brain, via the hypothalamus, is an important regulator of pituitary gland secretion. The hypothalamus collects and integrates information (e.g., pain, emotions, energy needs, water balance, olfactory sensations, electrolyte concentrations) from almost all parts of the body and uses this information to control the secretion of vital pituitary hormones.[6,7] Pituitary hormone secretion also is regulated by feedback control from peripheral target organ hormones or other target organ products. Some parts of the pituitary gland and hypothalamus have virtually no blood-brain barrier, allowing feedback products to exert potent effects.[8]

Functionally and histologically, the pituitary gland is divided into two distinct portions: the anterior lobe (adenohypophysis) and the posterior lobe (neurohypophysis).[6,7] The anterior pituitary lobe is embryologically derived from an upward invagination of pharyngeal epithelial cells (Rathke pouch). The posterior pituitary lobe develops from a downward outpouching of ectoderm from the brain.

Anterior Pituitary Lobe

The anterior pituitary lobe, which constitutes approximately 80% of the pituitary gland by weight, secretes six major peptide hormones.[7] Target sites for the anterior pituitary hormones are shown in Fig. 37.4. In addition to secreting the six "classic" hormones, the pituitary also secretes other hormones, including melanocyte-stimulating hormone, β-endorphins, substance P, and others.

1. Growth hormone (somatotropin) promotes skeletal development and body growth, stimulates insulin-like growth factor-1 (IGF-1) from the liver, and inhibits action of insulin on carbohydrate and fat metabolism.
2. Corticotropin or ACTH regulates the growth of the adrenal cortex and stimulates the release of cortisol and androgenic hormones from the zona reticularis and zona fasciculata of the adrenal gland. ACTH and its precursor proopiomelanocortin (POMC) contain a melanocyte-stimulating peptide sequence. As a result, increased ACTH is often associated with skin pigmentation.
3. Thyroid-stimulating hormone (thyrotropin) controls the growth and metabolism of the thyroid gland and the secretion of thyroid

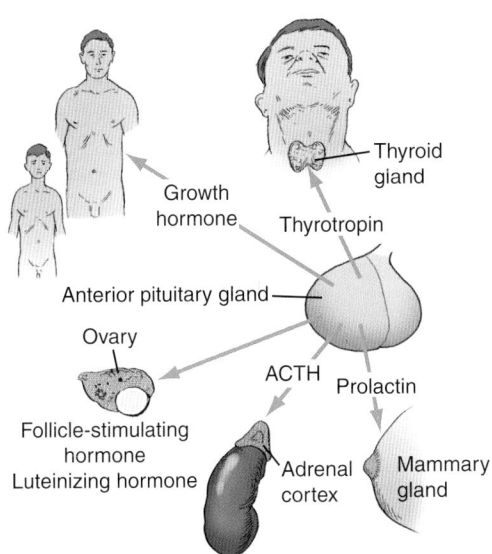

Fig. 37.4 Major target sites for anterior pituitary hormones. *ACTH,* Adrenocorticotropic hormone.

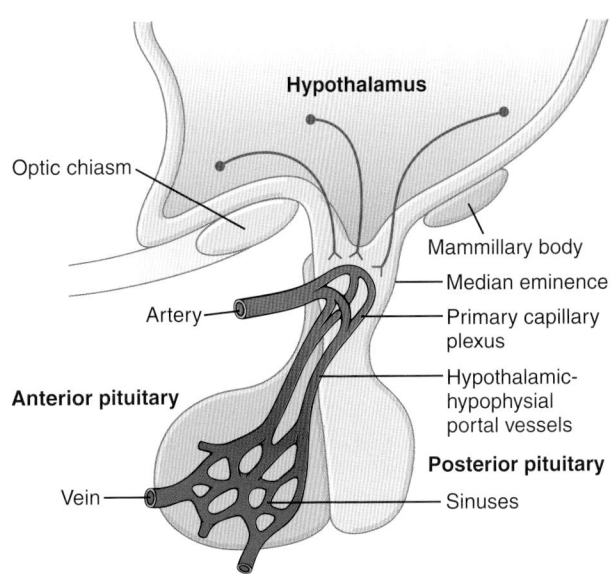

Fig. 37.5 Hypothalamic-hypophysial portal system. (From Hall JE, Hall ME. *Guyton and Hall Textbook of Medical Physiology.* 14th ed. Philadelphia: Elsevier; 2021:931.)

hormones (thyroxine and triiodothyronine), which regulate intracellular metabolic activity in virtually all cells of the body.

4. Follicle-stimulating hormone stimulates ovarian follicle development in females and spermatogenesis in males.

5. Luteinizing hormone induces ovulation and corpus luteum development in females and stimulates the testes to produce testosterone in males.

6. Prolactin promotes mammary gland development and milk production (lactogenesis) by the breasts. Prolactin also exerts an effect on reproductive function by inhibiting the synthesis and secretion of LH and FSH. Prolactin synthesis is markedly increased during pregnancy.

Anterior pituitary hormones are synthesized and secreted by five distinct endocrine cell types within the gland: somatotropes synthesize GH; gonadotropes synthesize the two gonadotropic hormones, LH and FSH; thyrotropes synthesize TSH; corticotropes synthesize ACTH; and lactotropes (mammotropes) synthesize prolactin.

Control of Anterior Pituitary Hormone Secretion

Synthesis of anterior pituitary hormones is controlled by signals from the hypothalamus. Neurosecretory cells in various hypothalamic nuclei respond to input from many sources in the body by synthesizing specific neurohormones that have corresponding anterior pituitary target cells.[7]

Hypothalamic neurohormones are released into a capillary bed of the hypothalamus in an area called the median eminence. The hypothalamic hormones travel from the capillary plexus of the median eminence, down the pituitary stalk, in a specialized vascular system called the hypothalamic-hypophysial portal vessels (Fig. 37.5). At the anterior pituitary lobe, the hypothalamic hormones are released in high concentrations into capillary sinuses located among the glandular cells.[7] The hypothalamic hormones then locate and bind to their specific target cell type.

Specific hypothalamic hormones have either an inhibitory or a stimulatory effect on their corresponding anterior pituitary target cells. Synthesis and release of most anterior pituitary hormones depend on a positive stimulatory signal from a given hypothalamic hormone. Some anterior pituitary cells are subject to both inhibitory and stimulatory control by more than one hypothalamic neurohormone.[6]

Synthesis of prolactin from anterior pituitary lactotroph cells is unique in that it is tonically restrained by inhibitory hormonal signals (dopamine) from the hypothalamus. These inhibitory signals serve as a physiologic brake for lactotroph growth and prolactin synthesis. The inhibitory effect of dopamine agonists, such as bromocriptine or cabergoline, is exploited therapeutically for suppressing pathologic production of prolactin from pituitary tumors.[6] Table 37.2 outlines the major hypothalamic releasing or inhibiting hormones (or factors) and their corresponding anterior pituitary target sites.

Anterior Pituitary Disorders

Disorders involving the anterior pituitary system may be due to a defect at the peripheral endocrine gland (primary disorder), the pituitary gland (secondary disorder), or the hypothalamus (tertiary disorder).[6] Pituitary tumors account for approximately 15% of all intracranial tumors.[9] Most pituitary tumors—both functional, secreting tumors and nonfunctional, nonsecreting tumors—are benign adenomas. Pituitary carcinoma is exceedingly rare.[9-11] The pituitary gland is highly vascular and therefore vulnerable to ischemia and infarction with head injury or shock.[5]

Hyposecretion. Anterior pituitary hormone deficiency states may occur when large, nonfunctional pituitary tumors (e.g., chromophobe adenoma, craniopharyngioma, Rathke pouch cysts) compress and destroy normal anterior pituitary cells. Postpartum hemorrhagic shock causing pituitary vessel thrombosis (Sheehan syndrome), bleeding into a pituitary tumor, irradiation, infections, trauma, damage to the pituitary stalk, and infiltrative disorders (e.g., sarcoidosis, amyloidosis) are other causes of pituitary hyposecretion. Generalized pituitary hypofunction (panhypopituitarism) involving all pituitary hormones (GH, TSH, ACTH, prolactin, gonadotropins) is more common than reduced output of a single anterior pituitary hormone.

Important effects of panhypopituitarism include decreases in thyroid function due to reduction in levels of TSH, depression of cortisol production by the adrenal cortex due to the lowering of ACTH levels, and suppression of sexual development and reproductive function due to deficient gonadotropic hormone secretion.[7] In addition, large pituitary tumors (macroadenomas >1 cm) may extend out of the sella turcica and compress the nearby optic chiasm and surrounding brain

TABLE 37.2   Hypothalamic Hormones and Corresponding Anterior Pituitary Hormones

Hypothalamic Releasing/ Inhibiting Hormones	Anterior Pituitary Target Cell Type	Anterior Pituitary Hormone Produced	Hormone Target Site	Primary Peripheral Hormone Involved in Negative Feedback
Thyrotropin-releasing hormone (TRH)	Thyrotrope	Thyroid-stimulating hormone (TSH, thyrotropin)	Thyroid gland	Triiodothyronine (T_3)
Corticotropin-releasing hormone (CRH)	Corticotrope	Adrenocorticotropic hormone (ACTH, corticotropin)	Zona fasciculata and zona reticularis of adrenal cortex	Cortisol
Gonadotropin-releasing hormone (GnRH)	Gonadotrope	Follicle-stimulating hormone Luteinizing hormone	Gonads (testes, ovaries)	Estrogen, progesterone, testosterone
Prolactin-inhibitory hormone (dopamine, PIH)	Lactotrope	Inhibits prolactin synthesis and secretion		None
Growth hormone–releasing hormone (GHRH)	Somatotrope	Growth hormone	All tissues	Growth hormone, insulin growth factor-1
Growth hormone–inhibitory hormone (somatostatin)	Somatotrope	Inhibits growth hormone secretion		Growth hormone, insulin growth factor-1

tissue, producing diplopia, visual loss, facial numbness, facial pain, or seizures.[12]

Surgical intervention may be implemented for decompression or removal of the pituitary tumor or to control bleeding. Surgical patients with acute hypopituitary disorders may require treatment of increased intracranial pressure and consideration of hormone replacement, especially thyroid and cortisol replacement.[13] Because of the possibility of diabetes insipidus (DI; low ADH) after removal of the tumor, vasopressin should also be available.

Hypersecretion. Most pituitary tumors are benign hypersecreting pituitary adenomas.[11,12] The three most common hypersecreting pituitary tumors are those that produce prolactin, ACTH, or GH. Tumors that secrete gonadotropin and thyrotropin hormones are rare. Pituitary tumors may also be inherited as part of multiple endocrine neoplasia (MEN) type 1, an autosomal dominant syndrome characterized primarily by a genetic predisposition to parathyroid, pancreatic islet, and pituitary adenomas.[9,11] (see Table 37.13).

Preparation pituitary surgery is guided by the results of preoperative neurologic and endocrine tests, hormone assays, and radiographic examination of the skull. Hypersecreting pituitary tumors are usually microadenomas. Less commonly, pituitary tumors become large and compress and destroy neighboring cells, producing a deficiency in hormones from surrounding anterior pituitary cells.

Hyperprolactinemia is the most common pituitary hormone hypersecretion syndrome in both men and women.[11] Prolactin-secreting tumors commonly produce symptoms of galactorrhea, amenorrhea, and infertility in women, and diminished libido and infertility in men.[12] Dopamine agonists (cabergoline, bromocriptine) are used to control prolactin levels, decrease tumor size, and restore normal gonadal function. Patients who have a suboptimal response to medical therapy benefit from microsurgical removal of the pituitary tumor.[12]

Specific anesthetic management implications for patients with excess ACTH (Cushing disease) and excess GH (acromegaly) are described in this chapter.

Growth Hormone

GH-secreting somatotrope cells constitute up to 50% of the total anterior pituitary cell population.[14] GH (somatotropin) is synthesized and secreted by somatotrope cells and is under complex control by the hypothalamus and peripheral factors.[7,14] GH-releasing hormone from the hypothalamus stimulates GH release, and GH-inhibiting hormone (somatostatin), also from the hypothalamus, is a powerful inhibitor of GH release.

Pulsatile fluctuations of the hypothalamic releasing and inhibiting hormones regulate somatotrope activity throughout the day.[6] In addition, GH secretion is stimulated by stress, trauma, hypoglycemia, strenuous exercise, and deep sleep.[6,7] The GH secretion rate is generally increased in childhood, followed by a further increase in adolescence, a plateau in adulthood, and declining values in old age. The normal physical decline associated with aging may be due in part to the age-related decline in GH production.[6,7]

Unlike other anterior pituitary hormones, GH does not exert its principal effects through a specific target gland but functions through all or almost all tissues of the body. It promotes the growth and development of most tissues capable of growing.[7] A major target of GH is the liver, where it stimulates the production of somatomedin C (also called IGF-1). Somatomedin C and other somatomedins mediate many of GH's effects.[7,9] Skeletal muscle, the heart, skin, and visceral organs undergo hypertrophy and hyperplasia in response to GH and somatomedins.[7,9,14,15]

The most obvious effect of GH is on the skeletal frame. It produces linear bone growth by stimulating the epiphyseal cartilage or growth plate at the ends of long bones. Throughout childhood, under the influence of GH, bone forming cells called osteoblasts are stimulated. Bones elongate at the epiphyseal plate, and the skeletal frame enlarges. After puberty, the growth plates unite with the shaft of the bone, bone lengthening stops, and GH has no further capacity to increase bone length.[7]

GH and IGF-1 support growth by increasing amino acid transport into cells and enhancing protein synthesis in the cell. GH also decreases the catabolism of existing proteins by stimulating lipolysis and mobilizing free fatty acids for energy use, a protein-sparing effect. In addition to its growth-promoting activities, GH is said to be a diabetogenic hormone. It increases blood glucose levels by decreasing the sensitivity of cells to insulin (promoting insulin resistance) and inhibiting glucose uptake into cells.[7,15]

As is true of other anterior pituitary hormones, GH secretion is subject to negative feedback control. GH, as well as IGF-1, exert negative feedback control on the pituitary and hypothalamus. GH release is also inhibited by hyperglycemia and increased plasma free fatty acids.

Hyposecretion. Deficient GH production in childhood can result in insufficient bone maturation and short stature, a condition known as dwarfism. Mild obesity, decreased lean body mass, and hypoglycemia are common in GH-deficient dwarfs. Puberty is usually delayed. Symptoms of GH deficiency may be the result of hypothalamic dysfunction, pituitary disease, failure to generate normal insulin growth factor hormones, or GH-receptor defects.[7]

The biosynthesis of human GH by recombinant DNA technology has enhanced the outlook for patients with GH deficiency. Treatment of GH-deficient dwarfs leads to a positive nitrogen balance, accretion of lean body mass, and an improvement in metabolic homeostasis.[7]

Hypersecretion. Approximately 15% of all pituitary tumors release excess GH. Hypersecretion of GH is usually caused by a GH-secreting pituitary adenoma (99% of cases), producing a highly distinctive syndrome in adults called acromegaly. Acromegaly is produced by the excessive action of GH and IGF-1 after adolescence, leading to anatomic changes and metabolic dysfunction.[12,15,16] If hypersecretion of GH occurs before puberty, that is, before closure of the growth plates, all body tissues grow and the individual grows very tall (8–9 ft), an extremely rare condition known as gigantism.

Because growth plates close with adolescence, the excessive production of GH associated with acromegaly does not induce bone lengthening but rather enhances the growth of periosteal bone by the stimulatory effects of GH on bone osteoblasts. Periosteal growth causes new bone to be deposited on the surface of existing bone. The unrestrained bone growth in patients with acromegaly produces bones that are massive in size and thickness. Bones of the hands and feet (acral) become particularly large, almost twice normal size.[9,11]

Acromegaly is diagnosed most often in adults in their 40s and 50s, but the disease is slowly progressive and is usually present for years preceding the diagnosis.[5] Soft tissue changes are also prominent with GH hypersecretion. The patient develops coarsened facial features (acromegalic facies) that include a large, bulbous nose, supraorbital ridge overgrowth, dental malocclusion, and a prominent prognathic mandible.[9] The changes in appearance are insidious, and many patients do not seek treatment until the diagnosis is obvious and the disease course is advanced.[9,17] Thick and course skin may become especially apparent when difficulty is encountered inserting an intravenous catheter.[5]

Overgrowth of internal organs is less apparent clinically but no less serious. The liver, heart, spleen, and kidneys become enlarged. Pulmonary function tests are consistent with increased lung volumes, but gas exchange is usually not grossly abnormal.[9] Exercise tolerance may be limited due to increased body mass and skeletal muscle weakness.

Cardiomyopathy and hypertension in patients with acromegaly can lead to symptomatic cardiac disease (e.g., diastolic dysfunction, heart failure).[11,17,18] Hypertension occurs in more than 40% of patients, and evidence of left ventricular hypertrophy is common.[11,12,15] Baseline echocardiography is indicated.[15]

The insulin-antagonistic effect of GH produces glucose intolerance in most patients and frank diabetes in up to 25% of patients with acromegaly.[11]

Clinical manifestations resulting from the local effects of the expanding tumor may include headaches and visual field defects.[11] Significant increases in intracranial pressure are uncommon. Compression or destruction of normal pituitary tissue by the tumor may eventually lead to panhypopituitarism. Common features of acromegaly are summarized in Box 37.1.

If untreated, acromegaly is associated with decreased life expectancy, with cardiac, cerebrovascular, and respiratory complications being the most common causes of death. Hormonal control has a beneficial impact on survival.[9,15,19,20] Lowering serum GH levels results in reduction of the mortality rate.

Treatment for acromegaly is aimed at restoring normal GH levels through surgical, pharmacologic, and radiotherapeutic approaches.[10,11,16]

> ## BOX 37.1 Common Features of Acromegaly
>
> - Skeletal overgrowth (enlarged hands and feet, prominent prognathic mandible)
> - Soft tissue overgrowth (enlarged lips, tongue, and epiglottis; distortion of facial features)
> - Visceromegaly
> - Hypertension
> - Osteoarthritis
> - Glucose intolerance
> - Peripheral neuropathy
> - Skeletal muscle weakness
> - Extrasellar tumor extension (headache, visual field defects)

The preferred initial therapy, especially for small, well-circumscribed adenomas, is microsurgical removal of the pituitary tumor, with preservation of the gland.[12] Surgery achieves biochemical cure in 70% to 90% of microadenomas (<1 cm) and approximately 50% remission for macroadenomas.[9,11]

The surgical approach to the pituitary tumor is most often via the transsphenoidal route, and this method is generally well tolerated by most patients.[9,13,21-23] (see Fig. 31.19). A transcranial surgical approach is usually reserved for very large tumors with suprasellar extension.[13]

For transsphenoidal pituitary surgery, the head of the bed is typically elevated 15 degrees to improve venous drainage. Venous air embolism is usually not a concern unless there is cavernous sinus invasion by the tumor and the patient is positioned in a steep head-up tilt. The approach and exposure of the tumor are not usually associated with significant blood loss.[9,22,23] An anesthetic technique that incorporates muscle relaxation and allows for smooth extubation and rapid neurologic assessment is desirable. The patient should be prepared preoperatively for awakening with nasal packing. Surgical complications are not common but may include epistaxis, transient DI, cranial nerve damage, hyponatremia, and cerebral spinal fluid leaks.[11,17,22,23] Surgical ablation is usually successful in rapidly reducing tumor size, inhibiting GH secretion, and alleviating some symptoms.[17,22]

Administration of octreotide or lanreotide (somatostatin receptor ligands), cabergoline (a dopamine agonist), pegvisomant (a GH-receptor antagonist), and gland irradiation may be used for tumor regression or as treatment options for patients who are not surgical candidates.[9,16,21] A more detailed discussion of anesthesia for pituitary surgery can be found in Chapter 31.

Anesthetic implications of acromegaly. Preanesthetic assessment of patients with acromegaly should include a careful examination of the airway. Facial deformities and the large nose may hamper adequate fitting of an anesthesia mask. Endotracheal intubation may be a challenge because of the patient's large and thick tongue (macroglossia), prognathism, enlarged thyroid gland, hypertrophy and distortion of the epiglottis, and general soft tissue overgrowth in the upper airway.[12,17,24-27] Subglottic narrowing and vocal cord enlargement may dictate the use of a smaller-diameter endotracheal tube. Nasotracheal intubation should be avoided or approached cautiously because of possible turbinate enlargement. The occurrence of Mallampati III and IV grades is higher in patients with acromegaly, and the incidence of difficult intubations may be four to five times higher than patients without acromegaly.[26] Preoperative dyspnea, stridor, or hoarseness should alert the anesthetist to airway involvement. Indirect laryngoscopy, lateral neck radiographs, and computed tomography (CT) of the neck may be performed for thorough assessment.[25-27] Airway adjuncts should be readily available during induction of anesthesia. If difficulties in maintaining an adequate airway are anticipated, optically guided intubation or fiberoptic-guided intubation in an awake patient is of proven value.[12,13,17] A surgeon should be on hand and equipment for tracheostomy available if airway changes are advanced.

Arthropathy affects approximately 75% of acromegaly patients.[15] Overgrowth of vertebrae may cause kyphosis and osteoarthritis and may make central neuraxial anesthesia a challenge.

More than 60% of patients with acromegaly have sleep apnea. The predisposition to airway obstruction in these patients makes assiduous perioperative monitoring of the patient's respiratory status an absolute precaution.[11-13,15,17]

The frequent occurrence of cardiomyopathy, coronary artery disease, and hypertension in acromegalic patients warrants a thorough preanesthetic cardiac evaluation. Hyperglycemia may complicate the perioperative period, mandating careful perioperative monitoring of blood glucose levels.[15,17]

Stress-level glucocorticoid therapy may be indicated to address any impairment of the adrenal axis.[12] Entrapment neuropathies, such as carpal tunnel syndrome, are common in patients with acromegaly. Hypertrophy of the carpal ligament may cause inadequate ulnar artery flow, which should be factored into any decision to place an arterial catheter.

Posterior Pituitary Lobe

The posterior pituitary lobe secretes two important peptide hormones: antidiuretic hormone (vasopressin) and oxytocin. Oxytocin and ADH are almost identical structurally. The two hormones have quite different actions at physiologic concentrations, but partial functional similarity may become apparent at supraphysiologic levels. ADH controls water reabsorption in the kidney and is a major regulator of serum osmolarity. It produces vasoconstriction at high levels, hence the name vasopressin. Oxytocin stimulates contraction of myoepithelial cells of the breast for milk ejection during lactation. It also powerfully stimulates uterine smooth muscle contraction during delivery of the baby at the end of gestation.[5] Oxytocin and its derivatives are used clinically for inducing labor and decreasing postpartum bleeding.

In contrast to the anterior pituitary lobe, which communicates with the hypothalamus via a vascular system, the posterior pituitary lobe communicates with the hypothalamus through a neural pathway. Also, unlike anterior pituitary hormones, posterior pituitary hormones are not synthesized within the pituitary gland itself but rather within two large nuclei of the hypothalamus, the supraoptic nucleus and the paraventricular nucleus. ADH is chiefly synthesized in the supraoptic nucleus and oxytocin in the paraventricular nucleus.[5,7] As shown in Fig. 37.6, nerve fibers arising from these hypothalamic nuclei transport ADH and oxytocin down the pituitary stalk by axoplasmic flow to the posterior pituitary lobe. There, the hormones are stored in secretory granules at the nerve terminals. With proper excitation, nerve impulses originating in the cell bodies of the supraoptic or paraventricular nucleus are transmitted down the pituitary stalk and stimulate the release of ADH or oxytocin from the posterior pituitary lobe. The hormones then diffuse into nearby blood vessels and are transported to their distant target sites.

Antidiuretic Hormone

ADH is the body's principal preserver of water balance. It acts on specific receptors on the distal tubule and medullary collecting ducts of the kidney to increase the absorption of solute-free water through water channels called aquaporins.[28] Without ADH, the collecting ducts are impermeable to water reabsorption, water loss in the urine is excessive, and serious dehydration and hypernatremia are provoked.[7]

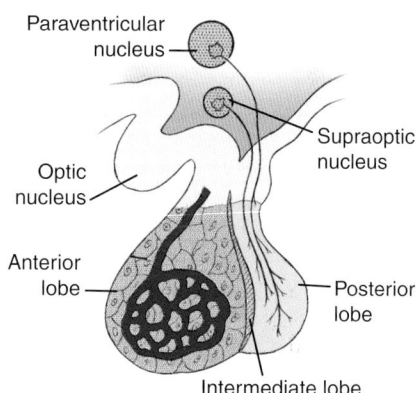

Fig. 37.6 Nerve fibers arising from the supraoptic nucleus and the paraventricular nucleus transport antidiuretic hormone and oxytocin to the posterior pituitary.

The integrated role of thirst, vasopressin, and renal response conserves water in the body and supports normal body fluid osmolarity. Plasma osmolarity is physiologically controlled within a small range (285–290 mOsm/L).[8]

Three major types of vasopressin receptors have been identified: V_1, V_2, and V_3. Activation of the V_1 receptor mediates vasoconstriction. V_2 receptors mediate water reabsorption in the renal tubules. V_3 receptors are found within the central nervous system, and their stimulation modulates corticotrophin secretion.[8,29]

ADH acts primarily to reabsorb water, increasing urine osmolarity, decreasing serum osmolarity, and increasing blood volume. Additionally, high levels of ADH stimulate V_1 receptors and cause potent systemic vasoconstriction, especially in splanchnic and renal vascular beds. ADH-induced vasoconstriction of vascular beds has been exploited therapeutically for control of catecholamine-resistant vasodilatory shock (vasoplegic syndrome), hemorrhage, and sepsis.[8,30,31] Desmopressin (1-deamino-8-D-arginine vasopressin [DDAVP]), a synthetic arginine analog of ADH and a selective V_2 agonist, increases circulating levels of von Willebrand factor and factor VIII. In addition to effectively treating ADH deficiency, DDAVP may be used to reverse coagulopathy associated with hemophilia A, the coagulopathy of renal failure, and platelet adhesion defects such as von Willebrand disease.[8]

Consonant with its role of maintaining normal fluid homeostasis, ADH is secreted in response to an increase in plasma osmolarity or plasma sodium ion concentration, a decrease in blood volume, or a decrease in blood pressure.[7]

The osmolarity of body fluids is the main variable controlling ADH secretion. Serum osmolarity changes are sensed by hypothalamic osmoreceptors, which in turn alter ADH synthesis and secretion. Although variable, one person to the next, the plasma osmotic threshold for ADH release is typically only 1% to 4% higher than normal plasma osmolarity.[5] Therefore, when the plasma tonicity increases even subtly, healthy individuals release ADH into the blood. The interplay between ADH and water is controlled by a delicate negative feedback loop. Water deprivation (increased plasma osmolarity) initiates signals in the hypothalamic osmoreceptors that cause ADH release from the pituitary gland to increase three- to fivefold. ADH, in turn, enhances renal tubular water reabsorption, dilutes the extracellular fluid, and restores normal osmotic composition.[7] Conversely, water ingestion (decreased plasma osmolarity) suppresses the osmoreceptor signal for ADH release. Thirst provides a second line of defense in water balance. The thirst threshold is set approximately 3% higher than the osmotic threshold for ADH.[28]

BOX 37.2   Stimulators of Antidiuretic Hormone Action or Release

- Increased plasma sodium ion concentration
- Increased serum osmolarity
- Decreased blood volume
- Decreased blood pressure
- Smoking (nicotine)
- Stress
- Nausea
- Vasovagal reaction
- Various medications (chlorpropamide, clofibrate, thiazide diuretics, carbamazepine, nicotine, cyclophosphamide, vincristine, morphine, high-dose oxytocin)
- Angiotensin II
- Positive pressure ventilation

A 10% to 20% decrease in blood volume or blood pressure also provokes ADH release.[28] Changes in blood volume are sensed in peripheral baroreceptors (especially the great veins and pulmonary vessels) and atrial stretch receptors. When these baroreceptors sense underfilling (volume depletion), they transmit afferent signals through vagal and glossopharyngeal nerves to the hypothalamus.[5,28] The hypothalamus responds by increasing ADH synthesis and stimulating ADH release, sometimes as high as 50 times the normal rate.[7]

ADH secretion also can be stimulated by nausea, vomiting, acute hypoglycemia, and glucocorticoid deficiency. Emetic stimuli are especially potent since they typically elicit an immediate increase (50- to 100-fold) in plasma ADH even when nausea is not associated with vomiting.[28]

The perioperative period is characterized by enhanced ADH secretion.[31,32] Common perioperative conditions, such as stress, nausea, hemorrhage, hypotension, and various drugs, can be strong stimuli to ADH release. Positive pressure ventilation enhances ADH release by reducing central blood volume. The mild hyponatremia sometimes observed postoperatively may be at least partly explained on the basis of ADH action.[33] Box 37.2 lists factors that stimulate ADH release or enhance the action of ADH at the renal tubules.

Deficient antidiuretic hormone and anesthetic implications. Inadequate ADH secretion from the posterior pituitary lobe or the inability of renal collecting duct receptors to respond to ADH (impaired receptor sensitivity) is called diabetes insipidus (DI). Decreased ADH synthesis, transport, or release from the posterior pituitary produces neurogenic or central DI.[34] Renal collecting duct resistance to vasopressin is termed nephrogenic DI.[28] Both forms of DI are characterized by the production of abnormally large volumes of dilute urine and continuous thirst.[5]

Common causes of neurogenic DI include surgery in or around the neurohypophysis, meningitis/encephalitis, infiltrating pituitary lesions, and brain neoplasms.[34] It is also a well-recognized complication associated with closed-head trauma.[35] Neurogenic DI that develops after pituitary surgery is usually transient and often resolves in about 5 days.[34] In about one-half of adult patients, neurogenic DI is idiopathic.[28]

Nephrogenic DI may be due to genetic mutations, drug induced, or acquired in association with disorders that damage the renal tubules or inhibit the generation of cAMP in tubular cells.[5] Hypercalcemia, hypokalemia, pyelonephritis, sarcoidosis, and amyloidosis can lead to nephrogenic DI.[28,35] Drugs that inhibit the action of ADH and induce a reversible form of nephrogenic DI include lithium, amphotericin B, cisplatin, rifampin, and demeclocycline.[5]

The hallmark of DI is the excretion of abnormally large volumes of dilute urine (polyuria). The inability to produce a concentrated urine results in dehydration and hypernatremia.[28,34] The syndrome is characterized by low urine osmolarity (<200 mOsm/L), low urine specific gravity (<1.010), and urine volumes up to 8 to 12 L/day.[5] The tremendous urinary water loss can produce serum osmolarities greater than 290 mOsm/L and serum sodium concentrations greater than 145 mEq/L. Neurologic symptoms reflect neuronal dehydration and include hyperreflexia, weakness, lethargy, seizures, and coma.[28]

The thirst mechanism assumes a primary role in maintaining water balance in awake patients with DI, preventing serious hyperosmolarity and life-threatening dehydration. In the anesthetized patient, intravascular volume must be carefully restored with intravenous fluids. Consequences of rapid correction include pulmonary and cerebral edema.[28,34]

Management of the patient with DI should be overseen by specialists (nephrologist, critical care specialists, or internal medicine specialists) practiced in this area of patient care. Most patients have incomplete DI and retain some capacity to concentrate their urine and conserve water. Treatment in general includes replacement of previous and ongoing fluid losses. In patients with central DI, DDAVP is the preferred agent in almost all cases. Administration of aqueous vasopressin to patients with coronary artery disease or hypertension risks unwanted arterial constrictive action.[28] DDAVP has less vasopressor (V_1) activity than vasopressin, a prolonged duration of action, and enhanced antidiuretic properties.[8,28,34] DDAVP can be administered nasally, intravenously, subcutaneously, or orally.

Therapy for symptomatic nephrogenic DI includes treatment of any reversible underlying disorder, correction of associated electrolyte disorders, and discontinuation of etiologic medications. Thiazide diuretics (hypovolemia-induced increase in proximal tubule sodium and water reabsorption) and nonsteroidal antiinflammatory drugs (NSAIDs; inhibit the renal synthesis of prostaglandins, which are ADH antagonists) also constitute effective treatment for nephrogenic DI.

Preoperative assessment of the patient with DI includes careful appraisal of plasma electrolytes (especially serum sodium), hydration status, renal function, and plasma osmolarity. Dehydration will make these patients sensitive to the hypotensive effects of anesthesia agents. Isotonic fluids can generally be administered safely during the intraoperative period in concert with hourly measurement of plasma osmolarity, urine output, and serum sodium concentration. Careful hemodynamic and laboratory monitoring should continue into the immediate postoperative period.

Hypersecretion of antidiuretic hormone and anesthetic implications. The syndrome of inappropriate antidiuretic hormone (SIADH) secretion is a disorder characterized by high circulating vasopressin levels with no relation to plasma osmolarity. The kidneys, under ADH stimulation, continue to reabsorb water from the renal tubules despite the presence of hyponatremia and plasma hypotonicity. Hormone-induced water reabsorption causes expansion of intracellular and extracellular fluid volumes and hemodilution. The urine is hypertonic relative to the plasma, and urine output is typically low.

Clinical features of severe SIADH reflect water intoxication, dilutional hyponatremia, serum hypoosmolality, and hypervolemia.[28,36-38] The following laboratory findings support the diagnosis of SIADH:

- Hyponatremia; plasma sodium level <135 mEq/L
- Plasma osmolarity <270 mOsm/L
- Concentrated urine relative to plasma (>100 mOsm/L)
- Low serum concentration of blood urea nitrogen (BUN), creatinine, and albumin (dilutional)
- Hypertension and peripheral edema are not common

The severity of symptoms with SIADH is related to the degree of hyponatremia and the rapidity of onset.[28,33,36-38] If the hyponatremia develops gradually, it may be without overt symptoms. However, if the hyponatremia develops acutely, it is usually accompanied by manifestations of water intoxication.[28] Signs and symptoms include headache, lethargy, mental confusion, anorexia, nausea, vomiting, seizures, and coma.[28,38] Severe acute hyponatremia is associated with swelling of brain cells and may be lethal.[28] Hyponatremia below 110 to 115 mEq/L is likely to cause severe, sometimes irreversible brain damage.[5]

Inappropriate hypersecretion of ADH can result from diverse pathologic processes, including exogenous administration of vasopressin, DDAVP, or large doses of oxytocin, hypothyroidism, pulmonary infection, head trauma, and meningitis.[28,36-38] Surgery can result in transient SIADH.[5] Secretion of ADH by neoplasms, especially small cell carcinomas of the lung, is a common cause of SIADH. The ectopic ADH produced by these tumors is identical to the ADH of hypothalamic origin. In addition, certain drugs are associated with enhanced ADH secretion or exaggerated response; these include sertraline, chemotherapeutic agents (e.g., cyclophosphamide, vincristine), narcotics, NSAIDs, quinolone antibiotics, chlorpropamide, nicotine, and clofibrate.[5,28] About 10% of the cases of SIADH are chronic, but in most patients the disorder is self-limited and remits spontaneously within 2 to 3 weeks.[28]

Most patients with mild to moderate SIADH are managed effectively with correction of the underlying cause and fluid restriction (800–1000 mL/day).[13,36] Patients with severe hyponatremia may require treatment with an intravenous infusion of hypertonic saline (3%).[28,36,37] A new class of drugs, ADH receptor antagonists or vaptans, has been approved for treating hospitalized patients with hyponatremia caused by excess ADH. Definitive treatment for SIADH is directed at the underlying disorder.

The management of hyponatremia depends on the severity and duration of symptoms. Management of the patient with SIADH should be overseen by specialists (nephrologist, critical care specialists, or internal medicine specialists) practiced in this area of patient care. Patients are at risk for acute loss of brain water and permanent neurologic damage (central pontine demyelination syndrome) with too rapid correction of hyponatremia.

Clinical assessment of the patient's volume status is an essential part of patient evaluation. Fluid management in the surgical patient with SIADH can usually be accomplished with fluid restriction that involves the use of isotonic solutions. Estimating central volume status based on central venous pressure measurements can help guide fluid replacement. Frequent determinations of urine output, serum sodium levels, plasma osmolality, and urine osmolarity can also help direct fluid management. Nausea and vomiting should be prevented because they are potent stimuli of ADH release.[28]

Table 37.3 compares important features of SIADH and DI.

PARATHYROID GLAND

The parathyroid glands are small (~3 mm wide × 6 mm long × 2 mm thick) oval bodies located on the posterior surface of the thyroid gland. Most individuals have four parathyroid glands, one on each pole of the thyroid, but some individuals have five glands and others have only three.[39]

Calcium Regulation

The adult human body contains approximately 1 to 2 kg of calcium. Approximately 99% of the calcium exists in the bony skeleton, about 1% in the cells and its organelles, and only about 0.1% is in the extracellular

	SIADH	DI
Serum osmolarity	<270 mOsm/L	>290 mOsm/L
Serum sodium	<135 mEq/L	>145 mEq/L
Urine volume	Low	High
Urine osmolarity	Hypertonic urine relative to plasma	Hypotonic urine relative to plasma
Treatment	Correction of underlying cause, fluid restriction; if patient symptomatic or serum Na⁺ <115–120 mEq/L, hypertonic saline may be considered	Correction of underlying cause, fluid replacement Central DI—DDAVP Nephrogenic DI—NSAIDs, thiazide diuretics

TABLE 37.3 Syndrome of Inappropriate Antidiuretic Hormone (SIADH) and Diabetes Insipidus (DI)

DDAVP, 1-deamino-8-D-arginine vasopressin.

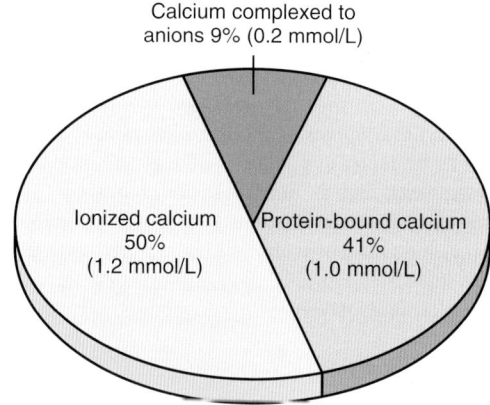

Fig. 37.7 Serum calcium exists in three different forms: ionized, bound to serum proteins, and bound to diffusible anions. Only the ionized form of calcium exerts physiologic effects. (From Hall JE. *Guyton and Hall Textbook of Medical Physiology.* 14th ed. Philadelphia: Elsevier; 2021:991.)

fluid.[39,40] Bone therefore serves as a large reservoir that can store or release calcium as needed.[41,42]

The concentration of the total serum calcium is tightly regulated within a range of approximately 8.5 to 10.5 mg/dL.[41] Serum calcium exists in three different forms (Fig. 37.7):

1. Approximately 9% exists complexed to anions such as citrate, bicarbonate, and phosphate and is diffusible across capillaries membranes.
2. Approximately 41% is combined with plasma proteins (primarily albumin) and is not diffusible across capillary membranes.
3. Approximately 50% exists in an ionized divalent cation form (normal level 4.3–5.2 mg/dL) and is diffusible across capillary membranes.

Only the free, ionized form of calcium exerts physiologic effects, hence measurement of serum ionized calcium levels provides a clinically relevant determination.[39,40] Ionized calcium performs a wide range of vital physiologic functions, including hemostasis (platelet aggregation, blood coagulation), hormone and neurotransmitter release, muscle contraction (skeletal, smooth, and cardiac muscle), bone formation, cell division, and many other aspects of cell function. Even small changes in calcium levels can cause extreme and immediate physiologic effects.[39,43]

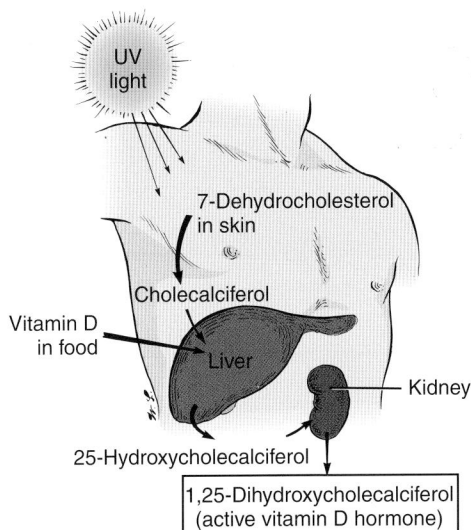

Fig. 37.8 Conversion of cholecalciferol or vitamin D to an active form (1,25-dihydroxycholecalciferol) involves hydroxylation in the liver and kidneys. Active vitamin D is important in transporting calcium across the gastrointestinal tract. *UV,* Ultraviolet.

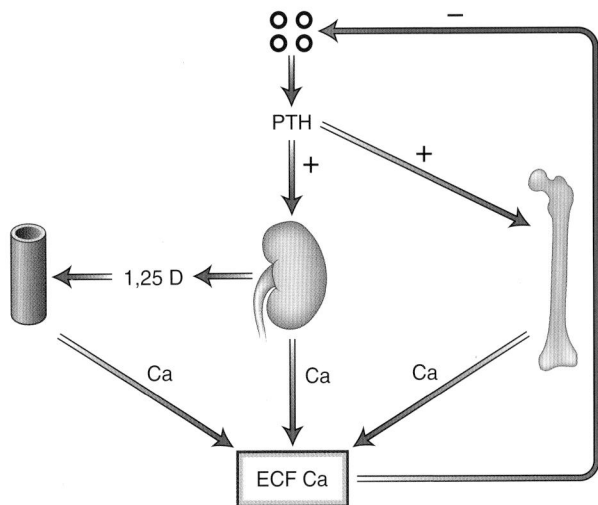

Fig. 37.9 Parathyroid hormone *(PTH)*–calcium feedback loop that controls calcium homeostasis. Four organs—the parathyroid glands, intestine, kidney, and bone—together determine the parameters of calcium homeostasis. –, Negative effect; +, positive effect; *1,25 D,* 1,25-hydroxyvitamin D; *ECF,* extracellular fluid. (From Melmed S, et al., eds. *Williams Textbook of Endocrinology.* 13th ed. Philadelphia: Elsevier; 2016:1256.)

Total blood calcium levels may not always reflect the ionized calcium status. Alterations in serum protein levels cause parallel changes in total blood calcium levels without modifying ionized calcium values. As an example, a decrease in serum albumin may cause an associated decrease in total serum calcium levels. Because of this, calcium levels may be reported as albumin-adjusted total calcium.

Alterations in the pH of blood affect ionized calcium levels. Plasma proteins are more ionized in an alkaline pH, providing an increase in the number of anion-binding sites for the positively charged calcium. Alkalosis decreases ionized serum calcium by increasing protein-calcium binding. Acidosis, on the other hand, increases ionized serum calcium by decreasing calcium-protein binding, as excess hydrogen ions bind to protein and displace calcium.[40-42]

Two principal hormones, vitamin D and PTH, operate in concert to regulate the plasma concentration of calcium. Both vitamin D and PTH raise serum calcium levels, but of the two, PTH has by far the strongest effect.

Vitamin D

Vitamin D compounds ingested from food or formed by the action of ultraviolet light on the skin are largely inactive prohormones.[40,42] Inactive vitamin D, called cholecalciferol, is converted by a series of reactions in the liver and kidneys to an active metabolite. The final step in the conversion of vitamin D to an active form is controlled in the kidneys by PTH.[42] The in vivo conversion of inactive vitamin D to the final active vitamin D product, 1,25-dihydroxycholecalciferol, is shown in Fig. 37.8.

Active vitamin D increases plasma calcium and phosphate ion concentrations by promoting their absorption across the intestinal epithelium. Inadequate vitamin D intake or absorption, or insufficient exposure to sunlight, can lead to poor intestinal absorption of calcium and phosphate. In children, the resulting calcium and phosphate deficiency leads to defective mineralization of bone, a condition known as rickets.[40,44] In adults, vitamin D deficiency, from for example renal disease or steatorrhea, results in impaired bone mineralization, a condition known as osteomalacia.[39]

Parathyroid Hormone

PTH is an 84–amino acid polypeptide hormone secreted from chief cells of the parathyroid gland in response to low serum ionized calcium concentrations. Hyperphosphatemia (indirect effect) also stimulates PTH secretion. PTH is the body's major hormonal regulator of calcium and phosphate metabolism. In general, PTH increases the extracellular calcium concentration and decreases the extracellular phosphate concentration.[42]

In PTH, the body possesses an extremely potent negative feedback agent for controlling serum calcium levels. A small decline in the level of circulating ionized calcium produces a rapid increase in PTH secretion from the parathyroid glands. A sustained deficit in serum calcium levels (e.g., lactation, pregnancy) may produce hypertrophy of the parathyroid glands, sometimes fivefold or greater, to maintain adequate PTH output.[39] High levels of extracellular calcium have a negative feedback to the parathyroid glands to decrease PTH release (Fig. 37.9).

Alternatively, an elevation in serum calcium ion concentration produces an abrupt decline in PTH synthesis and output. Conditions associated with chronic elevations of serum calcium (e.g., immobility, malignancy, Paget disease) blunt PTH output and provoke a diminution in gland size. Parathyroid gland function and PTH secretion may also be inhibited by chronic hypomagnesemia.[45]

The increase in serum calcium levels and decrease in serum phosphate levels in response to PTH secretion is the result of the hormone's effect on bone and the kidney and its indirect effect on the intestinal tract (Fig. 37.10).

Effect on bone. Bone is a living tissue that is constantly being remodeled.[40] In the healthy adult, bone-forming cells called osteoblasts are balanced by bone-destroying cells called osteoclasts.[39] Exchangeable calcium salts in bone serve as a large, rapid buffer that plays a vital role to keep calcium in the extracellular fluid stable. In addition to calcium, bone also provides an important reservoir for other ions such as magnesium and phosphorus.[39,41]

The most pronounced immediate control of blood calcium is due to PTH effects on bone.[42] When ionized serum calcium levels decline, PTH is released and it directs activity to mobilize skeletal calcium stores.[40]

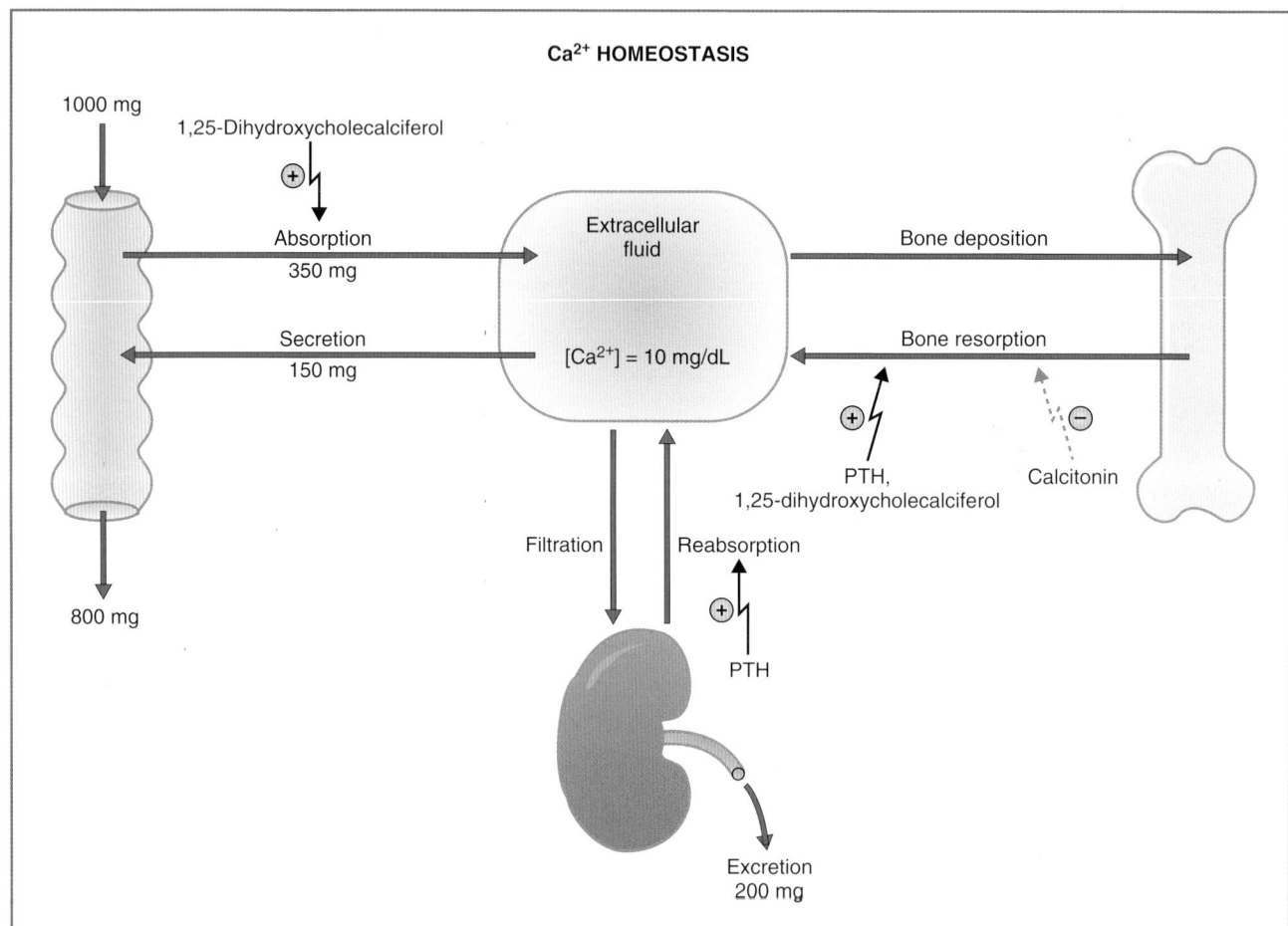

Fig. 37.10 Ca^{2+} homeostasis in an adult eating 1000 mg/day of elemental Ca^{2+}. Hormonal effects on Ca^{2+} absorption from the gastrointestinal tract, bone remodeling, and Ca^{2+} reabsorption in the kidney are shown. *PTH*, Parathyroid hormone. (From Costanzo LS. *Physiology*. 5th ed. Philadelphia: Elsevier; 2014;436.)

PTH promotes the activation and proliferation of osteoclasts, stimulating rapid resorption of calcium and phosphate from bone tissue to the extracellular fluid. Over time, abnormally high levels of circulating PTH can produce extensive absorption of calcium from the bone matrix.[39,42]

The reservoir of calcium in bone is approximately 1000 times greater than the amount of calcium in the extracellular fluid. Only after sustained PTH activation therefore does bone erosion and destruction become apparent. With protracted PTH stimulation, however, the bones eventually become severely depleted of calcium.[39]

Alternatively, an increase in extracellular fluid calcium causes PTH levels to decline via a negative feedback loop. Decreased PTH levels stimulate rapid deposition of calcium and phosphate bone salts, an effect that lowers serum calcium levels back to normal.

Effect on the intestinal tract. PTH indirectly enhances both calcium and phosphate absorption from the intestines by promoting formation of 1,25-dihydroxycholecalciferol, the active form of vitamin D. When the plasma calcium level is low, PTH stimulates 1α-hydroxylase, an enzyme in the kidney necessary for the formation of 1,25-dihydroxycholecalciferol. Active vitamin D in turn increases intestinal absorption of calcium and phosphate.[40]

In the absence of PTH, or in the presence of severe kidney disease, 1,25-dihydroxycholecalciferol is not formed, and the effect of vitamin D on calcium and phosphate regulation is lost. Patients with chronic renal failure often suffer from hypocalcemia in part because the diseased kidneys lose their ability to form active vitamin D. Consequently, these patients are unable to absorb enough calcium from the gastrointestinal tract.[42]

Effect on the kidney. PTH has two major effects on the kidney: It increases calcium reabsorption, and it increases phosphate excretion. PTH elevates serum calcium levels by augmenting the reabsorption of calcium from nephron distal tubules and collecting ducts to the extracellular fluid.[39,42] The decline in serum phosphate concentration caused by PTH-mediated renal phosphate excretion is generally strong enough to overcome any serum increases caused by PTH-induced phosphate absorption from bone and intestines.[39]

Calcitonin

Calcitonin is a hormone secreted from the thyroid parafollicular cells, or C cells, in response to elevated serum ionized calcium.[40] It has an effect opposite to that of the PTH system, lowering the serum ionized calcium concentration. Calcium levels are reduced by a calcitonin-mediated inhibition of bone osteoclasts, which shifts the balance toward osteoblasts and bone deposition.[40,42]

The serum calcium–lowering effect of calcitonin is weak, especially in adults. Its effect in lowering serum calcium is rapidly outweighed by the more powerful activity of PTH.[39] The rather weak effect of calcitonin is demonstrated by the observation that removal of the thyroid gland causes no significant alterations in bone density or long-term serum calcium levels.[39,40,42]

Parathyroid Gland Dysfunction

Hypoparathyroidism

Hypoparathyroidism is characterized by low PTH levels or a peripheral resistance to PTH effects.[42,46,47] It may be an inherited or acquired disorder. Patients with hypoparathyroidism typically have low plasma calcium levels (ionized calcium <4.5 mg/dL and total calcium <8.5 mg/dL). The serum phosphate concentration may be elevated because of decreased renal excretion of phosphate.

Inadvertent surgical removal of the parathyroid glands or damage to gland blood supply during parathyroid surgery, radical neck dissection, or thyroid surgery are the most common causes of hypoparathyroidism.[46,47] Hereditary or autoimmune hypoparathyroidism, parathyroid gland injury from irradiation or trauma, amyloidosis, and chronic severe magnesium deficiency (e.g., alcohol abuse, poor nutrition, malabsorption) are also causes of hypoparathyroidism.[45-47] Clinical signs of hypoparathyroidism depend on the degree of hypocalcemia and the rapidity of calcium decline. Like most electrolyte imbalances, a sudden drop in ionized calcium produces more severe symptoms than a slow decline.[43] Recommended treatment of chronic hypoparathyroidism includes activated vitamin D and calcium supplementation, as well as magnesium if indicated.[45-47] Use of recombinant human PTH (Natpara) can decrease supplemental calcium and vitamin D dosage requirements in patients with hypocalcemia caused by hypoparathyroidism, but current treatment recommendations restrict engineered PTH as only an adjunct treatment to calcium and active vitamin D.[47,48]

The decreased serum calcium ion concentration accompanying hypoparathyroidism produces hyperexcitability of nerve and muscle cells by lowering the threshold potential of excitable membranes. Cardinal features of neuromuscular excitability are muscle spasms and spontaneous nerve discharge. Symptoms vary in severity and may take the form of muscle cramps, perioral paresthesias, acral numbness, hyperactive deep tendon reflexes, and tetany. The patient may feel restless or hyperirritable. Life-threatening laryngeal muscle spasm may occur, producing stridor, labored respirations, and asphyxia.[39,42,46]

Two classic manifestations of latent hypocalcemic tetany are Chvostek sign and Trousseau sign. Chvostek sign is a contracture or twitching of ipsilateral facial muscles produced when the facial nerve is tapped at the angle of the jaw. Trousseau sign is elicited by the inflation of a blood pressure cuff slightly above the systolic level for 3 minutes. The resultant ischemia enhances muscle irritability in hypocalcemic states and causes flexion of the wrist and thumb with extension of the fingers (carpopedal spasm).[39] Fig. 37.11 illustrates some of the clinical manifestations of hypoparathyroidism and hypocalcemia.

Hyperparathyroidism

Primary hyperparathyroidism is a common endocrine disorder characterized by the presence of hypercalcemia and elevated serum levels of PTH.[49-51] It may result from a parathyroid adenoma, gland hyperplasia, or parathyroid cancer.[41,42] In approximately 80% of cases, primary hyperparathyroidism is caused by hypersecretion of a single parathyroid adenoma.[41,50-52] Multigland disease accounts for 10% to 15% of cases. Hyperparathyroidism may exist as part of a MEN syndrome (MEN-1, MEN-2A).[41,42] MEN includes endocrine syndromes that are familial and genetically linked (See section on pheochromocytoma later in this chapter). Carcinoma of the parathyroid gland is found in less than 1% of patients with hyperparathyroidism and is associated with particularly high serum calcium levels.[52]

There are many causes of hypercalcemia, but hyperparathyroidism and cancer account for 90% of all cases.[42] Primary hyperparathyroidism, with sustained overactivity of the parathyroid glands, is the most common cause of hypercalcemia in the general population. Most patients remain asymptomatic until the total serum calcium level rises above 11.6 to 12 mg/dL, but patient response is variable, and some patients remain asymptomatic even at this level.[39,42] Severe hypercalcemia, generally defined as greater than 14 mg/dL, can be a medical emergency and demands immediate attention.[42]

With the development of sensitive laboratory assays for calcium and PTH, today most patients with primary hyperparathyroidism are asymptomatic at diagnosis, with only a small fraction exhibiting classic signs and symptoms.[49,50] With advanced disease, sustained high levels of PTH lead to exaggerated osteoclast activity in bone, resulting in diffuse osteopenia, subperiosteal erosions, and elevated extracellular calcium levels. As osteoblasts attempt to reconstruct the ravaged bone, they secrete large amounts of the enzyme alkaline phosphatase.[39,40] An elevated serum alkaline phosphatase level therefore is a diagnostic feature of bone disease and hyperparathyroidism.[52] Despite an increased mobilization of phosphorus from bone, serum phosphate concentration usually remains normal or low as a result of increased urinary excretion.

The effect of hyperparathyroidism on bone becomes clinically apparent when osteoclastic absorption of bone overwhelms osteoblastic deposition. With severe and protracted disease, the entire skeleton may be involved, making bones painful and susceptible to fracture. Owing to early diagnosis, the destructive bone disease associated with severe hyperparathyroidism, osteitis fibrosa cystica, is not common today.

Symptoms caused by high PTH levels and hypercalcemia typically manifest insidiously over an extended time.[49,50] Many of the nonskeletal manifestations of primary hyperparathyroidism are related to the accompanying hypercalcemia.[49,51,52] Sustained and marked hypercalcemia may produce calcifications and other deleterious effects in the pancreas (pancreatitis), kidney (decreased response to ADH, polyuria, nephrolithiasis, nephrocalcinosis), blood vessels (hypertension), heart (shortened ventricular refractory period, increased ventricular excitability, bradyarrhythmias), and acid-producing areas of the stomach (peptic ulcer).[49,51,52] The classic mnemonic "stones, bones, and groans" summarizes renal, skeletal, and gastrointestinal features of advanced hyperparathyroidism.

Hypercalcemia raises the threshold of excitable cells and causes progressive depression of the nervous system.[39] Central and peripheral nervous system depressive effects begin to appear in many patients when blood calcium levels rise above approximately 12 mg/dL and

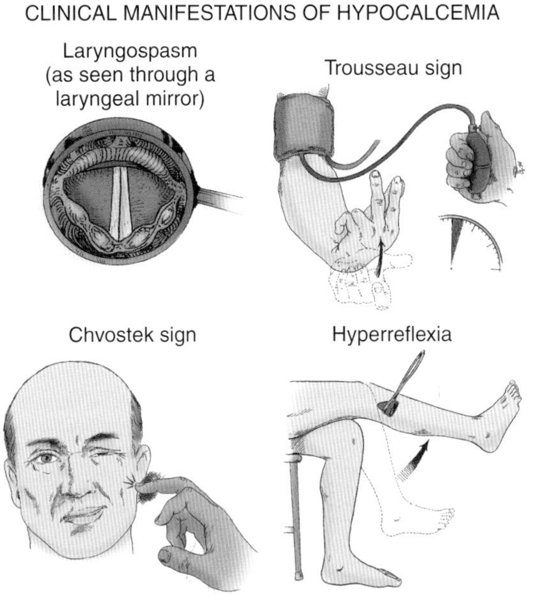

CLINICAL MANIFESTATIONS OF HYPOCALCEMIA

Laryngospasm (as seen through a laryngeal mirror)

Trousseau sign

Chvostek sign

Hyperreflexia

Fig. 37.11 Hypocalcemia produces hyperexcitability of nerve and muscle cells. Chvostek sign and Trousseau sign are two classic manifestations of hypocalcemic tetany. Deep tendon reflexes may be hyperactive. Laryngeal muscles are sensitive to tetanic spasm.

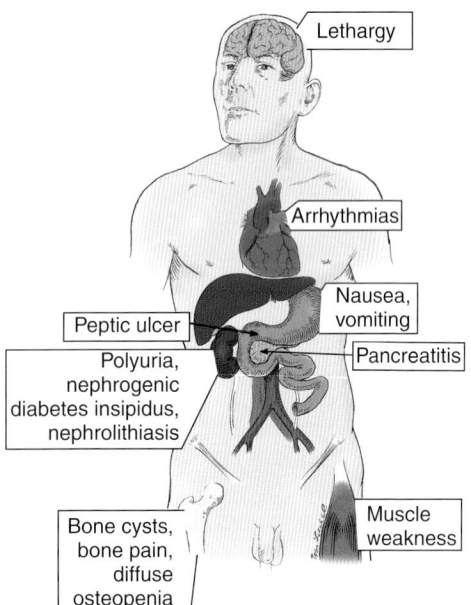

Fig. 37.12 The patient with hyperparathyroidism exhibits manifestations of hypercalcemia. With severe, protracted disease, skeletal destruction becomes evident.

TABLE 37.4 **Clinical Features of Hyperparathyroidism and Hypoparathyroidism**

System	Hyperparathyroidism	Hypoparathyroidism
Cardiovascular	Hypertension, cardiac conduction disturbances, shortened QT interval	Prolonged QT interval, hypotension, decreased cardiac contractility
Musculoskeletal	Bone pain, pathologic fractures, muscle weakness, muscle atrophy	Neuromuscular excitability; spasms; cramps
Neurologic	Somnolence, cognitive impairment, depression, hypotonia	Tetany, paresthesia, numbness in fingers and toes, seizures
Gastrointestinal	Anorexia, nausea, vomiting, constipation, abdominal pain, pancreatitis, peptic ulcer	Abdominal cramps
Renal	Tubular absorption defects, diminished renal function, kidney stones, polyuria	None significant

become marked as the calcium rises to 15 mg/dL.[39] Profound muscle weakness, confusion, nausea, vomiting, and lethargy are features of the disorder. Fig. 37.12 illustrates some of the clinical manifestations of hyperparathyroidism.

Secondary hyperparathyroidism develops in patients with chronically low levels of serum calcium, such as those with chronic renal failure. Vitamin D deficiency and gastrointestinal malabsorption of vitamin D can also lead to secondary increases in PTH activity in response to the resulting hypocalcemia. The clinical course is marked by the same PTH-mediated skeletal assault seen in the primary form of the disorder, but because it is an adaptive response secondary hyperparathyroidism is seldom associated with hypercalcemia. The bone disease seen in patients with secondary hyperparathyroidism associated with chronic kidney disease is termed renal osteodystrophy. Calcimimetic drugs are approved to treat patients with secondary hyperparathyroidism. These agents mimic calcium at PTH calcium-sensing receptors and subsequently promote decreased PTH release from the parathyroid gland.[42,50]

Hypercalcemia due to malignancy is common and occurs in as many as 20% of cancer patients.[42] Malignancy is the second most common cause of hypercalcemia in adults. The hypercalcemia may be due to local invasion of bone by cancer cells, but many cases are due to elaboration of a PTH-related peptide (PTHrP) from tumor cells. The overproduction of PTHrP by cancer cells mimics the effects of PTH, including bone destruction, hypophosphatemia, and hypercalcemia.[42]

Table 37.4 compares clinical features of hyperparathyroidism and hypoparathyroidism.

Anesthesia implications for hyperparathyroidism.
Parathyroidectomy is the only curative therapy for primary hyperparathyroidism.[49] Surgical removal of the culprit gland or glands is recommended for those younger than 50 years of age and those with bone disease, renal complications, or clinically significant hypercalcemia.[51] Among asymptomatic patients, parathyroidectomy halts progression of the disease, improves quality of life, and may decrease risk of fracture and adverse cardiovascular outcomes.[50]

Historically, parathyroidectomy was performed with bilateral neck exploration. The new standard for most surgeries involves preoperative imaging studies and intraoperative PTH monitoring to localize the abnormal tissue and permit directed and limited resection of only the hypersecreting gland.[53,54] General anesthesia is most often utilized, but this minimally invasive surgical approach may be performed with cervical plexus block anesthesia and monitored anesthesia care or even local anesthesia for excision of a single adenoma.[53-56]

The hypercalcemic patient may be dehydrated because of anorexia, vomiting, and the impaired ability of the kidneys to concentrate urine.[42] Special attention must be directed preoperatively to evaluating the patient's hydration status and restoring fluid balance if needed. Perioperative hydration aims to dilute serum calcium, maintain adequate glomerular filtration and calcium clearance, and ensure adequate intravascular volume. Vigorous hydration dictates the use of bladder catheterization and frequent determinations of serum electrolytes (calcium, sodium, magnesium, potassium, phosphorus).

Mild hypercalcemia (<12 mg/dL) preoperatively can usually be managed by saline infusion (150 mL/hr). Isotonic saline hydration decreases serum calcium levels by hemodilution, increased glomerular filtration, and enhanced excretion.[42]

Because elevated calcium levels depress the central and peripheral nervous systems, the use of preoperative sedatives in the hypercalcemic patient who appears lethargic or confused should be avoided.

Careful review of the patient's renal status is especially crucial in patients with secondary hyperparathyroidism. Associated complications of renal impairment (volume overload, anemia, electrolyte derangements) may affect anesthetic medication dosages and selection.

Cardiac conduction disturbances, a shortened QT interval, and a prolonged PR interval on the electrocardiogram (ECG) are observed with hypercalcemia.

Awareness of the effects of pH on the ionized portion of plasma calcium is important. Alkalosis shifts ionized calcium to the protein-bound form and decreases serum levels. Acidosis has the opposite effect, releasing calcium from protein binding and increasing serum ionized calcium levels.

The erosive effects of elevated PTH on bone and the systemic effects of chronic hypercalcemia should be considered in the anesthetic plan for patients with severe untreated disease. Patients with clinically significant bone disease are susceptible to fractures, and care must be exercised in positioning and padding.[49,51]

The response to neuromuscular blockade may be unpredictable. Muscle weakness, hypotonia, and muscle atrophy may increase the patient's sensitivity to nondepolarizing skeletal muscle relaxants. Careful titration of muscle relaxants in concert with neuromuscular blockade monitoring is prudent.

Parathyroid tissue resembles brown fat, and this can occasionally make it difficult for the surgeon to locate. Furthermore, parathyroid tissue is sometimes footloose and can be found in such ectopic places as the deep recesses of the mediastinum or the thymus gland.[40-42] The 5-minute half-life of PTH allows it to serve as a useful intraoperative marker.[53,56] The surgeon may use periodic intraoperative assays of serum PTH and ionized calcium levels to help guide surgical resection. PTH levels decline quickly after successful resection of the source. In most cases, the parathyroid gland is further confirmed histologically by frozen section.

Blood loss from parathyroid surgery is usually minimal, and advanced monitoring is not required based on the surgical procedure. Serum calcium, magnesium, and phosphorus levels should be monitored in the postoperative period until stable.

Temporary hypocalcemia may be observed even after successful parathyroid surgery for hyperparathyroidism.[42] In most cases, serum calcium levels start to decline within hours of surgery. Transient postoperative hypocalcemia may be the result of parathyroid gland suppression (by preoperative hypercalcemia) or rapid bone uptake of calcium ("hungry bone syndrome").[41,57] Inadvertent removal of all parathyroid glands or damage to parathyroid gland tissue may induce a marked decline in total serum calcium concentration. Even a small amount of remaining parathyroid tissue is usually capable of sufficient hypertrophy to preserve normal calcium-phosphate balance.[39]

After parathyroid surgery, monitoring of serum calcium and meticulous observation for signs of neuromuscular irritability should be performed. The threshold for the development of hypocalcemia-induced neuromuscular excitability is variable. Laryngeal muscles are especially sensitive to tetanic spasm, and laryngospasm may cause life threatening airway compromise in the hypocalcemic patient.[39] Patients with severe hypocalcemia, usually less than 7.5 mg/dL, or with cardiac arrhythmias, tetany, neurologic manifestations (seizures), or stridor (laryngospasm) should receive intravenous calcium.[43,58]

In addition to laryngeal muscle spasm, respiratory distress or stridor following parathyroid surgery may be secondary to edema, bleeding in the neck, or recurrent laryngeal nerve (RLN) injury. An expanding postoperative hematoma in the pretracheal space is potentially life threatening and demands immediate treatment. Incomplete RLN injury (paresis) produces vocal cord hypomobility. Patients present with hoarseness, dysphagia, or dyspnea and require close observation after surgery. Complete or bilateral RLN injury causes aphonia and requires immediate airway support and intubation.[39,59] Vocal cord function can be assessed pre- and postoperatively by asking the patient to phonate "E" or "moon." Electrophysiologic monitoring may be employed intraoperatively to help identify RLN nerve injury.[60]

Postoperative hypocalcemia may be apparent on ECG tracings as a prolonged QTc interval (normal, 0.35–0.44 second), reflecting delayed ventricular repolarization.[58] Cardiac dysrhythmias, decreased cardiac contractility, and hypotension may occur, and heart failure (although rare) is a danger.[42,58]

In addition to parathyroid surgery, circulating levels of ionized calcium can decline from other causes in the perioperative period. Precipitous increases in circulating levels of anions such as bicarbonate, phosphate, and citrate lower ionized calcium levels.[41,58] The rapid transfusion of citrated blood, or the rapid administration of bicarbonate, may induce overt tetany in a previously asymptomatic hypocalcemic patient. Hyperventilation and alkalosis decrease ionized calcium levels by increasing calcium binding to proteins. Vigorous diuresis can also augment calcium loss.[42,43,58]

As mentioned, patients with severe or symptomatic hypocalcemia require prompt therapy.[58] Acute hypocalcemia may be treated with an initial intravenous bolus of 10 mL of 10% calcium gluconate administered over 10 minutes, with ECG monitoring. Persistent hypocalcemia will require an intravenous infusion of calcium. Calcium, magnesium, phosphate, potassium, and creatinine levels should be monitored during calcium replacement. Magnesium deficiency can impair the secretion of PTH and should be corrected if low.[42,45,47]

PANCREAS

The pancreas is a flattened, elongated, retroperitoneal organ that has both exocrine and endocrine functions. Acinar cells, which make up the exocrine portion of the pancreas, account for approximately 98% of the gland's weight. Gastrointestinal enzymes and bicarbonate are synthesized in acinar cells and secreted into the pancreatic ducts to aid the digestive process.

Islets of Langerhans

The islets of Langerhans, which make up 1% to 2% of the pancreas's weight, constitute the endocrine pancreas. The islets are microscopic collections of cells organized around small capillaries and scattered throughout the gland. Each islet cell has an abundant blood supply. The islets produce hormones that do not enter ducts but rather are secreted directly into capillary blood vessels. Venous blood from the islets drains into the hepatic portal vein and then into the general circulation.[61]

At least four distinct cell types are found in the islets of Langerhans, identified as α (alpha), β (beta), δ (delta), and PP (pancreatic polypeptide) cells. Each cell type secretes a different peptide hormone. The β cells constitute approximately 60% of the islet mass and secrete the hormone insulin. Amylin is a hormone that is also secreted from the β cells parallel with insulin secretion. The α cells constitute approximately 25% of the islet cells and secrete the hormone glucagon. The δ cells represent approximately 10% of total cells and secrete the hormone somatostatin (the same hormone, GH-inhibiting hormone, that is released from the hypothalamus).[62]

Insulin and glucagon are crucial in regulating carbohydrate, fat, and protein metabolism. Their secretion is part of a hormonal regulatory system that accommodates repeated periods of feast and fasting throughout the day. Somatostatin has a paracrine role in suppressing the secretion of both insulin and glucagon.[62] Pancreatic peptide inhibits exocrine pancreatic secretion.

Energy Balance

Glucose is the body's most abundant circulating fuel. The breakdown of glucose into simpler compounds releases energy the body uses for cellular metabolism. The energy-yielding breakdown of glucose to pyruvate is called glycolysis or the Embden-Meyerhof pathway.

Despite daily fluctuations between feeding and fasting, plasma glucose concentration is maintained within an amazingly narrow range. This is accomplished by the counterbalancing effect of multiple hormones that control the storage of glucose and other nutrient fuels after meals and regulates fuel mobilization between meals. In healthy individuals, the liver is an important glucose buffer that stores enough glycogen to maintain a normal plasma glucose level during 8 to 12 hours of fasting.[63] An overnight fast usually lowers the blood glucose to 80 to 90 mg/dL. The blood glucose concentration increases briefly to 120 to 140 mg/dL after a meal before returning to control levels.[62] In a person with impaired glucose tolerance (prediabetic), the fasting plasma glucose (FPG) level is 100 to 125 mg/dL; in the diabetic patient, the FPG is equal to or greater than 126 mg/dL.[64]

Certain metabolic processes ensure the efficient storage of nutrients so they can be available for later use. Glycogenesis, or the storage of glucose as glycogen, occurs primarily in the liver and muscle. Lipogenesis, which represents the formation and storage of fat as triglycerides, occurs primarily in adipose tissue.

Other metabolic processes work in the opposite direction, providing adequate energy sources during times of fasting. Gluconeogenesis is the formation of glucose from lactate, pyruvate, amino acids, and glycerol; it is an important hepatic glucose production mechanism during fasting and starvation. Glycogenolysis, the breakdown of glycogen into glucose, occurs primarily in the liver. Lipolysis, the breakdown of stored triglycerides to free fatty acids and glycerol, is stimulated by the enzyme hormone-sensitive lipase.

The rates of glycogenesis, lipogenesis, gluconeogenesis, glycogenolysis, and lipolysis are determined largely by the actions of insulin and the opposing actions of the so-called counterregulatory hormones (GH, cortisol, epinephrine, and glucagon). Insulin plays an important role as an anabolic hormone. It promotes growth and the constructive phase of metabolism. The potent anabolic effects of insulin are balanced by the opposing catabolic actions of the counterregulatory hormones, which mobilize fuel substrates from protein, carbohydrate, and fat stores to meet the energy demands of various tissues in response to fasting or stress.[61]

The push-and-pull effect of these two hormone systems helps maintain normal glucose concentrations in the healthy individual. In type 1 DM, when insulin concentrations are low or absent, the unopposed counterregulatory hormones begin to exert more prominent metabolic effects.

Glucose Usage by the Brain

Different tissues have different glucose requirements. In addition, most tissues are able to adapt to alternative sources of fuel when glucose is scarce. Muscle and most tissues in the body use glucose for energy when it is available, but they can also shift to alternative sources of fuel (amino acids or fat) in the absence of glucose.

The brain is unique in that it is one of the few organs that uses only glucose for energy. It is said to be an obligate glucose organ. The retina and the epithelium of the gonads also depend on glucose as their sole source of energy.[62] Unlike most other tissues, obligate glucose organs cannot immediately switch to alternative fuels when glucose levels fall. The brain's absolute, uninterrupted requirement for glucose dictates that the blood glucose concentration always be maintained above a critical level. The central nervous system accounts for approximately 60% of total body glucose utilization, and normal cerebral function requires the delivery of approximately 125 to 150 g of glucose per day.[65] When blood glucose levels fall, neuroglycopenic symptoms (e.g., anxiety, irritability, nervousness, confusion, dizziness, headache) begin to occur (see Hypoglycemia, later).[63,66] During prolonged starvation, ketone bodies can substitute for glucose as cerebral fuel.

Insulin

Of the hormones secreted from the islet cells, insulin is of greatest physiologic importance. In 1922, the Canadian Frederick Banting and the American Charles Best first isolated this critical hormone from the pancreas in its pure form. The clinical importance of this event is demonstrated by insulin's history of lifesaving effects in those with DM, a previously uniformly fatal disease.

Insulin was also the first mammalian peptide hormone produced with the use of recombinant DNA techniques.

Storage and Release

Insulin is synthesized within the β cells of the pancreas, and it is packaged and stored in membrane-lined vesicles within the β-cell cytoplasm. Approximately 200 units of insulin are stored in the pancreas in this form. With stimulation, insulin is released via exocytosis from the β cell to the surrounding capillaries, where it enters the portal circulation. In the first pass through the hepatic circulation, the liver removes approximately 50% of the insulin delivered to it. Total daily insulin secretion is estimated to be approximately 60 units, but the total daily peripheral delivery is approximately 30 units.[61]

Insulin circulates almost entirely unbound to any carrier protein. The circulating half-life of insulin is approximately 6 minutes, and it is mainly cleared from the circulation in 10 to 15 minutes.[62] Almost all tissues in the body can metabolize insulin, but the major site of hormone degradation is the liver and, to a lesser degree, the kidney. Insulin is degraded by the enzyme insulinase.[62] As a result, patients with liver dysfunction or kidney disease may have prolonged effects of insulin with increased risk of hypoglycemia.

Effects of Insulin

Insulin is a hormone of energy or fuel storage. It is important to many cellular mechanisms related to growth, and it is intimately involved in the regulation of carbohydrate, fat, and protein metabolism.

Following ingestion of a meal, insulin levels increase sharply in response to stimulation by abundant circulating nutrient substrates. Insulin promotes the storage of carbohydrate, fat, and protein for future use when substrate supply is low.[62,64] Fig. 37.13 outlines the effects of insulin on nutrient substrates.

The cellular effects of insulin on target cells are initiated by reversible binding to specific cell membrane insulin receptors linked to the enzyme tyrosine kinase. Most cells in the body have insulin receptors, but the major targets of insulin action are the liver, muscle, and adipose tissue.[61,62,65]

Effects on carbohydrate metabolism Insulin is the body's key hormone controlling glucose removal from the plasma. It facilitates rapid uptake, storage, and use of glucose in almost all cells, but especially liver, muscle, and adipose cells. Neurons in the brain are

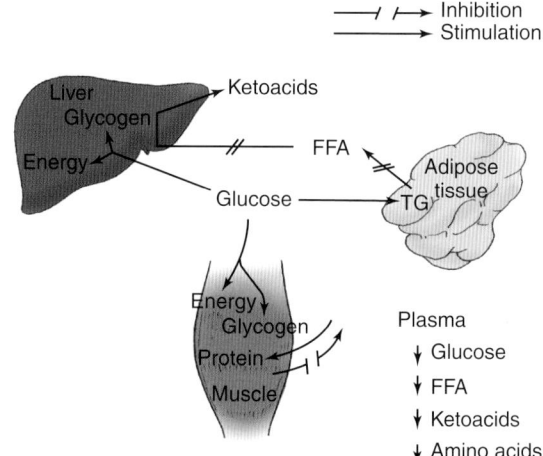

Fig. 37.13 The effect of insulin on the overall flow of metabolic substrates. Insulin promotes the uptake of glucose into insulin-responsive tissue to meet energy needs. In the liver and skeletal muscle, insulin promotes the storage of excess glucose as glycogen. In adipose tissue, excess glucose is stored as triglyceride *(TG)*. Insulin inhibits the breakdown of triglyceride into glycerol and free fatty acids *(FFA)*. Insulin promotes amino acid uptake into muscle for protein synthesis. Protein breakdown is inhibited.

some of the few cells in the body that do not require insulin for glucose transport.[62,65]

In the liver, and to a lesser extent in muscle cells, insulin promotes the efficient storage of excess glucose in the form of glycogen (glycogenesis).[61] Under normal circumstances, approximately 60% of the glucose ingested with a meal is stored in the liver as glycogen (~100 g of stored glycogen). In addition to promoting hepatic glucose storage, insulin limits hepatic glucose output by inhibiting enzymes responsible for gluconeogenesis.[61,62]

Between meals, when blood glucose levels fall, insulin secretion decreases, and glucose can be released back into the blood (glycogenolysis) and be made available for local energy use or delivery to the central nervous system. Glycogen content in the liver is limited and is largely depleted after an overnight fast. Therefore gluconeogenesis becomes the predominant source of glucose after prolonged fasting.[65]

Effects on protein metabolism. The actions of insulin on protein metabolism are also directed toward nutrient storage and growth (anabolism). Insulin stimulates the uptake of amino acids from the extracellular fluid to the cell. Once inside the cell, it promotes the synthesis of specific proteins. Insulin also conserves amino acids in existing proteins by inhibiting the breakdown of protein stores (inhibits catabolism), especially in muscle. Because insulin is required for protein synthesis, it is firmly established as an essential hormone for normal development, growth, and maintenance of healthy tissues.[62]

Effects on fat metabolism. The acute effects of insulin on fat metabolism are not as readily apparent as the effects on carbohydrate metabolism, but in the long run they are no less important.

Insulin favors fat storage. After a meal, carbohydrates not used for energy or stored as glycogen are converted, under the direction of insulin, to fatty acids and glycerol. Fatty acids and glycerol combine to form triglyceride, the storage form of fat. Insulin not only stimulates triglyceride storage in adipose tissue but also strongly inhibits the breakdown of stored triglyceride to free fatty acids and glycerol. Insulin blocks triglyceride hydrolysis and the liberation of free fatty acids into the circulating blood by suppressing the enzyme hormone-sensitive lipase.[62,67] Under ordinary conditions, insulin continually exerts a braking effect on free fatty acid release. A major consequence of lower concentrations of circulating free fatty acids is the decreased use of fatty acids for fuel.[61] In other words, insulin strongly suppresses fatty acid mobilization in the fed state when glucose is readily available to meet energy needs.

In the fasted state, when insulin levels are low, triglycerides release free fatty acids into the circulation, which provides metabolic fuel to most cells.[61,62] Organic acids called ketoacids or ketone bodies are generated in the liver from free fatty acid oxidation. Ketoacid production is increased in the fasted state when insulin levels are low. Conversely, ketoacid production is markedly reduced when insulin levels are high. Insulin is the body's major antiketogenic hormone.[62,65]

Effects on ion transport. Insulin stimulates the translocation of vital electrolytes from the extracellular compartment into cells. Potassium, phosphate, and magnesium uptake into cells is facilitated by an insulin mechanism.[61] Exogenous insulin administration may appreciably lower serum potassium, phosphate, and magnesium levels. Hypokalemia secondary to vigorous insulin treatment can be of great clinical significance.

Insulin's metabolic actions are complex and wide ranging. Overall, insulin promotes glucose transfer into cells and fosters glucose use for energy. When energy needs are met, insulin promotes glucose storage as glycogen or fat. Conversely, lack of insulin causes lipolysis and fat utilization for energy instead of glucose, except in neuronal cells.

Control of Insulin Secretion

Insulin synthesis and secretion are stimulated by feast or energy abundance. Ingestion of a meal increases the rate of insulin secretion four- to fivefold. Plasma insulin levels rise rapidly, reaching peak values 30 to 60 minutes after eating is initiated.[61] High insulin levels in turn direct nutrients to appropriate storage sites.[64]

Between meals, insulin levels drift downward, the storage process is reversed, and metabolic substrates are mobilized in the form of glucose, free fatty acids, and amino acids.

Plasma glucose is by far the most important regulator of insulin release. Elevated plasma glucose levels directly activate β cells of the pancreas, stimulating insulin synthesis and secretion. Low plasma glucose concentrations inhibit this response. Very little insulin is secreted at the normal FPG levels of 80 to 90 mg/dL and below.[61,62,67] As the blood glucose rises above 100 mg/dL, secretion of insulin rises rapidly. A maximal insulin response (10–25 times basal level) occurs at blood glucose concentrations of 400 to 600 mg/dL.[61,62] The dramatic rise in insulin secretion with increasing blood glucose is matched by the rapid turn-off of insulin when blood glucose is reduced.

Both adrenergic and cholinergic fibers of the autonomic nervous system innervate the islets. Parasympathetic vagal activity and sympathetic β-receptor stimulation increase insulin release.[62] Pancreatic insulin secretion, however, does not require intact autonomic innervation, as appropriate secretion responses occur in the transplanted pancreas as well.

Gastrointestinal (GI) hormones that accompany the digestive process potentiate insulin secretion. Food ingestion seems to send an "anticipatory" signal to the pancreas to discharge insulin in preparation for the absorption of glucose and amino acids.[62] The GI hormones glucose-dependent insulinotropic polypeptide (GIP) and glucagon-like peptide-1 (GLP-1), termed incretin hormones, help lower blood glucose levels by potentiating insulin production and decreasing glucagon secretion from the pancreas. GLP-1 is rapidly inactivated by the enzyme dipeptidyl peptidase-4 (DPP-4).[62] As discussed later in this chapter, drugs that mimic GLP-1 and inhibit DPP-4 have been developed to treat type 2 DM. Box 37.3 lists some of the factors that influence insulin secretion.

Glucagon

Glucagon is a polypeptide hormone produced by α cells of the pancreatic islets as a biologic antagonist to insulin.[61,62] The most important role of glucagon is to enhance hepatic glucose output (glycogenolysis and gluconeogenesis) and increase plasma glucose. A decrease in blood glucose concentration below 90 mg/dL increases

---

BOX 37.3 Factors That Influence Insulin Release

Stimulators
- Glucose, mannose, fructose
- Amino acids
- Gastrointestinal hormones
- Acetylcholine (parasympathetic stimulation)
- β-adrenergic stimulation

Inhibitors
- Hypoglycemia
- Somatostatin
- Glucagon, cortisol, growth hormone
- α-adrenergic stimulation

the plasma glucagon level by severalfold.[62] Thus hypoglycemia increases glucagon release and enhances glucose output from the liver. Hyperglycemia, on the other hand, decreases glucagon release from the α cells.

Insulin and glucagon have several biologic actions that are diametrically opposed. Whereas insulin is considered a hormone of energy storage, glucagon is considered a hormone of energy release.[62] Between meals, when blood glucose levels are low, the concentration of glucagon increases to maintain fuel production at a level that meets the energy needs of the individual, particularly the need for glucose delivery to the brain.[65]

Glucagon works in concert with other counterregulatory hormones to increase blood glucose concentration. These hormones are also secreted in response to various stresses such as injury and surgery.[61] Nondiabetic surgical patients may experience an increased plasma blood glucose, as much as 60 mg/dL above their preoperative levels, in response to surgical stress.[68,69]

Glucagon in high concentrations increases the heart rate and enhances cardiac contraction. It also causes GI smooth muscle relaxation and in some cases is used to facilitate colonoscopy.[70,71]

DIABETES MELLITUS

DM is a complex metabolic derangement caused by relative or absolute insulin deficiency. Carbohydrate, protein, and fat metabolism is markedly impaired. Diabetes has been called "starvation in a sea of food." Blood glucose may be present in abundance, but because of insulin lack or insulin resistance, it is unable to reach cells for energy provision. Criteria used to diagnose diabetes are outlined in Box 37.4. The FPG diagnostic level was reduced from a previous value of 140 mg/dL based on findings that patients with a FPG of 126 mg/dL or higher are at risk for diabetes-related complications.[66,72] The hemoglobin A_{1C} (HbA_{1C}), or glycosylated Hb level, provides an indirect estimate of the patient's overall plasma glucose control during the past 2 to 3 months. In patients with diabetes, maintaining a HbA_{1C} value of less than 6.5% to 7% is beneficial for preventing many complications such as retinopathy and nephropathy.[66,73]

There are two major categories of DM, designated as either type 1 or type 2 DM. Both types of diabetes are increasing worldwide, but the prevalence of type 2 DM is rising much more rapidly than type 1 DM. The rise in type 2 DM is attributed to a combination of three main factors: (1) an overweight population, (2) more sedentary lifestyles, and (3) a rise in the elderly population.[64,74] The prevalence of DM increases with age. As our population ages, the effect of the disease will become even more alarming. As outlined in Fig. 37.14, many pathophysiologic features of DM are directly attributable to a lack of insulin on carbohydrate, fat, and protein metabolism.

Today, diabetes affects over 34 million Americans or about 10.5% of the US population. In the United States, it is the leading cause of renal failure, nontraumatic lower extremity amputations, blindness in adults, and a major cause of hypertension and other cardiovascular diseases.[64,72,74]

Type 1 Diabetes Mellitus

About 5% to 10% of the diabetic population have type 1 DM.[72,74] This type of diabetes was formerly known as insulin-dependent diabetes or juvenile-onset diabetes. Individuals with type 1 DM have an absolute or near total deficiency of insulin and are therefore dependent on exogenous insulin therapy.[64,75,76] In the absence of sufficient exogenous insulin, the disease course may be complicated by periods of ketosis and acidosis.

In most cases, type 1 DM is caused by an unusually vigorous autoimmune attack on β cells of the pancreatic islets. Environmental factors, viral infections, or exposure to specific antigenic proteins are cited as possible initiators of the immune assault.[75,77] Patients with type 1 DM are also more likely to have other autoimmune diseases (hypothyroidism, hyperthyroidism, celiac disease).[75,77] A genetic predisposition for development of the disease may be involved.[64]

Type 1 DM usually develops before the age of 30 years, but it can develop at any age.[64] These patients tend to be nonobese and susceptible to the development of ketoacidosis. The classic symptoms of type 1 DM appear abruptly when β cells become nonfunctioning or are destroyed.[64,76] The lack of insulin has three major sequelae: (1) increased blood glucose levels, (2) increased utilization of fat for energy, and (3) depletion of the body's protein stores. Plasma glucose levels may rise to 300 to 500 mg/dL with severe untreated type 1 DM. In patients with type 1 DM, daily exogenous insulin therapy is essential for life.

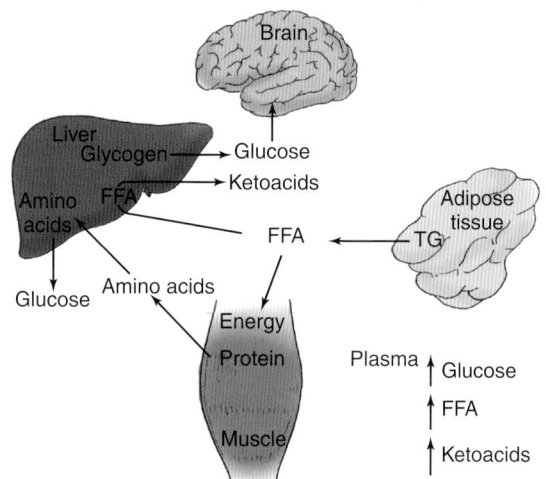

Fig. 37.14 The pattern of substrate flow in the diabetic state. Lack of insulin enhances hepatic glucose production because of increased gluconeogenesis and glycogenolysis. The diabetic state promotes protein breakdown, and the released amino acids are converted to glucose in the liver (gluconeogenesis). Lipolysis is augmented, and this increases free fatty acid supply to the liver, resulting in enhanced ketogenesis. Free fatty acids provide an energy source to muscle and other facultative tissue. Glucose uptake by the brain is sustained. *FFA,* Free fatty acids; *TG,* triglyceride.

BOX 37.4 Criteria for Diagnosing Diabetes: Four Options

1. A_{1C} ≥6.5%
   or
2. Fasting plasma glucose (FPG) ≥126 mg/dL
   Fasting defined as no caloric intake for at least 8 hr
   or
3. 2-hr plasma glucose ≥200 mg/dL during an oral glucose tolerance test
   75-g anhydrous glucose dissolved in water
   or
4. Random plasma glucose ≥200 mg/dL
   In a patient with classic symptoms of hyperglycemia or hyperglycemic crisis

From American Diabetes Association. Standards of medical care in diabetes—2019. *Diabetes Care.* 2019;42(S1).

Type 2 Diabetes Mellitus

Approximately 90% to 95% of the patients with diabetes have type 2 DM.[72,78] These patients consistently demonstrate three cardinal abnormalities[64,78]:

- Peripheral insulin resistance, particularly in muscle, fat, and liver
- Defective insulin secretion
- Excessive hepatic glucose production leading to hyperglycemia in the fasting state

Obesity is the major risk factor for type 2 DM, with over 80% of patients considered obese, primarily of the visceral or central type.[64] Type 2 DM was formerly known as noninsulin-dependent diabetes or maturity-onset diabetes.

Type 2 DM occurs in patients who have some degree of endogenous insulin production but produce quantities insufficient for sustaining normal carbohydrate homeostasis. Early in the disease process, insulin resistance contributes to an increase insulin secretion and subsequent hyperinsulinemia. The exact mechanism causing insulin resistance remains unclear, although it is present in several metabolic abnormalities classified as metabolic syndrome (obesity, insulin resistance, hyperglycemia, lipid abnormalities, hypertension). Eventually, a decline in insulin secretion occurs, which leads to an increase in hepatic glucose production and ultimately a hyperglycemic state. Insulin levels may be low, normal, or even elevated, but a relative (rather than absolute) insulin deficiency exists.[78] Typically, type 2 DM occurs in patients who are between the ages of 50 and 60 years and with a family history of the disease.[64] With the rise in childhood obesity there is an alarming rise in the number of young people with type 2 DM.[78]

There is a genetic predisposition to type 2 DM, but the genetics are not fully defined.[78] There is a strong association between nonalcoholic fatty liver disease (NAFLD) and hepatic insulin resistance. More than 90% of obese patients with type 2 DM have NAFLD.[79]

Type 2 DM has an insidious onset; indeed, it is estimated that half of those who have type 2 DM are not even aware of it. The disease course is rarely associated with ketosis or acidosis, but in poorly controlled patients it may be complicated by a nonketotic, hyperosmolar, hyperglycemic state.

Treatment for this class of diabetes consists primarily of oral glucose-lowering agents, exercise, and diet therapy. Weight reduction in the obese diabetic patient improves tissue responsiveness to endogenous insulin and, in many patients, restores normoglycemia.[80,81]

The distinction between insulin-treated diabetics and insulin-dependent diabetics is important. Some patients with type 2 DM benefit from exogenously administered insulin, especially during times of illness or stress. Patients with type 1 DM, on the other hand, are insulin dependent and require exogenous insulin daily to live.

Diabetes Associated With Other Conditions

Diabetes may result from other conditions such as pancreatitis, cystic fibrosis, polycystic ovary syndrome, Cushing syndrome, pheochromocytoma, and acromegaly. Gestational diabetes mellitus (GDM) is diabetes that is first diagnosed in the second or third trimester of pregnancy. In the United States, about 6% to 9% of pregnant women develop GDM.[82] Most women with GDM revert to normal glucose tolerance after delivery, but 35% to 60% go on to develop DM in the next 10 to 20 years.[64]

Insulin Deficiency

Effect of Insulin Deficiency on Carbohydrates

Insulin deficiency results in decreased uptake and use of glucose by insulin-sensitive cells. Glycogen storage is decreased, and gluconeogenesis is uninhibited with insulin lack, causing the liver to increase its glucose output. This produces an intracellular deficit and an extracellular surplus of glucose.[61] As the diabetic state evolves, glucose-deprived cells meet their energy requirements by drawing on fat and protein reserves.

The hyperglycemia produced by insulin lack has immediate adverse consequences. When the blood glucose concentration increases to a threshold level (~200 mg/dL), the amount of glucose filtered at the kidney glomerulus cannot be totally reabsorbed. The excess filtered glucose spills into the urine (glucosuria) and acts as an osmotic diuretic, pulling water with it. The increased urine output (polyuria) contributes to extracellular dehydration and electrolyte depletion. Intracellular dehydration also occurs because of the osmotic transfer of water out of cells and into the hypertonic extracellular fluid. To compensate for the hypovolemia, the diabetic patient may drink large quantities of water (polydipsia).

Effect of Insulin Deficiency on Fat

With insulin lack, all the insulin-mediated fat storage effects noted earlier are reversed.[62] The most important effect of insulin lack on fat metabolism is the activation of hormone-sensitive lipase, which causes uninhibited lipolysis of stored triglycerides, releasing free fatty acids and glycerol into the blood. This fat mobilization increases circulating lipids and may contribute to the atherosclerotic and angiopathic changes that complicate the disease.[62]

Insulin deficiency produces a shift from carbohydrate to fat metabolism. Free fatty acids become the main energy substrate for essentially all tissues (the brain excluded). With uncontrolled diabetes, the excess free fatty acids are converted in the liver to ketone bodies (acetoacetic acid, β-hydroxybutyric acid, acetone). This ultimately leads to greater circulating levels of ketoacids and an elevated hydrogen ion concentration in body fluids. In association with dehydration, this can cause serious acidemia (ketoacidosis). The ketone body acetone is a volatile acid and is excreted via the lungs. Consequently, one can frequently identify ketonemia in the patient with uncontrolled type 1 DM by detecting a fruity acetone breath.

Effect of Insulin Deficiency on Protein

The insulin deficiency of diabetes causes protein storage to halt and catabolism to ensue. Plasma amino acid concentration increases, and the excess circulating amino acids are converted in the liver to glucose (gluconeogenesis). The protein-wasting effects are among the most serious consequences of DM. Weight loss, weakness, and widespread organ dysfunction result. The diabetic may attempt to compensate for the protein loss and caloric drain by increasing food intake (polyphagia).

Many proteins, including hemoglobin and structural tissue proteins, become glycosylated in the presence of high circulating blood glucose levels. Glucose adducts can alter protein function and may contribute to the organ damage and functional derangements observed in individuals with diabetes.[61]

Long-Term Diabetic Complications

Diabetic patients are subject to long-term complications that confer substantial morbidity and premature mortality.[72,74,75]

The rates of diabetes-related complications have declined substantially in the past 2 decades, yet a large burden remains because the number of diabetic patients continues to increase.[83] These complications include microvascular and macrovascular disorders: retinopathy with potential loss of vision; nephropathy leading to renal failure; peripheral neuropathy with risk of foot ulcers and amputations; and autonomic neuropathy causing sexual dysfunction and GI, genitourinary, and cardiovascular aberrations. Hypertension and atherosclerosis in diabetics promote peripheral arterial, cardiovascular, and cerebral vascular disease.[66,84]

Cardiovascular disease is increased in patients with DM and is the leading cause of diabetes-related deaths.[72,74] Arterial thrombotic lesions in the diabetic population are widely distributed in the extremities, kidneys, eyes, skeletal muscle, myocardium, and brain. Owing to these diffuse lesions, diabetes, especially poorly controlled DM, carries a serious risk for the development of microvascular (e.g., nephropathy, retinopathy, neuropathy) and macrovascular (e.g., atherosclerosis, stroke, coronary artery disease, myocardial infarction [MI]) complications.[73,83-85] The incidence of circulatory insufficiency to the legs and feet is greater in diabetic men and women compared with their nondiabetic counterparts. As a result, most nontraumatic lower-limb amputations in adults occur in people with diabetes.[72,86]

Cardiomyopathy in diabetic patients is independent of coronary artery disease and often progresses to impaired myocardial relaxation and ultimately diastolic dysfunction.[87] Systolic dysfunction and decreased ejection fraction may occur with severe and longstanding disease. The risk of heart failure is two to three times higher in diabetic patients.[88]

Additionally, more than 70% of diabetic individuals have a medical history of hypertension, a rate of occurrence two to three times that for nondiabetic individuals. The risk of stroke is 1.5 times higher in people with diabetes, and their recovery rate after a stroke is poor.[72] Glucose-induced vasodilation complicates an organ's ability to autoregulate blood flow and defend against an increase in systemic blood pressure.

The eyes are vulnerable to vascular disease because of the dense network of capillary vessels in the retina. Individuals with DM are more likely to be legally blind than individuals without DM.[64] Diabetic retinopathy is characterized by microaneurysm formation, swelling and narrowing of retinal blood vessels, and neovascularization. These vascular lesions may result in vitreous hemorrhage and retinal scarring or detachment. Loss of vision from diabetic retinopathy is the leading cause of new cases of blindness in people aged 20 to 74 years in the United States.[72]

Diabetic renal disease affects patients with both type 1 and type 2 disease. Despite a plateauing or even decline in the incidence of diabetic nephropathy in recent years, diabetes remains the leading cause of kidney failure in the United States.[64,72,83,88] The nephropathy may be caused by hemodynamic alterations, inflammation, and thickening of the glomerular capillary basement membrane and other structural changes in the glomerulus.[64] Renal insufficiency or chronic renal failure is often the end result.

The diabetic process also interferes with normal nerve function. Diabetic neuropathy affects up to 50% of individuals with long-standing disease.[64,74] The peripheral and autonomic nervous systems may be involved. Both type 1 and type 2 diabetic patients are at increased risk for developing painless myocardial ischemia and infarction. Because myocardial ischemia may be painless, the possibility of an MI should be considered in the patient with a history of unexplained hypotension or dyspnea.[89-92]

Resting tachycardia is a common manifestation of cardiovascular autonomic neuropathy (CAN), and it occurs at a relatively early stage of the disease. A resting heart rate of 90 to 130 beats/min may be observed and is associated with vagal denervation. Blunted autonomic reflexes are components of CAN. Orthostatic hypotension occurs because of impairment of the sympathetic response to postural change and abnormalities in baroreceptor sensitivity.[88,90-92]

Other signs of autonomic neuropathy in the diabetic patient include early satiety, impaired bladder control, lack of sweating, impotence, and nocturnal diarrhea.[64,74,90] Impaired gastric emptying from autonomic neuropathy affects 30% to 50% of type 1 and type 2 diabetics.

> **BOX 37.5   Complications of Diabetes Mellitus**
>
> **Microvascular**
> - Retinopathy
> - Autonomic neuropathy
>   - Orthostatic hypotension, labile blood pressure, erectile dysfunction, loss of skin integrity, abnormal vascular reflexes, resting tachycardia, exercise intolerance, constipation, gastroparesis, diarrhea, impaired neurovascular response, hypoglycemic autonomic failure
> - Sensory neuropathy
>   - Paresthesia, numbness, burning sensation
> - Motor neuropathy
> - Nephropathy
>
> **Macrovascular**
> - Coronary artery disease
> - Peripheral vascular disease
> - Cerebrovascular disease
>
> **Other**
> - Infection
> - Cataracts
> - Stiff joint syndrome
> - Glaucoma
> - Poor wound healing

Patients who report anorexia, early satiety, bloating, nausea, vomiting, or abdominal pain may be at risk for gastroparesis and aspiration of stomach contents in the perioperative period.[88,93] Box 37.5 summarizes major complications of DM.

Anesthetic Management of the Diabetic Patient

Diabetes is the most common endocrine disorder encountered in surgical patients. Long-standing diabetes predisposes the patient to many disorders that may require surgical intervention. Cataract extraction, kidney transplantation, ulcer debridement, coronary artery bypass grafting, and vascular repair are some of the operations performed on diabetic patients.

Diabetic patients have higher morbidity and mortality in the perioperative period compared with nondiabetics of similar age. End-organ dysfunction associated with long-term DM and poor glycemic control are critical issues regarding perioperative risk and should be a focus of preoperative evaluation.[88]

Preoperative Considerations

The diabetic patient may come to the operating room with a spectrum of metabolic aberrations and end-organ complications that warrant careful preanesthetic assessment. Diabetes accelerates physiologic aging. A person with type 1 DM, even with good metabolic control, physiologically ages 1.25 years for every chronological year.[94]

The presence of hypertension, coronary artery disease, or autonomic nervous system dysfunction can result in a labile cardiovascular course during anesthesia. It is essential that the cardiovascular and volume status of the patient be thoroughly evaluated before surgery. A recent ECG is advised for all adult diabetic patients because of the high incidence of cardiac disease and the potential for painless myocardial ischemia.[88,90,92]

Autonomic nervous system dysfunction may result in delayed gastric emptying, making these patients prone to aspiration of stomach contents, nausea and vomiting, and abdominal distention. Preoperative aspiration prophylaxis with gastroprokinetic agents is recommended, especially for patients with a prolonged history of poor glycemic control.[85,93] The incretin mimetic agents prolong gastric emptying, and this effect may warrant additional considerations when determining preoperative gastric aspiration prophylaxis for patients on these drugs. Control of the airway with intubation is a safe choice for the patient with gastroparesis undergoing general anesthesia.

Patients with significant autonomic neuropathy may have an impaired respiratory response to hypoxia. These patients are especially sensitive to the respiratory-depressant effects of sedatives and anesthetics and warrant vigilance in the perioperative period. Autonomic neuropathy contributes to a diminished thermoregulatory response to hypothermia requiring careful monitoring of core temperature.[87] Peripheral neuropathies (e.g., paresthesias, numbness in the hands and feet) should be adequately documented in the preanesthetic evaluation. Their presence may affect the decision to use regional anesthesia.[95]

Glycosylation of tissue proteins and the development of periarticular thickening of the skin may produce a stiff-joint syndrome in diabetics, especially those with type 1 DM of long duration. Over 50% of patients with type 1 DM demonstrate restricted joint mobility.[96] Limited motion of the atlantooccipital and temporomandibular joints can make endotracheal intubation in diabetic patients more difficult compared with nondiabetic patients.[97,98] Demonstration of the prayer sign, an inability to approximate the palms of the hands and fingers, may help identify patients with tissue protein glycosylation and potentially difficult airways.

Evidence of kidney disease should be sought, and basic tests of renal function (urinalysis, serum creatinine, BUN) should be evaluated preoperatively. The presence of renal impairment may influence the choice and dosage of anesthetic agents, and potentially nephrotoxic drugs should be avoided.[99]

The anesthetist should examine the patient's history of glycemic control, including the FPG level on the morning of surgery, to ensure preoperative optimization of the patient's metabolic state.[100] Sustained hyperglycemia with attendant osmotic diuresis should alert the anesthetist to possible fluid deficits and electrolyte depletion. Preoperative electrolyte levels should be evaluated.

An important part of the preoperative evaluation is a review of oral hypoglycemic and insulin regimens. The goal of drug therapy for type 1 and type 2 diabetes is to eliminate symptoms related to hyperglycemia without inducing hypoglycemia and to reduce or eliminate the long-term microvascular and macrovascular complications of DM.[66,101]

Oral glucose-lowering agents. Oral glucose-lowering agents and insulin are used as adjuncts to diet therapy and exercise for treating type 2 DM. Currently available oral hypoglycemic agents fall into the following major classifications: (1) biguanides, (2) sulfonylureas, (3) meglitinides, (4) thiazolidinediones, (5) incretin mimetics (GLP-1 agonists and DPP-4 inhibitors), (6) α-glucosidase inhibitors, (7) sodium-glucose cotransporter-2 (SGLT-2) inhibitors, among others.[100-102] Most patients with type 2 DM require multiple drugs to achieve glycemic control. Table 37.5 outlines medications commonly used to treat type 2 DM.

Biguanides decrease hepatic glucose production, increase secretion of GLP-1, and increase peripheral glucose uptake. Metformin is the only remaining drug in this class. It is generally preferred as the first-line oral hypoglycemic agent and is available in fixed-dose combinations with

TABLE 37.5 Drugs for Type 2 Diabetes

Drug Class (A$_{1C}$ Reduction)	Mechanism	Adverse Effects
Biguanide (1%–1.5%) Metformin	Decreases hepatic glucose production, increases secretion of glucagon-like peptide-1 (GLP-1), and increases peripheral insulin sensitivity	Gastrointestinal upset; rare lactic acidosis; B$_{12}$ deficiency
GLP-1 Receptor Agonist (1%–1.5%) ("Incretin Mimetics") Exenatide Liraglutide Albiglutide Dulaglutide Lixisenatide	Potentiates insulin release, lowers serum glucagon levels, slows gastric emptying, and promotes satiety	Nausea, vomiting, diarrhea; acute pancreatitis; medullary thyroid C-cell cancer in animals and hyperplasia in humans
DPP-4 Inhibitor (0.5%–1%) Sitagliptin Saxagliptin Linagliptin Alogliptin	Inhibits metabolism of endogenously released incretin hormones. Potentiates insulin release, lowers serum glucagon levels, slows gastric emptying, and promotes satiety	Acute pancreatitis; fatal hepatic failure; possible worsening heart failure
Sulfonylurea (1%–1.5%) Glimepiride Glipizide Glyburide	Increases insulin production and secretion by pancreatic β cells	Hypoglycemia; weight gain; gastrointestinal upset
Meglitinide (0.5%–1%) Nateglinide Repaglinide	Increases insulin production and secretion by pancreatic β cells	Hypoglycemia; weight gain; multiple daily doses required
SGLT-2 Inhibitor (0.5%–1%) Canagliflozin Dapagliflozin Empagliflozin	Blocks the transport of glucose from the proximal renal tubule, decreasing renal glucose reabsorption and increasing glucose excretion	Volume depletion; hypotension; fractures; urinary tract infections, genital mycotic infection, ketoacidosis
Thiazolidinedione (1%–1.5%) Pioglitazone Rosiglitazone	Decreases hepatic glucose production and increases insulin sensitivity of adipose, muscle, and liver cells	Heart failure, possible decreased bone mineral density and fractures, hepatotoxicity, bladder cancer
Alpha-Glucosidase Inhibitor (0.5%–1%) Acarbose Miglitol	Blocks the intestinal enzymes that digest starches into absorbable monosaccharides, resulting in lower rise in postprandial plasma glucose	Abdominal pain; diarrhea; flatulence; contraindicated in patients with intestinal disease

DPP-4 inhibitor, Dipeptidyl-peptidase-4 inhibitor; *GLP-1*, glucagon-like peptide.
Modified from Drugs for Type 2 Diabetes. *Med Lett Drugs Ther.* 2019;61(1584):169–180.

many other glucose-lowering drugs.[101,102] It is associated with reduced risk of micro- and macrovascular complications. Lactic acidosis has been reported in surgical patients taking metformin, and some experts recommend that metformin be discontinued 24 hours or more prior to surgery.[103,104] Impaired renal function, liver failure, coadministration with radiocontrast material, major surgery, unstable heart failure, and alcoholism increase the risk of lactic acidosis.[101] Alternatively, perioperative administration of metformin has been reported without any increased risk of adverse outcomes.[105] Further, a Cochrane database systematic review concluded there was no evidence from prospective comparative trials or from observational cohort studies that metformin was associated with an increased risk of lactic acidosis, compared to other antihyperglycemic treatments.[106]

GLP-1 receptor agonists are approved for treatment of patients with type 2 DM. This class of drugs, called incretin mimetics, potentiates insulin release, lowers serum glucagon levels, slows gastric emptying, promotes satiety, and lowers blood glucose levels. Agents in this class do not cause hypoglycemia.[101] The first GLP-1 receptor agonist, exenatide, was derived from the saliva of the gila monster, a lizard that eats only 5 to 10 times a year in the wild. As a class, these drugs reduce the incidence of major adverse cardiovascular events.

DPP-4 inhibitors are oral agents that inhibit the destruction of incretin mimetics by blocking the DPP-4 enzyme responsible for GLP-1 degradation. Both GLP-1 receptor agonists and DPP-4 inhibitors are effective in lowering blood glucose levels but have been associated with acute pancreatitis.[101,102]

Sulfonylurea agents are the oldest class of oral hypoglycemic agents, first introduced in the 1950s. They increase the secretion of insulin from the pancreas and thus require the presence of functioning β cells. Long term, sulfonylureas effectively lower plasma glucose levels and decrease micro- and macrovascular complications.[107] Persistent and severe hypoglycemia is a possible adverse effect of sulfonylureas.

Meglitinides, or nonsulfonylurea secretagogues, increase insulin production by pancreatic β cells in a manner similar to the sulfonylureas.[102] Multiple daily doses are required. Hypoglycemia is a possible adverse effect of meglitinides.

SGLT-2 inhibitors lower blood glucose levels by blocking the transport of glucose from the proximal renal tubule, decreasing renal glucose reabsorption, and increasing glucose and water excretion. Because of their diuretic effect, these agents may lead to dehydration, hypovolemia, and hypotension, particularly in the elderly patient with renal dysfunction. Increased risk of fractures and risks of limb amputation have been reported with use of some SGLT-2 agents.[108] The US Food and Drug Administration (FDA) has warned that SGLT-2 inhibitors may lead to ketoacidosis and has therefore placed restrictions on use of these drugs in the perioperative period.[109,110]

Thiazolidinedione derivatives lower blood glucose levels in patients with type 2 DM by decreasing hepatic glucose production and by increasing the insulin sensitivity of adipose tissue, skeletal muscle, and the liver.[102] Thiazolidinediones have been associated with cardiac problems, liver failure, and possible risk of bone fractures. Restrictions that were placed on rosiglitazone in 2010 because of concern about its cardiovascular safety have been lifted by the FDA in November 2013.

α-glucosidase inhibitors block the intestinal enzymes that digest starches into absorbable monosaccharides resulting in a slower and lower rise in postprandial plasma glucose.

Insulin preparations. Insulin preparations are generated today by DNA recombinant technology, mimicking the amino acid sequence of human insulin. Most insulin formulations in the United States are prepared as U-100 (100 international units [IU]/mL), but U-200, U-300, and U-500 formulations are also available. For instance, the concentrated form of insulin glargine (Toujeo) contains 300 IU/mL

instead of insulin glargine (Lantus) at 100 IU/mL.[111] A rapid-acting inhaled insulin (Afrezza) was approved by the FDA in 2015 for treatment of patients with type 1 and type 2 DM. Afrezza has an onset of approximately 12 minutes and produces peak insulin activity in approximately 40 minutes.[75] Cough and throat irritation are side effects, and the long-term pulmonary safety of inhaling insulin is unknown.[75,101,112]

Insulin preparations differ in onset and duration based on delivery methods. In addition to subcutaneous bolus injections, insulin delivery devices (e.g., implantable pumps, mechanical syringes) are used to facilitate exogenous administration. The greatest risk with all forms of insulin is hypoglycemia.

Protamine is added to some insulins to prolong their effect. Protamine containing insulins (e.g., neutral protamine Hagedorn) may cause sensitization by stimulating antibodies against protamine sulfate. In patients taking protamine containing insulins, particular care must be exercised (slow and titrated doses) to monitor for hypersensitivity reactions when administering protamine sulfate to reverse the coagulation effects of heparin. The available insulins can be divided on a pharmacokinetic basis into four broad categories: rapid acting, short acting, intermediate acting, and long acting (Table 37.6).

It is imperative to know the surgical patient's normal insulin dosage regimen and treatment compliance. Many diabetic patients are on a regimen of long-acting insulin at bedtime and rapid-acting insulin analogues given with meals (basal-bolus regimen). Rapid-acting insulins, such as lispro, aspart, and glulisine have an onset of action of less than 1 hour and are used to reduce glycemia that occurs after

TABLE 37.6 Pharmacokinetic Properties of Insulin Preparations

Insulin Type	Onset	Peak	Duration
Rapid Acting			
Aspart *(Novolog)*	10–30 min	30–180 min	3–5 hr
Lispro (*Humalog* U 100, Humalog U-200, Admelog)			
Glulisine *(Apidra)*			
Aspart *(Fiasp)*	2.5 min	40–50 min	
Short Acting			
Regular U-100 (*Humulin R* U-100)	30–60 min	2–4 hr	U-100: up to 10 hr U-500: up to 24 hr
Regular U-100 (*Novolin R* U-100)			
Regular U-500 (*Humulin* U-500)			
Intermediate Acting			
NPH *(Humulin N)*	2-4 hr	4–8 hr	12–18 hr
NPH *(Novolin N)*			
Long Acting			
Detemir *(Levemir)*	2–4 hr	Minimal	Detemir: 12–24 hr
Glargine (*Lantus, Basaglar, Toujeo* U-300)			Glargine: up to 24 hr
Degludec (*Tresiba* U-100, Tresiba U-200)			Degludec: up to 48 hr

Time course is based on subcutaneous administration.
R, Regular; *NPH,* neutral protamine Hagedorn.
Adapted from Atkinson M, et al. Type 1 diabetes mellitus. In: Melmed S, Polonsky KS, Larsen PR, eds. *Williams Textbook of Endocrinology.* 10th ed. Philadelphia: Elsevier; 2020:1403–1437.

meal ingestion.[75,101] Long-acting insulins, including glargine, detemir, and degludec, have delayed absorption from subcutaneous tissue and prolonged effects. They are titrated to produce a steady, basal insulin level.[75,101,113]

Continuous subcutaneous insulin infusion (CSII) is increasingly used by motivated patients desiring an optimal physiologic regimen.[114] These infusion pumps administer rapid-acting insulin through a catheter that is usually inserted into the subcutaneous tissues of the anterior abdominal wall. These complicated pump delivery systems deliver a basal insulin infusion and can be programmed to increase and decrease at predetermined times of the day.[75,101]

Intraoperative Management

Diabetic patients represent a heterogeneous group requiring individualized perioperative care. The diabetic surgical patient's operation should be scheduled early in the day if possible to minimize disruptions in treatment and nutrition regimens. The specific approach to management depends on the type of diabetes (type 1 or type 2), the history of treatment and glycemic control, the presence of comorbidities, and the type and length of surgery. No specific anesthetic technique is superior overall for diabetic patients. Both general anesthesia and regional anesthesia have been used safely. Diabetes is not a contraindication to ambulatory surgery.[88]

Associated end-organ diseases are risks for the surgical diabetic patient and may include cardiovascular dysfunction, renal insufficiency, glycosylated joint proteins, and neuropathies. Focus on the cardiovascular system should be a major component of anesthesia care. Silent myocardial ischemia and infarction are more common in the diabetic patient. CAN contributes to hemodynamic instability and may complicate the anesthetic course. Indeed, the neurovascular compensatory mechanisms to anesthesia-induced vasodilation may be impaired, requiring the use of vasoactive drugs.[90,92]

Special care must be taken in positioning and padding the diabetic patient on the operating table. Decreased tissue perfusion and peripheral sympathetic neuropathy may contribute to the development of skin breakdown and ulceration.

Postoperative nausea and vomiting are common in many diabetics, and aggressive measures should be taken to prevent such incidences. If dexamethasone is used as an antiemetic it may increase blood glucose levels up to 20% and should be limited to 4 mg to prevent unwanted hyperglycemia.[115]

Surgery, particularly major surgery, produces a catabolic stress response and elevates stress-induced counterregulatory hormones.[68,69,116] In the diabetic patient, the hyperglycemic, ketogenic, and lipolytic effects of the counterregulatory hormones compound the state of insulin deficiency. For this reason, perioperative hyperglycemia and other metabolic aberrations are common in the surgical diabetic patient and may be more difficult to manage.[100,116] General anesthesia elicits a stronger counterregulatory hyperglycemic response than local or regional anesthesia.[117]

Frequent blood glucose determinations are an integral part of any diabetic management technique. An accurate and rapid means of monitoring blood glucose levels should be available. The practitioner should be aware that point-of-care testing devices using capillary blood measurement can vary by 20%, especially during periods of hypotension and poor tissue perfusion.[116,118,119] Point-of-care monitoring is sufficient for stable patients, but a higher threshold for hypoglycemia and more frequent monitoring may be indicated to ensure patient safety.[100] Arterial blood gas analysis and central laboratory measurement of blood glucose remain the gold standard, and aberrant glucose values should be verified by the central lab.[118] During a long surgical procedure or for major surgery, frequent (at

least hourly) intraoperative blood glucose measurement is the prudent course.

Preoperative hyperglycemia is an independent risk factor for perioperative morbidity.[88,100,120-123] Not surprisingly, high intraoperative blood glucose levels are associated with higher postoperative blood glucose levels.[120] Persistent hyperglycemia (preoperative HbA_{1C} >6.7, postoperative blood glucose >200 mg/dL) has been shown to impair wound healing and wound strength.[124] In addition, reports indicate that postoperative infection is more prevalent in diabetic patients with uncontrolled blood glucose levels.[117,125,126] Glucose-induced vasodilation disrupts autoregulation in target organs. Studies also provide evidence that hyperglycemia worsens the neurologic outcome after ischemic brain injury.[100,127-130]

Avoiding hyperglycemia in the perioperative period is warranted. The risks of intensive insulin therapy (IIT) were highlighted in the landmark international trial, Normoglycemia in Intensive Care Evaluation and Survival Using Glucose Algorithm Regulation (NICE-SUGAR), which questioned the safety of IIT.[131] Since then, several studies have demonstrated that aggressive glucose control, with near normal blood glucose targets, produced no survival benefit and a higher incidence of hypoglycemia and even death in surgical and critically ill patients.[132-136] Symptoms of hypoglycemia are difficult to recognize in the anesthetized or sedated surgical patient, and its presence can produce irreversible neurologic sequelae.

Various regimens have been tendered on how to best manage the metabolic changes that occur in the surgical diabetic patient.[116,132,137-142] The universal goal with all techniques is to avoid hypoglycemia and minimize metabolic derangements associated with marked hyperglycemia. Experts differ on optimal protocols for case management, but there is emphasis today on more moderate and individualized glycemic targets.[88,99,117,137-140]

It is clear that the tighter the glucose control, the greater the risk of hypoglycemia, but it is not clear what level of glycemic control is associated with the best risk-benefit ratio. With these caveats considered, many experts target a blood glucose range of 140 to 180 mg/dL.[63,117,141] Mild transient hyperglycemia prevents the poor outcomes associated with severe hyperglycemia and avoids the potentially catastrophic effects of hypoglycemia.[99,116,135,141,142] Frequent blood glucose determinations during surgery and in the immediate postoperative period are central to safe practice.[116,139,140]

Current recommendations regarding insulin use in the perioperative period include adjustments to the patient's usual insulin regimen based on the length of surgery, the type of surgery, and the degree of glycemic control.[100,116,141,143] Multidisciplinary groups within an institution can improve key measures of diabetic care by working together to establish appropriate perioperative blood glucose management protocols.

There is substantial variability in management techniques, but sample preoperative insulin protocols are outlined in Table 37.7. Patients should arrive to the preoperative area early enough to have their FPG level monitored and to determine needed adjustments in insulin dosage or the need for intravenous dextrose supplementation (5% dextrose in water, 75–200 mL/hour). For critically ill patients, long surgical procedures, and procedures with anticipated hemodynamic changes or temperature/fluid shifts, a separate and continuous intravenous insulin infusion can be used to meet basal metabolic requirements.[116,142,144,145] Effective insulin infusion protocols are assiduously titrated to frequent (at least hourly) blood glucose determinations.[117]

Sliding scale administration of bolus insulin as the sole glucose management technique is associated with roller coaster–like swings in blood glucoses levels, termed glucose variability, and correlates with poor outcomes in various populations.[100,141,142,145,146]

TABLE 37.7 Sample Management Techniques for Preoperative Insulin Therapy

Insulin Regimen	Day Before Surgery	Day of Surgery
Short and rapid acting	Usual dose	Hold dose
Intermediate acting	75% dose based on waking blood glucose (BG) level	50% of usual morning dose if BG >120 mg/dL; hold if BG <120 mg/dL
Long acting	75%–100% of night dose based on waking BG level evening before surgery	75%–100% of morning dose (if taken normally) on the morning of surgery
Insulin pump	No change	Basal "sleep" rate or discontinue and substitute with insulin infusion

Insulin regimens based on patient with normal diet until midnight and those permitted clear liquids until 2 hr before surgery.

For surgical patients having short, uncomplicated surgery, who are well controlled on CSII, their pump can be continued into the perioperative period and programmed to deliver a basal insulin dose, with adjustments based on frequent (at least hourly) serial blood glucose measurements.[147-150] For more complicated surgical procedures (lasting >2 hours), the pump should be discontinued and a continuous insulin infusion (with intravenous glucose) implemented for the perioperative period.[141,142,148]

Patients treated with oral hypoglycemic agents should be treated the same individualized perioperative management as those with type 1 DM, although their metabolic course is typically more stable. The duration of action of the patient's oral agent must be noted. Sulfonylurea and meglitinide agents stimulate insulin secretion, and hypoglycemia is a concern with these agents during periods of fasting.[116] For the well-controlled surgical patient with type 2 DM, most authors recommend holding the patient's oral hypoglycemic or noninsulin injectable medication the day of surgery.[100,116] Special consideration may focus on those patients receiving metformin and holding the drug 24 to 48 hours before surgery, particularly if the patient has renal dysfunction or will be receiving radiocontrast media.[100,116] Further, the FDA advises stopping SGLT-2 inhibitors before surgery because of the risk of ketoacidosis. Canagliflozin, dapagliflozin, and empagliflozin should be discontinued 3 days before scheduled surgery, and ertugliflozin should be stopped at least 4 days before. The SGLT-2 inhibitor may be restarted once the patient's oral intake is back to baseline and any other risk factors for ketoacidosis are resolved.[109]

Regardless of the technique chosen, central to any management plan is assessing plasma glucose frequently and regularly.

Acute Derangements in Glucose Homeostasis

Hypoglycemia

Hypoglycemia is encountered more often in the diabetic patient than in the nondiabetic patient, and it can develop insidiously during the perioperative period. Insulin and oral glucose lowering agents (especially sulfonylureas and meglitinides) are drugs that are potential causes of hypoglycemia in the surgical diabetic patient. Approximately 90% of all patients with DM who receive insulin have had a hypoglycemic episode.[151,152] Liver disease (impaired hepatic glucose output and impaired insulin metabolism), the altered physiology associated with

TABLE 37.8 Definitions of Clinically Relevant Hypoglycemia

Hypoglycemia Level	Definitions
Severe hypoglycemia	An event requiring assistance of another person to actively administer carbohydrates, glucagon, or take other corrective actions. Plasma glucose concentrations may not be available during an event, but neurologic recovery following the return of plasma glucose to normal is considered sufficient evidence that the event was induced by a low plasma glucose concentration.
Documented symptomatic hypoglycemia	An event during which typical symptoms of hypoglycemia are accompanied by a measured plasma glucose concentration ≤70 mg/dL.
Asymptomatic hypoglycemia	An event not accompanied by typical symptoms of hypoglycemia but with a measured plasma glucose concentration ≤70 mg/dL.
Probable symptomatic hypoglycemia	An event during which symptoms typical of hypoglycemia are not accompanied by a plasma glucose determination but that was presumably caused by a plasma glucose concentration ≤70 mg/dL.
Pseudohypoglycemia	An event during which the person with diabetes reports any of the typical symptoms of hypoglycemia with a measured plasma glucose concentration >70 mg/dL but approaching that level.

Seaquist ER, Anderson J, Childs B, et al. Hypoglycemia and diabetes: a report of a workgroup of the American Diabetes Association and the Endocrine Society. *Diabetes Care.* 2013;36:1384–1395.

gastric bypass surgery, or an insulin-secreting tumor of the islets of Langerhans (insulinoma) are conditions that are complicated by hypoglycemia. Renal failure may be associated with hypoglycemia due to prolonged insulin clearance.[143]

The threshold for hypoglycemia is defined by the American Diabetes Association as blood glucose values less than or equal to 70 mg/dL[66] (Table 37.8). The blood glucose concentration at which signs and symptoms of hypoglycemia appear varies widely from one person to the next, but blood glucose levels in the range of 50 to 70 mg/dL commonly produce symptoms (e.g., anxiety, irritability, nervousness, confusion, dizziness, headache) in the otherwise healthy patient.[62,151] Because the brain relies on glucose for energy requirements, it is most sensitive to glucose deprivation.[62,63,151] As the blood glucose level lowers, aberrant behavior, seizures, and loss of consciousness may occur. Other signs of hypoglycemia (e.g., tachycardia, diaphoresis, tremors, piloerection, pupillary dilation, and vasoconstriction) reflect sympathetic-adrenal hyperactivity.[62,153]

Acute treatment for the hypoglycemic surgical patient is administration of 25 g IV of 50% dextrose (50 mL). This treatment should raise the blood glucose level by 75 to 125 mg/dL, depending on the patient's weight. Blood glucose measurement should be repeated after

15 minutes with an additional glucose bolus if needed or with initiation of a glucose infusion of 5% dextrose.[63,100] Unconscious patients who do not have an intravenous line can be given 1 mg of glucagon subcutaneously. The goal is to achieve a blood glucose level greater than 100 mg/dL. Unless prompt glucose therapy is provided, irreversible brain damage may result.

Hypoglycemia is potentially catastrophic during surgery because most of the neurologic symptoms of glucose lack are masked by sedation and general anesthesia. Signs of sympathetic adrenal discharge also may be blunted by general anesthesia or severe diabetic autonomic neuropathy, making the diagnosis of hypoglycemia difficult. β-adrenergic receptor blocking agents can reduce the hyperglycemic effects of epinephrine, in addition to diminishing the symptomatic warning signs of hypoglycemia.[62,63,151] For these reasons, attention to detecting hypoglycemia, especially in the diabetic patient, must remain a critical focus. Careful determination of the patient's history, frequent blood glucose determinations, maintenance of mild hyperglycemia, and diligent monitoring help to avoid this feared complication during anesthesia.

Diabetic Ketoacidosis

Diabetic ketoacidosis (DKA) is a condition in which insulin deficiency leads to the biochemical triad of severe hyperglycemia, ketonemia, and acidemia.[75,101] DKA was formerly considered to occur only in patients with type 1 DM, but it is now recognized to also occur in patients with type 2 DM.[101] Hospitalizations for DKA have increased in the United States among all age groups.[154] It is triggered by a hyperglycemic event, and symptoms and physical signs usually develop over 24 hours.[101] Noncompliance with insulin treatment, critical illnesses (e.g., MI, trauma, cerebral vascular accident, burns), and infections are common precipitants of DKA.[153] As noted previously, SGLT-2 inhibitors can cause ketoacidosis in patients with type 2 DM.[109]

As described earlier, stressful events stimulate the release of hyperglycemic counterregulatory hormones (glucagon, cortisol, catecholamines, GH). Patients with diabetes are unable to secrete sufficient insulin to counterbalance the serum elevations of glucose, free fatty acids, and ketone bodies produced by these stress-induced hormones. Unless exogenous insulin is provided, the glycemic event may progress to severe ketoacidosis, dehydration, and acute metabolic decompensation.[101]

Patients with DKA classically present with hyperglycemia (blood glucose >250 mg/dL), metabolic acidosis (arterial pH <7.3), a calculated anion gap greater than 10 mEq/L, electrolyte depletion, serum hyperosmolarity (>300 mOsm/L), and abdominal tenderness and/or pain.[64] Nausea and vomiting are often prominent. Large fluid losses, on the order of 3 to 5 L, are common and lead to volume depletion, hypotension, and tachycardia.[101] Blood levels of ketone bodies (β-hydroxybutyrate, acetoacetate, and acetone) are elevated, and the patient's breath may have a fruity odor from excess acetone production. Plasma assays of β-hydroxybutyrate is preferred over urinary ketone determinations, which measure only acetoacetate and acetone.[101] Lactic acidosis secondary to poor perfusion may compound the ketoacidosis. Low pH generally improves with resolution of hypovolemia and hyperglycemia. Routine use of bicarbonate replacement is not recommended.[101] The respiratory center is typically stimulated by the low plasma pH, resulting in rapid, deep breathing (Kussmaul respiration). Acidosis, hyperosmolarity, and dehydration may depress consciousness to the point of coma.[75,101,153] Patients have decreased total-body potassium stores, but because of the acidosis and insulin lack, initial serum potassium levels (reported on laboratory results) are elevated. Patients require potassium replacement because as the acidosis is corrected and with insulin administration, potassium moves into cells and the serum levels can decline abruptly.[75] Fig. 37.15 outlines the pathophysiologic events leading to DKA.

Gangrene of an ischemic lower extremity is a surgical condition associated with DKA. Preoperative management of the emergency surgical patient with DKA requires a focused approach to restore intravascular volume, correct electrolyte abnormalities, improve acid-base balance, and treat insulin deficiency.[64,153] Early invasive hemodynamic monitoring should be considered.[75] The airway must be protected in the obtunded patient. Emergency surgery for a patient in an unstable metabolic state such as DKA is high risk; however, in a stabilized patient with DKA, once the surgical problem that initiated DKA (e.g., trauma, gangrene) has resolved, medical management is often more effective.

Hyperglycemic Hyperosmolar State

Hyperglycemic hyperosmolar state (HHS), or hyperosmolar nonketotic coma, is a life-threatening hyperosmolar condition triggered by a hyperglycemic event. This syndrome commonly occurs in elderly individuals with type 2 DM.[101] Like DKA, HHS is associated with insulin deficiency, volume depletion, and acid-base abnormalities. Patients with HHS generally have some endogenous insulin secretion, but the hyperglycemic episode overwhelms the pancreas and produces severe hyperglycemia and glucosuria.[153] The amount of insulin secreted is usually sufficient to prevent lipolysis and ketone production. Therefore, unlike DKA, this syndrome is not usually associated with significant ketoacidosis. But hypotension and poor tissue perfusion can result

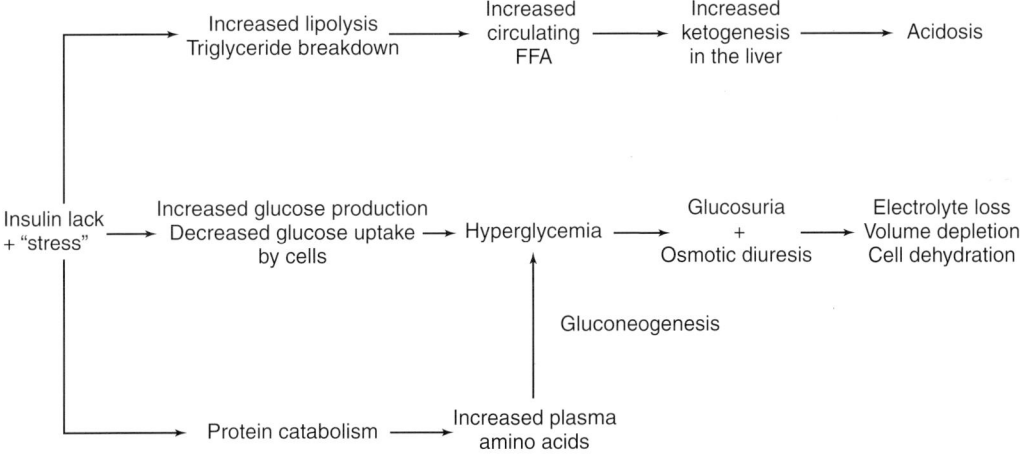

Fig. 37.15 Substrate flow with diabetic ketoacidosis. *FFA*, Free fatty acid.

TABLE 37.9 Representative Features of Diabetic Ketoacidosis (DKA) and Hyperglycemic Hyperosmolar Syndrome (HHS)

	DKA	HHS
Plasma glucose	250–600 mg/dL	600–1200 mg/dL
pH	6.8–7.3	>7.3
Serum bicarbonate	<15 mEq/L	Normal or slightly decreased
Serum osmolarity	300–320 mOsm/L	350–380 mOsm/L
Ketonemia	++++	+/-
Mental obtundation	Variable	Present
Hypovolemia	Present	Present
Serum potassium*	Normal or slight +	Normal
Arterial P_{CO2}	20–30 mm Hg	Normal

+, Increase; ++++, large increase.

*Plasma levels may be normal or high, but total body stores are usually depleted.

Adapted from Powers AC, Niswender KD, Rickels MR. Diabetes mellitus: management and therapies. In: Jameson J, Fauci AS, Kasper DL, et al., eds. *Harrison's Principles of Internal Medicine*. 20th ed. New York: McGraw-Hill; 2018.

in lactic acidosis. Table 37.9 compares common features of DKA and HHS.

Common precipitating factors of HHS include infection, sepsis, pneumonia, stroke, and MI.[64,153] Patients typically have a several week period of hyperglycemia, glucosuria, polyuria, poor oral intake, intravascular volume depletion, and weight loss. This culminates in mental confusion, lethargy, or coma.[101,153] Profound dehydration is present (average total body water deficit 9 L), resulting in increased plasma viscosity, hypotension, and tachycardia. Laboratory evaluation may reveal a biochemical profile of marked hyperglycemia, absent or minimal ketonemia, and serum hyperosmolarity (>350 mOsm/L).[101,153] Arterial and venous thromboembolic events are common. Unlike DKA, nausea, vomiting, Kussmaul respirations, and abdominal pain are not typically present. As with DKA, despite depleted total body potassium stores, the reported serum potassium levels at presentation may be normal or elevated due to acidosis and insulin deficiency. Even with appropriate treatment, the mortality figures for HHS are substantially higher (15%) than those for DKA (<1%) in part because HHS commonly affects an older patient population, often with accompanying comorbidities.[101]

Treatment for DKA and HHS are similar and include identification and management of the precipitating problem, careful isotonic fluid rehydration, correction of hyperglycemia with insulin, and electrolyte replacement.[64,153] Cerebral edema is the major nonmetabolic complication of DKA therapy, the result of overreplacement of free water and rapid normalization of serum glucose.[101] Problems inherent in aggressive fluid administration to the elderly patient with HHS include heart failure and pulmonary edema. Patients with DKA and HHS are critically ill and require an intensive care setting for careful assessment of fluid and renal status, continuous hemodynamic monitoring, and frequent determination of laboratory values.[101] Central hemodynamic monitoring is prudent in elderly patients during treatment.

ADRENAL GLANDS

The adrenal glands are located at the superior poles of each kidney and consist of two distinct anatomic and physiologic entities, the adrenal cortex and the adrenal medulla. The adrenal medulla comprises the central 20% of the adrenal gland and primarily secretes the

hormones epinephrine and norepinephrine. The adrenal cortex constitutes the outer part of the adrenal gland and secretes three main types of hormones: mineralocorticoids (e.g., aldosterone), glucocorticoids (e.g., cortisol), and androgenic precursor hormones (e.g., dehydroepiandrosterone).[155]

Adrenal Cortex

The adrenal cortex is composed of three layers, each having distinct properties. The zona glomerulosa is the outermost tissue of the cortex; it secretes mineralocorticoid hormones, primarily aldosterone. The zona fasciculata is the middle layer; it secretes primarily the glucocorticoid hormones, such as cortisol and corticosterone. The zona reticularis is the innermost layer of the adrenal cortex, and it secretes primarily adrenal androgenic hormones[155,156] (Fig. 37.16). The adrenal androgen precursor hormones, of which dehydroepiandrosterone is the most important, have effects similar to the male sex hormone testosterone and account for secondary sexual characteristics in females.[155] The glucocorticoids and mineralocorticoids are discussed in more detail in the following sections.

Hormones Secreted From the Adrenal Cortex

The adrenal cortex synthesizes more than 30 types of hormones, all of which have a steroidal structure and share a common cholesterol backbone. As a group, adrenocortical hormones are called corticosteroids. Corticosteroids have similar chemical structures but widely diverse functions.[157,158]

Glucocorticoid hormone production and release is controlled by ACTH from the anterior pituitary gland. Mineralocorticoids, on the other hand, are largely and separately controlled by the renin-angiotensin system and serum potassium. These distinct lines of control have important clinical consequences. Primary adrenal failure invariably produces cortisol and aldosterone deficiency, whereas ACTH deficiency from pituitary disease produces glucocorticoid deficiency but near normal aldosterone concentrations because its control systems are intact.[155]

Glucocorticoids. Cortisol (hydrocortisone) is the prototypical glucocorticoid, and it accounts for 95% of glucocorticoid activity from the adrenal cortex.[156] It is one of the few hormones essential for life. As previously stated, cortisol biosynthesis and secretion are controlled almost entirely by ACTH (corticotropin) from the anterior pituitary gland. ACTH, in turn, is controlled by corticotropin-releasing hormone (CRH) from the hypothalamus. Classic endocrine negative feedback loops are in place to control the secretion of both ACTH and CRH. When cortisol levels are high, the feedback system inhibits the release of ACTH from the anterior pituitary and CRH from the hypothalamus.[158] This powerful negative feedback circuit is known as the hypothalamic-pituitary-adrenal (HPA) axis. Fig. 37.17 summarizes the mechanisms regulating cortisol release.

ACTH stimulates glucocorticoid hormone synthesis by activating the cholesterol side-chain cleavage enzyme (cytochrome P450 side-chain cleavage enzyme [P450 11A1]), which catalyzes the conversion of cholesterol to pregnenolone, the first step in corticosteroid hormone synthesis (Fig. 37.18).[155] In addition to glucocorticoid hormone synthesis, ACTH controls adrenal gland growth, especially the zona reticularis and zona fasciculata. ACTH deficiency results in adrenal gland atrophy.

Daily cortisol production is about 20 mg, and most of this is produced and released in the morning. Secretion rates of CRH, ACTH, and cortisol follow a circadian rhythm: Levels are highest in the early morning, decline throughout the day, and reach a nadir in the evening.[155,156] After release from the adrenal cortex, cortisol circulates in the blood either as free cortisol (the physiologically active form)

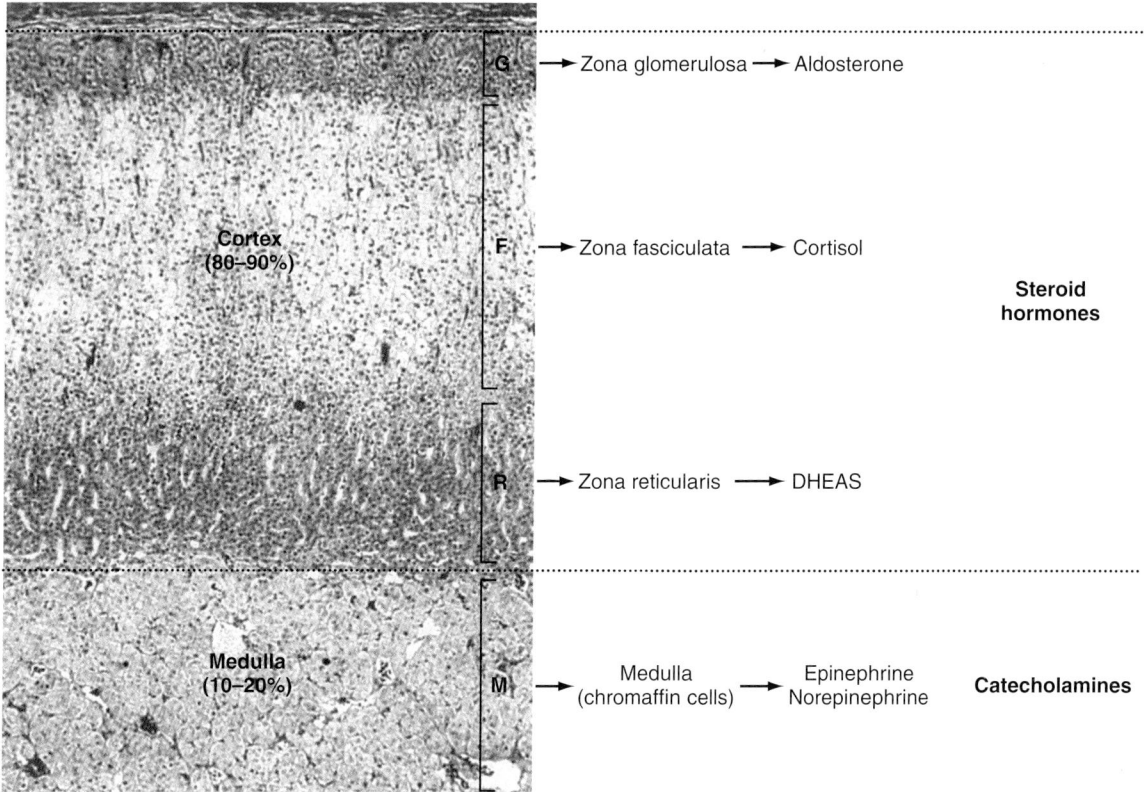

Fig. 37.16 Histology of the adrenal gland. Higher magnification clearly illustrating the zonation of the cortex. The corresponding endocrine function and the different zones of the cortex and the medulla are noted. *DHEAS,* Dehydroepiandrosterone sulfate. (In Koeppen BM, Stanton BA. *Berne and Levy Physiology (Updated).* 7th ed. Philadelphia: Elsevier; 2017:768. Modified from Young B, Woodford P, O'Dowd G. *Wheater's Functional Histology.* 6th ed. Philadelphia: Elsevier; 2014:328.)

or bound to cortisol-binding globulin (transcortin) or albumin.[155] Approximately 90% of cortisol is transported in the bound form. The circulating half-life of cortisol varies between 70 and 120 minutes, but it has a more prolonged end-organ effect.[158] Like other steroid hormones, cortisol exerts many of its effects by diffusion into the target cell, binding to intracellular receptors, and altering DNA transcription and protein synthesis. Most of the metabolic actions of cortisol therefore are not immediate but take several hours or days to fully develop. Cortisol is inactivated mainly in the liver and kidney and excreted in the urine as 17-hydroxycorticosteroids.[156]

Cortisol actions. Glucocorticoids have effects in virtually all cells in the body.[155] They are needed for the proper use of proteins, carbohydrates, and fats by the body. Furthermore, glucocorticoids have a permissive effect on catecholamine hormones from the adrenal medulla and help mediate their effects on the heart (contractility) and vascular tone. Cortisol is central to the body's response to stress.[155,156] Almost any stress, psychologic or physical, causes an immediate and marked increase in ACTH and cortisol production levels.[155-158]

Surgical stress is a potent stimulator of the HPA axis, and major surgery can increase the cortisol secretion to greater than 100 mg/day. Important perioperative stressors include pain, anxiety, trauma, infection, fever, and hypotension.[158] The type of surgery, degree of trauma, duration of the procedure, and depth of anesthesia affect the amount of cortisol released. Cortisol blood concentration may increase severalfold both during and after major surgery. Deep general anesthesia or regional anesthesia may blunt this stress response but does not eliminate it (Box 37.6). An inadequate cortisol response during critical illness and surgery can lead to hypotension, shock, and death.[155,157]

Glucocorticoids (cortisol, cortisone) have some mineralocorticoid (salt and water retention, loss of potassium and hydrogen ions) and androgenic activity that may become significantly apparent with hormone excess or supraphysiologic replacement dosages (cortisol, >30 mg/day).

Effect on carbohydrate metabolism. Overall, glucocorticoids enhance the production of high-energy fuel for metabolic needs.[155] Cortisol increases glucose production by the liver. A key function is their ability to stimulate gluconeogenesis (the formation of glucose from amino acids, lactate, glycerol, and other substances) in the liver. The rate of gluconeogenesis increases 6- to 10-fold in the presence of cortisol. Furthermore, cortisol mobilizes amino acids from extrahepatic tissues (mainly muscle), making them available for gluconeogenesis.[156] Cortisol antagonizes insulin's effects to inhibit gluconeogenesis in the liver and in most extrahepatic cells cortisol moderately decreases the rate of glucose uptake and utilization. Cortisol is called diabetogenic (adrenal diabetes) because these actions increase blood glucose concentrations.

Effect on protein and bone metabolism. Cortisol decreases protein synthesis and increases protein breakdown in should be treated all body tissue except the liver.[156] As such, high cortisol levels can impair wound healing.[159] In the presence of sustained cortisol excess, catabolic effects are marked. This is especially apparent in skeletal muscles, which become weak and atrophic, but also skin and connective tissue. Glucocorticoids inhibit osteoblast activity and inhibit intestinal calcium absorption. Both may account for the osteopenia and osteoporosis that characterize glucocorticoid excess.[158,160]

Effect on fat metabolism. Free fatty acids are mobilized from adipose tissue under cortisol's control. An increase in total circulating

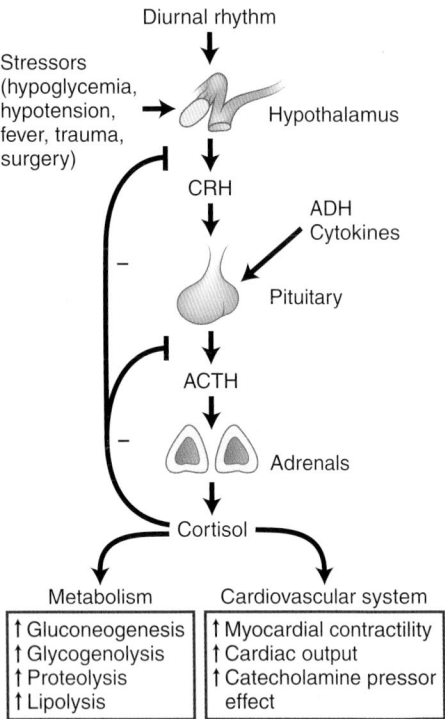

Regulation of cortisol secretion

Fig. 37.17 Normal negative feedback regulation of cortisol. Hypothalamic-pituitary-adrenal axis. Adrenocorticotropic hormone (ACTH) is secreted from the anterior pituitary under the influence of two principal secretagogues, corticotropin-releasing hormone (CRH) and arginine vasopressin; other factors, including cytokines, also play a role. CRH secretion is regulated by an inbuilt circadian rhythm and by additional stressors operating through the hypothalamus. Secretion of CRH and ACTH is inhibited by cortisol, highlighting the importance of negative feedback control. ADH, Antidiuretic hormone. (From Melmed S, et al., eds. *Williams Textbook of Endocrinology.* 13th ed. Philadelphia: Elsevier; 2016:497.)

triglycerides and cholesterol is observed.[158] The effects of cortisol help shift metabolic systems to the use of fatty acids instead of glucose for energy. Excess cortisol results in a distinctive obesity, with chest, abdominal, interscapular, and facial fat expansion, leading to a buffalo-like torso and moon facies.[155-157]

Effect on inflammation and immunity. Cortisol can diminish the body's inflammatory responses by suppressing all aspects of the inflammatory process. Migration of white blood cells into the inflamed area is decreased. At pharmacologic doses, cortisol stabilizes lysosomal membranes and decreases T-lymphocyte and antibody production.[155] These effects are the basis for therapeutic use of corticosteroids to reduce inflammatory responses associated with asthma, allergic reactions, and arthritis.

Cortisol decreases the number of eosinophils and lymphocytes in the blood. As mentioned earlier, T-lymphocyte and antibody output are decreased. The ability of cortisol to suppress immunity makes pharmacologic administration of glucocorticoids useful in treating a variety of autoimmune disorders. However, with pharmacologic doses of cortisol, the level of immunity to foreign invaders of the body is also reduced, and infection may ensue from disease that would otherwise not be pathologic.

Corticosteroids are used to treat a diverse variety of human diseases, primarily relying on their antiinflammatory and immune suppressive actions, and are given orally, parenterally, and by numerous topical routes (e.g., skin, inhalation).[158] Box 37.7 summarizes some of the therapeutic uses of corticosteroids.

Mineralocorticoids. In contrast to the diverse actions of glucocorticoids at numerous target sites, mineralocorticoids have a relatively restricted action, primarily at the renal distal tubules and collecting ducts (also salivary and sweat glands) to reabsorb sodium and water and excrete potassium or hydrogen. Mineralocorticoids are required for life as they play a major role in the regulation of extracellular sodium and potassium ion concentrations and total body fluid balance. With a total loss of mineralocorticoid secretion, death would ensue within days without treatment.[156,157] Aldosterone is the body's principal mineralocorticoid, accounting for 90% of all mineralocorticoid activity.[156] Daily secretion from the zona glomerulosa, the thin zone of cells on the surface of the adrenal cortex, is approximately 0.1 mg. As noted previously, in large part, the zona glomerulosa functions autonomously of the other two adrenal cortex zones. Most distinctly, control of aldosterone secretion from the zona glomerulosa is largely independent of ACTH control (Fig. 37.19). After secretion from the adrenal cortex, aldosterone circulates 60% bound to serum proteins. It has a relatively short half-life of approximately 20 minutes.[156]

Physiologic control mechanisms of aldosterone secretion are as follows[156]:

1. Increased serum potassium ion concentrations greatly increase aldosterone secretion—potent controller.
2. Increased angiotensin II (activation of the renin-angiotensin system) greatly increases aldosterone secretion—potent controller.
3. Increased serum sodium slightly decreases aldosterone secretion—minor effect.
4. Increased atrial natriuretic peptide (reflecting blood volume expansion) slightly decreases aldosterone secretion.
5. ACTH is necessary for adrenal cortex growth, but it has little effect on controlling aldosterone secretion under most physiologic conditions.

Aldosterone functions. One of the body's most significant protectors of volume status is the renin-angiotensin-aldosterone system. Renin is a proteolytic enzyme released from the juxtaglomerular cells of the kidney afferent arteriole in response to hypovolemia, sympathetic nervous system stimulation, hypotension, or hyponatremia.[158] Renin acts on the plasma protein angiotensinogen to form angiotensin I (a 10–amino acid decapeptide), which is acted on by angiotensin-converting enzyme (primarily in the lung) to form angiotensin II (an 8–amino acid octapeptide). Angiotensin II is an extremely powerful vasoconstrictor and a potent stimulus of aldosterone synthesis in the adrenal cortex.[155]

Aldosterone's primary target cells are called principal cells, located in the kidney distal convoluted tubules and cortical collecting tubules and ducts. Here, aldosterone causes the reabsorption of Na^+ from the tubular fluid in exchange for secretion of K^+ (or H^+) into the tubular fluid for excretion. Aldosterone's effect on the extracellular sodium ion concentration is limited because simultaneous with the Na^+ absorption is absorption of nearly equivalent amounts of water. Sodium and water reabsorption expand the extracellular fluid volume and elevate arterial blood pressure.[156]

Aldosterone's action on sweat glands and salivary glands is like that on renal tubules. The effect on sweat glands is important in hot environments where body salt conservation is needed.[156]

Disorders Associated With the Adrenal Cortex

An excess or deficiency of corticosteroids is associated with distinctive clinical syndromes.

Primary aldosteronism. J.W. Conn described the first case of primary mineralocorticoid excess (now known as Conn syndrome) in 1954, a

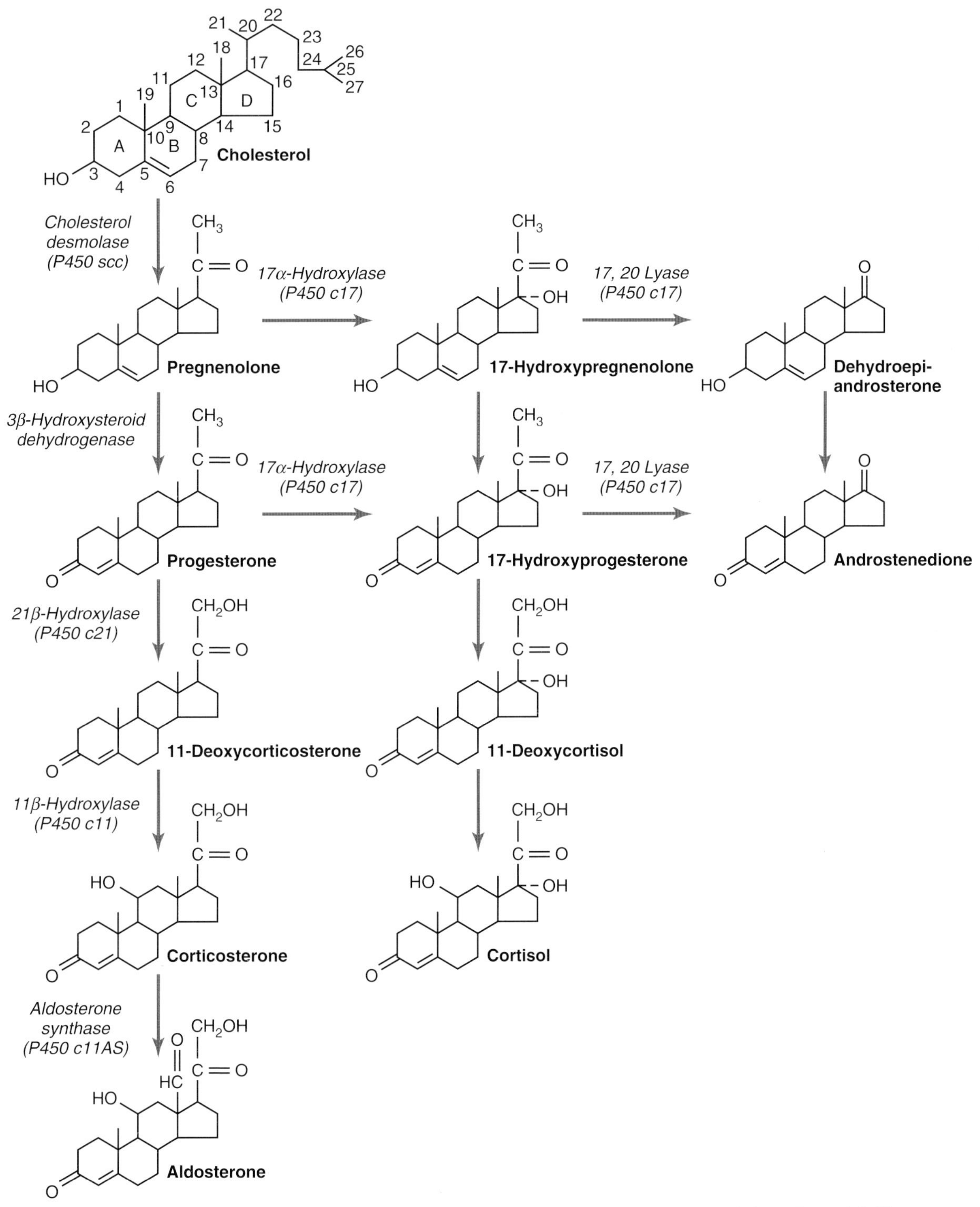

Fig. 37.18 Pathways for adrenal cortex steroidogenesis. The enzymes are shown in italics. (From Hall JE, Hall ME, eds. *Guyton and Hall Textbook of Medical Physiology.* 14th ed. Philadelphia: Elsevier; 2021:957.)

year after the biochemical composition of aldosterone was identified.[161] In most cases, Conn syndrome results from hypersecretion of aldosterone from an adrenal adenoma independent of stimulus. Primary aldosteronism may also be caused by adrenocortical hyperplasia or, rarely, carcinoma.[155] Systemic hypertension with coexisting spontaneous hypokalemia is pathognomonic of hyperaldosteronism.[155]

Manifestations of the syndrome reflect the exaggerated effects of aldosterone. Aldosterone's action of promoting renal excretion of K+ (or H+) in exchange for Na+ reabsorption results in hypokalemic

metabolic alkalosis. Hypertension associated with mineralocorticoid excess results from aldosterone-induced sodium retention and subsequent increase in extracellular fluid volume. Sodium levels tend to be modestly elevated or normal due to concurrent fluid retention.[155,158,162]

Primary aldosteronism is associated with low renin levels, a result of the elevated blood pressure's negative feedback to the juxtaglomerular cells.[155]

Treatment. Treatment of primary hyperaldosteronism involves surgical removal of the hypersecreting adenoma or medical management. Surgical intervention is more successful for primary aldosteronism caused by adrenocortical adenoma than for gland hyperplasia because adenomas are almost always unilateral. Posterior retroperitoneoscopic adrenalectomy or laparoscopic transperitoneal adrenalectomy are advocated as operations of choice for surgically remediable primary hyperaldosteronism.[163] When the affected adrenal gland is removed, the patient is cured in most cases. Medical management includes potassium supplementation and antihypertensive drugs. For patients with adrenal hyperplasia, pharmacologic antagonism of the mineralocorticoid receptor with spironolactone or eplerenone is often successfull.[155]

Management of anesthesia. Preoperative management of the patient with Conn syndrome includes correcting electrolyte imbalance and intravascular fluid volume levels and managing hypertension. Hypokalemia may produce muscle weakness and enhance nondepolarizing muscle relaxant responses, making neuromuscular blockade monitoring especially valuable. ECG signs of potassium depletion include prominent U waves and arrhythmias. Plasma electrolyte concentrations and acid-base status should be checked often during the perioperative period. Inadvertent hyperventilation may further decrease plasma potassium ion concentration.

Hypertension may be controlled preoperatively with sodium restriction and aldosterone antagonists such as spironolactone.[162] Spironolactone, 25 to 100 mg every 8 hours, slowly increases potassium levels by inhibiting the action of aldosterone on the distal convoluted tubule. Patients with primary aldosteronism have a higher incidence of left ventricular hypertrophy, albuminuria, and stroke than patients with essential hypertension.[155] Advanced hemodynamic monitoring of cardiac filling pressures may be needed to assess fluid volume status in the perioperative period.

Glucocorticoid excess (Cushing syndrome). Cushing syndrome is a diverse complex of symptoms, signs, and biochemical abnormalities caused by excess glucocorticoid hormones. Clinical features reflect glucocorticoid excess, either from overproduction of the adrenal cortex or exogenously administered corticosteroids. Understanding the normal physiologic effects of glucocorticoids, mineralocorticoids, and adrenal androgens is important for comprehending the clinical features of Cushing syndrome (Box 37.8).

Many of the abnormalities of Cushing syndrome can be ascribed to abnormal amounts of cortisol. The catabolic effects of excess cortisol

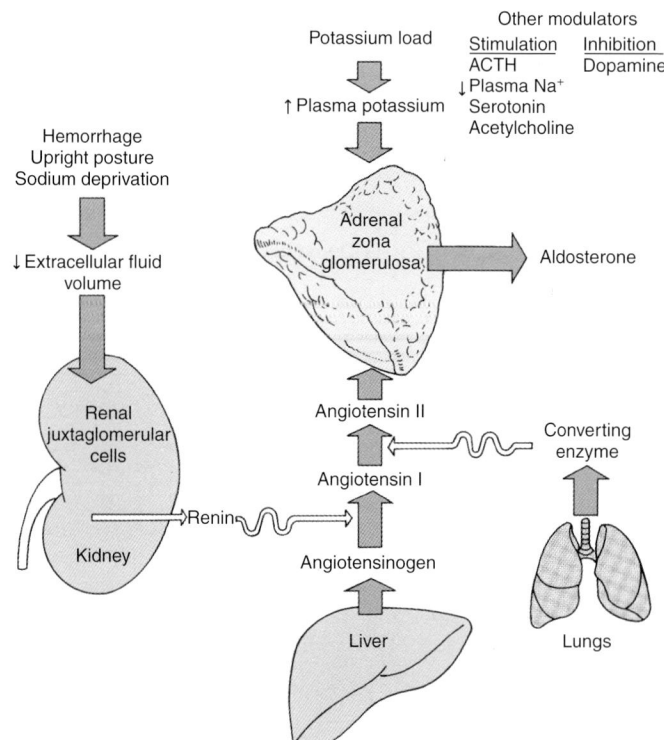

Fig. 37.19 Regulation of aldosterone secretion. Hyperkalemia and activation of the renin-angiotensin system in response to hypovolemia are the predominant stimuli to aldosterone production. Adrenocorticotropin hormone *(ACTH)* has only a minor tonic stimulatory effect. (From Berne RM, et al, eds. *Physiology.* 5th ed. St. Louis: Elsevier; 2004:905.)

result in proximal muscle atrophy and skin that is thin, atrophic, and unable to withstand the stresses of normal activity. The clinical picture of Cushing syndrome includes central obesity with thin extremities, florid complexion, moon facies, purplish skin striae, muscle weakness, and easy bruising.[155,156,164,165] Glucocorticoid-induced osteopenia or osteoporosis affects 50% of patients who are treated with corticosteroids for longer than 12 months.[158] Enhanced gluconeogenesis and decreased glucose utilization by tissues results in glucose intolerance.

BOX 37.8 Clinical Features of Glucocorticoid Excess (Cushing Syndrome)

- Hyperglycemia
- Systemic hypertension
- Weight gain; central obesity; fat pad on back of neck (buffalo hump); moon facies
- Increased susceptibility to infection
- Poor wound healing
- Hypokalemia
- Alkalosis
- Hirsutism; acne; loss of libido; menstrual disturbances
- Osteopenia; osteoporosis
- Skeletal muscle weakness (especially proximal muscle weakness)
- Cataracts
- Skin striae; spontaneous ecchymoses; facial plethora
- Depression; cognitive dysfunction; emotional lability

Overt DM is present in up to one-third of patients with Cushing syndrome.[158] Mineralocorticoid effects may be present (because of supraphysiologic concentrations of cortisol) and include fluid retention and hypokalemic alkalosis. Hypertension is a prominent feature of Cushing syndrome, occurring in up to 75% of cases.[158,165] Women manifest a degree of masculinization (e.g., hirsutism, thinning hair, acne, amenorrhea), and men manifest a degree of feminization (e.g., gynecomastia) due to androgenic effects of glucocorticoid excess.[155,156]

Causes of Cushing syndrome can be ACTH dependent (e.g., pituitary adenoma, ectopic secretion of ACTH by a nonpituitary tumor), ACTH independent (adrenal adenoma, adrenal carcinoma), or iatrogenic (e.g., supraphysiologic doses of administered glucocorticoids).

Cushing disease, first described by Harvey Cushing in 1932, specifically denotes an anterior pituitary tumor cause of the syndrome. The pituitary tumor, most often a microadenoma, produces excessive amounts of ACTH and is associated with bilateral adrenal hyperplasia.[155] Patients often develop skin pigmentation due to the melanocyte receptor stimulating properties of ACTH. The term *Cushing syndrome* is used to describe all causes of glucocorticoid excess, whereas *Cushing disease* is reserved for pituitary-dependent Cushing syndrome.[158]

Overall, the most common cause of Cushing syndrome today is the pharmacologic administration of glucocorticoids for various autoimmune and inflammatory conditions (e.g., asthma, arthritis).[155] Excluding iatrogenic causes, the most common cause of Cushing syndrome is Cushing disease (pituitary overproduction of ACTH), accounting for approximately 70% of cases.[158]

In about 15% of cases, Cushing syndrome is associated with autonomous ACTH secretion from nonpituitary tumors.[158] Tumors that are associated with ectopic ACTH production include lung carcinoma, medullary carcinoma of the thyroid gland, thymic or pancreatic carcinoids, and pheochromocytoma tumors.[155] Small cell lung carcinomas account for most of the cases of ectopic production of ACTH.[158,166]

Cushing syndrome may also be caused by autonomous cortisol production by an adrenal tumor, usually an adenoma, and most often unilateral.[155] This form of hyperadrenalism is associated with suppressed plasma ACTH levels due to cortisol feedback inhibition.[155-157] Adrenal tumors that are malignant are not common and are usually large by the time Cushing syndrome becomes manifest.

Diagnosis. There are several tests used to diagnose Cushing syndrome. A widely used initial test is the low-dose overnight dexamethasone suppression test, which measures plasma cortisol concentration in the morning after a 1-mg dose of dexamethasone.[158] Dexamethasone suppresses CRH, ACTH, and plasma cortisol secretion

in normal subjects but not in those with Cushing disease. Diagnosis of Cushing syndrome may also be based on salivary cortisol levels, urinary free cortisol excretion, and plasma ACTH.[155,167] Imaging studies of the adrenal glands and pituitary gland are performed in concert with biochemical evaluation.

Treatment. Treatment for Cushing syndrome depends on the cause.[168-170] For Cushing disease, selective removal of the pituitary corticotrope tumor (microadenomectomy), usually by a transsphenoidal approach, is the primary treatment option. Complications depend on the tumor size and therefore the extent of tissue removal and include hypopituitarism, transient DI, cranial nerve injury, and cerebrospinal fluid rhinorrhea.[158]

Management of Cushing syndrome caused by an adrenal tumor consists of surgical removal. A laparoscopic approach is the surgical treatment of choice for unilateral adrenal adenomas. Adrenalectomy for unilateral adrenocortical adenoma has a cure rate of 100%.[158,168,171] For larger tumors or those suspected of malignancy, an open laparotomy may be preferred.[155]

Plasma cortisol levels decline promptly with pituitary or adrenal tumor resection, therefore a continuous infusion of cortisol (hydrocortisone, 100–200 mg intravenously over 24 hours) is usually initiated intraoperatively and titrated postresection. Because the contralateral adrenal gland is preoperatively suppressed, glucocorticoid replacement may be necessary for several months after unilateral adrenalectomy until adrenal function returns.[155,158]

The treatment of choice for ectopic ACTH-secreting tumors is surgical removal, but this may not always be feasible because of the nature of the underlying process (e.g., metastatic carcinoma). If the tumor proves unresectable, ketoconazole, an antifungal drug that blocks the early stages of steroid synthesis, or metyrapone, an 11β-hydroxylase inhibitor, may be used to help lower cortisol levels. Mitotane, an agent that blocks steroidogenesis at several levels, is used to treat cancer of the adrenal gland that cannot be treated with surgery.[155,158,168-170]

Management of anesthesia. Important perioperative considerations for the patient with Cushing syndrome include normalizing blood pressure, plasma glucose levels, intravascular fluid volume, and electrolyte concentrations. The aldosterone antagonist spironolactone may be used to minimize extracellular fluid volume and correct hypokalemia.

Osteopenia is an important consideration in positioning the patient for the operative procedure. Pathologic fractures, even after minor trauma, are not uncommon.[158] Osteoporotic vertebral joints may render central neuraxial anesthesia more difficult. Special attention must be given to the patient's skin, which can easily be abraded and bruised by tape or minor trauma. NSAIDs should be used with caution due to the risk of peptic ulceration. Glucocorticoids are lympholytic and immunosuppressive, placing the patient at increased risk for infection and mandating enforcement of aseptic techniques when indicated.[155]

Obstructive sleep apnea is common in patients with Cushing syndrome, and the characteristic buffalo hump may complicate airway management by making supine positioning more difficult. The choice of drugs for induction and maintenance of anesthesia is not specifically influenced by the presence of hyperadrenocorticism. As a suppressor of cortisol synthesis, etomidate may transiently decrease plasma cortisol levels. Muscle relaxants may have a more exaggerated effect in patients with hypokalemia and preexisting myopathy, and a conservative approach to dosing is warranted when significant skeletal muscle weakness is present.

Thromboembolic phenomena occur more often in patients with Cushing syndrome, with an 11% incidence of deep venous thrombosis and a 2% to 3% incidence of pulmonary embolus postoperatively. The thromboembolic events are believed to be secondary to the prevalence of obesity, hypertension, elevated hematocrit, and increased factor VIII levels in these patients.[172]

Primary adrenocortical insufficiency (Addison disease). In 1855, the English physician Thomas Addison first described a relatively rare clinical syndrome characterized by wasting and skin hyperpigmentation and identified its cause as destruction of the adrenal glands. Primary adrenocortical insufficiency (Addison disease) becomes apparent when 90% of the gland is destroyed. Infectious diseases, including tuberculosis, acquired immunodeficiency syndrome, and fungal infections, are the most common causes of primary adrenocortical insufficiency worldwide.[173] In the Western world, most cases of primary adrenocortical insufficiency are the result of autoimmune destruction of the gland; 50% of these patients have an associated autoimmune disease, thyroid disease being the most common.[158] Less commonly, primary adrenal insufficiency is congenital or caused by adrenal hemorrhage, malignancy, or trauma.[155,173]

Clinical features of primary adrenocortical insufficiency reflect destruction of all cortical zones, resulting in adrenal androgen, glucocorticoid, and mineralocorticoid hormone deficiency.[158,173,174] The physiologic consequences of cortisol deficiency are extensive (Table 37.10). Weakness and fatigue are cardinal features. Reduced appetite with weight loss, vomiting, abdominal pain, and diarrhea are frequently reported. Hypoglycemia is often present.[174] Mineralocorticoid deficiency is manifested by hypovolemia, hypotension, hyponatremia, and hyperkalemia. Loss of glucocorticoid-mediated support of catecholamines compounds the low blood pressure. Azotemia and mild anemia are commonly revealed by laboratory screening.[156,174]

The adrenal-pituitary axis is intact in primary adrenal insufficiency, and ACTH concentrations are elevated because of the reduced production of cortisol. Increased melanin formation in the skin and hyperpigmentation of the knuckles of the fingers and toes, knees, elbows, and buccal mucosa are distinguishing features reflecting increased ACTH.

Treatment. Treatment for primary adrenal insufficiency aims to replace both glucocorticoid (antiinflammatory) and mineralocorticoid (salt retention) deficiency.[155,158,174] Table 37.11 outlines common steroid preparations and their glucocorticoid and mineralocorticoid potency. Replacement therapy typically includes hydrocortisone 15 to 20 mg on awakening and 5 to 10 mg in early afternoon. In primary adrenal failure, mineralocorticoid replacement is usually also required in the form of fludrocortisone.[158]

Patients with Addison disease are highly susceptible to the deteriorating effects of stress and may require supplementation of standard replacement dosages under stressful conditions.[156,158,174] (see Perioperative Steroid Replacement, later). Preparation of the surgical patient with a history of primary adrenal insufficiency should include correction of hypovolemia, hyperkalemia, and hyponatremia. Assiduous hemodynamic monitoring for manifestation of adrenal insufficiency should continue throughout the perioperative period (see Acute Adrenal Crisis, later). No specific anesthetic techniques are required when anesthetizing patients at risk for primary adrenal insufficiency, but the anesthetist should be mindful of the adrenal suppressive effects of the hypnotic etomidate. Etomidate blocks steroidogenesis by inhibiting the enzyme 11β-hydroxylase and P450 side-chain cleavage, inhibiting synthesis of cortisol and aldosterone.[175] Even a single dose of etomidate for induction of anesthesia can transiently decrease cortisol synthesis. Its administration should be avoided in patients susceptible to or with a diagnosis of adrenal insufficiency.[175-179]

Secondary adrenocortical insufficiency. Secondary adrenocortical insufficiency is caused by ACTH deficiency from two primary etiologies: (1) iatrogenic HPA axis suppression after exogenous glucocorticoid therapy, or (2) ACTH deficiency secondary to hypothalamic or pituitary gland dysfunction (e.g., tumor, infection, surgical or radiologic ablation). The most common cause of ACTH deficiency is suppression of hormone synthesis by the administration of exogenous steroids. Pharmacologic doses of steroids suppress secretion of ACTH, which leads to adrenal cortex atrophy and deficient adrenal cortex hormone production.

Up to 1% of the Western population is taking long-term glucocorticoid therapy.[158] In these patients, iatrogenic suppression of the HPA axis may occur, producing secondary adrenal cortical insufficiency.[158,174,180] HPA axis suppression by exogenous glucocorticoid has been described with topical, ocular, rectal, inhaled, and systemic therapy.[174,180-183] The longer the duration of treatment and the more potent the pharmacologic glucocorticoid, the greater the likelihood of HPA axis suppression. HPA axis suppression and adrenal atrophy may persist for several months to a year after cessation of therapy.[158,179]

Patients with HPA axis suppression may develop acute adrenal insufficiency during periods of stress (critical illness, surgery; see later). Interindividual variability to glucocorticoids is considerable, and there is no absolute dose, duration of treatment, or time since steroid withdrawal that will accurately predict adrenal suppression. The ACTH suppression test is a reliable predictor of HPA axis suppression, but it is often not available for review preoperatively. In general, sustained and clinically important adrenal suppression does not occur

TABLE 37.10 Clinical Features of Primary Adrenal Insufficiency

Feature	Frequency (%)
Symptoms	
Weakness, tiredness, fatigue	100
Anorexia	100
Gastrointestinal symptoms	92
Nausea	86
Vomiting	75
Constipation	33
Abdominal pain	31
Diarrhea	16
Salt craving	16
Postural dizziness	12
Muscle and joint pains	13
Signs	
Weight loss	100
Hyperpigmentation	94
Hypotension (<110 mm Hg systolic)	88–94
Vitiligo	10–20
Auricular calcification	5
Laboratory Findings	
Electrolyte disturbances	92
Hyponatremia	88
Hyperkalemia	64
Hypercalcemia	6
Azotemia	55
Anemia	40
Eosinophilia	17

From Newell-Price JDC, Auchus RJ. The adrenal cortex. In: Melmed S, Auchus RJ, Goldfine AB, et al., eds. *Williams Textbook of Endocrinology.* 14th ed. Philadelphia: Elsevier; 2020: 480–541.

TABLE 37.11 Steroid Preparations

Steroid	Glucocorticoid Potency (Antiinflammatory)*	Mineralocorticoid Potency (Salt Retention)	Approximate Equivalent Glucocorticoid Dose
Glucocorticoids			
Short Acting			
Cortisol (hydrocortisone)	1.0	1.0	20 mg
Cortisone	0.8	0.8	25 mg
Intermediate Acting			
Prednisone	4.0	0.25	5 mg
Prednisolone	4.0	0.25	5 mg
Methylprednisolone	5.0	0	4 mg
Triamcinolone	5.0	0	4 mg
Long Acting			
Dexamethasone	30	0	0.75 mg
Mineralocorticoids			
Fludrocortisone	12	125	

*Glucocorticoid and mineralocorticoid potencies are relative to cortisol, with cortisol being 1.0. When given at replacement doses, triamcinolone and dexamethasone have no clinically important mineralocorticoid activity.
Fludrocortisone is not used for antiinflammatory effect.
Wall RT. Endocrine disease. In: Hines RL, Marschall KE, eds. *Anesthesia and Co-Existing Disease.* 7th ed. Philadelphia: Elsevier; 2018:449–475.

with prednisone treatment of 5 mg/day or less.[179] Treatment periods long enough to provoke signs of Cushing syndrome are usually associated with adrenal suppression of clinical importance.[158,179,183,184]

Clinical manifestations of secondary adrenal insufficiency resemble the primary disease, except secondary insufficiency is less likely to be associated with severe hyperkalemia or hyponatremia because the renin-angiotensin-aldosterone system is intact, and mineralocorticoid secretion is usually preserved.[158] Hyperpigmentation is absent because ACTH levels are low.

Acute adrenal crisis (Addisonian crisis). Adrenal crisis is a life-threatening exacerbation or onset of severe adrenal insufficiency with an absolute or relative deficiency of cortisol. It is associated with high morbidity and mortality if allowed to progress unrecognized.[184-187] A patient with chronic adrenal insufficiency may deteriorate rapidly into an acute crisis state because of superimposed stress, such as infection, gastroenteritis, acute illness, emotional stress, or sepsis.[184-186] The stress of surgery or trauma in the patient with inadequate adrenal reserves can precipitate acute adrenal crisis in the perioperative period.[179,183,184,186]

Symptoms of adrenal crisis reflect acute deficiency of corticosteroids and include profound weakness, nausea, severe hypotension (systolic blood pressure <100 mm Hg), fever, marked acute abdominal pain (suggestive of early peritonitis), hyponatremia/hyperkalemia, and decreasing mental status.[173,184-186] In the surgical setting, adrenal crisis is manifest as hemodynamic instability or cardiovascular collapse. The index of suspicion for adrenal crisis should be particularly high in a patient with a history of Addison disease, exogenous steroid administration, progressive hyperkalemia, or hyponatremia.[174] Box 37.9 outlines clinical and laboratory features of adrenal crisis.

Acute adrenal crisis is a medical emergency requiring aggressive treatment of the steroid insufficiency and associated hypoglycemia, electrolyte imbalance, and volume depletion. Early recognition, urgent review by endocrinology specialists, and immediate interventions are crucial steps in altering the course of acute adrenal insufficiency.[185,186] Serum cortisol and ACTH levels should be sought, but treatment should not wait for assay results.[186] Volume deficits may be substantial

BOX 37.9 Clinical and Laboratory Features of Adrenal (Addisonian) Crisis

- Dehydration; hypotension or shock
- Nausea and vomiting; weight loss; anorexia
- Severe fatigue and weakness
- Abdominal pain (acute abdomen)
- Hypoglycemia
- Fever
- Hyponatremia, hyperkalemia (in primary adrenal disease), hypercalcemia
- Prerenal azotemia
- Hyperpigmentation (in primary adrenal disease)
- Delirium, obtundation, coma

From Newell-Price JDC, Auchus RJ. The adrenal cortex. In: Melmed S, Auchus RJ, Goldfine AB, et al., eds. *Williams Textbook of Endocrinology.* 14th ed. Philadelphia: Elsevier; 2020:480–541.

(2–3 L), and initial therapy begins with rapid intravenous administration of an isotonic sodium chloride solution (1000 mL in the first hour) with additional fluids guided by continuous cardiac monitoring.[184-186] Patients with hypoglycemia will require intravenous dextrose supplementation. Steroid replacement therapy typically begins with hydrocortisone, 100 mg bolus intravenously, followed by hydrocortisone, 200 mg as a continuous intravenous infusion over 24 hours.[184,185] Hydrocortisone (cortisol) is the preferred drug for treatment of an adrenal crisis as it provides balanced glucocorticoid-mineralocorticoid effects.[184-186] With treatment, clinical recovery within 24 hours is common. After the first day, steroid doses are reduced by 50% per day if the patient is stable.[184-186]

Perioperative steroid replacement. Case reports of perioperative cardiovascular collapse in surgical patients on pharmacologic doses of glucocorticoids were first reported in 1952.[187] These reports and subsequent knowledge regarding the stress response associated with surgery and suppression of the HPA axis with supraphysiologic doses of corticosteroids has led to the practice of administering perioperative glucocorticoids (stress doses) to patients who have taken steroids in the preoperative period.

Synthesis and secretion of cortisol can increase severalfold under conditions of severe stress, such as surgery, trauma, or infection. Major surgery of long duration produces a greater adrenal output response than minor surgery of short duration. For the adult patient who has received supraphysiologic doses of glucocorticoids, it may take up to 12 months from the time of discontinuation of steroids for the adrenal gland to recover full function.[188-191]

Debate exists regarding who should receive perioperative steroid coverage and what the appropriate steroid dose should be.[158,179,180,188-190,192] Some authors recommend that patients on therapeutic doses of corticosteroids undergoing surgery receive only their usual daily dose of glucocorticoid perioperatively. These recommendations are based on studies showing that glucocorticoid-induced adrenal insufficiency is uncommon and that surgical patients treated with their usual steroid dose do not routinely develop hypotension or any other perioperative signs of adrenal insufficiency.[183,184,190,191]

Other experts advise that surgical patients on chronic glucocorticoids may not be able to mount a sufficient increase in endogenous cortisol in the perioperative period, are at risk for acute adrenal insufficiency, and therefore require steroid supplementation. Many clinicians believe that because acute adrenal crisis is life threatening, even a small risk of adrenal insufficiency warrants supplemental steroid treatment. Based on this caveat, some experts assume that any patient who has taken steroids in the year preceding surgery is at risk for suppressed HPA function and requires perioperative supplementation.[192] Other experts consider the following conditions a requirement for stress dose coverage[179]:

1. The patient has taken pharmacologic doses of prednisone >20 mg/day (or its equivalent).
2. The period of treatment was for ≥3 weeks.
3. The treatment occurred during the immediate 12 months before surgery.

Under these conditions, supplemental intravenous administration of hydrocortisone may be needed to compensate for steroid the body is unable to produce in response to stress.

The precise amount of glucocorticoids required for adequate supplementation has not been established. Therapeutic aims are to tailor the steroid dose considering the patient's history and the length and severity of surgical stress, while administering the minimal dose that will fully protect the patient.[158,192] Guidelines for perioperative steroid supplementation are included in Table 37.12.

There is little risk of providing steroid coverage of hydrocortisone (100 mg/day) in the immediate perioperative period.[192] However, any benefits of perioperative steroid supplementation must be tempered by the potential negative effects of decreased glucose tolerance, fluid retention, immunosuppression, and impaired wound healing associated with steroids.

Adrenal Medulla

The adrenal medulla is a catecholamine-producing endocrine gland that is derived embryologically from neuroectodermal cells. Cells of the adrenal medulla are called chromaffin cells. Some chromaffin cells called paraganglia cluster outside of the adrenal medulla on either side of the aorta. The largest paraganglia is the organ of Zuckerkandl, which is a major source of catecholamines during the first year of life.[193,194]

The adrenal medulla is enervated by preganglionic cholinergic fibers of the sympathetic nervous system. Preganglionic fibers bypass the paravertebral ganglia and run directly from the spinal cord to the adrenal medulla. Catecholamine secretion from the adrenal medulla is stimulated by stress (e.g., anesthesia, surgery, hypoglycemia).

TABLE 37.12 **Guidelines for Perioperative Adrenal Supplementation Therapy**	
Type of Surgery Stress	**Additional Hydrocortisone Dose**
Superficial Surgery Dental Biopsies	None
Minor Surgery Inguinal hernia Colonoscopy	25 mg IV before induction of anesthesia
Moderate Surgery Colon resection Total abdominal hysterectomy Total joint replacement	50–75 mg IV before induction of anesthesia; taper by 50% per day, over 1–2 days
Major Surgery Cardiac Thoracic Liver	100–150 mg IV before induction of anesthesia; taper according to patient's postop condition

Additional Hydrocortisone Dose, Supplemental doses are administered in addition to the patient's daily maintenance dose if the surgical patient is undergoing treatment with glucocorticoids at the time of surgery; *IV,* intravenous.
Modified from Wall RT. Endocrine disease. In: Hines RL, Marschall KE, eds. *Anesthesia and Co-Existing Disease.* 7th ed. Philadelphia: Elsevier; 2018:449–475.

Epinephrine accounts for approximately 80% of the hormone secreted by the adrenal medulla, and norepinephrine accounts for 20%.[193] Norepinephrine is converted to epinephrine in the adrenal medulla by the enzyme phenylethanolamine-N-methyltransferase (PNMT). The ability of the adrenal medulla to synthesize epinephrine is probably influenced by the flow of glucocorticoid-rich blood from the adrenal cortex through the medulla. Fig. 37.20 outlines the biosynthetic pathway for catecholamines.

Catecholamines in the adrenal medulla are stored in chromaffin granules. Stimulation of the sympathetic nerves to the adrenal medulla causes large quantities of epinephrine and norepinephrine to be released into circulation, affecting many cardiovascular and metabolic processes. Catecholamines are short-lived signaling molecules and are removed from circulation by metabolism through two enzyme pathways. The enzyme catechol-O-methyltransferase (COMT) converts epinephrine to metanephrine and norepinephrine to normetanephrine. Metanephrine and normetanephrine are then oxidized to vanillylmandelic acid (VMA) by the enzyme monoamine oxidase (MAO). The byproducts of metabolism, VMA, normetanephrine, metanephrine, and free unchanged catecholamines are excreted in the urine.[193] Fig. 37.21 outlines major pathways of epinephrine, norepinephrine, and dopamine metabolism.

Norepinephrine stimulates α- and β-adrenergic receptors. It causes constriction of most blood vessels of the body and increases blood pressure through α_1-receptor stimulation. High circulating norepinephrine levels increase cardiac activity, inhibit gastrointestinal function, and dilate the pupils. Epinephrine has greater affinity for β-adrenergic receptors. Its actions are seen primarily in the heart, producing positive chronotropic and inotropic effects. Epinephrine causes less constriction of blood vessels than norepinephrine, and in fact it causes some vasodilation, mediated through its action on β_2-adrenergic receptors primarily in skeletal muscle vasculature. Norepinephrine and epinephrine

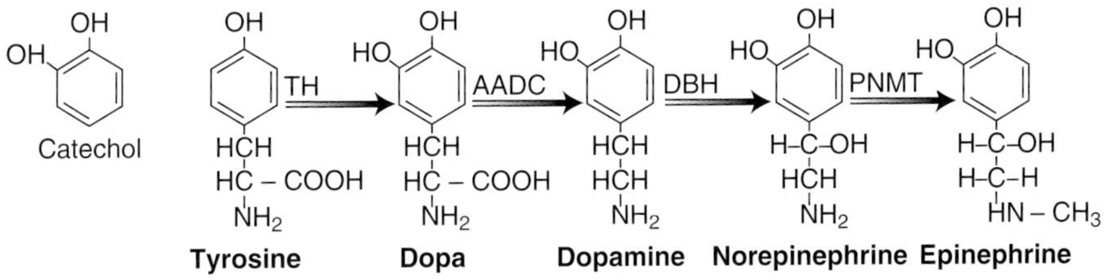

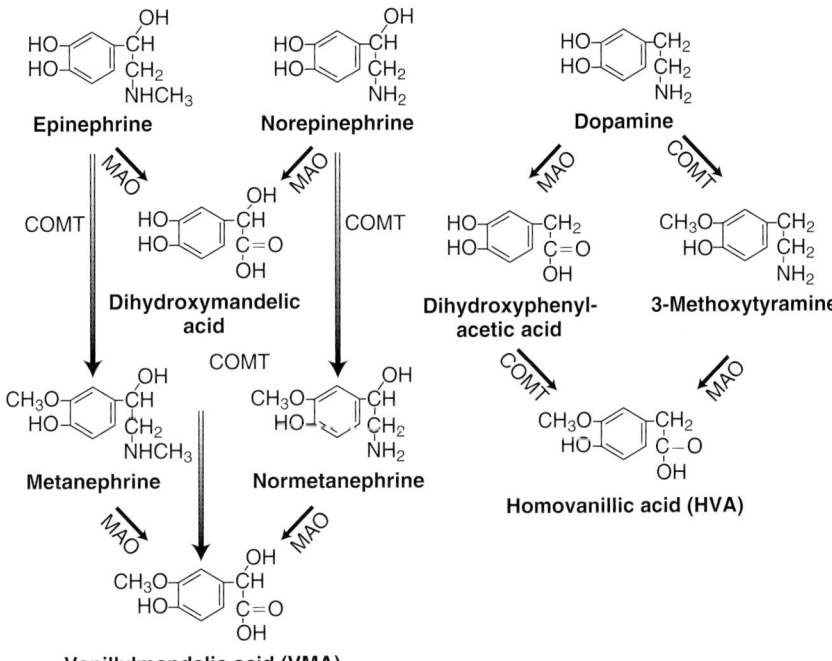

Fig. 37.20 Biosynthetic pathway for catecholamines. The term *catecholamines* comes from the catechol (ortho-dihydroxybenzene) structure and a side chain with an amino group—the "catechol nucleus" *(left)*. Tyrosine is converted to 3,4-dihydroxyphenylalanine (dopa) (rate-limiting step) by tyrosine hydroxylase *(TH)*; TH inhibitor, α-methyl-para-tyrosine (metyrosine). Aromatic L-amino acid decarboxylase *(AADC)* converts dopa to dopamine. Dopamine is hydroxylated to norepinephrine by dopamine β-hydroxylase *(DBH)*. Norepinephrine is converted to epinephrine by phenylethanolamine *N*-methyltransferase *(PNMT)*; cortisol serves as a cofactor for PNMT, which is why epinephrine-secreting pheochromocytomas are almost exclusively localized to the adrenal medulla. (From Melmed S, et al., eds. *Williams Textbook of Endocrinology.* 13th ed. Philadelphia: Elsevier; 2016:557.)

Fig. 37.21 Catecholamine metabolism. Metabolism of catecholamines occurs through two enzymatic pathways. Catechol-*O*-methyltransferase *(COMT)* converts epinephrine to metanephrine and converts norepinephrine to normetanephrine by meta-*O*-methylation. Metanephrine and normetanephrine are oxidized by monoamine oxidase *(MAO)* to vanillylmandelic acid (VMA) by oxidative deamination. MAO also may oxidize epinephrine and norepinephrine to dihydroxymandelic acid, which is then converted by COMT to VMA. Dopamine is also metabolized by MAO and COMT to the final metabolite homovanillic acid (HVA). (Modified and redrawn from Young WF. Endocrine hypertension. In: Melmed S, et al., eds. *Williams Textbook of Endocrinology.* 13th ed. Philadelphia: Elsevier; 2016:559.)

release from the adrenal medulla can increase the metabolic rate of the body by as much as 100% above normal.[193,194]

Pheochromocytoma

In 1905, the term *pheochromocytoma* was first used to describe the appearance of a tumor (cytoma) noted during autopsy resection to be a dusky (pheo) color (chromo) upon staining. Cesar Roux of Lausanne, Switzerland, and Charles Mayo of the United States were the first surgeons to successfully remove a pheochromocytoma.[194]

Pheochromocytomas are catecholamine-secreting tumors derived from chromaffin cells in the adrenal medulla. Approximately 85% of these tumors are found in the adrenal glands, and 95% are found in the abdomen and pelvis.[194] Extraadrenal catecholamine-secreting tumors

are called paragangliomas. Paragangliomas are found where there is chromaffin tissue along the paraaortic sympathetic chain, within the organ of Zuckerkandl near the aortic bifurcation and, less commonly, in the wall of the bladder or in the mediastinum.[194]

Most pheochromocytomas secrete both norepinephrine and epinephrine (and, less frequently, dopamine), but norepinephrine typically represents a higher fraction of the secreted catecholamines, compared to a normal gland.[195,196] In the majority of cases, it is impossible to predict the precise catecholamine secretion from clinical features alone.

Pheochromocytomas loosely adhere to what is known as the rule of 10. They involve both adrenal glands in approximately 10% of adult patients with the tumor, about 10% of the tumors are extraadrenal (paragangliomas), and at least 10% of the tumors are malignant.[197]

Biochemical testing and subsequent diagnosis of a catecholamine-secreting tumor includes elevated catecholamine and fractionated metanephrine levels in blood and urine.[198,199] CT or magnetic resonance imaging (MRI) of the abdomen and pelvis are the primary imaging modalities used for localization.[197]

Incidence and associated diseases. Pheochromocytomas are rare, occurring with an annual incidence of 0.6 cases per 100,000 people per year.[200] About 40% of patients with a pheochromocytoma have an inherited syndrome.[194] Major inherited syndromes that have been linked to pheochromocytoma include neurofibromatosis 1 (NF-1), previously known as von Recklinghausen disease, von Hippel–Lindau syndrome, and MEN-2A and MEN-2B.[194,201,202] Approximately 50% of patients with MEN-2A or -2B develop pheochromocytomas, and these tumors secrete predominantly epinephrine[194] (Table 37.13). It is recommended that patients with a family history of MEN syndrome be regularly screened for pheochromocytoma.

Pheochromocytomas can occur at any age, but usually occur within the third, fourth, or fifth decades of life, with equal frequency in both sexes in adults.[194]

Clinical manifestations. Signs and symptoms of a pheochromocytoma reflect the type of catecholamine released (predominately norepinephrine or epinephrine) and the amount of catecholamine secretion (activity of the tumor).[197] Manifestations vary in their intensity and may occur continuously or as paroxysms. Approximately 50% of intraadrenal pheochromocytomas are discovered as part of incidental radiographic findings or surgery performed for other reasons.[203,204]

Although less than 0.1% of hypertensive patients harbor a pheochromocytoma, the combination of diaphoresis, tachycardia, and headache in a hypertensive patient is a recognized and sensitive triad of symptoms for pheochromocytoma.[197,200,202] A catecholamine-mediated paroxysm or spell typically consists of a sudden and alarming increase in blood pressure, a severe throbbing headache, profuse sweating, a forceful heartbeat, tachycardia, anxiety, pallor, and nausea.[197,200,205] These hyperadrenergic spells are often followed by physical exhaustion. Clinical manifestations associated with pheochromocytoma are outlined in Box 37.10.

The typical duration of a pheochromocytoma spell is less than an hour, but it is variable.[197] Sustained hypertension between paroxysms occurs in 50% to 60% of patients.[206] The trigger for catecholamine release is unclear, and multiple mechanisms have been postulated.[194,197] The paroxysm may be spontaneous or triggered by abdominal pressure, exercise, surgery, change in posture, or lifting. Micturition may trigger symptoms if the pheochromocytoma is present in the urinary bladder

wall.[197] Various medications (e.g., tricyclic antidepressants, morphine, metoclopramide) can enhance the effects of paroxysms.[197] Mental or psychologic stress does not usually initiate a crisis.

Hyperglycemia may be present because of inhibition of insulin (α1 mediated) and enhanced hepatic glucose output. An overall increase in metabolism accelerates oxygen consumption. The cardiac output and heart rate may be significantly increased.

Owing to the usual predominance of norepinephrine secretion, the symptoms associated with many pheochromocytomas reflect primarily α-adrenergic activity. Vasoconstriction in the extremities may produce pain, paresthesias, intermittent claudication, or ischemia. Hypertension with a contracted blood volume is a distinctive manifestation of the disease; it is the result of norepinephrine causing arteriolar and venous constriction. As mentioned, the hypertension may be paroxysmal or sustained, and it is often severe.[196,197,206] Sustained hypertension is often resistant to conventional treatment. When pheochromocytomas are predominantly epinephrine or dopamine secreting, hypertension can alternate with periods of hypotension associated with syncope, particularly in the presence of a contracted vascular space.[207]

The catecholamine crises produced by a pheochromocytoma can lead to heart failure, pulmonary edema, arrhythmias, and intracranial hemorrhage.[197,208] ECG changes are common. Nonspecific ST segment and T-wave changes may be seen. The catecholamine storm induces sinus tachycardia, supraventricular tachycardia, and premature ventricular contractions. Ventricular tachycardia and sinus node arrest have been reported.[208]

Some pheochromocytomas may first present as a hypermetabolic state during anesthesia for unrelated surgery.[204,209-211] The hypertension, tachycardia, and hyperthermia of a pheochromocytoma spell may mimic light anesthesia, thyroid crisis, malignant hyperthermia, or sepsis.[205,210]

Surgery and preoperative management. The treatment of choice for pheochromocytoma is complete surgical resection. Most tumors can be completely excised, and hypertension cured.[194,212,213] The most common complications associated with surgical resection are intraoperative hypertension, blood pressure lability, and postresection hypotension.[194]

The effects of circulating catecholamines present major anesthetic challenges. Long-standing, uncontrolled catecholamine release can have serious and potentially lethal cardiovascular complications, such as severe dilated cardiomyopathy (catecholamine-induced cardiomyopathy), heart failure, and diastolic and systolic dysfunction.[214] A

TABLE 37.13 Manifestations of Multiple Endocrine Neoplasia*

Syndrome	Manifestations
MEN type 1 (Werner syndrome)	Hyperparathyroidism, pituitary adenomas, pancreatic islet cell tumors
MEN type 2A (Sipple syndrome)	Medullary thyroid cancer, primary hyperparathyroidism, pheochromocytoma, pigmented skin lesions (lichen amyloidosis)
MEN type 2B (Gorlin syndrome or mucosal neuroma syndrome)	Medullary thyroid cancer, pheochromocytoma, mucocutaneous neuromas (typically involving the tongue, lips, and eyelids), skeletal deformities (e.g., kyphoscoliosis, lordosis), intestinal ganglioneuromas

*Multiple endocrine neoplasia (MEN) is a group of rare diseases caused by genetic defects that lead to hyperplasia and hyperfunction of various components of the endocrine system.

BOX 37.10 Clinical Manifestations of Pheochromocytoma Listed by Frequency of Occurrence

1. Headaches
2. Profuse sweating
3. Palpitations and tachycardia
4. Hypertension, sustained or paroxysmal
5. Anxiety
6. Pallor
7. Nausea
8. Abdominal pain
9. Weakness
10. Weight loss
11. Paradoxic response to antihypertensive drugs
12. Polyuria and polydipsia
13. Constipation
14. Orthostatic hypotension
15. Dilated cardiomyopathy
16. Erythrocytosis
17. Elevated blood sugar

From Neumann HH. Pheochromocytoma. In: Jameson J, Fauci AS, Kasper DL, et al., eds. *Harrison's Principles of Internal Medicine*. 20th ed. New York: McGraw-Hill; 2018.

thorough cardiovascular examination is required, including ECG and echocardiography. Careful preoperative pharmacologic management is indicated for all surgical patients, even in those who are asymptomatic and normotensive.[209,215] Preoperative treatment aims to reverse the effects of excessive adrenergic stimulation. Antihypertensive therapy in concert with expansion of the intravascular fluid compartment before surgery greatly improves cardiovascular stability and has helped to decrease the surgical mortality rate for elective procedures from approximately 50% to the current rate close to 0% to 6%.[192,212,216] Combined α- and β-adrenergic blockade is a commonly used preoperative management approach to control blood pressure and heart rate and prevent intraoperative hypertensive crisis.[194,206,216] Table 37.14 outlines some of the drugs used in the preoperative management of pheochromocytoma.

α-adrenergic receptor blockade. Phenoxybenzamine is a frequently utilized drug for preoperative α-adrenergic blockade and blood pressure stabilization.[192,194,195,217,218] It is a nonspecific presynaptic (α_2) and postsynaptic (α_1) adrenergic receptor antagonist of long duration (24–48 hours). The initial oral dose is 10 to 30 mg/70 kg daily, and the dose is increased every 2 to 3 days as needed to control blood pressure and hypertensive spells preoperatively. Establishing normotension facilitates expansion of the intravascular fluid compartment.[214] Most adult patients with pheochromocytoma require an eventual oral dose between 60 and 250 mg/day.[192] Due to the long duration of phenoxybenzamine and a concern regarding hypotension after tumor resection, some practitioners discontinue the drug 12 to 24 hours before surgery or administer one-half to two-thirds of the normal oral dose on the morning of surgery.[214] Most patients require 7 to 10 days of α-adrenergic antagonist therapy to stabilize blood pressure and decrease symptoms.

Selective α_1-adrenergic receptor antagonists (doxazosin, terazosin) have also been used effectively for preoperative control of hypertension.[194,201,216] The appeal of selective α_1-receptor antagonists is that, in theory, they leave the α_2-receptor intact, thereby inhibiting the release of norepinephrine, allowing more effective management of blood pressure and heart rate, and resulting in less postresection hypotension.[201,206,216-219]

Labetalol, a mixed α- and β-receptor antagonist, is much less potent as an α-blocker than β-blocker. It has not been as effective as a first-line

drug in controlling the blood pressure response, but it may be used as an adjunctive agent.[220]

β-adrenergic receptor blockade. A β-adrenergic receptor antagonist is often introduced before surgery to control tachycardia, hypertension, and cardiac dysrhythmias. Caution must be exercised for the patient with a history of asthma, heart failure, and catecholamine-induced cardiomyopathy.[194] An additional important caveat is that β-adrenergic receptor antagonists should not be administered until after α-adrenergic blockade is established. Blocking β_2-receptor–mediated vasodilation without prior α-adrenergic blockade can increase the blood pressure even further in the patient with pheochromocytoma.[194,196,205,220] A helpful mnemonic for the reader is "a before b."

Other treatment regimens. Other strategies for preoperative blood pressure management include calcium channel blockers, clonidine, and magnesium sulfate. Calcium channel blockers have been used with variable success as monotherapy for the preoperative management of pheochromocytoma. Nicardipine is a commonly used calcium channel blocker in this setting.[194] In addition to their peripheral vasodilating effects, calcium antagonists also inhibit calcium-dependent norepinephrine release from the tumor. Some centers successfully use these agents alone or in conjunction with other vasodilating drugs.[221,222]

Roizen et al. in 1982 proposed objective end points of preoperative treatment for pheochromocytoma resection (often called the Roizen criteria):

- Normotension (no in-hospital blood pressure >160/90 for 24 hours before surgery)
- Orthostatic hypotension is acceptable as long as blood pressure is not <80/45 with standing
- No more than five premature ventricular contractions per minute
- No ST segment or T-wave abnormality on the ECG for 1 week prior to surgery[223,224]

Anesthetic management. Pheochromocytomas are excised by open laparotomy or minimally invasive adrenalectomy (laparoscopic, retroperitoneoscopic, robotic-assisted approaches) surgical techniques.[201,214,225-228] The minimally invasive surgical technique is considered the procedure of choice for resection of solitary intraadrenal tumors smaller than 6 to 8 cm diameter.[201,216] It is associated with better perioperative outcomes,

TABLE 37.14 Drugs Used for Preoperative Management of Pheochromocytoma

Drug	Action	Preoperative Blood Pressure Control	Comments
Phenoxybenzamine	Nonselective α-blocker	Initial oral (PO) dose 10–30 mg/day, daily dosage increased by 30 mg as needed	Long half-life; may accumulate; S/E postural hypotension, nasal congestion, diarrhea, retrograde ejaculation, miosis
Doxazosin	Selective α_1-antagonist	1 mg/day PO up to 8 mg/day PO	First-dose phenomenon; may cause syncope; dizziness; drowsiness
Propranolol	Nonselective β-blocker	40 mg/day PO up to 480 mg/day in divided doses to control tachycardia	Should not be administered without first creating α-blockade
Atenolol	Selective β_1-blocker	PO 50–100 mg/day	Long acting; eliminated unchanged by kidney; should not be administered without first creating α-blockade
Labetalol	α- and β-blocker	PO 200 mg, divided doses Up to 800 mg/day	A much weaker α-blocker than β-blocker; may cause pressor response with pheochromocytoma
Nicardipine sustained release	Calcium channel blocker	30 mg PO twice a day; up to 120 mg/day	Arterial vasodilator; edema; flushing; headache
α-methyltyrosine	Inhibitor of biosynthesis of catecholamines	Initial PO 1 g/day; up to 4 g/day in divided doses	For patients not amenable to surgery; may be nephrotoxic

Modified from Schwartz JJ, et al. Endocrine function. In: Barash PG, et al., eds. *Clinical Anesthesia.* 8th ed. Philadelphia: Wolters Kluwer; 2017:1341.

less postoperative pain, earlier mobilization, and faster recovery compared to open laparotomy.[226,228-231] During pneumoperitoneum for laparoscopy, significant catecholamine release has been reported and should be anticipated by the anesthetist.[232]

Effective anesthetic management of these challenging cases is based on (1) optimizing preoperative preparation of the patient, (2) selecting drugs that do not stimulate catecholamine release, (3) using monitors that facilitate early and appropriate interventions, and (4) responding cautiously but expeditiously to catecholamine-induced changes in cardiovascular function. Previously, 25% to 50% of hospital deaths in patients with pheochromocytoma occurred during surgery.[211] During our current era, these surgeries are increasingly performed in centers where surgical and anesthesia specialists are familiar with the complexity of this complicated management.

A number of drugs can precipitate hypertension in the surgical patient with pheochromocytoma. Dopamine antagonists (metoclopramide, droperidol), histamine-producing agents (radiographic contrast media, morphine), indirect-acting amines (ephedrine, methyldopa), and drugs that block neuronal catecholamine reuptake (tricyclic antidepressants, cocaine) may enhance the physiologic effects of tumor product.[197]

Pheochromocytomas are vascular tumors. Large-bore intravenous lines and a peripheral arterial catheter are required and should be established preoperatively. Advanced hemodynamic monitoring will help guide fluid management and intervention with inotropes or vasoactive drugs. Considerations should be given to rapid transfusion devices, especially for large tumors.[214] Intraoperative transesophageal echocardiography has the advantage of real-time monitoring of myocardial wall motion abnormalities and intravascular volume status, especially for patients with heart disease.[213,214] Arterial blood gases, electrolyte concentrations, and blood glucose levels should be assessed regularly during the anesthetic.

Critical intraoperative junctures are (1) during induction and intubation of the trachea (hypertension), (2) during surgical manipulation of the tumor (hypertension), and (3) after ligation of the tumor's venous drainage (hypotension).

A slow and controlled induction of general anesthesia is the aim. Maintenance with sevoflurane or isoflurane and short-acting opioids provides cardiovascular stability and possesses the ability to rapidly change anesthetic depth, which are attractive features in the anesthetic management of the patient with pheochromocytoma. The tachycardia and increased sympathetic stimulation associated with desflurane make it a less desirable choice for these cases. Ketamine is usually avoided due to its sympathomimetic effects.[213,214]

The use of selective α_2-receptor agonist dexmedetomidine may be useful in managing blood pressure and heart rate. Activating α_2-receptors results in sympathetic inhibition and has been shown to reduce the release of catecholamines resulting in decreased blood pressure and heart rate.[233-235]

The use of succinylcholine is controversial for patients with a pheochromocytoma because mechanical compression of an abdominal tumor by drug-induced skeletal muscle fasciculations may provoke catecholamine release.[236] Skeletal muscle paralysis with a nondepolarizing muscle relaxant devoid of vagolytic or histamine-releasing effects is desirable. Vecuronium and rocuronium is widely used and preferred at many centers.[214] Pancuronium should be avoided for its known chronotropic effect.

The anesthetist should anticipate a labile cardiovascular course during surgery, necessitating vasopressor and vasodepressor control (Table 37.15). Communication with the surgical team is important to anticipate dramatic changes in circulating catecholamine levels attendant with tumor manipulation and tumor vein ligation. Acute hypertension may be treated with intravenous sodium nitroprusside, nitroglycerine, clevidipine, nicardipine, magnesium sulfate, or other antihypertensives, as well as deepening the level of anesthetic.[195,210,214,237,238] Sodium nitroprusside is especially advantageous because of its rapid onset and short duration of action. Lidocaine, labetalol, or esmolol may be administered to decrease tachydysrhythmias. β-adrenergic receptor antagonists must be used cautiously in patients with catecholamine-induced cardiomyopathy because even minimal β-adrenergic blockade can accentuate left ventricular dysfunction. The short half-life of esmolol makes it the preferred choice for β-adrenergic blockade intraoperatively. Dysrhythmias associated

TABLE 37.15   Drugs Used in Intraoperative Management of Pheochromocytoma

Drug	Action	Intravenous Dosage	Comment
Phentolamine	Nonselective α-blocker	1 mg test dose, then 1–5 mg bolus every 5 min or infuse initially 0.5–1.0 mg/min as needed	Rapid onset; the response to bolus is maximal in 2–3 min and lasts 10–15 min; tachycardia; tachyphylaxis develops
Esmolol	Selective β_1-blocker	Loading dose 250–500 mcg/kg infused over 1 min, followed by maintenance infusion 25–250 mcg/kg per min	Ultrashort acting; elimination half-life approximately 9 min; may be used during anesthesia
Labetalol	α- and β-blocker	IV 10-mg bolus	A much weaker α-blocker than β-blocker; ratios of α- to β-blockade have been estimated to be approximately 1:3 (PO dose) and 1:7 (IV dose); may cause pressor response in pheochromocytoma if α-blockade inadequate
Nitroprusside	Direct vasodilator	IV infusion initially 0.5–1.5 mcg/kg/min Maximum 8 mcg/kg/min	Powerful vasodilator; short acting; monitor for cyanide toxicity; methemoglobinemia
Magnesium sulfate	Direct vasodilator	Initial loading dose of 50 mg/kg over 10 min followed by 15 mg/kg/hr	May potentiate neuromuscular blockade
Nicardipine	Dihydropyridine calcium channel blocker	1–2 mcg/kg/min initially and increased to 7.5 mcg/kg/min as needed	Arterial vasodilation; tachycardia common
Dexmedetomidine	Selective α_2-adrenergic receptor agonist	IV infusion: initially 1 mcg/kg over 10 min, then 0.5 mcg/kg/hr	

IV, Intravenous; *PO,* per os (oral).

Modified from Schwartz JJ, et al. Endocrine function. In: Barash PG, et al., eds. *Clinical Anesthesia.* 8th ed. Philadelphia: Wolters Kluwer; 2017:1341.

with hypertension may resolve by simply lowering abnormally high blood pressure.

After surgical ligation of the veins that drain a pheochromocytoma, the decrease in circulating catecholamines and the associated down-regulation of adrenergic receptors can precipitate an abrupt and marked drop in blood pressure.[237,239] Hypotension often responds to fluid and colloid administration, but intravenous administration of phenylephrine, norepinephrine, or vasopressin may be needed until the peripheral vasculature adapts to the decreased level of endogenous α-stimulation.[192,194,237,239] Adrenocortical insufficiency should be considered as a potential cause of postresection hypotension if both adrenal glands were manipulated or resected during surgery.[194,214]

Hyperglycemia is common before excision of the pheochromocytoma. With tumor removal, the sudden withdrawal of catecholamine stimulation can result in hypoglycemia. Blood glucose levels should be monitored at frequent intervals intraoperatively and postoperatively.

Postoperative management. Intensive monitoring must continue postoperatively as catecholamines withdraw. Hypertension persists in 50% of patients during the immediate postresection recovery period.[197,224] Fluid shifts, pain, hypoxia, hypercapnia, adrenergic instability, urinary retention, and residual tumor are all possible causes of postoperative hypertension.[240] Catecholamine levels decrease to normal over several days postoperatively, and most patients are normotensive by the time of hospital discharge.[194,197]

THYROID GLAND

The thyroid gland is one of the largest endocrine glands. It is located anterior to the trachea between the cricoid cartilage and suprasternal notch. The vascular supply to the gland is derived from the superior and inferior thyroid arteries. Blood flow is equivalent to approximately five times the weight of the gland, which is a blood supply as rich as almost any tissue in the body.[241] The gland consists of two lobes and an isthmus. The RLNs run along the lateral borders of each thyroid lobe, which is a consideration when surgery on the gland is performed. The gland produces and secretes two important hormones: triiodothyronine (T_3) and thyroxine (T_4).[241]

Microscopically, the thyroid is divided into lobules, each of which is composed of 20 to 40 follicles. The follicles are the functional units of the thyroid gland. They are lined by epithelial cells that surround central deposits of a proteinaceous substance called colloid. The major constituent of the colloid is a large glycoprotein called thyroglobulin, which serves as the backbone for the synthesis and storage of thyroid hormones.[241]

Synthesis of Thyroid Hormones

Iodide Trapping

Approximately 1 mg of ingested iodine is required each week to form normal quantities of thyroid hormones. Dietary iodine is reduced in the gastrointestinal tract to iodide. Common table salt is iodized with sodium iodide for the prevention of iodine deficiency.

The first stage of thyroid hormone formation is the transport of iodides from the extracellular fluid into the thyroid cells and follicles. Approximately one-fifth of the circulating iodide is removed from the blood by active transport into the thyroid cells and used for the synthesis of thyroid hormones, a process called iodide trapping. The iodide transport pump normally concentrates the intracellular iodide to approximately 30 times its concentration in the blood. Iodide trapping is the rate-limiting step in thyroid hormone synthesis and is under the control of TSH from the anterior pituitary. Once inside the thyroid gland, iodide ions are oxidized back to iodine.[241]

Thyroid Hormone Formation

Thyroid hormones are formed in the follicles of the thyroid gland under the control of TSH. Thyroglobulin contains the amino acid tyrosine, which combines with iodine to form various iodotyrosines, including the two major thyroid hormones. Thyroxine and triiodothyronine remain part of the thyroglobulin molecule, stored as colloid within the thyroid follicle until release. Enough hormone is synthesized and stored under basal conditions to supply the body with its normal hormone requirements for 2 to 3 months. As a result, if complete thyroid hormone synthesis ceases, the physiologic effects are not seen for several months.[241,242]

Although iodine is required for hormone synthesis, paradoxically, excess iodine (100 times the normal plasma level) can cause the gland to recede and inhibit production of thyroid hormone.

Release of Thyroxine and Triiodothyronine

TSH controls the release of hormones from the thyroid gland. On release, T_4 and T_3 are cleaved from the thyroglobulin molecule and secreted into the circulating blood. Thyroglobulin remains within the colloid.[241]

Under normal conditions, approximately 93% of the hormone released from the thyroid gland is T_4 and 7% is T_3.[241] The secretion of T_4 from the thyroid gland is 80 to 100 mcg/day. When thyroid hormones reach their target tissues, most of the T_4 is deiodinated to T_3, with T_4 serving largely as a hormone precursor. Triiodothyronine therefore is the primary thyroid hormone that stimulates target tissues and it is more potent and less protein bound than T_4.[242]

Transport of Thyroxine and Triiodothyronine to Tissues

Thyroid hormone exists in circulation in both free and bound forms. The amount of free hormone, which is the metabolically active fraction, is extremely small: less than 0.03% of total circulating T_4 and 0.3% of total circulating T_3. The majority of circulating hormone (99%) is bound to plasma proteins. Most of the thyroid hormones bind to the circulating protein thyroxine-binding globulin.[241,243]

Because of the very high amount of protein binding, free thyroid hormones are released to the tissue cells very slowly. The half-life of T_4 in circulation is 6 to 7 days, and the half-life of T_3 is approximately 24 hours.[242]

Functions of Thyroid Hormones

Increased Cellular Metabolic Activity

In large part, thyroid hormones work by binding to nuclear receptors in target cells (virtually all cells of the body) where they activate gene transcription and initiate protein formation (Fig. 37.22). Consequently, the level of enzymes, structural proteins, transport proteins, and other substances increases considerably under the direction of T_4 and especially T_3.[244] The net effect is increased metabolic activity, heat production, and oxygen consumption of all or almost all tissues in the body.[241,243] The basal metabolic rate can increase by as much as 60% to 100% above normal when large quantities of thyroid hormones are secreted. As a result, the rate and depth of respiration increase due to the enhanced metabolic rate and increased oxygen use and carbon dioxide formation by cells. The use of energy substrates is greatly accelerated. Protein synthesis is increased; however, protein catabolism is also increased. When the quantity of thyroid hormone is slightly increased, the muscles react with vigor; however, when the quantity is excessive, muscles become weakened from excess protein catabolism.[241]

Effect of Thyroid Hormone on Growth

Thyroid hormones are necessary for normal growth in infants and children. In a hypothyroid state, the rate of tissue growth is greatly reduced.

Thyroid hormone is required for normal growth and development of the brain during fetal life and for the first few years of postnatal life.[241]

Effect of Thyroid Hormone on Specific Systems

Thyroid hormones have direct and indirect effects on the excitability of the heart. The heart rate and the force of contraction are augmented with increasing thyroid hormone production. As such, the heart rate is a sensitive sign of excessive or diminished thyroid hormone production.[241] Vasodilation occurs from increased cellular oxygen consumption and results in increased blood flow to most tissues.[241]

Thyroid hormones increase the rate of hormone secretion from most endocrine glands, especially the pancreas. The heightened cellular requirement for glucose mandates higher insulin secretion. Thyroid hormones also enhance the secretion of digestive juices and the motility of the gastrointestinal tract, in addition to increasing an individual's appetite and food intake. In adults, thyroid hormones enhance the rapidity of cerebration.[241]

Regulation of Thyroid Hormone Secretion

Specific feedback mechanisms operate through the hypothalamus and anterior pituitary gland to precisely control the rate of thyroid hormone secretion. Thyrotropin-releasing hormone (TRH) from the hypothalamus causes cells of the anterior pituitary lobe to produce and secrete TSH. Potent stimuli to TRH and TSH release include low levels of T_3 and T_4 and exposure to cold.[241] TSH increases all known activities of thyroid gland cells, resulting in increased gland size and vascularity and increased hormone synthesis and release. These varied effects are mediated by activation of the second-messenger cAMP in thyroid cells. High circulating levels of primarily T_3, and to a lesser extent T_4, inhibit the secretion of TRH and TSH through a negative feedback effect on the hypothalamus and anterior pituitary. Fig. 37.22 summarizes the regulation of thyroid secretion.

Thyroid Gland Disorders

Hyperthyroidism

Hyperthyroidism is defined as thyroid gland hyperactivity. Thyrotoxicosis is defined as a state of thyroid hormone excess.[245] Today these terms are often used interchangeably.[246] The most common cause of thyrotoxicosis in the United States is Graves disease, affecting approximately 0.5% of the population and accounting for 60% to 80% of thyrotoxicosis cases.[245] Graves disease is an autoimmune disease in which TSH-receptor antibodies bind to and stimulate the thyroid gland, resulting in gland enlargement and excessive production and secretion of T_4 and T_3.[245-247] These unique immunoglobulin G (IgG) autoantibodies mimic the actions of TSH, but their effects last much longer and are not controlled.[248] Graves disease is four to five times more common in women than men, and the peak incidence occurs between 40 and 60 years of age. Potential risk factors for Graves disease include genetic susceptibility, stress, and cigarette smoking. There is an increase in Graves disease in the postpartum period.[245]

Other important causes of thyrotoxicosis include toxic nodular hyperthyroidism, due to the presence of autonomously functioning thyroid nodules, and thyroiditis, which results in the release of stored hormones.[245,246,248] A TSH-secreting pituitary tumor is a less common cause of thyrotoxicosis. Thyroid cancer is most often associated with a euthyroid state but may cause hyper- or hypothyroidism. Cancer of the thyroid gland is increasing at an alarming rate and is projected to replace colorectal cancer as the fourth leading cancer diagnosis by 2030.[249]

The antiarrhythmic agent amiodarone is iodine rich and may cause either hypo- or hyperthyroidism. Due to structural similarity with thyroid hormones, 14% to 18% of patients treated with amiodarone develop overt thyroid dysfunction.[250] Iodine

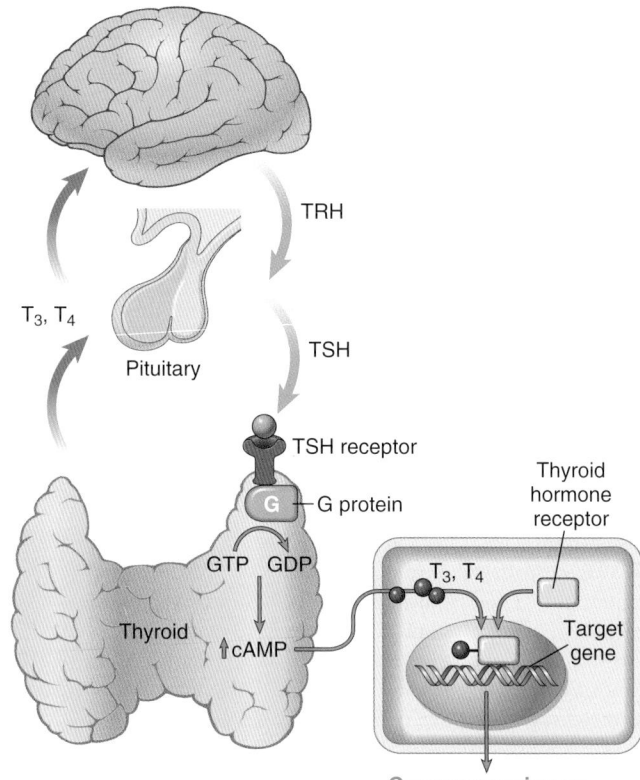

Fig. 37.22 Homeostasis in the hypothalamus-pituitary-thyroid axis and mechanism of action of thyroid hormones. Secretion of thyroid hormones (T_3 and T_4) is controlled by trophic factors secreted by both the hypothalamus and the anterior pituitary. Decreased levels of T_3 and T_4 stimulate the release of thyrotropin releasing hormone (TRH) from the hypothalamus and thyroid-stimulating hormone (TSH) from the anterior pituitary, causing T_3 and T_4 levels to rise. Elevated T_3 and T_4 levels, in turn, feed back to suppress the secretion of both TRH and TSH. TSH binds to the TSH receptor on the thyroid follicular epithelium, which causes activation of G proteins, and cyclic adenosine monophosphate (cAMP)–mediated synthesis and release of thyroid hormones (T_3 and T_4). In the periphery, T_3 and T_4 interact with the thyroid hormone receptor (TR) to form a hormone-receptor complex that translocates to the nucleus and binds to so-called thyroid response elements (TREs) on target genes to initiate transcription. (From Kumar V, et al. *Robbins and Cotran Pathologic Basis of Disease.* 9th ed. Philadelphia: Elsevier; 2015:1083.)

containing radiocontrast media contains at least 2000 times more iodine than the recommended daily allowance. This supraphysiologic amount of iodine has no major effects in euthyroid individuals but may cause either hyper- or hypothyroidism in susceptible individuals.[250,251]

Signs and symptoms. Clinical manifestations of thyrotoxicosis reflect the widespread hypermetabolic effects of excess thyroid hormones. The thyroid gland is usually enlarged two to three times its normal size. Physical manifestations include tachycardia, warm and moist skin, a fine hand tremor, diarrhea, osteopenia, and muscle weakness.[245,246,251-254] Despite extreme fatigue, sleep is often difficult. Weight loss (despite increased food consumption), anxiety, and intolerance to heat are additional clinical findings of thyrotoxicosis.[245-247]

The aberrant immunologic response associated with Graves disease targets primarily the thyroid gland but also other tissues, most notably extraocular muscles (Graves ophthalmopathy) and skin (thyroid dermopathy). Ophthalmopathy is observed in 30% to 50% of patients with Graves disease.[245-247,254,255] Thyroid-associated ophthalmopathy may cause exophthalmos (protrusion of the eyeballs), eye redness, and periorbital edema. Papilledema, diplopia, and loss of visual acuity may occur. Graves ophthalmopathy results from autoimmune-mediated inflammation and swelling of the periorbital connective tissue and extraocular muscles.[245-247] In many patients, the ophthalmopathy improves with treatment of the hyperthyroidism, but complete effective resolution remains a therapeutic challenge.[254]

The systolic blood pressure is typically elevated 10 to 15 mm Hg, and the diastolic pressure is reduced under the influence of excess thyroid hormone. The blood volume increases slightly due to vasodilation. Mean arterial pressure usually remains unchanged, but the pulse pressure increases. Blood flow to the skin increases in response to the increased need for heat elimination.[251-253]

The effects of thyrotoxicosis on the heart are pronounced.[251-253] Thyroid hormones have a direct effect on the excitability of the heart. Sinus tachycardia and cardiac dysrhythmias affect almost all patients.[251-253] The prevalence of atrial fibrillation is about 10%. The cardiac output increases with thyrotoxicosis, sometimes 50% to 300% above normal. However, with protracted disease, heart muscle strength may eventually become depressed because of protein catabolism.[251-253] Even patients with subclinical hyperthyroidism are at increased risk for cardiovascular conditions.[256]

Diagnosis of thyrotoxicosis is more difficult in the elderly because many of the hyperkinetic manifestations of hyperthyroidism are absent.[257] Elderly patients may feel constant fatigue and present with myocardial failure or atrial fibrillation.[245,246,257]

Diagnosis. The diagnosis of primary hyperthyroidism is established in most cases by the combined findings of abnormally high free serum T_4 and T_3 levels and low TSH levels.[246] Subclinical hyperthyroidism is defined as a low TSH but normal free T_4 and T_3. With Graves disease, the diagnosis may be supported by the presence of thyroid-stimulating immunoglobulins.[245,246] Serum alkaline phosphatase and calcium concentrations are elevated in approximately 20% of patients with Graves disease and reflect bone turnover.[258]

Other autoimmune diseases such as myasthenia gravis, rheumatoid arthritis, systemic lupus erythematosus, and type 1 DM are more common in patients with Graves disease.[245,246]

Treatment. A variety of treatment options are available for patients with thyrotoxicosis, but three common treatment options are radioactive gland ablation, surgery, and antithyroid drug therapy.[245,246,256,259,260] None of these options are ideal; drug-treated patients have a high relapse rate, and ablative therapies (total thyroidectomy, radioactive iodine) induce lifelong hypothyroidism.

Radioactive iodine. A common therapy for Graves disease in the United States is ablation of the thyroid gland with radioactive iodine (^{131}I). An injected dose of radioactive iodide is absorbed by the hyperplastic gland, and it slowly destroys most of the thyroid secretory cells. Two to 4 months is needed to reverse the hyperthyroidism with this approach. Hypothyroidism is common after treatment. Use of ^{131}I is contraindicated during pregnancy and breast feeding.

Thyroidectomy. Total thyroidectomy for treatment of Graves disease is an option, especially when antithyroid drugs are ineffective, if radioiodine treatment is refused, when malignancy is suspected, in children or pregnant women, or if the thyroid goiter is exceptionally large.[245,246] Patients should be treated preoperatively with antithyroid medication and rendered euthyroid prior to surgery.

Complications associated with thyroid surgery occur in less than 1% of cases and include damage to the RLN, hypoparathyroidism (hypocalcemia), and neck hematoma. Postoperative bleeding into the operative site can rapidly produce death by asphyxia and requires immediate evacuation. Thyroid carcinoma, reoperation for recurrent

goiter, nonidentification of the RLN, and total thyroidectomy are associated with a significantly increased risk of operative RLN injury.[259,261] As mentioned previously with parathyroid surgery, unilateral damage to the RLN causes postoperative hoarseness that usually improves in a few weeks. Bilateral RLN injury is much more serious because both vocal cords may assume a median or paramedian position and cause aphonia, stridor, and airway obstruction.[192,245,246,261] Immediate intubation and ventilatory support is required. Vocal cord function can be assessed pre- and postoperatively by asking the patient to phonate "E" to assess for adequate RLN function.[192] Additionally, various nerve integrity monitors may be used during thyroid surgery to help the surgeon identify the RLN.[262,263,264,265,266]

Thyroidectomy is most often performed under general endotracheal anesthesia.[266] The laryngeal mask airway has been used to facilitate laryngeal nerve monitoring using fiberoptic endoscopic examination of vocal cord movement.[267,268] Bilateral cervical plexus block can be used for those patients who pose a general anesthesia risk or in concert with general anesthesia for postoperative pain control.[269-271]

Antithyroid drugs and β-adrenergic receptor blockade. The main class of antithyroid medications is the thionamides, which include methimazole, carbimazole, and propylthiouracil (PTU). All thionamides inhibit thyroid hormone synthesis by interfering with the incorporation of iodine into tyrosine residues of thyroglobulin. A euthyroid state is usually obtained in 2 to 6 weeks. These agents block new hormone synthesis, but any already formed T_4 and T_3 stored in the colloid must be secreted and metabolized for clinical improvement to occur. PTU also inhibits conversion of T_4 to T_3.[260]

β-adrenergic blocking agents (propranolol, metoprolol, atenolol) are often included in an antithyroid regimen to reduce cardiovascular symptoms. Propranolol has the additional advantage of inhibiting the peripheral conversion of T_4 to T_3.[260] For patients with temporary forms of hyperthyroidism (e.g., thyroiditis), β-blockers may be the only treatment required. β-adrenergic blocking agents aggravate bronchospasm and therefore may be contraindicated in the patient with asthma or severe chronic obstructive pulmonary disease.

For the patient preparing for surgical thyroidectomy, preoperative pharmacologic management may include restoring the metabolic state to normal with antithyroid agents and then inducing involution of the gland with iodine.[246] Iodides in high concentration (100 times the normal plasma concentration) decrease all phases of thyroid activity and decrease the gland size and vascularity.

Preoperative preparation—hyperthyroidism. The key to successful preoperative preparation of the hyperthyroid surgical patient is a careful assessment of the extent and control of hyperthyroidism and the severity of end-organ manifestations. Thyrotoxicosis is associated with increased operative risk, so elective surgery should not proceed until the patient has been rendered euthyroid by medical management. In patients with untreated or poorly controlled hyperthyroidism, surgery can precipitate thyroid storm, a potentially life-threatening condition. Preoperative preparation of patients with Graves disease typically includes thionamides, β-blockers, and/or iodides. Medical management to achieve adequate control (normal free T_4 and T_3) may take 2 to 6 weeks. Antithyroid treatment should be continued through the morning of surgery.[245,246]

Hyperthyroid patients have increased blood volume, decreased peripheral resistance, and a wide pulse pressure. The cardiac output is increased due both to increased peripheral oxygen needs and increased cardiac contractility. The heart rate and systolic blood pressure may be increased.[251] Appropriate corrections of the patient's fluid volume and electrolyte status should be accomplished before surgery.

Only life-threatening emergency surgery should be performed in an untreated symptomatic hyperthyroid patient. In an emergency, the otherwise healthy patient can be expeditiously prepared for surgery with oral or nasogastric administration of thionamides followed by potassium iodide (saturated solution of potassium iodide [SSKI] or Lugol solution) at least 1 hour after thionamide administration. Carefully titrated intravenous propranolol or esmolol may also be utilized.[254,260,272] Central pressure monitoring may be necessary to guide therapy.

Preoperative assessment—goiter. A careful preoperative evaluation of the airway is mandatory in all hyperthyroid and hypothyroid patients undergoing surgery. Thyroid gland enlargement can be asymptomatic, while causing tracheal deviation and/or tracheoesophageal compression.[247,266] Chronic pressure on the trachea can result in tracheomalacia, a weakening of the thyroid cartilage that can cause tracheal collapse. In the postoperative period, its presence may necessitate a more prolonged intubation and vigilant observation after extubation. Immediate reintubation may be required due to loss of tracheal integrity.[192] Hoarseness, difficulty swallowing, sore throat, a feeling of pressure in the neck, coughing, orthopnea, or dyspnea suggests tracheal compression that can be caused by thyromegaly.[266] A bruit over the gland reflects increased vascularity. Imaging tests may be employed to evaluate thyromegaly. Ultrasonography is the most sensitive method for assessing gland architecture; CT is also used.[266]

Although an enlarged thyroid gland is not in itself a predictor of airway management problems, difficult intubation is reported in 5% to 8% of cases for goiter surgery.[273,274] A patient with a large goiter and an obstructed airway poses the same challenge as any other patient in whom airway management is problematic. An awake fiberoptic intubation with topical anesthesia is of proven value under these conditions.[247] Other suggested available equipment for management of an anticipated difficult airway include rigid bronchoscope, videolaryngoscopes, and laryngeal mask airways. There are situations where it may be beneficial to have a surgeon present in the room at induction for emergency airway access.[266]

Intraoperative management. No specific anesthetic agent or technique is required for the hyperthyroid surgical patient. Monitoring for early signs of thyroid storm is key to safe management, and so a general goal is prevention of sympathetic nervous system stimulation. This is accomplished by providing sufficient anesthetic depth and avoiding medications that directly or indirectly stimulate the sympathetic nervous system.

A preoperative anxiolytic medication is generally warranted. The antisialagogues, atropine and glycopyrrolate, should not be routinely administered because of their vagolytic effects and ability to impair sweating.

Induction of anesthesia may be achieved with several intravenous medications. Ketamine is generally not used because of the drugs sympathomimetic effects.

Because of the increased incidence of myasthenia gravis and skeletal muscle weakness in the hyperthyroid patient, precaution dictates careful titration of muscle relaxant doses with neuromuscular blockade monitoring. Pancuronium should be avoided because it has the potential to increase the heart rate. Respiratory failure has been described in surgical patients with uncontrolled hyperthyroidism.[275]

Isoflurane and sevoflurane are attractive choices for inhalation anesthetics because of their ability to offset sympathetic nervous system responses to surgical stimulation and because they do not sensitize the myocardium to catecholamines.

Monitoring of the hyperthyroid patient should focus on early recognition of increased thyroid gland activity suggesting the onset of thyroid storm. Core body temperature should be monitored closely. The ECG should be assessed for tachycardia or dysrhythmias. Hypotension occurring during surgery is better treated with direct-acting

vasopressors than with indirect-acting vasoactive drugs that stimulate the release of catecholamines.

Meticulous care of the eyes is required. The patient with exophthalmos is at risk for corneal exposure and damage, so special care should be taken to lubricate and protect the eyes intraoperatively. Box 37.11 summarizes key anesthesia implications for patients with hyperthyroidism.

Thyroid storm. A feared complication in the hyperthyroid surgical patient is thyroid storm or severe hyperthyroidism. Thyroid storm is an uncommon, life-threatening medical emergency that represents a severe exacerbation of hyperthyroidism in the previously undiagnosed or incompletely treated hyperthyroid patient.[245,246] Treatment with antithyroid medications helps protect the patient against thyroid storm. β-adrenergic blocking agents do not prevent thyroid storm. Precipitating events may include trauma, surgery (especially thyroid surgery), the peripartum period, acute illness, and infection.[276-278] Thyroid storm associated with surgery may occur any time in the perioperative period but has been reported most often 6 to 18 hours after surgery.[276-278]

The clinical manifestations of thyroid storm include striking alterations in consciousness, marked tachycardia, hyperpyrexia, hypertension, and arrhythmias (Box 37.12). Metabolic acidosis may be present secondary to increased lactate production from overactive metabolism. Similarities exist between the clinical features of thyroid storm and those of pheochromocytoma, neuroleptic malignant syndrome, and malignant hyperthermia, making clinical diagnosis challenging in some cases.[192,276-278] The clinical picture of severe hypermetabolism in a patient with a history of hyperthyroidism, exophthalmos, or goiter strongly supports the diagnosis.[245,246] To prevent substantial morbidity and mortality, emergency treatment should not await laboratory confirmation. Mortality rates are as high as 20% to 30%, even with early diagnosis and management.[245,246] The high mortality associated with

---

BOX 37.11   Anesthesia Implications for Thyroidectomy

- Determine the extent of thyrotoxicosis and end-organ complications.
- Ensure a euthyroid state prior to surgery.
- Evaluate the airway closely (goiter).
- Avoid sympathetic nervous system activation and sympathomimetic drugs.
- Titrate muscle relaxants carefully, considering possible myopathy.
- Position carefully (decreased bone density and predisposition to osteoporosis).
- Monitor core body temperature.
- Monitor closely for early signs of thyroid storm.
- Pad and protect the eyes.
- Postoperative hypocalcemia

BOX 37.12   Clinical Manifestation of Thyroid Storm

- Fever >38.5°C
- Tachycardia
- Confusion and agitation
- Tremor
- Weakness
- Dysrhythmias
- Nausea and vomiting
- Hypertension
- Heart failure

thyroid storm underscores the importance of achieving a euthyroid state before surgery.

Patients with thyroid storm are critically ill. Management in the perioperative period includes identifying and treating the precipitating cause, administering antithyroid medications, and providing continual monitoring and hemodynamic support. Carefully titrated β-adrenergic receptor blockers blunt adrenergic manifestations, and a short-acting agent like esmolol may be safer in this setting. Cautious administration is essential. Antithyroid drugs (PTU 200–400 mg orally or via nasogastric tube or rectally every 6 hours) block thyroid hormone synthesis.[235] PTU is preferable in this setting because it inhibits the generation of T_3 from T_4. Iodides (Lugol solution or SSKI) administered at least 1 hour after thionamides acutely retard the release of preformed hormone from the thyroid gland. Supplemental glucocorticoids (50–100 mg hydrocortisone intravenously) support the response to stress and inhibit the peripheral conversion of T_4 to T_3.[245,246,272,276-278]

Supportive measures include intravenous hydration with glucose-containing crystalloid solutions, correction of electrolyte and acid-base imbalances, and management of hyperthermia. Salicylates may displace T_3 and T_4 from carrier proteins, therefore acetaminophen is the recommended antipyretic for lowering body temperature in concert with a cold blanket or ice packs as required. Adequate oxygenation is of paramount importance during thyroid storm. Vasoactive medications and advanced hemodynamic monitoring may be necessary to help manage the labile cardiovascular course.[245,246,272,276-278]

Hypothyroidism

Hypothyroidism is a state of thyroid gland hypofunction. Laboratory findings show normal or decreased plasma free T_3 and T_4 concentrations and elevated TSH levels in patients with primary disease.[279-281] The spectrum of thyroid hormone deficiency can range from the asymptomatic patient with no overt physical findings to the classic myxedema coma patient with profound symptoms. Hypothyroidism is a common disease and the most common disorder of thyroid function. It occurs in approximately 5% of women and less commonly in men.[279]

Primary hypothyroidism accounts for 95% of all cases of hypothyroidism. An autoimmune-mediated inflammation and destruction of the thyroid gland, known as Hashimoto thyroiditis, is the most common form of hypothyroidism in the United States.[279,280] The disorder most often occurs during middle age and is associated with other autoimmune disorders such as myasthenia gravis, type 1 DM, and adrenal insufficiency.

In addition to autoimmune-mediated gland destruction, primary hypothyroidism may also be the result of severe iodine deficiency, colloid goiter, or iatrogenic causes (e.g., previous thyroid surgery, neck irradiation, radioiodine therapy).[279,280] As noted previously, the iodine-rich antiarrhythmic agent amiodarone can cause hyper- or hypothyroidism. Hypothyroidism is also associated with tyrosine kinase inhibitors, a class of anticancer drugs.[282,283] Lithium inhibits the release of thyroid hormone and causes hypothyroidism in some patients.

Rarely, secondary hypothyroidism is the result of pituitary or hypothalamic disorders. Secondary hypothyroidism is associated with decreased concentrations of both thyroid hormones and TSH. Regardless of the etiology, the clinical manifestations of hypothyroidism are similar.

Signs and symptoms.
Most cases of primary hypothyroidism today are subclinical, with laboratory findings of increased plasma TSH but T_3 and T_4 in the normal range.[281] Patients with more significant overt disease develop signs and symptoms that reflect a slowed metabolism and impaired cellular functions. Because of elevated TSH, the thyroid gland is usually enlarged (goiter), nontender, and firm. Patients with overt hypothyroidism have impaired body heat mechanisms with an intolerance to cold. Paresthesias, slow mental functioning, ataxia, a puffy face, and slow gastrointestinal function may be present. Dry skin and brittle hair and nails reflect failure of trophic functions. Lack of thyroid hormone causes the muscles to become weak. Extreme somnolence is characteristic of hypothyroidism with the risk of decreased ventilatory response to hypoxia and hypercarbia.[279,280] Accumulation of mucopolysaccharides and proteinaceous fluid in tissue and body cavities is a recognized feature of severe hypothyroidism. The tongue may be affected and enlarged. The most common sites of effusions associated with hypothyroidism are the pleural, pericardial, and peritoneal cavities. Inappropriate ADH secretion and impaired free water clearance can lead to hyponatremia. Accumulation of mucopolysaccharides and fluid imparts the characteristic edematous appearance called myxedema.[279,280]

Cardiovascular complications of hypothyroidism can be marked and include sinus bradycardia, dysrhythmias, cardiomegaly, impaired contractility, abnormal baroreceptor function, heart failure, and labile blood pressure. Symptoms of low exercise tolerance and shortness of breath with exertion may be partially the result of decreased cardiac function. Chronic vasoconstriction produces diastolic hypertension, a narrowed pulse pressure, and a contracted intravascular fluid volume. Overt hypothyroidism is associated with accelerated atherosclerosis and coronary artery disease, possibly owing to the higher incidence of hypercholesterolemia and hypertension.[252,279,280]

These classic clinical features of hypothyroidism are often lacking in the elderly hypothyroid patient, making the diagnosis of hypothyroidism more difficult.

Extreme hypothyroidism during fetal life, infancy, or childhood is termed cretinism. The condition is characterized by physical and mental growth retardation. In the newborn, unless cretinism is treated with adequate iodine or thyroxine within the first few weeks after birth, mental impairment remains permanent. For this reason, pregnant patients who are hypothyroid require treatment. Thyroid testing before and throughout pregnancy and neonatal screening (T_4 or TSH levels) have played a major role in preventing cretinism.[284]

Treatment.
Treatment of hypothyroidism requires replacement with thyroid hormone. The agent of choice is synthetic levothyroxine sodium (T_4) because of its long half-life (7 days), once-daily dosing, and its ability to attain physiologic levels of T_3.[284,285]

An area of particular concern during thyroid hormone replacement is the effect on the cardiovascular system. Initiation of thyroid hormone replacement in a patient with coexisting angina pectoris or underlying risk factors for coronary artery disease requires careful monitoring of both cardiovascular and thyroid status. Myocardial oxygen consumption is augmented by thyroid hormone, and a hypothyroid patient with deficient coronary artery circulation may not tolerate full replacement doses.[284,285]

Anesthetic management—hypothyroidism.
Ideally, all patients with hypothyroidism should have normal thyroid function restored prior to surgery. Patients with subclinical or mild hypothyroidism generally have low risk for serious complications.[192,286] A 2015 retrospective analysis of 800 hypothyroid patients having noncardiac surgery showed that hypothyroidism was not associated with worse postoperative mortality, wound infections, or cardiovascular complications compared to euthyroid patients.[286] Thyroid replacement therapy should be continued preoperatively, but postponing surgery to initiate levothyroxine therapy in patients with mild hypothyroidism is not supported.[286-289]

Patients with more severe or symptomatic hypothyroidism may be subject to a variety of complications with anesthesia and warrant heightened attention. Elective surgical procedures in these patients should be postponed to restore normal thyroid function.[287] Patients may require correction of plasma volume, electrolytes, and body temperature. Marked depression of myocardial function and abnormal baroreceptor function may be present.[192,252,287]

Slowed hepatic metabolism and renal clearance of injected drugs may prolong their effects and delay recovery.[287,288] Regional anesthesia is a prudent choice if the surgery permits it and there are no patient contraindications.

All patients with hypothyroidism should undergo careful preoperative evaluation of the airway. A large goiter can be asymptomatic, while causing airway compromise, tracheal deviation, or compression (see Preoperative Assessment—Goiter, earlier). Intubation may be challenged by an enlarged tongue and presence of a goiter. In addition to goiter, adequate air exchange may be compromised by myxedematous infiltration of the vocal cords.

Depression of the ventilatory responses to hypoxia and hypercarbia must be considered. Preoperative sedation should be avoided in the patient with macroglossia or impaired respiratory function. Hypothyroid patients may respond to opioids with increased central nervous and respiratory system depression, necessitating cautious dosing.[283] Although ketamine has been proposed as the ideal induction agent, even ketamine can produce cardiovascular depression in the absence of a robust sympathetic nervous system.

Supplemental (stress dose) cortisol is often considered in the perioperative period because of the potential for coexisting adrenal insufficiency.[192]

Body temperature should be monitored closely in hypothyroid patients, and mechanisms for warming the patient should be used during surgery. Box 37.13 summarizes anesthesia considerations for the patient with hypothyroidism.

Myxedema coma. Myxedema coma is a rare syndrome that reflects severe manifestations of untreated or insufficiently treated hypothyroidism. It is a medical emergency with a mortality rate greater than 50%. A critical insult (e.g., infection, surgery, cerebrovascular accident, pneumonia, gastrointestinal bleeding, cold exposure) can precipitate myxedema coma in a patient with hypothyroidism.[243,279,280,283]

Generally, the patient with myxedema coma is elderly, has severe clinical features of hypothyroidism, and is hypothermic, hypoventilating,

---

BOX 37.13   Anesthesia Implications for the Hypothyroidism

- Preoperatively, aim for euthyroid state for all patients.
- Evaluate the airway closely (macroglossia, goiter).
- Continue thyroid medication on the day of surgery.
- Monitor for exaggerated central nervous system depression with anesthetic agents.
- Consider decreased hepatic metabolism and renal elimination when dosing medications.
- Monitor core temperature; utilize patient warming devices.
- Titrate muscle relaxants carefully, considering possible coexisting muscle weakness.
- Monitor patient respiratory status closely, considering blunted ventilatory response to hypercarbia and hypoxia.
- Consider possible depressed myocardial function with anesthesia selection and dosing.
- Consider possible reduction in plasma volume when calculating fluid replacement.

---

hypotensive, and hyponatremic. The response to hypoxia and hypercapnia is measurably decreased, and mechanical ventilation may be required. The patient is typically lethargic or stuporous. The presence of coma is a marker of the patient's clinical deterioration rather than a primary effect of hypothyroidism. The skin is often pale as a result of cutaneous vasoconstriction.[243,279,280,283]

Therapeutic attention is paid to body temperature, shock, and respiratory failure. Treatment consists of hemodynamic and ventilatory support and the cautious administration of levothyroxine with continuous ECG monitoring for myocardial ischemia. Supplemental cortisol is appropriate because the myxedematous patient may have adrenal atrophy and decreased adrenal reserve. Because these patients may be vulnerable to water intoxication and hyponatremia, meticulous fluid replacement is important. Only lifesaving emergency surgery should proceed in a patient with myxedema coma.[243,279,280,283]

SUMMARY

The number and variety of patients with endocrine disorders presenting to surgery remains a consistent challenge for the practicing anesthesia provider. Our ability to diagnose and treat these disorders continues to evolve. Several advances in imaging and genetic profiling have yielded improved preoperative diagnostics. The increase in knowledge of the pathophysiology associated with each patient's individual condition will result in better anesthesia management.

REFERENCES

For a complete list of references for this chapter, scan this QR code with any smartphone code reader app, or visit the following URL: http://booksite.elsevier.com/9780323711944/.

38

Hematology and Anesthesia

Judith A. Franco, Mark H. Gabot

Disruptions within the endothelial lining of blood vessels can result from spontaneous plaque dislodging, trauma, or iatrogenic reasons such as venous access or surgical intervention. Any breach in the vessel wall initiates an extraordinary chain of events that cause the cessation of bleeding by the formation of a clot that allows the site of injury to heal. Clot formation is followed by clot dissolution. Hemostasis is the process by which the body maintains the delicate balance between bleeding and clotting. Were it not for this balance, hemorrhage or thrombosis would ensue.

The focus of this chapter is to review the normal and abnormal processes of hemostasis emphasizing the (1) vessel wall, (2) platelet, (3) coagulation cascade, (4) cell-based theory of coagulation, and (5) fibrinolytic system. An in-depth discussion surrounding the importance of hemostatic assessment and management, and care of the patient with hematologic pathologies during the perioperative period follows. A discussion concerning pharmacologic management concludes the chapter.

THE NORMAL VESSEL WALL

The normal blood vessel acts as a conduit maintaining a state of fluidity within the vascular system. Blood vessels are cylindric and consist of three distinct layers: the intima, the media, and the adventitia (Fig. 38.1).

The intima (the inner layer) is the lining separating the flowing blood from the vessel; it is made up primarily of endothelial cells. These endothelial cells play an important role in the modulation of hemostasis by synthesizing and secreting many procoagulants (initiators of coagulation), anticoagulants (inhibitors of coagulation), and fibrinolytics (dissolvers of clot) (Table 38.1). One of the important mediators, von Willebrand factor (vWF), is a necessary cofactor for the adherence of platelets to one another. Tissue factor (TF) (a cofactor from the coagulation cascade) activates the clotting cascade pathway when injury to the vessel occurs. Some mediators (e.g., thromboxane A2, adenosine diphosphate [ADP]) control blood flow by influencing vasoconstriction of blood vessels. Other mediators (e.g., nitric oxide [NO], prostacyclin) control blood flow by vasodilation of blood vessels. Endothelial cells can also suppress activation of the coagulation system by their expression of many coagulation inhibitors, such as TF pathway inhibitors.[1]

One of the most important yet simple functions of the endothelial lining on blood vessels is that of forming a barrier separating the fluid contents within the blood vessel (e.g., red blood cells [RBCs], white blood cells [WBCs], albumin, globulins, fibrinogen, and platelets) from the highly thrombogenic material (e.g., collagen and procoagulants) that lies beneath, within the subendothelial space. The smooth endothelial lining physically repels the blood components away from the vessel wall, preventing activation of the clotting mechanism. When the endothelial wall is damaged, the previously mentioned properties no longer apply.

The second layer of the vessel wall, the subendothelial layer, is extremely thrombogenic and very active. The subendothelial layer contains collagen, a potent and important stimulus for platelet attachment to the injured vessel wall. The subendothelial layer also contains fibronectin, which facilitates the anchoring of fibrin during the formation of a hemostatic plug.

The third layer, the adventitia, participates in the control of blood flow by influencing the vessel's degree of contraction. The endothelial cells produce NO and prostacyclin, which influence the adventitia. NO affects platelet function by inhibiting platelet adhesion, aggregation, and the binding of fibrinogen between glycoprotein IIb/IIIa (GpIIb-IIIa) pseudopods. Under the influence of nitric oxide synthetase (NOS), L-arginine is converted to NO, which then diffuses into the muscle cells and activates soluble guanylate cyclase, subsequently producing a second messenger, cyclic guanosine monophosphate, causing muscle relaxation.[1] Muscle relaxation then results in vascular vasodilation. Once the vessel vasodilates, the increase in blood flow limits the activity of procoagulant mediators by simply washing the procoagulant mediators away. This metabolic reaction occurs within the endothelial lining (Fig. 38.2). Prostacyclin, a lipid molecule produced in the endothelial cells from prostaglandin, also interferes with platelet formation and aggregation via prostacyclin's powerful vasodilating properties.

Platelets are an essential component of the thrombogenic response to bleeding. Platelets are round and disklike and circulate freely within the blood. They are formed in the bone marrow from megakaryocytes, maintain a concentration count of approximately 150,000 to 300,000/mm^3 and survive approximately 8 to 12 days.[2] Platelets are constantly working to "patch" thousands of minute vascular injuries that occur in perpetuity. Approximately 7.1×10^3 are used each day.[3]

The platelets flow along the vessel surface. Because they are smaller than some other constituents in fluid blood (e.g., RBCs, WBCs), they tend to be pushed aside, strategically positioned near the vessel-wall surface where they can then "react" in the event of injury (Fig. 38.3). The membrane surface of the platelet serves as a physical barrier between platelet cytoplasm and the surrounding plasma. Platelets contain mitochondria in their cytoplasm enabling them to participate in aerobic metabolism, and platelets have glycogen stores that allow for anaerobic metabolism.[4] Platelets also contain contractile proteins, store large amounts of calcium and various enzymes, and require the use of their phospholipid surface to promote cellular activity contain alpha (α) granules that store proteins (e.g., vWF, fibrinogen, fibronectin, platelet factor 4, and platelet growth factor), and dense granules that store nonproteins (e.g., serotonin, ADP, adenosine triphosphate [ATP], histamine, and epinephrine).[2] Many of these granules synthesize prostaglandins that enable the platelets to promote vascular and local tissue reactions.[2,4] Platelets also produce thrombin. In the platelet, thrombin's role is to activate some of the coagulation factors and to influence recruitment of platelets to the site of injury. All the contents in the cytoplasm of the platelet participate in regulating hemostasis.

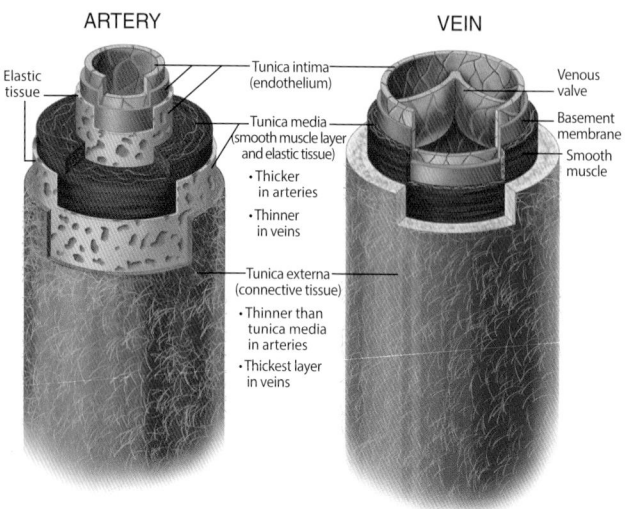

ARTERY   VEIN

Fig. 38.1 Artery and vein. Schematic drawings of an artery and a vein show comparative thicknesses of the three layers: the outer layer or tunica externa, the muscle layer or tunica media, and the tunica intima made of endothelium. Note that the muscle and outer layers are much thinner in veins than in arteries and that veins have valves. (From Patton KT, Thibodeau GA. *Structure & Function of the Body*. 16th ed. St. Louis: Elsevier; 2020:289.)

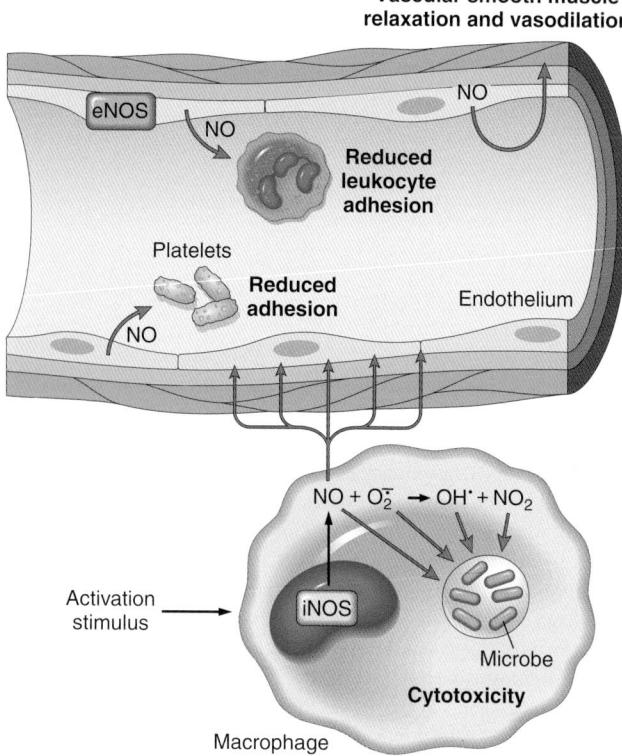

Vascular smooth muscle relaxation and vasodilation

Fig. 38.2 Functions of nitric oxide *(NO)* in blood vessels and macrophages. NO is produced by two NO synthase *(NOS)* enzymes. It causes vasodilation, and NO-derived free radicals are toxic to microbial and mammalian cells. (From Kumar V, et al. *Robbins and Cotran Pathologic Basis of Disease*. 10th ed. Philadelphia: Elsevier, 2021:115.)

Platelets do not contain a nucleus, ribonucleic acid (RNA), or deoxyribonucleic acid (DNA), so they do not reproduce.[2]

Platelets are largely inactive unless they become activated as a result of vascular trauma. Adequate hemostasis is not possible in the absence of an adequate quality or quantity of activated platelets. It is important to note that platelets do not work independently to achieve hemostasis. They work in conjunction with plasma proteins of the coagulation cascade (see Vessel Injury, next) to build a stable clot when injury to the vascular integrity occurs.

VESSEL INJURY

Clot formation in response to injury has traditionally been described to include the adherence of the platelet to the injured vessel wall and the response of the clotting cascade to form a stable clot and stop the progress of bleeding. When the endothelial lining is disrupted, as it might be by plaque dislodgement, surgical instrumentation, or trauma, an intricate process to maintain hemostasis and promote clot formation is initiated.

The vessel wall nearest the injury immediately contracts to cause a tamponade, decreasing blood flow. This contraction is a result of autonomic nervous system reflexes and the expression of thromboxane A2 and ADP.[2,5] The area adjacent to the injury vasodilates and distributes blood to the surrounding organs and tissues. Contraction is followed by three separate stages in the formation of a primary plug: adhesion, activation, and aggregation.

In the adhesion stage, vWF mobilizes from within the endothelial cells and emerges from the endothelial lining. Glycoprotein Ib (GpIb) receptors emerge from the surface of the platelet (Fig. 38.4).

TABLE 38.1	**Mediators Responsible for Procoagulant, Anticoagulant, and Fibrinolytic Activities**	
Property	**Mediator**	**Function**
Procoagulant	Coagulation factors	Coagulation
	Collagen	Tensile strength
	vWF	Adhesion
	Fibronectin	Mediates cell adhesion
	Thrombomodulin	Regulates anticoagulant pathway
Anticoagulant	Antithrombin III	Degrades factors XII, XI, X, IX, and II
	Protein C	
	Protein S	Degrades V and VII
		Cofactor for protein C
	Tissue pathway factor inhibitor	Inhibits tissue factor
Vasodilation	Nitric oxide	Vasodilates
	Prostacyclin	Vasodilates, inhibits aggregation
		Both promote smooth muscle relaxation
Vasoconstriction	Thromboxane A2	Vasoconstriction
	ADP	Vasoconstriction
	Serotonin	Vasoconstriction
Fibrinolytic	Plasminogen	Converts to plasmin
	tPA	Activates plasmin
	Urokinase	Activates plasmin
Antifibrinolytic	Plasminogen activator inhibitor	Inactivates tPA, urokinase
	α-antiplasmin	Inhibits plasmin

ADP, Adenosine diphosphate; *tPA*, tissue plasminogen activator; *vWF*, von Willebrand factor.

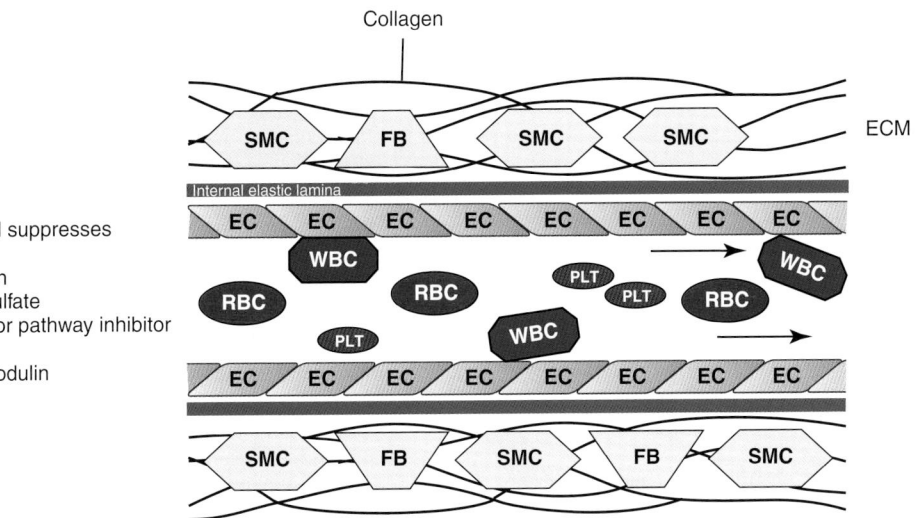

Fig. 38.3 Normal blood flow in intact vessels. Red blood cells *(RBCs)* and platelets flow near the center, and white blood cells *(WBCs)* marginate and roll. Endothelial cells and the extracellular matrix *(ECM)* provide several properties that suppress hemostasis. *EC,* Endothelial cell; *FB,* fibroblast; *PLT,* platelet; *SMC,* smooth muscle cell. (From Keohane EM, et al. *Rodak's Hematology.* 6th ed. St. Louis: Elsevier; 2020:185.)

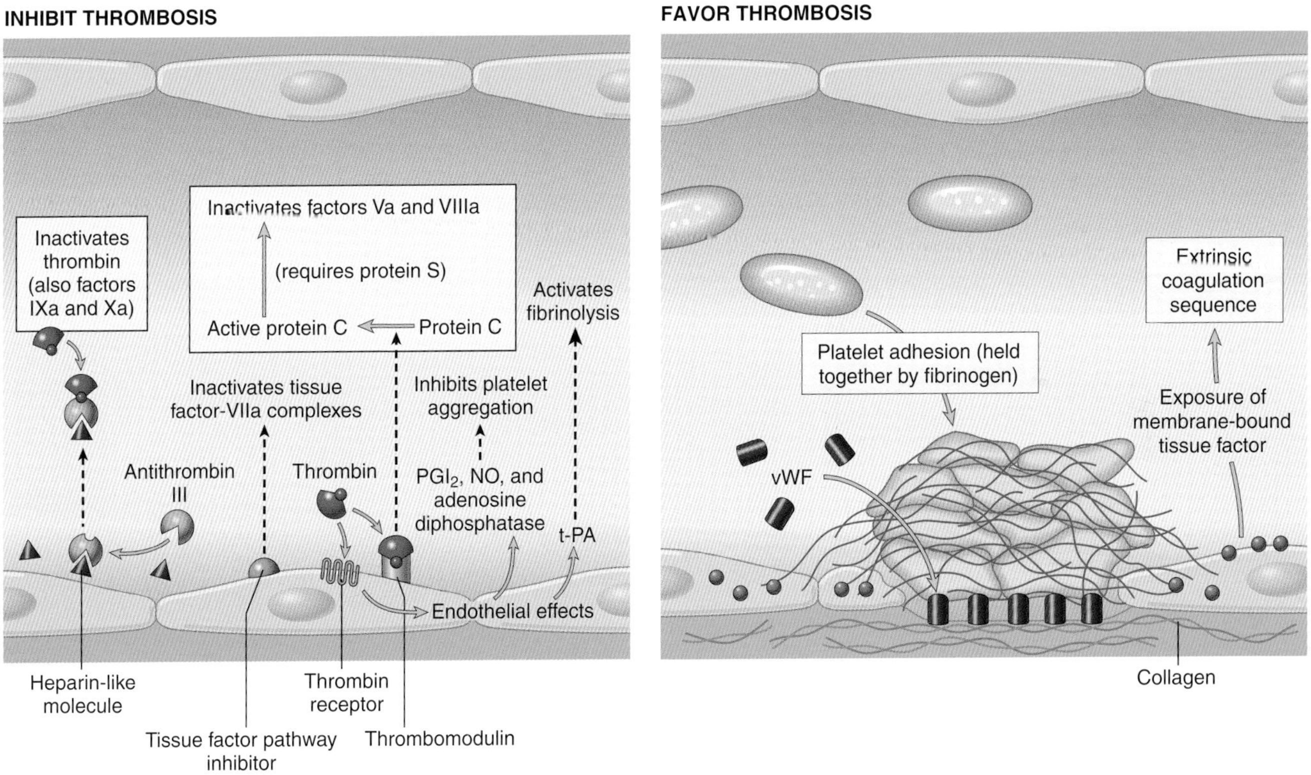

Normal ECM suppresses hemostasis:
• Prostacyclin
• Heparan sulfate
• Tissue factor pathway inhibitor
• Nitric oxide
• Thrombomodulin

INHIBIT THROMBOSIS

Inactivates factors Va and VIIIa

(requires protein S)

Active protein C ← Protein C

Inactivates thrombin (also factors IXa and Xa)

Activates fibrinolysis

Inactivates tissue factor-VIIa complexes

Inhibits platelet aggregation

Antithrombin III

Thrombin

PGI₂, NO, and adenosine diphosphatase

t-PA

Endothelial effects

Heparin-like molecule

Thrombin receptor

Tissue factor pathway inhibitor

Thrombomodulin

FAVOR THROMBOSIS

Extrinsic coagulation sequence

Platelet adhesion (held together by fibrinogen)

Exposure of membrane-bound tissue factor

vWF

Collagen

Fig. 38.4 Anticoagulant properties of normal endothelium *(left)* and procoagulant properties of injured or activated endothelium *(right)*. *NO,* nitric oxide; *PGI₂,* prostaglandin I₂ (prostacyclin); *t-PA,* tissue plasminogen activator; *vWF,* von Willebrand factor. Thrombin receptors are also called protease-activated receptors (PARs). (From Kumar V, et al. *Robbins Basic Pathology.* 10th ed. Philadelphia: Elsevier; 2018.)

The purpose of GpIb is to attach to vWF and attract platelets to the endothelial lining; vWF makes platelets "sticky" and allows platelets to adhere to the site of injury.

Under the influence of TF (a cofactor of the extrinsic clotting pathway), the platelet then undergoes a conformational transformation as it becomes activated (Fig. 38.5). The once disklike structure swells and becomes oval and irregular. From the platelet surface two other major

glycoproteins, IIb and IIIa (GpIIb/IIIa), project themselves outward. The purpose of the GpIIb-IIIa receptor complex is to link other activated platelets together in an effort to form a primary platelet plug. When this action is complete, the platelets form a mound whose only goal is to seal and heal the site of injury within the blood vessel.

As platelets undergo this metamorphosis, they release the α and dense granules, the contractile granules, thrombin, and many important mediators into the blood in an effort to promote procoagulant activity. All these mediators are responsible for platelet aggregation to form a primary unstable clot. When injury is minute and less threatening, this primary plug is enough to maintain hemostasis. When the injury is large, activation of the coagulation clotting cascade is required

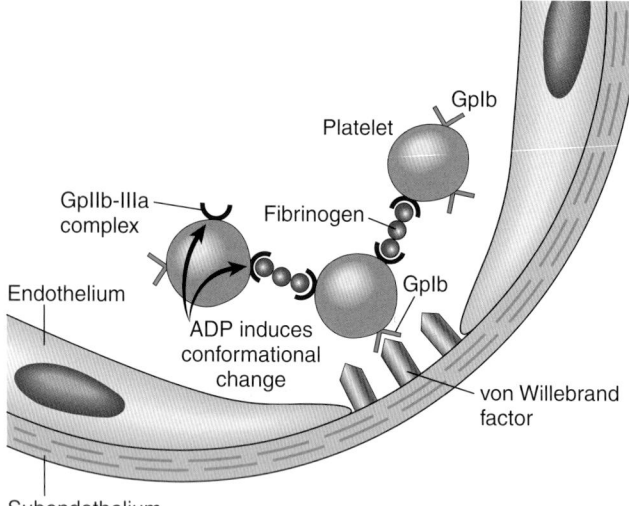

Fig. 38.5 Platelet adhesion and aggregation. Von Willebrand factor functions as an adhesion bridge between subendothelial collagen and the glycoprotein Ib *(GpIb)* platelet receptor. Platelet aggregation is accomplished by fibrinogen binding to platelet GpIIb-IIIa receptors on different platelets. Congenital deficiencies in the various receptors or bridging molecules lead to the diseases indicated in the colored boxes. *ADP,* Adenosine diphosphate. (From Kumar V, et al. *Robbins Basic Pathology.* 10th ed. Philadelphia: Elsevier; 2018:102.)

for permanent repair to create and stabilize a secondary clot to cease bleeding.[2]

The coagulation cascade illustrates the activation of cofactors (also referred to as zymogens) and their role in this process of hemostasis. Most cofactors are enzymes, with some exceptions (e.g., factors V and VIII). The coagulation factors circulate as inactive cofactors until they are activated to assist in the process of coagulation (Table 38.2). Activation of cofactors results from either tissue or organ damage and sets in motion a process that terminates in stabilization of hemorrhagic conditions in the absence of pathology. The factors are identified with Roman numerals for ease of interpretation.

The clotting pathways are thought to be two separate and distinct pathways (extrinsic and intrinsic) that worked independently of each other but in conjunction with platelet activity and the common coagulation pathway (Fig. 38.6). The extrinsic pathway (TF pathway) becomes activated by the release of TF when injury occurs outside the vessel wall (with organ trauma or crushing injuries). This section of the coagulation cascade consists of factor III (TF or thromboplastin) and factor VII (proconvertin).

When damage occurs outside of blood vessels, TF (factor III) activates proconvertin (factor VII), changing it to activated factor VII (VIIa). (When factor III activates factor VII, it is immediately inhibited by TF pathway inhibitor, so only a predetermined amount of factor VII is activated.) Once factor VII is activated, it in turn activates factor X (Stuart-Prower) of the common pathway. Factor X forms a complex with factor V (proaccelerin, a prothrombinase complex) activating factor II (prothrombin), which, when activated, becomes factor IIa (thrombin). Thrombin in turn activates factor I (fibrinogen) to form activated factor I (Ia, fibrin).

The intrinsic pathway (contact activation pathway) is initiated when damage occurs to the blood vessels themselves. The intrinsic pathway is initiated by prekallikrein, high molecular-weight kininogen (HMWK),

TABLE 38.2 Coagulation Factors

Factor	Factor Name	Synthesized	Vitamin K Dependent	Action
I	Fibrinogen	Liver	No	Form a clot
II	Prothrombin	Liver	Yes	When in active form, activates I, V, VII, XIII, platelets, and protein C
III	Tissue factor or thromboplastin	Vascular wall and extravascular cell membranes; released from traumatized cells	—	Cofactor of VII
IV	Calcium	Diet	—	Promotes clotting reactions
V	Proaccelerin	Liver	No	Cofactor of X; forms a prothrombinase complex
VI	(Unassigned)	—	—	—
VII	Proconvertin	Liver	Yes	Activates IX and X
VIII	Antihemophiliac	Liver	No	Cofactor to IX
vWF	von Willebrand	Endothelial cells	—	Mediates adhesion
IX	Christmas	Liver	Yes	Activates X
X	Stuart-Prower	Liver	Yes	Activates II, forms a prothrombinase complex with V
XI	Plasma thromboplastin antecedent	Liver	No	Activates IX
XII	Hageman	Liver	No	Activates XI
XIII	Fibrin stabilizing	Liver	No	Cross-links fibrin
Prekallikrein	Fletcher		—	Activates XII, cleaves HMWK
High-molecular-weight kininogen (HMWK)	Contact activation factor		—	Supports activation of prekallikrein, XII, XI

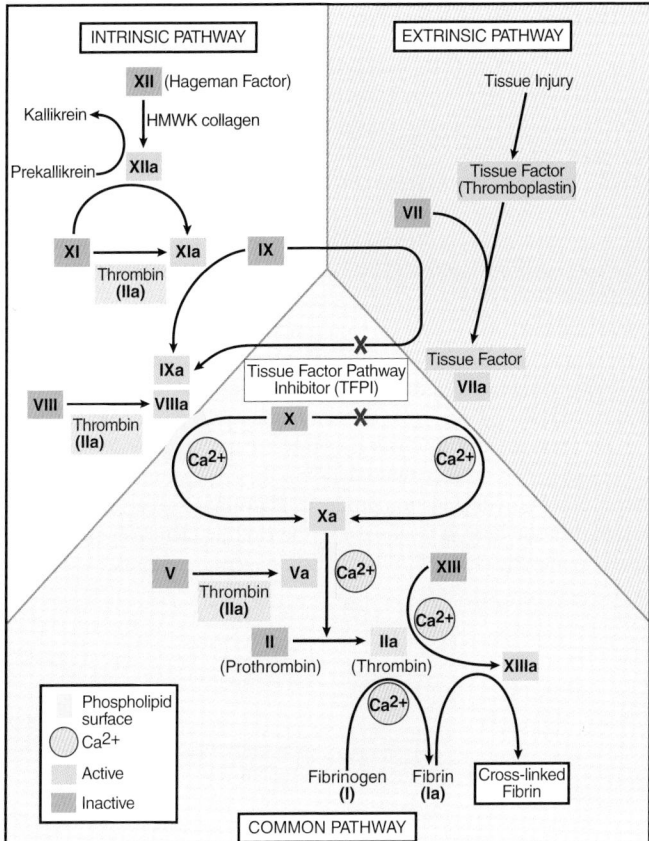

Fig. 38.6 The coagulation cascade. Factor IX can be activated by either factor XIa or factor VIIa. In laboratory tests activation is predominantly dependent on factor XIa, whereas in vivo, factor VIIa appears to be the predominant activator of factor IX. Factors in red boxes represent inactive molecules; activated factors, indicated with a lowercase *a*, are in green boxes. Note that thrombin (factor IIa) *(light blue boxes)* contributes to coagulation through multiple positive feedback loops. The red *X* denote points at which tissue factor pathway inhibitor (TFPI) inhibits activation of factor X and factor IX by factor VIIa. *Ca2+,* Calcium; *HMWK,* High-molecular-weight kininogen; *PL,* phospholipid. (From Kumar V, et al. *Robbins Basic Pathology.* 10th ed. Philadelphia: Elsevier; 2018:104.)

and by the activation of factor XII (Hageman). With the help of calcium (factor IV), the coagulation pathway initiates a domino effect. Each factor, once activated, affects its subsequent factor. Factor XII (Hageman) activates factor XI (plasma thromboplastin antecedent), which activates factor IX (Christmas), which then activates factor VIII (antihemophiliac factor), and ultimately (similar to the extrinsic pathway) merges at the common pathway and activates factor X. The result is the generation of fibrin from the activation of prothrombin to thrombin.

Conversion of prothrombin to thrombin is an important reaction for both coagulation pathways. Thrombin assists in activating factors V, VIII, I, and XIII and influences the recruitment of platelets to the injured area. Enough thrombin must be present to activate adequate fibrin to form a stable clot.

Thrombin also behaves as an anticoagulant. Thrombin (1) prevents runaway clot formation by releasing tissue plasminogen activator (tPA) from endothelial cells, (2) stimulates protein C and protein S to inhibit clot formation, and (3) forms a relationship with antithrombin III to interfere with coagulation.[1] The common pathway is the terminal pathway of the coagulation cascade. In the common pathway factor X has been activated by the intrinsic and extrinsic pathways. Factor

Cell-based theory of coagulation

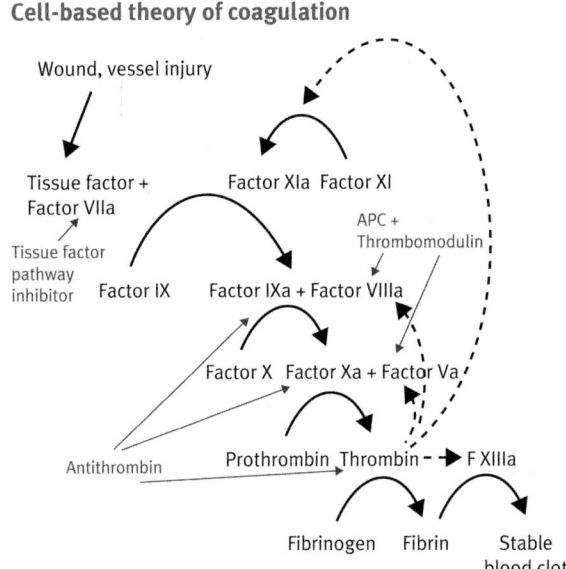

Tissue factor- Factor VIIa act as the initiation step on exposure to damaged endothelium.
The dotted arrows indicate amplification of cascade by thrombin.

The process of coagulation is regulated by antithrombin, tissue factor pathway inhibitor and activated protein C (APC).

Fig. 38.7 Cell-based theory of coagulation. (From Jobling L, Eyre L. Haemostasis, blood platelets and coagulation. *Anaesth Intensive Care Med.* 2013;41[2]:51–53.)

X requires the help of factor V (proaccelerin) and calcium to convert factor II (prothrombin) to its active-state thrombin (IIa). Thrombin then activates factor I (fibrinogen) to its active form, Ia (fibrin). Factor XIII (fibrin-stabilizing factor) is required to ensure the platelet plug will hold. Factor XIII helps form a cross-linked mesh within the platelet plug, increasing its strength. Fibrin (factor Ia) in conjunction with factor XIII finally secures a stable secondary plug, and bleeding stops. Once a clot is made, it retracts, eliminating its serum. As it retracts it weaves the edges of the vessel together, healing the site of injury.[2]

Most of the coagulation proteins are synthesized in the liver. Calcium, which is not a true factor, comes from diet; it is needed to "position" the coagulation factors on the surface of the platelet so clotting will ensue. vWF is synthesized in the endothelial cells, and factors II, VII, IX, and X are dependent on vitamin K for utilization.

CELL-BASED THEORY OF COAGULATION

The cell-based theory is a newer concept that hypothesizes *why* platelets and the extrinsic and intrinsic pathways of coagulation cascade do not work independently of one another but form a very interdependent relationship.[6] The theory posits that coagulation takes place on different cell surfaces that bear TF. These surfaces play a pivotal role in factor expression leading to hemostasis. The cell-based theory describes hemostasis as taking place in three phases: initiation, amplification, and propagation.

The initiation phase is triggered by injury to the endothelial surface (Fig. 38.7). When injury occurs, TF is exposed at the site of injury. In its presence, the endothelial surface of the blood vessel changes becoming acidic and making its phospholipid surface less repellent to platelets. TF down-regulates anticoagulants that reside in the subendothelial layer (e.g., antithrombin III, thrombomodulin) in an effort to promote coagulation.[7] This new medium enhances the many enzymatic processes that work to maintain hemostasis by encouraging aggregation and the activation of clotting factors to the site of injury. TF recruits platelets and activates factor VII.

In the cell-based theory, TF/VII reaction results in the activation of factors X (common pathway) and IX (intrinsic pathway). Factor X forms a complex with factor V, and together, these two activated factors are able to generate a small amount of thrombin for clot formation.[8] Only a small amount of thrombin is created because this reaction terminates almost immediately when tissue factor pathway inhibitor (TFPI) limits the amount of TF expressed. The activation of factor IX from the TF/VII complex does not participate in this initiation stage because IX does not act on TF-bearing cell surfaces.[7]

It is on the platelet cell surface that factor IX (generated from TF/VII) exerts its coagulation contribution to hemostasis. Factor IX attaches to the activated platelet cell surface and binds with a receptor, resulting in the activation of factor VIII, which in turn activates factor X. Additional thrombin is then produced.

As injury perpetuates and TF is expressed, platelets mobilize to the site of injury.[7] It is during the amplification phase that thrombin generation gains momentum and acceleration, and activation of clotting factors persists. Thrombin activates factors V, VIII, and IX.[6] Activated factor XI assists in generating even more factor IX on the platelet surface.[9] vWF promotes platelet aggregation through its adhesive properties with GpIb, and the expression of the GpIIb-IIIa pseudopods from the surface of platelets facilitates aggregation of additional platelets.

During the propagation phase, all coagulation factors are actively influencing one another, promoting coagulation, and activating prothrombin that results in a large burst of thrombin. Remember, enough thrombin must be present to convert fibrinogen to fibrin to form a stable secondary hemostatic plug. This burst of thrombin does just that.

The cell-based theory is a means of providing a more thorough understanding and an innovative interpretation of coagulation. It explains how cell surfaces do not just express coagulation factors; these surfaces participate in conjunction with platelets and the coagulation cascade pathways to maintain hemostasis. This theory also explains why certain deficiencies fail to cause bleeding, despite changes in laboratory values such as the prothrombin time (PT) or activated partial thromboplastin time (aPTT) indicative of coagulation problems.[6]

FIBRINOLYTIC SYSTEM

Once a disrupted vessel is sealed, there is no longer a need for a hemostatic plug. A counterbalance mechanism, the fibrinolytic system, exists to degrade fibrin. Initially, there is an increase in blood flow at the site of injury. This increase in blood flow washes away ADP and thromboxane A2 and other procoagulant mediators, which were initially present to encourage hemostasis and limit the size of the clot. Thrombin, which initially behaved as a procoagulant, now acts as an anticoagulant and activates additional anticoagulant mediators. TFPI stops the action of TF. Protein C and protein S inhibit coagulation factors III, V, and VIII. Antithrombin III inhibits thrombin activity by sequestering factors XII, XI, IX, and X. Antithrombin III is a mediator that corrals some of the factors present in the clotting cascade and takes them out of the clotting equation (Fig. 38.8). The clot manufactured is disrupted.

The process of fibrinolysis is highly regulated by plasma proteins (Fig. 38.9). A clot is composed primarily of plasminogen, plasmin, fibrin, and fibrin degradation products. Plasminogen is an enzyme synthesized in the liver. It is stored like the clotting factors in an inactive form. While the clot is forming, plasminogen incorporates itself into

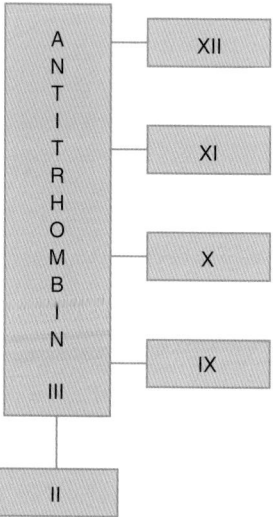

Fig. 38.8 Antithrombin III corrals clotting factors XII, XI, IX, and X. This influences factor II.

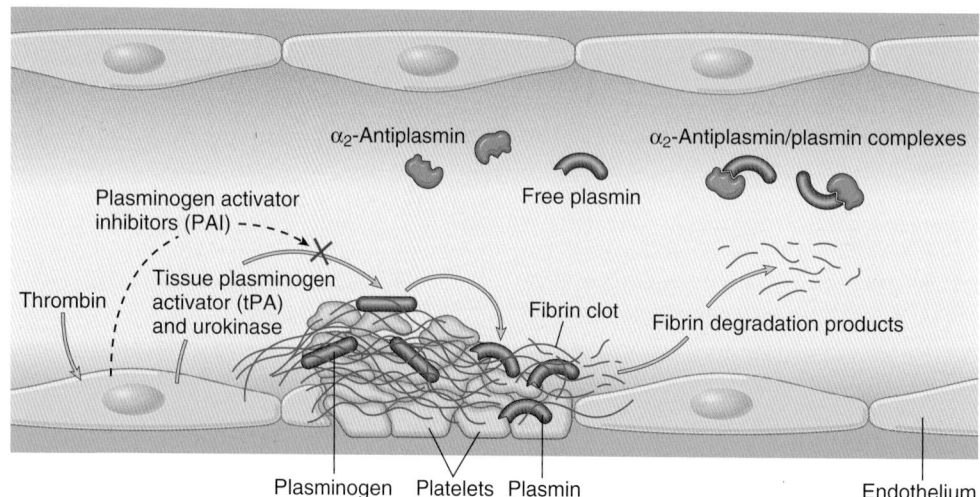

Fig. 38.9 The fibrinolytic system, illustrating various plasminogen activators and inhibitors. (From Kumar V, et al. *Robbins Basic Pathology.* 10th ed. Philadelphia: Elsevier; 2018:106.)

the clot. With the assistance of the body's own tPA and urokinase, plasminogen is activated to plasmin. Plasmin then acts on the fibrin causing fibrin to degrade into fibrin degradation products. The circulatory system removes the waste products of the clot. α-antiplasmin and tissue plasminogen activator inhibitor are important fibrinolytic mediators that stop the process of fibrinolysis when the clot has been digested.

Platelets, coagulation cofactors, and the fibrinolytic systems are dependent on each other to ensure a person does not bleed to death or clot to death at any given moment. This system of checks and balances maintains hemostasis when a breach in vascular integrity occurs.

ANESTHETIC IMPLICATIONS

Preoperative Considerations

The preoperative interview is the ideal time for the anesthesia provider to gather detailed information regarding the patient's health status. A thorough history and physical is the best way to identify patients at risk for surgical bleeding or those patients with thrombopoietic tendencies.[10] It is also during the interview that additional laboratory tests can be ordered to identify potential defects in hemostasis and to guide the decision regarding whether to order and/or administer blood products.

During the preoperative interview, it is important to ask questions directly related to bleeding: (1) Does the patient experience unusual bleeding or bruising (e.g., bleeding gums, epistaxis, mucous membrane bleeding, and bloody stools)? (2) Is there a history of previous bleeding with dental procedures? (3) Are there repeated spontaneous bleeding episodes or a history of excess bleeding that may have occurred after a minor procedure or childhood trauma? (4) Do familial bleeding tendencies exist? (5) Has there been a time when expected bleeding from a surgical procedure was more than anticipated?[4,11] These questions can reveal an undiagnosed inherited disorder of coagulation. Patients who have undiagnosed inherited coagulopathies may complain of hematomas, runaway bruising, and oozing even after the most minor injuries. An undetected preoperative bleeding tendency can lead to life-threatening blood loss during surgery.[4] Laboratory evaluation of platelets, coagulation, and fibrinolytic components can be screened with the commonly available coagulation tests.

When approaching the patient scheduled for surgery, a physical examination with a complete systems approach is necessary. The anesthesia provider must be alert to potential disruptions in hemostasis. Any overt physical sign of bleeding such as the appearance of bruising or petechial hemorrhages on the chest, abdomen, or upper extremities warrants further investigation. Small hemorrhages on the skin may also indicate the presence of small hemorrhages on other organs. Remember that the questionable coagulopathy can be related to any number of disruptions in the hemostasis process: a platelet problem, a factor deficiency, an inherited disorder of coagulation, the presence of circulating anticoagulants, or a disturbance in the fibrinolytic system.

During the physical assessment, disorders of malnutrition or liver insufficiency suggesting a vitamin K deficiency may be revealed. These disorders can influence coagulation and explain increased bleeding, even for the simplest surgery. Vitamin K is created from bacteria in the gut and is necessary for the formation of factors II, VII, IX, and X. When illness such as liver insufficiency, cirrhosis, absorption problems, and failure to secrete bile is present, the patient will be unable to form and use these factors for effective coagulation.

Patients with preexisting inherited disorders of coagulation must undergo an adequate preoperative workup prior to surgery. Consultation with a hematologist or transfusion specialist is strongly recommended. Patients with preexisting coagulation disorders require

considerable attention in the operating room. Damage to tissues may transpire during direct laryngoscopy, endotracheal intubation, peripheral or central line placement, and positioning or moving to and from the operating room table. If general surgery is anticipated, special attention must be made to ensure minimal damage to soft tissues occurs.

The preoperative use of many medications—prescribed, over-the-counter, and herbal remedies—can interfere with normal platelet function and coagulation (Box 38.1). The anesthesia provider must ascertain whether the patient regularly ingests medications that might interfere with normal coagulation. Additionally, the provider must be aware of the last time the patient ingested such medications. For example, many patients take aspirin for a number of reasons. Historically, it has been recommended that aspirin be held for 7 to 10 days prior to surgery. Current recommendations are discussed in detail later in this chapter. Aspirin directly affects the life of the platelet by irreversibly inhibiting cyclooxygenase resulting in decreased platelet function.[12] Nonsteroidal antiinflammatory drugs (NSAIDs) also inhibit cyclooxygenase, albeit reversibly, and the recommendation is to withhold NSAIDs for approximately 24 to 48 hours, depending on the drugs half-life, to avoid any bleeding effects in surgery[13,14] (Fig. 38.10).

A preoperative discussion between the patient, surgeon, and anesthesia provider must occur regarding transfusion requirements during surgery. Informing patients about the safety, screening measures, and

---

BOX 38.1 Frequently Encountered Medications That Influence Coagulation

Anticoagulants
- Unfractionated heparin
- Low-molecular-weight heparin
- Coumarin derivatives
- Direct thrombin inhibitors
- Direct factor Xa inhibitors

Procoagulants
- Vitamin K

Antiplatelets
- Nonsteroidal antiinflammatory drugs
- Persantine
- Thienopyridine

Antifibrinolytics
- Aminocaproic acid
- Tranexamic acid

Nonherbal Dietary
- Vitamin K
- Vitamin E
- Coenzyme Q10
- Zinc
- Omega-3 fatty acids

Herbal
- Garlic
- Ginger
- Ginkgo
- Feverfew
- Fish oil
- Flaxseed oil
- Black cohosh
- Cranberry

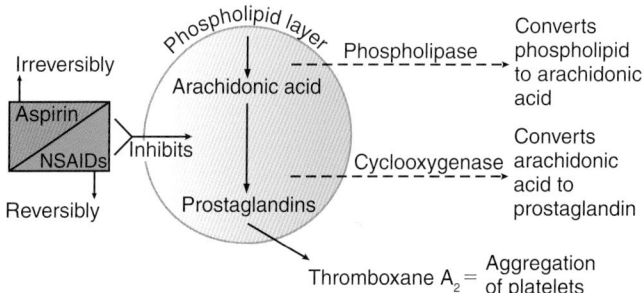

Fig. 38.10 Schematic illustration depicting the mechanism and site of action of aspirin and nonsteroidal antiinflammatory drugs (NSAIDs).

TABLE 38.3 Possible Causes and Treatment of Hemostatic Disorders

	CLINICAL COAGULATION TESTS						
BL	**aPTT**	**PT**	**BT**	**PC**	**Fib**	**Possible Cause**	**Treatment**
	Abn					Factor VIII, heparin, "lupus anticoagulant," poor sample	No treatment
+	Abn					Factors XI, IX, VIII, heparin therapy	FFP, protamine
+	Abn	Abn				Factors V, X, II, dysfibrinogenemia, heparin, coumarins	FFP, cryoprecipitate, protamine
+		Abn				Factor VII	FFP
+	Abn		Abn			von Willebrand disease	Desmopressin acetate, cryoprecipitate
+	Abn	Abn	Abn		Low	Hypofibrinogenemia	FFP, cryoprecipitate
+			Abn	Abn		Thrombocytopenia	Platelet concentrate (8–10 units)
+			Abn			Thrombocytopathy, aspirin, NSAIDs	Platelet concentrate
+	Abn	Abn	Abn	Abn	Abn	DIC, severe liver disease, dilutional coagulopathy	FFP, cryoprecipitate, platelet concentrate, whole blood

+, Increased clinical bleeding; *Abn*, abnormal result; *aPTT*, activated partial thromboplastin time; *BL*, bleeding; *BT*, bleeding time; *DIC*, disseminated intravascular coagulation; *FFP*, fresh frozen plasma; *Fib*, fibrinogen; *NSAIDs*, nonsteroidal antiinflammatory drugs; *PC*, platelet count; *PT*, prothrombin time.

TABLE 38.4 Coagulation Tests

Laboratory Test	Value*	Description
Bleeding time	3–7 min	Measures platelet function: adhesion, aggregation Not considered a routine test Modest prolongations do not predict surgical bleeding Altered by aspirin and NSAIDs*
Platelet count	150,000–350,000 mm^3	Thrombocytopenic: <100,000 mm^3 Surgical risk: <50,000 mm^3 Spontaneous bleeding: <20,000 mm^3
Prothrombin time (PT)	Normal: Control Average Normal: 12–14 sec	Value is reagent dependent Prolonged with: • Extrinsic pathway disorder • Common pathway disorder Altered by coumarin derivatives*
Activated partial thromboplastin time (aPTT) (intrinsic and common pathway)	Average normal: 25–32 sec	Prolonged with: • Intrinsic pathway disorder • Common pathway disorder Altered by heparin and Lovenox*
Thrombin time (common pathway)	8–12 sec	Measures fibrinogen-to-fibrin reaction
Activated clotting time (ACT)	80–150 sec	Guides anticoagulation dosing
Fibrinogen	>150 mg/dL; 200–350 mg/mL	Measures fibrinogen level
Fibrinogen (degradation products)	<10 mcg/mL	Measures byproducts from clot dissolution
D-dimer	<500 mg/mL	Measures degradation products secondary to fibrinolysis
Thromboelastogram		Measures global hemostasis
Antithrombin III	80%–120%	Measures antithrombin III levels; decreased level may explain subtherapeutic heparin. Severely depressed in DIC

*Values may vary among laboratories.
DIC, Disseminated intravascular coagulation; *NSAIDs*, nonsteroidal antiinflammatory drugs.

risks of blood administration cannot be ignored. A small percentage of patients will have to contend with the negative sequelae of transfusion therapy (e.g., hepatitis, human immunodeficiency virus [HIV], and bacterial transmission) despite careful screening and handling. In situations with emergent or trauma patients, many times a preoperative interview is unattainable, and the provider must rely purely on information supplied by family members (if present), physical assessment, and laboratory analysis.

Laboratory Tests

Routine laboratory tests must be evaluated preoperatively. They serve to guide the clinician in determining whether a coagulation disorder exists (Table 38.3). Laboratory tests should be ordered on an individual basis, considering the patient's history and planned surgical procedure.

The most frequently assessed tests are the bleeding time, platelet count, PT, and aPTT (Table 38.4). Together, these tests evaluate vascular contraction, platelet function, coagulation, and the fibrinolytic system. Results of these routine tests must fall within the normal range. If they are outside normal range, there must be a reasonable explanation, and adequate measures must be taken to correct or control hemostasis before bringing the patient into the operating room. For example, if the patient requires surgery but not emergently, vitamin K can be administered 4 to 6 hours prior to surgery. If the risk of bleeding is moderate, a type and crossmatch of the blood may be preferred to a type and screen. If the patient requires surgery emergently, ordering blood components such as packed RBCs (PRBCs), fresh frozen plasma (FFP), platelets, and cryoprecipitate may be advisable.

The bleeding time evaluates the capability of microvascular contraction and the function of platelets. When vascular injury occurs, the initial response from the blood vessels is to contract, and the response of the platelets is to adhere to the site of injury. If either of these two processes is compromised, prolonged bleeding will occur, resulting in inadequate hemostasis.

The bleeding time was once thought to be the best indicator of bleeding risk. The use of a bleeding time test, however, is open to much scrutiny, and there are many reasons to question its use and interpretation.[15] In the absence of drug ingestion a prolonged bleeding time suggests primary hemostasis abnormality, and further investigation is recommended. Although the bleeding time is a means of evaluating vascular integrity and platelet function, it is important to appreciate that a prolonged bleeding time is not a good predictor of bleeding or a sign that an abnormality is present.[16] In addition, an isolated prolonged value is not a reason to cancel or delay a surgical procedure.

The platelet count is the actual number of platelets present in blood per cubic millimeter. A normal platelet count does not imply normal platelet function exists, only how many platelets are present in plasma. It is used to evaluate patients who, when examined, have petechiae or unexplained spontaneous bleeding, and to monitor thrombocytopenia (low platelet count). The platelet's primary role is to maintain vascular integrity, aggregate when a plug is necessary to stop bleeding, and help initiate the clotting pathways. A normal platelet count is 150,000 to 300,000/mm³.[2] Patients are considered thrombocytopenic at counts less than 100,000 mm³. There are varying degrees of thrombocytopenia that must be considered preoperatively. Platelet counts greater than 100,000 are sufficient for hemostasis. When the platelet count declines to 50,000/mm³, spontaneous bleeding rarely occurs, but one should suspect prolonged bleeding under surgical conditions.[17] A platelet count less than 20,000 is considered a critical level, and spontaneous bleeding is likely to occur.[18,19]

The PT is used to evaluate the efficiency of the extrinsic factors (III and VII) and common coagulation pathway (factors X, V, II, I) in generating enough thrombin to form fibrin to create a stable clot. The PT is specific to the extrinsic pathway of the clotting cascade. It is the most commonly used test to monitor oral anticoagulant therapy (e.g., the coumarin derivatives). The PT will be prolonged when patients have abnormalities or are deficient in factors specific to the extrinsic and common clotting pathways (III, VII, X, IX, II, I).[5]

Despite the frequent assessment of the PT value preoperatively, this laboratory value has drawbacks. The PT is not a very sensitive test. The PT also fails to identify the specific factor defect in the hemostatic system. It only identifies an existing problem that may or may not cause bleeding.

The international normalized ratio (INR) evaluates the extrinsic and common pathway independently of various reagents used in different laboratory settings and in different areas of the world. The normal INR is 1.5 to 2.5. Many institutions report both PT and INR values.

The aPTT is a test used to evaluate the efficiency of the intrinsic coagulation pathway (factors XII, XI, IX, and VIII) and the common coagulation pathway (factors X, V, II, I, and ultimately XIII) to form

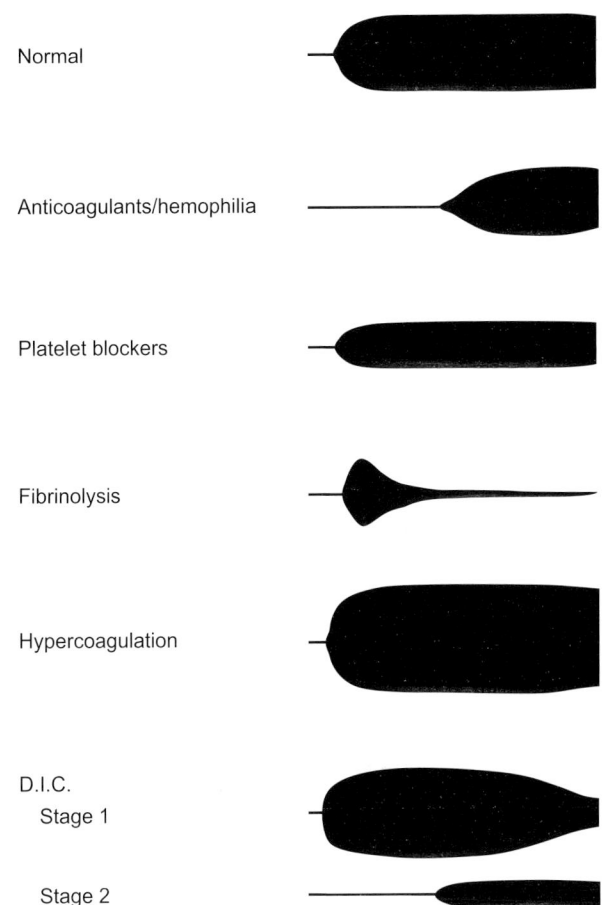

Fig. 38.11 Measurements taken by the thromboelastogram (TEG) determine the component that is required to treat coagulopathy. *DIC,* Disseminated intravascular coagulation. (From Cameron JL, Cameron AM. *Current Surgical Therapy.* 13th ed. Philadelphia: Elsevier; 2020:1251.)

fibrin and eventually a stable clot. The aPTT can identify abnormalities in all factors except III and VII. It is also used to monitor anticoagulation status when heparin therapy is used. The aPTT can be prolonged by abnormalities, deficiencies, or inhibitors of any intrinsic or common pathway defect. Factor concentration must be decreased 30% before evidence of a prolonged PT or an aPTT can be appreciated.[1,17]

Any factor deficiency in either limb of the clotting cascade can alter the PT and/or aPTT, but this does not imply that any prediction of an individual patient risk of bleeding can be anticipated.[7] For example, a decrease in factor XII will demonstrate an increase in aPTT but will not cause bleeding.[6] A decrease in factor XI may or may not cause abnormal bleeding. However, a decrease in either factor VIII or IX will definitely cause bleeding with injury. This is seen in hemophilia.

The activated clotting time (ACT) is a simple, quick test that can be used in surgery to monitor the ability of blood to clot. The ACT is also used to regulate heparin therapy. The normal ACT is 90 to 150 seconds. However, the ACT is not a sensitive test.

The thrombin time is a screening tool for assessing the ending phase of coagulation. Because fibrinogen can be assessed directly, analysis of the thrombin time is less emphasized.

The thromboelastogram (TEG) measures the process of clot formation over time (Fig. 38.11). The benefit of this test is its ability to evaluate (1) platelet reactions, (2) coagulation, and (3) fibrinolysis. A blood specimen is collected and placed in a machine that measures the speed at which a clot forms. The results of the TEG provide an indication of

TABLE 38.5   Blood/Coagulation Factor Replacements for Achieving Hemostasis

Resource	Dose and Effects	Product Content	Use
Packed red blood cells	1 unit (350 mL) increases hemoglobin level by 1 g/dL (10 g/L)	Red blood cells	Symptomatic anemia (guideline hemoglobin level < 6 g/dL if healthy), massive hemorrhage, decreased oxygen-carrying capacity
Platelets	1 unit (250 mL) increases the platelet count by 30,000–60,000/mm³	Platelets, clotting factors	Thrombocytopenia, massive hemorrhage, platelet function deficit
Fresh frozen plasma	1 unit (250 mL)	All coagulation factors, especially factors II, VII, IX, and X, proteins C and S, and antithrombin III	Reversal of warfarin therapy, massive transfusion, thrombotic thrombocytopenic purpura, coagulation factor deficiencies, antithrombin III deficiency
Cryoprecipitate	20 mL contains 200 mg fibrinogen, 70–80 units of factor VIII	Fibrinogen, VIII, and XIII	Hypofibrinogenemia, massive hemorrhage
Desmopressin	0.3–0.4 mcg/kg	Stimulates release of von Willebrand factor from endothelial cells	Uremic platelet dysfunction, von Willebrand disease
Vitamin K	Oral: 2.5–5 mg Parenteral: 10 mg	Stimulates production of factors II, VII, IX, and X	Liver dysfunction, reversal of warfarin therapy
Protamine sulfate	1 mg neutralizes 100 units of heparin	Heparin antagonist	Reversal of heparin therapy
Factor VII	50 mcg/kg (20–90 mcg/kg)	Recombinant factor VIIa	Massive hemorrhage, hemophilia A and B that have developed antibodies to traditional replacement therapy
Four-factor prothrombin complex concentrates	25–50 IU/kg	Factors II, VII, IX, X.	Reversal of warfarin or direct oral anticoagulants therapy
Activated prothrombin complex concentrates	50–100 IU/kg (max single dose)	Activated factor X Unactivated II, VII, IX, and X	Hemophilia A and B that have developed antibodies to traditional replacement therapy
Tranexamic acid	10–15 mg/kg loading dose Second dose 2–3 hr after loading dose or 1 mg/kg/hr infusion for 6–8 hr	Plasmin inhibitor	Fibrinolysis inhibitor
Aminocaproic acid	0.1 g/kg loading dose, followed by 1 g/hr infusion	Plasmin inhibitor	Fibrinolysis inhibitor

Adapted from Lawson JH, Bennett KM. Coagulopathy and hemorrhage. In: Cronenwett JL, et al., eds. *Rutherford's Vascular Surgery*. 8th ed. Philadelphia: Elsevier; 2014; Mayeux J, Alwon K, Collins S, et al. Tranexamic acid in anesthetic management of surgical procedures. *AANA J.* 2016;84(3):201–209.

(1) clot strength, (2) platelet number and function, (3) intrinsic pathway defects, (4) thrombin formation, and (5) the rate of fibrinolysis.[2]

Laboratory tests are only as good as the individual interpreting them and many times will not adequately reflect the potential to bleed or thrombose. The use of coagulation tests is best interpreted when patients are without pathology, are not on any medications that could disrupt the laboratory value measured, and are assessed in conjunction with physical assessment and clinical judgment. It is prudent to consult with a hematologist when there is any suspicion of the potential for abnormal bleeding in surgery or if a coagulation disorder exists. Coagulation tests can be performed in the operating room and may serve as a guide during critical volume loss and coagulopathic alterations.

Intraoperative Period

One important focus in the operating room is to recognize and efficiently control blood loss. Frequent evaluation of the patient's clinical status, surgical site, sponges, canisters, and the operating room floor cannot be overemphasized.[17] The surgeon and anesthesia provider are equally responsible in communicating that persistent oozing or frank bleeding is occurring. It is this open communication that helps the surgical team recognize problems and rapidly intervene by having blood components in the room, rechecking ABO compatibility, and anticipating the need for coagulation factor replacement if transfusion therapy is necessary.

The most commonly transfused blood components are RBCs, platelets, FFP, and cryoprecipitate (Table 38.5). The major reasons for transfusion therapy in the operating room are to replace volume and coagulation factors and improve oxygen-carrying capacity.[20] Each component carries its own concerns.

PRBCs are transfused to improve tissue oxygenation. Although the oxygen-carrying capacity of red cells decreases with the length of storage, it improves when 2,3-diphosphoglycerate (2,3-DPG) is regenerated once transfused. Platelets are provided to patients when a deficit is appreciated or when massive transfusion is required. Platelets can be given as a single-donor plateletpheresis pack or collected and pooled from multiple donors (random-donor platelets).

Platelet Infusion Guidelines

The recommended dose for platelet replacement is one plateletpheresis pack per each 10 kg of patient weight. This dose should increase the platelet count by approximately 5000 to 10,000 mm³.[5,17] Whereas the normal life span of a platelet is 7 to 10 days, the life span of a donated platelet is only 4 to 5 days.[9]

The American Society of Anesthesiologists Transfusion Task Force recommends[17] that (1) platelet transfusion may be indicated despite an apparently adequate platelet count or in the absence of a platelet count if there is known or suspected platelet dysfunction (e.g., the presence of potent antiplatelet agents, pulmonary bypass, congenital platelet dysfunction, and bleeding), and (2) in surgical or obstetric patients, platelet transfusion is rarely indicted if the platelet count is known to be greater than 100,00/μL and is usually indicated when the count is less than 50,000/μL in the presence of excessive bleeding.[17] Compatible plateletpheresis is recommended, but when matched platelets are unavailable, unmatched platelets can be given; however, this incompatibility shortens the life span of the platelet.[3,20] There are no high-quality data to guide plasma and platelet transfusions around the time of procedures. Current intensivist consensus expert opinion recommends administration of plasma in moderate- to high-risk procedures when INR is greater than 1.5. They recommend platelet transfusion in low-risk procedures when the platelet count is less than 20,000/μL for average-risk procedures when the platelet count is less than 50,000/mm[3], and for procedures involving the central nervous system when the platelet count is less than 100,000/mm[3].[21] When pooled platelets are administered to women of childbearing age, Rh sensitization can occur, and administration of RHO (D) immune globulin may be necessary prior to discharge.

Platelets carry the greatest risk of bacterial transmission.[21,22] Platelets are stored for 4 to 5 days at room temperature, providing an excellent medium for the growth and reproduction of bacteria. Standard protocols for blood banks and transfusion services require that a method be in place to detect bacterial contamination of platelets.[21,23]

Fresh Frozen Plasma Infusion Guidelines

FFP is the fluid portion of whole blood, separated, then frozen to preserve coagulation factors, and subsequently thawed on use. FFP contains all the clotting factors and naturally occurring inhibitors.[24] It does not provide platelet replacement. The average volume in a unit of FFP is 200 to 250 mL. FFP must be ABO plasma compatible whenever possible.

FFP is transfused for the following reasons: (1) correction of excessive microvascular bleeding (i.e., coagulopathy) in the presence of an INR greater than 2.0, and in the absence of heparin; (2) correction of excessive microvascular bleeding secondary to coagulation factor deficiency in patients transfused with more than one blood volume (~70 mL/kg) and when PT or INR and aPTT cannot be obtained in a timely fashion; (3) urgent reversal of warfarin therapy when PCCs are not available; and (4) correction of known coagulation factor deficiencies for which specific concentrates are unavailable. FFP is not indicated if (1) PT or INR and aPTT are normal or (2) solely for augmentation of plasma volume or albumin concentration. Administer FFP in doses calculated to achieve a minimum of 30% of plasma factor concentration. Four to five platelet concentrates, 1 unit single-donor apheresis platelets, or 1 unit fresh whole blood provide a quantity of coagulation factors similar to that contained in 1 unit of FFP.[17,20,24] Dilutional coagulopathies increase when blood is diluted to at least 30% or when a patient loses more than one volume of blood, indicating that only one-third of the coagulation factors are present.[25] This deficit is reflected in laboratory values. Laboratory analysis will reveal the need for FFP by a PT and aPTT prolonged more than 1.5 times normal. The use of FFP for volume replacement is contraindicated. Safety screening for FFP is the same as for RBCs.

Cryoprecipitate Infusion Guidelines

Cryoprecipitate is the precipitate collected off the top of FFP as it is thawed. Cryoprecipitate is then refrozen and thawed on use. It is rich in fibrinogen and contains factors VIII, XIII, and fibronectin. The current guidelines recommend cryoprecipitate for the following: (1) when a test of fibrinogen activity indicates a fibrinolysis; (2) when the fibrinogen concentration is less than 80 to 100 mg/dL in the presence of excessive bleeding; (3) as an adjunct in massively transfused patients

when fibrinogen concentrations cannot be measure in a timely fashion; and (4) for patients with congenital fibrinogen deficiencies. The guidelines also recommend that when possible, decisions regarding patients with congenital fibrinogen deficiencies should be made in consultation with the patient's hematologist. Transfusion of cryoprecipitate is rarely indicated if fibrinogen concentration is greater than 150 mg/dL in non-pregnant patients. Treat bleeding patients with von Willebrand disease (vWD) types 1 and 2A with desmopressin and subsequently with specific vWF/FVIII concentrate, if available. Cryoprecipitate should be administered if there is no response to or availability of desmopressin or vWF/FIII concentrate. Treat bleeding patients with vWD types 2B, 2M, 2N, and 3 with specific vWF/FVIII concentrate, if available. If vWF/FVIII concentrate is not available, cryoprecipitate is indicated.[17]

It is preferable to transfuse platelets, FFP, and cryoprecipitate with adherence to ABO compatibility to avoid hemolytic reactions, but there are times when this practice is impractical. When massive transfusion occurs, one should be alert to the risk of hemolytic reaction. In addition to viral screening for donor units, the institution of solvent detergents, psoralen derivatives, and methylene blue are being evaluated as a means to decrease emerging viral contaminations, especially when blood products are pooled. The effect of these additives on platelets, FFP, and cryoprecipitate is still under investigation.[21,23]

Transfusion Guidelines

There is no magic number or an absolute transfusion "trigger" for blood component administration. There are few if any fixed guidelines or practice standards for transfusion therapy. There are, however, many suggested guidelines and protocols that vary among individual institutions. Past literature recommends a hemoglobin (Hgb) of 10 g/dL as an indicator for RBC transfusion, but transfusion delivery based on one isolated laboratory value without regard to the patient's overall health status is irresponsible.[26] A Hgb value of 8 g/dL and even 6 g/dL may be acceptable when ischemia or risk factors for cardiovascular disease are not evident.[17,20] Strong randomized controlled trial evidence suggests the safety of restrictive transfusion triggers. As a consequence, a Hgb transfusion trigger of less than 7 g/dL is recommended for high-risk patients.[25]

There are also alternatives available to reduce or allay allogenic component replacement: preoperative autologous donation, acute normovolemic hemodilution, blood cell salvage, and recombinant factor VII.[27-29]

Recombinant factor VII was approved by the US Food and Drug Administration (FDA) in 1999 for hemophilia A (factor VIII) and B (factor IX), inhibitor disorders of factors VIII and IX, factor VII deficiency, and as a universal hemostatic agent.[8,30-32] Its off-label use has successfully treated coagulation insufficiencies associated with platelet dysfunction, intracranial hemorrhage, prostate surgery, and trauma.[33]

The exact mode of action of factor VII is undetermined. Both the classic coagulation cascade and the cell-based theory agree that factor VII enhances thrombin generation by augmenting TF/VII at the site of vessel injury and on the surface of the platelet.[6,30,31] Administration ultimately boosts thrombin to form fibrin for clot stabilization. The recommended dose of factor VII for hemophilia is 90 to 120 mcg/kg. There is no definitive dose for use in the operating room for patients without prior coagulation disorders, but 20 to 45 mcg/kg has been suggested.[8]

Factor VII will reverse prolonged INR, but it fails to replace all the clotting factors.[30] The anesthesia provider must remain vigilant intraoperatively, providing interventions that would prevent acidosis and hypothermia, both of which can interrupt the efficacy of the drug.[30,31,34] Patients have experienced cerebrovascular accidents, myocardial infarctions (MIs), pulmonary emboli, and arterial and venous thromboemboli. Factor VII should be used cautiously in any patient predisposed to thrombosis. The indications for the use of factor VII remain limited, and the treatment is very expensive.[17,24,32,33,35] An extensive discussion of transfusion management practices can be found in Chapter 22.

Postoperative Management

Patients should be reassessed in the postanesthesia care unit and again within 24 hours of surgery. Unrecognized bleeding can thus be identified and corrected before the patient deteriorates. Evaluations of (1) the patient's color and mentation, (2) trends in vital signs (with specific attention to tachycardia or hypotension), (3) urine output, (4) hypothermia, (5) hemodynamic values such as central venous pressure, (6) laboratory values, and (7) dressings and/or drain volume must be judiciously monitored.

SPECIFIC DISORDERS

Bleeding diathesis can result from any number of deficiencies in coagulation. A few disorders encountered in practice are described here, as well as points to consider when dealing with a patient requiring anticoagulant therapy. Commonly obtained tests to assess bleeding risk include PT, aPTT, and platelet count. PT and aPTT are tests that were developed to test the integrity of the coagulation pathway and do not predict perioperative bleeding. Abnormal platelet count, whether thrombocytopenia (<150,000) or thrombocytosis (>440,000), has been associated with a higher risk of perioperative bleeding. Other available tests include bleeding time, platelet function monitoring, thrombin time (TT), reptilase time, fibrinogen, and D-dimer.[36] INR is used to assess the effect of anticoagulants.

Von Willebrand Disease

vWD is a rare bleeding disorder that is inherited or may be acquired secondary to cardiovascular, malignant, or immunologic diseases. There are several subtypes. Acquired von Willebrand syndrome (AvWS) has similar laboratory findings: a decreased vWF antigen, vWF ristocetin cofactor activity, or factor VIII. Three mechanisms have been proposed[36]: (1) autoimmune clearance or inhibition of vWF for lymphoproliferative diseases, monoclonal gammopathies, systemic lupus erythematosus, other autoimmune disorders, and some cancers; (2) increased proteolysis of vWF caused by increased shear stress from ventricular septal defect, aortic stenosis, or primary pulmonary hypertension; and (3) increased binding of vWF to platelets or other cell surfaces. This large plasma glycoprotein mediates the adhesion of platelets at sites of vascular injury and binds and stabilizes factor VIII.

Inherited vWD patients are characterized by lifelong bleeding episodes, whereas a sudden onset of bleeding symptoms occurs in patients with acquired disease, which can induce acute bleeding episodes during critical surgical procedures.[37]

vWF is a heterogeneous multinumeric glycoprotein that serves two main functions: to facilitate platelet adhesion and to behave as a plasma carrier for factor VIII of the coagulation cascade.[36] Synthesis of vWF takes place in the endothelial cells and megakaryocytes.[37,38]

Similar to many coagulopathies, vWD has varying degrees of severity: mild, moderate, and severe. In the milder or moderate forms, regular or spontaneous bleeding is not evident but is likely after surgery or when trauma occurs.[10] In the more severe form of vWD, spontaneous epistaxis and oral, gastrointestinal, and genitourinary bleeding can be relentless.

As noted previously, most patients with vWD exhibit a prolonged bleeding time, a deficiency in vWF and factor VIII, decreased vWF activity measured by a ristocetin (an antibiotic) cofactor (RCoF) assay, and decreased factor VIII coagulant activity (VIII:C).[39]

BOX 38.2   Perioperative Treatment of von Willebrand Disease

- The treatment plan should be made according to the severity of disease and the type of surgery.
- *Major surgery:* Achieve 100% vWF preoperatively and maintain trough levels of 50% until adequate wound healing.
- *Minor surgery:* Achieve 60% vWF level preoperatively and trough daily levels of 30% until adequate wound healing.
- *Dental extractions:* Achieve 60% vWF level preoperatively.
- *Delivery and puerperium:* 80%–100% vWF level predelivery and trough levels of 30% for 3–4 days.
- In type 1 vWD with vWF level >10 IU/dL, desmopressin is the treatment of choice because it produces a complete or partial response in >90% of patients. Can be given within 40–60 min of surgery. Desmopressin increases endothelial cell release of factor VIII, vWF, and plasminogen activator. Goal vWF should be 80–100 IU/dL and to raise factor VIII. Dosing consideration for tachyphylaxis should be made as a result of depletion of endothelial stores.
- Types 2 and 3 require vWF concentrate administration.
- Tranexamic acid is also an important adjunctive therapy as either intravenous or oral therapy.
- Cryoprecipitate can be used; however, ristocetin cofactor activity level should not exceed >50% and should be monitored while bleeding is controlled.
- If properly corrected, pharmacologic antithrombotic prophylaxis should be considered postoperatively.

Adapted from Kim J, et al. Perioperative approach to anticoagulants and hematologic disorders. *Anesthesiol Clin.* 2016;34(1):101–125.

Treatment options to control acute hemorrhages or to prevent bleeding complications during surgery include desmopressin, FVIII/vWF concentrates, high-dose intravenous (IV) immunoglobulins, and plasma exchange. Desmopressin is a synthetic analogue of vasopressin that boosts plasma levels of factor VIII and vWF. As the half-life of vWF is reduced in AvWS, high doses of FVIII/vWF concentrates administered at frequent intervals may be necessary during bleeding episodes. Perioperative treatment of vWD is outlined in Box 38.2.[36]

Hemophilia

Hemophilia is an X-linked hematologic recessive disorder characterized by unpredictable bleeding patterns. Patients are either deficient in factor VIII (hemophilia A) or factor IX (hemophilia B). Hemophilia affects males almost exclusively, although females carry the gene for the disease. Patients with hemophilia A are grouped as mild (excessive bleeding after trauma or surgery), moderate (rarely have extensive, unprovoked bleeding), and severe (absence of factor VIII in the plasma). Hemophiliacs exhibit spontaneous bleeding, muscle hematomas, and pain at joint sites. Continued joint bleeding often results in decreased range of motion and progressive joint arthropathy and often requires orthopedic surgical intervention throughout life.[40]

In the past, the life expectancy for the hemophiliac was short. Because hemophiliacs were deficient in factors VIII and IX, they required blood component transfusion to replace the deficient or missing factors. The only factor components available were FFP and cryoprecipitate. Screening tests for donated blood units were unavailable, and patient mortality was high. Many hemophiliacs contracted transmissible diseases such as hepatitis and HIV and ultimately died from sequelae of blood transfusion therapy.[40] Furthermore, hemophiliacs were termed high risk for most surgical procedures and often turned down for many elective procedures. Today, blood components

Adapted from Kim J, et al. Perioperative approach to anticoagulants and hematologic disorders. *Anesthesiol Clin.* 2016;34(1):101–125.

BOX 38.3 Perioperative Management of the Hemophilic Patient

- No procedure is too minor for adequate hemostasis planning, including dental procedures, endoscopy with biopsy, arterial blood gas, or arterial lines.
- Preoperative assessment of inhibitor screening and inhibitor assay should be completed within 1 wk of surgery.
- Elective procedures should be scheduled early in the day and early in the week to ensure adequate laboratory support and availability of factor concentrates (or plasma).
- Adequate laboratory support is needed to have reliable clotting factor level and inhibitor monitoring.
- Treatment with viral inactivated plasma-derived or recombinant concentrates is preferred over cryoprecipitate or fresh frozen plasma (FFP). Cryoprecipitate, in turn, is preferred over FFP for hemophilia A because it is generally difficult to achieve high enough factor VIII levels with FFP alone; FFP can be used for treatment of hemophilia B. Other options include desmopressin, tranexamic acid, and epsilon aminocaproic acid.
- Desmopressin can be used for mild or moderate hemophilia A (particularly carriers) and some platelet disorders; however, it is of no value to hemophilia B because it does not affect factor IX. Individual response to desmopressin is varied and difficult to predict.

BOX 38.4 International Society of Thrombosis and Hemostasis Scoring System for Disseminated Intravascular Coagulation

1. Risk assessment: Does the patient have an underlying disorder known to be associated with overt DIC?
   If yes, proceed; if no, do not use this algorithm.
2. Order global coagulation tests (e.g., platelet count, prothrombin time, fibrinogen, soluble fibrin monomers, or fibrin degradation products).
3. Score global coagulation test results.
   _____ Platelet count (>100, 0; <100, 1; <50, 2)
   _____ Elevated fibrin-related marker (e.g., soluble fibrin monomers/fibrin degradation products) (no increase, 0; moderate increase, 2; strong increase, 3)
   _____ Prolonged prothrombin time (<3 sec, 0; >3 sec but <6 sec, 1; >6 sec, 2)
   _____ Fibrinogen level (>1 g/L, 0; <1 g/L, 1)
4. Calculate score
5. If ≥5, compatible with overt DIC; repeat scoring daily. If <5, suggestive (not affirmative) for nonovert DIC; repeat next 1–2 days.

DIC, Disseminated intravascular coagulation.
Adapted from Bakhtiari K, et al. Prospective validation of the International Society of Thrombosis and Haemostasis scoring system for disseminated intravascular coagulation. *Crit Care Med.* 2004;32(12):2416–2421.

undergo extensive screening, and newer and safer treatment modalities exist. Most surgeries are available to hemophiliacs, with a lower risk of uncontrolled bleeding.[41]

For patients with hemophilia or a family history of hemophilia, a preoperative assessment of hemostasis is imperative. Preoperative laboratory tests should include a platelet count and function, a coagulation panel (PT, aPTT, factor VIII, factor IX, and fibrinogen), in addition to an inhibitor test.[41] If the hemophiliac was given a test dose of factor VII preoperatively, the response to the test dose should be evaluated. The patient should be typed and crossmatched because even a low-risk procedure can be catastrophic for the hemophiliac.

A clearly defined anesthesia plan is essential for the hemophiliac, and close consultation with a hematologist is essential. Factor VIII concentrate can be given prior to surgery. Factor VII is administered intraoperatively to augment thrombin generation and deter bleeding. The dose should be precalculated and vial availability confirmed prior to going into the operating room. Desmopressin (0.3 mcg/kg) also can be administered to increase plasma levels of factor VIII and vWF for mild to moderate hemophiliacs.[36,42] There is no risk for viral transmission when either of these drugs is initiated. Perioperative management of the hemophilic patient is outlined in Box 38.3.

Disseminated Intravascular Coagulation

Disseminated intravascular coagulation (DIC) is a result of intravascular coagulation activation with microvascular thrombi formation, which causes thrombocytopenia and clotting factor depletion, leading to bleeding and end-organ complications.[36]

Clinical presentation of DIC may include thrombosis, hemorrhage, or both. Multiorgan system failure and hemorrhage is the result of widespread thrombotic microangiopathy and depletion of procoagulant factors (e.g., consumptive coagulopathy), respectively[43] (see Fig. 38.11).

The diagnosis of DIC is usually secondary to an underlying pathologic process. Acute DIC manifests as a complication of several disease processes, notably sepsis, the postoperative state, obstetric complications, blood transfusion reactions, and certain malignancies such as acute promyelocytic leukemia. Chronic DIC is seen in solid tumors and in large aortic aneurysms.[36]

Coagulation activation ranges from mild thrombocytopenia and prolongation of clotting times to acute DIC characterized by extensive bleeding and thrombosis.[44] Systemic activation of coagulation results in (1) intravascular deposition of fibrin, (2) thrombotic microangiopathy, (3) compromised blood supply to organs, and (4) multiorgan system failure. Systemic activation of coagulation also promotes the use and subsequent depletion of platelets and coagulation factors, which may induce severe bleeding from multiple sites.

Several factors play an important role in the pathogenesis of DIC. TF release is considered to play a central role in the development of hyperthrombinemia in DIC. Under normal conditions, mediators such as antithrombin and TFPI regulate the process of coagulation. During specific conditions, such as septicemia, liver impairment, capillary leakage, and the release of endotoxins and proinflammatory cytokines, the actions of these regulatory mediators are adversely altered. Experimental models of septicemia have shown increased fibrinolytic activity related to the acute release of tPA from the endothelium. The initial increased fibrinolytic activity is followed by the release of plasminogen activator inhibitor type 1 (PAI-1), which in turn impairs fibrinolysis and leads to accelerated thrombus formation in DIC. Finally, activated protein C mediates the release of inflammatory cytokines such as tumor necrosis factor and interleukins from endothelial cells. Complement activation and kinin generation increase the coagulation response leading to subsequent vascular occlusion.[45]

Diagnosis of DIC is made by evaluation of the patient's clinical presentation in conjunction with laboratory tests such as platelet count, aPTT, PT, fibrin-related markers (e.g., fibrin degradation products, D-dimer), fibrinogen, and antithrombin. Additionally, a scoring system developed by the International Society of Thrombosis and Haemostasis (ISTH) assists with the diagnosis[46] (Box 38.4). Acute (overt) DIC is characterized by ecchymosis, petechiae, mucosal bleeding, depletion of platelets and clotting factors, and bleeding at puncture sites. A score

---

BOX 38.5   Treatment of Disseminated Intravascular Coagulation

1. Identify and eliminate the underlying cause
2. No treatment if mild, asymptomatic, and self-limited
3. Hemodynamic support, as indicated, in severe cases
4. Blood component therapy
   - *Indications:* Active bleeding or high risk for bleeding
     1. Fresh frozen plasma
     2. Platelets
     3. In some cases, consider cryoprecipitate, antithrombin III
5. Drug therapy
   - *Indications:* Heparin for DIC manifested by thrombosis or acrocyanosis and without active bleeding; antifibrinolytic agents are generally contraindicated except with life-threatening bleeding and failure of blood component therapy

DIC, Disseminated intravascular coagulation.
From Shafer AI. Hemorrhagic disorders: disseminated intravascular coagulation, liver failure and vitamin deficiency. In: Goldman L, et al., eds. *Goldman Cecil Medicine.* 26th ed. Philadelphia: Elsevier; 2020:1147–1151.

BOX 38.6   Intraoperative Management of Patients With Sickle Cell Disease

- Provide adequate hydration (e.g., monitor hemodynamic status, urine output, central venous pressures when available)
- Transfusion of crossmatched red blood cells to replace surgical blood loss (e.g., avoid increasing the hemoglobin >10–11 g/dL)
- Avoid hypoxemia
- Maintain normothermia
- Maintain normal acid-base status
- Provide adequate perioperative pain management
- Caution using vasoocclusive devices such as tourniquets
- For younger, stable patients undergoing low-risk to intermediate-risk procedures, preoperative transfusion can be considered
- For patients with pulmonary disease or undergoing high-risk procedures, consideration should be made to decrease the hemoglobin S level to <30%, although some have suggested levels as high as 50%–60% could be equally as effective.

---

of 5 or greater indicates overt DIC. Chronic (nonovert) DIC is characterized by thromboembolism accompanied by evidence of activation of the coagulation system. A score less than 5 suggests nonovert DIC.

The management and treatment of DIC depends on identification of the underlying pathologic condition. In obstetric catastrophes, DIC may resolve as a result of prompt delivery. Treatment of sepsis with antibiotic therapy may halt the progression of DIC. Restoration of physiologic anticoagulant pathways with activated protein C in the treatment of sepsis with overt DIC holds promise.[45] Activated protein C inactivates factors Va and VIIIa resulting in decreased thrombin formation. Its use in treating DIC patients with severe sepsis has been approved by the FDA. For individuals requiring surgery who are bleeding or at risk for active bleeding, correction of coagulopathy with platelets, FFP, and/or cryoprecipitate must be used. Continued replacement of blood products should be based on the clinical presentation and reassessment of laboratory results.[5]

The use of antithrombotics for DIC remains controversial, especially in a patient who is prone to bleeding. Antithrombin administration for patients who have DIC associated with sepsis is useful not only for shortening the duration of DIC symptoms but also for improving the outcome. However, the optimum dose and dosing period still need to be determined. Bleeding may be exacerbated, and improvement of the outcome may be reversed by administration of antithrombin to patients who have DIC associated with sepsis and are concomitantly receiving heparin.[45] Suggestions for treatment of DIC are given in Box 38.5.

Sickle Cell Disease

Sickle cell disease (SCD) is a common hereditary hemoglobinopathy. Under normal circumstances the β-globin gene on chromosome 11 codes for the production of the β-globin chains of the protein hemoglobin A. However, in SCD there is an autosomal recessive genetic abnormality of the β-globin gene codes for the production of the variant hemoglobin, hemoglobin S. Patients may have sickle cell trait (SCT) or symptoms of SCD. There are several types, including hemoglobin SS, hemoglobin SC, hemoglobin SB+ (β) thalassemia, and β0-thalassemia.

SCT is a heterozygous disorder observed in 10% of the US black population.[36] Hemoglobin S levels range from 30% to 50%, and

erythrocyte sickling is observed with a partial pressure of oxygen (Po_2) of 20 to 30 mm Hg. In contrast, SCD is a homozygous disorder observed in 0.5% to 1.0% of blacks. The majority of the hemoglobin molecule is hemoglobin S, and sickling is observed with a Po_2 of 30 to 40 mm Hg. A sickle cell crisis may be triggered by hypoxemia, hypothermia, infection, dehydration, venous stasis, and acidosis. Sickle cell crisis may be characterized by chronic hemolytic anemia, recurrent episodes of intermittent vasoocclusion, severe pain, and end-organ damage. Although previous studies of SCD cite a perioperative morbidity and mortality greater than 50%, perioperative mortality has diminished steadily, which is attributed with overall improvements in anesthetic care.[47] Persons with SCD often require surgical intervention resulting from secondary conditions, which are directly related to their SCD. A cholecystectomy for gallstones is the most common operation required because of the excess bilirubin resulting from the rapid breakdown of sickle erythrocytes.

There is no universal method for caring for patients with a sickle cell disorder. The optimal percentage of hemoglobin S in patients receiving regular blood transfusions remains to be established, with clinical studies citing a range from 30% to 50%.[48,49] The benefit of preoperative blood transfusion is still open to debate. Providing preoperative transfusion supplementation always carries a risk of increasing the blood viscosity and causing end-organ damage. A conservative transfusion regimen has been shown to be as effective as an aggressive regimen in preventing perioperative complications and was associated with fewer transfusion-related adverse events.[8] Anesthesia management for a patient with SCD includes providing adequate hydration, promoting adequate oxygen saturation, ensuring normothermia, maintaining acid-base balance, and providing proper patient positioning. Supplying adequate analgesia may interrupt intraoperative and postoperative sickle cell crisis.[50] Suggestions for intraoperative management of patients with SCD are given in Box 38.6.

Heparin-Induced Thrombocytopenia

Heparin-induced thrombocytopenia (HIT) is an immune response to heparin that can progress to severe thrombosis, amputation, and in some cases death. HIT is recognized as the most important immunologic complication of heparin therapy and remains one of the few absolute contraindications for heparin use. Heparin continues to be used clinically because of its rapid onset, easy reversibility, and moderate therapeutic window with relatively few side effects. In the United States, approximately 30% of hospitalized patients or approximately 12

BOX 38.7 Heparin-Induced Thrombocytopenia (HIT) Type I and Type II

Type I
- Thrombocytopenia is mediated by direct heparin-induced platelet aggregation (e.g., nonimmune mediated)
- Onset is typically 1–4 days after start of heparin therapy
- Mild thrombocytopenia (e.g., <100,000/μL)
- Thrombocytopenia often resolves spontaneously even with continued administration of heparin
- Typically occurs with high-dose heparin administration
- Not associated with thrombosis and serious clinical sequelae

Type II
- Thrombocytopenia is mediated by the actions of the heparin, platelet factor 4, and immunoglobulin G expression (e.g., immune mediated)
- Onset is typically 5–14 days after start of heparin therapy
- Severe thrombocytopenia (e.g., <60,000/μL)
- Thrombocytopenia does not resolve spontaneously, therefore, heparin administration must be discontinued
- Occurs with any heparin dose and route
- Associated with thrombosis and serious clinical sequelae

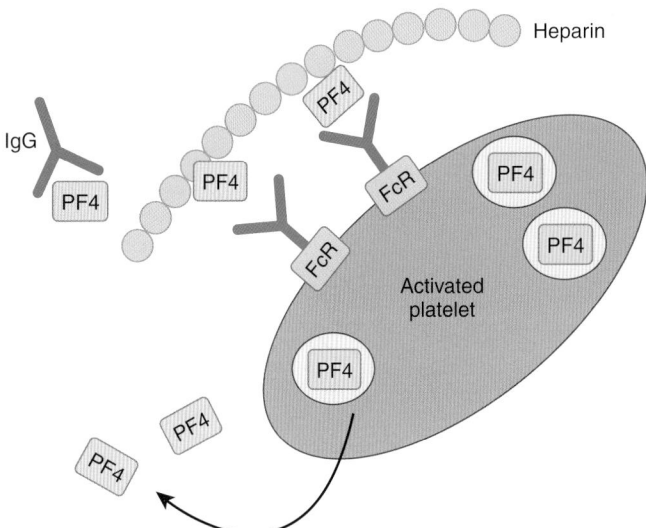

Fig. 38.12 Pathophysiology of heparin-induced thrombocytopenia (HIT) type II. *FcR*, Fc receptor; *IgG*, immunoglobulin G; *PF4*, platelet factor 4.

million people a year receive heparin. Approximately 5% of patients receiving heparin or low-molecular-weight heparin (LMWH) will develop immune reactions characteristic of HIT; of these patients, approximately 50% (or 300,000 people) will have clinically significant HIT thrombosis.[51] Overall, clinically symptomatic HIT develops in 1% of hospital patients receiving heparin in any form.[52]

HIT should be suspected in any patient on heparin or LMWH therapy who develops a decrease of greater than 50% in platelet count from baseline or total platelet count of less than 100,000 per mm³ with normal baseline counts. It occurs in 0.5% to 5% of heparin-treated patients, typically after 5 to 10 days, but in patients with previous heparin exposure HIT can have an earlier onset.[36]

The classic clinical presentation of HIT includes thrombocytopenia, resistance to heparin anticoagulation, thrombosis, and positive assay tests indicative of HIT. There are two classifications of HIT; Box 38.7 describes the defining characteristics of each type. Of the two classifications, type II is associated with the greatest clinical morbidity and mortality. HIT type II is caused by the formation of immunoglobulin G (IgG) antibodies directed against heparin-platelet factor-4 (H-PF4) immune complexes. The IgG antibody fixes to complements with H-PF4 and subsequently activates platelets via the Fc receptor causing platelet aggregation[52] (Fig. 38.12). Despite thrombocytopenia, patients clinically do not present with bleeding tendencies (e.g., spontaneous bleeding, hemorrhage, petechiae). Rather, HIT type II induces a clinically relevant hypercoagulable state with clotting and thrombus formation causing serious sequelae. Amputation and mortality associated with HIT type II is estimated to be 20% and 30%, respectively.[51]

Many tests are available with individual pros and cons; however, the current accepted gold standard test is the C-serotonin release assay.[14] Other useful tests include the heparin-induced platelet aggregation assay and antibody detection via an enzyme-linked immunosorbent assay.

Diagnosis and treatment of HIT should be based on clinical presentation and laboratory findings. Thrombocytopenia, cutaneous abnormalities (e.g., skin necrosis, ecchymosis, hematoma, purpura, blistering), and tachyphylaxis after heparin administration may indicate developing HIT. If HIT is suspected after heparin administration,

a hematologist should be consulted. In patients with high suspicion for HIT, heparin should be stopped immediately with an alternative anticoagulant administration even prior to the confirmatory test.[36] Treatment of HIT includes discontinuation of all sources of heparin (e.g., medications, heparin-coated invasive lines), administration of direct thrombin inhibitors (e.g., argatroban, lepirudin).[51,52] Arterial or venous thrombosis that compromises perfusion to distal sites may require prompt surgical intervention (e.g., embolectomy, vascular bypass).

OTHER CONSIDERATIONS

Perioperative Management of Patients Taking Antithrombotic Drugs

The advent of new antithrombotic medications within the last decade has garnered increasing interest regarding the perioperative management of these potent medications. Antithrombotic medications can be categorized based on their respective method of altering the normal physiologic process of hemostasis: antiplatelet, anticoagulant, and fibrinolytic medications (Figs. 38.13, 38.14, and 38.15)

Table 38.6 lists common antithrombotic medications.[53,57] Selection, dosing, and monitoring of antithrombotic therapy should be adjusted based on the patient's primary diagnosis, comorbidities, type of therapy (e.g., prophylaxis or therapeutic), and renal impairment. Classification of antiplatelet drugs are noted in Box 38.8.

The preoperative management of antithrombotic therapy is a pivotal topic in that the risk of disease exacerbation must be weighed against perioperative bleeding. Abruptly withholding antithrombotic medications places the patient at increased risk for arterial or venous thromboembolism (e.g., stroke or pulmonary embolism), MI, or death.[53-56] In contrast, excessive bleeding may occur if the anticoagulation medications are continued before surgery, which may lead to potentially serious intraoperative complications, adverse postoperative outcomes, and/or the need for blood product transfusion.

Situation-specific considerations are leading to new recommendations for perioperative management of patients on antithrombotic therapy (see Table 38.6). Table 38.7 outlines guidelines for neuraxial anesthesia in patients receiving antithrombotic therapy. For low-risk

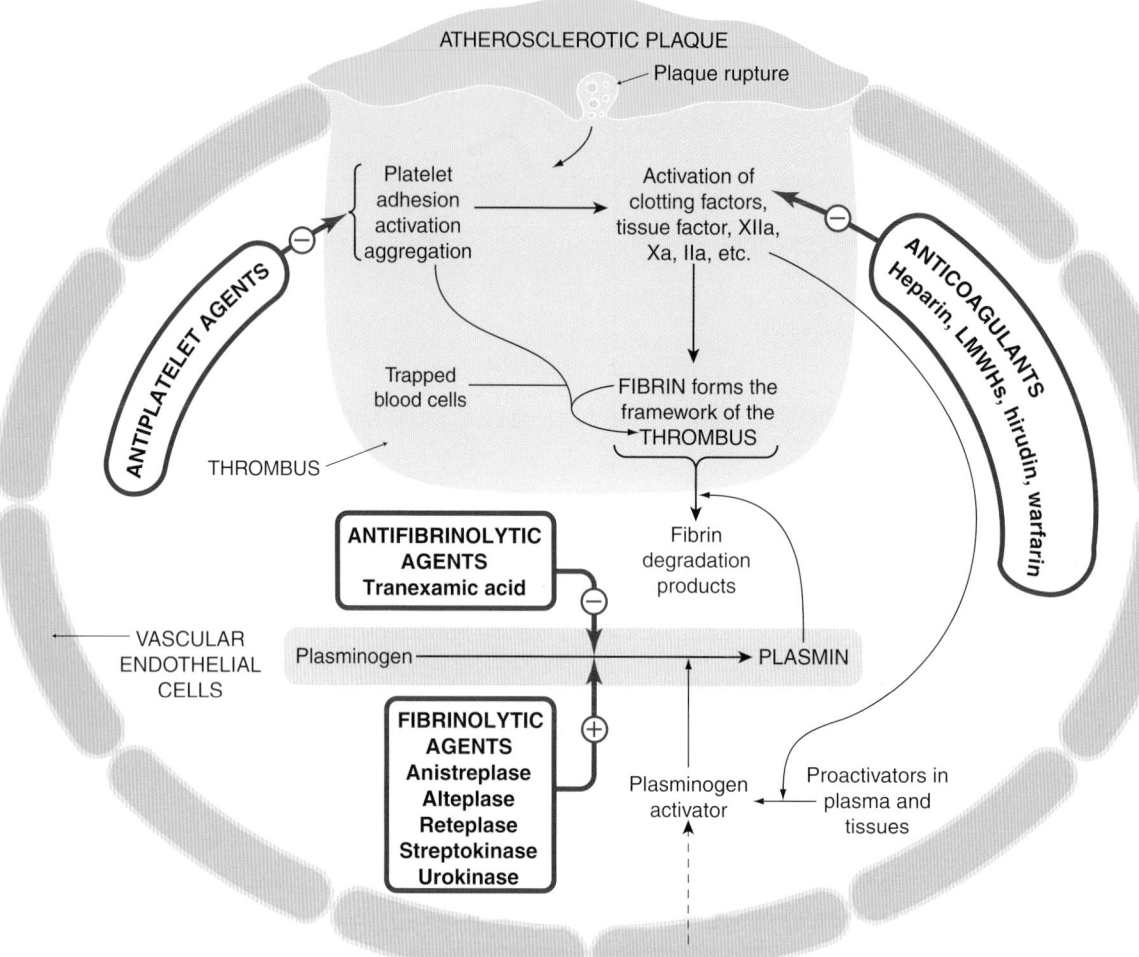

Fig. 38.13 Sites of action of various anticoagulant and antiplatelet drugs. *LMWH,* Low-molecular-weight heparin. (From Rang HP, et al. *Rang and Dale's Pharmacology.* 9th ed. London: Churchill Livingstone; 2020:332.)

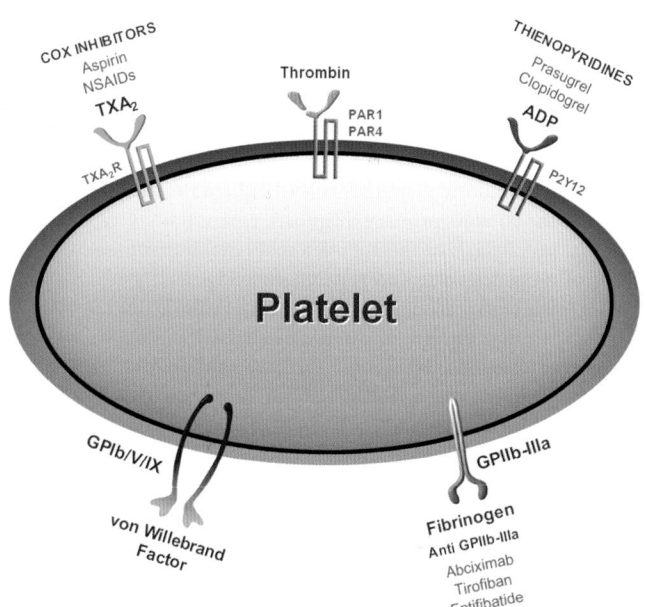

Fig. 38.14 Main platelet receptors, glycoproteins, and common inhibitors. *ADP,* Adenosine diphosphate; *COX,* cyclooxygenase; *GP,* glycoprotein; *NSAIDs,* nonsteroidal antiinflammatory drugs; *PAR,* protease-activated receptor. (From Albaladejo P, Samama CM. Patients under antiplatelet therapy. *Best Pract Res Clin Anaesthesiol.* 2010;24[1]:41–50.)

bleeding procedures such as minor ophthalmic, dental, dermatologic, gastrointestinal, orthopedic, and podiatric procedures, uninterrupted administration of anticoagulant therapy is generally safe (Box 38.9). For medium- to high-risk bleeding procedures, functional drug elimination (e.g., 5 half-lives) may be necessary between discontinuation of anticoagulant therapy and the start of the procedure. The risk for thromboembolism or MI, for both cardiac and noncardiac surgeries, must be evaluated thoroughly. This is to minimize complications that can lead to patient morbidity, mortality, prolonged hospitalization, and increased health care costs.[11] Lastly, careful consideration must be exercised when restarting these potent medications postoperatively. Once sufficient hemostasis has been obtained, the direct anticoagulant therapy may be restarted 24 hours after the procedure.[58] Longer wait times (up to 48–72 hours) may be necessary if larger initial doses are used.

Antiplatelet Drugs and Noncardiac Surgery: Patients With Coronary Stents

Coronary stents are placed to improve coronary artery flow in patients with stable but symptomatic coronary artery disease or acute coronary syndromes, including unstable angina, non-Q wave MI, and ST elevation acute MIs. Every year, more than 2 million patients undergo percutaneous coronary intervention (PCI). Of these 2 million patients, greater than 90% will require at least one intracoronary stent. Furthermore, approximately 5% of these patients will undergo noncardiac surgery within the first year after

INTRINSIC PATHWAY   EXTRINSIC PATHWAY

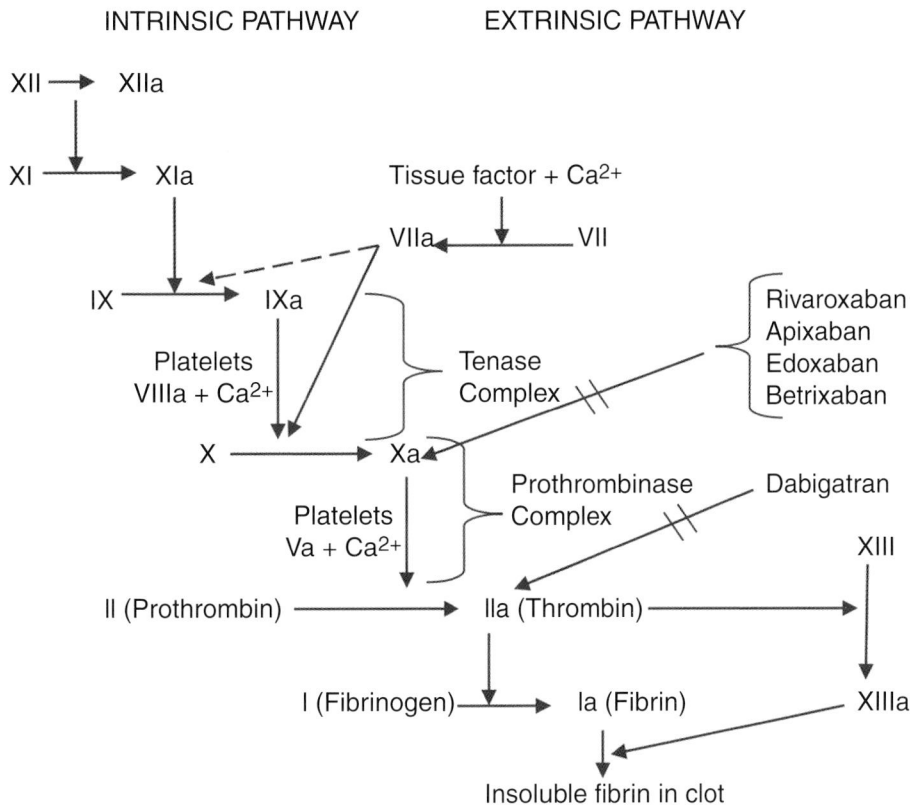

Fig. 38.15 Clotting cascade with targets of the direct oral anticoagulants. (From Dobesh PP, Bhatt SH, Trujillo TC, et al. Antidotes for reversal of direct oral anticoagulants. *Pharmacol Ther.* 2019;204:107405.)

stent placement, whereas many patients will continue to require surgery thereafter.[54]

There are two distinct complications associated with coronary stent placement: acute stent thrombosis and stent restenosis. Both complications result in major adverse cardiac events (MACEs), which include MI, the need for repeat revascularization, and death. These stent-related events accrue at a rate of approximately 2% per year between 1 and 5 years after PCI for all metallic coronary stents.[59]

Acute stent thrombosis causes abrupt occlusion of the coronary artery and increases the MI rate up to 64%, with a mortality rate between 20% and 45%. Stent thrombosis can occur any time after stent implantation, but most events of acute stent thrombosis occur within the first 30 days after stent placement. Box 38.10 outlines risk factors responsible for acute stent thrombosis. Patients are typically placed on long-term antiplatelet therapy to improve the efficacy of intracoronary stents and to mitigate the risk of stent thrombosis. In contrast, stent restenosis is a slowly developing occlusion directly related to excessive endothelial growth over time. In most cases, it peaks between 6 and 9 months after stent implantation. Restenosis can be insidious and lead to MACEs.[53-55] There are two types of stents available: bare-metal stents (BMS) and drug-eluting stents (DES).[60] For DES, sirolimus or paclitaxel is slowly released from the coronary stent to block endothelial growth proliferation.

It is common for anesthesia providers to encounter patients who have coronary stents and are on dual antiplatelet therapy. Aspirin is commonly combined with an ADP (P2Y12) receptor inhibitor such as clopidogrel or more recently ticagrelor (see Fig. 38.14). The most common cause of acute stent thrombosis is premature or abrupt discontinuation of dual antiplatelet therapy.[54] Abrupt discontinuation of

antiplatelet therapy can lead to a rebound effect, which is characterized by an inflammatory prothrombotic state. During this prothrombotic state there is increased platelet adhesion, platelet aggregation, and thromboxane A2 activity.[56] When this is combined with the inflammatory, prothrombotic surgical milieu, the risk of stent thrombosis significantly increases.[61] Current recommendations for management of perioperative antiplatelet therapy are given in Box 38.11. The risk of acute stent thrombosis is relatively low but may occur more commonly with DES because of the delayed or incomplete endothelialization process. Specific recommendations for managing patients on aspirin therapy are given in Box 38.12.[14]

This patient population requires special attention perioperatively. When considering discontinuing or modifying antiplatelet therapy, it is prudent to involve a multidisciplinary team, including the patient's cardiologist, surgeon, and anesthetist for guidance regarding preoperative and postoperative management of antiplatelet therapy. Important information should include the date of stent implantation, the type of stent deployed, and antiplatelet therapy if applicable. Additional points to consider are the type of operation planned and the risk of bleeding. The current medication regimen must be assessed because many patients have discontinued their antiplatelet medications preoperatively, whereas others continue them at the request of their cardiologist.

Surgery in which the risk of bleeding is low may not require discontinuation of antiplatelet therapy. The Perioperative Ischemic Evaluation (POISE-2) trial also evaluated the effectiveness of aspirin therapy in a cohort of patients without a recent stent. Administration of aspirin before surgery and throughout the early postoperative period had no effect on the rate of a composite of death or nonfatal MI, but it increased the risk of major bleeding. On the basis of

TABLE 38.6   Pharmacologic Properties of Common Antithrombotic Medications

	Type	Mechanism	Half-Life	Reversal Available	General Anesthesia Recommendations	Laboratory Monitoring
ASA	Antiplatelet	COX-1 inhibitor (irreversible)	20 min	Platelets	Stop 7 days	None
NSAIDs	Antiplatelet	COX-1 inhibitor (reversible)	2–10 hr	Platelets	Stop 24–48 hr	None
Clopidogrel	Antiplatelet	ADP receptor antagonist	7 hr	Platelets	Stop 5–7 days	None
Ticlopidine	Antiplatelet	ADP receptor antagonist	4 days	Platelets	Stop 7–10 days	None
Prasugrel	Antiplatelet	ADP receptor antagonist	7 hr	Platelets	Stop 7–10 days	None
Abciximab	Antiplatelet	Glycoprotein IIb/IIIa receptor antagonist	30 min	Platelets	Stop 48–72 hr	None
Eptifibatide	Antiplatelet	Glycoprotein IIb/IIIa receptor antagonist	2.5 hr	Platelets	Stop 8–24 hr	None
Tirofiban	Antiplatelet	Glycoprotein IIb/IIIa receptor antagonist	2 hr	Platelets	Stop 8–24 hr	None
Fondaparinux	Anticoagulant	Factor Xa antagonist (indirect*)	14–17 hr	None	Stop 2–4 days	Antifactor Xa assay
LMWH	Anticoagulant	Factor IIa and Xa antagonist (indirect*)	4.5 hr	Protamine (partial reversal)	Stop 12–24 hr	Antifactor Xa assay
Heparin	Anticoagulant	Factor IIa and Xa antagonist (indirect*)	1.5 hr	Protamine	Stop 6 hr	aPTT
Warfarin	Anticoagulant	Vitamin K epoxide reductase antagonist	25–60 hr	Vitamin K, FFP, PCC	Stop 4–5 days	PT
Dabigatran	Anticoagulant	Factor IIa antagonist (direct)	12–17 hr	Idarucizumab	Stop 1–4 days**	Dilute thrombin time, ecarin thrombin time
Rivaroxaban	Anticoagulant	Factor Xa antagonist (direct)	7–13 hr	Andexanet alfa	Stop 1–3 days**	Antifactor Xa assay
Apixaban	Anticoagulant	Factor Xa antagonist (direct)	8–15 hr	Andexanet alfa	Stop 1–2 days**	Antifactor Xa assay
Edoxaban	Anticoagulant	Factor Xa antagonist (direct)	10–14 hr	Andexanet alfa	Stop 1–2 days**	Antifactor Xa assay
Betrixaban	Anticoagulant	Factor Xa antagonist (direct)	19–27 hr	Andexanet alfa	Stop 3–4 days**	Antifactor Xa assay
t-PA	Fibrinolytic	Plasminogen activator	5 min	Antifibrinolytic	Stop 1 hr	PT/aPTT
Streptokinase	Fibrinolytic	Plasminogen activator	23 min	Antifibrinolytic	Stop 3 hr	PT/aPTT

*Antithrombin cofactor
**Dependent on renal insufficiency
ADP, Adenosine diphosphate; *ASA*, acetylsalicylic acid; *COX*, cyclooxygenase; *FFP*, fresh frozen plasma; *LMWH*, low-molecular-weight heparin, *NSAIDs*, nonsteroidal antiinflammatory drugs; *t-PA*, tissue plasminogen activator.
Adapted from Chen A, et al. Direct oral anticoagulant use: a practical guide to common clinical challenges. *J Am Heart Assoc.* 2020;9(13):e017559; Elisha S, et al. Venous thromboembolism: new concepts in perioperative management. *AANA J.* 2015;83(3):211–221; Kane TD, Tubog TD. Perioperative management of the direct-acting oral anti-coagulants. *AANA J.* 2019;87(4):325–331.

BOX 38.8   Classification of Antiplatelet Drugs

Arachidonic Acid Inhibitors
1. COX inhibitors: aspirin, ibuprofen, triflusal, nonsteroidal antiinflammatory agents, sulfinpyrazone
2. Phosphodiesterase inhibitors: dipyridamole, pentoxifylline, cilostazol, trapidil
3. Other: omega-3 fatty acids, eicosanoids (prostacyclin, prostaglandin analogues)

P2Y12 ADP Receptor Inhibitors
1. Thienopyridines (ADP antagonists): ticlopidine, clopidogrel, prasugrel
2. ATP derivatives: cangrelor
3. CPTPs: ticagrelor

Thrombin Protease-Activated Receptor-1 Inhibitors
1. Vorapaxar, E-5555

Platelet Glycoprotein IIb/IIIa Receptor Blockers
1. Intravenous: abciximab, tirofiban, eptifibatide

Drugs With Secondary Antiplatelet Activity
1. Direct thrombin inhibitors: bivalirudin, dabigatran
2. Direct factor Xa inhibitors: rivaroxaban, apixaban, edoxaban, betrixaban
3. Heparin, nitrates, fibrates, calcium channel antagonists, others

ADP, Adenosine diphosphate; *ATP,* adenosine triphosphate; *COX,* cyclooxygenase; *CPTPs,* cyclopentyltriazolopyrimidines.
Adapted from Wiviott SD, Guigliano RP. Non-ST segment elevation acute coronary syndromes. In: Antman EM, Sabatine MS, eds. *Cardiovascular Therapeutics: A Companion to Braunwald's Heart Disease.* 4th ed. Philadelphia: Elsevier; 2013:155; Knowles RB, Warner TD. Anti-platelet drugs and their necessary interaction with endothelial mediators and platelet cyclic nucleotides for therapeutic efficacy. *Pharmacol Ther.* 2019;193:83–90.

TABLE 38.7 Neuraxial Anesthesia in Patients Receiving Antithrombotic Therapy

Drug	Contraindications and Comments
Antiplatelet medications	Prior to neuraxial procedure: • NSAIDs: no contraindication • Thienopyridine (ticlopidine, clopidogrel, prasugrel): stop 5–10 days • Cangrelor: stop 3 hr • Ticagrelor: stop 5–7 days • GpIIb/IIIa antagonists (abciximab, eptifibatide, tirofiban): stop 8–48 hr • Cilostazol: stop 2 days • Dipyridamole: stop 24 hr
Unfractionated heparin (UFH), subcutaneous	• Neuraxial procedure 4–6 hr after low-dose prophylactic heparin administration (5000 units BID or TID) • Neuraxial procedure 12 hr after high-dose prophylactic heparin administration (7500–10,000 units BID or daily dose <20,000 units) • Neuraxial procedure 24 hr after therapeutic heparin administration >10,000 units per dose or daily dose >20,000 units) • Catheter removal 4–6 hr after last low-dose heparin administration • Delay UFH administration for 1 hr after needle placement or catheter removal
Unfractionated heparin (UFH), intravenous	• Neuraxial procedure 4–6 hr after heparin infusion discontinued and normal coagulation status verified • Catheter removal 4–6 hr after last heparin dose and normal coagulation status verified • Delay UFH administration for 1 hr after needle placement or after catheter removal • No mandatory surgical delay if traumatic insertion
LMWH	• Neuraxial procedure: 12 hr after a low (prophylactic) LMWH dose and 24 hr after high (therapeutic) LMWH dose • Catheter removal at least 12 hr after last LMWH dose • Delay LMWH administration 4 hr after catheter removal
Warfarin	• Normal INR (before neuraxial technique) • Catheter removal when INR ≤1.5 (initiation of therapy)
Fondaparinux	• Recommends single needle pass, atraumatic needle placement, avoidance of indwelling neuraxial catheters
Direct IIa inhibitors (intravenous): desirudin, bivalirudin, argatroban	• Recommends against neuraxial procedure
Factor IIa inhibitor (oral): dabigatran	• Contraindicated (per manufacturer) • Delay first dose 6 hr after needle placement or catheter removal
Factor Xa inhibitors: rivaroxaban, apixaban, edoxaban, betrixaban	• Neuraxial procedure 72 hr after last dose • Delay first dose 6 hr after needle placement or catheter removal
Herbal therapy	• No evidence for mandatory discontinuation before placement neuraxial procedure • Be aware of potential drug interactions with the three Gs: ginkgo biloba, garlic, and ginseng

For patients undergoing deep plexus or peripheral blocks, use these same recommendations.
ASRAPM, American Society of Regional Anesthesia and Pain Management; *GP*, glycoprotein; *INR*, international normalized ratio; *LMWH*, low-molecular-weight heparin; *NSAIDs*, nonsteroidal inflammatory drugs; *UFH*, unfractionated heparin.
Adapted from Horlocker TT, et al. Regional anesthesia in the patient receiving antithrombotic or thrombolytic therapy: American Society of Regional Anesthesia and Pain Medicine evidence-based guidelines (fourth edition). *Reg Anesth Pain Med.* 2018;43(3):263–309.

BOX 38.9 Procedures That May Be Performed Without Anticoagulant Discontinuation

Ophthalmic
• Cataract extractions
• Trabeculectomies

Dental
• Restorations
• Endodontics
• Prosthetics
• Uncomplicated extractions
• Dental hygiene treatment

Dermatologic
• Mohs micrographic surgery
• Simple excisions

Gastrointestinal
• Upper endoscopy and colonoscopy without biopsy
• Endoscopic retrograde cholangiopancreatography (ERCP) without sphincterotomy
• Biliary stent insertion without sphincterotomy
• Endosonography without fine-needle aspiration
• Push enteroscopy

Orthopedic or Podiatric
• Joint and soft tissue aspirations and injections
• Nail avulsions
• Phenol matrixectomies

BOX 38.10 Additional Risk Factors for Acute Stent Thrombosis

Coronary Anatomy Factors
- Site of stent placement (e.g., bifurcation stenting, side branch occlusion)
- Left main coronary artery stent
- Long stent length (>18 mm)
- Ostial stenting
- Overlapping stents
- Placement of multiple stents
- Small stent diameter (<3 mm)
- Suboptimal stent placement

Patient Risk Factors
- Advanced age
- Diabetes mellitus
- Gene polymorphism
- Hypercoagulable states (e.g., diabetes, malignancy, and surgery)
- Major cardiac adverse event within 30 days of percutaneous cardiac intervention

- Reduced left ventricular ejection fraction
- Prior brachytherapy
- Renal insufficiency

Stent Indication Factors
- Acute coronary syndrome
- Type C coronary lesion or total occlusion

Stent-Related Factors
- Type of stent placed
- Hypersensitivity to stent polymer

Pharmacologic Factors
- Abrupt discontinuation of antiplatelet therapy
- Diminished response or resistance to antiplatelet therapy

Adapted from Hall R, Mazer CD. Antiplatelet drugs: a review of their pharmacology and management in the perioperative period. *Anesth Analg.* 2011;112(2):292–318.

BOX 38.11 Perioperative Considerations for the Patient With a Coronary Stent

Stents
- Type of stent(s) (e.g., bare-metal stent [BMS], drug-eluting stent [DES])?
- When were stent(s) placed?
- Complications during the revascularization, such as malposition, longer length, overlapping?

Antiplatelet Therapy
- What is the antiplatelet regimen?
- What is the recommended duration of antiplatelet therapy?
- Consult patient cardiologist regarding antiplatelet management.

Elective Noncardiac Surgery
1. Elective noncardiac surgery should be delayed 30 days after BMS implantation and optimally 6 mo after DES implantation.
2. In patients treated with dual antiplatelet therapy (DAPT) after coronary stent implantation who must undergo surgical procedures that mandate the discontinuation of P2Y12 inhibitor therapy (clopidogrel or ticagrelor), it is recommended that aspirin be continued if possible and the P2Y12 platelet receptor inhibitor be restarted as soon as possible after surgery.
3. When noncardiac surgery is required in patients currently taking a P2Y12 inhibitor, a consensus decision among treating clinicians as to the relative risks of surgery and discontinuation or continuation of antiplatelet therapy can be useful.
4. Elective noncardiac surgery after DES implantation in patients for whom P2Y12 inhibitor therapy will need to be discontinued may be considered after 3 mo if the risk of further delay of surgery is greater than the expected risks of stent thrombosis.

5. Elective noncardiac surgery should not be performed within 30 days after BMS implantation or within 3 mo after DES implantation in patients in whom DAPT will need to be discontinued perioperatively.

Nonelective Surgery
1. *Determine risk for surgical bleeding:* If not at high risk, continue dual antiplatelet therapy. Discontinuation of dual antiplatelet therapy, in patients with incomplete stent endothelialization, markedly increases the risk of stent thrombosis, myocardial infarction, and death.
2. *High risk for bleeding:* Risk primarily associated with closed space surgeries (i.e., medullary canal spine surgery, intracranial surgery, posterior chamber eye surgery, and possibly prostate surgery) where increased tissue pressure would be deleterious. If dual antiplatelet therapy must be interrupted, aspirin should be continued, when possible. An evolving treatment option involves "bridging therapy" anticoagulation in which drugs of short duration (glycoprotein inhibitor [e.g., tirofiban, eptifibatide], direct thrombin inhibitor [e.g., bivalirudin], unfractionated heparin, low-molecular-weight heparin, nonsteroidal antiinflammatory drugs [e.g., flurbiprofen], cyclooxygenase-1 inhibitors) are administered for up to 6 hr during the surgery, with the goal of preventing stent thrombosis while dual antiplatelet therapy is interrupted. Restart dual antiplatelet therapy as soon as possible after the surgery.
3. Surgery should be performed in an institution where higher-acuity care and an interventional cardiologist are available when possible. Consult prior to surgery to determine procedural complexities and determine optimal antiplatelet therapy and requisite patient management.

Adapted from Levine GN, et al. 2016 ACC/AHA guideline focused update on duration of dual antiplatelet therapy in patients with coronary artery disease: a report of the American College of Cardiology/American Heart Association task force on clinical practice guidelines. *J Am Coll Cardiol.* 2016;68:1082–1115.

currently available literature, including the POISE-2 trial, aspirin should not be administered to patients undergoing surgery unless there is a definitive guideline-based primary or secondary prevention indication. The guideline also recommends strong consideration be given to the administration of aspirin for elective noncardiac surgery, without history of percutaneous coronary intervention and stenting, when the risk of myocardial ischemia exceeds the risk of surgical

bleeding. Aside from closed-space procedures, intramedullary spine surgery, or possibly prostate surgery, moderate-risk patients taking lifelong aspirin for a guideline-based primary or secondary indication may warrant continuation of their aspirin throughout the perioperative period.[62]

Patients who require emergent surgery should be evaluated on a case-by-case basis, weighing the risk of thrombosis against the

BOX 38.12 Recommendations for Perioperative Aspirin Management

- In the majority of patients using aspirin for **primary** cardiovascular (CV) disease prevention, preoperative aspirin cessation is safe. The drug may be safely discontinued 7 days preoperatively, and there should be full return of platelet function within this timeframe.
- For patients taking aspirin for **secondary** prevention but without a coronary stent, the data that do exist suggest that continuing aspirin might be prudent. Noncoronary stented patients with high CV disease risk should likely have aspirin continued throughout the perioperative period unless undergoing closed-spaced procedures such as medullary canal spine surgery, intracranial surgery, posterior chamber eye surgery, and transurethral urologic procedures.

- The overall dataset for the reduction of a major adverse cardiovascular events (MACE) by the continuation of antiplatelet agents in stable ischemic heart disease patients undergoing noncardiac surgery is negative. In the patient with a recent acute coronary syndrome the ideal is they be on dual antiplatelet therapy (DAPT) for 1 yr, but if surgery is urgent (i.e., cancer operation), it should proceed while continuing aspirin monotherapy at a minimum.
- For patients with cerebrovascular disease (CVD) and peripheral arterial disease (PAD) there is minimal prospective data, but recommendations suggest stopping preoperative aspirin is associated with significant risk, and it likely should be continued throughout the perioperative period.

Adapted from Gerstein NS, Albrechtsen CL, Mercado N, et al. A comprehensive update on aspirin management during noncardiac surgery. *Anesth Analg.* 2020;10.1213/ANE.0000000000005064.

TABLE 38.8 Risk Factors for Venous Thromboembolism

Major Risk Factors	Moderate Risk Factors	Low Risk Factors
Fracture (hip or leg)	Central venous lines	Prolonged bed rest
Hip or knee replacement	Congestive heart or respiratory failure	Immobility
Major general surgery	Paralytic stroke	Arthroscopic knee surgery
Major trauma	Malignancy	Laparoscopic surgery
Spinal cord injury	Postpartum period	Obesity
Advanced age	Drug therapy	Pregnancy
Previous VTE	Cancer chemotherapy	
Vascular disease or injury	Estrogen contraceptives or replacement therapy	Varicose veins
		History of unexplained or recurrent spontaneous abortion
Hypercoagulable state	Heparin-induced thrombocytopenia	Severe lung disease, including pneumonia (<1 mo ago)
	Sepsis or infection	Inflammatory bowel disease
	Erythropoiesis-stimulating agents	
	Blood transfusion	
History of VTE	Myeloproliferative disorders	Nephrotic syndrome

VTE, Venous thromboembolism.
Adapted from Heit JA, et al. The epidemiology of venous thromboembolism. *J Thromb Thrombolysis.* 2016;41:3–14; Zipes DP, et al. *Braunwald's Heart Disease: A Textbook of Cardiovascular Medicine.* 11th ed. Philadelphia: Elsevier; 2019:1822–1846; Horlocker TT, et al. Regional anesthesia in the patient receiving antithrombotic or thrombolytic therapy: American Society of Regional Anesthesia and Pain Medicine evidence-based guidelines (fourth edition). *Reg Anesth Pain Med.* 2018;43(3):263–309.

risk of bleeding. As a result of the lack of prospective studies and guidelines, a wide variety of potential approaches to the perioperative management of BMS, DES, and antiplatelet therapy have been proposed. In 2016 the American College of Cardiology/ American Heart Association (ACC/AHA) released their updated guidelines for management of patients with coronary stents[63,64] (see Box 38.11).

Outpatients Requiring Noncardiac Surgery

When determining the perioperative management of anticoagulation therapy, consideration must be given to a patient's risk for thromboembolism and the risk of bleeding as it relates to the type of surgery (Tables 38.8 and 38.9). When deemed necessary, warfarin therapy is typically discontinued 5 days before the elective procedure. This permits adequate time for in vivo production of functional vitamin K-dependent coagulation factors and waning of anticoagulant effects. During this period, bridging anticoagulant therapy with unfractionated heparin or LMWH can be used to minimize the time the patient lacks adequate anticoagulation, which minimizes the risk of thromboembolism. The last dose of unfractionated heparin or LMWH is administered 6 hours or 12 to 24 hours, respectively,

before the procedure. Warfarin therapy can be resumed 24 hours after the procedure and achievement of hemostasis. Unfractionated heparin or LMWH is necessary for near-term postoperative thromboprophylaxis as 5 to 10 days of warfarin treatment is required to obtain adequate anticoagulation. Warfarin, unfractionated heparin, and LMWH administration should be guided by PT, aPTT, and anti-factor Xa assay, respectively.

Recent trials suggest that the bleeding risk using perioperative unfractionated heparin or LMWH may be higher than previously thought. A 2015 study by Douketis et al. was a prospective, randomized, double-blind, placebo-controlled trial comparing bridge therapy with placebo or LMWH after perioperative interruption of warfarin therapy in patients with atrial fibrillation undergoing elective operation or other elective invasive procedure. Foregoing bridging anticoagulation (e.g., placebo arm) was noninferior to LMWH bridging for the prevention of arterial thromboembolism and decreased the risk of major bleeding.[65] To date, there lacks a robust volume of prospective, randomized, double-blind, placebo-controlled studies to evaluate perioperative bridge therapies for both warfarin and direct oral anticoagulant therapies. For these reasons, bridging anticoagulation should be approached cautiously.[66,67]

TABLE 38.9   Surgical Risk Factors for Venous Thromboembolism

Type of Surgery	Comments
Major general surgery	High risk; generally defined as abdominal or thoracic procedures under general anesthesia lasting ≥30 min; prophylaxis indicated
Orthopedic surgery	High risk; hip and knee replacements and other lower extremity procedures without prophylaxis show a VTE rate of approximately 4.3%; >90% of proximal thrombotic events occur on the operative side. LMWH reduces risk by two-thirds. Half of postoperative lower-extremity thrombi detected by scanning, develop in the operating room, and the remainder occurs over the next 3–5 days; prophylaxis indicated
Knee arthroscopy	Surgery is low to moderate risk. VTE prophylaxis optional
Most outpatient or same-day surgery	Low risk; prophylaxis not required unless patient has significant risk factors
Spinal surgery for nonmalignant disease	Low risk; prophylaxis not required unless patient has significant risk factors
Gynecologic noncancer surgery, cardiac and most thoracic surgery, spinal surgery for malignant disease	Moderate risk; prophylaxis indicated
Bariatric, gynecologic cancer surgery, pneumonectomy, spinal cord injury or other major trauma, major urology procedures	High risk; prophylaxis indicated
Intracranial, traumatic brain injury	High risk; anticoagulation relatively contraindicated because of bleeding risk; low-dose LMWH has been used
Laparoscopic procedures	Low risk; prophylaxis not required unless patient has significant risk factors

LMWH, Low-molecular-weight heparin.
Adapted from Horlocker TT, et al. Regional anesthesia in the patient receiving antithrombotic or thrombolytic therapy: American Society of Regional Anesthesia and Pain Medicine evidence-based guidelines (fourth edition). *Reg Anesth Pain Med.* 2018;43(3):263–309; Falck-Ytter YL, et al. Prevention of VTE in orthopedic surgery patients: antithrombotic therapy and prevention of thrombosis. 9th ed. American College of Chest Physicians evidence-based clinical practice guidelines. *Chest.* 2012;141(2):e278S-325S.

▌ SUMMARY

Each time patients consent to undergo a surgical or diagnostic procedure, the hemostatic system is challenged. An understanding of the normal hemostatic system, methods to prevent bleeding and decrease transfusion requirements, alternatives to blood transfusions, and an understanding of hemostatic pharmacology can only enhance patient care and safety when providing anesthesia care.

REFERENCES

For a complete list of references for this chapter, scan this QR code with any smartphone code reader app, or visit the following URL: http://booksite.elsevier.com/9780323711944/.

39

Anesthesia for Burn Patients

Valdor L. Haglund, Jessica Phillips

The individual who has sustained a burn injury and presents to the operating room for surgery requires clinician knowledge of the pathophysiologic processes that will impact almost every organ system. The American Burn Association (ABA) National Burn Repository of 2018 estimated approximately 486,000 individuals a year with burn injuries visited emergency departments in the United States (between 2011 and 2015).[1] Of these, approximately 40,000 individuals were hospitalized for acute burn injuries and 30,000 of those were admitted to 1 of the 128 specialized burn centers in the United States. These centers undergo a rigorous review by the ABA and the American College of Surgeons (ACS) to become verified ensuring high-quality, specialized care of burned patients, to maintain the necessary resources and medical services mandated by ABA guidelines.[2]

As a result of continuous improvement in the treatment of burns, the burn size—which was once lethal when the burn injury was 42% total body surface area (TBSA)—has now increased to more than 90% TBSA for young thermally injured patients. Increased survival is due to developments in critical care, advancements in resuscitation, control of infection through early excision, and pharmacologic support of the hypermetabolic response to burns.[3,4]

There has been a decline in the incidence of burn injury over the past 2 decades due in large part to the focus on burn prevention, including increased use of smoke detectors, fire and burn prevention education, decreased smoking, water temperature regulations, and regulation of consumer products and occupational safety. An improvement in all aspects of medical care of these patients has played a major role in improving survival. These include increased access to emergency medical care, advanced ventilation modalities and treatment of inhalation injuries, improved infection control practices, enhanced nutritional support, early burn wound excision and grafting, and the treatment of the hypermetabolic response. The development of evidence-based practice guidelines and multidisciplinary care models available at regional burn care centers have also contributed to survival.[5]

Nevertheless, during the period 2011–2015 in the United States, more than 1.25 million individuals sustained burn injuries annually with 486,000 receiving medical treatment.[6] Approximately 3390 die, from fire/smoke inhalation injury—2800 from residential fires and 355 from motor vehicle or aircraft crashes. Approximately 75% of deaths occur at the scene of the accident/injury or during initial transport.[7] Roughly 35% of all burn victims are younger than 17 years of age, with more than 15,000 children requiring hospitalization as a result of their burn injuries. Scald injuries predominate among small children, with a progressive increase in the frequency of burns in the elderly. Major causes of death in burn patients are multiple organ failure and infection. Major risk factors for mortality are older age (>60 years), a higher total percentage of burned surface area (>40% TBSA), and inhalation injury. The main causes of early death (<48 hours after injury) are shock and inhalation injury. Overall, multiorgan failure and sepsis are the most frequently reported causes of death. Death after a burn injury is not related to the pathologic effects on injured skin but to shock associated with metabolic and infectious consequences of a large open wound, sepsis, inhalation injury, and extensive malnutrition, which cumulatively set the stage for life-threatening bacterial sepsis.[8,9]

CLASSIFICATION OF BURN INJURY

Burn injuries, regardless of their etiology, are classified according to the depth and extent of skin and tissue destruction, as well as the surface area (TBSA) involved. First-degree (superficial) burns are limited to the epidermis, which is a thin, avascular layer, usually healing spontaneously and seldom requiring medical intervention. Second-degree burns, also known as deep and superficial partial-thickness burns, extend to the dermis. The dermis is very vascular and contains numerous blood vessels and nerves. Thus severity of the type of burn varies, depending on the amount and depth of the tissues involved. If the epithelial basement membrane of the dermis is intact, the skin will regenerate, and grafting may not be required. Third-degree burns, or full-thickness burns, extend to the subcutaneous tissue lying below the dermis. The entire skin thickness is destroyed with third-degree burns.[9] Skin grafting is required for these types of burns because the epithelium and the dermal appendages are destroyed. A fourth-degree burn classification is used by some to describe structures injured below the dermis, such as muscle, fascia, and bone. Table 39.1 classifies burns according to depth of skin layers affected. Fig. 39.1 illustrates the layers of burn injury.

The burn team will assess the extent of the burn injury and plan initial resuscitation efforts. Burn wounds can be readily quantified, but estimation of the burn size remains subjective and assessor dependent. The most widely used estimation is the rule of nines, which was first described by Lund and Browder (Fig. 39.2). The body is divided into regions that represent 9% or multiples of 9% of the TBSA. Specific modifications apply to children because the surface areas of the head and trunk are proportionally larger than the extremities.[10] The rule of nines is a quick method to visually estimate burn size; however, it may not be all inclusive. The extent of burn injury can be more specifically quantified using the Lund and Browder chart. Fig. 39.3 illustrates this method, which is more accurate in determining a burn victim's injury but is also more time consuming to use. This method is often used when determining the extent of burn in the pediatric patient.

According to the ABA, injury severity grading system, a major burn is (1) a second-degree burn involving more than 10% of the TBSA in adults or 20% at extremes of age, (2) a third-degree burn involving more than 10% of the TBSA in adults, (3) any electrical burn, or (4) a burn complicated by smoke inhalation. There has been much discussion about the use of mathematical models to predict outcome and mortality and which formulas are the most accurate.[11-13] Associated mortality estimates follow a burn formula derived from the National

Burn Registry: If the age of the patient plus percentage TBSA of burn exceeds 115, the mortality is greater than 80%. Additionally, clinical observations estimate the mortality of a burn victim is doubled if inhalation injury is sustained in conjunction with a thermal burn.[1]

ETIOLOGIES OF BURN INJURIES

On admission to a burn center, the cause and circumstances surrounding the injury are determined. This is important since specific pathophysiologic sequelae can be anticipated dependent on mechanism of injury. An individual burned in an enclosed space, such as in a house fire, should be suspected of having an inhalation injury as well. There are four types of burn injuries: chemical, electrical, thermal/heat (also referred to as flame or scald), and inhalation. The ABA National Burn Repository estimated the types of burns reported in 2018 included 43% flame or fire, 34% scalds, 9% contact, 4% electrical, 3% chemical, and 9% other.[2]

Chemical burns commonly occur in a laboratory setting or industrial environment when a noxious chemical substance comes into contact with skin. Tissue damage and destruction result from the reaction of the chemical with tissue proteins and cellular components. Skin disruption will continue until the chemical irritant is removed or neutralized. Initial treatment is the application of copious amounts of water or normal saline irrigation. Chemical burns are uncommon in children.[14,15]

Electrical burns can be the most damaging to skin and surrounding tissue. The extent of the burn depends on the amount of thermal energy conducted through the skin, based on the voltage and duration of contact with the electrical source. Significant tissue disruption can occur where electric current is most concentrated, at points of entry and exit, although two wounds are not always apparent. Initially, the extent of skin and underlying tissue involvement may be difficult to determine because surface damage may not reflect all tissue damage, and entrance wounds may appear superficially. Approximately 10% to 46% of individuals sustaining an electrical injury experience some form of cardiac arrhythmia and damage to the myocardium. Moreover, electrical burns can cause severe damage to bones, blood vessels, muscle, and nerves. If the amount of muscle damaged is significant, myoglobin can be released into the circulation causing myoglobinuria, which affects nephron and renal tubular function, placing the patient at risk for the development of renal failure.

TABLE 39.1	Degrees of Burn Injury	
Classification	**Tissue Level Involvement**	**Outcome and Treatment**
First-degree burn (superficial)	Epidermis	Skin appears red and slightly edematous; heals spontaneously; mild pain and no scarring; barrier preserved; sunburn or flash flame
Second-degree burn (partial thickness)		
Superficial dermal burn	Epidermis and upper dermis	Heals spontaneously; red and edematous; appears wet, hyperemic, and blistering; heals in 7–10 days; scar uncommon
Deep dermal burn	Epidermis and deep dermis	Requires excision and grafting for rapid return of function; heals in 2–8 wk; probable scar without surgery
Third-degree burn (full thickness)	Destruction of epidermis and dermis	Epidermal and complete dermal loss; wound excision and grafting required; limitation of function and scar formation; waxy white leathery appearance; no pain due to nerve damage
Fourth-degree burn	Skeletal muscle, fascia, bone	Complete dermal loss with injury down to tendon or bone; complete excision, limited function; muscle necrosis; electrical injuries; limb loss common

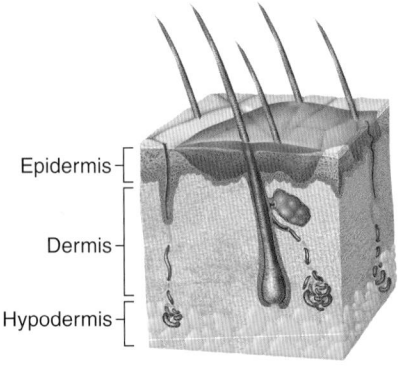
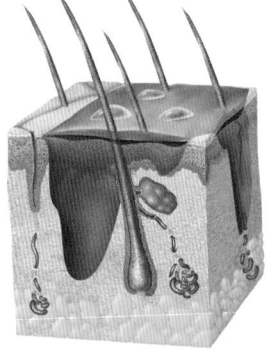
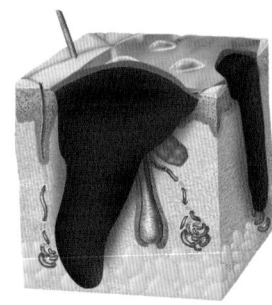

Epidermis		
Dermis		
Hypodermis		

| **Partial-thickness burns** | First-degree burn: Damaged epidermis and edema | Second-degree burn: Damaged epidermis and dermis | **Full-thickness burns** | Third-degree burn: Deep tissue damage |

Fig. 39.1 Classification of burns. Partial-thickness burns include first- and second-degree burns. Full-thickness burns include third-degree burns. Fourth-degree burns involve tissues under the skin, such as muscle or bone. (From Patton KT. *Anatomy & Physiology.* 10th ed. St. Louis: Elsevier; 2019:203.)

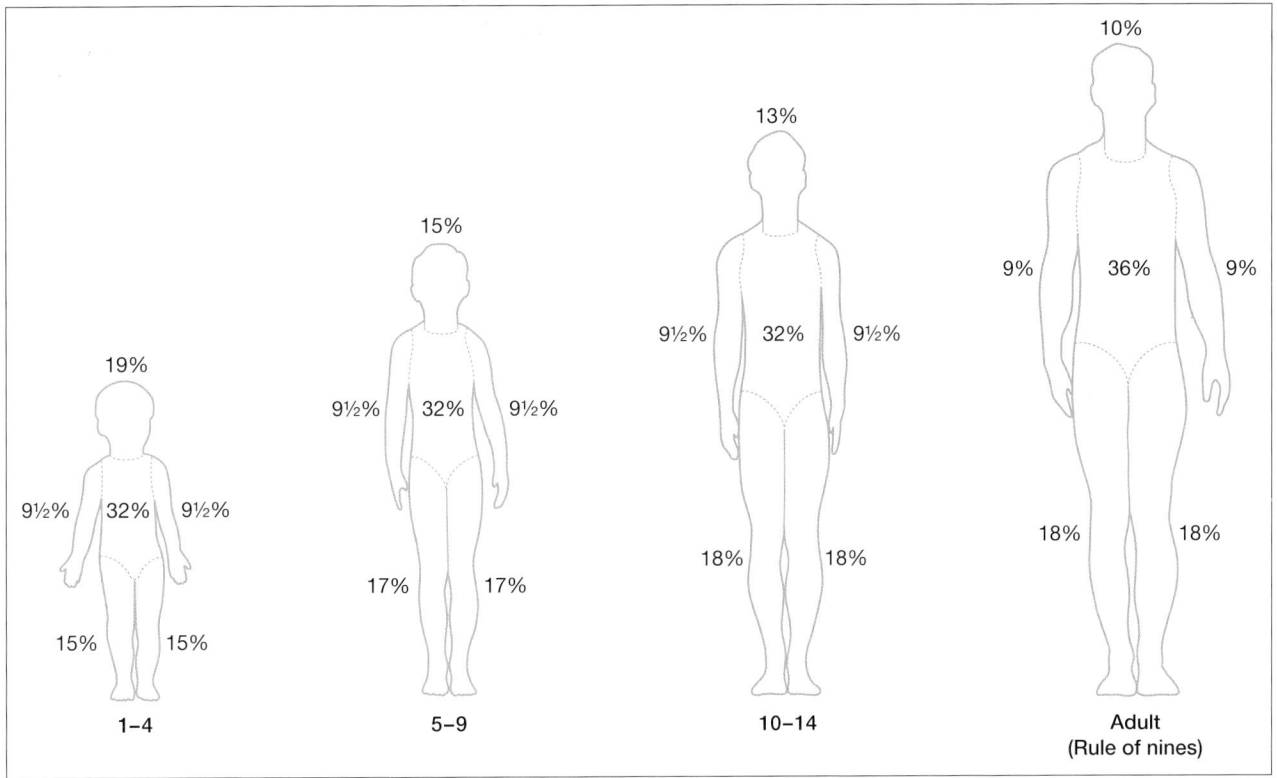

Fig. 39.2 Burn assessment chart with body proportions. Numbers under figures indicate age; other numbers indicate percent body surface. (From Herndon DN. *Total Burn Care*. 5th ed. Edinburgh: Elsevier; 2018:374.)

Thermal burns commonly occur in and around the home. Approximately 70% of burns sustained by those up to the age of 4 years are the result of scald injuries, whereas flame burns are the most common pattern among children aged 5 years and older. In general, younger children are at higher risk for sustaining burn injuries, where abuse or neglect may account for as much as 15% to 20% of these cases.[5]

Inhalation injuries may accompany a thermal burn and should be suspected until ruled out.[16-19] The extent of damage will depend on the where the fire occurred, its ignition source and temperature, and the concentration of the toxic gases. Inhalation injury is generally classified into four types based on anatomic location. The first type includes upper airway injuries caused primarily by thermal injury to the mouth, oropharynx, and larynx. The second type includes lower airway injuries to the trachea, bronchioles, and alveoli caused by chemical and particulate constituents of smoke. The third type includes pulmonary parenchymal injury, and the fourth type includes metabolic asphyxiation or systemic toxicity where smoke constituents such as carbon monoxide or hydrogen cyanide impair oxygen delivery or use by the tissues. All four types may coexist in the burned patient.

Damage to the airway can vary, depending on whether the upper airway or lower airway is affected. Upper airway injuries result from inhalation of superheated air or steam and toxic compounds found in smoke.[16] Brief exposure of the epiglottis or larynx to either dry air at 300°C or steam at 100°C can lead to massive edema and rapid airway obstruction. The addition of an inhalation injury to a cutaneous burn doubles the mortality rate[17] and is a greater determinant of death than size of the burn wound. Inhalation of heated air can result in direct injury to the face, oropharynx, and upper trachea, while sparing the lower airway. It is speculated that heat entrained is readily dissipated in the upper airway and reflex closure of the vocal cords to protect the lower airway. However, true thermal injury from exposure to live

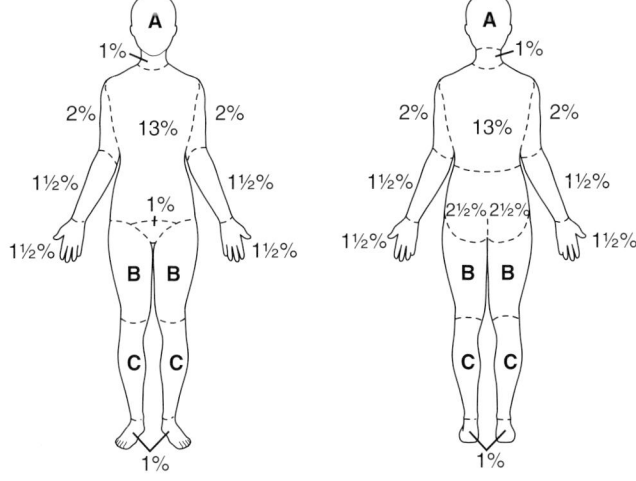

Area	Age 0	1	5	10	15	Adult
A - ½ of head	9½%	8½%	6½%	5½%	4½%	3½%
B - ½ of one thigh	2¾%	3¼%	4%	4¼%	4½%	4¼%
C - ½ of one leg	2½%	2½%	2¾%	3%	3¼%	3½%

Fig. 39.3 Lund-Browder chart.

steam can occur in the lower respiratory tract because heat-exchange mechanisms of the airway are unable to cool the gas sufficiently as it is inhaled. Obstruction of the upper airway is due to excessive edema, macroglossia, and swelling of the pharyngeal soft tissue. Lower airway injuries more commonly arise from the inhalation of soot particles

TABLE 39.2   Biphasic Organ System Response to Injury

Organ System	Early Change	Later Status
Cardiovascular	Shock	Hyperdynamic
Urinary	Oliguria	Diuresis
Gastrointestinal	Ileus	Hypermotility
Musculoskeletal	Hypoperfusion	Hyperperfusion
Pulmonary	Hypoventilation	Hyperventilation
Endocrine	Catabolism	Anabolism
Immunologic	Inflammation (SIRS)	Suppression (CARS)
CNS	Agitation	Obtundation

CARS, Compensatory antiinflammatory response syndrome; *CNS*, central nervous system; *SIRS*, systemic inflammatory response syndrome. From Anderson TA, Fuzaylov G. Perioperative anesthesia management of the burn patient. *Surg Clin North Am.* 2014;94(4):851–861.

TABLE 39.3   Grading Scheme for Flexible Scope Bronchoscopy Findings in Inhalation Injury

Grade	Findings	Mortality (%)
0	Normal (no inhalation injury)	0
B	Positive based on biopsy only	0
1	Hyperemia	2
2	Severe edema and hyperemia	15
3	Severe injury: ulcerations and necrosis	62

Adapted from Chou SH, et al. Fiber-optic bronchoscopic classification of inhalation injury: prediction of acute lung injury. *Surg Endosc.* 2004;18(9):1377–1379; Cancio LC. Airway management and smoke inhalation injury in the burn patient. *Clin Plast Surg.* 2009;36(4): 555–567.

and/or chemicals produced by a fire. In the lower airway, inhaled toxins react with the airway mucosa forming acidic and alkaline substances increasing capillary permeability. Extensive alveolar and epithelial damage can occur, with the trachea and bronchial tissue becoming necrotic. Warning signs of inhalation injury include hoarseness, sore throat, dysphagia, hemoptysis, tachypnea, the use of accessory muscles, wheezing, carbonaceous sputum, and elevated carbon monoxide levels.[16,20-22]

Treatment of the burn patient involves three distinct phases: the resuscitative phase, debridement and grafting, and the reconstructive phase. Each phase has its own set of challenges the anesthetist must consider when developing the anesthetic plan.

TREATMENT OF THE BURN PATIENT

Treatment of the burn patient will evolve as the patient progresses through the early resuscitative phase to the later hypermetabolic state. Data from the US Army Surgical Research Unit and the Army Burn Center characterize the biphasic organ system response to injury (Table 39.2).[23]

Resuscitative Phase

The resuscitative phase is the period of time postburn that encompasses the first 24 to 48 hours. Burn injury that affects more than 20% TBSA can result in burn shock, which leads to decreases in blood volume and cardiac output that inevitably impact perfusion to vital organs. Consequently, fluid resuscitation is critical to address ongoing burn shock in this early phase and the balance between overresuscitation and underresuscitation weighed.[24] Initial treatment of the burn patient involves attention to the airway, breathing, circulation, and any coexisting trauma, as well as previous health history. All burn patients must be considered at risk for pulmonary compromise, especially if the percentage of TBSA involved is significant, and signs of inhalation injury are present.

Airway Injury

Initially, it is essential to rule out upper airway injury in patients at risk (e.g., involving a fire that occurred in a closed space or the development of unconsciousness or stupor preventing the patient from protecting the airway). Diagnosis is made by history, the circumstances surrounding the burn injury, and physical examination. Burn injuries to the head and neck can produce inflammation causing decreased range

of motion, as well as edema of the tongue, oropharynx, and larynx, resulting in distorted anatomy that makes direct laryngoscopy almost impossible.[16] Heat rarely causes damage below the vocal cords because it is effectively dissipated. The other components of smoke such as particulate materials, systemic toxins, and respiratory irritants trigger a cascade of events, resulting in pulmonary edema and a ventilation/perfusion $(\dot{V}/\dot{Q})$ mismatch.[25] Airway examination is best accomplished by direct visualization of the airway with a laryngoscope or flexible intubation scope.[26] Flexible scope bronchoscopy is the gold standard for the diagnosis of severity of inhalation injury. Table 39.3 has a commonly used classification of flexible scope findings and associated mortality.[27] The chest radiograph may be normal in the early phase of inhalation injury (unless aspiration of gastric or pharyngeal contents occurred during the accident), becoming abnormal once pulmonary edema or infiltration develops. Chest computerized axial tomography (CT) may be more beneficial in determining the degree of pulmonary insult.[16] Treatment of upper airway injury involves early endotracheal intubation, even if the patient is not yet demonstrating signs of airway decompensation. Even in the absence of an inhalation injury, the lungs are at risk for compromise if the burn area is large.

Thermal damage to soft tissues of the respiratory tract and trachea can make endotracheal intubation difficult due to tissue swelling and bleeding. Intubation is much easier to perform earlier than later, when there may be glottic or facial edema, which worsens after fluid resuscitation.[20-30] Additionally, once sloughing off of tissue begins, mask ventilation may be difficult when unable to intubate the patient, making early intubation advisable in anticipated difficult airways. Depending on the area of the face and neck burned, many have moved directly to tracheostomy to avoid further airway difficulties as swelling increases. In the pediatric population, intubation should be performed with an uncuffed endotracheal tube, usually one size smaller than expected according to age and weight. Videolaryngoscopy, flexible scope intubation, or supraglottic airway-guided intubation techniques have all proven useful in securing the airway in the burned patient. Some have used a retrograde wire technique through the cricothyroid membrane as well.[31] Nasotracheal intubation in children may be preferred since it is better tolerated, and tube displacement with movement is less likely. Cuffed endotracheal tubes are traditionally used for pediatric patients older than 8 years of age. They are commonly used in pediatric burns because of the added flexibility of not requiring replacement that can be necessitated by decreasing edema and air leaks, which is the case with uncuffed tubes.[5,20]

In the absence of an airway abnormality, early tracheal intubation can usually be achieved using a routine technique with an intravenous induction agent and a rapid-acting muscle relaxant. There is general agreement that succinylcholine administration to patients more than 24 hours after burn injury is unsafe,[15,32] although some authors extend this safe period to 48 hours.[15] Cholinergic receptor up-regulation occurs after a burn injury, with proliferation of acetylcholine receptors throughout the muscle membrane. Succinylcholine can cause potassium (K^+) release from the entire muscle membrane rather than from discrete endplate junctions, leading to hyperkalemia and cardiac arrest.[33,34] The magnitude of K^+ elevation appears to be related to the size of the burn, and the process of receptor up-regulation takes days to develop, allowing an initial 24-hour window of safety if succinylcholine is considered. It is therefore wise to avoid the use of succinylcholine in a burn patient more than 24 hours after injury.[35]

Intubation with a nondepolarizing relaxant or without a relaxant via the techniques mentioned previously allow for safe airway control. Several factors produce an increased dose requirement of nondepolarizing relaxants in burn patients. These include up-regulation of acetylcholine receptors, massive fluid shifts producing significant changes in volume of distribution, and a qualitative decrease in receptor sensitivity. Plasma protein-binding alterations do not affect relaxants clinically because they are not highly bound. Rocuronium, for example, is only 30% protein bound, and the dose administered and serum concentrations required in the burn patient may be increased three- to fivefold to achieve the desired paralysis with a nondepolarizer.[36-38]

With an abnormal airway or upper airway obstruction, the safest way to secure the airway is with the patient awake. Effective topical anesthesia, patient positioning, and supplemental oxygenation will go hand in hand with incremental doses of ketamine or a dexmedetomidine infusion allowing the patient to breath spontaneously with airway reflexes intact while the airway is secured. Administration of sedatives may worsen airway obstruction and should be given judiciously. However, intravenous opioid administration may be appropriate for the alert patient in pain. To reiterate, methods to secure the airway include flexible scope intubation, direct or videolaryngoscopy, supraglottic airway-assisted intubation, blind nasal intubation, retrograde wire, or other video-assisted techniques. When the upper airway is badly damaged and endotracheal intubation is not possible, a direct surgical approach such as tracheotomy is indicated.

After the airway has been secured, the burn patient is taken to the intensive care unit and placed on ventilatory support.[39] Inspired gases should be humidified to aid clearing of tracheobronchial debris and prevent drying of secretions. The endotracheal tube must be kept in place until the surrounding laryngeal edema has subsided. A progressive air leak around the endotracheal tube, especially in uncuffed pediatric sizes, may be an indication that edematous tissue is returning to normal.[20,31,40]

Administration of nebulized heparin and N-acetylcysteine with massive burn and smoke inhalation injury results in a decreased incidence of reintubation for progressive pulmonary failure, decreased atelectasis, and reduced mortality. The Shriners Burn Hospital formula includes 5000 units of heparin and 3 mL of a 20% solution of N-acetylcysteine aerosolized every 4 hours for the first 7 days after the injury.[25]

Carbon Monoxide Poisoning

Any burn victim rescued from an enclosed-space fire should be considered at high risk for carbon monoxide poisoning. It is estimated that 50% to 60% of all fire victims die from carbon monoxide poisoning.[41] Symptoms depend on the carboxyhemoglobin (COHgb) level, although it is the tissue carbon monoxide level that determines the toxicity of carbon monoxide (Table 39.4).

Carbon monoxide binds to the hemoglobin molecule with 200 times greater affinity than oxygen, leading to a fall in oxyhemoglobin

TABLE 39.4 Carbon Monoxide Poisoning

Carboxyhemoglobin (%)	Symptoms
0–10	Normal
10–20	Headache, confusion
20–40	Disorientation, fatigue, nausea, visual changes
40–60	Hallucination, combativeness, convulsion, coma, shock state
60–70	Coma, convulsions, weak respiration and pulse
70–80	Decreasing respiration and stopping
80–90	Death in <1 hr
90–100	Death within a few minutes

From Einhorn IN. Physiological and toxicological aspects of smoke produced during the combustion of polymeric materials. *Environ Health Perspect.* 1975;11:163–189; Schulte JH. Effects of mild carbon monoxide intoxication. *Arch Environ Health* 1963;7:524–530.

saturation as tissues become unable to extract oxygen.[42] The end result is disruption in mitochondrial oxidative phosphorylation, producing metabolic acidosis at the cellular level. Arterial blood gas analysis reveals normal arterial oxygen tension but a decrease in total oxygen content due to markedly reduced hemoglobin oxygen saturation. Carbon monoxide increases the stability of the oxyhemoglobin molecule (COHgb), decreasing the release of oxygen to the tissues and producing a leftward shift in the oxyhemoglobin curve (see Fig. 18.8). Pulse oximeters do not detect COHgb in blood and therefore provide falsely elevated readings for oxygen saturation in its presence. The diagnosis of carbon monoxide poisoning requires measurement of arterial COHgb levels using a laboratory blood cooximeter, which measures concentrations of all hemoglobin moieties (i.e., oxyhemoglobin, deoxyhemoglobin, carboxyhemoglobin, and methemoglobin). The half-life of COHgb is variable in patients treated with 100% oxygen, ranging from 26 to 148 minutes. Treatment continues with 100% oxygen until the COHgb level is less than 5% or for 6 hours.[41-44]

Alternatively, hyperbaric oxygen therapy may be used as it accelerates the clearance of carbon monoxide, although debate continues over its effectiveness and availability.[45]

Cyanide Poisoning

Hydrogen cyanide (HCN) poisoning is another systemic poisoning that may occur when individuals succumb to a burn injury. It is produced by the combustion of materials such as plastics, foam, paints, wool, and silk producing tissue hypoxia by blocking the intracellular use of oxygen. Cyanide binds to the terminal cytochrome on the electron transport chain, causing hypoxia, lactic acidosis, and elevated mixed venous oxygen saturation. The half-life of HCN is approximately 1 hour. Signs and symptoms of poisoning include loss of consciousness, dilated pupils, seizures, hypotension, tachypnea followed by apnea, and high lactate levels. The main antidote, hydroxocobalamin (vitamin B_{12}) actively binds cyanide by forming cyanocobalamin, which is directly excreted via the kidney.

Hydroxocobalamin has a rapid onset of action, neutralizes cyanide without interfering with cellular oxygen use, and has a good safety profile. It is safe for use with smoke-inhalation victims, easy to administer, and is the preferred antidote to this type of cyanide poisoning. A hydroxocobalamin dose of 5 g over 15 minutes is recommended.

In addition, aggressive stabilization of cardiopulmonary function augments the hepatic clearance of cyanide via rhodanese and can resolve cyanide poisoning (blood levels, 5.6–9 mg/L), without the use of antidotes.[25,26,46]

Hypovolemic Shock Associated With Burn Injury

After the airway has been secured and other life-threatening injuries have been managed, the burn patient is aggressively resuscitated with large volumes of intravenous fluids. Fluid administration and restoration of blood volume are critical for patient survival and preventing renal failure. As mentioned previously, burns cause a form of hypovolemic shock, and changes are reflected in loss of circulating plasma volume, hemoconcentration, massive edema formation, decreased urine output, and depressed cardiovascular function.[30,47] Fluid losses are greatest in the first 12 hours after burn injury and then begin to stabilize after 24 hours. Fluid losses occur secondary to direct transudation of plasma and plasma proteins from the wound and from diffuse capillary leakage shifting fluid from the intravascular space to the interstitium of unburned tissue. Capillary leak results from the shedding of the endothelial glycocalyx, which normally supports the vascular wall.[102-104] Thus intravascular oncotic pressure is reduced, and plasma proteins are lost through the burn wound and what have become incompetent capillary beds. The result of changes in the microvasculature and disruption of barriers separating intravascular and interstitial compartments leads to an equilibration of these compartments. This causes severe depletion of plasma volume and a marked increase in extracellular fluid, clinically manifested as hypovolemia and burn-induced edema.[10,30,47]

Inflammatory mediators are released from burned tissues after injury, which causes localized inflammation and burn-wound edema. Localized mediators include oxygen radicals, arachidonic acid metabolites, histamine, prostaglandins, leukotrienes, products of platelet activation, and the complement cascade.[28,41,48] Most edema occurs locally at the burn site and is maximal at 24 hours after injury. The edema itself results in tissue hypoxia and increased tissue pressure with circumferential injuries. Aggressive fluid therapy can correct the hypovolemia but will also accentuate the edema process especially in nonburned areas. In minor burns, the inflammatory process typically remains sequestered in the wound area. However, in major burns, local injury signals the release of systemic circulatory mediators resulting in an overall systemic response.

Fluid Resuscitation

Immediately following an acute burn injury, massive fluid shifts begin to occur. Fluid resuscitation and airway management are the hallmarks of initial therapy and should be instituted by the first-response emergency medical providers. There are many formulas for calculating a burn patient's initial fluid resuscitation requirements. Crystalloid resuscitation often provides substantial volumes of fluid, often in excess of that predicted by current formulas, resulting in numerous edema-related complications. This phenomenon is coined "fluid creep," and fluid therapy after the initial 24 hours is constantly being refined. In most centers, two formulas are accepted as guidelines for the resuscitation of severely burned patients, the Parkland and modified Brooke formulas.[49,50] The need for blood transfusion is usually not a major concern during the immediate resuscitation phase in acutely burned patients unless other coexisting trauma exists. Transfusion management is a prominent issue during subsequent surgical intervention.

The current ABA consensus formula for fluid resuscitation and urine output in burn patients is given in Box 39.1. Table 39.5 lists other suggested fluid protocols. Common to all of these formulas is the patient's weight in kilograms and the percentage of TBSA

TABLE 39.5 Fluid Resuscitation Formulas for Burn Patients

Formula	First 24 Hr	Second 24 Hr
Modified Brooke		
Crystalloid	2 mL LR/% burn/kg, ½ in first 8 hr, ½ in next 16 hr	D₅W maintenance
Colloid	None	0.5 mL/% burn/kg
Parkland		
Crystalloid	4 mL LR/% burn/kg, ½ in first 8 hr, ½ in next 16 hr	D₅W maintenance
Colloid	None	0.5 mL/% burn/kg

D₅W, 5% dextrose in water; *LR*, lactated Ringer solution.

---

involved. The ACS Committee on Trauma has advocated only crystalloid formulas be used for burn resuscitation. Colloid solutions have historically not been advocated in the first 24 hours since capillary permeability is intensified, and colloids administered will theoretically extravasate into the interstitium. However, some burn centers are now reevaluating the use of colloids to decrease the total volume of crystalloids administered. In addition, recent studies have demonstrated administration of fresh frozen plasma ameliorating the endothelial (glycocalyx) dysfunction previously described. That said, isotonic crystalloid (Ringer lactate) is the most commonly used fluid for resuscitation in US burn centers. The modified Brooke formula reduces both the protein content and volume of the infused resuscitation fluid. That formula recognizes the findings of studies showing that in the first 3 hours after injury, burn wound edema is most strongly affected by intravascular pressure and later most strongly by capillary permeability. The initially increased capillary permeability decreases across time and establishes a new transcapillary equilibrium 24 hours after the burn, at which time the water and protein content of the burn wound peak.[51] The Parkland formula uses isotonic crystalloid solutions and estimates the fluid requirements in the first 24 hours to be 4 mL/kg per percentage TBSA burned. Crystalloid solutions generally provide adequate volume resuscitation, but the large volumes needed result in substantial tissue edema and

BOX 39.2 Criteria for Adequate Fluid Resuscitation

- Normalization of blood pressure
- Urine output (1–2 mL/kg/hr)
- Blood lactate (<2 mmol/L)
- Base deficit (<–5)
- Gastric intramucosal pH (>7.32)
- Central venous pressure
- Cardiac index (CI) (4.5 L/min/m²)
- Oxygen delivery index (DO₂I) (600 mL/min/m²)

From Woodsen LE, et al. Anesthesia for burned patients. In: Herndon DN, ed. *Total Burn Care*. 5th ed. Edinburgh: Elsevier; 2018:131–157.

hypoproteinemia. Consequently, complications of overresuscitation—including abdominal compartment syndrome (ACS), pleural and pericardial effusions, pulmonary edema, the need for fasciotomies, and conversion of partial-thickness lesions to full-thickness lesions—are more frequently observed.[50] It is important to remember that formulas for fluid guidelines are only that—guidelines. Individual factors must also be taken into account. It is crucial to resuscitate the patient with fluids according to patient response, hemodynamic variables, sensorium, and urinary output (0.5–1 mL/kg/hour in adults and 1 mL/kg/hour in children weighing <60 lb),[48] instead of by a fixed formula.[28] Fluid resuscitation in children requires extreme precision, owing not only to the individual's size but also their limited physiologic reserve. For example, infants and small children have high volume-to-surface-area ratios, and formulas that base fluid requirements on surface area burned and weight may underestimate the need. The ABA recommends that to counteract the rapid use of glycogen stores and prevent the development of hypoglycemia, a dextrose-containing intravenous solution be administered for maintenance purposes in burned children in the immediate postburn period.[15,52,53] Some clinical criteria to indicate adequate fluid resuscitation are noted in Box 39.2.

Intraabdominal hypertension (IAH) and ACS are increasingly recognized as causes of significant morbidity and mortality in critically ill burn patients. These are some of the most dangerous and frequently reported adverse outcomes of fluid creep in massive burn resuscitation. IAH is a continuum of progressively worsening organ dysfunction, whereas ACS is an all-or-none phenomenon resulting when IAH remains either unrecognized or untreated. IAH and ACS impact end-organ function within not only the abdominal cavity (e.g., kidneys, liver, intestine) but also throughout the body (e.g., brain, lungs, heart). The most recent consensus guidelines define IAH as an intraabdominal pressure (obtained by transduction of bladder pressure) greater than or equal to 12 mm Hg, and ACS as an intraabdominal pressure greater than 20 mm Hg with evidence of new-organ dysfunction. New-organ dysfunction typically manifests as oliguria, impaired mechanical ventilation with high peak airway pressures, worsening metabolic acidosis, and hemodynamic instability. ACS is fatal without treatment. Treatment includes the use of neuromuscular relaxants and increased sedation in mechanically ventilated patients, extension of escharotomies on any anterior trunk burns, judicious use of diuretics, and decompressive laparotomy.[54-59]

Invasive hemodynamic monitoring (central venous pressure, pulmonary artery catheter) is indicated in patients who do not respond to fluid resuscitation, have preexisting cardiopulmonary disease, or are at risk of IAH and ACS. Currently, the use of transpulmonary thermodilution via a radial artery catheter has replaced pulmonary artery catheters in many settings. This technology provides numerous cardiac indices through the analysis of pulsed-wave form. In addition, transesophageal echocardiography (TEE) has been more readily available to evaluate real-time ventricular function and volume in the transgastric short-axis view of the left ventricle.

Hypermetabolic or Hyperhemodynamic Flow Phase

Severe thermal injury with burns over 40% of TBSA is followed by a pronounced hypermetabolic response beginning 24 to 72 hours after injury and can persist for up to 1 to 2 years. During this phase, there are significantly increased metabolic rates, multiorgan dysfunction, muscle protein degradation, blunted growth, insulin resistance, and increased risk for infection. The initial stress response to severe injury lasts for the first 2 to 3 days postburn. The subsequent phase is characterized by an increase in metabolism and hyperdynamic flow. When left untreated, physiologic exhaustion ensues, and the injury becomes fatal.

Catecholamines and corticosteroids are the primary mediators of the hypermetabolic response after severe burns. There can be a 10- to 50-fold surge of plasma catecholamine and corticosteroid levels that can last up to 9 months postburn. Glucagon levels are also increased. Burn patients have increased resting energy expenditures, increased cardiac work, increased myocardial oxygen consumption, marked tachycardia, severe lipolysis, liver dysfunction, severe muscle catabolism, increased protein degradation, insulin resistance, and growth retardation.[60-62] Numerous efforts to control this response have been studied. Specific nutritional interventions and the use of anabolic agents, β-adrenergic receptor antagonists, and antihyperglycemic agents have successfully counteracted postburn morbidities, including catabolism, the catecholamine-mediated response, and insulin resistance. Early burn wound excision and complete wound closure, prevention of sepsis, the maintenance of thermal neutrality for the patient by elevation of the ambient temperature, and graded resistance exercises during convalescence are simple, nonpharmacologic effective treatment goals.[60-63]

Pathophysiologic Changes

As with any disease entity, certain pathophysiologic alterations occur after an acute burn injury (Table 39.6). It is important for the anesthetist to understand the basis for these changes as many must be managed intraoperatively and reflected in the anesthetic plan.

Cardiovascular system. The cardiovascular system is impacted greatly in the burn patient. Almost immediately after acute burn injury, intravascular fluid losses commence as a direct result of the loss of vascular and endothelial integrity (the glycocalyx) and the release of circulating mediators. The loss of plasma proteins within the intravascular compartment (due to disruption of the endothelium) persists up to 36 hours after the initial burn. Hypovolemia results, with subsequent hypotension and circulatory compromise. The size and extent of the burn determine the magnitude of this development, hence burn victims can develop burn shock within the first 24 to 36 hours after their injury. A reduction in cardiac output is a hallmark of burn shock and appears to occur within minutes after the injury. It is initially preserved through catecholamine responses, which cause tachycardia and vasoconstriction. However, with the progressive loss of intravascular fluids and proteins, left ventricular filling declines, leading to a reduction in cardiac output. Additionally, cardiac output is thought to be depressed from the release of myocardial depressant factor or proteins from burned tissues. The cardiovascular response to catecholamines is attenuated after burn injury as the result of reduced adrenergic-receptor affinity and decreased secondary-messenger production. Coronary blood flow can be reduced, further decreasing myocardial function. Systemic vascular resistance increases.

Aggressive fluid resuscitation in the first 24 to 36 hours is directed toward restoring intravascular volume and cardiac function. A systemic

TABLE 39.6 Pathophysiologic Effects of Major Burns

System	Considerations	System	Considerations
Respiratory Upper airway	Thermal damage to soft tissue and respiratory tract can require early endotracheal intubation; decreased chest wall compliance, functional residual capacity, and restricted chest wall expansion	Electrical burns and muscle necrosis damage renal tubules	Careful fluid resuscitation, renal function monitoring, and possible diuretic administration
Carbon monoxide poisoning	Considered in all victims of enclosed fires; treatment with 100% oxygen by mask, endotracheal intubation strongly advised until status can be evaluated	**Late** Increased renal blood flow	Variable drug clearance
		Nutrition Increased caloric requirements	Tight nutritional support mandatory
Neurologic Encephalopathy, seizures, increased intracranial pressure	Ongoing neurologic assessment mandatory because status frequently changes	**Hepatic** *Early* Decreased function and drug clearance	Hepatomegaly; hypermetabolism and enzyme induction during hypermetabolic phase; sepsis common
Hematology Anemia, thrombocytopenia, and coagulopathies	Coagulopathies, transfusion reactions, and infection are common	**Pharmacokinetics** Decreased albumin	Altered volume of distribution, protein binding; highly protein-bound drugs have a higher free fraction and thus a larger volume of distribution
Cardiac Burn shock phase (0–48 hr)	Hypovolemia is a major concern; fluid resuscitation mandatory; expect impaired cardiac contractility, initial myocardial depression, and decreased cardiac output	Increased α_1-acid glycoprotein	Usually minimal clinical effects of drugs in spite of the changes in protein levels
Hypermetabolic phase (>48 hr)	Increased blood flow to organs and tissues; manifested by hyperthermia, tachypnea, tachycardia, increased oxygen consumption, and increased catabolism	Denervation phenomenon with spreading of acetylcholine receptors	Succinylcholine avoided 24 hr after injury
Renal *Early* Reduced renal blood flow and glomerular filtration rate	Secondary to hypovolemia and decreased cardiac output; adequate fluid resuscitation and diuresis prevents renal failure; myoglobinuria and hemoglobinuria common, which alters urine-concentrating ability	Increased nicotinic acetylcholine receptors and decreased function	Requires a two- to threefold increased concentration of nondepolarizing muscle relaxant for clinical paralysis
		Skin Integrity Vulnerable to nosocomial infections	Strict adherence to aseptic individual patient rooms; wound care, including topical antimicrobial agents and early excision/grafting of the burn wound

inflammatory response syndrome is heralded by an increased cardiac output, tachycardia, and reduction in systemic vascular resistance. Thus the patient becomes hypermetabolic, with an increase in oxygen consumption and carbon dioxide production.[64]

Children with extensive burn injuries can become significantly hypertensive weeks after their injury. Heart rate, cardiac output, and cardiac index remain increased in burned children for up to 2 years when compared with normal ranges indicating vastly increased cardiac stress. Aggressive treatment of the hyperdynamic cardiac response may improve long-term morbidity.[65]

Pulmonary system. The pulmonary system can also be significantly impacted in burn patients. Pulmonary function may decrease significantly even in the absence of inhalation injury. For example, functional residual capacity is reduced, and lung and chest-wall compliance decrease, especially when the chest wall is circumferentially burned. With progressive fluid shift and interstitial edema formation in those individuals with eschar formation, the inability to adequately expand the lungs impairs ventilation. In these cases, escharotomies

are performed to alleviate the constrictive pressure of the chest wall to improve oxygenation and ventilation. The oxygen gradient between alveoli and arterial blood increases with minute ventilation increasing to as much as 40 L/min from what is normally 6 L/min.

Even without inhalational injury, the lungs are at risk for compromise. There are several mechanisms involved, including the effect of released mediators on the lung. In addition, plasma oncotic pressure is greatly reduced after burn injury, owing to the loss of plasma proteins in burned and unburned tissue. Impaired vascular and capillary permeability, combined with the amount of fluid resuscitation, can set the stage for the development of pulmonary edema.

Mechanical ventilation is often required after major burn injury, especially when the patient has concomitant inhalation injury. The term *acute lung injury* (ALI) is used to designate the acute onset of impaired oxygen exchange that results from lung injury, and the condition is characterized by a partial pressure of arterial oxygen/fraction of inspired oxygen (Pao_2/Fio_2) ratio of less than 300. Severe cases of ALI, categorized as acute respiratory distress syndrome (ARDS), are common as well. The risk for mortality from ALI and ARDS is due to respiratory failure and hypoxia or may result from associated multisystem organ failure or ventilator-associated pneumonia. New strategies for mechanical ventilation are currently being used to support burn patients who have respiratory insufficiency, ALI, and ARDS. These strategies include those changes associated with "protective ventilation" and the ARDS-Net protocol. Protective ventilation involves use of smaller tidal volumes (4–6 mL/kg) using ideal body weight and maintaining ventilatory plateau pressures less than 31 cm H_2O. These measures reduce overinflation, barotrauma, and atelectrauma.[66,67] Using ideal body weight is an important consideration in these since they have increases in body weight due to massive fluid resuscitation. Modest permissive hypercapnia is allowed.[68] Several nonconventional modes of ventilation have been proposed for the treatment of severe ARDS in patients with burn injury, including airway pressure release ventilation (APRV), pressure-regulated volume control (PRVC), volumetric diffuse respiratory ventilation (VDR), or even extracorporeal membranous oxygenation (ECMO).[69,70]

Immune system. The burn-injured victim is particularly susceptible to infection because the protective function that the skin provides has been breached, and the stage is set for microbial invasion. Within hours after an acute burn, altered immunologic responses become apparent. Leukocyte activity is depressed, as well as humoral and cellular responses. Burn eschar is a prime medium for bacterial growth. Colonization of gram-negative bacteria increases mortality. Patients often become septic and are vulnerable to pneumonia, particularly when prolonged endotracheal intubation is necessary. Strict asepsis is therefore required. Of those patients who die after sustaining a burn, infection is the leading cause of death in up to 100% of children and 75% of adults.[5,31,64]

Renal system. Renal function begins to decrease soon after burn injury as a result of myoglobinuria and hemoglobinuria. Myoglobinuria is most common after electrical injury, whereas hemoglobinuria is common after severe cutaneous burns of approximately 40% or greater. Acute kidney injury (AKI) is a common complication following major burns, and its incidence may be as high as 40%. Its development is dependent on the size and severity of the burn and the presence of an inhalation injury, which is a poor prognostic indicator. AKI is divided into early and late categories. Early AKI occurs within 5 days of burn injury and results from hypotension and myoglobinuria. Late AKI occurs after 5 days, and sepsis is the most common cause.[50] Patients may exhibit an inability to concentrate their urine. Elevated levels of stress hormones (e.g., aldosterone, angiotensin, catecholamines, and plasma renin) also contribute to renal dysfunction observed in the early postburn period. Several burn centers are using the RIFLE criteria to assess AKI. RIFLE is an acronym for *r*isk, *i*njury, *f*ailure, *l*oss, and *e*nd-stage kidney disease. It is often used in patients with renal disease in identifying the risk factors for occurrence of AKI, as well as analyzing the progression between stages of the RIFLE classification and the impact of progression of AKI on morbidity and mortality.[71,72]

Decreases in renal blood flow alter glomerular filtration. This is usually due to intravascular depletion, hypovolemia, decreased cardiac output, and increased levels of circulating plasma catecholamines. The renin-angiotensin-aldosterone system and the release of antidiuretic hormone are stimulated to conserve sodium and water.[73] Subsequently, alterations in electrolyte balance take place. Hourly urine output measurements remain the gold standard for assessing adequate fluid replacement and resuscitation (see Box 39.1). Delayed renal failure in children is rare.[74]

Gastrointestinal system/nutrition. Aggressive nutrition support is mandatory in the patient who has sustained severe burn injury. Metabolic rates may be increased by twice the normal rate secondary to the hypermetabolic state. Whole-body catabolism, muscle wasting, and severe cachexia occur with inadequate nutrition. Failure to meet the increased substrate requirements can result in impaired wound healing, multiorgan dysfunction, increased susceptibility to infection, and death.[75,76] In patients with extensive burns and a pronounced hypermetabolic response, carbohydrate is more effective than fat in maintaining body protein.[79] The burn-injured patient is resistant to the action of insulin in the liver and skeletal muscle, thus ongoing assessment of blood glucose with administration of insulin in a tight control protocol becomes necessary.

The need for continued adequate caloric intake during the preanesthetic period cannot be ignored. It is unwise to arbitrarily discontinue enteral feedings the evening before a scheduled surgical procedure. This action may result in an excessive loss of calories, especially if the patient is to undergo extensive burn excision and debridement. Preoperative nil per os (NPO) guidelines must be considered at a safe minimum to prevent the patient from reverting to a catabolic state. For example, intubated patients do not need enteral feedings discontinued before surgery, whereas unintubated patients may remain on nutritional support up to 4 hours before a scheduled surgical procedure.[77] This practice maintains preoperative nutrition without increasing the risk for aspiration. Upon admission to the operating room, a nonintubated patient's nasogastric tube (if present) should be suctioned and general anesthesia induced to ensure rapid protection of the airway. If the patient is not receiving enteral feedings, but rather parenteral feedings through a central venous catheter, the parenteral nutrition line should not be used for administering fluids or drugs during the course of the anesthetic. Parenteral hyperalimentation and lipid infusions should be continued intraoperatively. Monitoring of glucose levels in these patients is advised. The use of infusions pumps is recommended in children to avoid over- or underinfusions.[30,78]

Burn patients also demonstrate a decrease in overall gastrointestinal function. When the percentage of TBSA involved is greater than 20%, the development of ileus is common.[79] Other gastrointestinal sequelae include acute ulcerations of the gastric and/or duodenal mucosa known as Curling ulcers. Treatment of these stress ulcers includes the administration of acid suppressive therapy (AST), including H_2 blockers, proton pump inhibitors, and antacids.[26] Fortunately, with the use of AST, these ulcers have become less frequent.[80]

Hepatic effects of burn injury are variable. There may be an increase in liver function during the hypermetabolic phase followed by hypertrophy, hepatomegaly, and impaired protein synthesis. Hepatic dysfunction also may result from drug toxicity, sepsis, or blood transfusions. Preoperative assessment of liver function is advised.[81,82]

Burn Management: Debridement and Grafting

The goal of burn therapy is to rapidly restore skin integrity. After thorough cleansing, the burn wound is typically treated with antimicrobial agents to limit bacterial proliferation on the wound surface and to avoid bacterial wound invasion. Wounds have been shown to reepithelialize more rapidly with less pain and inflammation when they are covered and a thin layer of wound fluid is maintained in contact with the surface. Subsequent treatment involves surgical procedures such as amputation, grafting, and multiple debridements.[83] Early removal and excision of dead burn tissue with rapid closure of the burn wound has now become the standard in management of a severe burn. The early reestablishment of a physical skin barrier provides protection from bacteria, mechanical trauma, and insensible water loss improving long-term outcomes.[84]

Because most patients with extensive burns require multiple procedures, limiting a single procedure to 20% excision of body surface has been suggested; however, larger areas may be excised depending on the patient's preoperative and perioperative hemodynamic stability and coagulation status. Other surgical endpoints include a time of 2 to 3 hours if the patient's core temperature decreases to 35°C or if there has been blood loss requiring 10 units or more of packed red blood cells.[85] Generally, the burn patient may require surgical treatment every 2 to 3 days, with staging of burn wound excisions until full grafting has been completed. Significant blood loss during burn surgery continues to be a challenge. Implementation of blood-conserving protocols can decrease blood component requirements. Several options include tumescent epinephrine, thrombin, fibrin, and other systemic hemostatic agents. The best hemostatic protocol must be individualized.[86,87]

In patients with extensive burns and limited donor sites, the wound coverage may require a combination of skin grafts, cultured skin, and skin substitutes. Several temporary and permanent skin substitutes are available.[88]

Anesthetic Considerations

Preoperative evaluation. The burn patient requires a thorough and complete preoperative assessment in consultation with the burn team. Medical history, including laboratory studies, and physical examination with lung auscultation, assessment of chest compliance, and inspection of the neck and oral cavity to determine potential difficulties with airway management should be implemented. In addition, the clinician should be aware of any underlying trauma, mechanism of burn (electrical, inhalation), percentage of TBSA injured, location of the burn sites, and the type and extent of the planned procedure. This information may impact the selection of agents, appropriate monitoring, positioning, vascular access, and blood product requirements. A review of prior surgical procedures and anesthetics can be helpful in determining one's anesthetic plan, as these patients tend to have multiple procedures.

The setup and preparation. A successful anesthetic that facilitates surgical excision and grafting of a burn wound requires planning and preparation of all necessary equipment (Box 39.3). There are specific anesthetic interventions that should be considered prior to patient arrival in the operating room. Perioperative challenges in the acute burn patient are noted in Box 39.4.

Intraoperative management

Equipment and monitoring. Burn patients require all standard monitors intraoperatively, although this otherwise routine consideration may be challenging. Electrocardiogram (ECG) leads are often difficult to place due to a lack of intact skin. Alternatives include stapling lead electrodes to the skin, use of needle electrodes, or an atrial pacing-type esophageal stethoscope (Tapscope, CardioCommand, Tampa, FL) used for its ECG and temperature monitoring capability. Ideally, blood pressure cuffs should be placed on the unaffected limb or at a nonsurgical site. If the extent of surgical debridement is extensive or if movement of the patient's extremities intraoperatively limits accuracy of noninvasive cuff readings, the placement of an arterial line for blood pressure monitoring may be warranted, even in healthy patients. Large burns (i.e., >20%–30% TBSA) may necessitate invasive blood pressure monitoring after induction of anesthesia, if not in place preoperatively. Rapid and significant blood loss, potential for hemodynamic swings, and the need to verify intraoperative laboratory values more than validate this requirement.

Standard sites for monitoring pulse oximetry may not be available. Alternative sites include the nose, nasal alae or septum, ear, cheek, tongue, or toes. Any preexisting invasive monitors such as an arterial line, central venous catheter, or pulmonary artery catheter or transpulmonary thermodilution should be continued in the operating room. Noninvasive monitors for cardiac output, index, and stroke volume are also available.[89] Accurate temperature monitoring is essential as burn patients can become extremely hypothermic intraoperatively. Skin

temperature devices are highly inaccurate in these patients, and there may not be a suitable area to apply them. Temperature measurements are obtained from a properly positioned esophageal stethoscope (i.e., distal third of the esophagus) or other core temperature monitors. Because many of these patients are in intensive care units, they may already be benefiting from a urinary drainage catheter that supports bladder temperature monitoring.

Critically ill burn patients are usually transported by the anesthesia provider directly to the operating room from the burn intensive care unit (and vice versa, postoperatively). These patients are typically intubated or have a tracheostomy, are on continuous infusions of pharmacologic agents, and have invasive lines in place. Astute monitoring of the patient's vital signs during transport is mandatory. Extreme care and diligence should be taken during transport so that none of these become dislodged. Portable oxygen delivery system is another component of required transport equipment. Careful handling and vigilant guarding of the airway is crucial. Amnestic and analgesic drugs should be administered as needed to facilitate moving the patient.

Airway management. Acute airway problems are usually addressed immediately upon the patient's entry into the emergency department or once in the burn unit. In the nonintubated patient without an inhalation injury and whose airway is essentially normal, induction and intubation of the airway can proceed as with any other anesthetic apart from avoiding succinylcholine after the first 24 hours of injury.

The use of other airway methods discussed earlier may be considered if securing the airway is judged to be potentially difficult.

If the patient is already intubated, vigilance must be maintained to ensure the trachea does not become accidentally extubated. Edema of airway structures may make reintubation difficult if not impossible. Thus securing an endotracheal tube in these patients can be most challenging because tape does not readily stick to burned skin. Some clinicians have used soft straps, nasal septal ties, or sutures to secure the endotracheal tube. Cloth ties encircling the patient's head are frequently used as well.

Temperature regulation. Depending on the percentage of TBSA affected by a burn, temperature regulation can be problematic. There is a high risk for development of hypothermia secondary to evaporative heat loss and the body surface area exposed intraoperatively. The temperature in the OR should be between 28°C and 33°C (80°F and 100°F).[39,40,90] Intravenous solutions and skin preparations should be warmed. All methods of heat conservation should be employed while the patient is in the operating room. The use of inline circuit heat moisture exchangers or lower gas flows will reduce evaporative respiratory tract heat loss. Forced-air warming blankets are effective, but their use can be limited depending on the area of excision or surgical exposure. Over-body heating lamps have been used but need to be at a safe distance from the patient to prevent further burning. Plastic bags also can be helpful to insulate exposed body parts not requiring surgical access.

It has been suggested that keeping a patient warm is more beneficial than rewarming. When hypothermia ensues, deleterious effects of vasoconstriction occur, which may hinder any subsequent warming efforts. Moreover, slow rewarming in the postoperative period can lead to an increase in mortality.[91] If a patient becomes hypothermic despite efforts at prevention, the surgeon should be advised to conclude the procedure as quickly as possible. Heat loss in burn patients is characterized in Table 39.7.

Fluid and blood replacement. Surgical burn debridement procedures may be extraordinarily bloody operations. Surgical blood loss depends on the area to be excised (cm²), time since injury, type of excision planned, and the presence of infection. Surgical wound management involves removal of the eschar layer until brisk bleeding of the dermis is observed. The surgical team may remove eschar so rapidly that it becomes difficult to replace blood and intravenous fluid in a manner that parallels the loss, giving way to hypovolemia and hypotension. Some institutions have suggested stopping the surgical procedure after 2 hours if more than two blood volumes have been lost or if the body temperature falls to 35°C or by greater than 1.5°C from baseline.

There are several formulae used to approximate the extent of potential blood loss for a burn patient undergoing debridement. These vary from 200 to 400 mL of blood loss for each 1% of body surface area excised to as high as 4% to 15% of the patient's blood volume for every percentage of skin debrided.[31,40] After excision and debridement, several hemostatic therapies may be used, including tumescent epinephrine, phenylephrine thrombin, fibrin, and other systemic hemostatic agents. Gauze soaked in a vasoconstrictor preparation applied to the wounds may result in systemic absorption causing an undesired change in vital signs.[83] Table 39.8 lists a method for predicting surgical blood loss.

Preoperative anemia is another indicator for transfusion and is commonly seen in thermally burned patients with greater than 10% TBSA involvement.[92-94] There are several reasons for its development. The inflammatory process gives way to destruction of red blood cells that accumulate in thrombosed microcirculation of burned tissues, leading to an erythrocyte loss of up to 18% in full-thickness burns

greater than 15% TBSA.[95] Thus bone marrow suppression leads to a reduction in the production of erythropoietin after burn injury. Lastly, patients with extensive burns generally undergo numerous surgical procedures, resulting in blood loss and further anemia.

Adequate vascular access is critical before the initiation of surgical debridement. The size and extent of planned debridement will determine how much access is needed. One large-bore intravenous catheter is adequate for the induction of anesthesia in many burn patients, but at least two large-bore intravenous catheters are necessary before beginning a major excision. Obtaining sufficient intravenous access can be challenging and time consuming, depending on the extent and location of the burn. Critically ill patients or those with limited peripheral sites for intravenous access will often have a central venous catheter already in place. A large-bore catheter or a central line with multiple ports should be used whenever administration of large amounts of intravenous fluid and blood products is anticipated.

Availability of blood products should be confirmed before the patient is taken to anesthesia and operation. Ideally, blood products should have been checked and ready for administration at the outset of the procedure. This is particularly important in pediatric patients. Indeed, some clinicians initiate blood transfusion before the beginning of surgical debridement and apply compression dressings after excision and grafting.

Careful planning is essential when managing hemorrhage and potential complications associated with massive transfusion (e.g., citrate toxicity, loss of clotting factors, dilutional thrombocytopenia) during debridement. Visual estimation of blood loss is subjective at

TABLE 39.7 Heat Loss in Burn Patients

Source of Heat Loss	Amount	Methods to Decrease Heat Loss
Radiation	60	Warm operating room (OR)* (28°C–33°C) Heat lamps Reflective blankets
Evaporation	25	Warm OR
Convection	12	Place patient on insulated or warming blanket
Conduction	3	Cover patient with watertight material Humidify ventilator gases Intravenous fluid warmer Forced air warming blanket

*To decrease the difference in temperature between the patient and surrounding objects.
Modified from Anderson TA, Fuzaylov G. Perioperative anesthesia management of the burn patient. *Surg Clin North Am.* 2014;94(4): 851–861.

TABLE 39.8 Calculation of Expected Blood Loss

Surgical Procedure	Predicted Blood Loss
<24 hr since burn injury	0.45 mL/cm² burn area
1–3 days since burn injury	0.65 mL/cm² burn area
2–16 days since burn injury	0.75 mL/cm² burn area
>16 days since burn injury	0.5–0.75 mL/cm² burn area
Infected wounds	1–1.25 mL/cm² burn area

From Woodsen LE, et al. Anesthesia for burned patients. In: Herndon DN, ed. *Total Burn Care.* 5th ed. Edinburgh: Elsevier; 2018:131–157.

best and prone to miscalculation. Surgical suction is often not used during debridement, and surgical sponges are difficult to assess. Blood may leak onto the floor, be covered in the surgical drapes, or ooze beneath the patient. Thus proper monitoring of the patient's urinary output, hemoglobin, hematocrit, coagulation, and hemodynamic status is crucial during and after the surgical procedure.

Anesthesia Management

Induction. No single agent is preferred for intravenous induction of general anesthesia in the burn patient. As with all anesthetics, plans should be individualized and based on the patient's preoperative status and medical history. The acutely burned patient seldom comes to the operating room immediately after injury; generally, the patient is first admitted and stabilized in the burn unit. If requiring immediate surgery (e.g., escharotomy), the patient can be extremely labile within the first 24 hours of injury. The effects of anesthetic agents can be exaggerated, especially if fluid resuscitation is not adequate or has not been fully completed. The loss of intravascular volume coupled with the potential for a depressed myocardium can result in a hemodynamically unstable patient under general anesthesia. Careful, slow titration of anesthetic agents is vital. Appropriate premedication of stable patients with benzodiazepines or an opioid decreases anxiety and makes transfer to the operating room tolerable. Anxiety, depression, and pain are interrelated in patients with burns.[90,96] Intravenous induction of general anesthesia can be performed with the patient in bed so that subsequent movement onto the operating room table provokes little discomfort.

Regional anesthesia has been used for procedures confined to small areas, an extremity, or for surgery during the reconstructive phase. Advantages include prolonged postoperative analgesia, but variables in this patient population restrict its more general use. Performing a regional technique that requires passing a needle through burned tissue should be avoided due to the potential for spread of infection. The hypotension (hypovolemia) and vasodilation (with or without sepsis) that often accompany spinal or epidural anesthesia makes this choice undesirable until the burn wound has closed. In addition, coagulopathy and cardiorespiratory instability may be reasons to avoid a regional anesthetic technique. The greatest limitation to the use of regional anesthesia is the topographic extent of the surgical field where the anesthetized region must include both the area to be excised and the area to be harvested for skin graft.

In children, regional anesthesia is sometimes a viable option for postoperative analgesia. Caudal or epidural techniques have been used for debridement of the lower extremities or skin harvesting from the buttocks or thighs. Catheters can be used to extend the regional block for postoperative infusion analgesia.

After a burn injury, the pharmacokinetics and pharmacodynamics of the anesthetic drugs can be very different from those in nonburn patients.[97] Some pharmacokinetics and pharmacodynamics changes occurring in burn injured patients are noted in Box 39.5. All commonly used anesthetic induction drugs are acceptable. Propofol can be given if the patient is stable, and etomidate has been used as well (with special consideration of the patient's immunosuppression). Ketamine is an excellent alternative in unstable patients. Low doses of ketamine produce adequate amnesia and analgesia for the debridement of superficial burns; higher doses may be administered for more extensive procedures such as eschar excisions.[98] Postoperative emergence reactions can be minimized with the administration of benzodiazepines in small doses, and an anticholinergic prevents excessive pharyngeal and tracheobronchial secretions. In the pediatric burn patient, an inhalation induction with sevoflurane is certainly acceptable if the child does not

> ### BOX 39.5   Pharmacokinetic and Pharmacodynamic Changes in the Burn Patient
>
> - Fluid compartment alterations
> - Changes in cardiac output
> - Variability in organ perfusion
> - Decreased renal and hepatic function
> - Changes in serum protein levels
> - Hypermetabolism

From Anderson TA, Fuzaylov G. Perioperative anesthesia management of the burn patient. *Surg Clin North Am.* 2014;94(4):851–861.

have intravenous access prior to induction of general anesthesia and if the airway is otherwise normal.

Anesthesia in the burn patient can be maintained with opioids and/or inhalation agents if the hemodynamic status of the patient permits this. Volatile agents have been shown to be safe and effective, allowing rapid adjustment of anesthetic depth while permitting high oxygen concentrations. However, these patients may be sensitive to the cardiovascular depressant effects of inhaled anesthetics, especially if acute fluid resuscitation is incomplete. Inhaled agents do not provide analgesia in the postoperative period. Intubated burn patients who require intraoperative ventilation with specialized critical care ventilators (e.g., percussive ventilators), where standard anesthesia machine ventilators cannot be used, may require a total intravenous technique (TIVA).[99]

As discussed previously, succinylcholine should be avoided after the first 24 hours. The patient will exhibit resistance to nondepolarizing muscle relaxants due to the up-regulation of acetylcholine receptors, and higher and more frequent redosing is usually necessary. Other factors include massive fluid shifts producing significant changes in volume of distribution and a qualitative decrease in receptor sensitivity.[100]

Pain management. The necessity of proper pain management is well understood because almost every patient encounter may be associated with psychologic distress and physical pain. Establishment of pain treatment protocols for burn patients that address their anxiolytic and analgesic needs is essential. Intravenous (patient-controlled analgesia) is preferred early in the course of burn care because the absorption from intramuscular sites may be erratic or slow for rapid control of pain.

Opioids are an important adjunct in the care of burn patients. Pain from skin harvest sites frequently exceeds that from burned, debrided, and grafted areas. Morphine, fentanyl, and sufentanil all provide intra- and postoperative analgesia and are acceptable choices. Remifentanil, a short-acting opioid, may be used for dressing changes. Oftentimes, infusions of opioid will be used in the burn unit for pain control and/or sedation. One option is to continue these infusions during the operative procedure with bolus supplementation. Narcotic-based anesthetics provide the advantage of minimal cardiac depression. In addition, postoperative analgesia must be a vital constituent incorporated into the anesthetic plan.

Nonsteroidal antiinflammatory agents can be effective analgesics for smaller superficial burns. In larger burn injuries, the anticoagulant effects can lead to problems with hemostasis.

Painful procedures include dressing changes, debridements, nursing care, hydrotherapy, physiotherapy, and surgical procedures. The intensity of pain associated with treatments, together with the fact that they are inflicted repeatedly (sometimes twice a day or more) over long periods of time, explains the unique patient medication requirements in this population.[97,100,101]

Anesthetic emergence. The postoperative period should likewise be planned in advance. Critically ill and intubated burn patients should remain intubated postoperatively and transported directly to the burn unit. The anesthetist should safeguard the airway and be respectful of the patient's need for sedation and analgesia during this terminal phase of the anesthetic.

If extubation of the trachea is anticipated, opioids for postoperative analgesia can be titrated according to the need.

Reconstructive Phase

It is important to address the ongoing impact a burn injury can have on the individual. After numerous skin grafting and surgical procedures and some degree of healing has taken place, scarring may remain. To optimize function and prevent contractures and deformity, physical and occupational therapy are important considerations for these individuals. Months to years after hospital discharge, victims of major burns may return for reconstructive procedures to remove or reduce scar tissue. These procedures improve cosmetic and functional outcomes. Burn patients often experience anxiety, stress, and depression from prolonged hospital stays. The most important anesthetic concern is management of the airway, particularly if contractures of the face and neck are present. There are several options for airway management, as mentioned previously, from standard laryngoscopy, use of videolaryngoscope, or awake intubation using a flexible intubation scope. Intravenous access can be a problem as well when burn scars contract the extremities.

Invisible scars may remain as well in the patient who has suffered a burn injury. Psychologic issues should be explored while the patient is still in-hospital. This is especially important when dealing with children. Recreational therapists can help them work through their feelings and fears. Once the child is home and physically healed, group settings such as burn camps can offer opportunities to be with other children who have suffered similar injuries. In such an environment, the child can experience freedom from judgment and not feel ashamed of the burn scars.

SUMMARY

The anesthetic implications for the burn-injured patient can be numerous and extraordinarily challenging. As burn centers continue to evolve and improve their ability to treat and ultimately extend life after a burn injury, there is greater likelihood that an anesthesia provider will be involved in the care of such a patient. Clinicians should remember these patients are challenged both physically and emotionally. For many, the road to recovery is long and painful. As providers of anesthesia care and as patient advocates, it is important we take into account the unique aspects of the burn patient's overall care. As anesthetists, we play a significant role in helping these patients in their difficult journey to healing and recovery.

REFERENCES

For a complete list of references for this chapter, scan this QR code with any smartphone code reader app, or visit the following URL: http://booksite.elsevier.com/9780323711944/

40

Trauma Anesthesia

William O. Howie

ETIOLOGY OF TRAUMATIC INJURY

Traumatic injury is a unique condition. Unlike other diseases that have a biologic basis, trauma is the result of an external force that ultimately disrupts normal structure and function of the body. In most situations, the initial cause of injury is not attributable to genetics or environmental exposure, but circumstance and misfortune. Traumatic injury is a disease of human behavior. Although improvements to automobile safety and development of public policy have successfully reduced the annual number of traumatic injuries caused by motor vehicle collisions (MVCs), falls, and firearms by nearly one-third, traumatic injury still remains the leading cause of death for Americans age 1 to 44.[1] This translates to 214,000 deaths in the United States alone, or more simply put, one death every 3 minutes.[2] The mortality of injury is striking; however, it represents only a small fraction of those affected by trauma.

There is no exact number that can precisely quantify the effects and costs of trauma. Although figures vary by author, it has been estimated that the cost for medical care and lost productivity in the United States was more than $671 billion in 2013—of that amount, $75 billion resulted from MVCs in 2017.[3] These figures, although staggering, account only for expenses and do not account for the burden that injury places on utilization of scarce medical resources. Mortality is only the tip of the iceberg. Trauma accounts for nearly 40 million emergency department treatments per year in the United States.[4]

Improvements in prevention and treatment of trauma have been made in the United States; however, this is not the case for the incidence of trauma deaths outside of the United States. The World Health Organization (WHO) estimates there are 5 million injury-related deaths per year, accounting for 1.7 times more deaths globally than human immunodeficiency virus/acquired immunodeficiency syndrome, tuberculosis, and malaria combined.[5]

COORDINATED MANAGEMENT OF CARE

The acute management of a patient who has sustained a traumatic injury presents unusual challenges. In many instances, trauma requires immediate surgical intervention. Mechanism of action, multisystem injury, substance abuse, and preexisting medical conditions create complexities that all impact the management of the trauma patient.

A lack of time and complete preoperative information are important considerations when managing the critically unstable trauma patient. Frequently, surgical care takes priority over other preoperative exams and tests. Patients are often unable to provide a competent medical history as a result of injury or concurrent acute intoxication. Although every attempt should be made to ascertain a thorough history, it should not be done at the expense of delays in care.

Management of trauma in the United States has historically occurred at the municipal level, between the emergency medical system (EMS) and community hospital. Coordination between these stakeholders has varied widely across the United States, resulting in a range of outcomes. The evolution of modern trauma systems has challenged the community level care model—integrating prehospital, tertiary care providers, and public policy in the effort to direct trauma care—a multivariate phenomenon.

The implementation of the modern trauma system has resulted in significant improvement in patient outcomes. Pioneering examples of this paradigm shift can be seen throughout many cities in the United States and around the world; the impact of this shift on patient morbidity and mortality was formally recognized in 1998. The Skamania Symposium (Skamania Lodge, Oregon; Academic Symposium to Evaluate Evidence Regarding the Efficacy of Trauma Systems) was the first academic group to evaluate the efficacy of a trauma system.[6] This group systematically evaluated published data to determine the impact of trauma systems. Their findings indicated how care in a trauma center (vs a non–trauma center) was associated with fewer unnecessary deaths and less disability.[6,7] The results of this evidence have been supported by several other groups in the United States.

Risk of death is considerably lower among patients who require early surgical intervention if they are managed at a designated level I trauma center. Hass et al. studied all MVC occupants who presented to an emergency department in the Province of Ontario. They noted that 45% (n = 2003) were triaged from the scene of the injury directly to a level 1 trauma center. The remaining patients were triaged to a non–trauma center and were later transferred to the regional trauma center within 24 hours following their initial evaluation. The investigators concluded that initial triage to a non–trauma facility was associated with at least a 30% increase in mortality in the first 48 hours following injury. In addition to rapid trauma assessment and early intervention at the level 1 trauma centers, there are many other factors that contribute to the survival benefit of trauma center care.[6-8]

Studies in the United States show that mature, statewide trauma systems dramatically reduce unnecessary deaths and that they are more cost effective in managing more severely injured patients. For example, research by Hashmi et al. analyzed 1,949,375 adult trauma deaths in the United States between 1999 and 2016 and concluded that approximately 129,213 prehospital deaths might have been averted had they been transported to a level I/II trauma center within an hour of injury.[9]

Organization of trauma systems varies across the United States. Even though systems are not the same and may vary widely, the American College of Surgeons (ACS) Committee on Trauma has developed standards to which all trauma systems must adhere to become accredited.[10] Through these standards, a level (I, II, etc.) can be assigned to a particular center that enumerates the resources the center can provide to care for an injured patient. Fig. 40.1 describes the characteristics of

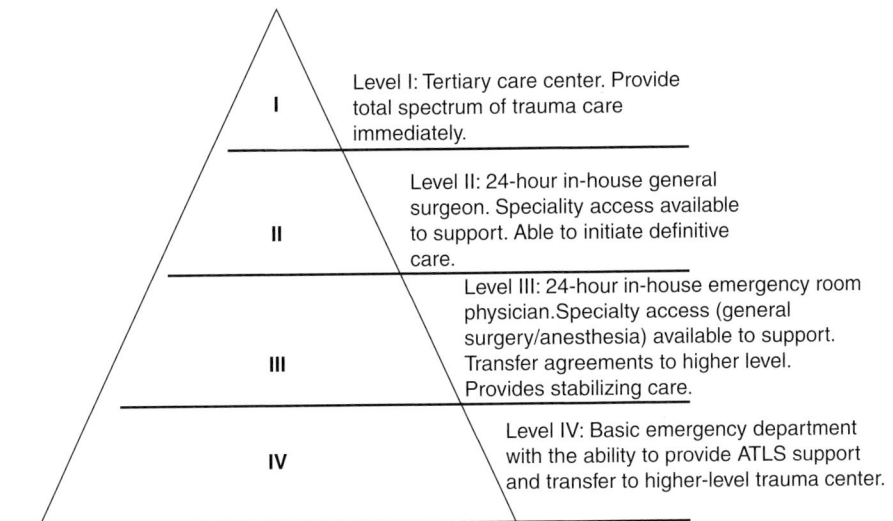

Fig. 40.1 The levels of trauma care as described in Advanced Trauma Life Support *(ATLS)*. Lower echelons of care provide stabilizing measures, and care sophistication increases with increasing levels.

the modern trauma system, requisite resources, and levels of trauma care. What we can take away from the conclusions of the Skamania Symposium and guidance of the ACS Committee on Trauma is that positive outcomes in patient care are directly related to experience and development of a trauma system. Trauma anesthesia is not just a skill that involves only massive fluid resuscitation but a specific set of clinical expertise where assessment, diagnosis, management, and therapy directly impact patient outcomes. In short, experience and proficiency matter.

EARLY EVALUATION OF THE TRAUMA PATIENT AND COMMON INJURY PATTERNS

Immediate Admission of the Trauma Patient

The Advanced Trauma Life Support (ATLS) course developed by the ACS provides a framework for the initial management and evaluation of the trauma patient from the prehospital setting through the hospital phase.[11]

Prehospital

The prehospital management of trauma patients has a deliberate pathway. The primary goals revolve around ensuring a patent airway and adequate ventilation, in addition to controlling external bleeding. Patients may be intubated in the field or treated with some other method of airway manipulation such as placement of a nasopharyngeal airway or chin-lift/jaw-thrust maneuver before arrival at the trauma center. There remains some controversy over the efficacy of rapid sequence induction in the prehospital setting; however, ensuring adequate oxygenation is essential. In the event a patient is intubated in the prehospital environment it is essential that the receiving facility immediately confirm correct placement of the endotracheal tube (ETT) using capnography and other means (i.e., chest x-ray, pulse oximetry, auscultation). All trauma patients should arrive at the hospital with some form of supplemental oxygen in place.

Contemporary research indicates that immediate causes of trauma-related death are brain injury and severe hemorrhage; late causes include infection, multisystem organ failure, brain injury, and hemorrhage. Postdischarge causes of trauma related death have been the result of a cardiovascular event, a second major traumatic injury, neurologic injury, and malignancy.[12]

Hemorrhage. Hemorrhaging blood from the circulatory system can spill into cavities throughout the body (e.g., thorax, abdomen, retroperitoneum [the pelvis], or fascial planes of long bones), and/or bleed into the environment (i.e., the street). Classically, hemorrhage has been managed using intravenous (IV) access and volume resuscitation in the prehospital setting. This practice, however, is going through a renaissance of sorts in an effort to determine what is best practice and management.

As discussed later in the chapter, early fluid resuscitation in the absence of surgical hemostasis may not be beneficial since it will likely increase bleeding and disrupt adequate blood clot formation. Without hemostasis, mortality increases. The concept of "injury first" has been further defined in the wars in Iraq and Afghanistan. Tactical Combat Casualty Care has replaced the ABC (airway-breathing-circulation) acronym with CABC (catastrophic bleeding–airway–breathing–circulation), emphasizing the immediate application of direct pressure or tourniquets to control exsanguinating hemorrhage.[13] The logic behind this change in priority initially focuses on control of bleeding because if it is not controlled, the patient will face certain death. Although civilian centers may not have to contend with the limited resources seen in austere environments, this change in approach exemplifies the important role hemorrhage control plays in hemorrhagic shock outcomes.

Primary Survey

Upon arrival to the hospital or trauma center, ATLS guidelines provide a logical and sequential treatment strategy for rapidly assessing the patient. This process is known as the primary survey and is commonly referred to as the ABCDEs of trauma care[11]:

Airway

Breathing

Circulation

Disability (neurologic status)

Environment/exposure (undress the patient to fully assess)

The goal of the primary survey is to identify and rapidly manage life-threatening conditions or injuries. This sequence of events will be abbreviated and discussed individually from the anesthesia perspective shortly. Generally, however, the primary assessment involves a rapid evaluation using physical examination techniques and American Society of Anesthesiologists (ASA) standard monitors. In addition, ultrasound and radiography are used to examine injuries and body cavities, with the initial goal of determining the extent of injury. During this time, initial blood samples and IV access are obtained. All aspects of the primary survey are done simultaneously, along with coordinating efforts from both surgical and anesthesia teams in the event the patient needs surgical intervention. If the injuries are beyond the management capabilities of the initial receiving facility, the primary survey provides the emergency team with enough information to stabilize and prepare the patient for transfer to a higher level facility.

Secondary Survey

The secondary survey begins after the completion of the primary survey and resuscitative and stabilization efforts have been initiated. The secondary survey is a more complete head-to-toe assessment that includes a neurologic examination.[11] This is a time where vigilance and thoroughness may determine if any patient injuries were not observed during the primary survey.

BLUNT VERSUS PENETRATING TRAUMA

Blunt Trauma

Direct impact, deceleration, continuous pressure, shearing, and rotary forces may all contribute to the resulting blunt trauma that a patient has incurred. These factors are associated with high levels of energy and result from high-speed collisions and falls from substantial heights. Newton's first law can explain how most traumatic injuries occur: An object tends to remain in motion until it is affected by an outside force. Abrupt deceleration creates negative gravitational forces. When the outside "shell" of the human body decelerates abruptly, the internal organs, which in a sense are separate from the exterior of the body, continue forward at the original velocity and are torn from their attachments by way of rotary and shearing forces. These forces often cause disruption of connective tissue, blood vessels, and nerves.[11]

Motor Vehicle Collision Trauma

Blunt trauma is most closely associated with MVCs and falls. Blunt trauma tends to cause damage beyond the obvious site(s) of injury. The five types of MVCs are classified as head-on, rear impact, side impact, rotational impact, and rollover. Injuries can be categorized as those above and those below the waist. The upper portion of the body may collide with the dashboard, steering wheel, or windshield, resulting in injuries of the head, neck, chest, abdomen, and upper extremities. Below the waist, injuries to the knees and femurs occur because of direct contact with the vehicle and lower dashboard. Acetabular fractures are typically a result of tensing the leg when bracing for impact. Blunt trauma rarely occurs in isolated body systems. As such, all blunt trauma victims should be suspected of and treated as if they have an unstable cervical spine until proven otherwise.[11] The greater the speed during the MVC is directly proportional to the amount of kinetic energy exerted on the person inside. This frequently translates to more severe injuries.

Thoracic Trauma

Blunt chest trauma is the third most common type of blunt injury, following traumatic brain injury (TBI) and extremity trauma. It is commonly associated with MVCs. Patients with blunt thoracic trauma present with unique concerns. These patients represent some of the most severely injured. Blunt thoracic injuries account for 20% to 25% of all deaths, and chest trauma has been named as a major contributor in another 50% of trauma-related deaths.[14,15]

Blunt thoracic trauma often results when drivers, who are not wearing safety belts, impact the steering wheel during a MVC. Additionally, direct trauma, rapid deceleration, and other mechanisms can lead to thoracic injuries. Both penetrating and blunt trauma to the chest may potentially injure several vital structures, which can have devastating consequences. Structures that may be injured include the chest wall, the lungs and airways, the heart and pericardium, nerves that innervate the airway, and/or the great vessels of the thorax. Injuries to these structures also compromise anesthesia care by affecting gas exchange and cardiac output. Trauma victims involved in high-energy blunt trauma events such as a fall over 10 feet or MVC at speeds greater than 40 mph are at an increased risk to sustain a blunt aortic injury (BAI). It is estimated that close to 80% of BAIs produce immediate death due to aortic transection at the scene.[16]

Pneumothoraces are present in as many as 40% of all blunt thoracic injuries. The size and location of the pneumothorax may vary throughout the lung field. It is estimated that as many as 50% of pneumothoraces are not detected on initial radiography.[15] This occurrence presents several clinical intraoperative issues since the identification of a pneumothorax may not be initially made. The use of positive pressure ventilation, increases in peak airway pressures, reduced tidal volumes, a general reduction in lung compliance, and a decreased oxygen saturation are all intraoperative signs of a developing pneumothorax. Nitrous oxide should be avoided in patients with suspected thoracic trauma.

A number of life-threatening injuries, described later, require immediate interventions in patients with thoracic/chest trauma.

Tension pneumothorax. Tension pneumothorax develops when the lung is punctured within the thoracic cavity, creating a one-way valve that traps air between the layers of the pleura. With each breath, more air becomes trapped within this space, increasing intrapleural pressure to the point that it eventually exceeds all other intrathoracic pressures. The enlarging pleural cavity then collapses the ipsilateral lung and shifts the structures of the mediastinum (e.g., trachea, great vessels, and heart) into the opposite hemithorax, thereby compressing the contralateral lung. The size of a pneumothorax will rapidly increase during positive pressure ventilation, especially if nitrous oxide is used.

Patients with a pneumothorax often present with symptoms of hypotension, subcutaneous emphysema of the neck or chest, unilateral decrease in breath sounds, diminished chest wall motion, hyperresonance to percussion of one hemithorax, distended neck veins, or tracheal shift. An upright expirational chest radiograph can provide definitive information if the problem is significant.

Massive pneumothorax can result in reductions in cardiac output and ultimately cardiopulmonary collapse. Under emergent situations a large-bore IV catheter (needle chest decompression) can be inserted into the second intercostal space just above the third rib, along the midclavicular line. An alternative site is the fourth intercostal space at the midaxillary line. A release of pressure allows for improved cardiac function. Initially the catheter can be temporarily attached to an IV line extension tube and placed under waterseal by putting it in a bottle of sterile water positioned beneath the level of the patient until proper chest tube thoracostomy can be performed. See Chapter 29 for a complete discussion of the diagnosis and management of a pneumothorax.

Pericardial tamponade. Acute pericardial tamponade that restricts filling of the cardiac chambers during diastole and produces a fixed low cardiac output is a life-threatening emergency that requires immediate drainage of fluid from the pericardial sack via a pericardiocentesis. Hypotension coupled with elevated venous pressure which causes jugular venous distention and muffled heart sounds are classic symptoms known as Beck triad. Additional signs and symptoms that reflect cardiac compressive shock include cool extremities, peripheral cyanosis, and a decrease in urine output. Pulsus paradoxus is a common finding in moderate to severe pericardial tamponade and is a result of both a decrease in left ventricular filling and a displacement of the intraventricular septum. It is observed when the systolic blood pressure (SBP) abnormally decreases (>10 mm Hg) on inspiration. Care should be taken when inducing anesthesia in patients with cardiac tamponade and transitioning from negative pressure breathing to positive pressure breathing because cardiovascular collapse can occur. Ketamine has been recommended as an induction agent in these patients.

Massive hemothorax. Massive hemothorax, which can be caused by bleeding from the heart and great vessels, requires immediate treatment and surgical intervention. Adequate fluid and blood resuscitation should be provided prior to placement of chest tubes. Chest tubes allow drainage of blood from the pleural cavity but can lead to more extensive bleeding and hypotension.

Cardiac rupture. Patients with cardiac rupture may present with a variety of symptoms related to the extent of cardiac injury. Most patients with a severe cardiac rupture will die in the prehospital setting before they reach definitive care. Efficient and rapid prehospital transportation coupled with a high index of suspicion and immediate surgical intervention may contribute to survival of patients who have suffered a cardiac rupture.

Traumatic aortic rupture. Traumatic aortic rupture, if complete, is usually fatal. However, the patient may be saved with an intimal tear that results in a dissecting aneurysm if the diagnosis and repair are performed promptly with concurrent well-managed fluid resuscitation and anesthesia care. Management of these cases requires rapid and accurate assessment and appropriate surgical and anesthesia intervention. Anesthetic management should include IV access with at least two large-bore cannulas, an arterial line, and hemodynamic control that targets a SBP less than 100 to 120 mm Hg and a heart rate less than 100 bpm. These hemodynamic goals are an effort to avoid extending the aortic injury and minimizing the chance of aortic rupture. Short-acting β-blockers, calcium channel blockers, and/or vasodilators (i.e., nitroprusside) are used to achieve these goals.[16,17] Surgical management will depend on the patient's presenting symptoms, the degree of injury, and the presence of comorbidities and other injuries. Surgical management may range from open repair to endovascular stent repair depending on the patient's hemodynamic stability, degree of vessel damage, and surgeon preference.

Tracheal injuries. Tracheal injuries represent a devastating and potentially lethal event after blunt thoracic trauma. Partial disruption of the trachea or major bronchi is often managed by securing the airway using intubation to bridge the transected tracheal parts or tracheostomy, and surgical correction. Total transection of the trachea is often fatal unless rapid surgical retrieval of the distal disrupted tracheal segment is accomplished to allow lifesaving mechanical ventilation. The majority of thoracic airway injuries are found below the carina and are often visible only during bronchoscopy or computed tomography (CT) examination.

Penetrating Trauma

Penetrating injuries can range from a simple pinprick to a high-velocity projectile injury. Damage depends on three interactive factors[18]:

1. The type of wounding instrument (e.g., knife; or projectile such as a bullet or fragment)
2. The velocity of the projectile at time of impact
3. The characteristics of tissue through which it passes (e.g., bone, muscle, fat, blood vessels, nervous tissues, and organs)

Low-velocity wounds (i.e., stab wound) inflict injury by lacerating and cutting tissue. Moderate- to high-velocity injuries (i.e., bullet) occur as a result of the deceleration of the object as it passes through tissue, causing kinetic energy to transfer to the surrounding tissue. Any one of these (i.e., penetration of low, medium, or high velocity) ultimately results in disruption of normal anatomy and physiology. Velocity of the projectile is the most significant determinant of wound potential. In other words, penetrating bullet wounds generally have a greater potential to inflict serious injury when compared with a knife or other handheld projectile.

Damage Control Surgery

Surgical management for the severely traumatized patient is often a multistep process. In many cases patients present to the trauma center with surgical emergencies. Early repair is often simply a lifesaving measure and is not intended to be a definitive repair but rather a stabilizing measure to reduce operating room time and morbidity. After stabilization, patients will be transported for further evaluation (secondary survey) or additional resuscitation measures in the intensive care unit. Often, patients will return to the OR several times because the surgical course involves several phases. This staged approach to surgical management is commonly known as damage control surgery (DCS).[19]

DCS is a concept that developed in the early 20th century. Its use fell in and out of favor until the 1970s and 1980s. Its utility in modern trauma care was rediscovered as advances in surgical technique, critical care medicine, and technology converged. DCS correlates with current concepts in trauma care that include damage control resuscitation with rapid surgical correction of bleeding and the prevention of the lethal triad of acidosis, hypothermia, and coagulopathy. Current research indicates that bleeding trauma patients should receive early blood and blood product administration in the form of fresh frozen plasma, platelets, and packed red blood cells (RBCs) at a ratio of 1:1:1.[20] Limiting the amount of crystalloids infused has also been recommended.[21] DCS is used in various surgical disciplines, from packing the abdomen after abdominal trauma to using external fixators to set complex orthopedic injuries.[21-23]

Damage Control Resuscitation in Trauma

Damage control resuscitation (DCR) is an overarching concept that combines DCS with techniques that prevent the trauma lethal triad (hypothermia, acidosis, and coagulopathy).[19-21] Historically, attempts to maintain normal blood pressure using primarily crystalloid solutions and PRBCs, along with definitive surgical repair of complex traumatic injuries, were keystones to trauma surgical care. DCR represents a significant shift in this approach and relies on (1) warming the patient, (2) early correction of coagulopathies, (3) avoidance of large amounts of crystalloid administration, (4) permissive hypotension until the bleeding is controlled, (5) reversal of metabolic acidosis, (6) early implementation of massive blood transfusion protocols (i.e., 1:1:1 ratios), and (7) utilization of antifibrinolytics (most notably tranexamic acid).[22-26]

One strategy is to focus on the SBP. As it starts to rise above 90 mm Hg during the early resuscitative phase of DCR, fentanyl may be titrated at a range of 50 to 150 mcg IV. This allows some degree of analgesia to the trauma patient. If there is a marked drop in the blood pressure below the targeted range of greater than 90 mm Hg, the patient requires additional fluid and blood resuscitation. Once the patient is able to tolerate a single bolus dose of fentanyl (up to 250 mcg) without a drop in blood pressure below the target of greater than 90 mm Hg, it is likely that the hypovolemic state has been corrected.[23,26]

It is critical that communication between the surgeon, anesthesia team, blood bank, laboratory, and intraoperative support personnel is maintained throughout all phases of the damage control process. It is additionally important to consider admission of the patient postoperatively to an intensive care unit to assist with further stabilization and monitoring of hemodynamic status.

Trauma centers that employ DCR techniques to the fullest capacity involve the use of point-of-care testing (i.e., thromboelastography [TEG] or rotational thromboelastometry [ROTEM]) to tailor blood product administration to the specific patient presentation and the use of hybrid angiography operating rooms that allow a patient to stay in the same location for interventional radiology and open repair, as needed. This concept has been termed RAPTOR (resuscitation with angiography, percutaneous techniques, and operative repair).[27] A newer procedure used to temporarily control noncompressible torso hemorrhage is termed REBOA (resuscitative endovascular balloon occlusion of the aorta). The REBOA devices are used as minimally invasive intravascular cross-clamps in patients with profound hypovolemia due to hemorrhagic shock. The device is inserted percutaneously or via a cut-down in the common femoral artery. Based on the area of injury the catheter can be placed in zone 1 (at the level of the diaphragm to help control intraabdominal hemorrhage) or zone 3 (at the bifurcation of the aorta) for pelvic hemorrhage. A primary goal of REBOA is to help maintain adequate cardiac and cerebral perfusion in a significantly hypotensive patient while the surgical team obtains effective hemostasis.[24]

Abdominal Trauma

Blunt abdominal trauma is a leading cause of morbidity and mortality among all age groups. Although diagnosis and treatment of penetrating trauma is easily determined, occult bleeding in blunt abdominal injury is often misdiagnosed.[26,28] Abdominal sonography such as the focused assessment with sonography for trauma (FAST) exam, CT scan, magnetic resonance imaging (MRI), or angiography may help in the diagnosis of specific injuries and various treatment modalities. However, extremely unstable patients will require immediate surgery. It is essential that multiple large-bore IV access or central venous access lines, along with arterial blood pressure monitoring, be in place above the diaphragm prior to surgical opening of the abdomen. The release of an intraabdominal tamponade can result in massive hemorrhage from a traumatic liver, spleen, or other intraabdominal organ injury.

THE ABCDS OF TRAUMA ANESTHESIA

Although the ATLS curriculum provides an organized framework for the management of traumatic injury, it is not specific to any one discipline. The following sections discuss the implications of the ABCDs of trauma anesthesia and provide an approach to clinical management.[11] A primary goal of the anesthesia team is to facilitate rapid surgical management. Trauma anesthesia and surgery is most often an emergency, and thus the objective should be to rapidly move the patient to the operating room for surgical correction of traumatic injury.

Airway

Endotracheal intubation poses significant risk and may be extremely challenging when caring for the acutely injured trauma patient. Difficult tracheal intubation is the third most common respiratory-related event leading to death and brain damage as reported in the ASA Closed Claims analysis.[29] Not all trauma patients will have a difficult airway; however, in trauma situations there are factors that increase airway difficulty that otherwise would not be present in elective cases. For example, the anesthetist may not have the opportunity or time to perform a thorough airway examination because of the urgency of airway management. In addition, airway management can be complicated by several variables such as facial injuries, airway foreign bodies, neck injuries, hypoventilation with hypoxemia, and apnea.

Common Indications for Airway Management

Patients with traumatic injury present with varying degrees of injury and may require emergent airway management. The most common indications for endotracheal intubation include (1) inadequate oxygenation/ventilation, (2) loss of airway reflexes, (3) decreased level of consciousness (Glasgow Coma Scale [GCS] <8), and (4) occasionally

the need for pain management and the ability to safely provide deep sedation during painful procedures.

Emergent intubation in the trauma patient may be required as a result of blunt or penetrating maxillofacial or neck injuries, smoke inhalation or facial burns, multisystem trauma, caustic ingestion, drowning, and/or massive hemorrhage.[30] Three assumptions should be made when approaching airway management in the trauma patient. First, trauma patients are assumed to have delayed gastric emptying and a full stomach. As such, they are at increased risk for aspiration and should receive either an awake intubation or rapid sequence induction. Second, cervical spine instability should be assumed in any patient with blunt trauma or penetrating injuries to the torso, neck, or face. Third, trauma patients many times arrive to the hospital in a decompensated state with significant hypotension and hypoxemia.

Rapid sequence intubation (RSI) is the standard method for traumatic airway management. One of the greatest differences between routine induction and RSI is the use of a muscle relaxant before confirmation of adequate ventilation. In trauma airway management, neuromuscular blockade is associated a higher overall success rate and provides the best conditions for rapidly securing the airway.[31,32]

Rapid Sequence Intubation

RSI in the trauma patient begins with appropriate planning and team practice. Sufficient personnel must be on hand to (1) provide manual inline stabilization (MILS) of the cervical spine after removing the front of the cervical collar, (2) provide cricoid pressure (Sellick maneuver), (3) oxygenate the patient with bag-valve-mask ventilation and perform direct laryngoscopy, and (4) administer medications.

MILS of the cervical spine is the preferred method in potentially unstable necks during laryngoscopy and intubation.[33] This technique has also be called manual inline axial traction. It is actively performed by a second individual (after the front of the cervical collar is removed) who stabilizes the head and neck by holding the head with both hands to counteract the movements exerted by the individual performing the laryngoscopy. An important consideration is the fact that both cervical spine injury and aspiration during intubation are moderately low-risk events when compared with the possible risks and injury from hypoxia. Therefore the priority during airway management is effective oxygenation. Inline stabilization and cricoid pressure should be relaxed if they are interfering with successful intubation.[31]

RSI is a procedure that is conducted to rapidly control a patient's airway while reducing the likelihood of gastric aspiration. RSI consists of five primary components: (1) preoxygenation, (2) cricoid pressure, (3) induction/muscle relaxation, (4) apneic ventilation, and (5) direct laryngoscopy. Each of these steps will be discussed in detail.[34]

Preoxygenation. Adequate preoxygenation should be performed prior to intubation to limit the possibility of hypoxia during airway management. Preoxygenation is accomplished using high-flow (10–15 L) oxygen via a nonrebreather facemask, bag-valve facemask, or anesthesia circuit. If out of the operating room, the addition of a nasal cannula to the nonrebreather facemask or bag-valve mask will increase the administered Fio_2. Although there is some debate, eight vital capacity breaths appear to provide superior preoxygenation when compared with 3 minutes of tidal breathing.[35]

Preoxygenation is challenging in patients who are unable to perform vital capacity breaths or follow commands when obtunded. In these circumstances, it is appropriate to provide controlled positive pressure mask ventilation throughout induction. The term *controlled* indicates that positive inspiratory pressure breaths will be monitored and kept below 20 cm H_2O in an effort to avoid gastric distention. An increased oxygen reservoir in the lung is likely to benefit the patient more than the (theoretic) increased risk of aspiration caused by ventilation during cricoid pressure.[36]

Cricoid pressure. Cricoid pressure is applied during the RSI and is intended to prevent both gastric insufflation during bag-valve-mask ventilation and passive reflux of gastric contents. Cricoid pressure was first described by Sellick in 1961.[36,37] The goal of this maneuver is to reduce the risk of pulmonary aspiration of gastric contents by compressing the esophagus against the cervical vertebra using the cricoid cartilage.[38] Cricoid pressure is maintained throughout the RSI and is not released until ETT placement has been confirmed. Determining the appropriate pressure to apply to the cricoid ring has been the subject of debate. Vanner and Pryle[38] have determined that 30 newtons (~3 kg or 10 lb of pressure) adequately occludes the esophagus.

Researchers have questioned the effectiveness of cricoid pressure since the foundations of its use were only demonstrated in cadaveric studies and case reports.[38] There is evidence to both support and refute the efficacy of cricoid pressure as an intervention to prevent pulmonary aspiration during RSI.[39] Much of the evidence has concluded that cricoid pressure does not show any increase in protection from pulmonary aspiration and that cricoid pressure may actually increase the difficulty of endotracheal intubation.[40] Despite the fact that some research questions the true effectiveness of cricoid pressure to prevent aspiration of gastric contents, it is still typically applied and modified to allow some degree of external laryngeal manipulation to potentially improve the airway view. Until convincing evidence emerges that definitively shows cricoid pressure is harmful, it is likely to continue to be routinely utilized. If at any time a clinician experiences difficulty during laryngoscopy while cricoid pressure is being performed, it should immediately be released in an effort to improve laryngeal viewing.

Rapid sequence induction agents. Anesthetic induction for RSI can be achieved by using a variety of agents. The evidence does not support the superiority of one agent over another. All induction agents will cause dose-dependent decreases in blood pressure in the hypovolemic, hemorrhaging patient. Dose-dependent hemodynamic instability can likely be attenuated by reductions in the induction dose. Although no formula can precisely predict the dose for a hemodynamically unstable patient, some authors suggest a dose that is one-tenth to one-half of the normal induction dose of propofol.[41] Ketamine or etomidate can be considered for RSI in the trauma patient, especially when hemodynamically unstable. A recent systematic review of etomidate and ketamine found no difference in mortality, length of hospital stay, or number of blood transfusions when either agent was used for induction of anesthesia in the hemodynamically unstable adult trauma patient.[42]

Ketamine is a dissociative agent that has a rapid onset when given IV and may be used intramuscular (IM) in uncooperative trauma patients who do not have adequate IV access or who require sedation for optimal preoxygenation. This drug indirectly increases cardiovascular stimulation through centrally mediated increased sympathetic tone and increased release of catecholamines. For a number of years, it was believed that ketamine may lead to increases in intracranial pressure (ICP) in patients with a TBI, but a recent systematic review indicated that any increase in ICP was not found to be clinically significant.[43] In addition, there is evidence to support the use of ketamine for induction in patients with TBI and hypovolemic shock. Ketamine has been shown to not only avoid increases in ICP but to cause it to decrease and improve cerebral perfusion pressure (CCP).[44]

A retrospective analysis of patients who received a single dose of etomidate to facilitate endotracheal intubation concluded that there was no difference in mortality as compared to patients who received other IV induction agents.[45] Etomidate is often used as the primary induction agent in the hemodynamically unstable trauma patient because of its ability to minimize significant hypotension.

Propofol is used frequently for RSI; however, if a patient is hemodynamically unstable the induction dose should be greatly decreased or another agent should be considered. Some providers consider reduction of the standard propofol intubating dose to a range of 0.5 to 1 mg/kg or less in patients with a potential for hemodynamic instability.[31,46] If the blood pressure decreases to an unacceptable level, a vasopressor such as phenylephrine can be used to maintain an acceptable mean arterial pressure (MAP) in hypovolemic patients.

Recall and awareness during induction are undesirable consequences; however, in the hemodynamically unstable trauma patient these issues are a secondary concern, especially when emergently managing the airway. Thus there may be situations where the use of an induction agent is considered too high risk because of severe hemorrhage and hypovolemic shock. In these situations, the use of a neuromuscular blocking agent only may be considered in an effort to avoid any decreases in blood pressure.

Succinylcholine (1.5 mg/kg) provides favorable and rapid muscle relaxation to facilitate intubation. It is generally the preferred agent for RSI for any patient who has no specific contraindication to its use. Succinylcholine administration may cause lethal hyperkalemia in patients with neurologic deficits from spinal cord injury (SCI) or massive crush injuries but usually not until 24 to 48 hours after injury.

Rocuronium (1.2 mg/kg) can be used for RSI. The onset time for high-dose rocuronium (1.2 mg/kg) is similar to that for succinylcholine (1 mg/kg), with only a slight delay in achieving complete relaxation.[47] Attention should be provided to the fact that prolonged paralysis will require sedation and will make any subsequent neurologic assessment more difficult.

Apneic oxygenation. Apneic oxygenation is the concept of pulmonary ventilation using high-flow oxygen. Its purpose is to reduce the potential risk of gastric distension and pulmonary aspiration from positive pressure ventilation. Apneic oxygenation is effective because of the diffusion of oxygen at the alveolar-capillary membrane. Higher and stable concentrations of oxygen in the pharyngeal spaces and tracheobronchial tree will flow to areas of lower concentrations inside the lungs (as long as there is no obstruction) as a result of the continuous diffusion of gas from the alveoli (and thus lower O_2 alveoli partial pressure) into the pulmonary capillary blood. To work appropriately, apneic oxygenation assumes that the airway is patent and that a high concentration of oxygen can be reliably administered. This is usually done with a nasal cannula using high flows (>15 L/min) during laryngoscopy and intubation.[48,49]

Direct and videolaryngoscopy. Both direct and videolaryngoscopy can be used for RSI in the trauma patient. No evidence indicates that a particular laryngoscope blade or size is optimal for RSI, although many emergency departments are primarily opting for videolaryngoscopy since standard geometry blades can be used for both direct and videolaryngoscopy while providing a video screen for team viewing. The choice is likely provider dependent.

Successful ETT placement is immediately confirmed by capnometry. If unsuccessful, a second laryngoscopy attempt should be attempted incorporating some change in technique (e.g., different provider, blade, or patient position). There are a variety of adjunctive tools available in the event of an unplanned difficult intubation. These include the intubating stylet or bougie and the more advanced flexible (fiberoptic) endoscopic equipment.

If intubation is again unsuccessful (third attempt), the next step should be an airway adjunct to support oxygenation using either a bag mask or a second-generation supraglottic airway device. In the situation of "cannot intubate and inadequate facemask ventilation," supraglottic airway device insertion should be the immediate next step.[32] At this point, if the provider cannot intubate and cannot ventilate/oxygenate, then a surgical airway should be considered as a final option.

The use of several devices in combination can be effective during laryngoscopy and intubation. For example, the bougie can be utilized to facilitate ETT delivery during videolaryngoscopy, or an intubating supraglottic airway device can be used in combination with a flexible intubating endoscope.

Emergency front of neck access. The need for an emergency surgical airway is increased in the trauma population, especially with trauma to the airway. Appropriate equipment, extra personnel, and (if available) surgical resources should be immediately available in the event a surgical airway is needed. Newer terminology such as *emergency front of the neck access* (eFONA) and *front of the neck access* (FONA) is being used to describe emergency cricothyrotomies. These procedures are performed in the "can't intubate and can't oxygenate (CICO)" situation, or when the upper airway is severely obstructed making intubation of the trachea through the mouth or nose impossible. For example, FONA may be performed in the case with potentially a difficult airway due to a distorting traumatic injury or a congenital deformity, whereas eFONA is the final lifesaving step to reverse profound hypoxia and avert cardiac arrest when confronted with a CICO scenario.[32]

Airway Management of Cervical Spine Injuries

Cervical spine injury remains a significant concern when facing airway management of the trauma patient. The incidence of cervical spine injury after trauma is relatively rare at 2% to 4% of all trauma; 20% of these are spinal cord injuries, 10% are reported as multilevel cervical spine injuries, and 10% are categorized as purely ligamentous injuries.[50] Cervical spine injury should be assumed until proven otherwise. Immobilization of the neck is essential. To that end, inline stabilization is essential because it allows for removal of the front of the cervical collar, allowing more area for jaw and mouth movement while limiting the risk for further injury.

The management and intubation of patients with suspected cervical spine injuries remains clinically controversial. Despite common belief, there is no evidence to suggest that flexible endoscopic intubation provides safer patient outcomes when compared with direct or videolaryngoscopy with inline stabilization. Ideally, the provider managing the airway should use the intubation device that is most familiar.[32] Management of a cervical spine injury may be done with the concepts of "emergent," which involves inline stabilization and RSI, versus "controlled," which involves an awake flexible intubating technique. Fig. 40.2 describes a logical management strategy for these two situations.

Airway Management for Contaminated Airways

Traumatic injury, especially trauma to the airway, may result in blood and vomit contaminating the airway. Initial suction attempts may not clear contaminants because of consistent massive regurgitation, emesis, and bleeding within the airway, consequently leading to a very difficult airway. These situations can be extremely stressful and time sensitive, requiring immediate decontamination of the airway and endotracheal intubation. One technique for airway decontamination being used in the prehospital and emergency room environments is the suction assisted laryngoscopy airway decontamination (SALAD) technique. It utilizes two suction setups with large-bore rigid suction devices (Fig. 40.3) paired with videolaryngoscopy. Fig. 40.4 shows the difference between the internal diameter openings of a SSCOR DuCanto suction device compared to a standard Yankauer suction

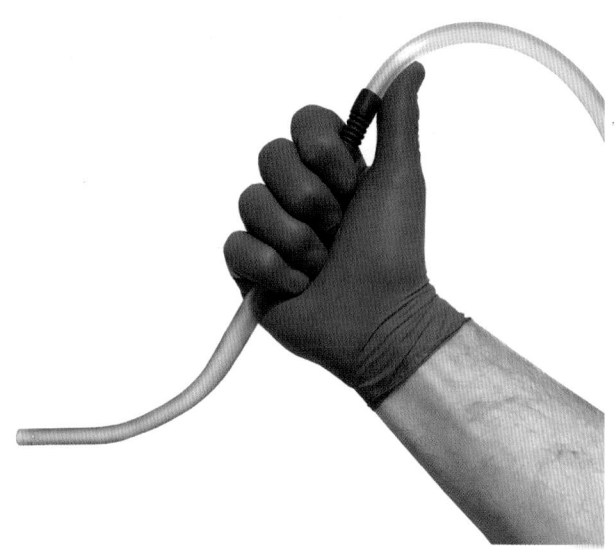

Fig. 40.3 The SSCOR DuCanto suction device held in an overhand dagger-like position for optimal tongue management and decontamination of the airway. This device has an internal diameter opening of 0.26 in. for suctioning of large particles and massive fluids within the airway. (Image courtesy SSCOR Inc.)

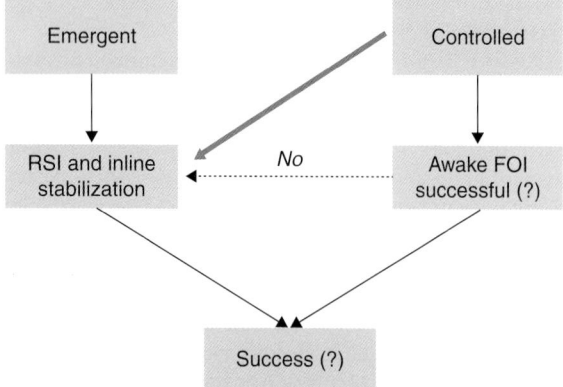

Fig. 40.2 A logical management algorithm for controlled versus emergent airway management for a patient with a cervical spine injury. *FOI*, Fiberoptic intubation; *RSI*, rapid sequence induction.

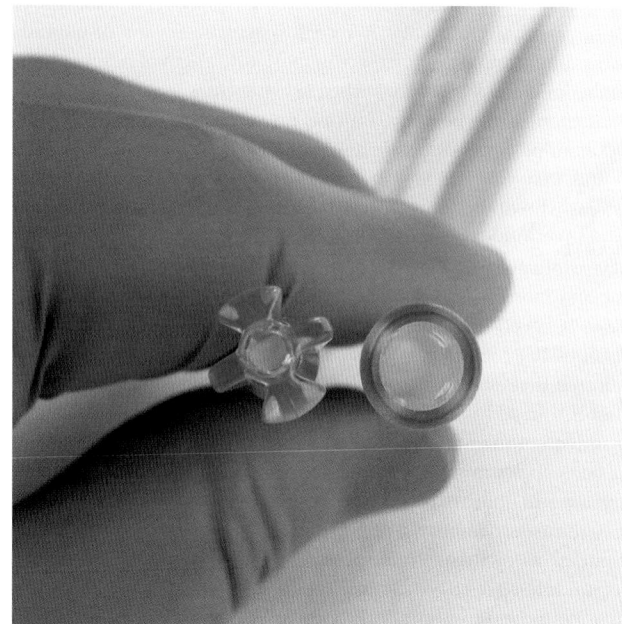

Fig. 40.4 The SSCOR DuCanto suction device compared to the standard Yankauer suction device. Note the SSCOR DuCanto large-bore opening and hyperangulated design. (Image courtesy SSCOR Inc.)

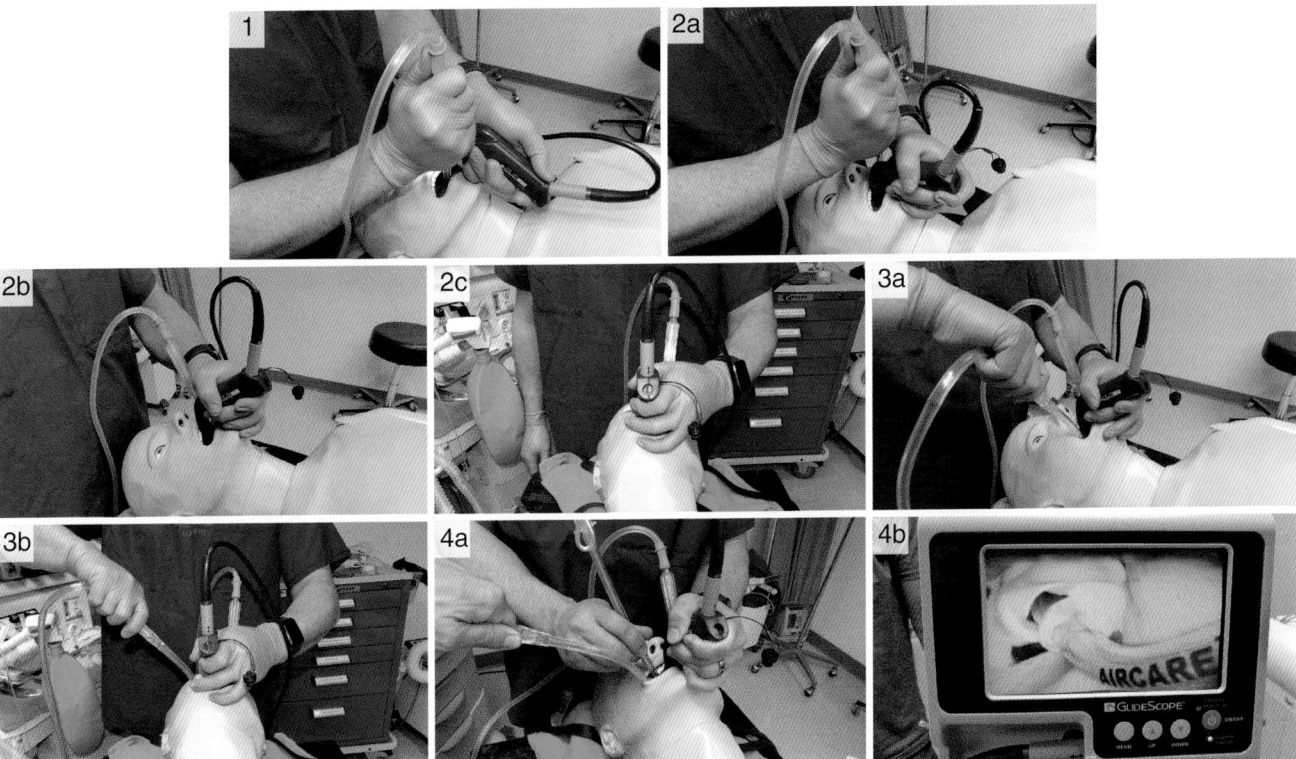

Fig. 40.5 Suction assisted laryngoscopy airway decontamination (SALAD). (1) The first step, which initially suctions the airway prior to advancing the videolaryngoscope. Note that the suction device is held like a dagger. (2a) Step 2 advances the suction down the tongue. The rigid suction device can also be used like a tongue blade to control and move the tongue out of the way. The videolaryngoscope is now slowly advanced into the airway. Avoid plunging the videolaryngoscope too deep into the airway since that risks immediate contamination of the optics. Essentially, the procedure is led with suction as the provider moves the videolaryngoscope down to the correct location for laryngeal visualization. (2b,c) Step 3 demonstrates how the primary suction device is left in place within the airway to continue to suction during videolaryngoscopy and positioned to the left of the videolaryngoscope handle securing it in place. (3a,b) Step 4 shows how a second rigid suction device can suction additional contaminate from the airway immediately prior to intubation. (4a) Step 5 is intubation of the trachea. First the airway provider passes the second suction to an assistant to allow for a free hand and intubation of the trachea. Note that the assistant can use the suction to move the lip to the side providing additional space to pass the endotracheal tube (ETT). (4b) A videolaryngoscopic view of the primary rigid suction device in place within the hypopharynx and successful passage of the ETT into the laryngeal opening.

device. If a large-bore suction device is not available, then a Yankauer suction device can be used. If an occlusion hole is present, it should be taped closed to provide continuous suction. Fig. 40.5 describes the SALAD technique.

Jim DuCanto, the developer of the SALAD technique, recommends that individuals who are likely to manage airways contaminated with blood or regurgitant practice the technique regularly in a simulated environment.[51]

Breathing (and Ventilation)

Regardless of the need to manage the airway, the adequacy of breathing and ultimately patient oxygenation is essential to survival and a primary goal. Pulse oximetry is a commonly used noninvasive method to continuously monitor oxygen saturation. Pulse oximetry is often employed as a surrogate measure of status. Although pulse oximetry provides a wealth of clinical information, this measurement may provide a false sense of security. For instance, an otherwise healthy patient breathing room air oxygen (21%) will have a partial pressure of arterial oxygen (Pao_2) level of approximately 100 mm Hg and an arterial oxygen saturation (Sao_2) of 100%. If the patient is placed on a

high-flow, nonrebreather mask of 100% oxygen, then the Pao_2 could be expected to be approximately 500 mm Hg and Sao_2 would remain at 100%. Patients who experience declining pulmonary function will have an Sao_2 of 100% over a wide range of Pao_2 readings. Supplemental oxygen, although necessary, can mask pulmonary injury and in some cases, respiratory decompensation. Therefore a saturation of 100% does not necessarily equate to a stable patient or the health of the pulmonary (breathing/ventilation) system.

Pulmonary contusions represent the most common lung injury. It is reported that as many as 70% of patients with blunt thoracic trauma present with some degree of pulmonary contusion.[52] Pulmonary contusions are injuries to the alveoli without gross disruption of pulmonary architecture. This injury is essentially a bruise to the lung tissue resulting in protein-rich fluid leaving ruptured pulmonary capillaries and settling into the alveolar membrane and interstitial space. As a result of the widening of the pulmonary membrane, pulmonary contusions result in varying degrees of reduced gas diffusion that may be clinically relevant. Pulmonary contusions can develop or "blossom" over a range of time and ultimately may advance into acute respiratory distress syndrome (ARDS).

ARDS is an acute diffuse inflammatory lung injury caused by a number of systemic or pulmonary insults.[53] It is a common problem in trauma care and may be the result of the initial traumatic injury or of the subsequent resuscitation efforts. In one study of 621 intubated trauma patients, 64% experienced hypoxemia, and 46% of these hypoxemic patients developed ARDS that was confirmed by chest radiography.[54] Pathologically, ARDS is a result of protein-rich fluid leaving the pulmonary capillaries and accumulating within the alveoli. As the disease progresses, the pulmonary capillary leakage is compounded by embolic events, which further increase intracapillary pressure and intensify interstitial leakage. Furthermore, the combination of intraalveolar edema coupled with the immune response causes surfactant dysfunction and the development of a hyaline membrane that prevents adequate gas exchange. ARDS culminates in hypoxia and decreased pulmonary compliance. Ventilating these patients is a challenge. Contemporary research indicates that patients with ARDS should be managed with low tidal volume ventilation, plateau pressures less than 30 cm H_2O, permissive hypercapnia, conservative fluid strategies in those without shock states, and prone positioning. Neuromuscular blockers may reduce mortality. Early management of ARDS is vital, and extracorporeal membrane oxygenation should be considered for those who do not respond to these aforementioned therapies.[53,54]

A variety of pulmonary techniques have been described for managing these patients. They range from high-frequency oscillation ventilation to cardiopulmonary bypass. Other than reduced tidal volume ventilation, no other technique appears to be superior. A target saturation of 90% to 94% is allowed in an effort to avoid oxygen toxicity. Positive end-expiratory pressure (PEEP) is another technique to recruit collapsed alveoli and improve ventilation. In patients with severe ARDS, the Fio_2 is increased as the PEEP increases.

Circulation

Up to 35% of prehospital trauma fatalities are attributable to hemorrhage, and 40% of trauma-related deaths within the first 24 hours result from hemorrhage and hemorrhagic shock. Hemorrhagic shock is the leading cause of early and late mortality after trauma.[51] Hemorrhagic shock is defined as a pathologic event that is triggered by the loss of circulating blood volume and results in a reduction in oxygen delivery to the tissue.

The physiologic response to hemorrhagic shock is a dynamic and complex process. Reductions in blood volume cause an immediate change in vascular tone and global systemic vascular resistance (SVR). Blood is shunted from low metabolic "ischemia-tolerant" vascular beds such as skin and bone, to highly metabolic tissues (e.g., brain, heart, gut) with the intent of maintaining cellular perfusion and aerobic respiration. Early shunting compensates for relative hypovolemia. If short lived, compensated shock has very few long-term sequelae.

Unfortunately, uncontrolled hemorrhage is a likely event in major trauma. As the degree of blood loss worsens, vascular shunting increases. In this state, patients rapidly progress from a compensated state to decompensated shock. Vascular shunting continues during decompensated shock. Blood is directed away from lower metabolic organs, such as the kidneys and gut, in an attempt to maintain perfusion in higher metabolic structures. During decompensated shock, changes to SVR are less likely to adequately maintain perfusion. The body attempts to further compensate a dwindling stroke volume and cardiac output by increasing heart rate and contractility.

Unfortunately, compensatory mechanisms are imperfect. Prolonged reductions in perfusion will result in cellular injury. During protracted shock events, venous oxygen reserves are extracted and used as the arterial oxygen supply declines. Metabolic imbalances between oxygen demand and delivery produce toxic metabolic byproducts such as lactic acid. As a result of this imbalance, cells are unable to maintain vital metabolic functions. Energy production falls. Intracellular energy-dependent pumps fail, reducing cell wall integrity.

In an attempt to maintain energy production, cellular mechanisms transition from aerobic to anaerobic respiration. The conversion to anaerobic respiration is made at a significant cost to the cell. In addition to vast reductions in energy production, lactic acid and free radicals are produced. These toxic cellular byproducts induce cellular injury, further reducing cellular function. At the tissue level, persistent and prolonged hypovolemia and vasoconstriction lead to hypoperfusion and end-organ damage, which will likely lead to multisystem organ failure in survivors. In extreme cases of hemorrhagic shock with exsanguination, hypoperfusion of the heart and brain yields cerebral anoxia and lethal pulseless arrhythmias within minutes.[55]

Despite vigorous resuscitation, hypovolemic hemorrhagic shock may result in patient death. Research by Newgard et al. examined outcomes of 778 shock patients and 2139 TBI patients, 28% of whom died within 28 days. Out of hospital time in excess of 60 minutes was not associated with worse outcomes after excluding confounding variables in the shock cohort. However, shock patients who required early critical hospital resources who were admitted after 60 minutes were approximately twice as likely to die.[56] This high mortality rate associated with the delayed treatment of hemorrhagic shock is the basis for the initiation of fluid resuscitation and hemostasis in the field.

The so-called golden hour was initially modeled from data collected from young, healthy males in military service during the Vietnam War. The golden hour represents a period of time (the initial 60 minutes after traumatic injury) in which selected patients will likely survive hemorrhagic shock if perfusion is restored.[56] This observation, however, cannot be extrapolated to the general population because, as stated, it was based on young, healthy men. It is likely, however, that when generalizing to the population at large, the golden hour is actually a nonspecific time that is age and health status dependent. The golden hour is likely an inverse relationship. As patients age, their ability to compensate during hypovolemic hemorrhagic shock decreases.

Hypovolemic hemorrhagic shock can progress through three stages over time if not corrected early. Stage I of shock is often called nonprogressive shock or compensated shock. A negative-feedback control mechanism of the circulation tries to return the cardiac output and arterial pressure to normal levels. This phenomenon is mediated through the baroreceptor reflexes, central nervous system (CNS) ischemic responses, contraction of blood vessels, release of vasopressin (antidiuretic hormone), formation of angiotensin, and compensation mechanisms that tend to return the blood volume back toward normal by mobilization of fluids from extravascular body spaces.

Stage II of shock is also known as progressive shock. A positive-feedback mechanism comes into play with this phase of shock. When shock becomes severe enough, components of the cardiovascular system start to deteriorate. This deterioration is associated with cardiac depression caused by ischemia, vasomotor failure, thrombosis of small vessels, increased capillary permeability, release of endotoxins by ischemic tissues, and generalized cellular degeneration.

Stage III of shock is also called irreversible shock. This stage occurs when adenosine triphosphate reserves are depleted and toxic substances are released from apoptotic cells. Death follows as the natural consequence of not successfully halting progressive shock.

A successful resuscitation will often leave patients in a temporary hypermetabolic and hyperdynamic state. This is caused by a "metabolic debt" for the period of ischemia. Patients often remain tachycardic despite appropriate resuscitation and sedation. Unfortunately, an apparent successful resuscitation does not mean survival. Morbidity as a result of hypovolemic hemorrhagic shock can be classified as early and late events. Acute irreversible shock presents as the classic massive hemorrhage and death. In this case the resuscitation attempt does not match the blood loss. Ongoing hemorrhage and hypoperfusion worsens, leading to acidosis, coagulopathy, and death.

Subacute irreversible shock appears clinically opposite to acute irreversible shock. In this instance, fluid volume is restored, hemorrhage is controlled, but the patient has suffered a significant dose of shock and cellular ischemia that cannot be overcome. Ultimately, the metabolic debit is too great. Over time, these patients succumb to multiorgan failure and related sequelae secondary to cellular hypoperfusion. Table 40.1 details ATLS classification of hemorrhagic shock.

Treatment of Hypovolemic Hemorrhagic Shock

Patients admitted for care with a traumatic injury often present with obvious signs of blood loss and have the potential to be in compensated shock with an unknown degree of hypovolemia. Quantifying or estimating potential blood loss is a challenging issue. Routine monitors are often inadequate in detecting losses until the late stages of shock when physiologic compensation begins to fail. Patients may have large blood volume losses and yet appear at first to be relatively normovolemic.

Blood loss can be unobservable in several locations in the body (e.g., the thorax, abdomen, pelvis, and lower extremities), thereby masking the blood loss and complicating the treatment plan. In addition, blood losses at the scene of injury are often not quantified. Blood loss to the environment (street) must be considered. The management of hypovolemic hemorrhagic shock from a traumatic injury follows a logical pathway as described in ATLS.[11]

Fluid resuscitation. The balance between the appropriate amounts of fluid is one of the greatest challenges of successful trauma resuscitation. Resuscitation is commonly seen from one perspective: blood pressure. Fluid resuscitation, however, should not only be viewed in terms of blood pressure (i.e., perfusion) but also in terms of the degree and state of repair of the injury. For limited injuries with little or no active bleeding, ATLS resuscitation guidelines advise brisk isotonic crystalloid infusion (up to 2 L) and component therapy for a larger resuscitation with greater blood loss.[11]

Unfortunately, therapy is not quite as simplistic in the case of ongoing or massive injury. The administration of fluid, in and of itself, may actually worsen the patient's clinical state if fluid administration is not timed appropriately. This necessary balance of body fluids is easily visualized when one considers a garden hose (vasculature), a water spigot (blood supply), and a sprinkler (perfusion). Imagine that a hose is connected to a water spigot and sprinkler. Water flows to the end of the hose and into the sprinkler in varying rates as the spigot is opened and closed causing variations of pressure. If the hose ruptures, water will move down the hose and exit at the tear. Depending on the amount of pressure, water may not reach the sprinkler at all. To maintain "normal" sprinkler function, water pressure would have to increase. Although this might seem advantageous, an increase in water pressure would also cause more water to exit at the tear in the hose. The additional loss of water or—in the case of a bleeding blood vessel—the additional loss of blood, would cause blood containing nutrients, coagulation factors, catecholamines, and oxygen-carrying capacity to be lost. This would of course be detrimental to the patient. In addition, the increase in pressure at the vascular injury is likely to prohibit effective coagulation and disrupt any existing clot that has formed.

For these reasons, some have advocated for hypotensive resuscitation. Hypotensive resuscitation is a controversial concept that is primarily used in the patient with penetrating trauma. It is a clinical methodology that guides fluid resuscitation in a manner that avoids excessive bleeding by maintaining a lower than normal SBP and limiting the amount of fluids administered. Even though targets may vary, most clinicians target SBP ≥ 85 to 90 mm Hg.[57] This reduction in systolic pressure reduces bleeding, allowing for improved surgical exposure and repair of vascular injury. As soon as the injury is repaired, resuscitative efforts should focus on increased blood and blood product administration with the goal of maintaining normotension. The evidence that supports hypotensive resuscitation is largely based on animal studies and one nonblinded semirandomized study in 1994.[58]

Hypotensive resuscitation was most notably described by Bickell et al.[58] in a research project commonly referred to as the Houston Trial. The Houston Trial enrolled 598 patients with penetrating thoracoabdominal trauma. The subjects were randomized in the field to a fluid administration or no fluid administration group. The research protocol continued through the primary evaluation and ended as patients were transported to the operating room. The Houston Trial found there was a significant difference in fluids administered between groups, and the resuscitation group had a higher mortality than the nonresuscitation group ($p = 0.04$). When possible, one can consider minimizing the initial fluid resuscitation until hemostasis occurs. After hemorrhage has been controlled, an SBP greater than 100 mm Hg and heart rate less than 100 bpm can be the goal. Hypotensive resuscitation should be avoided in patients with TBI since these patients frequently need higher MAPs to maintain cerebral perfusion.

Intravenous access. Appropriate IV access is a priority when managing a patient in hemorrhagic shock. The speed of IV fluid administration is directly related to the radial diameter of the catheter as described by Poiseuille's law. Larger catheters allow for increased flow by reducing turbulence. Patients should have access that has the least

TABLE 40.1   Advanced Trauma Life Support Classification of Shock

	Class 1	Class 2	Class 3	Class 4
Blood loss (%)	<15	15–30	30–40	>40
Heart rate (beats/min)	<100	>100	>120	>140
SBP (mm Hg)	Normal	Normal	Decreased	Decreased
Pulse pressure	Normal or increased	Decreased	Decreased	Decreased
RR (breaths/min)	14–20	20–30	30–40	>35
Mental state	Slightly anxious	Mildly anxious	Anxious, confused	Confused, lethargic
Base deficit	0 to −2 mEq/L	−2 to −6 mEq/L	−6 to −10 mEq/L	≤−10 mEq/L
Need for blood products	Monitor	Possible	Yes	Massive transfusion event

RR, Respiratory rate; *SBP*, systolic blood pressure.
Modified from American College of Surgeons Trauma Committee. *Advanced Trauma Life Support for Doctors.* 10th ed. Chicago: American College of Surgeons; 2018.

impediment to flow. In addition, catheter length should be minimized. As a rule of thumb, IV access should be "short and fat." Although central access is not necessary for resuscitation, patients suffering from significant hemorrhagic shock are often too vasoconstricted to cannulate large veins. Central venous access should be considered early in the management plan. Large-bore single- or double-lumen catheters should be used for central access.

In addition to size, location of the access is essential. IV access should be redundant and placed in locations that avoid circulation directly to an injured area. For instance, a femoral catheter should not be used when major abdominal, vascular, or pelvic injury has occurred. IV access above the diaphragm would provide the most assurance that the fluid would not dump or extravasate into the abdomen or retroperitoneum. In general, there should always at least two large-bore IV cannulas above the diaphragm.

Intravenous fluids. Isotonic crystalloid infusions expand plasma volume, increase cardiac output, and ultimately cause an increase in blood pressure. In addition, they may reduce vasoconstriction, hemodilute the blood, and induce immune dysfunction. As discussed earlier, vigorous fluid resuscitation must be tempered with the understanding that fluid increases blood pressure that can subsequently cause bleeding and disrupt blood clot formation. Bleeding causes recurrent hypotension and begins a vicious cycle of fluid—bleeding—hypotension. At the trauma center, RBCs should be replaced to provide adequate oxygen-carrying capacity. Lost blood is ideally replaced with a ratio of 1:1:1 volume of packed RBCs, plasma, and platelets.[20]

Serial electrolyte levels, hemoglobin and hematocrit levels, arterial blood gas analysis, and coagulation studies using TEG or ROTEM are obtained approximately every hour in severely injured, severely hemorrhagic, unstable patients in surgery until they are stable. Colloids usually allow rapid restoration of intravascular volume but can contribute to a later episode of pulmonary edema and increased bleeding if hemostasis has not been achieved. Balanced electrolyte solutions (isotonic solutions) are given to help maintain perfusion until blood products arrive.

Dextrose-containing solutions are generally undesirable for use in initial resuscitation fluid administration. Rapid determination of blood glucose levels is critical in patients with diabetes and in children. Although patients are more likely to become hyperglycemic than hypoglycemic after traumatic injury, hypoglycemia can occur. Significant hyperglycemia is associated with further neurologic injury.[59]

Stress-induced hyperglycemia is often associated with trauma and critical illness and is thought to be a consequence of many factors, including increased cortisol levels, catecholamines, glucagon, growth hormone, gluconeogenesis, and glycogenolysis.[60] Both hypoglycemia and hyperglycemia are implicated in worse outcomes in patients with TBI. Blood glucose levels of 170 mg/dL or greater upon admission to an intensive care setting have been shown to be an independent predictor of a worse neurologic outcome 5 days following admission. A target blood glucose range of 140 to 180 mg/dL (7.7–10 mmol/L) has been recommended to avoid significant hyperglycemia and iatrogenic injury produced by hypoglycemia in most trauma patients.[60]

Antifibrinolytic treatment. There is good evidence to support the early use of an antifibrinolytic agent, specifically tranexamic acid (TXA), in the trauma patient with severe hemorrhage. The CRASH2 trial evaluated over 20,000 bleeding trauma patients and determined that 1 g of TXA given within 3 hours of initial injury followed by 1 g administered over 8 hours significantly reduced the amount of bleeding and risk of death from bleeding.[61] TXA is a lysine analog that inhibits the conversion of plasminogen to plasmin and thus prevents the breakdown of the fibrin clot. It has been shown in many other studies to be particularly helpful at reducing surgical blood loss.

Coagulopathy and Trauma

A vast majority of patients that survive their initial injury and reach the hospital are coagulopathic when they die. It is estimated that between 25% and 35% of noncombat-related trauma admissions present with a biochemically evident traumatic-induced coagulopathy on admission.[62]

Once coagulopathy develops, patient morbidity and mortality drastically increase. Coagulopathy is an independent predictor of mortality. In otherwise healthy patients, an elevated prothrombin time (PT) on admission indicates rapid hemorrhage, massive injury, and a steadily worsening perfusion state.[62] In addition to the loss of life, coagulopathy indirectly levies a burden on society and the health care system. As such, management strategies to reduce the morbidity and mortality of trauma-induced coagulopathy have become of particular interest. Coagulopathy can also occur from (1) hypothermia and exposure to the elements and rapid administration cold IV fluids; (2) dilution of clotting factors from excessive crystalloid and/or packed RBC administration, and acidosis that results from hypoperfusion and/or hypoventilation, which causes a dysfunction of the clotting enzymes; and (3) hypovolemic hemorrhagic shock.

Clot formation. Hemostasis is a complex process involving proteins—cofactors and blood products that converge in a series of reactions intended to produce the fibrin and platelet network (with trapped RBCs) that is a clot. Clot formation begins with an initial vascular insult. Tissue injury immediately causes the release of tissue factor (TF) from the endothelium. At the same time vascular spasm causes platelets to migrate from the vascular lumen toward the site of injury. TF binds with activated, circulating factor VII (FVIIa). The interaction of FVIIa with TF begins the conversion of prothrombin (II) to activated thrombin (IIa) resulting in a "thrombin burst" on the surface of the platelet. Conversion of thrombin completes the coagulation process yielding fibrin (I) connections that stabilize clot formation.[62] Under normal conditions fibrinolytic pathways maintain appropriate clot size and location, limiting clot formation to the site of vascular injury.

Pathology and causes of coagulopathy. Massive injury can disrupt the clotting cascade at several points in the process, resulting in life-threatening consequences. As mentioned earlier, four mechanisms have been identified as primary causes of trauma-induced coagulopathy. These mechanisms are (1) dilution of factors, (2) hypothermia/acidosis, (3) severe TBI, and (4) hypovolemic hemorrhagic shock. Trauma-induced coagulopathy has both endogenous and exogenous components. Endogenous acute traumatic coagulopathy is associated with shock and hypoperfusion. Exogenous coagulopathy arises from effects of dilution resulting from fluid resuscitation and consumption through bleeding and loss of coagulation factors. Coagulopathy is present in 25% to 35% of injured patients, depending on injury severity, acidosis, hypothermia, and hypoperfusion.[62]

Dilution. Traumatic injury often requires massive resuscitation to replace blood volume and restore perfusion. ATLS guidelines advocate fluid administration but do not provide clear guidance on the administration of procoagulant products such as plasma, cryoprecipitate, and platelets.[11] Although required for initial resuscitation, crystalloid fluid administration dilutes coagulation factors and platelets and increases hydrostatic pressure. This ultimately leads to an inadequate clot and nonsurgical bleeding.

Resuscitation is a dynamic process. Treating one deficit, such as anemia, with RBCs will dilute coagulation factors and platelets leading to coagulopathy. The addition of crystalloid or nonblood colloids further exacerbates this tenuous situation.[62] Various authors advocate a balanced administration of RBCs, plasma, and platelets (1:1:1) for massive resuscitation.[20] Balanced administration of blood products functionally represents whole blood administration. Currently, the utilization of fresh whole blood has been limited to military settings. Although it is an improvement, balanced component therapy falls short of the ideal whole blood replacement by virtue of (1) dilution with anticoagulant and nutritive solutions as blood is collected and processed; (2) losses caused by centrifuging, separation, and readministration; and (3) losses over time in storage.[63]

Establishing clinical endpoints for correcting coagulopathy is challenging and historically has not been standardized. To rectify this, a consensus statement of the College of American Pathologists, the ASA, and the European Task Force for Advanced Bleeding Care in Trauma recommends administering procoagulant products to maintain an international normalized ratio (INR) 1.5 or less, and a platelet count above 50,000. In cases where a coagulopathy is suspected, viscoelastic assays (e.g., TEG and ROTEM) in addition to a platelet count are recommended. In the event the viscoelastic assays are not available, standard coagulation tests are obtained (e.g., INR, activated partial thromboplastin time [aPTT], fibrinogen concentration, platelet count).[64,65] Although these endpoints are helpful in creating a standard methodology of care, and for replacement of factors in stable patients, it must be acknowledged that acute care based on laboratory data may be unrealistic. Laboratory analysis is time consuming and may not provide information rapidly enough in an actively bleeding patient. The clinician is frequently required to make decisions about transfusion in anticipation of the patient's course, which is why authorities recommend empiric 1:1:1 therapy until the situation is stable enough to guide therapy based on laboratory values.

Hypothermia and acidosis. Occult hypothermia is an uncommon event. Less than 9% of trauma admissions are hypothermic on presentation.[66,67] Despite this, hypothermia remains an issue. Removal of clothing (*environment* in ATLS management), muscle relaxation, cold IV fluid administration (resuscitation), and frequent examination (removal of blankets) contributes to heat loss. Hypothermia may result in significant coagulopathy. The vast majority of patient hypothermia can be attributed to radiant heat loss caused by the gradient differences of patient and environmental temperature.[67]

Hypothermia induces a variety of physiologic changes. Although the precise mechanism is unclear, there is agreement that hypothermia alters platelet function and reduces fibrin enzyme kinetics.[68] Hypothermia and acidosis compromise thrombin-generation kinetics via different mechanisms. Hypothermia primarily inhibits the initiation phase of thrombin generation. In addition, hypothermia inhibits fibrinogen synthesis, leading to a potential deficit in fibrinogen availability. The clinical effect of hypothermia is a slowly formed and fragile clot that is unable to inhibit bleeding.[69]

Acidosis often accompanies massive injury, hemorrhage, and hypothermia. Acidosis in and of itself does not appear to have a significant impact on coagulation; however, in the presence of hypothermia, it can contribute to coagulopathy.[70,71] It is believed that acidosis impairs coagulation proteases and becomes clinically significant at a pH less than 7.1.[70,71] Unfortunately, administration of sodium bicarbonate to correct acidosis leads to increased carbon dioxide production and hypocalcemia, which are both direct myocardial depressants.[72]

The management of hypothermic and acidotic patients is fairly intuitive. The most efficacious management is to rewarm the patient and focus on restoring optimal perfusion to correct acidosis. Obviously, warming fluids as they are given and controlling the ambient room temperature of the resuscitation unit/operating room are essential. Hypothermia can be minimized when proper care is taken.

Activated protein C pathway. Trauma-induced coagulopathy is often thought of as a result of environmental or therapeutic interventions. Resuscitation necessitates large volumes of IV fluid to be administered causing hypothermia and dilution in the face of acidosis, leading to the lethal triad. In many ways, coagulopathy was a "cost of doing business." Recent research has challenged this belief.

The activated protein C (APC) pathway has been identified for decades. Although the role of the APC in fibrinolytic pathways has been well established, its pathologic role in trauma-induced coagulopathy is only now emerging.[73] It is believed that the APC pathway is initiated when thrombin binds with thrombomodulin. The thrombin-thrombomodulin (T-T) complex is a normally occurring anticoagulant that develops as a negative feedback during clotting to limit a clot to the area of injury.[68] APC is a vitamin K-dependent serine protease that induces anticoagulation by inhibiting factors V and VIII.[69,74] In a non-pathologic state, APC functions to limit clot propagation, ultimately maintaining blood flow in uninjured vessels. However, in the presence of damaged and hypoperfused tissue, it is believed that the APC pathway may lead to systemic coagulopathy.[70,73]

Traumatic brain injury–induced coagulopathy. TBI in isolation is self-limiting, often producing very little blood loss. Despite this, TBI continues to be a significant cause of morbidity and mortality, with TBI accounting for approximately 30% of all injury deaths. On a daily basis, approximately 138 people in the United States die as a result of injuries that include TBI.[75] Although the mechanism is not fully understood, it is believed that TBI causes a local release of TF and anionic phospholipid-rich microvesicles from injured neurons, activating the protein C pathway and triggering the release of anticoagulant mediators.[74]

Early management of TBI should include rapid administration of plasma. The endpoint of plasma administration should be to normalize the PT and INR. Because the plasma requirement needed to reverse TBI-induced coagulopathy is unpredictable, often requiring large quantities of plasma to reduce bleeding and normalize clot formation, administering plasma is recommended early, even before the initial PT or INR laboratory results return. The administration of low-dose recombinant FVIIa (rFVIIa) has been shown to be effective in improving the coagulation status of patients with TBI. In one study, the impact of rFVIIa at a dose of 20 mcg/kg improved the INR and coagulation status of patients without adverse effects.[76]

Shock and hypoperfusion-induced coagulopathy. Contemporary research suggests that hypoperfusion may be the sentinel step in trauma-induced coagulopathy. Like TBI, it is believed that hemorrhagic shock leads to activation of the protein C pathway, resulting in fibrinolytic coagulopathy.[77] Although the exact mechanism is unclear, it is believed that occult hemorrhage and hypoperfusion may increase T-T complexes, resulting in APC and clotting factor inactivation. This finding is consistent with observed clinical presentations. As previously noted, nearly half of all trauma fatalities are caused by coagulopathic patients in hemorrhage and hemorrhagic shock who have no sign of TBI, hypothermia, or significant prehospital resuscitation.[78]

Management strategies for these patients should include a vigorous yet controlled resuscitation. In addition to ATLS guidelines, warm fluids, and early blood product administration, the goal of the resuscitation team should be to maintain perfusion depending on the traumatic situation. If there is ongoing hemorrhage, then higher MAPs should be avoided until the hemorrhage is controlled. In contrast, those patients who have experienced a TBI should be allowed to maintain higher MAP values (i.e., >80 mm Hg) in an effort to promote cerebral perfusion.[79,80]

Management strategies aimed at avoiding secondary injury by maintaining CCP and optimization of cerebral oxygenation may be of tremendous benefit.[81] Research to date indicates that maintaining a CPP in the range 60 to 70 mm Hg is preferred.[71,72] Additionally, those patients whose CPP was maintained at levels at or above 70 mm Hg had decreased hospital mortality.[82]

Disability (Neurologic)

Neurologic assessment begins the moment the patient enters the hospital. Patient mentation, behavior, and response to stimuli all provide the clinician with a picture of any neurologic injury. A GCS score is assigned during the primary or secondary survey and reassessed throughout the hospital course. Head injuries are classified grossly as blunt or penetrating, and the severity of the injury is based on the GCS score.

The GCS evaluates the best eye response, best verbal response, and best motor response with a minimum score of 3 and maximum score of 15. A GCS of 13 or higher correlates with a mild brain injury, 9 to 12 a moderate injury and 8 or less a severe brain injury.[83] See Table 20.7 for the Glasgow Coma Scale.

Head Injury

Patients with head injury may sustain a primary TBI that cannot be anatomically corrected. The goal of care is the prevention of secondary brain damage resulting from intracranial complications that are aggravated by intracranial bleeding, edema, and resultant increases in ICP. The presence of hypotension on admission and the need for mechanical ventilation have been identified as potentially modifiable risk factors for morbidity and mortality following severe TBI.[84] Anesthesia management of head-injured patients includes early control of the airway and maintenance of cardiovascular stability.

Management of neurologic injury follows a similar treatment pathway as that for other trauma patients. A GCS of less than 8 necessitates endotracheal intubation. Goals for airway management should be to maintain blood oxygen saturation (SpO_2) greater than 90% and normoventilation to help reduce hypercarbia and hypoxemia, both of which contribute to elevated ICP.[81] Judicious use of induction agents and neuromuscular blocking agents can facilitate a straightforward intubation. Attempts to perform an awake intubation in an obtunded, semicomatose, head-injured patient may promote coughing, bucking, and thrashing about, along with concomitant increases in the ICP that carry the risk of tentorial herniation. Nasal intubation may be contraindicated in the head-injured patient because of possible basilar skull fractures that can facilitate contamination and ultimate sepsis from nasal microorganisms introduced into the cranial vault.[85] Late sepsis also can occur from a sinus infection caused by prolonged nasal tracheal intubation. Gastric tubes are placed orally in head-injured patients for the same reasons.[86]

Intracranial hemorrhage is a concern since it can rapidly increase the pressure within the cranial vault. Conditions such as subdural or epidural intracranial bleeds require surgical intervention. There is some evidence that TXA is beneficial for TBI patients with intracranial bleeds who have mild to moderate injuries. These would be patients with GCS scores of 9 or higher. The evidence suggests that early treatment with TXA is best and certainly within 3 hours of injury. The recommended dose of TXA is 1 g IV over 10 minutes followed by 1 g IV over 8 hours.[87]

Although hypotension is always a matter of concern, it is even more so for patients with neurologic injury. CPP describes the relationship between MAP (blood pressure) and ICP. SBP directly affects cerebral blood flow and should be allowed at higher levels to promote brain perfusion. It is recommended that a MAP greater than 80 mm Hg is maintained to allow for a CPP of greater than 60 mm Hg in the TBI patient with increased ICP.[79,80,82] Significant hypoxemia and hypotension are associated with increased morbidity and mortality. Thus primary management goals include support of the patient's cardiopulmonary status as well as strategies that reduce increased ICP.

Patients with a suspected open- or closed-head injury are placed in a head-up position to help promote venous drainage and reduce ICP. Management of ICP is a challenge. There is no exact treatment

threshold; however, most experts support treatment for ICP greater than 20 to 25 mm Hg.[88] No one technique (total intravenous anesthesia vs general anesthesia) has demonstrated superiority to another. Although some anesthetic agents may decrease cerebral metabolic demand, they also may reduce cerebral blood flow, which may not be a desired effect when trying to increase cerebral blood flow. Aggressive management of CPP has been correlated with improved patient outcome.[81,89] Patients with neurologic injury are more likely to die when their SBP falls below 90 mm Hg. Clinical targets should be to maintain a MAP at a minimum of 80 mm Hg to maintain a CPP of at least 60 mm Hg.[82,90] This gross target should be maintained until ICP monitoring can be initiated.

ICP monitoring is indicated for many instances of moderate and severe brain injury. Current ACS Committee on Trauma recommendations are for the placement of a ventriculostomy for ICP monitoring. It is the most accurate, cost-effective, and safe method for monitoring ICP.[91] Ventriculostomies allow for close monitoring of ICP, as well as treatment of elevated ICP by drainage of cerebrospinal fluid (CSF). Anesthetists should be familiar with this equipment and how to safely calibrate the drainage system, in addition to knowing how to open and close the system, as indicated, for the treatment of these patients.

The goal in treating intracranial hypertension is to promote adequate oxygenation and nutrient supply by maintaining CPP, oxygenation, and glucose supply without hyperglycemia.[92] The ACS recommends a three-tiered approach. Tier 1 interventions include elevation of the head of the bed to 30 degrees (reverse Trendelenburg), short-acting sedation and analgesia (propofol, fentanyl, midazolam), intermittent ventricular drainage, repeat neurologic exams, and repeat CT to exclude surgical mass lesions and to assist with management. If ICP remains greater than 20 to 25 mm Hg, proceed to tier 2. Tier 2 therapeutic measures include placement of an external ventricular drain to facilitate drainage of intermittent CSF and intermittent hyperosmolar therapy with mannitol (0.25–1 g/kg of body weight) or hypertonic saline (3% 250 mL IV infusion over 30 minutes or 23.4% 30 mL IV infusion over 10 minutes). If choosing mannitol, the serum osmolality level should be checked every 6 hours to avoid a serum osmolality greater than 320 mOsm/L. Also avoid mannitol administration if hypovolemia is suspected. The serum sodium (Na) and osmolality must be reviewed to ensure that Na levels remain less than 160 mEq/L. Additional neuromonitoring may include brain tissue oxygen partial pressure ($Pbto_2$), jugular venous oxygen saturation ($Sjvo_2$), and cerebral blood flow (CBF) to determine the ideal CPP. A partial pressure of carbon dioxide in arterial blood ($Paco_2$) of 30 to 35 mm Hg can be utilized as long as brain hypoxia is not suspected. Additional neurologic evaluation and head CTs should be considered to continue to exclude surgical mass lesions and as a guide to treatment. Neuromuscular blockade may be added if the aforementioned measures do not lower the ICP and restore the CPP to acceptable levels. Tier 3 is implemented in the event ICP remains greater than 20 to 25 mm Hg. Tier 3 interventions include surgical evacuation and control of the underlying pathology. Potential salvage therapies that are recommended include barbiturate- or propofol-induced coma and hypothermia (<36°C) in those cases of "rescue" or salvage therapy when reasonable efforts to reduce ICP using treatments prior to tier 3 have not been successful.[92]

Severe increases in ICP can result in impending brain herniation and death. This is a medical emergency that requires immediate intubation and surgical intervention. Signs that indicate impending brain herniation are hypertension, bradycardia, and irregular respirations. These are known as Cushing triad. Airway management during this crisis can be challenging and involves a balance between avoiding hypotension and decreases in CPP as well as avoiding severe increases in blood pressure that can exacerbate the herniating brain. Fentanyl can be used to manage the sympathetic response to intubation, and propofol can be used as an induction agent. Rapid paralysis can be achieved with the highest recommended intubating dose of rocuronium. Postintubation sedation should be considered to avoid severe increases in blood pressure.

Patients with significant head injury benefit from the placement of an arterial line in addition to the standard monitoring, which includes capnography and pulse oximetry. The placement of an ICP monitoring device facilitates the observation of changes in ICP dynamics that are influenced by drug administration and other manipulations. Intracranial hypertension exists when the ICP is at a sustained elevation of greater than 15 mm Hg. Again, therapeutic maneuvers are aimed at maintaining the CPP at approximately 60 mm Hg or greater and oxygen delivery SpO_2 at or above 90%. Of note, CPPs greater than 60 mm Hg have been linked to improved outcomes. Attempts to elevate the CPP to levels of greater than 70 mm Hg have been associated with increased pulmonary complications, including ARDS, as a result of volume overload.[92,93] Steroids have not been shown to improve outcome or reduce ICP.[92] The safety of isoflurane, desflurane, and sevoflurane has been demonstrated. Avoidance of nitrous oxide is recommended at least until the full extent of injuries is known because it may aggravate potential pneumocephalus and pneumothorax in the traumatized patient. Temporary reduction of ICP is often achieved using small incremental doses of propofol, moderate levels of hyperventilation (short term), mannitol and/or furosemide for diuresis, and elevation of the patient's head in relation to the heart for a beneficial gravitational influence.

Etomidate as an induction agent for an RSI has been advocated for use in trauma patients because of its minimal hemodynamic effects, thus minimizing a drop in CPP.[94] It is a sedative-hypnotic that stimulates γ-aminobutyric acid (GABA) receptors to block neuroexcitation and induce amnesia. It decreases the cerebral rate of oxygen ($CMRO_2$), CBF, and ICP, and is often employed for induction of anesthesia in the neurosurgical patient. To date, no studies have been published that have conclusively found a single dose of etomidate to facilitate endotracheal intubation has any significant impact on morbidity or mortality in the trauma patient.[43]

Ketamine is also an acceptable induction agent for RSI, especially in patients with normal to decreased blood pressure due to its propensity for sympathetic induced increases in MAP and CPP. Ketamine was removed as a relative contraindication for TBI in a 2011 update by the American College of Emergency Physicians (ACEP) clinical practice guidelines for ketamine sedation.[94]

Propofol is a frequently employed sedative-hypnotic that has a rapid onset, profound amnesia, short duration of action, and effective blunting of sympathetic outflow during laryngoscopy. Propofol decreases $CMRO_2$, CBF, and ICP, which makes this drug a preferred agent for hemodynamically stable TBI patients. Because propofol reduces SVR and has myocardial depressant effects, it must be used with extreme caution in patients with hemodynamic instability.

SPECIAL TOPICS IN TRAUMA ANESTHESIA

Spinal Cord Injury

The most common causes of SCI in the United States are MVCs (31.5%), falls (25.3%), and gunshot wounds (10.4%). MVCs are the primary mechanism of injury in victims until the age of 45 years; then, falls account for the majority of spinal cord injuries after age 45. The average age at the time of injury has increased from 29 years in the 1970s to 43 years since 2015.[95] It is estimated that the annual incidence of SCI is approximately 54 cases per million population, which translates to 17,810 new cases of SCI per year.[96] A coroner's analysis of 512 prehospital deaths from trauma indicated that the leading causes of

death in patients with SCI include head and spine injury (36%), hemorrhage (34%), asphyxia (15%), and combined neurotrauma/hemorrhage (15%).[97] It is estimated that males constitute approximately 80% of all new SCI cases. Of interest, the average age of those affected during the 1970s was 29 years, and the mean age at present is 43 years.[96] Few severe injuries have as devastating physical and psychologic effects as those caused by spinal cord trauma. Eventual outcome after an acute SCI depends on three factors: (1) the severity of the acute injury; (2) avoiding exacerbation of the injury during rescue, transport, and hospitalization; and (3) preventing hypoxia and systemic hypotension, which can further compromise neural function.[98] See Table 40.2 for the common mechanisms of spinal injuries.

Most SCIs involve the craniocervical junction (33%), which consists of the occiput and the first two cervical vertebrae.[99] Over 50% of all traumatic SCIs occur in the cervical region. The most common resulting injuries are incomplete tetraplegia (31%), complete paraplegia (25%), complete tetraplegia (20%), and incomplete paraplegia (19%).[100] SCIs can be categorized as complete or incomplete injuries. Complete injuries represent an absence of motor, sensory, bowel, and bladder function below the level of injury. There is some preservation of neurologic function with incomplete injuries.[100] SCI should be ruled out in any traumatized individual. The nature of the accident and the mechanism of injury should help guide the diagnosis and suspicion of

TABLE 40.2 Classification of Spinal Cord Injuries

Mechanism of Spinal Injury	Stability
Flexion	
Wedge fraction	Stable
Flexion teardrop fracture	Extremely unstable
Clay shoveler fracture	Stable
Subluxation	Potentially unstable
Bilateral facet dislocation	Always unstable
Atlantooccipital dislocation	Unstable
Anterior atlantoaxial dislocation with or without fracture	Unstable
Odontoid fracture with lateral displacement fracture	Unstable
Fracture of transverse process	Stable
Flexion Rotation	
Unilateral facet dislocation	Stable
Rotary atlantoaxial dislocation	Unstable
Extension	
Posterior neural arch fracture (C1)	Unstable
Hangman fracture (C2)	Unstable
Extension teardrop fracture	Usually stable in flexion; unstable in extension
Posterior atlantoaxial dislocation with or without fracture	Unstable
Vertical Compression	
Bursting fracture of vertebral body	Stable
Jefferson fracture (C1)	Extremely unstable
Isolated fractures of articular pillar and vertebral body	Stable

From Kaji A, et al. *Rosen's Emergency Medicine*. 8th ed. Philadelphia: Elsevier; 2014:385.

possible SCI. As mentioned earlier, MVCs are a major cause of morbidity and mortality. Half of those who are injured in a rollover collision sustain head, neck, and SCIs.[101] Cervical SCI should be assumed to be present in any patient who has sustained trauma to the head or face, in any unconscious trauma patient, and in any patient who complains of pain before or after careful palpation of the cervical spine. The clinician should be aware of the six conditions that are highly correlated with SCIs: paralysis, pain, position, paresthesias, ptosis, and priapism (Box 40.1). A comparison of cervical spine injuries and their acuity is noted in Table 40.2.

If an SCI is suspected, precautions should be taken for the prevention or further extension of actual or potential neurologic deficits. Spinal immobilization and a properly fitted cervical collar should be carefully placed before the patient is moved or extricated. The head should be stabilized in neutral alignment with no extension, flexion, or rotation. Stabilization can be accomplished by placing a cervical collar on the patient, splinting, and/or sandbagging the head in neutral alignment. The patient should be placed on a long spinal backboard before being moved.[100,102] All patients with suspected SCI must be assessed for adequacy of a patent airway. When managing and opening the airway, care should be used to avoid extension, flexion, or rotation of the neck. A gentle chin-lift maneuver may be adequate for securing a patent airway without disturbing the neutral neck position. Oxygen should be administered by mask immediately in the patient whose airway is secured at the scene.

Hypoxia and hypercarbia can further accentuate the damage sustained with SCIs. Injuries at the C1 or C2 level result in complete respiratory paralysis. Death follows within a few minutes if airway support with assisted ventilation is not commenced rapidly. In such patients, a laryngeal mask airway or a laryngeal tube airway may be placed in the patient at the scene by paramedics. Although these devices initially

---

BOX 40.1 **Six Signs and Symptoms Associated With Spinal Cord Injuries**

Paralysis
Inability to move the arms or legs should always raise suspicion of spinal cord injury.

Pain
Conscious patient may complain of pain localized at the site of the spinal injury.

Position
Patient holding the head upright or the neck with both hands may be indicating a Jefferson-type C1 fracture; the hold-up position (arms and hands held over the head as in a robbery) can indicate a C4-C5 fracture; the prayer position (arms folded across chest) indicates a possible C5-C6 fracture.

Paresthesias
Complaints of numbness, a pins-and-needles sensation, a burning sensation (dysesthesia), or a feeling of electric shock passing down the vertebral column or of water flowing down the back may indicate the presence of a spinal cord injury.

Ptosis
Drooping eyelid and myotic pupil, which are signs of Horner syndrome, may indicate a cervical spinal cord injury.

Priapism
Penile erection occurs in approximately 3% to 5% of spinal cord injuries. Its presence indicates that the sympathetic nervous system is involved.

---

may be adequate for allowing transport to a medical facility, they are replaced with an ETT as quickly as possible after the patient is admitted to a treatment facility.[11]

If the patient with a SCI is breathing spontaneously on arrival at the treatment facility, the adequacy of ventilation should be assessed immediately. If the patient is not able to self-protect the airway (because of being unconscious or semiconscious, having an absent or diminished gag reflex or cough, or having intraoral or facial injuries with significant edema, bleeding, or both), rapid intubation is needed. If ventilation appears to be reasonable, chest and cervical spine radiographic evaluation and neurologic examinations can be started while an arterial blood gas is completed. A lateral view of the cervical spine can be obtained quickly, and it reveals most unstable fractures. Multiple cervical x-ray films, a CT scan, or MRI may be required for a complete evaluation of the cervical spine. An adequate evaluation must include all seven cervical vertebrae; C7 is the most common site of injury.[103]

In children, uncooperative adults, or in patients in whom awake intubation fails, a carefully selected dose of propofol and a neuromuscular blocking agent is used for inducing general anesthesia for the intubation.[104] Orotracheal intubation can be safely performed with neck immobilization and inline stabilization. Although there is debate in the literature, it is preferable to intubate these SCI patients orally. SCI patients have the best chance of recovery if hypoxia, hypercarbia, and hypotension are avoided or rapidly corrected if encountered. Arterial blood gas values indicating that ventilation is suboptimal are corrected by intubation and mechanical ventilation. If there is a delay in establishing the airway, the patient is given ventilation by mask while cricoid pressure is maintained until the airway is secured. Severely traumatized patients who are hypoxic on arrival should undergo mask ventilation with application of cricoid pressure until intubation is completed. This method prevents further hypoxic insults that can occur during the apneic period between the administration of a muscle relaxant and the completed intubation. It is reasonable to consider a slight head-up position (reverse Trendelenburg) in patients at risk for aspiration as long as there are no significant concerns for hypotension. In addition, if preoxygenation or mask ventilation is anticipated to be difficult then apneic oxygenation with 15 L nasal oxygen may help to minimize clinically significant oxygen desaturation.[103,104]

Use of Muscle Relaxants in Patients With Spinal Cord Injury

As previously discussed, succinylcholine may precipitate cardiac arrest in patients with massive muscle injury or denervation that is seen in patients with SCIs, severe crush injuries, or burns. The basis for this problem involves up-regulation of acetylcholine receptors and massive potassium release as a result of the depolarizing effects of succinylcholine.[105] Normal depolarization results in a small potassium flux across the muscle cell membrane. If a muscle is crushed, burned, or denervated, acetylcholine receptors proliferate around the injured cell so that when the muscle is depolarized the flux of potassium is increased significantly.[106] The problem is thought to develop in response to succinylcholine several days after the injury. Therefore succinylcholine should not be administered to a patient after 24 hours from sustaining a SCI. Succinylcholine is also not recommended for intubation of the patient with acute SCI due to the muscle fasciculations that may exacerbate the SCI. It is also contraindicated for routine use in children.[107] A conservative approach to caring for patients with SCI is to use a nondepolarizing neuromuscular blocker such as rocuronium or avoiding paralysis altogether during airway management.[104]

Spinal Shock

A triad of hypotension, bradycardia, and hypothermia frequently results from a relative sympathectomy in SCI patients. The spinal shock is progressively intensified the more cephalad the SCI. Patients with SCIs at the T6 level or higher have severely impaired CNS function. Sympathetically mediated cardioaccelerator responses no longer oppose vagal innervation allowing the heart rate to slow dramatically. Loss of sympathetic tone allows vasodilation, pooling of the peripheral circulation, and decreased venous return to the heart. This situation results in a decreased cardiac output and hypotension. The SCI also interrupts sympathetic pathways from the hypothalamus (temperature control center) to peripheral blood vessels. The patient in spinal shock is unable to constrict vessels or shiver to produce heat or to dilate vessels to dissipate heat. The patient's body temperature has a tendency to migrate toward the environmental level.[103,104]

Treatment

Patients in spinal shock are hypotensive and bradycardic with warm, pink extremities. In contrast, patients in hemorrhagic shock tend to be hypotensive and tachycardic with cold, clammy skin. Use of invasive monitoring is critical for fluid resuscitation and appropriate intervention with vasoactive drugs, often norepinephrine infusion. An indwelling arterial catheter is mandatory in the acute phase of spinal shock for moment-to-moment control of arterial blood pressure, for the replacement of fluids, for the use of vasoactive drug therapy, and for arterial blood gas assessments.[108]

The SCI patient is frequently unable to maintain adequate cardiac filling pressures. However, overaggressive fluid therapy can precipitate pulmonary edema. For the maintenance of adequate arterial blood pressure and cord perfusion, various vasopressor therapies may be initiated.[108]

Other Considerations

Patients suffering from cervical SCI many times have associated intercostal muscle weakness, or complete paralysis depending on the degree and level of spinal injury. The amount of respiratory dysfunction correlates with the level of SCI. Vital capacity and the ability to protect the airway from secretions or even the ability to take a breath may be significantly decreased or absent. The primary muscles of respiration are located in the diaphragm, which are typically innervated by the C3, C4, and C5 nerves (these form the bilateral phrenic nerves) and the intercostal muscles that are in turn controlled by T2 through T11. SCI above C3 often leads to apnea, whereby survivors are typically rendered ventilator dependent.[109] There has been some success in weaning certain patients off the ventilator with significant SCI at higher levels with the use of exogenous pacing of the diaphragm via intramuscular diaphragmatic stimulation devices.[110]

Recent research by Jones et al. reviewed the records of all patients with an acute SCI from January 1998 through July 2012 at a level 1 regional trauma center. Records of 163 patients were analyzed, and 76 complete SCIs were identified. The investigators determined that 91% of these patients required more than 48 hours of mechanical ventilation. When the level of SCI was considered, mechanical ventilation was needed in 100% of patients with a C2 through C4 injury, 90% for a C5 injury, 79% for a C6 injury, and 80% for a C7 injury. It was concluded that all patients who suffered a complete CSI above C5 should undergo an elective tracheostomy. Additionally, the decision to perform a tracheostomy in a patient with an incomplete SCI should be based on the presence of associated intracranial and thoracic injuries.[110]

Patients who meet the appropriate guidelines should be extubated as soon as possible to avoid various pulmonary complications associated with mechanical ventilation and prolonged intensive care unit stays.[111] If the patient requires intubation because of associated pulmonary injuries or dysfunction, then a weaning program is started once the patient is able to tolerate. With frequent assessment of respiratory

status this weaning is usually begun within the first few days. Useful guidelines for assessing the adequacy of ventilation include measurement of the tidal volume (>5 mL/kg), negative inspiratory force (−20–25 cm H_2O pressure, needed for adequate cough), and vital capacity (>15 mg/kg). Patients with a high SCI often lose innervation of the intercostal and abdominal musculature.

Chest physiotherapy is initiated for all patients as soon as possible to reduce the risk of pulmonary congestion and infection. Oral or nasogastric tubes are placed for decompressing the stomach. This measure eases diaphragmatic excursion for improved ventilation and reduces the risk of aspiration. Peptic ulceration with loss of sympathetic innervation in the patient with a high SCI is a well-described complication, especially in patients receiving steroids.[108] Of note, treatment with high-dose steroids was common in patients with SCI in the past in an attempt to minimize secondary injury associated with inflammation and edema. Contemporary evidence-based recommendations caution against the use of routine steroid administration because of increased rates of gastrointestinal bleeding that may lead to death. Indeed, 15 medical societies have advocated against the use of steroids in those patients suffering a SCI.[112]

Two additional conditions associated with acute SCI include SCI without radiographic abnormalities (SCIWORA) and acute vertebral artery injury (VAI). SCIWORA refers to a patient who displays symptoms of a traumatic myelopathy or SCI despite the presence of a negative conventional x-ray or CT scan. MRI is considered the most accurate modality to diagnose this condition, and consequently an MRI is warranted in any patient suspected of having SCIWORA. Patients with SCIWORA may have a broad variety of neurologic deficits ranging from mild and transient paresthesia in the fingers to a complete quadriplegia. The primary treatment for SCIWORA is application of an external immobilization device such as a hard cervical collar for up to 12 weeks postinjury. It is critical that anesthesia providers consider this an unstable condition that requires the patient's neck to be kept in a neutral position for airway management and intraoperative positioning.[113]

It is estimated that the incidence of VAI in SCI patients is 53% to 88%.[114] MVCs are the most common cause of VAI, where a hyperextension injury of the neck, with or without lateral flexion or rotation, produces a closed injury to the vertebral artery. Additionally, VAI in the elderly is frequently attributed to falls from a standing position, which produces a C2 fracture.[115] The vertebral artery is most susceptible to injury at (1) its entry point into the C6 transverse foramen and (2) its exit point at the atlantoaxial junction. Patients suffering from a VAI may have strokelike symptoms. It is vital that the presence of a VAI be confirmed because the potentially devastating complications of a cerebrovascular accident leading to death can occur. The current standard diagnostic tool to detect the presence of a VAI is CT angiography. If a VAI is suspected, it is important to implement anticoagulant or antiplatelet therapy to reduce the likelihood of serve neurologic deficit or death.[115]

Surgical Intervention and Anesthesia Approach

Although external immobilization devices, including a halo vest, are sometimes used, many neurosurgeons believe that prolonged use of external fixation devices is contraindicated in patients with unsatisfactorily reduced spines. In addition, there is research indicating that use of a halo vest for older patients (those aged 60–73) may have higher rates of morbidity and mortality.[116] Frequently, spinal stabilization and/or decompression procedures are performed after initial resuscitation and diagnostic workup.

Contemporary investigation on the timing of surgical intervention after an initial SCI has not been definitive. There is some research indicating that early stabilization is associated with improved patient outcomes.[117] Conversely, in a study conducted by Liu that involved 595 patients, the investigators determined that early surgical intervention was linked to higher mortality and neurologic deterioration.[118] Research on military personnel experiencing an acute SCI in Afghanistan found that these patients fared better when surgical intervention was delayed until they were transported to a regional medical center. Specifically, those transferred to a regional medical center had half the rate of complications.[119] Yet additional research indicates that the optimal timing for surgery in patients with multisystem injuries involves balancing the risks of performing extensive spinal surgery with stabilization performed initially and deferring surgical intervention until such time as the patient is hemodynamically more stable.[120]

The patient's current neurologic status and any deficits should be documented before the start of anesthesia and intubation. In an awake intubation, the patient is assessed before and after ETT placement, as well as after the patient is positioned for surgery.

Whether an anterior or a posterior surgical approach is used for cervical stabilization after a SCI depends on the nature of the injury. Internal fixation devices are commonly placed in the acute phase for stabilization of lower SCIs. At times these procedures can be associated with significant surgical blood loss. Careful monitoring and replacement of blood loss are essential. Use of an autotransfusion device often saves considerable banked blood use in these procedures. Antifibrinolytic agents, most notably TXA, can be employed.[121]

In cooperative patients who are deferred for elective spinal stabilization procedures, awake fiberoptic intubations are often employed. In controlled conditions, this measure allows for the use of local, topical, and/or transtracheal anesthesia without the risk of pulmonary aspiration that is present in emergency procedures.[122] Glycopyrrolate is commonly given before administering local anesthesia to the airway in an effort to decrease secretions. Mild sedation can be considered and either nerve blocks using local anesthetics, topical anesthesia, or a combination of both can be utilized to anesthetize the airway.[123,124] At this point there is little research to suggest that nasal intubation is superior to oral intubation in all potential SCI patients. However, if possible, oral intubation should be considered to avoid potential complications typically associated with nasal intubation such as epistaxis and the rare instance of inadvertent avulsion of the turbinates.[124,125] Long-term use of nasal ETTs has been implicated as a cause of necrosis of the nasal alae. Sinusitis has been reported in both orally and nasally intubated patients.[125,126]

The choice of airway management technique with a SCI will depend to a great extent on the patient's injuries, level of cooperation, hemodynamic stability, and ability to protect the airway.[126] If the patient is cooperative and hemodynamically stable, an awake topicalized flexible intubation approach is considered the technique that produces the least amount of movement of the cervical spine.[123] This approach also affords an opportunity to perform a wake-up test, where the patient can respond to requests to test upper and lower extremities prior to induction of general anesthesia to confirm no change for the worse in neurologic status. Intraoperative neural monitoring that utilizes somatosensory-evoked potentials and electromyography should be employed throughout the entire operative period in an attempt to minimize secondary injury resulting from surgical manipulation or changes in spinal cord perfusion.[127,128]

In the case of a patient who is agitated, intoxicated, uncooperative, and/or hemodynamically unstable, any attempt to sedate and topicalize the airway may be ineffective and lead to airway obstruction, hypoxia, hypotension, or aspiration of gastric contents. These patients are best managed by a rapid sequence induction with direct or videolaryngoscopy using properly applied cricoid pressure and MILS of

the cervical spine as discussed earlier.[129] Some evidence indicates that video-assisted laryngoscopy may cause less distraction of the cervical spine and may offer better visualization of vocal cords than traditional laryngoscopy.[130]

There is controversy surrounding the issues of MILS, application of cricoid pressure, and the use of bag-valve-mask ventilation prior to intubation attempts during a traditional RSI in a patient with a potential cervical SCI. A Cochrane review examined the effect of applying cricoid pressure during an RSI and concluded that it may not be necessary to safely secure the airway, it may not prevent aspiration of gastric contents, and it may interfere with the clinician's view of the patient's airway.[131] It is currently recommended that if cricoid pressure is used and it interferes with the clinician's ability to provide adequate ventilation, identify airway structures, or pass ETT, then the cricoid pressure should be lessened or removed.[132]

The general consensus for MILS is that despite the fact that it may lead to a less than optimal view, it is still recommended under ATLS guidelines and current best practice recommendations to minimize the risk of secondary cervical SCI.[11,130,132] Although not an extensively studied topic, the use of a modified RSI technique that utilizes effective bag-valve-mask ventilation should be considered in appropriate patients to maximize the degree of oxygenation and to confirm that mask ventilation is indeed possible.[133] In addition, avoiding hypoxia is particularly important in patients who suffer from an acute TBI or SCI to minimize secondary injury.[104] Patients with high thoracic and cervical spine injuries should ideally have their blood pressure monitored with an intraarterial catheter that is placed prior to induction of general anesthesia to permit immediate response to changes in hemodynamic status.[134]

Opioids (i.e., fentanyl, sufentanil, remifentanil) and inhaled volatile anesthetic agents are commonly used during the intraoperative phase of repair. However, if spinal monitoring is being performed, volatile agents may need to be reduced or avoided. In such cases a propofol infusion can provide adequate anesthesia if the patient's cardiovascular status is stable. Neuromuscular blockade is generally used to secure the airway and then may be allowed to wear off if motor-evoked potentials are used. Succinylcholine can be used for rapid paralysis during RSI within the first 24 hours following an acute SCI. It may increase serum potassium levels by approximately 0.5 mEq/L in normal patients who have no contraindications to the drug such as a history of malignant hyperthermia or who have experienced a burn, stroke, or major crush injury 48 to 72 hours previously.[105]

Succinylcholine has been associated with life-threatening hyperkalemia when given to a patient with a SCI 48 hours postinjury. Research involving 131 patients who were intubated using succinylcholine noted that an additional risk of hyperkalemia was directly correlated with an increasing length of stay in an intensive care unit. The development of hyperkalemia at or above 6.5 mm/dL was highly significant after the 16th day in the intensive care unit. The investigators concluded that such levels were most likely related to decreased mobility and prolonged immobilization.[135]

Hemodynamic management of patients with an SCI is typically associated with sympathetic denervation and hypovolemia caused by concomitant injuries or a combination of the SCI and a secondary injury. The American Association of Neurological Surgeons guidelines for blood pressure controls include maintenance of a MAP range from 85 to 90 mm Hg for 5 to 7 days postinjury to optimize spinal cord perfusion.[136] To maintain this blood pressure, it may be necessary to administer IV fluids, blood products, vasopressors, and inotropes. A recent systematic review conducted by Saadeh et al. concluded that norepinephrine should be the initial vasopressor of choice for cervical and upper thoracic spinal cord injuries, and either phenylephrine or norepinephrine should be considered for mid- to lower thoracic injuries.[137]

Nitrous oxide is usually avoided in newly admitted trauma patients particularly if there is a chance the patient has a head injury, lung insult, or bowel obstruction. Nitrous oxide may increase the volume and pressure in any gas-filled spaces, leading to an increase in the size of a pneumothorax and/or pneumocephalus. Following injury to the chest wall, use of nitrous oxide with positive pressure can cause rapid expansion of a subclinical pneumothorax into a rapidly increasing and life-threatening pneumothorax with mediastinal shift.[138]

Induction agents most commonly used in the trauma setting for patients with SCI are etomidate, ketamine, and propofol. These have been discussed earlier under RSI and for TBI. Selection of the most appropriate agent is dependent on the hemodynamic stability of the trauma patient.

Autonomic Dysreflexia

Level 1 trauma centers are best equipped to manage neurologically injured patients during the initial hospitalization as well as for future related surgeries.[139] Patients who have sustained high thoracic and cervical SCI may require additional surgeries and can arrive in the operating room with several possible associated complications such as neurogenic shock, bradyarrhythmias, abnormal temperature regulation below the level of the lesion, and autonomic dysreflexia.[140] During the acute phase of a high-level SCI, patients often develop neurogenic shock. This is characterized by profound hypotension that requires inotropic support. From several weeks to 6 months post-SCI, up to 98% of these high paraplegics or quadriplegic patients will experience autonomic dysreflexia following a painful injury below the level of the spinal cord lesion. Autonomic dysreflexia is a potentially fatal clinical condition, is found in patients who suffer a SCI above T6, and is characterized by a sudden activation of sympathetic response as a result of a noxious stimuli. It could be triggered as a result of surgery or from colorectal or bladder distention. It often presents with severe hypertension and other life-threatening consequences, including seizures, pulmonary edema, myocardial infarction, acute renal injury, and intracranial hemorrhage.[141]

Management of an acute autonomic dysreflexia attack includes determining and correcting the noxious stimuli. Because bladder distention and fecal impaction are the most common triggers, bladder catheterization, exclusion of a urinary tract infection, and rectal disimpaction should be performed. The next step may involve positioning the patient in an upright position to produce an orthostatic reduction in blood pressure. If these measures fail to drop the SBP below 150 mm Hg, then pharmacologic intervention is required. Typical medications to reduce dangerous levels of blood pressure include nitrates, nifedipine, hydralazine, and labetalol.[140-142]

Orthopedic Injury and Trauma Anesthesia

Trauma to the extremities represents one of the most frequent injuries seen in emergency and orthosurgical practice. Civilian extremity injuries occur most often as a consequence of falls (43%) and MVCs (26%). In 2015, 345,558 lower extremity injuries and 272,845 upper extremity injuries were entered into the National Trauma Data Bank.[143] Despite the fact that many orthopedic injuries are not usually immediately life threatening and are considered during the secondary evaluation of the trauma patient, they can be associated with significant hemorrhage and other vascular problems such as fat emboli and thromboembolic hypoxic respiratory failure.[144]

During the primary survey, it is vital for the provider to recognize and control hemorrhage from all musculoskeletal injuries. Hemorrhage control is typically best accomplished with application of direct pressure followed by application and deployment of a tourniquet if pressure dressings are not effective.

It is also important to remember that bleeding from closed long-bone fractures can be extensive with significant loss of blood into the thigh.[11] Pelvic fractures can range from stable and benign to life threatening in terms of blood loss. A recent analysis by Huang et al. of 68 patients treated for severe pelvic fracture between 2006 and 2015 reported that the patients received blood transfusion volumes of 1200 to 10,000 mL with an average volume 2850 mL.[145] It is noteworthy that pelvic fractures are most often caused by high-energy mechanisms of injury and can frequently be associated with other severe injures (e.g., intraabdominal injuries, thoracic injuries, head injuries). Therefore providers should maintain a high index of suspicion for other potentially life-threatening injuries throughout the evaluation, diagnosis, and treatment phase of the trauma patient. If a significant pelvic injury is suspected and the patient is hemodynamically unstable, the pelvis can be "wrapped" with a simple bed sheet or a commercial pelvic binder. These expedient measures can create a tamponade effect to reduce hemorrhage from the fracture sites, stabilize the fractures, and improve patient level of comfort.[146,147]

Early fracture fixation with intramedullary nails often allows patients to ambulate within 24 hours of surgery and drastically reduces the incidence of pulmonary complications, including ARDS, fat emboli, and pneumonia.[144] In some instances, secondary neurovascular injury may occur in specific patterns because sharp edges of damaged bone may be forced into blood vessels and peripheral nerves at the fracture site. Furthermore, all providers should have a high index of suspicion for compartmental syndrome when high-energy trauma is responsible for the fractures.[144,145]

Despite some controversy regarding the optimal management of open fractures, recent evidence supports the initial debridement within 24 hours of injury with an appropriate surgical team. If there is significant vascular injury that compromises perfusion of the extremity, this should be addressed within 4 hours of loss of adequate perfusion to the limb.[146] Therefore timely communication between orthopedic surgery and vascular surgery is necessary to optimize patient outcomes. It is important to note that all patients taken to the operating room for emergency surgical repair are considered to have a full stomach. Consequently, steps should be taken to reduce the risk of aspiration and maintain adequate end-organ perfusion if general anesthesia is to be administered.[147]

Massive hemorrhage may be associated with pelvic fractures. Mortality rates can be as high as 70% with an open pelvic fracture.[148] Massive hemorrhage may be attributable to displaced pelvic bone fragments, which may cut arteries, veins, and nerves that exit the pelvis to the perineum and the lower extremities. Damage control resuscitative efforts and damage control surgical measures are critical to improve the outcome in such cases. Immediate care should include application of a pelvic binder as soon as possible following injury to help tamponade internal hemorrhage. External fixation, angiographic embolization, and application of pelvic packing have been used with some success as elements of DCS.[148,149] Primary intervention in these situations includes replacing blood loss using previously discussed principles of damage control resuscitation and maintaining adequate hemodynamic status. The use of REBOA as an early hemorrhage control strategy has been documented with increasing frequency as a potential lifesaving strategy to help improve survival of patients with serious traumatic abdominopelvic hemorrhage.[150]

Currently the primary endpoints to help ensure oxygenation and end-organ perfusion are relative normalization of serum lactate, base deficit, pH, early correction of clotting functions, and hemorrhage control.[151,152] Early identification and correction of coagulopathy in patients with significant bleeding is vital to optimize blood and blood product replacement therapies, to help guide fluid resuscitation and to prevent other consequences of significant hemorrhage. TEG analyzes real-time coagulation and helps determine which blood products are needed during the resuscitation.[153] TEG may prove useful by providing goal-directed targeted therapy to correct the coagulopathy of trauma since it allows management decisions to be individualized to the patient in a timely manner.[24]

Hypoxic respiratory failure in the orthopedic trauma setting is most commonly seen with pelvic and long bone fractures. Patients with one long bone fracture have approximately a 3% chance of developing fat emboli syndrome (FES). A patient with bilateral long bone fractures of the femur has a 33% chance of experiencing FES.[154] The hypoxia is attributable to seeding of fat cells from the disrupted bone marrow into the venous circulation. It is thought that these fat cells produce potent proinflammatory and prothrombotic reactions that can lead to rapid platelet aggregation and accelerated fibrin generation as they travel through the venous system to eventually lodge within the pulmonary arterial circulation. The resultant pulmonary capillary obstruction leads to diffuse interstitial edema, alveolar collapse, and subsequent reactive hypoxic pulmonary vasoconstriction. Massive fat emboli can produce macrovascular obstruction and profound shock.[154]

FES is typically seen 24 to 72 hours after the initial injury. Affected patients develop hypoxemia, neurologic impairment, and a classic petechial rash. Supportive care is the primary treatment for clinically evident FES, which may include endotracheal intubation and mechanical ventilation. There is some evidence that patients at high risk for the development of FES may benefit from low-dose methylprednisolone (1.5 mg/kg IV) every 8 hours for 6 doses.[154] It is likely that patients who experience long bone fractures will be taken to the operating room as soon as possible for surgical correction and stabilization of any long bone or pelvic fractures. This is thought to reduce the risk of FES in addition to other pulmonary complications such as pneumonia, pulmonary embolism, and ARDS.[155]

Continuum of Care

A dynamic and comprehensive trauma system is comprised of multiple integrated and coordinated components, with the goal of providing cost-effective services for injury prevention and optimal patient care. At the center of such a care system is what has been termed the continuum of care, which considers injury prevention, prehospital care, and posthospital rehabilitation care.[156] A recent analysis of 1,949,375 trauma-related deaths that occurred in the United States from 1999 to 2016 estimated that approximately 130,000 prehospital deaths could have been prevented over the 17-year period had the patients had more timely access to a designated trauma center.[157] The ACS Committee on Trauma has reported that application of a regionalized best practice approach, coupled with application of robust and rigorous disease management guidelines across the continuum of care improves patient outcomes.[158] This committee works on development and implementation of educational programs and legislation at the local and federal levels aimed at reducing the occurrence of preventable trauma-related deaths. Examples of these activities include laws and educational programs directed at eliminating distracted driver behaviors, intentional interpersonal violence, mandating use of seatbelts and motorcycle helmets, and implementation of the Stop the Bleed initiative.[159]

Realizing that military and civilian trauma systems have much to offer each other in terms of injury prevention, prehospital care, acute trauma care, and rehabilitation lessons learned, the US military has recently proposed a model for a national trauma care system.[163] Both military and civilian trauma leaders recognize that continued progress in trauma care requires lines of communication and collaboration along with a seamless exchange of knowledge between civilian and military sectors. The hope is that this partnership will provide improved outcomes for military and civilian victims of traumatic injury. The

far-reaching goal that this collaborative national trauma care system seeks to achieve is zero preventable deaths after injury and minimal trauma-related disability.[160]

Crisis management checklists are another tool to assist in the anesthesia care of the unpredictable and rapidly changing critically injured patient. Trauma-specific checklists review management protocols of patients prior to arrival, on arrival, intraoperatively, and postoperatively.[161] A recent systematic review concluded that application of a checklist during care of newly admitted trauma patients can improve adherence to ATLS guidelines and may result in improved survival rates of the most severely injured patients.[162]

Newer approaches to the continuum of care have recognized that pain management is often inadequately addressed. Consequently, contemporary research has placed greater emphasis on the utilization of regional anesthetics to reduce pain and diminish potential postoperative complications that may be associated with general anesthesia and systemic opioid use. Additionally, some experts are more strenuously advocating early use of regional anesthesia to increase a patient's self-care activities, such as coughing/deep breathing and earlier ambulation. More specifically, evidence supports the use of regional anesthesia for patients who have suffered rib, femur, and hip fractures and patients undergoing digital reimplantation in addition to free flaps.[163]

An area of increasing concern in health care is that of the global coronavirus pandemic. In late 2020, the total number of US-reported cases of Covid-19 was over 8 million, with a total death rate of over 233,000.[164] Throughout this recent pandemic, centers responsible for the care of trauma patients must remain open and ready to care for acutely injured patients who require immediate potentially lifesaving interventions and advanced critical care management to facilitate recovery. Recently, the ACS Committee on Trauma drafted a set of guidelines to advise trauma center medical directors on how to provide necessary patient care while maintaining optimal provider safety with regard to spread of Covid-19.[165]

Key elements of the ACS Committee on Trauma guidance plan include the following:

- Regional planning to engage coalitions with local and regional health departments for effective and timely triage of patients
- Hospital planning to optimize intensive care unit surge capability and capacity to care for anticipated increases in hospital admissions
- Policies and procedures to protect and support the trauma team in terms of personal protective equipment training and availability of necessary supplies
- Strategies to optimize point-of-care testing for Covid-19
- Strict enforcement of personal protective equipment (PPE) use as well as policies and procedures for airway management for potential Covid patients
- Operating room and intensive care unit policies to minimize the likelihood of Covid spread
- Development of strategies to manage scarce resources such as appropriated PPE, blood products, and availability of essential patient care providers

Finally, research concerning trauma anesthesia continues to grow exponentially, even outside the operating theater. For example, the R. Adams Cowley Shock Trauma Center in Baltimore, Maryland has implemented a Go-Team, which is deployed in circumstances where a trauma victim is unable to be extricated during a MVC, industrial accident, trench collapse, building collapse, or other situation. The Go-Team consists of a surgeon and a Certified Registered Nurse Anesthetist who are capable of advanced prehospital resuscitation and may implement such measures as fluid resuscitation, large-bore IV access, administration of blood products, IV anesthetics, and surgical procedures to facilitate extrication.[166]

SUMMARY

Despite development, innovation, and changes to public policy, traumatic injury continues to pervade modern society. Consequently, a comprehensive understanding of trauma care is important for modern anesthesia practice. Trauma management has moved away from the community-based care and has developed into a systems-based approach, coordinating prehospital care with larger centers, public policy, and a rational approach through the use of ATLS guidelines. The organization of trauma care in the United States has substantially improved survival and outcomes for severely injured patients.

Ideally, the anesthetist's involvement should begin as soon as the patient reaches the trauma facility. Care should follow the general ATLS algorithm. Anesthesia providers and the trauma team should focus on ensuring an adequate airway and breathing, while simultaneously diagnosing and controlling injuries. The principles of successful management of the trauma patient are based on organization and preparation, assessment of the patient's injuries, proper prioritization of therapeutic interventions, achievement and maintenance of a patent airway, fluid and blood resuscitation, damage control interventions when indicated, application of appropriate continuous invasive and noninvasive monitoring, correction of acid-base and electrolyte disturbances, correction of coagulopathy, and careful titration of anesthetic and adjunctive agents.

Trauma anesthesia can be a challenging specialty because patients often arrive with an unknown history and the inability to communicate comorbidities, allergies, drug/medication use, and myriad other pieces of information. Many such patients require immediate surgical intervention. Damage control resuscitation and DCS are primary interventions in the severely injured trauma patient. Frequently, these patients require multiple surgical procedures until definitive surgical correction is implemented. Consequently, anesthestic interventions are based on the patient's hemodynamic stability at any given point in time.

Current practice supports the use of fluids and blood products to restore adequate tissue level perfusion in hemorrhagic shock. The use of select vasopressors appears indicated when blood pressure cannot be maintained by fluids and blood products alone.[167]

The adequacy of end-organ tissue perfusion should be monitored throughout the initial intraoperative resuscitation phase by tracking arterial pH, base deficit, and lactate. It is also essential to consider the effect of citrate toxicity, frequently seen with administration of blood and blood products. Ionized calcium levels should thus be monitored and corrected when indicated.

Low doses of an inhaled anesthetic agent such as isoflurane are permissible to minimize the potential for recall and awareness in the early stages of intraoperative resuscitation, unless the SBP cannot be maintained at greater than 90 mm Hg. Intravenous fentanyl can also be administered for analgesia as long as the SBP is maintained above 90 mm Hg. Rapid sequence induction and intubation with MILS of the cervical spine is the recommended technique for securing the airway in the trauma patient. Adequate preoxygenation and even apneic oxygenation should be provided prior to RSI. Evidence supports the application of an intraoperative lung-protective strategy during mechanical ventilation with tidal volumes of 6 to 8 mL/kg. The use of nitrous oxide in the early stages of a trauma resuscitation should be avoided because it can expand any potential gas spaces and worsen pneumothoraces, small bowel obstructions, and pneumocephalus. Regional anesthetics in the form of peripheral nerve blocks as well as other nonopioid multimodal therapies offer advantages to help control pain without producing significant systemic hypotension, and their use is gaining popularity in the trauma anesthesia community.[163]

The degree of functional outcome of trauma patients is largely dependent on the early involvement of sound principles of anesthesia care in the resuscitation and overall anesthetic management during the perioperative period. In a well-managed team approach, assessment and treatment are carried out in rapid succession or even simultaneously. It is incumbent that those providing care to trauma patients regularly review emerging evidence to ensure the highest possible quality of care.

REFERENCES

For a complete list of references for this chapter, scan this QR code with any smartphone code reader app, or visit the following URL: http://booksite.elsevier.com/9780323711944/

Anesthesia for Transplant Surgery and Organ Procurement

Michael J. Anderson

HISTORY OF ORGAN TRANSPLANTATION

The number and types of organ transplants continue to increase to meet the demand in patients who are in need. This need is balanced by the supply of organs available and the severity of the patient's condition warranting transplant. Patients awaiting organ transplantation have sustained organ dysfunction and have exhausted other medical treatments and therapies. Organ transplantation can significantly improve and extend the quality of life.

The concept of organ transplantation has been in existence since the early 1900s and has evolved into a highly specialized and complex phenomenon. This is due to significant developments in medicine, surgery, anesthesia, pharmacology, and other entities. Alexis Carrel is recognized as a pioneer in the development of the concept of vascular anastomoses. It was this work that earned him the Nobel Prize for Medicine in 1912. His unique method of using fine needle and thread and experimentation on animals along with his publication, *The Transplantation of Veins and Organs*, granted him the title "father of transplant vascular surgery."[1] Many of the techniques developed by Carrel are still used today.

One of the major hurdles involved in organ transplantation was rejection by the recipient's immune system versus donor tissue. This led to catastrophic results. Ultimately the work of Peter Medawar, an immunologist who developed the theory of graft rejection as a result of an immunologic incompatibility, led to the idea of organ rejection and helped pioneer the use of immunosuppression medications to help prevent this from occurring.[2] This work led to Medawar receiving the Nobel Prize for Medicine and paved the way for further developments related to immunosuppressive therapies. Early on, either corticosteroids or whole-body radiation was used. In 1974 another major development occurred. Cyclosporine was introduced by Borel et al. and is still used today to prevent graft versus host rejection.[3]

These developments have paved the way for an evolution of care called organ transplantation. Today we have the technology and capability of transplanting kidney, liver, pancreas, heart, lungs, cornea, and stem cells. In this chapter, we discuss the types of organ donation, the anesthetic implications of organ transplantation, and anesthetic care for the organ donor.

Types of Organ Donation

Traditionally, organ donation has occurred once the donor is declared dead due to an absence of viable brain activity. This can be due to a variety of insults, and specific criteria have been developed to assess and determine if the patient meets the criteria for potential organ donation. This is termed organ donation after brain death (DBD). Brain death occurs when the brain is deemed irreversibly nonfunctional due to lack of blood supply and oxygen, which causes brain cells to die. This method remains the most common method of donation employed today. Another method has been introduced and is becoming more prevalent. This method is donation after cardiac death (DCD) and occurs when a patient meets specific criteria defined for DCD. Although this movement toward DCD was implemented due to a shortage of organs for transplantation, ethical considerations remain challenging and are a barrier to widespread acceptance.[4]

A third type of organ donation is living donor transplants. This occurs when a living person donates an organ to another person for transplantation. Living donors may be a family member, friend, or even strangers. Thousands of transplants each year are performed with organs from a living donor. In 2019 there were 7397 living donor transplants in the United States. This was a record for living donor transplants.[5,6]

Organ Transplantation Considerations

With the improvement of technology and medical advances, organ donation is considered an accepted medical treatment for patients with end-stage organ failure of various types. It is estimated that approximately 80 people receive organ transplants on a daily basis, but 20 people die each day while waiting for a organ transplant. The number of transplants and donors has steadily increased over the last 2 decades; however, the number of patients on the waiting list has grown at a staggering rate. In 2019 a record 39,718 transplants were performed in the United States, but that is in contrast to the more than 112,500 patients who remain on a national organ transplant waiting list.[5] The national organ transplant list is maintained by the United Network for Organ Sharing (UNOS), and strict standards are upheld for fair and ethical distribution of organs. Criteria considered include blood and tissue matching, organ size, medical urgency, wait time, and geographic location of the donor and recipient.[6] There are currently more than 120 million people in the United States alone who are identified as organ donors. One donor can save as many as eight lives through organ donation. Many of them will never have the chance to donate based on the original criteria for DBD. It is estimated that only 3 of 1000 people will die in a way that allows for organ donation. This has been the genesis for consideration and development of guidelines for DCD as well as living donor donation. Fig. 41.1 shows the number of people on the transplant waiting list compared to the number of transplants and the number of donors and how those numbers have increased over the years.[6]

RENAL TRANSPLANTATION

End-stage renal disease (ESRD) has a tremendous impact on our society in terms of cost and resource allocation. Patients often have many other comorbidities and ultimately may require hemodialysis as a lifesaving treatment regimen. The first kidney transplant was performed in 1954 when a living donor gave a kidney to his identical twin. Since then, renal transplantation has gained significant momentum with the development of immunosuppression in the 1960s.[7] The kidney is the most frequent solid organ transplanted today. Renal transplantation

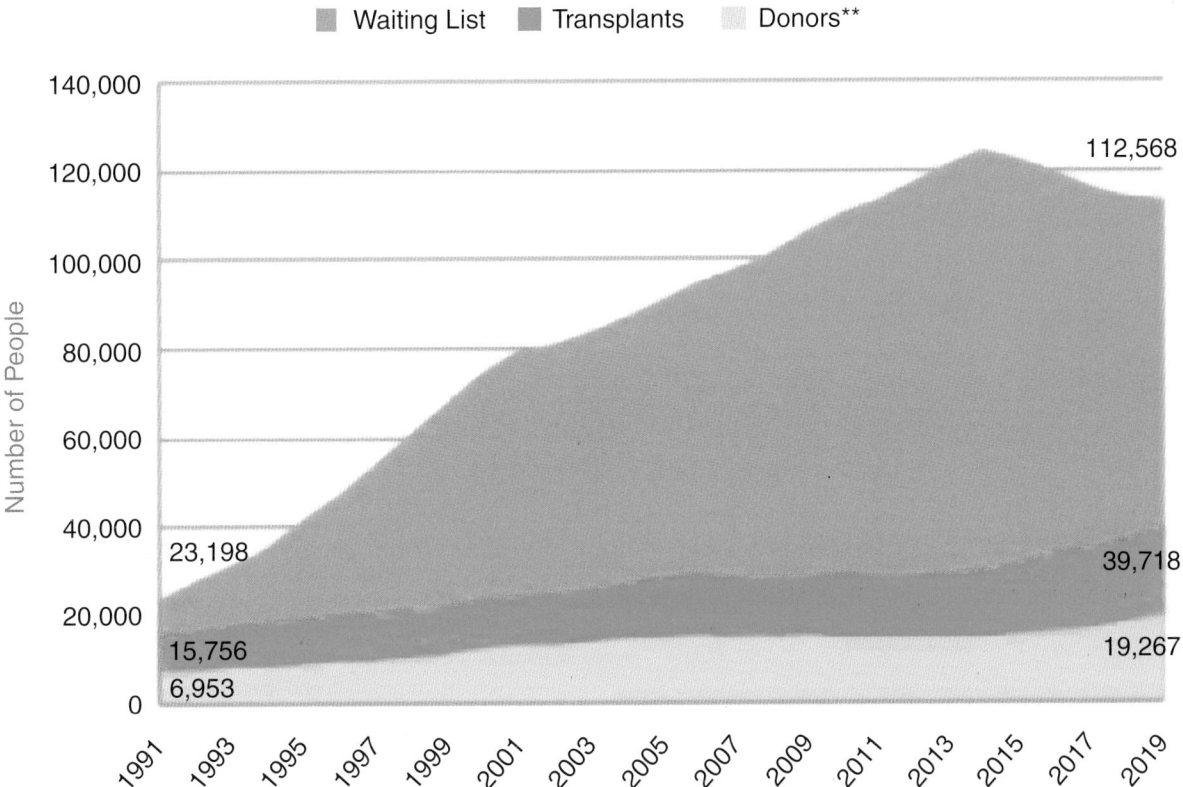

Fig. 41.1 Annual transplant data. (From Organ Procurement and Transplantation Network. https://optn.transplant.hrsa.gov. Accessed 2020.)

provides an improved quality of life and a longer survival rate than dialysis. Five-year posttransplantation survival rates are 91% for recipients of live donor grafts, 83% for standard non-ECD (extended criteria donor) deceased donor recipients, and 70% for recipients of grafts from ECDs.[8] After a steady increase in the incidence of ESRD from 1980 to 2001, the incidence rate has plateaued. The incidence is on the rise, however, in patients over the age of 65. Many factors have contributed to this increase, including diabetes and hypertension.[9]

Pathophysiology of End-Stage Renal Disease and Indications for Transplant

Kidney transplantation is a process by which a donated kidney is surgically attached and ultimately replaces the limited to nonfunctioning kidney. Kidney transplantation becomes necessary due to a variety of factors. It is commonly related to dysfunction and/or destruction of the kidney from glomerulonephritis, chronic interstitial nephritis, or congenital or hereditary disorders such as cystic disease. Kidney dysfunction related to hypertension and diabetes are now the most common indications for kidney transplantation in the United States.[8] ESRD is defined as a decline in kidney function to less than 10% of normal capacity. This decline in function is measured in glomerular filtration rate (GFR).[10] A GFR of less than 15% of normal capacity requires the patient to undergo chronic renal replacement therapy in the form of dialysis to adequately maintain fluid volumes, provide elimination of nitrogenous waste products, and maintain both plasma pH levels and production of erythropoietin.

ESRD has a significant impact on other organ systems, including the cardiac, cerebral, and peripheral vascular systems, as well as the gastrointestinal, hematologic, and central nervous systems. Careful preoperative assessment is crucial in patients with ESRD who are to undergo a surgical procedure requiring anesthesia, especially renal

TABLE 41.1 Classification and Staging of Chronic Kidney Disease (CKD) by the National Kidney Foundation*

Stage	Description	GFR (mL/min/1.73 m²)
1	Kidney damage with normal or ↑ GFR	≥90
2	Kidney damage with mild ↓ GFR	60–89
3	Moderate ↓ GFR	30–59
4	Severe ↓ GFR	15–29
5	Kidney failure	<15 or dialysis

*This widely adopted classification required evidence of kidney damage (such as increased proteinuria) above a glomerular filtration rate (GFR) level of 60 mL/min/1.73 m² for the diagnosis of CKD but not below this threshold. Chronic kidney disease is defined as either kidney damage or GFR <60 mL/min/1.73 m² for ≥3 months. Kidney damage is defined as pathologic abnormalities or markers of damage, including abnormalities in blood or urine test results, or imaging studies.
From Grams ME, et al. Epidemiology of kidney disease. In Yu ASL, et al., eds. *Brenner and Rector's The Kidney*. 11th ed. Philadelphia: Elsevier; 2020:616.

transplantation. Table 41.1 lists the classifications and stages of chronic kidney disease. Some recipient factors that may lead to rejection are listed in Box 41.1.

Preoperative Considerations for Renal Transplantation

Thorough preoperative evaluation is crucial in patients awaiting renal transplantation. Prior to transplantation, the patient will undergo a thorough, multidisciplinary evaluation to determine their eligibility for organ transplantation. The average time a patient is on the waiting list for a kidney is greater than 3 years; therefore careful medical management of their comorbidities, including hemodialysis, is crucial to their overall survival and bridge to transplantation.[11] Cardiovascular disease is a major factor in patients with ESRD. It can be manifested by ischemic heart disease (which may be silent, especially in diabetic patients), as well as congestive heart failure, untreated hypertension and chronic anemia. Congestive heart failure is most often caused by ischemic heart disease and is prevalent in approximately one-fourth of cases of chronic kidney disease.[12] Other significant sequelae include hyperlipidemia, peripheral vascular disease, hyperphosphatemia, and hyperkalemia. Preoperative optimization should focus on medical management of heart failure, as well as fluid and electrolyte abnormalities. Assessment of the patient's exercise tolerance and metabolic equivalent is also important. A baseline electrocardiogram (ECG) is an appropriate screening test for a patient who is scheduled to undergo kidney transplantation. Echocardiography may also be helpful to delineate specific cardiovascular abnormalities and assess the patient's ejection fraction and underlying heart rhythm. Ejection fraction is often affected due to heart failure and may improve after transplantation. A detailed cardiac exam should include the potential for coronary angiography and stress echocardiography, especially in those patients with a history of reversible ischemia and those patients who are deemed to be at high risk.[11]

Chronic anemia is a common occurrence in end-stage renal patients who are awaiting transplant. This is related to decreased erythropoietin production and hemolysis. The heart increases cardiac output to compensate for the anemia, which decreases oxygen-carrying capacity and can cause ischemia.[13] It is not uncommon for end-stage renal patients to have hemoglobin levels in the range of 5 to 8 g/dL. Administration of erythropoietin has the potential to increase the patient's hemoglobin levels over a period. Depending on the surgery and condition of the patient, blood transfusion with packed red blood cells (RBCs) may be warranted. Coagulopathies are also prevalent in this patient population due to a decrease in platelet adhesion. Treatment with desmopressin (DDAVP) or cryoprecipitate may be beneficial.

Electrolyte abnormalities are very common in patients with renal insufficiency and can lead to many untoward effects. These abnormalities can be of significant concern during transplant surgery. Hyperphosphatemia is common and is associated with hypocalcemia. This is caused by decreased calcium absorption due to the inability to activate vitamin D and can put the patient at risk for pathologic fractures. Care should be taken when positioning the patient for intubation and surgery. Hyperkalemia is the most hazardous electrolyte complication. Elevated potassium levels are common in end-stage renal patients, and dialysis is often needed to maintain the potassium levels in a safe range for the patient. Potassium levels of 5 to 5.5 mEq/L are generally considered acceptable in this patient population. Assessment of the patient's preoperative labs and review of their medication regimen and dialysis schedule is very important in the preoperative phase. Dialysis in the immediate preoperative phase may be beneficial prior to transplantation to ensure electrolyte levels are within the patient's homeostatic range; however, this may lead to decreased intravascular volume as well as other volume-related concerns intraoperatively. Patients undergoing kidney transplant surgery often have significant comorbidities. These factors should be identified during the preoperative evaluation not only for risk stratification but also for patient optimization and postoperative care (Table 41.2).

BOX 41.1   Recipient Risk Factors That May Lead to Acute Rejection

Previous blood transfusions, particularly if recent
Previous pregnancies, particularly if multiple
Previous allograft, particularly if rejected early
African ethnicity
cPRA >20%
Donor-specific antibody (current or historic)

cPRA, Calculated panel reactive antibody.
Adapted from Yu ASL, et al., eds. *Brenner and Rector's The Kidney.* 11th ed. Philadelphia: Elsevier; 2020:2254.

TABLE 41.2   Different Pathophysiologic Features of Transplant Recipients

Pathophysiologic Features		Preoperative Considerations	Intraoperative Considerations
Cardiovascular alterations	Hypertension Coronary artery disease Ventricular dysfunction Pulmonary hypertension Peripheral vascular status Decreased CSI	Repeated assessment Echocardiography	Use of intraoperative monitors Goal-directed therapy
Airway and lung considerations	↓ Lung volume ↓ Lung diffusion capacity Difficult airway	Prehabilitation	
Fluid and electrolyte disturbances	Fluid status Potassium overload Requirement of HD	Previous dialysis not mandatory	Nephroprotective strategies Goal-directed therapy
Blood and coagulation disturbances	Uremic thrombocytopenia HD-related heparin treatment Multifactorial anemia		Avoid epidural techniques Hb trigger: 7 g/dL 8 g/dL if previous cardiovascular disease

CSI, Cardiac stroke index; *HD,* hemodialysis; *Hb,* hemoglobin.
Adapted from Tena B, Vendrell M. Perioperative considerations for kidney and pancreas-kidney transplantation. *Best Pract Res Clin Anaesthesiol.* 2020;34(1):3–14.

Intraoperative Considerations for Renal Transplantation

Although there is an extensive assessment in the preoperative phase, once the patient is on the transplant list and a match is confirmed via the donor match system, the process speeds up extensively. Cadaveric donation is one method of organ donation in which the organ is procured from the donor via the DBD or DCD method described previously. Once the organ is procured, there is an urgency to implant the kidney as soon as possible. The cadaveric organ can only sustain viability with cold ischemia for a short period.

Another type of organ donation is where a living donor provides an organ to a matched recipient. This occurs more frequently with a family member or friend who is determined to be a match and offers to provide an organ, such as a kidney, to a recipient in need. In this setting, the donor will undergo general anesthesia, and the organ will be procured by the transplant team. Once this process is underway, the potential recipient will undergo general anesthesia in an adjacent room. The transplanted organ is generally placed in the right or left extraperitoneal fossa. The right side is generally most preferred.[7] The transplanted kidney is attached to the recipient's vasculature via vascular anastomoses of the external iliac artery and vein, and the ureter is anastomosed directly to the bladder[11] (Fig. 41.2).

General anesthesia with endotracheal intubation is the most common anesthetic method for kidney transplant surgery. The goals for anesthetic management include providing an appropriate depth of anesthesia and muscle relaxation to optimize the surgical conditions for the surgeon while maintaining hemodynamic stability. Patients with ESRD are at risk for aspiration due to gastroparesis, and care should be taken during induction to intubate the patient safely and effectively. Succinylcholine may be administered in this patient population, but care must be taken to ensure that potassium levels are within normal limits. Rocuronium may also be utilized for a rapid sequence induction (RSI) if hyperkalemia is a concern. Rocuronium is primarily excreted by the biliary system, and secondary metabolism is through the renal system. It should be noted that along with delayed plasma clearance of rocuronium, there is also a delayed plasma clearance of sugammadex in patients with severe renal impairment. In patients with severe renal impairment, sugammadex is under investigation but not yet recommended. Sources of concern include the possible instability of the rocuronium-sugammadex binding, different clearance times for these drugs, and difficult dosing for deep neuromuscular block (NMB).[14] Cisatracurium is an intermediate-acting muscle relaxant that is metabolized through Hofmann elimination. It produces the metabolite

laudanosine, which is partially eliminated through the kidneys. The duration of action may be slightly prolonged in renal patients; however, it is generally considered the muscle relaxant of choice in patients with ESRD.[15] Careful monitoring of neuromuscular blockade is important to ensure both an appropriate level and that the patient is adequately reversed at the end of the case.

Standard, noninvasive intraoperative monitoring may be adequate for young, healthier transplant recipients. Arterial blood pressure monitoring may be useful in patients with known coronary artery disease (CAD) and uncontrolled hypertension. Central venous pressure (CVP) monitoring is also beneficial in situations where assessment of CVP is indicated. Many transplant recipients require a central line because of the administration of immunosuppressive and vasoactive medications. In some circumstances, pulmonary artery catheter (PAC) and/or transesophageal echocardiography (TEE) may be useful in situations where heart failure and pulmonary hypertension are present. Large-bore peripheral intravenous (IV) lines are necessary to ensure the ability to administer adequate volume replacement, including blood transfusion(s) when necessary. This can prove difficult in this patient population due to the presence of one or more arteriovenous fistulas and the potential for venous thrombosis.

Induction of anesthesia can be carried out safely and effectively in this patient population with propofol. The pharmacokinetics and pharmacodynamics of propofol are unchanged in end-stage renal patients, and it is primarily metabolized in the liver.[13]

Maintenance of anesthesia is generally a combination of volatile inhalational gas and IV anesthetics. Inhalation anesthetics are titrated to provide an adequate level of anesthesia, and a combination of analgesics and neuromuscular blocking agents can assist with providing an optimal surgical environment. All inhalational anesthetics can be titrated appropriately to provide an optimal surgical environment. They all cause a dose-dependent reduction in renal blood flow and GFR. Desflurane, isoflurane, and sevoflurane are all safe to use in this patient population. Low-flow sevoflurane is a safe and effective agent and causes no nephrotoxic effects in patients with preexisting renal dysfunction.[16] Whether the inhalation agents are renoprotective is under investigation.

Pain management is an important part of transplant surgery. Analgesic medication should be used with caution in the perioperative period in patients with ESRD due to the potential for accumulation of their active metabolites. The effect of morphine is known to be prolonged in end-stage renal patients because of its metabolite, morphine-6-glucuronide. This can have negative untoward effects, therefore careful titration is necessary.[17] Meperidine should also be avoided due to its metabolite, normeperidine. Repeated doses of meperidine, resulting in metabolite accumulation, have been associated with central nervous system excitatory effects, including seizures.[18]

Other intraoperative pharmacologic considerations include the use of IV fluids. Maintenance of intravascular volume is vital to the performance and perfusion of the transplanted kidney. Fluids such as lactated Ringer are generally avoided due to the presence of potassium in that solution. More often, PlasmaLyte and normal saline are used, but care should be taken to avoid the development of a hyperchloremic metabolic acidosis from the administration of too much normal saline. This can ultimately cause worsening hyperkalemia.[13] Judicious use of colloids such as albumin can be helpful in maintaining intravascular fluid volume while avoiding a worsening acidosis related to normal saline. Vasoactive agents and other medications may be used to increase renal blood flow and urine output. Dopamine, dobutamine, and fenoldopam may be used intraoperatively to increase renal blood flow. Osmotic and loop diuretics have also been shown to increase kidney function once reperfusion is complete.[13] Mannitol and Lasix may be administered to

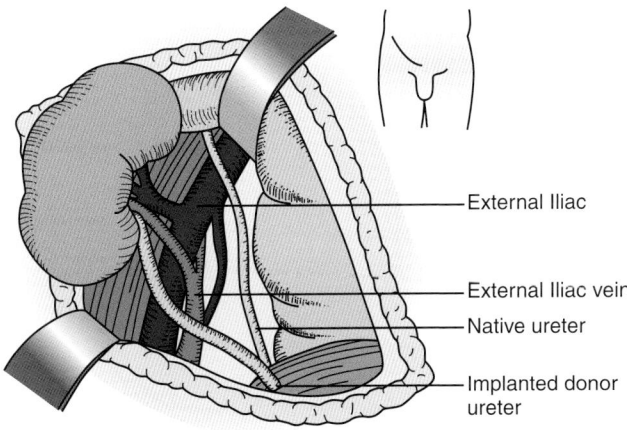

Fig. 41.2 Anatomy of a typical first kidney transplant. (From Yu ASL, et al. *Brenner and Rector's The Kidney*. 11th ed. Philadelphia: Elsevier; 2020:2244.)

- External Iliac
- External Iliac vein
- Native ureter
- Implanted donor ureter

assist with osmotic diuresis and should be on hand if requested. Anesthetic considerations for renal transplantation are noted in Box 41.2.

Immunosuppressive Therapy

Immunosuppressive strategies can also be divided into induction and maintenance therapy. Induction of immunosuppression is defined as the rapid achievement of profound immunosuppression, usually at the time of transplant, with the use of depleting agents. Maintenance immunosuppression is achieved by the combination of oral agents that take advantage of additive or synergistic immunosuppressive effects of different drug categories to minimize their nonimmunosuppressive side effects. Dosage is usually greater during the first 3 months after transplantation and decreases afterward. A combination of calcineurin inhibitor (CNI), antiproliferative agents, and corticosteroids is the most common regimen.

The vast majority of kidney transplant recipients in the United States are maintained on tacrolimus and mycophenolate mofetil (MMF), with approximately two-thirds of patients also treated with maintenance steroids. The greatest source of intraprogram variability in an immunosuppressive regimen is the choice of induction therapy and patient selection for and method of steroid withdrawal. When deciding on a regimen for a given recipient, the following factors are taken into consideration: (1) the patient's immunologic risk, (2) the baseline quality of the allograft, and (3) the anticipated vulnerability profile to specific side effects of immunosuppression. Familiarization with local challenges (e.g., regional distribution of patient risk factors, organ attribution scheme) is essential for successful optimization of immunosuppression protocols for any given patient.[19]

The specifics of the therapy are generally practiced and institutionally driven. Many institutions have protocols that are used to help guide the anesthetist regarding the specific immunotherapy agents for that particular case. There are two major regimens that are used: the more conventional high-dose regimen or the antibody induction regimen. The conventional regimen consists of either cyclosporine or tacrolimus, both of which are CNIs. These agents are used as prophylactic agents to prevent organ rejection. These agents must be administered concurrently with a corticosteroid and an antimetabolite agent such as MMF or azathioprine. The antibody induction regimen uses lower doses of these conventional medications but includes an antibody that is directed at T-cell antigens and antilymphocytic antibodies. These agents include thymoglobulin, alemtuzumab, and OKT3. Other antibody induction agents work on interleukin-2 (IL-2) receptor antagonists such as basiliximab (Simulect) or daclizumab (Zenapax). Studies have shown the antibody induction regimen to have better outcomes in terms of reduced graft rejection.[13] It should be noted that induction of immunosuppression should begin with administration of the corticosteroid and then an antilymphocyte immediately prior to reperfusion of the donated kidney. The common drugs used for immunosuppression and their mechanisms are listed in Table 41.3. Agents that may interact with transplant medications are noted in Table 41.4.

Postoperative Considerations for Renal Transplantation

After completion of the surgery and extubation, the patient will be monitored closely in the immediate postoperative period. Careful monitoring of the patient's hemodynamic parameters to include blood pressure and heart rate along with urine output is very important, and any acute changes in urine output should be evaluated to delineate the etiology and appropriate treatment. Aggressive fluid therapy should be initiated if the decreased urine output is deemed to be related to a prerenal etiology. Because of the reimplantation and surgical anastomosis of the ureter during transplantation, a kink in

---

BOX 41.2   Anesthesia for Renal Transplantation

I. Preoperative Assessment and Preparation
  A. Clinical evaluation
    1. Evaluate status of coexisting diseases
      a. Diabetes mellitus
      b. Hypertension
      c. Cardiac disease
      d. Hyperparathyroidism
      e. Pericardial tamponade
    2. Perform dialysis within 24 hr of transplantation; check weight.
    3. Evaluate tolerance to chronic anemia.
  B. Laboratory evaluation
    1. Complete blood count with platelet count
    2. Prothrombin time, partial thromboplastin time, bleeding time
    3. Blood urea nitrogen, creatinine, calcium, fluid balance
    4. Electrocardiography; chest radiography
  C. Type and crossmatch 2 units of washed, packed red blood cells
  D. Determine current drug regimen
  E. Premedication
    1. Benzodiazepines, narcotics
    2. Antacids, histamine-2 antagonist, metoclopramide
II. Monitors
  A. Electrocardiography
  B. Indirect or direct blood pressure measurement
  C. Precordial, esophageal stethoscope
  D. Neuromuscular blockade evaluation
  E. Foley catheter
  F. Central venous, transesophageal echocardiography, pulmonary capillary wedge pressure measurement, if required
III. Anesthetic Management
  A. Regional techniques
    1. Continuous spinal or epidural
    2. Advantages
      a. No need for muscle relaxants
      b. Potential respiratory tract infection from intubation is avoided
      c. Amount of local anesthetic required is small
      d. Patients awake and comfortable postoperatively
    3. Disadvantages
      a. Patient anxiety
      b. Uncomfortable surgical positions, especially for donor
      c. Coagulation abnormalities present
      d. Fluid management with sympathetic blockade a challenge
      e. Unprotected airway in patients with delayed gastric emptying
  B. General anesthesia
    1. Induction with propofol or etomidate
    2. Maintenance with volatile anesthetic (isoflurane, sevoflurane, or desflurane) or narcotic-based technique
    3. Neuromuscular blockers
      a. Succinylcholine
      b. Cisatracurium
      c. Rocuronium
IV. Miscellaneous Drugs
  A. Mannitol or furosemide
  B. Dopamine
  C. Calcium channel blockers
  D. Prednisone or methylprednisolone
  E. Patient-specific immunosuppressant therapy

TABLE 41.3   Drugs Used for Maintenance Immunosuppression

Drug	Mechanism of Action	Adverse Effects
Corticosteroids	Block synthesis of several cytokines, including IL-2; multiple antiinflammatory effects	Glucose intolerance, hypertension, hyperlipidemia, osteoporosis, osteonecrosis, myopathy, cosmetic defects; growth suppression in children
Cyclosporine	Inhibits calcineurin: synthesis of IL-2 and other molecules critical for T-cell activation thereby inhibited	Nephrotoxicity (acute and chronic), hyperlipidemia, hypertension, glucose intolerance, cosmetic defects
Tacrolimus	Similar to cyclosporine, although binds to different cytoplasmic protein (FKBP)	Broadly similar to cyclosporine; diabetes mellitus more common; hypertension, hyperlipidemia, and cosmetic defects less common
Azathioprine	Inhibits purine biosynthesis; lymphocyte replication therefore inhibited	Bone marrow suppression; rarely pancreatitis, hepatitis
Mycophenolate mofetil (MMF)	Inhibits de novo pathway of purine biosynthesis (relatively lymphocyte selective); lymphocyte replication therefore inhibited	Bone marrow suppression, gastrointestinal upset; invasive. CMV disease more common than with azathioprine
Sirolimus	Sirolimus-FKBP complex inhibits TOR blocking lymphocyte proliferative response	Bone marrow suppression, proteinuria, mouth ulcers, hyperlipidemia, interstitial pneumonitis; edema; enhanced nephrotoxicity of cyclosporine/tacrolimus
Belatacept	Blocks T-cell costimulation	PTLD in EBV seronegative, PML (rare), reactivation of TB

CMV, Cytomegalovirus; *EBV,* Epstein-Barr virus; *FKBP,* FK-binding protein; *IL-2,* interleukin-2; *PTLD,* posttransplant lymphoproliferative disorder; *TB,* tuberculosis; *TOR,* target of rapamycin.
From Yu ASL, et al., eds. *Brenner and Rector's The Kidney.* 11th ed. Philadelphia: Elsevier; 2020:2246.

TABLE 41.4   Agents That May Interact With Transplant Medications

Drugs That Interact With CNIs and Sirolimus		
Class of Drug	Increase Level	Decrease Level
Ca channel blocker	Diltiazem, verapamil	
Antibiotics	Erythromycin, azithromycin, clarithromycin	Nafcillin
Antifungals	Fluconazole, ketoconazole, itraconazole, voriconazole	
Antituberculin		INH, rifampin, rifabutin
Antiviral	Ritonavir, nelfinavir, saquinavir	Efavirenz, nevirapine
Antiseizure		Phenytoin, phenobarbital, carbamazepine, primidone
Antidepressant	Fluoxetine, nefazodone, fluvoxamine	
Foods and Herbal Preparations That Interact With CNIs		
Food	Grapefruit juice/ pomegranate juice	
Herbs		St. John wort

CNIs, calcineurin inhibitors.
From Yu ASL, et al., eds. *Brenner and Rector's The Kidney.* 11th ed. Philadelphia: Elsevier; 2020:2254.

BOX 41.3   Precautions for Procedures and Surgery in Kidney Transplant Recipients

- Caution with radiocontrast exposure.
- Maintain hydration.
- Avoid nephrotoxic antibiotics and analgesic.
- "Stress-dose steroids" not always necessary.
- If enteral route of medication is contraindicated, give CNI via IV route (one-third total oral dose).
- Monitor allograft function, plasma potassium, and acid-base balance daily.
- Consider wound-healing impairment.

CNI, Calcineurin inhibitor; *IV,* intravenous.
From Yu ASL, et al., eds. *Brenner and Rector's The Kidney.* 11th ed. Philadelphia: Elsevier; 2020:2244.

Other postoperative complications include wound infection, wound hematomas, and vascular thrombosis. Cardiac and respiratory complications are also possible, especially in higher risk patients with pre-existing cardiac and respiratory comorbidities. Box 41.3 notes some precautions when performing procedures and surgery in patients who have a kidney transplant.

Postoperative Pain Control

Pain management is highly variable and patient specific. The pain associated with kidney transplantation may be severe and very challenging in the immediate postoperative period. Most often, pain control is achieved by IV opioid analgesics via patient-controlled analgesia (PCA). Multimodal therapy may be beneficial, especially in patients with chronic pain history, and can include an IV ketamine and acetaminophen (Ofirmev) injection, and the addition of a transversus abdominis plane block prior to incision.[7] The use of thoracic epidurals for postoperative pain management is controversial due to the risk of coagulopathies and postoperative hypotension. Use of epidural anesthesia should be considered carefully and used sparingly.

the ureter or other technical problem may be the cause of a post-renal etiology of diminished urine output and may require surgical exploration and treatment. Intensive care unit (ICU) admissions in renal transplant patients are generally quite low. In a 10-year cohort study, Klouche et al. found the ICU admission rate was 6% in a single center where 1015 kidney transplants were performed.[20]

PANCREAS TRANSPLANTATION

Transplantation of the pancreas is a definitive treatment for patients with type I diabetes mellitus. Type I diabetics do not have the endogenous insulin required to sustain life. This is due to a variety of factors, including destruction of the pancreatic cells of the islets of Langerhans. Type II diabetics may also need pancreatic transplantation due to the severity of their disease. The pathophysiology of type II diabetes is based on resistance to the effects of insulin within the body. The end results of both type I and type II diabetes are chronic increased blood glucose concentrations and multisystem organ complications. Complications and multisystem effects of diabetes have a profound impact on the vascular system. It is widely known that diabetes plays a significant role in the development of atherosclerosis, CAD, and peripheral vascular disease (both at the microvascular and macrovascular levels). Diabetics are also prone to neuropathies of the peripheral and autonomic system that can cause paresthesias, gastroparesis, and other complications. Diabetic patients receive medical therapy during their wait for a transplant. This therapy includes oral hypoglycemic agents, insulin, or both, along with a prescribed exercise and weight loss program and strict dietary guidelines. The acute risks of diabetes manifest in conditions associated with extreme hyperglycemia. Diabetic ketoacidosis and hyperglycemic hyperosmolar nonketotic coma are severe complications of acute hyperglycemia, are associated with electrolyte abnormalities, and may be life threatening. Unfortunately, many patients who receive maximum medical therapy are still subject to uncontrolled diabetes and the risks associated with the disease. Early identification and management of diabetes is vital to an enhanced quality of life. Identification of uncontrolled diabetes and the need for transplant is an important step. Once a patient is identified, they go through the process of placement on the transplant list. The overall waiting list for pancreas transplant saw a steady decline between 2003 and 2013 but rose slightly again in 2014. The rationale for the overall decline during that time was related to enhancements in surgical techniques and improvements in immunologic therapies.[21]

Over the past 5 years, the pancreas transplant waiting lists have remained relatively stable. There has been a slight decrease noted in the solitary pancreas and pancreas transplant alone listings.[22]

Pancreas transplantation provides patients with an endogenous source of insulin that will restore normoglycemic conditions. There are several types of pancreas transplants, including pancreas alone (PTA), simultaneous pancreas and kidney (SPK), and pancreas after kidney (PAK). These are performed based on the needs of the patients and the allocation of the organs. There have been several key developments related to pancreas transplantation since 2014. A new organ allocation system specific to the pancreas was instituted in October 2014. This allowed a more streamlined process that combined all pancreas transplant types into one waiting list. Other key developments included revision of the criteria for type II diabetics relating to body mass index (BMI) and the development of a consistent definition relating to pancreas graft failure.[21]

Most often, the entire pancreas is transplanted into the recipient from a deceased donor. Occasionally, a living donor may donate the distal pancreas for transplantation, but that is less common.[7] There have been no documented living donor transplants in the United States over the past few years, and this is related to the relatively short wait times for donation. Alternative therapies are evolving to include transplantation of islet cells and the development of an artificial pancreas.[21]

Overall, the outcomes of pancreas transplantation are very good. Klouche et al. reported the 5-year patient survival rate for PTA is 78%, for SPK 93%, and for PAK 91%.[20]

In 2018 new definitions for pancreas graft failure were implemented. These include (1) a transplant recipient's pancreas is removed, (2) a transplant recipient is registered on the recipient list, (3) a recipient is registered on the islet transplant list after already receiving a pancreas, or (4) a pancreas transplant recipient dies. Since implementation of these new guidelines, there has not been an increase in early pancreas graft failure.[22]

Preoperative Considerations for Pancreas Transplant

As with any other type of transplant, the preoperative considerations for a patient who is to undergo a pancreas transplant starts with a thorough review of the history and physical exam. Understanding the patient's diabetic history and reviewing the comorbidities should be a top priority. This evaluation often includes a multidisciplinary team that reviews all aspects of the patient's condition to assess the extent of multisystem organ involvement. Due to the known risk of increase in micro- and macrovascular disease, a cardiac assessment should include assessment of the patient's exercise tolerance, as well as a 12-lead ECG to assess for previous myocardial infarction that may have gone undetected in the diabetic patient. Cardiac ischemia may be difficult to assess in this patient population due to the presence of neuropathies and silent ischemia. If CAD is suspected, a more thorough evaluation, including stress testing or coronary angiogram, should be considered. This may be performed during the assessment for placement on the transplant waiting list.

Pancreas transplant surgery is considered an urgent procedure, so the preoperative evaluation should focus on optimizing the patient's current status and assessing for any acute conditions that may impact the procedure. These can include the presence of ketoacidosis, electrolyte abnormalities, alterations in blood pressure, and volume status. Most often a pancreas transplant involves procurement of the organ from a deceased organ donor and thus there is a need to transplant the organ as soon as possible and within the 24-hour window for maximum cold ischemia time.

Close assessment of blood glucose measurements is important during the perioperative period, along with evaluation of the patient's insulin regimen and recent administration. Evaluation of fluid and electrolytes is also important to assess for renal function. Volume status is very important, especially if the patient has a history of ESRD and requires hemodialysis.

Immunosuppressive protocols for pancreas transplantation follow patterns similar to other solid organ transplants. Pancreas transplant recipients are believed to require higher levels of immunosuppression, possibly related to the increased immunogenicity of the composite pancreaticoduodenal graft, and/or underlying autoimmune status of the recipient. Currently, most centers use induction therapy with a T-cell–depleting antibody, such as antithymocyte globulin or alemtuzumab, or less often an IL-2 receptor blocking antibody such as basiliximab. For maintenance therapy, more than 80% of pancreas transplant recipients receive tacrolimus and MMF. Glucocorticoids are used in more than 60% of recipients. The standard regimen of antibody induction and maintenance with tacrolimus and MMF, with or without glucocorticoids, has ushered in an era of routine success in pancreas transplantation, with 1-year pancreas allograft survival near or exceeding 90%. Due to growing concern about the negative effects of steroids on β cells and the success of the Edmonton protocol for islet transplantation reported in 2000, the use of steroid-free regimens has now reached approximately 40% of the transplants. In addition to providing protection against alloimmune rejection and recurrent autoimmunity, modern dosing of tacrolimus-based regimens is not toxic to islet β cells, as evidenced by normal β-cell secretory capacity in pancreas transplant recipients.[23]

Intraoperative Considerations for Pancreas Transplantation

Pancreatic transplantation is performed under general anesthesia with endotracheal intubation and muscle relaxation. This holds true for all types of pancreas transplantation, including combined kidney and pancreas transplant. A combination of volatile anesthetic and narcotic agents works well in this patient population. Standard American Society of Anesthesiologists (ASA) monitoring is required, and invasive monitoring is often used and may be required, especially in patients where CAD is present and/or when closer hemodynamic monitoring is indicated. Advantages to invasive monitoring with an arterial line includes beat-by-beat blood pressure monitoring, as well as the ability to monitor arterial blood gases (ABGs), electrolytes, and blood glucose levels in an efficient manner. Placement of an arterial line prior to induction may assist in hemodynamic monitoring during the induction phase. Care should be taken during induction of anesthesia to prevent hypotension. A RSI should be considered due to the potential presence of gastroparesis and risk for aspiration during intubation. Administration of an oral nonparticulate antacid may also be considered in the immediate preoperative period. Adequate venous access is always a priority due to volume replacement and the potential for acute blood loss. A central line may also be necessary for administration of immunosuppressive and vasoactive medications.

A midline surgical incision is utilized for pancreas transplantation, as well as for combined kidney/pancreas transplants. As with other abdominal surgeries, the use of retraction is necessary to facilitate an optimal working environment for our surgical colleagues, and therefore muscle relaxation should be utilized to optimize that environment. The transplanted pancreas is placed in the iliac fossa, and arterial anastomosis is via the iliac artery, and venous anastomosis is via the iliac vein (Fig. 41.3). During the surgery, blood glucose levels should be monitored at least every hour to ensure that these levels are maintained at less than 200 mg/dL. Medications such as insulin, administered via subcutaneous route or intravenous infusion, may be necessary; a dextrose infusion may be needed if hypoglycemia occurs. Dextrose infusion may prevent the development of ketoacidosis and

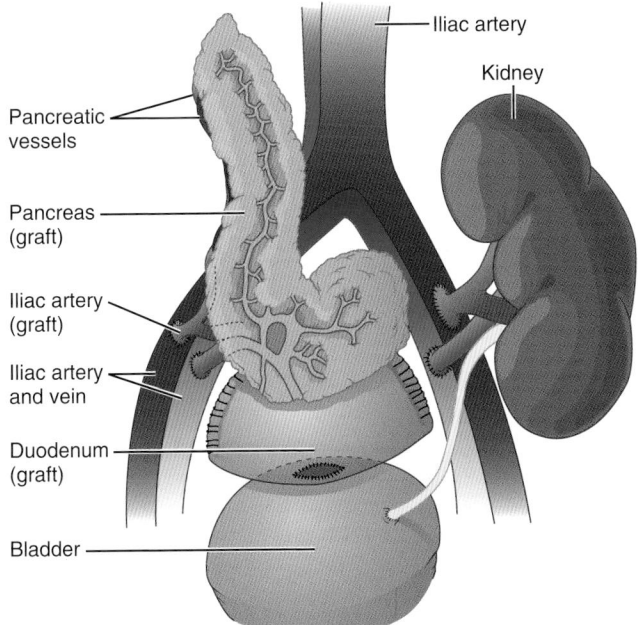

Fig. 41.3 Simultaneous kidney and pancreas transplant. (From Good VS, Kirkwood PL. *Advanced Critical Care Nursing*. 2nd ed. St. Louis: Elsevier; 2018.)

should be available throughout the procedure.[7] Volume replacement should be a priority, especially prior to unclamping the vascular anastomosis. Close hemodynamic monitoring is necessary during this time to prevent hypotension. During the reperfusion phase of the transplanted pancreas, it is imperative that blood glucose levels be monitored more frequently (every 15–30 minutes). This is due to the new pancreas releasing insulin within the circulation and for the prevention of hypoglycemia. Insulin infusions should also be weaned accordingly as the blood glucose normalizes. In some circumstances there may be a delay in the transplanted organ producing sufficient insulin. In these circumstances, the goal should be to maintain blood glucose levels less than 200 mg/dL; some of the literature even recommends keeping it in the 120 to 150 mg/dL range.[7,23,24] Tight glycemic control is required to reduce hyperglycemia but also to decrease stress on the newly transplanted β cells.

Postoperative Considerations for Pancreas Transplantation

Upon completion of pancreas transplantation, the patient is often extubated and transported to the postanesthesia care unit (PACU) or ICU. Regardless of the patient's postoperative disposition, they require vigilant postoperative monitoring. Frequent blood glucose monitoring, along with electrolytes and ABGs, is an essential component of the early postoperative period. Fluid therapy should be maintained with a goal for euvolemia. Monitoring the patient's hemoglobin and hematocrit may also be required. Pain control is another essential component of care in the immediate postoperative period. Multimodal IV analgesia works well for controlling the patient's pain, and transitioning them to a PCA pump is beneficial in the early postoperative period. Some institutions may use epidural analgesia for their transplant patients. Care should be taken to avoid hypotension associated with epidural infusions. Monitoring for graft complications is important in the early postoperative period. Early graft failure rates have decreased from 12.8% in 2005–2006 to 8.2% in 2013–2014.[7] Other complications can include intraabdominal bleeding, graft thrombosis, sepsis, and ultimately graft rejection. Anesthetic care of patients post pancreas transplant include reviewing the patient's transplant history and posttransplant care and complications if any. Close assessment of the patient's blood glucose should be performed. Other preoperative assessments should be made based on the overall condition of the patient and any other comorbidities that may be present.

Judging efficacy of immunosuppression regimens is more difficult with pancreas transplants than for other solid organ transplants such as liver or kidney, where functional tests are readily available. For SKP transplants, rejection of the pancreas may be followed using kidney function as a surrogate marker. Detection of rejection is more difficult for PAK and PTA procedures, and bladder drainage, which allowed monitoring amylase output, has fallen out of favor. Some centers have found percutaneous biopsies to be more valuable than ultrasound evaluation or measurement of circulating amylase and lipase.[23]

LIVER TRANSPLANTATION

The first successful liver transplant was performed in 1967. Limited amounts of liver transplants were performed in the 1970s; however, survival remained below 20%. The advent of immunosuppressive therapy, particularly the drug cyclosporine in the early 1980s, improved liver transplant survival to over 50% 1-year posttransplant and eventually lead to the adaptation of liver transplant as a viable solution for end-stage liver disease (ESLD) worldwide. Currently, 1-year survival data have climbed as high as 85% to 90%, with 5-year survival approximately 70% to 75%.[25] As with other organ transplants, the limiting factor for the overall number of liver transplantations performed is the wide disparity between available donors and patients needing transplant.[26] According to UNOS, 193,508 liver transplants were performed between 1988 and the beginning of 2020. There are currently more than 12,550 patients awaiting liver transplantation in the United States. This is in sharp contrast to the 9674 transplants performed during 2019.[27] Despite the progressive escalation in the severity of liver disease in recipients, graft survival continues to improve.[28] To increase the number of viable grafts for transplant into recipients, there has been increased discussion and experimentation with alternative organ donation efforts from the general heart-beating brain-dead donor. Some of these methods include using candidates that were previously considered marginal donors, such as non-heart-beating donors who have been infiltrated with a cold preservation solution via the femoral artery following cardiac standstill, extracorporeal membrane oxygenation (ECMO) support to facilitate organ perfusion after cardiac death, ex vivo perfusion of viable organs after cardiac death, and utilizing a split liver graft. Living donor liver transplantation has also been successfully performed utilizing a partial hepatectomy in place of a cadaveric liver. The liver is unique in that it can regenerate itself even after a large section is removed. In a healthy donor, up to 70% of the liver can be removed with the remaining section sufficiently functional to meet the metabolic needs of the donor. Benefits of living donor liver transplant include a shortened waiting period for recipients, elective nature of the surgery, high-quality graft as it is procured from a healthy donor with stable hemodynamics, and a very short cold/ischemic time made possible due to the planned nature of the case. A major factor that must be considered is the impact on the donor from the viewpoint that it is a major abdominal surgery with no personal benefit.[26] Due to the

concerns for complications with the donor, very few living donor liver transplants are performed (~300 per year).

Liver transplantation is the sole definitive treatment modality for patients with acute liver failure, ESLD, and primary hepatic malignancy. The etiology of ESLD can be categorized into seven primary categories (Table 41.5). The indications for liver transplantation are listed in Table 41.6.

Acute liver failure is defined as the development of severe acute liver injury with encephalopathy and impaired synthetic function (international normalized ratio [INR] >1.5) in the absence of preexisting liver disease or cirrhosis. These patients are given the highest priority for liver transplantation (UNOS status 1). Without transplantation, patients with acute liver failure will have either a complete recovery of function or die within days. These patients should be transferred to a liver transplant center as quickly as possible. Patients suffering from cirrhosis are not immediate candidates for liver transplant. However, the development of decompensation as evidenced by ascites, hepatic encephalopathy, and variceal bleeding are indications of significantly impaired survival and should lead to the patient being worked up for the transplant waiting list. The development of hepatorenal syndrome is an ominous sign and signals the need for immediate transplantation evaluation. The Model for End-Stage Liver Disease (MELD) score is a validated system that UNOS uses for prioritizing patients on the liver transplant waiting list.[29] Table 41.7 explains the MELD score. Although the most important aspect of successful organ donation is ABO compatibility, the MELD score is utilized to determine which patients have the greatest need for transplantation. There is some debate to its effectiveness, and some modifications have been proposed; it is utilized

TABLE 41.5   Chronic End-Stage Liver Disease: Etiologies

Category	Disease	Frequency
Hepatitis	(Hepatitis A)	Never chronic
	Hepatitis B	10%–15%
	Hepatitis C	40%
Noncholestatic	Laennec cirrhosis	
	Cryptogenic cirrhosis	
	Autoimmune hepatitis	
Cholestatic	Primary sclerosing cholangitis	
	Primary biliary cirrhosis	
Metabolic	Hemochromatosis	
	Wilson disease	
	α_1-antitrypsin deficiency	
Malignancies	Hepatocellular carcinoma	Adults
	Hepatoblastoma	Children
	Cholangiocarcinoma	Investigational
	Carcinoid/neuroendocrine	Rare
	Hemangioendothelioma	Rare
	Hemangiosarcoma	
Atresia: children	Biliary atresia	50%
Others	Budd-Chiari	Rare
	Cystic fibrosis	
	Congenital hepatic fibrosis	
	Benign tumors	

From Nissen NN, et al. Hepatic transplantation. In Yeo CJ, ed. *Shackleford's Surgery of the Alimentary Tract*. 8th ed. Philadelphia: Elsevier; 2019:1488–1507.

TABLE 41.6   Indications for Liver Transplantation

Indications	Examples
Acute hepatic necrosis	Viral hepatitis, drug toxicity, toxin, Wilson disease
Chronic hepatitis	Hepatitis B, hepatitis C, hepatitis D, autoimmune hepatitis, chronic drug toxicity or toxin exposure, cryptogenic cirrhosis
Cholestatic diseases	Primary biliary cirrhosis, sclerosing cholangitis, secondary biliary cirrhosis, biliary atresia, cystic fibrosis
Alcoholic cirrhosis	May be considered for transplant if abstinence of alcohol for 6 months and ongoing therapy and evaluation
Metabolic diseases	Wilson disease, cystic fibrosis hemochromatosis, α_1-antitrypsin deficiency, familial homozygous hypercholesterolemia, glycogen storage disease, tyrosinemia
Malignant diseases of the liver	Hepatocellular carcinoma, carcinoid tumor, islet cell tumor, epithelioid hemangioendothelioma
Chronic symptoms	Progressive hyperbilirubinemia, portal hypertension as evidenced by bleeding from esophageal or gastric varices, hypersplenism with thrombocytopenia, disabling portosystemic or hepatic encephalopathy, coagulation disorders, generalized wasting and failure to thrive
Acute symptoms	Acute liver failure, rapid decline in liver function, coagulopathy, jaundice, encephalopathy

TABLE 41.7 Three-Month Mortality According to MELD Score*

MELD Score	≤9	10–19	20–29	30–39	≥40
In hospital	4%	27%	76%	83%	100%
Outpatient	2%	6%	50%		

*The MELD score: 10 × (0.957 × $\log_e$ [creatinine] + $\log_e$ [bilirubin] + 1.12 × $\log_e$ [INR]).
MELD, Model for End-Stage Liver Disease.

BOX 41.4 Etiology of Liver Pathology

- Chronic viral hepatitis: B and C
- Hepatocellular cancer
- Alcohol
- Nonalcoholic fatty liver disease
- Autoimmune: autoimmune hepatitis, primary biliary cirrhosis, primary sclerosing cholangitis
- Hemochromatosis
- Drugs (methotrexate, amiodarone, acetaminophen)
- Cystic fibrosis, α_1-antitryptin deficiency, Wilson disease
- Vascular problems (portal hypertension with or without liver disease)
- Cryptogenic
- Others: sarcoidosis, amyloidosis, schistosomiasis

From Ramsay M. Anesthesia for liver transplantation. In: Busuttil RW, Klintmalm GB., eds. *Transplantation of the Liver.* 3rd ed. Philadelphia: Elsevier; 2015:611–631.

widely by transplant centers and UNOS for recipient-donor matching. The MELD score is a validated system that uses serum total bilirubin, serum creatinine, and the INR values to mathematically rank adult patients according to their expected survival rate without transplantation. Variations of the MELD score include the MELD sodium and MELD lactate.[29] There are many limitations to the MELD score that transplant centers are aware of; for instance, patients suffering from primary hepatocellular carcinoma may not have any, or minimal, increased markers measured by the MELD. Without a transplant, these patients face the risk of fulminant liver failure and metastasis that would preclude them from future transplant due to metastatic disease. To amend the MELD score for patients with conditions such as this, there are exception points. These are utilized to increase the MELD score for patients with conditions associated with chronic liver disease that may result in impaired survival but not directly accounted for in the MELD scoring system. These include hepatocellular carcinoma, hepatopulmonary syndrome (HPS), portopulmonary hypertension (must maintain mean arterial pressure [MAP] <35 mm Hg with treatment), familial amyloid polyneuropathy, primary hyperoxaluria, cystic fibrosis, hilar cholangiocarcinoma, and hepatic artery thrombosis (if within an appropriate time frame before transplant). Each transplant center has varying protocols for how to deal with these patients who do not conform to the MELD measurements. Other complicating conditions that could be related to a patient's liver disease that are not covered by official MELD exceptions points include recurrent cholangitis in patients with primary sclerosing cholangitis that is refractory to antibiotic therapy or needing repeated biliary interventions, refractory ascites, refractory hepatic encephalopathy, refractory variceal hemorrhages, and portal hypertensive gastropathy with chronic blood loss, among others. Each center has a protocol for dealing with patients of unique medical histories and prioritizing them on a case-by-case basis. Contraindications for a potential recipient to be listed for liver transplantation are often center specific. A generally accepted list of contraindications at most centers includes[30]:

- Cardiopulmonary disease that is uncorrectable
- Acquired immunodeficiency syndrome (AIDS)
- Untreated tuberculosis
- Malignancy not isolated to the liver that does not meet oncologic criteria for cure
- Hepatocellular carcinoma with metastatic spread
- Intrahepatic cholangiocarcinoma
- Hemangiosarcoma
- Anatomic abnormalities that preclude transplantation
- Uncontrolled sepsis
- Acute liver failure with intracranial pressure (ICP) greater than 50 mm/Hg or cerebral perfusion pressure (CPP) less than 40 mm/Hg
- Nonadherence to medical care
- Lack of social support system

Some relative contraindications include advanced age and human immunodeficiency virus (HIV) (not AIDS); however, there have been successful transplants in patients over age 65 with appropriate

evaluation of comorbid complicating factors.[31] Another factor that is very prevalent in the United States is class 3 obesity (BMI >40); many centers consider it a relative contraindication. However, patients will be encouraged to lose weight prior to transplantation, and some centers will even perform a gastric sleeve in an effort to optimize the potential recipient.[30] It is important to remember that these are generalities, and each liver transplant center will vary in what is and is not considered a contraindication. Patients who have a general contraindication are often assessed on a case-by-case basis to determine their appropriateness for transplant. The etiology of common liver problems is noted in Box 41.4.

Preoperative Considerations for Liver Transplantation

Patient demographics and disease severity are highly variable for liver transplantation. Age distribution has shifted toward older patients with liberalization of donor and recipient criteria, as well as advanced medical technologies, allowing patients to survive longer without transplant.[32] The detailed anesthetic preevaluation and planning is crucial due to the complex nature of comorbidities presented by liver failure patients. Careful planning and communication with the surgical team regarding their concerns and plan for approach (e.g., bicaval cross-clamp, piggyback, or venovenous bypass) has a large impact on anesthetic planning.[33] The primary goal of preanesthetic evaluation is to assess the patient's ability to tolerate surgery and posttransplantation care. A standard preanesthetic evaluation should include airway assessment, previous anesthetics, fasting (NPO [nil per os]) status, and an anesthesia-focused review of systems. In addition to the usual preanesthetic evaluation, the transplant anesthetist should concentrate extra efforts on the cardiopulmonary and hepatic systems. Further testing is indicated on a patient-specific basis if there is an abnormal result in initial screening or if the patient presents with abnormal signs and symptoms suspicious of undetected comorbidities. Standard laboratory panels should be done preoperatively, including ABO-Rh blood typing, liver biochemical/function tests (including INR), complete blood count, creatinine clearance, serum α-fetoprotein, calcium, viral and infective serologies, urinalysis, and urine drug screen. Liver disease can have significant cardiac comorbidities and needs an in-depth cardiopulmonary screening. The cardiac exam should include transthoracic echocardiography, 12-lead ECG, and noninvasive cardiac stress testing at a minimum. The 2013 practice guidelines from the American Association for the Study of Liver Diseases and the American Society of Transplantation recommend noninvasive stress (exercise or pharmacologic) testing for all pretransplantation patients.[30]

This is contrary to 2012 recommendations from the American Heart Association and the American College of Cardiology (ACC) Foundation suggesting noninvasive stress testing in patients with no active cardiac conditions if there are multiple risk factors for CAD present (diabetes, left ventricular hypertrophy [LVH], age >60 years, smoking, hypertension, hyperlipidemia).[34] One study found that utilizing submaximal cardiopulmonary exercise testing to calculate anaerobic threshold (which corresponds to cardiorespiratory reserve) positively predicted posttransplantation mortality.[35] Invasive cardiac catheterization and coronary angiography is recommended in patients with known CAD, diabetes, or more than two cardiovascular risk factors to assess the extent and severity of the CAD.[36] It is prudent to obtain preoperative pulse oximetry and ABG values to screen for HPS. The triad of liver disease, impaired oxygenation, and intrapulmonary vascular dilatations indicates the presence of HPS and worsens the prognosis for cirrhotic patients. Patients with HPS receive MELD exception points. It is important to rule out other pulmonary and cardiac etiologies that could cause low oxygen saturations via chest radiography, pulmonary function tests, and computed tomography (CT) scanning. A transthoracic echo is recommended preoperatively to assess for evidence of valvular heart disease, myocardial wall motion abnormalities, and portopulmonary hypertension. Other pulmonary diseases need to be assessed via pulmonary function testing when indicated with patient comorbidities such as chronic obstructive pulmonary disease (COPD), emphysema, and asthma. Cancer screening for patients with hepatocellular carcinoma should include CT and magnetic resonance imaging scanning to assess for metastases and determination of staging. It is also useful to assess the hepatic vasculature for anastomoses during the transplant procedure. Upper endoscopy should be performed in patients with cirrhosis and portal hypertension to evaluate for esophageal varices. A final and key portion is the psychosocial evaluation. It is utilized to identify major issues that may impair a successful outcome after transplantation. The major psychosocial problems include a lack of insight and knowledge into the nature of the transplant procedure, posttransplant care, and substance use disorders. Due to the fact that some liver transplant patients have a history of alcohol and drug abuse, it is of the utmost importance to provide pretransplant treatment to increase the likelihood of success posttransplantation.

There are many unique disease states that patients in liver failure may have that can have a profound effect on patient management. Typically, ESLD patients have high cardiac output, with high resting heart rates and relatively low blood pressures. Due to the hepatic cirrhosis reducing the metabolism of catecholamines, there are thought to be endogenous mediators in hepatic portal blood that "spill over" into the systemic circulation and cause profound splanchnic vasodilation and thus reduced systemic vascular resistance.[29] Due to the increased levels of circulation of catecholamines and generalized increased sympathetic activation, these patients are characterized as having a hyperdynamic circulation, which can fool the anesthetist into assessing cardiac function as adequate. The decreased afterload can actually mask cardiac dysfunction, and care needs to be taken not to overlook cardiac disease in otherwise "normal"-looking patients. Cirrhotic patients with ESLD often suffer from cirrhotic cardiomyopathy. This is characterized by increased cardiac output and a compromised ventricular response to stress. Cardiac performance declines, and the patient begins to suffer both diastolic and systolic dysfunction due to the activation of the cardiac renin-angiotensin system and impairment of the β-adrenergic receptor.[37] These patients have inotropic and chronotropic incompetence in conjunction with electrical and mechanical dyssynchrony. This is present in as many as 50% of patients undergoing liver transplant.[38] CAD is a significant risk factor and positive predictor for poor outcomes in liver transplantations.[29] It has been assessed that 25% of

ESLD patients have at least one coronary artery that can be classified as moderately or severely stenotic. Exercise stress testing can be difficult in ESLD patients due to their limited overall functional capacity; dobutamine stress and myocardial perfusion imaging can be done to detect ischemia successfully in these patients. In the presence of previously known or previous CAD and/or stable angina, the ACC recommends coronary angiography to assess for extent of stenosis. There are no definitive guidelines for revascularization, but in some high-volume centers there are case reports of combined liver transplant/cardiac surgery. Hemodynamically significant left ventricular outflow tract obstruction may be seen due to the combination of LVH and hyperdynamic systolic function found in patients with ESLD.[37] This can have a great impact on anesthetic management and precipitate intraoperative hypotension that would respond poorly to increased catecholamine administration.

Portopulmonary hypertension is defined as pulmonary hypertension syndrome with vascular obstruction in the presence of portal hypertension. It is characterized by a mean pulmonary artery pressure of greater than 25 mm Hg and is caused by an increase in pulmonary arterial flow due to varying degrees of pulmonary endothelial and smooth muscle proliferation with added vasoconstriction.[37] The development of intimal proliferation is a major reason that patients with portopulmonary hypertension have an increase in pulmonary vascular resistance (PVR). It must be differentiated from the 30% to 50% of patients with ESLD who have elevated pulmonary artery and venous pressures with normal PVR. This is a normal finding in an ESLD patient and not a contraindication to transplant.[29] A screening transthoracic echo can utilize tricuspid regurgitation to estimate right ventricular systolic pressure (RVSP); if the RVSP is greater than 50 mm Hg the patient should be recommended for a right heart catheterization to exclude other causes of pulmonary hypertension.[38] It is generally accepted that severe, untreated portopulmonary hypertension is a contraindication to transplantation.

HPS is characterized by arterial hypoxemia caused by intrapulmonary vascular dilatations. The classical triad of portal hypertension, hypoxemia, and pulmonary vascular dilatations characterizes HPS. An alveolar to arterial oxygen gradient of greater than 15 mm Hg and pulmonary vascular dilatation documented by delayed, contrast-enhanced echo with left heart detection of microbubbles greater than four cardiac cycles is considered diagnostic of HPS.[37] The classic hypoxic pulmonary vasoconstriction response to hypoxemia is impaired and leads to poor tolerance of gravitational effects on pulmonary blood flow leading to platypnea-orthodeoxia. This is a paradoxic increase in breathlessness and decrease in arterial partial pressure of oxygen; it occurs when a patient moves from supine to upright because of abnormal pulmonary vessel size. There is no known pharmacologic therapy to treat HPS. The outcome of patients with the syndrome who do not receive a transplant is poor. This is why UNOS recognizes it as a MELD exception status. Despite having outcomes after transplant that are less favorable than those who do not have HPS, it is an acceptable number and thus not a contraindication to transplant.[29]

A common and easily recognizable complication of liver disease and portal hypertension is the accumulation of ascites in the abdomen. Ascites can cause an increase in intraabdominal pressure, creating difficulty breathing; however, a more serious issue called hepatic hydrothorax can develop. This is a buildup of ascitic fluid in the thorax often on the right side. It is reasonable and appropriate to arrange preoperative drainage of larger hydrothoraces in patients with respiratory compromise.[29]

Hepatorenal syndrome is a severe form of acute kidney injury in patients with advanced ESLD. The international ascites club proposed diagnostic criteria for hepatorenal syndrome (Table 41.8). It is a form of prerenal failure that occurs in decompensated cirrhosis. The diagnostic criteria for hepatorenal syndrome are cirrhosis with ascites and a serum creatinine of greater than 1.5 mg/dL in the absence of parenchymal kidney disease, shock, or treatment with nephrotoxic drugs. Additional diagnostic confirmation is aided by no improvement of creatinine after a minimum of 2 days diuretic withdrawal and albumin intravascular volume expansion.[37] This is a form of prerenal failure precipitated by blood accumulating in the dilated splanchnic vasculature causing an effective depletion of arterial intravascular volume. This leads to the low systemic arterial pressure that follows, renin-angiotensin release, sympathetic system activation, renal vasoconstriction, low renal perfusion, and low GFR.[29] Two types have been identified: Type I is the more severe manifestation and is characterized by a rapid decline in GFR and a median survival of only 2 weeks, whereas type II is a more progressive and slower course of renal failure. It is important, as with other comorbidities related to ESLD, to differentiate hepatorenal syndrome from other causes of acute kidney failure.

Hepatic encephalopathy occurs when circulating neurotoxins, most commonly ammonia, accumulate in the brain and alter neurotransmission via glutamate or altered cerebral energy homeostasis.[37] The manifestations of hepatic encephalopathy range from mild apraxia and behavioral changes to decerebrate posturing and coma.[29] The actual pathophysiology of these changes is poorly understood but is thought to be related to poor metabolism of gut-produced ammonia and other byproducts. Treatment includes nonabsorbable disaccharides, which are thought to reduce encephalopathy by affecting bacterial function in the colon and thus reducing enteric production of ammonia. Other interventions aimed at reducing encephalopathy center around reducing nitrogen load in the gut, reducing dietary protein, correcting electrolyte and metabolic abnormalities, avoidance of benzodiazepines, and administration of metronidazole and rifaximin.[26]

In preparing the operating room for surgery, the anesthetist should have standard monitors, in addition to planning for an arterial line, large-bore IV access, central venous catheter, PAC, continuous invasive or noninvasive cardiac output/function monitoring, thromboelastogram (TEG), TEE, cell saver, rapid infuser devices, blood products in the operating room or immediately available (RBCs, fresh frozen plasma [FFP], platelets, and cryoprecipitate), and transfer to the ICU on mechanical ventilation afterward. PAC is the gold standard in hemodynamic monitoring during liver transplantation to which other monitors are compared.[38] It does have its limitations and dangerous side effect profile, which must be carefully considered when placing a PAC. Monitoring of central venous oxygen saturation and mixed venous oxygen saturation is of little value in liver transplant patients, and many of the newer noninvasive hemodynamic monitors can provide reliable cardiac function data.

Intraoperative Considerations for Liver Transplant

Careful monitoring and the availability of measures to maintain hemostasis, normothermia, and normovolemia are essential. Adequate assistance is necessary, as is access to point-of-service laboratory equipment or the presence of a "stat laboratory," so that current data are obtained. Rapid analyses of basic electrolytes, glucose, ABGs, ionized calcium and magnesium levels, as well as hemostasis profiles (hematocrit, prothrombin time, partial thromboplastin time, fibrinogen, platelet count, thrombin clot time, fibrin split products, and D-dimers), are required. The perioperative use of TEG or rotational thromboelastography allows an accurate assessment of the quality of the clotting system to be made in real time.[39] Coagulopathies that may occur during liver transplant procedures are listed in Table 41.9. After placement of a peripheral IV, preferably large bore, awake arterial access may be gained if the patient's condition allows it. It is prudent to limit the amount of sedative premedication, as patients with liver disease are particularly sensitive to it. There are no absolute contraindications to induction agents, and the anesthetist may choose midazolam, ketamine, propofol, or etomidate. Opioid choice depends on center preference and comfort of the anesthetist. Fentanyl, sufentanil, remifentanil, and alfentanil have all been used successfully.[33] Due to the reduced peripheral vascular resistance seen in patients with ESLD, it is common to encounter postinduction hypotension. Vasopressors such as phenylephrine are preferred for their α-adrenergic receptor specificity in the presence of an already hyperdynamic heart. Another vasopressor that should be immediately available is vasopressin. Due to its potent vasoconstricting ability, a vasopressin infusion during induction, and possibly in combination with a phenylephrine infusion and boluses, can help provide a stable MAP and ensure adequate organ perfusion. Any drugs primarily metabolized by the liver and cytochrome P-450 pathways will exhibit an altered pharmacokinetic and pharmacodynamic response in the

TABLE 41.8   International Ascites Club Proposed Diagnostic Criteria for Hepatorenal Syndrome

1	Cirrhosis with ascites
2	Serum creatinine >1.5 mg/dL
3	No improvement in serum creatinine after 2 days of volume expansion with albumin
4	Absence of shock
5	No recent treatment with nephrotoxic drugs
6	Absence of parenchymal kidney disease as indicated by proteinuria >500 mg/day

From Salerno F, et al. Diagnosis, prevention and treatment of hepatorenal syndrome in cirrhosis. *Gut.* 2007;56:1310–1318; Ramsay M. Anesthesia for liver transplantation. In: Busuttil RW, Klintmalm GB, eds. *Transplantation of the Liver.* 3rd ed. Philadelphia: Elsevier; 2015:611–631.

TABLE 41.9   Coagulopathy During Orthotopic Liver Transplantation

Stage	Coagulopathy
Dissection	Preexisting coagulopathy
	Dilution
	Fibrinolysis (mild)
	Ionized hypocalcemia
	Dilution
Anhepatic	Heparin effect (with venovenous bypass)
	Fibrinolysis (moderate)
	Hypothermia
	Ionized hypocalcemia
	Fibrinolysis (severe)
Early neohepatic	Heparin effect
	Intravascular coagulation
	Dilution
	Hypothermia
	Ionized hypocalcemia
Late neohepatic	Gradual recovery

From Kang Y, Audu P. Coagulation and liver transplantation. *Int Anesthesiol Clin.* 2006;44(4):19.

ESLD patient. Close care should be taken in aseptic technique when placing all invasive lines as the patient will be profoundly immunosuppressed on completion of transplantation. Induction of anesthesia should be undertaken using a RSI technique and succinylcholine with cricoid pressure, as the semiemergent nature of the surgery is likely to create a full-stomach situation. Preoperative potassium levels should be available to avoid succinylcholine-associated hyperkalemia. Utilization of nondepolarizing muscle relaxants is acceptable. The aminosteroid relaxants vecuronium and rocuronium undergo hepatic metabolism; however, due to the nature of the surgery in both duration and the high likelihood for prolonged recovery and mechanical ventilation in the ICU, careful dosage of both are appropriate.[29] Cisatracurium, which undergoes Hofmann elimination, is also an appropriate relaxant as it is not dependent on hepatic clearance. Quantitative neuromuscular monitoring is recommended regardless of the nondepolarizing muscle relaxant that is chosen. This will allow appropriate dosing and help prevent unnecessary overdosing of muscle relaxants leading to prolonged paralysis. After successful intubation, anesthesia via volatile anesthetics is maintained with age-adjusted minimum alveolar concentration equivalents titrated to the hemodynamic profile. It is useful to monitor entropy during the duration of the transplant to help ensure adequate anesthetic levels. After intubation the central venous catheter should be placed, and the PAC (if chosen) will be floated as well. Other large-bore peripheral access should be initiated as well as placement of an oral or nasogastric tube. A transesophageal echo probe may also be placed at this time, but discussion must take place with the surgical team prior to placing anything in the esophagus in case there are varices or the patient has altered coagulation factors that may increase the risk for bleeding. Intraoperative neurologic monitoring is crucial as patients with liver disease are at risk for a large range of neurologic complications, including cerebral edema, encephalopathy, seizures, hypoxia, and central pontine myelinolysis.[38] Increased ICP is especially common in patients with acute liver failure. This can be complicated by an increase in cerebral blood flow following hepatic reperfusion and thus higher ICP. In a 2016 study, it was shown that severe posttransplant brain injury occurred at a rate of 7.8% and was associated with severe pretransplant cerebral edema and a higher posttransplant INR.[37] ICP is classically monitored using an invasive catheter placed in the cranial vault and integrated with a pressure transducer. Due to the high likelihood of coagulopathies in liver transplant patients, there is a significant risk of intracranial hemorrhage with this technique. Moreover, this line must be placed as a separate surgical procedure by a neurosurgeon. When an ICP monitor was used in acetaminophen acute liver failure, there was no significant 21-day mortality benefit, and in nonacetaminophen acute liver failure, it was associated with worse outcomes. The use of transcranial Doppler, which measures CPPs noninvasively, has proven advantages, yet its use in the perioperative period has yet to be defined.[38] Transcranial Doppler has a diagnostic sensitivity of 67%.[37] Antibiotic dosages and timing, as well as immunosuppression administration, should be discussed with the surgery team and implemented as appropriate.

The liver transplantation is divided into three phases: preanhepatic, anhepatic, and neohepatic. Changes in physiologic parameters during each of the three phases are listed in Table 41.10. The preanhepatic phase includes the dissection and isolation of infra- and suprahepatic vena cava, as well as exposure of the porta hepatis and hilar structures of the liver. The anhepatic phase begins with clamping of the hepatic blood supply and venous drainage until reperfusion of the donor liver. Finally, the neohapatic phase begins at the reperfusion of the allograft. Patients receiving orthotopic liver transplants experience a wide variety of pharmacokinetic characteristics due to the amount of anesthetic drugs that are metabolized hepatically. There is a period of

no metabolism during the anhepatic phase, and certain medications will experience a complete cessation of metabolism. It is important to also understand that other factors, including massive blood loss and transfusion, can affect plasma concentrations of anesthetic drugs and must be taken into consideration when dosing.[40]

During the preanhepatic phase, the ascites is drained, and adequate exposure to the liver and surrounding vasculature is attained. It is very common to experience large fluid shifts during this phase of surgery, and the decreased intraabdominal pressure experienced by relieving the ascites can unmask intravascular volume depletion. Volume expansion should be accomplished with 5% albumin rather than large volumes of crystalloids.[33] Blood loss during this phase may be significant and is complicated by previous abdominal surgery, sepsis, coagulopathy, and peritonitis.[29] Maintaining a low to low-normal CVP will aid with reduction of blood loss but must also be balanced with transfusion of blood and coagulation factors. Preoperative INR has no predictive value on intraoperative blood loss; thus transfusion of FFP is debatable and could cause fluid volume overload.[37] Intraoperative clotting panels such as INR, fibrinogen, and platelet count can be useful to guide transfusion therapy; however, there are no defined laboratory values for an end goal of treatment. TEG is the gold standard for coagulation management in liver transplant due to the fact that it measures the viscoelastic properties of the blood during all stages of thrombus formation, as well as testing stability, firmness, and fibrinolysis of the clot. Usage of a TEG or derivative technology intraoperatively has been shown to reduce the transfusion requirements.[38] Large volumes of intravascular fluid boluses during this phase can cause hemodilution

TABLE 41.10 Relative Changes in Parameters During Liver Transplantation*

Variable	Preanhepatic	Anhepatic	Neohepatic
Glucose	+	–/+	+ +
Hemoglobin	–/– –	–	–/– –
Platelets	–	–	–
Urine output	+ +	– –	+/+ +
Cardiac index	+ +	+	+ + +
Systemic vascular resistance	– –	+ +	– – –
Peripheral vascular resistance	+	– –	+
Mean arterial blood pressure	–	– –	– – –/– followed by +
Lactate	+	+	+/+ +
Potassium (K)	+	+	+ + + followed by +
Calcium (Ca)	–	– –	–
Magnesium (Mg)	–	– –	–
Sodium (Na)	+	+	+
Temperature	–	– – –	+

*Increases: + = mild, ++ = moderate, +++ = marked; decreases: – = mild, – – = moderate, – – – = marked.
From Amand MS, et al. Liver transplant. In: Sharpe MD, Gelb AW, eds. *Anesthesia and Transplantation.* Boston: Butterworth-Heinemann; 1999:190; Robertson AC, et al. Anesthesia for liver surgery and transplantation. In: Longnecker DE, et al., eds. *Anesthesiology.* 3rd ed. New York: McGraw Hill; 2018:971–999; Wray CL, et al. Anesthesia for abdominal organ transplant. In: Gropper MA, et al., eds. *Miller's Anesthesia.* 9th ed. Philadelphia: Elsevier; 2020:1960–1992.

and hypothermia, which will worsen coagulopathies. When utilizing blood product transfusion, it is important to include packed RBCs, FFP, platelets, and cryoprecipitate clotting factors. The transfusion of too many RBCs can lead to a dilutional coagulopathy or thrombocytopenia. Another complication of blood product transfusion is hypocalcemia, as the citrate used to preserve the blood products will bind to calcium in the patient and cause a relative hypocalcemia. Complicating this factor is the reduced hepatic blood flow during surgery that further reduces citrate metabolism.[37] Intraoperative cell saver, or blood salvaging techniques, is a cost-effective and safe measure to limit transfusion and blood loss during the dissection phase. The primary contraindication for cell-saver usage is malignancy, although there are filters available that can effectively remove tumor load from the reperfused blood.

Once adequate exposure of the native liver is achieved, the second, or anhepatic, phase of the orthotopic liver transplant begins. The surgical approach to liver isolation that is used (bicaval clamp, piggyback, or venovenous bypass) will have a major impact on hemodynamic and fluid management during the anhepatic phase.[33] The bicaval clamp technique involves clamping the vena cava superiorly and inferiorly to the liver causing venous obstruction distal to the clamp and significantly dropping preload on the right side of the heart that can lead to profound hypotension and tachycardia. A secondary effect of this is the necessity of the anesthetist to treat this hypotension due to clamping by transfusing larger amounts of fluids leading to intravascular volume overload. A newer method is called the piggyback technique and involves only side clamping of the inferior vena cava (IVC) to preserve some degree of caval flow and limit the amount of decreased preload on the heart. This technique has many benefits in that it leads to shorter operative and warm ischemia times, as well as reduced blood/coagulation product use, while preserving similar graft function and survival outcomes. Venovenous bypass is seldom used since the development of the piggyback technique and its ability to preserve flow through the IVC. Although there is still debate among transplant surgeons, a reasonable approach is to try IVC side clamping to assess hemodynamic function; if there is profound hypotension associated with a reduced cardiac index unresponsive to inotropes and volume challenges, then venovenous bypass should be initiated. During the anhepatic phase, and especially in the face of hemodynamically significant IVC occlusion, fluid loading should occur with a target CVP of 10 to 20 cm H_2O (will vary among centers and surgeons). As the native liver is now excluded from systemic circulation, the metabolizing capacity of the liver, particularly on lactate with a corresponding rise in plasma lactate, is recognized. This will create a metabolic lactic acidosis that will worsen with reperfusion of the graft; thus it is good practice to treat acidosis during the anhepatic phase to help buffer against worsening acidosis after reperfusion.[29]

The last phase of the transplant involves reperfusion of the new liver. This occurs after caval and arterial anastomoses. Postreperfusion syndrome is the most significant anesthetic concern during the final phase of transplant. Postreperfusion syndrome is characterized by decreased cardiac output, systemic hypotension, bradyarrhythmias, asystole, pulmonary arterial hypertension, and raised pulmonary capillary wedge pressure in conjunction with increased CVP.[29] Clinically, it is defined as a decrease in systemic MAP greater than 30% below baseline for at least 1 minute during the first 5 minutes of hepatic reperfusion. The mechanisms that cause reperfusion syndrome and its associated hemodynamic instabilities are complex and not well understood. Recent analysis of postreperfusion syndrome indicates a 12% to 17% incidence rate and a high correlation with perioperative mortality and renal dysfunction. Preoperative echocardiograms demonstrated that left ventricular diastolic dysfunction was significantly associated with postreperfusion syndrome.[41] These findings emphasize the importance

of diastolic dysfunction and the importance of an adequate preoperative cardiovascular evaluation. Increasing age of the graft donor is the only other strongly predictive factor for graft postreperfusion syndrome. Key management techniques during reperfusion of the liver include prompt response to the actively moving physiologic parameters and optimizing graft perfusion conditions. The most important of these is maintenance of an adequate perfusion pressure to the new liver and avoidance of high CVPs. Increased CVP can cause graft venous congestion. Clear communication between the surgeon and anesthetist is again crucial as the color of the implanted liver can indicate to the surgical team that it may be at risk for venous congestion and require the anesthetist to lower CVP. Instituting diuresis may be appropriate at this stage of the procedure with care taken not to overdiurese and promote hemodynamic instability. Postreperfusion syndrome may be so acute and severe that it leads to cardiac arrest. Consideration must be taken for maintenance of the patient's core body temperature as cold preservative is used in the liver, and it is not uncommon for the recipient's temperature to drop 0.5°C to 1°C during the reperfusion time. A quick return of temperature can be utilized as a sign of good graft function. Stable glucose and acid-base status are also reassuring signs of adequate graft function.[29] After adequate hemostasis is assured and the surgical team has completed the anastomoses and graft function, closure of the fascia and skin will begin, and the anesthetist can prepare the patient for emergence and transport to the ICU. Some intraoperative complications that may occur and their management are listed in Table 41.11. Guidelines for anesthesia management of liver transplants are listed in Box 41.5.

Postoperative Considerations for Liver Transplant

The vast majority of liver transplant recipients are admitted to a specialized ICU after surgery because these patients are critically ill by definition. They have at least one major organ failure and often multisystem organ failure prior to transplant. Couple that with hemodynamic and cardiac instabilities, fluid shifts, coagulopathies, bleeding anastomoses, graft failure, and postoperative ventilation requirements, and the ICU is a necessity. In the near future, it is possible that there will be fast tracking of ideal liver transplant candidates. At this time, the focus for this lies primarily on patients with isolated hepatocellular carcinoma who have little to no comorbidities and are highly selectable for expedited recovery. Early extubation is warranted when appropriate and is beneficial in numerous ways. Early reduction of positive pressure ventilation can reduce intraabdominal pressures and help with graft perfusion.[29] Early extubation has been shown to reduce ICU stay and diminish resource use with a concomitant reduction in cost by as much as 13%.[32] Patient selection is key to successful early extubation and is performed in as many as 70% to 80% of cases in some centers. Pain control is often managed via PCA IV narcotic use and orally when the patient is able to take pills. Epidural pain management is often precluded in the presence of coagulopathic or suspected coagulopathic patients.

LUNG TRANSPLANTATION

Lung transplantation is the now accepted therapy for end-stage pulmonary and pulmonary vascular disease. The first human lung transplant was performed in 1963 by Hardy at the University of Mississippi. This patient died of renal failure 18 days after transplantation. Out of 40 transplants that followed in the next 20 years, only one patient survived more than 1 month.[42] The first series of successful lung transplants were achieved in 1983 by Joseph Cooper of Toronto University.[41] UNOS data as of 2020 report 41,550 successful lung transplants occurring in the United States since 1988. There are approximately 1000 patients on the lung transplant waiting list in the United States, as well as 50 awaiting heart/lung transplants. There has been a steady increase in the number of lung transplants every year. In 2019 there were 2755 performed in the United States.[43] Despite the similarity of these numbers the stringent exclusion criteria for lung transplantation leaves many patients on the list for extended periods of time. Thousands of patients have died while on the organ waiting list.

The history of lung transplantation has been plagued with difficulties such as high mortality and complication rates. Most early failures revolved around the bronchial anastomosis. Despite many technologic improvements along the way, the improvement of immunosuppression protocols has perhaps had the largest impact. Early immunosuppression consisted of high-dose corticosteroid therapy, which was a

significant contributor to the bronchial dehiscence.[44] The mortality rate for lung transplant still remains very high (20%–30%) with the main complication cited as primary graft dysfunction (PGD).[45] PGD presents as acute lung injury and/or acute respiratory distress syndrome that is propagated by a potent activation of inflammation pathways and localized inflammatory cytokine release. This often leads to prolonged mechanical ventilation and high fractions of inspired oxygen.

The most common indications for lung transplantation include COPD, cystic fibrosis, idiopathic pulmonary fibrosis, primary pulmonary hypertension, and α_1-antitrypsin deficiency. Other less common indications include congenital disease, retransplant (graft failure),

TABLE 41.11 Intraoperative Complications and Management During Liver Transplantation

Complication	Management
Hypothermia	Use heat exchanger, fluid warmer, warming blanket, forced-air units, postoperative ventilation, warm blood flush
Hyperkalemia	Elevated by massive transfusion
	Administer binding resins
	Perform diuresis, dialysis, hyperventilation
	Administer sodium bicarbonate, calcium chloride, insulin, or glucose
Hypocalcemia	Administer calcium chloride or gluconate by central line
	Citrate in blood may bind and thus lower calcium
Oliguria	Maintain adequate volume
	Increase renal perfusion pressure
	Administer mannitol, furosemide, and ethacrynic acid
	Renal replacement therapy
Hypotension	Maintain adequate volume
	Check calcium and magnesium
	Rule out cardiac dysfunction
	Administer vasopressors
	Transfuse blood products if anemia or coagulopathy is present
	Monitor for emboli
	Vena caval compression
Hypertension	Maintain adequate anesthetic depth
	Reduce filling pressures
	Avoid long-acting agents that are used to treat hypertension
Postreperfusion syndrome	Anticipate
	Ensure that volume loading is not excessive
	Administer calcium, vasopressors
Coagulation	Monitor coagulation status throughout massive transfusion
	Administer platelets, fresh frozen plasma and other antidotes as indicated

From Amand MS, et al. Liver transplant. In: Sharpe MD, Gelb AW, eds. *Anesthesia and Transplantation*. Boston: Butterworth-Heinemann; 1999:191; Robertson AC, et al. Anesthesia for liver surgery and transplantation. In: Longnecker DE, et al., eds. *Anesthesiology*. 3rd ed. New York: McGraw Hill; 2018:971–999; Steadman RH, Wray CL. Anesthesia for abdominal organ transplant. In: Gropper MA, et al., eds. *Miller's Anesthesia*. 9th ed. Philadelphia: Elsevier; 2020:1960–1992.

BOX 41.5 Anesthesia Guidelines for Liver Transplant

Preanhepatic Phase
- Modified rapid sequence induction
- Invasive monitors (central venous pressure catheter, arterial catheter, pulmonary catheter, transesophageal echocardiography)
- Forced air and rapid infusers with warmers
- IV antibiotics, baseline laboratory values
- Norepinephrine (or vasopressin) to keep mean BP >60 mm Hg
- Dopamine (or epinephrine) to keep CO at >5 L/min
- Maintain Hgb at >7 g/dL, platelets >40,000, MA (TEG) >45, fibrinogen >100 mg/dL
- Mannitol 0.5 g/kg IV over 1 hr, prior to anticipating clamping
- Just before clamping:
  - IV heparin if TEG is normal or hypercoagulable
  - Increase CVP to 10 cm H_2O with crystalloids
  - 25% albumin in severe hypoalbuminemia

Anhepatic Phase
- IV fluids to keep CVP at approximately 5 cm H_2O
- Crystalloids unless hematocrit is <21%, at which time blood transfusions should be considered
- Norepinephrine and/or vasopressin to keep mean BP >60 mm Hg and CO >5 L/min
- Bicarbonate infusion to correct base deficit
- IV calcium chloride to sustain normocalcemia

Neohepatic Phase
- When SVR is declining, IV vasopressin 1–5-unit bolus to keep mean BP at >60 mm Hg
- Epinephrine 20–100 mcg boluses if heart rate is <60/min
- Euvolemia: CVP of 5–10 cm H_2O
- Dopamine, epinephrine, norepinephrine, and/or vasopressin to keep CO at >5 L/min and mean BP at >60 mm Hg
- TEE if needed for detailed hemodynamic assessment
- Maintain Hgb at >7 g/dL, platelets at >40,000, fibrinogen at >100 mg/dL
- TEG:
  - Protamine 30 mg IV, if R is more than twofold compared to heparinase-R
  - Maintain MA at >45 mm with platelet transfusion
- If Ly30 is >8%, give IV EACA 5 g over 15 min:
  - Consider indication for postoperative mechanical ventilation per usual criteria
  - Transfer to critical care unit

BP, Blood pressure; *CO*, cardiac output; *CVP*, central venous pressure; *EACA*, ε-aminocaproic acid; *Hgb*, hemoglobin; *ICU*, intensive care unit; *Ly30*, the percentage of clot which has actually lysed after 30 min; *MA*, maximum amplitude; *OR*, operating room; *PACU*, postanesthesia care unit; *R*, reagent; *SVR*, systemic vascular resistance; *TEE*, transesophageal echocardiography; *TEG*, thromboelastography.

sarcoidosis, obliterative bronchiolitis, pulmonary vascular disease, occupational lung disease, rheumatoid disease, and bronchiectasis.[43] With advances, many of these indications for transplantation can be treated medically. This can often prevent the patient from being listed for transplant as the disease progress can be stymied. One such instance is primary and idiopathic pulmonary hypertension, which have responded well to new pulmonary vasodilators.

The surgical techniques for lung transplantation include single-lung transplant, en bloc double, sequential double, or heart-lung combined transplantation. The International Society for Heart and Lung Transplantation registry indicates that there has been an increase in double-lung transplants over the past years, whereas the number of single-lung transplants has remained fairly stable. The disease process of the recipient is a major determinant in whether the patient receives a single, bilateral-sequential, or heart-lung transplant. Patients whose transplanted lung will receive most of the ventilation and perfusion often undergo a single-lung transplant. These patients include those with COPD and idiopathic pulmonary fibrosis. This technique allows for an increased number of recipients from the limited donor pool. Patients who suffer from a disease that would contaminate a transplanted lung, such as those with cystic fibrosis, are indicated for a bilateral-sequential single-lung transplant. This technique utilizes bilateral bronchial anastomoses and often cardiopulmonary bypass. The double-lung transplant via a tracheal anastomosis has fallen out of favor as the bronchial anastomoses have fewer complications than the tracheal anastomoses.[46] Heart-lung transplants are generally reserved for those patients with primary cardiac disease complicated by pulmonary pathology, such as in primary pulmonary hypertension and unrepairable congenital defects.

Beginning in 2005, a new system for placing donor lungs with recipients was instituted. The Lung Allocation Score (LAS) allocates lungs primarily based on age, geography, and blood type (ABO) compatibility. The LAS is a score that reflects the waiting-list mortality while avoiding transplanting donor lungs into patients who have a very poor likelihood of survival posttransplant. The new LAS methodology deemphasized the time spent on the waiting list; this has prevented early listing of candidates simply to improve their probability of receiving a transplant. After implementation of the LAS waiting list, mortality initially decreased; however, it is now returning to pre-LAS baseline.[47] Patients who are older and sicker are also more likely to receive transplants than those on the previous lung allocation system. Guidelines developed by the International Society of Heart and Lung Transplantation for recipient selection include (1) patients who have clinically and physiologically severe disease for which medical therapy is ineffective or unavailable, (2) risk of death from lung disease without transplantation is greater than 50% within 2 years, (3) the likelihood of surviving 90 days posttransplantation is greater than 80%, (4) absence of nonpulmonary medical comorbidity that would be expected to limit life expectancy substantially in the first 5 years following transplantation, and (5) a satisfactory psychosocial profile and support system.[48] Guidelines for transplantation by the type of pulmonary disease are noted in Table 41.12.

Contraindications to lung transplantation include active mycobacterium tuberculosis infections, malignancy within the last 2 years, CAD that is not amenable to revascularization, uncorrectable bleeding disorders, BMI of 35 or greater, tobacco use, drug or alcohol dependency, advanced dysfunction of another major organ system (particularly renal, liver, and/or cardiac), progressive neuromuscular disease, noncurable chronic extrapulmonary infections (e.g., HIV, hepatitis B and C), and unresolved psychosocial problems or medical therapy noncompliance.[48] Recipient selection criteria are given in Box 41.6.

TABLE 41.12 Guidelines for Lung Transplantation by Pulmonary Disease

Pathology	Physical Findings
Chronic obstructive pulmonary disease	Patients with a BODE* index of 7–10 or at least one of the following: History of hospitalization for exacerbation associated with acute hypercapnia (P_{CO_2} >50 mm Hg) Pulmonary hypertension or cor pulmonale, or both, despite oxygen therapy FEV_1 <20% predicted and either DLCO <20% predicted or homogeneous distribution of emphysema
Cystic fibrosis and other causes of bronchiectasis	Oxygen-dependent respiratory failure Hypercapnia Pulmonary hypertension
Idiopathic pulmonary fibrosis and NSIP	Histologic or radiographic evidence of usual interstitial pneumonia and any of the following: DLCO <39% predicted ≥10% decrement in FVC during 6 mo of follow-up A decrease in pulse oximetry <88% during a 6-MWT Honeycombing on high-resolution computed tomography (fibrosis score >2) Histologic evidence of NSIP and any of the following: DLCO <35% predicted ≥10% decrement in FVC or 15% decrease in DLCO during 6 mo of follow-up
Pulmonary arterial hypertension	Persistent New York Heart Association class III or IV on maximal medical therapy Low (<350 m) or declining 6-MWT Failing therapy with intravenous epoprostenol or equivalent Cardiac index <2 L/min/m² Right atrial pressure >15 mm Hg

*BODE (Body-mass index, airflow Obstruction, Dyspnea, and Exercise) index is a multidimensional scoring system and capacity index used to test patients who have been diagnosed with chronic obstructive pulmonary disease and to predict long-term outcomes for them.
6-MWT, 6-minute walk test; *DLCO*, diffusing capacity of the lungs for carbon monoxide; *FEV₁*, forced expiratory volume in 1 sec; *FVC*, forced vital capacity; *NSIP*, nonspecific interstitial pneumonia; *P_CO₂*, partial pressure of carbon dioxide in arterial blood.
From Brown LM, et al. Lung transplantation. In: Sellke FW, et al., eds. *Sabiston and Spencer's Surgery of the Chest.* 9th ed. Philadelphia: Elsevier; 2016:240–266.

BOX 41.6 Recipient Selection Criteria

- Clinically and physiologically severe disease
- Medical therapy ineffective or unavailable
- Substantial limitations in activities of daily living
- Limited life expectancy
- Adequate cardiac function without significant coronary disease
- Ambulatory, with rehabilitation potential
- Acceptable nutritional status
- Satisfactory psychosocial profile and emotional support system

From Brown LM, et al. Lung transplantation. In: Sellke FW, et al., eds. *Sabiston and Spencer's Surgery of the Chest.* 9th ed. Philadelphia: Elsevier: 2016:240–266.

Donor selectivity has also changed over the decade. The original criteria were a patient less than 40 years of age, no smoking history, intubation of less than 3 days, no gram-negative rods or fungus on sputum stain, ratio of arterial oxygen partial pressure to fractional inspired oxygen (P:F ratio) of more than 350, and no infiltrates or pneumothorax on chest radiograph.[48] This strict donor selection criteria resulted in an 85% graft rejection rate, thus leading to longer waiting times and higher wait-list mortality.[44] Many centers have liberalized their donor acceptance criteria. Some of these liberalizations include no history of COPD, less than 5 days of intubation rather than 3 days, no fungus on Gram stain, P:F ratio of 250 instead of 350, and minimal chest infiltrates on radiograph.[46] Age of the donor is very case and center specific, with a recent trend of age in excess of 65 years as a relative contraindication only in the context of the other requirements. Ideal donor criteria are listed in Box 41.7.

Preoperative Considerations for Lung Transplantation

A thorough and recent preanesthetic evaluation is crucial for a patient prior to lung transplantation surgery. The preoperative evaluation should focus on the underlying diagnosis, the ventilation/perfusion scan, pulmonary artery pressures, four-chamber cardiac function, and baseline ABGs. These main areas will help the anesthetist direct therapy during transplantation and recovery. This process generally encompasses many specialties while the patient is initially worked up at a regional transplant center for listing. Right heart catheterization and transthoracic echocardiographic exams are crucial components of the preoperative evaluation.[44] Most patients are notified less than 6 hours before the lung transplant is scheduled.[46] Short notice in combination with the fact that many patients may have been on the waiting list for a significant amount of time since their last evaluations make preanesthetic evaluation a challenge in efficiency and prioritization. Depending on timing, repeat labs, radiography, and cardiac echocardiography may be performed with emphasis on not delaying the patient to the operating room. Two to four units of packed RBCs should be immediately available in the operative suite. FFP and platelets should be considered on a case-by-case basis. Anesthetic-specific evaluation should include routine details such as NPO status, previous anesthetic reactions, airway examination, and cardiovascular assessment. It is also important to discuss thoracic epidural analgesia as its use can provide pain relief and improve pulmonary function after transplantation. Epidural analgesia also benefits the patient by attenuating the stress response thereby decreasing chronic pain, pulmonary

complications, and overall patient mortality. Epidural placement can be limited depending on the likelihood of cardiopulmonary bypass (CPB) usage during the case. If CPB is planned, then epidural placement can occur immediately postoperatively once coagulopathies have been corrected. A prominent preoperative comorbidity associated with posttransplant mortality is mechanical ventilation prior to surgery.[49] The primary cause of this is patient deconditioning secondary to the requirement for sedation in order for the patient to tolerate invasive ventilation. There have been an increasing number of patients utilizing extracorporeal life support (ECLS) as a bridge to transplant in patients with pulmonary or cardiopulmonary failure.[48] A major benefit of ECLS (or ECMO) is that these patients can be awake undergoing physical therapy and have the ability to maintain an adequate nutritional status. An anesthetist receiving a patient to the operating room who is on bridge-to-transplant ECMO will still need to manipulate the airway for placement of the double-lumen endotracheal tube (ETT); however, mask ventilation would not be necessary due to oxygenation supplied through the ECMO circuit. Ventilation of the diseased lungs may prove near impossible and is also not required. IV induction and maintenance is preferred as the permeability of the inhalational anesthetics in the ECMO circuit, in particular the oxygenator, is unknown.[45] It is highly likely that patients about to undergo lung transplantation will be highly anxious; it is important, however, to administer anxiolytics sparingly with close monitoring of the patient's respiratory status. These patients often have a limited cardiopulmonary reserve, and overadministration of benzodiazepines and narcotics prior to induction could exacerbate preexisting hypercarbia and hypoxia. This can cause increased strain on the heart, which is likely to already have altered function. However, preoperative anxiety can also cause increased amounts of endogenous catecholamine release that can also worsen right heart function in a patient with some degree of pulmonary hypertension already present.[46] A unique perspective of preanesthetic evaluation in the lung transplant patient is that they are generally brought to the operating room without a guarantee that they will be receiving the donor lungs. It would be prudent to have a discussion outlining the possibility that they may arrive in the operating room, have monitors and lines placed, only to be informed that the donor lungs were not accepted for transplant. The patient will be brought to the operating room; a large bore peripheral IV will be initiated, standard monitors (ECG, noninvasive blood pressure [NIBP], and pulse oximeter oxygen saturation [SpO_2]) will be placed, oxygen will be delivered via nasal cannula, and an arterial line will be placed utilizing strict sterile technique. The donor team will be performing a visual and bronchoscopic inspection of the donor lungs prior to contacting the recipient team that everything is satisfactory to proceed with anesthetic induction and incision.[42]

Intraoperative Considerations for Lung Transplantation

Induction of anesthesia in the lung transplant recipient is complex and requires extreme vigilance. Mechanical ventilation combined with the administration of anesthetic drugs can lead to severe hypotension and even cardiac arrest. Due to patients' preoperative lung function, many will already have some degree of pulmonary hypertension, which makes them vulnerable to a sudden increase in PVR and subsequent right-sided heart failure. This—in combination with positive pressure ventilation, myocardial depressant, and vasodilation related to anesthetic administration, hypoxia, and hypercarbia secondary to apnea/hypoventilation—can cause significant hemodynamic instability during induction. A variety of vasoactive medications should be both available and prepared, including but not limited to phenylephrine, epinephrine, norepinephrine, dopamine, vasopressin, milrinone, and inhaled nitric oxide (iNO). It is prudent that both the surgeon and perfusion team be present in the operating room during induction in the event of profound hemodynamic instability and cardiac arrest.[42,44,45,50] Judicious preoxygenation should occur prior to induction of general anesthesia to optimize intubation. It is important to note that denitrogenation of a patient with end-stage lung disease will be slower because of increased ventilation/perfusion mismatching. It should also be noted that this same phenomenon will cause a greater time period for an amnestic level of inhaled anesthetic to be achieved, leaving the patient at a higher risk for recall immediately postintubation. Due to the emergent nature of these surgeries, the patients often arrive as "full stomachs," necessitating an RSI. Anesthetic agents should be chosen that optimize the patients' condition and have minimal cardiac depressant effects.[46] Induction with etomidate and narcotics, as well as hypnotics such as midazolam, ketamine, and propofol, can all be successfully used to induce general anesthesia. Slow titration of induction agents while closely monitoring the hemodynamic status is crucial. Optimization of hemodynamics through a combination of an inotrope (epinephrine), fluids, and a pulmonary vasodilator (milrinone or iNO) can help offset the detrimental effects of induction. Neuromuscular blockade with succinylcholine or rocuronium is acceptable depending on the need for RSI. There is no evidence that different anesthetic techniques or medications are superior to others. The goal of perioperative anesthetic management is constant maintenance of stable hemodynamics, oxygenation, ventilation, and tissue perfusion.[42] This can be achieved through diligent administration and slow titration of anesthetic drugs. Generally, the airway will be secured utilizing a left-sided double-lumen ETT due to the anatomy of the right upper lobe and the need for a more proximal bronchial anastomosis on the right compared with the left. Although it is technically more difficult, placing a left-sided double-lumen tube also eliminates the problem of obliterating the right upper lobe. A single-lumen ETT is acceptable with the use of a bronchial blocker. A secondary benefit of utilizing a bronchial blocker is that it precludes the necessity of removing a double-lumen tube and replacing it with a single-lumen ETT at the end of surgery. After the airway has been secured and appropriate positioning of the double-lumen ETT is confirmed fiberoptically, further invasive monitoring should be placed. This generally consists of an introducer with PAC and TEE. PAC placement allows for measurement of intracardiac and pulmonary pressures, as well as cardiac output. Some also allow for continuous mixed venous oxygen saturations and continuous cardiac output monitoring. TEE monitoring in combination with pulmonary artery pressures allows the anesthetist real-time assessment of right ventricular (RV) function. As stated previously, this is an area of major concern due to the high likelihood of pulmonary hypertension. iNO is the agent of choice for decreasing RV afterload due to its selective action on the pulmonary vasculature while having minimal effect on systemic vascular resistance.[42] It also allows for quick titration as the patient's condition warrants, whereas milrinone has a longer duration of action. One of the largest drawbacks of iNO is cost. At some institutions inhaled epoprostenol has replaced iNO because of its similar efficacy and cost effectiveness. Antibiotic and immunosuppression therapies are also being administered during this time, and careful communication with the surgical team regarding timing is crucial.

Maintenance of anesthesia can be achieved with either inhaled volatile anesthetics or IV anesthesia. Isoflurane has been implicated in improvement in ischemic preconditioning for multiple organs[44]; however, there is debate on the best maintenance drug. Mechanical ventilation should be tailored to each patient's preoperative pulmonary diagnosis. Preoperative ABG measurements should be utilized to guide ventilator management. Utilizing this technique can lead to permissive hypercapnia, allowing the patient's partial pressure

of arterial carbon dioxide ($Paco_2$) level to more closely correlate to preanesthetic level. The patient will likely tolerate this well, and it has been shown to reduce the risk of pulmonary barotrauma and dynamic hyperinflation.[42] Other methods for reducing barotrauma and hyperinflation include maximizing expiratory time through lower respiratory rates and tidal volumes, as well as intermittent circuit disconnection, to aid in complete exhalation. Dynamic hyperinflation can occur when gas trapping causes overinflation of the lungs, thus leading to an increase in intrathoracic pressure or auto–positive end-expiratory pressure (PEEP). Auto-PEEP impedes venous return to the right ventricle and may produce cardiac tamponade physiology by directly compressing the heart if it is not recognized and treated. PEEP must be administered carefully in these patients with constant attention paid to the hemodynamic effects. Extrinsic PEEP from the ventilator can compound intrinsic auto-PEEP while also compounding the effects of dynamic hyperinflation.[46] Compounding ventilator management will be needed for one-lung ventilation shortly after incision. Once single-lung ventilation is initiated the degree of intrapulmonary shunt will increase, as blood flow will continue to a varying degree to the nonventilated lung. Maintaining adequate ventilation during this time is achieved in the same manner it would in nontransplant thoracic anesthetics. Monitoring of serial ABGs for worsening of the ventilation/perfusion (V/Q) mismatch is important, and utilization of inotropic and vasoactive agents can aid in recovery. Shortly after this point, the surgeons will clamp the pulmonary artery, which may help improve the intrapulmonary shunt. At this point, the patient is on maximal vasoactive and mechanical support and, if still unstable, cardiopulmonary bypass should be discussed and possibly implemented. Some of the concerns with instituting CPB include increased blood loss, increased chance of the patient requiring a blood transfusion, increased V/Q mismatching, and graft dysfunction. Despite these increased risks there is no documented increase in overall mortality when CPB is used.[50] Patients with more severe pulmonary hypertension are more likely to need CPB. If the patient remains hemodynamically stable following pulmonary artery clamping, then CPB can be avoided. A secondary cause of cardiovascular instability is surgical manipulation and lifting of the heart by the surgeons for adequate exposure. Careful communication between the anesthetist and surgeon is required in the event of sudden hemodynamic changes. Ceasing in manipulation and allowing the patient time to recover before proceeding with the surgical dissection is crucial. During one-lung ventilation, several confounding factors affect the heart. One factor is hypotension from decreased RV preload in combination with RV dysfunction secondary to increased PVR. Fluid administration can improve preload while administering 100% fraction of inspired oxygen (Fio_2), and pulmonary vasodilators such as iNO can assist in reducing afterload (PVR).

After the bronchial and vascular anastomoses are complete, the remaining pneumoplegia is washed out using retrograde flow through the grafted lung. It is important that extreme care is taken during gentle reinflation of the donor lung. Rapid reexpansion can cause barotrauma with resulting pneumothorax. The anesthetist should be prepared for severe hypotension as the lung is reperfused due to the washout of metabolites from the ischemic lung. This can transiently require high doses of inotropic support. Coronary air embolus is not uncommon and must be monitored closely. Due to its anatomic location, the right coronary artery is particularly prone to air embolism. The right coronary artery supplies blood to the right ventricle, thereby compounding previous RV concerns. ST segment depression can occur, and these changes usually last less than 15 minutes.[50] If hypotension and cardiac dysfunction persist, the anesthetist and surgeon should search for a different etiology. The need for CPB or ECMO support is continuously monitored. If the patient is having a bilateral sequential lung transplant, then the process is repeated on the contralateral lung.

Reperfusion injury can also occur and lead to acute injury of the grafted lung. This is characterized by severe hypoxemia, pulmonary edema, impaired gas exchange, and increased pulmonary capillary permeability all generally occurring within the first 24 hours after transplant.[50] Causes of reperfusion injury have been postulated as poor preservation during transport, loss of lymphatic drainage, inflammatory mediators, and oxygen-related free radicals. Gentle ventilation with low-level PEEP to encourage alveolar recruitment and prevent atelectasis is important. iNO (if beneficial intraoperatively) should be maintained after reperfusion of the donor lung to aid in providing an optimal environment for reperfusion. Fluid management should be directed to maintain cardiac output while minimizing the risk of pulmonary edema. In general, it can safely be assumed that lung transplant teams will want their patients "dry," which has led to a general practice of limiting intraoperative crystalloid administration. Ventilation strategies should focus on minimizing peak inspiratory pressures while assuring adequate gas exchange. Ventilation with higher inflation pressures, but not necessarily higher tidal volumes, has been significantly associated with poorer outcomes after lung transplantation.[51]

Postoperative Considerations for Lung Transplantation

The patient will be taken directly from the operating room to the ICU and remain intubated and mechanically ventilated. Early postoperative care focuses on ventilator support and weaning, fluid and hemodynamic management, immunosuppression, detection of early rejection, and prevention/treatment of infection. Ventilation and weaning techniques are standard after single or bilateral lung transplantation except in certain circumstances. A patient post single-lung transplant for emphysema or COPD would not benefit from PEEP as it may cause overinflation of the native lung.[52] In many patients who do not experience difficulty with ventilation after transplant, weaning can proceed quickly during the first few hours to days post-ICU admission. After the patient is hemodynamically stable and able to be extubated, the primary focus of care shifts to pulmonary rehabilitation, toileting, pain management, physical therapy, immunosuppression, and infection prevention/treatment. Epidural pain management can be left in for days after surgery and is often an important aid in early extubation, inflammation control, and physical rehabilitation. The epidural catheter allows for titration of local anesthetic levels depending on each patient's individual pain response. Generally, it is pulled within a few days of transplant to limit the risk of infection. Acute rejection is a major cause of morbidity, especially in the first 100 days posttransplantation. During the first month postoperatively, most mortality is generally the result of primary graft failure, noncytomegalovirus (non-CMV) infections, cardiovascular complications, and technical problems.[50] Within 5 years of transplantation, 49% of patients develop bronchiolitis obliterans syndrome (BOS).[42] BOS is progressive and nonreversible. The hallmark clinical feature of BOS is the development of airway obstruction with a reduction of forced expiratory volume 1 (FEV_1) that does not respond to bronchodilators. Treatment involves augmenting the immunosuppressant therapy. Unfortunately, most patients either acquire progressive BOS or a lethal opportunistic infection as a result of the augmented immunosuppression.[53] Some risk factors for BOS are listed in Box 41.8. Patients are prone to infection due to immunosuppression, decreased mucociliary action, and decreased cough reflex. Anastomotic airway complications occur in approximately 20% of patients after lung transplantation and tend to be persistent, chronic problems that affect survival.

BOX 41.8   Risk Factors for Bronchiolitis Obliterans Syndrome After Lung Transplantation

Probable Role
- Acute rejection
- Cytomegalovirus (CMV) pneumonitis
- Human leukocyte antigen mismatching
- Lymphocytic bronchitis/bronchiolitis
- Noncompliance with medications
- Primary graft dysfunction

Potential Role
- *Aspergillus* spp. colonization of lower airways
- Aspiration
- CMV infection (without pneumonitis)
- Donor antigen-specific activity
- Epstein-Barr virus reactivation
- Etiology of native lung disease
- Gastroesophageal reflux
- Older donor age
- Pneumonia (gram negatives, gram positives, fungi)
- Prolonged allograft ischemia
- Recurrent infection other than CMV

From Hayes Jr D. A review of bronchiolitis obliterans syndrome and therapeutic strategies. *J Cardiothorac Surg.* 2011;6:92.

INTESTINAL TRANSPLANTATION

Intestinal transplantation is a complex surgery and is performed less frequently than other organ transplants. Intestinal transplant is indicated in treating patients who have endured intestinal failure and who have failed maximal medical therapy options, including total parenteral nutrition (TPN). The Intestinal Transplant Registry (ITR) has reported the three most common underlying disease states leading to transplantation in children as gastroschisis (21%), volvulus (17%), and necrotizing enterocolitis (12%). In contrast, the most common indications for intestinal transplantation in adults are ischemia (23%), Crohn disease (14%), and trauma (10%). Although the most common indications fall under the category of short bowel syndrome (SBS), children and adults may suffer from diseases that result in dysmotility or malabsorption, resulting in poor enteral function. For patients with SBS, the remnant intestinal length and presence or absence of an ileocecal valve have been identified as predictive factors as to whether rehabilitation will be successful. The main indication for transplantation in children and adults is TPN-dependent SBS complicated by progressive liver disease. Combined intestine-liver transplantation is the only alternative for patients in whom ESLD has developed. Isolated intestinal transplantation may be considered for patients with clinically significant liver disease that has not yet progressed to cirrhosis.[54] These patients have had previous extensive intestinal resections. Significant advances have been made in both medical treatment and surgical procedures, which has led to a decrease in the overall number of intestinal transplants over the past decade. There has also been a decrease in the number of patients on the intestinal transplant waiting list. Only 73 adults and 35 pediatric patients received intestinal transplants in 2013 according to the Scientific Registry of Transplant Recipients.[55] The vast majority of patients who remain on the waiting list are pediatric patients.

There are very few academic medical centers that perform intestinal transplantation. The care for these patients in the preoperative, intraoperative, and postoperative periods is similar to that of other abdominal organ transplant patients. Thorough preoperative assessment is the key to determining the patients' underlying condition and comorbidities and developing a comprehensive anesthetic plan. A midline incision is often performed. Invasive monitoring is helpful in terms of monitoring hemodynamics, as well as assessment of electrolytes, blood counts, coagulation, and ABGs. Close monitoring of the patients' volume status is very important in intestinal transplantation. There can be significant fluid shifts during these surgeries along with the potential for significant blood loss. Maintaining euvolemia with a combination of crystalloid and colloid is important as excess edema and fluid administration may cause graft edema and can cause deleterious effects, including abdominal compartment syndrome.[55] Although recipient survival rates have improved since the early days of intestinal transplantation (most notably 1-year survival), survival rates have plateaued, and a significant dropoff in survival is seen after 5 years, often related to chronic organ rejection.[54,55]

Postoperative pain management can be challenging and may include IV analgesia, PCA, and/or thoracic epidural analgesia. Care should be taken to ensure the patient does not have a coagulopathy prior to placement of the epidural. It should also be noted that psychological support is imperative and can improve overall patient outcomes.[55]

ANESTHETIC CONSIDERATIONS FOR THE ORGAN DONOR

Care of the organ donor is a very specialized process that requires knowledge of the patient's underlying condition and the plan for organ procurement. Each institution frequently has a protocol for management of the organ donor, and these protocols are often guided by the transplant surgeon and the transplant coordinators based on what organs are viable for procurement. Other factors include the type of donation, including DCD or DBD. As discussed previously, DBD is the more traditional method; however, DCD is becoming more prevalent based on the reasons described earlier in the chapter. Even with the evolution of DCD, there continues to be a significant discrepancy between the number of patients awaiting transplant and the number of organs available (see Fig. 41.1). As of 2020, there were nearly 121,000 patients awaiting an organ transplant. In 2019, 39,719 transplants were performed. The vast majority of transplants were from deceased donors (32,322). Of the 19,267 total donors, 11,870 were deceased and 7397 were living.[27]

Although very few publications describe anesthetic implications for this patient population, there is a significant body of literature available that describes management of these patients in the ICU prior to organ procurement. It is important for the anesthetist to understand the baseline condition of the patient and to be aware of the physiology and pathophysiology associated with the donor patient as it relates to the individual organs that may be procured. There are a multitude of physiologic changes that occur in the donor, and they can vary based on whether brain death has occurred as opposed to DCD. Pathophysiologic changes associated with brain death include complications at the cellular level and have a profound effect on all organ systems. Some of the significant signs and symptoms and pathophysiologic changes include hyper- or hypotension, bradycardia or other arrhythmias, pulmonary edema, disseminated intravascular coagulation (DIC), hyperglycemia, diabetes insipidus, and hypothermia.

DCD donors are a specialized category and do not meet the criteria for DBD. DCD donors often experience severe brain damage or spinal cord injury that is not reversible but is unlikely to progress to brain death. The likelihood of a meaningful quality of life is extremely poor. These cases are termed uncontrolled DCD versus controlled DCD and are further divided into five categories (Table 41.13). Categories 1, 2, and 5 are considered uncontrolled DCD due to the patient experiencing an unanticipated cardiac arrest.

It should be noted that the transplant team must not have any input on the discussion regarding withdrawal of life support. The medical team must discuss the situation with the potential donor's family, and after a decision is made to withdraw support, an independent physician who is not involved in transplantation must determine cessation of cardiac function. After confirmation of pulseless activity via physical examination and/or absence of arterial blood pressure waveform over a period of several minutes, death may be declared, and organ procurement may commence. Individual institutions may have other criteria that guide their practice for DCD, and the anesthetist should be familiar with that specific institution's guidelines.

Due to many physiologic alterations in patients awaiting organ procurement, management of these patients before and during the procurement phase can prove to be challenging. Hemodynamic stabilization is critical in providing an optimum environment for the transplant to occur and for preserving optimal function of the procured organs. Hypertension may be present and should be treated with a goal of maintaining MAP between 60 and 100.[27] Hypotension is more detrimental and may be more difficult to manage. Vasoactive medications may be used in either setting to ensure optimal blood pressure; however, they should be limited as much as hemodynamically possible. Care should be taken to ensure adequate fluid balance. Fluid therapy should be aimed at euvolemia as excessive fluid therapy may have detrimental effects, especially in lung transplant patients.[29] Invasive monitoring, including arterial line and monitoring CVP, may help guide volume therapy and allow for optimal monitoring of the patient's hemodynamics. Communication between the anesthetist, surgical team, and transplant coordinator is vital to ensuring efficiency and optimal quality of the organs. Once the aorta is cross-clamped and the organs are perfused with hypothermic solution, mechanical ventilation is ceased, and anesthetic management of the patient is stopped. The organ procurement coordinator is generally a resource during this time and can ensure appropriate measures are taken.[56-58]

Anesthetic Considerations for the Living Organ Donor

Another type of organ donation is where a living donor provides an organ to a friend or family member in a directed fashion. This type of donation is on the rise and has some advantages in that a thorough review of each patient's medical, social, and psychological history

TABLE 41.13   Categories of Controlled and Uncontrolled Donation via Cardiac Death

Category 1	Category 2	Category 3	Category 4	Category 5
Patient is dead on arrival to the hospital	Patient experiences devastating injury and has been unsuccessfully resuscitated	*Controlled DCD A patient where cardiac arrest is imminent	*Controlled DCD A brain death donor in cardiac arrest	Unexpected cardiac arrest in the intensive care unit

*Controlled DCD occurs when a planned withdrawal of life support occurs, and the transplant team is on standby and ready for rapid organ recovery.
DCD, Donation after cardiac death.

may be performed. It may be scheduled as an elective procedure and in a controlled and timely fashion to reduce the cold ischemia time related to organ procurement. The anesthetic considerations for each type of transplant are similar to those already discussed. The major difference is that most often the donor for living organ donation is generally in better health. Some of the concerns related to living donation include the potential decreased quality of life and medical risks associated with altered physiology from the donated organ. There is also a financial impact associated with donation that has to be considered. Overall, living donor organ donation can increase the number of donated organs and has shown to have some advantages over deceased donor transplantation, especially in liver transplant.[28]

Organ donation has evolved significantly over the years, and improved technology and pharmacology will continue to enhance transplantation. It should also be noted that increased awareness toward health prevention and maintenance may also continue to play an important role in potentially reducing the number of transplants needed.

SUMMARY

The ability to transplant organs has been a remarkable medical success story that has evolved over the past 100 years. Patients who previously had little hope can now lead active and near-normal lives thanks to these lifesaving procedures. Our understanding of the immune response to transplanted tissues and the development of successful strategies to control and prevent rejection are instrumental in this success. Surgical and anesthetic management of the transplant patient requires constant monitoring and adjustment for a successful outcome. Continued strategies to increase organ availability and decrease the risks of immunosuppression side effects and disease recurrence will be vital for continued enhancements in organ transplantation. The principles outlined in this chapter will educate the clinician on the current approach to management of these patients.

REFERENCES

 For a complete list of references for this chapter, scan this QR code with any smartphone code reader app, or visit the following URL: http://booksite.elsevier.com/9780323711944/

42

Outpatient Anesthesia

Robyn C. Ward

The concept of outpatient anesthesia (to facilitate outpatient surgery) is commonly used in todays anesthesia practice. The terms outpatient surgery or outpatient anesthesia is frequently used interchangeably with the terms ambulatory surgery or ambulatory anesthesia. It was first introduced in dental offices with the administration of nitrous oxide. Physician offices were next to offer this type of service for superficial procedures, which required at most the administration of local anesthesia. In 1909, Nicoll[1] first reported on 8988 outpatient surgical procedures performed at the Glasgow Royal Hospital for Sick Children. In 1916, in Sioux City, Iowa, Waters[2] opened the first freestanding unit designed for outpatient surgery.

The evolution of, and demand for, outpatient care has not slowed since first described by these pioneers. Surgical innovation, new anesthetic drugs and techniques, patient and provider preference, and changes in insurance carrier demands have increased the type and number of procedures performed at ambulatory care centers or traditional hospital operating rooms. The number of outpatient procedures in the United States has increased from an estimated 35 million outpatient surgical procedures in 2006 to 129 million in 2018. By 2023, outpatient surgical procedures are expected to increase to 144 million. Outpatient surgical procedures in the United States that are most common include dental, orthopedic, gastrointestinal, ophthalmic, ear/nose/throat, gynecologic, cosmetic, cardiovascular, and urologic surgeries.[3] In addition, difficult procedures performed even on patients with complex medical conditions are more routinely being performed on an outpatient basis. It is the responsibility of the attending anesthesia provider to ensure that these complex medical conditions are managed optimally before, during, and after the procedure.

It is expected that the patient will enter the outpatient surgical care facility, undergo the procedure, and then be released without needing an overnight stay. Outpatient surgery, in addition to office-based and freestanding ambulatory surgery centers, includes the "23-hour observation" patient, who may be admitted to the inpatient or overnight facility, yet is discharged before staying in the hospital 24 hours. Surgical procedures requiring the expertise of an anesthesia provider in the office setting are becoming increasingly popular. Office-based surgery can be performed more efficiently and at a lower cost than surgery performed in the hospital.[4] A trend from 2010 to 2019 shows a consistent percentage of operative procedures performed in office-based settings. Today, approximately 15% to 20% of operative procedures are completed in the office-based procedure category.[5-6] Optimal anesthesia and surgical techniques for office-based surgery are similar to ambulatory procedures performed at traditional ambulatory surgical centers. Although office-based surgery can be performed safely, it is not without risk. Current issues of discussion include patient and procedure selection, recovery, complication management, perioperative management, and facility requirements.[5,7] Office-based anesthesia practice standards and guidelines have been developed by the American Association of Nurse Anesthetists (AANA),[8] the American Society of Anesthesiologists (ASA),[9] and the Joint Commission.[10]

FEATURES OF OUTPATIENT SURGERY

Advantages

Financial

An advantage of ambulatory surgical settings has been the economic benefit for consumers, third-party payers, and medical facilities. Patients may benefit not only from reduced medical cost but also from minimized costs of outside child care and from resumption of normal living activities at an earlier time. Third-party payers concerned about cost containment are increasingly identifying procedures that may be performed only in the outpatient setting. Projected cost savings by the year 2022 range from $4.2 billion to $9.4 billion, compared to $2.3 billion in the year 2011.[11] Ambulatory centers, secondary to their design, facility layout, and patient selection, tend to operate more efficiently than hospital-based operating theaters in regard to surgical volume.

Medical

One medical advantage of ambulatory surgery is the increased availability of hospital beds for those patients who require hospital admission. For patients who are susceptible to infection (e.g., children, immunosuppressed patients, cancer patients, and transplant recipients), minimizing time and contact in the inpatient hospital setting may decrease the risk of nosocomial infections.[12]

Patient Satisfaction

Patients report greater satisfaction with outpatient procedures because of shorter waiting times and lower costs associated with less overnight admssions.[13,14] Delays secondary to lack of available beds, as seen with inpatient facilities, are less likely to occur. In addition, patients report satisfaction in the ease of scheduling and recovering in the comfort of their own home.

Social

Children benefit from outpatient surgery because it minimizes separation from parents and causes less disruption in a child's feeding schedule. The continued presence of and care offered by the parents is especially beneficial for children with mental or physical impairments.[15] Geriatric patients show better cognitive and physical capacity when separation from familiar surroundings and family is minimized. The elderly are better able to maintain their normal living routines (e.g., diet, medication, and sleep pattern). Postoperative cognitive dysfunction is decreased in geriatric patients undergoing outpatient procedures because they receive less medication and are returned to a familiar environment sooner than their inpatient counterparts.[16,17]

Staffing

The ambulatory surgery setting is more convenient than the inpatient surgery setting for the staff because it offers more efficient use of time, uniform work schedules, and more predictable surgical outcomes.

Disadvantages

The outpatient setting may have several disadvantages:

- Depending on the facility, the degree of patient privacy may be less than that in the inpatient setting.
- The patient may be required to make multiple trips to the physician's office or the ambulatory setting for evaluation and screening.
- Adequate home care must be ensured once the patient is discharged from the facility after surgery.
- Compliance and efficacy related to preoperative and postoperative instructions may not be as good as when the patient is admitted to the hospital before surgery.
- Because of the emphasis on efficiency, children have less time to adapt to the surgical setting than they would as inpatients.
- Observation time and monitoring for the occurrence of adverse events are decreased in the outpatient setting.
- Management of complications can be problematic at a freestanding ambulatory or office-based facility secondary to a lack of resources, and complications and emergencies will require transfer to a nearby hospital.

Demographic Considerations

Patient Age

Patients of any age can receive outpatient anesthesia; age should not be a limiting factor when determining appropriateness for ambulatory procedures. Approximately 6% of outpatients are younger than 15 years, and more than 14% are at least 75 years of age.[3] More than 60% of all anesthesia, administered for pediatric surgery, is performed on an outpatient basis.[15]

Surgical Time

Earlier guidelines recommended limiting the amount of time of an outpatient surgery to less than 1.5 to 2 hours.[18] The reasoning was that the longer surgery lasts, the more likely patients will experience severe pain or vomiting.[19,20] Surgical time exceeding 2 hours was also thought to be a strong predictor for delayed discharge and unplanned hospital admission postoperatively.[21] However, other factors such as the skill of the surgeon, the type of surgery performed, the patient's condition, and the anesthetic technique used must be considered. Arbitrarily limiting the length of surgery to less than 2 hours is no longer considered necessary; procedures exceeding 4 hours are routinely performed without complications in ambulatory centers.

Suitable Procedures

The list of procedures suitable for the ambulatory setting is constantly evolving. Endoscopy of the large and small intestine is the most common type of outpatient procedure, and ophthalmologic surgery is the second most common.[3] The outpatient surgical procedure should not involve extensive blood loss or physiologic shifts of considerable fluid volumes because these processes necessitate protracted patient observation and hydration. In the past, the potential for blood transfusion implied the need for the procedure to be conducted at an inpatient facility. Now, the increasing popularity of patient blood management for decreasing possible transfusion needs has facilitated outpatient surgery.[22]

The list of surgical procedures deemed acceptable for outpatient surgery is ever expanding. Facilities with a 23-hour observation area designed for extended patient assessment are often the desired locations for outpatient tonsillectomy and higher risk procedures.

Procedures requiring prolonged immobilization are best conducted on an inpatient basis. For procedures associated with postoperative discomfort, the appropriate inclusion of peripheral nerve block techniques and arrangements for parenteral opioid therapy in the home may be made, provided that adequate pain relief can be achieved with safe doses of opioids.

PATIENT SELECTION

Proper patient selection minimizes the number of hospital admissions that follow outpatient surgery. Primary predictors of unanticipated hospital admission (0.08% of all ambulatory cases) include age, frailty, and ASA status, as well as the type of surgical procedure and subsequent complications, such as nausea and vomiting, pain, or significant operative fluid shifts or blood loss.[7] Evaluation of patients to determine who is appropriate for outpatient surgery and anesthesia requires consensus and cooperation between the surgical and anesthesia staff. Factors to consider in determining the suitability of a patient for outpatient surgery include the following:

- *The anticipated surgical procedure for the patient.* The proposed surgery should have an insignificant incidence of intraoperative and postoperative problems and should not require intense postoperative patient management.
- *The physical and psychosocial health of the patient.* The patient is ideally in one's usual good health, or if ill, the condition should be well controlled. A reduction in postoperative complications has been shown if the patient's medical condition is stable for at least 3 months before surgery.[23] The patient and family should be receptive to the outpatient philosophy and the perioperative adaptations that will be required of them.
- *The surgeon's skills and cooperation.* Early referral to the anesthesia department for patients of questionable appropriateness helps streamline the outpatient process and minimize delays on the day of surgery.

Selection Criteria

Acute Substance Abuse

The patient with a history of substance abuse should be evaluated before the day of surgery. Counseling for such patients includes the warning that preoperative substance abuse will lead to cancellation of the surgery. A distinction between long-term and acute substance abuse must be made. A urinary drug screen should be performed in patients suspected of substance abuse. The patient with signs of acute substance intoxication is an inappropriate ambulatory surgery candidate because of the increased likelihood of impaired autonomic and cardiovascular responses. The surgery should be rescheduled after the patient is detoxified and treated. Patient management strategies should emphasize methods of minimizing postoperative pain because substance abusers are typically intolerant to pain. Regional or local anesthetic techniques, if their use is suitable to the surgeon and appropriate for the type of operation being performed, may be used if the patient wishes to abstain from sedatives and opioids. Postoperatively, pain may be minimized by using local wound infiltration, regional techniques, and the prophylactic use of nonsteroidal analgesics. Placing a catheter in the wound and instilling local anesthesia, either continuously or intermittently, has been shown to prolong pain relief and improve patient satisfaction and should be considered for this patient population.[24]

Age

Patient age by itself should not be the deciding factor for outpatient suitability. Meridy[25] retrospectively examined the charts of patients ranging in age from 9 months to 92 years and noted that most perioperative complications occurred in the 20- to 49-year age group. Children less than 2 years have a higher unanticipated hospital admission rate following surgery.[26] Patients older than 85 years, who required multiple hospitalizations within 6 months of the surgery, have been shown to have an increased risk of unanticipated hospitalization and death after outpatient surgery.[27] Although multiple medications and preexisting comorbidities (i.e., hypertension, cardiac disease, and diabetes) are more likely in the elderly, with proper care they may still undergo successful outpatient surgery.[28]

Premature infant. The premature infant (gestational age of ≤37 weeks at birth) is an inappropriate candidate for outpatient surgery because of potential physiologic aberrations. The premature infant may:

- Exhibit anemia
- Not have fully developed gag reflexes (and thus be more prone to aspiration of liquid or solid food)
- Have immature temperature control and be susceptible to the effects of hypothermia, which could contribute to postoperative apnea
- Demonstrate immature brainstem functioning, which predisposes the infant to pathologic respiratory conditions

The infant with a hemoglobin value less than the predicted normal value for that age will require additional evaluation before surgery. Hemoglobin values in the premature infant may drop to between 7 and 8 g/100 mL, at approximately 1 to 3 months after birth.[29] The presence of anemia (hematocrit <30%) may increase the incidence of apnea in the newborn.[30] Some investigators have recommended delaying elective surgery until the hematocrit is increased to greater than 30% through supplementation of iron intake.[31]

In the perioperative period, the preterm infant is at greater risk for developing respiratory complications, including apnea, than the full-term infant.[32] The preterm infant is susceptible to short apnea (6–15 seconds), prolonged apnea (>15 seconds), or periodic breathing (three or more periods of apnea of 3–15 seconds separated by <20 seconds of normal respiration). Short or prolonged apnea and periodic breathing predispose the infant to hypoxemia and bradycardia. An obstructive component that leads to quicker oxyhemoglobin desaturation appears to be part of postoperative apnea in these infants.[33] These infants have developed prolonged apnea as late as 12 hours after surgery.[32]

The older the infant, the less likely that respiratory complications such as apnea will occur. In evaluating the suitability of a former preterm infant for outpatient surgery, conservative measures are best; inpatient status should be assigned if significant concerns exist. These patients benefit from the intensive monitoring available in the inpatient setting. Much discussion has been held as to the postgestational age (gestational age plus postnatal age) at which the former preterm infant may safely undergo outpatient anesthesia. Healthy former premature infants whose postgestational age is less than 60 weeks should be admitted to the hospital for extended monitoring.[34,35] Postoperative apnea has been described even in the full-term infant.[36] The ability to exactly predict the susceptibility of an infant to postoperative apnea is lacking. Patients should be evaluated individually for appropriateness for outpatient surgery, and consideration should be given to growth and development, feeding problems, upper respiratory tract infections (URTIs), apneic history, and disorders of metabolic, endocrine, neurologic, or cardiac systems. All infants with a history of prematurity should be closely observed for signs of apnea and bradycardia. If any of these signs are evidenced in the postanesthesia care unit, patients should be admitted and observed. An infant with a history of apnea or bradycardia must be apnea free and without monitoring for at least 6 months to be considered for outpatient surgery. Efforts should be made to schedule surgery for these patients as early in the day as possible to allow for extended observation time.[37]

Beyond simply delaying surgery, attempts to minimize the likelihood of postoperative apnea in susceptible infants have been examined. Spinal anesthesia without sedation resulted in less prolonged apnea, oxyhemoglobin desaturation, and bradycardia than did general anesthesia or spinal anesthesia with ketamine sedation.[31] However, apnea and delayed respiratory failure have been reported in children who have had spinal or caudal anesthesia.[38] Infants treated with endotracheal intubation or mechanical ventilation (or both) for respiratory distress syndrome at birth have been shown to have abnormal arterial blood gas values and abnormal pulmonary function results as late as 1 year after treatment.[39] Infants exhibiting signs of bronchopulmonary dysplasia should not be considered for outpatient surgery,[40] as they are at risk of sudden infant death.[41]

Infants with a history of apneic events or who have siblings who developed sudden infant death syndrome (SIDS) are at risk for SIDS. The greatest at-risk age for the development of SIDS is between 1 month and 1 year of age.[42] In infants who have lost a sibling to SIDS, the risk of dying from the same syndrome is four to five times greater than that of the general population.[43] Patients at risk for the development of SIDS should not be considered for outpatient surgical procedures until they are at least 6 months to 1 year of age.[44]

Full-term infant. Healthy, full-term infants (>37 weeks of gestational age at birth) can be considered for minor outpatient surgery. Full-term infants with histories of apneic episodes, failure to thrive, and feeding difficulties are not suitable candidates for outpatient surgery. Infants with a history of respiratory difficulties at birth are not suitable outpatient candidates unless they are free of respiratory symptoms at the time of surgery and at the time of hospital discharge.[44] There are no formal practice guidelines from major anesthesia or pediatric organizations regarding outpatient surgery in infants. However, individual hospitals frequently establish a cutoff age of 60 weeks of postconceptual age in infants born before 37 weeks, and they consider factors such as anemia, prior apnea, and coexisting disease. Postoperative monitoring recommendations range from 12- to 24-hour admission for cardiorespiratory monitoring. Some facilities also restrict day surgery procedures for term infants to only those infants older than 50-52 weeks of postconceptual age. The facilities may also require a longer observation period (e.g., 4 hours) in phase II recovery.[45] Some evidence-based suggested guidelines are listed in Box 42.1.[45-47]

Geriatric patients. The decision of whether to perform ambulatory surgery on a geriatric patient (age ≥65 years) should be individualized and based on physiologic age rather than on chronologic age. Existing medical problems are a concern when considering the geriatric patient for outpatient surgery. There are more concomitant age-related diseases that should be optimally managed preoperatively in this group of patients. Patient age exceeding 80 years is a predictor of hospital admissions after outpatient surgery.[48,49] Thoughtful preoperative planning for the elderly patient's postdischarge care is paramount to ensure a safe and successful outpatient experience. The elderly population presenting for outpatient surgery has increased dramatically and will continue to increase as the population ages.[50] Appropriate home care and transportation to and from the outpatient center with a responsible caregiver must be ensured.

Special Considerations

Convulsive disorders. Surgery for patients with seizure disorders should be scheduled early in the day so patients can be observed for 4 to 8 hours after the operation before they are discharged. It is important to establish the patients' ability to maintain their schedule for anticonvulsant medications. Patients with uncontrolled seizure

BOX 42.1   Suggested Guidelines for Outpatient Surgery in Infants

- Preoperative evaluation is essential successful ambulatory anesthesia and surgery. Possible pediatric issues to consider include asthma, respiratory infections, prematurity, congenital syndromes, sleep apnea, congenital heart disease, and obesity.
- Identifying and managing risk factors helps to improve outcomes.
- Appropriate short-acting anesthetic agents may facilitate emergence and discharge.
- When possible, regional anesthetic techniques and nonopioid analgesics should be used instead of opioids.
- Former premature infants should be admitted for observation unless they are over 60 weeks of postconceptual age (depending on degree of prematurity) and are without anemia, ongoing apnea, or other significant medical problems. Infants meeting these criteria also need to have had an uneventful anesthetic and recovery room course before consideration of discharge. Full-term infants <50–52 weeks of postconceptual age who exhibit any respiratory abnormality should be observed overnight, as well as certain children with sleep apnea following a tonsillectomy.
- Term infants are acceptable for outpatient procedures providing they are otherwise healthy, the procedure is not likely to result in significant physiologic changes or postoperative pain requiring opioid medications, and the anesthetic proceeds uneventfully. It may be prudent to monitor these patients in the recovery area for several hours postoperatively.
- All infants should be cared for in a facility with adequate and appropriately sized equipment, with medical and nursing staff who have appropriate expertise in caring for this age group.

From Everett LL. How young is the youngest infant for output surgery? In: Fleischer LA, ed. *Evidence-Based Practice of Anesthesiology.* 3rd ed. Philadelphia: Elsevier Saunders; 2013:523–528; Butz SF. Pediatric ambulatory anesthesia challenges. *Anesthesiol Clin.* 2019;37(2): 289–300.

activity are not deemed appropriate for outpatient surgery by most institutions.

Cystic fibrosis. The extent of pulmonary involvement is the primary determinant of appropriateness for ambulatory surgery in patients with cystic fibrosis. Such patients should be evaluated several days before the proposed surgery; patients with symptomatic respiratory distress are better treated in an inpatient setting, where appropriate respiratory care management and hydration can be administered.[51] Protective airway measures should be instituted in the cystic fibrosis patient secondary to an increased risk of gastroesophageal reflux disease and pulmonary aspiration.[52]

Malignant hyperthermia susceptibility. Malignant hyperthermia (MH) susceptibility is impossible to predict because it occurs in phenotypically normal individuals.[53] A MH-susceptible patient is defined as having one or more of the following:[54-60]

1. A previous episode of MH
2. Masseter muscle rigidity with previous anesthesia
3. A first-degree relative with history of a MH episode or positive muscle biopsy
4. Diseases with known mutations on chromosome 19; these may include, but are not limited to, central core myopathy, King-Denborough syndrome, Native American myopathy, and hypokalemic periodic paralysis
5. Patients with heat-induced rhabdomyolysis

Diseases not associated with MH susceptibility include mitochondrial myopathies, Noonan syndrome, osteogenesis imperfect, and neuroleptic malignant syndrome.[53]

The MH-susceptible patient who has received a trigger-free uneventful anesthetic does not require overnight hospitalization based exclusively on being MH susceptible. The ambulatory facility should have a fully stocked emergency MH cart, the requisite monitoring and resuscitation capabilities, including a minimum of 36 vials of dantrolene sodium, for managing the MH patient.[60] Ryanodex is a form of dantrolene sodium that is easier and faster to mix with sterile water, and may be available is some facilities. An activated charcoal filter system (Vapor Clean) can be placed on the inspiratory and expiratory limbs of the anesthesia circuit to reduce the volatile anesthetic concentration to less than 5 parts per million (ppm) in as little as 2 minutes.[61,62] A point-of-care monitor (capable of measuring blood gases and electrolytes) and urinalysis with a dipstick (to detect myoglobinuria) are recommended monitoring devices used in the freestanding ambulatory center should symptoms of an MH event present.[63] Any patient who is known to be at risk for MH should be scheduled as early in the day as possible to allow for extended patient observation in the postanesthesia care unit (PACU) and phase 2 recovery. A lack of MH symtoms should be ensured before discharge is considered.[64] A patient who exhibits marked rigidity of the jaw muscles should not be discharged. Overnight observation is required for temperature rise, myoglobinuria, elevated creatine kinase levels, or progression to a MH episode. Patients who experience milder increases in jaw tension should be observed for signs and symptoms of MH for at least 12 hours. If there is evidence of myoglobinuria (i.e., dark, cola-colored urine), elevated temperature and pulse rate, or abnormality of acid-base balance, the patient should be emergently transferred and admitted to the nearest full-service facility and observed overnight.[62,64] Written discharge instructions should include (1) how to monitor the patient's temperature at home, (2) how to recognize the signs and symptoms of MH, and (3) contact information if emergency medical advice is required.[65]

Morbid obesity. The uncomplicated morbidly obese patient (now termed severely obese or class 3 obesity) may be scheduled for select outpatient surgeries.[66] Severely obese patients with significant preexisting cardiac, hepatic, pulmonary, or renal disease must be evaluated on an individual basis and may best be managed as an inpatient. Perioperative problems are more likely to occur when the body mass index (BMI) reaches 35 to 40 kg/m²; this was once considered to be the cutoff point for ambulatory surgery. With the introduction of select bariatric procedures into the outpatient setting, this exclusionary criterion has been reevaluated. A higher incidence of postoperative hypoxemia has been observed in patients with a BMI of 35 kg/m² or higher.[67] However, no increase in adverse postoperative outcomes, delayed discharge, or unanticipated hospital admission after ambulatory surgery was observed in obese patients with an average BMI of 44 kg/m².[68,69] Severely obese patients with high BMIs (BMI ≥50 kg/m²) may be at increased risk of exhibiting perioperative complications and should be considered with caution for ambulatory surgery.[66] The laparoscopic adjustable gastric banding procedure has allowed bariatric surgery to be performed on an outpatient basis because this procedure does not open the digestive tract.[70,71] Initial reports of outpatient laparoscopic Roux-en-Y procedures are being investigated for safety and appropriateness.[72] The ability to sufficiently manage postoperative pain and address postoperative ambulation should be discussed preoperatively by the surgeon and anesthesia provider. Again, the severely obese patient is at risk for persistent hypoxemia in the PACU, which may necessitate overnight supplemental oxygen therapy.

Preoperative airway evaluation (e.g., Mallampati classification, nuchal girth, redundant pharyngeal tissue) is especially important. A high Mallampati airway classification, reduced thyromental distance, and restricted mandibular mobility were predictive of difficult endotracheal intubation.[73]

Obstructive sleep apnea. Severe obesity is associated with an increased risk of obstructive sleep apnea (OSA); many obese patients present for ambulatory surgery with classic signs of OSA yet without formal sleep studies.[74] An assessment of intubating conditions in the patient with OSA found an increased incidence of difficult endotracheal intubation.[75] The likelihood of a difficult airway must be assessed preoperatively, and the ability to manage the difficult airway must be ensured.[76]

If continuous positive airway pressure (CPAP) is part of the patient's management of OSA, then the patient undergoing general anesthesia should be instructed to bring the CPAP machine into the surgery center for use in the immediate postoperative recovery phase. Intraoperative benzodiazepine and opioid usage, out of concern for worsening airway obstruction, should be minimized or avoided in these patients, and pain should be controlled with alternative techniques (e.g., nonopioid analgesics, regional anesthesia techniques, local wound infiltration with local anesthesia).[77,78] Moderate to severe OSA patients requiring postoperative opioids should not undergo ambulatory surgery.[79]

No increase in morbidity and mortality or unanticipated hospitalizations has been shown in OSA patients who are appropriately screened and deemed eligible to undergo ambulatory surgery.[16,80] The decision concerning whether to provide for the patient with OSA in the ambulatory setting should be contingent on certain criteria being met. The Society for Ambulatory Anesthesia has released a consensus statement on preoperative selection of adult patients with OSA scheduled for ambulatory surgery.[81] Patients with a known diagnosis of OSA and optimized comorbid medical conditions can be considered for ambulatory surgery. Adverse respiratory events are less likely if they are able to use a continuous positive airway pressure device in the postoperative period. Patients with a presumed diagnosis of OSA, based on screening tools such as the STOP-Bang questionnaire, with optimized comorbid conditions, can be considered for ambulatory surgery if postoperative pain can be managed predominantly with nonopioid analgesic techniques or with regional anesthesia techniques. On the other hand, OSA patients with nonoptimized comorbid medical conditions may not be good candidates for ambulatory surgery. All obese patients should be assessed with the STOP-Bang questionnaire as part of the preoperative evaluation (see Box 20.9). A score greater than 3 indicates a high suspicion for OSA. As noted previously, unless the patient's comorbid conditions are optimized and they are able to use CPAP after discharge and achieve postoperative pain relief without opiates, they are not candidates for outpatient surgery (Box 42.2).[81] Strict adherence to preoperative eligibility requirements and home care protocols is essential.[82] Consideration should be given to scheduling these patients early in the day to allow for prolonged observation of an additional 3 hours prior to discharge.[83] Three-hour observational time may not be necessary for patients with OSA receiving only moderate sedation.[16] Patients with OSA may be considered for discharge home if they are without (1) signs of moderate to severe OSA, (2) recurring PACU respiratory issues (i.e., apnea, bradypnea, oxyhemoglobin desaturation), and (3) potent postoperative opioids for analgesia.[84] A complete discussion of anesthesia and obesity can be found in Chapter 48.

Reactive airway disease. Before surgery is performed, the severity of reactive airway disease must be assessed, and optimal disease management should be achieved. A chest radiograph is indicated only if the patient is suspected of having an acute infiltrative process or if deterioration in the patient's physical condition has occurred. Likewise, arterial blood gases are indicated when signs and symptoms of chronic respiratory insufficiency are suspected. The patient may be best managed as an inpatient if indications for a chest radiograph or arterial blood gases are met. Consultation with the patient's internist may help in formulating therapeutic modalities and establishing baseline conditions for this patient. Patients receiving long-term medication therapy should continue to take their medications until the time of surgery. All parties involved must anticipate the possibility of admitting the patient to the hospital if the symptoms of the disease become exacerbated.

Sickle cell disease. Up to 8% to 10% of the African American population is diagnosed with the sickle cell trait (hemoglobin AS), and 0.2% are homozygous for sickle cell hemoglobin and have sickle cell anemia. Sickle cell trait is a heterozygous condition in which the individual has one βS globin gene and one βA globin gene. This results in the production of both hemoglobin S and hemoglobin A, with a predominance of hemoglobin A. Sickle cell trait is not clinically significant because hemoglobin AS cells begin to sickle only when the oxygen saturation of hemoglobin is less than 20%.[85]

The pathology of the different sickle cell states is attributable to three processes: the sickling or adhesion of cells in blood vessels, resulting in infarcts and subsequent tissue destruction secondary to tissue ischemia; hemolytic crisis secondary to hemolysis; and aplastic crises that occur with bone marrow exhaustion resulting in severe anemia. Patients currently in crisis should not undergo surgery except for emergencies, and then only after an exchange transfusion.[85]

Sickling is increased with lowered oxygen tensions, acidosis, hypothermia, and the presence of more desaturated hemoglobin S. Current therapy includes keeping the patient warm and well hydrated, administration of supplemental oxygen, maintaining high cardiac output, and avoiding areas of stasis with pressure or tourniquets.[85] The anesthesia management of sickle cell patients is discussed in Chapter 38.

The possibility of sickle cell hemoglobinopathy should be considered in every African American patient when obtaining the preoperative medical history. If individual or family history is suggestive of

---

BOX 42.2   The Society for Ambulatory Anesthesia Consensus Statement on Preoperative Selection of Adult Patients With Obstructive Sleep Apnea Scheduled for Ambulatory Surgery

- Patients with known OSA whose comorbid conditions are optimized and who are able to use CPAP after discharge are candidates for ambulatory surgery.
- Patients with known OSA whose comorbid conditions are not optimized are not candidates for ambulatory surgery and may benefit from further treatment.
- Patients with a presumptive diagnosis of OSA, optimized comorbid conditions, and postoperative pain that can be managed with nonopioid analgesics are candidates for ambulatory surgery.
- Patients with a presumptive diagnosis of OSA and nonoptimized comorbid conditions are not candidates for ambulatory surgery and may benefit from further treatment.

Adapted from Joshi GP, et al. Society for Ambulatory Anesthesia consensus statement on preoperative selection of adult patients with obstructive sleep apnea scheduled for ambulatory surgery. *Anesth Analg.* 2012;115(5):1060–1068.
All obese patients should be assessed via the STOP-Bang method for presumptive OSA (see Box 20.9).
Comorbid conditions include hypertension, arrhythmias, heart failure, cerebrovascular disease, and metabolic syndrome.
CPAP, Continuous positive airway pressure; *OSA,* obstructive sleep apnea.

the disease, a Sickledex may be obtained in children 6 months of age and older to determine the presence of sickle-shaped red blood cells.[86] The patient with sickle cell disease is at risk for crisis development if acidosis, dehydration, or hypoxia occur. These patients often present for cholecystectomy because cholelithiasis is a well-recognized complication of chronic hemolysis.[87]

The select patient diagnosed with sickle cell disease is an acceptable outpatient candidate with proper preparation and management.[88] Sickling of the red blood cells may occur when the patient with this trait is subjected to hypoxia.[89] If the patient with sickle cell anemia is to be cared for in the ambulatory setting, certain criteria must be satisfied:

1. The patient should have no major organ disease as a result of the sickle cell disease.
2. The patient should not have had a sickle cell crisis for at least 1 year.
3. The patient should be compliant with the prescribed medical care.
4. On discharge, the patient should have access to prompt medical care.
5. The patient should receive close follow-up postoperative care.

The procedure should not be a prolonged surgery that is associated with blood loss. The patient should arrive earlier than normal so adequate intravenous hydration can be established. The patient's surgery should be scheduled early in the day to allow for extended postoperative monitoring before being discharged from the ambulatory center.

Social Considerations

Factors other than physical condition must be weighed when considering a patient for outpatient surgery (Box 42.3). The lack of appropriate home support and care makes the outpatient option less desirable.

Unacceptable Patient Conditions for Ambulatory Surgery

Certain situations make ambulatory surgery impractical. Each patient must be considered individually for acceptability as an outpatient surgical candidate. Patients believed to be at increased risk for outpatient surgery and to be unacceptable candidates for such surgery are those with any of the following[23]:

- Unstable ASA physical status classification III or IV (e.g., cardiac, renal, endocrine, pulmonary, hepatic, or cancer diagnoses)
- Active substance/alcohol abuse
- Psychosocial difficulties (i.e., responsible caregiver not available to observe the patient on the evening of surgery) (see Box 42.3)
- Poorly controlled seizures
- Severe obesity with significant comorbid conditions (i.e., angina, asthma, OSA)
- Previously unevaluated and poorly managed moderate to severe OSA
- Ex-premature infants younger than 60 weeks of postconceptual age requiring general anesthesia with endotracheal intubation
- Uncontrolled diabetes
- Current sepsis or infectious disease necessitating separate isolation facilities
- Anticipated postoperative pain not expected to be controlled with oral analgesics or local anesthesia techniques

---

BOX 42.3   Social Considerations in Ambulatory Surgery

- Patient compliance
- Presence of responsible caregiver
- Discharge accommodations
- Access to assistance
- Financial and insurance considerations

PATIENT EVALUATION AND PREPARATION

To recognize anesthetic risks and determine the patient's suitability for the planned procedure, preoperative evaluation is mandatory for all patients preparing to undergo outpatient anesthesia and surgery. Challenges may include organizing and accomplishing all the necessary tests and evaluations, while causing the least amount of inconvenience to the patient. The preoperative interview elicits pertinent patient information and clarifies risk factors that may affect surgery and patient recovery, and may help to determine what further patient workup is required before surgery. A formalized preanesthesia assessment clinic is the most comprehensive and cost-effective process for preoperative evaluation and preparation.[90] Preoperative screening also allows the staff to communicate what will be expected of the patient in the perioperative phases.

Consultations, laboratory tests, and diagnostic procedures should be performed based on clinical findings rather than on a preestablished regimen of "standard" tests. Without any discoveries from the medical history and physical examination, the probability of observing a significant abnormality is negligible in diagnostic procedures, including electrocardiogram, chest radiograph, and laboratory tests. Abnormal test results obtained from routine testing potentially alter patient care only 0.22% to 0.56% of the time.[91] Routine preoperative laboratory screening is neither cost effective nor predictive of postoperative complications.[92-94]

Patient Interview

Patient screening should take place sufficiently in advance of the scheduled surgery to allow time for necessary risk assessment, preoperative testing, specialty consultations, and adjustments in patient care. Proper timing of the patient assessment, particularly for the patient with complex medical conditions, minimizes surgical delays and cancellations. The high-risk patient should be evaluated at least 1 week before the scheduled procedure. With respect to client convenience, the otherwise healthy individual who does not have the opportunity to visit the clinic can be evaluated on the day of surgery. In this circumstance, there is a higher potential for surgical postponement or cancellation with last-minute discovery (e.g., inappropriate fasting, suspected difficult airway).

Patient Orientation

The preoperative interview allows the staff to convey what is expected of the patient, and what the patient can expect perioperatively. Providing instructions to the patient, verbally and in writing, results in improved patient compliance. An information packet given to the patient at the interview is beneficial. It should detail specific instructions and concerns related to the procedure (Box 42.4).

Patients and family members should have the opportunity to become acquainted with the ambulatory surgery facilities and the anticipated sequence of events. This includes orientation to the laboratory and procedure areas, changing areas, waiting room, play areas, and the short-stay area, where the patient remains after surgery until discharge. This orientation is designed to reduce patient and family fear by providing relevant perioperative information (e.g., directions, anticipated schedule, instructions for physiologic preparation of the child, expected postoperative course, and discharge instructions), offering reassurance, and enhancing coping skills through familiarity. A variety of techniques may be incorporated to prepare the child for the operative procedure. Children can be oriented to equipment commonly used in the perioperative setting (e.g., anesthetic mask,

BOX 42.4   Preoperative Patient Instructions

Preoperative Instructions
- Inform the patient when and where laboratory tests, consultations, and diagnostic procedures will be completed.
- Clarify the appropriate time for the patient to be without food and drink.

Registration on the Day of Surgery
- Inform the patient where and the time to report for surgery, and mention that a wait can normally be expected.
- Describe the location of the parking areas.

Ambulatory Center Policies
- Inform the patient and family about expected conduct.
- Explain the ambulatory facility policies to the patient and family.
- Describe the family waiting area and services (e.g., dining areas).
- Review advance-directive information as required by law in some states.
- Review the patient's right-to-privacy policies.
- Outline the facility's cancellation policies: late arrival, nonadherence to fasting guidelines, inappropriate transportation home, lack of responsible person to help patient postoperatively, interim changes in patient's health status (e.g., upper respiratory tract infection [URTI]).

Personal Considerations
- Inform the patient to wear comfortable, loose-fitting clothing that may be easily stored.
- Instruct patient to wear no jewelry or makeup (remove nail polish from at least one nail).
- Instruct patient to bring personal toilet items (e.g., comb, brush, toothbrush) as required.
- Caution patient to leave valuables at home.
- Inform the caregiver to bring child's favorite toy, comforter, or pacifier, or light reading material for the older patient.

Postoperative Considerations
- Inform the patient and family of the discharge time, including the time spent in the postanesthesia care unit, and the customary length of stay until discharge.
- Instruct patient in the manner of discharge, the appropriate transportation arrangements, and the necessity for the presence of a responsible caregiver.
- Give the patient postoperative instructions: no driving, alcohol, or major decisions postoperatively for at least 24 to 48 hours after anesthesia (see Box 42.12 for additional information).
- Inform the patient where, how, and to whom complications should be reported. Supply telephone numbers.
- Indicate the possibility of hospital admission.

Considerations If the Patient's Physical Condition Changes
- Inform the patient to contact the surgeon.
- Inform the patient to contact the anesthesia department.
- Inform the patient to call regarding cancellations.

intravenous therapy equipment, the anesthesia machine and circuit, blood pressure cuff, thermometer, and postoperative oxygen therapy devices). Children can also be told when and where they will be reunited with their parents after surgery.

History and Physical

Results of a thorough medical history and physical examination performed by a member of the medical staff should be available in the patient's chart before the surgery is performed. A separate anesthesia history should be incorporated into a questionnaire specifically designed for preanesthetic evaluation; the anesthesia provider should review this history with the patient.

Such a review may be accomplished in a written format and would include a general review of the major systems, history of allergies, current medications, past and present medical problems, laboratory and diagnostic test results, and patient and family response to previous anesthetics. Prior anesthesia records should be examined for complications, response to anesthesia, and postoperative course. Patient evaluation should be conducted within 30 days of the scheduled surgery for medically stable patients and within 72 hours of the scheduled surgery for high-risk patients. The clinician should determine whether any changes might have occurred since the original history and physical examination were performed, and an update note should be made on the day of the procedure. A review of current vital signs, laboratory test results, diagnostic reports, and fasting status should be made.

Laboratory Evaluation

Each ambulatory center should have a consensus regarding the minimum testing requirement for surgery. These testing criteria depend on the proposed surgical procedure, the patient's medication history, and the patient's physical condition. Some states and regions have established minimum testing requirements. However, conducting a battery of preoperative laboratory tests, without specific indications, has not been shown to reduce patient morbidity, is not cost effective, and may even place the patient at increased risk.[92,93] Discriminate laboratory testing, based on findings from the history and physical examination, are indicated to help determine surgical and anesthetic risk. Normal laboratory tests and diagnostic procedure results are deemed current if the tests are performed within 6 months of surgery if the patient's physical condition remains stable.[94,95] Exceptions include serum potassium level determinations, which should be obtained within 7 days of surgery for patients receiving diuretics or digitalis, and blood glucose level determinations, which should be obtained on the same day of surgery for patients with diabetes controlled by medication. Physical conditions and systemic illnesses in which preoperative laboratory testing is appropriate are listed in Table 42.1.

Pregnancy Testing

The medical facility should have established guidelines delineating when testing for pregnancy is appropriate, and informed consent must be obtained. Anesthetic concerns include the effect of surgery and anesthesia on the developing fetus and the potential to trigger preterm labor. If the medical history and physical examination indicate that the patient may be pregnant, or if pregnancy might complicate the surgery, then pregnancy testing should be performed. It is important that the patient be educated as to the potential risks of exposing a fetus to an anesthetic. Whenever possible, especially in the adolescent population, a female staff member should question the patient in the absence of family members.[96] Suggested pregnancy testing guidelines are given in Table 42.2.

Diagnostic Procedures

Chest radiography. Performing routine preoperative chest radiography is not recommended without specific indications for the necessity of the test from the history and physical examination. Clinical findings obtained from the history and physical may be as efficient as a chest

TABLE 42.1 Preoperative (Noncardiac) Testing in Ambulatory Surgery Patients

Test	Indications
Electrocardiogram	Arrhythmias Acute ischemia Syncope
Complete blood count	Anemia Cirrhosis
Pregnancy test	May be offered to women of childbearing age for whom the result will alter management
Coagulation studies (prothrombin time [PT], international normalized ratio [INR], partial thromboplastin time, platelet count)	Personal/family history of bleeding diathesis Warfarin (PT, INR), or other anticoagulant use Cirrhosis Significant malnutrition
Polysomnography	At risk for sleep apnea (per screen, such as STOP-Bang), and result may affect candidacy for outpatient surgery or alter management
Chest radiograph	Investigation of new or active pulmonary symptoms
Type and screen	Anticipated blood loss >500 mL
Electrolytes	Diuretic use
Creatinine	Use of contrast dye
Glucose	When hypoglycemia, diabetic ketoacidosis, or hyperglycemic, hyperosmolar nonketosis is suspected

Patients having cataract surgery do not require preoperative testing.
Adapted from Okocha O, Gerlach RM, Sweitzer B. Preoperative evaluation for ambulatory anesthesia: what, when, and how? *Anesthesiol Clin.* 2019;37(2):195–213.

TABLE 42.2 Recommendations for Preoperative Pregnancy Testing

Population Type	Recommendations
Menstruating females age <13 yr	No pregnancy test unless history is either indicative of sexual activity or is inconclusive.
Patients of childbearing age (age >13 yr until 1 yr after last reported menses)	Preoperative pregnancy test should be offered to all patients regardless of history, except in patients with a history of hysterectomy or bilateral salpingo-oophorectomy.
Testing on the day of surgery	Urine pregnancy test is sufficient.
Testing within 1 wk of surgery	Serum pregnancy test is preferable.
All patients	Well-documented informed consent must be obtained from patients or their guardians.
All patients	There must be an established system involving an obstetric/gynecologic consultation for disclosing an unexpected positive result to the patient.
All patients	A thorough and detailed history should be obtained from all patients.

From Molov JL, Twersky RS. Is routine preoperative pregnancy testing necessary? In: Fleischer LA, ed. *Evidence-Based Practice of Anesthesiology.* 3rd ed. Philadelphia: Elsevier; 2013:26–30.

BOX 42.5 Risk Factors for Pulmonary Aspiration

- Age extremes (<1 yr or >70 yr)
- Anxiety
- Ascites
- Collagen vascular disease (e.g., scleroderma)
- Depression
- Esophageal surgery
- Exogenous medications (opioids or premedications [e.g., barbiturates] and anticholinergics)
- Failed intubation or difficult airway history
- Gastroesophageal junction dysfunction (e.g., hiatal hernia)
- Mechanical obstruction (e.g., pyloric stenosis, duodenal ulcer)
- Metabolic disorders (e.g., hypothyroidism, chronic diabetes, hepatic failure, hyperglycemia, obesity, renal failure, and uremia)
- Neurologic sequelae (e.g., developmental delays, head injury, hypotonia, seizures)
- Pain
- Pregnancy
- Prematurity with respiratory problems
- Smoking
- Type and composition of gastric contents (e.g., solid foods, milk products)

radiograph. A chest radiograph should be considered preoperatively if the patient (1) presents with new pulmonary signs or symptoms, (2) has end-stage renal disease, or (3) has decompensated heart failure. Patients with these symptoms might not be suitable candidates for ambulatory surgery, except for brief, minor procedures (e.g., ophthalmologic surgery).[94]

Electrocardiography. Few data support the routine performance of 12-lead electrocardiographic screening before elective surgery because it has not been shown to be cost effective, is a poor predictor of perioperative complications, and is of limited value in detecting ischemia in asymptomatic individuals. It has been proposed that routinely acquiring a preoperative electrocardiogram is not indicated in the patient undergoing ambulatory surgery.[95]

Fasting Status and Aspiration Risk

Part of the preoperative evaluation process identifies patients at risk for aspirating gastric contents into the lungs and developing aspiration pneumonitis. Factors associated with an increased risk of pulmonary aspiration of gastric contents are listed in Box 42.5. Recent ingestion of food and liquid before surgery contributes to an increased risk of aspiration. Solid foods must be digested to a bolus diameter of less than 2 mm before the food can pass through the pylorus. This process normally takes several hours for solids, whereas liquids pass through the pylorus in 1 to 2 hours. Historically, patients have been required to fast for extended periods to ensure an empty stomach. However, sustained fasting does not ensure that the stomach will be empty at the time of surgery. The traditional policy of fasting after midnight fails to address several variables that influence gastric emptying for surgery:

- The time of the scheduled surgery
- The time at which the patient retired for the night

- The variability of gastric emptying for solids and fluids across individuals

Several problems have been associated with prolonged fasting:
- Dehydration
- Hypoglycemia
- Hypovolemia
- Increased irritability
- Enhanced preoperative anxiety
- Reduced compliance with preoperative fasting orders
- Thirst and related discomfort (e.g., hunger, headache, unhappiness)

Data suggest that liquids (e.g., clear apple juice, clear broth, coffee, gelatin, Popsicles, pulp-free orange juice, water, and weak tea) may be given to healthy, unpremedicated patients up to 2 hours before surgery without placing them at increased risk for aspiration. There is no increase in gastric volume, nor is there a decrease in gastric pH, at the time of elective surgery. The studies that allowed patients to consume clear liquids until 2 to 3 hours before surgery demonstrated that although the patients appeared to be at no greater risk of aspirating gastric contents, the pH of the stomach contents remained less than 2.5. In light of these findings, recommended fasting guidelines for the otherwise healthy individual have been liberalized (Table 42.3).[97]

Special Considerations

Daily Medications

Patients should continue to take their prescribed medications on the morning of the surgery. The medications may be taken with a minimum of water (up to 150 mL in adults and up to 75 mL in children) up to 1 hour before anesthesia. Exceptions to this practice may include aspirin and antiplatelet drugs, diuretics, angiotensin-converting enzyme inhibitors, and angiotensin receptor blockers. Anesthesia departments and clinicians generally establish protocols for handling preoperative

TABLE 42.3 Preoperative Fasting Recommendations*

Ingested Materials	Minimum Fasting Period[†] (hr)
Clear liquids[‡]	2
Breast milk	4
Infant formula	6
Nonhuman milk[§]	6
Light meal**	6
Heavy meal; fried or fatty food	Additional fasting time (e.g., >8 hr may be needed)

*These recommendations apply to healthy patients who are undergoing elective procedures. They are not intended for women in labor. Following the guidelines does not guarantee complete gastric emptying.
[†]The fasting periods noted above apply to all ages.
[‡]Examples of clear liquids include water, fruit juices without pulp, carbonated beverages, clear tea, and black coffee.
[§]Since nonhuman milk is similar to solids in gastric emptying time, the amount ingested must be considered when determining an appropriate fasting period.
**A light meal typically consists of toast and clear liquids. Meals that include fried or fatty foods or meat may prolong gastric emptying time. From American Society of Anesthesiologists Task Force. Practice guidelines for preoperative fasting and the use of pharmacologic agents to reduce the risk of pulmonary aspiration. Application to healthy patients undergoing elective procedures. *Anesthesiology.* 2017;126(3):376–393.
Additional fasting time (e.g., ≥8 hr) may be needed in these cases. Both the amount and type of foods ingested must be considered when determining an appropriate fasting period.

medications. Management of preoperative antihypertensive medications is discussed in Chapter 13.

Warfarin sodium. Prior to surgery a consultation between the surgeon and the patients physician should determine whether the patient continues warfarin sodium therapy. If warfarin is discontinued then anticoagulation bridging may be accomplished with subcutaneous low-molecular-weight heparin or intravenous unfractionated heparin. The question of whether the disadvantages of stopping the administration of this medication before surgery outweigh any advantage must be addressed. If the decision to withhold warfarin is made, the drug should be discontinued approximately 5 days before the scheduled surgery, and an international normalized ratio (INR) should be determined on the day of surgery. With adequate hemostasis, warfarin should be resumed 12 to 24 hours after surgery.[98] A complete discussion on the perioperative management of anticoagulants can be found in Chapter 38.

Diabetes

Recommended care for the diabetic patient who is undergoing ambulatory surgery remains a subject of debate. Optimal goals for glucose level management and consensus guidelines are being actively studied.[80] The patient with diabetes is at increased risk for cardiovascular, pulmonary, and neurologic events and should receive an early and thorough preoperative evaluation, including electrocardiography, history, physical examination, and indicated laboratory analysis. The patient with insulin-dependent diabetes whose diabetes is not well controlled and whose serum glucose levels are prone to wide fluctuations may be best treated in the inpatient setting depending on the type of surgery. Considerations for care of the patient with diabetes who is undergoing ambulatory surgery include the following:[99-102]

- Schedule the patient's surgery for early in the day.
- Obtain baseline information regarding the patient's glycemic control (i.e., the frequency and severity of hypoglycemia, the blood glucose level when the patient becomes symptomatic and the manifestations, and whether the patient is hypoglycemic unaware).
- If available, review previous monthly trends for blood glucose and glycosylated hemoglobin A_{1C} (HbA_{1C}) to assess glycemic control. Patients with an HbA_{1C} greater than 6.9 mmol/L and those with significant comorbidities should receive consultation with the patient's internist for optimization prior to surgery.
- Determine type (e.g., oral antidiabetics and insulin), dose, and schedule of antidiabetic therapy.
- Obtain hospitalization history related to glycemic control issues.
- Instruct the patient in regard to fasting guidelines that are appropriate to the medications and glucose control.
- Monitor the patient's blood or serum glucose levels on arrival to the ambulatory center.
- Prevent hypoglycemia while maintaining blood glucose levels at less than 180 mg/dL.
- Manage preoperative oral antidiabetic and noninsulin injectable therapy.
- Manage preoperative insulin therapies (Table 42.4). Consider holding noninsulin therapies the morning of surgery.
- Return the patient to preoperative activities of daily living (e.g., baseline activity status, nutrition habits) as soon as possible.
- Make the patient aware that admission to the hospital is likely if persistent nausea and vomiting prevent resumption of normal dietary intake.

Heart Murmur

The surgical patient with a heart murmur requires further workup if the condition was previously undetected. Heart murmurs are

TABLE 42.4   Patient Instructions for Preoperative Insulin Administration

Insulin Regimen	Day Before Surgery	Morning of Surgery
Insulin pump (1% continuous infusion rate of rapid-acting insulin analog)	Usual basal rate	Usual basal rate (consider 20% dose reduction if basal rate is deemed inappropriately high)
Long-acting analog (glargine or detemir)	Morning dose NO change PM dose 80% of usual	85% of usual dose if patient uses twice daily injection, otherwise 100% (consider 20% dose reduction if usual dose is deemed inappropriately high)
Fixed combination insulins	No change	50%–75% of morning dose of intermediate-acting component
Short- and rapid-acting insulins	No change	Hold the dose

Adapted from Vogt AP, Bally L. Perioperative glucose management: current status and future directions. *Best Pract Res Clin Anaesthesiol.* 2020;34(2):213–224.

categorized as innocent or pathologic. Pathologic murmurs may be due to complex congenital malformations or heart disease and have accompanying physical dysfunction, whereas with innocent murmurs, the patient may be completely asymptomatic. Whether the murmur is benign, functional, or caused by organic heart disease, cardiologic assessment should be obtained before the induction of anesthesia.[103]

Rhinorrhea

Of all children, 20% to 30% display symptoms of rhinorrhea for a good portion of the year. Children younger than 2 years of age are prone to 5 to 10 viral respiratory infections annually.[104] For the child undergoing ambulatory surgery, individual patient evaluation is required for a runny nose. Both the history and physical examination are beneficial in determining the cause. The differential diagnosis of rhinorrhea should include the following:

- Allergic (seasonal) rhinitis
- Bacterial infection (early stages)
- Flu syndrome
- Upper respiratory tract infection (URTI)
- Vasomotor rhinitis
- Nothing found

The clinician obtaining the patient history should try to ascertain the allergic or acute nature of the runny nose and determine whether it is normal for the child, or if an illness has recently developed and worsened. Recently acquired (within 12–24 hours of surgery) rhinorrhea or chronic rhinorrhea in the otherwise fit child is not a contraindication to surgery. The differentiation between a noninfectious and an infectious runny nose might influence the decision of whether the procedure should be delayed (Box 42.6). Surgery might be delayed for 2 weeks in the child with localized infectious rhinorrhea.[105,106]

Considerations for Postponing Surgery

Lack of Drug Compliance

The patient with uncontrolled hypertension or diabetes who has wide swings in blood pressure or blood glucose levels may not be suitable for outpatient surgery; such conditions should be optimally managed before outpatient surgery and anesthesia are performed.

Fasting Status

For safety reasons, the patient not adhering to the fasting guidelines should not undergo surgery, and the rationale of not eating before surgery should be reinforced.

BOX 42.6   Differential Diagnosis of Rhinorrhea

Noninfectious Runny Nose
- Allergic rhinitis
- Seasonal
- Perennial
- Vasomotor rhinitis
- Emotional (crying)
- Temperature

Infectious Runny Nose
- Viral infections
- Nasopharyngitis (common cold)
- Contagious disease (e.g., chickenpox, measles)
- Acute bacterial infections
- Streptococcal tonsillitis
- Meningitis

Suspicion of Pregnancy

If the patient responds that she may be pregnant or if clinical signs are indicative of pregnancy, surgery should be delayed until determination of whether the patient is pregnant can be made. Decisions about whether surgery should be performed and what type of anesthesia should be used can be based on pregnancy test results.

Upper Respiratory Tract Infection

Acute respiratory infections are one of the leading medical causes for surgery cancellation in children. In patients with an acute infection, differentiating between a bacterial infection as causative of the URTI or lower respiratory tract infection (LRTI) and other causes—such as uncomplicated viral infection (afebrile, clear secretions) or allergic conditions—is important. Differentiating between a noninfectious process and an infectious process is paramount in the decision regarding whether the procedure should be performed. This differentiation may be difficult to make early in the course of the disease. Symptoms of URTI include the following:

- Possible elevated white blood cell count (>12,000 with a left shift)
- Mucopurulent nasal secretions
- Inflamed and reddened nasopharyngeal and oropharyngeal mucosa (with allergic rhinitis [e.g., nasal mucosa is ashen and boggy])
- Temperature of 37°C to 37.5°C (>37.5°C usually associated with lower respiratory tract involvement)
- Tonsillitis
- Viral ulcers in the oropharynx

Other accompanying symptoms may include conjunctivitis, coughing (nonproductive), fatigue, itching, laryngitis, malaise, myalgia, sneezing, headache, and sore throat. Laboratory and diagnostic testing in children with suspected URTI includes nasal or throat cultures

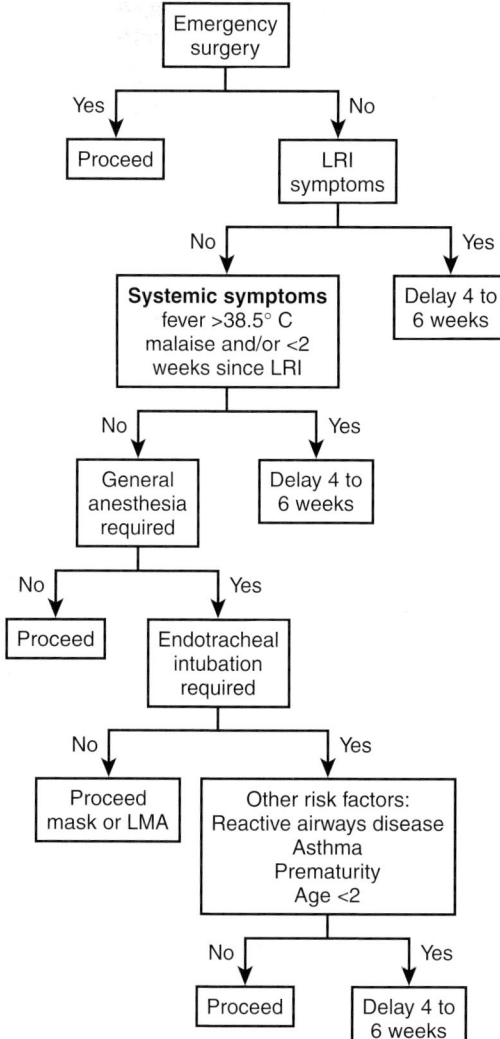

Fig. 42.1 Clinical decision tree for proceeding with surgery in children with respiratory tract infections. *LMA,* Laryngeal mask airway; *LRI,* lower respiratory tract infection. (From McKee CT, et al. Should a child with a respiratory tract infection undergo elective surgery. In: Fleischer LA. *Evidence-Based Practice of Anesthesiology.* 3rd ed. Philadelphia: Elsevier; 2013:534.)

if signs of an infectious process are observed. A chest radiograph is not warranted, especially if chest sounds are clear. Similarly, the value of obtaining a white blood cell count has been challenged because the results may be normal and typically do not influence whether to proceed with the surgery.[107]

As noted earlier, anesthetizing the patient who has a URTI or LRTI has been shown to increase the incidence of respiratory-associated complications two- to sevenfold. Bronchial reactivity may persist for 6 to 8 weeks after a viral LRTI. The anesthetized patient with a respiratory tract infection is more prone to experience breath holding, bronchospasm, coughing, desaturation, hypoxemia, increased secretions, laryngospasm, pneumonia, atelectasis, croup, and stridor. Risk factors for the development of perioperative adverse respiratory events include endotracheal intubation (<5 years of age), history of prematurity, history of reactive airway disease, exposure to secondhand smoke, surgery involving the airway, the presence of copious secretions, and nasal congestion.

A recent multicenter trial involving 16 centers and 621 children was performed in France. Children with a URTI who were allowed to proceed with anesthesia and surgery, had more adverse events and/or arterial desaturation. Predictors of adverse events included younger patient age, provider experience, premedication, and tracheal intubation. About 80% of pediatric patients with current or recent URTI symptoms proceeded with anesthesia; 20% of the surgeries were postponed. Factors associated with the decision to proceed with anesthesia included provider experience, emergency procedures, and type of URTI symptoms at presentation. They concluded that the risk of a respiratory adverse event in patients anesthetized in the presence of URTI was approximately 30%. Recommendations included a revision of the protocols for proceeding with surgery and for reducing adverse events in children with URTI.[108]

A minimum of 4 hours of postoperative observation is appropriate prior to discharge from the ambulatory setting. Each case should be reviewed individually. The decision to operate frequently depends on the urgency of the surgery, the duration and complexity of the surgery, and the need for instrumentation of the airway. Children with uncomplicated respiratory infection may undergo elective procedures without significantly increasing anesthesia complications.[106-109] Guidelines for assessment and anesthetic management of children with respiratory infections are given in Fig. 42.1.[107] Further discussion on the management of children with respiratory infection is in Chapter 53.

PREMEDICATION

Premedication should be provided on an individual basis and with minimally effective doses. The concern about giving anxiolytic and sedative medications is related to the potential for a prolonged patient stay in the PACU. Prophylactic drugs for postoperative nausea and vomiting (PONV) are commonly used in patients at risk. Oral nonsteroidal antiinflammatory drugs (NSAIDs), when indicated for analgesia, should be considered preoperatively. Preemptive analgesia may reduce postoperative pain by preventing surgically induced peripheral and central sensitization.[110] Lower postoperative pain scores and less opioid use have been seen when NSAIDs were given prior to surgery.[111] However, the use of premedication should not become routine; rather, the decision to administer these agents should be based on individual need and desired benefit.[112] Common indications for preoperative medication are as follows:

- To decrease patient anxiety and fear
- To facilitate smooth induction and emergence from anesthesia
- Pain management
- To supplement anesthesia and reduce the need for general anesthetic agents
- To reduce the volume and acidity of gastric contents
- Prophylaxis for PONV
- To provide a more pleasant stay in the PACU

Pulmonary Aspiration Prophylaxis

Patients at higher risk for aspirating gastric contents may be given medications before surgery to raise gastric pH and lower gastric volume, in order to minimize the risk for pulmonary aspiration. Pulmonary aspiration prophylaxis in patients who are not at risk is not recommended.[97]

Antacids

The value of oral antacids lies in their ability to rapidly reduce gastric acidity; they are effective in raising pH in 15 to 20 minutes.[113] This characteristic is useful in emergency situations, but it is of limited application in the ambulatory setting. Although oral antacids raise gastric pH, they have the disadvantage of increasing gastric volume. Clear, nonparticulate oral antacids (e.g., 2 tablets of Alka-Seltzer Gold in 30 mL of water; 30 mL [0.4 mL/kg pediatric dose] of 0.3 M sodium citrate [Bicitra]) are preferred over particulate antacids, such as Maalox or Mylanta, because particulate antacids may produce pulmonary injury if aspirated.[114]

Gastrokinetics

Reducing gastric fluid volume with a gastrokinetic agent such as metoclopramide (Reglan) helps minimize the risk of aspiration. Metoclopramide has been demonstrated to decrease gastric fluid volume by reducing gastric emptying time without increasing pH in adults and in children. Metoclopramide may also reduce the risk of pulmonary aspiration by increasing lower esophageal sphincter tone. It appears to exert a central antiemetic effect via dopamine receptor blockade of the chemoreceptor trigger zone.[115] The combination of metoclopramide with a histamine$_2$ (H$_2$)–receptor antagonist has been shown to be effective in raising gastric volume pH and decreasing gastric volume content.[116]

The intramuscular dose is 10 mg for adults (0.1 mg/kg for children) given at least 45 minutes before surgery. The intravenous dose is 10 to 20 mg for adults (0.15–0.2 mg/kg for children) given over the course of 3 to 5 minutes at least 20 to 30 minutes before surgery. These regimens allow sufficient time for the desired results to be achieved. The oral dose, 10 mg for adults (0.1 mg/kg for children), achieves peak plasma concentrations 40 to 120 minutes after administration.[23]

H$_2$-Receptor Antagonists

Selective and competitive H$_2$-receptor antagonists, such as cimetidine (Tagamet), famotidine (Pepcid), ranitidine (Zantac), and nizatidine (Axid), block hydrogen ion release by gastric parietal cells. These drugs do not alter the pH of gastric fluid already present in the stomach. All are available over the counter. These medications may be administered the night before surgery, on the day of surgery, or both, to reduce gastric acidity. Famotidine has a longer duration of action and exhibits a lower potential for side effects than cimetidine.[117] Ranitidine and nizatidine have recently been recalled by the US Food and Drug Administration (FDA) for manufacturing difficulties leading to possible carcinogens in some product formulation.[118]

Cimetidine. Although not commonly used, in one study, an adult of cimetidine 300 mg helped reduce the risk of pulmonary aspiration. The oral dose is 300 mg (3–4 mg/kg) for adults and 7.5 mg/kg for children, given from 1.5 to 3 hours before surgery.

Famotidine. The intravenous dose of famotidine is 20 mg for adults, given 15 to 30 minutes before surgery; this is effective in increasing gastric pH. Oral famotidine (40 mg) can also be administered the night before surgery and the morning of surgery. When compared with ranitidine, famotidine was slower in raising the gastric pH to safe levels.[119]

Gastric Proton-Pump Inhibitors

Omeprazole. Omeprazole (Prilosec) causes dose-dependent intracellular inhibition of gastric acid secretion in humans without affecting gastric volume. Omeprazole has a longer duration of action than the H$_2$-receptor antagonist agents in suppressing gastric acid secretion and appears to cause no significant side effects.

The intravenous dose of omeprazole is 40 mg, administered after the induction of anesthesia. This is as effective as ranitidine in raising gastric pH above 2.5.

The oral dose is 80 mg, given the evening before surgery. This has increased mean gastric pH to 4.56, compared with the pH of 2.05 that was achieved with the administration of a placebo. Orally administered omeprazole 40 mg was not found to be as effective as either famotidine 40 mg or ranitidine 300 mg in protecting against pulmonary aspiration in parturients.[117]

Lansoprazole, rabeprazole, and esomeprazole. Orally administered lansoprazole (Prevacid; 30 mg), rabeprazole (Aciphex; 20 mg), or esomeprazole (Nexium) administered 24 hours prior to surgery, and on the morning of surgery, were not as effective in raising pH and lowering gastric volume as a single morning-of-surgery dose of ranitidine 150 mg. Intravenous preparations of esomeprazole (20 and 40 mg) and lansoprazole (30 mg) are available.[117]

Pantoprazole. Pantoprazole (Protonix) is marketed as both an intravenous solution and as tablets, which may prove useful for perioperative use. Intravenously administered pantoprazole 40 mg was comparable with ranitidine 50 mg in increasing pH and reducing gastric fluid volume.[120]

A complete list of the proton pump inhibitors and their doses are listed in Table 33.8.

ANESTHETIC CONSIDERATIONS

Anesthetic techniques suitable for outpatient surgery include general anesthesia, regional anesthesia, and monitored anesthesia care. The goals for outpatient anesthesia, regardless of the type administered, are listed in Box 42.7, and factors influencing the choice of anesthesia are shown in Box 42.8. The ideal anesthetic agent for ambulatory anesthesia—whether it is administered inhalationally, intravenously, locally, or regionally—is one with the appropriate pharmacokinetic traits (i.e., rapid onset and offset, short duration, inert metabolites, and insignificant side effects).

General Anesthesia

General anesthesia is the most widely used anesthetic technique for ambulatory surgery. General anesthesia should be achieved with the less-soluble inhalation agents or with short-acting intravenous agents

BOX 42.7 Goals of Outpatient Anesthesia

- Minimize the physiologic changes associated with anesthesia.
- Provide a fast, smooth onset of anesthetic action.
- Promote intraoperative amnesia and analgesia.
- Afford suitable operating circumstances.
- Minimize perioperative anesthetic side effects.
- Allow rapid offset of anesthetic influence while maintaining patient comfort.

BOX 42.8 Considerations for Choice of Anesthetic

- Surgical requirements
- Skill of anesthesia provider
- Patient choice
- Patient age
- American Society of Anesthesiologists physical status classification
- Level of care available once patient is discharged from outpatient facility
- Risk of postoperative nausea and vomiting
- Postoperative analgesia requirements

that have the capability of reversal if required. A combination of potent rapid-onset and rapid-offset inhalation agents (e.g., desflurane, sevoflurane), along with intravenous agents (e.g., propofol, intravenous opioids, short-acting muscle relaxants, NSAIDs, and dexmedetomidine), comprise general anesthesia in contemporary practice. The popularity of general anesthesia in the ambulatory setting is related to its acceptance by the patient, the anesthesia provider, and the surgeon, and to the consistent pace that can be maintained with regard to achieving a satisfactory state of anesthesia.

Depth-of-Anesthesia Monitoring

Advances in depth-of-anesthesia monitoring technology have made their mark in ambulatory anesthesia. The data indicating that the routine use of bispectral index monitoring (BIS) during outpatient anesthesia improves outcomes is mixed. Some of the purported advantages of BIS monitoring in the outpatient setting include reducing the amount of anesthetic agent required, faster emergence from anesthesia, and a reduction in phase II vomiting.[121-126]

Airway Management

Issues regarding the use of general anesthesia with a facemask, a laryngeal mask airway (LMA), or an endotracheal tube in patients undergoing outpatient surgery are the same as those in patients undergoing inpatient surgery. The indications for intubating the trachea depend on the constraints of the surgery and the individual patient concerns (e.g., risk of regurgitation and aspiration, hypoventilation, access to the airway, use of muscle relaxants, and airway obstruction).

Drawbacks to endotracheal intubation specific to the outpatient setting must be considered. Irritation and trauma to the upper airway and trachea are a concern, especially in children. The development of postextubation croup is rare (0.1%), but the potential for its occurrence must be considered in the plan for discharge.[127] Strategies to help minimize the occurrence of post extubation croup in the young pediatric patient include (1) minimizing the potential trauma that can occur from laryngoscopy and intubation, (2) ensuring that an air leak is present at less than 20–25 cm H_2O, and (3) avoiding large diameter endotracheal tubes.

Supraglottic airway devices (such as the LMA) are effective airway management tools in the ambulatory setting. Patients tolerate LMAs at a lower anesthetic dose than that needed for endotracheal intubation. Neuromuscular blocking agents are rarely necessary for airway management, and the incidence of airway morbidity such as coughing and sore throat is lower with LMAs than with endotracheal tubes. These advantages may facilitate faster patient recovery and earlier discharge. Limitations include incomplete protection against aspiration of gastric contents, and a requirement for lower peak airway pressures during positive pressure ventilation.[129,130]

Intravenous Fluid Therapy

The optimum amount of perioperative fluid therapy remains unclear. The three most common total fluid regimens include restrictive, liberal, and hemodynamic goal directed. Each technique has its proponents.[131-134] Benefits of liberal fluid therapy include less thirst postoperatively, a lower incidence of sore throat, and a lower incidence of dizziness, drowsiness, and faintness on standing compared with patients for whom fluids were withheld perioperatively. Less PONV also has been reported.[135] Enhanced recovery after surgery (ERAS) was established to improve patient outcomes and reduce recovery times. ERAS protocols arose out of the need to decrease physiologic

and psychological surgical stress with an emphasis on recovery. Overall, ERAS aims to reduce adverse events, shorten the length of hospital stay, reduce costs, and improve patient recovery. Surgical subspecialties have embraced the philosophy of ERAS, creating unique protocols to meet their patients' needs. ERAS guidelines are available for nearly every specialty in ambulatory surgery.[136]

Perioperative fluids should be administered in the following situations:
1. *Procedures lasting longer than 30 minutes.* Longer surgical times increase the risk of hypothermia, increase the amount of anesthetics delivered to the patient, and result in a delay of resumption of normal diet.
2. *Procedures with an increased incidence of PONV.* Adequate hydration may influence the occurrence of PONV.
3. *Prolonged fasting before surgery.* If the child has been fasting for more than 15 hours, intravenous hydration is desirable for the maintenance of fluid and glucose homeostasis.
4. *Procedures associated with intraoperative and postoperative bleeding.*

Regional Anesthesia

The use of regional anesthesia in the ambulatory setting is well established. Uncontrolled postoperative pain delays recovery and increases the risk for chronic postsurgical pain. Regional anesthesia improves pain scores, decreases opiate use, lowers the incidence of PONV, shortens the recovery period, and reduces PACU stay.[80] Thus, more patients can be discharged home in less time with higher satisfaction.[137] The provider should assess the patient's appropriateness for regional anesthesia, which includes current medications, comorbidities, patient desire, and surgeon preference.

Local wound infiltration, peripheral nerve block, intravenous regional anesthesia, ophthalmic blocks (e.g., retrobulbar or periorbital), brachial plexus anesthesia, spinal anesthesia, and epidural anesthesia have all been used successfully during outpatient surgery. Although, both spinal and epidural anesthesia are not commonly used anesthetic techniques for ambulatory surgery. The proper application of outpatient regional anesthesia requires knowledge of the anticipated surgical procedure, anesthesia requirements, length of procedure, and appropriate patient selection. The shortest-acting agent capable of providing satisfactory central neuraxial blockade, in combination with a potent opiate (i.e., fentanyl), may be considered in the ambulatory setting if unreasonable delays in discharge are to be avoided. Lidocaine is a good agent for short procedures, yet some clinicians avoid its use secondary to concerns over transient neurologic symptoms (TNS). Low-dose bupivacaine (<6 mg) provides a low risk of TNS with the potential of a short discharge time, but with a high degree of variability and a limitation of adequate surgical anesthesia to the lower extremity and rectal area at the lower doses. The recovery from bupivacaine at doses of as little as 4 mg may take up to 240 minutes before discharge readiness is reached.[137] Prilocaine and preservative-free 2-chloroprocaine are popular short-acting agents approved for neuraxial use outside of the United States.[138,139] Potential risks and benefits of neuraxial agent selection should all be considered when used in the outpatient setting.

Ultrasound-guided, single-shot peripheral nerve blockade with longer acting local anesthetics can provide up to 24 hours of analgesia postoperatively. The use of ultrasound guidance has been shown to decrease the length of time needed to place a peripheral block, and to decrease the number of incomplete or failed blocks.[140] Peripheral nerve blockade in conjunction with general anesthesia has been found to reduce the incidence of unanticipated hospital admissions.[141-143]

Continuous peripheral nerve blocks may provide extended postoperative pain relief for outpatients for up to 7 days.[144] Continuous peripheral nerve blocks are also appropriate in pediatric and adolescent patients in the outpatient setting. Additional education and resources are required for patients who go home with continuous blocks.[145] Regional techniques may not provide reliable anesthesia when compared to general anesthesia, and may further delay surgery. Furthermore, other potential postoperative complications, may include postspinal headache, TNS after spinal anesthesia, and urinary retention.[146] The advantages and disadvantages of the use of outpatient regional anesthesia are listed in Box 42.9.[147]

Recommendations for the safe and effective use of regional anesthesia in outpatient surgery are noted in Box 42.10. Specific regional techniques are discussed in detail in Chapters 49 and 50.

POSTOPERATIVE CONSIDERATIONS

After the surgical procedure, care is provided in either the PACU (phase I) or the short-stay unit (phase II) until the patient is ready for discharge from the ambulatory setting. The location and the level of nursing care required vary according to the patient undergoing the procedure, the type of anesthesia used, and the surgical procedure. Properly addressing potential or realized complications in the most efficient manner possible expedites patient management and promotes a timely discharge process. Complications that might delay the patient's departure from the ambulatory facility include nausea, vomiting, and pain. Each outpatient facility has specific criteria for discharge that should be met before the patient is released from the facility.[148] A thorough discussion of the current practices in postanesthesia recovery is provided in Chapter 55.

Postoperative Complications and Management

With today's standard of anesthesia care, major morbidity and mortality after ambulatory surgery are extremely rare; however, a variety of adverse postoperative events may lead to unplanned hospital admission (Box 42.11).[149] PONV and pain are the most common reasons for hospitalization after ambulatory surgery. Certain procedures (e.g., laparoscopic inguinal herniorrhaphy; head and neck; ear, nose, and throat; urologic; orthopedic) are also associated with a higher incidence of unplanned hospital admissions. The hospital admission rate after ambulatory surgery is less than 2%.[150]

Nausea and Vomiting

Persistent nausea and vomiting are responsible for delays in discharge and for increases in patient cost, and are a common factor in unanticipated hospital admission after outpatient surgery. The reported incidence of PONV is approximately 30% on average and as high as 80% in high-risk patients. Postdischarge nausea and vomiting (PDNV) has been reported to occur in 37% of patients.[151] Many anesthetic- and nonanesthetic-related factors affect the susceptibility of patients to postoperative nausea and emesis. A complete discussion of PONV and PDNV and the antiemetic drugs can be found in Chapter 14.

Postoperative Pain

Appropriate postoperative pain management helps minimize the stress of surgery, thereby fostering a quicker convalescence. Uncontrolled postoperative pain causes triggering of the stress response, patient uneasiness, and neurohumoral responses, and increases nausea

---

BOX 42.9   Advantages and Disadvantages of Outpatient Regional Anesthesia

Advantages
- Peripheral nerve block recovery times are shorter than those of general anesthesia.
- Unanticipated admission to the hospital is reduced.
- Phase I recovery bypass (fast-track) eligibility is high.
- Provides excellent immediate postoperative pain relief.
- Improved postoperative pain scores compared to general anesthesia.
- Common side effects associated with general anesthesia (e.g., airway trauma, dizziness, "hangover," myalgia, nausea and vomiting, pharyngitis) are minimized.
- Patients who fear general anesthesia or "loss of control" have a satisfactory alternative.

Disadvantages
- Cooperation of both the patient and the surgeon is required.
- Regional anesthesia may require more time initially when compared to general anesthesia. Patient stays may be minimized by early placement of the proposed regional anesthetic if appropriate.
- Inherent problems associated with regional anesthesia, include the sympathetic block associated with spinal and epidural anesthesia, potential nerve injury, pneumothorax associated with interscalene and paravertebral blocks, fall risk with lumbar plexus blocks, as well as respiratory compromise that can come with phrenic nerve blockade.[158]
- Time to discharge may be delayed for slow recovery of neuraxial block.
- Additional education and resources may be necessary if patient is discharged following a single shot or continuous catheter peripheral nerve block.

BOX 42.10   Recommendations for the Use of Regional Anesthesia in Outpatient Surgery

- Local anesthesia is ideal and should be used whenever possible as the sole anesthetic regimen or be included for postoperative analgesia after any technique.
- Peripheral nerve blockade is highly effective in providing postoperative analgesia and rapid discharge when used for upper or lower extremity surgical procedures. It is also effective for truncal operations such as hernia repair. The use of continuous catheter techniques provides maximum benefit.
- Performance of a block in a separate induction room may reduce the additional time required for regional anesthesia.
- If neuraxial blockade is chosen, spinal anesthesia has the advantages of rapid onset and high reliability. Unfortunately, there appears to be a persistent risk of transient neurologic symptoms (TNS) with the current agents. Low-dose bupivacaine (<6 mg) provides a low risk of TNS with the potential of a short discharge time, but with a high degree of variability and a limitation of adequate surgical anesthesia to the lower extremity and rectal area.
- Excessive sedation should be avoided if the advantage of a high degree of alertness and rapid discharge is to be maintained.
- The addition of epinephrine to subarachnoid local anesthetics increases the potential for urinary retention and for prolonged discharge times. The use of fentanyl may be a better choice for intensifying local anesthetic effect without prolonging discharge due to urinary retention.
- Urinary retention after a short-acting spinal anesthetic in low-risk patients is not any more frequent than with general anesthesia, and these patients can be discharged without mandatory voiding.

Adapted from Alley EA, Mulroy MF. Is regional anesthesia appropriate for outpatient surgery. In: Fleischer LA, ed. *Evidence-Based Practice of Anesthesiology*. 3rd ed. Philadelphia: Elsevier; 2013:404–409.

and vomiting, psychologic distress, discharge delays, and unanticipated hospital admission. Nearly 12% of all ambulatory surgery cases reported inadequate pain control, with ophthalmology reporting the highest incidence of 19%.[27] Pain management should begin with the use of wound infiltration with local anesthesia such as bupivacaine or bupivacaine liposomes (Exparel); the use of peripheral or regional nerve block; perineural, incisional, or intraarticular local anesthesia catheters; and the administration of opioid and nonopioid (i.e., NSAIDs) analgesics preoperatively or intraoperatively, particularly in procedures associated with discomfort after emergence from anesthesia. These practices decrease analgesic requirements in the immediate recovery period, resulting in reduced pain scores and decreased PONV.[152]

The severity and onset of postoperative discomfort are influenced by previously administered analgesics. Immediate control of pain in the PACU can be achieved by incremental titration of small intravenous doses of a short-acting opioid analgesic such as fentanyl (12.5–75 mcg) or alfentanil (50–300 mcg) every 2 to 3 minutes until nociceptive pain relief has been achieved. Nonopioid analgesics should be considered to treat inflammatory pain or neuropathic pain. Advantages may include an improvement of overall analgesia, promotion of early mobilization, and a reduction of opioid-related side effects. Once patient discomfort has been controlled and the patient is tolerating oral fluids, early management of pain with oral analgesics (similar to those the patient will be taking after discharge) should be considered. This allows for evaluation of the analgesic's effect on pain

BOX 42.11 Reasons for Unplanned Hospital Admissions

Anesthetic
Inadequate pain control
Airway complication
Postoperative nausea and vomiting
Postoperative apnea
Aspiration
Prolonged emergence
Postoperative hypoxia

Medical
Exacerbation of preexisting medical condition
Treatment of new medical condition not defined elsewhere
Social factors
Parent or surgeon request
Surgery ends at a late time
No home support/escort

Surgical
Excessive bleeding or pain
More extensive surgery required
Subsequent procedure planned
Surgical complication or unanticipated surgical event
Inadequate pain control postdischarge
Malignancy
Nonsurgical site infections

Adapted from Teja B, et al. Incidence, prediction, and causes of unplanned 30-day hospital admission after ambulatory procedures. *Anesth Analg.* 2020;131(2):497–507; Whippey A, et al. Predictors of unanticipated admission following ambulatory surgery in the pediatric population: a retrospective case-control study. *Paediatr Anaesth.* 2016;26(8):831–837.

alleviation, and the patient's mental condition and respiratory drive. At home, postoperative analgesia should be safe and easily managed by the patient or caregiver.

Discharge Criteria

Before being discharged from the ambulatory facility, the patient must meet certain physiologic criteria-based scores of recovery from the effects of surgery and anesthesia. A consistent method of evaluating the patient for discharge readiness offers the advantages of reproducibility, standardization, and objectivity; however, no single universally accepted standard exists for determining discharge readiness. For discharge to occur, the patient must be clinically stable and able to continue the recovery process at a remote recovery location. The decision to discharge is best made on objective criteria outlined in the policies of each ambulatory surgical facility. Distinct objective discharge criteria must be addressed when assessing home readiness of the patient. (Note: Before discharge from phase I, the patient's vital signs will be stable, there will be no respiratory impairment, protective reflexes of swallow and cough will be present, and the patient will be oriented to the proper preoperative level. It is assumed that the status of these parameters will not deteriorate during the patient's stay in phase I.) Individually, the following clinical markers should be evaluated in an organized, concise manner:

1. Vital signs should be stable and age appropriate.
2. The patient should be oriented to person, place, and time or at a level appropriate for the patient's developmental and preoperative status.
3. Ambulation can be affected by the surgical procedure and the patient's developmental level. If assistance to ambulate is required, the home caregiver must be able to meet this need.
4. There should be no respiratory distress.
5. Swallowing and coughing protective airway reflexes must be present.
6. Bleeding should be minimal or appropriate for the surgical procedure.
7. Pain should be minimal or controlled with an appropriate analgesic regimen.
8. Nausea and vomiting should be minimal.
9. Oral intake prior to discharge is not necessary unless crucial to the patient's continued convalescence at home (e.g., diabetic patient, patient requiring oral analgesics).[153]
10. Voiding is not mandatory before discharge, except for patients at high risk for postoperative urinary retention (e.g., history of postoperative urinary retention, pelvic or urologic surgery, perioperative catheterization). In this high-risk population for urinary retention, a bladder scan should be employed prior to discharge to ensure overdistention is not an issue.[153]
11. A responsible caregiver should be available.

A complete discussion of postanesthesia discharge criteria can be found in Chapter 55.

Discharge Considerations

During the preparatory phase, the availability of a responsible person who will oversee the patient's care once the patient is discharged should be ascertained before surgery. In some cases, inpatient admission may be necessary if a responsible individual cannot be located. Postoperative care may be required for up to 48 hours in such cases, especially in elderly patients. The patient and responsible person should be provided with written instructions that are verbally

BOX 42.12   Key Education Points for Discharge Instructions

Medications

- Detail the name, purpose, and dosage schedule for each medication. Emphasize the importance of following the directions on the label.
- The patient should resume medications taken before surgery per the physician's order.
- If pain medication is not prescribed, nonprescription, nonaspirin analgesics (e.g., acetaminophen, ibuprofen) may be effective to treat mild aches and pains.
- Additional pain medication may be ordered by the physician after surgery. The patient should take these medications as directed, preferably with food to prevent gastrointestinal upset.
- Some centers provide necessary postoperative prescriptions during the preoperative visit. Reviewing medication instructions may be helpful.

Activity Restriction

- Caution the patient to exercise minimal exertion for the remainder of the day following surgery. Postoperative dizziness or drowsiness is not unusual after surgery and anesthesia, and may last several days.
- For the next 24 hours, the patient should not drive a vehicle, operate machinery or power tools, consume alcohol (including beer), make important personal or business decisions, or sign important documents.
- Describe the permissible activity level in specific behavioral terms (e.g., do not lift objects >20 lb); describe any limitation of activities.

Diet

- Explain any dietary restrictions or instructions.
- If no dietary restriction, instruct the patient to progress as tolerated to a regular diet.

Surgical and Anesthesia Side Effects

- Anticipated sequelae of surgery, such as bleeding and pain, should be delineated.
- Common side effects associated with anesthesia include dizziness, drowsiness, myalgia, nausea and vomiting, and sore throat.

Possible Complications and Symptoms

- Instruct the patient and responsible caregiver in pertinent signs and symptoms that could be indicative of postoperative complications.
- The patient should call the physician if any of the following develop:
  - Fever >38.3°C (>101°F)
  - Persistent, atypical pain
  - Pain not relieved by pain medication
  - Bleeding that does not stop or is prolonged, unexpected drainage from the wound
  - Extreme redness/swelling around the incision, drainage of pus
  - Urinary retention after 8 hr or as otherwise instructed
  - Unremitting nausea or vomiting

Treatment and Tests

- Provide instruction on procedures the patient or responsible caregiver are expected to perform, such as dressing changes, the application of warm, moist compresses, or other postoperative home treatments.
- Include a complete list of necessary supplies.
- If any postoperative tests are to be conducted, instructions as to the date, time, test location, and any previsit preparation should be listed.

Access to Postdischarge Care

- Provide the telephone number of the responsible and available physician.
- Provide the telephone number of the ambulatory center and the hours of operation.
- Provide the name, address, and telephone number of the appropriate emergency care facility.

Follow-Up Care

- Identify the date, time, and location of the patient's scheduled return visit to the clinic or surgeon.

Modified from Marley RA, Moline BM. Patient discharge from the ambulatory setting. *J Post Anesth Nurs.* 1996;11:41.

reinforced before the patient is discharged. This information should include the physician's telephone numbers and steps to be taken if questions or complications arise. Once the patient has satisfied the criteria for discharge from the outpatient facility, certain discharge instructions should be reviewed to expedite and streamline the discharge process (Box 42.12).

The period of patient recovery after discharge from the ambulatory facility until resumption of normal activities is termed phase III. This is an important and often forgotten aspect of postoperative ambulatory care. On patient discharge, it is important to convey that it may take several days before they begin to feel as they did before surgery.

▮ SUMMARY

The numbers and types of surgeries performed on an ambulatory basis will continue to increase, as will the ability of facilities to appropriately treat these patients. Anesthetic techniques and agents will continue to be refined and improved to increase patient safety and care efficiency,

allowing for newer groups of patients and surgical procedures to be conducted on an outpatient basis. These new groups will continue to challenge our resources for providing effective ambulatory anesthesia.

REFERENCES

For a complete list of references for this chapter, scan this QR code with any smartphone code reader app, or visit the following URL: http://booksite.elsevier.com/9780323711944/

43

Anesthesia for Ear, Nose, Throat, and Maxillofacial Surgery

Christopher J. Gill

The practice of anesthesia for the ear, nose, and throat (ENT) patient is both challenging and rewarding. The anesthesia practitioner is often required to make decisions regarding difficult airway management and must have the knowledge and skills to navigate abnormal and difficult anatomy. As a specialty, ENT presents specific concerns to the anesthetist in regard to the preparation and management of surgical procedures (Box 43.1). There are several essential goals when providing anesthesia for ENT and maxillofacial (i.e., plastics and dental) surgical procedures:

1. Possessing a thorough knowledge of the airway anatomy and function
2. Selecting and preparing for appropriate technique(s) and approach for airway management
3. Preventing and managing potential airway complications
4. Producing profound selective muscle relaxation during periods of extreme stimulation yet maintaining the potential for rapid recovery (e.g., suspension laryngoscopy)
5. Maintaining cardiovascular stability during periods of intense surgical stimulation
6. Omitting neuromuscular relaxation for surgical procedures that require isolation of nerves
7. Preventing or containing airway fires
8. Minimizing intraoperative and postoperative blood loss
9. Preventing adverse respiratory and cardiac responses resulting from manipulation of the carotid sinus and body
10. Taking the appropriate postoperative measures to prevent postoperative nausea/vomiting and treat postsurgical airway obstruction
11. Avoiding or limiting the use of nitrous oxide (N_2O) during tympanoplasty or other closed-space grafting

Surgical intervention for ENT procedures uses a variety of specialty equipment, including lasers, endoscopes, and specialized endotracheal tubes (ETTs) (e.g., laser and microlaryngeal tube). The basis of many ENT and maxillofacial surgical procedures includes endoscopic examination of the sinuses; tissue tumors of the head, neck, and oral cavity; abscesses; surgery to the middle ear; papillomas of the airway; hypertrophic tonsils and adenoids; acute epiglottitis; thyroid disorders; and traumatic or congenital facial deformities. Most of these procedures involve the nose, facial and frontal sinuses, larynx, oropharynx, nasopharynx, tongue, trachea, mandible, and maxilla, in addition to other supporting structures of the head and neck. These procedures necessitate sharing the airway with the surgeon and may lead to a tenuous airway and significant challenges perioperatively. Airway compromise in ENT patients may be subtle and can take several forms. Therefore good communication is essential in the preoperative period to ensure the safest approach to anesthesia.

This chapter describes the pertinent anatomy and physiology of the head and neck for the anesthetist, reviews specialized anesthetic considerations, reviews surgical and anesthesia equipment used during ENT procedures, analyzes some of the common pharmacologic agents used for ENT procedures, and discusses principles of anesthesia for ENT.

FUNCTIONAL ANATOMY OF THE HEAD AND NECK

A fundamental knowledge of the anatomic and physiologic function of the structures of the head and neck is essential for dealing with the myriad decisions arising perioperatively during these procedures. Commonly, ENT surgical procedures are performed because the anatomic structures are abnormal, distorted, or deviated. Having a working knowledge of the structures and their relationships before subjecting the patient to respiratory changes produced by anesthesia is imperative.

The anatomic structures of the head and neck and their relationships are complex (Fig. 43.1). The sensory and motor supply of the upper airway originates from cranial nerves and includes the trigeminal, glossopharyngeal, facial, and vagus nerves. Understanding the sensory supply is required to provide sufficient local and regional anesthesia. Likewise, motor function evaluated during and after surgical procedures may indicate trauma or damage to muscles. A thorough knowledge of which nerves control muscle function is essential to preventing such trauma.

The anatomic relationships regarding the nasopharynx, oropharynx, laryngopharynx, and lower airway structures such as the larynx, cricoid, thyroid, and vocal cords provide a basis for directing and providing care for the patient receiving ENT surgery. The nose is a major anatomic structure that is responsible for warming, filtering, and providing humidity to the air taken in during inspiration. The structures of the nose include the external nose, the nasal cavity, and frontal, maxillary, and ethmoid sinuses. The nares or nostrils are separated by the septum. The lateral margins of the nares are cartilaginous structures and extend posteriorly over the hard palate leading to a confluence at the soft palate, oropharynx, and base of the tongue. The oropharynx rests superior to the epiglottis, vocal cords, larynx, and trachea.[1-3]

Externally, the nose is composed largely of cartilage supported primarily by soft connective tissue and delicate mucous membranes, as is the nasal septum. The nasal cavities are hollow structures formed by a floor, roof, lateral wall, and the septum. The lateral aspects of the nasal cavities contain concha, or turbinates. The turbinates are highly vascular and are divided into three separate compartments: the superior, middle, and inferior. The turbinates greatly increase the surface area of the nasal cavities, aiding in filtration and humidification of inspired gases.

The extensive vascular supply of the turbinates may lead to severe bleeding if the nasal airway or nasoendotracheal tube is not inserted along the superior margin of the hard palate. Congestion of the mucosal veins in the turbinates of the nose causes swelling

BOX 43.1   Special Considerations for ENT Procedures

- Increased risk of unanticipated difficult airways
- Cannot intubate, cannot ventilate situation
- Use of specialized ventilation techniques
- Insufflation
- Intermittent apnea
- Apneic oxygenation
- Prevention of endotracheal tube fire
- Shared airway
- Surgical field avoidance
- Restricted use of nitrous oxide
- Restricted use of muscle relaxants
- Use of specialized equipment
- Use of laser for ablation
- High-frequency jet ventilation
- Transnasal humidified rapid-insufflation ventilatory exchange (or THRIVE)
- Potentially undiagnosed obstructive sleep apnea
- Potential for bleeding

ENT, Ear, nose, and throat.

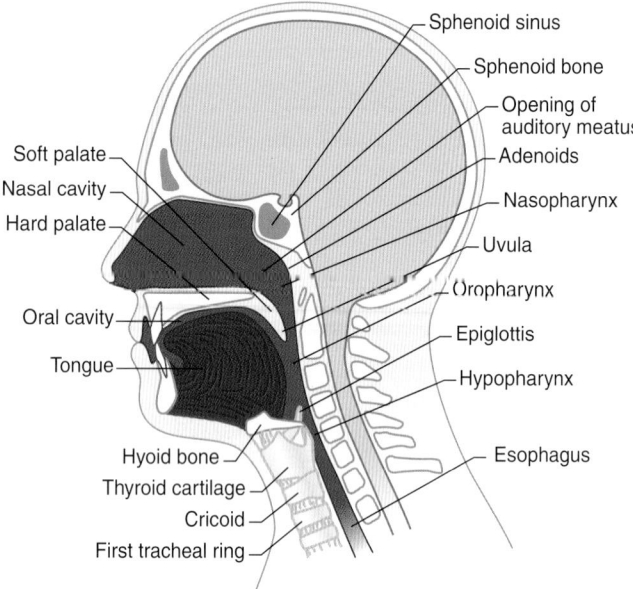

Fig. 43.1 Anatomy of nasal cavity, oral cavity, nasopharynx, oropharynx, and hypopharynx. (From Gropper MA, et al., eds. *Miller's Anesthesia.* 9th ed. Philadelphia: Elsevier; 2020.)

of these tissues, reducing the size of the nasal cavity (most notably, the paranasal sinuses), and thus creating the feeling of "congestion" during respiration. Inadvertent palatine submucosal insertion of the nasoendotracheal tube can lead to severe bleeding or infection in the perioperative period if entry of the tube is forced or tissues are engorged. These paired sinuses include the sphenoid, ethmoid, frontal, and maxillary sinuses. Turbinates filter, humidify, and warm the air during inspiration. These hollow structures are formed of low-density bone and are lined with a thin layer of mucous membranes, reducing the weight of the skull but making these bones more susceptible to fractures and cerebral spinal fluid leak secondary to facial trauma.[1-3]

The pharynx is composed of the terminal end of the nasopharynx, the oropharynx, and laryngopharynx or hypopharynx extending to the sixth cervical vertebra. The medulla oblongata inhibits respiration with swallowing; the pharynx then serves as a muscular tube that constricts, allowing the passage of food. The pharynx allows the smooth passage of air and functions as a modulator for the voice. The nasopharynx is continuous with the internal nasal cavities and extends to the soft palate. The nasopharynx communicates with the oropharynx and forms the posterior aspect of the throat. Major structures of the oropharynx include the base of the tongue, soft palate, uvula, and lymphatic structures (tonsils). The tonsils are the most sensitive areas of the oropharynx. Beginning with the anterior margin and progressing bilaterally and posteriorly, the oropharynx is defined by the soft palate, base of the tongue, uvula, palatine tonsils, and adenoids, forming Waldeyer tonsillar ring.[1-3]

Hypertrophy of the palatine and adenoid tonsils (exaggerated many times by chronic infection) and of the soft palate and uvula can pose serious airway compromise, particularly in young children. The generous blood supply to the tonsils from branches of the external carotid, maxillary, and facial arteries, and their close proximity to the facial and internal arteries, is a matter of concern regarding potential bleeding during "routine" tonsillectomy. The laryngopharynx includes the epiglottis, which provides protection for the vocal cords, and is the region shared by the esophageal orifice and larynx.

The complexity of the neuromuscular system, which controls the epiglottis, allows the isolation of the trachea from the esophagus during swallowing. Any interruption of this coordinated neuromuscular function of the epiglottis or of any other protective reflexes can provide a dangerous opportunity for the entrance of food or liquid into the larynx and lower airway. As food is squeezed posteriorly, an automatic swallowing reflex is initiated. The larynx is pulled superiorly allowing the epiglottis to cover and protect the opening of the larynx.[1] The epiglottis does not function as a movable lidlike structure that falls to close the larynx during swallowing, as is often claimed. Passage of food into the trachea can occur if the muscles and protective elevation of the larynx become rigid or are changed because of nerve interruption. A series of reflex and involuntary processes mediated by the superior laryngeal, recurrent laryngeal, and glossopharyngeal nerves coordinates and regulates glottic closure during swallowing.[1-3]

The larynx is a rigid organ composed of three paired and three unpaired cartilages (arytenoid, corniculate, and cuneiform; and thyroid, cricoid, and epiglottis, respectively) and is supported by the hyoid bone. This hollow structure forms a reservoir distal to Waldeyer tonsillar ring and provides the connection of the oropharynx to the trachea (Fig. 43.2). The primary functions of the larynx are vocalization and articulation; secondarily, it provides protection of the airway and allows respiration.[1] In the adult, the area of the vocal cords, or rima glottidis, is the narrowest portion of the larynx. In children, the cricoid ring has traditionally been regarded as the narrowest portion of the airway until approximately 10 years of age. Cuffed tubes were then generally recommended for those older than 8 to 10 years of age to allow for a better seal of the airway, prevent subglottic edema, and reduce the incidence of postoperative airway compromise.[4] However, studies have indicated no difference in the rate of postoperative complications, such as postintubation croup, between the use of cuffed and uncuffed ETTs. These studies instead support the use of a newer pediatric low-pressure cuffed tube called the Microcuff ETT (Microcuff GmbH, Weinheim, Germany, distributed by Kimberly-Clark USA).[5]

Specific nervous system structures of the head and neck are noteworthy because of their superficial location or proximity to operative sites. Surgeons may use audible or visual nerve-locating devices to find

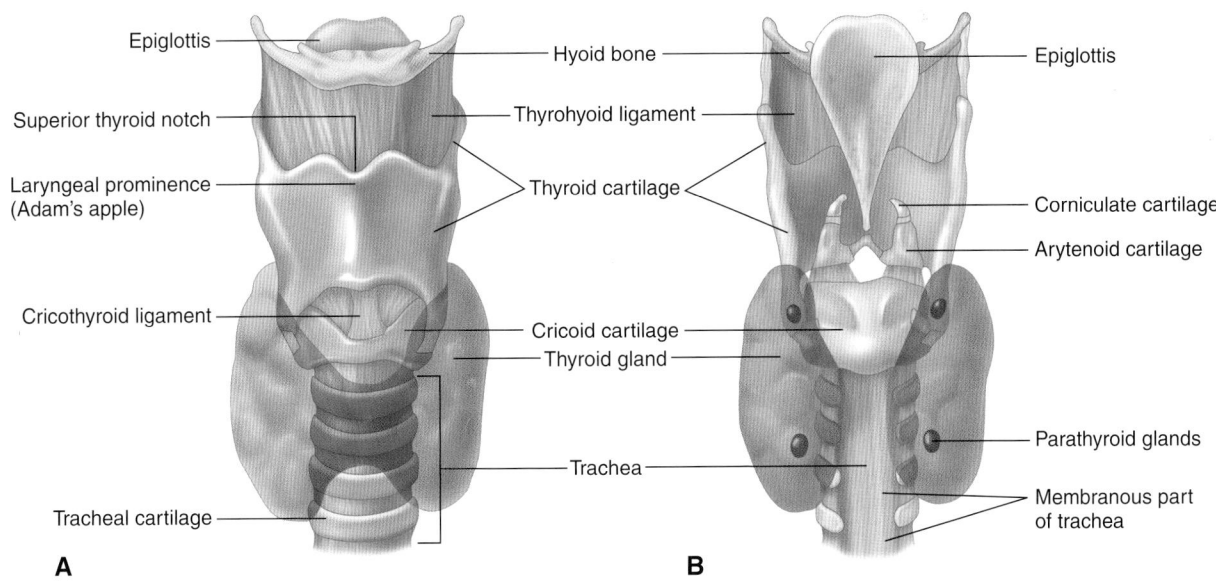

Fig. 43.2 Laryngeal cartilages. Some softer tissues of the larynx and surrounding structures have been removed to make it possible to see the cartilages of the larynx. Note the position of the nearby thyroid gland. (A) Anterior view. (B) Posterior view. (From Patton KT. *Anatomy & Physiology.* 10th ed. St. Louis: Elsevier; 2019:806.)

these nerves and their appropriate branches. To accurately locate these nerves, neuromuscular blocking agents may need to be avoided during the maintenance of certain general anesthetics.

The facial nerve (VII) has six major branches: four anterior (temporal, zygomatic, buccal, and mandibular), one inferior (cervical), and one posterior (posterior auricular) branch. The facial nerve located at the tragus of the ear is the motor and sensory supply to the muscles for facial expressions. The zygomatic branch exits the skull via the stylomastoid foramen and advances anteriorly over the maxilla. The chorda tympani branch of the facial nerve conveys taste from the anterior two-thirds of the tongue, and the more superficial tribranched facial nerve controls facial expression. The trigeminal nerve begins at the gasserian ganglion and divides into three branches: the ophthalmic (the first division, V_1), maxillary (the second division, V_2), and mandibular (the third division, V_3). All three divisions provide sensory and motor innervation to the nose, sinuses, palate, and tongue. They aid in the motor control of the face and in mastication.[1-3] The glossopharyngeal nerve provides motor and sensory innervation for the base of the tongue and nasopharynx and oropharynx. The glossopharyngeal nerve is responsible for eliciting the gag reflex during instrumentation of the posterior pharynx and vallecula.

The superior laryngeal nerve and recurrent laryngeal nerve (RLN) are both branches of the vagus (X). The superior laryngeal nerve descends to the hyoid bone and then branches into the internal laryngeal nerve, which passes through the thyrohyoid membrane, and the exterior laryngeal nerve, which descends over the lateral thyroid cartilage to the distal trachea. The RLN ascends from the vagus up the distal trachea, passing through the cricothyroid ligament into the proximal trachea and vocal cords. The RLN lies between the trachea and esophagus and supplies sensory innervation to the trachea and area below the vocal cords. This branch of the vagus nerve also affects vocal cord closure and sensory function up to the inferior aspect of the epiglottis. Stimulation of the epiglottis with the tip of a straight laryngoscope, blades, suction catheters, and placement of an ETT in the trachea can

produce a vagal response.[3] The paired and unpaired cartilages of the larynx are listed in Table 43.1. Nerve supply to the larynx is given in Table 43.2. The intrinsic muscles of the larynx, their nerve supply, and function are listed in Table 43.3. The extrinsic muscles of the larynx, their nerve supply, and function are listed in Table 43.4.[1-6]

TABLE 43.1   Paired and Unpaired Cartilages of the Larynx

Paired	Unpaired
Arytenoid	Thyroid
Corniculate	Cricoid
Cuneiform	Epiglottis

TABLE 43.2   Nerve Supply of to the Larynx

Nerve	Innervation
Sensory Nerves	
Superior laryngeal n. internal branch (vagus)	Laryngeal mucosa above vocal cords (inferior epiglottis)
Recurrent laryngeal	Laryngeal mucosa below vocal cords
Glossopharyngeal	Superior aspect of epiglottis and base of tongue
Motor Nerves	
Recurrent laryngeal	All intrinsic muscles except cricothyroid
Superior laryngeal n. external branch	Cricothyroid muscles

n, Nerve.

TABLE 43.3   Intrinsic Muscles of the Larynx

Muscle	Innervation	Function
Cricothyroid	Superior laryngeal nerve	Tension and elongates vocal cords
Thyroarytenoid	Recurrent laryngeal nerve	Relaxes vocal cords
Vocalis	Recurrent laryngeal nerve	Relaxes vocal cords
Posterior cricoarytenoid	Recurrent laryngeal nerve	Abducts vocal cords
Lateral cricoarytenoid	Recurrent laryngeal nerve	Adducts vocal cords
Transverse arytenoid	Recurrent laryngeal nerve	Adducts vocal cords
Aryepiglottic	Recurrent laryngeal nerve	Closes glottis
Oblique arytenoid	Recurrent laryngeal nerve	Closes glottis; approximates folds

TABLE 43.4   Extrinsic Muscles of the Larynx

Muscle	Innervation	Function
Sternohyoid	Cervical plexus; C1, C2, C3	Draws hyoid bone inferiorly
Sternothyroid	Cervical plexus; C1, C2, C3	Draws thyroid cartilage caudad
Thyrohyoid	Cervical plexus; hypoglossal nerve; C1 and C2	Pulls hyoid bone inferiorly
Thyroepiglottic	Recurrent laryngeal nerve	Inversion of aryepiglottic fold
Stylopharyngeus	Glossopharyngeal	Folds thyroid cartilage
Inferior pharyngeal constrictor	Pharyngeal plexus; vagus	Aids swallowing

PREPARATION AND CONSIDERATIONS FOR EAR, NOSE, AND THROAT PROCEDURES

The Shared Airway and Considerations for Positioning

Operative procedures involving the airway, mouth, or bony structures of the face involve a true sharing of the airway between the surgeon and the anesthetist. Therefore proper preparation requires planning and communication between the surgeon, surgical personnel, and the anesthetist prior to the surgical procedure. Sharing the airway also requires preparing and planning the use of the appropriate equipment. For example, during laryngoscopy, the ETT may have to be smaller in diameter and moved to the side opposite of the operative field to allow the surgeon ample room to work and to facilitate the surgery. The head of the table is often rotated 90 to 180 degrees away from the anesthetist, resulting in a vulnerable airway to which the anesthetist may have little or no access. Particular concerns are the maintenance of adequate ventilation and patency and security of the anesthesia circuit and ETT. Extubation, disconnects, and leaks must be prevented. Adequacy of ventilation is constantly assessed by observing chest movement, auscultation, pulse oximetry, end tidal CO_2, and blood gas analysis (if necessary). A sudden loss of breath sounds, rising inspiratory pressures, or a reduction in end tidal CO_2, particularly in the presence of a sharp reduction in inspiratory effort, may be caused by a deflation of the ETT cuff, obstruction of the ETT, dislodgment of the ETT, a disconnection of the anesthesia circuit, or severing of the ETT during surgical dissection.[6] When coupled with vigilance, precordial or esophageal stethoscopes are simple devices that should not be overlooked; these devices, in addition to more sophisticated mechanical devices, help the anesthetist maintain assessment of the airway.

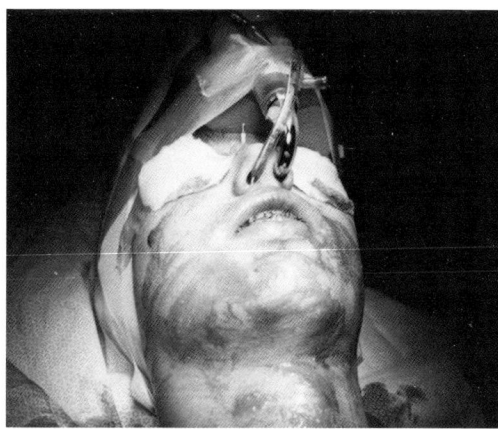

Fig. 43.3 Illustration of secured airway for a patient undergoing face, neck, or maxillofacial surgical procedures. Note that the tube is positioned to prevent pressure on the lip, nose, or forehead and secured with tape to prevent movement during surgery. The connection is covered by sterile surgical drapes and allows only limited access during the surgical procedure.

Assessment of the airway prior to induction is critical for all patients. Although the induction of anesthesia and securing of the airway are performed in the usual manner (with the anesthetist at the head of the table), the management of the airway can become questionable and difficult while at a distance. Obtaining a thorough history and performing an extensive evaluation of the airway for the ENT patient is crucial. A good examination of the airway will (1) allow for a careful and deliberate approach to airway management, (2) aid in evaluating the need for additional equipment and assistance, and (3) include alternative approaches for the difficult airway if the initial plan proves not to be successful. Once the induction is complete and the airway established, the anesthetist must be prepared to provide adequate ventilation, deliver necessary anesthetic and adjunct agents, place invasive lines, and safely monitor the patient while remaining at a distance and isolated from the airway.

Orchestrating how the patient is turned so that the patient's head is away from the anesthetist requires clear planning and preemptive discussion with the health care team. The ETT should be secured with tape or suture to prevent removal. Tape may require reinforcement of which transparent occlusive dressings are well suited. The invasive line tubing, intravenous (IV) access lines, monitoring devices, and breathing circuit typically require added length to extend distance from the patient without creating tension. This should be considered and placed before initial surgical draping. In addition to increasing line and tubing length, extra thought must be given to padding potential pressure points. The patient's entire head is frequently prepped and draped into the surgical field, limiting access to the ETT and breathing circuit connections (Fig. 43.3).

When repositioning of the head is necessary, communication between the surgeon and anesthesia provider is essential to reduce the possibility of extubation, position change, or occlusion of the ETT. Signs of air leaks around the ETT (e.g., bubbling, the sound of air escaping, or the smell of anesthetic agent) may well be more sensitive indicators than mechanical airway monitors. Occlusion of the ETT is best prevented but can be determined by good auscultation, watching chest wall motion, and monitoring inspiratory pressures and morphology of CO_2 waveforms. The thoughtful surgeon should communicate any changes in the surgical field, such as changing the position of a suspended or fixed laryngoscope, dark blood, manipulation of carotid bodies, or the need for a change in the patient's head position.[7] Increased inspiratory pressures or a rapid loss of inspiratory pressure, decreased oxygen saturation, changes in end tidal CO_2 measurements, or diminished breath sounds should in turn be communicated to the surgeon so that inspection of the airway and anesthesia circuit may be undertaken. If unable to arrive

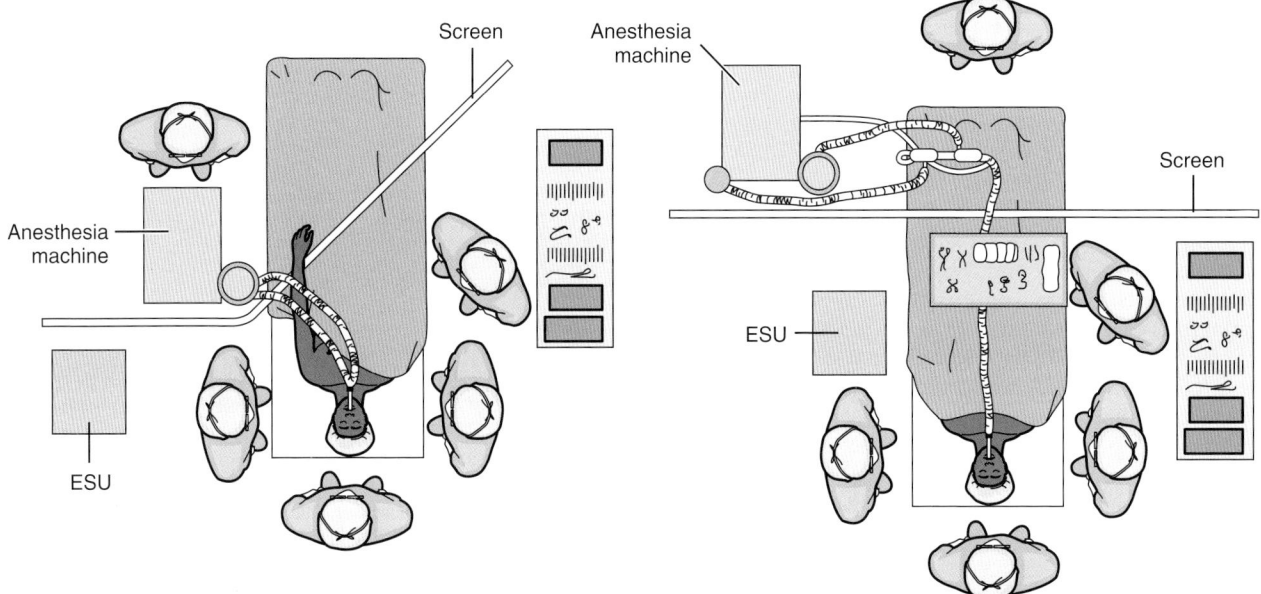

Fig. 43.4 Position of the anesthetist for surgery of the head and neck. The anesthetist is positioned at the side of the table and using a standard circle circuit *(left)*. The anesthetist is positioned at the foot of the bed and using a coaxial (Bain) circuit *(right)*. *ESU,* Electrosurgical unit. (From Phillips N, Hornacky A. *Berry & Kohn's Operating Room Technique.* 14th ed. St. Louis: Elsevier; 2021:851.)

at a cause, undraping the patient may become necessary for a thorough examination of tube placement and connections, or to find a leak in the anesthesia circuit that could compromise patient ventilation.

Procedures of the head and neck typically require access to all planes of the head by several members of the surgical team.[8] Because several problems can be encountered with the intubated patient during the surgical procedure, the surgeon may elect to perform a tracheostomy, then place and suture a flexible ETT in a fixed position during the procedure. A heightened state of vigilance must be maintained for occlusions from mucous plugs or blood, disconnects, ETT fires, and other problems that may arise during the anesthetic. During some ENT procedures, the surgical team may also need access to the chest, abdomen, or extremities for securing grafts for the esophagus or oral cavity. This often requires the anesthesia provider to take residence at either the side of the patient or at the foot of the operating table (Fig. 43.4). Providing a smooth transition while protecting the airway and preventing hypoxia are the primary concerns during movement of an operating table with an anesthetized patient.

The anesthesia circuit and other monitors should be temporarily and briefly disconnected before the bed is turned. This will prevent undue tension on the circuit and other lines that could lead to traumatic extubation or loss of access. Ventilation of the patient with 100% oxygen and adequate tidal volumes for 3 to 5 minutes before disconnection will denitrogenate the functional residual volume and provide an extra reservoir of oxygen during the turn, preventing even a short period of hypoxia. However, if a volatile agent is the primary source of anesthesia, the addition of IV anesthesia during this preoxygenation is necessary to maintain an adequate level of anesthesia and/or amnesia during this period. A saturation of 100% is a reasonable goal before the disconnection and table movement.

The degree of table movement should be discussed with the surgeon before any interruption in the anesthesia or the breathing circuit takes place. Turning of the operating table should be a well-organized procedure, understood by all members of the surgical team, and one that takes a minimum amount of time. After relocking the bed, reconnection of the anesthesia circuit must be immediate to reestablish oxygenation and/or anesthesia. Reevaluation and assessment of the tube placement,

breath sounds, chest expansion, oxygen saturation, anesthetic level, line and IV access, and end tidal CO_2 should be performed before prepping and draping is begun and throughout the case. Once adequate ventilation is established, the use of a heat moisture exchanging (HME) device or airway humidifier will help in decreasing insensible losses from the respiratory system during long periods of anesthesia.

Attention to simple practical points has significant potential to prevent inadvertent extubation or migration of the ETT into the mainstem bronchus. At least one large-bore IV line, in addition to arterial and central venous pressure (CVP) lines, should be started on the nonoperative side and if possible on the side of the patient that will be nearest to the anesthetist during the procedure. This will prevent obstruction of flow caused by the surgical procedure, afford easier access for drug administration and blood sampling, facilitate the manipulation or maintenance of lines during surgery, and allow the surgeon easy access to the operative field. If such lines must be placed on extremities opposite the anesthetist, adequate extensions should be placed before a change in position of the table to reduce the chance of lines being removed, infiltrated, or disconnected during movement. The calf of the leg may be used for noninvasive blood pressure measurements to prevent dampening of IV fluid flows in the upper extremities. Care must be taken to ensure that the measurement of the blood pressure takes into account variations in table changes from the horizontal position to prevent hypotension to vital organs. Monitoring of neuromuscular relaxation may be performed at locations other than the adductor pollicis. Stimulation of the tibial nerve produces flexion of the big toe and is similar to that of the adductor pollicis.[9] Since ENT procedures may take more than 3 hours and can require significant fluid administration, monitoring urinary output with a Foley catheter may be desirable.

SPECIALIZED EQUIPMENT FOR EAR, NOSE, AND THROAT PROCEDURES

Endotracheal Tubes Designed for ENT Surgery

Several ETTs are available for securing an airway. Standard ETTs equipped with flexible or straight connectors are appropriate for many

ENT procedures. The diameter and length of the ETT will affect ventilation and seal of the airway. Using a small-diameter ETT in a large adult airway will not only lead to less ventilation through increased resistance but also will allow only a small portion of the cuff to contact the trachea. Using specialized tubes with small diameters allows more even distribution of the cuff over the trachea during inflation. Several of these specially designed ETTs have found wide acceptance in ENT anesthesia. A variety of designs are used to limit encroachment of the ETT into the surgical field, prevent kinking of the ETT when severe angles are necessary, prevent fires in the airway during laser therapy, and provide maximal patient ventilation and safety.[10]

Several ETTs have been introduced for use in ENT anesthesia. The purpose for the evolution of these various types of ETT cuffs was to reduce cuff pressure on the tracheal wall allowing for improved tracheal perfusion, mitigate tracheal injury, and optimize airway access. Preformed right-angled ETTs, in cuffed and noncuffed types, are available for either oral or nasal intubation of adults or children. Oral RAE tubes (named after inventors Ring, Adair, and Elwyn) are an excellent choice for cleft palate repair, tonsillectomy, uvulopalatopharyngoplasty, and procedures of the eye or upper face. Nasal RAE tubes are particularly well suited to maxillofacial surgery that does not allow for oral intubation. The nasal RAE can be used for cosmetic procedures of the face, surgical procedures of the oral cavity and mandible, or to correct malocclusion. However, although the preformed bend in the RAE tube prevents the ETT from kinking in many instances, it may be too distal or proximal for an individual patient's airways. This may allow the tip of the ETT to rest well below or above the carina. A careful check of the breath sounds and inspiratory pressures is imperative after intubation with the RAE to ensure proper positioning. Nasal intubation and placement of a nasogastric tube in the unconscious patient with facial trauma is best avoided to prevent possible penetration of the brain. If available, a review of head CT should be undertaken during the preoperative anesthetic assessment.[11,12]

Armored or reinforced ETTs all have an embedded coiled wire or plastic coil strand to produce a tube with greater flexibility and memory. Armored tubes for oral or nasal intubation resist kinking and retain their original integrity. They are useful when acute neck flexion or severe angles of the ETT are required, as in procedures involving the base of the skull or posterior aspect of the neck. However, several reports suggest that even the edentulous patient can on occasion occlude a reinforced ETT.[13] Several varieties of metal-impregnated tubes are available for use with laser surgery; these are designed to reduce the occurrence of an airway fire (Figs. 43.5 and 43.6). The cuff of the laser tube is usually filled with saline to dampen or prevent ignition. In addition, it is recommended that the cuff be filled with methylene blue-dyed saline so that a cuff perforation is easily detected. Wrapping a standard ETT with reflective tape is not an adequate alternative to these commercially prepared tubes because the wrapped standard ETT will dry and lead to greater flammability.[14]

Although not classified as an ETT, the laryngeal mask airway (LMA) and the intubating LMA may be used to facilitate intubations, as well as control the airway. The LMA does not produce tracheal stimulation, which can be a considerable advantage in ENT procedures. The incidence of coughing on emergence is lower with the LMA than with the ETT. Another advantage of the LMA is the ability to insert the device without the use of neuromuscular blocking agents, or for airway rescue situations. Although LMA is contraindicated in some patients with laryngeal pathology, it is often the airway of choice when dealing with patients with pharyngeal pathology. Indications for LMA use in ENT surgery include a conduit for surgical access to the glottis and trachea, an aid to neurologic monitoring to avoid relaxant use, and as a means of isolating the glottis from bleeding from pharyngeal sources.[15]

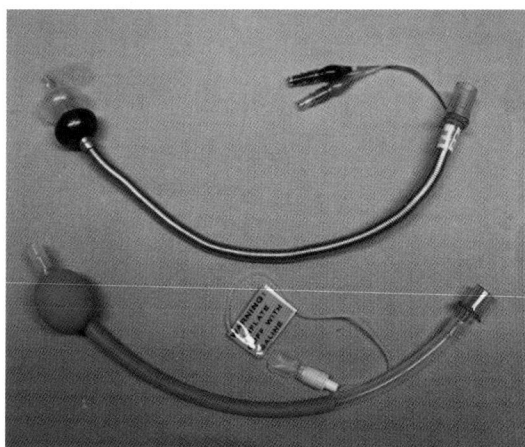

Fig. 43.5 Endotracheal tubes for laser surgery of the airway.

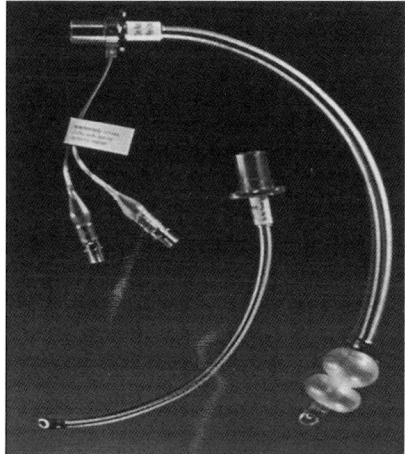

Fig. 43.6 The Laser Flex endotracheal tube comes with a double cuff or no cuff. The double cuff is typically filled with normal saline or blue dye to easily visualize cuff rupture. (Reprinted by permission from Nellcor Puritan Bennett LLC, Boulder, CO, part of Covidien.)

SPECIAL CONSIDERATIONS FOR EAR, NOSE, AND THROAT PROCEDURES

Pharmacologic Considerations

The use of local anesthetics is particularly prevalent during nasal and sinus surgery. The most commonly used local anesthetics for ENT surgery include the amide-based drugs. Though many procedures are performed using topical and local anesthesia as the sole agent, this may also occur in combination with IV sedation, monitored anesthesia care, or general anesthesia. Table 43.5 gives some topical local anesthetics commonly used in ENT surgery. Determination of doses of local anesthetics administered by injection and topically must be carefully calculated because more than one agent in various combinations is commonly used.

Additional information regarding local anesthetics for injection and topical use can be found in Table 10.8.

Vasoactive Drugs

The duration of action of a local anesthetic is proportional to the time the drug is in contact with nerve fibers. For this reason, epinephrine in varying concentrations (1:200,000 or 5 mcg/mL; 1:100,000 or 10 mcg/mL; and 1:50,000 or 20 mcg/mL) may be added to local anesthetic

TABLE 43.5   Topical Anesthetic Drugs

Drug	Concentration	Dose	Notable Features
Cocaine	4% solution	3 mg/kg	Only local anesthetic with vasoconstrictive ability; blocks reuptake of norepinephrine and epinephrine at adrenergic nerve endings
Lidocaine	2% and 4% solution; 2% viscous solution; 10% aerosol; 2.5% and 5% ointment; 10%, 15%, 20% cream	4 mg/kg plain; 7 mg/kg epinephrine 250–300 mg	Rapid onset; suitable for all areas of the tracheobronchial tree
Benzocaine	Cetacaine contains: 14% benzocaine, 2% butamben, and 2% tetracaine Hurricane, others		Short duration of action (10 min); can produce methemoglobinemia
Bupivacaine	0.25%, 0.5%, 0.75%	2.5 mg/kg plain	Slow hepatic clearance; long duration of action
Mepivacaine	1%, 2%	4 mg/kg	Intermediate potency with rapid onset
Dyclonine	0.5%, 1%	300 mg maximum	Topical spray or gargle; frequent use for laryngoscopy; absorbed through skin and mucous membranes

solutions to produce vasoconstriction. Vasoconstriction limits systemic absorption and maintains a higher drug concentration in the vicinity of the nerve fibers to be anesthetized, thus extending the effects of the local anesthetic. Addition of epinephrine to a local anesthetic prolongs the duration of blockade and decreases systemic absorption and plasma concentrations, thus decreasing toxicity.[16]

It is estimated that in the United States, topical cocaine (4%–10% solution) anesthesia is used in more than 50% of ENT procedures performed annually, specifically rhinolaryngology procedures.[16] Cocaine is a naturally occurring ester of benzoic acid that is hydrolyzed by plasma cholinesterase. Applied topically, it is an excellent local anesthetic and vasoconstrictor. The duration of action is approximately 45 minutes.[17] Cocaine produces vasoconstriction by blocking catecholamine reuptake into the adrenergic nerve ending resulting in vasoconstriction and shrinking of the mucosa. Epinephrine is also injected for ENT procedures and is usually injected shortly after the application of cocaine. This combination of cocaine and epinephrine will cause sympathetic nervous system stimulation. Caution must be exercised when combining use of both drugs as toxic levels of epinephrine may result.[18] This interaction can result in severe headaches, hypertension, tachycardia, and dysrhythmias.[19-21] Given these interactions, cocaine may be best omitted in the context of significant cardiac disease/risk factors for another vasoconstricting agent such as oxymetazoline.[19]

Anticholinergics

Anticholinergics were used liberally in the early days of anesthesia predominantly because of the excessive secretions caused by older volatile inhalation agents. With the advent of newer anesthetic agents, excessive secretions are not an issue, and the routine use of anticholinergics has diminished. The antisialagogue effects, however, may still be useful in certain intraoral procedures that require a drier operative field. Glycopyrrolate may be a better choice than atropine because it produces less tachycardia in comparison to atropine. Glycopyrrolate also does not readily cross the blood-brain barrier and thus lacks sedative effects.

Corticosteroids

Glucocorticoids may be administered preoperatively and intraoperatively to decrease laryngeal edema formation, reduce nausea and vomiting, and prolong the analgesic effects of local anesthetics. They should be administered as early as possible in the perioperative period to reach their peak effect prior to initiating surgery. The use of steroids may reduce the nausea and vomiting experienced after surgery.

Dexamethasone was also reported to prolong the analgesic effects of local anesthetics. It has been postulated that prostaglandins, histamine, and other mediators increase the permeability of local vessels, which changes nociception at the site of trauma and leads to the sensation of pain. Steroids inhibit the production of prostaglandins and therefore reduce pain. Although the use of steroids may be beneficial, they can also create sufficient immunosuppression to mask inflammation or infection.[22]

Postoperative Nausea and Vomiting

All patients are at risk for postoperative nausea and vomiting (PONV). ENT procedures, particularly of the middle ear, are associated with a high incidence of PONV.[22] PONV may cause discharge to be delayed from the postanesthesia care unit (PACU), or for severe cases, unscheduled hospital admission may be required. The accumulation of blood in the posterior oropharynx, which may drain into the stomach or be swallowed during the postoperative period, can lead to PONV. This frequently occurs during throat procedures such as tonsillectomy. Packing the back of the throat with surgical packs during the procedure can prevent some drainage into the stomach. Care must be taken that the patient is awake, all surgical packs are removed, and suctioning of the airway precedes the extubation process, producing a clear airway and ensuring the control of protective airway reflexes. A multimodal approach is advocated to attenuate PONV in ENT patients.[21-24] Antiemetic drugs are discussed in Chapter 14.

Special Anesthetic Techniques Associated With ENT Procedures

Deliberate Controlled Hypotension

Extensive dissection is required for many head and neck tumors with operative times extending to 12 or more hours. Considerable fluid replacement, blood loss, electrolyte imbalances, and cardiovascular and respiratory changes may occur during surgery. The surgeon may request deliberate controlled hypotension to reduce blood loss. Patients must be individually evaluated prior to controlled hypotension to determine a safe mean pressure. The effects of common IV controlled hypotensive techniques are compared in Table 43.6.[25] The practice of controlled hypotension focuses on reducing the mean arterial pressure (MAP) to some predetermined level related to the limits of cerebral and systemic autoregulation. Although the research is conflicting as to what values are best practice, the author's practice is to

TABLE 43.6   Common Intravenous Agents for Hypotensive Techniques

Drug and Dosage	Advantages	Disadvantages
Sodium nitroprusside: variable age- and anesthetic-dependent effects Young adults: 1–5 mcg/kg/min; children: 6–8 mcg/kg/min	Potent, reliable, rapid onset and recovery, cardiac output well preserved	Reflex tachycardia, rebound hypertension, pulmonary shunting, cyanide toxicity possible
Dexmedetomidine: 1 mcg/kg over 10 min then 0.2–0.7 mcg/kg/hr	Dose-dependent sedation and analgesia with associated hypotension, decreases intravenous/inhalational anesthetic requirements, smooth emergence	Bradycardia and hypotension most often seen with bolus, heart block
Esmolol: 200 mcg/kg/min to achieve 15% reduction of mean arterial pressure	Particularly useful to control tachycardia	Potential for significant cardiac depression
Nitroglycerin Adults: 125–500 mcg/kg/min; children: 10 mcg/kg/min	Preserves myocardial blood flow, reduces preload, preserves tissue oxygenation	Increases intracranial pressure, highly variable dosage requirements
Nicardipine: 5 mcg/kg/min	Ca^{++} channel blocker Preserves cerebral blood flow	
Remifentanil with propofol Remifentanil: 1 mcg/kg IV then continuous infusion 0.25–0.5 mcg/kg/min Propofol: 2.5 mg/kg IV, then infusion of 50–100 mcg/kg/min	Remifentanil reduces middle ear blood flow, creating a dry surgical field for tympanoplasty Propofol may help reduce PONV	No analgesic effect once remifentanil infusion discontinued, postoperative secondary hyperanalgesia

PONV, Postoperative nausea and vomiting.
Modified from DeGoute CS. Controlled hypotension: a guide to drug choice. *Drugs.* 2007;67(7):1053–1076; Jamaliya RH, et al. The efficacy and hemodynamic response to dexmedetomidine as a hypotensive agent in posterior fixation surgery following traumatic spine injury. *J Anaesthesiol Clin Pharmacol.* 2014;30(2):203–207.

not allow the mean pressure to fall below 50 to 60 mm Hg or a greater than 20% decrease of baseline MAP. Controlled hypotension requires achieving numeric goals while maintaining cerebral and renal autoregulation, in addition to adequate coronary artery blood flow. Patients with chronic hypertension may require a higher mean pressure to maintain adequate perfusion.[26] Regardless of the technique or medication chosen, it is imperative that urine output, mean arterial blood pressure, cerebral and cardiac perfusion pressure, and arterial blood gases be closely monitored and maintained. When using hypotensive anesthesia, an arterial line is required. Hypotensive techniques are also used with endoscopic sinus surgery. It has been noted that better operating conditions are achieved when moderate hypotension is produced with β-blocker, calcium channel blocker, or ultrashort-acting narcotic like remifentanil than when vasodilating agents are used alone.[25]

SELECT TECHNIQUES COMMONLY USED IN EAR, NOSE, AND THROAT PROCEDURES

Laser Surgery

Anesthesia and laser surgery is also discussed in Chapter 47; however, some specific issues concerning lasers are relevant to ENT surgery. Laser technology has been used in medicine for more than 30 years. The two most common lasers used in ENT surgery are the CO_2 and Nd:YAG (neodymium-doped yttrium-aluminum-garnet); recently, the argon laser has also become a popular choice.[27,28] Laser light is different from standard light. Standard light has a variety of wavelengths, whereas lasers have only one wavelength (monochromatic). Laser light oscillates in the same phase, or all the photons are moving in the same direction (coherent) and its beam is parallel (collimated). The wavelength of the Nd:YAG laser beam is shorter as it passes through the garnet than that of the CO_2 laser. The shorter wavelength allows less absorption by water and therefore less tissue penetration. For example, the shorter wavelength of the Nd:YAG allows the laser light to pass through the cornea, whereas the longer wavelength of the CO_2 laser

would burn the cornea. Laser light emits a small amount of radiation and can be infrared, visible, and ultraviolet in the spectrum. Lasers enable very precise excision, produce minimal edema and bleeding, and are favored by surgeons for resection of tumors and other obstructions of the airway. For operations in and around the larynx the CO_2 laser is frequently used because of its shallow depth of burn and extreme precision.[14] The CO_2 laser produces a beam with a relatively long wavelength that is absorbed almost entirely by the surface of these tissues, vaporizing cellular water. Intermittent bursts of the CO_2 laser produce intense, precisely directed energy that results in a clean cut through the target tissue with a minimal amount of penetration of surrounding tissue. A low-energy helium-neon laser is commonly used to aim or direct CO_2 laser beams.

The holmium yttrium-aluminum-garnet (Ho:YAG) laser is a relatively new laser. The Ho:YAG laser has a pulsed infrared output with a wavelength of 2.1 mm. The laser has excellent absorption in water-rich tissues, and in otolaryngology, it has been used for nasal surgeries and for tonsillectomies.

Laser light beams are primarily used for their thermal effect and can be used to cut, coagulate, or vaporize tissues. The exact tissue interaction of a laser is dependent on several variables, including the types of tissues being irradiated, the wavelength of the emitted beam, and the power of the beam.

Most surgical fires occur during head and neck surgery. This is caused by the presence of oxygen and the extensive use of lasers. The use of laser technology mandates taking measures to ensure the safety of the patient and operating room personnel (Box 43.2). Specific concerns include eye protection with appropriate colored glasses, avoidance of the dispersion of noxious fumes, and fire prevention. Stray or reflected beams of the Nd:YAG laser are capable of traversing the eye to the retina; therefore green-lensed eye protection for all personnel is mandatory during use of the Nd:YAG laser. All persons in the operating room must wear goggles specifically designed to absorb Nd:YAG laser beams. The required protective eyewear for CO_2 lasers can be any clear glass or plastic that surrounds the face. Orange-red eye protection

---

BOX 43.2 General Safety Protocol for Surgical Lasers

- Post warning signs outside any operating area: "WARNING: LASER IN USE."
- Patient's eyes should be protected with appropriate colored glasses and/or wet gauze.
- Matte-finish (black) surgical instruments reduce beam reflection and dispersion.
- Use the lowest concentration of oxygen possible ($\geq 30\%$).
- Avoid using nitrous oxide because it supports combustion.
- Lasers should be placed in STANDBY mode when not in use.
- Use an endotracheal tube specifically prepared for use with lasers.
- Inflate cuff of laser tube with methylene blue–dyed saline so that a cuff perforation is easily detected.
- All adjacent tissues should be shielded by wet gauze to prevent damage by reflected beams.
- Plume should be suctioned and evacuated from the surgical field.

BOX 43.3 Safety Measures for Preventing Fires During ENT Procedures

- Use only air for open delivery to the face if the patient can maintain a safe blood O_2 saturation without supplemental.
- If the patient cannot maintain a safe blood O_2 saturation without extra O_2, secure the airway with a laryngeal mask airway or tracheal tube.
- *Exceptions:* When patient's verbal responses may be required during surgery (e.g., carotid artery surgery, neurosurgery, pacemaker insertion) and when open O_2 delivery is required to keep the patient safe, do the following:
  - Deliver the minimum O_2 concentration necessary for adequate oxygenation at all times.
  - Begin with a 30% delivery O_2 concentration and increase as necessary.
  - For unavoidable open O_2 delivery above 30%, deliver 5–10 L/min of air under drapes to wash out excess O_2.
  - Stop supplemental O_2 at least 1 min before and during use of electrosurgery, electrocautery, or laser, if possible. Surgical team communication is essential for this recommendation.
  - Use an adherent incise drape, if possible, to help isolate the incision from possible O_2-enriched atmospheres beneath the drapes.
  - Keep fenestration towel edges as far from the incision as possible.
  - Arrange drapes to minimize O_2 buildup underneath.
  - Coat head hair and facial hair (e.g., eyebrows, beard, moustache) within the fenestration with water-soluble surgical lubricating jelly to make it nonflammable.
  - For coagulation, use bipolar electrosurgery, not monopolar electrosurgery.

During Oropharyngeal Surgery (e.g., Tonsillectomy)
- Scavenge deep within the oropharynx with a metal suction cannula to catch leaking O_2 and nitrous oxide.
- Moisten gauze or sponges and keep them moist, including those used with uncuffed tracheal tubes.

During Tracheostomy
- Do not use electrosurgery to incise the trachea.

During Bronchoscopic Surgery
- If the patient requires supplemental O_2, keep the delivered O_2 below 30%. Use inhalation/exhalation gas monitoring (e.g., with an O_2 analyzer) to confirm the proper concentration.

From Sheinbein DS, Loeb RG. Laser surgery and fire hazards in ear, nose, and throat surgeries. *Anesthesiol Clin.* 2010;28(3):485–496; Jones TS, Black IH, Robinson TN, et al. Operating room fires. *Anesthesiology.* 2019;130(3):492–501.

---

is required for the potassium titanyl-phosphate (KTP) laser, and orange glasses are required for the argon laser.

When tissues are cut by a laser, the smoke and vapors that are formed are called *laser plume*. This plume is an environmental concern and potentially toxic to operating room personnel. When the tissues vaporized by the laser are malignancies or viral papilloma, the concern arises as to whether these vapors are even more dangerous to operating room personnel if not removed from the environment. Current evidence shows that although actual environmental transmittance of these pathogens is low, the risk still exists, and encourages use of smoke evacuators at the site of laser vaporization.[29]

The prevention of combustion within the airway is of primary concern. Fire in the airway is relatively uncommon (0.4%), and it is usually the result of penetration of the laser through the ETT, which exposes the beam to a rich oxygen supply. N_2O, although not flammable, also supports combustion and can propagate the flame.[29] Positive pressure ventilation in the presence of intraluminal combustion produces a blowtorch effect that causes serious damage to the respiratory tract of the unfortunate patient.[30] Many important steps should be taken to minimize the risk of laser fires.[31,32] Box 43.3 lists safety measures for preventing fires during ENT procedures.[14] Operating room fires are discussed further in Chapters 47 and 59.

The ideal ETT for use with lasers remains a major discussion. However, several manufacturers have attempted to produce a laser-compatible ETT that allows for adequate ventilation during the laser procedure but reduces the risk of airway fire injury. The necessity of an inflatable cuff is a point of debate, although the ability to better ventilate the patient and keep the field free of combustible gases is an advantage. When filled with air, the cuff becomes a generous reservoir of combustion-supporting gas. If a cuffed tube is used, inflation with methylene blue-tinged normal saline is encouraged to make it possible to detect penetration. If a laser beam contacts the cuff, the colored liquid will absorb and disperse heat, alerting the operating team to the penetration; the liquid also will reduce combustion.[33]

Fire safety policies, procedures, and practice guidelines are now routine and observed in every modern operating room.[34] A further discussion of laser surgery and anesthesia is in Chapter 47.

Endoscopy

Endoscopic surgery includes panendoscopy, laryngoscopy, microlaryngoscopy (laryngoscopy aided by an operating microscope), esophagoscopy, and bronchoscopy. All these procedures can be performed using a rigid or flexible endoscope. If the rigid laryngoscope is used, the laryngoscope may be suspended from an arching support anchored to the patient's abdomen/chest or from a Mayo stand over the patient. One of the most common endoscopic procedures performed is endoscopic sinus surgery. Over 250,000 endoscopic sinus surgeries are performed yearly in the United States alone.[35,36] Endoscopic sinus surgery is often associated with recurrent and seasonal allergies leading to polyps. Patients undergoing endoscopic surgery are often also being evaluated for pathology responsible for hoarseness, stridor, or hemoptysis. Other possible reasons for endoscopic examination include foreign-body aspiration, papillomas, trauma, tracheal stenosis, obstructing tumors, or vocal cord dysfunction. Several complications can arise with endoscopic surgery: eye trauma, epistaxis, laryngospasm, and bronchospasm; excessive plasma levels of local anesthesia and epinephrine have also been reported. Preoperatively, the patient should be examined for any signs of airway obstruction, and proper measures should be taken to ensure safe and controlled airway management. Knowledge of the location and size of a mass is important, and discussion with the surgeon about chest radiography, magnetic resonance imaging (MRI), and computed tomography (CT) scan results can be invaluable.[36]

Special consideration should be given to whether administration of routine anxiolytic premedication is necessary in older children and adults with airway pathology as they may experience respiratory depression and worsening of airway obstruction. The airway must be protected from aspiration of gastric contents, especially during prolonged airway manipulation and deeper sedation. Premedication with an antisialagogue to dry secretions and a full regimen of acid aspiration prophylaxis in aspiration-prone patients may be indicated. An awake oral or nasal intubation with minimal sedation and topical anesthesia of the oral cavity, pharynx, larynx, and nasopharynx is common. In rare circumstances, an awake tracheostomy with local anesthesia may be safest. For shorter ENT procedures, anesthesia should be maintained with short-acting inhalation and IV agents to (1) avoid patient movement and vocal cord movement, and (2) control sympathetic nervous system response to brief periods of extreme stimulation, as in laryngoscopy.

Adequate muscle relaxation of the vocal cords is an essential part of anesthesia management for microsurgery of the larynx. A single-dose short-acting relaxant such as succinylcholine may be considered for brief cases. If the procedure is expected to last 30 minutes or more, use of an intermediate-duration neuromuscular-blocking drug such as vecuronium, cisatracurium, or rocuronium for the initial tracheal intubation allows the return of muscle strength and spontaneous respiration to meet extubation criteria at the end of the surgical procedure. In instances where the surgeon requests vocal cord immobility without neuromuscular blocking agents, use of remifentanil for the induction and maintenance may be useful. Emergence should include adequate oropharyngeal suctioning, humidified oxygenation, and observation in the PACU for laryngeal spasm, or postextubation croup or stridor.

One of the greatest management challenges during endoscopic procedures is that of sharing the airway continuously with the surgeon. Several methods have been used to provide oxygenation and ventilation during the procedures. One method is to control the airway by using a small cuffed ETT (5.0–6.0 for an adult) and 6.0 ETTs are designed for smaller patients, a better ETT selection might include the microlaryngeal endotracheal tube (MLT). The MLT in made similar sizes (5.0–6.0) has a cuff that is larger than the small standard ETTs allowing for a larger cuff distribution across the surface of the trachea and creating a wider field of pressure on the tracheal surface. Distinct advantages of an ETT include a secure airway with easily controlled ventilation, a cuff to protect the lower airway from debris, monitoring of end tidal CO_2, and the ability to administer inhalational anesthetics. Several disadvantages include the potential for extubation and loss of airway, complications during laser surgery, and interference with the operative field by the ETT.

Intermittent apnea is also used as a technique to ventilate patients in this shared space. The anesthetist or the surgeon repeatedly removes the ETT, operates during a brief period of apnea, and then allows the anesthesia provider to reintubate and ventilate the patient. One advantage of the technique is that no special equipment is needed to ventilate the patient. Many patients undergoing these procedures may have increased incidence of smoking exposure and alcohol use, which predisposes them to cardiovascular disease and labile vital signs. Some

of the disadvantages of this approach include difficulty in reintubation and the time allotment between ventilations while preventing desaturations. The procedure must be interrupted frequently to ventilate the patient, and the airway is unprotected while the ETT is removed. During this technique, the blood pressure and heart rate tend to fluctuate widely. The procedure resembles a series of stress-filled laryngoscopies and intubations, separated by varying periods of minimal surgical stimulation. Intravenous administration or topical application of agents such as lidocaine; small doses of alfentanil, remifentanil, sufentanil, or fentanyl; and/or adrenergic receptor-blocking drugs such as esmolol or dexmedetomidine may help mitigate the sympathetic response.[37]

Jet Ventilation

Jet ventilation has been used extensively for laryngeal surgery. When the trachea is not intubated, a metal needle mounted in the operating laryngoscope or passed through the cords can be used for jet ventilation. Jet ventilation may be performed manually, using a simple hand valve attached to an appropriate oxygen source, or together with various mechanical devices that allow for adjustment of rate and oxygen concentration. Because oxygen can support combustion, the lowest concentration of oxygen possible should be used. Many patients will tolerate a fraction of inspired oxygen (Fio_2) of 30% or less; however, oxygen requirements for each patient should be considered on an individual basis. Using lower levels of oxygen will decrease the likelihood of an airway fire.

High frequency is useful when access to the airway by the surgeon is limited by the ETT or the surgeon might interfere or ignite the tube. Jet ventilation does not require an ETT and requires only a narrow catheter with resistance to laser beams. There is no absolute contraindication to high-frequency jet ventilation (HFJV); however, it can be difficult maintaining oxygenation and/or CO_2 elimination in certain patients. These include patients who are morbidly obese, have a stiff thorax, or advanced forms of restrictive and/or obstructive lung disease, lung fibrosis, and reduced alveolar-capillary diffusion capacity, such as with pulmonary edema. Jet ventilation should be avoided in any situation in which an unprotected airway is a concern (e.g., full stomach, hiatal hernia, or trauma).[38]

Common types of HFJV include supraglottic, infraglottic, transtracheal, and via a rigid bronchoscope.[39] Fig. 43.7 shows the commonly used rigid bronchoscope technique. HFJV was originally used as a technique to provide adequate oxygenation and alveolar ventilation for rigid bronchoscopy and laryngeal surgery. HFJV is ventilation at

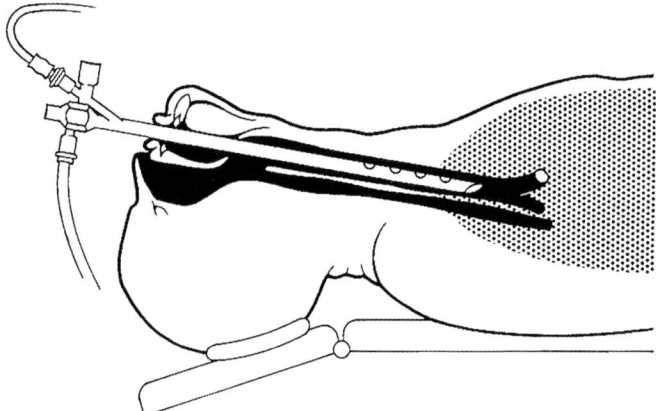

Fig. 43.7 Rigid bronchoscope connected at its proximal end through an oblique side port to the jet line of the ventilator. (From Biro P. Jet ventilation for surgical interventions in the upper airway. *Anesthesiol Clin.* 2010;28(3):397–409.)

low tidal volumes with high respiratory rates. A needle connected to a high-pressure hose with a regulator to adjust rate and volume is used to deliver the ventilation. With the tip of the needle either above or below the glottis, the anesthetist directs a high-velocity jet stream of oxygen into the airway lumen. The lungs are ventilated as the mixture of oxygen forces air into the lumen. Introduction of high-pressure (up to 60 psi) jet-injected oxygen entrains room air into the lung, allowing the jet stream of gases into the airway for ventilation.[39] Inspiration is accomplished by HFJV pressurizing gas into the airway, whereas the expiration is passive, and adequate exhalation should be constantly assessed both visually and mechanically. Some pauses in ventilation may be necessary to provide adequate time for expiration, particularly in patients with severe respiratory disease.

If an airway mass lies above the level of delivery of the gas jet, it may be easy to force the gas down the trachea during inspiration, but the gases will be trapped during expiration. This air trapping can lead to increased airway pressure, subcutaneous emphysema, and pneumothorax, particularly in patients with bullae. The anesthetist or surgeon also may find it difficult to aim the jet into the airway lumen, leading to hypoxia. If the jet is not accurately aimed, gastric distention, subcutaneous emphysema, or barotrauma may result. Patients with decreased pulmonary compliance or increased airway resistance from bronchospasm, obesity, or chronic obstructive pulmonary disease (COPD) are at high risk for hypoventilation with jet techniques. Adequacy of ventilation is assessed by observing chest movement, auscultation with the precordial stethoscope, and a pulse oximeter. IV anesthetic techniques are used with HFJV because environmental contamination by leaking volatile agents is a concern.[38]

Transnasal Humidified Rapid-Insufflation Ventilatory Exchange

Transnasal humidified rapid-insufflation ventilatory exchange (THRIVE) is an emerging mechanism by which patients are oxygenated and ventilated under anesthesia who have minimal or absent respiratory effort. This technique involves use of a noninvasive cannula, opposed to tracheal, which is utilized to provide passive apneic oxygenation. Oxygen is delivered at very high flows (10–12 L/min) with the addition of humidification and warmth to minimize trauma to nasal mucosa. This increases apneic times and may provide a more balanced risk profile when compared to jet ventilation.[40,41]

Foreign-Body Aspiration

Aspiration of foreign bodies is a common problem that carries high morbidity and mortality, particularly in children. Asphyxiation by an inhaled foreign body is a leading cause of accidental death among children younger than 4 years. Some common aspirants include peanuts, popcorn, jellybeans, coins, bites of meat, and hot dogs. Most aspirated items are food particles, with nuts and seeds being the most common. Aspiration of beads, pins, and parts of small toys are also not unusual. A common site of foreign-body aspiration is the right bronchus. If the patient is supine when the aspiration occurs, the object will most likely be found in the right upper lobe. If the patient is standing, the right lower lobe is most likely to be affected. Signs of aspiration include wheezing, choking, coughing, tachycardia, aphonia, and cyanosis. These signs indicate an obstructive, severe irritation and swelling in the airway. As a result of the swelling, air may be trapped in the lungs, not allowing adequate expiration. Although rigid bronchoscopy has been the traditional diagnostic gold standard, the use of CT, virtual bronchoscopy, and flexible bronchoscopy is increasing. Reported mortality during bronchoscopy is 0.42%. Although asphyxia at presentation or initial emergency bronchoscopy causes some deaths, hypoxic cardiac arrest during retrieval of the object, bronchial rupture, and unspecified

intraoperative complications in previously stable patients constitute contribute to significant in-hospital fatalities. Major complications include severe laryngeal edema or bronchospasm requiring tracheotomy or reintubation, pneumothorax, pneumomediastinum, cardiac arrest, tracheal or bronchial laceration, and hypoxic brain damage.[42]

Anesthetic management depends on the location of the airway obstruction, the size and location of the object, and the severity of the obstruction. If the foreign body is located at the level of the larynx, a simple laryngoscopy with Magill forceps should allow for easy removal of the object. Care must be taken not to dislodge the object and allow it to fall deeper into the airway. If the foreign body is in the distal larynx or trachea, the patient should have an inhalation induction performed in the operating room, maintaining spontaneous respiration. With the patient spontaneously breathing, the surgeon will most likely use a rigid bronchoscope for extraction of the foreign body. Usually a gentle mask induction without cricoid pressure or positive pressure ventilation is the preferred induction technique.[42] Attempts to assist respirations should not be made because that might cause the object to move farther into the airway and compromise ventilation with occlusion. Patients should be placed in the sitting position because it is known to produce the least adverse effect on airway symptoms. An antisialagogue, H_2 antagonist, and metoclopramide are often administered intravenously to decrease secretions and promote gastric emptying; the secretions may obscure the view through the bronchoscope. Patients with full stomachs who are induced with a rapid sequence must be prepared for complete occlusion of the airway.

Direct and sometimes rigid laryngoscopy is typically performed. A rigid bronchoscope is also used and inserted through the vocal cords into the trachea. Ventilation is accomplished through a side port of the laryngoscope or bronchoscope that can be attached to the anesthesia circuit. If a foreign body is present, the telescope eyepiece within the bronchoscope is removed and optical forceps are inserted through the bronchoscope for retrieval of the item. When the telescopic eyepiece is being changed a leak is present in the ventilation system, and protracted periods can lead to hypoxia. When an anesthesia gas machine circuit is used, high fresh gas flow rates, large tidal volumes, and high concentrations of inspired volatile anesthetic agents are often necessary to compensate for leaks around the ventilating bronchoscope. Coughing, bucking, or straining during instrumentation with the rigid bronchoscope may cause difficulty for the surgeon and result in damage to the patient's airway; these must be avoided. The best anesthesia technique for rigid laryngoscopy and bronchoscopy is total IV anesthesia, allowing greater control of cardiovascular stability and relaxation for short periods, as well as ventilation with 100% oxygen allowing longer periods of hypoventilation without hypoxia.

A rigid bronchoscopy can lead to several complications, including damage to dentition, gums, upper lips, and chipped or damaged teeth, all of which can be prevented to some degree with the use of a mouth guard and vigilance. A good range of motion of the cervical vertebra is also evaluated and necessary prior to insertion of a rigid scope. Vagal stimulation may be noted from the extreme head extension, and tracheal tears can occur with the introduction of the bronchoscope. Inadequate ventilation manifests as hypoxemia, hypercarbia, barotrauma, and dysrhythmias. The surgeon must be prepared to perform an emergency tracheotomy or cricothyrotomy if partial obstruction suddenly becomes complete.

At the end of the procedure patients can be intubated to provide ventilation until returning to consciousness. Allow the patient to return to consciousness and normocapnia as quickly as possible, with airway reflexes intact prior to extubation. Laryngeal and subglottic edema may occur for 24 hours after removal of a foreign body. To check for airway edema, the cuff of the ETT can be deflated, if not contraindicated, and the lumen of the ETT should be occluded for one or two breaths during inspiration and expiration while listening for air movement around the tube. If there is no air escaping around the ETT, postoperative sedation and ventilation might be considered. Close observation and use of humidified oxygen are suggested during the recovery period. Some additional supportive measures that can alleviate some of the postoperative complications that occur include racemic epinephrine, bronchodilators, and steroids.

PROCEDURES INVOLVING THE FACE, EAR, HEAD, AND NECK

Some of the common surgical procedures for the ear and face include myringotomy with insertion of tubes, mastoidectomy, acoustic neuroma, stapedectomy, and tympanoplasty. During ear surgery the anesthetist must be concerned with four major issues: (1) nerve preservation, (2) the effect of N_2O on the middle ear, (3) control of bleeding, and (4) PONV.

Nerve Preservation During Surgical Procedures

Surgical procedures of the ear and face require meticulous identification and preservation of the facial nerve and other cranial nerves especially during resection of a glomus tumor or an acoustic neuroma. Intraoperative neuromonitoring is a relatively recent advance in electromyography (EMG) applied to head and neck surgery. Its purpose is to allow real-time identification and functional assessment of vulnerable nerves during surgery. The nerves most often monitored in head and neck surgery are the motor branch of the facial nerve (VII), the recurrent or inferior laryngeal nerves (X), the vagus nerve (X), and the spinal accessory nerve (XI), with other lower cranial nerves monitored less frequently. Morbidity from trauma to these nerves is significant and obvious, such as unilateral facial paresis. Although functional restorative surgery can be performed, the importance of preventing nerve injury in head and neck surgery is obvious.

The identification of these nerves requires the surgeon to isolate and verify function by means of an electrical stimulation. One method used for nerve isolation is the brainstem auditory-evoked potential and electrocochleogram monitoring. Table 43.7 lists several types of intraoperative neurophysiologic monitoring used during ENT procedures and the effects of various anesthetic drugs on the monitoring modality.[43]

Patient movement during head and neck surgery must be prevented, especially if a positioning device is used for craniotomy. Muscle relaxants should only be used at induction and intubation to prevent interference with the nerve monitoring. The use of local anesthetics is also contraindicated because of their suppressant effects on muscle action potential amplitudes and muscle movement. Hemostasis during neck dissection is not as critical as during otologic or skull base neurosurgery, but the use of an opioid infusion such as remifentanil or sufentanil will help control blood pressure and aid hemostasis. The use of volatile anesthetic agents and N_2O is acceptable only if the N_2O is discontinued well before closing any cavity. Common anesthetic techniques include the use of remifentanil with short-acting volatile anesthetic agents with or without N_2O. Midazolam preoperatively helps assure amnesia and rapid emergence. Selected use of deep extubation helps prevent straining during emergence, as straining increases postoperative bleeding and may necessitate reexploration.[44]

Middle Ear Procedures

Middle ear procedures require a bloodless surgical field, specific head positioning, facial nerve monitoring, and management of PONV. The term *middle ear* refers to the air-filled space between the tympanic membrane and the oval window. It is connected to the nasopharynx by the eustachian tube and is in close proximity to the temporal lobe, cerebellum, jugular bulb, and labyrinth of the inner ear. The middle ear contains three ossicles—the malleus, incus, and stapes—which transmit sound vibration from the eardrum to the cochlea. This air-filled cavity is traversed by the facial nerve before it exits the skull via the stylomastoid foramen. The facial nerve provides motor innervation to the muscles of facial expression. Common surgeries in adults include tympanoplasty (reconstructive surgery for the tympanic membrane, or eardrum), stapedectomy or ossiculoplasty for otosclerosis, mastoidectomy for removal of infected air cells within the mastoid bone, and removal of a cholesteatoma. Common middle ear surgery in children includes tympanoplasty, mastoidectomy, myringotomy, grommet insertion, and cochlear implantation.[45]

Middle ear surgery can be accomplished with either local or general anesthesia depending on the patient's ability to cooperate. Local anesthesia with sedation requires the patient to remain still under surgical drapes for extended periods. The main advantages of performing middle ear surgery under local anesthesia are the ability to test hearing during surgery and less bleeding. Most middle ear procedures can be performed as outpatient surgery; thus rapid recovery, good analgesia, and avoidance of nausea and vomiting are essential. Pain is a primary problem at the beginning of surgery when multiple injections of local anesthetic with epinephrine are given. The use of a topical application of lidocaine and prilocaine (eutectic mixture of local anesthetics [EMLA]) may increase patient comfort. A bloodless surgical field is mandatory in microsurgery. A combination of physical and pharmacologic techniques is used to minimize bleeding. The patient's head is positioned to avoid venous obstruction and congestion.[45,46]

When general anesthesia is chosen, the airway can be maintained with a LMA or endotracheal intubation. Intubation may be more appropriate if extreme neck extension or rotation is required. A nerve stimulator is often employed for intraoperative monitoring of evoked facial nerve EMG activity to aid preservation of the facial nerve. Muscle relaxants are therefore avoided after intubation. A smooth recovery without coughing or straining is important to prevent prosthesis displacement, especially in patients who have undergone reconstructive middle ear surgery.

PONV, a common problem after middle ear surgery, can be minimized by the appropriate choice of anesthetic technique and antiemetic prophylaxis.[47] As noted previously, a bloodless operative field is essential. Physical and pharmacologic techniques are used to minimize bleeding. They include a head-up tilt of 15 to 20 degrees, avoidance of venous obstruction, normocapnia, and controlled hypotension. An ideal systolic blood pressure range is 80 to 90 mm Hg or a reduction of MAP to 20% of baseline in patients with hypertension. A slightly elevated position of the head reduces arterial and venous pressures in areas above the heart; however, it increases the risk of air embolism.

Pharmacologic agents used for controlled hypotension in ear, nose, and throat surgery include inhalation anesthetics, β-adrenoceptor antagonists (labetalol and esmolol), α_2-adrenergic agonists (dexmedetomidine), opioids (remifentanil), and more recently, magnesium sulfate.[44,48] Dexmedetomidine has several advantages as an adjunct to lower blood pressure. It produces sedation, analgesia, and a modest reduction in heart rate and blood pressure without respiratory depression. Dexmedetomidine has been used successfully to lower blood pressure during general anesthesia or as the primary sedative with supplementary low-dose propofol and midazolam for IV sedation.[49,50] At the completion of the surgical procedure the patient's head is lifted and usually wrapped with a bandage. The anesthetist will want to avoid excessive coughing and bucking of the patient during this period. Therefore using a technique that limits coughing is desirable. Provided there are no contraindications, a deep extubation might be considered.

TABLE 43.7   Types of Intraoperative Neurophysiologic Monitoring and the Effects of Various Anesthetic Drugs

Type or Modality of Neurophysiologic Monitoring	Surgery Examples	Region	Volatile Agents (e.g., Isoflurane)	Neuromuscular Blocking Agents*	TOTAL INTRAVENOUS ANESTHESIA		Local Anesthetics*	Nitrous Oxide
					Opioids	Propofol		
Brainstem auditory-evoked response	Acoustic neuroma, trigeminal neuralgia, facial nerve decompression, endolymphatic sac	Cerebellopontine angle, mastoid region, middle ear	1	0	0	1	0	0
Cortical somatosensory-evoked potentials	Spinal fusion, tumor, decompression	Spine (posterior columns)	2 (affect amplitude and latency of waveforms)	0	0	0	2	1 Nitrous oxide (affects amplitude only)
Neuromuscular junction monitoring	Neuromuscular blockade in anesthesia	Ulnar nerve, facial nerve, posterior tibial nerve	0	2	0	0	2	0
acIONM: spontaneous EMG†	Thyroid, parathyroid, parotid, neck dissection, skull base	Facial, vagal, recurrent laryngeal, other cranial nerves	0	2	0	0	2	0
pcIONM: evoked EMG†	Thyroid, parathyroid, parotid, neck dissection, skull base	Facial, vagal, recurrent laryngeal, other cranial nerves	0	2	0	0	2	0
MEP	Spinal fusion, tumor, decompression	Spine (anterior columns)	2	2	0	0	2	0
EEG† (BIS)	All	All	2	0	1	2	0	1
EEG†	Carotid endarterectomy	Carotid	2	0	2	2	2	2

*The two classes of drug to be avoided during monitoring of facial, recurrent laryngeal, vagal, and other cranial motor nerves are neuromuscular blocking agents and local anesthetics. Both may increase latency, decrease amplitude, and increase stimulus threshold of the evoked response, or may decrease the sensitivity of EMG to nerve injury.

†A conventional balanced anesthetic (opioid, nitrous oxide/oxygen, volatile agent) is suitable for surgery using EMG and EEG.

Scale: 0 = insensitive; 1 = somewhat sensitive; 2 = very sensitive.

acIONM, Active continuous intraoperative nerve monitoring; *BIS*, Bispectral electroencephalogram; *EEG*, electroencephalogram; *EMG*, electromyogram; *MEP*, motor-evoked potentials; *pcIONM*, passive continuous intraoperative nerve monitoring.

From Dillon FX. Electromyographic (EMG) neuromonitoring with otolaryngology-head and neck surgery. *Anesthesiol Clin.* 2010;28(3):434–442.

Nitrous Oxide and Middle Ear Surgery

Nitrous oxide is 34 times more soluble than nitrogen in blood and enters the middle ear cavity more rapidly than nitrogen leaves causing an increase in middle ear pressure if the eustachian tube is obstructed. Normally, pressure increases in the middle ear are vented via the eustachian tube into the nasopharynx. Yawning and swallowing actively open the eustachian tubes, but these equalizing maneuvers cannot occur in anesthetized patients. Additionally, pressure also may be increased in the middle ear with positive pressure ventilation by forcing air into the compartment through the eustachian tubes. During tympanoplasty the middle ear is open to the atmosphere; thus there is no buildup of pressure, but once a tympanic membrane graft is placed, the continued use of N$_2$O might cause displacement of the graft. At the end of surgery, when N$_2$O is discontinued, the remaining N$_2$O is rapidly absorbed, which may then result in negative pressure. This negative pressure may result in graft dislodgement, serous otitis media, disarticulation of the stapes, or impaired hearing. Some clinicians feel that discontinuation of the N$_2$O at least 15 minutes before closure of the middle ear is sufficient to ameliorate these adverse effects. Because N$_2$O is only a supplement to general anesthesia, avoiding it altogether during tympanoplasty is more reasonable. N$_2$O also may increase PONV, and its use in middle ear surgery may further increase the incidence of PONV above that already associated with this type of surgery.[44]

Myringotomy and Tube Placement

Most often patients scheduled for myringotomy are young, healthy patients. A myringotomy allows the pressure to equalize between the middle ear and the atmosphere, reducing the pressure in the middle ear compartment. Simple tubes with a lumen (grommets) are placed through the patient's tympanic membrane to alleviate the pressure created in the middle ear usually seen with chronic serous otitis media or recurrent otitis media. Chronic otitis media is manifested as fluid in the middle ear. Recurrent otitis media, a common pediatric disorder, is defined as either three or more acute infections of the middle ear cleft in a 6-month period or at least four episodes in 1 year. Untreated otitis media may lead to permanent middle ear damage and hearing loss, therefore appropriate treatment is necessary. Children with chronic otitis frequently have accompanying recurrent upper respiratory infections (URIs). Intervals between URIs may be brief, and the patient is usually on a regimen of antibiotics. Scheduling surgery during these interludes is often impractical. Frequently the eradication of middle ear fluid and inflammation resolves the URI, therefore surgery should not be delayed.

Bilateral myringotomies with tube insertions are typically very short operations. Sedative premedications may outlast the procedure and are usually not necessary. Mask or IV induction and maintenance using oxygen, N_2O, and a volatile inhalation agent such as sevoflurane is routine. If IV access is established, it is usually done after mask induction in children and may include fluid therapy or an injection cap for temporary access and administration of drugs. IVs are not usually necessary unless another procedure is performed at the same time.[46,51,52] N_2O is often avoided in surgeries that involve the middle ear, but given that the myringotomy surgical procedure is relatively short, and a tube will be placed through the tympanic membrane into the middle ear to relieve pressure, the effects of N_2O are not relevant. For bilateral procedures, the inhalation anesthetic is discontinued during the second myringotomy to facilitate prompt emergence. N_2O is continued until the completion of the surgery. Intubation is performed only if airway difficulties are anticipated or encountered, but airway equipment is always prepared and available. The procedure is typically without much risk of bleeding, but the patient's head must be held still, particularly when the myringotomy knife is being used.

The patient is supine with the head turned to expose the ear to the microscope. An ear speculum is inserted into the ear canal, cerumen is removed, and an incision is made in the tympanic membrane. Fluid is sometimes suctioned from the middle ear, and then a tympanostomy tube is inserted through the incision into the middle ear, straddling the tympanic membrane. Antibiotic and steroid eardrops are frequently inserted into the external auditory canal and pain medications given rectally, orally, intranasally or intravenously are administered in the perioperative period. The surgeon moves to the other side of the table, the microscope is repositioned, the head is turned, and the procedure is repeated in the other ear.[53,54]

Tonsillectomy and Adenoidectomy

The frequency of adenotonsillectomy in the United States has declined, although it remains a very common pediatric surgery.[55] The lateral tonsils, tonsillar tissue at the base of the tongue, and adenoids form a tonsillar "ring" around the oropharynx that can lead to significant airway challenges after surgical intervention. An adenotonsillectomy, although often considered a simple procedure, has the potential for significant airway challenges. Considerations of airway obstruction, shared airway, mechanical suspension of the airway, management of intubation and extubation, pain management, and the desire for a rapid awakening are all subtleties of anesthesia for this procedure. In adult patients, a tonsillectomy may also accompany a uvulopalatopharyngoplasty (UPPP) for Pickwickian syndrome or obstructive sleep apnea (OSA). OSA is typically seen with obesity and redundant pharyngeal tissue. OSA patients can also present with significant comorbid conditions, which may necessitate advanced postoperative planning.[56,57]

The patient undergoing a tonsillectomy and/or adenoidectomy will probably have a higher incidence of airway obstruction because of the hypertrophied tissues. Chronic obstruction and infections of the tonsils can lead to systemic involvement producing additional cardiac and respiratory anomalies. In the case of suspected airway obstruction, the clinician must choose wisely among routine IV induction, inhalation induction, awake intubation, or fiberoptic-assisted intubation before induction. Adult patients with severe OSA may require awake intubation before the induction of general anesthesia. Surgical approaches to tonsillectomy include coblation, cold steel, snare, monopolar cautery, and hot knife techniques. Techniques differ with respect to operative times, intraoperative blood losses, postoperative pain scores, or time to resumption of oral intake.[58]

In children, anesthesia is induced most commonly with sevoflurane, oxygen, and N_2O by mask depending on the age of the child and IV access. Some institutions allow parental presence in the operating room during induction to prevent separation anxiety in the child. LMA and ETT may both be used depending on the experience of the operating team.[59] A 2010 review noted that the use of the LMA during pediatric tonsil surgery does not appear to have any major disadvantages compared with use of the ETT. Analysis of safety, comfort, complications, and postoperative problems suggests that LMA may be superior for some outcome variables such as coughing and gagging. Use of spontaneous ventilation is more common among LMA patients.[60]

A cuffed tube is recommended in those older than 8 to 10 years of age,[4,5] with continued attention given to inflation pressures of the cuff. A properly sized pediatric ETT should allow a leak at 20 cm H_2O airway pressure, which reduces the likelihood of postoperative croup and edema. After the airway is secured, the mouth gag is inserted by the surgeon. An adequate depth of anesthesia is needed to facilitate gag insertion. The gag, designed to maintain an open mouth and tongue retraction, is equipped with a groove with which to seat the ETT or LMA (Fig. 43.8). The airway should be reevaluated at the time the gag is placed to ensure that the tube has not been moved from its original position and that occlusion of the tube has not occurred as a result of compression from the gag. The table is frequently turned 45 to 90 degrees away from the anesthetist just prior to incision.

The choice of maintenance techniques for anesthesia varies. Several goals need to be considered when choosing an anesthetic: (1) provide a depth of anesthesia adequate to blunt strong reflex activity elicited by the procedure, (2) a rapid return of protective airway reflexes, (3) good postoperative analgesia, (4) reduced postoperative

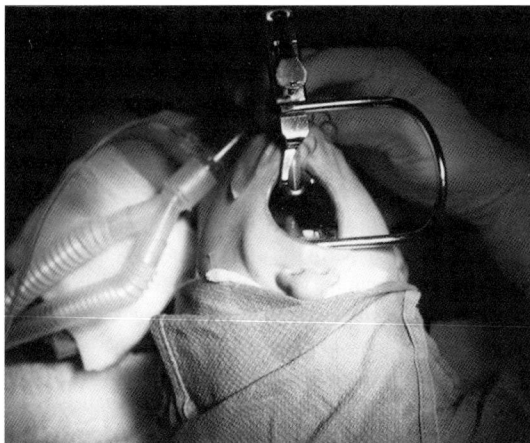

Fig. 43.8 Superior view of the suspension technique for tonsillectomy using the Crowe-Davis mouth gag. Note use of preformed RAE (Ring, Adair, and Elwyn) orotracheal tube.

bleeding, and (5) minimal PONV. The use of intermediate-acting muscle relaxants is acceptable; however, they are often unnecessary. Judicious narcotic supplementation will reduce the total amount of inhalation agent required and provide analgesia with minimal postoperative respiratory depression. Disadvantages of opiates include increased sensitivity, desaturation in sleep apnea patients, and PONV. Suggested techniques include modest opioids and IV acetaminophen doses for analgesia, dexamethasone and ondansetron for antiemetic prophylaxis, and deep extubation of the trachea to minimize coughing and airway stimulation when prudent.[60] Although an increase in postoperative bleeding has historically been a concern with the use of nonsteroidal antiinflammatory drugs (NSAIDs), a 2013 Cochrane review found that there was insufficient evidence to state whether NSAIDs increased bleeding risk posttonsillectomy. The review did note there was significantly less nausea and vomiting compared to use of opioid analgesics.[61,62]

Blood loss during tonsillectomy is difficult to assess but has been estimated to average 4 mL/kg or 5% of blood volume.[8] Average blood loss during UPPP is slightly higher because the procedure is frequently performed in conjunction with adenotonsillectomy. Although younger, healthier patients can tolerate greater volumes of blood loss, transfusion should be considered if blood loss, laboratory values, and patient factors indicate the need.

At the end of the surgical procedure the surgeon may release tension on the mouth gag to ensure that all bleeding has been controlled. The insertion of an orogastric tube and some irrigation may be used to remove blood and secretions from the stomach and oropharynx. This is thought to reduce the incidence of PONV. Suctioning of the oropharynx and nares should be done very gently and briefly, avoiding the surgical beds to prevent disruption and mucosal bleeding. Vigorous suctioning may induce laryngospasm and bronchospasm.

During emergence from anesthesia after tonsillectomy or UPPP the anesthetist should ensure that all protective reflexes have returned, the airway is free of blood and debris, and an adequate breathing pattern is present before the removal of the ETT. A topical spray of 2% lidocaine (maximum 3 mg/kg) on the glottic and supraglottic areas before intubation prevents postextubation stridor and laryngospasm after adenotonsillectomy. This approach has proved as effective as administering lidocaine (1–2 mg/kg IV) before extubation.[63]

The patient should be transported to the recovery in the "tonsil position"—that is, on one side with the head slightly down. This allows blood or secretions to drain out of the mouth rather than flow back onto the vocal cords. Adults, however, frequently prefer a middle- or high-Fowler position after UPPP. This position aids in ventilation and lessens the feeling of asphyxiation in the immediate postoperative period. Patients must be awake enough to manage their own airway. To hydrate the airway, 100% oxygen with a high-humidity mist is given by facemask or face tent. The pharynx should be rechecked directly for bleeding and edema before discharge.

Routine tonsillectomy is generally performed as an outpatient procedure. A small subset of children is observed overnight if there are sufficient age, comorbidity, or perioperative concerns. Although postoperative bleeding is the most serious complication, persistent vomiting, poor oral intake, and persistent desaturation are the most common reasons for unscheduled overnight admission after ambulatory surgery. The incidence of PONV can be as high as 70% during the first 24 hours after tonsillectomy.[64] This is the result of swallowed blood, opioid administration, or pharyngeal stimulation, and significantly increases the risk of overnight admission, delayed oral intake, and lower patient satisfaction.[57,63,64] As discussed previously, it is important to develop anesthetic techniques that incorporate the use of antiemetics to minimize episodes of nausea and vomiting. Codeine for postoperative pain

is contraindicated because of the potential for metabolic conversion to high levels of morphine (see Chapter 11).

Bleeding Tonsil

Posttonsillectomy hemorrhage (PTH) is the most common emergency pediatric airway surgery. Rates of PTH are between 0.5% and 7.5% and are most common in patients older than 15 years of age, male gender, patients with frequent infectious tonsillitis, and after hot (electrocautery) versus cold (scalpel) techniques. Approximately 75% of postoperative tonsillar hemorrhages occur within 6 hours of the surgical procedure. The remaining 25% of the postoperative bleeds occur within the first 24 hours postoperatively, although bleeding may be noted up until the sixth postoperative day.[65-67] Slow oozing of the tonsillar bed is far more common than profuse bleeding. Patients may swallow large volumes of blood before bleeding is discovered. The patient may have signs of hypovolemia evidenced by tachycardia, hypotension, and agitation. If the blood is swallowed, the patient may have nausea and vomiting. Appropriate laboratory tests, including hemoglobin, hematocrit, and coagulation profile, should be performed to determine patient status. Restoration of intravascular volume and/or blood based on the volume lost should precede induction. All patients should be assumed to have a significant amount of blood in the stomach and a rapid sequence induction is indicated. Care with laryngoscopy is necessary to prevent traumatic dislodgement of any clots. In some patients an awake intubation to maintain reflexes may be necessary. At induction of anesthesia an additional person should be available to provide suctioning of blood from the oropharynx. The patient should be placed in a slight head-down position to protect the trachea and glottis from aspiration of blood. Gastric decompression is performed to assess for occult blood loss and decrease the risk of subsequent pulmonary aspiration. The induction agent selected is based on the hemodynamics and condition of the patient. Emergence and extubation of the trachea should occur after return of protective laryngeal reflexes.[59]

Thyroid Surgery

A thorough knowledge of the specific issues related to anesthesia case management for thyroidectomy is essential to provide high-quality care. Airway management may be difficult despite a normal airway examination because of impingement of a thyroid mass on the laryngeal and tracheal structures. Since sympathetic nervous system hyperactivity is associated with increased amounts of thyroid hormone, it is essential that all patients having an elective thyroidectomy be rendered euthyroid prior to surgery. There are multiple preoperative antithyroid medication regimens that effectively treat thyroid hormone hypersecretion. Although it is a rare event, thyroid storm can still occur during the perioperative period.

The thyroid gland is butterfly-shaped and composed of two lobes that are connected by a median tissue mass named the thyroid isthmus. It is located on the anterior and anterolateral aspect of the trachea immediately inferior to the larynx. The thyroid gland is the largest endocrine gland in the body weighing 20 g in the healthy adult. Its major blood supply arises from the superior and inferior thyroid arteries, which are branches of the common carotid artery. Blood flow is approximately five times the weight of the gland, and therefore the thyroid receives one of the greatest blood supplies per gram of tissue measures in the body.[68]

Motor function associated with movement of the intrinsic muscles of the larynx that abduct, adduct, and tense the vocal cords is supplied by the RLN and the external branch of the superior laryngeal nerve. These nerves lie in close proximity to the lateral lobes of the thyroid gland. During surgical resection, if these nerves are temporarily or permanently damaged, then vocal cord movement can be adversely affected and may result in airway compromise after extubation. Anatomic representation of the thyroid gland and its associated structures are presented in Fig. 43.9.

Pathophysiology

Thyroid dysfunction can be treated medically or surgically. A thyroidectomy is performed as definitive treatment for thyrotoxicosis or malignancy. It can be performed open, minimally invasive video assisted, or robotic assisted.

Thyrotoxicosis refers to a condition in which excessive amounts of thyroid hormone are present in a patient's system, whereas hyperthyroidism (the most common cause of thyrotoxicosis) describes states in which the excessive thyroid levels are caused by a hyperactive thyroid gland.[69,70] Malignancies of the thyroid gland are the most common malignancies of the endocrine system and have been associated with prior exposure to radiation.[70,71] Thyrotoxicosis is a rare (2%) occurrence in thyroid malignancies. Surgery is the principal treatment used to treat thyroid malignancies both for purposes of excision of the tumor and staging. Most thyroid malignancies (>90%) are considered well differentiated and are categorized as papillary thyroid cancer (PTC) or follicular thyroid cancer (FTC). PTC accounts for 70% to 80% of thyroid cancer, usually presents at an early stage, and has an excellent prognosis (>95% 10-year survival). FTC accounts for 10% of thyroid cancer and tends to present at a later stage than PTC. The 10-year survival rate for FTC is 85%.[69]

Preoperative Assessment and Preparation

The primary goals during preoperative assessment are ensuring that the patient is euthyroid, assessing the degree of end-organ complications, and determining the extent of airway involvement. Thyroid tumors or large goiters can impinge upon the tracheal cartilages and esophageal tissues resulting in tracheomalacia and airway compromise. Preoperatively the patient will be taking a combination of antithyroid medications to decrease the synthesis and release of thyroid hormone, and to treat the hyperdynamic state associated with hyperthyroidism. The medical management of this condition often includes use of glucocorticoids and may require administration of a steroid stress dose preoperatively or intraoperatively. Patients should continue their regimen of antithyroid medications and β-blockade through the morning of surgery. Preoperative use of antithyroid drugs has greatly decreased morbidity from thyroid surgery and rendered thyroid storm a rare event. The aim of preoperative management is to restore a normal metabolic state prior to surgical interventions. Patients with hyperthyroidism have increased T_3 and T_4 values and decreased or normal thyroid-stimulating hormone (TSH) levels. β-blocking drugs are widely used as an adjunct to the antithyroid thionamides for symptomatic control. β-blockers are generally continued throughout the surgical period and may be incrementally withdrawn postoperatively. Drugs that are used to treat hyperthyroidism are listed in Table 43.8.[72]

All routine airway assessments should be performed in addition to a full visualization and palpation of the patient's neck for a thyroid

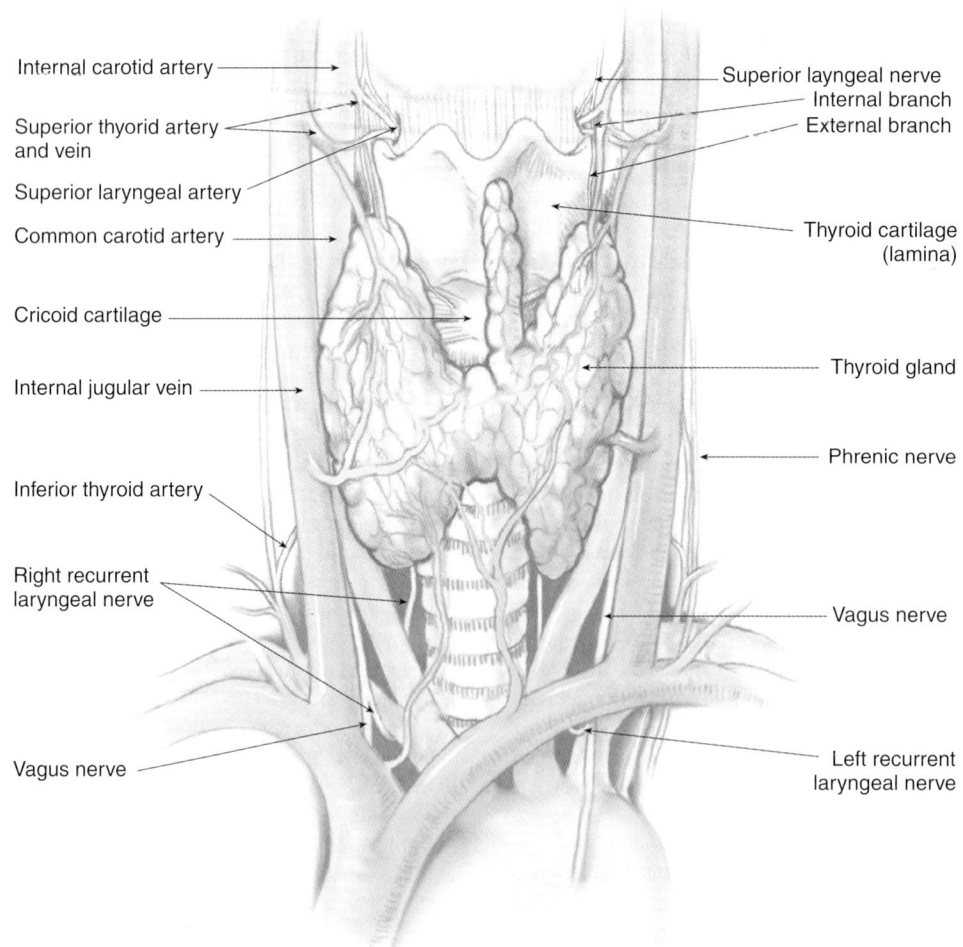

Fig. 43.9 Thyroid gland and surrounding anatomic structures.

TABLE 43.8	Oral Drugs Used to Treat Hyperthyroidism	
Drug	**Daily Oral Adult Dose**	**Comments**
Thionamides		
Methimazole (Tapazole), generic	Starting: 10–40 mg once or divided Maintenance: 5–15 mg once or divided	Methimazole is preferred because of ease of dosing and a better side effect profile; continue up to the morning of surgery
Propylthiouracil (PTU) (generic)	Starting: 100–450 mg divided bid or tid Maintenance: 100–150 mg divided bid or tid	
Iodide		Iodide therapy added 1 wk prior to surgery and continued through the day of surgery; decreases the production and release of thyroid hormone and reduces thyroid vascularity
SSKI	1–3 drops tid	
Lugol solution	5 drops tid (dissolve in a full glass of water)	
β-blockers		β-blockers without intrinsic sympathomimetic activity are preferred; also used in emergency thyroid surgery for adrenergic suppression
Propranolol (generic)	20–40 mg qid	
Propranolol (Inderal)—long acting	80–160 mg once	
Atenolol (generic and Tenormin)	25–100 mg once or bid	
Metoprolol (generic and Lopressor)	50–200 mg divided bid or tid	

bid, Twice a day; *qid*, four times a day; *SSKI*, saturated solution of potassium iodide; *tid*, three times a day.
Adapted from Elisha S, et al. Anesthesia case management for thyroidectomy. *AANA J.* 2010;78(2):151–160.

goiter. The patient's airway should be assessed in the supine position. If there is any indication of potential for airway compromise, a chest radiograph and a CT scan of the neck and chest should be performed and evaluated prior to induction of anesthesia. Preoperative testing may include an electrocardiogram if comorbid conditions/risk factors exist. Laboratory testing should be selected commensurate with findings in the preoperative evaluation. Patients with hyperthyroidism have a higher incidence of myasthenia gravis and may present with skeletal muscle weakness and an increased sensitivity to muscle relaxants.[72]

Intraoperative Anesthetic Management

General endotracheal anesthesia is the technique of choice for thyroidectomy, and the standard induction and maintenance drugs are used. Paralysis may inhibit the surgeon's ability to assess the integrity of the RLN, and relaxation is avoided after intubation if nerve testing is planned. Succinylcholine is chosen for intubation because of its short duration and spontaneous degradation. Intraoperative neural monitoring (IONM) during thyroid and parathyroid surgery has gained widespread acceptance as an adjunct to the gold standard of visual nerve identification.

A special ETT, the Medtronic nerve integrity monitor (NIM) EMG endotracheal tube (NIM 3.0 ETT), is frequently used to assess recurrent laryngeal and vocal cord function during surgery.[73] Injury during surgical procedures can lead to hoarseness, aphonia, and (although rare) difficulty with ventilation as a result of permanent adduction of the cords. The major advantage of using the NIM 3.0 ETT is that it allows the surgeon the capability of identifying the muscles innervated by the RLN prior to traction or severing the nerve. The NIM 3.0 ETT is a flexible silicone elastomer ETT with an inflatable cuff. The tube is fitted with four stainless-steel wire electrodes (two pairs) that are embedded in the silicone of the main shaft of the ETT and exposed only for a short distance, slightly superior to the cuff. The electrodes are designed to make contact with the patient's right and left vocal cords to facilitate EMG monitoring of the muscles innervated by the RLN when connected to a four-channel EMG monitoring device. If monitoring correctly, the EMG will display a consistent sound signal and an action potential tracing. The red wire pair of the NIM tube should contact the anterior and posterior portion of the right true vocal cord, and the blue wire pair should contact the anterior and posterior portion of the left true vocal cord (Fig. 43.10). Paralysis and laryngeal tracheal anesthesia with lidocaine both inhibit accurate EMG readings. Research is ongoing regarding the efficacy of EMG; however, some studies have shown no statistically significant difference in outcome between a standard ETT and a NIM tube.[72-75]

Maintenance of anesthesia can be provided by inhalational anesthetics with or without N_2O. A combined deep and superficial cervical plexus block may be considered for intraoperative and postoperative pain management; additionally, IV anesthesia may also be suitable and provide optimal conditions.[76] The patient should be constantly monitored for an increase in core body temperature and hyperdynamic response. If true hypotension occurs, it is best treated with a direct-acting vasopressor (phenylephrine) rather than an indirect-acting vasopressor (ephedrine), which stimulates the release of catecholamines.[72] Aberrant blood pressure readings should be investigated prior to pharmacologic treatment, as focused surgical colleagues have been known to inadvertently affect the cuff pressure. The patient is positioned supine with the head elevated 30 degrees and the neck extended using a roll behind the neck and shoulders (Rose position). The arms are tucked at the patient's sides with the ulnar nerves padded and protected. Hyperextension of the neck should be avoided in those patients with atlantoaxial joint instability and/or those with limited range of motion. Because there is limited access to the face, special care should be taken to protect the eyes from injury, especially in patients with exophthalmos.

Postoperative Management

The most common postoperative complications include hypocalcemia, RLN damage, and hematoma at the surgical site. A complete list

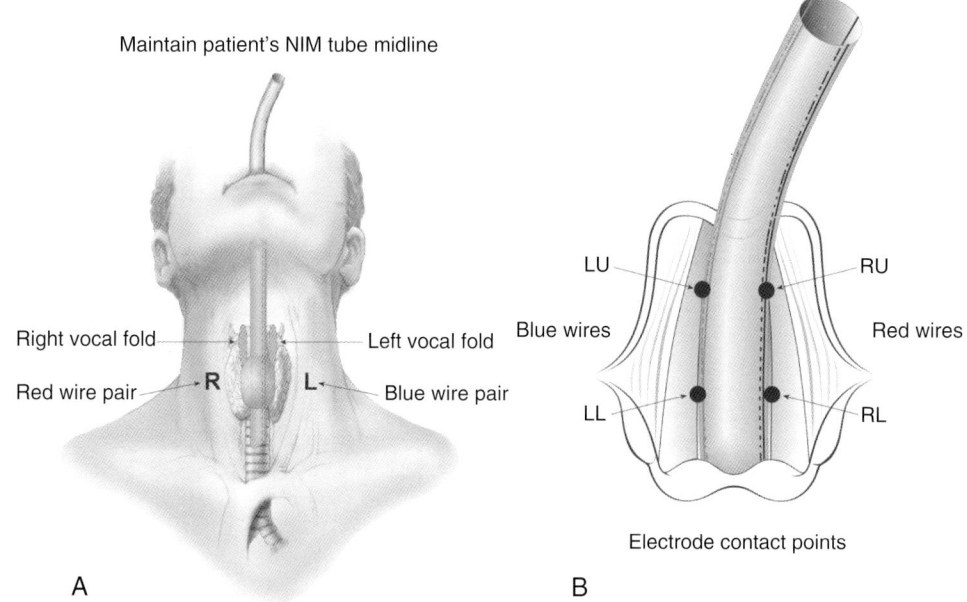

Maintain patient's NIM tube midline

Right vocal fold

Left vocal fold

Red wire pair   R   L   Blue wire pair

Blue wires   LU   RU   Red wires

LL   RL

Electrode contact points

A   B

Fig. 43.10 Nerve integrity monitor *(NIM)* endotracheal tube. (A) Proper placement of the NIM endotracheal tube in relation to the thyroid gland. (B) Four electrode contact points in relation to the vocal cords. *L,* left; *LL,* left lower; *LU,* left upper; *R,* right; *RL,* right lower; *RU,* right upper.

BOX 43.4   Complications Associated With Thyroidectomy

- Hypocalcemia-hypoparathyroidism
- Recurrent laryngeal nerve injury—unilateral or bilateral
- Neck hematoma
- Thyroid storm
- Superior laryngeal nerve injury
- Infection
- Pneumothorax
- Tracheomalacia

Adapted from Elisha S, et al. Anesthesia case management for thyroidectomy. *AANA J.* 2010;78(2):151–160.

---

of the potential postoperative complications is presented in Box 43.4. Postoperative hypocalcemia can result from hypoparathyroidism. The four parathyroid glands are located on the posterior aspect of the thyroid gland and produce parathyroid hormone, which increases serum calcium. Inadequate release of parathyroid hormone is caused by the inadvertent removal of the parathyroid glands during a total thyroidectomy. It can also occur secondary to parathyroid gland devascularization, injury, or "stunning" from dissection.[75,77]

Hypocalcemia causes neuronal excitability in sensory and motor nerves. Patients most commonly develop signs and symptoms associated with hypocalcemia 24 to 96 hours postoperatively. The degree of hypocalcemia coincides with the severity of the symptoms, which include perioral numbness and tingling, abdominal pain, paresthesias of the extremities, carpopedal spasm, tetany, laryngospasm, mental status changes, seizures, Q-T prolongation on the electrocardiogram, and cardiac arrest.[62,69,77] Neuromuscular irritability also can be confirmed by assessing for Chvostek sign (i.e., facial contractions elicited by tapping the facial nerve in the periauricular area) and Trousseau sign (i.e., carpal spasm on inflation of a blood pressure cuff). In addition, monitoring postoperative ionized calcium levels is recommended because these values are reflective of the physiologically active form of calcium.

Treatment for severe symptomatic hypocalcemia includes the administration of calcium gluconate or calcium chloride (10 mL of 10% solution) intravenously given over several minutes and followed by a continuous infusion (1–2 mg/kg/hr) until calcium levels normalize.[72]

Iatrogenic trauma to the RLN is estimated to occur in up to 14% of cases. The surgical identification and preservation of the RLN is essential to avoid injury. Damage to the RLN may be unilateral or bilateral; however, unilateral nerve injury is more common. Unilateral RLN damage causes the ipsilateral vocal cord to remain midline during inspiration resulting in hoarseness. Bilateral RLN injury results in dysfunction of both vocal cords, which remain midline during inspiration. After extubation, biphasic stridor, respiratory distress, and aphonia occur because of unopposed adduction of the vocal cords and closure of the glottic aperture. Unlike unilateral nerve injury, bilateral nerve injury necessitates immediate intervention requiring emergent reintubation or tracheotomy.[72]

Postoperative bleeding of the surgical site results in a neck hematoma, which causes airway obstruction and asphyxiation. This complication represents a true surgical emergency. Common symptoms of neck hematoma include neck swelling, neck pain and pressure, dyspnea, and stridor. Initial treatment includes the emergent evacuation of the neck hematoma followed by airway management.[72,77]

Cleft Palate and Lip

Cleft Palate (Hard Palate and Soft Palate)

Cleft lip and palate is one of the most common craniofacial abnormalities, occurring in approximately 1:700 births.[78] During fetal development, the bones of the face develop between the fifth and ninth weeks, and the growth of the palatal bones between the sixth and eleventh weeks. A cleft develops when the bones of the nasal and maxillary or the palatal bones fail to fuse. A fetus can develop both a cleft lip and palate or either alone. Up to 30% of these newborns have other congenital anomalies such as Down syndrome, Pierre Robin syndrome, and Treacher Collins syndrome.

The timing for surgery remains controversial. Generally, cleft lip repair with primary tip rhinoplasty is performed at age 3 months. This will enable the baby to feed and demonstrate normal facial expressions. The next repair involves closure of the posterior hard palate and the soft palate before the development of speech and is usually at 5 to 8 months of age depending on the exact defects. The patient's overall health status and the presence of other congenital anomalies are also considerations. Widely followed preoperative guidelines include the rules of 10: weight at least 10 lb, hemoglobin at least 10 g, white blood cell count less than 10,000/mm³, and age more than 10 weeks. Others advocate for earlier repair, and in utero techniques are under investigation.[79,80]

Intubation may sometimes be difficult if the laryngoscope blade slips into the cleft. However, packing the cleft with gauze assists in preventing this from occurring. An oral RAE tube or flexible connector is used and secured at the midline of the lower lip. A specialized mouth gag is used to hold the mouth open and the ETT in place during cleft palate surgery. All air bubbles should be carefully removed from IV lines to prevent air embolus because of the incidence of associated cardiac anomalies (e.g., atrioventricular defect) that may lead to air crossing from the venous to the arterial circulation. Congenital heart disease may influence which drugs are selected for maintenance of anesthesia and infiltration of the operative site, particularly if epinephrine is selected. Care must be implemented to protect the child's eyes because accidental damage may occur during the surgical procedure. Before emergence, a suture is often placed through the tip of the tongue and taped to the cheek. This suture eliminates the need for an oral airway and prevents damage to the palatal repair. If soft tissue obstruction occurs during emergence or recovery, traction on the suture can alleviate the problem. If edema occurs, a more aggressive and immediate airway management technique should be used. Copious secretions and blood may cause laryngospasm after extubation, and therefore a clear airway is imperative.

Cleft Lip

Management of unilateral cleft lip repair consists of routine induction followed by oral intubation using an RAE tube or a flexible connector. Secure the tube to the lower lip and midline via tape. To decrease tension on the surgical sutures at the end of the procedure, the surgeon may place a Logan bow across the upper lip of the patient.[81] When the Logan bow is placed, mask ventilation during emergence will become impaired or impossible. Extubation must be performed only with the patient fully awake and reflexes intact. The child's surgical site must also be protected from finger and hand manipulation. Some hospitals recommend the use of hand mittens or taping the extremities onto armboards during the postoperative period. Close monitoring of respiration must occur throughout the postoperative period.

Dental Restoration Procedures

Dental restoration procedures are performed under general anesthesia for a multitude of reasons. These include multiple cavities, history of cerebral palsy or Down syndrome, and an uncooperative patient who would not be an appropriate candidate for local anesthetic and an office procedure.

Developmentally delayed patients typically develop a close relationship with either a family member or a long-term health care worker. It is often suggested that this individual accompany the patient to decrease anxiety and communicate a health history to the anesthesia provider. A thorough airway assessment should be performed before considering induction. Midazolam (0.5 mg/kg by mouth [PO]) or ketamine (3–4 mg/kg intramuscularly [IM]) is most effective in sedating children in the preoperative arena. Many patients requiring dental restoration have congenital anomalies, and it is not uncommon to find a small oropharynx, enlarged tonsils, a large tongue, and increased secretions. Atlantoaxial instability and congenital heart disease should also be considered in the preoperative preparation and anesthetic management.[82-84] Preparation and appropriate airway management must be planned and implemented for these patients. Patients who receive phenytoin to control seizures may have gingival hyperplasia. Because the gingiva is highly vascular, any surgical manipulation during restoration may lead to significant blood loss.

In patients with normal airways a standard induction is appropriate, and a nasal intubation usually facilitates the dental procedure. The application of a topical vasoconstrictive nasal spray during the preoperative period reduces or prevents bleeding during the insertion of the nasotracheal tube. Following loss of consciousness, lubricated intranasal trumpets may be inserted into the most patent nasal airway. Starting with a smaller nasal trumpet, several are placed in increasing sizes to dilate the airway. When full dilation of the nares has occurred, a well-lubricated ETT is passed through the nose into the trachea, either blindly or assisted by Magill forceps under direct laryngoscopy. The nasal ETT is preferably placed on the side opposite where the surgeon will be working. The ETT is often sewn to the nasal septum by the surgeon. Throat packs may be placed to prevent blood from entering the stomach and causing nausea and vomiting; monitoring their removal is essential to preventing respiratory obstruction after extubation.

Sinus and Nasal Procedures

Nasal and sinus procedures for drainage of chronic sinusitis, polyp removal, repair of a deviated septum, or closed reduction of fractures generally involves the young and healthy patient population. Many patients who undergo sinus and nasal surgery have chronic environmental and drug allergies, therefore an increased incidence of reactive airway disease in these patients may be present. Nasal polyp removal, for example, may be necessitated by Samter syndrome. A patient with Samter triad has nasal polyps, asthma, and an aspirin allergy. The nasal polyps, if symptomatic, are removed surgically. The use of fiberoptics or functional endoscopic sinus surgery for nasal and sinus surgery has become a popular treatment for chronic sinusitis.

Nasal surgery may be successfully accomplished with local anesthesia, local combined with IV sedation, or general anesthesia. All three methods of anesthesia require vasoconstriction. The mucous membranes of the sinuses and nose are highly vascular, and blood loss may be significant if vasoconstriction is not used. The surgeon may select to control vasoconstriction with epinephrine or cocaine. Al Haddad et al.[85] found no difference in the quality of vasoconstriction when comparing topical cocaine to phenylephrine during septoplasty. A hypotensive technique or slight head elevation (i.e., 10–20 degrees) may be used during the procedure. Using general anesthesia has been associated with increased blood loss even with the use of an epinephrine injection. This exaggerated blood loss may be related to the vasodilatory properties of inhalation agents. Delivering general anesthesia for sinus surgery with propofol, as well as other IV anesthetic techniques for the maintenance of anesthesia, has been associated with less blood loss than occurs with the use of volatile agents for maintenance.[83] The removal of an oropharyngeal pack should be ensured prior to emergence. Suctioning of the stomach prior to extubation is desirable and may attenuate postoperative retching and vomiting; adequate depth of anesthesia must be present prior to this action. After all the packing is removed, extubation should be performed on the awake patient who has regained control of protective reflexes.[84] The use of IV or topical lidocaine may reduce some of the coughing prior to extubation, leading to less bleeding in the postoperative period.

Trauma

Initial Assessment

Traumatic disruption of the bony, cartilaginous, and soft tissue components of the face and upper airway require special consideration. It is imperative to create an anesthetic plan for securing the airway without promoting further damage or compromising ventilation. Possible mechanisms by which the upper or lower airway may become obstructed include edema, bleeding from the oral mucosa and palate, intraoral fracture sites, distortion of the nasal passages, injury of the pharynx and sinuses, open lacerations, and the presence of foreign bodies such as avulsed teeth, blood clots, or bony fragments.[86]

Initial management of the airway depends on the situation at hand. In the case of severe facial or neck trauma, alternative methods of tracheal intubation (e.g., fiberoptic laryngoscopy, retrograde wire placement, jet ventilation via cricothyrotomy, or emergent tracheostomy) may be necessary to secure the airway.[86]

Injuries of the head and neck may include cervical spine or cranial injury. Although a complete evaluation of all cervical vertebrae is ideal, inspection of radiographs of the cervical spine is judicious to determine the presence or absence of dislocations and fractures. All seven cervical vertebrae must be visible in such studies. The seventh cervical vertebra is the most common site of traumatic fracture of the spine.[87] Vertebral artery injury must be suspected with a cervical injury because these fractures can lead to vertebral artery tear or occlusion. If deteriorating respiratory function requires immediate airway management and intubation, the head should be maintained in a fixed position before any manipulation of the airway is performed. The use of manual axial inline stabilization and/or a rigid cervical collar in place is recommended. The removal of the anterior segment of the collar can facilitate intubation and manipulation of the soft tissues of the neck.[87,88]

Blunt trauma to the face or anterior neck may produce rapid airway occlusion from soft tissue edema or hematoma formation arising from injured vascular structures contained within the neck. The patient exhibiting smoke inhalation or blistering in the area of the mouth and nares or with a history of inhalation of toxic byproducts of combustion should be intubated immediately. Edema of the face and glottis, which may lack symptoms in the early stages, has the potential to produce serious airway compromise several hours after injury.

Maxillofacial Trauma and Orthognathic Surgery

Rene Le Fort[89] determined the common fracture lines of the maxilla and face by experimentation on cadavers in 1901. The Le Fort classification is based on his finding that blunt trauma tends to cause fractures along three particular lines of the face. Fractures occurring in 21st-century, real-life situations (in particular, in high-velocity motor vehicle accidents) often deviate from this classification system, and "pure" Le Fort fractures are rare. Nevertheless, the Le Fort classification system is widely known, and it provides a method for concise communication of fracture patterns between clinicians and radiologists.

The three types of Le Fort fractures, which describe a pattern of fractures involving multiple facial bones,[90,91] are divided into Le Fort I, II, and III (Fig. 43.11). The Le Fort I fracture is a horizontal fracture of the maxilla extending from the floor of the nose and hard palate, through the nasal septum, and through the pterygoid plates posteriorly. The palate, maxillary alveolar bone, lower pterygoid plate, and part of the palatine bone are all mobilized. The Le Fort II fracture is a triangular fracture running from the bridge of the nose, through the medial and inferior wall of the orbit, beneath the zygoma, and through the lateral wall of the maxilla and the pterygoid plates. The Le Fort III fracture totally separates the midfacial skeleton from the cranial base, traversing the root of the nose, the ethmoid bone, the eye orbits, and the sphenopalatine fossa.[89,92]

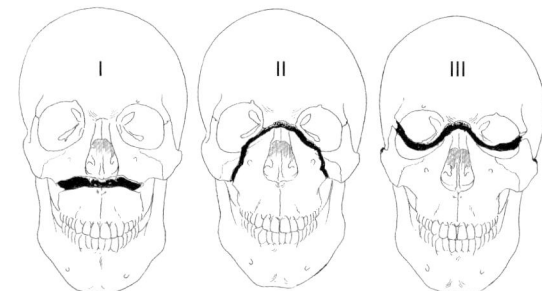

Fig. 43.11 Examples of Le Fort I, II, and III facial fractures (*left to right*).

A Le Fort I fracture generally causes little difficulty for the anesthesia provider. Patients may be intubated orally or nasally and the airway secured without a problem. The Le Fort II and III fractures are of particular concern when contemplating nasal intubation. In both these fractures, disruption of the cribriform plate may occur, opening the underside of the cranial cavity. The presence of cerebral fluid in the nose, blood behind a tympanic membrane, periorbital edema, or "raccoon-eyes" hematoma are indications that attempts to pass an ETT or nasogastric tube through the nares could lead to inadvertent intracranial placement.[92] Although the insertion of a nasal tube may aid the surgeon, an attempted nasotracheal intubation of a patient with a basal skull fracture involves the very serious risk of introducing the tube into the skull, bringing contaminated material into the subarachnoid space and causing meningitis. The tube may also inflict damage to the brain.[93]

The forces required to produce facial fractures are considerable and may be associated with other trauma. It is important that cervical spine injury, subdural hematoma, pneumothorax, and intraabdominal bleeding be investigated. Soft tissue injury to the airway and blood or debris in the oropharynx may make visualization impossible. If in doubt while in the emergency department, a tracheostomy under local anesthesia or an awake oral intubation with topical anesthesia should be considered. These patients should be treated with full-stomach precautions.

As with any trauma victim, attention is first directed toward maintaining the ABCs: airway, breathing, and circulation. The repair of the facial fracture itself is not an emergency and may be carried out later. Once the patient arrives in the operating room for surgery, it may be challenging to open the patient's mouth for intubation because of edema, pain, or trismus. It is necessary to differentiate the cause of the small mouth opening because it may be pain related or mechanical in nature. The administration of a short-acting narcotic or midazolam will sometimes assist the anesthesia provider in determining the cause of the restriction, which greatly influences the induction chosen. In mandibular or maxillary fractures, nasal intubation is usually best because the patient's teeth are brought together via wires or rubber bands at the conclusion of surgery (intermaxillary fixation). Anesthesia is induced with an IV agent and maintained with narcotics, muscle relaxants, and inhalation agents. Blood loss from facial fractures can be extensive. The patient's blood should be typed and crossmatched so that blood is immediately available. The fixation process closes the teeth in proper occlusion and prevents access to the oropharynx. Masking the patient at emergence requires that the patient be awake with intact reflexes at extubation. It also requires that wire cutters or scissors be available to cut the wire or rubber bands fixing the mandible to the maxilla in case an airway emergency occurs in the recovery area.[94]

Orthopedic orthognathic procedures often require sagittal splitting of the mandible to move the lower jaw either forward or back. A Le

Fort I or II osteotomy may be purposefully performed to move the maxilla in any direction to correct anomalies. Many of these patients have anomalies of the mandible and maxilla, small mouth openings, and appliances that make intubation difficult and airway management challenging. Because many of the malocclusions are treated orally, a nasal ETT is usually preferred over an oral intubation. Securing the nasotracheal tube away from the surgical field without causing necrotic injury of the nares is vital. Because blood loss during these procedures can be extensive, the patient is typed and crossmatched. Deliberate hypotensive anesthetic techniques are often used if the patient remains stable. Rigid metal or plastic external or internal fixation devices are used to maintain stability in both the mandible and maxilla postoperatively; therefore the proper cutting tools should be at the patient's bedside for emergency airway issues. Edema will often be extensive and progress over the first 24 hours after orthognathic surgery. To prevent postoperative respiratory problems, the patient may remain intubated for several days. If extubation is necessary, it should be done only when the patient is awake, in full command of protective reflexes, and can be carefully monitored in the postoperative period.

Radical Neck Dissection

Radical neck dissection is required when cancerous tumors have invaded the musculature and other structures of the head and neck. Neoplastic growths can occur anywhere within the upper airway and may achieve significant size with little evidence of airway penetration or obstruction. Such tumors are often friable and bleed readily. These patients may have a greater number of cumulative risk factors such as smoking, alcohol consumption, bronchitis, pulmonary emphysema, or cardiovascular disease. If the tumor interferes with eating, then associated weight loss, malnutrition, anemia, dehydration, and electrolyte imbalance can be significant. Patients who have had radiation treatments of the neck and jaw prior to surgical intervention will have soft tissues that are less mobile, making intubation more difficult. Many of these patients are older and have the comorbidities associated with age.[95,96] Attempted tracheal intubation can induce significant hemorrhage and edema, causing severe compromise of the airway.

Determining the appropriate techniques for airway management entails consultation with the surgeon as to the nature, extent, and location of the tumor; therapy administered (radiation or chemotherapy); CT results; history and physical examination; and relevant preoperative laboratory values.

Head and neck reconstruction is an integral part of surgical removal of head and neck tumors. Traditional methods of reconstruction include regional pedicle flaps with microvascular reconstruction. Flaps include the pectoralis major myocutaneous flap, trapezius flap, and local rotational flaps (e.g., forehead flap). Additionally, small bowel may be harvested to reconstruct the oropharynx and esophagus. Successful anesthesia plays an important role in maximizing the overall success rate of a free flap and microvascular flow of the flap.[97] The planned donor site should be determined to plan for any limitation on the available sites to place lines necessary for monitoring and venous access. Although the choice of monitoring is largely dependent on the general condition of the patient, the placement of a CVP line, a Foley catheter, and an arterial line (beat-to-beat and arterial blood gas trends) is suggested, particularly if deliberate hypotension during anesthesia is used. The internal jugular approach should be avoided because of proximity to the surgical site. Sites commonly used for the CVP placement when the internal jugular is not accessible are the subclavian and femoral veins, respectively.

Maintenance of anesthesia is often performed with an inhalation agent and supplemental narcotics. The use of a nondepolarizing muscle relaxant must be discussed with the surgical team preoperatively because a nerve stimulator is frequently used (by the surgeon) to locate nerves distorted by the tumor during the procedure. Significant blood loss can be a problem; sometimes, a controlled hypotension technique may be requested.[95,96] At least one and preferably two large-bore peripheral IV lines (14–16 gauge) should be in place. The patient's blood should be typed and crossmatched with blood readily available. It is important to replace blood loss but not to the point of fluid overload. Monitoring estimated blood loss and measuring the hematocrit may provide some guidelines for replacement of blood. A positive fluid balance in the postoperative phase can result in edema and congestion of the flap predisposing it to vascular compromise. Colloids may be used to help limit the amount of crystalloid required during the procedure. Patients undergoing a radical neck dissection are frequently hypovolemic and have electrolyte imbalances preoperatively. This requires judicious fluid replacement and electrolyte balance intraoperatively to maintain cardiovascular stability. Cerebral blood flow can be compromised by the tumor, retractors, or blood flow; therefore it is important to maintain adequate perfusion.

In preparation for a tracheostomy or total laryngectomy to be performed during the surgical procedure, the patient should be well oxygenated. The trachea will be transected by the surgeon, which requires that the anesthesia provider suction the airway and remove the ETT only to a level above the tracheal incision. Once the tracheostomy tube has been placed by the surgeon and ventilation validated, the ETT can then be completely removed. A reinforced tube is usually placed in the distal airway by the surgeon and connected to the anesthesia machine. A reassessment of the ventilation should be performed, including the entire procedure of listening to bilateral breath sounds, observing chest excursion, and checking end tidal CO_2 and positive inspiratory pressure or negative inspiratory pressure. After the anesthesia provider has validated tube placement, the ETT is sutured to the chest wall for the entire surgical duration. At the end of surgery, the reinforced tube may be switched for a tracheostomy cannula.

During radical lymph node dissection of the neck for carcinoma, manipulation of the carotid sinus may elicit a vagal reflex, causing bradycardia, hypotension, or cardiac arrest. Small doses of local anesthetic injected near the carotid sinus or administration of an anticholinergic may block vagal reflexes. Because of the long duration of the surgery and interruption of venous flow, venous thrombus is commonly seen in patients who are undergoing radical neck dissection. The head-up position and open neck veins during surgery may lead to venous air embolism. Careful monitoring with precordial Doppler sonography or transesophageal echocardiography provides the most precise detection of air embolism. Immediate removal of the air through the CVP is essential. Laryngeal edema, vascular occlusion, and obstruction can also occur as a result of the venous stasis that follows major disruptions in venous flow during surgery or with trauma. Continual review of complications and follow-up treatments are necessary.[94-96,98]

Postoperative considerations consist of tracheostomy care, controlled ventilation, chest radiography (to rule out pneumothorax, hemothorax, pulmonary edema), and monitoring for laryngeal edema induced by thrombosis. Postoperative characteristics of various surgical laryngectomy procedures are given in Table 43.9. It is suggested that these patients be admitted overnight to the intensive care unit because they have undergone major fluid and electrolyte shifts and altered ventilation-perfusion status and have spent an extensive time under the influence of anesthesia.[99,100]

TABLE 43.9   Laryngectomy

Structures Removed	Structures Remaining	Postoperative Conditions
Total Laryngectomy Hyoid bone, entire larynx (epiglottis, false cords, true cords), cricoid cartilage, two or three rings of trachea	Tongue, pharyngeal wall, lower trachea	Loses voice, breathes through tracheostomy, no problem swallowing
Supraglottic or Horizontal Laryngectomy Hyoid bone, epiglottis, false vocal cords	True vocal cords, cricoid cartilage, trachea	Normal voice; may aspirate occasionally, especially liquids; normal airway
Vertical (or Hemi-) Laryngectomy One true vocal cord, false cord, arytenoid one-half thyroid cartilage	Epiglottis, one false cord, one true vocal cord, cricoid	Hoarse but serviceable voice, normal airway, no problem swallowing
Laryngofissure and Partial Laryngectomy One vocal cord	All other structures	Hoarse but serviceable voice, occasionally almost normal voice, no airway problem, no swallowing problem
Endoscopic Removal of Early Carcinoma Part of one vocal cord	All other structures	May have a normal voice, no other problems

From Odom-Forren J. *Drain's Perianesthesia Nursing: A Critical Care Approach.* 7th ed. St. Louis: Elsevier; 2018:468.

▮ SUMMARY

Administering anesthesia for ENT and maxillofacial procedures requires knowledge in both basic and advanced anesthesia techniques. The usual tenets of safe practice must often be adhered to while remaining at a distance from the airway. Good preparation remains imperative. Cooperation and communication between the surgeon and anesthesia provider will improve the quality of care for patients having ENT surgery.

REFERENCES

For a complete list of references for this chapter, scan this QR code with any smartphone code reader app, or visit the following URL: http://booksite.elsevier.com/9780323711944/.

Anesthesia for Ophthalmic Procedures

Randolf R. Harvey

Ophthalmic anesthesia continues to be an exciting and challenging segment of anesthesia practice. Ophthalmologists recognize the value anesthesia practitioners provide to their patients and practice. Phacoemulsification and advances in intraocular lens technology have led to smaller incision cataract surgery, which is generally tolerated well under topical and intraocular anesthesia. Anesthesia practitioners have also taken a leading role in advancing safer orbital regional needle block techniques. Thanks to ophthalmic anesthesia educational programs, such as the Ophthalmic Anesthesia Society (OAS; eyeanesthesia.org), ophthalmologists, Certified Registered Nurse Anesthetists, and anesthesiologists have been meeting annually since 1987. The emergence of modified versions of Atkinson's original intraconal retrobulbar block technique has led to safer needle approaches to the intraconal space. The intraconal retrobulbar space remains the most effective area for anesthetic distribution throughout the orbit.[1] The extraconal peribulbar and the sub-Tenon block techniques are also being used to meet the growing demand of ophthalmic surgical procedures. Advances in retinal surgical techniques have increased the demand by surgeons for orbital regional injection eye blocks, replacing the use of general anesthesia except where clinically indicated such as pediatrics. This trend is also growing for corneal transplants, adult eye muscle, and glaucoma procedures. The use of regional blocks effectively provides anesthesia for both the surgical procedure and postop pain relief, reducing the need for opioids and the concomitant nausea/vomiting, which may result from pain and opioid administration.

Today, more than 1 million ocular blocks are performed annually for surgical procedures. As a result of anesthesia practitioners' active involvement in ophthalmic anesthesia, safer ocular blocks are being administered, and more efficient patient care is being provided. This expertise in ophthalmic blocks by anesthesia practitioners has spurred a high demand for such services in part because of the proliferation of ambulatory surgical centers (ASCs) to meet the increased demand for ophthalmic surgery.

OPHTHALMIC ANATOMY

Extraocular Muscles

The eye is surrounded by six extraocular muscles (Figs. 44.1, 44.2, and 44.3). The superior rectus muscle, located at the 12-o'clock position on the globe, moves the eye upward (i.e., supraducts the eye). The inferior rectus muscle, located at the 6-o'clock position on the globe, moves the eye downward (i.e., infraducts the eye). The medial rectus muscle, located 90 degrees medially to the 12-o'clock position on the globe, moves the eyeball nasally (i.e., adducts the eye). The lateral rectus muscle, located 90 degrees laterally to the 12-o'clock position on the globe, moves the eyeball laterally (i.e., abducts the eye). The superior oblique muscle, located on the superior aspect of the eye, rotates the eyeball on its horizontal axis toward the nose (i.e., intorts the eye and depresses

the eyeball). The inferior oblique muscle, located on the inferior aspect of the globe, rotates the eyeball on its horizontal axis temporally (i.e., extorts the eye and elevates the eyeball) (Table 44.1).

All the ocular muscles, except the inferior oblique, originate in the orbital apex around the annulus of Zinn (Fig. 44.4), which is a fibrinous ring that encircles the optic foramen. The four rectus muscles move forward in a conal pattern that forms the muscle cone around the globe. These muscles, which are approximately 40 mm long, insert into the globe just anterior to its equator.[2] The superior oblique muscle arises just superior to the annulus of Zinn and moves forward, becoming a tendon. This tendon passes through a cartilaginous ring called the trochlea, which is located on the medial supranasal orbital wall. After passing through the trochlea, the tendon is redirected in a posterolateral direction and inserts on the superolateral aspect of the globe under the superior rectus muscle. The inferior oblique muscle originates from the anterior nasal orbital floor and moves in a posterolateral direction along the globe, inserting inferior to the macula of the globe. The arching of both the inferior and the superior oblique muscles around the globe allows for the torsional movements of the eye.

Eyelid Muscles

The levator muscle of the upper eyelid is the primary muscle used for raising the upper eyelids. This muscle originates near the annulus of Zinn (see Fig. 44.1B). It moves forward just superior and slightly medial to the superior rectus muscle, inserting into the upper eyelid. Because the levator muscle only retracts and does not contract the eyelid, akinesia of this muscle is not necessary.

The orbicular muscle of the eye (Fig. 44.5) causes the eyelids to contract. This muscle has three divisions—orbital, palpebral, and tarsal—which are concentrically arranged around the eyelid. Akinesia of these muscles is generally desired for ocular procedures because if the muscles were allowed to contract around the globe, intraocular pressure (IOP) would increase. However, the recent success of cataract procedures performed with the use of topical and intraocular anesthesia has demonstrated that akinesia of the orbicular muscle of the eye is not always mandatory.

Cranial Nerves

The orbital portion of the optic nerve (cranial nerve II) (Fig. 44.6) is 25 to 30 mm long and travels anteriorly within the muscle cone, from the cranial cavity to insert into the posterior aspect of the globe. The optic nerve is actually longer than the distance from the posterior pole of the globe to the orbital apex, giving the optic nerve an S-shaped configuration. This shape allows free movement of the nerve so that the many positions of the eye are accommodated. The optic nerve is myelinated and is approximately 4 mm in diameter.[3] The optic nerve extends from the optic chiasm intracranially through the optic canal and continues until it inserts into the posterior pole of the globe. The optic chiasm is

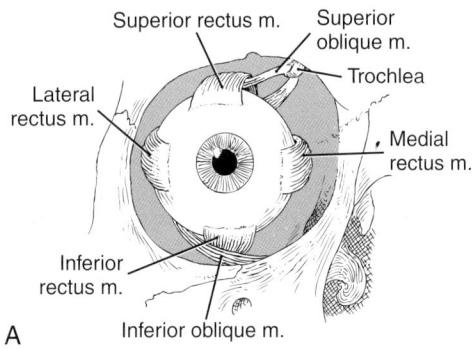

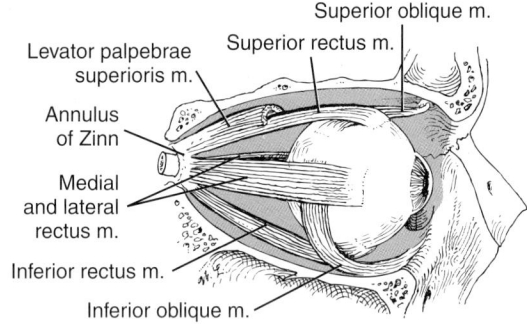

Fig. 44.1 (A) Frontal view of the orbit. (B) Lateral view of the orbit. *m.,* Muscle.

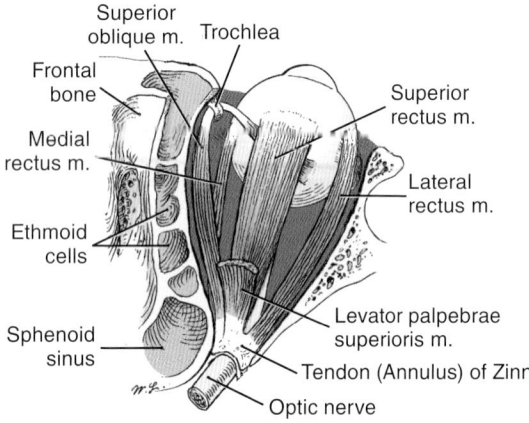

Fig. 44.2 Superior view of the orbit. *m.,* Muscle.

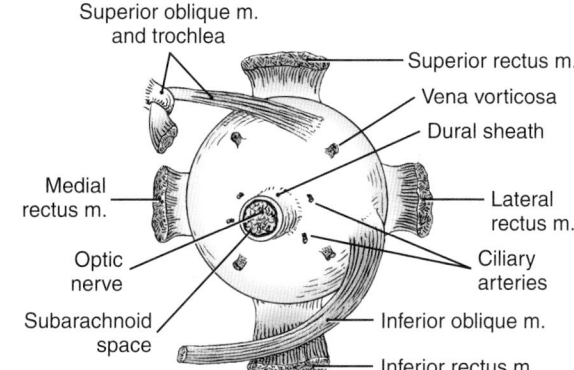

Fig. 44.3 Posterior view of the globe. *m.,* Muscle.

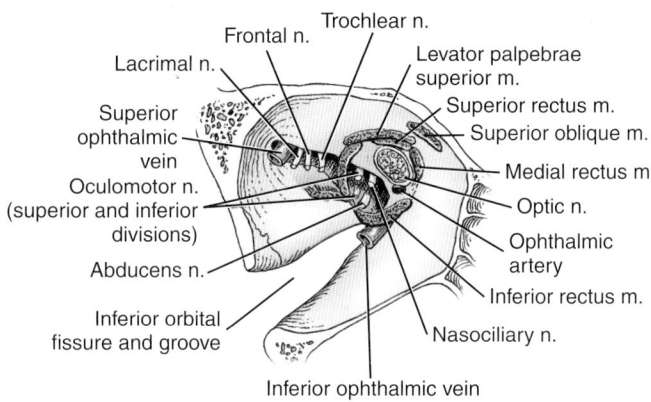

Fig. 44.4 View of the orbital apex. *m.,* Muscle; *n.,* nerve.

TABLE 44.1	**Orbital Muscles and Innervation**	
Muscle	**Function**	**Cranial Nerve**
Superior rectus	Supraduction	III
Inferior rectus	Infraduction	III
Medial rectus	Adduction	III
Lateral rectus	Abduction	VI
Superior oblique	Intorsion-depression	IV
Inferior oblique	Extorsion-elevation	III

the junction for both optic nerve tracts. Here, suspended in and surrounded by cerebrospinal fluid, the optic nerve fibers partially decussate, sending visual fibers to the contralateral eye.

The optic nerve is not a true cranial nerve but an outgrowth of the brain.[2] As a result, the optic nerve is also covered by the meninges, the fibrous wrappings of the arachnoid, dura, and pia mater, which envelop the central nervous system (CNS). Therefore any anesthetic agent injected into the optic nerve sheath can find its way back to the midbrain through the cerebrospinal fluid, resulting in CNS depression and respiratory arrest. The optic nerve also carries the central retinal artery and vein of the globe. The central retinal artery enters the optic nerve, and the central retinal vein exits the optic nerve approximately 8 to 15 mm posterior to the globe.[4]

The oculomotor nerve (cranial nerve III) innervates the following muscles of the orbit: the superior rectus muscle, the inferior rectus muscle, the inferior oblique muscle, the medial rectus muscle, and the levator

muscle of the upper eyelid. The oculomotor nerve is the primary motor nerve to the extraocular muscles of the orbit; this nerve branches superiorly and inferiorly (Fig. 44.7). The superior branch innervates the superior rectus muscle and the levator muscle of the upper eyelid. The inferior branch of the oculomotor nerve innervates the medial rectus muscle, the inferior rectus muscle, and the inferior oblique muscle. This nerve also sends parasympathetic fibers to the ciliary ganglion (Fig. 44.8), which is located adjacent to the optic nerve in the posterior portion of the orbit. The ciliary ganglion receives parasympathetic fibers from the oculomotor nerve and sympathetic fibers from the carotid artery plexus and a sensory branch from the nasociliary nerve, a branch of the ophthalmic nerve. The parasympathetic fibers move forward from the ciliary ganglion to innervate the iris sphincter muscles, which cause constriction of the pupil. The sympathetic motor fibers move forward to control the radial muscle of the iris for pupillary dilation.[2-4]

The trochlear nerve (cranial nerve IV) (see Fig. 44.7) provides the motor fibers for the superior oblique muscle. This nerve enters the orbit through the superior orbital fissure outside the muscle cone. It

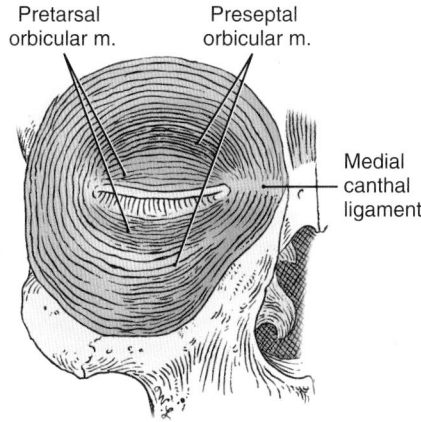

Fig. 44.5 Orbicularis oculi muscles. *m.*, Muscle.

is the only orbital cranial motor nerve that enters the orbit from outside the muscle cone. Once inside the orbit, the nerve root moves in a medial direction to innervate the superior oblique muscle.

The trigeminal nerve (cranial nerve V) (see Fig. 44.8) has sensory and motor components. In ocular anesthesia, the sensory component is of primary importance. The intracranial portion of the nerve forms the trigeminal ganglion, which has three main divisions: the ophthalmic, the maxillary, and the mandibular nerves. The ophthalmic branch provides for the sensation of pain, touch, and temperature to the cornea, ciliary body, iris, lacrimal gland, conjunctiva, nasal mucosa, eyelid, eyebrow, forehead, and nose. The maxillary branch provides for the sensation of pain, touch, and temperature to the upper lip, nasal mucosa, and scalp muscles.[5]

The ophthalmic nerve has three main branches: lacrimal, frontal, and nasociliary. The lacrimal nerve branch innervates the lacrimal gland in the superior lateral aspect of the orbit. The frontal branch is the largest branch of the ophthalmic nerve. This branch enters the orbit from outside the muscle cone through the superior orbital fissure and travels anteriorly outside the muscle cone superior to the levator muscle. The frontal nerve itself splits into two branches. The larger, supraorbital branch continues forward into the orbit and exits the orbit through the supraorbital notch; this branch innervates the

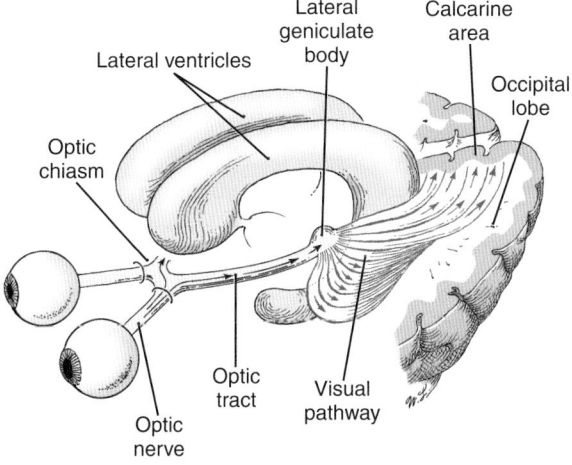

Fig. 44.6 Intraorbital and intracranial view of the optic nerve.

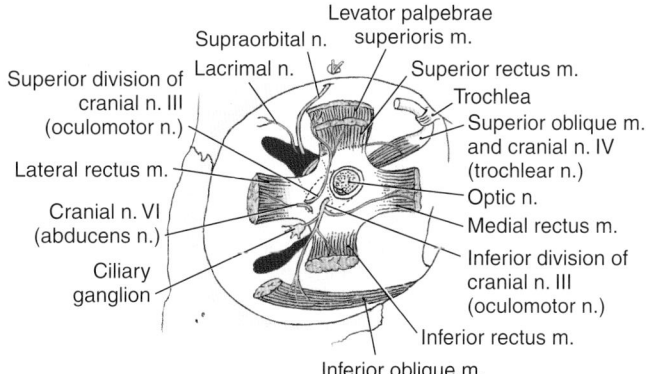

Fig. 44.7 Frontal view of the posterior orbit with its motor nerves and the extraocular muscles. *m.*, Muscle; *n.*, nerve.

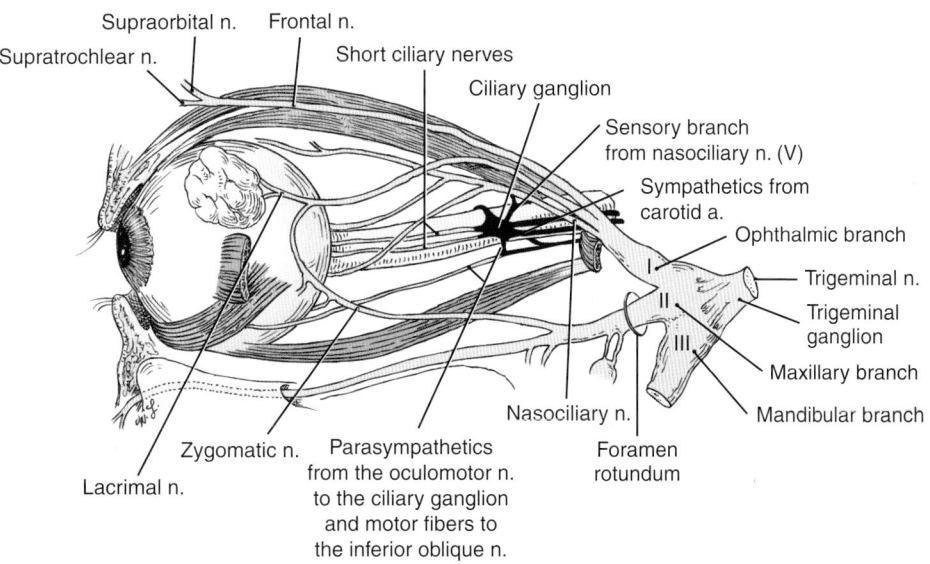

Fig. 44.8 Lateral orbital view of sensory nerves and ciliary ganglion. *a.*, Artery; *n.*, nerve.

forehead. The smaller branch is the supratrochlear nerve, which moves in a medial direction, supplying nerve roots to the forehead and the medial portion of the upper eyelid. The nasociliary nerve branch enters the orbit from inside the muscle cone and crosses over the optic nerve, sending nerve fibers medially and to the ciliary ganglion. The fibers to the ciliary ganglion form the short ciliary nerves, which continue anteriorly, penetrating the posterior portion of the globe near the optic nerve. The nasociliary nerve also gives rise to the long ciliary nerves, which continue anteriorly and enter the posterior portion of the globe supplying the ciliary muscle, iris, and cornea. The long ciliary nerves also carry sympathetic fibers to the dilator muscle of the iris from the superior cervical ganglion. The nasociliary nerve continues along the medial aspect of the orbit just superior to the medial rectus muscle until it passes through the orbital septum to become the infratrochlear nerve. The infratrochlear nerve provides sensory input to the side of the nose, the medial aspect of the eyelids, the medial conjunctiva, the caruncle, and the lacrimal sac.[2-5]

The abducens nerve (cranial nerve VI) (see Fig. 44.7) provides motor function to the lateral rectus muscle. The nerve enters through the superior orbital fissure within the muscle cone and continues along the conal surface of the lateral rectus muscle, eventually inserting in the posterior one-third of that muscle.

The facial nerve (cranial nerve VII) (Fig. 44.9) is predominantly a motor nerve for the muscles of the face. This nerve exits from the stylomastoid foramen. The facial nerve travels underneath the external auditory canal to the parotid gland, where it divides into an upper and a lower branch. Ocular anesthesia is more concerned with the upper branch of the facial nerve than with the lower. The upper branch further divides into the temporal and zygomatic branches, which innervate the orbicular muscle of the eye, the superficial facial muscles, and the scalp muscles.

The vagus nerve (cranial nerve X) provides motor function to the intrinsic muscles of the larynx and the heart; it provides major parasympathetic visceral innervation elsewhere. It is also the efferent pathway for the oculocardiac reflex, which can result in bradycardia and dysrhythmias.

Orbital Fossa

The orbital fossa has been described as pear shaped. The medial walls of the orbit extend almost straight back, whereas the lateral walls diverge at approximately a 90-degree angle to each other (Fig. 44.10). The superior and inferior orbital fissures are in the orbital apex, which is located in the posterior orbit. These fissures are the entry portals for the orbital nerves and vessels (Fig. 44.11). The optic foramen lies just medial to the superior orbital fissure and is the entry portal for the optic nerve and the ophthalmic artery from the intracranial to the intraorbital area. In the medial nasal aspect of the fossa, just behind the orbital rim, is the lacrimal bone, which is used as a landmark for the medial peribulbar block (Fig. 44.12). The ethmoid bone is just posterior to the lacrimal bone.[5]

The supraorbital nerve exits the orbit in the supraorbital notch, which is in the superior nasal aspect of the orbital rim. The infraorbital foramen, where the infraorbital nerve and artery exit, is just below the infraorbital rim at approximately the 6-o'clock position. The infraorbital nerve is the sensory branch of the maxillary nerve. The lacrimal,

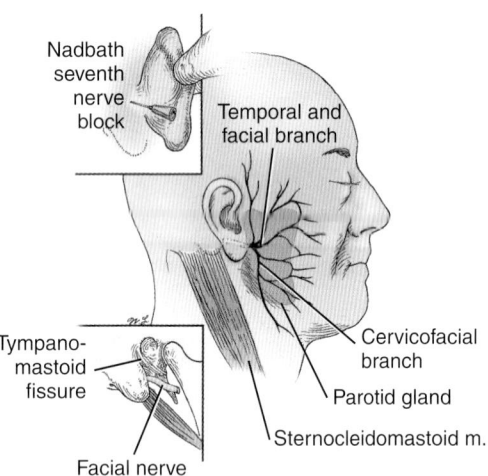

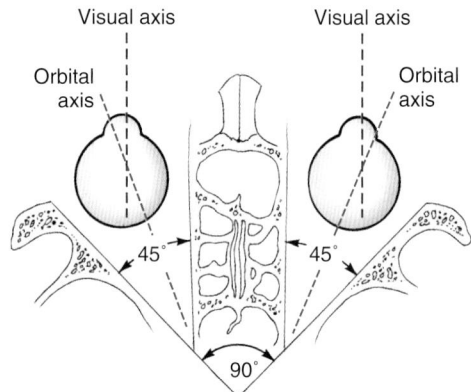

Fig. 44.9 The origin and branches of the facial nerve. *(Upper inset)* Needle placement for the Nadbath cranial nerve VII block. *m.,* Muscle.

Fig. 44.10 Superior view of the bony orbit, demonstrating the orbital and visual axes.

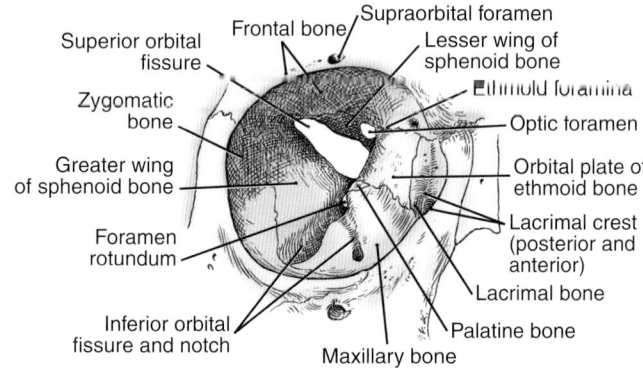

Fig. 44.11 Frontal view of the orbital.

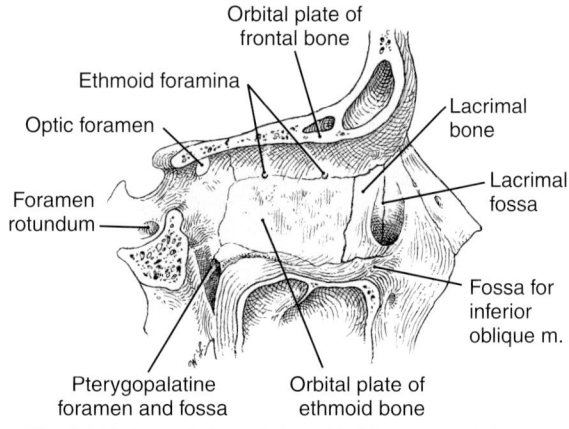

Fig. 44.12 Lateral view of the orbital bones. *m.,* Muscle.

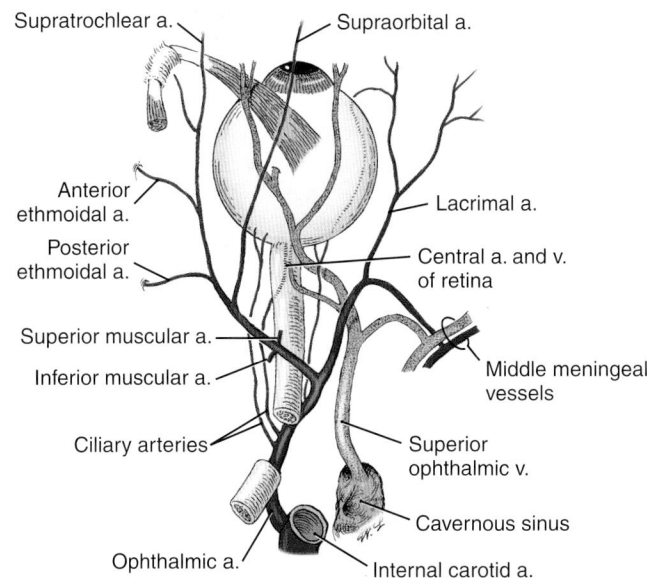

Supratrochlear a.

Supraorbital a.

Anterior ethmoidal a.

Posterior ethmoidal a.

Lacrimal a.

Central a. and v. of retina

Superior muscular a.

Inferior muscular a.

Middle meningeal vessels

Ciliary arteries

Superior ophthalmic v.

Cavernous sinus

Ophthalmic a.

Internal carotid a.

Fig. 44.13 Superior view of the orbital arteries and veins. *a.,* Artery; *v.,* vein.

frontal, and trochlear nerves all enter through the superior orbital fissure outside the muscle cone. The oculomotor, abducens, and nasociliary nerves all enter the orbit from inside the muscle cone.[5]

The ophthalmic artery (Fig. 44.13), which is the first branch of the internal carotid artery, passes into the orbit through the optic canal. The ophthalmic artery usually lies just inferolateral to the optic nerve. The artery extends along the optic nerve for a short distance, crossing over it in most cases, and continuing medially.[6] The first branch of the ophthalmic artery is usually the central retinal artery. The central retinal artery moves in an anterior direction underneath the optic nerve, usually entering the optic nerve on its inferomedial side 8 to 15 mm posterior to the globe.[4] The artery continues forward into the optic nerve head and branches into the retinal arteries. The ophthalmic artery gives rise to the long and short posterior ciliary arteries. The short posterior arteries move anteriorly and divide into many small branches that penetrate the globe close to the optic nerve and supply the choroid and the optic nerve head. The ophthalmic artery also provides branches to the optic nerve. The orbital branches of the ophthalmic artery include branches to the supraorbital arteries, the rectus muscles, and the lacrimal gland.[5]

The lacrimal artery moves anteriorly along the superior aspect of the lateral rectus muscle to the lacrimal gland. The supraorbital artery branches from the ophthalmic artery as it crosses over the optic nerve and extends just medial to the superior rectus and levator muscles. It continues forward on a superior nasal route and exits through the supraorbital notch or foramen.

The dorsal nasal artery is one of the terminal branches of the ophthalmic artery. It exits the orbital septum above the medial canthal tendon and joins with the angular artery, thus establishing communication between the internal and external carotid arteries.[2] The external carotid artery gives branches to the facial artery (the external maxillary artery). The facial artery originates near the angle of the mandible, extends toward the stylohyoid muscles, and then proceeds forward to the lower border of the mandible. The artery then turns upward and moves toward the nose, where it joins with the dorsal nasal artery in the medial canthal area. The inferior orbital fissure is the entrance site for the infraorbital artery. This artery moves anteriorly through the infraorbital canal and exits to the face through the infraorbital foramen.

The venous drainage system (see Fig. 44.13) for the orbit includes the superior and inferior ophthalmic veins, which drain into the cavernous sinus that is located intracranially. Radiographic studies have demonstrated a unique characteristic of the orbital vascular system: The orbital veins are independent of the orbital arteries. The venous system of the orbit is generally described as valveless, and blood flow in this area is determined by pressure gradients. The primary vein of the orbit is the superior ophthalmic vein. This vein travels posteriorly to the medial side of the superior rectus muscle, then beneath the superior rectus muscle inside a support hammock. The vein then emerges on the muscle's lateral aspect. The vein continues its posterior direction along the lateral aspect of the superior rectus, exiting the orbit through the superior orbital fissure and terminating in the cavernous sinus.[6]

Several veins enter the superior ophthalmic vein: the ciliary veins, the lacrimal veins, and the superior vortex veins, which are located on the posterior quadrants of the globe and drain the choroid, or second layer, of the globe. The inferior ophthalmic vein originates from a diffuse plexus on the floor of the orbit. This vein receives several branches, including the extraocular muscles and the inferior vortex veins located on the inferoposterior quadrants of the globe. The primary branch of the inferior ophthalmic vein also drains into the superior ophthalmic vein before its entrance into the cavernous sinus. The central retinal vein exits the globe inside the optic nerve. The central retinal vein then exits the optic nerve and enters the orbit between 8 and 15 mm posterior to the globe[4] and usually passes directly to the cavernous sinus.[2]

Orbit

An evaluation of the patient's orbit and globe size is important before ocular anesthesia is conducted. The usual volume of the orbit is 30 mL (Box 44.1). The volume of a typical globe (which has a diameter of ~25 mm) is 6.5 to 7 mL.[6] The balance of the orbital volume is approximately 23 mL and is composed of muscles, vessels, nerves, and fat. Katsev et al.[7] measured 120 orbits from 60 adult skulls and found an average orbital depth of 48 mm. The distance from the middle third and lateral third of the infraorbital rim to the superior aspect of the optic foramen was also measured and ranged from 42 to 52 mm. This distance should not be confused with the depth of the orbital floor. Because of the pear shape of the orbit, the orbital floor does not extend directly to the orbital apex. The orbital floor extends only to the posterior wall of the maxillary sinus, approximately two-thirds of the depth of the orbital apex.

Orbital fat is contained in both the extraconal and the intraconal areas. The orbital fat encircles and encapsulates all these areas of the orbit.

The orbital septum is a fibrinous tissue that defines the anatomic anterior boundary of the orbit and keeps the adipose tissue from protruding forward. The visual axis (also known as the optic axis or the geometric axis) is an imaginary line from the midpoint of the cornea (anterior pole) to the midpoint of the retina or macula (posterior pole) (Fig. 44.14). The horizontal (anteroposterior) diameter of the globe is an important consideration for ocular blocks. This measurement of the visual axis is referred to as the axial length. The axial length is measured preoperatively to determine the appropriate intraocular lens that should be placed in the eye after cataract removal. The axial length of the globe is only available when the ophthalmologist performs the measurement for an intraocular lens implant. Normal axial lengths range from 23 to 23.5 mm. In the hyperopic (farsighted) eye, the globe

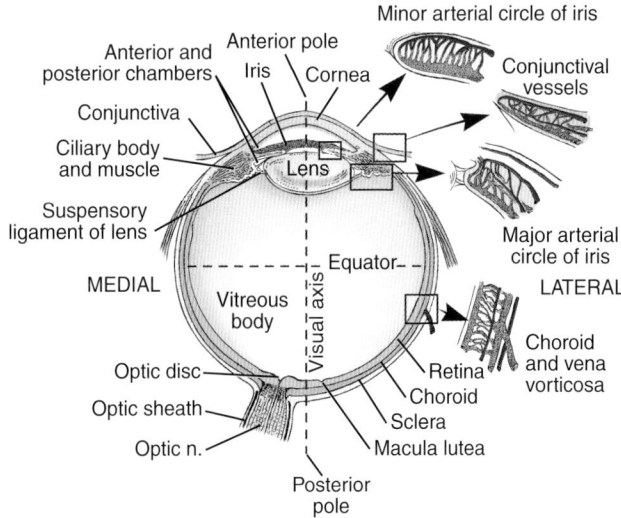

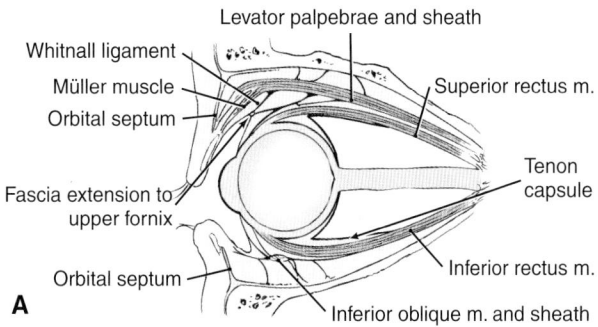

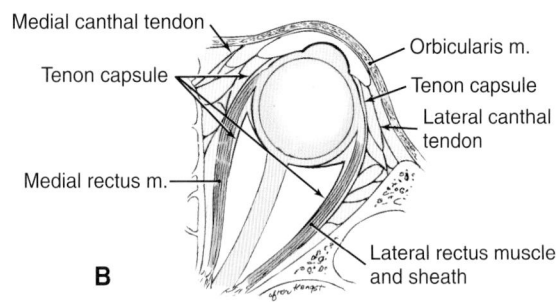

Fig. 44.14 Cross-sectional view of the globe. *n.,* Nerve.

Fig. 44.15 (A) Lateral view of the orbital connective tissue. (B) Superior view of the orbital connective tissue. *m.,* Muscle.

is less than 22 mm long. This shorter eye length may allow a little more working area behind the eye during an ophthalmic block; however, this advantage may be offset by a smaller overall orbit.[5,7]

The longer, myopic (nearsighted) eye, whose axial length is greater than 24 mm, presents a potential risk. The stretching of the globe is related to the extracellular matrix and biochemical properties of the sclera.[8] As the globe stretches, it is believed that the fibrinous scleral layer thins, making the globe easier to penetrate with a needle. This increased posterior length of the globe also increases the chance of puncturing the globe. Therefore because of a greater chance of contact in the posterior aspect of the orbit, the axial length of the eye, if this measurement is available, should be considered in the planning for the ocular block. If the axial length is unknown, which may be the case in glaucoma surgery, corneal transplants, retinal procedures, or muscle surgery, the practitioner's preoperative questions should include a history of nearsightedness or previous retinal procedures.

The separate coats, or tunics, of the eyeball (see Fig. 44.14) start with the sclera, which is the outer, fibrinous protective layer. The sclera is white and opaque and lies just posterior to the cornea. The cornea is the outer, fibrinous protective layer located anteriorly, and it is transparent and colorless. The middle, or vascular, layer is called the choroid. The retina is the inner layer of the posterior half of the eye. The limbal area is defined as the area at the junction between the cornea and the sclera.[2] The conjunctiva is a thin, transparent mucous membrane that covers the posterior surface of the eyelids and the anterior surface of the sclera.

A staphyloma is a bulging of the uvea, which comprises the iris, the ciliary body, and the choroid into a thin and stretched sclera. Staphylomas may occur in the anterior, equatorial, and posterior areas.[3]

Tissue Systems of the Orbit

Three connective tissue systems within the orbit have been defined by Koornneef.[9] They are the Tenon capsule, the orbital connective tissue, and the fascial sheaths of the extraocular muscles (Fig. 44.15).

Tenon capsule. The Tenon capsule (bulbar fascia) consists of fibrous connective tissue that covers the eyeball from near the corneal limbus, where it is fused to the conjunctiva, and extends behind the eye, with openings for the extraocular muscles and the optic nerve. The Tenon capsule serves primarily as a cavity in which the eye moves.

Orbital connective tissue. Koornneef demonstrated the presence of connective tissue attachments between both the globe and

the periorbital area. The connective tissue begins at the orbital apex and continues anteriorly, becoming more complex and more clearly defined at the level of the globe. Koornneef[9] also noted that the tissue septa are in a 360-degree encapsulation of the globe (see Fig. 44.15). These connective tissue septa encircle and support the globe within the bony orbit. Connective tissue septa were also noted between the superior and inferior oblique muscles, the Tenon capsule, the rectus muscles, and the ligaments stabilizing the globe within the orbit. This connective tissue septa meshwork limits displacement of the globe.

Fascial sheaths. The intermuscular membrane is a fibrous membrane that connects the four rectus muscle sheaths. Numerous extensions from these muscle sheaths form an intricate system of fibrinous attachments that interconnect the muscles into the orbit, support the globe, and check the ocular movements.

In the posterior orbit, the fascial sheaths of the extraocular muscles are not as well defined, as they are immediately behind the globe.[10] Koornneef was not able to identify a common muscle cone throughout the orbit (Fig. 44.16). The muscle sheaths themselves contribute fibrinous septa to the periorbit; these septa serve as ligaments for the extraocular muscles. These fascial extensions promote the efficiency of the extraocular muscle functions.[9-12]

PHARMACOLOGY: OCULAR MEDICATIONS AND ANESTHETIC AGENTS

A number of drugs are used in ophthalmology practice, including antibiotics, mydriatics, miotics, cycloplegics, antiinflammatory drugs, viscoelastics, and glaucoma therapies. Ocular medications are listed in Table 44.2.

Systemic Absorption of Eye Drops

The lacrimal apparatus includes the lacrimal gland, the puncta, the inferior and superior canaliculus, the common canaliculus, the lacrimal sac, and the nasolacrimal duct (Fig. 44.17). The lacrimal gland is located in a depression of the frontal bone in the superior temporal

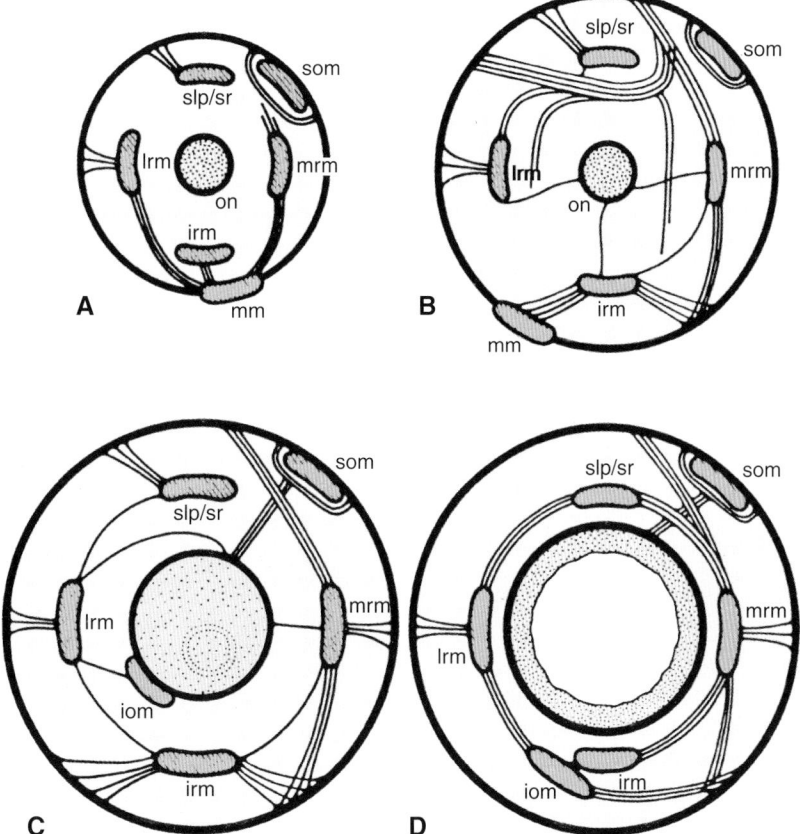

Fig. 44.16 Extraocular muscle connective tissue system. Highly schematic representation of the connective tissue system of the extraocular muscles. (A) Coronal section near the orbital apex. (B) Coronal section near the posterior portion of the globe. (C) Coronal section lying just anterior to the posterior portion of the globe. (D) Coronal section near the equator of the globe. *iom*, Inferior oblique muscle; *irm*, inferior rectus muscle; *lrm*, lateral rectus muscle; *m*, Müller muscle; *mrm*, medial rectus muscle; *on*, optic nerve; *slp/sr*, levator palpebrae superioris–superior rectus complex; *som*, superior oblique muscle. (From Koornneef L. Orbital septa: anatomy and function. *Ophthalmology*. 1979;86:876.)

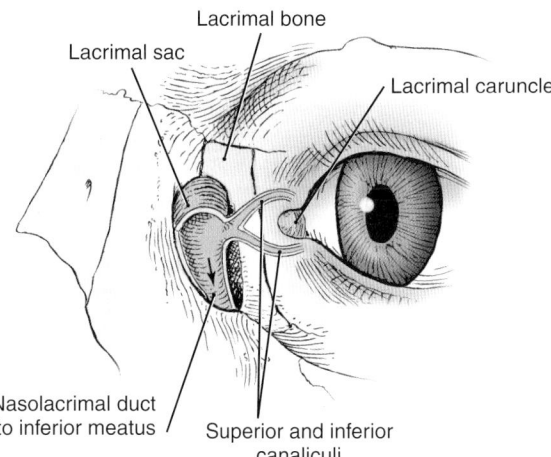

Fig. 44.17 Frontal view of the lacrimal drainage system.

orbit.[2,3] The gland has several ducts that lead to the conjunctival surface of the upper eyelid. Tears pass from the lacrimal gland through the ducts, over the cornea and conjunctiva, keeping the eye moist. Near the medial canthus, tears enter the puncta, travel through the canaliculus to the lacrimal sac, and drain into the nasolacrimal duct before entering the nasal mucosa.

Topical eye medications enter the bloodstream through the outer eye membrane and the lacrimal apparatus. The following measures reduce the amount of topical medications that enter the bloodstream:

- Have the patient close the eyes for 60 seconds after drops are instilled to encourage absorption by the eye and minimize drainage to the nasal mucosa.
- Have the patient avoid blinking, which rapidly moves the medication into the tear outflow canal and the systemic circulation.
- Block the tear outflow canal by placing the index finger over the medial canthus after the eye is closed.[3]

Patients may complain of a metallic taste after the administration of ocular anesthetics. This precursor to local anesthetic toxicity needs further evaluation. However, it is usually the result of the local anesthesia passing into the nasal mucosa.

SELECT OCULAR ANESTHESIA TECHNIQUES

Ophthalmic Block Techniques

Topical/Intraocular Anesthesia

Cataract and vitreoretinal surgeries are the most frequently performed intraocular surgical procedures.[13,14] Topical anesthesia for cataract surgery (e.g., 2% lidocaine) has proven to be effective in providing adequate analgesia for most patients during the surgical procedure and is commonly used with phacoemulsification. Topical anesthesia

TABLE 44.2   Ocular Medications

Class	Generic Name (Trade Name)	Comments
α_2-agonist	Brimonidine tartrate (Alphagan) Apraclonidine (Lopidine)	Glaucoma: reduces aqueous humor production Contraindicated with MAO inhibitors
Cholinesterase inhibitors	Echothiophate iodide (Phospholine Iodide)	Glaucoma: produces miosis by allowing acetylcholine to continually stimulate iris and ciliary muscles, improving uveoscleral outflow of aqueous humor; may prolong effects of succinylcholine, although rarely used
β-blockers	Timolol (Timoptic) Levobunolol (Betagan) Betaxolol (Betoptic) Metipranolol (OptiPranolol) Carteolol (generic)	Glaucoma: reduces aqueous humor production Use caution in patients with asthma, COPD, heart block, heart failure, and hypotension
Carbonic anhydrase inhibitors	Acetazolamide (Diamox) Dorzolamide (Trusopt) Brinzolamide (Azopt)	Glaucoma: reduces aqueous humor production
Cholinergic agonists	Pilocarpine, topical carbachol (Miostat)	Miotics; used to constrict pupil for surgical procedures
Cycloplegics	Atropine Homatropine Cyclopentolate	Pupillary dilators; cause temporary paralysis of ciliary muscle and muscles of accommodation
Intraocular gases	Sulfur hexafluoride Perfluoropropane	Retinal detachment: intravitreal insufflation to tamponade retina in place. *Avoid nitrous oxide for up to 3 mo*
Mydriatics	Phenylephrine Tropicamide Epinephrine	Pupillary dilators; cause either a direct or indirect effect on dilator muscle of iris
Nonsteroidal antiinflammatory agents	Flurbiprofen sodium (Ocufen)	Preserves pupillary dilation during surgical procedure by inhibiting prostaglandins, which cause miosis
Osmotic diuretics	Glycerin (oral agent) Mannitol	Reduce intraocular pressure
Prostaglandins	Latanoprost (Xalatan) Bimatoprost (Lumigan) Travoprost (Travatan) Tafluprost (Zioptan)	Glaucoma: promotes uveoscleral outflow of aqueous humor
Viscoelastics	Hyaluronate sodium (Healon, Amvisc)	Protect endothelial cells of cornea during surgical procedures
Rho kinase inhibitor	Netarsudil (Rhopressa)	Decreases resistance in the trabecular network outflow pathway.

COPD, Chronic obstructive pulmonary disease; *MAO*, monoamine oxidase.

is applied as drops or gels and may be supplemented by intracameral injection by the surgeon for better intraoperative pain control. Vitreoretinal surgery requires at least a sub-Tenon block and more frequently orbital regional injection anesthetic techniques.[14] Today's smaller-incision surgical techniques with foldable intraocular lenses provide a safer surgical experience for the patient and a more rapid recovery. Intraocular anesthesia can further enhance the analgesia for the surgical procedure; 1% lidocaine (preservative free) has been studied and recognized as safe for intraocular administration.[15] However, topical anesthesia may not be appropriate in all cases for the surgeon or the patient because it provides a lesser degree of analgesia and no akinesia of the ocular muscles or eyelids. There is wide variability in operative conditions, sensations, and pain relief, depending on the type of local anesthesia administered for intraocular surgery. Using data that present the strength of evidence as "strong evidence," "weak evidence," or "no evidence," the differences between local/regional anesthetic techniques for variables such as pain (during placement of the block and during the surgery), eye akinesia, eyelid sensation, and visual sensations were quantified on a + or − scale, and the conflicts of evidence are presented as a range in Table 44.3.[14]

TABLE 44.3   Comparisons of Local/Regional Anesthesia Techniques

	Topical	Sub-Tenon Block	Peribulbar Block	Retrobulbar Block
Pain on administration	0 or −	+ or ++	++ or +++	+++
Surgical pain prevented	− −	+++	++	++
Eye akinesia	− − −	0 or +	++	++
Eyelid sensation blocked	− − −	+	+	+
Visual sensations experienced	+++	++ or +	+	+

+Represents strength of affirmative evidence; 0 represents insufficient evidence; − represents strength of contrary evidence.

From Vann MA, et al. Sedation and anesthesia care for ophthalmologic surgery during local/regional anesthesia. *Anesthesiology.* 2007;107(3):502–508.

Sub-Tenon Block

The sub-Tenon block will produce a more profound analgesia; however, motor movement of the globe may still be present. The Tenon tissue, as described earlier, encapsulates the globe posteriorly and fuses with the conjunctiva anteriorly. Anteriorly it is inferior to the conjunctiva. The sub-Tenon block is a procedure performed between the rectus muscles of the globe. The conjunctiva is incised, the Tenon tissue is elevated and incised, and a short cannula is inserted into the sub-Tenon space. Local anesthetic is injected with the objective of a posterior spread of the agent. The dose is usually 3 to 4 mL to achieve analgesia; however, larger doses of up to 10 mL have been reported to achieve some degree of akinesia.[16]

OCULAR REGIONAL ANESTHESIA

The ocular regional needle block still remains the most common and effective way to consistently produce a profound analgesia and akinesia of the eye and eyelids.

The term *ocular local anesthesia* has been used to refer to retrobulbar or peribulbar blocks. More correctly, local anesthesia should be defined as superficial, topical, or cutaneous anesthesia, used, for example, when skin-laceration suturing is performed that poses minimal risks both to the body as a whole and to proximate vital organs.

Retrobulbar and peribulbar injections are categorized under regional anesthesia methods. These blocks are designed to anesthetize multiple cranial nerves (III, IV, V, VI, and VII). As described earlier, the optic nerve is a continuation of the brain. The dura mater divides at the entrance of the optic nerve into the orbit. The visceral layer of the dura covers the intraorbital part of the optic nerve, and the parietal layer blends into the periosteum of the orbit.[2] Therefore by anatomic definition, this procedure is performed in the orbital epidural space. As has been demonstrated in the anatomic reviews by Koornneef, no true muscle cone exists, especially in the posterior portion of the orbit.[9-12] Therefore old anatomic concepts such as the image of an intact muscle cone must be set aside in favor of concepts that illustrate a communication throughout the orbit.

Techniques and Modifications

The term *retrobulbar block* refers to an ophthalmic block technique originally described by Atkinson in 1936. The patient is instructed to look up and nasally (supranasal position). A 23-gauge retrobulbar (dull) needle is inserted through the skin in the infratemporal area, just above the inferior orbital rim and advanced toward the orbital apex 35 mm (1.38 in) deep into the muscle cone (retrobulbar space). After negative aspiration, 2 to 4 mL of anesthetic solution is injected into the muscle cone. After the injection is completed, the eyelids are closed, and digital pressure is applied over the globe to the orbit. A few minutes later, the eyelids are opened, and the globe is inspected for akinesia.[17] The popularity of the retrobulbar block for ophthalmic procedures grew, with more than 1 million blocks performed annually in the 1940s.[18] Unfortunately, so also did the complication rates.

The reported complications from retrobulbar anesthesia include trauma to the optic nerve, the blood vessels, and the globe, all of which can lead to loss of vision. Respiratory arrest may result when anesthetic agents enter the cerebrospinal fluid of the optic nerve. Seizures may occur when even small amounts of local anesthetic are injected intravascularly. As a result of the increasing number of complications being reported, practitioners began to alter the Atkinson retrobulbar technique in an effort to increase the margin of safety for ocular anesthesia.[19] Three major problem areas in the Atkinson technique are identified in this chapter, and technique modifications are discussed (Fig. 44.18).

Eye Position

The position of the eye during retrobulbar block anesthesia is an important consideration. When the patient looks upward and nasally, the optic nerve and blood vessels are placed in the path of the needle. Tension is created on the optic nerve and the surrounding vasculature, making the orbital structures more susceptible to trauma. In this position, the posterior pole of the globe also moves into the needle path. As a means of avoiding this problem, the following modification in technique has been recommended.

The primary gaze position, in which the patient is looking directly forward, allows the optic nerve to maintain its S-shaped curvature and releases the tension on the blood vessels. The down-and-out gaze position allows the optic nerve and vessels to rotate toward the optic foramen and farther away from the needle path. Both of these eye positions have the potential disadvantage of needle visualization by the patient. The upward-gaze position should only be used as described by Gills and Lloyd.[18] Their technique allows the use of the upward-gaze position because the needle is placed lateral and parallel to both the optic nerve and the vessels.

Needle Depth

A second problem is the depth of the needle insertion. The vital structures in the ocular anatomy are more crowded in the posterior orbit. Deep needle penetration in the orbit increases the likelihood of trauma to the optic nerve and vessels. If the depth of the needle insertion is decreased to approximately 25 mm (1 in),[19] the needle would lie just posterior to the globe, thereby reducing the risk of puncture of the vital structures. Studies have demonstrated that because of the wide variation in orbital and globe sizes, a needle depth of 19 to 31 mm (0.75–1.25 in) is safest.[7]

Needle Tip Shape

A pertinent issue debated in the literature is the use of sharp versus dull needles for ocular blocks. Dull or flat-grind needles made specifically for retrobulbar anesthesia are touted by some clinicians as the only safe needles for use in ocular blocks. It is not so much the type of needle but where the needle is placed that increases the risk.[20] Dull retrobulbar needles may not be tolerated as well by awake patients because of the sensation of pressure they create on insertion. Other needles proposed for ocular blocks include a curved retrobulbar needle[21] and a dull pinhead needle, in which the injection port is proximal to the head of the needle.[22]

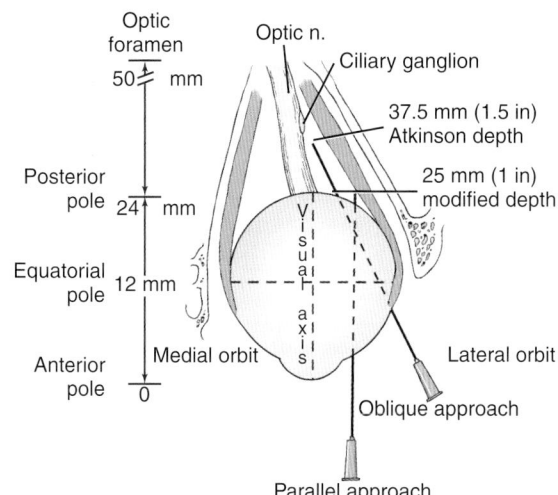

Fig. 44.18 Superior view of the parallel and oblique approach to retrobulbar anesthetic blocks. *n.,* Nerve.

Needle Angle

The angle of the needle is a third very important area that should be considered for modification. The original Atkinson technique uses an oblique approach; that is, the needle is inserted in the infratemporal area just above the inferior orbital rim and is directed toward the orbital apex, a pathway that tracts the needle tip toward the posterior pole of the globe, arteries, and the optic nerve.

Gills and Lloyd[18] developed a technique that takes into consideration not only the aforementioned changes but also the length and spherical shape of the globe. This technique changes the oblique approach to a parallel approach. The lateral limbic margin, corneoscleral junction, is identified, and the needle is inserted in the inferotemporal area transconjunctivally, just lateral and parallel to the lateral limbic margin. The needle is inserted to a depth of approximately 25 mm (1 in), entering the muscle cone just behind the globe. The advantages of this technique result from the needle position, which lies lateral and parallel to the optic nerve, the vasculature, and the posterior pole of the globe. However, the technique does not address the question, "When does the needle tip pass the equator of the globe?" The needle tip must pass the equator of the globe before it may be safely redirected cephalad and inserted into the intraconal space.

The original retrobulbar block technique described by Atkinson can be made safer by modification of the technique. Modifications that decrease the risk of adverse effects are as follows:

- Position the globe to decrease tension on the vital orbital structures and position them farther away from the needle (e.g., the primary gaze position).
- Use a depth of needle insertion of approximately 25 mm (1 in), which places the needle just behind the globe itself and avoids the structures deep in the orbit.
- Consider using a more lateral to parallel approach to the orbit than was originally demonstrated by Atkinson.

Some practitioners, in an effort to further improve the safety of ocular blocks, have advocated the use of extraconal peribulbar blocks.[23-27] The literature describes these techniques as directing the needle outside the muscle cone (i.e., extraconal). The anesthetic is injected, creating a positive extraconal pressure that spreads the agent inside the muscle cone to anesthetize the cranial nerves. To accomplish this, the needle is inserted parallel to, or is angled away from, the visual axis of the globe in an effort to remain outside the muscle cone. Peribulbar injections may be performed in the superior temporal, medial, and inferior temporal orbital areas. Peribulbar anesthesia requires larger volumes of anesthetic agents (8–12 mL). Owing to the many septal divisions of the orbit, the anesthetic flow may not adequately diffuse into the intramuscular cone. Therefore extraconal peribulbar anesthetic injections, as described in the literature, may not consistently produce adequate akinesia and may necessitate multiple repeat injections.[24]

Patients who may benefit from the extraconal peribulbar approach are those at increased risk for globe puncture, such as those with high myopia resulting in long axial lengths, significant enophthalmos, previous scleral buckling procedures, and staphylomas. However, peribulbar blocks have also resulted in globe punctures.[28]

The primary goal of extraconal peribulbar blocks is the avoidance of the muscle cone and its vital structures. With modified retrobulbar blocks, the goal is not only to avoid the vital structures but also to enter the muscle cone just posterior to the globe.

Koornneef and Kramer[11] have described the least vascular areas to perform ocular blocks (Fig. 44.19). The inferotemporal area can be used for both the intraconal modified retrobulbar and the extraconal peribulbar technique. The superior orbital area just lateral to the 12-o'clock position through the skin and the medial orbital area through the caruncle conjunctiva may be accessed for the extraconal peribulbar technique.

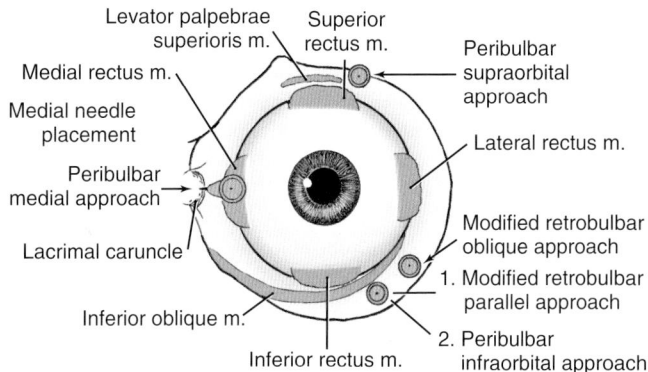

Fig. 44.19 Frontal view of needle placement for retrobulbar and peribulbar anesthetic blocks. *m.,* Muscle.

The most important considerations for ocular blocks are the position of the eye and the depth and angle of the needle. Needle placement should attempt to avoid the optic nerve, arteries, veins, extraocular muscles, and the globe itself. At what insertion depth does the needle tip reach the equator of the globe, a spherical tangential point beyond which it can be safely redirected into the retrobulbar space, is the question addressed in an abstract that was accepted and presented at the 23rd annual meeting of the Ophthalmic Anesthesia Society, "A Geometrical Method Applied to an Orbital Block." Harvey introduces the measurement of the dynamic orbital-globe relationship and uses the measured axial length to calculate the distance to the equator of the globe, beyond which the needle may be safely redirected cephalad and inserted into the retrobulbar space. The calculation mathematically demonstrated that a 0.5-inch (12.5-mm) needle insertion was usually beyond the equator of the globe but recommended calculating the distance to the equator on each patient for safety.[29]

The geometric method was further developed into a teaching video for practitioners. The American Academy of Ophthalmology accepted the video "Orbital Block Technique" in 2013 for their Network One website.[30]

Anesthesia Techniques

Gills-Lloyd Modified Retrobulbar Technique[18]

Equipment list
- One 3-mL syringe
- One 6-mL or 10-mL syringe
- One 25-gauge 1-in needle
- 1-in paper tape
- One 4 × 4 gauze pad

Description. Figs. 44.20 and 44.21 and Box 44.2 present valuable reference aids for the Gills-Lloyd modified retrobulbar technique.

The patient should be in a comfortable, reclining position. Anesthetic drops are placed in the conjunctiva, the eyelids are closed, and the outer eyelids are cleansed. The patient is asked to look directly overhead and to stare at a finger or other object. The eye should not look inward but may look somewhat outward. Needle insertion through the skin is preferably avoided in this technique so that patient discomfort is minimized. The lateral limbic margin, corneoscleral junction, is identified. The lower eyelid is everted and controlled with a finger. The needle is placed with the bevel toward the globe, just above the inferior orbital rim, just lateral and parallel to the lateral limbic margin. The needle is then inserted through the conjunctiva and directed toward the orbital floor until the orbital septum is penetrated. The needle is then redirected parallel to the visual axis of the globe to a depth of 25 mm (1 in). At this time, 1 to 1.5 mL of lidocaine, 1% to 2%, is injected

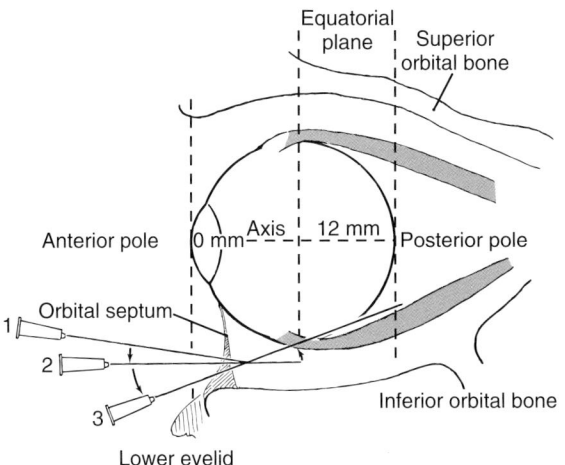

Equatorial
plane | Superior
orbital bone

Anterior pole | 0 mm Axis | 12 mm | Posterior pole

Orbital septum

1

2

3

Inferior orbital bone

Lower eyelid

Fig. 44.20 Lateral view of needle angles for a modified retrobulbar block.

BOX 44.2 The Gills-Lloyd Modified Retrobulbar Technique: Parallel Approach

- Insert the needle transconjunctivally or transcutaneously, with the bevel toward the globe, lateral to the limbic margin and angled away from the visual axis of the globe toward the orbital floor, until the orbital septum is penetrated (see Fig. 44.21A).
- After penetrating the orbital septum, redirect the needle parallel to the visual axis to a depth of approximately 12 mm (0.5 in) past the equatorial plane of the globe (see Fig. 44.21B).
- Past the equatorial plane of the globe, redirect the needle cephalad to a depth of approximately 25 mm (1 in), entering the muscle cone while remaining lateral to the lateral limbic margin, and inject the medications (see Fig. 44.21C).

---

after negative aspiration is performed. This initial extraconbular technique is effective in reducing the potential discomfort from the needle and the anesthetic injection of the modified retrobulbar block in the awake patient.

The eye is closed briefly in preparation for the modified retrobulbar injection. The lower eyelid is again everted and controlled with a finger. The needle is placed with the bevel toward the globe, just above the inferior orbital rim, just lateral and parallel to the lateral limbic margin. The needle is then inserted through the conjunctiva and directed toward the orbital floor until the orbital septum is penetrated. The needle is then redirected parallel to the visual axis of the globe past its equatorial plane, approximately 0.5 in (12.5 mm).[29] At this point, the needle is redirected cephalad between the lateral and inferior rectus muscles. Resistance may or may not be felt as the needle enters the muscle cone. The needle should be inserted approximately 25 mm (1 in), depending on the size of the orbit and the globe (range, 19–31 mm). After negative aspiration, the anesthetic agent is injected slowly, 1 mL/10 sec, until the orbit is filled. Orbital size governs the total amount of anesthetic injected; however, approximately 6 mL usually suffices. Once the orbit is full of anesthesia, as indicated by orbital tension, the needle is withdrawn. The eyelids are closed, a 4 × 4 gauze is placed over the eye, and positive digital pressure is applied. The pressure helps spread the anesthetic and detect any increasing orbital pressure, which might indicate a retrobulbar hemorrhage.

The initial needle insertion is directed away from the globe so that the risk of globe puncture is decreased. Resistance may or may not be

felt as the needle enters the muscle cone, depending on the presence or absence of the fibrinous connective tissue in the area behind the globe, as described by Koornneef and Kramer.[11] The sharper the needle, the less resistance felt by the practitioner and the less discomfort felt by the patient. By comparison, use of dull needles results in more resistance, potentially resulting in greater patient discomfort. Patients have described this resistance to the needle as pressure pain. Because a pop may or may not be felt as the needle enters the muscle cone, attention to needle depth is important for the avoidance of deep penetration into the orbit.

During injection, the patient is told to inform the practitioner if any discomfort, such as stinging or pressure, is experienced. If this occurs, the injection should be stopped to allow the agent to take effect. The pressure sensation appears to result from the spread of the local agent throughout the orbital area. The stinging is noticed more when the agent moves into the peripheral area along the upper and lower eyelids. This slow injection process is continued until the orbit is filled with the anesthetic agent. When the anesthetic is placed into the muscle cone, the effects are seen rapidly, and the block can be evaluated for akinesia after approximately 2 minutes.[1] Generous traction must be applied to the lower eyelid because this technique is performed before the orbicular muscles of the eyelids are anesthetized (i.e., seventh nerve block). Seventh nerve blocks can be very painful and are not well tolerated by patients. These blocks generally precede retrobulbar or peribulbar blocks but may not be necessary because the anesthetic agent from the modified retrobulbar or peribulbar block spreads randomly throughout the orbit and eyelids, providing adequate akinesia of the eyelids.[18,28]

Peribulbar Extraconal Techniques

Description. Figs. 44.22 and 44.23 and Box 44.3 serve as valuable reference aids for the peribulbar technique.

Extraconal peribulbar blocks may be performed using different techniques. One is a supraorbital-only technique of injecting a large volume (10–12 mL) of anesthetic agent, which should distribute throughout the orbit for completion of the block. An inferotemporal-only technique also involves injection of a large volume (10–12 mL) of anesthesia, which should distribute throughout the orbit and anesthetize the eye. A more reproducible approach to extraconal peribulbar anesthesia is the use of both the inferior and superior approaches. Each of these injections may be performed with a 6-mL syringe for a total volume of 10 to 12 mL. The combination technique generally provides a more consistent result.

Infraorbital and Supraorbital Extraconal Peribulbar Anesthesia

Equipment list
- One 10-mL syringe or two 6-mL syringes
- One or two 25-gauge needles
- One 4 × 4 gauze pad
- 1-in paper tape
- One alcohol or providone-iodine (Betadine) wipe

Description. For the infraorbital peribulbar technique, the lateral limbic margin is identified, and the patient is asked to look directly overhead. The lower eyelid is everted and controlled with a finger. The needle is placed, with the bevel toward the globe, just above the inferior orbital rim, lateral and parallel to the lateral limbic margin. The needle is then inserted through the anesthetized conjunctiva and directed toward the orbital floor until the orbital septum is penetrated. The needle is then redirected parallel to, or angled away from, the visual axis of the globe to a depth of approximately 25 mm (1 in). After the syringe is secured and negative aspiration is performed, 6 mL of the anesthetic agent is slowly (1 mL/10 sec) injected. The rate of injection

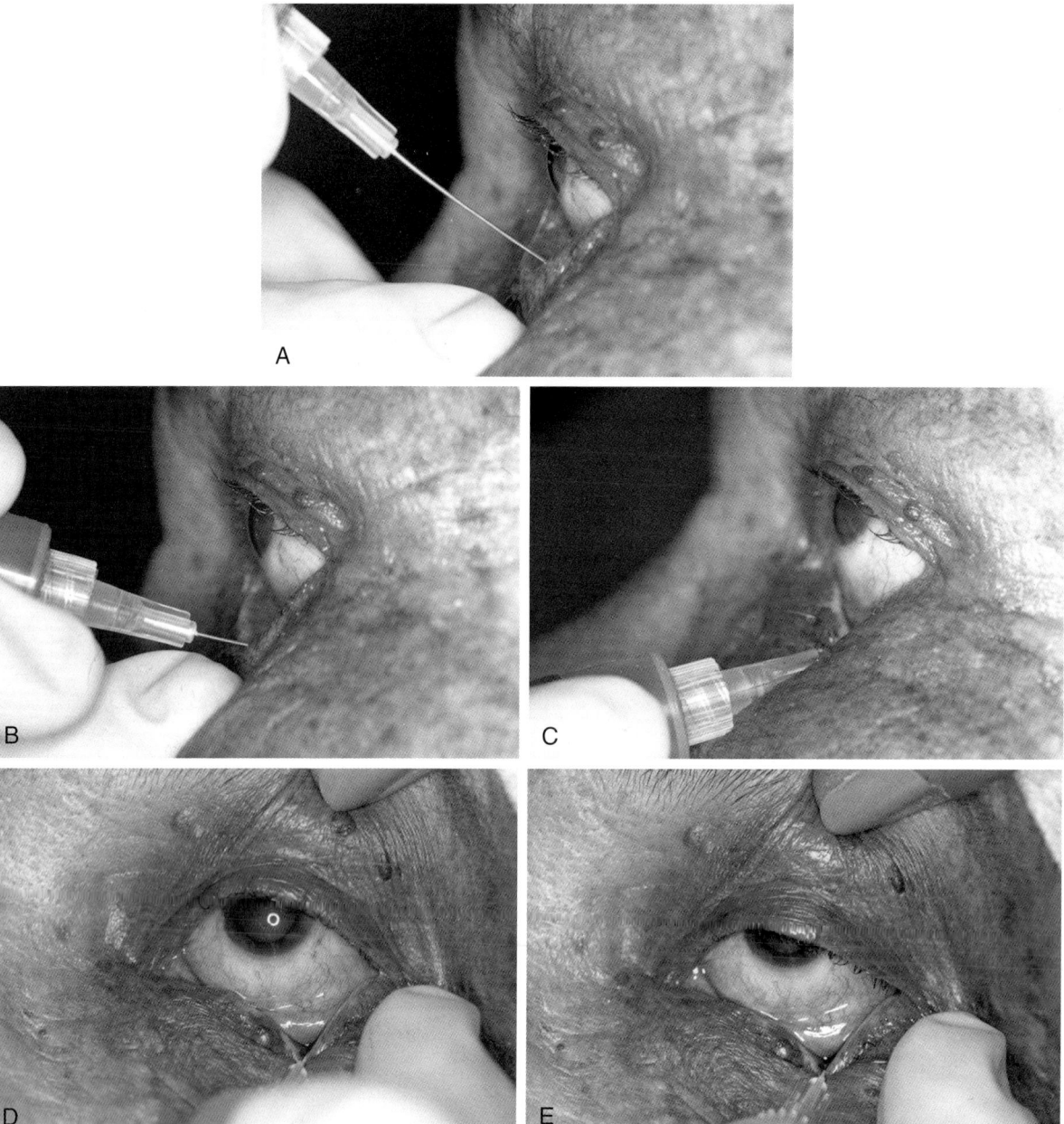

Fig. 44.21 (A) In the Gills-Lloyd modified retrobulbar technique, the needle should be inserted transconjunctivally or transcutaneously, angled away from the visual axis of the globe toward the orbital floor until the orbital septum is penetrated. (B) After penetrating the orbital septum, the needle should be redirected parallel to the visual axis to a depth of approximately 12 mm (0.5 in) passing the equatorial plane of the globe. (C) After passing the equatorial plane of the globe, the needle should be redirected cephalad to a depth of approximately 25 mm (1 in). At this point, the needle enters the muscle cone, and the medication is injected. (D) Needle placement, which is lateral and parallel to the lateral limbic margin. (E) Completion of the modified retrobulbar block. Some degree of globe proptosis and drooping of the upper eyelid should be expected.

is determined by patient comfort. After the injection, the eyelids are closed, and positive pressure is applied for dispersal of the medication.

The supraorbital peribulbar injection is performed just inferior to the supraorbital rim, just lateral to the 12-o'clock position and superior to the globe. The needle is inserted with the bevel toward the globe through the skin. This area is generally anesthetized from the original inferotemporal injection. The needle is inserted parallel to, or angled away from, the visual axis of the globe to a depth of approximately 25 mm (1 in). After negative aspiration is performed, the anesthetist may

begin a slow injection of 4 to 6 mL of anesthetic solution until a tense orbital area is observed. A tenser orbit should be expected to result from the extraconal peribulbar technique because of the increased extraconal pressure necessary to move the anesthetic intraconally.

Once this technique is completed, the eyelids are closed and taped shut. A 4 × 4 gauze pad is placed over the closed eye. A positive-pressure device is now placed over the eye to help distribute the agent throughout the orbit and achieve the desired analgesia and akinesia. The positive pressure device also decreases IOP to an acceptable surgical level. To avoid corneal abrasion, the eyelids must completely cover the eye. It may take up to 10 minutes for satisfactory surgical anesthesia to be established from an extraconal peribulbar block. If the peribulbar block fails to attain adequate akinesia within 10 minutes, the appropriate muscles must be reblocked by use of the inferior technique for the inferior rectus, inferior oblique, and lateral rectus muscles. The superior technique is used for the superior rectus, superior oblique, and medial rectus muscles. The supraorbital approach should not be attempted through the conjunctiva because of the potential for damage to the levator muscle of the upper eyelid; such damage may result in upper eyelid ptosis.

Medial Extraconal Peribulbar Block

Equipment list
- One 3-mL syringe
- One 30-gauge, 0.5-in needle

Description. Figs. 44.24 and 44.25 and Box 44.4 serve as valuable reference aids for medial peribulbar anesthesia.

The medial peribulbar area is a rather avascular, fatty compartment that lies just medial to the medial rectus muscle. This area narrows significantly as it approaches the posterior surface of the globe, with the medial rectus muscle lying next to the bony orbit. Superior to the medial peribulbar area is the supranasal area. This area contains a portion of

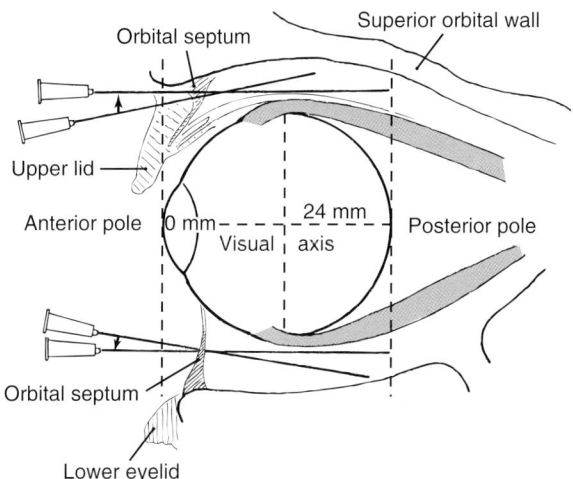

Fig. 44.22 Lateral view of needle angles for peribulbar block.

the superior ophthalmic vein and branches of the ophthalmic artery and should be avoided when ophthalmic blocks are performed.

The medial area also has herniated orifices within the connective tissue that communicate anteriorly to the posterior surface of the orbicular muscle of the eye. Therefore the anterior spread of the anesthetic agent blocks cranial nerve VII, resulting in satisfactory akinesia of the eyelids for surgery. The medial peribulbar technique can also be used with minimal discomfort to provide eyelid akinesia before a modified retrobulbar block is performed; in this case, proparacaine drops are applied to the caruncle before the block is administered. The anesthetic agent is injected into the periorbital space that exists between the medial wall of the bony orbit and the medial rectus muscle. The technique is very effective as a secondary block both for incomplete akinesia of the medial rectus muscle and the superior oblique muscle and as a primary block for the orbicular muscles of the eyelid.

To avoid needle injuries to the medial rectus muscle, a modified insertion site, needle length, and angle may enhance the ease of needle placement and safety. The landmark for the modified technique is the caruncle, a small mound at the inner canthus of the eye formed by a conjunctival fold at its junction with the skin. The needle is inserted through the caruncle conjunctiva, tangential to the globe, and is directed medially and posteriorly toward the lacrimal bone, which is just posterior to the lacrimal sulcus. Care must be taken to avoid trauma to the puncta, the lacrimal canaliculi, and the lacrimal sac. To avoid contact with the medial rectus muscle, it is important to keep the needle angled toward the lacrimal bone and away from the visual axis. Insert the needle, bevel toward the globe, to a depth of approximately 12 mm (0.5 in). After negative aspiration is performed, 3 mL or more of anesthetic agent may be injected for facilitation of the desired effect. After the block is completed, the eyelid should be closed and light pressure applied to reduce the incidence of bleeding.

Ocular Block Evaluation

After an ophthalmic block is performed, partial movement of one or more of the ocular muscles may occur. Residual movement should be assessed to determine which muscles are involved and whether additional anesthesia is required. Analgesia of the globe generally precedes akinesia of the eye muscles. Therefore analgesia of the globe may be assumed but not guaranteed in the presence of an akinetic muscle. The effectiveness of a modified intraconal retrobulbar block may be evaluated 2 minutes after it is administered, and an extraconal peribulbar

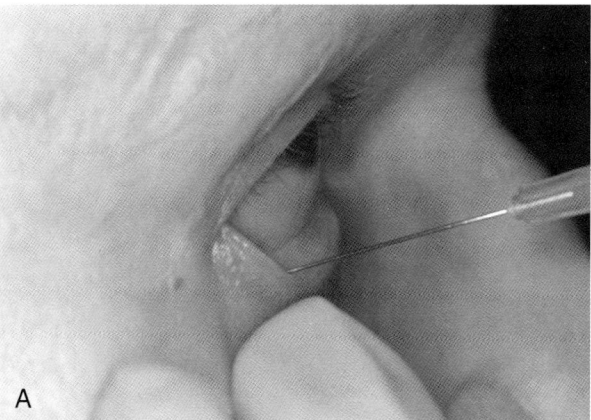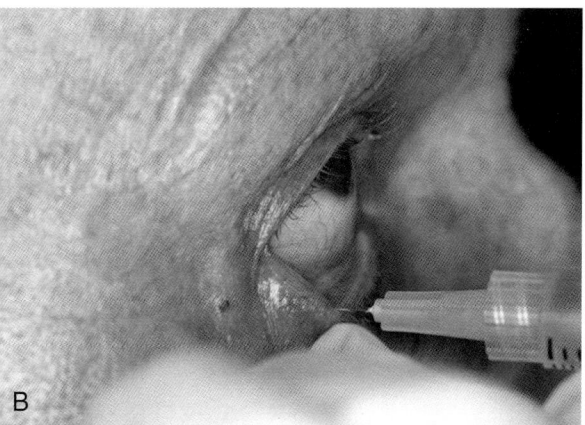

Fig. 44.23 (A) In the infraorbital approach, the needle is inserted transconjunctivally or transcutaneously and angled away from the visual axis of the globe toward the orbital floor to a depth of approximately 25 mm (1 in), and the medications are injected. (B) After penetration of the orbital septum, as shown in A, the needle is redirected parallel to the visual axis to a depth of approximately 25 mm (1 in), and the medications are injected.

Infraorbital Approach
- Insert the needle transconjunctivally or transcutaneously, with the bevel toward the globe, lateral to the lateral limbic margin and angled away from the visual axis of the globe toward the orbital floor, to a depth of approximately 25 mm (1 inch), and inject the medications (see Fig. 44.23A).
  or
- After penetrating the orbital septum, as described previously, redirect the needle parallel to the visual axis to a depth of approximately 25 mm (1 in), and inject the medications (see Fig. 44.23B).

Supraorbital Approach
- Insert the needle only transcutaneously, with the bevel toward the globe, just inferior to the supraorbital rim, just lateral to the 12-o'clock position and superior to the globe. Angle away from the visual axis of the globe toward the orbital ceiling, to a depth of approximately 25 mm (1 in), and inject the medications.
  or
- After penetrating the orbital septum, as described previously, redirect the needle parallel to the visual axis to a depth of approximately 25 mm (1 in), and inject the medications.

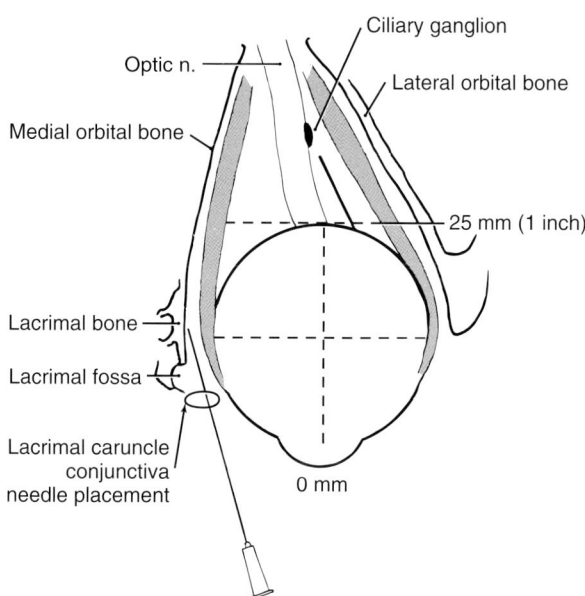

Fig. 44.25 Superior view of the needle angle for a medial peribulbar block. *n.,* Nerve.

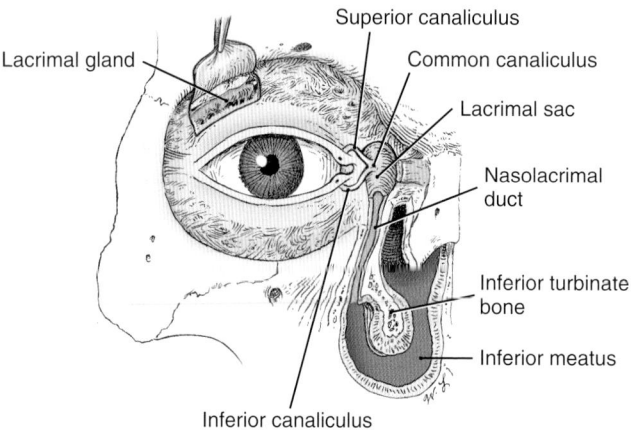

Fig. 44.24 Frontal view of the lacrimal drainage system.

Penetrate the caruncle conjunctiva with the bevel of the needle toward the globe and the needle angled toward the lacrimal bone, to a depth of approximately 12 mm (0.5 in), and inject the medications.

block, but it requires injections through the skin and has the potential for causing patient discomfort and eyelid ecchymosis. The preferred technique for eyelid akinesia remains the medial peribulbar block.

Orbicularis Oculi Block
Equipment list
- One 6-mL syringe
- One 30-gauge, 0.5-in needle
- One alcohol wipe

Description. Fig. 44.26 and Box 44.5 serve as valuable reference aids for the orbicularis oculi block.

This technique is performed after a modified retrobulbar or peribulbar block in which residual eyelid movement remains. The first injection is made inferotemporally in the lower eyelid. The needle is inserted bevel down, subcutaneously and tangentially to the lower eyelid, and 1 to 2 mL of the anesthetic agent is injected just under the skin of the eyelid. After the needle is removed, the local anesthesia should be digitally spread to the medial and the lateral canthi; this measure avoids running the needle across the lower eyelid. The second injection is made supranasally in the upper eyelid. A finger should be placed over the closed eyelid, slightly depressing the globe. The needle is again inserted, bevel down, subcutaneously and tangentially to the eyelid, and 1 to 2 mL of the agent is injected just under the skin of the eyelid. After the needle is removed, the local anesthetic is digitally spread to the medial and lateral canthi. Once the anesthetic is spread throughout the eyelids, light to moderate pressure is applied over the eyelids for prevention or reduction of superficial bleeding.

Van Lint Technique
Equipment list
- One 6-mL syringe
- One 25- or 27-gauge, 1.5-in needle

block 10 minutes after it is administered by observing for eye movement in all four quadrants.

Eyelid Block
Once satisfactory akinesia of the globe is established, evaluation for movement of the eyelids is necessary. Partial to complete akinesia of the orbicular muscle is generally found after the ocular block. If incomplete akinesia of the orbicular muscle persists, perform a medial peribulbar to complete the block of nerve VII. Several blocks of nerve VII are described in the literature, including those by Van Lint, O'Brien, Nadbath, and Hustead.[26,31]

The O'Brien and Nadbath techniques block cranial nerve VII proximally, resulting in unilateral facial paralysis. The O'Brien and Nadbath techniques are still used; however, their popularity is decreasing because of their systemic side effects and patient discomfort. The Van Lint technique more appropriately addresses the need for eyelid akinesia, with less potential for adverse effects, by blocking the temporal and zygomatic branches of the facial nerve to the orbicular muscles. However, it is very painful. A variation of these techniques may be used for orbicularis oculi block. This technique has the advantage of being safer, less painful, and better accepted by the awake patient than the Van Lint

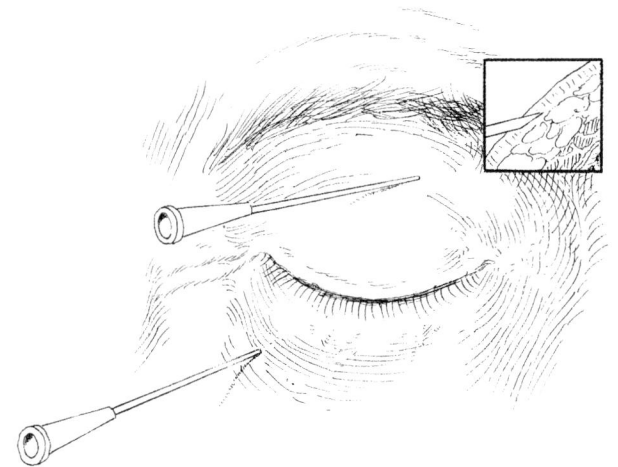

Fig. 44.26 Frontal view of the needle placement for an orbicularis oculi block.

BOX 44.5 Orbicularis Oculi Block

- *Lower lid:* Insert the needle subcutaneously, bevel down and tangential to the lid in the infratemporal area, and inject the medications.
- *Upper lid:* While slightly depressing the globe, insert the needle subcutaneously, bevel down and tangential to the lid in the supranasal area, and inject the medications.

- One alcohol or providone-iodine wipe
- One 4 × 4 gauze pad

Description. A 37.5-mm (1.5-in) needle is inserted inferotemporally into the subcutaneous tissue of the lateral canthus. The first injection of 1 to 2 mL of anesthetic agent is directed nasally along the lower margin of the orbit and then withdrawn to its origination point. The second injection of 1 to 2 mL of anesthetic agent is directed upward along the supratemporal margin of the orbit. After the block is completed, light pressure is applied over the closed eyelids to disperse the medication and decrease ecchymosis.

POSITIVE ORBITAL PRESSURE

The increased volume of local anesthetic required for both modified retrobulbar and peribulbar anesthetics causes an increase in orbital and IOPs. The anesthetic agent not only tracks along and penetrates the fascial sheaths behind the globe but also moves anteriorly underneath the conjunctiva, producing chemosis (i.e., subconjunctival edema) of the eye. Chemosis may not be preferred by some surgeons. However, the random diffusion of the orbital anesthetic cannot be controlled. The agent merely tracks along the path of least resistance. Clinically, chemosis can begin with the injection of as little as 1 to 2 mL of anesthetic. In other instances, chemosis has not been seen even after the injection of as much as 12 mL of anesthetic agent.

Positive-pressure devices are used to reduce increased intraocular/intraorbital pressures and chemosis. Such devices are placed directly over the globe and orbit to enhance the orbital spread of the anesthetic agent and return the orbital anatomy to a more normal state before surgery. Positive pressure devices deepen the anterior chamber by further reducing the IOP, thus allowing greater room for surgical intervention.

Positive Pressure Device
Honan Intraocular Pressure Reducer

The Honan IOP reducer, or Honan balloon, is an inflatable pneumatic device used to apply ocular compression after retrobulbar or peribulbar anesthetic injection. A rubber head strap is placed behind the head. The eye is taped closed, and a folded 4 × 4 gauze pad is placed over the eye. The Honan cuff is placed over the gauze pad and secured with the Velcro head strap. The pressure gauge is inflated to 30 mm Hg, a value marked in yellow on the gauge.

ANESTHESIA MANAGEMENT

Preoperative Preparation

Ophthalmic procedures are most commonly performed on young children and elderly persons. Each age group has a unique set of physical problems. For the young child, the questions regarding the patient's history should include any congenital, metabolic, and musculoskeletal abnormalities, such as malignant hyperthermia, that may affect anesthesia care. In the elderly patient, multisystem medical problems may be present, and drug interactions from multiple medication regimens may exist. Therefore a thorough patient history is paramount.

Admissions on the Day of Surgery

Anesthesia practitioners must remember how stressful a surgical procedure on the eye can be for patients. A kind and professional attitude on the part of all those providing care will help patients cope more effectively with personal stress. The proper use of progressive relaxation and hypnotic techniques further helps alleviate their anxiety. Establishing a good patient-provider relationship works synergistically with pharmacologic agents in promoting the best possible surgical environment. On admission, the patient's mental and physical status, vital signs, and electrocardiogram (ECG) should be reviewed for any changes that may require postponement.

Regional Versus General Anesthesia

Patients undergoing regional block, in which they are awake for the procedure, must be evaluated for claustrophobia, severe arthritis, tremors, restless leg syndrome, and any other physical derangements that may make it difficult for them to lie supine. Patients' mental status also must be evaluated so that their degree of cooperation and ability to follow commands can be determined.

Elderly patients often take multiple medications and may not remember all of them. Patients should be instructed to bring their medications on the day of surgery. A preoperative visit to the patient's primary care provider should be considered to confirm that the patient's overall medical condition is optimized for the planned surgical procedure.

The attending surgeon, in collaboration with the anesthesia practitioner, will make the final evaluation as to the patient's fitness on the day of surgery. An ECG performed within the past year is desirable with the medical evaluation. The preoperative ECG assessment furnishes a baseline of what is optimal for the individual patient. Comparing the baseline ECG against the patient's ECG on the day of surgery helps determine whether any further preoperative testing is warranted.[32] However, studies have questioned the value of a preop ECG in low-risk surgery.[33] For patients receiving regional anesthesia, routine laboratory tests are not ordered unless they are medically necessary. Appropriate laboratory data may be necessary when general anesthesia is planned.[34,35]

After the patient history and physical examination are completed, the appropriate anesthesia plan can be formulated. General anesthesia

BOX 44.6 **Indications for General Anesthesia**

- Pediatric patient
- Patient's lack of cooperation
- Severe claustrophobia
- Inability to communicate
- Inability to lie flat
- Open-eye injuries
- Procedures with durations >2 hr

BOX 44.7 **Disadvantages of General Anesthesia**

- Nausea/vomiting
- Retching/bucking
- Increased intraocular pressure
- Aspiration
- Complications secondary to other medical problems (e.g., cardiovascular disease)
- Time and expense

should be used for infants and young children. General anesthesia is also indicated for patients with severe claustrophobia, a history of uncontrolled acute anxiety attacks, or inability to cooperate, communicate, or lie flat (Box 44.6). It is also a consideration for procedures of greater than a duration of 2 hours.[36] Most adults tolerate ophthalmic procedures well when regional anesthesia is used. Given the potential risks associated with general anesthesia (Box 44.7), regional anesthesia should be considered the anesthetic of choice in adults, especially the elderly, for ophthalmic procedures.

Regional Anesthesia

Regional Block With Minimal Sedation

Nothing-per-mouth status. The views of anesthesia practitioners vary on the advisability of nothing-per-mouth (nil per os [NPO]) status prior to ocular procedures, especially cataracts. Some practices allow patients undergoing surgery in the morning to eat a light breakfast the day of surgery. Those undergoing surgery in the afternoon may be told to eat a light lunch.[37] Patients may also be encouraged to consume clear fluids until they are admitted to the facility.[38] However, practitioners also may mandate a strict NPO protocol.

Patients are requested to take their medications as prescribed on the day of surgery. An exception may be patients who complain of a frequent need to urinate after taking diuretic medications. Antiglycemic agents may be reduced or withheld when patients are NPO according to usual practice.[39] Evaluation and management of any anticoagulant medications are required for certain eye procedures to decrease the likelihood of bleeding. A medical consult with discontinuation several days prior to surgery may be necessary for certain anticoagulants. An increase in bleeding has been reported following vitreoretinal surgery in patients taking antiplatelet drugs.[40,41] Others note discontinuation is not necessary.[38] It is generally not required that antiplatelet drugs (e.g., aspirin, clopidogrel) and anticoagulants (e.g., warfarin [Coumadin]) be discontinued. The risk of systemic complications, such as cardiovascular accidents and myocardial infarctions, is potentially greater if administration of these products is discontinued. Continuing anticoagulant administration, however, requires consultation and agreement between the anesthesia practitioner and the surgeon.[19,42] If bleeding occurs, it may be more severe; therefore patients also need to be made aware of the risk and benefits

of continuing their anticoagulants. Patients who are receiving or have previously been treated with chemotherapy also may have prolonged bleeding times.

Regional Block Environment

Ocular blocks are commonly performed outside the operating room. This method facilitates a more efficient case flow and a more comfortable environment for the patient. The potentially life-threatening effects of orbital epidural blocks require that appropriate resuscitative equipment and trained personnel are available to monitor the patient. The area used for performing ocular blocks should have the following:

- Oxygen
- Bag-valve mask
- Suction
- Airways
- ECG equipment
- Blood pressure cuff
- Oxygen saturation monitor
- Capnography for deep sedation
- Canthotomy set
- Ammonia capsules
- Nitroglycerin tablets
- Atropine
- Glycopyrrolate

Additional resuscitative equipment and medications as recommended by advanced cardiac life support guidelines should be available.

Sedation for Regional Blocks and Ophthalmic Procedures

The goal of conscious sedation is to help patients gain and maintain control by reducing their heightened state of anxiety. This enhances their cooperation and ability to tolerate the awake surgical procedure.

Many techniques have been advocated to relax the patient prior to the ocular block and during the surgical procedure.[43,44] Sedation techniques have included the use of benzodiazepines, narcotics, and nonbarbiturates.[45] When these medications are properly tailored, they are tolerated well by the elderly patient. Sedation techniques should be designed to decrease anxiety (Box 44.8) and reduce the discomfort of the block (Box 44.9). When the block is less painful, patients require less sedation for comfort. The surgeon's preference for an awake, relaxed, or sleeping patient during the procedure also should be considered. Sleeping patients often snore and may have sudden head movements on awakening.

If the patient is to be asleep during the block, fasting before the procedure consistent with the facility's criteria for general anesthesia should be followed (Box 44.10). Propofol is an excellent choice for this technique because of its short duration of action.[46]

Sedation is typically effective and safe for ocular blocks and intraoperative use but necessitates provider vigilance and monitoring to recognize and treat any of the adverse medical events that may occur.

Monitoring for Regional Anesthesia

Communication is the cornerstone of interacting with the patient who is awake.[43] Informing the patient regarding what to expect and what to do if problems arise is mandatory. Questions and instructions must be clear and specific, especially if the patient is hearing impaired or if a language barrier exists.

The positioning of the patient is very important. Pillows may be used under the knees to decrease back strain. The patient with severe arthritis must be carefully padded and positioned. The patient's head and neck should be placed in a satisfactory surgical position. The practitioner should ensure that the patient is warm and as comfortable as possible. Nasally administered oxygen may be considered. Monitoring

BOX 44.8 Sedation Techniques

- Good rapport between patient and clinician—minimizes medications necessary
- Intravenous benzodiazepine administration
- Intravenous narcotic administration
- Intravenous propofol administration

BOX 44.9 Causes of Discomfort Resulting From Regional Blocks

- Needle injection through the skin
- Needle penetration of the conjunctiva
- Needle penetration of the orbital connective tissue
- Rapid injection of anesthetic
- Stinging from peripheral spread of anesthetic

BOX 44.10 Procedure for Patient Who Is Asleep During Regional Block

- Tilt head to maintain patent airway
- Open patient's eye in primary gaze position
- Administer regional block
- Administer incremental sedation as required

equipment should consist of the standard monitors used for all procedures. Observing the surgical procedure on a television monitor is preferable. This allows the anesthetist to follow the surgical progress and visualize critical points in the procedure at which patient movement would be most detrimental.

Carbon dioxide retention during ophthalmic surgery under MAC should be addressed.[47] The surgical draping placed over the patient's face should be tented, and high-flow air may be used to dissipate expired carbon dioxide more quickly. Claustrophobia can be a problem for patients who are awake. Techniques for dealing with claustrophobia include taping the nonsurgical eye or adjusting the drape so that the patient can see the room with the nonsurgical eye. If a patient experiences a claustrophobic attack, the surgical drapes should be tented away from the face immediately, while the sterile field is maintained, and verbal control of the patient is gained. At this point, the anesthetist must determine whether the patient can proceed with surgery under regional block. Rarely, the patient may experience incomplete ocular analgesia, even in the presence of muscle akinesia. This problem responds well to 2% lidocaine MPF (methylparaben free) drops or a subconjunctival anesthetic injection.

Acute increased IOP during the surgical procedure can be catastrophic and cause loss of ocular contents. Coughing or a choroidal hemorrhage can create this problem. The increased intrathoracic pressure created during coughing is reflected through the generally valveless orbital veins, resulting in an acutely increased IOP of 40 mm Hg or greater.[48] A choroidal hemorrhage occurs when a vessel in the vascular choroidal layer of the eye ruptures, bleeding into the closed cavity and creating an acute rise in IOP with potential expulsion of eye contents unless the eye is closed quickly. In the acute phase, medications that lower IOP may be of minimum benefit.

If the patient has a history of postnasal drip, vasoconstrictive nose drops may be given preoperatively. If the patient complains of a dry throat, small amounts of water may be given. These two remedies

are helpful in reducing the incidence of coughing intraoperatively. The patient must also be instructed to give notice before coughing. Instructing the patient to clear the throat effectively reduces the forcefulness of the cough. Quick, shallow breaths have been reported to help suppress the cough reflex.[48] Sedating the patient or using intravenous lidocaine to prevent further coughing can help but has minimal effect during an active coughing episode.[49]

After the surgery is completed, the patient is transported from the operating room to postanesthesia recovery (PAR). Postoperative recovery time should be in accordance with the individual patient's physical and mental status and the amount of medication administered.

In a meta-analysis of regional versus general anesthesia for ambulatory anesthesia, patients who received peripheral nerve blocks, such as orbital regional eye blocks, experienced less postoperative pain, nausea, and a decreased postanesthesia care time.[50] If postoperative nausea is noted immediately after surgery, it may result from the sedative medications, increased IOP, or ocular pain.[51] On the afternoon or evening after their surgery, patients are generally called at home to evaluate their status. A sudden onset of nausea at home after the procedure is more likely associated with increased IOP than anesthetic medications. Patients are usually examined the following day by the surgeon and are requested to fill out questionnaires regarding their experience on the day of surgery.

General Anesthesia

For general anesthesia, preoperative patient preparation should include the appropriate fasting guidelines for the patient's age and physical condition (e.g., diabetes). The patient should be reminded that the surgical eye will be patched upon awakening. Sedation should be administered as needed to help the patient relax. Benzodiazepines such as midazolam are effective in low doses. For reduction in the incidence of postoperative nausea, the use of a standard multimodal approach should be considered. Induction of general anesthesia with propofol or etomidate is recommended because they both decrease IOP. For infants and children, inhalation induction also decreases IOP. Due to the emetic effects, narcotics should be used in low doses. Other than during examinations under anesthesia or other shorter procedures, endotracheal intubation or laryngeal mask airways (LMAs) are indicated for maintenance of the airway.

Succinylcholine causes a transient increase in IOP; however, it can be used safely for ocular procedures. Some caveats include:
- The sustained contracture of the extraocular muscles after succinylcholine could cause an expulsion of the intraocular contents. This assumption is theoretical, and it is now felt that succinylcholine may be safely used in eye surgery. See full discussion later.
- In eye muscle surgery, the sustained contraction may interfere with the forced duction test used by the surgeon for the treatment plan.

Nondepolarizing muscle relaxants are satisfactory for induction and have the advantage of decreasing IOP.[52] Laryngoscopy, especially with light anesthesia, increases IOP, but intravenous lidocaine (1.5–2 mg/kg), given 1 to 1.5 minutes before laryngoscopy, helps attenuate this response. Inhalation anesthetics, which also decrease IOP, are commonly used for the maintenance of general anesthesia.

For intraocular procedures, the anesthesia provider will need to weigh the advantages and disadvantages of using or not using a nondepolarizing muscle relaxant for the anesthetic maintenance during the intraocular procedure. The anesthetist must be aware of the adverse ECG changes that may result from the oculocardiac reflex, which may be elicited when traction is exerted on the extraocular muscles and orbital structures. Patients undergoing eye muscle surgery have an increased incidence of malignant hyperthermia and postoperative nausea. In retinal procedures in which sulfur hexafluoride or perfluoropropane is used as an intraocular gas, the use of nitrous oxide should be discontinued 15 minutes before injection.

When spontaneous ventilation returns after neuromuscular blockade is reversed, the patient may be extubated while receiving deep anesthesia with 100% oxygen and placed in the lateral position until awakening. In the patient with a difficult airway, full stomach, or incompetent esophageal sphincter, gastric suction and intravenous lidocaine (1.5–2 mg/kg) may be given before the patient is extubated awake. This method helps reduce the incidence of coughing and vomiting, along with the deleterious effects.

The LMAs also have their respective place in ophthalmic procedures. They may be inserted without muscle relaxants and removed with less risk of coughing in the awake patient. Along with the usual risk assessment for gastric aspiration, the practitioner should also consider that the lack of access to the airway during the procedure, intraoperative malposition of the LMA, and light anesthesia in the absence of muscle relaxants may result in laryngospasm or coughing. The LMA is gaining popularity in extraocular procedures such as strabismus and scleral buckle surgeries.[53]

Postoperative care, with attention paid to the alleviation of pain and control of nausea, will help maintain a satisfactory IOP. The ophthalmologist should be made aware of continued postoperative nausea because it may be the result of acute increased IOP.[51]

Open-Eye Injury and the Use of Succinylcholine

Traumatic eye injuries can be categorized as either open- or closed-globe injuries. Open-eye injury in a patient with a full stomach is at best a difficult situation for the anesthesia provider. These injuries are commonly considered emergencies requiring general anesthesia. The clinician must protect the patient from aspiration and yet avoid increased IOP that could result in expulsion of intraocular contents. Authors have traditionally debated the risks and advantages of using succinylcholine for this procedure.[53,54] Normal IOP is 10 to 22 mm Hg, with slight diurnal and positional changes of 1 to 6 mm Hg. It is physiologically determined by aqueous humor dynamics, changes in choroidal blood volume, central venous pressure, and extraocular muscle tone. The most important determinant of IOP is the balance between production and elimination of aqueous humor, maintaining an average volume of 0.25 mL. Aqueous humor is formed in the ciliary process from capillaries by diffusion, filtration, and active secretion. It flows through the posterior chamber, around the iris, and into the anterior chamber. It is eliminated through the spaces of Fontana and canal of Schlemm at the iridocorneal angle, where it flows into the episcleral venous system. Any increase in venous pressure (e.g., cough, strain, head-down position) will increase IOP. Additionally, any decrease in cross-sectional area of the spaces of Fontana (e.g., mydriatic drugs) will increase IOP.[55-59] Administration of succinylcholine increases IOP within 1 minute and peaks at an increase of 9 mm Hg within 6 minutes after succinylcholine administration. The exact mechanism of this increase is unknown. Some feel that tonic contractions of the extraocular muscles may explain this IOP increase. It is now thought, however, that succinylcholine-induced IOP increase is a vascular event, with choroidal vascular dilation or a decrease in drainage secondary to elevated central venous pressure, temporarily inhibiting the flow of aqueous humor through the canal of Schlemm.[56]

It is clear that succinylcholine raises IOP. However, at induction of general anesthesia, there are many activities that raise IOP to a much greater degree than succinylcholine, including crying, Valsalva maneuver, forceful blinking, rubbing of the eyes, and coughing or bucking during poor intubating technique. Therefore the increase in IOP due to succinylcholine may be inconsequential if optimal intubating conditions are not provided.

Moreno wrote: "This observation, coupled with the lack of any documented cases of extrusion of intraocular contents in open globes of humans when succinylcholine is used, causes us to question the traditional teaching that succinylcholine should be avoided in all cases when open globe is suspected or known."[55]

Chidiac and Raiskin[56] have stated that two questions need to be asked before the decision about the use or avoidance of succinylcholine in open-globe surgeries is made: Is this an easy airway? and Is the eye viable? If the airway assessment shows that intubation should be easy, then regardless of the patient's aspiration risk, and regardless of the viability of the eye, succinylcholine can be avoided and replaced with rocuronium. If the airway assessment shows that this could be a difficult intubation, regardless of the patient's aspiration risk, then the second question becomes important (Is the eye viable?). If the ophthalmologist feels that the eye is viable, use of succinylcholine is recommended. Pretreatment with drugs that attenuate the IOP effect of succinylcholine, such as a small dose of nondepolarizing agent and lidocaine, should be used.

Choosing or avoiding succinylcholine is a matter of balance of risk. To control IOP at induction, there must be adequate dosing of drugs timed appropriately to coincide with the three potent stimuli: the administration of succinylcholine, the laryngoscopy, and the endotracheal intubation. It is clear that succinylcholine increases IOP, but this increase can be attenuated with various pretreatments, is less than increases seen with inadequate paralysis at the time of laryngoscopy and intubation, and is unimportant when weighed against the risk of loss of the airway. Therefore in the situation of "difficult airway, eye viable," one should use succinylcholine.

Closed-globe injuries require significant planning and preparation to prevent further damage to the eye by an increase in IOP. They also require smooth induction and emergence because patient coughing or bucking will cause a detrimental increase in IOP.[57]

OPHTHALMIC ANESTHESIA COMPLICATIONS

Anxiety coupled with underlying cardiovascular disease may promote marked hypertension, cardiac dysrhythmias, or angina in the patient before surgery. Vasovagal responses (e.g., fainting) secondary to anxiety are not unusual. Ammonia capsules are effective in preventing and treating fainting episodes.

Chronic coughing secondary to chronic obstructive pulmonary disease, asthma, or postnasal drip must be evaluated. Vasoconstrictive nose drops effectively decrease postnasal drip. Coughing and deep breathing before surgery help clear the lungs of excess mucus in patients with chronic pulmonary disease. Proper evaluation and treatment help reduce undesired perioperative systemic and ocular sequelae.

Most complications of regional ocular anesthetics can be attributed to direct traumatization of the orbital vessels, the globe, and the optic nerve. Trauma to these structures can result whenever a needle is placed near the eye. Frequently, the cause of complications during regional blocks and general anesthesia is patient movement.

Retrobulbar Hemorrhage

Retrobulbar hemorrhage results from trauma to an orbital vessel. The retrobulbar bleeding moves the eyeball forward (proptosis), and a subconjunctival hemorrhage is usually present. Venous hemorrhages are typically slow in onset, but arterial hemorrhage has a rapid onset and more pronounced proptosis and subconjunctival hemorrhage. Ecchymosis of the eyelids and orbit is usually present. The pressure caused by the bleeding in the bony orbital cavity produces increased orbital pressure on the optic nerve, vessels, and globe. This pressure usually resolves without problems but may result in an occlusion or spasm of

BOX 44.11 Canthotomy Procedure

Equipment
1 straight hemostat
1 plastic scissors

Procedure
1. If possible, inject lidocaine along the lateral canthus.
2. Place the hemostat in a temporal direction along the lateral canthus 4–6 mm, and clamp the hemostat.
3. Remove the hemostat.
4. Use the plastic scissors to incise only in the crush marks left by the hemostat.
5. Control local bleeding with the hemostat or with digital pressure.

BOX 44.12 Measures for Preventing Retrobulbar Hemorrhage

- Choose least vascular areas for needle placement.
- Avoid deep orbital injections.
- Avoid supranasal position of gaze.
- Use primary gaze position.
- Use upward-gaze position (Gills-Lloyd technique only).
- Insert needle slowly.

BOX 44.13 Measures for Preventing Seizures Resulting From Intravascular Injection

- Choose least vascular areas for needle placement.
- Avoid deep orbital injections.
- Avoid supranasal position of gaze.
- Insert needle slowly.
- Aspirate gently before injection; negative aspiration is no guarantee that you are not in a blood vessel.
- Avoid injection against resistance.
- Avoid forceful rapid injections.

BOX 44.14 Measures for Preventing Globe Puncture

- Use caution in patients with increased axial length.
- Avoid supranasal position of gaze.
- Direct needle away from axis of globe during insertion through the orbital septum.
- Observe globe movement with needle insertion.
- Insert needle slowly, with the bevel toward the globe.
- Never forcefully inject anesthetic.
- Use modified retrobulbar and peribulbar techniques (although globe punctures have also been reported with these).

the central retinal artery or vein, resulting in partial to complete loss of vision.[60] One may detect a progressively increasing orbital pressure when digital pressure is applied over the eye after an ocular block. Continuous digital pressure may be all that is required for stopping a venous hemorrhage.[19] If the orbital pressure continues to increase in the presence of digital pressure, a lateral canthotomy is indicated and may be performed by the ophthalmologist or the anesthesia practitioner, who should then notify the ophthalmologist. Canthotomy is a procedure performed to increase the orbital space by cutting the lateral canthus and reducing the orbital pressure that results from a retrobulbar hemorrhage.

A canthotomy set should be readily available when orbital blocks are being performed (Box 44.11). The ophthalmologist should examine the central retinal artery and vein for patency. Occlusion of these vessels may warrant further surgical intervention for reduction of elevated orbital pressure.

A localized episcleral hemorrhage also causes subconjunctival bleeding. In this situation, however, no proptosis of the globe or increase in orbital pressure is noted. These episcleral vessels are the same ones the ophthalmologist cauterizes after a conjunctival incision. The vessels break as a result of the spread of local anesthesia through the subconjunctival area and are of no consequence. However, the ophthalmologist should be notified of their presence before the procedure begins.

Retrobulbar hemorrhage remains the most common sequelae for ocular blocks (Box 44.12). Peribulbar injections also can cause orbital hemorrhages.[28] Retrobulbar hemorrhages have been reported to occur in 1% to 3% of cases.[61]

Intravascular Injection

Grand mal seizures have been reported to occur after retrobulbar injections with lidocaine, lidocaine-bupivacaine combinations, and ropivacaine.[62,63] Seizures may result from a less-than-toxic dose of local anesthesia by direct intraarterial injection, resulting in retrograde flow to the cerebral circulation (Box 44.13). Mathers[64] surveyed 200 ophthalmologists; 66 responded and reported three seizures occurring after retrobulbar injections. From these data, it appears that seizures after retrobulbar anesthesia may occur more frequently than reported in the literature. A reaction after an orbital vein injection has also been reported: The patient experienced uncontrolled shivering and rigor approximately 15 seconds after the retrobulbar injection. These symptoms resolved within 2 minutes of onset.[65]

Globe Puncture

Multiple reports have been published regarding globe perforations. Both sharp and dull needles have either penetrated or perforated the eye during retrobulbar and peribulbar injections. Although rare, globe punctures have occurred in the hands of experienced practitioners who have performed many thousands of ophthalmic blocks. The literature also notes that patients may or may not exhibit signs and symptoms of a puncture immediately, and the diagnosis has been made anywhere from 1 to 14 days after the event.[20,66-69] The most rare but devastating globe injury reported is an ocular explosion. The globe can rupture from the IOP exerted by the local anesthesia injection.[70,71]

The myopic eye has an increased axial length of greater than 24 mm. Scleral thinning may result from this increased anteroposterior diameter. A previous scleral buckling procedure also increases the anteroposterior diameter of the eye. Staphyloma, a bulging of the sclera, may also predispose the patient to globe puncture. The risk of puncture increases when this abnormality is located inferoposteriorly on the globe. Enophthalmos is a recession of the eyeball into the orbit. This condition decreases the distance between the posterior pole of the globe and the posterior orbital wall. The supranasal gaze position rotates the posterior pole of the globe in line and closer to the retrobulbar needle path. Multiple orbital injections have also been cited as a factor in globe punctures, along with unexpected patient movement (Box 44.14).

The choice of sharp versus dull retrobulbar needles is highly debated. The literature reviewed appears to draw conclusions based

BOX 44.15 Signs and Symptoms of Globe Puncture*

- Increased resistance to injection
- Immediate dilation and paralysis of the pupil
- Rapid increase in intraocular pressure with edematous cornea
- Hypotony of the globe
- Intraocular hemorrhage

*Patient may or may not exhibit signs and symptoms of a puncture immediately.

BOX 44.16 Measures for Preventing Optic Nerve Sheath Trauma

- Avoid supranasal eye position.
- Avoid deep orbital injection.
- Insert needle slowly.
- Avoid forceful injection of anesthetics.
- Use modified retrobulbar or peribulbar techniques.

BOX 44.17 Measures for Preventing Extraocular Muscle Trauma

- Avoid needle contact with extraocular muscles.
- Avoid deep orbital penetration.
- Avoid angling needle toward visual axis of the globe when parallel to an extraocular muscle.

more on opinion than on fact. A review of the literature confirmed a lack of safety with the use of blunt needles. Optic nerve penetration, ocular perforation, and CNS complications have resulted from the use of blunt needles.[20] The surgeon should be notified if a globe puncture is suspected (Box 44.15).

Optic Nerve Sheath Trauma

To review, the optic nerve sheaths surround the optic nerve and are composed of the meninges of the brain. The outer sheath contains the dura mater and the inner sheath consists of the arachnoid mater and pia mater. The subarachnoid space contains cerebrospinal fluid and is continuous with the optic chiasm. The dura splits into two layers at the optic foramen. The outer dural layer becomes continuous with the orbital periosteum. The inner layer forms the dural covering of the optic nerve, creating the orbital epidural space.[2] Anesthetic agents injected into the subdural or subarachnoid space may track back to the optic chiasm. Here, the anesthetic can affect the contralateral eye by blocking cranial nerves II and III as they proceed through the subdural or subarachnoid space; this block can result in contralateral amaurosis.[72-74] The condition can be a precursor to the continued migration of the anesthetic to the respiratory centers of the midbrain, resulting in respiratory arrest.[60,75,76]

The anesthetist should observe the contralateral pupil before an ocular block is performed. The pupil may be dilated from accidental administration of preoperative eye drops, a preoperative examination, or existing pathology. If the contralateral pupil is constricted before the ocular block and dilates after the ocular block contralateral amaurosis, one must assume that subarachnoid or subdural injection has occurred and be prepared to treat a respiratory arrest.

The onset of respiratory arrest is usually within 2 to 5 minutes after injection; however, it may occur as late as 10 to 17 minutes after injection. Spontaneous ventilation usually returns in 15 to 20 minutes but may take up to 55 minutes for complete recovery. Treatment includes appropriate ventilatory and cardiovascular support, supplemental oxygen with oxygen saturation monitoring, ECG monitoring for cardiac dysrhythmias, and blood pressure monitoring. The surgeon should be notified immediately so the eye can be examined for any optic nerve trauma that may require surgical intervention.

A retrobulbar hemorrhage resulting in increased extravascular pressure may result in occlusion of the central retinal artery or vein, or both. In addition, direct trauma to the ophthalmic artery or the optic nerve by the retrobulbar needle may cause artery or vein occlusion without causing retrobulbar hemorrhage[77] (Box 44.16).

Ocular Ischemia

Retinal vascular occlusion or thrombosis has been reported after ocular blocks.[78,79] Studies have also reported a decrease in the pulsatile ocular blood flow after ocular blocks, secondary to the pressure exerted by the volume of local anesthesia injected into the orbit. However, the same orbital injection volume did not cause a significant rise in the IOP. Even though not contraindicated, caution should be exercised in patients with

preexisting compromised ocular circulation.[80-83] Some authors have advocated not using epinephrine in the local anesthetic solution.[84,85]

Optic nerve atrophy has been reported after intraocular surgery with either regional block or general anesthesia.[60] Direct trauma to the optic nerve may result in transient symptoms, such as contralateral amaurosis or respiratory arrest, or it may result in vascular occlusion or thrombosis, or both, with partial to complete loss of vision.

Extraocular Muscle Palsy and Ptosis

Inferior rectus muscle palsy has been reported after retrobulbar anesthesia. Segmental inferior rectus muscle enlargement was noted posterior to the globe deep in the orbit.[86] The complication has not been reported to occur after general anesthesia.[87] The initial signs and symptoms of this problem manifest after surgery as persistent vertical diplopia. Surgical intervention may be indicated for correction of this condition. Trauma to the superior oblique tendon–trochlea complex also has been reported to occur with peribulbar anesthesia[88] (Box 44.17).

Carlson et al.[89] performed experiments on the rectus muscle of monkeys and humans and demonstrated minimal myotoxic damage to ocular muscles after retrobulbar administration of local anesthetics. Typically, after the injection of local anesthesia, the surface muscle fibers degenerate, then regenerate. However, direct injections of local anesthesia into the rectus muscle resulted in massive internal muscle lesions that were large enough to produce noticeable functional deficit. The myotoxicity of local anesthetics also may play a role in postoperative diplopia and/or ptosis,[90] especially in the elderly because regeneration of their muscle fibers may not be as complete as that in younger patients. However, ptosis is also associated with aging, the superior rectus stay suture, and the eyelid speculum. Postoperative ptosis may take as long as 6 months to resolve.

Facial Nerve Blocks

Patients commonly experience discomfort as a result of blocks of cranial nerve VII. Prolonged Bell palsy has been seen after Nadbath and O'Brien blocks, probably secondary to direct nerve trauma.[91] Several authors have reported cases of dysphagia, hoarseness, coughing, and respiratory distress after Nadbath blocks (Box 44.18). They noted that these symptoms were consistent with paresis of the vagus, glossopharyngeal, and spinal accessory nerves. These nerves exit the skull approximately 10 mm medial to cranial nerve VII. Therefore anesthesia injected for a cranial nerve VII block could also reach these nerves and result in unilateral vocal cord paralysis.[92,93]

Patients have also complained of jaw ache with movement for several weeks after a cranial nerve VII Nadbath block. Grand mal seizure

CHAPTER 44 Anesthesia for Ophthalmic Procedures 1029

BOX 44.18 Prevention and Treatment of Complications From the Nadbath Block

- Avoid using the Nadbath technique in patients weighing <45 kg.
- Avoid using large volumes of anesthesia and hyaluronidase.
- Avoid using the Nadbath technique when patients have a preexisting unilateral vocal cord dysfunction.
- Place the patient in seated or lateral position to maintain a patent airway and patient comfort.
- The patient with an unsatisfactory airway should be intubated.

has rarely occurred (1 report) when 3 mL of 2% lidocaine with epinephrine (1:200,000) was injected using the Nadbath technique.

Zaturansky and Hyams[94] reported an ocular perforation that occurred when a modified Van Lint procedure was performed after a retrobulbar block. The needle penetrated the proposed eye just under the insertion of the lateral rectus muscle.

Oculocardiac Reflex

The oculocardiac reflex is a trigeminal-vagal reflex that was first described in 1908 by Aschner. The stimulus for this reflex is generated by pressure on the globe, the orbital structures (e.g., the optic nerve), or the conjunctiva, or by traction on the extraocular muscles (particularly the medial rectus muscle). The afferent pathway for the stimulus is via the long and short ciliary nerves to the ciliary ganglion and then through the gasserian ganglion along the ophthalmic division of the trigeminal nerve, terminating in the main trigeminal sensory nucleus in the floor of the fourth ventricle. The efferent pathway consists of the vagus nerve to the cardioinhibitory center.

The reflex may be elicited during local infiltration anesthesia, retrobulbar or peribulbar blockade, and general anesthesia. The occurrence of the reflex in ocular procedures is variable, but it is commonly seen in muscle procedures performed in children. The oculocardiac reflex most often results in acute sinus bradycardia. However, it may also cause a wide variety of other cardiac dysrhythmias, such as nodal rhythms, atrioventricular block, ventricular ectopy, idioventricular rhythm, and asystole. Continuous ECG monitoring is essential for the diagnosis of dysrhythmias that result from the oculocardiac reflex. If cardiac dysrhythmias are observed, the surgeon must be instructed to immediately cease all pressure or traction on the orbit. Simultaneously, the patient should be assessed for adequate oxygenation and ventilation and for adequate anesthetic depth because one or more of these may be an underlying cause for the dysrhythmia. The aberrant rhythm usually resolves without intervention within a few seconds.

However, if the aforementioned measures are taken and the dysrhythmia continues, thus threatening to cause hemodynamic instability, intravenous atropine should be administered. Atropine, 2 to 3 mg, may be required for complete vagal blockade. Caution should be exercised with the administration of atropine because atropine itself may induce cardiac dysrhythmias. Glycopyrrolate may be given for less severe bradycardic episodes. The surgeon may proceed only after the dysrhythmia is resolved. If the reflex recurs, the aforementioned process should be repeated. The oculocardiac reflex, however, appears to fatigue with continued manipulations. The use of intravenous atropine or intravenous glycopyrrolate just before surgery may help reduce the incidence of the reflex, especially in children.[95,96]

Other Complications

Corneal abrasion is the most common injury occurring after general anesthesia. It is believed to result from the drying of the exposed cornea or from direct trauma, such as an anesthesia-mask injury. Ensuring that the eyelids are closed and secured with tape should provide satisfactory protection of the cornea. Movement during ocular surgery was identified as the single most common mechanism of injury. Movement was described as coughing and bucking, which resulted in poor visual outcome. In these reported cases, muscle relaxants were used less than 50% of the time, and nerve stimulators were omitted. Chemical injury can result from spillage of cleaning materials or preparatory solutions into the eye. In these cases, the eye should be flushed immediately with saline.[97]

Patient positioning for surgery under monitored anesthesia care and general anesthesia is important to reduce ophthalmic complications during the surgical procedure.[98] Central retinal artery occlusion may result from prolonged pressure on the eye.[99] This type of injury may result with the patient in the prone position. Attention to padding and periodic checks of the eyes is necessary, especially for long procedures. Eye protectors, along with foam headrests or gel donuts for the face, may help prevent eye trauma. It is prudent to request an ophthalmic examination immediately after surgery if the patient complains of any eye problems or if the anesthesia provider suspects a problem.

SUMMARY

Anesthesia management for ophthalmic procedures has changed rapidly in the last few years. As an anesthesia practitioner, you will be challenged with the increasingly complex comorbidities and multiple pharmacologic agents used in the care of the elderly patient. The pediatric patient also presents anesthetic challenges, many associated with the preterm infant and chronic upper respiratory infection. Newer surgical techniques for cataract surgery have increased the popularity of topical anesthesia for such procedures; however, the advances in retinal surgical techniques, corneal transplants, and adult eye muscle and glaucoma procedures are fueling an increased demand by surgeons for anesthesia practitioners to perform ophthalmic eye blocks versus general anesthesia. Orbital regional blocks have the further advantage of minimizing postoperative pain, requiring minimal to no opioid administration, with significant reductions in postoperative nausea and vomiting. General anesthesia will continue to be the technique of choice for the pediatric patient, patients with ocular trauma, and patients who are not candidates for topical or orbital regional blocks.

REFERENCES

For a complete list of references for this chapter, scan this QR code with any smartphone code reader app, or visit the following URL: http://booksite.elsevier.com/9780323711944/.

45

Anesthesia for Orthopedics

Daniel Frasca, Kevin Baker

Few surgical specialties encompass the procedural diversity associate with orthopedic surgery. On any given day in the orthopedic operating room, you might care for an infant undergoing Achilles tendon lengthening for talipes equinovarus (clubfoot), an adolescent with Duchenne muscular dystrophy scheduled for posterior spinal fusion, or an octogenarian who requires an intramedullary nail placement following a traumatic fall. This necessitates a strong command of the physiologic changes that occur across the lifespan along with a deep appreciation of the diverse spectrum of comorbidities encountered in these populations.

Many orthopedic procedures lend themselves to a variety of anesthetic techniques. The rapid evolution of ultrasound-guided regional anesthesia and proliferation of opioid-sparing techniques give us additional tools to provide safe passage for our patients throughout the perioperative continuum. As innovations in surgical and anesthetic methods accelerate, tomorrow's health care delivery system will be unrecognizable from our current vantage point. Therefore, it is incumbent upon clinicians to embark on the journey of lifelong learning, one that allows them to continuously develop their skill sets so they position themselves at the forefront of anesthetic practice in the years to come. In this chapter, we will elucidate the foundational anesthetic principles for orthopedic surgery.

The *Merriam-Webster Dictionary* defines orthopedics as "a branch of medicine concerned with the correction or prevention of deformities, disorders, or injuries of the skeleton and associated structures (as tendons and ligaments)."[1] Among the oldest surgical specialties, orthopedics is derived from the Greek words *orthos* and *paideia*, which mean "to straighten" and "nurturing of children," respectively. Historical evidence of orthopedic procedures dates back to ancient times. Egyptian artifacts demonstrate the use of splints, and some of the earliest documented orthopedic interventions came from the battlefields of gladiators. Although these initial encounters involved rather primitive anesthetic techniques, anesthesia for orthopedics has evolved into a sophisticated specialty that strives to provide individualized care to patients.

Much progress has been made in recent decades, including the development of better arthroscopic techniques, greater adoption of minimally invasive procedures, and the introduction of new devices that leverage biologics and three-dimensional (3D) printing. These advances could not come at a better time, as our aging population is poised to increasingly consume orthopedic services. To put this into perspective, in 2014, there were 370,770 primary total hip arthroplasties and 680,150 primary total knee arthroplasties performed in the United States. By 2030, it is estimated that these numbers will balloon to 635,000 to 909,900 primary total hip arthroplasties and 935,000 to 1.67 million primary total knee arthroplasties.[2] As more primary procedures are performed, one can logically deduce that the number of revision procedures will also rise. In 2014, there were 50,220 revision total hip arthroplasties and 72,100 revision total knee arthroplasties. Between 2014 and 2030, the number of revision total hip and total knee arthroplasties is expected to rise between 43% and 70%, and 78% and 182%, respectively.[3]

In the 21st century, we have seen many orthopedic procedures shift from inpatient to outpatient status. The advantages of today's surgical techniques are readily apparent. Smaller incisions result in less postoperative pain. Patients who have arthroscopic procedures experience faster recovery from surgery and anesthesia, have shorter lengths of stay, use fewer narcotics for pain relief, and return to work more quickly than those undergoing open procedures.[4] Although orthopedic techniques have improved over the years, these procedures predispose patients to a multitude of complications related to venous thromboembolism (VTE), bone cement implantation syndrome (BCIS), fat embolism, hemorrhage, positioning injuries, pneumatic tourniquet use, perioperative vision loss, and surgical site infection (SSI).

With a tremendous variety in patient populations and surgical options, the anesthetic plan can vary greatly. Options include general, regional, or local anesthesia or some combination of these. The choice of one anesthetic technique over another hinges on several factors: What is the nature of the patient's surgery? How long will the procedure last? What are the preferences of the patient and surgeon? Does the patient's anatomy complicate airway management or surgical positioning? What comorbidities are present? How are the speed and quality of recovery affected by a given anesthetic technique? Answers to these questions guide the decision-making process when formulating the anesthetic plan for orthopedic patients.

SELECTED COMORBIDITIES AND PRESURGICAL CONDITIONS

There are a myriad conditions that predispose patients to orthopedic complications. Osteoarthritis (OA) is the most prevalent.[5] Others include the family of inflammatory autoimmune rheumatoid diseases, such as rheumatoid arthritis (RA), systemic lupus erythematosus, and AS.[6] Arthritis is the leading cause of disability in the United States, affecting over 54 million people. These patients are twice as likely to fall and suffer a traumatic injury. Ninety-nine percent of all knee and hip replacements are due to arthritic symptoms. The annual cost of taking care of these patients is $81 billion,[5] and in many developed nations, this value approaches 1% to 2.5% of their gross domestic product.[7] Taking time to review some of these comorbidities will help your understanding of how to provide optimal care for patients undergoing orthopedic procedures.

Osteoarthritis

OA is the most common joint disease in the world and is the leading cause of joint replacement. Degenerative joint disease is sometimes used synonymously with OA; however, it is actually a misnomer because it fails to consider the local and systemic inflammatory processes inherent to OA.[7-9] OA is prevalent in individuals 60 years of age and older, and it more often affects women. Repetitive movements associated with activities of daily living culminate in the erosion of cartilage and bone. Chronic wear and tear of a susceptible joint leads to the loss of articular cartilage along with the formation of osteophytes. The most commonly affected joints include the hips, knees, hands, spine, and feet. Joint dysmorphia, poor quadriceps function, limb misalignment, limb length inequality, and high-intensity sports are all risk factors for OA. If these biomechanical factors were the only mechanism, however, we would see far fewer procedures. Indeed, other factors play a role as to whether an individual will need a joint replacement.[7]

Not only does aging impair the body's regenerative abilities, but it also brings with it a variety of comorbidities. Previous injury plays a role as well. These can lead to bone on cartilage activity and ligament tears. Obesity puts extra stress on the joints and favors the development of adipokines. In fact, weight loss and exercise aid in circumventing end-stage OA disease. As it often does, genetics also plays a pivotal role. Interestingly, genetics has a greater influence on OA of the spine and hip joints than in the hands and knees. While genetics has little effect on the presence or absence of OA, it does affect the severity of the disease.[7]

The joint capsule and surrounding tissue are made up of the cartilage, subchondral bone, and the synovium. OA affects all of these structures. The subchondral bone contributes to much of the pain associated with joint disease. The synovium produces lubricant and nourishes the bone and cartilage inside the joint.[7] Inflammation of the synovium, or synovitis, is often present throughout the disease process and contributes to pain and swelling of the joint.[8,9] Not only does OA consist of injury and inflammation of the affected joints, but it seems to contribute to systemic inflammation. Pain management for OA tends to be more reactive than proactive. In contrast to medical therapy for RA, there are no disease-modifying drugs for OA to date. Thus options for pain control are limited.[8] Arthroplasty is the procedure of choice for end-stage OA when other nonsurgical treatments have failed. Arthroscopic surgery, though once quite common for OA, has decreased in popularity as its efficacy is controversial.

Rheumatoid Arthritis

RA falls under the family of inflammatory autoimmune rheumatic diseases. These include, but are not limited to, systemic lupus erythematosus and AS. Eight percent of all women and 5% of all men will develop some form of inflammatory autoimmune rheumatic disease in their lifetime.[6] RA is the most common inflammatory disease of the joints in adults, where it leads to articular destruction, limited mobility, and chronic pain.[10,11] Close to 4% of all women and 2% of all men will develop RA. Most will not develop symptoms until after 60 years of age. Though modern therapeutics have improved patient outcomes over the years and our collective understanding of the disease has seen significant progress, there is no cure. It continues to negatively impact the patient's ability to perform activities of daily living and ultimately decreases their quality of life and longevity.[6,10-12]

Autoantibodies are the hallmark of autoimmune disease and therefore are found in patients with RA. Autoantibody production is initiated months to years before RA symptoms. Increases in cytokines, chemokines, and complement may also occur. These changes suggest subclinical systemic inflammation. As these autoantibodies reach their peak, symptoms begin to occur. Autoantibodies are found in 80% to 90% of RA patients. The presence of autoantibodies in patients with

early undifferentiated inflammatory disease can help lead to an early diagnosis of RA.[10]

RA is characterized by joint swelling, joint tenderness, and the destruction of synovial joints. In 2010, the American College of Rheumatology and the European League Against Rheumatism revised the classification criteria for RA. Criteria include the presence of synovitis in at least one joint (not otherwise explained), as well as confirmatory serologic testing. The updated scoring system allows for earlier detection and treatment of RA.[13]

The genesis of RA is not fully understood, but genetics and the environment both play a part.[12] They amplify events that lead to synovitis and chronic destructive arthritis. Environmental factors include smoking, obesity, periodontitis, and viral infections. A smoking habit of more than a 20 pack-year creates a high risk for developing RA. Interestingly, the risk returns to baseline 10 years after cessation. This may be a sign that, besides toxins introduced into the body, altered immunologic function related to smoking is also a contributing factor.[10]

Microbiomes of the gut and lungs may also play a significant factor by having a role in inflammation and autoimmunity. *Porphyromonas gingivalis*, which is associated with periodontitis, is one example. These bacteria may actually relocate from the digestive tract to the tissues.[10,12]

Of particular concern in clinical practice are the effects of RA on the cervical spine, temporomandibular joint, larynx, and pulmonary system. The deposition of rheumatoid nodules causes inflammation of the intervertebral discs and dura, which is expressed as atlantoaxial joint subluxation. The synovium of the temporomandibular joint is also affected by RA and can result in severe limitation of joint range of motion. The cricoarytenoid joints are common sites for rheumatoid nodule deposition. The resultant chronic synovitis may cause fixation of the vocal cords in adduction and airway obstruction.[13,14]

RA can also lead to cardiovascular disease, metabolic syndrome, osteoporosis, psychosocial detriments, and increased cancer rates. Interestingly, cardiovascular disease is the most common cause of death in patients with RA. On the surface, this does not seem to make sense. These patients are most often women who are treated with nonsteroidal antiinflammatory drugs (NSAIDs), which have antiinflammatory components and antiplatelet effects, all of which should confer protection against cardiovascular disease. Although the reasons are not fully understood, an association with atherosclerosis is likely a contributing factor. This could be related to the side effects of some antirheumatic medication such as glucocorticoid steroids and methotrexate. Another theory postulates chronic systemic inflammation of the vascular endothelium may be at play. Synovial inflammation may spread to the endothelial cells by mediators such as cytokines and other circulating immune moieties released into the circulation. A sedentary lifestyle due to physical limitations may also play a role.[6] Why is this information important? When interviewing a patient for joint reconstruction, consider risk factors associated with the primary diagnosis of RA. A potential history of smoking, poor oral hygiene, and cardiovascular disease is a good place to start and will help guide your anesthetic plan.

Ankylosing Spondylitis

AS belongs to the family of inflammatory autoimmune rheumatic diseases. As with RA, inflammatory processes, genetics, and environmental factors play a role in the etiology of AS.[15] Unlike rheumatoid disease, AS primarily affects the vertebral column and sacroiliac joints (though it can affect extraspinal joints as well).[16] Over the years, AS contributes to spinal column remodeling through ossifications, fusions, osteoporosis, and kyphosis. These pathologic changes weaken the vertebrae, setting the stage for pathologic fractures and a potential for spinal cord injury.

AS is a chronic condition that can start as early as the second or third decade of life and slowly progresses at a steady insidious state. Significant complications, such as spinal fractures, usually do not occur until later in life. In contrast to RA, AS is twice as predominant in men. The modified New York criteria help to identify patients with AS. It considers both radiographic and clinical factors (Table 45.1).

Inflammatory back pain is a hallmark of AS. It is differentiated from other types of back pain by the patient exhibiting at least two of the following four complaints: (1) morning stiffness lasting more than 30 minutes, (2) improvement of back pain with activity and not rest, (3) awakening due to back pain during the second half of the night, and (4) alternating buttock pain.[17] This inflammatory process leads to ossification within the affected spinal cord ligaments, intervertebral discs, and apophyseal structures. At the same time, bone is lost in other areas leading to osteoporosis and low bone mineral density. This contributes to a bamboo-like appearance of the vertebral bodies on x-ray. These changes can lead to a patient with a rigid hyperkyphotic vertebral column and impaired mobility. In combination with peripheral joint arthritis, these patients are at higher risk for falls and fractures.[18]

A potentially difficult airway may be present-from a small degree of limitation to limited mouth opening as a result of immobility of the temporomandibular joint to extreme cervical flexion and complete ankylosis. In the latter case, even slight manipulations of the neck may cause cervical fractures and injury. Proper positioning of these patients is of utmost importance, and awake intubation should be strongly considered.[16,19] For the less extreme airway, there are a host of airway options from which to choose. For example, videolaryngoscopes are viable alternatives.[20] These have a higher overall success rate of intubation with a shorter duration than direct visualization using a standard laryngoscope blade.[21]

AS is a systemic disease and which not only affects the vertebral column and joints. AS increases the risk of cardiovascular morbidity and mortality.[15,22] The most common cardiac sequelae are aortic insufficiency and conduction defects. Even in AS patients with no clinical signs of cardiac disease, global myocardial depression and stiffness in the aortic root can be found.[23] Inflammation seems to affect both the atrioventricular (AV) node and the interventricular wall with AV blockade being the most common arrhythmia.[15] Patients with a significant history of AS should have an extensive cardiac workup to detect cardiovascular disease.

Restrictive pulmonary disease occurs in advanced AS, as well as spontaneous pneumothorax and obstructive sleep apnea.[24] Interestingly, pulmonary function tests (PFTs) do not alter significantly in AS patients even with limited ribcage expansion because of compensatory changes in the diaphragm and abdominal muscles.[25]

TABLE 45.1 Modified New York Criteria for Ankylosing Spondylosis

Criteria	Description
Clinical	Inflammatory back pain
	Limited motion of lumbar spine in the sagittal and coronal planes
	Restriction of chest expansion relative to normal values correlated for age and sex
Radiologic	Sacroiliitis grade ≥2 bilaterally or grade 3–4 unilaterally

Ankylosing spondylosis is present if the radiologic criterion is associated with at least one clinical criterion.

From Rudwaleit M, et al. Inflammatory back pain in ankylosing spondylitis: a reassessment of the clinical history for application as classification and diagnostic criteria. *Arthritis Rheum.* 2006;54(2):569–578.

Anesthetic Management

The primary concern when caring for a patient with either RA or AS is the patient's airway. The mobility of the patient's cervical spine must be meticulously evaluated during the preoperative interview. Any neurologic symptoms that occur during movement of the cervical spine must be thoroughly documented at that time. As a result of RA or AS, cervical mobility may be severely restricted; therefore the patient may prove to be extremely difficult to intubate. Because of the high risk to these patients from cervical spine manipulation during direct laryngoscopy for tracheal intubation, awake fiberoptic or other intubation techniques may be the safer course of action. Airway management strategies may include positioning the patient such that neurologic symptoms remain absent before induction of general anesthesia. The cervical spine must be neutrally positioned throughout any surgical procedure, during emergence, and during transfer to the postanesthesia care unit. Regional anesthesia is a safe approach to extremity surgery for these patients.[26,27]

PREOPERATIVE CONCERNS

Frailty

By the year 2050, the number of people worldwide who are 65 years of age or older is expected to approach 2 billion. In the United States, there will be over 83 million citizens 65 years of age or older, double the number from 2012.[28] In fact, for the first time in history, there are more people 65 and older than children under 5. An aging population consumes a greater proportion of health care resources, and this population is at greater risk of perioperative complications that can lead to disability, loss of independence, inability to perform activities of daily living, and a higher rate of mortality.[29] Many elderly people have multisystem illnesses. Age-related diseases result from years of molecular and cellular damage as the body fights to preserve and repair its complex systems. For some, this steady decline erodes the mechanisms of homeostatic reserve until minor stressors become capable of triggering major adverse events. Frailty is a multifaceted syndrome that impacts physiologic, cognitive, social, and emotional well-being. A reduced homeostatic reserve makes frail patients more susceptible to poor health outcomes, such as falls, delirium, and disability[30] (Fig. 45.1; Table 45.2).

Not all elderly people are frail. Though frailty tends to increase with age (especially in women), there are plenty of exceptions to this rule. Indeed, many patients of extreme age are physiologically well. Studies show the incidence of frailty is seen in 10% to 27% of patients 65 and older and up to 48% in those 85 and older.[30] During the preoperative evaluation, it is extremely important to differentiate frailty from the normal effects of aging. Identification of frailty directs how to proceed

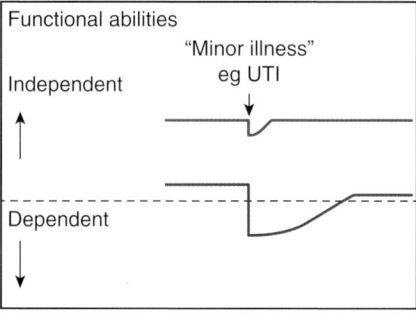

Fig. 45.1 Prevalence of frailty and factors associated with frailty in individuals aged 90 and older. (From Lee DR, et al. Prevalence of frailty and factors associated with frailty in individuals aged 90 and older: the 90+ study. *J Am Geriatr Soc.* 2016;64[11]:2257–2262.)

TABLE 45.2 Common Clinical Presentations Associated with Frailty

Nonspecific	Extreme fatigue, unexplained weight loss, frequent infections
Falls	Balance and gait impairment are core features of frailty and are important risk factors for falls. A hot fall is related to a minor illness that reduces postural balance below a critical threshold necessary to maintain gait integrity. Spontaneous falls occur in more serious frailty when vital postural systems (vision, balance, strength) are no longer consistent with safe navigation through undemanding environments. Spontaneous falls are typically repeated and are closely associated with the psychological reaction of "fear of further falls" so the person develops severely impaired mobility.
Delirium	Delirium (sometimes called acute confusion) is characterized by the rapid onset of fluctuating confusion and impaired awareness. It is related to a reduction in the integrity of brain function and is independently associated with adverse outcomes. Approximately 30% of older people admitted to a hospital will develop delirium, and the point prevalence estimate for delirium in long-term care is 15%.
Fluctuating disability	Day-to-day instability resulting in patients with "good" independent days and "bad" days in which professional care is often needed.

with the anesthetic plan.[30] There is a lack a universally agreed upon tool that both quantifies frailty-related risk and gives specific recommendations based on its result. The American Society of Anesthesiologists (ASA) physical status is subjective, and scores vary from user to user. It was also designed to garner information and rate comorbidities preoperatively, not postoperatively.[32] Some tools measure frailty by an index calculated from accumulated deficits, while others define phenotypes.[30] Thus, the modified frailty index is the most common validated clinical tool capable of predicting poor outcomes in frail patients. The modified frailty index includes several indices measuring 5 to 42 variables mined from the Canadian Study of Health and Aging (CSHA) frailty index. The CSHA is a 70-item index that can accurately predict poor outcomes in the elderly. A frailty score is derived by dividing the number of deficits by a total score of 70. A low ratio is indicative of a healthy, robust individual. An elderly patient with a ratio closer to 1 would be considered frail. As one can imagine, the CSHA would be a time-consuming questionnaire in the clinical arena, hence the modified versions.[32]

Frailty is nuanced, and sensory deficits, functional deficits, comorbidities, and cognitive function tests must be calculated into the equation. Various scales and questionnaires attempt to measure the phenotype of frailty. Phenotype is defined as a set of observable characteristics of an individual and their interaction with the environment. Frailty can be diagnosed if there is the presence of three or more of the following criteria: muscle weakness, slow walking speed, exhaustion, low physical activity, and unintentional weight loss. Both the phenotype of frailty and the frailty index equally predict adverse outcomes. Frailty is also associated with cardiovascular disease, insulin resistance, and female gender.[29,32] Women of color who are less educated and from a lower socioeconomic background are more apt to be labeled frail. Frail women were also strongly associated with an increase in hip fractures.[33]

There is evidence that inflammatory cytokines play a significant part in the pathophysiology of frailty. These include; interleukin, C-reactive protein, tumor necrosis factor-α, and CXC chemokine ligand-10.

Over time, a low-grade inflammatory response stimulates a hyperresponse that does not go away once the initial inflammatory stimulus is removed. These can lead to anorexia (nutritional compromise) as well as catabolism of skeletal muscle (muscle weakness) and adipose tissue (weight loss). Medications that show some promise in limiting the progression of frailty include angiotensin-converting enzyme (ACE) inhibitors, testosterone, and vitamin D.[31]

ARTHROSCOPY

Arthroscopy is a minimally invasive surgical procedure performed to examine and sometimes repair the damage of the interior of a joint using an arthroscope.[34] The concept was introduced in the United States in 1926.[35] However, without the availability of practical sources of illumination, arthroscopy languished. The development of fiberoptic light sources in the 1970s led to a resurgence of interest in the use of arthroscopy. Initially, arthroscopy was used to obtain a diagnosis of a patient's orthopedic malady so that a definitive, corrective surgical procedure could be performed. As interest in the procedure and technique increased and the necessary smaller surgical instrumentation was developed, previously open surgical procedures on the knee, such as partial or complete meniscectomy, loose-body removal, or ligament repair or reconstruction, were attempted and refined solely via the arthroscope.

Successful performance of arthroscopic procedures on the knee has several benefits for the patient, including reduced blood loss, less postoperative discomfort, and reduced length of rehabilitation. The success achieved with arthroscopic procedures on the knee led to the application of principles and techniques to other joints (e.g., the shoulder, elbow, wrist, hip, ankle, and phalangeal joints of the foot).[36-38] Many of these surgeries have become routine outpatient procedures. Through the mid-1990s, the application of arthroscopic procedures focused on the shoulder. Accordingly, shoulder arthroscopy procedures range from simple debridements to more complex rotator cuff repairs.[39] The development and refinement of shoulder arthroscopic procedures mirrored that of knee arthroscopic procedures; that is, as more skill and comfort were obtained with initial procedures, more traditionally open surgical treatments were attempted solely via the arthroscope.

Anesthetic Management

Patients undergoing arthroscopic procedures may be managed by almost any of the available anesthesia techniques (e.g., general anesthesia, regional anesthesia, combined regional and general anesthesia, or local blockade with sedation). Patient selection for a given anesthetic technique is crucial with arthroscopic procedures, as with all operative procedures. Reviewing the patient's chart and (more importantly) personally interviewing the patient, along with having an adequate understanding of the physiologic changes associated with various positions, assist in choosing the best care for each patient. Critical factors in the selection and presentation of the available anesthesia techniques appropriate for arthroscopic procedures are the patient positioning necessary to facilitate the proposed arthroscopic procedure and the overall state of health of the patient. The choice of position is determined in part by the nature and extent of the malady being surgically addressed. Patient positioning for arthroscopic procedures can encompass the entire gamut of possible operative positions. Most often, arthroscopic procedures for lower extremity joints use the supine position, as do most arthroscopic procedures on the upper extremities. Knee arthroscopy requires the supine position, with the foot of the operating room bed lowered (Fig. 45.2). The nonoperative leg should either be wrapped with an elastic bandage or have some form of compression stocking in place to reduce the pooling of blood and the potential for thrombus formation. Shoulder arthroscopy uses one of two positions to accomplish

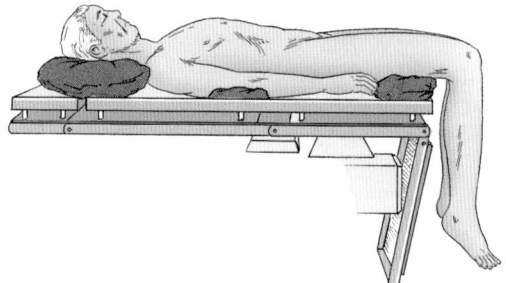

Fig. 45.2 Positioning for knee procedures.

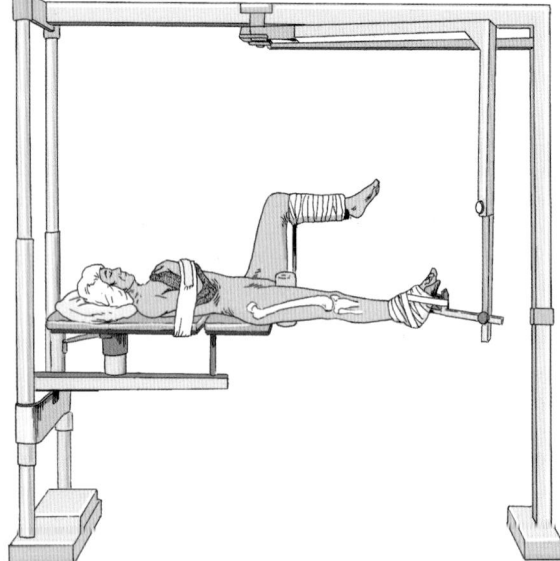

Fig. 45.3 Fracture table. Allows easy access for x-ray equipment.

BOX 45.1   **Signs and Symptoms of Tension Pneumothorax**

- Sudden, inexplicable hypoxemia
- Elevated central venous pressure
- Tachycardia
- Absent breath sounds on the affected side
- Cyanosis
- Diaphoresis
- Decreasing oxygenation
- Tracheal shift
- Agitation and anxiety (may be observed in patients receiving regional anesthesia)
- Hypotension
- Jugular vein distention
- Increased airway pressure
- Asymmetric chest wall movement
- Percussive hyperresonance over the affected side

the surgery: either the lateral decubitus or the modified Fowler (beach chair) position.[40] Patients undergoing elbow arthroscopy may be placed in the supine, lateral decubitus, or prone position; the position is dictated by operative necessity and surgeon preference. The prone position is advantageous primarily because of better limb stability during the procedure.[41] Hip arthroscopy is also typically accomplished via the lateral decubitus or the supine position, with the patient on a fracture table (Fig. 45.3). Detailed physiologic changes and complications relative to positioning can be reviewed in Chapter 23.

Complications

Complications associated with arthroscopic procedures occur in a small percentage of the total number of procedures performed.[42-45] They include subcutaneous emphysema, pneumomediastinum, and potentially life-threatening tension pneumothorax. The full range of potential anesthetic complications associated with patient positioning applies (e.g., inadvertent extubation, eye or corneal injury, visual loss from the prone position, and nerve injury from improper patient positioning). Blood loss is not generally a concern, but significant and sustained hypotension warrants immediate and thorough investigation. A pneumatic tourniquet may be used to provide a clear, bloodless surgical field. Trocar insertion sometimes results in inadvertent damage to vascular structures that may go undetected because of the tourniquet. In procedures that are performed proximally (i.e., hip or shoulder) and therefore without a tourniquet, vascular damage is discovered much earlier.

To provide optimal visualization of joint structures during arthroscopic procedures, the irrigating fluid used to distend the operative joint is instilled under pressure. This is achieved through gravity or mechanical pressurization. The typical irrigation setup uses large (3–5 L) bags of irrigating solution. The amount of fluid being infused in comparison with the outflow should be monitored. Even small differences can add up to a large volume for the patient, especially in the case of an extended procedure. This absorption could potentially lead to fluid volume overload, congestive heart failure, pulmonary edema, or even hyponatremia (if sterile water is used).[42-45]

Subcutaneous emphysema, tension pneumothorax, and pneumomediastinum have been reported during shoulder arthroscopy when subacromial decompression is used.[45] These complications appear to be associated in part with the use of mechanical irrigation pumps and power-saver suction. Careful assessment during this irrigation period is important. Box 45.1 lists the signs and symptoms associated with tension pneumothorax. Since tension pneumothorax is a potentially life-threatening event, early recognition and treatment are paramount.

ARTHROPLASTY

Arthroplasty is the surgical replacement of all (total arthroplasty) or part (hemiarthroplasty) of a joint to restore the natural motion and function of the joint, as well as restoring the controlling function of the surrounding soft tissues (i.e., muscles, ligaments, and tendons). The goals of arthroplasty are pain relief, stability of joint motion, and deformity correction. The original hip prosthesis was fabricated from stainless steel. Prostheses currently in use are stronger metal alloys based on nonferrous metals (generally cobalt or titanium). These alloys demonstrate greater tensile strength and are more resistant to fatigue than the original stainless steel. The search for stronger metals that can withstand greater amounts of abuse continues due to the increasing demand for these components to last longer. In fact, increasingly younger patients are presenting for joint replacements as people have become more active and athletic. The rigors of activities, such as running and skiing, are leading to the need for increased numbers of joint replacements in patients that are younger than ever before.[46]

Lower Extremity

Hip Arthroplasty

Several hundred thousand patients in the United States undergo some form of total hip arthroplasty (THA) each year. The mean age of patients undergoing THA is nearly 65 years, and most patients present with multiple comorbidities. Nearly 50% of these patients are obese.[47,48] THA is most often indicated for patients experiencing degenerative joint disease or arthritic damage. A report on outcomes noted that, in patients having total joint arthroplasty (TJA), younger age and male sex are associated with an increased risk of revision. Older age and male sex are associated with increased risk of postsurgical mortality, and older age is related to worse function, particularly among women. Age and sex do not influence the level of postsurgical pain. Despite these differences, all subgroups derived benefit from TJA.[49]

Anesthetic management. Several surgical approaches may be used for THA. The most common is the posterior approach, which requires a large incision extending from near the iliac crest across the joint to the midthigh level. More recently, the direct anterior approach (DAA) has gained in popularity, as it offers a minimally invasive alternative to THA. The DAA is a muscle-sparing procedure that involves a shorter incision, as well as less muscle and soft tissue dissection, resulting in shorter hospitalization and faster postoperative recovery. The DAA is technically more challenging than traditional approaches.[50,51] Regardless of the surgical approach, several large muscle groups must be incised and dissected through or separated to gain access to the joint, after which the joint is disarticulated. The muscle relaxation provided by a subarachnoid block makes this anesthetic technique ideal for facilitating the surgical process. The anesthetic plan for patients undergoing THA frequently involves the use of regional anesthesia. In the event of patient refusal or contraindication for spinal anesthetic, general anesthesia may be selected.

Patients undergoing THA utilizing an anterior approach are positioned supine on a specialized traction table. Patients being prepared for posterior THA are generally positioned in the lateral decubitus fashion. Placing the patient in a lateral decubitus position produces physiologic changes similar to those found in the supine patient.

Complications. During surgery, the femoral head and neck are excised, leaving the femoral canal open. After reaming of the femoral canal is complete, the canal is further cleaned with a sponge to prepare the surface for receipt of adhesive. Methyl methacrylate (MMA) cement may then be instilled into the femoral canal. For some procedures, usually in younger or very physically active patients, MMA is not used to secure the femoral prosthesis, and the prosthesis is referred to as being press-fit. In these cases, the femoral prosthesis is inserted into the canal and forcibly seated with a mallet. Physiologic changes (i.e., BCIS) are common with the instillation of the MMA.

There is no expert consensus as to the definition of BCIS, although it is characterized by a number of clinical features, including hypoxia, hypotension, cardiac arrhythmias, increased pulmonary vascular resistance, unexpected loss of consciousness when regional anesthesia is administered, and cardiac arrest. The etiology of these effects is poorly understood. Some theories involve the role of emboli formed during cementing and prosthesis insertion. Several mechanisms such as histamine release, complement activation, and endogenous cannabinoid-mediated vasodilation have been proposed. BCIS is most commonly associated with hip arthroplasty but may also occur during other cemented procedures, including knee arthroplasty and vertebroplasty. Although definitive studies are lacking, BCIS is estimated to occur in 2% to 17% of surgeries. It usually occurs at the following stages in the surgical procedure: femoral canal reaming, acetabular or femoral cement implantation, insertion of the prosthesis or joint reduction, and occasionally after limb tourniquet deflation.[52] Numerous patient-related risk factors have been implicated (Box 45.2).

An abrupt decrease in end tidal carbon dioxide concentration may be the first indication of clinically significant BCIS under general anesthesia. Early signs of BCIS in the awake patient undergoing

---

BOX 45.2 Significant Risk Factors for Developing Bone Cement Implantation Syndrome

- Preexisting cardiovascular disease
- Preexisting pulmonary hypertension
- American Society of Anesthesiologists class III or higher
- New York Heart Association class 3 or 4
- Canadian Heart Association class 3 or 4
- Surgical technique
- Pathologic fracture
- Intertrochanteric fracture
- Long-stem arthroplasty

Adapted from Donaldson A, et al. Bone cement implantation syndrome. *Br J Anaesth.* 2009;102(1):12–22.

---

regional anesthesia include dyspnea and altered sensorium. If BCIS is suspected, the inspired oxygen concentration should be increased to 100%, and supplementary oxygen should be continued into the postoperative period. It has been suggested that cardiovascular collapse in the context of BCIS be treated as right-sided heart failure. Aggressive fluid resuscitation is recommended, and hypotension should be treated with α-agonists.[52]

Communication between the surgical team and the anesthesia team is imperative at the time of cementing. Before cementing, the patient's blood pressure should be optimized, the patient should be placed on a 100% fraction of inspired oxygen (FiO_2), pressure bags should be available for rapid intravenous (IV) fluid administration, and IV fluid bags should be full or nearly full. It is also important to document the cement time on the anesthesia record. After cementing is complete, the acetabular component is secured in place with screws and bone grafting.

Knee Arthroplasty

Total knee arthroplasty (TKA) is the other frequently performed joint replacement procedure. The pneumatic tourniquet is placed circumferentially over the thigh to decrease blood loss and maintain a full view of the joint for the surgeon. Nevertheless, blood loss as a result of TKA can be greater than 1 L.[53] During the procedure, the articulating surfaces of the femur and tibia are excised via precise angular cuts, and the patellar articulating surface is shaved, all to conform the bones to surfaces of the prostheses. Both the femoral and tibial surfaces are covered with MMA cement, and the individual prosthesis components are forcibly seated with a mallet. The high-density polyethylene patellar component is cemented and seated with a viselike clamp. The medial and lateral menisci are replaced with a conforming wedge of high-density polyethylene. The same considerations related to MMA as discussed in hip arthroplasty apply for this procedure.[54]

Ankle Arthroplasty

Ankle arthroplasty is performed for several orthopedic problems. The most common intraarticular procedures are osteochondral lesion, ankle or subtalar debridement, subtalar fusion, and partial talectomy. The most common extraarticular procedures are os trigonum excision, tenolysis of the flexor hallucis longus tendon, and endoscopic partial calcanectomy. End-stage OA of the ankle is a major cause of pain and disability.[55] Arthroscopy is used not only to evaluate and treat intraarticular abnormalities but also to perform endoscopic and tendoscopic procedures.[56] A tourniquet may be used to facilitate a bloodless field. Deep vein thrombosis (DVT), pulmonary embolism (PE), and fat embolism are all associated with ankle arthroplasty.

Anesthetic management. Ankle arthroplasties can be performed with either a regional or a general anesthetic technique. Ankle procedures that require a tourniquet are commonly performed under spinal or epidural anesthesia. A combination of regional techniques may be used, such as spinal anesthesia for the surgical procedure followed by a popliteal, femoral, or combination of leg blocks for postoperative analgesia.[57,58] Regional anesthesia that combines sciatic and femoral nerve blocks is sufficient for all surgical procedures below the knee that do not require a thigh tourniquet. The femoral nerve innervates the medial leg to the medial malleolus, and the remainder of the leg below the knee (including the foot) is innervated by the common peroneal nerve and tibial nerve, both of which are branches of the sciatic nerve. The sciatic nerve is usually blocked high in the popliteal fossa to ensure anesthesia of the tibial and peroneal nerves.[59]

Upper Extremity Arthroplasty

The number of shoulder arthroplasties, particularly total shoulder arthroplasties (TSA), performed is rapidly increasing. The use of reverse total shoulder arthroplasty (RTSA), which was approved by the Food and Drug Administration in 2003, may be part of the reason for this increase, as it provides a better treatment option for more complex pathologies, rotator cuff tears, and revision of failed TSAs.[60,61]

The goals of TSA include pain reduction and improved range of motion. Indications for shoulder arthroplasty include posttraumatic brachial plexus injuries, paralysis of the deltoid muscle and rotator cuff, chronic infection, failed revision arthroplasty, severe refractory instability, proximal humerus fracture, and bone deficiency after resection of a tumor in the proximal aspect of the humerus.[60] TSA is performed with the patient in either the lateral decubitus or modified Fowler (beach chair) position (Fig. 45.4) Arthroscopy often represents an efficacious and less invasive option compared to arthroplasty, and it may be used for diagnostic purposes or to treat OA, impingement syndromes, and rotator cuff tears.[38] Because a pneumatic tourniquet cannot be used, shoulder arthroplasty is associated with higher amounts of blood loss.

Elbow arthroplasty is performed less frequently than shoulder arthroplasty. The goals for elbow arthroplasty are much the same as for shoulder arthroplasty: pain relief and improvement in joint function. The indications for elbow arthroplasty include RA, traumatic arthritis, and ankylosis of the joint.[38]

Elbow arthroplasty can be performed in any of three positions: supine (see Fig. 45.2), lateral decubitus, or prone (Figs. 45.5 and 45.6). The deciding factors on which position to use for this procedure are surgeon preference and health of the patient. Elbow arthroplasty can be managed by general anesthesia and/or supraclavicular, intraclavicular, interscalene, or brachial plexus blockade. During elbow arthroplasty, a pneumatic tourniquet is generally used to minimize blood loss and provide a clear surgical field. It is necessary to be prepared to treat the patient's tourniquet pain whenever regional anesthesia is used. Any time a pneumatic tourniquet is used, the risk of thromboembolism exists. This risk is increased in those patients with a history of VTE.[62]

Anesthetic Management

Patients undergoing TSA can be managed by general anesthesia, interscalene blockade, or supraclavicular blockade. Combined regional and general anesthesia is commonly used. It is important to be mindful of the ongoing potential for inadvertent extubation, which may occur as a result of patient positioning, as well as surgical manipulations close to the patient's head and neck. The patient's neck may be subjected to excessive stretch during the surgical manipulations, and, if the patient's head becomes dislodged from the supportive device used, there is the potential for cervical spine injury. It is essential to carefully monitor the patient's eyes for pressure throughout the surgery.

Complications

For patients undergoing shoulder surgery in the beach chair position, pulmonary function will more closely resemble normal function

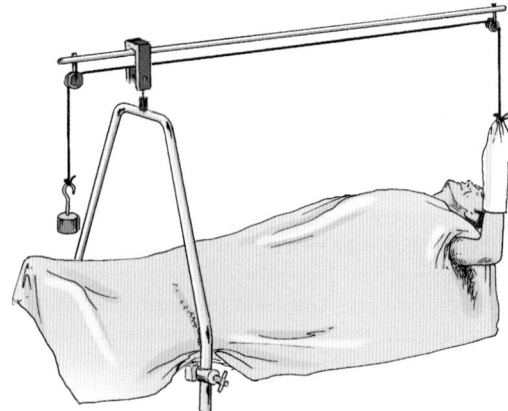

Fig. 45.5 Supine position for elbow surgery.

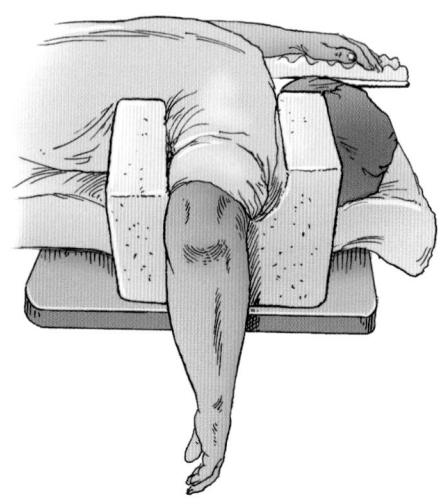

Fig. 45.6 Prone position for elbow surgery.

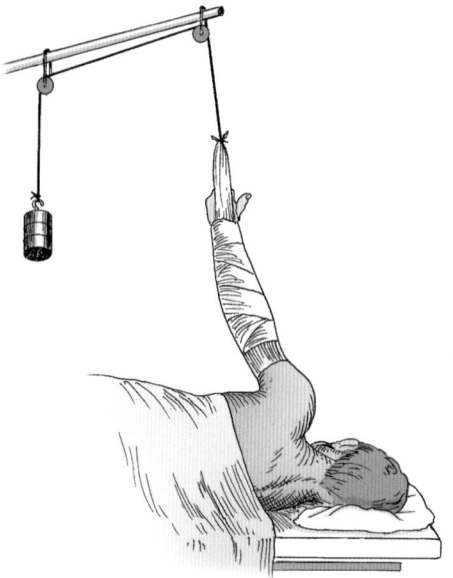

Fig. 45.4 Shoulder arthroscopy positioning.

than in the lateral position. The potential for venous air embolism is increased in this position. The risk of fat or bone marrow embolism and thromboembolism is incumbent with the required reaming of the shaft of the humerus. The potential cardiovascular effects of MMA cement also must be considered if the humeral component is cemented in place. The sitting position may result in cerebral ischemia in patients who develop hypotension.[63] Blood pressure measurements obtained on the arm are higher and not reflective of pressure within the circle of Willis. Complications during shoulder arthroscopy in the beach chair and lateral decubitus positions are compared in Table 45.3. Approaches for preventing position-related complications during shoulder arthroscopy are described in Table 45.4.

Postoperative visual loss may be especially problematic in patients having arthroscopic procedures that make deliberate use of hypotensive techniques. When intraoperative hypotensive techniques are used, cerebral perfusion and blood supply to the cranial nerves, including the optic nerve, are diminished. Intraoperative cerebral ischemia resulting from hypoperfusion has been reported. The decreased cerebral perfusion is likely due to several factors, including the decrease in blood pressure associated with anesthesia and an upright position. Other factors include failure to correct for the cerebral pressure being lower than the point of blood pressure measurement, and vascular compromise related to malpositioning of the head and neck, probably through changes in cerebral blood flow from a combination of postural hypotension and excessive head and neck manipulation. Pressure measurements must be assessed at the level of the brain because autoregulation occurs in the intracranial arterioles and capillaries. When the patient is seated upright, there is a significant hydrostatic gradient between the brain and the site of blood pressure measurement. The magnitude of the gradient is approximately 2 mm Hg per inch of height differential. When the cuff is on the upper arm, this difference can easily be 25 mm Hg. Failure to properly measure the blood pressure may lead to an inaccurate assessment of the patient's true cerebral perfusion.[64]

Hypotensive bradycardic episodes (HBEs) are a relatively common adverse effect of shoulder arthroscopy and may lead to potentially devastating complications. HBEs have been defined as a decrease in heart rate of at least 30 beats per minute within a 5-minute interval, any heart rate less than 50 beats per minute, and/or a decrease in systolic blood pressure of more than 30 mm Hg within a 5-minute interval or any systolic pressure below 90 mm Hg. These transient but profound hypotensive and/or bradycardic events have been reported in almost 30% of patients undergoing shoulder surgery in a semiupright position under an isolated interscalene block anesthetic. The etiology of these HBEs is unknown, but the most common proposed mechanism is the activation of the Bezold-Jarisch reflex (BJR).[65]

The BJR is a cardioinhibitory reflex mediated by intracardiac receptors responsive to volume, pressure, and chemical stimuli, as well as the heart's inotropic state. The afferent limb consists of unmyelinated vagal fibers, and the efferent limb augments vagal tone while simultaneously inhibiting sympathetic output. The net physiologic effect consists of vasodilation and bradycardia that, in some cases, may progress to asystole. In essence, activation of the BJR slows the heart to allow it adequate time to fill. Paradoxically, this occurs at the expense of cardiac output and systemic perfusion. In the case of surgical positioning with the patient in the beach chair position, pooling of blood in the lower extremities reduces venous return. Subsequent sympathetic activation, along with systemic absorption of epinephrine if it was included in a regional block, enhances the inotropic state of the heart. Taken together, an underloaded, hypercontractile ventricle may activate the BJR leading to vagally mediated bradycardia and hypotension that may be difficult to remedy.

The first descriptions of HBE, historically, were in patients receiving spinal anesthesia for a variety of surgeries. The mechanism clearly involves sympathetic blockade; however, decreased sympathetic tone to the heart with decreased cardiac filling is an important contributor. It has been proposed that epinephrine used with the local anesthetics for interscalene block may contribute to HBE by increasing cardiac hypercontractility, as well as exacerbating the position-related hypovolemic state.

It is possible that, when administered in a regional block, epinephrine is absorbed slowly, thereby physiologically mimicking low-dose IV administration. At such concentrations, epinephrine could predispose to HBE by increasing cardiac contractility, resulting in ventricular emptying, increasing heart rate (which reduces cardiac filling), and increasing peripheral vasodilation and pooling (decreased afterload); these factors ultimately create ventricular hypovolemia with hypercontractions.

TABLE 45.3 Position-Related Complications During Shoulder Arthroscopy

Beach Chair	Lateral Decubitus
Hypotensive bradycardic events with interscalene block (4%–29%)	Temporary paresthesia (10%)
Cervical plexus and hypoglossal nerve neurapraxias	Neurapraxias of the dorsal digital nerve of the thumb and the musculocutaneous, ulnar, and axillary nerves
Air embolism/pneumothorax	Permanent neurapraxia (2.5%)
Deep vein thrombosis	Risk of musculotendinous nerve injury (5-o'clock portal) (rare)
Unilateral vision loss and opthalmoplegia	Postoperative stroke
Cerebral hypoperfusion event	Deep vein thrombosis
	Fluid-related obstructive airway compromise

Adapted from Rains DD, et al. Pathomechanisms and complications related to patient positioning and anesthesia during shoulder arthroscopy. *Arthroscopy.* 2011;27(4):543–541; Li X, et al. A comparison of the lateral decubitus and beach-chair positions for shoulder surgery: advantages and complications. *J Am Acad Orthop Surg.* 2015;23(1):18–28.

TABLE 45.4 Prevention of Position-Related Complications During Shoulder Arthroscopy

Beach Chair	Lateral Decubitus
Reference systolic pressures at level of brain	Use of safe shoulder positions when arm is placed in traction 45 degrees of forward flexion with 90 degrees of abduction 45 degrees of forward flexion with 0 degrees of abduction
Attentive care to intraoperative head positioning	Placement of anterior inferior portal out of traction
Consider use of HBE prophylactic measures when using interscalene block	Consider use of general anesthesia for longer cases

HBE, Hypotensive bradycardic episodes.
From Rains DD, et al. Pathomechanisms and complications related to patient positioning and anesthesia during shoulder arthroscopy. *Arthroscopy.* 2011;27(4):543–541.

Prophylaxis to prevent HBE includes aggressive treatment of fluid deficits and blood loss. Minimize venous pooling in the upright position with support stockings. Avoid the use of local anesthetics containing epinephrine and consider the use of intraoperative β-blockade in select patients.[64]

FOOT AND ANKLE SURGERY

Each of us is acutely aware of any problems with our ankles or feet. They carry the weight of our body around, and we can feel any compromise in their integrity almost immediately. Patients may seek the care of an orthopedic surgeon for problems with their feet, or they may see a doctor of podiatric medicine. Both these specialists are highly skilled in the surgical correction of the multitude of problems that occur with the feet and ankles.[66]

The most commonly performed procedures on the ankle involve surgical repair of ankle fractures and fusion of the ankle joint. The Achilles tendon is also a frequent focus of surgery, particularly in more physically active individuals. The most widely known surgical procedures on the feet are bunionectomy (with or without fusion), correction of hammertoe deformities (with or without fusion), and plantar fasciotomy (either open or endoscopic).

Open repair of ankle fractures is usually accomplished using plates and screws to hold the bone fragment in proper alignment until the fragments grow back together. Ankle fusion (arthrodesis) is performed for a multitude of medical reasons and may involve two or three bones being fused to provide pain relief and greater joint stability. Incisions are usually made on both the medial and lateral aspects of the ankle joint to allow for optimal surgical access to the involved bones. The fracture is reduced, after which a plate is placed across the fracture site or sites. Holes are drilled with the plate acting as the template, and screws are placed into these holes. For ankle fusions, incisions are typically made across the medial and lateral aspects of the joint, and wires or screws are used to fuse the appropriate bones in place. The incisions are closed, and some type of inflexible stabilizing device is applied (e.g., cast, plaster splints, or ambulatory boot) while the patient is under anesthesia. Pneumatic tourniquets are almost always used to keep blood loss at a minimum and provide a clear surgical field.

Bunion deformity usually involves the first, or great, toe. The incision is made along the anterior surface from about midtoe across the metatarsophalangeal joint. The bony deformity is excised. Depending on the variation of the bunionectomy procedure chosen, excision of the bony deformity may be the totality of the procedure or the angular deformity may be corrected with a screw or wire fusion.

Hammertoe deformity correction involves incision of the anterior surface of the malformed toe or toes. The incision crosses the joint containing the bony deformity. The surgeon dissects down to the joint and excises the bony deformity. Depending on the severity of the deformity, the interphalangeal joint may be fused by inserting a wire.

Plantar fasciotomy is indicated for severe foot pain during or after ambulating or on arising after sleep. Pain results from chronic plantar fasciitis that has not responded to conservative therapy. Open fasciotomy is accomplished via a small incision along the posterior surface of the calcaneus. The plantar fascia is incised to relieve the tension across the plantar arch. Endoscopic plantar fasciotomy is accomplished via two "miniature" incisions, one medial and one lateral, at the beginning of the plantar arch. A small trocar is inserted through these incisions. The sheath of the trocar is slotted to allow visualization of the plantar fascia with the endoscope. The full thickness of the plantar fascia is incised, and the skin incisions are closed.

Anesthetic Management

Patients scheduled for foot or ankle surgery are excellent candidates for regional anesthesia. Most surgical procedures on the foot or ankle can be accomplished within a 2-hour time period, often on an outpatient basis. Spinal anesthesia provides sufficient surgical anesthesia to allow the completion of most procedures. However, the postanesthesia recovery phase may be long and require an overnight stay in the hospital or outpatient facility, which may be unacceptable to the patient.

Nerve blocks are especially effective for surgical procedures on the foot or ankle. IV sedation by either continuous infusion or intermittent bolus can provide amnesia and minimize or eliminate any anxiety the patient may have. The surgeon can inject the surgical site with long-acting local anesthetic (e.g., bupivacaine) to maintain the patient's comfort immediately and for several hours postoperatively.

FOREARM AND HAND SURGERY

Surgical procedures on the hand or forearm may be precipitated by trauma resulting in complex or dislocated fractures to the bones of the forearm, hand, or fingers, or may be performed to alleviate numbness of the hand resulting from compression of the nerves of the forearm or wrist, as in carpal tunnel syndrome. Procedures on the fingers and hand are often relatively quick, requiring 1 hour or less to complete, whereas surgical correction of complex or dislocated fractures of the forearm may require considerable instrumentation and time to complete. For virtually all surgical procedures of the hand and forearm, a pneumatic tourniquet is used.

Anesthetic Management

Patients scheduled for surgical procedures on the forearm or hand are good candidates for regional anesthesia. Ultrasound-guided brachial plexus blockade or an IV regional block (Bier block) provides excellent surgical anesthesia for most surgical procedures of the forearm and hand anticipated to last less than 1 hour. A Bier block is a simple and inexpensive regional technique, but it is associated with serious complications and even death. Local anesthetic systemic toxicity (LAST) is the leading cause of complications, with seizures and cardiac arrests being the most severe. As little as 1.4 mg/kg of lidocaine can lead to a seizure, and a dose of 2.5 mg/kg can lead to cardiac arrest. Symptoms can still be seen in some patients as late as 60 minutes of tourniquet time and in those individuals with tourniquet pressures set as high as 150 mm Hg above systolic blood pressure.[67] As with any procedure, it should be used only by those experienced with the technique. For more information on Bier blocks, see Chapter 50.

For procedures that may require considerable amounts of time to accomplish (e.g., those precipitated by traumatic injury such as complex, comminuted fractures or reconstruction of the vascular and nerve structures of the hand or forearm), the better anesthetic choice may be general anesthesia. Tourniquet pain becomes an issue with longer procedures if regional anesthesia is chosen. Also, for the patient requiring surgery caused by traumatic injury, the patient's nothing-by-mouth (NPO) status becomes important. Frequently, trauma patients have eaten or ingested liquids close to the time of the injury. For these reasons, rapid sequence induction of general anesthesia may be a more appropriate anesthetic course.

SPINAL SURGERY

Back injuries account for a large percentage of work-related injuries and are a leading cause of work absences. Occupational factors suspected of accelerating spinal degeneration include accident-related trauma; heavy physical loading, lifting, bending, and twisting; prolonged sitting, including while driving; and sustained nonneutral work postures.[68,69]

The most common indications for spinal surgery are intervertebral disc herniation and spinal stenosis. This pathology can occur anywhere along the spinal column from C2-C3 through the L5-S1 vertebrae. Bony decompression by laminectomy is considered the gold standard surgical approach for spinal stenosis. Surgical intervention via the posterior approach consists of a midline incision and tissue dissection to expose the disc herniation or stenotic areas. Surgery is undertaken to relieve the pressure on the nerve root that is causing the pain. Bony decompression may lead to spinal instability, and surgical lumbar interbody fusion (LIF) may be performed in addition to laminectomy.[70]

In addition to providing spinal stability, LIF may be used to treat spinal deformity and radiculopathy secondary to degenerative disc disease. Several techniques can be used to accomplish this fusion, including bone grafting via allograft or iliac autograft, the use of pedicle screws, or the use of cage devices. Approaches for LIF include anterior, lateral, posterior, and transforaminal. The posterior and transforaminal approaches are the most common. The fusion of two or more adjacent vertebrae through the disc space immobilizes the intervertebral joint and prevents painful movement. The goal of LIF is to prevent further degeneration and loss of the surgical correction achieved.[70-72] Cervical radiculopathy caused by nerve root compression may also be surgically managed. Surgical options include anterior cervical decompression and fusion, cervical disc arthroplasty, and posterior foraminotomy.[73]

Although surgical treatment of degenerative joint disease is most often achieved by fusion, some patients, particularly younger individuals, undergo total disc replacement.[74] Total disc replacement procedures are most commonly accomplished via an anterior approach. Anterior approaches to spinal surgery often require the assistance of a general surgeon to aid in the displacement of organs and vasculature.[72-75] A double-lumen tube may be used for lung isolation to facilitate surgical exposure. Fusion within the cervical spine is most often accomplished by initial discectomy followed by the insertion of a wedge-shaped bone graft (often cadaveric) or by fusion of the joint with a plate and screws.

Minimally Invasive Techniques

In the past, laminectomies required large incisions to afford the surgeon optimal visualization of the affected area of the spinal column. Currently, less invasive techniques that make use of the microscope afford the surgeon better visualization while eliminating the need for the large incisions that were commonplace in the recent past, even for straightforward, "simple" lumbar laminectomies. Also, the smaller incision results in reduced blood loss, faster wound healing, less trauma to surrounding soft tissues, shorter recovery, shorter length of hospitalization, and quicker return to a preinjury level of activity.[76]

Minimally invasive techniques are also being used for noncomplex spinal procedures. Percutaneous endoscopic lumbar discectomy is the technique of choice for minimally invasive spine surgery.[77] Other procedures that may be treated with minimally invasive techniques include vertebroplasty and kyphoplasty, cervical discectomy and foraminectomy, and intradiscal electrothermal therapy. The procedures are performed in an interventional radiology suite and usually require local anesthesia with IV sedation. General anesthesia is occasionally used for difficult procedures, and low-dose propofol, remifentanil, or dexmedetomidine infusions have all been used successfully for monitored anesthesia care.[78] The greatest anesthetic challenge may be positioning because these patients often have severe osteoporosis and other spinal deformities. They are often elderly and

have significant comorbidities, so thorough preoperative workup and preparation are essential.[79] Adequate postoperative analgesia improves recovery[80]

Complex Surgeries

Complex spinal surgery presents several anesthetic challenges, including airway control, positioning, fluid and blood transfusion management, hemodynamic control, and postoperative analgesia. Scoliosis is a good example of a complex case. With the large incision and complex dissection required for the multilevel spinal fusions and instrumentation, significant blood loss may occur. Procedures more likely to be associated with major blood loss are those involving the thoracic spine, particularly for malignancy or trauma. Autologous blood donation, the use of cell salvage devices, and serial monitoring of hemoglobin, hematocrit, and urine output are all used to manage fluid and transfusion therapy. Goal-directed fluid therapy based on stroke volume variation has been shown to reduce blood loss and the need for transfusion. Furthermore, it is associated with less postoperative pulmonary complications, a quicker return of bowel function, and shorter intensive care unit stays. The choice of anesthetic drugs is standard, with consideration for evoked-potential monitoring and postoperative analgesia included as part of the plan.

Scoliosis correction with large-scale instrumentation (e.g., Harrington instrumentation) is a major surgical intervention. Scoliosis is a lateral curvature of the spinal column by more than 10 degrees. Eighty percent of scoliosis cases are idiopathic. Other causes of scoliosis include congenital skeletal abnormalities, neuromuscular disease, neurofibromatosis, or irritative phenomena resulting from spinal cord compression from a tumor. If left untreated, scoliosis can lead to 3D structural deformities, including rotation in the transverse plane, curvature in the anterior-posterior plane, and angulation in the sagittal plane. Scoliosis may result in chronic pain, neurologic and cardiopulmonary compromise, and cosmetic concerns.[81] Treatment pathways are determined by the severity and cause of the deformity and may be nonsurgical or surgical.

Surgical intervention consists primarily of fusion of multiple joint spaces, with or without anterior release, and may include extensive instrumentation (e.g., Harrington rods or other instrumentation). Scoliosis repair may require anterior or posterior approaches or a combination of both. Any approach is a major surgical undertaking, but the anterior approach is more technically involved. The anterior approach to the thoracic spine is accomplished through a thoracotomy incision, so it requires the patient to be placed in the lateral decubitus position. Scoliosis of the lower thoracic to the upper lumbar spine may necessitate a thoracoabdominal incision and require the patient to be placed in a semilateral position.

Entry into the thoracic cavity necessitates placement of a double-lumen endobronchial tube so the ipsilateral lung can be deflated to facilitate visualization of the thoracic spine. Intubation may be difficult if the patient has a severe deformity. For surgical correction of scoliosis by spinal fusion with an anterior release, the patient is placed in the lateral decubitus position for the thoracotomy incision and will require endobronchial intubation. Depending on the direction of the curvature of the thoracic spine, the heart may need to be manipulated, which may produce cardiac dysrhythmias. In patients who are myelopathic or have cervical spine instability, a fiberoptic or other assisted device intubation, either awake or after the induction of general anesthesia, may be indicated. This may also be necessary for patients who have undergone previous spinal fusion with limitation of neck extension. In the anesthetized patient, evoked potentials can be measured before and after intubation, as well as before, during, and after positioning.[82]

BOX 45.3   Advantages of Laparoscopy for Anterior Spinal Surgery

- Enhanced visualization
- Decreased potential for infection
- Reduced trauma to surrounding soft tissues
- Shorter hospitalization
- Shorter rehabilitation period
- Decreased blood loss
- Improved intraoperative and postoperative ventilation
- Reduced intensive care unit time
- Better cosmetic appearance
- Reduced overall costs

In conjunction with the development of "cage" technology, the principles of laparoscopy/endoscopy are being adapted and applied to spinal surgery. The first use of laparoscopy for lumbar discectomy was documented by Obenchain[83] in 1991. Laparoscopic techniques were first used for thoracic spinal surgery by Mack et al.[84] in 1993. Application of laparoscopic principles and techniques offers numerous advantages to anterior vertebral joint fusion (Box 45.3), the most important being better respiratory function, diminished blood loss, and shorter length of stay, resulting in decreased medical costs. The major disadvantage of using laparoscopic techniques in spinal surgery is the time it takes for the surgeon to become proficient at the technique to avoid prolonged time in the operating room. Spinal fusion via laparoscopy provides the surgeon with enhanced visualization of the surgical site, reduces operative time once the surgeon and staff have acquired and are comfortable with the necessary skills, results in greatly reduced trauma to the surrounding soft tissues, produces dramatically less blood loss, reduces recovery and rehabilitation time, greatly reduces medical costs, contributes to an earlier return to preinjury level of activity, and is aesthetically more pleasing to the patient. It is important to compensate for any hypercarbia that may accompany the insufflation of carbon dioxide, particularly during long procedures.

Not all patients are good candidates for the laparoscopic approach. It is contraindicated for lumbar repair in patients with abdominal adhesions from inflammatory processes or previous abdominal surgery, and in abdominal trauma patients. Also, patients with marked cardiac or pulmonary disease processes may not be able to tolerate the hypercarbia that can result from abdominal insufflation with carbon dioxide. Laparoscopy is currently contraindicated for thoracic spinal surgery candidates who are unable to tolerate one-lung ventilation, as well as for those with severe or acute respiratory insufficiency, high positive airway pressures, and pleural symphysis. Patients who have had previous thoracotomy or chest tube placement must be more extensively evaluated preoperatively to determine whether thoracoscopic spinal surgery should be used. Additionally, at present, patients in need of internal fixation with extensive instrumentation of the anterior spine are not considered to be candidates for thoracoscopic spinal surgery.[85]

Positioning

Most patients having spinal surgery will be placed in a prone position for surgery. Patients in this position for prolonged periods present significant challenges. It is important to maintain an adequate venous return to maintain the hemodynamics of the patient. If the increased intraabdominal or intrathoracic pressures resulting from being prone reduce venous return, the cardiac output will be reduced. In addition, placing a patient in the prone position increases both systemic and pulmonary vascular resistance. These increases lead to decreases in stroke volume and cardiac index. Adequate volume resuscitation can help maintain normal hemodynamics. Use of a support system that allows a pressure-free abdomen, such as the Jackson spine table or longitudinal bolsters for prone positioning, will minimize the effect on cardiac output.[68,69]

Respiratory dynamics are greatly affected by placing the patient in the prone position.[86] Care is taken to prevent barotrauma through appropriate changes in ventilatory settings to maintain oxygenation and positive pressures within acceptable limits. The use of pressure-controlled versus volume-controlled ventilation may allow for lower peak airway pressure in the prone position.[87]

The prone position can alter central nervous system dynamics more than the supine position, which is of particular concern if head injury or closed head pathology is present or suspected.[88] The anterior neck is particularly supple and lacks considerable bony structural and protective support. Turning an unconscious patient or a patient under general anesthesia from the supine position to the prone position, and any head rotation undertaken during positioning, must be done with great care. If the patient's head is rotated 60 degrees, compression of the contralateral vertebral artery begins to constrain blood flow; if rotated 80 degrees, the contralateral vertebral artery becomes completely occluded.[89] The carotid artery and jugular vein on the upper side of the neck can become compressed by extreme degrees of head rotation, and those on the lower side of the neck may become compressed by inappropriate head support.[68] Optimal cerebral blood flow and cerebral venous drainage only occur when the head is in a centered position.[90]

Under general anesthesia, or with a patient whose level of consciousness is already altered, the alteration in arterial blood supply to the brain may not be easily recognized. Therefore it is prudent to maintain the patient's head in a neutral anatomic alignment while in the prone position. Even if no arterial or venous compression occurs, if the patient's head rests below the level of the heart, this creates an increased risk for postoperative visual loss (see later). Whether the head is rotated to the side or placed in a neutral sagittal position, careful attention must be paid to avoiding pressure on the orbit. This can be accomplished with soft surgical pillows or one of several commercially available foam supports. The use of a Mayfield (pinned) head holder or Gardner-Wells tongs for cervical spine traction provides an additional level of stability and eliminates pressure on the face or the eyes.[90,91]

When in the prone position, the patient's abdomen should not be compressed because this will displace the organs (and therefore the diaphragm) in the cephalad direction, producing reduced functional residual capacity, reduced tidal volume, and increased airway pressures. Abdominal compression also contributes to engorgement of the epidural venous network and can be a contributing factor to greater blood loss during the surgical procedure. To avoid abdominal compression, the abdomen must be elevated from the surface of the operating room bed.

Numerous methods and devices can be used minimize abdominal compression. The simplest method is the use of bilateral prone rolls or chest rolls, which are firm but compressible pads that extend from the shoulder to the iliac crest (Fig. 45.7). Other devices include the Wilson frame (Fig. 45.8), the Relton adjustable pedestal frame (Fig. 45.9), and the Andrews frame (also known as a spinal surgery table) (Fig. 45.10). Each of these positioning devices is designed to allow the abdomen to "hang" freely and reduce the possibility of compressing major vascular structures.

The Andrews spinal surgery table is the most complex of the positioning devices. With the Andrews table, as with the other positioning devices, the patient is induced and intubated on the transport stretcher, then lifted onto the table. On initial positioning on the Andrews table, the patient lies prone with the legs resting perpendicular to the plane of the table. A buttock support is securely attached to the framework of the table, and the bony prominences of the hips and especially the

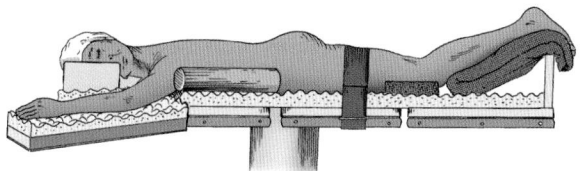

Fig. 45.7 Prone position using chest rolls.

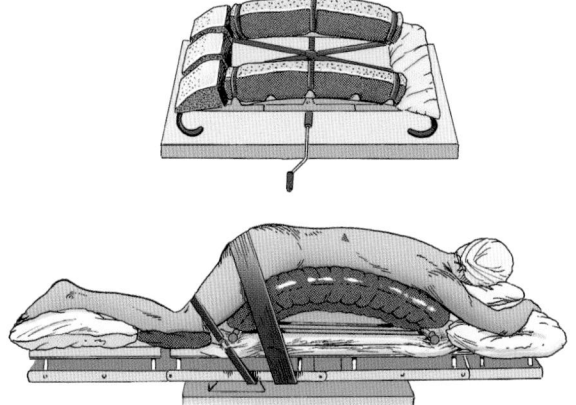

Fig. 45.8 Convex saddle frame (Wilson frame) used for spinal operations.

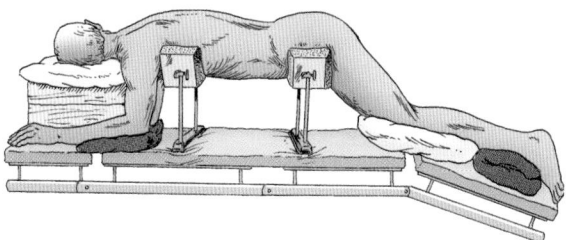

Fig. 45.9 The Relton adjustable pedestal frame.

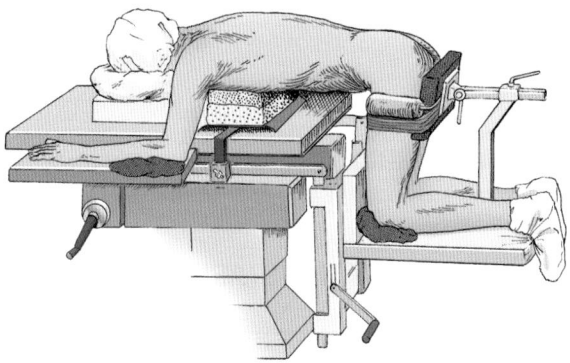

Fig. 45.10 The Andrews frame.

knees are adequately padded. The leg portion of the table is then lowered until the weight of the lower body rests on the knees, resulting in the patient's hips and knees being flexed at 90 degrees. This table produces a modified knee-chest position, allows the abdomen to hang freely, and greatly reduces the potential for compression of the major vascular structures of the lower abdomen and pelvic region (femoral arteries and veins). This position also maximizes the surgeon's visualization of the surgical site. Blood loss is decreased by using the Andrews spinal surgery table.[93,94] However, hypotension frequently occurs when this table is used as a result of blood pooling in the dependent lower

extremities. Antiembolic stockings may help counteract the tendency for blood to pool in the lower extremities, and any hypotensive event must be treated.

Anesthetic Management

General anesthesia provides the safest approach for spinal surgery. Not only is the airway secure, but muscle relaxants can be used (so long as motor-evoked potentials are not being monitored), preventing movement at critical times during surgery. Aspirin, antiplatelet drugs, and anticoagulants should be appropriately managed per institutional policy and patient status. Preoperative testing should include a complete blood count (CBC), platelet count, and coagulation studies. A preoperative chest x-ray, PFTs, electrocardiogram, and echocardiogram should be obtained, as appropriate. Evoked potentials will likely be monitored, and other neurologic testing may be performed, as indicated (see Chapters 19 and 31). The wake-up test may be performed if intraoperative neurophysiologic testing suggests unfavorable changes. First introduced in the 1970s, it was the gold standard for evaluating spinal cord injury, but its use has waned since the advent of intraoperative evoked potentials and electromyogram monitoring. Short-acting anesthetics and the ability to reverse any paralytic quickly will cut down on waiting time. If not, the patient wake-up might occur at the end of the case when everything is closed.[95]

While turning the patient, special attention must be given to the head and the endotracheal tube. Foam, gel pads, or head supports should be put in place before turning. Once the patient is turned, the first goal is to reconnect the breathing circuit and recheck the breath sounds to ascertain whether the tube is still in the correct place and has not migrated into the bronchus. The potential for eye or corneal injury is high in a prone position. Care must be taken to pad the extremities and prevent neural injury.

Complications

Postoperative Visual Loss

Postoperative vision loss (POVL) associated with general anesthesia and prone positioning in spinal surgery has increased over the past several decades. The ASA has developed a Postoperative Visual Loss Registry to better understand and evaluate this devastating operative complication. Over 93 incidents have been reported between 1999 and 2005.[82] The main causes of visual loss after nonocular surgery are retinal vascular occlusion and ischemic optic neuropathy (ION). Direct pressure to the periorbital region of the eye may cause increased pressure and blindness as a result of central retinal artery occlusion. The cause of ION is still unclear. Although it can occur in patients of any age, there is an increased incidence in patients less than 18 and greater than 65 years of age. The Postoperative Visual Loss Study Group has reported that obese and male patients have an increased risk of developing ION after major spinal surgery in the prone position. Increased intraabdominal, intrathoracic, and intraocular pressure in the prone position may lead to venous congestion and therefore contribute to the problem. Obesity, male sex, Wilson frame use, longer anesthetic duration, greater estimated blood loss, and lower percentages of colloid administration were significantly and independently associated with ION after spinal fusion surgery.[96,97] It has been speculated that estrogen has a protective effect on the optic nerve, which could explain why females are less likely to experience postoperative ION. The other five risk factors for ION are potentially related to increased venous pressure in the head with the development of interstitial edema (Box 45.4). Other researchers have also noted that significant risk factors include male sex, anemia from blood loss greater than 1 L, surgery lasting over 5 hours, and intraoperative hypotension. Volume replacement with colloid causes a smaller decrease in oncotic pressure and theoretically diminishes edema formation. This may explain why anemia alone was not identified as an independent risk factor in the multivariate analysis, as anemia may only be a surrogate marker for low oncotic pressure. Unlike corneal abrasion (the most common surgical eye injury), which is usually self-limiting, the prognosis for visual recovery from POVL is poor.[98,99]

Most cases of POVL occurring after spinal surgery are bilateral. Visual loss typically occurs within the first 24 to 48 hours postoperatively. There is usually painless visual loss, an afferent pupil defect or nonreactive pupil, and no light perception (or other visual field deficit). Color vision is decreased or absent. Elevated intraocular pressures greater than 40 mm Hg from prolonged prone positioning and fluids may be a factor. It is advisable to position a patient's head level with or above the heart, where possible, and in a neutral position.

A foam headrest should be used. Placing the head in pins is also acceptable but more invasive. For most patients in the prone position, the use of a commercial foam headrest is safe. The eyes should not be covered with goggles when using the square-shaped foam headrest. In addition, a foam headrest with a mirror attachment allows eyes to be observed easily during surgery. Ensure that the eyes are properly positioned and checked intermittently by palpation and visualization. Document eye checks at least every 20 minutes. A horseshoe headrest should not be used because of the greater risk of head movement caused by the surgeon, along with the resulting compression of the eye.[98,100-102] The ASA Task Force recommendations for the prevention of visual loss are provided in Box 45.5.[82,97,101,103] A complete discussion of postoperative visual loss can be found in Chapter 23.

Blood Loss

Sudden, dramatic, unanticipated, sustained hypotension requires rapid intervention and assessment of the cause. The surgeon should be informed, and a plan to rapidly determine the cause and initiate appropriate effective treatment measures may be instituted together. Because of the close proximity to the spinal column, injury to the aorta can occur during surgery on the thoracic or lumbar spine. In addition to aortic injury, the inferior vena cava, iliac vessels, and common femoral vessels may be damaged as a result of traction during laparoscopic spinal procedures.[85] Injury to these vascular structures can be a truly emergent situation. If the patient is in the prone position, rapid closure of the surgical wound is imperative so the patient can be repositioned, to facilitate repair of the damaged vessel. Volume resuscitation may be required in the event of an injury to a blood vessel. For this reason, it is advisable to have two large-bore IV access sites established, in addition to verifying the availability of blood. Venous air embolism can occur in certain procedures, and appropriate monitoring and vigilance are required (see Chapter 23).

The hemoglobin threshold at which red cell transfusion is warranted is controversial. Studies indicate there is no difference in

mortality, functional recovery, or postoperative morbidity between liberal and restrictive thresholds for red blood cell transfusion in people undergoing surgery for hip fracture.[104]

SPECIAL CONSIDERATIONS (ASSOCIATED CONCERNS)

Pneumatic Tourniquet

One of the methods in which blood loss can be decreased during extremity surgery is through the application of the pneumatic tourniquet. A bloodless field provides important advantages for the surgeon. Pneumatic tourniquets maintain a relatively bloodless field during extremity surgery, minimize intraoperative blood loss, aid identification of vital structures, and expedite the procedure.[105,106] The components of the pneumatic tourniquet consist of an inflatable cuff, connective tubing, a pressure device, and (usually) a timer. Specialized training and understanding of the application and management of the pneumatic tourniquet are required for proper intraoperative management of the device. Safety considerations for the use of a pneumatic tourniquet are noted in Box 45.6.

BOX 45.6 Safety Measures for Preventing Tourniquet Complications

- The tourniquet should be applied where the nerves are best protected in the underlying musculature.
- Proper functioning of the equipment should be tested before it is operated.
- The tourniquet should be used for no longer than 2 hr.
- The widest cuff possible should be chosen (wide bladders can occlude the blood flow with the use of a lower cuff pressure).
- A minimum of two layers of padding should be placed around the extremity. Check for the presence of loose fibers/lint that can become embedded in the contact closures. The best protection of the skin occurs with the use of an elastic stockinette.
- The tourniquet size should be half of the limb diameter. The cuff should overlap for 3–6 in. Large areas of overlap result in rolling and wrinkling of the underlying skin and increased pressure in that area.
- The tourniquet size chosen should allow placement of two fingers between the cast padding and the cuff.
- When possible, the extremity should be exsanguinated prior to inflation of the cuff. An Esmarch bandage is most commonly used.
- Only the minimally effective pressure should be used for occluding blood flow to the extremity. For the upper extremity, 70–90 mm Hg more than the patient's systolic blood pressure should be used. For the lower extremity, twice the patient's systolic pressure should be used. For Bier block anesthesia, a minimum standard tourniquet pressure of 250 mm Hg should be used unless the tourniquet is on the upper leg. In this instance, twice the patient's systolic pressure should be used unless that amount is <300 mm Hg.
- The pressure display must accurately reflect the pressure in the tourniquet bladder.

BOX 45.7 Physiologic Changes Caused by Tourniquets

Neurologic Effects
- Abolition of somatosensory-evoked potentials and nerve conduction occurs within 30 min.
- Application for >60 min causes tourniquet pain and hypertension.
- Application for >2 hr may result in postoperative neurapraxia.
- Evidence of nerve injury may occur at the skin level underlying the edge of the tourniquet.

Muscle Changes
- Cellular hypoxia begins to develop within 2 min.
- Cellular creatinine value declines.
- Progressive cellular acidosis occurs.
- Endothelial capillary leak develops after 2 hr.

Systemic Effects of Tourniquet Inflation
- Elevations in the arterial and pulmonary artery pressures develop. This is usually slight to moderate if only one limb is occluded.

Systemic Effects of Tourniquet Release
- Transient decrease in core temperature occurs.
- Transient metabolic acidosis occurs.
- Transient decrease in central venous oxygen tension occurs, but systemic hypoxemia is unusual.
- Acid metabolites (e.g., thromboxane) are released into the central circulation.
- Transient fall in pulmonary and systemic arterial pressures occurs.
- Transient increase in end tidal carbon dioxide occurs.

Tourniquets are most often applied after the initiation of anesthesia. The time of inflation should be documented in the anesthesia record and should match the time documented in the operating room record. The interruption of blood supply leads to tissue hypoxia and acidosis.[107] The degree of hypoxia and acidosis is partially influenced by the duration of insufflation. For this reason, the inflation device also comes with a built-in timer, generally set for 60-minute increments, with an alarm that will sound as a warning when the allotted time has been exhausted. A maximum of 2 hours is generally considered safe.[105,108] The pressure to which the tourniquet should be inflated depends on the patient's blood pressure and the shape and size of the extremity.

Deflation of the tourniquet results in the release of metabolic waste into the systemic circulation. The release of these substances can cause metabolic acidosis, hyperkalemia, myoglobinemia, myoglobinuria, and renal failure.[109,110] The deflation of the tourniquet may be marked by transient changes in the hemodynamics or pulse oximetry readings for the patient. Most of these changes resolve quickly, except in patients with extreme conditions related to their cardiac or vascular status. Box 45.7 lists common physiologic changes that occur with the release of a pneumatic tourniquet.

Nonpneumatic Tourniquets

A silicon ring tourniquet (SRT) may be used instead of a pneumatic tourniquet, particularly for brief procedures. The SRT consists of a silicone ring wrapped in a sleeve, with two pull handles connected by straps. The SRT is sterile and is rolled onto the extremity, resulting in exsanguination and occlusion of blood flow to the limb. SRTs come in various sizes and tensions based on systolic blood pressure. An appropriate model is selected based on patient size and the measured systolic

blood pressure. After surgery, the SRT is removed by cutting the silicone ring.[111] The exsanguination and tourniquet discomfort are similar to those induced by a pneumatic tourniquet, but the application time is more rapid.[112] Because these tourniquets are not electronic, they do not sound an alarm when a designated time is exceeded, so tourniquet time must be carefully monitored.

Tourniquet Pain

One of the greatest concerns when a tourniquet is in use is the patient perception of tourniquet pain. In 1944, Denny-Brown and Brenner[113] reported the first investigation into the cause of tourniquet discomfort. They listed characteristic anatomic changes associated with tourniquet ischemia that were due to acute compression of the nerves under the inflated cuff. The compression of the intraneural blood vessels caused secondary ischemia of the nerve fibers. Similar reports of "tourniquet discomfort" or "aching" despite adequate spinal anesthesia prompted the direction of considerable attention toward discovering ways to minimize subjective discomfort. Based on their discoveries and subsequent measurements of "occlusive pressure," in 1979, Klenerman and Hulands[114] suggested using tourniquet pressures of twice the patient's systolic blood pressure to minimize the subjective discomfort and destruction of tissues. Klenerman[115] modified this recommendation a year later to a value of 50 to 75 mm Hg greater than the patient's systolic blood pressure.

The ischemic pain associated with tourniquet application is similar to that of thrombotic vascular occlusion and peripheral vascular disease.[116] Approximately 45 to 60 minutes after tourniquet pressurization, patients report various symptoms that typically include dull aching, which progresses to burning and excruciating pain that may require general anesthesia. Once the pain begins, it is often resistant to analgesics and anesthetic agents, regardless of the anesthetic technique. Even with the use of a well-controlled general anesthetic at the time of tourniquet inflation, ischemic pain may begin during this same time interval and may increase the heart rate and blood pressure to the point that pharmacologic intervention is required.[117]

Although the specific neural and metabolic factors responsible for tourniquet pain are still unknown, several researchers have identified the nerve fibers that are responsible for transmitting the impulses. The burning and aching pain corresponds to the activation of the small, slow-conducting, unmyelinated C fibers. The pinprick, tingling, and buzzing sensations that frequently accompany tourniquet application often even after deflation correspond to activation of the larger and faster myelinated A-delta fibers.

Myelinated A-delta and unmyelinated C fibers differ in their sensitivity to local anesthetics. As the concentration of local anesthetic decreases, the activation of C fibers increases, but A-delta fiber activation is still suppressed. Thus C fibers may be more difficult to anesthetize than A-delta fibers, and tourniquet pain therefore seems more consistent with pain sensation carried by C fibers.[116] Other research has shown that certain local anesthetics enhance the effect of the blockade in the presence of increased stimulation of the isolated nerve fiber. For example, the potency of bupivacaine is enhanced by an increase in the rate of nerve stimulation and may offer an advantage by lowering the incidence of tourniquet pain.[118]

Regardless of the level of sensory blockade achieved in these patients, they still experience tourniquet pain. For leg surgeries, high-quality blockade of the sacral roots is more important than blockade at the thoracic sensory level for reducing the incidence of tourniquet pain because the intensity of pain may be due to ischemia of the entire leg as well as under the cuff.[119] The addition of opioids, ketorolac, melatonin, clonidine, or dexmedetomidine to local anesthesia solutions has shown some efficacy in reducing the incidence of tourniquet pain.[120-123]

Postoperative Tourniquet Paresthesia

Properly placed tourniquets inflated to appropriate pressures rarely cause injury. The use of excessive tourniquet pressure for a prolonged time may cause postoperative paresthesias that are frustrating to treat and very painful for the patient. Excessive tourniquet pressure causes deformation of the underlying nerves—the myelin may be stretched on one side of the node and invaginated on the other. Nerve damage due to the rupture of the Schwann cell membranes may also be present.[124] Use of proper padding, appropriate choice of tourniquet size, and adherence to recommendations for appropriate pressure and usage time minimize the incidence of this complication.

Thromboprophylaxis

Patients undergoing THA and TKA, as well as other orthopedic patients, are at risk for VTE, which includes DVT and PE. Most DVTs are asymptomatic, but they can lead to the same degree of long-term morbidity as symptomatic DVTs. Orthopedic surgery patients may exhibit unique coagulation factors that differ from those seen in patients undergoing other types of surgery.[125] The American College of Chest Physicians has developed evidence-based guidelines for preventing thromboembolism in orthopedic surgery. They recommend that patients undergoing major orthopedic surgery receive low molecular weight heparin; dabigatran, apixaban, and rivaroxaban (for THA or TKA, but not for hip fracture surgery); low-dose unfractionated heparin; adjusted-dose vitamin K antagonist; aspirin; or an intermittent pneumatic compression device (IPCD) for a minimum 10 to 14 days.

Thromboprophylaxis for up to 35 days is preferred. The guidelines recommend the use of low molecular weight heparin in preference to the other agents and suggest adding an IPCD during the hospital stay. In patients with an increased bleeding risk, the use of an IPCD alone with no pharmacologic prophylaxis is recommended.[126]

When planning a regional technique, great care should be given to patients on any antiplatelet or anticoagulant medications. Please refer to Chapters 14, 38, and 49. for more detail on appropriate timing of any regional technique.[127]

Surgical Care Improvement Project Protocol

SSI is a serious and potentially catastrophic complication after joint arthroplasty.[128] Hospital readmissions, additional surgical procedures, direct hospital costs, and additional care for patients both in the hospital and the rehab setting make SSIs in the orthopedic population extremely costly. Additional costs can add as much as $100,000 to the direct hospital costs per patient. Recent guidelines provide a standard approach to help prevent SSI using currently available clinical evidence.[129]

Initially, orthopedic surgeons evaluate their patients for the presence of infection before committing to joint replacement surgery.[130] Once in the operating room, all surgeons attempt to decrease the chance for SSI by the administration of appropriate preoperative antibiotics in a timely fashion. For cefazolin (a first-generation cephalosporin), the preoperative time allotment is within 1 hour of incision time; for vancomycin, it is within 2 hours of incision time (Table 45.5).[129]

Organisms commonly associated with orthopedic procedures include *Staphylococcus aureus*, gram-negative bacilli, coagulase-negative staphylococci (including *S. epidermidis*), and β-hemolytic streptococci. During arthroplasties, the additional concern of bacterial biofilms forming on implant devices can complicate antimicrobial coverage by assisting in antimicrobial resistance. Prophylactic antibiotics are not indicated in clean procedures such as diagnostic arthroscopic procedures and procedures not involving implantations. Spinal surgery with or without instrumentation should be covered by an antimicrobial agent.[129]

The Centers for Medicaid and Medicare Services introduced the program Surgical Care Improvement Project (SCIP). The goal of SCIP was to improve surgical care by defining common measures that can

TABLE 45.5 Antimicrobial Prophylaxis for Select Orthopedic Procedures		
Type of Procedure	Recommended Agents	Alternative Agents in Patients With β-Lactam Allergy
Orthopedic	None	None
Clean operations involving hand, knee, or foot not involving implantation of foreign materials	Cefazolin	Clindamycin, vancomycin
Spinal procedures with and without instrumentation	Cefazolin	Clindamycin, vancomycin
Hip fracture repair	Cefazolin	Clindamycin, vancomycin
Implantation of internal fixation devices (e.g., nails, screws, plates, wires)	Cefazolin	Clindamycin, vancomycin
Total joint replacement	Cefazolin	Clindamycin, vancomycin

From Bratzler DW, et al. Clinical practice guidelines for antimicrobial prophylaxis in surgery. *Am J Health Syst Pharm.* 2013;70(3):195–283.

be taken and providing appropriate guidelines for applying them that would decrease risks to patients when instituted. These risks may include SSI, postoperative thromboembolism, perioperative glucose management, and maintenance of normothermia. The items included on the list are constantly updated based on research findings and performance related to the measures.

Antifibrinolytic Drugs

A growing body of evidence supports the administration of tranexamic acid (TXA) to patients undergoing total joint replacement. The use of TXA has been shown to decrease perioperative blood loss and transfusion requirements with minimal risk of complications.[53,131,132] Developed in 1962, TXA is a synthetic analog of the amino acid lysine. TXA competitively blocks lysine receptors that activate plasminogen preventing the degradation of fibrin. In other words, it acts as an antifibrinolytic and maintains clot formation.[133,134]

TXA belongs to the family of antifibrinolytics that also includes ε-aminocaproic acid (EACA) and aprotinin. Aprotinin was removed from the market in 2008 because of its association with an increased mortality rate and an increased incidence in myocardial infarction (MI), stroke, and kidney failure. TXA is favored over EACA in orthopedics because it is significantly more potent, and it achieves a higher synovial concentration. Regardless of whether TXA or EACA is used, a decrease in allogeneic transfusion needs improves morbidity and saves the hospital money.[132,135]

Administering antifibrinolytics is associated with complications. These drugs have the potential to increase thromboembolic events in certain high-risk patients. Doctrine states TXA should be avoided in prothrombotic patients with a strong history of VTE, cerebrovascular accident (CVA), MI, or who have cardiac stents.[132] This belief is being challenged though, as there is increasing evidence that TXA is safe to give to high-risk patients undergoing total joint replacement and that there is no significant difference in adverse outcomes.[133,136] Theoretically, TXA increases the potential for thromboembolic complications, but multiple papers cite no clinical evidence of an increase in complications in high-risk patients receiving TXA. In fact, the clinical practice guidelines from the American Association of Hip and Knee Surgeons, American Society of Regional Anesthesia and Pain Medicine, American Academy of Orthopedic Surgeons, the Hip Society, and the Knee Society stated there was no evidence of an increased risk of thromboembolic events in patients with a history of VTE, MI, CVA, and vascular stent placement when TXA was employed, though they recognize more randomized clinical trials need to be done.[136] When making medical decisions in the real world, clinicians must balance the abovementioned statement with maintaining the safety of a patient with significant comorbidities that may include a complex prothrombotic and hypercoagulable state. At this point, TXA is still contraindicated in patients with subarachnoid hemorrhage, active intravascular clotting, and hypersensitivity to the drug. Interestingly, postoperative visual changes in acuity, color vision, and visual fields are signs of TXA toxicity. TXA is therefore contraindicated in patients with color blindness since the ability to differentiate color is required to assess for TXA toxicity in a postoperative ophthalmic exam.[137-139]

TXA (1–2 g) is administered perioperatively, either intravenously or topically at the surgical site.[53,131] In higher doses, TXA is associated with seizures, but this is mostly found in the cardiac surgical patient, where total TXA doses are typically higher.[140,141] In hip arthroplasty, Wei et al. suggest TXA should be given over 5 to 10 minutes at 5 to 20 minutes before incision. In knee arthroplasty, the best time is 5 to 20 minutes before tourniquet deflation or closure of the wound.[133] Sukeik et al. concluded that TXA given preoperatively reduced total blood loss in THA, decreased the need for transfusion, and did not increase complication rates.[142]

Fat Embolism

Fat embolism is a rare, yet deadly complication that can occur in the setting of orthopedic trauma and surgery. It is most common with single or multiple closed, long-bone fractures (particularly the femur) or pelvic fractures; however, it also can occur during THR, TKR, vertebroplasty, and procedures that require intramedullary reaming.[143-146]

Fat embolism is defined as the presence of fat globules in the systemic or pulmonary circulation. Symptoms can range from no apparent effect to mild respiratory distress to fat embolism syndrome (FES) or death.[147,148] Most occurrences of fat embolism are uneventful without noticeable sequelae.[149] The fat globules can often be visualized traveling through the heart via transesophageal echocardiography (TEE) during orthopedic surgery. Fat embolisms were found in up to 82% of blunt trauma patients during autopsy.[147]

FES occurs when a patient with a fat embolism experiences significant systemic manifestations that result in respiratory failure, neurocognitive insult, or death. Not all fat embolisms progress to FES. Consider FES at the end of the continuum of symptoms initiated by fat embolism.[147,148] The incidence has decreased significantly with changes in surgical techniques. While older literature cites an incidence of FES as high as 30%, more recent investigations note an incidence closer to 1%.[146] The International Classification of Diseases codes from the National Hospital Discharge Survey over a 26-year period that included 1 billion patients. It found among all patients with fractures the incidence was only 0.17%. Multiple fractures that included femur involvement had the highest incidence at 1.29%.[147,150]

FES typically affects the lungs, brain, and skin. More specifically, the clinical diagnosis includes the triad of hypoxemia, altered mental status, and a petechial rash.[147] Other signs include thrombocytopenia, anemia, and fever. Cardiovascular manifestations include hypotension, decreased cardiac output, and dysrhythmias.[148] Severe symptoms lead to acute respiratory distress syndrome-like distress, cerebral edema, and death.[144] In 1974, Gurd and Wilson established guidelines for the diagnosis of FES. A patient must have two of the three signs in the triad or one of the major signs in the triad and four of the following: fever, tachycardia, retinal changes, jaundice, renal changes, fat in urine or sputum, anemia, and thrombocytopenia.[151] Later, Lindeque et al. modified Gurd and Wilson's diagnosis with the addition of arterial blood gas criteria. Hypoxemia is now a major criterion. A PaO_2 of less than 60 mm Hg and hypocarbia commonly occur.[146,148]

Although the pathophysiology of FES is poorly understood, it can be explained by two hypotheses. The mechanical hypothesis posits that bone marrow intravasates into the bloodstream during trauma or reaming. Intramedullary pressures increase significantly during reaming and fractures forcing bone marrow fat into the bloodstream. These fat globules and bone fragments migrate to small pulmonary and systemic vessels, where the mechanical obstruction starves the distal tissue of oxygen and vital substrates.[143,148] The biochemical hypothesis refutes the existence of a mechanical blockage and, instead, asserts that fat in the bloodstream interacts with lipoprotein lipase to release free fatty acids. The toxic byproducts and inflammatory response that ultimately ensues cause direct injury to the parenchymal tissue leading to increased pulmonary permeability, alveolar edema, and respiratory failure.[143,147,148] Most likely, injury occurs from some combination of mechanical and biochemical causes (Fig. 45.11).[148]

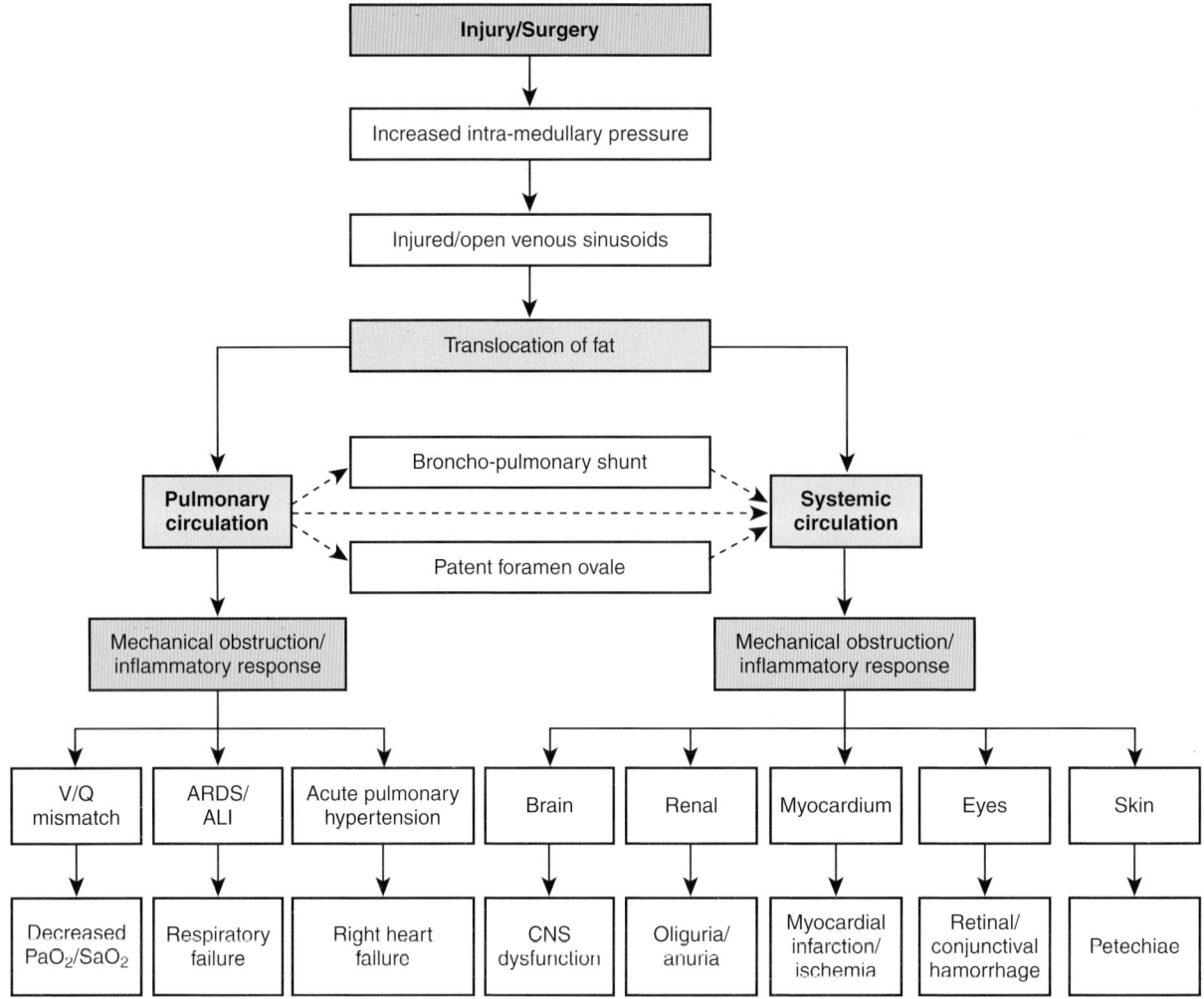

Fig. 45.11 Fat embolism. (From Akhtar S. Fat embolism. *Anesthesiol Clin.* 2009;27[3]. doi:10.1016/j.anclin. 2009.07.018.)

The diagnosis of FES is difficult.[147,148] Petechiae are only observed in 20% to 50% of patients. Interestingly, a petechial rash is usually identified on the chest, axilla, conjunctiva, and neck but never the back. This distribution occurs because most patients are supine. Fat floats to the top of the aortic arch (think oil and water) and embolizes to the nondependent portions of the body via the carotid and subclavian arteries.[146,147] Mental status changes occur in 86% of patients with FES, but these changes range from drowsiness to rigidity to convulsions and coma. Pulmonary effects usually occur first and are present in 75% of all FES patients. Actually, it is rare to encounter FES without a pulmonary component. Chest x-rays reveal diffuse evenly distributed interstitial and alveolar infiltrates.[144,148]

There are no definitive treatments or preventive measures for FES. Surgical modifications have improved the incidence of FES over the years, but anesthesia-related prophylaxis has been disappointing. Patient care with FES is supportive. There is no best anesthesia technique to decrease the possibility of FES or improve its outcome. General anesthesia and regional anesthesia are equally safe.[148] TEE during procedures has not shown to improve outcomes.[149] The renin-angiotensin pathway may play a role in FES. Besides being a potent vasoconstrictor, angiotensin II also initiates inflammation and is a profibrotic. In a recent study, a researcher treated rats with aliskiren, a renin inhibitor. Those rats treated with aliskiren displayed improved vessel diameter, decreased fibrosis, and lowered fat content. Though

not ready for clinical trials, this may have a future in providing prophylaxis against FES.[147]

Acute Extremity Compartment Syndrome

Acute compartment syndrome (ACS) is a condition in which increased pressure within a closed anatomic space compromises the local perfusion and function of the tissues within that space.[152,153] If not recognized quickly, irreversible damage can occur in the affected compartment, which can lead to infection, muscle necrosis, contractures, nerve injury, chronic pain, amputation, and death.[154] ACS can occur because of any number of conditions, but we will concentrate on how they relate to orthopedic injuries (Table 45.6).[153]

Two-thirds of all ACS diagnoses are related to fractures, and of all fractures, 75% of ACS cases occur in the lower leg. The tibial diaphysis is the most common fracture site associated with ACS because it is frequently injured and its fascial space is tight.[152,154] Other fractures associated with ACS include tibial plateau fractures, forearm diaphyseal fractures, and fractures of the distal radius.[154] As seen with the incidence of FES, closed fractures present a greater risk than open fractures.[153]

There are four muscle compartments in the lower leg: anterior, lateral, deep posterior, and superficial posterior. Soft tissue swelling and bleeding in any of these compartments can lead to compartment syndrome.[153,155]

TABLE 45.6	**Causes of Acute Compartment Syndrome**
Orthopedic	Fractures and surgical fractures
Vascular	Vascular injuries Reperfusion injury Hemorrhage Phlegmasia cerulea dolens
Soft tissue	Crushing injury Extensive burns Prolonged limb compression
Iatrogenic	Puncture in anticoagulated patients Employment of a pneumatic antishock garment (PASG) Casts and circular dressings Pulsatile irrigation
Miscellaneous	Snake venom Extreme muscle exertion

From: Köstler W, et al. Acute compartment syndrome of the limb. *Injury.* 2004;35(12):1221–1227.

Normal compartment pressures are below 10 mm Hg (Fig. 45.12A). The risk of significant injury occurs when the absolute intracompartmental pressure exceeds 30 to 50 mm Hg. More importantly, the mean arterial pressure [MAP] or diastolic blood pressure [DBP]—compartment pressure) should be above 70 to 80 mm Hg.[153] Depending on age, MAP or DBP is used. Conceptually, you can liken this pathophysiology to how cerebral perfusion pressure is critical in the setting of intracranial hypertension.[155]

Males less than 35 years of age are at the greatest risk of developing ACS. This might be explained by a higher degree of physical activity and greater muscle mass. The elderly have a lower risk because of a combination of sarcopenia (decreased muscle mass) and a higher incidence of hypertension. A higher driving pressure promotes better perfusion in the compartment, and sarcopenia allows for greater tissue expansion before the compartment pressure rises. The diagnosis and treatment of ACS are often delayed. Reasons for delayed treatment include the inexperience of the health care provider in assessing compartment syndrome, the use of general anesthesia or regional anesthesia that silences patient complaints, and multitrauma cases that can mask the specific pain caused by the compartment syndrome.[154]

ACS is difficult to diagnose with clinical signs alone. Sensitivity by this method is only 13% to 54%. Yet still, many health care providers rely solely on these.[154] The five *P*s of ACS include painful onset, pallor, paresthesia, paralysis, and pulselessness. Unfortunately, most of these are late signs.[154,155] Other major signs and symptoms include swelling and pain on passive stretch. Swelling is difficult to assess because casts may cover up evidence of swelling, or swelling is isolated in the actual compartment. Pain above expectation is usually the first and most common complaint of ACS but even this sign is not ubiquitous. Those who also experience local nerve injury or are under the influence of an anesthetic may not recognize the pain. Very young children or those patients with an inability to articulate their needs may not be able to communicate their pain. Inflammatory biomarkers may aid in the early diagnosis of ACS. Creatine, myoglobin, and fatty acid–binding protein biomarkers are released during cardiac and skeletal muscle injury. Though these markers are not specific to skeletal muscle, they can help guide the clinician toward a diagnosis of ACS when considered in context. Lactic acid is another nonspecific lab value that can be followed.[152] A delay in diagnosis can have devastating consequences. Without immediate treatment, a patient

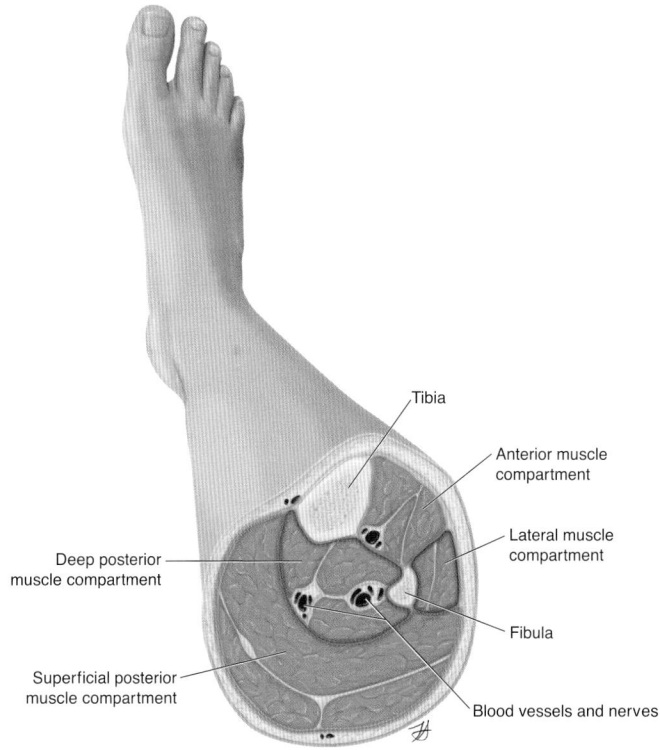

A   Compartment pressures are <10 mm Hg

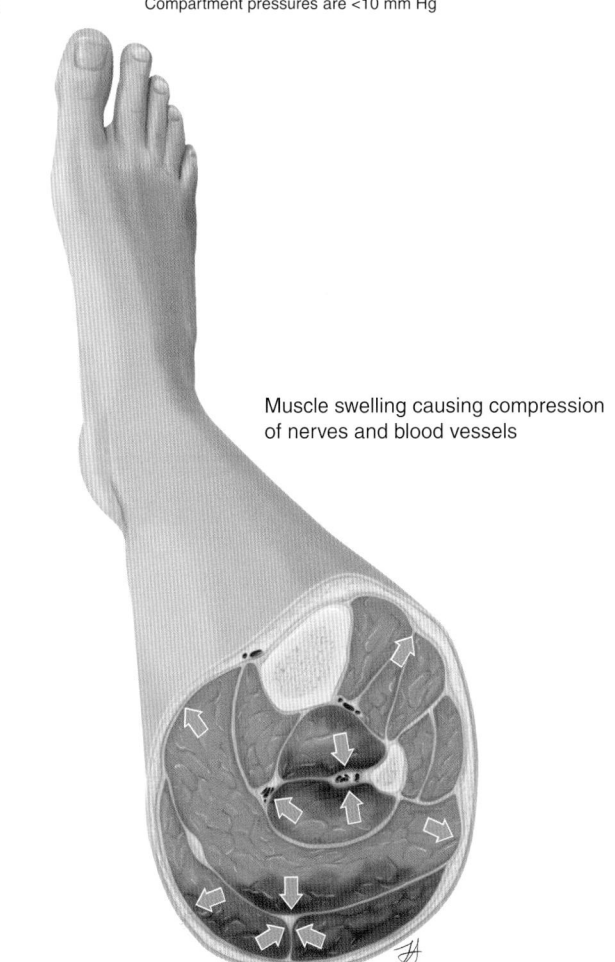

Muscle swelling causing compression of nerves and blood vessels

B   Compartment pressures are greater than 30 to 50 mm Hg absolute pressure or a delta P of <30 mm Hg for >2 hours

Fig. 45.12 (A) Healthy compartment. (B) Ischemic compartment.

could lose a limb or die. A delay that exceeds 12 hours contributes to irreversible tissue damage. Nerves are more sensitive than muscle and soft tissue.[153]

Intracompartmental pressure monitoring is the definitive diagnostic tool for ACS and is recommended for patients at risk. This should be the go-to monitor for unconscious patients or those who are unable to communicate.[152] Though its sensitivity and specificity are estimated as 94% and 98%, respectively, few institutions routinely employ this technique. This practice helps decrease the chance of irreversible ischemic changes and permanent disability.[154] There are conflicting thoughts on what absolute pressure is considered a critical threshold for morbidity and mortality. The range is relatively wide, and multiple variables play a role such as age and muscle mass. There now seems to be a consensus in using the delta P (differential pressure between the DBP and the compartmental pressure). A delta P of less than 30 mm Hg for greater than 2 hours indicates emergency fasciotomy[152-154] (see Fig. 45.12B).

Fasciotomy is the treatment of choice and should be performed to all compartments involved. The fasciotomy should remain open a minimum of 48 hours or until the pressure decreases to a safe level. In crush injuries, the addition of hyperbaric O_2 may be associated with improved recovery.[153]

SUMMARY

Orthopedic surgical procedures are varied and require a wide variety of anesthetic plans. The patient's health history, the acceptability of various anesthetic techniques to the patient, the proposed surgery and its duration, the patient's intraoperative position, and the need for postoperative pain management are important considerations in planning and preparing for a safe and comfortable outcome. In addition, many of these procedures carry a high risk for blood loss, so preoperative typing and crossmatching are indicated in nearly all these cases. The anesthetic plan must be adapted to the needs of the patient and the proposed surgery.

Developments in orthopedics over the last few decades have resulted not only in an increase in options and techniques but also in an improvement in patient outcomes. The invention of the arthroscope has diminished some of the severe consequences of certain repairs and has provided a diagnostic tool for surgeons. Coupled with this are a decreased length of stay and fewer side effects from anesthesia. Trauma and high-profile surgeries corresponding to the increasing geriatric population are challenging and require techniques that reduce complications and provide postoperative pain management.

REFERENCES

For a complete list of references for this chapter, scan this QR code with any smartphone code reader app, or visit the following URL: http://booksite.elsevier.com/9780323711944/.

46

The Immune System and Anesthesia

Bernadette T. Higgins Roche

The immune system, a combination of cells, chemicals, and physiologic processes, has evolved over time to protect the body from a wide variety of pathogenic microbes, including bacteria, fungi, protozoa, and viruses, as well as self cells with abnormal proteins. It is influenced by genetic and environmental influences, including age, gender, health status, seasonal circadian patterns, and exposure to symbiotic and pathogenic microbes.[1] A key characteristic of the immune system is the ability to distinguish between self and nonself; the ability to detect structural differences in pathogens and cells with abnormal proteins allows the immune system to effectively eliminate them without destroying normal cells.

The immune system is comprised of two subcategories, the innate (natural) immune system and the adaptive (acquired) immune system.[2-4] Together, they generate a humoral response and a cell-mediated response to pathogens. The term *humor*, a medieval term for body fluid, refers to the liquid, noncellular component of blood and lymphatic fluid. The humoral immune response is mediated by B-lymphocyte antibodies circulating in the lymph or blood. The cell-mediated response is provided by phagocytes, T lymphocytes, and cytokines. Cell-mediated immunity is directed primarily at microbes that survive in host cells. It also plays a major role in rejection of transplanted organs. Although the innate and the adaptive immune systems function differently and are historically presented as two different parts of the immune system, an effective immune response toward a pathogen requires a cooperative synergy between the two systems. The innate system generates the first line of defense; the adaptive system becomes dominant as it develops antigen-specific antibodies in response to activation by the innate system (Fig. 46.1).

THE IMMUNE SYSTEM

Innate Immune System

The innate immune system is inherited and constitutes the first line of defense to an invading pathogen.[5] It has a rapid response but lacks immunologic memory. Prior antigen exposure is not required for activation, and the response is always the same regardless of prior encounters with the same pathogen. It is not specific in its mechanism of defense and must rely on the adaptive immune system to mount a pathogen-specific response. Immune system cells are derived from hematopoietic stem cells that differentiate into a common myeloid stem cell and a common lymphoid progenitor, the precursor of the innate immune system cells. The lymphoid pathway produces lymphocytes, whereas the myeloid pathway produces granulocytes, monocytes, platelets, and red blood cells (RBCs) (Fig. 46.2). The major cellular components of the innate system include granulocytes (neutrophils, eosinophils, basophils), agranulocytes (monocytes and macrophages), dendritic cells (DCs), cytokines, and the complement system (Table 46.1).[2-5] Neutrophils, eosinophils, monocytes, macrophages, and DCs are responsible for phagocytosis, the process of ingesting and destroying pathogens such as bacteria, viruses, fungi, parasites, as well as tumor cells and apoptotic cells. Neutrophils have the fastest response to a pathogen; macrophages and DCs have a longer but sustained response. In addition to direct activation by pathogens, phagocytes are also activated by opsonization, a process where antibodies and complements (opsonins) bind to the pathogen and mark it for destruction by the phagocytes. The mononuclear phagocyte system (MPS), formerly known as the reticuloendothelial system, includes phagocytes located in reticular connective tissues, including the lymph nodes, lungs, liver, and spleen. The MPS is activated when it encounters a pathogen; in addition to phagocytosis of the pathogen, the MPS phagocytes secrete cytokines that promote the migration of neutrophils, monocytes, eosinophils, and basophils to the site of infection. They also secrete colony-stimulating factors that stimulate the production and release of additional phagocytes from the bone marrow. Erythrocytes and platelets also play a role in the innate immune response. Erythrocytes directly bind and scavenge pathogens; platelets activate the phagocytes of the innate immune system and modulate antigen presentation for an enhanced response of the adaptive immune system.[6-7] The innate system also includes surface barriers such as epithelial cell layers with tight junctions, which are present on the skin and mucous membranes of the gastrointestinal (GI), genitourinary, and respiratory tracts. The innate system is activated when a pathogen is first encountered on a surface barrier. Initial responses include sneezing, tearing, coughing, sweating, and maintenance of normal body temperature and gram-positive flora of the skin.

The cells of the innate immune system use intracellular or membrane pattern recognition receptors (PRRs) to recognize the molecular patterns of microbes.[2-5,8] The PRRs are specific for broad classes of infectious organisms, including bacterial lipopolysaccharides, peptidoglycans, bacterial deoxyribonucleic acid (DNA), and viral ribonucleic acid (RNA). The PRRs can recognize specific pathogen-associated molecular patterns (PAMPs) found exclusively on bacteria, fungi, parasites, and viruses. They also recognize danger-associated molecular patterns (DAMPs), also known as alarmins, on stressed host cells in response to infection, trauma, ischemia, and tissue damage. The Toll-like receptors (TLRs) were the first identified PRRs.[2-4,9] The TLR-2 receptor can identify gram-positive bacteria, and the TLR-4 receptor is responsible for recognition of gram-negative bacteria.[9] When a ligand binds to a TLR, the cell responds with increased production and secretion of cytokines and phagocytosis of the pathogen. Other PRRs include the Nod-like receptor (NLR), the RIG-I–like receptor (RLR), the cytosolic DNA sensor, and the C-type lectin receptor (CLR).

In addition to phagocytosis and direct destruction of microbes, phagocytes also act as antigen-presenting cells (APC) responsible for identifying and preparing a pathogen for presentation to cells of the adaptive immune system. Once the PPR receptor on the

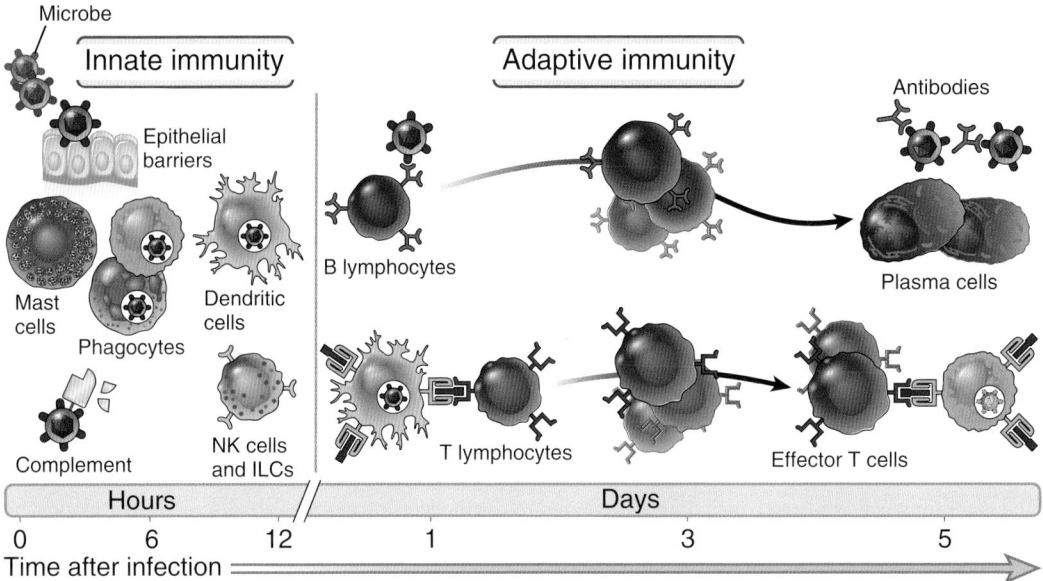

Fig. 46.1 Innate and adaptive immunity. An effective immune response toward a pathogen requires a cooperative synergy between the innate and adaptive immune systems. The innate system generates the first line of defense; the adaptive system becomes dominant as it develops antigen-specific antibodies in response to activation by the innate system. (From Abbas AK, Lichtman AH, Pillai S. *Basic Immunology: Functions and Disorders of the Immune System.* 6th ed. Philadelphia, PA: Elsevier; 2020:4.)

TABLE 46.1   Components of the Innate Immune System

Component	Type	Function
Granulocytes	Neutrophils	Prominent phagocyte of early inflammatory response; release of cytotoxic cytokines, phagocytosis; presentation of antigen to cells of adaptive immune system
	Eosinophils	Phagocytosis, release of cytotoxic cytokines, degradation of mast cell inflammatory mediators, destruction of parasites
	Basophils and mast cells	IgE receptors; release of histamine, leukotrienes, cytokines, prostaglandins, and other mediators of inflammation
Agranulocytes	Monocytes and macrophages	Prominent phagocyte of late inflammatory response; phagocytosis, release of cytotoxic cytokines
Dendritic cells		Phagocytosis, presentation of antigen to cells of adaptive immune system, release of cytotoxic cytokines
Cytokines	Interleukins	Regulation (activation and inhibition) of inflammatory response
	Interferons	Destruction of viral antigens
	Tumor necrosis factor	Mediation of inflammatory response
	Chemokines	Leukocyte chemotaxis, migration of phagocytes to site of infection, release of phagocytes from bone marrow
Complement		Opsonization of pathogens for destruction, cell lysis, leukocyte chemotaxis

phagocyte binds a pathogen, it processes it into short peptides and binds it with a self protein receptor called a major histocompatibility complex (MHC) molecule on the surface of the phagocyte.[2,4] Class I MHC proteins are essential for presenting viral antigens; they are found on nearly every cell type with the exception of RBCs. Class II proteins are only found on B cells, DCs, monocytes, and macrophages (Fig. 46.3). The T cells of the adaptive immune system can only recognize a nonself target after it has been processed and presented in combination with a MHC molecule by an APC of the innate immune system; this allows the T cells to ignore free extracellular antigens and focus on antigen-infected cells. Cytotoxic or killer T (Tc) cells only recognize antigens coupled to class I MHC molecules, whereas helper T (Th) cells and regulatory T (Treg) cells only recognize antigens coupled to class II MHC molecules. In humans, MHC molecules are classified as human leukocyte antigens (HLA). Class I MHC contains three genes (HLA-A, B, and C), and their proteins are expressed on most cells.[2,4] The proteins of class II MHC genes (HLA-DR, DQ, and DP) are expressed on APC macrophages, DCs, and B cells. Over 40 different diseases are associated with certain class I or II HLA alleles, including ankylosing spondylitis and type I diabetes mellitus. Similarities in MHC proteins allow donor and recipient matching between family members, which lowers the risk of transplant rejection.

Neutrophils

Neutrophils are the most numerous of the white blood cells (WBCs) and largely responsible for the elevated white cell count that occurs with infection (Table 46.2). They migrate rapidly to the site of bacterial infections, where they release cytotoxic cytokines and phagocytize and internally destroy microbes and particulate antigens through the production of reactive oxygen molecules that are cytotoxic to bacterial pathogens. Neutrophils have a half-life of only 6 hours and are sensitive to the acidic environment of infected tissues; dying neutrophils become part of the purulent exudate at the site of infection.

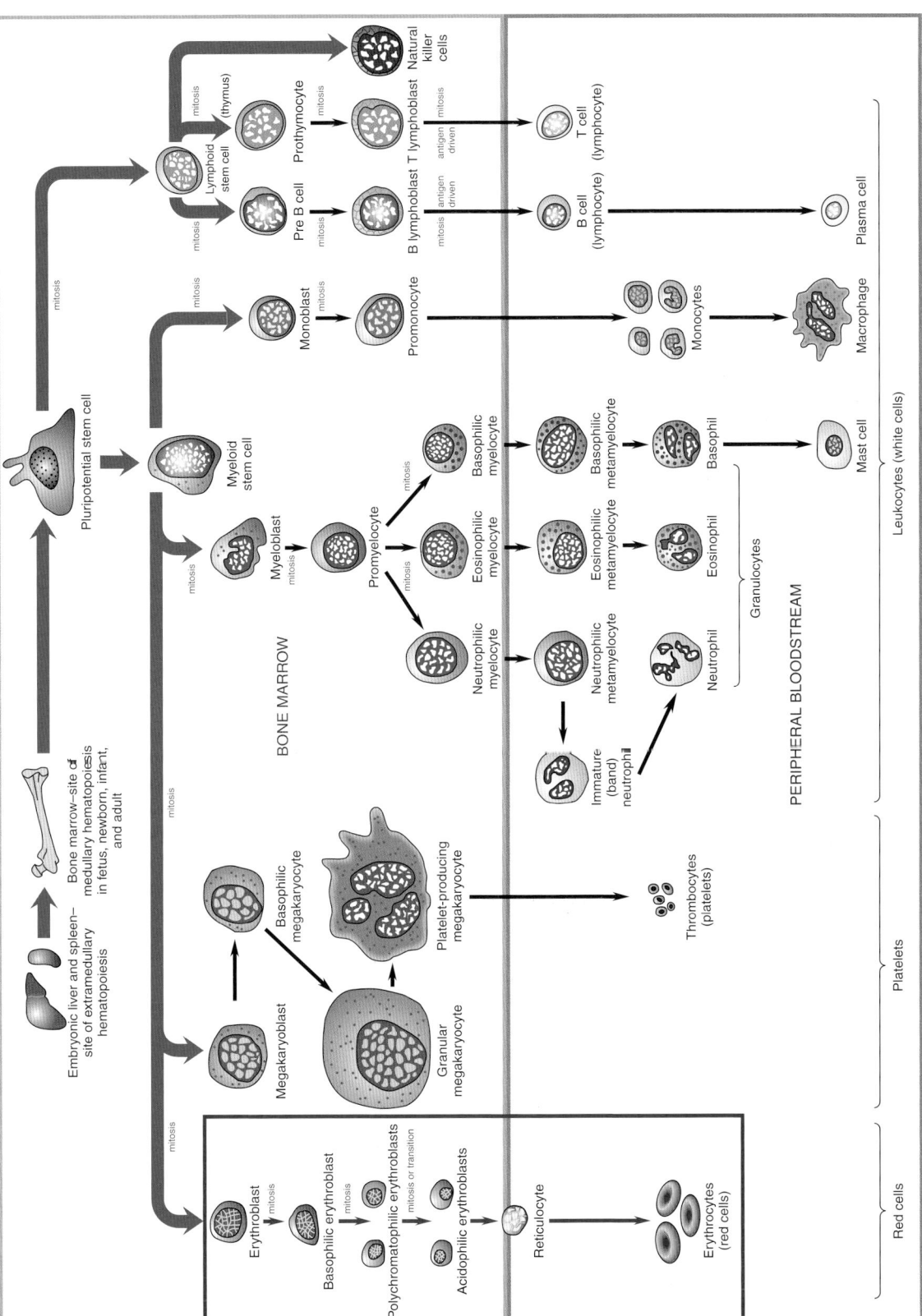

Fig. 46.2 Maturation of human blood cells showing pathways of cell differentiation from the pluripotent stem cell to mature granulocytes, monocytes, lymphocytes, thrombocytes, and erythrocytes. Production begins in embryo blood islands in the yolk sac. As the embryo matures, production shifts to the liver, spleen, and bone marrow. In an adult, nearly all hematopoiesis occurs in the bone marrow. The two major differentiation pathways are the myeloid pathway and the lymphoid pathway. The lymphoid pathway produces lymphocytes, whereas the myeloid pathway produces granulocytes, monocytes, platelets, and red blood cells. (From Copstead LE, Banasik J. *Pathophysiology*. 5th ed. St. Louis: Elsevier; 2013:160.)

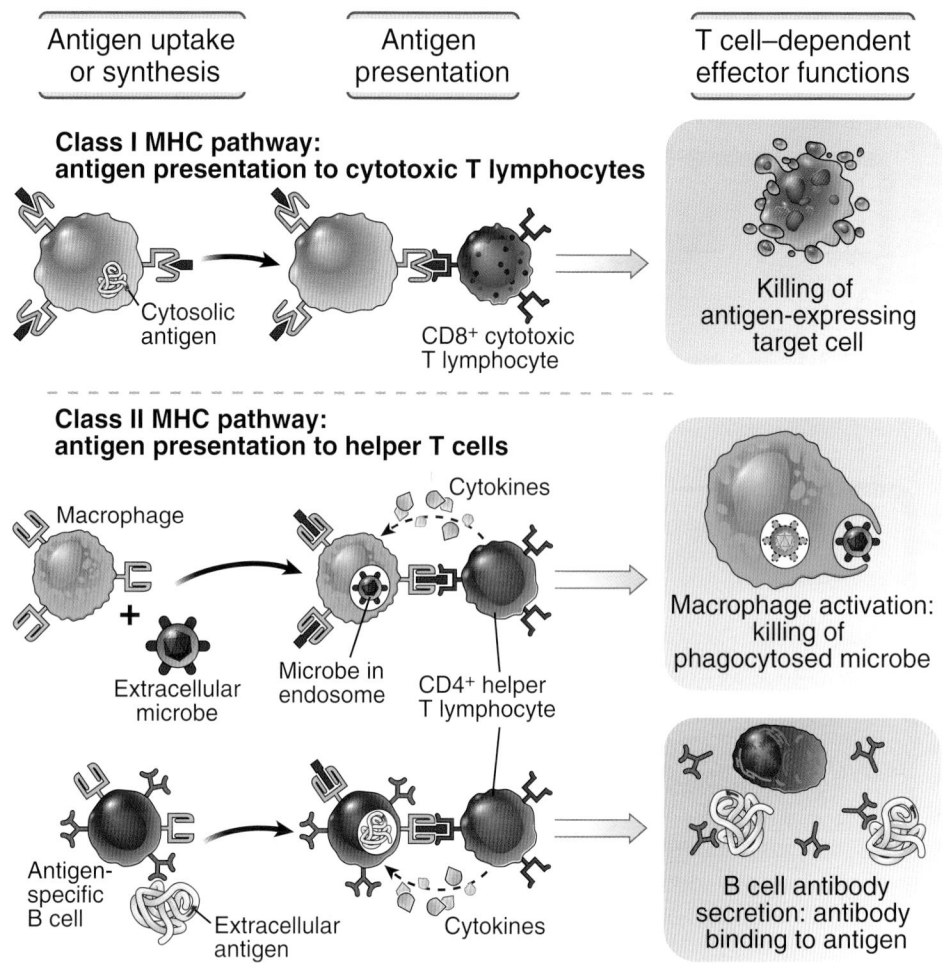

Fig. 46.3 Major histocompatibility complex *(MHC)* molecules. Phagocytes are antigen-presenting cells responsible for identifying and preparing a pathogen for presentation to cells of the adaptive immune system. Once the pattern recognition receptor on the phagocyte binds a pathogen, it processes it into short peptides and binds it with a self protein receptor called a MHC molecule on the surface of the phagocyte. Class I MHC proteins are essential for presenting antigens to CD8+ cytotoxic T lymphocytes. Class II MHC proteins present antigens to CD4+ helper T lymphocytes. (From Abbas AK, Lichtman AH, Pillai S. *Basic Immunology: Functions and Disorders of the Immune System.* 6th ed. Philadelphia, PA: Elsevier; 2020:70.)

TABLE 46.2	Normal Adult White Blood Cell (WBC) Count	
Cell	Plasma Count	% of WBC
WBC	$4.00–11.0 \times 10^9/L$	
Neutrophils	$2.5–7.5 \times 10^9/L$	40%–60%
Lymphocytes	$2.5–7.5 \times 10^9/L$	20%–40%
Monocytes	$0.2–0.8 \times 10^9/L$	2%–8%
Eosinophils	$0.04–0.4 \times 10^9/L$	1%–4%
Basophils	$0.01–0.1 \times 10^9/L$	0.5%–1%

Monocytes and Macrophages

Monocytes are the largest blood cells (see Table 46.2). They circulate in the blood before becoming tissue-specific macrophages, residing in Langerhans cells in the epidermis, Kupffer cells in the liver, alveolar cells in the lungs, and microglia cells in the central nervous system (CNS).[2,4] Macrophages are larger than monocytes and are more effective phagocytes. Monocytes and macrophages are mobilized shortly after the neutrophils and are responsible for phagocytic destruction of microbes and particulate antigens that have been marked by immunoglobulins (Ig) or complement proteins. They produce nitric oxide (NO) that destroys the microbe and cytokines that activate the adaptive immune system. Their presence is persistent at sites of chronic infection, and they play a major role in systemic granulomatous disorders.

Basophils and Mast Cells

Basophils are the least common blood granulocytes (see Table 46.2). Their tissue counterparts, the mast cells, reside in peripheral tissues, especially connective tissue close to blood vessels. Both cell types express cell surface high-affinity receptors for IgE and are key initiators of immediate hypersensitivity reactions through the release of histamine, leukotrienes, cytokines, and prostaglandins; they also stimulate smooth muscle contraction. They play a major role in atopic allergies such as hay fever, asthma, and eczema. They also respond directly to bacterial pathogens.

Eosinophils

Eosinophils are heavily concentrated in the GI mucosa, where they are the primary defense against parasites and the mucosa of the respiratory and urinary tracts (see Table 46.2).[2,4] Similar to neutrophils, they release cytokines capable of killing microbes. They also play a role in allergic reactions and asthma. Eosinophil lysosomes are responsible for degrading mast cell inflammatory mediators and limiting the vascular effects of inflammation.

Dendritic Cells

DCs are found throughout the body but are concentrated in secondary lymphoid tissue such as the spleen, lymph nodes, mucosa-associated lymphoid tissues, and tissues that have direct contact with the external environment, namely the skin and mucous membranes. DCs are the most potent APCs; they express class I and II MHC molecules that bind peptide fragments of antigens and display them on the cell surface for recognition by the appropriate T cell.[2,4] A second type of DC, the plasmacytoid DC (pDC), produces high levels of type I interferon (IFN) and is believed to play a role in antiviral host defense and autoimmune disorders.[10] Both myeloid stem cells and common lymphoid progenitor cells give rise to DCs and pDCs. After encountering a pathogen, the immature DC rapidly matures and migrates to the lymph tissue, where its MHC molecules present the pathogen peptide to the T-cell receptor (TCR) on the surface of Th and Tc cells. DCs are important for stimulating naive T cells that lack immunologic memory. The release of DC cytokines promotes B-cell activation and differentiation and contributes to B-cell memory. The DCs are also capable phagocytosis of pathogens (see Table 46.1).

Cytokines

Cytokines are small proteins with diverse functions that are secreted by immune cells, endothelial cells, neurons, glial cells, and other types of cells. They act as messengers in the immune system and modulate the response to pathogenic microbes, tumor cells, and apoptotic cells. They include interleukins, IFNs, tumor necrosis factor (TNF), and chemokines (Fig. 46.4). Interleukins are produced by lymphocytes and macrophages in response to microbes or products of inflammation.[2] Over 30 different interleukins are involved in the activation or inhibition of the inflammatory response (see Table 46.1). The major proinflammatory interleukins are IL-1 and IL-6; antiinflammatory interleukins include IL-10 and transforming growth factor-β (TGF-β). The IFNs are low molecular weight proteins necessary for destruction of viruses. They respond to viral RNA and viral PAMPs that are displayed by virally infected cells and prevent viral replication. Macrophages produce type I IFNs, which induce production of antiviral proteins in virally infected cells that cause viral resistance in the surrounding cells; this is the mechanism of action of therapeutic agents, such as IFN-α, in the treatment of melanoma. TNF-α is a proinflammatory cytokine, primarily secreted by macrophages in response to PAMP recognition by TLRs. Its primary role is regulation of proinflammatory effects, including induction of fever; it has also been implicated in tumor regression and septic shock. Chemokines are low molecular weight peptides produced by multiple cell types in response to proinflammatory cytokines. Their primary role is stimulation of leukocyte chemotaxis.

Complement

The complement system is so named because it complements the role of immune cells in both the innate and adaptive immune systems. Activated complement augments pathogen opsonization for destruction by phagocytes and antibodies. Its main function is to mark pathogens for permanent destruction and to recruit other immune cells to destroy the pathogens.[11] It includes over 30 plasma and cell surface proteins, most of which are produced in the liver. Many of the proteins are proteinases, and activation occurs in a cascade. The classic pathway for complement activation is initiated by an antigen-antibody complex that activates complement component 1 (C1). The alternative pathway

is activated by microbial cell wall components, mannans, which neutralize inhibitors of spontaneous complement activation and directly activate component C3. A number of immunologically active components are generated upon activation. Components C3 and C3b are deposited on the surface of the microbe (opsonization) to enhance phagocytosis of the microbe by phagocytes with C3 surface receptors (Fig. 46.5). Components C3a, C4a, and C5a cause degranulation of mast cells, and C5a attracts neutrophils to the area. Complement components C5b and C6 to C9 perforate and destroy the cell membrane of the microbe.[2,4,11]

Other Components of the Innate Immune System

Nucleotide-binding domain leucine-rich repeat proteins are found in the cytoplasm of immune cells; they recognize bacterial particles and signs of intracellular damage such as uric acid crystals. They initiate the inflammatory process through the activation of interleukin and recruit immune cells to the site to destroy the microbe and facilitate tissue repair.[2,4] Dectin-1, collectins, pentraxins, and ficolins are also pattern recognition proteins. They are responsible for opsonization of the microbe for phagocytosis, activation of proinflammatory cytokines, and production of antimicrobial reactive oxygen free radicals. The pentraxins include C-reactive protein (CRP) and serum amyloid P component (SAP). Binding of CRP to bacterial low-density lipoproteins and polysaccharides, and apoptotic host cells, activates the complement system and phagocytosis. Binding of SAP to microbial carbohydrates and amyloid fibrils activates complement; SAP is involved in autoimmunity and amyloidosis. The ficolins also bind microbial carbohydrates and activate the complement system.

Adaptive Immune System

The adaptive system is responsible for the proliferation of antibodies with specificity for different pathogens.[1-4] Initially, it has a slower response than the innate system but develops immunologic memory that allows it to respond more aggressively upon repeated exposure to the same pathogen (Table 46.3). Adaptive immune system cells are derived from hematopoietic stem cells that differentiate into a common lymphoid progenitor. The common lymphoid progenitor further differentiates into four types of mature lymphocytes: B lymphocytes (B cells), T lymphocytes (T cells), natural killer (NK) cells, and natural killer T (NKT) cells (see Fig. 46.2). Of the two major types of lymphocytes, B cells and T cells, 20% to 50% are circulating lymphocytes; the remainder reside in secondary lymph tissues, which includes lymph nodes, tonsils, spleen, Peyer patches of the intestines, appendix, and mucosa-associated lymphoid tissue (Fig. 46.6). Lymphocytes constitute 20% to 40% of the body's WBCs; approximately 80% are T cells, 15% are B cells, and the remainder are undifferentiated (see Table 46.3). First-time exposure to a pathogen requires a coordinated effort of both NKT and Th cells, as well as antibody-secreting B cells. Both memory T and B cells are responsible for stimulating a stronger and more rapid immune response to subsequent encounters with the same antigen.

B Cells

The major function of B cells is the production of antibodies, specialized glycoproteins that recognize and bind to foreign proteins of bacteria, viruses, and tumor cells (Table 46.4). Antibodies are large, Y-shaped proteins composed of two identical light chains and two identical heavy chains held together by disulfide bonds.[2,4] The N terminal or variable region (Fab) of each chain binds the antigen and is different for each class of immunoglobulin. The C terminal, or constant region (Fc), is composed of a relatively constant amino acid sequence that binds to Fc receptors on phagocytes (Fig. 46.7). The amino acid sequence of the Fc codes for five classes of Ig (G, M, A, E, and D) and the subclasses of G and A (see Table 46.4). The five Ig classes are distinguished by their heavy

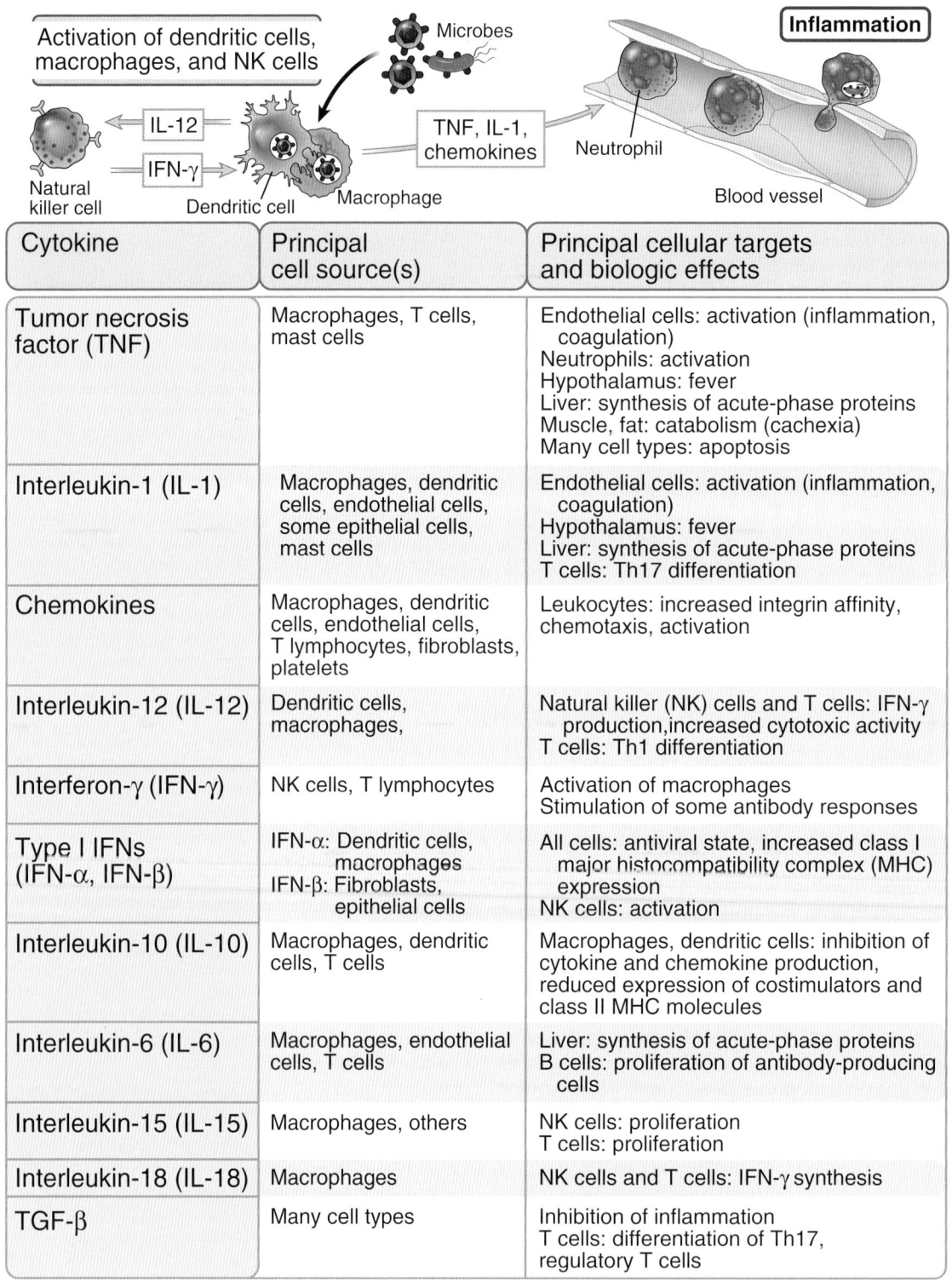

Fig. 46.4 Cytokines of innate immunity. **A,** Dendritic cells, macrophages, and other cells (such as mast cells and ILCs, not shown) respond to microbes by producing cytokines that stimulate inflammation (leukocyte recruitment) and activate natural killer (*NK*) cells to produce the macrophage-activating cytokine interferon-γ (*IFN-γ*). **B,** Some important characteristics of the major cytokines of innate immunity are listed. Note that IFN-γ and transforming growth factor beta (*TGF-β*) are cytokines of both innate and adaptive immunity. *TGF,* transforming growth factor. (From Abbas AK, Lichtman AH, Pillai S. *Basic Immunology: Functions and Disorders of the Immune System.* 6th ed. Philadelphia, PA: Elsevier; 2020:42.)

chains. The IgG molecule has gamma (γ) chains, IgM has mu (μ) chains, IgA has alpha (α) chains, IgE has epsilon (ε) chains, and IgD has delta (δ) chains.[2] The IgG and IgA antibodies are produced close to mucosal membranes and end up in secretions such as tears, saliva, and mucus, where they protect against GI and respiratory tract infections. The IgM antibodies are formed in response to infection; IgD is expressed with IgM on the surface of mature B cells and functions as a transmembrane antigen receptor. Allergic reactions are associated with IgE antibodies.

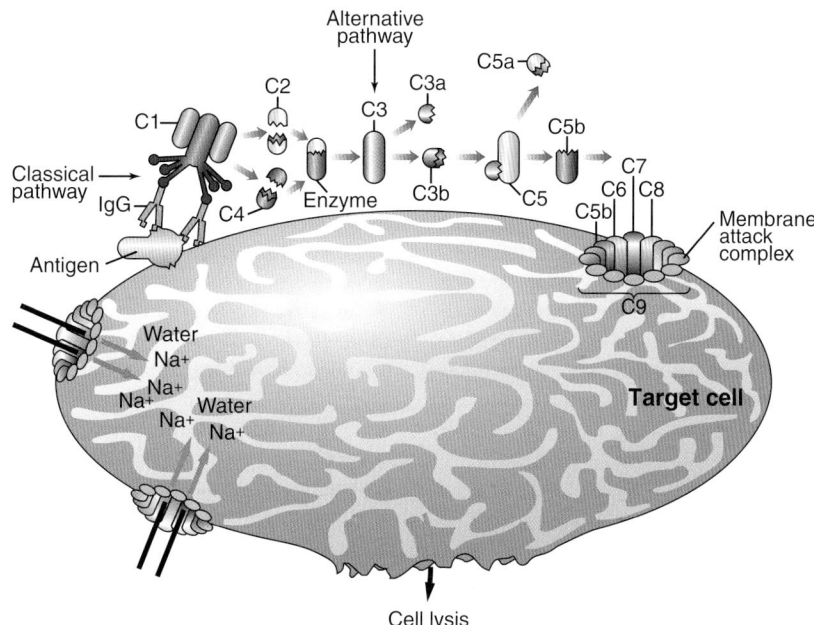

Fig. 46.5 Complement cascade. The cascade is activated by the first complement molecule, C1, which binds an antigen-antibody complex. This event begins a domino effect, with each of the remaining complement proteins performing its part in the attack sequence. The end result is a hole in the membrane of the offending cell and destruction of the cell. Activation of the complement cascade results in the formation of membrane attack complexes that insert in the cell membrane. These porelike structures allow sodium and water influx, which causes the cell to swell and rupture. (From Copstead LE, Banasik J. *Pathophysiology*. 5th ed. St. Louis: Elsevier; 2013:169; redrawn from Schindler LW. *Understanding the Immune System*. NIH Pub. No. 92–529. Bethesda, MD: US Department of Health and Human Services; 1991:11.)

TABLE 46.3 Components of the Adaptive Immune System

Component	Receptor	Function
B cells Surface markers: CD21, CD40	BCR	Antibody production (IgG, IgM, IgA, IgD, IgE). BCR is composed of a membrane-bound antibody that "tags" antigen for recognition by Th cells and destruction by complement and phagocytes.
T cells **Th1** Surface marker: CD4	TCR, binds class II MHC proteins	Secrete cytokines INF-γ and TNF-β that activate phagocytes and Tc, and induce B cells to produce antibodies. Effective against intracellular pathogens. Associated with many autoimmune diseases, including multiple sclerosis and arthritis.
Th2 Surface marker: CD4	TCR, binds class II MHC proteins	Secrete IL-4, IL-5, and IL-23 that stimulate isotype switching and production of IgE and IgG subset antibodies by B cells. Effective against extracellular bacteria. Involved with allergic responses.
Th17 Surface marker: CD4	TCR, binds class II MHC proteins	Secrete cytokines IL-17 and IL-23 that recruit phagocytes and stimulate inflammatory response in tissues with direct contact with external environment. Involved in pathogenesis of inflammatory disorders, such as Crohn disease.
Treg Surface markers: CD4, CD25	Distinct set of TCRs	Secrete cytokines IL-10 and TGF-β. Modulate immune response by suppressing effector T-cell proliferation in thymus and down-regulating Th cells to prevent excessive immune responses to self-antigens.
Tc Surface markers: CD8	TCR, binds class I MHC proteins	Secrete INF-γ, TNF-α, and cytotoxic substances that destroy infected cells: perforins damage cell membrane and granzymes cause intracellular destruction of the pathogen. Stimulate production of B-cell antibodies.
NK Surface markers: CD16, CD56	Lack TCR	Secretion of cytokines INF-γ, TNF-α for destruction of virus-infected self cells, tumor cells, and other abnormal cells that are missing MHC markers required for identification by other T and B cells.
NK T cells Surface markers: CD1d	Unique TCR-αβ binds MHC I–like molecules	Recognize lipid and glycolipid antigens presented by MHC I–like molecules; produce multiple cytokines, INF-γ, TNF-α, IL-4, IL-13, and MSF destroy bacterial and viral pathogens.

BCR, B-cell receptors; *CD*, cluster of differentiation; *IL*, interleukin; *INF*, interferon; *MHC*, major histocompatibility complex; *MSF*, macrophage-stimulating factor; *NK*, natural killer cells; *TCR*, T-cell receptor; *TNF*, tumor necrosis factor.

The IgG and IgD antibodies are anchored in the B-cell membrane where they function as B-cell receptors (BCRs) that are able to recognize a small region of the pathogen, called the antigenic epitope, that is bound to a MHC molecule on an APC, such as a DC.[2-4] The BCR can recognize and differentiate between the self MHC molecule and short peptide strands of the antigen. When an antibody binds with an MHC-antigen receptor complex, it activates other immune cells to destroy the pathogen. Clonal selection is initiated when a B cell has a receptor that can bind the invading antigen, resulting in a rapid increase in the number of plasma B cells with a high affinity and specificity for the antigen (plasma cells). Most immune responses are polyclonal because antigens can present with several different epitopes.[2] Multiple antibodies for a single antigen make it difficult for a pathogen to escape recognition, and the coating of an antigen with multiple antibodies also makes it easier for other immune cells to recognize and kill it. A number

of activated B cells become memory cells. Naïve B cells express IgM and IgD as BCRs; as they mature under the influence of Th cells, they undergo isotope switching to IgA, IgE, and subsets of IgG (Fig. 46.8).[2,4] At the same time, they undergo somatic mutations of the antigenic-binding portions of the heavy and light chains; the B cell will die if the mutation results in a loss of affinity for the antigen. If the mutations increase affinity, the cell continues to proliferate. Memory responses are characterized by production of specific IgG, IgA, or IgE antibodies, which allow the B cell to respond more quickly and aggressively upon repeated exposure to the same pathogen.

There are two types of B cells. The B1 cells produce IgM antibodies; although the IgM antibody can recognize several different antigens, it tends to have a low affinity for them. Most B cells are B2 cells and express both IgM and IgD antibodies. By the time the B2 cells have become memory cells, they have undergone class switching and produce IgG, IgA, or IgE antibodies (see Fig. 46.8). Plasma immunoglobulins are composed of 70% IgG, 20% IgA, 10% IgM, and small amounts of IgD and IgE (see Table 46.4). When an antigen is encountered for the first time, only B cells with a BCR that can identify the antigen are stimulated to differentiate and proliferate (clonal selection) into plasma cells. During initial exposure to the antigen there is a lag time of 5 to 7 days between recognition of the antigen and maturation and proliferation of B plasma cells and memory cells. In the initial response to the antigen, IgM is produced first, followed by IgG; antibody levels fall as the antigen is destroyed. A second exposure to the antigen produces a rapid response with IgG as the predominant antibody (Fig. 46.9).

T Cells

T cells originate in the bone marrow; they mature and differentiate in the thymus before migrating to the secondary lymphoid organs. Despite the partial degeneration of the thymus at puberty, T-cell

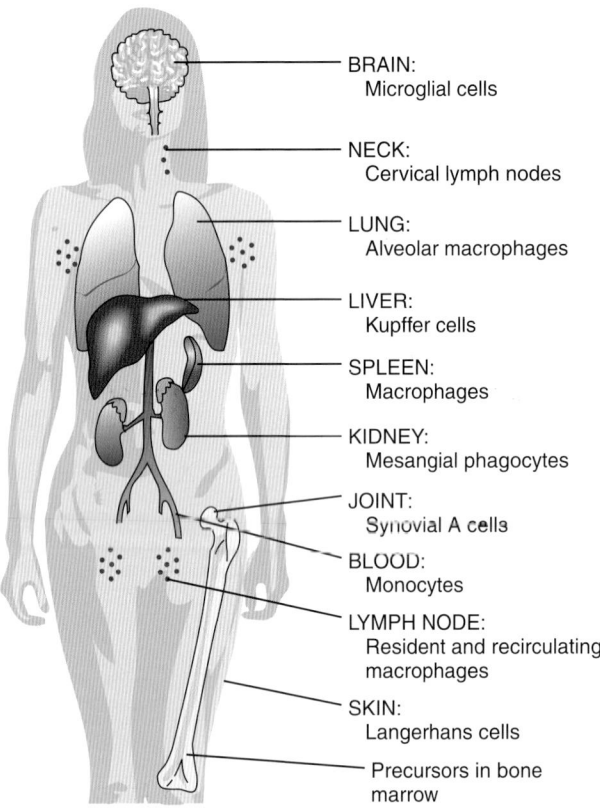

Fig. 46.6 Cells of the mononuclear phagocyte system. (From Copstead LE, Banasik J. *Pathophysiology*. 5th ed. St. Louis: Elsevier; 2013:159; redrawn from Schindler LW. *Understanding the Immune System*. NIH Pub. No. 92-529. Bethesda, MD: US Department of Health and Human Services; 1991:19.)

BRAIN:
Microglial cells

NECK:
Cervical lymph nodes

LUNG:
Alveolar macrophages

LIVER:
Kupffer cells

SPLEEN:
Macrophages

KIDNEY:
Mesangial phagocytes

JOINT:
Synovial A cells

BLOOD:
Monocytes

LYMPH NODE:
Resident and recirculating macrophages

SKIN:
Langerhans cells

Precursors in bone marrow

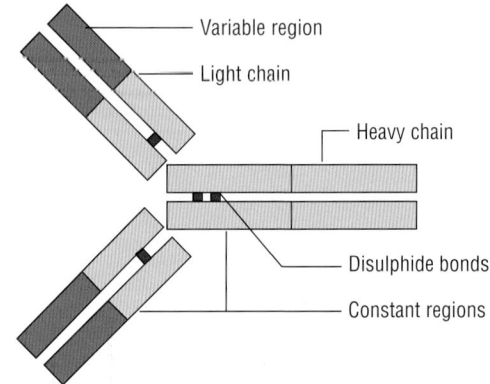

Variable region
Light chain
Heavy chain
Disulphide bonds
Constant regions

Fig. 46.7 Structure of immunoglobulin E. (From Parija SC. *Textbook of Microbiology and Immunology*. 3rd ed. Gurgaon, India: Elsevier India; 2016:91.)

TABLE 46.4   Properties of Immunoglobulins

Class	Heavy Chain	Subclass	Structure	Percent Total IG	Molecular Weight (kDa)	Plasma levels mg/dL (Adult)	Half-Life (Days)	Placenta/Milk Transfer
IgG	gamma (γ)	IgG-1, IgG-2, IgG-3, IgG-4	Monomer	70%	150	760–1590	23	+/+
IgM	mu (μ)		Pentamer	10%	900	37–286	5	–/–
IgA	alpha (α)	IgA-1, IgA-2	Dimer	20%	160	61–356	6–8	–/+
IgD	delta (δ)		Monomer	0.2%	180	0.3–3	2–8	–/–
IgE	epsilon (ε)		Monomer	0.002%	190	0.002–0.2	1–5	–/–

development in the thymus continues throughout life. Most T cells die in the thymus (apoptosis) because of failure to interact effectively with MHC molecules or because they react against self-components of host cells.[2-4] T cells that can recognize foreign antigens mature and migrate to lymphoid tissue. Two distinct types of T cells are produced in the thymus: Th and Tc cells (Fig. 46.10). Naïve Th cells (Th$_0$) continuously circulate in the blood and lymphoid tissues. They expand clonally and differentiate into several subsets after exposure to an antigen. Some T cells become memory T cells that have a quicker response the second time they encounter the antigen.

Mature T cells have transmembrane TCRs that can bind short antigenic epitopes bound to MHC molecules on APCs. Similar to the BCR on the B cells, the TCR can recognize and differentiate between self MHC and the antigenic epitope. The majority of T subsets are defined by their selective surface expression of the CD4 or CD8 proteins; these coreceptors are necessary for antigen recognition and T-cell activation. Immature T cells express both CD4 and CD8 proteins and can recognize antigen-derived peptides presented by either MHC class I or II molecules (see Fig. 46.10). As they mature in the thymus, they differentiate into CD4 and CD8 T cells that can recognize only MHC class II or I proteins, respectively.[2,4] The CD4 Th cells can recognize antigens presented by MHC class II molecules and are responsible for activating both humoral immune responses (B-cell antibodies) and cellular responses (delayed-type hypersensitivity reactions). The Th cells lack cytotoxic activity and do not kill pathogens or infected cells. A small number of Th cells become T memory cells that induce secondary cell-mediated immune responses. There are four major Th subsets: Th1, Th2, Th17, and Treg; differences in their production of cytokines, surface receptors, and internal adhesion molecules account for their different functionss.[2] The Th1 cells secrete cytokines that activate the phagocytes and Tc. The Th2 cells stimulate the secretion of antibodies by B cells (Fig. 46.11). The Th1 and Th2 cells display reciprocal inhibition and Th1:Th2 ratio is dependent upon the nature of the immune response. The Th17 cytokines stimulate the inflammatory response. The Treg

cells down-modulate the immune response, including suppression of effector T-cell proliferation in the thymus and down-regulation of Th cells when they are no longer needed, to prevent excessive T-cell activation and possible development of autoimmune disease. Destruction of helper CD4 T cells is seen with infection by the human papillomavirus (HPV). A loss of functional CD4 T cells leads to the symptomatic stage of human immunodeficiency virus (HIV) infection or acquired immunodeficiency syndrome (AIDS).

The Tc cells display CD8 proteins and can bind to antigens on MHC class I molecules (see Fig. 46.10). All nucleated cells have MHC class I molecules and can directly establish contact with CD8 Tc. The CD8 Tc can recognize and demonstrate direct cytotoxic activity toward virally infected cells, tumor cells, and transplanted organs. The Tc can destroy the abnormal cell in one of two ways: secretion of perforins and enzymes that penetrate the membrane and cause destruction of intracellular proteins, or secretion of a surface molecule that interacts with a surface proton on the target cell to induce apoptosis.[2,4] They can also down-regulate immune response (suppressor cells).

Natural Killer Cells

The NK cell is a large granular lymphocyte that lacks both a TCR and surface immunoglobulin and does not directly attack pathogens. The NK cells are activated when they do not see a normal self MHC on a virus-infected or tumor cell; they release perforin that damages the cell membrane and cytotoxic enzymes that enter the cell and destroy it. They can also recognize and destroy self cells that have down-regulated MHC class I molecular expression, which is a strategy that infected cells use to avoid detection by T cells. The NK and Tc cells complement each other. The Tc cells kill abnormal cells that express MHC class I proteins; the NK cells kill abnormal cells that have suppressed expression of MHC class I proteins. The NK cells also release cytokines that modulate the activity of other immune cells. Their cytotoxic activity is inhibited by self MHC molecules through inhibitory surface receptors that can recognize MHC class I molecules on healthy cells.

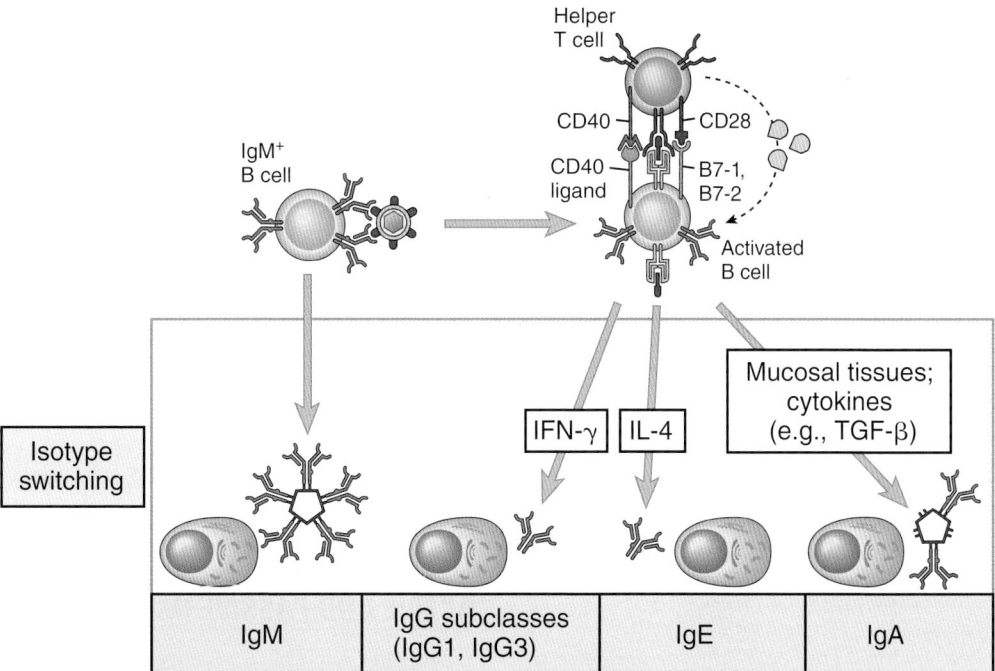

Fig. 46.8 Activated B cells undergo class switching from IgM to IgG, IgE, or IgA. Class switching is influenced by the presence of specific cytokines. *IFN,* Interferon; *IL,* interleukin; *TGF,* transforming growth factor. (From Copstead LE, Banasik J. *Pathophysiology.* 5th ed. St. Louis: Elsevier; 2013:187; redrawn from Abbas AK, et al. *Cellular and Molecular Immunology.* 7th ed. Philadelphia: Elsevier; 2012:257.)

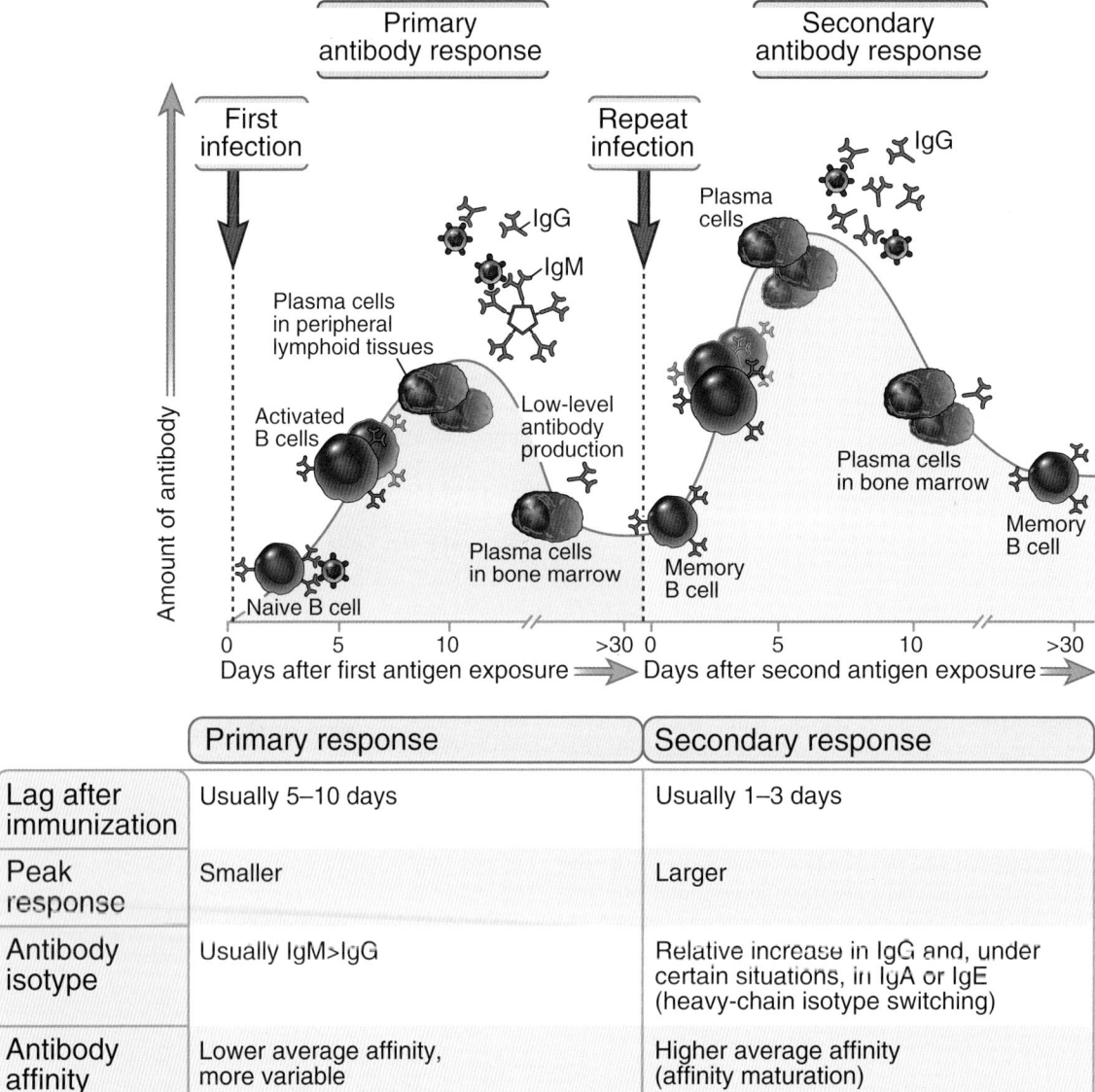

Fig. 46.9 Features of primary and secondary antibody responses. Primary and secondary antibody responses differ in several respects, illustrated schematically in (**A**) and summarized in (**B**). In a primary response, naive B cells in peripheral lymphoid tissues are activated to proliferate and differentiate into antibody-secreting plasma cells and memory cells. Some plasma cells may migrate to and survive in the bone marrow for long periods. In a secondary response, memory B cells are activated to produce larger amounts of antibodies, often with more heavy-chain class switching and affinity maturation. These features of secondary responses are seen mainly in responses to protein antigens, because these changes in B cells are stimulated by helper T cells, and only proteins activate T cells (not shown). The kinetics of the responses may vary with different antigens and types of immunization. *Ig,* Immunoglobulin. (From Abbas AK, Lichtman AH, Pillai S. *Basic Immunology: Functions and Disorders of the Immune System.* 6th ed. Philadelphia, PA: Elsevier; 2020:140.)

Natural Killer T Cells

The NKT cells are a specialized population of T cells with properties of both T cells and NK cells and account for 0.1% of peripheral T cells. They express both a unique T-cell alpha beta receptor (TCR αβ) that recognizes molecules presented by MHC I–like proteins and surface antigens typically associated with NK cells. The TCR αβ receptor recognizes lipid and glycolipid antigens presented by the MHC I–like molecule rather than protein peptides presented by MHC I or II molecules. Activated NKT cells rapidly produce multiple cytokines, including IFN, macrophage stimulating factor, interleukin, chemokines, and anti-trinitrophenol (TNP), which can destroy bacterial and viral pathogens. They can either contribute to immune surveillance or immunosuppression and can either inhibit or promote tumor growth and metastasis and development of autoimmune diseases.

ACTIVE AND PASSIVE IMMUNITY

The immune response to an antigen is a result of clonal expansion of B and T cells upon initial exposure to the antigen, which allows a rapid and vigorous response upon subsequent exposures to the antigen (see Fig. 46.9). Long-term immunity is acquired when B and T memory cells are activated in response to a pathogen. Vaccinations or immunizations also establish long-term immunologic memory.

Active Immunity

Active immunity is achieved when a pathogen is deliberately administered to an individual for the sole purpose of stimulating the immune system to produce antigen-specific antibodies. Upon repeat exposure to the antigen, the adaptive immune system is able to provide a quicker and more efficient response. Vaccines are composed of live attenuated or inactivated/killed viruses, inactivated bacterial toxins, bacterial toxins, or segments of the pathogen (subunit and conjugate).[12,13] Live, attenuated vaccines typically provide long-lasting immunity, but there are concerns for potential mutation or reversion of the vaccine virus to an active form capable of causing disease; consequently, live vaccines have been replaced by inactivated vaccines that provide a shorter length of protection and require booster vaccinations for long-term immunity. Toxoid vaccines are composed of inactivated bacterial toxin and are used for prevention of bacterial diseases, such as tetanus, that are caused by a toxin produced by the bacterium and not the bacterium itself. Recombinant vaccines are subunit vaccines that contain sections of a pathogen that the immune system can recognize as a foreign antigen. The hepatitis B virus (HBV) and HPV vaccines are recombinant, produced by the insertion of a segment of the viral gene into a yeast cell; the modified yeast cell produces HBV or HPV surface antigens that stimulate an active immune response in the recipient. Conjugate vaccines use a combination of a bacterial membrane protein that does not generate a strong immune response on its own and a carrier protein that elicits a strong immune response resulting in active immunity against future infections with the bacteria. The *Haemophilus influenzae* type B (Hib) vaccine is a conjugate vaccine (Table 46.5). The Centers for Disease Control and Prevention (CDC) has published immunization guidelines for children and adults.[14]

Passive Immunity

Passive immunity occurs when a person receives another individual's antibodies to help prevent or fight certain infectious diseases. The protection offered by passive immunization is immediate but short lived,

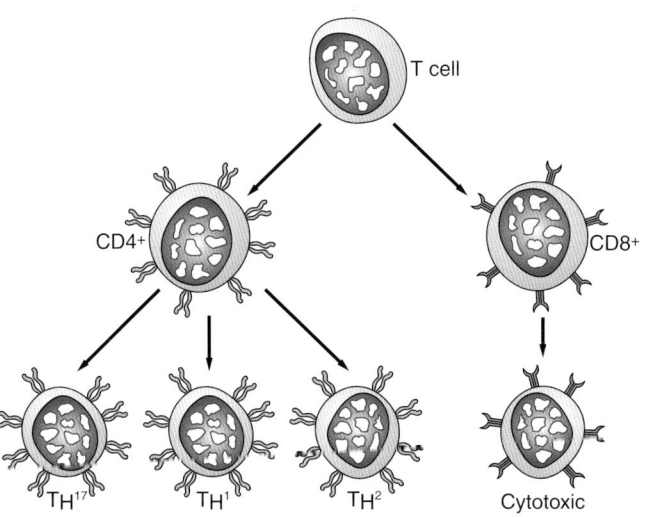

Fig. 46.10 Two major classes of T lymphocytes can be differentiated by CD markers on the cell surface. T helper cells have CD4 markers, whereas cytotoxic T cells have CD8 markers. CD4 cells can be further differentiated into Th1, Th2, and Th17, which secrete different cytokines. CD8 cells are cytotoxic T cells. (From Copstead LE, Banasik J. *Pathophysiology.* 5th ed. St. Louis: Elsevier; 2013:167.)

TABLE 46.5	Vaccine Types and Examples
Vaccine Type	**Examples**
Live, attenuated	Influenza (nasal spray)
	Measles, mumps, rubella (MMR combined vaccine)
	Rotavirus
	Shingles
	Varicella (chickenpox)
	Yellow fever
	Zoster (shingles)
Inactivated/killed	Hepatitis A
	Polio (IPV)
	Rabies
Toxoid (inactivated toxin)	Diphtheria, tetanus (part of DTaP combined immunization)
Subunit/conjugate	*Haemophilus influenza* type b (Hib)
	Hepatitis B
	Human papillomavirus (HPV)
	Influenza (injection)
	Meningococcal
	Pertussis (part of DTaP combined immunization)
	Pneumococcal

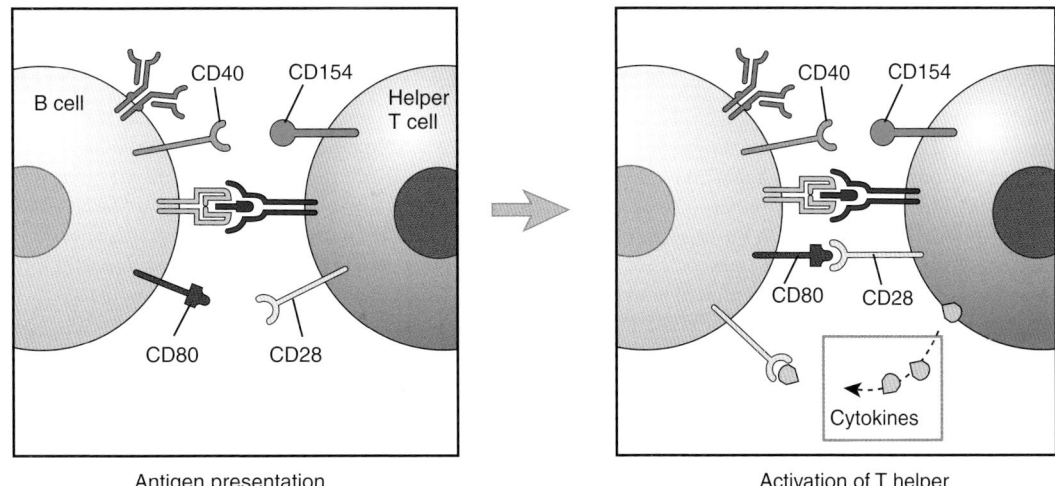

Antigen presentation to helper T cell

Activation of T helper to release cytokines

Fig. 46.11 Activation of a B cell requires T helper cell "help." This help is given through a number of cell-to-cell interactions via receptors, as well as through the secretion of cytokines that stimulate B-cell growth and differentiation. (From Copstead LE, Banasik J. *Pathophysiology.* 5th ed. St. Louis: Elsevier; 2013:185.)

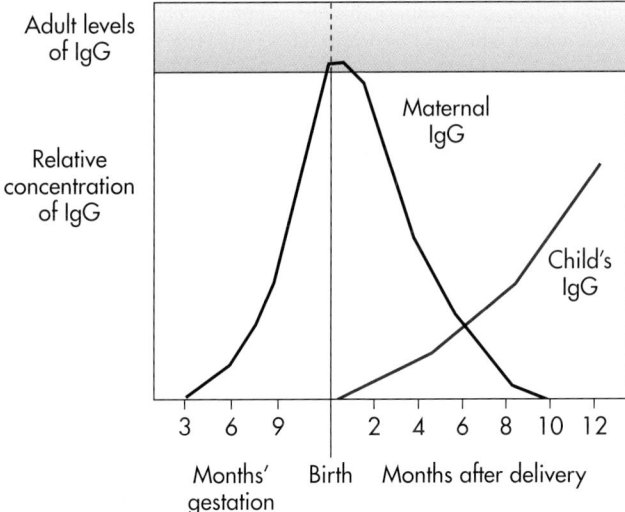

Fig. 46.12 Antibody levels in umbilical cord blood and in neonatal circulation. Early in gestation maternal IgG begins crossing the placenta and enters the fetal circulation. At birth, the fetal circulation may contain nearly adult levels of IgG, which is almost exclusively from the maternal source. The fetal immune system has the capacity to produce IgM and small amounts of IgA before birth *(not shown)*. After delivery, maternal IgG is rapidly catabolized and neonatal IgG production increases. (From McCance K, et al. *Pathophysiology: The Biologic Basis for Disease in Adults and Children*. 7th ed. St. Louis: Elsevier; 2014:257.)

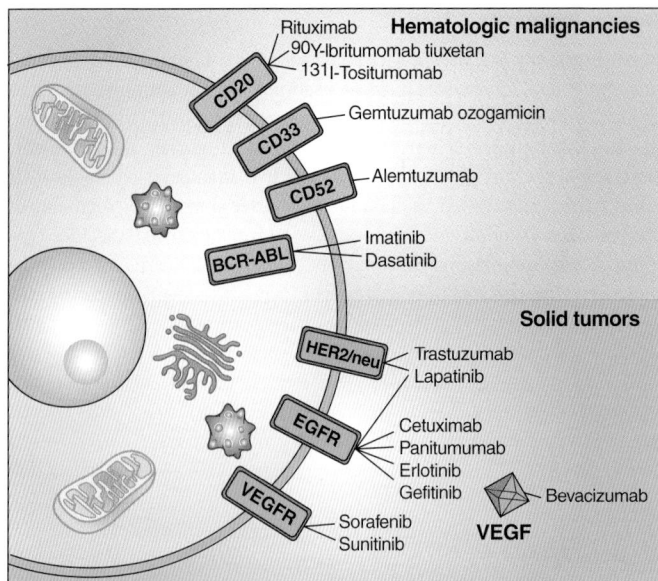

Fig. 46.13 Cancer cells express abnormal antigens (tumor-associated antigens) on their cell surface that can activate immune cells or be used as targets for monoclonal antibodies. Numerous medications are now available that use monoclonal antibodies to target cellular proteins relevant to several different types of cancer. *BCR*, B-cell receptors; *EGFR*, epidermal growth factor receptor; *HER2*, human epidermal growth factor receptor 2; *VEGF*, vascular endothelial growth factor. (From Copstead LE, Banasik J. *Pathophysiology*. 5th ed. St. Louis: Elsevier; 2013:137.)

usually lasting only a few weeks or months. During pregnancy, the fetus benefits from natural passive immunity provided by the mother's antibodies, specifically IgG, which has the same antigen specificity as the mother (Fig. 46.12).[15] After birth, neonatal IgG antibodies decline over time, and protection fades by 6 months of age; the maternal IgG can suppress vaccine-induced immune responses in the infant during the first 6 months of life. In contrast, maternal IgA antibodies are continuously supplied through breast milk; they enter the GI tract of the newborn and do not affect the immune response of the newborn to vaccination. Passive immunization is also used to temporarily boost a patient's immune system through the administration of immune globulins (IG) prepared from the pooled plasma of several thousand donors. Treatment with IG can be used for patients infected with diphtheria or the cytomegalovirus (CMV). It can also be used as a preventive measure in high-risk individuals with immune system deficiencies following exposure to the respiratory syncytial virus, measles, tetanus, hepatitis A, HBV, rabies, or chickenpox. Males with X-linked agammaglobulinemia who are unable to manufacture antibodies also benefit from IG administration. In special cases, the IG preparation may be harvested from individual donors who recently had a specific disease, such as rabies or tetanus. Similarly, patients exposed to TPA anthrax, a disease caused by the bacterium *Bacillus anthracis*, may receive IG from military personnel previously actively immunized with the anthrax vaccine. Other examples of passive immunity include administration of Rh immune globulin or RhoGAM, to Rh-negative mothers to prevent their immune system from developing antibodies to a fetal Rh antigen. As with natural passive immunity, IG conferred immunity is short lived and does not promote development of long-lasting memory cells in the adaptive immune system. Passive and active immunity may also be used together to protect the host. For example, an individual bitten by a rabid animal may receive IG rabies antibodies for an immediate response and a rabies vaccine to elicit a long-lasting immune response.

Monoclonal Antibodies

Monoclonal antibodies (MABs) are laboratory engineered molecules that mimic natural antibodies. They attach to abnormal cells and

mark them for identification and destruction by the immune system (immunotherapy); the surrounding healthy cells are unaffected by the MAB. A number of MAB drugs are currently used to treat different types of cancer (Fig. 46.13).[15,16] Rituximab (Rituxan) attaches to a specific protein (CD20) found only on B cells; it can mark lymphomas arising from these cells and make them visible for destruction by the immune system. Cetuximab (Erbitux) attaches to the receptor for epidermal growth factor (EGF) on cancer cells and slows or prevents the progression of certain cancers. Bevacizumab (Avastin) targets a vascular endothelial growth factor (VEGF) that cancer cells secrete to develop new blood vessels. Ado-trastuzumab emtansine (Kadcyla), a MAB combined with a chemotherapeutic drug, is used to treat human epidermal growth factor receptor 2 (HER-2)-positive breast cancers. Radioimmunotherapy combines a MAB with a radioactive isotope (e.g., ibritumomab [Zevalin]), which attaches to cancer cell receptors and destroys the cancer cell through radiation. Originally developed for the treatment of cancers and to prevent rejection of transplanted organs, MABs are also used in the treatment of autoimmune diseases; adalimumab (Humira) and etanercept (Enbrel) interfere with TNF and are used in the treatment of rheumatoid arthritis (RA) and Crohn disease. Although MABs exert selective immunomodulation by targeting specific cells expressing a specific antigen, they are associated with a widespread perturbation of the immune system and a possible increased risk of infections and cancer progression.

HYPERSENSITIVITY

A hypersensitivity reaction or intolerance refers to an immune system response to a foreign environmental antigen that causes an altered T-cell and antibody response upon reexposure to the antigen. It requires prior sensitization to the antigen, and it can be immediate or delayed. Common antigens include environmental allergens such

Type of hypersensitivity	Pathologic immune mechanisms	Mechanisms of tissue injury and disease
Immediate hypersensitivity (Type I)	Th2 cells, IgE antibody, mast cells, eosinophils	Mast cell–derived mediators (vasoactive amines, lipid mediators, cytokines) Cytokine-mediated inflammation (eosinophils, neutrophils)
Antibody-mediated diseases (Type II)	IgM, IgG antibodies against cell surface or extracellular matrix antigens	Complement- and Fc receptor–mediated recruitment and activation of leukocytes (neutrophils, macrophages) Opsonization and phagocytosis of cells Abnormalities in cellular function, e.g., hormone or neurotransmitter receptor signaling
Immune complex–mediated diseases (Type III)	Immune complexes of circulating antigens and IgM or IgG antibodies deposited in vascular basement membrane	Complement- and Fc receptor–mediated recruitment and activation of leukocytes
T cell-mediated diseases (Type IV)	1. CD4+ T cells (cytokine-mediated inflammation) 2. CD8+ CTLs (T cell–mediated cytolysis)	1. Macrophage activation, cytokine-mediated inflammation 2. Direct target cell lysis, cytokine-mediated inflammation

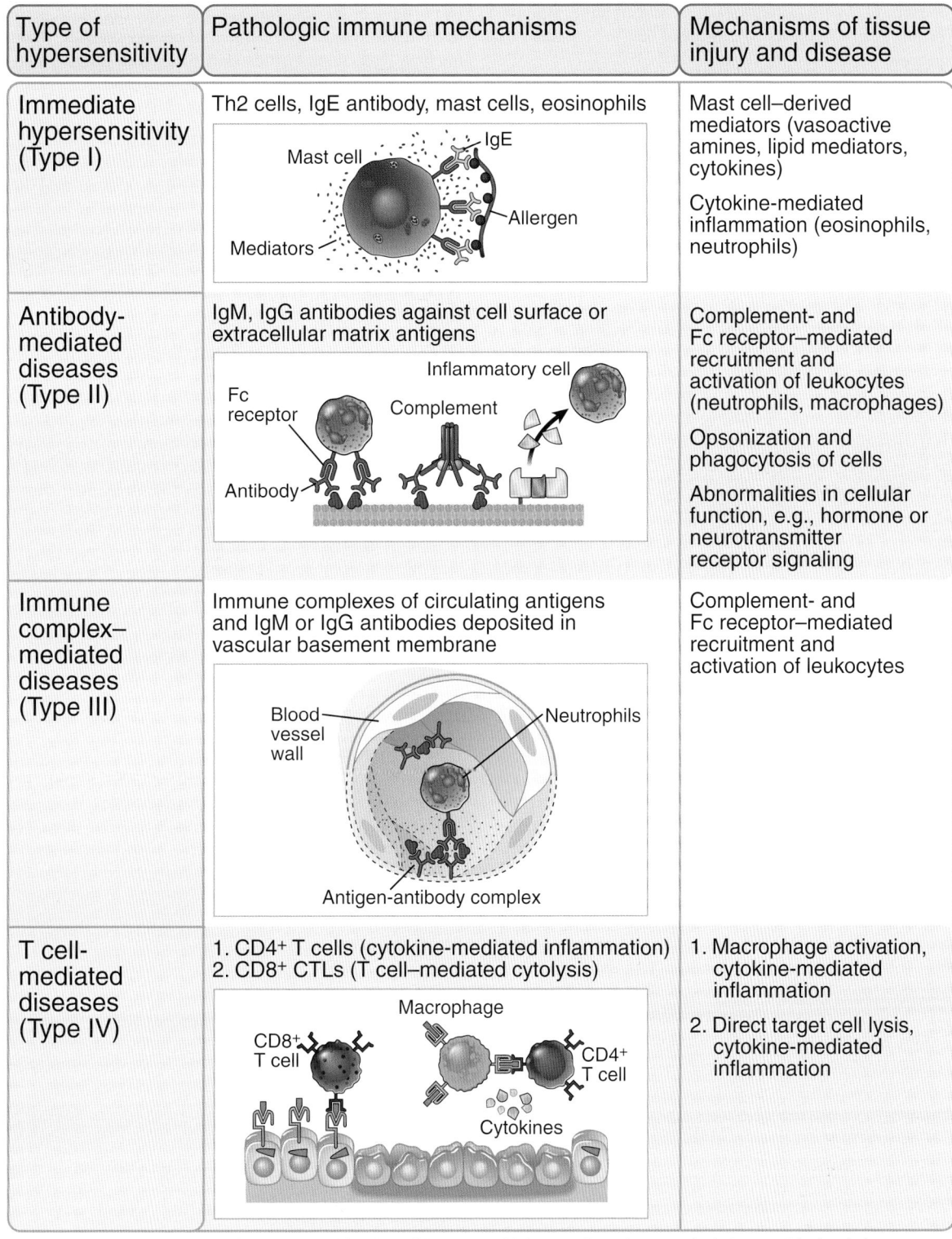

Fig. 46.14 Gell and Coombs classification of hypersensitivity reaction; does not include type V stimulating autoantibodies. (From Abbas AK, Lichtman AH, Pillai S. *Basic Immunology: Functions and Disorders of the Immune System.* 6th ed. Philadelphia, PA: Elsevier; 2020:220.)

as grass, pollen, and animal dander; topical allergens such as latex; food allergens such as gluten and nuts; and medications. Drugs are the most common cause of anaphylaxis in adults. Nonsteroidal antiinflammatory drugs (NSAIDs) are the most frequent trigger of anaphylaxis followed by β-lactams and non-β-lactam antibiotics, and proton pump inhibitors (PPIs).[17,18] The reaction to the allergen varies; it may

be physically uncomfortable, damaging to organ function, or fatal to the individual. The Gell and Coombs classification system divides hypersensitivity reactions into four types based on the mechanisms involved and time required for the response (Fig. 46.14).[2,4] However, a fifth class, stimulatory hypersensitivity, involving autoantibodies is now recognized. In addition, some conditions or diseases may involve more than one type of hypersensitivity reaction. The immune response may be the primary cause of the tissue damage or may be secondary to the disease process.

Type I Hypersensitivity

A type I hypersensitivity reaction, also known as an immediate hypersensitivity, occurs within 15 to 30 minutes of exposure to the antigen. Following initial exposure, T cells stimulate the B cells to produce antigen-specific IgE antibodies that bind to IgE receptors on mast cells and basophils. Upon a second exposure to the antigen, cross-linking of two IgE receptors on the mast cells and basophils by the antigen increases calcium (Ca^{++}) influx. The increased intracellular Ca^{++} is responsible for degranulation of the cells and release of preformed mediators, including histamine, heparin, proteolytic enzymes, and chemotactic factors. Degranulation also increases the production of other mediators responsible for modulating the inflammatory response, including bradykinins, leukotrienes, interleukins, slow-reacting substance of anaphylaxis, serotonin, prostaglandins, and thromboxanes. Histamine is the most important mediator of type I reactions. Binding of histamine to H$_1$ receptors triggers bronchoconstriction, increased vascular permeability, vasodilation, urticaria, pruritus, increased gut permeability, and increased mucous production. Binding of the H$_2$ receptors increases gastric acid secretion and decreases histamine release from mast cells and basophils. Histamine also activates other cells of the immune system, including complement via the alternate pathway. Tryptase is released from mast cells and is significantly elevated during an allergic response in approximately 70% of individuals. Serial serum total mast cell tryptase (MCT) is the gold standard for differential diagnosis of anaphylaxis.[19] Postmortem MCT evaluation is used in forensic medicine when anaphylaxis is a possible cause of death. Newly discovered biomarkers associated with anaphylaxis include platelet activation factor (PAF), chymase, carboxypeptidase A3, dipeptidyl peptidase I (DPPI), basogranulin, and Chemokine ligand-2 (CCL-2). Immediate hypersensitivity reactions that are IgE mediated require prior exposure to the offending agent.[17] Manifestations of a type I reaction vary in onset, severity, and intensity; they are graded I to V depending on their presenting signs and symptoms, which can range from mild cutaneous or GI manifestations to cardiovascular collapse and death (Table 46.6).

Treatment of type I reactions includes antihistamines to prevent systemic effects of histamine; cromolyn sodium to inhibit mast cell degranulation; and bronchodilators for treatment of bronchospasm, including β$_2$-adrenergic receptor agonists (albuterol), leukotriene receptor blockers (Singulair, Accolate), and inhibitors of the cyclooxygenase pathway (zileuton). In addition, IgG antibodies against the

Fc portions of IgE that binds to mast cells can block mast cell sensitization and is used in treatment of certain allergies. Diagnostic tests for type I reactions include skin (prick and intradermal) tests with suspected allergens and immunoassays that measure plasma total IgE and specific IgE antibodies. Increased IgE response to skin tests or elevated IgE levels is indicative of an atopic condition; however, IgE can be elevated in nonatopic diseases such as myelomas and helminthic (parasitic) infections. Hypersensitization (immunotherapy or desensitization), requiring injections of small amounts of the allergen over a period of months to years, may be used to treat allergies to insect venoms and pollens.

Type II Hypersensitivity

Type II hypersensitivity, also known as cytotoxic hypersensitivity, is primarily mediated by IgM or IgG antibodies and the complement system, with secondary activation of macrophages, in response to endogenous antigens on host cells. In addition, exogenous antigens, including drugs, may bind to the membranes of specific cells and cause a type II reaction. The antibody–cell complex is recognized by APCs of the innate immune system, which activate the B cells to produce antibodies against the cells containing the antigen, such as circulating RBCs and the basement membrane of certain tissues (see Table 46.6). The reaction time can take minutes to hours. Examples of type II reactions include type I diabetes mellitus, myasthenia gravis, drug-induced hemolytic anemia, granulocytopenia, thrombocytopenia, transfusion reactions, and Goodpasture nephritis. Diagnostic tests include positive antibody titers against the involved tissues and presence of antibody and complement in the biopsied tissue. Treatment includes antiinflammatory and immunosuppressive agents.

Type III Hypersensitivity

Type III hypersensitivity, also known as immune complex hypersensitivity, is a result of failure of the immune system to effectively rid the body of antibody-antigen complexes. It is also mediated by IgG and IgM antibodies, but the antigen is soluble and not tissue fixed; it may be exogenous (bacteria, virus, or parasite) or endogenous (see Table 46.6). The antibody-antigen complexes are deposited in joints and various tissues, including the kidneys, skin, and eyes, where they activate complement (C3a, 4a, and 5a) and stimulate the release of inflammatory mediators; the inflammatory response is directed toward the antibody-antigen complex and is not tissue specific. Type III reactions can take hours to weeks to develop. Examples include serum sickness, systemic lupus erythematosus (SLE), and RA. Confirmatory diagnosis includes tissue biopsies of Ig complexes, macrophages, and complement; depletion in complement level is

TABLE 46.6   Hypersensitivity Reactions

Type	Mediator	Antigen	Mechanism	Conditions
I: immediate, (anaphylactic)	IgE, mast cells, basophils	Exogenous	IgE binding to mast cells, and basophils release reactive substances	Drug allergy, hay fever, asthma
II: cytotoxic	IgG, IgM, compliment	Cell surface or tissue antigen	Antigen-antibody complex activates complement and destroys target cell	Erythroblastosis fetalis, blood transfusion, acute transplant rejection, myasthenia gravis
III: immune complex	IgG, IgM, neutrophils, compliment	Soluble	Antigen-antibody complex deposited in tissue stimulates inflammation	Systemic lupus erythematosus, rheumatoid arthritis
IV: delayed	T cells, monocytes, macrophages, cytokines	Tissues	Antigen activates Tc that kills target tissue	Poison ivy, transplant rejections
V: stimulatory	Humoral antibodies	Cell surface receptor	Antibody binding mimics receptor-ligand interaction	Graves disease

also diagnostic. Treatment includes antiinflammatory and possibly immunosuppressant agents.

Type IV Hypersensitivity

Type IV hypersensitivity, also known as cell-mediated or delayed-type hypersensitivity, is characterized by a delayed cellular response to an antigen taking anywhere from 24 hours to 14 days. The primary mediators are T lymphocytes and monocytes and macrophages, and it does not involve antibodies (see Table 46.6). The Th cells secrete cytokines, which activate Tc and recruit and activate monocytes and macrophages. Localized mast cell degranulation occurs prior to the local invasion of the monocytes and macrophages. Examples of type IV reactions include contact hypersensitivity (poison ivy) and granulomatous sensitivity (tuberculosis and leprosy). Treatment of type IV reactions is symptomatic. The Mantoux or purified protein derivative (PPD) reaction is a classic example of a type IV reaction that is used as a diagnostic test for exposure to the tuberculin bacilli (TB). Greater than a 10-mm induration in 48 to 72 hours following an intradermal injection of 0.1 mL PPD is confirmatory of TB exposure. However, there may be a false-negative result (anergy) in individuals with low T cells, especially CD4, including the elderly and individuals with HIV infections. Skin patch testing is used for diagnosis of contact dermatitis. Antiinflammatory and immunosuppressive agents are used for treatment of type IV reactions.

Type V Hypersensitivity

Although less understood, a type V hypersensitivity is a result of IgG class autoantibodies that bind and stimulate specific cell targets (see Table 46.6). Graves disease is a type V reaction in which autoantibodies stimulate the thyroid-stimulating hormone (TSH) receptor on the thyroid gland, leading to excessive secretion of thyroid hormones. Maternal stimulating antithyroid IgG antibodies can also cross the placenta and cause neonatal hyperthyroidism.

Anaphylaxis

Anaphylaxis is a severe type IV hypersensitivity with a lifetime prevalence of approximately 5% and less than 1% of total mortality rate.[20] Risk factors for severe or fatal anaphylaxis include cardiovascular disease, asthma, advanced age, mast cell disorders, and β-blockers and angiotensin-converting enzyme inhibitor (ACEI). In adults, drugs and insect venom are the leading causes of anaphylaxis, and foods and insect venom are the most common causes of anaphylaxis in children.[21,22] Uniphasic reactions account for 80% to 90% of anaphylactic reactions. The reaction occurs immediately upon the second exposure to the allergen; it typically resolves within hours with or without treatment. Biphasic anaphylaxis can occur in 4% to 5% of patients.[21] It is a secondary anaphylactic episode that occurs following an asymptomatic period and without a second exposure to the allergen. It predominantly occurs within 8 hours of the initial exposure to the allergen but can be delayed for as long as 72 hours. A severe initial anaphylactic response that required multiple doses of epinephrine and a delayed administration of epinephrine are risk factors for a second episode. Treatment of biphasic anaphylaxis is similar to that for the initial event and requires a longer observation period; antihistamines and/or glucocorticoids do not appear to prevent a biphasic event.[21] Anaphylaxis is characterized by angioedema, systemic vasodilation, hypotension, extravasation of protein and fluid, bronchospasm, and dysrhythmias.[2,23,24] Clinical manifestations of anaphylaxis occur within minutes of exposure to the precipitating antigen, especially in sensitive individuals. Untreated severe anaphylaxis can rapidly progress to pulseless electrical activity (PEA) and cardiac arrest. Epinephrine is the definitive treatment for anaphylaxis (Box 46.1).[21,23,24] Epinephrine decreases degranulation of mast cells and basophils and its vasoactive properties—α_1 stimulatory

---

BOX 46.1 Treatment of Intraoperative Anaphylaxis in the Adult Patient

Assessment
Grade 1: Cutaneous signs: generalized erythema, urticaria, angioedema
Grade II: Cutaneous signs, hypotension, tachycardia, cough, difficult ventilation
Grade III: Hypotension, tachycardia or bradycardia, arrhythmias, bronchospasm
Grade IV: Cardiac and/or respiratory arrest, pulseless electrical activity

Initial Treatment
Discontinue triggering agent
Trendelenburg position
Ventilation with 100%

Epinephrine
Grade II: 10–20 mcg SC/IM
Grade III: 100–200 mcg SC/IM/IV q 1–2 min; 1–4 mcg/min
Grade IV: 1 mg IV repeat as needed: 0.05–0.1 mcg/min

Fluids
Normal saline/lactated Ringer: 10–30 mL/kg or colloid: 10 mL/kg

Secondary Treatment
Epinephrine unresponsiveness: vasopressin: 2–10 units IV; norepinephrine: 0.05–0.1 mg/kg/min
Bronchospasm: albuterol or ipratropium inhalants, terbutaline 0.25 mg SC (may be repeated in 15–30 min)
Preoperative β-blockade: glucagon 1–5 mg IV every 5 min; 5–15 mcg/min
Antihistamines: diphenhydramine or hydroxyzine: 0.5–1.0 mg/kg IV; ranitidine: 50 mg IV
Airway edema: hydrocortisone 250 mg IV

Postresuscitation
Serum tryptase <120 min
24-hr monitoring for recurrence
Patient/family notification of reaction
Referral to allergist

---

effects support the blood pressure, β_1 stimulation increases the inotropic and chronotropic response of the myocardium, and β_2 stimulation causes bronchodilation. Rapid administration of IV fluids is necessary to counteract the loss of intravascular volume into extravascular space, a consequence of altered vascular permeability. Arginine vasopressin is indicated for hypotension that is unresponsive to epinephrine; it decreases NO production via the nonadrenergic vasopressin-1 receptor. Similarly, methylene blue, a selective inhibitor of guanylate cyclase, prevents NO-mediated vascular smooth muscle relaxation.[23] Glucagon directly activates adenyl cyclase and is indicated for continuing hypotension and bronchospasm in patients on β-blockers. Second-line treatment includes antihistamines, H_1 antagonists (diphenhydramine and hydroxyzine), and H_2 antagonists (ranitidine/famotidine). Bronchodilators, β_2-agonists, albuterol, terbutaline, and anticholinergic ipratropium bromide are used to treat bronchospasm. Corticosteroids may be indicated for airway edema.

Non-IgE-mediated type I reactions, previously called anaphylactoid reactions, can occur upon first exposure to an antigen and are a result of direct degranulation of mast cells and basophils and complement activation. The presenting signs and symptoms may be indistinguishable from IgE-mediated anaphylaxis, and treatment is the same. Elevated plasma total tryptase and β-tryptase levels confirm the degranulation of mast cells and basophils but cannot differentiate between IgE and non-IgE-mediated reactions. Tryptase has a short half-life, and blood samples must be obtained within 120 minutes of the anaphylactic event.[19] Individuals should be referred for skin testing for potential allergens. However, skin prick testing will only identify an IgE-mediated hypersensitivity, and a negative skin test does not necessarily exclude a drug as a non-IgE-mediated allergic trigger.

Intraoperative Anaphylaxis

During anesthesia the patient is exposed to multiple agents with the potential for producing a potentially fatal anaphylactic or anaphylactoid reaction, including anesthetics, antibiotics, antiseptics, contrast dyes, and blood products.[17,18,25] The estimated incidence of a hypersensitivity reaction in anesthetized patients is 1 in 3500 to 20,000 depending on the reporting country, with a mortality rate of 3% to 10%.[23,24,26] Approximately 60% to 70% of anesthesia-related reactions are IgE-mediated type I reactions.[27,28] Neuromuscular blocking agents (NMBA) are the most frequently incriminated drugs, accounting for 50% to 70% of the reactions. Neuromuscular blockers are the anesthetic drugs associated with the highest incidence of anaphylaxis. Succinylcholine and rocuronium account for the highest incidence of type I reactions, followed by vecuronium and pancuronium; atracurium, mivacurium, and cisatracurium have the lowest incidence of type I reactions.[29] The quaternary ammonium structure of NMBA is believed to be responsible for the reaction. The majority of NMBA reactions occur upon first exposure, a result of prior exposure to shampoos, detergents, and toothpaste, and metabisulfite food preservatives that include the same quaternary ammonium group. Cross reactions are also noted between iodinated contrast agents, NMBAs, penicillin, and first-generation cephalosporins. Females are three times more likely to be affected by a type I reaction; however, there is no sex difference in adolescence, suggesting a role for sex hormones in the increased incidence observed in adult females. The use of sugammadex has been proposed as a possible treatment of rocuronium-induced anaphylaxis. However, there have been multiple reports of sugammadex type I reactions that meet the World Anaphylaxis Organization (WAO) criteria for anaphylaxis and were confirmed by skin testing.[30,31] In a 3-year retrospective study of 15,479 patients who received sugammadex, the incidence of anaphylaxis associated with sugammadex was 0.039%, an incidence approaching that of succinylcholine or rocuronium.[32] The second and third leading causes of anaphylaxis in anesthetized patients are antibiotics and latex.[27,28] However, the incidence of latex-associated anaphylaxis is rapidly decreasing as a result of prevention policies.[26] Less commonly implicated agents include opioids, hypnotics, colloids, dyes, and antiseptics.[25] Paralleling their increased use in the general population, the occurrence of type I reactions to NSAIDs is increasing. Allergic reactions to local anesthetics are uncommon; cardiovascular reactions to local anesthetics generally result from an inadvertent intravascular injection of the drug rather a hypersensitivity reaction.

Intraoperative type I drug reactions occur within minutes of IV drug administration, frequently occurring during induction; skin or mucosal reactions to chlorhexidine occur in 15 to 30 minutes, and reactions to latex can take 30 to 60 minutes.[26,28] In the anesthetized patient covered by surgical drapes, the cutaneous signs of a type I reaction frequently go unrecognized. The primary presenting symptoms of anaphylaxis in anesthetized patients include hypotension, tachycardia, and bronchospasm followed quickly by hypovolemia, shock, and hypoxemia; left untreated, it rapidly progresses to PEA and cardiac arrest. Epinephrine is the definitive treatment for intraoperative anaphylaxis (see Box 46.1). Refractory anaphylaxis is a rare but potentially fatal reaction characterized by a lack of response to at least two doses of epinephrine.[33] Histamine activation of signaling pathways increases production of NO, which in turn activates guanylate cyclase resulting in an increased synthesis of the endogenous vasodilator cyclic guanylate monophosphate (cGMP). Refractory anaphylaxis is associated with drug-induced anaphylaxis, especially if allergens were administered intravenously; the mortality rate (26.2%) is significantly higher than the mortality rate of severe anaphylaxis (0.353%).[33] Perioperative drugs, especially IV medications, are most frequently associated with refractory anaphylaxis; a delay in recognition and delayed administration of epinephrine may contribute to the incidence of refractory cases. Use of methylene blue to competitively inhibit guanylate cyclase and reduce cGMP production, and dopamine to support cardiac output, may improve the outcome of perioperative refractory anaphylaxis.[23,33]

ALLOIMMUNITY

Alloimmunity, or isoimmunity, is the response of the immune system toward nonself antigen of other members of the same species, called alloantigens or isoantigens. Two major types of alloantigens are blood group antigens and histocompatibility antigens. Blood group alloantigens are responsible for thrombocytopenia, and rejection of solid organ transplantations is due to histocompatibility alloantigens.

Neonatal Alloimmune Thrombocytopenia

Neonatal alloimmune thrombocytopenia (NAIT) presents as transient neonatal thrombocytopenia, a result of maternal antibodies against paternal antigens expressed on fetal platelets. Fetal antigens (inherited from the father) cross the placenta and stimulate IgG alloantibody production in the mother; the antibodies cross the placenta and produce alloimmune disease in the fetus. The mother lacks the antigens and will have no symptoms of the disorder. NAIT is the most common cause of neonatal thrombocytopenia. It can present with petechiae, purpura, unexpected severe thrombocytopenia without overt bleeding or severe thrombocytopenia (<50,000/μL) intracranial hemorrhage (ICH), and fetal demise.[34] Thrombocytopenia is seen as early as the 16th week of gestation, and up to 75% of ICH cases occur in utero. Diagnosis is confirmed with a platelet antigen incompatibility and presence of maternal antibodies. Most cases of NAIT resolve within 7 days; a platelet count greater than 50 × 109/L is desirable for neonates who experience ICH. Prenatal and postnatal intravenous immunoglobulin (IVIG) and corticosteroids may be considered.

Transfusion Reaction

Transfusion reactions occur in response to surface antigens on donor RBCs.[35] There are over 80 different RBC antigens, but the strongest humoral alloimmune response is to the A, B, and Rh antigens. The A and B antibodies, isohemagglutinins, are IgG antibodies. The A and B antigens are codominant and may be expressed simultaneously; consequently, individuals can have one of four blood types: A, B, AB, or O, which lacks both the A and B antigen. Considered universal recipients, type AB individuals can receive A, B, AB, and O blood because they lack both anti-A and anti-B antibodies. In contrast, type O recipients can only accept type O blood; they are considered universal donors because they lack both A and B antigens. The Rhesus (Rh) blood group includes over 50 different antigens on RBCs; five antigens (D, C, c, E, and e) are the most important. The Rh factor refers to the RhD antigen, which determines if the individual is Rh positive (Rh+) or negative (Rh−). Approximately 15% of North Americans are Rh−. During the first pregnancy, a Rh− female develops IgG anti-RhD alloantibodies in response to fetal Rh+ RBCs. The antibodies cross the placenta where they have minimal effect on the fetus; in subsequent pregnancies, however, the maternal antibodies to the RhD antigens on fetal RBCs can cause erythroblastosis fetalis, which may be fatal for the fetus. Maternal antibody titers should be monitored throughout pregnancy in Rh- individuals. Regardless of fetal blood type, they should receive

Rh immune globulin (RhIG) to prevent maternal sensitization and development of RhD antibodies at 28 weeks of gestation and within 72 hours after delivery of a RhD-positive neonate. Individuals who are Rh⁻ should also receive RhIG following a miscarriage or abortion.

Transplant Rejection

Transplant rejection is a response to antigens, primarily HLA antigens, on the donor organ. Hyperacute rejection occurs immediately following transplantation and is due to preexisting antibodies in the recipient from a prior graft or blood transfusion of platelets and leukocytes that contained HLA antigens. It can be avoided by preoperative screening for antigraft antibodies. Acute rejection is a cell-mediated immune response that can occur weeks to months after transplant; it is caused by recipient DCs responding to unmatched HLA subgroups and inducing Th1 and Tc to directly attack the donor cells. Acute antibody-mediated rejection is mediated by antibody and complement and takes approximately 2 weeks to occur. Long-term maintenance with immunosuppressive agents is necessary to prevent acute rejection. Chronic rejection, a cell-mediated response to minor histocompatibility antigens, is characterized by graft arterial occlusions from increased proliferation of smooth muscle cells and production of collagen and progressive failure of the donor graft; it may take months or years to occur.

AUTOIMMUNITY

The ability of the immune system to recognize and avoid destruction of host cells is called self-tolerance. Central self-tolerance develops during the embryonic period; autoreactive lymphocytes are destroyed in the primary lymphoid organs during differentiation and proliferation of immature T and B cells. Peripheral tolerance continues in the secondary lymphoid tissue and is controlled by Treg cells and APC DCs that suppress maturation of lymphocytes with self antigen receptors.[2] Autoimmunity is an abnormal response to self antigens resulting in production of self antibodies or autoantibodies and damage to self tissues due to dysfunction of the innate and/or adaptive immune systems. Some individuals may have a genetic predisposition toward developing an autoimmune disorder; not infrequently, more than one autoimmune disorder can occur in the same individual. The HLA alleles and non-MHC genes that encode for cytokines and other costimulatory factors have been implicated in a large number of autoimmune diseases. It is hypothesized that microorganisms, such as bacteria or viruses, or drugs may trigger immune system dysfunction. Chronic inflammation is the classic sign of an autoimmune disease. There is a higher incidence of autoimmune disease in females, especially females of childbearing years. There are over 80 different types of autoimmune disorders that can affect almost any tissue of the body. The six most common autoimmune diseases include Graves disease, Hashimoto thyroiditis, multiple sclerosis (MS), RA, SLE, and type 1 diabetes mellitus (Box 46.2).

Graves Disease

The most common cause of hyperthyroidism, Graves disease affects 3% of adult females and 0.5% of adult males between 30 and 60 years of age. It is a type V hypersensitivity caused by autoantibodies to the TSH receptor on thyroid follicular cells.[36] The thyroid-stimulating antibody (TSAb) stimulates the thyroid gland, causing excessive production of thyroxine (T_4) and triiodothyronine (T_3). Symptoms of excessive thyroid hormone production include tachycardia, palpitations, tremor, heat intolerance, and anxiety. Physical symptoms include thyroid enlargement (goiter) and weight loss. Ophthalmopathy changes (exophthalmos) are a distinguishing characteristic of the disease and believed to be a result of TSI binding to TSH retroorbital

---

> ## BOX 46.2 Autoimmune Disorders
>
> *Multiple organ systems:* systemic lupus erythematous
> *Eye:* acute anterior uveitis, Sjögren syndrome
> *Skeletal system:* ankylosing spondylitis, reactive arthritis or Reiter syndrome, rheumatoid arthritis
> *Endocrine organs:* diabetes mellitus type, autoimmune pancreatitis, adrenal 21—hydroxylase deficiency, Hashimoto disease, Graves disease
> *Skin, connective tissue:* scleroderma, dermatomyositis, psoriasis, vitiligo, alopecia areata
> *Nervous system:* multiple sclerosis, myasthenia gravis
> *Blood and blood vessels:* polyarteritis nodosa, antiphospholipid antibody syndrome, hemolytic anemia, idiopathic thrombocytopenic purpura
> *Gastrointestinal system:* autoimmune hepatitis, celiac disease, inflammatory bowel disease (Crohn disease and ulcerative colitis), primary biliary cirrhosis

tissues. Graves disease is diagnosed by elevated plasma levels of T_3 and T_4, low or absent TSH, radioactive iodine (RAI) uptake, and thyroid ultrasound. Treatment includes antithyroid medications (methimazole and propylthiouracil) to normalize production of T_3 and T_4. Thyroidectomy and RAI destruction of the thyroid are also treatment options but typically require replacement therapy. Another thyroid autoantibody, the TSH stimulation blocking antibody (TSBAb), blocks TSH stimulation of the thyroid resulting in hypothyroidism.

Hashimoto Thyroiditis

Hashimoto thyroiditis, also known as chronic lymphocytic thyroiditis and autoimmune thyroiditis, is the most common thyroid disorder in the United States. Females are seven times more likely to suffer from the disease than males. Thyroglobulin (Tg), a major thyroid-specific protein, is normally not secreted into the systemic circulation. Along with other antigens, such as thyroid peroxidase (TPO), Tg can enter the circulation during acute thyroid inflammation, hemorrhage, or rapid disordered growth of thyroid tissue and stimulate the production of Tg and TPO antibodies (TgAb and TPOAb). Diffuse lymphocytic infiltration of the thyroid and activation of the other components of the immune system cause follicular destruction of the thyroid. A unique subtype of Hashimoto thyroiditis, IgG-4 thyroiditis, characterized by high plasma levels of IgG-4, is associated with rapid progression of hypothyroidism and higher levels of circulating antibodies. Symptoms of Hashimoto thyroiditis include goiter and hypothyroidism. Confirmatory diagnostic tests include low plasma levels of total T_4 and elevated TSH levels. The presence of TgAb and TPOAb and biopsy of Hurthle cells, large follicular cells with extensive granular eosinophilic cytoplasm, are confirmatory for the diagnosis. Hashimoto thyroiditis is treated with thyroid hormone replacement (levothyroxine sodium).

Multiple Sclerosis

MS is the most prevalent demyelinating disorder of the CNS. It primarily affects young adults between the ages of 20 and 40 years, and females are affected two times more than males. MS is an immune-mediated inflammatory disease that attacks the myelin, oligodendrocytes (myelin producing cells), and the underlying nerve fibers, producing significant physical disability within 20 to 25 years.[37] In addition to the proinflammatory CD4 Th1/Th17 cell subsets, B-cell antibodies, NK cells, CD8 Tc, microglia/macrophages, and complement also contribute to the demyelination and neurodegeneration. Symptoms include fatigue, tingling, numbness, muscle weakness, ataxia, vertigo, tremor, spasticity, bladder and bowel dysfunction, pain, and heat intolerance. The disorder is initially characterized by periods of relapse due to a new influx of immune cells into the CNS, and periods of remission characterized by remyelination. Diagnosis of MS includes MS lesions on magnetic resonance imaging (MRI), elevated IgG in the cerebrospinal fluid (CSF), and decreased conduction velocity on evoked response studies (visual, auditory, and somatosensory). Treatment with immunomodulatory agent is directed toward reducing the formation of new lesions and decreasing the incidence of relapse.[38] The Food and Drug Administration (FDA) has approved a number of disease-modifying agents for MS (DMAMS), including IFN-β1b (Betason), IFN-β1a (Avonex, Rebif), and glatiramer acetate (Copaxone). Treatment of acute relapses may include corticosteroids and plasma exchange (plasmapheresis) whereas antineoplastic agents, including cyclophosphamide (Cytoxan) and mitoxantrone (Novantrone), are used for severe progressive MS.

Rheumatoid Arthritis

RA is an inflammatory autoimmune disease characterized by synovial inflammation and hyperplasia, cartilage and bone destruction, and systemic features, including cardiovascular, pulmonary, psychological, and skeletal disorders. It initially affects the smaller joints of the hand and feet but spreads to the larger joints as the disease progresses. It has a peak incidence between the ages of 35 and 50 years; females are affected three times more often than males. The disorder involves both the innate and the adaptive immune systems and a complex interaction of many proinflammatory cytokines, especially TNF-α and IL-6.[39] The T cells play a pivotal role in the initiation of RA, especially the CD4 Th cells, which activate macrophages and synovial fibroblasts, the main producers of TNF-α, IL-6, and IL-1. The APCs (DCs, macrophages, and activated B cells) are responsible for activating the T cells, and there is an abnormal production and regulation of both proinflammatory and antiinflammatory cytokines.[7] In addition to their APC role, B cells produce rheumatoid factor (RF) and anticyclic citrullinated peptide (anti-CCP) antibodies. Approximately 60% of RA patients have a HLA-antigen D–related (DR)–4 cluster for certain HLA-DR molecules associated with RA. However, the concordance rate is only 12% to 15% for identical twins, which supports the theory that nongenetic factors play an important role in the disease. Environmental triggers can trigger an autoimmune response and can increase proinflammatory gene expression. Infection may also play a role, especially periodontopathic bacteria; the synovial fluid of RA patients has been found to contain high levels of oral anaerobic bacterial antibodies. Extraarticular involvement is more common in patients with RF and/or the *HLA-DR4* gene. Systemic manifestations include vasculitis and accelerated atherosclerosis, pericarditis, pulmonary fibrosis, visceral nodules, anemia, leukopenia, and Sjögren syndrome. Diagnostic tests for RA include an elevated erythrocyte sedimentation rate (ESR) and CRP, and the presence of RF and anti-CCP antibodies. Synovitis, bone erosion, and destruction of cartilage are evident on x-ray and MRI. Disease-modifying antirheumatic drugs (DMARDs) are used to control pain and inflammation and reduce joint damage. Methotrexate (MTX), the most commonly used first-line DMARD, inhibits cytokine production, blocks lymphocyte and monocyte proliferation, and prevents osteoclast formation.[40] Biologics, a subset of DMARDs, target specific immune mediators of the inflammatory process and are frequently combined with MTX. NSAIDs and corticosteroids are effective in early or mild cases. Surgical procedures include synovectomy, tendon repair, joint fusion, and total joint replacement.[39-41]

Systemic Lupus Erythematosus

SLE is an autoimmune inflammatory disease with widespread effects, including cardiovascular, hepatic, pulmonary, renal, joints, and skin. It occurs in young adults; approximately 20% develop the disease before the age of 20 years, and it is 10 times more common in females.[42]

Early diagnosis of SLE is difficult because of widespread and nonspecific symptoms. It is characterized by a large variety of autoantibodies, including but not limited to antibodies against coagulation proteins, erythrocytes, lymphocytes, nucleic acids, platelets, and phospholipids. The American College of Rheumatology has identified 11 common findings in SLE; a minimum of four symptoms are required for a diagnosis of SLE. These include a butterfly-shaped rash on cheeks/red rash with raised round or oval patches/rash on skin on exposure to sun, mouth sores, arthritis, pleuritic or pericarditis, renal impairment, CNS involvement (seizures, strokes, or psychosis), and abnormal blood tests. Laboratory abnormalities includes anemia, leukopenia, or thrombocytopenia, elevated ESR and/or CRP levels, and presence of antinuclear antibodies (ANA). Confirmatory diagnostic tests include anti–double-strand DNA (anti-dsDNA), anti-Smith (anti-Sm) or antiphospholipid antibodies, lupus anticoagulant (LA), IgG and IgM anticardiolipin (aCL), IgG and IgM anti-β$_2$-glycoprotein, elevated C3 and C4 or CH50 complement levels, and a false-positive blood test for syphilis. Treatment is dependent on the severity of the symptoms. Avoidance of triggers such as viral infections, sunlight, cigarette smoking, and certain drugs and the use of NSAIDs are effective in mild cases; corticosteroids or immunosuppressants (azathioprine, mycophenolate, mofetil, MTX) are necessary for severe cases. In combination with steroids and DMARDs, the MAB belimumab (Benlysta) B-lymphocyte stimulator–specific inhibitor reduces the number of severe flareups when used in combination with steroids and DMARDs.[42]

Type 1 Diabetes Mellitus

Type 1 diabetes mellitus accounts for less than 10% of diabetes cases; type 1A diabetes (T1AD) is a result of autoimmune destruction of the insulin-producing β cells of the pancreatic islets of Langerhans.[43] In contrast, type 1B (T1BD), idiopathic diabetes, is characterized by almost complete insulin deficiency with a strong hereditary component but no evidence of autoimmunity. The pathogenesis of type 2 diabetes involves both decreased insulin release and insulin resistance.

The majority of individuals with T1AD are diagnosed between 5 and 7 years of age or around puberty; females and males are affected equally. Latent autoimmune diabetes of adulthood (LADA) is a form of T1AD that occurs later in adults. The onset of the clinical symptom correlates with the end stage of β-cell destruction. Approximately 1 in 20 siblings of patients with T1AD will develop the disease; 60% of monozygotic twins have T1AD. The increased incidence of T1AD over the last 50 years supports the influence of unidentified environmental factors. The major genetic determinants of T1AD are three classes of HLA genes, specifically class II genes HLA-DQ and HLA-DR, which are expressed on APCs responsible for presenting antigens to CD4 Th cells. The great majority of individuals with T1AD have HLA-DR3 or DR-4 class II antigens. Immune markers are detectable after the onset of the autoimmune process and long before clinical presentation of the disease. The pathogenesis of T1AD involves T-cell infiltration, specifically CD8 Tc cells and macrophages, of the islets that results in insulitis and destruction of β cells, decreased insulin production, and insulin-dependent diabetes. Four autoantibodies are involved in destruction of the β cells: islet cell antibodies (ICAs), glutamic acid decarboxylase (GAD-65), insulin autoantibodies (IAAs), and protein tyrosine phosphatase (IA-2A). Pancreatic α-cell function is also abnormal in T1AD, resulting in excessive secretion of glucagon. Relatives with two or more antibodies have a 90% predictive incidence of T1AD. Insulin replacement therapy is the mainstay treatment of T1AD, but despite insulin therapy, the disease is associated with nephropathy, retinopathy, neuropathy, and cardiovascular disease. To date, MAB therapy and vaccinations have proved to be disappointing in the treatment of T1AD.

IMMUNODEFICIENCY DISORDERS

Primary immunodeficiency disorders (PIDDs) are a result of a genetic defect in cells of the immune system, including lymphocytes, antibodies, phagocytes, and complement proteins. Secondary deficiencies are a consequence of disease, such as cancer, infections, malnutrition, and medications. Immune function decreases in old age as a result of reduced production and diminished function of mature lymphocytes in secondary lymphoid tissues. The hallmark of both primary and secondary immunodeficiency is an increased susceptibility to infection.[44]

Primary Immunodeficiency Disorders

There are over 200 different forms of PIDD that are caused by a defect in the immune system and are often sex linked.[45] They are characterized by low antibody levels, defective antibodies, or defective cells of the immune system, including T cells, B cells, neutrophils, and complement (Table 46.7). In the United States, approximately 500,000 people have a PIDD; most present at birth or in early childhood but can present at any age. Increased susceptibility to repeated infections is characteristic of PIDD, including recurrent, unusual, or difficult to treat infections, especially pneumonia, ear infections, and sinusitis. Other symptoms include poor growth patterns or weight loss, recurrent deep abscesses of organs or skin, enlarged lymph glands or spleen, and a coexisting autoimmune disease. Classification of PIDDs is based on the genetic defect, laboratory findings, and associated features of the disorder. PIDDs result from defective genes coding for the immune system.[45] Historically, treatment was largely supportive, with the exception of bone marrow transplantation. Recent advances in immunobiology, genetics, and availability of biologic modifiers represent new therapeutic options in PIDDs.[42]

Common Variable Immune Deficiency

Common variable immune deficiency (CVID) is one of the most common types of PIDD; it is also known as acquired agammaglobulinemia, adult-onset agammaglobulinemia, or late-onset hypogammaglobulinemia. It occurs in 1 in 25,000 to 50,000 individuals, is most commonly diagnosed between ages 20 and 40, and affects females and males equally. It is characterized by low or absent antibody levels. The number of B cells may be normal, but they fail to differentiate into plasma cells that produce antibodies. Low levels of antibodies in the blood, including IgG, IgA, and IgM, are diagnostic of the disorder, especially in response to a challenge with vaccines such as tetanus, diphtheria, and pneumococcal polysaccharide. Recurrent infections are common, especially respiratory infections. Of individuals with CVID, 25% also have an autoimmune disorder, most commonly immune thrombocytopenia, autoimmune hemolytic anemia, and RA, and they have an increased incidence of malignancies, especially cell lymphomas.

Treatment for CVID is immunoglobulin replacement therapy, administered intravenously (IVIG) or subcutaneously (SCIG); antibiotics are indicated for acute infections and steroids for autoimmune disorders.

X-Linked Agammaglobulinemia

X-linked agammaglobulinemia (XLA), also called Bruton agammaglobulinemia and congenital agammaglobulinemia, is caused by a gene mutation of Bruton tyrosine kinase (BTK) on the X chromosome, an enzyme that is crucial for normal B-cell development. The lack of B cells causes a severe antibody deficiency. Approximately 1 in 250,000 males have XLA; diagnosis is usually not made until 9 to 12 months of age because of passive maternal IgG protection. Females can present with an immunodeficiency called autosomal recessive agammaglobulinemia (ARA) with an antibody deficiency that is similar to XLA. In addition to frequent infections, patients with XLA have underdeveloped secondary lymphoid organs, including small tonsils, lymph nodes, and spleen, which is an indication of low or absent B lymphocytes. The diagnosis of XLA is confirmed by low or absent plasma B cells and IgG, and no detectable IgM or IgA; a low B-cell count is the most reliable indicator of both XLA and ARA. A confirmatory diagnosis test is absence of the *BTK* gene. Treatment includes prophylactic antibiotics and passive immunotherapy with IVIG or SCIG every 3 to 4 weeks. Hematopoietic stem cell transplantation (HSCT) may also be used for correction of B-cell and myeloid deficiencies. Live vaccines should be avoided in patients with XLA.

X-Linked Hyper-IgM Syndrome

The X-linked hyper-IgM syndrome (XHIGM) is a rare form of PIDD caused by a genetic mutation of the CD40L gene that codes for the CD40 ligand. An X-linked recessive trait, XHIGM is only found in males. When the CD40 ligand binds to the CD40 receptor on B cells, it triggers the B cells to undergo class-switching from IgM to IgG, IgA, and IgE. Individuals with XHIGM have normal or elevated IgM and low levels of IgG, IgA, and IgE. The CD40 ligand also plays a key role in T-cell differentiation and activation of macrophages. Symptoms of XHIGM are present in the first or second year of life. In addition to recurrent infections, approximately 50% of the patients develop neutropenia, which is associated with inflammation or ulceration of mucosal membranes and skin infections. Other symptoms include enlargement of the lymph nodes and spleen; enlarged tonsils and adenoids may cause snoring and obstructive sleep apnea. A rare form of XHIGM, ectodermal dysplasia, is characterized by sparse body hair, conical teeth, and recurrent infections. Diagnosis of XHIGM is confirmed with normal or elevated levels of IgM and low or absent IgG, IgA, and IgE. DNA tests may be used to confirm the CD40L gene mutation. Treatment includes antibiotics and IVIG or SCIG. Granulocyte-colony stimulating factor (G-CSF) is indicated for patients with severe neutropenia. HSCT may be considered for patients with severe symptoms. Patients with XHIGM have an increased susceptibility to *Pneumocystis jirovecii* pneumonia, and prophylactic treatment with trimethoprim-sulfamethoxazole is initiated as soon as the diagnosis of XHIGM is confirmed.

Selective IgA Deficiency

Selective IgA deficiency (SIgAD) is the most common type of PIDD, affecting 1 in 700 to 2000 individuals, especially those of European descent. The exact cause of selective IgA deficiency is unknown. In affected individuals, B cells are normal, but they lack a response to interleukins and fail to become plasma cells that produce IgA; production of other immunoglobulins is normal. IgA antibodies are transported in secretions to mucosal surfaces that come in contact with the environment, including the mouth, ears, sinuses, nose, throat,

TABLE 46.7	Primary Immunodeficiency Disorders	
B-cell deficiencies	IgA deficiency
	Common variable immunodeficiency
	X-linked immunodeficiency with hyper-IgM syndrome
	X-linked agammaglobulinemia
T-cell deficiencies	Wiskott-Aldrich syndrome
	DiGeorge syndrome
Combined B- and T-cell deficiency	Severe combined immunodeficiencies
Macrophage deficiency	Chronic granulomatous disease

respiratory tract, GI tract, eyes, and genitals, where they play a major role in protecting those sites from infection. People with selective IgA deficiency are at risk for repeated infections of the ears, sinuses, GI, genitourinary, and respiratory tracts. Allergies are more common in individuals with selective IgA deficiency. Over 30% of patients with selective IgA deficiency have an autoimmune disorder, especially RA and SLE. An absence of IgA and normal levels of IgG and IgM are confirmatory of the disorder. Treatment includes antibiotics for infections; unlike other PIDD, IVIG or SCIF is not indicated unless the individual also has a concomitant IgG subclass deficiency. Some individuals with selective IgA deficiency have anti-IgA antibodies and are at risk of an anaphylactic reaction if they receive blood products, including IVIG, which contain IgA. In these individuals, washed RBCs or irradiated blood and IgA-depleted IVIG are indicated.

IgG Subclass Deficiency

IgG is divided into four subclasses: IgG-1, IgG-2, IgG-3, and IgG-4. Circulating IgG is 60% to 70% IgG-1, 20% to 30% IgG-2, 5% to 8% IgG-3, and 1% to 3% IgG-4. An IgG subclass deficiency is a result of a lack of or very low levels of one or two IgG subclasses; IgG-4 and IgG-2 deficiency frequently occur together. The IgG subclasses have different protective roles, and lack of a specific IgG subclass is associated with specific types of infections. The IgG-1 and IgG-3 subclasses are effective against serious bacterial infections such as diphtheria and tetanus, as well as viral infections. The IgG-2 antibodies are effective against the polysaccharide coating of bacteria that cause ear and sinus infections, pneumonia, and meningitis. Diagnosis of IgG subclass deficiency is confirmed by low plasma levels of one or more IgG subclass antibodies and normal levels of total IgG, IgA, and IgM. An additional subset of patients has normal levels of IgG and IgG subclasses but are unable to produce antibodies in response to infections or vaccines. The IgG subclass deficiency tends to improve over time without medical intervention. Antibiotics may be needed to treat recurring infections; IVIG or SCIG may be used in limited circumstances for serious infections.

DiGeorge Syndrome

DiGeorge syndrome, also known as 22q11.2 d deletion syndrome, is due to a genetic defect on chromosome 22. It is the most common microdeletion syndrome, occurring in 1 in 4000 live births, and affects females and males equally. The genetic mutation causes a wide variety of abnormal cell and tissue growth during fetal development. Defects in cardiac and major vessels, poor immune system function, cleft palate, hypoparathyroidism, hypothyroidism, esophageal atresia, urogenital anomalies, and unusual facial features, including mandibular hypoplasia, heavy eyelids, and abnormal ear lobes, are associated with DiGeorge syndrome. Patients with DiGeorge syndrome have a higher incidence of autoimmune disease. Hypoplasia of the thymus is associated with a decreased production of T cells; B cells are normal, but their production of antibodies is inhibited by the absent or low number of mature T cells. Diagnosis of the syndrome is primarily based on DNA testing for the chromosome 22 deletion present in 90% of individuals with DiGeorge syndrome. Individuals lacking the genetic defect are diagnosed by clinical features and exclusion of other syndromes. Treatment of the immune presentations of the disease includes antibiotics, IVIG or SCIG, thymic tissue transplant, and steroids.

Wiskott-Aldrich Syndrome

The Wiskott-Aldrich syndrome (WAS) is caused by a mutation of the *WAS* gene that codes for WASP, an important signaling protein found on the surface of all blood cells. It is a recessive gene mutation on the X chromosome and only affects males. Both the T and B lymphocytes

are affected; WAS is associated with decreased IgM, low to normal IgG, and elevated IgA and IgE. Classic symptoms of WAS include thrombocytopenia purpura; recurring bacterial, viral, and fungal infections; and eczema. There is also a higher incidence of autoimmune disorders in individuals, including hemolytic anemia and idiopathic thrombocytopenia purpura (ITP). Cancer is also more common, especially B-cell lymphomas and leukemia. Microthrombocytopenia, a decreased number and size of platelets, is unique to WAS and characteristic of the disorder. Absence of the WAS protein in blood cells, or a mutation within the *WAS* gene, may be used for confirmatory diagnosis. Treatment of WAS includes antibiotics and IVIG or SCIG. A HSCT offers a curative option for patients with WAS.

Severe Combined Immunodeficiency

Severe combined immunodeficiency (SCID), also known as alymphocytosis, Glanzmann-Riniker syndrome, severe mixed immunodeficiency syndrome, and thymic alymphoplasia, refers to a rare group of PIDDs considered to be the most serious form of PIDD. Numerous genetic mutations are responsible for the absence of functional T and B lymphocytes and the heterogeneous clinical presentations.[46] Approximately 50% of the mutations are sex linked to the X chromosome. The majority of SCID are characterized by a genetic mutation in the IL-2 receptor gamma *(IL2RG)* gene or JAK3, an important signaling molecule for *IL2RG*. In other forms of SCID, a genetic deficiency of enzyme adenosine deaminase causes an accumulation of adenosine that is toxic to immature lymphoid cells of the immune system. Infants with SCID have a high rate of serious and life-threatening infections, including pneumonia, especially *P. jirovecii*, meningitis, CMV infection, and septicemia. They are also susceptible to vulnerable fungal infections and chronic diarrhea, which can lead to growth failure and malnutrition. Protective isolation of the infant is necessary to decrease the risk of infection. Diagnosis includes low levels of plasma lymphocytes and low T-cell function. Curative therapy includes HSCT; there is greater than a 90% success rate if it is undertaken during the first 3 months of life. Other treatment includes IVIG or SCIG, enzyme replacement, and gene therapy.[46]

Chronic Granulomatous Disease

Chronic granulomatous disease (CGD), also known as Bridges-Good syndrome, chronic granulomatous disorder, and Quie syndrome, is a diverse group of immune disorders due to inability of phagocytes to kill ingested pathogens. CGD is a rare and potentially fatal disorder of neutrophil function. In the phagocyte, nicotinamide adenine dinucleotide phosphate (NADPH) oxidase is responsible for oxidizing NADPH and reducing molecular oxygen to produce reactive oxygen compounds (superoxide radical and hydrogen peroxide) that destroy ingested bacteria. The rapid release of reactive oxygen compounds is called a respiratory burst. In CGD, phagocytes lack or have a defective NADPH oxidase and are unable to produce the reactive oxygen compounds that are necessary to kill ingested microorganisms. The incidence of CGD is 1 in 250,000, and the most common form is X linked; however, there are other autosomal recessive forms of the disease. The majority of children with CGD are diagnosed before the age of 5 years. Individuals with CGD suffer from recurrent infections at epithelial surfaces such as the skin, GI tract, respiratory tract, and organs with a large number of phagocytes, such as the liver. Granulomatous lesions are frequently found throughout the GI tract, causing dysphagia, dysmotility, or obstruction. Defective neutrophil uptake of dihydrorhodamine, a fluorescent dye, is diagnostic of the disorder. In addition to antibiotics for recurrent infections, treatment includes glucocorticoids, IFN, anti-TNF, and cyclosporine. Surgery may be required for GI granulomata; an allogeneic HSCT offers the only cure for CGD.[47]

Acquired Immune Deficiency Disorders

Approximately 90% of immune deficiencies are acquired. One of the most recognized forms of acquired immune deficiency (AID), also known as secondary immune deficiency, is acquired immune deficiency syndrome (AIDS). However, the most prevalent cause of AID worldwide is severe malnutrition. Other causes of AID include human T-cell lymphotropic virus type 1 (HTLV-1) infection, lymphoid cancers such as leukemia and lymphoma, autoimmune disease such as T1AD, splenectomy, aging, malnutrition, and immunosuppressant drugs, including corticosteroids, chemotherapy, and DMARDs. Secondary immunodeficiency affects both the innate and the adaptive immune systems; treatment of the primary condition usually results in improvement of the associated AID.

Acquired Immune Deficiency Syndrome

AIDS is the final stage of infection caused by HIV, a retrovirus that was first identified in 1983. According to the CDC, approximately 1.2 million people in the United States were HIV positive in 2018, including 37,968 individuals who received a new HIV diagnosis.[48] There are two forms and many subtypes of HIV. Over 90% of HIV-1 infections belong to the HIV-1 group M. Although it also affects monocytes and macrophage, the T cells, specifically the CD4, are the central targets of attack by HIV. A retrovirus, HIV is a single-stranded RNA molecule; through the process of reverse transcription, the infected CD4 cell makes a DNA double-stranded helix that contains all the viral genetic information. The infected cells produce viral progeny at a slow, steady rate for an indefinite period. The CD4 protein normally helps Th cells activate other immune cells; cytokines from Th cells induce B cells to become activated and undergo clonal expansion to form mature plasma cells that secrete HIV antibody. Infected cell membranes display viral glycoproteins that contain several regions that are highly antigenic and can be recognized by APCs for presentation to NK, Tc, and B cells for destruction. However, HIV is capable of changing the amino acid sequences of the antigenic regions of their glycoproteins; the new version is not recognized by the existing antibodies and escapes destruction. The virally infected cells continue to multiply until the immune system is able to produce new, virus-specific antibodies. In contrast, the smallpox, polio, and measles viruses are not antigenically variable, and immunity established against one form of those viruses provides lifelong protection against other forms of the same virus. Acute HIV infection is characterized by flulike symptoms, a result of increased release of inflammatory mediators, including IL-1 and TNF-α, and transient decline in circulating CD4. During this stage, viral levels in the blood are high, and the individual is very contagious. A variable asymptomatic period follows, as HIV antibodies destroy the infected T cells. However, HIV reproduction continues at very low rates, and there is a gradual, progressive fall in CD4 Th cells concomitant with a gradual increase in the plasma viral load; the individual is still contagious. Over time, the immune response is unable to control viral replication and mutation, the CD4 cell count falls below 200 cells/mm, and the individual moves into the final stage of infection, AIDS. Common symptoms of AIDS include chills, fever, sweats, swollen lymph glands, weakness, weight loss, and heightened risk of severe opportunistic infections and diseases.

Diagnostic tests for HIV include plasma HIV antigen and HIV antibodies; a CD4 T-cell count less than 200/mL (normally 600–1500/mL) is diagnostic of AIDS. The HIV viral load (HIV RNA) measures the number of HIV virus particles, called copies, in a milliliter of blood. The goal of treatment is to suppress the viral load to an "undetectable" level; the lower limit of HIV detection varies from 20 to 75 copies/mL depending on the laboratory performing the test. High viral loads are associated with faster disease progression. Genotyping of HIV is necessary to determine if the particular virus is resistant to any of the anti-HIV medications.

Individuals diagnosed with HIV should be immediately started on antiretroviral therapy (ART) regardless of the stage of their infection. FDA-approved antiretroviral drugs (ARVs) include fusion inhibitors that interfere with the HIV's ability to fuse with a cellular membrane; entry inhibitors that interfere with the ability of HIV to bind to external cell receptors; nucleoside/nucleotide reverse transcriptase inhibitors (NRTIs); faulty DNA building blocks that interfere with HIV DNA synthesis; nonnucleoside reverse transcriptase inhibitors (NNRTIs) that bind to reverse transcriptase (RT) and prevent the conversion of HIV RNA into HIV DNA; protease inhibitors (PIs) that interfere with HIV protease, which is essential for cutting long chains of HIV proteins into smaller individual proteins; and integrase strand inhibitors (InSTI) that block the HIV enzyme integrase that is responsible for the integration of viral RNA into the DNA of the infected cell.[49] The recommended initial ART regimen consists of two NRTIs and an InSTI. An optional regimen includes a NNRTI or boosted PI combined with two NRTIs.[50]

Preexposure prophylaxis (PrEP) is recommended for individuals at risk for HIV infection through sex or injection drug use. It includes a daily two-drug combination of emtricitabine, a nucleoside reverse transcriptase inhibitor, and tenofovir alafenamide, a nucleotide reverse transcriptase inhibitor. The risk of getting HIV from sex is reduced 99% with PrEP, and the risk of drug injection is reduced by 74%. Clinical trials of HIV vaccines have produced mixed results in part due to the ability of HIV to undergo multiple mutations.

CANCERS OF THE IMMUNE SYSTEM

According to the Leukemia & Lymphoma Society, 178,520 individuals in the United States are diagnosed with leukemia, lymphoma or myeloma, cancers of the WBCs, and lymphatics each year.[51] Their distribution is often age related. New cases account for 10% of new cancer cases and 9.4% of all cancer deaths (Box 46.3).

Leukemia

Leukemia is a result of uncontrolled clonal proliferation of malignant, dysfunctional leukocytes that grow rapidly and prevent the development of normal hematopoietic cells in the bone marrow. The incidence is higher in males and increases with age.[4] Down syndrome and neurofibromatosis, environmental exposure to radiation treatments and benzene, cigarette smoking, and a family history of leukemia are associated with an increased risk of leukemia. Survivors of leukemia have an increased risk of other cancers, possibly an effect of leukemic chemotherapy and radiation treatments. Childhood survivors are at increased risk for osteonecrosis of the large joints and endocrine abnormalities. Signs and symptoms are dependent upon the type of leukemia. Malignant lymphoblasts replace the normal marrow elements, significantly

---

BOX 46.3   Cancers of the Immune System

Leukemia
Acute lymphocytic leukemia
Acute myelogenous leukemia
Chronic lymphocytic leukemia
Chronic myelogenous leukemia

Lymphoma
Non-Hodgkin lymphoma
Hodgkin lymphoma

Myeloma
Multiple myeloma

Localized Myeloma
Extramedullary myeloma
Plasmacytoma

decreasing production of normal blood cells; consequently, anemia, thrombocytopenia, and neutropenia occur to varying degrees in all leukemias. The abnormal lymphoblasts also proliferate in lymphoid organs, including the liver, spleen, and lymph nodes. Common symptoms include fever or chills; fatigue; weakness; frequent or severe infections; weight loss; enlarged lymph nodes, liver, and spleen; bruising; recurrent nosebleeds; petechiae; and bone pain. A bone marrow biopsy with immunophenotyping is necessary for accurate diagnosis. Classification of the leukemia is based on the abnormal cell origin, lymphoid or myeloid, and the rate of the progression, acute or chronic. Lymphoid cells are precursors of lymphocytes, and lymphocytic leukemia affects lymphocytes of lymphoid or lymphatic tissue. Myeloid cells are immature blood cells that are precursors of granulocytes or monocytes; myelogenous leukemia affects the myeloid cells of the bone marrow. Acute leukemia involves immature blood cells that multiply aggressively and rapidly. Chronic leukemia involves mature blood cells that multiply slowly and can go undetected for years. Rare forms of leukemia include hairy cell leukemia, myelodysplastic syndromes, and myeloproliferative disorders.

Acute Lymphocytic Leukemia

Approximately 50% of acute lymphocytic leukemia (ALL) in the United States occurs in children and teenagers. It is the most common cancer and most frequent cause of cancer death before 20 years of age; it is also the second most common acute leukemia in adults. The incidence of ALL presents as a bimodal distribution, first peaking in childhood with a second peak occurring at age 50. Approximately 85% of ALL is classified as precursor B-cell and 15% has precursor T-cell lineage.[52] There are distinct genetic mutations associated with ALL; the increased incidence of T-cell ALL among males suggests a Y chromosome–related mutation. Symptoms of ALL include thrombocytopenia, anemia, and neutropenia. The cancer progresses rapidly as leukemia cells spread to the brain, liver, lymph nodes, and testes, where they continue to grow and divide, causing a wide array of symptoms. Patient age and initial WBC count are strong predictors of treatment outcomes. A standard risk is seen with children ages 1 to 9 and WBCs of 50,000/mL or less; children 10 years or older and WBCs of 50,000/mL or greater are considered high risk. Poorer outcomes are associated in children diagnosed before the age of 1 year. The time required to reach undetectable levels of leukemic cells is the single most powerful prognosticator of successful treatment in children with ALL. Treatment includes an intensive induction and consolidation regimen that is associated with an 85% 5-year event-free survival rate and an overall 90% survival rate. Survival rate among teenagers with ALL is less than younger children. Induction of remission includes 4 to 6 weeks of prednisone, vincristine, anthracycline, cyclophosphamide, and/or L-asparaginase. However, relapse is inevitable within 6 to 8 weeks, and consolidation therapy is necessary to prevent development of overt CNS leukemia. This includes repeated courses of methotrexate and folinic acid, followed by 18 to 30 months of antimetabolic therapy with mercaptopurine, thioguanine, daunorubicin, cytosine arabinoside (Ara-C), and methotrexate, and possibly 5- to 7-day "pulses" of prednisone and vincristine. There is a 15% to 20% relapse rate for ALL, and cure rates are lower after relapse. Treatment with an allogenic HSCT is more common after relapse. Other treatment options include immunotherapy. A cell surface antigen receptor, CD19, is present on most ALL B cells. Blinatumomab, a monoclonal anti-CD19 antibody, binds to the CD19 receptors on T-cell receptors and activates them to recognize and destroy B cells with the CD19 surface antigen. Patients with ALL frequently require blood transfusion therapy, a result of both an inability to produce normal blood cells and the effects of chemotherapy. All blood products must be irradiated.

Acute Myelogenous Leukemia

Acute myelogenous leukemia (AML), also known as acute myeloblastic leukemia, acute granulocytic leukemia, or acute nonlymphocytic leukemia, is the most common type of acute leukemia and accounts for 98% of acute adult leukemias; the median age at diagnosis is 64 years. It is associated with abnormal myeloid stem cells, which have the potential to produce different cell types; consequently, there are eight different AML subtypes that can present in a variety of ways.[53] Acute granulocytic leukemia is the most common AML subtype. Similar to ALL, the onset of AML is abrupt, but the survival rate is poorer (<50% for children, 35%–40% for individuals age <60 years, and 5%–15% for patients age >60 years). Relapse occurs within 3 years in the majority of patients. Treatment of AML includes induction and consolidation therapy; as with ALL, an allogenic HSCT is reserved for patients with relapsed AML. Individuals who relapse again after transplant may receive repeat induction therapy and supplemental donor lymphocytes. Individuals ineligible for HSCT may be treated with cytarabine and hypomethylating agents, decitabine, and azacitidine.

Chronic Lymphocytic Leukemia

Chronic lymphocytic leukemia (CLL) accounts for 30% of leukemias. The average age at diagnosis is 67 years, and it is rarely seen in children. A malignant B-cell precursor is responsible for 95% of CLL cases. It is a slow-growing disease; approximately 70% of individuals with CLL are asymptomatic, and the disease is discovered on a routine blood test (neutropenia, anemia, and thrombocytopenia). Lymphadenopathy and splenomegaly, a result of malignant lymphocyte invasion of lymphoid tissue, are usually the presenting symptoms. The CLL B cells do not produce normal antibodies, and patients are susceptible to infection. Diagnosis is confirmed by the clonal expansion of plasma B lymphocytes and confirmed by immunophenotyping; a bone marrow biopsy is not necessary for diagnosis of CLL. The disease may be monitored without treatment in individuals with indolent disease; chemotherapy and allogenic HSCT may be used to induce remission in individuals with rapidly progressing disease.

New pharmacologic therapies have been developed to improve life expectancy and decrease the toxicity associated with older chemotherapeutic agents. BTK inhibitors (ibrutinib, acalabrutinib) decrease cancer cell proliferation. Monoclonal antibodies (obinutuzumab) bind to and activate immune effector cells and directly activate intracellular death signaling pathways. Lastly, venetoclax inhibits antiapoptotic B-cell lymphoma-2 (Bcl-2) protein, causing programmed cell death of CLL cells.

Chronic Myelogenous Leukemia

Chronic myelogenous leukemia (CML) accounts for approximately 15% of leukemia; the highest incidence is in adults aged 40 to 50 years. Approximately 95% of patients with CML have an abnormal shortened chromosome 22, called the Philadelphia chromosome, a result of reciprocal translocation between chromosomes 9 and 22. The Philadelphia chromosome is responsible for stimulating cell proliferation and decreasing apoptotic cell death. In addition to the common symptoms of leukemia, CML usually presents with an increased granulocyte count and splenomegaly. Its categorization as chronic is an indication that CML grows slowly. However, it can change from a slowly progressing form of cancer into a rapidly growing, acute form that can spread to almost any organ in the body. Tyrosine kinase inhibitors (TKIs), such as imatinib, targets the enzyme responsible for the uncontrolled cell proliferation in the bone marrow. Although not curative, TKIs can provide long-term control of the disease; HSCT is reserved for younger patients or patients who fail to respond to TKIs.

Lymphoma

Lymphomas are a diverse group of neoplasms that are a result of proliferation of malignant lymphocytes in the lymphoid tissue. Lymphoma can occur at any age but is the most common cancer in young adults. Lymphomas are divided into two groups, non-Hodgkin lymphoma (NHL) and Hodgkin lymphoma (HL); classification is based on a range of pathologic and clinical features. Both HL and NHL arise in the head and neck regions; extranodal disease, with or without lymph node involvement, occurs more frequently in NHL. Approximately 90% of lymphomas are NHL and 10% are HL. Lymph node biopsies are mandatory for the diagnosis and classification of lymphoma. Computed tomography (CT), MRI, positron emission tomography (PET), bone marrow biopsy, and CSF analysis are used to stage the lymphoma. The stages of lymphoma identify the degree of cancer spread. The tumor is localized in stage I, and there is limited spread confined to one side of the diaphragm in stage II. Regional spread to either side of the diaphragm or to an area near the primary lymph node tumor is observed in stage III, and in stage IV there is distal spread beyond the lymphatic system. Lymphoma is further divided into A or B according to the associated symptoms; B-denoted lymphoma is more advanced and characterized by unexplained weight loss of 10% or greater, unexplained fever, and night sweats.

Non-Hodgkin Lymphoma

Most of the NHLs are B-cell lymphomas; the remainder are T-cell and NK lymphomas. The two most common types of NHL are diffuse large B-cell lymphoma, which accounts for 30% to 40% of lymphoma, and follicular lymphoma.[54] Although it commonly occurs in the lymph nodes, NHL can originate in any lymphoid tissue. It is more common in individuals 60 years of age and older. Overall, the risk of NHL is higher in males, but some types are more common in females. The symptoms of NHL are very similar to common viral illnesses, including painless swelling of the lymph nodes, and the disease is usually in stage III or IV when diagnosed. The tumors often arise in disparate lymph nodes, and extranodal involvement occurs early in the disease, including infiltration of the GI tract, bone marrow, testes, liver, and skin. The prognosis varies among the different types of NHL, but the overall survival rate is approximately 50%. Risk factors include environmental chemical exposure (benzene, herbicides, and insecticides), prior chemotherapy, radiation exposure, immune system deficiency or suppression (organ transplantation or autoimmune disease), infections (HIV, HTLV-1, human herpesvirus 8 [HHV8], and Epstein-Barr virus [EBV]), autoimmune disease (RA, SLE, Sjögren disease, and celiac sprue), and chronic immune stimulation (*Helicobacter pylori*, HBV, hepatitis C [HCV], and *Chlamydophila psittaci*). Radiation can be curative for early stages of indolent NHL. Chemotherapy with CHOP protocol (*c*yclophosphamide, *h*ydroxydaunorubicin, vincristine [*O*ncovin], and *p*rednisone) and/or MABs (rituximab) is used for advanced states. Aggressive NHL is treated with CHOP chemotherapy and radiation or rituximab; HSCT may be indicated for relapsed forms of NHL. Biologic drugs, such as IFN, and immunomodulating agents (thalidomide and lenalidomide) may be used if all other treatments have failed.

Hodgkin Lymphoma

The average age of HL diagnosis is 64 years, with two peaks occurring in the mid-20s and mid-60s. Prior EBV infection appears to be a risk factor for HL. Reed-Sternberg (RS) cells, malignant B lymphocytes, are characteristic of HL.[55] There are two main forms of HL. The majority of cases are classic HL, which presents earlier and has a longer survival rate. Nodular lymphocyte-predominant HL can transform into diffuse B-cell lymphoma. The RS cells secrete cytokines and TGF-β, which induce infiltration and proliferation of inflammatory cells that result in large, painless lymph nodes. In contrast to NHL, the spread of HL occurs in a predictable sequential fashion to local contiguous lymph nodes. The cervical, axillary, inguinal, and retroperitoneal lymph nodes are most frequently affected. Confirmatory diagnosis of HL requires an RS-positive lymph node biopsy. Treatment of HL includes chemotherapy, doxorubicin (Adriamycin), bleomycin, vinblastine, and dacarbazine (ABVD protocol), followed by radiation therapy. Brentuximab vedotin has FDA approval for the treatment of HL. An antibody-drug conjugate containing MAB and antimitotic drug, it binds to CD30 proteins found on HL cells. It has a high overall response rate in patients with refractory HL. One of the most curable forms of cancer, the 5-year relative survival rate for HL is 94% for individuals diagnosed before the age of 45 years. The survival rate is also dependent upon the disease stage at time of diagnosis; it is 90% to 95% for stages I and II, 80% to 85% for stage III, and 75% for stage IV

Multiple Myeloma

Approximately 103,500 people in the United States have myeloma. The 5-year relative survival rate is 48.5%. Multiple myeloma (MM), also known as Kahler disease, is the most common type of myeloma, accounting for over 90% of myelomas and 10% of hematologic malignancies. It is most common in individuals over the age of 50 and is rarely seen in children and young adults. It is more common in males, and blacks are nearly twice as likely as whites to develop myeloma. A mutation of plasma B cells results in rapid proliferation of abnormal myeloma cells that crowd out the normal stem cells in the bone marrow and interfere with the production of WBCs, RBCs, and platelets.[56] The myeloma cells produce monoclonal proteins or M protein microglobulins. The M proteins accumulate into plasmacytomas that erode the cortex of the bone resulting in osteoporosis and bone fractures. The abnormal proteins are also deposited in organs throughout the body. When present in the urine, they are called Bence Jones proteins. Anemia, bleeding, bone lesions and pain, hypercalcemia, and renal failure are common. The disease is staged as I, II, and III depending on the degree of anemia, number of M proteins, and renal damage. A bone marrow biopsy diagnosis requires at least 10% of clonal plasma cells or plasmacytoma plus evidence of associated end-organ damage. In addition to chemotherapy and glucocorticoids, treatment includes targeted drug therapy with proteasome inhibitors (bortezomib) that induce cell death, immunomodulating drugs (thalidomide, lenalidomide, pomalidomide) that enhance the immune system's ability to recognize and destroy the myeloma cell, and MABs (daratumumab, elotuzumab) that target receptors on myeloma cells. IFN can also slow the growth of myeloma. Bisphosphonates (alendronate, zoledronic acid), MABs (denosumab), and recombinant parathyroid hormone (teriparatide) are used to increase bone density. Autologous or allogeneic HSCT following high-dose chemotherapy may be used for advanced stages.

SURGERY AND THE IMMUNE SYSTEM

Immune surveillance is provided by the coordinated activity of NK cells of the innate immune system and the cytotoxic CD8+ T cells of the adaptive immune system to destroy cancer cells and infectious organisms. Surgery and anesthesia provoke a variety of metabolic and endocrine responses that decrease normal immune surveillance. The resulting state of immunosuppression is associated with surgical site infections (SSIs), postoperative sepsis, and tumor migration and metastasis.[57] In the immediate postoperative period, an initial proinflammatory phase is quickly followed by a period of immunosuppression. The immune suppression appears to be primarily related to the surgical stress activation of the sympathetic nervous system (SNS) and the hypothalamic-pituitary-interrenal (HPI) axis. Increased circulating inflammatory mediators, hyperglycemia, hypothermia, blood transfusions, and anesthetic agents contribute to postoperative immunosuppression. A number of patient factors contribute to perioperative immune system dysfunction, including but not limited to a preexisting immune deficiency, immune suppression therapy for autoimmune diseases or organ transplantation, increasing age, preexisting diseases such as diabetes mellitus, and preoperative sepsis (Box 46.4).[58,59] The innate immune system has an earlier recovery from postoperative immunosuppression than the adaptive system.[63]

Surgical Site Infections

The CDC defines SSI as an infection that occurs at or near the surgical incision within 30 or 90 days of the procedure depending on the type of surgery.[60,61] Of nearly 30 million inpatient and outpatient surgical procedures performed annually in the United States, up to 5% will have an associated SSI, the third most frequently hospital-acquired nosocomial infection. SSIs are associated with prolonged hospitalizations and increased patient morbidity and health care costs. The most commonly implicated organisms are *Staphylococcus aureus, Staphylococcus epidermidis,* aerobic streptococci, and anaerobic cocci. Causes of SSIs are multifactorial; they include patient age, comorbidities, smoking habits, obesity, nutritional status, immunosuppression, malignancies, and postsurgical wound contamination.[62]

The innate immune system is activated during surgery and, in response to the tissue damage and blood loss, a sterile systemic inflammatory response occurs within hours of the procedure.[58,59] The DAMPs released from injured tissue promote neutrophil and macrophage migration to the site of injury for removal of tissue debris. They also provide a link between the innate and adaptive immune systems by activating APCs, including monocytes and DCs. Inflammatory cytokines, chemokines, and antimicrobial peptides are released by immune cells to enhance eradication of injured cells and microbes. Surgery is associated with an increased release of Th1 cytokines (IL-6 and TNF); postoperatively Th1 cytokines decrease and Th2 cytokines increase (IL-10 and TGF). Following surgery, there is also a decrease in T cells that correlates with the duration of the procedure and intraoperative blood loss. Laparoscopic surgery is associated with a decreased immune suppression, and it attenuates the cytokine cascade of a decrease in lymphocytes and shift toward a Th2 dominance. If the acute inflammatory response to surgery is not tempered by homeostatic antiinflammatory mechanisms, it can result in excessive death of phagocytes and increased susceptibility to infection by invading pathogens. The invading microbes contain PAMPs, which further stimulate the immune effector cells. The TLRs are responsible for identifying DAMPs released from stressed cells and PAMPs from invading microbes. A vicious cycle ensues, with surgical trauma causing inflammation and immunosuppression, and subsequent infection from invading microbes increasing the inflammatory response. The end result is tissue injury and potential organ failure.

Surgery also causes profound changes in the neuroendocrine system. Stress hormones (specifically epinephrine, norepinephrine, and cortisol) are elevated in the postoperative period, a direct result of the activation of the HPA axis and the SNS. The result is an increase in the number of Th2 and Treg, an altered Th1/Th2 balance, and decreased function of NK and IL-12. Cortisol interferes with the production of cytokines and prostaglandins, impedes aggregation of macrophils and neutrophils, induces apoptosis in T cells, promotes Th2 dominance

(which decreases NK function), and suppresses phagocytosis at the surgical site. Immunomodulating diets (IMD) containing supplemental arginine and omega-3 fatty acids, and β-blockade, reverse the Th1/Th2 imbalance and may be beneficial in reducing the immunosuppression associated with surgical trauma.

Cancer Recurrence

Approximately 80% of cancer patients require anesthesia and analgesia for a variety of diagnostic and therapeutic procedures. Paradoxically, surgical excision of tumors may actually stimulate proliferation and metastasis of tumor cells. Surgical excision disrupts the blood vessels supplying the tumor and allows tumor cells to enter the systemic circulation. The immune and inflammatory processes that are activated in response to surgery can promote the survival and proliferation of cancer cells that persist after surgery contributing to the development of metastatic disease.[55] The postoperative period is the most vulnerable period for metastasis of cancer cells. This can be attributed to the surgical suppression of cell-mediated immunity, which can last several days after the procedure and is proportional to the extent of the surgical trauma.[55]

Immune control of tumor cells is carried out predominantly through cell-mediated immunity and is dependent on the normal function of Tc, NK and NKT cells, DCs, and macrophage inflammatory mediators, including INF, interleukins, and Th1 cytokines, which increase the cytotoxic activity of Tc and NK cells. The Th2 cytokines increase humoral immunity and suppress the Th1 response. The surgical induced activation of the HPA axis and SNS increases release of cortisol and catecholamines, which inhibit the proliferation of NK cells and CD8+ T cells that are necessary to destroy cancer cells. It also promotes proliferation of protumor Treg and Th2, which contributes to tumor growth and metastasis. Tumor cells express adrenergic β-receptors that regulate multiple cellular processes necessary for the initiation and progression of cancer; β-receptor activation suppresses NK activity and supports metastasis. The increased epinephrine and norepinephrine released in the HPA stress response bind to the β-receptors on tumor cells and increase their proliferation and survival. Current research involves the use of β-blockers to reduce the progression rate of solid tumors. Immune-suppressive agents intended to prevent rejection of transplanted organs also allow cancers to grow and depress the ability of the immune system to target and kill viruses associated with cancer, including HPV and HCV. Transplant recipients of solid organs have an increased risk for cancer and are almost three times more likely to die from cancer than the general population, especially lung cancer and NHL. The risk for cancer is significantly higher among young adults who had transplant surgery during childhood.[64,65]

Trauma to normal tissue during surgical resection of a tumor stimulates an inflammatory response necessary for normal wound healing at the surgical site. This includes release of humoral factors, such as prostaglandins, cytokines, TNF, and chemokines. In turn, these factors activate macrophages, neutrophils, and fibroblasts to release additional cytokines and growth factors. Unfortunately, the factors that promote normal tissue healing also stimulate residual cancer cell proliferation and migration. When combined with the hypothalamic-pituitary-adrenal (HPA) axis inhibition of NK cells and CD8+ T cells, this inflammatory response supports invasion of surrounding normal tissue by tumor cells as well as inflammatory oncotaxis (i.e., metastasis of tumor cells to distant sites).[66]

Perioperative Blood Transfusion

Blood transfusions are associated with a depression of the immune system and metastasis and recurrence of cancer. A perioperative blood transfusion is an independent correlate of a poor outcome following cancer surgery.[67-70]

Transfusion-related immunomodulation (TRIM) was first recognized in the early 1970s when it was noted that kidney transplant recipients who received allogenic blood transfusions had better allograft survival rates. The mechanism of TRIM involves donor leukocyte suppression of monocytes, altered lymphocyte function, release of immunosuppressive prostaglandins, inhibition of IL-2, increased suppressor T-cell activity, and a shift toward protumor Th2 cells. In addition to higher allograft survival rates, TRIM is associated with an increased risk of postoperative infections, increased tumor recurrence after surgical resection, activation of latent viral infections, and improvement in autoimmune disease.[67] Irradiated or leukocyte-depleted blood products are recommended for cancer patients to offset the depression of the immune system by donor leukocytes. However, the increased risk for cancer metastasis appears to be similar for recipients of allogenic, autogenic, or leukocyte reduced transfusions. In vivo studies suggest that the cancer-stimulating effects of transfusion increase with increasing product storage duration.[66] Use of intraoperative cell savers may also contribute to cancer recurrence as the surgical blood can contain tumor cells. Transfusions are discussed in Chapter 22.

Perioperative Hyperglycemia

Diabetes mellitus is associated with an increased susceptibility to bacterial, fungal, and viral infections secondary to depression of both the innate and adaptive immune systems.[71] In a similar manner, perioperative hyperglycemia is associated with an increased incidence of SSI and poor patient outcomes. Hyperglycemia is associated with decreased neutrophil proliferation and function. It decreases mobilization and adherence of monocytes at the site of infection, impedes their bactericidal activity, and limits their ability to stimulate apoptosis in pathogenic cells. Hyperglycemia decreases the complement response; it inhibits opsonization by binding to the C3 receptor and preventing it from attaching to the microbe and activating phagocytosis. Hyperglycemia is associated with increased synthesis and release of cytokines, specifically IL-6, TNF, and CRP. It also suppresses vasodilation during acute tissue inflammation, effectively reducing blood flow to infected tissue and limiting the migration of phagocytes to the site.[71] Even transient episodes of hyperglycemia can depress immune function, and tight glycemic control reduces nosocomial infections in critically ill patients and SSIs. To attenuate the effects of hyperglycemia on the immune system, intraoperative glycemic control should be implemented to ensure a target blood glucose that is less than 200 mg/dL.[60]

ANESTHESIA AND THE IMMUNE SYSTEM

A large number of cancers are amenable to surgery; approximately 80% of cancer patients will require anesthesia for diagnostic, therapeutic, or palliative interventions.[72] In addition to the immunosuppression and enhanced inflammatory response impact of surgery, anesthetic agents may also act as immunologic modulators and influence wound infection and cancer recurrence. While it is difficult to separate the effects of surgery and anesthesia on the immune system, anesthetic agents are associated with impaired immune function, including depressed function of NK cells, neutrophils, macrophages, DCs, and T cells. Most of the research on the direct effect of anesthetic agents has been performed in vitro; in vivo research is complicated because of multiple contributing factors, but the evidence suggests that the choice of anesthetics can contribute to poor long-term cancer outcomes.[72-77]

Inhalation Anesthetics

Inhalation anesthetics suppress the cytotoxicity of NK cells and macrophages; induce apoptosis of T cells; decrease IL-2 and restrict proliferation of T cells; up-regulate tumorigenic growth factors, hypoxia-inducible factor, and IGF; and enhance angiogenesis.[75-80] Inhalation anesthetics impair adhesion of phagocytes and inhibit the respiratory burst necessary for destruction of pathogens. There is conflicting research on the impact of inhalation anesthetics on tumor cells. In some cases, volatile agents appear to stimulate cancer cell activity and prometastatic processes and inhibit NK activity while in other cases they inhibit cancer cells and decrease the risk of metastasis. The differing effect on metastasis may be dependent on the specific cancer; sevoflurane stimulates renal cancer cells and increases risk of metastasis but inhibits non-small cell lung carcinoma cells.[81]

Intravenous Agents

Midazolam decreases IL-8 necessary for migration and adhesion of neutrophils but does not appear to affect cytotoxic T lymphocytes.[76] Ketamine and thiopental depress NK cell activity and induce T-lymphocyte apoptosis.[76] Propofol appears to be the one IV agent that protects against immunosuppression by promoting the proliferation and cytotoxicity activity of NK cells, decreasing proinflammatory cytokines and inhibiting prostaglandin E_2 (PGE$_2$) and cyclooxygenase (COX) activity.[82-86] Propofol may also inhibit oncogenes and angiogenesis.[66]

Opioids

Uncontrolled postoperative pain, a potent stimulant of the HPA axis and SNS, contributes to perioperative immune suppression. Effective pain control attenuates the surgery-induced stress response that promotes metastatic susceptibility, and opioids are commonly used throughout the perioperative period. Opioids suppress NK cells that are vital for the eradication of tumor cells and viruses, increase regulatory T cells, promote angiogenesis, and suppress apoptosis.[87]

The immune modulatory effects of opioids appear to be mediated by the mu (μ) opioid receptor (MOR) on lymphocytes.[2] Inflammatory cytokines regulate the expression of the *MOR* gene, which regulates opioid and growth factor-induced receptor signaling, leading to the proliferation and migration of cancer cells. MOR is overexpressed in some types of cancers; this can result in direct opioid stimulation of tumor growth, angiogenesis, and metastasis. Methylnaltrexone (MNTX), a selective peripheral MOR antagonist, significantly reduces opioid-induced tumor growth and metastasis. However, in some cases, opioids appear to paradoxically suppress tumor migration and proliferation and induce apoptosis in cancer cells. Morphine inhibition of the migration and adhesion of colon cancer cells has been demonstrated, as well as induction of apoptosis in lung carcinoma and some leukemias.

Opioids differ in their ability to modulate the immune response. Morphine and fentanyl suppress NK cell cytotoxicity, increasing the risk for metastasis; tramadol increases NK cell cytotoxicity, reducing metastasis; and buprenorphine has no effect on NK cell cytotoxicity.[66,87,88] Morphine is associated with the greatest depression of the immune system. Codeine, methadone, remifentanil, and fentanyl demonstrate strong immune modulation; weaker modulation is seen with hydromorphone, oxycodone, tramadol, and hydrocodone. Buprenorphine has minimal or no effect on the immune system, and remifentanil increases antiinflammatory cytokines (IL-10) with antitumor activity. Poorly controlled pain and increased opioid requirements are associated with lower survival rates in patients with advanced lung cancer.[66] However, it is difficult to discern the cause of immune suppression, as poorly controlled pain may increase opioid requirements.

NSAIDs have beneficial anticancer effects due to inhibition of prostaglandin synthesis.[89,90] Postoperative immunosuppression causes excess release of prostaglandins, which promote cancer cell adhesion, migration, and invasion; prostaglandins also inhibit the activity of Tc and DCs, down-regulate antineoplastic cytokines (TNF-α and INF-γ), and up-regulate immunosuppressive cytokines (IL-10, IL-4, and IL-6).

COX converts procarcinogens to carcinogens and can initiate cancer cell growth. COX-2 is overexpressed in some breast and colorectal cancers; the product, PGE_2, is believed to contribute to the metastatic potential of these cancers.[66] NSAIDs attenuate prostaglandin synthase by COX inhibition. Administration of COX-2 inhibitors, alone or in conjunction with morphine, prevents induced tumor growth and metastasis, as well as angiogenesis. The opioid-sparing analgesic effects of NSAIDs may also play a role in disease progression.[66] Long-term use of COX inhibitors, especially COX-2 inhibitors, is associated with a reduced risk of cancer.

Regional Anesthesia

By blocking afferent neural transmission, regional anesthesia attenuates the surgical stress response and supports preservation of normal immune function. It is associated with decreased cortisol levels, normal NK cell function, and preservation of normal Th1/Th2 balance. In addition, regional anesthesia decreases the use of opioids and volatile anesthetics and is associated with a lower incidence of SSI compared to general anesthesia. Local anesthetics, especially the amides, are associated with cytotoxic effects on cancer cells. Bupivacaine directly inhibits cancer cell viability, proliferation, and migration, and lidocaine increases NK activity and decreases tumor size and metastasis.[66] A combination of general anesthesia and epidural anesthesia may mitigate the surgical-induced immune suppression. In combination with general anesthesia or alone, regional anesthesia is associated with a longer cancer-free time interval and a lower incidence of breast, colon, prostate, and melanoma cancer reoccurrence. Patients who received propofol and paravertebral anesthesia for breast cancer surgery had increased infiltration of their tumors by NK and Th cells.[66] Anesthetics such as propofol and local or regional anesthesia, which decrease surgery-induced neuroendocrine responses through HPA axis and SNS suppression, may cause less immunosuppression and recurrence of certain types of cancer compared to volatile anesthetics and opioids.[66] A combination of propofol, COX antagonists, and regional anesthesia is associated with decreased immunosuppression.

ANESTHETIC MANAGEMENT OF THE IMMUNOCOMPROMISED PATIENT

Up to 1.5% of the US population may have a defective immune system, and an unknown number may be immunocompromised because of underlying disease and medical interventions. Patients with immunodeficiency syndromes and iatrogenic induced immune suppression for treatment of autoimmune diseases and prevention of organ transplant rejection have an increased risk for SSIs, as well as migration and proliferation of cancer cells. Preoperative tests for immunosuppression include complete blood counts with a differential smear, serum immunoglobulins, complement assays, T-cell function (skin testing), and B-cell function (antibody titers).

Central and peripheral vascular catheters account for 15% to 30% of all nosocomial bacteremias, and central venous catheters (CVCs) are more frequent sources of bacteremia.[89] The risk of CVC-associated bacteremia is dependent on catheter choice, insertion site, insertion technique, and catheter maintenance. Infections are higher for multilumen catheters compared to single-lumen catheters. Coagulase-negative staphylococci occur most frequently with CVCs, whereas *S. aureus* and

BOX 46.5   Anesthetic Management of the Immunocompromised Patient

- Assessment of preoperative immune status
- Regional anesthesia/combined general and regional anesthesia
- Antibiotic administration 30–40 min prior to incision
- Nonopioids for pain management
- Active patient warming for long cases
- Tight blood glucose control
- Leukocyte poor or irradiated blood transfusion if warranted
- Strict aseptic technique during insertion of central venous lines
  - Frequent glove use and hand cleansing during provision of patient care
  - Cleaning of anesthesia workstations between surgical cases

Enterobacteriaceae species are more frequent with peripheral catheters.[91,92] Strict aseptic technique and maximum barrier precautions are mandatory for placement of a CVC. Antibiotic or antiseptic impregnated catheters, sutureless securement devices, chlorhexidine impregnated dressings, and disinfection caps can reduce the infection rate associated with intravascular catheters.[92]

Three-way stopcocks are associated with a higher incidence of catheter-related bloodstream infections than needleless connectors (NC).[93] However, NCs are frequently left open to the environment and provide an immediate portal of entry for bacteria into the bloodstream; contamination of the NC is responsible for approximately 50% of catheter-related infections.[95] Aseptic technique is mandatory when accessing NCs as deviation from the standard of care places the immunocompromised patient at a high risk for postoperative infection. According to CDC guidelines for prevention of intravascular catheter-related infections, the NC hub should be disinfected with greater than 0.5% chlorhexidine with alcohol, 70% alcohol, or 10% povidone-iodine prior to access. Antiseptics should be allowed to dry for maximal effect.[94,95] Use of alcohol chlorhexidine disinfection caps creates a physical and chemical barrier between the lumen and the environment.

The inclusion of a neuraxial block in the anesthetic plan will blunt the surgical-induced HPA axis and SNS response associated with immune suppression and a heightened risk of infection. Prophylactic antibiotics should be administered at least 30 minutes before skin incision. Prevention of intraoperative hypothermia mandates the use of active warming modalities for long surgical cases. Intraoperative hyperglycemia must be avoided, and an insulin infusion may be warranted. Leukocyte poor and irradiated blood should be used when transfusion is unavoidable. Postoperative pain is best controlled with a combination of neuraxial anesthesia and nonopioid agents.

Standard precautions that reduce the risk of SSIs include good hand hygiene, safe injection practices, and targeted cleaning of the anesthetizing workstation between cases. The operating room environment is not conducive to frequent physical hand washing with soap and water during case management. Use of single and double gloves that are removed after contamination and frequent hand cleaning with an alcohol-based product are both mandatory when caring for patients with compromised immune function (Box 46.5).

SUMMARY

An effective immune response requires a cooperative synergy between the innate and the adaptive immune system to protect the body from a wide variety of pathogens. The innate system generates the first line of defense, and the adaptive system provides antigen-specific antibodies

for future encounters with the same antigen. Both the innate and adaptive immune systems include a cell-mediated response that is carried out by phagocytes, T lymphocytes, and cytokines in response to antigens in host cells; a humoral response is mediated by B-lymphocyte antibodies. Passive immunity with administration of IG can temporarily increase a patient's immune system. Active immunity, achieved with prior antigen exposure or immunizations, establishes long-term immunologic memory in the adaptive immune system.

Abnormalities of the immune system include hypersensitivity reactions, alloimmunity and autoimmunity, primary and secondary immune deficiencies, and malignancies of the immune cells and lymphoid tissue and organs. Surgery causes a generalized state of immunosuppression in the immediate postoperative period that is associated with a reduced resistance to infection, development of postoperative septic complications, and tumor metastasis. Confounding factors include cancer type, allogeneic blood transfusions, and intraoperative hypothermia or hyperglycemia or administration of glucocorticoids. Anesthesia is also associated with depressed immune function, but it is difficult to separate the effects of surgery and anesthesia on the immune system. There is some evidence of an association between anesthesia and cancer recurrence, but overall results from retrospective studies on SSI and cancer recurrence are conflicting, and there are no randomized controlled trials that support the selection or exclusion of a specific technique or agent. The decreased

cortisol levels and preservation of Th1/Th2 balance that is associated with regional anesthesia may be due to a direct effect of the regional anesthesia, attenuation of the surgery-induced stress response, and/or a reduced use of opioids. Whereas there is no evidence to support the use of regional anesthesia over general anesthesia, the combination of the two techniques will blunt the surgery-induced stress response and provide postoperative pain control in combination with nonopioid agents such as NSAIDs and acetaminophen. Surgical patients can exhibit a wide array of immune system dysfunction as a result of primary or secondary immune deficiency syndromes, chronic immune suppression therapy, increasing age, preexisting disease, and preoperative sepsis. Consequently, they have an increased risk for SSIs and postoperative migration and proliferation of cancer cells. Appropriate anesthesia care includes the issue of strict aseptic technique for invasive procedures, administration of prophylactic antibiotics 30 to 60 minutes prior to skin incision, prevention of intraoperative hypothermia and hyperglycemia, immediate removal of contaminated gloves, NC disinfection prior to access, targeted cleaning of the anesthetizing workstation, and frequent hand cleansing throughout the perioperative period.

REFERENCES

For a complete list of references for this chapter, scan this QR code with any smartphone code reader app, or visit the following URL: http://booksite.elsevier.com/9780323711944/.

47

Anesthesia and Laser Surgery

Bernadette T. Higgins Roche

INTRODUCTION

In 1900, Max Planck identified the relationship between energy and frequency of radiation; he proposed that energy is emitted, transferred, and absorbed in discrete amounts of energy or "quanta" that is related to the frequency of radiation (Planck's constant). In 1905, Einstein identified the quantum particles of energy as photons and theorized that atoms move from the ground-energy state (E_0) to higher energy levels when energy is added to them and release energy as they fall back to their ground state. Years later, he introduced the concept of stimulated emission where a collision between a photon and an excited atom stimulates the emission of a photon from the atom that possesses the same frequency, phase, and direction as the stimulating photon. The first laser was developed by Arthur Schawlow and Charles Townes in the late 1950s; and the term *laser*, an acronym for *l*ight *a*mplification by the *s*timulated *e*mission of *r*adiation, was proposed by Gordon Gould in 1959. In 1960, Theodore Maiman built the first functioning laser using a mixture of helium and neon, and in rapid succession a number of lasers were developed: the yttrium-aluminum-garnet (YAG) laser treated with 1% to 3% neodymium (Nd:YAG) in 1961, then the argon (Ar) laser in 1962. The ruby laser, the first medical laser, was introduced in 1963, followed by the carbon dioxide (CO_2) laser in 1964. Medical lasers were first used in retinal surgery. The development of smaller and more powerful lasers expanded the use of lasers to all surgical specialties.[1-4] Capable of making incisions as small as 0.5 microns, the laser scalpel offers definite advantages over traditional surgery, including improved access to operative sites, greater precision in tissue destruction and removal, and controlled hemostasis. Lasers have hard and soft tissue applications in dentistry and continue to play a major role in ophthalmology. In large part because of the introduction of the excimer laser in the 1980s, laser-assisted in situ keratomileusis (LASIK) is one of the most common surgical procedures in the United States. Surgical lasers have revolutionized the field of dermatology and esthetic surgery. Lasers are also used in spas and beauty salons for laser hair removal (LHR) by cosmetologists and estheticians. Medical use of lasers also includes photodynamic therapy (PDT) in which laser-activated drugs are used to destroy abnormal cells. Medical lasers can only be used by licensed practitioners; states regulate the practitioners authorized to use medical lasers.

BASIC PRINCIPLES OF LASERS

Electromagnetic Spectrum

Electromagnetic (EM) radiation is a broad spectrum of heat energy that travels in waves; it includes radio waves, microwaves, infrared waves, visible light waves, ultraviolet (UV) waves, x-rays, and gamma rays (Fig. 47.1). The wavelength decreases and the frequency increases as the EM spectrum moves from radio waves to gamma waves. The optical portion of the EM spectrum includes infrared, visible, and UV waves with a wavelength range of 200 to 1000 nm. Infrared waves are invisible to humans, and infrared radiation is perceived as heat. Visible light includes a rainbow of colors—red, orange, yellow, green, blue, indigo, and violet—with a very narrow wavelength range of 400 nm (violet) to 700 nm (red).[1-4] UV radiation is also invisible to humans and causes a chemical reaction in human skin with little heat production.

Light can be described as both a wavelength and a particle of energy called a photon. The energy of an EM wave is proportional to its frequency and inversely proportional to its wavelength. UV radiation possesses a short wavelength and high-frequency, intense energy that can damage the skin. The energy of a photon refers to the energy emitted when an electron falls from an excited orbit to one of lower energy; the energy between the two orbits defines the wavelength of the emitted photon. The relationship between the energy and the wavelength of light is:

$$E = hc/\lambda$$

where E is energy in joules, h is Planck's constant (6.63×10^{-34} J-s), c is the speed of light (2.998×10^{-8} m/s), and λ is wavelength in meters.[1,3]

Spontaneous and Stimulated Absorption and Emission of Energy

In an atom, electrons exist in specific orbits or orbitals with each orbital representing a specific level of energy. The ground state or orbital closest to the nucleus has the lowest energy; the higher orbitals, located farthest from the nucleus, have the greatest energy. Energy is required for movement of an electron to a higher orbital and must equal the difference in energy between the two orbitals. Conversely, an electron will lose energy if it falls to a lower orbit. Electrons tend to return to the ground state spontaneously, releasing a photon of light energy in the process, a spontaneous emission of radiation. The energy of the released photon and therefore its wavelength is dependent on the energy difference between the two orbits. The light produced by fluorescent lights or incandescent bulbs is a result of electrons changing orbits and returning to ground state. Both the energy of the released photon and the wavelength of the light are proportional to the energy difference between the excited state and the ground state of the atom. Light produced by spontaneous emission of radiation is composed of different wavelengths and frequencies; consequently, the photons oscillate randomly (noncoherence), and the light disperses as it travels.

In contrast to spontaneous emission of radiation, an electron can be pumped from a ground state to a higher orbital by a stimulating photon with energy equal to the energy difference between the two orbitals. A stimulating photon can also cause an atom in an excited state to fall to a lower orbital and release energy. When struck by a stimulating photon, an excited atom decays back to its ground state and emits a second photon. If the energy of the stimulating photon is equal to the

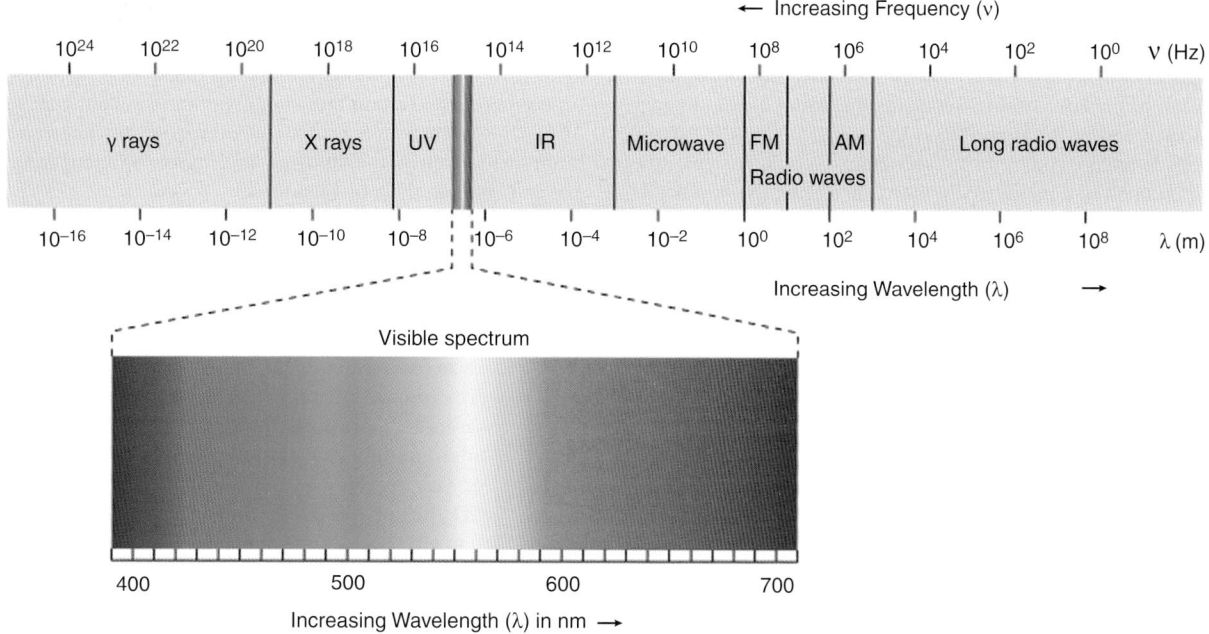

Fig. 47.1 The electromagnetic spectrum. (From https://commons.wikimedia.org/wiki/File:EM_spectrum.svg.)

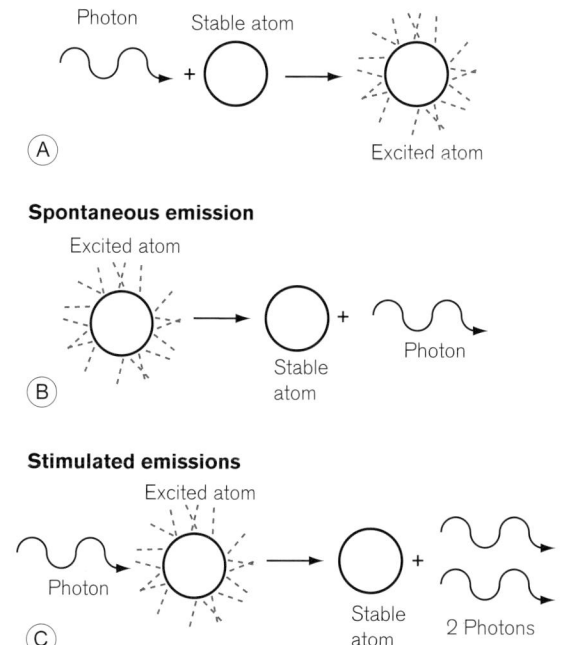

Absorption

Photon   Stable atom

Excited atom

(A)

Spontaneous emission

Excited atom

Stable atom

Photon

(B)

Stimulated emissions

Excited atom

Photon

Stable atom

2 Photons

(C)

Fig. 47.2 The interaction of light (a photon) with an atom. Three processes are shown: (A) the absorption of a photon by an atom in a low-energy state, (B) the spontaneous emission of a photon from an atom in an excited state, and (C) the stimulated emission of a photon by a second photon of the same wavelength from an excited-state atom. (From Davey A, Diba A. *Ward's Anaesthetic Equipment.* 6th ed. Philadelphia: Elsevier; 2012:476.)

energy difference between the excited and ground states of the atom, the emitted photon will have the same wavelength, energy, frequency, and direction as the stimulating photon. This process is known as stimulated emission of radiation (Fig. 47.2). The two photons, the stimulating photon and the emitted photon, can strike other excited atoms

and stimulate additional emissions of photons resulting in a burst of coherent radiation as all the atoms return rapidly to ground state.

Coherence, directionality, and monochromaticity differentiate laser light from fluorescent or incandescent light.[2] Laser beam photons have the same wavelength and oscillate synchronously in identical phase with one another (coherence). Laser light moves in a parallel, narrow beam (spatial coherence) over long distances and displays minimal dispersion. This spatial coherence, known as collimation, allows the laser light to be focused on a very small area. Reflection of a laser beam can reduce the collimation and increase the dispersion, especially if the reflecting surface has a matte or dull finish; however, the reduction in collimation and increased dispersion of a reflected laser beam is insignificant if the reflecting surface is smooth and shiny. The distance between the earth and the moon is calculated by the length of time it takes for a laser light to return to earth from reflectors placed on the moon. Laser light is composed of specific and discrete wavelengths; consequently, the light emitted is monochromatic and specific for each laser. Just as white light is composed of multiple colors, some lasers are tunable and can emit light at several different wavelengths. However, tunable lasers can only emit one color or wavelength at a time. A typical lightbulb is more powerful than a laser, but its light is not collimated, and the dispersion of the light reduces its intensity. In contrast, the intensity of a 1-milliwatt (mW) laser is six times greater than a 100-watt (W) incandescent bulb. Although a typical laser emits only a few milliwatts of power, from a distance of 100 ft lasers can produce a highly intense beam of 1 to 2 mm that can be 1 million times more concentrated than light from an incandescent source.

Laser Physics

A laser unit requires an external energy source, optical resonating cavity, and laser medium (Fig. 47.3).[2] The external energy source pumps up the energy of the laser medium and allows the electrons to move to a higher energy state or orbital. External energy sources include flash lamps, continuous light, high-voltage discharge, diodes, or another laser. Electric current is used to excite gas lasers, such as CO_2 and Ar lasers. Liquid and solid-state lasers, such as the potassium-titanyl-phosphate (KTP) laser, require energy from a flash lamp or another laser.

The optical resonating cavity, a tubelike structure, provides optimal amplification of the laser beam. It contains the lasing medium and a mirror at each end of the tube. When the lasing medium is excited by the outside energy source (e.g., flash lamp, electric current), the atoms are pumped to a higher energy level increasing the number of atoms in the excited state. Population inversion is necessary for stimulated emission of radiation, and it occurs when more atoms are in an unstable excited state than the resting state.[2] When one of the atoms spontaneously decays back to its ground state, it releases a photon that stimulates other excited atoms to decay back to ground state, releasing additional photons. The wavelength, frequency, phase, and direction

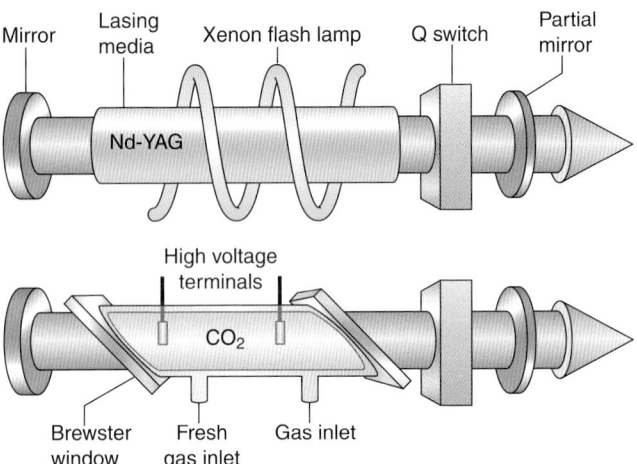

Fig. 47.3 A laser system consists of several components, regardless of whether the laser is a solid-based, liquid-based, or gas-based device. The central component is the laser medium itself, which may be a solid crystal of yttrium-aluminum-garnet *(YAG)* with a small concentration of neodymium *(Nd)* as dopant, or it may be a tube containing carbon dioxide *(CO₂)*. The energy pump (xenon flash lamp or an electric spark generator) provides the means of obtaining a population inversion of orbital electrons. A pair of axial mirrors permits repeated passes of collimated photons through the laser medium allowing maximum amplification by stimulated emission. The mirror on the right is not 100% reflective and allows the beam to escape. The optional Q switch increases the efficiency of pulsed lasers by allowing a small delay to increase the pumping. (From Miller RD, et al. *Miller's Anesthesia*. 7th ed. Philadelphia: Elsevier; 2010:2408.)

of the secondary photons are identical to those of the first photon. The mirrors reflect the excited photons back into the resonating cavity at approximately 186,000 miles per second, where they travel back and forth in a parallel fashion, stimulating the release of more photons from other excited atoms and amplifying the resultant laser light (Fig. 47.4). One of the mirrors is partially transparent and allows a very thin beam of the coherent, collimated, and monochromatic laser light to exit and focus on the target tissue.[2]

The laser medium can be a solid, gas, liquid, or semiconductor that is stimulated to a metastable state when pumped with an external energy source. Lasers are commonly named after the medium that determines the wavelength output of the laser. Solid-state lasers such as the Nd:YAG laser, use a solid matrix fabricated into a rod approximately the size of a cigarette. The rod is doped with a small amount of Nd impurity (dopant) that provides the energy source for the laser. Solid-state lasers are more powerful than gas lasers and require optical pumping with white light for a flashlamp, or monochromatic light from another laser. Gas lasers use a variety of gases as lasing media, including argon, CO_2, helium (He), helium-neon (He-Ne), and krypton (Kr), and require an electrical source of energy for pumping. Liquid lasers utilize complex dyes dissolved in a liquid such as methanol; optically pumped, they are tunable over a broad range of wavelengths, mostly in the visible spectrum. Excimer lasers are gas lasers that use a mixture of chlorine or fluorine and an inert gas such as argon, krypton, or xenon. Electrical stimulation is used to produce a dimer of the halogen; the resultant dimer is unstable and quickly decomposes into its constituent atoms releasing energy in the form of light. Semiconductor lasers or diode lasers are composed of semiconductor crystals that are pumped by a high-intensity current. They are commonly used in compact disc players, laser printers, and laser pointers. The gallium-arsenide laser is an example of a semiconductor laser.

Laser Operation

Laser effect on tissue is dependent on the wavelength of the laser light, which in turn is determined by the laser medium. Consequently, laser selection is based on the desired effect of the laser on the targeted tissue.[4,5] The majority of medical lasers deliver only one wavelength. In addition to selecting the appropriate wavelength, the surgeon must use the appropriate exposure time and energy density (power setting) to achieve the intended photomechanical, photo thermolysis, or photochemical effect.

A laser beam can be delivered in a continuous wave (CW), pulsed wave, or Q-switched mode. In the CW mode, the laser continues to emit a steady beam as long as the laser medium is excited. Output is

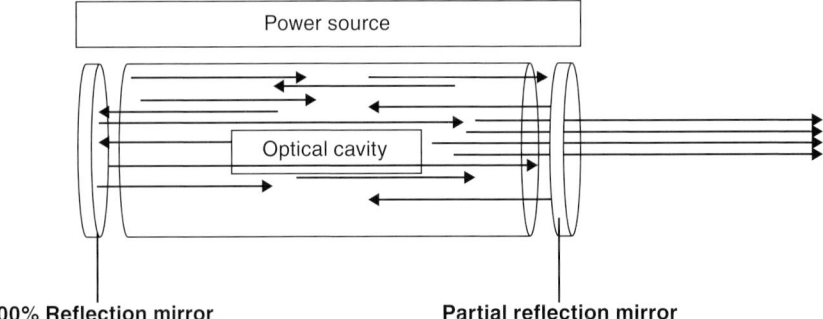

Fig. 47.4 Basic components of a laser. The optical cavity contains the lasing medium (e.g., solid, liquid, gas). The power source (e.g., flash lamp, electric current, other laser) pumps up the electrons in the lasing medium to a higher energy state. Two mirrors reflect the photons back into the cavity, where they stimulate other excited atoms to emit identical photons. One mirror is partially transparent and allows a portion of the laser beam to exit the cavity in a narrow beam.

BOX 47.1 Laser Output

Energy: Proportional to the number of photons, measured in joules (J)
Power: Rate of delivery of the energy, measured in watts (W) (1 W = 1 J/sec)
Fluence: Energy delivered per unit area, measured in J/cm^2
Irradiance (or flux): Power per unit area, measured in W/cm^2

BOX 47.2 Laser-Tissue Interactions

Photomechanical reaction: Mechanical energy creates a shock wave that causes explosive tissue expansion and destruction.
Photothermal reaction: Rapid increase in temperature causes tissue vaporization and coagulation.
Photochemical reaction: Destruction of molecular bonds or stimulation of cellular molecules into a biochemically reactive state.
Photodynamic reaction: Laser light activates photosensitizing medications that cause cytotoxicity by producing a biologically reactive form of oxygen (singlet oxygen).

measured in watts and can vary significantly among lasers; for example, the power of the helium-neon laser is measured in milliwatts, whereas the output of the more powerful CO_2 laser is measured in kilowatts. Power density of the beam (irradiance or flux) varies from a few watts per square centimeter to hundreds of watts per square centimeter (Box 47.1). In the pulsed mode, the laser emits peak energy levels in individual pulses from femtoseconds (quadrillionths of a second) to seconds. The power of a pulsed laser is measured in joules, and energy intensity is expressed as joules per square centimeter. In the Q-switched mode, the laser emits high-energy, ultrashort pulses (~10–250 nsec). A shutter is placed in the optical path to allow the buildup of a large population inversion. After release of the shutter, the electrons fall rapidly to ground state releasing a large amount of energy that is measured in megawatts.

The mode of delivery determines the effect of the laser on the tissue. For example, the Nd:YAG laser utilizes the CW mode for coagulation of tumors, the pulsed mode for hair removal, and the Q-switched mode for tattoo removal. In the CW mode, the CO_2 laser can be focused very tightly and used for incision, much like a scalpel, whereas the defocused mode can be used to vaporize a larger area of tissue. When delivered through a scanning device, the CO_2 laser beam can remove a predetermined thickness of skin. Fiberoptic cables are used for delivery of laser beams with visible and near infrared wavelengths. Articulated arms with reflecting mirrors mounted in tubes are used to direct the beam of a far infrared laser (CO_2). Additional attachments include slit lamps for use on the eye, operating microscopes, and insulated fibers for use with endoscopes. Contact laser probes (sapphire) on the distal end of a fiberoptic bundle transform the light energy into heat for precise cutting and reduced penetration.

LASER EFFECTS ON BIOLOGIC TISSUES

Lasers are associated with rapid and precise vaporization or coagulation of tissues and are commonly used in a variety of unrelated diagnostic and therapeutic procedures.[4,5] Collateral tissue damage occurs when the laser beam is held on tissue longer than the thermal relaxation time, the time for 50% of the laser energy to be thermally conducted to surrounding tissue. Pulsing the laser beam or scanning a continuous beam concentrates the energy, limits the exposure time, and minimizes thermal damage. The duration of laser beam exposure is controlled by computerized scanning of the beam in a preset pattern prior to delivery of the laser beam to the tissue.

Laser light is monochromatic, and it has very selective effects on biologic tissues. The degree of laser light transmission, scattering, reflection, or absorption is dependent on the tissue and the wavelength of the light.[1,4] Absorption of the light is necessary for the laser to be effective; if the tissue transmits, reflects, or scatters the light, the laser will have little or no effect on the tissue. A specific wavelength may be absorbed by one type of tissue and transmitted by another. Biologic tissues can be thought of as an aqueous solution of light-absorbing molecules. Chromophores, such as hemoglobin and melanin, and water are the main absorbing components, and they determine the reaction of the tissue to the laser light. To be effective, the laser light must match the absorptive property of the tissue. If light absorption occurs, the laser light is converted to

heat; vaporization or ablation of the tissue occurs when the temperature reaches 100°C. As the tissue is vaporized, the thermal energy of the laser beam cauterizes capillaries and provides immediate hemostasis. Tissue coagulation or denaturation rather than ablation occurs at lower temperatures. The reaction of tissue to light absorption is dependent on the wavelength, intensity, and exposure time of the light. Laser-tissue interactions include photomechanical, photothermal, photochemical, and photodynamic reactions (Box 47.2). Photomechanical effects are caused by powerful, short pulses of laser light that are converted into mechanical energy in the form of a shock wave causing explosive tissue expansion and destruction. Photothermal reactions occur when low-power, long pulses of laser cause a rapid increase in temperature resulting in tissue vaporization and coagulation. When applied for longer durations, low-power lasers can cause a photochemical reaction that either breaks molecular bonds in cells or excites cellular molecules into a biochemically reactive state. In a photodynamic reaction, the laser light activates photosensitizing medications that are selectively absorbed by a specific tissue. The photosynthesizing drug causes cytotoxicity by producing a biologically reactive form of atomic oxygen after stimulation with light of an appropriate wavelength. Biostimulation lasers, also called low-level laser therapy (LLLT), cold lasers, soft lasers, and laser acupuncture devices, have Food and Drug Administration (FDA) approval for the temporary relief of pain.[6]

Laser Absorption

Biologic tissue absorption of laser energy is a function of light wavelength. Absorption depth is defined as the tissue depth at which the intensity of the laser beam is reduced by 63%.[2] Water absorbs infrared wavelengths and allows transmission of visible wavelengths. Hemoglobin gives blood its red color because it reflects red wavelengths. Deoxygenated blood absorbs more red wavelengths and consequently appears darker than oxygenated blood. Hemoglobin absorbs blue and green wavelengths, and lasers with blue and green wavelengths, such as the Ar and Nd:YAG lasers, are very effective in well-perfused tissues.[2,5] Melanin in the skin absorbs all visible wavelengths, but absorption is greatest with UV wavelengths. The best absorption of xanthophyll, a retinal pigment, is at 460 nm. Collagen, a structural component of most tissues, readily absorbs infrared laser energy. Atherosclerotic plaques are made of fat and collagen deposits; they do not absorb visible or near infrared light, and pulsed midinfrared and UV lasers are required to ablate arterial plaques.

Tissue absorption is greatest with longer wavelengths such as the far infrared wavelength of the CO_2 laser (10,600 nm). The CO_2 laser beam is completely absorbed by water in the first few cellular layers, resulting in explosive vaporization of the top layer, but little or no damage to the underlying tissues. Excimer lasers (UV) are associated with an even more superficial effect because of their strong absorption by water. Light from lasers with visible wavelengths, such as the ruby, Ar, and Kr lasers, is transmitted by water and absorbed by cells that contain dark pigment. It can penetrate the skin and the cornea to coagulate pigmented or vascular lesions. Near infrared laser light has greater tissue penetration and is transmitted rather than absorbed by water; near infrared lasers (e.g., Nd:YAG) are suitable for deeper procedures such as tumor debulking. Advantages of lasers include precision, access to remote sites in the body, reduced blood loss, reduced damage to adjacent tissue, and improved patient satisfaction. A disadvantage of laser therapy may be a delay in wound healing.

SURGICAL LASERS

The major types of lasers used in medicine are far infrared (CO_2), midinfrared (erbium [Er]:YAG, holmium [Ho]:YAG, Nd:YAG), near infrared (diode), visible (ruby, krypton, argon, copper, and gold vapor), and UV (excimer) (Table 47.1).

TABLE 47.1 Common Surgical Lasers

Laser	Wavelength	Applications
Far Infrared		
CO_2	10,600 nm	Multiple uses: general surgery, orthopedics, gynecology, urology, otolaryngology, plastic surgery
Midinfrared		
Nd:YAG	1064 nm	Multiple uses: gastroenterology, pulmonology, urology, ophthalmology, dermatology
Ho:YAG	2070 nm	Orthopedics, urology
Er:YAG	2940 nm	Dermatology
Near Infrared		
Diode	800-900 nm	Multiples uses: ophthalmology, otolaryngology, periodontics, cosmetic surgery, pain management. Multiple nonmedical applications
Visible		
Argon	488 and 514 nm	Multiple uses: ophthalmology, plastic surgery, dermatology, gynecology, otolaryngology
Krypton	476, 521, 568 nm	Dermatology
Copper bromide	511 and 577 nm	Dermatology, photosynthesizer
KTP	532 nm	Dermatology
Pulsed dye	577–585 nm	Dermatology
Gold	578–628 nm	Oncology
Ruby	694 nm	Dermatology
Alexandrite	755 nm	Dermatology
Ultraviolet (Excimer)		
Argon-fluoride	193 nm	Multiple uses: ophthalmology, dermatology
Krypton-fluoride	249 nm	Dermatology
Xenon-chloride	308 nm	Multiple uses: dermatology, ophthalmology, dermatology
Xenon-fluoride	351 nm	Multiple uses: angioplasty, ophthalmology, dermatology

Er:YAG, Erbium: yttrium-aluminum-garnet; *Ho:YAG,* holmium:YAG; *KTP,* potassium-titanyl-phosphate; *Nd:YAG,* neodymium:YAG

Carbon Dioxide Laser

The CO_2 laser, the most commonly used surgical laser, has wide application in all surgical specialties. The infrared light of the CO_2 laser (10,600 nm) is invisible to the human eye, and a low-power helium-neon (He-Ne) laser (633 nm) is incorporated to provide a visible red beam for surgical aim. It is a powerful laser that emits light in the infrared region of the EM spectrum that basically melts whatever is in the path of its beam, including steel. A very precise laser, the lateral zone of damage is less than 0.5 nm from the area of incision. The laser beam is not transmitted by quartz, glass, or other transparent material; it must be delivered as a free beam or through a rigid endoscope with a mirrored, articulated arm. The CO_2 laser light is strongly absorbed by water, and vaporization of cells occurs within the first 100 to 200 mcm of the irradiated surface. It can be used in both the CW and pulsed-wave mode. Focused into a tight beam, the CO_2 laser can be used for cutting tissue. Defocusing the beam decreases the power density and causes tissue vaporization or ablation. The laser has extensive applications in general surgery, orthopedics, gynecology, urology, and otolaryngology and is associated with minimal blood loss (see Table 47.1). Thin layers of skin are ablated for cosmetic skin resurfacing when used with a scanning device.

Yttrium-Aluminum-Garnet Lasers

The lasing medium of the YAG laser is a YAG crystal rod doped with atoms of rare earth minerals, which account for the different properties of YAG lasers. These lasers can be used in the CW, pulsed-wave, or Q-switched mode.

Neodymium: Yttrium-Aluminum-Garnet Laser

The Nd:YAG laser emits a near infrared invisible light at 1064 nm and requires the addition of a visible aiming beam. The Nd:YAG laser-tissue interaction produces a scattering effect, which decreases the penetration of the laser beam, typically limited to 5 to 7 mm. The decreased penetration results in a slower heating of tissues making the laser ideal for coagulation and debulking of gastrointestinal and tracheobronchial tumors and genitourinary lesions.[1]

The pulsed and Q-switched Nd:YAG laser is used in ophthalmology (see Table 47.1). In the Q-switched mode, the laser removes black tattoo ink and hair. Since the energy of the Nd:YAG beam is widely dispersed, damage to adjacent tissues may not be evident for hours after the laser procedure.

Holmium: Yttrium-Aluminum-Garnet Laser

When doped with Ho, the YAG laser emits a midinfrared beam at 2070 nm that is strongly absorbed by water. Output in the midinfrared spectrum requires a coincident aiming beam. The Ho:YAG laser is used to vaporize, cut, coagulate, and sculpt avascular tissue with a minimal amount of thermal necrosis. The primary applications of the Ho:YAG laser are in endoscopic orthopedic procedures (bone and cartilage ablation) and urology (stone removal and transurethral resection of the prostate [TURP]) (see Table 47.1).

Erbium: Yttrium-Aluminum-Garnet Laser

When a YAG laser is doped with Er, it emits a midinfrared beam at 2940 nm (peak absorption of water). Because the infrared beam is not transmitted by quartz or glass, the Er:YAG can be used only as a free beam or through a rigid endoscope. It has limited penetration and excellent precision. It is used extensively in laser resurfacing of the skin and vaporization of fibrous tissue, cartilage, and bone (see Table 47.1). The Er:YAG laser has widespread application in dentistry.

Diode Lasers

Diode lasers are semiconductors that emit a near infrared light (800–900 nm) when pumped with a high-intensity electric current. Medical uses include ophthalmology, dermatology (hair removal), and periodontal surgery. Diode lasers are also used to pump other laser media such as YAG rods (see Table 47.1).

Visible Lasers

Argon Laser

In an Ar laser, the gas has lost one or more of its electrons, and the positive ions are excited by a large electrical discharge. The Ar ion laser emits visible blue-green light with wavelengths of 488 nm and 514 nm simultaneously. The light is transmitted by water and absorbed by hemoglobin and melanin, where the main effect is photocoagulation. Penetration is approximately 1 to 2 mm, but this can vary depending on the degree of pigmentation. The beam can be passed through quartz optical fibers, allowing the laser to be used with a microscope or endoscope. The Ar laser is used in ophthalmology, plastic surgery, dermatology, gynecology, and otolaryngology (see Table 47.1).

Krypton Laser

The active medium, Kr, is also a rare gas with one or more electrons removed, and the Kr ions are excited by an electrical discharge. The laser produces visible green and blue light at 476, 521, and 568 nm. It is absorbed by hemoglobin and used for photocoagulation of vascular or pigmented lesions. Primary application of this laser is in dermatology (see Table 47.1).

Ruby Laser

The ruby laser uses a synthetic ruby crystal of aluminum oxide doped with chromium (Cr). It emits a red light with a wavelength of 694 nm and has a penetration greater than 1 mm. The light is absorbed by melanin and blue, green, and black pigment. It is very effective for removal of tattoos, hair, and pigmented lesions such as freckles, liver spots, and nevi (Q-switched mode) (see Table 47.1). Although it was one of the first medical lasers, its use in surgery has declined in favor of newer and more powerful lasers.

Alexandrite Laser

Named after Czar Alexander II, the solid-state alexandrite laser contains a rod of synthetic chrysoberyl doped with Cr. It emits a deep red light at 755 nm, but frequency doubling can produce a tunable laser output of 360 to 400 nm. Blue and black pigments absorb the beam, with a lesser degree of absorption by melanin. It is used for tattoo removal and treatment of some pigmented lesions (see Table 47.1).

Metal Vapor Lasers

The active medium of metal vapor lasers is a neutral metal heated beyond its vapor point. A pulsed electrical discharge is used for excitation of the vapor. Vaporized copper bromide ($CuBr_2$) emits green light at 511 nm and yellow light at 577 nm, which is used to treat vascular lesions. It also has applications for facial resurfacing. The gold (Au) vapor laser (578–628 nm) is used in photodynamic treatment of cancer (see Table 47.1).

Potassium-Titanyl-Phosphate Laser

The wavelength of the Nd:YAG laser is halved when it is passed through a KTP crystal. A solid-state laser, the KTP laser is similar to the Ar gas laser. The beam is transmitted by water and absorbed within 1 to 2 mm of vascular or pigmented tissue. A bright green light (532 nm) delivered through fiberoptics, scanners, or microscopes is used to cut tissue (CW mode) and remove vascular lesions (pulsed mode) and red-orange and black tattoo ink (Q-switched mode) (see Table 47.1). Although the power density of the KTP laser is sufficient to cut vascular tissue, it does not provide effective hemostasis.

Dye Lasers

Organic fluorescent materials are dissolved in a solvent such as methanol and are typically pumped with a flashlamp or another laser. The energy levels of the dyes are very close to one another and allow the lasers to release a wide range of wavelengths. In the CW and pulsed mode, dye lasers have wavelengths of 400 to 1000 nm. They can produce extremely short pulses (measured in trillionths of a second [picoseconds]). The major advantage of the dye laser is the ability to tune the wavelength to maximize the laser-tissue interaction. Dye lasers are used in dermatology for excision of vascular and pigmented lesions, in urology for treatment of urinary calculi, and in oncology for PDT. The pulsed dye laser uses a rhodamine dye to emit a yellow laser beam at 577 to 585 nm (peak absorption of hemoglobin). It is the laser of choice for treatment of port-wine stains and thick red scars (see Table 47.1).

Excimer Lasers

Derived from the terms *excited* and *dimer,* excimer lasers use a medium composed of a reactive noble gas (chlorine or fluorine) and an inert halogen gas (argon, krypton, or xenon). When the medium is electrically stimulated, an unstable pseudomolecule (dimer) is produced. As the dimer breaks down to its constituent atoms, it releases light in the UV range that is strongly absorbed by water. Excimer lasers have a photochemical effect on targeted tissues (pulsed mode), with minimal thermal effect on the underlying tissue. The very short wavelength (UV) is capable of high resolution and has applications in microscopic surgery. Examples of excimer lasers include the argon-fluoride (193 nm), krypton-fluoride (249 nm), xenon-chloride (308 nm), and xenon-fluoride (351 nm) lasers (see Table 47.1). They are currently used in ophthalmology for photorefractive keratectomy (PRK) and LASIK. Other uses include removal of arterial plaques and treatment of psoriasis.

Cold Lasers

Cold lasers, also called LLLT and soft lasers, use diodes to produce visible to infrared light. The laser beam can penetrate up to 2 in without damaging tissues or producing a significant amount of heat. Through biostimulation of cellular metabolism, cold lasers speed up the healing process and reduce pain. They are used for treatment of carpal tunnel syndrome and other soft tissue injuries.

Photodynamic Therapy

PDT, also known as photochemotherapy, involves the administration of photosensitizers, chemical entities that absorb light and induce a change in another chemical. They are used in the diagnosis and treatment of cancer because of their tendency to accumulate in cancer cells. Approximately 72 hours after intravenous administration, when the photosensitizer has left normal cells but remains in cancer cells, the tumor is exposed to laser light with a red wavelength. The photosensitizer absorbs the light and reacts with oxygen to produce free oxygen radicals that destroy cancer cells (phototoxicity). Currently, PDT is used to treat bladder, esophageal, pulmonary, and skin cancer. It is also used in dermatology (local application) for treatment of acne, psoriasis, and skin cancer. Its use in antimicrobial therapy is promising because of its ability to target and destroy viral, fungal, and bacterial pathogens. Patients must avoid direct exposure to sunlight during treatment because of photosensitization of the eyes and skin, a side effect of the treatment.

LASER SAFETY

Lasers are divided into four classes according to their potential for causing biologic damage (Table 47.2). Class I lasers are incapable of producing damaging radiation and are exempt from radiation hazard controls. This classification includes CD players and laser printers; supermarket laser scanners are classified as IA. Class II lasers emit radiation in the visible portion of the EM spectrum, but their radiant power is less than 1 mW. The human aversion reaction to bright light will protect the eyes, but injury can occur if the beam is viewed directly for an extended period. Class II lasers include laser pointers and scanners. Class III lasers, which include spectroscopy and light shows, can cause eye injury if viewed directly. The direct and reflected beams of class IV lasers are hazardous to the eye and are potential fire and skin hazards. Reflected laser beams are specular and maintain the beam coherence; diffuse beams are scattered when they are reflected from a rough or matte surface. Most medical lasers are class IV; these lasers also create hazardous airborne contaminants and require a high-voltage power supply.

The US FDA regulates the manufacturing and marketing of lasers used in medicine.[6] The American National Standards Institute (ANSI) addresses medical laser safety and control measures for the four laser classifications.[7] The ANSI recommends the appointment of a laser safety officer (LSO) who is responsible for overseeing education, operation, maintenance, safety, and servicing of medical lasers at institutions that utilize class IIIB or class IV lasers. However, institutional compliance with the ANSI guidelines is voluntary. The Occupational Safety and Health Administration (OSHA) has identified the hazards associated with the use of medical lasers and developed safety standards to protect patients and operating room personnel.[8] The Association of Perioperative Registered Nurses (AORN) and other professional organizations have also developed standards and recommendations for laser safety (Box 47.3).[9,10]

When not in use, lasers should be disabled and stored in a secure location. Licensed health care providers who use lasers should have appropriate training and institutional privileges for laser use. An aiming beam should be used for lasers that do not produce a visible light. A warning sign must be posted inside and outside of all entrances; it should include the type and wavelength of the laser in use and the specific laser safety eyewear (LSE) required for everyone entering the laser area (Fig. 47.5). When a laser is in use, entrance to the lasing area should be restricted to personnel assigned to the procedure. The use of a safety interlock system, a trigger shutoff device, will disable the laser if the door is unexpectedly opened during laser use. All other optical paths (windows) should be covered to prevent the transmission of a misdirected laser beam. A variety of laser-absorbing glass, plastics, laser safety curtains, and screens are available that attenuate the laser energy. Window coverings are not

TABLE 47.2 Laser Classification

Class	Laser Description
I	Do not emit hazardous radiation and are exempt from radiation hazard controls. Typically, continuous wave of 0.4 μW at visible wavelengths. *Examples:* CD players and laser printers, CD-ROM devices, geologic survey equipment, and laboratory analytic equipment.
IA	Includes lasers that are not intended for viewing. Maximum power is 4.0 mW. *Example:* supermarket laser scanners.
II	Do not cause ocular injury unless viewed directly for an extended period. The normal aversion response to bright light protects the eye from a brief exposure. Class II lasers only operate in the visible range (400–700 nm). Maximum power is ≤1 mW. *Examples:* helium-neon lasers and some laser pointers.
IIA	Special-purpose lasers not intended for viewing. Power output is <1 mW. Ocular injury can occur if viewed directly for >1000 seconds over an 8-hr day, not continuous exposure. *Examples:* scanners and bar-code readers.
IIIA	Do not pose a serious eye hazard unless viewed through optical instruments (e.g., microscopes). Power outputs for continuous wave (CW) lasers operating in the visible range are between 1 and 5 mW. *Examples:* solid-state laser pointers.
IIIB	Direct beam viewing or specular reflections result in ocular injury. Power output is between 5 and 500 mW for CW lasers and <0.125 J within 0.25 sec for a pulsed laser. Do not produce a hazardous diffuse reflection and are not considered fire hazards. *Examples:* spectroscopy, stereolithography, and entertainment light shows.
IV	Significant ocular injury can result from direct beam viewing, specular reflections, and diffuse reflections. These lasers require significant controls. Power output is >500 mW for a CW laser and >0.125 J within 0.25 sec for a pulsed laser. Skin and fire hazards are also present with class IV lasers. *Examples:* medical lasers and industrial lasers (drilling, cutting, and welding).

BOX 47.3 Laser Safety Precautions

- Restrict laser use to qualified personnel.
- Restrict access to laser area during laser operation.
- Close all doors and cover windows.
- Post laser warning signs inside and outside the laser area.
- Use appropriate laser safety eyewear (LSE) for operating room personnel and awake patients.
- Provide eye protection for anesthetized patients.
- Provide skin protection for patients and operating room personnel.
- Minimize the potential for specular reflections by removal of unnecessary shiny surfaces.
- Maintain room lights as bright as possible to constrict the pupils.
- Adjust brightness of patient monitors to ensure appropriate degree of visibility with LSE.
- Require surgeon to warn of activation of laser and to keep the beam path above or below normal eye level (<4.5 ft or >6.5 ft).
- Use an aiming beam or operational warning devices for lasers with invisible beams.
- Avoid looking into the primary beam at all times.
- Place laser in standby mode when it is not in active use.
- Do not leave an active laser unattended.
- Restrict maintenance of laser to authorized individuals who are trained in laser maintenance.

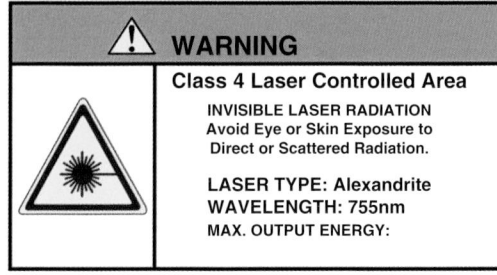

Fig. 47.5 Laser warning sign indicating laser procedure in progress. (From https://www.lasertraining.org/DangerSigns.html)

necessary for CO_2 lasers because glass absorbs their laser energy (10,600 nm). Specular reflections from flat, shiny surfaces have the potential to cause significant ocular or skin trauma. Surgical cabinets and large surgical instruments should have a matte or dull surface to avoid reflection of a misdirected laser beam. Curved mirrorlike surfaces, such as surgical instruments or jewelry, provide a diffuse surface that will reflect the laser beam in many directions. Specular and diffuse reflections from a given surface are dependent upon the laser wavelength; a surface that causes diffuse reflections of a visible laser with minimal tissue impact may cause harmful specular reflections of an infrared laser beam. While associated with less tissue trauma, the diffuse reflections from high-powered class IV lasers are capable of initiating a fire.

The majority of laser-related injuries are primarily the result of inappropriate use of the laser or intentional use of malfunctioning equipment. The most common hazards of medical lasers include thermal trauma, eye injury, perforation of organs or vessels, gas embolization, electrical shock, air contamination, and fire. Beam injuries are caused by the direct effects of the laser on the eye, skin, and other tissues; nonbeam injuries are secondary and caused by laser-generated air contaminants (LGACs), fire, and electrical shock.

Thermal Trauma

The most common cause of tissue damage during laser use is thermal in nature; exposure to high-energy beams for an extended period results in increased tissue temperature and protein denaturation. Tissue damage can range from mild reddening of the skin to blistering and charring. The risk of thermal trauma (burns) is greatest with laser exposure times greater than 10 mcs and wavelengths ranging from near UV to far infrared (315–10,300 nm) (see Table 47.2); the thermal effects of pulsed or scanning lasers are additive. Longer wavelengths have a deeper skin penetration than shorter wavelengths, which are absorbed

TABLE 47.3   Effect of Lasers on Eyes and Skin

Laser	Eye Effect	Skin Effect
Ultraviolet C (200–280 nm)	Photokeratitis	Erythema (sunburn)
Ultraviolet B (280–315 nm)	Photokeratitis	Increased pigmentation
Ultraviolet A (315–400 nm)	Photochemical cataract	Darkening/burn
Visible (400–700 nm)	Photochemical and thermal retinal injury	Darkening/burn
Infrared A (700–1400 nm)	Cataract, retinal burn	Burn
Infrared B (1400–3000 nm)	Cataract, corneal burn, aqueous flare	Burn
Infrared C (3000–10,000 nm)	Corneal burn	Burn

in the first 4 mm of the skin. UV A wave (315–400 nm) exposure causes hyperpigmentation and erythema, but the greatest skin damage is caused by UVB radiation (280–315 nm). In addition to thermal trauma, carcinogenesis is a potential risk of UVB exposure. Exposure to UVC waves (200–280 nm) is less harmful to the skin because they are predominantly absorbed in the outer dead layers of the epidermis. The CO_2 and other infrared lasers have deeper tissue penetration and are associated with first-degree (reddening), second-degree (blistering), and third-degree (charring) burns. Lasers also may precipitate the development of or exaggerate existing skin lesions, including reactivation of viral infections.

In addition to restricted access to the lasing area, safety interventions to prevent thermal trauma include application of saline-soaked towels to the skin surrounding the path of the laser beam, and use of long-sleeved jackets, gloves, and face shields by operating room personnel (see Box 47.3). Topical sunblock cream will protect against UV radiation for patients undergoing repeat laser treatments.

Ocular Trauma

Since their light beam is not coherent, incandescent and fluorescent lights do not pose a hazard for eyes. However, the human eye is extremely vulnerable to laser radiation because the light beam is coherent, and all of its energy can be focused on a very small portion of the cornea or retina. Eye trauma from laser light is dependent on the power and wavelength of the laser beam, exposure duration, pupil size, retinal pigmentation, and location of the injury (Table 47.3). Pulsed-mode lasers present an additional hazard to the eye because they induce shock waves that rupture tissue, resulting in a larger area of permanent retinal damage.

UV (200–400 nm) and midinfrared (1400–3000 nm) radiation is absorbed by the cornea and can cause corneal photokeratitis (Fig. 47.6). Visible lasers and near infrared lasers (400–1400 nm) are associated with retinal injury. Midinfrared wavelengths greater than 1400 nm are absorbed by water; they can damage the cornea and increase the opacity of the lens resulting in traumatic cataracts. They are also associated with aqueous flare, an increased turbidity of the aqueous humor. Far infrared radiation (3000–10,000 nm) is absorbed by the cornea and can result in corneal burns and potential loss of vision. Inadvertent exposure to the invisible CO_2 laser beam (10,600 nm) causes burning pain of the cornea or sclera. There are no immediate signs of exposure to UV radiation, but severe eye pain and a sensation of sand in the eye presents later. After minor injury, regeneration of the epithelium occurs without any permanent abnormality, but corneal scarring and cataract formation may result with more extensive injury.

Two types of photoreceptors, rods and cones, comprise the retina. Rods make up over 95% of the retina; they are sensitive to light but not color. Less than 5% of the retina is composed of cones, which are responsible for detecting color and fine detail. They are heavily concentrated in the fovea centralis, an area associated with the sharpest and

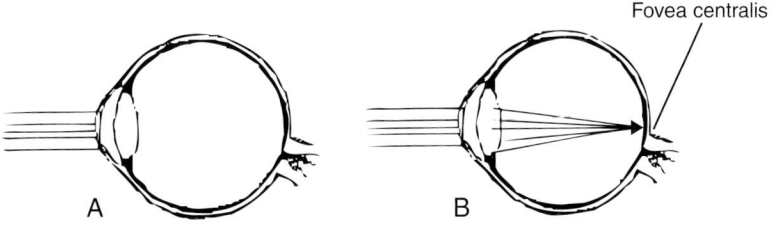

Fig. 47.6 Laser-associated eye injury. (A) Midinfrared and far infrared wavelengths (<400 nm and >1400 nm) are absorbed by the cornea and associated with corneal injury. (B) Retinal injury is associated with visible and near infrared (400–1400 nm) wavelengths.

most brilliantly colored vision. Retinal damage is associated with visible and near infrared (400–1400 nm) lasers. The beam is transmitted by the cornea and focused by the lens to produce an intense concentration of light energy on a small portion of the pigmented retina. Focusing of the laser by the lens amplifies the irradiance on the retina 100,000 times (see Fig. 47.6). One milliwatt of visible laser radiation entering the eye deposits 100 W/cm^2 at the retina. The conversion of the light energy to heat can cause retinal burns, partial visual loss, or total blindness. Wavelengths less than 400 nm and greater than 1400 nm are not associated with retinal damage.

A visible laser beam produces a bright color flash of the emitted wavelength followed by an afterimage of its complementary color (e.g., a green, 532-nm laser light would produce a green flash followed immediately by a red afterimage). If the cones are damaged by a green laser light, the individual may have difficulty discriminating between blue and green colors thereafter. The Q-switched Nd:YAG laser beam (1064 nm) is especially hazardous to the eye because the beam is invisible, and the retina lacks sensory innervation. Visual disorientation resulting from retinal damage may not be apparent until considerable thermal damage has occurred. Unlike corneal injuries, laser damage to the retina is permanent. Acute and chronic loss of color sensitivity has been reported by ophthalmologists who frequently use surgical lasers.

All medical lasers are class IV lasers (see Table 47.2), and LSE is required to prevent injury from the direct laser beam or reflected beam from surgical instruments, cabinets, lights, watches, jewelry, and other smooth reflective surfaces in the operating room.[9,10] Although LSE will protect against accidental exposure to a laser beam, it will not protect against direct viewing of a laser beam. The eye aversion or blink response of 0.25 second is triggered by bright, visible light but will not prevent ocular injury caused by invisible laser beams and provides no protection against lasers with a wavelength of 700 to 1400 nm. The aversion response is absent or sluggish under general anesthesia and deep sedation; in operating rooms darkened for video and microscope use, the pupils of the eyes will dilate increasing the risk for laser exposure for both surgical personnel and awake patients. During laser procedures, operating room personnel and awake patients must wear LSEs specific for the type of laser in use (see Box 47.3). Anesthetized patients should have the eyes covered with saline-moistened eye pads and laser shields. Petroleum-based eye ointments should not be used during laser procedures because they may cause severe burns if ignited by a misdirected laser beam.

The maximum permissible exposure (MPE) is the level of laser radiation exposure not associated with biologic changes in the eye. It is directly related to the wavelength and inversely related to the exposure time and expressed as radiant exposure (J/cm^2) or irradiance (W/cm^2). The ANSI standard identifies acceptable MPE levels for medical lasers.[7,8] The nominal hazard zone (NHZ) refers to the physical space in which the direct, reflected, or scattered laser radiation exceeds the MPE. During laser procedures, the entire operating room is considered to be within the NHZ; however, it may extend beyond transparent windows for certain lasers.

During laser procedures, LSE must be worn by everyone in the room (see Fig. 47.5 and Box 47.3). The LSE must have the appropriate optical density (OD) and reflective properties for the laser wavelength, the beam intensity, and the expected exposure conditions; it must also have side shields and allow transmission of visible light. The OD refers to the ability of a material to attenuate or absorb energy of a specific wavelength to a safe level below the MPE while allowing transmission of sufficient ambient light for safe visibility. The definition of OD is the $\log_{10} (E_i / E_t)$ where E_i is the incident beam irradiance (W/cm^2) or worst-case scenario, and E_t is the transmitted beam irradiance (MPE limit in W/cm^2).[7-9] LSE with an OD of 2 will allow transmission of

1/100 of the laser energy; in contrast, LSE with an OD of 4 will allow transmission of only 1/10,000 of the laser energy. The OD is rated for a specific wavelength or range of wavelengths; use with a different wavelength will result in a completely different OD value. Because LSE is laser specific, the wavelength and OD are imprinted on the LSE, and users must ensure they are wearing the appropriate LSE for the laser in use. For example, LSE for the Nd:YAG laser has an OD of 6 at 1064 nm, whereas the LSE for the CO_2 laser has an OD of 7+ at 10,600 nm. In addition, LSE with an OD of 4 and a wavelength of 755 nm will not protect against a laser beam that requires LSE with an OD of 6 and a wavelength of 755 nm. Lasers may also operate at different wavelengths; for example, doubled Nd:YAG lasers, and tunable lasers, such as the titanium-doped sapphire laser, require different levels of protection at each wavelength and may require the use of two different types of LSE. Certain lasers require amber, green, or red filters, but the color of the LSE lens should not be used for LSE identification. Vision correction glasses may attenuate the effect of the CO_2 laser beam but do not completely protect the eye from direct or reflected laser beams because they lack protective side shields. Medical lasers generally require LSE of 4 to 7 OD. There are no laser glasses available that protect against all types of laser beams; LSE that covers several wavelengths would require very dark filters, which would interfere with visual acuity.

Vessel and Viscus Perforation

Operator error, such as a misdirected laser beam or failure to check for proper laser function before use, accounts for the majority of laser perforations of a viscus or vessel.[8-10] A pneumothorax can be a life-threatening complication of a misdirected laser beam, especially during the administration of nitrous oxide (N_2O). Lasers cannot photocoagulate blood vessels larger than 5 mm, and unexpected or excessive bleeding may accompany an accidental perforation with a misdirected beam. Perforation with a Nd:YAG laser beam is associated with delayed tissue damage because of its greater tissue penetration and dissemination; perforation, bleeding, or edema may not be apparent for hours to days. Patients undergoing Nd:YAG laser surgery of the airway should be monitored for 24 to 48 hours after the procedure.

Gas Embolism

Some lasers require a coolant to prevent the tip of the quartz fibers from overheating. The coolant may be air, CO_2, or a liquid. Although a rare event, venous gas embolism is a potential fatal hazard of laser procedures, especially with the gas-cooled Nd:YAG laser. Coronary and cerebral embolisms have occurred during endobronchial Nd:YAG therapy, and transmyocardial laser revascularization is also associated with cerebral microembolization. Fatal venous air embolism has been reported during Nd:YAG hysteroscopies. A liquid coolant will reduce the risk of air embolism. A CO_2 embolus appears to be less damaging than air or nitrogen emboli because of its faster absorption.

Air Contamination

Thermal destruction of tissue with a laser or electrosurgical unit (ESU) creates a smoke plume of LGACs.[11] Ninety-five percent of the LGACs are water; the remainder are particulate matter, volatile gases, and microorganisms. Approximately 150 chemical LGACs have been identified, including fatty acid esters, hydrocarbons, phenols, nitriles, and volatile organic compounds such as acetone, ethanol, and formaldehyde (Box 47.4).[11-13] Viable bacteria and viruses have been retrieved from the laser smoke plume. The smoke plume contains fine particulates (0.3 mcm) that can be deposited in the lower airways. In addition to ocular and respiratory irritation, the smoke plume has the potential for causing cellular mutations.[12,13] The CO_2 laser produces the greatest amount of LGAC; smoke produced from 1 g of tissue is equivalent to

BOX 47.4 Select Laser-Generated Air Contaminants (LGAC)

Acetonitrile	Formaldehyde
Acetone	Methane
Acetylene	Nitriles
Alkylbenzene	Phenol
Butane	Polycyclic aromatic hydrocarbons
Carbon monoxide	Propane
Cresol	Pyrrole
Ethane	Styrene

smoke from three to six cigarettes. The LGACs have the potential to cause respiratory, ocular, dermatologic, and other diseases, including cancer, in patients and operating room personnel. There has been no documented transmission of infectious disease through LGACs; however, there is potential for the LGAC to contain infectious material and viral deoxyribonucleic acid from vaporization of viral lesions, such as genital warts.

There are no specific OSHA standards addressing the hazards of the surgical smoke plumes other than expecting employers to advise employees of the hazards of surgical smoke.[11] The AORN has recommended practices for laser safety that are based on the ANSI recommendations.[14,15] In addition to the mandatory minimum of 20 air exchanges/hour in the operating room, the National Institute for Occupational Safety and Health (NIOSH) recommends the use of a local exhaust ventilation (LEV) system such as a portable smoke evacuator as the most efficient method to control laser-generated smoke.[16] It should contain a high-efficiency particulate air (HEPA) filter or equivalent for trapping particulates, and the suction nozzle should be kept within 2 in of the surgical site to effectively capture the LGAC. Evacuation tubing, filters, and absorbers are potential sources of infectious waste and should be replaced between patients. A triple filtration smoke evacuator is indicated for evacuation of a large smoke plume. Three-stage disposable filter systems include a HEPA filter that can filter 0.3-mcm particulate matter, a layer of activated charcoal for odor absorption, and an ultralow-penetration air (ULPA) filter that can filter particulate matter as small as 0.01 mcm. Fit-tested high-filtration masks, such as the surgical N95 particulate filtering facepiece respirator, should be worn by operating room personnel to prevent exposure to particulate matter and noxious odors. Despite the support from professional organizations such as the AORN for active smoke evacuation during laser procedures, the lack of a regulatory OSHA mandate continues to place many operating room personnel at risk for exposure to LGAC.[16] Noncompliance with current recommendations includes an institutional lack of smoke evacuation equipment and staff education on health risks of surgical smoke and surgeon refusal to use LEV equipment.

Electrical and Other Hazards

Lasers require a high-power source with a potential for electrical injury. Electrocution is the leading cause of laser-related injury and death in all industries; laser repair technicians appear to have the highest risk in the health care community. Contributing factors for electrical shock and electrocution include damaged electrical cords, inadequate grounding, inadequate safeguards, lack of compliance with safety procedures, and use by unqualified personnel. Older laser models that use an external water-cooling system present a great electrical hazard. Liquid gases that are used to cool some laser mediums, especially liquid nitrogen, pose additional health hazards if accidentally spilled on the skin. Some of the chemicals used in dye lasers are toxic and hazardous to handle.

SURGICAL FIRES

A surgical fire is a rare but preventable hazard of surgery that can have devastating effects on patients, including disfiguring or disabling injuries and death. Surgical fires can also have devastating consequences for the operating room staff and the reputation of the health care facility. The actual number of surgical fires is difficult to discern as many states do not have mandatory reporting requirements. Historically, surgical fires were associated with the use of explosive or flammable anesthetics, but currently, surgical fires are primarily associated with the use of electrosurgical units (ESUs) and surgical lasers; ESUs account for 90% of the fires, and lasers are responsible for the remaining 10%. Unlike ESUs, lasers do not require direct contact for ignition of a fuel source. According to the Emergency Care Research Institute (ECRI), there are approximately 90 to 100 surgical fires annually in the United States, a significant decrease from the 2007 estimate of 550 to 650 per year.[17] This aligns with the Pennsylvania Patient Safety Authority that reports a 44% reduction in surgical fires since 2011 and a 71% reduction since 2004.[18] The decreased incidence can be attributed to the prevention initiatives of health care institutions and professional organizations.

The great majority of surgical fires (85%) occur during high-risk procedures, which involve the head, neck, or upper chest.[19-22] The airway is the most common site of surgical fires (34%), followed by head and face (28%).[22,23] Immediate recognition and management of a surgical fire can limit patient injury, whereas delayed recognition and response can be fatal for the patient. In addition to burns, patient injuries include inhalation of toxic products of combustion, including carbon monoxide, ammonia, hydrogen chloride, and cyanide, that can cause significant airway and pulmonary damage (see Box 47.4). The Joint Commission considers a surgical fire to be a sentinel event.

Fire Triangle

Three components of the fire triangle must be present for a fire to occur: a fuel source, an oxidizer, and an ignition source (Fig 47.7). All three components are present in surgical areas, and operating room personnel must understand the fire hazards presented by all three sides of the fire triangle, including those not under their direct control. Vigilance is key, and communication among all members of the surgical team is mandatory. It is imperative that surgical personnel are aware of the hazards of fire during laser procedures and know how to prevent and respond to operating room fires (Box 47.5).[19,20]

Fuel Sources

Fuel sources are abundant in the operating room; they include surgical preparation solutions, petroleum-based ointments, facial hair, surgical drapes, gloves, ointments, sponges, dressings, endotracheal tubes, laryngeal mask airways (LMAs), breathing circuits, nasogastric tubes, suction catheters, pneumatic tourniquet cuffs, silastic stents, suction catheters, and tracheostomy tubes (see Fig. 47.7).[19] Bowel gas, which contains methane and hydrogen, also provides a fuel source during intraabdominal laser procedures. Volatile organic chemicals such as alcohol, acetone, and ether are common components of skin preparations, tinctures, degreasers, suture pack solutions, and liquid wound dressings. Alcohol and alcohol-based solutions are very volatile and pose a significant fire hazard in the operating room if adequate drying time is not provided.[19] Care must be taken to ensure that the surgical preparation solution does not pool under the patient or saturate the drapes. Alcohol-based hand sanitizers may also release alcohol vapor, which is flammable and

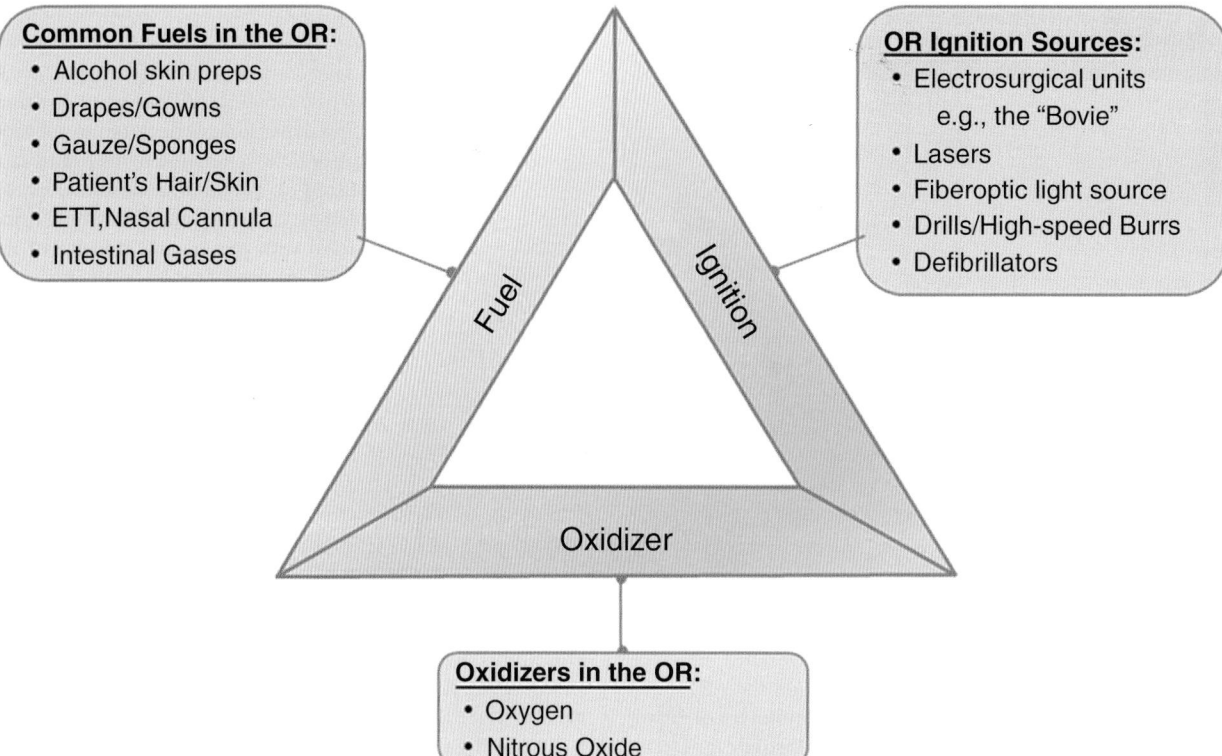

Fig. 47.7 Surgical components of the fire triangle. (From Jones TS, Black IH, Robinson TN, et al. Operating room fires. *Anesthesiology*. 2019;130:492–501.)

poses an additional fire hazard in the operating room. Although they resist ignition and slow the spread of a flame in room air, fire-retardant drapes and materials are not fireproof and may ignite and burn quickly at a higher temperature when exposed to an oxidizer-enriched environment.

Endotracheal tubes (ETTs) are a fuel source during airway surgery if the laser beam or reflected laser light comes into direct contact with them.[19,23] Localized thermal trauma occurs when the fire is contained to the outside of the ETT. Rupture of the ETT cuff allows leakage of anesthetic gases into the path of the laser beam, increasing the risk of an ignition. If the fire burns through to the inner side of the tube, an intraluminal fire occurs fed by the anesthetic gases and the volatile products of combustion of the ETT. The intraluminal flame will travel toward the source of the oxidizer, and a secondary flame can shoot out of the distal end of the ETT like a blowtorch and cause extensive lower airway damage.

Oxidizers

Common oxidizers in the operating room include air, O_2, and N_2O; these are under the control of the anesthetist (see Fig. 47.7). Oxygen is the oxidizer in 95% of surgical fires.[19] Heavier than air, it tends to accumulate around and under surgical drapes. In an oxygen-rich environment, materials ignite faster, burn more quickly with greater intensity, release more heat, and are more difficult to extinguish.

Ignition Source

The surgeon controls the sources of ignition, including ESUs, fiberoptic light sources or cables, high-speed drills, and lasers (see Fig. 47.7). However, electrical sparks from malfunctioning equipment not under the surgeon's control, including monitors and defibrillators, can also result in a fire. Desiccated anesthesia soda lime is another possible source of ignition in the breathing circuit.

Prevention of a Surgical Fire

All operating room personnel must be educated on the fire triangle, be able to identify the procedures that present a risk of fire, understand their role in preventing a surgical fire, and know how to respond to a surgical fire (Box 47.6).[24] They should be aware of the fire hazards present in the laser area, including anesthetic gases, skin preparation solutions, adhesive plastic tape, and surgical drapes (see Fig. 47.7). In collaboration with the Anesthesia Patient Safety Foundation (APSF), the ECRI developed a surgical fire prevention algorithm (Fig. 47.8), and the AORN has a fire safety tool kit that includes an assessment of fire risk.[25] The American Society of Anesthesiologists (ASA) has a management algorithm for both airway and nonairway fires (Fig. 47.9). Fire posters are available on the ECRI website, and a free video, in both English and Spanish, on the prevention and management of operating room fires, is available on the APSF website.[26]

All operating room personnel must be familiar with the location and function of fire alarms, fire extinguishers, and emergency exits and should know how to shut off electrical and medical gas supplies (see Box 47.6). A CO_2 fire extinguisher (class BC) is appropriate for extinguishing surgical fires. The BC fire extinguisher leaves no residue and will not damage human tissue. Dry powder extinguishers (class ABC) are inappropriate as the first response because the powder (ammonium phosphate) is a respiratory irritant and may interfere with visibility during a fire. All surgery practice sites should have a fire safety plan in place that includes mandatory fire drills for all operating room personnel, including anesthesia providers and surgeons. Simulation of a surgical fire scenario in a high-fidelity simulation center provides an excellent opportunity for team training in the prevention and management of a surgical fire.

Anesthetic Gases

An O_2 concentration less than 30% reduces the risk of a rapid and wide-spread propagation of fire (Table 47.4). Pulse oximetry can differentiate

BOX 47.5 Prevention of Surgical Fires

- Educate surgical personnel on the fire triad and common sources of fuels, ignition, and oxidizers in the operating room (OR).
- Schedule annual mandatory fire drills for the entire OR team and include evacuation of anesthetized patients in the event of an uncontrolled surgical fire.
- Identify location of fire alarms and extinguishers and shutoff valves for pipeline gases.
- Encourage good communication among surgical staff.
- Conduct a preoperative fire risk assessment prior to every surgery.
- Alert surgical team members to potential sources of fire: oxidizers, fuels, and source of ignition.
- Avoid open administration of supplemental oxygen (O_2), administer only through an endotracheal tube (ETT) or laryngeal mask airway.
- Limit supplemental O_2 to <30%.
- If possible, discontinue supplemental O_2 at least 1 min before and during laser use for head and neck surgery, and especially surgery of the airway.
- Avoid pooling of preparation solutions and allow adequate drying time before draping patient.
- Coat facial hair with a water-soluble surgical lubricant during head and neck surgery.
- Use flame-retardant drapes and moistened sponges and towels in the area of the laser.
- Use laser-resistant ETTs during laser surgery of the upper airway. Inflate the cuffs with saline and dye to allow early recognition of cuff rupture.
- Use moistened sponges to prevent air leaks, especially when using uncuffed tubes during airway surgery. Surgical sponges and pledgets should also be moistened to resist ignition.
- Use a properly applied incise drape to help isolate head, neck, and upper-chest incisions from an O_2-enriched atmosphere and anesthetic gases.
- Use continuous suction to minimize the buildup of O_2 in the oropharynx during airway surgery and beneath the drapes during monitored anesthesia care for head and neck surgery.
- Have a container of water immediately available to extinguish burning materials. Two syringes of sterile saline should be available during laser surgery of the airway.
- Have fire extinguishers available in the room or immediately accessible.

BOX 47.6 RACE Response to Fire

Rescue the patient.
Alert other staff and **a**ctivate the fire alarm system.
Confine the fire by shutting doors, closing off gas supplies and electrical power, and using fire extinguishers.
Evacuate the room.

between a patient who may require supplemental O_2 and a patient who can tolerate ventilation with room air. Mild drug-induced respiratory depression following low-dose sedatives and narcotics that results in a stable decrease in O_2 saturation (Sao_2) as low as 92% does not require supplemental oxygen, but a Sao_2 of 90% or less is undesirable. If supplemental oxygen is necessary, the airway should be secured with a LMA or ETT, and O_2 concentration should be the lowest possible to support acceptable patient oxygenation but should not exceed 30%.[19,24-26] The anesthetist must be alert to the possibility of trapping of O_2 and anesthetic gases under the drapes.[19] Buildup of oxygen should be minimized by scavenging the operative site with suction; the oropharynx should be suctioned throughout the airway procedures.

If unanticipated supplemental O_2 (<30%) via a mask or nasal cannula becomes necessary during a monitored anesthesia care (MAC) case, it should be discontinued at least 1 minute before and during laser use; this will require close communication between the anesthetist and the surgeon, who must give adequate notice of their intent to activate the laser. N_2O readily supports combustion and should be avoided in cases with potential for fire. Suitable gas mixtures for laser procedures include O_2 and air, O_2 and nitrogen, and O_2 and helium. Helium has a high thermal conductivity and is more resistant to ignition. In addition, its lower viscosity can help overcome the increased resistance from the requisite smaller internal diameter (ID) endotracheal tubes during airway surgery. Inhalation anesthetics are nonflammable, but their use is not recommended during airway laser procedures because of their potential to deteriorate into toxic compounds in the presence of a fire.

Airway Management Devices

Polyvinyl chloride (PVC) nasal cannulas, masks, oral and nasal airways, and ETTs ignite easily and produce toxic materials that can increase the amount of damage to the airway. The breathing circuit attached to the patient airway poses an additional fire hazard. The PVC ETT is susceptible to damage by the CO_2 laser; however, presence of blood on the ETT also makes it susceptible to damage by the Nd:YAG laser. In addition, the radiopaque barium sulfate strip found on most PVC tubes has a faster ignition rate than the PVC. Red rubber tubes appear to be more resistant to initial ignition, have a slower rate of burn, and produce less toxic smoke. However, they tend to melt and can produce carbon monoxide. Although silicone tubes are also less combustible, inhalation of silica ash may produce pulmonary damage.

Laser-Resistant Endotracheal Tubes

Laser-resistant ETTs should be used during laser surgery of the airway (see Box 47.6). Historically, application of a metallic foil wrap (aluminum or copper) or a thin metal-coated plastic tape has been used to protect PVC and red rubber ETTs during laser surgery of the airway. Recognized problems with foil wrappings include tissue damage from reflected laser beams, potential areas of exposed tube, unprotected cuff, need for a smaller size ETT, and airway damage from the sharp edges of the foil wrap. Only the Merocel Laser-Guard ETT wrap (Medtronic) has FDA approval for ETT protection. The Laser-Trach (Kendall/Sheridan) is a red rubber tube with an embossed copper foil for use with CO_2 and KTP lasers. The Laser-Flex tracheal tube (Nellcor) is a flexible stainless-steel tube with a matte finish that is resistant to the CO_2 and KTP lasers. In the event of a proximal-cuff rupture with a laser beam, the distal cuff will maintain a tracheal seal and prevent anesthetic gases from leaking into the path of the laser beam. The LaserTubus (Rüsch) is a soft, white rubber tube that is resistant to the argon, Nd:YAG, and CO_2 lasers. The lower 17 cm of the tube is covered with a Merocel Laser-Guard wrap that dissipates the laser light and prevents backscatter. Soaking the tube in water will reduce ignition potential. The LaserTubus has two high-volume cuffs, one inside the other. Manufactured from natural rubber latex, it should be avoided in latex-sensitive individuals. The Bivona Fome-Cuf (Portex), a silicone and aluminum spiral tube, is designed for use with the CO_2 laser. It has a polyurethane self-inflating foam cuff covered with silicone that is designed to maintain a tracheal seal in the event of a cuff rupture. Inability to deflate the foam after cuff rupture is a recognized problem with this tube.

Laser-resistant ETTs are not laserproof and carry an inherent risk of ignition. Cuff rupture is often the prelude to an airway fire, and cuffs should be inflated with normal saline; addition of methylene blue will alert the surgeon to cuff rupture. The ETT cuff should be fully inflated, and absence of an air leak should be confirmed before the laser is used.

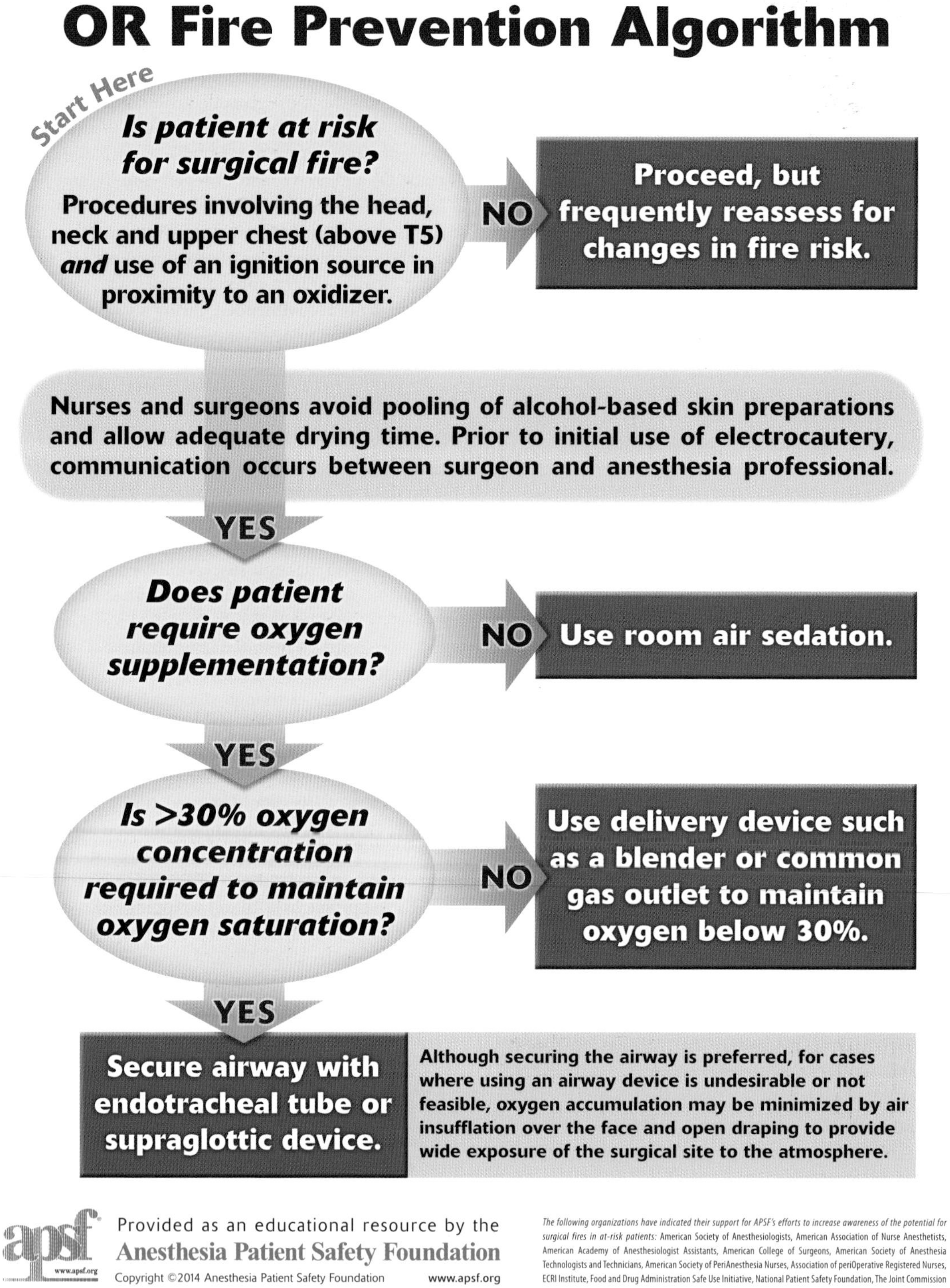

OR Fire Prevention Algorithm

Start Here

Is patient at risk for surgical fire?
Procedures involving the head, neck and upper chest (above T5) *and* use of an ignition source in proximity to an oxidizer.

NO → Proceed, but frequently reassess for changes in fire risk.

Nurses and surgeons avoid pooling of alcohol-based skin preparations and allow adequate drying time. Prior to initial use of electrocautery, communication occurs between surgeon and anesthesia professional.

YES

Does patient require oxygen supplementation?

NO → Use room air sedation.

YES

Is >30% oxygen concentration required to maintain oxygen saturation?

NO → Use delivery device such as a blender or common gas outlet to maintain oxygen below 30%.

YES

Secure airway with endotracheal tube or supraglottic device.

Although securing the airway is preferred, for cases where using an airway device is undesirable or not feasible, oxygen accumulation may be minimized by air insufflation over the face and open draping to provide wide exposure of the surgical site to the atmosphere.

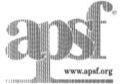

Provided as an educational resource by the
Anesthesia Patient Safety Foundation
www.apsf.org   Copyright ©2014 Anesthesia Patient Safety Foundation   www.apsf.org

The following organizations have indicated their support for APSF's efforts to increase awareness of the potential for surgical fires in at-risk patients: American Society of Anesthesiologists, American Association of Nurse Anesthetists, American Academy of Anesthesiologist Assistants, American College of Surgeons, American Society of Anesthesia Technologists and Technicians, American Society of PeriAnesthesia Nurses, Association of periOperative Registered Nurses, ECRI Institute, Food and Drug Administration Safe Use Initiative, National Patient Safety Foundation, The Joint Commission

Fig. 47.8 Operating room fire prevention algorithm. (From Cowles C, Lake C, Ehrenwerth J. Surgical fire prevention: a review. *APSF Newsletter*. 2020;35(3):82–84.)

Saline-moistened cotton gauze should be placed proximal to the ETT cuff; the gauze and the attached cotton strings should be constantly remoistened. At least 1 minute should elapse before a laser is used after reinflation of an ETT cuff or repositioning of the ETT for correction of a leak.

Laryngeal Mask Airways

The tube of the standard silicone LMA is more resistant to laser beams than the disposable PVC LMA, but the PVC cuff is more resistant to laser beams than the silicone cuff. The intubating LMA (silicone and steel) is more sensitive to the KTP laser. The presence of blood increases the vulnerability of all LMAs, especially with the KTP laser. Similar to ETTs, precautions for use of an LMA during laser procedures include inflation of the cuff with saline and methylene blue and protection of the cuff with moistened gauze. The use of 5 to 10 cm H_2O positive end-expiratory pressure (PEEP) has been advocated during laser surgery of the airway to prevent hot, toxic gases from reaching the lower airways.

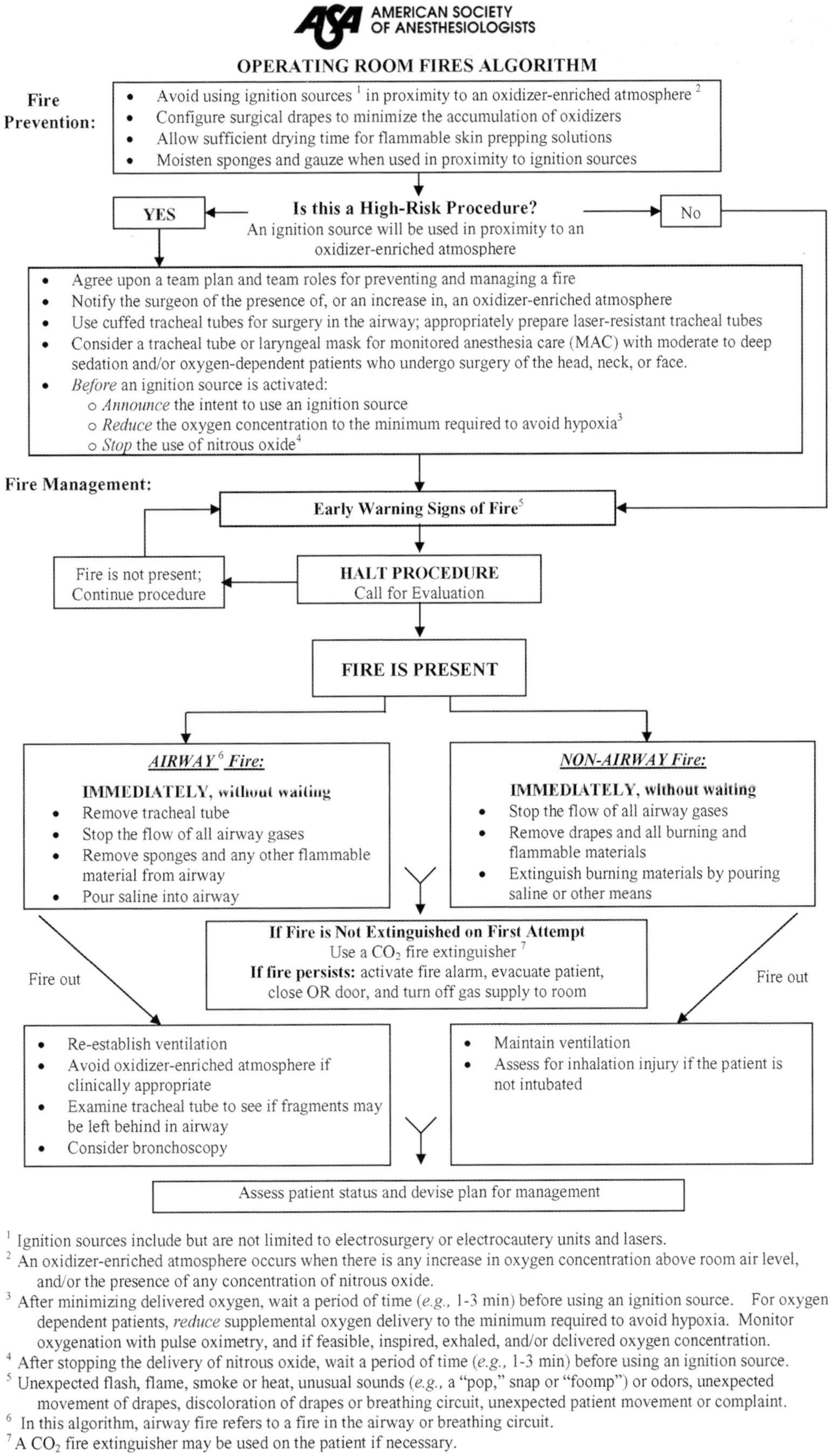

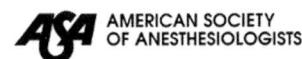

AMERICAN SOCIETY
OF ANESTHESIOLOGISTS

OPERATING ROOM FIRES ALGORITHM

Fire Prevention:

- Avoid using ignition sources [1] in proximity to an oxidizer-enriched atmosphere [2]
- Configure surgical drapes to minimize the accumulation of oxidizers
- Allow sufficient drying time for flammable skin prepping solutions
- Moisten sponges and gauze when used in proximity to ignition sources

Is this a High-Risk Procedure?
An ignition source will be used in proximity to an oxidizer-enriched atmosphere

YES ◄— | —► No

- Agree upon a team plan and team roles for preventing and managing a fire
- Notify the surgeon of the presence of, or an increase in, an oxidizer-enriched atmosphere
- Use cuffed tracheal tubes for surgery in the airway; appropriately prepare laser-resistant tracheal tubes
- Consider a tracheal tube or laryngeal mask for monitored anesthesia care (MAC) with moderate to deep sedation and/or oxygen-dependent patients who undergo surgery of the head, neck, or face.
- *Before* an ignition source is activated:
  - *Announce* the intent to use an ignition source
  - *Reduce* the oxygen concentration to the minimum required to avoid hypoxia [3]
  - *Stop* the use of nitrous oxide [4]

Fire Management:

Early Warning Signs of Fire [5]

Fire is not present; Continue procedure ◄—

HALT PROCEDURE
Call for Evaluation

FIRE IS PRESENT

AIRWAY [6] _Fire:_

IMMEDIATELY, without waiting
- Remove tracheal tube
- Stop the flow of all airway gases
- Remove sponges and any other flammable material from airway
- Pour saline into airway

NON-AIRWAY Fire:

IMMEDIATELY, without waiting
- Stop the flow of all airway gases
- Remove drapes and all burning and flammable materials
- Extinguish burning materials by pouring saline or other means

Fire out

If Fire is Not Extinguished on First Attempt
Use a CO_2 fire extinguisher [7]
If fire persists: activate fire alarm, evacuate patient, close OR door, and turn off gas supply to room

Fire out

- Re-establish ventilation
- Avoid oxidizer-enriched atmosphere if clinically appropriate
- Examine tracheal tube to see if fragments may be left behind in airway
- Consider bronchoscopy

- Maintain ventilation
- Assess for inhalation injury if the patient is not intubated

Assess patient status and devise plan for management

[1] Ignition sources include but are not limited to electrosurgery or electrocautery units and lasers.
[2] An oxidizer-enriched atmosphere occurs when there is any increase in oxygen concentration above room air level, and/or the presence of any concentration of nitrous oxide.
[3] After minimizing delivered oxygen, wait a period of time (*e.g.,* 1-3 min) before using an ignition source. For oxygen dependent patients, *reduce* supplemental oxygen delivery to the minimum required to avoid hypoxia. Monitor oxygenation with pulse oximetry, and if feasible, inspired, exhaled, and/or delivered oxygen concentration.
[4] After stopping the delivery of nitrous oxide, wait a period of time (*e.g.,* 1-3 min) before using an ignition source.
[5] Unexpected flash, flame, smoke or heat, unusual sounds (*e.g.,* a "pop," snap or "foomp") or odors, unexpected movement of drapes, discoloration of drapes or breathing circuit, unexpected patient movement or complaint.
[6] In this algorithm, airway fire refers to a fire in the airway or breathing circuit.
[7] A CO_2 fire extinguisher may be used on the patient if necessary.

Fig. 47.9 Operating room fire algorithm. (From Committee on Standards and Practice Parameters. Practice advisory for the prevention of operating room fires: an updated report by the American Society of Anesthesiologists Task Force on Operating Room Fires. *Anesthesiology.* 2013;118:271–290.)

TABLE 47.4   Gas Mixtures That Deliver ≤30% Oxygen

Air (L/min)	Oxygen (L/min)	Total Gas Flow (L/min)	O₂ Concentration
0.90	0.10	1	28.9%
1.80	0.20	2	28.9%
2.70	0.30	3	28.9%
3.60	0.40	4	28.9%
4.50	0.50	5	28.9%

Management of a Surgical Fire

Fire must be anticipated during any laser procedure (see Figs. 47.7 and 47.8). Communication among all members of the surgical team is vital for the prevention of and coordinated response to a surgical fire. Fire management includes early recognition, procedure termination, fire extinguishment, room evacuation if necessary, and appropriate postoperative care of the patient.[25,26] For a nonairway fire, all gases should be discontinued and all drapes and burning material removed from the patient and extinguished with saline, water, or by smothering. The patient should be immediately assessed for thermal trauma or smoke inhalation. In the event the fire spreads, the acronym RACE refers to the necessary steps required of operating room personnel: **r**escue the patient; **a**lert other staff and **a**ctivate the fire alarm systems; **c**onfine the fire by shutting doors, closing off gas supplies and electrical power, and using fire extinguishers; and **e**vacuate the room (see Box 47.6).

In the event of an airway fire, the anesthetist has approximately 6 seconds for recognition and removal of a burning ETT or LMA. Signs of an airway fire include darkening of the ETT, LMA, or breathing circuit with soot; an orange or red glow to the ETT or LMA; and the presence of flames in or around the ETT or LMA. The ETT and LMA act like a blowtorch, with high concentrations of O_2 adding to the intensity of the fire. Within seconds, the flames can reach a height of 5 to 10 in. Intraluminal fires will spread toward the proximal end of the tube, the source of the O_2. Severe thermal or chemical trauma is unlikely to occur if the flame is vented through the tube or oropharynx. Downstream gases contain the products of oxidation and a low concentration of O_2; however, a free-end fire can occur if the products of oxidation ignite in the O_2-rich alveoli.

In rapid succession, the ETT should be removed, all flammable and burning material removed from the airway, all gases discontinued, and saline poured into the patient's airway to extinguish any residual smoldering material and cool the tissues (Box 47.7). Ventilation should be resumed, but an O_2-enriched gas mixture should be avoided until all risk of reignition is eliminated. The ETT or LMA should be examined for intactness, and direct visualization of the tracheobronchial tree with a rigid bronchoscope is recommended for assessment of thermal injury and removal of foreign material, including ETT fragments. A flexible bronchoscope may be necessary for evaluation of distal airways, and tracheobronchial lavage with saline solution should be considered. If reintubation is indicated, a smaller ETT should be used; a chest x-ray and arterial blood gases are indicated to guide postoperative management. Carboxyhemoglobin levels are needed for assessment of smoke inhalation.

After an airway fire, 24-hour observation of the patient is indicated. A patient with minor burns should be monitored for development of laryngeal-tracheal edema. A patient with severe airway burns should remain intubated and receive 30% to 60% humidified O_2; a tracheostomy and mechanical ventilation with PEEP may be

BOX 47.7   Management of Airway Fires

- Discontinue use of laser.
- In rapid succession, remove ETT or LMA, turn off all gases, remove sponges and any flammable material, and pour saline into airway.
- Extinguish burning ETT/LMA in basin of water.
- Resume ventilation with air. Ventilate with 100% O_2 only when the fire is extinguished.
- Examine airway and remove residual debris with rigid bronchoscope. Consider lavage with normal saline. Examine small and distal airways with flexible fiberoptic bronchoscope.
- Administer humidified O_2 by mask if airway damage is minimal and risk of laryngeal edema is low.
- If indicated, reintubate with a smaller ETT.
- Assess extent of thermal trauma with ABG, carboxyhemoglobin levels, and CXR.
- Keep patient intubated and administer 40% to 60% humidified O_2 if airway burn is present or suspected.
- Consider tracheostomy and mechanical ventilation for postoperative management.
- Consider administration of steroids.
- Admit patient to ICU for a minimum 24-hr observation.
- Retain all equipment and materials involved in the fire for further inspection.
- Reassemble surgical team to identify the sequence of events that led to the surgical fire.
- Report fire as a sentinel event to The Joint Commission, ECRI, and FDA.

ABG, Arterial blood gas; *CXR*, chest x-ray; *ECRI*, Emergency Care Research Institute; *ETT*, endotracheal tube; *FDA*, Food and Drug Administration; *ICU*, intensive care unit; *LMA*, laryngeal mask airway; *O₂*, oxygen.

warranted. Corticosteroids have been recommended for the treatment of both smoke inhalation and bronchospasm that may be precipitated in patients with irritable airways. Additional treatment is dependent on the extent of the injury and the response of the patient. Complications may be delayed, and tracheal stenosis can occur months after an airway fire. A monthly laryngoscopy or bronchoscopy may be indicated for up to 6 months. All equipment and materials involved in a surgical fire should be retained for further inspection; all surgical fires should be reported to The Joint Commission as sentinel events.

ANESTHESIA FOR LASER PROCEDURES

Anesthesia is frequently required for laser procedures, and most anesthetic techniques are suitable for these procedures. Although they may appear to be less invasive, laser procedures have complications similar to those of traditional surgery. Continuous use of LSE by operating room personnel and awake patients is mandatory during laser surgery. The lenses of CO_2 LSE are usually clear and do not affect color perception, but tinted or colored LSE required for some lasers can affect color perception. Some Nd:YAG LSE can significantly dim the green color on monochrome monitors, tempting the anesthesia provider to remove the LSE while the laser is in use. Prior to anesthetizing a patient for a laser procedure, the anesthetist should observe the monitors through the LSE to ascertain the effect of the tinted LSE on the visibility of the displayed parameters. Display lights and alarms of patient monitors should be set to maximum brightness or otherwise adjusted to compensate for the color restriction. Audible alarms should be adjusted to the loudest setting.

Major anesthetic concerns exist when the airway is shared between the anesthetist and the surgeon during a laser procedure. The proximity of the endotracheal tube and anesthetic gases to the laser beam creates a very real hazard of airway fire.[20,23] Communication between the surgeon and the anesthetist is paramount to ensure patient safety, maximize surgical access, and avoid complications. Ventilation techniques during laser procedures of the airway are dependent on surgeon preference and the site of the laser application.

Supplemental oxygen is indicated for patients with less than or equal to 90% O_2 saturation (SaO_2) on room air; the airway should be secured with a LMA or ETT, and O_2 concentration should not exceed 30%. Use of an air/O_2 blender will allow delivery of the desired O_2 concentration. The anesthetist can also deliver less than 30% O_2 directly from the flowmeters, but the exact O_2 concentration delivered to the patient can vary, especially with manual flowmeters, and demands the continuous use of an O_2 analyzer (see Table 47.4). A sudden, unexpected need for supplemental O_2 during a MAC case, as evidenced by a SaO_2 less than 90%, mandates continuous communication between the surgical team. Continuous scavenging of the operative site with suction is necessary to prevent buildup of O_2. The supplemental oxygen should be discontinued 1 minute before and during laser use. During airway procedures, small-sized ETT are necessary to maximize surgical view and access for airway procedures, and the anesthetist must be prepared to deal with the associated increase in resistance to ventilation. Even when the airway is secured with a LMA or ETT, the oropharynx should be continually suctioned throughout an airway procedure. Use of excessive tape to secure the ETT should be avoided to allow easier removal of the tube in the event of an airway fire. Two syringes filled with normal saline should be readily available to extinguish an airway fire (see Box 47.6). Some surgeons may prefer an apneic technique, in which case the airway is alternately shared between the surgeon and the anesthetist. The patient is hyperventilated by mask with less than 30% O_2 after brief intermittent periods of laser application. The SaO_2 must be monitored closely and ventilation immediately resumed if oxygenation decreases 2% to 3% below the patient's initial saturation, or when 1.5 to 2 minutes have elapsed. However, this technique is to be discouraged because high O_2 concentrations can build up in the upper and lower airways during the apneic periods and are susceptible to ignition by the laser beam. Inhalation anesthetics are best avoided during laser surgery of the airway because of their potential to deteriorate toxic compounds in the presence of a fire. A basin of water or normal saline should be available during laser procedures to extinguish a sudden fire.

SUMMARY

Lasers have numerous applications in all surgical specialties because of their ability to cut, coagulate, vaporize, and selectively destroy abnormal tissue. Anesthetists provide care for patients undergoing a wide variety of laser procedures in hospital operating rooms and off-site locations, ambulatory surgeries and clinics, and private practice offices. Safe provision of anesthetic care requires an understanding of laser physics and recognition of the potential hazards associated with the use of lasers. Use of eye and skin protection for both the patient and health care providers, high filter surgical masks, and continuous use of a smoke evacuator is mandatory. The anesthetist must be acutely aware of the risk of fire during laser procedures, especially during high-risk procedures of the airway, head, neck, and upper chest. Fire safety education is the most effective way to both prevent and manage surgical fires. Fire drills with mandatory involvement of all members of the surgical team, including anesthesia providers and surgeons, should be held annually.

REFERENCES

For a complete list of references for this chapter, scan this QR code with any smartphone code reader app, or visit the following URL: http://booksite.elsevier.com/9780323711944/.

48

Obesity and Anesthesia Practice

Mary Anne Krogh

OVERVIEW

Obesity is a complex, multifactorial, chronic disease that develops from an interaction between an individual's genotype and the environment.[1-6] It is the second leading cause of preventable death in the United States.[1] Obesity is associated with an increased incidence of a wide spectrum of medical and surgical conditions and morbidity. As a result, anesthetists can expect to encounter overweight and obese patients frequently in their practices. These patients may present a considerable challenge due to the multiple pathophysiologic changes associated with obesity. A thorough understanding of the pathophysiology, pharmacology, and specific anesthetic considerations associated with obesity will promote optimal anesthesia care.

Statistics

The prevalence of obesity around the world continues to rise, and in the United States, millions of Americans are considered to be severely obese.[7] Current estimates are that over 210 million, or 75%, of US adults are classified as overweight or obese. The age-adjusted prevalence of obesity in 2017–2018 was 42% for adults (43% men and 42.1% women). The corresponding values for severe obesity (body mass index [BMI] ≥40) were 6.9% for men and 11.1% for women.[8]

There are an estimated 26 million people in the United States with a BMI of at least 35 kg/m², and 15 million with a BMI of 40 kg/m² or higher.[1,4] There has been an increase in the proportion of obese persons aged 20 years and older from 23% in 1994 to approximately 42.4% presently (Fig 48.1).

Obesity is not confined to the United States; it is a health problem that is increasing at an alarming rate throughout the world. Globally, there are approximately 2 billion individuals documented as overweight (BMI 25–29.9 kg/m²).[9,10] It is estimated that there were more than 650 million obese people worldwide in 2016, and three countries report more than 50% of their population is obese. According to the World Health Organization (WHO), the global obesity incidence has nearly tripled since 1975.[11] Concerns about the global obesity crisis are growing, and WHO reports that obesity accounts for more than 400,000 deaths annually, making it second only to tobacco-related disease as a cause of preventable and premature death.[12]

In the United States, individuals who are obese have a 10% to 50% greater risk of death from all causes compared with healthy-weight individuals (BMI 18.5–24.9). Obesity is associated with approximately 112,000 preventable deaths per year.[13] Most of the increased risk is due to cardiovascular causes.[14]

Cost of Obesity

More than $315 billion was spent in 2014 for health care costs related to obesity.[15] This does not take into account the additional dollars spent annually on weight-reduction programs, exercise equipment, low-fat diet products, pharmacologic agents, advertising, and marketing related to obesity.[4] Obesity is a major health concern, and obese patients admitted for surgery may exhibit one or more medical conditions in addition to the primary underlying problem.[16] Clearly, identification of obesity-related conditions is vital to the safe administration of an anesthetic.

Definitions

BMI is the accepted measure of body habitus that describes adiposity normalized for height.[1] BMI can be calculated according to the following formulas:

- BMI = weight (in kilograms)/height (in meters)²
- BMI = (weight [in pounds]/height [in inches]²) × 703

Overweight is defined as a BMI of 25 to 29 kg/m², and obesity as a BMI of 30 kg/m².[1-3] Historically, individuals with a BMI greater than 30 kg/m² had higher mortality rates for a number of conditions, especially those associated with cardiovascular disease. However, evidence suggests that modern screening has limited the excess mortality related to obesity, particularly in obese patients with a BMI less than 35 kg/m².[17] A person's degree of obesity is commonly defined using BMI (Table 48.1). A BMI greater than or equal to 25 kg/m² is considered overweight, and a BMI greater than or equal to 30 kg/m² is considered obese. Obesity can be subcategorized into class I (30–34.9 kg/m²), class II (35–39.9 kg/m²), and class III (>40 kg/m²). The term *morbid obesity* has been abandoned due to its negative connotations, and the term *extreme obesity* is used instead.[17] Some sources have abandoned the classification system for a more simplified description, with obesity defined as greater than 30 kg/m² and severe obesity defined as greater than 40 kg/m².[8] Ideal body weight (IBW) is a term used interchangeably with both normal weight and desirable weight.[1-3] IBW is a measurement of height and body mass that exhibits the lowest morbidity and mortality for a given population.[2] Determination of IBW is especially useful in calculating drug and intravenous infusion doses in morbidly obese patients. Certain drugs, if administered according to actual body weight, can produce toxicity, renal damage, or hemodynamic instability. Conversely, some drugs must be given according to actual body weight if therapeutic effects are to be achieved. The lean body mass increases by approximately 30% in obese individuals due to the increased muscle developed to carry extra body weight. As a result, lean body weight (LBW) is 30% higher than IBW. Simplified weight calculations for IBW and LBW are as follows:

- For men: IBW = Height (in centimeters) – 100
- For women: IBW = Height (in centimeters) – 105
- LBW = IBW × 1.3

Risk Factors

Obesity is associated with an increase in the incidence of many medical conditions (Box 48.1). The risk for cardiovascular disease, certain cancers, diabetes, and overall mortality is linearly related to weight gain.

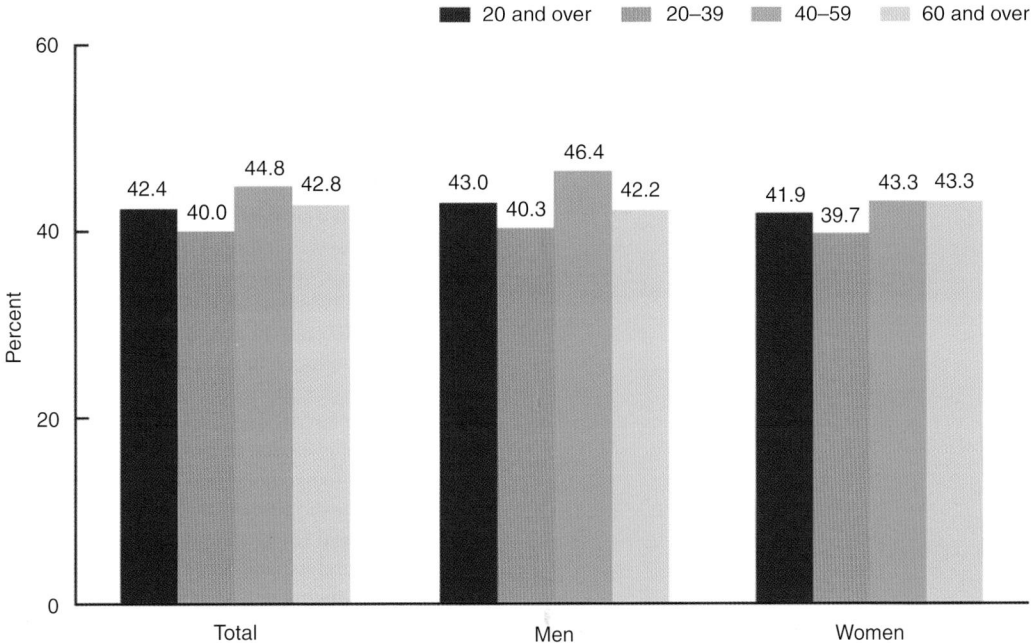

Fig. 48.1 Prevalence of obesity among adults aged 20 and over, by sex and age: United States, 2011–2014. NOTES: Totals were age-adjusted by the direct method to the 2000 U.S. census population using the age groups 20–39, 40–59, and 60 and over. Crude estimates are 36.5% for all, 34.5% for men, and 38.5% for women. (From Ogden CL, et al. Prevalence of Obesity Among Adults and Youth: United States, 2011–2014. *NCHS Data Brief*. 2015;219:1–8. Source: CDC/NCHS, National Health and Nutrition Examination Survey, 2011–2014.)

TABLE 48.1   Classification of Overweight and Obesity by Body Mass Index

	Obesity Class	Body Mass Index (kg/m²)
Underweight	—	Less than 18.5
Normal	—	18.5–24.9
Overweight	—	25–29.9
Obesity	I	30–34.9
	II	35–39.9
Extreme obesity	III	>40

Type 2 diabetes, coronary heart disease, hypertension, and hypercholesterolemia are common conditions in overweight and obese patients.[1-3] With increasing weight gain and increased adiposity, glucose tolerance deteriorates, blood pressure rises, and the lipid profile becomes more atherogenic.[2] Using BMI, age, and gender as independent variables, a multiple logistic regression model established that males (P = 0.021), those with higher BMI (P < 0.0001), and older individuals (P < 0.0001) tend to have higher cardiovascular risk than those who are younger, thinner, and female. These data suggest that male gender, the extent of obesity, and age are risk factors because they are markers for sicker patients.[18] Hormonal and nonhormonal mechanisms contribute to the greater risk of breast, gastrointestinal, endometrial, and renal cell cancers.[6]

ADIPOSE TISSUE

Adipose tissue has major integrative physiologic functions, secretes numerous proteins, and is considered an endocrine organ.[2] Its major functions as an organ are to provide a reservoir of readily convertible and usable energy and to maintain heat insulation.[2,3,19] Functions associated with liver fat metabolism include degradation of fatty acids into usable units of energy, synthesis of triglycerides from carbohydrates and proteins, and synthesis of other lipids from fatty acids, particularly cholesterol and phospholipids.[19] The ability of the liver to desaturate fatty acids is tremendously important because all cells contain some unsaturated fats synthesized by the liver.

Body fat is also important in heat regulation and insulation. Fat cells, which arise from modified fibroblasts, enlarge and fill with liquid triglycerides to nearly 95% of their storage capacity.[19,20] When the skin is exposed to cold conditions (over several weeks), the fatty acid chains of the triglycerides shorten or become more unsaturated.[3] This phenomenon lowers their melting point, which allows the fat in the fat cells to maintain a liquid state. Metabolically, this is significant, as only liquid fat can be hydrolyzed and transported from the cells to be used for energy.[3]

Body Fat Distribution

In early childhood, fat cell formation occurs rapidly.[2] Overfeeding during this time accelerates fat storage and triggers hyperproliferation of fat cells. During adolescence, the number of fat cells stabilizes and remains constant throughout adult life. Children become obese through an increase in fat cell numbers, whereas adults become obese through hypertrophy of existing fat cells.[2,3] The distribution of body fat, however, is a clearer indicator of increased health risk.[19]

Central, android, or abdominal visceral obesity (apple shape), with a waist:hip ratio greater than 0.85 in women and greater than 0.92 in men, is correlated with a higher risk of comorbidities in obese patients[2,21] (Fig. 48.2A). The waist:hip ratio is calculated by dividing the narrowest waist measurement by the broadest hip measurement, taken while the patient is standing.[2] Waist circumference is the newly established marker for abdominal obesity. A waist circumference greater than 102 cm (40 in) in men or a waist circumference greater than 88 cm (35 in) in women denotes an increased risk for ischemic heart disease, diabetes mellitus, hypertension, dyslipidemia, and death.[1-3,19]

Peripheral gynoid or gluteal femoral obesity (pear shape), with a waist:hip ratio below 0.76, is associated with varicose vein development,

BOX 48.1   Conditions Associated With Obesity

Cardiovascular System
- Coronary heart disease
- Hypertension
- Dyslipidemia
- Cerebrovascular disease
- Thromboembolic disease
- Cardiomegaly
- Congestive heart failure
- Pulmonary hypertension

Endocrine System
- Type 2 diabetes
- Thyroid disorders

Respiratory System
- Restrictive lung disease
- Obesity hypoventilation syndrome
- Obstructive sleep apnea

Gastrointestinal System
- Hiatal or inguinal hernia
- Gallbladder disease
- Nonalcoholic fatty liver disease: steatosis, cirrhosis, hepatomegaly
- Gastroesophageal reflux disease (GERD)

Other Systems
- Gout
- Infertility
- Impaired immune response
- Wound infections
- Osteoarthritis
- Malignancy: esophageal, gallbladder, colon, breast, uterine, cervical, prostate, renal
- Urinary incontinence
- Pancreatitis
- Low back pain
- Obstetric complications

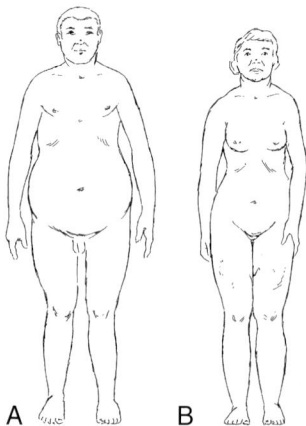

Fig. 48.2 Obesity. (A) Central, android, or abdominal visceral. (B) Peripheral, gynoid or gluteal.

joint disease, and a reduced incidence of non–insulin-dependent diabetes mellitus (see Fig. 48.2B). Medical risks are decreased in individuals with gynoid fat distribution compared to those with the android pattern.[1,22]

Differences in morbidity between android and gynoid fat distribution are attributable to the metabolic characteristics of the adipose tissues and adjacent tissues. Gynoid repositories of fat, found primarily in women, are metabolically static and are proposed to function as energy depots for pregnancy and lactation.[3,22] Android fat distribution, typically seen in males, is metabolically active with regard to free fatty acid (FFA) release.[2] When elevated levels of FFAs are mobilized from adipose tissue, portal venous drainage delivers high concentrations of FFAs to the liver. Continual delivery of excessive FFAs stimulates hepatic synthesis of very low-density lipoproteins (VLDLs) and circulation of low-density lipoproteins (LDLs). Hepatic exposure to high concentrations of FFAs also increases gluconeogenesis and inhibits insulin uptake, which induces the development of non–insulin-dependent diabetes mellitus. Although VLDLs, LDLs, and hyperglycemia are catalysts for the formation of associated cardiovascular and cerebrovascular disease, evidence from some studies supports the possibility that hyperinsulinemia alone may cause hypertension.[2,3] Additionally, patients with android fat distribution have an increased risk of visceral and retroperitoneal fat, which increases the compression of renal veins, lymph vessels, ureters, and renal tissues. This increased pressure has been linked to a higher risk of hypertension.[23]

CAUSES OF OBESITY

Body size is dependent on genetic and environmental factors. Genetic predisposition, believed to be a primary factor in the development of obesity, explains only 40% of the variance in body mass.[6] The significant increase in the prevalence of obesity has resulted from environmental factors that result in increased calorie intake and reduced physical activity.[6,19] Other factors such as socialization, age, sex, race, and economic status affect the progression of obesity. In the United States, food consumption has risen as a result of the "super-sizing" of portions and the availability of high-fat fast food and snacks. Physical activity has been reduced as a result of modernization (e.g., television and computers), as well as sedentary lifestyles and work activities. Cultural and lifestyle variations play an important role in the development of obesity.[6]

A link between systemic inflammation and obesity has long been recognized. Adipocytes are known to produce and store several inflammatory mediators, including leptin,[24] tumor necrosis factor-α, monocyte chemotactic protein,[24] and interleukin-6.[24,25] Weight loss results in a reduction in both the inflammatory mediators and comorbidities associated with obesity.[25] Continued investigation into genetic-environmental interactions may provide further understanding of and treatment for obesity.[21,22]

PATHOPHYSIOLOGY OF OBESITY

A number of pathophysiologic changes occur as a result of overweight and obesity.[26] These changes involve all of the major body organ systems, leading to an increase in morbidity and premature death. The risk of many of the medical conditions associated with obesity increases linearly with increasing BMI.[2-4]

Cardiovascular Considerations

Cardiovascular considerations are predominantly a reflection of the progressive compensatory processes that evolve to meet the increased metabolic demands of the fat organ.[27,28] Cardiovascular disease is the primary cause of the morbidity and mortality associated with obesity and manifests in the form of ischemic heart disease, hypertension, and cardiac failure.[15] Development and sustenance of the fat mass necessitates the formation of extra blood vessels and increased circulatory, pulmonary, central, and peripheral blood volume.[2-4] For every 13.5 kg of fat gained, an estimated 25 miles of neovascularization is generated to provide blood flow at a rate of 2 to 3 mL/100 g of tissue per minute. This represents an increased cardiac output of 0.1 L/min for each kilogram of fat acquired.[3] An expanded blood volume, stimulated by hypoxia-induced chronic respiratory insufficiency, is seen in severe obesity. Accelerated renin-angiotensin activity and the perfusion requirements of the fat organ further increase the vascular fluid compartment.[2-4,27,28]

Movement of the expanded blood volume through extensive vascular tissue, under compression by adipose tissue, places greater demand on the myocardium. The increased workload caused by elevation of the basal metabolic rate is reflected in an increased cardiac output, increased oxygen (O_2) consumption, increased carbon dioxide production, and normal or slightly abnormal arteriovenous O_2 difference.[2,29] Chronically elevated cardiac output precedes increased left-sided heart pressures and left ventricular hypertrophy. Because the heart rate usually remains the same, cardiac output must be augmented by an increase in stroke volume. Therefore, cardiomegaly, atrial and biventricular dilation, and biventricular hypertrophy ensue. These contribute to the development of hypertension and eventual congestive heart failure.[2-4,30]

Hypertension is defined as a systolic blood pressure greater than 140 mm Hg, a diastolic pressure greater than 90 mm Hg, or both.[3] The prevalence of hypertension in obese patients is more than twice as high as in lean men and women.[30,31] Blood pressure has been shown to increase 6.5 mm Hg for every 10% increase in body weight.[32] In severely obese individuals who are not hypertensive, decreased systemic vascular resistance may serve to facilitate forward blood flow through the doubled body habitus.[2,4] Hypertension is precipitated by increased blood viscosity, altered catecholamine kinetics, and possibly increased estrogen concentrations. Hyperinsulinemia, elevated mineralocorticoids, and abnormal sodium reabsorption have also been implicated as causes of hypertension.

Renal mechanisms are also associated with the development of obesity-related hypertension. Causes of renal-induced hypertension include visceral compression of the kidneys from fat deposits in and around the kidney, impaired sodium excretion, activation of the renin-angiotensin-aldosterone system, and increased sympathetic nervous system activity.[23]

Hypercholesterolemia (i.e., cholesterol levels >240 mg/dL) often coexists with hypertension, thereby predisposing obese patients to atherosclerosis and cerebrovascular accident.[29,31] Arrhythmias may occur as a result of hypoxemia, hypercapnia, electrolyte disorders, sleep apnea, ventricular hypertrophy, hypertension, and coronary artery disease (CAD).[27,28]

CAD is frequently associated with obesity but is an independent risk factor. It appears with or without hypertension, hypercholesterolemia, diabetes mellitus, hyperlipidemia, or a sedentary lifestyle.[2-4,33] Obesity coincident with CAD results in frequent angina, congestive heart failure, acute myocardial infarction, and sudden death.[15,29,30] Ischemic heart disease is more common in obese individuals with a central fat distribution.[29]

Respiratory Considerations

Compromise of respiratory function results from the compression of fat on abdominal, diaphragmatic, and thoracic structures. Over time, thoracic kyphosis and lumbar lordosis develop, resulting in impaired rib movement and fixation of the thorax in an inspiratory position.[1,3] As a result, chest wall, lung, parenchyma, and pulmonary compliance are reduced to 35% of predicted values.[33,34] The metabolic needs of the fat organ and the greater mechanical work of breathing stimulate increased myocardial O_2 consumption. Increases in carbon dioxide production and retention, coupled with decreased ventilation, coincide with reduced respiratory muscle efficiency.[2] A restrictive pattern of respiration results from reductions in both chest wall

and lung compliance.[35] Lung inflation is inhibited, which causes declinations in functional residual capacity (FRC) to less than closing capacity. Premature airway closure increases dead space and causes carbon dioxide retention, ventilation-perfusion mismatch, shunting, and hypoxemia.[1,21] Extreme obesity is associated with reductions in FRC, expiratory reserve volume (ERV), and total lung capacity.[33-36] FRC declines exponentially with increasing BMI.[2] In a 2006 study of pulmonary function in morbidly obese patients, forced vital capacity varied inversely with BMI, and patients with a very high BMI, even when asymptomatic, had major reductions in lung function.[37]

Concomitant diminution of vital capacity, total lung capacity, ERV, and inspiratory capacity are demonstrated by rapid, shallow breathing. These ventilation patterns are characteristic of restrictive lung disease.[2,34,36] Eventual hypoventilation, hypercarbia, and acidosis result from the depression of central nervous system responsiveness to chronic hypoxia.[3] Recurrent hypoxemia leads to secondary polycythemia and is associated with an increased risk of CAD and cerebrovascular disease.[19] Respiratory muscle dysfunction has also been reported with obesity,[35,38] and it may result from inefficiency secondary to changes in chest-wall compliance or the lower lung volumes found in obese individuals. These abnormalities predispose obese patients to respiratory failure in the setting of even mild pulmonary or systematic insults.[39]

Obesity has been closely linked to the development of asthma-like symptoms, with weight loss resulting in an improvement in shortness of breath. However, in a 2016 study, obese patients were found to be no more likely to have airflow obstruction than the general population. The study identified possible causes of the asthma-like symptoms in the obese population, including increased perception of dyspnea, systemic inflammation, and increased work of breathing.[40] Inactivity has been linked with these asthma-like symptoms.[24]

Obstructive Sleep Apnea

Obesity is a well-established risk factor for sleep apnea, with the incidence of obstructive sleep apnea (OSA) increasing in direct proportion with the level of obesity. Patients with OSA tend to have a BMI greater than 30 kg/m^2, abdominal fat distribution, and a large neck girth (>17 in for men and >16 in for women).[2] For patients with clinically severe obesity (BMI ≥35 kg/m^2) who present for bariatric surgery, the incidence of sleep apnea ranges from 71% to 77%.[41-43]

OSA is characterized by excessive episodes of apnea (10 seconds) and hypopnea during sleep that are caused by complete or partial upper airway obstruction.[35,44] Up to 25% of all surgical patients are at risk of OSA.[45] OSA is characterized by intermittent closure or narrowing of the upper airway during sleep, which leads to episodes of apnea-hypopnea, arousal, and O_2 desaturation.[46] This disorder is pervasive and affects nearly 18 million Americans.[47] It is estimated that as many as 80% to 95% of persons with OSA are undiagnosed.[48]

Apnea is the cessation of airflow at the nose and mouth for more than 10 seconds.[24,49] Apnea is considered obstructive if there is continued respiratory effort despite airflow cessation. Hypopnea is defined as a 50% reduction in airflow for 10 seconds that occurs 15 or more times per hour of sleep and is associated with snoring and a 4% decrease in O_2 saturation. It connotes a transient reduction in airflow caused by increased upper airway resistance.[48] OSA syndrome is diagnosed by polysomnography (PSG) using an apnea-hypopnea index (AHI).[50] There are different definitions of OSA. The AHI is the number of abnormal respiratory events per hour of sleep. Classically, the accepted minimal clinical diagnostic criteria for OSA are an AHI of 10 plus symptoms of excessive daytime sleepiness. The American Academy of Sleep Medicine defines mild OSA as an AHI between 5 and 15, moderate OSA as an AHI between 15 and 30, and severe OSA as an AHI greater than 30. Medicare guidelines recognize the presence of OSA with an AHI of 15, or an AHI of 5 with two comorbidities.[41]

Patients with obesity hypoventilation syndrome (OHS) may have elevated bicarbonate levels.[35]

The pathogenesis of OSA is likely multifactorial.[51] Contributing factors include airway anatomy, the state-dependent control of the upper airway dilator muscles, and ventilatory stability. The site of upper airway obstruction typically lies in the pharynx. The pharyngeal luminal area during inspiration reflects a balance between collapsing intrapharyngeal negative suction pressure and dilating forces provided by the pharyngeal muscles.[52] In awake human subjects, the patency is maintained by continual mediation of the contraction of the tensor muscles by the central nervous system. These dilator muscles oppose the negative collapsing force developed during inspiration.[48] This activation of muscle tone is typically reduced during sleep, and in many individuals leads to compromised patency of the upper airway with turbulent airflow and snoring. In obese patients, the presence of more adipose tissue in the pharyngeal structures increases the likelihood that relaxation of the upper airway muscles will cause collapse of the soft-walled oropharynx between the uvula and the epiglottis. Extraluminal pressure is increased by superficially located masses, and the upper airway is compressed externally.[46,48,53,54]

While sleeping, any and all of these mechanical, neural, and structural factors may contribute to upper airway collapse that either interferes with or eliminates ventilation, which results in a surge of pharyngeal dilator muscle activity that subsequently opens the airway. A period of hyperventilation then follows, which reverses hypercarbia, and the central respiratory drive is then reduced correspondingly. The process can repeat itself continually throughout the night, causing intermittent hypoxia and hypercarbia, fragmenting sleep, and triggering adrenergic output with each cycle.[48,49,52] Five or more clinically significant apneic episodes per hour or more than 30 episodes per night result in hypoxia, hypercapnia, systemic and pulmonary hypertension, and cardiac arrhythmias.[22,34,36,44]

Holter-monitored patients with OSA have a higher incidence of nocturnal paroxysmal asystole, episodic bradycardia, and sinus node dysfunction.[55] A study of OSA patients with permanent pacemakers demonstrated that subjects had fewer episodes of OSA if their pacemakers were set to increase their heart rate during the night. It is hypothesized that the increased vagal tone accompanying bradycardia also affects airway patency.[56]

Patients with OSA also have a higher incidence of comorbidities. Approximately 50% to 60% of patients with OSA are hypertensive, and an estimated 50% of hypertensive patients have sleep apnea.[57] Since up to 80% to 95% of all patients with OSA are undiagnosed and untreated, the disorder will not be identified in the medical records of many patients who present for surgery. During preanesthetic evaluation, patients should be asked about their sleeping patterns, and anesthesia providers should have a high index of suspicion for OSA in all obese patients.[58] Some advocate that all obese patients, or those who observe obese patients while they sleep, be routinely asked about nocturnal snoring or apnea, arousals, and diurnal sleepiness.[59] Overnight PSG is the gold standard test used in the diagnosis of OSA, as well as many other sleep disorders. Costly, time-consuming, and labor intensive, PSG involves the simultaneous recording of multiple physiologic variables while the patient sleeps.[60] Several screening tools have been developed for preoperative use. The STOP-Bang screening tool (Box 48.2) is easy to use and has a sensitivity of up to 93%.[45,60-62]

Before patients at increased perioperative risk from OSA are scheduled to undergo surgery, a determination should be made regarding whether a surgical procedure is most appropriately performed on an inpatient or outpatient basis. Factors to be considered in determining whether outpatient care is appropriate include (1) sleep apnea status, (2) anatomic and physiologic abnormalities, (3) status

of coexisting diseases, (4) nature of surgery, (5) type of anesthesia, (6) need for postoperative opioids, (7) patient age, (8) adequacy of postdischarge observation, and (9) capabilities of the outpatient facility. The availability of difficult airway equipment, respiratory care equipment, radiology facilities, clinical laboratory facilities, and a transfer agreement with an inpatient facility should be considered in making this determination.[58]

The safety of performing surgery on an outpatient basis in patients with OSA is controversial. The American Society of Anesthesiologists (ASA) guidelines recommend against discharge of the OSA patient undergoing any ambulatory procedure, except those performed under straight local anesthesia on the day of surgery. Subsequent data from Johns Hopkins challenged this position with a study that suggested that ambulatory surgery for appropriately selected patients was not associated with unplanned admission, readmission, or serious respiratory or cardiovascular adverse events.[58,62] The Society for Ambulatory Anesthesia issued a consensus statement addressing the appropriate patient selection for adult patients scheduled for ambulatory surgical procedures. In this document, the authors advised that OSA patients with controlled comorbidities may be reasonable candidates for ambulatory procedures if their pain can be appropriately managed with minimal or no postoperative opioids.[45,51]

Suggestions for the management of OSA patients are listed in Table 48.2.

Obesity Hypoventilation (Pickwickian) Syndrome

OHS, or Pickwickian syndrome, is a complication of extreme obesity characterized by OSA, hypercapnia, daytime hypersomnolence, arterial hypoxemia, cyanosis-induced polycythemia, respiratory acidosis, pulmonary hypertension, and right-sided heart failure. At its extreme, patients develop nocturnal episodes of central apnea (apnea without respiratory efforts), which reflects progressive desensitization of the respiratory centers to nocturnal hypercarbia.[34,36,44,53]

OHS is defined as obesity (BMI >30 kg/m^2), daytime hypoventilation with awake partial pressure of arterial carbon dioxide (P_{CO_2}) greater than 45 mm Hg, and sleep-disordered breathing in the absence of other causes of hypoventilation. Approximately 90% of patients with OHS also have OSA. The prevalence of OHS in patients with OSA is uncertain but is estimated to be between 4% and 20%.[35,63]

BOX 48.2 STOP-Bang Scoring Model for Screening for Obstructive Sleep Apnea

1. **S**noring: Do you snore loudly (loud enough to be heard through closed doors)? — Yes No
2. **T**ired: Do you often feel tired, fatigued, or sleepy during daytime? — Yes No
3. **O**bserved: Has anyone observed you stop breathing during your sleep? — Yes No
4. Blood **P**ressure: Do you have or are you being treated for high blood pressure? — Yes No
BMI: >35 kg/m^2? — Yes No
Age: >50 yrs old? — Yes No
Neck circumference: >40 cm? — Yes No
Gender: Male? — Yes No
High risk of OSA: Answering yes to ≥3 items
Low risk of OSA: Answering yes to <3 items

BMI, Body mass index; OSA, obstructive sleep apnea.
Adapted from Chung F, et al. STOP questionnaire: a tool to screen patients for obstructive sleep apnea. *Anesthesiology.* 2008;108(5):812–821.

TABLE 48.2 Perioperative Anesthetic Management of Obstructive Sleep Apnea

Phase	Anesthetic Concern	Principles of Management
Preoperative period	Cardiac arrhythmias and unstable hemodynamic profile	Indirect evidence advocating the usefulness of PAP to reduce cardiac arrhythmias, stabilize variable blood pressure, and decrease myocardial oxygen consumption
	Multisystem comorbidities	Preoperative risk stratification and patient optimization
		Individualized intraoperative anesthetic management tailored to comorbidities
	Sedative premedication	Minimal or no sedation; α_2-adrenergic agonist (dexmedetomidine) premedication may reduce intraoperative anesthetic requirements and have an opioid-sparing effect
	OSA risk stratification, evaluation, and optimization	Preoperative anesthesia consults for symptom evaluation of obstructive sleep apnea, obesity hypoventilation syndrome and metabolic syndrome, airway assessment, polysomnography if indicated, and formulation of anesthesia management and postoperative plan
Intraoperative period	Regional anesthesia	Consider regional block when appropriate
	Difficult intubation	Ramp from scapula to head
		Adequate preoxygenation
		Use CPAP during preoxygenation
		ASA difficult airway algorithm
	Opioid-related respiratory depression	Opioid avoidance or minimization
		Use of short-acting agents such as remifentanil
		Regional and multimodal analgesia (e.g., nonsteroidal antiinflammatory drugs, acetaminophen, tramadol, ketamine, gabapentin, pregabalin, dexamethasone)
	Carryover sedation effects from longer acting intravenous sedatives and inhaled anesthetic agents	Use of propofol for maintenance of anesthesia
		Use of insoluble potent anesthetic agents (sevoflurane and desflurane)
	Excessive sedation in monitored anesthetic care	Use of capnography for intraoperative monitoring
Reversal of anesthesia	Postextubation airway obstruction and desaturations	Verification of full reversal of neuromuscular blockade
		Ensure patient is fully conscious and cooperative before extubation
		Semiupright posture for recovery
Immediate postoperative period	Respiratory	Use CPAP and supplemental oxygen
		Avoid opiates
		Use intensive respiratory monitoring
	Suitability for outpatient surgery	Prophylaxis for venous thromboembolism
		Lithotripsy, superficial, or minor orthopedic surgeries using local or regional techniques may be considered for outpatient surgery
		No requirement for high-dose postoperative opioids
		Transfer arrangement to inpatient facility should be available
	Postoperative respiratory event in known and suspected high-risk patients with OSA	Longer monitoring in the PACU
		Continuous oximetry monitoring and PAP therapy may be necessary if recurrent PACU respiratory events occur (e.g., desaturation, apnea, bradycardia)

ASA, American Society of Anesthesiologists; *CPAP,* continuous positive airway pressure; *OSA,* obstructive sleep apnea; *PACU,* postanesthesia care unit; *PAP,* positive airway pressure.
Adapted from Seet E, Chung F. Obstructive sleep apnea: preoperative assessment. *Anesthesiol Clin.* 2010;28(2):199–215; Bluth T, et al. The obese patient undergoing nonbariatric surgery. *Curr Opin Anaesthesiol.* 2016;29(3):421–429.

OHS, which occurs in 8% of the obese population, is clinically distinct from simple obesity.[36] With simple obesity, the P_{CO_2}, pH, and pulmonary compliance are within normal ranges.[33] Hypoxia may be present, but no evidence of cardiac failure or differences in arterioalveolar O_2 exists. In contrast, OHS is diagnosed when the morbidly obese patient exhibits inappropriate and sudden somnolence, sleep apnea, hypoxia, and hypercapnia.[3] A P_{CO_2} greater than 45 mm Hg during wakefulness with compensatory metabolic compensation and hypoxemia (partial pressure of oxygen [P_{O_2}] <70 mm Hg) is suggestive of OHS.[63] Alveolar ventilation is reduced because of shallow and inefficient ventilation related to decreased tidal volume, inadequate inspiratory strength, and inadequate elevation of the diaphragm. Cardiac enlargement, cyanosis, polycythemia, and twitching also are evident on physical examination.[4] In the early stages of OHS development, patients will maintain normocapnia during wakefulness but have increased bicarbonate and base excess due to chronic hypercapnia during sleep.

It has been suggested that early diagnosis of OHS may be facilitated by screening obese individuals at risk for the development of the disorder for increased bicarbonate levels and base excess.[64] Activities of daily living are altered by the somnolent episodes. Operating machinery or driving a vehicle may cause injury or death in these individuals.

Gastrointestinal Disease

The incidence of gastroesophageal reflux disease, gallstones, and pancreatitis increases with obesity. Patients with excess visceral fat are much more likely to develop dyspeptic symptoms.[65] Obesity is associated with a number of liver abnormalities referred to as nonalcoholic fatty liver disease (NAFLD).[66] NAFLD includes steatosis, steatohepatitis, fibrosis, cirrhosis, hepatomegaly, and abnormal liver biochemistry. Patients with NAFLD are at risk for developing cirrhosis, hepatic decompensation, and hepatocellular carcinoma. The pathogenesis of NAFLD is not fully understood, although researchers have found that a combination of environmental, genetic, and metabolic factors lead to advanced disease. There have been improvements in the use of noninvasive radiographic methods to diagnose NAFLD, especially for advanced disease; however, liver biopsy is still the standard method of diagnosis for NAFLD.[67]

NAFLD affects up to 30% of individuals in developed countries and nearly 10% of individuals in developing nations, making NAFLD the most common liver condition in the world. The pathogenesis of NAFLD is related to insulin resistance, and it is frequently found in individuals who have central obesity or diabetes. Insulin resistance and excess adiposity are associated with increased lipid influx into the liver and increased hepatic triglyceride accumulation. Defects in mitochondrial oxidation of lipids and lipid export may also contribute to hepatic lipid buildup. Clinically, NAFLD is commonly asymptomatic and usually detected incidentally by liver function tests or imaging performed for other reasons. Subjects with NAFLD have a higher mortality rate than the general population and are at increased risk of developing cardiovascular disease and diabetes.[66] In obese patients, the mortality rate from liver cirrhosis is 1.5 to 2.5 times higher than in nonobese persons.[20]

Gallstones

Gallstones are 30% more prevalent in obese than nonobese women, and this prevalence increases linearly with BMI.[4] Higher concentrations of cholesterol in the bile and an increased ratio of bile salts to lecithin are responsible for the development of gallstones.[68] Jaundice may also accompany bile duct obstruction. Laparoscopic and open cholecystectomies are commonly performed in this group of patients because of the increased incidence of gallbladder disease in the obese. Although technically more difficult for both surgical and anesthesia teams, the benefits of laparoscopic gallbladder removal (e.g., reduced postoperative pain, shorter hospitalization, earlier return to activities of daily living) outweigh the risks.

Endocrine and Metabolic Disease

Obesity is seldom the result of primary endocrine dysfunction. Thyroid, adrenocortical, and pituitary function should be investigated in obese patients who manifest atypical symptoms.[3] Menstrual problems such as oligomenorrhea, amenorrhea, menorrhagia, and the presence of hirsutism may signal hypothalamic-pituitary abnormalities. Obese men may experience decreased libido or impotence indicative of hypogonadism, and low serum follicle-stimulating hormone and testosterone levels are frequently evident.[22]

Eighty percent of individuals with type 2 diabetes mellitus are obese. The risk of type 2 diabetes increases linearly with BMI.[22,69] There is a 35% to 40% prevalence of metabolic syndrome in the US population. Patients with obesity and metabolic syndrome may have complicated medical histories that include diabetes, heart disease, and OSA. Central or android fat distribution is strongly linked to metabolic syndrome; Weight gain with visceral obesity is a major predictor of the metabolic syndrome.[70] Metabolic syndrome consists of an array of conditions, including glucose intolerance and/or type 2 diabetes mellitus, hypertension, dyslipidemia, and cardiovascular diseases. Patients with metabolic syndrome have an increased risk of developing CAD, stroke, peripheral vascular disease, and type 2 diabetes mellitus, and are at greater risk of mortality from coronary disease and other causes. These patients also exist in a proinflammatory and prothrombotic state. Whether this syndrome is a disease itself or is composed of discrete disorders is the subject of much investigation and controversy. Individuals with metabolic syndrome have a cardiovascular risk that is 50% to 60% higher than normal. The definition and characteristics of metabolic syndrome are noted in Box 48.3.[70,71]

BOX 48.3   Metabolic Syndrome Defined

The American Heart Association and the National Heart, Lung, and Blood Institute define metabolic syndrome as the presence of three or more of the following criteria:

1. Elevated waist circumference
   - Men: ≥40 in (102 cm)
   - Women: ≥35 in (88 cm)
2. Elevated triglycerides
   - ≥150 mg/dL
3. Reduced HDL cholesterol
   - Men: <40 mg/dL
   - Women: <50 mg/dL
4. Elevated blood pressure
   - ≥130/85 mm Hg
5. Elevated fasting glucose
   - ≥100 mg/dL

HDL, High-density lipoprotein.
Adapted from Levin PD, Weissman C. Obesity, metabolic syndrome, and the surgical patient. *Anesthesiol Clin.* 2009;27(4):705–719.

Orthopedic and Joint Disease

Obese persons often develop osteoarthritis from continued mechanical stress on weight-bearing joints. There is a linear relationship between weight and the degree of arthritis.[2-4] Ankles, hips, knees, and the lumbar spine are frequently burdened. Bone resorption secondary to limited physical activity also may reduce bone density and contribute to the development of stress fractures. Weight reduction can curb orthopedic injury and lessen discomfort in the back and lower extremities.

PEDIATRIC OBESITY

It is currently estimated that 42 million children are obese worldwide, and another 18 million are overweight.[72] The prevalence of childhood obesity was 6.7% in 2010 and is expected to be 9.1% in 2020.[72] Adolescents are more overweight than preschool children.[73-75] These adverse trends in obesity have potentially profound effects on children's health now and for their long-term health outlook.

Pediatric obesity is recognized as a BMI greater than the 95th percentile on the Centers for Disease Control and Prevention growth chart.[72,74] Evidence-based guidelines and expert committee recommendations have repeatedly stressed that the BMI for age should be the basis of our definitions of pediatric overweight and obesity.

Studies document links between early childhood and adolescent obesity and adult obesity:

- Obese adolescents have a 70% to 80% chance of being obese adults.[76]
- Childhood obesity is associated with a higher chance of premature death and disability in adulthood, particularly in urban areas.[77]
- Childhood and adolescent overweight and obesity are linked with adult cardiovascular and endocrine problems.[78]
- Obese children are three to five times more likely to suffer a heart attack or stroke before they reach the age of 65.[78]
- Being overweight as young as 18 could be the strongest predictor of future hip replacement due to osteoarthritis.[79]

Determinants of obesity are multifactorial and include genetics, biology, and social and environmental behaviors that may begin in early childhood. The escalating national and global epidemics of obesity and sedentary lifestyles warrant increased attention by physicians and other health care professionals. The health goals for obese children and adolescents should be to develop healthy eating habits, maintain weight or reduce the rate of gain, and be active rather than sedentary.[80]

Some specific problems obese children face related to the health care community are the following:

- Pediatric obesity is more common than diabetes, human immunodeficiency virus, cystic fibrosis, and all childhood cancers combined.
- Primary hypertension in children has become increasingly common in association with obesity and risk factors such as a family history of hypertension and an ethnic predisposition to hypertensive disease. Obese children are at approximately a threefold higher risk for hypertension than nonobese children.[81]
- Most children with type 2 diabetes are overweight or obese at diagnosis and usually have a family history of type 2 diabetes. Americans of African, Hispanic, Asian, and Native American descent are disproportionately represented in this population.[82]
- OSA occurs more often in obese children and increases as the BMI percentile increases.[74] Bariatric surgery may be useful, but only in carefully selected obese children with serious comorbidities and unresponsiveness to interventions. The biggest barrier to performing child bariatric surgery is the psychosocial aspect, although complications include leaks, deep vein thrombi, micronutrient deficiency, bleeding, and infection.[83]

Unfortunately, children with long-standing obesity (especially class II and III obesity) develop medical problems previously seen only in adulthood. The medical effects of obesity that were previously reserved for adults, such as hypertension, insulin resistance, CAD, and metabolic syndrome, are on the rise in children and adolescents.[74,84,85]

The prevalence of metabolic syndrome is high among obese children and adolescents, and it increases with worsening obesity. Diagnosis of metabolic syndrome in children and adolescents is only now receiving greater attention, and there does not seem to be consensus on precise standards of treatment. As with adults, the dominant underlying risk factors for this syndrome appear to be abdominal obesity, insulin resistance, hypertriglyceridemia, hypertension, and proinflammatory and prothrombotic states.[85]

Studies show that obesity increases the burden of disease for children and adolescents, and special attention has been given to clinical complications for that population. These include cardiovascular disease (dyslipidemia and hypertension), respiratory disease (sleep apnea, snoring, asthma), orthopedic conditions (Blount disease, slipped capital femoral epiphysis), gastrointestinal disease (gallbladder, steatohepatitis), and endocrine disease (insulin resistance, hyperinsulinism, impaired glucose tolerance, and type 2 diabetes, which is normally reserved for adults). Other conditions in adolescent females include polycystic ovarian syndrome and menstrual irregularity. Studies also include psychosocial conditions such as depression, eating disorders, and social isolation.[86]

MATERNAL OBESITY

Obstetric complications of maternal obesity correlate more with pregravid obesity than with excessive weight gain during gestation. Maternal obesity, not diabetes, seems to be the most important link to the nation's increase in mean birthweight. The mean increase in birthweight at 37 to 41 weeks of gestation in the past 30 years was 116%.[87] Prepregnancy obesity significantly increases the parturient risk for cesarean delivery.[88]

Both the first and the second stages of labor are prolonged in obese women. Neonatal outcomes for obese women are comparable to those for women with normal prepregnancy BMI.[89]

The National Institutes of Health recognizes many risk factors associated with maternal obesity. Outcomes in pregnancy complicated by obesity include gestational diabetes,[88,89] preeclampsia,[88,89] preterm labor,[89] cesarean delivery,[88,89] postpartum hemorrhage, infection, pregnancy-induced hypertension (PIH),[88] and macrosomic infants.[87] The American College of Obstetricians and Gynecologists (ACOG) reports that the risk of spontaneous abortion and miscarriage in the first 6 weeks of pregnancy is almost doubled in obese women compared to nonobese women.[87] Metabolic syndrome in pregnancy manifests as preeclampsia, gestational hypertension, insulin resistance, and diabetes. The risk of preeclampsia increases further in obese women with gestational diabetes mellitus (GDM) that is poorly controlled, a previous history of GDM, a family history of type 2 diabetes, and history of a macrosomic fetus.[84] Obese parturients are at increased risk of instrumental and cesarean deliveries, difficult neuraxial placement, difficult intubation, and postoperative complications.[88]

Bariatric Surgery for Obese Women: Gestational Considerations

Many women of reproductive age undergo bariatric procedures as an alternative to lifestyle changes. One study showed an increased risk of complications during pregnancy after these malabsorptive procedures, including an increase in premature rupture of membranes, small bowel ischemia, nutrient deficiencies, and fetal abnormalities. Cesarean delivery rates also increased in women who had previous bariatric surgery. Gestational diabetes and PIH disorders were significantly reduced in women who had undergone laparoscopic adjustable gastric banding procedures. There were no significant differences in placental abruption and previa, labor dystocia, or perinatal complications with bariatric surgery prior to conception.[87]

TREATMENT OF OBESITY

A multimodal approach in the treatment of obesity includes dietary intervention, increased exercise, behavior modification, drug therapy, and surgery. Weight-loss programs should be individualized to each patient based on the degree of obesity and coexisting conditions. Drug therapy is initiated in patients with a BMI greater than 30 kg/m^2 or a BMI between 27 and 29.9 kg/m^2 with a coexisting medical condition.[2-4]

Surgical Treatment

Besides common surgeries performed within the general population, obese persons undergo additional procedures to ameliorate obesity-related diseases (Box 48.4). The four most common bariatric procedures at present are the Roux-en-Y gastric bypass (RYGB), laparoscopic adjustable gastric bypass (LAGB), laparoscopic sleeve gastrectomy (LSG), and biliopancreatic diversion with duodenal switch (BPD with DS). Recent advancements in endoscopic technologies and techniques have opened a new field of minimally invasive endoscopic treatment options for combatting obesity, both as a first-line and an adjunctive therapy. Presently, two endoscopic space-occupying devices (intragastric balloons) have received FDA approval for 6-month implantation in patients within a BMI range of 30 to 40 kg/m^2. Furthermore, full-thickness suturing has led to the development of primary endoscopic sleeve gastroplasty and RYGB revision as viable endoscopic alternatives to surgical approaches. These techniques have the potential to reduce adverse events, cost, and recovery times.[90-94] The mechanisms of various bariatric procedures are shown in Box 48.5. Despite the technically demanding nature of the RYGB procedure, it has become the procedure of choice for clinically severe obesity. LAGB is greatly increasing in frequency in the United States.[90-94]

TABLE 48.3   Some FDA-Approved Drugs for the Long-Term Treatment of Obesity

Drug	Usual Adult Dosage	Mean Weight Loss
Sympathomimetic amines		
Benzphetamine	Generic	For short-term use only, <1 lb/wk weight loss
Diethylpropion	Generic	
Phendimetrazine	Generic	
Phentermine	Generic	
Sympathomimetic amine/antiepileptic combination Phentermine/topiramate ER (Qsymia)	7.5/46–15/92 mg once/day	4.1–10.7 kg
Lipase inhibitor Orlistat (Xenical) (Alli)	102 mg tid 60 mg tid	2.5–3.4 kg
Serotonin receptor agonist Lorcaserin (Belviq)	10 mg bid	2.9–3.6 kg
Opioid antagonist/antidepressant combination Naltrexone/bupropion (Contrave)	16/180 mg bid	3.7–5.2 kg
GLP-1 receptor agonist Liraglutide (Saxenda)	3 mg SC once/day	5.8–5.9 kg

ER, Extended release; GLP-1, glucagon-like peptide-1; SC, subcutaneous.
Adapted from Diet, drugs, and surgery for weight loss. Med Lett Drugs Ther. 2018;60(1548):91–98; Heymsfield SB, Wadden TA. Mechanisms, pathophysiology, and management of obesity. N Engl J Med. 2017;376:254–266.

BOX 48.4   Obesity-Related Diseases Requiring Surgery

- Cholelithiasis
- Thromboembolism
- Peripheral vascular disease
- Urolithiasis and urinary incontinence
- Osteoarthritis-related orthopedic procedures
- Varicose veins
- Hiatal and abdominal wall hernias
- Cancer (endometrial, breast, prostate, colorectal, renal)
- Uterine fibroma
- Ovarian cysts
- Increased risk of fetal distress requiring cesarean section

BOX 48.5   Mechanism of Action of Bariatric Operations

Restrictive
- Vertical banded gastroplasty (VBG; historic purposes only)
- Laparoscopic adjustable gastric banding (LAGB)
- Laparoscopic sleeve gastrectomy (LSG)

Largely Restrictive, Mildly Malabsorptive
- Roux-en-Y gastric bypass (RYGB)

Largely Malabsorptive, Mildly Restrictive
- Biliopancreatic diversion (BPD)
- Duodenal switch (DS)

Adapted from Richards WO. Morbid obesity. In: Townsend CM, et al., eds. Sabiston Textbook of Surgery: The Biological Basis of Modern Surgical Practice. 20th ed. Philadelphia: Elsevier; 2017:1168.

BOX 48.6   Indications for Bariatric Surgery

Patients must meet the following criteria for consideration for bariatric surgery:
- BMI >40 kg/m^2 or BMI <35 kg/m^2 with an associated medical comorbidity worsened by obesity
- Failed dietary therapy
- Psychiatrically stable without alcohol dependence or illegal drug use
- Knowledgeable about the operation and its sequelae
- Motivated individual
- Medical problems not precluding probable survival from surgery

BMI, Body mass index.
Adapted from Richards WO. Morbid obesity. In: Townsend CM, et al., eds. Sabiston Textbook of Surgery: The Biological Basis of Modern Surgical Practice. 20th ed. Philadelphia: Elsevier 2017:1165.

BOX 48.7   Pharmacokinetic Changes Associated With Obesity

- Increased fat mass
- Increased cardiac output
- Increased blood volume
- Increased lean body weight
- Changes in plasma protein binding
- Reduced total body water
- Increased renal clearance
- Increased volume of distribution of lipid-soluble drugs
- Abnormal liver function
- Decreased pulmonary function

Advances in laparoscopic surgery have significantly improved surgical procedure times, as well as the morbidity and mortality related to bariatric surgery. Pneumoperitoneum can have a negative impact on respiratory system mechanics and oxygenation during laparoscopy. LAGB is associated with a shorter length of stay, lower morbidity, lower mortality, and lower hospital costs compared with an open procedure. Overall, the use of laparoscopic techniques has reduced morbidity related to bariatric surgery.[95-98] Indications for bariatric surgery are noted in Box 48.6.

PHARMACOLOGIC CONSIDERATIONS

Obesity causes physiologic changes that can affect the pharmacokinetics and pharmacodynamics of anesthetic agents. An overview of these changes is shown in Box 48.7. The common approach to anesthetic drug administration is to give water-soluble drugs according to IBW and lipid-soluble drugs according to total body weight (TBW). Lean body mass increases approximately 20% to 40% in obesity, so adding 30% to the IBW is a convenient dose adjustment to account for this change. Contradictory results from individual drug studies in small patient groups are common; therefore specific recommendations are frequently conflicting. A few general observations can be made. Postoperative respiratory depression is especially problematic in obese patients, therefore most clinicians favor short-acting drugs that allow for fast recovery. The newer inhalation agents desflurane and sevoflurane produce excellent recovery profiles in obese patients. Although desflurane

TABLE 48.4 Guidelines for Dosages of Intravenous Anesthetics in Obese Patients

Drug	Dose Recommendation	Comments
Propofol	Induction dose based on LBW Maintenance dose based on TBW	Increased fat mass does not affect initial distribution/redistribution during induction; cardiac depression at high doses is a concern
Succinylcholine	Intubating dose based on TBW	Increased fluid compartment and pseudocholinesterase levels require higher doses to ensure adequate paralysis
Rocuronium Vecuronium Cisatracurium	All doses based on IBW	Hydrophilic drugs given according to IBW will ensure shorter duration and a more predictable recovery in this respiratory-challenged population
Fentanyl Sufentanil	Loading dose based on TBW Maintenance doses based on LBW and response	Increased distribution volume and elimination time correlate with degree of obesity
Remifentanil	Infusion rates based on IBW	Distribution volumes and elimination rates are similar to normal-sized individuals; fast offset requires planning for postoperative analgesia
Dexmedetomidine	Infusion rates of 0.2 mcg/kg/min	Useful as an adjunct; lower than usual infusion rates are recommended to minimize adverse cardiac side effects
Sugammadex	Reversal doses based on TBW	No change from usual dosing required

IBW, Ideal body weight; LBW, lean body weight; TBW, total body weight.

is less soluble than sevoflurane, clinical differences are minimal. Nitrous oxide can be safely used in patients where a requirement for high O_2 concentrations does not preclude its administration. Nitrous oxide is being increasingly used in extremely obese patients as a volatile-sparing adjunct. The second gas effect of nitrous oxide at induction and emergence can accelerate uptake and elimination of the volatile agent. Nitrous oxide may also have the potential of reducing chronic postoperative pain, which occurs even after laparoscopic surgery. Appropriate antiemetic prophylaxis should be administered when anesthetic gases, and especially nitrous oxide, are used. Succinylcholine doses for intubation are given according to TBW to ensure excellent intubating conditions, whereas the nondepolarizing muscle relaxants used for operative maintenance are given according to IBW. Use of a nerve stimulator to guide relaxant administration is necessary to minimize residual paralysis and reversal concerns. Remifentanil infusion is an especially popular analgesic due to its titratability and rapid offset and is administered according to IBW. Dexmedetomidine is also a useful adjunct for sedation, amnesia, and analgesia. Sugammadex is given in the usual doses. Specific dosing recommendations for some common anesthetic agents in obesity are listed in Table 48.4.[89,99]

ANESTHETIC MANAGEMENT: PREANESTHETIC EVALUATION

The goals of the preanesthetic evaluation are to obtain pertinent data regarding the patient's medical or surgical history, to optimize current physiologic functioning, and to determine an appropriate anesthetic plan (see Chapter 20). Of paramount importance is the need to establish a nonjudgmental and trusting relationship with the patient. Explanations of anticipated events during preoperative preparation (e.g., multiple venipunctures, central and arterial line insertions, awake intubation, pain management) and protection of the patient's privacy will allay anxiety.

Medications

Obese persons must be questioned regarding the use of weight-reducing substances, herbal supplements, and anorexiant drugs. Patients who take over-the-counter drugs, including herbal medications, often forget or are afraid to reveal that they are taking these preparations, which can have deleterious consequences on induction. The patient's usual medications should be continued until the time of surgery, with the exception of insulin and oral hypoglycemics.[100] Recommendations for preoperative management of antidiabetic drugs are given in Chapters 20 and 37. Antibiotic prophylaxis is important because of an increased incidence of wound infections in the obese.[101] Venous thromboembolism (VTE) prophylaxis should be planned with the surgeon and administered as appropriate.[99]

Laboratory Tests

Only the laboratory tests appropriate in light of the patient's history, physical examination, and planned surgery should be ordered.[15] Baseline studies that may be directly affected by associated medical conditions such as metabolic syndrome should be considered. Preoperative testing should focus on comorbid disease states such as renal, hepatic, cardiovascular, and endocrine states related to obesity.[102] Because obese patients have a high risk of cardiovascular disease and diabetes mellitus, electrocardiogram (ECG) and glucose should be considered routine. All other tests should be guided by the patient's underlying condition, medications, or surgical procedure.[102,103]

Cardiac Assessment

Evaluation of cardiac function is essential in overweight and obese patients undergoing surgery. Investigation of prior myocardial infarction and the presence of hypertension, angina, or peripheral vascular disease is crucial. Limitations in exercise tolerance, history of orthopnea, and paroxysmal nocturnal dyspnea may indicate left ventricular dysfunction.[89] A careful elicitation of drug history is invaluable in garnering clues about the patient's coexistent diseases. When possible, cardiac medications should be continued up to and including the morning of surgery.

An ECG is essential for determination of resting rate, rhythm, and ventricular hypertrophy or strain. Because of the increased incidence of CAD and myocardial infarction in this population, the preoperative ECG is also helpful in providing a reference for comparison in the event that myocardial ischemia develops in the perioperative period. Beyond this, there is no reason to believe that extensive preoperative testing to detect CAD is indicated based solely on a patient being obese.[103] The ECG may be of low voltage because of the excess overlying tissue, and therefore might result in underestimation of the severity of ventricular hypertrophy. Axis deviation and atrial tachyarrhythmias are relatively common in this population.[4]

QT-interval prolongation, discovered retrospectively in severely obese patients who died from refractory dysrhythmias, is a marker for sudden cardiac arrest.[3] In addition, sudden cardiac death is more prevalent in morbidly obese patients with left ventricular hypertrophy and ventricular ectopy.[5] If ventricular hypertrophy or cardiomyopathy is suspected, echocardiography is useful. Tricuspid regurgitation on echocardiography is the most confirmatory test of pulmonary hypertension when combined with clinical evaluation.[104]

Respiratory Evaluation

Careful preoperative evaluation of the patient's respiratory function assists in the identification of potential problems. A patient who becomes dyspneic and desaturates when recumbent will experience the same symptoms during induction in the supine position. The patient must be asked about the presence or absence of OSA, orthopnea, wheezing, sputum production, or smoking history. They must also be assessed for OHS. Recent upper respiratory infection, snoring, or sleep disturbances may signal obstructive processes. The potential for difficult mask ventilation also should be considered during the preoperative visit. Obese patients have a high risk for difficult mask ventilation.[35] The presence of a beard, lack of teeth, and snoring history compound this risk in the obese patient.[105] Room air pulse oximetry saturations and arterial blood gases obtained in supine and upright positions may reflect disturbances in cardiac compensation.[106]

Airway Evaluation

A thorough airway evaluation is warranted for determination of the optimal airway management technique in overweight and obese patients.[35] A variety of assessment criteria have been evaluated for prediction of difficult intubation in obese patients. Most practitioners use evaluation of multiple patient physical characteristics to identify potential airway problems indicative of the unanticipated difficult airway. These include measurement of interincisor distance, thyromental distance, head and neck extension, Mallampati classification, body weight, and, most importantly, a history of difficult airway management.[107-109] Inspection of the oropharynx is necessary to determine the Mallampati classification for intubation difficulty.[107] The value of oropharyngeal Mallampati classification alone is low. Evaluation of the length of upper incisors, visibility of the uvula, shape of the palate, compliance of the mandibular space, and length and thickness of the neck provide further criteria for assessment.

Opinions differ about the use of a patient's weight (BMI) as an independent predictor of difficulty in intubation. Some have demonstrated that difficult intubation is more common in obese patients.[110] Others have demonstrated that increased BMI per se is not a predictor of difficult intubation.[111] Variables that are likely to predict difficulty in intubation of the obese patient include increased neck circumference, Mallampati classification greater than 3, increased age, male sex, temporomandibular joint pathology, a history of OSA, and abnormal upper teeth.[35,111,112] Of these, a high Mallampati score (≥3) with a large neck circumference and a history of sleep apnea were, in the aggregate, found to be good predictors of difficulty in intubation.[35,107]

Excessive tissue around the neck (restricting neck motion) and fat in the airway (decreasing glottic opening) together increase the difficulty of successfully intubating the trachea. The larger the neck circumference, the more difficult the laryngoscopy and intubation.[113] A neck circumference of 40 cm was associated with a 5% probability of difficult intubation, and a neck circumference of 60 cm or greater was associated with a 35% probability of difficult intubation. A normal neck circumference in a 70-kg man is approximately 35 cm. Other researchers, using ultrasound to quantify the amount of anterior neck soft tissue, produced data that support these findings.[114]

Anatomic aberrations of the upper airway induced by severe obesity include reduced temporomandibular and atlantooccipital joint movement. Unsatisfactory mouth opening, presence of neck or arm pain, or an inability to place the head and neck into sniffing position may indicate the need for awake fiberoptic intubation. Extreme airway narrowing in conjunction with a shortened mandibular-hyoid distance (less than three fingerbreadths) can complicate mask ventilation and intubation. The presence of a short, thick neck, pendulous breasts, hypertrophied tonsils and adenoids, or a beard can contribute to a difficult airway. Marginal room air pulse oximeter saturations, abnormal arterial blood gases, and a history of complicated airway management also indicate a potentially difficult intubation (see Chapter 24 for a full description of the assessment and management of a difficult airway).[107-109] Airway management techniques should be explained to the patient, with emphasis on awake intubation and the need for postoperative ventilation.[115,116]

Vascular Access

Venipuncture can be challenging in overweight and obese patients with excessive fat that obscures blood vessels from visualization and palpation.[16] Central cannulation of vessels is impeded by distortion of the underlying anatomy by adipose tissue.[117] Hemorrhage, hypothermia, and trauma further reduce the likelihood of accessing vessels with ease. Use of a portable ultrasound machine may improve central and peripheral venous catheter placement. As in all patients, iatrogenic pneumothorax must be avoided. Morbidly obese patients are less able than nonobese patients to tolerate the ensuing respiratory impairment.

ANESTHETIC MANAGEMENT: PREPARATION

Operating Room Equipment

In preparation for either emergent operating room procedures or nonemergent hospital admission, appropriate equipment must be readied. The anesthesia provider should always verify the weight limit on the operating room table when caring for obese patients. In cases of extreme obesity, hydraulic beds should be obtained and used in the operating room. Heavy-duty stirrups, extra-large retractors, elongated instruments, arm sleds, doubled arm boards, gel pads for positioning, and extremity tourniquets must be obtained. Sometimes, a sanitized engine crane or other hoisting device must be used to suspend the panniculus adiposus for optimal surgical exposure.

Extra-large thigh cuffs can be used on the upper arm or the lower leg (over the posterior tibial artery). A regular-size or large blood pressure cuff can be used on the forearm over the radial artery until arterial cannulation for blood pressure monitoring can be performed. Bed-warming devices, fluid warmers, and warm airflow blankets should be used to prevent hypothermia, which can occur rapidly when large areas of body surface are exposed.

Airway Equipment

An equally important part of airway assessment is the preparation of equipment and personnel necessary to ventilate and intubate the morbidly obese patient. An assortment of blades, laryngoscopy handles, endotracheal tubes, masks, oral and nasopharyngeal airways, and stylets should be assembled. Laryngeal mask airways (LMAs), intubating laryngeal mask airways (ILMA), videolaryngoscopes, fiberoptic and bronchoscopic devices, Eschmann introducers, a jet ventilator (or Venturi apparatus), and emergency tracheotomy and cricothyrotomy kits must be available in the event that ventilation by mask or endotracheal tube is unsuccessful. Most departments have a difficult-airway cart that has all of the available equipment that should be placed in the operating room.[118,119]

Monitoring

Intraoperative monitoring, both basic and advanced, should address the specific needs of the patient. Selection of ECG leads, when possible, should enhance detection of myocardial ischemia and pathology (leads II and V_5). Needle electrodes may be useful for obtaining a better tracing. Cuffs with bladders that encircle a minimum of 75% of the upper arm circumference (but preferably the entire arm) should be used. Forearm measurements with a standard cuff overestimate both systolic and diastolic blood pressures in obese patients.[120] Placement of an arterial catheter is appropriate for monitoring hemodynamic status and is advocated for all but the most minor procedures in the morbidly obese.[20] The use of central venous catheters is not standard but should be considered in patients undergoing extensive surgery or in those with serious cardiorespiratory disease.[117,121]

Aspiration and Postoperative Nausea and Vomiting Prophylaxis

Anesthesia providers have traditionally considered obese patients to be "full-stomach" patients and at risk for regurgitation and subsequent pulmonary aspiration.[122-124] It is known that gastroesophageal reflux and hiatal hernia are more prevalent in the obese, and this may predispose them to esophagitis and pulmonary aspiration. However, data obtained in 1998 demonstrated that obese patients (with a BMI >30 kg/m²) may have a lower volume of stomach contents compared with lean patients.[125] The actual incidence of clinically significant aspiration in these patients has not been conclusively determined but is likely quite low. The airway should be secured expeditiously, but use of a rapid sequence induction should be reserved for patients with a known aspiration risk.[121] Ultrasonography of the stomach has been proposed as a tool for clinicians to identify obese patients at risk for aspiration. Gastric ultrasonography has been used to assess preoperative gastric volume in obese patients with a BMI of 35 kg/m² and greater. The data showed that obese individuals have a larger antral size and gastric volume than their nonobese counterparts.[126] If the gastric volume is less than 1.5 mL/kg, then the risk of aspiration can be considered low. Patients who have recently undergone gastric banding are at increased risk for pulmonary aspiration of esophageal contents.[99]

There is no consensus on whether obese patients have delayed, normal, or accelerated gastric emptying.[127,128] Current recommendations suggest that obese patients should follow the same fasting guidelines as nonobese patients. All patients should be allowed to drink as much as 300 mL of clear liquids until up to 2 hours before elective surgery; that volume has been demonstrated to have no adverse effect on the pH and volume of gastric contents at induction of anesthesia.[35,129]

Historically, obesity has been linked to the presence of gastroesophageal reflux disease (GERD).[130,131] Although increased body mass has been shown by some researchers to correlate directly with an increased incidence of reflux symptoms,[132] others have demonstrated the opposite, and question the routine use of rapid-sequence induction on all patients who present with a diagnosis of GERD.[133]

Due to more recent and favorable data, some advocate avoiding rapid sequence induction in obese patients as standard protocol, citing that it is a common misperception that all obese patients should be viewed as "full-stomach" patients, and in the event of failed intubation, obese patients may have poorer outcomes.[134,135] Although obese patients and patients with sleep apnea syndrome (SAS) are prone to GERD, and both groups may also have an increased risk of difficult intubation, in the case of elective surgery in a fasted patient with no risk factors other than obesity or SAS, the requirement for rapid sequence induction is debatable.[35,136]

If reflux symptoms are present in obese patients with GERD, the potential increased risk of aspiration should be discussed with the patient, and prophylactic measures (e.g., cricoid pressure, H_2 blockers, and proton-pump inhibitors) should be considered.[137] Although rapid sequence induction may be safe for some obese patients, its safety in extremely obese patients has been questioned. For patients with a BMI greater than 50 kg/m², or those with a lower BMI who have risk factors such as OSA or a large neck circumference, either an awake intubation (with local anesthesia) with spontaneous respiration of the patient or intubation without relaxants (after only propofol administration) is suggested.[138]

Nausea following bariatric surgery is very common and is probably largely mechanical in origin, related to staple lines and pressure on the stomach tissues. The incidence of nausea is highest after gastric sleeve surgery and lowest after gastric banding. Standard multimodal antiemetics are recommended. The use of an opioid-sparing technique for bariatric surgery may be helpful for reducing postoperative nausea and vomiting.[121]

Patient Positioning for Induction

Obese patients are more difficult to intubate in the sniffing position, but when placed in the ramped position there is no evidence that this risk is greater than in members of the general population.[70] It is essential that optimal patient positioning for laryngoscopy is ensured prior to induction of anesthesia. This includes placing towels under the patient's shoulders and head, and putting the patient in the reverse Trendelenburg position to increase the patient's FRC.[35] The acronym HELP (*h*ead *e*levated *l*aryngoscopy *p*osition) reminds clinicians of the importance of patient positioning for successful laryngoscopy.[139] This position generally improves the view during laryngoscopy and contributes to increasing the safety period until patients demonstrate signs of O_2 desaturation. This is also a better patient position for using rescue ventilation techniques, such as bag-valve-mask ventilation or insertion of a LMA, should they be required.

In one study, the proper positioning for morbidly obese patients included elevating the head, upper body, and shoulders significantly above the chest, such that an imaginary horizontal line could connect the patient's sternal notch with the external auditory meatus. Positioning patients in this manner resulted in successful intubation in 99 of 100 morbidly obese patients, with all having a Cormack grade I view.[140]

Others have concluded that the ramped position (with blankets used to elevate both the upper body and head of the patient) improves laryngeal view in obese patients compared with patients who were intubated with a conventional 7-cm cushion placed under the head (i.e., in the sniffing position) (Fig. 48.3).[35,141] Without proper support and alignment of the oropharynx and trachea (see Fig. 24.5), ventilation may be obstructed, and visualization of the laryngeal structures may be obscured.

The importance of proper positioning and the difficulty of repositioning morbidly obese patients during failed intubation can be underestimated by practitioners who are not experienced in airway management in obese patients. If direct laryngoscopy is unsuccessful, LMAs can be effective for establishing ventilation and should be immediately available.[115,129] In one study, the use of an intubating laryngeal mask resulted in better patient oxygenation compared with intubation through direct laryngoscopy in morbidly obese patients.[119]

If a patient is at risk for aspiration, a rapid sequence induction may be performed with application of cricoid pressure while the patient's trachea is intubated. There is much discussion regarding the effectiveness of cricoid pressure and the advantages and risks associated with the technique.[142]

ANESTHETIC MANAGEMENT: MAINTENANCE

Intubation

For airway management to be facilitated, obese patients should be positioned with the head elevated (reverse Trendelenburg position) on the operating room table. This position promotes patient comfort,

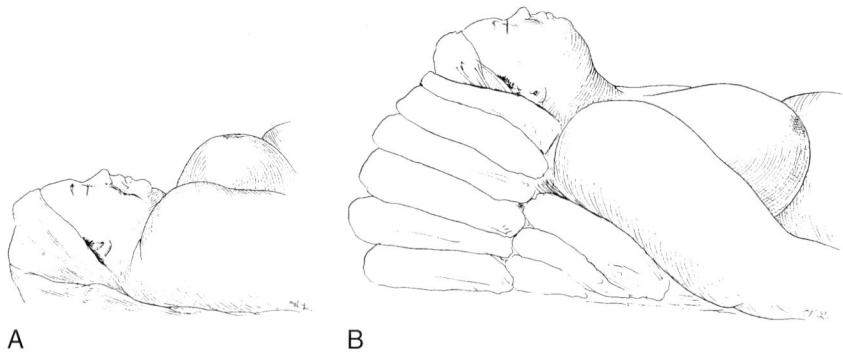

Fig. 48.3 (A) Supine position. (B) Sniffing position.

reduces gastric reflux, provides easier mask ventilation, improves respiratory mechanics, and helps maintain FRC. The reduced FRC in obese patients contributes to the rapid desaturation that occurs with induction of general anesthesia.[143,144] To attenuate desaturation and maximize O_2 content in the lungs, patients should be preoxygenated with a 100% mask O_2 for at least 3 to 5 minutes with continuous positive airway pressure (CPAP), as tolerated.[35,144,145] Adequate preoxygenation is vital in obese patients because of rapid desaturation after loss of consciousness secondary to increased O_2 consumption and decreased FRC. Application of positive pressure ventilation during preoxygenation decreases atelectasis and improves oxygenation in morbidly obese patients. In a study of morbidly obese individuals, the administration of CPAP during the preoxygenation period and gentle ventilation with positive end-expiratory pressure (PEEP) during anesthetic induction significantly reduced atelectasis, as documented by chest computed tomography scans.[146] An associated benefit to the reduced atelectasis was a significantly increased average partial pressure of arterial oxygen (Pao2) (457 ± 130 pascals [Pa] vs 315 ± 100 Pa, P = 0.035) in those subjects who received CPAP-PEEP versus the control subjects. Theoretically, the increase in Pao2 would increase the apneic time to O_2 desaturation if an airway event were to occur.[147] Alternatively, high-flow nasal oxygen has been found to be helpful in reducing oxygen desaturation during anesthesia induction.[144]

Many clinicians advocate the use of a modified rapid sequence induction when aspiration is a concern.[148] This technique employs preoxygenation and cricoid pressure as usual, but the lungs are lightly ventilated prior to securing the airway. This approach avoids the rapid desaturation that frequently occurs in the obese patient, with no risk or a minimal increased risk of aspiration.

The surgeon and another skilled anesthesia provider also must be in attendance during induction. Muscle hypotonus in the floor of the mouth, followed by rapid occurrence of soft tissue obstruction and hypoxia, requires one person to support the mask and airway while another person bag ventilates the patient. In the case of inability to ventilate or intubate, the ASA's difficult airway algorithm should be followed (see Chapter 24). Intubation of the obese patient can be safely accomplished with careful assessment and planning and use of modern airway techniques.

Effects of General Anesthesia on Respirations

General anesthesia depresses respiration in normal subjects, so any preexisting pulmonary dysfunction is exaggerated by anesthesia.[20] The type of surgery, positioning, and underlying disease pathology further compound the undesirable respiratory responses caused by obesity and anesthesia.[149-154] General anesthesia causes a 50% reduction in FRC in the obese anesthetized patient, as compared with a 20% reduction in anesthetized nonobese patients.[155] Airway collapsibility is likely due to the decreased lung volume associated with deeper anesthesia, as the

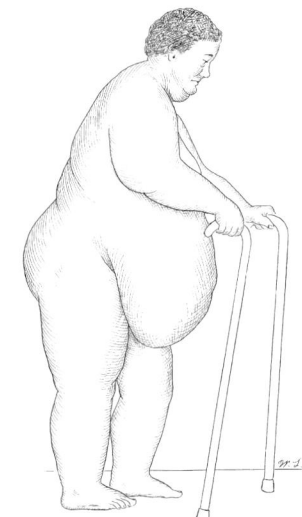

Fig. 48.4 Panniculus in a standing patient.

end-expiratory esophageal pressure is reduced with lighter planes of anesthesia.[155] FRC can be increased by ventilating with large tidal volumes (15–20 mL/kg), although this has been shown to improve arterial O_2 tension only minimally.[90,149] In contrast, the addition of PEEP achieves an improvement in both FRC and arterial O_2 tension, but only at the expense of cardiac output and O_2 delivery.[151,152] Current ventilation recommendations include using tidal volumes of 6 to 10 mL/kg of IBW to avoid barotrauma.[90]

Prolonged (>2–3 hours) and extensive procedures (those involving the abdomen, thorax, and spine) negatively influence respiratory function. Subdiaphragmatic packing, cephalad displacement of organs, and surgical retraction cause decreased alveolar ventilation, atelectasis, and pulmonary congestion.[149,150] Recumbent or Trendelenburg positioning further reduces diaphragmatic excursion, which is already impaired by the weight of the panniculus (which can be very large) (Fig. 48.4). Trendelenburg positioning also causes elevated filling pressures, which then increase right ventricular preload. Subsequently, myocardial O_2 consumption, cardiac output, pulmonary artery occluding pressures, peak inspiratory pressures, and venous admixtures are increased above upright-sitting values.[151] In robotic procedures requiring steep Trendelenburg, obese patients exhibit decreased lung compliance and increased peak inspiratory pressures along with declining oxygen saturation to a greater degree than nonobese patients.[156]

In a severely obese patient, positive pressure ventilation (which impedes venous return) and an inability to increase cardiac output may result in cardiopulmonary decompensation.[152,153] This is exhibited intraoperatively by hypoxia, rales, ventricular ectopy, congestive heart failure, and hypotension.[154] Bag ventilation by hand may be useful to attenuate hypotension resulting from positive pressure ventilation.

Use of ventilators powerful enough to inflate the morbidly obese thorax is critical to minimizing hypoxia. Pressure- or volume-controlled ventilators can be used to maintain adequate oxygenation and normocapnia. Avoidance of prolonged prone, Trendelenburg, or supine positioning also decreases ventilation-perfusion mismatch. Optimization of oxygenation by using at least 50% flow of inspired O_2 is emphatically recommended.[20,36,90] The intermittent manual application of large volume "sighs" can also augment the FRC.

Application of PEEP can reduce venous admixture and support adequate arterial oxygenation. Large amounts of PEEP, however, can impair arterial oxygenation in some patients when it is superimposed on large tidal volumes.[153] For these reasons, PEEP that exceeds 15 cm H_2O is not recommended.

Other intraoperative events, such as hemorrhage or hypotension, further impair ventilatory homeostasis and result in hypoxemia that may extend into the postoperative period.[34] A vertical abdominal incision, compared with a horizontal (transverse) incision, also prolongs postoperative hypoxia.[35] Pain causes further reductions in diaphragmatic excursion and vital capacity, leading to atelectasis and ventilation-perfusion mismatch.[20,90] For these reasons, 24-hour postoperative admission to a monitored bed is prudent for severely obese patients, who already exhibit higher morbidity and mortality even in the absence of anesthesia and surgery. Some suggested ventilatory strategies are listed in Table 48.5.

Choice of Anesthetic Technique

Selection of the anesthetic technique is dependent on the patient history, planned surgical procedure, and anesthetist and patient preference. Diverse anesthetic techniques have been described for use with obese patients undergoing surgical and diagnostic procedures.[70,121,157,158] Anesthetic management of obese patients can include local or monitored anesthesia, general anesthesia, regional blocks, or a combination of techniques.

No demonstrable difference in emergence from inhalation versus narcotic anesthetic technique has been discerned in the obese patient.[20] The use of short-acting anesthetic agents facilitates smooth anesthetic induction, maintenance, and emergence from anesthesia. Objectives for maintenance of anesthesia in the obese patient include strict maintenance of airway, adequate skeletal muscle relaxation, optimum oxygenation, avoidance of the residual effects of muscle relaxants, provision of appropriate intraoperative and postoperative tidal volume, and effective postoperative analgesia. Depending on the patient's condition and the type of surgery, these can be achieved by either general or regional anesthesia, or a combination of the two.

Volume Replacement

Despite the augmentation of circulatory fluid that accompanies extreme obesity, the estimated blood volume is actually diminished.[26] Fat, which contains only 8% to 10% water, contributes less fluid to total body water (TBW) than equivalent amounts of muscle. The normal adult percentage of TBW is 60% to 65%.[20] In the severely obese, TBW is reduced to 40%; therefore calculation of estimated blood volume should be 45 to 55 mL/kg of actual body weight rather than the 70 mL/kg apportioned in nonobese adults.[19] Use of reduced parameters for volume replacement and avoidance of rapid rehydration reduce the risk of cardiopulmonary compromise. Fluid management should be guided by the usual clinical parameters such as blood pressure, heart rate, and urine output measurements. Fluid requirements for bariatric procedures may be greater than anticipated to maintain renal

TABLE 48.5 Ventilator Management for Morbidly Obese Patients

Goal/Recommendation	Rationale/Additional Information
Prevent Hypoxemia During Induction	
HOB elevated (backup Fowler or reverse Trendelenburg) 30 degrees	May increase the safe apnea period during induction and intubation
Preoxygenate with 100% O_2	
Use of CPAP during induction	
Consider high-flow nasal cannula for apneic oxygenation during intubation	
If O_2 saturation is ≤95%, perform a blood gas analysis for diagnosis of OHS	
Prevent/Reverse Atelectasis	
Restrict the use of Fio_2 to <0.8 during maintenance of anesthesia	Use of a high Fio_2 concentration during anesthesia accelerates the onset and the amount of atelectasis
Recruitment ("vital capacity") maneuver after intubation by using sustained (8–10 sec) pressure of 35–40 cm H_2O	Monitor for adverse effects (bradycardia, hypotension)
Maintain Lung Recruitment	
Use PEEP (10–12 cm H_2O)	Monitor for hypotension or decreasing arterial oxygenation (PEEP-induced increase in pulmonary shunt fraction)
Prevent Reoccurrence of Atelectasis	
Intermittent intraoperative re-recruitment	Monitor highest oxygenation and respiratory system compliance achieved after recruitment: a decline may be a sign of redeveloping atelectasis or a pulmonary shunt
Avoid Lung Overdistension	
Use tidal volume 6–10 mL/kg of ideal body weight	Increase the ventilation rate to control excessive hypercapnia instead of using large tidal volumes or high ventilatory pressures
Keep plateau pressures <30 cm H_2O	
Consider mild permissive hypercapnia if necessary	
Maintain Postoperative Lung Expansion	
Use CPAP or BiPAP immediately after tracheal extubation	
Administer supplemental O_2	
Keep the upper body elevated	
Maintain adequate pain control	
Use incentive spirometry	
Encourage early ambulation	

BiPAP, Bilevel positive airway pressure; *CPAP*, continuous airway pressure; *Fio₂*, fractional inspired oxygen concentration; HOB, head of bed; OHS, obesity hypoventilation syndrome; PEEP, positive end-expiratory pressure.

Adapted from Thompson J, et al. Anesthesia case management for bariatric surgery. *AANA J.* 2011;79(2):147–160; Bluth T, et al. The obese patient undergoing nonbariatric surgery. *Curr Opin Anaesthesiol.* 2016;29(3):421–429.

perfusion. Although rare, acute renal failure occurs in approximately 2% of patients undergoing bariatric procedures. Predisposing factors to renal compromise include hypovolemia, a BMI greater than 50 kg/m^2, prolonged surgery time, intraoperative hypotension, and preexisting renal disease.[159] Adequate intraoperative fluid replacement also helps reduce postoperative nausea and vomiting after bariatric procedures.[160] Volume expanders such as hetastarch (Hespan) should not be administered at greater than recommended volumes per kilogram of IBW (20 mL/kg). Dilutional coagulopathy, factor VIII inhibition, and decreased platelet aggregation can result from excessive administration. Albumin may be used as indicated to support circulatory volume and oncotic pressure. No difference in the criteria between the administration of blood products in normal-weight patients versus severely obese patients has been identified.

Intraoperative Positioning

Surgical positioning of morbidly obese patients necessitates extra precautions for the prevention of nerve, integumentary, and cardiorespiratory compromise. The type of surgery, combined with inordinate stretching or compression of nerve plexuses and prolonged immobility, cause local tissue ischemia and damage, which begins at the cellular level. Hypothermia, hypotension, table positioning, and the pressure the adipose tissue places on orthopedic or cardiopulmonary structures potentiate impairment.[161]

Although many peripheral nerves are subjected to possible ischemia or necrosis, the ulnar, brachial plexus, radial, peroneal, and sphenoid nerves are the most vulnerable to injury in any anesthetized patient. In morbidly obese patients, the incidence may be increased because of excessive weight on the anatomic structures.[162] Care must be taken when positioning obese individuals' extremities in slings, draping them on Mayo stands, or securing them in lithotomy stirrups. Excess weight and loose skin may strangle or macerate tissues on the dangling ankle or wrist. Draping of heavy upper extremities atop poorly secured Mayo stands can cause cuts, bruises, or abrasions of the arm, breast, or abdomen, as well as obscure early signs of skin breakdown or circulatory compromise.

Prolonged hyperextension, external rotation, or abduction greater than 90 degrees overstretches the brachial plexus and can cause postoperative muscle pain, nerve palsies, or paralysis. Often, obese patients do not have the range of motion that nonobese individuals possess; therefore it may be necessary to restrict the amount of flexion, abduction, and rotation of hips, legs, and arms. Frequent palpation of pulses, generous padding, correct alignment, and repeated inspection of extremities for color and temperature can help diminish the incidence of positioning-related injuries.[161,163]

Lower back pain can be aggravated by both spinal and general anesthesia because of ligamentous relaxation that results in loss of lumbar curvature. Surgical towels placed under the lumbar spine before induction will enhance lordosis and reduce postoperative discomfort.[162]

Treatment of the panniculus is often a major concern for both the anesthetist and the surgeon. Extra-long straps and wide adhesive tape can secure the panniculus and reduce shifting when the operating table is changed. If Trendelenburg positioning is anticipated, some means to prevent the panniculus from sliding cephalad must be devised. The head-down position, coupled with the crushing weight of the thorax and panniculus, compresses the brachial neurovascular bundle between the clavicle and first rib. If the patient requires a fracture table, ensure that sufficient padding encircles the pole adjacent to the patient's vulva or penis.[163] Genital and pudendal nerve injury can be profound if adipose tissue surrounding the thigh is not carefully distracted to reveal proper placement of the padding.

Integumentary Concerns

Decubitus ulcers, skin infection, and wound dehiscence are exceedingly common in the severely obese. Decubitus ulcers arise from prolonged immobility and compression of fat on bony prominences and vessels. Traction, external fixation devices, and straps may cause injury. Skin creases are subject to erosion and ulceration from sweat and constant friction with opposing skin surfaces. Inability to perform hygiene under the breasts, between neck folds, or beneath the abdominal pannus promotes organism proliferation. Concomitant diabetes further accelerates the growth of bacterial or fungal infections. As a result, wound dehiscence, particularly in the abdomen, can occur after suboptimal surgical closure of compromised skin. A poorly vascularized panniculus and torsion on the wound by the weight of the fat apron also contribute to malunion of the tissue.[163] Although atelectasis and hypoxia are less frequent with a horizontal laparotomy, a vertical laparotomy approach is often preferred by the surgical team. Compression of abdominal contents on superficial wound layers is lessened during ambulation and may therefore reduce the occurrence of dehiscence.[92]

Extubation

The risk of airway obstruction after extubation is increased in obese patients.[35,164] A decision to extubate depends on evaluation of the ease of mask ventilation and tracheal intubation, the length and type of surgery, and the presence of preexisting medical conditions, including OSA. Criteria for extubation must include all standard objective and subjective criteria used by every clinician. Patients are usually placed with the head up or in a sitting position prior to extubation. If doubt exists regarding the ability of the patient to breathe adequately, the endotracheal tube is left in place, and extubation over an airway exchange catheter or via a fiberoptic bronchoscope may be performed.[35,164,165]

Regional Anesthesia

Regional anesthesia can be used as the primary anesthetic in selected cases or as an accompaniment to postoperative pain and mobility management.[20,29,88,163] However, difficulties are frequently encountered in severely obese patients. Anatomic landmarks used to guide conduction blockade are not easily visible, palpable, or identifiable with ultrasound. Brachial plexus anesthesia can be hampered by adipose tissue in the axillary region, an inability to position the arm, and an undetectable pulse. Full-term pregnancy, obesity, and the coincident discomfort of active labor further inhibit the discernment of spinous processes and posterior iliac crests. Redundant rolls of fat, unsatisfactory ventilation, and the inability of the patient to sustain optimal positioning make neuraxial anesthesia even more challenging.

For subarachnoid or epidural anesthesia, it is recommended that the patient sit upright so that landmarks such as C7 or L3-L4 can be more easily identified.[93] In addition, skin-fat folds will fall toward the operating table, and respiratory ventilation will be enhanced. A selection of longer needles (7 in) should also be available before anesthetic administration is begun. Generous infiltration with local anesthetic will provide greater patient comfort during insertion of the "finder," Tuohy, or spinal needle. The importance of generous administration of local anesthetic cannot be overemphasized because repeated insertions and repositioning of the needle or introducer may be required before access to the epidural (or subarachnoid) space is achieved.

Another consideration regarding subarachnoid or epidural anesthesia in severely obese pregnant or surgical patients is the lack of predictability of the spread of the local anesthetic. Epidural anesthetics in obese patients have a higher rate of failure and difficulty of placement.[88] Obese patients will also experience a greater incidence of respiratory complications from a high regional block than normal-weight patients.[166] Successful laparotomy procedures after epidural anesthesia have been described.[167]

In obese parturients, a cesarean section can be performed under spinal or epidural anesthesia. A significant correlation exists with increased body mass and rostral spread of epidural subarachnoid anesthetics when a patient is in a supine position. Undesirable cephalad spread of local anesthetics can be obviated by reducing the volume and increasing the patient's upright sitting time.

ANESTHETIC MANAGEMENT: POSTOPERATIVE CARE

Pain Management

Optimal postoperative pain management is facilitated by the use of oral analgesics, nonsteroidal antiinflammatory drugs, patient-controlled analgesia, local infiltration of the surgical site, and epidural anesthesia. Obese patients are more sensitive to the respiratory-depressant effects of opioid analgesics, therefore caution and close monitoring are warranted.[168] Supplemental O_2 and pulse oximetry monitoring are mandated. If the patient was on CPAP (nasal or facemask) preoperatively, CPAP should be applied at all rest times in the early post-general anesthetic period. CPAP protects the patient with OSA against airway obstruction during sleep by pneumatically splinting the oropharynx.[35,49,169,170] Postoperative opioids must be used judiciously.[99]

Postoperative Complications

Morbidity and mortality rates are higher in obese patients than in normal-weight patients; however, various studies have reported that the mortality rate during the perioperative period has decreased among morbidly obese patients in recent years.[35,171] Older age, a high BMI, and male gender have been confirmed as increased surgical risk factors for morbidity in obese patients undergoing gastric bypass surgery.[172,173] Other factors that have been shown to increase mortality risk include hypertension, diabetes, postoperative leak with bariatric procedures, and thromboembolism.[174] Patients with major comorbid diseases had a higher BMI, a higher mortality, a greater leak rate, and a higher rate of surgical site infections.[175] Ventilation abnormalities are exacerbated in obese patients with OSA and OHS, and may last for several days. The maximum decrease in PaO_2 occurs 2 to 3 days postoperatively.[33] Blouw et al.[176] investigated factors influencing the frequency of respiratory failure in patients with morbid obesity and found that a higher rate of respiratory failure is associated with individuals having a BMI greater than 43 kg/m^2.

Rhabdomyolysis (RML) is a complication that occurs in approximately 1.4% of bariatric surgeries, owing to high pressures exerted on deep tissues. Measurement of serum creatinine phosphokinase (CPK) pre- and postoperatively aids in early diagnosis and treatment, and can help reduce further complications such as myoglobinuric acute renal failure, which occurs in up to 30% of patients with serum CPK greater than 5000 units/L.[177] RML and subsequent acute renal failure can be serious problems following bariatric operations. Risk factors of developing RML include male gender, elevated BMI, and prolonged operating time. Early diagnosis and treatment are important to avoid the complications of RML. Recognition of the signs and symptoms, physical evaluation, and laboratory findings may aid diagnosis. Elevation of CPK levels is the most sensitive diagnostic evidence of RML. Treatment of RML is geared toward preserving renal function by avoiding dehydration, hypovolemia, tubular obstruction, aciduria, and free radical release. Early recognition allows prompt treatment, including the administration of fluids, bicarbonate, and mannitol.[177-179]

The risk of VTE wound infections, and atelectasis is amplified in patients with increased BMI.[33,165] Thromboembolism is facilitated by immobility (venous stasis), increased blood viscosity (polycythemia, hypovolemia), increased abdominal pressure, and abnormalities in serum procoagulants and anticoagulants.[6] Obesity is an independent risk factor for development of VTE.[180] Thromboembolism is reported to be the most common cause of postoperative mortality after bariatric surgery, accounting for as many as 50% of all deaths.[181]

Four important risk factors, namely venous stasis disease, BMI of 60 kg/m^2 or more, truncal obesity, and OHS or SAS, are significant in the development of postoperative VTE, and if present, preoperative prophylactic placement of an inferior vena cava filter should be considered. Venous stasis disease, BMI greater than 60 kg/m^2, truncal obesity, OHS, OSA, a previous incidence of pulmonary embolism, and hypercoagulable states have been suggested as factors that increase the baseline risk of perioperative pulmonary embolism in obese patients after bariatric surgery.[182] Administration of minidose heparin (5000 units administered subcutaneously twice per day), administration of low molecular weight heparin, antiembolic stockings, and correctly fitting pneumatic compression boots can lessen the occurrence of deep vein thrombosis in the early postoperative period. Early ambulation and maintenance of vascular volume further attenuate the likelihood that clots will develop. The incidence of wound infections and pulmonary embolism is 50% higher in obese patients than in normal-weight patients.[183-185]

Post-Gastric Bypass Anastomotic Leaks

In a series of more than 3000 gastric bypass patients from four centers, the anastomotic leak rate was 2.1%.[186] The most common signs and symptoms of a leak were tachycardia (72%), fever (63%), and abdominal pain (54%). An upper gastrointestinal series was positive in 17 of 56 patients. Tachycardia is the most sensitive sign of an anastomotic leak, and a heart rate greater than 120 beats per minute should prompt an investigation, even if the patient looks and feels well. Tachypnea or decreasing O_2 saturations can also signal early sepsis from a leak and may be clinically indistinguishable from pulmonary embolism. Signs and symptoms of an anastomotic leak are shown in Box 48.8.[187-189]

In general, morbidly obese patients have higher rates of postoperative and intensive care unit (ICU) complications, and they may require more intensive care and increased staffing.[190] Investigations in surgical/trauma ICU patients universally report an adverse effect of obesity on

---

BOX 48.8 Signs and Symptoms Associated With Anastomotic Leak

- Unexplained tachycardia (sustained heart rate >120 bpm)
- Shoulder pain (usually left)
- Abdominal pain
- Pelvic pain
- Substernal pressure
- Shortness of breath
- Fever
- Increased thirst
- Hypotension
- Unexplained oliguria
- Hiccups
- Restlessness

Adapted from Thompson J, et al. Anesthesia case management for bariatric surgery. *AANA J.* 2011;79(2):147–160.

outcomes. In a surgical ICU, investigators reported that morbid obesity conferred elevated odds of death after 4 days of ICU stay,[191] and among blunt-trauma patients, obese patients suffered more frequent complications (e.g., multisystem organ failure, acute respiratory distress syndrome, myocardial infarction, and renal failure), including the need for more vasopressors, additional days of ventilator support, and more frequent extubation failure. Among survivors, obese patients had a longer ICU and hospital length of stay.[192]

SUMMARY

Obesity is a complex and multifactorial disease, and its incidence is continuing to increase in the US patient population. Through an understanding of the implications of conditions associated with obesity, the anesthetist can promote more favorable anesthetic outcomes.

Consideration of the physiologic and pharmacologic changes in obese patients and their implications for optimal anesthetic management guides clinical practice.

REFERENCES

For a complete list of references for this chapter, scan this QR code with any smartphone code reader app, or visit the following URL: http://booksite.elsevier.com/9780323711944/.

49

Regional Anesthesia: Spinal and Epidural Anesthesia

Joseph E. Pellegrini, Richard P. Conley

Spinal and epidural blocks are known collectively as central neuraxial blockade (CNB) because they involve the placement of local anesthetic solution onto or adjacent to the spinal cord. Both spinal and epidural blocks share much of the same anatomy and physiology but are distinct from one another due to their unique anatomic, physiologic, and clinical features.

The persons most credited with introducing spinal anesthesia are Augustus Bier and Théodore Tuffier, who in 1898 described the injection of cocaine into the spinal column and its potential for use as a surgical anesthetic technique. When cocaine was introduced into the subarachnoid space, anesthesia lasted approximately 1 hour. With the development of newer and safer anesthetic drugs, needles, and techniques, regional anesthesia expanded to include many neural blocks for the enhancement of surgery and obstetrics and the management of pain.[1,2] Modern procedures have simplified, refined, and increased the safety and success of regional anesthesia techniques.[2]

APPLIED ANATOMY AND PHYSIOLOGY OF THE CENTRAL NEURAXIS

Knowledge of anatomic landmarks and underlying structures aids the anesthetist in forming a three-dimensional mind's-eye picture. This picture, coordinated with the feel of the structures and tissues against the needle and a steady, sensitive hand, facilitates accurate placement of the needle tip and administration of appropriate techniques and medications. Although anatomy is the oldest of medical sciences (with detailed descriptions of the spinal column dating from the 19th century), modern imaging methods such as computed tomography (CT), magnetic resonance imaging (MRI), and endoscopic examination have permitted in vivo investigations that further our understanding of spinal anatomy. The following is a current review of applied anatomy of the central neuraxis.

The sequential interconnectivity of the 33 bones called vertebrae form the spinal, or vertebral, column, which is used as a bony reference during the placement of various anesthetics or analgesics. This column is located in the posterior midline of the trunk and allows for truncal flexibility because movable joint surfaces and cartilaginous vertebral bodies exist between 24 of the 33 vertebrae (Fig. 49.1). The vertebral column extends from the base of the skull and the foramen magnum to the tip of the coccyx. The vertebral bodies are stacked on top of one another, separated by fibrocartilaginous intervertebral disks that provide support for the cranium and trunk. The anterior, cylindrical portion of the vertebra, called the body, is solid. This heavier portion of the vertebra forms the anterior portion of the vertebral arch. The body of each vertebra is contiguous with two pedicles that stretch in a posterior and slightly lateral direction, joining to two laminae that stretch posteriorly and medially to complete an arch, creating an oval-triangular foramen. This foramen, known as the vertebral foramen, allows for

the passage and protection of the spinal cord. Transverse processes on both sides of the pedicles allow for muscular attachments and the control of movement. A spinous process projects along the median plane from the union of the laminae in a posterior inferior direction. The spinous process is the long, slender, bony prominence that can often be seen and felt along the midline of the back. The spinous process also provides a place for muscular attachment and movement control. In addition, the inferior angle of the bone creates an overlap that further protects the spinal cord (Fig. 49.2).[3]

The pedicles and processes of each vertebra have superior and inferior articular surfaces and lateral notches. The superior notch is shallow when compared with the deeper inferior notch. When the vertebrae are stacked, the notches and the articulating surfaces, known as zygapophyseal or facet joints, form the intervertebral foramina. The intervertebral foramina provide safe passage for spinal nerves passing from the spinal cord to the rest of the body. The articular surfaces of the facet joints are covered with hyaline cartilage, which permits a gliding motion between the vertebrae. Because the facet joints are innervated by branches from closely associated spinal nerves, these joints often become clinically important. When the joint is injured, the associated spinal nerves may also be affected, leading to pain along associated dermatomes or muscle spasm along associated myotomes.[3]

The size and shape of vertebral lamina and spinous processes differ among the thoracic, lumbar, and sacral regions, and variation exists within each region. Knowledge of these variations is important in the practice of regional anesthesia and in selection and administration of spinal and epidural anesthesia. For instance, cervical and thoracic vertebrae have spinous processes that angle acutely in a caudal direction such that the process of the superior vertebra overlaps the inferior vertebra and its process. This construction adds protection to the spinal cord when an individual stands erect. When attempts are made to insert a needle into the cervical or thoracic regions, the tight construction and angles of the vertebral column must be considered.

In the lumbar region the vertebrae are larger, and the spinous processes become shorter and broader and have a posterior orientation with less overlap than in other vertebrae. Relatively large gaps, bridged by ligaments, exist between the spinous processes in the lumbar area. This provides the anesthesia practitioner easier access for needle placement, catheter passage, and the instillation of anesthetic into the epidural or subarachnoid space for surgical or obstetric procedures.

The sacrum is a triangle-shaped section of fused bodies of vertebrae. The broader portion is the base, which tapers as it approaches the coccyx. The sacrum is shaped so the weight of the body forces the base of the sacrum downward and forward. It is wedged tightly between the two iliac crests by the downward forces exerted on the spinal column. The lamina of the last sacral vertebra is incomplete and bridged only by ligaments. This area is known as the sacral hiatus (Fig. 49.3). The coccyx is composed of four small segments of bone that become fused into two bones as an individual ages; between the ages of 25 and 30 years,

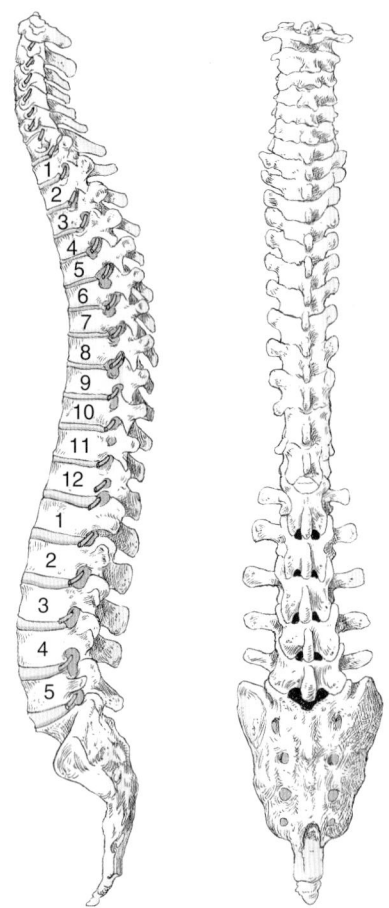

Fig. 49.1 The spinal, or vertebral, column with its 33 vertebrae.

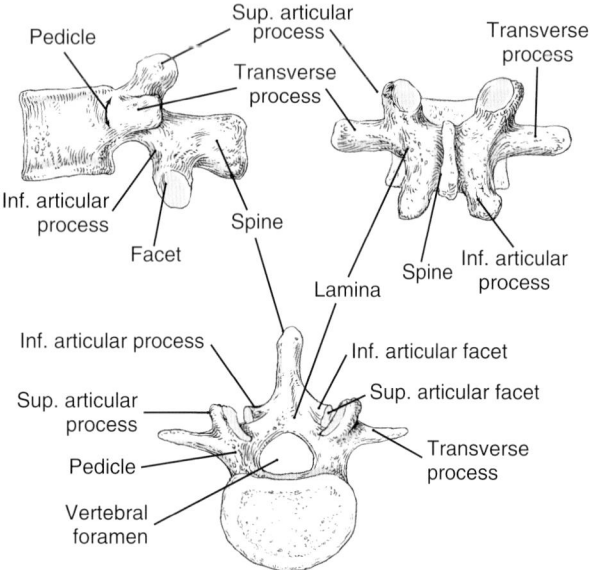

Fig. 49.2 Articular surfaces, transverse processes, and spinous process. *Inf,* Inferior; *Sup,* superior.

fusion is complete. The bodies of the vertebrae can be identified with the transverse processes and articular processes. No pedicles or spinous processes are present. The last, or fourth, bone is small and resembles a nodule. The changing size of the bone from the first to the fourth vertebra gives the coccyx the appearance of a triangle. The projections

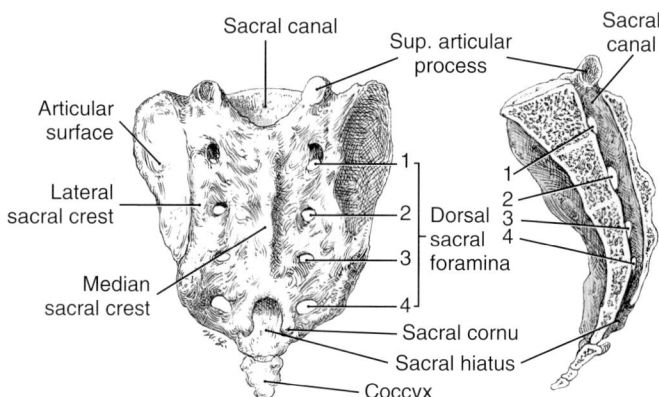

Fig. 49.3 Sacrum and coccyx.

of the rudimentary articular processes are known as the cornua, and the superior pair is the most pronounced. These sacral cornua are the "horns" or bony protuberances that guard the area of the sacral hiatus.[3] Because they can be easily palpated in children and in most adults, they are important surface anatomic landmarks for the performance of a caudal anesthetic procedure.

Of the more than 35 pairs of muscles and ligaments in the back, the supraspinous ligaments, the interspinous ligaments, and the ligamentum flavum (yellow ligaments) are of special significance to the anesthesia practitioner. These three structures act as landmarks that help in identification of and access to the epidural and subarachnoid spaces. The supraspinous ligament is a strong, cordlike ligament that connects the apices of the spinous processes; it is thick and serves as the major ligament in the cervical and upper thoracic regions. The supraspinous ligament consists of three layers: The superficial layer extends over several vertebral spinous processes, the middle layer connects two or three spinous processes, and the inner layer connects only the neighboring spinous processes. The ligament blends at all levels with the thin interspinous ligaments that run between adjacent spinous processes. The interspinous ligaments are usually absent or of poor quality in the cervical region and can be exceptionally thin in the lumbar area, even in young people. The ligamenta flava are the strongest of the posterior ligaments. These broad elastic bands join the vertebral arches through vertical extensions from adjacent lamina. The ligamenta flava are paired flat ligaments that run caudad from the inferior border of one lamina to the upper border of the lower lamina on both sides of the midline. The two ligaments almost fill the space, leaving only a separation in the midline and thereby creating a V or wedge that points posteriorly to align with the interspinous and supraspinous ligaments. The V is thin on the lateral edge and thickest midline; in an adult it is approximately 3 to 5 mm at the L2-L3 interspace. The ligaments extend from each lamina with an overlapping of fibers that creates the appearance of a contiguous ligament from one vertebral body to the next. The ligament is thicker in the lumbar area than in the cervical area and is responsible for maintenance of upright posture. The ligament color comes from the high content of yellow elastic tissue.[4]

The spinal cord itself is a cylindrical structure extending from the medulla oblongata through the spinal foramen to the level of the L2 vertebra in most adults and ranges from 42 to 45 cm in length (Fig. 49.4). Because the vertebral column grows more rapidly than the spinal cord, the spinal cord in children extends initially to the level of the third lumbar vertebra. In approximately 1% of adults, the spinal cord may extend below L2 and rarely to the level of L3. The spinal cord tapers to the conus medullaris, and nerve pathways continue in a collection of rootlets called the cauda equina or horse's tail, which extends from L1 to S5. The spinal cord is enlarged in two regions. The first,

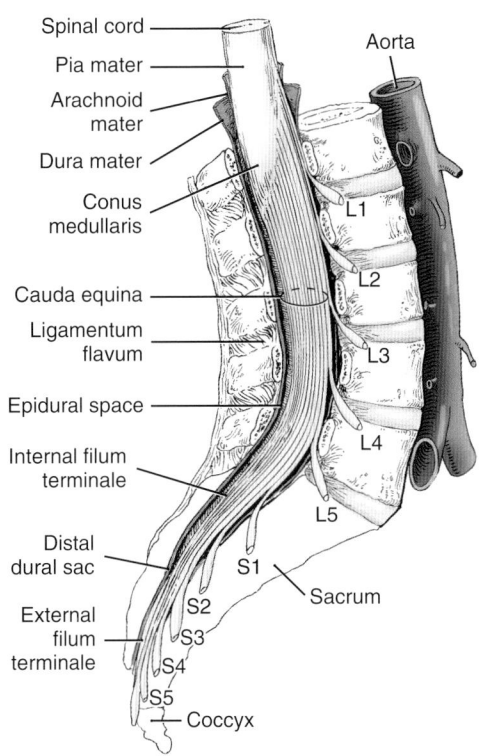

Fig. 49.4 Extension of the spinal cord to the second lumbar vertebra.

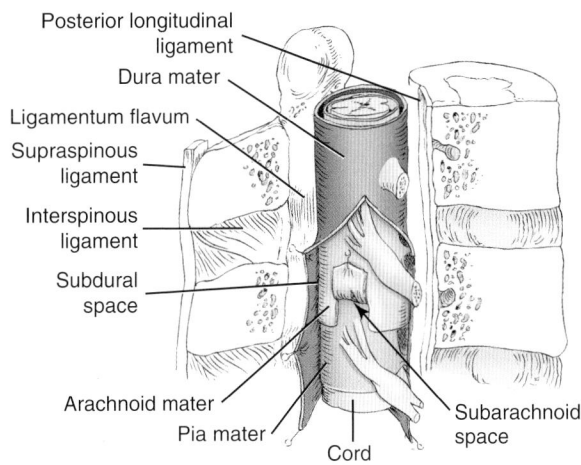

Fig. 49.5 The linings of the spinal cord and the posterior ligaments of the spinal column.

called the cervical enlargement, extends from the spinal segments C4 to T1. The ventral rami of the spinal nerves in this enlargement form the brachial plexus of nerves that innervates the upper limbs. The second enlargement stretches from segments L2 to S3. This lumbosacral enlargement contributes corresponding nerves to create the lumbar and sacral plexuses. It is important to note that the spinal cord levels do not directly correspond with vertebral levels. For example, in adults the lumbosacral enlargement (L2-S3) usually extends from the body of the T11 vertebra to the body of the L1 vertebra.[3]

The spinal cord is enveloped by the same three membranes that line the cranium, and they are collectively called the meninges. The meninges are nonnervous support tissues that provide a protective covering for the cord and nerve roots from the foramen magnum to the base of the cauda equina. The linings are identified as the dura mater, the arachnoid mater, and the pia mater. The dura mater is the outermost layer. It is a thick, tough membrane that provides most of the protection for the central cord structures. The nerve roots are covered with dura mater while inside the spinal canal. As the roots exit the canal via the intervertebral foramen, the dura blends into the root at a junction referred to as a dural cuff or root sleeve. The arachnoid mater is a thin, spiderweb-like covering that forms the middle layer. Beneath the arachnoid mater is a space that is continuous with the central canal of the cord and the ventricles. This space, which is filled with cerebrospinal fluid (CSF), is known as the subarachnoid space. This mater and the fluid protect the spinal cord from shock injuries and are the medium for the interaction with local anesthetics and opioids that occurs during the administration of regional anesthesia. The innermost layer, the pia mater, is thin and is in direct contact with the outer surface of the spinal cord (Fig. 49.5).[3]

The epidural space is a potential space outside the dural sac but inside the vertebral canal and is continuous from the base of the cranium to the base of the sacrum at the sacrococcygeal membrane and is typically only 5 mm wide. The epidural space is classified as a potential space because much of the dura is in contact with the walls of the vertebral canal. The epidural space contains epidural veins, fat, lymphatics, segmental arteries, and nerve roots. Fat in the epidural spaces is physiologically fluid, acting as a pad and lubricant for the movement of neural structures within the canal. The posterior epidural space, as it is approached by the anesthetist's advancing needle, is protected by the ligamenta flava, the lamina, and the spinous processes. It is easy, but inaccurate, to depict the epidural space as a uniform column surrounding an equally uniform and tapering spinal cord. A better mental picture is provided by a look along the longitudinal axes. The epidural space can be envisioned as a series of lateral, posterior, and anterior compartments existing among the vertebral body, lamina, and pedicles. The compartments, occupied mostly by fat but also by nerves and fibrous tissue, repeat at each segment in a metameric fashion. Of greatest interest to the anesthetist, the posterior epidural space is a series of fat-filled tripodial pads shaped like a three-sided sand dune. The pad stretches and narrows in a caudad direction as it approaches the next inferior lamina. In areas of the vertebral canal surrounded by bone, the dura contacts bone, leaving only a potential epidural space that physically separates the epidural fat-containing compartments. The posterior epidural space therefore is a discontinuous group of tapering fat pads that repeat throughout the length of the spinal canal and are separated by a potential space that allows the passage of fluids or small catheters.[4-7]

The distance from the skin to the epidural space and the depth of the epidural space, or the distance to the dura, is of interest to one wishing to avoid needle injury of neural and vascular tissues. The distance to the epidural space varies with vertebral level and is loosely correlated with patient weight. The distance from skin to the lumbar epidural space using a midline approach varies between 2.5 and 8 cm, with an average of 5 cm. Because the space itself is not uniform in shape, the depth of the epidural space from the ligamenta flava to the dura varies considerably. Given the tripodial, dunelike shape of the epidural space, expect the space to narrow considerably when approaching laterally to the midline and in more caudad areas in the space. The depth of the epidural space is also relative to the vertebral level of approach and angle of needle entry, but some clinical generalizations can be made. The epidural space is largest (posterior to anterior) in the midline of the midlumbar region, at 5 to 6 mm. The midline thoracic region epidural space width varies between 3 and 5 mm deep but is only about 1 to 2 mm wide in the lower cervical region.[5]

In addition to a larger epidural space in the midline of the vertebral column, another reason to use a midline approach is it helps avoid

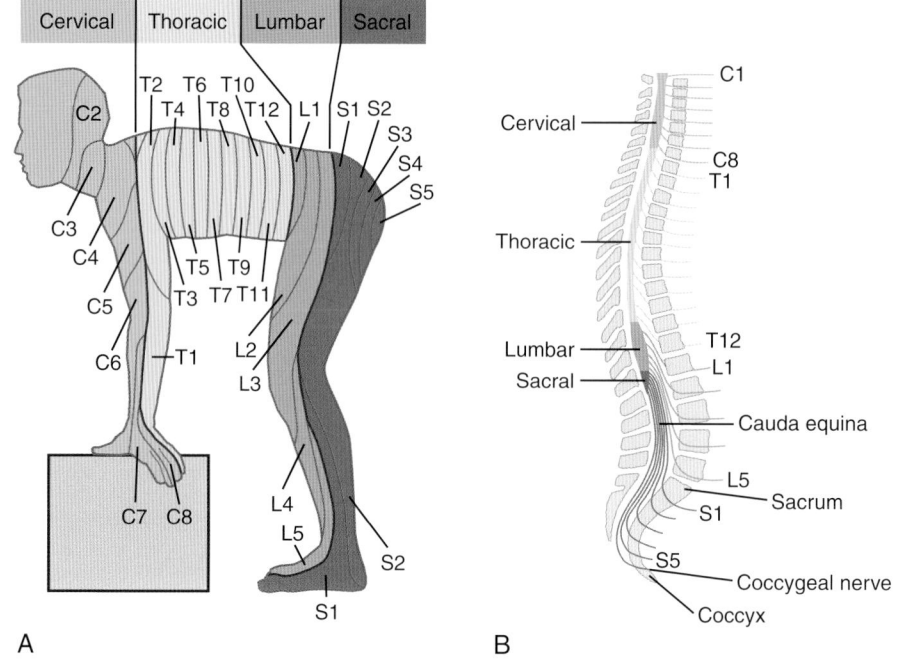

Fig. 49.6 A. Dermatomes. B. Spinal cord divisions. (From Koeppen B, Stanton B. *Berne & Levy Physiology.* 6th ed. Philadelphia, PA: Mosby; 2008.)

contact with epidural veins. As compared to most veins the epidural veins are valveless and form a plexus that drains the blood from the spinal cord and the linings of the cord. The plexus is most prominent in the lateral portion of the epidural space. In pregnant or obese patients, the epidural veins become engorged and swollen as increased intraabdominal pressure results in venous congestion of the lumbar and sacral vessels. The potential for injury or accidental cannulation of these vessels is increased because of this physiologic compensation.[3,4,6]

A final anatomic consideration for neuraxial anesthesia is the existence of normal and abnormal curvatures of the spinal column. A median-plane longitudinal view of the vertebral column reveals four curvatures in the normal adult. The thoracic and sacral curvatures have posterior curvatures (concave anteriorly), whereas the cervical and lumbar regions have anterior curvatures (concave posteriorly). In a supine patient, the apex of the lumbar curve is usually at L3-L4, and the trough of the thoracic curve is at T4.[8] Scoliosis, the most common abnormal curvature, is a lateral curvature of the spine; kyphosis is an excessive posterior curvature or hump, usually of the thoracic region. Excessive lordosis, or hollowing of the back, may occur as a result of obesity as the body attempts to restore the center of gravity. A temporary lordosis may also occur during pregnancy. Changes in these anatomic curves will challenge the anesthesia practitioner during the performance of epidural or spinal anesthetic techniques. Clear knowledge of the curves is also important when anticipating the spread of local anesthetics in the subarachnoid space relative to the site of injection and the patient's position.[9]

Neuroanatomic Mapping and Evaluation of Neuraxial Anesthesia

The goal of neuraxial anesthesia is to block pain transmission from areas of injury, disease, or surgical intervention. Therefore it is clinically useful to have knowledge of the innervations of body structures being operated on in relation to spinal nerve location within the vertebral column. Anatomic maps have been generated based on cutaneous sensation alone. These sensation maps are referred to as dermatomal maps, charts, or levels. A dermatome is the area of cutaneous sensation

supplied by a spinal nerve that is anatomically identified as it passes through an intervertebral foramen. For example, the umbilical area is directly anterior to the L3 vertebra but receives cutaneous innervations from T7-T11, depending on the dermatomal map consulted (Fig. 49.6).

For the practical clinician, use of accepted anatomic landmarks and test methods is perhaps the best method for documenting the functional level of blockade or the level of the loss of sensation achieved. The level of anesthetic can be evaluated in many ways, and tests can be used to evaluate several components of the neuraxial anesthetic. For motor function, a straight-leg raise or plantar flexion of the foot (ask the patient to "step on the gas") works well as a clinical measure. Cutaneous sensation can be evaluated through use of a Wartenberg pinwheel, a Semmes-Weinstein monofilament aesthesiometer, or (more practically and simply) with the stylet from the spinal or epidural needle, a portion of a broken wooden tongue blade, or even a peripheral nerve stimulator. Such pressure or scratch tests are done using two surface-anatomy points for comparison. Inform the patient that the sensation on a normal area, such as the skin surface of the shoulder, is scratchy or sharp. Next, scratch or press an area expected to be numb, such as the lateral thigh. Gradually work cephalad in 2- or 3-in bands until the patient notices a change in sensation. Note the level of the change in sensation relative to a dermatomal map (see Fig. 49.6). This approximates the upper level of sensory loss. Skin refrigerant, ice cubes, and alcohol pads can be used in a similar manner to identify changes in temperature sensation that correlate to sensory block level.

Physiology and Mechanisms of Action

Despite decades of experience with spinal and epidural anesthesia, much speculation remains regarding the exact cellular locations and molecular mechanisms involved when local anesthetics, opioids, and other pharmacologically active agents bind to produce spinal analgesia and anesthesia.[10,11] What is known and clinically important about spinal and epidural anesthesia is that the primary site of action for local anesthetics is on the nerve roots within the spinal cord. When

TABLE 49.1	**Classification of Nerve Fibers**			
		CONDUCTION		
Nerve Fiber	Myelination	Diameter (μm)	Velocity (m/sec)	Function
A-α	Heavy	6–22	70–120	Motor
A-β	Moderate	6–22	30–70	Touch and pressure
A-γ	Moderate	3–6	30–70	Proprioception
A-δ	Light	1–5	12–30	Pain and temperature
B	Light	1–4	3–15	Preganglionic, autonomic
C	None	0.5–1	0.5–2	Pain and temperature

a drug is injected directly into the CSF, the drug distributes through the subarachnoid space based on the physical and chemical properties of the injectant and the characteristics of the space in which it must spread. When the drug concentration reaches a minimal effective concentration, neuronal transmission is altered in a manner that clinically provides anesthesia. Neurons—some myelinated, others not; some relatively large, others smaller—differ in susceptibility to drugs such as local anesthetics, and these pharmacodynamic relationships are not easily explained (Table 49.1). The processes involved at the cellular level are complex, and *blockade* is perhaps a confusing term. It is more accurate to say that anesthetic drugs alter nerve transmission, predominantly by affecting sodium ion channels and inhibiting the units of information that are transferred along the spinal cord. Complete blockade or a chemical transection of the cord is an oversimplification. For example, somatosensory-evoked potentials have been recorded in individuals made functionally insensate from lidocaine epidural anesthesia. This suggests that neural transmissions are reaching the brain without causing sensory perceptions.[4,12]

When a local anesthetic interrupts nerve transmission of autonomic nerves but not sensory nerves or motor nerves (because of a variation in susceptibility), a "differential block" is said to have occurred. A differential block is seen in the more rostral spinal segments of a spinal anesthetic. As the spinal anesthetic spreads from the epicenter of injection, the distal reaches of drug distribution are presumably of lesser concentrations. A differential block is clinically important when sensory anesthesia is desired at a specific level; however, sympathetic blockade could be deleterious in a patient with coexisting disease. The level of sympathetic blockade could be as high as six or more dermatomal levels above the level of sensory blockade and therefore contributes to hypotension and bradycardia.[11]

Drug injected into the epidural space is distributed to the same sites of action as a spinal anesthetic but in a slightly different manner. The drug must first distribute along the epidural space then diffuse through the meninges and dural cuffs to reach the nerve roots or reach the spinal cord through absorption into the radicular arteries. It has been noted that when a substance is injected into the epidural space it travels primarily by bulk flow rather than diffusion and spreads more in a noncircumferential spread, suggesting a possible rationale for one-sided analgesic distribution.[11,13] Data exist to support the clinical impression that spinal anesthesia is generally more effective or complete from the patient's perspective than epidural anesthesia and therefore referred to as a more dense anesthetic. Epidural local anesthetics first act at sites such as the dural cuffs, at which spinal nerves pass through the peridural spaces. This is consistent with the segmental onset often associated with epidural anesthesia. If the concentration and volume of the anesthetic agent are increased, or if time is allowed for the drug to

diffuse into the CSF or pass via radicular arteries into the spinal cord, the epidural anesthetic can become denser.[4,8]

Central Neuraxial Blockade: Indications and Preoperative Considerations

Spinal and epidural anesthesia (central neuraxial blocks) can be used successfully for a variety of inpatient or ambulatory surgical procedures involving the lower extremities, perineum, and abdomen. In addition, spinal and epidural anesthesia or analgesia is used for the treatment of acute and chronic pain syndromes, can be used for obstetric procedures and labor analgesia, and can be applied in patients at the extremes of age.[14] Spinal anesthesia techniques may also be used in combination with other techniques, such as epidural catheter techniques, general or intravenous (IV) anesthetic techniques, or localized nerve blocks to facilitate during surgery. Such combinations, or balanced techniques, minimize the side effects of any one anesthetic technique, maximize the benefits, and offer options in the selection of anesthesia or analgesia for surgical or obstetric procedures.[15]

As with any anesthetic plan, proper preparation, patient selection, education, and collaboration with surgeons and nurses are keys to success. Often the best time to obtain a truly informed consent is during the preoperative visit. It is important to establish rapport with patients to gain their trust and cooperation. Patients eager to be involved in their own care often have the emotional maturity to understand the benefits of their anesthetic options and make rational choices. Anticipate patient fears and anxieties; they are often easily dealt with through education and the reassurance provided by the calm voice of a confident and competent anesthetist.

Before presenting the option of a regional anesthetic to the patient, the anesthesia practitioner should answer the following three important questions about the procedure:
1. Will the patient be comfortable having this surgical procedure performed with the proposed regional anesthetic technique?
2. Will the patient be able to remain in the required position without difficulty for the length of the procedure?
3. Does this regional anesthetic technique outweigh the risks of performing this procedure using an alternate anesthetic technique?

The answers to these questions directly affect the choice of anesthetic techniques offered to the patient. When recommending any anesthetic technique to the patient, the practitioner has a responsibility to educate the patient, the patient's family, and other interested parties about the anesthesia procedure and the potential outcomes. One can then garner the trust of the patient and the family before obtaining the informed consent.

Studies have shown that when compared with general anesthesia, regional anesthesia is associated with a reduction in surgical time, perioperative blood loss, deep surgical site infection, hospital length of stay, and rates of pulmonary and cardiovascular complications.[16,17] Other potential advantages of neuraxial anesthesia as compared to general anesthesia include a reduction in postoperative nausea, vomiting, length of hospital stay, and overall cost and an increase in mental alertness. In addition, neuraxial anesthesia techniques offer preemptive analgesia, which could result in decreased analgesic requirements throughout the perioperative and postoperative periods. In addition, studies have shown neuraxial anesthetics to decrease intraoperative blood loss, lower the incidence of postoperative thromboembolic events and postoperative ileus, increase patency of vascular grafts, and improve respiratory function and cardiac stability.[16,18-21] Although headache remains a small concern, this risk is greatly reduced because of the more frequent use of blunt-tipped spinal needles.[22]

Another group of patients well known to benefit from the use of CNB techniques are patients those who require anesthesia for obstetric procedures. The administration of an epidural analgesic for the parturient in labor is a primary example. No other modality can provide the parturient with relative relief from the severe discomfort of labor with minimal risk of respiratory distress, and still permit the newborn baby mother to interact immediately after delivery. In addition, epidural techniques in labor allow a safe conversion of the analgesia to a surgical anesthetic if a cesarean section becomes necessary.[23,24]

Patient safety may be increased with spinal or epidural anesthesia. Urologic procedures such as cystoscopy examinations and transurethral resections of the prostate (TURP) are most often performed with the use of spinal anesthesia. When awake and anesthetized to the level of the dome of the bladder (T10), the patient may verbally respond to bladder overdistention, thereby helping the urologist minimize the potential for bladder rupture. In addition, the mental status and sensorium of a responsive patient can easily be monitored for the development of conditions associated with TURP syndrome, such as hypervolemia, hyponatremia, and ammonium toxicity.[20,25]

Safety is also an issue when the patient is placed in the prone or jackknifed position as for perianal procedures. A patient in such a position under general anesthesia is at risk for inadvertent extubation and positioning injury. A hypobaric spinal anesthesia technique offers several advantages. The anesthetic procedure can be performed after the patient is positioned and has verbalized being comfortably padded. With hypobaric spinal anesthesia, the spread of the local anesthetic is controlled, and spontaneous ventilation is maintained.

Pain in the postoperative period is often expressed as a primary concern of patients.[26] A distinct advantage of spinal anesthesia is that long-term analgesia can be provided by administration of an intrathecal adjunct, such as long-acting opioids, or α_2-agonists, such as clonidine. An epidural catheter is better suited for long-term postoperative analgesia because it allows for administration of an opioid with or without a low-concentration local anesthetic agent. The use of a low-dose, low-concentration epidural analgesic regimen in the postoperative period has been shown to be highly effective in promoting a shorter length of stay and an earlier return of normalized function.[4,8] However, the use of long-acting opioids or indwelling epidural catheters is not considered appropriate for most outpatient surgery, and a risk-benefit analysis will need to be done in conjunction with both surgeon and patient.

The patient's right to be fully informed also necessitates a discussion of the disadvantages of CNB. Consider the patient's perspective, and keep in mind that the disadvantages and risks inherent in any anesthetic plan are relative only to those of another anesthetic option. For example, patients with a history of headaches or backaches are at increased risk of experiencing these problems after spinal and epidural analgesia, but they also may have exacerbations of these problems after a general anesthetic. Such patients should be evaluated and counseled regarding this potential problem before the administration of any anesthetic. A thorough history of the patient's previous pattern of headaches or backaches is essential when faced with the challenge of evaluating similar symptoms in the postoperative period.

To many patients, the risk of paralysis is the most important concern despite the extreme rarity of any neurologic sequela. Multiple studies have reported that the incidence of any neurologic injury is between 0.03% and 0.1%, or 1:240,000 cases, but few of these could be directly linked to the CNB.[4,27-30] Common patient questions may also include the following:

- "Will the injections hurt?"
- "How long will I be numb?"
- "I am afraid of hearing (or smelling or feeling) the surgery. Can I be asleep?"

Patient perceptions and fears can be diminished with thoughtful explanation and discussion of the clinician's expectations regarding

the patient's case. Additional discussion should include the topic of intraoperative risks such as the inability to obtain adequate anesthesia, paresthesia, hypotension, dyspnea, high or total spinal anesthesia, nausea and vomiting, use of additional sedation, and allergic reactions. Postoperative complications may include backache, postdural puncture headache (PDPH), hearing loss, transient neurologic symptoms, infection, and peridural abscess or hematoma formation.[5,30-34]

Before administration of any anesthetic, a thorough preoperative history and physical examination must be conducted, and any concerns regarding administration of neuraxial anesthesia can be identified. Often the terms *absolute* and *relative contraindications* are used; the definition of these categories varies, and their use is controversial. Many practitioners will include a list of controversial contraindications when discussing the use of a CNB. For the purposes of this text these terms are defined as follows: Absolute contraindications are indicated when placement of a CNB is absolutely inadvisable since it may result in a greater risk to the patient. A relative contraindication is when the anesthetist, patient, and surgeon deem the risk is acceptable because the benefits outweigh the risk. Controversial contraindications include those areas where it is difficult to determine if the use of a CNB will result in greater risk to the patient. A list of the most cited contraindications are found in Table 49.2.

It is more important to think of the anesthetic risks and associated complications relative to the possible benefits of the proposed anesthetic technique. Other preoperative concerns include increased intracranial pressure, significant preexisting or therapeutic coagulopathy, skin infection at the site of injection, hypovolemia, spinal cord disease, an anticipated lengthy surgical time, and patients with a fixed-volume cardiac anomaly, such as hypertrophic cardiomyopathy or severe aortic valve stenosis. Finally, if a difficult airway is anticipated, the plan of care must be discussed with both patient and surgeon.

Neurologic diseases are often listed as potential, absolute, or relative contraindications for neuraxial anesthesia. Prior to performance of

TABLE 49.2   Contraindications to Central Neuraxial Blockade

Absolute Contraindications
Patient refusal
Coagulopathy or bleeding diathesis
Increased intracranial pressure
Severe aortic or mitral stenosis
Ischemic hypertrophic subaortic stenosis
Severe hypovolemia
Infection at the site of injection

Relative Contraindications
Preexisting neurologic complications
Peripheral neuropathies
Sepsis
Hypertrophic obstructive cardiomyopathy
Uncooperative patient
Severe spinal deformity
Demyelinating lesions

Controversial Contraindications
Prior back surgery
Prolonged operation
Major blood loss
Complicated surgery
Maneuvers that compromise respiration

any CNB the anesthetist needs to ascertain the risk and benefits for the patient, including possible exacerbation of disease symptoms. In patients with a preexisting increase in intracranial pressure, the risk of brain herniation is increased, which can be catastrophic if an inadvertent dural or subarachnoid puncture should occur. A dural puncture by a spinal needle or a larger epidural needle creates a rent or hole in dural tissue that may or may not leak CSF. This dural rent/hole may be undetected by the anesthetist at the time of placement but could result in a PDPH or, in the case of persons with increased intracranial pressure, a catastrophic event. Therefore, it is important that the anesthetist do a thorough evaluation of all patients in receipt of a neuraxial procedure in the postprocedural period. If a PDPH is noted either from a dural rent/hole or from a witnessed puncture, treatment may require injection of blood into the epidural space, which could result in an increase in intracranial pressure; therefore a complete neurologic examination is required prior to the placement of any treatment using an epidural blood patch for PDPH.[4,8]

Musculoskeletal deformities such as severe kyphoscoliosis, arthritis, osteoporosis, or fusion and scarring of the vertebrae are considered relative contraindications to neuraxial anesthesia. Secondary to these abnormalities it can make proper placement of the spinal or epidural needle more challenging and can result in an alteration of the anesthetic agent spread and distribution.[27,35] It has been suggested that prior to placement of a CNB it may be prudent to do a preprocedural ultrasound examination of the spine to identify the best level to place the epidural or spinal needle.[36]

Peripheral neuropathies are often the result of metabolic, autoimmune, infectious, or hereditary etiologies. The resultant abnormal tissues may not respond to pharmacologic agents in predictable ways, and the preexisting neural compromise is more susceptible to and less able to recover from injury when exposed to a secondary insult. This secondary insult might stem from needle or catheter trauma, ischemic injury from the use of vasoconstrictors, or direct local anesthetic neurotoxicity. For example, diabetes mellitus is the most prevalent cause of peripheral polyneuropathy, with most patients having some abnormalities in nerve conduction. The frequency of subclinical neuropathy in diabetic patients ranges between 47% and 77%, thereby presenting significant challenges to the anesthesia provider because regional anesthesia can precipitate a double-crush phenomenon.[37] Double-crush phenomena is a state where the axons that are vulnerable at one site become especially susceptible to damage at another site. For example, a compression that occurs in the lumbar region of the spine can result in a worsening of a lower extremity radiculopathy. The double-crush phenomenon has been attributed to factors such as mechanical trauma by the needle, ischemia from injection of epinephrine-containing solutions, or a toxic reaction from the local anesthetic solution.[38] Patients who have a demyelinating lesion condition are also susceptible to double-crush syndrome, and the risk of further neurologic injury is possible along the same conduction pathway. The most common demyelinating disease is Guillain-Barré syndrome (GBS). In patients with GBS, neuraxial anesthesia is a relative contraindication as these patients have an increased sensitivity to local anesthetics, and a postoperative neurodeficit is possible secondary to an interaction between the local anesthetic and myelin, which may cause direct damage to the nerve roots.[39] If a neuraxial block is the appropriate anesthetic choice, then precise documentation of the patient's preexisting disease state must be carried out, and neurophysiologic studies to help identify subclinical neuropathy to minimize the risk of neurologic injury should be considered.[4,8,27,29,30,38,40]

The existence of a significant preexisting or therapeutic coagulopathy increases the risk of spinal or epidural hematoma formation in a patient receiving a CNB. Spinal or epidural hematoma is a rare but devastating complication, possibly resulting in permanent neurologic injury. Central neuraxial anesthesia should be avoided in any patient with a known coagulopathy. Insufficient data are available to quiet the controversy surrounding absolute laboratory values in which the practitioner should avoid CNB. To determine whether a CNB technique should be avoided, it has been suggested that the following arbitrary values be used as a guide: platelet counts of less than 100,000 and prothrombin time (PT), activated partial thromboplastin time (aPTT), and bleeding times that are greater than two times normal values. For a spinal anesthetic, this is perhaps an overly conservative guide.[41] However, severe bleeding with or without symptomatic hypovolemia or the potential for severe bleeding is a possible contraindication to the administration of a regional anesthetic because the sympathectomy caused by CNB further aggravates severely contracted volume states.

Much discussion has arisen regarding the use of spinal and epidural anesthesia when coagulopathy for thromboprophylaxis or therapeutic treatment of coexisting disease has been initiated, planned, or is ongoing because the therapies, timing, and effects on coagulation are highly varied. Many surgical patients take drugs that impair coagulation, and this is a concern in patients receiving a CNB with the risk of a compressive vertebral canal hematoma (VCH). The incidence of VCH is extremely low but increases in patients who are taking anticoagulation drugs.[42-46]

Even planned intraoperative anticoagulation with heparin is reasonably safe after atraumatic dural puncture if the patient presents with a normal coagulation profile. Traditionally, a patient's bleeding time was obtained prior to administration of neuraxial anesthesia, but the predictive value of bleeding time has not been established in patients taking aspirin and nonsteroidal antiinflammatory drugs (NSAIDs).[29,42,43] In addition, with the increased use of natural and herbal medicines, anesthetists must be alert to the possibility of drug interactions. Alone, herbal supplements do not appear to increase the risk of spinal hematoma; however, data on combinations of herbal and other anticoagulants are not available.[44] Herbal medications that affect hemostasis and some perioperative concerns are listed in Table 49.3. If basic precautions are followed, many thromboprophylaxis strategies have had an extensive safety record when coadministered with neuraxial anesthetics. The surgeon and anesthesia practitioner should consider the potential benefit versus risk before neuraxial intervention for patients who have been or will be anticoagulated for thromboprophylaxis. The number, variety, and indications for the use of anticoagulants and thrombolytics continue to increase.

The incidence of neurologic dysfunction resulting from hemorrhagic complications resulting from neuraxial blockade is unknown. Overall, the risk of clinically significant bleeding increases with age, associated abnormalities of the spinal cord or vertebral column, the presence of an underlying coagulopathy, difficulty during needle placement, and an indwelling neuraxial catheter during sustained anticoagulation, particularly with standard heparin or low molecular weight heparin (LMWH).[43,44] The American Society of Regional Anesthesia and Pain Medicine (ASRA) convened its Fourth Consensus Conference on Regional Anesthesia and Anticoagulation in 2018, where practice guidelines on regional anesthesia in the patient receiving antithrombotic or thrombolytic therapy were formulated. The Society for Obstetric Anesthesia and Perinatology (SOAP), in collaboration with ASRA, formulated guidelines on the anesthetic management specifically for the pregnant and postpartum woman receiving thromboprophylaxis or high-dose anticoagulants.[41] These newer guidelines indicate that even in doses as low as 10,000 units/day neuraxial anesthesia should be postponed for at least 4 hours following heparin injection. In regard to LMWH, it is recommended that at least 12 hours should have elapsed to administer a neuraxial anesthetic. For intermediate- and high-dose LMWH, it is recommended that neuraxial anesthesia not be administered from 12 to

TABLE 49.3 Herbal Medications Affecting Hemostasis*

Herb	Important Effects	Perioperative Concerns	Time to Normal Hemostasis After Discontinuation
Garlic	Inhibition of platelet aggregation (may be irreversible) Increased fibrinolysis Equivocal antihypertensive activity	Potential to increase bleeding, especially when combined with other medications that inhibit platelet aggregation	7 days
Ginkgo	Inhibition of platelet-activating factor	Potential to increase bleeding, especially when combined with other medications that inhibit platelet aggregation	36 hr
Ginseng	Lowers blood glucose Increased prothrombin (PT) and activated partial PTs in animals Other diverse effects	Hypoglycemia Potential to increase risk of bleeding Potential to decrease anticoagulant effect of warfarin	34 hr

*At this time it is not deemed necessary to discontinue herbal medications and allow resolution of their effects on hemostasis before surgery or anesthesia.
Adapted from Horlocker TT, et al. Regional anesthesia in the patient receiving antithrombotic or thrombolytic therapy: American Society of Regional Anesthesia and Pain Medicine evidence-based guidelines (fourth edition). *Reg Anesth Pain Med.* 2018;43(3):263-309.

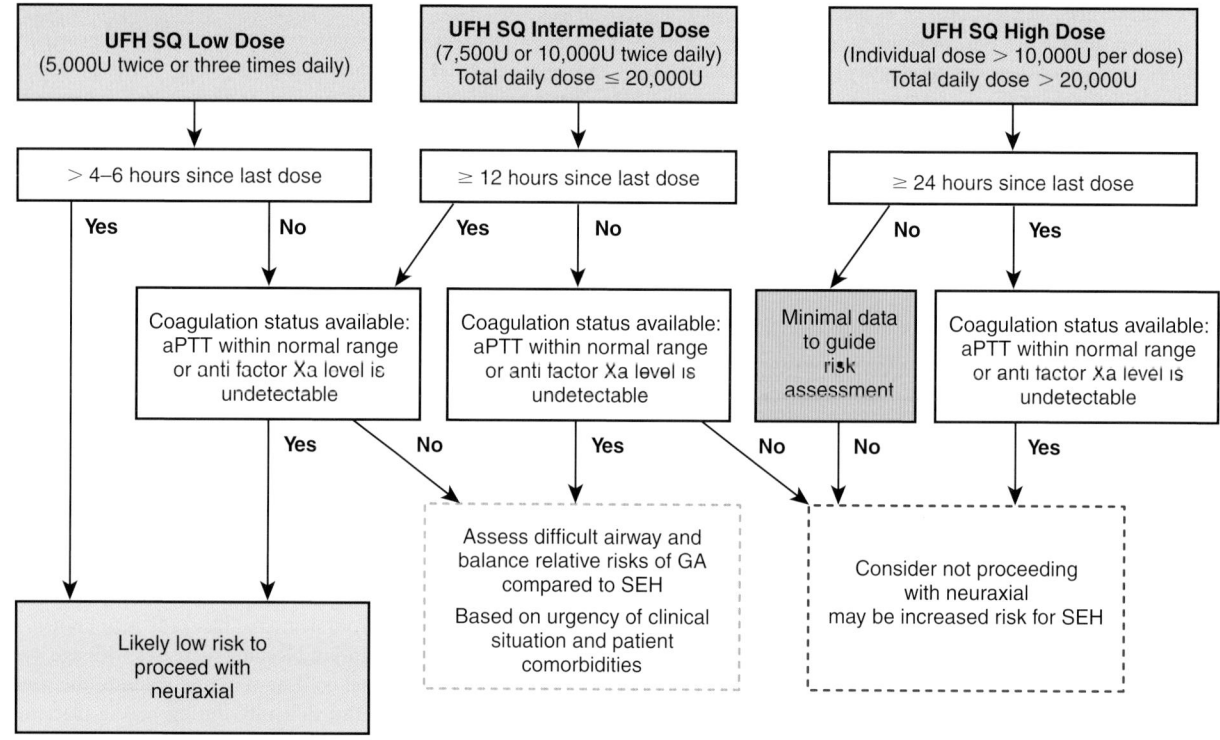

Fig. 49.7 Decision aid for patients receiving unfractionated heparin and central neuraxial blocks. (From Leffert L, Butwick A, Carvalho B, et al. The Society for Obstetric Anesthesia and Perinatology consensus statement on the anesthetic management of pregnant and postpartum women receiving thromboprophylaxis or higher dose anticoagulants. *Anesth Analg.* 2018;126[3]:928-944 [fig 3].)

24 hours following administration. Always check product labeling to ensure an adequate time interval has elapsed prior to placement of any neuraxial anesthetic (Figs. 49.7 and 49.8). Many international anesthesia societies have also issued guidelines for the use of regional blocks in patients receiving thromboprophylaxis[44-46] (Table 49.4).

Neurologic complications are extremely rare from neuraxial anesthesia. For example, in over 1.7 million neuraxial anesthetics performed in Sweden in the 1990s there were only 127 serious complications reported, with 85 resulting in permanent injury.[35] Similar findings were reported in a meta-analysis by Brull et al.[47] where they reported the risk of permanent neurologic injury as 1 to 4.2 per 10,000 after spinal anesthesia and 0 to 7.6 per 10,000 after epidural anesthesia. To minimize permanent nerve injury, scrupulous postoperative nursing surveillance is required to support patient safety. Any complaint of a new-onset weakness or sensory deficit to the lower limbs, alteration in bowel and bladder dysfunction, or complaint of new-onset back or lower extremity pain needs to be investigated. Permanent nerve injury is more likely to occur if assessment and intervention do not occur within 8 hours of the initial injury. Therefore, immediate recognition is important.[29,35,47]

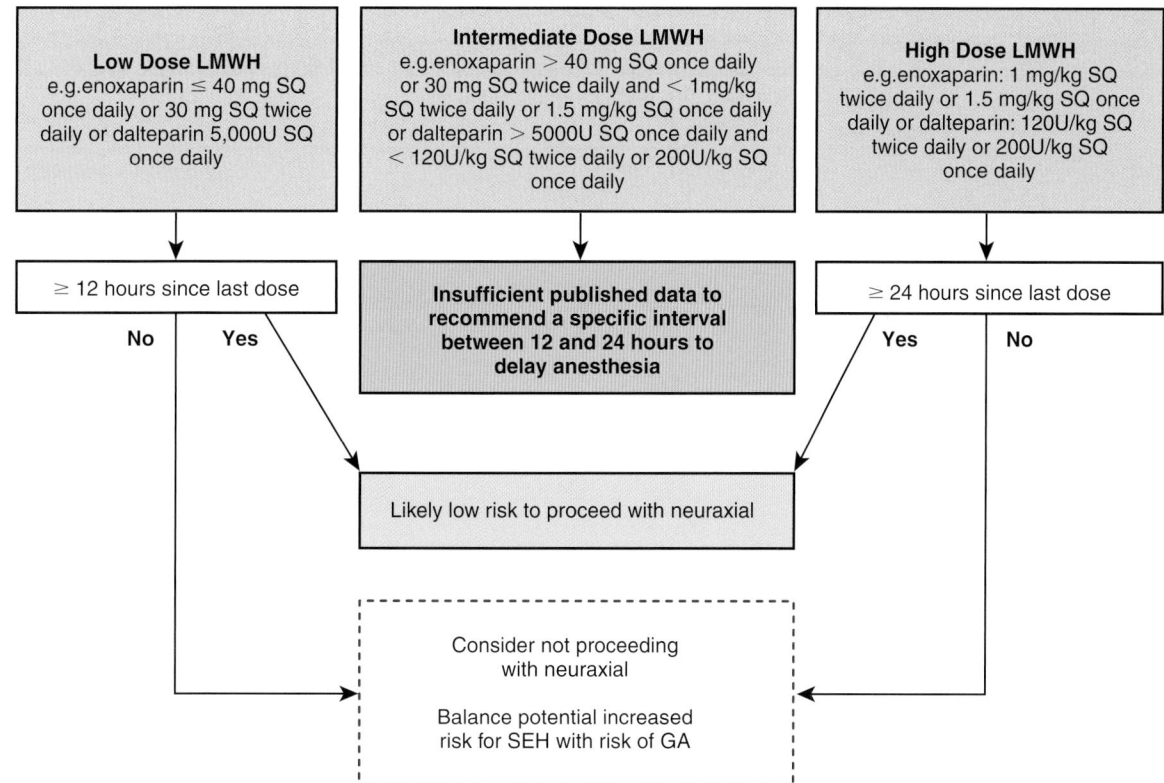

Fig. 49.8 Decision aid for patients receiving low molecular weight heparin and central neuraxial blocks. (From Leffert L, Butwick A, Carvalho B, et al. The Society for Obstetric Anesthesia and Perinatology consensus statement on the anesthetic management of pregnant and postpartum women receiving thromboprophylaxis or higher dose anticoagulants. *Anesth Analg.* 2018;126[3]:928-944 [fig 4].)

Neurologic injury can also occur secondary to infection. The etiology of neuraxial infection is based on the theory that needle placement disrupts the body's physiologic protective mechanisms and deposits infectious or noxious agents beyond the skin into underlying tissues and the peridural space and past the blood-brain barrier into subarachnoid spaces. Indeed, skin infection at the site of injection increases the risk of meningitis or epidural abscess formation. Infectious complications include but are not limited to epidural, spinal, or subdural abscess; paravertebral, paraspinous, or psoas abscess; meningitis; encephalitis; sepsis; bacteremia; viremia; fungemia; osteomyelitis; or discitis. Although colonization of the catheter may be considered a precursor to infection, colonization per se is not considered an infection.

It is extremely important that the anesthetist maintain strict aseptic technique during the preparation and administration of any CNB to minimize the potential for infection. Septic meningitis or epidural abscess due to bacterial contamination, and the consequences of persistent neurologic deficits such as loss of bowel and bladder control, chronic pain, and lower extremity weakness or paraplegia, can be devastating. Other factors that increase the risk of infection include dermatologic conditions such as psoriasis that prevent aseptic skin preparation, underlying sepsis, diabetes, immunologic compromise, steroid therapy, and the preexistence of chronic infections such as human immunodeficiency virus (HIV) or herpes simplex virus (HSV). Because meningitis after spinal or epidural anesthesia is so rare, it has been difficult to directly attribute causality to the anesthetic or to identify significant risk factors. In fact, based on the limited data available, it would appear all forms of regional anesthesia are safe in cases of secondary HSV infection and reasonable for patients in the early stages of HIV infection. All patients should be monitored for signs of meningeal irritation, fever, increasing back pain, neurologic changes, and local tenderness to injection sites. Although classic

symptoms such as high fever, nuchal rigidity, and severe headache may be present, less alarming symptoms can occur, resulting in misdiagnosis. It is not uncommon to find α-hemolytic streptococci in spinal block meningitis, whereas *Staphylococcus aureus* is the most common causative organism in epidural abscesses. This can be especially problematic since the overall incidence of methicillin-resistant *S. aureus* infection rates for US facilities was approximately 1% in 2015.[48] Epidural abscess, like epidural hematomas with evidence of neurologic deficit, can best be diagnosed by MRI. Early, aggressive surgical intervention and antibiotic administration are vital.[4,27,35,49-51] A 2017 advisory committee published guidelines noting several factors to consider to minimize infections. They included conducting a history and physical examination, reviewing all preprocedure laboratory evaluations, using prophylactic antibiotic therapy as indicated, and using strict aseptic techniques, including proper antiseptic solution. Other standard of care interventions include the use of sterile occlusive dressings at the catheter insertion site, placement of a bacterial filter during continuous epidural infusion, limiting disconnection and reconnection of neuraxial delivery systems, and limiting the duration of catheterization.[34]

In addition to infection, arachnoiditis and aseptic meningitis can occur when foreign substances are introduced causing an irritation to the meninges. It is imperative precautions are taken to ensure glass or metal particles, highly concentrated local anesthetics, detergents or antiseptics, or a core of epidermis is not introduced into the subarachnoid space. Indwelling catheters, previous myelography, and hemorrhages into the subarachnoid or epidural space also have been associated with meningeal irritation and scarring. To minimize the overall risk, standard CNB techniques incorporate the use of disposable equipment, needles with matched stylets, filter needles, and improved pharmacologic agents that make these complications rare.[52]

TABLE 49.4 **European Society of Anaesthesiology's Recommended Time Intervals Before and After Neuraxial Puncture or Catheter Removal***

	Time Before Puncture/Catheter Manipulation or Removal	Time After Puncture/Catheter Manipulation or Removal	Laboratory Tests
Unfractionated heparin (UFH) (for prophylaxis, ≤15,000 IU/d)	4–6 hr	1 hr	Platelets during treatment for >5 days
UFH (for treatment)	Intravenous 4–6 hr Subcutaneous 8–12 hr	1 hr 1 hr	Activated partial thromboplastin time (aPTT), Activated clotting time (ACT) platelets
Low molecular weight heparin (LMWH) (for prophylaxis)	12 hr	4 hr	Platelets during treatment for >5 days
LMWH (for treatment)	24 hr	4 hr	Platelets during treatment for >5 days
Fondaparinux (for prophylaxis, 2.5 mg/day)	36–42 hr	6–12 hr	Antifactor Xa, standardized for specific agent
Rivaroxaban (for prophylaxis, 10 mg/day)	22–26 hr	4–6 hr	Antifactor Xa, standardized for specific agent
Apixaban (for prophylaxis, 2.5 mg twice daily)	26–30 hr	4–6 hr	Antifactor Xa, standardized for specific agent
Dabigatran (for prophylaxis, 150–220 mg)	Contraindicated according to the manufacturer	6 hr	Thrombin time (TT)
Coumarins	International normalized ratio (INR) ≤1.4	After catheter removal	INR
Hirudins (desirudin)	8–10 hr	2–4 hr	aPTT, Ecarin clotting time (ECT)
Argatroban	4 hr	2 hr	aPTT, ECT, ACT
Acetylsalicylic acid	None	None	
Clopidogrel	7 days	After catheter removal	
Ticlopidine	10 days	After catheter removal	
Prasugrel	7–10 days	6 hr after catheter removal	
Ticagrelor	5 days	6 hr after catheter removal	
Cilostazol	42 hr	5 hr after catheter removal	
Nonsteroidal antiinflammatory drugs	None	None	

*All time intervals refer to patients with normal renal function. Prolonged time interval in patients with hepatic insufficiency.
Adapted from Horlocker TT, Vandermeuelen E, Kopp SL, et al. Regional anesthesia in the patient receiving antithrombotic or thrombolytic therapy: American Society of Regional Anesthesia and Pain Medicine evidence-based guidelines (fourth edition). *Reg Anesth Pain Med.* 2018;43(3):263–309 (table 7).

Shock and severe uncorrected hypovolemia are absolute contraindications to spinal or epidural anesthesia because both techniques can cause a significant sympathetic blockade. Sudden changes in the form of profound hypotension and cardiovascular collapse may occur. This hemodynamic instability is due to the massive vasodilation preventing physiologic compensation that normally occurs (i.e., vasoconstriction, increase in cardiac output). Management of shock and hypovolemia often requires aggressive fluid therapy and multisystem treatments that can be physiologically and psychologically uncomfortable for the aware patient.[4,8,27]

Patients with a fixed-volume cardiac state such as hypertrophic cardiomyopathy or severe aortic valve stenosis do not tolerate bradycardia or tachycardia, decreases in systemic vascular resistance, or decreases in venous return and left ventricular filling, all physiologic changes that can be anticipated with neuraxial block by local anesthetics. In these patients, even transient episodes of hypotension can cause serious coronary hypoperfusion and cardiac arrest. Therefore spinal and usually epidural anesthesia are contraindicated; however, few things in anesthesia are truly absolute. For example, epidural administration of opioids has been used to provide obstetric analgesia and may provide cardiac benefit for these patients. Precautions in such a scenario might include close hemodynamic monitoring with an arterial line and pulmonary artery catheter, careful titration of the anesthetic, intravascular volume expansion, and use of ephedrine or phenylephrine to treat hypotension.[29]

Spinal anesthesia is typically a singular deposit of local anesthetic and provides anesthesia for a fixed duration. If uncertainty exists about the anticipated length of surgery, epidural catheter placement is more appropriate to allow for the additional administration, or continuous infusions, of anesthetic agents. If the extent of the surgery is unknown, a neuraxial anesthetic may be initiated only to be converted later to a general anesthetic when the surgeon exceeds the limits of the anesthetic block. This is rarely an ideal situation; the patient may experience discomfort, albeit brief, and the anesthesia practitioner must contend with less-than-ideal intubating conditions. Despite the advantages of neuraxial anesthesia, many patients such as the elderly and those with arthritis or musculoskeletal limitations of the neck and upper extremities poorly tolerate prolonged immobility. The judicious use of conscious sedation can quickly lower the patient's ability to maintain adequate ventilation secondary to hypoventilation, resulting in hypoxia and hypercarbia. To avoid such circumstances, combined neuraxial and general anesthetic techniques are advocated and offer advantages by minimizing the total dose of general anesthetic used. Such techniques lower the risk of secondary effects of general anesthesia (e.g., nausea and vomiting) while gaining the advantages associated with neuraxial anesthesia, such as attenuation of the stress hormone response and improved postoperative pain relief.[8]

When spinal or other regional anesthesia is instituted, the reticular activating centers in the brain receive less input. This often results in somnolence in a normal patient but can result in unconsciousness in the overly sedated or inebriated patient. In addition, spinal or epidural anesthesia may reach an undesirably high level that is physically and psychologically intolerable for the patient, which could evolve into a total spinal. A total spinal is characterized by unresponsiveness accompanied by cardiac and respiratory compromise. In such situations, airway support is required, and the emergent management of any airway can severely compromise patient safety. Therefore regional anesthesia is not an alternative to a secure airway. For patients identified as potentially difficult to intubate, equipment should be immediately available to secure the airway in a safe manner. Advances in airway management such as the laryngeal mask airway, improved fiberoptics, videolaryngoscopes, and adjunct airway equipment may tip the risk-benefit scale in favor of regional anesthesia.[8,11,52]

SPINAL ANESTHESIA

Spinal anesthesia became popular after the discovery of the local anesthetic properties of cocaine, the invention of the hollow needle and syringe, and the written descriptions of the first lumbar puncture. The first clinical application of the technique was reportedly performed in the late 1890s. However, spinal anesthesia's prominence was short lived. The introduction of specific, reversible neuromuscular blocking drugs and concurrent improvements in inhalation agents for general anesthesia soon displaced its popularity. It has regained popularity in large part because of the introduction of newer agents, equipment, and techniques to employ it safely in the ambulatory setting.

Equipment and Techniques

Preparation for spinal anesthetic procedures, like for any other regional technique, requires the immediate availability of emergency equipment and supplies should emergent resuscitation be required. Usually spinal anesthetics are administered in the operating room where the minimal requirements—functional laryngoscopes, endotracheal tubes, induction agents, cardiovascular drugs (including atropine and ephedrine or phenylephrine), suction, oxygen and ventilation equipment, a noninvasive blood pressure monitor, pulse oximetry, and electrocardiographic monitoring equipment—are readily available.

The original spinal technique, performed by August Bier in 1898, has been continually examined and modified in hope of reducing the incidence of complications, primarily that of PDPH. The goal of needle design has been to create a needle that minimally rends, tears, or cuts dural tissues. As technology has improved, the use of sterile, disposable procedure trays containing needles, syringes, catheters, and drugs has virtually eliminated problems previously associated with dull needles or contaminated equipment and has allowed for the development of innovative needles. Spinal anesthesia can be administered using either a cutting or a noncutting needle. Examples of a cutting needle include the Quincke-Babcock, Greene, or Pitkin needle with matching stylets to minimize tissue coring and beveled tips with cutting edges. Examples of a noncutting pencil-point needle include the Sprotte, Whitacre, and Pencan needle with a pencil-point tip and rounded edges. Several of the more popular types of spinal needles are shown in Fig. 49.9. Spinal needles also have matched stylets and are marketed for spinal anesthesia use in sizes ranging from 22 to 29 gauge and in lengths of approximately 3.5 to 5 in (88–120 mm). Most blocks are performed using needles of 25 to 27 gauge, 3.5 in (88 mm).[27,52]

Data support the use of noncutting needles over cutting needles for several reasons.[27] Cadaver lumbar punctures performed with sharp cutting needles show piercing of the cauda equina roots without resistance, thereby practitioners do not appreciate the dural puncture at their fingertips. Pencil-point needles pierce the dura with a clearly

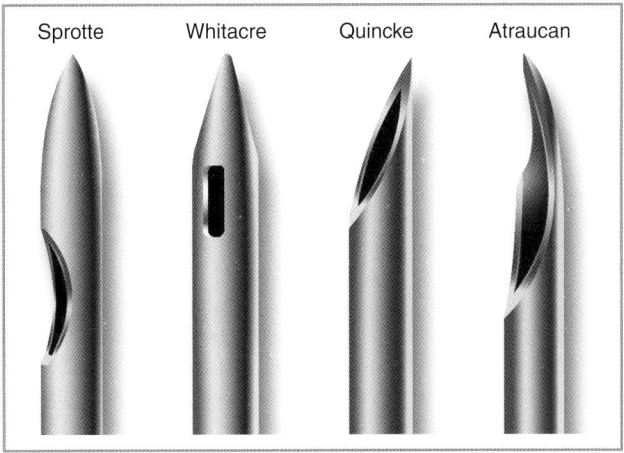

Fig. 49.9 Spinal needle assortment often used in parturients. The Sprotte and Whitacre needles have cone-shaped bevels, whereas the Quincke and Atraucan needles have cutting bevels. (Other sizes are available in some of these needle designs.) (From Chestnut DH, Wong CA, Tsen LC, et al. *Chestnut's Obstetric Anesthesia Principles and Practice.* 6th ed. Philadelphia, PA: Elsevier; 2020.)

perceptible click or pop not as easily noticed with cutting needles. Newer, thin-walled noncutting needles have improved CSF flow rates without compromise to strength. This allows for their use for CSF diagnostic procedures and helps simplify the identification of the intrathecal space by permitting quick return of CSF after stylet removal. It was also noted that the bevel of cutting-tip needles often would deviate on insertions, whereas symmetric noncutting needles routinely remained midline. Another significant difference was that when a noncutting needle is used, the bevel of the needle must be oriented parallel to the dural fibers to avoid cutting across; conversely, when using a noncutting needle, the bevel orientation is not a concern since the blunt tip tends to separate the fibers without cutting. This is important because cutting across the dural fibers increases the risk of PDPH. In a 2017 meta-analysis by Xu et al., they reported the overall incidence of PDPH from a cutting spinal needle was 6.6% as compared to a 2.6% incidence when a noncutting or pencil-point spinal needle is used.[8,27,53,54]

After the patient arrives in the surgical or obstetric preoperative area, the consents for surgery and anesthesia should be verified, and any further patient questions or concerns should be addressed. Review of the anesthetic preoperative history and physical examination should include the addition of any last-minute changes in patient status and notation of recently obtained diagnostic results. IV access is achieved, and a continuous crystalloid infusion is begun. Preoperatively, most patients benefit from low-dose anxiolysis. With the increased emphasis on same-day admission, surgery, and discharge, long-acting agents are avoided. A rapid-acting benzodiazepine with a relatively short duration, such as midazolam, is highly titratable in 0.5- to 1-mg increments given intravenously and minimally alters the patient's hemodynamic status when used in low doses. The drug's effects can be reversed with flumazenil.

Monitors appropriate to the patient's physical status should be applied and at minimum include blood pressure monitoring, a continuous electrocardiogram, and pulse oximetry. For baseline comparisons, vital signs must be assessed with the patient in both the supine position and the position in which the block will be administered.

The surgical or obstetric procedure to be performed helps determine the patient's position for the administration of the block. For example, if vaginal or urologic surgery is planned, a saddle block with the patient in a sitting position may be indicated. The prone position is useful for rectal surgery because the patient can be placed in position before the block is implemented (if a hypobaric local anesthetic is used). This reduces the time required for positioning by permitting the patient to move with minimal assistance and to personally verify comfort and adequacy of padding. A lateral position favors spinal drug spread for right- or left-sided extremity or abdominal procedures when a hyperbaric local anesthetic solution is used. When the patient is in the lateral position, a pillow placed under the head and perhaps shoulders helps maintain neutral alignment of the spinal column. Surgical table height or patient position may need to be adjusted to compensate for variations in anatomic structure or physiologic limitations and to maximize anesthetist ergonomics. To maximize the space between spinous processes, the patient should arch the back (with assistance from the clinician) into a C shape or "like a Halloween cat." Once the patient is positioned, anatomic surface landmarks are used to identify the lumbar region of the back to be used for dural puncture below the end of the spinal cord (L2). The line formed between the tops of the iliac crests, called the intercristal line or Tuffier line, crosses the vertebral column as high as the L3-L4 disk or as low as the L5-S1 disk (Fig. 49.10). The accuracy of predicting the precise level of needle insertion is at best 50%. This fact may account for variability in the spinal anesthesia level ultimately achieved, yet this landmark has been clinically useful since the advent of spinal anesthesia.[7] The skin overlying a prominent spinous process at this level is marked for easy identification after the skin is prepared and draped. A surgical skin-marking pen is useful for this purpose, with caution exercised to avoid scratching the skin surface and predisposing the patient to infection.

Next, the spinal anesthesia tray is opened, and sterile gloves are donned. The patient is prepared with an antiseptic solution such as Betadine, a povidone-iodine solution that releases a concentration of 1% free iodine as it dries on a surface. The solution must remain in contact with the skin for at least 1 minute to be effective, and then the dry residue can be wiped away with sterile gauze to help prevent a chemical arachnoiditis. Do not use alcohol to remove residue because alcohol neutralizes the iodine solution and minimizes its antiseptic effect. Historically povidone-iodine solution has been used as an antiseptic skin prep solution but is quickly being replaced with alcohol-based solutions such as DuraPrep (iodine povacrylex [0.7%] and isopropyl alcohol [74%]) or ChloraPrep (0.5%–2% chlorhexidine gluconate and isopropyl alcohol [70%]). ChloraPrep is used in many practices to provide skin disinfection. Routinely ChloraPrep is available in concentrations of 0.5% and 2%, and the concentration of 0.5% is recommended if a dural puncture is possible. Reports of meningeal irritation have occurred in rare cases when the 2% solution is used. A concentration of 0.5% has been shown to be just as effective in skin disinfection as the 2% solution.[34,55] Following antisepsis an aseptic technique needs to be maintained, and the sterile drape must be applied to the back. Many spinal and epidural drapes have a circular window that is placed over the area of anticipated injection and adhesive strips to simplify application to the patient's back. Avoid touching the adhesive because this has been shown to create small holes in gloves, which increases the risk of infection in both the patient and anesthesia practitioner.[56]

A rapid-acting local anesthetic such as 1% lidocaine is used for local infiltration of the area just caudal to the identified spinous process. Approach the skin of the back with the bevel of the needle facing away from the skin and at a 15- to 30-degree angle from the skin. Start injecting as the bevel of the needle enters the skin and raise a skin wheal placing the local anesthetic into the subdermal tissues that contain the dermal nociceptors. Deep tissues, including the supraspinous ligament, can be anesthetized by spreading 3 to 5 mL of local anesthetic through the tissues using a fanlike injection technique.[8,27]

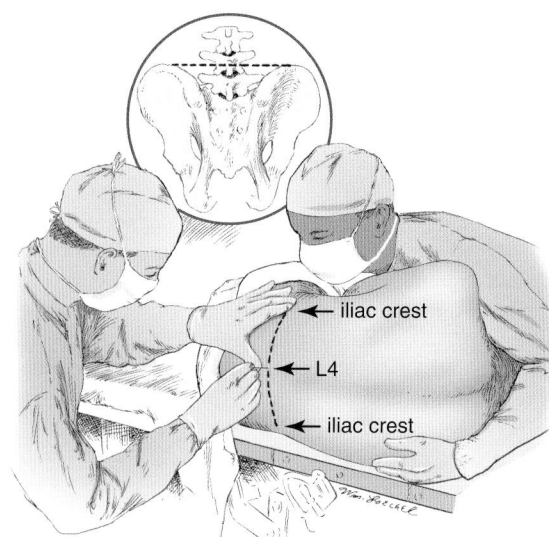

Fig. 49.10 Patient positioning and identification of landmarks in the lumbar region of the back.

Larger, 22-gauge spinal needles have tensile strength sufficient to permit introduction of the needle without additional support. However, spinal needles smaller than 22 gauge often require an introducer needle to help stabilize the needle during insertion and minimize infection from the surrounding dermis. The introducer needle is typically 18 or 20 gauge, which is matched to the spinal needles. The introducer is inserted through the skin and supraspinous ligament and into the interspinous ligament. Care must be taken, especially in thin individuals, not to enter the subarachnoid space with the introducer needle because the dura can be very shallow in the thin patient. An introducer needle placed into the subarachnoid space would likely cause a PDPH. The average depth from the skin to the subarachnoid space is 4.5 cm (1.8 in) in the male and 4.18 cm (1.67 in) in the female.[4,8,15,27]

Several common spinal anesthesia techniques can be used, including a straight midline approach. With this easy-to-learn technique, the anesthesia practitioner inserts the needle directly midline between the spinous processes and toward the umbilicus perpendicularly to all planes or at the lumbar level with a slight cephalad angle (Figs. 49.11 and 49.12). If bone is encountered early, the needle is withdrawn into the introducer and subcutaneous tissue. The introducer and spinal needle are then redirected in small angular increments in a cephalad direction. If bone is encountered when the needle is deeply inserted, the needle should be withdrawn and redirected caudad. If bone is still encountered, it is recommended that the introducer and spinal needle be completely withdrawn and reintroduced into the same interspace or at another vertebral interspace either above (assuming needle placement is not above L2) or below the predesignated site. As the tip of the spinal needle passes through the ligament flavum, the sensation is similar to that felt when a needle is passed through a pencil eraser. As the needle tip passes through the dura, the anesthesia practitioner may sense a pop or click. The stylet is removed, and several seconds are given for CSF to return through the small-gauge needle. Once CSF return is confirmed, some authors recommend rotating the needle 360 degrees in 90-degree increments to ensure that the needle tip is seated well within the subarachnoid space (see Fig. 49.12). Other authors suggest that such needle manipulation risks a larger dural rent/hole or needle dislodgement. Whichever method is used, secure needle handling is important. As shown in Fig. 49.13, firmly place the dorsum of one's nondominant hand against the patient's back and below the spinal needle. Grasp the needle hub between the thumb and index finger.

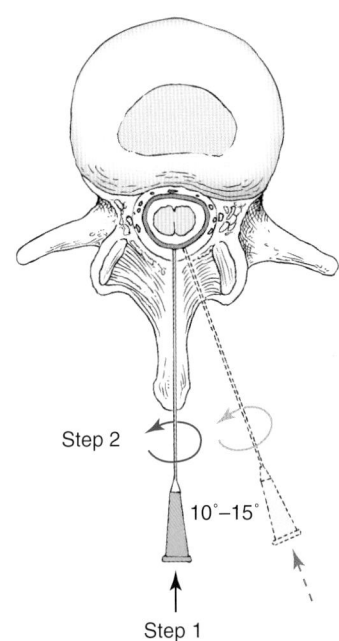

Fig. 49.11 Insertion of the needle between the spinous processes and toward the umbilicus.

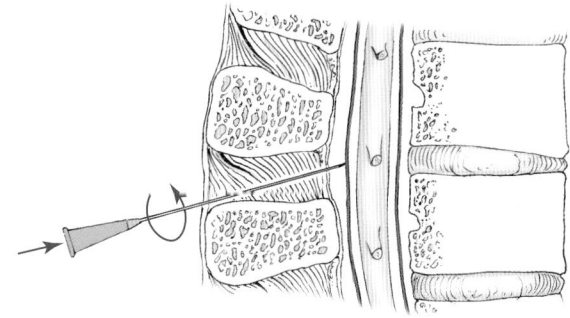

Fig. 49.12 Spinal needle rotated 360 degrees to aid evaluation of tip location within the subarachnoid space.

With this Bromage type of grip, the patient's body then acts as a firm support for the needle-stabilizing hand and helps prevent advancement or withdrawal of the needle tip from the subarachnoid space when the syringe is applied to inject the anesthetic agent.

A second technique is called the paramedian approach. With this technique, the needle is inserted 1 cm or approximately one fingerbreadth lateral and 1 cm caudal to the desired vertebral interspace. The needle is directed toward the spinal canal and angled slightly cephalad and then medially approximately 10 to 20 degrees (see Fig. 49.12). Elderly and arthritic patients may have decreased back flexibility and degenerating, calcified ligaments. For such patients, this approach may be the only possible means of entering the subarachnoid space because it aims for the largest area between processes and avoids calcified interspinous ligaments. It has been reported the paramedian approach allows for faster onset on epidural and spinal anesthesia than a conventional midline insertion.[57] A third approach to the subarachnoid space, known as the Taylor approach, takes advantage of the largest vertebral interspace located between L5 and S1. This approach uses a paramedian approach between L5 and S1 and is useful in the elderly because it tends to be less affected by degenerative changes than the other lumbar spaces. A point 1 cm medial and 1 cm caudad to the

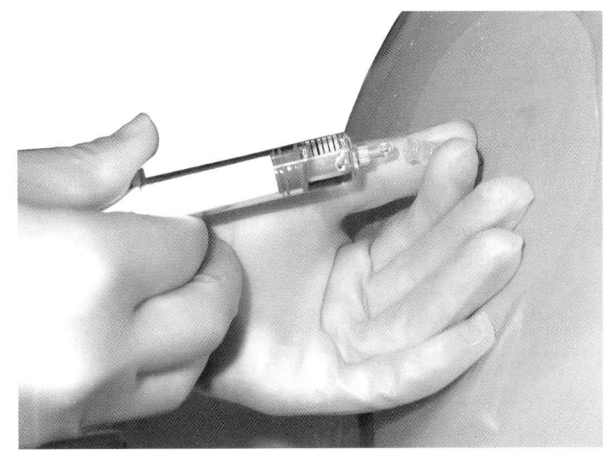

Fig. 49.13 The Bromage grip, showing needle control and syringe connection.

posterior superior iliac spine is located, and the needle is angled medially and cephalad at a 55-degree angle toward the fifth lumbar interspace. The Taylor approach is best used for pelvic and perineal surgical procedures.[4,7,8,15,27]

Intrathecal Drugs, Spread, and Block Levels

Once the anesthetic solution is delivered into the CSF, the distribution of its active molecules through the subarachnoid space is dependent on the chemical and physical characteristics of the solution in relation to the chemical and physical characteristics of the patient's CSF and the subarachnoid space. In adults, approximately 500 mL of CSF is produced each day, predominantly by the choroid plexuses of the cerebral ventricles. Much of the CSF is reabsorbed by arachnoid granulations along the sagittal sinus to regulate CSF pressure to 10 to 20 cm H_2O. At any given time, approximately 140 mL of CSF flows by bulk through the subarachnoid spaces, the central canal of the cord, and the ventricles of the brain. It is estimated that only 30 to 80 mL of the total CSF is present in the spinal canal. However, this quantity is difficult to measure, variable among individuals, and uncontrollable by the clinical anesthetist.[3,4,58]

The density of a substance compared with the density of water is a ratio known as specific gravity. The specific gravity of CSF is 1.004 to 1.009 and can vary depending on variations in temperature and location of the fluid within the subarachnoid space. For example, the specific gravity of CSF sampled from the lumbar area is slightly greater than that of CSF from the ventricles. This difference is directly dependent on the protein in the CSF as well as on the effects of gravity and the position of the patient. The specific gravity of CSF also tends to increase as patient age increases, correlating to increases in glucose and protein. Hyperglycemia and uremia increase the specific gravity of CSF, whereas jaundice and related liver problems may decrease its specific gravity. The change in specific gravity is related to the presence of bilirubin within the CSF. An increase in a solution's temperature decreases its specific gravity. This decrease averages a fall of approximately 0.001 for each degree rise in Celsius temperature. Although all these factors influence the distribution of an anesthetic solution injected into the CSF, they are usually beyond the control of the anesthetist.[4,8,15,27,58]

A closely related concept, baricity refers to the resting position of two fluids with differing specific gravities when the fluids are mixed in a single container, such as CSF and an anesthetic agent in the subarachnoid space. The baricity of the injected solution is compared with that of the CSF. Knowledge about the baricity of an injected solution provides the practitioner with information that helps determine the potential spread of the anesthetic mixture in the subarachnoid space. Therefore, when several medications are combined, the specific gravity of the combined solution at body temperature should be considered when the spread of the medication is anticipated. Unfortunately these bedside mixtures are rarely controlled or measured, and use becomes reliant on practical experience. When baricity (i.e., the ratio of specific gravity of local anesthetic to patient CSF) equals 1, the solution is referred to as being isobaric. Because the specific gravity of CSF is variable, it is not possible to prepare a solution that is precisely isobaric. Near-isobaric solutions remain and act in approximately the same location in which they are injected. A hyperbaric solution has a specific gravity that is greater than that of CSF. The solution would fall or sink to the lowest anatomic point at which CSF is contained within the subarachnoid space in relation to gravity and the patient's position (presuming drug preparations are corrected for body temperature). Hypobaric solutions that are less dense than CSF rise or float to the highest anatomic position possible when injected into the subarachnoid space.

Because the normal range for the specific gravity of CSF is variable, local anesthetics, opioids, or other solutions injected into the CSF must be predictably hypobaric or hyperbaric. By tradition, hypobaric solutions are defined as having a baricity of less than 0.999, and hyperbaric solutions have a baricity of greater than 1.0015. Clinically this is accomplished by dissolving the drug in either sterile water to create a hypobaric solution or 5% to 8% dextrose solutions to create a hyperbaric solution. If CSF or normal saline is added to the medications, the specific gravity of the solution is similar to that of CSF, and the drugs remain approximately where injected.[4,8,15,27,58]

More than 23 factors, including CSF density and local anesthetic baricity, have been thought to affect the spread of local anesthetics in CSF and therefore affect the level and quality of the anesthesia achieved. Less than half of these factors have been found to have clinical significance, and an even smaller number are controllable by the anesthetist performing the anesthetic procedure.[27] Clinically the most important factors are those that can be manipulated by the anesthesia practitioner. These are the total dose of the local anesthetic, the site of injection, the baricity of the drug (drug choice), and (when nonisobaric solutions are used) the position or posture of the patient during and after injection.[58]

The duration of a spinal anesthetic is based primarily on local anesthetic choice and total dose. Highly protein-bound drugs, such as tetracaine, bupivacaine, and ropivacaine, have long durations of action compared with less protein-bound drugs such as lidocaine and mepivacaine. Vasoconstrictors such as 0.1 to 0.2 mL of 1:1000 (1 mg/mL) epinephrine solution are sometimes added to the local anesthetic solution to prolong the duration of action. Epinephrine is thought to prolong the duration of spinal anesthesia by causing vasoconstriction, thereby delaying normal uptake of local anesthetics, by direct antinociceptor action, or by a combination of these effects. The effect of added epinephrine on the prolongation of anesthesia is greatest with tetracaine, less with lidocaine, and minimal with bupivacaine. In addition, local anesthetic solutions may include opioids (10–25 mcg fentanyl, 2.5–10 mcg sufentanil, or 100–250 mcg preservative-free morphine) or an α_2-agonist (clonidine 150 mcg or dexmedetomidine 5 mcg) to prolong duration. These agents act at opioid and α_2-adrenergic receptors, respectively. The exact nature of the synergistic effect among opioids, α_2-agonists, and the local anesthetics is not clear, but the result is again prolonged spinal anesthesia. It has been noted that the addition of opioids or an α_2-agonist to the spinal anesthesia admixture prolongs the duration of spinal anesthesia and improves postoperative analgesia without a significant impact on overall hemodynamics or motor

blockade.[59] Increasing the total dose of a spinal local anesthetic will increase its duration of action and affect the sensory level achieved. Duration of sensory and motor blockade for local anesthetics has been shown to be predictable. For example, increasing the dose of hyperbaric bupivacaine from 10 mg to 15 mg prolongs the duration of sensory block by 50% and increases the maximum sensory level achieved. Based on these principles, Table 49.5 offers medication administration suggestions to achieve an approximate sensory level and duration of spinal anesthesia in a typical clinical setting.[58,60]

Selecting the precise site of injection, as mentioned, is technically inaccurate at the clinical level.[7] The higher the site of injection, obviously, the higher the level of sensory block, but this is limited by the anatomy of the spinal cord and the anesthetist's desire to approach the subarachnoid space below the termination of the spinal cord. Theoretically, if a patient is administered a hyperbaric solution at the L3 level and placed supine, the local anesthetic would flow both cephalad and caudad from the relative peak of the lumbar lordosis to the troughs of the thoracic kyphosis and sacral regions. If a hyperbaric drug is placed below L3 with the patient in a sitting position, and the patient is left sitting for 5 minutes, a lumbar and sacral-root anesthetic known as a saddle block will occur. However, even under experimental conditions using the second to fifth lumbar interspace, the data on the ability to control the maximum sensory block level achieved are inconsistent. Therefore the site of injection can be a poor predictor of the final level of sensory anesthesia achieved.[58]

Several authors suggest the level of the anesthetic can be adjusted or modified by use of position changes within the first few minutes after injection or until the medication becomes fixed on the nerve roots and the spinal cord. Some have even found that changes in position as late as 60 minutes after injection can alter the level of block achieved. For example, one of the suggested methods used to modify the level of the anesthetic is to raise a supine patient's legs 45 degrees. This position is thought to increase blood flow through the epidural venous plexus, indirectly altering CSF pressures. Such a position also flattens the lumbar lordosis, altering flow of hyperbaric local anesthetic within the subarachnoid space. The combined effects result in further cephalad spread of local anesthetic solutions. If one uses a similar line of thought, morbid obesity and third-trimester pregnancy also are associated with epidural venous engorgement when the patient is supine, and a slightly higher level of spinal anesthesia is found when compared with controls. With traditional hyperbaric solutions, the block achieved may range from T3 to T6. Therefore, the anesthetist's ability to precisely control the level of sensory anesthesia through baricity and changes in posture is associated with great variability and low predictability from patient to patient.[27,58,61] Once achieved, the final level of sensory blockade should be determined, as discussed previously, and then documented.

Continuous spinal anesthetics are administered with the same techniques used to establish a spinal or epidural anesthetic. A small epidural needle is used for the procedure, with the bevel turned parallel to dural fibers to help minimize the risk of PDPH. After the needle is inserted into the subarachnoid space, the bevel of the needle is turned either caudad or cephalad to facilitate passage of an epidural catheter into the subarachnoid space. The catheter is inserted only 2 to 3 cm into the subarachnoid space. Further insertion could result in advancement of the catheter along a nerve root or in curling of the catheter. The incidence of headache is minimal in elderly patients or when the catheter can remain in the subarachnoid space for at least 40 hours. Because of reports of cauda equina syndrome, in 1992 the Food and Drug Administration (FDA) removed small needles and microcatheters designed to further reduce the risk of PDPH from the

TABLE 49.5 Choice of Medication for Spinal Anesthesia Used for Surgical Procedures

Procedure	Medication*	Dosage	Duration Without Epinephrine	Duration With Epinephrine
Vaginal delivery	Tetracaine	5 mg	1–1.5 hr	2.5–3 hr
	Bupivacaine	5–7 mg	1 hr	1.5 hr
	Lidocaine	25 mg	15–25 min	45 min–1 hr
Cesarean section	Tetracaine	8 mg	1–1.5 hr	2.5–3 hr
	Bupivacaine	10 mg	1–1.25 hr	1.5–2 hr
	Lidocaine	50–75 mg	30–45 min	1–1.25 hr
Anorectal surgery	Tetracaine (hyperbaric)	6 mg	1–1.5 hr	3 hr
	Tetracaine (hypobaric)	6 mg	1 hr	3 hr
	Bupivacaine	8 mg	1 hr	1.5–2 hr
	Lidocaine	25–50 mg	15–30 min	45 min
Genital or lower-extremity procedure	Tetracaine	6–10 mg	1.5 hr	2–3 hr
	Bupivacaine	8–12 mg	1.5 hr	2 hr
	Lidocaine	75–100 mg	45–60 min	1.25–1.5 hr
Hernia, pelvic procedure	Tetracaine	10–12 mg	1.5 hr	2–3 hr
	Bupivacaine	12–15 mg	1.5 hr	2 hr
	Lidocaine	100 mg	45–60 min	1.25–1.5 hr
Intraabdominal surgery	Tetracaine (by patient height)	5 ft to 5 ft, 5 in = 12 mg; 5 ft, 6 in to 6 ft = 15 mg; >6 ft = 18 mg	1.5 hr	2–3 hr
	Bupivacaine (by patient height)	5 ft to 5 ft, 5 in = 15 mg; 5 ft, 6 in to 6 ft = 18 mg; >6 ft = 20 mg	1.5 hr	2 hr
Back and spine surgery	Tetracaine	10–15 mg	1–1.5 hr	2–2.5 hr
	Bupivacaine	15–20 mg	1–1.5 hr	1.5–2 hr

*Local anesthetic solutions administered to intrathecal or epidural spaces must be sterile and preservative free.

US market. Cauda equina syndrome, or persistent paralysis of the nerves of the cauda equina with resultant lower extremity weakness and bowel and bladder dysfunction, has subsequently been attributed to the deposition pooling and possibly repeat dosing of neurotoxic concentrations of hyperbaric local anesthetics, particularly 5% lidocaine.[4,8,35,60]

This same solution of lidocaine in varying concentrations has been associated with transient neurologic syndrome. Symptoms are usually described as pain originating in the gluteal region that radiates to both lower extremities. Symptoms appear within a few hours up to 24 hours after recovery and spontaneously disappear in virtually all cases in 10 days. The symptoms range from mild to severe radicular back pain in up to 30% of patients, and although NSAIDs are the usual treatment, opioids may be required. Symptoms include a burning, aching, cramp-like, and radiating pain in the anterior and posterior aspects of the thighs. Pain radiates to the lower extremities, and lower back pain is common. Other anesthetics have been implicated, but it is much more prevalent after spinal lidocaine.[62] Surgical positioning may be a factor as well.[63,64] The exact mechanism is unclear. Newer techniques and agents other than lidocaine are being used now, and that has diminished this problem as a clinical issue. Treatment is supportive and should include NSAID agents when possible.[65,66]

Physiologic Alterations and Their Management

Spinal anesthesia causes several physiologic changes that are predictable and can usually be readily managed through anticipation and prevention or with minimal intervention. Physiologic changes include effects on the central nervous system, cardiovascular system,

respiratory system, and gastrointestinal (GI) system. In addition, physiologic alterations caused by central neural blockade affecting neuroendocrine, renal, and hepatic function are mentioned.

The obvious central nervous system effect of spinal anesthesia is the inhibition of nerve impulse conduction resulting in spinal anesthesia. This occurs when the local anesthetic concentration exceeds the minimal blocking concentration of the particular nerve exposed to the drug. Neurons have different levels of susceptibility to local anesthetics, and this partially explains the differential block seen with spinal and epidural anesthesia. As a local anesthetic spreads from the epicenter of its injection site, the concentration of molecules decreases. As the local anesthetic spreads rostral and the concentration gradient lessens, only the most susceptible neurons will be blocked, and a differential block occurs. With spinal anesthesia, kinesthetic sense is typically inhibited at a dermatomal level higher than light touch or cold sensation, which in turn is inhibited at a more rostral dermatomal level than pinprick anesthesia. Therefore a differential blockade among the levels of sympathetic, somatic sensory, and somatic motor fibers can be identified. Attempts to demonstrate the numbers of segments between areas of differential blockade have found that sympathetic fibers are blocked two to six dermatomes beyond the level of the sensory block.[10,11]

The reticular excitatory area in the brainstem is responsible for the brain's overall state of alertness or arousal. The primary determinant of the activity of the reticular excitatory area is the amount of sensory input from the body. Because spinal anesthesia greatly decreases the number of sensory impulses to the reticular excitatory area, normal patients often experience somnolence. Caution must be taken during administration of spinal anesthesia to a patient in pain and already under the influence of central depressants such as alcohol or opioids. The pain caused by the injury may be the only stimulus for consciousness, and when spinal or other regional anesthesia is instituted, unconsciousness may ensue.[11]

Spinal or epidural techniques using local anesthetics block sympathetic nerve transmission in addition to blocking sensory and motor fibers. Therefore the sum effect of neuraxial anesthesia on the cardiovascular system depends primarily on the overall degree of sympathetic blockade in terms of the rostral spread of the anesthetic and partially on the degree of patient sedation and central sympathetic inhibition. Blockade of the sympathetic nervous system causes arterial vasodilation, decreased systemic vascular resistance, venous pooling, and a reduction in venous return. These changes cause a redistribution of blood that often results in hypotension. If the block is high enough, the sympathetic nerve fibers that innervate the heart, known as the cardiac accelerators (T1-T4), become anesthetized, which can result in bradycardia and thus further exacerbate hypotension. Following administration of spinal anesthesia, hypotension is caused from a massive sympathetic blockade, which can initiate a parasympathetic overdrive and alteration of volume receptor reflexes. Another causative factor is the initiation of a paradoxic reflex called the Bezold-Jarisch reflex (BJR). The BJR is an inhibitory reflex induced by simulation of mechanoreceptors and chemoreceptors in the heart, which promotes parasympathetic activity leading to bradycardia, vasodilation, and hypotension. The BJR is elicited because spinal anesthesia decreases the venous return to the heart secondary to the sympathetic blockade, causing a fall in the blood pressure. This drop in blood pressure is sensed by the carotid baroreceptors and causes a sympathetic activation that promotes a rapid contraction of the ventricles. This rapid contraction of the underfilled ventricles results in activation of the serotonin (5-HT$_3$) receptors present in the ventricle wall, which can result in profound hypotension, bradycardia, and vasodilation from vagal activation. Studies have shown that the administration of a 5-HT$_3$ antagonist such as ondansetron (4 mg) given at the time of spinal anesthesia injection significantly reduced the overall incidence of spinal-induced hypotension (SIH).[67,68] Other baroreceptor reflexes, volume receptor reflexes, and the overall decreased central sympathetic outflow all contribute to the complexity of the cardiovascular response to neuraxial anesthesia. The overall result is loss of normal cardiovascular homeostatic reflexes and the ability to compensate for minor cardiovascular stresses.[70-72] Rapid changes in position, changes in skeletal muscle tone caused by relaxation, decreased venous return, low preoperative volume status, reflex surgical stimulation, preoperative medications (especially opioid and sedative hypnotics), and concurrent conditions such as pulmonary embolism, pregnancy, and systemic reactions to medications have all been implicated in increased severity of perioperative hypotension.[11,69,70]

Hypotension is immediately relevant to the perfusion of critical organs such as the heart and brain and is important to all organs in maintaining near homeostasis. Although normotensive patients have been shown to maintain cerebral blood flow despite a moderate decrease in blood pressure, hypertensive subjects may have altered cerebral blood flow autoregulation and are less tolerant of changes in mean arterial pressures.[11] A similar situation exists with elderly patients and patients with known coronary disease. With these caveats in mind, most clinicians allow a decrease in blood pressure of 20% from a patient's baseline before initiating treatment.

Clinicians continue to debate the optimal treatment of SIH and bradycardia. The most used techniques include pelvic tilting, administration of crystalloid and colloid solutions, administration of vasopressor agents, positioning during spinal anesthesia placement, and the use of

serotonin (5-HT$_3$) antagonists. The treatment is often dependent on coexisting disease, but some general recommendations can be made. In addition to the use of 5-HT$_3$ antagonism, practitioners will often administer crystalloid solution using either a preload or coload strategy. The traditional preload technique involves the administration of 15 to 20 mL/kg of crystalloid solution given over 20 minutes before injection of a spinal anesthetic, whereas the coload involves administration of the same volume over 20 minutes initiated at the time of the spinal injection. Studies have shown that using the coload technique resulted in less hypotension and a decrease in the incidence of bradycardia and need for vasopressors.[69,70,72] Infusions of α-adrenergic vasoconstrictors and sympathomimetic agents have also been shown to help reduce the incidence of cardiovascular side effects requiring treatment. Should the treatment of hypotension become necessary, the ongoing administration of IV solution is often the first response; however, excessive fluid therapy can lead to fluid overload and urinary retention, especially in the elderly.[69,70]

Continued treatment is guided by the patient's presenting symptoms and coexisting disease. The heart rate can be used to help guide pharmacologic intervention. Ephedrine (a mixed α- and β-agonist) in 5 to 10 mg IV boluses is the agent of choice in patients with symptomatic bradycardia. The indirect effects of ephedrine cause an increase in peripheral vascular resistance and heart rate. If the heart rate is normal or elevated, incremental injections of an α-agonist, such as 50 to 100 mcg of IV phenylephrine, causes increased systemic vascular resistance without further increasing the heart rate. The use of phenylephrine may therefore be more efficacious in the elderly. Bradycardia is treated with IV atropine of 0.4 to 0.8 mg. Severe hypotension should be managed aggressively with medication and fluids because mortality from rare cardiac arrests increases when treatment is delayed.[4,10,15,69,70]

Most studies demonstrate that midthoracic levels of either spinal or epidural anesthesia have minimal effects on tidal volume, respiratory rate, minute ventilation, and arterial blood gas tensions in otherwise healthy individuals. The phrenic nerve is rarely paralyzed, even when sensory levels reach the cervical dermatomes. However, the accessory abdominal and intercostal muscles for ventilation are impaired, and the ability to cough and clear secretions is inhibited. With the loss of perception of intercostal and abdominal wall muscle movement and the inability to cough, the patient may begin to feel dyspneic. Caution must be exercised if the accompanying anxiety is treated with large doses of sedatives or opioids. They may worsen ventilation and result in hypoxia. Although regional techniques have been shown to have minimal effects, adequate ventilatory ability during surgery is dependent on multiple factors, and improved pulmonary outcomes have not been clearly demonstrated. Some of the factors that affect ventilatory ability under spinal or epidural anesthesia include the presence of coexisting disease, depressant medications, patient position, type and location of the surgery and incision, and presence of hypotension and hemorrhage. The anesthetic plan must be adapted to the patient and the operation.[10,11]

The GI tract is regulated by the parasympathetic and sympathetic nervous systems. The parasympathetic innervation of the GI tract is primarily via the vagus nerves and is composed of both afferent and efferent fibers. Parasympathetic afferent nerves transmit sensations of satiety, distention, and nausea, whereas efferent outflow generally increases GI activities such as tonic contractions, sphincter relaxation, peristalsis, and secretion. Sympathetic innervation of the GI tract stems from the T5-L2 spinal cord segments and via prevertebral ganglia. Sympathetic afferent nerves are responsible for transmitting pain information; efferent nerves inhibit peristalsis and gastric secretion and cause sphincter contraction and vasoconstriction. When spinal and epidural anesthesia cause a sympathetic blockade, the result is unopposed or dominant parasympathetic activity. The neuraxial sympatholysis results in a generalized constriction of the bowel, normal to increased peristalsis, increased intraluminal pressure, and increased GI blood flow.[10,11,15] The combination of abdominal muscle relaxation and a contracted bowel offers improved operating conditions for intraabdominal procedures, but because gastric motility can be increased, some clinicians have questioned the risk of wound disruption. Several studies have reported that the intraoperative and postoperative use of neuraxial anesthesia does not increase the risk of wound breakdown. A 2017 review by Carmichael et al.[73] reported that the use of thoracic epidural analgesia was beneficial in open colorectal procedure recovery as compared to conventional systemic analgesia but not for routine use in laparoscopic colorectal surgeries.

Nausea and vomiting are associated with neuraxial block in up to 20% of patients. Nausea and vomiting are primarily related to the GI hyperperistalsis of parasympathetic dominance, although other contributing factors may include hypoxemia, hypotension, systemic medications (opioids or rapidly infused antibiotics), and psychological stimuli. A cardiac mechanism associated with spinal anesthesia, as proposed by some authors, also may lead to nausea and vomiting. Theoretically, cardiac vagal afferent nerves can be activated in response to a decrease in venous return via ventricular mechanoreceptors, especially with high block levels. Therefore the vagolytic properties of atropine provide indirect-acting antiemetic effects in the treatment of the nausea and vomiting associated with high spinal anesthesia.[11,15]

The neuroendocrine stress response is a combination of responses of the body to tissue trauma (such as surgery) or critical illness. The response includes components of neural, immune, endocrine, metabolic, and inflammatory systems that are closely integrated through a complex mechanism of hormones, neurotransmitters, and receptors that affect cells throughout the body. These systems are activated in proportion to the level of critical illness or tissue injury experienced by the body.[11] The stress response is usually associated with increases in blood concentrations of adrenocorticotropins, cortisol, insulin, growth hormone, aldosterone, and glucose. Initially a protective response, the stress response can lead to tachycardia, hypertension, catabolism, immunosuppression, and hypercoagulability.[10] Regional blocks such as spinal and epidural techniques moderate the stress response to surgery. Although spinal anesthesia blocks this response only for the duration of the anesthetic administration, the use of continuous epidural analgesia well into the postoperative period has the potential to improve perioperative outcome.

Renal blood flow and function are well preserved during spinal anesthesia when blood pressure is maintained. Hepatic blood flow is directly proportional to the mean arterial pressure and therefore depends on the treatment of any hypotension associated with the spinal or epidural anesthetic.[10] Spinal and epidural anesthetics block sympathetic fibers, thereby increasing the tone of the internal urethral sphincter; in addition, neuraxial opioids cause a decrease in detrusor contraction and an increase in bladder capacity. These changes in the genitourinary system can result in the rare complication of urinary retention.

Complications of Spinal Anesthesia

Postdural Puncture Headache

PDPH is perhaps the most discussed and managed complication of neuraxial anesthesia, with a documented incidence that has varied over the years from 0.2% to 24%. Theoretically PDPH is caused by a decrease in the CSF available in the subarachnoid space through a leak created by the dural puncture from an intruding needle. The medulla and brainstem, having lost their hydraulic support, drop into the foramen magnum, stretch the meninges, and pull on the tentorium. This

pulling, further irritated by movement and the upright position, causes a characteristic headache.[4,27,31,74] A contributing theory suggests that cerebral vasodilation may result from low CSF pressure. This theory is supported by the beneficial effects of vasoconstrictor drugs such as caffeine and theophylline.[74]

Several factors are known to increase the incidence of PDPH. The use of large, non–pencil-point needles or a cutting-needle bevel direction that is perpendicular to the long axis of the body will make larger holes in the dural fibers and create larger CSF leaks. In fact, the risk of PDPH is 70% when the dura is punctured with a 16-gauge Touhy epidural needle, 5.2% when a 26-gauge Quinke (cutting needle) is used, and only 1.2% when a 25-gauge Whitacre (noncutting needle) is used.[74,75] Therefore it is recommended that only a noncutting (pencil-point tipped) needle should be used for spinal anesthesia, especially in those predisposed to PDPH. Other factors predisposing a patient to PDPH are multiple punctures, female gender, and age. There is extensive evidence showing PDPH is relatively uncommon in those over the age of 60 and more prevalent in those less than 40 years of age. This is thought to occur because in the elderly the dura may be more inelastic and less likely to remain open following a dural puncture. Patients with a history of PDPHs are also predisposed to another headache after a subsequent spinal anesthetic procedure. One should keep in mind that not all headaches following spinal anesthetic procedures are PDPHs. It is common for patients to experience headaches after surgery and even after general anesthetics. Factors contributing to headaches may include anxiety, interrupted sleep, dehydration, hypoglycemia, and even the lack of normal morning caffeine intake. A differential diagnosis approach should be taken to identify serious complications such as subdural hematoma, subarachnoid hemorrhage, meningitis, sinusitis, or subarachnoid hemorrhage.[15,27,31,74,76]

Fortunately, PDPHs have several characteristic features that aid in diagnosis. They usually occur within several hours to the first or second postoperative day. Historically, bed rest was thought to help prevent PDPH, but subsequent studies found avoiding early ambulation simply postponed the onset. The headache is described as a mild to incapacitating bilateral frontal headache radiating from behind the eyes and across the head toward the occiput and often into the neck and shoulders. The headache is considered positional because it is relieved when the patient is lying down. The only other form of headache with this positional component is caused by pneumocephalus, therefore it may be beneficial to use normal saline as your medium when placing an epidural as opposed to air. Other symptoms associated with PDPH include nausea and vomiting, appetite loss, blurred vision or photophobia, a sensation of a plugging of the ears and loss of hearing acuity, tinnitus, vertigo, and depression.[8,27,31,74]

Although PDPHs are self-limiting and often resolve in less than 10 days, early identification and prompt treatment are essential if complications of immobility, depression, and patient dissatisfaction (a potential reason for litigation) are to be avoided. Conservative management includes a horizontal position, adequate hydration, oral analgesics, and the administration of 500 mg IV caffeine benzoate, 300 mg of oral caffeine, or theophylline. Caffeine has shown effectiveness for treating PDPH, decreasing the proportion of participants with PDPH persistence and those requiring supplementary interventions. Gabapentin, theophylline, and hydrocortisone also have shown a decrease in pain severity scores when compared with placebo or conventional care. There is a lack of conclusive evidence for the other drugs such as sumatriptan.[77,78] The horizontal position is impractical for most patients, especially mothers of newborns, and encourages further complications of immobility.[74] Abdominal binders, thought to increase epidural venous plexus blood flow and therefore CSF pressure, are uncomfortable and often impractical. Increasing fluids during the evaluation and early management period was thought to increase the central volume and increase the secretion of CSF from the choroid plexus, but this is not well supported in the literature. However, adequate hydration should be maintained in all patients.[27] Caffeine and theophylline are both methylxanthine derivatives that cause cerebral vasoconstriction and central nervous system stimulation. Caffeine therapy, both oral and parenteral, is the most used pharmacologic treatment modality. Caffeine has been shown to eliminate headache in up to 70% of patients, but this effect may be transient.[74] In a 2014 review by Baysinger[79] it is reported caffeine is frequently used and shows efficacy as do some newer treatment regimens that include administration of adrenocorticotropic hormone (ACTH), gabapentinoids, and repeated doses of hydrocortisone, with mixed results.

A treatment regimen being used to treat PDPH is the transnasal sphenopalatine ganglion block (SPGB). The SPGB is a noninvasive treatment first used in 1908 for the treatment of nasal headaches.[80] The sphenopalatine ganglion (SPG) is an extracranial neural structure located in the pterygopalatine fossa that has both sympathetic and parasympathetic components with somatic sensory roots. Blockade of the SPG has been used in the treatment of migraine headaches, trigeminal neuralgia, and PDPH in surgical, obstetric, and emergency room patients.[75,81,82]

An epidural blood patch is considered the definitive treatment for PDPH. Thought to work via clot formation that seals the dural puncture and increases CSF pressure, the epidural blood patch is associated with a greater than 90% cure rate. Clinically an epidural blood patch is performed in a manner similar to that of placing an epidural catheter. First, the availability of IV access is identified, usually in the antecubital fossa, and informed consent is obtained. Both the patient's back and IV access site are prepared and draped in an aseptic manner. An insertion site at or below the level of the lowest initial needle insertion is chosen because blood has been shown to spread in a predominantly cephalad direction within the epidural space. The epidural space is typically identified using a loss-of-resistance technique using normal saline or air as the medium (see Epidural Anesthesia, later). Autologous venous blood (~20 mL) is withdrawn from the vein and then slowly injected through the epidural needle into the epidural space. The injection proceeds until the patient senses pressure in the back, buttocks, or legs. Typically this occurs at a volume of 12 to 15 mL, which is a sufficient blood volume to patch most patients. Following injection, the needle is removed, and the patient is placed in a supine position for at least 30 minutes to 1 hour before being allowed to ambulate. Many patients will complain of low back pain, and placing a pillow under the knees while in the supine position will often help decrease their lower back discomfort. Relief of the headache is often instantaneous. In the rare case in which an epidural blood patch fails, a repeat blood patch may be attempted in 24 hours, with a similar success rate.[27,31,74]

The success rate and excellent safety record of the epidural blood patch encourage the use of this therapeutic option early in the treatment of PDPH, but it has been shown that success rates for its use in treating PDPH increase exponentially if placed greater than 24 hours after the dural puncture. Some risks, although minor or rare, are associated with this more invasive procedure. Backache, often associated with the administration of general, spinal, or epidural anesthetic techniques, occurs in up to 35% of patients after an epidural blood patch. Although rarely as debilitating as a PDPH, backache risk should be explained to the patient. The most common cause of backache is relaxation of the muscles of the back and flattening of the normal lordotic curve. As the muscles stretch, injury to tendons and ligaments can occur. The position of the patient might increase the severity of the problem. An exaggerated lithotomy position or a completely supine position can further increase tension on tendons, resulting in increased trauma to both the muscles and the tendons. Trauma from multiple punctures, hemorrhage, infections, use of large needles/retractors/forceps, extremes of positions, preexisting diseases such as arthritis and osteoporosis, and prolonged labor can contribute to backaches that may persist well into the postoperative period.[27,74]

Management of backache includes the use of antispasmodics and NSAIDs to reduce discomfort, permit ambulation, and promote a more rapid recovery. In addition, authors have reported a 5% incidence of transient (24- to 48-hour) temperature elevation, a 1% incidence of neck ache, radicular pain, nerve root irritation, cranial nerve palsy, and meningitis, although the cause of meningitis was unproven.[22,27,74]

Several caveats regarding the treatment of PDPH are worth mentioning. Systemic infection, perhaps indicated by fever, presents a relative contraindication to epidural blood patch and warrants a trial of pharmacologic intervention. The risk of neurologic sequelae after epidural blood patch in the presence of HIV infection or sepsis is controversial because few data are available, leading some authors to suggest alternative therapies such as epidural 0.9% sodium chloride or dextran or using the SPGB.[15,50,74] Prophylactic epidural blood patch placement has not been shown to be consistently successful.[31] In light of the relatively low incidence of PDPH and the effectiveness of the epidural blood patch, treatment should not begin until the problem exists. Finally, an alternative diagnosis should be sought if two epidural blood patches fail to resolve the patient's symptoms.[27,74]

Nausea

As with general anesthesia, intraoperative and postoperative nausea and vomiting (PONV) associated with CNB is a complex issue. Although it is believed PONV is less common with regional anesthesia techniques than general anesthesia techniques, agents such as propofol have considerably narrowed the incidence gap. Although not life threatening, PONV remains a significant concern for patients and clinicians. General strategies can be implemented to help reduce the incidence of this unpleasantness.

Nausea immediately after the initiation of CNB is often considered a sign of significant hypotension and an increasing block level. It is thought the nausea is secondary to the sudden onset of hypotension resulting in cerebral ischemia affecting the vomiting centers of the medulla, triggering nausea. Others posit gut ischemia leads to the release of emetogenic substances such as serotonin from enterochromaffin cells in the GI mucosa that pass into the systemic circulation and act directly on the central serotonin receptors in the vomiting center in the brain. Treatment for this SIH nausea is typically treated with fluid and sympathomimetic drug administration. Another contributing element may result from the sympathectomy caused by the onset of CNB. The resulting unopposed parasympathetic activity in the GI tract results in hyperactivity, possibly contributing to nausea. Evidence this may be the case is vagolytic agents such as atropine are efficacious in treating this nausea.[83]

Avoiding hypotension, providing adequate hydration, and supporting perfusion with supplemental oxygen are the basis of an antiemetic plan for CNB. Premedication and intraoperative sedation can significantly affect the incidence of intraoperative nausea and PONV. Clonidine does not influence the incidence of PONV, and evidence supports propofol has antiemetic effects. The addition of epinephrine to local anesthetics administered intrathecally for spinal anesthesia increases the incidence of nausea. Additionally, a dose-dependent increase in PONV occurs when intrathecal morphine is used. However, the addition of 20 mcg fentanyl or 2.5 to 5 mcg of sufentanil to spinal bupivacaine results in less intraoperative nausea compared with placebo. Similar strategies apply to epidural anesthesia, although opioid use must be matched to patient and case type to maximize analgesia while minimizing secondary effects.[83] Multimodal approaches that have been widely adapted should also be applied to PONV after regional anesthesia.[84]

Urinary Retention

Urinary retention is common after anesthesia and surgery with a reported incidence of between 5% and 70%. Spinal or epidural anesthetics block sympathetic fibers and increase the tone of the internal urethral sphincter. However, other factors often contribute to the risk of urinary retention after surgery and anesthesia. These include the type of surgical procedure, bladder distention from the administration of large volumes of IV fluids, bladder trauma, prolonged hypotension, incision pain, urethral edema caused by prolonged labor, benign prostatic hypertrophy, and the use of neuraxial or intraoperative opioids, anticholinergics, sympatholytics, and other drugs. Comorbidities, type of surgery, and type of anesthesia influence the development of postoperative urinary retention (POUR). The risk of retention is especially high after anorectal surgery, hernia repair, and orthopedic surgery and increases with advancing age. Certain anesthetic and analgesic modalities, particularly spinal anesthesia with long-acting local anesthetics, adding epinephrine and epidural analgesia, promote the development of urinary retention. Reasonable fluid administration with less than 1000 mL helps avoid bladder overdistention. Portable bladder ultrasound provides rapid and accurate assessment of bladder volume and aids in the diagnosis and management of POUR. Catheterization is recommended when bladder volume exceeds 600 mL to prevent the negative sequelae of prolonged bladder overdistention. Urinary retention and subsequent catheterization can lead to complications such as urinary tract infections and urethral strictures. Low-risk patients with less than 600 mL bladder volume may be sent home with instruction to return if they cannot void.[84-88]

Neurologic Risk

Patients greatly fear the perceived risk of paraplegia resulting from neuraxial anesthetics, and the seriousness of such complications warrants concern. Several very large series have shown the incidence of persistent motor paralysis is exceedingly rare (<1/10,000). Because neurologic sequelae are rare, the knowledge base of complications comes from case studies, and often the cause is not proved but rather inferred by association. Direct needle or catheter nerve injury, drug-related neurotoxicity, anterior spinal artery syndrome, undiagnosed neurologic disease, intraneural or intramedullary injections, the presence of blood in the CSF, patient positioning, hematomas, and abscesses are associated with permanent neurologic deficits. Therefore good clinical practice depends on (1) the use of appropriate anesthetic techniques minimizing risk and (2) conducting postoperative assessments in a manner that promotes early detection, diagnosis, and treatment, especially because reversibility of complications is often time dependent.[15,27,29,88,89]

Unexpected Cardiac Arrest

Cardiac arrest associated with neuraxial anesthesia is often sudden and unexpected and can result in severe neurologic injury and death. Additionally, this undesired complication occurs in a significant number of young, previously healthy patients. Estimates of occurrence are 7:10,000 for spinal anesthesia and 1:10,000 for epidural anesthesia. This suggests cardiac arrest is not such a rare event in neuraxial anesthesia. How then might it be differentiated from arrests under general anesthesia (3:10,000)?[90]

Because unexpected cardiac arrest with spinal anesthesia has been reported in previously healthy patients, some authors consider this a physiologic response to neuraxial blocks.[91] Other authors suggest a pattern of presentation with a gradual downward trend in heart rate followed by an abrupt onset of severe bradycardia or asystole.[11,92] Spinal anesthesia cardiac arrest can occur well after the onset of spinal blockade. Large recent retrospective studies note arrests can occur 20 to 60 minutes after the onset of spinal blockade and are frequently associated with intraoperative events such as significant blood loss and orthopedic cement placement.

The etiology of cardiac arrest during spinal block anesthesia is related to cardiocirculatory factors, mainly a reduction of preload resulting from sympathetic blockade. These decreases in preload may initiate reflexes causing severe bradycardia. Three reflex responses have been suggested. The first involves the pacemaker stretch. The rate of firing of these cells within the myocardium is proportional to the degree of stretch. Decreased venous return results in decreased stretch and a slower heart rate. The second reflex may be attributable to the firing of low-pressure baroreceptors in the right atrium and vena cava. The third is the paradoxic BJR reflex, in which mechanoreceptors in the left ventricle are stimulated and cause bradycardia.[92] Other factors increasing the risk of developing cardiac arrest include changes in patient positioning and hypovolemia.

Maintaining preload should be a priority, and prophylactic preloading or coloading with a bolus of IV fluid should not be omitted before initiating spinal anesthesia. It is important to institute treatment as soon as possible. Standard regimens for volume preloading may not be sufficient to maintain adequate preload, so a low threshold for administering additional fluid boluses, using vasopressors or repositioning the patient to augment venous return, may be appropriate. For patients with bradycardia during spinal anesthesia, the stepwise escalation of treatment of bradycardia with atropine (0.4–0.6 mg), ephedrine (25–50 mg), and, if necessary, epinephrine (0.2–0.3 mg) may be appropriate. For severe bradycardia or cardiac arrest, full resuscitation doses of epinephrine should be promptly administered.[91-94]

Auditory, Ocular, and Facial Complications

Unexpected complications or complications a patient may not ascribe to anesthesia may be unreported or underreported, especially if they are transient in nature and not life threatening. The complications of transient hypoacusis or hearing loss and retinal hemorrhage are thought to be caused by changes in CSF pressure, either from postdural puncture leaks or increases in pressure from the epidural administration of a large volume of solution. Epidural injection of 8 to 16 mL of fluid can increase CSF pressure by 85 cm H_2O for several minutes before compensation occurs. Horner syndrome (i.e., ptosis, miosis, anhidrosis, and enophthalmos) and trigeminal nerve palsy probably result from a high spread of local anesthetic to the sympathetic fibers of the head and neck and to cranial nerve V, respectively. These problems are usually self-limiting; however, knowledge of their previous occurrence enables the compassionate anesthetist to provide counsel and reassurance to anxious patients.[32,94]

EPIDURAL ANESTHESIA

Epidural anesthesia is a central neuraxial block that can be used for a wide variety of procedures. Unlike spinal anesthesia that results in an all-or-none block, epidural anesthesia can be titrated to deliver either analgesia or anesthesia for a wide variety of surgical and analgesic procedures. Epidural anesthesia allows the anesthesia practitioner better control of the extent of sensory and motor blockade than is offered by spinal anesthesia. The luxury of placing an epidural catheter that can be used before, during, and for an extended period after any surgical procedure is another advantage. The general indications for epidural anesthesia are the same as those outlined for spinal anesthesia, with the distinct difference that an epidural allows for continuous anesthesia secondary to placement of an epidural catheter. This makes epidural anesthesia more suitable for procedures of long duration and for extended use in the postoperative period to deliver long-term, titratable analgesia.

Local anesthetics or other analgesic solutions injected into the epidural space spread anatomically. Horizontally, medication spreads to the regions of the dural cuffs, where it can diffuse into the CSF and leak into the intravertebral foramen and paravertebral spaces to achieve analgesia/anesthesia. Longitudinally, medication spreads in a cephalad direction, with possible sites of anesthetic action along the paravertebral nerve trunks, intradural spinal roots, dorsal and ventral spinal roots, the dorsal root ganglia, the spinal cord, and the brain. Initial blockade is probably a result of anesthetic blockade at the spinal roots within the dural sleeves.[4] The dural cuffs or sleeves have a proliferation of arachnoid villi and granulations that effectively reduce the thickness of the dura mater, permitting rapid diffusion of anesthetics from the epidural space through the dura and into the CSF. Differences in physicochemical properties of anesthetics (e.g., lipid solubility) may account for the differences in diffusion rates across the dura, which contributes to the variances seen in sensory, motor, and sympathetic blockade.[5] Because epidural anesthesia is diffusion dependent, relatively large volumes (20 mL) of local anesthetics must be used to achieve anesthesia as compared with spinal anesthesia, which routinely only requires 1 to 2 mL. In addition, because epidural anesthesia requires the medication be delivered to the subarachnoid space by the process of diffusion and spread, anesthesia takes significantly longer to achieve than spinal anesthesia. Given these caveats, any procedure that can be done with the patient under spinal anesthesia can also be done under epidural anesthesia.[4] However, epidural techniques allow for the placement of a continuous catheter, which is especially useful in cases of unpredictable duration, for prolonged postoperative analgesia, and for chronic pain control. In addition, labor epidural analgesia is the only method currently available that can relieve most of the discomfort of labor while minimally affecting maternal or fetal physiology. Labor epidural analgesia is highly satisfactory in these patients because it permits their participation in a comfortable delivery and allows maternal-infant bonding after delivery. Labor analgesia also satisfies obstetricians and anesthesia practitioners in that its flexibility allows quick conversion from an analgesic technique to a surgical anesthetic technique for cesarean section.

Equipment and Techniques

Patient preparation, positioning, and the availability of emergency equipment and monitors are similar to the preparation for a spinal anesthetic. With a spinal anesthetic, the practitioner seeks CSF by piercing the dura, while the tip of the epidural needle seeks the fat-filled space deep to the ligamentum flavum and shallow to the dura. The standard epidural needle is typically 16 to 18 gauge and 3.5 in long, with a blunted bevel and gentle curve of 15 to 30 degrees at the tip. This blunt bevel and curve allow the needle to pass through the skin and ligamentum flavum and abut against the dura, rather than penetrate through the dura. The two most common epidural needles used in clinical practice with a curvature at the blunt bevel are the Tuohy and Hustead needle designs. The Tuohy needle has the most pronounced curvature (30 degrees) at the tip and is often cited as the easiest for beginning practitioners to place because it allows directional placement of the epidural catheter into the space, and the curved, blunt tip is less likely to penetrate into the subarachnoid space. However, it has also been noted that placement of the Tuohy needle can be more difficult because the tip's exaggerated curvature is too blunt, inhibiting penetration through the skin and ligamentum flavum as compared with

other needle tips. The Hustead needle is an intermediate needle with a less-pronounced 15-degree curvature that can more easily pass though skin and ligamentum flavum.

A third epidural needle is the Crawford needle. It is a thin-walled epidural needle that does not have the curvature of the Tuohy or Hustead needle. The straight tip may allow easier access through the skin into the epidural space. The Crawford needle is preferred by practitioners when catheter advancement into the epidural space is difficult or the angle of approach is steep, as encountered with thoracic epidural catheter placement. Because the Crawford needle lacks the curvature at the bevel end, it has also been implicated in a higher ratio of accidental dural punctures and is typically not used by beginning practitioners. These three common epidural needles are shown in Fig. 49.14. Smaller-gauge (20–22) epidural needles are available in each needle design for pediatric catheter techniques, regional blocks, and specialty use. Many needle designs incorporate wings near the base or hub. The wings provide a grip for the practitioner that permits distribution of pressure equally over the needle during insertion. The wings and notches in the hub also align with the stylet and needle tip to indicate the direction of the needle tip's bevel and lumen. Needles also may have clear hubs to allow early detection of blood or CSF, plastic stylets to prevent coring, and 0.5- or 1-cm depth markings along the needle shaft.

Epidural catheters also come in a variety of materials and designs. Typically, catheter diameter is 2 gauges smaller than the needle. For example, a 20-gauge catheter would be used with an 18-gauge Tuohy needle. Catheters are constructed of physiologically inert materials designed to resist kinking, compression, and stretching and should be radiopaque. The two most common epidural catheters used in clinical practice are the single-holed, open-ended (uniport) and the lateral-holed, closed-tip (multiport) epidural catheters. Each catheter design is reported to offer several advantages and disadvantages. Studies that have compared the differences in catheter designs show a significantly lower incidence of inadequate analgesia with stiff multiport catheters but a higher incidence of inadvertent IV cannulation.[95] The flexible uniport and multiport epidural catheters show no differences in analgesia success rate or complication rate.[96] Catheters have markings that identify the tip of the catheter to help verify removal of the catheter and identify when the catheter is at the tip of the needle, with 1-cm markings to measure depth of catheter placement. The depth that a catheter should be threaded beyond the needle tip and into the epidural space is often a controversial topic. Manufacturers of epidural catheters recommend that a catheter should be threaded 1 to 3 cm into the epidural space to avoid possible migration into an epidural vein or through an intravertebral foramen.[15,97] However, in clinical practice practitioners noted that when an epidural catheter was only threaded 1 to 3 cm, a higher incidence of epidural catheter failure could result. Many practitioners reported anecdotally that when the catheter was threaded 3 to 5 cm into the epidural space, a higher success rate without a resultant increase in migration into an epidural vein or intravertebral foramen occurred. This routine clinical practice was validated by Beilin et al.[97] They reported that a catheter insertion of less than 3 cm resulted in a higher incidence of inadequate analgesia, and an insertion depth of more than 5 cm resulted in an increase in inadvertent IV cannulation. They recommended that optimal catheter insertion should be 3 to 5 cm into the epidural space.

Proper patient positioning is important to ensure successful catheter placement. Epidural anesthesia is most often instituted with the patient in the sitting or lateral decubitus position and the landmarks, aseptic preparation, draping, and localization are similar to those for a spinal anesthetic. The spine should be in proper alignment, using pillows or pads if necessary, and intervertebral spaces should be identified and marked prior to preparation of the patient's back (see Fig. 49.10).

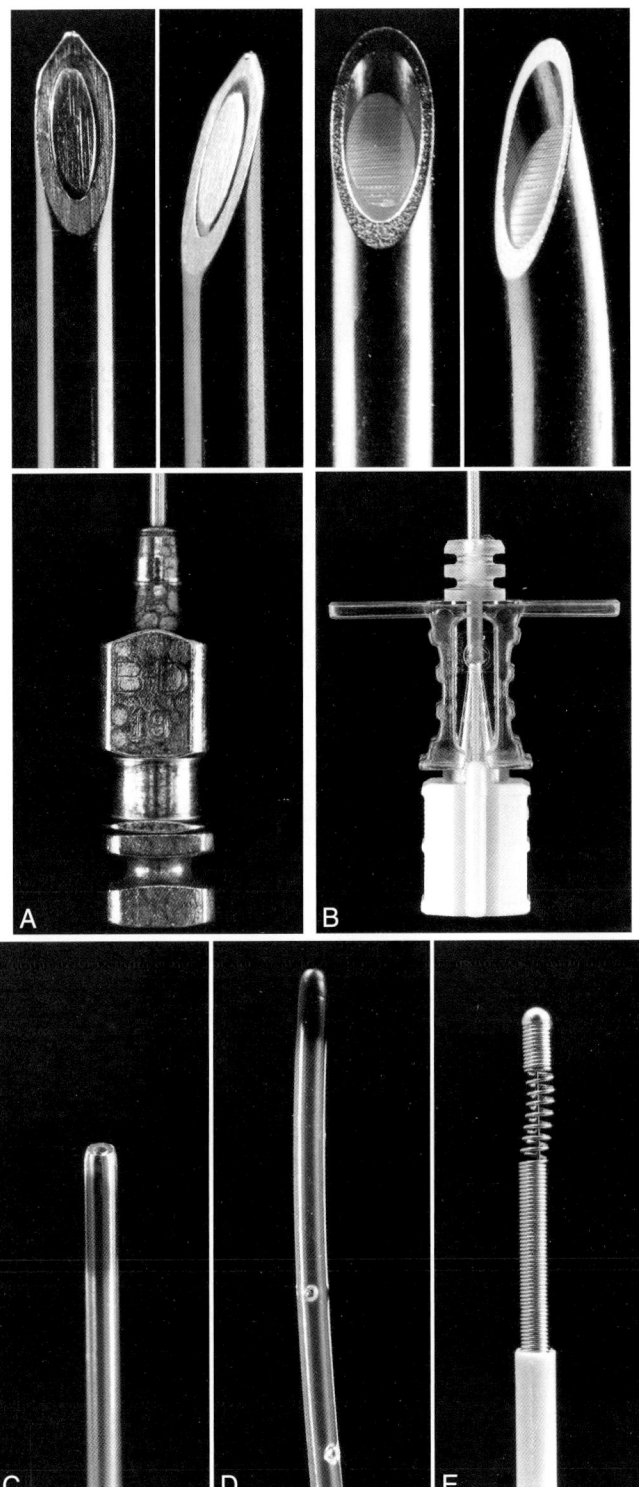

Fig. 49.14 Epidural needles with catheter assortment. (A) A 19-gauge reusable Crawford epidural needle. (B) A 19-gauge disposable Tuohy needle. (C) Single–end-hole epidural catheter. (D) Closed-tip, multiple–side-hole catheter. (E) Spring wire–reinforced, polymer-coated epidural catheter. (From Gropper MA., et al. *Miller's Anesthesia.* 9th ed. Philadelphia: Elsevier; 2020:1435.)

In contrast to thin, flexible spinal needles, epidural needles are larger and more rigid. Therefore, placement of the epidural needle does not require an introducer needle and offers better directional control; however, all needle-handling techniques must anticipate patient movement. Whether inserting a spinal or epidural needle into a patient, a similar controlled grip is used to accommodate for potential patient movement. This grip, described earlier as the Bromage grip (see Fig. 49.13), allows the patient's body to act as a firm support for the needle-stabilizing hand and helps prevent advancement or withdrawal of the needle tip from its position (1) if the patient should move, (2) when the syringe is applied, and (3) as a catheter is passed into the epidural space. The needle is placed bevel tip cephalad through the supraspinous ligament and seated in the interspinous ligament before the stylet is removed. After the stylet is removed, the needle is slowly advanced by use of either the hanging-drop technique or the loss-of-resistance technique into the epidural space.[5]

After the needle is seated in the interspinous ligament, the hanging-drop technique is accomplished by filling the hub of the needle with saline. The surface tension of the saline creates a droplet hanging on the needle hub. The needle is then advanced slowly in a slight cephalad orientation toward the epidural space. As the needle is advanced through the ligamentous structures, the drop should not move; however, as the tip of the needle enters the epidural space, the negative pressure within the space will cause the drop of fluid to be drawn into the needle. This aspiration of the hanging drop into the needle signifies that the needle has successfully entered the epidural space. It should be noted that if the needle becomes plugged or the negative pressure in the epidural space is very low, the drop will not be drawn into the hub of the needle and passage into the epidural space will not be recognized. A dural puncture could result. Therefore the hanging-drop technique is not recommended for the novice practitioner.[5]

The loss-of-resistance technique is the most common method used to enter the epidural space. The epidural needle is placed through the dermis into the interspinous ligament or ligamenta flava, at which time the stylet of the epidural needle is removed. Once the needle has been firmly seated into the ligament, a loss-of-resistance syringe (plastic or glass) containing 2 to 3 mL of normal saline or air and a freely movable plunger is attached. If the needle is properly seated in the ligament, it should be difficult to inject the normal saline or air, and slight pressure on the syringe plunger should result in the plunger springing back to its original position. Some practitioners use a combination of saline and air in the syringe during the loss-of-resistance technique, using approximately 3 mL of normal saline and a small air bubble (0.1–0.3 mL). They report this provides them with a more compressible feel for entry into the ligamentum flavum. If the air bubble cannot be compressed without injecting the normal saline, the needle is most likely not seated into the ligamentum flavum and may still be in the interspinous ligament or off midline into the paraspinous muscles. The needle is advanced toward the epidural space by application of pressure to the needle, not the syringe or syringe plunger. If normal saline is used, constant pressure may be applied to the syringe plunger. Contact with the needle or needle wings is maintained to control needle advancement. As the needle passes through the ligamentum flavum, resistance increases, and it is very difficult to inject either saline or air. Once the bevel of the needle completes passage through the ligamenta flava and enters the epidural space, an immediate loss of resistance occurs. The contents of the syringe can then be injected gently and without resistance. After the syringe is removed from the needle, an outward rush of a small amount of air or fluid may occur. Penetration of the dura with a large epidural needle usually results in profuse return of CSF; the needle should be removed immediately to minimize CSF loss.

The loss of resistance experienced by a beginning practitioner, or by the experienced practitioner in a patient with difficult anatomy, may not be easily discerned. Sometimes it may be necessary to further evaluate the needle tip's location. For example, several milliliters of air can be injected through the needle while the soft tissue lateral to the spinous process is palpated. If crepitus is felt, the needle is most likely located in the tissues adjacent and shallow to the spinous process. If fluid returns from either the needle or catheter, CSF can be distinguished from normal saline or local anesthetic. CSF is warm to the forearm, compared with recently administered room-temperature fluids. Glucose test paper will detect the glucose in CSF. Multiple tests should be used to achieve the most accurate confirmation of fluid type.

Once the practitioner is reassured of the needle tip's position, an epidural catheter is threaded through the needle and into the epidural space to a depth of 3 to 5 cm. As the catheter is passed into the epidural space, a paresthesia (i.e., funny-bone sensation down one or both legs) may indicate the catheter has brushed by a nerve root as it was passing into the epidural space or perhaps even lodged into the nerve root. If the paresthesia is persistent prior to or after needle removal, the catheter must be withdrawn and replaced. Injection of medication into a patient complaining of persistent paresthesia can result in nerve root damage or even nerve root death and cause long-term morbidities. If the catheter is being replaced secondary to a persistent paresthesia, it is best to move to a new interspace to avoid oversensitized nerve roots. It is important that the needle remain stabilized during catheter advancement. Often if a patient experiences a paresthesia during threading of the catheter, the patient will move reflexively. Unanticipated movement and an uncontrolled needle could result in inadvertent subarachnoid puncture. Once the catheter is threaded approximately 3 to 5 cm, the needle is withdrawn slowly over the catheter. It is common practice to note the depth of the catheter at the level of the skin (by noting the centimeter depth mark on the catheter) both prior to and after removal of the epidural needle. Once the epidural needle is removed, the catheter depth should be noted and documented. If the catheter was inadvertently threaded deeper than desired into the epidural space, it should be slightly withdrawn to the desired depth as noted at the level of the skin. If the catheter migrated out of the epidural space, again the depth should be observed and recorded. Finally, if the depth into the epidural space is less than 1 cm, replacement of the catheter should be considered before any attempts are made to inject through the catheter. Never attempt to withdraw the catheter through the needle! This can shear the catheter tip and embed foreign material in the patient's back. Surgical intervention may be required for catheter remnant removal.

Once a catheter is placed and the needle removed safely, a catheter-to-syringe adapter is placed on the free catheter end. Observe the clear catheter as it enters the back. Look for backflow of CSF or blood. Owing to the greater resistance of a long and narrow catheter compared with a needle, gravity flow alone may not reveal the presence of blood or CSF. Therefore gentle syringe aspiration is applied to the catheter via the adapter. Because tissue at the catheter tip may create a ball-valve effect, CSF or blood may not flow out; therefore a negative aspiration test does not guarantee that the catheter tip is in the epidural space. Only if fluids do return does this test confirm that the catheter tip is placed into either an epidural vein or the subarachnoid space. The return of CSF or blood indicates that the catheter should be removed and replaced at a different interspace. To avoid this ball-valve effect or to dislodge any skin or tissue that may have lodged at the catheter tip, some practitioners advocate injection of 1 to 2 mL of normal saline solution through the catheter to confirm catheter patency before injection of medications. After needle removal, the catheter should be taped away from the midline of the back to avoid spinous processes and

minimize the risks of catheter displacement from the epidural space or pressure injuries over bony prominences.

Prior to injection of a large amount of medication into an epidural space, a test dose of a small amount of medication is administered to determine whether the catheter or needle has inadvertently entered the subarachnoid space or possibly threaded into an epidural vein. A test dose of 3 mL of a rapid-acting, low-toxicity local anesthetic agent with or without a small concentration of epinephrine is most typically used. A lidocaine 1.5% with 1:200,000 epinephrine solution provides 45 mg of lidocaine with 15 mcg of epinephrine per 3-mL dose. If the needle or catheter tip is in the subarachnoid space, this dose will result in spinal anesthesia within 3 minutes. If the same test dose is injected into a blood vessel, the 15 mcg of epinephrine will result in a 20% rise in heart rate and systolic blood pressure within 30 seconds. The patient also may experience sensations from the intravascular lidocaine, describing symptoms such as tinnitus, a metallic taste, circumoral numbness, or a rushing sound in the ears. The duration of these test-dose effects is less than 5 minutes. After the test dose is injected, vital signs are reassessed. Additionally, 100 mcg of undiluted fentanyl can be injected as a test dose to avoid potential complications caused by even low doses of epinephrine. If the needle or catheter is intravascular, the patient will experience immediate dizziness and sleepiness from the opioid. Despite all efforts to avoid them, systemic toxic reactions can still occur. Be vigilant, be cautious, and be prepared to handle emergencies.[99-102]

Epidural anesthesia also can be administered by direct injection through the needle once it has been placed into the epidural space. This is called a single-shot epidural anesthesia technique, and the same contraindications and safety precautions apply as those already reported for catheter insertion. Once the needle is placed into the epidural space, the end of the open needle is observed for the presence of blood or CSF. Allow a few seconds for gravity flow of fluids to detect blood or CSF when the single-shot technique is used, then attach a syringe for medication administration using needle control techniques previously discussed.

Epidural anesthesia can be performed at any of the four segments of the spine but is most typically performed at the lumbar level. As with spinal anesthesia, there are two approaches (midline and paramedian), which are used to facilitate placement of the epidural needle into the epidural space. The most common approach is the midline because it is the easiest to perform and helps place the catheter in the medial region of the epidural space. The paramedian approach is usually selected when surgery or degenerative joint disease contraindicate the midline approach. Using the paramedian approach is more difficult for the beginner because advancement into the interspinous ligament does not occur. The needle advances primarily through paraspinous muscle mass, and resistance is only felt when entering the ligamentum flavum. The technique for paramedian placement involves identification of the desired interspace and the spinous process. The skin surface area approximately 3 cm lateral to the lowest aspect of the spinous process is prepped and anesthetized. The epidural needle is then placed through the anesthetized region and directed toward the midline using a slight cephalad orientation. Once the dermal levels are penetrated and the paraspinous muscle mass encountered, the needle stylet is removed and a syringe containing either air or normal saline (or both) is attached, and the epidural needle is advanced. The midline of the spine should be encountered approximately 3 to 5 cm from the entry point. The needle is advanced slowly using the incremental approach described earlier through the ligamenta flava and then into the epidural space. When a paramedian approach is required by difficult surface anatomy or a steep approach to the thoracic levels is anticipated, the Crawford needle may be preferred. The Crawford needle's straight, blunt bevel allows the catheter to pass directly through the end of the needle, thus facilitating threading of the catheter.

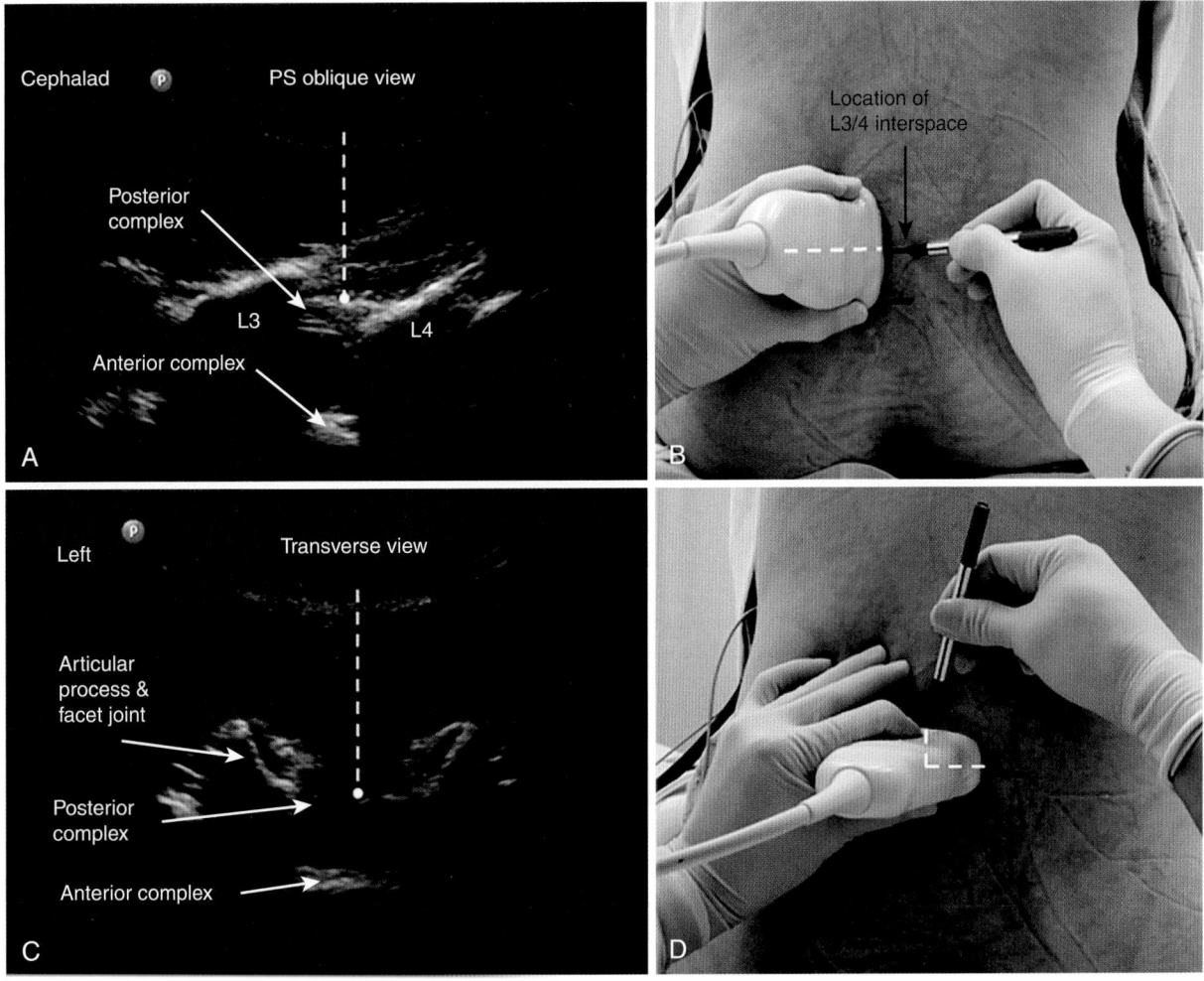

Fig. 49.15 Orientation of ultrasound probe and identification of underlying structures. A. Paramedian Sagittal (PS) ultrasound view of the L3/L4 interspace. B. PS or longitudinal ultrasound probe placement at the skin identifying the L3/L4 interspace. C. Transverse ultrasound view of the spinal midline at the lumbar level. D. Transverse ultrasound probe placement at the skin identifying the lumbar interspace midline. (From Chin KJ, Karmakar MK, Peng P. Ultrasonography of the adult thoracic and lumbar spine for central neuraxial blockade. *Anesthesiology.* 2011;114[6]:1459-1485 [fig 8]. [Article states permission was from www.usra.ca].)

Ultrasound Epidural Placement

The loss of resistance technique using air, normal saline, or a combination of air/normal saline is the gold standard method used by anesthesia practitioners to identify the entry into the epidural space. Traditionally epidural needle placement at a desired interspinous level is determined by palpation of anatomic landmarks; however, appreciating these landmarks can be extremely difficult in some patients. This difficulty could be secondary to obesity and/or scoliosis of the spine, which often require multiple passes with the epidural needle before proper placement or completely abandoning attempted placement secondary to an inability to find the epidural space. Despite considerable improvement in the quality of needles and epidural catheters within the last 30 years, the techniques for identification of the epidural space have remained the same, and, as described previously, using these techniques to identify the epidural space can be impossible in some individuals.

Ultrasound can now be used to facilitate placement of spinal and epidural analgesia/anesthesia. It has been found to be particularly useful in determining the spinous and transverse processes, thereby facilitating easier placement.[36,102,103] In addition, ultrasonography also allows the anesthesia provider to adequately determine the distance from the skin to the epidural space, which may result in a lower

incidence of accidental dural punctures. Two useful acoustic windows can be used to assess lumbar spine anatomy. One of these windows is assessed using a transverse midline approach, whereas the other is assessed using a paramedian longitudinal approach (Fig. 49.15). The transverse midline approach allows the anesthetist to adequately identify the midline, whereas the paramedian longitudinal approach allows for assessment of the interspace. In addition, the depth to the epidural space can be determined using ultrasound equipment.

In contrast to the ultrasound machines used for peripheral nerve blocks, which operate using a high-frequency linear probe (10–15 MHz), the ultrasound probe used for spinal and epidural placement needs to be low frequency (2–5 MHz). These low-frequency probes are traditionally curvilinear or convex probes, and of the same type used routinely on pregnant women in labor and delivery to assess fetal function. The ultrasound can be used to identify the epidural space, depth, and position, or it can be used to facilitate real-time viewing of epidural needle placement into the epidural space. The technique of using one or two operators is well described in the literature.

Technique

An ultrasound machine that is capable of deep scans and equipped with a low-frequency (2- to 5-MHz) curvilinear probe should be used to facilitate the scan. Two different approaches (longitudinal paramedian and transverse midline) are used to help identify spinous processes, articular processes, ligamentum flavum, anterior dura mater, posterior dura mater, and depth to epidural and subarachnoid space.[104] The patient is placed in a lateral position with flexed knees and hips or in a sitting position with the back curved, as described for the landmark technique. After proper positioning of the patient, the low-frequency ultrasound probe is placed over the sacral area, 3 cm left of midline and slightly angled toward the center of the spine. The hyperechoic (white) line of the sacrum is identified, and then the probe is moved slowly cephalad until hyperechoic sawlike images are seen (see Fig. 49.15A). These sawlike projections are the verterbral lamina, and between the sawlike images are the interlaminar space. Next the ligamentum flavum, posterior dura mater, and vertebral body are identified, and the exact level of each interspace. The spinous process is centered in the screen, and a mark is placed on the skin at the center of the ultrasound probe. The probe is then placed horizontal along the midline of the spine at the marked levels of the interspaces and spinous processes. The hyperechoic spinous process is identified using the long triangular hypoechoic (darker) shadow. The probe is moved caudad or cephalad to capture the best view of the interspace, ligamentum flavum, and dorsal dura mater. The midline is marked on the skin at the center of the ultrasound probe. The insertion point is determined by the intersection of the extensions of the two marks on the skin in the vertical and horizontal planes. One mark identifies the midline and the other identifies the interspace (see Fig. 49.15D). Once a clear image is obtained, the screen is frozen, and depth to the epidural or subarachnoid space is obtained using the ultrasound machine calipers; one prong of the calipers is placed at the skin and the other at the inner side of the ligamentum flavum.[105]

Epidural Drugs, Spread, and Block Levels

As with any anesthetic technique, the clinical success of epidural anesthesia is often dependent on experience because multiple factors must be managed and balanced to provide safe patient care. Two of these factors, dose and the site of injection, are the most important factors in determining the extent of dermatomal blockade. It should be remembered that the size of the segmental epidural space increases down the spinal cord as the spinal cord occupies less and less space. For example, when a very small volume of local anesthetic is injected into the cervical region, it will spread across a larger number of segments as compared to when the same volume is injected into the thoracic region. This is also true when comparing the dermatomal spread between the thoracic and lumbar or caudal regions. The suggested dose of local anesthetic is dependent on the location of the catheter tip as it lies in the epidural space. Common clinical practice is to insert the epidural needle at a vertebral interspace such that the catheter tip falls near the middle of the spinal dermatomes of the proposed surgical incision. For example, an epidural catheter placed for labor or lower abdominal anesthesia would be placed at the L2 or L3 interspace. Placement would be at T8-T10 for upper abdominal surgery, T4-T5 for thoracic surgery, and C7-T1 for chronic pain treatments or surgeries of the arms, shoulders, or upper chest. This has several advantages. The catheter tip, being at the relative center of the spread of the local anesthetic, creates an area of high concentration at the spinal nerves specific to the site of the operation with the least amount of local anesthetic. This high concentration at a specific location results in rapid block onset and greater block density, which often creates a differential blockade that can be controlled by dose.

Dose is described as volume multiplied by concentration. The concentration of the local anesthetic generally affects the density of the block, whereas the volume, within limits, affects the spread from the

needle or catheter tip throughout the epidural space. Successful analgesia can be achieved with relatively small volumes and relatively low concentrations of local anesthetics. To achieve anesthesia, larger volumes with higher concentrations are typically necessary. Clinically useful doses are based on volumes that permit an even filling of the anterior and posterior epidural spaces at the level of insertion. For example, the suggested volumes per segment at the cervical and thoracic levels are 0.7 to 1 mL per segment, remembering that the spread will occur in both a cephalad and caudad fashion. Therefore an initial total dose, usually less than 10 mL, will achieve a 10- to 14-dermatomal spread of local anesthetic. In contrast, when the local anesthetic is injected at the lumbar level, the volume of local anesthetic required is 1.25 to 1.5 mL per segment. A typical initial volume of 15 to 20 mL is required to ensure adequate anesthesia by blocking a total of 12 to 16 segments (6–8 segments above and below the catheter tip). It should also be remembered that spread of blockade tends to occur faster in the cephalad direction from the catheter tip, possibly because thoracic nerve roots are smaller in diameter than large lumbar and sacral nerve roots.[4,5,8]

Other factors thought to affect the level of blockade achieved with epidural anesthesia include height, weight, age, patient position during injection, pregnancy, and the speed or mode of injection. However, the clinical significance of these factors has been challenged. Correlations between patient height and weight and the spread of the epidural block are clinically insignificant, except perhaps in the extremely tall, short, or morbidly obese patient. Studies have examined patients in the sitting and lateral positions during administration of epidural anesthetics and found small differences in spread and onset that favor the dependent portion of the patient's body. Therefore, provision of anesthesia to the sacral roots might be facilitated by having the patient sit up during the injection. In addition, leaving the patient on the operative side after the solution is injected may speed onset. However, these are clinically small differences and may not always be effective.

Drugs should be injected slowly into the epidural space to avoid rapid increases in CSF pressure, headache, and increased intracranial pressure. A rapid speed of injection has not been shown to increase the spread of anesthetic. In addition, incremental or bolus injection modes appear to have no influence on spread. The spread of epidural anesthetics may be 3 or 4 dermatomes greater in elderly patients due to age-related tissue changes creating a less compliant and less leaky epidural space. Although conflicting data exist, some studies suggest that the epidural spread of anesthetics is greater in pregnant patients.[4,5,8] It is recommended that the volume of anesthetic solution administered to pregnant patients and elderly patients should initially be limited to 0.5 to 1 mL per segment when injected at lumbar levels.

The density of block is more dependent on the concentration of local anesthetic used. The lower the concentration, the lower the effect the local anesthetic will have on the degree of sensory and motor blockade. Routinely a lower concentration of local anesthetic is used to facilitate analgesia (as in laboring analgesia) or to provide a sympathectomy. If the primary purpose of the epidural is to provide complete surgical anesthesia, higher concentrations must be used. Table 49.6 lists recommended volumes of local anesthetic to achieve anesthesia based on the position of the catheter and the location of the intended surgical intervention. All solutions should be injected in increments of 3 to 5 mL every 3 minutes and titrated to the desired anesthetic level. With loading doses and intermittent injections, aspiration of the catheter should occur before any injection. This gradual administration of the medication slows the rate of onset of the anesthetic level and controls the development of the sympathetic blockade. After a loading dose is given, the anesthetic is maintained with either intermittent dosing or a continuous infusion technique.

TABLE 49.6 Recommended Doses for Epidural Anesthesia

Procedure	Position of Catheter	Dose (mL)
Chest	T12–L2	8–12
Upper Abdomen		
Cholecystectomy	L2	12–16
Gastric resection	L2	12–16
Incisional pain	L2	7–10
Lower Abdomen		
Colon resection	L2	12–16
Repair of aortic aneurysm	L2	12–16
Retropubic prostatectomy	L3	12–16
Herniorrhaphy	L3	8–12
Incisional pain	L3	8–12
Pancreatic pain	L3	5–7
Hysterectomy	L3	10–14
Lower Extremities		
Anesthesia	L4	10–14
Sympathetic block	L2	5–7
Perineum		
Transurethral resection of prostate	L4	8–12
Vaginal hysterectomy	L4	8–12
Back and Flank		
Nephrectomy	L2	10–14
Vaginal Delivery		
First-stage labor	L3	5–7
Second-, third-stage labor	L3	10–12

Intermittent injections are most often used when high concentrations of local anesthetic (2% lidocaine or 0.5% bupivacaine) are administered. A continuous infusion is more appropriate when the goal of the epidural is to provide a consistent level of analgesia. Continuous infusions typically use a lower concentration of local anesthetic solution (0.0625%–0.125% bupivacaine or 0.1%–0.2% ropivacaine), and the level of block is monitored at regular intervals. A continuous opioid infusion may also be used either as a sole agent or as an admixture with low concentrations of local anesthetic. Typical infusion rates range from as low as 2 mL/hour for concentrated hydrophilic opioid solutions, such as preservative-free morphine, up to 20 mL/hour for dilute solutions of local anesthesia (0.125% bupivacaine or 0.1% ropivacaine) used for postoperative or labor analgesia. Often continuous infusions will contain a dilute concentration of local anesthetic solution with an admixture of a low-dose lipophilic opioid such as fentanyl (1–5 mcg/mL) or sufentanil (1–1.5 mcg/mL). Epidural infusions of these mixtures augment the quality and duration of analgesia while limiting the side effects of any one drug.

Epidural Opioids

Opioids placed into the epidural space may undergo uptake into the epidural fat, systemic absorption, or diffusion across the dura into the CSF.[106] When administered via the epidural route, opioids produce considerable CSF concentrations of drug. Penetration of the dura from the epidural space into the subarachnoid space is influenced by lipid solubility and molecular weight. The administration of an epidural opioid by either an intermittent or continuous infusion has become common in many anesthesia practices. When an opioid is administered epidurally, it needs to cross from the epidural space through the dura to reach the opioid receptors located in the substantia gelatinosa in the spinal cord. Besides the physical barrier of the dura, epidural opioids also may be deposited in the fat and connective tissues in the epidural space, which may significantly increase the opioid dose required to achieve analgesia. In fact, to achieve adequate analgesia from epidurally administered opioids, the dose is increased by approximately 10 times the opioid dose administered intrathecally. The epidural space is also highly vascularized, and there is significant absorption of the opioids into the systemic circulation; however, the rate of absorption is dependent on individual pharmacokinetics and lipid solubility of the opioid. For example, epidural administration of fentanyl and sufentanil (highly lipid-soluble opioids) results in a serologic level of opioid similar to that produced when the drugs are administered intravenously. When an opioid is administered by the epidural route, the onset of action and the duration are dependent on the type of drug used. A faster onset and analgesic peak effect is achieved when a more lipophilic opioid is used versus an opioid that is more hydrophilic. Epidural opioids can be administered by either a single bolus dose or a continuous infusion. A continuous infusion provides easier analgesic titration to patient requirements, which is especially important when a shorter-acting opioid such as fentanyl is used. Epidural opioids can also be administered using patient-controlled (assisted) epidural analgesia (PCEA), which is a hybrid of continuous infusion and patient-assisted boluses to titrate analgesic requirements based on individual patient needs. The goal is to establish a continuous or basal rate infusion to optimize the analgesic effect. The PCEA bolus component can then be preset by the anesthesia practitioner to meet individual patient requirements and used in the event of breakthrough pain.[106] Table 49.7 lists the opioids and dosages most commonly used to achieve epidural-based analgesia.

Extended-release epidural morphine (DepoDur). A sustained-release formulation of morphine sulfate (DepoDur) is available for use in the treatment of acute postoperative pain. DepoDur consists of microscopic spherical particles with integral aqueous chambers separated by lipid membranes containing an encapsulated dose of morphine. DepoDur is unique in that it delivers standard morphine sulfate using DepoFoam technology. DepoFoam is a drug-delivery system composed of multivesicular lipid particles containing nonconcentric aqueous chambers that encapsulate the morphine sulfate, allowing the morphine to be released over an extended period of time (up to 48 hours) without a requirement for subsequent dosing.[107-109] The half-life of DepoDur is dose dependent, but the DepoFoam technology allows for larger doses to be administered than could be given when conventional epidural injection is used. For example, a study done by Carvalho et al.[107] compared analgesia and side effects in groups of cesarean section patients receiving either a single epidural injection of 5 mg of preservative-free morphine or 5, 10, or 15 mg of DepoDur. After cord clamp, the authors noted that patients who received the 10- and 15-mg doses of DepoDur had significantly lower pain scores and analgesic requirements for the first 48 hours after cesarean delivery. A prospective audit of patients undergoing open and laparoscopic colorectal procedures demonstrated that the use of DepoDur, as part of an enhanced recovery program, resulted in 81% of patients at 24 hours and 62% of patients at 48 hours requiring only nonopioid analgesics postoperatively.[109]

TABLE 49.7   Recommended Doses of Epidural Opioids

| Agent | ANALGESIA | | | | CONTINUOUS INFUSION RATE | | | |
	Bolus Dose	Onset (min)	Peak (min)	Duration (hr)	Range (mL/hr)	Basal Rate (mL/hr)	PCEA Bolus (mL)	Interval (min)
Morphine	3–5 mg	20–30	30–60	12–24				
Morphine 0.05%–0.1% solution					1–6			
Morphine 0.05%–0.1% + bupivacaine 0.0625%–0.125%					3–6	3–4	1	20
Morphine 0.05%–0.1% + ropivacaine 0.08%–0.2%					2–4	3–4	10	20
Meperidine	25–100 mg	5–10	10–30	4–6				
Meperidine 0.1%–0.25% bupivacaine 0.0625%–0.125%					2–10	5	1	12
Hydromorphone	1 mg	10–15	20–30	8–15				
Hydromorphone 0.05%					0.8			
Fentanyl	50–100 mcg	5–10	20	2–6				
Fentanyl 0.001%–0.002%					4–12			
Fentanyl 0.001% + bupivacaine 0.0625%–0.1%					4–10	5	1	12
Sufentanil	10–60 mcg	5–10	20–30	4–6				
Sufentanil 0.0001%					10			

DepoDur is intended to be used as a sole agent and cannot be administered concomitantly with a local anesthetic solution. Because DepoDur is encapsulated by DepoFoam technology, studies have shown that administration of any local anesthetic solution may elicit a physicochemical interaction and cause a reduction in the sustainability of the DepoFoam to release the morphine over an extended period. This can result in an increase in the quantity of the encapsulated morphine released to the systemic circulation and place the patient at increased risk for respiratory depression and hypotension. This recommendation for not mixing with local anesthetics does not preclude the anesthetist from testing the epidural catheter for possible subarachnoid or intravascular migration preceding injection, and it is recommended that a routine test dose be performed prior to injection of the DepoDur, with some added precautions. The manufacturer recommends that the test dose be administered using prescribed techniques, then the catheter should be flushed with at least 1 mL of 0.9% NaCl solution a minimum of 15 minutes prior to injection of the DepoDur. If a large dose of local anesthetic is administered via the epidural, such as 20 mL of 2% lidocaine with epinephrine for a cesarean section, it is recommended that the administration of DepoDur should be delayed for at least 1 hour to prevent mixing.[110] It has also been recognized that sustained levels of analgesia from DepoDur require a minimum dose of 10 mg. Current research shows that when a dose of 5 mg of DepoDur is administered, the terminal half-life of the morphine is comparable to a similar 5-mg dose of standard morphine.[107]

Management of Epidural Anesthesia

After epidural administration of local anesthetic, the spread of the dermatomal block will continue and peak in an amount of time dependent on the factors previously mentioned and the local anesthetic solution used. Typically, the time to maximal spread is between 10 and 25 minutes, and the level of the block will regress over time; therefore consistent monitoring of sensory dermatomal level should be performed. When the sensory level of the block has diminished by 1 or 2 dermatomes, as detected by the scratch or ice test used to denote dermatomal level, then another dose, 30% to 50% of the initial dose, is given to reestablish the initial level of anesthesia. It is important to perform consistent monitoring of the anesthetic level because tachyphylaxis, or the need for an increase in the dosage required to maintain an adequate level of blockade, may occur if the regression is allowed beyond two dermatomal segments. The phenomenon of tachyphylaxis is poorly understood but is more likely to occur with short-acting amides such as lidocaine or mepivacaine. It can be avoided by using longer-acting agents (e.g., bupivacaine, ropivacaine, and tetracaine) or using a continuous infusion device.

One of the most frustrating problems that can occur with epidural anesthesia is the phenomenon of an inadequate block, a one-sided block, or single-sensory dermatome segment that fails to achieve adequate anesthesia. A variety of techniques are used to deal with these phenomena. Some anesthetists will attempt to increase the spread of the local anesthetic to the area of missed dermatomes by repositioning the patient with the unblocked side down (dependent) or by administering more local anesthetic solution. An inadequate block could be secondary to coiling of the epidural catheter or an anatomic abnormality. A unilateral block can occur when the catheter is located in the lateral aspect of the epidural space. This can sometimes be improved by withdrawing the catheter 1 to 2 cm, with the aim of positioning the catheter midline in the posterior epidural space. Inadequate anesthesia during epidural placement may be secondary to the technique used during identification of the epidural space. Studies have shown that using air during the loss-of-resistance technique may be a contributing factor in missed dermatomal spread of the local anesthetic. Studies by Beilin et al.,[111] Segal et al.,[112] and Shenouda and Cunningham[113] report that when air was used during a loss-of-resistance technique, a significant number of patients experienced missed dermatomal spread of the local anesthetic solution. They recommend using normal saline during catheter placement to minimize this complication.

Rarely, an epidural catheter passes through dura without penetrating the arachnoid membrane. This is sometimes thought of as intradural placement. Spread of the injected anesthetic in this situation can be very unpredictable. Anesthesia can range from a patchy, inadequate block to a rapid and high level of anesthesia requiring ventilatory support similar to the total spinal anesthetic complication. Fortunately, intradural catheter placement is rare, and complications can be avoided by the careful use of test doses, maintained vigilance, and a high index of suspicion. If an intradural catheter placement is suspected, the catheter needs to be removed and replaced after resolution of any side effects (e.g., hypotension, bradycardia). Additionally, it is recommended that the catheter be replaced at a dermatomal level more cephalad to the interspace previously attempted.[5,14]

Complications of Epidural Anesthesia

As with spinal anesthesia, the hemodynamic changes seen with epidural anesthesia are attributed to sympathetic blockade and subsequent arterial and venous dilation. Use of plain local anesthetic solutions in the epidural space to create a high level of blockade will decrease the mean arterial pressure, cardiac output, stroke volume, heart rate, and peripheral vascular resistance. The addition of epinephrine (usually a 1:200,000–1:400,000 solution) to the epidural local anesthetic solution diminishes and slows systemic uptake, resulting in lower plasma levels of the local anesthetic and prolongation of its duration of action. However, the epinephrine is thought to be absorbed systemically in low levels, thereby causing β_2-adrenergic vasodilation. The result is lower arterial pressure and peripheral resistance when compared with spinal anesthesia. Treatments of these hemodynamic alterations are very similar to those used for effects of spinal anesthesia. They include ephedrine 5 to 10 mg, phenylephrine 50 to 100 mcg, or a low- to moderate-rate infusion of dopamine, keeping in mind the caveats for use of these potent vasopressors. Atropine or glycopyrrolate is also useful for the treatment of bradycardia.[4,8]

One complication that is more prevalent with epidural anesthesia than spinal anesthesia is backache. The incidence of back pain after epidural anesthesia is between 30% and 45%, especially in the obstetric patient.[15] Several studies have identified various techniques used to decrease the incidence and severity of back pain after epidural anesthesia. For example, Todd et al.[114] analyzed what effect the addition of ketorolac to the dermal anesthesia solution would have on the overall incidence and severity of back pain after laboring epidural placement and delivery. These authors reported that the addition of 6 mg ketorolac to 3 mL 1% lidocaine dermal anesthetic solution resulted in a decrease in the incidence and severity of back pain in the postpartum period as compared with a similar group receiving 1% lidocaine solution alone for dermal anesthesia prior to entry of the epidural needle through the skin.[114]

Other complications associated with epidural catheters are similar to those associated with spinal anesthesia and have already been discussed. As with spinals, the overall risk of PDPH is low. For placement of epidural catheters, the PDPH rate is 1% to 2% due to the larger diameter compared to spinal needles. An inadvertent dural puncture created by a 17-gauge Tuohy is a rather large dural perforation, and is referred to as a "wet tap" because of the brisk free flow of CSF that can escape through the needle. With such a rent in the dura, the incidence of PDPH can be as high as 75% in young patients. Epidural catheters are also more likely to place a patient at risk for neuraxial anesthesia complications than the single passage of a smaller-gauge spinal needle because the catheter acts as a foreign body that remains within the patient. The catheter causes mechanical tissue disruption, acts as a physical irritant, may provide a path for infection, and will cause tissue trauma on removal, perhaps as much trauma as that associated with catheter placement. Therefore, although complications are rare overall, patients must be followed closely in the postoperative period for signs and symptoms of neurologic compromise such as spine ache, nerve root pain, weakness, and bowel or bladder dysfunction.

COMBINED SPINAL AND EPIDURAL ANESTHESIA

First described in 1937, the combined spinal epidural (CSE) anesthesia technique has risen in popularity and is used successfully for orthopedic, urologic, and gynecologic surgeries and for providing postoperative pain relief. It also has gained favor in the obstetric suite for providing anesthesia and analgesia for labor and delivery and for cesarean section.[116-120]

CSE anesthesia and analgesia offers the advantages of both spinal and epidural techniques while reducing or eliminating the associated disadvantages.[5,60] The CSE technique is appropriately used in any setting in which the practitioner plans a spinal or epidural anesthetic and desires to exploit the advantages of each technique, usually the quicker onset of the spinal anesthetic combined with the flexibility of an epidural catheter.

History and Development

In 1937 Soresi described the sequential injection of local anesthetic, first into the epidural space, then into the subarachnoid space, using the same small-gauge spinal needle. Soresi described placing an epidural needle (without a stylet) into the epidural space using a hanging-drop technique and injecting 7 to 8 mL of procaine, then advancing the needle into the subarachnoid space, where he injected 2 additional mL of procaine. He reported that the anesthesia lasted between 24 and 48 hours. His experience using this technique in more than 200 patients led him to state "by combining the two methods many of the disadvantages of both methods are eliminated and their advantages are enhanced to an almost incredible degree."[120]

In 1979 Curelaru reported application of the CSE technique in 150 patients. He used a two-puncture technique; he placed an epidural catheter first, using a standardized epidural needle, followed by a subarachnoid puncture, using a spinal needle one or two interspaces below the level of the epidural puncture. Advantages of the technique included "the possibility of obtaining a high-quality conduction anesthesia, virtually unlimited in time, the ability to extend over several anatomic regions the surgical field, minimal toxicity, the absence of postoperative pulmonary complications, and the economy." Disadvantages included "the need for two vertebral punctures, the longer induction time of anesthesia, and some difficulty in finding the subarachnoid space after catheterization of the epidural space."[121]

Finally, in 1982 Coates[117] used a single-space technique in which a long spinal needle was inserted through the epidural needle to provide the spinal component of the CSE technique.[116] Coates stated the technique was "simple, reliable and quick to perform." He was, however, concerned that "the theoretical hazards of this technique include the possible passage of the epidural catheter through the hole in the dura mater and the possibility of subarachnoid effects from epidurally injected drugs by passage through the hole in the dura." Eldor[118] described finding metallic particles while using the needle-through-needle technique, supposedly formed by abrasion of the inner surface of the epidural needle by the passage of the spinal needle. They were concerned these particles might be introduced into the epidural space. In addition, they were concerned uneven distribution of the spinal local anesthetic was possible. The delay, they theorized, inherent in introducing the epidural catheter after intrathecal administration of local anesthetic could affect the spread of the anesthetic. These concerns led to the development of a combined spinal-epidural needle with two separate conduits to allow the epidural catheter to be placed first, followed by the spinal puncture. Because the needle had two conduits, it allowed both techniques to be performed with one puncture at one interspace. This innovation led to the development of several needle types, each of which sought to improve on the others.

A recent technique that is different than the CSE technique is the dural puncture epidural (DPE) technique. The DPE technique is a method in which a dural puncture is created prior to placement of the epidural catheter. This technique is based on the early work by Suzuki et al.,[122] where they reported the effect of a dural puncture (with no drug injected) as compared to a group receiving conventional epidural anesthesia. They reported that those receiving the dural puncture with a 26-gauge spinal needle (using the needle-through-needle technique) prior to placement of an epidural catheter achieved significantly greater caudal anesthesia and no differences in cranial spread. These investigators also reported no differences in adverse effects between the groups.[122] Subsequent studies have validated these initial findings in which they reported using the DPE technique results in a faster onset of analgesia/anesthesia and a better quality of labor analgesia when used in the obstetric population.[123,124]

Equipment and Techniques

Two-Level Technique

The two-level technique is unique in that each component is performed separately at two different interspaces. An epidural catheter is inserted first, followed by a spinal anesthesia needle placed one or two interspaces lower. The primary advantage of this technique is the ability to insert and test the epidural catheter first, then place the spinal anesthetic needle. Once the spinal needle is placed, no delay occurs in positioning the patient, which may be an important factor when using a hyperbaric spinal anesthetic solution. Prior placement of the epidural catheter is not entirely benign. Potential problems include the inability to distinguish the epidural test dose from the spinal block, inability to differentiate the epidural test dose from CSF, epidural catheter laceration by the spinal needle, misdirection of the spinal needle by the catheter, inability to obtain CSF because of compression of the dural sac by the test dose, and an increased risk of dural puncture by the epidural catheter.[113] Other disadvantages include increased discomfort, tissue trauma, and morbidity associated with multilevel interspinous space penetration (e.g., backache, epidural venous laceration, hematoma, infection, and technical difficulties).[119]

Single-Level Technique: Needle Through Needle

First described in 1982, the needle-through-needle technique involves insertion of an epidural needle at the appropriate interspace and then using the epidural needle as a guide for the spinal needle.[114,115] A small (25-, 27-, or 29-gauge) pencil-point spinal needle is inserted through the epidural needle into the subarachnoid space, and local anesthetic is injected. The spinal needle is removed, and an epidural catheter is threaded into the epidural space. The epidural needle is removed, and the catheter is secured. The main advantages are related to performance of a single interspace insertion (e.g., less tissue trauma,

backache, and associated morbidity). Disadvantages include the possibility of inadequate spinal block if catheter placement is delayed, potential for increased nerve root trauma if paresthesias occur during catheter insertion, and the inability to reliably test the catheter with a preexisting spinal block. Inability to obtain CSF because of inadequate spinal needle length is a risk avoided by using the appropriate specialized needles.

Dural Puncture Epidural Technique

The DPE technique is a modification of the conventional epidural and the combined spinal-epidural techniques. The DPE is typically performed using the needle-through-needle approach, but instead of administering any medication through the subarachnoid needle, the needle is withdrawn following dural puncture, and the epidural catheter is threaded into the epidural space. Following placement of the epidural catheter, the epidural needle is removed, and conventional epidural anesthesia/analgesia is done using the epidural catheter (Fig. 49.16).

Specialized Needles

Eldor[118] was the first to develop and patent a combined spinal-epidural needle with two channels, one for the epidural catheter and the other for the spinal needle. The needle is placed at the selected interspace, the epidural catheter is inserted through its designated conduit, and then the spinal needle is placed through its conduit. Once CSF is obtained, the chosen local anesthetic is injected, and the needle is removed. The catheter is taped in place, and the patient is positioned. Purported advantages and disadvantages are similar to those described for the single-level technique. Although the risk of metallic particle formation may be reduced, the risk of trauma to the interspinous ligaments is increased because of a larger needle diameter.

Several other needles have been developed, all seeking to minimize or eliminate potential problems.[118] To reduce external size, decrease needle abrasion, and allow for a direct angle of approach to the dura, a Tuohy needle was modified with a separate back-eye at the bend of the needle, thereby permitting straight passage of the spinal needle. These needles are subject to their own limitations and failure rates as well. The spinal needle can miss the back-eye hole and exit the epidural needle through the main orifice, as occurs in the needle-through-needle technique.

Sequential Technique

Rawal et al.[116] described a single-level sequential technique that was developed to minimize the hypotensive effects of the spinal component of CSE anesthesia for cesarean section. An epidural needle is placed at the selected interspace, and a low-dose (7.5 mg of hyperbaric bupivacaine) spinal anesthetic is placed using the needle-through-needle technique. The spinal needle is removed, the catheter is inserted and

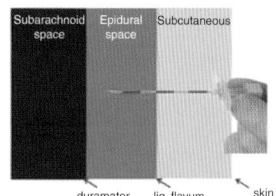
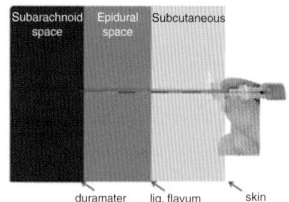
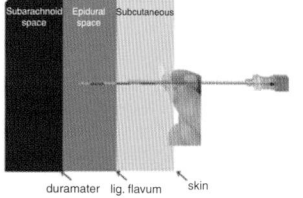
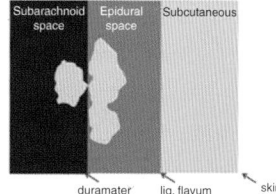

Step 1. Performing standard epidural block

Step 2. Introducing the long spinal needle with needle through needle technique like in CSE.

Step 3. Withdrawing the spinal needle without administering any subarachnoid drug and then placing the epidural catheter into epidural space.

Step 4. Most of the drug solution distribute within the epidural space while some of it translocate from the dural hole created with the spinal needle to the subarachnoid space.

Fig. 49.16 Schematic display of performing dural puncture epidural. (From Gunaydin B, Erel S. How neuraxial labor analgesia differs by approach: dural puncture epidural as a novel option. *J Anesth.* 2019;33:125–130 [fig 1].)

taped in place, and the patient is placed in the supine position with a left lateral tilt. After 15 minutes, the block is extended by titrating epidural local anesthetic until the desired level is achieved (1.5–2 mL for each unblocked segment). Although this technique takes longer to perform, it has been shown to decrease the frequency and severity of the hypotension seen with spinal anesthesia. This technique has also been applied in other types of surgery.

Agents

As discussed previously, local anesthetic agents and their concentration are chosen depending on the effects desired. Appropriate anesthetics for the spinal component include isobaric or hyperbaric 5% lidocaine with or without epinephrine, hyperbaric 0.75% (spinal) bupivacaine, and isobaric or hyperbaric 1% tetracaine. Appropriate anesthetics for the epidural component include 2% lidocaine with or without epinephrine, 0.5% bupivacaine, 2% or 3% 2-chloroprocaine, and 1% ropivacaine. The concentration of these agents may be adjusted to provide postoperative analgesia in combination with opioids such as morphine and fentanyl. All agents should be preservative free to reduce or eliminate any neurotoxic effects. Note the bupivacaine liposome injectable suspension (Exparel) is not listed as it is approved only for infiltration or use in an interscalene nerve block and not for central neuraxial administration.

Management of CSE Anesthesia

Although the CSE technique may be used in any type of surgical procedure in which a spinal or epidural would be acceptable, this technique may be particularly well suited to providing analgesia and anesthesia in obstetric patients. The CSE technique offers the following potential advantages over conventional epidural anesthesia and analgesia.[115]

- Rapid onset of the intrathecal component for women who are in the later stages of labor and in significant pain and distress
- The use of intrathecal opioids (e.g., fentanyl, sufentanil, morphine, and meperidine) in early labor; the minimal-to-absent motor block associated with intrathecal opioids allows the patient to ambulate while in labor

The CSE technique for the laboring patient usually involves the placement of an epidural needle at the selected (usually lumbar) interspace, followed by the placement of the spinal needle using the needle-through-needle technique. Intrathecal opioids (5–10 mcg sufentanil or 10–25 mcg fentanyl) may be given alone or in combination with a small dose (2.5 mg bupivacaine) of local anesthetic, saline, or both. The spinal needle is withdrawn, and the epidural catheter is inserted. The epidural needle is removed, and the catheter is taped in place. The catheter can be activated at any time if supplemental analgesia or anesthesia is required. Standard testing of the epidural catheter before use is always recommended.

The CSE technique also can be used to provide anesthesia for cesarean section if required. If the patient already has an epidural catheter in place, a test dose (3 mL 1.5% lidocaine with 1:200,000 epinephrine) is given to rule out intrathecal and intravascular placement. After a negative test dose, incremental administration of 2% lidocaine, 0.5% bupivacaine, or 3% 2-chloroprocaine can be given 2 to establish a level of surgical anesthesia.

If a catheter has yet to be placed, and if time allows, the anesthetist can proceed as with any new patient. After the spinal needle is placed, an intrathecal dose of local anesthetic (12–15 mg 0.75% bupivacaine) with or without opioid (10–15 mcg fentanyl, 0.2–0.3 mg preservative-free morphine, or both) is given. The catheter is inserted and taped in place. The spinal anesthetic will set up quickly and allow for urgent (but maybe not emergent) delivery.

Despite the utility and flexibility of the CSE technique, several concerns related to its use exist. The first of these concerns is related to the use of intrathecal sufentanil and its associated hypotension.[125] Controversy exists with regard to whether intrathecal sufentanil causes clinically significant changes in blood pressure and fetal heart rate (fetal bradycardia). Purported mechanisms include pain relief, mild sympatholysis, and uterine hypertonus.[127-129] Studies show no differences in outcome between CSE using intrathecal sufentanil and epidural anesthesia.[129,130]

A second concern with CSE analgesia is the ability to ambulate after receiving intrathecal narcotics. The concern is related to possible motor weakness if low-dose local anesthetic is added and regarding the effects on blood pressure.[131] Hypotension appears within the first 30 minutes after intrathecal fentanyl but remains stable through ambulation and follow-up doses of epidural local anesthetic. Studies demonstrate the safety of allowing ambulation with no apparent deleterious effects.[132]

A third concern with CSE technique in laboring patients is related to complications. Overall, the complications of itching and hypotension, although bothersome, do not appear to significantly affect outcome or patient satisfaction.[111] CSE anesthesia is associated with faster onset, denser motor block, lower anxiety, lower preoperative and intraoperative pain scores, and greater patient satisfaction preoperatively. There were no significant differences in the incidence or severity of hypotension or nausea, the need for supplemental analgesics, or the postoperative assessments of intraoperative pain, anxiety, and satisfaction.[133] However, certain data indicate that when a CSE technique is used where intrathecal bupivacaine (3.125 mg) plus 5 mcg fentanyl is injected preceding epidural placement, CSE provides better first-stage analgesia and less requirement for supplemental bolus epidural injections.[134]

Complications of CSE Anesthesia

Spinal and epidural anesthesia both have their own associated complications as discussed. The CSE technique has the same complications and some additional unique complications. Therefore, as always, vigilance is prudent.

Failure to Obtain a Subarachnoid or Epidural Block

The failure rate for subarachnoid block alone ranges from 3.1% to 17%. With the single-level CSE technique for anesthesia the range is 0% to 24.5%, and for the two-level technique the range is 1.6% to 4%.[136-138] Failure with the single-level CSE technique may occur because the epidural needle is not in the epidural space, because the epidural needle is off midline, because the spinal needle is too short (or dull) and does not penetrate the dura, or because the angle of approach of the spinal needle is too oblique to puncture the dura. The overall failure rate of the epidural catheter has also been shown to be lower when the CSE technique is used as compared to when a conventional catheter is used. In a 2016 study by Groden et al.[136] they noted that catheter failure was approximately two times higher in the conventional epidural placement group compared to when the CSE technique was used. These same investigators noted that mean time to replacement between the groups was also significantly prolonged in the CSE group.

One of the most important considerations is the length of the spinal needle, specifically the length of needle that extends beyond the tip of the epidural needle.[119] Studies have shown an increased success rate when the tip of the spinal needle extends 7 to 15 mm beyond the tip of the epidural needle.[137,138] The angle at which the spinal needle approaches the dura may also be important. As the spinal needle exits a standard epidural needle tip, the angle caused by the epidural needle's curve may be 4 to 5 degrees or more.[139] This factor, combined with inadequate needle length, may result in failure to obtain CSF.

This situation has led to the development of a modified Tuohy needle that has a separate back-eye at the bend of the needle to allow for a straight-on approach to the dura. Pan[140] determined the success rate for the needles exiting the correct hole ranged from 50% to 67%. The success rate can be improved to 81% to 94% by bending the spinal needle slightly in the direction of the epidural needle bevel and to 91% to 96% by orientating the epidural needle bevel upward.

Failure rates may also be directly related to level of experience with the technique and are not easily correctable. The problem of spinal needle displacement during connection of the syringe, aspiration, or injection of the local anesthetic has led to the development of locking devices that fix the spinal needle in the epidural needle once the dura has been punctured. Their efficacy has not yet been confirmed.

Catheter Migration

Another problem with the needle-through-needle technique is the possibility of catheter migration through the dural puncture caused by the introduction of the spinal needle.[139] Studies assessing the risk of catheter migration through a dural puncture site demonstrated little to no risk if the dural puncture was made with a 25-gauge or smaller spinal needle but an increased risk if the dural puncture was made by a larger (18-gauge) Tuohy needle.[142-144] Many factors may result in catheter placement in, or migration into, the subarachnoid space, including patient movement, undetected dural puncture with the epidural needle with subsequent catheter placement, and (least likely) diffusion of local anesthetic from the epidural space into the subarachnoid space through the dural puncture. The prudent practitioner is advised to adopt a conservative approach that includes a high index of suspicion and frequent aspiration and testing of the catheter.

However, even the question of when to test the epidural catheter can be problematic. The purpose of the epidural catheter test dose is to rule out inadvertent placement or migration of the catheter into the subarachnoid space or into an epidural vein. A preestablished subarachnoid block may preclude the ability to reliably test for subarachnoid catheter placement and mask intravascular placement. To date, no published studies have demonstrated reliable detection of inadvertent subarachnoid catheter placement in someone with a preexisting spinal block.

Increased Spinal Level After Epidural Administration

The CSE technique is known to cause an increased spread of spinal anesthesia after injection of solutions through the epidural catheter. Although controversial, several theories may help explain this phenomenon. First, the volume effect theory states that the volume of fluid injected into the epidural space compresses the subarachnoid space and the CSF within it, thereby increasing the spread of the intrathecal local anesthetic. This effect has been documented clinically and by use of contrast media and radiography. The second theory presupposes a leak or flow of local anesthetic from the epidural into the subarachnoid space through the dural puncture. This effect also has been demonstrated clinically and by radiography.[144,145] Other radiographic studies have been unable to confirm these results.[143,146]

Metallic Particles

Eldor and Levine[135] noted the production of metallic particles when passing a spinal needle through a Tuohy epidural needle. Subsequently, Eldor[147,148] has implied that scratches in the spinal needle and metallic particles may be associated with an increase in aseptic meningitis and cancer in patients who have received CSE anesthesia via the needle-through-needle technique. No studies have been published to support these assertions, but several studies have examined the issue of metallic

particle formation.[149] These studies used electron microscopy, atomic absorption spectroscopy, photomicrography, and microscopy; none were able to detect metallic particle formation.[143,150]

Postdural Puncture Headache

Conflicting evidence exists regarding whether a greater risk of PDPH is associated with the CSE technique compared with conventional epidural anesthesia and analgesia. Both techniques involve the placement of an epidural needle, with its attendant risk of dural puncture. In addition, the CSE technique involves a dural puncture, usually with a small-gauge, pencil-point spinal needle. Because this type of spinal needle is associated with an extremely low incidence of PDPH, one would expect an equally low incidence with the CSE technique. A review of the literature on the CSE technique shows a PDPH rate between 0% and 2.3% in laboring patients.[151] Theoretic reasons for a low incidence with the CSE technique include the following:

- The epidural needle serves as an introducer for the smaller-gauge spinal needles and allows for a straight approach at the dura.
- CSF leakage through the dural puncture is abated because of the presence of the epidural catheter and fluids, which increases pressure in the epidural space.
- The spinal needle penetrates the dura at a slight angle, which may help dural fibers seal the hole on withdrawal.

Studies suggest that the use of intrathecal opioids as part of the CSE technique may offer a protective effect from PDPH.[152,153] In addition, the success rate in obtaining CSF may be higher when the patient is in the sitting position, rather than in the lateral position. The sitting position allows for correct midline placement of the epidural needle and makes it more likely that CSF will be obtained with the spinal needle (higher hydrostatic pressure). Both these factors contribute to minimization of the number of dural punctures and may decrease the risk of PDPH.

Infection

The incidence of infectious complications associated with epidural and spinal anesthesia has always been considered to be very low, in the range of 0% to 0.04%.[29,154,155] However, perhaps because of close monitoring of this newer technique, an increase has occurred in the number of case reports of patients who have developed complications that may be associated with the use of the CSE technique. Bouhemad et al.[156] cite cases (three between 1994 and 1998) of bacterial meningitis associated with the use of CSE. The authors believed that potentially infectious skin matter was first introduced into the epidural space during the insertion of the epidural needle and was then introduced into the CSF by the passage of the spinal needle into the subarachnoid space. Because the CSE technique requires invasion of both the epidural and subarachnoid spaces, strict aseptic technique should be practiced. As with other complications associated with the use of CSE, further study of this area is warranted.

Neurologic Injury

Neurologic injury associated with spinal and epidural anesthesia is also very low, ranging from 0.02% to 0.1%, and is usually transient in nature.[5] Although there does not appear to be any increased risk inherent in the CSE technique as compared with either spinal or epidural anesthesia alone, there have been several case reports of cauda equina syndrome in patients who underwent CSE anesthesia.[157,158] In each of these cases the cause was never identified. Possible causes include preexisting spinal deformity (present in one case), use of lidocaine (present in one case), and an intrathecal catheter (never proved or disproved).

A final concern with the use of the CSE technique is paresthesia on epidural catheter insertion. A preexisting spinal block may mask a significant paresthesia on catheter insertion and result in neurologic injury. Paresthesias during epidural catheter placement range in frequency from 20% to 44%.[159] However, studies show no significant difference in the frequency of paresthesias reported for either technique.[137,159]

CAUDAL ANESTHESIA

Caudal anesthesia can be thought of as a distal approach to the epidural space. Therefore anesthetics administered or catheters placed via the caudal route will act as epidural administered anesthetics but first on the sacral dermatomes. A caudal technique is useful for perirectal surgery, urologic surgery, and orthopedic surgery of the lower extremity. Caudal techniques are especially useful in pediatrics but also can be used for labor and delivery and for chronic pain states. With the success of lumbar epidural catheters for labor and delivery, caudal anesthesia is rarely used in this population currently and is less likely to be used in the adult population in general. After the age of 12, sacral anatomy changes and bone growth make identification of the epidural space by this approach difficult and the spread of anesthesia less reliable.[8] Caudal anesthesia is most often used in combination with a light general anesthetic to augment postoperative analgesia in preadolescent pediatric patients.

Equipment and Techniques

The patient can be placed either prone or in a lateral position. The posterior iliac spines and the sacral hiatus are identified. Positioning the patient prone with the legs slightly apart, the heels rotated outward, and a pillow under the buttocks facilitates the palpation of the cornua of the sacral hiatus. In the lateral, Sims, or knee-chest position, identification of the cornua can be enhanced by adjusting the amount of hip flexion. Excess flexion can stretch the skin, making landmark identification difficult. An assistant is often useful when one is positioning patients who are anesthetized.

In pediatric patients, general anesthesia is usually induced, the airway and IV access secured, and the patient turned prone or placed in a lateral decubitus position. After aseptic preparation is performed, the index and second fingers of one hand are placed on the cornua of the sacrum, with the hand cephalad and against the patient's back. A 22- to 25-gauge short needle attached to a 10-mL syringe filled with local anesthetic is inserted midline between the cornua at a steep angle to the skin into the sacral hiatus. Alternatively, a 20-gauge over-the-needle IV catheter is sufficiently long enough for the block, and the catheter can be passed into the epidural space while the needle is removed. This allows the anesthetist better control when administering the local anesthetic. The needle is inserted with the bevel of the needle directed toward the sacrum. As the membranes are penetrated and the ventral canal of the sacrum is entered, a popping sensation can be felt. At this point the needle angle is lowered parallel to the sacrum and the spinal canal. The needle is advanced into the epidural space for a distance of 1 to 3 cm, but no farther than the second sacral interspace. The second sacral interspace lies 1 to 2 cm below a line drawn between the posterior iliac spines. The needle position is evaluated for entrance into the subarachnoid space or epidural veins via gentle aspiration and examination for CSF or blood return through the needle. Once the appropriate location of the needle is verified, the anesthetic is incrementally injected as with an epidural. During injection, the skin area above the end of the needle is palpated. Bulging over the needle tip indicates subcutaneous or superficial injection rather than injection into the epidural space. If the needle is in the subperiosteal area, resistance to injection is felt, and the needle must be repositioned.

Agents

In children, 0.5 to 1 mL of solution per kilogram of body weight is injected to reliably achieve a level of analgesia to the umbilicus. Bupivacaine or ropivacaine, in concentrations of 0.125% to 0.5%, are usually administered with epinephrine 1:200,000 to a maximum dose of 2.5 mg/kg body weight. These dosing regimens have been shown effective for children undergoing subumbilical surgical procedures, providing analgesia or anesthesia for the lower extremities and the abdomen, urogenital surgery, inguinal hernia repair, or orthopedic procedures with analgesia that lasts 3 to 5 hours postoperatively.[8,160,161] Clonidine 1 mcg/kg of body weight added to the local anesthetic has been shown to be comparable with opioids added to enhance analgesia. Clonidine has fewer side effects than caudal opioids (e.g., delayed recovery, respiratory depression, and nausea).[162] Some patients may be unable to tolerate the loss of lower-extremity motor control. These patients should be identified before the anesthetic is administered and be offered another technique. For example, infants too young to walk greatly benefit from caudal analgesia, but toddlers may be frightened by their inability to move their legs. Ropivacaine may have benefits over bupivacaine because analgesia in the postoperative period is equivalent, but ropivacaine offers shorter duration of motor blockade and less risk of CNS and cardiotoxicity.[8,161-164]

In adults, the principles of epidural drug administration should be followed, with use of a 3-mL test dose and incremental injections and aspiration. Only 12 to 15 mL is necessary for sacral anesthesia, and up to 20 to 30 mL offers sufficient spread for lower-extremity procedures to approximately the 10th thoracic dermatome. The spread of drug, duration of anesthesia, and desired level of anesthesia are less predictable than with epidural anesthesia because of the variability in the volume, content, and leakage of the caudal canal. The maximum recommended dose of lidocaine or mepivacaine is 10 mg/kg of body weight and 2.5 mg/kg of body weight for bupivacaine.[8] All agents injected into the epidural or subarachnoid spaces should be preservative free.

Management of Caudal Anesthesia

Caudal anesthesia, like epidural anesthesia, is adaptable to a continuous catheter technique. However, if a Tuohy needle is used, the angle of the tip must be kept in mind when one attempts to pass the catheter into the epidural space. Management is similar to that with an epidural catheter.

Complications of Caudal Anesthesia

Caudal anesthesia has complications very similar to those of epidural anesthesia. The caudal canal has a sacral epidural venous plexus with vessels that can be unintentional recipients of a needle or catheter tip, with subsequent IV injection of local anesthetic. Dural puncture is also possible, although the dural sac usually ends, in adults, at the lower border of L2, and in infants the sac can extend to S4. High spinal punctures are less likely but have been reported. In addition, the anatomy of caudal anesthesia is variable enough, especially in adults, to cause a high failure rate (10%–15%) as the needle is unintentionally inserted into false passages. The proximity of the caudal canal to the rectum theoretically makes infection a potential risk, although clinically significant infection is rarely reported.[8,164] The risk of infections, perhaps, will best be shown to be minimized with the use of chlorhexidine solutions instead of povidone-iodine solutions.[165]

SUMMARY

In 1899 Alice Magaw described the job of an anesthetist and best summarized the reality of the practice of regional anesthesia. She stated, "While one should be competent in the theoretical part of this important work, there is nothing so helpful to the anesthetist as the hard school of practical experience."[166] Regional anesthesia techniques are a vital part of modern anesthesia practice. Our ability to understand and apply neuraxial anesthesia continues to evolve. These techniques are increasingly being used for all types of anesthetics, including many outpatient procedures. Their utility in providing for perioperative pain management has greatly enhanced our ability to provide comfort to our patients.

REFERENCES

For a complete list of references for this chapter, scan this QR code with any smartphone code reader app, or visit the following URL: http://booksite.elsevier.com/9780323711944/.

50

Regional Anesthesia: Upper Extremity, Lower Extremity, and Truncal Blocks

Christian R. Falyar

Peripheral nerve blocks are an essential component of many enhanced recovery after surgery (ERAS) protocols that aim to reduce or eliminate opioid administration. The incorporation of ultrasound, peripheral catheter techniques, and newer, long-acting local anesthetics such as Exparel afford providers numerous options for perioperative management. Regional anesthesia offers several benefits to the patient, including reduced postoperative nausea and vomiting (PONV), improved pain scores, reduced opioid consumption, decreased length of hospital stay, and improved patient satisfaction.[1] It is important for the anesthetist to possess a comprehensive understanding of the functional anatomy and sonoanatomy, as well as a mastery of the techniques required to perform the multitude of regional anesthesia options available, to improve patient outcomes while limiting risks and complications.

The goals of this chapter are to present basic functional anatomy and sonoanatomy, as well as indications and techniques for performing many of the landmark/nerve stimulation and ultrasound-guided peripheral nerve blocks common in current anesthetic practice.

SELECTION OF REGIONAL ANESTHESIA TECHNIQUES

There are many factors to consider when determining the most appropriate regional anesthetic for a surgical procedure. Peripheral nerve blocks are used as either the primary anesthetic or as part of a multimodal postoperative pain management plan. Additionally, certain blocks are used to treat chronic pain syndromes. Important considerations include the proposed surgery, its anticipated length and associated pain, and patient factors, including allergies, comorbidities, and nil per os (NPO) status. When a regional anesthetic is proposed for a case, the technique should be thoroughly discussed with the patient. As part of the informed consent process, the anesthetist must explain the risks and benefits of the procedure as well as potential complications and alternative treatment options.

Peripheral nerve blocks are appropriate for numerous surgical procedures involving the extremities, chest, and trunk. They are routinely used in combination with intravenous or general anesthesia allowing the practitioner to customize the anesthetic plan based on the patient's condition and comorbidities. For example, when a patient presents with a difficult airway or full stomach, the addition or supplementation of a peripheral nerve block can provide surgical anesthesia while allowing the patient to maintain upper airway and pharyngeal reflexes. Fig. 50.1 relates common peripheral nerve blocks to surgical sites.

Contraindications

There are few contraindications for performing peripheral nerve blocks. Absolute contraindications include patient refusal, uncorrected coagulation deficiencies, and infection at the block site. Patient refusal is the most significant absolute contraindication to performing a peripheral nerve block. However, this is often related to misconceptions regarding regional anesthesia. Patient education regarding the proposed procedure, the advantages and disadvantages of the technique, risks and complications, as well as other anesthetic options provides the patient with the information needed to make an informed decision. Patients who have difficulty understanding the procedure or are unable to cooperate should undergo an alternative type of anesthesia.

The puncture of a vessel with subsequent bleeding is a potential complication. Unlike the catastrophic consequences of spinal hematoma due to bleeding in a noncompressible space, the bleeding risks in anticoagulated and coagulopathic patients undergoing a deep plexus or peripheral nerve block are less clear. Despite the benefits afforded by a regional anesthesia, peripheral nerve blocks are often not performed because of the fear of bleeding. While case reports detail significant morbidity related to bleeding following peripheral nerve blockade, there is a lack of evidence identifying the frequency and severity of peripheral nerve blocks in anticoagulated patients.[2] The American Society of Regional Anesthesia and Pain Medicine (ASRA) suggests following the same guidelines as those pertaining to neuraxial techniques for patients undergoing perineuraxial, deep plexus, or deep peripheral block. These recommendations can be found in Chapter 38, Table 38.7.[2]

An active infection at the site of the proposed procedure is a contraindication for needle placement for a peripheral nerve block, and an alternative anesthetic plan should be selected. In addition to potentially spreading or seeding the infection, an acidic environment will reduce local anesthetic effectiveness and block efficacy. Sepsis and systemic infection are considered relative contraindications.[3]

True local anesthetic allergies are rare.[4] Patients with a history of an adverse local anesthetic reaction should undergo further evaluation in a controlled situation by an allergist, as these are often the result of epinephrine, vasovagal syncope, or toxicity.[5] Allergies to ester local anesthetics are more common because hydrolysis by cholinesterase results in the metabolite paraaminobenzoic acid (PABA), a known allergen. Although extremely rare, there have been documented cases of amide local anesthetic allergies.[6] Additionally, additives such as methylparaben and metabisulfite cause an allergic reaction as they are chemically similar to PABA.

Regardless of the etiology, patients with chronic neurologic compromise are at increased risk for further neurologic injury.[7] The double-crush phenomenon first described by Upton and McComas theorized that patients with preexisting neurologic disease are susceptible to further injury if exposed to a secondary insult.[8] Theoretically, performing a regional anesthetic on a patient with preexisting neurologic disease places the patient at increased risk of experiencing the double-crush phenomenon. Due to the infrequency of these disease processes and

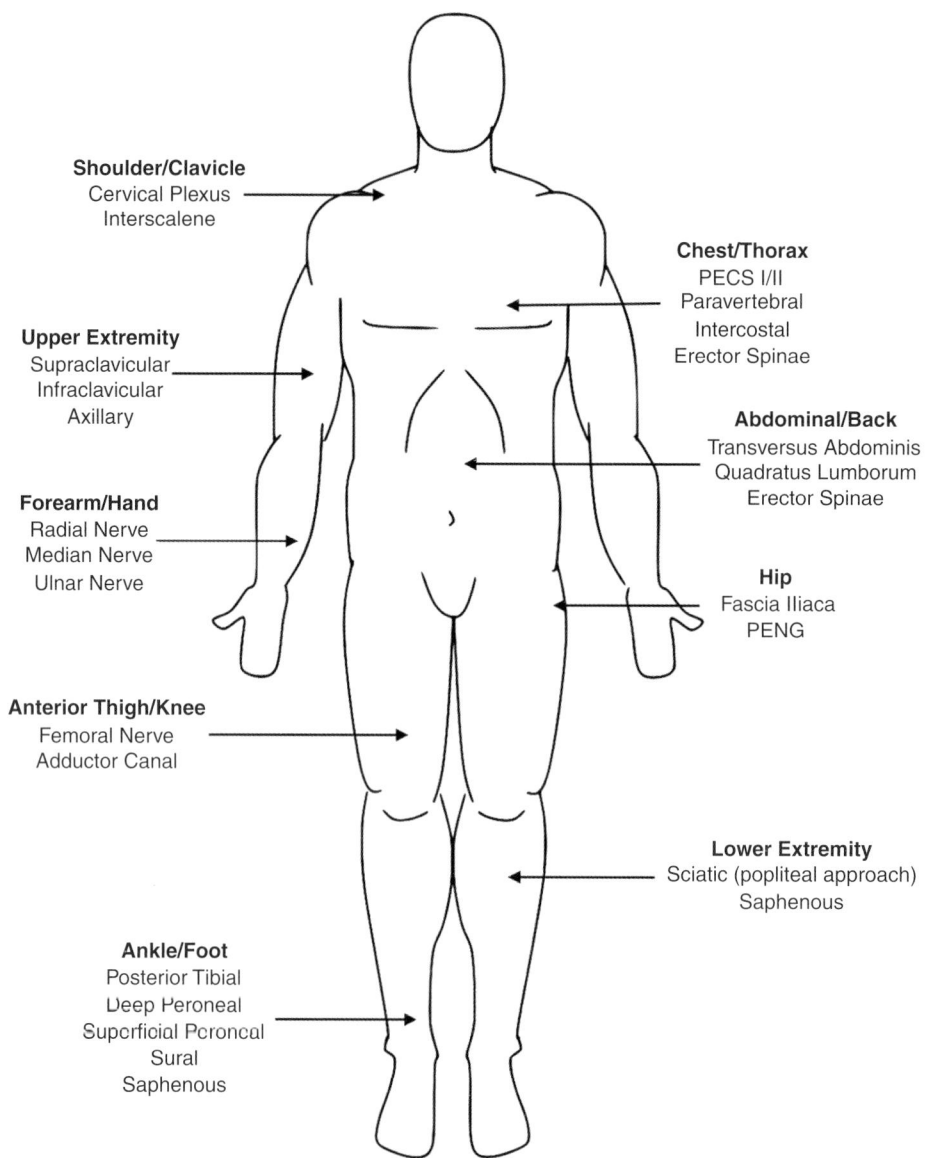

Shoulder/Clavicle
Cervical Plexus
Interscalene

Chest/Thorax
PECS I/II
Paravertebral
Intercostal
Erector Spinae

Upper Extremity
Supraclavicular
Infraclavicular
Axillary

Abdominal/Back
Transversus Abdominis
Quadratus Lumborum
Erector Spinae

Forearm/Hand
Radial Nerve
Median Nerve
Ulnar Nerve

Hip
Fascia Iliaca
PENG

Anterior Thigh/Knee
Femoral Nerve
Adductor Canal

Lower Extremity
Sciatic (popliteal approach)
Saphenous

Ankle/Foot
Posterior Tibial
Deep Peroneal
Superficial Peroneal
Sural
Saphenous

Fig. 50.1 A list of common peripheral nerve blocks related to their appropriate area of surgery. *PENG,* Pericapsular nerve group

lack of sufficient clinical outcome information, it is difficult to make recommendations from the current scientific literature.[7] Patients must be well informed as to the potential risks of the proposed regional technique. Documenting a baseline neurologic and functional exam is essential. Regional anesthesia rarely results in changes to the patient's baseline examination; however, if neurologic deficits increase or persist, the regional anesthetic technique cannot be ruled out as the cause.

COMPLICATIONS OF PERIPHERAL NERVE BLOCKADE

Documented complications associated with regional anesthesia include direct and indirect nerve injury, local anesthetic systemic toxicity (LAST) events, vascular injury, hematoma, and infection.[9,10] Each peripheral nerve block has specific risks and complications that are discussed in later sections of the chapter.

The overall incidence of severe or permanent peripheral nerve injury (PNI) following a block is extremely low, with a reported long-term injury rate of approximately 2 to 4 per 10,000 blocks.[11] However,

it is not uncommon in the early postoperative period for as many as 15% of patients to complain of paresthesia, also known as postoperative neurologic symptoms (PONS).[10] Over time there is a steady and significant reduction in symptoms, with the latest estimates suggesting an incidence of 0% to 2.2% at 3 months, 0% to 0.8% at 6 months, and 0% to 0.2% at 1 year.[9]

Nerve injury resulting from a peripheral nerve block may be direct or indirect in nature. Direct nerve injury results from either needle trauma or placement of a peripheral nerve catheter. The type of needle used also plays a role, as a smaller gauge, short-beveled needle is less likely to damage the nerve as less force is required to advance it, and the nerve fascicles tend to migrate away from the tip.[12,13] The lack of motor response when using peripheral nerve stimulator (PNS) does not guarantee that intraneural needle placement has not occurred, and confirming nerve stimulation when apparent intraneural needle position is noted on ultrasound can lead to unnecessary nerve trauma.[14] Indirect nerve injury refers to nerve injury occurring from local anesthetic toxicity, ischemia, or inflammation. All local anesthetics used in clinically relevant concentrations are potentially neurotoxic. While the exact cause is not known, the site of administration appears to be an important factor with intrafascicular injections being more toxic than intra- or extraneural placement of local anesthetic.[15] Ischemia may occur from vascular occlusion, hemorrhage, edema compression, or direct injury. Inflammation also appears to play a role in nerve injury. For example, adhesions, fascial thickening, vascular changes, and scar tissue have led to compression of the phrenic nerve, resulting in diaphragmatic paralysis after the placement of an interscalene block.[16]

Patients receiving peripheral blocks are at increased risk of LAST because potentially toxic volumes of local anesthetic are frequently injected into vascular areas. Although the risk of LAST has been significantly reduced with the use of ultrasound, serious LAST events still occur at a rate 2.5 per 10,000 blocks.[17] A complete discussion of the management of LAST can be found in Chapter 10. All patients should have a functional intravenous line, and blocks should be performed only in areas where patient monitoring, equipment, and drugs to treat LAST are immediately available.[10]

Significant bleeding events from vascular puncture are uncommon in patients without known bleeding diathesis or those receiving therapeutic anticoagulation. A meta-analysis concluded the incidence of unintended vascular puncture was reduced with ultrasound when compared to other measures.[10]

The incidence of local infection, abscess formation, and sepsis caused by peripheral nerve blocks is rare. The largest retrospective study analyzing over 7000 single-shot nerve blocks over a 10-year period found no incidence of infection that could be related to the regional procedure.[18] In a study looking at continuous peripheral nerve block catheters, the authors noted that while bacterial colonization rates of the catheter were high, clinically relevant infection was rare.[19] Despite the low incidence of infection, the use of strict aseptic technique remains essential.[10]

Local Anesthetic Considerations

Local anesthetics are an essential component of peripheral nerve blockade. Selection is dependent upon numerous factors, including onset of action, duration, and the desired density of the block (pain management vs primary anesthetic). Anesthetists must recognize the potential for LAST when performing any regional procedure and be prepared to expeditiously manage this complication. Chapter 10 contains a detailed discussion of pharmacokinetics and pharmacodynamics of local anesthetics.

Although the rates of LAST and PONS due to peripheral nerve blocks are low, multiple strategies can be used to improve the safety profile of these procedures. LAST is often the result of an inadvertent intravascular injection, although excessive injection of local anesthetic at an appropriate site has been implicated as well.[20] Local anesthetic absorption and duration of action vary according to injection site. In general, the highest concentrations of local anesthetic in the blood are found after intercostal blockade, followed by caudal, epidural, brachial plexus (BP), and lower extremity blocks. Newer fascial plane blocks, such as the transversus abdominis plane (TAP) block, have an increased rate of absorption possibly related to the compact area between the fascia in which the local anesthetic is injected.[21] For shorter acting local anesthetics, such as lidocaine, epinephrine (1:200,000–1:400,000) may be added to induce vasoconstriction, reducing systemic absorption while also increasing block duration. When properly used, ultrasound guidance can also help reduce inadvertent vascular injection. In addition to visualizing needle movements in real time and observing the spread of local anesthetics, color Doppler can determine the presence or absence of blood vessels within the injection plane.

Nerve injury due to local anesthetic toxicity is a rare complication related to regional anesthesia and peripheral nerve blocks. Patients with preexisting conditions such as diabetes or peripheral neuropathy appear to be at greater risk for the double-crush phenomenon, where the compromised nerve is exposed to a secondary insult resulting in permanent injury.[7,22] The type of local anesthesia may also have a role in the development of neurotoxicity, with esters being more toxic than amides; ropivacaine appears to have the lowest potential for toxicity.[9] The degree of neurotoxicity from local anesthesia has been demonstrated to be concentration (or dose) dependent.[23,24]

Exparel

Despite advances in peripheral nerve block techniques with ultrasound and the use of peripheral nerve catheters, pain management in the postoperative period is a challenge for any clinician. Uncontrolled pain can have a significant impact on recovery and rehabilitation, and if not properly treated it may lead to chronic pain syndromes. Exparel is a newer generation of local anesthetic that can provide pain relief for up to 72 hours. It uses DepoFoam multivesicular liposome technology that encapsulates liposomal bupivacaine in a particle suspension of an isotonic aqueous saline solution that consists of tiny lipid-based particles containing discrete water-filled chambers through a lipid matrix.[25] This formulation results in a delayed release of the encapsulated bupivacaine resulting in a sustained drug delivery while avoiding LAST from high plasma levels.[26] Originally approved in 2011 by the US Food and Drug Administration for use as a local anesthetic infiltration for hemorrhoidectomies and bunionectomies,[27] Exparel is now used for a variety of peripheral nerve blocks. The maximum approved dosage is 266 mg. Because of its delayed onset, it is not uncommon to mix Exparel with standard bupivacaine to reduce the onset effect time of the block. Current manufacturer recommendations state that liposomal bupivacaine should not be administered for at least 20 minutes following any injection of lidocaine. Furthermore, other formulations of bupivacaine should not be given for at least 96 hours after a procedure using Exparel.[28] In addition, it should not come in contact with common antiseptics such as chlorhexidine or povidone-iodine solution since contact with these solutions may cause the liposomes to degrade, releasing toxic amounts of bupivacaine into the plasma.[28] If a topical antiseptic is used it must be allowed to dry before any injection of Exparel.

Equipment and Preparation

Regional procedures can be performed in the preoperative holding area, postanesthesia care unit, operating room, or dedicated peripheral nerve block area (Fig. 50.2). Optimally, this area is large enough to monitor the patient, enable the staff to safely and ergonomically perform the procedure with the patient in a comfortable position, and (if required) allow for resuscitation efforts. Additionally, a central location allows for the immediate availability of all equipment and supplies needed to perform the procedure (Table 50.1) and treat any unanticipated side effects or complications.

All patients who receive a regional anesthetic should have standard hemodynamic monitoring, including pulse oximetry, electrocardiogram (ECG), and noninvasive blood pressure monitoring. If the patient receives preprocedure sedation, administer oxygen via nasal canula or simple face mask and monitor end tidal carbon dioxide ($ETCO_2$). Short-acting benzodiazepines and opioids are often given for anxiolysis and comfort during the procedure. Anesthetists administering titratable doses must ensure the patient remains cooperative and is able to communicate any inadvertent events, such as nerve contact, immediately to the provider. Strict sterile technique should always be observed throughout the procedure. To maintain cleanliness, a sterile sheath is often placed over the transducer, especially when peripheral nerve catheters are placed. Conduction gel placed inside the sheath ensures optimal transmission of the ultrasound beam.

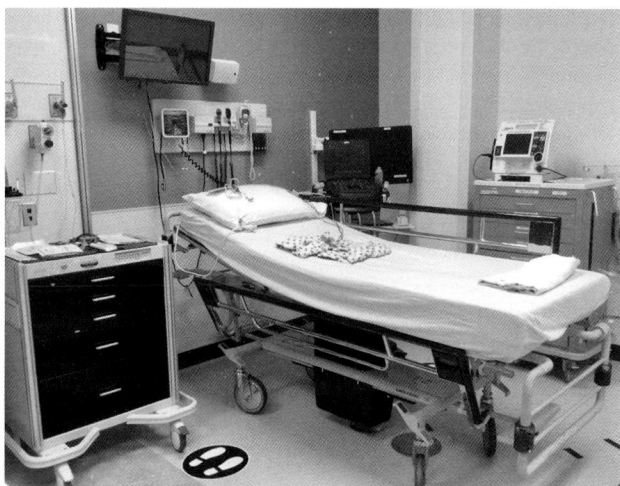

Fig. 50.2 A dedicated block room with ultrasound, regional supplies, and emergency equipment provides a central location with all necessary equipment to treat unanticipated side effects or complications.

TABLE 50.1 Block Room Supplies and Equipment
Patient Monitoring
• Electrocardiogram, blood pressure, and pulse oximetry
• Oxygen (end tidal carbon dioxide monitoring)
Block Specific
• Ultrasound system
• Nerve stimulator
• Block needles
• Local anesthetic
• Patient cleaning supplies
• Equipment cleaning supplies
Emergency Equipment
• Airway/intubation
• Crash cart
• Emergency medications
• Intralipid

Following the procedure, the patient should be observed for at least 30 minutes for potential signs of LAST or other adverse outcomes as blood levels peak.

Discharge Information

A useful tool for patients who have received a regional anesthetic is a discharge information sheet (Box 50.1). This sheet provides information about the nature of the anesthetic and what to expect as the block wears off. Most importantly, it should alert the patient about certain symptoms after discharge that indicate potential complications. If any negative consequences should occur there is also information on how to contact the anesthetist.

BLOCK TECHNIQUES 1

Nerve Stimulation and Peripheral Nerve Blocks

Historically, peripheral nerve blocks were performed under the dictum "no paresthesia, no anesthesia," in which blocks were placed based on anatomic knowledge with the goal of eliciting a response by contacting the targeted nerve with the block needle. However, these techniques were associated with an increased risk of nerve trauma.[29] When first

---

BOX 50.1   Regional Anesthesia Discharge Information Sheet

What Is Regional Anesthesia?
Regional anesthesia is the injection of local anesthetic (such as lidocaine) near nerves that sense pain in the area where you had surgery. This is very similar to a dentist injecting local anesthesia into your mouth—it numbs an area of your body so the procedure doesn't hurt.

What Should I Expect After Regional Anesthesia?
Following regional anesthesia, the area where you had surgery will be numb for several hours. Depending on the local anesthetic used, it can be numb for up to 72 hours. The block will wear off slowly, and your first sensations will be a tingling feeling in the area that was numb.

What Should I Do When the Block Starts to Wear Off?
As soon as you develop any feeling, start taking your prescribed pain medication. It is much easier to treat pain before it begins than try to catch up after it has started.

What Should I Be Careful About After Regional Anesthesia?
Because part of your body is numb, you won't know if you injure it. Be sure to protect that part of your body from being bumped, cut, and otherwise harmed. Look at it frequently to make sure you haven't accidently injured it. Finally, avoid lying on the numb area when you sleep.

What Complications Should I Watch for After Regional Anesthesia?
The site of your body where the injection was made will be sore for a few days. This pain should be controlled with over-the-counter pain relief medicine (e.g., Tylenol, Advil). It is common to have strange sensations (e.g., mild numbness, tingling) for a days after the block. In rare cases these sensations can last as long as 6 months.
It you experience any of the following, immediately notify your health care provider:
• Sensation doesn't begin to return in 24 hr
• Numb area regained sensation but becomes numb again
• Skin in the numb area turns blue or feels cool
• Persistent pain in the area that was numb, several days after the surgery

---

described in the literature over 50 years ago, the listed benefits of nerve stimulation included the ability to reduce the volume and dose of local anesthetic agents, increase block efficacy, and locate difficult to find nerves.[30] Today, most providers perform peripheral nerve blocks using only ultrasound; however, nerve stimulation remains a valuable tool in the practice of regional anesthesia. For the practitioner new to ultrasound, it provides a means to verify correct needle placement. In addition, recent studies demonstrate nerve stimulation can increase the safety profile of certain nerve blocks.[31] Understanding basic principles and functions facilitates optimal use.

Peripheral nerve stimulators provide a controlled pulse of variable amplitude through a conducting device. The location of neural fibers can be determined without eliciting repeated paresthesia. Specialized, insulated needles have been designed to localize the distribution of the stimulating charge to the tip of the needle. This property reduces confusion from wide-field stimulation of the area around the nerve, isolating the desired nerve fibers.[32]

The negative lead is attached to the skin with an ECG electrode, and the positive lead is attached to the needle. Most electrical devices are equipped with an adjustable amplitude from 0 to 5 mA. The needle is advanced slowly, allowing the amplitude of the unit to be adjusted as the needle approaches the nerve[29,32] (Fig. 50.3).

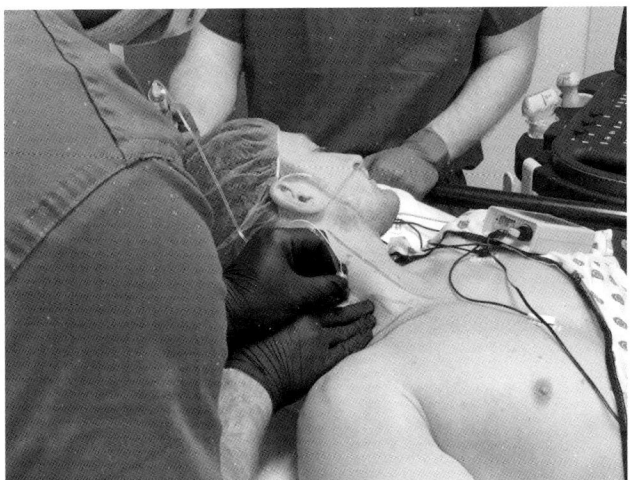

Fig. 50.3 Anesthetists perform a landmark-guided interscalene block using nerve stimulation.

The stimulator should not be turned on until the needle has entered the skin. This reduces patient discomfort during initial advancement. The patient is instructed to identify discomfort verbally and not to move as the needle is advanced. Premedication with titratable short-acting benzodiazepines and/or opioids helps maintain patient alertness and cooperation in response to nerve stimulus. As the needle comes within close contact of the desired nerve, the current will elicit a motor response. The amplitude is continuously decreased, and the needle is adjusted so that motor response is maintained. The lower amplitude enhances the ability to accurately identify the neurovascular bundle while decreasing patient discomfort. The goal is to elicit a motor response with minimal amplitude (i.e., 0.3–0.5 mA), which approximates the needle tip to the target nerve. If motor response is elicited with less than 0.2 mA, it is possible that the tip has penetrated the nerve's epineurium, and the practitioner should not proceed with injection.[29]

Patients may complain of soreness and/or weakness along the path of the stimulated nerve following the procedure. Severe or prolonged discomfort occurs when the stimulus is delivered over a long period or at a high current. Placement of the negative electrode in close contact to the target nerve can result in electrotranslocation enhancement. If the nerve fiber is located under the negative electrode, an exaggerated response may occur.[29,32]

Ultrasound-Guided Regional Anesthesia

Ultrasound has revolutionized the practice of regional anesthesia. Ultrasound technology and our clinical understanding of anatomic sonography has evolved immensely over the past 15 years. In anesthesia departments across the United States, ultrasound-guided regional anesthesia (UGRA) has become routine, and some argue it is the gold standard for performing nerve blocks.[33,34] The use of ultrasound affords the provider three distinct advantages over the landmark/nerve stimulation technique: (1) imagery and identification of anatomic structures beneath the skin, (2) visualization of needle movements in real time, and (3) observation of local anesthetic distribution.[35] These advantages translate into faster block onset, more efficacious blocks, fewer failed blocks, less complications such as LAST, fewer side effects, and improved patient satisfaction.[17,36,37] Advantages of using ultrasound-guided techniques are listed in Box 50.2. It should be noted that the incorporation of ultrasound into regional anesthesia has not resulted in the decreased incidence of nerve injury. The frequency of reported long-term neurologic

symptoms following an ultrasound-guided block is nearly identical to previous reports where nerve stimulation was used as the identification tool.[11]

As with any anesthesia-related skill, ultrasound is user dependent and not something learned quickly. Providers wishing to add this expertise to their anesthesia skillset should follow a regimented plan that includes attending educational meetings that offer didactic and hands-on training, learning sonoanatomy and needle insertion techniques using repeated practice, and spending time observing and learning ultrasound-guided regional techniques with an experienced individual.[38] A study investigating novice trainee performance in performing ultrasound-guided blocks on cadavers found that on average 28 supervised procedures using deliberate practice techniques were required before competency was achieved.[39]

What Is the "Sound" in Ultrasound?

Sound is a pressure wave created when a vibrating object sets a medium into motion, resulting in pressure variations. This causes the medium to vibrate back and forth. Sound is a longitudinal and mechanical wave that moves in a series of compressions and rarefactions. Longitudinal waves travel, or propagate, in their direction of movement. Mechanical waves require a medium. When a sound wave is generated, it compresses the medium it travels in as it moves forward, creating an area of high pressure called a compression. As the wave continues along its path, the medium is stretched, generating an area of low pressure known as a rarefaction. Fig. 50.4 details the important properties of a sound wave. A single compression and rarefaction form a cycle. The number of cycles that occur in 1 second is a called a Hertz (Hz). Human hearing can detect sound frequencies from 20 to 20,000 Hz. By comparison, diagnostic ultrasound operates at frequencies between 2 and 15 million cycles/second, or megahertz (MHz). In general, high-frequency ultrasound (>7 MHz) creates high-resolution images; however, these waves degrade (attenuate) quickly, which limits visualization to structures at shallow depths (≤4 cm). Low-frequency ultrasound (2–5 MHz) can image deeper structures but with decreased resolution[40] (Fig. 50.5).

Sound travels at different speeds through different medium, known as propagation velocity. In diagnostic ultrasound, human tissue is the medium in which sound travels. The standardized propagation velocity of sound through tissue is approximately 1540 m/second, which is derived by averaging the different velocities of soft tissues in the body. By comparison, the propagation velocity of air is quite slow at 440 m/second and in bone it is 5000 m/second.[40] A list of various propagation velocities can be found in Table 50.2.

The impedance (Z) of tissue describes its stiffness, or resistance against the propagation of sound. It is equal to density (p) multiplied

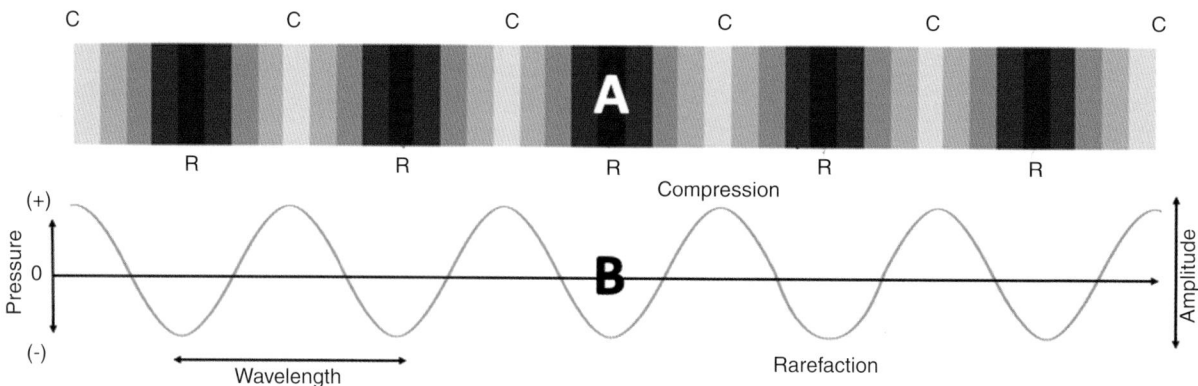

Fig. 50.4 Although sound is often drawn as a transverse wave (B), it is in actuality a longitudinal mechanical wave (A) that travels parallel to its propagation. *C*, Compression; *R*, rarefaction.

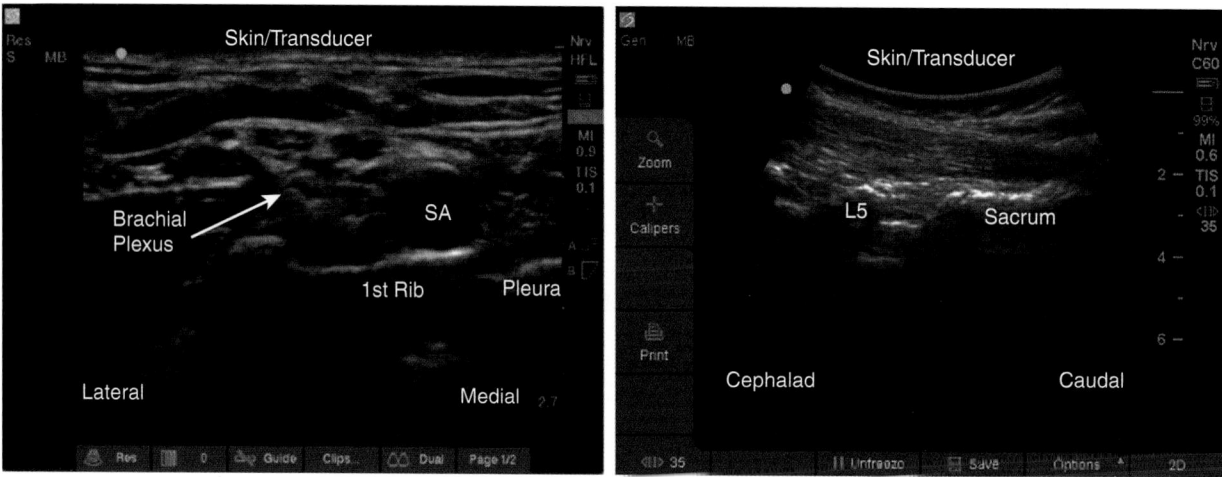

Fig. 50.5 Comparison of high-frequency ultrasound image of the brachial plexus (left) and low-frequency ultrasound image of the L5-S1 spinous interspace (right). *SA*, subclavian artery.

TABLE 50.2   Propagation Velocities

Medium	Velocity
Air	331 m/sec
Brain	1541 m/sec
Kidney	1561 m/sec
Liver	1549 m/sec
Muscle	1585 m/sec
Fat	1450 m/sec
Soft tissue (average)	1540 m/sec
Bone (different densities)	3000–5000 m/sec

by propagation velocity (*v*), where $Z = p \times v$.[41] Differences in impedance along tissue borders result in reflection, refraction, scattering, and ultimately attenuation.

Reflection of an ultrasound wave is the basis of all diagnostic imaging. Reflection occurs when a sound contacts the borders of two tissues with different densities (acoustic impedances), where part of the beam is reflected back to the transducer and part continues through the tissue. The amount of reflection of the incidence beam is proportional to the difference of the impedance between the two tissues. If the two tissues have the same acoustic impedance, their boundary will not produce an echo. Conversely, if the impedance between the two boundaries is significant, the majority of the wave will be reflected back to the transducer. Large, smooth surfaces, such as bone, are called specular reflectors. Soft tissue is classified as a diffuse reflector, as adjoining cells create an uneven surface, and reflections return in various directions in relation to the transmitted beam. However, due to the multiple surfaces, sound is reflected back to the transducer in a relatively uniform manner.

Refraction refers to the reflection of sound when a wave strikes the border of two tissues at an oblique angle. The echoes do not return directly back to the transducer. The angle of refraction is dependent on two things: the angle at which the sound wave strikes the boundary between the two tissues and the difference in their propagation velocities. Ultrasound systems assume that sound travels in a straight line; since the reflection is returning at an oblique angle, the image may be distorted or potentially altered.

Scattering occurs at interfaces involving structures of small dimensions. This is common with red blood cells (RBCs), where the average diameter of an RBC is 7 μm, and an ultrasound wavelength may be 300 μm (5 MHz).[41] When the wave is greater than the structure it contacts, it generates a uniform, low amplitude reflection in all directions. Scattering is dependent on four different factors: (1) the dimension of the scatterer, (2) the number of scatterers present, (3) the extent to which the scatterer differs from surrounding material, and (4) the ultrasound frequency.[40]

The culminating effect of tissue on sound as it travels through the body is attenuation. As sound passes through a medium, energy is absorbed, and the intensity of the wave decreases. The reflection and

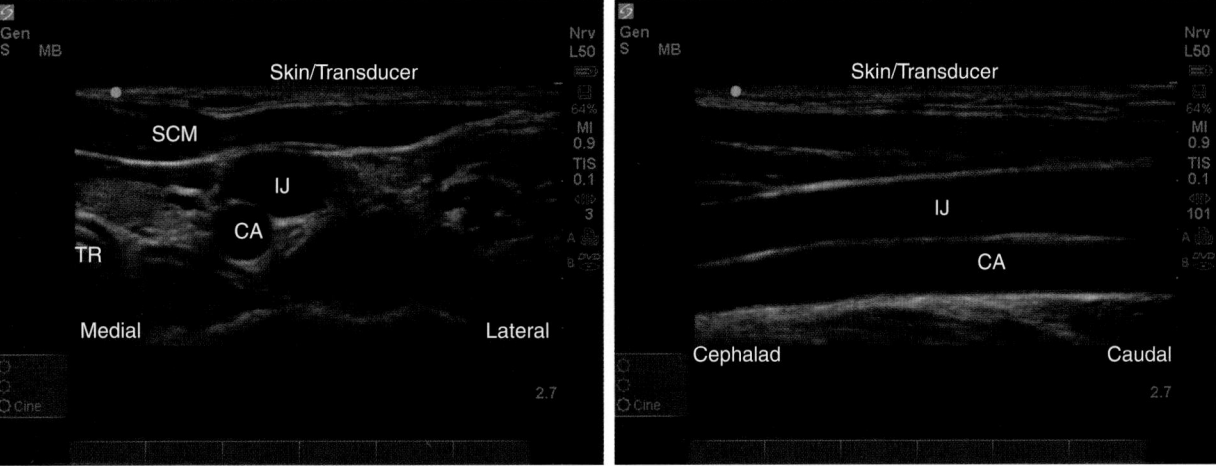

Fig. 50.6 Comparison of cross-sectional *(left)* and longitudinal *(right)* B-mode ultrasound images of the carotid artery and internal jugular vein in the neck. *CA,* Carotid artery; *IJ,* internal jugular vein; *SCM,* sternocleidomastoid muscle; *TR,* tracheal rings.

scatter that occur between tissue borders also contribute to this phenomenon. The deeper into the tissue sound travels, the weaker the wave becomes, reducing image quality. Ultimately, the sound wave becomes so degraded that returning echoes are not capable of generating an image. Attenuation is high in muscle and skin, and low in fluid-filled structures. High-frequency waves are attenuated to a greater extent than low-frequency waves.

Diagnostic ultrasound uses a pulse-echo technique in which a handheld transducer emits short pulses of ultrasound into the body and then waits for returning echoes created by the interaction of sound at tissue borders. By knowing the velocity at which sound travels through tissue, the depth at which the echo occurs can be determined. This can be calculated as $2s = v \times t$, where $2s$ is the distance between the transducer and the reflector, v is the velocity of sound in tissue, and t is the elapsed time.[40] The computer then processes these echoes based on their strength and the time they were received, displaying them on a screen in a two-dimensional slice of tissue centered beneath the transducer, similar to an individual image on a computed tomography (CT) scan. This is known as a B-mode (brightness mode) or grayscale image. The on-screen vertical axis represents the distance an anatomic structure or block needle is from the ultrasound transducer, whereas the horizontal axis represents the distance to the right or left of the center of the transducer. B-mode images are obtained in either cross-sectional or longitudinal views. The cross-sectional view is the short-axis representation of anatomy, similar to a slice of bread, whereas longitudinal views are long-axis depictions of the anatomy.

The differences in acoustic impedance at tissue borders create the ability to identify specific anatomy. In general, the denser a structure is, the brighter (whiter) it will appear on the screen. Tissue is described as hyperechoic, hypoechoic, or anechoic. Hyperechoic structures are dense structures that generate strong echoes. They appear bright on the ultrasound image. Specular reflectors such as bone, fascia, and block needles are common examples. Diffuse reflectors such as soft tissue are hypoechoic structures and appear as varying shades of gray. Additionally, soft tissue can be described as either homogenous or heterogeneous. Homogenous is used to describe specialized cells that make up organs, such as the thyroid gland or liver, and the cells appear very uniform on ultrasound. Heterogeneous tissue, such as muscle, looks less uniform because of the different densities in the cells interspaced with fascial planes.

Nerves can appear either hyper- or hypoechoic depending on their location in the body.[42] Proximal nerves, such as the roots of the BP, are pure fascicle, which is less dense than the surrounding connective tissue, making them appear hypoechoic on ultrasound. Conversely, peripheral nerves, such as the tibial and peroneal nerves in the popliteal fossa, appear hyperechoic because they are mixed nerves created from multiple nerve roots held together by connective tissue. At this level, the nerve composition is denser than the surrounding muscle so they appear brighter on the ultrasound image.

Fluid-filled structures, such as blood vessels and cysts, do not reflect sound waves. Since an echo is not generated, they are called anechoic and appear black on the ultrasound image. Although arteries and veins are both anechoic on ultrasound, veins appear ovoid and are easily compressible, whereas arteries are round and pulsatile in nature. In a short-axis or transverse orientation, vessels appear as circles. Rotating the transducer 90 degrees creates a long-axis view, which makes the vessels appear tubular (Fig. 50.6).

Although not used to create a picture, Doppler is an essential component in ultrasound imaging. The central tenant of the Doppler effect is that the frequency of a sound wave is perceived to change when either the source or detector is moving.[40] The change in pitch of a siren as an ambulance travels down the street is a familiar example. In diagnostic imaging, Doppler is used to detect and measure blood flow. When Doppler ultrasound is oriented over a blood vessel so that blood is flowing toward the transducer, the reflected wave will have a higher frequency than the incident or originating signal. This is a positive Doppler shift. Conversely, if blood is flowing away from the transducer, a lower frequency wave will be reflected, resulting in a negative Doppler shift. The angle between the receiver and the transmitter plays an important role in determining the amount of shift. Doppler shifts calculated by an ultrasound system use the cosine of the angle between the axis of the ultrasound beam and the direction of flow. A maximum Doppler shift occurs at 0° (cosine of 0° = 1) when flow is either directly toward or away from the transducer.[40] When blood flow is perpendicular to the ultrasound beam, no shift is detected (cosine of 90° = 0).[40] Color-flow Doppler technology assigns a color to the blood flow based on its direction in relation to the transducer. Contrary to what is written in some texts, the red and blue colors used in color-flow Doppler do not represent arterial or venous blood, only the direction in flow.[40]

Transducer orientation is another important aspect of ultrasound-guided procedures. Proper transducer placement in relation to the

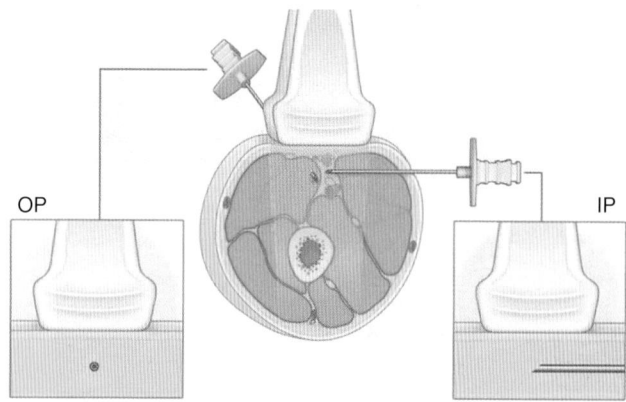

Fig. 50.7 An illustration of a cross-sectional image of an extremity comparing in-plane *(IP)* and out-of-plane *(OP)* needle insertion techniques.

patient's position is key in determining an accurate image. All transducers have an orientation indicator that corresponds to an icon on the ultrasound screen. In diagnostic ultrasound imaging, proper orientation is achieved when the orientation indicator is aligned to the provider's left in a transverse view or toward the patient's head in a sagittal view. When done consistently, the anesthetist can predict where needle insertion will occur and the direction of any adjustments required during the procedure.

Needle orientation to the transducer during a block is typically described by its relationship to the image plane. During the in-plane approach, the entire length of the needle is visualized within the plane of the ultrasound image; in the out-of-plane approach, the cross section of the needle is seen as a hyperechoic dot where it crosses the plane (Fig. 50.7). The in-plane approach is generally preferred since it allows for visualization of the entire needle throughout the procedure; however, the anatomy associated with certain blocks may necessitate use of the out-of-plane approach.[43]

In 1999 the American Institute of Ultrasound in Medicine (AIUM) published guidelines for describing basic movements when scanning with the ultrasound transducer[44] (Fig. 50.8):

- *Sliding* the transducer along the skin allows the practitioner to determine the best window to perform the procedure.
- *Rotating* the probe clockwise or counterclockwise allows for viewing structures in both cross-sectional and longitudinal views.
- *Rocking* the transducer allows for centering the area of interest or extending the field in one direction or another. It is also used to optimize transducer to skin contact, reducing air artifact. It is sometimes called in-plane motion.
- *Tilting* allows for other planes to be identified in the same axis with sliding the transducer. It is also referred to as cross-plane motion.
- *Compressing* is used to optimize contact between the transducer face and scanning surface, and decrease the distance between the transducer and target organ.

CLINICAL ANATOMY

A fundamental knowledge of the functional anatomy of the major nerve plexi, as well as their terminal branches, is essential when performing regional anesthesia. This section reviews the important anatomic structures of the spine, upper extremity, trunk, and lower extremity.

Spine

A complete anatomic and physiologic description of the neuraxis can be found in Chapter 49. For the purposes of this chapter, we review only the important aspects of the central nervous system, such as the

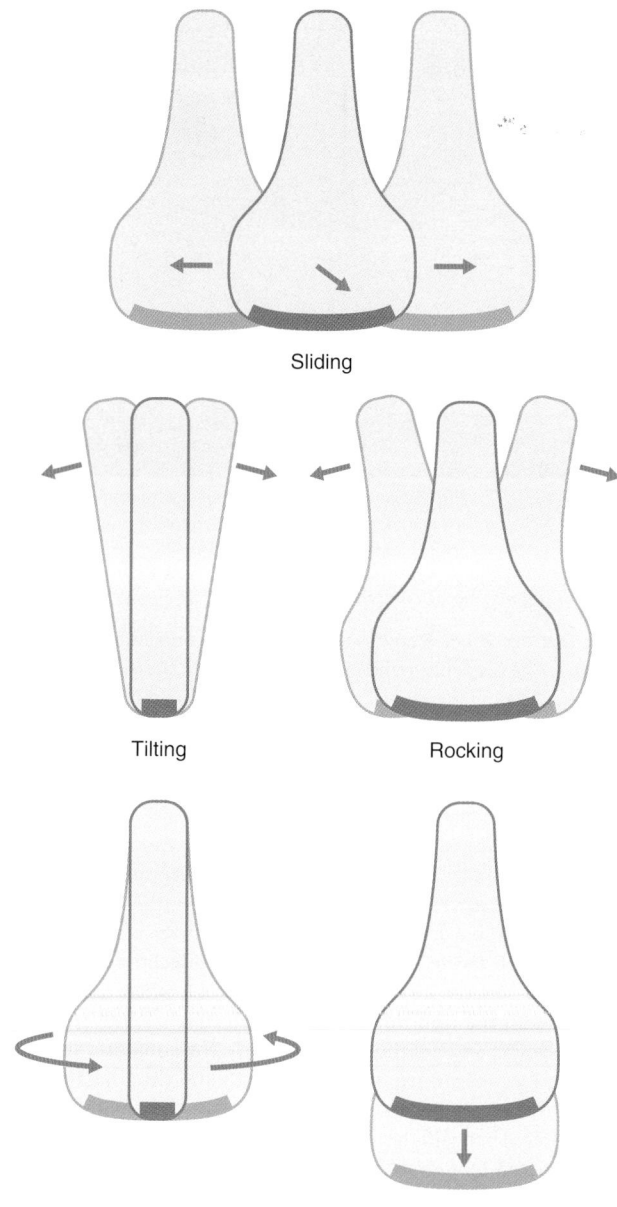

Fig. 50.8 Basic transducer movements established by the American Institute of Ultrasound in Medicine (AIUM): sliding, tilting, rocking, rotating, and compressing. (Modified from Smith CF, Dilley A, Mitchell B, et al. *Gray's Surface Anatomy and Ultrasound.* Philadelphia: Elsevier; 2018:11.)

spinal nerves and important vertebral structures, that are key to performing certain blocks.

Spinal Nerves

Spinal nerves are an integral part of the peripheral nervous system. There are 31 pairs of spinal nerves: 8 cervical, 12 thoracic, 5 lumbar, 5 sacral, and 1 coccygeal. Each of the spinal nerves are formed by both ventral and dorsal nerve fibers from the spinal cord. Spinal nerves contain sympathetic fibers that innervate blood vessels, smooth muscle, and glands of the skin. After exiting the vertebral foramen, the spinal nerve divides into dorsal and ventral rami (branches). The ventral rami are larger and travel lateral and anterior innervating the tissues of the head, neck, trunk, and upper and lower extremities. The dorsal rami innervate the paravertebral muscles and subcutaneous tissues of the back.

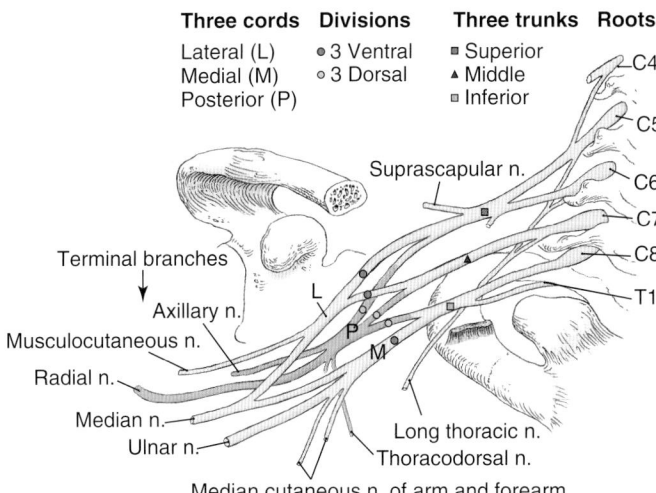

Three cords	Divisions	Three trunks	Roots
Lateral (L)	● 3 Ventral	▪ Superior	
Medial (M)	○ 3 Dorsal	▲ Middle	
Posterior (P)		▫ Inferior	

Fig. 50.9 Derivation of the brachial plexus from the cervical spine. *n.,* Nerve.

The first 8 spinal nerves exit at the level above its corresponding vertebrae (e.g., spinal nerve C7 exits above the seventh cervical vertebrae). This changes at the first thoracic vertebrae (because of the eighth spinal nerve), where all spinal nerves then exit below the level of the corresponding vertebrae (e.g., spinal nerve L1 exits below the first lumbar vertebrae).

Paravertebral Space

The paravertebral space (PVS) is an area created at the borders of each vertebrae that allow spinal nerves to pass along the entire vertebral column. It is a wedge-shaped area formed medially by the posterolateral aspect of the vertebral body, disc, and intervertebral foramen; posteriorly by the superior costotransverse ligament; laterally by the posterior intercostal membrane; and anteriorly by the parietal pleura. The PVS is contiguous with the epidural space medially. The sympathetic ganglia lie close to the somatic nerves, and both are frequently blocked when local anesthesia is injected into this space.

Vertebral Body Process

Vertebral anatomy varies along the spinal column—in particular, the relationship between the spinous process and specific functional anatomy, and the spinous and the transverse processes. The differences between the vertebral processes can influence the manner in which various truncal blocks are performed.

Prominent spinous process landmarks relevant to regional anesthesia include T7, which aligns with the distal edge of the scapula, and L4, which approximates the level of the iliac crests (i.e., Tuffier line). In the thoracic spine, the spinous processes angle in an inferior direction, creating a protective ridge. As a result, the transverse processes move progressively superior in relation to their corresponding spinous process. For example, the transverse process of T1 is nearly lateral to the T1 spinous process, whereas the transverse process of T7 is lateral to the spinous process of T6. The spinous processes of the lumbar vertebrae are relatively straight, and the corresponding transverse process is at the same level.

Upper Extremity

Brachial Plexus

Knowledge of the BP is essential for proper administration of regional anesthesia in the upper extremities. Generations of nurse anesthesia students have drawn and learned a variety of acronyms to describe this plexus, which supplies innervation to nearly all of the shoulder and upper extremity. However, being proficient in the various BP blocks requires

an understanding of not only the network of nerves that comprise the plexus but also the relationships of the surrounding muscle, fascia, and vasculature. The plexus originates from the ventral rami of five spinal nerve roots (C5-C8 and T1) in the neck and extends through the axilla, innervating the upper extremity (Fig. 50.9). In a small number of individuals there are contributions from the ventral rami of the fourth cervical (C4) and/or second thoracic (T2) spinal nerves. As it courses distally, the five roots of the plexus converge and diverge to form three trunks (upper, middle, and lower), six divisions (three anterior and three posterior), three cords (medial, posterior, and lateral), and five terminal branches (axillary, radial, musculocutaneous, median, and ulnar). The supraclavicular portion of the BP (roots, trunks, and divisions) lies in the posterior triangle of the neck, and the infraclavicular portion of the plexus (cords and terminal branches) is located in the axilla. Obtaining a basic knowledge of the BP shown and described in only two dimensions and without the associated bone, muscle, and vascular structures can lead to a difficulty in understanding how it is applied in the clinical setting. Augmenting didactic learning with hands-on practice that is mentored by experienced anesthetists will improve the understanding and performance of the various BP blocks.[45-47]

The roots of the BP pass between the anterior scalene muscle (ASM) and middle scalene muscle (MSM) as they exit their respective vertebral foramen. As the roots pass the lateral border of the scalene muscles, they converge into three trunks. The C5 and C6 spinal nerves combine to form the superior or upper trunk, the C7 spinal nerve becomes the middle trunk, and the C8 and T1 spinal nerves form the inferior or lower trunk. The trunks are surrounded by a fascial sheath, which originates from the posterior fascia of the ASM and the anterior fascia of the MSM. Variations in individual anatomy occur, and it is possible for the nerves to be isolated during a procedure, resulting in an incomplete block.[48]

At the lateral border of the first rib and posterior to the clavicle, the trunks divide into anterior and posterior divisions. These divisions are clinically important with regard to the evaluation of BP blocks as the anterior divisions generally supply the ventral (and flexor) areas of the upper extremity, while the posterior divisions supply the dorsal (and extensor) regions of the upper extremity. As these divisions enter the axilla, the three posterior divisions merge, forming the posterior cord. The anterior divisions of the superior and middle trunks combine to form the lateral cord, and the anterior division of the inferior trunk becomes the medial cord. The cords are named according to their position in relation to the axillary artery. At the lateral border of the pectoralis minor muscle, the cords diverge into the five terminal branches that form the peripheral nerves of the upper extremity. The median nerve arises from branches of the lateral and medial cords, the musculocutaneous nerve is a continuation of the lateral cord, and the ulnar nerve extends from the medial cord. The axillary and radial nerves both arise from the posterior cord.[48]

Understanding the anatomic relationships and innervation of the terminal nerve branches is of paramount importance in the clinical application, evaluation, and supplementation of the various BP blocks. The branches of the lateral and medial cords (median, ulnar, and musculocutaneous nerves) predominantly supply the ventral portions of the upper extremity, while the branches of the posterior cord (radial and axillary nerve) predominantly supply the dorsal portions. However, in certain areas of the upper extremity, such as the posterior portion of the hand and digits, there is considerable cutaneous innervation by the median and ulnar nerves.[45-48]

Terminal Nerves of the Upper Extremity

The radial nerve (C5-C8 and T1) is the major nerve supply to the dorsal extensor muscles, such as the triceps, of the upper limb below the shoulder. It supplies sensory innervation to the extensor region of the arm, forearm, and hand. The musculocutaneous nerve (C5-C7) supplies the flexor muscles, such as the biceps, brachialis, and coracobrachialis, of the ventral upper arm. It supplies sensory innervation to the lateral aspect of the forearm between the wrist and elbow as the lateral antebrachial cutaneous nerve. The median and ulnar nerves pass through the arm and provide sensory and motor innervation to the forearm and hand. The median nerve (C6-T1) is better represented than the ulnar nerve in the forearm, where it supplies most of the flexor and pronator muscles. It also supplies sensory innervation to the ventral portion of the thumb, the first and second fingers, the lateral half of the third finger, and the palm of the hand. The ulnar nerve (C8 and T1) has greater representation than the median nerve in the hand. It supplies motor innervation to the majority of the small flexor muscles. The ulnar nerve does not supply sensory innervation to the forearm. In the hand, it supplies sensation to the medial part of the third finger, the entire fourth finger, and the remainder of the palm of the hand.[45-47]

Truncal

The trunk can be divided into the chest and abdomen. The ventral rami of spinal nerves T1-T6 supply the chest wall, while the abdomen is supplied from the ventral rami of T6-L1. Important anatomic landmarks include the nipple line (T4), the xiphoid process (T6), the umbilicus (T10), and the pubis (T12). At the thoracic level, the ventral rami of each spinal nerve enter a neurovascular bundle with a corresponding artery and vein, traveling in the intercostal groove along the anterior aspect of the caudal rib border. The fascial borders of the innermost internal and external intercostal muscles provide the border for the intercostal groove. In the abdomen, the intercostal nerves course anteriorly past the midaxillary line and enter the fascial plane between the transversus abdominis muscle (TAM) and internal oblique muscle (IOM). They then continue to the midline, piercing the rectus abdominis muscles. At the midaxillary line, a lateral cutaneous branch pierces the external oblique muscle (EOM), supplying innervation to the skin of the flanks and back. As the lower intercostal nerves course anteriorly, they enter the rectus sheath at the posterolateral border of each muscle body and terminate in the rectus abdominis muscle.[49-51] The tendinous intersections at the rectus abdominis muscle create segmented intercostal nerve distributions; however, there may be some overlapping in innervation. The anterior rectus sheath is dense and fibrous, extending from the xiphoid to the pubis. The posterior sheath is easily identifiable down to the umbilicus and provides a wall when injecting local anesthetic. Below the umbilicus it becomes a thin sheath of transversalis fascia (TF) that adheres tightly to the peritoneum.

While the ventral rami of T1-T6 supply the cutaneous innervation of the chest/breast and intercostal muscles, branches of the BP innervate much of the other muscles of the chest. The lateral pectoral nerve (C5-C7) and medial pectoral nerve (C8-T1) innervate the majority of the pectoralis major and minor muscles. The long thoracic nerve (C5-C7) and the thoracodorsal nerve (C6-C8) are two other important branches of the BP.[52] The long thoracic nerve innervates the chest wall superficial to the serratus anterior muscle, and the thoracodorsal nerve innervates the latissimus dorsi muscle.[53]

The lumbar triangle of Petit describes the neurovascular plane of the lateral abdominal musculature, where the IOM can be localized directly.[54] In most individuals it is found just beyond the peak of the iliac crest. The base of the triangle is formed by the iliac crest; at this point the transversus abdominis attaches to the inner lip of the crest, while internal oblique attaches to the intermediate area. The external oblique and latissimus dorsi muscles attach to the external lip and form the apex of the triangle as they course superiorly.

Inguinal Nerves

The iliohypogastric and ilioinguinal nerves arise from the lumbar plexus and are classically described as terminal branches of L1. There is occasional innervation from T12 (often referred to as the subcostal nerve); however, variation from person to person is significant, and as many as 20% of individuals may have contribution from L2-L3 spinal nerves. Both nerves exit the psoas major and course inferolaterally along the anterior surface of the quadratus lumborum muscle (QLM) and TAM parallel and superior to the iliac crest. The iliohypogastric nerve enters the TAP at the anterior third of the iliac crest and divides into anterior and lateral cutaneous branches that innervate the skin over the hypogastrium and gluteal regions. The ilioinguinal nerve enters the TAP very close to the anterior superior iliac spine (ASIS), rising through the IOM and EOM on its course to the inguinal canal. It supplies innervation to the lower abdominal wall, upper thigh, and pubic areas.[51,55]

Lower Extremity

The lower extremity is innervated by two separate and distinct plexi, the lumbar plexus and sacral plexus (Fig. 50.10). The lumbar plexus is formed from the ventral rami of the first, second, third, and fourth lumbar spinal nerves. There is occasional contribution from the 12th thoracic nerve. The lumbar plexus provides sensory and motor innervation to the skin and muscle of the lower anterior wall and part of the genitalia, to the anterior and medial aspects of the thigh and knee, as well as sensory innervation along the medial aspect of the lower extremity distal to the knee. The lumbosacral trunk is formed by the union of a branch of the L4 spinal nerve with the ventral rami of the L5 spinal nerve. This trunk combines with the ventral rami of the S1-S4 spinal nerves that exit through the anterior sacral foramina to form the sacral plexus. The nerves converge at the greater sciatic foramen on the pelvic wall, anterior to the piriformis muscle.

Lumbar Plexus

The lumbar plexus originates anterior to the QLM and posterior to the psoas major muscle. There are three terminal branches: the femoral

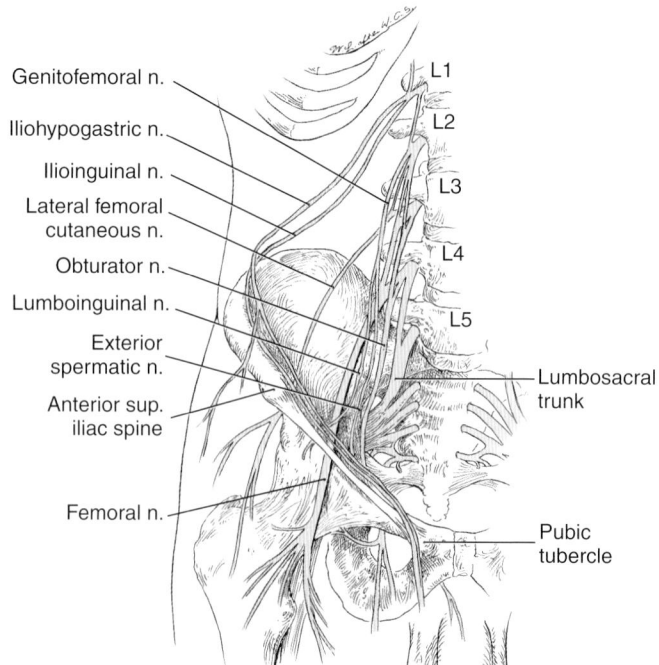

Fig. 50.10 Origin and position of the nerves of the lower extremity. *n.*, Nerve.

nerve (FN), lateral femoral cutaneous nerve (LFCN), and the obturator nerve (ON). These nerve branches are tightly bound to muscle bodies and the connecting fascia as they course distally within the leg.

The FN is the largest of the three branches. It is formed from contributions of the second, third, and fourth lumbar spinal nerves. It forms and appears at the middle to lower third of the psoas major muscle. It remains within the groove of the psoas major and the iliac muscles as it courses deep to the inguinal ligament, where it lies anterior to the iliopsoas muscle, beneath the fascia lata and iliaca, and lateral to the femoral artery.

As the FN passes under the inguinal ligament it forms into anterior and posterior branches. The anterior branch provides innervation to the anterior surface of the thigh and the sartorius muscle. The saphenous nerve (SphN) also arises from the anterior branch. The posterior branch provides innervation to the quadriceps muscles, the knee joint, and its medial ligament. The FN is bound by several structures above and below the inguinal ligament. Proximal to the inguinal ligament, the FN is encapsulated by the fascia iliaca laterally, the psoas fascia medially, and the transverse fascia anteriorly. The bony structure of the pelvis makes up the posterior border of this capsule or sheath.[45,56,57] At the level of the inguinal ligament, the FN joins the femoral artery and enters the lower extremity. The FN is bordered by the iliopsoas fascia posterolaterally, the inguinal ligament anteriorly, and the femoral vessels border it medially. The femoral nerve and vessels course distally along the proximal thigh in the femoral triangle, which is a space created by the inguinal ligament proximally (base of the triangle), the sartorius muscle laterally, and the adductor longus medially.[58] The floor of the triangle consists of the iliopsoas muscle laterally and the pectineus and adductor longus muscles medially.[59] The apex of this triangle, created by the intersection of the sartorius and adductor longus, is the origin of the adductor canal (AC). The location of the AC is described just distal to the midpoint between the ASIS and the base of the patella.[58] It is a musculoaponeurotic tunnel formed by the vastus medialis muscle anterolaterally and the adductor longus and magnus muscles posteromedially. The canal is roofed by the vastoadductor membrane. The terminal branch of the FN, the SphN, and the nerve to the vastus medialis are consistently found within the AC.[59,60]

The LFCN is formed from the ventral rami of the second and third lumbar spinal nerves and is the first to leave the compartment. It emerges from the lateral border of the psoas major at its midpoint. The nerve then traverses the iliac muscle obliquely toward the anterior iliac spine. The LFCN passes under the lateral border of the inguinal ligament and provides sensory innervation to the lateral aspect of the thigh.[45,56,57]

The ON arises from the ventral rami of the second, third, and fourth lumbar spinal nerves. It emerges from the medial border of the psoas major at the level of the sacroiliac joint and is covered by the external iliac artery and vein. The ON passes into the pelvis minor and runs anteroinferiorly to the obturator canal, which it traverses near the obturator vessels. Due to the proximity of the nerve to the external iliac artery, it can be injured in patients undergoing extensive pelvic surgery.[45,56,57] The ON is primarily a motor nerve to the adductor muscles in the medial thigh. In addition, it provides mixed sensory fibers to the hip, medial aspect of the femur, as well as the skin and soft tissue along the medial aspect of the thigh proximal to the knee.[45,56,57]

Sacral Plexus

There are two major branches of the sacral plexus: the sciatic nerve, which is a continuation of the plexus, and the pudendal nerves. In addition, several smaller branches provide both sensory and motor innervation to the gluteal region and posterior thigh. The sciatic

nerve is formed by the L4-S3 nerve roots, is the continuation of the upper division of the sacral plexus, and is the largest nerve in the body. It supplies the posterior muscles and skin of the upper leg and the lower leg and foot. The sciatic nerve passes through the pelvis via the great sacrosciatic foramen, below the piriform muscle, and descends between the major trochanter and the tuberosity of the ischium to the lower third of the thigh. Proximal to the popliteal fossa, the sciatic nerve bifurcates into the tibial nerve (TN) and common peroneal nerve (CPN).[46] The TN is the larger of the two branches and courses medially in the popliteal fossa beneath popliteal fascia and between the gastrocnemius muscles. The CPN courses laterally over the head of the fibula (hence the CPN is often referred to as the common fibular nerve) and then divides into the deep and superficial peroneal nerves.

Nerve Innervation of the Foot

Five nerves innervate the foot. Terminal branches of the sciatic nerve include the PTN, deep peroneal nerve (DPN), superficial peroneal nerve (SPN), and sural nerve (SN). The only terminal branch of the FN within the foot is the SphN.

The PTN provides the greatest innervation to the foot. At the level of the medial malleolus, it branches into the medial and lateral plantar nerves, which provide innervation to the sole of the foot, and the calcaneal nerve that provides sensation to the heel (Fig. 50.11).[61] The DPN travels distally between the anterior tibial muscle and the long extensor muscle of the great toe into the ankle (Fig. 50.12). At the level of the distal tibial, it lies lateral to the anterior tibial artery and long-extensor muscle of the great toe.[61] The DPN innervates the short extensors of the toes and provides sensory innervation to the lateral aspect of the great toe and the medial aspect of the second digit. The SPN courses laterally along the lower leg in a groove created by the peroneus brevis longus and the extensor digitorum longus muscles that lead to the lower fibula. It provides sensation to the dorsum of the foot and toes (see Fig. 50.12).[61] The SN is formed by the union of branches from both the TN and CPN. The medial SN is a branch of the TN that courses distally between the heads of the gastrocnemius muscle, before becoming superficial at the midcalf where it joins the sural communicating nerve, a branch of the CPN. At this point the SN takes a superficial course behind the lateral malleolus (Fig. 50.13). It provides sensation to the posterior heel, lateral portion of the foot, as well as part of the Achilles tendon above the ankle.[61] Distal to the knee, the SphN courses along the medial aspect of the lower leg in the subcutaneous tissue. At the level of the ankle, it travels alongside the saphenous vein, anterior to the medial malleolus (see Fig. 50.12). The SphN provides only sensory innervation to the medial aspect of

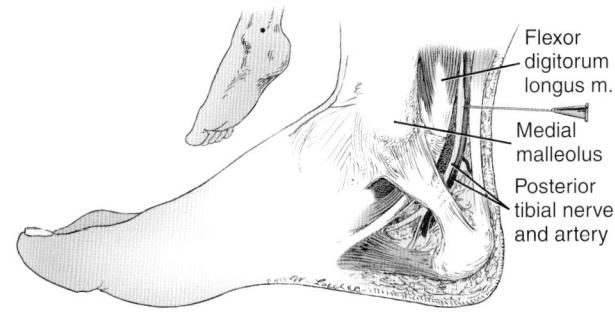

Fig. 50.11 Path of the posterior tibial nerve in the ankle in relation to the posterior tibial artery and Achilles tendon. *m.,* Muscle.

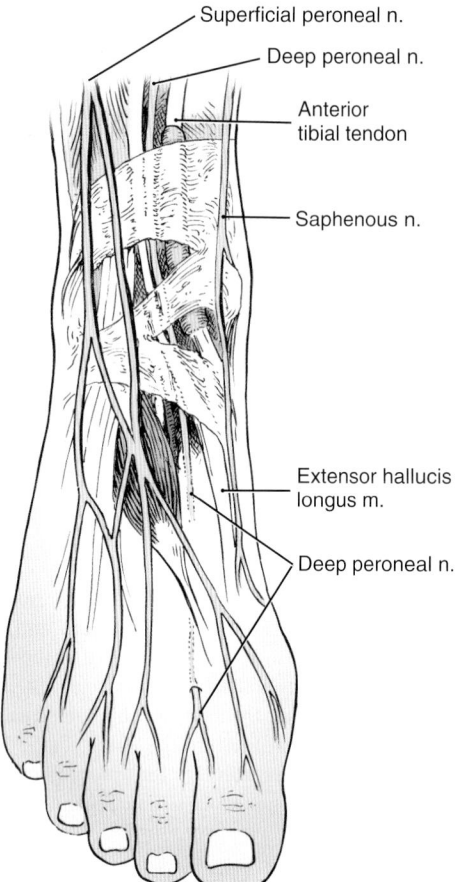

Fig. 50.12 Anatomic course of the nerves innervating the ankle. *n.,* Nerve

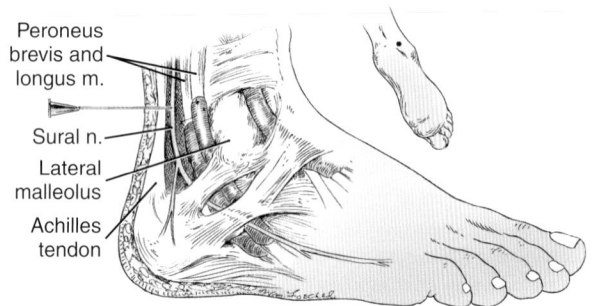

Fig. 50.13 Path of the sural nerve behind the lateral malleolus into the ankle. *m.,* Muscle; *n.,* nerve.

the lower extremity below the knee, ankle, and medial aspect of the forefoot.[61]

BLOCK TECHNIQUES 2

The remainder of this chapter focuses on the indications, approaches, local anesthetic considerations, and potential risks and complications of performing single-injection nerve blocks on the upper extremity, truncal regions, and lower extremity of the body. Both landmark/nerve stimulation and ultrasound-guided techniques are discussed, with the differences and similarities between the two approaches detailed. Since

ultrasound-guided technique has become commonplace in current anesthesia practice, the majority of images and references presented are dedicated to those procedures. A brief review of catheter techniques is given at the end of the chapter.

Upper Extremity Peripheral Nerve Blocks

With few exceptions, the BP innervates the entire upper extremity. Depending on the proposed surgery, local anesthetics can be placed at four different levels to achieve the desired coverage: (1) the interscalene groove where the roots pass between the anterior and middle scalene muscles, (2) the supraclavicular fossa posterior to the clavicle at the level of the first rib, (3) the infraclavicular fossa inferior to the clavicle and medial to the coracoid process, and (4) the proximal upper arm at the level of the axilla. Additional factors, such as patient considerations (body habitus, coexisting disease nature, and location of the injury) and anesthesia provider skill and experience, should be considered when determining the potential risks and complications associated with the proposed approach.[62] Additionally, the terminal branches of the plexus can be blocked distally at the elbow or wrist joints. The incorporation of ultrasound into regional anesthesia has greatly expanded the available options while decreasing potential complications, especially when targeting the nerves in highly vascular areas or near the pleura.[17,36,37] A review of BP anatomy can be found in Clinical Anatomy, earlier.

Interscalene Approach

Interscalene brachial plexus blocks (ISBPBs) are commonly performed for surgical procedures involving the shoulder and proximal upper arm. In 1970 Alon Winnie popularized this approach using anatomic landmarks to estimate the location of cervical roots 5 to 7 as they passed between the anterior and middle scalene muscles in the neck.[63] Variations of Winnie's technique have been described over the years, including the incorporation of nerve stimulation to locate nerves and changes to the needle insertion angle to better approximate nerve location.[63] Chan was one of the first to describe an ultrasound guided ISBPB.[64] It is not indicated for procedures below the level of the elbow, as spinal nerve roots C8-T1 (lower trunk), which innervate part of the forearm and hand, are often spared.

- Landmark/Nerve Stimulation Technique[63]
  - The provider stands on the side of the procedure, and (according to Winnie) the patient is placed in the supine (or dorsal) recumbent position, with the head turned to the nonoperative side. The C6 level of cervical vertebra is determined by extending a line laterally from the cricoid cartilage. This line passes over Chassaignac tubercle (the transverse process of C6), which is avoided because applying pressure causes considerable discomfort. The patient is instructed to elevate the head slightly to bring the clavicular head of the sternocleidomastoid muscle into prominence. The palpating finger is placed immediately behind this muscle, and the patient is instructed to relax. The finger now rests on the belly of the ASM. When the finger is moved to the lateral edge of this muscle, the groove between the anterior scalene and middle scalene muscles (interscalene groove) is identified. The index and middle fingers straddle the cricoid line in the groove, indicating the point of needle insertion (see Fig. 50.3).[63] The external jugular vein often overlies the interscalene groove at the level of C6 and should be identified prior to the procedure.[62,65]
  - If nerve stimulation is used, once the patient is appropriately prepped and draped, a skin wheal of local anesthetic is made at the needle insertion point. A 22-gauge, 5-cm B-bevel insulated needle is inserted through the skin wheal perpendicular

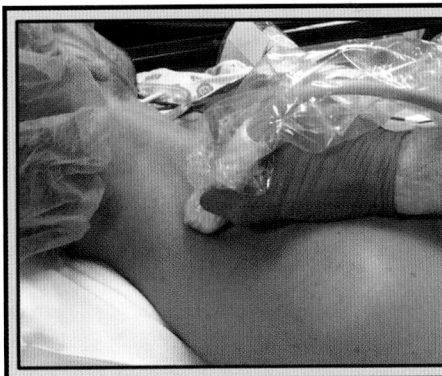
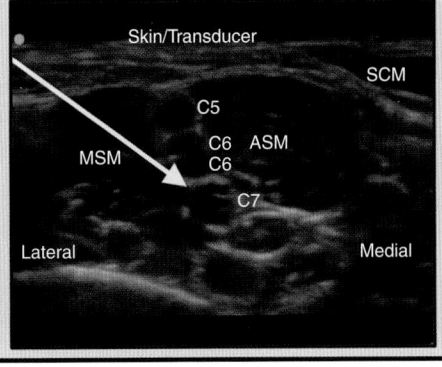

Interscalene block
- High frequency linear array transducer
- Root level brachial plexus block
- Surgical procedures of the shoulder and proximal upper arm
- Needle inserted lateral to medial
- 15-20 mL local anesthetic around roots

ASM   Anterior scalene m.
MSM   Middle scalene m.
SCM   Sternocleidomastoid m.
C   Cervical nerve roots
—   Needle approach

Skin/Transducer
SCM
C5
C6 ASM
MSM   C6
C7
Lateral   Medial

Fig. 50.14 Transducer position and corresponding image for an ultrasound-guided interscalene block.

to the skin on all planes. The negative lead is attached to the patient and the positive lead to a nerve stimulator. The needle is slowly advanced until a motor response is elicited. The current is decreased as the needle is advanced to ensure optimal needle position (usually a depth of 1–2 cm) and to minimize discomfort to the patient. Following negative aspiration for blood or cerebrospinal fluid, a test dose of 1 mL of local anesthetic solution is injected. If the needle is within close proximity of the BP, the quality of the motor twitch will diminish, or fade, and the patient is assessed for signs of LAST. Following each negative aspiration for blood, incremental injections of 5 mL of local anesthetic are administered up to 25 mL total.[65,66]

- Ultrasound Guidance
  - The patient is placed supine or in the lateral position with the head of the bed slightly elevated. The area is prepped and draped in an appropriate manner. With the patient's head turned to the nonoperative side, a high frequency (10–12 MHz) linear array transducer is placed in the supraclavicular fossa and directed slightly caudal. The trunks/divisions of the BP appear as a series of small hypoechoic circles, lateral to the pulsating, circular subclavian artery and superior to the hyperechoic first rib. This is also the image for performing a supraclavicular block. Once the BP is identified, the transducer is slid cephalad until the cross sections of the roots, visualized as a series of small hypoechoic circles, are identified between the ASM and MSM (Fig. 50.14). A small skin wheal is placed at the lateral edge of the transducer. Using an in-plane approach, a 22-gauge, 5-cm B-bevel block needle is placed through the skin wheal in a lateral to medial direction, passing through the MSM to the base of the hypoechoic roots. Following negative aspiration, 20 mL of local anesthetic delivered in increments of 5 mL is deposited until circumferential spread is observed under direct ultrasound visualization.
- Pearls
  - The hypoechoic roots stacked between the ASM and MSM are often referred to as either the snowman or stoplight sign. Early literature often identified these roots as C5-C7. However, recent studies have demonstrated there is significant variation among individuals, and the three hypoechoic circles identified between the scalene muscles are often combinations of C5 and C6.[67] Given that the BP innervation of the shoulder comes primarily from these two roots, blocking the plexus at this level is sufficient to achieve adequate anesthesia coverage for surgical procedures of the shoulder.

- Risks and Complications
  - Unilateral phrenic nerve blockade can occur due to its close proximity to the injection site, resulting in ipsilateral diaphragmatic hemiparesis.[68] While in healthy patients this rarely results in respiratory compromise, the provider should use caution when caring for patients with severe pulmonary disease, such as chronic obstructive pulmonary disease (COPD). The resultant phrenic nerve paralysis may result in severe dyspnea, hypercapnia, and hypoxemia. The stellate ganglion (cervicothoracic ganglion), located at C7, can also be blocked, resulting in Horner syndrome (ptosis, miosis, and anhydrosis).[69] Injection of large volumes of local anesthetics has resulted in recurrent laryngeal paralysis, which presents as hoarseness. As little as 1 mL of local anesthetic inadvertently injected into the vertebral artery or subarachnoid space may induce seizures.[70] Due to the close proximity of the pleura, pneumothorax is possible (Fig. 50.15).[71] When performing an ultrasound guided ISBPB, the needle approach is lateral and inferior when compared to the landmark technique,[35] with the needle passing through the MSM to reach the BP. The dorsal scapular nerve and long thoracic nerve, branches of C5 and C6, often pass through the MSM. Case reports of injury to these nerves due to needle trauma have been reported.[72] Several authors recommend using nerve stimulation to alert the provider when the needle is in close proximity to the nerve.[72,73] As an alternative to the ISBPB, some authors have advocated the upper trunk block as it reduces the incidence of phrenic nerve paralysis and injury to the long thoracic nerve and dorsal scapular nerve.[74,75]

Supraclavicular Block

The supraclavicular block targets the trunks/divisions of the BP. The exact level of plexus blockade is variable depending on the patient's anatomy and the site of injection. It is not considered an optimal approach for surgical procedures of the shoulder as the suprascapular nerve, which arises from the proximal upper trunk, is often missed. The supraclavicular approach creates a dense block for surgeries of the arm because the nerves are most compact at this level as they travel under the clavicle and over the first rib. Many practitioners prefer to perform this block under ultrasound guidance due to the close proximity of the pleura and subclavian artery and their associated risks.

- Landmark/Nerve Stimulation Technique
  - The patient is placed with the head of the bed elevated 30 to 45 degrees with the head turned to the nonoperative side. The major landmarks for this block are the patient's midline, the

clavicle, and the lateral (clavicular) attachment of the SCM. The patient is instructed to drop the shoulder and flex the elbow so that the forearm in resting in the lap. The wrist is supinated so that the palm faces the patient. This assists the provider in identifying forearm or hand movements during nerve stimulation. The outline of the clavicle and SCM are drawn to aid in visualization. The lateral border of the SCM is followed distally to its insertion point on the clavicle. Medial to this point, there is increased risk of pneumothorax, and the provider may draw a parasagittal line (parallel to midline) to appreciate the risk. The anesthetist places an index finger approximately 2.5 cm lateral from the SCM insertion point, directly above the clavicle. After the patient is appropriately prepped and draped, a skin wheal of local anesthetic is placed at the needle insertion site. A 22-gauge, 5-cm B-bevel needle, attached to a nerve stimulator, is advanced perpendicularly into the skin directly above the palpating finger, then directed caudal and under in a plane parallel to midline until stimulation (preferably finger flexion or extension) is elicited. The nerve stimulator current is lowered as the needle is advanced to minimize excessive current to the patient and to ensure proper needle position. Following negative aspiration for blood, a test dose of 1 mL of local anesthetic solution is injected. If the needle is properly placed, there will be fade in the motor response. If there are no signs of LAST, incremental injections of 5 mL of local anesthetic are administered following each negative aspiration. In adult patients, the typical volume is 25 to 35 mL.

- Ultrasound Guidance
  - The ultrasound-guided supraclavicular block is best obtained with the patient in the supine position, with the head slightly elevated and turned to the nonoperative side (Fig. 50.16). The clavicle and surrounding areas are prepped and draped in an appropriate manner. As the trunks/divisions are typically less than 2 cm from the skin at this level, a high-frequency (10–12 MHz) linear array transducer is placed in the midclavicular fossa and directed slightly caudal. At this level, the BP appears as a small cluster of hypoechoic circles lateral to the hypoechoic pulsating subclavian artery and superior to the first rib. Doppler ultrasound can be used to confirm flow through the artery. Once all anatomic structures are identified, the transducer is tilted so the first rib is aligned under the nerves and over the pleura, creating a protective barrier during needle insertion. A 22-gauge, 5-cm B-bevel needle is passed in-plane from lateral to medial, immediately adjacent to the subclavian artery and superior to the first rib. Following negative aspiration, incremental injections of 5 mL are deposited between the inferior border of the plexus, superior to the first rib, pushing the plexus upward. The needle is then redirected to the superior aspect of the plexus, and, following negative aspiration, incremental injections of 5 mL are delivered until circumferential spread of local anesthetic is observed around the plexus. A total of 20 mL is normally sufficient to achieve an efficacious block.

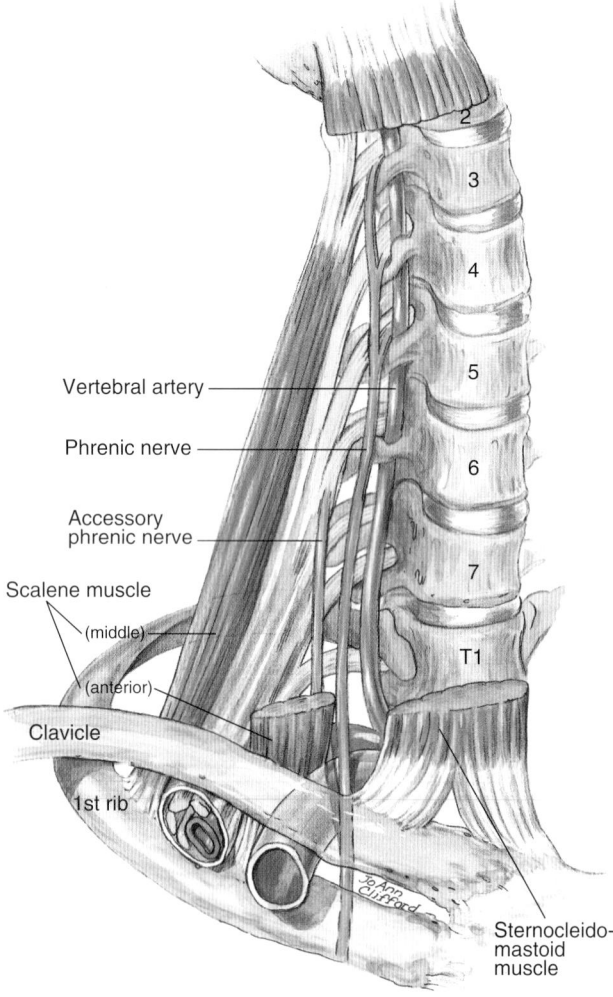

Fig. 50.15 Note the proximity of both the phrenic nerve and the vertebral artery to the location of the interscalene block. (From Farag E, Mounir-Soliman L. *Brown's Atlas of Regional Anesthesia*. 5th ed. Philadelphia: Elsevier; 2017:30.)

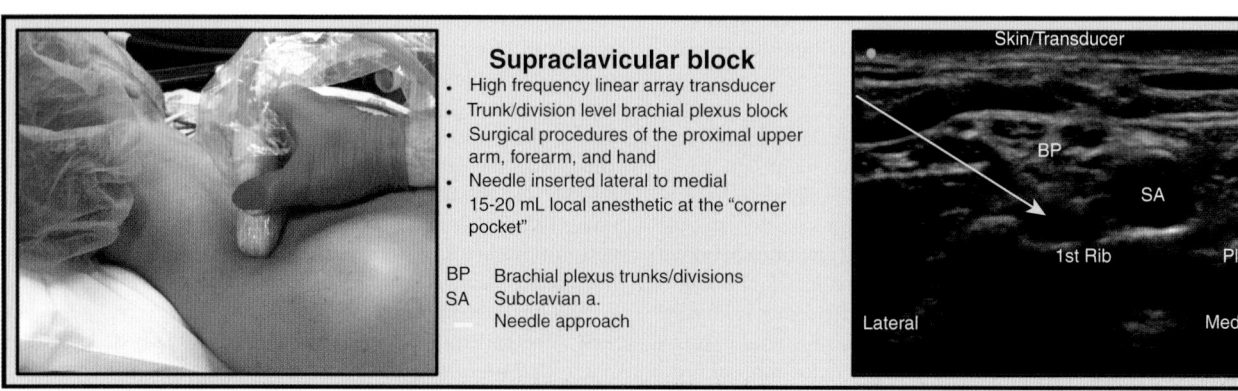

Fig. 50.16 Transducer position and corresponding image for an ultrasound-guided supraclavicular block. Note the position of the first rib between the brachia plexus and pleura.

- Pearls
  - Tilting the transducer caudal to ensure the first rib is positioned between the BP and pleura will reduce the incidence of pneumothorax, which is greater in taller individuals.
- Risks and Complications
  - The greatest risk is pneumothorax, as the pleura is immediately inferior to the first rib.[76,77] Careful needle placement, as previously described, is imperative. The risk of pneumothorax is greater when landmarks are difficult to identify, the patient is very thin, or if the dome of the lung is unusually high. As with the interscalene block, Horner syndrome and diaphragmatic hemiparesis can occur. Negative needle aspiration prior to the injection of local anesthetic is key for assessing for potential subclavian artery puncture. The development of a hematoma after an unintentional subclavian artery puncture may be difficult to compress and must be closely observed.

Infraclavicular Block

The infraclavicular block targets the cords of the BP medial to the coracoid process at the shoulder. The cords are named according to their anatomic relationship with the axillary artery. The lateral cord lies superior and lateral to the artery, the posterior cord is posterior, and the medial cord is posterior and medial. This approach may be used as an alternative to the supraclavicular block in patients with COPD, abnormal subclavian pathology, or localized infection. Because the pectoris major and pectoris minor must be traversed to perform this block, it can be uncomfortable for some patients.

- Landmark/Nerve Stimulation
  - Various approaches are described in the literature; here we describe the lateral approach because of the reduced risk of axillary artery puncture and pneumothorax. The patient is positioned supine with the arm adducted at the side or with the hand on the abdomen. The head is either neutral or turned to the nonprocedural side. The skin is prepped and draped in a sterile manner. The anesthetist identifies the medial aspect of the coracoid process and 2 cm caudad and 2 cm medial from this location makes a skin wheal for needle insertion. The anesthetist inserts a 22-gauge, 9-cm B-bevel insulated block needle in vertical parasagittal plane (cephalad to caudal). The first motor response elicited is elbow flexion, from stimulation of the musculocutaneous nerve. Either flexion or extension of the wrist is required to successfully achieve complete anesthesia of the hand.[78] Examination of the fifth digit when using nerve stimulation has been described in the literature as a means of determining approximate needle location during the block. When the block needle stimulates the lateral cord, the fifth digit will move

laterally; when the medial cord is stimulated, the fifth digit will flex; and when the posterior cord is stimulated, the fifth digit will extend.[78,79] Following negative aspiration, incremental 5-mL doses of local anesthetic are injected for a total of 30 mL.

- Ultrasound Guidance
  - Since the cords are located deep in the tissue compared to the supraclavicular approach, they may be more difficult to visualize with ultrasound. A 7-MHz linear array transducer allows for greater penetration into the tissue and should be considered when performing this block. Some authors have advocated the use of PNS in conjunction with ultrasound to identify nerves.[80] The patient is positioned in a similar fashion to the landmark technique, laying supine with the head turned to the nonoperative side and the arm adducted, flexed at the elbow with the hand resting on the abdomen. The area of the distal clavicle and coracoid process is prepped and draped in the appropriate manner. Depending on body habitus, either a high-frequency (6–10 MHz) linear array transducer or a low-frequency (2–5 MHz) curvilinear array transducer is placed in a sagittal orientation just distal to the clavicle and medial to the coracoid process. The resultant image is a cross-sectional view of the cords of the BP and axillary vessels (Fig. 50.17). The lateral cord of the plexus is often visualized as a hyperechoic oval structure cephalad to the axillary artery. The medial and posterior cords are more difficult to identify as the medial cord often lies between the axillary artery and vein and the posterior cord lies deep to the axillary artery. Unlike the interscalene and supraclavicular blocks, the nerves at this level appear hyperechoic rather than hypoechoic. This is most likely due to the increased amount of connective tissue surrounding the nerve fascicles as they move distal into the extremity. A skin wheal is placed just cephalad to the transducer. A 22-gauge, 9-cm B-bevel needle is passed in-plane caudally and posteriorly. Because there is high variability in the location of the cords, nerve stimulation can also be used in conjunction with ultrasound. The goal is to place the needle posterior to the axillary artery. Following negative aspiration, local anesthetic is injected in 5-mL increments, up to 30 mL. A complete block is obtained when local anesthetic spreads from the area of the posterior cord cephalad and caudally, forming a semicircle around the axillary artery.
- Pearls
  - Compared to the interscalene and supraclavicular approaches, the risk of phrenic nerve and stellate ganglion block is greatly reduced with the infraclavicular approach, making it a desirable block for upper extremity surgery in patients with severe respiratory compromise.[48] Due to the steep needle angle required

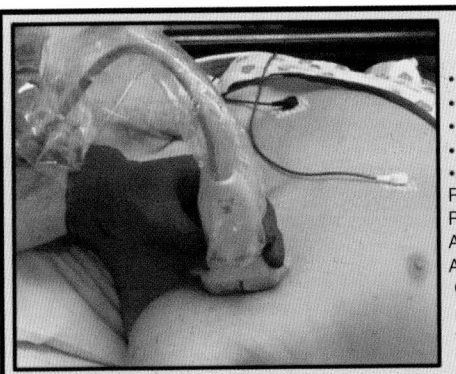
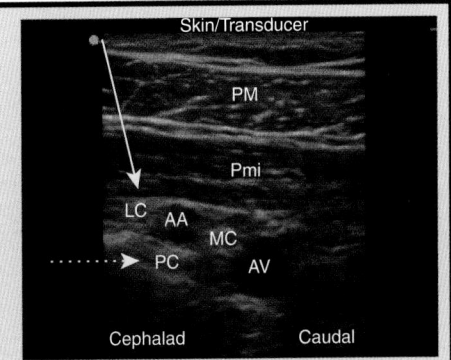

Infraclavicular block
- High frequency linear array transducer
- Cord level brachial plexus block
- Surgeries of the elbow, forearm, and hand
- Needle inserted cephalad to caudad
- 15-30 mL local anesthetic around AA

PM   Pectoralis major m.
Pmi   Pectoralis minor m.
AA   Axillary a.
AV   Axillary v.
C   Cords (L-lateral, M-medial, P-posterior)
     Needle approach
     RAPTIR approach

Fig. 50.17 Transducer position and corresponding image for an ultrasound-guided infraclavicular block.

to perform this block, abducting the arm displaces the clavicle allowing the provider to insert the needle more cranial to the transducer, improving needle imaging.[81]

- An ultrasound-guided *retro*clavicular *ap*proach to *the infra*-clavicular *region* (RAPTIR) has been popularized over the past several years as a way to better visualize needle insertion. When performing the RAPTIR, the needle insertion point is between the clavicle and trapezius in the supraclavicular fossa, with the needle passing underneath the clavicle entering the ultrasound image parallel to the transducer (see Fig. 50.17).[82,83] However, the RAPTIR is not without risks because the suprascapular nerve and vein are vulnerable to injury as they are not identifiable in the acoustic shadow created by the clavicle.[84]

- Risks and Complications
  - The infraclavicular block is the most painful of the BP approaches because the needle must pass through both the pectoralis major and minor muscles. Additional subcutaneous local anesthetic is often required when performing this block. Additionally, since the cords pass deep beneath the skin, obtaining a consistent needle image is challenging, and inadvertent vascular puncture is a potential complication. Therefore careful aspiration should precede every incremental injection to reduce the chance of intravascular injection and possible local anesthetic toxicity. Insertion of the needle slightly lateral, away from the chest wall, decreases the risk of pneumothorax.[48]

Axillary Block

The axillary block targets four terminal branches of the BP as they course distally with the axillary artery and vein along the humerus from the apex of the axilla. It provides anesthesia to the upper extremity distal to the elbow. The primary nerves are the radial, median, and ulnar branches, which are located around the axillary artery, and the musculocutaneous branch, which is positioned outside the axillary sheath. The course of the terminal nerves in relation to the axillary artery is as follows: The median nerve is located anterior and medial, the musculocutaneous nerve lies anterior and lateral, the ulnar nerve lies posterior and medial, and the radial nerve lies posterior and lateral (Fig. 50.18). Because the musculocutaneous nerve exits the axillary sheath proximal to this area and travels through the coracobrachialis muscle, it must be blocked separately. There are few contraindications to the axillary block.

- Landmark/Nerve Stimulation
  - Prior to UGRA, the axillary block was the most frequently used technique for anesthesia of the forearm and hand because of its ease of performance, relatively high success rate, and low incidence of complications. With the patient in the supine position, the arm is abducted and the forearm flexed to 90 degrees resting parallel to the long axis of the body. The anesthetist uses the index and middle fingers to identify the axillary artery in the groove between the coracobrachialis muscle and the pectoralis major muscle high in the axilla (see Fig. 50.18). Injecting below this point in the mid to lower axilla reduces the chance local anesthetic will reach the musculocutaneous nerve before it leaves the sheath. A well-defined, localized pulsation of the axillary artery is more important for an efficacious block than the point at which needle insertion occurs within the axilla. Following prepping and draping of the skin, a skin wheal is raised just proximal and superior to the palpating index finger. A 22-gauge, 5-cm B-bevel needle is inserted through the skin wheal. During needle insertion, moderate digital pressure should be applied to the artery to minimize the distance between the skin and subcutaneous tissue. With nerve stimulation, it is desirable to

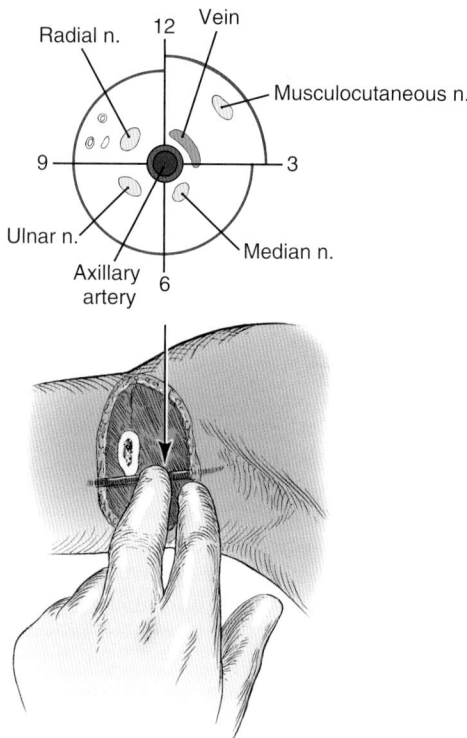

Fig. 50.18 Identification of the axillary artery in preparation for the axillary block. *n.,* Nerve.

block the nerves innervating the proposed surgery first. For the median and musculocutaneous nerves, the needle is directed slightly superior the artery, and for the radial and ulnar nerves the needle is directed slightly inferior. Because of its location within the coracobrachialis muscle, direct nerve stimulation of the musculocutaneous nerve (elbow flexion) is desirable for localization but not required for the other nerves. Approximately 10 to 15 mL of local anesthetic is deposited at each nerve. If the axillary artery is punctured prior to any nerve stimulation, convert to the transarterial technique.

- The transarterial technique uses intentional penetration of the axillary artery and aspiration of blood as the end point for determining that the needle is within the neurovascular sheath. Once the axillary artery is located, a skin wheal is raised directly above the artery at the planned point of needle insertion (see Fig. 50.18). A 22-gauge needle is inserted perpendicularly to the skin and advanced slowly until blood is aspirated by an assistant. The needle is then advanced along the same plane until blood can no longer be aspirated, indicating the needle bevel has exited the posterior wall of the artery. Prior to injection, the patient is instructed to inform the anesthetist of any symptoms of LAST. The needle is held fixed in position, and an assistant gently aspirates the syringe while the operator observes for blood, indicating the needle has reentered an axillary vessel. Once negative aspiration is confirmed, a 3- to 5-mL test dose of the local anesthetic is injected, and the patient is observed for at least 1 minute and assessed for any symptoms of LAST. If none occur, the remainder of the local anesthetic is injected in 5-mL increments, with each injection preceded by aspiration and observation for blood. Injection of each 5 mL of local anesthetic should be considered a test dose because unrecognized penetration of the artery or rapid uptake of the local anesthetic is possible

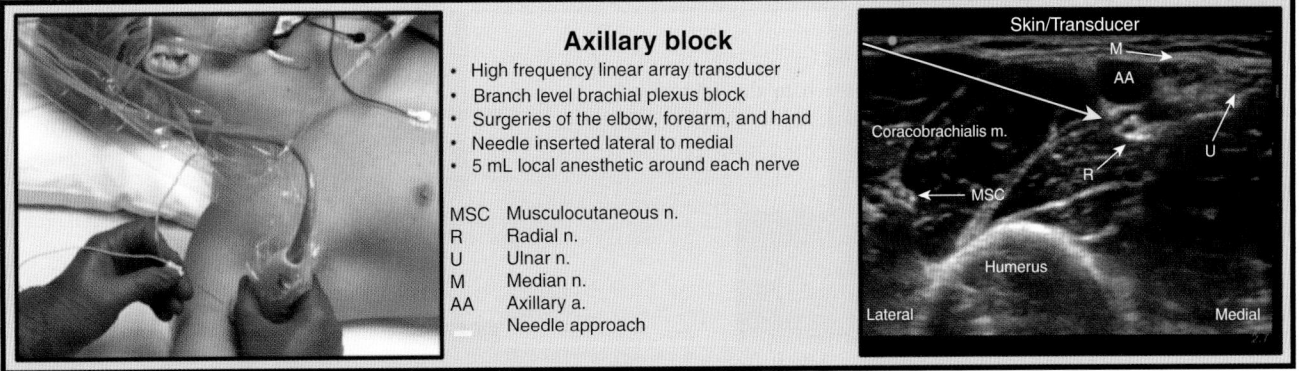

Fig. 50.19 Transducer position and corresponding image for an ultrasound-guided axillary nerve block.

throughout the procedure. When 40 mL of local anesthetic solution has been injected, the needle is withdrawn to the level of the skin in preparation for a separate block of the musculocutaneous nerve, as well as subcutaneous injections of the medial brachial cutaneous and the intercostobrachial nerves, which do not arise from the BP.

- Ultrasound Guidance
  - The ultrasound-guided axillary nerve block targets the radial, ulnar, median, and musculocutaneous branches of the BP. Failure to block one of the nerves may result in an unsuccessful procedure. For this reason, the ultrasound-guided approach is often considered more technically challenging than other approaches to the BP. The patient is placed in the supine position, with the head facing the nonoperative side, and the arm is abducted and rotated 90 degrees. A high-frequency (10–12 MHz) linear array transducer is placed in the axilla at the crease formed by the pectoralis major and biceps muscles with the ultrasound beam positioned perpendicular to the axillary artery in the proximal upper arm (Fig. 50.19). An in-plane approach is used to achieve circumferential spread around each branch. Because the MCN is surrounded by muscle, it is the easiest to identify of the four branches. Confirmation of this nerve can be made by scanning proximally and observing it join the lateral cord in the axilla. The median, radial, and ulnar nerves can be confirmed by following each distally along the arm. The median nerve travels alongside the brachial artery as it courses distally to the elbow. The radial artery will move posterior and lateral as it travels along the distal upper arm. The ulnar nerve continues medially along the upper arm as it travels into the medial epicondyle of the humerus. Once confirmed, each branch is traced back proximally to the axilla where all nerves are visualized in the same plane. Then 5 to 10 mL of local anesthetic is injected around each nerve.[48,85]
- Pearls
  - Because of the distance between the branches, the anesthetist must circumvent the axillary artery and veins to ensure adequate local anesthetic is deposited around each nerve. Sliding the transducer proximal and distal during a preprocedure scan will identify the location where all nerves are visualized in the same plane. This single view allows for blockade of all nerves with one needle insertion, reducing trauma.
- Risks and Complications
  - Complications during an axillary block are not common. Depending on the technique utilized, systemic uptake of local anesthetic and subsequent toxicity appear to be the most

concerning and frequent complications.[86] In addition, there is risk of local infection, nerve injury, and bleeding.

Selective Blocks at the Elbow

Selective blocks at the elbow and wrist permit the surgeon to complete a procedure while minimizing the amount of anesthesia required. Blocks at the elbow and wrist are primarily sensory blocks. The patient retains the ability to move the hand during the procedure. Reducing the anesthetized area and amount of sedation required decreases the potential for complications and minimizes the patient's stay in an outpatient center. These selective nerve blocks of the upper extremity are often used as a rescue when the regional anesthetic technique fails to provide adequate surgical coverage and avoids the conversion to a general anesthetic.[87-89]

Each nerve supplying sensory branches to the arm can be blocked at the elbow and wrist. When performing landmark technique, the use of a nerve stimulator at the elbow (for the median and radial nerves) and wrist (for the ulnar and median nerves) can improve block success.

When a tourniquet is required for the procedure, the intercostobrachial and brachial cutaneous nerves should be blocked along the medial aspect of the upper arm in the axilla. These blocks provide anesthesia against possible tourniquet pain. In addition, blocking the coracobrachial muscle at the shoulder has also been shown to be beneficial.[87]

- Landmark/Nerve Stimulation Technique
  - As the ulnar nerve traverses the ulnar sulcus of the humerus, it is tightly fixed within the groove. Performing a regional anesthetic technique in this location increases the risk of nerve entrapment. Limiting the volume of local anesthetic will reduce the amount of pressure exerted on the nerve and the ischemia that could develop from injection of a large volume (avoid volumes >3 mL).[90]
  - The technique should be performed 1 to 2 cm proximal to the sulcus. The patient's elbow is flexed 90 degrees, and the medial condyle of the humerus is identified. A finger is placed in the ulnar sulcus, extending approximately 1 cm proximal to the condyle (Fig. 50.20). The insertion point for the needle is between the medial condyle of the humerus and the olecranon process of the ulna. A 22-gauge, 5-cm B-bevel needle is inserted at a 45-degree angle to the skin and perpendicularly to a line drawn between the medial condyle and the olecranon process. If a paresthesia is elicited on introduction of the needle, the needle is slightly withdrawn, and 2 to 3 mL of local anesthetic is injected. If a paresthesia is not elicited, the volume of the solution can be increased. The total volume of the local anesthetic solution is 3 to 5 mL. The onset of action is determined by the

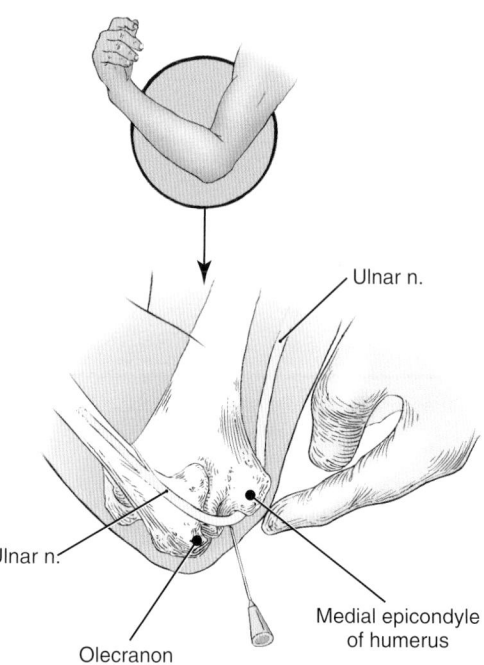

Fig. 50.20 Technique of ulnar block at the elbow. The patient's elbow is flexed 90 degrees, and the medial condyle of the humerus is identified. *n.*, Nerve.

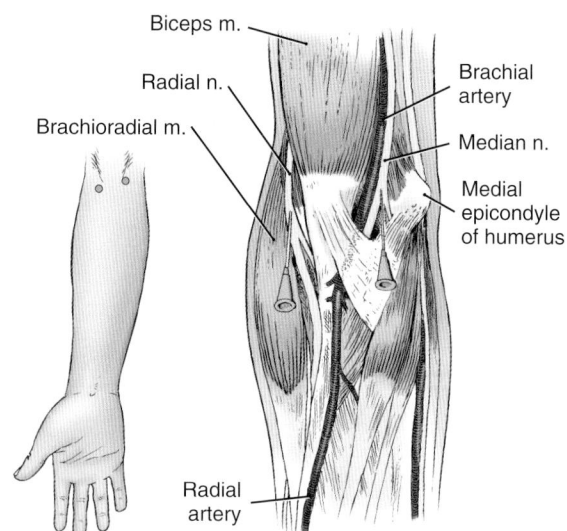

Fig. 50.21 Performance of median nerve block, positioning the patient's arm on a stable surface with the elbow slightly flexed. After the brachial artery is identified, a short B-bevel needle is inserted slightly medial to the brachial artery. *m.*, Muscle; *n.*, nerve.

local anesthetic selected for the procedure. Epinephrine can be used at this level; however, this agent delays the onset.[87-89]

- Anesthesia of the forearm and hand can be achieved by blocking the median and ulnar nerves as an adjunct to another technique or as the primary anesthetic. This combination provides adequate anesthesia for procedures on the cutaneous portions of the lower forearm, the hand, and the second, third, and fourth digits. The median nerve block can be used to supplement an incomplete BP block. It should be avoided in patients with carpal tunnel syndrome, neuritis, or when the artery is perforated. If the median and ulnar nerves are blocked, the patient will still retain limited function of the hand.[88,89]

- The median nerve block is accomplished by positioning the patient's arm on a stable surface with the elbow slightly flexed. A line is drawn from the medial to the lateral condyle of the humerus along the anterior surface of the elbow. The brachial artery is then identified as it crosses this line (Fig. 50.21). A 22-gauge, 5-cm B-bevel needle is inserted slightly medial to the brachial artery to a depth of 5 to 7 mm. Identification of the median nerve is necessary to ensure an efficacious block. A nerve stimulator can aid the performance during the procedure as stimulus from a low amplitude will elicit a motor response. Once the nerve is located, 3 to 5 mL of local anesthetic is injected. As the needle is withdrawn through the fascia, an additional 1 to 2 mL of local anesthetic is injected to block cutaneous branches of the nerve.[91,92]

- The radial nerve is adjunct to axillary perivascular techniques. This block is also indicated for surgery of the forearm and hand within the distribution of the radial nerve or in conjunction with other nerve blocks. With the elbow extended and stabilized on a firm surface, the brachioradialis muscle and biceps tendon are identified. The radial nerve is located in the groove formed by the fascial border of the brachioradialis muscle (see Fig. 50.21) on the lateral edge and the biceps tendon medially.

A line is drawn between the medial and lateral condyles. A 22-gauge, 5-cm B-bevel needle is inserted along the medial border of the brachioradialis muscle toward the lateral condyle at the point at which the line between the condyles crosses the facial groove. The needle is directed toward the anterior aspect of the lateral condyle so that gentle contact occurs. After contact with the condyle, the needle is slightly withdrawn, and 3 to 5 mL of local anesthetic is injected. This procedure is repeated two or three times while the needle is moved slightly more proximally with each injection. As the needle is withdrawn subcutaneously, an additional 3 to 5 mL of local anesthetic is injected.[91,92]

- An alternative approach to the radial nerve requires identification of the lateral border of the brachioradialis muscle. Measuring 3 to 5 cm proximal from the lateral condyle along the border of the brachioradialis muscle enables palpation of the radial nerve as it parallels the humerus. The nerve is adherent to the bone at this level and can be easily injured during the performance of the block. Applying slight pressure to this area will elicit a paresthesia to the nerve. A 22-gauge, 5-cm B-bevel needle is inserted in a plane perpendicular to the humerus and advanced to the proximity of the identified radial nerve. Because of its fixation against the humerus, the needle must be advanced slowly and the position evaluated to avoid injury to the nerve.[91,92]

Selective Nerve Blocks at the Wrist

- Landmark/Nerve Stimulation
  - With the wrist slightly flexed and stabilized on a firm surface, the ulnar flexor muscle of the wrist is identified. A line is then drawn across the forearm at the level of the styloid process of the ulna. A 22-gauge, 5-cm B-bevel needle is inserted perpendicularly to the skin on the radial side of the ulnar flexor muscle of the wrist, where it is traversed by the line. At this point, the needle is slightly lateral to the ulnar artery, and medial deviation can position the needle over the artery. While the ulnar artery can be palpated with moderate wrist extension, severe extension results in artery collapse. Following the needle insertion, 2 to 4 mL of local anesthetic is injected. An additional 2 mL is

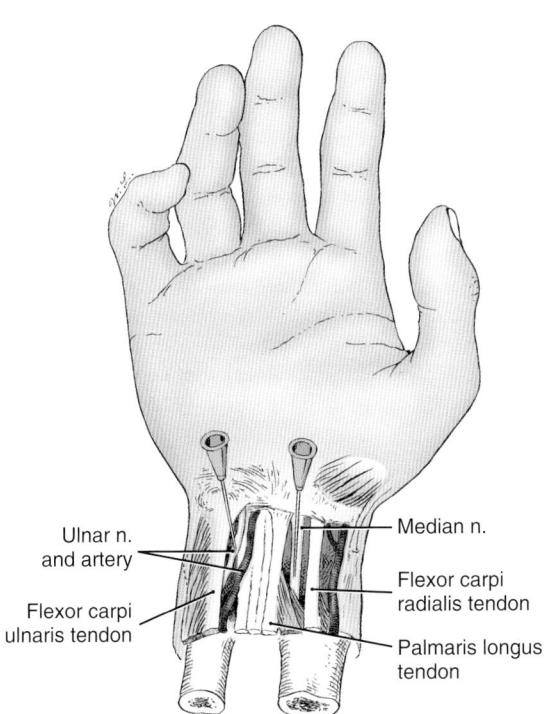

Fig. 50.22 With the patient's wrist slightly flexed and stabilized on a firm surface, the ulnar flexor muscle of the wrist is identified. A short B-bevel needle is inserted perpendicular to the skin on the radial side of the ulnar flexor muscle of the wrist. *n.,* Nerve.

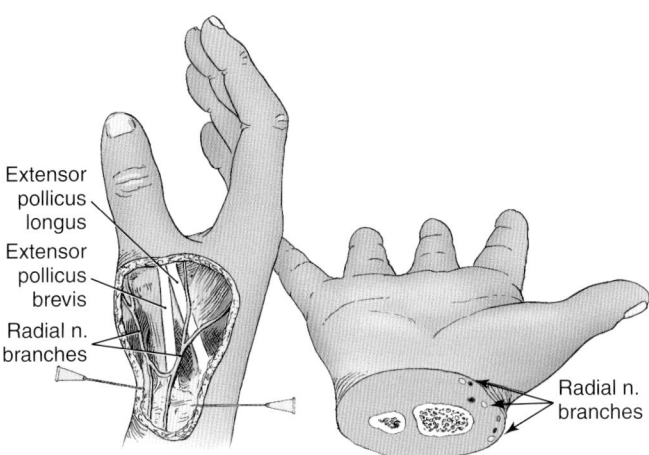

Fig. 50.23 Anesthesia of the radial nerve is achieved by injecting a subcutaneous ring of local anesthetic solution at the radial flexor muscle of the wrist, extending to the dorsal surface of the ulnar styloid. *n.,* Nerve.

injected as the needle is withdrawn from the deep fascia. The dorsal branch of the ulnar nerve is blocked by injecting 3 to 5 mL of local anesthesia in a half-ring around the ulnar aspect of the wrist. The needle is placed subcutaneously at the radial margin of the ulnar flexor muscle of the wrist and advanced to the midportion of the dorsal aspect of the wrist.[91,92]

- The wrist is stabilized on a firm surface and slightly flexed against resistance. When the wrist is flexed, the long palmar muscle and the radial flexor muscle of the wrist are easily identified (Fig. 50.22). A line is drawn across the wrist that parallels the proximal crease. A 22-gauge, 5-cm B-bevel needle is inserted approximately 0.5 to 1 cm perpendicularly to the skin between the two tendons. The carpal tunnel is a tightly confined space, and the nerve is located superficially. If a persistent paresthesia is elicited during needle insertion, it must be withdrawn and repositioned. Up to 5 mL of local anesthetic is injected in the carpal tunnel, and another 2 to 3 mL is injected as the needle is withdrawn from the fascia.[91,92]

- The superficial branches of the radial nerve at the wrist supply sensory innervation to the hand. A subcutaneous ring of local anesthetic, beginning at the radial flexor muscle of the wrist and extending to the dorsal surface of the ulnar styloid, is sufficient to block these branches (Fig. 50.23). When an ulnar nerve block is also performed, a contiguous ring of local anesthetic around the wrist should be avoided because circulation to the hand could be compromised.

- The radial nerve can also be blocked by identifying the brachioradialis muscle proximal to the wrist. Between 6 and 8 cm proximal to the wrist, 5 to 7 mL of local anesthetic is injected under the brachioradialis muscle. However, this technique is the least well tolerated of all the supplemental blocks, and it is associated with limited success.[91,92]

Intravenous Regional Anesthesia (Bier Block)

Intravenous regional anesthesia (IVRA), also known as the Bier block, is still performed at many facilities. First described by famed German surgeon Augustus Bier in 1908 and re-popularized by Holmes in 1963, this technique is a simple and relatively safe procedure to perform. It is best suited for soft tissue surgeries of the upper extremity that are short in duration (<1 hour) and minimally invasive, such as carpal tunnel release and foreign-body removal. In addition, they have been used for surgeries involving the foot and ankle and have been successfully used to treat certain chronic pain syndromes.[93] This technique is limited to surgeries lasting 1 hour or less because of tourniquet pain, which is required to initiate and maintain the block. The necessity for intravenous access, manipulation of the affected extremity, the prerequisite of a tourniquet, as well as block density and duration of surgery all influence the application of this technique.[94,95]

When performing IVRA for upper extremity surgery, the patient is placed in the supine position, with the operative extremity abducted. A small-bore (22–25 gauge) peripheral intravenous catheter with a heparin lock is inserted in a dorsal vein of the operative hand and flushed with saline. The proximal upper arm is padded, and a dual tourniquet is placed on the upper arm. Passive exsanguination is first accomplished by elevating the extremity. An Esmarch bandage is then tightly wrapped at close intervals, starting distally at the fingertips and moving proximally over the tourniquet, to achieve complete exsanguination (Fig. 50.24). The proximal cuff of the double tourniquet is inflated to 250 mm Hg (or 100 mm Hg greater than the systolic blood pressure). Following cuff inflation, the Esmarch bandage is removed, and 50 mL of 0.5% preservative-free lidocaine is administered over several minutes through the heparin lock. The patient should be carefully monitored during the injection for signs of toxicity. Ketorolac has been added to the local anesthesia and appears to be the only agent to offer any significant clinical benefit. Studies show 15 to 30 mg of ketorolac added to the local anesthetic provides some postoperative analgesia without increasing the risk of bleeding.[96]

Anesthesia onset usually occurs within 5 to 10 minutes and can last as long as 60 minutes. Tourniquet pain typically develops within 20 to 30 minutes. When this occurs, the distal cuff is inflated, then the proximal cuff is deflated. Patients are able to tolerate the tourniquet for an additional 15 to 20 minutes since the area under the distal cuff is anesthetized. Following a very short procedure (i.e., 5–10 minutes),

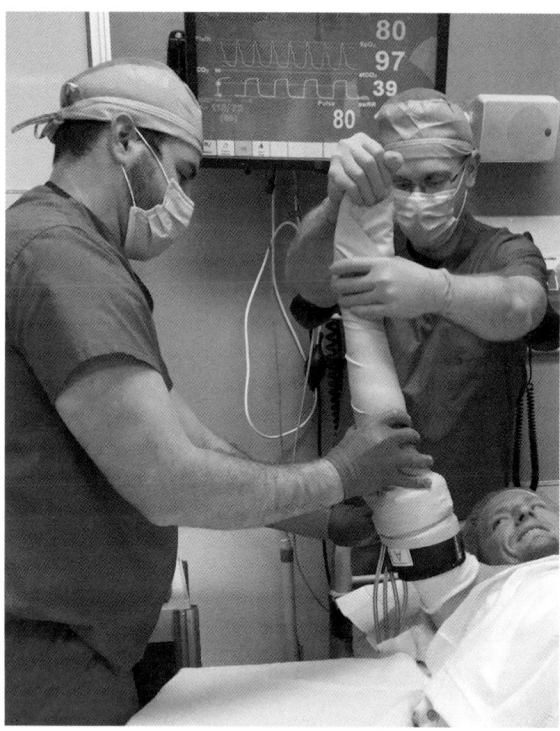

Fig. 50.24 Anesthetists exsanguinate the right upper extremity with an Esmarch bandage prior to tourniquet inflation for an intravenous regional anesthetic.

the cuff must remain inflated for at least 20 minutes.[93] This is important to avoid a LAST event from premature tourniquet cuff deflation. The amount of local anesthesia released to central circulation can be limited by intermittent cuff deflation followed by immediate inflation. The patient is evaluated every 2 to 3 minutes for signs of toxicity until adequate time is reached and the risk of LAST is decreased.

Although not as common, IVRA is also utilized for procedures involving the lower extremity. In general, the procedure is the same; however, greater volumes of local anesthetic (100 mL 0.5% lidocaine) are required to fill the vasculature from the distal IV catheter in the foot to the proximal cuff on the thigh. Additionally, authors have noted a greater chance of local anesthetic leakage under the cuff when IVRA is performed on the lower extremity compared to the upper extremity. This increases the risk of a LAST event and the possibility of an inadequate block.[93]

As noted earlier, the greatest risk associated with IVRA is a rapid transfer of local anesthetic to the central circulation due to improper cuff fitting and inadequate cuff inflation or cuff failure, which precipitates a LAST event. Although rare, documented complications of IVRA include neurologic injury, compartment syndrome, phantom pain, and even limb amputation. Prior to 1999, three cases of either brain injury or death were attributed to IVRA in the American Society of Anesthesiologists, closed claims analysis.[97] As with every regional anesthetic, the procedure should be performed using standard hemodynamic monitoring in an area where emergency and resuscitation equipment is readily available.

Truncal Blocks

Traditionally, truncal blocks, like other peripheral nerve blocks, were performed using anatomic landmark technique. Paravertebral and intercostal blocks provided anesthetists with unilateral pain management options for patients suffering from chest trauma or undergoing thoracic surgery when an epidural was either contraindicated or not

possible. In modern anesthesia practice, the majority of truncal blocks are performed using ultrasound, offering the anesthetist a plethora of options for pain management of the chest, abdomen, and back. There are few indications for using a truncal block as the primary anesthetic. These blocks differ from most upper and lower extremity blocks in that local anesthetic is placed in fascial planes where the nerves course, rather than identifying and blocking specific nerve roots or branches. The advantages of fascial plane blocks, such as the Pecs I, Pecs II, and serratus plane blocks, over paravertebral and thoracic epidural include the ability to use ultrasound, perform them on patients receiving anticoagulant therapy, and the lack of sympathectomy making them a desirable analgesic option for patients undergoing surgeries of the anterior and anterolateral chest.[52] A review of nerve innervation of the chest and abdomen can be found in Clinical Anatomy, earlier.

Paravertebral Nerve Block

Paravertebral blocks (PVBs) are commonly referred to as unilateral epidurals because they target the spinal nerves on the side of the injection. PVBs can be performed at both the thoracic and thoracolumbar levels. These blocks are indicated for anesthetic/analgesic management of thoracic surgery, breast surgery, cholecystectomy, herniorrhaphy, and appendectomy, as well as acute pain management for rib fractures, flail chest, and blunt abdominal trauma. In addition, PVBs have been used to reduce chronic pain syndromes, including osteoporotic vertebral fractures, and herpes zoster. Both somatic and sympathetic fibers are blocked; however, the hemodynamic response is less significant as compared to epidurals.

- Landmark Technique
  - The patient is placed in the sitting or lateral position with the head dropped in the low position and the thoracic region flexed. The provider determines the sensory levels to be anesthetized and identifies the corresponding spinous processes (refer to vertebral anatomy section). To achieve adequate analgesia at least three segments are blocked to account for sensory overlap of the nerves. At each level, a line is drawn 2.5 cm laterally from the spinous process and marked. This approximates the transverse process. Following proper prepping and draping, skin wheals are placed at the marked transverse process locations. A 22-gauge, 5- to 9-cm B-bevel needle is inserted through the skin wheal and directed slightly cephalad. Contact with the transverse process typically occurs 2 to 4 cm at the thoracic level and 5 to 8 cm at the lumbar level. The depth of the needle at contact should be noted. The needle is redirected either cephalad or caudal over the transverse process approximately 1 to 1.5 cm further into the PVS. A subtle click may be noted as the needle penetrates the costotransverse ligament. Nerve stimulation can assist in locating the PVS. Once the needle is inserted into the skin, the current is set to 2 to 5 mA, and the needle is advanced until motor stimulation of the appropriate muscles is noted. The current is slowly decreased to 0.5 mA to localize the nerve. When performing a loss of resistance technique, a 22-gauge Tuohy needle is used. The needle is walked off the transverse process, and a pop or loss of resistance using a syringe occurs when entering the PVS. Following negative aspiration, up to 7 mL can be injected.
- Ultrasound Guidance
  - Ultrasound-guided PVBs are an advanced technique associated with serious complications if done improperly. They are performed using either a sagittal or transverse approach. Here we will describe the transverse approach. The patient is placed in the lateral decubitus position with the block side up. A high-frequency (10–12 MHz) linear array transducer is placed just

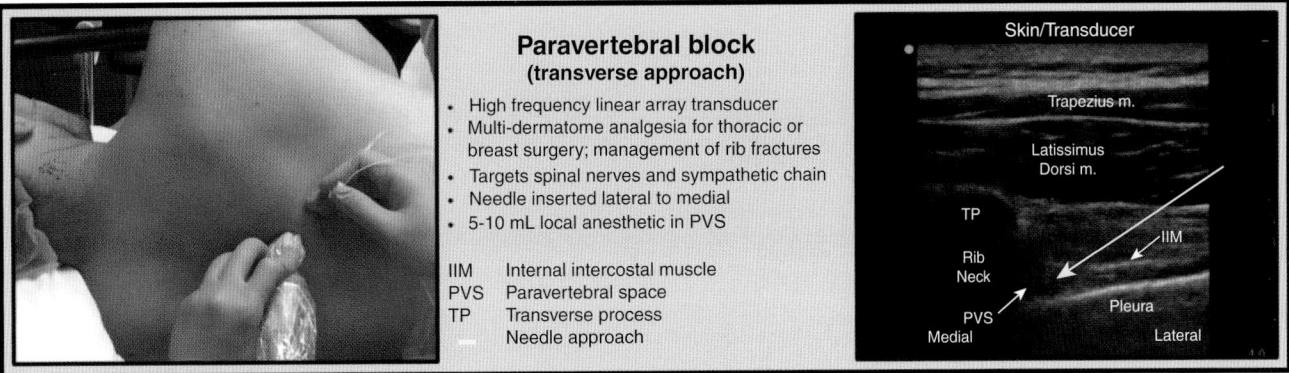

Paravertebral block
(transverse approach)
- High frequency linear array transducer
- Multi-dermatome analgesia for thoracic or breast surgery; management of rib fractures
- Targets spinal nerves and sympathetic chain
- Needle inserted lateral to medial
- 5-10 mL local anesthetic in PVS

IIM   Internal intercostal muscle
PVS   Paravertebral space
TP   Transverse process
—   Needle approach

Fig. 50.25 Transducer position and corresponding image for an ultrasound-guided paravertebral block.

lateral to midline at the desired level of anesthesia/analgesia. Once the thin hyperechoic border of the rib is identified (by the acoustic shadowing beneath it) the transducer is slid caudally to identify the intercostal space and then moved slightly medial to identify the PVS. It is characterized by the hyperechoic pleural line below the internal intercostal membrane (IIM), which is a continuation of the internal intercostal muscle that is contiguous with the costotransverse ligament (Fig. 50.25). After the patient is prepped and draped appropriately, a 22-gauge, 5-cm B-bevel block needle is inserted in-plane lateral to medial through the IIM. Following negative aspiration, 5-mL incremental injections of local anesthetic are administered, up to 20 mL.

- Pearls
  - Local anesthetic should be injected slowly and in small volumes. Avoid high pressures to reduce the possibility of epidural spread. The PVS is highly vascularized, and frequent aspiration is recommended to avoid inadvertent vascular injection. To reduce the incidence of pneumothorax when performing landmark technique, the needle should be directed slightly medial and never more than 2 cm past the transverse process. When using ultrasound guidance, real-time downward displacement of the pleura during injection of local anesthetic indicates proper needle placement.
- Risks and Complications
  - Pneumothorax is a potentially serious complication of this block. Cadaveric studies show that up to 40% of ultrasound-guided PVBs result in epidural spread of local anesthetic.[98] If bilateral spread does occur, hemodynamic changes similar to those seen with epidural anesthesia are possible. In addition to vascular injection, epidural and subarachnoid injections are possible. Postdural puncture headache has been reported following PVB.[99]

Intercostal Nerve Block

Intercostal nerve blocks provide analgesia for postoperative pain control when epidural analgesia is not desired or possible. They provide single dermatome level sensory and motor blockade from the xiphoid to the pubis. Intercostal nerve blocks are indicated for numerous acute and chronic pain conditions affecting the chest and thorax, including rib fractures, herpes zoster, cholecystectomy, and chest-tube insertion. Landmarks are easily identifiable in most patients. The procedure can be performed with the patient in either the prone or lateral position. Intercostal nerve blocks facilitate normal ventilation and deep breathing in the postoperative period, while reducing the amount of opioid pain medication associated in respiratory depression. Since these blocks provide coverage for only one dermatome level, the procedure

must be performed at each level where anesthesia is desired. If blockade of intercostal nerves at any of the five upper ribs is required, this is best accomplished using the paravertebral approach.

- Landmark Technique
  - Once the patient is placed in the lateral position with the block side up, the rib at the desired block level is palpated posterior to the midaxillary line to facilitate the identification of landmarks. The lateral border of the sacrospinalis muscle (~7–10 cm from midline) must be identified prior to attempting the block. After the patient is prepped and draped appropriately, a skin wheal is raised over the point chosen for the injection using a small 25- to 27-gauge needle. A 22-gauge, 5-cm B-bevel needle is then inserted perpendicularly to the rib through the skin wheal and advanced until it contacts the bone. The needle is slowly walked off the rib in a caudal direction. As the edge of the rib is cleared, the needle is advanced another 2 to 3 mm. Following negative aspiration, 3 to 5 mL of the local anesthetic is injected. If resistance is encountered during the injection, the injection should be stopped and the needle repositioned. If the patient begins to cough or move, reevaluate the needle position prior to injecting. Advancing the needle even a few more millimeters can result in nerve puncture by the needle, causing severe pain and possible nerve injury.
- Ultrasound Guidance
  - The patient is placed in the lateral or prone position. A high-frequency (10–12 MHz) linear array transducer is placed in a sagittal orientation 5 to 7 cm lateral to midline at the desired dermatome level to be blocked. The ribs appear as a short hyperechoic line with shadowing beneath them. The intercostal space appears as a gutter between the ribs, with the thin hyperechoic pleura located at its base (Fig. 50.26). The presence of lung sliding during ventilation provides confirmation of the location of the lung. The patient is prepped and draped in the usual manner, and a skin wheal is placed 1 to 2 cm caudally from the transducer. A 22-gauge, 5-cm B-bevel block needle is inserted through the skin wheal and directed in-plane, caudal to cephalad. The slightly distal insertion point improves needle visualization as the trajectory is flattened, optimizing needle reflection. The needle is advanced until it passes through the costotransverse ligament caudal to the inferior border of the superior rib. Following negative aspiration, 3 to 5 mL of local anesthetic is injected. Proper needle placement is verified by real-time visualization of downward displacement of the pleura.
- Pearls
  - In the obese population, landmark identification is better accomplished in the sitting position with the upper body supported

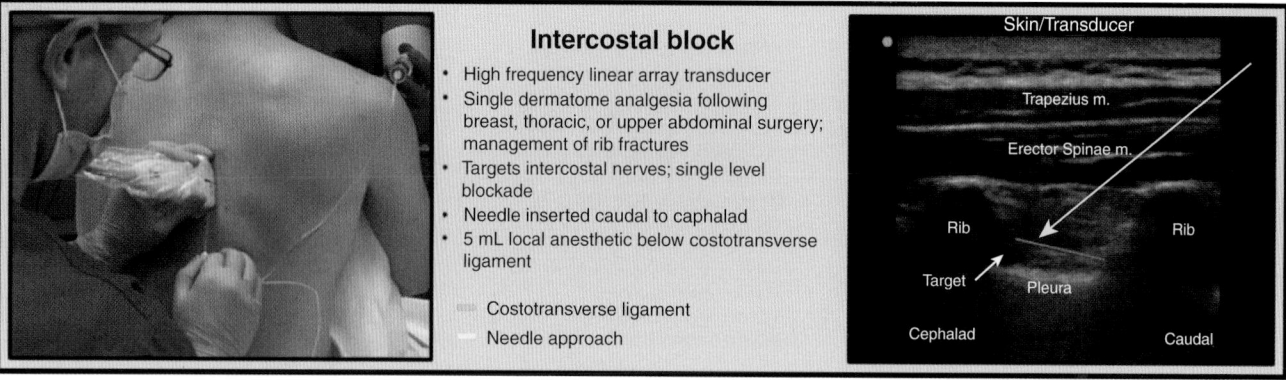

Intercostal block

- High frequency linear array transducer
- Single dermatome analgesia following breast, thoracic, or upper abdominal surgery; management of rib fractures
- Targets intercostal nerves; single level blockade
- Needle inserted caudal to caphalad
- 5 mL local anesthetic below costotransverse ligament

Costotransverse ligament
Needle approach

Skin/Transducer
Trapezius m.
Erector Spinae m.
Rib
Rib
Target
Pleura
Cephalad
Caudal

Fig. 50.26 Transducer position and corresponding image for an ultrasound-guided intercostal block.

over a table or a stand. The likelihood of complications, such as pleural injection and pneumothorax, can be reduced by use of a short B-bevel needle. To avoid an intraneural injection, the needle is directed cephalad as it passes over the ridge of the rib. The use of a free block needle (not directly attached to a syringe), as used with BP blocks, increases maneuverability and control during the procedure.

- Risks and Complications
  - In most patients a small leak of air does not cause a symptomatic pneumothorax. Most patients are able to compensate for any reduced ventilatory capacity, and the pneumothorax resolves without intervention. In a small percentage of patients, intervention is needed for relief of the discomfort and dyspnea. Radiologic studies should be performed after completion of the procedures so that the status or occurrence of a pneumothorax can be established. The studies can be used during follow-up evaluations and therapy if required.[49] Because the intercostal space is highly vascularized, local anesthetics can be absorbed quickly resulting in toxicity if large volumes are injected.

Transversus Abdominis Plane Block

The TAP block is a fascial plane block in which local anesthetic is deposited in the fascial plane deep to the IOM and superficial to the TAM, providing somatic coverage of the abdominal wall and the parietal peritoneum.

It does not provide coverage to the abdominal viscera. TAP blocks are a multimodal analgesic alternative for mid to low abdominal wall surgery when spinal or epidural anesthesia and/or intrathecal opioids are contraindicated or refused. A single injection is required for a unilateral incision, while bilateral injections are required for midline or transverse abdominal incisions. Common procedures include cesarean section, laparoscopic abdominal procedures, open appendectomy, radical prostatectomy, gynecologic surgeries, and hernia repair. Originally described by Rafi in 2001 as a landmark technique,[54] TAP blocks are now mostly performed under ultrasound guidance.[100]

- Landmark Technique
  - The patient is placed in the supine position. The ASIS is identified, and the crest is followed posterior to the point where it dives slightly inward. Further posterior movement will abut against muscle, which is assumed to be the lateral border of the latissimus dorsi. The area is marked, and the skin is prepped and draped appropriately. A skin wheal of local anesthetic is placed at the planned insertion site. A 22-gauge, 5-cm B-bevel needle is inserted perpendicularly until it contacts bone. The needle is then advanced over the crest until a definite pop or giving way is felt. At this point, the needle is located between the IOM and TAM. Following negative aspiration, 5-mL incremental

injections of local anesthetic are administered for a total of 20 mL. When local anesthetic is deposited using this technique, the lower intercostal, iliohypogastric, and ilioinguinal nerves will be blocked.[54]

- Ultrasound Guidance
  - Hebbard et al. first described the ultrasound-guided TAP block in 2007. They demonstrated how the transducer can be transversely oriented on the anterolateral abdominal wall allowing easy identification of the EOM, IOM, and TAM. After the TAP is located, the transducer slides posterolaterally across the midaxillary line just superior to the iliac crest.[100] Several authors have demonstrated differences in local anesthetic spread due to the complex course of the thoracolumbar nerves and the variations between the muscle layers and aponeurotic layers.[51,101,102] Three approaches are currently described in the literature: the subcostal, lateral, and posterior. Depending on the extent of the abdominal procedure, these blocks can be performed individually or in combination to provide optimal coverage. Needle insertion for all three approaches is either medial to lateral or ventral to dorsal, using an in-plane technique until the tip of the needle is visualized piercing the fascia between the IOM and TAM. Local anesthesia is injected in 5-mL increments, after negative aspiration, up to a total volume of 20 to 30 mL.
  - When performing the subcostal approach, the transducer is placed lateral to the xiphoid and parallel and inferior to the costal margin.[103] The rectus abdominis, an elliptical appearing structure, is noted medially (Fig. 50.27). Scanning laterally, it abuts the linea semilunaris (LS) fascia, which is the posterior rectus sheath. The LS gives rise to the EOM and IOM. The needle is inserted medial to lateral in the plane between the LS fascia (posterior rectus sheath) and the superior border of the TAM. Following negative aspiration, a small amount of local anesthetic is injected to confirm its placement in the fascial plane. The needle is then slowly advanced into the space created.[102]
  - The lateral approach begins with the transducer placed at the midaxillary line, superior to and parallel with the iliac crest where the EOM, IOM, and TAM are identified parallel to each other.[100,103] The needle tip is guided to the midaxillary line to ensure the lateral cutaneous branches of the thoracolumbar nerves are blocked.[100]
  - When performing a posterior approach, the transducer is initially placed along the midaxillary plane, as in the lateral approach.[100] It is then slid posterior of the midaxillary line until the aponeurosis of the tensor fascia latae (TFL), a series of aponeuroses and fascial layers that encapsulate the deep muscles of the back, are imaged (Fig 50.28). The needle is inserted ventral to dorsal at the point where the IOM and TAM taper off into the TFL.

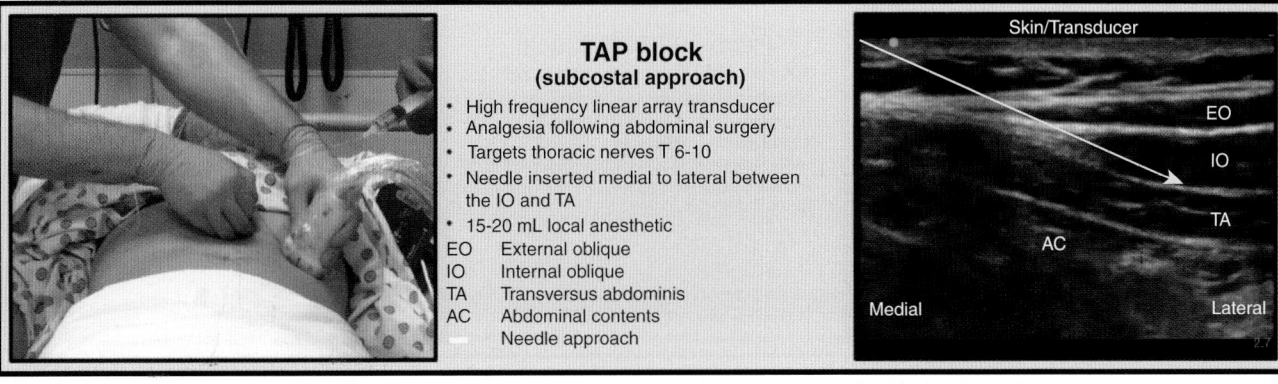

Fig. 50.27 Transducer position and corresponding image for an ultrasound-guided subcostal transversus abdominis plane block.

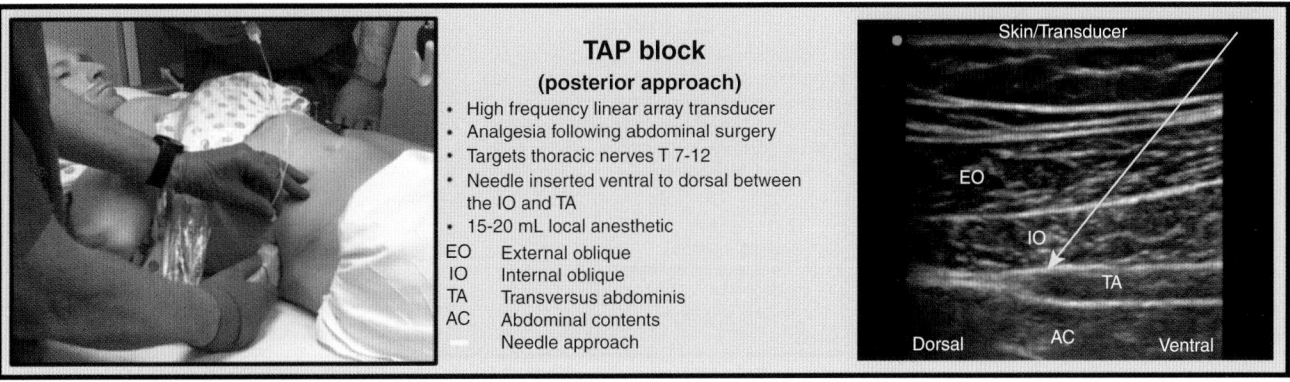

Fig. 50.28 Transducer position and corresponding image for an ultrasound-guided posterior transversus abdominis plane block.

- Pearls
  - Børglum et al. demonstrated how the spread of local anesthetic varied depending on the ultrasound-guided approach used.[102] Subcostal TAP blocks are indicated for surgical procedures requiring supraumbilical analgesia. Lateral and posterior TAP blocks provide reliable analgesia for procedures below the umbilicus. Blunt-tip block needles are recommended to increase tactile feel during the procedure and minimize the possibility of visceral injury if the needle is advanced past the TAM into the peritoneum.
- Risks and Complications
  - Block failure will occur when local anesthetic is injected into the incorrect plane. Local anesthetic systemic toxicity is a potential complication following placement of TAP blocks.[104] When bilateral injections are performed, careful adherence to maximum local anesthetic dose limits should be maintained because of the risk of LAST. Additionally, fascial plane blocks, such as the TAP block, have been shown to have an increased rate of absorption, possibly related to the compact area between the fascia in which the local anesthetic is injected.[105]

Rectus Sheath Block

Rectus sheath blocks provide postoperative analgesia following abdominal surgery requiring a midline incision. It is indicated for the management of incisional pain following umbilical hernia repair and is commonly used in pediatric patients. Additional uses include cesarean section when midline incision is used and postpartum laparoscopic tubal ligation.

- Landmark Technique
  - The patient is placed in the supine position. The anesthetist stands on either side of the patient. Depending on the area to be anesthetized, as many as six injection sites may be required. Following appropriate sterile preparation with draping, several skin wheals are placed in the rectus muscle bellies between the tendinous intersections. A 22-gauge, 5-cm B-bevel needle is inserted through the skin and advanced until stiff resistance from the anterior rectus sheath is felt. The needle is then passed through the sheath; if puncture of the sheath is not a definite snap, the procedure should be stopped. Once confirmed, the needle is advanced through the less dense muscle belly until the anesthetist feels the firm resistance of the posterior sheath, at which point the needle is no longer advanced. Following negative aspiration, incremental injections of 5 mL (up to a total of 10 mL) are administered. This process is repeated at each injection site.
- Ultrasound Guidance
  - The patient is placed in the supine position and prepped and draped in the appropriate manner. A high-frequency (10–12 MHz) linear array transducer is placed in transverse orientation at the level to be blocked (Fig. 50.29). A skin wheal is raised at the lateral border of the transducer, and a 22-gauge, 5-cm B-bevel needle is inserted in-plane lateral to medial until the tip is positioned between the muscle belly and posterior rectus sheath. Following negative aspiration, 10 mL of local anesthetic is placed in incremental injections of 5 mL.
- Pearls
  - When performing landmark technique, blocks above the umbilicus should be performed first, and the depth of needle insertion noted.

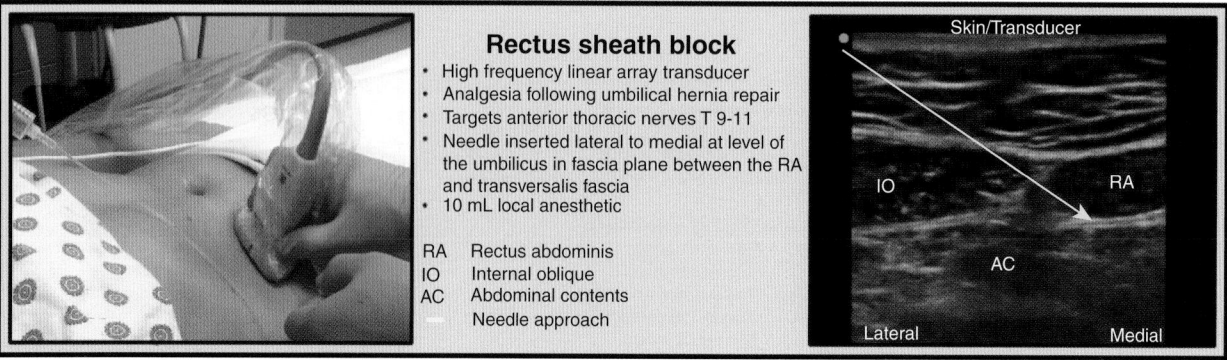

Fig. 50.29 Transducer position and corresponding image for an ultrasound-guided rectus sheath block.

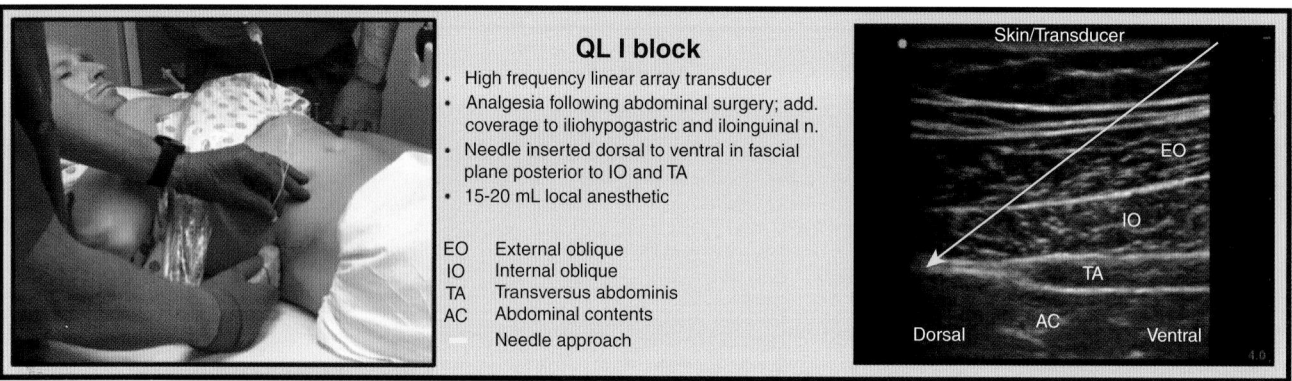

Fig. 50.30 Transducer position and corresponding image for an ultrasound-guided quadratus lumborum (QL) I block.

- Risks and Complications
  - Inadvertent vascular injection is possible within the intercostal arteries and superior and inferior epigastric arteries since these vessels course within the rectus sheath.[55] Below the umbilicus, the posterior rectus sheath becomes thinner and less dense, and it may be difficult to appreciate puncture through the sheath into the peritoneum.

Quadratus Lumborum Block

Quadratus lumborum (QL) blocks are newer ultrasound-guided regional techniques for the management of postoperative pain following abdominal and hip surgeries. While some authors consider it an indirect PVB, there are several theories as to the exact mechanism of action as local anesthetic spread varies according to the approach.[106,107] The lack of consensus regarding the mechanism of spread may be partly the result of the varying approaches used in performing the block. Here we will describe only the QL I and QL III techniques. The QL block is seen by some as a time-consuming, advanced block that is technically challenging to perform and has made little impact on the practice of nonregional anesthesia practitioners in the management of patients having abdominal surgery.[108]

- Ultrasound Guidance
  - Originally described as a variant of the posterior ultrasound-guided TAP block, the QL I approach targets the TF at the point where the IOM and TAM taper off posteriorly and abut the lateral border of the QL muscle. The patient is placed in the supine position, and a high-frequency (7–12 MHz) linear array transducer is placed in transverse orientation at the midaxillary just above the iliac crest (Fig. 50.30). After the patient is prepped and draped appropriately, a skin wheal is placed on the medial border of the transducer. A 22-gauge, 9-cm B-bevel needle is inserted ventral to dorsal in-plane and advanced between the posterior aponeurosis of the TAM and the TF just lateral to the QL muscle. Following negative aspiration, up to 20 mL of local anesthetic is injected in 5-mL increments.
  - The QL III, or shamrock sign, transmuscular QL technique was first described by Børglum.[109] When using this approach, the patient is placed in the lateral decubitus position, and a low-frequency (2–5 MHz) curvilinear array transducer is placed in a transverse orientation above the iliac crest at the midaxillary line. The transverse process of the L4 lumbar vertebrae is identified as an anechoic projection (Fig. 50.31), which represents the stem of the shamrock; the erector spinae, QL, and psoas muscles comprise the leaves. After the patient is prepped and draped appropriately, a skin wheal is raised at the dorsal side of the transducer. A 22-gauge, 9-cm B-bevel block needle is passed dorsal to ventral through the QL muscle to the interfascial plane between the QL and psoas muscles.[110] Following negative aspiration, up to 20 mL of local anesthetic is injected in 5-mL increments.
- Pearls
  - As a fascial plane block, the QL techniques require large volumes of low-concentration local anesthetic to obtain a reliable block. Some authors believe the QL III reduces the risk of unintentional peritoneal cavity injection as it avoids the recess between the abdominal wall and psoas major.[110] Color Doppler may be useful in identifying abdominal branches of lumbar arteries that may course through the path of the needle. Following the injection of local anesthetic, rotating the transducer longitudinally can confirm cephalad spread.

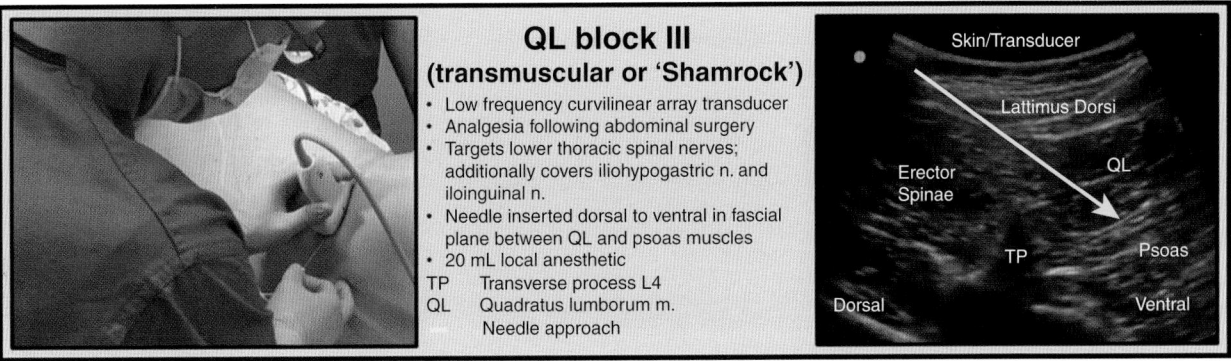

Fig. 50.31 Transducer position and corresponding image for an ultrasound-guided quadratus lumborum (QL) III block.

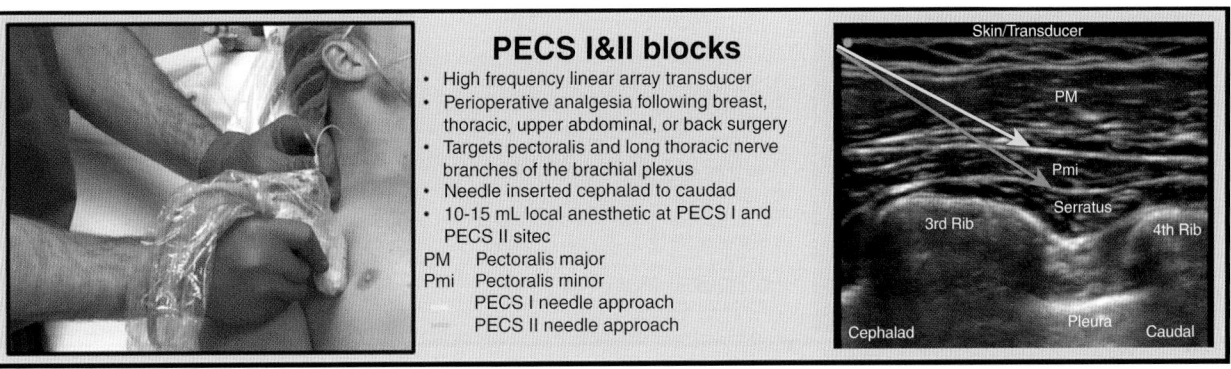

Fig. 50.32 Transducer position and corresponding image for an ultrasound-guided Pecs I and Pecs II block.

- Risks and Complications
  - Due to its close proximity there is increased risk of inadvertent peritoneal puncture. It is common to visualize the lower pole of the kidney and the lower lobes of the liver and spleen. Care must be taken to avoid visceral injury.

Pectoralis Blocks

The pectoralis or Pecs blocks are newer ultrasound-guided approaches designed to provide anesthesia/analgesia to the anterior upper chest wall without the risks and complications associated with neuraxial or thoracic paravertebral techniques. They are indicated for breast surgeries, insertion of portacaths or pacemakers, or subpectoral prothesis.[52] When combined with a thoracic PVB, Pecs blocks have been used to perform breast surgeries under propofol sedation.[111] Blanco first described the Pecs block as a technique in which local anesthetic was injected in the plane between the pectoralis major and pectoralis minor muscles, adjacent to the pectoral branch of the thoracolumbar artery.[112] This procedure (i.e., Pecs or Pecs I block) targeted the medial and lateral pectoral branches of the BP.[53,113] The Pecs block was later modified to provide additional coverage by adding a second injection in the plane between the pectoralis minor and serratus anterior muscles at the level of the third and fourth ribs. This modification (i.e., Pecs II block) targeted the long thoracic nerve and lateral cutaneous branches of the thoracic intercostal nerves and is indicated for more extensive procedures involving the chest wall and axilla.[52,111,113,114] The Pecs block terminology has led to some confusion, as some authors have erroneously used "Pecs II" to describe only the deep injection.[53]

- Ultrasound Guidance
  - To perform a Pecs I block, the patient is positioned supine with the arms resting at the side. A high-frequency (7–12 MHz)

linear array transducer is placed in a sagittal orientation beneath the clavicle as if performing an infraclavicular block. The transducer is slid slightly lateral and caudal to identify the pectoralis minor and serratus anterior muscles at the level of the third and fourth ribs. Once identified, the probe is rotated slightly infero-laterally (Fig. 50.32). After the patient is prepped and draped appropriately, a skin wheal is placed on the cephalad side of the transducer. Using an in-plane technique, the needle is inserted cephalad to caudad to the interfascial plane between the pectoralis major and pectoralis minor muscles. Following negative aspiration, 10 mL of local anesthetic is injected in 5-mL increments. To perform the Pecs II block, the transducer remains in the same position, and the needle is redirected to the interfascial plane between the pectoralis minor and serratus anterior muscles. Following negative aspiration, up to 20 mL local anesthetic is injected in 5-mL increments.

- Pearls
  - A serratus plane block is a variation of the Pecs block that aims to increase the amount of intercostal nerve coverage from T2 to T9.[53] The block is performed more lateral and distal than the Pecs II block, overlying the fifth rib at the midaxillary line. Under ultrasound guidance, local anesthetic can be placed either superficial or deep to the serratus anterior muscle.[53] As with the Pecs II block, this block does not provide coverage to the pectoralis muscles, and a Pecs 1 block must be performed when anesthesia of the medial chest is desired.

- Risks and Complications
  - The large volume of local anesthetic required to achieve analgesic spread places the patient at risk of LAST. The pectoral branch of the thoracolumbar artery lies within the interfascial plane of the Pecs I injection, increasing the risk of inadvertent vascular

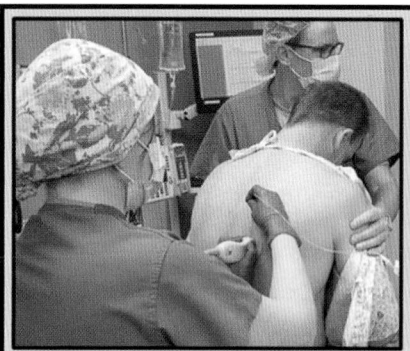
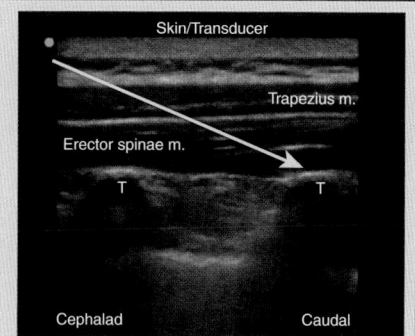

Erector Spinae block
- High frequency curvilinear array transducer
- Perioperative analgesia following breast, thoracic, upper abdominal, or back surgery
- Targets the dorsal rami with potential spread to ventral rami
- Needle inserted cephalad to caudad until contact with TP
- 10-15 mL local anesthetic between erector spinae m. and TP

TP   Transverse process
      Needle approach

Fig. 50.33 Transducer position and corresponding image for an ultrasound-guided erector spinae block at the thoracic level.

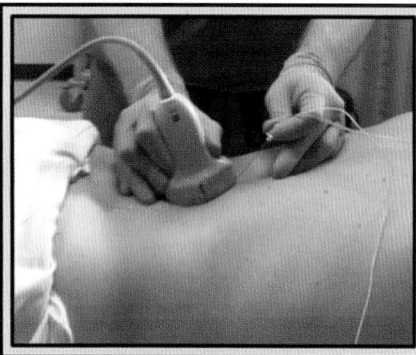
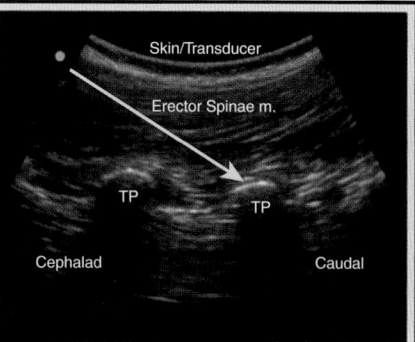

Erector Spinae block
- Low frequency curvilinear array transducer
- Perioperative analgesia following breast, thoracic, upper abdominal, or back surgery
- Targets the dorsal rami with potential spread to ventral rami
- Needle inserted cephalad to caudad until contact with TP
- 10-15 mL local anesthetic between erector spinae m. and TP

TP   Transverse process
      Needle approach

Fig. 50.34 Transducer position and corresponding image for an ultrasound-guided erector spinae block at the lumbar level.

injection. Pneumothorax is a potential complication since the intercostal space and pleura lie just inferior to the serratus anterior muscle when performing a Pecs II block.

Erector Spinae Block

The erector spinae (ESP) block is an ultrasound-guided interfascial plane technique that targets local anesthetic injection superficial to the transverse process and deep to the erector spinae muscles of the back. The goal is to block the dorsal and ventral rami of the thoracic spinal nerves at the level of the injections.[115,116] Ueshima et al. demonstrated spread to the thoracic PVS following the placement of ESP catheters in three subjects.[117] However, Ivanusic et al. reported in a cadaver study that despite significant craniocaudal spread, dye did not reliably spread anteriorly to the PVS or to the ventral or dorsal origins of the thoracic spinal nerves. Dye spread was consistent only around the dorsal ramus.[118] First described in 2016 as a means to treat severe thoracic neuropathic pain,[115] numerous case reports have demonstrated its utility for a variety of surgical procedures, including lumbar spine surgery, video-assisted thoracic surgery, breast surgery, rib fractures, bariatric surgery, and various abdominal procedures.[119-128]

- Ultrasound Guidance
  - When placing an ESP block at the thoracic level, the patient can be placed in the sitting, lateral, or prone position, and a high-frequency (10–12 MHz) linear array transducer is placed in a parasagittal orientation at the T5 spinous process. Following the appropriate prepping and draping, a skin wheal is placed at the cephalad edge of the transducer, and a 22-gauge, 5-cm B-bevel needle is passed cephalad to caudad where the erector spinae muscles abut the transverse process. Following negative aspiration, up to 20 mL of local anesthetic is injected in 5-mL increments, observing for the separation of

the erector spinae muscle off the bone (Fig. 50.33). When performing an ESP block for lumbar back surgery, the patient is placed in the prone position, and a low-frequency (2–5 MHz) curvilinear array transducer is placed at the anticipated level of surgery in a parasagittal orientation over the transverse process (Fig. 50.34). After the patient is prepped and draped appropriately, a skin wheal is placed at the cephalad edge of the transducer. A 22-gauge, 9-cm B-bevel block needle is inserted cephalad to caudad to the area where the erector spinae muscles meet the transverse process. Following negative aspiration, administer a total of 20 mL of local anesthetic in 5-mL increments, observing for separation of the erector spinae muscles from the bone.

- Pearls
  - When performing the ESP block at the thoracic level, the trapezius muscle is often seen superficial to the erector spinae muscle as seen with an ultrasound-guided intercostal block (see Fig. 50.33). Numerous authors have demonstrated significant craniocaudal spread when performing this block, so a single injection generally provides sufficient coverage to multiple dermatome levels.[127] As the ESP block provides single-sided analgesia, bilateral injections are required for midline procedures such as ventral hernia repairs.

- Risks and Complications
  - The ESP block is simple to perform, with readily identifiable landmarks. Due to the distance of the pleura from the injection site, there are few risks associated with this procedure.

Lower Extremity Peripheral Nerve Blocks

Lower extremity peripheral nerve blocks are well described in the literature and provide anesthesia for lower extremity surgical procedures

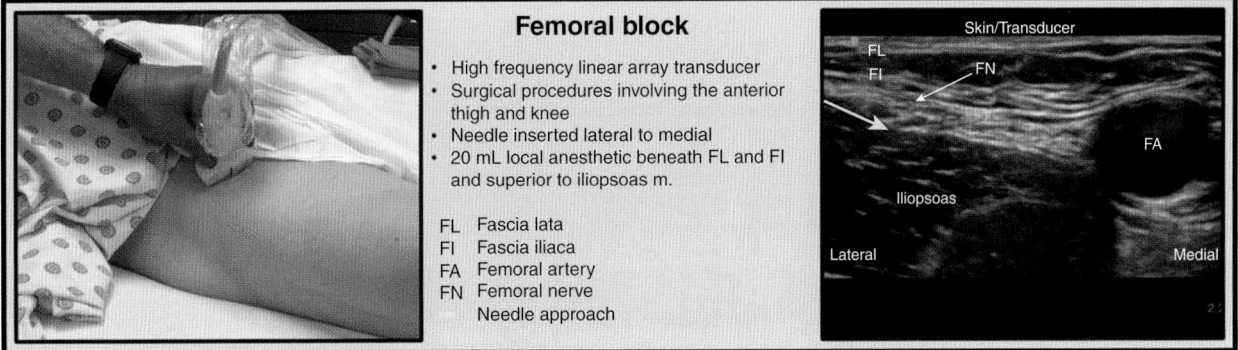

Fig. 50.35 Transducer position and corresponding image for an ultrasound-guided femoral nerve block.

as either the primary anesthetic or part of a multimodal pain management plan. The lower extremity receives innervation from the lumbar and lumbosacral plexi. Thus the proposed procedure should provide the appropriate coverage based on the surgical procedure, duration, and postoperative pain requirements. A review of lower extremity innervation can be found in Clinical Anatomy, earlier.

Femoral Nerve Block

The femoral nerve block (FNB) has many clinical applications in anesthesia and pain management. Once considered the mainstay of anesthesia/analgesia for total knee arthroplasty, the block is still commonly used for surgical procedures of the femur, patella, quadriceps surgery, and analgesia following hip fracture. When combined with the sciatic nerve block, the FNB provides complete coverage of the lower extremity. Whether performed using the landmark technique or under ultrasound guidance, FNB is effective and easy to perform with minimal risk.

- Landmark Technique
  - The patient is positioned supine with slight external rotation of the extremity. At the level of the inguinal ligament, a line is drawn from the pubic tubercle to the ASIS. The femoral artery is palpated. The injection site is marked 1 cm lateral to the artery and 1 cm inferior to the inguinal ligament. After the area is appropriately prepped and draped, a skin wheal of local anesthetic is placed at the needle insertion site. A 22-gauge, 5-cm B-bevel needle is advanced perpendicularly into the skin. The nerve stimulator is set at 1 mA and advanced until quadriceps contraction or patellar snap is elicited. Stimulation is decreased to a motor response at 0.3 to 0.5 mA to ensure proper needle location. Following negative aspiration, up to 20 mL of local anesthetic is injected in 5-mL increments. Gentle but firm pressure can be applied caudal to the needle to limit the distal spread of local anesthetic.[129,130] There is no sciatic distribution when performing this technique. If the surgical procedure requires anesthesia along the sciatic distribution, a separate procedure must be performed.[130]
- Ultrasound Guidance
  - The patient is placed in the supine position, with slight external rotation of the lower extremity. A high-frequency linear array transducer (10–12 MHz) is usually sufficient, but in patients with a large body habitus a lower frequency (7 MHz) may be required. The transducer is placed in transverse orientation at the inguinal crease, and the major anatomic landmarks are identified (Fig. 50.35). If the femoral artery has bifurcated, the transducer is slid cephalad until the common femoral artery is identified proximal to the bifurcation of the superficial femoral and profunda femoris arteries. The skin is prepped

and draped in the appropriate manner, and a skin wheal is placed along the lateral edge of the transducer. A 22-gauge, 5-cm B-bevel needle is inserted using an in-plane approach under ultrasound guidance through the fascia lata and fascia iliaca, just lateral to the femoral artery. The posterior division of the FN innervates the quadriceps muscles. It is generally found on the inferolateral aspect of the nerve, and the needle should be directed there. A PNS can be used in conjunction with ultrasound to verify proper needle placement and muscle response prior to injection of local anesthetic. Hydrolocation, the process of injecting a small amount of fluid (1–3 mL) while advancing the needle through the tissue, can be used to determine the exact location of the tip. Injecting D5W when performing hydrolocation will enhance nerve stimulation.[131] Following negative aspiration, 20 to 30 mL of local anesthetic is injected in 5-mL increments.

- Pearls
  - The mnemonic NAVL (nerve, artery, vein, lymph) is often used when going lateral to medial to remember the relationship of the FN to the other structures at the inguinal crease. With either technique (landmark or ultrasound guidance) the needle tip must penetrate both the fascia lata and fascia iliaca to ensure an efficacious block. Studies demonstrate that the local anesthetic volumes greater than 20 mL are not associated with improved block rates.[132]
- Risks and Complications
  - Although not common, inadvertent vascular puncture and nerve injury are complications associated when performing this block.[132] Because of the associated quadriceps weakness with this block, it has been speculated that peripheral nerve blockade contributes to the rate of falls following lower extremity total joint surgery. However, contrary to these concerns, a study examining 190,000 records found that peripheral nerve block did not alter the risk of inpatient falls of 1.6% in this group.[133]

Adductor Canal Block

The adductor canal block (ACB) was first described by Kirkpatrick et al. as a means to identify the SphN in the proximal to midthigh using the superficial femoral artery as an anatomic reference.[134] More recent studies have demonstrated that the medial vastus nerve also provides significant innervation to the knee capsule, through intramuscular, extramuscular, and deep genicular nerves.[60,135] Because it spares quadriceps strength, the ACB is commonly used as part of multimodal pain management for total knee arthroplasties. It is also indicated for any surgery involving the anteromedial knee, including anterior

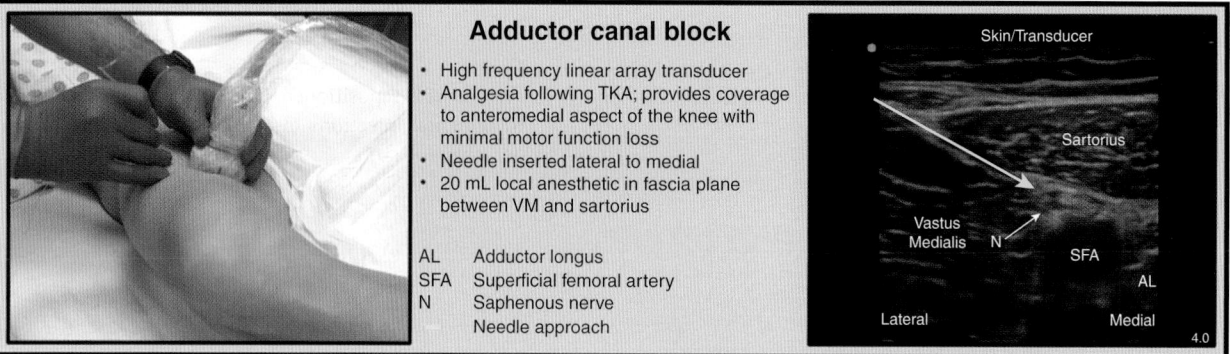

Fig. 50.36 Transducer position and corresponding image for an ultrasound-guided adductor canal block.

cruciate ligament/medial collateral ligament repairs and patella fractures. Although this block has been described being performed blindly with nerve stimulation,[136] it is normally performed under ultrasound guidance.

- Ultrasound Guidance
  - The patient is placed in the supine position with slight external rotation of the leg. A high-frequency linear array transducer (>7 MHz) is placed in transverse orientation on the medial aspect of the middle and distal third of the thigh (Fig. 50.36). The superficial femoral artery is identified inferior to the sartorius muscle; color Doppler can assist in locating the artery if it is not readily identifiable. After the patient is appropriately prepped and draped, a skin wheal is placed at the lateral edge of the transducer. A 22-gauge, 9-cm B-bevel needle is inserted lateral to medial and advanced to the edge of the artery into the fascial plane separating the sartorius and adductor longus muscles. Once the needle tip is located anterolateral to the artery, 1 to 2 mL of local anesthetic is injected following negative aspiration. Separation of the fascial plane between the muscles and artery will further define the SphN. After confirming proper placement 10 to 20 mL of local anesthetic is injected in 5-mL increments, confirming negative aspiration of blood prior to each injection.
- Pearls
  - To accomplish a sensory nerve block of the SphN, the transducer is slid distally until the artery is noted to pass through the adductor hiatus, at the most distal area where the nerve still lies beneath the sartorius muscle.[137]
  - Visualization of the nerve is not necessary for this block; in certain individuals the saphenous or branches may lie anteromedial to the artery. If this is recognized during a preprocedure scan, local anesthetic is deposited on both sides of the artery.
- Risks and Complications
  - Proximal injections and large volumes of local anesthetic (20–30 mL) are associated with increased risk of quadriceps weakness.

Lumbar Plexus (Psoas Compartment) Block

After emerging from the intervertebral foramina, the L2-L4 nerve roots form the lumbar plexus within the psoas muscle. Also known as the three-in-one block, this approach attempts to block the plexus as it lies in the fascial plane bordered medially by the vertebral column, dorsally by the QLM, and ventrally by the psoas major muscle. Blockade of the plexus as a unit can be accomplished by injecting local anesthetic into the fascial sheath surrounding the plexus. This block is an advanced regional technique and not commonly performed today because ultrasound-guided procedures provide greater efficacy and less risk to the patient.

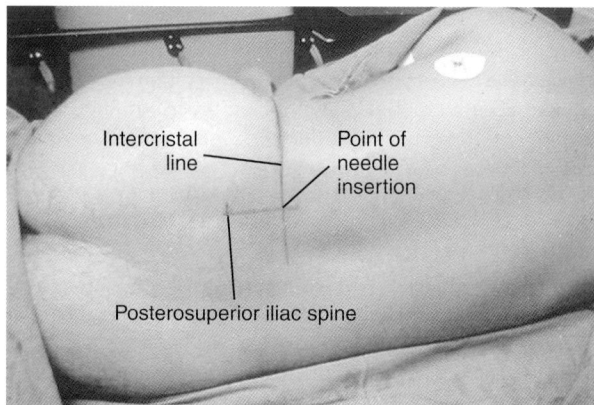

Fig. 50.37 Anatomic landmarks for a lumbar plexus (psoas compartment) block.

- Landmark Technique
  - The patient is placed in the lateral decubitus position with a slight forward tilt. The patient should be in a relaxed but curled position similar to that used for spinal or epidural anesthesia, lying on the nonoperative side with the extremity to be blocked positioned over the dependent leg so motor response can be easily noted.[138] The patient is prepped and draped in the appropriate manner. From the spinous process of L4, a line is drawn caudally approximately 3 cm. A 5-cm line is drawn perpendicularly and laterally from this point toward the side to be blocked. This perpendicular line will typically end at the medial edge of the iliac crest. This spot identifies the point of needle insertion (Fig. 50.37). A skin wheal is raised, and a 21-gauge, 12-cm B-bevel block needle is inserted perpendicularly on all planes and advanced until contact with the transverse process of L5, usually at a depth between 5 and 10 cm. The needle is then withdrawn, redirected slightly cephalad, and advanced until it slides over the transverse process of L5. Using the loss-of-resistance technique, the psoas compartment is usually encountered at the depth of 8 to 12 cm. The tip of the needle now lies in the psoas compartment. When using nerve stimulation, quadriceps contraction is used to verify proper needle location. Needle placement can also be confirmed by advancing the needle slightly into the psoas muscle and reconfirming a loss of resistance while withdrawing the needle slightly into the psoas compartment. Following negative aspiration, 25 to 35 mL of local anesthetic is injected in incremental doses of 5 mL.
- Pearls
  - To limit the spread of local, the patient should remain in the lateral decubitus position for several minutes following injection.

- Risks and Complications
  - The lumbar plexus block is an advanced technique. Numerous complications have been described, including epidural spread of local anesthetic (most common), spinal anesthesia, LAST, hypotension, and renal hemotoma.[138]

Fascia Iliaca Block

The fascia iliaca block (FIB) is an anterior approach to the lumbar plexus with a puncture point much further from its origin. The FIB has been described as a low-tech alternative to the FN or lumbar plexus block.[139] Since the FN, ON, and LFCN lie deep to the fascia iliaca, injecting a large volume of local anesthetic beneath the fascia should result in sufficient spread cephalad, medially, and laterally to anesthetize all three nerves. When performing this procedure using landmark technique, nerve stimulation is not required. Initially described in children in 1989, the fascia iliaca compartment block has been widely used for postoperative analgesia following hip, femoral shaft, or knee surgery. Compared with the landmark technique three-in-one block, it provides a faster and more consistent simultaneous blockade of the LFCN and FN.

- Landmark Technique
  - The patient is placed in the supine position. At the level of the inguinal ligament, a line is drawn from the pubic tubercle to the ASIS and trisected. The puncture site is marked 1 cm caudal to the point separating the lateral and middle third of the inguinal line. After the patient is appropriately prepped and draped, a skin wheal with local anesthetic is made at the needle insertion site. A 22-gauge, 5-cm B-bevel needle is inserted perpendicular to the skin. An initial loss of resistance is felt as the needle tip punctures the fascia lata. The needle is advanced until a second loss of resistance is felt as the fascia iliaca is pierced. Following negative aspiration, 30 to 40 mL of local anesthetic is injected in increments of 5 mL.[140-142]
- Ultrasound Guidance
  - The two approaches commonly described are the transverse and longitudinal suprainguinal. When performing the transverse approach, the patient is positioned supine with slight external rotation of the extremity (if tolerated). This provides optimal access to the inguinal region and visualization of key anatomic structures. The skin is prepped and draped in an appropriate manner, and the transducer is placed in a transverse orientation at the inguinal crease. It is slid medially or laterally until a single hypoechoic femoral artery and vein are identified. The FN lies just lateral to the artery and superior to the large dark, hypoechoic iliopsoas muscle. The nerve should appear as a bright, hyperechoic oval structure (see Fig. 50.35). If the nerve is not easily identifiable, tilting the transducer slightly cephalad or caudad will help distinguish it from the muscle and the more superficial subcutaneous tissue. The thin bright fascia iliaca covers the iliopsoas muscle, separating it from the subcutaneous tissue above it. The fascia lata rests superiorly within this tissue. Sliding the transducer laterally several centimeters brings the sartorius muscle into view, which is covered by its own fascia and the fascia iliaca (Fig. 50.38). Once all pertinent structures are identified, a small skin wheal is placed at the lateral edge of the transducer. A 22-gauge, 5-cm B-bevel needle is inserted through the skin wheal and advanced in-plane under ultrasound guidance beneath the fascia lata and iliaca, lateral (near but not adjacent) to the FN. To achieve the optimal spread of local anesthetic, the needle must pass through both fascia. Following negative aspiration for blood (indicating the needle is likely not within a blood

vessel), 1 to 2 mL of local anesthetic is injected, observing for separation of the fascia iliaca from the iliopsoas muscle. If local anesthetic is observed above the fascia or in the muscle itself, the needle is repositioned. Once correct placement is verified, incremental injections of 5 mL are achieved following each negative aspiration. Local anesthetic spread should be noted medially and laterally from the injection point. Additional needle repositions may be required. A total of 30 to 40 mL of dilute local anesthetic is usually required to achieve the spread medially toward the FN and laterally toward the sartorius muscle. When properly performed, the FN is reliably blocked 100% of the time and the LFCN greater than 80% of the time.[139] The ON is not reliably blocked. Levente et al. showed block efficacy up to 48 hours when an ultrasound-guided FIB was placed in the emergency department.[143]

- When performing the longitudinal suprainguinal approach, the patient is appropriately prepped and draped, and a high-frequency (10–12 MHz) linear array transducer is placed in a sagittal plane to obtain an image of the ASIS. The transducer is slid medially, and the fascia iliaca, sartorius, iliopsoas, and internal oblique muscles are identified (Fig. 50.39). After identifying the bowtie sign formed by the fascia of the sartorius and internal oblique muscles, a skin wheal is placed at the caudal edge of the transducer. A 22-gauge, 9-cm B-bevel needle is inserted 1 cm cephalad to the inguinal ligament in-plane to the fascia iliaca. Hydrolocation can be used to separate the fascia from the muscle. In the space created, the needle is advanced slightly in a cranial and dorsal direction. Following negative aspiration, up to 40 mL of local anesthetic is injected in 5-mL increments.[144]
- Pearls
  - The FIB is a large-volume block (30–40 mL). If the spread of local anesthetic does not appear adequate, or it pools toward one location, the needle should be repositioned. Additional injections may be required to ensure adequate spread.
  - The deep circumflex artery lies just superior to the fascia iliaca, and an upward movement on injection is used as a marker for successful penetration of the fascia iliaca.[144]
- Risks and Complications
  - Due to the large volumes of local anesthetic and the proximity of the FN during injection, quadriceps weakness often occurs, limiting postoperative mobility.
  - Because of the large volume of local anesthetic injected, rapid absorption or inadvertent intravascular injection can result in LAST.

Pericapsular Nerve Group Block

The pericapsular nerve group (PENG) block is a single-injection technique recently described for analgesia following hip fracture and arthroplasty.[145] This block targets the articular branches of the FN, as well as the accessory obturator and obturator nerves, while sparing the FN and its associated quadriceps innervation.[146,147] Several small case studies have demonstrated significant pain relief without quadriceps weakness.[148-150] However, currently there are no cadaveric studies demonstrating dye spread of local anesthetic or randomized controlled trails establishing efficacy, safety, or advantages over other procedures.

- Ultrasound Guidance
  - The patient is placed supine, and a low-frequency (2–5 MHz) curvilinear array transducer is placed in a transverse orientation parallel to the inguinal ligament at the level of the ASIS. The transducer is then slid caudally until the anterior inferior iliac spine and pubic ramus are visible. At this level, the FN,

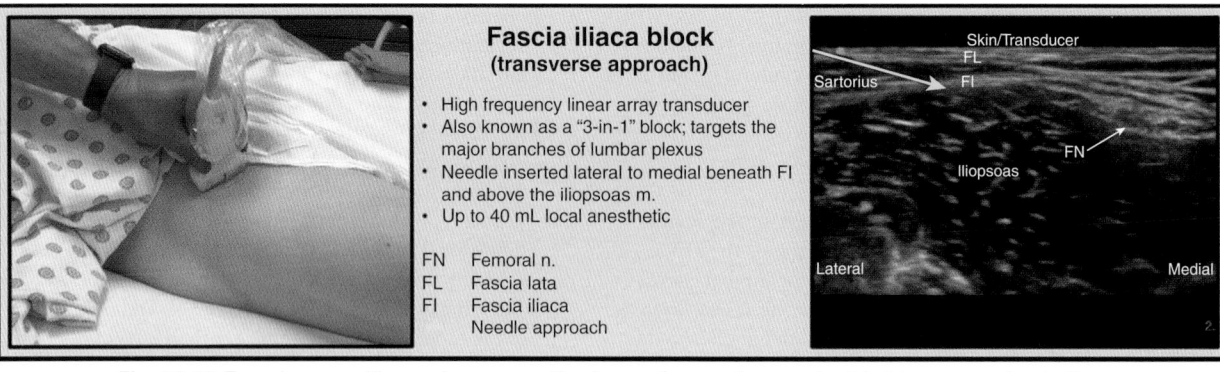

Fig. 50.38 Transducer position and corresponding image for an ultrasound-guided transverse fascia iliaca block.

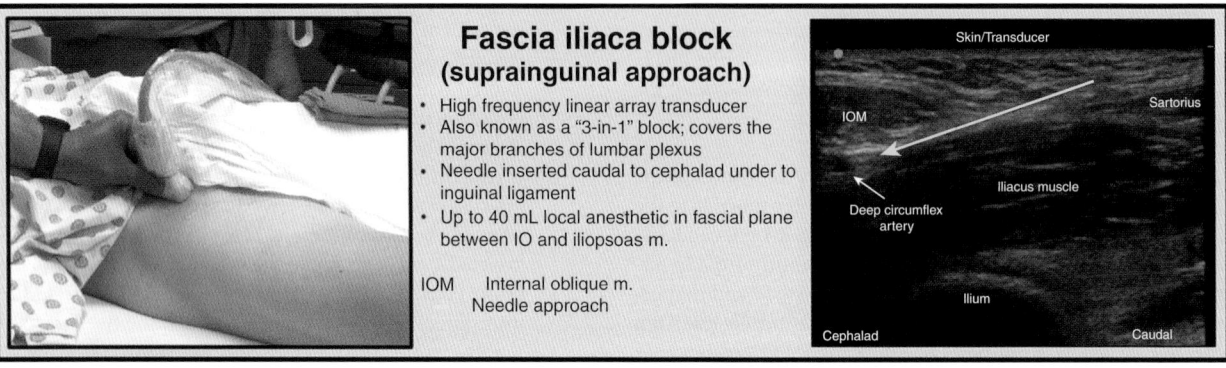

Fig. 50.39 Transducer position and corresponding image for an ultrasound-guided suprainguinal fascia iliaca block.

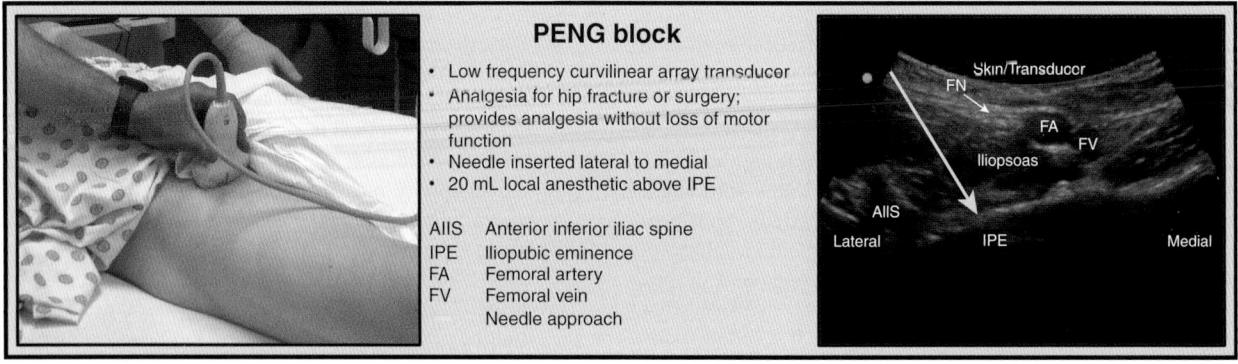

Fig. 50.40 Transducer position and corresponding image for an ultrasound-guided pericapsular nerve group (PENG) block.

artery, and vein are identified. The iliopubic eminence, created by the junction of the ilium and pubis, is also identified (Fig. 50.40). After the patient is prepped and draped appropriately, a skin wheal is raised at the lateral edge of the transducer. A 22-gauge, 9-cm B-bevel block is inserted in-plane, lateral to medial between the psoas muscle with prominent tendon and the pubic ramus, medial to the anterior inferior iliac spine. Following negative aspiration, up to 20 mL of local anesthetic is injected in 5-mL increments.[149,150]

- Pearls
  - Because the PENG is an analgesic block, it does not require large volumes of high-concentration local anesthetics.
- Risks and Complications
  - Because the ureter in the pelvis is within close proximity of the ON, advancing the needle too far medially places it and other vital structures at risk for injury.

Sciatic Block—Subgluteal

Although posterior and lateral popliteal approaches to the sciatic nerve are performed most commonly for ankle and foot surgery, and higher approaches to the sciatic nerve are performed more commonly for surgery above and at the knee, there is no clinical evidence to support one particular sciatic approach over another. The classic landmark approach to the sciatic nerve will be described here. The indications for a given approach are based on the specific surgical requirements.[151-153]

- Landmark Technique
  - When performing the classic posterior approach, the patient is positioned in the Sims position with the operative leg positioned superiorly and flexed at the knee. A line is drawn from the posterior superior iliac spine to the greater trochanter of the femur. A second line is drawn from the sacral hiatus to the greater trochanter, and a third line is drawn perpendicular to

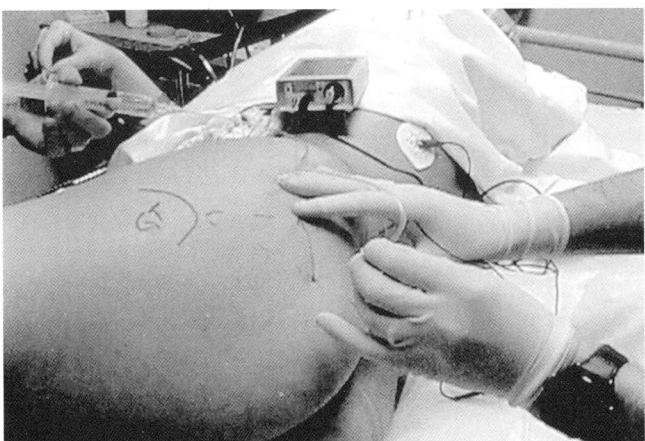

Fig. 50.41 Landmark/nerve stimulation for a sciatic nerve block.

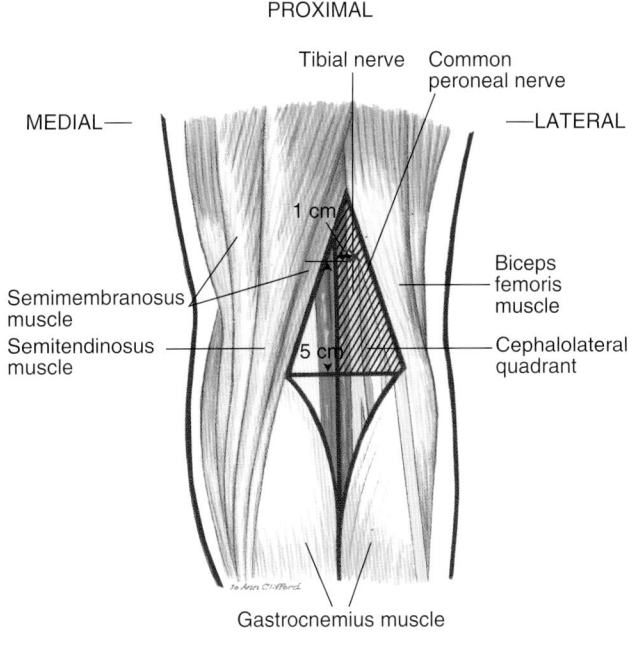

PROXIMAL

Tibial nerve | Common peroneal nerve

MEDIAL —

— LATERAL

1 cm

Biceps femoris muscle

Semimembranosus muscle

Semitendinosus muscle

5 cm

Cephalolateral quadrant

Gastrocnemius muscle

DISTAL

Fig. 50.42 Landmark/nerve stimulation for a sciatic nerve block in the popliteal fossa.

and bisecting the first line. The needle entry point is the intersection of the second and third lines (Fig. 50.41). The patient is prepped, draped appropriately, then infiltrated with 2 to 3 mL of 1% lidocaine solution subcutaneously at the insertion site. A 22-gauge, 9-cm B-bevel block needle is inserted perpendicularly to the skin. Nerve stimulation is set to 2 Hz at an intensity of 1 mÅ, and the needle is advanced until either a PTN distribution (plantar flexion) or peroneal nerve distribution (dorsal flexion) motor response is elicited. The intensity level is then decreased to 0.3 to 0.5 mÅ, and the needle is redirected as needed to maintain the appropriate motor response. Following negative aspiration, 20 mL of local anesthetic is injected in 5-mL increments.[153]

- Pearls
  - If contraction of the gluteal muscle is seen, the needle must be advanced further. If the needle is advanced and nerve localization is not detected, withdraw the needle and redirect slightly caudal from the initial angle. If this fails to elicit a response, the needle should be withdrawn and redirected in a slightly cephalad direction. Failure to obtain a response may indicate inappropriate placement and alert the anesthetist to reassess the landmarks and patient position.
- Risks and Complications
  - Because of the unique course of the sciatic nerve, there is an increased risk for mechanical and pressure injury. Due to the proximity of pelvic vessels and the increased volumes usually associated with this block, there is increased risk of hematoma and LAST. If the needle is advanced too far medially, perforation of pelvic organs is possible.[154]

Sciatic Nerve Block—Popliteal

The popliteal block targets the sciatic nerve in the proximal popliteal fossa. It is indicated for surgical procedures of the lower extremity distal to the knee, including the ankle, Achilles tendon, and foot. The block has relatively few complications and can be easily performed using either landmark technique with nerve stimulation or ultrasound guidance. At this location the sciatic nerve is posterior and lateral to the popliteal artery and vein. The popliteal fossa is defined by three anatomic structures: the popliteal crease, the medial border of the femoris biceps muscle laterally, and the tendon of the semitendinosus muscle medially.[151,155]

- Landmark Technique
  - A line is drawn joining the medial border of the femoris biceps muscle laterally and the lateral border of the semitendinous muscle medially at the level of the popliteal crease. At the midpoint

of this line, a perpendicular line is extended approximately 8 to 10 cm cephalad. The needle insertion point is 1 cm lateral to this. The patient is prepped and draped appropriately, and a skin wheal is raised. A 22-gauge, 9-cm B-bevel needle connected to a nerve stimulator is introduced through a skin wheal at a 45- to 60-degree anterosuperior angle. Nerve stimulation is set to 2 Hz at an intensity of 1 mÅ, and the needle is advanced until either PTN distribution (plantar flexion) or peroneal nerve distribution (dorsal flexion) motor response is elicited, usually at a depth of 1 to 3 cm in an adult. Following negative aspiration, up to 30 mL of a local anesthetic is injected in 5-mL increments (Fig. 50.42).[151,155]

- Ultrasound Guidance
  - The ultrasound-guided sciatic block in the popliteal fossa can be performed in the supine, lateral, or prone position. Here we discuss the supine approach. A high-frequency (10–12 MHz) linear array transducer is placed in transverse orientation at the popliteal crease where the artery and vein are initially identified. The TN is typically visualized at this level superficial to the popliteal vessels. Lateral to the nerve lies the biceps femoris muscle. Medial to the nerve lie the semimembranosus and semitendinosus muscles. Once the TN is identified, the transducer is slowly slid cephalad to the point where the TN is joined by the CPN (Fig. 50.43). The lateral thigh is prepped in the appropriate manner, and a 22-gauge, 9-cm B-bevel block needle is inserted lateral to medial using an in-plane approach and advanced until the needle tip is between the bifurcation of the two nerves. Following negative aspiration, 5 mL of local anesthetic is injected to confirm needle tip placement between the two nerves. The needle is then advanced further to the medial border of the TN. Following negative aspiration, 10 mL of local anesthetic is injected to create a circumferential spread around the TN. The needle is then withdrawn until it is positioned at the lateral edge of the peroneal nerve. Following negative aspiration, 10 mL of local anesthetic is deposited observing for circumferential spread around the nerve. Nerve stimulation

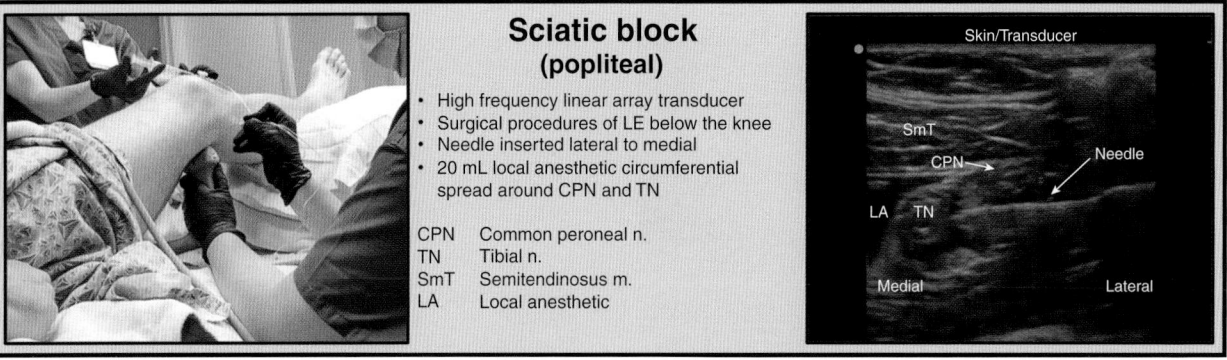

Fig. 50.43 Transducer position and corresponding image for an ultrasound-guided sciatic nerve block in the popliteal fossa.

can be used in conjunction with ultrasound to confirm appropriate muscular movement.[151,155]

- Pearls
  - The sciatic nerve divides into the TN and CPN at varying locations along the popliteal fossa, making it important to scan the region proximally and distally to determine the area that offers the greatest chance of success.
  - The practitioner should also note the point at which the sciatic nerve begins to divide as it is the desired location for local anesthetic placement.
  - It is important to note that when one performs the block with the patient in the supine position, the ultrasound image is inverted, and the transducer should be reversed to produce the proper orientation.
- Risks and Complications
  - Although uncommon, inadvertent vascular injection from an unrecognized puncture can result in a LAST event. Hematoma and nerve injury are also possible.

Ankle Blocks

Ankle blocks are routinely performed for both surgical anesthesia and postoperative analgesia for procedures involving the foot. Some authors describe ankle blocks as simple to accomplish, effective, and devoid of systemic complications; others perceive them as difficult and unreliable.[156,157] Historically, ankle blocks have been performed using an infiltration technique based on anatomic landmarks. Depending on the surgery, some or all of the nerves in the ankle may need to be blocked. With the exception of the superficial peroneal, these nerves course near vascular structures, placing the patient at increased risk for local anesthetic toxicity due to inadvertent intravascular injection.

- Landmark Technique
  - The approach to the SN and PTN can be enhanced by placing the patient in the prone position. However, the patient should be placed in the most comfortable position that permits sufficient mobility of the foot. The posterior tibial artery is palpated at the superior portion of the medial malleolus. Once the artery is located, the needle is inserted lateral to the artery in a line drawn from the superior portion of the medial malleolus to the lateral malleolus across the Achilles tendon (see Fig. 50.11). If the artery is not palpated, the needle is inserted lateral to the Achilles tendon at the level of the superior portion of the medial malleolus. The needle is advanced toward the medial malleolus and lateral to the position of the posterior tibial artery. As the needle is advanced toward the outer aspect of the medial malleolus, a paresthesia may be elicited. If this occurs, the needle is slightly withdrawn. Following negative aspiration, 5 mL of the

anesthetic solution is injected; an additional 3 mL is injected as the needle is withdrawn. If a paresthesia is not elicited, the medial malleolus is gently contacted with the needle tip and then withdrawn from the bone. Following negative aspiration, the local anesthetic is slowly injected at this position, and the location is gently massaged after the injection.[158,159]

- To block the SN, the patient remains in the same position, and a line is drawn from the medial malleolus across the Achilles tendon to the lateral malleolus. The needle is inserted under the skin along the lateral border of the Achilles tendon in the plane with the line that is between the medial and lateral malleoli. The needle is advanced subcutaneously toward the superior edge of the lateral malleolus (see Fig. 50.13). Following negative aspiration, 5 mL of solution is injected in the subcutaneous tissues as the needle is withdrawn. The solution must reach the superior edge of the lateral malleolus to anesthetize all the fibers of the SN.
- To block the DPN, the patient is placed in the supine position, and the anterior aspect of the ankle is prepped and draped. A line is drawn from the superior edge of the medial malleolus to the superior border of the lateral malleolus across the anterior aspect of the ankle. The tendons of the anterior tibial muscle and the long muscles of the great toe are identified by having the patient flex the foot against resistance. Where the line crosses the midpoint between the two tendons, the needle is inserted toward the tibia (Fig. 50.44). As the needle advances through the fascia, a paresthesia may be elicited. If the paresthesia is not obtained, the needle is slowly advanced until it gently contacts the tibia. The needle is then slightly withdrawn, and 5 mL of local anesthetic is injected after negative aspiration. The needle is then withdrawn through the fascia, and an additional 3 mL is injected.[158,159]
- Without removing the needle, the SPN is blocked by inserting the needle subcutaneously toward the inferior border of the lateral malleolus. At this level, the nerve is located in subcutaneous tissue. As the needle is withdrawn, 5 mL of anesthetic solution is slowly injected, creating a subcutaneous ring (see Fig. 50.44).[158,159] The needle is withdrawn to the midpoint, and the needle direction is again changed and redirected to the inferior border of the medial malleolus. The SphN is in the subcutaneous tissue, superficial to the saphenous vein. If the needle is not superficial, the saphenous vein could be pierced. Following negative aspiration, 5 mL of local anesthetic is injected toward the medial malleolus. As the needle is withdrawn, an additional 3 mL is injected. The DPN and the PTN are the only nerves of the ankle that do not exist within the subcutaneous tissue (see Fig. 50.44).[158,159]

- Ultrasound Guidance
  - The five nerves of the ankle can all be blocked under ultrasound guidance. This presents some challenges as it requires identification and specific injection of local anesthetic at multiple sites.

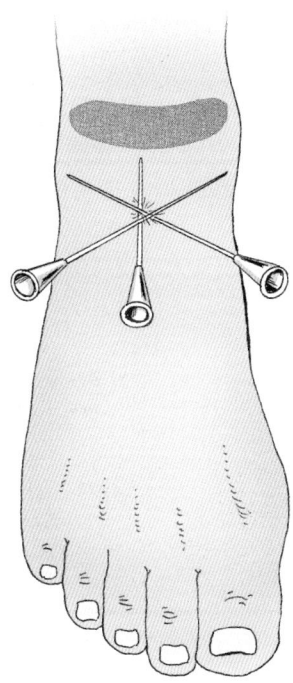

Fig. 50.44 Landmark technique to block the deep peroneal, superficial peroneal, and saphenous nerves.

A high-frequency (10–12 MHz) linear array transducer is used when performing ultrasound-guided ankle blocks, as the nerves are usually superficial (<2 cm) to the skin. Because of the limited surface area at the ankle, a small-footprint transducer is often preferred to reduce air artifact.[61] In addition, with the exception of the SPN, the remaining nerves are all in close proximity to blood vessels, increasing the potential for an inadvertent vascular puncture and injection. As with all ultrasound-guided blocks, observing circumferential spread around the nerve during injection ensures an efficacious block.[61]

- The PTN is the most prominent and easy to identify nerve with ultrasound at the ankle. With the patient in the supine position, the transducer is placed just above the medial malleolus on the medial aspect of the leg. The nerve will appear as a hyperechoic circle just behind the posterior tibial artery (Fig. 40.45). A high-frequency (10–12 MHz), small-footprint linear array transducer is ideal for performing this block. The TN is larger as the transducer is slid cephalad. Once all anatomic structures are identified and the ultrasound image is optimized, the patient is prepped in the appropriate manner, and a 22- to 25-gauge needle is inserted in-plane deep to the nerve and vessels. Following negative aspiration, 5 mL of local anesthetic is injected.

- The DPN is identified by placing a high-frequency (10–12 MHz) linear array transducer 1 to 2 cm above the superior border of the medial malleolus at the level of the extensor retinaculum.[61] The hypoechoic pulsating dorsalis pedis artery is used as a reference point to identify the nerve, which appears as a small hyperechoic circle just lateral to the artery (Fig. 50.46). Once the ultrasound image is optimized, the patient is prepped in the appropriate manner, and a 22- to 25-gauge needle is inserted in-plane from lateral to medial. Following negative aspiration, 5 mL of local anesthetic is injected deep to the nerve, elevating it off the bone.

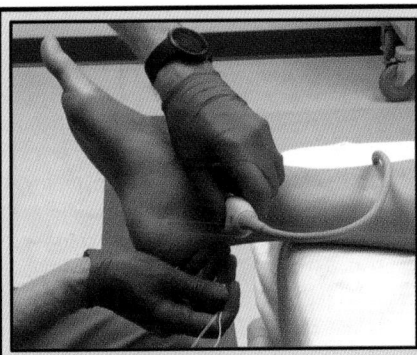

Posterior tibial nerve block

- High frequency linear array transducer
- Indicated for surgery of the lower ankle/foot
- Needle approach is dorsal to ventral
- 5 mL local anesthetic around PTN posterior to PTA

PTN   Posterior tibial nerve
PTA   Posterior tibial artery
PTV   Posterior tibial vein
         Needle approach

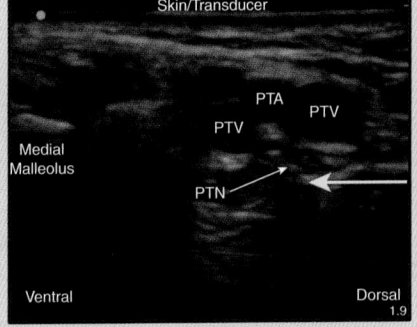

Fig. 50.45 Transducer position and corresponding image for an ultrasound-guided posterior tibial nerve ankle block.

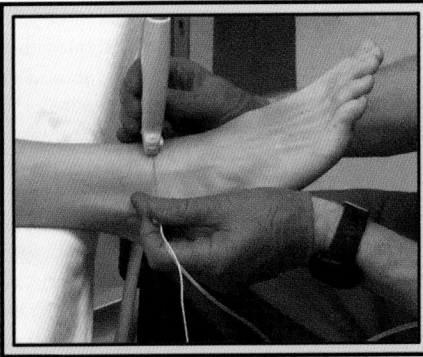

Deep peroneal nerve block

- High frequency linear array transducer
- Indicated for surgery of the great toe and second digit
- Needle approach is lateral to medial
- 5 mL local anesthetic lateral to ATA

DPN   Deep peroneal n.
ATA   Anterior tibial a.
ATV   Anterior tibial v.
         Needle approach

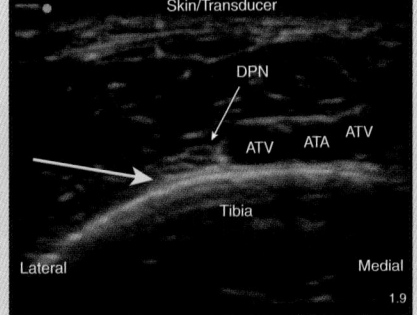

Fig. 50.46 Transducer position and corresponding image for an ultrasound-guided deep peroneal nerve ankle block.

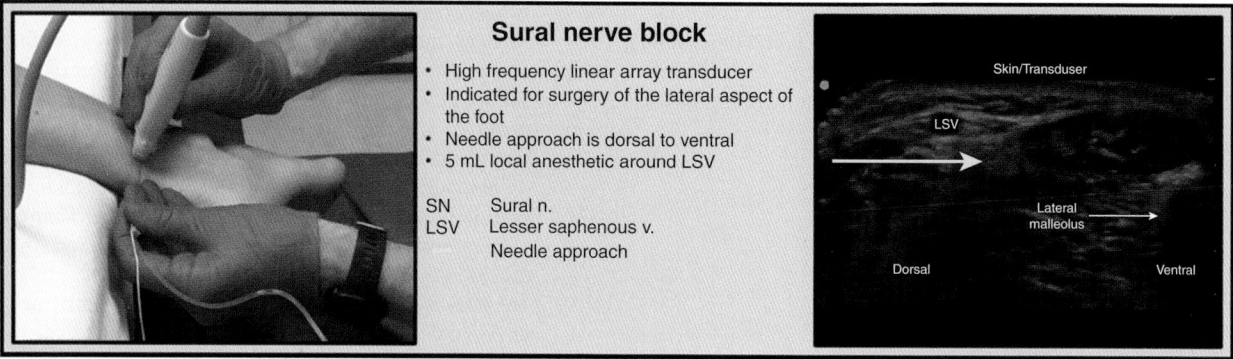

Fig. 50.47 Transducer position and corresponding image for an ultrasound-guided sural ankle nerve block.

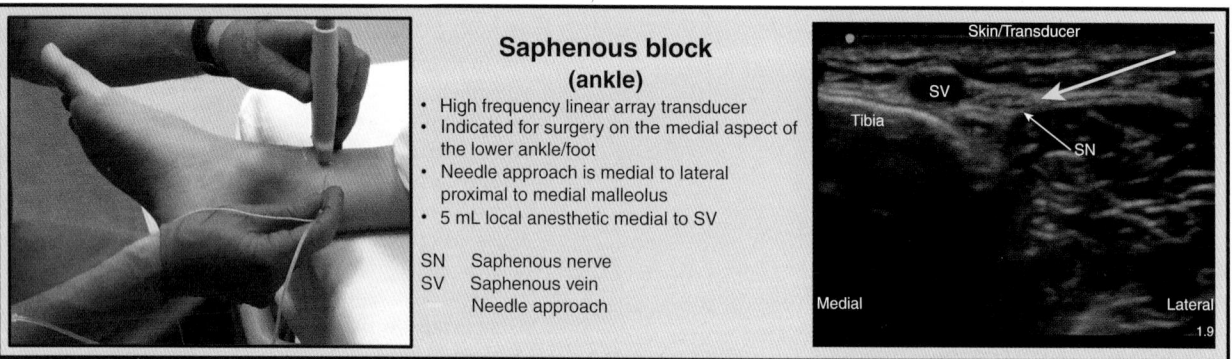

Fig. 50.48 Transducer position and corresponding image for an ultrasound-guided saphenous nerve ankle block.

- The SN is the least studied nerve in anesthesia-related litera ture.[160] Redborg et al. created a protocol for blocking the SN at the ankle with ultrasound.[161] The patient is placed in the prone position, and a tourniquet is applied around the proximal tibia, to distend the lesser saphenous vein (LSV). A high-frequency (10–12 MHz) linear array transducer is placed in a transverse orientation approximately 1 cm proximal to the lateral malleolus (Fig. 50.47), and the LSV is imaged in cross-sectional view. No attempt is made to locate the SN. The needle is inserted using an out-of-plane technique with the primary goal being to achieve circumferential spread with 5 mL of local anesthetic around the LSV. However, as the SN offers only a small contribution to the forefoot, it is procedure specific. Coe and Sundaram completed a series of 30 ankle blocks that excluded the SN, finding that in patients having surgery medial to the third toe, excellent pain relief was achieved in all cases.[162]
- The SphN is often blocked in conjunction with the sciatic nerve at the popliteal fossa for surgeries of the ankle or foot. Below the knee, the SphN is within close proximity to the saphenous vein, as it courses along the medial aspect of the tibia. The patient is placed in the supine position with slight external rotation of the lower extremity, and the transducer is placed in a transverse orientation approximately 10 cm cephalad to the medial malleolus using the greater saphenous vein as a landmark. A tourniquet can be placed on the proximal calf to better visualize the vein. The SphN appears as a small hyperechoic structure medial to the vein (Fig. 50.48). The needle is inserted either medial or lateral when using an in-plane technique. Following negative aspiration, 3 to 5 mL of local anesthetic is injected until circumferential spread is achieved.[61] As with the SN, the SphN provides

limited sensory innervation to the foot and can be excluded for certain procedures. In a prospective study using ultrasound-guided ankle blocks for hallux valgus surgery, Lopez et al. examined the contribution of the SphN and found that 97% of patients would not have benefited from a SphN block.[163]
- The SPN provides cutaneous innervation to the dorsum of the foot and five toes. It is a branch of the CPN and courses laterally along the tibia to the ankle. The transducer is placed in a transverse orientation approximately 5 cm proximal to the lateral malleolus. The SPN appears as a small hyperechoic structure in the subcutaneous tissue superficial to the fascia in the prominent groove created by the peroneus brevis longus and extensor digitorum longus muscles that lead to the fibula (Fig. 50.49). Since it is not located near vascular structures and the nerve is small, imaging with ultrasound is not always possible.[156]
- Pearls
  - Ankle blocks are performed with the patient in either the supine or prone position. The lower extremity can either be supported under the calf or positioned off the stretcher to provide greater access to the ankle required when blocking the SN and PTN.
  - Support the scanning hand to use as little pressure as possible when scanning to prevent collapse of vessels.
- Risks and Complications
  - Inadvertent vascular puncture may result in bleeding and hematoma. Because individual injection volumes are small, risk of LAST is minimal.
  - Nerves such as the deep peroneal lie within tight spaces between ligaments, tendons, and bone, thus increasing the risk for ischemia from hydrostatic pressure created by the injection of local anesthetic.[61]

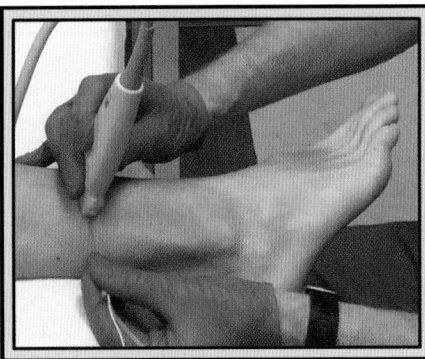
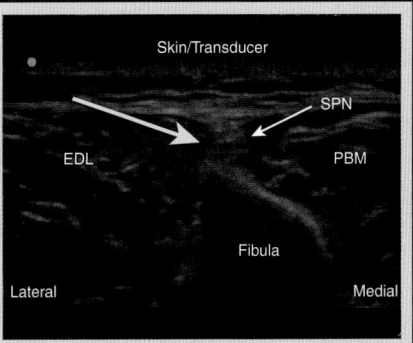

Superficial peroneal nerve block

- High frequency linear array transducer
- Indicated for surgery of the lateral aspect of the foot
- Needle approach is lateral to medial
- 5 mL local anesthetic in groove between PBM and EDL

SPN   Superficial peroneal n.
EDL   Extensor digitorum m.
PBM   Peroneus brevis m.
      Needle approach

Fig. 50.49 Transducer position and corresponding image for an ultrasound-guided superficial peroneal nerve ankle block.

Special Considerations

Continuous Catheter Techniques

Depending on the amide or ester anesthetics used, a single-injection nerve block lasts for approximately 8 to 24 hours.[164] Early mobilization following surgery is instrumental to recovery; however, this must be balanced with the ability to assess neurologic function. The administration of low-concentration local anesthetics through catheters as part of a multimodal pain management plan can have significant benefits by reducing postoperative analgesic requirements, including superior control of incident pain, and facilitating postoperative rehabilitation.[165] The advent of cheaper and more reliable pump technologies has given rise to a significant growth in the use of continuous peripheral nerve blocks.[165]

Regardless of the block technique, catheters are placed within the tissue compartment that contains the nerves of interest. There are some special anesthetic considerations when placing catheters. Because a larger block needle (17–18 gauge) is required to facilitate passage of the catheter, sufficient local anesthetic should be placed in the subcutaneous tissue at the anticipated injection site. Additionally, when Tuohy-style block needles are used, a cutting-tip needle is often first inserted at the skin in an effort to decrease the force required to pass the block needle into the tissue. As with all peripheral nerve blocks, complaints of pain during needle insertion or injection suggest intraneural penetration. In this event, the needle should be withdrawn and redirected. Following negative aspiration, an initial bolus of local anesthetic (5–10 mL) is injected slowly after negative aspiration for blood, to facilitate passage of the catheter. It is then threaded 3 to 5 cm beyond the needle tip (insertions >5 cm have been associated with catheter knotting).[164] The catheter is then secured by one of several mechanisms, such as a securing device, or the catheter may be secured using a suture and/or a clear dressing applied over the catheter. Once secured, it is again aspirated to ensure migration into a vessel has not occurred. A continuous infusion of local anesthetic is initiated immediately after the bolus injection at a rate of 4 to 6 mL/hour. Ropivacaine 0.2% and bupivacaine 0.25% are the most common local anesthetics and concentrations used.

With any block it is important to maintain strict aseptic techniques during placement and maintenance of the catheter, and it has been recommended that the catheter be removed after 48 hours. The patient should be counseled to immediately report any extended loss of sensation and/or motor control of the extremity, as well as any other potential complications (see Box 50.1).

SUMMARY

Regional anesthesia is an invaluable tool that can be used as a primary anesthetic or for providing pain relief during the perioperative period. There are a wide variety of techniques available, including subarachnoid, epidural, caudal, BP, lumbar plexus, selective block of the upper and lower extremity nerves, intravenous infusion, intercostal nerve block, and specialized trauma techniques. Placement of these blocks can be facilitated by technology such as the PNS and ultrasonographic nerve location. Regional anesthesia may be used alone or in combination with general anesthesia and offers patients and surgeons excellent options for safe, effective anesthesia and analgesia.

REFERENCES

For a complete list of references for this chapter, scan this QR code with any smartphone code reader app, or visit the following URL: http://booksite.elsevier.com/9780323711944/.

51

Obstetric Anesthesia

Lee J. Ranalli, Greg A. Taylor

Parturients who request or require obstetric anesthesia services represent a unique challenge to anesthesia providers. Techniques for providing pain relief during labor and delivery are continuously being refined in an effort to provide the best care possible to this uniquely vulnerable patient population. A thorough understanding of the anatomic and physiologic changes that occur during pregnancy and the anesthetic considerations associated with such changes are necessary for a safe and effective anesthetic course.

ANATOMIC AND PHYSIOLOGIC CHANGES DURING NORMAL PREGNANCY

The physiologic changes that occur during pregnancy are the result of increased metabolic demands and hormonal and anatomic changes. These changes begin early in pregnancy and continue into the postpartum period. These marked changes have significant implications for the anesthesia provider.

Cardiovascular Changes

Cardiovascular changes begin as early as the fourth week of pregnancy and continue into the postpartum period.[1] Maternal heart rate (HR) is increased by 20% to 30% at term. This increase begins in the first trimester and peaks by 32 weeks of gestation.[2] Normal HR variability does not appear to be changed until late in pregnancy, when tachyarrhythmias are more common.[3] Cardiac output increases by approximately 40% over nonpregnant values.[4] This increase in cardiac output begins in the fifth week of pregnancy and results from an increase in stroke volume (SV) (20%–50%) and, to a lesser extent, HR.[5] Cardiac output increases consistently throughout pregnancy.[6] Some studies previously indicated cardiac output decreases in the third trimester, but these results were likely due to aortocaval compression from studying subjects in the supine position.[7] At term, approximately 10% of the cardiac output perfuses the gravid uterus.[8,9] When a woman is in labor, cardiac output increases during uterine contractions as a result of autotransfusion from the contracting uterus to the central circulation.[10]

Immediately after delivery, cardiac output increases as much as 80% above prelabor values. This occurs because of the autotransfusion of blood into central circulation from the contracting uterus and increased venous return from aortocaval decompression. As a result, patients with preexisting cardiac anomalies are at an increased risk for decompensation in the immediate postpartum period. Cardiac output gradually returns to baseline within 14 days as HR and SV normalize.[11]

During pregnancy, the diaphragm is displaced cephalad, shifting the heart up and to the left, making the cardiac silhouette appear enlarged on x-ray examination. The ventricular walls thicken and end-diastolic volume increases. A physical examination of the pregnant patient may appear to elicit abnormal findings. A benign grade 1 or 2 systolic murmur or a third heart sound may be heard on auscultation.[12] These findings are common; however, if the systolic murmur is greater than grade 3 or accompanied by chest pain or syncope, further evaluation is necessary. Diastolic murmurs and cardiac enlargement are considered pathologic. Normal pregnancy may also result in signs of cardiac abnormality such as exercise intolerance, shortness of breath, and edema.

Total blood volume increases 25% to 40% throughout pregnancy, in part to prepare for the normal blood loss associated with delivery. Plasma volume increases 40% to 50%, whereas red blood cell (RBC) volume increases by only 20%.[13] As a result, a relative or dilutional anemia is commonly seen as the plasma volume increases to a greater extent relative to the actual RBC volume. The increased plasma volume is likely caused by circulating levels of progesterone and estrogen resulting in enhanced renin-angiotensin-aldosterone activity.[14] RBC volume increases as a result of elevated erythropoietin levels seen after the eighth week of gestation.[15] Normal blood loss for vaginal delivery is less than 500 mL, and for an uncomplicated cesarean delivery the blood loss is 500 to 1000 mL. Normal blood losses at delivery are generally well tolerated in the healthy parturient as a result of these compensatory mechanisms. During labor, each contraction moves 300 to 500 mL of blood from the contracting uterus to the central circulation.[16] Pregnant women have greater baroreflex-mediated changes in HR at term than at 6 to 8 weeks postpartum.[17] In the presence of adequate neuraxial analgesia, there is often a corresponding decrease in maternal HR during uterine contractions due to the transiently increased preload.

Systemic vascular resistance (SVR) decreases as much as 21% by the end of a term pregnancy, owing in large part to decreased resistance in the uteroplacental, pulmonary, renal, and cutaneous vascular beds.[18,19] At term gestation 10% of the cardiac output perfuses the low resistance intervillous space of the uterus. Baseline central sympathetic outflow is twice as high in normal, term pregnant women as in nonpregnant women.[20] The venous capacitance system loses tone, allowing pooling of the larger blood volume. This decrease in SVR results in minimal overall systolic blood pressure change during normal pregnancy, despite the increased blood volume.[21] A decrease in diastolic blood pressure of up to 15 mm Hg may occur, resulting in a decrease in mean pressure.

Aortocaval Compression

In the early 1950s, a syndrome involving supine hypotension was identified in term or near-term pregnant women.[22,23] This syndrome is caused by compression of the vena cava and aorta by the gravid uterus, which restricts venous return to the heart when the parturient lies in the supine position. Compression can be more severe when the abdomen is tense or when the uterus is larger than normal, as in polyhydramnios or multiple gestation pregnancies. This decreased venous return results in a significant reduction in SV and, ultimately, cardiac output. Hypotension can be severe enough to cause loss of consciousness in some women. Maximal decreases in

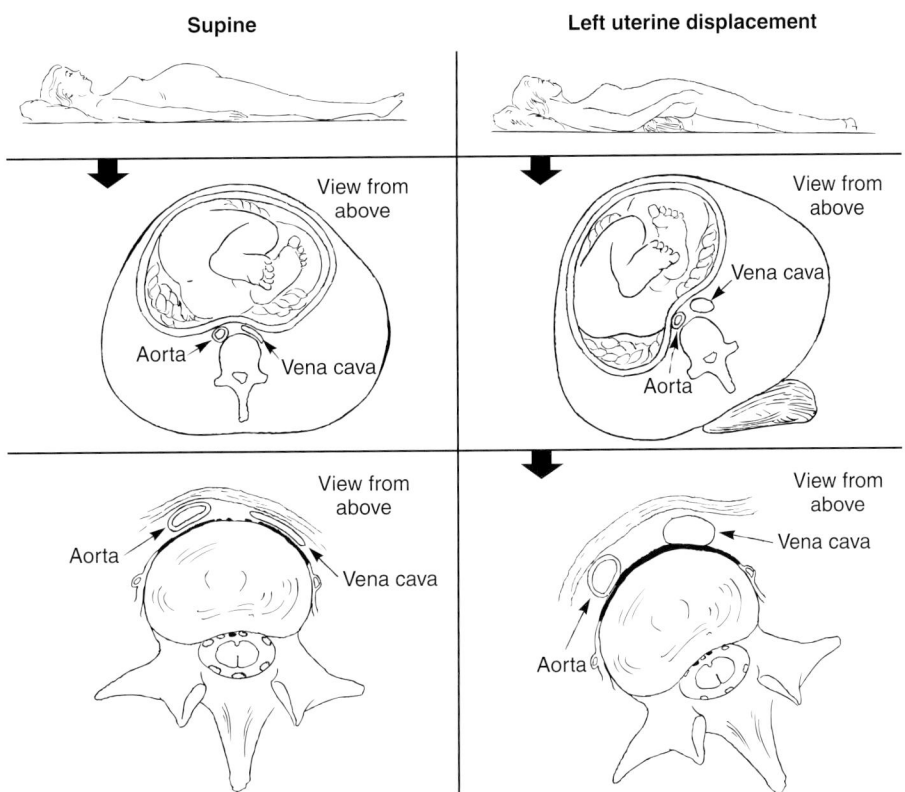

Fig. 51.1 Effects of left uterine displacement on the diameter of the abdominal aorta and vena cava.

blood pressure may require up to 10 minutes to develop; however, some women experience the decrease almost immediately. The normal physiologic responses to aortocaval compression are tachycardia and vasoconstriction of the lower extremities. Despite this attempted compensation, uterine blood flow and therefore fetal oxygenation are reduced.[24] Fig. 51.1 depicts changes in aortocaval compression with changes in position.

In addition to compressing the vena cava, the gravid uterus may compress the abdominal aorta. For this reason, supine hypotensive syndrome is more correctly referred to as aortocaval compression. When the abdominal aorta is compressed, upper-body blood pressure remains relatively normal, whereas blood pressure distal to the site of aortic compression (uterus and lower extremities) may be significantly reduced.

Compression of the aorta and vena cava can usually be relieved by shifting the uterus to the left (left uterine displacement) or by lying on the side.[25] Left uterine displacement can be accomplished by rotation of the operating room table 15 degrees to the left or by placing a 15-cm-high wedge under the parturient's right hip and back (see Fig. 51.1). Most anesthetists have been shown to underestimate the angle of tilt they provide, so care should be taken to ensure adequate left uterine displacement.[26] In women with an exceptionally large uterus, greater displacement may be necessary to be effective.

There has been much debate regarding the optimal position for performing neuraxial anesthesia for labor analgesia and cesarean delivery. Many clinicians feel that the lateral position is optimal to facilitate both maternal and fetal hemodynamics. Researchers have found that cardiac index is improved in both the left and right lateral positions when compared to the sitting flexed position in healthy pregnant women. However, when umbilical Dopplers were monitored in the same group as a surrogate for healthy fetal blood flow, no differences were identified.[27] Although positioning for neuraxial anesthesia may influence maternal hemodynamic variables, there were no differences in healthy fetal blood flow indices among positions, suggesting that these changes are not clinically significant.

Hematologic Changes

Due to the parturient's hypercoagulable state, concentration of factors I (fibrinogen), VII, VIII, IX, X, and XII increase through pregnancy and peak at term. Additionally, vWF significantly increases by upward to 400% at term. Alternatively, factors XI and XIII tend to decrease during pregnancy.[28] In the nonpregnant state, fibrinogen levels average from 200 to 400 mg/dL. Late in pregnancy, fibrinogen levels are normally at least 400 mg/dL and may be as high as 650 mg/dL. These increased levels place the parturient at risk for thromboembolic events, which remain one of the leading causes of maternal mortality. The platelet count remains stable or is decreased slightly in the third trimester. The prevalence of maternal thrombocytopenia (platelet count $<150 \times 10^9$/L) in normal pregnancy has been shown to be 11.6%[29] and is not associated with increased morbidity or mortality. The pathogenesis is not well understood but may involve factors such as hemodilution and/or accelerated platelet clearance.[30,31] Overall, the white blood cell count tends to rise in pregnancy. In the third trimester, the mean is 10,500/mm[3], and in labor, it may increase to 20,000 to 30,000/mm[3].[32]

Respiratory Changes

The respiratory changes that accompany normal pregnancy are of particular importance to the anesthesia provider. Capillary engorgement in the upper airway results in a narrowed glottic opening and edema in the nasal and oral pharynx, larynx, and trachea. These changes carry over into labor, as has been shown by the Mallampati score changing as labor progresses.[33] Airway tissues are susceptible to damage and bleeding during placement of airway adjuncts. For this reason, nasal intubation in the parturient should generally be avoided. A 6.5- to 7-mm cuffed oral endotracheal tube is recommended when intubation is necessary. Obese patients with enlarged breasts may benefit from the use of a short-handled laryngoscope.

Term pregnancy is accompanied by an increase in oxygen (O_2) consumption by up to 33% at rest and 100% or more during the second stage of labor. Minute ventilation at term is increased by 50%. This is primarily due to a 40% increase in tidal volume, whereas the respiratory rate remains unchanged or increases by only 10%.[34] By 12 weeks of gestation, the normal arterial partial pressure of carbon dioxide ($Paco_2$) decreases to approximately 30 to 32 mm Hg and remains in this range throughout pregnancy.[35] Metabolic alkalosis is rarely seen because there is a compensatory decrease in the serum bicarbonate from 26 to 22 mEq/L. The normal arterial partial pressure of O_2 is greater than 100 mm Hg.

The functional residual capacity (FRC), expiratory reserve volume, and residual volume are decreased primarily as a result of upward pressure on the diaphragm, with results functionally similar to restrictive lung disease. The FRC plays an important role in preserving O_2 saturation during periods of hypoventilation or apnea. The decrease in FRC (20%) combined with the increase in O_2 consumption in pregnancy commonly results in rapid arterial desaturation in the apneic pregnant patient.[36] Morbid obesity, labor, and sepsis exaggerate this effect. For this reason, preoxygenation with 100% O_2 prior to induction of general anesthesia is important. Closing capacity (CC) does not change, which results in a decreased FRC:CC ratio, often leading to small-airway closure before the tidal volume has been exhaled. This mechanism may explain the reduction in O_2 saturations seen in parturients during natural sleep. When compared with nonpregnant controls, whose average oxygen saturation during sleep was 98.5%, healthy near-term pregnant women averaged only 95.2%, with temporary desaturations below 90% not being uncommon.[37] The increased cardiac output and a shift to the right in the oxyhemoglobin dissociation curve help to maximize oxygen delivery.

Minute ventilation can increase to 300% during contractions and cause maternal $Paco_2$ to drop below 15 mm Hg. This alkalemia can cause hypoventilation between contractions, resulting in hypoxemia. Some evidence indicates that hyperventilation may cause a decrease in uterine blood flow. However, in animal studies, this finding has usually been associated with stressful events such as intubation and invasive procedures. In pregnant, laboring human volunteers, hyperventilation to a $Paco_2$ of 20 mm Hg does not appear to harm the fetus. Specifically, the fetus does not develop hypoxia or acidosis as determined by analysis of a scalp blood sample. However, in the presence of a complicated labor with preexisting fetal compromise, the effects could be detrimental.[38]

Nervous System Changes

Beginning in the first trimester, pregnant women have an increased sensitivity to local and general anesthetic medications.[39] The exact mechanism remains unclear, but animal studies have demonstrated a variable reduction in the minimum alveolar concentration (MAC) of inhalation agents in rabbits chronically exposed to progesterone.[40] In pregnant rats, the effects of endorphins on pain thresholds are also demonstrated, which may also be an important factor.[41] Additionally, research and clinical experience have demonstrated an increase in the sensitivity of nerves to local anesthetics during pregnancy.[42] Mechanical changes within the epidural space may also play a role in the increased block height seen in pregnancy.[43] Epidural veins become engorged as a result of increased intraabdominal pressure and cause a decrease in the volume of both the epidural and subarachnoid spaces.

Gastrointestinal Changes

The parturient is at increased risk for regurgitation and aspiration of gastric contents because of anatomic and physiologic changes associated with pregnancy. A significant number of pregnant women, and women immediately postpartum, have gastric volumes in excess of 25 mL and gastric pH below 2.5.[44] Ultrasound has demonstrated solid food in the stomach of almost two-thirds of women in whom neuraxial analgesia had been instituted and in the stomach of more than 40% of laboring women who had not eaten in 12 to 24 hours.[45] Increased levels of gastrin during pregnancy result in greater gastric volume and lower pH. Upward displacement of the stomach by the gravid uterus may result in mechanical obstruction to outflow through the pylorus, delayed gastric emptying, and increased intragastric pressure. Elevated levels of progesterone, a smooth-muscle relaxant, also decrease gastric motility and cause a reduction in lower esophageal sphincter tone. This explains the heartburn frequently experienced by pregnant women. Gastrointestinal changes do not completely normalize until several weeks postpartum.

The onset of labor is accompanied by a further reduction in the rate of gastric emptying in part due to pain and the use of parenteral opioids. American Society of Anesthesiologists (ASA) guidelines allow for the ingestion of a moderate amount of clear fluids in uncomplicated laboring patients. Uncomplicated patients undergoing elective cesarean delivery may have modest amounts of clear liquids up to 2 hours prior to induction of anesthesia. The same guidelines state that patients with additional risk factors for aspiration (e.g., morbid obesity, diabetes, difficult airway) or patients at increased risk for operative delivery (e.g., nonreassuring fetal heart rate [FHR] pattern) may have further restrictions of oral intake. Administration of nonparticulate antacids, H_2-receptor antagonists (to increase gastric pH), and metoclopramide (to promote gastric emptying, reduce nausea and vomiting, and increase lower esophageal sphincter tone) may be beneficial prior to cesarean delivery and should be considered. Additionally, ondansetron should be considered prior to the administration of spinal anesthesia for cesarean delivery for purposes of hypotensive prophylaxis.[46] The use of these drugs is also advocated when a general anesthetic becomes necessary. When general anesthesia is used, a rapid sequence induction with cricoid pressure using a cuffed endotracheal tube is necessary from the 20th week of gestation extending to the immediate postpartum period.

Hepatic Changes

During pregnancy, levels of aspartate aminotransferase, alanine aminotransferase, lactate dehydrogenase, and alkaline phosphatase increase to the upper limits of nonpregnant normal levels. Serum albumin concentration decreases and may result in increased free fractions of highly protein-bound drugs. Serum cholinesterase activity decreases by 30% or more during the first or second trimester. Although activity recovers slightly by term, it remains reduced compared with prepregnant values. Despite these decreases in cholinesterase activity, clinically relevant prolongation of the duration of action of drugs that depend on cholinesterase for elimination, such as ester local anesthetics, succinylcholine and remifentanil, is uncommon in women with genotypically normal cholinesterase enzymes.

Renal Changes

During pregnancy, increased cardiac output leads to increased renal plasma flow and increased glomerular filtration rate (GFR). Creatinine clearance rises to 140 to 160 mL/min. As a result, the level of blood urea nitrogen decreases to approximately 8 mg/dL and creatinine decreases to approximately 0.5 mg/dL. Urinary excretion of glucose is common in the absence of disease and is attributable to increased GFR and reduced renal absorption. The urinary excretion of protein in normal

BOX 51.1 Summary: Physiologic Changes in Pregnancy

- Cardiac output increases mostly because of an increase in stroke volume and, to a lesser extent, an increase in heart rate.
- Blood volume is markedly increased and prepares the parturient for the blood loss associated with delivery.
- Plasma volume is increased to a greater extent than red blood cell volume, resulting in a dilutional anemia.
- Minute ventilation increases 45%, and this is due mostly to an increase in tidal volume.
- Oxygen consumption is markedly increased; carbon dioxide production is similarly increased.
- Pregnant women have an increased sensitivity to local anesthetics and a decreased minimum alveolar concentration for all general anesthetics.
- Platelet count remains stable or decreases slightly; coagulation factors and fibrinogen are increased, resulting in a hypercoagulable state in pregnancy.
- Aortocaval compression results in profound hypotension and can be relieved by left uterine displacement.
- All pregnant women are at increased risk of aspiration because of the anatomic and physiologic changes to the gastrointestinal system and should be considered to have a full stomach after week 12 of gestation.
- Pregnancy and labor are associated with significant airway changes that can result in a difficult intubation. This highlights the importance of a comprehensive airway evaluation prior to general anesthesia.

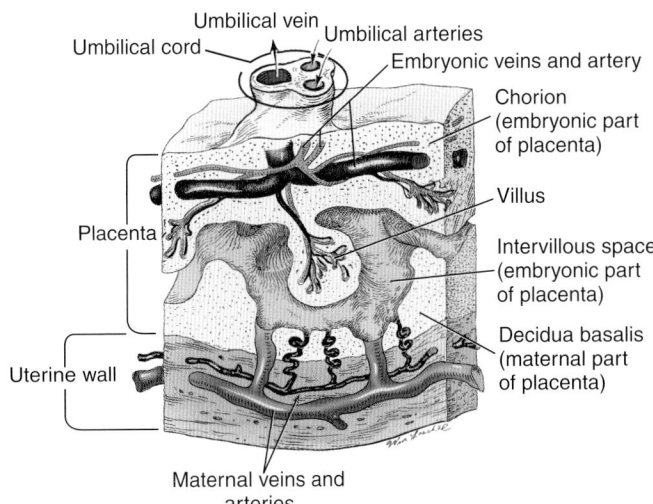

Fig. 51.2 Cross section of the uteroplacental interface and the maternal and fetal blood supply.

TABLE 51.1 Summary of the Physiologic Changes in Pregnancy at Term

Parameter	Change	Amount
Heart rate	↑	20%–30%
Stroke volume	↑	20%–50%
Cardiac output	↑	40%
Systemic vascular resistance	↓	20%
Total blood volume	↑	25%–40%
Plasma volume	↑	40%–50%
Red blood cell volume	↑	20%
Coagulation factors	↑↑	
Platelets	No change or ↓	
Minute ventilation	↑	50%
Tidal volume	↑	40%
Respiratory rate	↑	
Functional residual capacity	↓	20%

blood from the intervillous space and return it to the general circulation. Uterine blood flow at term increases to a maximum of 800 mL/minute, accounting for approximately 10% of maternal cardiac output. Of this, approximately 150 mL/minute supplies nutritive flow to the myometrium, and 100 mL/minute flows to the decidua (the lining of the uterus); the remainder flows to the intervillous space.

Deoxygenated blood flows from the fetus to the uterus via two umbilical arteries. These vessels perfuse capillary networks within placental villi that protrude into the pool of maternal blood. Placental villi are small, fingerlike projections, the purpose of which is to maximize the placental surface area in contact with maternal blood. Each villus contains a capillary network that exchanges respiratory gases, nutrients, and wastes with maternal blood (Fig. 51.2). Both O_2 and CO_2 diffuse through placental tissue readily and are considered to be perfusion limited, meaning their transfer to the fetus is limited only by the perfusion of the placenta, not by the rate of diffusion of the gases. Therefore decreases in maternal uterine artery blood flow or increases in placental vascular resistance decrease fetal oxygenation.

Autoregulation of intervillous blood flow does not seem to occur. Thus the uteroplacental perfusion is solely dependent on maternal blood pressure. The spiral arteries, however, do constrict in response to α-agonists (e.g., phenylephrine). However, human studies indicate phenylephrine does not appear to be harmful to the fetus when used at clinically relevant doses.[47] Unlike patients who receive neuraxial anesthesia, patients receiving inhalation anesthesia seem to maintain adequate placental blood flow, despite somewhat reduced blood pressure; this may be a function of altered uterine blood flow, altered fetal O_2 requirements, or both.

Placental Transfer and Fetal Effects of Drugs

Placental transfer of free (non–protein-bound) drug is dependent on the magnitude of the concentration gradient, the molecular weight, lipid solubility, and state of ionization. Drugs with molecular weights greater than 1000 daltons (Da) cross the placenta poorly, whereas drugs with weights less than 500 Da cross easily. Most drugs that are administered to the parturient are relatively small compounds and are thus able to cross to the placenta readily. However, size is only one of the determinants of permeability.

Transfer of drugs from the maternal circulation to the fetal unit is determined primarily by diffusion. Factors that favor diffusion include low molecular weight, high lipid solubility, low degree of ionization,

pregnancy is slightly elevated toward the upper limits of normal. The gravid uterus may occasionally produce mechanical obstruction of a ureter. A summary of the physiologic changes in pregnancy at term appears in Box 51.1 and Table 51.1.

Uterine Blood Flow

The uterus undergoes tremendous changes during pregnancy. The uterus enlarges, and its blood flow increases to meet both uterine and fetal metabolic demands. Uterine blood flow is supplied by two uterine arteries that are thought to be maximally dilated throughout pregnancy. Placental blood flow on the uterine side is supplied via the maternal arcuate, radial, and spiral arteries. The spiral arteries expel blood into the intervillous space. The maternal venous sinuses receive

and low protein binding. Cell membranes consist primarily of phospholipids such that a drug's degree of lipid solubility favors its passage through a cell membrane. Highly lipid-soluble drugs such as fentanyl cross readily. On the other hand, ionized drugs are polar and water soluble, which inhibits diffusion through lipophilic cell membranes. Local anesthetics are examples of variably ionized basic compounds, whereby the degree of ionization is dependent on the ambient pH; the more alkaline the pH, the greater the degree of nonionization. It is the nonionized portion that crosses phospholipid membranes readily. Nondepolarizing muscle relaxants are an example of large, ionized drugs that are not affected by ambient pH because of the quaternary groups in their structure and are inhibited from crossing the placenta.

When a drug enters the fetal circulation, a variety of factors minimize the effects on the fetus. First among them is dilution. Before reaching the fetus, a drug is diluted in intervillous blood, absorbed by the placenta, further diluted in placental blood, and then circulated to the fetus. Once in the fetus, the drug is distributed within the fetal intravascular volume and redistributed to fetal tissues. Umbilical venous blood from the placenta must first pass through the liver on the way to the fetal heart. The resultant increase in maternal hepatic enzyme activity likely reduces serum drug levels before entering the general fetal circulation. Other factors limit the effects of maternally administered drugs on a fetus. Approximately one-fifth of the fetal cardiac output returns directly to the placenta because of shunt flow through the foramen ovale and ductus arteriosus. This shunted blood does not circulate, and any drug it contains does not have a systemic fetal effect.

The acid-base status of the fetus may affect the accumulation of a drug. A fetus who has become acidotic will alter the degree of ionization of a drug, potentially resulting in ion trapping leading to accumulation. For a complete discussion of fetal ion trapping see Chapter 10.

LABOR AND DELIVERY

Pain in Labor and Delivery

First-stage labor pain is primarily the result of cervical distension, stretching of the lower uterine segment, and (possibly) myometrial ischemia. The resultant nonspecific nociceptor visceral stimulation is carried to the central nervous system (CNS) by afferent unmyelinated C fibers that enter the cord at the T10, T11, T12, and L1 segments (Table 51.2 and Fig. 51.3). Thus, the pain of first-stage labor is frequently described as nonlocalized aching or cramping. Second-stage labor begins when cervical dilation is complete, and the presenting part descends into the pelvis. Compression and stretching of the pelvic musculature and perineum produce pain that is mediated by somatic afferent fibers carried via the pudendal nerves that enter the spinal cord at the S2, S3, and S4 levels. After administration of neuraxial anesthesia, sensory blockade that extends from T10 to S4 nerve roots can be effective in relieving the pain of both first- and second-stage labor.

The experience of pain is a highly individualized phenomenon, and pain tolerance varies widely among patients. Many factors outside a parturient's control are also related to the perception of pain; these range from the presence or absence of social support to physical factors such as fetal presentation. Labor and vaginal delivery can be described as a process in which three essential components must work in concert. First, the fetus must be properly positioned and of an appropriate size to ensure passage through the bony pelvis, dilating cervix, and vagina. Second, the uterus must contract regularly and effectively. Third, the pelvic outlet itself must be configured in a way that the fetus can pass. A flaw in any of these three elements can result in a difficult, painful, and prolonged labor. A few women are able to tolerate labor and delivery without significant discomfort; others experience pain in excess of their ability to cope. When women choose labor analgesia, it can make

| TABLE 51.2 | **Pain Pathways During Labor** | |
Area	Innervation	Comments
Uterus and cervix	T10–L1	Pain impulses carried by visceral afferent type C fibers
Perineum	S2–S4	Pain impulses carried by somatic nerve fibers; pudendal nerves

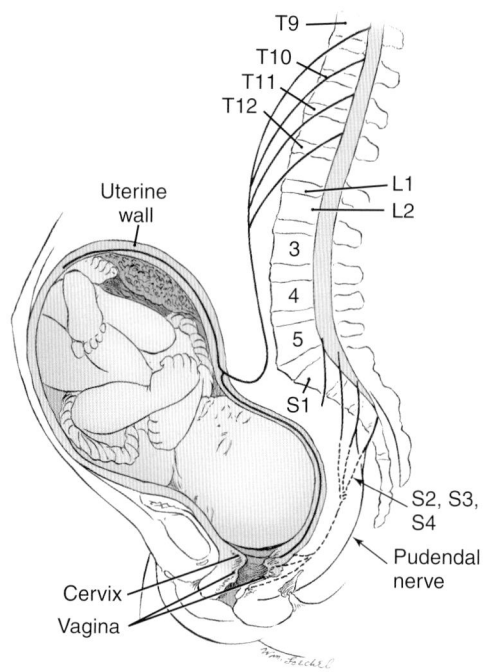

Fig. 51.3 Lower thoracic, lumbar, and sacral regions of the spine showing spinal cord, nerve roots, and sensory innervation to the uterus, cervix, and vagina.

the birthing process more enjoyable and provide the opportunity to better control their body and environment, thereby allowing them to maintain personal dignity.

Stages of Labor and Delivery

Labor is defined as progressive dilation of the cervix in response to uterine contractions. Although sporadic and irregular third-trimester contractions are common, labor is not said to begin until those contractions are regular and result in a change to the cervix. Labor is generally divided into three stages. First-stage cervical changes consist of effacement and dilation. The first stage is further divided into at least the latent and active phases. The latent phase is of variable duration and is defined as the period between the onset of labor and the point at which the cervix begins to rapidly change. Active phase usually begins at 2 to 3 cm dilation and is the period during which the cervix undergoes its maximum rate of dilation.

The second stage begins at full cervical dilation (10 cm) and ends with delivery of the fetus. The third stage encompasses the delivery of the placenta. The length of time it takes to progress through these stages is dependent on parity, effective uterine contractions, the size and type of pelvis, and fetal presentation. The Friedman curve is used to track the normal progress of labor (Fig. 51.4). Cervical dilation normally progresses 1 to 1.2 cm/hour during the active phase of labor for nulliparous parturients. When labor progress no longer follows the normal pattern, it is considered a dysfunctional labor and may require the use of oxytocin to augment contractions.

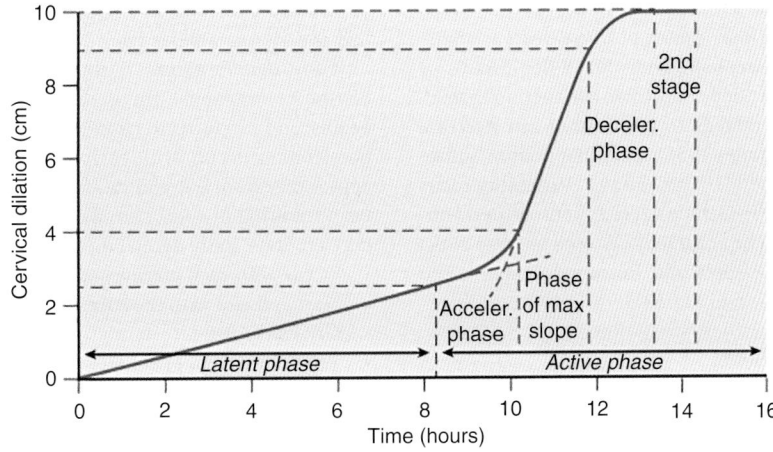

Fig. 51.4 Curve representing average dilation for nulliparous patients in labor. *accel.*, Acceleration; *decal.*, deceleration; *sec.*, second. (Redrawn with modifications from Miller RD, et al. *Miller's Anesthesia*. 9th ed. Philadelphia: Elsevier; 2020:2014.)

Intrapartum Fetal Evaluation

Intrapartum FHR monitoring is now used routinely in the United States. Although continuous or intermittent FHR monitoring is not a specific predictor of fetal well-being, it is the most readily available method for the assessment of fetal condition. Intermittent monitoring can be performed using a manual stethoscope known as a fetoscope. Continuous FHR monitoring is accomplished using either external Doppler ultrasonography or an internal fetal electrocardiography (ECG) electrode. The internal method requires ruptured amniotic membranes and a partially dilated cervix through which the electrode can be inserted. The continuous FHR is recorded in a two-channel format with the FHR displayed directly above a graphic representation of the uterine contractions. In this way, it is possible to relate FHR changes to uterine activity. The most commonly used scaling is a paper speed of 3 cm/minute on the horizontal axis and 30 beats/minute per centimeter of paper for the FHR (vertical axis).[48] Each sequential vertical line is 10 seconds apart, and every sixth vertical line (bold) represents a period of 1 minute.

Uterine contractions are monitored either externally via a tocodynamometer or internally with an intrauterine pressure catheter attached to a transducer placed between the fetus and uterine wall. Data obtained from external contraction monitoring is limited to temporal elements such as contraction duration and interval, which cannot be used to estimate contraction strength. External monitoring is subject to a great deal of artifact from maternal movement and errors in transducer placement. Internal contraction monitoring is more reliable and allows for precise determination of intrauterine pressure and thus contraction strength. Its use is also predicated on ruptured amniotic membranes and a partially dilated cervix. Internal pressure monitoring is commonly utilized with high-risk parturients or those in whom labor augmentation with oxytocin is being used. Most commercially available intrauterine pressure catheter systems also allow for the infusion of fluids into the amniotic space (amnioinfusion), which is thought to reduce the risk of fetal aspiration of meconium-stained amniotic fluid.[49]

Fetal pulse oximetry has been introduced but is largely investigational. A wide range in normal values has been reported, and use of oximetry has not been shown to decrease overall cesarean delivery rates, making its ultimate benefit questionable.[50]

Information about the baseline status of a fetus should be obtained during the preanesthetic assessment. The FHR can also reveal information about the fetal response to anesthetic interventions. This information is useful before neuraxial anesthetic placement, for assisted or operative delivery, and for nonobstetric surgery during pregnancy. Current American Association of Nurse Anesthetists (AANA) and ASA obstetric practice guidelines state that fetal status should be monitored prior to and following a neuraxial analgesic intervention.[46,51]

Changes in Fetal Heart Rate

The individual components of the FHR pattern do not occur alone, and changes generally evolve over time. Therefore, a full description of a FHR tracing requires a qualitative and quantitative description of baseline rate, variability, presence of accelerations or decelerations, and trends over time.[32] In the presence of a normally functioning uteroplacental unit, fetal oxygenation is limited primarily by uterine blood flow. As stated, uterine arteries are maximally dilated in pregnancy, which results in the inability of the uterus to autoregulate blood flow. Decreases in maternal blood pressure and uterine artery blood flow ultimately compromise placental blood flow. The reduction in placental blood flow can result in fetal hypoxia and acidosis, which can be manifested as FHR changes. The normal FHR ranges from 110 to 160 beats per minute (bpm). An immature fetus has a higher HR as compared to a term fetus. Tachycardia is defined as a HR greater than 160 bpm in a term fetus. Tachycardia can result from fetal asphyxia, fetal arrhythmias, maternal fever, chorioamnionitis, and maternally administered drugs such as terbutaline and atropine. Ephedrine can increase both FHR and variability if given to the parturient in large enough doses.[53] Fetal bradycardia is present when the FHR is less than 110 bpm. Bradycardia can be caused by maternally administered drugs, compression of the fetal head, compression of the umbilical cord, or hypoxia (fetal or maternal).

Variability

FHR variability is thought to be the single best indicator of fetal wellbeing because it likely indicates adequate fetal oxygen reserve. Variability is the result of interaction between the fetal sympathetic and parasympathetic autonomic nervous systems. Baseline variability is defined as fluctuations in the FHR of two cycles per minute or greater that are irregular in amplitude and frequency.[52] It is quantified by measuring the amplitude from peak to trough in beats per minute. Variability is described as absent, minimal (<5 bpm), moderate (6–25 bpm), and marked (>25 bpm). In general, baseline FHR variability increases with advancing gestational age. Variability represents an intact CNS and normal cardiac function. Hypoxia causes fetal CNS depression, which results in decreased variability. Other causes of decreased variability include fetal sleep, acidosis, anencephaly, drugs (CNS depressants or autonomic agents), and defects of the fetal cardiac conduction system. For example, administration of opioids to the mother can decrease FHR variability for up to 30 minutes.[54] Maternal magnesium sulfate administration may also attenuate FHR variability.[55] Variability refers to the baseline FHR and does not include accelerations or decelerations. Beat-to-beat variability can be accurately assessed only by direct FHR monitoring with a fetal scalp electrode. Examples of absent and moderate FHR variability are shown in Fig. 51.5.

Accelerations and Decelerations

An acceleration is an abrupt increase in the FHR above baseline. Accelerations occur in response to fetal movement and indicate adequate oxygenation. The FHR pattern is said to be reactive when there are two or more accelerations in a 20-minute period. Decelerations are classified as early, variable, or late.

Early decelerations. Early decelerations occur in concert with uterine contractions. The deceleration begins when the contraction begins, and it returns to baseline when the contraction ends. An early deceleration occurs with each uterine contraction and has the same appearance from one contraction to the next. Compression of the fetal head resulting in vagal stimulation is thought to be the cause of early decelerations. Early decelerations have the following characteristics:

- Occur with each uterine contraction
- Start and end with the contraction
- Gradually decrease in rate and then end in a return to baseline
- Are uniform in appearance
- Are associated with a mild decrease in FHR (≤20 bpm)
- Are accompanied by a loss in beat-to-beat variability during the deceleration

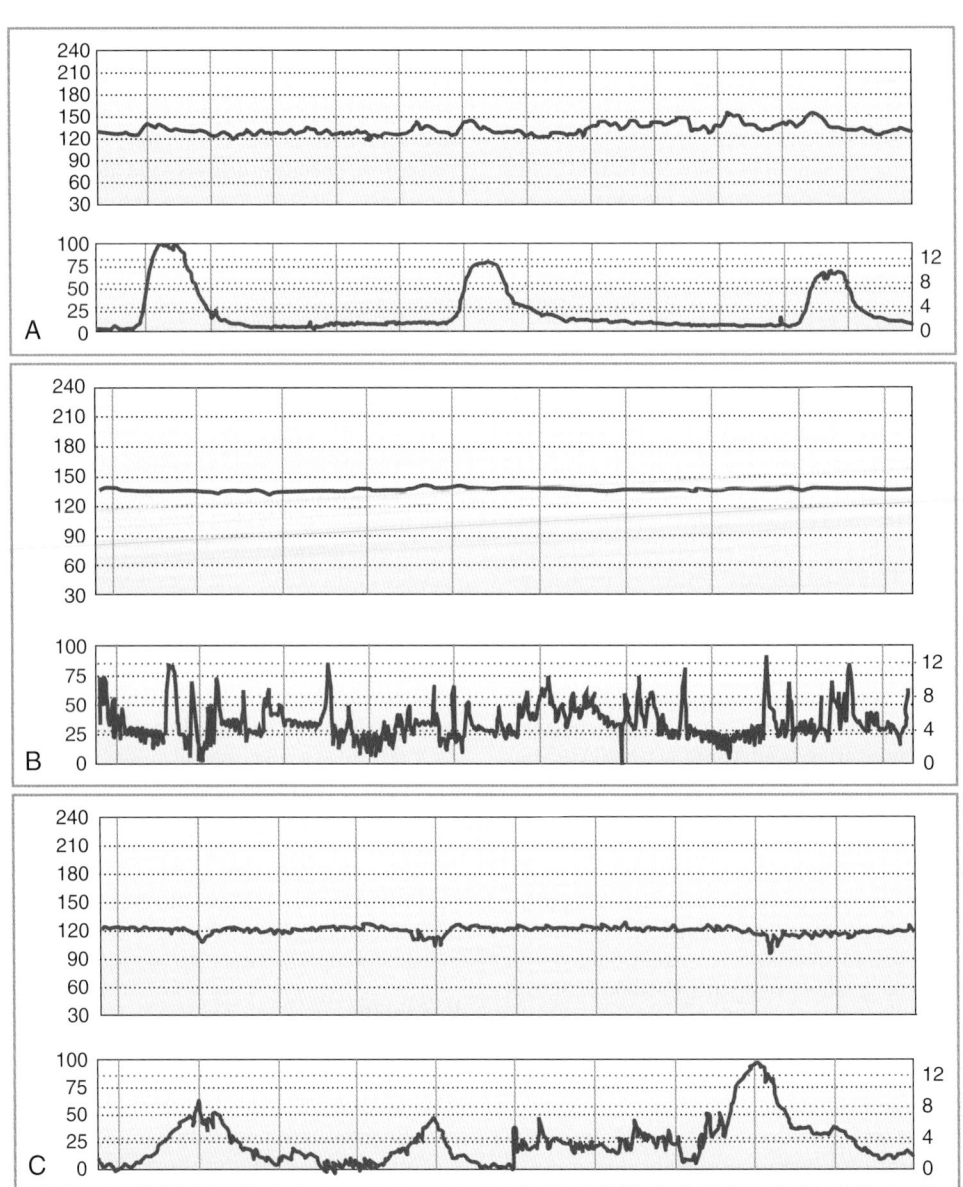

Fig. 51.5 (A) Normal intrapartum fetal heart rate (FHR) tracing. The infant had Apgar scores of 8 and 8 at 1 and 5 minutes, respectively. (B) Absence of variability in a FHR tracing. Placental abruption was noted at cesarean delivery. The infant had an umbilical arterial blood pH of 6.75 and Apgar scores of 1 and 4, respectively. (C) Early FHR decelerations. After a normal spontaneous vaginal delivery, the infant had Apgar scores of 8 and 8, respectively.

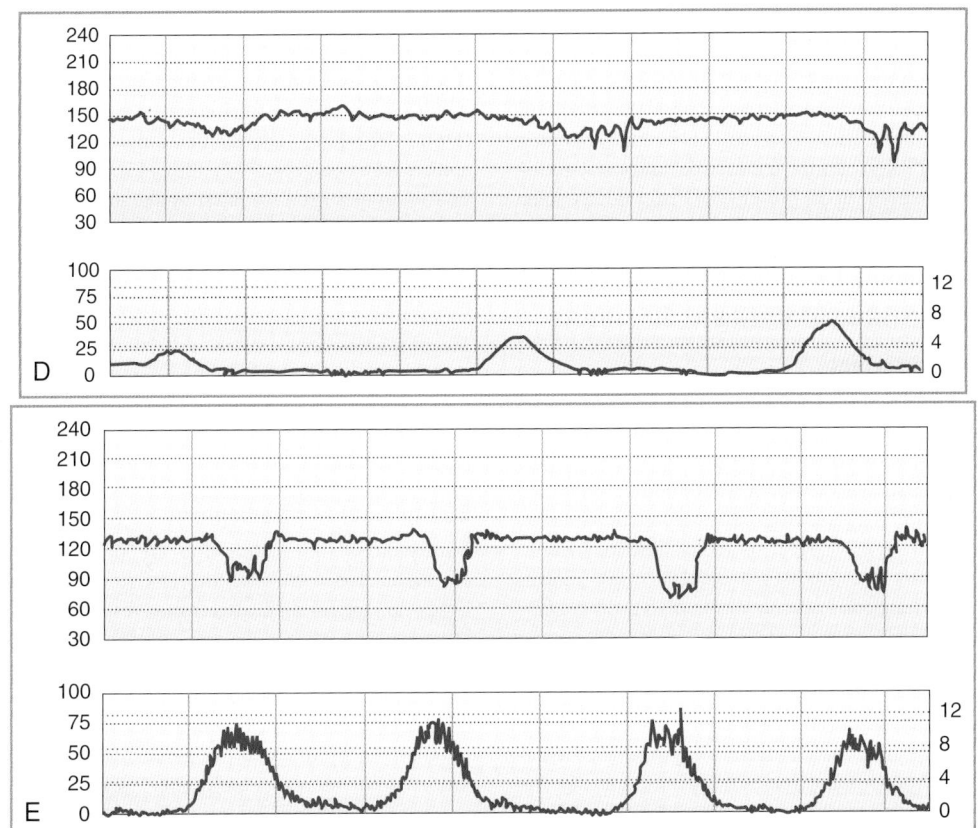

Fig. 51.5 cont'd (D) Late FHR decelerations. The amniotic fluid surrounding this fetus was meconium stained. Despite the late FHR decelerations, the variability remained acceptable. The infant was delivered by cesarean delivery and had an umbilical venous blood pH of 7.30. Apgar scores were 9 and 9, respectively. (E) Variable FHR decelerations. A tight nuchal cord was noted at low-forceps vaginal delivery. The infant had Apgar scores of 6 and 9, respectively. Numerical scales: *Left upper panel margin,* FHR in beats per minute; *left lower panel margin,* uterine pressure in mm Hg; *right lower panel margin,* uterine pressure in kilopascal (kPa). (From Chestnut DH, et al. *Chestnut's Obstetric Anesthesia.* 6th ed. Philadelphia: Elsevier; 2020:159–160.)

Variable decelerations. Variable decelerations are the most frequent FHR changes related to labor and are described as a sudden decrease in FHR that occurs irrespective of uterine contractions.[56] Variable decelerations are abrupt in both onset and recovery and vary in occurrence, onset, depth, duration, and appearance. Beat-to-beat variability is normally present during the decelerations. Variable decelerations are thought to be caused by a baroreceptor-mediated response to umbilical cord compression and are often considered to be a nonominous sign for neonatal outcome. Alternatively, if the fetus is compromised, then the recovery phase of the deceleration may be delayed. Variable decelerations have the following characteristics:

- Vary in appearance, duration, depth, and shape
- Demonstrate abrupt onset and recovery
- Maintain beat-to-beat variability with the deceleration

Late decelerations. Late decelerations begin late in the contraction and represent uteroplacental insufficiency. The lowest point of the deceleration occurs after the peak of the contraction. Like early decelerations, they are smooth in both onset and recovery. Late decelerations are normally repetitive. Beat-to-beat variability may or may not be present during the deceleration, depending on the degree of fetal hypoxia and myocardial depression. Late decelerations are nonreassuring and should be investigated for potential causes.[57] Fig. 51.5 shows a FHR tracing that depicts late decelerations and minimal variability.

Late decelerations have the following characteristics:

- Occur with each uterine contraction
- Low point of the deceleration after the peak of the contraction
- Gradually decrease in rate and end in a return to baseline
- Are uniform in appearance
- Vary in depth according to the strength of the uterine contraction
- May or may not be accompanied by beat-to-beat variability

Categories for the Evaluation of Fetal Heart Rate

The American College of Obstetricians and Gynecologists (ACOG) recommends a three-tiered system to evaluate FHR tracings. Category I FHR tracings are considered normal and include normal baseline HR and moderate variability with absent variable and late decelerations. Category I tracings predict normal acid-base balance. Category II FHR tracings include all tracings that are not classified as category I or III. Category II tracings do not predict abnormal acid-base status and warrant continued observation. Category III tracings include those with fetal bradycardia or absent variability accompanied by recurrent late or variable decelerations. Category III tracings predict abnormal acid-base status and require prompt intervention.[58]

Anesthetic Considerations in the Presence of Nonreassuring FHR Tracings

If the FHR tracing recorded during the preanesthesia assessment suggests hypoxia, caution should be used in making the decision to proceed with neuraxial analgesia. Careful consideration must be given to the severity of the fetal compromise and to the possibility that it may be worsened by anesthetic intervention. However, the obstetric team may request a neuraxial anesthetic for a patient with a nonreassuring FHR tracing in anticipation of a possible urgent and unplanned operative vaginal delivery or cesarean delivery.

Intrauterine resuscitation describes interventions that can be used by the obstetric staff and anesthesia provider to improve the condition of a compromised fetus in utero. These interventions include changing maternal position, rapid infusion of intravenous (IV) fluids, discontinuing oxytocin, IV pressor support in the presence of maternal hypotension, the use of tocolytic agents, and maternal oxygen administration to correct maternal hypoxia.[59]

ANALGESIA FOR LABOR AND VAGINAL DELIVERY

IV Analgesia in the Parturient

Although less effective than neuraxial analgesia, systemic medications can be used for labor pain relief when neuraxial analgesia is unavailable, refused, or contraindicated. However, the use of systemic medications presents several disadvantages. The pain relief they afford is often inadequate, and both fetal and maternal respiratory depression, nausea, vomiting, and decreased lower esophageal sphincter tone may result. Controlled, randomized trials investigating neuraxial versus IV analgesia in labor are difficult to design and execute due to high protocol failure rates. In a systematic review of studies involving over 9600 women that compared neuraxial analgesia to opiates, neuraxial techniques offered better pain relief and a reduced risk of fetal acidosis. On the contrary, epidural analgesia was associated with a longer first and second stage labor while also being more likely to receive oxytocin augmentation. However, epidural administration does not appear to increase the risk of cesarean delivery or long-term backache. The administration of an epidural also does not appear to adversely impact neonatal status, as evidenced by Apgar scores or neonatal intensive care admissions.[60]

Since opioids are lipid soluble and relatively small (<500 Da), they rapidly cross the placenta to gain access to the fetal circulation and may result in fetal depression. A neonate's blood-brain barrier is less developed, and its ability to metabolize narcotics is less mature when compared to an adult. Opioids can be administered by IV bolus or patient-controlled analgesia (PCA). The advantage of PCA is it allows the parturient greater control over drug dosing and has resulted in greater patient satisfaction. However, in one study, PCA was compared with nurse-administered boluses, and there was no difference in pain scores or maternal and fetal side effects.[61] The use of parenteral narcotics in early labor has declined as the practice of obstetric anesthesia has evolved to include those patients in early labor as acceptable candidates for neuraxial analgesia.

Meperidine

Meperidine is administered as a parenteral opioid for labor analgesia. A typical dose is 50 to 100 mg intramuscular (IM) and can be repeated every 4 hours. Meperidine crosses the placenta easily and has been recovered from the fetus within 2 minutes of IV administration. The maternal half-life of meperidine is 2.5 to 3 hours. Like all opioids, it can cause neonatal respiratory depression, although less so than morphine. Because of differences in pH and protein binding, the level of meperidine in the fetus is likely to be higher than the maternal blood level. Normeperidine is an active metabolite of meperidine with an elimination half-life of 30 hours. Normeperidine remains in the neonate for several days after delivery and may lead to depression of neonatal behavioral assessment scores. Both meperidine and normeperidine can be antagonized by naloxone.

The overall analgesic effect of meperidine in labor is marginal. In a random trial of 102 women, acetaminophen 1000 mg IV was found to provide similar analgesia when compared to meperidine 50 mg IV. The incidence of maternal side effects was 64% in the meperidine group and 0% in the acetaminophen group.[62]

Fentanyl

Fentanyl's high potency and short duration of action make it a reasonable choice for labor. It is highly lipid soluble and protein bound, and it can be detected in fetal circulation after 1 minute of IV administration. Depressant effects, including a reduction in beat-to-beat variability, have been seen.[63] Fentanyl can be administered IV, IM, or via PCA. Dosages used for labor analgesia range from 25 to 100 mcg IV in hourly increments[64] or by PCA bolus 25 to 50 mcg with a lockout interval of 3 to 6 minutes and a 4-hour limit of 1 to 1.5 mg.[65]

Morphine

Morphine has been used in early labor to provide analgesia and sedation but is no longer widely accepted due to high rates of maternal sedation, neonatal depression, and an undesirable prolonged duration.[66] Morphine crosses the placenta easily and, in animal studies, crosses the fetal blood-brain barrier more readily than in adults.[67]

Butorphanol and Nalbuphine

Butorphanol and nalbuphine are opioid agonist-antagonists that are associated with a ceiling effect, whereby incrementally higher doses do not result in increasing respiratory depression. They may also result in less nausea and vomiting than pure opioids. Agonist-antagonists have typically been used in first-stage latent-phase labor to provide sedation and a period of maternal rest. A typical butorphanol dose for labor is 1 to 2 mg IV or IM. Butorphanol is five times as potent as morphine and has a half-life of 3 hours. Unlike morphine, butorphanol increases pulmonary artery pressure and myocardial work.[64] Butorphanol has no active metabolites. The nalbuphine dose in labor is 5 to 10 mg IV, IM, or subcutaneous (SC) and is equivalent to morphine 10 mg. Nalbuphine results in a greater reduction in FHR variability compared with meperidine.[68] Because these compounds possess significant antagonist properties, their use in opioid-dependent patients should be avoided.

Remifentanil

Remifentanil is an ultrashort-acting opioid receptor agonist. It is rapidly hydrolyzed by plasma and tissue esterases to an inactive metabolite. The context-sensitive half-life remains short (3.2 min) regardless of prolonged administration times.[69] This unique pharmacokinetic profile makes it suitable for PCA use in labor. Remifentanil crosses the placenta readily but is rapidly redistributed and metabolized by the fetus.[70] Douma et al.[71] compared remifentanil, fentanyl, and meperidine PCAs in labor and found that remifentanil PCA was associated with the greatest reduction in pain scores; however, the relief was described as mild to moderate. The same group has found that remifentanil PCA is less effective when compared with standard epidural labor analgesia.[72] A PCA bolus of 0.25 mcg/kg with a lockout interval of 2 minutes and a background infusion of 0.025 to 0.05 mcg/kg/min is common.[63,73,74] Use of remifentanil during labor is a relatively new technique that appears to have an acceptable safety profile. However, its use mandates careful monitoring due to the potential for adverse maternal events.[75]

Ketamine

Ketamine is a derivative of phencyclidine and an N-methyl-D-aspartate (NMDA) receptor antagonist that produces a dissociative anesthetic effect. It produces profound analgesia at subhypnotic doses. Its use as a labor analgesic is limited, however, by its short duration of action and high incidence of amnesia. Low-dose ketamine preserves airway reflexes while causing somatic analgesia, sedation, and occasionally a dreamlike state. Satisfactory labor analgesia has been described by using a continuous infusion of ketamine at 0.2 mg/kg/hr.[76] Small intermittent IV doses of ketamine can be used to supplement a suboptimal neuraxial anesthetic when replacement or adjustment is not possible. Ketamine doses of 0.2 to 0.5 mg/kg produce rapid analgesia with a dose-dependent duration of action of approximately 5 to 15 minutes.

Ketamine has sympathomimetic properties that result in increased HR, blood pressure, and cardiac output, which may be desirable in a hypovolemic parturient. The hyperdynamic effects, however, may be problematic in the parturient with hypertension or preeclampsia. It is the agent of choice for induction in the patient with acute asthma requiring general anesthesia for urgent cesarean delivery. The emergence delirium and hallucinations limit the effectiveness of ketamine for routine use in obstetrics. Uterine arterial blood flow does not decrease after ketamine administration. Ketamine is lipid soluble and readily crosses the placenta. Neonatal depression has not been demonstrated after maternal ketamine doses of up to 1 mg/kg. Doses larger than 1 mg/kg may result in neonatal respiratory depression, uterine hypertonicity, and lower Apgar scores.[77]

Nonpharmacologic Methods

A multitude of nonpharmacologic techniques are currently in use, but Wong states the effectiveness of these techniques generally lacks rigorous scientific study, and conclusions regarding their efficacy cannot be made.[78] Nonpharmacologic alternatives include hydrotherapy, hypnotherapy, massage, movement, and positioning. Although maternal satisfaction is without a doubt influenced by the degree of pain endured, it is influenced to a greater extent by whether the actual birth event met the mother's personal expectations.[79] The role of an obstetric anesthesia provider is to support laboring women such that they can make informed choices that meet their individual expectations, while at the same time ensuring the safety of both the mother and infant.[80]

Neuraxial Analgesia for Labor and Vaginal Delivery

Neuraxial analgesia is currently the best method of pain relief for labor and delivery. When properly placed and dosed, a neuraxial anesthetic is the only modality available that can provide complete relief from labor pain with minimal depression of the parturient or fetus. Common neuraxial anesthetics include epidural, combined spinal-epidural (CSE), and spinal techniques. ACOG has stated that, absent medical contraindications, maternal request is sufficient reason to provide labor analgesia.[81] However, labor is a prerequisite for neuraxial analgesia and is defined as regular uterine contractions that result in cervical dilation and effacement.

Early initiation of neuraxial anesthesia may be considered for those parturients at increased risk of experiencing anesthetic or obstetric complications during labor.[82] These patients include those with morbid obesity, severe scoliosis, or known difficult airway. Obstetric indications for early placement include multiple gestation pregnancies and severe preeclampsia. Early initiation allows for better cooperation with positioning during placement and adequate time to confirm proper block function. An indwelling epidural catheter can be dosed to provide surgical anesthesia if a cesarean delivery becomes urgently necessary, reducing the need for a general anesthetic.

Absolute contraindications to neuraxial anesthesia include patient refusal, inability to cooperate, uncorrected severe hypovolemia, uncorrected coagulopathy or pharmacologic anticoagulation, elevated intracranial pressure secondary to a mass, or infection at the site of insertion. There are many relative contraindications, which include but are not limited to stable preexisting CNS disease, chronic severe headaches or back pain, untreated bacteremia, and severe stenotic valvular lesions. Patients with these and other preexisting conditions should undergo careful preanesthetic evaluation and consultation that takes into consideration the risks and benefits of the proposed procedure. With recognition and proper optimization of these preexisting conditions, patients can often safely receive neuraxial anesthesia.

Historically, the platelet count at which a neuraxial anesthetic could be safely administered has been considered to be greater than 100,000/µL. However, contemporary practice surveys indicate that most practitioners are comfortable providing a regional anesthetic with the platelet count as low as 75,000 to 80,000/µL.[83] Careful consideration of thrombocytopenic parturients should include a thorough history and physical examination for signs and symptoms of coagulopathy with an emphasis on previously administered medications, including herbal supplements. A review of laboratory findings should include all prior platelet counts (to establish any trends) as well as other relevant laboratory findings.

Patients receiving prenatal and/or intrapartum antithrombotic or thrombolytic therapy require special consideration. Normal pregnancy is associated with a hypercoagulable state that, alone or in combination with certain pathologic conditions, can predispose parturients to thromboembolic events. Conditions that may require anticoagulation therapy in the obstetric population include deep vein thrombosis, antiphospholipid antibody syndrome, factor V Leiden mutations, and protein S and C deficiencies. The major concern with conducting a neuraxial anesthetic is the potentially catastrophic complication of epidural hematoma. Epidural hematoma results from uncontrolled bleeding in the nondistendable epidural space, which, if untreated, can cause ischemic injury to the cord resulting in persistent neurologic dysfunction. Epidural hematoma is a rare complication that is estimated to occur in less than 1 in 150,000 epidural and 1 in 220,000 spinal anesthetics.[84] The American Society of Regional Anesthesia and Pain Medicine (ASRA) has published consensus statements in an effort to guide practitioners in the management of these complex patients.[85]

Preprocedure Preparation

History and physical. It is optimal to complete the history and physical for every patient whose plan includes a neuraxial anesthetic early in the labor process, often before the regional anesthetic is indicated. An early history and physical allows for recognition of potential problems and provides time for additional workup if necessary. Valuable time can also be saved with a previously completed history and physical if an anesthetic intervention becomes urgently necessary.

The history should include questions regarding pertinent systemic diseases, as well as the obstetric history and course of the current pregnancy. Particular attention should be directed toward problems with previous pregnancies, deliveries, or anesthetics. A review of the patient's medical record to include previous analgesic interventions, such as IV narcotics, should be performed. The physical examination should include an inspection of the back, heart, and lungs, as well as an airway examination. It has been demonstrated that the airway examination can change during labor.[32] Therefore a repeat examination is indicated immediately before administering anesthesia in labor regardless of prior examination results.

The maternal vital signs and fetal condition should be documented. This includes dilation, effacement, station, FHR, membrane status, and variability. The obstetric history includes gestational age and the parturient's gravidity (i.e., number of conceptions) and parity (i.e., number of live births). Obtaining a platelet count before the institution of neuraxial anesthesia in healthy patients with uncomplicated pregnancies has not been shown to reduce overall complication rates.[86] However, in the presence of hypertensive disorders or coagulopathies with anesthetic implications, the elective anesthetic should generally be delayed until appropriate laboratory results are available (e.g., coagulation studies, platelet count). In the absence of comprehensive prenatal care, obtaining baseline laboratory values may be indicated due to the possibility of undiagnosed medical conditions.

Informed consent. Those who provide anesthesia for laboring women have an obligation to obtain informed consent prior to the procedure. The elements of informed consent include a description of the procedure, the risks, benefits, potential complications, and alternatives. However, there are several issues unique to obstetric anesthesia that can complicate informed consent. The first involves capacity and whether a woman in great pain and distress has the ability to understand and reason.[87] There is evidence to indicate that women retain the ability to assimilate information and make informed decisions despite the pain of labor. Jackson et al.[88] found that most women in active labor were able to voluntarily consent and that their ability to understand was not affected by pain, premedication, or duration of labor. Affleck et al.[89] determined that recall of risks by parturients is similar to the recall of risks by other patients and does not appear to be affected by parity or the reported level of pain.

A second confounding issue with regard to informed consent is caring for the pregnant minor. Competence describes the legal authority to make a decision and is recognized in the United States as occurring at age 18 years. However, various state laws make exceptions (emancipation) for minors who are free of parental care, control, and custody. This may occur when a minor is married, a member of the military, or a high school graduate. Pregnancy does not necessarily constitute emancipation. With respect to obstetric anesthesia, it is best to include the legal guardian of a minor patient in the informed consent process. Anesthesia providers must have a working knowledge of various local, state, and federal guidelines, as well as their institutions' applicable policies and procedures.

Informed consent should include those risks that are reasonably foreseeable, but it does not have to include every possible risk. Material risks are those that a reasonable person would want to be made aware of before deciding on a recommended therapy.[90] They include risks that commonly occur, as well as those risks that are rare but may result in severe morbidity and mortality. There exists no distinct and inclusive list of potential risks and complications; however, several surveys of practitioners demonstrate some consensus regarding what should be disclosed.[91,92]

Drugs and equipment. It is the provider's responsibility to ensure that the anesthesia equipment available in the obstetric area is consistent with other anesthetizing locations in the facility.[93] An oxygen source, a positive pressure apparatus capable of delivering 100% oxygen, and an appropriate suction assembly must be present at every location where neuraxial anesthesia is provided. Emergency airway supplies such as face masks, oral and nasal airways, laryngeal mask airways, laryngoscope handle/blades, endotracheal tubes and stylet, and an Eschmann intubating stylet need to be immediately available. Carbon dioxide monitoring can be accomplished with a qualitative carbon dioxide detector. Emergency drugs include propofol (for terminating a local anesthetic–induced seizure), succinylcholine, ephedrine, epinephrine, phenylephrine, naloxone, atropine, calcium chloride (for treating magnesium sulfate overdose), and sodium bicarbonate. The equipment should be checked prior to each anesthetic.

As services are often provided at each bedside in a labor and delivery unit, an epidural cart that contains routine supplies, as well as emergency equipment and drugs, is preferred. A standard crash cart with a defibrillator and a supply of intralipid 20% to treat intravascular injection of local anesthetics should be readily available (see Chapter 10 for a complete discussion of local anesthetic toxicity). Noninvasive automatic blood pressure monitoring and pulse oximetry are required in each labor and delivery room. In addition to proper drugs and equipment, a knowledgeable assistant is essential for the safe insertion of a neuraxial anesthetic. An obstetric nurse who can assist with FHR

monitoring and positioning is desirable. IV access is required prior to initiating a neuraxial anesthetic and should be maintained throughout its duration. IV insertion sites should take into consideration the vigorous arm movement that can occur during second-stage labor. The dilute concentrations of local anesthetic commonly used in labor analgesia today result in significantly less sympathetic blockade and hypotension compared with traditional high-dose blocks.[94] As a result, the administration of a fixed volume of IV fluid is not required before neuraxial analgesia is initiated.[86]

Local Anesthetics

Bupivacaine. Bupivacaine is an amino-amide local anesthetic with a relatively long duration of action and the ability to produce a differential block whereby sensory fibers are blocked more readily than motor fibers. When compared with lidocaine, there is less tachyphylaxis during long-term administration. In lower doses, it has limited placental transfer, as well as minimal neonatal effects. These characteristics have made it the most commonly used local anesthetic in obstetric anesthesia. Bupivacaine is marketed as a racemic mixture of the S− and R+ isomers. Refractory cardiac arrest has been associated with high concentrations of bupivacaine inadvertently administered intravascularly. It is more difficult to resuscitate patients who experience bupivacaine-induced cardiac arrest when compared with other local anesthetics. The exact cause remains unclear; however, evidence suggests that toxicity occurs primarily at sodium channels, and there may be qualitative differences in cardiotoxicity caused by low- and high-potency local anesthetics.[95] The epidural administration of 0.75% bupivacaine has been prohibited for use in obstetric anesthesia due to its increased potential for toxicity. Clinical techniques to reduce the incidence of cardiac toxicity include fractional dosing (<5 mL), frequent aspiration for blood during injection, and use of a test dose. The use of low concentrations for continuous epidural infusion and low doses (<15 mg) for spinal anesthesia are not associated with cardiac toxicity.[96]

Lidocaine. Lidocaine is an amino-amide local anesthetic that has been used extensively in obstetric anesthesia for decades. It has a rapid onset and an intermediate duration of action. When given in the epidural space, it produces a dense motor block when combined with epinephrine, which makes it well suited for epidural anesthesia for cesarean delivery. This dense motor block, however, makes it less desirable for labor analgesia. Lidocaine administered in the subarachnoid space is potentially neurotoxic.[97] In 1991, four cases of cauda equina syndrome were reported after the use of lidocaine in small-diameter catheters designed for continuous spinal anesthesia (CSA). In all four cases there was initial evidence of a focal sensory block, and to achieve adequate analgesia, a dose of local anesthetic was given that was greater than that usually administered with a single-injection technique. The authors postulated, and subsequent data substantiated, that the combination of maldistribution and a relatively high dose of local anesthetic resulted in neuronal injury.[98] Transient neurologic symptoms consisting primarily of lower extremity pain also have been attributed to 5% hyperbaric lidocaine.[99]

2-Chloroprocaine. Chloroprocaine is an amino-ester local anesthetic that is rapidly metabolized by ester hydrolysis. As such, its potential to produce cardiac and CNS toxicity after inadvertent IV administration is low. It has a rapid onset and brief duration of action. Chloroprocaine is used primarily in obstetric anesthesia to rapidly produce a surgical block in the presence of a preexisting epidural in the case of an emergency cesarean delivery. However, the epidural administration of chloroprocaine has been shown to reduce the effectiveness of subsequently administered epidural morphine, possibly by antagonism at the opioid receptors.[100] Neurotoxicity has been reported after inadvertent spinal administration of large doses intended for the epidural space but was likely a result of the low pH and/or the preservatives.[101]

Ropivacaine. Ropivacaine is an amino-amide local anesthetic that is produced as the pure levorotatory enantiomer and is structurally similar to bupivacaine. It has a propyl group attached to the aromatic ring as opposed to bupivacaine, which has a butyl group attached to the ring. Ropivacaine was developed largely to address the cardiac toxicity associated with bupivacaine, and when equivalent masses of drug are compared, it appears to be less toxic. Both levobupivacaine and ropivacaine have a clinical profile similar to that of bupivacaine, and the minimal differences observed are mainly related to different anesthetic potency, with bupivacaine > levobupivacaine > ropivacaine.[102,103] When clinical dosing is adjusted for the decreased potency, the toxicity advantage of ropivacaine is diminished.[104] Although equipotent doses of ropivacaine have been shown to produce less motor block when compared with bupivacaine, it has not been shown to influence the mode of delivery, the duration of labor, or neonatal outcome.[105]

The potential cardiotoxicity of ropivacaine is limited to animal models and in vitro preparations, and they have found either an advantage for ropivacaine in regard to toxicity or no difference between ropivacaine and bupivacaine. It is possible that ropivacaine is less cardiotoxic than bupivacaine at high doses, but at the more dilute concentrations clinically relevant to obstetric anesthesia, this difference is less likely to be important.[106]

Synthetic opioids increase the potency of amide local anesthetics. Significantly longer labor analgesia can be achieved with ropivacaine-sufentanil and levobupivacaine-sufentanil, and ropivacaine is associated with comparatively less motor blockade. Labor duration after epidural analgesia has been found to be shorter when bupivacaine-sufentanil combinations are used and there is a low incidence of instrumental delivery.[107]

Neuraxial Anesthetic Placement

Strict aseptic technique must always be used during the insertion of neuraxial anesthetics. This includes preprocedural hand hygiene; wearing of sterile gloves, cap, and mask (new for each case); removal of rings and watches; and sterile draping of the back. A newly opened single-use container of preparation solution should be used for skin surface disinfection. Chlorhexidine gluconate in an alcohol-based solution should be considered the antiseptic of choice. When compared with other commonly used antiseptic solutions, it is effective against a wider array of pathogens, has a greater degree of potency, shows a more rapid onset of action with an extended duration of effect, and has fewer and less severe localized skin reactions.[108] In addition, the efficacy of chlorhexidine gluconate is maintained in the presence of protein-based organic compounds such as blood and other body fluids. Whether chlorhexidine gluconate or povidone-iodine solution is utilized for skin surface disinfection, the agent needs to be allotted enough time to dry prior to starting the neuraxial procedure. Upon completion of the procedure, a sterile occlusive dressing should then be placed over the catheter insertion site.

Baseline blood pressure and pulse oximetry should be obtained prior to the procedure and then measured at regular intervals once neuraxial dosing has begun. Typically, blood pressure is monitored every 2 minutes for 15 minutes, then every 5 minutes for another 15 minutes, thereby enabling the early detection and treatment of neuraxial anesthesia–induced hypotension. It is preferable to remain in the anesthetizing location during this time to monitor the proper onset and progression of the neuraxial block and to enable prompt recognition and treatment of potentially catastrophic complications

such as with total spinal anesthetic or local anesthetic systemic toxicity (LAST).

The sitting position is often easiest for the laboring parturient to assume and maintain and normally offers the anesthetist the maximum interspace width. On the other hand, use of the lateral position has been found to reduce the incidence of intravascular catheter placement.[109] The lateral position can make identification of the midline more difficult due to skin shifting and requires meticulous attention to shoulder position. The upper shoulder naturally rotates anteriorly resulting in a concomitant rotation of the vertebral column that, if not corrected, can result in anatomic distortion. The lateral position may also help limit movement if the patient is having a difficult time with positioning. Occasionally, obstetric emergencies such as fetal head entrapment, prolapsed umbilical cord, and footling breech presentation may preclude the use of the sitting position for neuraxial anesthesia placement.

It has long been observed that the failure rate associated with epidural anesthetics is greater in the obese patient. At the same time, neuraxial anesthetics are particularly desirable in obese parturients because of their increased cesarean delivery rates and concerns surrounding potential airway difficulty. The distance between the skin and the epidural space increases as the body mass index (BMI) increases, which can make epidural insertion more difficult.[110] However, morbid obesity, when considered alone, is not a predictor of difficult block placement. In a study of 427 morbidly obese patients receiving neuraxial anesthetics, four variables were evaluated to determine whether they could predict difficult insertion. The authors found that only the ability to palpate bony landmarks and the patient's ability to flex the back were significant predictors of difficulty, whereas BMI and the practitioner's experience level were not predictive.[111] Prelabor consultation for women with a BMI greater than 50 kg/m² should be considered where an anesthesia plan can be made after a focused history and physical exam. Neuraxial anesthesia for the morbidly obese parturient should include a thorough check of equipment for appropriate size, consideration of early placement and anticipation of difficulty with prolonged labor, and the increased likelihood of cesarean delivery. Frequent evaluation of the block and communication with all caregivers is paramount.[82]

The use of ultrasound imaging as an aid in the placement of neuraxial anesthetics is a relatively new and growing technique. The placement of neuraxial anesthetics relies primarily on palpation of underlying anatomy and visualization of surface landmarks and is therefore an essentially blind technique. Preprocedural imaging may ultimately improve clinical practice and the ability to teach these techniques.[112] Ultrasound imaging is particularly useful in determining the skin to epidural space depth, the location of the midline, and the precise interspace. Palpation alone, regardless of BMI, is a relatively ineffective method for determining vertebral interspace, which is of particular importance when performing neuraxial techniques.[113] Morbidly obese patients or those with a history of difficult block placement may benefit from this technique.[114]

The type of epidural catheter used influences the anesthetic. Spiral wire-embedded flexible polyurethane catheters with a soft tip have been shown to result in fewer paresthesias and intravascular placements when compared with nylon catheters.[115] Previous comparisons between multiple- and single-orifice catheters focused on standard nylon (stiff) designs and found an advantage favoring multiple-orifice catheters. A study comparing both versions (single orifice and multiple orifice) of soft catheters has found no difference.[116] Multiple-orifice closed-end catheters are less prone to obstruction and likely result in better spread of local anesthetic in the epidural space.[117]

Historically, when larger doses of local anesthetic were used, a bolus of IV fluids was administered prior to placement of the regional analgesic in an effort to reduce the incidence and magnitude of hypotension. However, when dilute concentrations of local anesthetics combined with lipid-soluble narcotics are used to initiate neuraxial analgesia for labor and are combined with efforts to reduce aortocaval compression, the incidence of hypotension is approximately 5%.[118] Zamora et al.[119] found that a 1-liter preload did not provide added protection against hypotension but likely resulted in decreasing contraction frequency and was associated with delays in providing analgesia.

Test Doses

High cephalic spread of a neuraxial block remains one of the most common causes of anesthesia related maternal mortality in obstetrics.[120] A test dose is intended to identify epidural catheters that are inadvertently inserted into either the subarachnoid space or an epidural vein. First, it is essential to aspirate for blood or cerebrospinal fluid (CSF) after placement of the epidural catheter and before every manually administered dose. However, negative aspiration does not conclusively indicate that the catheter is not in the subarachnoid or intravascular space. Therefore the epidural test dose is designed to reveal inadvertent subarachnoid or intravascular injection of local anesthetic without producing systemic toxicity or widespread subarachnoid block. The test dose is the minimum amount of drug required to produce a modestly detectable effect when injected either intrathecally or systemically. A commonly administered test dose is 3 mL of lidocaine 1.5% with epinephrine 1:200,000. This 45-mg dose of lidocaine, if unexpectedly administered in the subarachnoid space, will produce a noticeable but manageable spinal anesthetic within 3 to 5 minutes while having no appreciable effect when given in the epidural space.

When administered intravascularly, lidocaine 45 mg will often result in early signs and symptoms of modest systemic toxicity such as circumoral numbness, lightheadedness, or auditory changes. The previously mentioned test dose also includes 15 mcg of epinephrine that, when given intravascularly into an epidural vein, has been shown to reliably increase HR in nonpregnant patients. The maternal HR should be monitored continuously using either pulse oximetry or ECG during administration of the test dose to detect these HR changes. In the laboring parturient, increases in HR are a less specific indicator of intravascular injection because of the changes in HR that normally occur during uterine contractions. Even when a test dose is carefully timed to be administered between contractions, it lacks both sensitivity and specificity. As a result, it is not universally accepted for use in obstetric anesthesia. Furthermore, concern exists that epinephrine may cause significant uterine artery constriction in a small number of patients, resulting in a decrease in fetal O_2 delivery.[121]

Some practitioners believe that by using multiple-orifice catheters in combination with incrementally administered (every 3–5 min) small doses (<5 mL) of dilute (<0.125%) local anesthetic, an epinephrine-containing test dose is unjustified for labor analgesia. Careful aspiration of the epidural catheter for blood or CSF alone, without the administration of a test dose, may be effective in revealing an intrathecal or intravascular catheter.[122] If a parturient receiving a continuous epidural infusion of dilute local anesthetic remains comfortable, the catheter must, by default, be in the epidural space. However, if the catheter was intravascular, the parturient would have inadequate analgesia, and, if it were intrathecal, a significant motor block would ensue.[123]

Observing for blood or CSF while aspirating from the epidural catheter had a 0% false-positive rate and a 0.2% false-negative rate in over 1000 women in whom 60 intravascular or subarachnoid catheter placements were performed.[124] However, a test dose with epinephrine is necessary when administering larger and more concentrated doses such as those given in an epidural for cesarean delivery.[122] Ideally, the administration of every epidural dose should be considered a test dose

in which the catheter is carefully aspirated and incrementally injected. In summary, every precaution to ensure proper placement of the epidural catheter should be employed, including the use of minimum effective doses, careful aspiration, and incremental injection, coupled with the use of intravascular markers when large doses are used. Epinephrine remains the most widely used and studied marker, but its reliability is impaired in the face of β-blockade, advanced age, and active labor. As an alternative, the use of subtoxic doses of local anesthetics themselves can produce subjective symptoms in patients. Fentanyl has also been confirmed to produce sedation in pregnant women when used as an alternative. The use of ultrasound observation of needle placement and injection may be useful. Constant vigilance and suspicion are still needed along with a combination of as many of these safety steps as practical.[125,126]

Anesthetic Effects on the Progress of Labor

It is likely that women who request early labor analgesia have more pain than women who do not, and pain is a marker for risk of cesarean delivery.[127] In a systematic review of 10 trials that enrolled over 2300 patients in which the effects of epidural versus parenteral opioids in labor were examined, Halpern et al.[128] found that epidural labor analgesia was not associated with increased rates of instrumented vaginal delivery or cesarean delivery. Not surprisingly, patient satisfaction and neonatal outcomes were better after epidural when compared with parenteral opioid analgesia. Another systematic review of seven existing trials found that epidural analgesia using low concentrations of bupivacaine and fentanyl was unlikely to increase the risk of cesarean delivery but may increase the risk of instrumented vaginal delivery.[129] Although women in those studies had a longer labor, they had better pain relief. It could be argued that the increased risk of instrumented vaginal delivery was the result of obstetricians choosing this method more frequently because of the presence of a functioning epidural.[130] It has been postulated that early initiation of neuraxial analgesia (<4 cm) may increase the incidence of labor dystocia and cesarean delivery. However, a 2009 large study from China involving almost 13,000 patients found no difference in the duration of labor or cesarean delivery rate when primiparous women were randomized to receive epidural analgesia at 1 cm dilation versus 4 cm or more dilation.[131] Overall, the use of epidural analgesia does not appear to increase the risk of cesarean delivery. It may affect the incidence of forceps delivery, but it depends on the medications used. Epidural analgesia does appear to prolong labor, although the clinical significance of this prolongation has not been shown.[132]

Epidural Analgesia for Labor

Epidural analgesia remains a popular, safe, and effective means of providing analgesia for labor. The use of an indwelling epidural catheter gives the anesthetist the ability to produce a segmental block of varying density that can be adapted to the patient's changing requirements. This is accomplished by changing the volume and concentration of local anesthetic administered. Dosing an epidural with dilute concentrations of local anesthetic often results in satisfactory labor analgesia without producing significant motor block. When necessary, the same labor epidural can be converted to a surgical anesthetic that includes a dense motor and sensory block by administering a larger volume of a more concentrated local anesthetic.

Combining a lipid-soluble opioid allows a decrease in concentration of local anesthetic without compromising analgesia while at the same time preserving motor function. Decreasing the dose of both drugs minimizes the potential complications and side effects of each. An epidural for labor analgesia is optimally inserted at the L2-L3 or L3-L4 interspace to allow for effective blockade of the T10-L1 dermatomes necessary for analgesia in first-stage labor. Analgesia for second-stage labor and subsequent repair, if needed, requires an extension of the block to include the S2-S4 dermatomes that innervate the perineum and vagina. Adequate analgesia must be balanced against loss of the sensation of labor, which is not desirable during the second stage, and motor block, which is bothersome to the mother during labor and prevents effective pushing during the second stage.

Although the small amount of epinephrine present in a test dose should be safe for a healthy fetus, the larger amounts present in the volume of local anesthetic used in epidural infusions carry some risk of umbilical artery constriction in some parturients.[133] Epinephrine-containing local anesthetics also result in significantly enhanced motor block. For these reasons, routine use of epinephrine-containing solutions for labor analgesia is not recommended, especially in the pre-eclamptic patient.

To avoid aortocaval syndrome, after epidural analgesia has been instituted, the patient should be instructed to avoid the supine position. A hip roll, wedge, or pillow should be used to maintain a left or right lateral position. Following the initial and all subsequent doses, the patient should not be left unattended for at least 20 minutes. The anesthetist should remain aware of cervical dilation and the progress of labor after the epidural catheter has been placed. Communication with the obstetric personnel is important to prevent the use of a drug, dose, or concentration of local anesthetic that is inappropriate for the patient's circumstances.

Maintaining Epidural Analgesia for Labor and Delivery

Although it is possible to maintain epidural analgesia with intermittent bolus administration, this technique is associated with periods of analgesia alternating with periods of pain, as well as frequent provider interventions. Hypotension occurs less often when a continuous infusion is used as a result of fewer changes in the level of sympathetic blockade. Continuous infusion results in less total local anesthetic administered (when compared with intermittent boluses), more effective analgesia, and significantly reduced workload. There is also no need for the careful incremental administration of local anesthetic associated with bolus doses.

The parturient's analgesia level and degree of motor block should be frequently assessed and changes in the infusion rate and/or concentration made as needed. An epidural catheter originally sited in the epidural space can potentially migrate into the subarachnoid or intravascular space. If the epidural catheter migrates into the subarachnoid space after placement while receiving a continuous infusion, the resulting gradual increase in motor block should be easily recognized. Alternatively, if the catheter enters the intravascular space, the patient will have a loss of analgesia without overt symptoms of systemic toxicity.

Infusions of bupivacaine (0.0625%–0.125%) or ropivacaine (0.1%–0.2%) with fentanyl (1–3 mcg/mL) or sufentanil (0.3–0.5 mcg/mL) at infusion rates of 8 to 12 mL/hour are commonly used. Lower concentrations may be effective as long as adequate spread is achieved. However, maintaining an adequate sensory level with lower concentrations may necessitate an increased infusion rate of 10 to 15 mL/hour. In most women, this dilute concentration is associated with minimal motor block, although the block will become denser as the infusion is maintained over time. A higher concentration may be needed as labor intensifies or in women who experience greater pain.

The epidural infusion should be maintained as the parturient transitions to second-stage labor provided the block is stable and effective while preserving adequate motor function. The ideal block provides effective analgesia for uterine contractions, dense analgesia of the perineum for delivery, and little motor block. If motor block hinders pushing or if sensory block prevents the parturient from sensing contractions and therefore effectively prevents pushing, the epidural infusion may be decreased or changed to a more dilute solution. Additionally, the block can be supplemented during second-stage labor if additional perineal analgesia is required. This can be accomplished by injecting a relatively large 6- to 10-mL volume of bupivacaine 0.25%, lidocaine (1%–2%), or 2-chloroprocaine 2%. Fentanyl (50–100 mcg) can be added to the aforementioned bolus to further enhance analgesia. Instrumented vaginal delivery generally requires a denser block, in which case lidocaine 2% with epinephrine 1:200,000 can be used with or without the addition of fentanyl.

Patient-Controlled Epidural Analgesia

Patient-controlled epidural analgesia (PCEA) is an alternate technique that allows the parturient to self-administer bolus doses as needed. It is normally initiated after analgesia has been established with an epidural. When compared with continuous epidural infusion, PCEA has several distinct advantages.[134] It reduces the number of unscheduled interventions required by the anesthetist, the total dose of drug used, and lower extremity motor block, all without sacrificing effective analgesia. Maternal satisfaction would be expected to increase due to enhanced control, but this has not been consistently shown to be the case. The best combination of variables (e.g., background infusion rate, bolus dose, and lockout interval) has yet to be established. The use of a background infusion likely reduces breakthrough pain but has been shown to result in an increase in total local anesthetic used.[135] Background infusion rates of bupivacaine (0.125%) or ropivacaine (0.2%) between 2 and 10 mL/hour have been used effectively. Bolus doses greater than 5 mL may provide superior analgesia compared with smaller boluses.[134] PCEA may also presumably limit the number of epidural catheter disconnections and reconnections necessary to manually bolus a catheter, hence reducing the potential exposure to pathogens and catheter contamination.

Programmed Intermittent Epidural Boluses

There is evidence to indicate that there may be more widespread distribution of local anesthetic solution within the epidural space when large volumes are injected as a bolus compared with a slow infusion.[136] Automated epidural infusion pumps capable of administering programmed intermittent boluses have been recently introduced. With this technique, a bolus dose is automatically administered at regular intervals as opposed to a continuous infusion. Optimal dosing regimens are being studied at this time, but some evidence indicates that larger boluses timed more widely apart appear to increase effectiveness. Wong et al.[137] found that extending the programmed intermittent bolus interval and volume from 15 minutes to 60 minutes, and 2.5 mL to 10 mL, respectively, decreased overall bupivacaine consumption without decreasing patient comfort or satisfaction.

Combined Spinal-Epidural

The combined spinal-epidural (CSE) is a commonly used technique that many practitioners feel provides superior analgesia for labor and vaginal delivery. A CSE combines positive attributes from both techniques while minimizing their respective disadvantages. Analgesia obtained from the spinal component is uniformly effective and has a rapid onset. The epidural catheter allows the analgesia to be prolonged as required and provides the ability to convert the block to a surgical level if operative delivery is indicated.

Several methods have been described for performing the block, including the early technique of spinal needle insertion and removal immediately followed by epidural insertion at the same or different level. Most practitioners now use the needle-through-needle technique in which the epidural space is identified with an epidural needle

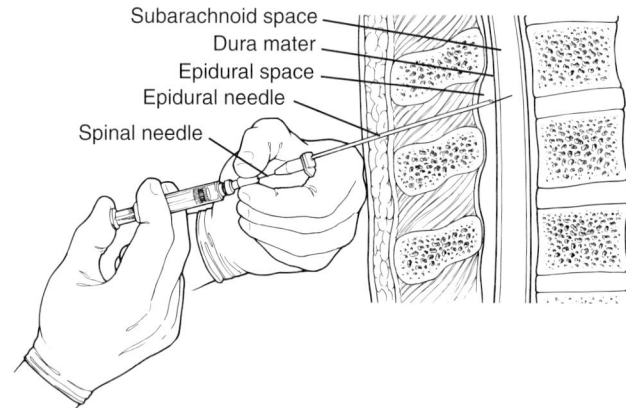

Fig. 51.6 The proper orientation of both the spinal and epidural needles during the needle-through-needle combined spinal-epidural (CSE) technique. (From Birnbach DJ, et al. *Textbook of Obstetric Anesthesia.* Philadelphia: Churchill Livingstone; 2000:166.)

followed by placement of a longer small-gauge spinal needle through the existing epidural needle. Care must be taken to avoid displacing the spinal needle during injection. The spinal needle is then withdrawn completely, and an epidural catheter is then inserted. The needle-through-needle technique provides the additional benefit of confirming proper epidural needle location. If the epidural needle is not inserted in the midline of the epidural space, the subsequently placed spinal needle will not likely penetrate the dura and CSF flow will not be obtained. Fig. 51.6 shows the proper orientation of both the spinal and the epidural needles during a CSE technique.

The spinal component of a CSE can be dosed with either a lipid-soluble narcotic alone or in combination with isobaric bupivacaine. Narcotics are commonly used alone in early first-stage labor. For example, fentanyl (15–25 mcg) or sufentanil (10 mcg) in the subarachnoid space can provide analgesia for up to 2 hours with no motor block. Local anesthetic is often combined with the narcotic in late first-stage labor to produce a rapid-onset analgesia with minimal motor block. Off-label intrathecal administration of isobaric bupivacaine 0.25% 1 mL (2.5 mg) combined with fentanyl or sufentanil provides a denser analgesia than narcotic alone. Consideration should be given to initiating an epidural infusion before resolution of the spinal component to avoid the need for bolus dosing the epidural catheter.

An additional approach that has gained popularity among anesthesia personnel is the dural puncture epidural (DPE) technique. This approach is similar to the aforementioned CSE; however, there is no subsequent intrathecal dosing after confirmed puncture of the dura with a 25-gauge spinal needle. Following puncture of the dura, the spinal needle is removed, and the epidural catheter is subsequently threaded into the epidural space via the Tuohy needle. The epidural catheter is then dosed in standard fashion. Chau et al.[138] found that the DPE technique provided enhanced block quality versus the standard epidural resulting in significantly less provider top-up boluses, decreased incidence of unilateral blockade, and improved sacral coverage. Additionally, compared to the CSE technique, there were significantly decreased incidence of side effects that included maternal hypotension, pruritus, and uterine hypertonus.[138]

Spinal Analgesia

In contemporary practice, a single-shot spinal is rarely an appropriate anesthetic choice for a patient in labor due to its finite duration and lack of flexibility. The technique can often be performed rapidly, and it is generally reserved for multiparous patients in advanced second-stage

labor when delivery is clearly imminent or for those exhibiting poor control who can then have an epidural placed with better cooperation. It is also suitable in parturients who have labored without anesthesia and require an instrumented vaginal delivery or those who have delivered without anesthesia and require an extensive perineal repair. In rare cases, multiple single-shot spinal anesthetics, placed every 2 to 3 hours, have been used in parturients with conditions that preclude epidural placement such as a previous history of spinal surgery in which the epidural space has been surgically obliterated.

CSA using a macrobore epidural catheter is an option in certain high-risk patients such as the extremely morbidly obese, those with previous spinal surgery or deformity, or those whose dura has been inadvertently punctured with the epidural needle. A CSA may be particularly indicated in a high-risk parturient after failed attempts at a conventional neuraxial anesthetic due to the increased morbidity and mortality associated with general anesthesia. The morbidly obese parturient is at greater risk for both cesarean delivery and failed regional technique. To perform a CSA, an epidural needle is used to identify the subarachnoid space, and the epidural catheter is then intentionally threaded into the subarachnoid space. This spinal catheter can then be dosed as a spinal anesthetic using isobaric bupivacaine (0.25%) in 0.5- to 1-mL increments for labor analgesia. A CSA is not considered a first-line technique because it is clearly associated with an increased risk of postdural puncture headache (PDPH). There is evidence to indicate that a catheter left in situ in the subarachnoid space for at least 12 hours results in fewer cases of PDPH.[139] It is postulated that the epidural catheter creates a localized inflammatory response where it passes through the dura, which results in decreased CSF leakage when the catheter is ultimately removed. However, in a subsequent trial of 97 patients with accidental dural puncture (ADP) who were randomized to either a CSA or a repeat of the block, no difference in the incidence of headache or blood patch was found.[140] If a CSA is used, block level must be carefully monitored and all caregivers in contact with these patients should be notified that the epidural catheter is actually subarachnoid to prevent accidental overdose. It is also necessary to clearly label the catheter as a spinal catheter.

Microcatheters (27–32 gauge) were developed for use in the early 1990s specifically for this purpose but were found to result in an unacceptably high incidence of cauda equina syndrome.[97] The low-flow velocity through the very small-diameter catheter resulted in poor mixing of the lidocaine local anesthetic that was used at the time, creating a pool of concentrated local anesthetic in close proximity to the nerve roots. Microcatheters were subsequently removed from the market by the Food and Drug Administration (FDA).[141]

Regional Opioids for Labor Analgesia

The combination of dilute local anesthetics with low-dose opioids allows for the reduced dose of both agents that ultimately results in decreased motor block while preserving acceptable analgesia and minimizing side effects. The agents work by binding to separate and distinct receptors. Local anesthetics work at the nerve axon, whereas neuraxial opioids bind to receptors in the substantia gelatinosa within the dorsal horn of the spinal cord. These receptors are stimulated by the administration of opioids via the subarachnoid or epidural routes. Epidurally administered opioids are believed to be absorbed into the CSF, and ultimately the spinal cord, to exert their action on spinal opioid receptors. When opioids are administered within the epidural or subarachnoid space, they are known to possess a ceiling effect, whereby increasing the dose beyond conventional regimens does not result in an increased duration or quality of analgesia. Common side effects are, however, more severe and prolonged at the increased dose levels.

Side effects of epidural and subarachnoid opioid administration include respiratory depression, itching, urinary retention, nausea, and vomiting. IV doses of an opioid antagonist (naloxone) or agonist-antagonist (nalbuphine) are effective at reducing or eliminating the undesirable effects without antagonizing the analgesia and are often more effective against pruritus than an antihistamine.

Fentanyl. When used in combination with local anesthetics, fentanyl in epidural doses of 50 to 100 mcg and subarachnoid doses of 10 to 25 mcg produces good to excellent analgesia in 5 to 10 minutes. Administration of these doses, repeated as often as every 90 minutes in women in labor, has been shown not to affect Apgar scores, umbilical cord blood analysis, or neurobehavioral test results for up to 24 hours after delivery.[142-144] Fentanyl 100 mcg in the epidural space has been shown to be undetectable in breast milk.[145] When opioids are used alone, much higher doses are needed to provide labor analgesia, and even these higher doses are not entirely effective during the second stage of labor. When analgesia from fentanyl administration is at its peak, serum fentanyl levels are lower than those known to produce equivalent analgesia after IV administration. In fact, most women have undetectable plasma fentanyl levels after receiving 100 mcg of epidural fentanyl.[146]

The duration of action of fentanyl in the epidural space is 60 to 140 minutes. Because fentanyl is so much more lipid soluble than morphine, it is absorbed into neural tissue faster, therefore it has a faster onset and shorter duration of action when compared with morphine. As a result, the cephalad migration of fentanyl is much less than that of morphine and is associated with a significantly lower incidence of CNS side effects. This is likely why respiratory depression has rarely been reported following subarachnoid or epidural administration of fentanyl in conventional doses.

For continuous epidural infusion, fentanyl concentrations up to 2.5 mcg/mL of local anesthetic can be used without adversely affecting neonatal respiration or neurobehavioral scores.[147] Bupivacaine (up to 0.125%) or ropivacaine (up to 0.2%) with 1 to 2 mcg/mL of fentanyl is a widely used combination.[148]

Sufentanil. Sufentanil (5–10 mcg) can be combined with bupivacaine or ropivacaine to initiate analgesia for first-stage labor. When added to a continuous epidural infusion the concentration is normally 0.3 to 0.5 mcg/mL. Because sufentanil is commercially prepared in a concentration of 50 mcg/mL and clinically relevant doses used in neuraxial anesthesia are significantly lower, care must be taken when using sufentanil to avoid medication errors.

Morphine. Morphine is more ionized and therefore less lipid soluble as compared with fentanyl or sufentanil. When administered in the epidural or subarachnoid space it has a slow onset of action of 30 to 60 minutes and, when used alone for labor analgesia, is not associated with a high degree of maternal satisfaction. It is this pharmacologic profile that makes it a poor choice for use in labor analgesia. However, morphine is uniquely suited for use as a postoperative analgesic when neuraxial anesthesia is utilized for cesarean delivery (see next section). Optimal analgesia and less pruritis are produced with an intrathecal dose of 0.15 mg.

ANESTHESIA FOR CESAREAN DELIVERY

Birth by cesarean delivery now accounts for over 30% of all deliveries, and it is performed over 1.5 million times annually in the United States.[149,150] Common indications include cephalopelvic disproportion, nonreassuring fetal status, arrest of dilation, malpresentation, prematurity, prior cesarean delivery, and prior uterine surgery. The choice of anesthesia depends on maternal status, urgency of the surgery, condition of the fetus, and the patient's desires. This fact highlights the need

for strong communication between the obstetrician, nursing staff, and anesthesia provider. The use of neuraxial anesthesia for cesarean delivery has increased dramatically along with a commensurate decrease in the use of general anesthesia.[151] Neuraxial anesthesia has significant advantages, including decreased risk of mortality from failed intubation and aspiration of gastric contents, better neonatal outcomes from the use of less depressant agents, and the ability of the mother to be awake for the delivery. Evidence also suggests that general anesthetic agents are associated with apoptosis of fetal brain neurons in animal models.[152]

Regardless of the anesthetic technique used, left uterine displacement should be provided as soon as possible. The table should be rolled to the left or a wedge placed under the right hip of the patient to shift the uterus off the inferior vena cava and abdominal aorta, thereby preserving fetal oxygenation. Fetuses delivered of mothers with left uterine displacement have a lower incidence of CNS depression and acidosis than those delivered of mothers in the supine position.[153] In an awake parturient with a neuraxial anesthetic, it is not a requirement to secure the upper extremities to the armboards. The lower extremities, however, should be secured to prevent unintentional movement from the table.

Blood loss during cesarean delivery is usually between 500 and 1000 mL. However, the reported range of blood loss is great—in one study, from 164 to 1438 mL.[154] Many factors affect the volume of blood lost during cesarean delivery, including surgical time, surgical technique, blood pressure, fetal lie, fetal size, placental implantation, maternal coagulation status, and the ability of the uterus to contract after the placenta has been delivered. Visual estimation of blood loss is inaccurate and often complicated by the presence of large volumes of amniotic fluid and variably saturated sponges. Normal amniotic fluid volume is approximately 700 mL (range 300–1400 mL) and should be accounted for when estimating blood loss.[155]

Neuraxial Anesthesia for Cesarean Delivery

A dermatome level of T4 is required to provide effective anesthesia for cesarean delivery. This level of block can result in profound sympathectomy that frequently causes maternal hypotension and, if untreated, fetal compromise. Common measures to minimize hypotension include left uterine displacement, IV fluid administration, and vasopressor use.

A nonparticulate antacid should be administered preoperatively for aspiration prophylaxis. An H_2-receptor antagonist and metoclopramide can also be used preoperatively to increase gastric pH and enhance emptying. Prior to conducting spinal anesthesia for cesarean delivery, ondansetron administration should be considered for hypotensive prophylaxis and for the prevention of intraoperative nausea.[46] Anxiolytics are normally not administered preoperatively to minimize fetal depression. Prophylactically administered antibiotics have been traditionally withheld until cord clamping in an effort to prevent fetal transmission and the obscuring of any subsequent neonatal sepsis workup. However, antibiotics administered preincision have been shown to decrease the surgical site infection rate from 6.4% to 2.5%, making the practice much more common.[156] Requirements for standard monitoring remain the same as with any anesthetic; however, blood pressure should be assessed at least every minute for the first 20 minutes or until the patient's condition has stabilized. Left uterine displacement is an essential aspect of positioning to preserve maternal cardiac output and uteroplacental exchange.

The routine supplemental use of oxygen in the absence of preexisting fetal compromise or maternal hypoxemia has not been shown to be of any maternal or neonatal benefit in spite of its common practice.[157] Although supplemental oxygen may reduce postoperative nausea and vomiting after general anesthesia, its administration during cesarean delivery with neuraxial anesthesia does not decrease the incidence or severity of intraoperative or postoperative nausea or vomiting.[158] Oxygen administration during elective cesarean delivery appears to increase oxygen-free radical activity in both the mother and fetus. However, the intervention was neither beneficial nor harmful to the neonate's short-term clinical outcome as assessed by Apgar scores.[159] Consideration, however, should be given to the use of end tidal CO_2 monitoring made possible by the use of sampling nasal cannula for those patients susceptible to intraoperative respiratory compromise or those who have been administered IV sedation.

Spinal Anesthesia for Cesarean Delivery

Single-shot spinal anesthesia has become the most commonly used anesthetic technique for cesarean delivery because it offers many distinct advantages. This technique has a rapid onset of action, provides a more dense block, and requires less local anesthetic when compared with epidural anesthesia. Its simplicity and rapid onset make it suitable for all but the most emergent cesarean deliveries when compared with general anesthesia. It is considered an economical anesthetic as its rapid onset functions to decrease overall operating room times. Drawbacks include its fixed duration of action and rapid onset of sympathectomy with resultant hypotension. Hyperbaric bupivacaine (0.75% 13 mg) is effective in 95% of patients (ED_{95}) and provides 90 to 120 minutes of surgical anesthesia. In practice, neither the patient's height, weight, nor BMI correlates to the ultimate block level obtained.[160] The compound curvature of the spine in the supine position serves to limit the upward spread of the block when hyperbaric local anesthetics are used. A series of studies has determined that decreasing the bupivacaine dose results in less hypotension but is associated with an increased risk of intraoperative pain, a shorter duration of effective anesthesia, and a slower onset.[161]

When a spinal anesthetic is used to produce the T4 block needed for cesarean delivery, hypotension has been shown to occur in up to 80% of patients despite left uterine displacement.[162] Maternal hypotension results mainly in nausea and vomiting but, if severe and untreated, may lead to a decreased level of consciousness, uteroplacental hypoperfusion, and cardiovascular collapse. The goal should be to prevent and effectively treat hypotension before these complications arise.

Administering crystalloids to increase intravascular volume has traditionally been used in an effort to prevent hypotension but has been shown to be minimally effective, possibly due to its rapid redistribution from the intravascular space.[163,164] A multicenter, randomized, double-blinded CAESARean delivery surgical techniques (CAESAR) trial demonstrated the efficacy of a mixed 500-mL 6% hydroxyethyl starch (HES) 130/0.4 + 500 mL Ringer lactate (RL) preload in significantly reducing hypotension, compared to a 1 liter of RL preload, without adverse effects on coagulation and neonatal outcomes in healthy parturients undergoing caesarean delivery under spinal anaesthesia.[165] Despite these findings, the routine use of HES continues to be debated because of its disadvantages, including cost, potential allergic reactions, and pruritus.

The timing of the fluid administration has also been investigated comparing preloading (prior to anesthetic placement) with coloading (given rapidly at the time of intrathecal injection). It appears that crystalloid coloading is somewhat effective compared with crystalloid preloading, provided the infusion rate and volume are high enough during the first 5 to 7 minutes after spinal injection when the sympathetic block is being established.[166] On the contrary, the timing of a colloid administration does not appear to change its degree of effectiveness.[167] Current evidence suggests that combining a prophylactic vasopressor regimen with crystalloid coloading is the best method of

preventing maternal hypotension after the initiation of spinal anesthesia. Crystalloid preloading is clinically ineffective and thus should no longer be used.

Ephedrine and phenylephrine are vasopressors commonly used to treat maternal hypotension. Ephedrine is a synthetic, nonselective, noncatecholamine sympathomimetic. Doses of 5 to 15 mg IV are used to treat acute decreases in blood pressure. The duration of ephedrine's cardiovascular effects varies with the dose given. The effect of a 5- or 10-mg IV dose usually persists for 5 minutes. Tachyphylaxis can occur with repeated administration of small doses, resulting in a noticeably reduced clinical effect after subsequent dosing. Ephedrine is metabolized in the liver, and up to 40% is excreted unchanged by the kidneys. It has an elimination half-life of 3 hours.

Ephedrine causes direct β-stimulation and indirect α-stimulation through the release of endogenous norepinephrine. It has long been used in obstetric anesthesia because it was thought to impact uterine artery blood flow less than direct-acting vasoactive drugs in pregnant ewes.[168] However, evidence suggests that ephedrine crosses the placental barrier and stimulates fetal β-adrenergic receptors, raising the fetal metabolic rate and results in a depression of fetal acid-base status.[169] Although the ultimate clinical relevance of this effect has yet to be defined, many practitioners may administer phenylephrine as a first-line vasopressor to treat maternal hypotension.[47] Hypotension is a primary cause of intraoperative nausea and vomiting in the early period after spinal anesthesia. Hypotension may lead to cerebral hypoperfusion, which is thought to activate the vomiting center. It has also been suggested that hypotension results in gastrointestinal hypoperfusion with the subsequent release of emetogenic substances such as serotonin. Optimum use of vasopressors to prevent hypotension significantly reduces the incidence of intraoperative nausea and vomiting.[170]

Phenylephrine is a direct-acting α_1-adrenergic agonist that results in vasoconstriction and increased peripheral vascular resistance. It can result in a reflex bradycardia with a subsequent decrease in cardiac output. Based on early animal studies, α-agonists were thought to decrease uterine artery blood flow,[168] but phenylephrine has been shown to be safe for the treatment of maternal hypotension during regional anesthesia when given in the conventional dose range.[171] Neonatal blood gas values and Apgar scores remain within normal limits in all healthy subjects after the administration of 80-mcg or 100-mcg bolus doses of phenylephrine.[172] Phenylephrine can be administered by either bolus dosing or continuous infusion; however, the optimal regimen for each has yet to be determined. Many practitioners select their vasopressor based on the assessment of the parturient's HR. There is evidence to indicate that during phenylephrine infusion there is a dose-dependent decrease in cardiac output that parallels a decrease in HR.[173] When the HR is at baseline or above, phenylephrine may be used. When the HR is below baseline, ephedrine will increase the blood pressure and HR without further reductions in cardiac output. A 2012 systematic review supports the favorable effects of phenylephrine over ephedrine as for treating maternal hypotension for parturients undergoing cesarean delivery.[174]

Maternal complaints of nausea, vomiting, and visceral pain occur occasionally even in the presence of an adequate T4 block. It is common practice to add opioids to hyperbaric bupivacaine for cesarean delivery spinal anesthesia to provide additional intraoperative and postoperative analgesia without affecting the block height. Intraoperative block quality can be significantly improved with the addition of fentanyl (10–20 mcg) or sufentanil (2.5–5 mcg). The onset of these lipid-soluble opioids is 5 to 10 minutes with an effective duration of 60 to 90 minutes. In addition to either fentanyl or sufentanil, preservative-free morphine can be added to provide long-acting postoperative analgesia. Morphine has an onset of action of 60 to 90 minutes that coincides with the effective duration of fentanyl or sufentanil such that, when used in combination, the patient has uninterrupted opioid analgesia intraoperatively and for 12 to 18 hours postoperatively.

After the placenta has been delivered, oxytocin should be given as directed by the obstetrician. Pitocin is the clinically available synthetic equivalent of oxytocin, a naturally occurring hormone synthesized in the supraoptic and paraventricular nuclei of the hypothalamus. In the mature uterus of a pregnant woman, oxytocin causes an increase in the frequency and strength of uterine contractions. Endogenous oxytocin release occurs with stimulation of the cervix, vagina, and breasts.

The half-life of oxytocin varies from 4 to 17 minutes. It is metabolized by liver, kidney, and plasma enzyme pathways in the parturient. Commercially available preparations of oxytocin contain a preservative that may cause systolic and especially diastolic hypotension, flushing, and tachycardia when infused at high doses.[175] The amount of oxytocin added to the IV solution should be tailored to the volume of solution remaining in the bag, the flow rate of the IV, and the patient's condition. If an unusually large blood loss results in hypotension, and fluid resuscitation is required, it may be helpful to infuse the oxytocin at an appropriate rate and to start a second IV line for administering fluid volume at a rapid rate. If the solution with the added oxytocin is infused rapidly enough to replace intravascular volume, it is possible that the high dose of oxytocin may cause further hypotension. In some cases, the obstetrician may choose to administer oxytocin directly into the uterine muscle to maximize its effect.

Transversus abdominis plane blocks or quadratus lumborum blocks can be successfully administered to provide postoperative analgesia in patients who are not candidates for intrathecal morphine, when neuraxial anesthesia is contraindicated, or in those who receive general anesthesia. Blanco et al. found that patients in the quadratus lumborum block group received significantly less postoperative morphine at 12, 24, and 48 hours postpartum as compared to the transversus abdominis plane block group.[176] Regarding transversus abdominis plane blocks, sensory nerves that supply the anterior abdominal wall course through the fascial plane between the internal oblique and the transversus abdominis muscles. Local anesthetics injected into this plane anesthetize sensory impulses from the anterior abdominal wall and are effective in relieving pain associated with a Pfannenstiel incision.[177] A suggested technique for spinal anesthesia for cesarean delivery is outlined in Box 51.2.

BOX 51.2 Spinal Anesthesia Management for Cesarean Delivery

- Consider timely administration of a nonparticulate antacid, H_2-receptor antagonist, and/or metoclopramide preoperatively
- Administer an intravenous preload (colloid) or coload (crystalloid or colloid)
- Apply standard monitors and record preprocedure vital signs
- Record preprocedure fetal heart tones
- Consider oxygen administration
- Perform lumbar puncture at L3-L4
- Sitting or lateral position
- Small-gauge (24- or 25-gauge) noncutting needle (e.g., Sprotte, Whitacre, Pencan)
- Hyperbaric bupivacaine 15 mg in 8.25% dextrose (12–15 mg)
  - Add fentanyl 10–20 mcg for intraoperative analgesia
  - Add preservative-free morphine 150 mcg for postoperative analgesia
- Supine position with left uterine displacement
- Monitor blood pressure every 1 min at least until birth
- Confirm block level (T4) prior to surgical start
- Treat hypotension (e.g., phenylephrine, ephedrine)
- Administer oxytocin as directed at delivery

Epidural Anesthesia for Cesarean Delivery

An epidural inserted in the operating room for an elective cesarean delivery is not often the technique of choice because it has a slower onset and requires a higher milligram dose of local anesthetic to achieve a surgical level of anesthesia when compared with a spinal anesthetic. However, an epidural catheter does provide the flexibility to extend the duration of the anesthetic when a prolonged surgical time is anticipated. The slower onset sympathectomy associated with an epidural may make treating the resultant hypotension easier and can be of value in patients who are particularly susceptible to abrupt changes in blood pressure. Attention to correct catheter placement and dosing safety is required when this technique is used due to the increased volume and concentration of local anesthetic needed to obtain a surgical block. After a negative test dose and careful aspiration for blood and CSF, lidocaine 2% with epinephrine 1:200,000 can be used when dosed in 3- to 5-mL increments. A total volume of approximately 15 to 20 mL is required to obtain a T4 level.

When a parturient with an epidural in place for labor analgesia requires a cesarean delivery, the indwelling epidural catheter should be used to provide surgical anesthesia. Because larger volumes of more concentrated local anesthetic are required to produce surgical anesthesia, and unrecognized epidural catheter movement into either the intrathecal or intravascular space is always a possibility, careful aspiration and incremental dosing is again important. The selection of local anesthetic is largely determined by the urgency required for delivery. The addition of sodium bicarbonate 1 mEq/10 mL to lidocaine 2% with epinephrine 1:200,000 will hasten the onset of anesthesia when a rapid conversion to surgical anesthesia is necessary. Commercially prepared lidocaine containing epinephrine has a low pH to preserve the epinephrine. The addition of sodium bicarbonate immediately prior to use increases the biologically active nonionized fraction of drug.[178] This combination normally results in approximately 90 to 120 minutes of surgical anesthesia. Sodium bicarbonate cannot be added to bupivacaine as it results in precipitation when the pH is raised. 2-chloroprocaine is rapidly metabolized by ester hydrolysis and, as a result, is associated with a very low incidence of toxicity; it can be used to rapidly convert a labor epidural to a surgical anesthetic with little concern of toxicity but will likely require intraoperative augmentation because it has an effective duration of approximately 45 minutes. The efficacy and duration of epidural morphine analgesia is diminished when administered after 2-chloroprocaine. The precise mechanism of this interaction is unknown but may be the result of opioid receptor antagonism.[100]

In the presence of a well-functioning epidural used for labor analgesia, the total volume required to raise the block level from the existing T10 to the required T4 is approximately 10 to 15 mL. Conversion of a labor epidural to a surgical anesthetic can be initiated in the labor room in an emergency. Careful attention should be directed toward the existing analgesia level, incremental dosing, and maternal vital signs while in the labor room. On arrival to the operating room, the block level can be assessed, and additional doses provided as required during the surgical preparation.

Breakthrough pain in labor requiring multiple epidural doses is a significant predictor of subsequent failure of surgical anesthesia and highlights the need to replace inadequately functioning epidural catheters before an unplanned cesarean is required.[179] Efforts should be directed toward avoiding the situation of a failed epidural in the operating room. This includes early recognition and replacement of poorly performing labor epidurals. However, if an inadequate epidural is identified in the operating room, and the fetal status allows, consideration

BOX 51.3 Converting an Epidural in Use for Labor Analgesia to Cesarean Anesthetic

- Consider timely administration of a nonparticulate antacid, H_2-receptor antagonist, and/or metoclopramide preoperatively
- Discontinue continuous epidural infusion
- Administer an intravenous coload (crystalloid)
- Apply standard monitors and record preprocedure vital signs
- Record preprocedure fetal heart tones
- Consider oxygen administration
- Place in supine position with left uterine displacement
- Carefully aspirate epidural catheter for blood and cerebrospinal fluid
- Administer lidocaine 2% with epinephrine 1:200,000 and sodium bicarbonate 1 mEq/10 mL local anesthetic (total dose 10–15 mL)
- Administer 3 mL and observe maternal heart rate for 60 seconds and level of block for 3–5 min
- If no sign of subarachnoid or intravascular injection, administer 3–5 mL and observe for 3–5 min
- Treat hypotension (e.g., phenylephrine, ephedrine)
- Confirm block level (T4) prior to surgical start
- Administer 3 mg preservative-free morphine via the epidural catheter after the umbilical cord is clamped for postoperative analgesia
- Administer oxytocin as directed at delivery

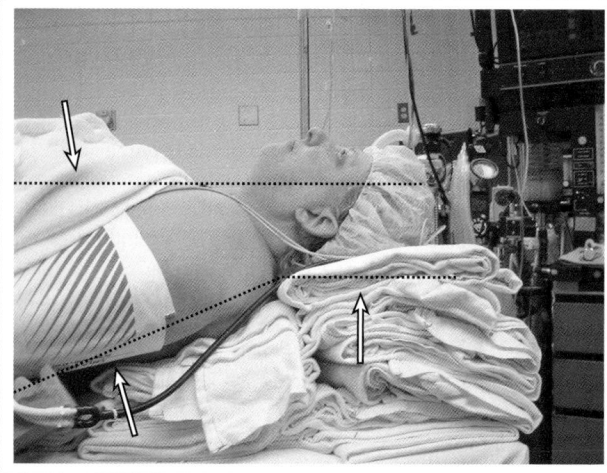

Fig. 51.7 Positioning for the obese parturient for laryngoscopy. (From Chestnut DH, et al. *Chestnut's Obstetric Anesthesia.* 6th ed. Philadelphia: Elsevier; 2020:701.)

should be given toward replacing the epidural to a different interspace or replacing the epidural with a CSE technique in which local anesthetic medication is injected with a reduced dose and the epidural is subsequently used to augment the level as needed. In the scenario of a recently dosed inadequate epidural, a superimposed conventionally dosed single-shot spinal anesthetic can often produce an unpredictable, and frequently higher than expected, block level. Alternatively, the inadequate epidural can be given time to absorb and resolve before a single-shot spinal. Ultimately, a general anesthetic may be required in select circumstances. A suggested technique for converting an epidural that is used for labor analgesia to one that provides anesthesia for cesarean delivery is provided in Box 51.3.

Combined Spinal-Epidural for Cesarean Delivery

As with labor analgesia, the CSE technique for cesarean delivery can provide several advantages over either technique when used alone. A lower spinal dose can be used, resulting in a decreased incidence of hypotension, whereas the epidural can be augmented to increase the block height or prolong the duration if necessary. The technique, however, is not without its disadvantages. Because the spinal component is injected prior to placement of the epidural catheter, if difficulty is encountered with catheter placement, the patient could remain in the sitting position for a prolonged time, resulting in lower block height. The presence of a dense spinal blockade makes evaluating subsequent test doses for subarachnoid injection less reliable. If a lower spinal dose is used and the block is not adequate for surgery, subsequent epidural dosing will delay the start of surgery. Some practitioners advocate the CSE technique after attempts with a spinal have been unsuccessful. An epidural needle has a larger diameter and may be less likely to deflect from its intended direction around dense ligaments or bone.

General Anesthesia for Cesarean Delivery

General anesthesia may be indicated despite the numerous disadvantages of the technique when compared with regional anesthesia. General anesthesia allows for better control of the airway and

improved hemodynamic control, making it useful in cases of existing or expected hypovolemic shock or maternal cardiac disease. General anesthesia is a necessary choice when a neuraxial anesthetic is not in place and a surgical delivery is urgent enough to preclude its placement or when contraindications, such as patient refusal or coagulopathy, are present. It is also an alternative when a failed neuraxial technique occurs. Neuraxial techniques have progressively eclipsed general anesthesia for use in cesarean delivery primarily in an effort to reduce maternal mortality resulting from airway complications.[151] However, general anesthesia is likely safer today compared to the 1970s and 1980s due to the use of supraglottic airway devices, videolaryngoscopes, and difficult airway algorithms.[180] Practical steps to decrease the use of general anesthesia include referral and evaluation of high-risk parturients early in pregnancy to optimize their medical condition and plan for anesthetic management, considering early neuraxial anesthetic placement to ensure proper functioning, and promptly replacing epidural catheters that are providing suboptimal labor analgesia.[181]

The difficult airway. An airway evaluation is an important part of the preparation for anesthesia in any patient and even more so in the parturient. Airway problems occur with more frequency in obstetric patients compared to nonpregnant patients; failure to intubate has been reported to occur as frequently as 1 in 250 obstetric patients.[182] This is true in part because of the soft tissue edema often present in the hypopharynx. A patient's airway may also significantly change during her labor and, as such, should be evaluated again prior to an operative delivery. Breast enlargement and cephalad displacement of the thorax can make maneuvering the laryngoscope into the mouth difficult, necessitating the use of a short-handled laryngoscope. Placement of a rolled towel along the thoracic spine or under the shoulders helps to elevate the chest off the operating table. This makes it possible to extend the neck and position the head more optimally, facilitating insertion of the laryngoscope blade and improving visualization of the glottis. The external auditory meatus can be aligned with the sternal notch by utilizing a ramp built with blankets. This position can facilitate oral tracheal intubation in the obese parturient. Positioning of the obese parturient for laryngoscopy is shown in Fig. 51.7.

Airway difficulties resulting in a failure to oxygenate and ventilate remain an avoidable cause of anesthesia-related mortality in the obstetric population.[183] Although rapid sequence induction is the technique most commonly used to minimize the risk of gastric

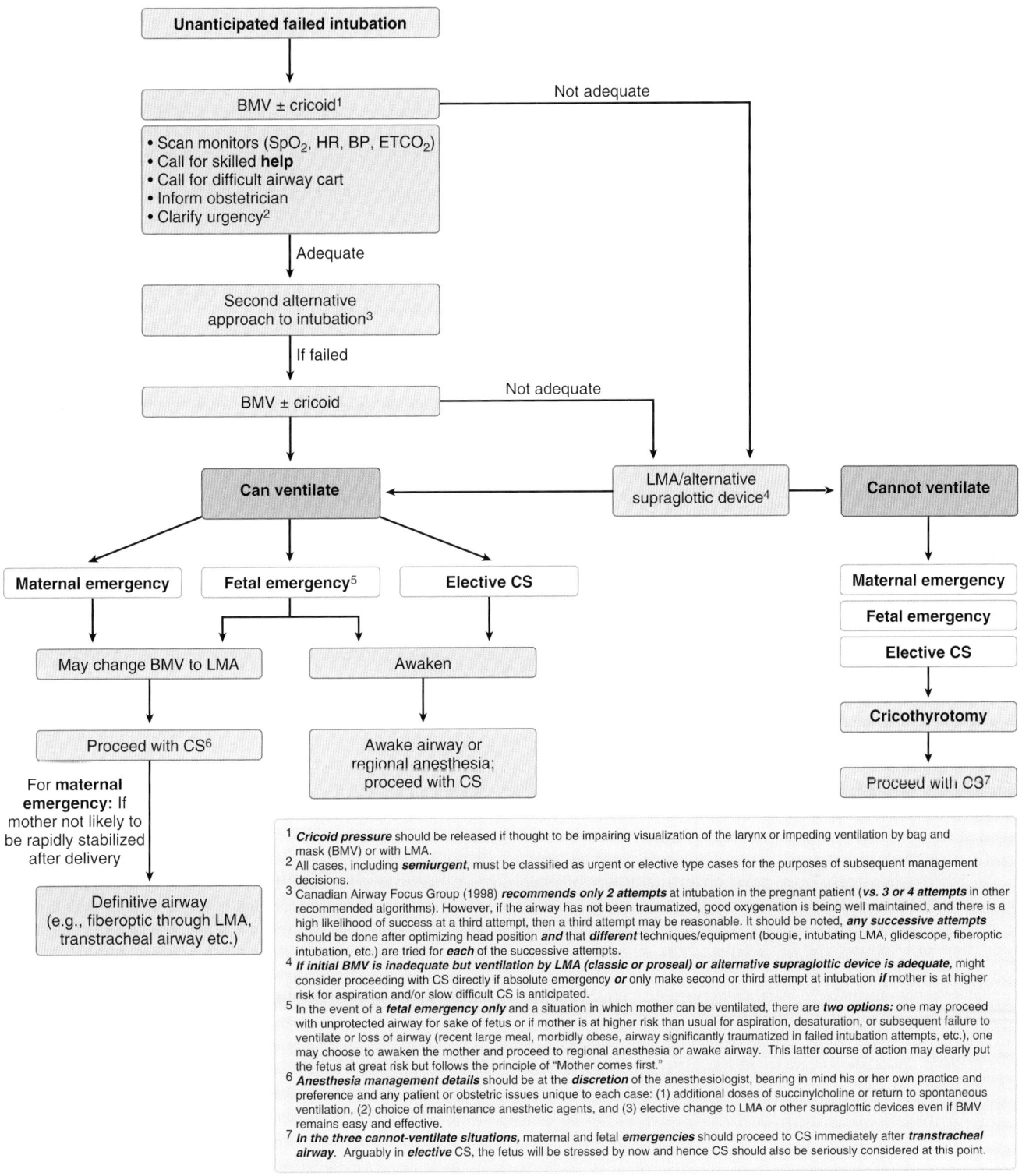

Fig. 51.8 Algorithm for management of unanticipated difficult airway in obstetric patients. *BMV,* Bag-mask ventilation; *BP,* blood pressure; *CS,* cesarean section; *ETCO2,* end tidal carbon dioxide; *HR,* heart rate; *LMA,* laryngeal mask airway; *SpO2,* oxygen saturation. (From Miller RD, et al. *Miller's Anesthesia.* 9th ed. Philadelphia: Elsevier; 2020:2024.)

aspiration during induction of general anesthesia, it is *not* normally indicated if the laryngoscopist has doubts about being able to intubate the patient. In such a case, an alternative method, such as awake intubation, may be necessary. Blind nasal intubation should be performed cautiously, if at all, in the parturient, who commonly has swollen nasal mucosa that are prone to bleeding. The anesthetist should be familiar with and be able to perform interventions as outlined in the algorithm in Fig. 51.8.

Induction. Induction of general anesthesia requires a rapid sequence technique using cricoid pressure after denitrogenation and preoxygenation has occurred, which takes an estimated 3 minutes. The standard induction agent in the healthy parturient is propofol (2–2.5 mg/kg). As expected, propofol produces neonatal depression but is rapidly redistributed and cleared from the neonate, resulting in a rapid emergence.[184,185] Etomidate (0.3 mg/kg) can be considered for patients who present with unstable hemodynamics. Ketamine (1 mg/kg) is especially useful in patients who have active airway disease or patients presenting hemodynamically unstable. Ketamine has been associated with lower analgesic demands during the first 24 hours postoperatively.[186] The indirect sympathomimetic effects of ketamine help to support blood pressure until adequate intravascular volume can be replaced.

The induction of anesthesia should be delayed until all preparation for surgery is complete and the surgical staff indicates they are ready. The operating surgeon should be instructed to delay incision until confirmation of correct endotracheal tube placement is made. The incision is only made after verification by capnography, auscultation of breath sounds over the chest, and bilateral chest expansion. The reasoning behind delaying induction until the surgical team is ready is to minimize the total fetal exposure to depressant drugs.

Succinylcholine (1–1.5 mg/kg) remains the muscle relaxant of choice during induction of general anesthesia in the parturient. When succinylcholine is contraindicated, a fast-acting nondepolarizer such as rocuronium (0.6–1.2 mg/kg) can be administered, or an awake intubation may be attempted. Although intubation can be accomplished quickly with a fast onset nondepolarizing muscle relaxant, the duration of action will be longer than with succinylcholine. Pregnancy is associated with fewer fasciculations and less succinylcholine-related muscle pain; therefore a defasciculating dose of a nondepolarizing muscle relaxant is not recommended.

Maintenance of anesthesia. General anesthesia can be maintained with a volatile inhalational agent with or without nitrous oxide. The predelivery goal of at least 0.80 MAC should be delivered with a relatively high fresh-gas flow rate consisting of 50% oxygen/50% nitrous oxide to ensure adequate anesthesia and minimize intraoperative awareness. If fetal distress is present or if maternal O_2 saturation is below 97%, high concentrations of O_2 may be used without nitrous oxide. Administering 100% O_2 does result in improved fetal oxygenation compared with 50% O_2, but questions have been raised about the danger of free radical activity in neonates born to women administered greater than 50% O_2.[187] Comparisons of Apgar scores, umbilical venous O_2 tension, time to breathing, and resuscitation efforts in neonates has revealed that infants born to women given 100% O_2 before delivery have slightly better outcomes.[188] Maternal hyperventilation should be avoided during mechanical ventilation because a $PaCO_2$ less than 20 mm Hg can result in decreased uterine blood flow and a shift of the oxyhemoglobin dissociation curve to the left. Maternal $PaCO_2$ should ideally be maintained at the normal term pregnancy range of 30 to 32 mm Hg.

The use of bispectral index (BIS) monitoring remains controversial in that even the most rapid application before an emergency cesarean delivery takes some time, and its use has not been shown to conclusively prevent recall in all cases.[189] When used, a target BIS score of 40 to 60 can be obtained at a MAC of approximately 0.8 or above.

Volatile inhalational agents are tocolytic and result in decreased uterine contractility and tone that can result in increased postdelivery blood loss. The uterus continues to contract in response to oxytocin provided the MAC is less than 1.0.[190] In the presence of uterine atony and hemorrhage, their concentration can be decreased at delivery and anesthesia supplemented with narcotics and benzodiazepines as needed. The routine use of intraoperative muscle relaxation is generally not necessary and can be left to the surgeon's preference.

Immediately after delivery, the recently distended abdominal musculature is quite flaccid, and the surgical team should be accustomed to performing cesarean deliveries on spontaneously ventilating patients. In the absence of neuromuscular relaxation, the anesthetic depth can be better adjusted to the patient's requirements according to respiratory rate and depth. Intraoperative awareness from inadequate anesthesia may be less likely to occur in a patient who is not surgically relaxed.

Infants delivered by cesarean delivery under general anesthesia are more likely to be depressed and to require active resuscitation compared with those delivered with a neuraxial anesthetic, and therefore an individual other than the anesthesia provider who is trained in neonatal resuscitation should be present at delivery.[191] The length of time from uterine incision to delivery has been shown to correlate with the degree of neonatal acidosis.[192] The interval should be recorded. An interval of 3 minutes seems to be the critical value as neonates delivered later than 3 minutes after uterine incision are more likely to be depressed.[193] At the completion of surgery, the patient is extubated awake (i.e., following commands) after full recovery of neuromuscular function has been confirmed and extubation criteria have been met. A suggested method for providing general anesthesia for cesarean delivery is given in Box 51.4.

COMPLICATIONS OF REGIONAL ANESTHESIA

Hypotension

Hypotension is a frequent complication associated with obstetric neuraxial anesthesia and results from a rapid onset sympathectomy and subsequent decreased venous return and decreased cardiac output. Hypotension commonly manifests as maternal nausea and vomiting and can impair uterine perfusion. Maternal hypotension of sufficient magnitude and duration results in uteroplacental hypoperfusion and fetal acidemia. It has been defined as a 20% decrease from baseline or a systolic pressure less than 100 mm Hg. Blood pressure should be monitored at least every 2 minutes following the initiation of neuraxial anesthesia until stabilized. Efforts to reduce the incidence of hypotension include left uterine displacement, IV fluid administration, and use of vasopressors. Additionally, administration of a 5-hydroxytryptamine 3 (5-HT_3, serotonin) receptor antagonist, such as ondansetron, prior to spinal anesthesia may reduce the occurrence of the Bezold-Jarisch reflex that can present as hypotension and bradycardia following spinal anesthesia. Heesen et al.[194] found that 5-HT_3 antagonists significantly reduced the incidence of hypotension and bradycardia in the subgroup of patients undergoing cesarean delivery with spinal anesthesia.

Nausea and Vomiting

Nausea and vomiting are a common occurrence during labor and delivery. The causes are often multifactorial and include pain, delayed gastric emptying, administration of parenteral opioids, visceral traction with exteriorization of the uterus, and motion during transport. The aggressive treatment of hypotension can prevent nausea and vomiting from occurring. Some clinicians believe that a sympathetic block results in unopposed gastrointestinal vagal stimulation, which predisposes the patient to nausea. Opioids administered in either the epidural or subarachnoid space improve block quality and do not appear to increase intraoperative nausea.

Multimodal approaches combining antiemetics with different mechanisms of action may be more effective than single drugs when treating nausea and vomiting. Metoclopramide (10 mg IV) is a prokinetic that likely reduces the incidence of intraoperative nausea and vomiting. It can be given preoperatively or at cord clamp.[195] The

BOX 51.4 General Anesthesia for Cesarean Delivery

- Discuss the operative plan with the multidisciplinary team
- Perform preanesthetic assessment and obtain informed consent
- Prepare necessary medications and equipment
- Place patient supine with left uterine displacement
- Secure 16- or 18-gauge intravenous access; send blood specimen for baseline laboratory measurements; consider type and screen (or crossmatch) if risk factors for peripartum hemorrhage are present
- Consider timely administration of a nonparticulate antacid, H_2-receptor antagonist, and/or metoclopramide preoperatively
- Administer antibiotic prophylaxis if necessary (with 60 min prior to incision)
- Initiate monitoring
- Perform a team "time-out" to verify patient identity, position, and operative site; procedure to be performed; and availability of special equipment, if needed
- Provide 100% oxygen with a tight-fitting face mask for ≥3 min, when possible, for denitrogenation/preoxygenation; otherwise, instruct patient to take four to eight vital-capacity breaths immediately before induction of anesthesia
- After abdomen has been prepared and operative drapes are in place, verify surgeon and assistant are ready to begin surgery
- Initiate rapid sequence induction
- Cricoid pressure 10 newtons while awake; increase to 30 newtons after loss of consciousness
- Propofol 2–2.5 mg/kg and succinylcholine 1–1.5 mg/kg; wait 30–40 sec then perform tracheal intubation; confirm correct placement of endotracheal tube
- Provide maintenance of anesthesia
- Use isoflurane, sevoflurane, or desflurane (~1 minimum alveolar concentration [MAC]) in 100% oxygen, or oxygen/nitrous oxide (up to 50%)
- Treat hypotension (e.g., phenylephrine, ephedrine)
- If additional muscle relaxant (e.g., rocuronium, vecuronium) is necessary, titrate dose according to response to peripheral nerve stimulator
- Observe delivery of infant
- Initiate infusion of oxytocin; consider other uterotonic agents (e.g., methylergonovine, 15-methyl prostaglandin $F_{2\alpha}$, misoprostol) if uterine tone is inadequate; monitor blood loss and respond as necessary
- Adjust maintenance technique after delivery of the infant
- Administer a reduced concentration of a volatile halogenated agent (0.5–0.75 MAC)
- Supplement anesthesia with nitrous oxide and an intravenous opioid
- Consider administration of a benzodiazepine (e.g., midazolam)
- Perform extubation when neuromuscular blockade is fully reversed and the patient is awake and responds to commands
- Evaluate postoperative issues (e.g., pain, nausea)

Modified from Tsen LC, Bateman BT. Anesthesia for cesarean delivery. In: Chestnut DH, et al, eds. *Chestnut's Obstetric Anesthesia: Principles and Practice.* 6th ed. Philadelphia: Elsevier; 2020:590.

serotonin receptor antagonist ondansetron (4 mg IV) may be more effective compared with metoclopramide in preventing intraoperative nausea.[196] Granisetron 1 mg IV appears to be ineffective reducing the incidence of intraoperative nausea and vomiting during elective cesarean delivery.[197] Scopolamine transdermal patches have been shown to significantly reduce the incidence of post-cesarean delivery nausea and vomiting resulting from regional anesthesia.[198] Transdermal scopolamine begins to be effective in 2 to 4 hours. Although this onset time is long, the duration of action (≥48 hours) and simplicity of the scopolamine patch make it an attractive choice for parturients with a strong history of postoperative nausea and vomiting. Side effects include dry mouth and dizziness, which may outweigh the benefits of scopolamine for some patients.

Postdural Puncture Headache

PDPH is a significant source of morbidity among parturients who receive neuraxial anesthesia.[199] PDPH most commonly results from ADP with a large bore (16- to 18-gauge) epidural needle during attempted epidural placement. ADP has been reported to occur in 1% to 2% of epidural placements and subsequently results in a PDPH in 80% to 86% of women.[200] The resulting large dural defect provides a source for CSF to leak from the subarachnoid space to the epidural space. The loss of intracranial pressure causes caudad displacement of the cranial contents and traction on meningeal structures when the patient assumes a head-up position. The hallmark of a PDPH is this postural component. The headache is relieved when the patient is supine and returns upon sitting or standing. Cerebral venous dilation also occurs in response to intracranial hypotension and contributes to the PDPH symptoms. PDPH symptoms commonly include frontal and occipital pain radiating to the neck or shoulders. Nausea, vertigo, and low back pain are also seen. Ocular dysfunction as a result of a cranial nerve VI (abducens nerve) palsy is less common and can result in double vision and a deviated gaze.[201]

PDPH is not the only cause of significant headache after regional anesthesia in the obstetric patient. In a retrospective review of 95 women who experienced a headache more than 24 hours after delivery, Stella et al.[202] found that tension/migraine and preeclampsia/eclampsia accounted for over 70% of reported headaches, whereas a diagnosis of PDPH was made in 16%. More serious causes of postpartum maternal headache include meningitis and intracranial pathology such as cortical vein thrombosis and subarachnoid hemorrhage.

The incidence of PDPH is inversely related to age and seen infrequently in those older than 70 years. Women appear to be slightly more susceptible than men, and pregnancy may increase the incidence. In general, large-diameter needles are more likely to be associated with PDPH when compared with small-diameter needles.

With spinal anesthesia, the incidence of PDPH is significantly reduced with the use of pencil-point needles (e.g., Pencan, Sprotte, Whitacre) compared with beveled cutting needles (e.g., Quincke) (Fig. 51.9). In a retrospective study of 366 obstetric patients, the incidence of PDPH after the use of a Sprotte needle was 1.5%, compared with 9% after the use of a beveled Quincke needle of similar gauge.[203]

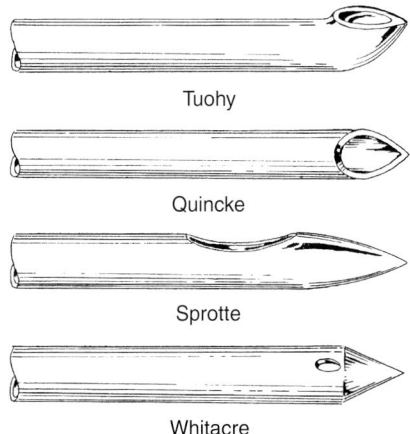

Tuohy

Quincke

Sprotte

Whitacre

Fig. 51.9 Physical characteristics of four different types of spinal and epidural needles. Needle diameters are not to scale.

Some evidence indicates that the bevel orientation relative to the dural fibers plays a role. Electron microscopy has confirmed that the collagen fibers composing the dura are primarily oriented longitudinally.[204] Penetrating the dural fibers along their vertical axis may result in less CSF leakage compared with horizontal bevel orientation. The angle at which the needle approaches the dura may also modify the amount of CSF leakage and therefore the incidence of PDPH; however, the angle of approach is most often dictated by anatomy, and therefore it is difficult for the anesthetist to modify effectively.

When ADP occurs during epidural placement, there has been some evidence to indicate that placing a subarachnoid catheter reduces the incidence of PDPH and the requirement for epidural blood patch (EBP).[139,205] However, in a 2012 study of 97 women randomly assigned to either a repeat of the epidural procedure or converting to continuous spinal analgesia there was no difference in the incidence of PDPH or the requirement for EBP.[140] Interestingly, those in the repeat epidural group experienced a 9% ADP as a result of the second attempt. Based on these results, it would appear prudent to move forward with spinal analgesia to provide rapid and reliable labor analgesia and to avoid the significantly increased chance of a second ADP.

The use of air as opposed to saline in the loss of resistance technique may also be associated with greater PDPH rates. Aida et al.[206] studied 3700 patients who received epidural anesthesia and found that 100 experienced an ADP. PDPH occurred in 67% of the patients in the air group as opposed to 10% in the saline group. A head computed tomography (CT) scan was done in all 100 PDPH patients and identified supraspinal intrathecal air bubbles in 78% of those with PDPH indicating that intraventricular air plays a role in PDPH symptoms.

Treatment

Patients should be given a choice of treatments ranging from conservative to aggressive. PDPH can be a mild irritation for a few days, or it may become debilitating. Conservative treatment is appropriate for mild headaches and includes bedrest, caffeine, and oral analgesics. Although aggressive hydration is not contraindicated, there is little evidence to indicate increased fluid intake affects CSF production.[207] Caffeine is a cerebral vasoconstrictor that can be transiently effective in relieving the symptoms of PDPH that result from cerebral vasodilation. An additional treatment modality for PDPH is the administration of a topical sphenopalatine ganglion block (SPGB). Cohen et al.[208] found no significant differences regarding headache relief at 24 hours, 48 hours, and 1 week posttreatment when compared to an EBP. Cohen et al.[208] concluded that a SPGB carries less procedural risk and should be considered prior to the administration of an EBP.

Patients with a debilitating PDPH who are unresponsive to conservative therapy for 24 hours post-ADP should be evaluated for an EBP. This procedure has an estimated treatment success rate of 75%.[209] After resolution of the neural blockade has been confirmed, an EBP is performed by placing an epidural needle in the epidural space, preferably at the same interspace as the dural puncture or one interspace below. When viewed under fluoroscopy, an autologous blood/dye combination spreads one spinal segment below and 4 spinal segments above point of injection.[210] Once the needle is in place, an assistant performs a peripheral venipuncture and draws 20 mL autologous blood using strict aseptic technique. The blood is then slowly injected into the epidural space. The ideal volume for injection appears to be between 15 and 20 mL.[211] If back pain develops, the injection is temporarily stopped. If the discomfort passes quickly, slow injection of the target volume of 15 to 20 mL may continue until discomfort returns. After the desired volume is injected, the Tuohy needle is withdrawn, and the patient should remain at rest for at least 1 hour.[212]

The mechanism of action of an EBP appears to be twofold. First, the epidural blood covers the dural defect with a fibrin clot. Secondly, the injected volume of blood applies pressure to the dura, decreasing the relative total volume of CSF necessary to relieve the postural headache.

Prophylactic blood patch is a technique in which autologous blood is injected through the epidural catheter following delivery and immediately prior to its removal. However, its use is controversial for several reasons. Immediately after delivery, the patient likely has yet to develop a headache and thus may receive an unnecessary treatment. In addition, the absolute sterility and precise location of an indwelling epidural catheter cannot be determined. Lastly, prophylactic blood patches do not appear to consistently influence the incidence or severity of PDPH.[213]

Local Anesthetic Systemic Toxicity

LAST during epidural anesthesia can result from inadvertent intravascular injection into an epidural vein or accumulation from repeated dosing. The signs and symptoms of LAST are directly related to the serum concentration and increase in severity as the concentration rises. Early signs of systemic toxicity include circumoral numbness, lightheadedness, along with visual and auditory disturbances; however, neurologic and cardiovascular signs may occur simultaneously. Unconsciousness, seizures, and cardiovascular depression/collapse follow as plasma concentrations increase further.

Necessary measures to prevent LAST during epidural anesthesia include aspiration of the catheter for blood prior to injection, use of an appropriate test dose, fractionated dosing, and vigilance for clinical signs of toxicity. The incidence of venous cannulation with an epidural catheter is approximately 6% in the obstetric population.[214] In a review of randomized controlled trials, Mhyre et al.[215] identified effective strategies to reduce the incidence of venous cannulation that included insertion in the lateral as opposed to the sitting position, using single-orifice rather than multiorifice catheters, using wire-embedded polyurethane (soft) rather than nylon (hard) catheters, and limiting the depth of insertion to less than 6 cm.

The initial intervention when any signs or symptoms of LAST occur is discontinuation of the injection of local anesthetic. Early recognition of a positive response to a test dose often halts the progression of symptoms. If signs and symptoms of LAST escalate to seizure activity, both mother and fetus are at risk for hypoxia. Rapid response involves the administration of medications such as benzodiazepines to end the seizure and support of ventilation and oxygenation. Emergency drugs and airway equipment should be on all epidural insertion carts. Advanced cardiac life support is provided symptomatically per guidelines. Careful evaluation of the maternal and fetal status should dictate decisions regarding obstetric management. ASRA has issued a practice advisory on LAST, and it is presented in detail in Chapter 10.[216]

Rescue treatment with 20% lipid emulsion has been shown to be effective in treating local anesthetic-induced cardiotoxicity. The precise mechanism of action remains unknown but may involve the exogenous lipid providing an alternate binding site for the lipid-soluble local anesthetic, often referred to as the lipid sink theory. Although the timing, dose, and duration has yet to be firmly established, its low cost, simplicity of use, and apparent lack of significant side effects leads to the recommendation that 20% lipid emulsion be available wherever regional anesthesia is used.[217] Guidelines for lipid use and a checklist for managing LAST should be readily available.[218]

Total Spinal Block

Total spinal anesthesia is a complication that results from the excessive and unintended cephalic spread of local anesthetic within the subarachnoid or epidural space. It can follow the inadvertent injection of a large epidural dose of local anesthetic into the subarachnoid space after unrecognized subarachnoid catheter placement or by migration of a previously placed epidural catheter into the subarachnoid space. Unintentionally high or total spinal block also can result from a single-shot spinal anesthetic performed after a failed epidural block. It is thought that the large amount of previously placed epidural local anesthetic migrates through the dural hole made by the spinal needle. A total spinal block is normally rapid in onset and preceded by complaints of dyspnea, difficult phonation, and hypotension. Bradycardia can occur resulting from blockade of the sympathetic innervation to the heart, which is located at the T1-T4 spinal cord segment. In the presence of these symptoms, consideration should be given to alternative diagnoses that include anaphylactic shock, eclampsia, or amniotic fluid embolus.

Accidental Subdural Injection

Rarely an epidural catheter may be inadvertently placed in the subdural space between the dura and arachnoid membranes.[219] Subdural injection presents as an excessively high sensory block with little motor involvement and is normally unilateral and delayed in onset by 10 to 25 minutes.[220] The magnitude of the block is significantly greater than would be anticipated if the catheter were located in the epidural space. Hypotension caused by extensive sympathetic block is usually the primary problem and is treated with vasopressors as needed. If the block is sufficiently extensive to compromise respiration or airway maintenance, endotracheal intubation may be necessary. This complication is uncommon and likely unpreventable. The possibility of delayed respiratory compromise emphasizes the necessity for close monitoring after epidural administration.

Cardiac Arrest in Pregnancy

Cardiac arrest in pregnancy has been estimated to occur in less than 1:20,000 women and presents specific challenges to the obstetric care team. In a consensus statement from the Society of Obstetric Anesthesia and Perinatology, several important recommendations were made to improve resuscitation in maternal cardiac arrest.[221]

In addition to standard American Heart Association (AHA) advanced cardiac life support (ACLS) guidelines, it is recommended for patients in the third trimester that hand placement during compressions be 2 to 3 cm higher on the sternum than in nonpregnant patients.[222] Manual left uterine displacement is necessary when the uterus is palpable above the umbilicus and is best performed by using two hands from the patients left and pulling leftward and up. Resuscitation drugs should be administered consistent with standard ACLS guidelines as none are contraindicated during maternal cardiac arrest.[223]

A perimortem cesarean delivery is required to improve maternal and fetal survival if return of spontaneous circulation does not occur within minutes of the arrest.[224] This makes direct oxygenation of the neonate possible and has resulted in substantially improved venous return in the mother, ultimately allowing for improved success of resuscitation.[225] The goal of a perimortem cesarean delivery during cardiac arrest is uninterrupted chest compressions and delivery no more than 5 minutes after the onset of cardiac arrest.[226] Because transport to the operating room is time consuming and impairs quality chest compressions, it is recommended the procedure be performed in the labor room.[227]

Neurologic Injuries

Neurologic complications following labor and delivery are uncommon and may be associated with labor, delivery, positioning, or

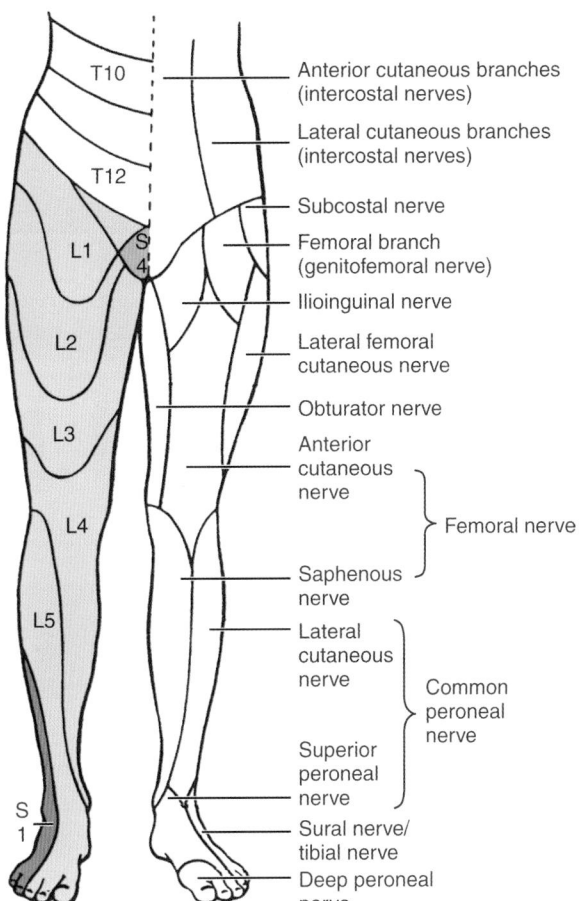

Fig. 51.10 The dermatomal *(right leg)* and peripheral *(left leg)* sensory nerve distributions useful in distinguishing central from peripheral nerve injury. (In: Chestnut DH, et al. *Chestnut's Obstetric Anesthesia: Principles and Practice.* 6th ed. St. Louis: Elsevier; 2020:756; from Redick LF. Maternal perinatal nerve palsies. *Postgrad Obstet Gynecol.* 1992;12:1–6.)

neuraxial anesthesia.[228] In a retrospective review of observational studies, Ruppen et al.[229] found the incidence of persistent neurologic injury in obstetric patients who received epidural anesthesia to be 1 in 240,000 and the rate of transient (<1 year duration) neurologic injury to be 1 in 6700. Obstetric nerve injuries related to childbirth involve pressure and stretching of peripheral nerves by the descending fetus and are identified by the appearance of a single peripheral neuropathy. Alternatively, neuraxial anesthesia-related injuries involve a spinal nerve root and follow a dermatomal distribution. Although neuraxial anesthesia is often cited as the cause of postpartum nerve injuries, careful identification and evaluation of the defect can indicate otherwise. ASRA has published a practice advisory on neurologic complications that discusses this topic further.[230] Fig. 51.10 illustrates both peripheral nerves conducting sensory innervation and spinal dermatome distribution.

OBSTETRIC COMPLICATIONS

Postpartum Hemorrhage

Approximately 4% of all parturients who deliver vaginally experience postpartum hemorrhage (PPH), and the incidence appears to be increasing.[231,232] Aggressive recognition and treatment has the potential to prevent the development of serious PPH.[233]

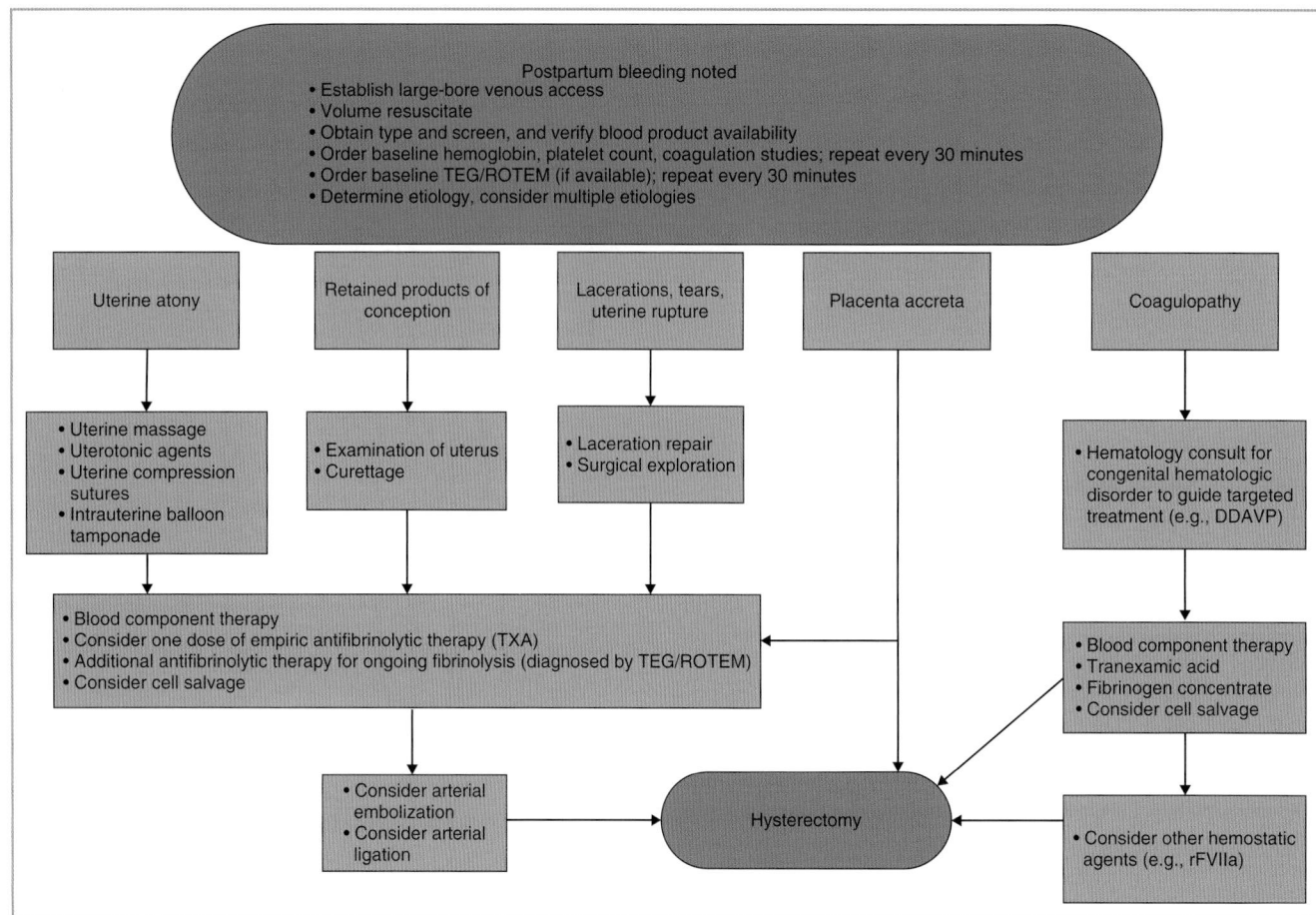

Fig. 51.11 Management options for postpartum hemorrhage. *DDAVP*, 1-desamino-8-D-arginine-vasopressin; *rFVIIa*, recombinant factor VIIa; *ROTEM*, rotational thromboelastometry; *TEG*, thromboelastography; *TXA*, tranexamic acid. (From Chestnut DH, et al. *Chestnut's Obstetric Anesthesia*. 6th ed. St. Louis: Elsevier; 2020:908.)

ACOG defines early PPH as an estimated blood loss that meets or exceeds 1000 mL or symptomatic hypovolemia resulting from blood loss that occurs within 24 hours of the birthing process (including intrapartum loss) regardless of vaginal versus cesarean delivery.[234] This differs from more traditional definition, which defined PPH as an estimated blood loss greater than 500 mL after vaginal delivery or greater than 1000 mL with cesarean delivery.[235] ACOG continues to advise vigilance for potential intervention in cases resulting in an estimated blood loss of 500 to 999 mL.[234] PPH may occur as a result of uterine atony (accounting for 70%–80% of all PPH), placental retention, abnormalities of the uterus, lacerations of the cervix or vaginal wall, uterine inversion, and abnormalities of coagulation. Uterine atony is associated with multiparity, prolonged infusions of oxytocin before delivery, polyhydramnios, and multiple gestation.[235]

ACOG has made recommendations for the prevention and treatment of PPH that includes the use of uterotonic agents such as oxytocin followed by methylergonovine, prostaglandins, and misoprostol when oxytocin is ineffective.[235] A sample flow chart for managing obstetric hemorrhage is shown in Fig. 51.11.

When oxytocin does not adequately stimulate uterine contraction, another uterotonic, an ergot alkaloid (Methergine) can be used. Because of their potent vascular effects, ergot alkaloids are not administered IV. Ergot alkaloids normally cause an increase in blood pressure, central venous pressure, and pulmonary capillary wedge pressure. An IM dose of Methergine 0.2 mg is commonly administered for stimulating uterine contractions and can be administered every 2 to 4 hours. Methergine is contraindicated with hypertension, preeclampsia, cardiovascular disease, or hypersensitivity to ergot alkaloids.[235]

Following the use of oxytocin and ergot alkaloids, prostaglandin F_{2a} (e.g., carboprost [Hemabate], 250 mcg) can be administered either IM or directly into the uterine muscle. The 250-mcg dose can be repeated every 15 to 90 minutes up to an eight-dose maximum. Prostaglandins are potent stimulators of uterine contractions but may cause nausea, bronchospasm, and increased pulmonary vascular resistance. Due to its potential to cause bronchospasm, prostaglandin F_{2a} is contraindicated in asthmatics. If uterine atony continues, misoprostol 600 to 1000 mcg can be administered rectally, vaginally, or orally as a one-time dose. An adverse reaction with misoprostol is the potential to cause a transient hyperthermic response.[235]

Antifibrinolytic agents such as tranexamic acid strengthens fibrin clots by inhibiting enzymatic fibrinolysis, and they have shown promise when used in combination with uterotonic agents. ACOG does not recommend the administration of tranexamic acid prophylactically; however, it does recommend the consideration of tranexamic acid administration during obstetric hemorrhage in which traditional modalities have failed.[235] A large international, double-blinded, randomized, placebo-controlled study was put forth by the WOMAN Trial Collaborators,[236] which consisted of 20,060 study participants that compared tranexamic acid administration versus placebo in the event of PPH. A dose of 1 g tranexamic acid IV was administered within standard PPH care and readministered after 30 minutes if bleeding continued or stopped and restarted within 24 hours. Overall mortality due to bleeding was significantly reduced in the tranexamic acid group. Adverse effects, such as thromboembolic events, were not significantly different from the tranexamic acid group versus placebo. The authors concluded that tranexamic acid administration should not be delayed once a PPH is recognized.[236]

Institution-specific massive transfusion protocols and policies can be invaluable in coordinating communication between anesthesia, blood bank, and intensive care staff. Regardless of the approach, planning for the management of PPH should be an integral part of an obstetric anesthesia practice.[237] Although historically controversial due to the risk of amniotic fluid embolus and Rh incompatibility, the use of intraoperative cell salvage is now accepted and should be considered in the setting of massive intraoperative obstetric hemorrhage. Cell salvage should start after delivery of the placenta, and use of a leukocyte depletion filter improves safety.[238,239]

A retained placenta or placental fragments can precipitate PPH and are often removed manually. Nitroglycerin, a potent uterine relaxant with a relatively short duration of action, can be administered IV or sublingual as an alternative to terbutaline or general anesthesia with volatile agents to provide sufficient uterine relaxation necessary for placental extraction.[51,240] Regarding dosing, low-dose nitroglycerin administration (e.g., 40 mcg IV) should be considered to aid in the extraction of retained placenta according to AANA obstetric practice guidelines.[46]

When hemostasis is not achieved despite the use of pharmacologic adjuncts, the obstetric staff may place an intrauterine balloon. The device is specifically designed for this purpose, and it is placed in the uterine cavity and filled with saline to exert a tamponade effect. Balloon tamponade is a minimally invasive and rapidly applied approach that can be used alone or as a temporizing measure while other resources are being mobilized.[241]

Anesthetic Implications

Anesthesia for uterine exploration can be accomplished with a variety of methods, including the use of an epidural catheter, a single-shot spinal saddle block, or a general anesthetic. The choice of technique is dependent on the patient's condition and the urgency of the proposed procedure. Under normal circumstances, the continuous epidural infusion is routinely discontinued at completion of delivery and repair; however, the epidural catheter should remain in place until the maternal patient is stable. In this manner, if a postpartum surgical intervention becomes necessary, reestablishing epidural anesthesia is an option.

Preeclampsia

Description

Preeclampsia is a pregnancy-specific multisystem disorder of unknown etiology. The disorder affects approximately 5% to 7% of pregnancies, and it is a significant cause of maternal and fetal morbidity and mortality.[242] The incidence of preeclampsia has increased by 25% in the United States over the last 20 years.[243] The pathophysiology appears to involve deranged placental angiogenesis leading to constricted myometrial arteries with exaggerated vasomotor responsiveness, superficial placental implantation, and placental hypoperfusion.[244] Mediators

secreted by the placenta cause widespread endothelial dysfunction resulting in multisystem organ dysfunction.[245]

Diagnostic criteria for preeclampsia include assessment of a systolic blood pressure of 140 mm Hg or higher or diastolic blood pressure of 90 mm Hg or higher on two separate occasions greater than 4 hours apart after 20 weeks of gestation in a patient that was previously normotensive. Additionally, these blood pressure readings would be accompanied by proteinuria as evidenced by 300 mg or greater in a 24-hour urine collection, protein/creatinine ratio of 0.3 or greater, or a dipstick reading of 2+. In the absence of proteinuria, preeclampsia can meet diagnostic criteria if new-onset hypertension is accompanied by thrombocytopenia ($<100 \times 10^9$/L), renal insufficiency, impaired liver function, pulmonary edema, or a new-onset headache that is unresponsive to medication or attributable to alternative diagnoses.[246]

The primary cause of hypertension related maternal mortality is cerebral hemorrhage. Pulmonary edema, renal failure, hepatic rupture, cerebral edema, and disseminated intravascular coagulation (DIC) are also associated with preeclampsia. Eclampsia is the onset of seizures in a patient with signs and symptoms of preeclampsia.

Pathophysiology

The precise pathogenesis of preeclampsia is complex and not well understood but likely involves a failure in normal placental angiogenesis resulting in decreased placental perfusion. Placental function worsens as the pregnancy progresses, often resulting in intrauterine growth restriction. The hypoperfused placenta releases factors into the maternal circulation that damage the maternal endothelium, resulting in systemwide manifestations.

The upper airway edema normally associated with pregnancy can be more pronounced in the preeclamptic patient. The decreased colloid osmotic pressure associated with urinary protein loss combined with increased vascular permeability predisposes the parturient to pulmonary edema. CNS effects include headache, hyperexcitability, and hyperreflexia. Thrombocytopenia occurs in up to 20% of women and is related to the severity of the disease process. Increased vascular tone results from hypersensitivity to endogenous catecholamines. SVR is increased, which can result in end organ ischemia. Plasma volume is normal in mild disease but may be severely reduced in severe disease.[246] Hepatocellular necrosis results in hepatic enlargement, which ultimately can lead to hepatic capsule rupture. Proteinuria occurs as a result of glomerular capillary endothelial destruction. There is now evidence to indicate that a woman who has had preeclampsia during pregnancy is at an increased risk of later-life cardiovascular disease.[247]

Obstetric Management

Delivery is, at present, the only definitive way of ending the disease process of preeclampsia. The obstetric decision to deliver is based on the presence of complicating factors such as uncontrolled severe hypertension, eclampsia (seizures), pulmonary edema, placental abruption, or evidence of nonreassuring fetal status. For preeclamptic parturients, the mode of delivery (cesarean delivery or vaginal) is determined by fetal gestational age, fetal presentation, cervical status, and maternal and fetal condition.[247] In the absence of severe features, a 24- to 48-hour trial of corticosteroids may be administered to enhance fetal lung maturity.

Obstetric treatment is directed toward preventing eclampsia (seizures), avoiding decreases in uteroplacental blood flow, and maximizing organ perfusion. ACOG recommends magnesium sulfate as the drug of choice for prophylaxis and treatment of eclampsia in patients with gestational hypertension with severe features or preeclampsia with severe features in the intrapartum and postpartum periods. ACOG states that ideal dosing of magnesium sulfate is not consistent within the literature but that the therapeutic range is typically between 5 and 9 mg/dL for the prevention of eclampsia. According to ACOG, the preferred dosing in the United States of magnesium sulfate for severe preeclampsia includes a loading dose of 4 to 6 g over 30 minutes followed by an infusion of 1 to 2 g/hour followed by routine lab draws. Regular assessment needs to be conducted regarding the patient's urine output, respiratory status, and tendon reflexes. Regarding symptoms of toxicity, the loss of patellar reflexes occurs at levels greater than 9 mg/dL, respiratory paralysis greater than 12 mg/dL, and cardiac arrest greater than 30 mg/dL.[246] Magnesium sulfate (which is also used as a tocolytic) causes venous dilation, mild CNS depression, a decrease in the rate of hepatic fibrin deposition, and a reduction in uterine activity. Decreasing fibrin deposition prevents further decay in organ perfusion and often greatly decreases liver pain. Hypertension can be treated to prevent maternal complications such as intracranial hemorrhage and hypertensive myocardial ischemia. There is no evidence to indicate that treating the hypertension changes the underlying maternal disease process.

Anesthetic Implications

Regional analgesia and anesthesia are generally preferred for both spontaneous vaginal delivery and cesarean delivery in the preeclamptic patient when neuraxial techniques are not otherwise contraindicated. Historically, there was concern that neuraxial techniques, especially spinal anesthesia, would result in severe hypotension refractory to fluids and vasopressors due to the chronic volume depletion associated with preeclampsia. In reality, prospective studies have shown that parturients with preeclampsia experience less severe and less frequent hypotension compared to normotensive controls.[248,249] These findings indicate that spinal anesthesia can be safely administered to severely preeclamptic patients and that spinal-induced hypotension can generally be treated safely.[244]

Early epidural placement for labor analgesia is encouraged in severely preeclamptic patients because it provides a means for rapid anesthesia if an urgent cesarean delivery is required, thereby avoiding the potential use of general anesthesia. Although the use of epidural anesthesia for cesarean delivery in preeclampsia likely results in a lower requirement for vasopressors when compared to spinal,[249] the difference is small and of little clinical significance. Therefore, when no epidural catheter is present, a spinal anesthetic is generally preferred for the severely preeclamptic parturient if there are no contraindications because of its rapid onset may be of value in an urgent setting.

Uncontrolled hypertension in response to laryngoscopy is a major cause of hemorrhagic stroke in severely preeclamptic parturients.[250] Airway edema normally associated with pregnancy is exaggerated and can add to the risk of failed or difficult intubation. Labetalol is generally considered to be the first-line drug in treating hypertension during anesthesia. Treatment of systolic blood pressures above 160 mm Hg should be a guide to avoid intracranial bleeding.[251] Opioids administered prior to delivery are normally avoided because they can result in undesirable neonatal and maternal respiratory depression.[252] Maternal respiratory depression can become a significant issue in the event of a failed intubation. Control of blood pressure during induction of general anesthesia demands both careful planning and skill.

Nondepolarizing muscle relaxants are markedly potentiated in women with preeclampsia who have therapeutic levels of magnesium. Magnesium sulfate reduces the onset time of rocuronium and prolongs the total recovery time by approximately 25%.[253] If a nondepolarizing muscle relaxant is indicated, a decreased dose should be administered, and the response should be carefully monitored with a peripheral nerve stimulator.

Thrombocytopenia in preeclampsia is common and results from endothelial dysfunction that stimulates excess platelet activation and consumption. There is no universally accepted platelet count for a safe neuraxial anesthetic, but practice guidelines and expert opinion indicate most practitioners require a platelet count of 75,000 to 80,000/μL[85,254] (see Neuraxial Analgesia for Labor and Vaginal Delivery, earlier). In the setting of severe preeclampsia complicated by thrombocytopenia it may also be advantageous to confirm normal partial thromboplastin (PTT) and prothrombin (PT) times prior to initiating neuraxial anesthesia.

HELLP Syndrome

HELLP syndrome is a complication of preeclampsia, which consists of *h*emolysis, *e*levated *l*iver enzymes, and a *l*ow *p*latelet count. An estimated 5% to 10% of women with preeclampsia develop HELLP syndrome, and it is associated with a progressive and often sudden deterioration in maternal and fetal condition. Clinical signs of HELLP syndrome include epigastric pain, upper abdominal tenderness, proteinuria, hypertension, jaundice, nausea, and vomiting. Rarely, HELLP syndrome may result in hepatic rupture. Some experts believe that a degree of compensated DIC is present in all patients with HELLP syndrome. Due to increased maternal morbidity and mortality, the presence of HELLP syndrome is generally considered to be an indication for immediate delivery.[246]

Obesity

Obesity affects over 20% of pregnancies and is associated with significant increases in obstetric- and anesthesia-related morbidity.[255] Obese parturients are more likely to experience prenatal hypertensive and hyperglycemic disorders. Labor is often complicated by fetal macrosomia, prolonged duration, failed induction, and increased cesarean delivery rates.[82] Cesarean deliveries are also characterized by increased complication rates such as prolonged operative times, infectious complications, and thromboembolic events.[256]

Neuraxial catheter techniques are clearly indicated for labor analgesia because they can offer complete pain relief without respiratory depression while providing a ready option for anesthesia if cesarean or instrumented delivery becomes necessary. They are, however, associated with more difficult insertion and higher complication rates.[257] Early placement of the anesthetic may be considered to allow for enhanced maternal cooperation and adequate time for troubleshooting thereby reducing the possibility of a general anesthetic and related potential airway difficulties. Early prenatal consultation and examination is advised, and effective communication between all members of the care team is of great importance.

Abnormal Placental Implantation

Placenta Previa

Placenta previa is present when the placenta has implanted on the lower uterine segment and either partially or completely covers the opening of the cervix. Placenta previa has an incidence of up to 1%, and the mortality rate for those with it approaches 1%. Risk factors include uterine scars from prior uterine surgery, prior placenta previa, and advanced maternal age. It most often results in painless vaginal bleeding prior to the onset of labor that can result in hemodynamically significant blood loss. The risk of bleeding increases if the placenta is disturbed by manual examination of the cervix. Postpartum bleeding is often increased as well because the lower uterine segment, where the placenta previa was implanted, does not contract to the same extent as the remainder of the uterus. Three variations of placenta previa are shown in Fig. 51.12. The diagnosis of placenta previa is made by ultrasound and normally indicates cesarean delivery.

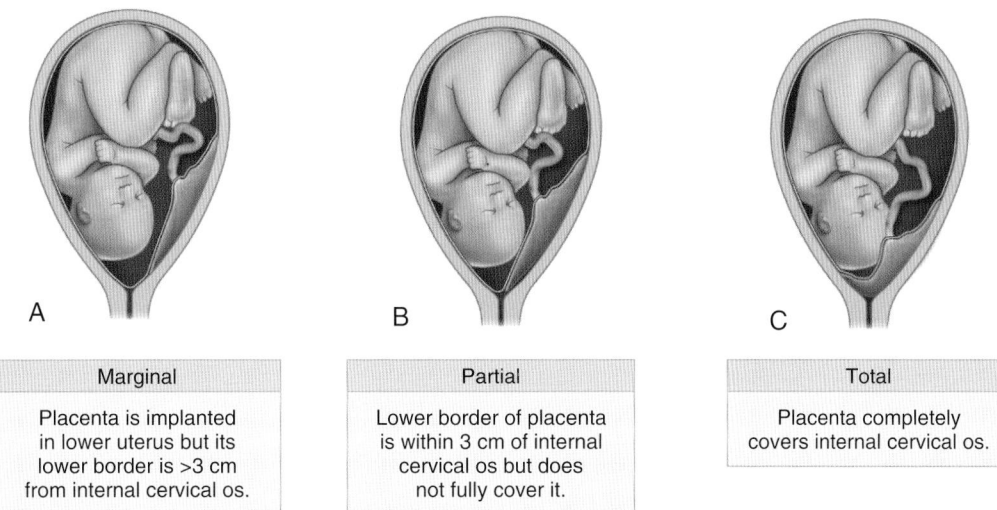

Fig. 51.12 Three variations of placenta previa. (From Silvestri LA, Silvestri AE. *Saunders Comprehensive Review for the NCLEX-PN Examination.* 8th ed. St. Louis: Elsevier; 2022: 285.)

Marginal	Partial	Total
Placenta is implanted in lower uterus but its lower border is >3 cm from internal cervical os.	Lower border of placenta is within 3 cm of internal cervical os but does not fully cover it.	Placenta completely covers internal cervical os.

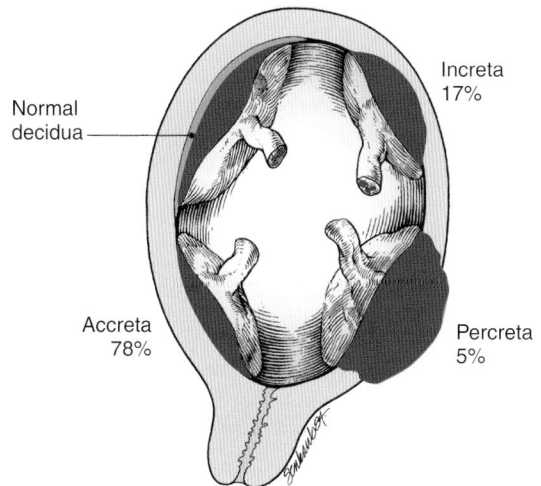

Fig. 51.13 An example of placenta increta, percreta, and accreta. (From Landon MB, et al. *Gabe's Obstetrics: Normal and Problem Pregnancies.* 8th ed. Philadelphia: Elsevier; 2021:351.)

Placenta Accreta

The placenta normally implants into the endometrium. Placenta accreta is the abnormal growth of the placenta onto the myometrium, and placenta increta describes abnormal placental growth into the myometrium. In placenta percreta the placenta grows completely through the myometrium into the surrounding structures such as bowel, bladder, or ovaries (Fig. 51.13). Overall, rates are directly related to the number of prior uterine scars (cesarean deliveries) and the presence of placenta previa. In patients with known placenta previa, placenta accreta was found to be present in 3% (first), 11% (second), 40% (third), 61% (fourth), and 67% (fifth) or more for repeat cesarean deliveries.[258] Delivery of patients with placenta accreta is often complicated by massive intraoperative hemorrhage. Treatment at the time of delivery can include surgical techniques such as uterine artery embolization, and preoperative planning should include the possibility of cesarean hysterectomy.

Placental Abruption

Placental abruption occurs when the placenta begins to separate from the uterus before delivery. This allows bleeding to occur behind the placenta and jeopardizes fetal blood supply. Placental abruption results in hemorrhage, uterine irritability, abdominal pain, and fetal hypoperfusion. Open venous sinuses in the uterine wall may allow amniotic fluid to enter the maternal circulation, resulting in an increased incidence of DIC. The reported incidence of abruption in the general population varies widely but is much higher in women with hypertension (up to 23% among women with preeclampsia).

In cases of placental abruption without fetal distress, vaginal delivery may still be possible. Because fetal distress can occur without warning, the anesthetist should be prepared to administer anesthesia for an emergency cesarean delivery. Performing a preanesthetic evaluation as soon as the diagnosis of placental abruption becomes known and confirming adequate IV access is recommended. If the mother is unstable or if fetal distress is present, operative delivery is necessary. Although placental abruption does not usually result in sudden blood loss, a large volume of trapped blood may become apparent at delivery. Consideration should be given to the parturient's existing volume status and potential for increased intraoperative blood loss.

Amniotic Fluid Embolus

Amniotic fluid embolism (AFE) is rare and may occur during labor, vaginal, or operative delivery and it is occasionally associated with placental abruption. A classic triad of AFE symptoms include acute respiratory distress, cardiovascular collapse, and coagulopathy that occur during the labor process. Additional AFE symptoms include hypotension, fetal distress, frothing from the mouth, uterine atony, loss of consciousness, and convulsions. Clinical management is supportive and includes airway management, hemodynamic resuscitation, and appropriate treatment of coagulopathy.[259] Based on case report data, Rezai et al.[259] advocate for the consideration of atropine 1 mg IV (vagolytic), ondansetron 8 mg IV (antiserotonin), and ketorolac 30 mg IV (antithromboxane) administration in addition to the traditional therapy during AFE resuscitation (A-OK regimen).

Prematurity

Premature delivery is a significant cause of fetal morbidity and mortality, and it is implicated in more than 50% of all perinatal deaths. Premature labor and delivery occur before 37 weeks of gestation. Late preterm births, defined as those of 34 to 36 weeks of gestation, compose approximately 70% of all preterm births. Fetal birthweight below 1500 g is considered very low birthweight and is associated with the greatest risk of long-term complications.[260] Severe morbidity associated with preterm delivery includes respiratory distress syndrome, intracranial hemorrhage, and hyperbilirubinemia. A diagnosis of preterm labor can be facilitated by measuring fetal fibronectin, which is a protein normally undetected before 35 weeks of gestation.[261]

The ability to stop premature labor can allow the fetal lungs additional time to mature. Delaying delivery for 24 to 48 hours can allow for the administration of corticosteroids and antibiotics that promote fetal lung maturation and decrease maternal chorioamnionitis. Drugs used to prevent and suppress preterm labor include magnesium sulfate, calcium channel blockers, and β-sympathomimetics.

There is evidence to indicate that bacterial colonization of fetal membranes and amniotic fluid triggers an inflammatory response in the mother and fetus that leads to preterm labor and associated long-term neurologic and respiratory complications in the neonate. This raises questions about the desirability of prolonging pregnancy in this context. Combined with 2012 meta-analyses that failed to demonstrate improvements in neonatal outcome with tocolytic therapy, as well as a poor maternal/fetal side effect profile, the case for continued use of these drugs needs to be questioned.[262]

Neuraxial analgesia is indicated when a vaginal delivery is planned as it provides excellent relaxation of the pelvic musculature, thereby reducing the incidence of intracranial trauma. Deliveries involving infants with very low birthweight (<1500 g) or those in the breech position are normally performed via cesarean delivery. The choice of anesthetic technique is directed toward avoiding fetal trauma and maintaining uteroplacental perfusion.

ANESTHESIA FOR THE PREGNANT PATIENT UNDERGOING A NONOBSTETRIC PROCEDURE

Occasionally, anesthetists must provide anesthesia care for a pregnant woman having nonobstetric emergency procedures. Approximately 1% to 2% of pregnant women will require a surgical procedure. The most common procedures are appendicitis, ovarian cysts, trauma, and cervical cerclage. Although there are theoretical concerns involving the teratogenicity of anesthetic agents as a result of animal studies, there is no clear information applicable to humans regarding the toxicity of specific agents. Animal studies involving multiple exposures to anesthetic agents suggest CNS neuronal apoptosis and associated expressed abnormalities.[263] Anesthesia management issues in pregnancy include appreciating the alterations in maternal physiology, maintenance of uterine perfusion, and prevention of premature labor. Goals for intraoperative management include maintaining maternal oxygenation, avoiding hyperventilation, and hypotension. Virtually all anesthetic agents rapidly cross the placenta and exhibit fetal effects except for muscle relaxants, which cross the placenta with difficulty due to their charged status. If steroidal nondepolarizing muscle relaxants are administered for the facilitation of nonobstetric surgery during pregnancy, the Society of Obstetric Anesthesia and Perinatology[264] provided a statement that encourages anesthesia personnel to avoid sugammadex in early pregnancy due to the potential binding to progesterone. Furthermore, avoidance or caution of sugammadex administration is recommended at term due to its unknown impact on lactation. Routine neuromuscular blockade reversal should continue to be administered by utilizing a combination of a cholinesterase inhibitor and anticholinergic agent. In select circumstances, the benefit of sugammadex administration may outweigh the potential risks (e.g., unanticipated difficult airway or inadequate reversal with cholinesterase inhibitors).[264]

It is realistic to monitor FHR after approximately 20 weeks of gestation. If the fetus is previable, it is generally sufficient to obtain a FHR via Doppler before and after the procedure. If the fetus is considered viable, simultaneous electronic FHR with contraction monitoring should be assessed before and after the procedure at the minimum. Intraoperative electronic fetal monitoring may be indicated if the fetus is viable, type of procedure provides intraoperative monitoring physical feasibility, obstetric provider is available to intervene, consent for emergency cesarean delivery is obtained, and the potential exists for safe interruption of the planned surgery. When monitored intraoperatively, the FHR normally displays decreased variability and likely does not reflect poor acid-base status. Alternatively, intraoperative fetal bradycardia is a more ominous sign and should be investigated for treatable causes. Organogenesis occurs in the first trimester, during which surgical procedures are avoided if possible. Whereas premature labor becomes the primary concern during the third trimester. Therefore nonemergent procedures that can be timed for the second trimester may be most optimal.[265] The maternal airway changes that accompany normal pregnancy favor regional anesthesia techniques when possible.

Cervical cerclage is a surgical intervention used to prevent second trimester fetal loss due to cervical incompetence and is generally performed between 12 and 26 weeks of gestation. Sutures are placed in the cervical os to prevent further dilation and ultimately premature delivery. The superficial nature of the procedure often makes a spinal anesthetic a suitable choice. Key points are noted in Box 51.5.

NEONATAL RESUSCITATION

All labor and delivery personnel, including anesthetists, should be trained in basic neonatal resuscitation. The anesthetist in clinical practice may participate in neonatal resuscitation, but the primary responsibility is attending to the care of the mother. An individual other than the anesthetist should be assigned responsibility for care of the newborn at every delivery.

Approximately 10% to 15% of newborns require resuscitation, but this can generally be predicted from known risk factors. Tactile stimulation of the newborn will often result in spontaneous respiration. If spontaneous respiration is delayed after stimulation, initiation of assisted ventilation should begin.

The Apgar scoring system is widely used to assess newborns. The score is derived from five parameters, including HR, respiratory rate, muscle tone, reflex irritability, and color. The assessment is performed at 1 minute and again at 5 minutes. The score is used to guide resuscitation. A score of 8 to 10 is considered normal, 4 to 7 indicates moderate distress or impairment, and 0 to 3 indicates the need for immediate resuscitation.

If the parturient has received prenatal care, there may be previous knowledge or suspicions of a congenital anomaly that can be used to guide resuscitation. In the event of little or no prenatal care, this information may be unavailable.

Most newborns do not require neonatal resuscitation. However, approximately 10% of newborns require some type of resuscitative assistance at birth. The vast majority will require assisted ventilation only. Approximately 1% will require major interventions such as intubation, chest compressions, or emergency medications. AHA guidelines for neonatal resuscitation are summarized in Box 51.6.

BOX 51.5 Key Points for the Pregnant Patient Undergoing Nonobstetric Procedure

- A significant number of women undergo anesthesia and surgery during pregnancy for procedures unrelated to delivery.
- Maternal risks are associated with the anatomic and physiologic changes of pregnancy (e.g., difficult intubation, aspiration) and with the underlying maternal disease.
- The diagnosis of abdominal conditions often is delayed during pregnancy, which increases the risk of maternal and fetal morbidity.
- Maternal catastrophes involving severe hypoxia, hypotension, and acidosis pose the greatest acute risk to the fetus.
- Other fetal risks associated with surgery include increased fetal loss, increased incidence of preterm labor, growth restriction, and low birth-weight. Clinical studies suggest that anesthesia and surgery during pregnancy do not increase the risk of congenital anomalies.
- It is unclear whether adverse fetal outcomes result from the anesthetic, the operation, or the underlying maternal disease.
- No anesthetic agent is a proven teratogen in humans, although some anesthetic agents, specifically nitrous oxide, are teratogenic in animals under certain conditions.

- Many anesthetic agents have been used for anesthesia during pregnancy, with no demonstrable differences in maternal or fetal outcome.
- The anesthesia management of the pregnant surgical patient should focus on the avoidance of hypoxemia, hypotension, acidosis, and hyperventilation.
- When performing a maternal laparoscopy, the use of an open technique or a Veress needle to enter the abdomen is desirable.
- Monitor maternal end tidal carbon dioxide to avoid fetal hypercarbia and acidosis.
- Low pneumoperitoneum pressures (between 10 and 15 mm Hg) should be used.
- Limit the extent of Trendelenburg or reverse Trendelenburg positions and initiate any position slowly.
- Monitor fetal heart rate and uterine tone preoperatively and postoperatively.
- Tocolytic agents should not be used prophylactically but should be considered when evidence of preterm labor is present.

Adapted from Van de Velde M. Nonobstetric surgery during pregnancy. In: Chestnut DH, et al. *Chestnut's Obstetric Anesthesia: Principles and Practice.* 5th ed. St. Louis: Elsevier; 2014:375; Reitman E, Flood P. Anaesthetic considerations for non-obstetric surgery during pregnancy. *Br J Anaesth.* 2011;107(suppl 1):i72–i78.

BOX 51.6 Neonatal Resuscitation Guidelines

- Initial evaluation of the newborn with emphasis on heart rate and respirations. Pulse oximetry should be used for evaluation of oxygenation because assessment of color is often unreliable.
- The temperature for nonasphyxiated infants should be maintained between 36.5°C and 37.5°C.
- In infants born <32 weeks of gestation, consider radiant warmers, plastic wrap with a cap, increased room temperature, thermal mattress, and/or warmed humidified resuscitation gases.
- Ventilatory resuscitation should begin with air rather than 100% oxygen in term infants receiving resuscitation at birth with positive pressure ventilation (PPV). If, despite effective ventilation, there is no increase in heart rate or if oxygenation, best guided by pulse oximetry, remains unacceptable, a higher concentration of oxygen should be considered. Oxygen saturation during labor and just after birth is approximately 60% and will increase to ±90% after 10 min.
- PPV is an extremely important and effective intervention that should be initiated if the infant is apneic or gasping or if the heart rate is <100 bpm after 30 sec of administering the initial steps of resuscitation. Prompt improvement in heart rate is the best indicator of adequate ventilation. The T-piece resuscitator is specifically used for neonatal resuscitation and is the device of choice.
- In births with meconium-stained amniotic fluid, suctioning of the oropharynx and nasopharynx before delivery of the shoulders is no longer recommended. In babies born through meconium-stained fluid, available evidence does not support or refute the routine endotracheal intubation and suctioning, even if they are depressed at birth, and the current practice should not be changed.
- Detection of exhaled carbon dioxide, in association with clinical assessment (e.g., increasing heart rate) is the most reliable method for confirming endotracheal tube placement in infants with spontaneous circulation. Colorimetric exhaled CO_2 detectors are useful in identifying airway obstruction during facemask ventilation in preterm infants.

- Chest compressions are indicated when the heart rate is <60 bpm despite adequate ventilation for 30 sec. In the newly born infant, the standard compression:ventilation ratio is 3:1.
- If the arrest is clearly due to a cardiac etiology, a higher compression:ventilation rate (e.g., 15:2) may be considered. Compressions should be delivered on the lower third of the sternum at a depth of one-third of the anteroposterior diameter of the chest. The two thumb-circling hands method is recommended because this process allows for better control of the depth of compressions.
- The use of drugs is rarely indicated because the most important and effective step is establishing adequate ventilation. If emergency drugs are required, they can be given by three possible routes: venous (e.g., umbilical vein), endotracheal tube, and intraosseous. If the heart rate remains <60 bpm despite adequate assisted ventilation for 30 sec and chest compression for an additional 30 sec, then the administration of epinephrine at the dose of 0.01–0.03 mg/kg, intravenously or 0.05–0.1 mg/kg via the tracheal route.
- The use of therapeutic hypothermia, both whole-body hypothermia and selective head-cooling, may reduce the risk of death and disability in infants with moderate-to-severe hypoxic-ischemic encephalopathy. Hypothermia is recommended as a treatment for neonates with suspected asphyxia. Hypothermia should be induced, lowering temperature to 33.5–34.5°C within 6 hr of birth, continuing it for 72 hr, and then rewarming over at least 4 hr. Treated infants should be followed up on a long-term basis.
- Health care providers may consider not initiating neonatal resuscitation when there are factors associated with almost certain infant death or unacceptable morbidity, or both. The parents must be included in the decision-making process regarding initiating or withholding resuscitation of their infant, particularly in situations when the prognosis is uncertain and morbidity rate is very high. Discontinuing continuous and adequate resuscitation after 10 min, if there are no signs of life, is justifiable.

Adapted from Wyckoff MG, et al. Part 13: neonatal resuscitation: 2015 American Heart Association guidelines update for cardiopulmonary resuscitation and emergency cardiovascular care. *Circulation.* 2015;132(2):S543–S560.

SUMMARY

Nurse anesthetists play a major role in providing obstetric anesthesia care. The practice of obstetric anesthesia has the additional challenge of assuring the safety of the newborn. Advances in monitoring and prenatal care have allowed for continuous refinements in regional and general anesthesia management of these patients. A thorough knowledge of the physiologic changes associated with pregnancy, anesthetic techniques, and potential complications associated with labor and delivery will help the anesthetist to make calculated decisions to help ensure the highest quality of care.

REFERENCES

For a complete list of references for this chapter, scan this QR code with any smartphone code reader app, or visit the following URL: http://booksite.elsevier.com/9780323711944/.

52

Neonatal Anesthesia

Andrew Miller, Sass Elisha

The neonatal period is defined as the first 28 days of extrauterine life. Anesthesia for the neonate may be required as the result of a life-threatening illness or medical conditions requiring surgical intervention, and may be palliative, staged, or corrective in nature. The neonate is particularly vulnerable to internal and external stressors, and the anesthetic plan must be tailored to help mitigate physiologic stress, which serves to improve neonatal morbidity and mortality. The differences between neonatal and adult anatomy and physiology are clearly greatest during this transitional period, especially when birth occurs before term. Term neonates may possess a poor ability to physiologically compensate during times of stress, and this is even further accentuated in premature neonates. It is important to note that there is an inverse relationship regarding physiologic compensation and gestational age of the neonate. The anesthetist must have a thorough understanding of the transition from intra- to extrauterine life, normal growth and development, the anatomic and physiologic differences during various stages of maturation, how immature organ systems affect anesthetic pharmacokinetics and pharmacodynamics, and how prematurity further affects each of these. Anesthetic management of the neonate, term and premature, requires integration of specialized knowledge regarding these delicate patients, extreme vigilance, and refinement of acquired technical skills.

Neonatal anesthesia has become increasingly safe since advances have been made in their care within the hospital setting, particularly in the intensive care units. In the past, neonates, and in particular those born preterm or deemed sick or unstable, were anesthetized with the Liverpool technique, which consisted of oxygen, possibly nitrous oxide, and curare. Volatile anesthetics and opioids were not used, and the "stable" state that resulted was due to a sympathetic system stimulation. Eventually, it was discovered that this method resulted in increased levels of endogenous cortisol and catecholamines causing metabolic acidosis as well as increased morbidity and mortality. Since 1987, our understanding of neonatal physiology, particularly neurobiology, has led to an active program of research in the field of neonatal anesthesia leading to the current consensus that neonates, term and preterm, respond to painful stimuli.[1] Signs of distress are evident when neonates are exposed to painful stimuli. The behavioral, physiologic, and humoral signs are similar to those seen in older children and adults.[2] Therefore, all neonates require general or regional anesthesia to blunt and control the sympathetic response associated with pain. It is important to note that in hemodynamically unstable neonates, amnesia may not be a key component to the anesthetic plan, and an opioid plus neuromuscular blocking agent anesthetic plan may be necessary.

There is a 10-fold increased incidence of morbidity and mortality in neonates as compared with older pediatric patients.[3] Neonates and infants younger than 12 months exhibit the highest rate of adverse events during the postoperative period. Preterm neonates are more prone to developing respiratory complications. Respiratory control centers are not fully mature until roughly 44 weeks of gestation. Postoperatively, apnea is a common occurrence in young infants who are less than 60 weeks postconceptual age, or earlier if they have comorbid conditions or prematurity, and observation for 24 hours is necessary.[4,5] It is important to note that each pediatric institution has its own policies in place regarding age restrictions, factoring in comorbidities and prematurity, for postoperative admission for apnea monitoring. In pediatric medicine, the term *postmenstrual age* (PMA) is preferred as compared to postconceptual age to describe the child's age during the perinatal period. A description of terms related to the perinatal period are listed in Box 52.1.

DEVELOPMENTAL CONSIDERATIONS

Fetal Circulation

Understanding fetal circulation, and the changes that occur immediately after birth, are extremely important to the anesthetist. The following discussion on fetal blood supply, fetal shunts, and fetal circulation is depicted in Fig. 52.1. The fetus relies on the mother's placenta, not the fetal lungs, for delivery of oxygen and transport of carbon dioxide (CO_2). The chorionic villus is the functional unit of the placenta. Normally, fetal blood is separated from the maternal blood in the placenta by a thin layer of cells known as syncytial trophocytes. Oxygen, CO_2, and small nonionized particles readily pass through this layer, whereas substances with a larger molecular weight are prevented from diffusing across the syncytial trophocytes. Fetal circulation is characterized by high pulmonary vascular resistance (PVR) (uninflated atelectatic lungs and hypoxic vasoconstriction) and low systemic circulatory resistance (high flow and low impedance of the placental vessels). Oxygenated blood originating from the placenta travels to the fetus via a single umbilical vein. This oxygenated blood bypasses the lungs by flowing through extracardiac (ductus arteriosus [DA], ductus venosus [DV]) and intracardiac (foramen ovale [FO]) shunts, forming a parallel circulation. Most of the oxygenated blood is shunted past the essentially unnecessary liver sinusoids via the DV and enters the right atrium via the inferior vena cava (IVC). It is important to note that the partial pressure of arterial oxygen (Pao_2) in the IVC blood is approximately 26 to 28 mm Hg. From here, blood is directed toward the atrial septum via the eustachian valve and across the FO, to the left atrium and ventricle, and out of the fetal aorta. This ensures that blood with the highest Po_2 is delivered to the head, neck, brain, and coronary arteries. Of note, this is one reason why the neonatal head is quite large in comparison to the rest of the body. After delivering oxygen to the head and brain, the less oxygenated (Pao_2 12–14 mm Hg) blood returns to the right atrium via the superior vena cava (SVC), where it is directed to the right ventricle and exits the fetal heart via the pulmonary artery. Since gas exchange and oxygenation occur in the mother's placenta, the fetal lungs display high PVR and exhibit minimal gas exchange. Blood is then shunted across the DA. Only 5% to 10% of the combined ventricular output flows through the pulmonary circulation. The less oxygenated blood (deoxygenated) travels through the aorta suppling oxygen needed in the abdominal organs and lower extremities before continuing through the fetal iliac arteries and entering the placenta through a pair of umbilical arteries. The umbilical arteries divide, forming the arterioles,

capillaries, and venules of the intervillous placental space. Combined cardiac output for the fetal right and left ventricles is approximately 450 mL/kg/min, which decreases to approximately 200 to 250 mL/kg/min in the newborn period.

Transitional Circulation

The transitional circulation is established at the time of birth. With the cessation of placental blood flow, aortic pressure increases. Clamping of the umbilical vein cuts off the blood supply from placenta to fetus, and the clamping of umbilical arteries acts to increase systemic vascular resistance (SVR) twofold. PVR falls with lung expansion, and increasing Pao_2 produces pulmonary vasodilation resulting in further decreases in PVR. These changes in systemic and pulmonary blood flow produce corresponding changes in intracardiac pressure. Decreases in right atrial pressure, with accompanying increases in left atrial pressure, change the direction of blood flow through the FO, resulting in the functional closure of the FO. The FO may reopen if right atrial pressure is greater than left atrial pressure (e.g., pulmonary hypertension [PHN], neonatal distress, and certain congenital

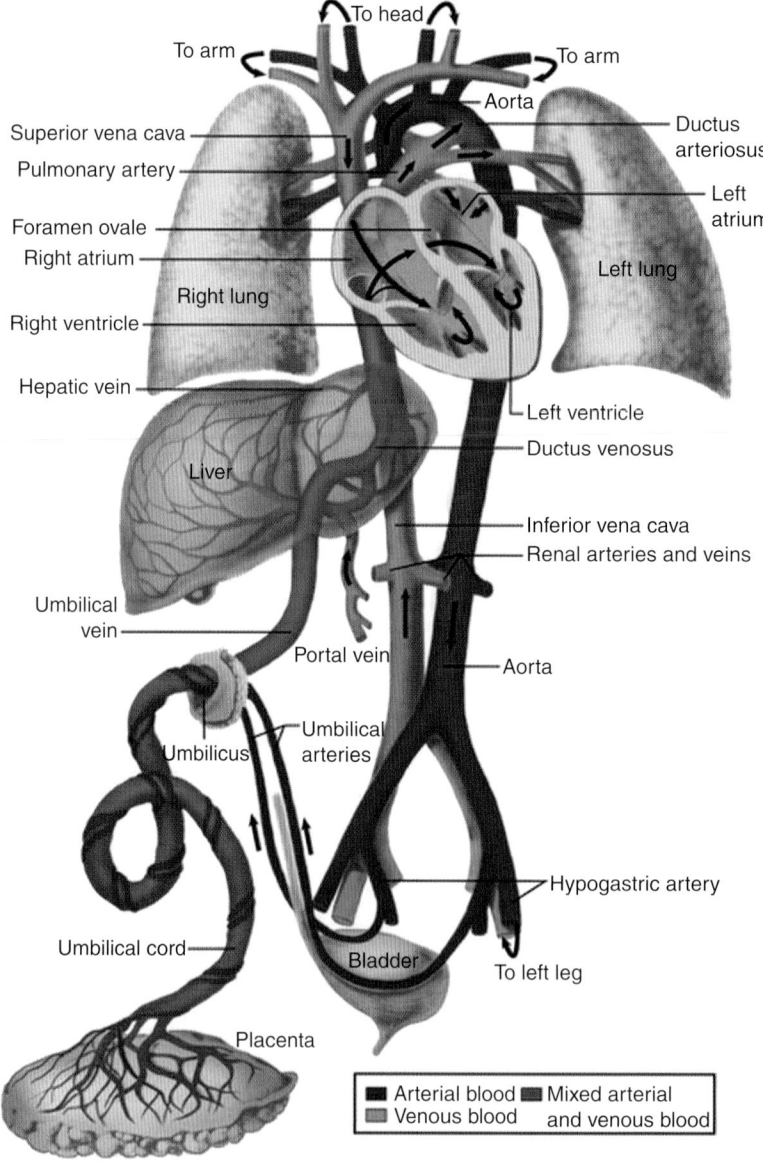

Fig. 52.1 Schematic representation of fetal circulation depicting fetal blood supply, fetal shunts, and fetal blood flow. (From Gropper MA, et al. *Miller's Anesthesia.* 9th ed. Philadelphia: Elsevier; 2020:2461.)

diaphragmatic hernias [CDHs] relying on mixing), permitting venous blood to flow from the right heart to the left heart. Though this chapter does not focus on congenital heart disease, it is important for the anesthetist to be familiar with congenital heart defects that rely on mixing of oxygenated and deoxygenated blood (generally at the atrial level) for survival and those defects that require surgical or interventional atrial septostomy (i.e., single ventricle physiology). Within a period of 2 to 3 months, though usually sooner, the FO will undergo permanent closure, which is also known as anatomic closure. Up to 25% of adult patients may demonstrate a probe patent FO at autopsy.[4] It is important to always adhere to strict bubble precautions in all neonates when administering intravenous fluids or blousing medications through ports or stopcocks.

Closure of the DA is precipitated in part by the increase in SVR and decrease in PVR. In utero, prostaglandins maintain the patency of the DA, but the supply of prostaglandins is reduced when the placenta is no longer providing blood supply to the fetus (i.e., clamping of the umbilical cord and delivery of the placenta). Within a few hours after birth, the muscular wall of the DA constricts, preventing retrograde blood flow from the aorta into the pulmonary artery. This functional closure (thrombosis) occurs within 1 to 8 days. Anatomic closure (fibrosis of the DA) requires 1 to 4 months. Closure of the DA is influenced by elevations in the systemic Pao_2, or increases in oxygen tension, that occur after birth. It is important for the anesthetist to again be familiar with the congenital heart defects that require a patent ductus arteriosus (PDA) for systemic or pulmonary blood flow (e.g., interrupted aortic arch, hypoplastic left or right heart). Infusion of prostaglandins may be needed to maintain patency of the DA until a more permanent solution can occur. A persistent PDA produces a left-to-right shunt and requires closure by either pharmacologic, surgical, or interventional means (see later section). Placement of the a pulse oximeter on the preductal extremity (right hand) as well as the postductal extremity (all other limbs) when providing neonatal anesthesia is recommended. A large discrepancy between oxygen saturation values can warn the anesthetist that the child may have a certain degree of PHN is returning to fetal circulation, or has a right-to-left intracardiac shunt. The majority of portal blood flow continues to enter the DV after interruption of umbilical vein blood flow. Although the cause of the initiating mechanisms of DV closure is unknown, the muscular wall of the DV begins to constrict within 1 to 3 hours of birth. Blood flow is directed into the liver, and portal venous pressure increases. During transitional circulation, there is a decrease in PVR with accompanying increases in SVR as the child is born and the placental blood supply ceases. Of note, PVR remains slightly elevated over the first few months of life as the pulmonary vasculature undergoes remodeling. This is slight but still accounts for right ventricular hypertrophy seen on neonatal electrocardiogram (ECG) tracings, and it is the reason why many patients with ventricular septal defects (VSDs) are not symptomatic until the child reaches several months of age when PVR decreases, leading to left-to-right shunting and symptoms of congestive heart failure.

Persistent Pulmonary Hypertension of the Newborn

Persistent pulmonary hypertension (PPHN) of the newborn is the result of an abnormal early adaptation to the perinatal circulatory transition. PPHN is characterized by a sustained elevation of PVR, decreased perfusion of the lungs, and continued right-to-left shunting of blood through the DA. When PVR remains high after birth, right (and sometimes left) ventricular function and cardiac output are depressed. Moderate or severe PPHN is believed to affect up to 2 to 6 per 1000 live births and complicates the course of 10% of all infants admitted to neonatal intensive care units (NICUs). These circulatory abnormalities are also responsible for an 8% to 10% risk of death and

a 25% risk of long-term neurodevelopmental morbidity. Significant PHN may also develop in neonates and young infants as a result of bronchopulmonary dysplasia (BPD) or cardiac disease, though this often occurs over time. When the neonate's cardiovascular and/or pulmonary system is stressed, the infant can revert to fetal circulation with high PVR and right-to-left shunting of blood through the DA. PHN affects roughly one-third of infants with moderate-to-severe BPD.[5-7] BPD is common in premature neonates due to early life exposure to high oxygen concentrations and mechanical ventilatory support leading to lung inflammation, scarring, and damage to alveoli. Though mechanical ventilation may be unavoidable in premature neonates, due to underdeveloped and immature lungs, the concentration of oxygen delivered should be appropriately titrated based on gestational age of the premature baby. Umbilical vein Po_2 is generally around 30 mm Hg with an oxygen saturation in the low 70% range. When these babies are born prematurely and high oxygen concentrations are administered, they are potentially exposed to hyperoxia, thus placing them at risk for developing retinopathy of prematurity (ROP) and BPD. It is important to note that it is not current practice to allow Po_2 and oxygen saturation of premature neonates to remain this low.

During fetal development, PVR is high but rapidly decreases at birth and continues to decline to near-normal levels over the first few months of life as the pulmonary vasculature remodels. This allows the lungs to become a gas-exchanging organ. Before anatomic closure of the DA and FO, fetal circulation may be reestablished and persist during times of stress. PPHN manifests as increases in PVR and accompanying PHN, which produces a right-to-left shunt across the FO and the DA, with resulting systemic cyanosis and hypoxemia. The presence of various congenital cardiovascular or pulmonary diseases may inhibit functional and anatomic closure of the fetal shunts, and it may even be necessary to maintain these shunts to maintain life. Persistent fetal circulation is common in preterm neonates and infants with metabolic derangements (e.g., asphyxia, sepsis, meconium aspiration, and CDH). Hypoxemia, acidosis, pneumonia, and hypothermia are primary precipitating factors of PPHN. Oxygenation, ventilation, correcting acidosis, and maintenance of normothermia will attenuate the increase in PVR. It is also important to be mindful of ventilation during neonatal resuscitation to prevent barotrauma with possible pneumothorax, resulting in further increases in PVR. Continual increases in pulmonary vascular pressure and resistance will precipitate the development of right ventricular hypertrophy (cor pulmonale). Although pulmonary vasodilators may have some utility in decreasing PVR, concurrent reductions in SVR can occur and may worsen intracardiac shunting. Inhaled nitric oxide causes less reduction in SVR when compared to intravenous epoprostenol. Milrinone is another important therapy for neonates with PHN due to its ability to lower PVR while also supporting a struggling right ventricle through inhibition of phosphodiesterase-3. This inhibition leads to a reduction in cyclic adenosine monophosphate (cAMP), ultimately leading to increases in intracellular calcium concentrations resulting in vascular relaxation (reductions in SVR and PVR) and accompanying increases in cardiac contractility. Milrinone does not appear to affect SVR in neonates as much as it does in adults. If a vasoactive medication is needed to counteract low blood pressure states with PHN, or reductions in SVR from drug therapy such as that seen with milrinone, vasopressin may be the drug of choice as it does not increase PVR to the degree that medications that agonize α-1 may (i.e., phenylephrine). Low blood pressure states associated with low cardiac output are generally treated with medication that causes positive inotropic properties (i.e., epinephrine).

The primary aim of PPHN therapy is selective pulmonary vasodilation. Treatment of PHN includes optimization of lung function, oxygen delivery, and support of cardiac function. Optimal lung inflation is essential because PVR is increased when the lungs are underexpanded (i.e., atelectasis) or overexpanded, independent of lung disease. The use of lung recruitment strategies, such as high-frequency ventilation and exogenous surfactant administration, is particularly important in infants with PPHN associated with parenchymal disease, but it has limited impact in infants with primary vascular disease. Correction of severe acidosis and avoidance of hypoxemia are important because they both stimulate pulmonary vasoconstriction. Maintaining a normal hematocrit is also important to ensure adequate oxygen-carrying capacity while avoiding polycythemia because hyperviscosity can increase PVR. Alternately, a low hematocrit reduces oxygen carrying capacity. The threshold for blood transfusions in these patients is lower than that of the healthy neonate. The anesthetist must always be familiar with factors that lead to increases in PVR, including but not limited to hypercapnia, hypoxemia, acidosis, hypothermia, high positive end-expiratory pressure (PEEP), high peak inspiratory pressure (PIP), atelectasis, unpalliated pain with sympathetic stimulation, and vasoactive medications that affect PVR (e.g., phenylephrine). Treatment includes inhaled nitric oxide, epoprostenol, phosphodiesterase-5 inhibitors sildenafil/tadalafil, phosphodiesterase-3 inhibitor milrinone, endothelin receptor antagonist bosentan, and prostanoids such as prostacyclin, iloprost, or treprostinil.[5,7]

GROWTH AND DEVELOPMENT

Cardiovascular System

During embryologic and fetal development, the heart undergoes a very specific set of looping and septation to become the four-chambered structure that we see in normal neonatal cardiac structures. Many congenital heart defects are a result of inappropriate looping or septation during embryologic development. The myocardium of the newborn is structurally and functionally immature. The neonatal heart contains the essential architectural elements of the adult heart; however, there is cellular disorganization and fewer myofibrils. Although the ventricles are of equal size and shape, the contractile components (sarcoplasmic reticulum and T-tubule system) are immature. Accordingly, the neonatal heart is less capable of generating a response to an increase in resistive load (increase in stroke volume [SV]) and is dependent on free ionized calcium for contractility. Thus neonatal SV is relatively fixed making cardiac output heavily dependent on heart rate (CO = HR × SV). Despite this immaturity, the neonatal heart is capable of very limited increases in SV up to left atrial pressures of 10 to 12 mm Hg when afterload remains low. This information suggests that the neonatal heart is operating near the peak of the Frank-Starling curve, and there is limited reserve in the face of increases in both preload and afterload. The neonatal myocardium is incredibly sensitive to changes in calcium levels, and calcium is vital for neonatal myocardial performance. Calcium administration in the form of calcium chloride or calcium gluconate may be considered in the hypotensive neonate that is not responding to an appropriate fluid bolus.

During maturation, the left ventricle will hypertrophy through an increase in the number and size of myofibrils. This maturation is a consequence of left ventricular contraction against a higher postnatal systemic pressure. Acute increases in afterload (i.e., acidosis, hypothermia, and pain) will produce further reductions in cardiac output. In the immediate postnatal period, left ventricular compliance is low. The neonate may develop congestive heart failure because the stiff left ventricle will not stretch to accommodate large fluid loads. Left ventricular distention from volume overload compresses the adjacent right ventricle, producing additional reductions in cardiac output. Likewise, ventilation with high peak pressure will produce left ventricular dysfunction

and progressive overload of the right ventricle. The left and right ventricles show interdependence. The right ventricle receives perfusion during diastole and systole, but when systolic pressures approach aortic pressures, as seen in neonates with PPHN, there is a reduction in right ventricular coronary perfusion. As right ventricular strain increases, end-diastolic pressure rises leading to further reductions in diastolic coronary perfusion. The right ventricle is susceptible to failure with prolonged exposure to high pulmonary pressures, and the ventricular septum will eventually start bowing into the left ventricle as the right ventricle continues to distend. This bowing reduces left ventricular preload, cardiac output, and coronary blood flow, which further reduces blood supply to the failing right ventricle and perpetuates this downward spiral for these neonates.

Due to the immaturity of the contractile elements of the neonatal myocardium, the belief is that pediatric cardiac output is highly dependent on heart rate. Atropine may be administered to decrease the potential of bradycardia, especially when vagal stimulation may occur (i.e., suctioning and intubation). However, marked increases in heart rate fail to a large extent to produce further increases in cardiac output. Although the neonatal myocardium is not as compliant as in an older child or adult, increased preload does not increase SV to the same degree. However, volume expansion (VE) remains important, albeit to a smaller extent than in the adult, in increasing SV. The combination of hypovolemia and bradycardia produces dramatic decreases in cardiac output that threaten organ perfusion. Epinephrine rather than atropine increases contractility and heart rate and is warranted for the treatment of bradycardia and decreased cardiac output in pediatric patients. The baroreceptor reflex is not completely developed, limiting the neonate's ability to compensate for hypotension with the reflexive tachycardia that would be expected in the older child and adult. Baroreceptor dysfunction is more pronounced in the premature neonate, and the heart rate may seem fixed despite intervention or changes in the neonate's physiology. This is quite important when providing anesthesia and choosing appropriate interventions for these patients.

Autonomic innervation of the neonatal heart is predominantly controlled by parasympathetic nervous system predominance; the sympathetic nervous system is immature at birth. Parasympathetic predominance produces bradycardia that may occur with minor clinical interventions such as pharyngeal suctioning and laryngoscopy. Marked variation in the newborn heart rate and rhythm occurs secondary to changes in autonomic tone. The ECG recording in the newborn reflects the immaturity of the conduction system. The ECG axis is shifted to the right as a result of higher PVR in the neonate. The axis shifts to the left as the pulmonary vasculature remodels, and the left ventricle undergoes hypertrophy with increasing SVR. The P wave is evident; the PR interval is less than 0.12 second and increases until adolescence. T waves are upright in the recorded chest leads reflecting right ventricular domination. The newborn heart rate generally ranges from 100 to 160 beats per minute (bpm), but averages 120 bpm during the first day of life. Heart rate may increase close to 160 bpm at 1 month of age, then steadily decreases to an average of 75 beats by the adolescent period. Sleep may produce heart rates lower than 100 bpm, whereas pain can increase the heart rate up 200 bpm.

Blood pressure increases immediately after birth, rising to a mean systolic pressure of 70 to 75 mm Hg within the first 48 hours. As the heart rate decreases with maturation, there is an accompanying increase in blood pressure. Blood pressure is lower in the preterm infant, and severely premature neonates often have mean arterial pressures approximately equaling their gestational age. A premature neonate at 25 weeks will display a mean arterial pressure of 25 to 30 mm Hg. The American Heart Association defines pediatric hypotension in relation to the systolic blood pressure as shown in Box 52.2. Table 52.1 shows general values for heart rate and blood pressure at various ages.

Fetal hemoglobin is the predominant hemoglobin species in the newborn, contributing between 70% and 90% of the total hemoglobin. A normal hemoglobin range at birth is approximately 18 to 20 g/dL. Fetal hemoglobin has a lower P-50 and shifts the oxyhemoglobin dissociation curve to the left, which causes a higher affinity for oxygen than adult hemoglobin. In utero, this increased oxygen affinity facilitates oxygen uptake as fetal blood circulates through the placenta, increasing the binding of oxygen to fetal hemoglobin and allowing the fetus to exist in an environment with a relatively low PaO_2. There is a rapid change in the fetal hematopoietic physiology due to increased oxygen concentrations after birth. The increased arterial oxygen content results in a decrease in erythropoietin activity, in combination with a decrease in the rate of hematopoiesis. A decrease in erythropoiesis and a decreased life span of the newborn's red blood cells (RBCs) produce a progressive decrease in hemoglobin, which peaks approximately between 3 and 4 months of age. The period of "physiologic anemia of infancy" does not compromise the oxygen delivery to tissues because the oxyhemoglobin dissociation curve shifts to the right, and RBC concentrations of 2,3-diphosphoglycerate (DPG) increase (Fig. 52.2). Adult hemoglobin has two alpha chains and two beta chains, whereas fetal hemoglobin consists of two alpha chains and two gamma chains. This is relevant because 2,3-DPG only binds to beta chains. During a blood transfusion, there is a shifting toward the adult oxygen dissociation curve, allowing hemoglobin to not only carry more oxygen but also release more oxygen to the tissues. Fetal hemoglobin is replaced by adult hemoglobin during the first 3 to 6 months, producing a rightward shift of the oxyhemoglobin dissociation curve as compared to the neonatal period.

It is important to note that premature neonates may experience a dramatic fall in hemoglobin because of insufficient body stores of iron. Premature infants should receive iron and vitamin K prophylaxis because the concentration of vitamin K-dependent clotting factors (II, VII, IX, and X) are 20% to 50% of adult levels.[8] Premature infants have lower levels of vitamin K dependent clotting factors. Full liver maturation may take up to 2 years for the child. Maternally ingested drugs

such as warfarin and isoniazid may precipitate the development of a coagulopathy.

The newborn's blood volume is dependent on the time of cord clamping (transfusion from the placenta). Delaying umbilical cord clamping in premature neonates for 30 seconds stabilizes transitional circulation, decreases the need for inotropic medications, and reduces blood transfusions, necrotizing enterocolitis (NEC), and intraventricular hemorrhage (IVH).[9] Blood volume is approximately 80 to 90 mL/kg but may be as high as 100 mL/kg in the premature neonate. The intravascular volume decreases 25% in the immediate postnatal period with the loss of intravascular fluid. It is common for newborns to lose 10% of their body weight within the first 24 hours of life. Blood volume increases over the next 2 months, peaking at 2 months of age. Table 52.2 provides an estimate of circulating blood volume development.

Respiratory System

In utero, fetal lung development beings with the formation of lung buds, which occurs during the first few weeks after conception. During organogenesis, which occurs in the second trimester, creation of distinct bronchi and bronchopulmonary segments extends downward to the terminal bronchioles. There are 10 to 20 million terminal sacs, which, after elongation, begin to develop into alveoli after birth. The neonate's alveoli surface area is approximately one-third that of the adult. The process of alveolar formation is accelerated between 12 and 18 months postnatally and rapidly increases to 200 to 300 million between 8 and 10 years of age.

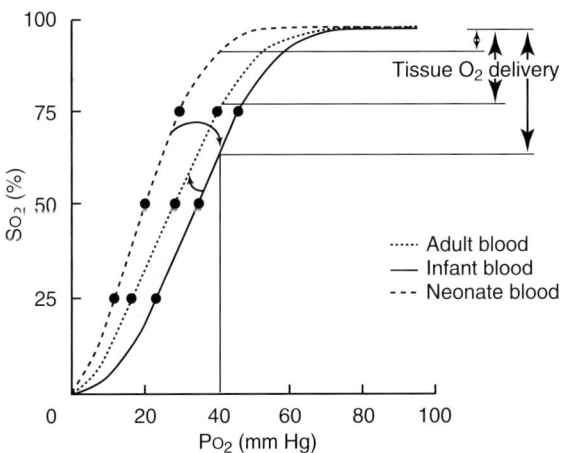

Fig. 52.2 Schematic representation of oxyhemoglobin dissociation curves with different oxygen affinities. *(Top arrows)* Direction of rightward shifting of the oxyhemoglobin dissociation curve (and P-50) after birth. By 10 weeks of age, the adult position of the curve is reached. *Pao₂*, Partial pressure of oxygen; *Spo₂*, oxygen saturation. (From Davis PJ, Cladis FP. *Smith's Anesthesia for Infants and Children.* 9th ed. Philadelphia: Elsevier; 2017:60.)

TABLE 52.1 Age-Related Changes in the Cardiovascular System

Age	Heart Rate	Systolic BP	Diastolic BP
Neonate	140	70–75	40
12 mo	120	95	65
3 yr	100	100	70
12 yr	80	110	60

BP, Blood pressure.

TABLE 52.2 Estimated Blood Volumes by Age

Age Group	Volume (mL/kg)
Premature	90–100
Newborn (age <1 mo)	80–90
Infants age 3 mo–3 yr	75–80
Children age >6 yr	65–70
Adults	65–70

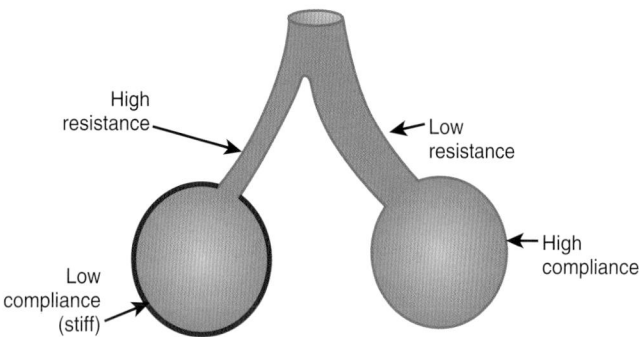

Fig. 52.3 An idealized state showing the reciprocal relationship between resistance and compliance; gas flow is preferentially delivered to the most compliant regions, regardless of the rate of inflation. Static and dynamic compliance are equal. (From Davis PJ, Cladis FP. *Smith's Anesthesia for Infants and Children.* 9th ed. Philadelphia: Elsevier; 2017:359.)

Surfactant is produced and secreted by type II pneumocytes, which generally begins between 22 and 26 weeks, with concentrations peaking between 35 and 36 weeks of gestation. Surfactant is responsible for decreasing surface tension within the alveoli to decrease alveolar collapse and maintain alveoli patency during low lung volume states. This relationship can be explained by the law of Laplace (see upcoming equation). In the absence of adequate pulmonary surfactant such as in a premature neonate, or with secondary surfactant dysfunction, alveoli become stiff and noncompliant (Fig. 52.3). Severe atelectasis decreases alveolar surface area available for oxygen and carbon dioxide exchange. Increased physiologic dead space and ventilation perfusion mismatch cause hypoxia and hypercarbia, necessitating mechanical ventilation. The treatment for infantile respiratory distress syndrome (RDS) includes synthetic surfactant, continuous positive airway pressure (CPAP), and mechanical ventilation.[10] It is important to monitor blood gases shortly after surfactant administration and adjust ventilator settings, as lung compliance can change drastically shortly after administration. As lung compliance changes over the first few hours, it is vital to adjust mechanical ventilation and take measures to prevent underventilation (atelectasis) or overventilation (barotrauma, volutrauma). Surfactant may also be administered prophylactically to premature neonates, especially extremely premature neonates (age varies across facilities), and during conditions that can potentially lead to surfactant dysfunction (e.g., pulmonary hemorrhage, neonatal sepsis, meconium aspiration during birth, and pneumonia).

$$P = 2T/R$$

P = pressure within a sphere, T = surface tension,
R = radius of the sphere

Anatomy

At birth, the neonatal larynx is small compared with the mouth and pharynx. The epiglottis of the neonate takes on a more U shape, is stiffer than that of an adult's, and the vallecula is shallow so that the tongue approximates the epiglottis. The larynx is pointed toward the nasopharynx, facilitating nasal breathing, and infants are obligate nasal breathers until roughly 5 months of age. Obligate nasal breathing allows the neonate and infant to feed and breath at the same time, but neonates can transition to mouth breathing if nasal passages are blocked. It is important for the anesthetist to understand the severity of obstructed nasal breathing in the face of oral obstruction to breathing (e.g., bilateral choanal atresia). The arytenoids are large in proportion to the lumen of the larynx. The subglottic region is smaller than the glottic opening, with the cartilages telescoping into one another,

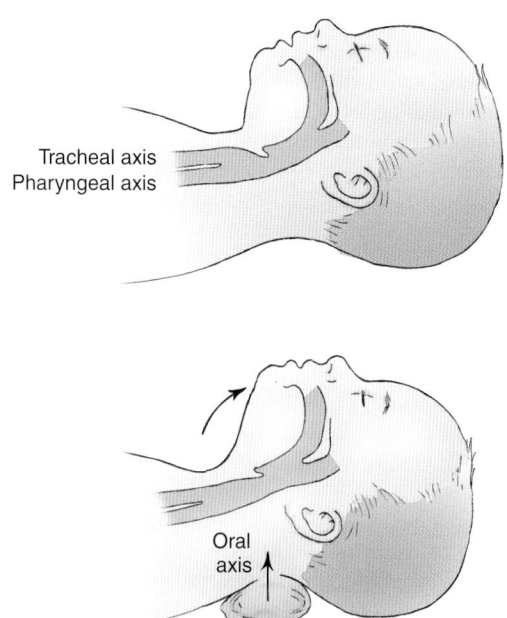

Fig. 52.4 Alignments of visual, oral, and laryngeal axes during laryngoscopy.

forming a conical shape.[11] The cricoid cartilage is believed to be the narrowest portion of the airway, and the cricoid lumen is not round but mostly an ellipsoid structure. It is lined with a pseudostratified epithelium that can be easily injured during laryngoscopy and can result in airway edema, stridor, and bleeding. The pediatric airway is more cylindric than funnel shaped.[12] The implication for clinical practice is that an endotracheal tube (ETT) that may pass through the vocal cords during insertion may not easily advance due to the narrowed cricoid cartilage. The vocal cords may be displaced or stretched to fit a certain size ETT, but the ETT may not pass through the cricoid cartilage making this fixed structure the narrowest portion of the pediatric airway. To this day there remains some debate regarding the narrowest portion of the pediatric airway.

The newborn tongue is large and difficult to manipulate because of the position of the hyoid bone. In addition, a smaller potential submental space is present, meaning there is less space to displace the tongue during laryngoscopy. The anterior position of the larynx, in conjunction with the large tongue, can increase the potential for airway obstruction and the difficulty of mask ventilation. It is important to always be mindful of hand position during mask ventilation of the neonate, as it is quite easy to obstruct the airway with minimal pressure on the submental space. The neonatal tongue may also stick to the hard/soft palate, making mask ventilation difficult. Placement of an appropriately sized oral airway will alleviate this problem.

The larynx is located more cephalad and anterior, extending from the second to the fourth cervical vertebrae (C2-C4), when compared to the adult laryngeal position of C5-C6. Not only is the larynx located higher and more anterior, but the neonate's occiput is larger and more prominent in relation to the rest of the body. The anesthetic implication of the more cephalad location of the larynx, in combination with a larger head, is that placing a neonate in the so-called sniffing position for laryngoscopy and intubation will only move the larynx in an anterior direction, potentially increasing the difficulty of intubation. A shoulder roll aids in the visual alignment of the oral, pharyngeal, and tracheal axes during laryngoscopy (Fig. 52.4 and Table 52.3).

TABLE 52.3 Differences: Adult Airway and Pediatric Airway

	Pediatric	Adult
Laryngeal location	C2–C4	C3–C6
Narrowest location of airway	Cricoid cartilage	Glottis
Shape of epiglottis	Longer, more narrow	V shaped
Right mainstem bronchus	Less vertical	More vertical

Once the ETT passes the vocal cords into the trachea, it is important for the anesthetist to consider the size and anatomy of the trachea and bronchi. The right bronchus is much straighter in the neonate and remains this way until roughly 3 years of age. Mainstem intubation is much more common in the right bronchus and must be recognized immediately in this patient population. It is also important to understand the effects of even the slightest head movement on ETT position within the small trachea of the neonate. The ETT movement follows the position related to the patient's nose. Even minimal flexion of the neck following intubation can lead to mainstem location of the ETT, and mild neck extension may lead to inadvertent extubation of the neonate. If the head is going to be manipulated during the procedure, the anesthetist must test head movement when deciding where the ETT should be safely secured to avoid a mainstem ETT location or inadvertent extubation.

Mechanics of Breathing

The neonate's chest wall is pliable due to a lack of developed musculature and a skeletal structure primarily composed of cartilage. The ribs are horizontal in orientation, providing minimal assistance in the expansion of the chest wall with inspiration. During inspiration, the compliant chest wall tends to collapse inward (paradoxic breathing). To maintain negative intrathoracic pressure, despite having a compliant chest wall, the neonate and infant actively recruit accessory muscles of respiration (i.e., intercostal muscles). Additionally, exhalation is limited by the adductor muscles of the larynx, which contract and serve as an expiratory valve, or brake, to maintain end-expiratory pressure. These structural differences are responsible for the decrease in functional residual capacity (FRC) with administration of general anesthesia in the neonate and infant. The previously cited muscular activity responsible for maintaining FRC is diminished with the administration of sedatives, inhalation anesthetics, and neuromuscular blocking agents. Rapid hypoxemia can occur with the loss of FRC. The neonate also has a high oxygen consumption, nearly two times higher than adults, and this in conjunction with a reduced FRC leads to rapid desaturation with apnea. FRC may be restored with the application of CPAP or controlled ventilation. The premature neonate displays even more chest wall pliability, and paradoxic chest movement may occur with breathing at rest.

The diaphragm contributes to the differences in respiratory function of the neonate and infant. Unlike the adult diaphragm, which is dome shaped, the diaphragm of the neonate and infant is relatively flat. Accordingly, its anterior insertion on the chest wall fails to contribute any mechanical advantage with contraction. Primarily the diaphragm and, to a lesser extent, the intercostal muscles allow for expansion of the thoracic cavity and the associated increase in negative intrathoracic pressure. As a result, during inspiration, air is drawn into the lungs, and air passively exits the lungs due to the elastic recoil with relaxation of these muscles. Two types of muscle fibers are present in muscle tissue: the diaphragm and intercostals. Type 1 muscle fibers are slow-twitch muscle fibers and are resistant to fatigue. These fibers are essential for

sustained ventilatory activity. Type 2 muscle fibers, also known as fast-twitch muscle fibers, are built for short bursts of activity but fatigue rapidly. A newborn's diaphragm is composed of 25% type 1 muscle fibers as compared to 55% type 1 muscle fibers in the adult diaphragm. In addition, type 2 muscle fibers are predominant within the intercostals. Therefore newborns and young infants are at risk of muscle fatigue, respiratory distress, and respiratory arrest. The anesthetist must assess for airway obstruction and respiratory compromise resulting from the depressant effects of residual anesthetic agents, airway obstruction, and postoperative pain. Assisting with respirations and relieving airway obstruction during the perioperative period will promote adequate gas exchange and decrease the degree of atelectasis.

Control of Breathing

Respiratory maturation and control of breathing occurs around 42 to 44 weeks of gestation. The control of breathing is dependent on the Pao_2 sensed via the peripheral chemoreceptors (carotid and aortic bodies), the partial pressure of arterial CO_2 ($Paco_2$), and pH, which influence the central chemoreceptors within the respiratory control center of the medulla. Increases in $Paco_2$ produce corresponding increases in tidal volume (Vt) and respiratory rate, although this response is not as vigorous as in the adult. Increases in Pao_2 will depress the ventilatory response in the newborn, whereas a decreased Pao_2 will increase the ventilatory response. It is important to note that before maturation of the respiratory centers and control of breathing, hypoxemia will depress ventilation, whereas increases in ventilation in response to hypoxemia occur following maturation. The ventilatory response to hypoxemia produces two distinctly different responses. Initially, hypoxemia produces an increase in ventilation for the first minute but produces ventilatory depression for the next 3 to 5 minutes. Due to the newborn's lack of ability to compensate for physiologic stress, rapid ventilatory depression and arrest are possible if hypothermia, acidosis, or hypercarbia occurs. Hypoglycemia may also reduce ventilatory effort in the neonate, so the anesthetist must be mindful of this and take steps to reduce hypoglycemia.

Respiratory depression and/or apnea may develop in the newborn after stimulation of the carina and/or the superior laryngeal nerve, following upper airway obstruction or following sustained lung inflation (Hering-Breuer reflex). The newborn may exhibit periodic breathing with inspiratory pauses lasting 10 seconds, followed by abrupt increases in ventilation. Periodic breathing is more common in the premature neonate and occurs more often during rapid eye movement sleep. Apneic episodes are not uncommon in premature neonates; such episodes can produce rapid arterial desaturation. If apnea is not rapidly resolved, bradycardia and cardiac arrest may occur. The suspected causes of apnea in premature neonates include immature responses of the respiratory control centers to hypercarbia or hypoxic stimuli and respiratory fatigue.

Lung Volumes

The mean values for pulmonary function in the newborn and adult are shown in Table 52.4. The neonate's metabolic rate and oxygen consumption are approximately twice that of the adult. The decreased reservoir for oxygen (i.e., decreased FRC), coupled with the increased demand for oxygen (i.e., increased metabolic rate), results in rapid desaturation when ventilation is interrupted, as seen with intubation. Preoxygenation prior to induction and intubation will help lengthen the time before desaturation, but not to the extent seen in adults. Airway closure produces a mismatching of ventilation and perfusion. The volume of poorly ventilated alveoli that contributes to intrapulmonary shunting is greater in neonates than in adults. In addition, increased PVR can produce a right-to-left shunt through the FO or a PDA,

TABLE 52.4 Mean Values for Normal Pulmonary Function in the Newborn and the Adult

	Newborn	Adult
Body weight (kg)	3	70
Tidal volume (mL/kg)	6	6
Respiratory rate (bpm)	35	15
Alveolar ventilation (mL/kg/min)	130	60
Oxygen consumption (mL/kg/min)	6.4	3.5
Total lung capacity (mL/kg)	63	86
Functional residual capacity (mL/kg)	30	34
Vital capacity (mL/kg)	35	70
Residual volume (mL/kg)	23	16
Closing capacity (mL/kg)	35	23
Arterial pH	7.38–7.41	7.35–7.45
$Paco_2$ (mm Hg)	30–35	35–45
Pao_2 (mm Hg)	60–90	90–100
Sao_2 (%)	95–100	95–100

$Paco_2$, Partial pressure of arterial carbon dioxide; Pao_2, partial pressure of arterial oxygen; Sao_2, oxygen saturation.

resulting in the rapid development of hypoxemia. Hypercapnia and hypoxemia increase PVR, which will perpetuate this cycle of hypoxic pulmonary vasoconstriction (HPV), right-to-left shunting, further hypoxia and hypercapnia, and potential respiratory and/or cardiac arrest in neonates.

Airway Dynamics

Airway resistance is greater in neonates and declines markedly with growth from 19 to 28 cm H_2O/L/sec to less than 2 cm H_2O/L/sec in adults.[13-15] According to Poiseuille's law, airway resistance is inversely proportional to the fourth power of the radius of the airway during laminar flow. A neonate must overcome the resistance to airflow, as well as the elastic recoil of the lungs and chest wall, so changes in either of these factors can have drastic effects on the newborn. Mild reductions in airway diameter, as seen with airway edema, can be very detrimental to the neonate. Airway resistance changes with age. Although the larger airway resistance remains constant, airway resistance in the smaller airways is increased. The increase in airway resistance increases the work of breathing in the neonate. Small airway disease (e.g., pneumonia) produces additional increases in the work of breathing as the lungs become stiff and noncompliant. There is an increase in airway resistance from small distal airways, increased propensity of ventilation perfusion mismatch, and high metabolic rate potentially leading to barotrauma and rapid hypoxemia. Ventilation strategies utilizing pressure-limited ventilation and volume-targeted ventilation in preterm and term neonates have shown to be effective at avoiding these complications.[17]

The metabolic energy expenditure of breathing in the neonate is approximately 0.5 mL per 0.5 L of ventilation, which is similar to that of an adult. This is equivalent to 1% of the metabolic energy. The premature neonate's metabolic expenditure of breathing is 0.9 mL per 0.5 L, almost double the metabolic price. If the neonate has pulmonary comorbidities, as seen in premature neonates and those with CHD, the energy expenditure can increase.[16] There are many modes available on ICU ventilators and the ventilators seen on current anesthesia machines, and the mode selected may depend on the procedure being performed, respiratory status of the neonate, and the anesthetist's preference.

Nervous System

The central nervous system (CNS) in the newborn differs from the older child in relation to the degree of myelination, muscle tone and reflexes, and development of the cerebral cortex. In the peripheral nervous system, myelination begins in the motor roots and progresses to the sensory roots. In contrast, the myelination in the cerebral sensory systems precedes that of the central motor systems. This incomplete myelination is associated with those reflexes that are used to measure neural development, the Moro and grasp reflexes. Myelination of the nervous system is not complete until approximately age 3 years.

Development of Neuromuscular Junction

The neuromuscular junction (NMJ) undergoes developmental changes during the first 2 months of life. During the maturation process, the NMJ differs in several ways. There is a difference in the maturity, density, sensitivity, and distribution of the postsynaptic acetylcholine (Ach) receptors; in the rapidity of neuromuscular transmission; and in muscle fiber type.[18] The functional difference between immature Ach receptors as compared to those that are fully developed is a prolonged opening of the ionic channels. This prolonged channel opening allows the immature muscles to be more easily depolarized. These Ach receptors also have a greater affinity for depolarizing agents and a lower affinity for nondepolarizing muscle relaxants (NDMRs). The clinical implication of these maturational changes is that neonates can have a greater variability in response to NDMRs. Monitoring for neuromuscular function after NDMR administration via a peripheral nerve stimulator is critical. Neuromuscular immaturity may be demonstrated with the appearance of fade after tetanic stimulation in the absence of neuromuscular blocking drugs (NMBDs). It is also worth noting that the type 1 fibers are more sensitive to NDMRs when compared with type 2 fibers. The clinical relevance of this difference is that the diaphragm of a neonate has fewer type 1 fibers as compared to the diaphragm of a toddler or an adult. This makes the diaphragm of a neonate more responsive to NDMRs than the peripheral musculature, so larger doses may be needed to facilitate peripheral paralysis.[19] The use of intermediate acting neuromuscular blocking agents during anesthesia has been associated with an increased risk of clinically significant postoperative respiratory complications.[20] It has not been scientifically determined if assessment of neuromuscular blockade via an accelerometer is a more effective measure of residual neuromuscular blockade in pediatric patients. Neonates have a higher percentage of total body water (TBW) and thus a larger volume of distribution (Vd) for water-soluble drugs, such as NDMRs and depolarizing muscle relaxants (succinylcholine).

Pain Sensitivity

Pathways required for pain perception can be traced from sensory receptors in the skin to sensory areas in the cerebral cortex of newborns and infants. These pain pathways have been demonstrated in the perioral area as early as 7 weeks of gestation. With positron emission tomography (PET) scans, neonates demonstrate maximal metabolic activity in the regions associated with sensory perception, such as the cortex, thalamus, and midbrain-brainstem regions. Pediatric anesthetists have seen newborns exhibit signs of increased sympathetic activity (i.e., tachycardia and hypertension) in response to surgical stimulation with inadequate anesthesia. When the neonate is exposed to noxious stimulation with inadequate or absent pain control, there can be significant physiologic consequences, including poor control of physiologic stress response, increased levels of catecholamines and cortisol, poor healing conditions, and higher morbidity and mortality. Additional consequences in the presence of abnormal cerebral autoregulation could result in IVH. Because the neonate already has increased PVR, and the pulmonary vasculature is still undergoing change and proliferation, PHN can occur secondary to increased endogenous catecholamine levels with unpalliated pain.[21]

The neonate has immature inhibitory descending pain pathways, which may increase the intensity and duration of the painful stimulus. It has been suggested that newborns and infants may develop prolonged responses to painful procedures that far outlast the stimuli by hours or days. This is illustrated by the following examples. Premature infants mount a metabolic stress response that can be blocked with opioids, increased crying, and interrupted sleep patterns; behavioral changes have been shown to occur for days after circumcision[22]; and with repeated heel lancing, there appears to be a hyperalgesic response to injury.[23] Other physiologic alterations that have been demonstrated are increased right-to-left shunting, hypoxemia, acidosis, and IVH.[21]

Sensory nerve distribution is formed by 20 weeks of gestational age. Pain pathways and receptors are present within the CNS at birth. Physiologic stimulation from anesthesia management and surgery dramatically increase circulating catecholamines and other stress hormones. As in adults, during the perioperative experience, pediatric patients exhibit tachycardia and hypertension if light anesthesia is coupled with significant surgical stimulation. Due to the lack of cerebral vascular autoregulation, increased blood pressure can cause intracerebral bleeding, especially in premature neonates. The pain threshold for infants and children may be lower than in older children and adults, possibly due to increased pain sensitivity, behavioral factors, or both. Preoperative and postoperative signs of pain in patients who are preverbal include tachycardia, elevated blood pressure, crying, restlessness, and grimacing.

In recent years, the safety of anesthetic medications and their effect on the developing brain have been questioned. In animal studies, agents that either antagonize N-methyl-D-aspartate (NMDA) receptors or potentiate the neurotransmission of γ-aminobutyric acid (GABA) agents have been implicated, and no safe doses or durations of exposure of these agents have been defined.[24] One proposed mechanism of action for these effects is through inhibition of brain-derived neurotrophic factor, which stimulates neural development.[25] Neurotoxicity resulting in neuroapoptosis, interference with nerve pathway, and nerve cell development can result in long-term neurocognitive deficits.[24,26-28] Most damage occurs during maturation periods when synaptogenesis rapidly occurs.[29] The Food and Drug Administration (FDA) is addressing this issue by forming a public-private partnership with the International Anesthesia Research Society called SmartTots (Strategies for Mitigating Anesthesia-Related Neuro-Toxicity in Tots). This partnership will seek to mobilize the scientific community, stimulate dialogue among thoughtful leaders in the anesthesia community, and work to raise funding for the necessary research. The topic of effects of anesthesia on the developing brain is an ongoing discussion.

Until the risks related to neurocognitive development and anesthetic agents are definitively determined, recommendations to minimize the potential for iatrogenic effects include (1) attempting to minimize the duration of anesthesia and surgery and (2) using short-acting drugs and/or a combination of general anesthesia and multimodal pain therapy (including systemic analgesics) and local or regional anesthesia to reduce the overall drug dosage.[30,31] It is important to note that opioids do appear to be safe in regard to neurodevelopment and the neonatal brain. For an in-depth discussion of pediatric pain and its management, refer to Chapter 56.

Cranium and Spinal Column

The most significant neurologic growth and development occur in utero. The neural tube is nearly completely formed by 3 to 4 weeks of gestational age. It further differentiates over the next 4 to 12 weeks to create other anatomic structures that include the forebrain, facial bones, and spinal cord. Neurogenesis proceeds during weeks 12 to 20, followed by synaptogenesis and increased myelination. Increased density of synaptic connections and glial cells continues to develop until 2 years of age and is estimated to be 50% greater than that of the adult brain.[32]

After birth, there is a rapid continuation of functional and structural brain development. The brain doubles in weight within the first 6 months of life and triples in weight within a year. At 1 year of age, maturation of the cerebral cortex and brainstem is nearly complete. Myelination of nerve cells continues until 3 years of age. By 2 years of age, the child's brain is 80% of the adult weight and 90% by age 5 years. Due to the rapid neuronal development and growth, fontanelles and supple cranial bones allow the skull to accommodate increases in cerebral volume without increasing intracranial pressure (ICP). There are two major fontanelles, anterior and posterior (Fig. 52.5). In 96% of children, the anterior fontanelle closes by 2 years of age. The posterior fontanelle closes at approximately 4 months. The anterior fontanelle can be used to assess increased ICP (bulging anterior fontanelle) as well as dehydration (sunken anterior fontanelle).

The blood-brain barrier (BBB) is immature until approximately 1 year of age. Therefore higher concentrations of medications and toxins that would be impermeable to the adult brain can result in higher cerebral concentrations throughout infancy.[33] With neonates having lower body fat, especially premature neonates, the brain may be the area of highest fat concentration in the body and become the major storage for fat-soluble drugs. Nerve cells within the spinal cord continue to mature until 6 to 7 years of age. As the pediatric patient grows, the conus medullaris and the dural sac migrate cephalad. Although the exact vertebral level of these structures varies slightly, the conus medullaris terminates between L2 and L3 in neonates. The dural sac ends between S2 and S3 until approximately 6 years of age. Being mindful of this information is imperative to providing safe anesthesia during placement of a spinal or caudal anesthetic. By age 8 years, the spinal cord approximates the adult and ends at L1.[33] Fig. 52.6 illustrates the comparison between the adult and infant spinal anatomy.

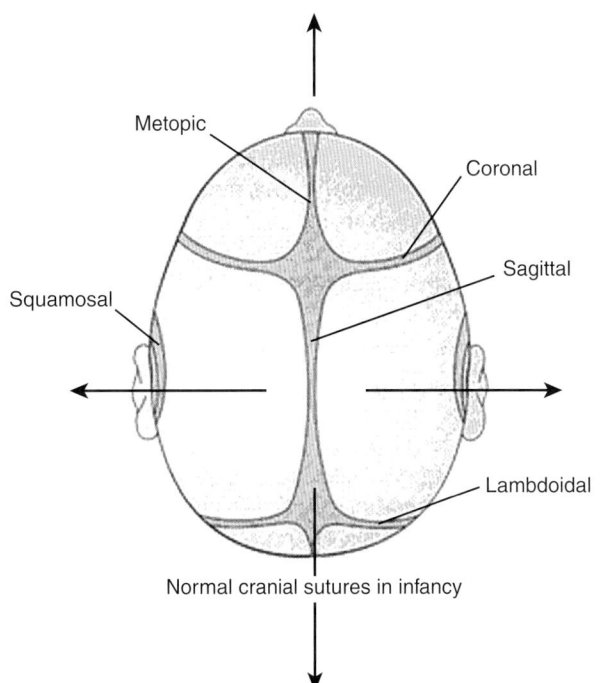

Fig. 52.5 Cranial sutures and fontanelles in neonates and infants. (Modified from Davis PJ, Cladis FP. *Smith's Anesthesia for Infants and Children*. 9th ed. Philadelphia: Elsevier; 2017:745.)

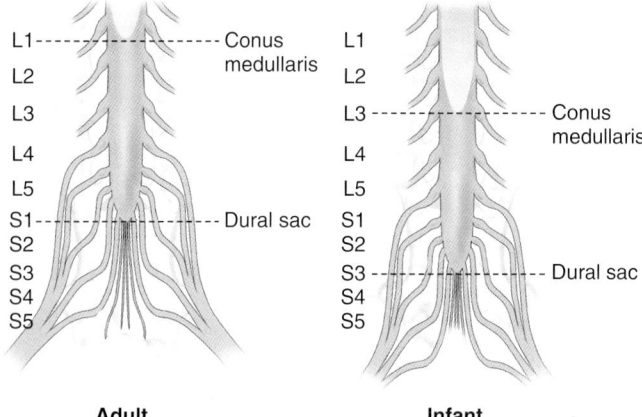

Fig. 52.6 Comparison of levels of the conus medullaris and the dural sac in the infant and the older child or adult. (From Davis PJ, Cladis FP, Motoyama EK. *Smith's Anesthesia for Infants and Children.* 8th ed. Philadelphia: Elsevier; 2011:463.)

Cerebral Metabolic Requirement

Due to the rapid maturation of the CNS during infancy and that continues throughout childhood, proper nutrition is essential to ensure normal development. With maturation there is an increase in the metabolic demands of the CNS. The primary fuel for the brain is glucose, and in the neonate there are decreased stores of glycogen making hypoglycemia a major source of morbidity causing apnea, hypotension, bradycardia, convulsions, and brain injury. Thus it is important to consider dextrose-containing solutions during surgical intervention based on type and length of procedure as well as comorbidities of the neonate.

Cerebral Blood Flow

Cerebral blood flow (CBF) is closely coupled with cerebral metabolic rate of oxygen consumption (CMRO$_2$). CBF in the premature infant is 40 mL/100 g/min, and in older children approaches the adult level of 100 mL/100 g/min. Autoregulation of CBF refers to the ability of the CNS to regulate CBF over a wide range of cerebral perfusion pressures. It is currently believed that CBF autoregulation is present in the neonate, but the specific limits are unknown. Complete loss of cerebral autoregulation may occur with hypoxia, severe hypercapnia (>80 mm Hg), BBB disruption after head trauma, subarachnoid or intracerebral hemorrhage, cerebral ischemia, or after the administration of high concentrations of potent inhalation anesthetics and vasodilators (nitroprusside). Remember that the neonatal BBB is immature and may already be disrupted. Changes in CBF will parallel changes in cerebral blood volume, except when cerebral perfusion decreases and autoregulation produces vasodilation to maintain a constant flow. The cerebral vessels are very fragile in preterm and low birthweight (LBW) infants, and this fragility predisposes neonates to intracranial hemorrhage. Intracranial hemorrhage may be precipitated by hypoxia, hypercarbia, hyperglycemia, hypoglycemia, hypernatremia, and wide swings in arterial or venous pressure. It is important for the anesthetist to assess for the presence of IVH preoperatively. The intravenous administration of hypertonic solutions may damage these fragile vessels. Therefore concentrations of sodium bicarbonate that would be administered to an adult should not be administered to neonates

Autonomic Nervous System Immaturity

At birth, the autonomic nervous system is developed but not mature as in an adult. The sympathetic nervous system innervation to the heart and vasculature is less responsive compared with parasympathetic nervous system innervation. As a result, physiologic stress can cause

severe and rapid cardiovascular collapse. It is important for the anesthetist to consider times when vagal stimulation may be increased (i.e., laryngoscopy and suctioning). As the pediatric patient ages, the child's sympathetic responsiveness becomes pronounced, and the child can compensate for stress by increasing heart rate and blood pressure. If bradycardia occurs, the anesthetist should focus first on hypoxia as a possible cause, but secondary causes should be in the back of the anesthetist's mind. Rapid assessment and treatment are essential. Specific causes that could lead to bradycardia and cardiac arrest are included in Box 52.3.[3]

Renal System

In utero, fluid and electrolytes equilibrate across the placenta in response to fetal growth and metabolic demands. The fetal kidneys make urine that passes into the amniotic cavity to compose one-half of the amniotic fluid, which is then swallowed and absorbed in the gut. Assessment of amniotic fluid volume represents an important tool for evaluating fetal kidney function and development. Structurally, the kidney is different in the neonate. Nephrons are still being formed at up to 35 weeks of gestation. The resulting glomerular filtration rate (GFR) is much lower in a preterm (0.55 mL/min/kg) than a full-term baby (up to 1.6 mL/min/kg) or a 2-year-old child (2 mL/min/kg). Decreased systemic arterial pressure, increased renal vascular resistance, and decreased permeability of the glomerular capillaries contribute to the low GFR. The stiff, noncompliant myocardium of the neonate cannot tolerate fluid overload, and this is further accentuated by lower GFR. GFR reaches adult levels by 6 to 12 months of age. The renal medulla is not completely mature, and the potential effect of antidiuretic hormone (ADH) is diminished. However, all the hormones that affect the kidney are active even in a very immature neonate, albeit with reduced potency. Neonates are called obligate sodium excreters because of their inability to conserve sodium, even in cases of severe sodium depletion. The renin-angiotensin-aldosterone system (RAAS) acts to reduce sodium loss from the distal tubule, but the immature renal tubules fail to respond as well as children and adults. In addition, the renal tubules have a limited ability to reabsorb glucose. Increasing plasma glucose concentrations may elicit osmotic diuresis, depleting intravascular volume. Table 52.5 lists the daily electrolyte requirements for the newborn. Renal tubular function is immature until the age of 2 to 3 years. The neonate has a limited ability to concentrate urine compared with an adult (700 vs 1200 mOsm/L). Assessment of serum osmolality is an important tool for the anesthetist to determine fluid status of the neonate. Atrial natriuretic peptide is present, but its effects are blunted. In effect, the neonatal kidney is able to excrete water and sodium but cannot conserve these as well as the kidney of an older child.[34] By the end of the first month of life, renal function is approximately 70% of adult levels, and by the end of the first year, renal function reaches adult levels.

Fluid Balance

Due to their high metabolic rate and increased composition of body water as compared to a child, the neonate's fluid requirements are substantial. After the first week of life, a neonate requires 150 mL/kg/day of fluid (equivalent to 20 pints/day for an adult). Neonates also have high insensible losses, particularly from evaporation, as a result of a high surface area/body weight ratio (four times higher than an adult) and immature skin. These problems are accentuated for the preterm neonate. There is a fine balance, however, and fluid administration of greater than 150 mL/kg/day may precipitate fluid overload and congestive heart failure in the neonate. This value may be as low as 125 mL/kg/day in premature neonates. Thirst mechanisms are poorly developed and are affected by sepsis or RDS. Also, a surge of ADH at birth causes oliguria over the first few days. Table 52.6 summarizes indicators of fluid balance.

Hepatic System

The liver begins to develop at 10 weeks of gestation, and by 12 weeks of gestation it has already begun to function. Gluconeogenesis and protein synthesis are under way, and by 14 weeks of gestation glycogen is found in liver cells. The fetal liver possesses the ability to synthesize glycogen. Glycogen storage capacity is greatly increased just before birth. Approximately 98% of this stored glycogen is released from the liver within the first 48 hours of life, and glycogen levels are not restored to adult levels until the third week of life. Glycogen stores are further limited in preterm or small-for-gestational-age (SGA) infants. Therefore preterm and SGA infants should be monitored for hypoglycemia, and

TABLE 52.5 Daily Electrolyte Requirements of the Newborn

Electrolyte	Daily Requirement
Sodium	2–3 mEq/kg
Potassium	1–2 mEq/kg
Calcium	149–200 mg/kg

TABLE 52.6 Indicators of Fluid Balance

Parameter	Normal Range
Sodium	133–144 mmol/L
Body weight	Should fall by up to 10% below birth by 1 wk, then increase
Hematocrit	Increases (without transfusion) suggest dehydration
Creatinine	Should fall from maternal levels to <50 µmol/L after 5 days

the administration of dextrose-containing solutions during anesthesia care should be considered.

The function of the liver is decreased, and the capability for biotransformation is decreased, with oxidative activities approximating one-quarter to one-half of adult values.[35] The capacity to enzymatically break down proteins is depressed at birth as a result of a decrement in quantity and quality of hepatic enzymes. Albumin, an essential protein that regulates colloidal osmotic pressure, is produced beginning at 3 to 4 months of gestation, approaching 75% to 80% of adult levels at the time of birth. Plasma concentrations of albumin (which predominately binds acidic drugs) and α-acid glycoprotein (AAG) (which predominately binds basic drugs) are lower in newborns and even lower in premature neonates. The lower ability of the newborn to bind drug to plasma proteins results in greater levels of free drug. Unbound or free drug is active, and increased levels of free drug can lead to toxicity in these delicate patients. At approximately 1 year of age the concentrations of plasma proteins approximate adult levels.

Glucuronyl transferase activity within the neonatal liver is depressed as compared to a child. This enzyme is responsible for the metabolic breakdown of bilirubin. Hyperbilirubinemia may develop in term infants within the first days of life and may occur with increased frequency in the preterm neonate. Bilirubin production as a result of the breakdown of RBCs and enterohepatic circulation is increased due to the aforementioned depressed activity of glucuronyl transferase, which is required for hepatic conjugation. Bilirubin levels of 6 to 8 mg/100 mL are not uncommon in term infants; however, premature infants may have levels as high as 10 to 12 mg/mL on the third day of life. Phototherapy and, in rare cases, exchange transfusion are used to avoid the development of encephalopathy (kernicterus). In neonates with hyperbilirubinemia, it is imperative that a determination of physiologic versus pathologic jaundice be determined. Bilirubin can also compete with drugs for binding sites on plasma proteins. With high bilirubin levels, in conjunction with an already decreased concentration of plasma proteins, the amount of free drug can be even higher in term and premature neonates.

Concentrations of clotting factors in the premature neonate and the term newborn are low; however, hepatic synthesis of essential clotting factors reaches adult levels during the first week after birth. In utero, the liver is the organ responsible for hematopoiesis, but by 4 to 6 weeks after birth, this function is assumed by the bone marrow. Neonates have incredibly little vitamin K at the time of birth, which is required for certain clotting factors (II, VII, IX, and X). Without administration of vitamin K at birth, the neonate is predisposed to bleeding and intracranial hemorrhage, and 1 mg of vitamin K is often administered.

Temperature Regulation

The neonate lacks the ability to precisely regulate body temperature. Large surface area, lack of subcutaneous tissue as an insulator, and the inability to shiver all contribute to inadequate thermoregulation.

The neonate has minimal ability to shiver, so sympathetic nervous system stimulation enhances the metabolism of brown fat to increase heat production, a process known as nonshivering thermogenesis (NST). It is a metabolically driven heat production that does not involve muscular work. Brown fat stores located in the scapulae, axillae, mediastinum, and the retroperitoneal space surrounding the kidneys are metabolically active and contain a high density of mitochondria. Hypothermia stimulates the release of norepinephrine, which acts on brown fat to uncouple oxidative phosphorylation.[36] Heat production follows an increase in the basal metabolic rate stimulated through the release of anterior pituitary hormones. The result of NST is ultimately heat production, but there is also an increase in metabolic byproducts of brown fat metabolism: acetone, acetoacetic acid, and β-hydroxybutyric acid. Metabolic acidosis can rapidly lead to bradycardia and cardiac arrest in a neonate. Therefore it is especially important to maintain body temperature during surgery and anesthesia in pediatric patients.

Perioperative hypothermia has many contributing causes, including a cold operating room environment, anesthetic-induced vasodilation, the infusion of room-temperature intravenous fluids, evaporative heat loss from opened body cavities, use of cool irrigating solutions, and the inspiration of cool/dry anesthetic gases. During laparoscopic surgery, the temperature of the carbon dioxide gas used for insufflation is 21°C. So despite having less direct exposure of the intraabdominal cavity to the environment, patients remain at risk for developing hypothermia.

Neonates are at risk for rapid heat loss, leading to hypothermia and bradycardia, which can result in cardiac arrest. When cold blood is administered there is a risk for cell lysis accompanied by increases in serum potassium levels. So when the neonate becomes cold, it is not uncommon that coagulopathies occur resulting in increased hemorrhage. Administration of cold blood products in this situation may not only further this vicious cycle of coagulopathy and hypothermia but may also precipitate cardiac arrest from either hypothermia, hyperkalemia, or acidosis.

It is well recognized that the thermoregulatory response is inhibited by anesthetic agents. Core body temperature may decrease by as much as 1°C to 3°C. Heat loss occurs as a result of the internal redistribution of heat, reduced metabolism and heat production, increased heat loss to the environment, and the effects of anesthetic agents on thermoregulatory control. Heat loss occurs more rapidly in neonates because of their increased body surface to body weight ratio. The skin (particularly of the premature neonate) is thinner and has less subcutaneous tissue, increasing the rate of evaporative heat loss.[37-40]

Radiant heat loss is responsible for the majority of heat loss during anesthesia.[34] It occurs with the transfer of heat to the environment and is dependent on the temperature differences between the neonate and the environment. Radiant heat loss may be minimized by wrapping the neonate in a warm blanket and isolating the skin from the cold operating table, effectively decreasing the transfer of heat. Radiant heat lamps may be used to maintain temperature during surgical positioning and preparation but are ineffective during the surgical procedure. Radiant heat lamps increase the temperature of the air between the neonate and the lamps, thereby minimizing radiant heat loss. However, radiant heat lamps are ineffective when operating room personnel or large objects are placed between the lamp and the patient. In addition, the placement of a radiant heat lamp near the neonate may produce thermal injury.

An example of conductive heat loss includes placing the neonate on a cold operating table, resulting in heat transfer from the neonate to the table and thereby causing a decrease in core body temperature. Conductive heat loss is minimized with the use of warmed irrigating solutions, the use of warm blankets or heated forced-air blankets to cover the nonoperative areas of the patient, and the preoperative warming of the operating room. Underbody warming devices during induction of anesthesia, positioning, and time leading up to surgical prep and incision can help reduce heat loss in the neonate. Covering the head with a stockinet or reflective cap dramatically decreases conductive heat loss. Blood flow to the neonate's head is high, and the neonate's head may account for up to 60% of the total heat loss during the perioperative period. The use of warm prepping solutions can also help with preserving heat.

Convective heat loss is precipitated by moving air currents. The operating room air circulation is changed 6 to 12 times per hour and, in conjunction with cool ambient temperatures, increases heat loss.

The air surrounding the body is warmed and subsequently rises, being replaced by the cooler ambient air. To minimize convective heat loss, the ambient air temperature must be increased. Prudent practice is to preheat the operating room to 26°C (78.8°F) for premature and neonatal surgical patients. This may be even higher in severely premature neonates or burn children. The premature infant or neonate arrives in the operating room in a heated Isolette and is immediately covered with a warm blanket before being transferred to the operating table. Convective heat loss may be increased when wet clothes are in contact with the neonate. Wet diapers and blankets soiled with preparation solutions must be replaced and not allowed to remain in contact with the skin.

Evaporative heat loss occurs through the vaporization of liquid from body cavities and the respiratory tract. Evaporative heat loss is either sensible loss (the evaporation of sweat) or insensible loss (the evaporation of water through the skin). The thin-skinned premature neonate is particularly susceptible to insensible evaporative heat loss. Sensible evaporative heat loss may be prevented by removing wet clothing or blankets and thoroughly drying the neonate. Insensible evaporative heat loss may be mitigated by increasing the relative humidity of the operating room, covering the patient with a plastic barrier, and using warmed irrigating solutions. Insensible respiratory tract evaporative heat loss may be prevented with humidification of the inspired gases, which requires attentive temperature monitoring to avoid superheating of airway gases and subsequent airway burns. The addition of in-line humidifiers to the patient breathing circuit adds to the complexity and weight, perhaps increasing the likelihood of unintended tracheal extubation. These humidifiers may also contribute to unintended increases in core body temperature during lengthy surgical procedures. When using active humidification on neonatal circuits it is important to monitor the temperature of gases entering the neonate's lungs. The use of a passive heat and moisture exchanger, added between the patient circuit and ETT, has been of questionable efficacy.[41,42] It is always important to examine the recommended Vt for a given humidification filter and to choose an appropriate one based on patient size to prevent CO_2 retention and rebreathing. NICU ventilators generally deliver much more precise Vt for these delicate patients, and ventilatory maintenance can be accomplished with NICU ventilators throughout the procedure, with anesthesia provided via intravenous route.

Iatrogenic increases in core body temperature may occur. Attentiveness to the patient's core temperature is essential. Covering the neonate may result in progressive increases in core temperature during prolonged surgical procedures.

ANESTHETIC PHARMACOLOGIC CONSIDERATIONS IN THE NEONATE

Physiologic characteristics that modify the pharmacokinetic and pharmacodynamic activity in the neonate include differences in TBW composition; immaturity of metabolic degradation pathways; reduced protein binding; immaturity of the BBB; greater proportion of blood flow to the brain, heart, liver, and lungs; reduced GFRs; smaller FRC; and increased minute ventilation.

Pharmacokinetics

Several age-related differences in absorption, distribution, metabolism, and elimination affect pharmacologic responses in the neonate. Absorption and distribution are increased due to an increased cardiac output on a per kilogram of body weight basis, decreased protein concentration and binding capabilities, body composition, and the immaturity of the BBB. Elimination is decreased due to immature metabolic pathways and renal immaturity. It is important to consider the following components of drug pharmacology when selecting appropriate drug interventions in the neonatal population: protein binding, half-life ($t_{1/2}$), elimination $t_{1/2}$, metabolism, elimination, and water versus fat solubility.

Cardiac Output

Resting cardiac output in the neonate at birth is approximately 400 mL/kg/min, in the infant is approximately 200 mL/kg/min, and in the adolescent is approximately 100 mL/kg/min. Therefore, the circulation time in neonates and infants is faster when compared to the adult, assuming normal ventricular function and the absence of intracardiac or intrapulmonary shunts. For this reason, after hepatic and renal maturity occur, drug delivery and metabolism of medications from their sites of action are at a more rapid rate compared to the adult.

TBW and extracellular fluid (ECF) are increased, and intracellular fluid (ICF) is decreased, in neonates and fall proportionately with postnatal age. The premature neonate has a TBW of roughly 85% to 90%, with 60% being represented by ECF and 25% represented by ICF. In term neonates TBW is approximately 75%, of which 40% is ECF and 35% is ICF. For comparison, the adult TBW is roughly 60% (20% ECF and 40% ICF). The percentage of body weight contributed by fat is 3% in a 1.5-kg premature neonate and 12% in a term neonate. The proportion of fat doubles by 4 to 5 months of age. These body component changes affect the Vd of drugs. Water-soluble drugs such as NDMRs distribute rapidly into the ECF but enter cells more slowly. The initial dose of water-soluble drugs is consequently higher in the neonate than in the child or adult. With NDMRs, a larger initial dose is needed to fill this larger Vd for these water-soluble drugs, but subsequent doses may be smaller owing to the immaturity of the nicotinic cholinergic receptors (nAChR) at the motor endplate and decreased biotransformation.

Delayed awakening occurs because CNS concentration of drugs remains higher than that observed in older children as a consequence of this reduced redistribution.[43] It is important to note that neonates, and especially preemies, may be very sensitive to lipophilic drugs as they have very little peripheral fat stores, and the most lipophilic area of the body may be the brain. Table 52.7 illustrates the changes in TBW, ICF, and ECF during stages of maturation.

Protein Binding

Protein binding of parenterally administered drugs is diminished in the neonate due to lower concentrations of plasma proteins. Drugs that are highly protein bound in an adult can have a greater free fraction of the drug and therefore a greater pharmacologic effect. Albumin and AAG concentrations are reduced in neonates but are similar to those in adults by 5 to 6 months. Plasma albumin concentrations approximate adult values by 5 months of age and are lowest in preterm neonates. Binding capacity approaches adult values by 1 year of age.

Blood-Brain Barrier

The BBB restricts diffusion of compounds between blood and brain. It is immature in neonates, which can have clinical consequences. BBB function improves gradually, possibly reaching maturity at term. Until maturation, small molecules access the fetal and neonatal brain more

easily than adult brains. Drugs bound to plasma proteins will not normally cross the BBB; however, unbound lipophilic drugs passively diffuse across the BBB to achieve rapid equilibrium. This may contribute to the tendency of drugs such as local anesthetics to produce seizures in neonates. Specific active transport systems across the BBB can be affected by CNS pathology, thereby changing the clinical effects of opioids and other compounds.[43,44] This is more important in the neonatal population, especially in preemies, as plasma proteins are already low, and hyperbilirubinemia may further displace drugs leading to higher unbound drug concentration reaching the brain.

Metabolism

Generally, due to a large proportion of the cardiac output that traverses the liver in the pediatric patient, there is a more rapid clearance of drugs. However, phase I cytochrome P-450 (CYP) dependent reactions (e.g., oxidation, reduction, hydrolysis) are not fully developed during the neonatal and early infancy periods, thereby decreasing metabolism of anesthetic drugs that are dependent on hepatic metabolism. These processes begin to mature within the first week of life, with remaining cytochrome-dependent metabolic pathways continuing to increase during the first 3 months of life.[45] Phase II reactions (conjugation reactions) increase water solubility to promote renal excretion, and this process is underdeveloped in neonates. Certain cytochrome-dependent reactions can be induced prior to delivery when the mother is exposed to certain drugs and cigarette smoke.[46,47]

The neonate lacks the capacity to effectively conjugate bilirubin (decreased glucuronyl transferase activity) and metabolize medications such as acetaminophen, chloramphenicol, and sulfonamides. Although the necessary enzyme systems are present at birth, enzyme activity is reduced, increasing drug elimination half-lives.[48-52] The anesthetist must always consider the $t_{1/2}$ of drugs administered to the neonate. Phase I, phase II, and glucuronyl transferase activity are further reduced in the premature neonate.

Excretion

Most anesthesia-related drugs are eliminated by the kidney. In the neonate, GFR and tubular function is reduced, particularly in those neonates born at less than 34 weeks. However, renal function reaches adult levels by 8 to 12 months of age. Healthy preterm and full-term neonates have relatively normal renal drug clearance by 3 to 4 weeks of age. Reductions in drug excretion must be considered in neonates requiring surgery in the early neonatal period.

Pharmacodynamics

Pharmacodynamics describes how the pharmacologic actions of drugs affect human physiology. The actions of a drug and its receptor are influenced by the number and type of receptors present and the action of the drug in the receptor population. Neonates can have significant differences in their dynamic response to drugs as compared with adults, due to receptor immaturity.

Nicotinic Cholinergic Receptors

In its fetal form, the nicotinic Ach receptor remains open longer after binding Ach, protecting or increasing the safety factor of neuromuscular transmission, and this could account for the neonate's resistance to muscle relaxants.[53] As it transitions into its adult form, the duration that the receptor remains open is decreased after binding. This results in less propensity for generation of an action potential, manifesting as less resistance to muscle relaxants. There is also a reduction in Ach release in the NMJ in the neonate, which could account for the increased sensitivity to NDMRs.[54] These opposing factors make a neonate's response to a neuromuscular blocking agent unpredictable.

TABLE 52.7	Fluid Compartment Volumes			
	Premature	**Infant**	**Child**	**Adult**
Total body water	80%–90%	75%	65%–70%	55%–60%
Extracellular fluid	50%–60%	40%	30%	20%
Intracellular fluid	60%	35%	40%	40%

Opioid Receptors

The mu and kappa receptors are responsible for the respiratory depression associated with opioids. In the neonate, changes in the number and affinity of these receptors may account for the increased respiratory depression that results when opioids are used. Respiratory control centers are also immature, generally not showing maturation until 42 to 44 weeks of gestation, making the neonatal population more sensitive to apnea following opioid administration. The anesthetist must also be cognizant of the $t_{1/2}$ of opioids being administered, as well as the presence of active metabolites. Though it is a popular drug in NICU and PICU neonates, morphine does have an active metabolite (morphine-6-glucuronide [M6G]). The $t_{1/2}$ of morphine is approximately 6 to 12 hours in preemies, compared to approximately 6 to 9 hours in term neonates, and the $t_{1/2}$ of M6G in this population is even longer.

γ-Aminobutyric Acid Receptor

The action of general anesthetics may be associated with activation of GABA receptors.[55,56] The number of $GABA_A$ receptors in the neonate is only one-third that of the adult, and half of these receptors have a high affinity for binding with benzodiazepines and other anesthetics.[57] The potency of anesthetics and benzodiazepines in neonates could be explained by the high affinity of these receptors. This explains why minimum alveolar concentration (MAC) for volatile anesthetics may be lower in the neonate and then increase steady around 1 month of life.

DRUGS USED TO PROVIDE NEONATAL ANESTHESIA

Inhalation Agents

Inhaled anesthetic agents equilibrate more rapidly in neonates due to increased minute ventilation, increased cardiac output, which is directed mainly to the vessel-rich group of tissues, and reduced solubility of the inhaled anesthetics in blood. In addition, their decreased distribution and amount of adipose tissue, as well as decreased muscle mass, affect the rate of equilibration among the alveoli, blood, and brain. The MAC of the inhalation anesthetics is less in neonates than in infants. Neonates have a slightly lower MAC, which peaks at approximately 30 days of age and decreases thereafter (Fig. 52.7). The anesthetic implication of this is that induction is more rapid, and the development of cardiovascular side effects can occur in seconds and with greater frequency. The margin of safety between adequate anesthesia and significant cardiopulmonary depression is very narrow. Elimination of inhalation agents, and therefore recovery, is also rapid, provided that cardiopulmonary function is not depressed.

In the neonatal period, during transitional circulation, both left-to-right and right-to-left intracardiac shunting occur. In the presence of a left-to-right intracardiac shunt there is a minimal increase in inhalation anesthetic uptake; however, when there is a right-to-left intracardiac shunt, there is a slowing of the rate of rise of the alveolar concentration of inhaled agents due to decreases in the anesthetic concentration in arterial blood of the arterial system. The clinical implication of right-to-left intracardiac shunting results in inhalation induction requiring more time until loss of consciousness to occur.

Potent inhalation agents depress ventilation in a dose-dependent manner and increase the risk of apnea. Likewise, they readily depress the myocardium and blood pressure because of immature compensatory mechanisms. Inhalation anesthetics are myocardial depressants, and this effect is amplified in neonates. An immature heart cannot increase contractility or SV due to decreased preload, and neonatal cardiac output is extremely reliant on adequate preload and heart rate. This reduction in inotropy and chronotropy, combined with a reduction in

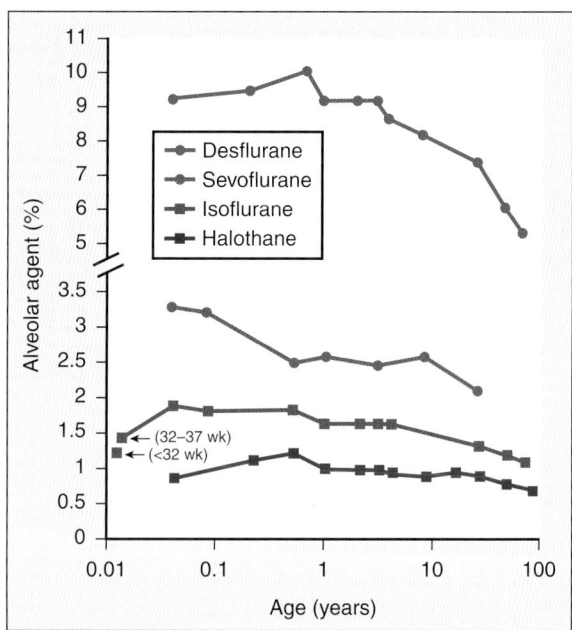

Fig. 52.7 Effect of age on minimum alveolar concentration (MAC) of anesthetic gases. MAC is higher at birth than in adults and increases until peaking at 3 to 6 months. The values at 1 year of age are closer to the adult values. (From Greeley WJ. Pediatric anesthesia. In Miller RD, ed. *Atlas of Anesthesia*. Vol 7. Philadelphia: Elsevier; 1999:55.)

SVR from volatile anesthetics and immature baroreceptors compensatory mechanisms, can lead to rapid deterioration especially with high concentrations of inhalation anesthetics. Inhalation anesthetics cause a dose-dependent reduction in SVR leading to a reduction in preload, which exacerbates the negative effects in neonates. It is important to note that critically ill neonates, especially the extremely premature, frequently do not tolerate the effects of inhalation anesthetics, and anesthesia may be administered using a combination of benzodiazepine, opioid, and NDMRs.

Intravenous Agents

Neonates and infants have a higher proportion of cardiac output delivered to vessel-rich tissues (e.g., heart, brain, kidneys, and liver). Intravenous anesthetic agents are readily taken up by these tissues and are subsequently redistributed to tissues less well perfused (muscle and fat). Intravenously administered drugs may have a prolonged duration of action in neonates and infants due to decreased percentages of muscle and fat. The CNS effects of opioids may also be prolonged due to the immaturity of the BBB.[50] The CNS affects can also be explained because peripheral fat stores are low and the brain may be the area of highest fat concentration, making it the main storage area of opioids in neonates. Anesthetists have historically been hesitant to use opioids because of their perceived toxicity profile in neonates, particularly morphine. Fentanyl is well tolerated even in the most critical neonates. It is now understood that appropriate anesthetic drugs are necessary for neonatal procedures.[58] Significant amounts of anesthetic drugs may be required for complex neonatal procedures.[59,60] Although some pharmacodynamic evidence suggests that intravenously administered anesthetic doses should be reduced, one must also recall the effect of increased body water. Neonates requiring major or frequent surgical procedures, especially those born prematurely, have probably been exposed to benzodiazepines and opioids and will develop tolerance leading to higher dose requirements. Increased doses of propofol are required because of increased metabolic rate and a greater Vd.[43,44,61]

In most circumstances, when a neonate requires surgical intervention, intravenous access is established prior to arrival in the operating room.

Neuromuscular Blocking Drugs

Neonates have an increased sensitivity to the effects of NMBDs. The reason is the result of varied pharmacokinetic and pharmacodynamics profiles as compared to the adult. The increased Vd causes single doses of NMBDs for a neonate to be similar to that of the older infant, but due to reduced clearance, immature receptors, and increased sensitivity, also prolonged duration. NMBDs are highly ionized and possess a low lipophilicity, which limits their ability to cross the BBB. This pharmacologic property restricts the distribution of NMBDs to the ECF compartment, which is larger in the neonate and infant than in the child and adult (see Table 52.7). Increases in ECF volume and the ongoing maturation of neonatal skeletal muscle and Ach receptors affect the pharmacokinetics and pharmacodynamics of neuromuscular blockers. Table 52.8 references the effective doses of NMBDs in various age groups.

The NMJ is incompletely developed at birth. The presynaptic release of Ach is slowed at birth compared with that in the adult, which explains the decreased margin of safety for neuromuscular transmission in the neonate. The Ach receptors of the newborn are anatomically different from the adult receptors, which may explain the sensitivity of the neonate to NMBDs. Maturation of the NMJ occurs over the first few months of life.

Neonates are more resistant to the effects of succinylcholine as compared to children and adults. This is illustrated by the intravenous effective dose (ED$_{95}$) for neonates (620 mcg/kg), infants (729 mcg/kg), children (423 mcg/kg), and adults (290 mcg/kg) (see Table 52.8). The increase in dose requirement is in part a result of the increased Vd within the large extracellular compartment. Plasma cholinesterase activity is reduced in neonates; however, the duration of action after a single dose of succinylcholine is 6 to 10 minutes. A prolonged duration of action after a single bolus dose of succinylcholine would suggest the presence of an inherited deficiency of plasma cholinesterase activity. The FDA recommends that the use of succinylcholine in pediatric patients be limited to airway emergencies due to the increased risk of severe hyperkalemia in patients with undiagnosed myopathies.[62] It is important to note that this hyperkalemic response is not necessarily linked to malignant hyperthermia but is associated with a response called anesthesia-induced rhabdomyolysis. Succinylcholine-induced hyperkalemia is more frequent in males and in children less than 8 years old.

The selection of NMBDs should take into consideration the desired degree and duration of skeletal muscle paralysis, the immaturity of

organ systems, and the associated side effects of the selected relaxant. The variability in response to these drugs is significant, particularly in premature neonates and infants. Monitoring of neuromuscular function must be used to guide repeated administration of these drugs in all neonatal patients, just as it should be used in any patient requiring neuromuscular blockade.

Reversal of Neuromuscular Blockade

The neonate is extremely vulnerable to rapid hypoxemia if respiration is impaired due to residual muscle weakness caused by paralytic agents. Neuromuscular blockade should always be reversed unless mechanical ventilation in the postoperative period is planned. The safest treatment of prolonged muscle weakness is to provide sedation and controlled ventilation until the neuromuscular blocking agent is eliminated.

It can be difficult to determine the adequacy of reversal in neonates. Observing flexion of the elbows and hips, knee to chest movements, return of abdominal muscle tone, and presence of facial grimacing are important signs. Another measurement is the ability to generate a maximum negative inspiratory force (MIF) greater than −25 cm H$_2$O or a crying capacity of more than 15 mL/kg.[63] Neonates are capable of generating an MIF of −70 cm H$_2$O with the first few breaths after birth.[64] An MIF of at least −32 cm H$_2$O has been found to correspond with leg lift, which is indicative of the adequacy of ventilatory reserve required before tracheal extubation.[65] If a peripheral nerve stimulator is used, the train-of-four should demonstrate the standard 90% recovery, though placement of these monitors may be difficult given the small size of the neonate.[66]

The two anticholinesterase drugs used for reversal of neuromuscular blockade are neostigmine (0.05–0.07 mg/kg) and edrophonium (0.5–1.0 mg/kg). Neostigmine is routinely administered as it is more potent, and therefore it has a greater efficacy for inhibiting cholinesterase. An anticholinergic agent, atropine (0.02 mg/kg) or glycopyrrolate (0.01 mg/kg), should be given prior to the anticholinesterase in neonates to prevent cholinergic side effects such as bradycardia and bronchospasm. Due to similarities in time to onset and duration of action, glycopyrrolate is usually combined with neostigmine and atropine with edrophonium. The selective muscle relaxant binding agent sugammadex (Bridion) has not currently received FDA approval for administration to patients less than 18 years old.

Drug Preservatives

Premature neonates have a reduced ability to metabolize the preservatives benzyl alcohol and sodium benzoate. Numerous anesthetic and nonanesthetic medications contain preservatives such as benzyl alcohol. This accumulation of benzoic acid can result in benzyl alcohol gasping syndrome and can manifest as gasping respirations, metabolic acidosis, and multiple organ system failure. These agents can produce severe CNS toxicity, seizures, and permanent brain damage. The use of preservative-free drugs and solutions is essential when possible.[67]

FLUID MANAGEMENT

Neonatal fluid management varies based on gestational age, birthweight, rate of caloric expenditure and growth, ratio of evaporative surface area to body weight, the degree of renal functional maturation and reserve, and TBW.[68] TBW accounts for approximately 75% of body weight in term neonates and 90% in preterm neonates. This high percentage of TBW results from expansion of the ECF compartment, which may account for 50% of the TBW. In the first few days of life, a term neonate can lose 5% to 15% of its body weight. Urine output is low, and if the neonate is kept warm, fluid requirements are relatively low, as little as 40 to 60 mL/kg/day.[69,70] Box 52.4 shows the common

TABLE 52.8 Effective Doses (ED$_{95}$) of Neuromuscular Blocking Drugs (mcg/kg)

Neuromuscular Blocking Drugs	Neonate	Infant	Child	Adult
Succinylcholine*	620	729	423	290
Atracurium	120	156–175	170–350	110–280
Cisatracurium	—	43	41	50
Vecuronium	47	42–47	56–80	27–56
Rocuronium	600	600	600	300
Pancuronium	—	55	55–81	49–70

*Should only be used for emergency airway stabilization in children <8 yr. Not for routine intubation.

BOX 52.4 Common Intravenous Fluid and Electrolyte Requirements in the Newborn

Glucose
- Most newborns require 2–4 mg/kg/min.
- SGA/LGA infants may require >15 mg/kg/min on days 1–3 of life.
- Glucose tolerance may fluctuate significantly in very low and extremely low birthweight (VLBW and ELBW) infants.

Sodium
- Most neonates require no sodium for the first 24 hr of life.
- On day 2 and beyond, most newborns receive 2–4 mEq/kg/day.
- Sodium requirement may change dramatically in response to gastrointestinal, genitourinary, or transcutaneous losses or drug or metabolic effects.
- The ELBW infant may have huge transcutaneous losses, requiring meticulous monitoring and replacement.

Potassium
- Requirements for potassium are minimal for the first 24–48 hr of life.
- Subsequently, maintenance delivery is approximately 1–3 mEq/kg/day, always in the presence of a normal urine output.
- Serum levels in the newborn, especially VLBW and ELBW, are higher than in older infants.
- Replace gastrointestinal, genitourinary, or iatrogenic losses cautiously.

Calcium
- Requirements for calcium range between 200 and 400 mg/kg/day (calcium gluconate).
- Requirements for calcium vary with gestational age, history of asphyxia, and growth disturbances (e.g., SGA, LGA).
- Serum levels can be obtained for total Ca^{2+} and/or ionized Ca^{2+}.

LGA, Large for gestational age; *SGA,* small for gestational age.
From Gregory GA, Brett C. Neonatology for anesthesiologists. In: Davis PJ, Cladis FP, eds. *Smith's Anesthesia for Infants and Children.* 9th ed. Philadelphia: Elsevier; 2017:517.

TABLE 52.9 Clinical Signs and Symptoms for Estimation of Severity of Dehydration in Infants

Clinical Signs	DEGREE OF DEHYDRATION		
	Mild	Moderate	Severe
Weight loss (%)	5	10	15
Behavior	Normal	Irritable	Hyperirritable to lethargic
Thirst	Slight	Moderate	Intense
Mucous membranes	May be normal	Dry	Parched
Tears	Present	±	Absent
Anterior fontanelle	Flat	±	Sunken
Skin turgor	Normal	±	Increased

From McClain CD, McManus ML. Fluid management. In: Cote CJ, et al, eds. *A Practice of Anesthesia for Infants and Children.* 5th ed. Philadelphia: Elsevier; 2013:170.

TABLE 52.10 Water Requirements of Newborns

Birth Weight (g)	WATER REQUIREMENT (ML/KG/24 HR) BY AGE		
	1–2 Days Old	3–7 Days Old	7–30 Days Old
<750	100–250	149–300	120–180
749–1000	80–150	100–150	120–180
1000–1500	60–100	80–150	120–180
>1500	60–80	100–150	120–180

From Merves MH. Neonatology. In: Tschudy MM, Arcara KM, eds. *The Harriet Lane Handbook.* 19th ed. Philadelphia: Elsevier; 2012:455–475.

electrolyte requirements in the newborn. Traditional NICU practice may be to limit fluids to less than 120 mL/kg/day to prevent congestive heart failure in sick and premature neonates, but there is variability in practice.

Assessing Fluid Requirements

In the neonatal period, several physiologic and physical factors can affect fluid requirements. The smaller the neonate, the larger the percentage of body water to total body weight. With smaller amounts of body fat, the major part of the neonate's body weight is water. The combination of renal loss and a large insensible water loss makes the neonate prone to dehydration and hemodynamic instability. There are physical observations that can assist in estimating the fluid status of the pediatric patient (Table 52.9).[71]

Anesthesia and surgery have a significant effect on fluid homeostasis and renal function. The combination of vasodilation and myocardial depression may result in blood pressure fluctuation that alters fluid compartment dynamics, vascular capacitance, and/or organ blood flow. The RAAS is generally inhibited as a result of anesthesia.

Water Requirements

Holliday published a seminal work identifying caloric requirements of the "average" hospitalized infant based on body weight.[69] A secondary finding showed that the water requirement in milliliters was equivalent to the total energy expended in calories. Table 52.10 gives the water requirements of newborns.

Several considerations in planning the fluid management in the neonatal surgical patient are warranted:
- Degree of dehydration present before preoperative nil per os (NPO) guidelines
- Fluid deficit due to NPO guidelines
- The presence of intravenous fluid administration during NPO time leading up to surgery
- Maintenance requirements during anesthesia/surgery
- Estimated third-space loss
- Alterations in body temperature
- Blood loss during procedure
- Risk for hypoglycemia (e.g., receiving dextrose-containing fluids on floor/PICU/NICU, diabetic mother, long procedure)

Due to the nature of the surgical interventions required the neonate, most will have had their fluid status managed in a neonatal unit. If that is not the case, during the time of the preoperative evaluation, deficits should be determined, and dehydration or electrolyte imbalances should be reversed. Other issues such as acidosis, low hemoglobin, poor urine output, and poor perfusion should be resolved.[21] It is important to assess serum and urine osmolality as well. The anesthetist must investigate the causes of deficits and ensure that these are corrected with the proper types of fluid or blood products prior to surgery.

There is no evidence that children who are denied oral fluids for more than 6 hours preoperatively benefit in terms of decreased intraoperative gastric volume and gastric acidity as compared with children permitted unlimited fluids up to 2 hours preoperatively. Children permitted fluids have a more comfortable preoperative experience in terms of thirst and hunger. Current guidelines for healthy infants (<2 years), children (2–16 years), and adults state that continued fasting from the intake of clear liquids at least 2 hours before elective procedures requiring general anesthesia, regional anesthesia, or sedation/ analgesia (i.e., monitored anesthesia care) should occur. Examples of clear liquids include but are not limited to water, fruit juices without pulp, carbonated beverages, clear tea, and black coffee. The volume of liquid ingested is less important than the type of liquid ingested. It is important to fast from intake of breast milk at least 4 hours and infant formula at least 6 hours before elective procedures. Fasting from intake of a light meal or nonhuman milk should be 6 hours or more. Fried, fatty foods or meat may prolong gastric emptying time. Additional fasting time (i.e., ≥8 hours) may be needed in these cases. Both the amount and type of food ingested must be considered when determining an appropriate fasting period.[72,73]

Knowledge of the caloric requirements for a neonate can be used to estimate the maintenance fluid requirements. The classic 4-2-1 rule takes the caloric expenditure into consideration because it is calculated by body weight. A neonate weighing less than 10 kg will require 100 mL/kg/day or 4 mL/kg/hour. Dextrose should be added in most neonates, especially those at increased risk for developing hypoglycemia.

Fluid deficits are generally a result of preoperative fasting or excessive gastrointestinal (GI) losses. Neonates receiving adequate preoperative maintenance will have no deficit and will require no deficit replacement calculated into their fluid management plan. If there has not been adequate maintenance, the fluid deficit can be calculated by multiplying the hourly maintenance rate by the number of hours without feeding. Total deficit restoration may require several hours or even days in the smallest babies. Current Pediatric Advanced Life Support (PALS) guidelines recommend an isotonic crystalloid fluid bolus of 10 to 20 ml/kg for severe hypovolemia. The goal is to restore and preserve the cardiovascular stability and renal perfusion. Fluid boluses should not be given with dextrose-containing solutions or parenteral nutrition.

If total parenteral nutrition (TPN) is being administered, the amount of glucose/kg/min, as well as other components such as sodium, potassium, and calcium currently being administered, should be noted. If possible, the TPN should be maintained without interruption. If it must be discontinued, glucose must be monitored vigilantly, and dextrose should be added to the fluid management plan as acute hypoglycemia can occur. When TPN is discontinued, D_{10} is frequently the fluid of choice, and blood glucose should be monitored.

Third-space losses need to be replaced with a solution that does not contain glucose (e.g., normal saline, lactated Ringer, or PlasmaLyte). In those patients with abdominal lesions such as gastroschisis or NEC, the third-space losses can be exceptionally large. These patients may need as much as 25 to 100 mL/kg/hour to replace fluid loss. It is important to monitor signs and labs for hypovolemia, inadequate tissue perfusion, and hemodynamic instability to guide fluid administration during these situations.

Urine osmolality, urine specific gravity, and serum osmolality are important indices in managing intraoperative fluids in neonates. They provide information as to the need for fluid, solute, and electrolyte replacement. Normal urine osmolality in the neonate ranges from 49 to 800 mOsm/L, with an average of 270 mOsm/L. Osmolality should be maintained between 200 and 400 mOsm/L and specific gravity between 1.006 and 1.012. Serum osmolality ranges between 270 and 280 mOsm/kg.[74] Hyperosmolar states can result in IVH or kidney damage.

Fluid Management of the Premature Infant

Proper fluid management of the premature neonate requires an understanding of several variables: the extensive variability in body fluid composition, renal maturation, neuroendocrine control of intravascular fluid status, and insensible fluid loss with age.[75] Renal tubular function develops after 24 weeks of gestation, and nephrons mature by week 36.[68] The premature infant has a lower GFR and immature tubular function. The immature kidneys are unable to excrete sodium and excess fluid. The inability to concentrate urine, secondary to the inability to reabsorb sodium, leads to the excretion of large quantities of dilute urine. Therefore underestimation of fluid requirements may lead to more serious consequences than overestimation of fluid requirements.[70,76]

Blood glucose can be highly variable in the premature neonate. Hypoglycemia can be attributed to inadequate glycogen stores and the inability of the immature liver to perform gluconeogenesis. Symptoms of hypoglycemia are jitteriness, cyanosis, apnea, lethargy, hypotonia, and seizures. These signs may be masked by general anesthesia, making this difficult to assess without direct blood glucose measurement. If not treated rapidly, hypoglycemia in the preterm neonate can lead to neurologic damage. Preterm and SGA neonates often have a glucose requirement of 5 to 10 mg/kg/min to prevent hypoglycemia, compared to term neonates whose glucose requirements are generally 2 to 4 mg/ kg/min. Glucose as a D5 or D10 solution followed by a 10% to 15% dextrose solution can be titrated to maintain a serum glucose level greater than 40 mg/dL.[21] It is equally important to avoid hyperglycemia, which can result in IVH, osmotic diuresis, dehydration, and release of insulin, leading to hypoglycemia.

Electrolyte abnormalities are often seen in preterm neonates. Hypernatremia may result if water loss is greater than sodium depletion combined with abnormal renal tubular function. Hypokalemia can result from respiratory alkalosis or aggressive diuresis. Hyperkalemia can be caused by infusion of large amounts of potassium-containing fluids, as well as large quantities of banked blood.

Blood Replacement

Over the first 6 months of life, many physiologic changes are occurring that can complicate the decision to replace blood in the neonatal surgical patient. Fetal hemoglobin (HgbF), which has a higher affinity for oxygen than adult hemoglobin, can range from 70% to 80% of the neonate's total hemoglobin at birth and can be as high as 97% in the preterm neonate.[77] The clinical implication is that the younger the patient, the higher the fraction of HgbF thus lowering the oxygen-carrying capacity and oxygen delivery to the tissues. Of note, the P-50 of the neonate is approximately 19 mm Hg as compared to that of the adult at 26.5 mm Hg. When the neonate is transfused, the oxyhemoglobin dissociation curve shifts to the right, allowing Hgb to give up oxygen more readily to the tissues.

Replacement of blood loss is critical in the surgical neonate, especially in the face of prematurity. Blood volume is extremely small in this patient (85–100 mL/kg), and a loss of 10 mL could be approximately 10% of total blood volume. This becomes even more critical in the extremely premature neonate, or micro-preemie population, where 5 mL of blood loss may be 10% of the blood volume. The clinical indication for blood administration should not be based on a predetermined percentage of total blood volume. Maintaining oxygen-carrying capacity, oxygen delivery to peripheral tissues, and improving coagulation are the primary concerns. The transfusion trigger in this age group will need to be at higher hemoglobin and hematocrit levels than the older infant or child. Rapid blood loss in neonates can result in cardiovascular complications quicker than in the adult, therefore transfusion may be required sooner. Low Hgb values at birth (<12 g/dL) show significant association with mortality in preterm neonates born at or before 32 weeks of gestation.[78] The decision to transfuse should be based on the underlying and current cardiopulmonary status, ongoing blood loss, anticipated further blood loss, and baseline hemoglobin. Another concern is the presence of congenital heart disease or lung disease, resulting in a decreased ability to oxygenate blood, thus leading to a lower threshold for transfusion. These patients may require blood to aid in oxygen-carrying capacity and not necessarily due to excessive surgical bleeding.

The accurate measurement of blood loss in neonates and infants is crucial to any replacement regimen. The margin of safety is reduced in the neonate, and because oxygen consumption is twice that of the adult a smaller percentage of blood loss will result in cardiovascular instability. A major cause of cardiac arrest in pediatric surgical patients is associated with hypovolemia from blood loss and hyperkalemia from transfusion of stored blood.[79] It is mandatory to monitor blood loss through the weighing of sponges, the use of small calibrated suction containers, and vigilant visual estimation of ongoing blood loss. When saturated, every 4 in by 4 in of a surgical sponge is equal to approximately 10 mL of blood loss.

As noted earlier, VE in neonates or infants during anesthesia may lead to fluid overload and can be difficult to assess. New techniques to evaluate transfusion effects include the use of transesophageal Doppler (TED), a noninvasive cardiac output monitoring technique, which can provide a comprehensive estimation of the volume status. TED-derived indexed SV measurement is useful to predict and follow VE responsiveness in neonates and infants without myocardial dysfunction.[80]

Estimating Allowable Blood Loss

The estimated blood volume (EBV) and allowable blood loss (ABL) must be calculated prior to induction of anesthesia for any procedure in which blood loss is expected. EBV is calculated based on age and body weight (see Table 52.2).

A predetermined acceptable low hematocrit is identified based on the clinical situation and the neonate's health. Maximum allowable blood loss (MABL) can be calculated with the following formula in which Hct_0 is the beginning hematocrit, Hct_l is the lowest acceptable hematocrit, and Hct_a is the average hematocrit, $(Hct_0 + Hct_l)/2$:

$$MABL = wt\ (kg) \times EBV \times (Hct_0 - Hct_l)/Hct_a$$

Example: A surgical neonate who weighs 4 kg is going to have an abdominal procedure. Beginning hematocrit is 42%. The lowest acceptable hematocrit is 30%. The MABL for this patient is 106 mL.

$$MABL = 4 \times 320 \times (42 - 30)/(42 + 30)/2 = 106$$

When the blood loss equals or exceeds the calculated allowable loss, transfusion should be considered. The volume of packed RBCs to be infused may be determined by the following formula:

$$Packed\ RBCs\ (mL) = \frac{(Blood\ loss - ABL) \times Desired\ hematocrit\ (30\%)}{Hematocrit\ of\ PRBCs\ (75\%)}$$

Using the previous example of a 4-kg infant, with a total blood loss of 175 mL, the volume of packed RBCs (PRBCs) would be 175 − 106 × 30/75 = 27.6 mL.

The administration of PRBCs can lead to a significant increase in the plasma potassium concentration and cardiac arrest. Hyperkalemia associated with massive transfusion has been reported to be the most common cause of arrest in noncardiac procedures.[81] Rapid administration of PRBCs stored for less than 2 weeks via handheld syringes and small-gauge catheters (≤23 gauge) has also been reported to result in

hyperkalemia.[82] Hypocalcemia and cardiovascular instability can result from the rapid administration of blood due to the amount of citrate contained in the stored blood. The neonatal myocardium is extremely sensitive to changes in calcium, and the anesthetist should have a low threshold for administering calcium to the neonatal patient receiving PRBCs. Often with multiple transfusions, an intravenous fluid bolus will be given, and if the blood pressure does not increase then hypocalcemia should be considered. It is important to note that calcium chloride contains approximately three times the amount of elemental calcium when compared to calcium gluconate. Whole blood should not be used, and irradiated blood should be given only to immunocompromised patients. Irradiation accelerates the leakage of potassium from RBCs into serum. To reduce the risk of hyperkalemia, washed or fresh (i.e., <7 days old) PRBCs should be used.[77]

ANESTHETIC EQUIPMENT

Anatomic differences in the face and upper airway of neonates affect the design and fit of the masks, laryngoscopes, and ETTs. Physiologically, the need to minimize the resistance and dead space has design implications for breathing systems, connectors, and tubes. Disposable, humidified pediatric circle systems are more commonly used in neonates for some important reasons. These systems have low compliance, are lightweight, and, with the addition of plastic valves, have eliminated the high resistance associated with older systems. Resistance and increased work of breathing can be detrimental to the neonatal population. These circuits also offer a more reliable method of monitoring end-tidal carbon dioxide ($ETco_2$). Ventilation is most often controlled in these patients, reducing the deleterious effects of increased work of breathing in the spontaneously ventilated neonate.

The anesthesia machine should be equipped to deliver air when nitrous oxide is not desirable, for example, in the neonate undergoing an abdominal procedure or when it is necessary to reduce the inspired oxygen concentration to avoid the potential for ROP, or when maintenance of fetal circulation is desirable (i.e., unrepaired cardiac defects necessitating ductal blood flow for pulmonary blood flow or cardiac output). The newest anesthesia machines have ventilators designed to deliver pressure ventilation modes that are reflective of the Vt that is desired. It is also possible to adapt and use the ventilators in the NICU, as these ventilators often deliver more precise Vt to small neonatal patients. In some pediatric centers, with the most critically ill neonates, certain operative procedures are performed in the NICU to avoid disturbing the delicately balanced ventilation patterns, prevent heat loss during transport, and preserve cardiorespiratory stability.

Due to the stiff epiglottis and short neck, a straight blade may be preferable. However, in one study in children ages 1 to 24 months, the Miller and the Macintosh blades provided similar laryngoscopy views and intubating conditions.[83] The blade is placed along the right side of the mouth, sweeping the tongue to the left. With a straight laryngoscope blade, the epiglottis is lifted with the tip of the blade and tracheal inlet exposed. The ETT is inserted with the convex side to the left. The advantage of one over another is the characteristic that allows the large tongue of the neonate to be manipulated out of the visual field. There are also modifications of straight blades that allow insufflation of oxygen into the pharynx during intubation. The use of videolaryngoscopy for pediatric patients has become popular especially in those patients who are suspected to have a difficult airway. Presently there is no evidence to suggest that videolaryngoscopy is superior or inferior to tradition laryngoscopy.[84]

Oral endotracheal tube (OETT) size for neonates cannot be calculated by formula because of the rapid growth during the immediate postnatal period. It can be determined from a table based on the child's

TABLE 52.11 Recommended Endotracheal Tube Sizes

Neonatal Age	Endotracheal Tube Size
Preterm neonate	2.0–3.0
Full-term neonate	3.0–3.5
Age 3 mo–1 yr	3.0–4.0

weight in kilograms (Table 52.11). It is common for the full-term neonate to accommodate a 3-mm ETT and a premature infant (<2 kg) to need a 2.5-mm or smaller ETT. Selecting an ETT that will result in an air leak at 20 to 30 cm H_2O pressure to avoid postextubation airway edema is advisable. It may be advantageous to have multiple-sized ETTs available in the event the neonate has congenital subglottic stenosis, and the predicted ETT size will not pass into the trachea. If the neonate has had a chest x-ray, it is possible to measure the tracheal size, and this should become part of the pediatric anesthetist's practice during the preoperative evaluation to help guide ETT sizes for these small patients.

The length of the trachea (vocal cords to carina) in neonates and infants up to 1 year varies from 5 to 9 cm. Insertion distance of an ETT should be less than 10 cm, falling within the 8 to 10 cm range. It is important for the anesthetist to be cognizant of the head and neck position during the surgical procedure. Extension of the neck will pull the ETT from the trachea toward the vocal cords leading to potential inadvertent extubation, whereas neck flexion will advance the ETT leading to potential inadvertent mainstem intubation. If the neck is going to be flexed or extended during the surgical procedure (e.g., neurosurgery and certain otolaryngologic procedures), the anesthetist should check the ETT location with a fiberoptic scope with the head and neck position simulated for the procedure prior to ETT securement.

Traditionally, the use of an uncuffed ETT was the accepted method for endotracheal airway management in pediatric patients younger than 8 years old, primarily due to a perceived decrease in the incidence of postextubation croup. The current standard practice in neonatal anesthesia has been the use of uncuffed ETTs for reasons of airway resistance and tracheal damage from inflated cuffs. The proper use of specially made cuffed ETTs under certain clinical situations is considered acceptable. Indications include the use of a cuffed ETT in certain thoracic or abdominal procedures or when high-pressure or complex ventilator modes are planned. The advantages include decreased operating room contamination with the inhalation anesthetic agent, the use of lower fresh gas flow rates (more economic), the possible avoidance of repeated laryngoscopy and intubation to assess and seal leaks, more accurate capnography readings, and better control of ventilation.[85-87] It is important to note that the use of uncuffed ETTs is a standard of practice that comes from NICU management strategies and may not be the best solution for neonates presenting to the operating room. Term neonates are generally intubated with 3-mm cuffed ETTs without issues. The use of a low-volume, low-pressure cuffed ETT (e.g., Microcuff ETT) can help prevent airway edema and postextubation stridor. Smaller neonates, particularly preemies, may need smaller ETTs, and an uncuffed tube may be the best option.

Monitoring of the neonate during anesthesia is important in detecting small changes that can be incredibly significant because of their smaller physiologic margin of safety. The precordial or esophageal stethoscope, as the case allows, is a simple means of assessing heart rate, rhythm, sound, ETT position, and secondarily extrapolating vascular volume. Continuous ECG monitoring is used for monitoring of not only heart rate but also for detection of arrhythmias, particularly in the baby that has electrolyte imbalances and/or preexisting CHDs. Pulse oximetry is standard of care for all patients in a critical care or surgical environment. The other standard monitoring parameters are blood pressure, inspired oxygen concentration, $ETco_2$ and inhalation agent concentration, and peak airway and end-expiratory pressure monitoring. Neuromuscular monitoring is technically difficult in the neonate, particularly preterm and very low birthweight (VLBW) babies, owing to their small muscle mass and large size of monitor compared to the size of the child.

PREOPERATIVE ASSESSMENT

The perioperative management of any neonate is determined by the nature of the surgical procedure, the gestational age at birth, the postgestational age at surgery, and any associated medical conditions. A comprehensive preanesthetic assessment is essential to completely determine a specific plan of care. Increased perioperative mortality associated with pediatric anesthesia include children less than 1 year of age, increased American Society of Anesthesiologists (ASA) physical status (III-V), emergency surgery, cardiac or vascular surgeries, and multiple surgeries performed under the same anesthetic technique.[88] It is also important for the anesthetist to examine prematurity, with its associated issues and comorbidities, and the presence of syndromes.

Gestational Age and Postgestational Age at Surgery

The gestational age, postgestational age, and birthweight are critical to the determination of the physiologic development of the neonate. The history of the delivery and the immediate postdelivery course can influence the choice of anesthetic technique and assist in anticipating possible postoperative complications.

Preterm neonates are classified as borderline preterm (36–37 weeks of gestation), moderately preterm (31–36 weeks of gestation), and severely preterm (24–30 weeks of gestation).[89] Neonates can be classified according to their weight and their gestational age. Full term is 37 to 42 weeks of gestation. Large for gestational age (LGA) is defined as weight above the 90th percentile at gestational age, and SGA refers to weight below the 10th percentile at gestational age. Low birthweight is defined as a weight below 2500 g, whereas VLBW is defined as a weight below 1500 g, and extremely low birthweight (ELBW) is below 1000 g. Full-term neonates that are SGA often present with conditions requiring surgical intervention. SGA neonates have different pathophysiologic problems as compared to preterm infants (<37 weeks of gestation) of the same weight.[90] Immaturity, as determined by gestational age, increases the potential for neonatal comorbidities. It is important to note that maternal health problems can have significant implications for all neonates. It is vital to examine the birth history, health during pregnancy, as well as overall health of the mother. Table 52.12 lists several common maternal problems and the possible associated neonatal sequelae. Some of the common issues that accompany the premature neonate are BPD, ROP, apnea of prematurity (AOP), IVH, PDA, and hernias.

Prematurity

Due to the advances in neonatal medicine, many preterm babies born at exceptionally early gestational age and ELBWs are surviving, and in turn they are challenged with a plethora of unique diseases that pose anesthetic challenges. Prematurity presents its own set of complications, including anemia, IVH, periodic apnea accompanied by bradycardia, and chronic respiratory dysfunction. Some of the associated issues associated with premature neonates are a result of their

TABLE 52.12   Maternal History With Commonly Associated Neonatal Problems

Maternal History	Anticipated Neonatal Sequelae
Rh-ABO incompatibility	Hemolytic anemia, hyperbilirubinemia, kernicterus
Toxemia	Small for gestational age and its associated problems. Muscle relaxant interaction after magnesium therapy
Hypertension	Small for gestational age and its associated problems
Drug addiction	Withdrawal and small for gestational age
Infection	Sepsis, thrombocytopenia, viral infection
Hemorrhage	Anemia, shock
Diabetes	Hypoglycemia, birth trauma, large or small for gestational age and associated problems
Polyhydramnios	TE fistula, anencephaly, multiple anomalies
Oligohydramnios	Renal hypoplasia, pulmonary hypoplasia
Cephalopelvic disproportion	Birth trauma, hyperbilirubinemia, fractures
Alcoholism	Hypoglycemia, congenital malformation, fetal alcohol syndrome, small for gestational age and associated problems

TE, Transesophageal.
Adapted from Ghazal EA, et al. Preoperative evaluation premedication and induction of anesthesia. In: Cote CJ, et al, eds. *A Practice of Anesthesia for Infants and Children.* 5th ed. Philadelphia: Elsevier; 2013:31–63.

physiologic immaturity (i.e., NEC due to PDA) or from therapies they receive as a consequence of being born prematurely (i.e., mechanical ventilation and oxygen administration leading to lung damage and the development of BPD and ROP). It is beyond the scope of this chapter to address all pathologic conditions regarding preterm neonates and anesthetic implications.

Premature neonates are challenging to evaluate, and considerable controversy exists regarding the appropriateness of elective surgical intervention and proper postoperative care. Postgestational age (gestational age + postnatal age) should be determined at the time of the anesthetic evaluation. Premature infants of less than 60 weeks of postgestational age have the greatest risk of experiencing postanesthetic complications as well as postoperative ventilatory issues and apnea. The manifestations of prematurity are thought to occur as a result of the inability of the neonate to adequately compensate during periods of physiologic stress. Inadequate development of respiratory drive and immature cardiopulmonary responses to hypoxia and hypercapnia have been implicated. Therefore premature infants have a significant risk of postoperative apnea and bradycardia during the first 24 hours after general anesthesia.[91-93] Box 52.5 lists contributing factors that may influence the occurrence of apnea in premature infants. Each facility has its own policies regarding admission of neonates following anesthesia administration based on age, presence of prematurity, and comorbidities. It is not uncommon to see all neonates with a postgestational age of 44 weeks or younger requiring overnight monitoring following anesthesia. This also applies to patients who are less than 60 weeks of postgestational age in ex-preemies and those infants with comorbidities. It is important to note that this postanesthesia monitoring applies to sedation (e.g., procedural sedation for magnetic resonance imaging, endoscopies).

BOX 52.5   Factors Contributing to Increased Incidence of Apnea in the Premature Infant

Physiologic Contributors
- Inadequate development of respiratory centers
- Incomplete myelination of central nervous system
- Incomplete cardiovascular development leading to altered responses to stress

Metabolic Contributors
- Hypothermia
- Hypoglycemia
- Hypocalcemia
- Acidosis
- Respiratory instability

Anesthetic Contributors
- Residual anesthetics, opiates, relaxants, sedatives
- Prolonged intubation and ventilation

Apnea in the Premature Infant

Apnea associated with prematurity is a significant clinical problem manifested by an unstable respiratory rhythm, reflecting the immaturity of respiratory control centers. The ventilatory response to hypoxia and hypercarbia is impaired, and inhibitory respiratory reflexes are exaggerated in the neonate. Treatment strategies attempt to stabilize the respiratory rhythm. Caffeine and CPAP remain the primary treatment modalities; methylxanthines such as caffeine are presumed to work through blockade of adenosine receptors, as adenosine inhibits respiratory drive. Caffeine is initially loaded at a dose of 20 mg/kg, and maintenance therapy is generally 5 mg/kg/day. AOP typically resolves with maturation suggesting increased myelination of the brainstem.[94,95]

Apnea occurs in 7% of babies born between 34 and 35 weeks of gestation, 14% born between 32 and 33 weeks, 54% between 30 and 31 weeks, and 80% of neonates born earlier than 30 weeks. Although most apneas resolve by the time the infant reaches 37 weeks of postconceptional age, 80% of VLBW infants, in one study, still had significant apneas at 37 weeks. There are a variety of conditions that predispose an infant to apnea, including CNS lesions, infections and sepsis, ambient temperature fluctuations, cardiac abnormalities, metabolic derangements, anemia, upper airway structural abnormalities, NEC, drug administration (including opiates and general anesthetics), and possibly gastroesophageal reflux. Various monitoring techniques are used to detect apneic episodes, although pulse oximetry and abdominal-pressure transduction are the most common. As noted previously, standard therapy is with caffeine 5 to 10 mg/kg.[94-96]

Preventing and treating apnea. Anesthesia and surgery for neonates is indicated only when significant pathology exists, at which time general anesthesia and airway management are most often used. General anesthesia with desflurane (maintenance only) or sevoflurane is preferred due to the rapid emergence. It is important to note that neonates with PHN may have increases in PVR with desflurane administration owing to sympathetic stimulation and airway irritation, and thus its use should be avoided. To reduce the risk of perioperative complications related to inadequate ventilation, the use of nonopioid medications such as acetaminophen are preferable. Spinal or caudal anesthesia can also be performed, as well as transversus abdominis plane (TAP) blocks to decrease the incidence of postoperative pain and decrease the postoperative need for opioids.[97] Due to the decreased hepatic metabolism and renal excretion of intravenous medication in the neonate, the dose of local anesthetic administered must be calculated to avoid local anesthetic toxicity. There is significant risk of local anesthetic toxicity in neonates after a TAP block or other regional techniques.[98]

Intubation provides the greatest airway control and provides the safest ventilation method for neonates. Extubation should occur when the infant is awake, shows adequate respiratory effort, and demonstrates vigorous purposeful movement. All infants under 62 weeks of PMA should be monitored postoperatively with an oxygen saturation monitor, at the minimum. It is important to note that there are policies for postoperative monitoring of neonates that vary among various organizations. Infants over 62 weeks of PMA with a significant history of apnea or respiratory disease should also be monitored. Infants over 62 weeks of PMA can be discharged following minor surgery after an appropriate period of recovery (minimum 4 hours) if they are stable, vital signs have returned to baseline, postanesthesia care unit (PACU) time was uneventful, and they are otherwise healthy. Higher risk infants require 24 hours of monitoring based on the procedure and comorbidities present in the child.[94-96,99]

Preanesthetic Assessment and Neonatal Anesthetic Implications

One of the most important parts of the anesthetic for a neonate is the preoperative evaluation because having an understanding of the problems a child has coming into a procedure can help the anesthetist avoid complications. The information gathered during the preoperative assessment will allow the anesthetist to develop an individualized anesthetic plan based on the patient's pathology and the surgical and anesthetic implications. Table 52.13 gives the characteristics of the body system and the anesthetic implications. A thorough review of the birth history such as gestational hypertension, preeclampsia, or gestational diabetes is important. Maternal use of cigarettes, alcohol, or drugs use should also be ascertained, and the anesthetist should review the effects of each of these on the neonate, both long and short term.

System Review and Examination

The two body systems that are of primary interest in a preanesthetic system review are the respiratory and cardiovascular systems. However, there are other important metabolic and structural problems that can have a significant impact on the anesthesia plan. When performing a physical assessment, the anesthetist should assess for the presence of congenital anomalies. These problems occur most often in SGA and LGA neonates (Box 52.6).

Head and Neck Abnormalities

Any abnormality of the head and/or neck should raise concerns regarding airway management. The shape and size of the head, with or without the presence of pathology, can make airway management difficult. The small mouth and large tongue can obstruct the airway during mask ventilation, in healthy neonates. This becomes more concerning in the presence of syndromes affecting the mouth and tongue (e.g., trisomy 21 and Beckwith-Wiedemann). Neonates have very small nares, and when obstructed by an anesthesia facemask, airway obstruction can occur particularly if the mouth is being held closed. A small and/or receding chin, as seen in Pierre Robin and Treacher Collins syndromes, may make direct laryngoscopy and visualization of the glottis impossible, requiring airway adjunctive equipment. It is important to have a comprehensive airway plan prior to the planed procedure. An intubating laryngeal mask airway (LMA) is an important tool to have readily available for these patients. The pediatric anesthetist must take the time to become familiar with the more common syndromes associated with airway and cardiac abnormalities (Table 52.14). Cleft lip, with

or without cleft palate, may complicate intubation. Anomalies such as cystic hygroma or hemangioma of the neck can produce upper airway obstruction, making mask ventilation and intubation more challenging. In the case of a preterm neonate, it should also be determined whether the patient has ROP, cataracts, or glaucoma because atropine administration could result in significant increases in intraocular pressure and further damage to the eye.

Respiratory System Abnormalities

The incidence of RDS and BPD is inversely related to gestational age at birth. The onset of RDS can be as early as 6 hours after birth, and symptoms include tachypnea, retractions, grunting, and oxygen desaturation. BPD manifests as a need for supplemental oxygen, lower airway obstruction and air trapping, carbon dioxide retention, atelectasis, bronchiolitis, and bronchopneumonia. Oxygen toxicity, barotrauma of positive pressure ventilation on immature lungs, and endotracheal intubation have been reported as causative factors due to lung scarring and damage. Mechanical ventilation will lead to abnormal growth and development of the lungs and pulmonary vasculature. When examining the Pao_2 in utero, the approximate value is 30 mm Hg. When premature babies are born, they receive oxygen and their Pao_2 may become 40 to 50 mm Hg. This may or may not be significant in the development of lung disease. Careful monitoring of the acid-base status, the use of increased PIP, and PEEP may be needed to maintain oxygenation during surgery.

Cardiovascular System Abnormalities

During the evaluation of the neonate's cardiovascular system, several variables should be examined: heart rate, blood pressure patterns, skin color and temperature, intensity of peripheral pulses, capillary filling time, and baseline oxygen saturation. Presence of a murmur or abnormal heart sound, low urine output, metabolic acidosis, dysrhythmias, sluggish capillary refill, dusky extremities, weak peripheral pulses, or cardiomegaly, alone or in combination, raises the concern of some type of congenital heart defect. These patients should be further evaluated by chest x-ray, ECG, echocardiogram, and other indicated cardiac tests or labs as appropriate. The results of these diagnostic tests will allow for effective planning of the anesthetic plan, decreasing the possibility of complications (Table 52.15). It is important for the anesthetist to understand how to manipulate intracardiac shunts for children with congenital heart defects by increasing and decreasing SVR and PVR. A classic example of understanding cardiac shunt manipulation, as well as understanding the child's history, is the neonatal patient with a PDA, which generally has a left-to-right intracardiac shunt. Mild hyperventilation can lower PVR and increase this shunt, putting the neonate into pulmonary overcirculation and possible congestive heart failure.

It is beyond the scope of this chapter to discuss all anesthetic implications associated with congenital heart disease in the neonate; however, important information includes the following[100]:

- Direction and flow through any shunt, which can be bidirectional and manipulated by manipulating SVR and PVR
- Presence of single ventricle physiology and what has been done for palliation
- Baseline oxygenation to determine presence or degree of shunting and/or mixing of oxygenated and deoxygenated blood
- Dependence of the systemic or pulmonary circulation on flow through the DA
- Presence and size of any obstruction to blood flow, where this obstruction is located, and presence of collateral circulation
- Heart failure (high output, low output, or hypoxic)
- Drug therapy
- Antibiotic prophylaxis (i.e., bacterial endocarditis)

TABLE 52.13   Preanesthetic Assessment and Neonatal Anesthetic Implications

System	Characteristics	Anesthetic Implications
Central Nervous System	Incomplete myelination	Judicious use of muscle relaxants
	Lack of cerebral autoregulation	Cerebral perfusion pressure control
	Cortical activity	Pain relief/adequate level of anesthesia
	Retinopathy of prematurity (ROP)	Oxygen saturation (94%–98%, maybe even as low as 88%–94%)
	Birth history	A review of the pregnancy, including complications such as pregnancy-induced hypertension, preeclampsia, gestational diabetes, vaginal bleeding, infections, and falls; also any cigarette, alcohol, or drug (prescription, herbal, illicit) use
Respiratory		
Birth History		Weeks of gestation, neonatal intensive care unit admission, history of intubation or oxygen requirement, maternal complications including infection with herpes simplex virus or human immunodeficiency virus, and prenatal smoke exposure
Mechanical	↓ Lung compliance	Assist or control ventilation during general anesthesia
	↓ Elastic recoil	
	↓ Rigidity of chest wall	
	↓ $\dot{V}/\dot{Q}$ due to lung fluid	
	↑ Fatigue of respiratory muscles	
	↓ Coordination, nose/mouth breathing	Do not obstruct nasal passages
Anatomic	Large tongue	
	Position of larynx, epiglottis, vocal folds, subglottic region	
Biochemical	Response to hypercapnia not potentiated by hypoxia	Avoid hypoxia
		Maintain normothermia
Reflex	Hering-Breuer reflex	Apnea/no desaturation/stimulation
	Periodic breathing	Stimulation/airway support
	Apnea	
Cardiovascular	↓ Myocardial contractility/↓ myocardial compliance	Maintain adequate intravascular volume
		Maintain heart rate
		Myocardium sensitive to calcium levels
	CO rate dependent	Use vagolytic agents
	Vagotonic	
	Limited sympathetic innervation	
	Reactive pulmonary vasculature	Avoid hypoxemia and hypercapnia resulting in ↓ PBF and possible shunting
	PDA/FO shunting	Strict bubble precautions with intravenous fluids and medication blousing at stopcocks
Renal	↓ GFR	Maintain intravascular volume/CO
	↓ Tubular function	Avoid overhydration
	Low glucose threshold	Avoid excess glucose (0.5–1 g/kg)
Hepatic	Depressed hepatic enzymes	Judicious use of drugs metabolized by liver
	↓ Metabolism and clearance of drugs	
	Decreased protein (albumin, α-acid glycoprotein)	Increased free drug for highly protein bound drugs
	Hypoglycemia due to ↓ glycogen stores	
	Low prothrombin levels	Vitamin K (1 mg) before surgery
Hematologic	Fetal hemoglobin (does not readily release O_2 to tissues)	Avoid hypoxia
	Oxyhemoglobin dissociation curve shifted left	Lower P-50
		Transfusion shifts neonate toward adult oxygen dissociation curve allowing O_2 to be released more readily at tissues

CO, Cardiac output; *GFR*, glomerular filtration rate; *PBF*, pulmonary blood flow; *PDA/FO*, patent ductus arteriosus/foramen ovale; *V/Q*, ventilation/perfusion ratio.

BOX 52.6 Common Metabolic and Structural Problems in SGA and LGA Infants

Small for Gestational Age (SGA)

- Congenital anomalies
- Chromosomal abnormalities
- Chronic intrauterine infection
- Heat loss
- Asphyxia
- Metabolic abnormalities (hypoglycemia, hypocalcemia)
- Polycythemia/hyperbilirubinemia

Large for Gestational Age (LGA)

- Birth injury (brachial, phrenic nerve, fractured clavicle)
- Asphyxia
- Meconium aspiration
- Metabolic abnormalities (hypoglycemia, hypocalcemia)
- Polycythemia/hyperbilirubinemia

From Gregory GA, Brett C. Neonatology for anesthesiologists. In: Davis PJ, Cladis FP, eds. *Smith's Anesthesia for Infants and Children.* 9th ed. Philadelphia: Elsevier; 2017:517.

TABLE 52.14 Syndromes Associated With Difficult Airway

Syndrome	Airway Implication
Pierre-Robin sequence	Micrognathia, glossoptosis, cleft palate, micrognathia (unilateral), cervical dysfunction
Treacher Collins syndrome	Micrognathia, small oral opening, zygomatic hypoplasia
Apert syndrome	Limited cervical motion, macroglossia, micrognathia, midface hypoplasia
Hunter and Hurler syndrome	Cervical dysfunction, macroglossia
Beckwith-Wiedemann syndrome	Macroglossia
Freeman-Sheldon syndrome	Circumoral fibrosis, microstomia, limited cervical motion
Down syndrome	Atlantooccipital abnormalities, small oral cavity, macroglossia
Klippel-Feil syndrome	Cervical fusion
Hallermann-Streiff syndrome	Microstomia
Arthrogryposis	Cervical dysfunction
Cri-du-chat syndrome	Micrognathia, laryngomalacia
Edwards syndrome	Micrognathia
Fibrodysplasia ossificans progressiva	Limited cervical motion

Adapted from Harless J, Ramaiah R, Bhananker SM. Pediatric airway management. *Int J Crit Illn Inj Sci.* 2014;4(1):65–70.

Central Nervous System Abnormalities

An assessment of the CNS should include the status of the infant's ICP and intracranial compliance. IVH is almost exclusively seen in preterm neonates, and there can be spontaneous bleeding into and around the lateral ventricles of the brain. The hemorrhage is usually the result of RDS, hypoxic-ischemic injury, and/or episodes of acute blood pressure fluctuation that rapidly increase or decrease CBF. This is due to an immature cerebral autoregulation seen in premature neonates. Laryngoscopy and intubation in the presence of inadequate anesthesia can

precipitate IVH.[101] The symptoms of IVH include hypotonia, apnea, seizures, loss of sucking reflex, and a bulging anterior fontanelle. It is important for the anesthetist to assess for the presence and grade of IVH present preceding surgical intervention to understand the child's baseline and avoid precipitating IVH or worsening preexisting IVH. Evaluation of the neonate with myelomeningocele (spina bifida) is discussed subsequently.

Preoperative Laboratory Values

Premature neonates (<60 weeks of postgestational age), those with concurrent cardiopulmonary disease, and those undergoing procedures associated with major blood loss should at minimum have a complete blood count and electrolyte panel, but they may also need blood gases and serum osmolality measured. A type and screen should also be completed, as neonates have a lower threshold for transfusion in procedures with significant anticipated blood loss. The test values will assist in fluid, electrolyte, and blood replacement during the surgical procedure. Other testing will be dictated in accordance with the history and physical findings.

Preoperative Treatment of Significance for Anesthesia

Many of the preexisting conditions in the neonate will require medical treatment. Table 52.16 illustrates some of the preoperative drugs and their anesthetic implications. Parental preparation with psychosocial support is important. It is imperative that the parents be prepared and the informed consent for anesthesia be obtained. The anxiety of the parents of a newborn with a serious illness requiring surgical intervention is frequently high, especially when repeat and numerous procedures have been or will be completed. The anesthetist should foster trust and confidence through being understanding and explaining the anesthetic experience.

Regional Anesthesia in the Neonate

Regional anesthesia in the neonate can be a useful option when the risks of complications from general anesthesia and endotracheal intubation are exceedingly high. These techniques have allowed surgical procedures to be done on critically ill neonates under minimal general anesthesia, with considerable reduction in the need for CNS depressant drugs. The use of regional techniques must be associated with sufficient knowledge about the various techniques, as well as adherence to adequate dosage guidelines and other safety precautions. Regional anesthesia may offer advantages in these patients, although opinions differ on which techniques are appropriate.[102,103] An additional benefit to the use of regional anesthesia in this age group is postoperative pain control. Unpalliated or poorly palliated pain can lead to abnormal breathing patterns, or restricted breathing and guarding, which can affect minute ventilation and predispose the child to atelectasis and poor pulmonary outcomes. The two most common techniques used in the neonate are spinal and caudal epidural blocks.

Anatomic differences in the neonate must be considered, particularly the location of the terminal end of the spinal cord, the dural sac, and the volume of cerebrospinal fluid (CSF). The spinal cord extends as far as L3 in the newborn and does not reach the adult position of L1 until 1 year of age. The dural sac extends from S3 to S4 in these babies and does not reach the adult position of S1 until approximately 1 year of age (see Fig. 52.6). The volume of CSF is twice that of the adult (4 mL/kg vs 2 mL/kg). This dilutes the local anesthetics injected and could explain the higher dose requirements and shorter duration of analgesia for spinal anesthetics.

Patients in this age group have been reported to have a fairly stable cardiovascular response to regional anesthesia. It is believed that this may be due to the immature sympathetic nervous system or the

TABLE 52.15 Pathophysiology and Clinical Picture of Congenital Heart Defects

Lesion Type	Pathophysiology	Clinical Signs and Symptoms
Shunt Lesion Without Outflow Tract Obstruction		
Atrial septal defects	Intracardiac L-R shunt	CHF (systemic and pulmonary vascular congestion); no
Ventricular septal defects	Increased pulmonary blood flow	cyanosis (unless high pulmonary blood flow leads
Atrioventricular canal defects		to increased left atrial pressure, pulmonary edema,
Patent ductus arteriosus		and intrapulmonary $\dot{V}/\dot{Q}$ mismatch and shunt)
Aortopulmonary window		
Shunt Lesions With Right Ventricular Outflow Tract Obstruction		
Tetralogy of Fallot	Intracardiac R-L shunt	Cyanosis
Ebstein anomaly	Decreased pulmonary blood flow	
Pulmonary stenosis with atrial or ventricular septal defects		
Eisenmenger syndrome		
Transposition Physiology (Intercirculatory Mixing)		
Dextrotransposition of the great arteries	Intracardiac L-R and R-L shunts are equal	Cyanosis
Single-Ventricle Physiology		
One-Ventricle Lesions		
Hypoplastic left heart syndrome	Mixing of systemic and pulmonary venous blood	CHF (systemic and pulmonary vascular congestion);
Tricuspid atresia	Parallel distribution of pulmonary and systemic blood	cyanosis
Double-inlet left ventricle	flow determined by relative circuit resistances	
Two-Ventricle Lesions		
Truncus arteriosus		
Tetralogy of Fallot with pulmonary atresia		
Severe neonatal aortic stenosis		
Left Ventricular Outflow Tract Obstructive Lesions		
Mitral Stenosis		
Valvular cor triatriatum		
Aortic Stenosis		
Valvular	Left ventricular pressure overload from aortic lesions	CHF (if high left atrial pressure leads to pulmonary
Subvalvular (subaortic membrane)	Increased left atrial pressure from left ventricular	vascular congestion); no cyanosis (unless high
Supravalvular (Williams-Beuren syndrome)	systolic and diastolic dysfunction; OR obstruction to	left atrial pressure leads to pulmonary edema and
	left atrial emptying	intrapulmonary $\dot{V}/\dot{Q}$ mismatch and shunt)
Coarctation		
Shone syndrome (mitral stenosis, aortic stenosis, coarctation)		
Mixing of Systemic and Pulmonary Venous Blood With Series Circulation		
Partial anomalous pulmonary venous return (PAPVR); total anomalous pulmonary venous return (TAPVR)	Mixing of systemic and pulmonary venous blood	*CHF:* Systemic and pulmonary vascular congestion;
	Increased pulmonary blood flow	pulmonary vascular congestion is severe if pulmonary venous obstruction; no cyanosis
		PAPVR: Cyanosis
		TAPVR: Exacerbated if pulmonary venous obstruction leads to pulmonary edema and intrapulmonary $\dot{V}/\dot{Q}$ mismatch and shunt

CHF, Congestive heart failure; *L-R,* left to right; *R-L,* right to left; *V/Q,* ventilation/perfusion ratio.
From Davis PJ, Cladis FP. *Smith's Anesthesia for Infants and Children.* 9th ed. Philadelphia: Elsevier; 2017:634.

proportionally small blood volume in the lower limbs, decreasing the amount of venous pooling.[104,105] The ventilatory response to the regional anesthetic is related to the level of the block. With a level as high as T2-T4, there could be intercostal muscle weakness that requires the dependence on diaphragmatic movement for tidal breathing, but Vt and respiratory rate may not be affected.[106]

There are pharmacologic considerations when regional anesthesia is used in neonates. The ECF volume is greater when compared to the adult, and the initial dose of local anesthetic will be diluted into a larger Vd resulting in a lower initial plasma peak concentration. Local anesthetics, particularly amides, are metabolized more slowly in neonates due to immature hepatic degradation. The major elimination pathway

TABLE 52.16 Preoperative Treatment of Significance for Anesthesia

Drug	Implication
Diuretics for heart failure bronchopulmonary dysplasia (BPD)	Hypokalemia Increased bicarbonate levels: neonate sensitive to hyperventilation with intracardiac shunts
Digoxin for heart failure	ECG abnormalities
Steroids for BPD	Hyperglycemia
Immunocompromised	
Anticonvulsants	Cardiac arrhythmia Potent inducer of hepatic enzymes: increased NDMR metabolism
Indomethacin	Increases risk of bleeding Displaces bilirubin from protein-binding sites Transient hyponatremia
Renal Impairment	
Theophylline or caffeine	Significant toxic side effects; convulsions, tachycardia, tremor
Prostaglandins E_1 or E_2	Ventilatory depression and apnea Hypotension, cerebral irritability, seizures, tachycardia, pyrexia, cardiac irritability, transient oliguria, increased gastric acid
Prostacyclin	Hypotension Inhibition of platelet aggregation, rebound PPHN with withdrawal

PPHN, Persistent pulmonary hypertension of the newborn.

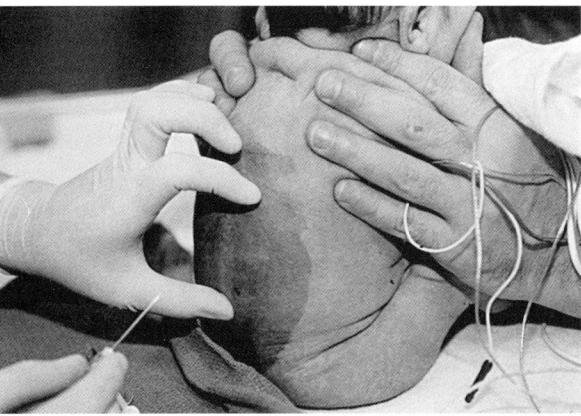

Fig. 52.8 Spinal block performed in sitting position. Note that the head is in neutral position to prevent airway obstruction. (From Suresh S, et al. Regional anesthesia. In: Cote CJ, et al, eds. *A Practice of Anesthesia for Infants and Children.* 5th ed. Philadelphia: Elsevier; 2013.)

for ester local anesthetics is hydrolysis via plasma cholinesterase, which is decreased in a neonate. In total, the metabolism and elimination of all local anesthetics may be prolonged in the neonate.

Most neonates will have a regional technique performed after the induction of general anesthesia due to the age of the patient and the possibility of agitation and continuous movement affecting the placement and success of the block.[107] The use of ultrasound-guided blocks has decreased the risk of complications associated with the placement of spinal and epidural needles and catheters and have allowed the anesthetist to monitor the spread of local anesthetics.[108]

Spinal Anesthesia

The use of spinal anesthesia in neonates and infants was common in the early part of the 20th century, but its use declined with the advent of safer general anesthesia in this delicate age group. There has been a renewed interest in various regional techniques in select patients such as those at risk for AOP. It is also useful in neonates and infants undergoing surgical procedures of the lower abdomen. Caudal blocks are common in neonatal anesthesia because of their simplicity and ability to provide excellent analgesia, which helps avoid large amounts of opioid analgesics with potential side effects that may impair recovery. Spinal anesthesia via catheters in the younger infant, neonate, and even preterm neonate remains controversial.[109]

Spinal anesthesia can be performed in the sitting or lateral position; however, the neck should be extended to prevent airway obstruction (Fig. 52.8). The lumbar puncture is performed at the L3-L4 or L4-L5 interspace because the spinal cord ends at L3 in the neonate. A 1.5-in, 22-gauge needle is inserted, and even with this small

needle resistance can be felt when the needle enters the ligamentum flavum, and the characteristic "pop" occurs when the needle enters the subarachnoid space. This distance is approximately 1 cm.[110] Large amounts of local anesthetics are necessary to produce an adequate block (0.14 mL/kg of bupivacaine 0.5%). When the local anesthetic is injected, the neonate should be immediately placed in the supine position, and the legs should be secured with tape to prevent them from being raised.

Caudal Anesthesia

Caudal anesthesia is the most commonly used regional anesthetic technique in pediatric anesthesia. It can be used for any procedure involving innervation from the sacral, lumbar, or lower thoracic dermatomes.[103] In the youngest patients, the caudal block can be used as an adjunct to general anesthesia or solely for postoperative analgesia. In the neonate, it is most often placed after induction of general anesthesia prior to the beginning of the surgical procedure.

With ultrasound, it is now possible to visualize the injection of local anesthetics in the caudal space, as well as monitor the cranial spread. The use of ultrasound is highly recommended in neonates who receive concomitant general anesthesia.[103,105] The patient is placed in the lateral position with the knees flexed (Fig. 52.9). The landmarks are identified: the tip of the coccyx to fix the midline, and the sacral cornu on either side of the sacral hiatus. These landmarks form the points of an equilateral triangle with the tip resting over the sacral hiatus. A 22-gauge needle is placed bevel up at a 45-degree angle to the skin. When the sacrococcygeal membrane is punctured, a distinctive loss of resistance is felt, and the angle of the needle is reduced and advanced cephalad. Saline should be used with the loss of resistance technique because the use of air has been reported to cause both intravascular air embolism and permanent spinal cord injury. After aspiration, and the absence of CSF or blood, the local anesthetic can be administered. Any local anesthetic can be used. The volume of the local anesthetic determines the height of the block. Volumes of 1.2 to 1.5 mL/kg provide analgesia and anesthesia to the T4-T6 dermatome, but 1 mL/kg is generally the dose used for lower procedures. The choice of local anesthetic is determined by the practitioner's preference; however, the concentration is adjusted to deliver no more than 2.5 mg/kg. The addition of epinephrine (1:200,000), clonidine (1–2 mcg/kg), or fentanyl will prolong the block significantly. Clonidine 1 mcg/kg can be used; however, side effects (including hypotension, bradycardia, and sedation) can occur.[111]

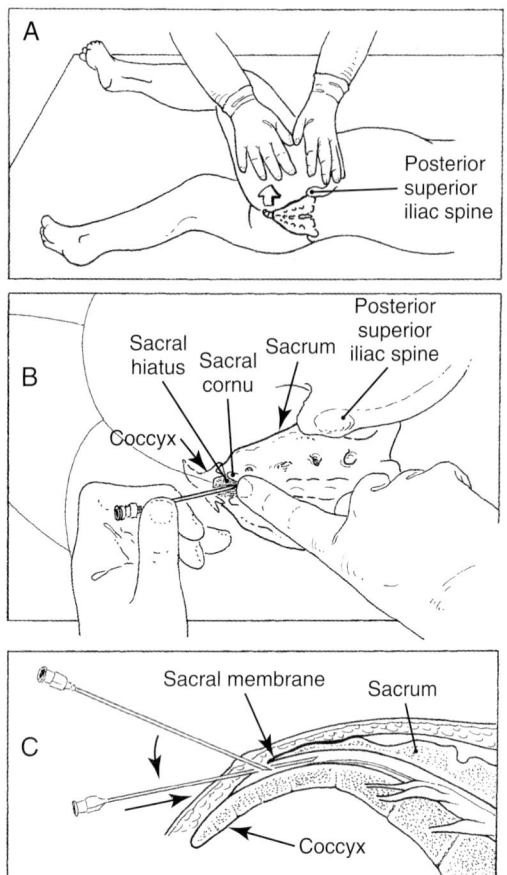

Fig. 52.9 Performing a caudal block. (A) Identification of the posterior superior iliac spine. (B) Palpation of the sacral hiatus. (C) Puncture of the sacrococcygeal or sacral membrane. (From Suresh S, et al. Regional anesthesia. In: Cote CJ, et al, eds. *A Practice of Anesthesia for Infants and Children.* 5th ed. Philadelphia: Elsevier; 2013.)

Anesthesia for the Micro-Preemie

Most individuals define a micro-preemie as a premature neonate that weighs less than 1000 g and is born before approximately 28 weeks of gestation. These delicate neonates encompass a patient population that is one of the most difficult to manage during anesthesia. The morbidity and mortality are positively correlated to the age of the neonate when born, as well as associated conditions and maternal factors. This population generally accounts for the highest percentage of neonatal morbidity and mortality. The common problems the anesthetist may see these patients for is PDA, NEC, BPD, PDA, ROP, retinal detachment, IVH, sepsis, and hyperbilirubinemia.

The mean arterial blood pressure of a micro-preemie should be roughly equal to the gestational age. This means that a 23-week old micro-preemie may have a mean arterial pressure around 25 mm Hg, with systolic blood pressure in the 30s. We truly do not know what the cerebral perfusion pressure is in these tiny neonates, but cerebral autoregulation is often abnormal in this patient population.

Many of these children have, or will develop, chronic lung disease. This is a result of lung tissue being exposed to mechanical ventilation and oxygen administration from an incredibly young age, for prolonged periods. Exposing these neonates' lungs to mechanical ventilation will cause scarring and prevent normal growth and development of the lungs and pulmonary vasculature, predisposing them to the development of BPD. Severely premature neonates are also exposed to oxygen concentrations that they would not otherwise be exposed to in

utero, contributing to BPD and the potential for ROP. The anesthetist should deliver only enough oxygen to maintain an oxygen saturation of 88% to 94%.

The preoperative assessment for this population should focus on preexisting conditions, intravascular access, goals of management in the NICU, fluid status, trending laboratory values, and birth history. It is important to understand preexisting conditions, and their severity, to avoid exacerbation when constructing an anesthetic plan. Many of these neonates may have umbilical vein catheters (UVC) and/or umbilical artery catheters (UAC) but may also require peripheral intravenous access and/or peripherally inserted central catheters (PICC). It is important for the anesthetist to assess and plan vascular access accordingly. The anesthetist should discuss the neonate's care with the neonatologists as well as the nurses in the NICU. There are extremely important pieces of information that can be obtained by the neonatologists and NICU nurses such as the neonate's response to drugs and position changes; fluid status and goals for intake and output; changes being made in intravenous alimentation based on blood glucose and electrolytes; glucose requirements; history of blood transfusions; hemodynamic changes and support; and oxygen and ventilatory needs and goals.

The micro-preemie's fluid status involves assessment of the anterior fontanelle, peripheral pulses, capillary refill, urine output, urine specific gravity, and hematocrit. Fluids are generally limited in the NICU, and significant amounts of fluid may need to be administered depending on the procedure that is being performed. Distal peripheral pulses should be palpable in even the most severely premature neonate, and absence or weakness of these pulses can be an important indication of hypovolemia. The skin overlying the fontanelle should be even with the outer table of the skull; if it is even with the inner table or lower, the neonate may be approximately 5% to 10% down in volume. Capillary refill may be delayed at 3 to 4 seconds in micro-preemies.

Hematocrit for term neonates may be around 55%, whereas the hematocrit of a micro-preemie may be closer to 45%. The anesthetist must be extremely vigilant with fluid administration in the micro-preemie and should understand that the MABL is quite small. For example, the circulating blood volume for these neonates is often 90 to 100 mL/kg, meaning that a 500-g micro-preemie has an approximate circulating blood volume of 50 mL. This would mean that a 5-mL blood loss is a 10% reduction in blood volume. Fluid bolus administration must be accomplished slowly to avoid rapid overload of the micro-preemie myocardium. If intravenous hyperalimentation is infusing, the anesthetist should continue this as the neonate's maintenance infusion and third space and surgical losses should be replaced with crystalloid, colloid, and/or blood products. Capillary leaking can occur when capillary junctions are not tight, and severely premature neonates may have an increased incidence of capillary leak. Albumin may be quite useful, especially during intraabdominal procedures, to reduce the amount of fluid lost from the intravascular space thus reducing edema formation. This becomes especially important in intraabdominal cases during abdominal closure.

ANESTHETIC CONSIDERATIONS FOR SELECTED CASES

Gastrointestinal

The acuity of intraabdominal procedures is variable and can range from a hernia repair to a complex abdominal/thoracic procedure. Implications such as increased intraabdominal pressure causing ventilation perfusion mismatch, initiation of the celiac reflex, heat loss, and hemorrhage are always concerns. With the advent of laparoscopic surgery, complications such as CO_2 gas embolism, intraabdominal organ damage, and ventilation strategies must also be considered.

Pyloric Stenosis

Pyloric stenosis is an obstructive lesion characterized by an olive-shaped enlargement of the pylorus muscle. It is a common GI anomaly, particularly in males, and many times seen in the first born. It is usually diagnosed between 2 and 12 weeks of life, and clinical symptoms include nonbilious postprandial emesis that becomes more projectile with time, a palpable pylorus, and visible peristaltic waves. A pyloromyotomy is performed to relieve the gastric outlet obstruction.

Pyloric stenosis is considered a medical emergency, and initial management is focused on correcting hypovolemia, acid base disorders, and electrolyte abnormalities. The use of laparoscopy has become standard and has greatly facilitated the surgical course.[111] Due to difficulty with feeding and regurgitation, optimization of fluid and electrolyte imbalance is essential in the preoperative period. Fluids, electrolytes, and acid-base balance should be corrected prior to anesthesia. The metabolic disorder that is most associated with pyloric stenosis is hypochloremic, hypokalemic, metabolic alkalosis. It is important to always ensure these labs have normalized, and hydration status is assessed prior to bringing the child to the operating room.

Prior to induction, all quadrants of the neonate's stomach are suctioned via a multiorifice orogastric tube. This is accomplished by placing the orogastric tube and suctioning the neonate's stomach in the supine, right lateral, and left lateral positions. Some anesthetists will irrigate the stomach via the orogastric tube with warm normal saline until the aspirate is clear and minimal. Infants having a pyloroplasty are considered at increased risk of gastric aspiration due to their disease process.

After preoxygenation, a rapid-sequence induction with cricoid pressure is completed. Some anesthetists opt for gentle positive pressure ventilation via mask, but many abstain from mask ventilation. An awake oral intubation can also be performed. Oral endotracheal intubation is mandated to protect the airway from any gastric contents that may be residual. Maintenance of anesthesia may be accomplished using inhalation anesthetics or in combination with intravenous anesthetic agents. Extubation should occur when the infant's airway reflexes are intact.

Postoperatively, these patients, particularly a preterm or SGA neonate, could exhibit drowsiness, lethargy, or apnea. This could be attributed to electrolyte abnormalities, postgestational age, or residual anesthetics.

Inguinal Hernia

The presence of an inguinal hernia is prevalent in the preterm neonate. This surgical problem is associated with the possibility of incarceration of the small bowel within the hernia defect, resulting in potential colon ischemia and tissue death. Another concern is potential injury to the ipsilateral testicle. The surgical approach can be accomplished with an open procedure via standard abdominal incision or by laparoscopic technique. In most situations, the contralateral side is explored to rule out the presence of another defect due to the high incidence of bilateral involvement.

The choice of anesthetic is based on practitioner preference. The most frequent indication for placing a caudal block while the neonate is awake is for inguinal hernia repair.[103] Inhalation or intravenous induction is acceptable, as is airway management with the LMA or ETT. The use of the laparoscopic approach will necessitate an ETT. Maintenance can be accomplished solely with inhalation anesthetics or in combination with intravenous drugs. Small neonates who are at risk for postoperative apnea may benefit from spinal anesthesia.[112]

Omphalocele and Gastroschisis

Omphalocele and gastroschisis anomalies are both defects in the abdominal wall that occur during gestation when the visceral organs fail to move from the yolk sac back into the abdominal cavity. It is more common to encounter omphalocele in term newborns and gastroschisis in preterm newborns. There are several differences between the two defects that are noted in Table 52.17. These are often associated with other anomalies. Some of those anomalies might be cardiac, genitourinary (bladder exstrophy), metabolic (e.g., Beckwith-Wiedemann syndrome with macroglossia, hypoglycemia, organomegaly, and gigantism), malrotation, Meckel diverticulum, and intestinal atresia. When the omphalocele is in the epigastric region, cardiac and thoracic pathology is more prevalent. If the omphalocele is located in the hypogastric area, cloacal anomalies and exstrophy of the bladder are seen more often.[113] These abdominal wall defects have quite different surgical management techniques and outcomes. Gastroschisis outcomes have improved dramatically over the past 4 decades but still encompass the largest group of patients needing bowel transplant. Omphalocele outcomes remain poor overall despite many advances in care. Large omphaloceles are difficult conditions to manage in pediatric surgery, and there is no standardized closure technique.[120] Both GI anomalies, although different in presentation, are similar as far as the anesthetic management.

A newborn with an omphalocele or gastroschisis is brought to the operating room soon after birth to minimize the possibility of infection, loss of fluid and heat, and the potential for death of bowel tissue. A thorough preoperative evaluation must be done to identify the presence of any of the previously mentioned comorbidities. Historically, the surgical approach was an immediate attempt at primary closure of the defect. This entailed placing a large amount of abdominal contents into a cavity that was not generally large enough, and the result was a significant increase in intraabdominal pressure. This impeded ventilation and caused profound hypotension secondary to aortocaval compression. Over the past decade, surgeons have opted for a staged closure, using a Silastic silo as a temporary housing for the bowel. This silo is sutured to the defect, and over the next 3 to 7 days the silo is reduced to accommodate the gastric contents and allow abdominal wall stretching. The neonate is usually then brought to surgery for complete closure of the defect.[120-122]

The choice of anesthetic agents and technique is determined by several guiding principles: severe dehydration and massive fluid loss from exposed viscera and internal third spacing of fluid due to bowel obstruction, hypothermia, the potential for sepsis,

TABLE 52.17 Differences Between Gastroschisis and Omphalocele

	Gastroschisis	Omphalocele
Covering membrane	No	Yes
Location of defect	Right of umbilicus	Midline, including umbilicus
Umbilical cord insertion	Body wall at normal location	Omphalocele membrane
Herniated abdominal organs	Bowel	Bowel and sometimes liver
Associated anomalies	Uncommon	Very common
Prognostic factors	Condition of bowel	Associated anomalies

From Ledbetter DJ. Congenital abdominal wall defects and reconstruction in pediatric surgery: gastroschisis and omphalocele. *Surg Clin North Am.* 2012;92(3):714.

associated anomalies, and postoperative ventilation requirements. It is not uncommon for the anesthetist's choice to be an opioid and NDMR technique; however, even with the use of muscle relaxants, the abdominal wall may not allow primary closure. Ventilatory compromise and decreased organ perfusion are major problems as intraabdominal pressure increases. It is imperative to have adequate intravenous access and be prepared to infuse large amounts of fluid quickly. The administration of colloids is important to help reduce the amount of fluid loss from the intravascular space and ensuing formation of bowel and abdominal wall edema. Invasive monitoring of arterial pressure is advantageous to guide fluid replacement and allow for sampling of blood for the trending of laboratory values. A pulse oximeter probe placed on a lower extremity will indicate whether there is compromise in the perfusion to the lower extremities due to obstruction of venous return.

Postoperative ventilation is mandatory on each of these neonates, requiring the continued use of paralytics and sedation with an opioid infusion until their clinical status stabilizes and abdominal closure can be accomplished.

Necrotizing Enterocolitis

NEC is an intestinal inflammatory condition that is a life-threatening emergency. It occurs primarily in preterm babies with a gestational age less than 32 weeks and a weight less than 1500 g. The etiologic factors associated with NEC are reported to be secondary to bowel ischemia and immaturity, probable bacterial invasion, and premature oral feeding.[113,116] NEC is also more common and associated with premature neonates with PDAs, especially in the face of early feeding. Neonates with a PDA generally have a left-to-right shunt leading to pulmonary overcirculation at the expense of systemic perfusion. This leads to undercirculation of the GI tract, which in the presence of oral feeding stasis can lead to bacterial load, ischemia, and ultimately bowel perforation and sepsis. The origin of infection may also be the umbilical cord stump, infection due to circumcision, and similar lesions.[128] Box 52.7 lists the common symptoms of NEC. Diagnosis is confirmed by imaging studies that commonly show fixed dilated intestinal loops, pneumatosis intestinalis, portal vein air, ascites, and pneumoperitoneum. Accompanying laboratory values may show hyperkalemia, hyponatremia, metabolic acidosis, hyperglycemia, hypoglycemia, and, in the most serious cases, signs of disseminated intravascular coagulation.

The primary initial intervention revolves around medical management and focuses on ensuring oxygenation and the resolving of hypovolemia and acidosis. When medical management is unsuccessful, surgical intervention consists of an exploratory laparotomy or laparoscopy with resection of dead bowel, usually a colostomy, and peritoneal lavage.

Neonates with NEC may be septic and frequently come to the operating room already intubated and on ventilator support. In many institutions, bedside exploratory laparotomies are more commonly performed in the NICU, especially in severely premature neonates, as they are often quite unstable and require immediate intervention. Neonates with NEC and sepsis will generally not be able to tolerate volatile anesthetics. Nitrous oxide must be avoided due to the potential for bowel extension. If cardiac output is low and renal perfusion is below normal, inotropes may be indicated. Assessment of the neonate's blood pressure and pulmonary pressures, in combination with comorbid conditions, can help the anesthetist determine what type of inotrope and/or vasopressor to choose. It is important to monitor the neonate's hydration status by assessing urine output, serum and urine osmolality, hemoglobin and hematocrit, lactic acid, palpation of peripheral pulses, assessment of capillary refill, and palpation of the anterior fontanelle. The amount of third-space loss in these patients is exceptionally large and may require multiple blood volumes of crystalloid and colloid combinations to replace intravascular volume. RBCs, fresh frozen plasma (FFP), and platelets may also be required to increase oxygen-carrying capacity or to treat factor deficiency.[113,116] Blood administration should be considered very early during these procedures, especially in the presence of extreme prematurity and comorbid conditions. Most of these neonates are pervasively premature and have much lower circulating blood volumes (90–100 mL/kg) meaning that a smaller blood loss leads to a much greater compromise (i.e., low MABL). It is important to remember that large quantities of PRBCs alone can lead to dilutional coagulopathy, and the addition of FFP and platelets may be considered after a few PRBC transfusions. Postoperative care should focus on continuation of the fluid resuscitation, cardiopulmonary support, and mechanical ventilation.

Malrotation and Midgut Volvulus

Intestinal malrotation in the newborn is usually diagnosed after signs of intestinal obstruction occur, such as bilious emesis, and can be corrected with the Ladd procedure.[127] As the intestine is developing and migrating into the abdominal cavity during the first trimester of gestation, it can become twisted, compromising superior mesenteric artery and intestinal blood flow. The ensuing ischemia can cause bowel strangulation, bloody stools, peritonitis, and hypovolemic shock. When this occurs, it is called volvulus, which is generally an emergent procedure.[116]

Many of these neonates are diagnosed in the first week of life when the neonate presents with bilious vomiting, a tender and distended abdomen, and increasing hemodynamic instability. The surgical procedure relieves the obstruction by reducing the volvulus, dividing the fixation bands between the cecum and the duodenum or jejunum, and widening the base of the mesentery.

The major concerns for these neonates include airway management, fluid and electrolyte replacement, treatment of sepsis, and postoperative pain management. Any neonate or infant with intestinal obstruction will likely have abdominal distention, which could impede diaphragmatic movement, placing the infant at a higher risk for aspiration of gastric or intestinal contents. This necessitates the use of a rapid sequence induction with the proper application of cricoid pressure. If there is concern for difficult airway, an awake intubation should be considered. Altered fluid status resulting in hypovolemia can be caused by inadequate feeding, regurgitation, peritonitis, ileus, bowel manipulation, and sepsis. It is necessary to have adequate intravenous access, and it may be desirable to have a central line and an arterial line. Fluid replacement with a combination of crystalloid and colloid may help reduce the amount of fluid lost from the intravascular space to the interstitial space, thus helping reduce edema formation and facilitate abdominal closure. When the

---

BOX 52.7	**Common Symptoms of Necrotizing Enterocolitis**
• Increased gastric residuals with feeding	• Hypothermia
	• Abdominal mass
• Abdominal distention	• Oliguria
• Bilious vomiting	• Jaundice
• Lethargy	• Apnea and bradycardia
• Occult or gross rectal bleeding	• Fever
• Fever	

neonate has a "tight" abdomen, and closure is difficult, ventilation can be affected and become exceedingly difficult unless exceedingly high PIPs are used.

Imperforate Anus

During the first few days after birth, when there is no passage of meconium, the diagnosis of imperforate anus is considered. The degree of this anomaly can range from a mild stenosis to complete anal atresia that may be associated with other anomalies. The VACTERL association (see following section on tracheoesophageal fistula [TEF]) represents other potential associated conditions.[129] In male neonates, the operative procedure may be urgent to allow the passage of meconium via a colostomy. In female newborns, owing to the common presence of a rectovaginal fistula, the procedure can be delayed for a few weeks. The anesthetic considerations for these neonates are based on the existence of associated anomalies, as well as fluid and electrolyte balance.

Thoracic

Congenital Diaphragmatic Hernia

A CDH is a defect of the diaphragm that allows extrusion of the abdominal contents into the thoracic cavity. This disorder has an incidence of 1 in 2500 live births.[113,114] The herniated abdominal contents act as a space-occupying lesion and prevent normal lung growth and development. The diagnosis of CDH should be made prenatally in virtually all cases where routine maternal ultrasonography is available. Prognosis can be predicted based on whether the diaphragmatic hernia is isolated, as well as the degree of pulmonary and/or intraabdominal organ involvement. Prenatal intrauterine surgical intervention may be offered in fetuses that have a predicted poor outcome. The aim of this procedure is to reverse pulmonary hypoplasia. Percutaneous fetal endoscopic tracheal occlusion by a balloon is a minimally invasive procedure that has been shown to be safe and yields a 50% survival rate in severe cases. Outcomes can be predicted by the gestational age at birth, the lung size before and after balloon placement, and whether the balloon has been removed prenatally.[115] Nearly 80% of CDH patients experience herniation of the abdominal contents through the left side of the diaphragm through the foramen of Bochdalek. The lung most affected is on the ipsilateral side, but the contralateral lung can be affected as well. The lungs demonstrate reduced size of the bronchi, less bronchial branching, decreased alveolar surface area, and abnormal pulmonary vasculature. There is a thickening of the arteriolar smooth muscle extending to the capillary level of the alveoli. This results in increased pulmonary artery pressure and causes right-to-left shunting.[116]

Neonates with CDH present immediately after birth with dyspnea, tachypnea, cyanosis, absence of breath sounds on the affected side, and severe retractions. Their physical appearance includes a scaphoid abdomen and a barrel chest. It is estimated that nearly half of neonates with CDH have other anomalies, particularly heart lesions.

The emergent nature of the repair has been reexamined in the past decade, and more emphasis is now placed on stabilizing PHN and other medical comorbidities. A review of these cases noted that the median age at operation was 4 days and the median weight was 3800 g. Laparotomy, thoracoscopic repair, and a laparoscopic approach may be used.[117]

Studies published by Azarow et al.[118] and Jona[119] in the late 1990s demonstrated that the ventilation parameters were a major factor in survival of these babies. Permissive hypercarbia with high-frequency, oscillatory ventilation was most successful in improving outcomes. Care must still be taken to not allow carbon dioxide levels to get too high as this can further increase PVR, worsening pulmonary hypertensive conditions and precipitating increases in right-to-left shunting through a PFO, leading to further hypoxia. This makes controlling

other factors that affect PVR that much more important and avoiding increasing hypoxia, hypothermia, and acidosis. PIP should ideally be maintained less than 25 to 30 cm H_2O, as barotrauma with resulting pneumothorax of the one good lung could prove catastrophic in these neonates. Listening to breath sounds will assist in evaluating the degree of ventilation on each side of the chest after intubation. Due to the increased incidence of respiratory complications, most of the patients will already be intubated and have intravenous access and an arterial line in place when they arrive in the operating room

It is important to administer an anticholinergic (atropine 0.02 mg/kg) intravenously just prior to induction to prevent bradycardia during induction and intubation. If an awake intubation is planned, some type of analgesia should be used to decrease the stress response of airway instrumentation. Ventilation should be delivered gently to avoid inflating the stomach with air, which would increase the potential for passive gastric regurgitation and further decrease pulmonary compliance. Extreme care must be taken to avoid volutrauma or barotrauma to the one good lung.

The patient's hemodynamic stability should determine the anesthetic drugs that are administered. The use of inhalation agents and narcotics are guided by the cardiovascular stability.

If cardiopulmonary instability prevents the neonate from being transported to the operating room, the anesthetist might be required to administer anesthesia in the NICU while the baby is still on extracorporeal membrane oxygenation (ECMO). Under these circumstances, the recommended anesthetic choice is to administer an opioid and nondepolarizing muscle relaxant instead of an inhalation agent. Postoperative ventilation is required, with the goal of keeping the arterial oxygenation greater than 150 mmHg and slowly weaning to lower oxygen concentrations over a 48- to 72-hour period.[116]

Tracheoesophageal Fistula and Esophageal Atresia

The development of the upper respiratory and GI tracts takes place between the 21st day and the 5th week of gestation. Esophageal atresia (EA), with or without TEF, can be suspected prenatally by the presence of polyhydramnios and finding a stomach bubble on ultrasound. It is normally diagnosed immediately after birth when an orogastric tube cannot pass into the stomach, when there is coughing and choking after the first feeding, or after recurrent pneumonia associated with feedings.[113] In the past, this condition was often lethal. Today, there is an expectation of approximately 100% survival.[123] There are five types of TEF (A, B, C, D, E, and F), of which type C is most common.

There is a significant association between TEF and other serious congenital anomalies. Some sources report that as high as 30% to 50% of newborns with EA and TEF have other anomalies. The VACTERL association can be used to recall the most common developmental pathologic conditions:

- Vertebral anomalies
- Anal atresia (imperforate anus)
- Cardiac anomalies
- TEF and EA
- Renal anomalies
- Limb malformation

Preoperative echocardiography is necessary to exclude both associated cardiac defects and a right-sided aortic arch, which occurs in 2.5% of cases. An identified congenital heart defect may need to be managed preoperatively after consultation with a pediatric cardiologist, although surgical correction is almost always performed after the TEF/EA surgery. In the case of a right-sided aortic arch, surgical access to the esophagus and the TEF via the typical right thoracotomy is associated with the potential for massive rapid hemorrhage, making a left-sided thoracotomy more common in these situations.[123]

EA with a distal fistula is the most common presentation of TEF in approximately 80% to 90% of patients.[113] The esophagus ends in a blind pouch, and the distal esophagus forms a fistula with the trachea, usually above the carina. There are other configurations of this anomaly, varied by the location of the fistula and the presence or absence of EA, of which type C is the most common (Fig. 52.10). The morbidity and mortality of TEF are directly related to the resulting pulmonary complications caused by gastric aspiration.[124] The focus of the preoperative preparation should be to minimize the pulmonary complications by discontinuing oral feedings, placing a balloon-tipped catheter to suction nasopharyngeal secretions that accumulate in the blind esophageal pouch and prevent further aspiration, maintaining the infant in a semirecumbent position to minimize aspiration of secretions, and placing of a gastrostomy tube to prevent excessive gastric distention resulting in impaired ventilation. The surgical procedure is performed via a right-sided thoracotomy. The sequence of the repair is the ligation of the fistula and then anastomosis of the two ends of the esophagus if possible. Complete surgical correction may also be accomplished in several stages.

Standard monitors should be used. The cardiopulmonary condition of the neonate should dictate the use of more invasive monitoring techniques such as an arterial line commonly placed either in the umbilical or the radial artery. Preductal and postductal oximeter probes should be used to assess the degree of shunting that can occur in times of stress in these neonates.[21] Unknown features and potential problems with airway management in TEF leads some clinicians to perform bronchoscopy intraoperatively before intubation and thoracotomy. Bronchoscopy has been used effectively to assess the presence, type, number, size, and location of fistulas, while also determining or excluding additional fistulas that may otherwise be unidentified. This may leave the neonate with a continued source of aspiration.

The induction technique should be based on the clinician's evaluation of the airway. Some clinicians feel that inhalation induction with spontaneous respiration avoids overventilation and reduces the physiologic stress associated with airway manipulation. This technique minimizes gastric distention from anesthetic gases passing through the fistula and allows proper placement of the ETT without positive pressure ventilation. Gastric distention can impede ventilation leading to rapid desaturation, hypoxia, bradycardia, and eventual cardiac arrest. If this technique is used, care must be taken to avoid hypoxemia that will result from the respiratory depression produced by high concentrations of inhalation agents. With any of the described techniques, once the ETT is placed, proper position must be verified. A common method of verifying the correct position is to intubate the right mainstem bronchus and then withdraw the ETT until breath sounds are heard on the left side of the chest. The tip of the ETT is likely between the fistula and the carina at this point (Fig. 52.11). If a gastrostomy is in place, an alternative method is to submerge the gastrostomy tube in water and, if there are bubbles on ventilation, the fistula is being ventilated and the tube must be repositioned. The bevel of the ETT should be turned anteriorly to allow the posterior surface of the ETT to occlude the fistula. In one configuration of TEF, the fistula is located remarkably close to the carina. In this case, the ETT may need to be placed in the bronchus of the nonoperative lung until the fistula can be ligated. After ligation, the tube can be withdrawn above the carina.

During the procedure it is essential to monitor ventilation to ensure adequate oxygenation and to minimize PIP. Airway obstruction can occur if the trachea is compressed or if secretions or blood block the openings of the ETT.

The neonate who does not have significant preoperative pulmonary pathology and who meets extubation criteria may be extubated in the operating room. If there is any concern about airway obstruction or impaired ventilation, mechanical ventilation should be continued. It is possible that bag-mask ventilation or reintubation can potentially place undue stress on the suture lines of the repair, with laryngoscopy and neck extension resulting in damage to the esophagus necessitating additional procedures. Another problem that can occur with early extubation in smaller neonates is an inability to maintain the work of breathing due to preoperative lung disease. Always err on the side of caution. If postoperative mechanical ventilation is needed, the ETT should be positioned 1 cm away from the fistula repair to allow for healing of the suture line. A suction catheter should be clearly marked with a distance for insertion that approximates the distance just above the anastomotic repair.[125] Postoperative pain can be managed with opioids and/or an epidural, placed intraoperatively.

Complications may occur later that could influence anesthetic management. Neonates who have had EA/TEF repair early in life can develop a diverticulum at the site of the old tracheal fistula. This could present problems in the future if inadvertent intubation of the diverticulum occurs. Esophageal stricture could develop at the site of esophageal anastomosis requiring repeated dilation or possible resection.[126]

Patent Ductus Arteriosus

During transitional circulation of the neonate, the DA begins to close due to the reasons discussed early in this chapter. A PDA leads to a left-to-right shunting of blood leading to pulmonary overcirculation and symptoms of congestive heart failure. The stealing of systemic blood

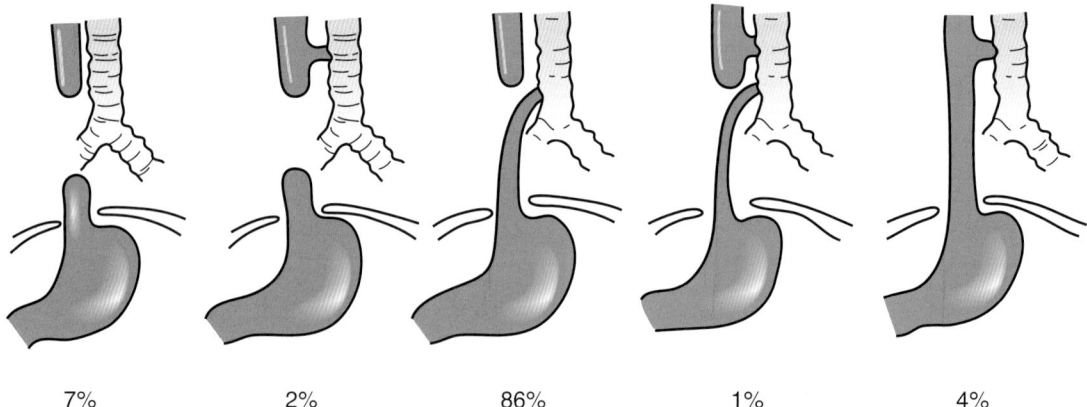

7%   2%   86%   1%   4%

Fig. 52.10 Anatomic variants and incidence of esophageal atresia with tracheoesophageal fistula. (From Townsend CM, et al. *Sabiston Textbook of Surgery: The Biologic Basis of Modern Surgical Practice.* 19th ed. Philadelphia: Elsevier; 2012:1838.)

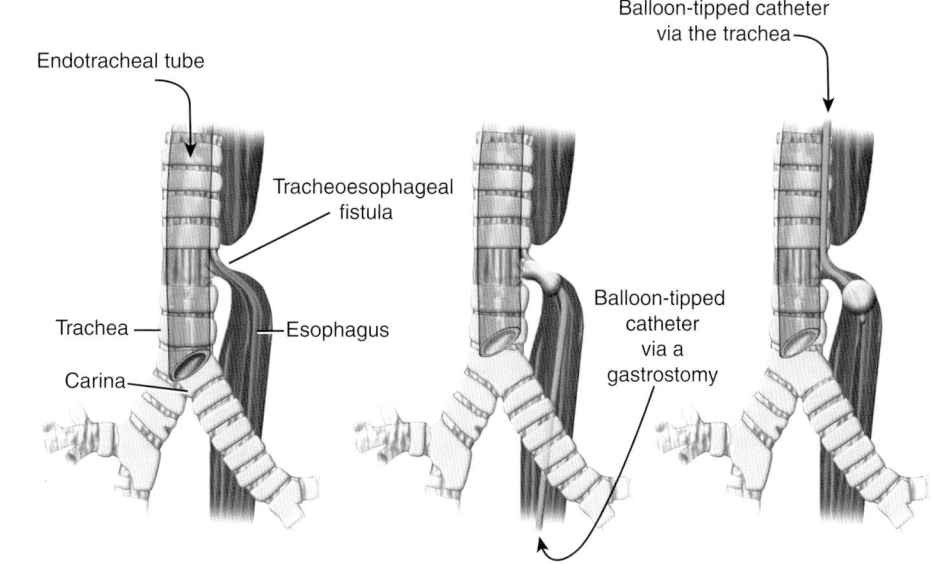

Fig. 52.11 Methods for minimizing gastric insufflation in infants with a tracheoesophageal fistula. (From Cote CJ, et al. *A Practice of Anesthesia for Infants and Children.* 5th ed. St. Louis: Elsevier; 2013.)

flow becomes important when examining NEC. Traditionally these defects have been ligated at the bedside, or in the operating room, with a surgical team via thoracotomy. There is an increased risk for recurrent laryngeal nerve injury using thoracotomy approach for PDA ligation, and pain control may be more difficult as well.

These defects can be repaired in the pediatric cardiac catheterization (PCC) lab. Access is obtained through the femoral vessels. The closure of the PDA is a wire driven, fluoroscopic-guided approach that uses transthoracic echo for placement confirmation. Closure in the PCC lab can be accomplished on premature neonates as small as 600 to 700 g, and the child may be on jet ventilation for the procedure. It is important to note that ventilation must be stable prior to closure, regardless of the approach for a given facility. If a child is transitioned from jet ventilation to conventional ventilation, there should be evidence of stable blood gases for several hours before ductal ligation or closure.

Whether the PDA is ligated or occluded, the anesthetist should realize the changes in blood pressure that occur following closure, particularly regarding diastolic blood pressure and pulse pressure. Postligation cardiac syndrome (PLCS), which contributes to systemic hypotension with poor cardiac output and accompanying increases in pulmonary artery pressure is associated with increased morbidity and mortality. Between 30% and 45% of PDA closures suffer from PLCS. PLCS often does not begin to manifest until at least 2 hours postligation and may be prolonged up to 24 hours following ligation. Many centers are pretreating these neonates with steroids prior to ligation (i.e., 1 mg/kg hydrocortisone every 6 hours). Treatment of PLCS revolves around hemodynamic support with fluid administration, milrinone, and/or epinephrine, and ventilatory support with mechanical ventilation. The premature neonate has a stiff, noncompliant left ventricle that may not tolerate PDA ligation. The neonate is prone to diastolic dysfunction, which may be worsened when the ductus is closed/ligated leading to pulmonary venous congestion.

Neurosurgical

Neonatal Hydrocephalus

Hydrocephalus is most often the result of an existing pathologic process, and it is a consequence of obstructed CSF flow within the brain. As a result, ICP increases. With emergent CSF accumulation, and

worsening neurologic and/or hemodynamic symptoms, a ventriculostomy may be performed to drain the excessive CSF. The standard treatment, however, includes placement of a drainage catheter into the ventricles of the brain to decrease ICP by means of shunting the fluid outside of the cranium. This is termed a ventriculoperitoneal (VP) shunt. Most often, the shunt is placed from the ventricle to the peritoneal cavity, but occasionally the catheter is placed into the right atrium or pleural cavity. In the neonate, if the hydrocephalus develops slowly, the cranial vault will expand to accommodate the increase in brain bulk. This occurs because the cranial sutures have not fully formed and fontanelles have not closed yet, and the skull can accommodate swelling and fluid accumulation to a certain degree. When intracranial volume is at capacity, ICP begins to increase and results in cerebral ischemia and cerebral herniation. The signs and symptoms associated with increasing ICP are bulging anterior fontanelle (when child is not crying), irritability, somnolence, vomiting, loss of consciousness, and/or cardiovascular collapse.

Anesthetic management is directed at controlling the ICP and relieving the obstruction. The urgency of the procedure is determined by the preanesthetic assessment of the ICP and associated symptoms present in the neonate. The major risk associated with delay is the possibility of herniation of the brain due to increasing pressure in the cranial vault. Herniation has associated cardiopulmonary consequences. Comorbidities such as prematurity, in combination with all its associated problems, must be addressed.

Intubation in the presence of increased ICP is frequently accomplished with rapid sequence induction. A variety of anesthetic agents are acceptable for maintenance, with the goal being to extubate the patient at the end of the procedure. Inhalation agents, which cause cerebral vascular dilation at MAC of greater than 1 vol %, can result in greater increases in ICP. The preoperative neurologic status, in combination with the intraoperative surgical and anesthetic course, will guide the decision to extubate following surgery or if mechanical ventilation and sedation should continue.

Myelomeningocele

Myelomeningocele, a form of spina bifida, is the most common CNS defect that occurs during the first month of gestation. This is

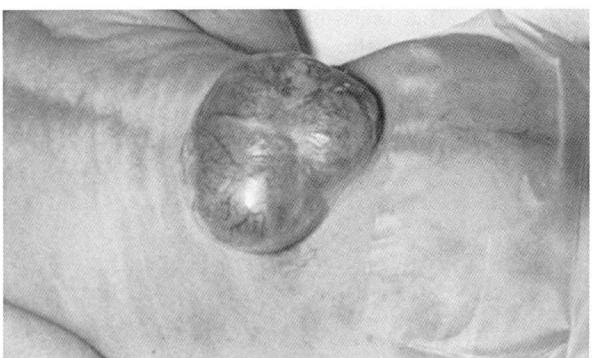

Fig. 52.12 A lumbar myelomeningocele is covered by a thin layer of skin. (From Kliegman RM, et al. *Nelson Textbook of Pediatrics*. 19th ed. Philadelphia: Elsevier; 2011:2001.)

a consequence of failure of the neural tube to close, resulting in herniation of the spinal cord and meninges through a defect in the spinal column and back. If the herniation only contains meninges, it is termed a meningocele, whereas herniation containing meninges and neural elements is termed a myelomeningocele. These lesions most often occur within the lumbosacral region, but it can occur at any level of the neuroaxis. Repair of the defect is considered urgent, and it is usually undertaken within the first 24 hours of life to avoid increasing risk of bacterial contamination of the spinal cord and further deterioration of neural and motor function (Fig. 52.12). Most newborns with a myelomeningocele do not have other associated anomalies or congenital heart disease. These neonates, however, may have Arnold-Chiari malformation, which is the result of the hindbrain displacing downward into the foramen magnum, leading to hydrocephalus. This will necessitate the placement of a VP shunt, usually during the myelomeningocele repair. There are usually significant neurologic deficits below the level of the lesion, and evaluation of the degree of deficit is important during anesthetic decision making. Preoperative assessment should include a thorough review of all other organ systems to rule out additional congenital anomalies. Laboratory testing should at minimum include a complete blood count and a type of screen.

Routine neonatal monitoring is necessary, and the use of invasive monitoring techniques should be based on the neonate's status. Positioning and airway management are big challenges for the anesthetist. Most of these neonates can be induced and intubated in the supine position with the lumbosacral defect supported in a donut-shaped ring or with strategically placed towels to avoid direct pressure on the dural sac. If the defect is quite large, or if there is accompanying severe hydrocephalus, it may be necessary to place the neonate in the lateral position for induction and intubation. The anesthetist may opt for videolaryngoscopy if the neonate is to be intubated in the lateral position. If there is a suspicion of a difficult airway, the ETT may be placed with the patient awake. Adequate intravenous access is essential because of the possibility of significant blood loss during the procedure, and arterial access should be considered for strict hemodynamic monitoring. If the defect is large, the surgeon may be required to undermine a large amount of tissue for closure, resulting in a large blood loss.

Anesthesia can be induced with an inhalation or intravenous technique. After the ETT is placed, the procedure is performed in the prone position with appropriate protection of all body parts. Anesthesia can be maintained with a variety of drugs, keeping in mind the goal of extubation at the end of the procedure and the possibility of postoperative apnea.

These patients are prone to developing hypothermia, and conservation of body heat should include warming the operating room to at least 27°C before the procedure and until the patient is draped. Radiant heat lamps should be used during line placement, induction and intubation, during surgical preparation, and during positioning of the patient. A forced-air warmer also should be placed underneath the neonate to maintain body temperature. Anesthetic gases should be humidified to prevent heat loss and minimize pulmonary complications. The anesthetist should also consider using fluid warming devices to deliver warm fluids. An increased sensitivity to latex in these neonates has been reported. As a precaution, they should be treated as latex allergic, avoiding all products that contain latex.[130,131]

SUMMARY

Despite the advances in neonatal medicine, surgery, and particularly anesthesia, the anesthetic management of critically ill neonates continues to be a challenge. A thorough knowledge of developmental physiology, in combination with knowledge of neonatal disease states and their treatment, is imperative for providing safe anesthesia. Providing neonatal anesthesia requires the anesthetist to be intensely vigilant to ensure perioperative safety.

REFERENCES

For a complete list of references for this chapter, scan this QR code with any smartphone code reader app, or visit the following URL: http://booksite.elsevier.com/9780323711944/.

53

Pediatric Anesthesia

Paula J. Belson, James S. Furstein

Pediatric subspecialty practice requires mastery of the foundations associated with pediatric growth and development, the anatomic and physiologic differences during various stages of maturation, and the influence of anesthetic medications on immature and developing organ systems. Anesthetic management for the pediatric patient requires integration and application of this specialized knowledge, in addition to refinement of the acquired technical skills employed during adult anesthetic management.

This chapter provides an extensive discussion of the essential aspects of care requisite for safe, effective pediatric anesthetic management. The foundation of anesthetic management is developed through an understanding of the pharmacologic and physiologic differences between infants, children, and adults; a clinical strategy for anesthetic management; and the morbidity and mortality associated with pediatric anesthesia.

PEDIATRIC ANATOMY AND PHYSIOLOGY

A thorough understanding of the anatomic and physiologic differences between pediatric and adult patients is of paramount importance when providing safe anesthesia care. The psychological and physical stress of surgery, the effects of anesthetic medications, and related pathology all play an integral role in determining patient outcomes. In addition, the immaturity of organ systems through 2 years of age affects anesthetic pharmacokinetics and pharmacodynamics. Pediatric patients are commonly subdivided by age based on physiologic and developmental milestones. Categoric groupings include the following: neonates (birth–1 month), infants (1 month–1 year), toddlers (1–3 years), preschool (4–6 years), school age (6–13 years), and adolescents (13–18 years).

A thorough discussion of anatomy and physiology for the pediatric patient is presented in Chapter 52.

PEDIATRIC PHARMACOLOGIC CONSIDERATIONS

Immature organ systems are largely responsible for the pharmacologic differences that exist between infants, children, and adults. Physiologic characteristics that modify pharmacokinetic and pharmacodynamic activity include differences in total body water (TBW) composition, immaturity of metabolic degradation pathways, reduced protein binding, immaturity of the blood-brain barrier, a greater proportion of blood flow to the vessel-rich organs (i.e., brain, heart, liver, and lungs), reductions in glomerular filtration, a smaller functional residual capacity, increased minute ventilation, and immature receptor responses.

Water freely diffuses across cell membranes and is essential for the transport of cellular nutrients and substrates that support metabolic reactions. TBW is the water content throughout the entire body and is represented as a percentage of total body weight expressed in liters (1 L of water weighs 1 kg). Gender and body habitus impact TBW and increases in age result in steadily decreasing TBW. TBW is distributed into the intracellular fluid (ICF) and extracellular fluid (ECF) compartments. With maturation, there is an accompanying decrease in the relative volumes of TBW and ECF during the first year of life, followed by additional decreases in ECF later in childhood. Table 53.1 illustrates the changes in TBW, ICF, and ECF during maturation.

Volume of Distribution

Drug distribution from the blood to various tissues throughout the body is heavily influenced by the volume of distribution, which is calculated by dividing the dose of the administered drug by the resulting plasma concentration. Gross differences between infant and adult compositions result in alterations in plasma drug concentrations following drug administration. Infants have a larger ECF compartment and a greater TBW content. Due to a dilutional effect, lower plasma drug concentrations occur rapidly after administration of water-soluble drugs. Accordingly, a larger drug loading dose is required to achieve the desired plasma concentration in this patient population. The fat, muscle, and fluid volume compartments of neonates and adults are compared in Table 53.1. Higher plasma concentrations occur for lipid-soluble drugs when administered according to weight due to the decreased fat and muscle volume of infants as compared with adults.[1]

Protein Binding

Protein binding refers to the degree that medications bind to a subset of proteins found in the blood. Accordingly, alterations in protein binding will impact the amount of free fraction of highly protein-bound drugs that is readily available. Reductions in plasma proteins such as albumin and α_1-acid glycoprotein (AAG) increase the free-drug fraction, which may increase the availability of active drug. Total plasma protein levels are lower in infants, reaching equivalent adult concentrations by 5 to 6 months of age. Albumin, the predominant plasma protein found in the body, is responsible for the binding of primarily acidic pharmacologic compounds, while AAG and other proteins are responsible for the binding of basic drugs. Although albumin and AAG concentrations are diminished at birth, with mean plasma concentrations of AAG in infants about 50% of that seen in healthy adults, adult levels are reached by 5 to 6 months of age. Albumin binding capacity approaches fully functional adult levels at approximately 1 year of age. Albumin concentrations may fluctuate, decreasing in chronic disease states. While protein binding of many anesthetic drugs is lower in infants and toddlers relative to adults, there is little clinical consequence. Comparatively, the reduced clearance of drugs exerts a much larger effect on drug action.

Metabolism and Excretion

Drug metabolism takes place in a host of locations throughout the body, including the liver, gastrointestinal tract, gastric mucosa, and lungs. In most instances, metabolism reduces drug activity; however, metabolism may activate the metabolite, as with a prodrug. The

TABLE 53.1   Body Composition During Growth

	Preterm Newborn (1.5 kg)	Full-Term Newborn (3.5 kg)	Adult (70 kg)
Muscle mass as % of BW	15	20	50
Fat as % of BW	3	12	18
Total body water	90%	80%	60%
Extracellular fluid	50%	40%	20%
Intracellular fluid	40%	40%	40%

BW, Body weight.

ultimate goal of drug metabolism is the production of a water-soluble compound that can be more easily excreted.

Drug metabolism occurs in two phases. Phase I metabolism consists of three enzymatic reactions (oxidation, reduction, and hydrolysis) catalyzed by the cytochrome P-450 (CYP450) enzyme system. Enzyme systems within the red blood cells, plasma, and other extrahepatic tissues are capable of hydrolyzing a variety of pharmacologic agents, including local anesthetics, the depolarizing relaxant succinylcholine, and nondepolarizing relaxants atracurium and cisatracurium. Esmolol is hydrolyzed by esterases in red blood cells. Phase I reactions introduce polar hydroxyl, amino, sulfhydryl, or carboxyl groups to produce a water-soluble metabolic product for excretion in the bile or urine. Phase II reactions, which are immature at birth, consist of conjugation or synthesis. Conjugation couples the drug with an endogenous substrate (i.e., via glucuronidation, methylation, acetylation, and sulfation) to facilitate excretion. The newborn lacks the capacity to efficiently conjugate bilirubin due to decreased glucuronyl transferase activity.

Although the necessary enzyme systems are present at birth, enzyme activity is reduced, thereby increasing drug elimination half-lives. Many medications have a prolonged effect in newborns and young infants. Some medications that have a prolonged plasma half-life in the pediatric patient include bupivacaine (25 hours),[2] mepivacaine (8.5 hours),[3] diazepam (up to 100 hours),[4] indomethacin (15–20 hours),[5] meperidine (22 hours), and phenytoin (21 hours).[6]

Absorption and Routes of Drug Administration

Most drugs used in anesthesia are given by the inhalation or intravenous (IV) routes. Routine medications are also administered orally and rectally during the preoperative and postoperative phases of care. Most drugs are formulated as liquid preparations for oral administration in children. Midazolam may be administered orally or intranasally for premedication, and the rectal route may be selected for the administration of acetaminophen, opioids, and benzodiazepines.[7] Both routes rely on passive diffusion for drug absorption, although the pharmacologic effect of drugs administered by the rectal route can be highly variable. The resulting plasma drug concentration is dependent on the molecular weight, degree of drug ionization, and lipid solubility.

The degree of ionization of orally administered drugs is dependent on gastric and intestinal pH levels. Acidic drugs are nonionized and are favorably absorbed in an acidic environment such as the stomach. Basic drugs are more favorably absorbed in the alkaline medium of the intestine. Most oral medications are absorbed in the intestine. The rate of absorption of many orally administered drugs is slower in neonates and young children because of a delayed gastric emptying time, which prolongs the time it takes for the medication

to reach the intestines. Gastric emptying time reaches the adult range by 6 months of age.[8-10]

Rectal drug absorption is directly affected by drug formulation and rectal blood flow. The superior (upper third of the rectum), middle, and inferior rectal veins carry blood away from the rectal mucosa. The superior rectal vein empties into the portal system, whereas the middle and inferior rectal veins empty into the systemic circulation by way of the inferior vena cava. For example, the administration of acetaminophen to the upper third of the rectum results in a lower plasma concentration because of first-pass metabolism with drug transport to the liver. Opioids and midazolam undergo first-pass metabolism, and their administration to the upper third of the rectum should be avoided.

Acetaminophen is a commonly prescribed antipyretic and analgesic administered to children during the perioperative period. It is capable of inducing dose-dependent hepatocyte injury, which is directly related to the dose and the duration of administration. Acetaminophen is metabolized by the hepatic microsomal enzyme system, and approximately 80% of the parent drug is conjugated with glucuronic acid and sulfate (phase II metabolism). Animal data suggest that a small amount of the parent drug is metabolized by the CYP450 enzyme system (phase I metabolism), producing an intermediate metabolite that undergoes conjugation with glutathione and is excreted in the urine. High doses of acetaminophen may deplete glutathione, increasing the accumulation of this intermediate metabolite, which is thought to be responsible for acetaminophen-induced liver necrosis. Glutathione depletion may develop with continued administration of high doses of acetaminophen.[11] Doses used in anesthesia rarely approach toxic levels.

Types of Agents

Inhalation Agents

The rapid increase in the alveolar concentration of an inspired anesthetic is quantified by the ratio of the alveolar concentration divided by the inspired concentration (F_A/F_I). Factors that affect the F_A/F_I ratio include the delivered inspired anesthetic concentration, the blood-gas partition coefficient of the inhalation agent, alveolar ventilation (V_A), cardiac output (Q_t), and the distribution of Q_t to the vessel-rich organs (i.e., heart, brain, kidneys, and liver). Tidal volume is similar between children and adults (5–7 mL/kg). Neonates and children have significantly greater minute ventilation and a higher ratio of tidal volume to functional residual capacity (5:1) compared to adults (1.5:1) due to their greater metabolic rate. The greater minute ventilation and higher Q_t in infants and children are responsible for rapid inhalation anesthetic uptake and rapidly increasing alveolar anesthetic concentrations. In addition, their decreased distribution of adipose tissue and decreased muscle mass affect the rate of equilibration among the alveoli, blood, and brain. The percentage of blood flow to the vessel-rich organs in children is greater than in the adult resulting in lower blood-gas partition coefficients in infants and children.[12,13]

The minimum alveolar concentration (MAC) of inhalation anesthetics is an indicator of dose and anesthetic requirements and varies with age. The MAC of sevoflurane is higher in neonates and infants and decreases after 6 months of age (Fig. 53.1). This differs from other inhalational agents (isoflurane, halothane, and desflurane) where MAC increases with age from the neonatal period to age 6 months and then decreases with increasing age.[14,15] The rationale for why the MAC of sevoflurane varies from the other halogenated agents remains undetermined. In general, however, age-related alterations in MAC requirements are believed to be secondary to maturation of the CNS, as well as hormonal factors.

Myocardial depression may be exaggerated when inhalation anesthetics are administered to pediatric patients.[16,17] A more rapid rise in the F_A/F_I ratio, the greater percentage of blood flow to the vessel-rich

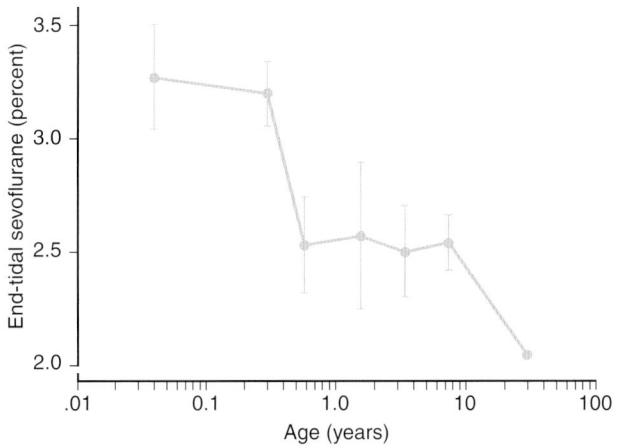

Fig. 53.1 Effects of age on maximum alveolar concentration. (Data from Lerman J, et al. The pharmacology of sevoflurane in infants and children. *Anesthesiology*. 1994;80:814–824.)

organs, and higher inhaled anesthetic concentration requirements are central to the cause of myocardial depression. To summarize, inhalation induction is more rapid in pediatric patients because of increased minute ventilation; however, the incidence of hemodynamically compromising myocardial depression in this population is greater than in an adult because of the structural and functional immaturity of the pediatric heart.

Sevoflurane. The MAC of sevoflurane in oxygen is 3% for infants up to 6 months of age, decreasing to 2.5% to 2.8% up to 1 year of age.[18,19] Sevoflurane produces a rapid induction and emergence due to its low blood-gas partition coefficient.[20] Unlike other inhalation anesthetic agents, sevoflurane is not a potent airway irritant and as a result is the preferred agent for inhalation inductions. Additionally, sevoflurane is nonpungent in nature making it more readily accepted. Sevoflurane depresses minute ventilation and, at higher cerebral concentrations, the respiratory rate. At high inspired concentrations, apnea will occur.[21,22]

Sevoflurane metabolism may produce concentration-dependent elevations in serum fluoride levels that decline when it is discontinued.[23] Concerns regarding fluoride-induced renal damage, however, have not proven to be clinically significant. Sevoflurane does not sensitize the myocardium to the effects of endogenous and exogenous catecholamines. As with any inhalation agent, the degree of myocardial depression is dependent on the concentration—higher concentrations cause a greater degree of inhibition of myocardial contractility and peripheral vascular dilation.

Isoflurane. The MAC of isoflurane in oxygen is 1.6% in infants and children. Isoflurane is more pungent than sevoflurane and can be an irritant to the airway at doses greater than 1.0 MAC and subsequently more likely to produce adverse respiratory events (i.e., breath holding, coughing, and laryngospasm with copious secretions) when compared to sevoflurane. Administration of isoflurane to adults produces dose-dependent decreases in peripheral vascular resistance, whereas an increased heart rate maintains blood pressure. This compensatory advantage (i.e., the maintenance of blood pressure by the increased heart rate) does not occur in infants due to the immature receptors and inability to produce a response to stimuli. Anesthetic induction in infants with isoflurane produces significant dose-dependent decreases in heart rate, blood pressure, and mean arterial pressure.[24]

Desflurane. The MAC of desflurane in oxygen is 9% for infants and 6% to 10% for children. Desflurane has the lowest blood-gas partition coefficient of all the inhalation anesthetics (0.42), which facilitates a rapid induction, rapid alterations in anesthetic depth, and rapid

emergence. Like isoflurane, desflurane is pungent, and it is associated with more adverse respiratory events during inhalation induction, including breath holding, laryngospasm, coughing, and increased secretions with accompanying hypoxia. After inhalation induction with sevoflurane, desflurane is appropriate for the maintenance of general anesthesia with facemask, endotracheal tube (ETT), or a laryngeal mask airway (LMA). As in the adult population, rapid increases in inhaled concentrations of desflurane may induce sympathetic stimulation, as evidenced by tachycardia and hypertension.[25,26] Due to its low solubility and faster washout, desflurane provides a more rapid and predictable recovery for obese pediatric patients.[27] Return to protective airway reflexes is prolonged with increased body mass index, a relationship that is more pronounced with sevoflurane when compared to desflurane. The comparatively more rapid return of protective airway reflexes following administration may make desflurane the inhaled anesthetic of choice with obese patients as this patient population is at an inherently increased risk for respiratory events during the recovery from anesthesia.

Nitrous oxide. Nitrous oxide has very limited solubility in the blood with a blood-gas partition coefficient of 0.47. The MAC of nitrous oxide in adults is 104%. (MAC of nitrous oxide in children has not been determined.) Simultaneous administration of nitrous oxide with sevoflurane during pediatric inhalational induction increases the uptake of sevoflurane. This is known as the second-gas effect. This increase in speed of onset is beneficial in decreasing the amount of time the patient is in the second stage of anesthesia. The second-gas effect also occurs during emergence where the rapid elimination of nitrous oxide from the tissues accelerates the removal of the accompanying volatile agent.

Inhaled anesthetics and the developing brain. There are concerns about the potential long-term impact of inhaled anesthetics on neural development in the young child. Although animal research has demonstrated both structural and functional changes following exposure to anesthesia early in life, this is a retrospective association and not proof of definitive causation. Furthermore, cell death observed in young animals has not consistently predicted future disability. In humans, epidemiologic studies are inconclusive largely due to the host of confounding variables that make it challenging to discern the exact impact anesthetic exposure truly has on neural development.

Current literature suggests that general anesthesia for a surgical procedure in early childhood may be associated with long-term diminution of language abilities and cognition, as well as regional volumetric alterations in brain structure. The issue of causation, however, remains unresolved. Unfortunately, current animal research has not clearly identified a particular age after which anesthetic exposure causes structural abnormalities, hence no age for postponing "elective" procedures can be recommended. Should the family express concerns, it would be wise to share what has been repeatedly reported in the literature: Untreated pain is deleterious to the developing nervous system and delaying or not performing vital surgeries may be more deleterious than the theoretic risk of anesthetic exposures.

Intravenous Anesthetics

As discussed previously, a higher proportion of cardiac output is delivered to vascular-rich tissues (i.e., heart, brain, kidneys, and liver) in infants and children. IV-administered drugs are rapidly delivered and absorbed by these tissues, and they are subsequently redistributed to muscle and fat, tissues that are less well perfused. IV-administered drugs may have a prolonged duration of action in infants due to decreased hepatic degradation and renal excretion. The central nervous system (CNS) effects of opioids may also be prolonged because of the immaturity of the blood-brain barrier.[28,29] Increased doses of propofol and ketamine are required when compared to adult patients presumably because of a greater volume of distribution and a greater metabolic rate.[30]

Propofol. Propofol has a rapid onset and a short duration of action, and it is the most popular IV agent in pediatric anesthetic management for induction and maintenance of general anesthesia and unconscious sedation. It may also be combined with an opioid or ketamine to provide total IV anesthesia. Propofol may be delivered as a continuous infusion for short diagnostic and radiologic procedures and is used as a primary sedative when planning extubation of intensive care patients who have been ventilated for a prolonged period of time. Additionally, the drug's antiemetic properties may reduce the incidence of postoperative nausea and vomiting (PONV) in children.[31] Infants require larger induction doses (2.5–3 mg/kg) than children (2–2.5 mg/kg).[32,33] These induction doses may produce decreased systolic blood pressure due to direct myocardial depression and vasodilation.[34,35] The pain that accompanies IV administration may be reduced with the addition of lidocaine or ondansetron. Additional strategies used to decrease the pain during injection include a slower injection of propofol into a rapid-running IV line or injection into larger IV catheters placed in the antecubital space.[36]

In 1992, Parke et al. reported the deaths of five children who received long-term, high-dose propofol infusions.[37] The large doses were administered by continuous infusion in critical care units with long-term sedation over several days; however, this phenomenon was not associated with short-term anesthesia use. Additional case reports followed, further characterizing this serious reaction, which is referred to as propofol infusion syndrome. Propofol infusion syndrome causes severe lactic acidosis, hypertriglyceridemia, fever, hepatomegaly, dysrhythmias, rhabdomyolysis, and heart failure. It frequently results in cardiovascular collapse and death. The likely mechanism involves propofol inhibiting mitochondrial function and uncoupling oxidative phosphorylation. Children with mitochondrial defects may have an increased risk of developing this syndrome.[38,39] Propofol infusions at doses of greater than 4 mg/kg/hour for greater than 48 hours increase the risk of this syndrome. However, propofol infusion syndrome can also develop with infusions less than 4 mg/kg/hour. When prolonged administration is planned, algorithms have been proposed to help prevent this adverse drug effect.[40]

Etomidate. Etomidate is a hypnotic IV anesthetic that maintains cardiovascular stability. It can be utilized for the induction of children with congenital heart disease, cardiomyopathy, or hypovolemic shock. The recommended induction dose is 0.2 to 0.3 mg/kg. The suppression of adrenal cortical function following a single dose has limited the use of etomidate, especially when sepsis is a concern.[41]

Ketamine. Ketamine is a dissociative anesthetic commonly used in pediatrics. When used for induction of anesthesia, ketamine can be administered either IV or intramuscularly (IM). The induction dose is 1 to 2 mg/kg IV or 4 to 6 mg/kg IM. It is useful for children with cardiovascular instability and/or hypovolemia as it maintains systemic vascular resistance. However, ketamine can act as a myocardial depressant, decrease systemic blood pressure, and lead to cardiovascular collapse in children with depleted endogenous catecholamine stores due to its direct negative inotropic effects.[42]

Neuromuscular Blocking Agents

Neuromuscular blocking drugs are highly ionized and have a low lipophilicity, restricting their distribution to the ECF compartment. Since the ECF compartment is larger in neonates and infants than in children and adults, a dilutional effect occurs, ultimately increasing the volume of distribution for neonates and infants. Variance in ECF volume and the ongoing maturation of both neonatal skeletal muscle and

acetylcholine receptors impact the pharmacokinetics and pharmacodynamics of neuromuscular relaxants. Table 52.8 references the effective doses of neuromuscular blocking drugs for various age groups.

The neuromuscular junction is incompletely developed at birth, maturing after 2 months of age.[43] Skeletal muscle, acetylcholine receptors, and the accompanying biochemical processes essential in neuromuscular transmission mature during infancy and continue to develop throughout childhood.

The presynaptic release of acetylcholine is slow in children compared with adults, which decreases the margin of safety for neuromuscular transmission in the neonate. The acetylcholine receptors of the newborn are anatomically different from adult receptors, with the fetal form of the receptor containing a gamma subunit (composition alpha 2, beta, gamma, delta), which is gradually replaced by the epsilon subunit-containing adult form (alpha 2, beta, epsilon, delta), which may explain the sensitivity of the neonate to nondepolarizing neuromuscular relaxants.[44,45] This neuromuscular immaturity may be demonstrated with the appearance of fade after tetanic stimulation in the absence of neuromuscular blocking drugs.[46,47]

Succinylcholine. In the early 1990s, a series of unexpected cardiac arrests were reported after the routine administration of succinylcholine to children thought to be otherwise healthy in which less than 40% of the patients were successfully resuscitated. It was determined that the patients had Duchenne muscular dystrophy but were undiagnosed. Duchenne muscular dystrophy is associated with ongoing muscle atrophy resulting in hyperkalemia. Succinylcholine administration produces massive hyperkalemia and subsequent cardiac arrest in children with Duchenne muscular dystrophy.[48] Ultimately, the US Food and Drug Administration (FDA) relabeled succinylcholine, restricting its use to emergency airway management in children.[49,50] It is used primarily as an emergency medication in the treatment of laryngospasm and for rapid sequence induction in the case of a full stomach. Most clinicians avoid routinely using this medication for patients through the early teen years and in patients with muscle disorders. Its use is contraindicated in patients with malignant hyperthermia (MH).[51,52]

Nondepolarizing neuromuscular blocking agents. Infants and children are more sensitive than adults to the effects of nondepolarizing neuromuscular blocking drugs (see Table 52.8). A lower plasma concentration of the selected neuromuscular relaxant is required to achieve the desired clinical level of neuromuscular blockade. This does not imply that the selected dosage should be decreased as infants have a greater volume of distribution. The larger volume of distribution and slower drug clearance, however, results in longer elimination half-life, decreasing the need for repeated drug dosing (longer dosing intervals). Neuromuscular function must be monitored to guide repeated administration of these drugs in all pediatric patients. The degree of neuromuscular blockade should be assessed using physical signs (e.g., strength of movement, spontaneous respirations with adequate tidal volume) and neuromuscular monitoring (i.e., train-of-four and sustained tetanus). Neuromuscular function should be checked by assessing the adductor pollicis muscle on the forearm because function in this region is more reflective of diaphragmatic activity as compared with the orbicularis oculi (temporal region). The selection of a nondepolarizing neuromuscular relaxant should take into consideration the desired degree and duration of skeletal muscle paralysis, the immaturity of the organ systems, and the associated side effects of the selected relaxant.[53,54]

Antagonism of neuromuscular blockade. Residual neuromuscular blockade places the infant and child at risk of hypoventilation and the inability to independently and continuously maintain a patent airway. Due to the increased basal oxygen consumption, impaired respiratory function will lead to arterial oxygen desaturation and CO_2 retention. The detection of residual neuromuscular blockade requires the integration of clinical criteria and the assessment of neuromuscular blockade via a peripheral nerve stimulator. Conventional doses of the anticholinesterase inhibitors (50–60 mcg/kg of neostigmine; 500–1000 mcg/kg of edrophonium) combined with appropriate doses of atropine (0.02 mg/kg) or glycopyrrolate (0.2 mg for each 1 mg of neostigmine) are acceptable for antagonism of nondepolarizing neuromuscular blockade. Because bradycardia is a consequence of administering an anticholinesterase drug, some anesthesia providers will administer the anticholinergic drug prior to the anticholinesterase drug to avoid this complication.

Presently, sugammadex is not FDA approved for the antagonism of neuromuscular blockage in patients younger than 18 years of age. However, research has shown that sugammadex is well tolerated in pediatric patients.[55] A recent study reported no significant association between sugammadex administration in pediatric patients and anaphylaxis.[56] The use of sugammadex in a "cannot intubate cannot ventilate" scenario after administration of rocuronium or vecuronium adds another safety option to the pediatric difficult airway algorithm.[57]

Voluntary clinical assessments, such as sustained head lift or response to verbal questions, are most often not able to be obtained from the infant and young child. Useful clinical signs of successful antagonism of neuromuscular blockade include the ability to flex the arms, lift the legs, and flex the thighs upon the abdomen, providing evidence of the return of abdominal muscle tone in addition to the return of a normal response to nerve stimulation.[58] Neonates are capable of generating a negative inspiratory force (NIF) of −70 cm H_2O with the first few breaths after birth.[59] A NIF of at least −32 cm H_2O has been found to correspond with leg lift, which is indicative of the adequacy of ventilatory reserve required before tracheal extubation.[60,61]

PREOPERATIVE ASSESSMENT

Preoperative assessment and preparation are often completed shortly before scheduled surgery in the preoperative anesthesia clinic or in the patient's room in the hospital. Patients who are acutely ill or medically unprepared should be assessed in the preoperative area to ensure optimization of chronic diseases and to create a comprehensive individualized anesthetic plan.

Parents or caretakers offer valuable insight into the history of their child. It is important to establish open communication and gain the trust of the patient and family members. Parental preparation is equally as important and is an opportunity to allay fears and answer questions. A thorough preoperative assessment will foster trust and confidence through a courteous and understandable explanation of the anesthetic experience. Parental anxiety may be driven by negative personal past anesthetic experiences, such as painful intravenous catheter placement, coerced mask induction, or postoperative pain, nausea, and vomiting. When the child appears for a repeat surgical procedure, the parents may have important information that is helpful in detailing a successful plan of care for their child.

Review of Systems

Reviewing the medical record can answer many questions before approaching the patient/parents for information. Understanding congenital history can help preparation and development of a plan of care. If available, previous anesthetic records can also provide valuable information. Table 53.2 lists the anesthetic implications of the review of systems and history.

- *Birth and development.* Was the child born prematurely or at term? Did the child experience any neonatal complications or spend any time in the neonatal intensive care unit? Was the child discharged home without issues or additional monitoring? Does the child have any history of apnea or bradycardia? Is there any history of sudden infant death syndrome in the child's family? Are there any developmental or learning setbacks? Is the child achieving developmental milestones as anticipated?
- *Neurologic disorders.* Has the child experienced any neurologic symptoms such as seizures?
- *Heart disease.* Does the patient play at school without severe shortness of breath or syncope? Does the child have a heart murmur?
- *Pulmonary disorders/disease.* Does the child have asthma, bronchitis, or pneumonia? If the child has asthma, what are the triggers, does the child use daily inhalers, and are there any recent changes in medication need? Does the child currently receive, or has the child received in the past, supplemental oxygen therapy? Has the child had a recent cold, cough, or respiratory infection? It should be noted that children often present with persistent nasal drainage secondary to an inner ear infection. It is important to ask the parent about the color, consistency, and duration of drainage.
- *Does the child have a history of diabetes or endocrine disorders?*
- *Bleeding disorders.* Does the child have sickle cell anemia? Does the child bleed or bruise easily?
- *Liver disease.* Has the child had jaundice or liver problems?
- *Urology disorders.* Has the child had problems with the kidneys, ureters, or bladder? Any urinary tract infections?
- *Gastrointestinal disorders.* Has the child had gastric acid reflux or a hiatal hernia? Has the child experienced problems with diarrhea or vomiting?
- *Muscle or joint deformities?*
- *Any skin related concerns? Eczema or rashes?*
- *Has the child ever been in the emergency room or hospitalized for any reason?*
- *Obstetric history.* Could the patient possibly be pregnant (controversial topic)? When was the patient's last menstrual period?
- *Airway assessment.* Does the patient have a history of a difficult intubation? Does the child have trouble opening the mouth? Are there any chipped, missing, or loose teeth? Is there a history of snoring/apnea? If so, how often and how long are the pauses?
- *Other concerns.* Does the child have any other medical conditions or concerns we have not yet discussed?
- *Medications.* Is the child currently on any medications, or taken any within the last 3 months? Has the child taken steroids within the last year? If so, for what condition?
- *Allergies.* Is the patient allergic to any medication or food? Are there any problems with latex or other environmental items?

Fasting Status

The risk of pulmonary aspiration in the pediatric patient is extremely low (1 in 10,000).[62] Although the goal of preoperative fasting is to ensure an empty stomach at the time of anesthetic induction, prolonged fasting may produce irritability as a result of thirst and hunger. Prolonged fasting may also alter fluid balance, producing preinduction hypovolemia and hypoglycemia. Hypoglycemia is especially problematic in premature infants. Preoperative access to clear fluids (e.g., apple juice, water) 2 hours before anesthetic induction has been shown to have a minimal impact on gastric volume. Current recommendations by the American Society of Anesthesiologists (ASA) are 2 hours of fasting for clear liquids; 4 hours for breast milk; 6 hours for infant formula, nonhuman milk, and a light meal; and 8 hours for a

TABLE 53.2	Medical History and Review of Symptoms: Anesthetic Implications	
System	**Factors to Assess**	**Possible Anesthetic Implications**
Respiratory	Cough, asthma, recent cold Croup Apnea/bradycardia	Irritable airway, bronchospasm, medication history, atelectasis, infiltrate Subglottic narrowing Postoperative apnea/bradycardia
Cardiovascular	Heart murmur Cyanosis History of squatting Hypertension Rheumatic fever Exercise intolerance	Septal defect, avoid air bubbles in intravenous line Right-to-left shunt Tetralogy of Fallot Coarctation of the aorta; renal disease Valvular heart disease Congestive heart failure, cyanosis
Neurologic	Seizures Head trauma Swallowing incoordination Neuromuscular disease	Medications; metabolic derangement Elevated intracranial pressure Aspiration, esophageal reflux, hiatal hernia Neuromuscular relaxant drug sensitivity, malignant hyperthermia
Gastrointestinal and hepatic	Vomiting, diarrhea Malabsorption Black stools Gastroesophageal reflux Jaundice	Electrolyte abnormality; dehydration; full stomach Anemia Anemia, hypovolemia Possible need for full stomach precautions Altered drug metabolism; risk of hypoglycemia
Genitourinary	Frequency Frequent urinary tract infections	Urinary tract infection, diabetes, hypercalcemia Evaluate renal function
Endocrine and metabolic	Abnormal development Hypoglycemia, steroid therapy	Endocrinopathy, hypothyroid, diabetes Hypoglycemia, adrenal insufficiency
Hematologic	Anemia Bruising, excessive bleeding Sickle cell disease	Transfusion requirement Coagulopathy, thrombocytopenia Possible transfusion; hydration
Allergies	Medication history	Drug reactions; drug interactions
Dental	Loose or carious teeth	Dental trauma; aspiration of a loose tooth; bacterial endocarditis prophylaxis

Modified from Ghazal EA, et al., eds. In: Coté CJ, et al., eds. *A Practice of Anesthesia for Infants and Children.* 6th ed. Philadelphia: Elsevier; 2019:40.

regular meal, including fatty foods (see Table 42.2 NPO guidelines). The guidelines can be referred to as the "2-4-6-8 rule."[63] These parameters are suggested for healthy patients undergoing elective surgery. No gum is to be chewed after midnight; prescribed medications can be taken with a sip of water or as a prescribed liquid mixture. For patients scheduled for elective surgery who have not achieved the appropriate fasting time, the best decision is most often to postpone surgery until the proper NPO status has been achieved. If the procedure is urgent or necessary, a rapid sequence induction should be performed.

As the tenets of enhanced recovery after surgery (ERAS) have gained popularity in pediatric anesthesia practice, the concept of preoperative carbohydrate loading has been introduced into practice. While definitive guidelines have not yet been determined, early literature supports the notion that oral carbohydrates are safe, well tolerated, and do not increase the incidence of perioperative adverse events. Additionally, it has been reported that oral carbohydrates reduce preoperative discomfort with elective surgery, improve postoperative pain management (especially with cardiac surgery), reduce PONV, and improve postoperative metabolism by decreasing insulin resistance. The period of greatest relevance when developing preoperative fasting recommendations is the terminal phase of clearance, which has been reported to be approximately 3 to 3.5 hours following ingestion of clear carbohydrate drinks. Therefore, it has been offered that while many of these drinks are clear in nature, due to their protein content they should not be considered a clear liquid and perhaps should require a 6-hour window to prevent untoward events.[64]

Upper Respiratory Infection

Upper respiratory infections (URIs) are common in pediatric patients, are frequently seasonal, and may be accompanied by cough, pharyngitis, tonsillitis, and croup. The child with an active or resolving URI will have increased airway reactivity with a propensity for the development of atelectasis and mucous plugging of the airways, as well as the potential to experience postoperative arterial hypoxemia.[65] In addition, bronchial reactivity may persist for 6 to 8 weeks after a viral lower respiratory tract infection. The presence of chronic respiratory disease (asthma or bronchopulmonary dysplasia) requires a thorough assessment and medication review to ensure that the disease is well controlled and that the child is not currently experiencing an exacerbation. A history of steroid use necessitates consideration of steroid supplementation throughout the perioperative period.

Healthy children who are scheduled for placement of tympanostomy tubes frequently present with otitis and rhinitis. When determining whether to proceed with anesthesia and the surgical procedure, additional patient history must be obtained to differentiate between a chronic allergic or an acute infectious presentation. It is also imperative to determine whether there is lower airway involvement. Assessment of the color and duration of nasal drainage will assist in deciding whether rhinorrhea is chronic or acute. Purulent nasal discharge associated with pharyngitis, cough, or fever may be indicative of a bacterial or viral URI. Additional information may be obtained by questioning the parents regarding their assessment of the child's current health. Helpful questions include: Does your child appear ill? Is your child eating, sleeping, and playing normally? Is there anyone in the family (including siblings) who is currently ill? Children with chronic allergic rhinorrhea who exhibit a clear nasal drainage without accompanying signs of illness (e.g., no cough, pharyngitis, wheezing, or associated fever) are less likely to experience untoward events during the course of general anesthesia, although there remains an imposed increased risk.

Lower respiratory tract dysfunction typically accompanies viral or bacterial URI. This combination may be associated with a greater frequency of laryngospasm (5-fold greater incidence) and bronchospasm (10-fold greater incidence) during anesthetic management, particularly when endotracheal intubation is performed.[66] Although a mild URI may be inconsequential during the intraoperative period, significant problems may develop in the immediate postoperative period. Multiple studies have reported an increase in the incidence of postintubation croup, hypoxemia, and bronchospasm in patients with URIs compared with asymptomatic children.[66-68]

Multiple factors must be considered when deciding whether to cancel an elective procedure. Children with signs and symptoms of acute airway dysfunction should have further medical evaluation performed by a pediatrician. Elective surgery should be postponed for children who have a cough and pharyngitis accompanied by fever and wheezing. Whether symptoms are acute versus chronic needs to be determined prior to postponing the procedure. Children with a fever of 38.0°C and higher, malaise, wheezing, dyspnea, rhonchi, nasal congestion, and a productive cough are signs of an acute infection necessitating the postponement of surgery.[69,70] Evidence-based recommendations are given in Box 53.1.

Laboratory Testing

Laboratory testing should be ordered preoperatively based on the patient's medical history and physical examination and the type of surgical procedure planned. Indications for preoperative laboratory testing are listed in Box 53.2. The American Academy of Pediatrics states that routine laboratory tests do not need to be performed in healthy patients undergoing outpatient surgery.[71] However, in patients presenting with an abnormality, preoperative testing is imperative to guide surgical and anesthetic care.

Preoperative laboratory tests should be ordered based on abnormal findings from the medical history and physical examination. A definitive "adequate" hemoglobin (Hgb) concentration that is essential for oxygen delivery is 7 to 8 g/dL for most hospitalized adult patients. However, there have been few studies to quantify these transfusion triggers in the pediatric population. Red blood cell transfusion therapy varies between medical service specialties and institutions; however, using a restrictive transfusion threshold of 7 g/dL may result in reduced transfusion rates and lowered associated risks and costs.[72]

The determination of an acceptable preoperative Hgb level requires an understanding of the child's current medical history, the proposed surgical procedure, and global oxygen transport and use. The value of routine Hgb screening has been questioned for some time and has been found to rarely affect the anesthetic management of children. Children who benefit from preoperative Hgb determinations include premature infants less than 60 weeks of postconceptional age, children with concurrent cardiopulmonary disease, children with known hematologic dysfunction (e.g., sickle cell disease), and children in whom major blood loss is anticipated during the surgical procedure. Anemia of prematurity is not uncommon, with Hgb levels declining in the first 8 to 10 weeks of life. This is secondary to a decline in red blood cell counts in response to an increase in the availability of oxygen and downregulation of erythropoietin, which will continue until oxygen delivery is inadequate for metabolic demand and erythropoietin production is stimulated.[73]

BOX 53.1 Recommendations for Patients With Upper Respiratory Tract Infections

When feasible, efforts should be made to make parents aware of the problems with respiratory tract infections and anesthesia, and parents should be encouraged to call before the day of surgery to discuss the symptoms and possible need for delay. There may be a role for pediatricians and other primary care practitioners to play in the process of perioperative evaluation and education.

First, an emergency case mandates judicious airway management and logically must proceed regardless of the presence or absence of respiratory symptoms. In patients undergoing elective nonurgent surgery, initial consideration should be with respect to the severity of respiratory tract symptoms. Often, careful questioning of parents can differentiate acute from chronic symptoms. Patients with severe symptoms such as fever >38.4°C, malaise, productive cough, wheezing, rhonchi, or recent emesis should be considered for delay of elective surgery. A reasonable period of delay would be 4–6 wk. If mild symptoms are present, such as nonproductive cough, sneezing, or mild nasal congestion, surgery could proceed for those having regional or general anesthesia without endotracheal tube (ETT) placement. The intraoperative plan should include early use pulse oximetry, decision of facemask or laryngeal mask airway use, and careful suctioning of the nasopharynx and oropharynx under deep anesthesia before emergence. Additional management considerations for patients with upper respiratory tract infection (URI) or lower respiratory tract (LRI) undergoing anesthesia include hydration status, use of airway humidification, and the potential benefit of pharmacologic agents such as anticholinergics and bronchodilators to help with airway secretions and airway hyperreactivity.

However, for those patients who require ETT placement for anesthesia, especially children <1 year of age, it is important to identify risk factors such as passive smoke exposure and underlying conditions (e.g., asthma, chronic lung disease) because these children may benefit from a slight delay of 2–4 wk. Finally, those patients with resolving respiratory tract infections with severe symptoms or mild symptoms should have the same relative waiting periods fulfilled (i.e., 2–4 wk after resolution of minor URI and 4–6 wk after resolution of severe URI or LRI) to minimize the risks of proceeding with surgery.

Modified from McKee CT, et al. Should a child with a respiratory tract infection undergo elective surgery? In: Fleisher LA, ed. *Evidence-Based Practice of Anesthesiology*. 3rd ed. Philadelphia: Elsevier; 2013:529–536.

Premedication

The selection and administration of premedication for the pediatric patient requires an understanding of the desired goals, the planned surgical procedure (inpatient or outpatient procedure), the familiarity and previous experiences with the particular drug, and the availability of nursing staff to monitor the child after administration of the drug (Box 53.3). The ideal premedication should be predictable, have a rapid and reliable onset and offset, and should have minimal side effects.[74] Table 53.3 lists commonly prescribed pediatric premedicants. Premedication must be individualized to account for differences in maturation and development and for the child's previous surgical experiences, as well as the potential impact on perioperative outcomes.

A thorough anesthetic plan should include preoperative assessment of patient anxiety. Children who are highly anxious preoperatively have been reported to have significantly higher postoperative pain, delayed discharge, higher incidence of emergence delirium, sleep disturbance, and maladaptive behaviors postoperatively. The reliance on pharmacologic premedication in preparing the child for

BOX 53.2   Indications for Preoperative Laboratory Testing

Complete Blood Count
- Hematologic disorder
- Vascular procedure
- Chemotherapy
- Unknown sickle cell syndrome status

Hemoglobin and Hematocrit
- <6 mo of age (<1 yr of age if born premature)
- Hematologic malignancy
- Recent radiation or chemotherapy
- Renal disease
- Anticoagulant therapy
- Surgical procedures with potential for large blood loss
- Coexisting systemic disorders (e.g., cystic fibrosis, prematurity, severe malnutrition, renal failure, hepatic disease, congenital heart disease)

White Blood Cell Count
- Leukemia or lymphomas
- Recent or concurrent radiation or chemotherapy
- Suspected infectious process
- Aplastic anemia
- Hypersplenism
- Autoimmune collagen vascular disease

Blood Glucose
- Diabetes mellitus
- Current corticosteroid use
- History of hypoglycemia
- Adrenal disease
- Cystic fibrosis

Serum Chemistry
- Renal disease
- Adrenal or thyroid disease
- Previous or concurrent hemotherapy
- Pituitary or hypothalamic dysfunction
- Body fluid loss or shifts (e.g., dehydration, bowel preparation)
- Central nervous system disease

Potassium
- Digoxin or diuretic therapy

Creatinine and Blood Urea Nitrogen
- Hypertensive cardiovascular disease
- Renal disease
- Adrenal disease
- Diabetes mellitus
- Digoxin or diuretic therapy
- Body fluid loss or shifts (e.g., dehydration, bowel preparation)
- Administration of intravenous radiocontrast material

Liver Function Tests
- Hepatic disease
- Exposure to hepatotoxic agents

Coagulation Studies
Prothrombin Time
- Activated partial thromboplastin time (aPTT)
- Leukemia
- Hepatic disease
- Known coagulation disorder (e.g., hemophilia, Christmas disease)
- Concurrent anticoagulant therapy
- Severe malnutrition or malabsorption

Platelet Count or Bleeding Time
- Known coagulation disorder (e.g., hemophilia, Christmas disease)
- Purpura (increase in bruising)

Pregnancy Test
- Serum human chorionic gonadotropin (HCG) in menstruating, sexually active patient

Electrocardiogram
- Family history of prolonged QT interval
- Congenital heart disease
- History of sleep apnea or chronic airway obstruction (adenotonsillar hypertrophy)
- Possible previously undiagnosed heart murmur

Chest Radiograph
- Suspected intrathoracic pathology (e.g., tumors, vascular ring)
- Congenital heart disease
- History of prematurity with residual bronchopulmonary dysplasia
- Obstructive sleep apnea with cardiomegaly

Cervical Spine Radiograph
- Down syndrome (subluxation of atlantooccipital junction)

the surgical experience should not be routine; rather, it should be individualized to the patient's age, anxiety level, surgical procedure, and physical history. While this can be performed a multitude of ways, determining if the patient is experiencing state- or trait-related anxiety can help guide the use of preoperative anxiolytics. Anxiolytics and sedatives may prolong the time to discharge, thereby increasing patient care costs.[75] Additionally, some anxiolytics may impact airway to a lesser degree than others, which should be a consideration when determining selection of premedication. Midazolam is the most commonly used premedication in the pediatric patient for anxiolysis. This short-acting benzodiazepine produces amnesia and anxiolysis and in sufficient dosages may produce sleep (hypnosis). Other medications that have been used preoperatively include dexmedetomidine, ketamine, clonidine, and pregabalin.[76] Oral acetaminophen

BOX 53.3   Goals for Premedication

- Anxiolysis (especially in children undergoing repeat procedures)
- Amnesia (insertion of intravenous access)
- Analgesia (children in pain)
- Antisialagogue effects (airway manipulation, but rarely needed)
- Increased gastric pH
- Reduction of gastric volume
- Reduced anesthetic requirements
- Blunting of central nervous system reflex responses
- Prevention of subacute bacterial endocarditis
- Prevention of allergic reactions (latex)
- Minimize postoperative nausea and vomiting
- Decreased incidence of infectious processes

TABLE 53.3 Commonly Prescribed Pediatric Premedicants

Drug Name	Pediatric Dose
Opioids	
Morphine sulfate	0.1–0.3 mg/kg IM
	0.05–0.1 mg/kg IV
Fentanyl	0.5–1.0 mcg/kg IV
	10 mcg/kg oral transmucosal
Benzodiazepines	
Midazolam	0.05–0.1 mg/kg IM
	0.2 mg/kg nasally
	0.025–0.05 mg/kg IV
	0.25–1.0 mg/kg PO
	0.5–1 mg/kg rectally
Ketamine	5–10 mg/kg PO
	2–10 mg/kg IM
	1–2 mg/kg IV
Clonidine	2.5–5.0 mcg/kg PO
	1–2 mcg/kg IV
Dexmedetomidine	0.5–1.0 mcg/kg intranasally
	2–5 mcg/kg PO
	0.4–0.6 mcg/kg IV infusion in 100 mL saline
Anticholinergics	
Atropine	0.02 mg/kg PO, IV, IM
Glycopyrrolate	0.01 mg IV

IM, Intramuscular; *IV,* intravenous; *PO, per os.*

BOX 53.4 Manipulation of the T-Piece (Open Circuit)

Manipulation to Increase Pao_2
- Increase inspired oxygen delivery
- Increase fresh gas flow (decreases entrainment of room air from reservoir tubing)
- Increase length of reservoir tubing (increases oxygen storage capacity)

Manipulation to Decrease $Paco_2$
- Increase fresh gas flow (wash out expired air from reservoir tubing)
- Decrease length of reservoir tubing (decreases volume of expired air; also decreases Fio_2)

Fio_2, Fraction of inspired oxygen, *Pao_2,* partial pressure of arterial oxygen, *$Paco_2$,* partial pressure of arterial carbon dioxide.
From Litman RS, ed. *Pediatric Anesthesia: The Requisites.* Philadelphia: Mosby; 2004:102.

can be given preoperatively to patients undergoing short, minimally painful procedures such as myringotomy tube placement. Nonpharmacologic interventions that can decrease preoperative anxiety in the pediatric patient include playing videos of the child's choice during induction, low sensory stimulation, and handheld videogames.[77] Allowing patients to use a handheld interactive device or tablet preoperatively has been associated with lower preoperative anxiety and emergence delirium scores and earlier discharge times than with those given oral midazolam.[78] The use of virtual reality goggles is a newer technique to help decrease preoperative anxiety although results have been mixed.[79]

Parental Presence During Anesthetic Induction

In addition to administering preoperative medication, various anesthetic departments allow a parent to be present for anesthetic induction. The frequency with which parents are allowed to accompany a child during anesthesia induction varies widely among institutions and even among individual clinicians. Anesthesia departments may have age limitations, not allowing parental presence for children less than 12 months of age, for example. Studies examining the efficacy of parental presence are mixed, though parental presence has been demonstrated to reduce the child's anxiety, precluding the need for premedication.[80] However, an evidence-based review noted no advantage, and oral midazolam was found to be more effective for the control of the child's preoperative anxiety than parental presence.[81] Parents who are motivated to be present in the operating room during the induction of anesthesia may be very anxious, and their children are likely to have high anxiety levels during anesthetic induction. Before entering the operating room

with parent and child, a thorough explanation of the expected behavior of the child during anesthetic induction (e.g., excitement, spontaneous involuntary movements, snoring, uncoordinated breathing pattern, unconsciousness) should be provided to the parent or guardian. It is important that there be a clear line of communication between the anesthetist and the parent. In addition, the parent should agree to leave the operating room, accompanied by an escort, when the child has lost consciousness.

ANESTHETIC MANAGEMENT

Pediatric Breathing Circuits

In the United States, standard pediatric breathing circuits utilizing a circle system are used to provide pediatric anesthesia. An ideal pediatric breathing circuit is lightweight, minimizes dead space, provides low resistance and a low compressible volume, is capable of providing humidification and warming of inspired gases, and permits the collection and scavenging of exhaled anesthetic gases.

Prior to modern advances in anesthesia machines and ventilator capacity, open circuit breathing systems were used during anesthesia. Open circuits are still used today in developing countries. Pediatric breathing circuits can be characterized by the number of valves within the circuit.[82] A circuit without valves, such as the Ayre T-piece, is an open circuit (Box 53.4). The Ayre T-piece was first used for the delivery of anesthesia to infants undergoing cleft lip and palate repair and continues to be commonly used throughout hospitals to provide supplemental oxygen during patient transport.[83] The T-piece, which is in a T configuration, is formed by an inspiratory limb for the delivery of oxygen and anesthetic gas, a limb directed to the patient for connection to a facemask or ETT, and an opposite expiratory limb that is open to the atmosphere for the removal of exhaled gas. This expiratory limb also may serve as a reservoir for oxygen that may be rebreathed. There are no valves within the breathing circuit, and therefore the inspired air is drawn from both the inspiratory limb and the expiratory limb. The rebreathing of expired CO_2 can be prevented with the administration of fresh gas flows at least twice the patient's minute ventilation. The T-piece can be configured to increase oxygen delivery or decrease arterial partial pressure of carbon dioxide.

Modification of the Ayre T-piece with the addition of a single valve allows the delivery of positive pressure ventilation. A variety of modifications of the Ayre T-piece have been classified by Mapleson. The

Mapleson A circuit is best employed for a patient who is spontaneously breathing. The Mapleson D system contains an expiratory valve at the distal end of the expiratory limb and is used for controlled ventilation. The Mapleson E system was modified by Jackson-Rees with the addition of a reservoir bag with an adjustable valve at the tail of the bag. Spontaneous ventilation is permitted with the opening of the adjustable valve, whereas closing the valve fills the reservoir bag, and repeated manual compression allows the delivery of continuous positive airway pressure (CPAP), or positive pressure ventilation. With an expiratory pause of sufficient duration and sufficient fresh gas flows, exhaled CO_2 is washed from the reservoir tube, preventing the inhalation of exhaled CO_2 with subsequent inspiration. Fresh gas flows of two to three times the child's minute ventilation are required to prevent rebreathing of exhaled gases. Due to the high fresh gas flow rates, this circuit is not economical for children who weigh more than 20 kg. Mapleson C circuits, also known as the Water circuit, allow for fresh gas flow entry with expiratory valves located at the patient end of the circuit and reservoir bag at the end of the circuit. These circuits are commonly used for transport and may be used to facilitate emergency resuscitation.

The circle breathing system is the standard for anesthetic gas delivery for pediatric patients in the United States. Advances in the anesthesia machine design have decreased the resistance imparted by the absorbent canisters and the one-way inspiratory and expiratory valves. Overall, system compliance is greater as compared to open breathing circuits. The breathing tubing for pediatric circle systems is a smaller diameter than the adult tubing and has a lower compression volume, allowing accurate delivery of desired tidal volumes. The circle system is characterized by the presence of CO_2-absorbent canisters and a total of three valves (a one-way inspiratory valve, a one-way expiratory valve, and a pop-off or adjustable pressure-limiting [APL] valve) that directs exhaled gas to the scavenging system. Advantages of the circle system include the conservation of potent inhalation agents, the ability to retain both heat and humidity, and the ease of collecting and scavenging waste gases.

The reservoir bag serves as a visual and tactile monitor to assess the presence and adequacy of ventilation. Reservoir bags are shaped to allow compression with one hand, and they are constructed of rubber and latex, although latex-free bags are most commonly used within the United States. Commonly employed reservoir bags in pediatric practice range in size from 0.5 to 2 L. The selected reservoir bag must be appropriate for the patient's size (i.e., capable of containing a volume in excess of the child's inspiratory capacity). The use of an inappropriately small reservoir bag may restrict respiratory efforts, and the use of a large reservoir bag inhibits the ability to use the reservoir bag as a ventilation monitor.[84-86]

Anesthetic Induction

Inhalation (Mask) Induction
Anesthetic induction may be accomplished in a variety of ways dependent on the child's age, current state of health, level of anxiety, the proposed surgical procedure, and the parents' agreement with regard to the proposed anesthetic plan. Inhalation induction, which is commonly called mask induction, is the most popular technique for otherwise healthy infants, toddlers, and school-age children and is easily accomplished in children less than 8 years of age, as well as in older children who do not have initial IV access.

Sevoflurane is the volatile agent of choice for inhalation inductions, as it has minimal airway irritant properties. Oxygen or a nitrous oxide–oxygen mixture is used during the induction. It is the anesthesia provider's choice as to the initial concentration of sevoflurane to be administered. Some anesthetists will begin with lower concentrations (e.g., 2%) and then increase the concentration incrementally to avoid excessive myocardial depression and vasodilation. Others will begin with high concentrations of sevoflurane (e.g., 8%) to increase the speed of induction. Following loss of consciousness and prior to intubation, nitrous oxide (if used) is discontinued, and sevoflurane is administered in 100% oxygen.

Prior to establishing IV access and intubation, it is desirable for the patient to breathe spontaneously while the anesthetist manually assists ventilation. As the concentration of sevoflurane increases in the brain, respiratory depression and arrest can occur. Continued delivery of high concentrations of sevoflurane via controlled respiration, as opposed to spontaneous respiration, during the induction process increases the likelihood of respiratory depression and cardiac arrest. Once the anesthetist deems that the child is adequately anesthetized, the inspired anesthetic concentration of sevoflurane should be decreased. During assisted ventilation, IV access should be established. For procedures that do not require an IV, it is imperative the anesthetist has the ability to rapidly gain vascular access. Additionally, it is essential to have calculated doses of emergency medications ready to be administered IM. An example of a surgical procedure that may not require IV access is the placement of myringotomy tubes.

Establishing IV access in children prior to laryngoscopy and endotracheal intubation is recommended. For elective surgical procedures, neonates may be managed with a 24-gauge catheter, infants with a 22-gauge catheter, and children with a 20- or 22-gauge catheter. Surgical procedures that are expected to produce large third-space fluid loss or blood loss require an additional IV catheter. Preferred sites for IV access include the nondominant upper extremity (dorsum of the hand, antecubital fossa) and the lower extremity (dorsum of the foot, or the saphenous vein). The advent of ultrasound-guided vascular access techniques has made the basilic and cephalic veins common sites of IV insertion as well. The deep saphenous vein is most easily accessed with a 20- or 22-gauge catheter. This vein can be identified by placing the thumb over the medial malleolus and moving it toward the anterior portion of the tibia. By extending the foot, piercing the skin parallel to the tibia, and passing subcutaneously, the saphenous vein may be cannulated. To prevent the child from dislodging the catheter, a sterile transparent dressing can be applied. The extremity can be secured to a padded board to decrease the chance of catheter kinking or dislodgement, especially during the postoperative period. Prior to establishing IV access, the anesthetist should ensure that the patient is adequately anesthetized to avoid the potential for laryngospasm and bronchospasm.

Following the establishment of IV access, the airway device should be placed, unless the anesthetic will be managed by mask airway. Laryngeal mask airway placement can be accomplished with deep inhalational anesthesia or with the administration of supplemental propofol (1–2 mg/kg). Endotracheal intubation may be accomplished with or without muscle relaxation. Without muscle relaxation, the exhaled anesthetic agent levels should be at least 1.0 MAC to prevent response to intubation. Propofol (2–3 mg/kg) with or without fentanyl can also be administered prior to ETT placement. The administration of a neuromuscular relaxant prior to intubation decreases the potential for the cardiovascular depression that accompanies the administration of high concentrations of inhalation and/or intravenous anesthetic agents that may be required to facilitate laryngoscopy and intubation. The inspired concentration required for acceptable intubating conditions with sevoflurane in children aged 1 to 8 years is $3.54 \pm 0.25\%$. The addition of 66% nitrous oxide decreases the required concentration by 40%.[87] A survey of members of the Society of Pediatric Anesthesia found that inhalation agent administration without neuromuscular blockade was used to facilitate endotracheal intubation 38% of the time in infants (0–12 months old) and 43.6% of the time in children (1–7 years old).[88,89] Whichever method is selected to facilitate intubation, the inhalation agent should be discontinued immediately before laryngoscopy. This practice minimizes the contamination of the operating room with free-flowing inhalation agent from the patient breathing circuit, and the delivery of high inspired anesthetic concentrations is avoided immediately after intubation during the confirmation of ETT placement. Following confirmation that the ETT is in the proper position, it should promptly be secured to avoid unintentional displacement.

Intravenous Induction

An IV induction may be clinically indicated when the child has a full stomach or a history of gastroesophageal reflux. IV inductions are routinely performed in children older than 10 years of age. IV induction is a rapid and dependable means of ensuring unconsciousness and facilitating prompt securement of the airway. Venipuncture can be a frightening and traumatic experience for children. Oral premedication with midazolam before IV insertion in the preoperative area can be given to decrease the child's anxiety and gain cooperation. The eutectic mixture (equal quantities as measured by weight) of local anesthetic (EMLA cream) is a combination of lidocaine (2.5%) and prilocaine (2.5%) that can be applied to the skin causing numbness to help facilitate IV catheter placement. The medication should be applied well in advance (30–60 minutes) to achieve an adequate effect. Methemoglobinemia is a rare side effect that is associated with prilocaine toxicity.[90] Alternate devices such as the J-Tip can also be employed to facilitate IV cannulation in the awake child. The J-Tip is a needleless injection device that uses carbon dioxide gas to create a fine stream of liquid anesthesia, which passes through the skin and into the subcutaneous tissue. Ethyl chloride spray and mechanical stimulation devices can also be used.

Intramuscular Induction

On rare occasions, an IM administered drug may be required in children who are uncooperative and who refuse alternative routes (i.e., oral, nasal, or rectal) for premedication. Ketamine is an excellent induction agent in these situations. With appropriate IM dosing, a catatonic state will quickly be induced following administration. Parents who witness the administration of ketamine should be warned that their child might exhibit spontaneous involuntary movements and nystagmus. The psychogenic effects such as emergence delirium may be decreased with the concomitant administration of a benzodiazepine. Ketamine administered via the IM route in a dose of 4 to 6 mg/kg facilitates inhalation induction in children who are reluctant to be subjected to inhalation induction or venipuncture.

Pediatric Airway Equipment

The child's age, weight, medical history, and proposed surgical procedure guide the selection of essential pediatric anesthesia airway equipment. This includes but is not limited to a variety of sizes of anesthesia masks, oral and nasal airways, LMAs, laryngoscope blades, ETTs, and ETT stylets.

Airway Equipment

The pediatric facemask is designed to fit the smaller facial features of the child and eliminate mechanical dead space. Contemporary masks are manufactured from transparent plastics, have a soft inflatable cuff that sits on the face, and do not contain latex. The transparent body of the mask allows continuous observation of skin color and the appearance of gastric contents if vomiting occurs. Appropriately sized oral airways must be readily available. The relatively large infant tongue predisposes to airway obstruction after the induction of general anesthesia. Oral airways that are too small or too large may produce airway obstruction. The oral airway should be inserted while displacing the tongue toward the floor of the mouth to allow smooth insertion of the airway. The anesthetist must be aware of the possibility of dislodging loose deciduous teeth. Nasal airways are infrequently used in children less than 1 to 2 years of age. The internal diameter of the nasal airway may unnecessarily increase the work of breathing. Adenoid hypertrophy may make nasal airway placement difficult and produce severe epistaxis.

Endotracheal tubes. Since the 1960s it has been common practice to use an uncuffed ETT in infants and children less than 8 years of age to minimize the potential for postextubation croup. Although this practice is still widely accepted, recent literature suggests that this belief is not universally applied, is empirical rather than scientifically based, and is a perpetuated myth of pediatric anesthesia. The age-old argument against the use of a cuffed ETT in infants and children is quite logical; the narrowest portion of the infant and child airway is the cricoid cartilage, and the diameter of the pediatric trachea is small compared to the adult. Thus a small amount of tracheal edema can cause increased work of breathing and possibly respiratory distress. Cuffed ETTs have been shown to be effective for use in the pediatric population. There is no significant difference in the incidence of airway injury and postextubation croup when comparing cuffed and uncuffed ETTs.[91] Additionally, cuffed ETTs have been associated with a decreased incidence of sore throat.[92] The differences associated with the adult and pediatric airway are summarized in Table 52.3.

Sizing the endotracheal tube. Early detailed accounts of the laryngeal framework suggested that the larynx is shaped as a cone, with the apex at the level of the cricoid cartilage.[93,94] Compression of the tracheal mucosa at the level of the cartilaginous cricoid ring by an oversized ETT may therefore produce mucosal edema. This traditional understanding has been challenged. Magnetic resonance imaging of sedated newborns to children 14 years of age has demonstrated that the lumen of the cricoid cartilage is not round but elliptical in shape, with the narrowest dimension in the transverse plane at the level of the vocal cords.[95] Evidence that disputes this claim was obtained by studying videobronchoscopic images and magnetic resonance spectrographs from 135 children aged 6 months to 13 years. The laryngeal dimensions, including the cross-sectional area and the anteroposterior and transverse diameters at the level of the glottis and the cricoid, were measured. This study found that the glottis rather than the cricoid was the narrowest portion of the pediatric airway. The authors also noted that, as in adults, the pediatric airway is more cylindric than funnel shaped.[96] Accordingly, the pressure exerted upon the laryngeal and tracheal mucosa with the use of an uncuffed ETT is in the posterior lateral position. This has been verified, as evidenced by the associated pathologic lesions found posteriorly in the subglottic region. In addition, trauma that appears within the trachea occurs anteriorly from the impingement of the distal end of the ETT upon the anterior tracheal wall. The goal of ETT selection is the placement of an appropriately sized tube that allows controlled ventilation but minimizes laryngeal or tracheal injury. Due to anatomic variability, many formulas exist for the determination of the correct ETT size and for the depth of insertion. There is no consensus related to a standard formula. In addition, many practitioners fail to appreciate the differences in the internal diameter of small ETTs. ETTs for neonates are sized by the internal diameter, yet the external diameters may differ by as much as 0.9 mm among manufacturers in tubes with identical internal diameters.[97]

TABLE 53.4 Airway Device Details

	Preterm Neonate	Full-Term Neonate	INFANT		CHILD										Adult
			6mo	1yr	2yr	3yr	4yr	5yr	6yr	8yr	10yr	12yr	14yr	
Average weight (kg)		3.5	7	10	12	14	16	18	20	25	30	40	50	70
Approx.BSA (m^2)		0.25	0.38	0.49	0.55	0.64	0.74	0.76	0.82	0.95	1.18	1.34	1.5	1.73
ETT size (age + 16)/4	2.5–3	3–3.5	3.5–4	4	4.5	4.5	5	5	5.5	6	6.5	7	7	7.5–8
Teeth to midtrachea (cm)	7–8	9	11	12	13	14	14	15	15	16	17	18	20	20
Nare to midtrachea (cm)	8–9	10	12	14	15	16	17	18	19	20	21	22	23	24
Laryngeal mask airway		1	1.5	1.5	2	2	2	2	2.5	2.5	2.5	3	3	4

Calculations for estimating the internal diameter of an endotracheal tube:
   (16 + age in years)/4
   (Age in years/4) + 4
Calculations for estimating the length required for an orotracheal tube:
   Height (in cm)/10 + 5
   Weight (in kg)/5 + 12
Advance the endotracheal tube:
   3 times the internal diameter from the alveolar ridge
   (Age in years/2) + 12
Insert the endotracheal tube to the first or second black line marked on the tube.
Advance the endotracheal tube into a bronchus, then withdraw it 2 cm.
BSA, Body surface area; *ETT,* endotracheal tube.
From Holzman RS. Airway management. In: Davis PJ, et al., eds. *Smith's Anesthesia for Infants and Children.* 9th ed. Philadelphia, Elsevier; 2017:349–369.

Several formulas have been developed to estimate appropriate ETT size in children. One formula commonly used for uncuffed ETT size (mm ID) for patients older than 2 years, is as follows:

$$(\text{Age in years} + 16)/4$$

For cuffed ETT size, the following formula can be used:

$$(\text{Age in years}/4) + 3$$

To accommodate the variability in patient airway size, ETTs a half size larger and a half size smaller should be immediately available.

The depth of ETT insertion from the lips/teeth may be estimated using the "1, 2, 3, 4/7, 8, 9, 10" rule. For example, the ETT is inserted to a depth of 7 cm in a neonate weighing 1 kg and to a depth of 8 cm in a 2-kg neonate. Another approximate method is to insert the ETT to a depth in centimeters three times the internal diameter of the ETT in millimeters. For example, a 3-mm ETT should be inserted to a depth of 9 cm. Uncuffed ETTs are marked distally with a double black line that provides a visual indication of the depth of the ETT. During intubation, the ETT is passed until the intubation depth mark has reached the level of the vocal cords.[98]

An optimally sized ETT is one that easily passes through the glottis and subglottic regions without resistance. Once placed, auscultating for an audible air leak between peak inspiratory pressures of 15 to 30 mm Hg helps confirm appropriate size and determine the need for cuff inflation. This pressure range maintains tracheal mucosal perfusion while limiting a large anesthetic gas leak. The provider can place a stethoscope over the patient's mouth or neck to check for a leak during manual ventilation. Intracuff pressure can change with changes in head and neck position and the use of nitrous oxide. One study suggests checking cuff pressure for long surgical procedures to decrease the incidence of edema and tracheal damage.[99]

Confirmation of proper ETT placement is imperative. Positive end tidal carbon dioxide ($ETCO_2$), chest rise, and bilateral breath sounds are checked. Lung auscultation helps confirm proper ETT position. As the ETT is secured, it is important not to dislodge or inadvertently extubate the trachea, which would necessitate reintubation. Table 53.4 lists specific airway devices and details regarding their use.[100] Alignment of the head and its effect on the airway are depicted in Fig. 52.3.

Laryngeal mask airway. The original LMA was intended as an alternative method of securing the airway compared to endotracheal intubation. The LMA can be used for surgical procedures that do not require endotracheal intubation. Relative contraindications for use of an LMA include increased risk of gastric aspiration, abnormal airway anatomy, laparoscopic surgery, and emergency resuscitation. The LMA can be used as an emergency airway device in a "cannot ventilate, cannot intubate" scenario. The LMA is available in sizes specific for the neonate, infant, child, and adolescent (Table 53.5). Many alternative designs for special uses are available. The inflation of the pharyngeal cuff can produce undue pressure on pharyngeal structures. Like the ETT cuff, the LMA cuff may be expanded during the course of the anesthetic procedure with the administration of nitrous oxide. The initial volume of air injected into the laryngeal cuff may be regulated by identifying the amount of air and airway pressure that produces an audible leak. This pressure is generally between 15 and 25 cm H_2O. The LMA cuff should be inspected before each use, the volume of air required for cuff inflation should not exceed the manufacturer's recommendation, and the LMA cuff should be periodically checked during the administration of nitrous oxide to prevent overinflation.[101]

The LMA has traditionally been removed in the adult when airway reflexes return. Removal of the LMA in the pediatric patient can be associated with biting, severe laryngospasm, pulmonary edema, and separation of the tube from the pharyngeal mask.[102,103] Several studies

LMA Size	Patient Weight (kg)	Suggested Inflation Volume
1	<5	up to 4 mL
1.5	5–10	up to 7 mL
2	10–20	up to 10 mL
2.5	20–30	up to 14 mL
3	30–50	up to 20 mL
4	50–70	up to 30 mL
5	70–100	up to 40 mL

TABLE 53.5   Laryngeal Mask Airway Sizes

LMA, Laryngeal mask airway.
From Teleflex-North America, Wayne, PA.

have examined the appropriate time for LMA removal in children. In one study, oxygen desaturation was more prevalent (31.3%) after awake removal, compared with removal in a deep anesthetic plane (4.5%), whereas airway obstruction occurred more frequently (20%) with deep removal.[104] Researchers have reported a 10% incidence of severe laryngospasm with awake removal, compared to 5% with deep removal.[105]

Special airway equipment. Specialized uncuffed and cuffed oral and nasal ETTs may be chosen for otolaryngologic, ophthalmologic, and dental procedures. The oral right angle endotracheal (RAE; Mallinkrodt; Argyle, New York) tube is premolded, with the acute angle of the tube designed to be positioned over the lower lip. The nasal RAE tube is premolded with a 180-degree bend that directs the tube toward the top of the head. These tubes facilitate the routing of the breathing circuit away from the surgical field. RAE tubes are longer than straight ETTs and place the distal end of the tube in closer proximity to the carina, thereby minimizing the chance of inadvertent extubation with neck extension. The RAE tube is designed with two Murphy eyes located at the distal end of the tube to facilitate uninterrupted ventilation if the tube migrates in a caudal fashion. However, proper ETT placement must be determined with confirmation of bilateral breath sounds after intubation and repositioning of the head. The use of a precordial stethoscope placed over the left anterior area of the chest will aid in the detection of right bronchial migration of the RAE tube.

The clinical application of laser technology to treat airway pathology necessitates the use of a specialized ETT. ETT ignition may occur in as many as 1.5% of patients during CO_2 laser laryngeal procedures.[106] Modern polyvinylchloride ETTs absorb infrared light and may be ignited with a direct hit from a CO_2 laser or as a result of burning material in close proximity to the tube. Laser-resistant or "laser-safe" ETTs are available from several manufacturers, and are marketed for specific laser applications (e.g., CO_2, neodymium-doped:yttrium-aluminum-garnet [Nd:YAG], and potassium titanyl phosphate [KTP]). An alternative is wrapping the external surface of a polyvinylchloride ETT with a metallic foil (see Chapter 43).

Maintenance of a Patent Airway

A variety of anatomic and neurologic interactions are essential for the maintenance of a patent airway. The larynx is innervated by a variety of receptors that, when stimulated, can initiate intense physiologic reactions. Airway patency is dependent upon lung stretch reflexes, central and carotid body chemoreceptor reflexes, and CNS arousal mechanisms. Pharyngeal patency is established and maintained through a delicate balance of CNS-derived dilating and collapsing forces upon the pharyngeal airway.[107,108] The pharynx may be conceptualized as a collapsible tube within a box, bordered by the tongue and soft palate, and enveloped by the bony elements of the mandible anteriorly and

the cervical vertebra posteriorly. Pharyngeal patency is a function of the overall size of this box and the amount of soft tissue between the bony elements and the pharynx. An increase in the amount of soft tissue within the box (e.g., obesity, hypertrophy of adenoids and tonsils, large tongue), or a decrease in the size of the bony elements (e.g., small craniofacial structures or craniofacial deformity) will limit the content of the box, resulting in compression of the pharyngeal airway. In effect, the pharyngeal airway functions as a Starling resistor.[109]

Airway Management of the Infant and Child

In an awake infant or child, the tongue, the upper airway muscles (i.e., genioglossus, geniohyoid, sternohyoid, and sternothyroid) interact to tent the pharynx, preventing collapse. Anesthetic agents inhibit the neural activity of these airway muscles, resulting in pharyngeal narrowing or collapse secondary to loss of tone.[110,111] The young infant depends upon compensatory mechanisms to maintain pharyngeal patency, but is disadvantaged because of an anatomic imbalance (i.e., small maxilla and mandible, large cranium, large tongue).[112] Steadily increasing the anesthetic depth during inhalation induction will depress these compensatory mechanisms, leading to pharyngeal narrowing and collapse.

Incomplete airway obstruction may be clinically evident early in the inhalation induction process, as audible inspiratory or expiratory sounds are evident through the precordial stethoscope. As the obstruction increases, a tracheal tug becomes notable with attempted inspiration. The infant has a compliant chest wall, and because of forceful diaphragmatic contraction the chest will collapse with inspiratory efforts against partial pharynx collapse. With continued inspiratory attempts, a paradoxic movement of the chest and abdomen (i.e., the contraction of the chest with abdominal expansion) also occurs. This thoracoabdominal asynchrony is an important clinical sign of upper airway obstruction. With complete pharyngeal collapse, the audible signs of obstruction are no longer observed, and thoracoabdominal asynchrony continues.

Due to the immaturity of the CNS, the regulation of the pharyngeal dilator muscles is ineffective in opening the pharyngeal airway in the infant.[113] The application of CPAP at 5 to 10 cm H_2O is essential in the reestablishment of a patent pharyngeal airway until the patient is sufficiently anesthetized to allow the placement of an oral airway. The application of CPAP accompanied by airway opening maneuvers (jaw thrust with anterior displacement of the mandible forcing the tongue away from the palate) will reverse the anatomic imbalance, increase tidal volume, and diminish thoracoabdominal asynchrony.[114] The triple airway maneuver, which is a combination of mouth opening, chin lift and head extension, and jaw thrust is an important airway maneuver because it widens the anteroposterior diameter (at the epiglottis) and the transverse diameter (at the level of the soft palate) of the pharyngeal airway in children without adenotonsillar hypertrophy (ATH).[115] However, in children with ATH, chin lift with CPAP is more effective at decreasing upper airway obstruction.[116]

General anesthesia causes depression of CNS compensatory mechanisms for the maintenance of a patent pharyngeal airway, so tracheal extubation in infants should be undertaken when the infant is awake and has adequate respirations. Thoracoabdominal asynchrony appearing immediately after extubation is indicative of upper airway obstruction and is not accompanied by traditional sounds of upper airway obstruction (i.e., snoring), as it is in the adult. Following extubation, the lateral decubitus position may be advantageous, as it has been shown to decrease the compressive effects of the soft tissue that surrounds the pharynx in individuals with obstructive sleep apnea.[117]

Pharyngeal patency improves during the first year of life as the anatomic imbalance is lessened (due to continued growth of the maxilla and mandible) and CNS regulation matures. However, when airway obstruction develops during inhalation induction, the obstruction is generally easily managed with the previously cited maneuvers used to improve airway patency.

Airway Complications

Two common airway complications with a pediatric patient are laryngospasm and bronchospasm. The larynx is the superior portion of the airway that protects the lungs from aspiration of foreign material. This function is most evident during swallowing, when the glottic closure reflex is initiated by stimulation of the superior laryngeal nerve, facilitating sphincteric closure of the airway. Laryngospasm is a hyperresponsive glottic closure reflex to noxious stimuli of the superior laryngeal nerve and may persist despite the immediate removal of the stimulus. Laryngospasm can precipitate serious complications, including complete airway obstruction, gastric aspiration, postobstruction pulmonary edema, cardiac arrest, and death.[118]

The frequency of laryngospasm is greatest in patients with a URI (95.8/1000).[119] Children exposed to secondhand tobacco smoke have a 10-fold increase in the relative risk of laryngospasm (0.9% with no exposure vs 9.4% with exposure).[120] Although laryngospasm may be self-limiting, the clinical importance of proper management is exemplified by the fact that 5 of every 1000 children who experience laryngospasm have a subsequent cardiac arrest.[121]

The incidence of laryngospasm may be greater in the pediatric population because of specific practices that are used in the anesthetic management of infants and children. Several factors are generally associated with the development of laryngospasm (Box 53.5). The risk of laryngospasm is increased when airway instrumentation is attempted before an adequate depth of anesthesia has been achieved, without the benefit of neuromuscular blocking drugs, and in infants and children with residual effects of resolving upper respiratory tract infections.

The precise pathophysiologic mechanism responsible for laryngospasm remains elusive. To expand our understanding of laryngospasm and its clinical management, it is best to revisit the original description provided by Fink in 1951.[122] The basic execution of laryngeal closure follows superior laryngeal nerve stimulation. It has been theorized that stimulation on airway structures causes an afferent sensory impulse mediated via the internal branch of the superior laryngeal nerve. The efferent response that causes the vocal cords to close is via the external branch of the superior laryngeal nerve, resulting in cricothyroid muscle contraction. The mechanism resembles a shutter, where the laryngeal inlet is closed by the action of the supraglottic folds, the false vocal cords, and the true vocal cords. Fink suggested that glottis closure is a dual mechanism, in which the first response is the closure of the vocal cords (a shutter effect) followed by a ball-valve effect with closure of the false cords and the subsequent rounding of the supraglottic tissue after the shortening of the thyrohyoid muscle. This produces an envelopment of the laryngeal inlet by the supraglottic tissue with continued inspiratory effort, producing complete airway obstruction.

Box 53.6 lists measures that can be used to prevent laryngospasm. Prompt recognition and management are imperative to prevent hypoxemia, bradycardia, and cardiac arrest.

Incomplete airway obstruction (Fig. 53.2) may be evident as grunting or audible inspiratory and expiratory phonation as heard through a precordial stethoscope, accompanied by tracheal tug and thoracoabdominal asynchrony. Management consists of three essential processes. First, the noxious stimuli should be discontinued if possible (e.g., surgical stimulation, attempted airway instrumentation during light anesthesia). Next, anesthetic depth should be increased by the delivery of an increased concentration of an inhalation agent or IV administration of a small dose of propofol. Third, gentle positive pressure ventilation using 100% oxygen should be attempted using a properly applied

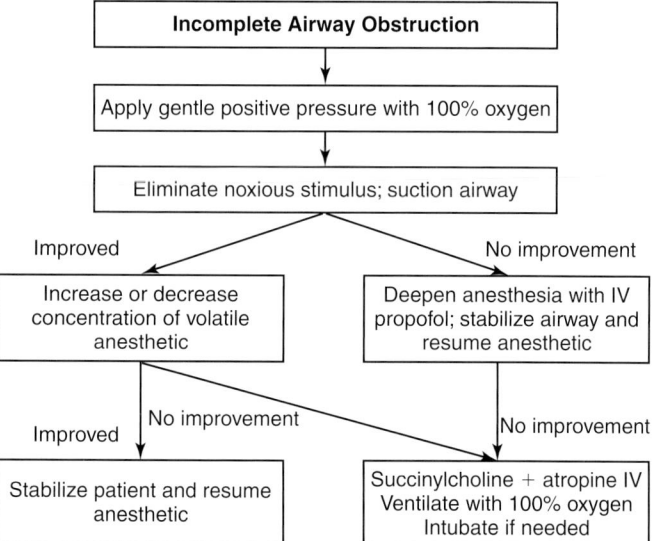

Fig. 53.2 Incomplete airway obstruction algorithm. (From Wittkugel E. Pediatric laryngospasm. In: Atlee JL, ed. *Complications in Anesthesia.* 2nd ed. Philadelphia: Elsevier; 2007:601.)

facemask with concurrent airway opening maneuvers (i.e., slight head extension, chin lift, and jaw thrust).

The transition to complete airway obstruction (Fig. 53.3) becomes evident with the absence of inspiratory and expiratory sounds, as well as the inability to deliver positive pressure ventilation. The application of positive airway pressure for treating complete airway obstruction may not be successful. Further deterioration of arterial oxygen saturation with accompanying bradycardia may occur despite the continued application of positive pressure ventilation. The administration of succinylcholine will then be required to relieve the laryngospasm.

The application of firm and direct bilateral pressure toward the skull base produces an anterior displacement of the mandible. In addition

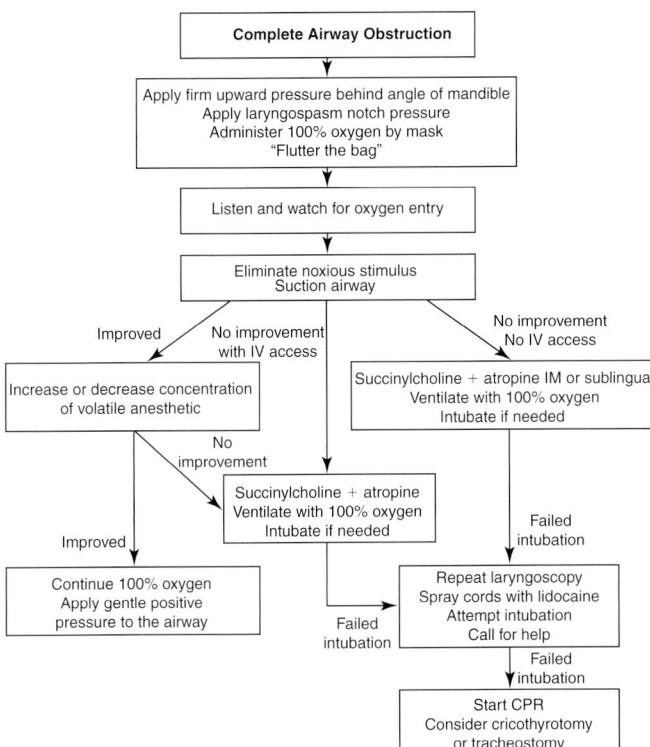

Fig. 53.3 Complete airway obstruction algorithm. *CPR,* Cardiopulmonary resuscitation; *IM,* intramuscular. (From Wittkugel E. Pediatric laryngospasm. In: Atlee JL, ed. *Complications in Anesthesia.* 2nd ed. Philadelphia: Elsevier; 2007:600.)

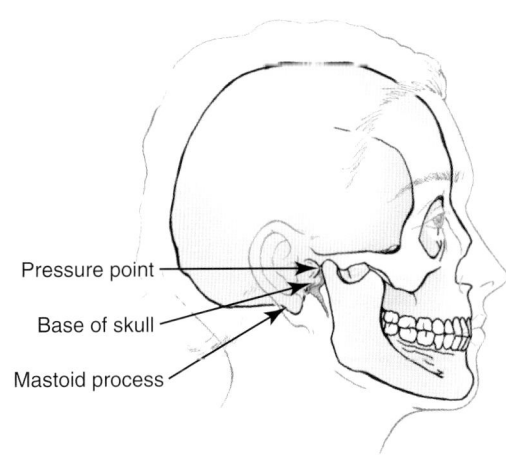

Fig. 53.4 The laryngospasm notch.

to producing a jaw thrust, the intense stimulation with postcondylar pressure in the lightly anesthetized patient often produces a ventilatory sigh.[123] This maneuver may be successful for the treatment of laryngospasm. Fig. 53.4 shows the laryngospasm notch.

If complete airway obstruction continues unabated, atropine and succinylcholine should be administered intravenously without delay. In the absence of IV access, IM succinylcholine (4 mg/kg) should be administered in the deltoid muscle. Following IM administration, the vocal cords will relax within 30 to 60 seconds, permitting positive pressure ventilation and endotracheal intubation. With continued deterioration in arterial oxygen saturation, intubation may be required prior to the onset of skeletal muscle relaxation. Severe hypoxia and hypercarbia inhibit skeletal muscle function and decrease laryngospasm.[124]

BOX 53.7 **Physical Examination of the Pediatric Airway**

- Note the size and shape of the head
- Facial features—size and shape of mandible and maxilla
- Oral examination—size of tongue, loose or missing dentition, prominence of upper incisors
- Range of motion of jaw and cervical spine

Bronchospasm causes increased airway resistance that eventually resolves spontaneously or with pharmacologic intervention. It is a disorder of the smooth muscle. It is known that airway resistance increases after instrumentation of the airway. This only rarely results in bronchospasm (0.4%); however, in children with known asthma or a current URI, the incidence is increased (4.1%).[125-127]

Bronchospasm may manifest as an audible wheeze. The anesthetist may notice a prominent slope on the expiratory portion of the $ETco_2$ waveform that is indicative of prolonged expiration, a rise in $ETco_2$, decrease in oxygen saturation, increased peak inspiratory pressures, decrease in tidal volume, and difficulty ventilating. Before the diagnosis of bronchospasm is confirmed, the anesthetist must consider other causative factors such as anaphylaxis, fluid overload, airway manipulation, pharyngeal irritation and/or secretions, esophageal intubation, pneumothorax, and inadequate anesthetic depth.[128] Physical signs that are associated with bronchospasm include but are not limited to hypoxemia, hypercarbia, wheezing, increased peak airway pressures, inability to ventilate, chest retraction during spontaneous respirations, and altered $ETco_2$ waveform (as described previously).

When ventilation is compromised, the first intervention is to administer 100% oxygen. Auscultation of the lungs may reveal wheezing. If the problem is severe, the surgeon should be informed to stop the surgery. The anesthetic depth should be assessed and deepened as needed, and the patient should be manually ventilated. A bronchodilator medication, such as albuterol, can be given via ETT.

In pediatric patients, the respiratory reserve is limited, and when coupled with an increased metabolic rate, rapid hypoxia can occur. Epinephrine (5–10 mcg/kg) should be administered subcutaneously if an IV has not been established.[129] In life-threatening emergencies, dilute a 1-mg vial of epinephrine in a 10-mL syringe and give 1 to 2 mL (100–200 mcg) IV push, in increments, for a maximum dose of 0.5 mg of a 1:1000 solution.[130] Another treatment for bronchospasm includes corticosteroids. IV steroids help to decrease inflammation but are not considered to be immediately effective in an acute airway emergency due to their prolonged onset of action.

Difficult airway. A difficult airway may be defined as difficulty in accomplishing mask ventilation and/or endotracheal intubation. The identification of the difficult pediatric airway begins with a thorough history followed by physical examination of the mouth, head, and neck. The physical examination should focus on the assessment of facial skeletal features, specifically the size and shape of the mandible and maxilla, the size of the tongue in relation to the oral cavity, an absence of dentition, the presence of loose dentition, and the range of motion of the neck. Box 53.7 lists some features of pediatric airway physical examination. Box 53.8 lists pathologic conditions that impact pediatric airway management.

A history of snoring, difficulty breathing with feeding, current or recent upper respiratory tract infection, and past history of croup should be identified. Previous anesthetic records are a valuable resource for determining whether a history of difficult airway management exists. However, a prior uneventful anesthetic does not preclude the possibility of difficult airway management with succeeding anesthetics.

BOX 53.8   Pathologic Pediatric Airway Conditions

Nasopharynx
- Choanal atresia
- Cleft lip, cleft palate
- Foreign body/tumors
- Adenoid hypertrophy

Tongue
- Hemangioma
- Angioedema
- Down syndrome
- Beckwith-Wiedemann syndrome
- Mucopolysaccharidosis
- Cystic hygroma
- Lacerations

Skeletal Structure
- Pierre Robin syndrome
- Treacher Collins syndrome
- Goldenhar syndrome

- Fractures
- Juvenile rheumatoid arthritis
- Cervical spine injury
- Mandibular ankylosis
- Arnold-Chiari malformation

Pharynx and Larynx
- Laryngeal web
- Laryngeal stenosis
- Laryngomalacia
- Laryngeal papillomatosis
- Laryngotracheobronchitis
- Tracheomalacia
- Foreign body
- Postextubation croup
- Epiglottitis
- Peritonsillar abscess
- Retropharyngeal abscess

If there is any indication from the history and physical examination of a potentially difficult airway, these guidelines should be followed:
1. Do not give neuromuscular blocking agents.
2. Prepare a variety of laryngoscope blades, ETTs, and oropharyngeal airways.
3. Plan for different induction options: awake fiberoptic; sedation, anesthetizing spray, and awake fiberoptic; inhalation induction.
4. After a deep plane of anesthesia is achieved, administer 100% oxygen.
5. Establish IV access (if not established preoperatively) and consider atropine or glycopyrrolate to decrease oral secretions.
6. Always maintain spontaneous respirations.
7. Use external manipulation of the trachea when possible to facilitate visualization of the glottis.
8. Use and/or have available adjunct airway equipment: videolaryngoscopy, fast-track LMA, blind nasal intubation, light wand, Eschmann stylet, cricothyrotomy.
9. Follow the standardized difficult airway algorithm (see Chapter 24).

Emergence and Extubation

Emergence delirium. A variety of terms are used interchangeably when referring to postoperative agitation. These include *emergence delirium*, *emergence agitation*, and *postanesthetic agitation*. These terms describe altered behavior in the immediate postoperative period that manifest as restlessness, crying, moaning, incoherence, and disorientation.[131,132] These episodes can be very upsetting to the parents and caregivers. Emergence delirium, fortunately, is self-limiting but may manifest for as long as 45 minutes. The incidence of emergence delirium ranges from 10% to 80% in the pediatric population.[133] It occurs during the early stage of emergence during initial wakening. No single factor has been identified as the cause of emergence agitation; it appears to be a composite of biologic, pharmacologic, psychological, and social components.[134] One hypothesis as to why this phenomenon occurs is that the rapid emergence associated with novel low-solubility anesthetic agents, such as sevoflurane and desflurane, may create a dissociative state in which children awaken with altered cognitive perception. The speed of emergence as a cause of emergence delirium is not universally accepted though, as it does not fully explain the variance

in incidence between inhalational agents.[135] There is conflicting research as to the incidence of emergence agitation with the slower emergence that occurs with the use of isoflurane.[136,137] An alternative explanation is the dose-dependent effect of sevoflurane on neuroexcitability, as sevoflurane increases seizurelike electroencephalogram activity in a dose-dependent fashion.[138]

Proposed causes also include rapid awakening in unfamiliar settings, pain, stress during induction, hypoxia, airway obstruction, a noisy environment, anesthesia duration, the child's personality, premedication, and the type of anesthesia used. It has been determined that propofol, fentanyl, dexmedetomidine, and preoperative analgesia have a prophylactic effect in preventing agitation and treating acute episodes. Midazolam and serotonin (5-HT$_3$) antagonists do not appear to significantly decrease the incidence of emergence delirium.[139]

Extubation. Similar to adults, the end of surgery in the pediatric patient involves the return of spontaneous breathing and weaning of anesthetic agents. It is important to have airway equipment readily available in case of the need to reestablish a patent airway after extubation. The incidence of critical airway events has been found to occur more often during emergence and extubation than induction and intubation.[140] The decision to extubate deep versus awake has long been a matter of debate in pediatric anesthesia. The choice depends on many factors, including the patient's medical history and type of surgical procedure.

Awake extubation is recommended in children with a history of difficult airway and full stomach, while deep extubation is preferred in children with reactive airway and when postsurgical coughing and bucking should be avoided. For awake extubation, the child should show signs of alertness such as facial grimacing, spontaneous eye opening, and purposeful movement. It is vital that the patient not be in the second stage of anesthesia during extubation as this increases the chance of airway complications, including laryngospasm.

Deep extubation can be performed after prudent suctioning of the oropharynx and stomach in patients with a normal airway and an empty stomach. It should be carefully decided whether the patient is appropriate for a deep extubation. In addition, the anesthetist must be aware of the level of care in the postoperative care unit where the patient will be recovering. Patients who were difficult to ventilate or intubate, those with a full stomach, and neonates and young infants should be fully awake prior to extubation. In a recent meta-analysis, deep extubation was found to increase the risk of upper airway obstruction compared to awake extubation but decrease the risk of overall airway complications, including cough and desaturation.[141]

All standard monitoring should continue until extubation is complete and the patient is stable. When breathing remains satisfactory, the patient can be transported to the postanesthesia care unit (PACU). Placing the patient in a lateral position can help decrease the risk of airway obstruction and pulmonary aspiration if vomiting occurs. The use of supplemental oxygen is recommended for all pediatric patients.

Fluid Management

The maintenance of euvolemia is essential during the comprehensive intraoperative care of the pediatric patient. The restoration and maintenance of pediatric intravascular volume are crucial if cardiac output is to be optimized and tissue oxygen delivery ensured.

The intravascular fluid balance is influenced by a number of preoperative and perioperative circumstances. Preoperative IV fluid administration minimizes the degree of dehydration that accompanies the period of fasting. Unless there is a compelling reason to place an IV catheter preoperatively, IV therapy is generally avoided in the pediatric patient under the age of 10 until general anesthesia has been induced via inhalation.

Perioperative fluid homeostasis is altered by several factors, including inhalation agent administration, the environmental temperature of the operating room, iatrogenic hyperventilation, and surgical stress. Potent inhalation agents produce peripheral vasodilation and varying degrees of myocardial depression, decreasing systemic blood pressure and end-organ perfusion. Dehydration after prolonged preoperative oral fluid abstinence aggravates these decreases in systemic blood pressure. The delivery of cold, dry anesthetic gases via an ETT bypasses normal anatomic humidification, increasing the loss of fluid from the respiratory tract. These insensible respiratory fluid losses can be minimized by the use of active or passive humidification systems during the intraoperative period. The operating room temperature also influences fluid balance. Basal caloric and water requirements are increased in a cold environment. A 1°C increase in core body temperature may increase caloric expenditure by 12% to 14%.

General anesthesia modifies the neuroendocrine control of fluid balance in a multitude of ways. Surgical stress increases plasma glucose levels. Hyperglycemia results in an osmotic-induced renal loss of free water. Anesthetic agents modify the neuroendocrine regulation of fluids and electrolytes. Opioids increase the release of antidiuretic hormone (ADH) from the posterior pituitary.[142] ADH stimulates the release of aldosterone to conserve water through the renal reabsorption of sodium and water and the excretion of potassium. Decreased glomerular filtration, which parallels the decrease in renal perfusion, alters the kidneys' ability to handle administered fluid loads. Decreased renal perfusion stimulates the release of renin, which cleaves angiotensin I to form angiotensin II, a powerful vasoconstrictor that acts to increase systemic blood pressure. In turn, renin stimulates the release of aldosterone.

Surgical trauma modifies the fluid balance to a degree that is dependent on the invasiveness of the surgical procedure. IV fluids are used to replace intraoperative blood loss and fluid loss resulting from evaporation and third spacing. Physiologic parameters such as temperature, heart rate, blood pressure, capillary refill time, urine output, and ongoing blood loss are continually assessed. The rate of intraoperative fluid administration is continuously modified to maintain circulatory homeostasis. Peripheral surgical procedures (extremity procedures) have minimal evaporative or third-space fluid losses. However, intracavitary procedures (intraabdominal or intrathoracic procedures) are associated with greater blood loss, third-space fluid loss, and substantial evaporative fluid losses that approach 10 to 15 mL/kg of body weight per hour.

Pediatric Fluid Compartments

The growth of the newborn is accompanied by a decrease in the relative TBW and ECF volumes during the first year of life, followed by additional decreases in ECF later in childhood. The TBW of the premature infant is as high as 80% of total body weight, whereas the TBW of the term infant is approximately 70% to 75% of total body weight. The adult value of TBW (55%–60%) is reached between 6 months and 1 year of age. Knowledge of body fluid distribution is important when selecting specific fluids and volumes for administration. The differences in TBW, as well as in the ICF and ECF compartments in the premature infant, term infant, child, and adult, can be found in Table 52.7.[143]

Maintenance-Fluid Calculation

The most direct and widely accepted method for determining IV fluid requirements is based on body weight. Holliday and Segar proposed a formula for the calculation of hourly maintenance fluids based on caloric expenditure studies in children. The hourly maintenance fluid level is determined by the "4-2-1" formula, calculated as follows (Table 53.6)[144]: For the first 10 kg of body weight, 4 mL of crystalloid IV fluid

TABLE 53.6 **Hourly Fluid Requirements: The "4-2-1" Formula**	
Weight (kg)	**Fluid**
0–10	4 mL/kg/hr for each kg of body weight
10–20	40 mL + 2 mL/kg/hr for each kg >10 kg
>20	60 mL + 1 mL/kg/hr for each kg >20 kg
Sample Calculated Fluid Requirements	**Maintenance Fluid/HR**
4 kg	16 mL
9 kg	36 mL
15 kg	50 mL
30 kg	70 mL

(e.g., lactated Ringer) is administered for each kilogram of body weight per hour. The hourly maintenance fluid requirement of a child who weighs 10 kg would be calculated as 10 kg × 4 mL/kg/hour = 40 mL/hour. Children weighing more than 10 kg but less than 20 kg would receive an additional 2 mL/kg/hour for body weight in excess of 10 kg, thus a child weighing 14 kg would receive 4 mL/kg/hour for the first 10 kg (40 mL) plus an additional 2 mL/kg/hour for a total of 48 mL/hr. Children weighing more than 20 kg would receive an additional 1 mL/kg/hour in hourly fluid. This hourly maintenance fluid calculation serves as a basic guideline and does not take into account fluid deficits that develop during the NPO period and additional fluid losses (such as blood and third-space losses) that occur during the perioperative period.

Preoperative fluid deficits develop during the period of time in which the child has not received oral or IV maintenance fluids. This time should be kept to a minimum to avoid dehydration. The preoperative fluid deficit is calculated by determining the hourly maintenance fluid rate and multiplying this rate by the number of hours the child has been without IV or oral intake. The following calculations are used to determine the preoperative fluid deficit of an 8-kg child who has been NPO for 6 hours:

$$\text{Maintenance fluid} = 8 \text{ kg} \times 4 \text{ mL/kg/hr} = 32 \text{ mL/hr}$$

$$\begin{aligned}\text{Deficit} &= \text{NPO hours} \times \text{maintenance fluid rate} \\ &= 6\text{hr} \times 32 \text{ mL/hr} = 192 \text{ mL}\end{aligned}$$ [145]

The calculated fluid deficit is replaced following the guidelines of Furman et al.[146]: Half the fluid deficit is replaced during the first hour, with the remainder divided in half and replaced in the subsequent 2 hours. Using the calculations just presented, the following plan for IV fluids is developed.

Weight = 8 kg	**Hour 1**	**Hour 2**	**Hour 3**
Maintenance fluid (mL/hr)	32	32	32
Deficit (mL/hr)	96	48	48
Hourly total (mL/hr)	128	80	80

In addition to the calculated maintenance and deficit fluids necessary to replace insensible fluid losses, additional IV fluid is required to replace third-space fluid losses that occur with surgical trauma. Lactated Ringer solution, 0.9% normal saline, and PlasmaLyte are acceptable for the replacement of insensible and third-space fluid losses at a rate of 1 to 2 mL/kg/hour. Expected third-space fluid losses can be categorized as minimal surgical trauma (an additional 3–4 mL/kg/hour), moderate

TABLE 53.7   Fluid Replacement for Third-Space Fluid Losses

Expected Surgical Trauma	Administration Rate (mL/kg/hr)	Recommended Intravenous Fluid
Minimal	3–4	Lactated Ringer 0.9% NS, PlasmaLyte
Moderate	5–6	Lactated Ringer 0.9% NS, PlasmaLyte
Severe	7–10	Lactated Ringer 0.9% NS, PlasmaLyte

NS, Normal saline.

surgical trauma (5–6 mL/kg/hour), and major surgical trauma (7–10 mL/kg/hour). Table 53.7 lists an approximation for fluid replacement and third-space losses.

Glucose-Containing Solutions

Historically, glucose was administered during the perioperative period to prevent hypoglycemia, provide free water to replace the insensible water lost during the NPO period, conserve protein, and avoid ketosis by preventing gluconeogenesis.[147] Surgical stress (e.g., surgical incision) elicits a neuroendocrine response, increasing plasma glucose levels. Despite extended periods of fasting, studies have noted that healthy pediatric patients infrequently become hypoglycemic.[148,149] However, very critically ill infants and those weighing less than 10 kg may develop hypoglycemia with prolonged periods of fasting. Routine dextrose administration is no longer advised for otherwise healthy children receiving anesthesia.[150] Most clinicians administer a glucose-free IV solution (e.g., lactated Ringer) for maintenance and replacement of third-space fluid loss and intraoperative blood loss. If the child has had an extended NPO period, glucose level may be determined intraoperatively, and appropriate adjustments in therapy can be made. Although the CNS is totally dependent on a continuous supply of exogenous glucose for the maintenance of cellular energy requirements, the continuous administration of glucose or elevated plasma glucose levels may worsen neurologic outcome in the event of an ischemic or hypoxic event, as glucose is converted to lactate during anaerobic metabolism. This association between hyperglycemia and worsened neurologic outcome has been well established.[151,152]

Hypoglycemia is likely to develop in a variety of clinical circumstances. Examples include infants who are premature, infants of diabetic mothers, children with diabetes who have received a portion of daily insulin preoperatively, and children who receive glucose-based parenteral nutrition. A glucose containing IV solution is administered to these patients as a controlled secondary infusion, with frequent plasma glucose determinations performed to avoid hyperglycemia. Infants born to mothers with diabetes and infants of mothers who receive glucose-containing solutions during labor may require a continuation of these solutions for the prevention of rebound hypoglycemia. Premature infants, who have had less time to store glycogen in the liver than term infants, are more susceptible to hypoglycemia. For this reason, premature infants may receive an infusion of 10% dextrose.

Crystalloid Intravenous Fluids

Crystalloid IV fluids contain water, various concentrations of electrolytes, and varying amounts of glucose. These solutions move freely between the intravascular and interstitial fluid compartments.

Crystalloid IV solutions are advantageous for perioperative administration because they are the least expensive of the available IV solutions and are acceptable for the replacement of preoperative, intraoperative, and postoperative isotonic fluid deficits. Unlike colloid solutions, crystalloid solutions do not produce allergic reactions. Crystalloid IV solutions can be further subdivided by their tonicity in relation to plasma (i.e., hypotonic, isotonic, or hypertonic). Tonicity is a measurement of the comparative osmolarity of solutions, which is determined by the sodium chloride content. For example, a hypotonic solution (e.g., 0.45% normal saline) has a lower sodium concentration (<130 mEq/L) and an osmolarity of less than 280 mOsm/L; an isotonic solution (e.g., lactated Ringer) has a sodium concentration between 130 and 155 mEq/L and an osmolarity between 280 and 310 mOsm/L; a hypertonic solution (e.g., 3% normal saline) has a sodium concentration greater than 155 mEq/L and an osmolarity in excess of 310 mOsm/L. These sodium-containing solutions move freely about the extracellular space, whereas sodium-free IV solutions, such as 5% dextrose in water (D_5W), will be distributed throughout all fluid compartments. Table 53.8 lists the physical constituents and the osmolarities of popular crystalloid solutions. An isotonic solution does not need to be equivalent to plasma in exact physical constituents (e.g., sodium, chloride, potassium) to be considered an isotonic solution because it is the number of particles dissolved in solution (principally sodium) that determines the osmolarity.

Estimation of Blood Volume

The goal of perioperative blood administration is to maintain acceptable oxygen-carrying capacity. Pediatric patients have a relatively low intravascular volume compared with adults, therefore vigilance and an accurate determination of intraoperative blood loss are fundamental to quality patient care. The intravascular volume may be estimated by multiplying the child's weight by the estimated blood volume (EBV). The EBVs are as follows: premature infant, 90 to 100 mL/kg; full-term newborn, 80 to 90 mL/kg; infants 3 months to 3 years, 75 to 80 mL/kg; children 3 to 6 years, 70 to 75 mL/kg; and children older than 6 years, 65 to 70 mL/kg. For example, the EBV of a 6-month-old infant who weighs 7 kg is 525 mL (7 kg × 75 mL/kg = 525 mL).

The determination of intraoperative blood loss can be difficult. Subjective estimates of blood loss are grossly inaccurate. Blood collected from the surgical field in suction canisters can be easily measured, but up to one-half of blood lost during surgery can be contained in items such as surgical drapes, sponges, and towels, which is difficult to measure. These items need to be weighed to obtain an accurate account of surgical blood loss. Every 1 g of weight is approximately equivalent to 1 mL of blood loss. Ongoing surgical blood loss requires frequent reassessment of the child's blood pressure, heart rate, urine output, and hematocrit (Hct).

Mild dehydration is associated with a decrease in body weight of less than 5%. Signs and symptoms are blood pressure, heart rate, and capillary refill all within normal limits. Dry mouth and malaise can possibly be seen preoperatively; however, they are not evident if the patient is under general anesthesia. Urinary output of less than 1 mL/kg/hour should be maintained. Moderate dehydration is associated with a 5% to 10% decrease in the patient's body weight. Significant hypotension and tachycardia may not be present in mild dehydration due to physiologic compensation. Severe decreases in intravascular volume are associated with a greater than 10% decrease in body weight. Signs and symptoms are tachycardia, hypotension, narrowed pulse pressure, low urine output, decreased central venous pressure, pallor, slow capillary refill, lethargy, thick and/or dry mucous membranes, and depression of the anterior fontanelle. The patient will have a decreased level of consciousness, mottled and cool skin, and may be

TABLE 53.8 Physical Characteristics of Popular Intravenous Crystalloid Solutions

	Sodium (Na) (mEq/L)	Chloride (Cl) (mEq/L)	Potassium (K) (mEq/L)	Calcium (Ca) (mg/mL)	Glucose (mg/dL)	Osmolality mOsm/L
0.45% normal saline	77	77	0	0	0	154
5% dextrose in water	0	0	0	0	5	278
0.9% normal saline	154	154	0	0	0	310
Lactated Ringer	130	109	4	3	0	273
Ringer acetate	130	112	5	2	0	276
PlasmaLyte A	140	98	5	0	0	294
5% sodium chloride	855	855	0	0	0	1700
7.5% sodium chloride	1283	1283	0	00		2400

Adapted from Ellis D, Moritz M. Regulation of fluids and electrolytes. In: Davis PJ, et al., eds. *Smith's Anesthesia for Infants and Children.* 9th ed. Philadelphia: Elsevier; 2017:108–144.

anuric. A sudden decrease in blood pressure in neonates and infants is indicative of significant intravascular volume depletion. Fluid management for dehydrated patients includes a 10 to 20 mL/kg fluid bolus over 10 to 30 minutes. After evaluation of fluid bolus response, subsequent boluses may be required.

Permissible Blood Loss

This transfusion trigger has been redefined considering the risks of bloodborne pathogen transmission, transfusion-related lung injury, and other related conditions that increase morbidity and mortality. Permissible blood loss must be defined individually for each patient based on current medical condition, surgical procedure, and cardiovascular and respiratory function. Children with normal cardiovascular function may tolerate a lower Hct and may compensate with an increased cardiac output if a higher inspired oxygen concentration is provided to improve oxygen delivery. An exception is the premature infant. The incidence of apnea is higher in neonates and premature infants with Hct levels below 30%. A definitive adequate Hgb concentration that is essential for oxygen delivery has been determined to be 7 to 8 g/dL for most hospitalized adult patients.[153] Maximum allowable blood loss (MABL) may be calculated with the following formula[108]:

$$MABL = EBV \times (Starting\ Hct - Target\ Hct) / Starting\ Hct$$

Blood loss may be replaced with suitable crystalloid solutions (e.g., 0.9% normal saline, lactated Ringer) by administering 3 mL for each 1 mL of blood loss. Recall that the intravascular volume is one-third of the ECF volume. Accordingly, one must administer 3 mL of an IV crystalloid solution to replace each 1 mL of blood loss. A blood loss of 100 mL therefore requires replacement with 300 mL of a crystalloid solution. Blood loss that is less than the calculated permissible blood loss may be replaced with colloid (1 mL for every 1 mL of blood loss).

When the blood loss equals or exceeds the calculated allowable loss, transfusion should be considered. Before transfusion is performed, a current Hgb and Hct should be obtained. The surgeon should be included in the decision process. These discussions and the resultant Hgb and Hct are recorded in the anesthetic record. The volume of packed red blood cells (PRBCs) to be infused may be determined by the following formula:

$$Volume\ of\ PRBCs = (Desired\ Hct - Current\ Hct) \times EBV/Hct\ of\ PRBCs$$

The Hct of the PRBCs can be approximated at about 60%.[108] Once the blood loss exceeds one blood volume, coagulopathy can ensue. This occurs because of dilutional thrombocytopenia and a reduction in circulating clotting factors. Platelets, fresh frozen plasma, and cryoprecipitate transfusions become necessary. See Chapter 22 for blood transfusion guidelines.

Blood Transfusion

Before blood component therapy is initiated, the proper equipment (e.g., filters, infusion devices, blood warming devices) should be obtained and tested. Blood is usually warmed before infusion. The American Association of Blood Banks has published standards for the use of blood-warming devices. Blood warmers must have a visible thermometer and an audible warning indicating excessive heating (>42°C). Warming devices for adult transfusions (e.g., in-line water baths, countercurrent heating with water through large-bore tubing) are cumbersome to use for the small volumes to be transfused in the pediatric patient. The selected blood component containers may be placed under the forced-air warming blanket, or the measured aliquot of blood drawn into a syringe may be warmed with the hand.

Blood used for neonatal transfusion is preferably less than 1 week old, to preserve 2,3-diphosphoglycerate levels, and irradiated to prevent graft-versus-host disease. When PRBCs are transfused, the blood should not be diluted prior to transfusion; this may contribute to hypervolemia. As a rule, 4 mL/kg of PRBCs will be required to raise the Hgb level by 1 g/dL.[154]

POSTOPERATIVE CARE

Similar to an adult patient, standard monitoring is continued when the pediatric patient arrives in the PACU. Although all the parameters are important, special attention to oxygenation is crucial. Postoperative hypoxia may be the result of several factors, but postextubation croup and laryngospasm are more likely in children compared to adults.[155] Airway obstruction, obstructive sleep apnea, postextubation croup, and apnea of prematurity can all occur and need to be recognized with prompt intervention. Airway obstruction can be due to inadequate positioning of the patient's head or by the tongue. Simply repositioning the head can sometimes relieve this problem. Positioning and adequate oral suctioning can help prevent obstruction and possible laryngospasm.

The incidence of postextubation croup has been reported to be 1.6% to 6%. Prevention of tracheal irritation is the best way to prevent this problem. Using the correct ETT size with a leak near 20 cm H_2O, prevention of friction of the tube in the trachea by proper securement, and prevention of unplanned extubation are ways to help decrease the risk of developing postextubation croup.[156]

Readiness for discharge from the PACU is typically evaluated using a scoring system that includes blood pressure, heart rate, respirations, temperature, pain, nausea/vomiting, physical activity, and level of consciousness. The goal is for the patient to return to preprocedural hemodynamic and respiratory levels before discharge. One common method that is used is the modified Aldrete scoring (see Chapter 55). When evaluating a patient in the ambulatory surgery center to be fast-tracked, a score of 12 or higher is needed.[157] When fast-tracking is anticipated, the anesthetic can be planned to allow for short PACU times and quick discharge to home.

REGIONAL ANESTHESIA

Over the past 10 years, the use of regional anesthesia with pediatric patients has grown exponentially, largely due to the advent of ultrasound-guided techniques. Regional anesthesia provides perioperative analgesia (minimizing the reliance on opioids and subsequently the risk of respiratory depression), modifies the metabolic responses to anesthesia and surgery, and may improve patient outcomes.[158,159] In pediatrics, regional anesthesia is typically performed with the child under general anesthesia. Though there have historically been concerns that the detection of inadvertent intravascular injection, and/or local anesthetic toxicity, would be masked during general anesthesia, several studies have reported the safety of performing regional anesthesia under general anesthesia in children.[160] Nonetheless, there remains limited ability to properly assess the sensory level of block in the child under general anesthesia, and the consequences of accidental dural puncture are more challenging to assess and treat.

Unlike the adult patient, the pediatric patient will most often receive a peripherally or centrally administered regional anesthetic after the induction of general anesthesia. The child's inherent fear of needles and pain, the fear of neurologic injury in a combative child, and the difficulty in providing adequate sedation to ensure patient immobility during the introduction of the block often necessitate the execution of the regional anesthetic during general anesthesia. The risk of neurologic injury may be lower in the anesthetized child who is not resistant and combative during attempted epidural or caudal anesthesia now that the use of ultrasound-guided blocks is routine.[161] See Chapter 52 for a complete description of caudal anesthesia in children.

OUTPATIENT ANESTHESIA

Outpatient surgery is the mainstay of modern surgical and anesthesia practice.[162] Many specialties are performing procedures in the ambulatory surgery center, including otolaryngology, ophthalmology, general surgery, urology, plastic surgery, orthopedics, radiology, dentistry, and others. The postoperative goals are the same for all surgeries: hemodynamic stability, minimal pain and nausea, and the return of a preoperative level of consciousness. However, with ambulatory surgery, the discharge criteria are more rigid due to the fast-paced nature of the perioperative process. It is of the utmost importance that the patient be able to take oral medications without nausea and vomiting when leaving the surgery center.

There are few absolute contraindications to ambulatory surgery for the pediatric patient. Infants who were born premature at less than 35 weeks of gestation or those who are less than 60 weeks of postconceptual age are at risk for postoperative apnea.[163,164] These children require an overnight stay in the hospital for observation. Patients who

have a personal or family history of MH may undergo outpatient surgery as long as the nontriggering anesthetic has been uneventful and they are monitored postoperatively for a period of 1 to 2 hours. If the patient develops MH in the surgery center, immediate administration of dantrolene followed by emergency transfer to a higher level of care is necessary.

Induction, airway management, and maintenance of anesthesia are similar when giving anesthesia in the hospital and in the surgery center. When the patient is spontaneously breathing, the anesthetist can decide to extubate the patient deep or awake. Other factors that influence procedures and patient selection for a surgery center are the need for postoperative analgesia and minimizing PONV. Local anesthesia injection by the surgeon or regional anesthesia is imperative, if applicable, for multimodal pain management. Patients may also be given acetaminophen before or during surgery. Nausea can be managed by using multimodal pharmacologic treatment and by prophylactically identifying high-risk patients and then tailoring the anesthetic with agents that are not considered to be emetogenic.[165,166]

PEDIATRIC ANESTHETIC MORBIDITY AND MORTALITY

Anesthetic morbidity and mortality differ between the pediatric patient and the adult patient. Accordingly, children require individualized and specialized anesthetic care. When compared with adults, children often present for surgery with unique symptoms. Their lack of ability to communicate effectively further complicates proper diagnosis and interventions. Fortunately, with a well-conducted history and physical examination and effective caregiver communication, a safe anesthetic may be planned and executed.

The Pediatric Perioperative Cardiac Arrest Registry (POCA), an ongoing database of pediatric cardiac arrests established in 1994, is a self-reporting, voluntary registry recording institutional cardiac arrests in children up to 18 years of age from as many as 80 participating institutions in Canada and the United States. The POCA data provide a retrospective assessment of contributing factors rather than determining causation of cardiac arrest. The initial registry results for the years 1994 to 2005 found 373 cardiac arrests in more than

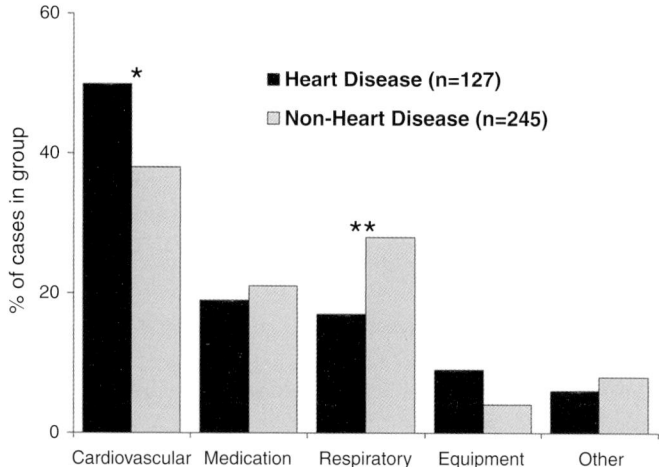

Fig. 53.5 Causes of anesthesia-related cardiac arrest associated with heart disease (n = 127) versus non–heart disease (n=245). *P = 0.03, **P = 0.01. (From Ramamoorthy C, et al. Anesthesia-related cardiac arrest in children with heart disease: data from the Pediatric Perioperative Cardiac Arrest (POCA) registry. *Anesth Analg.* 2010;110(5):1376–1382.)

1 million pediatric anesthetic experiences; 193 arrests (49%) were judged to be anesthesia related.[167] When cardiac arrest occurred, children with congenital or acquired heart disease were more likely to progress to cardiac arrest as compared with those without heart disease (50% vs 38%).[168] The patients with heart disease had higher ASA classifications (ASA III or above) and were more difficult to successfully resuscitate. Hyperkalemia from blood transfusions and hypovolemia were additional cardiovascular-related causes for cardiac arrest. Other reasons for cardiac arrest included respiratory-related causes (most often laryngospasm) and vascular injuries from central line placement. The incidence of medication-induced cardiac arrest has decreased since sevoflurane replaced halothane as the inhalation agent of choice during perioperative management. Fig. 53.5 shows the causes of anesthesia-related cardiac arrest specifically associated with heart disease as compared to patients without cardiac pathology.

SUMMARY

Anesthetic morbidity and mortality are greater in the pediatric patient, and the causes are multifactorial. Pediatric subspecialty practice requires the anesthetist to have a working knowledge of the foundations of pediatric growth and development, the anatomic and physiologic changes that occur with maturation, and the influence of anesthetic agents upon immature organ systems. Anesthetic management of the pediatric patient requires integration of this specialized knowledge, refinement of the acquired technical skills of adult anesthetic management, and the ability to apply this knowledge when caring for pediatric patients.

REFERENCES

For a complete list of references for this chapter, scan this QR code with any smartphone code reader app, or visit the following URL: http://booksite.elsevier.com/9780323711944/.

54

Geriatrics and Anesthesia Practice

Sandra K. Bordi

The number of people in the world who are 65 years and older has increased by 300% over the last 50 years. It is projected that the United States will have approximately 73 million people aged 65 years and older by 2030 and 83 million by 2050, almost double its estimated population in 2012. By 2050, the surviving baby boomers will be the oldest old (≥85 years), which is estimated to triple in number and place the United States as the largest population of oldest old among the developed countries. For the first time in history, the number of individuals 60 years of age and older will exceed the number of younger adults. The population of older adults will become more racially and ethnically diverse; the number of blacks over the age 65 years will double, and the number of those of Asian and Hispanic descent will triple.[1] The aging population will also affect hospital utilization, surgical services, and health care costs. The National Hospital Discharge Survey reported that those over 65 years of age have higher rates of inpatient and outpatient surgical and nonsurgical procedures as compared to other age groups, with the oldest old having significantly higher rates of hospitalization as compared to adults 84 years and younger.[2] It is inevitable that surgical services and hospitalizations for older adults will increase as its population increases. Therefore the increased aging of the United States, and its diversity, will have significant implications for anesthesia practitioners and their approach to the anesthetic management of the geriatric patient.

Definitions of aging are often subjective and place an arbitrary marker on chronologic age; however, this section will operationally define "older adults" or "elderly" as persons 65 years or older. Although aging is not routinely associated with surgical risk, the challenges related to anatomic and physiologic changes that occur with aging impact every aspect of the perioperative course.

The intent of this chapter is to provide a targeted review of the anatomic and physiologic changes that occur with aging and identify how these changes affect anesthesia. In addition, this information might offer practitioners additional evidence to be considered in their current practice, thus providing a foundation for modifying the current options to improve perioperative outcomes if required.

PREOPERATIVE ASSESSMENT

Preoperative evaluation is thoroughly discussed in Chapter 20; however, the preoperative assessment of older adults warrants some special considerations. Older adults are prone to progressive decline of baseline functions, age-related comorbid disease(s) causing an increase in American Society of Anesthesiologists (ASA) physical status classification; these place older adults at greater risk for perioperative complications that are directly related to increased morbidity and mortality in the postoperative period. Most postoperative complications in the elderly are related to cardiac, pulmonary, and neurologic dysfunction.[3,4] Factors that influence perioperative outcomes in older adults include emergency surgery, the number of comorbidities, and the type of surgical procedure. There is an array of risk assessment tools used in the clinical setting. These vary from assessing operative risk and overall physical status in relationship to type of surgery and organ-specific indices (i.e., cardiac, neurocognitive).[3,4] Risk assessment and stratification is also important to assist in determining a multidisciplinary team approach to perioperative management. Moreover, patients and anesthesia providers use this information as part of their surgical and anesthesia informed consent. Depending on the risk(s) deemed, a different surgical and/or anesthetic approach may be necessary, or surgery may not be performed at all. Therefore identifying perioperative risk is part of the preoperative assessment and is preferably performed prior to the day of surgery.

To provide high-quality care for the older adult surgical patient, a comprehensive and thorough preoperative evaluation is essential. The American College of Surgeons (ACS) National Surgical Quality Improvement Program (NSQIP) and the American Geriatrics Society (AGS) developed Best Practice Guidelines for Optimal Preoperative Assessment for the elderly surgical patient.[5] Based on these guidelines, in addition to conducting a complete and thorough history and physical examination, there are specific assessment categories that are highly recommended to provide guidance for perioperative management of this complex patient population (Table 54.1). These specific assessment categories will be discussed within the age-related physiologic body system changes of this chapter.

AGE-RELATED PHYSIOLOGIC CHANGES IN THE OLDER ADULT

Aging can be defined as a time-dependent biologic continuum that begins with birth and persists with gradual impairments of organ subsystems and ultimately causes an organism to become more susceptible to illness and death. By the age of 30 years, most age-related physiologic functions in humans have peaked and gradually decline thereafter. Aging is not synonymous with poor physiologic function. Because chronologic age (age in years since birth), which is often used in clinical practice, and biologic age (functional status) differ, chronologic age alone is no longer a reliable indicator of morbidity or of mortality. The degree of functional status that remains with increasing age varies. For example, a 75-year-old patient who bicycles 3 miles every day, has no evidence of coexisting diseases, and lives a healthy lifestyle is considered "physiologically young." Whereas a 75-year-old patient who is sedentary, has a history of hypertension and diabetes mellitus, and is a chronic smoker may be deemed as "physiologically old." In addition, changes in organ function manifest as decreased margins of reserve. Aging patients may be able to maintain homeostasis but become increasingly less able to tolerate changes or restore homeostasis when exposed to surgical stress, trauma, or diseases.

TABLE 54.1 ACS NSQIP/AGS Assessment Categories

Assessment Category	Screening Tool
Cognitive ability capacity	Mini-Cog 3 Item Recall and clock draw
Decision-making capacity	Legally relevant criterion: 1. Understanding 2. Appreciation 3. Reasoning 4. Choice
Depression	Patient Health Questionnaire-2 (PHQ-2)
Risk for postoperative delirium	Review: Cognitive and behavioral disorders Coexisting diseases/illnesses Metabolic disturbances Functional impairments Other: polypharmacy, history of UTI, constipation or presence of Foley catheter
Alcohol and substance abuse	Modified CAGE
Cardiac	ACC/AHA algorithm for patients undergoing noncardiac surgery; METs
Pulmonary	Review: Patient-related risk factors Surgical procedure risk factors
Frailty	Slowness Weight loss Grip weakness Exhaustion Decrease in physical activity
Functional status	Proxy report TUGT
Nutritional status	BMI Serum albumin Unintentional weight loss
Medications	Review prescribed, herbal, and OTC *Beer's Criteria* addressed
Patient counseling	Perioperative goals Assistance needs Advanced directives DNR status Social support

ACC/AHA, American College of Cardiology/American Heart Association; *BMI,* body mass index; *DNR,* do-not-resuscitate; *METs,* metabolic equivalent of tasks; *OTC,* over the counter; *TUGT,* The Timed Up and Go Test; *UTI,* urinary tract infection.
From American College of Surgeons. Optimal perioperative management of the geriatric patient: best practices guideline from ACS NSQIP/American Geriatrics Society. https://www.facs.org/quality-programs/acs-nsqip/geriatric-periop-guideline. Accessed 2020.

Cardiovascular System

Age-related changes in the cardiovascular system involve structural and functional changes in the heart, vessels, and autonomic nervous system. In the older adult, the heart and vascular system is less compliant, leading to a faster propagation of the pulse pressure waveform, increase in afterload, and an increase in systolic blood pressure, leading to ventricular thickening (hypertrophy) and prolonged left ventricular ejection times. The combination of ventricular hypertrophy and slower myocardial relaxation often results in late diastolic filling and diastolic dysfunction. When these changes occur, atrial contraction becomes important in the maintenance of adequate ventricular filling. Even though the elderly have higher amounts of circulating catecholamines, they exhibit decreased end-organ adrenergic responsiveness. Therefore the older adult has a reduced capacity to increase heart rate in response to hypotension, hypovolemia, and hypoxia. Prolonged circulation time causes a faster induction time with inhalation agents but delays the onset of intravenous drugs. There is calcification of the conducting system with loss of sinoatrial node cells, which predisposes the elderly to atrial fibrillation, sick sinus syndrome, first- and second-degree heart blocks, and arrhythmias. Hence a higher proportion of elderly patients may have or require permanent pacemakers and/or automatic internal cardiac defibrillators. Calcification is not limited to the conducting system but may be present in the heart valves (primarily aortic and mitral), predisposing elderly patients to stenosis or regurgitation.

Hypertension is a risk factor for perioperative complications, with the risk doubling for every 20-mm Hg systolic/10-mm Hg diastolic increase in blood pressure. With aging, the pulse pressure widens because of a greater proportionate increase in systolic blood pressure compared with diastolic blood pressure. Decreased venous compliance can lead to decreased preload and reduced atrial filling. Likewise there is decreased sensitivity of baroreceptors in the aortic arch and carotid sinuses in response to blood pressure changes, which results in increased episodes of hypotension. Age-related changes in the cardiovascular system of the older adult also include changes in the heart's regulation of calcium, which causes the myocardium to generate force over a longer period after excitation and prolongs the systolic phase of the cardiac cycle.[6]

The myocardium in older adults has decreased sensitivity to β-adrenergic modulation, physiologically evident as decreased heart rate and lower cardiac dilation at the end of diastole and systole. In general, older adults may have higher blood pressures caused by increased peripheral vascular resistance, decreased arterial elasticity, both which increase myocardial workload. Other cardiac changes include decreased cardiac output and stroke volume because of decreased conduction velocity and reduction in venous blood flow. Age-related cardiovascular changes and their anesthetic implications are noted in Table 54.2. The combined effect of decreased cardiac reserve and decreased maximum heart rate adversely affects the compensatory mechanisms of the older adult under the stress of anesthesia and surgery.

The elderly are significantly more vulnerable to adverse perioperative cardiac events. Myocardial infarction is the most common cardiac complication and the leading cause of death in the postoperative period. Therefore a complete cardiac assessment of the cardiovascular system in the older adult undergoing noncardiac surgery is essential and should be based on guidelines according to the American College of Cardiology/American Heart Association (ACC/AHA) as discussed in Chapter 20. Other risk stratification tools that are highly recommended in the older adult by the ACS NSQIP/AGS include measuring the patient's functional capacity via metabolic equivalents (METs) and the perioperative cardiac risk calculator, an interactive web-based tool, which replaces the Revised Cardiac Risk Index. The interactive perioperative cardiac risk calculator quantifies risk according to the type of surgical procedure, functional status, creatinine level, ASA classification, and age.[7,8] It provides a probability for perioperative cardiac events (i.e., myocardial infarction, cardiac arrest), which can assist in guiding perioperative management and informed consent. The most frequently associated cardiovascular coexisting diseases in the older adult are hypertension, hyperlipidemia, coronary artery disease (ischemic heart disease), and congestive heart disease (heart failure) (Fig. 54.1).

TABLE 54.2 Age-Related Cardiovascular Changes and Anesthetic Implications

Age-Related Change	Mechanism	Consequences	Anesthetic Implications
Myocardial hypertrophy	Apoptotic cells are not replaced and there is compensatory hypertrophy of existing cells; reflected waves during late systole create strain on myocardium leading to hypertrophy	Increased ventricular stiffness; prolonged contraction; and delayed relaxation	Failure to maintain preload leads to an exaggerated decrease in CO; excessive volume more easily increases filling pressures to congestive failure levels; dependence on sinus rhythm and low-normal HR
Myocardial stiffening	Increased interstitial fibrosis; amyloid deposition	Ventricular filling dependent on atrial pressure	—
Reduced LV relaxation	Impaired calcium homeostasis; reduced β-receptor responsiveness; early reflected wave	Diastolic dysfunction	—
Reduced β-receptor responsiveness	Diminished coupling of β-receptor to intracellular adenylate cyclase activity; decreased density of β-receptors	Increased circulating catecholamines; limited increase in HR and contractility in response to endogenous and exogenous catecholamines; impaired baroreflex control of BP	Hypotension from anesthetic blunting of sympathetic tone; altered reactivity to vasoactive drugs; increased dependence on Frank-Starling mechanism to maintain CO; labile BP, more hypotension
Conduction system abnormalities	Apoptosis; fibrosis; fatty infiltration; and calcification of pacemaker and His-bundle cells	Conduction block; sick sinus syndrome; AF; decreased contribution of atrial contraction to diastolic volume	Severe bradycardia with potent opioids; decreased CO from decrease in end-diastolic volume
Stiff arteries	Loss of elastin; increased collagen; glycosylation cross-linking of collagen	Systolic hypertension; arrival of reflected pressure wave during end-ejection leads to myocardial hypertrophy and impaired diastolic relaxation	Labile BP; diastolic dysfunction; sensitive to volume status
Stiff veins	Loss of elastin; increased collagen; glycosylation cross-linking of collagen	Decreased buffering of changes in blood volume impairs ability to maintain atrial pressure	Changes in blood volume cause exaggerated changes in cardiac filling

AF, Atrial fibrillation; *BP,* blood pressure; *CO,* cardiac output; *HR,* heart rate; *LV,* left ventricular.
From Sanders D, et al. Diastolic dysfunction, cardiovascular aging, and the anesthesiologist. *Anesthesiol Clin.* 2009;27(3):497–517.

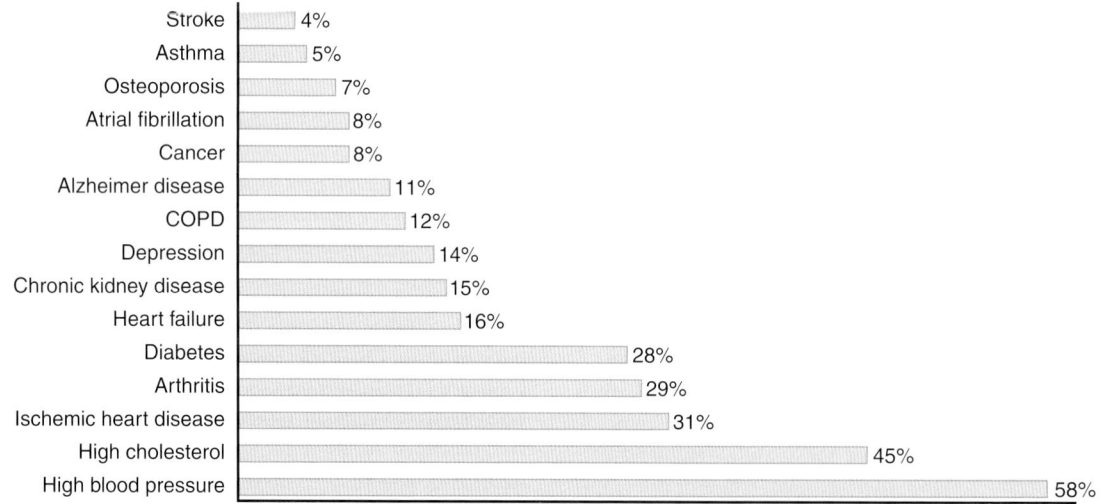

Fig. 54.1 Percentage of Medicare fee-for-service beneficiaries with 15 selected chronic conditions: 2010. *COPD,* Chronic obstructive pulmonary disease. (In: Goldman L, Schafer AI, eds. *Goldman-Cecil Medicine.* Vol. 1. 25th ed. Philadelphia, PA: Elsevier; 2016:100–121. From Centers for Medicare and Medicaid Services. Chronic conditions among Medicare beneficiaries, chartbook: 2012 edition. Based on 2010 Centers for Medicare and Medicaid Services administration claims data for 100% of Medicare beneficiaries enrolled in the fee-for-service program.)

Respiratory System

There are various age-related alterations of the respiratory system that have an impact on oxygenation in the elderly patient. Aging causes calcifications to form on the chest wall, intervertebral joints, and intercostal joints. These factors, along with decreased intercostal muscle mass, contributes to a decrease in chest wall compliance. In addition, there is a flattening of the diaphragm, a loss of intervertebral disc height, and changes in spinal lordosis, which further diminishes

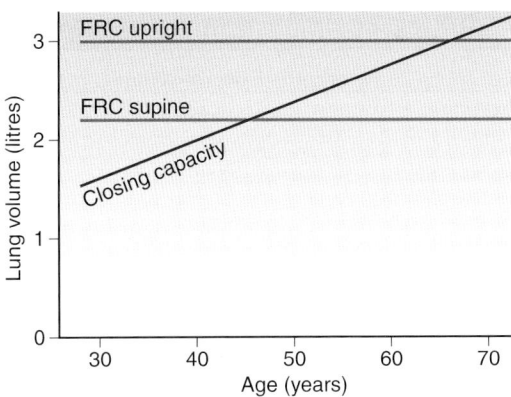

Fig. 54.2 Functional residual capacity *(FRC)* and closing capacity as a function of age. (In: Lumb AB. *Nunn's Applied Respiratory Physiology*. 8th ed. Philadelphia, PA: Elsevier; 2017:29. Data from Leblanc P, et al. Effects of age and body position on 'airway closure' in man. *J Appl Physiol*. 1970;28:448–453.)

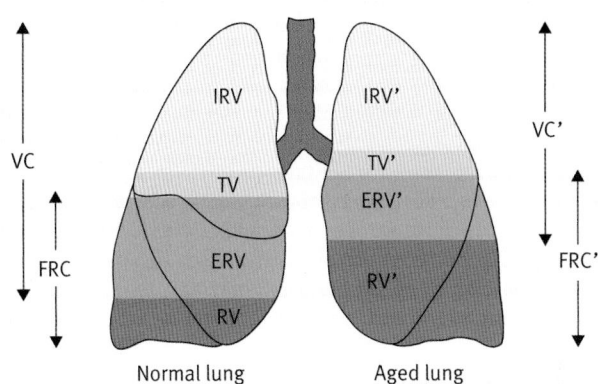

Fig. 54.3 Schematic representation of lung volume changes associated with aging. Note that with senescence, there is a decrease in the inspiratory reserve volume *(IRV')*, the expiratory reserve volume *(ERV')*, and the vital capacity *(VC')*. There is a corresponding increase in residual volume *(RV')* and functional residual capacity *(FRC')* such that the total lung capacity remains approximately the same. *TV'*, Tidal volume. (In Maguire SL, Slater BMJ. Physiology of aging. *Anaesthesia & Int Care Med*. 2010;11(7):290–292. From Chan ED, Welsh CH. Geriatric respiratory medicine. *Chest*. 1998;114(6):1704–1733.)

chest wall compliance. Changes also occur with the lung parenchyma. There is a generalized loss of elastic tissue recoil of the lung. Consequently, there is reduced functional alveolar surface area available for gas exchange. In elderly patients, even in the absence of disease, an increase in lung compliance impairs the matching of ventilation and perfusion, increases physiologic shunt, and results in the reduction of oxygen exchange at the alveolar level. Elastic recoil is necessary for maintaining patency of small distal airways, and increased lung compliance causes small airway diameter to narrow and eventually increases the closing volume (i.e., lung volume at which small airways in the dependent parts of the lung begin to close). The closing volume exceeds functional residual capacity (FRC) at approximately 65 years of age in the erect position and at age 45 years in the supine position (Fig. 54.2). Other dynamic and static lung volume changes include a decrease in vital capacity, an increase in residual volume, and an increase in FRC with decreases in inspiratory reserve volume and expiratory reserve volume. Total lung capacity remains unchanged or may slightly decrease because of its correlation with height. There is also a decrease in forced expiratory maneuvers. The forced vital capacity (FVC) and the forced expiratory volume in 1 second (FEV_1) are both decreased as a result of the loss of lung elastic recoil, decrease in small airway diameter, and subsequent airway collapse with forced expiration (Fig. 54.3). Impaired oxygenation is reflected by a decline in resting arterial oxygen tension (PaO_2), which remains somewhat stable at approximately 83 mm Hg, after 75 years of age. This decline in PaO_2 is attributed to the premature closing of small airways and the reduction in the alveolar surface area.[9]

Regulation of breathing is also affected with aging. The central (medulla) and peripheral (carotid and aortic bodies) chemoreceptors affect ventilation with changes in pH, PaO_2, and partial pressure of CO_2 in arterial blood ($PaCO_2$). In the elderly, the ventilatory response to hypoxemia and hypercarbia is decreased, predisposing them to increased episodes of apnea. Another challenge associated with oxygenation is the progressive decrease in laryngeal and pharyngeal support that accompanies aging, which can result in airway obstruction. In addition, protective airway reflexes (i.e., coughing and swallowing) are decreased, which increases the risk for pulmonary aspiration. Age-related pulmonary changes and their anesthetic implications are noted in Table 54.3.

Similar to other organ systems, pulmonary changes in the elderly are extremely variable among individuals. Age alone and prevalence of coexisting pulmonary diseases, (i.e., chronic obstructive pulmonary disease [COPD] and asthma) increase the risk for postoperative

pulmonary complications (PPCs) in the older adult. PPCs include atelectasis, bronchospasm, exacerbation of an underlying chronic lung disease, pneumonia, prolonged mechanical ventilation, and postoperative respiratory failure.[10] Therefore preoperatively assessing the elderly for their risk of developing PPCs is strongly recommended by the ACS NSQIP/AGS. Additional risk factors for PPCs include patient-related and surgical-related factors (Box 54.1). Of the modifiable risk factors, strategies should be implemented to minimize risks and prevent PPCs. For example, smoking cessation at least 8 weeks prior to surgery, implementing inspiratory muscle training and lung expansion maneuvers via incentive spirometry, and medically optimizing patients with COPD and/or asthma.

Renal Function

Age-related changes in renal function are particularly significant because of the many roles of the kidneys. Older adults have a significant baseline decrement in renal function relative to their younger counterparts. Progressive atrophy of kidney parenchymal tissues, deterioration of renal vascular structures, and decreased renal blood flow cause an overall decrease in renal mass. The cumulative effect is a decrease in the glomerular filtration rate (GFR) resulting in decreased renal drug clearance and decreased renal blood flow from age 20 years to age 90 years (approximately a 25%–50% decline). The combined effect is particularly apparent with diminished renal clearance of hydrophilic agents and hydrophilic metabolites of lipophilic agents.

The vital role that the kidneys play in the maintenance of fluid and electrolyte balance, their contribution to acid-base balance and to the excretion of drugs and their metabolites, affects anesthetic management. The decrease in GFR and impairment of the nephron can easily predispose the patient to fluid overload if overzealous intravenous fluid is administered. The production of renin and aldosterone is decreased with age, causing impairment of sodium conservation. Sodium conservation and hydrogen ion excretion are decreased, resulting in an impaired ability of the kidneys to respond to changes in electrolyte concentrations, intravascular volume, and free water.[11] The kidneys do not respond to nonrenal loss of water and sodium, and as a result,

TABLE 54.3   Age-Related Pulmonary Changes and Anesthetic Considerations

Structural Changes	Consequences	Anesthetic Considerations
Chest wall	Impaired gas exchange	Risk for respiratory failure
Stiff/decreased compliance	Increased WOB	Careful use of NDMRs, opioids, and benzodiazepines
Flattened diaphragm		
Lung parenchyma	Impaired gas exchange	Risk for respiratory failure
Increased lung compliance	Increased V̇/Q̇ mismatch	Avoid high pressure/large TV
		Consider longer I:E ratio
Increased small airway closure	Increased anatomic dead space	Consider alveolar recruitment maneuvers (PEEP)
	Decreased alveolar surface area	Limit high inspired oxygen
	Decreased PCBF	Maintain $Paco_2$ near normal preoperative value
	Decreased Pao_2	Consider regional/local with sedation
Muscle strength		Risk for respiratory failure
		Risk for aspiration
Decreased	Increased WOB	Adequate hydration
	Decreased protective airway reflexes	Consider RSI with GA
		Ensure fully reversed prior to extubation
		Consider postoperative CPAP or BiPAP
		Vigilant monitoring
		Encourage cough/deep breathing postoperatively
Control of breathing		Risk for respiratory failure
Decreased central/peripheral chemoreceptor sensitivity	Increased hypoventilation	Consider postoperative CPAP or BiPAP
	Increased apnea	Vigilant monitoring
	Decreased ventilator responses	Encourage cough/deep breathing postoperatively
		Supplemental oxygen postoperatively

BiPAP, Bilevel positive airway pressure; *CPAP*, continuous positive airway pressure; *GA*, general anesthesia; *I:E*, inspiratory/expiratory; *NDMRs*, nondepolarizing muscle relaxants; *Pao₂*, resting arterial oxygen tension; *Paco₂*, partial pressure of CO_2 in arterial blood; *PCBP*, pulmonary capillary blood flow; *PEEP*, positive end-expiratory pressure; *RSI*, rapid sequence induction; *TV*, tidal volume; *V̇/Q̇*, ventilation-perfusion; *WOB*, work of breathing.

dehydration can occur. The serum creatinine is often unchanged in the absence of renal failure because of decreased creatinine production from the overall declining skeletal muscle mass associated with aging. Creatinine clearance is the best indicator of drug clearance. The Cockroft-Gault equation is a common formula for estimating creatinine clearance, which in turn estimates GFR (eGFR) in the healthy older adult.[12]

$$eGFR \ (mL/min) = \frac{(140 - age \ in \ yrs) \times (weight \ in \ kg)}{72 \times (serum \ creatinine \ in \ mg/dL)}$$

$$(\times 0.85 \ for \ female \ patients)$$

When this formula is applied to the critically ill or to patients taking medications that directly affect renal function, caution must be employed, as it overestimates creatinine clearance. Therefore older patients with renal impairment may be at increased risk for (1) fluid overload, (2) accumulation of metabolites and drugs that are excreted by the kidneys, (3) decreased drug elimination, which can prolong the effects of a wide range of anesthetic drugs and adjuncts, and (4) electrolyte imbalances, which can lead to arrhythmias by affecting cardiac conduction.[11,12] The elderly are at higher risk for chronic kidney disease (CKD) because of the aforementioned physiologic and functional kidney changes, the prevalence of coexisting diseases that are associated with CKD (i.e., COPD, hypertension, vascular disease), and with coinciding frailty, complex medical regimens, and polypharmacy. All, or a combination, may induce CKD in the presence of marginal renal function in the elderly patient.

Hepatic Function

The aging adult liver decreases in mass by approximately 20% to 40% and may be attributed to the decrease in its blood flow. Age-related functional hepatic changes primarily affect drug metabolism and protein binding. The age-related physiologic changes in hepatic function may cause decreased metabolism, prolonged half-life, and either increased or decreased distribution of medications. Generally, hepatic functioning is well preserved in the healthy older adult; it is the combination of coexisting diseases (i.e., hepatitis, drug-induced liver injury, cirrhosis) and lifestyle habits (i.e., smoking, alcohol consumption, poor nutrition) that affect liver function more so than the physiologic aging liver. Even so, as with other organ systems, there is a decrease in functional hepatic reserve in the elderly patient.

Phase 1 hepatic degradation reaction of a drug involves oxidation, reduction, and hydrolysis; it is primarily mediated by the cytochrome P-450 system. Phase 2 drug metabolism involves conjugation reactions, sulfonic acid, or acetylation. Age has been identified as an insignificant factor during phase 2 drug metabolism.

The liver produces key proteins such as albumin and α_1-acid glycoprotein (AAG). In the elderly, serum albumin decreases and AAG increases. Serum albumin primarily binds acidic drugs (i.e., benzodiazepines, opioids), and AAG binds basic drugs (i.e., local anesthetics). The effects of these alterations depend on the type of protein the medication is bound to and the resultant concentration of the unbound drug. Theoretically this may result in adverse drug effects especially when malnutrition is present. However, protein binding changes with aging do not routinely require alterations in drug dosing as the protein

BOX 54.1   Risk Factors for Postoperative Pulmonary Complications

Patient-Related Factors
- Age >60 yr
- Chronic obstructive pulmonary disease
- ASA class II or greater
- Functional dependence
- Congestive heart failure
- Obstructive sleep apnea
- Pulmonary hypertension
- Current cigarette use
- Impaired sensorium
- Preoperative sepsis
- Weight loss >10% in 6 mo
- Serum albumin level <3.5 mg/dL
- Blood urea nitrogen level ≥7.5 mmol/L (≥21 mg/dL)
- Serum creatinine level >133 mol/L (>1.5 mg/dL)

Surgery-Related Factors
- Prolonged operation (>3 hr)
- Surgical site
- Emergency operation
- General anesthesia
- Perioperative transfusion
- Residual neuromuscular blockade after an operation

ASA, American Society of Anesthesiologists.
Adapted from Chow WB, et al., American College of Surgeons National Surgical Quality Improvement Program, American Geriatrics Society. Optimal preoperative assessment of the geriatric surgical patient: a best practices guideline from the American College of Surgeons National Surgical Quality Improvement Program and the American Geriatrics Society. *J Am Coll Surg.* 2012;215(4):455.

binding on free plasma concentration is rapidly counteracted by clearance.[13] In the presence of concomitant diseases that affect liver function, the dosing of drugs dependent on hepatic metabolism must be considered.

Endocrine System

The endocrine system also undergoes age-related changes that have widespread effects on other body systems and processes. Nevertheless, few of these changes affect anesthetic management. The most notable endocrine organ to impact the aging adult patient and postoperative morbidity is the pancreas. There is a decline in number and function of the pancreatic islet beta cells that results in decreased insulin secretion. Furthermore, insulin resistance occurs peripherally, which contributes to increased hepatic production of glucose and impaired breakdown of fats and proteins making the elderly glucose tolerant or diabetic. Diabetes is a major risk factor for cardiovascular disease, which increases the risk for perioperative and postoperative complications (i.e., stroke, myocardial infarction, ketoacidosis, infection). Patients with long-term diabetes often have compromise in one or more organ systems.[14] Diabetes and its associated complications (i.e., microvascular disease, cardiovascular disease, and hypertension) place the older adult patient with diabetes at increased risk for developing complications during the perioperative and postoperative period. There are also a number of diabetic complications that have plausible relationships with the aging adult, which may have an impact on perioperative management. For example, diabetes has an effect on brain aging and is associated with playing a role in impaired cognition and Alzheimer dementia.[15,16]

Assessment of the older patient with diabetes includes identification of the type of diabetes, diabetes control (hemoglobin A_{1C}), length of disease, and complications from diabetes. Patients with a history of diabetes for greater than 10 years are particularly at increased risk for complications.[17] Perioperative assessment of the degree of endocrine dysfunction is essential, along with ongoing monitoring and timely intervention when appropriate.

Body Composition and Thermoregulation

Body composition and metabolism changes occur during the aging process. There is a decrease in the basal metabolic rate (BMR) as a result of decreased physical activity and/or decreases in serum testosterone and growth hormone levels. The decreased BMR may have an effect on muscle mass and thermoregulation. Skeletal muscle mass and strength declines with aging with 50% of skeletal mass being lost by the age of 80 years. The loss of skeletal muscle tissue (sarcopenia) is one of the causes of functional decline and independence in the elderly.[18] There is also a significant loss in body protein because of a decrease in skeletal muscle mass and alterations in carrier proteins (e.g., albumin and AAG). At the same time, body fat increases with the aging adult; it is distributed more so in the viscera, subcutaneous abdominal area, and intramuscular and intrahepatic areas. In addition to changes in lean mass and body fat there are changes in total body water. Blood volume decreases approximately 20% to 30% by age 75 years. As a result of decrease in total body water, older adults are more vulnerable to hypotension, and they have difficulty compensating for positional changes. Overall, the body composition changes primarily affect the pharmacokinetics of medications in the elderly and are described later in this chapter.

Thermoregulation in the elderly is also impaired. In the older adult, there is a decrease in the function of the hypothalamus. Hypothermia is more pronounced and lasts longer because of a lower basal metabolic rate, a high ratio of surface to body area mass, and less effective peripheral vasoconstriction in response to cold.[19] It is particularly detrimental in the elderly patient because it slows the elimination of anesthetic medications, prolongs recovery from anesthesia, impairs coagulation, impairs immune function, blunts the ventilatory response to CO_2, and increases the chance that the patient will shiver.[20] Shivering drastically increases oxygen consumption, which can lead to hypoxia, acidosis, and cardiac compromise. It is also known that inhaled anesthetics inhibit the temperature-regulating centers in the hypothalamus. Thermoregulatory vasoconstriction can cause significant peripheral vasoconstriction, predisposing older adults to produce less heat per kilogram of body weight. As a result, older adults may be unable to maintain their heat in the cooler environment of the operating room. Moreover, once temperature decreases in the elderly patient, it is difficult to restore normal body temperature. Methods to maintain normothermia in the older adult patient should involve prevention of heat loss and active warming initiated in the preoperative area and continued perioperatively.[20] Warning strategies include the administration of all fluids and blood transfusions through a warming device, a thermal mattress or forced air warmer, and an environmental humidity higher than 50%.

The elderly have a decrease in dermal and epidermal thickness of the skin, which is caused by a loss of collagen and elastin. Because there is a decrease in subcutaneous fat and thinness of the skin, the aging adult is prone to skin tears and nerve injuries with positioning.

Central Nervous System

Age-related physiologic changes of the central nervous system (CNS) are characterized by a progressive loss of neurons and neuronal substance, decrease in neurotransmitter activity, and decreased brain volume. These losses are most prominent in the cerebral cortex, particularly the frontal lobes. The associated physiologic changes cause a decrease in cerebrospinal fluid, a decrease in nerve conduction velocity, and degeneration of peripheral nerve cells. In addition, there is a decreased number of myelinated nerve fibers. The regulation of brain function, including neuronal membranes, receptors, ion channels, neurotransmitters, cerebral blood flow, and metabolism, is affected by general anesthetics at all levels. Consequently, there are changes in mood, memory, and motor function. In addition, cellular processes that participate in neurotransmitter synthesis and release such as intraneuronal signal transduction and the second messenger system, may be altered.[21] These CNS changes result in an increased sensitivity to anesthetic agents; as a result, there may be an increased risk for postoperative delirium (POD) or cognitive dysfunction.[22] Brain function monitoring (bispectral index monitoring) may be beneficial in the elderly surgical patient. It may assist in guiding the titration of medications and inhalation agent, thus speeding recovery times and perhaps decreasing the incidence of POD and postoperative cognitive dysfunction (POCD).[23-25]

Older patients may experience increased sensitivity to drugs due to receptor downregulation. The blood-brain barrier becomes more permeable, which may also contribute to the sensitivity of medications in addition to neurocognitive disorders such as Alzheimer dementia and delirium.[26,27] Older patients frequently experience an exaggerated response to CNS-depressant drugs with particular sensitivity to general anesthetics, hypnotics, opioids, and benzodiazepines.[22] The dose of induction agents should be decreased by as much as 50% in older patients, arguing for very meticulous titration. Benzodiazepines should be used with caution and (if necessary) in small doses in older adults because they contribute to adverse events (i.e., falls, confusion, POD).[28,29]

CNS changes in the elderly also affect neuraxial anesthesia. The number of myelinated nerve fibers are decreased, and this poses a risk for neural damage with regional anesthetics. Anatomic changes such as decreased intervertebral disc height, narrowing of the intervertebral foramina, decreased space between the posterior spinous processes, presence of calcifications, and changes in normal lordosis contribute to difficulties associated with patient positioning and spinal or epidural needle placement. It is also postulated that the dura is more permeable to local anesthetics and that the CSF specific gravity increases, whereas its volume decreases. All these alterations in the nervous system may produce a more enhanced spread of local anesthetics within the subarachnoid space.[30] Severe hypotension that is refractory to vasopressors may result from sympathectomy following neuraxial anesthesia. This could potentially be detrimental in the presence of impaired cardiac function. There is also an enhanced spread of local anesthetics with epidural blockade. In addition, the use of an epinephrine test dose for identification of intrathecal injection is less reliable in the elderly because of the decreased end-organ adrenergic responsiveness.[31] Therefore a decreased dose of local anesthetic is recommended for subarachnoid and epidural blockade. Overall, subarachnoid and epidural blockades are generally not contraindicated in the elderly patient. A plan of anesthesia should be developed based on patient history and surgical procedure while considering the risks and benefits in an effort to decrease postoperative morbidity and mortality.

ISSUES OF SPECIFIC IMPORTANCE IN THE OLDER ADULT PREOPERATIVE ASSESSMENT

Cognitive Ability/Capability and Decision Making

As there is an increasing rate of neurocognitive disorders in older adults, it is highly recommended by the ACS NSQIP/AGS that their cognitive ability, capacity for decision making, and risk factors for

---

> **BOX 54.2** **Cognitive Assessment**
>
> 1. Get the patient's attention, then say:
>   - "I am going to say three words that I want you to remember now and later. The words are *banana, sunrise, chair*. Please say them for me now."
>   - Give the patient three tries to repeat the words. If unable after three tries, go to the next item.
> 2. Say all the following phrases in the order indicated:
>   - "Please draw a clock in the space below. Start by drawing a large circle. Put all the numbers in the circle and set the hands to show 11:10 (10 past 11)."
>   - If the patient has not finished clock drawing in 3 minutes, discontinue and ask for recall items.
> 3. Say: "What were the three words I asked you to remember?"

In: Chow WB, et al., American College of Surgeons National Surgical Quality Improvement Program, American Geriatrics Society. Optimal preoperative assessment of the geriatric surgical patient: a best practices guideline from the American College of Surgeons National Surgical Quality Improvement Program and the American Geriatrics Society. *J Am Coll Surg.* 2012;215(4):455. From Mini-Cog, copyright S. Borson [soon@uw.edu].

POD be assessed. A preoperative neuropsychiatric assessment establishes a clinical baseline if changes are observed postoperatively and guides perioperative management. The guidelines recommend that a screening tool be used. Several screening tools are available, but the Mini-Cog can be rapidly administered, is highly sensitive and specific for dementia, and is unbiased by variances in education or language. It consists of a three-item recall and a clock draw algorithm (Box 54.2 and Fig. 54.4).[8]

Determining one's decision-making capacity is important to provide informed surgical consent. It is recommended that the surgeon identifies the decision-making ability of the patient during the informed consent. However, it is also the anesthesia provider's responsibility to ensure that the patient is able to make sound decisions. The four legally relevant criteria for decision-making capacity are (1) understanding treatment options, (2) appreciating and acknowledging medical condition and likely outcomes, (3) exhibiting reasoning and engaging in a rational discussion of surgical treatment options, and (4) clearly choosing a preferred treatment option.[5,8]

Frailty

Frailty is a perioperative risk factor for complications and mortality. Estimated frailty rates of 25% to 40% have been reported in surgical patients.[32,33] Frail older adults are more likely to have complications postoperatively, are at increased risk for longer length of hospital stay, and are more likely be discharged to a skilled or assisted living facility.[32,33]

There is no uniform definition of frailty. This may be related to the complexity of the syndrome and the fact that frailty often overlaps with other syndromes. However, most agree that frailty is a biologic state associated with increased vulnerability to adverse outcomes that result from decreased resistance to stressors as a result of deterioration in multiple physiologic systems. Frailty is classified as primary or secondary. Primary frailty occurs as part of the intrinsic process of aging. Secondary frailty is related to the end stage of chronic illnesses and is caused by inflammation and wasting (e.g., heart failure, COPD, inflammation, and wasting associated with cancer). Because frailty serves as an indicator for adverse outcomes and mortality in older adults, ACS NSQIP/AGS guidelines recommend that elderly surgical patients be

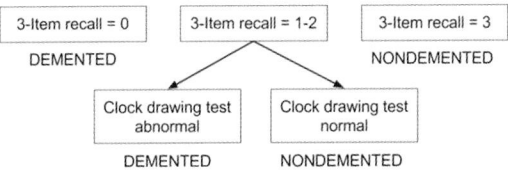

Fig. 54.4 Mini-Cog scoring algorithm. (In: Nakhaie M, Tsai A. Preoperative assessment of geriatric patients. *Anesthesiol Clin.* 2015;33[3]:471–480. Adapted from Borson S, et al. The Mini-Cog: a cognitive "vital signs" measure for dementia screening in multi-lingual elderly. *Int J Geriatr Psych.* 2000;15[11]:1024. With permission.)

> **BOX 54.3   Functional Status Assessment Proxy**
>
> Questions to ask the older adult:
> Can you...
> 1. Get out of bed or the chair by yourself?*
> 2. Dress or bathe yourself?*
> 3. Make your own meals?*
> 4. Do your own grocery shopping?*
>
> If "no" is answered to any of the questions it warrants further in-depth screening and appropriate referrals for perioperative interventions (i.e., physical therapy, social services).

* The answer may not be reliable when neurocognitive disorders are present.
From American College of Surgeons. Optimal perioperative management of the geriatric patient: best practices guideline from ACS NSQIP/American Geriatrics Society. https://www.facs.org/quality-programs/acs-nsqip/geriatric-periop-guideline. Accessed 2020.

assessed for frailty via a validated screening tool. Whereas there are multiple frailty screening tools, Fried et al. created an operational frailty score based on the physiologic parameters of grip strength, weight loss, walking speed, as well as energy level and physical activity. The total scores are categorized as frail, intermediate/prefrail, or nonfrail.[4,34] However, this tool does not include mental health or psychosocial status, which can be a part of frailty. Frailty has also been operationalized as a frailty index.[34] The frailty index defines frailty as the proportion of accumulated deficits over time, including diseases, disability, geriatric syndromes, psychosocial risk factors, and physiologic and cognitive impairment. It is suggested that the frailty index may be more sensitive to the identification of adverse outcomes than Fried's frailty phenotype. Overall, there are many frailty instruments utilized in determining risk of adverse outcomes in individuals. Due to a variation in agreement among frailty instruments, no single instrument has been identified as the gold standard.

Nutritional Status

A nutritional assessment is imperative in the older adult surgical patient. There is no uniform definition for malnutrition in the older adult. Most definitions include specific laboratory indices and body mass index (BMI). However, malnutrition in older adults is common, frequently overlooked, and results in postoperative complications, increased hospital cost, and death. Malnutrition, and protein deficiency (PD) in particular, are key factors for sarcopenia, frailty, and osteoporosis; all can result in disability, loss of independence, falls, fractures, and death in the elderly population.[35] Undernutrition and/or malnutrition is common in the elderly as a result of changes in taste, smell, a reduced ability to purchase and/or prepare food, and decreased functional status.[36] Other factors that may directly influence dietary intake changes include coexisting diseases, cognitive and physical decline, emotional and social changes, and depressive symptoms. Aging is associated with decreases in all the senses, thus it is speculated that the decrease in smell and taste may cause foods to be less appetizing. Practitioners must be vigilant because disease and aging cause decreased lean body mass that may mimic or be confused with malnutrition. Even so, malnutrition should not be discounted in the aging patient because it may contribute to decreased albumin levels that can affect protein binding of medications and impair wound healing. For the older adult surgical patient, decreases in caloric intake combined with illness depletes body caloric reserves necessary to withstand the stress of anesthesia and surgery. Regrettably, no clearly beneficial preoperative medication has been identified that stimulates the appetite in older adults. Multiple validated screening tools exist for identifying risk factors for malnutrition. However, there is no consensus as to which tool should be used for screening. Per the ACS NSQIP/AGS guidelines, if an older adult surgical patient exhibits any one of the following criterion: (1) a BMI less than 18.5 kg/m, (2) serum albumin less than 3 g/dL without evidence of renal or hepatic dysfunction, or (3) unintentional weight loss within the past 6 months of greater than 10% to 15%, then this person

is deemed to be at severe nutritional risk.[5] Those at severe nutritional risk should undergo further in-depth nutritional screening by a dietician with a plan for optimization. Postponement of the surgery may be indicated until nutritional status has improved because malnutrition and PD are associated with increased risk of postoperative complications (i.e., surgical site infection, pneumonia), increased length of hospital stay, and mortality.

Functional Status

The assessment of functional status identifies the older adult's ability to perform self-care tasks, or activities of daily living (i.e., bathing, dressing, toileting), and instrumental activities of daily living (i.e., preparing meals, handling finances, driving, or using public transportation).[4] A preoperative functional status assessment serves as a baseline in physical capacity and assists in determining reasonable and individualized postoperative goals. Impaired preoperative functional status is a predictor for longer postoperative recovery time with poor postoperative outcome, increased risk for POD, and increased length of hospitalization.[37] Functional status can be assessed through proxy report (Box 54.3). In addition, assessing falls through inquiry, and visualizing gait and mobility, assists in identifying the risk for falls. The Timed Up and Go Test (TUGT) can be implemented to establish mobility and gait. This entails having the older adult patient rise from a standard chair, walk approximately 10 ft, turn back, and return to the chair and sit down again. If it takes longer than 20 seconds to complete the test, the patient is determined to be at risk for falls. Longer TUGT times are associated with increased postoperative complications and 1-year mortality among older adult surgical patients.[38] Deficits in vision and hearing can also contribute to fall risk and should be included in the mobility assessment. The most important goals in the perioperative care of older adults are the avoidance of functional decline and maintenance of independence postoperatively.

Review of Medications and Polypharmacy

A thorough review of all medications (i.e., prescription, over the counter [OTC], dietary supplements, herbals) that the older adult is currently taking is critical in identifying medications that should be discontinued prior to surgery, those to consider starting prior to surgery, and those to avoid administering perioperatively. In a 2016 study, it was determined that from 2010 to 2011, 15% of older adults were at risk for a potential major drug-drug interaction as compared to 2005 to 2006, which was approximately 8%.[39] The use of prescription medications, dietary supplements, and concurrent use of five or more medications or supplements also increased in older adults.[39] Polypharmacy, or multiple medication use, is common in older adults and is associated with adverse drug reactions (ADRs) or unwanted side effects. ADRs may be caused by prescribing error (e.g., large dose prescribed without considering decreased renal and/or hepatic clearance) or not taking into account CNS sensitivity.

To help prevent prescribing errors, medication side effects, and ADRs, the American Geriatric Society developed guidelines (*Beer's Criteria for Potentially Inappropriate Medication Use in Older Adults*) for safe prescribing of drugs to older adults. *Beer's Criteria* includes a list of medications that should be avoided or have their dose adjusted based on the older adult's renal function and select drug-drug reactions.[29] Per ACS NSQIP/AGS guidelines, the preoperative review of medications should consist of (1) discontinuing or substituting medications that have potential drug reactions with anesthesia, (2) discontinuing nonessential medications that increase surgical risk, (3) identifying medications that should be discontinued based on *Beer's Criteria*, (4) continuing medications with withdrawal potential, (5) avoiding starting new benzodiazepines and reducing the dose prescribed to patients at risk for POD, (6) avoiding administering meperidine for analgesia, (7) using caution with antihistamines and medications with strong anticholinergic effects, (8) considering starting medications that decrease perioperative cardiovascular adverse events per ACC/AHA guidelines for β-blockers and statins, and (9) adjusting dosing of medications that undergo renal excretion based on estimated GFR.[5]

A medication history may be difficult to obtain or inaccurate if the older adult suffers from cognitive or hearing impairment. Medication compliance and use of OTC, dietary supplements, and herbal supplements may be difficult to ascertain. The preferred approach to the preoperative medication review and perioperative management of the older adult is appreciation for individualized physiologic aging, pharmacokinetic and pharmacodynamics changes with aging, presence of coexisting diseases, and respect for decreased functional reserve.

AGE-RELATED PHARMACOLOGIC IMPLICATIONS IN THE OLDER ADULT

Exaggerated responses to anesthetic drugs and a prolonged duration of action are often seen in the elderly. These differences in drug response are the result of both pharmacokinetic and pharmacodynamic changes associated with aging. Pharmacokinetic alterations occur in the volume of distribution, renal and hepatic clearance rates, compartmental redistribution, and elimination half-lives. A decreased blood volume results in a smaller volume of distribution, which produces a higher-than-expected initial concentration of drug with an intravenous bolus injection. Changes in steady-state volumes of distribution (Vd_{ss}) vary. In aging patients who have an increase in body fat, decrease in lean body mass, and decrease in total body water, there is an increased Vd_{ss} for lipophilic drugs and a decrease for hydrophilic drugs.[22] Decreased plasma protein binding in the elderly theoretically results in an increase in the free plasma concentration for drugs that are highly protein bound. A decrease in renal function resulting from lower renal blood flow, glomerular filtration, and tubular secretion leads to increased serum concentration and prolonged effects of drugs dependent on renal elimination. The elimination of hepatic-dependent drugs varies. Phase I metabolism may be reduced, but phase II metabolic pathways are not affected by age.[13,22]

Pharmacodynamic changes in the elderly include altered receptor density and binding, changes in signal transduction, and impaired cellular responses. Drug-induced changes tend to be prolonged and require a greater length of time for recovery to preanesthetic steady

TABLE 54.4 Recommended Dosing for Perioperative Medications

Agent	Anesthetic Considerations	Dose
Propofol	Hypotension; prolonged recovery; increased brain sensitivity	↓ bolus and infusion by 50% (manufacturer recommends 1–1.5 mg/kg bolus for induction)
Etomidate	Increased brain sensitivity; greater hemodynamic stability	↓ bolus by 50%
Opioids	Increased brain sensitivity; profound physiologic effects; slower onset and delayed recovery; consider route of metabolism and metabolites; avoid meperidine	↓ bolus by 50%
Midazolam	Increased brain sensitivity; avoid per *Beer's Criteria*	Avoid or ↓ dose by 75%
Nondepolarizing MRs	Slower onset and delayed recovery; consider route of metabolism and metabolites; avoid long-acting NDMRs	No significant changes with intubating dose; maintenance dose per PNS twitch response
Depolarizing MR	Slower onset and delayed recovery	No dose adjustment

↓, Decreased; *MRs*, muscle relaxants; *NDMRs*, nondepolarizing muscle relaxants; *PNS*, peripheral nerve stimulator.

state. The minimal alveolar concentration (MAC) of inhalational agents decreases roughly 6.7% per decade from the MAC value of 40-year-old adults.[40,41]

In elderly patients, pharmacokinetics are significantly altered. For all neuromuscular blocking drugs, the onset of action may be prolonged.[22] Most of the nondepolarizing neuromuscular blockers are metabolized by the liver and excreted via the kidney, and in the presence of coexisting hepatic or renal disease there may be a prolonged effect. This residual neuromuscular blockade, in combination with the loss of pharyngeal and muscular support that is required to protect the airway, increases the risk for postoperative respiratory failure and/or aspiration. The neuromuscular blocking medication of choice for the older adult is cisatracurium due to Hoffman elimination and ester hydrolysis.

Currently, there are no specific medication dosing guidelines for anesthesia medications for the older adult patient. Suggested dosing adjustments for perioperative medications are found in Table 54.4. Postoperative pain control and analgesics in the elderly surgical patient are discussed in Chapter 56.

COMORBIDITY IN THE OLDER ADULT

The definitions for *comorbidity* and *multimorbidity* are unclear in the literature. Therefore this section will use both terms interchangeably. It is defined as two or more chronic medical conditions within one person.[42,43] In the United States, multimorbidity has increased with advanced age, even though mortality rates have declined. It is associated with an increased risk for death, disability, poor functional status, ADRs, and increased length of hospitalization and health care costs.[44,45] Multimorbidity increases steeply with older adults. The prevalence of multimorbidity in those 65 to 74 years of age is approximately

62%, at ages 75 to 84 years it is 75%, and 81% in those who are 85 years of age and older.[44,46] The most common multimorbidities in the older adult include hypertension, hyperlipidemia, diabetes, and ischemic heart disease. Prevalence varies by sex; women have more arthritis than men, and men have more heart disease than women. Prevalence also varies by race, with older adult Hispanics and blacks having higher rates of hypertension, diabetes, and metabolic syndrome as compared to whites.[4,46]

Multimorbity in the older adult is common, and it is strongly associated with frailty and poor postoperative outcomes.[43] Even so, older age and presence of multimorbidities should not be limiting factors for surgical treatment. Compared with younger surgical patients, the older adult is at relatively increased risk for morbidity and mortality after elective surgery but is at 30% higher risk for postoperative complications and mortality with emergency surgery.[47-50] Therefore a multidisciplinary approach to individualized preoperative care and optimization is essential with the goal of avoiding postoperative complications and returning the older adult patient to the same presurgical state.

ETHICAL ISSUES IN THE TREATMENT OF THE OLDER ADULT

The advances in medical treatment, changes in the health care system, and aging of US residents have given rise to specific ethical dilemmas that anesthesia providers encounter in the older adult. The older adult patient often has other complicating factors (i.e., coexisting diseases, impaired cognition, impaired decision-making capacity, insufficient social support), which adds to the complexity in ethical issues. Examples of ethical issues in the older adult surgical patient include informed consent, advanced directives (ADs), and perioperative do-not-resuscitate (DNR) orders. The basic principles in ethical decision making that apply to the older adult are the same as those that apply to all patients. In health care, the most common principles are (1) autonomy, (2) beneficence, (3) nonmaleficence, and (4) justice. Ethical principles are defined in Box 54.4. Certified Registered Nurse Anesthetists (CRNAs) follow the American Nurses Association Nursing Code of Ethics in their daily practice and abide by the American Association of Nurse Anesthetists (AANA) Code of Ethics in guiding ethical decision making. As professionals we base our decisions on "ethics of obligation," yet personally we base them on "ethics of the good."[51] Unfortunately, difficult and complex situations arise that challenge the anesthesia providers. Personal values and biases must be recognized while acknowledging, appreciating, and upholding the patient's desires and decisions regarding health care.

Informed consent is the cornerstone for upholding the practice of autonomy. However, all the ethical principles are involved when a patient makes an informed decision regarding health care. Older age alone is not an obstacle to practicing autonomy. An important aspect of the informed consent is assessing and ensuring that the patient has the cognitive ability/capability for decision making. Informed consent is discussed in Chapter 20, and assessing cognitive capability/ability for decision making during the preoperative assessment is vital. Legally and ethically, anesthesia providers and other practitioners must disclose factual, truthful information while being objective and free of personal bias.

Autonomy is also exercised through an AD. This legal document enables a surrogate or agent to act on the patient's behalf when the patient is unable to make health care decisions. The patient has communicated one's beliefs and values about health care decisions and life-sustaining treatment and appoints a surrogate. In 1991, legislation enacted the Patient Self-Determination Act (PSDA), which requires hospitals and other health organizations that receive Medicare funds

> ### BOX 54.4 Ethical Principles
> - *Autonomy:* Patient's right to self-determination
> - *Beneficence:* An obligation or responsibility to help the patient; "to do good"
> - *Nonmaleficence:* To not intentionally harm the patient; "do no harm"
> - *Justice:* To treat the patient fairly

to provide information to patients regarding their right and refusal of care (i.e., ADs). Since its inception, completion rates of ADs have risen; only 50% of older adults have ADs, however.[52] As ADs are legislated at the state level there may be differing standards and laws for each state. Unlike an AD, a living will (LW), or directive to physicians, are death with dignity declarations, which provide specific instructions to the attending physician(s) stating the patient's desired treatment for care when the patient's decision-making capacity is lost because of a terminal or end-stage illness. LWs primarily direct resuscitation and withdrawal of life-sustaining treatment.[53] Unfortunately, this document is limited to delineated medical situations and does not account for unforeseen circumstances. Regardless of which legal document the patient has, a review of the document and a conversation should take place between the practitioner(s) and patient concerning health care wishes/goals during the perioperative period.[51]

Informed consent is not limited to surgical procedures and anesthetic technique; it is also applicable to the perioperative DNR order. Health care providers are taught that it is their duty to provide care that is beneficial to the patient. Hence, in the presence of a patient who is undergoing surgery with a DNR status, health care providers may feel compelled to suspend the DNR in the event that heroic measures are needed. From the perspective of anesthesia providers, it is their responsibility to ensure that the patient has a positive anesthetic outcome. Even though anesthesia providers view that suspending the DNR status will inevitably help the patient in the event that cardiopulmonary resuscitation is needed, the DNR suspension may not be aligned with the patient's view of beneficence or desires. Therefore anesthesia providers cannot assume what is best for the patient; the patient or surrogate needs to have informed consent regarding the alternatives of the DNR status while in the operating room to make an informed decision based on personal wishes, values, and beliefs. Because of this circumstance, the ASA suggests that specific resuscitation alternatives during the surgical procedure be presented and discussed with the patient. These three alternatives include (1) the full suspension of the DNR status intraoperatively and postoperatively, (2) the acceptance or refusal of specific resuscitative interventions (i.e., chest compressions, defibrillation, vasopressor administration) with full documentation of these in the medical record, and (3) resuscitation procedures will be determined by the anesthesia provider and the surgeon based on clinical judgment, while keeping in mind the patient's values and wishes.[54,55] The AANA also developed practice guidelines that address the reconsideration of ADs prior to surgery, which are similar to the ASA and are found in Box 54.5.

Facility policy is also used as a resource in guiding the practitioner in addressing DNR status of a patient undergoing surgery. Each patient and accompanying surgical procedure should be addressed on a unique case-by-case matter. After an informed discussion, an agreement should be made on the DNR status by the patient or surrogate, surgeon, and anesthesia provider. Lastly, the perioperative DNR status should be documented in the medical record to substantiate the agreement and to inform all health care providers of the designated plan.

It is widely accepted that chronologic age is possibly an independent risk factor for anesthesia and surgery; its specific role as a risk factor is difficult to ascertain. Each patient should be treated fairly, regardless of age. The ethical principle of social justice is not providing the greatest good for the greatest number of people; it is treating people equally, regardless of their age, race, cultural beliefs, religion, disease processes, or resuscitation status.[51] Every patient should be informed, at a comparable level, of all the alternatives regarding resuscitation when undergoing any surgical procedure. It is a matter of justice to ensure adequate and equitable informed anesthesia consent to all surgical patients. Therefore age, as an independent factor, should not be regarded as a reason to exclude an older adult for any procedure.

POSTOPERATIVE DELIRIUM

POD and POCD are the most frequently occurring neurologic phenomena in older adults. POD and POCD are distinct conditions, with age over 65 years being the predominant risk factor for both.

POD is characterized by disruption of perception, thinking, memory, psychomotor behavior, sleep-wake cycle, consciousness, and attention.[56,57] Its clinical presentation varies with hypoactive symptoms (e.g., decreased motor activity and depression), hyperactive symptoms (e.g., aggression and agitation), or a combination thereof. In some instances, hypoactive symptoms are unrecognizable, which results in misdiagnosis of POD.[5,58] Symptoms typically manifest acutely within the first few days after surgery and can last for several days or weeks. The exact cause of POD is not known but is likely multifactorial. Risk factors that have been associated with the development of POD are older age, male gender, dementia, history of alcohol abuse, depression, duration of anesthesia, poor functional status, abnormal electrolytes and glucose, Parkinson disease, cardiovascular disease, dehydration, metabolic diseases (e.g., diabetes, hyperthyroidism), anticholinergic drugs used intraoperatively, patients requiring admission to the intensive care unit, inadequate pain control, ASA greater than or equal to 3, low serum albumin, and type of surgery.[59-66] Depending on the type of procedure, the rate of POD ranges from 9% to 50% with a high incidence occurring in aortic and orthopedic procedures.[5,67] POD is associated with increased risk of postoperative adverse reactions (i.e., pulmonary and cardiac), increased length of hospital stay, increased health care cost, poor functional and cognitive recovery, and death.[63,68,69]

The treatment of POD begins with prevention. Preoperatively, health care providers should identify patients who are at high risk for POD, including age over 65 years, chronic cognitive decline or dementia, poor hearing or vision, presence of infection, current hip fracture, or severe illness. In combination with the risk factors, the physiologic stress of surgery, which is determined by the extent of the operation, may cumulatively contribute to the development of POD. Once POD

is diagnosed, treatment is dependent on the identifying cause. After treating the underlying cause it is recommended that health care providers use multicomponent nonpharmacologic interventions (i.e., frequent reorientation, calm environment, eliminating restraint use, and ensuring the use of hearing aids/glasses). The use of pharmacologic interventions (i.e., haloperidol, lorazepam) should be reserved for those who are highly agitated and are threatening harm to self and/or others.[5,56,70] Other recommendations for anesthesia providers include (1) administering regional anesthesia for postoperative pain control thereby potentially preventing delirium, (2) intraoperative electroencephalogram (EEG) monitoring during intravenous sedation or general anesthesia as EEG suppression has been identified as an independent risk factor for POD, and (3) conducting a thorough review of medications preoperatively while avoiding medications per *Beer's Criteria.*[20,25,71] Furthermore, it is suggested that the perioperative administration of dexmedetomidine may decrease the incidence of POD.[72-74]

POSTOPERATIVE COGNITIVE DYSFUNCTION

POCD is often reported as being part of the same continuum as POD. Even though they are both neurocognitive disorders that contribute to increased hospital costs, morbidity, and mortality, there are differences. POCD is characterized by an array of cognitive impairments such as memory deficits, difficulty with concentration, impaired comprehension, and delayed psychomotor speed. Unlike POD, the onset of POCD is subtle, and neurocognitive deficits may not present themselves until weeks to months after surgery. This ultimately results in the inability to work, a decline in activities of daily living, and perhaps a need for assisted care.[57]

Currently, there are no universally accepted diagnostic criteria for POCD, nor is there a standard definition. To diagnose POCD, a battery of time-consuming and sophisticated neurocognitive tests must be done preoperatively and postoperatively in identifying cognitive decline after surgery and anesthesia. Establishing baseline cognitive function is critical because preoperative cognitive impairment may be present prior to surgery. However, preoperative test timing, specific test(s), and test interpretations remain inconsistent and debatable. Risk factors for POCD are also controversial, with advanced age being the most agreed upon. Other risks may include lower educational level, longer duration of anesthesia, preoperative depression, preoperative cognitive decline, postoperative infection, and second operation[57] (Box 54.6).

The cause of this neurocognitive postoperative complication is still unknown and appears to be multifactorial. However, several theories have been postulated. Common theories include cerebral hypoperfusion (severe hypotension and embolic events), the inflammatory process associated with surgery, and general anesthetics.[25,57,75-77] Similar to POD, the physiologic mechanisms responsible for POCD are yet to be elucidated. However, potential mechanisms include neuroinflammation, dopamine excess and acetylcholine deficiency, and central cholinergic deficiency.[75-79] An array of human biomarkers reflective of these mechanisms are being investigated. However, currently the diagnosis of POD or POCD is not supported by any specific biomarkers.

Presently, there is no known cure for POCD, and patients who suffer from it may not recover to their preoperative cognitive state. The pathogenesis of POCD is multifactorial and unclear, and strategies should be aimed at prevention. Unfortunately, there are no proven effective strategies. However, based on the knowledge that the elderly have decreased nervous system function and decreased cognitive reserve, efforts should consist in identifying risk factors and tailoring anesthetic management to minimize them. Recommendations are aimed at maintaining oxygenation and cerebral perfusion.[76] It has been speculated that POCD may be caused by general anesthesia and/or surgery. Therefore it is only prudent that short and minimally invasive surgical procedures are desirable. Overall, there is no consensus in the literature regarding the most appropriate anesthetic technique for the elderly surgical patient.

SUMMARY

The United States is on the cusp of a very racially and ethnically diverse aging population surge. Health care providers will face many challenges in keeping pace with a more comprehensive preoperative elderly assessment, which will identify perioperative risks, assist with optimizing the older adult, and improve postoperative outcomes. The goal of anesthesia for the older adult is the same as for any other patient. However, the physiologic changes, multimorbidities, and functional decline in all organ systems of the older adult affect every aspect of the perioperative course. Anesthesia for the elderly patient is no longer an empiric specialty; the practice of anesthesia for elderly patients is a multidisciplinary team approach built on evidence-based quality care.

REFERENCES

For a complete list of references for this chapter, scan this QR code with any smartphone code reader app, or visit the following URL: http://booksite.elsevier.com/9780323711944/.

55

Postanesthesia Recovery

Jan Odom-Forren, Joni M. Brady

The term *perianesthesia patient care* reflects a continuum of care because the patient is moved from the preanesthesia holding or admitting area to the surgery suite (operating room [OR]) and then to the postanesthesia care unit (PACU). The term *postanesthesia recovery* refers to those activities undertaken to manage the patient after completion of a surgical or nonsurgical procedure in which anesthesia, analgesia, or sedation was administered. The primary purpose of postanesthesia recovery is the critical assessment and stabilization of patients after these procedures, with an emphasis on prevention and detection of complications.[1] Care in the postanesthesia phase I unit centers on providing immediate postanesthesia nursing care and transitioning the patient to the intensive care setting, the inpatient setting, or phase II outpatient care.[2] The focus of this chapter is on the postanesthesia care of patients with the goals of improving postanesthetic safety and quality of life, reducing postoperative adverse events, providing a uniform assessment of recovery, and streamlining postoperative care and discharge criteria.

POSTANESTHESIA CARE UNIT ADMISSION

Before the patient is transferred, PACU personnel should be notified not only to expect the transfer but also to have any necessary equipment (e.g., ventilator, nebulizer, invasive monitoring equipment, pharmacologic infusions, and capnograph) ready and waiting. Knowledge of the patient's acuity enables the PACU staff to best plan the patient's care and assign that care to an appropriately experienced practitioner.

Both the anesthesia provider and the PACU nurse (and OR nurse, if available) should collaborate in the patient's admission to the PACU. The immediate priority is evaluation of respiratory and circulatory adequacy. During this initial assessment, any signs of inadequate oxygenation or ventilation are identified, as well as the cause (Boxes 55.1 and 55.2). Although many of the signs of respiratory compromise could have multifactorial explanations, assessment of the adequacy of oxygenation and ventilation ensures that respiratory inadequacy is not contributory. Any evidence of respiratory compromise requires immediate correction.

Electrocardiographic (ECG) monitoring is initiated for determination of cardiac rate and rhythm. Any deviation from preoperative or intraoperative findings is noted and evaluated. In addition, blood pressure is measured, and adequacy of organ perfusion is determined. Any necessary invasive monitoring, such as an arterial line, is initiated. Any evidence of cardiocirculatory compromise requires immediate correction.

The anesthesia provider should be active during the patient's transfer and stabilization in the PACU. Assistance in the initiation of oxygen therapy, maintenance or verification of airway adequacy, and assessment of circulatory status familiarizes PACU personnel with the patient and fosters a smooth transfer of care. After initially stabilizing the patient, the anesthesia provider can communicate relevant preoperative and intraoperative data to the PACU nurse.

ANESTHESIA REPORT

To ensure patient safety and continuity of care, the anesthesia provider must give a verbal handoff report to the PACU nurse that specifies the details of the surgical and anesthetic course, the preoperative conditions that warrant or influence the surgical and anesthetic outcome, and the PACU treatment plan, including suggested interventions and endpoints. Transfer of the patient from the OR to the PACU is a critical patient handoff and should include an opportunity for the PACU nurse to ask questions and the anesthesia provider to respond. Communication errors can occur during the process of a handoff. Proper handovers have been hampered by inadequate preparation on how to perform handovers, a lack of a standardized process, inadequate communication skills, lack of time for transfer of information, information loss, distractions, interruptions, and limited opportunity to ask questions or voice concerns.[3,4] To decrease these communication errors, handoff information needs to be standardized and communicated in a logical and meaningful manner.[3,4] The use of a checklist will improve the information that is transferred from one health care provider to another and decrease omission of important elements of care.[3] A logical order for the presentation of this information is presented in Box 55.3. There should also be an opportunity for questions and answers.

The importance of the handoff and anesthesia report is reflected in the American Association of Nurse Anesthetists (AANA) *Postanesthesia Care Practice Considerations*: "Evaluate the patient's status and determine when it is appropriate to transfer the responsibility of care to another qualified healthcare provider. Communicate the patient's condition and essential information for continuity of care."[5] AANA also states "the handoff should be a two-way interaction, preferably face-to-face."[5] The American Society of Anesthesiologists (ASA) points to the importance of a verbal report to the responsible PACU nurse but also goes on to state, "The member of the Anesthesia Care Team shall remain in the PACU until the PACU nurse accepts responsibility for the nursing care of the patient."[6] Anesthesia personnel must assist in management of the patient until PACU providers secure admission vital signs and attach appropriate monitors. To optimize safety, the anesthesia provider cannot shift responsibility to PACU personnel until the patient's airway status, ventilation, and hemodynamics are appropriate.[5,6]

INITIAL POSTANESTHESIA CARE UNIT ASSESSMENT

Accurate and vigilant nursing assessment is vital because of how quickly a patient's condition can change in the PACU. Many postanesthesia assessment approaches (e.g., head to toe, major body systems assessments, and scoring systems) are currently used in PACUs, and each approach has its benefits and limitations. The assessment approach should accomplish the following:

BOX 55.1 Signs and Symptoms of Hypoxia

Respiratory
- Shallow, rapid respirations or normal, infrequent respirations
- Tachypnea
- Dyspnea
- Oxygen saturation <90%

Neurologic
- Anxiety, restlessness, inattentiveness
- Altered mental status, confusion
- Dimmed peripheral vision
- Seizures
- Combativeness, late
- Unresponsiveness, late

Skin
- Diaphoresis
- Cyanosis

Cardiac
- *Early:* Tachycardia
- Increased cardiac output
- Increased stroke volume
- Increased blood pressure
- *Late:* Bradycardia, hypotension
- Dysrhythmias

From Grape S, et al. Postoperative cognitive dysfunction. *Trends Anaesth Crit Care.* 2012;2:98–103; Mondor E. Assessment: respiratory system. In: Hardin M, et al. *Lewis' Medical-Surgical Nursing.* 11th ed. St. Louis, MO: Elsevier; 2020.

BOX 55.2 Causes of Hypoxemia

- *Hypoventilation*—Alveolar ventilation is abnormally low in relation to oxygen uptake or carbon dioxide output; causes a raised arterial P_{CO_2} and arterial hypoxemia
- *Diffusion limitation*—Oxygen, carbon dioxide are affected as they cross the blood-gas barrier by simple passive diffusion
- *Shunt*—The entry of blood into the systemic arterial system without going through ventilated areas of lung
- *Ventilation-perfusion relationships*—A mismatch of ventilation and blood flow

P_{CO_2}; Partial pressure of carbon dioxide.
Modified from Powell, et al. Ventilation, blood flow, and gas exchange. In: Mason RJ, et al. *Murray and Nadel's Textbook of Respiratory Medicine.* 6th ed. Philadelphia: Elsevier; 2016:44–75.

- Determine the patient's physiologic status at the time of admission to the PACU.
- Allow the periodic reexamination of the patient so that physiologic trends become obvious.
- Establish the patient's baseline level so that the effect of previous medical conditions can be assessed and predicted as they affect current physiology.
- Assess the ongoing status of the surgical site and its effect on any preexisting conditions and recovery.
- Assess the patient's recovery from anesthesia and note residual effects.

BOX 55.3 Anesthesia Admission Report

General Information
- Patient name
- Patient age
- Surgical procedure
- Name of surgeon and anesthesia provider(s)
- Type of procedure

Patient History
- Acute (indication for surgery)
- Chronic (medical history, medication use, allergies, obstructive sleep apnea, cognitive issues)
- Sensory devices and location, if appropriate

Intraoperative Management
- Anesthetic agents, including dose and technique
- Time of last opioid administration
- Administration of reversal agents
- Intraoperative medications (antibiotics, antiemetics, vasopressors)
- Estimated blood loss
- Fluid and blood administration
- Urine output

Intraoperative Course
- Unexpected response to anesthetic administration
- Unexpected surgical course
- Laboratory results (arterial blood gas, glucose, hemoglobin)

Postanesthesia Care Unit Plan
- Potential and expected problems
- Pain and comfort management interventions
- Other suggested interventions
- Limits of acceptability of laboratory tests
- Any cultural considerations
- Discharge criteria
- Responsible contact person

- Prevent or immediately treat complications that occur.
- Provide a safe environment for the patient who is impaired physically, mentally, or emotionally.
- Allow the compilation and trend analysis of patient-specific characteristics that relate to discharge or transfer criteria.[1,7]

Assessment Scoring Systems

The most commonly used assessment approach is a combination of a scoring system and a major body systems assessment. The Aldrete postanesthetic scoring system[8] is the most widely used scoring system in PACUs, although its predictive value in determining recovery from anesthesia has not been studied prospectively (Box 55.4). No consensus exists to date regarding the variables any scoring system instrument should contain. In a systematic review conducted to investigate assessment criteria of adult patients, the key recommendations were that pain, conscious state, blood pressure, and nausea/vomiting should be assessed before discharge.[9] The use of urinary output and oral fluid intake as criteria need further research. The American Society of Peri-Anesthesia Nurses (ASPAN) does not require a scoring system nor recommend any one scoring system while recognizing that a postanesthesia scoring system may be a component of the facility's discharge criteria.[2]

BOX 55.4   Postanesthesia Recovery Score

Activity
0 = Unable to lift head or move extremities voluntarily or on command
1 = Moves two extremities voluntarily or on command and can lift head
2 = Able to move four extremities voluntarily or on command. Can lift head and
    has controlled movement. *Exceptions:* Patients with a prolonged block such
    as with bupivacaine (Marcaine), who may not move an affected extremity
    for as long as 18 hr; patients who were immobile preoperatively

Respiration
0 = Apneic; condition necessitates ventilator or assisted respiration
1 = Labored or limited respirations; breathes by self but has shallow, slow
    respirations; may have an oral airway
2 = Can take a deep breath and cough well; has normal respiratory rate and
    depth

Circulation
0 = Has abnormally high or low blood pressure; blood pressure within
    50 mm Hg of preanesthetic level
1 = Blood pressure within 20–50 mm Hg of preanesthetic level
2 = Stable blood pressure and pulse. Blood pressure 20 mm Hg of prean-
    esthetic level (minimum 90 mm Hg systolic). *Exception:* Patient may be
    released by anesthesia provider after drug therapy

Neurologic Status
0 = Not responding or responding only to painful stimuli
1 = Responds to verbal stimuli but drifts to sleep easily
2 = Awake and alert; oriented to time, place, and person

O$_2$ Saturation
0 = O$_2$ saturation <90%, even with O$_2$ supplement
1 = Needs O$_2$ inhalation to maintain O$_2$ saturation >90%
2 = Able to maintain O$_2$ saturation >92% on room air

Modified from Ead H. From Aldrete to PADSS: reviewing discharge criteria after ambulatory surgery. *J Perianesth Nurs.* 2006;21:259–267.

BOX 55.5   Criteria for Initial Assessment: Phase I Postanesthesia Care Unit

Initial assessment and documentation include:
1. Integration of data received at transfer of care
   a. Pertinent medical history, including allergies, devices
   b. Surgical/procedural status (reason for surgery, procedure performed)
   c. Anesthesia/sedation technique and agents
   d. Length of time anesthesia/sedation administered
   e. Pain and comfort interventions and plan
   f. Medications administered
   g. Estimated fluid deficit/blood loss and replacement
   h. Complications during course of anesthesia and response to treatment
   i. Emotional status preprocedure
2. Vital signs
   a. Respiratory status—airway patent, breath sounds, type of artificial
      airway, mechanical ventilatory settings, oxygen saturation, end tidal
      CO$_2$ (if indicated)
   b. Blood pressure—noninvasive or arterial line
   c. Pulse—apical, peripheral
   d. Continuous cardiac monitoring, rhythm documented
   e. Temperature/route
   f. Hemodynamic pressure readings: central venous, pulmonary artery,
      and wedge; intracranial pressure as indicated
   g. Pregnancy related assessments (e.g., fetal heart tones)
3. Pain and comfort level
4. Sedation level
5. Neurologic function to include level of consciousness; presence of delirium,
   pupillary response as indicated
6. Sensory and motor function as appropriate
7. Position of patient
8. Condition and color of skin
9. Patient safety needs (e.g., medication reconciliation, fall risk assessment)
10. Neurovascular: peripheral pulses and sensation of extremity(ies) as applicable
11. Condition of dressings and visible incisions
12. Type and patency of drainage tubes, catheters, and receptacles; effec-
    tively secured
13. Amount and type of drainage
14. Fluid intake (e.g., intravenous, oral, feeding tube)
15. Intravenous assessment: location of lines, condition of intravenous site,
    type of solution infusing
16. Procedure-specific assessment (i.e., firmness of abdomen)
17. Medication management
18. Nursing actions with outcome
19. Inclusion of family in physical, spiritual, emotional care as indicated
20. Postanesthesia scoring system if used (not required—facility-developed
    discharge criteria that may include a scoring system as a component of
    the assessment)

Modified from American Society of Perianesthesia Nurses (ASPAN). *Perianesthesia Nursing Standards and Practice Recommendations 2019–2020.* Cherry Hill, NJ: ASPAN; 2018.

Major Body Systems

The major body systems assessment systematically evaluates the body systems that are most affected by anesthesia and the surgical procedure. After the patient is admitted to the PACU, an assessment of cardiorespiratory stability and a more in-depth cardiac assessment are performed. Respiratory assessment comprises rate, depth of ventilation, auscultation of breath sounds, oxygen saturation level, and end tidal carbon dioxide, if appropriate. Type of oxygen delivery system and presence of any artificial airway should be noted.[10] The heart is auscultated, and the quality of heart sounds, the presence of any adventitious sounds, and any irregularities in rate or rhythm are noted. Unexpected findings are compared with preoperative data. Arterial pulses are evaluated for strength and equality. An ECG strip is obtained on admission to the PACU and compared with the preoperative ECG. Alarms are on and audible.[7] In addition, body temperature and skin color and condition are assessed and the findings documented.

After respiratory and cardiac assessments are completed, the neurologic system is evaluated, with a focus on the level of consciousness, orientation, sensory and motor function, and pupil size, equality, and reactivity. The patient is assessed on ability to follow commands and move extremities purposefully and equally.[7]

The renal system assessment focuses on fluid intake and output (e.g., blood, crystalloids, and colloids), as well as on volume and electrolyte status. The anesthesia provider relates intraoperative fluid totals in the verbal report, and the PACU nurse notes and documents all intravenous lines, irrigation solutions, and infusions that enter the patient. All output devices, including drains, catheters, and tubes, are inspected, and the color and consistency of any drainage are noted.

The surgical site is examined. The amount and color of any drainage on the bandage are noted. The patient is also assessed for pain or discomfort, such as nausea, with appropriate interventions administered.

All data obtained in the admission assessment should be documented in a manner that facilitates data collection, trend analysis, and retrieval. Recommended criteria for the initial assessment of a patient in the PACU are included in Box 55.5.

ONGOING ASSESSMENT

Perioperative and postanesthetic management of the patient includes ongoing assessment and monitoring of the following[2,11]:

- Respiratory function (e.g., obstruction, hypoxemia, hypercarbia)
- Cardiovascular function (e.g., hypotension, hypertension, dysrhythmias)
- Neuromuscular function (e.g., inadequate reversal of neuromuscular blockade)
- Mental status (e.g., delayed awakening, emergence delirium)
- Pain
- Temperature (e.g., hypothermia)
- Nausea and vomiting
- Fluids
- Urine output and voiding

Respiratory Function

The most common cause of airway obstruction in the immediate postoperative phase is the loss of pharyngeal muscle tone in a sedated or obtunded patient. The loss of pharyngeal muscle tone immediately after surgery is mainly due to the lasting effects of the anesthetic agents, neuromuscular blocking drugs, and opioids.[12]

Obstruction

In postanesthesia patients, the tongue causes most upper airway obstructions. Obstruction occurs when the tongue falls back into a position that occludes the pharynx and blocks the flow of air into and out of the lungs.

Signs and symptoms of an upper airway obstruction include snoring and activation of accessory muscles of ventilation. Intercostal and suprasternal retractions may be noted. However, patients are usually somnolent and may be difficult to arouse. Risk factors for an upper airway obstruction include anatomy (e.g., obesity, large neck, or short neck), poor muscle tone (secondary to opioids, sedation, residual neuromuscular blockade, or neuromuscular disease), or swelling (secondary to surgical manipulation, edema, or anaphylaxis).

The goal for the relief of a tongue obstruction is a patent airway. Treatment consists of a series of interventions. The initial intervention may be as simple as stimulating the patient to take deep breaths, or it may require repositioning of the airway via a jaw thrust or a chin lift. Placement of an oral or a nasal airway may be required. The nasal airway is tolerated much better by patients emerging from general anesthesia, and, unlike the oral airway, it is unlikely to cause gagging or vomiting. A jaw thrust with continuous positive airway pressure (CPAP; 10–15 cm H_2O) is often enough to open the upper airway.[12] If the obstruction remains unrelieved, reintubation may be required, with or without adjunctive mechanical ventilation.

Laryngeal obstruction may occlude the airway as a result of partial or complete spasm of the intrinsic or extrinsic muscles of the larynx. Laryngospasm may be the result of a reflex closure of the glottis (intrinsic muscles) or the larynx (extrinsic muscles). Glottic closure usually manifests as intermittent obstruction; laryngeal closure manifests as complete obstruction. Airway irritation that predisposes a patient to laryngospasm may be the result of laryngoscopy, secretions, vomitus, blood, artificial airway placement, coughing, bronchospasm, or frequent suctioning. Symptoms that suggest laryngospasm include agitation, decreased oxygen saturation, absent breath sounds, and acute respiratory distress. Incomplete obstruction may manifest as a crowing sound or stridor.

Treatment of laryngospasm must be immediate. A jaw thrust maneuver in conjunction with CPAP (up to 40 cm H_2O) is often sufficient to disrupt the laryngospasm. If this intervention is ineffective, a subparalytic dose of intravenous succinylcholine (0.1–1 mg/kg) or 4

---

mg/kg intramuscularly) may be given by the anesthesia provider.[12] If succinylcholine is administered, assisted ventilation for 5 to 10 minutes is required, even if the obstruction has been relieved. Reintubation is undesirable and should be used only if severe airway edema is present or if the obstruction persists despite treatment interventions. During the crisis, the anesthesia provider should consider medication for sedation, such as midazolam, to alleviate the possibility of an awake or partially awake patient.

Steroids and topical or intravenous lidocaine have been included in the prevention and management of airway irritability. Other preventive strategies include obtaining meticulous hemostasis during surgery, suctioning the oropharynx before extubation to clear any retained blood or secretions, and extubating when the patient is in either a very deep plane of anesthesia or the awake state. When obstruction occurs, rapid intervention is imperative.

Obstructive sleep apnea. Obstructive sleep apnea (OSA) is associated with diminished muscle tone in the airway, which leads to airway obstruction during sleep.[13] There is a high prevalence of diagnosed OSA and an estimated 12 to 18 million adults undiagnosed. OSA is associated with an increased incidence of complications, including difficult intubation, length of stay in the PACU, unplanned admission, and other respiratory and cardiovascular complications.[14] The ASA and the ASPAN have practice recommendations/guidelines for care of the patient with OSA during the perioperative period.[13,15] Box 55.6 includes an overview of the ASPAN practice recommendations. Use of standardized screening improves preoperative diagnosis of OSA. The screening instrument with the highest validity and ease of use is the STOP-Bang clinical scale (http://www.stopbang.ca).[13] Patient management includes a well-planned anesthetic, including regional anesthesia with minimal sedation when appropriate. Postoperative management includes analgesia, positioning, oxygenation, and monitoring concerns.[16] When a patient has a known diagnosis of OSA, plans should be made preoperatively to provide CPAP in the immediate postoperative period, and those patients should be asked to bring their CPAP machines with them on the day of surgery.[12,16] Each institution should have a multidisciplinary guideline that addresses the needs of this patient population.

Hypoxemia

Hypoxemia, defined as low arterial oxygen pressure PaO_2 <60 mm/Hg is characterized by nonspecific signs and symptoms ranging from agitation to somnolence, hypertension to hypotension, and tachycardia to bradycardia. Pulse oximetry may confirm low oxygen saturation (<90%); arterial blood gas analysis may confirm a PaO_2 of less than 60 mm Hg. Hypoxemia, if untreated, can result in organ ischemia.

Hypoxemia can be the result of a delivered airway obstruction, low concentration of oxygen, hypoventilation, impaired alveolar-capillary diffusion, ventilation-perfusion mismatches, or increased intrapulmonary shunting.[12,17] The most common causes of hypoxemia in the PACU include atelectasis, pulmonary edema, pulmonary embolism, aspiration, bronchospasm, and hypoventilation. A brief explanation of these pathologic states follows.

Clinical issues with pulse oximetry have to be considered when used to determine oxygen saturation levels. The relationship between percent of hemoglobin saturated with oxygen (SaO_2) and the partial pressure of oxygen in the blood (PaO_2) is symbolized by the oxyhemoglobin dissociation curve. Shifts in the oxyhemoglobin dissociation curve are caused by abnormal values of pH, temperature, partial pressure of carbon dioxide, and 2,3-diphosphoglycerate. The patient's level of hemoglobin must also be considered because if it is too low even fully saturated hemoglobin is not adequate to meet the tissues metabolic needs.[1]

Atelectasis

Atelectasis is the most common cause of postoperative arterial hypoxemia and can lead to an increase in right-to-left shunt. Atelectasis may be the result of bronchial obstruction caused by secretions or decreased lung volumes. Hypotension and low cardiac output conditions can also contribute to the development of decreased perfusion and atelectasis. Treatment includes the use of humidified oxygen, coughing, deep breathing, postural drainage, and increased mobility. Incentive spirometry and intermittent positive pressure ventilation also may be used. Smoking cessation 6 to 8 weeks before surgery is beneficial to decrease atelectasis. Preventative strategies include adequate pain control and cautious use of nasogastric tubes.[18]

Pulmonary Edema

Pulmonary edema, which is caused by fluid accumulation within the alveoli, may be the result of an increase in hydrostatic pressure, a decrease in interstitial pressure, or an increase in capillary permeability.

An increase in hydrostatic pressure is usually the result of fluid overload, left ventricular failure (especially in the presence of systolic hypertension), mitral valve dysfunction, or ischemic heart disease. Increased capillary permeability may be the result of sepsis, aspiration, transfusion reaction, trauma, anaphylaxis, shock, or disseminated intravascular coagulation and is frequently referred to as adult respiratory distress syndrome.[17]

A decrease in interstitial pressure is often seen after prolonged airway obstruction, such as laryngospasm. Acute pulmonary edema that occurs shortly after relief of severe upper airway obstruction is called postobstruction or negative pressure pulmonary edema or noncardiogenic pulmonary edema. The airway obstruction causes extreme negative intrapleural pressure that increases the pulmonary transvascular hydrostatic pressure gradient. The rapid movement of fluid from pulmonary vasculature to interstitium exceeds the clearing capacity of the pulmonary lymphatic system, and the alveoli become flooded.[19] Patients who are muscular are at an increased risk of postobstruction pulmonary edema because of the ability to produce substantial inspiratory force.[12] Other causes of noncardiogenic pulmonary edema are

bolus dosing with naloxone, incomplete reversal of neuromuscular blockade, or a significant period of hypoxia.[20]

Pulmonary edema is characterized by hypoxemia, cough, frothy sputum, rales on auscultation, decreased lung compliance, and pulmonary infiltrates seen on chest radiography. Treatment of pulmonary edema is directed toward identification of the cause and reduction of hydrostatic pressure within the lungs. Oxygenation must be maintained (particularly in the presence of profound hypoxemia) via oxygen mask, CPAP with mask, or (if necessary) intubation, mechanical ventilation, and the addition of positive end-expiratory pressure (PEEP) ventilation. Diuretics (most commonly furosemide) and fluid restriction are a part of treatment. Dialysis may be used if the fluid retention results from renal failure. Preload and/or afterload reduction, which is achieved through the use of nitroglycerin or sodium nitroprusside, may be used to decrease myocardial work.[17] Patients with noncardiogenic pulmonary edema usually recover quickly after the acute phase and have no permanent sequelae.[20] Resolution of symptoms usually occurs within 12 to 48 hours when immediately treated.[12]

Pulmonary Embolism

Pulmonary embolism is a leading cause of morbidity and mortality, accounting for 60,000 to 100,000 deaths annually in the United States. Most cases of pulmonary embolism are not fatal; however, sudden death is the first symptom in approximately 25% of people who have one.[21] Patients are considered to be at risk for pulmonary embolism if three conditions, known as Virchow triad, exist: venous stasis, hypercoagulability, and abnormalities of the blood vessel wall. These conditions are accentuated in the presence of obesity, varicose veins, immobility, malignancy, congestive heart failure, increased age, and after pelvic or long-bone surgery or injury. However, 90% of all pulmonary emboli arise from deep veins in the legs.[22] Thrombosis in postoperative patients seems to be related to surgical tissue trauma and liberation of tissue factor that leads to thrombin formation.

A pulmonary embolism should be suspected in a patient who complains of or whose presenting signs include acute-onset tachypnea, dyspnea, and tachycardia, particularly when the patient is already receiving oxygen therapy. Classic presenting symptoms are pleuritic chest pain and dyspnea at rest.[23] Signs and symptoms also may include dyspnea, chest pain, hypotension, hemoptysis, dysrhythmias, and congestive heart failure. Multidetector computed tomography (CT) pulmonary angiography has largely replaced ventilation-perfusion lung scanning for pulmonary embolism diagnosis and pulmonary angiography, and can provide rapid results.[22,23] Pulmonary angiography is infrequently performed because of its high risk and associated mortality. See Table 55.1 for pretest likelihood of pulmonary embolism.

Treatment of a pulmonary embolism is directed toward the correction of hypoxemia and support of hemodynamic stability. Preventive measures may include the use of antiembolic stockings or sequential compression devices. Subcutaneous heparin therapy also may be initiated. Once the occurrence of a pulmonary embolism has been confirmed, intravenous heparin therapy is started for the prevention of further clot formation. The goal of heparin therapy is an activated partial thromboplastin time that is 1.5 to 2 times the control value. Early anticoagulation has been associated with decreased mortality for patients with acute pulmonary embolism.[23] Subcutaneous low molecular weight heparin or fondaparinux or oral rivaroxaban can be used for intermediate- or low-risk pulmonary emboli patients and do not require coagulation monitoring. However, heparin is the drug of choice in the case of renal disease.[22]

TABLE 55.1 Wells's Clinical Prediction Rule for Likelihood of Pulmonary Embolism

Variable	Points
Predisposing Factors	
Previous VTE	1.5
Recent surgery or immobilization	1.5
Cancer	1
Symptoms	
Hemoptysis	1
Signs	
Heart rate >100 beats/min	1.5
Clinical signs of DVT	3
Clinical Judgment	
Alternative diagnosis less likely than PE	3

Clinical Probability	Total Points
Low	<2
Moderate	2–6
High	>6

DVT, Deep vein thrombosis; *PE,* pulmonary embolism; *VTE,* venous thromboembolism.
From Weitz JI, Ginsberg JS. Pulmonary embolism. In: Goldman L, Schafer AI. *Goldman-Cecil Medicine.* 26th ed. Philadelphia: Elsevier; 2019:74, 476-486.e3.

Aspiration

Aspiration is a potentially serious airway emergency that can compromise patient safety and stability on the induction of, or the emergence from, anesthesia. Aspiration may occur in the OR, in the PACU, or at any time during transfer. Patients may aspirate foreign matter (e.g., a tooth), food, blood, or gastric contents. Each type of material is associated with a characteristic clinical presentation.

Foreign matter aspiration may result in cough, airway obstruction, atelectasis, bronchospasm, and pneumonia. A profound reflex sympathetic nervous system (SNS) response might also cause hypertension, tachycardia, and dysrhythmias. In the absence of complete upper airway obstruction, complications are often localized and treated with supportive care once the foreign matter has been expelled or removed by bronchoscopy.[24]

Aspiration of blood may result from trauma or surgical manipulation and may also cause minor airway obstruction that is rapidly cleared by cough, resorption, and phagocytosis. Massive blood aspiration interferes with gas exchange through mechanical blockage of airways and leads to chronic fibrinous changes in air spaces or pulmonary hemochromatosis from iron accumulation in phagocytic cells. Aspiration of blood may result in infection, particularly if particles of soft tissue are aspirated along with the blood. Treatment involves correction of hypoxemia, maintenance of airway patency, and initiation of antibiotic therapy, if indicated.[20]

Aspiration of gastric contents is the most severe form of aspiration and may result in a chemical pneumonitis. Patients have diffuse bronchospasm (secondary to reflex airway closure), hypoxemia (compromised alveolar-capillary membrane), atelectasis (loss of surfactant), interstitial edema (loss of capillary integrity), hemorrhage, and adult respiratory distress syndrome. Gastric aspiration also may cause laryngospasm, infection, and pulmonary edema.

For this reason, the prevention of gastric aspiration, rather than its treatment, is the goal. Patients who are at risk for gastric aspiration (e.g., obese or pregnant patients or those with a history of hiatal hernia, peptic ulcer, or trauma) may be given histamine-2 (H_2) blockers, gastrokinetic agents, nonparticulate antacids, or anticholinergics before anesthesia induction. Prophylactic medications are not recommended for those patients who are not at risk, although antiemetics may be given.[25] Rapid sequence induction is likely used. Intraoperatively, a nasogastric tube may be inserted and is usually then removed to decrease gastric volume and decompress the stomach. Postoperatively the patient should be left intubated until airway reflexes return.

Treatment of gastric aspiration is directed toward correction of hypoxemia and maintenance of hemodynamic stability. Antibiotics are indicated only if signs of infection (e.g., fever, leukocytosis, positive culture results) are present. No beneficial effect of corticosteroids has been determined. Administration of corticosteroids produces no positive effects, but may contribute to bacterial superinfections.[24]

If aspiration causes hypoxemia, increased airway resistance, atelectasis, or pulmonary edema, institution of support with supplemental oxygen, PEEP, or CPAP and mechanical ventilation is often necessary. Pulmonary edema is usually secondary to increased capillary permeability, so diuretics should not be used to decrease intravascular volume. Bacterial infection does not always occur, so prophylactic antibiotics might merely promote colonization by resistant organisms. If evidence of secondary bacterial infections appears, specific antibiotic therapy is instituted, based on sputum samples obtained for Gram stain and culture or on prevailing colonization experience within the institution.[20,24]

Bronchospasm

Bronchospasm results from an increase in bronchial smooth muscle tone, with resultant closure of small airways. As a result of the strong increase in inspiratory force against these narrowed airways, airway edema develops, causing secretions to build up in the airway. Clinically, the patient demonstrates wheezing, dyspnea, use of accessory muscles, and tachypnea. Airway resistance is increased, and increased peak inspiratory pressures are noted if the patient is receiving mechanical ventilation.

Bronchospasm may result from aspiration, pharyngeal or tracheal suctioning, endotracheal intubation, histamine release secondary to medications, or an allergic response, and it may be seen in greater frequency in patients with a history of asthma or chronic obstructive pulmonary disease.[26]

Treatment of bronchospasm requires confirmation and removal of the precipitating cause. Pharmacotherapy is instituted, with the goals of decreasing airway irritability and promoting bronchodilation. Medications used in the management of bronchospasm include inhalation anesthetic agents, β_2-agonists such as albuterol (Proventil, Ventolin), the long-acting agent salmeterol (Serevent), and (if the condition is life threatening) intravenous epinephrine. Anticholinergics such as atropine sulfate, glycopyrrolate, and ipratropium have been given via nebulization to decrease secretions. Use of intravenous lidocaine is controversial but more beneficial than intratracheal lidocaine, which can attenuate histamine-induced bronchospasm.[26] Steroids have been used if the underlying cause is an inflammatory disease such as asthma.[20,26] The potential benefit of sevoflurane as rescue therapy for severe, refractory bronchospasm has been reported.[27]

Hypoventilation

Hypoventilation is a common, easily recognizable complication in the PACU. It is manifested clinically by a decrease in respiratory rate that results in an increase in $Paco_2$ secondary to a decrease in alveolar ventilation. This may occur because of a decrease in central respiratory drive, poor respiratory muscle function, or a combination of both.[12]

Physiological factors:

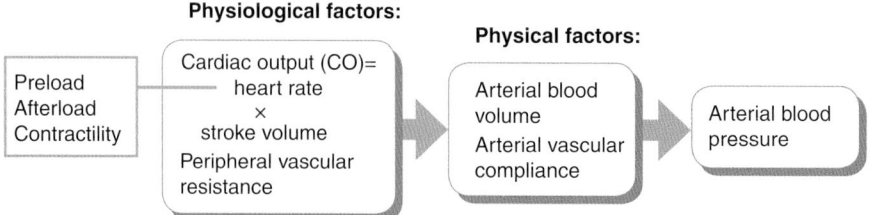

Fig. 55.1 Both physiologic and physical factors affect arterial blood pressure. Cardiac output is the result of heart rate × stroke volume. Heart rate is affected by preload, afterload, and contractility. (From Seifert PC, Wadlund DL. Crisis management of hypotension in the OR. *AORN J*. 2015;102:67; originally in Pappano AJ, Wier WG. *Cardiovascular Physiology: Mosby Monograph Series*. 10th ed. St. Louis: Elsevier; 2013:236.)

Depression of central respiratory drive can occur with both intravenous and inhalation anesthetics. Central respiratory depression is most profound on admission to the PACU, although the time and route of anesthetic administration may suggest otherwise. For example, an intravenous dose of fentanyl given just before the patient emerges from anesthesia may not peak until later in the PACU. An intramuscular dose of an opioid takes substantially longer to peak than does an intravenous dose.[24]

Patients also may demonstrate a secondary stage of respiratory depression once certain stimuli are removed. For example, a patient may be admitted awake and breathing to the PACU with an endotracheal tube in place. After extubation, because of the loss of stimulation from the endotracheal tube, the patient may become hypercarbic secondary to residual opioid effects and hypoventilation. Verbal and tactile stimulation, deep breaths, and repositioning the patient may increase ventilatory function and decrease carbon dioxide.[12] Pulse oximetry monitors oxygenation but does not reflect the adequacy of ventilation. Capnography measuring end tidal CO_2 is of use in patients at risk.[1,20]

Poor respiratory muscle function can result from many conditions. Some of the most common situations are inadequate reversal of neuromuscular blocking agents, surgery involving the upper abdomen, positioning, obesity, OSA, and diseases involving the neuromuscular system.

Inadequate reversal of neuromuscular blocking agents can result in hypoventilation secondary to respiratory muscle weakness. Factors that can adversely affect neuromuscular blockade and reversal include certain medications, hypokalemia, hypermagnesemia, hypothermia, and acidosis[28] (see Chapter 12).

Medications that have been associated with prolongation of blockade include the aminoglycoside antibiotics (e.g., gentamicin, clindamycin, and neomycin), as well as magnesium and lithium. Hypermagnesemia and hypothermia may potentiate neuromuscular blockade. Hypokalemia and respiratory acidosis inhibit reversal.[28]

Upper abdominal surgery also can affect respiratory muscle function. Hypoventilation occurs because of a reduced vital capacity secondary to poor diaphragmatic function. A reduction in vital capacity of up to 60% has been noted on the first postoperative day.[12] Obesity, especially when combined with upper abdominal surgery, further contributes to hypoventilation because of the increased intraabdominal pressure in obese patients.

Diseases of the neuromuscular system can also affect ventilation. Patients with muscular dystrophy, myasthenia gravis, Eaton-Lambert syndrome, Guillain-Barré syndrome, or other muscle diseases can exhibit postoperative muscle weakness (see Table 12.9). Patients with severe scoliosis also exhibit poor respiratory muscle function. It is often in the best interests of patients with these disorders that they remain intubated in the PACU until complete return of function occurs and any residual anesthetic effects are absent.

Cardiovascular Function

Hypotension

The term *hypotension* has been defined as a fall in arterial blood pressure of more than 20% below baseline, or an absolute value of systolic blood pressure (SBP) below 90 mm Hg, or of mean arterial pressure (MAP) below 60 mm Hg.[29] However, the clinical signs of hypoperfusion, rather than numeric values, should be the indicators of compromise. Since the autonomic nervous system preferentially maintains blood flow to the brain, heart, and kidneys, signs of hypoperfusion to these organs (including disorientation, nausea, loss of consciousness, chest pain, oliguria, and anuria) reflect the failure of physiologic compensation. Hypoxia, which results from hypoperfusion, may cause lactic acidosis. Intervention must be implemented in a timely fashion so that cerebral ischemia, cerebrovascular accident (CVA), myocardial infarction or ischemia, renal ischemia, bowel infarction, and spinal cord damage do not develop.[30]

Hypotension in the PACU is most commonly caused by hypovolemia secondary to inadequate replacement of intraoperative fluid and blood loss (decreased preload) (Fig. 55.1). Hypovolemia may be due to volume depletion as a result of inadequate fluid replacement during surgery, blood loss during surgery, or ongoing blood loss postoperatively.[31] As a result, initial treatment should focus on restoring circulating volume. The patient should be assessed for active bleeding, and a 300 to 500 mL fluid bolus of physiologic saline or lactated Ringer solution should be given. If no response is noted, myocardial dysfunction should be considered the cause of hypotension.

Cardiogenic hypotension (intrinsic pump failure), as is the case with myocardial infarction, tamponade, or embolism, results in an acute fall in ventricular emptying and cardiac output. Secondary cardiac dysfunction occurs as a result of the negative chronotropic and negative inotropic effects of medications. The surgical procedure and the patient's preoperative cardiac risk and medical condition are important indicators in a differential diagnosis.[12]

Decreased afterload or low systemic vascular resistance (SVR) also can contribute to hypotension. Numerous anesthetic agents cause histamine release with subsequent vasodilation (e.g., morphine, atracurium), whereas others cause vasodilation by directly relaxing arterial smooth muscle (e.g., volatile inhalation anesthetics, local anesthetics used for producing spinal anesthesia). Sensitivity to vasodilators such as hydralazine, sodium nitroprusside, and nitroglycerin also can produce profound hypotension. Table 55.2 lists medications associated with a hypotensive crisis. Sepsis may be another cause of low SVR.

Dysrhythmias that interfere with cardiac conduction and subsequently compromise cardiac output also can produce hypotension. Tachydysrhythmias prevent optimal ventricular filling and emptying. Conduction blocks compromise myocardial effectiveness, resulting in

TABLE 55.2 Medications Associated With a Hypotensive Crisis

Medication	Mechanism of Action
Anesthetic agents[1]	May cause a drop in blood pressure as a result of the release of histamine during an anaphylactic reaction to anesthetic medications, which occurs most commonly with neuromuscular blocking agents
Antibiotics[1,2,3]	Cause- an allergic reaction as a result of a release of histamine that is characterized by flushing and hypotension; antibiotics are the most common class of medications to cause allergic reactions
Antihypertensive agents[4]	May cause refractory hypotension in the hypertensive patient who is taking angiotensin-converting enzyme inhibitors
Hypnotics[2]	Cause- hypotension through vasodilation
Induction agent—propofol[2]	May cause an allergic reaction in patients allergic to eggs and soybeans
Inhalation agents[5]—isoflurane, sevoflurane, desflurane	Decrease mean arterial pressure (MAP) in a dose-dependent manner related to a decrease in systemic vascular resistance; sevoflurane has less impact on hemodynamics
Intravenous contrast agents[1,2]	May cause a hypotensive event in 5%–8% of patients who experience intravenous contrast—related reactions, which is a result of anaphylaxis or release of vasoactive substances
Latex products (allergic reaction)[2]	Cause- a delayed anaphylactic reaction when an allergic patient is exposed to latex products; hypotension and vascular collapse occur approximately 40 min after exposure
Local anesthetics[6]	Cause- a toxic central reaction if systemic or inadvertent intravascular injection occurs—a later sign
Methyl methacrylate[7]	May cause hypotensive episode from 30–60 sec up to 10 min after placement of the cement as a result of: • Tissue damage secondary to the exothermic reaction that occurs within the cement • Release of vasoactive substances when the cement is hydrolyzed to methacrylate acid • Embolization as the bone is reamed • Vasodilation caused by absorption of the volatile monomer
Opioids[2]	Cause- hypotension as a result of decreasing sympathetic tone, which then causes bradycardia
Neuromuscular blocking agents[2]	Cause- the release of histamine with resultant hypotension after rapid injection; sugammadex is one of the newest causes of perioperative anaphylaxis, which can result in hypotension
Regional anesthetics[5,8]	Cause- vasodilation with subsequent hypotension, which occurs below the level of the regional block secondary to the blockade of sympathetic conduction fibers

[1]Patton K, Borshoff, DC. Adverse drug reactions. *Anaesthesia.* 2018;73(1):S76–S84.
[2]Volcheck GW, Hepner DL. Identification and management of perioperative anaphylaxis. *J Allergy Clin Immunol Pract.* 2019;7:2134–2142.
[3]Blumenthall KG, Peter JG, Trubiano JA, et al. Antibiotic allergy. *Lancet.* 2019;393(10167):183–198. https://doi.org/10.1016/S0140-6736(1832218-9).
[4]Berg SM, Braehler MR. The postanesthesia care init. In: Gropper MA, Cohen NH, Eriksson, et al., eds. *Miller's Anesthesia.* 9th ed. Philadelphia, PA: Elsevier; 2020:2586–2613.
[5]Eis S, Krame J. Anesthesia inhalation agents cardiovascular effects. StatPearls. https://www.ncbi.nlm.nih.gov/books/NBK541090. Accessed December 2020.
[6]Cherobin ACFP, Tavares GT. Safety of local anesthetics. *Anais Brasileiros de Dermatol.* 2020;95(1):82–90.
[7]Hines CB, Collins-Yoder A. Bone cement implantation syndrome: key concepts for perioperative nurses. *AORN J.* 2018;109(2):202–213.
[8]Fitzgerald JP, Fedoruk KA, Jadin SM, et al. Prevention of hypotension after spinal anaesthesia for caesarean section: a systematic review and network meta-analysis of randomised controlled trials. *Anaesthesia.* 2020;75:109–121.
Modified from Seifert PC, Wadlund DL. Crisis management of hypotension in the OR. *AORN J.* 2015;102:67.

a lowered cardiac output and hypotension. Box 55.7 provides a differential diagnosis of hypotension in the postoperative patient.

Intervention should always include supplemental oxygen therapy and elevation of the legs while the cause of the hypotension is being investigated.[20] Volume status should be evaluated, and preoperative and intraoperative fluid administration should be considered. Hypotension caused by artifact of the measurement system also should be considered (e.g., a blood pressure cuff that is too large or too small or an inappropriate transducer height).[31] The presence of hypotension secondary to myocardial dysfunction suggests the need for coronary vasodilators, inotropic therapy, and afterload reduction (e.g., through nitroglycerin therapy, dobutamine therapy, or both). Secondary myocardial dysfunction may require that administration of the causative medications be discontinued. Vasodilation resulting in lower SVR and symptomatic hypoperfusion can be treated with vasoconstrictive agents, either by intravenous bolus (ephedrine [5–50 mg], epinephrine [10–100 mcg], phenylephrine [50–200 mcg], or vasopressin [1–4 units]) or by infusion (dopamine or epinephrine).[29]

Hypertension

The term *hypertension* is defined as a rise in arterial blood pressure of more than 20% above baseline or an absolute value of arterial blood pressure above age-corrected limits.[29] Hypertension is a common finding in the PACU and can be caused by stimulation of the SNS, as well as pain, respiratory compromise, visceral distention, and significant increases in plasma catecholamine levels that produce vasoconstriction (Box 55.8). Pain remains the leading cause of hypertension and tachycardia in the PACU and results in stimulation of the somatic afferent nerves, producing a pressor response known as the somatosympathetic reflex.[30] The use of analgesics attenuates the sympathetic response, thereby normalizing blood pressure.

Hypoxemia and hypercarbia cause direct stimulation of the vasomotor area of the medulla, resulting in increased vasomotor tone, increased arteriolar constriction, and increased blood pressure.[30] Correction of the respiratory compromise should result in normalization of blood pressure.

Distention of the bladder, bowel, or stomach causes stimulation of afferent fibers of the SNS, producing an increase in plasma catecholamine levels. Catheterization of the bladder and decompression of the bowel or stomach remove the offending stimulus.

Hypertension also may develop as a sequela of hypothermia. Increased catecholamine secretion is an important endocrine response to cold.[30] As cooling occurs, blood vessels become more sensitive to catecholamines, resulting in arteriolar and venous constriction. Rewarming reverses the process. As vasodilation occurs, reperfusion of the extremities and skin decreases systemic elevations in pressure.

Preexisting hypertension exists in many of the patients who develop hypertension in the PACU; 30% of the general population in the PACU have preexisting hypertension. The degree of elevation in pressure is greater if preoperative antihypertensive medications are withdrawn suddenly. Preoperatively, all antihypertensive medications should be continued, except angiotensin-converting enzyme (ACE) inhibitors or angiotensin II antagonists, for which no clear consensus exists.[32] Hypertension also may be seen secondary to revascularization and baroreceptor stimulation after vascular or cardiac surgery, including carotid endarterectomy. Pharmacologic intervention is required for the protection of graft sites and the prevention of hemorrhage. Sodium nitroprusside and nitroglycerin are agents of choice for vasodilation.

A significant number of patients, especially those with a history of essential hypertension, will require pharmacologic blood pressure control in the PACU.[12] Agents that may be used for the reduction of blood pressure include hydralazine (2–4 mg) and labetalol hydrochloride (5–10 mg). Hydralazine relaxes vascular smooth muscle, preferentially favoring the arteriolar circulation. Labetalol is both an α- and a β-blocking agent, causing peripheral vasodilation and slowing of the heart rate. Other β-blockers used postoperatively include metoprolol (1–2 mg) and esmolol (10–50 mg).[29] β-blockers assist in controlling the sympathetic responses of patients during recovery. α$_2$-agonists also can be used postoperatively to assist when needed. Many other agents are available and may include the patient's usual prescription antihypertensive for mild increases. Patients who were on β-blockers prior to surgery should have them continued throughout the perioperative period.

Dysrhythmias

Dysrhythmias seen in the PACU are often transient and most commonly have an identifiable cause that is not an actual myocardial injury. The major postanesthetic and surgical factors that lead to a relatively high incidence of perioperative dysrhythmias include hypokalemia, excess fluid administration, anemia, hypoventilation with subsequent hypercarbia, altered acid-base status, substance withdrawal, and circulatory instability.[12] Medications commonly administered in the perioperative period have been linked to significant prolongation of the QT interval. Although the rationale for and clinical relevance of this relationship are not well defined, an associated risk for torsades de pointes development related to prolonged QT interval should be considered post general anesthetic administration.[33]

Arterial desaturation is a common postoperative complication that may result from obstruction or hypoventilation[12] and less commonly from pulmonary embolism, pulmonary edema, or aspiration. A direct consequence of hypoxia is myocardial ischemia and depression of cardiac contractility. Signs of cardiac irritability may be manifested by atrial and ventricular dysrhythmias, conduction delays, and heart block.

Hypercarbia caused by reduced alveolar ventilation results in elevation of the arterial carbon dioxide tension, which in turn stimulates the SNS and sensitizes the myocardium to the arrhythmic effects of endogenous catecholamines. Among the earliest signs of hypercarbia are tachycardia and hypertension, which may progress to ventricular dysrhythmias.

Hypokalemia may occur secondary to hyperventilation, respiratory alkalosis, gastric suctioning, insulin administration, and diuretic use. The ECG may demonstrate widening of the QRS complex, U waves, and ST segment abnormalities that may progress into premature ventricular complexes, ventricular tachycardia, and ventricular fibrillation.

Acid-base disturbances may occur as a result of alterations in ventilation, gastrointestinal losses, and lactic acid production during hypotension or shock. The cardiovascular effects include increased cardiac excitability and irritability.

Hypotension may result in impaired oxygen transport and compromised coronary circulation, leading to myocardial ischemia with associated conduction deficits.[29] The use of vasoconstrictive medications designed to treat the hypotension also may contribute to the development of dysrhythmias. Patients with preexisting heart disease, particularly those who have a history of myocardial infarction or pulmonary hypertension, are at continued risk for myocardial ischemia throughout the perioperative period. Myocardial ischemia is rarely accompanied by chest pain in postanesthesia patients. All PACU patients who do complain of chest pain should have a 12-lead ECG and troponin level done.[12]

Hypothermia resulting from general and neuraxial anaesthesia[34] prolongs the refractory period, contributing to the development of sinus bradycardia and atrial fibrillation. Conduction deficits may progress to atrioventricular block and eventually to ventricular fibrillation.

Vagal reflexes are usually transient and are produced by the Valsalva maneuver or direct eye, vagal nerve, or carotid sinus pressure. Severe sinus bradycardia with possible ventricular escape beats may occur. Vagotonic medications such as neostigmine also can produce these dysrhythmias.

The presence of residual anesthetics in both blood and tissue in patients admitted to the PACU may contribute to dysrhythmias. Ketamine may contribute to sympathetic stimulation, resulting in tachyarrhythmias and hypertension, as can vagolytic drugs such as atropine and glycopyrrolate. Opioids such as morphine, fentanyl, and sufentanil may result in the indirect development of dysrhythmias. Opioid-induced ventilatory impairment, a potential side effect of opioids, may result in hypoxemia and hypercarbia,[35] each known to be dysrhythmogenic. Anticholinesterase agents may produce severe bradyarrhythmias or heart block.[29]

Surgical stress and pain can significantly increase plasma catecholamine levels. Although this sympathetic response may be mitigated by anesthetic administration, norepinephrine and epinephrine concentrations are consistently elevated in PACU patients who are experiencing acute pain. Administration of analgesic medications may blunt this sympathetic response; however, cardiac irritability, tachycardia, and conduction dysrhythmias may occur.

Neuromuscular Function

Reversal of Neuromuscular Blockade

Incomplete reversal of neuromuscular relaxation can lead to postoperative pulmonary complications, including obstruction and hypoventilation. Patients who received a reversal agent often exhibit signs of residual neuromuscular blockade in the PACU, particularly the elderly.[36] Therefore objective monitoring measures (e.g., train-of-four ratio <0.90) should be performed regularly in the early postanesthesia phase to determine depth of residual blockade and prevent pulmonary complications.[37] (See Chapter 12 for a complete discussion of residual neuromuscular agent paralysis.)

Residual paralysis compromises cough, airway patency, ability to overcome airway resistance, and airway protection. Intraoperative use of shorter-acting relaxants might decrease the incidence of residual paralysis but does not eliminate the problem. Reversal agents such as neostigmine and edrophonium chloride will be given in conjunction with either atropine or glycopyrrolate.[28] Sugammadex, a newer generation reversal agent, is specifically designed to reverse rocuronium. The main advantage of sugammadex is reversal of neuromuscular blockade without relying on inhibition of acetylcholinesterase, and earlier spontaneous postoperative ventilation.[38] Marginal reversal can be more dangerous than near-total paralysis because an agitated patient exhibiting uncoordinated movements and airway obstruction is more easily identified. A somnolent patient exhibiting mild stridor and shallow ventilation from marginal neuromuscular function might be overlooked. Insidious hypoventilation leading to respiratory acidemia or regurgitation with aspiration can occur later into recovery. Patients

with coexisting neuromuscular abnormalities such as myasthenia gravis,[32,37] Eaton-Lambert syndrome, or muscular dystrophies exhibit exaggerated or prolonged responses to muscle relaxants. Even without muscle relaxant administration, such patients can exhibit postoperative respiratory insufficiency from inadequate neuromuscular reserves (see Table 12.9).

Residual neuromuscular blockade is associated with increased mortality,[36,39] and therefore, its assessment and management are essential in the early postanesthesia phase. Simple bedside tests help evaluate mechanical ability to ventilate. Forced vital capacity of 10 to 12 mL/kg and inspiratory pressure more negative than −25 cm H_2O imply that strength of ventilatory muscles is adequate to sustain ventilation. Sustained head elevation in a supine position, hand grip, and ability to bite down, swallow, and stick out the tongue are easily assessed parameters. These measures, along with tactile train-of-four and double-burst stimulation assessment, more accurately predict a patient's ability to maintain sustained ventilation.

Mental Status

Postoperative mental status changes may be associated with poor anesthetic outcomes, therefore periodic mental and behavioral status assessments are recommended from the time of emergence and throughout the early postanesthesia recovery period.[6]

Emergence Delirium

Postoperative emergence delirium is the alteration in neurologic functioning that causes the most concern to the practitioner. Emergence delirium has been associated with a risk of bodily injury to the patient and caregiver, increased resource utilization, and an extended PACU length of stay. The term *delirium* is defined as a condition characterized by extreme disturbances of arousal, attention, orientation, perception, intellectual function, and affect. It is most commonly accompanied by fear and agitation.[40,41]

Attempts have been made to differentiate emergence delirium from agitation,[42] with the term *agitation* defined as mild restlessness and mental distress. Agitation can be due to pain, physiologic compromise, or anxiety. Delirium can be confused with agitation or be the source of agitation, and the two conditions can be very difficult to differentiate. Adding further to confusion is lack of differentiation between emergence delirium and postoperative delirium. Emergence delirium is most common in healthy pediatric and younger adult patients; postoperative delirium is usually observed in older patients with multiple comorbidities.[41] Hypoactive emergence is related to delayed recovery and is characterized by depressed mental status and reduced arousal. The presence of hypoactive emergence may go undetected.[42]

The incidence of postoperative emergence delirium has been reported to occur in 4% to 31% of the general surgery patient cohort, with the incidence as high as 50% to 80% in children.[40,43] Emergence delirium also appears to occur with greater incidence among combat veterans compared with the general military population of the same age.[44] Preexisting psychiatric disorders, use of psychotropic drugs, and substance abuse can also predispose adults to emergence delirium.[40]

Confusion and agitation are common during recovery from inhalation anesthetics. Sevoflurane in particular has been associated with emergence delirium in children.[45] Benzodiazepines have been related to adult emergence delirium, but no pediatric cases.[40] Procedure severity has been identified as a significant factor for a patient to experience delirium postsurgery.[41] Other causes of postoperative delirium include pain, visceral distention (bowel and bladder), anxiety (including separation anxiety in children), hyperthermia, and hypothermia.[43,45] Again, treatment is directed at correction of the cause. Common causes of emergence delirium include presence of an endotracheal tube, pain, and anxiety. In children, both the determination of cause and the treatment of delirium are complex, with pain and anxiety more easily recognized and treated than other anesthetic-related causes.[45]

Several instruments have been studied in the pediatric population, but the most widely used and validated is the Pediatric Anesthesia Emergence Delirium (PAED) scale.[43,46] In the adult population, the Confusion Assessment Method in the Intensive Care Unit (CAM-ICU) has been used with success. The CAM-ICU has not been validated for emergence delirium, but is the only instrument used in the past few years in studies for emergence delirium.[42] Another instrument is the Richmond Agitation-Sedation Scale (RASS). If the RASS score is zero and the CAM-ICU is positive, the results can help identify hypoactive emergence.[42,43]

Management of emergence delirium focuses on prevention and alleviation of risk factors. Preoperative education can alleviate anxiety, which is correlated with emergence delirium. Evaluation of the anesthesia plan is important, and consideration of intravenous anesthesia (propofol) should be considered. Dexmedetomidine has been shown to be effective preoperatively as well as during anesthesia.[43,47] Ketamine was first related to emergence delirium, but current studies point to low-dose ketamine during induction of anesthesia to improve both emergence agitation and postoperative pain.[40] Postoperatively, it is important to determine the cause of the emergence delirium. Optimization of pain control is important. Treatment of postoperative nausea, vomiting, and hypothermia is needed. Catheters or other items that are no longer needed should be removed. Parental presence may be warranted if appropriate; it has been related to decreasing emergence delirium in children. Byun et al. determined that use of the mother's voice versus a stranger's voice replayed on a recorder reduced emergence delirium scores and the incidence of emergence delirium in pediatric patients.[48]

Once hypoxemia has been eliminated as a cause of postoperative delirium, and all known causes have been evaluated, sedation may prove useful in controlling the agitation and providing for patient safety. Fig. 55.2 summarizes an algorithm that can be useful for severe emergence agitation or delirium in children.

Delayed Awakening

Delayed awakening is a common, often easily explained postoperative finding and can be defined as a clinician's expectation in a specific circumstance that the patient "should be awake by now" but is not.[49] Although delayed awakening may slow turnover of PACU beds and delay patient discharge from the PACU,[12] the causes and consequences of delayed awakening are rarely serious. The most common causes of delayed awakening are as follows:

- Prolonged action of anesthetic drugs
- Metabolic causes
- Neurologic injury

Prolonged action of anesthetic drugs is the most common cause of delayed awakening.[12] This may occur secondary to alterations in drug pharmacokinetics and pharmacodynamics. Pharmacokinetic alterations include changes in drug distribution secondary to mobilization of drugs from body tissue stores, redistribution, or decreased protein binding; changes in metabolism; and excretion secondary to renal or hepatic dysfunction. Pharmacodynamic alterations include increased patient sensitivity to drug effects because of extremes of age, hypothermia, or concomitant alcohol and drug use.[20] Other patients at risk for delayed awakening are those with preexisting cognitive or psychiatric disorders, patients who chronically take sedative medications, patients who were intoxicated with alcohol or illicit drugs at the time of anesthesia, and those who were physically exhausted prior to surgery.

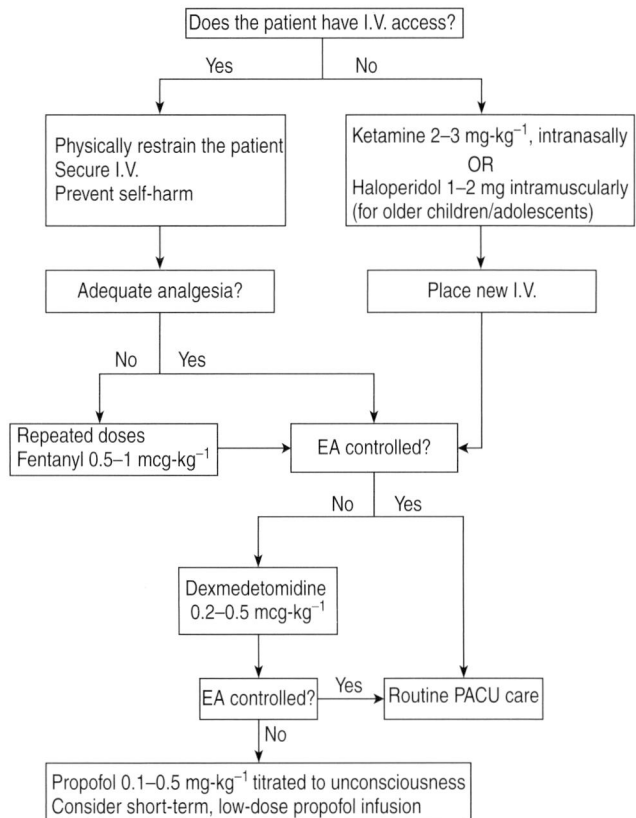

Fig. 55.2 Treatment of severe emergence agitation/delirium. (From Olds T, Weldon C. Emergence agitation and emergence delirium. In: Fleisher LA, Rosenbaum SH, eds. *Complications in Anesthesia*. 3rd ed. Philadelphia, PA: Elsevier; 2018:730.)

Prolonged effects of inhalation anesthetics may be seen secondary to alterations in ventilation. Hypoventilation limits exhalation and prolongs elimination of inhalation agents.[24] Retention of carbon dioxide contributes to narcosis, particularly in the presence of inhalation agents, and compounds the problem.

The potentiating effects of combining inhalation agents with intravenous anesthetics and opioids can also contribute to delayed awakening.[12] Premedications, particularly the long-acting benzodiazepines diazepam and lorazepam, may contribute to delayed awakening, especially in the elderly. Prolonged effects of inhalation and intravenous agents also may occur secondary to multiple drug interactions. Prolonged neuromuscular blockade may mean the patient is awake but unable to move. Some herbal supplements, especially kava kava, St. John's wort, and valerian, have the potential to interact with anesthetic medications and cause delayed awakening.[50]

Metabolic causes contributing to delayed awakening include hypoglycemia, hyperglycemia, electrolyte disturbances, and hypothyroidism.[20,51] Diabetic patients have an increased risk of postoperative hypoglycemia. Taking the usual insulin dose (or half the dose) on the morning of surgery, the patient's nil per os (NPO) status, and the stress of surgery all contribute to the development of hypoglycemia.[51,52] It is important to monitor serum glucose levels intraoperatively and postoperatively. Central nervous system changes may occur as blood glucose levels fall below 50 mg/dL. It is prudent to obtain a baseline blood glucose level of all diabetic patients before they are admitted to surgery. Procedures requiring general anesthesia lasting longer than 2 hours will have greater glucose variations and require more frequent monitoring and treatment. Blood glucose levels of greater than 600 mg/dL can produce hyperosmolar, nonketotic, hyperglycemic coma. Approximately half of these patients have type 2 diabetes, but the syndrome can occur with severe dehydration (especially in the elderly), uremia, pancreatitis, sepsis, pneumonia, CVA, and large surface burns. Minimizing blood glucose variability during the perianesthesia period should be part of any glycemic control strategy.[20,51]

Electrolyte disturbances, specifically alterations in sodium, calcium, and magnesium, can prolong awakening. Dilutional hyponatremia, occurring secondary to water intoxication, may develop after transurethral prostate resection surgery, producing sedation, coma, or even hemiparesis. Hypocalcemia, seen after parathyroidectomy and occasionally thyroidectomy, may delay awakening. Hypermagnesemia, which may occur after prolonged administration of magnesium sulfate to women with eclampsia or preeclampsia, may result in sedation and muscle weakness after general or regional anesthesia for cesarean section.[20,52]

Neurologic injury is a rare cause of delayed awakening of the non-neurosurgical patient. Potential causes of neurologic injury include CVA, intracranial hemorrhage, increased intracranial pressure, uncontrolled extreme hypertension (especially in the anticoagulated patient), air or fat emboli, and uncontrolled hypotension (especially in patients with hypertension or occlusive carotid disease).[12,50]

Evaluation of the patient who fails to awaken begins with an assessment of the patient's preoperative status and a review of intraoperative events.[20] Oxygenation and gas exchange must be assessed and verified with pulse oximetry, physical assessment, and arterial blood gas analysis. When prolonged drug effects are suspected as the cause of delayed awakening, care must be taken to ensure the adequacy of ventilation and oxygenation through appropriate patient monitoring.[6,12]

Residual drug effects should be considered. If possible and not contraindicated, reversal of medications should be attempted. A residual neuromuscular blockade can be reversed with neostigmine/glycopyrrolate or sugammadex. Flumazenil 0.1 to 0.2 mg every 1 minute up to 1 mg can be given to reverse benzodiazepines. Naloxone given in small increments of 40 mcg every 2 minutes up to 200 mcg reverses opioids.[12,20] Central anticholinergic syndrome is also a possibility. Cholinergic transmission can be increased by a trial of physostigmine 0.03 to 0.04 mg/kg repeated at 10- to 30-minute intervals[52] or 1 to 2 mg given intravenously.[12]

If other contributing factors are found, intervention should be initiated. Hypothermia necessitates rewarming, and electrolyte disturbances require correction. Hypoglycemia and hypocalcemia are treated with the intravenous administration of glucose and calcium, respectively. Hyperglycemia is treated with intravenous insulin to lower blood glucose levels and 0.5% normal saline to correct dehydration. Carbon dioxide narcosis can be corrected with hyperventilation.

A neurologic cause of delayed awakening is usually either a diagnosis that is initially expected because of patient status or known because of intraoperative events or a diagnosis of exclusion (i.e., suspected after all other causes have been ruled out). At this point, a CT scan and neurologic consultation are warranted for a more in-depth evaluation.[12]

Serotonin Syndrome

The age, comorbidity status, and number of surgical patients undergoing treatment with combination medication therapy are increasing, particularly in those diagnosed with chronic pain. These patients are at greater risk for developing serotonin syndrome, a possibly fatal condition that can affect patients across the lifespan. The condition is associated with medication treatment-related serotonin level elevation.[53,54]

Serotonin syndrome may be precipitated by the concurrent administration of two or more serotonergic medications, such as the monoamine oxidase inhibitors, tricyclic antidepressants, selective serotonin reuptake inhibitors, and serotonin and norepinephrine reuptake inhibitor agents. Concomitant fentanyl administration has been associated with serotonin syndrome development in several documented cases.[53,54]

Symptom onset occurs quickly, and severity of this syndrome varies. The triad of symptoms commonly linked to serotonin syndrome includes autonomic hyperactivity, neuromuscular abnormalities, and changes in mental status.[53,54] This triad is difficult to recognize intraoperatively and postoperatively. In the mild form, the patient may exhibit dilated pupils, diaphoresis, myoclonus, tachycardia, anxiety, and restlessness. In its worst form, the patient may present with a fever, mental status changes, muscle rigidity, and multiple organ failure.

Serotonin syndrome can be difficult to diagnose because its symptoms may mirror other concerning postanesthetic conditions, such as malignant hyperthermia and delayed awakening.[53] Diagnostic criteria available (i.e., Hunter Serotonin Toxicity and Sternbach) have limited application in the early postanesthesia period.[53,55]

Differential diagnosis is made through direct clinical observation and by ruling out other possible causes. Therefore, knowledge of the patient's medication history and its related potential to precipitate serotonin syndrome is very important. Future expansion of cytochrome P-450 2D6 (CYP2D6) genetic testing can better support the preemptive identification of patients at greatest risk for developing serotonin syndrome.[54]

Treatment is based on the severity of symptoms with early intervention desirable to mitigate further complications. Prudent PACU measures include cardiac monitoring, intravenous fluid resuscitation, oxygen administration, discontinuation of serotonergic medications, and stabilization of vital signs. Benzodiazepine administration may help to control tremors and support physical safety for the agitated patient across the syndrome severity spectrum. Active teamwork, specialty consultation, and provision of supportive care often resolve concerning symptoms within 1 day of onset but may require continued vigilance for patients taking serotonergic medications having a longer duration of action. A further discussion of serotonin syndrome can be found in Chapter 14.

Pain

Relief of surgical pain with minimal side effects is a primary goal of PACU care and a very high priority for both the anesthesia provider and patient. Patients should be assessed on admission to PACU and at frequent intervals using a verbal rating scale, visual analog scale, or an appropriate assessment tool based on cognitive function, age, and developmental age to assess for severity of pain (Fig. 55.3).[10,56,57] When prioritizing pain assessment, the patient's self-report is the most important measure of pain. Other measures used to assess pain intensity include the patient's exposure to painful procedures, behavioral signs such as crying or agitation, a proxy pain rating by someone who knows the patient well, and physiologic indicators such as elevated vital signs.[57] Genetic factors can interfere with pain perception and the effectiveness of medications used to treat pain, although preoperative genetic testing is limited at this time.[58] Inadequate postoperative analgesia is a major source of preoperative fear. Postoperatively, pain often impedes mobility and recovery and is a major source of dissatisfaction in surgical patients. Whereas clinicians have increasingly adopted the use of preemptive and coordinated multimodal opioid-sparing strategies to promote comfort and allay opioid side effects,[59,60] profound nationwide variations in practice have been identified.[61] Over 80% of postoperative patients experience acute pain, with two-thirds of those patients reporting pain described as moderate, severe, or extreme.[62,63] In addition to minimizing distress and improving patient comfort, relief of pain reduces SNS response and helps avoid hypertension, tachycardia, and dysrhythmias (Table 55.3).

Pain Intensity Scales
Simple descriptive pain intensity scale*

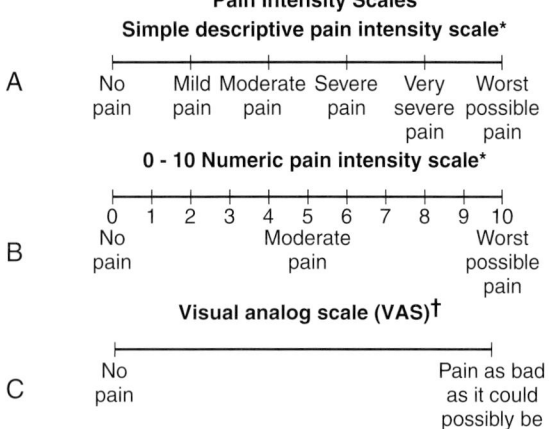

A

| No pain | Mild pain | Moderate pain | Severe pain | Very severe pain | Worst possible pain |

0 - 10 Numeric pain intensity scale*

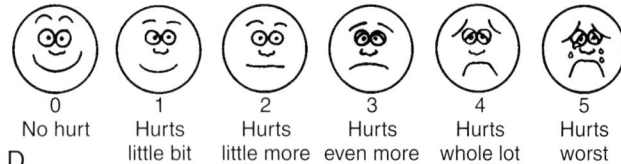

B

0 1 2 3 4 5 6 7 8 9 10
No pain   Moderate pain   Worst possible pain

Visual analog scale (VAS)†

C

No pain ———————————————— Pain as bad as it could possibly be

* If used as a graphic rating scale, a 10-cm baseline is recommended.
† A 10-cm baseline is recommended for VAS scales.

Which face shows how much hurt you have now?

D

| 0 No hurt | 1 Hurts little bit | 2 Hurts little more | 3 Hurts even more | 4 Hurts whole lot | 5 Hurts worst |

Fig. 55.3 Pain intensity scales. (A-C from Acute Pain Management Guideline Panel. *Acute Pain Management in Adults: Operative Procedures: Quick Reference Guide for Clinicians* [AHCPR Publication No. 92-0019]. Rockville, MD: Agency for Health Care Policy and Research; 1992; from Hockenberry MJ, et al. *Wong's Essentials of Pediatric Nursing.* 10th ed. St. Louis: Elsevier; 2017. Used with permission.)

A multiple logistic regression model determined that severe postoperative pain occurred significantly more often in patients with the CYP2D6 poor metabolizer (PM) genotype and smokers.[64] Advances in genomic testing can provide specific information on the rate at which a patient metabolizes an opioid based on individual variability in genetic makeup and may increasingly support more effective procedural pain treatment interventions.[57,58,65]

Incisional pain may be effectively treated with careful titration of intravenous opioids with frequent cardiorespiratory assessments.[66] Short-acting intravenous opioids are useful to expedite discharge and minimize nausea in ambulatory settings. Nonsteroidal antiinflammatory drugs (NSAIDs) and acetaminophen are effective analgesics with antiinflammatory characteristics that can be administered via the most appropriate patient-specific route[67] to lower opioid requirements and reduce the risk for opioid-induced respiratory depression.[35,68,69]

Other analgesic modalities interfere with nociception at multiple levels along the neural pathway to promote effective pain relief beyond the PACU. Intravenous opioid loading in the PACU is helpful for smooth transition to patient-controlled analgesia (PCA). Reduction in the demand for postoperative analgesics has been shown when intravenous administration of magnesium[70] or dexmedetomidine[71] is included during general anesthesia. Continuous lidocaine or ketamine infusion in the early postoperative period has been shown to be effective in the chronic pain patient population.[72] Use of a continuous subcutaneous local anesthetic device or peripheral nerve catheter promotes early ambulation and opioid-sparing goals. Injection of opioids into the epidural or subarachnoid space during anesthesia or in the PACU often yields prolonged postoperative analgesia. Epidural opioid analgesia is effective after thoracic and upper abdominal procedures and helps wean patients with obesity or chronic obstructive

TABLE 55.3	Physiologic Effects Associated with Unrelieved Pain
Domains Affected	**Specific Responses to Pain**
Endocrine	↑ ACTH, ↑ cortisol, ↑ ADH, ↑ epinephrine, ↑ norepinephrine, ↑ GH, ↑ catecholamines, ↑ renin, ↑ angiotensin II, ↑ aldosterone, ↑ glucagon, ↑ interleukin-1, ↓ insulin, ↓ testosterone
Metabolic	Gluconeogenesis, hepatic glycogenolysis, hyperglycemia, glucose intolerance, insulin resistance, muscle protein catabolism, ↑ lipolysis
Cardiovascular	↑ Heart rate, ↑ cardiac workload, ↑ peripheral vascular resistance, ↑ systemic vascular resistance, hypertension, ↑ coronary vascular resistance, ↑ myocardial oxygen consumption, hypercoagulation, deep vein thrombosis
Respiratory	↓ Flows and volumes, atelectasis, shunting, hypoxemia, ↓ cough, sputum retention, infection
Genitourinary	↓ Urinary output, urinary retention, fluid overload, hypokalemia
Gastrointestinal	↓ Gastric and bowel motility
Musculoskeletal	Muscle spasm, impaired muscle function, fatigue, immobility
Cognitive	Reduction in cognitive function, mental confusion
Immune	Depression of immune response
Developmental	↑ Behavioral and physiologic responses to pain, altered temperaments, higher somatization, infant distress behavior, possible altered development of the pain system, ↑ vulnerability to stress disorders, addictive behavior, and anxiety states
Future pain	Debilitating chronic pain syndromes: postmastectomy pain, postthoracotomy pain, phantom pain, postherpetic neuralgia
Quality of life	Sleeplessness, anxiety, fear, hopelessness, ↑ thoughts of suicide

↓, decreased; ↑, increased; *ACTH,* adrenocorticotrophic hormone; *ADH,* antidiuretic hormone; *GH,* growth hormone.
From Pasero C, McCaffery M. *Pain Assessment and Pharmacologic Management.* St. Louis: Elsevier; 2011. Copyright Pasero C, McCaffery M. Used with permission.

pulmonary disease from mechanical ventilation. Epidural analgesia may also improve surgical outcomes after orthopedic and urologic procedures. With epidural or intrathecal opioid administration, immediate and delayed ventilatory depression can occur[73] along with other side effects, such as nausea and pruritus.

PCA allows patients to administer their own pain medication. The most commonly used methods of PCA are intravenous or epidural. Patient therapy should be initiated in the PACU after the patient's initial pain level is under control. Oral opioids are often used with outpatients and have been studied in appropriate orthopedic patients with success.[74] Nonopioids available in an intravenous format include acetaminophen, ketorolac, and ibuprofen. Inclusion of opioid-sparing medications should always be considered for use with the postoperative patient when developing a multimodal plan for pain management.[73]

Placement of long-acting regional analgesic blocks reduces pain, controls SNS activity, and often improves ventilation,[75] particularly when analgesic requirements surpass a single injection's efficacy. For example, an interscalene block yields almost complete pain relief from shoulder or upper extremity procedures, with only moderate inconvenience from motor impairment. Paralysis of the ipsilateral diaphragm can impair postoperative ventilation in patients with marginal respiratory reserve. The adductor canal and/or femoral nerve block promote pain relief for total knee replacement surgery.[73] Caudal analgesia is effective in children after inguinal or genital procedures, whereas infiltration of local anesthetic into joints, soft tissues, or incisions decreases the intensity of pain. Other uses of local anesthesia include continuous wound infusion, in which the catheter is inserted at the end of the case by the surgeon, and perineural infusions, in which the anesthesia provider inserts the catheter near the affected peripheral nerves or a nerve plexus.[76] Deposition of long-acting liposomal formulations of bupivacaine to the surgical site can provide pain relief postdischarge.

Opioid treatment for postoperative or chronic pain is frequently associated with adverse effects, the most common being dose-limiting and debilitating bowel dysfunction. Postoperative ileus, although attributable to surgical procedures, is often exacerbated by opioid use during and after surgery.[77] Postoperative ileus is marked by increased inhibitory neural input, heightened inflammatory responses, decreased propulsive movements, and increased fluid absorption in the gastrointestinal tract. The current management of opioid-induced bowel dysfunction among patients receiving opioid analgesics consists primarily of nonspecific ameliorative measures. Several drugs for opioid-induced constipation are available, including alvimopan (Entereg), naloxegol (Movantik), and methylnaltrexone (Relistor), which can normalize bowel function without blocking systemic opioid analgesia.[78] They are opiate receptor antagonists, which are not absorbed systemically so they do not interfere with systemic analgesia. Their action is confined to the bowel. A chloride channel activator called lubiprostone (Amitiza) is also approved for opioid-induced constipation. Nonpharmacologic interventions may include positioning for comfort, verbal reassurance, touch, applications of heat or cold, massage, transcutaneous electrical nerve stimulation, relaxation techniques, imagery, biofeedback-controlled breathing, and use of the patient's support system (e.g., parent or significant other), particularly in children. Nonpharmacologic interventions should supplement and not replace pharmacologic therapy.[10]

Guidelines for pain management may be generalized and thus lack specific application for different types of surgery. An excellent resource for evidence-based guidelines in the field of pain management is the procedure-specific guidelines offered via a web-based program called PROSPECT (Procedure-Specific Postoperative Pain Management). An international panel of surgeons and anesthesiologists reviews procedure-specific pain research and grades the evidence. Then clinical practice guidelines and recommendations are developed after consensus by the working group and presented in a comprehensive web-based platform. The PROSPECT website offers current procedure-specific guidelines for managing pain associated with various surgical procedure patient cohorts.[79] These recommendations are typically incorporated into enhanced recovery after surgery (ERAS) protocols.

Hypothermia

Hypothermia is a condition marked by an abnormally low internal body temperature (<36°C) that occurs when systemic heat loss exceeds heat production.[80] The majority of unwarmed surgical patients experience hypothermia.[81] Patients admitted into the PACU with hypothermia can experience prolonged recovery, compromised physiologic stability, and greater postoperative morbidity.[82] The patient's interaction with the environment determines the degree of heat loss.[81] Heat loss may occur via radiation, convection, conduction, or evaporation.

Radiant heat loss involves the loss of heat from a warm or hot surface (the body) to a cooler one (the environment). It does not require that the two surfaces be in direct contact with each other. Radiant heat loss accounts for 40% to 60% of heat loss to the environment. It is especially profound in the elderly, debilitated, and neonatal populations.[83]

Convective heat loss depends on the existence of a temperature gradient between the body and the ambient air. This type of heat loss may occur in the OR, particularly in laminar flow rooms, and accounts for 25% to 50% of heat loss.[83]

Conductive heat loss involves loss of heat from a warm surface that comes into contact with a cooler one; it accounts for as much as 10% of heat loss in the OR, where patients lose heat to cooler OR tables, sheets, drapes, skin preparation fluids, and intravenous fluids or irrigants.[83]

Evaporative heat loss involves transfer of heat during the change from a liquid to a gas. Evaporative heat loss occurs via perspiration, respiration, or exposed viscera during surgery. Evaporation accounts for as much as 25% of heat loss in the OR.[66]

Patients at high risk for developing hypothermia can be identified.[81] Elderly patients are at risk because of their decreased subcutaneous fat and alterations in their hypothalamic function. Neonates are at risk because of their immature thermoregulatory center and their high surface-to-volume ratio. Intoxicated individuals are at risk because of vasodilation and depression of their heat regulatory center. Patients taking vasodilators, NSAIDs, and phenothiazines have alterations in thermoregulation that are caused by either vasodilation or suppression of the thermoregulatory center.[34] Other risk factors are female gender, decreased ambient room temperature, length and type of surgery, preexisting conditions such as peripheral vascular disease or burns, use of cold irrigants, and use of general or regional anesthesia.[83]

General anesthetics depress the thermoregulatory center, with a usual temperature drop of 1°C to 3°C. General anesthesia reduces the vasoconstriction threshold; general anesthesia and regional anesthesia both cause peripheral vasodilation, which results in a core-to-peripheral redistribution of heat. Opioids and muscle relaxants depress voluntary shivering as a mechanism for the generation of heat. Any patient in whom a body cavity is entered may lose heat via convection and evaporation. Irrigation solutions used in genitourinary procedures or with cardioplegia in cardiac surgery cause internal cooling.[34]

Physiologically, hypothermia results in decreased oxygen availability by shifting of the oxyhemoglobin dissociation curve to the left. Shivering may increase oxygen demand by 400% to 500%. Metabolically dependent processes slow, thereby decreasing drug biotransformation. Renal transport processes are slowed, thereby decreasing glomerular filtration. Cardiac rate and rhythm disturbances, including bradydysrhythmias and premature ventricular contractions, may occur. Central nervous system depression may be profound.[84] Other adverse effects of perioperative hypothermia include patient discomfort, increased adrenergic stimulation, coagulopathy, increased blood loss, impaired wound healing, surgical site infection, and increased hospital costs.[34,81,85]

Treatment of hypothermia should ideally be focused on prevention.[85] Assessment of the patient's need for prewarming begins preoperatively, and active warming measures can be instituted for hypothermic patients.[10,85] The patient's temperature should be monitored throughout the perioperative period. During the surgical procedure, warming methods should be used to prevent hypothermia. Passive, active, or a combination of warming methods may be used during surgery based on patient needs or procedure requirements. Passive warming methods, such as blankets, are used as an adjunct for prevention of heat loss.[86]

As a result of positioning, operating time, and anesthetic exposure, therapeutic intervention most often begins in the PACU. Every patient in the PACU should be assessed for hypothermia with care initiated to restore normothermia when indicated.[81] ASPAN's multidisciplinary

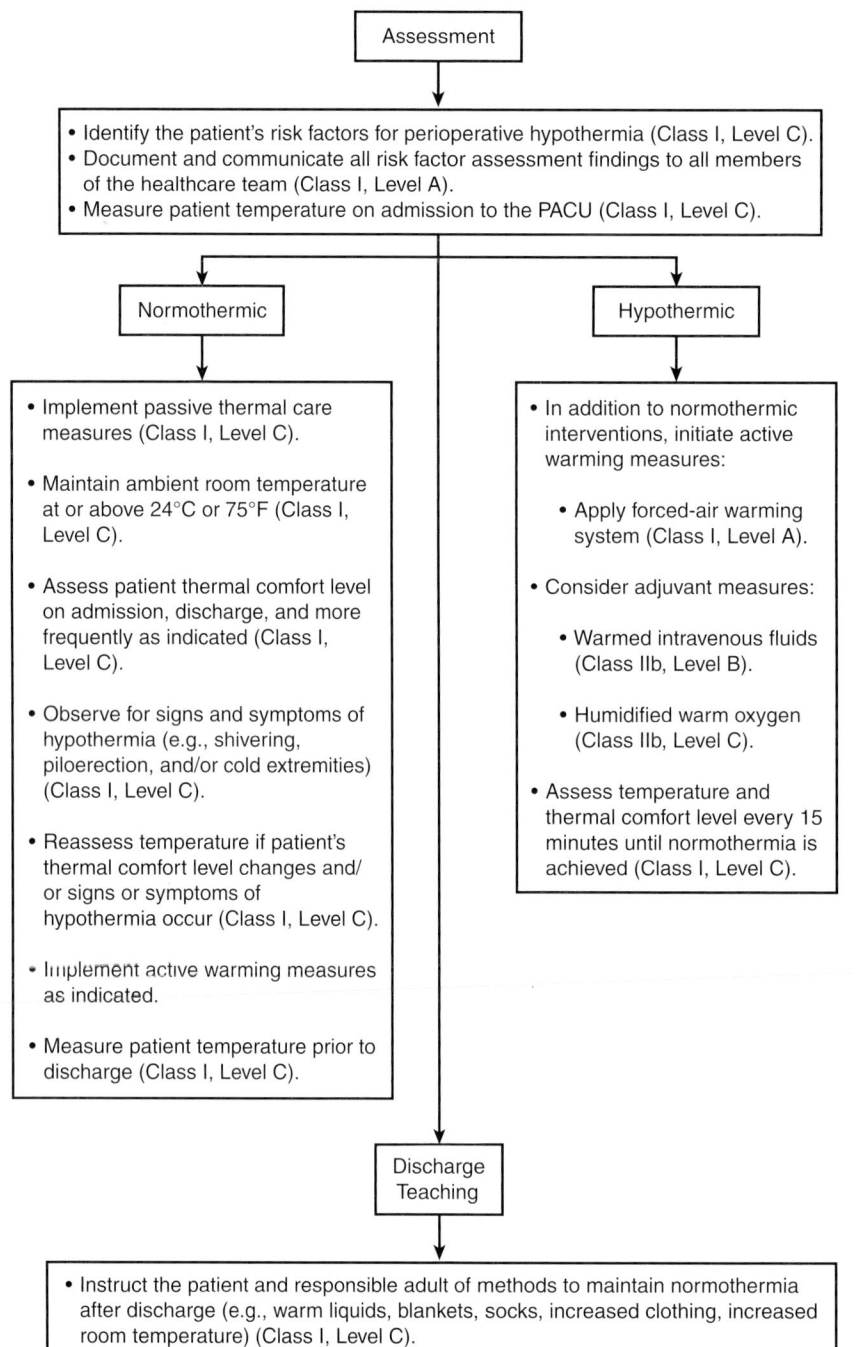

Fig. 55.4 Preoperative, intraoperative, and postoperative patient management recommendations for promotion of normothermia. *PACU,* Postanesthesia care unit. (From Hooper VD, et al. ASPAN's evidence-based clinical practice guideline for the promotion of perioperative normothermia. 2nd ed. *J Perianesth Nurs.* 2010;25:346–365.)

evidence-based clinical practice guideline for the promotion of perioperative normothermia provides an algorithm to guide maintenance of normothermia in surgical patients (Fig. 55.4).[80] Passive rewarming is designed to maximize basal heat production. Active rewarming consists of the use of external rewarming techniques and may include the use of heated blankets, heated water blankets, and radiant warmers. Madrid et al.[84] determined that single strategies such as forced-air warming were more effective than passive warming; however, combined strategies, including using prewarming preoperatively, using warmed fluids plus forced-air warming, as well as other active strategies, were more

effective in vulnerable groups. Forced-air rewarming systems are the most effective method for treating hypothermia.[6] Warming the patient in phase I and phase II PACU can increase patient satisfaction and decrease opioid requirements.[85] Active warming decreases the amount of time required for the patient to reach normothermia and thus can decrease length of stay in the PACU.

Postoperative shivering consists of muscular tremor and rigidity. It is often associated with body heat loss, although hypothermia alone does not fully explain the occurrence of shivering. Shivering is self-limiting, never becomes chronic, and is rarely associated with major

BOX 55.9 Evidence-Based Risk Factors Associated With Postoperative Nausea and Vomiting

Patient Specific
- Female gender
- Age <50 years
- Nonsmoker
- History of PONV
- History of motion sickness

Anesthetic Related
- Use of volatile anesthetics
- Duration of anesthesia
- Use of nitrous oxide
- Postoperative opioid use

Surgery Related
- Type of surgery, especially laparoscopy, gynecologic, cholecystectomy

PONV, Postoperative nausea and vomiting.
Data from Apfel CC, et al. Who is at risk for postdischarge nausea and vomiting after ambulatory surgery? *Anesthesiology.* 2012;117(3):475–486; Apfel CC, et al. Evidence-based analysis of risk factors for postoperative nausea and vomiting. *Br J Anaesth.* 2012;109:742–753; Gan T, et al. Fourth consensus guidelines for the management of postoperative nausea and vomiting. *Anesth Analg.* 2020;131:411–448.

morbidity. However, it affects the comfort of patients and may sometimes lead to more serious complications.[34] Treatment is rewarming; however, when clinically indicated during recovery, small opioid doses can be effective within 3 minutes in the treatment of shivering.[87]

Nausea and Vomiting

In 1914, the first journal devoted solely to the topic of anesthesia featured an original article titled, "Prophylaxis of Postanesthetic Vomiting."[88] More than 100 years later, postanesthetic vomiting is still one of the major problems faced in the PACU. Postoperative nausea and vomiting (PONV) affects 20% to 30% of all surgical patients, and the chance for PONV can be as high as 70% to 80% for high-risk patients.[89] Postdischarge nausea and vomiting (PDNV) is still considered an equally troublesome and all-too-frequent patient complication. The incidence of vomiting is lower than nausea.[90] The evidence-based risk factors for adults listed in Box 55.9 are positive overall for PONV. Females experience PONV two to three times more often than males, although these differences do not show up until after puberty. Being a nonsmoker and having a history of motion sickness or PONV are also independent predictors of PONV. One theory is that smoking may be protective because of functional changes in neuroreceptors from chronic exposure to nicotine and that the smoker's susceptibility to PONV is reduced due to nicotine withdrawal.[91] Use of volatile anesthetics is dose dependent and typically is only associated with PONV 2 to 6 hours after surgery.[92] There is conflicting evidence for some risk factors, including ASA physical status, menstrual cycle, level of experience of anesthesia provider, and preoperative fasting. Anxiety, obesity, use of a nasogastric tube, history of migraines, and supplemental oxygen have been disproven or not clinically relevant as predictors.[92]

When examining anesthetic-related risk factors, the use of volatile anesthetics is the strongest predictor of PONV. The risk of PONV decreases with use of total intravenous anesthesia or regional anesthesia that is free of opioids, multimodal pain medication, perioperative use of α_2-agonists, and β-blockers. The duration of surgery contributes

to the incidence of PONV. Longer procedures are associated with a longer exposure to inhalation agents and possibly a larger dose of opioids during the surgery. In particular, cholecystectomy, laparoscopic, and gynecologic surgeries have been associated with PONV.[92] Interestingly, one study of 203 adult ambulatory surgery patients over 5 days postoperatively found significantly more PDNV in patients with a high level of pain than those with lower levels of pain, even when controlling for opioid use.[93]

Simplified risk-assessment instruments are available that identify patients' risk for PONV. The use of risk assessment tools decreases the incidence of both PONV and PDNV. The two tools most commonly used are the Koivuranta score and the Apfel score. The Apfel risk assessment tool[89,91] scores the patient based on four risk factors: gender, smoking status, history of PONV or motion sickness, and postoperative use of opioids. A patient's risk increases with the number of risk factors present. The Koivuranta score includes the four risk predictors in the Apfel score but adds length of surgery greater than 60 minutes as an additional predictor.[94] An assessment of risk factors should be done preoperatively, and the management of patients at risk should be guided by the number of risk factors and chance of PONV. An ambulatory surgery patient can be further assessed for the development of PDNV. The Apfel risk assessment for PDNV includes female gender, history of motion sickness and/or PONV, age less than 50 years, the use of postoperative opioids, and PONV in the PACU.[90] The expected incidence of PONV and PDNV based on the number of risk factors is noted in Table 55.4.

The risk factors for children include age older than 3 years, a history of PONV or motion sickness, family history of PONV, and females who are postpuberty. Other intraoperative risk factors for children are eye surgeries, tonsillectomies, otoplasty, surgery greater than 30 minutes, volatile anesthetics, and use of anticholinergic medication. A postoperative risk factor is the use of long-acting opioids.[90] A simplified risk score to predict postoperative vomiting (POV) in children was developed by Eberhart et al.[95] and includes the following four variables: duration of the surgical procedure greater than or equal to 30 minutes, age older than or equal to 3 years, strabismus surgery, and a personal history of POV or PONV in immediate relatives.

The Society for Ambulatory Anesthesia (SAMBA) offers clinical practice guidelines and recommendations for antiemetic prophylaxis and treatment of PONV and PDNV. Twenty-four professional organizations, including AANA and ASPAN, have endorsed the Fourth SAMBA consensus guidelines for PONV and PDNV.[92]

Management of nausea and vomiting should originate from a prophylactic rather than a therapeutic approach, particularly in patients identified as at risk. To decrease the risk of PONV in all patients, an individualized plan of care should be developed. Strategies recommended are using multimodal analgesic regimens with less opioids, using regional anesthesia when possible, avoidance of inhalational anesthetics, use of propofol as the primary anesthetic, and use of adequate hydration in day-surgery patients.[92] Two other recommendations are to use sugammadex instead of neostigmine for reversal of neuromuscular blockade and to avoid use of nitrous oxide when the surgery will last longer than 1 hour. One important difference in the current SAMBA guidelines from their past guidelines is to administer multimodal prophylaxis in patients with one or more risk factors. Fig. 55.5 provides an algorithm for management of PONV.

The patient who experiences PONV may begin with nausea, a subjective feeling of discomfort, or the need to vomit. Nausea can be rated on a verbal descriptor scale or numeric rating scale to determine its severity. Commonly, antiemetic prophylaxis will be given to patients at risk. The number and variety of agents administered will be increased according to the number of risk factors present in a

TABLE 55.4 Incidence of PONV and PDNV Based on the Number of Risk Factors With Apfel Scoring Systems

Number of PONV Risk Factors	Incidence %
1	10–20
2	40
3	60
≥4	80

PONV risk factors include female gender, age <50 years, history of motion sickness and/or PONV, nonsmoking, and the use of postoperative opioids.

Number of PDNV Risk Factors	Incidence %
0	10
1	20
2	30
3	50
4	60
5	80

PDNV risk factors include female gender, history of motion sickness and/or PONV, age <50 years, the use of postoperative opioids, and PONV in the PACU.

PACU, Postanesthesia care unit; *PDNV*, postdischarge nausea and vomiting; *PONV*, postoperative nausea and vomiting.
Data from Gan T, et al. Fourth consensus guidelines for the management of postoperative nausea and vomiting. *Anes Analg.* 2020;131:411–448; Apfel CC, et al. A simplified risk score for predicting postoperative nausea and vomiting. *Anesthesiology.* 1999;91:693–700; Apfel CC, et al. Who is at risk for postdischarge nausea and vomiting after ambulatory surgery? *Anesthesiology.* 2012;117:475–486.

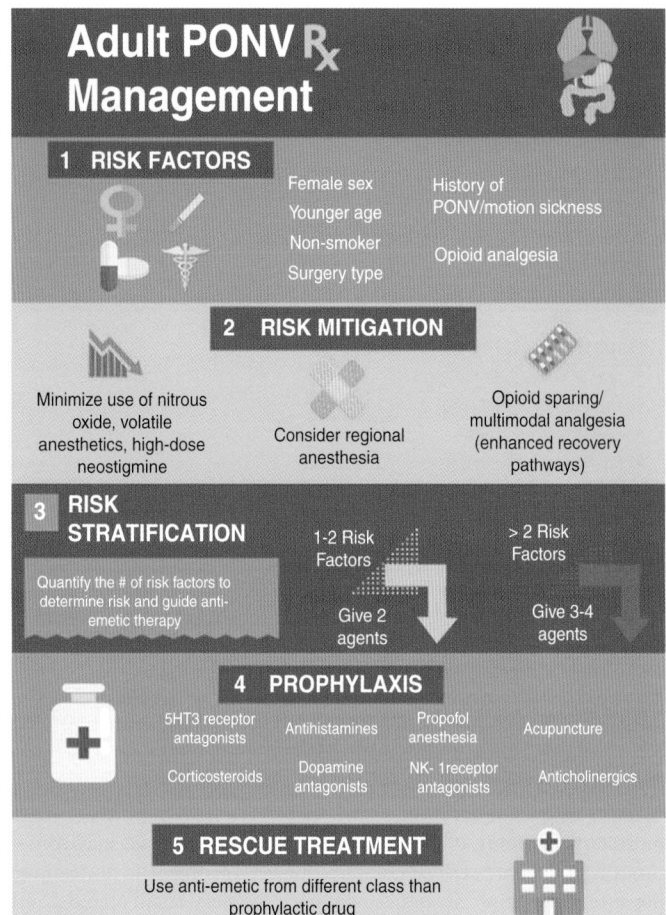

Fig. 55.5 Algorithm for postoperative nausea and vomiting *(PONV)* management in adults. Summary of recommendations for PONV management in adults, including risk identification, stratified prophylaxis, and treatment of established PONV. Note that two antiemetics are now recommended for PONV prophylaxis in patients with one or two risk factors. *5HT3*, 5-hydroxytryptamine 3. (Figure reused with permission from the American Society for Enhanced Recovery.)

multimodal approach. Smaller doses of drugs with differing mechanisms are chosen to allow for a broader array of potential coverage. If a patient experiences PONV and has already received an antiemetic, a rescue drug or drugs with a different mechanism are chosen.[92,96] Other rescue interventions should be implemented, including verification of adequate hydration, as supplemental intravenous crystalloids or colloids are associated with a lower incidence of several PONV outcomes.[92] Drugs that block the serotonin receptors (5-HT₃) are ondansetron, granisetron, and palonosetron. Dolasetron, tropisetron, and ramosetron are not available in the United States but are used in other countries.[92,96] Ondansetron, granisetron, and dolasetron should be administered at the end of surgery.[92] Due to a 40-hour half-life, palonosetron should be administered at the beginning of surgery.[96] Antidopaminergics include a recently approved drug for PONV, amisulpride, which is a dopamine D_2, D_3 receptor antagonist. An antiemetic dose was not associated with sedation, extrapyramidal side effects, or QTc prolongation. Droperidol blocks the dopamine (D_2) receptor sites. Although the Food and Drug Administration (FDA) black box warning about QT prolongation and required ECG monitoring must be kept in mind, recent studies have shown that an antiemetic dose of 0.625 mg is effective and safe.[92] Haloperidol in low doses is sometimes used as an alternative to droperidol, but the half-life is longer. Haloperidol is not FDA approved for PONV. Other D_2-blocking agents are perphenazine and metoclopramide. Perphenazine has limited data that suggest it is effective at a dose of 5 mg intravenously. Metoclopramide can be used if no other dopamine antagonists are available. Studies suggest that the 10-mg dose is not as

effective as the 25- or 50-mg dose, but extrapyramidal symptoms are more common with higher doses. Substance P is another neurotransmitter that belongs to the neurokinin family of neurotransmitters. Substance P has affinity for neurokinin 1 (NK-1) receptors. Aprepitant, which has a half-life of 40 hours, is available in oral and parenteral (fosaprepitant) forms. Other NK-1 receptor antagonists are available but not approved for PONV use.[92,96] The NK-1 receptor antagonists reduce the incidence of postoperative vomiting more effectively than postoperative nausea.[91] For histamine receptors, promethazine or diphenhydramine can be used. Diphenhydramine is more effective with the 50-mg dose than the 25-mg dose. Promethazine preferably should be administered deep intramuscular rather than intravenous because of the damage it can cause to surrounding issue if it extravasates. If given intravenously, it should be in a concentration of 25 mg/mL or less and should not exceed 25 mg/min, or be diluted in 50 mL of saline.[92,96] Dexamethasone, a corticosteroid, is as effective as ondansetron in incidence of PONV. An added advantage is that dexamethasone has reduced the need for analgesics in some studies, and when given in a single dose it has few side effects.[92]

Transdermal scopolamine, an anticholinergic, is effective in the PACU and for 24 hours postoperatively. Side effects can include dry mouth, blurry vision, and dizziness. The patch can be applied behind the

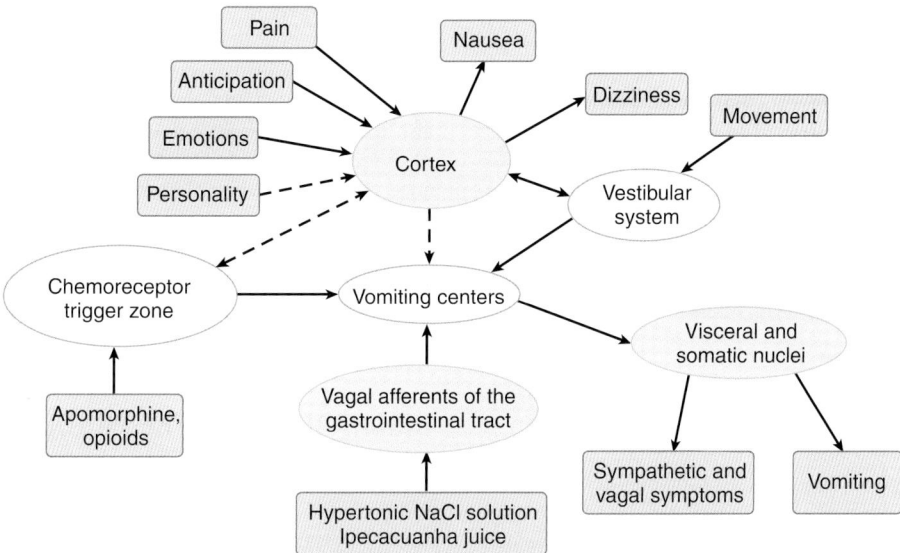

Fig. 55.6 Pathways for nausea and vomiting. Dotted lines are hypothetic pathways with only indirect evidence. *NaCl,* Sodium chloride. (Created by Christian Apfel, MD, PhD.)

ear the night before surgery or 2 to 4 hours before surgery. It is contraindicated in older adults and patients with narrow angle glaucoma.[92,96]

Other drugs used include gabapentinoids (gabapentin and pregabalin). Gabapentin has been effective in reducing PONV and opioid consumption when given orally 1 to 2 hours before surgery; however, it was associated with respiratory depression. Increased attention should be given to patients who have also received opioids.[97] Ephedrine 0.5 mg/kg can reduce PONV for 3 hours postoperatively when given near the end of surgery.[92] Caution should be taken with those at risk for myocardial ischemia.

Nonpharmacologic interventions also may be appropriate for the patient with PONV in addition to pharmacologic interventions.[24,92,96] Acupuncture, transcutaneous electrical nerve stimulation, acupoint stimulation, and acupressure have been shown to be effective in reducing the incidence of PONV and need for rescue medication. P6 stimulation has been shown to be effective, as well as Korean hand acupoints.[92,96] Aromatherapy (e.g., isopropyl alcohol, peppermint oil) has been used to treat PONV.[92,96,98] However, a Cochrane review found that aromatherapy did not reduce the incidence or severity of PONV. It did, however, reduce the need for rescue antiemetics. Isopropyl alcohol decreased the severity of nausea but not the need for rescue antiemetics.[99] Controlled breathing has been shown to be as effective alone as in combination with isopropyl alcohol in the treatment of PONV.[100] Adequate hydration can also reduce the risk of PONV. Supplemental crystalloids (10–30 mL/kg) can reduce early and late PONV and the need for rescue antiemetics.[101] Some commonly used antiemetics for PONV and PDNV are listed in Table 14.7. Colloids reduced PONV more effectively in surgeries lasting more than 3 hours but not in surgeries less than 3 hours.[102] Dextrose infusions were not effective in reducing risk of PONV.[103,104]

Side effects (e.g., agitation, restlessness, drowsiness) may be associated with the use of some antiemetics. Prophylaxis using a combination of antiemetic drugs and/or nonpharmacologic methods has been suggested as an effective strategy for minimizing PONV. The effectiveness of combination antiemetic therapy versus single therapy for high-risk patients is clear.[92] Combination therapy should consist of medications from different classes. ERAS pathways include PONV management as an important part of patient care. Multimodal PONV prophylaxis is recommended within each pathway.[92]

Pathways for nausea and vomiting are shown in Fig. 55.6.

Fluids

The goal of fluid management during the perioperative period is to maintain adequate intravascular fluid volume, left ventricular filling pressure, cardiac output, systemic blood pressure, and oxygen delivery to tissues. Appropriate concentrations of body fluid and electrolytes in the perioperative patient are essential to normal physiologic function of all body systems.[105] According to ASA practice guidelines,[25] routine perioperative assessment of patients' hydration status and fluid management reduces adverse outcomes and improves patient comfort and satisfaction. Crystalloid solutions begin to exit the intravascular space in just minutes. This factor limits hemodynamic support. Crystalloids accumulate in body tissue to include incision sites and lungs, which promotes weight gain, edema, and a prolonged recovery.[106]

The principles of goal-directed fluid therapy (GDFT), particularly in the high-risk surgical population, support prevention of postoperative fluid overload. Implementation of ERAS pathways that incorporate euvolemia versus traditionally liberal perioperative fluid administration has been positively linked to lower cardiopulmonary complications and overall postoperative morbidity, and a decreased length of stay.[75,107] When the patient can safely ingest fluids, ERAS pathway adoption of early postoperative oral hydration in the PACU has been shown to prevent ileus and promote early recovery from surgery.[108]

Upon the patient's admission to the PACU, intravascular volume is estimated with consideration given to preoperative status, type and duration of surgery, estimated blood loss, fluid replacement, and hemostasis. Monitoring urine output as an index of intravascular volume can be misleading. Surgery and anesthesia impair renal tubular concentrating ability, and glycosuria causes osmotic diuresis, each falsely indicating that intravascular volume is adequate. Central venous pressure, pulmonary arterial pressure, or transesophageal ultrasound monitoring can help clarify volume status. Symptoms such as poor skin perfusion (e.g., cool, pale, and clammy skin) particularly in the feet, oliguria, hypotension, tachycardia, and tachypnea can indicate hypovolemia.[12,105]

A reduction in circulating intravascular volume decreases ventricular filling and cardiac output. SNS-mediated tachycardia, increased SVR, and venoconstriction might compensate for a 15% to 20% loss of intravascular volume. Greater deficits can cause hypotension. Failure to replace preoperative fluid deficit and fluid or blood lost during surgery frequently causes hypovolemia. In the PACU, ongoing hemorrhage, sweating, and exudation of fluid into tissues (i.e., third-space losses) exacerbate hypovolemia. Blood loss is often occult, as with retroperitoneal bleeding, diffuse oozing related to coagulopathy, or hemorrhage into muscle after trauma or orthopedic procedures. Third-space losses can continue for up to 48 hours after surgery and can be massive during high-permeability pulmonary edema or accumulation of ascites. In a hypothermic, vasoconstricted patient, a low intravascular volume might maintain cardiac output on PACU admission but cause hypotension when venous capacity increases during rewarming.[34]

Urinary Output and Voiding

Monitoring kidney function during recovery reduces morbidity in patients with marginal cardiovascular or renal status. The ability to void after spinal or epidural anesthesia should be assessed because autonomic effects of regional anesthetics or opioids interfere with sphincter relaxation and promote urine retention.[109] Intrathecal anesthetic administration impacts the lower urinary tract at a higher rate and thus increases the threat of urine retention. Opioids, ketamine, general anesthetics, and NSAIDs may also increase the risk of postoperative urine retention (POUR) because they impede lower urinary tract function.[110] Diabetes can decrease sensation and contractility in the bladder and increase bladder capacity, therefore assessment is important because diabetic patients frequently develop POUR.[111]

Urinary retention is common after urologic, inguinal, and genital surgery and frequently delays discharge. It is reasonable to discharge inpatients to a surgical floor and selected ambulatory surgical patients from the facility before they void.[6] However, it is important to ensure that urine output is monitored after discharge from the PACU to avoid urinary retention. A predictor of POUR was the presence of greater than 400 to 500 mL of urine in the bladder immediately after spinal anesthesia.[110] The amount of urine retained in the bladder can be assessed with use of a bladder scanner.[109,112] Accurate bladder volume assessment informs clinical decisions regarding the appropriateness of in-and-out catheterization to drain the urine and prevent complications.[112] It is prudent to give ambulatory patients who are discharged without voiding a specific time interval in which to void (e.g., 6–8 hours after discharge). If retention persists, the patient should be instructed to contact a health care facility. Patients with indwelling catheters should have urinary output recorded hourly.

Urine color is not useful for assessment of renal tubular function such as concentrating ability, but color can signal hematuria, hemoglobinuria, or pyuria. Urine osmolarity is a more reliable index of tubular function than specific gravity, which is affected by molecular weight.

Oliguria (<0.5 mL/kg/hour) occurs frequently during recovery and usually reflects an appropriate renal response to hypovolemia or systemic hypotension.[12] Low urine output may also result from intentional GDFT, which should be considered as an intended causative factor.[113] However, a decreased urine output might indicate abnormal renal function. The acceptable degree and duration of oliguria vary with underlying renal status, the surgical procedure, and the anticipated postoperative course. If events related to the surgical procedure could jeopardize renal function (e.g., aortic cross-clamping, severe hypotension, massive transfusion), oliguria must be aggressively evaluated. In patients without catheters, bladder volume and interval since last voiding should be checked to help differentiate between oliguria and inability to void. Urinary catheters should be checked for kinking and obstruction by blood clots or debris. Patient position might also place the catheter tip above the urinary level in the bladder.[109]

Polyuria, a state of profuse urine output, usually reflects generous intraoperative fluid administration. Osmotic diuresis caused by hyperglycemia and glycosuria is another cause, particularly if glucose-containing crystalloid solutions have been infused. Polyuria might also reflect intraoperative diuretic administration. Sustained polyuria (4–5 mL/kg/hour) can indicate abnormal regulation of water clearance, especially if urinary losses compromise intravascular volume and systemic blood pressure. Polyuria related to diabetes insipidus occurs secondarily to intracranial surgery, pituitary ablation, head trauma, increased intracranial pressure, and inadvertent omission of preoperative vasopressin. The diagnosis is made by comparing urine and serum electrolytes and osmolarity. High-output renal failure also should be considered as a cause.[24]

DISCHARGE FROM THE POSTANESTHESIA CARE UNIT

The patient leaving the PACU may be discharged to home, an ambulatory surgical unit, a surgical inpatient unit, or an intensive care unit. The choice of a discharge facility should depend on the patient's need and physical status and the availability of appropriate resources.

When possible, before discharge, each patient should be sufficiently oriented to assess one's own physical condition and be able to summon assistance. Airway reflexes and motor function must be adequate to prevent aspiration. Ventilation and oxygenation should be acceptable and demonstrate sufficient reserve to safely cover minor deterioration in unmonitored settings. To detect hypoxemia, oxygen saturation should be monitored for an appropriate period after discontinuation of supplemental oxygen. Before discharge, patients should be observed for a period after the last intravenous opioid or sedative is administered to assess peak effects and side effects. Hemodynamic measurement and indexes of peripheral perfusion should be relatively constant. Achievement of normal body temperature (>96.8°F) should occur before discharge home or to a medical floor; the ICU staff can continue an active warming process. Resolution of shivering is important. Acceptable analgesia must be achieved and vomiting appropriately controlled. Likely surgical complications must be determined (e.g., bleeding, vascular compromise, pneumothorax, complications of coexisting diseases such as coronary artery disease, diabetes, hypertension, or asthma). The results of postoperative diagnostic tests should be reviewed. The routine requirement for urination before discharge should not be part of a discharge protocol and may be necessary only for selected day-surgery patients. Likewise, the requirement of drinking clear fluids should not be part of a discharge protocol and may be necessary only for selected patients (e.g., diabetic patients) and determined on a case-by-case basis.[6]

Outcome indicators applied to discharge criteria should be written with a patient focus (e.g., "Before discharge, the patient will maintain vital signs within the preoperative range"). Examples of discharge criteria are found in Box 55.10. The patient's ability to meet these criteria constitutes clearance for discharge from the PACU but does not imply readiness for discharge to home. Two scoring systems designed to evaluate patients for outpatient discharge have been piloted by clinicians Aldrete[8] and Chung et al.[114] The Aldrete modified postanesthesia recovery (PAR) score is a modification of the original Aldrete score for PAR (Table 55.5). This modification of the scoring system changed assessment of "color" to assessment of "oxygen saturation." This scoring system is for use when patients are discharged from PACU phase I. A further modification of the Aldrete scoring system for outpatients' street fitness is given in Table 55.6.

Chung et al.[114] developed the Postanesthesia Discharge Scoring system as a simple, objective tool to assess the readiness of patients to be

BOX 55.10 Postanesthesia Care Unit Discharge Criteria

- Regular respiratory pattern
- Respiratory rate appropriate for age
- Absence of restlessness and confusion
- Vital signs within preoperative range
- Pulse oximetry indicates 95% saturation* or value equal to preoperative saturation
- Arterial blood gas values within normal limits[†]
- Ability to maintain patent airway
- Surgical stability of operative site or system
- Pain status controlled
- Postoperative nausea and vomiting addressed
- Temperature within normal limits

* Unit policies may dictate another number needed for oxygen saturation on discharge. There is no known accepted saturation level for discharge; most units require at least 92%.
[†] Not routinely obtained before discharge.

TABLE 55.5 Aldrete Postanesthesia Scoring System

			Admit	15 min	30 min	45 min	60 min
Activity	Able to move voluntarily on command	Four extremities	2	2	2	2	2
		Two extremities	1	1	1	1	1
		No extremities	0	0	0	0	0
Respiration	Able to breathe deeply, cough freely		2	2	2	2	2
	Dyspnea or limited breathing		1	1	1	1	1
	Apnea		0	0	0	0	0
Circulation	BP ± 20 mm Hg of preanesthesia level		2	2	2	2	2
	BP ± 20–50 mm Hg of preanesthesia level		1	1	1	1	1
	BP ± 50 mm Hg of preanesthesia level		0	0	0	0	0
Consciousness	Fully awake		2	2	2	2	2
	Arousable on calling		1	1	1	1	1
	Not responding		0	0	0	0	0
O_2 saturation	Able to maintain O_2 saturation >90% on room air		2	2	2	2	2
	Needs O_2 inhalation to maintain O_2 saturation >90%		1	1	1	1	1
	O_2 saturation <90% even with O_2 supplementation		0	0	0	0	0

BP, Blood pressure; O_2, oxygen.
From Marshall S, Chung F. Assessment of 'home readiness' discharge criteria and post-discharge complications. Curr Opin Anesthesiol. 1997;10.445–480.

TABLE 55.6 Modified Postanesthesia Recovery Score for Outpatients' Street Fitness

Parameter	Description	Score	Parameter	Description	Score
Activity	Able to move four extremities voluntarily on command	2	Dressing	Dry	2
	Able to move two extremities voluntarily on command	1		Wet but stationary	1
	Able to move no extremities voluntarily on command	0		Wet but growing	0
Respiration	Able to breathe deeply and cough freely	2	Pain	Pain free	2
	Dyspnea or limited breathing	1		Mild pain handled by oral medications	1
	Apneic	0		Pain requiring parenteral medications	0
Circulation	BP ± 20 mm Hg of preanesthetic level	2	Ambulation	Able to stand up and walk straight*	2
	BP ± 21–49 mm Hg of preanesthetic level	1		Vertigo when erect	1
	BP + 50 mm Hg of preanesthetic level	0		Dizziness when supine	0
Consciousness	Fully awake	2	Fasting and feeding	Able to drink fluids	2
	Arousable on calling	1		Nauseated	1
	Not responding	0		Nausea and vomiting	0
O_2 saturation	Able to maintain O_2 saturation >92% on room air	2	Urine output	Has voided	2
	Needs O_2 inhalation to maintain O_2 saturation >90%	1		Unable to void but comfortable*	1
	O_2 saturation <90% even with O_2 supplement	0		Unable to void and uncomfortable	0

*May be replaced by Romberg's test or picking up 12 clips in one hand.
From Aldrete JA. The postanesthesia recovery score revisited. J Clin Anesth. 1995;7:89–91.

BOX 55.11   Postanesthesia Discharge Scoring System

Vital Signs

2 = Within 20% of preoperative value

1 = 20%–40% of preoperative value

0 = >40% of preoperative value

Activity and Mental Status

2 = Oriented three separate times and a steady gait

1 = Oriented three separate times or a steady gait

0 = Neither

Pain, Nausea, Vomiting

2 = Minimal

1 = Moderate, requiring treatment

0 = Severe, requiring treatment

Surgical Bleeding

2 = Minimal

1 = Moderate

0 = Severe

Intake and Output

2 = Postoperative fluids and void

1 = Postoperative fluids or void

0 = Neither

From Chung F, et al. A post-anesthetic discharge scoring system for home-readiness after ambulatory surgery. *J Clin Anesth.* 1995;7:500–506.

discharged to home (Box 55.11). A score of 9 is needed for the patient to be discharged. Although studied retrospectively, the scoring system has yet to be tried as a predictive index in a widespread clinical trial. Regardless of the method used to assess readiness for discharge, the assessment should be documented in an objective manner using criteria agreed upon by the departments of anesthesia, nursing, and surgery.

More research to support PACU patient discharge criteria is needed.[115] Fixed PACU discharge criteria must be used with caution because variability among patients is tremendous. Scoring systems that quantify physical status or establish thresholds for vital signs are useful for assessment[11] but cannot replace individual evaluation. Hawker et al. have pointed out the need for an evidenced-based, psychometrically tested discharge scoring instrument.[116]

Fast-tracking outpatients after general anesthesia has assumed increased importance in ambulatory anesthesia because of the cost-saving potential when patients are transferred directly from the OR to the less labor-intensive phase II recovery area. Given the inherent risks of complications associated with bypassing the PACU, effective and reliable fast-track criteria that allow anesthesia providers to rapidly assess a patient's postoperative alertness, physiologic stability, and comfort level immediately before transferring the patient from the OR are clearly needed. An outpatient should be discharged to a responsible adult, who will accompany the patient home and able to report any postprocedure complications. In addition, outpatients should be provided with written instructions regarding postprocedure diet, medications, activities, and a phone number to call in case of emergency.[1]

Ideally, each patient should be evaluated for discharge by a qualified anesthesia provider using a consistent set of criteria[117] that take into consideration the severity of the underlying disease, the anesthetic and recovery course, and the level of care at the destination, especially for ambulatory patients.

▮ SUMMARY

PACUs are vital to the safe recovery of patients from surgery and anesthesia. Nurses provide the skillful bridge to ensuring a successful perioperative experience. They assess and monitor patients for residual anesthetic effects and surgical complications and reinstitute care for preexisting medical problems. Integrating care provided by the nurse with that of the anesthesia and surgical teams is essential in advancing optimal team-based postoperative patient outcomes.

REFERENCES

For a complete list of references for this chapter, scan this QR code with any smartphone code reader app, or visit the following URL: http://booksite.elsevier.com/9780323711944/.

56

Acute Pain: Physiology and Management

Sandra K. Bordi

Pain is well recognized as a public health concern and is associated with emotional, personal, and societal costs. In the United States, it is estimated that approximately 50 million adults suffer from chronic pain, and 19.6 million of those experience high-impact chronic pain, which limits quality of life and work activities.[1] In an era burdened with an opioid crisis, health care providers are challenged with alleviating patients' pain while reducing the risk of opioid misuse/abuse. Multiple clinical practice guidelines (CPGs) exist for pain management. However, the degree to which they are adopted and implemented are unknown. Therefore several professional and regulatory groups have proposed standards, responsibilities, and outcome measures to improve pain management. The Joint Commission (TJC) published new and revised pain assessment and management standards that were implemented in 2018[2] (Box 56.1). The implementation and clarification of these standards are momentous steps in the improvement of pain management.

As providers of anesthesia care in the United States, Certified Registered Nurse Anesthetists (CRNAs) are integral to the research and management of acute and chronic pain. CRNAs practice both autonomously and in collaboration with other health providers to deliver high-quality, holistic, evidence-based anesthesia and pain care services.[3] CRNAs are recognized as experts in the area of pain management, and their knowledge and skills are essential in pursuing effective pain management modalities.

PAIN

Definition

Pain remains a very complex and multidimensional experience. It was defined by the International Association for the Study of Pain (IASP) as "an unpleasant sensory and emotional experience associated with actual or potential tissue damage or described in terms of such damage."[4] The inherent context of this definition is that pain is a physiologic, emotional, and behavioral experience.[5] Commonly used pain terminology is listed in Box 56.2.

Classification of pain is primarily based on longevity (acute vs chronic) and/or the underlying pathophysiology (nociceptive or nonnociceptive). Nociceptive pain is associated with the stimulation of specific nociceptors and can be either somatic or visceral. Somatic pain refers to pain that has an identifiable locus as a result of tissue damage causing the release of chemicals from injured cells that mediate pain. Somatic pain is well localized, sharp in nature, and generally hurts at the point or area of stimulus. Conversely, visceral pain is diffuse, can be referred to another area, and is often described as "dull," "cramping," "squeezing," or vague in nature. Visceral pain is often associated with the distention of an organ capsule or the obstruction of a hollow viscus. It is also often accompanied with autonomic reflexes such as nausea, vomiting, and diarrhea.[6] In contrast, nonnociceptive pain can be categorized as being neuropathic. Neuropathic pain is caused by damage to peripheral or central neural structures resulting in abnormal processing of painful stimuli.

It is a dysfunction of the central nervous system (CNS) that allows for spontaneous excitation in chronic pain states. Neuropathic pain is often described as "burning," "tingling," or "shocklike."[7] Lastly, unlike neuropathic pain, inflammatory pain is a result of sensitization of the nociceptive pathway from multiple mediators being released at the site of tissue inflammation without neural injury. Patients in chronic pain states often exhibit more than one type of pain.[8]

Anatomy and Physiology

Somatic nociceptive pain is most commonly defined in terms of four processes: transduction, transmission, perception, and modulation. Transduction is the transformation of a noxious stimulus (chemical, mechanical, or thermal) into an action potential. A noxious stimulus is detected by pain receptors, or nociceptors, which are free nerve endings. These peripheral nociceptors that conduct noxious stimuli to the dorsal horn of the spinal cord are categorized according to morphology (diameter, myelination, and conduction velocity). The myelinated A-delta (Aδ) primary afferent neurons conduct action potentials at velocities between 6 and 30 m/s and elicit fast-sharp pain. They are responsible for the initial mechanical or thermal pain that is felt and alert an individual of tissue damage, thereby resulting in the reflex withdraw mechanism. The smaller nonmyelinated C fibers conduct at velocities significantly slower, between 0.5 and 2 m/s. Because C fibers respond to mechanical, thermal, and chemical injuries, they are also known as polymodal fibers. As a result of their slow conducting velocity, a delayed, slow, second pain is elicited by C fibers.[8] Slow pain is commonly described as "dull," "burning," "throbbing," and "aching."

Consequently, when peripheral tissues (skin, bone, and viscera) receive chemical, thermal, or mechanical stimuli or are traumatized by either surgery or injury, a series of biochemical events takes place in peripheral pain transduction. These events include the release of chemical mediators from the inflammatory response and the release of neurotransmitters from nociceptive nerve endings (Fig. 56.1). The chemical mediators and neurotransmitters released are extensive, with the more prominent substances in the following list:

- Substance P is a peptide found and released from the peripheral afferent nociceptor C fibers and is involved with slow, chronic pain. It acts via the G protein–linked neurokinin-1 receptor, resulting in vasodilation, extravasation of plasma proteins, degranulation of mast cells, and sensitization of the stimulated sensory nerve.[9]
- Glutamate is a major excitatory neurotransmitter released in the CNS and from the Aδ and C primary afferent nerve fibers. Its effects are instantaneous, producing initial, fast, sharp pain.[9]
- Bradykinin is a peptide released during the inflammation process and is notably algesic. It has a direct stimulating effect on peripheral nociceptors via specific bradykinin receptors (B1/B2).
- Histamine is an amine released from mast cell granules, basophils, and platelets via substance P. It reacts with various histamine receptors to produce edema and vasodilation.

BOX 56.1   The Joint Commission Pain Management Standards

The Joint Commission pain management standards require organizations to:

- Identify pain assessment and pain management, including safe opioid prescribing, as an organized priority
- Actively involve the organized medical staff in leadership roles in organization performance improvement activities to improve quality of care, treatment, and services and patient safety
- Assess and manage the patient's pain and minimize the risks associated with treatment
- Collect data to monitor its performance
- Compile and analyze data

From The Joint Commission. Pain assessment and management standards for hospitals. https://www.jointcommission.org/-/media/tjc/documents/standards/r3-reports/r3_report_issue_11_2_11_19_rev.pdf. Accessed 2020.

BOX 56.2   Pain Terminology

Algesia: Increased sensitivity to pain
Algogenic: Pain producing
Allodynia: A normally nonharmful stimulus is perceived as painful
Analgesia: The absence of pain in the presence of a normally painful stimulus
Dysesthesia: An unpleasant painful abnormal sensation, whether evoked or spontaneous
Hyperalgesia: A heightened response to a normally painful stimulus
Neuralgia: Pain in the distribution of a peripheral nerve(s)
Neuropathy: An abnormal disturbance in the function of a nerve(s)
Paresthesia: An abnormal sensation, whether spontaneous or evoked

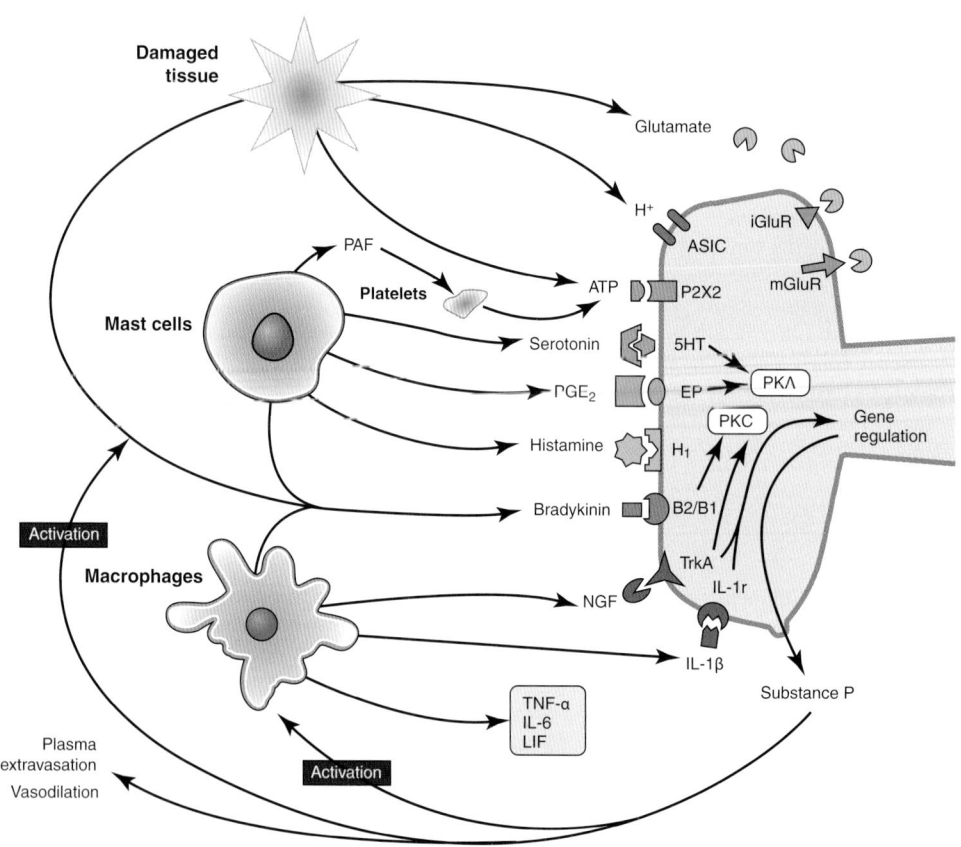

Fig. 56.1 Inflammation and peripheral nociception. After tissue injury, mast cells, macrophages, and neutrophils are activated and/or recruited to the area. In addition, small nociceptor nerve endings are triggered. A variety of algogenic substances are released as a result of the inflammatory response and from the nociceptor nerve endings. These algogenic substances contribute to the pain process either directly (i.e., increasing excitability of nerves) or indirectly via second messenger (i.e., PKA, PKC) responses. *5HT*, 5-Hyroxytryptamin receptor; *ATP*, adenosine triphosphate; *B2/B1*, bradykinin 1 and bradykinin 2 receptor; *EP*, prostaglandin E receptor; *H+*, excess free hydrogen ion; *H₁*, histamine-1 receptor; *iGluR*, ionotropic glutamate receptor; *IL-6*, interleukin-6; *Il-1β*, interleukin-1β; *Il-1r*, interleukin 1 receptor; *LIF*, leukemia-inhibiting factor; *mGluR*, G protein–coupled metabotropic glutamate receptor; *NGF*, nerve growth factor; *P2X2*, primary receptor family for ATP; *PAF*, platelet-activating factor; *PGE₂*, prostaglandin E₂; *PKA*, protein kinase A; *PKC*, protein kinase; *TNF-α*, tumor necrosis factor-α; *TrkA*, tyrosine kinase receptor A. (Modified from Nouri KH, et al. Neurochemistry of somatosensory and pain processing. In: Benzon HT, et al., eds. *Essentials of Pain Medicine.* 4th ed. Philadelphia: Elsevier; 2018:11–20.)

- Serotonin (5-hydroxytryptamine [5-HT]) is an amine stored and released from platelets after tissue injury. It reacts with multiple receptor subtypes and exhibits algesic effects on peripheral nociceptors. Like histamine, serotonin can potentiate bradykinin-induced pain.
- Prostaglandins (PGs), along with thromboxanes and leukotrienes, are a metabolite of arachidonic acid. PGs, specifically, are synthesized from cyclooxygenase-1 (COX-1) and COX-2. They are associated with chronic pain; PGs sensitize peripheral nociceptors, causing hyperalgesia.
- Cytokines are released in response to tissue injury by a variety of immune and nonimmune cells via the inflammatory response. Cytokines, including interleukin-1β (IL1β), IL6, and tumor necrosis factor-α (TNF-α) can lead to the increased production of PGs, thereby exciting and sensitizing nociceptive fibers.[10]
- Calcitonin gene-related peptide (CGRP) is a peptide found and released from the peripheral afferent nociceptor C fibers. It is responsible for producing local cutaneous vasodilation, plasma extravasation, and sensitization of the stimulated sensory nerve.

These chemical mediators and neurotransmitters stimulate the peripheral nociceptors, causing an influx of sodium ions to enter the nerve fiber membranes (depolarization), and a subsequent efflux of potassium ions (repolarization). An action potential results, and a pain impulse is generated.

Transmission is the process by which an action potential is conducted from the periphery to the CNS. There are multiple pathways that carry noxious stimuli to the brain. The spinothalamic (anterolateral) system, which carries pain signals from the trunk and lower extremities, will be discussed here. The primary afferent neurons (Aδ and C fibers) have cell bodies located in the dorsal root ganglia of the spinal cord. Upon entering the dorsal cord these fibers segregate and ascend or descend several spinal segments in the tract of Lissauer. After leaving the tract of Lissauer, the axons of the primary afferents enter the gray matter of the dorsal horn, where they synapse with second-order neurons and terminate primarily in Rexed laminae I, II, and V (Fig. 56.2). Two types of second-order neurons exist: (1) nociceptive neurons, which receive input solely from primary afferent Aδ and C fibers, and (2) wide-dynamic-range (WDR) neurons that receive input from both nociceptive (Aδ and C fibers) and nonnociceptive (Aβ) primary

afferents. WDR neurons are therefore activated by a variety of stimulants (innocuous and noxious) (Fig. 56.3).

Second-order neurons then cross the midline of the spinal cord through the anterior commissure and ascend in the anterolateral pathway of the spinothalamic tract to the thalamus. In the lateral thalamus and the intralaminar nuclei, second-order neurons synapse with third-order neurons, which then send projections to the cerebral cortex. Perception of pain occurs once the signal is recognized by various areas of the brain, including the amygdala, somatosensory areas of the cortex, the hypothalamus, and the anterior cingulate cortex.

Modulation of pain transmission involves altering neural afferent activity along the pain pathway; it can suppress or enhance pain signals. Suppression of pain impulses occurs through local inhibitory interneurons and descending efferent pathways. The descending efferent modulatory pathways from the brain are considered the body's analgesia system or pain control system.[9] It is proposed that the descending dorsolateral efferent pathway is activated via a noxious stimulus. Descending axons from the cerebral cortex, hypothalamus, thalamus, periaqueductal gray area (PAG), nucleus raphe magnus, and locus coeruleus (LC) via the dorsolateral funiculus (DLF) synapse with and suppress pain transmission to the brainstem and the spinal cord dorsal horn. Several neurotransmitters and their receptors play critical roles in the inhibitory modulation of pain, including the inhibitory

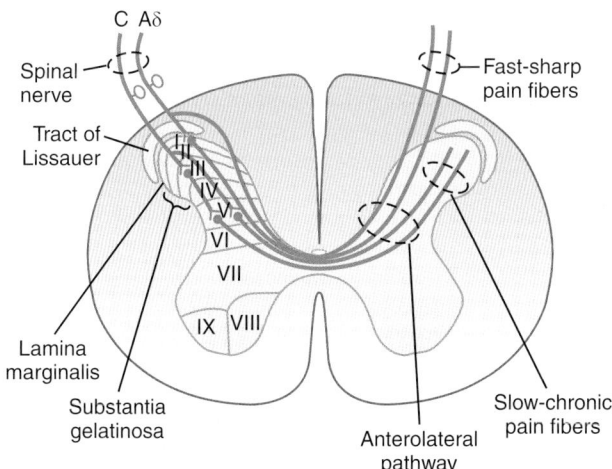

Fig. 56.2 Transmission of both fast-sharp and slow-chronic pain signals into and through the spinal cord on their way to the brain. Aδ fibers transmit fast-sharp pain, and C fibers transmit slow-chronic pain. (From Hall JE, Hall ME, eds. *Guyton and Hall Textbook of Medical Physiology.* 14th ed. Philadelphia: Elsevier; 2021:615.)

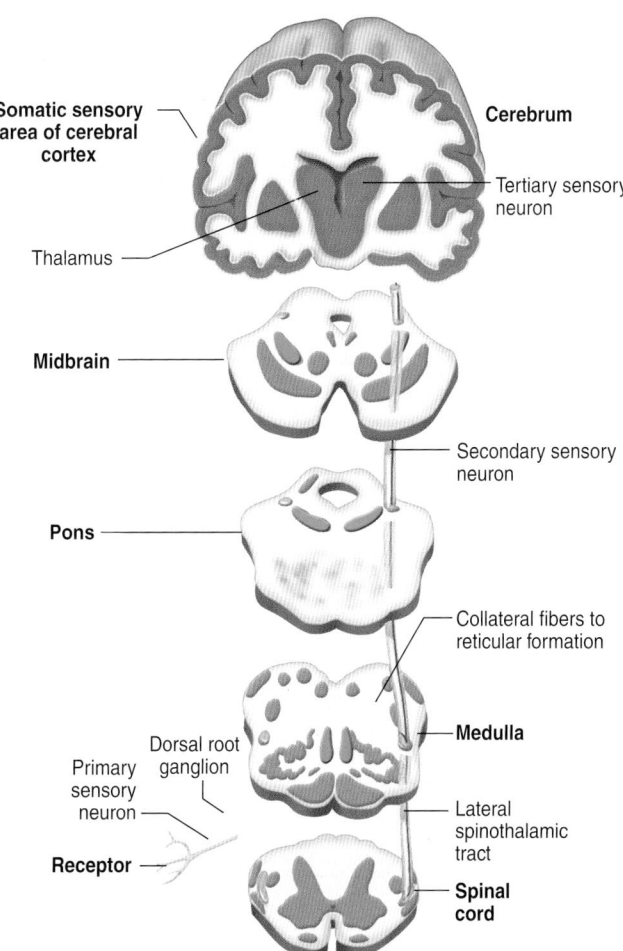

Fig. 56.3 Ascending lateral spinothalamic tract. (From Patton KT, ed. *Anatomy and Physiology.* 10th ed. St. Louis: Elsevier; 2018:439.)

TABLE 56.1 Pain-Modulating Neurotransmitters

Neurotransmitters	Receptor
Excitatory Neurotransmitter	
Substance P	Neurokinin 1 (NK-1), neurokinin 2 (NK-2)
Glutamate	NMDA, AMPA, kainite, mGluRs
Inhibitory Neurotransmitter	
Glycine	Chloride linked (GlyR)
GABA	$GABA_A$, $GABA_B$, $GABA_C$
Enkephalin	μ, δ
Serotonin	5-HT ($5\text{-}HT_{1\text{-}3}$)
Norepinephrine	α_2 adrenergic

5HT, 5-Hydroxytryptamine; *AMPA,* α-amino-3-hydroxy-5-methyl-4-isoxazolepropionic acid; *GABA,* γ-aminobutyric acid; *GlyR,* glycine receptor; *mGluRs,* metabotropic glutamate receptors; *NMDA,* N-methyl-D-aspartate.

endogenous opioids (enkephalin/dynorphin). Action potentials arrive at the substantia gelatinosa via the DLF and activate enkephalin-releasing neurons. Enkephalin then binds to the opiate receptors on presynaptic first-order or postsynaptic second-order afferent fibers, which decrease substance P release, thereby suppressing ascending pain transmission. Other inhibitory neurotransmitters released via the descending pathway include glycine, norepinephrine, serotonin, and γ-aminobutyric acid (GABA) (Table 56.1). Pharmacotherapies for pain control are aimed at many of these neurotransmitters and their receptors.

PHYSIOLOGIC CONSEQUENCES

Acute pain is caused by noxious stimulation resulting from traumatic injury (chemical, thermal, or mechanical), surgery, or acute illness. Generally, the intensity of acute pain diminishes over the course of healing; however, social, cultural, and personality factors may affect this. Its duration is usually self-limited and resolves within healing of the underlying injury, which may take from 1 day to 6 months. Acute pain is responsive to pharmacotherapy and treatment of the precipitating cause. Unfortunately, poorly controlled acute pain may lead to chronic pain states. Therefore optimal pain management is crucial in expediting the healing process and for the prevention of chronic pain.

It is well documented that acute pain causes adverse physiologic consequences involving multiple organ systems, which can contribute to morbidity and mortality in surgical patients. Neuroendocrine responses that are triggered primarily by the sympathetic nervous system (SNS) in response to surgical stress and pain initiate these effects. Factors such as the extent of the surgical field, the number of pain receptors involved in the area, bleeding, infection, anxiety, and presence of coexisting diseases may accelerate the endocrine stress response.

The activation of the SNS in response to the stress of pain from surgery or trauma results in many cardiovascular responses. The increased release of catecholamines from the SNS and adrenal glands, along with cortisol, produces an increased heart rate, increased vascular resistance (peripheral, systemic, and coronary), increased myocardial contractility, and increased arterial blood pressure. These ultimately increase the myocardial demand and myocardial oxygen consumption. Additionally, in the presence of coexisting cardiovascular disease, atherosclerotic

plaque from vascular walls may rupture, thereby decreasing oxygen supply further. This may lead to dysrhythmias, angina, myocardial ischemia, and myocardial infarction. Overall, the incidence of increased myocardial oxygen demand and decreased myocardial oxygen supply can have deleterious effects in those patients with coexisting cardiovascular disease. Therefore aggressive pain management is essential in reducing the incidence of postoperative cardiac complications.[11]

The presence of pain can have significant effects on the respiratory system. These effects are most pronounced in those patients having surgery or trauma in the upper abdominal area and thorax. Inadequate pain management causes a measurable decrease in tidal volume because of limited thoracic and abdominal movement. Specifically, there are decreases in vital capacity, inspiratory capacity, and functional residual capacity (FRC), in addition to a decreased physical ability to clear the airway because of unrelieved pain. Additionally, muscle spasm below and above the site of injury caused by the noxious stimuli promotes limited movement of the respiratory muscles. Patients often voluntarily decrease the movement of the thorax and abdomen (splinting) and are reluctant to breathe deeply or cough in an attempt to limit pain, which can lead to atelectasis and pneumonia.[12,13] These pulmonary alterations may be aggravated in those patients with preexisting pulmonary dysfunction (e.g., asthma, chronic obstructive pulmonary disease) or in those with decreased FRC (e.g., morbidly obese, elderly). Consequently, those affected by postoperative respiratory compromise as a result of inadequate pain management also may be at risk for deep venous thrombosis and subsequent pulmonary embolism caused by a decrease or delay in mobilization. Table 56.2 provides physiologic consequences of acute pain.

The physiologic effects and the consequences of inadequate pain management have been reported to have an impact in prolonging postoperative stay and patient recovery, and an overall increase in health care costs.[14] It also negatively impacts the patient's surgical/hospitalization experience, resulting in reduced patient satisfaction.

Acute Pain Assessment

To devise a plan for intraoperative and postoperative surgical pain management, a preoperative pain assessment and discussion with the patient should be conducted. A thorough preoperative assessment should involve a physical and medical history assessment, including laboratory and diagnostic tests that are patient and surgery specific. Inquiries specific to preoperative pain also should be addressed (Box 56.3). Part of the preoperative pain assessment process also should consist of identifying those at high risk for increased postoperative acute pain. Predictors of acute postoperative pain after elective surgery include (1) the presence of preoperative pain, (2) patient fear regarding the outcome of the surgery, (3) patients who catastrophize pain, and (4) expected postoperative pain.[15-19] Overall, goals for pain management should be based on patient physical/medical assessment, history, invasiveness of the surgical procedure, an individual's pain response, and prediction of identifying those who are at high risk for developing increases in acute pain postoperatively. The patient should be informed of the varying modalities for postoperative pain control, and a unique pain management plan should be implemented by both the patient and care providers. Furthermore, realistic expectations for postoperative pain control should be discussed.

As discussed earlier, adequate postoperative pain control is essential in the recovery process. Assessing the adequacy of postoperative pain control through vigilance and by using simple assessment tools is vital. Because pain is subjective, the most reliable pain assessment tool is primarily via self-report. Pain assessment scales, which are both clinically valid and used in research, are available and are based on measuring pain intensity. The common pain intensity scales include

TABLE 56.2 Physiologic Effects of Acute Pain

Organ System	Physiologic Effect	Adverse Outcome
Cardiovascular	Increased heart rate Increased PVR Increased ABP Increased myocardial contraction Increased myocardial work	Dysrhythmias Angina Myocardial ischemia Myocardial infarction
Pulmonary	Decreased VC Decreased TV Decreased TLC Muscle spasms (respiratory/abdominal) Decreased ability to cough/deep breathe	Ventilation/perfusion mismatch Atelectasis Pneumonia Hypoventilation Hypoxia Hypercarbia
Gastrointestinal	Decreased gastric emptying Decreased intestinal motility Increased smooth muscle sphincter tone	Nausea/vomiting Paralytic ileus
Coagulation	Increased platelet aggregation Venostasis	Thrombosis DVT/PE
Immunologic	Decreased immune function	Increased risk of infection
Genitourinary	Increased urinary sphincter tone	Oliguria Urinary retention
Psychological		Fear Anxiety Depression Feelings of helplessness Anger

ABP, Arterial blood pressure; *DVT*, deep vein thrombosis; *PE*, pulmonary embolism; *PVR*, peripheral vascular resistance; *TLC*, total lung capacity; *TV*, tidal volume; *VC*, vital capacity.
Adapted from Joshi GP, Ogunnaike BO. Consequences of inadequate postoperative pain relief and chronic persistent postoperative pain. *Anesthesiol Clin North Am.* 2005;23(1):21–36.

BOX 56.3 Preoperative Pain Assessment

- Determine the existence of chronic pain
- Current medications (prescription and OTC)—continuous or prn for pain
- Inquiry regarding previous injuries
- Location of pain
- Quality of pain
- Intensity of pain
- Adjunctive therapies (e.g., acupuncture, TENS, injection therapy, SCS)
- Exacerbating factors
- Alleviating factors
- Limitations in movement
- Coexisting psychological diseases

OTC, Over the counter; *prn*, as needed; *SCS*, spinal cord stimulator; *TENS*, transcutaneous electric nerve stimulation.

the visual analog scale (VAS), the numerical rating scale (NRS), and the Wong-Baker FACES scale. Even though these scales are available and are used in the clinical setting, they are not all inclusive. The NRS, VAS, and Wong-Baker FACES scales assign a numeric value to an individual's pain, which is subjective and multidimensional. In addition, they do not take into consideration the patient's age or variations in cognitive level. The NRS is most often used by practitioners in assessing pain by asking the patient, "What is your pain level on a scale of 1 to 10, with 10 being the worst pain you have ever experienced and 0 being pain free?" Although this is a quick tool used to assess pain, it lacks the depth of determining the quality of pain or exacerbating factors that affect pain. Inevitably it is the provider's responsibility to investigate the patient's pain, be it surgical or nonsurgical, and intervene with a treatment modality. Key to successful acute pain control is

vigilant reassessment and evaluation of the patient's response to a given treatment and changing treatment modalities, if necessary, in an effort to alleviate pain.

Preventive Analgesia

Preemptive analgesia is a concept first postulated approximately 100 years ago. It was asserted that by administering analgesics prior to noxious stimulation a decreased pain response would result. The premise is that peripheral and central sensitization results from noxious stimulation, thereby causing an increase in postoperative pain. Therefore the term *preemptive* analgesia refers to the administration of analgesics preoperatively. The term *preventive* analgesia is defined as the attenuation of noxious stimuli pre-, intra-, and postinsult, thereby preventing central sensitization. Preventive analgesia refers to the administration of analgesics throughout the perioperative course.[20] It consists of a multimodal approach to acute pain management. Multimodal pain management utilizes a combination of analgesics that work on a variety of receptors with different mechanisms of action, both peripherally and centrally, resulting in additive or synergistic effects in an effort to improve pain control (Fig. 56.4). Preventive analgesia that institutes multimodal approaches is a common component of enhanced recovery after surgery (ERAS) pain protocols that are currently being used to decrease opioid consumption and opioid side effects, decrease postoperative pain scores, and reduce hospital stay.[21]

PHARMACOLOGY

Nonsteroidal Antiinflammatory Drugs

Nonsteroidal antiinflammatory drugs (NSAIDs) are best known for their use in the management of mild to moderate postoperative pain and pain related to inflammatory conditions. They are the most common analgesic adjuvants used in multimodal analgesia remedies. When using NSAIDs and opioids together, a synergistic effect results in analgesia along with an overall decreased dose of opioids and decreased opioid side effects. NSAIDs vary in chemical structure but all possess antiinflammatory, antipyretic, and analgesic properties. They produce their therapeutic effects by inhibiting COX and thereby preventing conversion of arachidonic acid to prostaglandins (Figs. 56.5 and 56.6). Prostaglandins (primarily PGE_1 and PGE_2) are responsible for sensitizing and amplifying peripheral nociceptors to the inflammatory mediators (substance P, bradykinin, and serotonin), which are released when tissue is traumatized. Therefore prostaglandins do not directly produce pain but instead contribute to hyperalgesia. Centrally, prostaglandins mediate pain by enhancing the release of substance P and glutamate in first-order neurons, increasing nociceptive transmission at

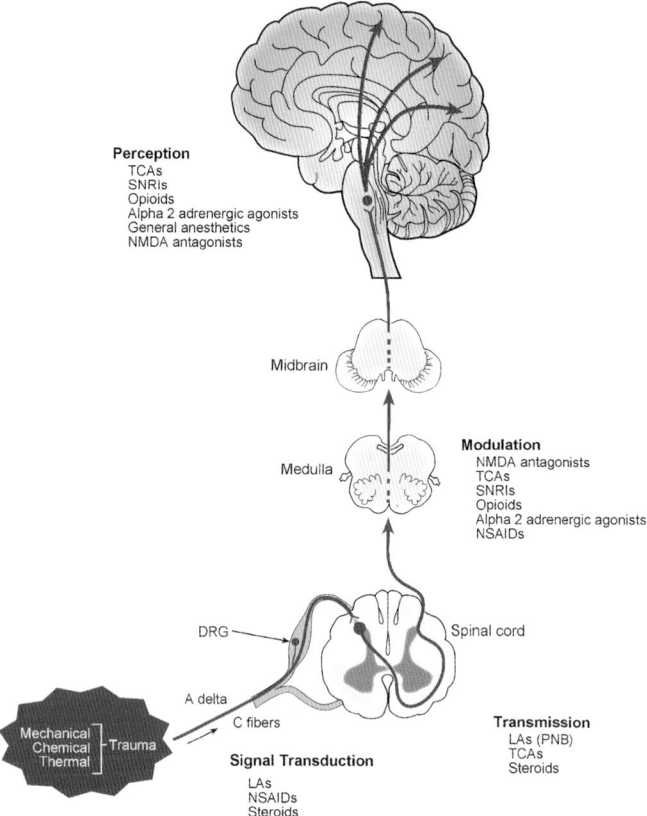

Fig. 56.4 Pharmacotherapy and pain processing targets. The four processes of somatic nociceptive pain are signal transduction, transmission, modulation, and perception. Pharmacotherapy has an overall inhibitory effect on these processes. Modulation occurs primarily in the dorsal horn of the spinal cord but also takes place in supraspinal structures. The endogenous descending inhibitory modulating pathway is also involved in pain inhibition *(not present in this illustration)*. *LA,* Local anesthetic; *NMDA,* N-methyl-D-aspartate antagonist; *NSAIDs,* nonsteroidal antiinflammatory drugs; *PNB,* peripheral nerve block; *SNRI,* selective serotonin-norepinephrine reuptake inhibitor; *TCA,* tricyclic antidepressant.

second-order neurons, in addition to inhibiting the release of descending inhibitory neurotransmitters. For a further description of NSAIDs, see Chapter 11.

Ketorolac

Ketorolac, a nonselective COX inhibitor, is also available for short-term acute postoperative pain, administered either alone or in combination with other analgesic modalities. Ketorolac can be administered orally, intravascularly, intramuscularly, and intranasally. Comparatively, the analgesic potency of ketorolac 30 mg intramuscular (IM) is equivalent to approximately 12 mg of morphine IM.[22] Because of the potential adverse effects caused by the inhibition of COX-1, ketorolac should not be administered beyond 5 days.[23] Contraindications for administering ketorolac include coagulopathies, renal failure, active peptic ulcer disease, gastrointestinal bleeding, history of asthma, hypersensitivity to NSAIDs, and surgery that involves a high risk for postoperative bleeding. In addition, controversy exists regarding bone healing and NSAID administration.[24,25] NSAID inhibition of COX-1, COX-2, and prostaglandin synthesis interrupts normal prostaglandin effects on osteoblast and osteoclast functioning that promotes bone healing.[26] However, there are currently no recommendations regarding NSAID administration and orthopedic procedures.

Acetaminophen

Even though it is not a true NSAID, acetaminophen reduces prostaglandin synthesis by an uncertain mechanism. It has minimal antiinflammatory effects with mainly analgesic and antipyretic properties. It is suitable for acute, mild to moderate postoperative pain and fever. Oral acetaminophen is frequently combined with weak opioids (e.g., oxycodone, hydrocodone, codeine) for the treatment of moderate postoperative pain and chronic pain syndromes. Because it lacks the negative effects of typical NSAIDs (e.g., platelet inhibition, gastrointestinal irritation, renal toxicity), acetaminophen is an ideal drug for multimodal analgesia for surgical pain. Acetaminophen is metabolized primarily by the liver and is therefore contraindicated in patients with liver failure. The Food and Drug Administration (FDA) has limited the strength of acetaminophen to 325 mg per tablet, capsule, or other dosage unit, when combined with weak opioids, thereby limiting severe reactions related to acetaminophen. Parenteral acetaminophen (Ofirmev) is also available for the treatment of acute, mild to moderate pain and is effective in treating moderate to severe pain with adjunctive opioid analgesics.[27] Dosing for adults weighing over 50 kg is 1000 mg every 6 hours or 650 mg every 4 hours infused over 15 minutes to a maximum of 4000 mg/day. Dosing in children over 2 years of age and under 50 kg is 15 mg/kg every 6 hours or 12.5 mg/kg every 4 hours to a maximum of 75 mg/kg/day. Onset of action is approximately 10 minutes with a duration of action of 4 to 6 hours. Adverse effects of intravenous (IV) acetaminophen are rare when dosed accordingly, with more common side effects being nausea, vomiting, headache, and insomnia.[28]

Opioids

Opioid analgesics remain the most widely used treatment of moderate to severe pain in the early postoperative period. Opioids produce analgesia by binding to and activating G protein-coupled opioid receptors (GPCRs) peripherally and in the CNS. Centrally, opioid receptors are predominantly found in the dorsal horn of the spinal cord, specifically Rexed lamina II of the substantia gelatinosa, and supraspinally in the PAG, medial thalamus, amygdala, and limbic cortex. Peripherally, they are found on afferent sensory nerve fibers, as well as in the gastrointestinal tract, lungs, and joints.[29] There are several subtypes of opioid receptors with the principal ones being mu (μ), delta (δ), and kappa (κ). When bound by opioids presynaptically, these GPCRs cause a biochemical change that decreases adenylate cyclase activity, thus inhibiting calcium channels and resulting in a decreased release of excitatory neurotransmitters such as substance P. Postsynaptically, there is an increase in outward potassium conductance with a subsequent hyperpolarization and an inhibition of excitatory neurotransmission.[30]

A thorough understanding regarding opioid pharmacodynamics and pharmacokinetics is essential when choosing a specific opioid. This is discussed in Chapter 11. Perioperatively, the more common opioids used for acute pain are fentanyl, morphine, and hydromorphone. These are predominantly administered parenterally but can be administered in a variety of routes depending on the opioid (e.g., oral, epidural, intrathecal, intraarticular, and transdermal). Common side effects found with most opioids are dose dependent and include respiratory depression, pruritus, urinary retention, constipation, and nausea and vomiting.

Fentanyl

Intravenously, fentanyl's analgesic potency is approximately 80 to 100 times more than morphine. Its short onset of action (2–5 minutes) makes it an ideal opioid for treating acute pain. The duration of action of fentanyl is approximately 20 to 40 minutes because it is metabolized by the liver via *N*-dealkylation into inactive metabolites

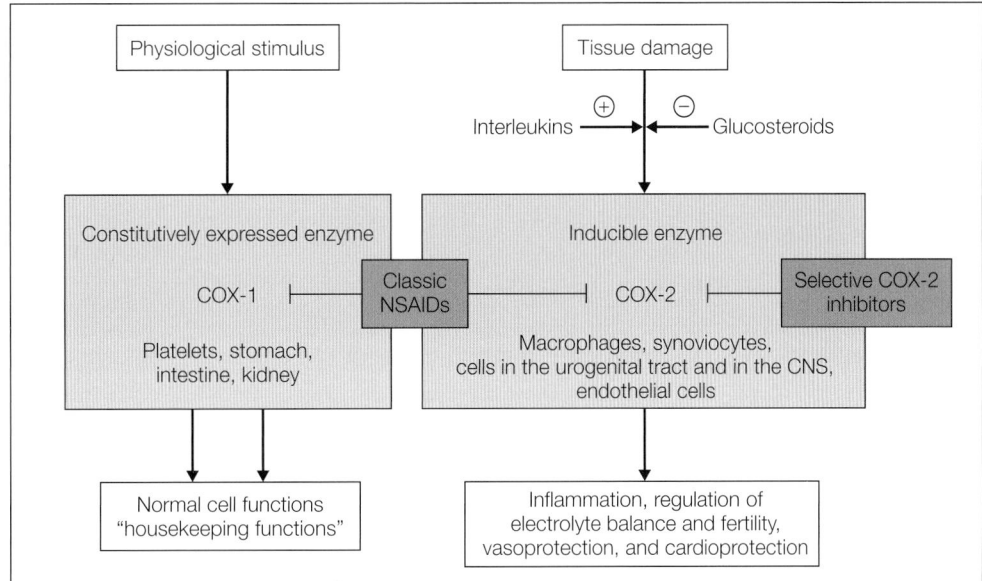

Fig. 56.5 Simplified description of the physiologic and pathophysiologic roles of cyclooxygenase-1 *(COX-1)* and COX-2. COX-1 is expressed constitutively in most tissues and fulfills housekeeping functions by producing prostaglandins. COX-2 is an inducible isoenzyme that is expressed in inflammatory cells (e.g., macrophages and synoviocytes) after exposure to proinflammatory cytokines and is down-regulated by glucocorticoids. In the kidney (macula densa) and other areas of the urogenital tract and in the central nervous system *(CNS)*, COX-2 is already significantly expressed even in the absence of inflammation. Induction of expression of COX-2 in peripheral and central nervous tissues appears to be most prominent in connection with inflammatory painful reactions. Both enzymes are blocked by classic acidic antipyretic analgesics (nonsteroidal antiinflammatory drugs *[NSAIDs]*). (From McMahon S, et al. *Wall and Melzack's Textbook of Pain.* 6th ed. Philadelphia: Elsevier; 2013:445.)

and excreted by the kidneys. Fentanyl can be administered intrathecally, epidurally, and intravenously via postoperative patient-controlled analgesia (PCA). It is also available transdermally for the treatment of chronic pain. Because fentanyl is highly lipophilic, its administration intrathecally is limited because of its short duration of action, with a single dose lasting 2 to 4 hours.[31,32] The duration of action for a single dose of epidural fentanyl (50–200 mcg) will be approximately 2 to 3 hours.[33] Intrathecal and epidural fentanyl can be given as a single dose or a continuous infusion and is discussed in Chapter 49.

Morphine

Morphine is the prototypical opioid by which all others are compared and is the most widely used for acute and chronic pain management. Metabolism of morphine is via hepatic glucuronidation resulting in the metabolites morphine-3-glucuronide (M3G) and M6G, with the latter being the active metabolite. Both metabolites are excreted via the kidneys; however, in patients with renal failure M6G may result in prolonged effects.

Morphine is commonly used to treat moderate to severe perioperative and postoperative pain. Morphine can be administered intravenously, intrathecally, epidurally, or orally. When administered IV, the onset of analgesia is approximately 20 minutes with duration of action being approximately 4 to 5 hours depending on the dose administered. Unlike fentanyl, morphine is hydrophilic, making penetration of the blood-brain barrier and spinal cord more difficult. This results in a delayed onset of action (20–30 minutes) and a prolonged duration of action (8–24 hours) for single-dose intrathecal or epidural morphine. Similar to fentanyl, morphine can be given in a single dose or continuous intrathecal or epidural infusion. PCA intravenously is also an option for morphine administration.

Hydromorphone

Hydromorphone is a derivative of morphine and is approximately seven to eight times more potent. Metabolism of hydromorphone is via hepatic conjugation; however, unlike morphine, it lacks the active metabolite M6G. Therefore administration in renal patients is considered safe. IV administration results in analgesia in approximately 15 minutes with a duration of action equivalent to morphine, approximately 4 to 5 hours. Hydromorphone is an ideal opioid for moderate or severe acute perioperative pain and is used for chronic pain management. Modes of administration include oral, intrathecal, epidural, intraarticular, and intravenous PCA. When administered via single dose intrathecally or epidurally, onset of action is more rapid than morphine (approximately 15 minutes), with a duration of action of approximately 10 to 16 hours.[34] The common side effects associated with morphine administration remain similar to hydromorphone when equivalent doses are administered. However, histamine release is less likely to occur with hydromorphone compared to morphine.[35]

Analgesic Adjuncts
N-Methyl-D-Aspartate Antagonists

Ketamine, a noncompetitive N-methyl-D-aspartate (NMDA) antagonist and a phencyclidine derivative, is primarily used as an anesthesia induction agent. It is also used as part of a multimodal approach for perioperative pain control in conjunction with other medications. Ketamine prevents the activation of the NMDA receptor, which has been associated with the development of "wind-up" or central sensitization and chronic pain states along with the AMPA (α-amino-3-hydroxy-5-methyl-4-isoxazolepropionic acid) receptor. The NMDA receptor remains closed at rest because of a magnesium plug. Activation of the receptor involves the simultaneous binding of the excitatory

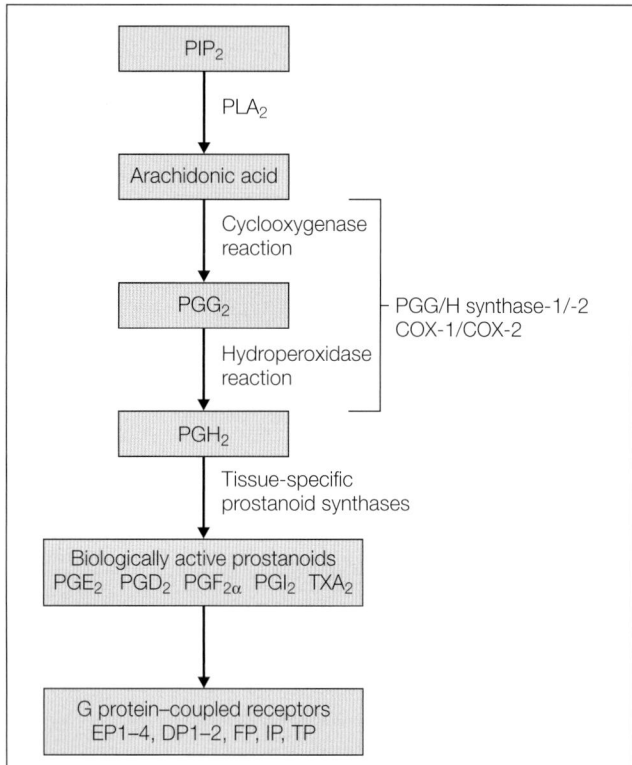

Fig. 56.6 Classic prostanoid biosynthesis pathway. Prostanoid biosynthesis starts with the release of arachidonic acid from cell membranes, mainly through cytosolic phospholipase A_2 (PLA$_2$)–dependent hydrolysis. Arachidonic acid is subsequently metabolized by the either one of the two cyclooxygenases (COX-1, COX-2). Prostaglandin H$_2$ (PGH$_2$) is biologically largely inactive but serves as a substrate for tissue-specific prostaglandin synthases, which produce the different biologically active prostanoids. These prostanoids exert their biologic action through binding to specific G protein–coupled receptors. PIP$_2$, Phosphatidylinositol 4,5,-bisphosphate; TXA$_2$, thromboxane A$_2$; PG, prostaglandin; EP, DP, FP and IP, prostaglandin receptors; TP, thromboxane receptor. (From McMahon S, et al. *Wall and Melzack's Textbook of Pain.* 6th ed. Philadelphia: Elsevier; 2013:445.)

neurotransmitter glutamate, which causes an influx of calcium, resulting in an increase in second messengers. The up-regulation of second messengers produces a hyperexcitability of the NMDA receptors, which causes neuronal plasticity, excitability, and wind-up. In addition, research suggests that ketamine may exhibit antiinflammatory effects.[36]

Ketamine is rapidly acting; an anesthetic IV dose response is seen in 30 to 40 seconds with a duration of 80 to 180 minutes. In addition to IV administration, it can be administered intramuscularly, nasally, rectally, via epidural, and intrathecally. Metabolism of ketamine is predominantly by the liver and produces norketamine.

Because ketamine exhibits both anesthetic and analgesic effects, its use has drawn more interest in the perioperative setting. Its administration at higher doses and as the sole anesthetic is less desirable because of psychotomimetic adverse effects. Ketamine has been used in low doses either as a single dose administered on induction of anesthesia and/or as a continuous infusion for acute perioperative pain. There is no conclusive, consistent consensus in regard to what is considered low-dose ketamine. Studies report minimal adverse effects with subanesthetic doses of ketamine, in addition to decreased perioperative opiate consumption.[37-39] However, randomized controlled trials and reviews have noted mixed results regarding efficacy of low-dose ketamine and postoperative analgesia.[37-43]

α$_2$-Adrenergic Agonists

Clonidine and dexmedetomidine are α$_2$-adrenergic agonists that are used as analgesic adjuncts for multimodal anesthesia. They exhibit their analgesic effect by interacting with the G protein-coupled α$_2$ receptors, both centrally (dorsal horn of the spinal cord) and peripherally. Activation of the α$_2$ receptor results in inhibition of adenyl cyclase and decreased cyclic adenosine monophosphate (cAMP) levels. It also activates postsynaptic potassium channels while inhibiting presynaptic voltage-gated calcium channels, thus reducing neurotransmitter release. In addition, it is suspected that activation of central α$_2$ adrenoreceptors in the LC are responsible for supraspinal analgesia.[44,45]

Clonidine, a centrally acting selective partial α$_2$-adrenergic receptor agonist, can be administered orally, intravenously, rectally, transdermally, intrathecally, epidurally, and via an intraarticulate route. For acute pain management, clonidine is administered primarily intrathecally or epidurally. Its half-life is approximately 5 to 13 hours. Metabolism of clonidine is via the liver with the remainder of the drug being excreted unchanged in the urine. Because clonidine exerts its effects on both α$_2$ and α$_1$ receptors (400:1 α$_2$ to α$_1$), side effects such as sedation, hypotension, and bradycardia can occur.[46] Clonidine has been reported to decrease postoperative opioid requirements and prolong the duration of analgesia when administered via epidural with local anesthetics.[47-49] When combined with local anesthetics in peripheral nerve blocks, it is reported to prolong postoperative analgesia.[50-52]

Dexmedetomidine is a highly selective α$_2$-adrenergic agonist. It is approximately 7 to 10 times more selective for the α$_2$ receptors (1600:1 α$_2$ to α$_1$) when compared with clonidine.[46] Like clonidine, it exhibits sedative, anxiolytic, analgesic, sympatholytic, and vagomimetic effects with little or no respiratory depression. Dexmedetomidine is most commonly administered intravenously; however, it can be administered intramuscularly, transdermally, or intranasally. It has a rapid onset of action (approximately 5 minutes), with a short duration of action and an elimination half-life of approximately 3 hours. Metabolism of dexmedetomidine occurs via extensive hepatic glucuronide conjugation with the absence of active metabolites. Hepatic clearance may be decreased in the presence of liver disease. Dexmedetomidine is often used for procedural sedation in nonintubated patients, sedation for intubated and mechanically ventilated patients, as well as a general anesthesia adjunct. In a Cochrane review, it was reported that when dexmedetomidine was administered perioperatively for acute pain in abdominal surgery patients, there were some opioid-sparing effects. However, there were no significant differences in postoperative pain when compared to placebo.[53]

Local Anesthetics

Unlike the previous analgesics whose actions are targeted at specific receptors on primary nociceptors and in the CNS, resulting in reduced presynaptic transmitter release and decreased postsynaptic excitability, local anesthetics inhibit conduction of action potentials along a nerve fiber. Local anesthetics block sodium channels in both afferent and efferent neuronal membranes, thereby inhibiting pain transmission. They are often given as the sole anesthetic; however, for optimal postoperative analgesia, local anesthetics should be administered with adjuvant medications.

Nerve morphology (diameter and myelination) affects the sensitivity of nerve blockade achieved. An understanding of local anesthetic properties such as potency, onset of action, and duration of action is crucial in choosing a specific local anesthetic. These are addressed in Chapter 10. Metabolism of local anesthetics is determined by the chemical class. Amide local anesthetics are metabolized primarily by

TABLE 56.3 Methods of Administering Local Anesthetics

Route	Technique	Mode of Delivery
Topical		SS
Local infiltration	Subcut, subdermal	SS
	Intraarticular	SS, C
Neuraxial	Subarachnoid	SS, C, PC
	Epidural	
	Caudal	
Peripheral nerve blocks	*Lower extremity*	SS, C, PC
	Lumbar and sacral plexus	
	Femoral	
	Sciatic	
	Popliteal	
	Ankle	
	Upper extremity	
	Brachial plexus	SS, C, PC
	Cervical plexus	SS, C
	Intercostal	SS, C, PC
	IV regional (Bier block)	SS
	Digit	SS
Systemic	IV	SS
Diagnostic/interventional	Trigger point injection	SS
	Somatic nerve blockade	SS
	Sacroiliac injection	SS
	Facet injection	SS
	Epidural steroid injection	SS
	Selective sympathetic blockade	SS
	Intervertebral disc injection	SS
	Differential nerve blockade	SS

C, Continuous; *IV*, intravenous; *PC*, patient-controlled; *SS*, single shot; *Subcut*, subcutaneous.

the liver, whereas ester local anesthetics are metabolized via plasma cholinesterase. Conditions that alter liver function (hepatic disease) and/or decrease plasma cholinesterase levels will inevitably reduce the rate of metabolism.

Methods for administering local anesthetics are listed in Table 56.3. The most common techniques for acute pain management are local infiltration of the operative area, peripheral nerve blocks, as well as epidural and subarachnoid blocks with adjuvant medications (primarily opioids). Prior to surgical incision, a local anesthetic can be injected intradermally or subcutaneously near the incisional area to decrease the inflammatory response; local anesthetic infiltration reduces up-regulation of peripheral nociceptors. Common local anesthetics used for operative area infiltration include bupivacaine or ropivacaine because of their longer duration of action.

Peripheral nerve blocks can be administered as a single injection or via a continuous catheter technique. Chapters 49 and 50 provide a thorough description of regional techniques and peripheral nerve blocks. Most peripheral nerve blocks consist of a bolus dose of local anesthetic injected to infiltrate an area or a peripheral nerve site. These techniques are primarily used for minor surgical procedures that provide analgesia in the immediate postoperative period. The use of continuous catheters or continuous peripheral nerve blocks (CPNBs) involves an initial bolus dose of local anesthetic followed by a continuous infusion near the surgical site and adjacent to a nerve. CPNBs are increasing in popularity; they provide prolonged

analgesia in those patients who are expected to have moderate to severe postoperative pain lasting more than 24 hours and are commonly used for the brachial plexus, intercostal, femoral, and sciatic nerves.

Both subarachnoid and epidural blockade (primarily epidural) have been found to be useful in the management of postoperative pain. The primary site of action of local anesthetics when injected in the subarachnoid or epidural space is the nerve roots of the spinal cord. Because neuraxial anesthesia (local anesthetic with or without opioids) provides profound analgesia, some clinicians use the epidural technique with light general anesthesia during the surgical procedure; at the end of the procedure, the epidural catheter is left in place for postoperative pain management. Medications (e.g., local anesthetics, opioids, and adjuvant medications) can then be administered as bolus injections, continuous infusion, or via a patient-controlled device. The continuous epidural technique can be used for thoracic, abdominal, and lower extremity surgery.

IV infused lidocaine, as a component of a multimodal analgesia, should be considered in patients undergoing open and laparoscopic abdominal surgeries.[54] Studies involving these surgical procedures reported a decrease in postoperative pain scores when compared to placebo. In addition, patients had a shorter duration of ileus postoperatively.[55,56] Conversely, in a Cochrane review it was reported that when lidocaine was infused perioperatively it was uncertain if lidocaine was beneficial in decreasing pain scores, gastrointestinal recovery, postoperative nausea, or opioid consumption.[57]

Local anesthetics are used not only for acute postoperative pain management but also commonly used in the diagnosis and treatment of several chronic pain states. Examples of diagnostic and interventional uses include facet joint injection, sacroiliac injection, selective sympathetic blockade, and trigger point injection. Therapeutic injections and nerve blocks for chronic pain are discussed in Chapter 57.

Patient-Controlled Analgesia

PCA was developed in the early 1970s with the advent of microprocessor technology. This administration technique has changed the face of acute pain management and has become a standard technique for postoperative pain control. Intravenous PCA involves self-administration of predetermined doses of analgesics. This ideally results in the patient's ability to self-medicate to one's own pain needs and allows for more effective pain control while avoiding peaks (opioid side effects) and troughs (pain) in plasma concentrations that are commonly present with as-needed IV administration. Current PCA models have different variables for administration allowing for selective dosing. These variables include (1) an initial loading dose, (2) a demand dose or bolus dose, (3) a lockout interval, (4) a basal continuous infusion rate, and (5) 1-hour and 4-hour maximal dose limits.[58,59] The initial loading dose is administered by the programmer or postanesthesia care nurse for initial setup in titrating the analgesic and/or for breakthrough pain. The demand or bolus dose is the quantity of analgesia administered to the patient on activation of the PCA demand button. The length of time after a demand dose is given by the patient, during which another demand dose will not be delivered, is the lockout interval. The lockout interval prevents overdosage with continual demand, with lockout intervals between 5 and 10 minutes being optimal.[58,59] A basal or continuous infusion is the administration of analgesics at a constant given rate regardless of the patient using the demand button. Continuous infusion rates are predominantly only administered in chronic opioid-dependent patients because continuous infusion in opioid-naïve patients may result in overdose and increased risk for respiratory depression/arrest. For chronic opioid-dependent patients, a continuous infusion may suffice their daily equivalent dose of opioid

TABLE 56.4   Intravenous Patient-Controlled Analgesia Regimens

Drug Concentration	Size of Bolus	Lockout Interval (min)	Continuous Infusion
Agonists			
Morphine (1 mg/mL)			
Adult	0.5–2.5 mg	5–10	—
Fentanyl (0.01 mg/mL)			
Adult	10–20 mcg	4–10	—
Hydromorphone (0.2 mg/mL)			
Adult	0.05–0.25 mg	5–10	—
Methadone (1 mg/mL)	0.5–2.5 mg	8–20	—

Adapted from Gropper MA., et al. *Miller's Anesthesia.* 9th ed. Philadelphia: Elsevier; 2020:2618.

with demand doses assisting with their postoperative analgesia. However, extreme caution and vigilance should be used in monitoring these patients. A maximal dose limit of 1-hour or 4-hour intervals is proposed to be another safety mechanism against overdose. Nevertheless, this remains controversial because opponents argue that if a patient reaches the 1-hour or 4-hour demand dose limit, then the patient probably requires more analgesia.

Because PCA requires the patient to control the delivery system, candidates for PCA must be cooperative, be able to understand the concept, follow the directions of use, and be able to push the demand button. In addition, education should be provided to the patient and family members regarding the PCA delivery system.

The medications most often used for PCA are morphine, hydromorphone, and fentanyl. Meperidine is not recommended because of its neurotoxic metabolite, normeperidine. The neurotoxic side effects that are not reversible with naloxone include shakiness, tremor, twitches, multifocal myoclonus, and grand mal seizures.[60,61] Other medications that can be used via IV PCA include local anesthetics, ketamine, and clonidine. Dosing guidelines for specific medications are institution specific. A sample IV PCA dosing guideline for opioid-naïve patients is found in Table 56.4.

ACUTE PAIN MANAGEMENT IN SPECIAL POPULATIONS

Acute Pain in a Patient With Chronic Pain

Because millions of Americans are affected with chronic pain, it is inevitable that anesthesia providers will be faced with challenges in providing acute surgical pain management for those who have a chronic pain condition. The IASP defines chronic pain as pain that has no apparent biologic value and lasts longer than 3 months in duration or beyond the normal course of healing. It is often associated with insomnia, lost workdays, impaired mobility, and emotional distress (i.e., anxiety, depression, anger, and fear). Management of the chronic pain patient is complex with cultural, emotional, biologic, and social influences all needing to be addressed. Chronic pain physiology and treatment are discussed in Chapter 57. Medical regimens can be very complex in this patient population and warrant an in-depth review preoperatively. In addition to the

acute pain analgesics previously presented, other common analgesics used for the treatment of chronic pain syndromes are discussed here.

Chronic Pain Analgesics and Adjuncts

Anticonvulsants. Anticonvulsants or antiepileptics are commonly used in certain neuropathic pain syndromes when treatment is refractory to traditional analgesics. First-generation anticonvulsants such as carbamazepine and phenytoin have been used for many years for neuropathic pain; however, more recently the second-generation anticonvulsants gabapentin (Neurontin) and pregabalin (Lyrica) are the most widely used. Anticonvulsants inhibit neuronal excitation and stabilize nerve membranes in an effort to decrease repetitive neural ectopic firing, which is common in neuropathic pain.

Gabapentin and pregabalin are used for the management of postherpetic neuralgia, diabetic neuropathy, trigeminal neuralgia, and other neuropathic pain and chronic pain syndromes. Their mechanism of action is similar; it is believed that both block the alpha 2 delta ($\alpha_2\delta$) subunit of the presynaptic voltage-gated calcium channels in the CNS, thereby preventing excitatory neurotransmitter release.[62] Pregabalin and gabapentin are structural analogs of GABA, which lack affinity to the GABA receptors. Both exhibit anticonvulsant, anxiolytic, and antihyperalgesic effects.[62-64] When compared with gabapentin, pregabalin displays a pharmacokinetic profile that requires less dosing with fewer side effects.[62,64]

Common side effects are dose dependent and include dizziness, somnolence, peripheral edema, and weight gain. Currently pregabalin and gabapentin are available in the oral form only. Because neither drug undergoes hepatic metabolism, drug-drug interactions are minimal. The unchanged form of the drug is excreted by the kidneys, therefore patients with compromised renal function may require dose modifications.[62,64] Pregabalin and gabapentin use is not limited to chronic pain syndromes. They are also being effectively used in multimodal techniques for acute postoperative pain management, which has resulted in lower reported pain scores and lower opioid consumption.[65-69] Lastly, patients scheduled for surgery who are routinely taking anticonvulsants as part of a chronic pain syndrome treatment regimen should continue taking their medication throughout the perioperative period because this will optimize their pain management.

Antidepressants. Several antidepressants are being used for chronic pain syndromes. Similar to anticonvulsants they are effective in the treatment of neuropathic pain syndromes. Common antidepressants include the tricyclic antidepressants (TCAs), selective serotonin reuptake inhibitors (SSRIs), and selective norepinephrine and serotonin reuptake inhibitors (SNRIs) (Table 56.5). In the presence of central sensitization, the descending inhibitory pathway, which uses inhibitory neurotransmitters (i.e., serotonin and norepinephrine), is altered. It is believed that antidepressants may exert their analgesic effects by blocking the reuptake of serotonin and norepinephrine in the CNS, thereby increasing their availability. They may also act at other sites via (1) blocking of sodium and calcium channels, (2) decreasing PGE_2 and TNF-α, (3) blocking NMDA receptors, and (4) enhancing opioid receptors, which may account for additional analgesic effects. Analgesic dosage is much lower than the recommended antidepressive dose, and their analgesic effects may not occur until 4 to 10 days after initiating treatment.

TCAs (amitriptyline and nortriptyline) tend to have more side effects than the SSRIs and SNRIs because they antagonize other receptors, including muscarinic (e.g., dry mouth, blurred vision, and urinary retention), histaminergic (e.g., sedation, appetite stimulation with subsequent weight gain), and adrenergic (e.g., orthostatic

TABLE 56.5 Common Antidepressants Used for Chronic Neuropathic Pain

Drug Class	Generic Name	Trade Name
TCAs	Amitriptyline	Elavil
	Nortriptyline	Pamelor
	Imipramine	Tofranil
SNRIs	Venlafaxine	Effexor
	Duloxetine	Cymbalta
	Milnacipran	Savella
SSRIs	Fluoxetine	Prozac
	Citalopram	Celexa

SNRI, Selective serotonin-norepinephrine reuptake inhibitors; *SSRI*, selective serotonin reuptake inhibitors; *TCA*, tricyclic antidepressant.

BOX 56.4 Systemic Effects of Steroids

Endocrine
- Adrenal-pituitary insufficiency
- Hypercortisolism
- Hyperglycemia
- Cushing syndrome

Cardiovascular
- Hypertension
- CHF
- DVT
- Cardiomyopathy

Musculoskeletal
- Muscle weakness
- Osteopenia/osteoporosis
- Avascular necrosis of bone
- Pathologic fractures
- Truncal obesity

Dermatologic
- Skin thinning
- Alopecia

- Petechiae
- Facial flushing
- Striae
- Hirsutism

Renal
- Sodium and water retention

Gastrointestinal
- Peptic ulceration
- Gastritis
- Hyperacidity

Neurologic/Psychological
- Headache
- Vertigo
- Euphoria
- Restlessness
- Insomnia
- Mood swings
- Depression

CHF, Congestive heart failure; *DVT*, deep vein thrombosis. Adapted from Baqai A, Bal R. The mechanism of action and side effects of epidural steroids. *Tech Reg Anesth Pain Mgmt.* 2009;13(4):205–211.

hypotension, prolonged QT interval). They are contraindicated in patients with a history of a recent myocardial infarction, prolonged QT interval, cardiac dysrhythmias, or unstable congestive heart failure. Drug levels can be monitored to ensure unintentional overdose. The metabolism of all antidepressants is primarily hepatic. TCAs are commonly used for the treatment of postherpetic neuralgia, headaches, and fibromyalgia.[70,71]

SNRIs (duloxetine, venlafaxine) are generally better tolerated than the TCAs because of the lack of affinity for the adrenergic, histaminergic, and cholinergic receptors. Therefore they are preferred for those patients with cardiac disease. Both drugs (duloxetine and venlafaxine) have similar side effects: nausea, dry mouth, somnolence, headaches, and sexual dysfunction.[70,71] Likewise, the concomitant use of SNRIs with SSRIs or triptans is not recommended because this may precipitate a serotonin syndrome. Serotonin syndrome is an acute toxicity of serotonin manifesting as anxiety, agitation, delirium, seizures, hyperthermia, diaphoresis, tachycardia, hypertension or hypotension, hyperreflexia, myoclonus, and muscle rigidity. Symptoms vary from mild to life threatening, and diagnosis is based on patient medication history, physical examination, and exclusion of other neurologic disorders.[72,73]

SSRIs for the treatment of chronic pain are still under investigation because very few clinical trials have been done. They are primarily used for the treatment of depression, and their analgesic effects, thus far, are relatively weak.[70,71] Regardless of the type of antidepressant being taken for chronic pain, they should be continued throughout the perioperative period.

Corticosteroids. Exogenous corticosteroids (glucocorticoids) are administered in a variety of routes (e.g., oral, intravenous, epidural, caudal, and intraarticular) as adjunct analgesics for multiple types of acute onset and chronic pain syndromes. They exert multiple effects on the body, including autoimmune, antiinflammatory, antiedema, and antiallergic. Typical disease processes and pain syndromes that are treated with corticosteroids include rheumatoid arthritis, osteoarthritis, herpetic neuralgia, chronic low back pain, and chronic neck pain. In the treatment of acute and chronic pain syndromes, corticosteroids exert their effects in several ways. They are primarily known for their antiinflammatory effect because they prevent the release of arachidonic acid by inhibiting phospholipase A2 on cell membranes (see Fig. 56.6). Through this mechanism they decrease inflammatory cytokines (Il6, IL1, TNF-α) and prostaglandins. When corticosteroids are injected epidurally, it is also purported that they exhibit nociceptive properties by blocking C fiber transmission. In addition, they suppress ectopic firing of nociceptors in the presence of nerve injury, which produces a direct membrane-stabilizing effect.[74,75]

Side effects of corticosteroids are reflective of supraphysiologic doses that usually exceed the rate of endogenous steroid production, which is approximately 20 mg/day of hydrocortisone or its equivalent for more than 3 weeks.[76] Many organ systems can be affected with long-term steroid use (Box 56.4). These effects are variable among patients and are dependent upon the degree of hypothalamic-pituitary-adrenal (HPA) axis suppression, which is attributed to the type of steroid, duration of use, frequency of ingestion, route of administration, and dosage. However, when corticosteroids are administered as an intermittent injection (e.g., epidural, intraarticular, caudal) versus chronic daily use, side effects are usually mild and transient. It has been purported by Kay et al.[77] that weekly epidural steroid injections given over 3 weeks caused dramatic HPA axis suppression with normal cortisol levels returning within 1 month. Similarly, it has been found that a single epidural steroid injection can cause HPA axis suppression from 7 days following injection and lasting up to 5 weeks.[78] Currently, there is no consensus among pain management specialists on the dosing, frequency, or total number of repeated steroid injections. Regardless, in the event of a major surgical procedure after the recent administration of an epidural steroid, it may be prudent to administer a dose of exogenous steroid.

Methadone. Methadone is a synthetic opioid historically used for the treatment of opioid addiction in detoxification or medication-assisted treatment (MAT) programs. Recently, its use is increasing for the treatment of severe acute pain in addition to chronic cancer and noncancer pain management. Structurally, methadone is a racemic mixture of two enantiomers, D-isomer (S-methadone), and L-isomer (R-methadone). The D-isomer is responsible for antagonizing the NMDA receptor and inhibiting serotonin and norepinephrine uptake, which possibly contributes to its benefits in the treatment of neuropathic pain, along with the prevention of opioid tolerance and hyperalgesia.[79] The L-isomer is responsible for binding to opioid receptors thereby giving its analgesic effects.

Methadone is a viable option for chronic pain patients who have tolerance (intolerable side effects or inadequate analgesia) to current opioids. It can be administered orally, intravenously, rectally, and subcutaneously. As a result of its high degree of lipid solubility, it is well absorbed via the gastric mucosa with peak analgesic effects in 30 to 60 minutes. When given intravenously, the drug has peak effects that are seen in 15 to 20 minutes. Unlike other opioids, methadone has a long half-life of approximately 15 to 60 hours. This long half-life is ideal for maintenance programs and preventing withdrawal symptoms. However, when methadone is administered for chronic pain states, it is difficult to initiate, to titrate, and to convert from another opioid, which makes dosing a challenge.[80,81] Even so, methadone's lack of active metabolites, long half-life, and low cost make it desirable for chronic nonmalignant pain management.

Metabolism of methadone is primarily via the CYP450 enzyme, specifically CYP3A4 and CYP2B6, into inactive metabolites that are excreted in the urine.[82] Therefore any medications that inhibit (e.g., phenytoin, carbamazepine) or induce CYP450 may dramatically alter methadone metabolism.[83]

Side effects of methadone are similar to other opioids, including respiratory depression and excessive sedation; respiratory depression peak effects occur later than the analgesic peak effects. A unique side effect of methadone includes QT interval prolongation, which could lead to potentially lethal ventricular tachyarrhythmias and torsades de pointes. Patients taking methadone on a continuous basis should be carefully monitored with a cardiac evaluation. An electrocardiogram (ECG) should be obtained pretreatment and periodically thereafter depending on dose changes, baseline ECG findings, and other risk factors for QT prolongation. A QT interval that exceeds 500 ms is deemed a risk factor for lethal arrhythmias, and discontinuation of methadone or a dose reduction is advisable.[83]

As a result of methadone's long half-life, its use in acute pain management is limited but effective. In complex surgical procedures it has been reported that methadone administered intraoperatively decreased postoperative pain scores and reduced postoperative opioid requirements.[84,85] In the event that methadone is chosen as an analgesic for perioperative pain management, an ECG is warranted preoperatively with identification of those at risk for prolonged QT interval. These risk factors include the concomitant use of antiarrhythmic agents, some TCAs and calcium channel blockers, the presence of hypokalemia, and a history of prolonged QT interval. Furthermore, chronic pain patients are often taking a combination of medications such as benzodiazepines and other CNS depressants, which poses an added risk for respiratory depression and sedation.[83]

Buprenorphine. Buprenorphine is used to treat moderate to severe acute pain as well as chronic pain. However, it is primarily used as an alternative to methadone maintenance therapy for the treatment of opioid use disorder or MAT programs. Buprenorphine is a semisynthetic opioid derivative that acts as a partial agonist at the mu-opioid receptor and a full antagonist at the kappa-opioid receptor. It has an extremely high affinity (50 times greater than morphine) to the mu-opioid receptor with a much slower dissociation as compared to full opioid agonists, allowing for its prolonged duration of action and resistance to antagonism with naloxone.[30] Likewise, this displaces and prevents binding of the mu receptor by concurrently administered full opioid agonists, thereby reducing the effectiveness of other opioids. Due to the receptor affinity properties it is suggested that there is a ceiling effect for respiratory depression but no ceiling for analgesia.[30] However, respiratory depression and arrest can still occur especially in patients with reduced respiratory reserve or when buprenorphine is coadministered with benzodiazepines or other CNS depressant medications.

Buprenorphine is available in a variety of routes (intravenous, intramuscular, subcutaneous, oral, sublingual, epidural, buccal, transdermal patch, and subdermal implant) and formulations (alone or in combination with naloxone and extended release/long acting). The preparations containing buprenorphine with naloxone are most widely used in MAT programs as this combination is an abuse deterrent. When administered for acute pain management, the intravenous, intramuscular, sublingual, and transdermal routes are most widely utilized. The analgesic effect of 0.3 mg of parenteral buprenorphine is equivalent to approximately 10 mg of morphine.[30] Currently in the United States, transdermal buprenorphine is supplied as a patch (5, 7.5, 10, 15, and 20 mcg/hour) that delivers the medication for 7 days.[86] The transdermal buprenorphine patches are predominantly used in treating moderate to severe chronic pain. However, studies have revealed that transdermal buprenorphine can be safely used for postoperative analgesia.[87,88]

Buprenorphine is metabolized via the CYP450 3A4 hepatic system through N-dealkylation to the active metabolite norbuprenorphine. Norbuprenorphine can further undergo glucuronidation and is eliminated via the urine and feces. The excretion of buprenorphine is not affected by the presence of renal disease and appears to be safe to administer in those receiving dialysis.[89,90] Likewise, liver function should be monitored when initiating buprenorphine and when hepatic disease is suspected during treatment. Patients with liver dysfunction or those on concomitant medications that induce or inhibit the CYP 3A4 enzyme should be monitored for alterations in buprenorphine plasma concentrations.[91] Caution is advised in those who have a history of prolonged QT and/or taking antiarrhythmics as the concomitant administration of buprenorphine, especially at high doses, could result in prolonged QT interval.[86,91] As with other opioids, prolonged use of buprenorphine and/or methadone for the treatment of chronic pain is associated with the risks of dependence, tolerance, addiction, and (rarely) misuse.

Dependence can be either physiologic or psychologic in nature. Physiologic dependence is a pharmacologic property of opioid drugs defined by the manifestation of a withdrawal syndrome after abrupt discontinuation of the opioid or after the administration of an opioid antagonist (naloxone) or a mixed agonist-antagonist. Because opioids inhibit cAMP, any abrupt discontinuation of the opioid can cause a rebound disinhibition of cAMP and subsequent withdrawal symptoms. Withdrawal symptoms include autonomic nervous system responses such as increased irritability, restlessness, tremors, chills, muscle cramps, sweating, mydriasis, abdominal pain, diarrhea, and tachycardia.[30] Physiologic dependence should always be assumed to exist after repeated administration of an opioid for more than a few days.[30,92] To prevent opioid withdrawal syndrome, opioids should always be tapered before being discontinued, and daily scheduled opioids should be continued perioperatively.

Psychological dependence is defined by the American Society of Addiction Medicine (ASAM) as a "subjective sense of need for a specific psychoactive substance, either for its positive effects or to avoid negative effects associated with its abstinence."[93] Psychological dependence is inappropriately referred to as "addiction" and is more accurately described as a component of addiction.

In contrast, the term *addiction* is defined by the ASAM as a "primary, chronic disease of brain reward, motivation, memory, and related circuitry. Dysfunction in these circuits leads to characteristic biological, psychological, social, and spiritual manifestations. This is reflected in an individual pathologically pursuing reward and/or relief by substance use and other behaviors."[93] Features of addiction include cravings, obsessive thinking over a drug, impaired behavioral control, compulsive drug taking, and the inability to recognize one's problems with interpersonal relationships and one's own behaviors.[93,94] Unlike physical dependence and tolerance, the incidence of addiction among patients taking chronic opioids for noncancer pain is rare.[94] However, those with preexisting vulnerabilities (i.e., history of substance abuse, younger age, concurrent mental health disorders) may be at increased risk.[95,96]

Pseudoaddiction is often confused with psychological dependence because the behavior of the patients can be the same. Patients with both these conditions exhibit what appears to be drug-seeking behavior. However, in the patient who has pseudoaddiction, the origin of the behavior is inadequate analgesia. When these patients receive adequate analgesia, they no longer demonstrate drug-seeking behavior.

Tolerance refers to a change in the dose-response relationship induced by repeated exposure to the drug and manifested as a need for a higher dose to maintain an analgesic effect. Tolerance may be the result of several mechanisms such as enzyme induction caused by continued opioid administration or down-regulation of opioid receptors.[97] Other mechanisms involved with tolerance continue to be debated and include changes in drug-receptor interactions, cellular alterations, and long-term adaptations in gene expression.[98,99] The development of tolerance to an opioid is a normal physiologic response. When tolerance to an opioid occurs, opioid rotation is suggested. Opioid rotation involves switching from one opioid to another in an effort to improve analgesia and decrease side effects.

Opioid-induced hyperalgesia (OIH) is a phenomenon that usually occurs with chronic opioid therapy, which attributes worsening pain to high, escalating doses of opioids. OIH has been reliably demonstrated in animal studies.[100-102] However, there is limited research documenting the development of OIH in humans. Even so, case reports corroborate that OIH may be clinically significant in chronic opioid-dependent patients.[103-107] Manifestations of OIH include complaints of pain in locations different from the original pain area, whole-body hyperesthesia, allodynia, agitation, multifocal myoclonus jerks, and seizures.[106,108] OIH is often improved by reducing or discontinuing the opioid. The exact mechanism of action of OIH is not fully understood. However, there are many proposed theories. For instance, central activation of NMDA receptors via glutamate may play a role in OIH[109] and a shifting of the pain modulation system from a descending inhibitory pathway to a facilitating pronociceptive pathway.[110] It has also been suggested that neuroinflammation (via astrocytes and microglia) may contribute to the development of OIH.[111-113] Diagnosing OIH is difficult because it resembles opioid tolerance. Once diagnosed, treatment strategies consist of weaning the patient from high-dose opioids and starting nonopioid analgesics (e.g., NMDA receptor antagonists, NSAIDs, COX-2 inhibitors).[114-117]

Opioid Tolerance

Chronic opioid therapy (COT) for the treatment of chronic nonmalignant pain and for drug maintenance programs for opioid addiction is escalating in the United States. COT patients who require elective or emergent surgery present many challenges for the anesthesia provider in regard to perioperative analgesia. Patients taking COT are at risk for higher than normal levels of postoperative pain, slower pain resolution, longer hospital stay, and increased likelihood of readmission than those not on COT.[118,119] Thus it is imperative to collaborate with the patient and the surgical team to develop a unique and realistic perioperative pain management plan. As with treating patients in acute pain, a multimodal approach to pain management should be implemented.

Perioperative Management

Preoperative management. Preoperatively, preferably prior to the day of the surgical procedure, an investigation regarding the types of medications, dosages, and duration of therapy is helpful in determining the extent and severity of the chronic pain syndrome. Inquiries specific to preoperative pain and the patient's chronic pain state should be addressed (see Box 56.3). If the patient is on an opioid maintenance program for addiction, methadone or buprenorphine dosage should be verified by the prescribing physician/clinic. Chronic opiate therapy, including methadone, should be continued throughout the perioperative period because this will provide uninterrupted dosing for the patient's baseline opioid requirement and avoid withdrawal. If the patient has not taken the daily scheduled opioid, an equivalent dose of opioid should be administered preoperatively. Currently, there is no consensus or high-level evidence for the optimal perioperative management of patient's chronically taking buprenorphine. Clinical recommendations have been developed using a Delphi approach, with the major recommendation being to continue buprenorphine throughout the perioperative period, with careful consideration for discharge planning. In the event the patient has a transdermal fentanyl patch,[20] it should remain on throughout the perioperative period unless a collaborative decision has been made based on the invasiveness of the surgical procedure to remove it. If the patch is removed, a continuous IV infusion of fentanyl should be initiated and maintained perioperatively. Alternatively, equipotent morphine also can be administered. If a patient has an implanted intrathecal or epidural opioid infusion system, it should continue perioperatively.[120] Other medications taken for chronic pain (e.g., antidepressants, anticonvulsants, α_2 agonists) should be continued on the day of surgery.

The preoperative assessment is the ideal setting in which to establish a positive rapport with the patient, especially in the presence of a chronic pain state or a maintenance program. Chronic opiate therapy patients can be highly anxious, fearful, or depressed, and reassurance that their pain will be aggressively treated is paramount. Furthermore, realistic expectations regarding pain control should be discussed. Administering a benzodiazepine, along with initiating multimodal analgesia with adjuvant analgesics, is optimal and should be started within 1 to 2 hours prior to surgery.[81] This is also the time to discuss options for regional anesthesia/analgesia techniques. These techniques would be of great benefit for intraoperative and postoperative analgesia in the COT patient.

Intraoperative management. There are no data supporting a specific opioid for pain control intraoperatively for COT patients, nor have any specific dosing guidelines been established. The specific opioid selected is an anesthesia provider preference with patient coexisting diseases and surgical procedure dictating one versus another. The intraoperative opioid selected should provide adequate baseline opioid requirements and render intraoperative and postoperative analgesia. Intraoperative opioids may need to be increased 30% to 100%[121] when compared with the opioid-naïve patient because of receptor down-regulation and/or tolerance. Titration of opioids to heart rate and blood pressure response, in addition to pupil size, may be useful for estimating adequate analgesia with general anesthesia. Respiratory rate and depth may also be monitored in the spontaneously breathing, awake, or anesthetized patient to estimate adequate analgesia. In the event that a specific opioid is not efficacious, opioid rotation is recommended.[122] Cross tolerance among opioids may be incomplete, hence a specific opioid will not produce a similar degree of tolerance as a different opioid within the same class. Opioid antagonists and agonist-antagonists should be avoided because these will precipitate an acute withdrawal syndrome.

Nonopioid analgesic adjuncts (ketamine, clonidine, and dexmedetomidine) should also be a part of the multimodal approach to perioperative pain management. Several studies corroborate that when ketamine is administered intraoperatively at a continuous infusion in COT patients, there is a decrease in postoperative opioid requirements[123,124] and pain scores.[125]

TABLE 56.6 Recommendations for Perioperative Management of the Chronic Opioid Therapy Patient

Preoperative	Intraoperative	Postoperative
Pain assessment	Continue baseline opioid (oral, transdermal, IV, intrathecal pump)	Multimodal analgesic techniques
Precise opioid use (dose/type)—continue DOS	Increases in intraoperative opioids because of tolerance—titrate or continuous infusion	Maintain baseline opioid
Adjuvant medications for CP—continue DOS	Consider opioid rotation	Titrate opioids aggressively to achieve adequate pain control
Reassurance and address fears/anxiety	Multimodal approach	PCA—primary or supplementary for epidural/regional
Multimodal pain plan—consider NSAIDs, acetaminophen, 1–2 hr prior to surgery, anxiolytics	Consider regional, LA wound infiltration, PNB, CPNB, epidural/SAB	Continue applicable regional techniques
Consult with addiction specialist/clinic if indicated—continue methadone maintenance	Consider adjuvants—ketorolac, ketamine, clonidine, dexmedetomidine	Continue ketamine or low-dose ketamine infusion, if started in the operating room
Plan for postoperative analgesia	Anticipate increases in inhalation agent Avoid opioid antagonists and mixed agonists	Monitor for respiratory depression Continued assessment of analgesia Implement nontraditional comfort measures

CP, Chronic pain; *CPNB,* continuous peripheral nerve block; *DOS,* day of surgery; *IV,* intravenous; *LA,* local anesthetic; *NSAIDs,* nonsteroidal anti-inflammatory drugs; *PCA,* patient-controlled analgesia; *PNB,* peripheral nerve block; *SAB,* subarachnoid blockade.

Lastly, it is recommended that regional anesthesia with local anesthetics and opioids be a part of the anesthetic plan whenever possible in COT patients; this will reduce opioid requirements and provide analgesia. If regional anesthesia is used, intrathecal and/or epidural opioid administration is not adequate for baseline opioid therapy. Equipotent IV opioids should be given as the baseline therapy for the prevention of withdrawal.[126] Another option for perioperative analgesia includes peripheral nerve blocks with a continuous catheter infusion of local anesthetic.

Postoperative management. If the patient is not a candidate for regional anesthesia/CPNB or did not benefit from it, then intravenous PCA should be considered. Setting appropriate parameters for the PCA in the COT patient can be very challenging. A basal continuous infusion is suggested to replace the daily dose of opioid with demand doses varying among individuals.[126,127] When COT patients are able to resume oral intake, dosing is variable among individuals with gradual weaning to their presurgical therapy regimen. Consultation with a pain specialist regarding PCA dosing and opioid conversion for various routes of administration for COT patients is highly recommended. Other recommendations for perioperative pain management for the patient on COT are found in Table 56.6.

Elderly

In the United States, 20% of the population will be 65 years of age and older by 2030.[128] With the advances in medical technology older adults are undergoing surgical procedures to improve functionality, quality of life, and are thus living longer. Common surgical procedures include joint replacement surgery, emergent orthopedic procedures for fall-related injuries, coronary artery bypass grafting, aneurysmal repairs, and surgeries for cancer. All these are associated with significant postoperative pain, which, when not adequately treated, can alter the postoperative outcome and increase morbidity and mortality in the older adult. Acute surgical pain management in the older adult is challenging. As described in Chapter 54, the physiologic changes, multimorbidities, changes in pharmacokinetics and pharmacodynamics, and functional decline in organ systems all have an effect on analgesics administered in the elderly patient.

Specific to pain physiology, the aging adult has alterations in pain processing and perception. Peripherally there is a decrease in nociceptive processing via the C and Aδ fibers that results in a decrease in the older adult's ability to sense and respond to initial fast-sharp pain. There are also decreases in concentrations of substance P and calcitonin gene-related peptide, which results in loss of integrity or cellular elements of the nociceptive pathway. In the CNS there are reductions in neurotransmitters (i.e., GABA, serotonin, norepinephrine, acetylcholine, and endorphins) that may cause inadequate pain signal transmission and/or neuromodulation. It is also suggested that there is a dysfunction of the descending inhibitory pathway in the older adult.[129-131] Pain perception is altered in the elderly; the pain threshold increases and pain tolerance decreases. Generally the threshold for pain varies based on the stimulus (i.e., increases with heat, decreases with mechanical pressure and ischemia). Unfortunately, this has led health care providers to assume that the elderly do not experience pain.[130]

Another challenge with pain management in the older adult includes the increased risk for adverse side effects from analgesics compared to younger counterparts. This is the result of the increased incidence of polypharmacy, altered drug metabolism, presence of comorbidities and end-organ function, and increased sensitivity to medications. There is also the incidence of frailty and malnutrition that may predispose the older adult to drug toxicity.

Pain assessment in the older adult is a component of any preoperative assessment, therefore any preexisting pain prior to surgery should be extensively queried. According to the National Health and Aging Trends Study, the overall prevalence of bothersome pain in the last 30 days afflicts approximately half of the older aged (≥65) adult population.[132] Chronic pain in the elderly is addressed in Chapter 57. As discussed earlier, multiple pain assessment scales are utilized to assess pain with patient self-report being the gold standard. Because the elderly have a decrease in all the senses, it is suggested that when presenting the chosen pain assessment tool, it should be in large, clear letters or numbers. In addition, the elderly may require repeated explanations and more time for responses to questions during the pain assessment. Pain assessment via self-report in

TABLE 56.7	Pain Assessment Tools for Cognitively Impaired	
Visual Analog Scale	Marks a score on a graded line representing no pain to severe pain	Cognitively intact patients; difficulty speaking
Numeric Rating Scale	0–10 score for no pain to severe pain	Cognitively intact patients; validated in mild to moderate cognitive impairment. Preferred
Verbal Descriptor Scale	Ranks "mild, moderate, severe pain"	Cognitively intact patients; validated in mild to moderate cognitive impairment. Preferred
Faces Scale	Ranks pain on a series of smiling to frowning faces	Validated in mild to moderate cognitive impairment
Pain Assessment Checklist for Seniors with Limited Ability to Communicate Pain Assessment in Advanced Dementia Doloplus-2	—	Validated in severe cognitive impairment
Visual scales, assistive hearing devices	—	Hearing impairment

In McKeown JL. Pain management issues for the geriatric surgical patient. *Anesthesiology Clin.* 2015;33:563–576. Data from Falzone E, et al. Postoperative analgesia in elderly patients. *Drugs Aging* 2013;30(2):81–90; Gagliese L, Katz J. Age differences in postoperative pain are scale dependent: a comparison of measures of pain intensity and quality in younger and older surgical patients. *Pain* 2003;103(1–2):11–20.

the older adult with neurologic disorders such as dementia might be compromised and insufficient. In advanced dementia, self-report may be unobtainable because of impaired communication, cognitive, and memory function. Those with dementia are at increased risk of having pain and for being undertreated.[133-135] Therefore undertreated pain can lead to chronic pain, which will adversely affect the older adult's ability to function and quality of life. Several pain assessment tools have been validated for the older adult who is cognitively impaired (Table 56.7).

A multimodal approach to perioperative pain management should be instituted while making a risk-to-benefit assessment for each patient. Analgesics used in healthy younger adult surgical patients may present risks to the older adult. Some considerations for medication selection include comorbidities, renal and hepatic functioning, current medication regimen, type of surgery, frailty, and nutritional status. In addition, the safe prescribing guidelines (*Beer's Criteria for Potentially Inappropriate Medication Use in Older Adults*) developed by the American Geriatric Society should be considered.[136] *Beer's Criteria* includes a list of medications that should be avoided or have their dose adjusted based on the older adult's renal function and select drug-drug reactions. Regional and neuraxial analgesic techniques are also an option in the elderly population. In some instances these may be a safer approach than opioid analgesia because of their adverse effects and increased risk for postoperative respiratory depression. However, opioid analgesics are the first-line treatment for major surgery. Because the elderly have an increased sensitivity to medications, it is prudent to administer the lowest dose and titrate more as needed. Similar to healthy younger adults, intravenous PCA with an opioid is the mainstay treatment for acute moderate to severe postsurgical pain. However, the use of nonopioid analgesics (i.e., NSAIDs, acetaminophen), regional nerve block techniques with local anesthetics, in combination with opioids is optimal, thereby minimizing opioid side effects (i.e., sedation, respiratory depression), and in some instances, postoperative delirium.[137,138] Postoperatively once the older adult surgical patient is able to resume taking fluids by mouth, oral opioids and/or nonopioids should be substituted for the intravenous route.

Pediatric

Acute pain management is equally important in the neonatal and pediatric populations. Pain physiology in the neonate is also discussed in Chapter 52. Nociceptive pathways are well developed in premature and full-term infants. However, the maturation of the descending pathway precedes that of the ascending neural pathway. Therefore pain perception and the stress response may be more exaggerated in the premature neonate. Neonates are subjected to painful procedures within the first few days of life with immature newborns receiving the highest number of painful events (i.e., heel lancing, suctioning, venous catheter placement). The repeated exposure to untreated painful stimuli early in life can result in central sensitization, an increase in stress-related markers, and elevated free radicals after simple procedures,[139,140] which can have short- and long-term consequences on future pain perception and behavioral and neurologic outcome. For example, in a systematic review, infants who were born at 29 weeks of gestation or earlier received the greatest number of painful procedures, and this was associated with delayed postnatal growth, poor quality of cognitive and motor development at 1 year of age, and altered brain development (cortical thickening) at 7 years of age.[141]

In neonates, several pain assessment tools are utilized at the bedside that primarily assess pain through physiologic monitoring (i.e., changes in heart rate, respiratory pattern, blood pressure, oxygen saturation) and behavioral responses (i.e., crying, body movements, facial expressions). Tools commonly used in the neonatal intensive care unit for assessing procedural pain include the Premature Infant Pain Profile (PIPP), Neonatal Facial Coding System, and the Behavioral Infant Pain Profile.[140] Neonatal tools that assess postoperative pain include the CRIES scale (*c*rying, *r*equires increased oxygen administration, *i*ncreased vital signs, *e*xpression, *s*leeplessness) and PIPP.[140,142] Confounding factors, such as mechanical ventilation, pharmacologic interventions, physical restraint, and gestational age, can alter the behavioral and physiologic responses in the neonate. Unfortunately there is no reliable or specific physiologic or behavioral indicator for demonstrating the presence of pain in the preterm neonate. Generally, a combination of physiologic and observational pain assessment tools is used to assess pain in infants and toddlers (up to 3–4 years of age). Children 5 years of age and older can self-report pain with use of several validated visual or faces scales (FACES, VAS); standard adult pain assessment tools are instituted at approximately 7 to 8 years of age.[143,144]

Neonatal acute pain management consists of reducing the number of painful procedures performed, decreasing the number of bedside disruptions as this may increase pain responses, and integrating nonpharmacologic and pharmacologic approaches. Nonpharmacologic approaches to acute pain management consist of swaddling, facilitated

TABLE 56.8   Intravenous Patient-Controlled Analgesia Dosing Regimens for Pediatrics

Drug	Continuous Basal Infusion* mcg/kg/hr (Range)	Demand Dose mcg/kg (Range)	Lockout Interval min (Range)	Number of Demand Doses per Hr (Range)	4-Hr Limit mcg/kg
Morphine (standard 1 mg/mL; younger patients 0.2 mg/mL; tolerant or high-need patients 10 mg/mL)	20 (10–30)	20 (10–30)	8 (6–15)	5 (1–10)	250–400
Fentanyl (>30 kg 0.02 mg/mL; 10–29 kg 0.01 mg/mL; <10 kg 0.005 mg/mL; tolerant or high-need patients 0.05 mg/mL)	0.5 (0.2–1)	0.5 (0.2–1)	15 (6–15)	4 (1–10)	7–10
Hydromorphone (standard 0.2 mg/mL; tolerant or high-need patients 1 or 5 mg/mL)	4 (2–6)	4 (2–6)	8 (6–15)	5 (1–10)	50–80

*A basal infusion is not always used. It may increase the risk of respiratory depression and excessive sedation.
From Davis PJ, Cladis FP, eds. *Smith's Anesthesia for Infants and Children.* 9th ed. Philadelphia: Elsevier; 2017:437.

tucking (holding the infant in a flexed position and supporting the hands or feet while allowing the infant to control own movements), kangaroo care or maternal skin-to-skin contact, massage therapy, acupuncture, and nonnutritive sucking. Nonpharmacologic therapies are beneficial for minor pain and as adjuncts to pharmacologic therapy in moderate to severe pain.[145] In older children, nonpharmacologic therapies include guided imagery, relaxation techniques, hypnosis, and distraction techniques (i.e., cartoon videos, videogames). In addition, a multimodal approach to acute surgical pain management in pediatrics is recommended. This may include opioids, nonopioid analgesics (i.e., NSAIDS, acetaminophen), local anesthetics, α_2-adrenergic agonists, and NMDA antagonists being administered via different routes and at varying times perioperatively in an effort to maximize postoperative analgesia and minimize adverse effects. The pharmacodynamics and pharmacokinetics of analgesics vary with the neonate and pediatric patient and are discussed in Chapters 52 and 53. Similar to acute pain management in adults, opioids are the first-line agent for moderate to severe postoperative pain. Routes of administration are similar to adults and are discussed earlier in this chapter. Opioid administration via IV PCA is an option for the pediatric patient. Children as young as 5 to 6 years of age can safely use IV PCA as long as there is the mental capacity/understanding, manual dexterity, and ability (muscle strength) to initiate a demand dose. In those who cannot administer the PCA independently, the use of nurse-controlled or parent-controlled analgesia is common in pediatrics. However, the activation of a PCA by an unauthorized agent (i.e., parent) is not endorsed by TJC because of safety issues.[146] Even so, health care providers must continuously monitor the patient who is receiving PCA, whether nurse or parent controlled, and be anticipatory to the risk of opioid overdose, respiratory depression, and suboptimal analgesia. Therefore continuous monitoring via pulse oximetry and/or capnography is prudent in this vulnerable population. Morphine, hydromorphone, and fentanyl are the most commonly used opioids for PCA. Depending on the surgical procedure and analgesic requirements, a basal infusion of opioid may be required postoperatively for pain control. However, extreme vigilance is warranted as this may increase the risk of respiratory depression and sedation. A sample IV PCA dosing guideline for pediatric patients is found in Table 56.8.

Regional anesthesia, when used in combination with general anesthesia or alone, is another technique for intraoperative and postoperative analgesia in the pediatric patient. Anesthesia providers must be familiar with the physiologic and pharmacologic differences in the pediatric patient versus the adult. Developmental, physiologic, and anatomic differences are explained in Chapters 52 and 53. Regional anesthesia techniques in pediatric patients include caudal block, subarachnoid block,

TABLE 56.9   Peripheral Nerve Blocks and Indications in Pediatrics

Block	Indications
Head and Neck	
• Infraorbital	Cleft lip/palate repair; nasal septal surgery
Upper Extremity	
• Interscalene	Shoulder and upper arm surgery
• Supraclavicular	Upper extremity procedures
• Infraclavicular	Distal upper extremity procedures
• Axillary	Forearm and hand procedures
• Digital	Finger procedures
Lower Extremity	
• Lumbar plexus	Low abdominal, groin, and upper leg surgeries
• Femoral	
• Sciatic	Above-the-knee (thigh) surgeries; Below-the-knee (foot/knee) surgeries
Truncal	
• Transverse abdominis plane (TAP)	Abdominal wall surgeries
• Ilioinguinal/iliohypogastric	Groin and hernia surgeries

Adapted from Suresh S, et al. Common peripheral nerve blocks in pediatric patients. *Anesthesiol News.* 2010:19–26.

lumbar and thoracic epidural blocks (with and without continuous catheters), and peripheral nerve blocks (with and without continuous catheters). Various peripheral nerve blocks and potential surgical uses are described in Table 56.9. A thorough description of regional techniques and peripheral nerve blocks is beyond the scope of this chapter, but can be found in Chapters 49 and 50. Local anesthetics possess pharmacokinetic and pharmacokinetic differences in the pediatric patient compared to the adult; these are discussed in Chapters 10, 52, and 53. The decision to administer a regional anesthetic should be based on the type of surgical procedure (i.e., duration, invasiveness, anticipated pain area), patient criteria (i.e., absence of coagulopathies, infection), parental consent, and skill and comfort level of the anesthesia provider performing the regional technique. For safety reasons regional anesthetic techniques are usually performed in the pediatric patient under general anesthesia. However, in older children who are able to cooperate, regional anesthesia can be administered with mild sedation.

SUMMARY

Pain is a complex, multidimensional, and personal experience that requires an interdisciplinary approach for treatment. If acute pain is left undertreated or mismanaged, it can progress to chronic pain, which can affect an individual's quality of life and well-being. As an integral component of the interdisciplinary team, it is essential that nurse anesthetists are knowledgeable and current with the advances in pain physiology, assessment, management, and treatment modalities. Acute pain management no longer consists of monotherapy; a multimodal and individualistic approach to pain management across the lifespan is required. Likewise, adequate pain management is equally important in special populations because they possess inherent and distinctive challenges. Overall, CRNAs are in a unique position to provide effective, innovative, high-quality, and holistic pain management across the continuum in an effort to improve the health and well-being of patients.

REFERENCES

For a complete list of references for this chapter, scan this QR code with any smartphone code reader app, or visit the following URL: http://booksite.elsevier.com/9780323711944/.

57

Chronic Pain: Physiology and Management

Steven R. Wooden

Pain is a subjective term that is individually defined, and there is great variability in one's perception of its intensity. Its purpose is integrally tied to the human central nervous system (CNS) and the human response to physical threats. However, when pain persists and no longer serves as a survival response, it can cause damage to the nervous system, decrease productivity, and result in physical and psychological disabilities. Persistent pain is defined in a variety of ways but is universally recognized as containing negative physical, psychological, and quality of life components.[1] At the same time, it financially impacts health care in the United States to a greater degree than either cancer, heart disease, or diabetes.[2]

Chronic pain is characterized by persistent pain, associated with a distinct period of uninterrupted pain of 3 months or more, that includes a negative sensory and emotional experience.[3] Other definitions of chronic pain often contain a category (psychogenic, inflammatory, or neuropathic) and a time period, which ranges from 2 to 6 months. The categories of chronic pain are important to understand since each type demonstrates unique characteristics related to spinal cord and sensory neuron changes.[4] In addition, understanding the neurochemical markers related to the generation of chronic pain in each category may be important in helping to identify treatment options for chronic pain patients. However, chronic pain is a complex phenomenon, which often contains inflammatory, neuropathic, and emotional components.

Chronic pain has been linked to divorce, poverty, homelessness, despair, and sometimes suicide.[5] The management of chronic pain can be challenging since the source is not always clearly understood. Assessment and treatment require an understanding of how the physical, psychological, and social aspects affect the multidimensional nature of chronic pain. Advanced practice nurses are particularly well suited to address this problem using nursing theory, evidenced-based intervention, multidisciplinary collaboration, and their unique skill as nurses.

ANATOMY AND PHYSIOLOGY OF PAIN

The body is under constant sensory stimulation (i.e., excitation). Pain inhibitory transmission systems are important physiologic mechanisms that help to regulate the body's response to sensory stimulation, and pain transmission is dependent upon a normal balance between sensory transmission and inhibition. It is important to identify the need for an appropriate amount of sensory information to respond to potential harm.

There are three subdivisions of painful stimulation: (1) painful stimulation without tissue damage, (2) tissue damage without nerve damage, and (3) nerve damage.[6] An understanding of each of the subdivision's response to painful stimulation is helpful when developing and implementing individualized treatment plans.

Perceived pain without tissue damage normally illicits a withdrawal from the stimulation. This withdrawal terminates the sensation and

response. Under normal circumstances, the painful stimulation is specific to the site of potential injury and does not radiate beyond that site.

If tissue injury occurs, pain would then persist after removal of the stimulus. The area of injury will then exhibit an intensified response to tactile stimulation, and the sensation of pain will spread beyond the local area of injury. The local and extended responses are intended to protect the body and promote healing. Tissue damage causes the release of a number of substances that activate and support the body's physiologic response to pain. These substances include potassium, red cells, white cells, clotting factors, peptides, prostaglandins, inflammatory substances (which cause vascular leaking and swelling), and other substances that promote neurotransmission through nerve membrane channel activation.

The final subdivision of pain stimulation is damage that includes nerve injury. This can be caused by a disease state that invades and damages nerves, trauma to tissues involving nerve fibers, or the unintentional or unavoidable transection of a nerve. The extent of nerve injury can be classified into demyelinating or axonal injury. The type of nerve injury may indicate the probability of return to normal function with treatment.[7] Peripheral myelin injury will often regenerate while axonal injury to the nerve will likely result in permanent injury.[8]

Normal activation of neurotransmission is an important part of recognizing injury and limiting further damage. Once stimulated, Aδ and C nociceptive fibers produce an action potential mediated by the release of substance P and other excitatory amino acids appropriate to the intensity and duration of stimulation. The sensory stimulation proceeds through the afferent nervous system to the dorsal horn of the spinal cord. At this point, inhibitory mechanisms play an important role in modulating sensation and response. If the stimulation is sufficient to overcome the inhibitory mechanisms of the spinal neuroanatomy, then the sensory information proceeds to the pain perception centers in the brain. This information is used to provide a motor response to pain, in addition to building experience, expectation, and mood.

PAIN PHYSIOLOGY

There are four major aspects of pain physiology:
1. Transduction
2. Transmission
3. Perception
4. Modulation

Transduction

Transduction is a physiologic process where a noxious mechanical, chemical, or thermal stimulus is converted into an electrical impulse called an action potential. It occurs at specialized nerves called nociptors. These nerves are a subpopulation of primary sensory neurons that are activated by intense stimuli such as pressure, heat, or mechanical insults. Stimulation of nociceptors cause the release of neurochemicals.

Some of these chemicals, such as bradykinin, cholecystokinin, and prostaglandins, activate or sensitize nearby nociceptors.

Once released, these chemicals bind and activate specific receptors on the nerve endings of small-diameter nerve fibers, increase the excitability of the cell membrane, and lead to the creation of action potentials. Secondary messengers are then released and activated, leading to a state of peripheral sensitization. The primary treatment of pain includes reducing transduction through the inhibition of chemicals released during painful stimulation.

Transmission

After transduction, action potentials are transmitted to the central nervous system through two types of primary afferent neurons: (1) thinly myelinated, faster conducting Aδ fibers and (2) unmyelinated, slowly conducting C fibers. Action potentials result from activation of specific sodium channels. Nociceptive impulses travel along these primary afferent peripheral nerve fibers to the dorsal horn of the spinal cord where they synapse with second-order neurons. Here, the impulse is further transmitted via neurons, which cross the spinal cord and ascend to the thalamus and brainstem. The nociceptive impulses are then relayed to multiple areas of the brain.

Perception

Perception is the process where potential or actual tissue trauma is recognized as pain by a conscious person. Multiple areas of the brain are involved. Discriminative capabilities in the brain allow identification of the type, intensity, and bodily location of the traumatic event. The affective-emotional response to the stimulus is mediated by the limbic system.

All pain has an emotional component that influences future behavioral responses. Cognitive-behavioral therapies such as distraction, relaxation, and imagery operate at this level of the pain pathway. Some patients have a dominant affective emotional component and present with increased pain behaviors, anxiety, and depression that must be treated to achieve effective pain control.

Modulation

Input from the brainstem influences central transmission in the spinal cord. This creates modulation that results in inhibition of painful perception through the release of neurotransmitters such as serotonin, norepinephrine, and endogenous opioids. Psychological factors such as fear and anxiety exert contrary influences through these modulatory systems.[9-11]

PAIN PATHOPHYSIOLOGY

As described previously, pain is not just a localized phenomenon. There are three anatomic regions that are associated with every pain response. The peripheral, spinal, and cerebral areas contribute to various aspects of pain recognition and response. When pain is present for an extended time, it can create dysfunctional changes in these three areas that may become irreversible. This dysfunctional activity is the basis for chronic pain. To treat chronic pain, it is not always sufficient to simply remove the source of the pain. We must address the source of the pain, which generally is located outside of the CNS and created by soft tissue or nerve tissue damage. If the pain has become chronic, inhibitory mechanisms in the peripheral and spinal nervous systems may have become ineffective. Thus a singular focus that corrects the original source of pain is insufficient, and negative sensations will likely continue. For that reason, the dysfunctional inhibitory mechanism in the peripheral and spinal nervous system must also be addressed. Finally, pain perception in the cerebrum is normally a protective

mechanism that allows us to anticipate painful stimulation and avoid it. However, chronic pain can interfere with these perceptive functions; therefore an important part of chronic pain management is addressing the dysfunction within this area.

Treatment of chronic pain must include all three areas involved in pain transmission and perception. A return to normal function includes addressing and/or removing the cause of pain, assisting the peripheral system with the blockade of noxious stimulation, facilitating a return to balance within the spinal ascending inhibitory system, and helping to normalize the forebrain's perception of stimulation.[12] Cerebral processes in the development and treatment of pain are often overlooked. The human forebrain has significant involvement in the nociceptive process. Pain is a conscious experience that includes discrimination, motivational, and cognitive components that produce the unified sensation of pain. The components are mediated through separate mechanisms that reside in the cerebral forebrain. A broad range of environmental influences, such as attention, fear, and the placebo effect on the perception of pain, suggests that cortical association areas and their subcortical connections are critical participants in mediating the cognitive aspects of pain.

Pain perception is critically determined by expectations and is modified through learning. Traumatic experiences can often create unrealistic perceptions of chronic pain. This can lead to exaggerated and unexpected social behavior, substance-seeking activity, and depression. Addressing the impact that chronic pain has on an individual's perceptions is part of a comprehensive treatment plan that must not be ignored.[13]

TYPES OF CHRONIC PAIN

Psychogenic

Although the term *psychogenic pain* is still used, many pain practitioners feel it is a meaningless term because all pain experiences have a psychological component. The fact that a physical cause cannot be identified does not indicate that the pain is psychosomatic (i.e., that the physical pain originated purely from a psychological component). Psychosomatic pain is thought to exist by some groups of practitioners, but the phenomenon appears to be rare and difficult to validate. Using such a description in the absence of any physical evidence related to pain may only stigmatize the patient and perhaps ignore the real possibility that an occult physical condition has contributed to some sort of psychopathology.[14]

Noceceptive (Inflammatory)

Tissue damage in the human body results in a cascade of neurochemical responses. These responses involve the peripheral and central nervous systems and are both local (at the site of injury) and systemic. The localized response serves as a protective mechanism to help prevent further tissue damage, initiates a healing process, and begins a sensory response through the peripheral and central nervous systems to create the perception of pain and trigger further protective mechanisms.[15] The localized response includes the release of inflammatory mediators that produce capillary vasodilatation, smooth muscle contraction, and promote synaptic transmission of pain impulses to the CNS. These mediators include histamine, bradykinin, and substance P.[16] Increases in substance P, and substance P receptors, are specifically associated with inflammatory pain. These increases appear to be diminished or absent in neuropathic and cancer pain.[4]

The sensory portion of the inflammatory response is often called nociception. Nociception is a neural process that translates and then processes injurious stimuli to something the brain can understand. It begins in the peripheral nervous system at the point of injury with the stimulation of nociceptors. The signals created by these nociceptors, as a result of inflammation and tissue damage, generate an action potential that is carried to the dorsal horn of the spinal cord. The impulse then ascends to the thalamus where the perception of pain occurs.[16]

Neuropathic

This type of pain is caused by a disease, lesion, or damage to the somatosensory nervous system (i.e., sensory nervous system). The somatosensory nervous system innervates the skin, muscles, joints, and tissue facias and is involved with the perceptions of touch, temperature, pain, pressure, movement, position, and vibration. It includes several types of sensory receptors (chemoreceptors, mechanoreceptors, nociceptors, thermoreceptors, etc.) that send signals to the spinal cord and then to the brain for sensory processing. Thus when nerves are injured, pain can radiate within the somatosensory nervous system and result in abnormal sensations such as dysesthesia or a condition called allodynia.[17] Allodynia is the triggering of a pain response from stimuli that do not normally provoke pain. Individuals with allodynia often have an intense burning sensation, with small changes in temperature or light touch, typically along the dermatome of the injured nerve.

Pain and the pain response to a normal inflammatory process differs from neuropathic pain in three ways. First, the pain associated with tissue injury improves within a reasonable period of time, and the inflammatory response resolves. In contrast, neuropathic pain is persistent and is often accompanied by an apparent or occult inflammatory response, even when there is evidence of tissue healing. The second difference is the presence of allodynia with neuropathic pain, which is absent with normal inflammatory response. The third difference suggests that neuropathic pain is inadequately managed with nonsteroidal antiinflammatory agents.[18]

The Unique Problem of Chronic Postsurgical Pain

Chronic postsurgical pain (CPSP), sometimes called persistent postsurgical pain, is a particularly troublesome type of chronic pain that has a reported incidence of between 5% and 50% depending on the particular type of surgical procedure.[19] Large gaps in the evidence exist precluding the ability to effectively identify all the reasons for CPSP.[20] However, pain sensitization, which is influenced by inflammation and nerve injury and can lead to long-term synaptic plasticity within the brain, is a well-recognized contributor to CPSP. The International Association for the Study of Pain defines CPSP as "a persistent pain state that is apparent more than 2 months postoperatively that cannot be explained by other causes such as recurrence of disease, apparent inflammation, or others." This very simplistic and obscure definition does little to help identify and treat the causative factors.

Much of the research into CPSP has been focused on specialty surgical procedures, but a compilation of studies related to CPSP reveals a grouping of the most common surgical procedures related to CPSP and various attempts to predict and prevent it. Although CPSP appears to be neuropathic in nature, it is not always associated with an identifiable nerve injury.[21,22]

The most common surgical procedures associated with CPSP are those that require a thoracotomy or thoracic penetration. These procedures include mastectomy, thoracotomy, cholecystectomy, nephrectomy, sternotomy, and other chest and upper abdominal procedures. Other common types of surgery that report a high incidence of CPSP are amputation and inguinal surgical procedures such a hernia repair. Nearly one of four patients who undergo thoracic surgery develop CPSP, but only one-third of them have an identifiable nerve injury.[23] This evidence suggests that multiple factors are likely responsible for CPSP. Certainly, a recurrence of the initial operative problem and nerve injury to the affected body area should be investigated. Finally,

even if nerve injury is not the causative factor, other nerve problems, such as nerve compression, entrapment, and/or other types of nerve involvement, can be considered as potential causes of CPSP.

Predictors of CPSP can help identify likely candidates but do little to distinguish a treatable source of pain. Some studies suggest that CPSP is functional,[24] whereas others identify psychological factors.[25] Preoperative pain appears to be a predictor of CPSP, and in at least one study, it was the most significant clinical predictor of CPSP.[26] Still others indicate multiple predictive factors such as thyroid function, occult wound infection, psychological influences, or nociceptive pain as possible contributors to CPSP.[27] There are a few factors that predict a low incidence of CPSP, which include young age,[28] and immunosuppressant therapy. The latter suggests that autoimmune issues may play a role in CPSP because those who are immunosuppressed postoperatively have a significantly lower incidence of CPSP for identical surgical procedures when compared with those who are not immunocompromised.

Treatment of CPSP is currently not standardized; however, some researchers have identified significant benefits using preventative measures such as reducing central sensitization through the use of regional anesthesia, preoperative doses of antiinflammatory agents, and administration of antihyperalgesia medications (i.e., ketamine, esmolol, lidocaine, dexmedetomidine).[29-31] Aggressive postoperative intervention appears to be important in the treatment of recognized CPSP. Antidepressants, short-term opioid use, the selective use of anticonvulsants, topical agents, and N-methyl-D-aspartate (NMDA) antagonists are options for the management of CPSP.[32-34]

It is apparent that CPSP is complex and that successful treatment can be difficult and prolonged. An understanding of the different types of chronic pain, and the anatomic, physiologic, and pathophysiologic mechanisms that influence the development of chronic pain, can help in the development of effective and reasonable management strategies for CPSP.

Evolution of Chronic Pain (Wind-Up)

Repetitive stimulation from chronic inflammation or nerve damage can lead to a condition referred to as wind-up. Wind-up is a cyclical response to pain that leads to an abnormal pain response and chronic pain sensation. It can contribute to physical and psychological debilitation. Preventing wind-up is critical to the prevention of chronic pain. Addressing patient symptoms and focusing on treatment of the underlying cause of pain is an important part of preventing wind-up. It is possible to falsely label those who complain about chronic pain as "drug seekers," "chronic complainers," or even "crazy." These types of statements indicate a lack of understanding of the patient's history and physical issues, the chronic pain pathophysiologic process, and the fact that living with chronic pain has left the patient in a position to find any means to stop the pain. Chronic pain is not a psychological condition, but it can lead to psychological dysfunction.[6]

The wind-up phenomenon is a chronic discharge of neurons that overwhelms the inhibitory neuropathways. A simple example of one pathway that is associated with chronic pain cyclic wind-up is as follows:
1. Chronic repetitive stimulation
2. Increased cellular calcium
3. Release of inflammatory substances
4. Cyclooxygenase production
5. Synthesis of prostaglandins, which are responsible for a reduction in neuropathway inhibition
6. Increased neurologic pathway excitability
7. Formation of hyperalgesia, which then leads back to point number 1

The pathway to chronic pain can be complex and pervasive. The systems that contribute to chronic pain and hyperalgesia include:

Neuronal Adaptation With Repetitive Noxious Stimuli

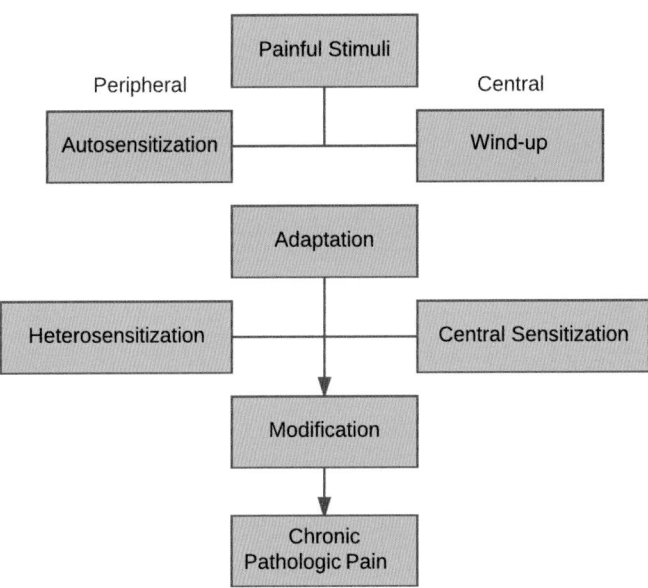

Fig. 57.1 Neuronal plasticity changes of the somatosensory system with exposure to repeated noxious stimuli.

I. Interneuronal networks
   a. Glutamate release—activating of NMDA receptors
   b. Loss of γ-aminobutyric acid (GABA) and glycine inhibition
II. Bulbospinal systems
   a. Serotonergic (5-hydroxytryptomine) pathway and receptor dysfunction
III. Nonneuronal cells
   a. Glial cell (toll-like receptor) dysfunction

Neuronal plasticity transforms as a result of chronic exposure to noxious stimuli and leads to changes in the somatosensory system (Fig. 57.1).

TREATING CHRONIC PAIN

Treatment goals for chronic pain should be multifaceted in an attempt to manage the complexity of the disease. Goals include the removal of the primary stimulus (typically located in the peripheral area), improving the function of inhibitory mechanisms (located within the central spinal area), and management of the psychological impact of chronic pain (located in the prefrontal cerebral area).

The focus of pain treatment is often directed toward one or more of the major aspects of pain physiology. Transduction can be addressed through inhibition of chemicals released during painful stimulation.

Several pain management strategies address transmission:
- Local anesthetics and some antiepileptic drugs block sodium channels and inhibit the production of action potentials along the nociceptive afferents.
- Opioids bind to presynaptic receptors in the dorsal horn and decrease release of neurotransmitters such as glutamate.
- Peripheral and spinal nerve blocks interfere with propagation of action potentials and pain transmission into the central nervous system.
- Epidural and intrathecal analgesics may provide both presynaptic and postsynaptic inhibition of receptors at the level of the dorsal horn neurons and can affect the transmission of nociceptive impulses.

While transduction and transmission can be addressed pharmacologically, perceptions often require cognitive-behavioral therapies such as distraction, relaxation, or other nonchemical treatments. Pain modulation can be manipulated in an effort to reduce the perception of pain. Drugs and therapies such as antidepressants, spinal cord stimulation, and epidural/intrathecal drug delivery systems can be used alone or in combination to modulate the perception of pain.[10,11]

Peripheral Nerve Pathways

Potential trauma or exposure to harmful stimuli in the peripheral areas elicits a normal response to withdraw. This response is initiated by the transmission of sensory impulses through the afferent peripheral nervous system, to the spinal nervous system, and into the perceptive centers of the brain that initiate a motor response. The peripheral fibers responsible for this quick response are myelinated, fast, and moderate-acting nociceptors called A fibers. These fibers are responsible for sensations that mediate cold temperature, pressure, and sharpness. The unmyelinated afferent peripheral C fibers are slow acting and are responsible for secondary sensations such as warmth, burning, itching, and touch. Neuropathic pain is thought to involve dysfunctional activity of both A and C fibers.

Stimulation of A and C fibers causes the release of substance P and excitatory amino acids which then activate neurokinins. Neurokinins generate an action potential, which carries sensory impulses up the afferent nerve pathways within the spine to the CNS. Once in the CNS, the impulse is interpreted according to its intensity and duration of stimulation. Under normal conditions, NMDA receptors remain inactive because of magnesium stability. However, pathologic chronic pain causes the displacement of magnesium leading to NMDA receptor activation and an exaggerated release of substance P and excitatory amino acids. The dysfunctional activation of NMDA receptors is a primary contributor in the transmission of pain within the peripheral pathway.[35]

Spinal Nerve Pathways

The spinal neuroanatomy has many complex features with similar cross-sectional structures at all levels of spinal cord. Ascending spinal nerve pathways relay sensory information from the periphery to the CNS via afferent fibers. Motor neurons in the ventral horn of the spinal cord project their axons toward peripheral skeletal and smooth muscles to mediate voluntary and involuntary reflexes at the level of stimulation without the need for CNS control. Descending spinal nerve pathways contain neurons whose descending axons provide the autonomic control for most visceral functions.

Various substances reside in the spinal anatomy and play a role in neurotransmission. For example, galanin is a neuropeptide that functions as a cellular messenger. One of its primary protective functions is to inhibit action potentials. Galanin is also implicated in many dysfunctional physiologic activities that may be connected with chronic pain such as depression and eating disorders.[36,37] Chronic pain may trigger the inappropriate activation of neuropeptides, within the spinal nerve pathways, creating negative consequences.

Cerebral Nerve Pathways

One of the least understood but most important areas of pain activity are the cerebral nerve pathways. Various regions of the brain are involved in pain modulation. The human brain is capable of recognizing prior pain experiences, developing attention and expectations related to those experiences, and creating anticipatory responses that are not always proportional to the situation. Pain experiences and cerebral responses to painful activity affect mood, create anxiety, and can lead to depression.[38]

An intriguing aspect of pain modulation related to cerebral activity is the placebo effect. What was once thought to be a purely psychological event now appears to be associated with neurophysiologic responses.[39] The effects of placebo analgesia are prompted by both verbal instruction and previous pain relief experiences that lead the individual to an anticipatory benefit and expectation of analgesia. Placebo analgesia is a prime example of cognitive modulation of pain.[38] This cognitive modulation includes the release of endogenous opioids, which may imply that placebo activity is actually a neurochemical event. It is evident that cerebral involvement in pain modulation is a complex system of events that includes both psychologic and physiologic activities resulting in the promotion of protective mechanisms when functioning properly. However, these protective mechanisms can be altered in conditions that are associated chronic pain.

Interestingly, it appears that an individual's perception of another's pain responses may be a factor related to that individual's experiences with pain. Empathy, which is the ability to understand and share the feelings of another, is influenced by cerebral mechanisms involved with neuroprotection. Studies suggest that firsthand emotional experiences with pain are an important aspect of empathetic development. One study found that opioid analgesics and opioid antagonists may have the unwanted effect of reducing empathy and concern for others.[40]

PHARMACOLOGY

Several pharmacologic agents are used in the management of various mechanisms involved with chronic pain. Some agents help promote a return to normal function after the development of chronic pain, while others simply treat pain perception and do little or nothing to reduce the dysfunctional cycle of chronic pain.

Nonsteroidal Antiinflammatory Drugs

Nonsteroidal antiinflammatory drugs (NSAIDs) contain properties well suited to help reduce the development of chronic pain and to treat ongoing chronic pain symptoms. Drugs in this category have antipyretic, antiinflammatory, and analgesic properties. Their primary mechanism of action is the acetylation of cyclooxygenase (COX), which prevents the synthesis of prostaglandins from arachidonic acid. Arachidonic acid is present in cellular tissue, and it is released when the cellular membranes are disrupted by injury or disease. Prostaglandins are localized hormones that are responsible for inflammatory activity (vasodilation, erythema, edema, and fever) and nociceptor sensitization, among other things.[41,42] Elevated levels of prostaglandins, consistent with the intensity of tissue damage, are related to trauma and surgery.[43]

There are two types of COX enzymes in the human body (Table 57.1). The first is COX-1, which is a constitutive enzyme continually produced to protect gastric mucosa, reduce gastric acid secretions and pepsin content, and promote platelet aggregation. The other enzyme, COX-2, is activated or induced by tissue damage and is responsible for inflammation, fever, some anticoagulation activity, modulation of cell proliferation, and pain sensation.[44,45]

Understanding the pharmacokinetics of NSAIDs is critical to a long-term treatment plan. Distribution and elimination of any drug play important roles in effectiveness, side effects, and toxicity. Oral NSAIDs are absorbed in the stomach and small intestines. Peak plasma concentrations of NSAIDs occur in 1 to 4 hours and are delayed by food consumption; however, taking NSAIDs with food does not reduce the negative gastric mucosa effects. This class of drugs is weakly acidic, highly plasma bound, and lipophilic, and only the unbound portion of the drug is effective. Elimination is accomplished primarily through hepatic oxidation and conjugation. Less than 10% is eliminated through

TABLE 57.1	**Cyclooxygenase Activity**
COX-1 Activity	**COX-2 Activity**
1. Hemostasis	1. Inflammatory response
2. Gastric mucosa protection	2. Fever
	3. Pain sensation
	4. Anticoagulation
	5. Modulation of cell proliferation
COX-1 Inhibition Benefits	**COX-2 Inhibition Benefits**
1. Possible reduced neuroinflammation targeted at microglia	1. Reduced inflammation
2. Cardioprotective anticoagulation	2. Reduced fever
	3. Reduced pain sensation
	4. Possible reduction in cancer progression
COX-1 Inhibition Risks	**COX-2 Inhibition Risk**
1. Can cause bleeding	1. Increase risk of thrombotic activity
2. Increased risk of gastric irritation and ulcers	

TABLE 57.2	**Side Effects—Nonsteroidal Antiinflammatory Drugs**
Side Effect	**Observed Frequency**
Gastric mucosa degradation	30–40%
Dyspepsia	15%
Decreased renal function	18%
Hepatic side effects	3%

renal activity. Some of these drugs have active metabolites. Generally, NSAIDs have similar targets of action, but their therapeutic profiles are different. Some are more COX selective than others, peak plasma times differ, distribution profiles vary, and elimination profiles may differ depending on an individual with kidney and/or liver disease.

NSAIDs are the most widely used analgesics in the United States, with over 30 million users. They are reasonably safe when used as intended, but serious side effects still exist. The most significant side effects of long-term NSAID use include nephrotoxicity, thrombotic events, peptic ulceration, and bleeding. The antiinflammatory effects of NSAIDs make them ideal for back pain related to neuraxial inflammation, but their distribution profile requires maximum recommended doses to be effective. Ibuprofen, for example, has an over-the-counter (OTC) dosing recommendation of 6 tablets (1200 mg) in a 24-hour period, but some studies indicate that an effective minimum dose of ibuprofen in a 24-hour period for the treatment of inflammatory back pain is 1600 mg (8 tablets). Even at doses of 1600 mg/day, the risks associated with ibuprofen are limited.

Acetylsalicylic acid (ASA) is a nonselective COX inhibitor. It has excellent long-term antipyretic and antiinflammatory properties, but unlike other NSAIDs ASA causes irreversible COX inhibition. The irreversibility may contribute to more serious side effects that cannot be limited by discontinuation of the drug. ASA has a significant impact on platelet aggregation that may be prolonged. In small doses ASA has been shown to help reduce cardiothrombotic events. Its effectiveness to decrease pain is tempered by its potential side effects and irreversibility.

The side effect profile of NSAIDs is relatively safe but not inconsequential (Table 57.2). Higher doses and long-term therapy necessary for the treatment of chronic inflammation and chronic pain can lead to significant side effects, which need to be considered when designing a chronic pain plan of care. Select NSAIDs and their dosing are given in Chapter 11.

Acetaminophen

Acetaminophen is not classified as an NSAID since it lacks significant antiinflammatory properties. Acetaminophen does inhibit COX activity, but it is thought to provide this inhibition in the CNS rather than peripherally. This explains the lack of antiinflammatory activity. The exact mechanism of acetaminophen is not fully understood; however, pain relief is thought to be provided by a reduction in nociceptor activity in the CNS.[46]

Due to the fact that acetaminophen does not have antiinflammatory activity, it is not well suited for treatment of chronic pain related to inflammatory processes. Studies indicate that acetaminophen used for back pain was no more effective than a placebo.[47] However, unlike opioids, acetaminophen is not addictive and it has a reasonably safe therapeutic profile when doses are limited to less than 1 g/dose or 4 g/day.[48] Because the action of acetaminophen is thought to be the inhibition of prostaglandin production in the CNS rather than peripherally, many hematologic side effects associated with other NSAIDs do not occur. For this reason, it is a safe alternative in reduction of pain symptoms for those patients who are at high risk for hematologic or cardiovascular problems.

Acetaminophen can cause acute liver failure from accidental overdose.[49] Accidental overdoses are often related to the fact that acetaminophen is combined with many common prescription and OTC drugs. Careful monitoring of total acetaminophen intake for chronic pain patients is essential in prevention of liver toxicity.

Opioids

Similar to acetaminophen, opioids act in the CNS and do not have peripheral effects. This prevents opioids from being effective in decreasing pain at its source, but they are valuable for short-term relief of operative and traumatic injury. Their mechanism of action includes binding to opioid receptors within the CNS that inhibit nociception. Table 57.3 describes the primary receptor site activity of opioids.

Many of the side effects associated with opioids are caused by metabolites. Some metabolites can produce hyperalgesia. Opioid-induced hyperalgesia (OIH) can be a significant problem with long-term opioid use. It is characterized by a paradoxic response to opioid therapy where patients become more sensitive to painful stimulation. Elimination of opioid therapy resolves the hyperalgesia.[50]

Morphine is the prototype opioid to which all other opioids are compared.[51] It acts at the mu and delta receptors. Oxycodone, one of the most widely prescribed semisynthetic opioids, has significant kappa activity, making it highly addictive. Oxymorphone has more mu receptor activity, some delta activity, and less kappa activity. Hydromorphone is primarily a mu agonist with significant kappa activity. Hydrocodone produces mu activity and some delta activity. Methadone is an interesting synthetic mu agonist. It is also an NMDA antagonist like ketamine, a mu receptor agonist like morphine, and does not have any metabolites. The unique properties of methadone have generated renewed interest in its use for chronic pain. However, it does have a complicated dosing profile, and because it has potential cardiotoxic effects it is inappropriate for most outpatient applications.

Opioid therapy for chronic pain treatment is an inadequate long-term solution because of the substantial negative side effects and lack of value in treating the source of pain. In addition to potentially fatal side effects, tolerance develops over time, which reduces the therapeutic value and increases risk.

In consideration of the use of opioids for patients with chronic pain, it is important to understand their limited value in such situations, the

TABLE 57.3 Opioid Receptors and the Effects of Receptor Stimulation

Receptor	Positive Effects	Negative Side Effects
Mu	Analgesia, euphoria	Respiratory depression, sedation, decreased gastrointestinal motility, pruritus
Kappa	Spinal analgesia	Respiratory depression, dysphoria, sedation, dyspnea, dependence
Delta	Dopamine release	Psychomimetic effects, dysphoria

TABLE 57.4 Opioid Side Effects and Related Frequency

Opioid Side Effect	Observed Frequency	Notes
Constipation	40–95%	Caused by opioid receptors in the gut Does not resolve over time
Nausea	25%	Direct stimulation of the chemotactic trigger zone, gastric distention, and increased vestibular sensitivity
Pruritus	10%	Some histamine release, but more significantly a direct stimulation of mu receptors
Sedation	60%	Transient
Respiratory depression	Dose dependent	Long-term opioid use may lead to sleep apnea
Endocrine	52–74%	Amenorrhea and low testosterone
Immunologic	?	Inhibition of cellular immune response

need to develop individualized opioid treatment plans, and the need to use dosing strategies that minimize use and maximize the value of such drugs. Dosing strategies include the use of nonopioid drugs that help to reduce the frequency of opioid-related side effects (Table 57.4). Rotation of opioids improves analgesia and reduces side effects. Close monitoring of opioid use and effectiveness can help minimize dependence and reduce opioid-related deaths.

Pharmaceutic research continues to pursue development of a pain medication that provides analgesia without the unwanted side effects and dependence.[52,53] The pursuit of such a drug is elusive. In the meantime it seems prudent, safer, and less costly to find ways to reduce opioid use for chronic pain. Opioids are discussed in detail in Chapter 11.

Antidepressants for Chronic Pain

Antidepressants can play a very important role in treating chronic pain. Pain perception is a chemically mediated event and can often be addressed with the addition of antidepressants to the chronic pain treatment plan. Antidepressants can also improve mood, increase treatment compliance, and reduce opioid use. Some of the older tricyclic antidepressants are effective for the treatment of chronic pain but have significant side effects that make them unacceptable in many cases. The serotonin-norepinephrine reuptake inhibitors (SNRIs) are effective and produce more tolerable side effects. Selective serotonin reuptake inhibitors (SSRIs) can also be useful but appear to be less effective in most cases than SNRIs.

Antidepressants can take days or weeks before they reach effective levels, which limits their ability to manage acute pain. Extended-release compounds appear to be most effective for chronic pain management. The SNRIs and SSRIs are generally well tolerated. Antidepressants are sometimes rejected by patients as a treatment for chronic pain because they may feel taking this class of drugs will label them as psychologically impaired. It may be helpful to explain how these medications provide valuable effects beyond their original intent. Select antidepressants and their doses are listed in Chapter 11.

Anticonvulsants for Neuropathic Pain

The use of anticonvulsants for chronic neuropathic pain is controversial. Some studies have found little to no value in using anticonvulsants for chronic nociceptive pain, whereas others have demonstrated some efficacy for specific neuropathic pain.[54] Anticonvulsants that have been found to provide some value are gabapentin and pregabalin. In a 2013 Cochrane review, both drugs were found to be associated with modest pain reduction when used for diabetic neuropathy and postherpetic neuralgia when compared with a placebo.[55,56] Pregabalin has become a widely prescribed drug for use in patients with chronic pain and has shown efficacy for the treatment of diabetic neuropathic pain, fibromyalgia, postherpetic neuralgia, and trigeminal neuralgia.[57]

The Role of N-Methyl-D-Aspartate Receptors in Chronic Pain

Evidence indicates a significant role of NMDA receptors in the development of chronic pain.[58] NMDA receptor systems are believed to be involved in the development of chronic pain wind-up, and preemptive treatment may be effective in the prevention of postoperative pain hypersensitivity. The mechanisms behind the development of postoperative pain hypersensitivity are poorly understood. However, NMDA receptors are thought to support synaptic plasticity, CNS pain processing, and modulation of central pain sensitization induced by incision and tissue damage.[59] NMDA receptor antagonists, such as ketamine, have been available for many years.

Ketamine blocks NMDA receptor site activity and may be useful in the treatment and prevention of chronic pain. Further study is necessary to support such a conclusion, but low-dose ketamine (0.1–0.5 mg/kg) has been used successfully as an adjunct to general anesthesia while reducing postoperative opioid requirements. Side effects associated with ketamine have concerned providers, but research on low-dose and postoperative infusion of ketamine in surgical patients does not support these concerns. A meta-analysis indicated that low-dose intravenous ketamine resulted in a reduction in nausea, small improvements in postoperative analgesia, and a reduction in opioid requirements, while other adverse events, such as hallucinations and vivid dreams, were not reported.[60]

Muscle Relaxants and Pain Treatment

Many patients with chronic back pain are routinely given muscle relaxants; however, these drugs are not without risk and should not be routinely prescribed. Muscle relaxation does not provide source treatment, and such drugs become ineffective within a few weeks. Furthermore, they should only be used for short-term symptomatic relief of muscle spasms. One of the most commonly prescribed muscle relaxants is cyclobenzaprine (Flexeril). It is chemically related to the antidepressant amitriptyline, and its effectiveness begins to decline within 4 days of therapy. When used alone for back pain, it is less effective than ibuprofen. Cyclobenzaprine is best used as an adjunct to NSAIDs. Other muscle relaxants that have been prescribed for chronic back pain such as carisoprodol (Soma) have a high potential for dependence, tolerance, and mental impairment. Carisoprodol has been taken off the market in some countries because of its high potential for abuse and

dependence.[61] There have also been some efforts to reclassify the drug in the United States as a controlled substance because of the potential for abuse.[62] Other drugs developed for muscle spasms such as baclofen should never be used for muscle spasms related to acute or chronic pain. Baclofen was designed for extreme spasmodic conditions such as cerebral palsy, tetanus, and multiple sclerosis. Withdrawal from baclofen can cause respiratory failure, hemodynamic changes, seizures, and delirium. It is highly toxic, and the benefits do not outweigh the risks in most situations.

Topical Anesthetics for Pain

Topical NSAIDs and topical anesthetic agents are important adjuncts for the treatment of chronic pain. Some patients and providers confuse topical agents with drugs that are delivered systemically through a dermal delivery system. Topical agents work without significant systemic absorption, their therapeutic benefit is high, and their safety profile is more favorable than oral comparisons when used in therapeutic doses.[63] The most common side effect of topical agents is skin irritation. One of the reasons that these drugs have not be used more frequently in the past is because of their relative high cost. Recently, topical agents such as 4% lidocaine have become much more affordable and available OTC.

Topical anesthetic agents are uniquely suited for some chronic pain conditions since these types of conditions require continued peripheral nerve stimulation. Application of anesthetic agents to the source of pain may help restore normal peripheral nociceptive inhibitory systems. Select topical agents and their doses are listed in Chapter.

Sleep Aids and Pain Management

Sleep is essential to the healing processes because it plays an important part of cellular regulation and regeneration.[64] Chronic pain disrupts sleep, which in turn impairs cellular regeneration. Lack of sleep can also lead to depression, which also complicates the treatment of chronic pain.[65] Sleep deprivation resulting from chronic pain can become a vicious cycle. For this reason, promotion of quality sleep is an important part of chronic pain therapy. Current sleep aids are not without risk. Some pharmacologic sleep aids can lower the quality of sleep by disrupting rapid eye movement sleep. Thus treatment of sleep deprivation associated with chronic pain should start with mechanical aids such as better pillows, stretching before bed, proper positions, and white noise.

Withdrawal, Tolerance, and Dependence

Most of the medications used for chronic pain management can create dependence, require increased concentrations over time because of tolerance, and have adverse physiologic and psychological responses when withdrawn.[66,67] These issues need to be considered as part of a long-term care plan with chronic pain patients. Strategies to reduce dependence and tolerance include multimodal therapy, alternating drug classes, and implementation of psychological and social support systems. Withdrawal of any therapeutic agent can have potentially devastating consequences under some circumstances. It is usually not advisable to completely withdraw any long-term medication without considering tapering the dose over time. Patients should be monitored closely for withdrawal symptoms when medication is discontinued or modified and treated appropriately. Some multimodal treatment options for chronic pain therapy are listed in Table 57.5.

Polypharmacy in Pain Management

Multiple prescription and nonprescription drugs are often necessary for the treatment of chronic pain. Use of multiple pharmaceutic agents, often called polypharmacy, has the inherent risk of negative medication

TABLE 57.5 Multimodal Treatment Options for Chronic Pain Management

Multimodal Treatment Modalities	Types
Medications	Antiinflammatory medications (NSAIDs, tylenol), muscle relaxants, opioids, neuropathic medications (anticonvulsants, TCA, SNRI), SSRI, NMDA antagonist, α_2 agonist, topical medications
Rehabilitation	Physical therapy, occupational therapy, TENS, bracing
Psychology	Cognitive behavioral therapy, biofeedback, relaxation therapy, support groups
Interventional pain management	Epidural injections, facet joint injections, peripheral nerve block, major joint/bursa injections
Implantable therapies	Spinal cord stimulator therapy and intrathecal pumps
Complementary and alternative treatments	Acupuncture, chiropractic manipulation, massage, craniosacral therapy
Nutrition counseling	Weight loss, bone density
Vocational counseling	Return to work

NMDA, N-methyl-D-aspartate; *NSAIDs*, nonsteroidal antiinflammatory medications; *SNRI*, selective norepinephrine reuptake inhibitor; *SSRI*, selective serotonin reuptake inhibitor; *TCA*, tricyclic antidepressant; *TENS*, transelectrical nerve stimulation.
From Dinakar P. Principles of pain management. In: Daroff RB, et al. eds. *Bradley's Neurology in Clinical Practice.* 7th ed. London: Elsevier; 2016:723.

interaction, unnecessary duplication of medication, toxicity, disruption of important physiologic functions, and an increased mortality rate.[68,69] The risk of negative drug interactions can range from 13% with two medications to 82% with seven or more medications.[70]

Among medications common to chronic pain and used in combination with other drugs are anticonvulsants, antidepressants, and NSAIDs. Anticonvulsants present a higher incidence of toxicity secondary to competition for metabolic pathways with other drugs. Some antidepressants increase warfarin levels, whereas those that inhibit the reuptake of serotonin pose a risk of fatal serotonin syndrome when combined with monoamine oxidase inhibitors used to treat atypical depression. Some drugs can inhibit hepatic enzyme activity and increase the risk of elevating other drugs to toxic levels because of diminished hepatic degradation. Adequate renal clearance is critical for many drugs, and competition for renal clearance is maximized when multiple drugs are administered. The competition for renal clearance also increases the blood levels of active metabolites found in many pain medications.

TARGETED PAIN MANAGEMENT

Imaging and Radiation Safety

The use of radiation for imaging during the diagnosis and treatment of chronic pain is not only common but also necessary to identify pathology, to validate treatment plans, and to safely provide interventional treatment.

There are two general categories of radiation. The first is nonionizing radiation such as visible light, infrared, microwave, radio waves, ultrasound, and magnetic resonance. Nonionizing radiation

is thought to be harmless to human tissue. The second category of radiation is ionizing radiation, which can cause cellular damage. Examples of ionizing radiation are alpha and beta particles, gamma waves, and x-rays. The most common type of ionizing radiation used in imaging is x-ray. Whenever x-ray radiation is used, it poses a risk to health care providers and patients; thus precautionary measures should be taken to reduce the risk of exposure when this type of radiation is used.[71]

Due to improvements in modern radiographic equipment and strict regulation, radiation exposure is limited. However, it must be kept in mind that the effects of ionizing radiation are cumulative, and multiple exposures over time will increase the risk of cellular damage. Damage to organic cells is called the stochastic effect. The stochastic effect can take place at any dose; therefore there is no known minimum safe dose of ionizing radiation. Although the Occupational Safety and Health Administration has established standards for maximum acceptable doses of ionizing radiation, these standards could be based on inaccurate assumptions.[72] The best course of action is to use the concept of "as low as reasonably achievable" (ALARA) when using ionizing radiation. It is also important to understand and use techniques that help shield health care providers and patients from the potential hazardous effects of ionizing radiation. The main principles of ALARA are reduced time and dose, shielding all body parts as much as practical, and being aware that rapidly reproduced cells are at highest risk of stochastic effect.[73] Rapidly reproduced cells include reproductive, thyroid, cornea, hair, and skin cells.

Fluoroscopy is the most common form of imaging used during the treatment of chronic pain. It provides detailed images of bony landmarks, quick identification of needle placement, and real-time visualization of injection. Fluoroscopy does not allow for the visualization of soft tissue, which can pose a risk of inadvertent needle placement within a nerve or vascular structure. However, the use of a contrast agent does allow for the visualization of vasculature. Another risk of fluoroscopy is the high ionic radiation exposure over time to patients and health care providers.

Computed tomography (CT) scanning is used by some practitioners for interventional treatment of chronic pain. The use of CT can render the procedure more technically complex; however, the images of bony landmarks are very detailed. Three-dimensional technologies for CT are emerging that will allow better visualization of structures, especially during cases of difficult needle placement. Disadvantages of the use of CT during interventional procedures include increased time, limited real-time injection capabilities, positioning that is often uncomfortable for patients, and level of ionizing radiation exposure that is significantly higher as compared to fluoroscopy.

Ultrasound is emerging as an alternative to ionizing radiation for some, but not all, interventional techniques. There is no ionizing radiation risk, and proximal bony landmarks can help guide the initial needle approaches for therapy. Ultrasound cannot reliably provide real-time injection images so the risk of vascular injection is increased with this imaging modality. Ultrasound imaging is limited when dense tissue is observed (e.g., bone).

Magnetic resonance imaging (MRI) is more helpful for diagnosis than it is for interventional purposes. It provides excellent soft tissue imaging, which aids in the identification of inflammation and other pain generators. There is no ionizing radiation risk, but special equipment is required if interventional therapy is provided with MRI assistance because of the image distortion created by metal objects such as needles.[74]

The risks and benefits of using imaging must be considered for both the patient and provider, and maintaining radiation safety is of utmost importance in an effort to limit exposure.

Interventional Treatment

The global management of chronic and acute pain issues that are not related to expected postsurgical pain management is referred to as non-surgical pain management (NSPM). Interventional pain management is more narrowly defined within the area of NSPM as the use of special techniques, equipment, implanted devices, and injections to diagnose and treat pain-related disorders. Common interventional approaches are to treat the occult inflammatory processes by injecting therapeutic substances to reduce pain and inflammation. The goals of these techniques are to improve sensory and motor function, promote healing, and may help to reset inhibitory pathways and processes that were damaged by chronic pain dysfunction. Long-term and more invasive interventional treatments include the implantation of electrical nerve stimulators or high-concentration opioid pumps. Table 57.6 lists some commonly used interventional pain management techniques and their indications.

Therapeutic Injections

A variety of spinal, soft tissue, and joint conditions are associated with nerve irritation and inflammation, which often respond well to interventional treatments. The conditions in the spinal column include disc herniation, spondylosis, nonspecific radiculopathy, spinal stenosis, disc degeneration, and postlaminectomy syndrome. Facet and sacroiliac joints also respond well to therapeutic treatment when the nerves within the joints become inflamed. Injections of therapeutic agents into tendon sheaths, along ligaments, around intercostal and cranial nerves, into ganglion cysts, or into carpal and tarsal tunnels can provide therapeutic or diagnostic results.

Placement of a needle near spinal nerve roots and injecting therapeutic substances remains controversial. Some evidence suggests epidural steroid injections provide no better pain relief than a placebo, whereas other evidence indicated that injections tailored toward specific conditions have therapeutic value.[75]

Lumbar epidural injections are the most common interventional pain management procedure for lower back pain. There are two common approaches for placing therapeutic medication (usually a combination of corticosteroids and local anesthetic agents) around the injured spinal nerve root. One approach is placing a needle through the intervertebral lamina and into the epidural space near the affected nerve root, and the other is placing the needle into the neuroforamen of the affected nerve root. The former is called an interlaminar epidural steroid injection (IESI), whereas the latter is often described as a transforaminal epidural steroid injection (TESI). The TESI is thought to have better therapeutic outcomes because it provides more precise placement of concentrated medication to the affected nerve root.[76] However, IESI is technically easier and safer to accomplish in most circumstances.

Specific lumbar conditions that are thought to respond best to either type of ESI include disc degeneration, disc herniation, spinal nerve root compression, spinal nerve root inflammation, postherpetic neuralgia, and spinal stenosis.[77-80]

Spinal nerve root inflammation is not isolated to the lumbar region. Although less common, interventional therapy is also effective in the sacral, thoracic, and cervical regions. However, there are a number of anatomic and safety considerations that need to be considered when injecting at various levels in the spinal column.

Anatomically the sacral epidural space is easy and relatively safe to access through the sacral hiatus. This approach is called a caudal ESI and may be just as effective for lower back pain as a lumbar ESI in some situations; it may also help many patients avoid surgical intervention.[81]

Thoracic ESIs are useful for postherpetic neuralgia and discogenic pain associated with inflammation. However, needle placement is often

TABLE 57.6	**Commonly Used Interventional Pain Management Techniques and Indications**
Name of Procedure	**Indication**
Celiac plexus block	Pancreatic cancer, chronic pancreatitis
Diskography	Diagnosis of anatomic localization of discogenic pain
Epidural corticosteroid injection	Lumbar, cervical, or thoracic radiculopathy
Facet joint block/medial branch block	Lumbar, cervical, or thoracic facet joint syndrome
Facet joint rhizotomy/ radiofrequency lesioning	Lumbar or cervical facet joint syndrome
Gasserian ganglion block Maxillary nerve block	Trigeminal neuralgia
Greater occipital nerve block Lesser occipital nerve block Superficial cervical plexus block	Occipital neuralgia
Intravenous regional block	Complex regional pain syndromes
Lumbar sympathetic block	Complex regional pain syndromes of the legs
Percutaneous disk decompression	Lumbar or cervical disk herniation
Sacroiliac joint injection	Sacroiliac joint pain
Sphenopalatine ganglion block	Headache and facial pain
Spinal cord stimulator	CRPS, PVD, low back pain, angina
Stellate ganglion block	CRPS of arm, neck, and head; headache
Suprascapular nerve block	Shoulder pain
Vertebroplasty	Vertebral fracture
Motor cortex stimulation	Neuropathic pain
Deep brain stimulation	Neuropathic pain

CRPS, Complex regional pain syndrome; *PVD,* peripheral vascular disease.
From Dinakar P. Principles of pain management. In: Daroff RB, et al. *Bradley's Neurology in Clinical Practice,* 7th ed. London: Elsevier; 2016.

more difficult because of the increased angulation of the vertebra at this level, and the risk of arterial injury is higher with a TESI because of the proximity of the artery of Adamkiewicz.[82]

The cervical ESI has a high therapeutic value but also a high risk. The anatomic and pathologic conditions involving the cervical spine create conditions that present a very narrow space. Very small vertebral arteries travel along the transverse foramen from C6 to C1, creating the possibility of arterial damage or thrombosis, which could lead to catastrophic complications. The risks of TESI in the cervical region have prompted a call for elimination of that approach to interventional treatment, and some recommend that all steroid injections within the epidural space be eliminated.[83,84]

Contraindications to interventional therapy are dependent on location, injectate, and other patient factors. Patient factors include refusal, known hypersensitivity to agents, local or systemic infection, local malignancy, certain hematologic therapies, or disorders that may predispose a patient to bleeding risks, congestive heart failure, and uncontrolled diabetes mellitus. Risks associated with interventional therapy include infection, bleeding, nerve injury, transient numbness or weakness, paralysis, contrast agent reactions, adrenal suppression, fluid retention, pneumothorax, and/or total spinal blockade.

Regardless of technique and location, interventional pain management should be provided by practitioners with adequate education and training, who are prepared to identify and treat possible complications. A well-planned and executed approach to interventional treatment is important for success. This begins with a thorough evaluation, identification of a target point, proper patient positioning, proper use of imaging, verification of needle placement, and use of a minimum effective dose and volume of the therapeutic agent.[85]

Other Therapeutic Nerve Blocks for Chronic Pain

An often underdiagnosed and poorly treated chronic pain condition is occipital neuritis. This condition is caused by chronic irritation of the occipital nerve as it travels along the superior nuchal angle at the base of the skull. It causes neck pain and cluster headaches and responds well to anesthetic agents and steroid injections near the greater occipital nerve at the base of the skull. Occipital injections do not effectively treat migraine headaches.[86]

Zygapophyseal joints, which are often called facet joints, are synovial joints between and along the lateral aspect of each vertebra. They help to limit movement and resist excessive biomechanical forces. These joints sometimes become dysfunctional and inflamed causing localized back pain and muscle spasms. Chronic inflammation of the facet joint can also affect the medial branch of the spinal nerve that corresponds to the particular anatomic facet. Diagnosis and short-term treatment of facet joint pain can be accomplished by injecting the joint with anesthetic agents and steroids.[87] Once a definitive diagnosis is made by diagnostic block, a long-term therapeutic remedy is denervation by radiofrequency ablation.[88]

Intercostal blocks can provide pain relief to the torso when epidural injections are difficult or contraindicated. Clinical applications for chronic pain management include chronic postsurgical pain, cancer, costochondritis, postherpetic neuralgia, and localized torso pain. The risks specific to intercostal blocks include pneumothorax, intravascular injection, and local anesthetic systemic toxicity secondary to rapid uptake of local anesthetic medication.

The sacroiliac joint is the largest joint in the human body. It supports the spine, and it acts to transfer weight and decrease stress to the pelvis and spine. Like the facet joint, the sacroiliac joint can become dysfunctional, inflamed, and painful. Injecting local anesthetic agents and steroids into the joint can be both diagnostic and therapeutic.[89]

Radiofrequency and Cryoablation for Chronic Pain

Long term (but temporary) elimination of sensory nerve pain impulses can be accomplished using heat (radiofrequency ablation) or cold (cryoablation). The goal of each modality is the destruction of the nerve myelin covering while leaving the axon reasonably intact. This allows for regeneration of the nerve over time while reducing the risk of permanent complications that sometimes accompany chemical or surgical nerve destruction. In addition to providing long-term pain relief for many conditions, these techniques help reduce or eliminate the use of opioid analgesics and the long-term detrimental effects of opioid therapy.[8]

Sympathetic Blocks for Chronic Pain

Targeted sympathetic nerve blocks to treat chronic pain are a controversial approach to short- and long-term treatment of many conditions. The sympathetic chain travels from the cervical spine to the coccyx along the lateral aspect of vertebral column. As it travels down the spinal column, it branches off at nerve bundles, or ganglion, and supplies targeted organ systems. The major sympathetic ganglions, which can be blocked for short- and long-term treatment of chronic pain, include the sphenopalatine (facial pain), stellate (upper extremity and thoracic pain, hyperhidrosis, angina, postherpetic neuralgia), celiac (abdominal pain caused by cancer or chronic pancreatic), and hypogastric (chronic pelvic pain).[90-95] There has also been some promising research in the use of stellate ganglion blocks for the treatment of posttraumatic stress syndrome.[96]

Evidence exists that has demonstrated little use for sympathetic blocks for most complex chronic pain issues.[97] However, specific conditions and some blocks have shown promise. Specific conditions include pain from vascular spasms such as Raynaud disease, hyperhidrosis, and terminal cancer pain. The procedure includes a diagnostic short-term block, followed by a therapeutic long-term block. After a diagnostic block with local anesthetic provides successful resolution of the unwanted symptoms, without unwanted side effects, a longer term or permanent block can be performed with alcohol, phenol, or radiofrequency ablation. The risk of such long-term blocks includes partial or incomplete sympathectomy. These blocks should only be performed after a thorough informed consent with the patient and only by experienced providers.[98]

Steroids and Local Anesthetics

Corticosteroids and local anesthetic agents are the most common medications used for the interventional treatment of chronic pain. Local anesthetic agents are beneficial for the immediate reduction or elimination of pain symptoms, as well as identifying proper placement of steroids in the targeted area. Research has indicated that local anesthetic agents alone may provide long-term pain relief for certain chronic pain conditions,[99] which suggest that blocking pain responses for even short periods of time may help to reset inhibitory nociceptor mechanisms.

Corticosteroids are thought to support release of antiinflammatory proteins and repress proinflammatory proteins. They are also known to suppress COX activity, which reduces the formation of prostaglandins and decreases pain. The most common steroids used in interventional therapy are moderate- to long-acting particulate steroids such as triamcinolone (Kenalog), betamethasone (Celestone), and methylprednisolone (Depo-Medrol). Betamethasone contains the smallest particles, triamcinolone's are intermediate in size, and methylprednisolone has the largest particles. Dexamethasone is classified as a nonparticulate corticosteroid. The vehicle, which contains particles, helps to provide localized long-acting antiinflammatory action. However, the particles contained within these solutions can lead to serious complications if accidently injected into the vascular system. The theory explains that if the particulates enter an artery they could block blood flow to the spinal cord at the level they were injected. This risk is especially pronounced in the cervical spine region where arteries are small, and infarction with accidental injection of particulate material is a stronger possibility.

Contrast Agents

To reduce the risk of inadvertent vascular injection and provide assurance that the needle is properly placed, radiographic imaging is essential for most interventional injections. Because ionizing radiation does not provide an image of soft tissue, contrast agents are used to enhance the visibility of soft tissue under ionizing radiation. This can help identify needle placement in joints and near nerves, and demonstrate expected therapeutic flow patterns in spaces. Most importantly, it can identify inadvertent intravascular needle placement before a particulate steroid is accidentally injected.

There are two types of contrast agents commonly used in pain management: iodinated agents and nonionic agents. The nonionic agents are safer because they have less free iodine, which has been implicated in serious allergic reactions. Both agents are excreted by the kidneys, therefore it is imperative that adequate renal function is present before contrast agents are used. There are many potentially negative adverse reactions associated with contrast agents. The most common include nausea, hypotension, bronchospasm, hives, and anaphylactic reactions.

Implantable Devices

In the absence of chronic pain and when the nervous system is functioning properly, inhibitory systems in the dorsal horn of the spinal cord prevent continuous pain sensation. For individuals with chronic pain, this mechanism appears to be dysfunctional. In theory, this inhibitory mechanism can be stimulated by electrical impulses applied to the dorsal column of the spinal cord producing changes within the ascending sensory fibers that modulate the sensation of pain.[100] An external device called a transcutaneous electrical nerve stimulator (TENS) unit accomplishes this through nonpainful stimulation that competes with nociceptive fibers in the dorsal horn, resulting in an inhibition of painful sensory perceptions through the same inhibitory pathways. Implantable devices that directly stimulate the spinal cord have been attempted with varying success.[101-103]

Another highly invasive method for treating chronic pain is the use of implanted intrathecal drug delivery systems. These devices can be surgically implanted in the body and programmed to deliver continuous doses of highly concentrated microdoses of medication into the CNS. The reservoir is typically implanted in the abdomen, and an infusion catheter is tunneled to the intrathecal space. The value of intrathecal drug delivery systems is the ability to better manage side effects and tolerance.[104] These devices are most useful for those with chronic pain related to terminal illness and failed back surgery where conservative methods are ineffective at providing the patient with an adequate quality of life.[105]

Complications and Management

Complications of interventional therapy are uncommon when proper technique and precautions are followed. However, even in the best of hands and with the safest techniques, complications still occur. Follow-up, recognition of complications, and the ability to manage and treat patients who develop complications are all important parts of the care plan.

One of the most common complications includes persistent pain from a traumatic injection or failure to respond to the therapeutic agent. Occasionally, needle placement can disrupt the dural membrane and create a temporary leakage of spinal fluid, leading to a postural headache. The headache that develops, usually within 24 to 48 hours, is often debilitating. Dural punctures most often heal spontaneously with rest and without necessary intervention. The symptoms related to dural puncture generally resolve within 1 to 3 days since the choroid plexuses and lateral and fourth ventricles within the brain produce 600 to 700 mL of cerebral spinal fluid per day. If symptoms do not resolve or are particularly severe, an epidural blood patch can be performed. This involves placing approximately 20 mL of the patient's blood in the epidural space at the puncture site under sterile conditions, which can immediately and permanently treat the postural headache.

In rare circumstances, a subdural or epidural hematoma may cause spinal compression, paralysis, and possibly death if left unrecognized and untreated. This is a potential complication in patients being treated with medications that can increase bleeding. Spinal cord trauma, injection into spinal arteries, anaphylaxis, and arachnoiditis are among other rare but possible complications of interventional pain management.

AGE-RELATED CONSIDERATIONS

There are significant physiologic differences between various age groups. These differences are more pronounced in the pediatric and geriatric populations. There are physical and functional implications that can create significant barriers to proper assessment, diagnosis, and treatment. It is important to recognize and incorporate age-related physiology into any plan of care.[106]

Pediatric Patients

Pediatric patients have specific physiologic differences that must be considered when treating pain. One of the more challenging aspects of pain management in the very young is identification. Pain is often ignored in this age group because of their inability to vocalize discomfort.

Alternative assessment methods for infants and young children are necessary. The most sensitive and reliable method for pain assessment is facial expression. Infants who are in pain do not always cry. Body motion, facial expression, and vital signs are all part of a comprehensive assessment necessary to accurately determine if an infant is in pain. Relying on vital signs alone may yield inaccurate information, leading to mismanagement of pain. Limited neurologic development and illness may also be factors that influence the infant's and the young child's responses to pain and complicate assessment.

The most common treatments for pain in infants are topical and local anesthetics, opiates, and acetaminophen. Alternative treatments are often a more effective and safer approach. They include nonnutritive sucking that stimulates the orotactile centers in the brain, increasing endorphins, which naturally relieves pain. Breast feeding can also reduce painful sensations through the same mechanism. Swaddling, holding, rocking, skin-to-skin contact, and auditory stimulation are all mechanical methods for treating pain. The olfactory centers of infants are very effective in dealing with painful stimulation. The smell of amniotic fluid, mother's milk, and baby oil have all been shown to reduce pain in infants.

The negative psychological and physical impacts of untreated and undertreated pain on the very young can have serious consequences. There is evidence that chronic painful stimulation in infants can lead to permanent changes in the CNS and, as a result, alterations in responsiveness of the neuroendocrine and immune systems to stress as they mature.[107]

Geriatric Patients

Aging is an inconsistent and complex phenomenon that involves the progressive degeneration of organ systems.[108] It involves changes in cellular homeostasis, organ function, and functional reserve, which impair an individual's ability to cope with stress, pain, and other health care challenges.[109]

Aging adults report a greater incidence of chronic pain, and studies indicate a reduced tolerance to pain.[110] One theory recognized that the increase in pain and reduced tolerance in older adults may be related to aging nerve fibers that show damage similar to younger tissue that develops neuropathic pain.[111] In addition to progressive tissue damage with aging, chronic inflammatory responses play a key role in increased pain, pain perception, and development of chronic pain.[112]

Elderly patients feel and sense pain; however, pain responses may be altered because of changes in cognitive, communication, and motor functions. In addition, the elderly may be reluctant to report pain because of fears of pathology or negative social issues related to acknowledgement of pain.[113]

Assessment and management of pain in this patient population can be difficult. One reason may be a limitation in treatment options based on multiple health issues. Therapeutic options can also be restricted by potential interactions with other medications being taken for chronic conditions that do not include pain. Opioids may be considered for short-term pain relief, but their use should be limited due to potential side effects, which include dysphoria, respiratory depression, drug interactions, and constipation. Immobility contributes to painful conditions and limits options for physical therapies. Conventional treatment that is effective in a younger population is not always an appropriate choice for the elderly.

An understanding of how comorbidities, polypharmacy, communication, as well as functional and cognitive impairments is necessary when developing elderly plans of care. Treatment of acute and chronic pain can be challenging, but it is a critical component to improving the quality of life of individuals in the geriatric population.

PATIENT-CENTERED APPROACH

Nurses bring a unique philosophic and theoretic approach to patient care and pain management. Nursing care plans often bring in strategies that include effective communication, partnership, and health promotion.[114]

Patient-centered care is especially important when treating the multidimensional problems associated with chronic pain. A patient-centered approach allows for a foundation for creating an assessment and treatment plan based on the physical, psychological, and social needs, while working to avoid constraints often found in more traditional medical models.[115]

Utilizing the expertise from multiple health care resources and incorporating a variety of philosophies and various treatment regimens are important aspects of a patient-centered approach. Reasonable therapeutic goals should include functional improvement in activities of daily living, psychological improvement, rational pharmacologic

management of ongoing pain, and return to productive activities. Treatment teams can work with patients to develop a joint plan of care based on unique needs of that patient. Primary goals for the joint plan of care can include the identification of resources available, primary and secondary treatment plans, support systems, and spiritual resources as requested by the patient.

A one-size-fits-all approach is seldom effective. Consumer and health care providers tend to compartmentalize their health care problems by seeking a "specialist." This kind of approach often narrowly focuses the treatment and excludes complimentary therapies that may enhance, rather than interfere with, each other. One example of a cooperative approach is the combination of interventional therapy with physical therapy or chiropractic care. Evidence exists that this multidisciplinary approach to pain care is often more successful than a single discipline or treatment.[116]

FAILURE TO TREAT PAIN

Many of the barriers involved in the prevention of timely and appropriate chronic pain management are patient related. The most common issues include lack of access to adequate health care, fear of treatment, misinformation, and cultural barriers. However, provider issues can also create barriers. Sometimes preconceived notions play a role in mismanagement of chronic pain. Such misplaced notions can hinder judgment and lead to erroneous assumptions.[117] Empathy without preconceived judgment is essential for building patient rapport and can assist with the development of effective chronic pain management plans.[118]

▮ SUMMARY

Unlike the story of *Androcles and the Lion* depicted in Aesop's fable, treatment of chronic pain is far more complex than simply "removing a thorn from the paw" and addressing a single source of pain. Identification and treatment of the original source of injury is the beginning to the overall goals of pain management. Chronic pain is a complex disease that involves a vicious cycle of dysfunction and leads to a breakdown in homeostasis. Returning homeostasis requires addressing peripheral, spinal, and cerebral mechanisms that have become dysfunctional

because of repetitive nociceptive stimulation. Absent or inappropriate treatment of chronic pain can result in debilitation, lower quality of life, depression, unemployment, bankruptcy, homelessness, divorce, or suicide. The longer proper treatment is delayed, the more likely that the problem can become irreversible or unmanageable. Chronic pain management often requires a significant time commitment from both the patient and the provider to identify a pathway to functional improvement and return to homeostasis.

REFERENCES

For a complete list of references for this chapter, scan this QR code with any smartphone code reader app, or visit the following URL: http://booksite.elsevier.com/9780323711944/.

58

Non–Operating Room Anesthesia

Renata Sobey, Andy Tracy

Considering the evolving patient population and dynamic needs of a health care system under redesign, it should come as no surprise that the world of anesthesia is also under reconstruction. Although most anesthetics were traditionally administered in the operating room (OR), it is no longer unusual for services to be provided outside the operating suite in a variety of locations that are far from the traditional setting. Estimates today indicate that up to 55% of the procedures that require anesthesia services are taking place outside the conventional OR.[1] These include diagnostic, interventional, and traditional surgery involving cardiology, vascular, emergency department, gastroenterology, gynecology, hematology, oncology, thoracic, neurologic and neurosurgical, plastic, ophthalmology, orthopedic, psychiatric, radiology, and other diagnostic and dental procedures.[2] Studies indicate that the mean age of patients undergoing non-OR procedures was 3.5 years older than those undergoing traditional OR procedures. Older patients tend to be more medically complex with numerous comorbidities, and many patients are poor surgical candidates.[3,4]

Patients treated in these remote settings require the same safe and vigilant attention, anesthetic administration, and recovery care as those patients treated in the operating suite. The key for the anesthesia provider is to ensure that the therapeutic and diagnostic environment where anesthesia is to be performed is as familiar, as well equipped, and as safe as it is in the OR.

Although certain therapeutic and diagnostic procedures are sometimes performed without anesthesia, the patient's condition, or the requirements of the test or procedure, may necessitate administration of an anesthetic. Anesthesia could range from local anesthetic infiltration and regional anesthesia techniques to monitored anesthesia care (MAC) involving enteral minimal sedation, parenteral moderate sedation/analgesia, deep sedation/analgesia, or general anesthesia. Patients can range in age from pediatric to geriatric. In remote locations, patients who require anesthesia may be confused or disoriented, uncooperative, unwilling or unable to understand the requirements of the procedure, claustrophobic, anxious, or mentally disabled.

Several challenges to deliver anesthesia exist that are unique to remote locations. These include working with support staff who are unfamiliar with anesthetic management and who may not recognize an impending critical situation. Variation of the physical setup of the procedure room and monitoring equipment may result in decreased familiarity by the anesthesia provider. Equipment may be poorly maintained, availability of necessary supplies may be inadequate, and scheduling of the procedure utilizing anesthesia services may be inefficient resulting in expeditious patient preparation. Lastly, remote positioning of the patient during a potentially lengthy procedure creates unique challenges that are exacerbated in unfamiliar locations. Given the rapid advances in medical knowledge and technology, coupled with a strong societal impetus to reduce health care costs, more therapeutic and diagnostic procedures will be performed in remote locations.[1,3]

ADMINISTRATION OF ANESTHESIA IN REMOTE LOCATIONS

Special Considerations

The OR provides an ideal environment for the administration of anesthesia and the performance of surgical procedures because of the familiarity of the physical layout; the rapid availability of anesthesia equipment, medications, and supplies; and the accessibility of well-trained adjunct personnel. The anesthesia setting in a remote location must possess the same level of safety and high standards. Many considerations and plans must be executed before a patient can safely receive anesthesia for a therapeutic or diagnostic procedure in a remote location. Box 58.1 provides a comprehensive checklist of the requisites that will facilitate planning and assembling necessary equipment, supplies, and medications.

A policy must be developed that outlines the organization of emergency services for non-OR facilities. Office-based facilities should have a plan for regular emergency training of personnel, interoffice communication during an emergency, communication with emergency medical personnel, and transportation to the nearest hospital emergency department.

An anesthesia machine and portable anesthesia cart with the listed equipment, supplies, and medications should be dedicated strictly for use in remote locations. This can save preparation time whenever a procedure is required. It also increases patient safety and decreases the risk of a mishap resulting from lack of necessary equipment and materials.

As part of the planning process before patient treatment, it is important to familiarize oneself with the personnel and the work area environment. The workplace allotted for anesthesia care may be small, crowded, and different from the usual OR setting. Preplanning is vital to make this unique location familiar to the anesthetist and safe for the patient. All remote locations should have the ability to manage a variety of anesthetic procedures and include equipment, medications, supplies, positive pressure ventilation, resuscitation, and suction as a means to provide safe patient care.

The American Association of Nurse Anesthetists (AANA),[5,6] the American Society of Anesthesiologists (ASA),[7-9] and The Joint Commission (TJC)[10] have established written standards and professional commentary to provide for the basic rights and safety of patients along with the safety of anesthesia providers and ancillary personnel. As technology advances, these standards are adapted and new recommendations made.

Licensed registered nurses, who are not qualified anesthesia providers, have become involved in the monitoring of patients and the administration of medications for procedural sedations involving therapeutic and diagnostic procedures, in addition to certain surgical procedures.

BOX 58.1   Requisites for Administration of Anesthesia in Remote Locations

Utilities

- Adequate workspace
- Adequate overhead lighting
- Adequate number of and current-carrying capacity of electrical outlets
- Electrical service with either isolated electric power or ground fault circuit interrupters, including backup generator power
- Adequate communication pathway, within the department and outside the department
- Suitable area for postprocedure recovery (All building codes, fire codes, safety codes, and facility standards must be met.)

Equipment

- Patient chair, cart, or operating surface that can be quickly placed into Trendelenburg position
- Regularly serviced and functioning equipment
- Patient monitors
- Pulse oximeter
- Electrocardiograph
- Blood pressure monitor with a selection of adequate-sized cuffs
- Capnography
- Body temperature monitor
- Oxygen supplies
- Minimum of two oxygen sources must be available with regulators attached (compressed oxygen should be the equivalent of an E cylinder)
- Positive pressure ventilation sources, including a self-inflating resuscitator bag capable of delivering at least 90% oxygen and a mouth-to-mask unit
- Defibrillator—manual biphasic or automatic external defibrillator (AED) (charged, ready, and easily accessible)
- Suction source or a suction machine (electric-powered suction, battery-powered suction, or foot pump suction devices are available), tubing, suction catheters, and Yankauer suctions
- Lockable anesthesia cart to permit organization of supplies, including endotracheal equipment, laryngeal mask airways, tube of water-soluble lubricating jelly, an assortment of various-sized disposable facemasks, nasal cannulas, oral and nasal airways, syringes (1 mL tuberculin syringe, 3 mL, 5 mL, 10 mL, 20 mL, 60 mL), needles, intravenous catheters, tourniquet, intravenous fluids and tubing, alcohol pads, adhesive tape, sterile intravenous site covers, disposable gloves, stethoscopes, precordial stethoscope with monaural earpiece and extension tubing, precordial stethoscope adhesive disks, and appropriate anesthetic medications
- Battery-powered flashlight for the illumination of the patient, the anesthesia machines, and the monitors along with spare batteries
- Syringe pump, wall plug/transformer, and spare batteries
- Warm blankets, electric blanket (check with hospital policy before using an electric blanket), or forced-air warming devices with the appropriate blanket, towels, or hat to cover the patient's head to preserve body warmth
- Blankets, towels, or foam for padding for protection of skin integrity, bony prominences, and body extremities

- Emergency medications may include atropine, dextrose 50%, diphenhydramine, ephedrine, epinephrine, flumazenil, hydrocortisone, lidocaine, naloxone, nitroglycerin, phenylephrine, succinylcholine, vasopressin, and a bronchial dilator inhaler such as albuterol or nebulized epinephrine (Note that some anesthetic medications must be kept refrigerated until ready for use.)
- Preoperative anesthesia evaluation forms
- Anesthesia consent form

Additional Requirements for General Anesthesia

- Oxygen fail-safe system
- Oxygen analyzer
- Waste gas exhaust scavenging system
- End tidal carbon dioxide (ET_{CO_2}) analyzer, extra ET_{CO_2} filter, and extension sample tubing
- Vaporizers—calibration and exclusion system
- Respiratory monitoring apparatus (for the anesthesia circuit reservoir bag)
- Alarm system
- In addition to the emergency medications listed previously, consider the following:
  - Premedication drugs—midazolam, ketamine, nitrous oxide, diazepam, chloral hydrate
  - Induction drugs—propofol, etomidate, ketamine
  - Maintenance drugs—bottles of sevoflurane, isoflurane, desflurane, propofol, ketamine, dexmedetomidine
  - Narcotics—fentanyl, alfentanil, sufentanil, remifentanil
  - Muscle relaxants—succinylcholine, rocuronium, cisatracurium, vecuronium
  - Muscle relaxant reversal agents—neostigmine, atropine, glycopyrrolate, sugammadex
  - Cardiovascular drugs—labetalol, esmolol, verapamil, hydralazine, vasopressin
  - Narcotic reversal drugs—naloxone
  - Antiemetic drugs—ondansetron, dolasetron, metoclopramide, scopolamine
- Emergency cart and equipment
- Laryngoscope handle with assorted blades, laryngeal mask airways in assorted sizes, and endotracheal tubes (adult and pediatric)
- Self-inflating resuscitator bag (Ambu bag)
- Difficult airway equipment, including an emergency cricothyrotomy kit
- Malignant hyperthermia emergency drugs, equipment, and the phone number for the Malignant Hyperthermia Association of the United States (MHAUS) for live help during the treatment of malignant hyperthermia onsite (United States and Canada: 1-800-MH HYPER or 1-800-644-9737; outside the United States and Canada: 001-1-315-464-7079). More information is available at the MHAUS website (http://www.mhaus.org).

The AANA and the ASA, separately and together, have issued statements in regard to criteria (Box 58.2) that must be met by nonanesthesia providers to protect the safety and well-being of the patient.[11,12]

Standards for the Delivery of Anesthesia in a Remote Location

A. Perform a Complete Preanesthesia Assessment

The patient, parent(s), or legal guardian(s) must be thoroughly interviewed and assessed before the performance of any anesthetic procedure. The preanesthesia assessment should be performed in consideration of patients' right to privacy and confidentiality, and which safeguards their dignity and respects aspects of their psychological, cultural, and spiritual values. During this assessment, information is obtained regarding the patient's medical history (prior allergy must be assessed), anesthesia history (noting any prior complications and responses to prior anesthetic experiences), surgical history, medication history (including tobacco, alcohol, and any substance abuse), as well as the patient's exercise tolerance capacity. A complete physical assessment of the patient is made, along with inspection of the head,

---

BOX 58.2 Criteria for the Management and Monitoring of Patients Undergoing Sedation Delivered for Therapeutic or Diagnostic Procedures by Nonanesthesia Providers

- Guidelines for patient monitoring, drug administration, and protocols are available for dealing with potential complications or emergency situations, developed in accordance with accepted standards of anesthesia practice.
- A qualified anesthesia provider or attending physician selects and orders the agents to achieve sedation and analgesia.
- Registered nurses who are not qualified anesthesia providers should not administer agents classified as anesthetics, including but not limited to ketamine, propofol, etomidate, nitrous oxide, and muscle relaxants.
- The registered nurse managing and monitoring the patient receiving an analgesia sedation shall have no other responsibilities during the procedure.
- Venous access shall be maintained for all patients having sedation and analgesia.
- Supplemental oxygen shall be available for any patient receiving sedation and analgesia and when appropriate, in the postprocedure period.
- Documentation and monitoring of physiologic measurements, including but not limited to blood pressure, respiratory rate, oxygen saturation, cardiac rate and rhythm, and level of consciousness, should be recorded at least every 5 min.
- An emergency cart must be immediately accessible to every location where analgesia sedation is administered. This cart must include emergency resuscitative drugs, airway and ventilatory adjunct equipment, defibrillator, and a source for administration of 100% oxygen. A positive pressure breathing device, oxygen, suction, and appropriate airways must be placed in each room where analgesia sedation is administered.
- Backup personnel who are experts in airway management, emergency intubations, and advanced cardiopulmonary resuscitation must be available.
- A qualified professional capable of managing complications is present in the facility and remains in the facility until the patient is stable.
- A qualified professional authorized under institutional guidelines to discharge the patient remains in the facility to discharge the patient in accordance with established criteria of the facility.

BOX 58.3 Specific Patient Conditions That Warrant Anesthesia-Care Vigilance

- Mental impairment with an inability to cooperate
- Severe gastroesophageal reflux; delayed gastric emptying; aspiration risk
- Orthopnea; obstructive sleep apnea
- Decreased level of consciousness; depression of airway protection reflexes
- Increased intracranial pressure
- Difficult airway; oral, dental, craniofacial, cervical, or thoracic abnormalities that could preclude airway access and maintenance
- Respiratory tract infection
- Morbid obesity
- Therapeutic or diagnostic procedures that impede access to the airway
- Therapeutic or diagnostic procedures that are complex, lengthy, painful, or invasive
- Positioning that is complex, atypical, painful; prone position
- Patient suffering acute trauma
- Patients with extremes of age
- Prematurity
- Physical status 3 or 4

---

neck, mouth, and airway. The patient's nil per os (NPO) status must be assessed in addition to any recent change in condition that may complicate or prohibit the delivery of anesthesia for a nonemergent procedure. Review of diagnostic data such as patient laboratory values, radiographs, and electrocardiogram (ECG) is completed, and important findings are noted in the patient's anesthesia record. A physical status classification is then assigned to the patient. Box 58.3 outlines specific patient conditions that alert the anesthetist to the need for special attention related to the delivery of anesthesia during therapeutic and diagnostic procedures.

B. Obtain Informed Consent for the Planned Anesthetic Intervention From the Patient or Legal Guardian

The anesthesia provider should discuss the course of the anesthetic plan of care and enumerate the following in understandable terms appropriate for the patient or guardian:

- How the anesthetic procedure will be performed
- Possible risks of the anesthetic procedure
- Pertinent possible reactions or complications the patient might expect while receiving a typical anesthetic, along with informing the patient or guardian that the anesthetist has permission to make changes or adjustments as deemed necessary according to professional judgment

- Possible options to the type of anesthetic to be received by the patient
- The ability for the patient/parent(s)/guardian(s) to have any concerns addressed and questions answered

At times, anesthesia for therapeutic and diagnostic procedures will require only minimal, moderate, or deep sedation, which by definition may not include patient amnesia. Only general anesthesia ensures amnesia as a standard of care. Therefore discussion of what the patient can reasonably expect should take place at this time.[13] It is far easier to discuss these points with the patient before the anesthetic procedure than to explain these issues postprocedure.

C. Formulate a Patient-Specific Plan for Anesthesia Care

The art and science of anesthesia mandate that the safest and least invasive anesthetic technique be administered to the patient to avoid complications for the patient and promote positive patient outcomes while practicing at a remote setting.

D. Implement and Adjust the Anesthesia Care Plan Based on the Patient's Physiologic Response

Immediately before implementation of anesthesia, reassess the patient (e.g., vital signs, airway status, and response to preprocedure medications given) and document a reassessment note in the anesthesia record. TJC mandates a preanesthetic evaluation on all patients receiving anesthesia and defines "immediately" as the moments just before the sedation is administered. Ensure that all anesthesia equipment, supplies, and medications are checked and immediately available should the patient status require a change in the anesthetic plan.

E. Properly Prepare, Dispense, and Label All Medications to Be Used for the Patient

All medications drawn up prior to the case must be labeled with the drug name, concentration, amount (if not apparent from the container), and expiration date (if not used within 24 hours), the time, and initials of the individual drawing up the medication. To reduce the risk of infections, the AANA, along with other health care organizations, now recommends the Centers for Disease Control and Prevention (CDC) guidelines for the use of single-dose vials, single-use needles, and single-use syringes.

F. Adhere to Appropriate Safety Precautions and Protocols, as Established by the Institution, to Minimize Risks to the Patient and Ancillary Staff

This standard is important for the patient, the anesthesia provider, and ancillary personnel for the prevention of accidents and injury related to fire, explosion, electrical shock, and equipment malfunction. These issues are also a consideration from a medicolegal perspective. The anesthesia provider is also an integral part of the team involved with protocols for preventing wrong site, wrong procedure, and wrong person surgery, also known as the Universal Protocol established by TJC.[11,14,15] Anesthesia services must be consulted for scheduling consideration of patients in remote locations, as these therapeutic and diagnostic procedures are often complex when compared to anesthesia delivery in the operating room and may require additional staffing resources.

G. Monitor and Document the Patient's Physiologic Condition as Appropriate for the Type of Anesthesia and Specific Patient Needs[6,7]

- *Perform a complete anesthesia equipment safety check daily and document in the patient's medical record.* An abbreviated check of all equipment is acceptable before each subsequent anesthetic is administered.
- *Monitor ventilation continuously.* Ventilation may be monitored in the patient undergoing mild, moderate, or deep sedation with a precordial stethoscope or by direct auscultation of the patient's ventilatory effort. Verify intubation of the trachea by auscultation, chest excursion, and confirmation of carbon dioxide in the expired gas. In cases of moderate or deep sedation, the AANA and ASA mandate the measurement of end tidal carbon dioxide ($ETco_2$) unless the patient, procedure, or equipment interferes or precludes monitoring. Continuously monitor $ETco_2$ during controlled, assisted, or spontaneous ventilation, including any anesthesia or sedation technique requiring artificial airway support. Use spirometry and ventilatory pressure monitors as indicated.[9]
- *Monitor oxygenation continuously* by clinical observation and pulse oximetry. Cerebral oximetry and/or arterial blood gas analysis may be indicated.
- *Monitor cardiovascular status continuously* via ECG and heart sounds. Record blood pressure and heart rate at least every 5 minutes.
- *Monitor body temperature continuously* in all patients when clinically significant changes in body temperature are intended, anticipated, or suspected. Maintenance of normothermia must be an integral part of the anesthetic plan to preserve essential body functions and to prevent complications leading to patient morbidity and mortality. Temperature monitoring is a standard of care when delivering general anesthesia to the patient and optional while performing mild, moderate, or deep sedation.[9]
- *Monitor neuromuscular function and status* prior to the procedure and recovery when neuromuscular blocking agents are administered.
- *Monitor and assess patient positioning and protective measures* at frequent intervals. Periodic assessment of eye protection, skin, bony prominences, and extremities is mandatory.

H. Precautions Shall Be Taken to Minimize the Risk of Infection to the Patient, the Operator, and Ancillary Personnel

Clean equipment regularly; maintain sterility of supplies until ready for use and ensure that medications are not expired, opened, or tampered with before use. Protective eyewear for the anesthesia provider should be readily available in addition to an assortment of sterile and nonsterile gloves.

I. There Must Be Complete, Accurate, and Time-Oriented Documentation of Pertinent Information on the Patient's Anesthesia Record

Document baseline patient vital signs before the anesthetic procedure and the therapeutic or diagnostic procedure have begun. Documentation must be made of all vital signs: heart rate, blood pressure, pulse oximeter readings, patient temperature, and the presence of $ETco_2$. Documentation that includes names and quantities must be made of all fluids and medications administered. Compliance to institutional-specific anesthesia documentation practices applies to remote locations in addition to the OR.

J. After the Anesthetic Treatment for Therapeutic or Diagnostic Procedures, Transfer the Responsibility for Care of the Patient to Other Qualified Personnel in a Manner That Ensures Continuity of Care and Patient Safety

Anesthesia care does not end with the completion of the therapeutic or diagnostic procedure. The patient may receive postanesthesia care at the site of the therapeutic or diagnostic procedure or may be transported to a separate area for postanesthesia care by fully trained recovery staff or the anesthesia provider, utilizing appropriate monitoring devices. A comprehensive report is given to the recovery personnel, and the transfer of care is documented, including the receiving staff member. The anesthesia provider thoroughly assesses stability of the patient and airway maintenance before exiting the recovery area. The patient's condition is evaluated continually in the recovery area, and the patient may be discharged from the recovery area once discharge criteria are achieved.[16] Table 58.1 provides a non-OR anesthesia safety checklist.

K. Summary

The standards listed in this section describe the minimum requirements for treatment and monitoring of any patient who requires anesthesia care. These guidelines are established to maintain patient safety and facilitate positive patient outcomes. The omission of any monitoring standard should be documented and the reason for such omission stated on the patient's anesthesia record. Any anesthetic procedure, including those performed in a remote location, should not begin until the anesthetist feels sufficiently comfortable, safe, and well prepared to deliver the anesthetic treatment required for the patient.

Guidelines for Sedation

Therapeutic and diagnostic procedures can be performed with various methods of sedation. Sedation is possible with enteral, rectal, parenteral (intravenous [IV]), and inhaled medications. It is important to remember that the depth of sedation in a patient is a continuum of progressive alterations in cognition, respirations, and protective reflexes. Many anesthetic agents are synergistic and potentiate the effects of one another when a multimodal approach is used, and consequently the patient may quickly progress from one level of sedation/anesthesia to another. It is essential that the anesthesia provider be able to respond to all depths of anesthesia and have quick access to vital equipment, supplies, and trained and qualified ancillary personnel who are familiar with anesthesia delivery, emergencies, and monitoring.

Sedation exists as a continuum, and it is not always possible to predict the individual responses of each patient to a particular level of anesthesia. Consequently, the anesthesia provider must be able to intervene when the depth of anesthesia exceeds expectations. Table 58.2

TABLE 58.1 Nonoperating Room Anesthesia Safety Checklist

Before Induction of Anesthesia	Before Procedure Start	Before Patient Leaves Procedure Room
Has the patient confirmed his or her identity, site (if applicable), procedure, and consent? ☐ Yes Is the site marked? ☐ Yes ☐ Not applicable	Confirm all team members have introduced themselves by name and role Confirm the patient's name and procedure	Nurse verbally confirms: The name of the procedure Completion of instrument counts (if applicable) Specimen labeling (read specimen labels aloud, including patient name) Whether any equipment problems need to be addressed
Is the anesthesia machine and medication check complete? ☐ Yes Does the patient have a: Known allergy? ☐ No ☐ Yes Difficult airway or aspiration risk? ☐ No ☐ Yes, and equipment and assistance are available Risk for >500 mL blood loss (7 mL/kg in children)? ☐ No ☐ Yes, and two intravenous lines or central access and fluids planned Is the pulse oximeter on the patient and functioning? ☐ Yes	Has antibiotic prophylaxis been given within the last 60 min? ☐ Yes ☐ Not applicable Anticipated critical events: *To proceduralist:* What are the critical or nonroutine steps? How long will the case take? What is the anticipated blood loss? *To anesthetist:* Are there any patient-specific concerns? *To nursing team:* Has sterility (including indicator results) been confirmed? Are there any equipment issues or concerns? Is essential imaging displayed? ☐ Yes ☐ Not applicable	To the proceduralist, anesthetist, and nurse: What are the key concerns for recovery and management for this patient?

From Lane-Fall M. Engineering excellence in non-operating room anesthesia care. In: Weiss M, Fleisher LA, eds. *Non-Operating Room Anesthesia*. Philadelphia: Elsevier; 2015:3.

TABLE 58.2 The Continuum of Depth of Sedation: Definition of General Anesthesia and Levels of Sedation/Analgesia

	Minimal Sedation Anxiolysis*	Moderate Sedation/ Anxiolysis ("Conscious Sedation")**	Deep Sedation/ Analgesia***	General Anesthesia****
Responsiveness	Normal response to verbal stimuli	Purposeful response to verbal or tactile stimulation	Purposeful response following repeated or painful stimulation	Unarousable even with painful stimulation
Airway	Unaffected	No intervention required	Intervention may be required	Intervention often required
Spontaneous ventilation	Unaffected	Adequate	May be inadequate	Frequently inadequate
Cardiovascular function	Unaffected	Usually maintained	Usually maintained	May be impaired

*Minimal sedation (formerly known as anxiolysis) is a drug-induced state during which patients respond normally to verbal commands. Although cognitive function and coordination may be impaired, ventilatory and cardiovascular functions are unaffected.

**Moderate sedation/analgesia (formerly conscious sedation) is a drug-induced depression of consciousness during which patients respond purposefully to verbal commands, either alone or accompanied by light tactile stimulation. No interventions are required to maintain a patent airway, and spontaneous ventilation is adequate. Cardiovascular function is usually maintained. (NOTE: Reflexive withdrawal from a painful stimulus is not considered a purposeful response.)

***Deep sedation/analgesia is a drug-induced depression of consciousness during which patients cannot be easily aroused but respond purposefully after repeated or painful stimulation. The ability to independently maintain ventilatory function may be impaired. Patients may require assistance in maintaining a patent airway, and spontaneous ventilation may be inadequate. Cardiovascular function is usually maintained.

****Anesthesia (general anesthesia) consists of general anesthesia and spinal or major regional anesthesia. It does not include local anesthesia. General anesthesia is a drug-induced loss of consciousness during which patients are not aroused, even by painful stimulation. The ability to independently maintain ventilatory function is often impaired. Patients often require assistance in maintaining a patent airway, and positive pressure ventilation may be required because of depressed spontaneous ventilation or drug-induced depression of neuromuscular function. Cardiovascular function may be impaired.

Modified from American Society of Anesthesiologists. Continuum of depth of sedation: definition of general anesthesia, and levels of sedation/analgesia, 2019. https://www.asahq.org/standards-and-guidelines/continuum-of-depth-of-sedation-definition-of-general-anesthesia-and-levels-of-sedationanalgesia. Accessed 2020.

lists definitions of the four levels of sedation and physiologic responses associated with each category as described by the ASA. From these definitions, standards are provided to practitioners for the administration of safe and high-quality care to patients.[17]

Accepted standards for moderate sedation/analgesia and deep sedation/analgesia state the following[10,17,18]:

1. The process from minimal sedation (anxiolysis) to general anesthesia is a continuum, and individuals vary in their responses to medications.
2. Qualified individuals with appropriate credentials (e.g., nurses, Certified Registered Nurse Anesthetists [CRNAs], anesthesiologists, and dentists) who are trained in professional standards and techniques do the following:
   a. May administer pharmacologic agents to achieve a desired level of sedation.
   b. Must monitor patients carefully to maintain the patient's vital functions at the desired level of sedation. Appropriate equipment must be available for monitoring heart rate via ECG, respiratory rate and adequacy of pulmonary ventilation, oxygenation via pulse oximetry, and blood pressure measurement at regular intervals (at least every 5 minutes).
   c. Must be competent to evaluate the patient before performing the moderate sedation/analgesia and deep sedation/analgesia.
   d. Must be competent to support the patient's psychological functions and physical comfort.
   e. Must be competent in the administration of sedatives, analgesics, hypnotics, and other medications to produce and maintain moderate sedation/analgesia and deep sedation/analgesia.
   f. Must be competent to rescue the patient who unavoidably or unintentionally moves into a deeper than desired level of sedation and analgesia. In addition, for patients undergoing deep sedation/analgesia, one must also have competency to manage cardiovascular compromise.
   g. Must properly document the patient's response to care.
   h. Must supervise recovery of the patient after the sedation postanesthesia recovery area or until transfer of care to another qualified health care provider.
   i. Must discharge the patient once discharge criteria have been achieved and in conjunction with the proceduralist.
3. Adequate numbers of qualified and competent personnel must be present during the performance of moderate sedation/analgesia, deep sedation/analgesia, and general anesthesia to serve as a skilled second pair of hands if necessary. This should include not only qualified anesthesia providers as described earlier but also nurses, assistants, technicians, and other office staff to meet the needs of the patient.[17,18]

Pain Management

Pain control after surgery remains challenging despite an improved understanding of the mechanism of pain. This also applies to non-OR anesthesia cases, where one of the most common minor adverse events is inadequate pain control. Anesthesia providers are equipped with a varied toolbox to help patients in managing pain in the perioperative period. Traditional pharmacotherapy works by affecting the transduction, transmission, modulation, and perception of pain. Multimodal analgesia has been shown in multiple clinical situations to have strong efficacy in the treatment of postoperative pain. This form of pain control works by targeting different pain pathways to produce a synergistic effect at lower analgesic doses. In addition to the use of opioids in pain control, multimodal analgesia utilizes acetaminophen, gabapentinoids, nonsteroidal antiinflammatory drugs (NSAIDs), and ketamine to augment analgesia.[4]

The Pediatric Patient

The pediatric population can pose complex challenges for the delivery of anesthesia. Pediatric patient behavior and degree of cooperation can range from very helpful to extremely anxious and even combative. Pediatric sedation and anesthesia improve the patient care experience by greatly reducing anxiety and eliminating movement while providing for safe patient outcomes for therapeutic or diagnostic procedures. The primary considerations in the practice of anesthesia are patient safety and guardianship of patient welfare. Children under the age of 5 years seem to be at the greatest risk for adverse events even with no underlying disease. Adverse events have occurred more commonly with the use of multiple drugs, especially sedative medications.[19-23] The problems encountered most often are respiratory events: respiratory depression, respiratory obstruction, and apnea.[20-22]

Adverse events can be reduced by proper adherence to patient selection and a comprehensive preoperative assessment, proper dosage of medications to minimize unexpected responses, proper monitoring, skilled administration of anesthesia, and proper recovery time. The anesthesia provider must be prepared to alter anesthetic plans based on the patient response to anesthetic agents.[20-23] Consideration must be made for the type of procedure to be performed, past medical history, past sedation/anesthesia history, current medication therapy, allergies, and respiratory or airway difficulties. Questions regarding the degree of patient stimulation expected throughout the procedure, amount of anticipated blood loss, ability to maintain normothermia, and ability to have close proximity in which to monitor the patient are all necessary for the anesthesia provider to address. Length of procedure is critical information as adverse reactions are reduced with procedures that last less than 1 hour.[23] Clear communication with the adjunct medical staff is essential to clarify the requirements for the patient to be safe and properly anesthetized for the procedure.

The pediatric patient and the parent or legal guardian must be properly prepared for the planned therapeutic or diagnostic procedure. Clear explanation of the entire anesthetic process to the parent or guardian is based on the developed treatment plan and is offered in age-appropriate terms for the pediatric patient.[19] Discussion with the parent/guardian about separation from the patient, where the parent/guardian will wait during the procedure, and the ability to be reunited postprocedure will alleviate anxiety.

Box 58.4 identifies some relevant pediatric safety considerations and specific preprocedural assessments of the pediatric patient. It is particularly important to assess any recent upper respiratory infections, fever, cough, snoring, and sputum production, which could result in an airway compromise during sedation. Additional attention must be paid to the airway to assess for any loose dentition or anatomic aberrancies.

Knowledge of the most common causes of adverse pediatric anesthesia events can help the anesthetist plan for and avoid these events (Box 58.5).[20,21,23] Most adverse anesthesia events are caused when multiple anesthetic agents are used.[24]

The Geriatric Patient

As a result of a number of factors, including better nutrition, more physical activity, less tobacco and alcohol use, and improved medical care and medical technologies, more Americans are living longer. In 2016, the US Census Bureau released population projections stating that the population of people within the United States currently over the age of 65 is 15.2% and will reach 78 million by 2035 with the continued increased life expectancy.[25] The increasing elderly population is placing, and will continue to place, many demands on the health care system. Medical technology is advancing, and therefore more procedures requiring anesthesia will be performed on elderly patients. It is estimated that approximately 55% of anesthesia cases are being performed outside of the traditional OR and that the elderly population accounts for a large percentage of those anesthetics.[1] Perioperative complications can increase with age, and consequently special considerations related to the physiology of aging are necessary for the safe delivery of anesthesia.

Aging is associated with a progressive loss of functional reserve in all organ systems. However, there is considerable individual variability in the onset and extent of these changes. The elderly have a greater prevalence of comorbidities such as atherosclerosis, infections, autoimmune diseases, chronic disorders, and cancer. The immune system gradually and slowly diminishes in function with age. Therefore the ability to heal and fight foreign bacteria, viruses, and malignant cells diminishes. Additional components of the aging process include an increase in the ratio of adipose tissue to aqueous body tissue resulting in greater storage of lipid-soluble anesthetic agents. Basal metabolic rate along with liver and kidney functions all decrease with age causing a prolonged effect of anesthetic agents due to a decrease in metabolism and excretion. Cerebral atrophy occurs with aging resulting in an overall loss of neurons in the neocortex, which suggests increased sensitivity to anesthetic medications. The elderly are at an increased risk for perioperative delirium and postoperative cognitive dysfunction. Therefore the dosage requirements for anesthetic drugs are usually decreased.[26]

The geriatric patient's level of activity is one indicator of cardiovascular function, and this generally decreases with age; this decrease in activity usually correlates with limited physiologic reserves. Patients may be restricted in their activity because of arthritis or other debilitation. Circulation time is decreased, and skeletal muscle diminishes with a decline in physical activity, which decreases total oxygen consumption and blood-flow needs to the muscles, resulting in decreased cardiac output. The ability of the cardiovascular system to respond to the effects of anesthetic drugs, fluid administration, and the stresses of therapeutic and diagnostic procedures can cause decreased cardiac function, resulting in hemodynamic instability and reduced circulation to vital organs.[26]

Tissue oxygenation can decrease because of changes in ventilation ability and lung tissue. Lung compliance is decreased, resulting in ventilation-perfusion mismatch. Aging itself brings on the increasing inability to respond to hypoxia and hypercapnia, especially when experiencing the effects of anesthesia. Therefore the anesthetist must always ensure and constantly monitor the supply of adequate amounts of oxygen to the elderly patient and be ready to offer ventilatory support. The ability to thermoregulate is also decreased with age.[26]

Several electroencephalography (EEG) processing monitors are available that help in assessment of patient responses to anesthetic medications. These devices monitor anesthesia awareness, level of consciousness, depth of sedation, and response to anesthetic medications, which allows for more precise titration of anesthetic medications according to patient needs. Care must be taken to preserve body warmth and ensure the continual delivery of adequate warmth when necessary. Protection of the eyes, skin, and the extremities, both while moving the patient and during the procedure, by skin padding of bony prominences must also be ensured.[26] These variables are a component of the anesthetic plan when administering care to the geriatric patient. Finally, consider verbal and written postoperative instructions to both the elderly patient and caregivers/significant others who will accompany the patient and be present to both monitor and care for the elderly patient after a therapeutic or diagnostic procedure.

ANESTHESIA FOR SPECIFIC PROCEDURES IN REMOTE LOCATIONS

Cardiology Procedures

Automatic Implantable Cardiac Defibrillator and Cardiac Pacemaker

See Chapter 27 for a complete discussion of cardiac devices.

Cardioversion

Procedure overview. Cardioversion is the discharge of electrical energy, synchronized to the R wave of the QRS complex of the ECG, to convert hemodynamically unstable supraventricular rhythms such as atrial flutter, atrial fibrillation, or hemodynamically stable ventricular tachycardia (VT). These rhythms can be life threatening if left untreated. Atrial flutter and atrial fibrillation are associated with the development of congestive heart failure and with the formation of thromboemboli, which can lead to stroke. Cardioversion is usually a scheduled and planned procedure unless the patient's condition warrants otherwise. Patient optimization may not be possible if there is urgency for cardioversion as a result of hemodynamic instability. Much less electrical energy is required to synchronously cardiovert a patient when compared with asynchronous defibrillation.[27,28] Defibrillation is an unplanned and usually emergent application of unsynchronized electrical energy. Cardioversion is believed to be therapeutic because it closes an excitable gap in the myocardium, which causes currents to reenter and excite the electrical system of the heart.[29]

Anesthetic considerations. Because cardioversion is usually a nonemergent and planned procedure, patient conditions can usually be optimized. Proper NPO status must be observed unless the cardioversion is deemed urgent or emergent. Standard monitors are applied, with special attention paid to the ECG. A monitor of anesthesia awareness/level of consciousness/depth of sedation via EEG processing can be used to assess consciousness during cardioversion.[30] IV access is necessary. The energy required for cardioversion is measured in joules (watt-seconds). The cardiologist uses a cardioverter-manual monophasic or biphasic defibrillator for the procedure. The optimal shock dose for cardioversion of atrial flutter and other supraventricular tachycardias is 50 to 100 J.[27,28,31-33] The operator applies cardioversion-defibrillator paddles with conduction gel or defibrillator pads to the patient's skin. One paddle or pad is placed parasternally over the second and third intercostal space. The other paddle or patch is placed over the area of the apex of the heart.[27,28,31,32] The cardioverter-defibrillator is set to the synchronized (sync) mode. Visible synchronization marks are placed by the cardioverter atop the tallest R waves of the ECG. Energy shocks are delivered initially at 50 to 100 J, then titrated progressively to 360 J as necessary after observation of the effectiveness of the synchronized shock.[27,28,33]

Midazolam may be administered as both a sedative and amnestic agent before cardioversion. Oxygen via nasal cannula or facemask is administered to the patient. Moderate sedation is often acceptable to counter the intense and brief pain of cardioversion. Because of the intense and brief pain of cardioversion, an ultrashort-acting general anesthetic such as propofol or etomidate is administered.[30] After the administration of anesthesia to the appropriate level, an "all-clear" signal is given by the operator. Then the synchronized shock or shocks are administered. Muscle relaxation is not necessary. As always, an assortment of oral airways, nasal airways, laryngeal mask airways (LMAs), endotracheal tubes (ETTs), and laryngoscopes with blades and suction should be readily available in case complications occur. If cardioversion is required in a patient who has not fasted, general anesthesia with tracheal intubation is necessary to prevent aspiration of gastric contents.[33]

Postanesthesia care. It is expected that the patient's heart is now beating in a desirable cardiac rhythm and that the patient's blood pressure is stable. Spontaneous respirations return, along with swallowing and coughing reflexes. The patient is observed for any reactions to the anesthetic, and care is turned over to the nurse accompanying the patient or the person who will be providing the postanesthesia care.

Radiofrequency Catheter Ablation

Procedure overview. Radiofrequency catheter ablation (RFCA) uses a catheter with an electrode at its tip, which is guided under fluoroscopy to an area of heart muscle that has demonstrated accessory electrical conductive pathways.[34-36] RFCA has all but replaced arrhythmia surgery and is now considered the foremost therapy for the treatment of many arrhythmias in pediatric and adult patients.[36,37] Supraventricular tachycardia is the most common tachyarrhythmia in children, and symptomatic supraventricular tachydysrhythmias are most often treated by RFCA.[34] Accessory electrical conductive pathways are distributed unevenly along the right and left atrioventricular (AV) valve annuli. Left-sided accessory pathways are most common, but both right- and left-sided accessory electrical pathways can be accessed and ablated.[34,35] Other treatments possible with RFCA include modification of the sinus node or AV node, ablation of atrial flutter and atrial tachycardia, and ablation of focal atrial fibrillation and VT foci.[34-36] Patients must undergo electrophysiologic studies to determine the origin and pathway of the arrhythmia, in addition to the mechanism of action, before RFCA can be chosen as a therapy.

Cryoablation is now being used prior to RFCA or in place of RFCA. Liquid nitrous oxide is circulated through the catheter tip to cause temperatures at the tip of $-22°C$ to $-75°C$. At a higher temperature ($-22°C$ or lower), tissue can be temporarily "ice mapped," which is a trial to see whether this nonpermanent freezing of the tissue will successfully eliminate the dysrhythmia. If the ice mapping is successful, then the probe is further cooled, causing permanent destruction of the arrhythmogenic tissue. Cryoablation causes less discomfort and has been found to be safer to use in cases of dysrhythmias in the area of the AV node where iatrogenic complete AV heart block can be caused. Iatrogenic AV block is relatively common and may require placement of a transvenous pacemaker.[37,38]

RFCA is safe with success rates of 95% overall. Many patients no longer need their antiarrhythmic medications soon after therapy.[33,34] RFCA is now being used as treatment for liver metastases from colorectal cancer. RFCA is providing a new treatment option for those patients with high risks for surgery but who would be at a lesser risk for the less-invasive RFCA.

Anesthetic considerations. Electrophysiologic studies conducted before RFCA are time-consuming procedures that may require moderate sedation in adults or general anesthesia in children. RFCA can be performed in the OR, in a special cardiac procedure room, or in the cardiac catheterization suite by a cardiologist. The electrode catheter is guided via the femoral artery and vein to the area of the accessory electrical pathway or an area of arrhythmogenic focus.[34,37] The internal jugular vein also may be used. The electrode is then energized with radiofrequency energy, and cells within the path of the electrode are obliterated. The procedure can produce brief periods (<1–2 minutes) of mild to moderate retrosternal, angina-like pain.[37]

RFCA is a short procedure where patients must remain perfectly still, except for respiratory movement, during the procedure.[36,37,39] Many adults can be anesthetized with moderate sedation/analgesia along with a local anesthetic applied by the operator.[39] Children may be best treated with general anesthesia using either a LMA or ETT to secure the airway. If general endotracheal anesthesia is used, the patient may be held apneic for a short period of time while the catheter is accurately directed and the ablation procedure performed.[37] Full monitors and an IV catheter are necessary. Total IV anesthesia (TIVA) is often used because, during the cryoablation, 25% of cardiac output is transiently lost when the pulmonary artery is occluded. Patients can develop significant hemodynamic instability. Pulmonary artery occlusion also interferes with uptake and distribution of volatile anesthetics making TIVA technique ideal. TIVA with propofol and ondansetron has a much lower rate of nausea (postoperative nausea and vomiting [PONV]) than use of an inhaled anesthetic and an antiemetic. Careful attention must be paid to the ECG because the patient must stop taking any antiarrhythmic drugs before the electrophysiologic study and RFCA are performed.[34-37,39]

Possible thermal injury to the esophagus is a concern during RFCA of the left atrium resulting in esophageal ulcerations or an atrioesophageal fistula, which is an extremely rare but often fatal complication of RFCA. Insertion and use of an esophageal temperature probe during general anesthesia is essential, as is the position of the probe. The probe should be inserted so that it is alongside the esophageal tissues with no space in between. Constant monitoring and communication with the procedural team are necessary for prevention, identification, and treatment of complication.[40] Electrophysiology procedures, anesthesia techniques, and estimated anesthesia times are listed in Table 58.3.

Postanesthesia care. Patients must be observed for possible RFCA procedural complications such as bleeding, ECG changes, cerebrovascular accidents, cardiac tamponade, or damage to the aortic valve.[34-37]

Percutaneous Coronary Intervention

Procedure overview. Percutaneous coronary intervention (PCI) encompasses a wide variety of procedures performed in the cardiac catheter laboratory (CCL). PCI is being performed on adults and is now more commonplace on younger and sicker patients. The CCL is generally located remotely from the ORs and the blood bank. It consists of a large procedural area with a small control room. PCI procedures use x-radiation/fluoroscopy doses "as low as reasonably achievable" (the ALARA principle), in addition to the use of IV radiocontrast media. The heart is commonly accessed via the femoral artery, although the brachial or radial artery can be used. The right side of the heart and pulmonary circulation are commonly accessed via the femoral vein.[41,42]

Anesthetic considerations. PCI necessitates access to major blood vessels and the heart itself. Box 58.6 lists possible PCI complications that affect the safety of the anesthetic and may require interventions from the anesthetist. Consideration for rapid access to competent anesthesia assistance has to be prepared well in advance of PCI anesthesia. Anesthesia techniques can range from IV moderate sedation/analgesia, or deep sedation/analgesia, to general anesthesia, aided with local anesthetic infiltration at the insertion site and alongside the major vein used for insertion of the PCI armamentaria.[41,42]

Postanesthesia care. Care of the patient undergoing PCI usually does not end with completion of the PCI procedure. Arrangements can be made for observation and ongoing care of the patient in a telemetry environment or in the intensive care unit, depending on how critical the patient remains. Immediate postanesthesia concerns are continuing dysrhythmias, hypothermia, current fluid status, changes in fluid status, PONV, hemodynamic status related to hemorrhage, and analgesia.[42]

TABLE 58.3 Electrophysiology Procedures, Anesthesia Techniques, and Estimated Anesthesia Times

Category	Procedure	Usual Anesthetic Technique	Time
MAC in recovery unit	Cardioversion	A short period of deep sedation usually using a bolus dose of propofol (or etomidate if the ejection fraction is low)	15 min
	TEE	Deeper sedation may be required for some patients undergoing TEE who are unable to tolerate the procedure with conscious sedation by the cardiology team	60 min
	NIPS	Deep sedation may be required for cardioversion or defibrillation	30–45 min
MAC in electrophysiology laboratory	Pacemaker placement or battery change	Fentanyl/midazolam or infusions of propofol/remifentanil/midazolam	3–4 hr
	ICD or biventricular ICD placements or battery changes	Fentanyl/midazolam or infusions of propofol/remifentanil/midazolam (defibrillator threshold testing will require a short period of deeper anesthesia similar to that in a cardioversion)	3–4 hr
	Loop recorder placement in superficial anterior chest wall	Fentanyl/midazolam or infusions of propofol/remifentanil/midazolam	2–3 hr
	Atrial flutter radiofrequency ablation	Infusions of propofol/remifentanil/midazolam	6–10 hr
	Ventricular tachycardia or ventricular fibrillation or premature ventricular contraction radiofrequency ablation	Usually infusions of remifentanil only; discuss additional sedatives with cardiologist	6–10 hr
General anesthesia in electrophysiology laboratory	Atrial fibrillation radiofrequency ablation	General endotracheal anesthesia using jet ventilation and TIVA, which predominantly involves propofol and remifentanil infusions Radial arterial lines commonly placed	6–10 hr
	Lead extraction (especially using laser)	General endotracheal anesthesia	3–4 hr
	Ventricular tachycardia or ventricular fibrillation radiofrequency ablation using an epicardial approach	General endotracheal anesthesia	6–10 hr

ICD, Implantable cardioverter-defibrillator; *MAC,* monitored anesthesia care; *NIPS,* noninvasive programmed stimulations; *TEE,* transesophageal echocardiography; *TIVA,* total intravenous anesthesia.
From Tanner JW, et al. Anesthesia for electrophysiology procedures. In: Weiss M, Fleisher LA, eds. *Non-Operating Room Anesthesia.* Philadelphia: Elsevier; 2015:92; Fritz MA, Speroff L. *Clinical Gynecologic Endocrinology and Infertility.* 8th ed. Baltimore: Lippincott Williams & Wilkins; 2011:1331–1382; Tsen LC. Anesthesia for assisted reproductive technologies. *Int Anesthesiol Clin.* 2007;45:99–113.

BOX 58.6 PCI Complications That May Affect the Delivered Anesthetic and Require Anesthetist Intervention

- Supraventricular dysrhythmias
- Ventricular dysrhythmias
- Severe and rapid hemorrhage
- Pain
- Anaphylaxis related to administration of intravenous contrast media
- Vasovagal response
- Cardiac arrest
- Thromboembolic events
- Hypotension/hypertension
- Respiratory instability

PCI, Percutaneous coronary intervention.
Adapted from Buja LM, Schoen FJ. The pathology of cardiovascular interventions and devices for coronary artery disease, vascular disease, heart failure, and arrhythmias. In: Butany J, Buja ML. *Cardiovascular Pathology.* 4th ed. London: Elsevier; 2016:577–610.

BOX 58.7 Indications for Colonoscopy, Esophagogastroduodenoscopy, and Endoscopic Retrograde Cholangiopancreatography, With Anesthetic Implications

Colonoscopy
- Routine screening
- Gastrointestinal bleeding and occult bleeding
- Evaluation of an abnormality on barium enema
- Polypectomy
- Unexplained iron deficiency anemia
- Significant diarrhea
- Chronic inflammatory bowel disease
- Malignancy
- Dilation of stenotic lesions
- Foreign body removal

Esophagogastroduodenoscopy
- Persistent and recurrent dyspepsia (heartburn)
- Persistent nausea or vomiting
- Dysphagia (difficulty swallowing)
- Chest pain with a negative cardiac evaluation
- Iron-deficiency anemia
- Suspected small bowel malabsorption
- Malignancy
- Stomach or esophageal ulcer
- Control of bleeding
- Ligation or sclerosis of varices
- Dilation of strictures
- Percutaneous gastrostomy
- Polypectomy
- Removal of foreign body

Endoscopic Retrograde Cholangiopancreatography (ERCP)
- Suspected biliary ductal disorder
- Suspected pancreatic ductal disorder
- Biliary drainage
- Pancreatic drainage
- Biopsy
- Bile or pancreatic juice collection
- Mapping of the pancreatic duct before intended surgery
- Manometry of the sphincter of Oddi or other ductal mapping

Data from Rubin PH, et al. Colonoscopy and flexible sigmoidoscopy. In: Podolsky DK, et al. *Yamada's Textbook of Gastroenterology.* 8th ed. Wiley Blackwell; 2015; Arain MA, Freeman ML. Endoscopic retrograde cholangiopancreatography. In: *Yamada's Textbook of Gastroenterology.* 8th ed. Hoboken, NJ: Wiley Blackwell; 2015; James TW, Baron TH. Endoscopic and radiologic treatment of biliary disease. In: Feldman M, et al, eds. *Sleisenger and Fordtran's Gastrointestinal and Liver Disease.* 11th ed. Philadelphia: Elsevier; 2021:1113–1128.

Gastroenterology Procedures

Colonoscopy, Esophagogastroduodenoscopy, and Endoscopic Retrograde Cholangiopancreatography

Procedure overview. Endoscopy came into popular use in the early 1960s with the invention of a snare for retrieving intestinal polyps for biopsy. Endoscopy for gastrointestinal procedures is the use of a flexible fiberoptic endoscope that transmits brilliant, coherent, high-resolution, magnified, direct visual images to the operator. The operator may then examine, biopsy, dilate, or cauterize portions of the gastrointestinal tract. The endoscopist may pass accessory devices down the endoscope such as biopsy forceps, dilation devices, cytology brushes, measuring devices, needles for injection, Doppler probes, ultrasound probes, and probes to measure electrical activity and pH. Even foreign bodies may be removed with the aid of a snare passed through an endoscope. Endoscopes are available in different diameters for use in pediatric to adult patients.[43]

An upper endoscopy, such as an esophagogastroduodenoscopy (EGD), is an accurate way for the operator to evaluate the mucosa of the esophagus, stomach, and duodenum. A colonoscopy allows total diagnostic visualization of the mucosa of the tortuous colon from the anus to the cecum. Endoscopic retrograde cholangiopancreatography (ERCP) is used for the diagnosis of obstructive, neoplastic, or inflammatory pancreatobiliary structures. The use of ERCP is decreasing because of the availability of less-invasive and noninvasive techniques. Box 58.7 provides a brief list of indications for colonoscopy, EGD, and ERCP.[43] Use of endoscopic ultrasound (EUS) has been growing since its inception in the 1980s and continues to broaden possibilities for the patient and practitioner. Once used solely for diagnostic and cancer staging purposes of the pancreas, periluminal structures, and biliary tract, it is now being used for therapeutic modalities such as cyst drainage, celiac plexus neurolysis for pain, and fine-needle injection of therapeutic medication.[44,45]

Endoscopy for gastrointestinal procedures may be performed by a gastroenterologist, general surgeon, family practitioner, or proctologist. The endoscope is passed into the gastrointestinal tract with the aid of lubricant. The endoscope has controls to change the direction of the flexible tip, allow flushing with water, application of suction, or insufflation of air or carbon dioxide within the portion of the gastrointestinal tract being observed.[43]

Anesthetic considerations. Endoscopic procedures often cause discomfort and require the patient to remain relatively motionless during the procedure. Consequently, anesthesia services have been utilized with more frequency to enhance the patient experience and improve patient outcomes. A proper preanesthetic assessment of the patient must be performed, focusing on the areas of age, ability to cooperate, level of anxiety, mental disability, allergies, fluid status, laboratory electrolyte values, cardiac history, hypertension, bleeding history, clotting status, respiratory status, obesity, drug and alcohol abuse, gastroesophageal reflux, esophageal abnormalities, and pregnancy.[9,17]

Endoscopy has been safely performed in pregnant patients; however, elective procedures should be reconsidered and performed only after consultation with the patient's obstetrician. Urgent endoscopic procedures must be performed. None of the common sedative drugs such as propofol or the opioid fentanyl have been demonstrated to cause teratogenic changes in the fetus. Midazolam has also been shown to cross the placenta and cause neonatal central nervous system (CNS) depression.[46] Studies of the obstetric effect of anesthetic drugs are limited because of the infrequent requirements for surgery during pregnancy and the ethical difficulties associated with performing controlled trials.

Patients must adhere to proper NPO guidelines, and these procedures have a greater risk of aspiration because of the pathology of the gastrointestinal tract and the introduction of the invasive endoscopy. Preemptive analgesia with gargled viscous lidocaine may help reduce the patient's gag reflex making an endoscopy of the upper gastrointestinal tract more feasible. Moderate sedation/analgesia is usually accomplished with short-acting sedatives such as midazolam or propofol and analgesics such as remifentanil, alfentanil, or fentanyl. Deep sedation can be achieved with titration of propofol until effective, along with an analgesic medication.[47-50] Upper endoscopy may necessitate the use of an antisialagogue such as glycopyrrolate.[48,49]

Colonoscopy requires thorough cleansing of the lumen of the colon to remove fecal material. The colon may be partly prepared with a cleansing enema. Full preparation of the colon is accomplished commonly with orally administered balanced electrolyte solutions. Other types of bowel preparations are also available.[43] Patients often find this preparation the most distressing portion of the procedure. The bowel preparation can lead to abdominal cramping, diarrhea, weakness, and nausea. Patients who arrive for the procedure require reassessment and the insertion of an IV catheter with IV fluid, usually lactated Ringer solution or normal saline.

Conventional monitors, including pulse oximeter, noninvasive blood pressure monitor, and ECG, are attached. The patient is supplied with oxygen through a disposable nasal cannula or disposable facemask. Ideally with ETco₂ monitoring as discussed previously. Patients are usually asked to assume a left lateral decubitus position and will typically remain on the transport stretcher for the procedure duration. It is optimal for the body to be flexed, the head and back bent downward toward the knees, and for the patient's legs to be bent toward the abdomen to optimize visualization of the gastrointestinal tract. Patient anxiety, distention related to insufflation, and acute discomfort during the maneuvering of the endoscope usually necessitate the administration of deep sedation or a general anesthetic in some cases. Strong vagal nerve stimulation can occur as a result of distention of the colon. This may cause hypotension, bradydysrhythmias, and ECG changes.[43,51,52]

EGD and EUS require a patient assessment with special emphasis on any cardiac history, hypertension, bleeding disorders, nausea, dysphagia, and gastroesophageal reflux. The patient must be NPO according to guidelines. Occasionally patients require moderate sedation or deep sedation as topical anesthesia and even hypnotic sedation may be less effective.[47-50] An IV catheter is inserted, with fluids such as lactated Ringer or normal saline attached. The patient is connected to standard monitors. Oxygen can be supplied through a disposable nasal cannula or a disposable facemask, preferably with ETco₂ monitoring. EGD is generally performed with the patient positioned supine or in a left lateral decubitus position. After the patient is adequately sedated, the operator inserts a hollow oral airway gently into the patient's mouth, and the endoscope is advanced through this airway, allowing direct visualization of the larynx, hypopharynx, esophagus, and stomach, and through the pylorus into the duodenal bulb.[43,50]

ERCP requires thorough assessment of the patient, including a review of laboratory values of a complete blood count, serum liver chemistries, and amylase or lipase levels to evaluate liver function, and clotting studies. Patients also must be evaluated for anticoagulant medications, bleeding history, and prosthetic heart valves.[43,53] Allergies must be evaluated, especially those to iodinated contrast media.[54] Patients who require ERCP are usually more ill than patients seen routinely for colonoscopy or EGD. The patient must be NPO according to AANA and ASA guidelines. IV access is obtained, and fluid is administered. Standard monitors are applied, and oxygen is supplied to the patient via a disposable facemask or nasal cannula, or as appropriate for anesthesia plan. The procedure requires that the patient be in a prone, semiprone, or slightly left lateral decubitus position. Often the extreme lateral patient position compromises airway access and prohibits airway rescue should the patient require ventilatory assistance. An appropriate anesthetic plan should be discussed prior to positioning the patient to determine if general anesthesia with a protected airway is required; otherwise, deep sedation will be necessary to facilitate the procedure.[53-56]

Pediatric endoscopy has been performed with patients under deep IV sedation with agents such as propofol, midazolam, and alfentanil (when the patient will allow placement of the IV catheter) and under general endotracheal anesthesia.[49] Propofol provides anterograde amnesia during the procedure but little retrograde amnesia.[48,49] The use of a eutectic mixture of local anesthetics lidocaine and prilocaine (EMLA cream) facilitates the placement of the IV catheter. EMLA must be applied to undamaged skin under an occlusive dressing for a period of 45 to 60 minutes before the IV catheter is inserted. When general anesthesia is administered, a secured ETT should be considered because of relative inaccessibility to the airway, the patient position required for pediatric colonoscopy or for EGD, and because of the shared airway with the proceduralist.[49]

These procedures can cause vomiting, aspiration, laryngospasm, bleeding, severe bradycardia, hypotension, bowel rupture, or duct rupture. The anesthetist must be ready with immediate airway intervention, hemodynamic support as necessary, and monitored emergency transport to the operating room for surgical intervention if necessary.[43]

Postanesthesia care. Postprocedure morbidity differs with each of the described procedures. All patients must be monitored in a postanesthesia care area until they have recovered from the sedation or general anesthetic and meet discharge criteria. Colonoscopy patients have intestinal distention, which is relieved with encouragement to pass flatus. Rectal bleeding, nausea, hypotension, dehydration, and vomiting may also be seen. Administration of a bolus of IV fluids along with an IV antiemetic agent may help alleviate some of the symptoms. EGD morbidity relates to bleeding, nausea, vomiting, aspiration, dysphagia, and hypotension. Treatments such as those used for colonoscopy may be indicated.[57,58]

ERCP morbidity relates to possible reactions to iodinated contrast media. Patient reactions can be mild (such as nausea, vomiting, pruritus, diaphoresis, flushing, or mild urticaria), moderate (such as faintness, severe vomiting, profound urticaria, mild bronchospasm, mild hypotension, mild tachycardia, or bradycardia), or severe (hypotensive shock, angioedema, respiratory arrest, cardiac arrest, convulsions, or death).[57] Postprocedure bleeding, pain, nausea, and vomiting (PONV) are possible and can be treated as described previously.

Gynecology Procedures
Assisted Reproductive Technologies
Procedure overview. Assisted reproductive technologies (ARTs) refer to all techniques used to retrieve and fertilize the human oocyte. In vitro fertilization (IVF) is the most common technique used to artificially fertilize the human oocyte. Research by reproductive endocrinologists has advanced technology since the first "test-tube

baby" was born in 1978 and continues to result in new and more effective techniques. Based on the CDC 2018 Fertility Clinic Success Rates Report, there were 306,197 ART cycles performed during 2018 resulting in 81,478 live born infants. Approximately 1.9% of all infants born in the United States every year are conceived using ART.[59-61]

IVF encompasses a series of procedures that involve ultrasound-guided oocyte retrieval, fertilization of the egg in a laboratory, and subsequent transfer of the embryo back into the uterus through the cervix. The oocyte is retrieved transvaginally, transabdominally, or via laparoscopy with an ultrasonically guided probe. Typically, repeated attempts are necessary for a successful procedure. Although IVF is a relatively simple procedure for the reproductive endocrinologist to perform, especially outside the operating room, IVF is an uncomfortable procedure and requires that patients do not move while the probe is guided for retrieval and later reimplantation. The vaginal wall must be pierced for the desired ovary to be accessed. In addition, major blood vessels are present in the proximity of the ovaries, and their injury could lead to complications.[62] Thus it is important to maintain a comfortable setting and minimize a patient's pain and anxiety while undergoing oocyte retrieval.

Anesthetic considerations. Oocyte retrieval for IVF is usually performed transvaginally under ultrasound guidance, which is a relatively brief (20- to 30-minute) outpatient procedure. It necessitates a short-acting anesthetic approach with minimal side effects. The various anesthetic modalities used for transvaginal oocyte retrieval include MAC, conscious sedation, general anesthesia, regional anesthesia, local injection as a paracervical block, epidural block, subarachnoid block, TIVA, patient-controlled analgesia (PCA).[60]

Anesthetic agents have been found in the follicular fluid, and these drugs may have adverse effects on oocyte fertilization and embryonic development. Most of the anesthetic agents being used in general anesthesia have been identified in the follicular fluid; however, the uterus becomes more relaxed under general anesthesia making it is easier for the clinician to aspirate a large number of ovarian follicles, unlike sedation where a contracted myometrium may interfere with oocyte retrieval. The duration of general anesthesia should be kept minimum to avoid detrimental effects of these drugs on oocytes.[59]

MAC is relatively easy to deliver; drugs are well tolerated and best suited in outpatient settings, and it avoids the potentially harmful effects of general anesthetic drugs on oocytes. Different methods of conscious sedation and analgesia have been used for oocyte recovery for IVF techniques. Drugs used for these procedures are selected by the quality of sedation and analgesia and their deleterious effects on reproductive outcomes. The optimal method should be individualized based on the preferences of both the women and the clinicians and resource availability; however, moderated sedation is usually sufficient for most women.[59]

Techniques with quick onset and a short duration are preferred. Propofol is being used extensively in IVF with added advantages of the antiemetic property along with faster recovery. No data from human trials have ever condemned the use of local anesthetic agents for oocyte retrieval. Morphine has been shown to adversely affect fertilization of sea urchin eggs in vitro by allowing more than one sperm to enter the oocyte in 30% of cases; therefore it is not used because of the existence of safe alternatives such as fentanyl, alfentanil, and remifentanil. Midazolam, when titrated in small doses to provide mild to moderate sedation and anxiolysis, is safe, with no accumulation in follicular fluid or indication of being a teratogen. Ketamine (0.75 mg/kg) with midazolam (0.06 mg/kg) used as moderate sedation/analgesia is safe as an alternative to general anesthesia with isoflurane. Sevoflurane and desflurane are avoided because of possible negative effects to ART outcomes.[63] NSAIDs may be avoided because of inhibition

---

BOX 58.8 Anesthetic Agents That May Cause Problems With Assisted Reproductive Technologies

- Morphine
- Sevoflurane
- Desflurane
- Nonsteroidal antiinflammatory drugs—ibuprofen, indomethacin, ketoprofen, ketorolac, meloxicam, naproxen, oxaprozin
- Metoclopramide
- Postanesthesia care: As in all cases of anesthetic administration, the patient is assessed in a postanesthetic recovery area. Vital signs and pulse oximetry are assessed and must be stable. If intrathecal anesthesia was used, the patient must have a recovery of sensorium, be able to ambulate, and be able to void. All patients must be free of nausea.

---

of prostaglandin synthesis and possible effects on embryo implantation.[62,63] Metoclopramide is known to induce rapid hyperprolactinemia and should also be avoided. Box 58.8 lists common anesthetic agents that could cause problems with ART.[62,63]

Hysteroscopy

Procedure overview. Currently, hysteroscopy can be considered the gold standard for examination of the uterine cavity thus bypassing the significant limitations of dilatation and curettage (D&C). Modern hysteroscopy allows for the diagnosis and treatment of uterine pathology. Traditionally, hysteroscopy was performed in a conventional OR under general anesthesia as an inpatient procedure. In the early 1990s, the use of low-viscosity fluid and technologic advances permitted the reduction of the hysteroscope diameter making hysteroscopy less painful and invasive, thus allowing it to be performed in an ambulatory setting. Consequently, the number of ambulatory outpatient hysteroscopy procedures has increased.[64]

In outpatient hysteroscopy, saline solution and CO_2 are the most common media for intracavity distention. Although CO_2 is generally well tolerated, uterine distension with saline solution is preferable. Distension with fluid is a cost-effective approach associated with less patient discomfort and clearer hysteroscopic vision in the occurrence of intrauterine bleeding. For the vaginoscopic approach, liquid distension with a watery medium is required. This medium can be administered at atmospheric pressure, by means of a pressure cuff or employing an automated microprocessor with flow and pressure control. The newest generation of fluid pumps has contributed to the improvement of patient comfort by measuring and controlling the intrauterine pressure. In the vaginoscopic approach, passage through the internal cervical os and the intrauterine pressure created by the distention medium (and in case of CO_2, the irritation of the peritoneum when gas is passing the fallopian tubes) can provoke pain. Compared to traditional methods such as D&C, hysteroscopy offers multiple advantages. It allows for visualization of focal abnormalities suggestive of endometrial hyperplasia inside the uterine cavity and the ability to perform targeted hysteroscopic biopsy withdrawal under visualization in the presence of infertility and intrauterine abnormalities. Possible risks with hysteroscopy include pain, nausea, bleeding, infection, and (rarely) uterine perforation.[64]

Anesthetic considerations. Cervical dilatation generally requires administration of local cervical anesthesia. Standard protocols regarding the type, maximum dosage, and route of administration of anesthesia should be developed and implemented to help both recognize and prevent rare but potentially serious adverse effects resulting from systemic vascular absorption. Instillation of local anesthetic into the cervical canal does not reduce pain during diagnostic outpatient hysteroscopy but may reduce the incidence of vasovagal reactions. Paracervical local anesthetic blocks are often combined with IV sedation techniques, and in some instances a general anesthetic may be required to control pain, alleviate anxiety, and maintain immobility during the procedure. A combination of preoperative anxiolytics and a low-dose oral narcotic may improve patient comfort and reduce anxiety. Pretreatment with NSAIDs is recommended to reduce pain in the immediate postoperative period. Postprocedure monitoring of the patient for a minimum of 30 to 60 minutes to assess for bleeding is recommended.[64]

Office-Based Surgery

General Dental Procedures

Procedure overview. Anesthesia for dental procedures and dental surgery can present many challenges. The demand for dental care and visits from patients are increasing. Dentistry has changed from a role of therapeutic treatment of dental disease to a role of prevention. Historically, only 50% of the population ever visited a dentist, and typically that intervention was for treatment of extreme pain or an emergency. The most recent demographic statistics show that this percentage has improved. More women see dentists annually than men, and, as employment status, income, and educational levels increase, so do the number of annual visits to the dentist. Children ages 6 or younger and adults ages 65 or older are seeing dentists more frequently than in the past.[65-67] These numbers are expected to increase as the US government's *Healthy People Initiative* has added oral health to the objectives for the current and coming years.[66]

Dental procedures may be performed in an OR, a specially equipped hospital suite, an ambulatory surgical center, or a dental office operatory (dental surgical area).[68] Anesthesia may be required for dental procedures in the following areas of dentistry[69]:

- *Pediatric dentistry*—an age-defined specialty that provides primary and comprehensive preventive and therapeutic oral health care for infants and children through adolescence, including those with special health care needs.
- *Oral and maxillofacial surgery (OMS)*—the specialty that includes the diagnosis, surgical, and adjunctive treatment of diseases, injuries, and defects involving both the functional and esthetic aspects of the hard and soft tissues of the oral and maxillofacial region.
- *Periodontics*—the specialty that encompasses the prevention, diagnosis, and treatment of diseases of the supporting and surrounding tissues of the teeth, or their substitutes, and the maintenance of the health, function, and esthetics of these structures and tissues.
- *Endodontics*—the specialty that is concerned with the etiology, diagnosis, prevention, and treatment of diseases and injuries of the pulp and associated periradicular (concerning the root of the tooth) conditions.
- *Prosthodontics*—the dental specialty involved with the diagnosis, treatment planning, rehabilitation, and maintenance of oral functions, comfort, appearance, and patient health associated with clinical conditions of missing or deficient teeth, and/or oral and maxillofacial tissues along with biocompatible substitutes.
- *General dentistry*—encompasses the etiology, diagnosis, and treatment of conditions of oral, head, and neck tissues; the general dentist may perform procedures that encompass any or all of the dental specialty areas; this depends on the training, abilities, and experiences of the general dentist.
- *Dental hygienist*—a licensed oral health professional trained to treat patients by the removal of dental plaque and calculus (tartar) above or below the gingiva.[68,69]

> ### BOX 58.9   Considerations Related to Anesthesia in the Dental Setting
>
> - Anesthesia may be administered in an unfamiliar area. Carefully plan, equip, and set up the operatory so that it is as familiar and comfortable as in an operating room.
> - The established airway will be shared with the dental surgeon.
> - The potential exists for heavy bleeding because of the vast blood supply to the head and neck region.
> - There could be the use of small instruments, burs (dental drill bits), files, implants, and filling materials in the mouth, with the potential of falling into the oropharynx, or being aspirated.
> - Patients may be receiving dental prosthetic devices such as crowns, bridges, or full or partial dentures, which can also affect the airway.
> - There exists the possibility of intense pain, transmitted primarily by the maxillary and mandibular divisions of the trigeminal nerve.
> - Patients usually display a high level of anxiety, and adequate time must be incorporated into the schedule to allow for safe anesthetic treatment.

Anesthetic considerations. Important considerations that must be part of the anesthesia treatment plan for the dental setting are outlined in Box 58.9. The patient may require minimal sedation, moderate sedation/analgesia, deep sedation/analgesia, or general anesthesia for dental surgery. The anesthesia required depends on the patient-related factors of fear, anxiety, age, medical condition, level of cooperation and behavior, gagging, ineffective local anesthesia in the past, mental impairment, and physical disability. A thorough, documented patient assessment along with appropriate laboratory studies and possible physician consultation regarding patient clearance for physically and/or psychologically stressful dental surgery are necessary.[70,71] In pediatric dentistry, a comprehensive and personalized discussion with the parent or guardian (with or without the patient present) of what the anesthetic procedure will entail, coupled with an opportunity for the parent or patient to engage in dialogue and ask questions, can alleviate the stress of the upcoming procedures for all parties.[70]

The dental operatory must be of adequate size for both access and egress of the patient and personnel. Proper considerations and advanced planning must be made to accommodate patients according to the Americans with Disabilities Act.[72,73] The anesthetist must have full and rapid access to both the patient and all required equipment and supplies. Full monitors are necessary. Consider the use of the anti-sialagogue glycopyrrolate, as dental surgery can stimulate the flow of saliva. Excess salivation can lead to coughing, choking, laryngospasm, or aspiration in the sedated patient. Delivery of anesthesia in the dental operatory should be as familiar as if it were in an OR. Postoperative problems in dentistry are generally minimal but can involve pain, swelling, bleeding, nausea, vomiting, the vasovagal response, airway problems, hypoxemia, or hypothermia as a result of anesthetic procedures other than local anesthesia administered. Hypothermia can be addressed by the use of an electric blanket; forced-air warming may or may not be feasible for the dental operatory.

General dentists and board-certified dental specialists are also trained to administer intraoral local anesthesia, which is a cardiac depressant and may cause either CNS depression or excitation. Local anesthesia for dentistry is commonly administered in conjunction with a vasoconstrictor to minimize bleeding. Dental specialists and specially trained general dentists can be licensed by state dental boards to administer the continuum of anesthesia, from minimal sedation to general anesthesia, while performing the dental surgery.[74-76] Each dental specialty has particular anesthetic considerations, which are discussed in the following sections.

Pediatric dentistry. Pediatric dental patients can require the continuum of anesthesia from enteral minimal sedation to parenteral moderate sedation/analgesia, deep sedation/analgesia, or general anesthesia if the patient is behaviorally uncooperative, immature, frightened, mentally disabled, or because of the necessity to perform all necessary dental surgery in one session. Pediatric dentists may have a patient immobilization device available, commonly called a papoose board, to safely restrain the patient until anxiolytic anesthesia can be administered. Anesthetic choices such as oral or IV ketamine; a mixture of oral chloral hydrate, narcotics, and midazolam; and propofol have been used with success. Premedication with orally administered midazolam dissolved in a small amount of the liquid forms of acetaminophen, ibuprofen, aspirin, or low-sugar clear juice is commonly used. For the liquid forms of acetaminophen, ibuprofen, or aspirin, the anesthesia provider should refer to the package insert for the proper dosing based on the patient's weight. Intranasal or rectal midazolam can be used alone or given before general endotracheal anesthesia and has proved as effective as nitrous oxide for sedation.[74,76,77] After an inhaled mask or IV induction, endotracheal intubation via either the oral or nasal route can be performed to allow the pediatric dentist full access to the mouth. Pediatric dentists typically are, and should be, very cognizant of the importance of sharing the airway during surgery. Typical pediatric dental procedures include restorative dentistry, such as fillings of amalgam or composite, and placement of stainless-steel crowns for posterior teeth, polycarbonate crowns, composite crowns, or stainless-steel crowns with porcelain for anterior teeth, pulpotomies, tooth extractions, and space maintainers. Successful treatments can be provided along with stress reduction for the patient, parents or guardians, and health care providers, with appropriate airway maintenance under deep sedation or general anesthesia.[74-77]

Oral and maxillofacial surgery. Procedures performed within the specialty of OMS are among the most invasive in dentistry. Oral surgeons perform uncovering of teeth for orthodontic treatment; extraction of impacted, severely carious, and multiple teeth; insertion of dental implants; treatment of infections of the head and neck; surgical remodeling of maxillary and mandibular alveolar bone; facial cosmetics; and removal of soft tissue or bony tumors, in addition to many other procedures. These procedures can produce both severe pain and heavy bleeding. Many OMS procedures are performed within the office setting. Oral and maxillofacial surgeons receive 6 years of postdoctoral training and become licensed by the state dental board to perform the continuum from minimal sedation to anesthesia (general anesthesia) care. Patients can have challenging physical and mental conditions, therefore a thorough preanesthetic assessment is necessary.[78] The patient's airway is shared with the oral surgeon, therefore nasal intubation may be necessary. It may be possible to perform some oral surgical procedures while carefully working around an unsecured tube or with a standard or reinforced LMA. Local anesthesia in combination with IV sedation (propofol, midazolam), inhalation sedation (nitrous oxide), inhaled potent endotracheal anesthetics, and total IV general anesthesia are techniques available for office-based OMS.[70,78] Remifentanil has become a useful adjunct with the techniques listed to counteract the intense stimulation of OMS.[79] An anesthesia awareness/level of consciousness/depth of sedation monitor is also useful for careful anesthetic titration.[77]

Periodontics. Periodontal procedures can involve painful stimulation. Periodontists generally work in a particular quadrant of the patient's mouth and administer local anesthetic for the particular area of surgery. Periodontal treatment involves surgery of the teeth, gingiva,

connective tissue, periodontal ligament, and alveolar bone, in addition to insertion and maintenance of dental implants. Local anesthetics are administered in conjunction with epinephrine concentrations that may be greater than normal concentrations to ensure hemostasis. Periodontal surgery can involve lengthy procedures with moderate amounts of hemorrhage and can be well managed with minimal sedation (both enteral or with inhalation sedation) or moderate sedation/analgesia.[70,78] As with all procedures requiring MAC, use of standard monitoring is necessary. Midazolam with a propofol infusion helps achieve the goals of safety and comfort for periodontal surgical patients.[70]

Endodontics. Anesthesia for endodontic procedures is similar to that described for periodontal surgery. Local anesthesia provides adequate comfort, but in the presence of patient anxiety related to the length of endodontic procedures, minimal sedation (both enteral or with inhalation sedation) or moderate sedation/analgesia can make the procedure tolerable and less anxiety producing for the patient. A dental dam is usually applied around the tooth and held in place with a special clamp to prevent aspiration of dental burs and endodontic files.

General dentistry and prosthodontics. General dentistry can encompass all procedures from all of the dental specialties, depending on the interest and training of the general dentist. Anesthesia can be delivered along the continuum of care to ensure safety for the patient and to fill the requirements of the particular dental procedure.[67,70,71]

Dental hygiene. Dental hygienists are also involved with providing dental care to patients who may require anesthesia along the continuum from minimal sedation/analgesia to deep sedation/analgesia with combinations of inhalation nitrous oxide/oxygen, local anesthesia, and IV medications. Thorough treatment can generate tooth or gingival sensitivity and pain. Even in the absence of pain, special populations such as pediatrics, the mentally handicapped, and those with severe anxiety disorders may require some degree of anesthesia for even routine dental care. Procedures range from routine hygiene to deep scaling and root planing of teeth with heavy dental accretions.

Postanesthesia care. Patients should be allowed to recover in a quiet, monitored environment. IV access allows the titration of additional analgesia or antiemetics as necessary. Fortunately, patient morbidity from general anesthesia for dental procedures is low.[80] Patients who receive inhaled sedation are less stressed postoperatively than those who receive general anesthesia, but TIVA procedures with proper airway maintenance and supplemental oxygen have also demonstrated significant success with good patient outcomes.[69,71,80]

Invasive dental procedures can be a source of distress in children, which can lead to crying, nausea, vomiting (PONV), and bleeding postoperatively. The addition of a potent long-acting opioid, ketorolac, or both greatly aids patient comfort in the postsurgical anesthesia recovery area. The use of oral minimal to moderate sedation in pediatric patients ages 2 to 34 months has been found to have no effect on behavior when the individual requires treatment later.[69,76]

Psychiatric Procedures

Electroconvulsive Therapy

Electroconvulsive therapy (ECT) is the intentional inducement of a generalized seizure of the CNS for an adequate duration of time to treat patients with certain severe neuropsychiatric disorders.[81-84] The American Psychiatric Association continues to support ECT as a safe and evidence-based medical treatment when administered by trained, qualified personnel.[81-83] ECT in general, however, continues to be a topic of controversy. Research studies differ in the effectiveness of ECT. Most studies agree that the short-term effects of ECT are substantial; however, they argue about the long-term benefits, with current research supporting the effectiveness of maintenance ECT.[85,86]

BOX 58.10   Possible Physiologic Effects of Electroconvulsive Therapy

Cardiovascular

Parasympathetic Response During Tonic Phase of Seizure
- Bradycardia
- Hypotension
- Bradydysrhythmias

Sympathetic Response During Clonic Phase of Seizure
- Tachycardia
- Hypertension
- Tachydysrhythmias

Cerebral
- Increased cerebral blood flow (increases of 100%–400% above baseline are possible)
- Increased intracranial pressure

Other
- Increased intraocular pressure
- Increased intragastric pressure
- Hypoventilation

Adapted from Reti IM, et al. Safety considerations for outpatient electroconvulsive therapy. *J Psychiatr Pract.* 2012;18(2):130–136; Matsumoto N. Circulatory management, especially blood pressure and heart rate. In: *Anesthesia Management for Electroconvulsive Therapy.* Japan: Springer; 2016:79–99.

TABLE 58.4   Anesthetic Medications Used for Electroconvulsive Therapy

Drug	Dose
Anticholinergics	
Atropine	0.4–1 mg IV or IM
Glycopyrrolate	0.005 mg/kg IV or IM
Anesthetics	
Etomidate	0.15–0.3 mg/kg IV
Ketamine	0.5–1 mg/kg IV
Methohexital	0.5–1 mg/kg IV
Propofol	0.75–1.5 mg/kg IV
Muscle Relaxants	
Depolarizing	
Succinylcholine	0.5–1 mg/kg IV (onset 30–60 sec)
Nondepolarizing	
Cisatracurium	0.15–0.25 mg/kg IV (onset 1–2 min)
Rocuronium	0.3–0.9 mg/kg IV (onset 1–2 min)

IM, Intramuscular; *IV,* intravenous.
Modified from Kadoi Y. Selection of anesthetics and muscle relaxants for electroconvulsive therapy. In: Saito S. *Anesthesia Management for Electroconvulsive Therapy.* Japan: Springer; 2016:49–66; Mirzakhani H, Kopman AF, Naguib M. Neuromuscular blockers and electroconvulsive therapy: how much is enough? *Anesth Analg.* 2016;123(4):1059–1060.

Antidepressant medication administration, along with ECT, is well tolerated by patients, and both therapies can be beneficial. ECT may be performed as an inpatient or outpatient procedure. Acute patients receive three treatments per week and can undergo multiple treatment continuing on into maintenance ECT.[81-84] When clinical improvement is seen, it typically occurs within the first few treatments, and positive response to treatment is seen in 70% to 90% of patients, even those who had been treatment resistant.[85,86] ECT is also used in certain patients who experience mania, catatonia, vegetative dysregulation, inanition, suicidal drive, and schizophrenia with affective disorders, and it has begun to be used for patients with Parkinson disease.[81-86]

ECT is one of the most controversial and invasive treatments in medicine. The first documented use of ECT was in 1938.[81,82] Early ECT was performed without anesthesia, resulting in the occurrence of many adverse effects such as bitten tongues, broken bones, and broken teeth. Treatment involves placement of electrodes with a conducting gel, either right unilateral, bitemporal (bilateral), or bifrontal.[83] An alternating current of electricity is passed through the electrodes. Theories for the mechanism of ECT are related to profound changes in brain chemistry such as enhancement of dopaminergic, serotonergic, and adrenergic neurotransmission. Another theory postulates the release of hypothalamic or pituitary hormones, which have antidepressant effects. Finally, ECT produces anticonvulsant effects that raise the seizure threshold and decrease seizure duration exerting a positive effect on the brain.[81,82] Some physiologic effects of electroconvulsive therapy are given in Box 58.10.

Anesthetic considerations. Anesthesia for ECT involves the administration of an ultrabrief general anesthetic to provide lack of consciousness to the patient for the procedure (Table 58.4).

A thorough preanesthetic assessment must be performed, with consideration given to the possible critical physiologic hemodynamic responses generated by the induced seizure activity. Box 58.11 lists possible physiologic effects as a result of ECT.

BOX 58.11   Absolute and Relative Contraindications to Electroconvulsive Therapy (ECT)

Absolute Contraindications to ECT
- Pheochromocytoma
- Recent myocardial infarction (<4–6 wk ago)
- Recent cerebrovascular accident (≤3 mo ago)
- Recent intracranial surgery (≤3 mo ago)
- Intracranial mass lesion
- Unstable cervical spine

Relative Contraindications to ECT
- Angina
- Congestive heart failure
- Cardiac rhythm management device (pacemaker, automatic internal cardiac defibrillator)
- Severe pulmonary disease
- Major bone fracture
- Glaucoma
- Retinal detachment
- Thrombophlebitis
- Pregnancy

Modified from Reti IM, et al. Safety considerations for outpatient electroconvulsive therapy. *J Psychiatr Pract.* 2012;18(2):130–136; Yamahuchi S, Takasusuki T. Pre-procedural assessments and consideration. In: *Anesthesia Management for Electroconvulsive Therapy.* Japan: Springer; 2016:1–16.

Few absolute and relative contraindications to ECT exist (see Box 58.11).[81,82,87,88] Patients may have results of laboratory studies, a pharmacologic regimen, and ECG readily available because of their psychiatric hospitalization. Informed consent is obtained whenever possible from the patient or legal guardian. An IV catheter is inserted in a peripheral vein. Patients undergoing chronic ECT may have a long-term subcutaneous injection port placed, which may be used for IV access. The patient is monitored with a pulse oximeter, ECG, noninvasive blood pressure monitor, temperature-monitoring device, and peripheral nerve stimulator. Use of $ETco_2$ monitoring has been suggested because hypercarbia and hypoxia shorten seizure duration. Suction, oxygen, a positive pressure Ambu bag and facemask, and rubber bite protectors must be present in addition to necessary airway and cardiovascular resuscitation equipment, medications, and supplies. ECT is usually performed in a dedicated psychiatric suite or special treatment room.[87]

The patient is preoxygenated before induction. Anticholinergics may be administered as an antisialagogue or to prevent asystole.[89,90] The induction agent is administered intravenously. Methohexital, propofol, or etomidate may be used without compromise of the therapy.[87,89-93] Ketamine is used, although an enhanced hemodynamic response and increased intracranial pressure are possible after using ketamine. After loss of consciousness, positive pressure ventilation is applied to the patient via the breathing bag and a facemask and is continued until after treatment is completed and spontaneous respirations resume. To assess the duration of the induced convulsion the psychiatrist usually applies a tourniquet, or manual blood pressure cuff inflated to slightly greater than the systolic blood pressure, above a lower extremity so that the muscle relaxant cannot reach the skeletal muscle in the extremity. A reusable rubber or disposable foam bite block is gently placed in the patient's mouth to prevent biting of the teeth, lips, and tongue, and a short-acting muscle relaxant is administered. Succinylcholine is typically the muscle relaxant of choice for ECT because of its rapid onset, short duration, and independent reversibility.[94-97] Succinylcholine IV injection after the induction of anesthesia attenuates the potentially dangerous skeletal muscle contractions produced with seizure activity. Nondepolarizing agents can be used; however, induction dosage is typically adjusted to create a shorter duration of neuromuscular blockade.[87,89,94] With the addition of sugammadex, a new reversal agent for steroidal nondepolarizing neuromuscular blocking agents, nondepolarizing agents may be used at higher than previous doses. A nerve stimulator must be used, and appropriate neuromuscular blockade reversal agents such as sugammadex should be administered as necessary. The electrodes are applied, the proper waveform and current level are selected, and the electroconvulsive seizure is induced. The seizure lasts from 30 to 90 seconds; the motor seizure is shorter than the seizure duration as seen on an EEG. Use of an anesthesia awareness/level of consciousness/depth of sedation monitor correlates with the EEG, and it can be a useful tool for the anesthetist and the psychiatrist. The level of sedation displayed by this monitor correlates with the proper point to induce seizure, the duration of seizure, and the potential for awareness during the ECT procedure.[88] At the end of the seizure spontaneous respirations resume, and the patient is transferred to a postanesthesia recovery area where vital signs are continually monitored until the patient is determined to be stable and able to be safely discharged.[81,87,88] Certain anesthetic medications and techniques such as hyperventilation can affect seizure duration (Box 58.12).

Adult patients about to undergo ECT should follow fasting guidelines of at least 6 hours for solids and 2 hours for liquids. Necessary bronchodilators may be taken. Oral medications, such as antihypertensives, cardiac medications, anticoagulants, and thyroid medications, may be taken with a sip of water up to 2 hours before the procedure.[87,88] Rapid sequence induction of general anesthesia with endotracheal intubation can be performed for patients at high risk for gastrointestinal reflux or hiatal hernia. One must take into consideration the total

---

BOX 58.12 Effects of Common Medications and Conditions on Seizure Duration

Medications That Can Prolong Seizure Duration
- Alfentanil with propofol
- Aminophylline
- Caffeine
- Clozapine
- Etomidate
- Ketamine (a proconvulsant)

Conditions That Can Prolong Seizure Duration
- Hyperventilation/hypocapnia

Medications That Can Shorten Seizure Duration
- Diltiazem
- Diazepam
- Fentanyl
- Lidocaine
- Lorazepam
- Midazolam
- Propofol
- Sevoflurane

Medications With No Apparent Effect on Seizure Duration
- Clonidine
- Dexmedetomidine
- Esmolol (may possibly shorten seizure duration)
- Labetalol (may possibly shorten seizure duration)
- Nicardipine
- Nifedipine
- Nitroglycerin
- Nitroprusside

Modified from Kadoi Y. Selection of anesthetics and muscle relaxants for electroconvulsive therapy. In: Saito S. *Anesthesia Management for Electroconvulsive Therapy.* Japan: Springer; 2016:49–66; McTague A, Cross JH. Treatment of epileptic encephalopathies. *CNS Drugs.* 2013;27:175–184.

---

number of ECT treatments to be received weighed against the necessity for repeated intubations and the fact that most patients, even obese patients, have rarely been found to aspirate as a result of ECT.[87]

Postanesthesia care. The intentional creation of CNS convulsions has profound effects on the patient's physiology. Patients usually experience multiple types of temporary cognitive and memory impairment after ECT. The first type of impairment that may be seen is postictal confusion, in which the patient is transiently restless, confused, and agitated immediately after the convulsive episode and for approximately 30 minutes following the treatment. The agitation can be difficult to manage for the recovery nurse and staff. Some patients require physical restraint or sedation with a benzodiazepine, antipsychotic medication, or propofol to treat postictal agitation.[95] One theory postulates that the postictal agitation or anxiety is a result of increased plasma lactate levels possibly caused by inadequate neuromuscular blockade, and that increasing the dose of muscle relaxant is necessary with the next treatment.[94] A second type of cognitive impairment that may be seen later is anterograde memory dysfunction, in which the patient may rapidly forget new information. The patient may not remember recent facts or information in the days after ECT. Anterograde amnesia usually subsides within a few days or weeks; however, it can be frightening to the patient. A third cognitive impairment is retrograde memory dysfunction, which is the loss of memories from several weeks to several months before the ECT treatment. No evidence suggests that ECT neither causes any brain damage nor impairs the long-term ability for the patient to learn and retain new information. The cognitive effects described vary depending on the frequency and the number of ECT treatments the patient has received. The quantities of energy used to elicit the convulsions and the placement of the electrodes are also considered factors for cognitive dysfunction, in addition to the type of anesthetic drugs used.[81,82]

Cardiovascular stimulation also occurs with ECT. The sympathetic and parasympathetic nervous systems are stimulated sequentially. Therefore the patient may experience an increase in heart rate and blood pressure followed by a period of bradycardia or even asystole. This can lead to increases in myocardial oxygen demand, arrhythmias, and transient ischemic changes in susceptible individuals. Transient cardiac changes can be managed before ECT with anticholinergics, IV local anesthetics such as lidocaine, or IV narcotics such as remifentanil.[81,82,87-99] Changes after ECT can be managed with β-blockers such as esmolol, labetalol, calcium channel blockers, or other antihypertensives.[97]

Finally, patients may also experience headache, muscle aches, or nausea as a result of ECT treatments. Symptoms of headache or muscle ache respond well to acetaminophen, aspirin, or NSAIDs such as IV or intramuscular ketorolac, or oral ibuprofen. Nausea can be caused by the stress and anxiety before the ECT treatment, the anesthetic agents used, the seizure itself, or air in the stomach from assisted ventilation. Nausea can be treated with agents such as ondansetron, dolasetron, granisetron, or metoclopramide.[86,87]

New Therapies for Major Depressive Disorders

Two new therapies for severe major depressive disorders are now available, which often require anesthetic treatment: repetitive transcranial magnetic stimulation (rTMS) and vagus nerve stimulation (VNS).[100,101] Neuroanatomic studies have suggested that patients with major depressive disorder (MDD) have dysfunction within the frontal cortical-subcortical-brainstem neural network, specifically the dorsolateral prefrontal cortices. ECT and antidepressant medications do not act in these discrete areas of the brain, but new therapies stimulating these focal areas of the brain are now approved and in use in the United States.

Repetitive transcranial magnetic stimulation and magnetic seizure therapy. rTMS uses electric current passing through an electromagnetic coil that has been placed on the scalp. The coil delivers brief, rapidly changing magnetic field pulses to specific areas of the brain. These bursts of pulses are called a train of stimuli. Multiple trains of rTMS may be delivered in one session. The scalp and skull are transparent to magnetic fields, an advantage over ECT, in which the scalp and skull are resistors to the electrical stimulation. To produce antidepressant effects, a convulsion must be initiated by trains of rTMS, because subconvulsive trains of rTMS are ineffective.[99,101,102]

Convulsive magnetic energy levels are determined by the use of motor threshold (MT). MT is the point at which a single pulse of magnetic energy begins to elicit an electromyographic response (i.e., twitch) usually of the abductor pollicis brevis muscle of the thumb or first dorsal interosseous muscle of the index finger.[99,101] Treatment with rTMS is safe and well tolerated, with reduced cognitive side effects when compared to ECT. Patients are found to recover much more rapidly from rTMS or magnetic seizure therapy (MST) compared to ECT.[101,103]

MST uses a higher intensity, more frequent, and longer duration magnetic seizure-inducing dose when compared with the magnetic dose required for rTMS. MST can stimulate tonic-clonic seizures in more localized and focal regions of the prefrontal cerebral cortex when compared with ECT and generalized tonic-clonic seizures that resemble ECT.[103-105] MST does not produce the rigid bilateral masseter muscle contractions noted during ECT but can produce elevations in blood pressure and heart rate similar to ECT.[101-103]

After rTMS some patients experience mild headache, disorientation and inattention (although patients become reoriented much more quickly than with ECT), retrograde amnesia, some anterograde amnesia, transient auditory threshold increases as a result of the high-frequency clicking sound heard during coil discharge (which can be alleviated with the use of foam earplugs), and (rarely) generalized seizure.[101,102] A single TMS treatment may be all that is necessary for treating certain severe MDD nonpsychotic patients along with their medications, although rTMS may be necessary.[99]

The anesthesia requirements for rTMS or MST range from none needed to ultrabrief general anesthesia as for ECT.[99,101-103] A patent and secure IV catheter is established, and full monitors are applied. Glycopyrrolate 0.004 mcg/kg is administered as an antisialagogue, along with ketorolac 0.4 mg/kg, 2 to 3 minutes prior to induction of ultrabrief general anesthesia. Methohexital 0.5 to 1 mg/kg may be used for induction in addition to propofol 1 to 2.5 mg/kg.[89] Succinylcholine 0.5 to 1 mg/kg can be used as the muscle relaxant after isolation of a lower extremity for observation of seizure duration.[89,94] The anesthetist must use the smallest amount of muscle relaxant necessary to enable recovery from paralysis prior to the return of consciousness. The anesthetist can then manually hyperventilate the patient's lungs with a facemask to an $ETco_2$ value of 30 to 34 torr. At this point, the magnetic stimulus may be applied.[101-103]

Vagus nerve stimulation. VNS requires surgical implantation of a programmable battery-powered electrical stimulator that connects with the patient's left vagus nerve (cranial nerve X). The stimulator is usually implanted in the patient's chest with minimal sedation, moderate sedation/analgesia, deep sedation/analgesia, or under general anesthesia. Because of the delicacy of the surgery and its proximity to vital structures, no extraneous patient movement is permitted. Although originally approved for treatment-resistant epilepsy, the VNS is now approved for major depressive episodes that have not responded to four antidepressant medication trials.[100,104,105]

Radiologic and Diagnostic Procedures

Medical science has been able to use the sciences of physics, chemistry, and computers to produce remarkably accurate images of the internal structure and function of the body to aid medical diagnosis. Energy is transmitted to the patient and interacts with patient tissues. This energy is then detected, processed, and displayed on a computer console, which allows images to be selected for further investigation and diagnosis. Some medical images are created in real time and allow observation of flow or changes in tissue resulting from treatment.

Procedure Overviews

Computed tomography. Computed tomography (CT) uses x-rays generated from a rotating anode x-ray generator. The patient is placed supine on a flat, wooden, wheeled platform and moved inside the scanning gantry. X-rays are then projected through the patient at different angles, penetrating tissues differently according to the atomic numbers of the atoms within the tissue. Dense tissue such as bone attenuates (reduces the energy of) the x-ray beam more than less dense tissue such as muscle, yielding high-resolution images of the scanned tissue. The patient images are then detected, and the computer acquires the image data. Finally, an image analyzer projects the analyzed data in the form of a tomogram or body section slice onto an operator console and a physician-viewing console. CT is excellent for imaging bone.

The diagnostic quality of a CT scan is enhanced with the injection of IV contrast media (ICM). Contrast media containing iodine may be administered to the patient enterally or parenterally to further attenuate the x-ray beam to enhance the images for CT vascular or gastrointestinal studies.[106,107]

Magnetic resonance imaging. Magnetic resonance imaging (MRI) uses the dipole moment (i.e., the ability of the atomic nucleus to behave as a magnet) of the hydrogen atom. The patient is placed supine within the scanning gantry or bore of the magnet. The magnet used for MRI can be a permanent magnet or a powerful superconducting electromagnet cooled with liquid helium to 4° Kelvin. Magnetic strength is measured in teslas (T); 1 T is equivalent to 10,000 gauss or oersted. MRI magnets can generate field strengths of 0.15 to 4 T, although MRI magnetic field strength generally ranges from 0.15 to 2 T. The quality of the MRI image is directly related to the strength of the magnetic field.[106,108] The spin of the electron in hydrogen will align the hydrogen atoms parallel to this powerful magnetic field. The patient's water-containing tissues are then excited with variable radiofrequency pulses. After the proton in hydrogen receives this radiofrequency energy, it emits radiofrequency energy with three-dimensional (3D)–appearing spatial information. MRI technology now allows its use within the OR with an open-bore, portable, 0.12-T, low-intensity magnet to assist the neurosurgeon with diagnostic decisions.[106,109] Contrast media are also used in MRI studies to enhance the patient's tissues and allow the scan to provide further diagnostic information. MRI contrast is most commonly gadopentetate dimeglumine, which contains the element gadolinium bound as a chelated structure and administered primarily parenterally but rarely enterally.[106,109,110]

The FDA classifies the MRI as a class II device. Class II devices require special labeling, mandatory performance standards, and post-market surveillance by the FDA. The electromagnetic energy greatly drops off just outside the margins of the bore of the electromagnet. This is called the fringe field. There are no known reports of harmful physiologic effects from magnetic fields.[106,107]

Because of the potential danger of the powerful electromagnetic attraction of ferromagnetic objects to both the patient and health care personnel, the American College of Radiology divides the MRI suite into four zones as noted in Box 58.13.[111]

Interventional radiology (vascular and nonvascular), and radiotherapy or radiosurgery. Interventional radiology (IR) involves minimally invasive procedures and therapies performed by radiologists, especially in patients at high medical risk.[112,113] Major IR therapies include angiography, the embolization of blood vessels such as arteriovenous malformations or for epistaxis, the delivery of chemical or physical vascular occlusive devices, the removal of thrombi, ablation of aneurysms, and angioplasty of blood vessels with stent placement.[112,114] Box 58.14 lists indications for endovascular embolization procedures. See Chapter 28 for a discussion of interventional vascular surgery and Chapter 31 for interventional neuroradiology (INR) procedures.

Radiation is a treatment itself for both benign tumors (e.g., low-grade astrocytoma, meningioma, pituitary adenoma, craniopharyngioma, schwannoma, pineocytoma, chemodectoma, and low-grade papillary neoplasms) and aggressive tumors (e.g., germinoma, primitive neuroectodermal tumor, chordoma, intermediate-grade pineal tumor, immature teratoma, undifferentiated sarcoma, anaplastic oligoastrocytoma, and metastatic tumors). Radiation surgery is the delivery of a single massive dose of radiation to the target tissue. Radiation therapy is the delivery of smaller doses of radiation over several sessions.[115]

Gamma radiation is used for radiotherapy and radiosurgery. The gamma radiation is introduced to the patient by the use of either a Gamma Knife or a CyberKnife. Each uses beams of gamma rays

obtained from the radioactive decay of cobalt 60 or from a linear accelerator. The CyberKnife is used by first obtaining stereotactic 3D images, which then allow computer-controlled robot arm guidance of the CyberKnife. The CyberKnife therapy delivers a sequence of many hundreds of gamma beams to the cancerous tumor from many different directions. Gamma Knife therapy delivers gamma radiation to the cancerous tumor simultaneously in a single dose.[114,115]

Interventional neuroradiology. INR is the diagnosis and treatment of CNS diseases endovascularly to deliver therapeutic medications or devices. INR was first used in the early 1980s when digital subtraction angiography was developed. Digital subtraction angiography first uses an original angiograph of the blood vessels to be studied. Then a contrast medium is injected into the same blood vessels, and opaque structures such as bone and tissues can be digitally subtracted or removed from the angiographic image, leaving a clear picture of the blood vessels.[116]

BOX 58.13 Magnetic Resonance Suite Zones

Zone	Activity
Zone I	All areas freely accessible to the general public. This is the area through which personnel and patients access the MRI area.
Zone II	The area between the uncontrolled zone I and the strictly controlled zone III. This is the area where patients are greeted, histories obtained, and questions answered. Movement by non-MRI personnel and patients is under the supervision of MRI personnel.
Zone III	This is a restricted area. Movement in this area is strictly controlled by MRI personnel. Access to this area is only after screening for the presence of ferromagnetic material. Ferromagnetic objects may produce a serious hazard if brought into this area.
Zone IV	This is the MRI scanner room itself. By definition it is within zone III.

MRI, Magnetic resonance imaging.
From Phillips MC. Room setup, critical supplies and medications. In: Weiss M., Fleisher LA, eds. *Non-Operating Room Anesthesia.* Philadelphia: Elsevier; 2015:21.

BOX 58.14 Indications for Endovascular Embolization

- Arteriovenous malformation
- Arteriovenous fistula
- Intracranial aneurysm
- Recurrent epistaxis
- Hemoptysis
- Traumatic solid organ hemorrhage
- Preoperative major organ tumor embolization for blood loss reduction
- Gastrointestinal hemorrhage
- Uterine leiomyoma (fibroid)
- Uterine hemorrhage
- Pelvic fracture hemorrhage
- Postoperative hemorrhage after prosthetic hip or knee replacement
- Varicocele

Modified from Temple M, Marshalleck FE. *Pediatric Interventional Radiology: Handbook for Vascular and Non-vascular Interventions.* New York: Springer; 2014.

Improvements in vascular access techniques, new thin and flexible catheters and guidewires, and the development of innovative coils and therapeutic medications have made new treatments possible. Conditions that once required extensive surgery, with accompanying patient morbidity and mortality, can now be performed less invasively.[112,114] Some major procedures performed with INR are mechanical or chemical removal of emboli or thrombi that cause stroke, the physical occlusion of malformed vascular structures such as arteriovenous malformations with chemicals or flow-directed balloons, dilation of stenotic blood vessels, and embolization (blocking blood flow) of cerebral vascular aneurysms using catheter-deployed coils.[112,114,116]

Box 58.15 lists some current uses for each of the previously mentioned radiologic and diagnostic procedures. As technology advances, more uses will be seen.

Anesthetic Considerations

Computed tomography. CT scans require that the patient remain as motionless as possible for several minutes to an hour. Patient motion can produce artifacts in the diagnostic images to be read by the radiologist. Patients must lie on a flat, lightly padded wheeled platform, which is rolled into the short-bore scanning gantry of the CT scanner. Although the majority of patients are able to cooperate and tolerate CT, others may not be able because of extremes in age, concurrent medical conditions, or mental disability. The CT scan is neither physically invasive nor painful. Patients enter the CT scanner without precautions for ferromagnetic objects as for an MRI scan. CT is more rapidly performed than an MRI scan, especially if a spiral CT scanner is used.

The patient may require anesthesia anywhere along the continuum from minimal sedation to general anesthesia. Use of ferromagnetic anesthesia equipment and supplies around the CT scanner is not a concern. A standard anesthesia machine, laryngoscope and blades, and IV infusion pumps can be used as if in the OR. A LMA is an appropriate alternative choice as a minimally invasive and secure airway in the patient without contraindications to its use. A LMA is contraindicated in patients with gastroesophageal reflux disease or a full stomach. Attention must be paid to securing the airway, and the anesthesia breathing circuit, the leads for the ECG, the noninvasive blood pressure cuff, the IV line, and the pulse oximeter must extend into the scanning gantry. The anesthetist must allow for extra lengths of anesthesia circuitry and electrical monitoring leads because of patient movement that will occur during intermittent repositioning of the mechanized table that positions the patient within the scanning gantry.[88,107]

Sedation can be performed with a variety of agents, including midazolam or propofol. General anesthesia can be performed with TIVA, such as with IV propofol, or with potent inhaled agents.

All personnel must be aware of the use of ionizing radiation during the CT scan and should take precautions to be shielded from any exposure to the radiation. Radiation exposure is cumulative over a lifetime, and every precaution must be made to protect oneself from any unnecessary doses of radiation, which can cause genetic mutation and may lead to cancer. Protection can be accomplished with the use of a lead-glass barrier, a lead apron, a lead thyroid collar, and lead-glass safety glasses. Radiation dose badges are available that attach to clothing. The badge monitors the dose of radiation received and is evaluated monthly. Federal technical information and guidelines for working in conjunction with radiation is available from the US Environmental Protection Agency.[116]

ICM can cause an unexpected allergic reaction in some patients, varying from itching with hives to severe, life-threatening anaphylactoid and anaphylactic reactions.[110,117,118] Adverse reactions to ICM are more likely to develop in patients with asthma, a history of allergy, or

---

BOX 58.15   Some Indications for Radiologic and Diagnostic Procedures

Computed Tomography
- Assessment of the airway with neck or thoracic tumors
- Assessment of bony trauma, especially the spine
- Assessment of head trauma
- Assessment of increased intracranial pressure
- Assessment of neoplasms
- Imaging of brain tumors
- Imaging of intracerebral hemorrhage

Magnetic Resonance Imaging
- Central nervous system imaging
- Imaging of the blood-brain barrier
- Kidney imaging
- Liver imaging
- Urinary bladder imaging

Interventional Radiology (Vascular and Nonvascular), Radiotherapy, and Radiosurgery
- Angiography
- Catheterization of ducts, and vascular lesions for drainage of cysts or hemangiomas (e.g., liver hydatid cyst, renal cyst, soft tissue hemangiomas)
- Catheterization of tumors for delivery of chemotherapy directly to tumors (e.g., liver tumors)
- Embolization, embolectomy, or thrombofragmentation of vascular lesions and tumors (pulmonary thrombi or emboli)
- Radiosurgery
- Stereotactic radiosurgery
- Radiotherapy
- Transluminal dilation, angioplasty, and stent insertion for vascular stenosis, biliary stenosis, or tracheal malacia

Interventional Neuroradiology
- Angioplasty and stent placement for an atherosclerotic lesion
- Angioplasty or endovascular ablation of cerebral vasospasm from aneurysmal subarachnoid hematoma
- Balloon angioplasty of cerebral vasospasm
- Brain arteriovenous malformation embolization
- Carotid artery stenting
- Carotid cavernous fistula and vertebral fistula treatment
- Carotid test occlusion
- Dural arteriovenous malformation embolization
- Embolization of highly vascularized intracranial tumors
- Glomus tumor treatment
- Intracranial aneurysm ablation
- Juvenile nasopharyngeal angiofibroma treatment
- Meningioma treatment
- Sclerotherapy of venous angiomas
- Spinal cord lesion embolization
- Therapeutic carotid occlusion
- Thrombolysis of acute thromboembolic stroke
- Trigeminal nerve rhizotomy or glycerol injection
- Vein of Galen malformation treatment
- Vertebroplasty for back pain/vertebral body fractures

---

with multiple morbidities. These reactions can be divided into renal or general, then subdivided into acute and delayed. Fatal reactions are rare. Contrast-media-induced renal impairment can be reduced with the use of low-osmolality contrast media and extracellular volume

BOX 58.16 Considerations and Treatment Protocols for Preventing Intravenous Contrast Medium Extravasation

Considerations

- Use intravenous catheters (as opposed to metal needles or butterfly needles).
- Avoid use of the same vein if the first attempt at intravenous catheterization was missed.
- Ensure the intravenous catheter is patent and is free flowing.

Treatments

- Attempt to aspirate as much ICM as possible.
- Elevate the affected limb.
- Apply ice packs for 20–60 min until swelling resolves.
- A heating pad may be necessary in place of ice for swelling.
- Observe the patient for possible tissue damage related to continual contact with ice or heat.
- Observe the patient for 2–4 hr before discharge; consider medical/surgical consultation if necessary.
- Follow up with patient assessing for residual pain, increased or decreased temperature, hardness, change in sensation, redness, or blistering.

ICM, Intravenous contrast medium.
Modified from American College of Radiology. Extravasation of contrast media. In *ACR Manual on Contrast Media.* Version 10.1; 2020. https://www.acr.org/-/media/ACR/Files/Clinical-Resources/Contrast_Media.pdf#page=21; Reynolds PM, et al. Management of extravasation injuries: a focused evaluation of noncytotoxic medications. *Pharmacotherapy.* 2014;34(6):617–632.

expansion.[118,119] ICM also can cause local tissue sloughing and necrosis if the ICM extravasates from the vein into the surrounding tissue.[117,119] Clinicians should be familiar with treatment protocols to minimize patient morbidity (Box 58.16).

ICM is typically a water-soluble, iodine-containing solution of two available types: media that can dissociate into ions in solution and media that will remain in a neutral state in solution. ICM is also formulated as high-osmolar contrast media (HOCM), which contain few dissolved particles and iodine atoms, and low-osmolar contrast media (LOCM), which contain greater numbers of dissolved particles with iodine. A HOCM solution causes fluid shift from the cell to the vein with the ICM, whereas a LOCM solution is closely isoosmolar, inducing less fluid shift from the cell. Nonionized LOCM is a more costly contrast media for the patient. Some advocate that it should be the only contrast media used for CT with dye studies.[110,118]

Reactions are possible with either type of ICM solution, although fewer reactions occur with LOCM.[117,118] Some reactions may occur anywhere from 30 minutes to 1 week after the administration of the ICM. Reactions to ICM are theorized to be caused by the ICM molecule's serving as an antigen and affixing itself to either mast cells or basophils. This causes release of mediators such as histamine and tryptase, which can inhibit coagulation, dilate blood vessels, release complement, or even stimulate an immunoglobulin E (IgE)–modulated immune reaction.[110,117,118] A new ICM using gold nanoparticles is available and undergoing tests prior to use in humans. It has many advantages over iodinated ICM, such as higher radiation absorption, yielding better images with lower x-ray dose, low allergenic response, and longer imaging times because of its nanoparticle size.[119,120]

A thorough preanesthetic assessment for a patient about to undergo CT should include questions pertaining to asthma, allergies, and any previous reactions to contrast media. Diabetic patients taking metformin must withhold the medication because of the risk of lactic acidosis. This problem is mainly observed in patients with diabetic nephropathy. Other patients at risk for reactions to ICM are patients with multiple medical problems, especially those with cardiac disease or with preexisting azotemia, patients of advanced age, and patients being treated with nephrotoxic agents such as the aminoglycoside antimicrobials gentamicin, tobramycin, streptomycin, amikacin, kanamycin, and neomycin, or NSAIDs. ICM is contraindicated in pregnant patients.[110,118]

Clinicians may use preventive measures in patients who may be at risk for a reaction to ICM. The radiologist should use the smallest amount of contrast agent necessary. To safeguard against the possibility of renal failure, the patient should be adequately hydrated beginning 1 hour before the procedure and continuing for another 24 hours. Patients who are at risk for possible anaphylactoid reactions should be pretreated with corticosteroids, such as methylprednisolone, or prednisone administered by mouth or intravenously. In cases of moderate or severe previous ICM reactions, a histamine-1 (H_1) blocker such as diphenhydramine and an H_2-blocker such as cimetidine or ranitidine should be given together either intravenously or by mouth. ICM is probably the most frequently used agent that causes anaphylactoid reactions. Anaphylaxis recognition and treatment are outlined in Chapter 46; as little as 1 mL of ICM can initiate these reactions.[110,117,118]

Magnetic resonance imaging. MRI can take up to 1 hour or longer. During this time, the patient must remain extremely still to reduce motion artifacts. These artifacts can cause unfaithful representations of the tissues being studied. The motions of breathing, the heart, blood flow, swallowing, and even cerebral spinal fluid flow produce artifacts in a highly sensitive MRI scan. Patients must remain within the bore of the magnet for an MRI scan for longer periods of time than for a CT scan. During this time the MRI suite's ambient temperature is cold.

The patient is exposed to varying magnetic fields of up to 4 T, along with additional exposure to variable radiofrequency radiation. Blood flow is decreased by strong magnetic fields, and blood pressure compensates by rising. Patients have also reported symptoms of vertigo, nausea, headache, and visual sensations.[108,109]

The MRI machine produces loud vibratory and knocking noises as coils are switched on and off during the course of the study. The size of the MRI magnet bore may preclude the morbidly obese or claustrophobic patient from MRI scanning, although a more open-bore MRI is available. Most patients are content with an explanation of what to expect during the procedure and with reassurance. Some patients need minimal or moderate sedation. Patients with claustrophobia or those who cannot, or will not, remain motionless during the study, in addition to critically ill patients, may require deep sedation or general endotracheal anesthesia.[106,108,109,111] MRI is not painful so opioids are not usually required. Sedation has been performed with oral and IV midazolam, ketamine, pentobarbital, or propofol.[106-109,111] Minimal sedation requires full monitoring. Deep sedation or general anesthesia requires IV access and full monitoring. The LMA has served as an excellent, relatively noninvasive airway for MRI. Some anesthesia providers prefer general endotracheal intubation. Children who cannot, or will not, cooperate experience better MRI scans with general endotracheal anesthesia in shorter periods of time, despite longer recovery times when compared with sedation.[112,114]

Because of the intense magnetic field always present in the MRI suite, anesthesia providers must be aware of every item on their person and every item that is to be used in conjunction with anesthesia administered to the patient. Ferromagnetic (iron-containing) substances are attracted at astonishing rates of speed into the bore of the magnet. Personal items such as pens, certain types of eyeglasses, jewelry, watches, pagers, personal computers, calculators, name badges, coins, audiotapes, videotapes, and credit cards are some of the items that should never enter the MRI suite, in addition to any ferromagnetic anesthesia equipment, medication vials, and supplies. If a patient were present within the bore of the MRI, injury or death could be possible from the missile created. As newer and more powerful 3-T MRI scanners become more prevalent, previously "safe" items could cause injury. Metals known to be safe within the proximity of the MRI bore are stainless steel, nonferrous alloys, nickel, and titanium. Materials and equipment constructed of plastic are safe.[107,109]

Patients possessing certain medical therapeutic devices may be prohibited from an MRI scan. MRI lists devices or metal that patients may possess that could be affected by the MRI and cause patient morbidity or mortality (Box 58.17).[107-111] Further investigation by the anesthetist in concert with the radiologist or MRI technician regarding the metal content and MRI compatibility of these metal items is necessary.

Cardiac pacemakers may be affected several ways by the electromagnetic field: Reprogramming may occur, the pacemaker may be inhibited, it may revert to an asynchronous mode, the reed switch may close, the pacemaker may become dislodged, or it may become heated by the magnetic field.[108,109,111]

Manufacturers have developed a host of MRI-compatible anesthesia equipment and supplies (Box 58.18). This host of equipment and supplies allows performance of the anesthetic procedure directly within the MRI suite. Be aware that some equipment designated by the manufacturer as MRI compatible may not be compatible as magnet strengths increase.[111]

Facilities that cannot afford MRI-compatible equipment and supplies can provide anesthetic services to their patients by inducing anesthesia outside the MRI suite. The patient is placed on an MRI-compatible cart or a detachable MRI scanning table that fits within the bore of the electromagnet, where anesthesia may be then induced. With the aid of extralong circuits, extension IV tubing, and properly insulated monitor cables, the anesthesia can be maintained with full monitors and a standard anesthetic machine outside the MRI suite. The patient is then carefully moved on a flat, relatively hard, wheeled platform into the bore of the electromagnet. Attention should be paid to isolate any monitor leads or IV tubing from touching the skin of the patient. Any monitor leads and IV tubing should be kept in straight alignment because the intense magnetic fields in the MRI suite can induce current flow in coiled leads or tubing and severely burn the patient. Flexible LMAs and ETTs that contain wire windings can also be sources of burns. The American College of Radiology recommends strong attention to and the elimination of induced current, which can be large tissue loops such as the loop created by the hand touching the hip or thigh or the loop created when the feet or calves of the legs touch.[111]

Consideration must be given to the MRI contrast media administered to patients. Fortunately, the dyes used for MRI contrast are nonionic gadolinium chelates and have extremely low allergy rates.[110,118,119] Nausea is a common side effect. Urticaria (hives) and anaphylactoid reactions occur in less than 1% of patients.[112,118] The risk of a reaction to MRI dye is increased in patients with a history of asthma or other allergies or drug sensitivities, especially to iodinated contrast dyes.[118] Proper equipment, medications, and supplies must be immediately available for management of a reaction if one occurs. Treatments for anaphylactoid and anaphylactic reactions are discussed in Chapter 46.

Although MRI does not use ionizing radiation, patients and personnel are exposed to constant levels of magnetic force while in the MRI suite. Acute exposure to magnetic fields under 2.5 T has not been shown to have adverse effects in humans. All care providers must make their own determinations regarding how much magnetic exposure they will accept during a patient's MRI scan. Doses both to the patient

> ### BOX 58.17 Potentially Harmful Items When in Proximity to MRI
>
> - Automatic implantable cardiac defibrillators
> - Cardiac pacemakers
> - Certain mechanical heart valves
> - Cochlear implants
> - Deep brain neurostimulators
> - Dorsal column stimulators
> - Pacing wires
> - Penile implants
> - Permanent eyeliner or tattoos
> - Prostheses (including dental prostheses)
> - Implanted pumps (such as baclofen, narcotic, or insulin pumps)
> - Internal plates, wires, or screws
> - Metallic aneurysm clips (clips manufactured after 1995 and certified MRI compatible can be scanned)
> - Certain metallic implants (history of recent orthopedic implants inserted within 3 mo, dental implants)
> - Metallic sutures
> - Shrapnel and metal fragments (especially intraocular metal shrapnel)
> - Tissue expanders with metallic ports
>
> *MRI,* Magnetic resonance imaging.

> ### BOX 58.18 List of Available MRI-Compatible Equipment and Supplies
>
> - MRI-compatible anesthesia machine
> - Pulse oximeter
> - Intravenous bag pole
> - Liquid crystal temperature monitoring strip
> - Thermocouple temperature probe with radiofrequency (RF) filter
> - Respiratory rate monitor
> - Noninvasive blood pressure monitor
> - Pulse oximeter
> - Electrocardiograph
> - Electrocardiograph patches
> - Electrocardiograph cable
> - Capnograph
> - Laryngoscope with lithium batteries and aluminum spacers
> - Laryngoscope blades
> - Nerve stimulator
> - Intravenous infusion pump
> - Oxygen tanks
> - Precordial stethoscope
> - Esophageal stethoscope
> - Patient carts
> - Tables and trays
>
> *MRI,* Magnetic resonance imaging.

and to all personnel should be minimized.[107,111] Pregnant anesthesia personnel have no restrictions on presence in the MRI scanner room during all of the required anesthesia preparations necessary to treat the patient, but the American College of Radiology recommends that personnel not be present in the MRI scanner room during the scan. Pregnant patients should discuss risks and benefits with their physician.[111]

If the anesthesia provider is away from the patient during the procedure, it should be ensured that all airway circuitry, monitoring leads, and IV connections are secure and tight. A respiratory monitoring apparatus (RMA) built into the anesthesia circuit reservoir bag will soon be available to monitor respiration with both visual and audible signals pertaining to movement of the RMA relative to the patient's respiratory rate and tidal volume.

When the environment could pose physical danger, anesthetists must be cognizant of their own safety and physical well-being while administering anesthesia for patients, especially during repeated exposures of radiation and/or chemicals. Therefore a means for remote observation and monitoring either via a clear window, a camera, or telemetry must be available, although controversies regarding the traditional standards of physical presence during the conduct of anesthesia exist.[107,111] In conjunction with recognized standards of safety, the anesthetist must use monitors with both audible and visual alarms and have a clear and continual view of the patient and the anesthesia monitors. Consideration must be made for safe and rapid access to the patient should the need exist.[107,109,111]

The functional MRI (fMRI) is a tool used to better differentiate residual pathologic tissue from normal healthy tissue to perform higher quality tumor resection. An fMRI scan requires the patient to remain motionless and cooperative to avoid artifact. It is known that anesthetic agents can alter cerebral blood flow and cerebral oxygen metabolism, which can affect the interpretation of the fMRI scan. Therefore fMRI use for uncooperative or pediatric patients may preclude its use in this cohort of patients. Anesthesia research will provide the anesthetist tools to enable this population to receive both an anesthetic and needed fMRI.[109-111]

Positron emission tomography scan. A positron emission tomography (PET) scan is used for the imaging and detection of malignant disease, neurologic function, and cardiovascular disease. The isotope fluorodeoxyglucose (FDG) is injected and is then absorbed into metabolically active cells. The absorbed isotope emits minute amounts of positron antimatter, which are detected and produce high-resolution images of diseased tissue. The patient must remain still for approximately an hour after the injection of FDG to minimize the amount of the muscle uptake of this glucose-like molecule. The patient must have fasted to minimize blood glucose levels. Any sedation medications containing sugar should also be avoided.[120-123]

Interventional radiology (vascular and nonvascular), radiotherapy, stereotactic radiosurgery, and interventional neuroradiology. As skills, techniques, and technology progress, more procedures will be performed with radiation or under radiologic guidance.[112] These procedures all require the absolute immobility of the patient, with periods of controlled apnea, which assist in the viewing or treatment of the targeted area of the patient, especially during whole-body therapeutic radiation treatment.[112,114-116] These procedures are also time consuming, taking up to several hours to complete. Procedures may be necessary in patients of various age groups from infants to geriatrics and in all states of health.[114,116] A thorough preanesthetic assessment is imperative to ensure patient safety.

With the exceptions of angiography or radiotherapy, procedures for IR are painful, physically invasive to the patient, and may need to be accomplished over several treatment sessions. Treatment may be required electively or urgently.[112] Patients may require anesthesia along the continuum from minimal or moderate sedation/analgesia, local or regional anesthesia, with the trend moving toward general anesthesia because of the superior image quality obtained in a motionless patient, especially if the patient is held apneic for a brief period of time by the anesthetist.[113,114] Studies have shown patients with acute ischemic strokes undergoing intraarterial therapy may have worse outcomes with general anesthesia compared with conscious sedation.[113] Full monitors and IV access are required. Additional catheterization and monitoring of arterial pressure and central venous pressure may be necessary.[114,116]

Certain procedures require monitoring of the patient's neurophysiologic status for changes. The patient also may need to be assessed awake and then resedated at times during the procedure.[118] Anesthetics that can be used are midazolam, propofol, ketamine, dexmedetomidine, and the other potent inhaled general anesthetics.[112,114,115] Dexmedetomidine, a selective α_2-adrenoreceptor agonist, is being used for its reduction of intraprocedural and postprocedural anesthetic requirements.[114,118] Rapid recovery from anesthesia to assess and monitor the patient's neurologic functioning at the end of the case is ideal.

It may be necessary to manipulate or manage normal systemic blood flow, normal cerebral blood flow, or other regional blood flow. The anesthetist may be called on to control deliberate hypertension or deliberate hypotension, manage anticoagulation, and manage unexpected procedural complications.[114-116]

Intraoperative radiation therapy (IORT) is the delivery of radiation to the patient via a linear accelerator, at times in conjunction with tumor surgery. If surgery is performed coincidental to the dose of radiation, normal tissues may be able to be moved away from the ionizing radiation beam. Normal tissues and organs can be shielded with lead beforehand. Some facilities use a dedicated IORT suite, whereas others use an OR with transport of the patient to the radiation oncology suite. General anesthesia is performed if the surgical and radiation procedures are concurrent. All personnel must leave the room during IORT and stereotactically guided Gamma Knife or CyberKnife surgery so that high-dose radiation can be delivered to the patient while protecting personnel from the scattered radiation. The radiation oncology suite is heavily shielded and has a lead or iron door that can take from 30 to 60 seconds to open. The patient is monitored via closed-circuit video and hands-off anesthesia delivery during treatment.[115]

Complications can occur rapidly and be life threatening. Foremost is the possible complication of hemorrhage. A sedated patient experiencing hemorrhage may show sudden signs of headache, nausea and vomiting, and vascular pain. A patient under general anesthesia may experience sudden bradycardia. The airway must be secured first if necessary, followed by support of the cardiovascular system, discontinuation of heparin, and administration of protamine (1 mg/100 units of total heparin dose administered). Other possible complications are radiocontrast reactions, embolization of particles or tissue, perforation of an aneurysm, and unintended obliteration of physiologically necessary arteries. Patient safety necessitates skilled and competent staff assistance in treatment of complications. Complications may necessitate the safe transfer of the patient to the OR.[114-116]

Postanesthesia Care

Physiologic stability is the goal in any patient undergoing a radiologic or diagnostic procedure. The patient must be observed for possible reactions to dyes administered by the radiologist. The patient must be relieved of pain. Cardiovascular status must be stable. Hospital admission may be necessary for observation after any complication experienced by the patient or suspected to have occurred. One should always err on the side of patient safety and patient welfare.

REMOTE ANESTHETIC MONITORING USING TELECOMMUNICATION TECHNOLOGY

Telecommunications technologies are being implemented to improve access and optimize care. First used in primary care over 30 years ago to gain specialty consultation from a distance, telecommunication technologies are now advancing throughout health care disciplines and specialties.[123] Communication technology, in conjunction with reliable and accurate electronic monitoring (telemonitoring), has made it possible to provide anesthetic monitoring and consultation with the anesthetist in one location while the therapeutic or diagnostic proceduralist is in another physically remote, geographically isolated, or environmentally extreme environment. The anesthetist may be involved with communication and monitoring through a variety of synchronous communication methods involving land-line telephone, cellular telephone, computer/monitor interlinks, and internet audio-videoconferencing.

The purposes of telemonitoring are the benefits to patients requiring therapeutic or diagnostic procedures with the added safety of available expert specialty care to assist the anesthetist in performing anesthesia in a challenging environment. Anesthetists can collaborate and use their combined skills during the entire anesthetic procedure, from preoperative planning to postprocedure care and eventual discharge.

SUMMARY

New procedures and patient treatments are evolving and moving out of the traditional OR and into non-OR anesthesia environments. This demands evolution of anesthesia providers, equipment, and techniques for the provision of anesthesia services to patients in need of such services. Although anesthesia providers are required to be flexible to adapt to these dynamic changes in the health care world, this should never be at the cost of patient safety. The same standards of care that apply in the OR setting should always be adhered to outside of the traditional operating suite. Clinicians must be absolutely comfortable that all required equipment, medications, and supplies are available, as would be true in a typical, fully equipped OR. It is easier and safer to prepare beforehand than to gather the items needed for safe anesthesia delivery later or to go without them. Where cases of "minor" surgery or patient intervention may exist, cases of "minor" anesthesia do not.

REFERENCES

For a complete list of references for this chapter, scan this QR code with any smartphone code reader app, or visit the following URL: http://booksite.elsevier.com/9780323711944/.

59

Anesthesia Complications

M. Roseann Diehl

Every day, health care professionals practice within enormously complex environments, and unexpected patient outcomes or complications can occur at any time. Public interest regarding patient safety has increased significantly over the past decade, largely as a result of the staggering number of preventable deaths cited in the Institute of Medicine's 1999 landmark report.[1] The results of this report have led to implementation of a broad range of improvement efforts concentrating on the prevention and detection of errors in health care. Complications can arise as consequences of another concurrent disease or of mishap. Often, these complications appear unexpectedly, and they have been experienced by well-intentioned health care professionals who are surrounded by complex clinical conditions, poorly designed processes, and suboptimal communication patterns.[2,3]

The goal of this chapter is to provide more insight into common and emerging types of anesthetic complications and to introduce organizational concepts that often surround complications in anesthesia. This chapter will discuss how to deal with complications systematically and examine the underlying human factors and lapses in communication involved in the development of these complications.

MORTALITY IN ANESTHESIA

Risks related to anesthesia have declined over the past several decades. However, the exact cause of this decline is unclear.[4,5] Anesthesia has had a 10-fold decrease in mortality since the 1980s and is often cited as reaching a Six Sigma defect rate (99.99966% of end products are statistically free of defects, or 3.4 defects per million).[4,6] Today, anesthesia-related mortality is about 1.1 persons per million per year in the United States. Outcome measures studied related to the risk of anesthesia include mortality, morbidity, patient satisfaction, and quality of life.[7] Perioperative risk related to anesthesia is multifactorial and depends on several interactions between anesthesia type, surgical procedure/location, and patient health.[5] The dramatic improvement in anesthesia patient safety over the last 30 years was not initiated by electronic monitors. It was largely by a set of behaviors known as safety monitoring that were then made decidedly more effective by extending the human senses through better monitoring practices (e.g., capnography, pulse oximetry) and improved understanding of anesthetic-related deaths, improved airway management tools, sharing of safety knowledge, and peer review.[8-10]

Mortality data are difficult to use when extrapolating conclusions about anesthesia safety because no standard definition of anesthesia mortality has been established. There is a lack of consensus related to the period postanesthesia that should define anesthesia-related mortality. In addition, significant morbidity involving patients who do not die has not been considered in regard to safety. Depending on which studies are referenced, this time frame can vary from 24 hours to 30 days postanesthesia.[5,6,11]

Another issue that clouds morbidity and mortality outcome data is the fact that older patients with multimorbidities are now considered operable (e.g., less invasive procedures) resulting in skewed perioperative surgical and anesthetic risk.[8] Actual data are difficult to analyze because most studies use coroner registries, voluntary reports, surveys, and malpractice claims as primary data sources for perioperative death. As a result, prevalence data available for anesthesia-related mortality are approximate estimates as documented in Table 59.1.

Over 60% of surgical procedures are now performed in an ambulatory setting. Procedures associated with greater perioperative risk are increasingly being performed on an outpatient basis, and the use of regional techniques has increased.[12] As a result, claim areas in which a reported mortality increase has occurred over the years include regional anesthesia (16% of all claims), chronic pain management (18% of all claims), and acute pain (9% of all claims).[7] By contrast, claims related specifically to surgical anesthesia have declined from 80% during the 1980s to 65% as compared to all anesthesia malpractice claims since 2000.[7]

The American Society of Anesthesiologists (ASA) classifies patient physical status related to incidence of mortality on a scale of 1 to 5 based on comorbid conditions, 1 being the healthiest individual with no comorbidities and 5 being the individual that will likely die if surgery is not performed within 24 hours. The most current incidence of anesthesia mortality in a patient with an ASA physical status of 1 is 0.04 per 10,000 (0.0004%) anesthetics. Patients with comorbid conditions have higher risk. For example, an ASA physical status 2 risk is 0.5 per 10,000 (0.005%) anesthetics, an ASA physical status 3 risk is 2.7 per 10,000 (0.027%) anesthetics, and an ASA physical status 4 risk is 5.5 per 10,000 (0.055%) anesthetics.[12] Death still remains the leading outcome in the ASA Closed Claims Project database representing 26% of the most common complications from 1990 to 2007.[7]

MORBIDITY IN ANESTHESIA

The term *morbidity* is indicative of disease, incorporating any complication, excluding death, occurring during the perioperative period (Box 59.1). The most common events leading to injury in anesthesia claims included regional blocks (20% of claims), respiratory problems (17% of claims), cardiovascular events (13% of claims), and equipment problems (10% of claims)[7,9] (Box 59.2).

Trends in anesthesia practice leading to morbidity claims have changed considerably over the last 2 decades. Acute pain claims have increased to 8% within the last decade, with no claims present 20 years ago. Chronic pain claims have also increased from less than 5% to 18% during the same time period. Monitored anesthesia care (MAC) claims have also increased from 2% to 10% over the decades. Obstetric claims trends have decreased, and regional anesthesia claims have remained steady at 20% to 25% over the last 20 years.[7]

BOX 59.1 Morbidity Classification

Minor morbidity: Moderate distress without prolonging hospital stay. No permanent complications (e.g., postoperative nausea and vomiting).
Intermediate morbidity: Serious distress prolonging hospital stay or both. No permanent complications (e.g., dental injury).
Major morbidity: Permanent disability or complication (e.g., spinal cord injury; anoxic brain injury).

From Haller G, et al. Morbidity in anaesthesia: today and tomorrow. *Best Pract Res Clin Anaesthesiol.* 2011;25(2):123–132.

TABLE 59.1 Anesthesia-Related Deaths by Type of Complication (United States 1999–2005)

Type of Complication	Number of Deaths	%
Complications of anesthesia during pregnancy, labor, and puerperium	79	3.6
Cardiac complications	60	2.7
Overdose of anesthetics	1030	46.6
Inhaled anesthetics	233	10.5
Intravenous anesthetics	419	19.0
Other and unspecified general anesthetics	254	11.5
Local anesthetics	86	3.9
Unspecified anesthetics	38	1.7
Adverse effects of anesthetics in therapeutic use	940	42.5
Opioids and related analgesics	439	19.9
Benzodiazepines	42	1.9
Opioids and related analgesics	40	1.8
Local anesthetics	137	6.2
Unspecified anesthetic	257	11.6
Other complications of anesthesia	162	7.3
Malignant hyperthermia	22	1.0
Failed/difficult intubation	50	2.3
TOTAL	2211	100.0

Adapted from Haller G, et al. Morbidity in anaesthesia: today and tomorrow. *Best Pract Res Clin Anaesthesiol.* 2011;25(2):123–132; Li G, et al. Epidemiology of anesthesia-related mortality in the United States, 1999–2005. *Anesthesiology.* 2009;110(4):759–765.

The incidence of adverse outcomes with minor morbidity is quite high (18%–22%). For example, hoarseness has been cited to occur in 14% to 50% of patients and may accompany a traumatic lesion in the larynx or hypopharynx in 6.3% of patients. Drug errors (0.1%), equipment malfunction (0.23%), postoperative nausea and vomiting (10%–79%), and accidental dural perforation (0.5%–0.6%) are all fairly common anesthesia-related morbidities. Therefore, if morbidity is included in the definition of harm caused by anesthesia and linked to anesthesia safety within the framework of Six Sigma, then anesthesia remains far from being 99.99966% free of defects (Fig. 59.1).[4]

Several areas within anesthesia continue to possess risk even today, including perioperative airway control during general anesthesia, perioperative management of hemorrhage, and circulatory perturbations associated with regional anesthesia. It is difficult to quantify human error related to morbidity, and more research should be conducted in this area.

BOX 59.2 Complications of Anesthesia Identified by ASA Closed Claims Database

- Aspiration of gastric contents
- Failed intubation
- Esophageal intubation
- Other problems with the induction of general anesthesia
- Inadequate ventilation
- Airway obstruction
- Respiratory failure
- High spinal or massive epidural
- Neuraxial cardiac arrest
- Local anesthetic toxicity
- Drug reaction
- Anaphylaxis
- Overdose of sedatives
- Prolonged hypotension or hypertension
- Intraoperative cardiac arrest during anesthesia of undetermined etiology

ASA, American Society of Anesthetists.
From Metzner J, et al. Closed claims' analysis. *Best Pract Res Clin Anaesthesiol.* 2011;25:263–276.

EMERGING AREAS OF ANESTHETIC MORBIDITY AND MORTALITY

Perioperative Human Error

Human error contribution to morbidity is a significant concern identified in 51% to 77% of anesthesia-related deaths.[4,9] Teamwork and communication represent human factors that cause adverse outcomes, contributing to 43% to 65% of sentinel events occurring in the operating room (e.g., wrong side/site, medication error, transfusion error). Communication breakdown (oral 36%, written 20%) and absence of help (44% of failures) when needed also contribute to morbidity.[4] Newer anesthetic medications are safer than ever before; however, drug errors occur relatively frequently, 1 of every 113 to 450 anesthetics administered.[13] Human factors related to complications are discussed in more detail later in this chapter.

The Parturient and Neonatal Resuscitation

Anesthetic complications in the parturient are the seventh leading cause of pregnancy-related mortality in the United States, accounting for 1.6% of all pregnancy-related deaths. Parturients are approximately 17 times more likely to die from general anesthesia than neuraxial anesthesia.[10] An 18-year retrospective study of maternal mortality was conducted in the state of Michigan. Eight anesthesia-related and seven anesthesia-contributing maternal deaths were cited, and the pattern of deaths illustrates three key points. First, all anesthesia-related deaths from airway obstruction or hypoventilation took place during emergence and recovery, not during induction of general anesthesia. Second, system errors contributed to the majority of deaths, for example, lapses in standard postoperative monitoring or missed diagnoses (e.g., cardiomyopathy, ischemic heart disease, sleep apnea). Third, obesity and African descent were important risk factors associated with anesthesia-related maternal mortality.[14]

Closed claims for newborn death and severe brain damage formed 20% of 263 obstetric anesthesia malpractice claims from 2000 to 2010 as a result of anesthesia provider "Good Samaritan" resuscitation intervention. In contrast, 71% of obstetric anesthesia claims were for maternal injuries, consistent with the anesthesia

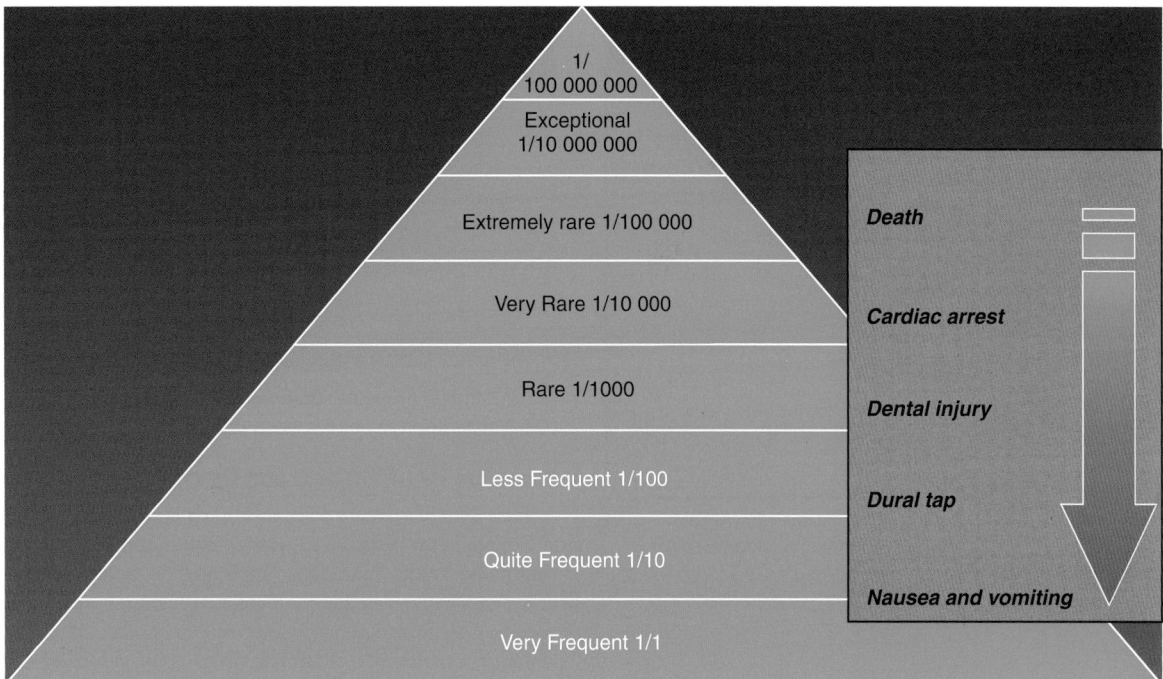

Fig. 59.1 Anesthesia morbidity. (From Haller G, et al. Morbidity in anaesthesia: today and tomorrow. *Best Pract Res Clin Anaesthesiol.* 2011;25[2]:123–132.)

provider's primary responsibility. Anesthesia care was thought to have contributed to some extent in only one-third (n = 25) of claims for newborn death/brain damage. Anesthesia delays, poor communication, and substandard care occurred more frequently when anesthesia care may have contributed to the newborn outcome. Anesthesia delays (15–67 minutes) were due to anesthesia provider being outside of the hospital or unavailable inside of the hospital, or inappropriate choice of regional rather than a general anesthesia. Thirty minutes or less decision-to-incision time for emergency cesarean section is controversial; however, failure to adhere to this interval is important in medical malpractice and contributes to the assessment of substandard care. Miscommunication was involved related to the level of urgency of the cesarean section and has been identified as the most frequent preventable cause of newborn death/brain damage. Other anesthetic causes contributing to newborn death/brain damage were maternal hypoxia due to difficult intubation or severe hypotension and hypoxia due to high block/total spinal.[15]

Acute and Chronic Pain

Future morbidity/mortality issues will likely include more acute and chronic pain issues, and regional anesthesia. Analysis of these rare events is imperative and can improve practice and ultimately patient safety. The proportion of anesthesia malpractice claims associated with chronic pain management has increased in 1980–2011 from 3% to 18%, reflecting an increased shift in chronic pain intervention. The three most common procedures cited in closed claims from 2000 to 2012 related to chronic pain were cervical injections (44%), lumbar injections (29%), and device implantation/maintenance/removal (27%). Claims related to cervical procedures were out of proportion to the frequency with which they are performed. These findings suggest that pain specialists should aggressively continue to search for safer and more effective strategies.[16,17]

Elderly (>70 Years of Age)

Several large studies using worldwide databases have been published with an attempt to identify elderly patient risk factors that could predict postoperative mortality. The most important resource available to date related to exploring complications and mortality after surgery is the National Surgical Quality Improvement Program (NSQIP) database in the United States. The NSQIP was established in the early 1990s as part of the US Veterans Health Administration, is now run by the American College of Surgeons, and contains data on millions of surgical patients. The database has been associated with hundreds of publications centered on perioperative risk.[18]

One such study from the NSQIP database extracted data on 25,000 patients aged 80 years or more and 550,000 patients aged less than 80 years, who had noncardiac surgery under general, spinal, or epidural anesthesia. In the cohort over 80 years of age, the top five variables associated with 30-day mortality were (1) ASA physical status, (2) preoperative plasma albumin concentration, (3) emergency surgery, (4) preoperative functional status, and (5) preoperative renal impairment.[18,19]

The Australian and New Zealand College of Anaesthetists Trials Group has published the Research into Elderly Patient Anaesthesia and Surgery Outcome Numbers (REASON) study, which is a prospective observational study of 4100 patients in 23 hospitals.[19,20] Patients 70 years and older undergoing noncardiac surgery and expected to stay at least 1 night in the hospital were included. The major findings of this study are that 1 in 20 patients (5%) died within 30 days of surgery, and 1 in 5 (20%) had at least one major complication within 5 days of surgery. Four preoperative factors emerged predicting postoperative mortality similar to the results of the NSQIP database study: age, ASA physical status, albumin, and those patients who had an accident and needed emergency surgery were at increased risk. A useful statistic from the REASON study is that patients aged 70 years, who were an ASA physical status 1 or 2, had a 30-day mortality of 1% for inpatient surgery. Patients 80 to 89 years had an odds ratio for 30-day mortality

TABLE 59.2 Factors Associated With Increased 30-Day Mortality

Factors	Odds Ratio Compared With Healthy 70-Year-Old Patients
Age 80–89	2.1
Age 90	4.0
ASA 3	3.1
ASA 4	12.4
Plasma albumin <30 g/L	2.8
Emergent surgery	1.8
Thoracic surgery	2.6
Systemic inflammation	2.5
Acute renal impairment	3.3
Unplanned ICU admission	3.1

ASA, American Society of Anesthetists; *ICU,* intensive care unit.
From Story DA, et al. Complications and mortality in older surgical patients in Australia and New Zealand (the REASON study): a multicentre, prospective, observational study. *Anaesthesia.* 2010;65(10):1022–1030.

of 2.1, meaning that this age group is twice as likely to die when compared with healthy patients 10 years younger. Additionally, patients who were 90 years of age had an odds ratio for 30-day mortality of 4.0 or are 4 times as likely to have postoperative mortality when compared with healthy patients in their 70s (Table 59.2). The most important postoperative complications were systemic inflammation, acute renal impairment, and unplanned critical care admission.[19,20]

One emerging area in the care of older patients is the attempt to define and quantify frailty and risk of postoperative complications. Five domains of frailty have been described as depicted in Box 59.3. They include age, sex, comorbidities, physical status, and type of surgeries. Patients with two or three domains are considered to have intermediate frailty, and those having four to five domains are classified as frail. The odds ratio is 2.0 for postoperative complications in those who are considered to have intermediate frailty and 2.5 for frail patients.[21] Frailty is the new addition to this paradigm. Risk assessment should begin with patient factors that are more strongly associated with outcome than type of operation. Preoperative albumin should be measured regularly in patients over 70 years of age.

Postoperative cognitive changes after anesthesia have been reported in the elderly for over a century, and more recently in children displaying behavioral and developmental disorders after anesthesia.[22] Postoperative cognitive problems can be categorized as postoperative cognitive dysfunction (POCD), delirium, dementia, confusion, learning, and memory problems. The two most common postoperative cognitive disorders in the elderly are delirium and POCD, and both can be difficult to diagnose. A comparison of these two disorders can be found in Table 59.3. The incidence of delirium is approximately 20% in hospitalized elderly patients, and 80% in sedated intensive care unit (ICU) patients. Delirium is independently associated with increased hospital stay and mortality. Recent randomized controlled trials (2016) suggest that pain management and depth of general anesthesia are important modifiable factors for postoperative delirium after hip fracture surgery. Regional anesthesia with light propofol sedation compared with deep sedation was associated with a 50% decrease in postoperative delirium.[23] Another study reported a 35% reduction in postoperative delirium after hip arthroplasty using a multifactorial approach. Perioperative interventions consisted of supplemental oxygen, systolic blood pressure greater than 90 mm Hg, transfusion for hemoglobin less than 10 g/dL, adequate pain relief, intravenous

BOX 59.3 Domains of Frailty Measurements

1. Unintentional weight loss
2. Exhaustion measured by assessing effort and motivation
3. Decreased grip strength
4. Slowed walking speed
5. Low physical activity

Poh AWY, Teo SP. Utility of frailty screening tools in older surgical patients. *Ann Geriatr Med Res.* 2020;24(2):75–82.

fluid supplementation, normothermia, avoidance of polypharmacy, spinal anesthesia, propofol sedation, and use of paracetamol (acetaminophen) in addition to opioids as needed.[24,25]

Pediatric Brain Growth and Development

A great deal of concern has recently emerged regarding the safety of anesthesia in the pediatric population and continues to be hotly debated. Anesthetic agents have been implicated in pediatric developmental delays in patients who have undergone prolonged and/or multiple procedures.[26] A growing body of evidence in animals suggests that under certain circumstances, anesthetic drugs could adversely affect neurologic, cognitive, and social development of neonates and young children.[26,27] Exposure to certain anesthetic agents during sensitive periods of brain development in animal studies has been postulated to result in widespread neuronal apoptosis and functional deficits later in development. So far, N-methyl-D-aspartate (NMDA) receptor antagonists and γ-aminobutyric acid (GABA) agonists have been implicated; however, no safe doses of these agents or safe duration of administration of these agents has been defined.[26,28] For example, 5-day-old nonhuman primates exposed to ketamine for either 9 or 24 hours experienced neuroapoptosis. A similar neurologic damaging effect was observed in the fetuses of pregnant rhesus monkeys (third trimester) exposed to ketamine for 24 hours. No effect was seen when ketamine exposure duration was 3 hours. Neuroapoptosis has also been demonstrated in primates given isoflurane on postnatal day 6.[27] The Food and Drug Administration and others are currently conducting more studies to address the neurocognitive and neurobehavioral aspects of anesthetic-induced apoptosis.

Studies in children have attempted to assess the effect of anesthetics on the developing human brain. A retrospective cohort analysis followed a birth cohort of 383 children who underwent inguinal hernia repair during the first 3 years of life and compared them with 5050 children in a control sample who had undergone no hernia repair before the age of 3 years. The children who underwent hernia repair were twice as likely as those who did not to have a developmental delay or behavioral disorder.[27] Another study (2011) retrospectively examined children (age <4 years) who were exposed to a single anesthetic (n = 449), two anesthetics (n = 100), or more (n = 44) and how this related to the development of learning disabilities. No increased risk of learning disabilities was found with a single anesthetic. However, significant increased risk of learning disabilities was associated with two or more anesthetics and increased with greater cumulative exposure to anesthesia.[28]

It appears that windows of anesthetic vulnerability exist that are dependent on the exposure time, amount, and type of anesthesia. However, no definitive conclusions can be drawn on the basis of these nonrandomized studies in humans because of the substantial potential for confounding and bias. Interpretation is difficult because of the retrospective nature of the studies; lack of precise information in terms of age, agent, duration, and dose of anesthetics; specific agents used; variable outcome endpoints used; and method outcomes that were assessed.[27] Although withholding anesthesia in children who

TABLE 59.3 Characteristics of Postoperative Cognitive Problems in the Elderly

Postoperative Cognitive Problem	Onset	Symptoms	Anesthetic Issues
Delirium	Acute: hours/days	Decreased awareness of environment Fluctuating course Hyperactive state • Increased psychomotor activity • Rapid speech • Irritability • Restlessness • Disruptive to others Hypoactive state • Calm appearance • Inattention • Decreased mobility • Difficulty answering simple orientation questions • May be confused with depression/fatigue	Avoid polypharmacy and long-acting sedatives (e.g., benzodiazepines) Use propofol, paracetamol, opioids as needed Regional techniques better Schedule surgery early after injury or illness Early geriatric consultation Effective pain management
POCD	Weeks/months (usually not detectable during first days after surgery)	Affects wide variety of cognitive domains • Memory • Information processing • Executive functionDifficult to manage job Impaired attention Normal consciousness	Recognize risk factors Anesthetic issues undefined

POCD, Postoperative cognitive dysfunction.
Adapted from Monk TG, Price CC. Postoperative cognitive disorders. *Curr Opin Crit Care.* 2011;17(4):376–381; Björkelund KB, et al. Reducing delirium in elderly patients with hip fracture: a multifactorial intervention study. *Acta Anaesthesiol Scand.* 2010;54(6):678–688.

need surgery is unreasonable, obtaining more information about safe use is imperative. If anesthetic agents are found to affect the developing brain, strategies for mitigating and managing such risks can be implemented.[26-29]

Adults With Congenital Heart Disease

A rapidly growing population of adults with congenital heart disease (CHD) is at increased risk of perioperative morbidity and mortality. A recent closed claims analysis revealed that over half of the damaging events in noncardiac cases occurred outside of the operating room, and less than half (48%) of all adverse events were directly related to the CHD. Over half of call adverse events were associated with cardiac surgery, compared with noncardiac procedure groups (orthopedic ambulatory surgery most common). Although many cases involved common anesthetic complications (e.g., awareness, positioning, postoperative respiratory complications), a lack of comprehensive expertise in CHD and poor recognition of implications of care were thought to be major contributors to poor patient outcomes.[30]

Intraoperative Cardiac Arrest

Currently cardiac arrest during anesthesia is usually a concomitant and not a causative factor. Incidence of intraoperative cardiac arrest has been cited as 0.2 to 1.1 per 10,000 adults and 1.4 to 2.9 per 10,000 children. The largest group of arrests were cited to occur between 51 and 70 years of age and with ASA physical status 3 and 4. Males comprised 61% of the cardiac arrest cases. Cardiac arrest during neuraxial anesthesia is less frequent compared to general anesthesia, with an incidence of 0.04 to 1.8 per 10,000 anesthetics.[31] Causative factors can be grouped into categories: preoperative complications (65%), surgical procedures (24%), intraoperative pathologic events (9%), and those attributable to anesthetic management (2%).[32,33] Excessive surgical bleeding can be identified in

70% of surgical procedure-related deaths, in addition to major causes of intraoperative pathologic events (e.g., myocardial ischemia, pulmonary embolism, and severe dysrhythmias). Most anesthesia-related cardiovascular complications included myocardial infarction, hypotension, ST segment depression, bradycardia, ventricular fibrillation, or myocarditis. Anesthesia-related cardiac arrest data from a large academic medical center reported a 70% mortality rate. This is the same mortality rate found for perioperative cardiac arrests not related to anesthesia.[31] Perioperative cardiac arrest is multifactorial in origin, including factors such as patient comorbidities, inadequate risk estimation, inappropriate anesthetic management, and human error or misjudgment.[32,33]

Supraglottic Devices and Endotracheal Intubation

Perioperative pulmonary complications are common, often equal to or outnumbering cardiac events. Pulmonary/respiratory events account for 17% of closed claims outcomes with brain damage and death being the most serious. There is no unifying definition of what constitutes a postoperative pulmonary complication (POPC). Commonly cited POPCs are listed in Box 59.4.[34] This discussion highlights the complications associated with manipulation and management of the airway.

Supraglottic Devices

Airway mortality does not happen because of failure to intubate. Airway mortality occurs as a result of failure to ventilate. A major challenge for any evidence-based evaluation of airway management techniques is the extremely low incidence of severe adverse events directly attributed to inadequate ventilation.

Incidence of difficult mask ventilation has been cited to be 1.4% to 5%.[35-37] A 2009 study of 94,630 anesthetics reported impossible mask ventilation in 0.2% of patients, and within this group 25% were also difficult to intubate.[37] Combined difficult mask ventilation and difficult intubation was encountered 0.4% of the time. Finally, the incidence of cannot ventilate–cannot intubate is a very small but devastating 0.008%.[38] Complications related to mask ventilation are underappreciated and underestimated (Box 59.5).

BOX 59.4 **Commonly Cited Postoperative Pulmonary Complications**

- Laryngospasm
- Bronchospasm
- Airway obstruction
- Desaturation
- Pneumonia
- Pulmonary embolism
- Clinically significant atelectasis
- Reintubation/mechanical ventilation for >48 hr
- Severe coughing
- Stridor
- Pleural effusion
- Pneumothorax
- Respiratory infection not otherwise specified
- Aspiration pneumonitis
- Worsening of obstructive sleep apnea
- Acute or worsening respiratory failure

From Johnson DC, Kaplan LJ. Perioperative pulmonary complications. *Curr Opin Crit Care.* 2011;17(4):362–369; Diaz-Fuentes G, Hashmi HR, Venkatram S. Perioperative evaluation of patients with pulmonary conditions undergoing non-cardiothoracic surgery. *Health Serv Insights.* 2016;9(1):S9–S23.

Many airway devices exist today to assist with difficult or cannot ventilate and/or difficult to intubate situations. A considerable body of evidence exists regarding successful use of the classic laryngeal mask airway (cLMA) in patients with difficult-to-manage airways.[39] The intubating LMA has also been used successfully 97% to 100% of the time for ventilation in both the anticipated and unanticipated difficult airway. Level 4 evidence of successful ventilation in patients with difficult airways was described for many other supraglottic devices in a 2011 review: LMA ProSeal, Supreme LMA, i-gel, Ambu Aura-I and air-Q intubating laryngeal airways, Cobra perilaryngeal airway, Cobra-PLUS, and Laryngeal Tube.[40,41] However, even with current evidence of successful use of various supraglottic devices in difficult airways, there is still not enough evidence to judge one individual device superior.

As useful as these devices are, they are not without complications. The LMA has been associated with inadequate seal, induced laryngospasm, and aspiration of gastric contents. Failed placement has been documented to occur in 1% to 5% of patients, although this decreases with operator experience. Other supraglottic device complications tend to be similar to those found with the LMA and result from cuff overfilling, dislodgment, trauma during insertion, and insufficient anesthesia depth during insertion.[38]

Endotracheal Intubation

The phrase "cannot intubate" represents an infrequent but serious challenge for the provider, but it also represents increased anesthetic risk to the patient. There is a close relationship between difficult intubation and traumatic intubation. Difficult intubation has been documented as a significant factor in 27% of all airway injury claims.[10] Eighty-seven percent of these were temporary, and 8% resulted in death. In 21% of claims, the standard of care was not performed.[38]

BOX 59.5 **Airway Management Complications**

Mask Ventilation
- Mucosal, skin irritation, conjunctivitis caused by cleansing agents
- Soft tissue damage from excessive pressure
- Corneal abrasion, retinal artery occlusion, blindness
- Damage to mandibular branch of facial nerve causing transient facial nerve paralysis
- Damage to mental nerves causing lower lip numbness
- Broken teeth, mucosal tears
- Worsening obstruction from malposition of tongue
- Subluxation of the temporomandibular joint
- Gastric distention increasing risk for aspiration
- Gastric rupture
- Subcutaneous emphysema

Laryngeal Mask Airway
- Folding of epiglottis tip causing labored breathing, coughing, laryngospasm, and obstruction
- Excess lubricant that causes coughing or laryngospasm
- Lack of protection from aspiration of gastric contents
- Laryngospasm, coughing
- Sore throat
- Increased intracuff pressures with prolonged procedures using nitrous oxide and carbon dioxide
- Dysarthria
- Edema of epiglottis, uvula, posterior pharyngeal wall
- Hypoglossal nerve paralysis
- Postobstruction pulmonary edema
- Tongue cyanosis

Endotracheal Intubation
- Damage to teeth
- Mucosal injuries
- Lip injuries
- Swelling tongue
- Sore throat
- Trauma to larynx/vocal cords
- Arytenoid dislocation/subluxation
- Tracheobronchial trauma
- Barotrauma
- Nerve injury
- Cervical spine injury
- Vocal cord paralysis
- Temporomandibular joint injury
- Laryngospasm
- Bronchospasm
- Hemodynamic perturbations

Extubation
- Hemodynamic perturbations
- Laryngospasm
- Laryngeal edema
- Bronchospasm
- Negative-pressure pulmonary edema
- Aspiration
- Airway compromise
- Difficult/accidental extubation

From Hagberg C, et al. Complications of managing the airway. *Best Pract Res Clin Anesthesiol.* 2005;19(4):641–659.

Inside the operating room, 67% of difficult intubations are encountered at induction of general anesthesia and are unanticipated.[10] Airway management plans when dealing with difficult airways must have backup plans that require the same level of thought as the primary airway plan. All airway plans can fail. Early recognition by the anesthesia provider that the current plan is not working and good communication throughout the procedure are both crucial. This may seem obvious, but unless all plans have been thought out, the clinical situation can quickly deteriorate. To date, fiberoptic intubation of the spontaneously breathing patient is the gold standard for elective intubation in the anticipated difficult airway.[42]

Video laryngoscopy has emerged as an alternative for anticipated difficult airway cases and has become widely available.[43] These devices may seem like a panacea for difficult airway management, but they have several limitations. Most devices are primarily designed for orotracheal intubation and require some mouth opening to allow the device to pass. Several case reports cite pharyngeal mucosal perforation and trauma from GlideScope use.[44-46] This complication could be minimized by increased vigilance and visual observation when passing the rigid stylet because there is a potential blind spot in the oropharynx when attention is focused on the GlideScope monitor. Care should be taken to cautiously pass the endotracheal tube and not use unnecessary force during insertion or a too-large laryngoscope blade. The introduction of sugammadex for neuromuscular blockade reversal as become an adjunct for difficult airway management, especially for the "cannot intubate, cannot ventilate" (CICV) scenario and should be actively sought out as an intervention early in CICV. After 5 minutes of apnea and several intubation attempts followed by sugammadex administration, patient outcomes still may be adversely affected.[10]

Complications of endotracheal intubation encompass both hemodynamic pathophysiologic effects and associated anatomic injuries (see Box 59.5). Fifty percent of dental trauma occurs during laryngoscopy; sore throat occurs as often as 40%, and occurs greater than 65% when blood is noted on airway instruments. Trauma to the larynx, although not as common, has been documented in 6.2% of cases, 4.5% of which developed vocal cord hematomas. Granulations of the laryngeal area can occur as a result of long-term intubation, and vocal cord paralysis can cause long-term hoarseness. Supraglottic complications induced by long-term intubation may be prevented by early tracheostomy.[38] For a more comprehensive list see Box 59.5.

INTRAOPERATIVE AWARENESS

Awareness during general anesthesia with explicit recall has been reported to occur in 1 to 2 per 1000 patients during general surgery when the Brice methodology/questionnaire is utilized for case identification[47,48] (Box 59.6). High-risk cases (e.g., trauma, obstetric, cardiovascular) possess 10 times the risk for awareness with an incidence of 1 case in 100[49,50] (Box 59.7). Patient movement has been cited in approximately one of every seven awareness case reports, and development of tachycardia and hypertension occurs in approximately one of every five episodes of awareness.[51,52]

MAC is an emerging concern in a surprising number of cases. Mashour et al.[49,50] examined 22,885 patients receiving MAC and found that 1 in every 3269 (0.03%) experienced awareness. Awareness was not related to pain but was a source of distress. Several patients reported hearing unwanted conversations and remembered bright lights during their procedure inconsistent with their expectations, making them distraught. Therefore it might be prudent to spend more time preparing patients for such experiences to avoid

BOX 59.6 Assessing Incidence of Awareness

Modified Brice Interview
- What was the last thing you remember before going to sleep?
- What is the first thing you remember after waking up?
- Do you remember anything between going to sleep and waking up?
- Did you dream during your procedure?
- What was the worst thing about your operation?

From Mashour GA, et al. Protocol for the Michigan Awareness Control Study: a prospective, randomized, controlled trial comparing electronic alerts based on bispectral index monitoring or minimum alveolar concentration for the prevention of intraoperative awareness. *BMC Anesthesiol.* 2009;9:7.

BOX 59.7 Risk Factors for Awareness

- Female sex
- Age (younger adults, but not children)
- Obesity
- Clinician experience
- Previous awareness
- After normal hours operations
- Emergency procedures
- Type of surgery (obstetric, cardiac, thoracic)
- Use of nondepolarizing relaxants

From Pandit JJ, et al. 5th National Audit Project (NAP5) on accidental awareness during general anaesthesia: protocol, methods, and analysis of data. *Br J Anaesth.* 2014;113(4):540–548.

disparities in expectations that could lead to complications of awareness, posttraumatic stress disorder (PTSD), future surgery apprehension, and enhanced medicolegal risks associated with anesthesia. The B-Aware trial (2004), a randomized controlled trial studying awareness, reported a 71% incidence of postawareness PTSD.[53] Not all patients who have documented intraoperative awareness develop PTSD, but initial emotional distress and the experience of paralysis have been cited as most predictive of developing PTSD. Postoperative sequelae reported related to PTSD include sleep disturbances (19%), nightmares (21%), fear of future anesthetics (20%), and daytime anxiety (17%).[52]

OPIATE-INDUCED RESPIRATORY DEPRESSION

Most opiate-related respiratory events were heralded by somnolence in 62% of written cases.[10,54] Of events resulting in death or permanent brain damage, 97% were thought to have been preventable with better monitoring/surveillance. Opiate-induced respiratory depression occurs in patients with obstructive sleep apnea (OSA), older individuals, premature infants (<60 weeks of postconceptual age), renal disease, cardiac disease, and pulmonary disease (e.g., COPD). Different opiates can pose variable risk such as the accumulation of active metabolites or long clearance half-lives (e.g., morphine/morphine-6-glucuronide). Hydromorphone has a delayed onset time, allowing for potential overdosing when patient-controlled analgesia settings are used. Closed Claims Project data examining opiate-induced respiratory depression additional patient risk factors included female gender (57%), obesity (66%), ASA physical status 1 and 2 (63%), age over 50 years (44%), lower extremity surgery (41%), and diagnosed OSA (16%).[54] Pulse oximetry combined with CO_2 monitoring with true respiratory rate monitoring provides the best recognition of incipient opiate respiratory depression.[10,54]

SEDATION AND ANESTHESIA OUTSIDE OF THE OPERATING ROOM

Administration of sedation/anesthesia outside of the operating room is expanding with little outcome data regarding complications and adverse events. Some out of operating room locations, increasingly utilizing anesthesia services, include gastroenterology and interventional radiology. Additionally, short, uncomfortable procedures (e.g., bone marrow biopsies, cardioversions) and procedures where the patient must lie still or can experience claustrophobia (magnetic resonance imaging, computed tomography scan) often require sedation and/or general anesthesia.[55] A survey of 5000 gastroenterologists' sedation practices revealed that 79% of endoscopy patients had sedation performed by nurses under the supervision of a gastroenterologist, whereas an anesthesia provider only administered 29% of all sedation within the endoscopy suite.[56]

Closed claims from anesthesia care outside of the operating room had a higher proportion of death that was primarily attributed to adverse respiratory events (44%). Respiratory depression secondary to oversedation and polypharmacy (propofol combined with other sedatives/analgesics) accounted for over one-third of the claims. Capnography was only employed in a minority of claims associated with oversedation (15%), and no respiratory monitoring was used in 15% of these claims.[55]

PREANESTHESIA SHARED DECISION MAKING AS COMPLICATION PREVENTION

Patients often have preferences for their health care, including anesthesia options, yet may feel intimidated or vulnerable when discussing their plans with anesthesia providers. The Picker Institute conducted a multiyear survey of patients' perceptions regarding most important health care delivery characteristics specifically related to quality and safety. Patients identified respect for individual values, preferences, and expressed needs and provision of high-quality information/education as two of the eight most important principles. Shared decision making has emerged as a method of communication with patients to encourage engagement related to treatments that have options. Shared decision making is best utilized when there is no medically "best" choice and any medical decisions are preference sensitive. Decision aids are evidence-based patient education tools often used in shared decision making related to a particular anesthetic choice or issue discussing anesthetic options and risks/benefits as well as probabilities of outcomes (e.g., peripheral nerve blocks, epidural and spinal anesthesia). Decision aids can take various forms, including computerized programs, videos, pamphlets, or checklists. A Cochrane review found that the use of decision aids led to enhanced patient knowledge, more accurate perceptions of risks, and more decisions that correlated with patients' values. Washington State legislature has incorporated medical legal protections for health care providers if shared decision making with use of decision aids is used.[57]

MANAGEMENT OF COMPLICATIONS

The aftermath of critical incidents and complications is equally as important as the incident itself because incident investigation is a prerequisite for learning about the actions and events surrounding the critical incident and for prevention.[58,59] It is important to view the critical incident from an organizational point of view after it has occurred. A critical incident is defined as an undesirable event during patient care that could have led to harm; an adverse event is an unintended injury to a patient as a result of health care management rather than the disease process, sufficiently serious to prolong hospital admission or to cause disability persisting after discharge or to contribute to death.[60] Patients, their families, supporting individuals, and health care professionals involved are all affected. Taking care of both the patient and the families is an important element of handling adverse events. Every health care organization should have a framework for handling critical events and complications embedded in effective communication between all parties involved, while also supporting the health care provider in the process.[58,59] There are many systematic approaches for handling critical incidents. Root cause analysis (RCA) is discussed in this chapter. It would be helpful for anesthesia providers to explore each institution's approach for handling critical incidents.

Incident Reporting

When a critical incident occurs, the anesthesia provider's first obligation is to protect the patient from further harm, providing the care required, and mitigating further injury. Continuation of patient care by the same team, at least for a short period of time, is up to the individuals involved in the critical incident.[58,59,61,62] After the critical incident has been stabilized, actions to secure the area, debrief the team, and analyze the incident should be taken. First, secure implicated drugs, equipment, and records for further investigation. Debrief all members of the care team as soon as possible so all members are fully aware of the issues and all subsequent communications are consistent with the patient and family. Decide immediately who will have primary responsibility for communicating with the patient and family about the event. Determine the circumstances surrounding the adverse events and factors contributing to it as quickly as possible while memories of those involved are fresh. This information can be crucial to the immediate clinical treatment plan for the patient, as well as for analysis of the situation. Report the event to the appropriate institutional officer.[62] A recent national study of nurse anesthetists' and student nurse anesthetists' experiences with a catastrophic perioperative event reported three emotional impact items: reliving the event (72%), guilt (70%), and anxiety (67%). Anger, depression, excessive sleepiness, and perceived loss of reputation were also statistically significant findings especially in those CRNAs with less than 5 years of experience.[63]

Root Cause Analysis

A retrospective analysis of the critical incident should ensue. One common methodology utilized is RCA, which is based on the premise that critical incidents and adverse events are caused, not by individual human errors, but by combinations of factors linked to organizational processes and structures, by which errors are missed and adverse events are not prevented.[64] The objective of an RCA is to systematically uncover multiple factors or causal chains that contribute to a critical incident, developing systems changes to make it less likely that the incident will recur. During this process, the importance of unbiased investigation and blame avoidance is important. The RCA process is organized in sequential steps, including (1) identifying the incidents/problem statement, (2) organizing a multidisciplinary team to conduct the RCA, (3) exploring processes involved, (4) collecting facts and written statements from all involved, (5) performing an evidence-based literature review, (6) identifying possible causes, (7) analyzing the data, (8) proposing possible actions, (9) writing a report, and (10) reevaluating actions taken.[65-67] There is also broad consensus that RCA represents various approaches rather than a single method. A commitment to using some sort of systematic and disciplined approach should remain.[67]

The first vital step in any RCA process is to identify the problem. Okes[66] has five components that should be answered when developing a problem statement (Table 59.4). The problem statement should represent cogent thinking and contain definitive, straightforward terminology that is well recognized and not misunderstood.

The second step calls for assembling a multidisciplinary group that will facilitate the process.

TABLE 59.4   Components of a Problem Statement When Conducting a Root Cause Analysis

What	What happened or should not have happened, or what change in performance is desired?
Where	Where specifically was the problem? This can be geographic, where in a process, and/or location on a piece of equipment.
Who	Who does this problem directly affect, either individual or group?
When	When was the problem first found or when did it begin?
How much	The frequency or magnitude of the problem: numbers provided should be absolute values plus percentages.

From Okes D. *Root Cause Analysis: The Core of Problem Solving and Corrective Action.* Milwaukee: American Society for Quality: Quality Press; 2009.

The third step seeks to understand the processes involved in and around the critical event. Why focus on process? Because everything individuals do on a daily basis is a process. Understanding the process is about stepping back and taking a broad view of the problem before jumping to possible causes. This step is especially important if the problem is thought to have been solved previously but has recurred.[66] Keep the process boundaries internal to the organization and limit them to those circumstances over which there is control. A flowchart diagram can be helpful for understanding the steps.

An example of a scenario would be a 48-year-old male undergoing a redo three-level laminectomy, who awakened with bilateral blurry vision, only able to see shadows. It was concluded that that patient had developed postoperative vision loss. Previous medical history included secondary hypertension and dyslipidemia. Vital signs included blood pressure 145/88 mm Hg, heart rate 78 beats/minute, respiratory rate 14 breaths/minute, and room air saturation 96%. Recent laboratory results included sodium 136 mEq/L, chloride 108 mEq/L, potassium 3.8 mEq/L, hemoglobin 14.3 g/dL, hematocrit 44%, and platelets 240 K/μL. The surgical procedure lasted 5.5 hours, and the total anesthesia time was 6.2 hours. Estimated blood loss was 850 mL. Fig. 59.2 shows a sample flowchart diagram related to the postoperative visual loss.

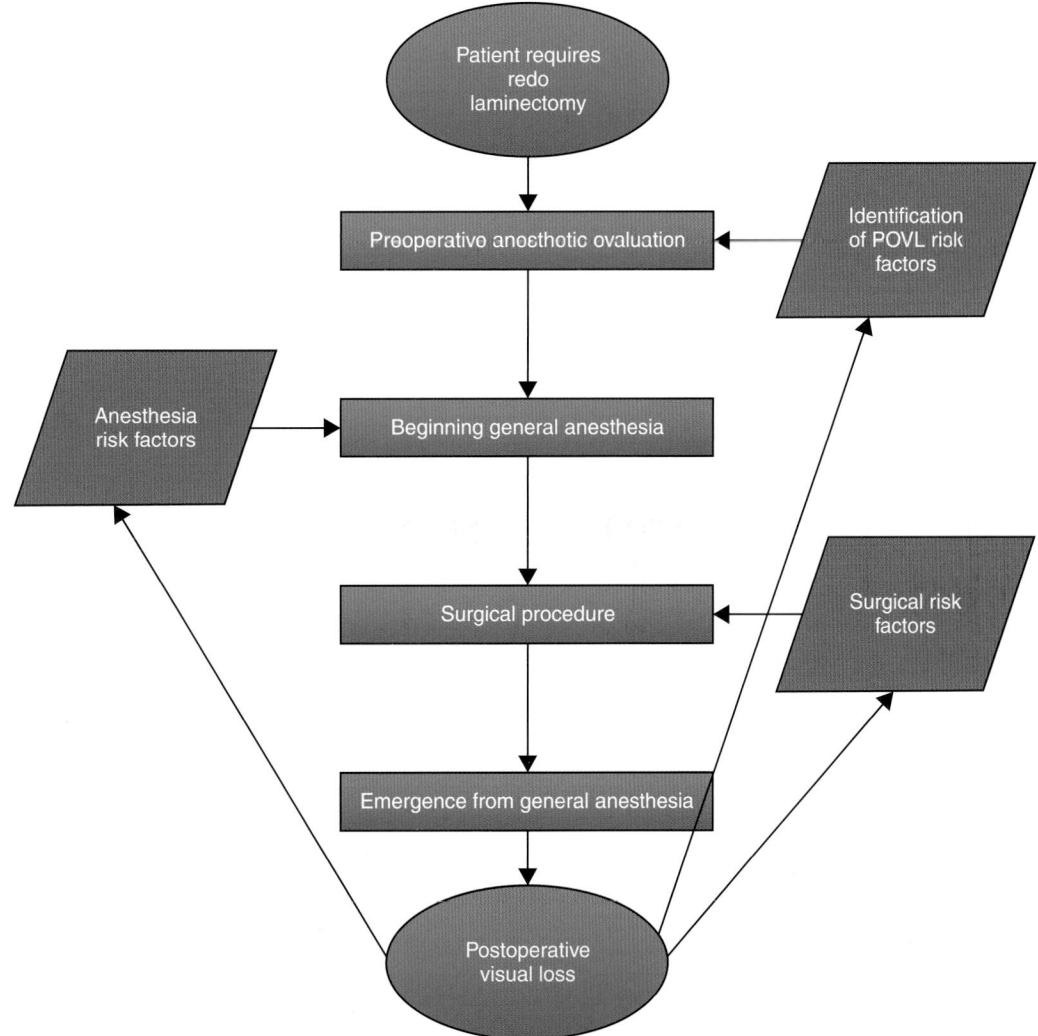

Fig. 59.2 Sample flowchart diagram for step 3, understanding the process, in a root cause analysis. *POVL,* Postoperative visual loss.

The fourth step entails collecting factual information and perspectives from individuals involved. This should be performed by one individual and compiled for future use by the multidisciplinary group.

The fifth step involves developing a search strategy using large databases to locate meaningful, best-available evidence to support, refute, or reveal new information related to the critical event being studied. The essence of evidence-based decision making includes locating the latest and highest quality information, combined with practitioner experience and skill, and incorporating the patient's desires as much as possible.[68]

Once all pertinent data have been accumulated, brainstorming for all possible causes occurs in the sixth step. Each brainstormed cause from the multidisciplinary group should ask the question "Why?" to form a connection to the critical event. A logic tree is helpful for depicting this thought process and for formulating relationships between each potential cause. An example of a logic tree related to the topic of postoperative visual loss in the scenario described earlier is shown in Fig. 59.3.[66] Notice that the tree is hierarchic. The top level of the logic tree is the problem statement (or shorter description), and the next level lists potential causes across

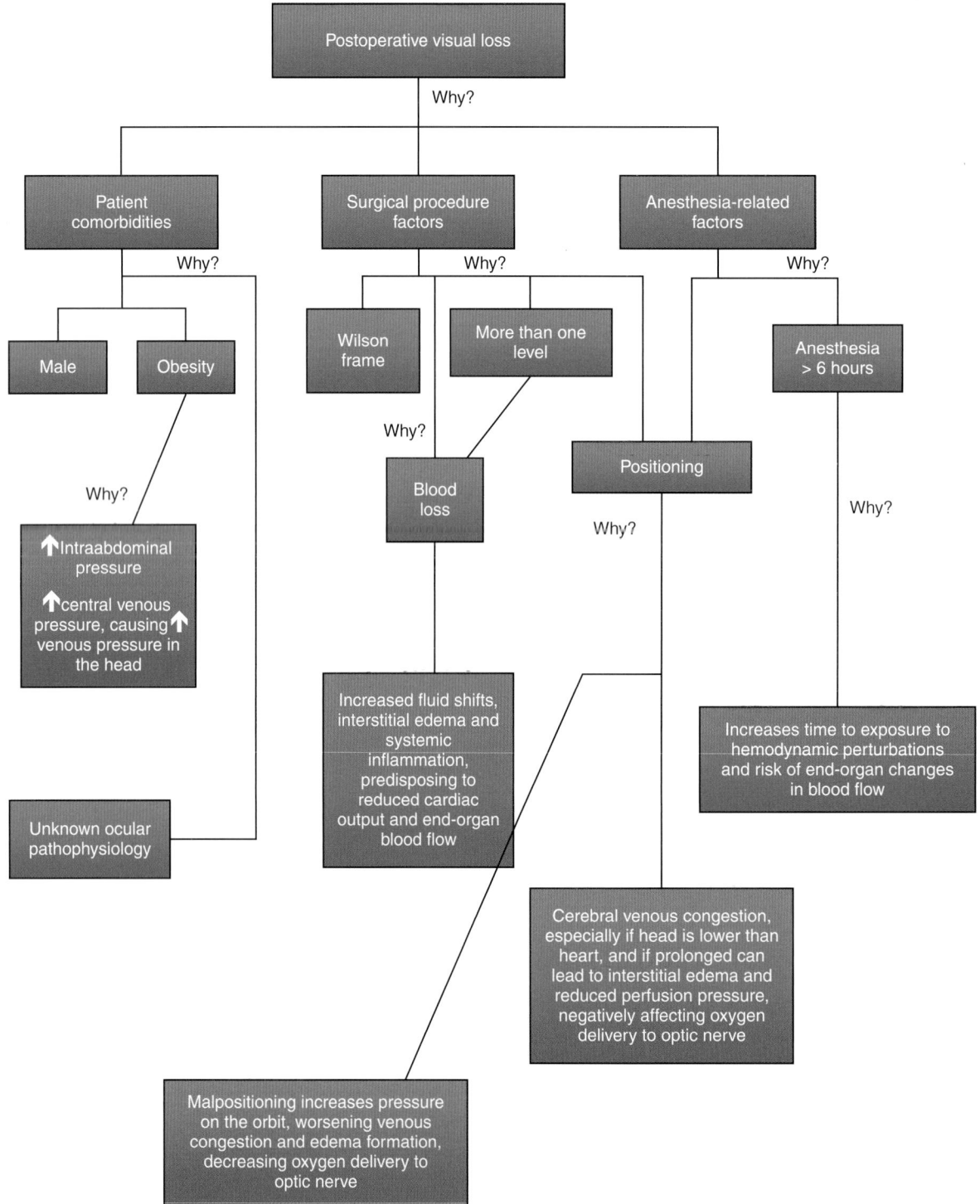

Fig. 59.3 Sample logic tree diagram for step 6, identifying potential cause, in a root cause analysis.

on the same level. Then each level below that should describe the causes. Each level of the tree is developed by asking "Why?" or how the previous step could have occurred. There is a recommendation to ask "Why" a minimum of five times to fully develop and ask the right question.[69]

The seventh step, data analysis, examines which of the causal theories appear plausible and which do not. Being clear about the theory (problem) to be tested and the data acquired to test for truth is important in analyzing each of the potential causes. Ask questions such as the following: What would the data look like if the theory (problem) were true? Do data collected support or deny the theory (problem) being tested? It is important to consider other conclusions the data might support, other ways to look at the same data, and other data that might confirm or deny the same conclusions. This is where the multidisciplinary group becomes very helpful. There are many ways to analyze data using a variety of diagrams and tools that are beyond the scope of this chapter. Please consult the References section of this chapter to view excellent sources for a more detailed approach to data analysis.[66]

The eighth step involves proposing possible actions related to the incident, event, or complication. This step should be embraced with caution as a tendency exists to formulate and accept only one idea or action that everyone thinks will work and then immediately implement it. Many tend to think that doing otherwise wastes time, but what is likely to happen is that the institution misses the opportunity to identify and implement breakthrough ideas. If a central idea has emerged, create a concept map expanding on that idea. The central idea is in the center of the diagram with lines connecting it to expanded or related concepts.[66,68,70]

Writing a formal report related to the RCA process is vital for a successful ninth step. There are many methods for constructing a report, but primarily, the report must be logical, cogent, and factual, and devoid of emotion or blame (Box 59.8).

The tenth step calls for reevaluation of actions taken within a certain predetermined time frame. Taking action without checking to see whether the process improvement worked is like shooting in the dark.[66]

A vital aspect of RCA is that during discussions of adverse events, focus on the individual is removed. Therefore it is less likely that defensive behavior will occur and more likely that reflection on

practice will occur openly. RCA can be used to reinforce good practice, support individuals involved in incidents so that they can come to terms with the event, and to explain to patients and families why care was suboptimal and what staff will do to prevent the event from recurring.[64]

Disclosure

Open disclosure of a critical incident and timely communication with patients and families is increasingly being emphasized and is largely responsible for decisions regarding legal action.[58,59] Open disclosure includes accurate information about the critical incident, immediate consequences and remedial action, expression of regret, and other information about preventing such an incident from occurring again. A survey of 958 adults (31% reported experience with medical errors involving either themselves or another family member) revealed that not disclosing information was associated with lower patient satisfaction, less trust, and stronger negative emotional responses. Patients and families have interpreted health care provider silence as hiding information, covering up errors, or showing a lack of respect. Patients and families who take legal actions related to critical incidents do so in an effort to prevent that incident from ever happening again; they want an explanation and often feel abandoned. Patients and family members desire to make the physicians/health care providers realize what they have done.[58,59] A recent interview study (n = 23) using open disclosure after a critical incident supported the positive aspects of open disclosure. All interviewees appreciated the opportunity to meet with staff to receive an explanation of the incident.[70] More research needs to be conducted in this area related to the full impact and techniques of open disclosure on patients, families, and health care providers. It is imperative that anesthesia providers comply with state law and/or institutional policies regarding disclosure and not view disclosure as an individual endeavor (Box 59.9).

THE SECOND VICTIM

Complications, from the healthcare providers perspective have been described as the darkest hour of their professional career.[71] Involvement of health care providers in critical incidents and the emotional turmoil that ensues is often regarded as taboo and to be avoided at all costs. No one wishes to be involved in the drama. Psychological stress and negative emotional responses can engulf the practitioner, creating serious health and performance deficits.[58,59,71,72] This practitioner is called the second victim: a health care provider involved in an unanticipated adverse patient event who becomes victimized. The second victim is often traumatized by the critical/adverse event. Frequently

---

BOX 59.8 Elements of a Root Cause Analysis Report

Executive Summary
- Incident description and consequences
- Preinvestigation risk assessment
- Background and context
- Terms of reference
- Members of the investigation team
- Scope and level of investigation
- Involvement and support of patient and relatives
- Involvement and support for staff involved

- Information and evidence gathered
- Chronology of events
- Detection of incident
- Notable practice
- Care and service delivery problems
- Contributory factors
- Root causes
- Lessons learned
- Recommendations
- Arrangements for shared learning
- Distribution

From Nicolini D, et al. Policy and practice in the use of root cause analysis to investigate clinical adverse events: mind the gap. *Soc Sci Med.* 2011;73(2):217–225.

BOX 59.9 Process for Effective Disclosure

- Continuation of care
- Acknowledgement of incident and patient consequences
- Information on what happened and what to expect
- Apology (when appropriate)/expression of regret
- Advice about necessary treatment
- Information about preventing recurrence
- Tangible support regarding physical, psychological, social, and financial consequences

From Iedema R, et al. Practising open disclosure: clinical incident communication and systems improvement. *Sociol Health Illn.* 2009; 31(2):262–277.

these individuals feel personally responsible and believe they have failed their patients and begin second-guessing their clinical skills and knowledge.[58,59,71] Some health care providers even report developing PTSD, sleep disturbances, and problems with irritability. As a result, it becomes harder to work clinically and have job satisfaction. Published evidence addressing emotional and health-related effects of critical incidents on health care providers have looked only at short-term outcomes. However, a 2006 prospective longitudinal study examining medical errors by residents (n = 184) over a 3-year period found that self-perceived errors were common among trainees. These errors were associated with significant personal distress, burnout, loss of empathy, and increased risk of making another error[73] Time to recovery from these symptoms lasted for several months.[72]

Stages of Recovery

Health care providers who have been involved in a critical incident often develop their own unique way of coping. Six stages of recovery have been identified (Box 59.10).[71] The moment the critical incident occurs, the involved clinician can usually describe chaotic and confusing scenarios of external and internal turmoil that ultimately lead to a realization about what happened. There is a period immediately after the incident of rapid inquiry to verify exactly what happened. Additional clinicians are summoned to provide support. The victim is frequently distracted, immersed in self-reflection, while also trying to manage a patient in crisis. The second stage is characterized by haunted reenactments, often accompanied by feelings of internal inadequacy. The victim reevaluates the situation repeatedly with "what if" questions. The third stage begins when the victim seeks support from a trusted individual, usually a colleague or supervisor, friend, or family member. One of the biggest challenges in this stage is an inability to move forward. Relentless introspection lingers related to "what others will think of me" and "if I will ever be trusted again." Then in the fourth stage, the individual wonders what the ramifications from the institution will be and "if I will ever practice again." Second victims in the fifth stage seek out respected and safe colleagues again to confide in, often related to litigation issues. The sixth stage is unique in that it describes the second victim as moving on—dropping out, surviving, or thriving.[71]

What do practitioners need emotionally and professionally after a critical incident involvement? Little evidence exists to address this issue, but four primary needs have been identified after a critical incident involvement: (1) talking to someone about what happened, (2) validation of the decision-making process, (3) reaffirmation of professional competence, and (4) personal reassurance.[58,59] Colleagues and supervisors are perceived as being the most helpful people with whom to discuss the situation. However, evidence suggests that little support is obtained at an organizational level. This lack of support after a critical incident often causes the negative emotional responses and psychological stress to be sustained.[71] Along with emotional needs there are definite professional needs that should also be met.

BOX 59.10   Stages of Second Victim Recovery

1. Chaos/accident response
2. Intrusive reflections
3. Restoring personal integrity
4. Enduring inquisition
5. Obtaining emotional first aid
6. Moving onward

From Scott SD, et al. Caring for our own: deploying a systemwide second victim rapid response team. *Jt Comm J Qual Patient Saf.* 2010; 36(5):233–240.

The anesthetist should consider speaking with the appropriate hospital administrators and possibly an attorney if there is litigation or expected litigation.[74]

THE HUMAN FACTOR IN COMPLICATIONS

Human Error

The term *human factors* describes human performance and behavior related to interaction with the environment.[75] Human factors have been identified in 51% to 77% of anesthesia-related deaths.[11] Many cases are related to a lack of experience or competence observed in 89% of human failure–related deaths. Less frequently, errors of judgment or analysis have been detected in 11% of these deaths.[4]

The topic of human error is rich in myths such as error is intrinsically bad, bad people make bad errors, and errors are random and highly variable. Errors are not intrinsically bad, but instead are essential for coping with trial-and-error learning in novel situations. One of the basic rules of error management is that the best people can make the worst errors. Errors do not occur "out of the blue" but can take on recurrent and predictable forms. Different errors occur in different situations. Errors can happen when individuals know what they are doing, but actions do not go as planned, taking the form of absentminded slips and memory lapses. Errors also can happen when individuals think they know what they are doing, as in dealing with what appears to be a trained-for problem but then misapply a normally good rule, apply a bad rule, or fail to apply a good rule. Errors are certain to occur when individuals are not sure what they are doing.[61]

Past concepts related to human error in health care have not embraced the statement that human error is inevitable, but tried to avoid or prevent human error, doing so without success.[76] It has been argued that judgments of human error should form the starting point of accident investigations, not be the explanation for the failure.[76,77] Human involvement in complex systems is necessary and beneficial because of our ability to adapt, our creativity, and our ability to be flexible.[76] This relevance of human factors in improving safety cannot be overstated. Even though we cannot change the human condition, we can change the conditions under which humans work.[61]

The aviation industry realized, embraced, and acted upon optimizing human factors to decrease human error more than 20 years ago. A systematic approach to safety at an organizational level is currently in practice in the aviation industry and recommended as an approach to dealing with human factors in anesthesia. This type of safety culture possesses certain features such as standard operating procedures, operations manuals, and checklists that could be incorporated into anesthetic practice; however, there is a certain amount of reluctance to embrace these tools, perhaps for fear of being constrained in exercising clinical judgment and critical thinking in addition to being forced to forego practical long-standing techniques.[76]

A key concept related to human factors is the concept of resilience. *Resilience* is an everyday word synonymous with *buoyant*, *elastic*, and *flexible*, and it can describe an individual's ability to recover readily from illness, depression, or some other life adversity. The human factor perspective of resilience refers to the ability to understand how failure is avoided and how to learn from successes and error avoidance rather than simply conduct a reactive search for causes and remedies. It offers a systems-based approach to understanding how to stay safe proactively. Resilience is a positive human attribute that can be used to bounce back from errors made, learn from mistakes, and move forward. Resilience has the potential to provide significant advances in patient safety by shifting focus from an emphasis on human error and error counting to preventing these errors from being repeated.[77-79]

Human factors that contribute to complications often include nontechnical skills and behaviors. Lack of communication and teamwork contribute up to 80% of sentinel events occurring in the operating room (e.g., wrong side, transfusion error). The specialty of anesthesia has made huge strides in identifying human factors that lead to adverse events by examining the aviation industry. For example, poor flight team performance and a series of plane crashes in the 1980s became the trigger for the development of aviation's crew resource management (CRM).[80] Subsequently in the mid-1990s CRM was adapted to anesthesia practice in the form of anesthesia crisis resource management (ACRM) by Gaba et al.[81] Subsequently, the development of a behavioral marker system framework identifying and describing daily behaviors of good and poor anesthesia practice has been developed, called Anaesthetists' Non-Technical Skills (ANTS).[82] A rating tool also exists utilizing this ANTS framework (Fig. 59.4).[83]

Communication is fundamental in ACRM and ANTS to foster workplace efficiency and safety. Elements of good communication are not just verbal but also nonverbal (Box 59.11). Good communication is a major part of good teamwork. Teamwork represents a distinguishable set of two or more people who interact dynamically, interdependently, and adaptively toward achieving a common goal, who have each been assigned specific roles or functions to perform, and who have a limited life span of membership (Box 59.12). Effective teamwork and communication do not happen alone but must be developed through training. Training individuals working in a team is based on developing competence, knowledge, skills, and attitude of individuals in addition to training objectives. Teams should develop identity, in which team members learn their own roles and tasks and understand those of other team members.[61,82] Simulation provides a teaching and learning methodology that allows team members to practice ACRM and develop nontechnical skills and behaviors to improve teamwork and communication.[4]

Distractions in the Anesthesia Work Environment

All types of perioperative distractions affect vigilance, situational awareness, and the ability to respond promptly to adverse effects, posing additional patient safety risks. Externally imposed distractions include interruptions from the environment, other operating room team members, or technology. Internally motivated distractions are under complete control of the anesthesia provider and include looking up patient information on the electronic medical record (EMR) and locating health care information on the internet; distractions can also be nonpatient related (e.g., texting, checking emails).[84] Limited data exist on the role of distracted behavior causing patient harm. Closed claims data report 10 (of 5822) injury claims related to distraction in the operating room.[85] The majority of these claims included reading printed materials, phone calls, and loud music. Recommendations from the Anesthesia Patient Safety Foundation include using the "sterile cockpit" approach during critical periods, prioritizing alarms, and defining what is not permitted on facility-provided computers. Table 59.5 provides a complete list of recommendations.[84]

Fatigue

Fatigue is the largest identifiable and preventable cause of accidents. The aviation industry estimates that fatigue may involve 4% to 7% of civilian aviation accidents and anywhere between 4% and 25% of military aviation accidents.[82,86] Fatigue, anesthesia, and complications have not traditionally been discussed together but are an expanding science of interest and a significant safety concern. Anesthesia care

is a 24/7 profession, and consequently, this can require long working hours, sustained vigilance, unpredictability of stressful situations, and production pressure.[82] Currently, no quantitative data exist regarding the incidence of complications in anesthesia related to the fatigued provider. Reducing work hours and allowing 24 hours of sleep time between shifts significantly impacted attentional failures (i.e., intrusion of slow rolling eye movements into confirmed episodes of wakefulness during work hours) in a small prospective study with interns.[86] The Joint Commission has published evidence-based actions that health care organizations can incorporate to help mitigate the risks of fatigue (Box 59.13).[87]

Stress

Every anesthesia provider knows what it feels like to be under stress, both professionally and personally. Stress can have both acute and chronic effects. Acute stress in humans can be related to the classic fight, flight, or freeze response.[75,83] Chronic stress is related to conditions in the workplace and the individual's reaction to these over a period of time. Stress has been linked to safety outcomes such as accident involvement. Because stress has been linked to accident involvement and safety outcomes, the ability to recognize and manage stress in self and others is an important nontechnical skill. Job demands, control over work activities, support, or lack thereof from managers or coworkers, poor relationships, uncertain work roles, uncertainty about change, and family-personal problems are all considered stressors. How each individual handles these with the resources available to them using prior experience, training, personality, fitness, social support, and coping strategies will indicate whether the stress will have a positive or negative effect on the individual. The effects of stress on behavior are generally the most readily observable by work colleagues (Table 59.6). For example, a normally peaceful coworker becomes irritable, or a colleague who generally has a neat appearance begins to take less interest in one's self.

Patient Handoff/Communication

Communication issues and breakdowns in communication have been estimated to contribute between 15% and 67% to the development of critical incidents.[88] In particular, communication at organizational interfaces (e.g., care transitions, shift changes) with changing responsibility for care is a key target for improvement.[89] A surgical patient undergoing elective surgery can have direct patient care change a minimum of at least four times (e.g., admission area, to surgery/anesthesia, to postanesthesia care area, to unit/floor).

A clinical handover/handoff or transfer of care is by definition "the transfer of professional responsibility and accountability for some or all aspects of care for a patient, groups of patients to another person or professional group on a temporary or permanent basis."[58,59,89-91] The Joint Commission defines handoffs as the real-time process of passing patient-specific information from one caregiver to another or from one team of caregivers to another for the purpose of ensuring the continuity and safety of patient care.[92]

Historically, patient handover has not been studied systematically, which is in stark contrast to other high-risk industries where handovers have received considerable attention. Qualitative studies and surveys across different health care settings cite that handover processes are highly variable with widespread dissatisfaction among physicians and nurses.[58,59,88] As a result, patient handover has been recognized as a safety initiative by the World Health Organization (WHO) Alliance for Patient Safety and the WHO Collaborating Center for Patient Safety and is listed as one of the National Patient Safety Goals by The Joint Commission.[92] There has been a substantial increase in research

ANTS System –Observation and Rating Sheet

Consultant:_____
Trainee:_____
Date: _____

Categories	Elements	Observations	Element Rating	Debriefing notes and category rating
Task Management	Planning & preparing			
	Prioritising			
	Providing & maintaining standards			
	Identifying and utilising resources			
Team Working	Co-ordinating activities with team			
	Exchanging information			
	Using authority & assertiveness			
	Assessing capabilities			
	Supporting others			
Situation Awareness	Gathering information			
	Recognising & understanding			
	Anticipating			
Decision Making	Identifying options			
	Balancing risks & selecting options			
	Re-evaluating			

ANTS System –Observation and Rating Sheet

Additional Notes

Rating Options	Descriptor
4 – Good	Performance was of a consistently high standard, enhancing patient safety; it could be used as a positive example for others
3 – Acceptable	Performance was of a satisfactory standard but could be improved
2 – Marginal	Performance indicated cause for concern, considerable improvement is needed
1 – Poor	Performance endangered or potentially endangered patient safety, serious remediation is required
Not observed	Skill could not be observed in this scenario

ANTS System-Observation and Rating Sheet. 2004. (Accessed May 1, 2006, at
http://www.abdn.ac.uk/iprc/papers%20reports/Ants/ANTS%20System%20Observation%20Rating%20Sheet.doc.)

Fig. 59.4 Anaesthetists' Non-Technical Skills (ANTS) system observation and rating sheet. (From University of Aberdeen. Anaesthetists' Non-Technical Skills [ANTS] System Handbook. V1.0. Framework for Observing and Rating Anaesthetists' Non-Technical Skills. 2015. https://www.abdn.ac.uk/news/8202/. Accessed August 1, 2020.)

activity and literature reviews across health care disciplines focusing on a specific type of handover in a specific clinical setting (e.g., nursing, physicians, perioperative care area)[88,93,94] (Fig. 59.5).

Certain handoff attributes contribute to potential complications such as truncated handoffs and omission of information resulting from work demands or time constraints, unfinished diagnostic and care activities, or a perceived lack of trust or familiarity with the participating individual.[95,96] A self-reporting survey among 133 residents found that 31% had experienced an issue for which the handover had not prepared them.[97] Another study (2010) reviewing 2729 critical incidents found that the most frequent type of handover incident reported, besides an incomplete handover (45.2%), was no handover at all (29.3%).[98]

Information transfer and communication (ITC) across the entire surgical care pathway in patients undergoing major gastrointestinal procedures was assessed. Most ITC failures were observed during the preoperative phase (61.7%) and postoperative handover (52.4%). Seventy-five percent of patients had clinical incidents or adverse events because of ITC failures.

So what constitutes a handover that contributes to the quality and safety of patient care? Quality of the handover depends on the perception as to what is the primary function of the handover (e.g., information or responsibility transfer, shared decision making).[58,59,89,90] Handover quality measures can be grouped into five areas: (1) information delivery or transfer, (2) responsibility/accountability, (3) context and environments, (4) the handover process, and (5) handover outcome.[79,88] For a conceptual model of handover elements, see Fig. 59.5.

Measures of handover content appear to be straightforward, but which items should be included in a list for a quality handoff can vary depending on the clinical setting, timing, and individual perceptions and experience.[58,59] The list can often become lengthy and generate heated discussions. Most handover content should concentrate on

---

BOX 59.11 Elements of Effective Communication

- Send information clearly and concisely
- Include context and intent during information exchange
- Receive information, especially by listening
- Identify and address barriers to communication

From Flin R, et al. *Safety at the Sharp End: A Guide to Non-Technical Skills*. Burlington, VT: Ashgate Publishing Ltd; 2008.

BOX 59.12 Elements of Effective Team Work

- Supporting others
- Solving conflicts
- Exchanging information
- Coordinating activities

From Flin R, et al. *Safety at the Sharp End: A Guide to Non-Technical Skills*. Burlington, VT: Ashgate Publishing Ltd; 2008.

BOX 59.13 The Joint Commission Action Suggestions for Health Care Provider Fatigue

1. Assess organizational fatigue-related risks (e.g., shift hours)
2. Assess patient handoff processes
3. Invite staff input for schedule design to promote less fatigue
4. Create and implement a fatigue management plan to help fight fatigue
   a. Conversation
   b. Strategic caffeination
   c. Short naps (<45 min)
5. Educate staff about sleep hygiene and effects on patient safety
6. Provide opportunities for expressing concerns about fatigue
7. Encourage teamwork as a strategy to support staff working extended hours
8. Consider fatigue potentially contributing to adverse events

From Jeffcott SA, et al. Improving measurement in clinical handover. *Qual Saf Health Care.* 2009;18(4):272–277.

TABLE 59.5 Anesthesia Patient Safety Foundation Recommendations With Associated Potential Interventions

Recommendation	Potential Interventions
Eliminate unnecessary clinical distractions and minimize unavoidable distractions	Use "sterile cockpit" approach during critical periods, prioritize alarms, and define clearly what is not permitted on facility-provided computers
Minimize avoidable distractions	Create and follow a well-defined, risk-stratified policy for acceptable and unacceptable use of personal electronic devices
Reduce environmental noise	Modulate music volume in clinical environment
Address factors that can worsen effects of distraction	Develop and promote best practice stress and fatigue/sleep deprivation management strategies
Apply human factors engineering to improve technologies	Distraction should be considered in design and implementation of all medical technology in perioperative area
Foster a culture of high reliability and safety	Use teamwork, communication, conflict resolution via simulation-based methods
Utilize professional society guidelines and tool kits	Disseminate materials already developed by AANA, ACS, AORN, ASA
Develop/implement local policies/guidelines	Create local guidelines and policies derived from national guidelines and best practices
Prioritize compliance and accountability	Increase local measurement, reporting, and appropriate consequences for deviation from local distraction management
Intensify research	Conduct more research on impact of local interventions on distraction occurrence and effect
Learn more from other industries	Formulate and explore multidisciplinary collaborations to facilitate research, education, and policy development

AANA, American Association of Nurse Anesthetists; *ACS,* American College of Surgeons; *AORN,* Association of Perioperative Registered Nurses; *ASA,* American Society of Anesthesiologists.
From Van Pelt M, Weinger J. Distractions in the anesthesia work environment: impact on patient safety. Anesthesia Patient Safety Foundation Newsletter. www.apsf.org/wp-content/uploads/newsletters/2017/Oct/pdf/APSF201710.pdf. Accessed August 1, 2020.

TABLE 59.6	Indicators of Chronic Stress			
Behavioral	**Emotional**	**Somatic**	**Thinking**	**Organizational**
• Absenteeism	• Anxiety	• Decline in physical appearance	• Lack of concentration	• High staff turnover
• Abuse of drugs	• Hopelessness	• Chronic fatigue	• Reduced attention	• Absenteeism
• Hostile behavior	• Cynicism	• Frequent infections	• Difficulty in remembering	• Poor timekeeping
• Apathy	• Resentfulness	• Health complaints (e.g., headache, stomach)	• Impaired decision making	• Decreased productivity
• Reduced productivity	• Depression		• Failures in planning	• Increased client complaints
• Distracted	• Irritability			• Increased employee compensation claims
• Careless errors				• More near-misses and accidents

From Flin R, et al. *Safety at the Sharp End: A Guide to Non-Technical Skills.* Burlington, VT: Ashgate Publishing Ltd; 2008.

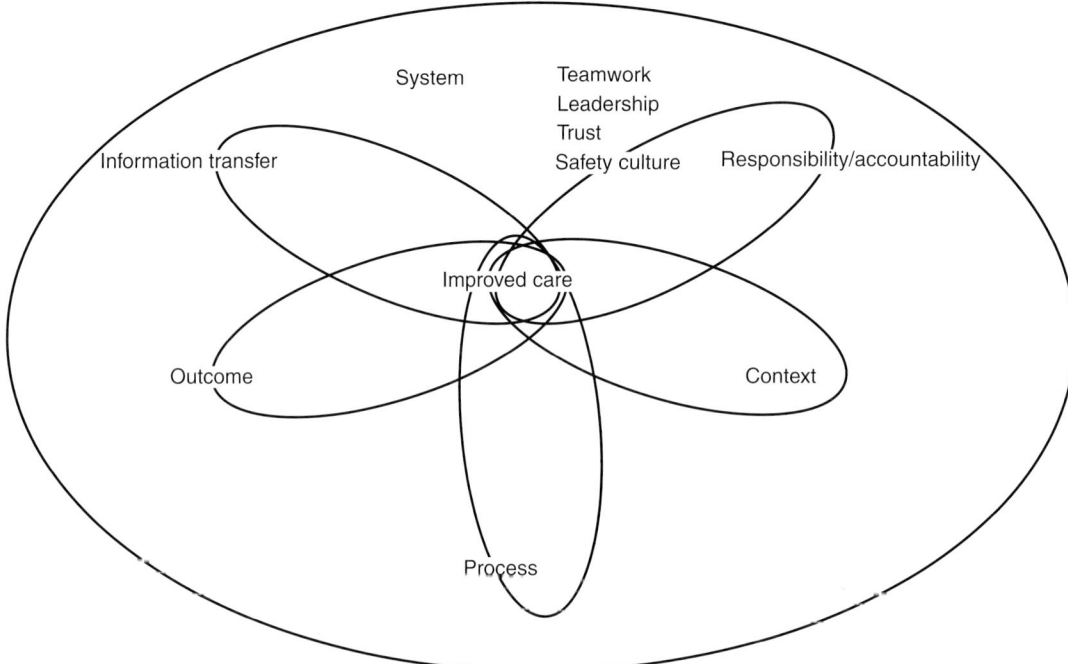

Fig. 59.5 Conceptual model of handover elements. (From Jeffcott SA, et al. Improving measurement in clinical handover. *Qual Saf Health Care.* 2009;18[4]:272–277.)

completeness and accuracy of information and related errors. Purely verbal handovers have been found to be the most incomplete when compared with information available in the patient record or located in a predefined protocol[89,90,95] A noisy operating room and an anesthetist that is in a hurry may not create the optimal handover process, leaving a gap for crucial information to be missed. The generation of evidence in this area is extremely limited, and there is still an open question regarding how various process measures translate into safe care.[58,59,89,90]

Handover outcome measures usually include health care provider satisfaction. An observational study conducted in three different clinical settings (e.g., paramedic to emergency room, anesthetist to postanesthesia care unit (PACU), and PACU to floor/unit nurse) found that although information transfer was the key characteristic, overall handover quality was predicted by three factors: information transfer, shared understanding, and working atmosphere.[58,59,89,90]

Professional organizations have published guidelines for handover communication, and standard approaches do exist that can improve handover communication. Study outcomes evaluating adherence to a protocol for handovers demonstrated statistically significant improvement in handover quality and improved teamwork.[99] Another

approach focuses on general interaction structures and does not define actual content but instead focuses on an order of topics to be covered. Both approaches have demonstrated improvements in teamwork and communication, which are factors that have translated into a significant reduction in morbidity and mortality in surgical patients.

An emerging area related to communication and handovers is incorporating a shared understanding among a health care team during a handover so that a handover is not a one-person–one-way process. An ideal patient handover conducted as a team-based activity would comprise an episode of shared cognition and understanding among health care providers and an opportunity for collaborative cross-checking. In this view, handovers represent a source of resilience for health care systems.

Standardized handovers in anesthesia have been proposed. One approach to handover content defines specific content to be included and also an order in which the information should be presented using a checklist-type format. A second approach focuses on the environment and general interaction structures without any defined content.[58,59]

The EMR system has been proposed as one solution that provides a handover sheet that can easily be extracted to improve completeness of handover information. Arora et al.[89,90] systematically reviewed studies reporting interventions for improving patient handovers and found that technology solutions were associated with a reduction in preventable adverse events and improved satisfaction with handoff quality, and they improved provider identification. Technology, however, ignores behavioral and cultural aspects of communication and does not necessarily improve communication.

SUMMARY

Perioperative complications will occur. It is important not only to recognize and understand how and why complications arise but also to systematically deal with postcomplication issues. It is important to recognize the effect of local culture as a key underpinning for process improvement. A culture of blame is no longer acceptable and should not be supported.[58,59] Learning from a critical incident can be both prospective (deliberating in advance of process changes and how they might affect safety) and retrospective (learning from events that have already transpired). It should be reinforced that errors are not always the cause of accidents, and blaming an individual may hinder uncovering a latent error or problem in the system. If reporting is safe and provides useful information from expert analysis, then it can measurably improve safety.

REFERENCES

For a complete list of references for this chapter, scan this QR code with any smartphone code reader app, or visit the following URL: http://booksite.elsevier.com/9780323711944/.

60

Crisis Resource Management and Patient Safety

Cormac O'Sullivan, Heather Bair

In 1999, the Institute of Medicine shocked the public when they informed Americans that medical errors were responsible for between 44,000 and 98,000 deaths annually in the years just prior to 1999.[1] *To Err Is Human* and *Crossing the Quality Chasm,* published in 2001, started the greatest push for increased patient safety in the history of the US health care system. Despite the immense efforts to improve patient safety and health care outcomes, a 2013 study estimated that health care errors may be responsible for upwards of 200,000 to 400,000 preventable deaths per year.[2] Considering that in the current health care environment there is an increased number of surgeries, higher acuity of patients, time pressures to accomplish more with less, and a global pandemic, it is possible that the rates of adverse events in various health care settings increases.

Health care providers are more likely to make critical decisions and manage crises on a regular basis than almost any other professional except maybe front-line emergency responders. A crisis can be defined as "an unstable, crucial time or state of affairs in which a decisive change is impending…one with a distinct possibility of a highly undesirable outcome."[4] This definition could be expanded to envision a perioperative crisis as the point during a surgical procedure where a decisive change occurs, leading to recovery, disability, or death. Many, if not all, of the decisions made by anesthesia providers during their daily work could result in a life and death situation. Daily actions of Certified Registered Nurse Anesthetists (CRNAs) such as induction, intubation, extubation, conscious sedation, central neuraxial blockade, or peripheral nerve blocks have the potential to cause significant patient injury or even mortality. A crisis may occur due to a cannot intubate/cannot ventilate situation, or something as simple as administering a medication that results in a severe allergic reaction. Any crisis situation could result in an undesirable outcome if not properly and efficiently managed. This is the nature of anesthesia practice. A primary goal of this chapter will be to discuss crisis resource management and its relationship to patient safety. The latter half of the chapter will discuss interdisciplinary team crisis simulations focused on appropriate management, with the goal of improving patient outcomes.

HEALTH CARE CRISES EVENTS

Health care crises, also referred to as adverse patient events, happen during surgery and anesthesia (Fig. 60.1). Malignant hyperthermia (MH) occurs in 1:30,000 to 1:100,000 pediatric or adult anesthetics.[5] The incidence of local anesthetic systemic toxicity (LAST) is estimated at 0.27 to 1.8 times per every 1000 peripheral regional anesthesia blocks.[6] Intraoperative cardiac arrest is reported to occur 0.2 to 1.1 times per 10,000 surgeries in adults and 1.4 to 4.6 times per 10,000 surgeries in children.[7] The rates of perioperative cardiac arrest rise for elderly patients and for emergent surgery.[7] There is up to a 70% mortality (within 30 days) for those patients who experience a perioperative cardiac arrest. For the remaining 30% who slighlty less than half of those have a functionally good outcome 90 days after surgery.[8,9] A comprehensive discussion of anesthesia complications, risks, related factors, and analysis of health care outcomes can be examined in Chapter 59. Events such as anaphylaxis, MH, LAST, massive hemorrhage, cardiac arrest, or a cannot intubate/cannot ventilate airway are uncommon, however, when they occur, even when managed well, may result in a poor (permanent disability) or even catastrophic (death) outcome. The rarity of such events leads to a lack of experience treating these emergencies, and increases the likelihood of providers making errors during management.[10] To further complicate matters, it is unlikely the team that is assembled to perform the surgery has ever encountered such an emergency together as a group. The team members may not even work together regularly. How a crisis is managed, how quickly it is recognized, how rapidly help is summoned, how efficiently evidence-based interventions are applied, and the effectiveness of team communication throughout the emergency each have a significant impact on patient outcome.[3,11,12] Lack of experience, lack of competence, and errors of judgment lead to human errors, which were identified in 51% to 77% of anesthesia-related deaths in a French study.[13] Teamwork and communication errors, written and oral communication breakdowns, and an absence of help have all been identified as significant factors during crises and sentinel events.[12]

CRISIS RESOURCE MANAGEMENT

The collective actions of a team during a health care crisis is referred to as crisis resource management (CRM). CRM began in the aviation industry as cockpit "crew" resource management in the 1970s.[14] Analysis of aviation accidents by the National Transportation Safety Board and the National Aeronautics and Space Administration concluded the majority of "errors" were due to deficiencies in communication, workload management, delegation of tasks, situational awareness, leadership, and the appropriate use of resources. Throughout the 1970s and 1980s, military and commercial airlines throughout the world combined research from psychology, human factors, business management, and aviation to develop programs in simulation-based training for flight crews. The program replicated flights from start to finish and included debriefing sessions with videos of the simulated scenario. Simulation training has been used for military, commercial, and recreational pilots to obtain flight skills since the 1920s.[15] Simulation training for pilots and flight crews is widely credited for improving flight safety, more than any other method of transportation available today.[16]

CRM first appeared in health care literature in the 1990s and is described as the combination of behaviors of individuals and crews that focus on dynamic decision making, interpersonal behavior, and teamwork during crises.[17] David Gaba and colleagues were the first to study the relationship between patterns of behavior, knowledge and skill

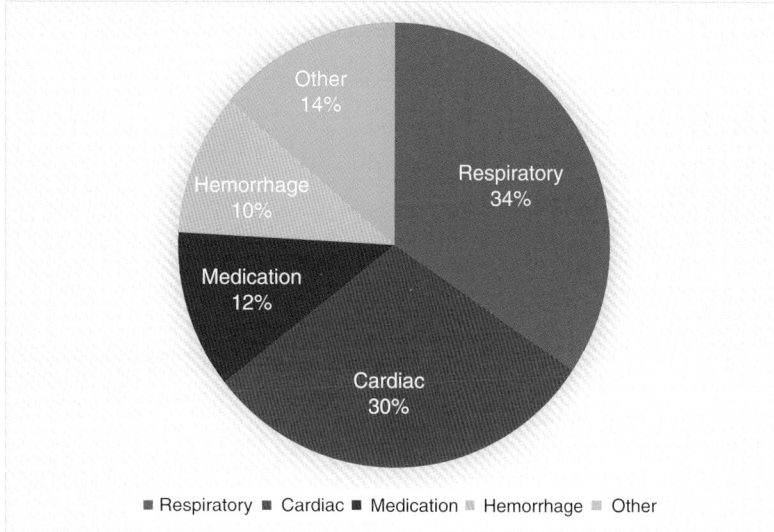

Fig. 60.1 Categories of perioperative crisis events that led to death in anesthetized patients. (From Hranchook AM, Jordan L, Geisz-Everson M, et al. A content and thematic analysis of closed claims resulting in death. Poster presentation at the 2018 Nurse Anesthesia Annual Congress in Boston, MA.)

gaps, and performance in anesthesia crisis situations.[18] CRM is part education, part training, part assessment, and part refinement at the individual and team levels. It must be supported throughout the institution by individuals, team leaders, departmental chairs, and senior leadership to have an impact on patient safety. It should also focus on systematic change, equipment, processes, procedures, resource availability, and individual and team behaviors.[18] CRM has been increasingly incorporated into undergraduate and graduate health care educational programs, continuing educational programs (such as the American Association of Nurse Anesthesiologists Annual Congress in 2018 and 2019), and used as an incentive to reduce malpractice insurance premiums for those who have completed CRM education.[19]

Core Principles of Crisis Resource Management

The four core principles of CRM are team management, resource allocation, awareness of the environment, and dynamic decision making.[18] Within each of these core principles are multiple areas of importance (Fig. 60.2 and Table 60.1). The core principle of team management includes the required step of establishing a leader and the role of followers by other participants responding to the crisis situation. Closely related is the principle of role clarity. Not everyone can be the leader, but a leader needs to be identified and it is important for everyone to know who's the leader and who's following. This can be established by someone simply asking, "Who is the leader?" or stating, "I am going to be the leader." Some institutions have the crisis leader wear a red hat or brightly colored vest to be clearly identified by anyone arriving to the crisis.

Once established, the leader is responsible for appropriately distributing the workload, requesting additional help in a timely manner, and ensuring effective communication between all team members. Distributing the workload through the use of red lanyards with preidentified role placards has shown to improve outcomes for code situations.[20] To ensure effective communication, a closed-loop style may be used where the leader specifically identifies a team member and assigns them an action. Next, the team member acknowledges the communication or direction and repeats it, with the initial leader verifying the communication as correct. This type of communication avoids non-specific statements such as "Someone start an IV!" or "Call the pharmacy!" that could result in the task not

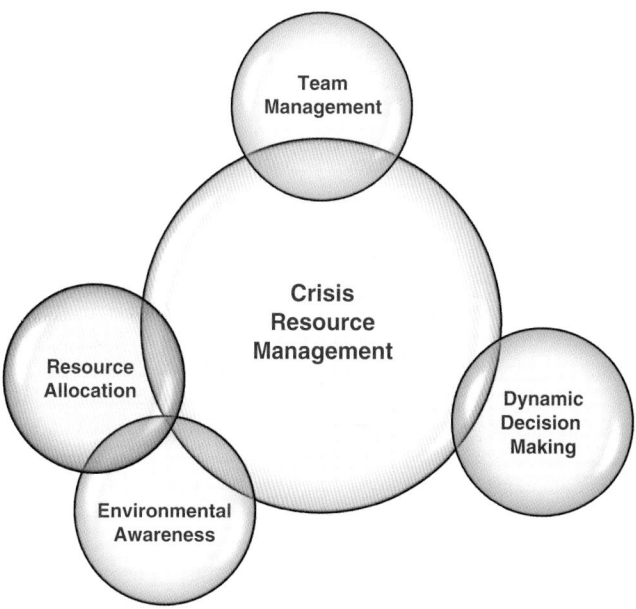

Fig. 60.2 Core principles of crisis resource management. (Adapted from Fanning RM, Goldhaber-Fiebert SN, Udani AD, et al. Crisis resource management. In: Levine AI, DeMaria Jr S, Schwartz AD, et al., eds. *The Comprehensive Textbook of Healthcare Simulation.* New York: Springer Science+Business Media; 2013.)

being completed or multiple people performing the same task unnecessarily. Closed-loop communication decreases medical errors and improves time-to-task completion.[21,22] The important step of having the follower report back to the leader when tasks are completed allows the leader to maintain awareness of the situation and gives the leader a chance to assign a new task to the team member or release the team member from any further tasks.

A primary responsibility of the leader is to manage the team during the crisis. If another health care provider with greater leadership ability, or more knowledge and experience about the current situation arrives, it is acceptable for the leader to transfer leadership to the newly arrived individual. However, the leadership role should not be a rotating position

TABLE 60.1   Critical Aspects of Crisis Resource Management Core Principles

Team Management	Resource Allocation/Environmental Awareness	Dynamic Decision Making
• Leadership/followership • Role clarity • Workload distribution • Requesting timely help • Effective communication	• Know the environment • Anticipate and plan • Resource allocation and mobilization	• Situational awareness • Use all available information • Avoid fixation errors • Use cognitive aids

Adapted from Fanning RM, Goldhaber-Fiebert SN, Udani AD, et al. Crisis resource management. In: Levine AI, DeMaria Jr S, Schwartz AD, et al., eds. *The Comprehensive Textbook of Healthcare Simulation.* New York: Springer Science+Business Media; 2013.

within a given crisis. Furthermore, leadership is not necessarily assigned according to seniority, title, rank, or the simple fact that one has previously been a leader in another crisis. There may be organizational, personal, or unavoidable issues that precipitated the crisis; however, treating the patient and managing the crisis is paramount, and all other extraneous issues should be discussed at a later time. Another responsibility of the leader is to facilitate a debriefing session after the crisis is complete.

The next two principles overlap significantly and include, resource allocation and environmental awareness. Understanding the environment during a crisis is critical to a successful outcome. An intimate knowledge of the environment generally comes with experience, however, it is not uncommon for an anesthesia provider to be called to other areas of the hospital (such as the intensive care unit or emergency department) to manage a crisis. In these situations a lack of knowledge about that environment may occur, and clear communication with team members is essential to manage resources and complete needed tasks. Next, a prope knowledge of resource allocation and the ability to mobilize those resources effectively is crucial to a successful outcome. For example, a Level 1 trauma center has significantly more resources available and deployable than a rural critical access hospital (CAH). Either facility might receive a gunshot wound to the chest; however, the trauma center would likely order a blood type and crossmatch upon arrival, have a full team in hospital, and be able to mobilize to the operating room (OR) rapidly. In contrast, the rural CAH may not keep blood products in the facility, the surgeon may not be readily available, and the OR team may need to be called in from home. The anesthesia provider responding to these patient situations in the two different hospitals would need to provide the team with vastly different tasks based on the availability of resources and the skill set of the team members. Trauma center leadership would focus on preparing the patient for surgery rapidly and transporting to the OR as soon as possible. In the rural hospital, leadership would focus on stabilizing the patient, ensuring a patent airway, and establishing intravenous access for transport to the nearest trauma facility. Appropriate decision making by the leader, based on awareness of the local environment and proper allocation of available resources, may be the difference between life or death for a patient.

A very important core principle in CRM is dynamic decision making. The leader is responsible for making decisions about the current crisis situation affecting the current patient, with the available resources and information within the current environment. The key concept *dynamic,* signals that the situation and environment are in a state of change or fluctuation. This means the correct decision path may change dramatically from hour to hour based on the available personnel and equipment resources. All decisions affect patient outcomes. For example, it is possible there was an initial misdiagnosis of the problem and a different course of action is necessary. Followers should speak up if they are questioning a decision or identifying a mistake. Creating a culture of safety and trust among team members is vital. Situational awareness is key when making decisions as the particulars of a given patient, surgery, and anesthetic will

TABLE 60.2   Common Fixation Errors and Examples of Thought Processes Involved

Fixation Error	Thought Process Examples
Cognitive tunnel vision	"Intubation is the only way to ventilate." "An arterial line is the only way to get an accurate blood pressure." "Intravenous route is the only way to give a medication."
Avoidance error	"This just couldn't be a myocardial infarction, this patient is so healthy." "It can't be anaphylaxis, that reaction is so rare."
Artifact error	"It's just the surgeon leaning on the blood pressure cuff." "It must be artifact from the electrocautery."

change the course of action significantly. A patient who develops cardiac arrest due to anaphylaxis requires different interventions compared to a patient who develops asystole due to delayed LAST secondary to a nerve block. The leader must ensure that the entire team has what is termed a shared mental model, meaning the team is on the "same page" having a shared understanding of what the working diagnosis is and what their anticipated next actions will be.[23] One major problem when making decisions in a crisis is a fixation error, which occurs when the decision maker continues down a given path of treatment despite the presentation of evidence to the contrary. In this situation, the followers must continue to present evidence as often, and in as many different ways as possible until the leader makes the change. If the leader refuses and the evidence is obvious, one of the followers must speak up and possibly even assume leadership in order to make the necessary change in treatment. Fixation errors are typically easier to identify when reviewing an incident after the fact but very hard for the team to see during the crisis (Table 60.2). One type of fixation error, cognitive tunnel vision, occurs when the team focuses on a given treatment plan and literally cannot see any other course of action because they are convinced they are on the correct path. A second type of fixation error is an avoidance error. This occurs when the team refuses to believe the cause of the crisis event could be what it most likely is, because the outcome would be devastating or highly unlikely. In this type of fixation error the team simply refuses to consider, and even avoids, a recommended course of action. One of the more concerning fixation errors is the artifact error, where every sign or symptom of an impending crisis is attributed to artifact or an inaccurate observation, leading to a noneffective course of action, and a potential exacerbation of the crisis. For example, hypotension displayed on a patient monitor is attributed to someone leaning on the noninvasive blood pressure cuff, or the low pulse oximetry reading is due to artifact, or a lack of end tidal carbon dioxide is due to a faulty $ETco_2$ monitor. These types of errors result in a failure to recognize and appropriately manage the crisis, call for help, and may elevate whatever is happening to emergency status. There are definitive ways a team can build capacity to limit fixation errors. One useful technique to avoid fixation errors is the 10 seconds for 10 minutes principle.[24] Using this method, the team takes a brief (10-second) pause in activity to review the key points and treatment thus far, while second opinions are sought about the appropriateness of the interventions. Care must be taken to avoid an extended pause and continue managing the ongoing emergent situation. Another useful adjunct that may help to limit fixation errors is the use of cognitive aids such as Advanced Cardiac Life Support (ACLS) cards, emergency manuals, or operating room crisis checklists.

Cognitive Aids in Crisis Resource Management

A survey of health care providers revealed that only 34% feel comfortable when dealing with a crisis situation.[25] Other evidence has found that the use of cognitive aids during a crisis situation reduces errors up to 75%, improves task performance, increases adherence to evidence-based care, and increases provider satisfaction with performance.[26-28] A cognitive aid is a tool to help one remember the correct steps to be performed in the correct order during a crisis to maximize the possibility of a positive outcome. Cognitive aids do not replace knowledge, are not a crutch for information that is unknown, and should not be viewed as a recipe to adhere to without conscious thought. Effective use requires expert clinical knowledge and skills (Fig. 60.3). Cognitive aids are quite literally an aid to cognition for practitioners to remember the that assists them in remembering the correct steps in the right order, to help provide optimal care, and avoid fixation errors during a stressful crisis situation.[18] Multiple different cognitive aids are available for use during perioperative emergencies. Table 60.3 lists some of the more common cognitive aids for use in anesthesia and for perioperative crises. Most are free for download to print and are available electronically for integration with an electronic medical record. Most cognitive aid websites ask for an email address to provide updated versions in the future. Most manuals were developed under a creative commons license, and users are encouraged to adapt/edit the manual to their environment/facility. A fairly comprehensive listing of manuals available for free download is available from the Emergency Manuals Implementation Collaborative (EMIC) website (https://www.emergencymanuals.org/tools-resources/).[29]

Once a cognitive aid is downloaded and placed around the facility in both procedural and anesthetizing locations, the work of implementation begins. Without an implementation and eduction plan, proper use of these cognitive aids is unlikely.[30] Implementation of cognitive aids is one facet of CRM, if their use is not practiced, they may become a distraction during a crisis event.[31] Ariadne Labs, EMIC, and Stanford teamed up to create a toolkit for successful emergency checklist implementation, available at https://www.implementingemergencychecklists.org/. During implementation of the Stanford Emergency Manuals throughout multiple facilities, including several rural CAHs, the authors found successful implementation requires three Ps: careful placement, perception, and lots of practice. Careful placement is key, as the aid can only be used if it can be easily accessed; cultural perception states that it is okay and even expected to use a cognitive aid during crisis management. The use of simulation to gain familiarity with and practice using the cognitive aid improves practitioner acceptance. Once cognitive aids are actually utilized in practice, anesthesia providers have reported decreased stress, better teamwork, and a calmer atmosphere which allowed for decreased errors of omission.[32]

DEVELOPING A CRISIS RESOURCE MANAGEMENT PROGRAM

The key to a successful CRM program is the assessment of available resources and development of a process to ensure resources are present and available in a sufficient quantity. Two concepts from business theory are helpful when designing a CRM program. First is the concept of reaching for the low-hanging fruit: Is there an obvious crisis that seems to be occurring with some level of regularity, or was there a recent crisis that is still fresh in people's mind? During the Covid-19 crisis, early simulations were used to test new protocols and to prepare clinicians to care for patients with a highly contagious airborne disease.[33] As the Covid-19 crisis continued, simulations transitioned to safe intubation techniques, beneficial ventilation modes, and safe

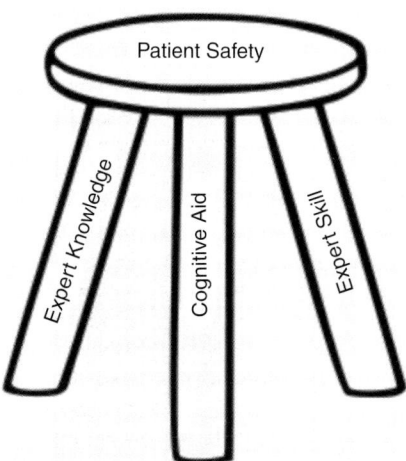

Fig. 60.3 The three legs of expert knowledge, expert skill, and cognitive aid use support improved patient safety during perioperative crises.

TABLE 60.3	Partial List of Cognitive Aids for Use During an Anesthesia/Perioperative Crisis	
Cognitive Aid	**Description**	**Access at:**
Stanford Emergency Manual	Created by the Stanford Anesthesia Cognitive Aid group. Free to download and adapt to any institution. Available in several different languages.	https://emergencymanual.stanford.edu/
OB Stanford Emergency Manual	Obstetric-specific emergency manual produced by the Stanford Group.	http://med.stanford.edu/cogaids/obanesem.html
Pedi Crisis 2.0 Critical Events Checklists Mobile App	The Society for Pediatric Anesthesia created this free downloadable app to help clinicians respond to pediatric perioperative life-threatening critical events. It features weight-based dosaging and access to critical resources.	Available for the iPhone and iPad on the Apple App Store and for Android on the Google Play Store
Operating Room Crisis Checklists—Ariadne Labs	Developed by the team at Ariadne Labs with the goal of improving care during 12 of the most common operating room crises.	https://www.ariadnelabs.org/areas-of-work/surgery-or-crisis-checklists/

transportation of pateints with the virus. The first crisis simulated should focus on eliminating the most pressing institutional issues, since this is likely to have rapid beneficial results, and improve buy-in for future changes within the facility.

The second principle related to developing a CRM program is the diminishing rate of return on investment. As more resources are devoted to any project, the additional benefit from each infusion of resources is less, and may even cause harm. Think of the Frank-Starling curve and preload for the heart. If a patient's blood pressure increases after a fluid bolus, the patient was on the steep upward slope of the curve, and the added fluid was beneficial. If another bolus is given, and there is no additional increase in blood pressure, the patient is likely on the upper, flat part of the curve. At this point additional fluid boluses may push the patient into fluid overload and pulmonary edema. Determining which crises events to initially address requires data gathering and analysis. Alternatively, one could review the latest anesthesia closed claims studies related to anesthesia. These are published regularly in the American Association of Nurse Anesthetists (AANA) and other anesthesia journals.[34-37] Table 60.4 summarizes themes from closed claims studies in anesthesia/surgery, which usually show the most common crises revolve around airway management, cardiac complications (cardiac arrest, bradycardia, myocardial infarction), medication errors, hemorrhage, and other issues. A common theme that regularly appears in closed claims analyses is that communication errors between team members during the crisis management lead to the poor outcome.[36]

All of the major adverse events summarized in a closed claims analysis would benefit from application of the principles of CRM and provide a solid foundation for a CRM simulation program. The best way to improve CRM and team communication during a crisis is through simulation practice of the events surrounding the crisis.[17] A well-designed simulation allows a group to experience a crisis situation without the risk of a real-life patient morbidity or mortality. During the debriefing after the simulation, the facilitator (simulationist) will ask the team to review and reflect upon the scenario, actions taken and treatments chosen. The ensuing discussion is always enlightening for participants and facilitators. Debriefing is a skill that takes frequent and dedicated practice. This chapter will provide some debriefing tips and includes a simple debriefing tool to aid the novice simulationist. Upon the completion of the debriefing after the first simulation, the group is frequently allowed to repeat

the same scenario with the opportunity to apply their newfound understanding of each other's performance and communication idiosyncrasies. Immediately repeating the scenario helps to reinforce the learning principles and increases participant satisfaction.[38] This is followed by a second debriefing where final learning points are summarized and solidified. Most commonly the outcome is improved, and the group leaves with a feeling of accomplishment and an ability to function better in a future crisis situation—not necessarily the one simulated, but any crisis situation. This is especially true when the simulation design is based on developing better CRM skills and not focused on the specific treatment or technical skills. Technical skills can be practiced at another time utilizing task trainers or other modes of education if deficiencies are revealed. Medical mismanagement and inefficiencies in care should be remedied, and may be corrected by the use of evidence-based cognitive aids during simulation education.

Designing Crisis Resource Management Simulations

Improving CRM skills involves developing interpersonal behaviors and actions that cannot typically be learned in a classroom. Didactic knowledge of CRM principles should serve as a base, followed by simulation, expert feedback and continued practice in an effort to develop mastery. Indeed, studies have shown that team CRM simulation improves provider reaction time, correct implementation of evidence-based treatments, and patient outcomes.[40-44] CRM simulation involves the practice of deliberately preparing for and practicing nontechnical skills required for effective teamwork in a crisis situation, and is key to any CRM program.[45] Most comprehensive CRM programs involve a multimodal educational technique, utilizing didactic techniques such as lectures or presentations combined with simulation.

The Society for Simulation in Healthcare (SSH) defines simulation as a "technique that creates a situation or environment to allow persons to experience a representation of a real event for the purpose of practice, learning, evaluation, testing, or to gain understanding of systems or human actions." CRM simulation involves creating an experience for the team members that allows them to practice CRM skills. It does not have to be complicated or high fidelity. Simulation can be used for formative (recommended) or summative (not recommended) assessment. Formative assessment aims to foster professional growth and learning; summative assessment focuses on achieving a set outcome (e.g., assigning a pass/fail score).[46] If participants believe their performance will be evaluated in any way that could affect their job, salary, promotion, or organizational status, they will limit their participation for self-preservation.[47] If they believe their participation will lead to improved patient care without retribution, they will fully participate, be engaged in the learning, and be part of improving patient care at the facility.

The most important part of designing a quality CRM simulation experience is to design the simulation around objectives based on CRM principles described earlier in this chapter (see Fig. 60.1). Often, time is limited so it is best to focus on up to three simple measurable objectives. Including the use of a cognitive aid, such as the Stanford Emergency Manual as an objective, can take the place of an objective to ensure that that the correct treatment measures are sought or performed (Table 60.5). Several assessment tools have been created to evaluate team performance and nontechnical skills that are key to CRM. These tools can be used to help create objectives and formatively evaluate team performance.[48,49] The TeamSTEPPS Team Performance Observation Tool (https://www.ahrq.gov/teamstepps/instructor/reference/tmpot.html) and the Team Emergency Assessment (TEAM) tool (https://nexusipe.org/advancing/assessment-evaluation/team-emergency-assessment-measure-team) are easy-to-use resources that help to guide objective

TABLE 60.4 Crisis Events Leading to Death in Anesthetized Patients

General	Specific Issue	n	%
Respiratory issues	Airway loss	23	34.5%
	Aspiration	7	
Cardiac issues	Cardiac arrest	15	29.9%
	Bradycardia	8	
	Myocardial infection	3	
Medication issues	Narcotic only	6	11.5%
	Other medications	4	
Hemorrhage		9	10.3%
Other		12	13.8%
Total events		87	100%

Adapted from Hranchook AM, Jordan L, Geisz-Everson M, et al. A content and thematic analysis of closed claims resulting in death. Poster presentation at the 2018 Nurse Anesthesia Annual Congress in Boston, MA.

TABLE 60.5   Sample Simulation Objectives for Each of the Crisis Resource Managment (CRM) Core Principles

CRM Principle	Simulation Objective Examples: *By the end of this simulation the team will:*
Team Management	• Clearly identify a team leader • Establish clear roles and responsibilities based on appropriate abilities • Clearly identify the working diagnosis to establish a shared mental model • Avoid thin-air statements • Utilize closed-loop communication • Foster an environment where all members feel free to speak up • Check and cross-check information • Act with composure and control
Resource Allocation/ Environmental Awareness	• Call for help early • Mobilize special equipment or teams • Eliminate or reduce distraction • Distribute workload evenly • Seek information from all available sources • Maintain situational awareness
Dynamic Decision Making	• Use cognitive aids • Avoid fixation errors • Follow approved standards and guidelines

development and assessment of team performance.[50] The low-hanging fruit that seems to be an issue for most teams includes establishing a clear leader, establishing clear roles and responsibilities, use of effective communication, and the use of cognitive aids. It is also very important to involve multiple specialties of the team in either the development or approval of the team simulation scenario objectives and design. Rarely is a surgery performed with only four nurses or four surgeons and no other providers in the operating room, yet simulations are often conducted with a single group of providers due to ease of scheduling or budgeting. To achieve the greatest benefits from CRM education, the simulations must be interprofessional, which requires budget support from upper-level administration.

Developing realistic scenarios, collecting all the required equipment, and finding the time to implement the program does not need to be challenging. A sample simulation script and supply list is included at the end of this chapter for use and adaptation (see Appendix A). The simulation script provided focuses on the use of the Stanford Emergency Manual in practice. The participants receive presimulation education via an email, which contains the objectives of the simulation, a copy of the Stanford Emergency Mannual, and educational videos on the use of cognitive aids in practice, including Stanford's "Why and How to Implement Emergency Manuals" (https://www.youtube.com/watch?v=shc1BBzsIyI).[51]

Multiple other scenarios are also available, and many simulationists share their scenarios with others to improve patient outcomes. MedEdPORTAL is an online open-access medical teaching and learning journal that publishes teaching and learning modules that include simulation scenarios and designs. It is easily searchable and accessed at https://www.mededportal.org. Simulationists are often eager to share simulation scenarios and scripts through simulation societies such as the SSH (https://simconnect.ssih.org/home) simconnect group or the

AANA (https://connect.aana.com/home) AANAconnect group. Further education and credentialing in health care simulation can also be sought through the SSH. Many simulation applications and programs are also available for purchase through simulation companies, and most academic medical centers have simulationists who are available to help.

Components of a Crisis Resource Managment Simulation Program

When developing a program of simulation for your facility, it is critical to include the administrative team to gain their buy-in and resource allocation. When administrators realize that crisis simulation can reduce adverse events, reduce adverse outcomes, and possibly reduce insurance premiums, they are frequently supportive. Most organizations have a multidisciplinary quality and safety committee whose support is also beneficial.

A crucial step is finding a reasonable time to conduct simulations when a multidisciplinary team of providers can be assembled. Surgeries involve an interprofessional team providing care to the patient and managing any adverse events that may occur. Each professional discipline (surgeon, anesthesia, nursing, technologists, assistants, pharmacy, etc.) has its own strengths and weaknesses in CRM, which can be recognized during the simulation. Most facilities have a day of the week and a time of the day when the patient volume is lower or when time is protected for educational meetings. These are perfect times to conduct a simulation. It is best if a regular simulation time is prioritized and scheduled. Quarterly or bimonthly simulation is recommended. It is especially effective if the simulations can be done in situ or in the actual environment where the crisis may occur. This helps to improve realism, and it can identify systems issues that are not noticed in the simulation center. This could be an empty operating room or a late-start room. The Foundation for Healthcare Simulation Safety provides free toolkits to assure in situ simulation safety, including a pre– and post–in situ simulation safety checklist (https://healthcaresimulationsafety.org/tool-kit-resources/).

Cost is another great reason to conduct simulations within regularly scheduled work hours. The simulations must be designed to fit within the given time frame, starting on time and ending on time. Effective team simulations can be conducted within a 30-minute to 1-hour time frame. This strategy requires simply designed scenarios with standardized simulation toolkits that can be performed whenever time permits.

Planning simulations requires planning, time and effort. Complications with simulation administration are not uncommon where something is forgotten, equipment does not work the day of the simulation, and/or the participants do unexpected things. CRM simulations are not focused on technical skills, so they can be done with minimal equipment use. The simulation can be divided into two distinct events, the preeducation and the actual simulation activity. The first is more of an educational presentation giving the participants information on CRM that they will need to be successful during the hands-on portion. It provides the knowledge base. The education can be presented in a lecture format, prerecorded and watched asynchronously, sent out electronically, or read as handouts to be reviewed prior to the simulation. It is best to provide the educational materials far enough in advance of the simulation (3–5 days) to give the participants time to review, but not too far where they may forget the content. Providing the educational materials in advance reduces the time commitment during the simulation, and possibly the cost if participants are being paid for their time. A simulation confidentiality contract can also be sent with the education material to save time.

The simulation activity can be broken down into three parts. The prebrief, the actual simulation experience, and the debrief. The prebrief establishes a safe confidential learning environment and explains to the participants everything they will need to know to engage in a successful simulation experience.[52] Because too much stress hinders learning, the prebrief should aim to bring the stress level to an area where optimal learning can occur (Fig. 60.4).[53] The objectives of the simulation are reviewed so the participants do not need to guess why they are present and it gives them the opportunity to perform their best during the simulation. It also reminds the debriefer what objective observations to note for discussion in the debriefing. As part of the prebrief participants are given a chance to review the physical layout of the simulation, touch equipment, and look for required medications. The instructor will tell the participants the "rules of engagement" for the simulation, what is expected and tolerated, what equipment will and will not work, how to obtain additional help or equipment if needed. The prebrief is also a time when the instructor asks the participants to suspend their disbelief and fully participate in the simulation for their educational benefit, and the benefit of other participants. The participants are asked to sign a simulation contract stating they will not discuss the activities of simulation with anyone outside the simulation and to verify the simulation is a safe environment where everyone is expected to show respect for others. Lastly, a statement is typically made referring to the assumption that everyone is competent and doing their best and that mistakes will occur, are expected, and will be part of the learning that is about to happen.[52] Once the prebrief is completed, participants are asked to quickly introduce themselves, and team roles are assigned or self-selected. It is best to have the participants play the actual role or a similar role that they would play during a real crisis event.

The simulation is allowed to continue for a predetermined length of time, until the objectives are met, or a desired outcome is achieved. If the participants are having difficulty during a particular point in the simulation, the instructor may elect to verbally announce a specific piece of unnoticed information or action that needs to be taken to make sure there is an opportunity to meet the objectives within the limited simulation time frame. The instructor may also elect to stop the simulation, review specific pertinent information, and then restart the simulation. The simulation script will have specific alterations in vital signs and patient status related to scenario objectives. Frequently there are two or more divergent pathways the scenario will take based on participant intervention. Care must be taken to avoid scenarios that are too complicated since this may make it difficult to determine which pathway has been taken and which outcome is realistic. Most CRM simulations can be done with simple vital sign changes related to participants' actions and treatments. Display of vital signs can be as simple as using a simulation application on a tablet computer device. The instructor determines when the simulation is complete and announces "the simulation now is over." Once the simulation is completed, participants and instructor can relocate and debrief as someone else resets the simulation scenario for a second attempt. If time does not allow for movement to another location or if another location is not available, debriefing can occur in the simulation environment. When participants return for the second attempt, the instructor can give a shortened prebrief, and the simulation is conducted again. The second simulation is conducted similar to the first with the goal of participants correcting errors made during the first simulation. Even the most efficient, properly completed simulation has areas for improvement that are frequently related to team interaction and communication. It is also

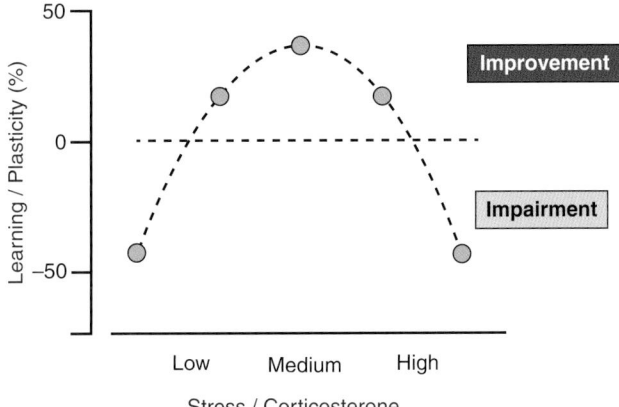

Fig. 60.4 Stress and learning. A medium amount of stress is associated with optimal learning. (From Sandi C. Glucocoticoids act on glutamatergic pathways to affect memory processes. *Trends Neurosci.* 2011;34[4]:165–176.)

important to reinforce good behaviors and see them continue in the second simulation. A simple simulation activity outline in shown in Fig. 60.5.

Debriefing is an extremely important part of any simulation, and many experts believe it is where most learning occurs.[54] Complete coverage of this topic is beyond the scope of this chapter, and there are a number of very good resources for the interested reader, including "Pocket Book for Simulation Debriefing in Healthcare" by Oriot and Alinier.[55] Simplistically, debriefing is a discussion of the simulation that is facilitated by the instructor with the goal of improving actions and behaviors to make patients and environments safer. The debriefing process does not simply inform the participants about what they did wrong or well. The key to debriefing is to get learners to have their own "aha" moments, which lead to a change in their thought patterns, which then may drive their future actions.[56] The goal of the debrief is to lead to behavioral change and action. Debriefing consists of three phases: (1) gathering reactions, (2) analyzing or understanding what happened, and (3) summarizing the findings.[57] Debriefing starts with a reflective question (e.g., "How did that go?"). Participants usually discuss the simulation, congratulate each other on good performances, frequently self-identify major mistakes, and summarize what they perceived happened during the simulation. If there was a major issue, it is usually good to discuss the participants' concerns at the beginning of the debriefing period. The debriefer can discuss behaviors and actions that were observed based on the objectives and then asks the participants for their viewpoints. This technique is referred to as the advocacy and inquiry approach and allows each participant the opportunity to explore the reasons behind their behaviors.[57] A review of the objectives of the simulation may help to keep participants on track and let the group discuss and decide whether or not the objectives were met. This ensures that learning is centered around the purpose of the simulation. It is never appropriate during a debrief to assign blame for a poor simulation outcome or make fun of any participants' actions. The debriefer often completes the debriefing by allowing each participant to verbalize what they learned (takehome points) and/or what could be done differently in the future. Using a debriefing tool or script has been shown to be effective for the novice debriefer.[58,59] Phrampus and O'Donnell created the GAS (corresponding goals, actions, sample questions and time frame) debriefing tool, which can be adapted to any simulation

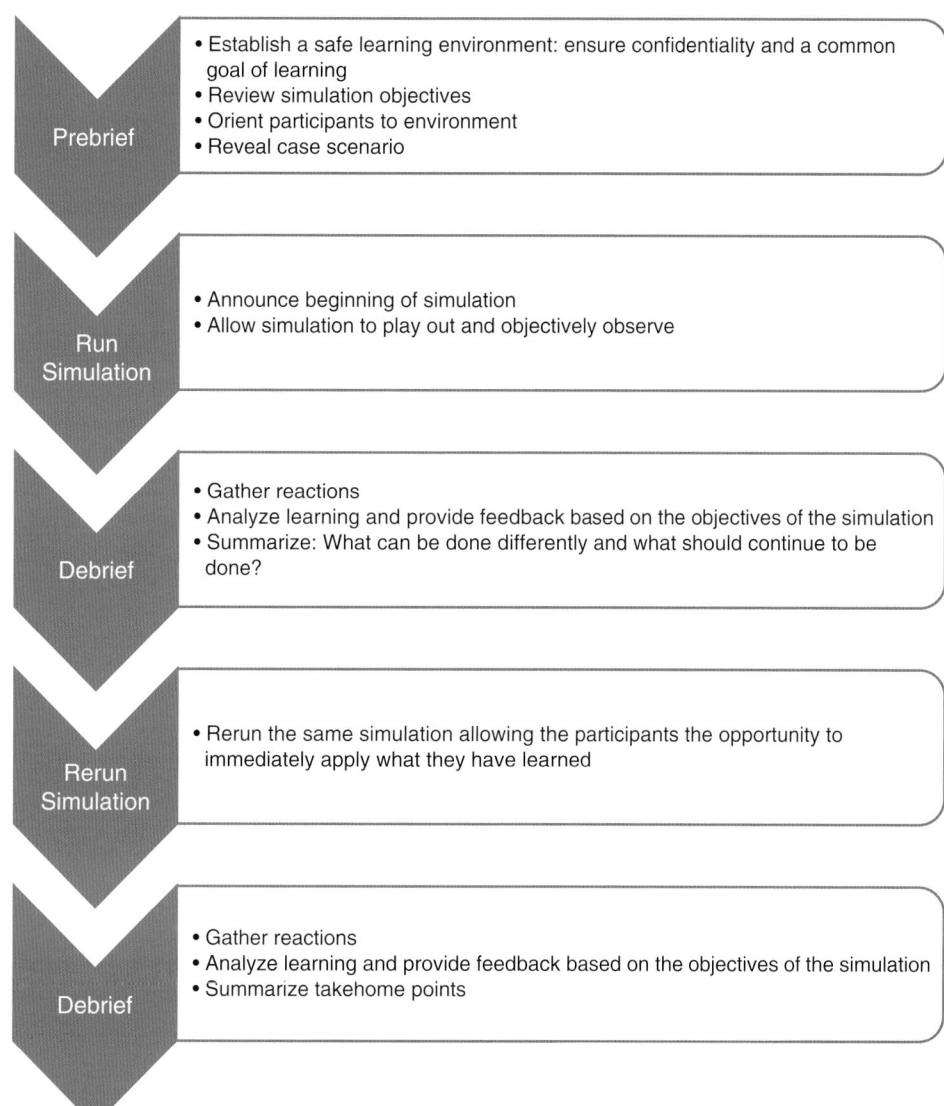

Prebrief
- Establish a safe learning environment: ensure confidentiality and a common goal of learning
- Review simulation objectives
- Orient participants to environment
- Reveal case scenario

Run Simulation
- Announce beginning of simulation
- Allow simulation to play out and objectively observe

Debrief
- Gather reactions
- Analyze learning and provide feedback based on the objectives of the simulation
- Summarize: What can be done differently and what should continue to be done?

Rerun Simulation
- Rerun the same simulation allowing the participants the opportunity to immediately apply what they have learned

Debrief
- Gather reactions
- Analyze learning and provide feedback based on the objectives of the simulation
- Summarize takehome points

Fig. 60.5 Sample outline for crisis resource management simulation.

(Fig. 60.6) as it outlines the three phases of debriefing (Gather, Analyze, Summarize).[60] This GAS tool is based on simulation education best practice standards and can be used in real time to guide discussion and learning.[61]

Implementing a Crisis Resource Management Simulation Program

Implementing a comprehensive crisis simulation program is difficult to achieve because it requires commitment from multiple disciplines to participate in the simulations. This process usually requires more time to coordinate than the actual education and simulations. It also requires a commitment from facility administration to provide space, resources for equipment and training, and salary support for the simulation instructor and possibly for participating staff. For participants to learn and benefit during simulations, the education does not need to be complicated, difficult, or high fidelity. The majority of the issues related to poor outcomes in crises situations involve communication and team dynamics. CRM is designed to address those issues. The main focus of

the crisis simulation program should be to facilitate the participants to work through a crisis situation as a team, and then debriefing to elicit feedback from the participants about the simulation in an effort to improve performance.

A comprehensive crisis management program will ideally address the specific needs of the facility, staff, and community. If not previously discussed, the very topic of crisis resource management will need to be presented and discussed before simulating a crisis. This is an optimal time to inform participants about how the simulation program will be used to improve care, interpersonal and team communication, and team dynamics. Staff may have preferences for certain types of simulations in which they would like to participate, but the educational content and simulations should be chosen based on facility data or published literature. It has been shown a significant percentage nurses could not pass the Basic Life Support (BLS) assessment 12 months after certification, and that ACLS skills degrade even faster. These are skills commonly used in most health care crises, and should therefore, be part of any crisis simulation program. A sample schedule of a 3-year CRM simulation program is shown in Table 60.6. The schedule

Phase	Goal	Actions	Sample Questions	Time
Gather	Listen to participants to understand what they think and how they feel about session	• Request narrative from team leader • Request clarifying or supplemental information from team	All: How do you feel about the simulation (assess readiness)? Team Leader: Can you tell us what happened? Team members: Can you add to the account?	25%
Analyze	Facilitate participants' reflection **on** and analysis **of** their actions	• Review of accurate record of events •Report observations (correct and incorrect steps) •Ask a series of questions to reveal participants' thinking processes •Assist participants to reflect on their performance •Direct/redirect participants to assure continuous focus on session objectives	•I noticed… •Tell me more about… •How did you feel about… •What were you thinking when… •I understand, however, tell me about "X" aspect of the scenario… •Conflict resolution: •Let's refocus- "what's important is not who is right but what is right for the patient…"	50%
Summarize	Facilitate identification and review of lessons learned	•Participants identify positive aspects of team or individual behaviors and behaviors that require change •Summary of comments or statements	•List two actions or events that you felt were effective or well done •Describe two areas that you think you/team need to work on…	25%

Fig. 60.6 GAS (corresponding goals, actions, sample questions and time frame) debriefing tool. (Used with permission from Phrampus PS, O'Donnell JM. Debriefing: using a structured and supported approach. In: Levine AL, Bryson EO, DeMaria S, et al., eds. *The Comprehensive Manual of Healthcare Simulation.* New York: Springer; 2013.)

TABLE 60.6   Sample Schedule for a Crisis Resource Management (CRM) Simulation Program

	Year 1	Year 2	Year 3
		ACTIVITY	
January	Presentation on CRM Core Principles	CRM review	CRM review
February		Education: Cardiac	Education
March	Education on Crises Event: Airway	Cardiac Simulations	Simulation
April	Airway Crisis Simulations	Education: Airway	Education
May	Education on Crises Event: Hemorrhage	Airway Simulations	Simulation
June	Hemorrhage Simulations	No Events	Education
July	No events	Education: Malignant Hyperthermia (MH)	Simulation
August	Education on Crises Event: Cardiac	MH Simulations	Education
September	Cardiac Simulations	Education: Pediatric	Simulation
October	Education on Crises Event: Pediatric	Pediatric Simulations	Education
November	Pediatric Simulations	Education Trauma	Simulation
December	No events	Trauma Simulations	No events

alternates educational presentations and related simulation throughout the year. The goal is to complete four sets of education-simulation each year. Since respiratory and cardiac events account for 64% of deaths in closed claims analysis (see Table 60.4), simulations focusing on airway management and BLS/ACLS skills should be performed annually at a minimum. The exact order of the education and specific simulations does not matter as long as the topics are appropriate to the facility and

staff educational needs are rotated. Ideally, the simulation education coordinator collaborates with the quality assurance and risk manager to track data about the facility over time. What is hopefully sen after successful implementation of a CRM program is an improvement in crisis event outcomes. It may be difficult to show a definitive improvement since crisis events are rare; however, the prevention of one bad outcome may result in a life saved.

SUMMARY

The majority of poor perioperative outcomes are due to inadequate communication and team dynamics. Crisis resource management is a valuable tool that improves outcomes during perioperative emergencies. CRM is a health care adaptation of crew resource management in the military, which occurred in the 1990s. The core principles of CRM are team management, resource allocation, environmental awareness, and dynamic decision making. Cognitive aids reduce errors, increase adherence to evidence-based practices, improve outcomes, and improve practitioner satisfaction during perioperative crises. Simulation of perioperative crises results in improved teamwork and patient outcomes. Conducting the simulations in the actual location where the crisis may occur will identify system issues that affect patient outcomes. Regular practice of the principles of CR with a multidisciplinary team, using perioperative crisis simulation and a cognitive aid to guide interventions, should become a regular part of every anesthesia provider's practice.

REFERENCES

For a complete list of references for this chapter, scan this QR code with any smartphone code reader app, or visit the following URL: http://booksite.elsevier.com/9780323711944/.

61

Infection Control and Prevention

Michael Anderson, Charles Griffis, Marjorie Everson, Lynn Reede, Leslie Jeter

INTRODUCTION

Infection control and prevention is a core patient safety concept known for centuries and not always widely embraced. It began with Ignaz Semmelweis, a physician from Hungary who observed that women who had their babies delivered by physicians and medical students had a much higher incidence of puerperal fever (13%–18%) than women who were delivered by midwife trainees or midwives (2%).[1] This observation led to him to review the delivery process and outcomes. It was noted that the physician and medical students performed the autopsies and delivered babies. The midwives and midwifery students did not. This led Semmelweis to hypothesize that the exposure to the corpses was the reason for the increased risk of puerperal fever and that simply washing their hands between duties could decrease that risk.[2-4] Shortly thereafter, Semmelweis developed a handwashing study to assess this hypothesis and saw a decrease in the physician and medical student cohort to 2% or the same as the midwife cohort (Fig. 61.1).[5] This breakthrough allowed Semmelweis to earn the title "father of infection control" as the first to identify the importance of handwashing in infection control.[1]

Infection control, although vital to health and safety, has often taken a back seat to other issues as it relates to health care providers' perceptions and practice. This is especially true for anesthesia providers in the operating room environment. Numerous studies have and have called into question anesthesia providers' priorities as it relates to infection control. Hospital-associated infections (HAIs) are a significant economic burden to our health care system and society. The average range of direct medical costs related to HAIs in the United States is between $28.4 and $33.8 billion per year.[3] This is a staggering number considering the improvements in medical, surgical, and pharmaceutic care and technology. There are numerous challenges related to HAIs, especially the operating room environment. Some of those challenges include the following[4]:

1. There is a lack of a universal policy and procedures related to anesthesia infection control among health care facilities.
2. Infection control has not been a priority, thus there is a lack of data from infection control audits within institutions.
3. There is a significant amount of variation related to the cleaning and disinfecting of anesthesia workspaces in the operating room between cases, thus the risk of cross-contamination remains high.
4. Use of multidose vials for more than one patient, lack of use of double gloving during airway manipulation, and lack of frequent hand hygiene during anesthesia care all lead to HAIs.

There has been a shift in prioritization toward infection control amidst the Covid-19 pandemic that required health care providers to prioritize infection control. This focus highlighted many gaps in infection control preparedness at the facility level, including the supply chain for infection control-related items. To control the spread of contagion, infection control and prevention has permeated practice to prevent viral spread to patients, health care providers, friends, and family. In the early stages of this pandemic, it has become apparent that infection control practices (ICPs) are paramount in the mitigation of pandemics with many unknowns as to what the new normal will be moving forward.

This chapter offers fundamental anesthesia infection control and prevention practices to provide a framework to continuously improve and optimize patient and provider safety.

BIOLOGY OF DISEASE TRANSMISSION AND THE ANESTHESIA WORK ENVIRONMENT

Understanding the biologic mechanisms of disease transmission supports best practice for anesthesia personnel to protect themselves and their patients from infectious disease. Three elements are necessary for human disease transmission. First is a reservoir of infectious agent.[6] Second, three types of microorganisms are responsible for most infectious disease (viruses, bacteria, fungi) as well as parasitic organisms and prions (proteinaceous particles with abnormal conformations rendering them infectious)[7-9] These microorganisms may be found in an infected human host, or contaminated equipment, environmental setting, or animal host. Each microbe uses a particular route or mode or method of transmission. Finally, there must be a susceptible human host—in the current context, this would be the nurse anesthetist in a clinical environment.[7]

In anesthesia settings, often the reservoir is an infected patient who may be difficult to identify due to presenting as asymptomatic and untested. High touch areas of the clinical environment can also be reservoirs of infection-causing microbes residing on surfaces (Fig. 61.2).[10,11] The movement of equipment in and out of the operating room creates the potential for equipment to carry microbes from one area and patient to another.

Direct Contact Transmission

There are recognized mechanisms or routes of transmission by which infectious microbes move from host to host.[7] The first to be considered is the contact route, which may be either direct or indirect. Direct contact transmission in the clinical care setting refers to transmission of an infectious microbe from an infected person to another person by direct contact with the body, or broken or damaged skin, or mucous membrane of the susceptible host, without any intermediary object. Anesthesia care requires frequent touching of the patient, potentially providing a means of contact transmission. There may be direct contact with infectious secretions or blood on the patient's skin or body, or splashes might occur during care measures or procedural interventions. Intact, nondamaged skin presents a complex and effective barrier to pathogens.[12] Some infectious organisms may enter the body through contact with damaged, nonintact skin or mucous membrane present in

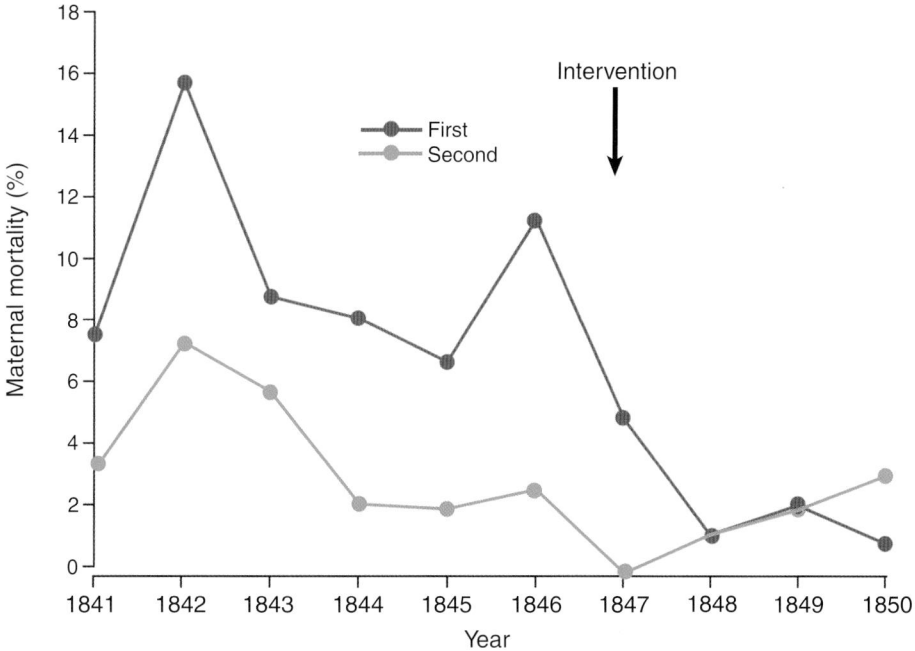

Fig. 61.1 1847 maternal mortality prior to hand hygiene introduction.

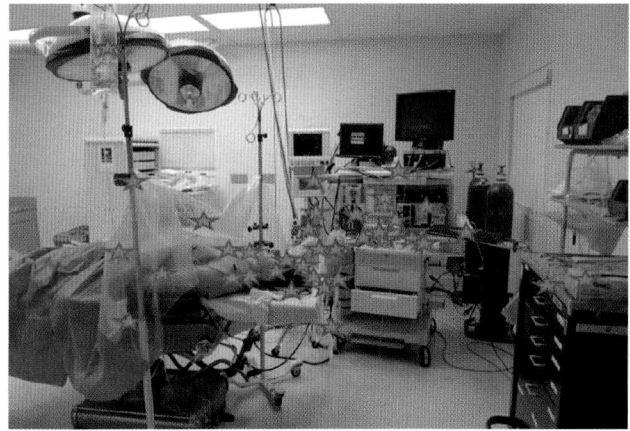

Fig. 61.2 Anesthetizing location touch contamination. (Reproduced and modified with permission. Birnbach DJ, Rosen LF, Fitzpatrick M, et al. Double gloves: a randomized trial to evaluate a simple strategy to reduce contamination in the operating room. *Anesth Analg.* 2015;120:848–852.)

the eyes, mouth, or nose, thus avoiding the host protections of intact.[13] It should be noted that mucosal surfaces are complex environments with innate immune defenses against microbial invasion, including innate and adaptive immune cells. The efficacy of the intact skin and mucous membrane as barriers to prevent infection is related to the overall status of the host's immune system.

Indirect Contact Transmission

Indirect contact transmission involves an intermediary object serving as a connecting bridge between an infected human reservoir and susceptible host.[7] The most common bridge is the contaminated hands of health care workers that move from an infected patient or environment and then make contact with another patient or health care worker without performing hand hygiene, transferring infectious material by touch. Health care equipment that is not decontaminated between patients can transfer infectious material to health care workers or patients. Equipment that presents multiple surfaces difficult to clean, such as close

connector fittings or keyboards, may be at increased risk of contamination as infectious materials and particles become trapped and are not eliminated by disinfection procedures. Common to the anesthesia environment is the use of intravenous equipment and parenteral therapy, and invasive procedures requiring insertion of needles, and intravascular and regional anesthesia catheters. If not maintained sterile, these objects can infect susceptible patients by breaching the protective skin barrier. Likewise, airway equipment that contacts mucous membrane can transfer infectious materials to patients if not sterile, whether a single-use device or decontaminated prior to next use.

The droplet mode of transmission refers to small liquid particles (>5 microns in size) of infected saliva or mucus expelled from an infected person's mouth and/or nose during coughing or sneezing, which eventually are inhaled into the airway of an uninfected host, usually requiring close contact.[7] Microbes are absorbed by the mucous membrane of eyes, mouth, or nose into the host. The distance such droplets can travel depends on multiple factors such as the force with which the particles are expelled, the viscosity and weight of the material, air currents, and surrounding temperature and humidity. Therefore the critical distance over which such particles might cause infection is a matter of debate, though current recommendations for donning facial protection have increased from within 3 to 6 feet of an infected individual, based on epidemiologic data.[14,15]

Microbes may also infect human hosts by traveling long distances through the air as very fine (<5 microns in size) airborne particles of infectious material.[7,14,15] Such microparticles, if inhaled by susceptible hosts, can infect them at long distances from the infected person when the microbes come in contact with the mucous membranes of the upper and lower respiratory tracts. The distance of spread depends on the material exhaled by the infected person, air currents, and environmental conditions. Airway procedures may influence these factors and produce droplets and aerosols or suspensions of microscopic infectious particles.

Host Susceptibility

Host susceptibility to infection is determined by multiple factors. As humans age, both innate and adaptive immune cell function begins to wane, and there are sex-specific differences to some diseases.[16,17] By affecting immunity and resistance to disease, factors such as comorbid conditions, medication therapies, and nutritional status also play a role. Finally, susceptibility to infection is dependent on preventive factors and actions taken by the potential host, such as engaging in recommended preventive procedures (discussed later) and having undergone effective vaccination.

THE CHAIN OF INFECTION

There are six distinct links in the chain of infection and related definitions at which a pathogen's course can be interrupted to block infecting a health care provider or patient (Fig. 61.3 and Table 61.1).[18] Each type of pathogen has unique transmission characteristics that allow it to produce disease.[7] Factors that determine whether a pathogen will cause an infection include the organism's virulence (the ability to grow and multiply), its invasiveness (the ability to enter tissue), and pathogenicity (the ability to cause disease). The links that are most susceptible

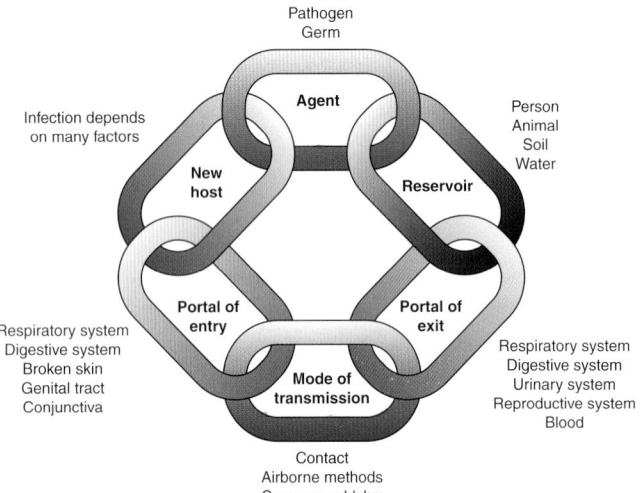

Fig. 61.3 Links in the chain of infection. Infection prevention and you: Break the chain of infection. apic.org. Infectionpreventionandyou.org. https://professionals.site.apic.org/protect-your-patients/break-the-chain-of-infection/#:~:text=The%20six%20links%20include%3A%20the,of%20entry%2C%20and%20susceptible%20host.&text=The%20way%20to%20stop%20germs,this%20chain%20at%20any%20link. Published 2016. Accessed December, 2020.

to interventions include controlling or eliminating the pathogen at its source, protecting portals of entry, and supporting the host's defenses.[19] Health care workers, by practicing frequent hand hygiene, being up to date on vaccinations, staying at home while sick, following recommendations for standard and contact isolation, utilizing appropriate personal protective equipment (PPE), cleaning and disinfecting the environment, sterilizing medical equipment, and following safe injection practices, can work together to strengthen the links of the chain of infection.[18]

In summary, infectious organisms may be transmitted by a single route or by a combination of mechanisms. The ease of inactivation of organisms by disinfectant methods varies, and appropriate measures (transmission precautions) are necessary to prevent transmission (discussed later).

STANDARD AND TRANSMISSION-BASED PRECAUTIONS

Standard precautions constitute a group of infection control and prevention (ICP) measures that are integrated into patient care to reduce the risk of transmission of infectious agents and microorganisms among patients and health care providers.[7,20] The practice of standard precautions is grounded in the science that all blood, bodily fluids, secretions, excretions (except for sweat), nonintact skin, and mucous membranes may harbor transmissible infectious pathogens.[7] Standard precautions include but are not limited to hand hygiene and the use of PPE.

PPE includes protective clothing and equipment devised to protect from injury or contamination.[21] Proper use of PPE is vital for protection. The Centers for Disease Control and Prevention (CDC) recommends health care organizations provide human and fiscal resources to meet occupational health needs related to infection control and to provide necessary supplies and equipment for consistent observance of Standard Precautions.[22] PPE examples and guidelines are provided in Table 61.2.[20,23-26]

HAND HYGIENE

Hand hygiene is a general term describing the physical removal of visible soil, organic matter, or transient microorganisms from the hands by means of washing the hands with soap and water or utilizing an

TABLE 61.1   The Chain of Infection

Term	Definition	Sources of Transmission
Infectious agent	Pathogen capable of causing infection	All links in the chain must be in place for an infection to occur. Infectious agents include bacteria, viruses, fungi, protozoa, and prions
Reservoir	Optimal environment for a pathogen to live, grow, and reproduce (may be a person or object carrying the disease)	Sources include places in the environment where pathogens exist: people, medical equipment, insects, animals, soil
Portal of exit	The way the pathogen exits the reservoir (open wounds, aerosols, splatter/splash of body fluids, coughing, or sneezing)	Respiratory, alimentary, genitourinary tracts, transplacental, skin
Mode of transmission	The way in which the infectious agent is passed on (may be direct or indirect, inhalation, etc.)	Contact (direct or indirect) Droplet Airborne Bloodborne
Portal of entry	The way in which the infectious agent enters a new host	Three primary portals include the respiratory system, digestive system, and breaks in skin; also mucous membranes of eyes, nose, mouth
Susceptible host	Any person/complex relationship between a potential host and infectious agent	Any person who can get sick when exposed to a disease-causing microorganism

TABLE 61.2   Indications for Hand Hygiene

Before	After
Patient Contact	***Patient Contact***
• Patient contact	• Contact with patient's intact skin
• Between tasks/procedures on the same patient	• Contact with blood, body fluids, excretions, mucous membranes, wound
• Accessing intravenous catheters, handling invasive devices	dressings, nonintact skin
• Performing an invasive procedure, clean, or aseptic procedure	• Contact with a patient's airway
Personal Protective Equipment (PPE)	***PPE***
• Donning PPE	• Removing gloves and other PPE
Environment	***Environment***
• Between patients	• Contact with the floor or anything that has been in contact with the floor
• Entering the operating room	• Contact with inanimate objects/medical equipment/monitors
	• Exiting the operating room

TABLE 61.3   Hand Hygiene Definitions and Best Practice

Term	Definition	Protocol
Antiseptic handwash	Washing hands with water and an antiseptic agent, (e.g., soap, hand rub)	• Wet hands with water, apply antiseptic soap, and rub hands together for at least 20 sec.
Alcohol-based hand rub	Rubbing nonvisibly soiled hands with a product that contains alcohol to decontaminate hands	• Apply manufacturer recommended amount to palm. • Rub hands together covering all surfaces and fingernails until dry. • Refrain from contact until hands are completely dry.
Surgical hand antisepsis	Washing hands with an antiseptic agent before a surgical procedure[2,7,8]	• Remove jewelry (e.g., rings, bracelets, wristwatches) prior to performing surgical hand hygiene. • Follow manufacturer guidelines for scrub time. • Clean under fingernails using a nail cleaner. • Keep natural nail length to less than 0.25 in. • Do not wear artificial nails or nail extenders.

alcohol-based hand rub (ABHR).[24] Hand hygiene interrupts the transmission of pathogens between health care providers, patients, and contaminated fomites found in the environment or patient surroundings.[25]

Hand Disinfectants

The two primary categories of hand disinfectants are (1) soap and water and (2) alcohol-based products. Antimicrobial soaps contain active ingredients such as iodophors, chlorhexidine, chloroxylenol, hexachlorophene, triclosan, and quaternary ammoniums. An alcohol-based hand rub is an alcohol-containing preparation designed to reduce microorganisms and typically contains 60% to 95% of volume of ethanol, n-propranolol, or isopranolol. The n-propranolol preparation is the most efficacious, and ethanol is the least active alcohol preparation.[27] Alcohol-based hand rub products are available in foams, liquids, and gels.[23]

If hands are visibly soiled with blood, bodily fluids, or proteinaceous material, they should be washed with either a nonantimicrobial or antimicrobial soap and water. When hands are not visibly soiled, an ABHR should be used. ABHRs should be the primary method for decontaminating hands in most clinical settings.[20] ABHRs demonstrate a broader antibacterial range than the use of soap and water against gram-positive and gram-negative bacteria, oral tuberculosis, and fungi.[27] Alcohol-based hand rub offers virtually no protection from spores (e.g., *Clostridium difficile*).[23]

Benefits of an alcohol-based hand rub are as follows:
- Eliminates most bacteria and viruses
- Reliably reduces bacterial counts to a greater degree than antiseptic soaps

- Short time required for action (approximately 20 seconds)
- Faster onset
- Availability of product at point of care
- Improved skin tolerability

Microorganisms, including *Staphylococcus aureus, Streptococcus pyogenes,* and Vancomycin-resistant *Enterococcus,* are spread by the hands of health care providers.[24] The hands of health care providers become increasingly colonized with potential pathogens during patient care. The higher the degree of hand contamination, the more likely that microbial transfer will occur.[28] Hand bacterial contamination is a modifiable risk factor for cross-contamination between the health care provider and patients. Hand hygiene definitions and best practices are listed in Table 61.3[23,27] and Fig. 61.4.[26]

Hand hygiene compliance is defined as behaviors consistent with accepted guidelines such as from the World Health Organization (WHO) and CDC. For nonanesthesia settings, hand hygiene should be performed according to WHO's five moments for effective hand hygiene (Fig. 61.5).[26] However, there exists no specific hand hygiene guidelines or recommendations for anesthesia care locations.[11] Studies have demonstrated that the overall hand hygiene compliance rate among anesthesia providers is poor.[10,11,29] In a study by Munoz-Price et al., the mean number of hand hygiene events per 100 opportunities was 4 during induction and 9 during maintenance.[30]

Anesthesia Infection Control and Prevention During Urgent/Emergent Care

Anesthesia providers are often challenged to comply with the WHO guidelines due to the multitude of anesthesia tasks performed, the fast-paced operating or procedure environment, the need to respond quickly to changes in a patient's hemodynamic status, and frequent repeated contact with the patient.[31] In addition, anesthesia providers must exercise their best clinical judgment to balance appropriate ICPs with management of urgent and life-threatening patient needs.[32]

According to the Society for Healthcare Epidemiology (SHEA) guidance, hand hygiene should at a minimum be performed prior to aseptic procedures/tasks, after removing gloves, when hands are visibly soiled/contaminated, before touching items on the anesthesia cart, and when entering and exiting the operating room.[4] Suggestions to improve hand hygiene compliance include performing hand hygiene every 5 to 10 minutes regardless of any specific contact and strategic placement of alcohol-based hand sanitizer dispensers in the vicinity of the anesthesia work area.[30] Strategies for maintaining infection control during urgent and emergent anesthesia care are provide in Table 61.4.[32]

Gloves and Alcohol-Based Hand Rub

Due to the large number of tasks performed by anesthesia providers during certain key portions of anesthesia (such as induction and emergence), performing timely hand hygiene may not be a viable option. When it is challenging to change exam gloves or perform hand hygiene, using an ABHR directly on nonsterile nitrile gloves is an option. Multiple applications of ABHR on gloves has been used as a temporizing measure when treating patients with Ebola virus. While anesthesia providers are encouraged to perform hand hygiene in accordance with recommended guidelines, when necessary, limited repeat use of ABHR on gloves does not impair glove integrity, impede tactile sensation, and is an alternative when performing hand hygiene or changing gloves is not possible. Additional studies are needed to determine how many ABHR applications can occur without compromising glove integrity.[4]

How to Handrub?

RUB HANDS FOR HAND HYGIENE! WASH HANDS WHEN VISIBLY SOILED

Duration of the entire procedure: 20-30 seconds

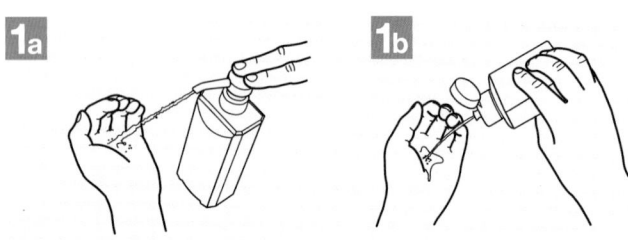

Apply a palmful of the product in a cupped hand, covering all surfaces;

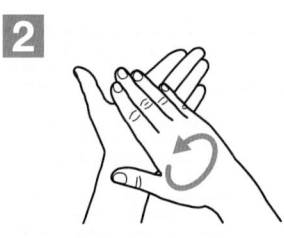

Rub hands palm to palm;

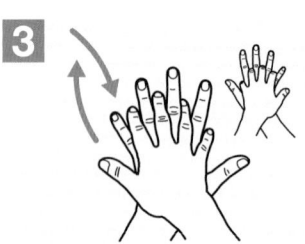

Right palm over left dorsum with interlaced fingers and vice versa;

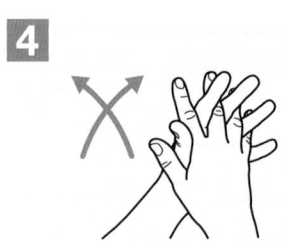

Palm to palm with fingers interlaced;

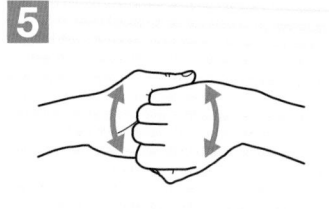

Backs of fingers to opposing palms with fingers interlocked;

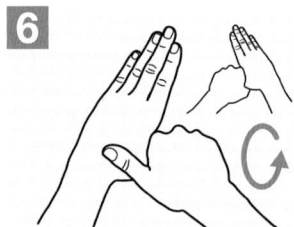

Rotational rubbing of left thumb clasped in right palm and vice versa;

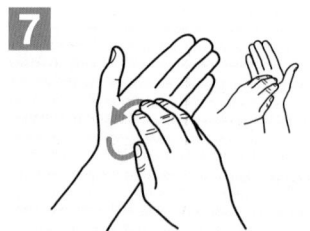

Rotational rubbing, backwards and forwards with clasped fingers of right hand in left palm and vice versa;

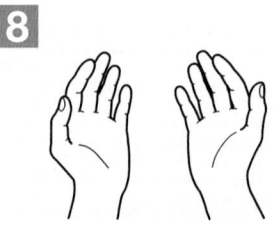

Once dry, your hands are safe.

A

Fig. 61.4 Hand rub (A) and handwash (B) procedures. (From the World Health Organization.)

HOW TO HANDWASH?

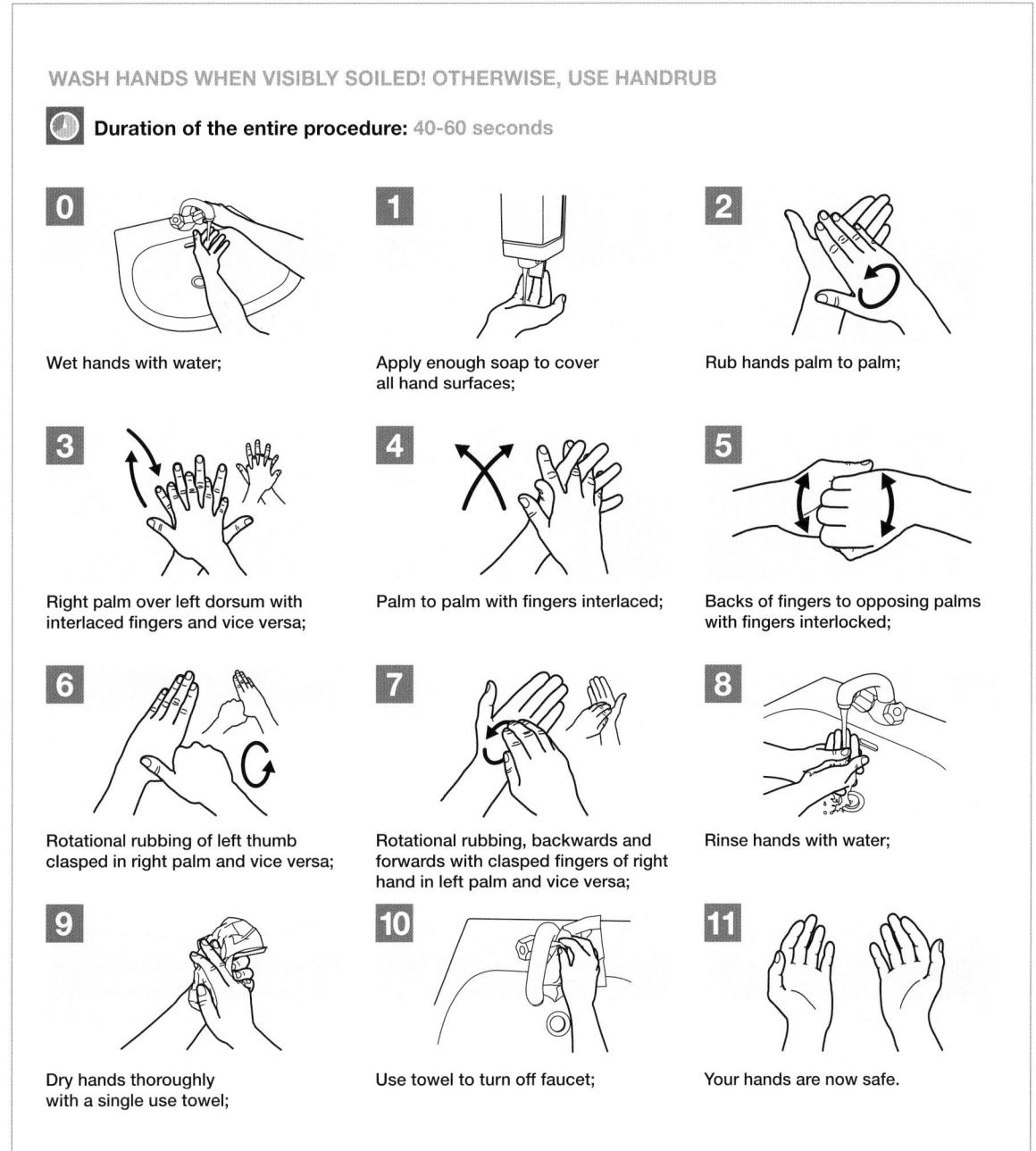

WASH HANDS WHEN VISIBLY SOILED! OTHERWISE, USE HANDRUB

Duration of the entire procedure: 40-60 seconds

0 Wet hands with water;

1 Apply enough soap to cover all hand surfaces;

2 Rub hands palm to palm;

3 Right palm over left dorsum with interlaced fingers and vice versa;

4 Palm to palm with fingers interlaced;

5 Backs of fingers to opposing palms with fingers interlocked;

6 Rotational rubbing of left thumb clasped in right palm and vice versa;

7 Rotational rubbing, backwards and forwards with clasped fingers of right hand in left palm and vice versa;

8 Rinse hands with water;

9 Dry hands thoroughly with a single use towel;

10 Use towel to turn off faucet;

11 Your hands are now safe.

B

Fig. 61.4–contd

PERSONAL PROTECTIVE EQUIPMENT

In addition to the practice of hand hygiene, another fundamental component of standard precautions is the utilization of PPE, which is essential to prevent exposure to potentially infectious pathogens, reduce the transmission of bloodborne or other microorganisms, and prevent cross-contamination during patient care. PPE refers to a variety of barriers used alone or in combination to protect the respiratory tract, mucous membranes, skin, and clothing from contamination with potentially infectious microorganisms. Examples of PPE include gloves, gowns, goggles, safety glasses, face shields, masks, and respirators. Determinants of the type of PPE to be worn include the likely mode of transmission of the infectious pathogen and the type of interaction between the health care provider and the patient.[7]

Personal Protective Equipment Respirator Use During Covid-19

Respirators, including fit-tested N95, elastomeric, or powered air-purifying respirators (PAPR), reduce the health care provider's risk of inhaling droplet and aerosolized infectious materials. These respirators should be worn during aerosol generating procedures (AGP) (Table 63.5).[7,20,33] N95 respirators should be fit-tested for individual providers. N95 respirators filter at least 95% of aerosolized particles less than 5 microns and droplet size of 5 to 50 microns.[7,20] PAPRs with high-efficiency particulate air (HEPA) filters will filter at least 99.7% of particles 0.3 micron in diameter.[7,20] PAPRs should be worn by health care workers who are not N95 fit-tested, fail N95 fit testing, or have facial hair.[33]

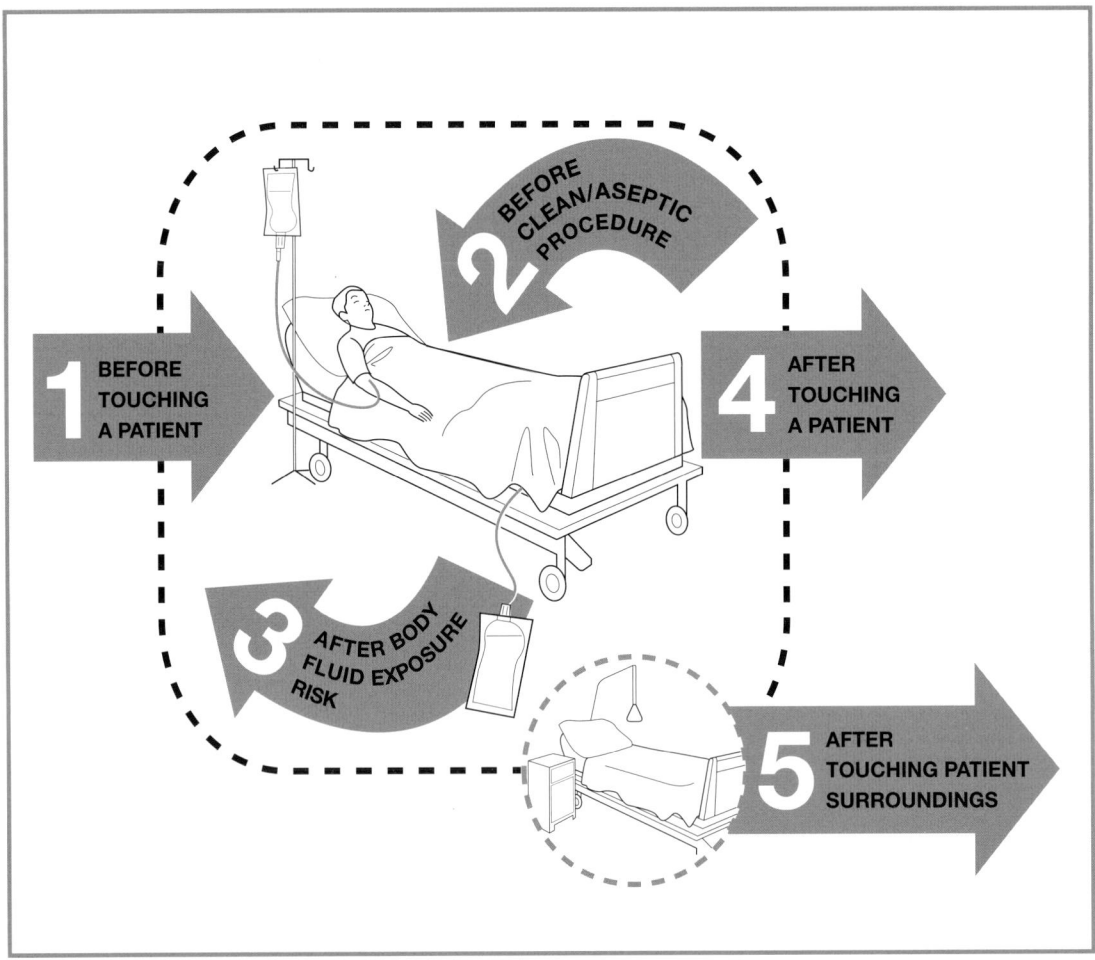

Fig. 61.5 Moments for hand hygiene. (From the World Health Organization.)

TABLE 61.4	**Strategies for Maintaining Infection Control During Urgent/Emergent Care**
1.	Plan ahead, anticipating emergency situations that will or might arise in each clinical situation, using anesthesiology and critical care training and simulation training to appropriately prioritize and plan for associated infection control practices.
2.	During emergency care, prioritize life-protecting and sustaining interventions, but include infection control activities as permitted without increasing risk of patient injury.
3.	Ensure immediate availability of all infection control supplies—personal protective equipment, alcohol-containing intravenous (IV) port caps, sterile needles/syringes and angiocatheters/IV infusion sets, alcohol-based hand rubs.
4.	Keep uncontaminated supplies clean, covered (e.g., in the anesthesia cart), and segregated from contaminated materials until needed.
5.	Keep all IV and arterial line ports covered with alcohol-containing IV port caps.
6.	Keep syringes covered with sterile tip caps when not in use.
7.	Keep prepackaged sterile saline syringes immediately available for drug dilution and flushes.
8.	In emergencies, consider double-gloving, removing outer gloves as these become contaminated, and removing inner gloves followed by hand hygiene as soon as possible.
9.	If feasible, appoint an "infection control officer" colleague during emergencies to help choose and prepare uncontaminated supplies, and identify and safely store contaminated equipment for later disinfection.
10.	Clean and disinfect the patient and environment as soon as situation stabilizes.
11.	Consider consult with infectious disease service if contamination and exposure is considered to have occurred.
12.	Prepare stat rooms (e.g., trauma rooms) as close to the time of use as possible, label all supplies with date and time of preparation, ensure all supplies are kept clean and covered as allowed by the resuscitation requirements of the anticipated situation. Devise department policies governing the protection, care, and length of time such supplies may remain unused before being discarded.

TABLE 61.5   Aerosol Generating Procedures

- Endotracheal intubation, extubation, suctioning
- Tracheostomy care
- Ventilation, airway suctioning
- Bronchoscopy
- Endoscopy
- Transesophageal echocardiogram
- High-frequency jet ventilation
- Bilevel positive airway pressure/continuous positive airway pressure
- Nebulizer treatments
- Aerosolizing procedures of the airway, lung, sinus oropharynx, skull base surgery
- Cardiopulmonary resuscitation

Donning and Doffing Personal Protective Equipment

The use of PPE reduces but does not eliminate the risk that health care providers may contaminate their skin and clothing with infectious microorganisms. Contamination contributes to dissemination of pathogens increasing the risk for infection. Despite wearing gowns and gloves, Tomas et al. found that 2% to 24% of providers caring for patients with multidrug-resistant organisms (MDROs) and *C. difficile* pathogens self-contaminated and acquired those microorganisms on their hands following removal of gloves.[34] One strategy to decrease the likelihood of contamination during donning (putting on) and doffing (taking off) PPE is to educate the provider on the proper technique based on CDC recommended protocols.[35]

How to Don Personal Protective Equipment

More than one donning method may be acceptable.[36] Training and practice using your health care facility's procedure is critical. Following is one example of donning.

1. *Identify and gather the proper PPE to don.* Ensure choice of gown size is correct (based on training).
2. *Perform hand hygiene using hand sanitizer.*
3. *Put on isolation gown.* Ensure all ties on the gown are tied. Assistance may be needed by other health care personnel.
4. *Put on National Institute for Occupational Safety and Health (NIOSH)–approved N95 filtering facepiece respirator or higher (use a facemask if a respirator is not available).* If the respirator has a nosepiece, it should be fitted to the nose with both hands, not bent or tented. Do not pinch the nosepiece with one hand. Respirator/facemask should be extended under the chin. Both the mouth and nose should be protected. Do not wear respirator/facemask under the chin or store in scrubs pocket between patients.*
   - *Respirator:* Respirator straps should be placed on crown of head (top strap) and base of neck (bottom strap). Perform a user seal check each time you put on the respirator.
   - *Facemask:* Mask ties should be secured on crown of head (top tie) and base of neck (bottom tie). If mask has loops, hook them appropriately around the ears.
5. *Put on face shield or goggles.* When wearing an N95 respirator or half facepiece elastomeric respirator, select the proper eye protection to ensure that the respirator does not interfere with the correct positioning of the eye protection, and the eye protection does not affect the fit or seal of the respirator. Face shields provide full face coverage. Goggles also provide excellent protection for the eyes, but fogging is common.
6. *Put on gloves.* Gloves should cover the cuff (wrist) of gown.
7. *Health care personnel may now enter patient room.*

How to Doff Personal Protective Equipment

More than one doffing method may be acceptable. Training and practice using your health care facility's procedure is critical. Following is one example of doffing.

1. *Remove gloves.* Ensure glove removal does not cause additional contamination of hands. Gloves can be removed using more than one technique (e.g., glove-in-glove or bird beak).

2. *Remove gown.* Untie all ties (or unsnap all buttons). Some gown ties can be broken rather than untied. Do so in gentle manner, avoiding a forceful movement. Reach up to the shoulders and carefully pull gown down and away from the body. Rolling the gown down is an acceptable approach. Dispose in trash receptacle.*
3. *Health care personnel may now exit patient room.*
4. *Perform hand hygiene.*
5. *Remove face shield or goggles.* Carefully remove face shield or goggles by grabbing the strap and pulling upwards and away from head. Do not touch the front of face shield or goggles.
6. *Remove and discard respirator (or facemask if used instead of respirator).* Do not touch the front of the respirator or facemask.*
   - *Respirator:* Remove the bottom strap by touching only the strap and bring it carefully over the head. Grasp the top strap and bring it carefully over the head, and then pull the respirator away from the face without touching the front of the respirator.
   - *Facemask:* Carefully untie (or unhook from the ears) and pull away from face without touching the front.
7. *Perform hand hygiene after removing the respirator/facemask and before putting it on again if your workplace is practicing reuse.*

SAFE INJECTION PRACTICES

Preventable harm to patients, health care providers, and the community can be avoided by exercising safe injection practices.[4,23,37-39] There were 33 outbreaks of hepatitis B or C viral infection in nonhospital settings between 1998 and 2008. Several of these outbreaks occurred directly related to anesthesia medications in settings such as pain clinics, endoscopy clinics, and private physician offices. Unsafe injection practices may have legal consequences for anesthesia providers. For example, in Michigan, it is a felony offense to reuse a single-use device.[38] A summary of current safe injection practice guidelines and recommendations from the American Association of Nurse Anesthetists (AANA), the WHO, CDC, and SHEA is provided in Table 61.6.[4,23,37-39]

ANESTHESIA EQUIPMENT AND ENVIRONMENT DISINFECTION

The role of anesthesia providers in keeping an environment clean is vital to ICPs. Ensuring that work surfaces are properly cleaned and disinfected is a major factor in reducing the risk of cross-contamination for an optimal work environment. The anesthesia work area and patient-specific equipment are cleaned between cases and terminally at the end of the day following each facility's infection control policies and procedures that include a method for monitoring for compliance. Using Environmental Protection Agency (EPA)–approved disinfectant wipes is recommended for ensuring that the surfaces are properly disinfected.[40]

---

*Facilities implementing reuse or extended use of PPE will need to adjust their donning and doffing procedures to accommodate those practices.

TABLE 61.6 Safe Injection Practice Guidelines

Item	Guideline
Aseptic technique	Should be maintained during preparation and administration of medications
Needles	Do not recap; are considered single use
Syringes	• Are considered single use • Do not use on more than one patient even if needle is changed • Do not refill even if being used on same patient • Needleless syringes should be recapped with sterile cap when being used to administer multiple doses to the same patient
Injection port	• Disinfect injection ports with a sterile alcohol-based disinfectant prior to use • Consider isopropyl alcohol caps • Replace sterile cap on stopcock after use
Fluid administration set	Single-patient use
Intravenous solution	• Single-patient use • Do not use as a diluent source for multiple patients
Single-dose medication vial	• Single-patient use • Scrub the vial diaphragm with 70% alcohol prior to accessing • Do not access vial with a used needle and/or syringe
Multidose medication vial	• Single-dose medication vial • Store outside of patient treatment area • Discard within 28 days of opening (unless manufacturer expiration date precedes the 28 days • Discard if sterility is questionable
Medication ampule	Scrub the ampule with 70% alcohol prior to opening the ampule and accessing

Spaulding Disinfection and Sterilization Classification Scheme

The Spaulding disinfection and sterilization classification scheme is used to classify (from critical to noncritical) disinfection and sterilization methods for medical equipment (Table 61.7).[23]

Breathing Circuit Filter Application

Care is taken to minimize contamination of the anesthesia delivery system (ADS). Contamination may be caused by pathogens entering the ADS via the circuit and the gas analysis sampling line into the ADS and/or gas monitor and potentially to another patient. The single patient use of high-quality heat and moisture exchange filter(s) (HMEFs) on the distal end of the anesthesia circuit can significantly reduce the risk of contamination of the anesthesia machine and the gas sample line and protect the patient from ADS contamination (Fig. 61.6).[41] Adding another filter on the expiratory limb protects the machine and provides backup for any particles that may pass through the airway filter (per Anesthesia Patient Safety Foundation [APSF] guidelines). This is especially effective and necessary with the Covid-19 pandemic and the risks associated with that virus. This includes the secondary filter if one is in use. The type of circuit filter needed to prevent contamination from a patient with Covid-19 to the anesthesia machine is unknown as no data are yet available regarding the efficacy of breathing circuits for prevention of Covid-19 transmission. A filter with a viral filtration efficiency (VFE) of 99.99% should be used to provide the best protection available. The APSF compiled a list of breathing circuit filters for use with various anesthesia machine breathing circuits (Table 61.8).[41] If at any time it is suspected that the anesthesia machine may be contaminated, then the machine should be removed from use, and the manufacturer or technical manual should be consulted regarding cleaning and/or sterilization. Each manufacturer may have specific recommendations for cleaning and decontamination of the ADS. Federal and state regulations, as well as individual facility policies, should be used for guidance.

AIRWAY MANAGEMENT: CONSIDERATIONS SPECIFIC TO ANESTHESIA CARE

Airway management is an integral part of patient safety and anesthesia practice. The physical location of the anesthesia provider near the airway and the maneuvers required to ensure airway patency during sedation, general anesthesia, and the insertion of airway devices pose three unique risks. First, unaddressed or undermanaged patient ventilation could result in injury or death from hypoxia. Second, the anesthesia provider risks exposure to pathogens from airway secretions and aerosols generated during positive pressure ventilation, airway manipulation, instrumentation, and airway reflex activity such as coughing, gagging, or sneezing. The third risk is that subsequent patients may be exposed to pathogens from environmental contamination. The following practice considerations may mitigate the infection risk for the patient, anesthesia provider, and environment.

Risk to Patient

- Oxygenation and ventilation are top priorities during airway manipulation, balanced with infection control activities when possible.[42]
- Immediate ventilation is indicated prior to hand hygiene following airway device placement to oxygenate and assess airway patency.[42] This sequence is in conflict with CDC recommendations of immediate hand hygiene following airway intervention but is in accordance with standard of care for airway instrumentation and maintenance, and patient physiologic and safety needs.[7,42]

Risk to Certified Registered Nurse Anesthetists

If the patient is suspected or confirmed to be positive for a disease transmitted by aerosol or droplet production, in addition to Standard Precautions, the Certified Registered Nurse Anesthetist (CRNA) should don appropriate transmission-based PPE (described later) prior to patient contact, including gloves, gown, cap, eye goggles, face shield, and N95 respirator or PAPR as indicated.

TABLE 61.7   Spaulding Disinfection and Sterilization Classification Scheme

Device Classification	Device Example(s)	Process	Recommendation
Critical *Contact sterile tissue or the vascular system.*	Surgical instruments	Sterilization	• Sterilize devices with sterilant that destroys all vegetative bacteria, nonlipid viruses, and bacterial spores. • Rinse with sterile water. • Medical devices can be sterilized using chemical or physical properties depending on degree of contact with the patient. • Chemical germicides should be used rationally and in accordance with manufacturer recommendations and facility policy.
Semicritical *Contact mucous membranes or nonintact skin.*	Anesthesia and respiratory therapy equipment, breathing circuits, endotracheal tubes, endoscopes, laryngoscopes, fiberoptic scopes, Magill forceps, cystoscopes Laryngoscope blades	High-level disinfection	• Clean and disinfect devices with high-level disinfectants to destroy all vegetative bacteria and nonlipid viruses. • Rinse with sterile water. • Dry all equipment surfaces to prevent humidity from encouraging microorganism growth. • Wrap laryngoscope blades individually. • If high-level disinfection is used, a closed plastic bag may be used for storage. If steam sterilized, a peel pack may be used for storage.[40] • Partially remove the blade from the package, attach to light source, and test, or keep the blade covered—manipulation of the blade onto the light source/handle can be tested without removing the blade from the bag or pack without touching the blade itself. • Following testing, insert the blade back into the package and return to a clean storage location. This protocol applies to disposable blades as well.
	Laryngoscope handles		• At a minimum, wipe the handle with an intermediate-level disinfectant after use. This protocol applies to disposable handles as well.
Noncritical *Contact intact skin.*	Patient care items: electronic devices, stethoscopes, blood pressure cuffs, arm board, nametags, pulse oximeter sensors, head straps, monitor cables, blood warmers, medication administration pumps, carts, beds, and monitors	Intermediate or low-level disinfection	• Clean all equipment between patients and when visibly soiled in accordance with manufacturer recommendations and facility policy. • Low and intermediate-level disinfection differs by disinfectant type, concentration, and exposure to pathogen. • Stethoscopes may be washed with water and wiped with alcohol. • Use protective covering for noncritical surfaces that are difficult to clean (e.g., keyboard covers). • Hydrogen peroxide gas decontamination is an effective sterilization method for reusable items that are difficult to clean.
	Environmental surfaces: bed rails, food utensils, bedside furniture, computer keyboards, floors, mobile devices	Low-level disinfection (unless otherwise noted)	• Clean all equipment between patients and when visibly soiled in accordance with manufacturer recommendations and facility policy. • Use protective covering for noncritical surfaces that are difficult to clean (e.g., keyboard covers).

• If time allows, consider head-to-toe application of chlorhexidine wipes, povidone iodine nasal swabs to nares, and gargle with oral chlorhexidine solution to reduce microbial load.[43]

• The patient should wear a face mask at all times until induction of anesthesia.[23,44,45]

• As indicated by the patient's airway status, consider avoiding positive pressure ventilation to prevent aerosol formation. Intubation should perform rapid sequence induction and intubation

using a videolaryngoscope in an effort to avoid any unnecessary airway manipulation and aerosol production.[44,45]

• If a supraglottic airway device is placed, consider covering mouth, nose, and face with transparent film dressing to prevent aerosol escape. Continuous suction via appropriate catheter may be placed under the transparent film dressing to evacuate any escaped aerosol.

Consider preoperative testing (for infection spread by droplet and aerosol) of patients scheduled for elective procedures. For patients known to be free of upper airway infectious pathogens, the CRNA may consider the use of Standard Precautions, and Droplet Precautions (described as follows), as indicated by patient assessment and institutional policy.

- The anesthesia provider uses double-glove technique for all airway management.[11,23,46,47] Following insertion of airway device(s), remove outer gloves and discard safely, then connect the anesthesia circuit to the airway device and confirm correct device placement with clean inner gloves. Once device is secured, remove inner gloves and perform hand hygiene and don clean gloves.
- Double-gloving and infection control actions as described should also be used during airway device removal.

Risks to Environment

- Airway manipulation contaminates the environment around the patient.
- When the patient is stable following airway management, the CRNA should perform environmental cleaning as permitted by available supplies and patient status targeting all areas that were potentially contaminated.[23]
- Following completion of a case, the care environment is appropriately decontaminated using EPA-approved disinfectants and following institutional and manufacturer-recommended protocols.[23]

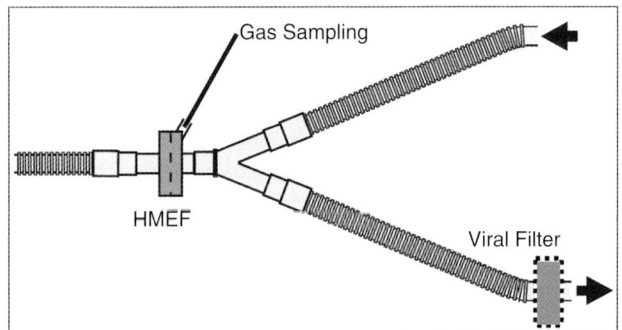

Fig. 61.6 Preferred filter configuration. Viral filtration efficiency is greater than 99.99% for each filter. Gas sampling on machine side of filter. (Courtesy Draeger Medical.)

TRANSMISSION-BASED PRECAUTIONS

In addition to standard precautions, transmission-based precautions should be employed for patients with suspected or documented infection with a highly transmissible or epidemiologically significant organism for which added precautions are warranted to prevent transmission.[7,20]

Modes of Transmission

There are four routes of infectious transmission: contact, droplet, airborne, and bloodborne.

Contact

Contact is the most common mode of transmission and includes both direct and indirect routes.[7] Direct contact occurs when there is physical contact between an infected person and a susceptible individual. Diseases spread through direct contact are unable to survive extended periods of time away from the host. Indirect contact occurs when there is no person-to-person contact, but the disease is transmitted through contaminated objects/patient environment.[48] Extensive environmental contamination increases the risk of disease transmission.[20] Contaminated surfaces (fomites) include but are not limited to medical instruments, computer keyboards and mice, handrails, hospital bed/operating room table, doorknobs, pens, and phones.[7] Special precautions should be taken with patients experiencing extensive wound drainage and fecal incontinence (norovirus, *C. difficile*). The CDC recommends contact precautions for patients with MDROs, including Methicillin-resistant *Staphylococcus aureus* (MRSA) and Vancomycin-resistant *Enterococcus*. Appropriate PPE includes gowns, gloves, and a mask with eye protection if contact with bodily fluids is expected.

Droplet

Some diseases can be transferred by respiratory droplets contacting surfaces of the mouth, nose, and eyes.[49] Droplets may also be inhaled into the lungs by individuals in close proximity.[50] Droplets containing infectious pathogens can be generated when an infected person coughs, sneezes, talks, or during procedures such as suctioning and bronchoscopy. In general, these pathogens do not remain infectious over long distances. Droplets range from 30 to 50 microns in diameter compared to aerosolized droplet nuclei, which are often <5 microns.[49] PPE includes masks, goggles, and safety glasses with side

TABLE 61.8 Breathing Circuit Filters by Recommended Application—For Use With Anesthesia Machine Breathing Filters	
Filter	**Location in the Breathing Circuit**
Airway heat and moisture exchange filter (HMEF)	For use at the patient's airway between the airway and the breathing circuit.
Airway filters—no humidification	For use at the patient's airway and may be suitable alternative to HMEF during low-flow anesthesia, short procedures, or with an active humidifier. All of these filters include a port for sampling gases for analysis.
Breathing circuit filters	For use between the expiratory limb and the anesthesia machine. Adult or pediatric applications. Patient size irrelevant. While airway filters without humidification (above) are suitable, devices without a sampling port are desirable to reduce the risk of an undesired leak if the sampling port is not completely closed.
Water trap filter (breathing circuits and nasal cannulas)	These filters are internal to the water traps used to prevent water from entering gas analyzers. When the gas sampling line is connected to an HMEF or airway filter, there is already one level of protection. If sampled gases are returned to the breathing system or enter the room, effective viral filtering at the water trap adds an important measure of protection. If sampled gases are directed to a suction or scavenging system, high-level filtration in the water trap is not as important.
Note: Sampling lines can also be protected by adding a 0.2-micron hydrophilic drug filter used to eliminate pathogens and contaminants from injected medications. An example is the filter used in the epidural drug tray.	

Adapted with permission

TABLE 61.9 Transmission-Based Precautions

Precaution	Protocol	Examples
Contact: Prevent transmission of infectious agents spread by contact with patient, inanimate object, or environment	Wear a gown and gloves for all patient contact or contact with environment.	Includes but not limited to: • *Clostridium difficile*[a] • Norovirus[a] • Scabies • Patient with multidrug-resistant organisms
Droplet: Prevent transmission of infectious agents spread by close contact with respiratory secretions	• Wear gown, gloves, and respirator for all contact with the patient and patient's environment. • Place facemask on the patient during transport.	Includes but not limited to: • Covid-19 (SARS-CoV-2) • SARS • Bacterial meningitis • Influenza • Pertussis • Mumps • Rubella
Airborne: Prevent transmission of infectious agents suspended in the air	• Place patient in an airborne infection isolation room designed with monitored negative pressure, 12 air exchanges per hour, and air exhausted directly to the outside or recirculated through high-efficiency particulate air filtration. • Isolate patient with N95 or higher level masked patients in a private room when airborne precautions cannot be achieved. • Health care workers don gloves, gowns, eye protection, N95 or powered air-purifying respirator when entering patient's room or for aerosol generating procedure. • Immune health care workers are the preferred providers for infectious patients with airborne diseases.	Includes but not limited to: • *Mycobacterium tuberculosis* • Measles • Varicella • Chickenpox • Anthrax • Smallpox
Bloodborne: Prevents transmission of infectious agents in the blood	Personal protective equipment includes gloves. For anticipated exposure due to sprays, splatters, and splashes, don a gown, eye protection (goggles or glasses with solid side shields) or face shield.	Includes but not limited to human immunodeficiency virus, hepatitis B virus, hepatitis C virus High-risk body fluids include: • Blood • Semen, vaginal secretions • Cerebrospinal fluid • Synovial, amniotic, pericardial, and pleural fluid Low-risk body fluids include[b]: • Urine, feces • Tears, saliva, vomitus • Nasal secretions

[a]Recommended environmental cleaning with use of a hypochlorate solution.
[b]Unless blood stained.

shields and/or face shields. Special air handling/room ventilation is not required for droplet transmission prevention.[7]

Airborne

Airborne-based precautions are required when entering a patient's room/environment or providing care to a patient who has been diagnosed or suspected of harboring a respirable infectious agent that is <5 microns in size. Airborne pathogens remain infectious over long distances and facilitate the transmission and dissemination of the airborne droplet nuclei into the upper and lower respiratory tracts.[49] Aerosol generating procedures necessitate airborne precautions.

Bloodborne

Bloodborne pathogens are microorganisms that reside in an infected person's bloodstream. These pathogens include human immunodeficiency virus (HIV), hepatitis B virus (HBV), and hepatitis C virus (HCV). Most bloodborne diseases acquired by health care workers are due to percutaneous injuries (needle sticks, cuts, punctures).[49] The CDC estimates that 385,000 percutaneous injuries occur annually in US hospitals. Transmission of HIV, HBV, and HCV have been reported following mucous membrane or nonintact skin exposure, though the risk of bloodborne pathogens is considered lower than the risk associated with percutaneous exposure. The risk of exposure to the health care worker is dependent on a variety of factors, including patient factors (titer of the virus in patient's blood or body fluid), type of injury, quantity of blood/body fluid transferred to the health care worker, and health care worker's immune status.[50] If exposed to blood-containing products/fluids, immediately wash the affected area with soap and warm water and obtain an infectious disease history from the patient. Postexposure prophylaxis for HBV and HIV should be considered.

The summary of transmission-based precautions and related protocol is presented in Table 61.9.[7,19,23,49,50]

ANESTHESIA CARE AND INFECTION CONTROL FOLLOWING THE COVID-19 PANDEMIC

On March 11, 2020, deeply concerned about the rapid spread of the devastating Covid-19 caused by a novel coronavirus discovered in

December 2019, the WHO declared the outbreak a world pandemic.[51] Shortly thereafter, the United States responded by closing nonessential businesses and public venues and issuing stay-at-home orders around the country. The virus spread rapidly in areas of high contact and dense population, filling intensive care units and morgues, overwhelming numerous health care institutions, exhausting supplies, and forcing health care workers—many of whom became infected and succumbed—to provide care to infected patients without proper or reused PPE. As the entire population donned masks, infection control and prevention were the new top priorities for all health care providers and the American public.

It is anticipated that this will change infection control practices during anesthesia care. In the short term, all patients are screened for viral illness and vaccination history. Longer term changes will likely include requiring vaccination (and possibly antibody titers of health care providers), treating all patients as potentially infected with airborne illness unless tested negative immediately prior to induction, routine use of protective HEPA filters on all anesthesia circuits, stricter enforcement of PPE use rules (including donning and doffing training), even more use of disposable equipment, stricter rules about keeping equipment not intended for immediate use confined and protected from contamination, and much stricter enforcement of fastidious cleaning and disinfection of the care environment between cases.[14,33,43,44]

INVASIVE PROCEDURE INFECTION CONTROL AND PREVENTION

Invasive procedures are a vital part of any anesthetic that carry with them significant infection risk for the patient and the provider. It is important that proper infection control measures be taken in an effort to minimize the risk of adverse events and reduce surgical site infections, central line-associated bloodstream infections, and catheter-associated urinary tract infections. All anesthesia providers should perform thorough hand hygiene prior to any invasive procedures and after the procedure is complete. Washing hands is the most effective manner of hand hygiene and should be employed when possible and especially when hands are visibly soiled. Alcohol hand sanitizing solutions are an effective alternative.

TABLE 61.10 Aseptic Technique Guidelines

Precaution	Guidelines
Equipment	May include some or all of the following items depending on the procedure: • Sterile gloves, gown, mask • Sterile drapes
Preparation	• Antiseptic skin preparation of patient prior to procedure • Consult manufacturer product instructions for directions and warnings regarding the proper use and application of specific skin antiseptics such as chlorhexidine-alcohol or povidone-iodine. • Confirm that all instruments, equipment, and devices are sterile.
Environmental Controls	• Close doors during operative procedures. • Minimize unnecessary staff traffic in/out of operating room.
Contact	• Precautions should be taken to mitigate contact with nonsterile surfaces and objects.

Aseptic Technique

Aseptic technique protects the patient and the health care provider from transmission of microorganisms in an environment. Aseptic technique guidelines are listed in Table 61.10.[23,39]

Skin Preparation

Preparing the patient's skin prior to performing any invasive procedures will reduce the risk of infection. Although there are many skin preparation agents on the market, the goal of the agent is to reduce the number of microorganisms on the skin in an efficient and effective manner and ultimately reduce the regrowth of microorganisms over time. Each of the skin preparation agents has specific advantages and disadvantages when selecting the agent for the procedure and patient. Patients may have allergies or skin conditions that may warrant consideration when choosing the appropriate skin preparation agent. Examples of skin preparation agents as well as advantages and disadvantages of their use are listed in Table 61.11.[23]

TABLE 61.11 Skin Preparation Agent Examples, Descriptions, and Recommendations

Agent	Description and Recommendations
Chlorhexidine gluconate	• Preferred skin prep agent due to immediate action, residual activity, and persistent effectiveness against a wide range of microorganisms. • Strong tendency to bind to tissue, contributing to extended antimicrobial action. • Highly effective in the presence of blood and organic material. • Addition of alcohol to the disinfectant provides more rapid and effective germicidal activity. • Limited sporicidal activity. • Not recommended for use on eyes, ears, brain and spinal tissues, mucous membranes, or genitalia. • Concentrations >0.5% not recommended for procedures such as epidurals and other neuraxial procedures due to neurotoxicity.
Povidone-iodine	• Suitable alternative when chlorhexidine is contraindicated. • Highly effective against a broad range of microorganisms and acts immediately. • Safe to use on face, head, mucous membranes, vaginal area, and during other neuraxial procedures. • Minimally persistent compared to chlorhexidine. • Limited residual activity. • Decreased effectiveness in the presence of blood and organic material.
Parachoroxylenol	• Less effective than chlorhexidine gluconate and povidone-iodine at eliminating microorganisms. • Moderately effective against a broad range of microorganisms. • Moderate persistent/residual activity. • Nontoxic with no tissue contraindications. • Remains effective in the presence of blood and organic material and in the presence of saline solution.
Iodine-base with alcohol	• Highly effective against a broad range of microorganisms. • Acts immediately. • Highly flammable.

Considerations for Ultrasound-Guided Procedures

Ultrasound guidance for procedures[23] such as vascular access and catheter placement has been shown to reduce infection rates and improve patient satisfaction. Considerations include identification of any adjacent pathology near the needle insertion. In addition to hand hygiene, PPE, skin preparation, and drape, the use a sterile sheath, sterile probe covers, and sterile ultrasound gel will mitigate the risk of site contamination. Following the procedure, the ultrasound probe must be disinfected using a manufacturer-approved cleaning process to prevent transducer damage.

Considerations for Epidural Catheters and Continuous Peripheral Nerve Block Catheters

Adherence to strict aseptic technique and use of single-use sterile gel to prevent contamination during catheter placement is necessary.[23] It is vital to don maximal sterile barriers, especially surgical masks, during the procedure.

- Prepare patient skin with an appropriate agent.
- Dress the insertion site with a sterile transparent, occlusive dressing.
- Use chlorhexidine-impregnated dressings at insertion sites to reduce epidural skin entry-point colonization.
- Check the insertion site and overall patient status at least daily for early identification of superficial infection (e.g., erythema, tenderness, itching at the site), deep infection (e.g., fever, back pain, lower limb weakness, headache), and sensory motor status.
- Remove once no longer clinically indicated.

Disconnected Catheters

The use of an epidural catheter for a prolonged time increases the risk of becoming disconnected from the insertion site, heightening the risk of infection. The choice to reconnect or remove the catheter is at the discretion of the anesthesia professional if not addressed in facility policy. Factors to be considered include the potential of contamination and patient-specific risk-benefit ratios. When a disconnected catheter is discovered and static fluid has moved more than 5 in from the disconnected end, the catheter should be removed.

Considerations for Central Venous Catheter Maintenance and Procedures

Central venous catheters (CVC), also known as central lines, are used to administer medications, intravenous fluids, blood products, and

TABLE 61.12 Examples and Descriptions of Central Venous Catheters

Catheter	Description
Tunneled catheter (e.g., Hickman, Groshong)	• Surgically inserted for extended use (months to years). • Catheter and attachments emerge from underneath the skin.
Non-tunneled catheter (e.g., Quinton)	• Percutaneously inserted for shorter use (1–2 wk). • Catheter attachments protrude directly.
Peripherally inserted central catheter	• Inserted into a peripheral vein in the arm.
Implanted port	• Inserted entirely under the skin. • Medications administered through blunt needle (e.g., Huber needle) placed through the skin to the catheter.

hemodynamic monitoring. Manufacturer recommendations and facility policies should be followed for specific care and maintenance of CVC. Several CVC descriptions are noted in Table 61.12.[23]

Central Venous Catheter Insertion[23]

To reduce the incidence of infections such as central line-associated bloodstream infections, it is important to consider the risks and benefits of placing a central line at various sites (e.g., subclavian, peripheral, jugular, femoral) before insertion. As with all invasive procedures, perform hand hygiene and don sterile gloves, sterile gown, surgical cap, and surgical mask, and cover the patient's entire body with a large sterile drape prior to insertion. Prepare patient skin using appropriate agent.

Additional considerations include the use of an antibiotic-impregnated catheter if the catheter is to remain in place for longer than 5 days. Replace catheter when adherence to aseptic technique cannot be ensured (e.g., catheters inserted during a medical emergency). Otherwise, do not routinely replace CVC. Remove any intravascular catheter once it is no longer indicated. For complete guidance, refer to the CDC's *Guidelines for the Prevention of Intravascular Catheter-Related Infections*.

Central Venous Catheter Access[23]

When accessing CVC, closed access systems are preferred in addition to scrubbing the injection cap or port (e.g., needleless connector) with an appropriate antiseptic agent and allowing it to dry according to manufacturer recommendations. Povidone-iodine is the recommended agent for children under 2 months of age.

Central Venous Catheter Flushing Technique[23]

The type of flush (e.g., saline, heparin, dilute heparin), concentration, volume, and frequency of flushing is in accordance with manufacturer indications for use as noted in the facility policy and per the treating clinician's orders. Individualized patient needs should also be considered.

Use a single-use flushing system with a minimum 10-mL syringe and flush (e.g., prefilled syringe, single-dose vial). Flush the catheter vigorously using a positive pressure technique, and maintain pressure on the syringe plunger at the end of the flush to prevent reflux prior to clamping or closing the line.

Heparin Flush[23]

Flushing a CVC with heparin solutions is a recommended practice in many guidelines despite the lack of conclusive evidence of efficacy and safety compared with 0.9% normal saline flush. A higher concentration heparin flush is appropriate for maintaining patency of CVC for dialysis. It is important that the injected volume of the heparin flush not exceed the internal volume of the catheter and that any catheter aspirate be discarded and not readministered to the patient. Higher concentrations of heparin may also be indicated for patients who have evidence of occlusion or thrombosis.

Specimen Collection[23]

- Access the catheter as outlined earlier, maintaining aseptic technique.
- Draw the first 3 to 5 mL of blood, dispose in an appropriate biohazardous waste receptacle, or return to the patient in accordance with the procedure or as indicated by the patient.
- Before specimen is collected, flush catheter in accordance with facility policy and per the treating clinician's orders.
- Discard 1.5 to 2 times the volume of the internal catheter lumen before drawing the specimen.

- Collect the specimen.
- Flush the catheter as directed by the procedure and facility policy and per treating clinician's orders.
  - Clamp the catheter as flushing is completed and promptly dispose of used syringe(s).

Changing the Injection Cap[23]

Maintaining the sterility of line injection and stopcock ports cannot be overemphasized. Change an injection port cap (e.g., needleless connector, Luer lock) immediately if suspected to be contaminated or when there are signs of contamination (e.g., blood, precipitate) or damage has occurred (e.g., leaks, septum destruction). Scrub the injection cap and catheter hub with appropriate agent (e.g., chlorhexidine, isopropyl alcohol); clamp the catheter if necessary, as cap is removed. Attach a new cap to catheter hub using aseptic technique.

Site Dressing[23]

According to facility policy, central lines in the anesthetizing area must be dressed in the same manner as any central venous catheter in the facility.

Considerations for Implanted Ports

In addition to the following recommendations, always discuss with the patient the best approach or technique for accessing and deaccessing the patient's port.

Port Access Procedure[23]

Don clean gloves and examine the port site for any swelling, erythema, drainage, or leakage, or assess for presence of pain, discomfort, or tenderness. Palpate the outline of the port to identify insertion diaphragm. Mark location on patient skin for blunt needle insertion. Remove gloves, perform hand hygiene, and don new sterile gloves. Cleanse port site with appropriate agent prior to entry. Stabilize port with one hand and insert blunt, noncoring needle (e.g., Huber needle) until port backing is felt. Aspirate blood to ensure patency by return. Stabilize needle/port with tape, securement device, or stabilization device. Apply gauze and tape for short-term use (e.g., outpatient treatment).

Port Deaccess Procedure[23]

Don clean gloves. Flush device in accordance with facility policy and per the treating clinician's orders. Stabilize port with one hand and remove needle with the other hand.

Maintain positive pressure technique on the syringe while deaccessing by flushing the catheter while withdrawing the needle from the septum. Apply dressing.

Considerations for Arterial Catheters and Pressure Monitoring Devices[23]

Catheters that need to be in place for longer than 5 days should not be routinely changed if no evidence of infection is observed. Maintain sterility of stopcocks by placing sterile cap when not in use and cleansing cap and stopcock with 70% alcohol prior to removing sterile cap.

HEALTH CARE–ACQUIRED INFECTIONS

Approximately 2 million hospitalized patients will develop a health care–acquired infection (HCAI) annually in the United States resulting in 90,000 deaths.[52-55] Examples of HCAI include ventilator-associated pneumonia (VAP), central line–associated bloodstream infection (CLABSI), catheter-associated urinary tract infection (CAUTI), and surgical site infection (SSI). HCAI exacts both human and economic tolls on society and health care systems, including increased length of hospital stay (LOS), long-term disabilities, morbidity, and mortality.[52] Common pathogens causing HCAI include bacteria, fungi, and viruses. A major cause of HCAI is a lack of consistency in observing basic ICP.[23]

SURGICAL SITE INFECTION

The term *surgical site infection* was established in 1992 and replaces the original term *surgical wound infection*.[53] A SSI is acquired by a patient in a heath care facility following surgery, which was not present or incubating at the time of admission. The infection occurs at or near the surgical site within 30 days of the procedure or within 90 days of a prosthetic implantation.[54] Common signs and symptoms of SSI include redness and pain surrounding the surgical site, drainage from the surgical site, and fever.

The CDC National Healthcare Safety Network (NHSN) is the most widely utilized tracking system for HCAI.[55] The NHSN's Patient Safety Component Manual lists the three types of SSI. SSI is classified by the depth and the tissue spaces affected.[56] SSI may be superficial incisional, involving the skin and subcutaneous tissue surrounding the incision; deep incisional, affecting fascia and/or muscle layers; or organ/space, involving any part of the surgically manipulated tissue below the muscle/fascia layers (Fig. 61.7).[57]

Scope of the Problem

Although the majority of SSI are preventable, these infections are the most common and costliest of all HCAI.[58] SSI accounts for 20% of all HCAI, and 3% of patients who develop SSI will die from the infection.[56] The severity of SSI can range from a superficial skin infection to life-threatening conditions, including sepsis. SSI rates range from 2% to 5% of all inpatients undergoing surgical procedures.[59] The incidence of SSI in the ambulatory surgical setting is less common but still contributes to patient morbidity in that setting.[60]

On average, SSI increases hospital stay by 9.7 days, increases risk of mortality by 2- to 11-fold, and costs the US health care system $3.5 to $10 billion annually.[56] It is estimated that over half of SSI is deemed preventable by the use of evidence-based measures. As such, SSI has

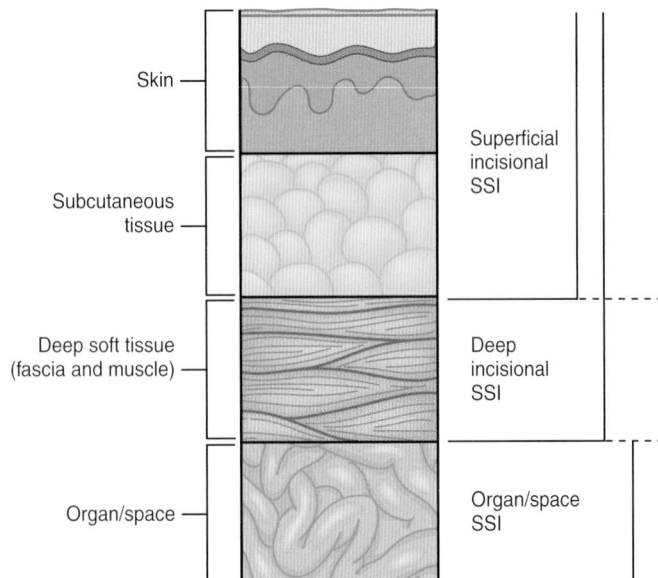

Fig. 61.7 Center for Disease Control and Prevention's National Healthcare Safety Network classifications of SSIs (Horan, et al., 1992).

become a pay-for-performance metric and an incentive for quality improvement and patient safety projects.[61] Since 2008, the Centers for Medicare and Medicaid Services (CMS) no longer reimburses hospitals for HCAI, including SSI.[55]

Pathophysiology

The pathogenesis of developing SSI is dependent on the following factors: microbial characteristics, including the degree of contamination and the virulence of the pathogen; patient characteristics, including but not limited to immune status and comorbid conditions; type of surgery; introduction of a foreign material; and amount of tissue damage.[32]

The risk of SSI can be calculated as follows[19]:

$$\text{Risk of SSI} = \frac{\text{Dose of bacterial contamination} \times \text{virulence}}{\text{Resistance of the host}}$$

Surgical incision exposes tissue to endogenous skin flora contamination, including *Staphylococcus aureus* and coagulase-negative *Staphylococci* species.[62,63] Specifically regarding the *S. aureus* pathogens, 49.2% were classified as MRSA, resulting in extended hospital stay, higher costs to the health care facility, and higher mortality rates.[58,63] In clean-contaminated procedures, including abdominal, heart, kidney, and liver transplants, the most common organisms isolated included gram-negative rods, enterococci, and skin flora.[58,64] External bacteria from the operating room staff, equipment, implanted materials, and the operating room environment may also contribute to the development of SSI.[64]

Role of the Anesthesia Provider in Surgical Site Infection Control

The anesthesia provider is positioned to play a vital role in reducing the risks of HCAI and SSI by complying with basic ICPs.[23,58] Prevention of HCAI should be a priority of anesthesia providers as they are responsible for processes impacting patient care and the risk of development of HCAI.[65] Studies have demonstrated the transmission of pathogens, including Vancomycin-resistant enterococci, *C. difficile*, and *Acinetobacter* species in a contaminated health care environment. These pathogens are shed by patients and operating room personnel, where they can contaminate surfaces for days.[66]

Intraoperatively, the contaminated hands of anesthesia providers can transmit pathogens to patients. Hand hygiene is integral to the prevention of HCAI. Loftus et al. found that anesthesia provider hand contamination was responsible for transmission of enterococcal and staphylococcal transmission to anesthesia work areas.[67] They also demonstrated that transmission of bacteria in the work area was associated with 30-day postoperative infections, which affected up to 16% of patients undergoing surgical procedures.[68]

The combination of horizontal transmission of pathogens from one individual to another coupled with inefficient disinfection of work surfaces and a lack of consistent hand hygiene among anesthesia providers places patients at risk for SSI. In a study by Loftus et al., 66% of providers' hands were contaminated with one or more pathogens prior to patient contact.[69]

Specifically, contamination of the anesthesia work area, stopcocks and intravenous tubing, syringes, touchscreens, computer keyboards, and mouse are implicated in the transmission of HCAI.[70] The anesthesia computer mouse is one of the most highly contaminated objects in the operating room, followed by the operating room table, nurse computer station mouse, the operating room door, and the anesthesia cart.[4,71]

It has been shown that even following routine terminal cleaning that 17% of operating room surfaces remain contaminated with bacterial pathogens.[72] Anesthesia work surfaces may be contaminated with pathogenic bacteria, including coagulase-negative *Staphylococcus*, *Bacillus* species, *Streptococcus*, *S. aureus*, *Acinetobacter*, and other gram-negative bacilli.[4,73]

Loftus et al.[74] demonstrated that pathogenic organisms, including multidrug-resistant bacteria, can be transmitted to patients during the immediate intraoperative patient environment during routine cases of general anesthesia. A significant increase in patient mortality secondary to the increased bioburden of workspaces was associated with an increased risk of patient contamination by stopcock sets.[74]

Four ICPs have been recommended by SHEA to reduce SSI rates. These include hand hygiene, safe injection practices of intravenous drugs, airway management, and environmental cleaning.[4,75]

1. Hand hygiene: Practice consistent and appropriate hand hygiene. Anesthetizing sites should have alcohol-based hand sanitizers conveniently located. Anesthesia providers should perform hand hygiene as follows:
   a. Prior to aseptic interventions
   b. After glove removal
   c. When hands are soiled
   d. Before and after touching anesthesia cart/machine
   e. Upon room entry and exit
2. Safe injection practices: one syringe, one patient, at one time.
   a. Use single-dose vials.
   b. Stopcocks should be covered with sterile caps.
   c. All syringes, even if unused, should be discarded at the end of the case.
   d. Injection ports and vial stoppers should be disinfected prior to accessing.
3. Airway management: Double-glove so that one layer can be removed when contamination is likely (e.g., following intubation).
   a. Disinfection of reusable laryngoscope handles or utilizing single-use laryngoscopes is recommended.
   b. Flexible and rigid laryngoscopes (blades and handles) are semi-critical devices due to contact with mucous membranes and must undergo high-level disinfection or sterilization.
4. Environmental disinfection: Disinfect frequently touch surfaces on anesthesia machines/carts, keyboard, monitors, computer mouse between surgeries.

ASSESSING PATIENT RISKS DURING THE PERIOPERATIVE PHASE

Numerous factors have been implicated in the development of SSI following surgery. These factors are categorized as intrinsic (patient) factors that are either modifiable or nonmodifiable and extrinsic (procedure, facility, preoperative, and operative) factors (Table 61.13).[56,76]

COMMON SURGICAL SITE INFECTION CARE BUNDLES AND THE ROLE OF ANESTHESIA PROVIDERS IN PREVENTING/REDUCING PERIOPERATIVE SURGICAL SITE INFECTIONS

Although the prevention of SSI is a multidisciplinary team effort, the anesthesia provider has at hand a number of interventions to reduce SSI through dynamic SSI prevention bundles. A bundle is a set of evidence-based strategies that can be consistently implemented by anesthesia personnel to reduce the incidence of SSI in all patients. The

TABLE 61.13 Surgical Site Infection Risk Factors

Risk Factors*

Modifiable	Nonmodifiable
Alcohol use	Increased age
Tobacco use	Recent irradiation of surgical site
Obesity	History of skin/soft tissue infection
Blood glucose	Specific diseases, including cancer
Diminished respiratory status	
Preoperative album in <3.5 mg/dL	
Total bilirubin >1 mg/dL	
Compromised immune status	
Presence of infection at remote site	
Prolonged hospital admission time prior to surgery	

Extrinsic Risk Factors*

Procedure related	Type, length, complexity of surgical procedure
	Emergency
	Wound classification
Preoperative	Preexisting infection
	Inadequate skin prep
	Hair removal
	Antibiotic choice, timing of administration
Intraoperative	Duration of surgical procedure
	Blood transfusion
	Maintenance of asepsis
	Poor hand scrubbing/gloving technique
	Hypothermia
	Poor glycemic control
	Degree of tissue trauma/microenvironment of wound
	Degree of microbial wound contamination/ pathogenicity of wound microorganism
	Blood transfusion
	Lack of appropriate antibiotic redosing
Facility related	Inadequate operating room ventilation, humidity, temperature
	Appropriate equipment sterilization

efficacy of care bundles relies on consistent compliance of the elements to realize substantial benefits.[56,77] Current SSI prevention guidelines and recommendations are provided in Table 61.14.[78]

Anesthesia Surgical Site Infection Prevention Bundle

Parenteral Antibiotic Prophylaxis

One of the most important roles that the anesthesia provider can play in the prevention of SSI is the timing of antibiotic prophylaxis. The efficacy of antibiotic prophylaxis for the prevention of SSI was first demonstrated as early as 1961.[65] Selection of appropriate antimicrobial agents is dependent on the type of surgery planned and the most common pathogens anticipated to be encountered during the procedure as well as wound classification (clean, clean-contaminated). Antibiotic administration should be timed to establish bactericidal concentrations of the drug in the blood and tissue at the time of incision or

prior to tourniquet inflation.[61] Most guidelines recommend antibiotics be administered within 60 minutes prior to surgical incision and 120 minutes for vancomycin or fluoroquinolones. In the case of cephalosporins, some studies recommend administration 30 minutes prior to surgical incision.[78] Patients known to be colonized with MRSA should receive vancomycin preoperatively.[65] Anesthesia providers should use weight-based dosing of antibiotics, especially in obese patients. Antibiotics should be administered prior to tourniquet inflation. For cesarean section procedures, antibiotic prophylaxis should be administered prior to incision. Redosing of antibiotics to maintain adequate tissue levels is based on the length of the procedure, the two half-lives of the drug, or for every 1500 mL of blood loss occurring during the surgical procedure.[76] Antibiotics should be discontinued at the end of the surgical procedure. Exceptions to this would include breast implant surgery, joint arthroplasty, and cardiothoracic procedures.

Maintenance of Normothermia

Hypothermia is defined as a core temperature below 35°C. Prevention of intraoperative hypothermia has been shown to reduce the incidence of SSI significantly.[65] Hypothermia occurs intraoperatively due to the impairment of thermoregulation caused by anesthesia-induced vasodilation and the often cold temperature in the operating room. Hypothermia triggers vasoconstriction and tissue hypoxia, which contribute to impaired wound healing. Additionally, hypothermia can impair the function of neutrophils, reducing the body's protection against infection.[58] Multiple guidelines recommend maintaining normothermia (35.5°C–36°C) perioperatively and utilizing warming devices to maintain core temperature of 36°C. Preoperative warming of patients has also been recommended.

Strict Glycemic Control

During the perioperative period, short-term blood glucose control has been shown to be more important than long-term blood sugar management. There is some movement to expand perioperative glucose control to all patients regardless of diabetic status.[56] Hyperglycemia is associated with a higher risk of contracting SSI.[76] Surgical stress triggers the release of cortisol. Hyperglycemia impairs neutrophil function, resulting in immune dysfunction.[58] Recommendations range from blood glucose levels less than 200 mg/dL to as low as 110 to 150 mg/dL. For cardiac patients, the target is 180 mg/dL or lower.[76]

Supplemental Oxygen

The American College of Surgeons and Surgical Infection Society SSI Guidelines recommend the administration of supplemental oxygen (80% FiO_2) during surgery as well as in the immediate postoperative period for patients undergoing general anesthesia. The CDC guidelines for the prevention of SSI recommend that patients with normal pulmonary function having a general anesthetic with endotracheal tube (ETT) be administered an increased FiO_2 during surgery and in the immediate postoperative period.[54] A meta-analysis of several randomized controlled studies demonstrated a lower risk of SSI if supplemental oxygen was administered at an FiO_2 of 80% versus an FiO_2 of 30%.[79]

Fluid Management/Normovolemia

Perioperative fluid therapy helps to prevent tissue hypoxia by improving arterial oxygenation and maximizing cardiac output during surgery; however, both hypervolemia and hypovolemia in surgical patients can result in impaired wound healing and the development of SSI.[80] Specifically, hypovolemia can cause vasoconstriction and a reduction in perfusion, resulting in decreased oxygen delivery to organs and peripheral tissues. Organ dysfunction may result. Hypervolemia may result in tissue edema, local inflammation, and impairment of collagen regeneration. This in turn can result in wound infection

TABLE 61.14 Current Guidelines and Recommendations for the Prevention of Surgical Site Infections

Recommendation	American College of Surgeons and Surgical Infection Society	World Health Organization	Centers for Disease Control and Prevention
Parenteral antibiotic prophylaxis	Antibiotics should be given 60 min of incision (redosing should be based on the half-life of the antibiotic and blood loss) Antibiotics should stop at closure of incision, with few exceptions Cardiac and orthopedic patients colonized with *Staphylococcus aureus* should be decolonized	**Moderate-quality evidence** Antibiotics should be given prior to incision (within 120 min of incision, with half-life of the antibiotic taken into consideration) Antibiotics should not be given after operation Nasal carriers of *S. aureus* should be decolonized prior to surgery	**High-quality evidence** Antibiotics should be given so that bactericidal concentration of agent is present during incision Antibiotics should stop at closure of incision for clean/clean-contaminated incisions
Alcohol-based skin preparation	Alcohol-based preparations should be used unless contraindicated	**Moderate- to low-quality evidence** Alcohol-based solutions should be used rather than aqueous solutions	**High-quality evidence** Alcohol-based preparations should be used unless contraindicated
Perioperative glucose control	Target blood glucose levels should be between 100 and 150 mg/dL	**Low-quality evidence** Protocols for patients with and without diabetes should be used before the operation (timing and glucose targets are not defined)	**High- to moderate-quality evidence** Target blood glucose levels should be <200 mg/dL
Temperature regulation	Preoperative and intraoperative warming is recommended	**Moderate-quality evidence** Warming devices should be used during the surgical procedure	**High- to moderate-quality evidence** Perioperative normothermia is recommended
Tissue oxygenation	80% supplemental oxygen should be given before the operation	**Moderate-quality evidence** 80% fraction of inspired oxygen should be used intraoperatively 80% fraction of inspired oxygen should be given for 2–6 hr postoperatively	**Low-quality evidence** Unclear risk vs benefit for supplemental perioperative oxygenation

Adapted from Fields AC, Pradarelli JC, Itani KMF. Preventing surgical site infections: looking beyond the current guidelines. *JAMA.* 2020;323(11):1087–1088.

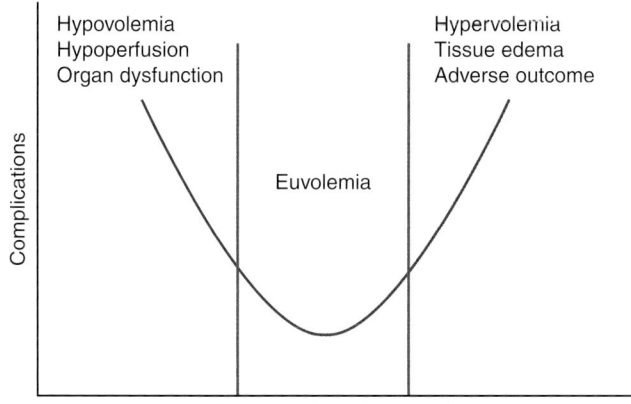

Fig. 61.8 Goal-directed fluid therapy: Bellamy curve.

and dehiscence. Current recommendations include adherence to "goal directed fluid therapy" protocols and euvolemia, rather than standard fluid management calculations as described in the Bellamy curve (Fig. 61.8).[81]

Blood Loss Prevention

Blood transfusions have been shown to increase the risk of SSI due to immunosuppressive effects. It is important for the anesthesia provider to take steps to reduce the need for blood transfusion; however, blood products should never be withheld if indicated.

CDC Guidelines on Preventing Surgical Site Infections in Patients Undergoing Joint Arthroplasty

Avoid withholding necessary blood products in an attempt to prevent SSI in a patient undergoing a prosthetic joint arthroplasty. For those patients undergoing prosthetic joint arthroplasty procedures and who have received systemic corticosteroids or immunosuppressive therapy, no additional antibiotics should be administered following closure of the surgical wound in the operating room, irrespective of drain placement.[54]

Enhanced Recovery After Surgery

Enhanced recovery after surgery (ERAS) bundles incorporating SSI guidelines include recommendations for parenteral antibiotic prophylaxis, strict glycemic control, and goal-directed fluid therapy.[77]

HEALTH CARE WORKER VACCINATIONS AND SCREENING

The CDC recommends that health care workers should receive various vaccines for prevention of contracting and spreading disease.[82] These recommendations include influenza, hepatitis B, meningococcal, measles-mumps-rubella (MMR), tetanus-diphtheria-pertussis (Tdap), and varicella vaccinations. Influenza vaccination annually is recommended. A three-dose hepatitis B vaccination is recommended for health care workers who have not previously completed the series or who have no documented immunity to hepatitis B. One dose of the meningococcal vaccine is recommended for those who have routine exposure to *Neisseria meningitidis*. The MMR vaccine is recommended for those born after 1957 and either never had the MMR vaccine or have no serologic evidence of immunity. The Tdap vaccination is recommended for those who have never had the vaccine to be followed up with a Td booster every 10 years. Pregnant health care workers should receive a Tdap vaccination during each pregnancy. Varicella vaccination is recommended for those who have never had chickenpox or who have no serologic evidence of immunity. The CDC updated its tuberculosis (TB) screening and testing of health care workers recommendations in 2019.[83] The CDC recommends all health care workers be screened for TB upon hire and prior to working in the facility. However, annual TB testing is not recommended unless there is a known exposure or ongoing transmission.

HEALTH CARE WORKER POSTEXPOSURE PROPHYLAXIS

Health care workers have the potential of being exposed to infectious diseases while providing services to patients. The CDC has recommendations for postexposure prophylaxis related to HBV, HIV, and TB.[84] When a health care worker is exposed to hepatitis B, the CDC recommends washing the exposed skin site with soap and water, flushing exposed mucous membranes with water, and administering the hepatitis B vaccine and, in some circumstances, adding hepatitis B immune globulin. Antiretroviral drugs should be administered as soon as possible (within 72 hours of exposure) and should be continued for a 4-week period after exposure to HIV. Follow-up testing and monitoring are recommended for 4 to 6 months after exposure. Regarding TB exposure, health care workers should be screened for symptoms and tested for TB.[83]

SUMMARY

In this chapter, a comprehensive review of infection control guidelines and recommendations for the CRNA to observe during clinical care. The AANA Infection Prevention and Control Guidelines were used to identify and prioritize important areas of clinical practice for which to address infection control considerations. Special attention was given to the effect of the coronavirus pandemic upon ICPs. Infection control will continue to be of paramount concern to CRNAs during clinical practice. It is our hope that this foundational knowledge will play a key role in keeping patients and practitioners safe in the course of receiving and administering anesthesia care.

REFERENCES

For a complete list of references for this chapter, scan this QR code with any smartphone code reader app, or visit the following URL: http://booksite.elsevier.com/9780323711944/

Page numbers followed by "f" indicate figures, "t" indicate tables, and "b" indicate boxes.